COLOR ATLASES

I. ATLAS OF DERMATOLOGY

Stephen F. Templeton / Thomas J. Lawley

A. Common Skin Diseases and Lesions

IA-1 Acne vulgaris **IA-2** Acne rosacea **IA-3** Psoriasis **IA-4** Atopic dermatitis **IA-5** Dyshidrotic eczema **IA-6** Seborrheic dermatitis **IA-7** Statis dermatitis **IA-8** Allergic contact dermatitis **IA-9** Lichen planus **IA-10** Pityriasis rosea **IA-11** Vitiligo **IA-12** Alopecia areata **IA-13** Urticaria **IA-14** Epidermoid cysts **IA-15** Seborrheic keratoses **IA-16** Keloids **IA-17** Cherry hemangiomas

B. Cutaneous Neoplasms

IB-18 Actinic keratoses **IB-19** Keratoacanthoma **IB-20** Basal cell carcinoma **IB-21** Squamous cell carcinoma **IB-22** Kaposi's sarcoma **IB-23** Mycosis fungoides **IB-24** Non-Hodgkin's lymphoma **IB-25** Metastatic carcinoma

C. Pigmented Lesions—Benign and Malignant

IC-26 Nevus **IC-27** Dysplastic nevi **IC-28** Superficial spreading melanoma **IC-29** Lentigo maligna melanoma **IC-30** Nodular melanoma **IC-31** Acral letiginous melanoma

D. Infectious Disease and the Skin

ID-32 Impetigo contagiosa **ID-33** Folliculitis **ID-34** Erysipelas **ID-35** Herpes simplex **ID-36** Varicella **ID-37** Herpes zoster **ID-38** Spread of herpes zoster with chemotherapy **ID-39** Verrucae **ID-40** Molluscum contagiosum **ID-41** Oral hairy leukoplakia **ID-42** Pseudomembranous oral candidiasis **ID-43** Tinea corporis **ID-44** Tinea cruris **ID-45** Tinea versicolor **ID-46** Scabies **ID-47** Erythema chronicum migrans **ID-48** Rocky Mountain spotted fever **ID-49** Disseminated gonococcemia **ID-50** Fulminant meningococcemia **ID-51** Primary syphilis **ID-52** Secondary syphilis **ID-53** Secondary syphilis **ID-54** Condylomata lata **ID-55** Chancroid **ID-56** Condylomata acuminata **ID-57** Skin lesions of neutropenic patients

E. Immunologically Mediated Skin Disease

IE-58 Systemic lupus erythematosus **IE-59** Discoid lupus erythematosus **IE-60** Dermatomyositis **IE-61** Dermatomyositis **IE-62** Scleroderma **IE-63** Scleroderma **IE-64** Erythema multiforme **IE-65** Erythema nodosum **IE-66** Vasculitis **IE-67** Pemphigus vulgaris **IE-68** Dermatitis herpetiformis **IE-69** Bullous pemphigoid

F. Skin Manifestations of Internal Disease

IF-70 Acanthosis nigricans **IF-71** Pretibial myxedema **IF-72** Sarcoid **IF-73** Neurofibromatosis **IF-74** Coumarin necrosis **IF-75** Pyoderma gangrenosum

II. ATLAS OF ENDOSCOPIC FINDINGS

II-1 Normal esophagus **II-2** Peptic regurgitant esophagitis **II-** Ulcerated squamous cell carcinoma **II-4** Moniliasis of the esophagus **II-5** Barrett's metaplasia of the esophagus with an adenocarcinoma **II-6** Normal body of the stomach with rugal folds **II-7** Large, benign, lesser curve gastric ulcer **II-8** Gastric polyp **II-9** Arteriovenous malformation of the gastric mucosa **II-10** Normal pylorus **II-11** Normal duodenal bulb **II-12** Duodenal ulcer **II-13** Normal papilla of Vater **II-14** Periampullary carcinoma **II-15** Endoscopic papillotomy **II-16** Normal colon **II-17** Colonic adenomatous polyp **II-18** Multiple, small, colonic adenomatous polyps **II-19** Colon adenocarcinoma **II-20** Crohn's colitis **II-21** Severe ulcerative colitis **II-22** Kaposi's sarcoma involving the colon **II-23** Colonic varices **II-24** Ileal pouch

III. ATLAS OF FUNDUSCOPIC EXAMINATION

III-1 Cytomegalovirus **III-2** Hollenhorst plaque **III-3** Hypertensive retinopathy **III-4** Central retinal vein occlusion **III-5** Anterior ischemic optic neuropathy **III-6** Retrobulbar optic neuritis **III-7** Optic atrophy **III-8** Papilledema **III-9** Optic disc drusen **III-10** Retinal detachment **III-11** Glaucoma **III-12** Age-related macular degeneration **III-13** Diabetic retinopathy **III-14** Retinitis pigmentosa **III-15** Melanoma **III-16** Kayser-Fleischer ring

IV. ATLAS OF HEMATOLOGY

IV-1 Normal blood smear **IV-2** Megaloblastic anemia **IV-3** Liver disease **IV-4** Iron-deficiency anemia **IV-5** β Thalassemia intermedia **IV-6** Sickle cell anemia **IV-7** Traumatic hemolysis **IV-8** Spur cell anemia **IV-9** Uremia **IV-10** Hereditary spherocytosis **IV-11** Immunohemolytic anemia **IV-12** Leukoerythroblastic smear **IV-13*A*.** Normal granulocyte **IV-13*B*.** Normal monocyte and lymphocyte **IV-14*A*.** Normal eosinophil **IV-14*B*.** Basophil **IV-15** Normal granulocyte precursors in marrow **IV-16** Neutrophils with toxic granulation **IV-17** Band with Döhle body **IV-18** Hypersegmentation **IV-19*A*** Chédiak-Higashi anomaly **IV-19*B*** Pelger-Hüet anomaly **IV-20** Reactive lymphocytes **IV-21** Chronic granulocytic leukemia **IV-22** Promyelocytic leukemia **IV-23** Chronic lymphocytic leukemia **IV-24** Leukemia cells in acute lymphoblastic leukemia **IV-25** Hodgkin's disease, mixed cellularity **IV-26** Follicular lymphoma **IV-27** Multiple myeloma **IV-28** Diffuse large B cell lymphoma **IV-29** Burkitt's lymphoma **IV-30** Acute myelocytic leukemia **IV-31** Auer rod **IV-32** Normal bone marrow biopsy **IV-33** Aplastic anemia **IV-34** Marrow fibrosis **IV-35** Erythroid hyperplasia **IV-36** Granulocytic hyperplasia **IV-37** Megaloblastic erythropoiesis **IV-38** Marrow iron stores **IV-39** Ringed sideroblast

14TH EDITION

Harrison's PRINCIPLES of INTERNAL MEDICINE

EDITORS OF PREVIOUS EDITIONS

T.R. Harrison
Editor-in-Chief, Editions 1, 2, 3, 4, 5

W.R. Resnick
Editor, Editions 1, 2, 3, 4, 5

M.M. Wintrobe
Editor, Editions 1, 2, 3, 4, 5
Editor-in-Chief, Editions 6, 7

G.W. Thorn
Editor, Editions 1, 2, 3, 4, 5, 6, 7
Editor-in-Chief, Edition 8

R.D. Adams
Editor, Editions 2, 3, 4, 5, 6, 7, 8, 9, 10

P.B. Beeson
Editor, Editions 1, 2

I.L. Bennett, Jr.
Editor, Editions 3, 4, 5, 6

E. Braunwald
Editor, Editions 6, 7, 8, 9, 10, 12, 13
Editor-in-Chief, Edition 11

K.J. Isselbacher
Editor, Editions 6, 7, 8, 10, 11, 12
Editor-in-Chief, Editions 9, 13

R.G. Petersdorf
Editor, Editions 6, 7, 8, 9, 11, 12
Editor-in-Chief, Edition 10

J.D. Wilson
Editor, Editions 9, 10, 11, 13
Editor-in-Chief, Edition 12

J.B. Martin
Editor, Editions 10, 11, 12, 13

A.S. Fauci
Editor, Editions 11, 12, 13

R. Root
Editor, Edition 12

D.L. Kasper
Editor, Edition 13

14TH EDITION

VOLUME 2

Harrison's PRINCIPLES of INTERNAL MEDICINE

EDITORS

Anthony S. Fauci, MD
Chief, Laboratory of Immunoregulation; Director, National Institute of Allergy and Infectious Diseases, National Institutes of Health, Bethesda

Eugene Braunwald, AB, MD, MA (Hon), MD (Hon), ScD (Hon)
Distinguished Hersey Professor of Medicine, Faculty Dean for Academic Programs at Brigham and Women's Hospital and Massachusetts General Hospital, Harvard Medical School; Vice-President for Academic Programs, Partners HealthCare System, Boston

Kurt J. Isselbacher, AB, MD
Mallinckrodt Professor of Medicine, Harvard Medical School; Physician and Director, Massachusetts General Hospital Cancer Center, Boston

Jean D. Wilson, MD
Charles Cameron Sprague Distinguished Chair and Clinical Professor of Internal Medicine, The University of Texas Southwestern Medical Center, Dallas

Joseph B. Martin, MD, PhD, FRCP (C), MA (Hon)
Dean of the Faculty of Medicine; Caroline Shields Walker Professor of Neurobiology and Clinical Neuroscience, Harvard Medical School, Boston

Dennis L. Kasper, MD, MA (Hon)
William Ellery Channing Professor of Medicine, Harvard Medical School; Director, Channing Laboratory; Co-Director, Division of Infectious Diseases; Executive Vice-Chairman, Department of Medicine, Brigham and Women's Hospital, Boston

Stephen L. Hauser, MD
Chairman and Betty Anker Fife Professor, Department of Neurology, University of California San Francisco, San Francisco

Dan L. Longo, AB, MD, FACP
Scientific Director, National Institute on Aging, National Institutes of Health, Gerontology Research Center, Bethesda and Baltimore

McGraw-Hill
HEALTH PROFESSIONS DIVISION

New York St. Louis San Francisco Auckland Bogotá Caracas Lisbon London Madrid Mexico City Milan Montreal New Delhi San Juan Singapore Sydney Tokyo Toronto

A Division of The McGraw-Hill Companies

Note: Dr. Fauci and Dr. Longo's works as editors and authors were performed outside the scope of their employment as U.S. government employees. These works represent their personal and professional views and not necessarily those of the U.S. government.

Harrison's
PRINCIPLES OF INTERNAL MEDICINE
Fourteenth Edition

4567890 DOWDOW 0403020100
ISBN 0-07-020291-5 (COMBO)
0-07-020292-3 (VOL 1)
0-07-020293-1 (VOL 2)
0-07-912013-X (SET)

FOREIGN LANGUAGE EDITIONS
Arabic (Thirteenth Edition)—McGraw-Hill Libri Italia srl (est. 1996)
Chinese (Twelfth Edition)—McGraw-Hill Book Company–Singapore © 1994
Croatian (Thirteenth Edition)—McGraw-Hill Libri Italia srl (est. 1996)
French (Thirteenth Edition)—McGraw-Hill Libri Italia srl © 1995
German (Thirteenth Edition)—McGraw-Hill Libri Italia srl © 1995
Greek (Twelfth Edition)—Parissianos © 1994
Italian (Thirteenth Edition)—McGraw-Hill Libri Italia srl © 1995
Japanese (Eleventh Edition)—Hirokawa © 1991
Portuguese (Thirteenth Edition)—McGraw-Hill/Nueva Editorial Interamericana © 1995
Spanish (Thirteenth Edition)—McGraw-Hill Interamericana de España © 1994
Turkish (Thirteenth Edition)—McGraw-Hill Libri Italia srl (est. 1996)

This book was set in Times Roman by Monotype Composition Company. The editors were J. Dereck Jeffers, Martin J. Wonsiewicz, and Mariapaz Ramos Englis; editorial assistants were Rose Derario and Daniel J. Green. The production director was Robert Laffler. The index was prepared by Irving Tullar. The text and cover designer was Marsha Cohen/Parallelogram Graphics.

R.R. Donnelley and Sons, Inc., was the printer and binder.

Library of Congress Cataloging-in-Publication Data

Harrison's principles of internal medicine.—14th. ed./editors,
Anthony S. Fauci . . . [et al.]
p. cm.
Includes bibliographical references and index.
ISBN 0-07-020291-5 (1 vol. ed.).—ISBN 0-07-912013-X (2 vol. ed.
: set).—ISBN 0-07-020292-3 (2 vol. ed. : bk 1).—ISBN
0-07-020293-1 (2 vol. ed. : bk 2)
1. Internal medicine. I. Harrison, Tinsley Randolph.
II. Fauci, Anthony S.
[DNLM: 1. Internal Medicine. WB 115 H322 1998]
RC46.H333 1998
616—dc21
DNLM/DLC
for Library of Congress 97-14184

CONTENTS

Names of contributors and their affiliations are listed in Volume 1, pages xv–xxiv.

PREFACE

The first edition of *Harrison's Principles of Internal Medicine* was published nearly 50 years ago, and subsequent editions have incorporated advances that have occurred in biomedical research and clinical practice in the interim. In the 14th edition, the text has been revised to reflect further understanding of the biology and pathophysiology of disease and at the same time to retain those facts that, while not new, remain clinically useful and important. Virtually every chapter in the 14th edition has been completely or substantially rewritten, and major new chapters have been added. In this preface, we cannot describe all of these changes; however, we would like to call to the reader's attention those that are particularly noteworthy.

Part One, "Introduction to Clinical Medicine," contains new chapters dealing with the influence of environmental and occupational hazards on health. Disease prevention is becoming more important in the current era, and both general principles of prevention and specific guidelines for primary care physicians are presented in a new chapter on preventive medicine. Chapters on medical ethics, women's and adolescent health, geriatric medicine, medical complications of pregnancy, and cost awareness and quantitative aspects of medicine have been revised and updated.

Part Two, "Cardinal Manifestations and Presentation of Diseases," serves as a comprehensive introduction to clinical medicine. Major symptoms are reviewed by organ system and are correlated with specific disease states—the basis of differential diagnosis. New chapters have been added on fever and rash; hypothermia; faintness, syncope, and dizziness; weakness, abnormal movements, and imbalance; coma and acute confusional states; aphasia and other focal cerebral disorders; memory loss and dementia; heart murmur; hypertension; voiding dysfunction, incontinence, and other common urologic complaints; manifestations of cancer; and breast masses in women and men. For the first time in *Harrison's*, a comprehensive approach to the diagnosis and treatment of common eye disorders is presented. The chapter on diarrhea and constipation has been extensively revised, with a focus not only on etiology but also on acute and chronic treatment. The chapter on gastrointestinal bleeding has been rewritten to focus on early diagnosis and the latest approaches to treatment.

Part Three, "Genetics and Disease," has been extensively updated and includes a new formulation of the role of classic and molecular genetics in health and disease and a major revision of the chapter on cytogenetics.

Part Four, "Clinical Pharmacology," contains a new chapter on nitric oxide. Nitric oxide or its inhibition may be important in the management of coronary insufficiency, septic shock, erectile impotence, primary pulmonary hypertension, and the adult respiratory distress syndrome.

Part Five, "Nutrition," covers nutritional considerations related to clinical medicine, including nutritional requirements, assessment of nutritional status, protein-energy malnutrition, and diet therapy.

The core of *Harrison's* encompasses the disorders of the organ systems and is contained in Parts Six through Fifteen. These sections include succinct accounts of the pathophysiology of the major systems and emphasize disease manifestations, diagnostic procedures, differential diagnosis, and treatment strategies. The treatment sections of virtually every chapter have been amplified, supplemented by the liberal use of algorithms, and clearly highlighted.

Part Six, "Oncology and Hematology," has been completely reorganized and extensively rewritten under the direction of our newest editor, Dr. Dan L. Longo, who brings to the textbook a wealth of experience at the bench and bedside in both hematology and oncology. He has called upon a distinguished group of contributors to reorganize this section. The oncology chapters that were distributed among several sections in previous editions have been brought together in a single section on neoplastic disorders (with the exception of tumors of the thyroid, central nervous system, and heart). There are eight new chapters, including those on the approach to the patient with cancer, cancer prevention and early detection, cancer cell biology, invasion and metastasis, sarcomas and bone tumors, and oncologic emergencies. Twenty-seven additional chapters have new authors. An effort was made to organize the chapters in a more uniform fashion and to include molecular and genetic mechanisms involved in tumors (and their clinical correlations) where that information is known. The chapter on lymphoid malignancies includes the novel classification scheme of the International Lymphoma Working Group. Where appropriate, diagnostic and management algorithms have been incorporated.

Changes in Part Seven, "Infectious Diseases," include a greater emphasis on the treatment of infections and infestations. Specific, current recommendations for therapy are made against a background of up-to-date information on the etiology, epidemiology, diagnosis, and prevention of infectious diseases. Special care has been taken to update and expand the information presented on the biology of microorganisms, microbial resistance to therapeutic agents, and emerging and reemerging infections, including mycobacterial infections, recently identified viral infections, and infections due to other newly recognized pathogens such as *Helicobacter pylori.* The revised chapter on the laboratory diagnosis of infectious diseases is complemented in this edition by the inclusion (as Appendix B) of comprehensive instructions for the collection and transport of specimens for culture. New and expanded chapters cover the health risks to travelers, the approach to patients with parasitic infections, and recommendations for the administration of standard and special-use vaccines. The chapter on the human retroviruses has been revised and expanded, as have the chapters on the biology of viruses and antiviral therapy. This edition's chapter on *Pneumocystis carinii* infection appears in Section 15, "Fungal Infections," reflecting the change in the classification of this pathogen from a protozoan to a fungus.

In Part Eight, "Disorders of the Cardiovascular System," a new chapter on atherosclerosis focuses not only on the importance of traditional risk factors but also on factors that influence plaque stability and instability. The current approach to the prevention of atherosclerosis is clearly delineated. An understanding of prevention of plaque instability is of critical importance, since it is now clear that plaque rupture can cause acute coronary syndromes (unstable angina and acute myocardial infarction) and sudden death.

Despite major advances in its diagnosis and therapy, acute myocardial infarction is the most common cause of death in industrialized nations. The new chapter on acute myocardial infarction provides important information on myocardial reperfusion therapy—thrombolysis and primary coronary angioplasty—and summarizes guidelines for acute coronary care and for risk stratification in the postinfarct patient.

Pulmonary thromboembolism is a major complication of the postoperative state and of a variety of illnesses. In Part Nine, "Disorders of the Respiratory System," major advances in prevention and therapy are presented in a new chapter that includes a useful algorithm for the work-up of patients with suspected pulmonary embolic disease. Enormous strides have been made in the use of lung transplantation for selected patients with end-stage, irreversible, pulmonary parenchymal and vascular disease, and a new chapter on this topic focuses on patient selection for this therapy.

In Part Ten, "Disorders of the Kidney and Urinary Tract," there has been considerable revision. In Part Eleven, "Disorders of the Gastrointestinal System," the new chapter on peptic ulcer and gastritis focuses on the role of *Helicobacter pylori,* with particular attention to its diagnosis and treatment. This chapter can be viewed as *the* definitive chapter on peptic ulcer and gastritis. The chapters on irritable bowel syndrome and diverticular diseases are also new, and the chapters on acute hepatitis and complications of cirrhosis have been extensively revised, the latter with a specific focus on the treatment of hepatic coma, ascites, and portal hypertension.

In Part Twelve, "Disorders of the Immune System, Connective Tissue, and Joints," the updating focuses on therapy. The chapter on "Introduction to the Immune System" has been completely rewritten and provides a comprehensive review of the human immune system. The chapter on HIV disease and AIDS is comprehensive and up-to-date and includes coverage of the natural history, epidemiology, and immunopathogenic mechanisms of HIV disease. In addition, the chapter contains both an organ system by organ system approach and a delineation of the major complications of HIV disease. The sections on therapy include a state-of-the-art discussion of the treatment of HIV infection with combinations of antiretroviral agents.

In Part Thirteen, "Endocrinology and Metabolism," there are new chapters on the hyperlipoproteinemias, lysosomal storage diseases, and glycogen storage disease. The chapter on diabetes mellitus includes a discussion of the impact of tight control on the development of diabetic complications.

As a new editor, Dr. Stephen L. Hauser, Chairman of the Department of Neurology at the University of California San Francisco, joins Dr. Joseph Martin in providing a comprehensive neurology section applicable to general internal medicine. Dr. Hauser's contributions to Part Fourteen, "Neurologic Disorders," have been substantial, including chapters on multiple sclerosis, disorders of the spinal cord, and stroke. The entire section on neurology has been extensively revised and updated. New or extensively rewritten chapters on neuroimaging, epilepsy, stroke, Alzheimer's disease, Parkinson's disease, ataxia, spinal cord disease, tumors, and chronic meningitis provide an up-to-date summary of this rapidly changing field. The traditional focus of *Harrison's* textbook—providing an in-depth review of the pathophysiologic basis of each neurologic disorder—has been retained, and important advances in molecular pathogenesis and treatment have been included. When possible, diagnostic and therapeutic algorithms have been prepared that standardize and simplify the approach to different neurologic problems. A major effort has been made to expand the neuroimaging figures throughout the section. The anatomic figures have also been expanded and improved.

Finally, Part Fifteen, "Environmental and Occupational Hazards," has been expanded and reorganized.

Beginning with the 12th edition of *Harrison's,* the editors decided to provide laboratory values expressed in two ways: according to the International System (SI) and according to the conventional laboratory terminology used by hospitals in the United States. We felt that this was important because, although the SI units are used in many scientific and medical journals in the United States and elsewhere and in hospitals in many parts of the world, there remains considerable resistance to their adoption from some hospitals and some medical journals. Thus, it is apparent that physicians in many parts of the world will have to live indefinitely with two systems of laboratory values—one for the practice of medicine and another for access to large parts of biomedical science. Consequently, in this edition we continue to list the SI units first and the conventional units in parentheses for all measurements except blood pressure, which is given only in millimeters of mercury, and for those measurements in which the values are the same in both systems, as in the case of serum sodium measurements (expressed in meq/L and mmol/L). In most instances, the interconversion between SI and conventional units is straightforward. However, it is imperative that readers consult their own laboratory for normal values. Perhaps the greatest potential danger inherent in the existence of the two systems is in the interpretation of plasma glucose and plasma calcium levels, but caution should be observed in the interpretation of all laboratory values.

In view of the requirements for continuing education for licensure and relicensure, as well as the emphasis on certification and recertification, a revision of the *Pre-Test Self-Assessment and Review* will be published with this edition. It consists of several hundred questions based on *Harrison's,* along with answers and explanations for the answers. The *Companion Handbook* that was pioneered as a supplement to the 11th edition of *Harrison's* has been updated and will appear shortly after the publication of this edition. The 13th edition of *Harrison's* has been available in a CD-ROM version. An expanded CD-ROM version of the 14th edition will be available and will be regularly updated.

We wish to express our appreciation to our many associates and colleagues, who, as experts in their fields, have helped us with constructive criticism and helpful suggestions. We acknowledge especially the contributions of Gary Abrams, David Acker, Robert Alpern, Donna Ambrosino, Joseph Antin, Karen Antman, James Armitage, Cameron Ashbaugh, Tamar Barlam, Arthur L. Beaudet, Richard Blumberg, Timothy Brewer, Bruce Chabner, Paul Choi, Hal Churchill, Jeffrey Cohen, Oren Cohen, George Curlin, Richard T. Davey, Jr., Margo A. Denke, Judith Falloon, Christopher Fanta, Mark Feinberg, Paul Fitzgerald, Lawrence Friedman, Joseph L. Goldstein, Daryl Gress, Rachel Haft, Helen H. Hobbs, Stephanie James, Clay Johnston, Keith Joiner, Stephen Kohl, Catherine Lachenauer, John LaMontagne, H. Clifford Lane, James Maguire, James Mastrianni, Carol Mendelsohn, Kirk Miller, James Murtagh, Thomas Nutman, Mario Ostrowski, David Ozonoff, Jeffrey Parsonnet, John Reilly, Elizabeth Robbins, David Rosenthal, John Rutherford, Richard Schwartzstein, Robert Seder, Ellen Seely, Julian Seifter, John Spengler, Ray Swanson, Jorge Tavel, Scott Thaler, Kenneth Tyler, Mark Udey, Sasha Vinogradov, C. Fordham von Reyn, Ronald Walls, Fred Wang, Arnold Weinberg, Michael Weinblatt, Scott Weiss, Peter Weller, Michael Wessels, and Stephen Zucker.

This book could not have been edited without the dedicated help of our co-workers in the editorial offices of the individual editors. We are especially indebted to Pat Duffey, Caroline Figoni, Christy K. Gonzales, Terry Jones, Leslie LaPiana, Julie McCoy, Pamela Oliver, Jaylyn Olivo, Kathryn Saxon, Marie Scurti, and Elin Woodger.

Finally, we continue to be indebted to three outstanding members of the McGraw-Hill organization: Mariapaz Ramos Englis, Managing Editor; J. Dereck Jeffers, Editor-in-Chief; and Martin J. Wonsiewicz, Editorial Director. They are an effective team who have given the editors constant encouragement and sage advice and have been of enormous help in bringing this edition to fruition in a timely manner.

The Editors

PART NINE

DISORDERS OF THE RESPIRATORY SYSTEM

SECTION 1
DIAGNOSIS

249

Jeffrey M. Drazen, Steven E. Weinberger

APPROACH TO THE PATIENT WITH DISEASE OF THE RESPIRATORY SYSTEM

Patients with disease of the respiratory system generally present because of symptoms, an abnormality on a chest radiograph, or both. A set of diagnostic possibilities often is suggested by the initial problems at presentation, including the particular symptom(s) and the appearance of any radiographic abnormalities. The differential diagnosis is then refined on the basis of additional information gleaned from physical examination, pulmonary function testing, additional imaging studies, and bronchoscopic examination. This chapter will consider the approach to the patient based on the major patterns of presentation, focusing on the history, the physical examination, and the chest radiograph. Pulmonary function testing is covered in Chap. 250, and other diagnostic studies are discussed in Chap. 251.

CLINICAL PRESENTATION

HISTORY Dyspnea (shortness of breath) and cough are the primary presenting symptoms for patients with respiratory system disease. Less common symptoms include hemoptysis (the coughing up of blood) and chest pain, often with a pleuritic quality.

Dyspnea (See also Chap. 32) When evaluating a patient with shortness of breath, one should first determine the time course over which the symptom has become manifest. Patients who were well previously and developed *acute* shortness of breath (over a period of hours to days) can have acute disease affecting the airways (an acute attack of asthma), the pulmonary parenchyma (acute pulmonary edema or an acute infectious process such as a bacterial pneumonia), the pleural space (a pneumothorax), or the pulmonary vasculature (a pulmonary embolus). A *subacute* presentation (over days to weeks) can suggest an exacerbation of preexisting airways disease (asthma or chronic bronchitis), a parenchymal infection or a noninfectious inflammatory process that proceeds at a relatively slow pace (*Pneumocystis carinii* pneumonia in a patient with AIDS, mycobacterial or fungal pneumonia, Wegener's granulomatosis, eosinophilic pneumonia, bronchiolitis obliterans with organizing pneumonia, and many others), neuromuscular disease (Guillain-Barré syndrome, myasthenia gravis), pleural disease (pleural effusion from a variety of possible causes), or chronic cardiac disease (congestive heart failure). A *chronic* presentation (over months to years) often indicates chronic obstructive lung disease, chronic interstitial lung disease, or chronic cardiac disease. Chronic diseases of airways (not only chronic obstructive lung disease but also asthma) are characterized by exacerbations and remissions. Patients often have periods when they are severely limited by shortness of breath, but these may be interspersed with periods in which symptoms are minimal or absent. In contrast, many of the diseases of pulmonary parenchyma are characterized by a slow but inexorable progression.

Other Respiratory Symptoms *Cough* (Chap. 33) indicates the presence of lung disease, but cough per se is not useful for the differential diagnosis. The presence of sputum accompanying the cough often suggests airway disease and may be seen in asthma, chronic bronchitis, or bronchiectasis.

Hemoptysis (Chap. 33) can originate from disease of the airways, the pulmonary parenchyma, or the vasculature. Diseases of the airways can be inflammatory (acute or chronic bronchitis, bronchiectasis, or cystic fibrosis) or neoplastic (bronchogenic carcinoma or bronchial carcinoid tumors). Parenchymal diseases causing hemoptysis may be either localized (pneumonia, lung abscess, tuberculosis, or infection with *Aspergillus*) or diffuse (Goodpasture's syndrome, idiopathic pulmonary hemosiderosis). Vascular diseases potentially associated with hemoptysis include pulmonary thromboembolic disease and pulmonary arteriovenous malformations.

Chest pain (Chap. 13) caused by diseases of the respiratory system usually originates from involvement of the parietal pleura. As a result, the pain is accentuated by respiratory motion and is often referred to as *pleuritic*. Common examples include primary pleural disorders, such as neoplasm or inflammatory disorders involving the pleura, or pulmonary parenchymal disorders that extend to the pleural surface, such as pneumonia or pulmonary infarction.

Additional Historical Information Information about risk factors for lung disease should be explicitly explored to assure a complete basis of historical data. A history of current and past smoking, especially of cigarettes, should be sought from all patients. The smoking history should include the number of years of smoking, the intensity (i.e., number of packs per day), and, if the patient no longer smokes, the interval since smoking cessation. The risk of lung cancer falls progressively with the interval following discontinuation of smoking, and loss of lung function above the expected age-related decline ceases with the discontinuation of smoking. Even though chronic obstructive lung disease and neoplasia are the two most important respiratory complications of smoking, other respiratory disorders (e.g., spontaneous pneumothorax, eosinophilic granuloma of the lung, and pulmonary hemorrhage with Goodpasture's syndrome) are also associated with smoking. A history of significant secondhand (passive) exposure to smoke, whether in the home or at the workplace, should also be sought as it may be a risk factor for neoplasia or an exacerbating factor for airways disease.

The patient may have been exposed to other inhaled agents associated with lung disease, which act either via direct toxicity or through immune mechanisms (Chaps. 253 and 254). Such exposures can be either occupational or avocational, indicating the importance of detailed occupational and personal histories, the latter stressing exposures related to hobbies or the home environment. Important agents include the inorganic dusts associated with pneumoconiosis (especially asbestos and silica dusts) and organic antigens associated with hypersensitivity pneumonitis (especially antigens from molds and animal proteins). Asthma often is exacerbated by exposure to environmental allergens (dust mites, pet dander, or cockroach allergens in the home or allergens in the outdoor environment such as pollen and ragweed) or may be caused by occupational exposures (diisocyanates). Exposure to particular infectious agents can be suggested by contacts with individuals with known respiratory infections (especially tuberculosis) or by residence in an area with endemic pathogens (histoplasmosis, coccidioidomycosis, blastomycosis).

A history of coexisting nonrespiratory disease or of risk factors for or previous treatment of such diseases should be sought, as they may predispose a patient to both infectious and noninfectious respiratory system complications. Common examples include systemic rheumatic diseases that are associated with pleural or parenchymal lung disease (Chap. 313), metastatic neoplastic disease in the lung, or impaired host defense mechanisms and secondary infection, which occurs in the case of hematologic and lymph node malignancies. Risk factors for AIDS should be sought, as the lungs not only are the most common site of AIDS-defining infection but also can be involved by nonfectious complications of AIDS (Chap. 308). Treatment of nonrespiratory disease can be associated with respiratory complications, either because of effects on host defense mechanisms (immunosuppressive agents, cancer chemotherapy) with resulting infection, or because of direct effects on the pulmonary parenchyma (cancer chemotherapy, radiation therapy, or treatment with other agents, such as amiodarone, that cause interstitial lung disease), or on the airways (beta-blocking agents causing airflow obstruction, angiotensin converting enzyme inhibitors causing cough) (Chap. 253).

Family history is important for evaluating diseases that have a genetic component. These include disorders such as cystic fibrosis, α_1-antitrypsin deficiency, and asthma.

PHYSICAL EXAMINATION The general principles of inspection, palpation, percussion, and auscultation apply to the examination of the respiratory system. However, the physical examination should be directed not only toward ascertaining abnormalities of the lungs and thorax, but also toward recognizing other findings that may reflect underlying lung disease.

On *inspection*, the rate and pattern of breathing as well as the depth and symmetry of lung expansion are observed. Breathing that is unusually rapid, labored, or associated with the use of accessory muscles of respiration generally indicates either augmented respiratory demands or an increased work of breathing. Asymmetric expansion of the chest is usually due to an asymmetric process affecting the lungs, such as endobronchial obstruction of a large airway, unilateral parenchymal or pleural disease, or unilateral phrenic nerve paralysis. Visible abnormalities of the thoracic cage include kyphoscoliosis and ankylosing spondylitis, each of which can alter compliance of the thorax, increase the work of breathing, and cause dyspnea.

On *palpation*, the symmetry of lung expansion can be assessed, generally confirming the findings observed by inspection. Vibration produced by spoken sounds is transmitted to the chest wall and is assessed by the presence or absence and symmetry of tactile fremitus. Transmission of vibration is decreased or absent if pleural liquid is interposed between the lung and the chest wall, or if an endobronchial obstruction alters sound transmission. In contrast, transmitted vibration may increase over an area of underlying pulmonary consolidation.

The relative resonance or dullness of the tissue underlying the chest wall is assessed by *percussion*. The normal sound of underlying air-containing lung is resonant. In contrast, consolidated lung or a pleural effusion sounds dull, while air in the pleural space sounds hyperresonant.

On *auscultation* of the lungs, the examiner listens for both the quality and intensity of the breath sounds and for the presence of extra, or adventitious, sounds. Normal breath sounds heard through the stethoscope at the periphery of the lung are described as *vesicular breath sounds*, in which inspiration is louder and longer than expiration. If sound transmission is impaired by endobronchial obstruction or by air or liquid in the pleural space, breath sounds are weaker or absent. When sound transmission is improved through consolidated lung, the resulting *bronchial breath sounds* have a more tubular quality and a more pronounced expiratory phase. Sound transmission can also be assessed by listening to spoken or whispered sounds; when these are transmitted through consolidated lung, *bronchophony* and *whispered pectoriloquy*, respectively, are present. The sound of a spoken E becomes more like an A, though with a nasal or bleating quality, a finding that is termed *egophony*.

The primary adventitious (abnormal) sounds that can be heard include crackles (rales), wheezes, and rhonchi. *Crackles* represent the sound created when alveoli and small airways open or close during respiration, and often they are associated with interstitial lung disease, microatelectasis, or filling of alveoli by liquid. *Wheezes*, which are generally more prominent during expiration than inspiration, reflect the oscillation of airway walls that occurs when there is airflow limitation, as may be produced by bronchospasm, airway edema or collapse, or intraluminal obstruction by neoplasm or secretions. *Rhonchi* is the term applied to the sounds created when there is free liquid in the airway lumen; the viscous interaction between the free liquid and the moving air creates a low-pitched vibratory sound. Other adventitious sounds include pleural friction rubs and stridor. The gritty sound of a pleural friction rub indicates inflamed pleural surfaces rubbing against each other, often during both inspiratory and expiratory phases of the respiratory cycle. Stridor, which occurs primarily during inspiration, represents flow through a narrowed upper airway, as occurs in an infant with croup.

A summary of the patterns of physical findings on pulmonary examination in common types of respiratory system disease is shown in Table 249-1.

A meticulous *general physical examination* is mandatory in patients with disorders of the respiratory system. Enlarged lymph nodes in the cervical and supraclavicular regions should be sought. Disturbances of mentation or even coma occur in patients with acute carbon dioxide retention and hypoxemia. Telltale stains on the fingers point to heavy cigarette smoking; infected teeth and gums may occur in patients with aspiration pneumonitis and lung abscess.

Clubbing of the digits can be found in lung cancer, interstitial lung disease, and chronic infections in the thorax, such as bronchiectasis, lung abscess, and empyema. Clubbing can also be seen with congenital heart disease associated with right-to-left shunting and with

Table 249-1

Typical Chest Examination Findings in Selected Clinical Conditions

Condition	Percussion	Fremitus	Breath Sounds	Voice Transmission	Adventitious Sounds
Normal	Resonant	Normal	Vesicular (at lung bases)	Normal	Absent
Consolidation or atelectasis (with patent airway)	Dull	Increased	Bronchial	Bronchophony, whispered pectoriloquy, egophony	Crackles
Consolidation or atelectasis (with blocked airway)	Dull	Decreased	Decreased	Decreased	Absent
Asthma	Resonant	Normal	Vesicular	Normal	Wheezing
Interstitial lung disease	Resonant	Normal	Vesicular	Normal	Crackles
Emphysema	Hyperresonant	Decreased	Decreased	Decreased	Absent or wheezing
Pneumothorax	Hyperresonant	Decreased	Decreased	Decreased	Absent
Pleural effusion	Dull	Decreased	Decreased*	Decreased*	Absent or pleural friction rub

* May be altered by collapse of underlying lung, which will increase transmission of sound.

SOURCE: Adapted from Weinberger.

a variety of chronic inflammatory or infectious diseases, such as inflammatory bowel disease and endocarditis. A number of systemic diseases, such as systemic lupus erythematosus, scleroderma, and rheumatoid arthritis, may be associated with pulmonary complications, even though their primary clinical manifestations and physical findings are not primarily related to the lungs. Conversely, other diseases that most affect the respiratory system, such as sarcoidosis, can have findings on physical examination not related to the respiratory system, including ocular findings (uveitis, conjunctival granulomas) and skin findings (erythema nodosum, cutaneous granulomas).

CHEST RADIOGRAPHY

Chest radiography is often the initial diagnostic study performed to evaluate patients with respiratory symptoms, but it can also provide the initial evidence of disease in patients who are free of symptoms. Perhaps the most common example of the latter situation is the finding of one or more nodules or masses when the radiograph is performed for a reason other than evaluation of respiratory symptoms.

A number of diagnostic possibilities are often suggested by the radiographic pattern. A localized region of opacification involving the air spaces is usually characterized as having an alveolar, an interstitial, or a nodular pattern. In contrast, increased radiolucency can be localized, as seen with a cyst or bulla, or generalized, as occurs with emphysema. The chest radiograph is also particularly useful for the detection of pleural disease, especially if manifested by the presence of air or liquid in the pleural space. An abnormal appearance of the hila and/or the mediastinum can suggest a mass or enlargement of lymph nodes.

A summary of representative diagnoses suggested by these common radiographic patterns is presented in Table 249-2.

Additional Diagnostic Evaluation Further information for clarification of radiographic abnormalities is frequently obtained with computed tomographic scanning of the chest (see Chap. 251). This technique is more sensitive than plain radiography in detecting subtle abnormalities, can suggest the presence of certain diseases based on the pattern of abnormality, and is very useful as a means of gathering quantitative information about specific radiographic findings. The use of other imaging studies, including magnetic resonance imaging, scintigraphic studies, ultrasound, and angiography, are discussed in Chap. 251.

Alteration in the function of the lungs as a result of respiratory system disease is assessed objectively by pulmonary function tests, and effects on gas exchange are evaluated by measurement of arterial blood gases or by oximetry (Chap. 250). As part of pulmonary function testing, quantitation of forced expiratory flow assesses the presence of obstructive physiology, which is consistent with diseases affecting the structure or function of the airways, such as asthma and chronic obstructive lung disease. Measurement of lung volumes assesses the presence of restrictive disorders, seen with diseases of the pulmonary parenchyma or respiratory pump and with space-occupying processes of the pleura.

Bronchoscopy is useful in some settings for visualizing abnormalities of the airways and for obtaining a variety of samples from either the airway or the pulmonary parenchyma (Chap. 251).

Table 249-2

Major Respiratory Diagnoses with Common Chest Radiographic Patterns

Solitary circumscribed density—nodule (<6 cm) or mass (≥6 cm)
Primary or metastatic neoplasm
Localized infection (bacterial abscess, mycobacterial or fungal infection)
Wegener's granulomatosis (one or several nodules)
Rheumatoid nodule (one or several nodules)
Vascular malformation
Bronchogenic cyst
Localized opacification (infiltrate)
Pneumonia (bacterial, atypical, mycobacterial, or fungal infection)
Neoplasm
Radiation pneumonitis
Bronchiolitis obliterans with organizing pneumonia
Bronchocentric granulomatosis
Pulmonary infarction
Diffuse interstitial disease
Idiopathic pulmonary fibrosis
Pulmonary fibrosis with systemic rheumatic disease
Sarcoidosis
Drug-induced lung disease
Pneumoconiosis
Hypersensitivity pneumonitis
Infection (*Pneumocystis*, viral pneumonia)
Eosinophilic granuloma
Diffuse alveolar disease
Cardiogenic pulmonary edema
Acute respiratory distress syndrome
Diffuse alveolar hemorrhage
Infection (*Pneumocystis*, viral or bacterial pneumonia)
Sarcoidosis
Diffuse nodular disease
Metastatic neoplasm
Hematogenous spread of infection (bacterial, mycobacterial, fungal)
Pneumoconiosis
Eosinophilic granuloma

INTEGRATION OF THE PRESENTING CLINICAL PATTERN AND DIAGNOSTIC STUDIES

Patients with respiratory symptoms but a normal chest radiograph most commonly have diseases affecting the airways, such as asthma or chronic obstructive pulmonary disease. However, the latter diagnosis is also commonly associated with radiographic abnormalities, such as diaphragmatic flattening and attenuation of vascular markings. Other disorders of the respiratory system for which the chest radiograph is normal include disorders of the respiratory pump (either the chest wall or the neuromuscular apparatus controlling the chest wall) and occasionally interstitial lung disease. Chest examination and pulmonary function tests are generally helpful in sorting out these diagnostic possibilities. Obstructive diseases associated with a normal or relatively normal chest radiograph are often characterized by findings on physical examination and pulmonary function testing that are typical for these conditions. Similarly, diseases of the respiratory pump or interstitial diseases may also be suggested by findings on physical examination or by particular patterns of restrictive disease seen on pulmonary function testing.

When respiratory symptoms are accompanied by radiographic abnormalities, diseases of the pulmonary parenchyma or the pleura are usually present. Either diffuse or localized parenchymal lung disease is generally visualized well on the radiograph, and both air and liquid in the pleural space (pneumothorax and pleural effusion, respectively) are usually readily detected by radiography.

Radiographic findings in the absence of respiratory symptoms often indicate localized disease affecting the airways or the pulmonary parenchyma. One or more nodules or masses can suggest intrathoracic malignancy, but they also can be the manifestation of a current or previous infectious process. Patients with diffuse parenchymal lung disease present on radiographic examination may be free of symptoms, as is sometimes the case with pulmonary sarcoidosis.

In approaching the patient with pulmonary disease, consideration must be given to the observation that substantial changes in the relative incidence of disease affecting the respiratory system have taken place in the United States during the past three decades. The prevalence of chronic infectious disorders such as lung abscess and bronchiectasis has decreased. Tuberculosis declined only to undergo resurgence when two susceptible populations, patients with AIDS and immigrants from Southeast Asia, increased in number. Patients with chronic bronchitis and with emphysema now survive longer and form an increasing fraction of patients with chronic respiratory disease, as do patients with environmental lung disease and with drug-induced pulmonary disease. Modern intercontinental travel has increased the appearance in the western world of parasitic infestations of the lung. Also, the reduction of immune competence that occurs in patients with AIDS and in diabetics as well as in patients being treated for a variety of malignancies and those receiving immunosuppressive drugs has led to an increasing incidence of opportunistic infections of the lungs with a variety of microorganisms that were rarely pathogenic in the past.

BIBLIOGRAPHY

DeGowin R et al: *DeGowin & DeGowin's Diagnostic Examination*, 6th ed. New York, McGraw-Hill, 1994

Ebi-Kryston KL: Respiratory symptoms and pulmonary function as predictors of 10-year mortality from respiratory disease, cardiovascular disease, and all causes in the Whitehall Study. J Clin Epidemiol 41:251, 1988

Godden DJ et al: Outcome of wheeze in childhood. Symptoms and pulmonary function 25 years later. Am J Respir Crit Care Med 149:106, 1994

Weinberger SE: *Principles of Pulmonary Medicine*, 2d ed. Philadelphia, Saunders, 1992

Welty C et al: The relationship of airways responsiveness to cold air, cigarette smoking, and atopy to respiratory symptoms and pulmonary function in adults. Am Rev Respir Dis 130:198, 1984

250

Steven E. Weinberger, Jeffrey M. Drazen

DISTURBANCES OF RESPIRATORY FUNCTION

The respiratory system includes the lungs, the central nervous system (CNS), the chest wall (with the diaphragm and intercostal muscles), and the pulmonary circulation. The CNS controls the activity of the muscles of the chest wall, which constitute the pump of the respiratory system. Because these components of the respiratory system act in concert to achieve gas exchange, malfunction of an individual component or alteration of the relationships among components can lead to disturbances in function. In this chapter we consider three major aspects of disturbed respiratory function: (1) disturbances in ventilatory function, (2) disturbances in the pulmonary circulation, and (3) disturbances in gas exchange. Disorders relating to CNS control of ventilation are discussed in Chap. 263.

DISTURBANCES IN VENTILATORY FUNCTION

Ventilation is the process whereby the lungs replenish the gas in the alveoli. Measurements of ventilatory function in common diagnostic use consist of quantification of the gas volume contained in the lungs under certain circumstances and the rate at which gas can be expelled from the lungs. Two measurements of lung volume commonly used for respiratory diagnosis are total lung capacity (TLC) and residual volume (RV). The former is the volume of gas contained in the lungs after a maximal inspiration, whereas the latter is the volume of gas remaining in the lungs at the end of a maximal expiration. The volume of gas that is exhaled from the lungs in going from TLC to RV is called the *vital capacity* (VC) (Fig. 250-1).

Common clinical measurements of airflow are obtained from maneuvers in which the subject inspires to TLC and then forcibly exhales to RV. Three measurements are commonly made from a volume-time recording—i.e., a spirogram—obtained during such a forced expiratory maneuver: (1) the volume of gas exhaled during the first second of expiration (forced expiratory volume in 1 s, or FEV_1), (2) the total volume exhaled (forced vital capacity, or FVC), and (3) the average expiratory flow rate during the middle 50 percent of the vital capacity (forced expiratory flow between 25 and 75 percent of the vital capacity, or $FEF_{25-75\%}$, also called the maximal midexpiratory flow rate, or MMFR) (Fig. 250-2).

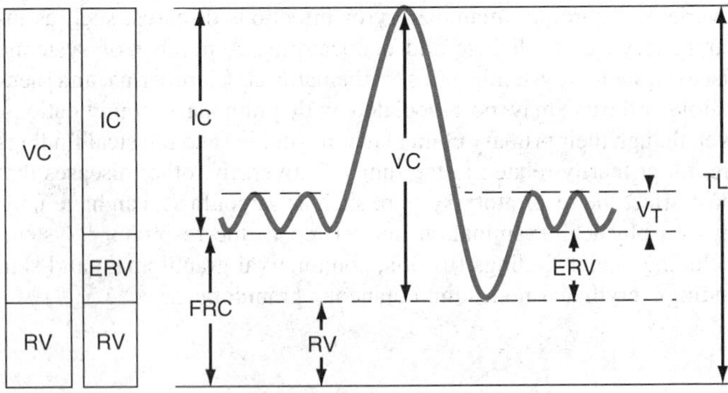

FIGURE 250-1 Lung volumes, shown by block diagrams *(left)* and by a spirographic tracing *(right)*. TLC, total lung capacity; VC, vital capacity; RV, residual volume; IC, inspiratory capacity; ERV, expiratory reserve volume; FRC, functional residual capacity; V_T, tidal volume. *(From Weinberger, with permission.)*

PHYSIOLOGIC FEATURES The lungs are elastic structures, containing collagen and elastic fibers that resist expansion. For normal lungs to contain air, they must be distended either by a positive internal pressure—i.e., by a pressure in the airways and alveolar spaces—or by a negative external pressure—i.e., by a pressure outside the lung. The relationship between the volume of gas contained in the lungs and the distending pressure (the transpulmonary pressure, or P_{TP}, defined as internal pressure minus external pressure) is described by the pressure-volume curve of the lungs (Fig. 250-3*A*).

The chest wall is also an elastic structure, with properties similar to those of an expandable and compressible spring. The relationship between the volume enclosed by the chest wall and the distending pressure for the chest wall is described by the pressure-volume curve of the chest wall (Fig. 250-3*B*). For the chest wall to assume a volume different from its resting volume, the internal or external pressures acting on it must be altered.

At functional residual capacity (FRC), defined as the volume of gas in the lungs at the end of a normal exhalation, the lungs are partially inflated, so their elastic recoil exerts a force tending to empty the lungs. At the same time, chest wall volume is such that its elastic recoil promotes outward expansion. Functional residual capacity oc-

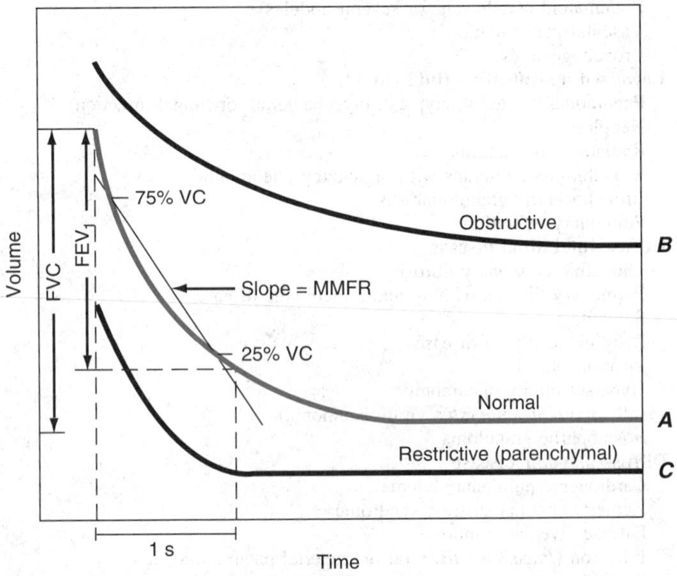

FIGURE 250-2 Spirographic tracings of forced expiration, comparing a normal tracing *(A)* and tracings in obstructive *(B)* and parenchymal restrictive *(C)* disease. Calculations of FVC, FEV_1, and $FEF_{25-75\%}$ are shown only for the normal tracing. Since there is no measure of absolute starting volume with spirometry, the curves are artificially positioned to show the relative starting lung volumes in the different conditions.

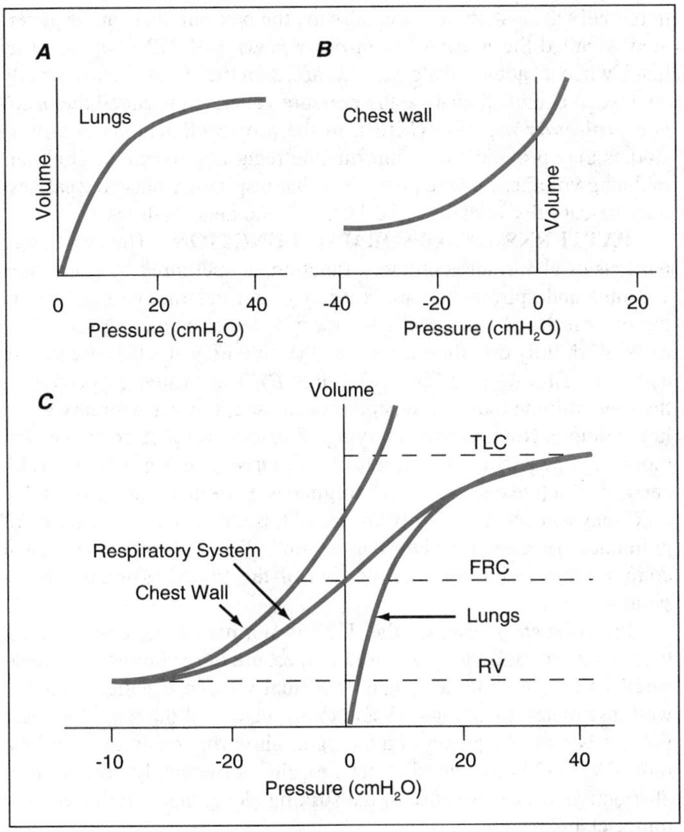

FIGURE 250-3 *A.* Pressure-volume curve of the lungs. *B.* Pressure-volume curve of the chest wall. *C.* Pressure-volume curve of the respiratory system, showing the superimposed component curves of the lungs and the chest wall. RV, residual volume; FRC, functional residual capacity; TLC, total lung capacity. *(From Weinberger, with permission.)*

curs at the lung volume at which the tendency of the lungs to contract is opposed by the equal and opposite tendency of the chest wall to expand (Fig. 250-3*C*).

For the lungs and the chest wall to achieve a volume other than the resting volume (FRC), either the pressures acting on them must be changed passively—for example, by a mechanical ventilator that delivers positive pressure to the airways and alveoli—or the respiratory muscles must actively oppose the tendency of the lungs and the chest wall to return to FRC. During inhalation to volumes above FRC, the inspiratory muscles actively overcome the tendency of the respiratory system to decrease volume back to FRC. During active exhalation to volumes below FRC, expiratory muscle activity must overcome the tendency of the respiratory system to increase volume back to FRC. At TLC, the maximal force applied by the inspiratory muscles to expand the lungs is opposed mainly by the inward recoil of the lungs. As a consequence, the major determinants of TLC are the stiffness of the lungs and inspiratory muscle strength. If the lungs become stiffer—i.e., less compliant—TLC is decreased. If the lungs become less stiff (more compliant), TLC is increased. If the inspiratory muscles are significantly weakened, they are less able to overcome the inward elastic recoil of the lungs, and TLC is lowered.

At RV, the force exerted by the expiratory muscles to decrease lung volume further is balanced by the outward recoil of the chest wall, which becomes extremely stiff at low lung volumes. Two factors influence the volume of gas contained in the lungs at RV. The first is the ability of the subject to exert a prolonged expiratory effort, which is related to muscle strength and the ability to overcome sensory stimuli from the chest wall. The second is the ability of the lungs to empty to a small volume. In normal lungs, as P_{TP} is lowered, lung volume decreases. In lungs with diseased airways, as P_{TP} is lowered, flow limitation or airway closure can limit the amount of gas that is expired. Consequently, either weak chest wall muscles or intrinsic airways disease can result in an elevation in measured RV.

Dynamic measurements of ventilatory function are made by having the subject inhale to TLC and then perform a forced expiration to RV. If a subject performs a series of such expiratory maneuvers using increasing muscular intensity, expiratory flow rates will increase until a certain level of effort is reached. Beyond this level, additional effort will not increase the forced expiratory flow rate; this phenomenon is known as the *effort independence* of forced expiratory flow. The physiologic mechanisms determining the flow rates during this effort-independent phase of forced expiratory flow have been shown to be the elastic recoil of the lung, the airflow resistance of the airways between the alveolar zone and the physical site of flow limitation, and the airway wall compliance at the site of flow limitation. Physical processes that decrease elastic recoil, increase airflow resistance, or increase airway wall compliance decrease the flow rate that can be achieved at any given lung volume. Conversely, processes that increase elastic recoil, decrease resistance, or stiffen airway walls increase the flow rate that can be achieved at any given lung volume.

MEASUREMENT OF VENTILATORY FUNCTION Ventilatory function is measured under static conditions for determination of lung volumes and under dynamic conditions for determination of forced expiratory flow rates. VC, expiratory reserve volume (ERV), and inspiratory capacity (IC) (see Fig. 250-1) are measured by having the patient breathe into and out of a spirometer, a device capable of measuring expired or inspired gas volume while plotting volume as a function of time. Other volumes—specifically, RV, FRC, and TLC—cannot be measured in this way because they include the volume of gas present in the lungs even after a maximal expiration. Two techniques are commonly used to measure these volumes: helium dilution and body plethysmography. In the helium dilution method, the subject repeatedly breathes in and out from a reservoir with a known volume of gas containing a trace amount of helium. The helium is diluted by the gas previously present in the lungs and is not absorbed into the pulmonary circulation. From knowledge of the reservoir volume and the initial and final helium concentrations, the volume of gas present in the lungs can be calculated. The helium dilution method may underestimate the volume of gas in the lungs if there are slowly communicating airspaces, such as bullae. In this situation, lung volumes can be more accurately measured with a body plethysmograph, a sealed box in which the patient sits while panting against a closed mouthpiece. Because there is no airflow into or out of the plethysmograph, the pressure changes in the thorax during panting cause compression and rarefaction of gas in the lungs and simultaneous rarefaction and compression of gas in the plethysmograph. By measuring the pressure changes in the plethysmograph and at the mouthpiece, the volume of gas in the thorax can be calculated using Boyle's law.

Lung volumes and measurements made during forced expiration are interpreted by comparing the values measured with the values expected given the age, height, sex, and race of the patient (see Appendix A). Regression curves have been constructed on the basis of data obtained from large numbers of normal, nonsmoking individuals without evidence of lung disease. Predicted values for a given patient can then be obtained by using the patient's age and height in the appropriate regression equation; different equations are used depending on the patient's race and gender. Because there is some variability among normal individuals, values between 80 and 120 percent of the predicted value have traditionally been considered normal. Increasingly, calculated percentiles are used in determining normality. Specifically, values of individual measurements falling below the fifth percentile are considered to be below normal.

The normal value for the ratio FEV_1/FVC is approximately 0.75 to 0.80, although this value does fall somewhat with advancing age. The $FEF_{25-75\%}$ is often considered a more sensitive measurement of early airflow obstruction, particularly in small airways. However, this measurement must be interpreted cautiously in patients with abnormally small lungs (low TLC and VC). These patients exhale less air during forced expiration, and the $FEF_{25-75\%}$ may appear abnormal rela-

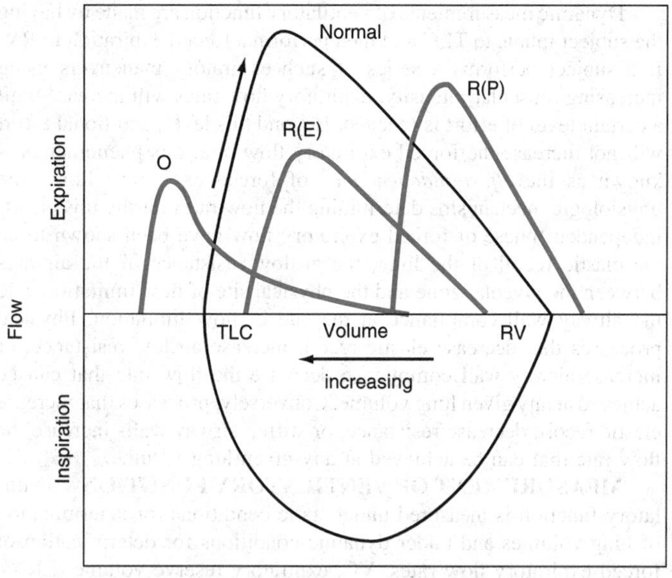

FIGURE 250-4 Flow-volume curves in different conditions: O, obstructive disease; R(P), parenchymal restrictive disease; R(E), extraparenchymal restrictive disease with limitation in inspiration and expiration. Forced expiration is plotted in all conditions; forced inspiration is shown only for the normal curve. TLC, total lung capacity; RV, residual volume. By convention, lung volume increases to the left on the abscissa. The arrow alongside the normal curve indicates the direction of expiration from TLC to RV.

tive to the usual predicted value, even though it is normal relative to the size of the patient's lungs.

It is also a common practice to plot expiratory flow rates against lung volume (rather than against time); the close linkage of flow rates to lung volumes produces a typical *flow-volume curve* (Fig. 250-4). In addition, the spirometric values mentioned above can be calculated from the flow-volume curve. Commonly, flow rates during a maximal inspiratory effort performed as rapidly as possible are plotted as well, making the flow-volume curve into a *flow-volume loop*. At TLC, before expiratory flow starts, the flow rate is zero; once forced expiration has begun, a high peak flow rate is rapidly achieved. As expiration continues and lung volume approaches RV, the flow rate falls progressively, in a nearly linear fashion as a function of lung volume for a person with normal lung function. During maximal inspiration from RV to TLC, inspiratory flow is most rapid at the midpoint of inspiration, so the inspiratory portion of the loop is U-shaped or saddle-shaped. The flow rates achieved during maximal expiration can be analyzed quantitatively by comparing the flow rates at specified lung volumes with the predicted values or qualitatively by analyzing the shape of the descending limb of the expiratory curve.

Assessing the strength of respiratory muscles is an additional part of the overall evaluation of some patients with respiratory dysfunction. When a patient exhales completely to RV and then tries to inspire maximally against an occluded airway, the pressure that can be generated is called the *maximal inspiratory pressure* (MIP). On the other hand, when a patient inhales to TLC and then tries to expire maximally against an occluded airway, the pressure generated is called the *maximal expiratory pressure* (MEP). In the proper clinical setting, these studies may provide useful information regarding the cause of abnormal lung volumes and the possibility that respiratory muscle weakness may be causally related to the lung volume abnormalities.

PATTERNS OF ABNORMAL FUNCTION The two major patterns of abnormal ventilatory function, as measured by static lung volumes and spirometry, are restrictive and obstructive patterns. In the *obstructive pattern*, the hallmark is a decrease in expiratory flow rates. With fully established disease, the ratio FEV_1/FVC is decreased, as is the $FEF_{25-75\%}$ (see Fig. 250-2, line *B*). The expiratory portion of the flow-volume loop demonstrates decreased flow rates for any given lung volume. Nonuniform emptying of airways is reflected by a coved (concave upward) configuration of the curve (see Fig. 250-4). With early obstructive disease, which originates in the small airways, FEV_1/FVC may be normal; the only abnormalities noted on routine testing of pulmonary function may be a depression in $FEF_{25-75\%}$ and an abnormal configuration in the terminal portion of the forced expiratory flow-volume curve.

In *obstructive* disease, the TLC is normal or increased. When helium equilibration tests are used to measure lung volumes, the measured volume may be less than the actual volume if helium was not well distributed to all airways and to all regions of the lung. Residual volume is elevated owing to trapping of air during expiration, and the ratio RV/TLC is increased. Vital capacity is frequently decreased in obstructive disease because of the striking elevations in RV with only minor changes in TLC.

A *restrictive pattern* can be broadly divided into two subgroups, depending on the location of the pathology—pulmonary parenchymal and extraparenchymal. For extraparenchymal disease, dysfunction can be predominantly in inspiration or in both inspiration and expiration (Table 250-1). The hallmark of a restrictive pattern, found in all these subcategories, is a decrease in lung volumes, primarily TLC and VC. In pulmonary parenchymal disease, RV is also generally decreased, and forced expiratory flow rates are preserved. In fact, when FEV_1 is considered as a percentage of the FVC, the flow rates are often supranormal, i.e., disproportionately high relative to the size of the lungs (see Fig. 250-2, line *C*). The flow-volume curve may graphically demonstrate this disproportionate relationship between flow rates and lung volumes, since the expiratory portion of the curve appears relatively tall (preserved flow rates) but narrow (decreased lung volumes), as shown in Fig. 250-4.

In the extraparenchymal pattern characterized by *inspiratory dysfunction*, caused either by inspiratory muscle weakness or a stiff chest wall, inadequate distending forces are exerted on an otherwise normal lung. As a result, TLC values are less than predicted, RV is often not significantly affected, and expiratory flows are preserved. If inspiratory muscle weakness is the cause of this pattern, then MIP is decreased. In the extraparenchymal pattern characterized by *inspiratory and expiratory dysfunction*, the ability to expire to a normal RV is also limited, because of either expiratory muscle weakness or a deformed chest wall that is abnormally rigid at volumes below FRC. Consequently, RV is often elevated, unlike the pattern observed in the other restrictive subcategories. The ratio FEV_1/FVC is variable and depends on expiratory muscle strength. If expiratory muscle strength is significantly decreased, then MEP is decreased, the ability to expire rapidly is impaired, and FEV_1/FVC may be decreased even though there is no airflow obstruction. If expiratory muscle strength is normal but the chest wall is abnormally stiff below FRC, then FEV_1/FVC is normal or increased.

Table 250-1

Alterations in Ventilatory Function

	TLC	RV	VC	FEV_1/FVC	MIP	MEP
Obstructive	N to $\uparrow$	$\uparrow$	$\downarrow$	$\downarrow$*	N	N
Restrictive						
Pulmonary parenchymal	$\downarrow$	$\downarrow$	$\downarrow$	N to $\uparrow$	N	N
Extraparenchymal—inspiratory	$\downarrow$	N to $\downarrow$	$\downarrow$	N	$\downarrow$/N†	N
Extraparenchymal—inspiratory + expiratory	$\downarrow$	$\uparrow$	$\downarrow$	Variable	$\downarrow$/N†	$\downarrow$/N†

* Mild obstructive (small airways) disease may have $FEF_{25-75\%}$ with normal FEV_1/FVC.
† Reduced if due to respiratory muscle weakness; normal if due to chest wall stiffness.
NOTE: N = normal; for other abbreviations, see text.

Table 250-2

Common Respiratory Diseases by Diagnostic Categories

Obstructive	
	Asthma
	Chronic obstructive lung disease (chronic bronchitis, emphysema)
	Bronchiectasis
	Cystic fibrosis
	Bronchiolitis
Restrictive—Parenchymal	
	Sarcoidosis
	Idiopathic pulmonary fibrosis
	Pneumoconiosis
	Drug- or radiation-induced interstitial lung disease
Restrictive—Extraparenchymal	
	Neuromuscular
	Diaphragmatic weakness/paralysis
	Myasthenia gravis*
	Guillain-Barré syndrome*
	Muscular dystrophies*
	Cervical spine injury*
	Chest wall
	Kyphoscoliosis
	Obesity
	Ankylosing spondylitis*

* Can have inspiratory and expiratory limitation (see text).

CLINICAL CORRELATIONS Table 250-1 summarizes the expected alterations in ventilatory function as indicated by pulmonary function testing. One reason to establish a ventilatory diagnosis is to categorize the functional disorder. This information can be useful in diagnosis, as outlined in Table 250-2. Note that lung disease can be present without abnormal ventilatory function, but the presence of specific diagnostic findings is an aid in differential diagnosis.

DISTURBANCES IN THE PULMONARY CIRCULATION

PHYSIOLOGIC FEATURES The pulmonary vasculature must handle the entire output of the right ventricle, approximately 5 L/min in a normal adult at rest. The comparatively thin-walled vessels of the pulmonary arterial system provide relatively little resistance to flow and are capable of handling this large volume of blood at perfusion pressures that are low compared with those of the systemic circulation. The normal mean pulmonary artery pressure is 15 mmHg, as compared to approximately 95 mmHg for the normal mean aortic pressure. Regional blood flow in the lung is dependent on hydrostatic forces. In an upright person, pulmonary arterial pressure is lowest at the apex of the lung and highest at the lung base. As a result, in the upright position, perfusion is least at the apex and greatest at the base. When cardiac output increases, as occurs during exercise, the pulmonary vasculature is capable of recruiting previously unperfused vessels and distending underperfused vessels, thus responding to the increase in flow with a decrease in pulmonary vascular resistance. In consequence, the increase in mean pulmonary arterial pressure, even with a three- to fourfold increase in cardiac output, is small.

METHODS OF MEASUREMENT Assessment of circulatory function in the pulmonary vasculature depends on measuring pulmonary vascular pressures and cardiac output. Clinically, these measurements are commonly made in intensive care units capable of invasive monitoring and in cardiac catheterization laboratories. With a flow-directed pulmonary arterial (Swan-Ganz) catheter, pulmonary arterial and pulmonary capillary wedge pressures can be measured directly, and cardiac output can be obtained by the thermodilution method. Pulmonary vascular resistance can then be calculated according to the equation

$$PVR = 80(PAP - PCW)/CO$$

where PVR = pulmonary vascular resistance (dyn·s/cm^5); PAP = mean pulmonary arterial pressure (mmHg); PCW = pulmonary capillary wedge pressure (mmHg); and CO = cardiac output (L/min).

The normal value for pulmonary vascular resistance is approximately 50 to 150 dyn·s/cm^5.

MECHANISMS OF ABNORMAL FUNCTION (See also Chap. 260) Pulmonary vascular resistance may increase by a variety of mechanisms. Pulmonary arterial and arteriolar vasoconstriction is a prominent response to alveolar hypoxia. Pulmonary vascular resistance also increases if intraluminal thrombi or proliferation of smooth muscle in vessel walls diminishes the luminal cross-sectional area. If small pulmonary vessels are destroyed, either by scarring or by loss of alveolar walls, the total cross-sectional area of the pulmonary vascular bed diminishes, and pulmonary vascular resistance increases. When pulmonary vascular resistance is elevated, either pulmonary arterial pressure rises to maintain normal cardiac output or cardiac output falls if pulmonary arterial pressure does not increase.

CLINICAL CORRELATIONS Disturbances in the function of the pulmonary vasculature as a result of primary cardiac disease, either congenital heart disease or conditions that elevate left atrial pressure, such as mitral stenosis, are beyond the scope of this chapter and are discussed in Chaps. 235 and 237, respectively. Instead, the focus will be on the pulmonary vasculature as its function is affected by diseases primarily involving the respiratory system, including the pulmonary vessels themselves.

All diseases of the respiratory system causing hypoxemia are potentially capable of increasing pulmonary vascular resistance, since alveolar hypoxia is a very potent stimulus for pulmonary vasoconstriction. The more prolonged and intense the hypoxic stimulus, the more likely it is that a significant increase in pulmonary vascular resistance producing pulmonary hypertension will result. In practice, patients with hypoxemia caused by chronic obstructive lung disease, interstitial lung disease, chest wall disease, and the obesity hypoventilation–sleep apnea syndrome are particularly prone to developing pulmonary hypertension. If there are additional structural changes in the pulmonary vasculature secondary to the underlying process, these will increase the likelihood of developing pulmonary hypertension.

With diseases directly affecting the pulmonary vessels, a decrease in the cross-sectional area of the pulmonary vascular bed is primarily responsible for increased pulmonary vascular resistance, while hypoxemia generally plays a lesser role. In the case of recurrent pulmonary emboli, parts of the pulmonary arterial system are occluded by intraluminal thrombi originating in the systemic venous system. With primary pulmonary hypertension (Chap. 260) or with pulmonary vascular disease secondary to scleroderma, the small pulmonary arteries and arterioles are affected by a generalized obliterative process that narrows and occludes these vessels. Pulmonary vascular resistance increases, and significant pulmonary hypertension often results.

DISTURBANCES IN GAS EXCHANGE

PHYSIOLOGIC FEATURES The primary functions of the respiratory system are to remove the appropriate amount of CO_2 from blood entering the pulmonary circulation and to provide adequate O_2 to blood leaving the pulmonary circulation. For these functions to be carried out properly, there must be adequate provision of fresh air to the alveoli for delivery of O_2 and removal of CO_2 (ventilation), adequate circulation of blood through the pulmonary vasculature (perfusion), adequate movement of gas between alveoli and pulmonary capillaries (diffusion), and appropriate contact between alveolar gas and pulmonary capillary blood (ventilation-perfusion matching).

A normal individual at rest inspires approximately 12 to 16 times per minute, each breath having a tidal volume of approximately 500 mL. A portion (approximately 30 percent) of the fresh air inspired with each breath does not reach the alveoli but remains in the conducting airways of the lung. This component of each breath, which is not generally available for gas exchange, is called the *anatomic dead space component*. The remaining 70 percent reaches the alveolar zone, mixes rapidly with the gas already there, and can participate in gas exchange. In this example, the total ventilation each minute is approximately 7 L, composed of 2 L/min of dead space ventilation and 5 L/min of alveolar ventilation. In certain diseases, some alveoli are ventilated but not perfused, so that some ventilation in addition to the anatomic dead space component is wasted. If total dead space ventilation is increased but total minute ventilation is unchanged, then alveolar ventilation must fall correspondingly.

Gas exchange is dependent on alveolar ventilation rather than total minute ventilation, as outlined below. The partial pressure of CO_2 in arterial blood (Pa_{CO_2}) is directly proportional to the amount of CO_2 produced per minute ($\dot{V}_{CO_2}$) and inversely proportional to alveolar ventilation ($\dot{V}_A$), according to the relationship

$$Pa_{CO_2} = 0.863 \times \dot{V}_{CO_2}/\dot{V}_A$$

where $\dot{V}_{CO_2}$ is expressed in mL/min, $\dot{V}_A$ in L/min, and Pa_{CO_2} in mmHg. At fixed $\dot{V}_{CO_2}$, when alveolar ventilation increases, Pa_{CO_2} falls, and when alveolar ventilation decreases, Pa_{CO_2} rises. Maintaining a normal level of O_2 in the alveoli (and consequently in arterial blood) also depends on provision of adequate alveolar ventilation to replenish alveolar O_2. This principle will become more apparent from consideration of the alveolar gas equation below.

Diffusion of O_2 and CO_2 Both O_2 and CO_2 diffuse readily down their respective concentration gradients through the alveolar wall and pulmonary capillary endothelium. Under normal circumstances, this process is rapid, and equilibration of both gases is complete within one-third of the transit time of erythrocytes through the pulmonary capillary bed. Even in disease states in which diffusion of gases is impaired, the impairment is unlikely to be severe enough to prevent equilibration of CO_2 and O_2. Consequently, a diffusion abnormality rarely results in arterial hypoxemia at rest. If erythrocyte transit time in the pulmonary circulation is shortened, as occurs with exercise, and diffusion is impaired, then diffusion limitation may contribute to hypoxemia. Exercise testing can often demonstrate such physiologically significant abnormalities due to impaired diffusion. Even though diffusion limitation rarely makes a clinically significant contribution to resting hypoxemia, clinical measurements of what is known as *diffusing capacity* (see below) can be a useful measure of the integrity of the alveolar-capillary membrane.

Ventilation-Perfusion Matching In addition to the absolute levels of alveolar ventilation and perfusion, gas exchange depends critically on the proper matching of ventilation and perfusion. The spectrum of possible ventilation-perfusion ($\dot{V}/\dot{Q}$) ratios in an alveolar-capillary unit ranges from zero, in which ventilation is totally absent and the unit behaves as a shunt, to infinity, in which perfusion is totally absent and the unit behaves as dead space. The P_{O_2} and P_{CO_2} of blood leaving each alveolar-capillary unit depend on the gas tension (of blood and air) entering that unit and on the particular $\dot{V}/\dot{Q}$ ratio of the unit. At one extreme, when an alveolar-capillary unit has a $\dot{V}/\dot{Q}$ ratio of 0 and behaves as a shunt, blood leaving the unit has the composition of mixed venous blood entering the pulmonary capillaries, i.e., $P\bar{v}_{O_2} \approx$ 40 mmHg and $P\bar{v}_{CO_2} \approx$ 46 mmHg. At the other extreme, when an alveolar-capillary unit has a high $\dot{V}/\dot{Q}$ ratio, it behaves almost like dead space, and the small amount of blood leaving the unit has partial pressures of O_2 and CO_2 ($P_{O_2} \approx$ 150 mmHg, $P_{CO_2} \approx$ 0 mmHg while breathing room air) approaching the composition of inspired gas.

In the ideal situation, all alveolar-capillary units have equal matching of ventilation and perfusion, i.e., a ratio of approximately 1 when each is expressed in L/min. However, even in the normal individual, some $\dot{V}/\dot{Q}$ mismatching is present, since there is normally a gradient of blood flow from the apices to the bases of the lungs. There is a similar gradient of ventilation from the apices to the bases, but it is less marked than the perfusion gradient. As a result, ventilation-perfusion ratios are higher at the lung apices than at the lung bases. Therefore, blood coming from the apices has a higher P_{O_2} and lower P_{CO_2} than blood coming from the bases. The net P_{O_2} and P_{CO_2} of the blood mixture coming from all areas of the lung is a flow-weighted average of the individual components, which reflects both the relative amount of blood from each unit and the O_2 and CO_2 *content* of the blood coming from each unit. Because of the sigmoid shape of the oxyhemoglobin dissociation curve (see Fig. 107-1), it is important to distinguish between the partial pressure and the content of O_2 in blood. Hemoglobin is almost fully saturated at a P_{O_2} of 60 mmHg, and little additional O_2 is carried by hemoglobin even with a substantial elevation of P_{O_2} above 60 mmHg. On the other hand, significant O_2 desaturation of hemoglobin occurs once P_{O_2} falls below 60 mmHg and onto the steep descending limb of the curve. As a result, blood coming from regions of the lung with a high $\dot{V}/\dot{Q}$ ratio and a high P_{O_2} has only a small elevation in O_2 content and cannot compensate for blood coming from regions with a low $\dot{V}/\dot{Q}$ ratio and a low P_{O_2}, which has a significantly decreased O_2 content. Although $\dot{V}/\dot{Q}$ mismatching can influence P_{CO_2}, this effect is less marked and often is overcome by an increase in overall minute ventilation.

MEASUREMENT OF GAS EXCHANGE **Arterial Blood Gases** The most commonly used measures of gas exchange are the partial pressures of O_2 and CO_2 in arterial blood, i.e., Pa_{O_2} and Pa_{CO_2}, respectively. These partial pressures do not measure directly the quantity of O_2 and CO_2 in blood but rather the driving pressure for the gas in blood. The actual quantity or content of a gas in blood also depends on the solubility of the gas in plasma and the ability of any component of blood to react with or bind the gas of interest. Since hemoglobin is capable of binding large amounts of O_2, oxygenated hemoglobin is the primary form in which O_2 is transported in blood. The actual content of O_2 in blood therefore depends both on the hemoglobin concentration and on the Pa_{O_2}. The Pa_{O_2} determines what percentage of hemoglobin is saturated with O_2, based on the position on the oxyhemoglobin dissociation curve. Oxygen content in normal blood (at 37°C, pH 7.4) can be determined by adding the amount of O_2 dissolved in plasma to the amount bound to hemoglobin, according to the equation

$$O_2 \text{ content} = 1.34 \times [\text{hemoglobin}] \times \text{saturation} + 0.0031 \times P_{O_2}$$

since each gram of hemoglobin is capable of carrying 1.34 mL O_2 when fully saturated, and the amount of O_2 that can be dissolved in plasma is proportional to the P_{O_2}, with 0.0031 mL O_2 dissolved per deciliter of blood per mmHg P_{O_2}. In arterial blood, the amount of O_2 transported dissolved in plasma (approximately 0.3 mL O_2 per deciliter of blood) is trivial compared with the amount bound to hemoglobin (approximately 20 mL O_2 per deciliter of blood).

Most commonly, P_{O_2} is the measurement used to quantitate the adequacy of oxygenation of arterial blood. Direct measurement of O_2 saturation in arterial blood by oximetry is also important in selected clinical conditions. For example, in patients with carbon monoxide exposure, carbon monoxide preferentially displaces O_2 from hemoglobin, essentially making a portion of hemoglobin unavailable for binding to O_2. In this circumstance, carbon monoxide saturation is high and O_2 saturation is low, even though the driving pressure for O_2 to bind to hemoglobin, reflected by P_{O_2}, is normal. Measurement of O_2 saturation is also important for the determination of O_2 content when mixed venous blood is sampled from a pulmonary arterial catheter to calculate cardiac output by the Fick technique. In mixed venous blood, the P_{O_2} is normally about 40 mmHg, but small changes in P_{O_2} may reflect relatively large changes in O_2 saturation.

A useful calculation in the assessment of oxygenation is the alveolar-arterial O_2 difference ($PA_{O_2} - Pa_{O_2}$), commonly called the *alveolar-arterial O_2 gradient* (or A − a gradient). This calculation takes into account the fact that alveolar and, hence, arterial P_{O_2} can be expected to change depending on the level of alveolar ventilation, reflected by the arterial P_{CO_2}. When a patient hyperventilates and has a low P_{CO_2} in arterial blood and alveolar gas, alveolar and arterial P_{O_2} will rise; conversely, hypoventilation and a high P_{CO_2} are accompanied by a decrease in alveolar and arterial P_{O_2}. These changes in arterial P_{O_2} are independent of abnormalities in O_2 transfer at the alveolar-capillary level and reflect only the dependence of alveolar P_{O_2} on the level of alveolar ventilation.

In order to determine the alveolar-arterial O_2 difference, the alveolar P_{O_2} ($P_{A_{O_2}}$) must first be calculated. The equation most commonly used for this purpose, a simplified form of the alveolar gas equation, is

$$P_{A_{O_2}} = F_{I_{O_2}} \times (P_B - P_{H_2O}) - P_{a_{CO_2}}/R$$

where $F_{I_{O_2}}$ = fractional concentration of inspired O_2 (≈0.21 when breathing room air); P_B = barometric pressure (approximately 760 mmHg at sea level); P_{H_2O} = water vapor pressure (47 mmHg when air is fully saturated at 37°C); and R = respiratory quotient (the ratio of CO_2 production to O_2 consumption, usually assumed to be 0.8). If the preceding values are substituted into the equation for the patient breathing air at sea level, the equation becomes

$$P_{A_{O_2}} = 150 - 1.25 \times P_{a_{CO_2}}$$

The alveolar-arterial O_2 difference can then be calculated by subtracting measured $P_{a_{O_2}}$ from calculated $P_{A_{O_2}}$. In a healthy young person breathing room air, the $P_{A_{O_2}} - P_{a_{O_2}}$ is normally less than 15 mmHg; this value increases with age and may be as high as 30 mmHg in elderly patients.

The adequacy of CO_2 elimination is measured by the partial pressure of CO_2 in arterial blood, i.e., $P_{a_{CO_2}}$. A more complete understanding of the mechanisms and chronicity of abnormal levels of P_{CO_2} also requires measurement of pH and/or bicarbonate (HCO_3^-), since P_{CO_2} and the patient's acid-base status are so closely intertwined (see Chap. 50).

Pulse Oximetry Because measurement of $P_{a_{O_2}}$ requires arterial puncture and provides intermittent rather than continuous data about the patient's oxygenation, it is not ideal for close monitoring of unstable patients. Over the past several years, an alternative method for assessing oxygenation, pulse oximetry, has become readily available in many clinical settings. The pulse oximeter measures oxygen saturation (rather than $P_{a_{O_2}}$) using a probe usually clipped over a patient's finger. The device measures absorption of two wavelengths of light by hemoglobin in pulsatile, cutaneous arterial blood. Because of differential absorption of the two wavelengths of light by oxygenated and nonoxygenated hemoglobin, the percentage of hemoglobin that is saturated with oxygen, i.e., the $S_{a_{O_2}}$, can be calculated and displayed instantaneously.

Although the pulse oximeter has been a major advance in the noninvasive, continuous monitoring of oxygenation, there are several issues and potential problems concerning its use. First, the clinician must be aware of the relationship between oxygen saturation and tension as shown by the oxyhemoglobin dissociation curve (see Fig. 107–1). Because the curve becomes relatively flat above an arterial P_{O_2} of 60 mmHg (corresponding to $S_{a_{O_2}}$ = 90 percent), the oximeter is relatively insensitive to changes in $P_{a_{O_2}}$ above this level. In addition, the position of the curve and therefore the specific relationship between $P_{a_{O_2}}$ and $S_{a_{O_2}}$ may change depending on factors such as temperature, pH, and the erythrocyte concentration of 2,3-diphosphoglycerate (2,3-DPG). Second, when cutaneous perfusion is decreased, for example owing to low cardiac output or the use of vasoconstrictors, the signal from the oximeter may be less reliable or even unobtainable. Third, other forms of hemoglobin, such as carboxyhemoglobin and methemoglobin, are not distinguishable when only two wavelengths of light are used. The $S_{a_{O_2}}$ values reported by the pulse oximeter are not reliable in the presence of significant amounts of either of these forms of hemoglobin. In contrast, the device used to measure oxygen saturation in samples of arterial blood, called the CO-oximeter, uses at least four wavelengths of light and is capable of distinguishing oxyhemoglobin, deoxygenated hemoglobin, carboxyhemoglobin, and methemoglobin. Finally, the clinician must remember that the often-used goal of $S_{a_{O_2}} \geq 90$ percent does not indicate anything about CO_2 elimination and therefore does not ensure a clinically acceptable P_{CO_2}.

Diffusing Capacity The ability of gas to diffuse across the alveolar-capillary membrane is ordinarily assessed by the diffusing capacity of the lung for carbon monoxide ($D_{L_{CO}}$). In this test, a small concentration of carbon monoxide (0.3%) is inhaled, usually in a single breath that is held for approximately 10 s. The carbon monoxide is diluted by the gas already present in the alveoli and is also taken up by hemoglobin as the erythrocytes course through the pulmonary capillary system. The concentration of carbon monoxide in exhaled gas is measured, and $D_{L_{CO}}$ is calculated as the quantity of carbon monoxide absorbed per minute per mmHg pressure gradient from the alveoli to the pulmonary capillaries. The value obtained for $D_{L_{CO}}$ depends on the alveolar-capillary surface area available for gas exchange and on the pulmonary capillary blood volume. In addition, the thickness of the alveolar-capillary membrane, the degree of $\dot{V}/\dot{Q}$ mismatching, and the patient's hemoglobin level will affect the measurement. Because of this effect of hemoglobin levels on $D_{L_{CO}}$, the measured $D_{L_{CO}}$ is frequently corrected to take the patient's hemoglobin level into account. The value for $D_{L_{CO}}$, ideally corrected for hemoglobin, can then be compared with a predicted value, based either on age, height, and gender or on the alveolar volume (V_A) at which the value was obtained. Alternatively, the $D_{L_{CO}}$ can be divided by V_A and the resulting value for $D_{L_{CO}}/V_A$ compared with a predicted value.

Approach to the Patient

Arterial Blood Gases Hypoxemia is a common manifestation of a variety of diseases affecting the lungs or other parts of the respiratory system. The broad clinical problem of hypoxemia is often best characterized according to the underlying mechanism. The four basic mechanisms of hypoxemia are (1) a decrease in inspired P_{O_2}, (2) hypoventilation, (3) shunting, and (4) $\dot{V}/\dot{Q}$ mismatching. Hypoxemia due to decreased diffusion occurs only under selected clinical circumstances and is not usually included among the general categories of hypoxemia. Determining the underlying mechanism for hypoxemia depends on measurement of the $P_{a_{CO_2}}$, calculation of $P_{A_{O_2}} - P_{a_{O_2}}$, and knowledge of the response to supplemental O_2. A flowchart summarizing the approach to the hypoxemic patient is given in Fig. 250-5.

A decrease in the inspired P_{O_2} and hypoventilation both cause hypoxemia by lowering $P_{A_{O_2}}$ and therefore $P_{a_{O_2}}$. In each case, gas exchange at the alveolar-capillary level occurs normally, and $P_{A_{O_2}} - P_{a_{O_2}}$ is not elevated. Hypoxemia due to decreased inspired P_{O_2} can be diagnosed from knowledge of the clinical situation. Inspired P_{O_2} is lowered either because the patient is at a high altitude, where barometric pressure is low, or, much less commonly, because the patient is breathing a gas mixture containing less than 21% O_2. The hallmark of hypoventilation as a cause of hypoxemia is an elevation in $P_{a_{CO_2}}$. This is associated with an increase in $P_{A_{CO_2}}$ and a fall in $P_{A_{O_2}}$. When hypoxemia is due purely to a low inspired P_{O_2} or to alveolar hypoventilation, $P_{A_{O_2}} - P_{a_{O_2}}$ is normal. If $P_{A_{O_2}} - P_{a_{O_2}}$ and $P_{a_{CO_2}}$ are both elevated, then an additional mechanism, such as $\dot{V}/\dot{Q}$ mismatching or shunting, is contributing to hypoxemia.

Shunting is a cause of hypoxemia when desaturated blood effectively bypasses oxygenation at the alveolar-capillary level. This situation occurs either because a structural problem allows desaturated blood to bypass the normal site of gas exchange or because perfused alveoli are not ventilated. Shunting is associated with an elevation in the $P_{A_{O_2}} - P_{a_{O_2}}$ value. When shunting is an important contributing factor to hypoxemia, the lowered $P_{a_{O_2}}$ is relatively refractory to improvement by supplemental O_2.

Finally, the largest clinical category of hypoxemia is $\dot{V}/\dot{Q}$ mismatching. With $\dot{V}/\dot{Q}$ mismatching, regions with low $\dot{V}/\dot{Q}$ ratios contribute blood with a low P_{O_2} and a low O_2 content. Corresponding regions with high $\dot{V}/\dot{Q}$ ratios contribute blood with a high P_{O_2}. However, because blood is already almost fully saturated at a normal P_{O_2}, elevation of the P_{O_2} to a high value does not significantly increase O_2 saturation or content and therefore cannot compensate for the reduction of O_2 saturation and content in blood coming from regions with a low $\dot{V}/\dot{Q}$ ratio. When $\dot{V}/\dot{Q}$ mismatch is the primary cause of hypoxemia, $P_{A_{O_2}} - P_{a_{O_2}}$ is elevated, and P_{CO_2} generally is normal. Supplemental O_2 corrects the hypoxemia by raising the P_{O_2} in blood coming from regions with a low $\dot{V}/\dot{Q}$ ratio; this response distinguishes hypoxemia due to $\dot{V}/\dot{Q}$ mismatching from that due to true shunt.

The essential mechanism underlying all cases of hypercapnia is alveolar ventilation that is inadequate for the amount of CO_2 produced. It is conceptually useful to characterize CO_2 retention further, based on a more detailed examination of the potential contributing factors. These include (1) increased CO_2 production, (2) decreased ventilatory drive ("won't breathe"), (3) malfunction of the respiratory pump or increased airways resistance, which makes it more difficult to sustain adequate ventilation ("can't breathe"), and (4) inefficiency of gas exchange (increased dead space or $\dot{V}/\dot{Q}$ mismatch) necessitating a compensatory increase in overall minute ventilation. In practice, more than one of these mechanisms is commonly responsible for hypercapnia, since increased minute ventilation is capable of compensating for increased CO_2 production and for inefficiencies of gas exchange.

Diffusing Capacity Although abnormalities in diffusion are rarely responsible for hypoxemia, clinical measurement of diffusing capacity is frequently used to assess the functional integrity of the alveolar-capillary membrane, which includes the pulmonary capillary bed. Diseases that affect solely the airways generally do not lower $D_{L_{CO}}$, whereas diseases that affect the alveolar walls or the pulmonary capillary bed will have an effect on $D_{L_{CO}}$. Even though $D_{L_{CO}}$ is a useful marker for assessing whether disease affecting the alveolar-capillary bed is present, an abnormal $D_{L_{CO}}$ does not necessarily imply that diffusion limitation is responsible for hypoxemia in a particular patient.

CLINICAL CORRELATIONS Useful clinical correlations can be made with the mechanisms underlying hypoxemia (see Fig. 250-5). A lowered inspired P_{O_2} contributes to hypoxemia if either the patient is at high altitude or if the concentration of inspired O_2 is less than 21%. The latter problem occurs if a patient receiving anesthesia or ventilatory support is inadvertently given a gas mixture to breathe containing less than 21% O_2 or if O_2 is consumed from the ambient gas, as can occur during smoke inhalation from a fire. The primary feature of hypoventilation as a cause of hypoxemia is an elevation in arterial P_{CO_2}. The clinical correlations with hypoventilation are discussed in Chap. 263.

Shunting as a cause of hypoxemia can reflect transfer of blood from the right to the left side of the heart without passage through the pulmonary circulation, as occurs with an intracardiac shunt. This problem is most common in the setting of cyanotic congenital heart disease, when an interatrial or interventricular septal defect is associated with pulmonary hypertension so that shunting is in the right-to-left rather than the left-to-right direction. Shunting of blood through the pulmonary parenchyma is most frequently due to disease causing absence of ventilation to perfused alveoli. This can occur if the alveoli are atelectatic or if they are filled with fluid, as in pulmonary edema (both cardiogenic and noncardiogenic) or with extensive intraalveolar exudation of fluid due to pneumonia. Less commonly, vascular anomalies with arteriovenous shunting in the lung can cause hypoxemia. These anomalies can be hereditary, as found with hereditary hemorrhagic telangiectasia (Osler-Rendu-Weber syndrome), or acquired, as in pulmonary vascular malformations secondary to hepatic cirrhosis, which are similar to the commonly recognized cutaneous vascular malformations ("spider hemangiomas").

Ventilation-perfusion mismatch is the most common cause of hypoxemia clinically. Most of the processes affecting either the airways or the pulmonary parenchyma are distributed unevenly throughout the lungs and do not necessarily affect ventilation and perfusion equally. Some areas of lung may have good perfusion and poor ventilation, whereas others may have poor perfusion and relatively good ventilation. Important examples of airways diseases in which $\dot{V}/\dot{Q}$ mismatch causes hypoxemia are asthma and chronic obstructive lung disease. Parenchymal lung diseases causing $\dot{V}/\dot{Q}$ mismatch and hypoxemia include interstitial lung disease and pneumonia.

Clinically important alterations in CO_2 elimination range from excessive ventilation and hypocapnia to inadequate CO_2 elimination and hypercapnia. These clinical problems are discussed in Chap. 263.

Diffusing Capacity Measurement of $D_{L_{CO}}$ may be useful for assessing disease affecting the alveolar-capillary bed or the pulmonary vasculature. In practice, three main categories of disease are associated with lowered $D_{L_{CO}}$: interstitial lung disease, emphysema, and pulmonary vascular disease. With interstitial lung disease, scarring of alveolar-capillary units diminishes the area of the alveolar-capillary bed as well as pulmonary blood volume. With emphysema, alveolar walls are destroyed, so the surface area of the alveolar-capillary bed is again diminished. In patients with disease causing a decrease in the cross-sectional area and volume of the pulmonary vascular bed, such as

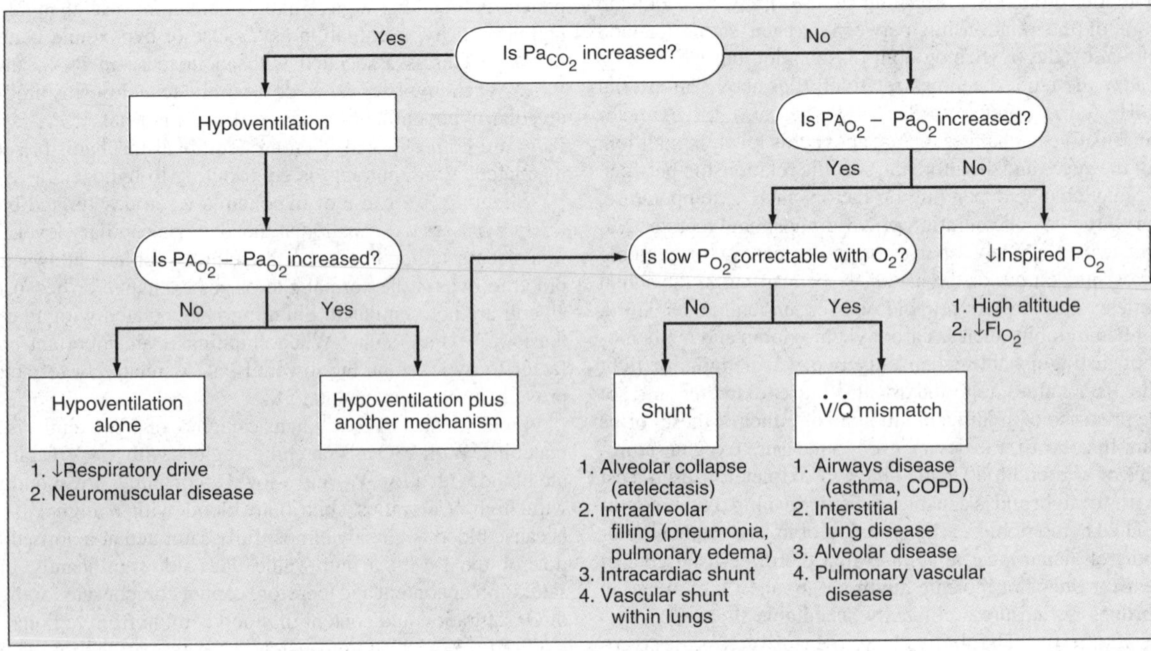

FIGURE 250-5 Flow diagram outlining the diagnostic approach to the patient with hypoxemia (Pa_{O_2} < 80 mmHg). $PA_{O_2} - Pa_{O_2}$ is usually < 15 mmHg for subjects ≤30 years old and increases by ~3 mmHg per decade after age 30.

recurrent pulmonary emboli or primary pulmonary hypertension, DL_{CO} is commonly diminished.

Diffusing capacity may be elevated if pulmonary blood volume is increased, as may be seen in congestive heart failure. However, once interstitial and alveolar edema ensue, the net DL_{CO} depends on the opposing influences of increased pulmonary capillary blood volume elevating DL_{CO} and pulmonary edema decreasing it. Finding an elevated DL_{CO} may be useful in the diagnosis of alveolar hemorrhage, as in Goodpasture's syndrome. Hemoglobin contained in erythrocytes in the alveolar lumen is capable of binding carbon monoxide, so the exhaled carbon monoxide concentration is diminished and the measured DL_{CO} is increased.

BIBLIOGRAPHY

American Thoracic Society: Lung function testing: Selection of reference values and interpretative strategies. Am Rev Respir Dis 144:1202, 1991

Clark JS et al: Noninvasive assessment of blood gases. Am Rev Respir Dis 145:220, 1992

Crapo RO: Pulmonary-function testing. N Engl J Med 331:25, 1994

———, Forster RE II: Carbon monoxide diffusing capacity. Clin Chest Med 10:187, 1989

Gibson GJ: Standardised lung function testing. Eur Respir J 6:155, 1993

Quanjer PH et al: Lung volumes and forced ventilatory flows. Report Working Party Standardization of Lung Function Tests, European Community for Steel and Coal. Official Statement of the European Respiratory Society. Eur Respir J [Suppl] 16:5, 1993

Society of Critical Care Medicine: A model for technology assessment applied to pulse oximetry. Crit Care Med 21:615, 1993

Weinberger SE: *Principles of Pulmonary Medicine*, 2d ed. Philadelphia, Saunders, 1992

West JB: *Respiratory Physiology: The Essentials*, 5th ed. Baltimore, Williams & Wilkins, 1995

251

Steven E. Weinberger, Jeffrey M. Drazen

DIAGNOSTIC PROCEDURES IN RESPIRATORY DISEASE

The diagnostic modalities available for assessing the patient with suspected or known respiratory system disease include imaging studies and techniques for acquiring biologic specimens, some of which involve direct visualization of part of the respiratory system. Methods used to characterize the functional changes developing as a result of disease, including pulmonary function tests and measurements of gas exchange, are discussed in Chap. 250.

IMAGING STUDIES

ROUTINE RADIOGRAPHY Routine chest radiography, which generally includes both posteroanterior and lateral views, is an integral part of the diagnostic evaluation of diseases involving the pulmonary parenchyma, the pleura, and, to a lesser extent, the airways and the mediastinum. Common radiographic patterns and their clinical correlates are reviewed in Chap. 249. Lateral decubitus views are often useful for determining whether pleural abnormalities represent freely flowing fluid, whereas apical lordotic views can often visualize disease at the lung apices better than the standard posteroanterior view. Portable equipment, which is often used for acutely ill patients who either cannot be transported to a radiology suite or cannot stand up for posteroanterior and lateral views, generally yields just a single radiograph taken in the anteroposterior direction.

COMPUTED TOMOGRAPHY Computed tomography (CT) offers several advantages over routine chest radiography. First, the use of cross-sectional images often makes it possible to distinguish between densities that would be superimposed on plain radiographs. Second, CT is far better than routine radiographic studies at characterizing tissue density, distinguishing subtle differences in density between adjacent structures, and providing accurate size assessment of lesions. As a result, CT is particularly valuable in assessing hilar and mediastinal disease (which is often poorly characterized by plain radiography), in identifying and characterizing disease adjacent to the chest wall or spine (including pleural disease), and in identifying areas of fat density or calcification in pulmonary nodules (Fig. 251-1). Its utility in the assessment of mediastinal disease has made CT an important tool in the staging of lung cancer (see Chap. 90), as an assessment of tumor involvement of mediastinal lymph nodes is critical to proper staging. With the additional use of contrast material, CT also makes it possible to distinguish vascular from nonvascular structures, particularly important in distinguishing lymph nodes and masses from vascular structures.

Helical CT scanning allows the collection of continuous data over a larger volume of lung during a single breath-holding maneuver than is possible with conventional CT. With high-resolution CT (HRCT), the thickness of individual cross-sectional images is approximately 1 to 2 mm, rather than the usual 10 mm, and the images are reconstructed using high-spatial-resolution algorithms. The detail that can be seen on HRCT scans allows better recognition of subtle parenchymal and airway disease, such as bronchiectasis, emphysema, and diffuse parenchymal disease (Fig. 251-2). Certain nearly pathognomonic patterns have now been recognized for many of the interstitial lung diseases, such as lymphangitic carcinoma, idiopathic pulmonary fibrosis, sarcoidosis, and eosinophilic granuloma; at present it is not yet clear in what settings these patterns will obviate the need for obtaining lung tissue.

MAGNETIC RESONANCE IMAGING The role of magnetic resonance imaging (MRI) in the evaluation of respiratory system disease is less well defined than that of CT. Because MRI generally provides a less detailed view of the pulmonary parenchyma as well as poorer spatial resolution, its usefulness in the evaluation of parenchymal lung disease is limited at present. However, MRI has advantages over CT in certain clinical settings. Because its images can be reconstructed in sagittal and coronal as well as transverse planes, MRI may be better for imaging abnormalities near the lung apex, the spine, and the thoracoabdominal junction. In addition, vascular structures can be distinguished from nonvascular structures without the need for contrast. Flowing blood does not produce a signal on MRI, so vessels appear as hollow tubular structures. This feature can be useful in determining whether abnormal hilar or mediastinal densities are vascular in origin and in defining aortic lesions such as aneurysms or dissection.

SCINTIGRAPHIC IMAGING Radioactive isotopes, administered by either intravenous or inhaled routes, allow the lungs to be imaged with a gamma camera. The most common use of such imaging is ventilation-perfusion lung scanning performed for evaluation of

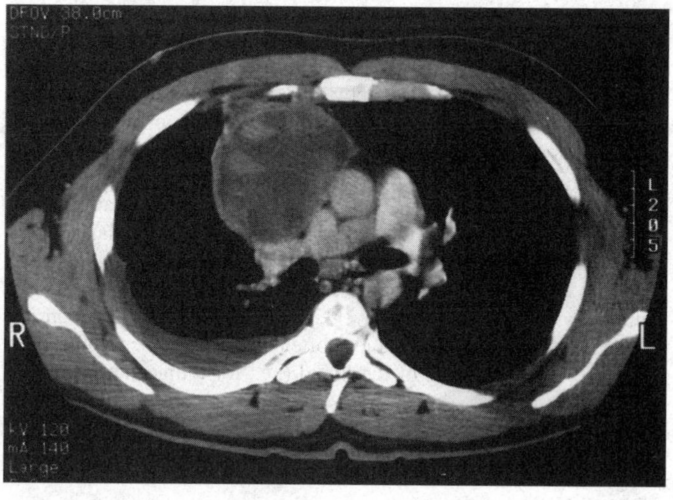

FIGURE 251-1 CT scan demonstrating a mediastinal mass of heterogenous density. CT is superior to plain radiography for the detection of abnormal mediastinal densities and the distinction of masses from adjacent vascular structures.

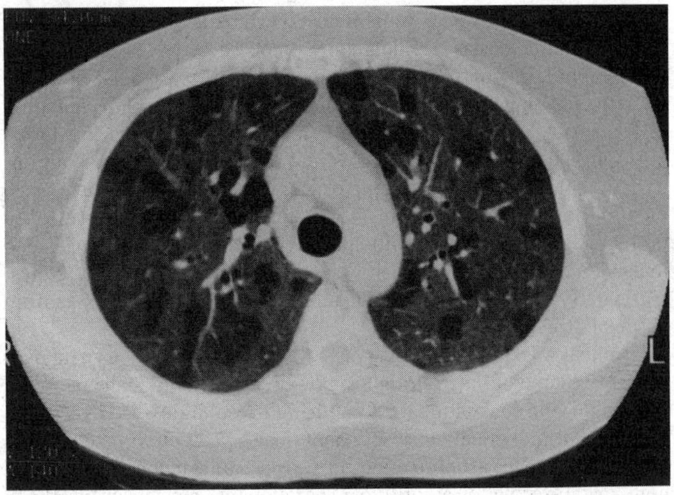

FIGURE 251-2 High-resolution CT scan demonstrating pulmonary parenchyma with a heterogeneous appearance. Most of the parenchyma has a subtle "ground-glass" pattern of increased density, best recognized by comparison with the intervening areas of normal lung, which have irregular but well-defined borders. The ground-glass pattern in this patient was due to hypersensitivity pneumonitis.

pulmonary embolism. When injected intravenously, albumin macroaggregates labeled with technetium 99m become lodged in pulmonary capillaries; therefore, the distribution of the trapped radioisotope follows the distribution of blood flow. When inhaled, radiolabeled xenon gas can be used to demonstrate the distribution of ventilation. For example, pulmonary thromboembolism usually produces one or more regions of ventilation-perfusion mismatch—that is, regions in which there is a defect in perfusion that follows the distribution of a vessel and that is not accompanied by a corresponding defect in ventilation (see Chap. 261). Another common use of such radioisotope scans is in a patient with impaired lung function who is being considered for lung resection. The distribution of the isotope(s) can be used to assess the regional distribution of blood flow and ventilation, allowing the physician to estimate the level of postoperative lung function.

Another scintigraphic imaging technique, gallium imaging, has been of diagnostic value in patients with *Pneumocystis carinii* pneumonia and other opportunistic infections. Use of gallium imaging may provide clues to sort out the differential diagnosis of pulmonary infiltrates in immunosuppressed patients, especially patients with AIDS.

PULMONARY ANGIOGRAPHY The pulmonary arterial system can be visualized by pulmonary angiography, in which radiopaque contrast medium is injected through a catheter previously threaded into the pulmonary artery. When performed in cases of pulmonary embolism, pulmonary angiography demonstrates the consequences of an intravascular clot—either a defect in the lumen of a vessel (a "filling defect") or an abrupt termination ("cutoff") of the vessel. Other, less common indications for pulmonary angiography include visualization of a suspected pulmonary arteriovenous malformation and assessment of pulmonary arterial invasion by a neoplasm.

ULTRASOUND Because ultrasound energy is rapidly dissipated in air, ultrasound imaging is not useful for evaluation of the pulmonary parenchyma. However, it is helpful in the detection and localization of pleural liquid and is often used as a guide to placement of a needle for sampling of the liquid (i.e., for thoracentesis).

TECHNIQUES FOR OBTAINING BIOLOGIC SPECIMENS

COLLECTION OF SPUTUM Sputum can be collected either by spontaneous expectoration or after inhalation of an irritating aerosol, such as hypertonic saline. The latter method, called *sputum induction*, is used routinely to obtain sputum for diagnostic studies. Knowledge of the appearance and quality of the sputum specimen obtained is especially important when one is interested in Gram's staining and culture. Because sputum consists mainly of secretions from the tracheobronchial tree rather than the upper airway, the finding of alveolar macrophages and other inflammatory cells is consistent with a lower respiratory tract origin of the sample, whereas the presence of squamous epithelial cells in a "sputum" sample indicates contamination by secretions from the upper airways.

Besides processing for routine bacterial pathogens by Gram's staining and culture, sputum can be processed for a variety of other pathogens, including staining and culture for mycobacteria or fungi, culture for viruses, and staining for *P. carinii*. In the specific case of sputum obtained for evaluation of *P. carinii* pneumonia in a patient infected with human immunodeficiency virus (HIV), for example, sputum should be collected by induction, rather than spontaneous expectoration, and an immunofluorescent stain should be used to detect the organisms. Cytologic staining of sputum for malignant cells, using the traditional Papanicolaou method, allows noninvasive evaluation for suspected lung cancer. Traditional stains and cultures are now also being supplemented in some cases by immunologic techniques and by molecular biologic methods, including the use of polymerase chain reaction amplification and DNA probes.

PERCUTANEOUS NEEDLE ASPIRATION A needle can be inserted through the chest wall into a pulmonary lesion for the purpose of aspirating material for analysis by cytologic or microbiologic techniques. The procedure is usually carried out under CT guidance, which assists in the positioning of the needle and assures that it is localized in the lesion. Although the potential risks of this procedure include intrapulmonary bleeding and creation of a pneumothorax with collapse of the underlying lung, the low risk of complication in experienced hands is usually worth the information obtained.

THORACENTESIS Sampling of pleural liquid by thoracentesis is commonly performed for diagnostic purposes or, in the case of a large effusion, for palliation of dyspnea. Diagnostic sampling, either by blind needle aspiration or after localization by ultrasound, allows the collection of liquid for microbiologic and cytologic studies. Analysis of the fluid obtained for its cellular composition and chemical constituents, including glucose, protein, and lactate dehydrogenase, allows the effusion to be classified as either exudative or transudative (Chap. 262). In some cases, particularly in the setting of possible tuberculous involvement of the pleura (tuberculous pleuritis), closed biopsy of the parietal pleura is also performed, using a cutting needle (either an Abrams or a Cope biopsy needle) to sample tissue for histopathologic examination and culture.

BRONCHOSCOPY Bronchoscopy is the process of direct visualization of the tracheobronchial tree. Bronchoscopy with a rigid bronchoscope is generally performed in an operating room on a patient under general anesthesia. The development of a flexible fiberoptic bronchoscope has revolutionized the diagnostic use of bronchoscopy. Although bronchoscopy is now performed almost exclusively with fiberoptic instruments, rigid bronchoscopes still have a role in selected circumstances, primarily because of their larger suction channel and the fact that the patient can be ventilated through the bronchoscope channel. These situations include the retrieval of a foreign body and the suctioning of a massive hemorrhage, for which the small suction channel of the bronchoscope may be insufficient.

Flexible Fiberoptic Bronchoscopy This is an outpatient procedure that is usually performed in an awake though sedated patient. The bronchoscope is passed through either the mouth or the nose, between the vocal cords, and into the trachea. The ability to flex the scope makes it possible to visualize virtually all airways to the level of subsegmental bronchi. The bronchoscopist is able to identify endobronchial pathology, including tumors, granulomas, bronchitis, foreign bodies, and sites of bleeding. Samples from airway lesions can be taken by several methods, including washing, brushing, and biopsy. Washing involves instillation of sterile saline through a channel of the bronchoscope and onto the surface of a lesion. A portion of the liquid is collected by suctioning through the bronchoscope, and the recovered material can be analyzed for cells (cytology) or organisms (by standard stains and cultures). Brushing or biopsy of the surface of the lesion, using a small brush or biopsy forceps at the end of a long cable inserted through a channel of the bronchoscope, allows recovery of cellular material or tissue for analysis by standard cytologic and histopathologic methods. The bronchoscope may provide the opportunity for treatment as well as diagnosis. For example, an aspirated foreign body may be retrieved with an instrument passed through the scope, and bleeding may be controlled with a balloon catheter similarly introduced.

The bronchoscope can be used to sample material not only from the regions that can be directly visualized (i.e., the airways) but also from the more distal pulmonary parenchyma. With the bronchoscope wedged into a subsegmental airway, aliquots of sterile saline can be instilled through the scope, allowing sampling of cells and organisms even from alveolar spaces. This procedure, called *bronchoalveolar lavage*, has been particularly useful for the recovery of organisms such as *P. carinii* in patients with HIV infection.

Brushing and biopsy of the distal lung parenchyma can also be performed using the same instruments that are used for endobronchial sampling. These instruments can be passed through the scope into small airways, where they penetrate the airway wall, allowing biopsy of peribronchial alveolar tissue. This procedure, called *transbronchial biopsy*, is used when there is either relatively diffuse disease or a localized lesion of adequate size. With the aid of fluoroscopic imaging, the bronchoscopist is able to determine not only whether and when the instrument is in the area of abnormality, but also the proximity of the instrument to the pleural surface. If the forceps are too close to the pleural surface, there is a risk of violating the visceral pleura and creating a pneumothorax; the other potential complication of transbronchial biopsy is pulmonary hemorrhage. The incidence of these complications is less than several percent.

A relatively new procedure involves use of a hollow-bore needle passed through the bronchoscope for sampling of tissue adjacent to the trachea or a large bronchus. The needle is passed through the airway wall, and cellular material can be aspirated from mass lesions or enlarged lymph nodes, generally in a search for malignant cells. This procedure can facilitate the staging of lung cancer by identifying mediastinal lymph node involvement and in some cases obviates the need for a more invasive procedure.

VIDEO-ASSISTED THORACIC SURGERY Recent advances in video technology have allowed the development of thoracoscopy, or video-assisted thoracic surgery (VATS), for the diagnosis and management of pleural as well as parenchymal lung disease. This procedure, done under general anesthesia, involves the passage of a rigid scope with a distal lens through a trocar inserted into the pleura. A high-quality image is shown on a monitor screen, allowing the operator to manipulate instruments passed into the pleural space through separate small intercostal incisions. With these instruments, the operator can biopsy lesions of the pleura under direct vision, which provides an obvious advantage over closed pleural biopsy. In addition, this procedure is now used commonly to biopsy peripheral lung tissue or to remove peripheral nodules, for both diagnostic and therapeutic purposes. Because this procedure is much less invasive than the traditional thoracotomy performed for lung biopsy, it has largely supplanted "open lung biopsy."

THORACOTOMY Although frequently replaced by VATS, thoracotomy remains an option for the diagnostic sampling of lung tissue. It provides the largest amount of material, and it can be used to biopsy and/or excise lesions that are too deep or too close to vital structures for removal by VATS. The choice between VATS and thoracotomy needs to be made on a case-by-case basis, and the relative indications for each are still evolving as more experience is being gained with VATS.

MEDIASTINOSCOPY AND MEDIASTINOTOMY Tissue biopsy is often critical for the diagnosis of mediastinal masses or enlarged mediastinal lymph nodes. Although CT is useful for determining the size of mediastinal lymph nodes as part of the staging of lung cancer, confirmation that enlarged lymph nodes are actually involved with tumor generally requires biopsy and histopathologic examination. The two major procedures used to obtain specimens from masses or nodes in the mediastinum are mediastinoscopy (via a suprasternal approach) and mediastinotomy (via a parasternal approach). Both procedures are performed under general anesthesia by a qualified surgeon. In the case of suprasternal mediastinoscopy, a rigid mediastinoscope is inserted at the suprasternal notch and passed into the mediastinum along a pathway just anterior to the trachea. Tissue can be obtained with biopsy forceps passed through the scope, sampling masses or nodes that are in a paratracheal or pretracheal position. Left paratracheal and aortopulmonary lymph nodes are not accessible by this route and thus are commonly sampled by parasternal mediastinotomy (the Chamberlain procedure). This approach involves either a right or left parasternal incision and dissection directly down to a mass or node that requires biopsy.

BIBLIOGRAPHY

DICHTER JR et al: Approach to the immunocompromised host with pulmonary symptoms. Hematol Oncol Clin North Am 7:887, 1993

ETTINGER NA: Invasive diagnostic approaches to pulmonary infiltrates. Semin Respir Infect 8:168, 1993

HARRIS RJ et al: The diagnostic and therapeutic utility of thoracoscopy. A review. Chest 108:828, 1995

MCELVEIN RB: Procedures in the evaluation of chest disease. Clin Chest Med 13:1, 1992

MURRAY JF, NADEL JA: *Textbook of Respiratory Medicine*, 2d ed. Philadelphia, Saunders, 1994

NAIDICH DP et al: *Computed Tomography and Magnetic Resonance of the Thorax*, 2d ed. New York, Raven Press, 1991

WANG K-P, MEHTA AC: *Flexible Bronchoscopy*, Cambridge, MA, Blackwell, 1995

WEINBERGER SE: *Principles of Pulmonary Medicine*, 2d ed. Philadelphia, Saunders, 1992

SECTION 2

DISEASES OF THE RESPIRATORY SYSTEM

252

E. R. McFadden, Jr.

ASTHMA

DEFINITION Asthma is a disease of airways that is characterized by increased responsiveness of the tracheobronchial tree to a multiplicity of stimuli. It is manifested physiologically by a widespread narrowing of the air passages, which may be relieved spontaneously or as a result of therapy, and clinically by paroxysms of dyspnea, cough, and wheezing. Asthma is an episodic disease, acute exacerbations being interspersed with symptom-free periods. Typically, most attacks are short-lived, lasting minutes to hours, and clinically the patient seems to recover completely after an attack. However, there can be a phase in which the patient experiences some degree of airways obstruction daily. This phase can be mild, with or without superimposed severe episodes, or much more serious, with severe obstruction persisting for days or weeks, a condition known as *status asthmaticus*. In unusual circumstances, acute episodes can cause death.

PREVALENCE AND ETIOLOGY Asthma is very common; it is estimated that 4 to 5 percent of the population of the United States is affected. Similar figures have been reported from other countries. Bronchial asthma occurs at all ages but predominantly in early life. About one-half of cases develop before age 10, and another third occur before age 40. In childhood, there is a 2:1 male/female preponderance, but the sex ratio equalizes by age 30.

From an etiologic standpoint, asthma is a heterogeneous disease. It is useful for epidemiologic and clinical purposes to classify asthma by the principal stimuli that incite or are associated with acute episodes. However, it is important to emphasize that this distinction may often be artificial, and the response of a given subclassification usually can be initiated by more than one type of stimulus. Further, the application of molecular and cell biologic techniques to asthma pathogenesis is also beginning to blur this type of classification. With these reservations in mind, one can describe two broad types of asthma: allergic and idiosyncratic.

Allergic asthma is often associated with a personal and/or family history of allergic diseases such as rhinitis, urticaria, and eczema, with positive wheal-and-flare skin reactions to intradermal injection of extracts of airborne antigens, with increased levels of IgE in the serum, and/or with a positive response to provocation tests involving the inhalation of specific antigen.

A significant fraction of asthmatic patients present with no personal or family history of allergy, with negative skin tests, and with normal serum levels of IgE, and therefore have disease that cannot be classified on the basis of defined immunologic mechanisms. These patients are said to have *idiosyncratic asthma*. Many develop a typical symptom complex upon contracting an upper respiratory illness. The initial insult may be little more than a common cold, but after several days the patient begins to develop paroxysms of wheezing and dyspnea that can last for days to months. These individuals should not be confused with persons in whom the symptoms of bronchospasm are superimposed on chronic bronchitis or bronchiectasis (Chaps. 256 and 258).

Many patients have disease that does not fit clearly into either of the preceding categories but instead falls into a mixed group with features of each. In general, asthma that has its onset in early life tends to have a strong allergic component, whereas asthma that develops late tends to be nonallergic or to have a mixed etiology.

PATHOGENESIS OF ASTHMA The common denominator underlying the asthmatic diathesis is a nonspecific hyperirritability of the tracheobronchial tree. When airway reactivity is high, symptoms are more severe and persistent, and the amount of therapy required to control the patient's complaints is greater. In addition, the magnitude of diurnal fluctuations in lung function is greater, and the patient tends to awaken at night or in the early morning with breathlessness.

In both normal and asthmatic subjects, airway reactivity rises following viral infections of the respiratory tract and exposure to oxidant air pollutants such as ozone and nitrogen dioxide (but not sulfur dioxide). Viral infections have more profound consequences, and airway responsiveness may remain elevated for many weeks after a seemingly trivial upper respiratory tract infection. In contrast, airway reactivity remains high for only a few days after exposure to ozone. Allergens can cause airway responsiveness to rise within minutes and to remain elevated for weeks. If the dose of antigen is high enough, acute episodes of obstruction may occur daily for a prolonged period following a single exposure.

A number of causes have been postulated for the increased airway reactivity of asthma, but the basic mechanism remains unknown. The most popular hypothesis at present is that of airway inflammation. Increased numbers of mast cells, epithelial cells, neutrophils, eosinophils, and lymphocytes have been found in the bronchoalveolar lavage fluid of patients with asthma, as have a variety of mediators. An active inflammatory process is frequently observed in endobronchial biopsy specimens even from asymptomatic patients. The airways can be edematous and infiltrated with eosinophils, neutrophils, and lymphocytes, with or without thickening of the epithelial basement membrane. There may also be glandular hypertrophy. The most ubiquitous finding is a generalized increase in cellularity associated with an elevated capillary density. Occasionally, denudation of the epithelium may also be observed.

Although the translation of these histologic observations into a disease process is still incomplete, it is widely believed that the physiologic and clinical features of asthma derive from an interaction among the resident and infiltrating inflammatory cells in the airways and the surface epithelium. The cells thought to play important roles are mast cells, eosinophils, macrophages, neutrophils, and lymphocytes. The mediators released—histamine; bradykinin; the leukotrienes C, D, and E; platelet-activating factor; and prostaglandins (PGs) E_2, $F_2\alpha$, and D_2—produce an intense, immediate inflammatory reaction involving bronchoconstriction, vascular congestion, and edema formation. In addition to their ability to evoke prolonged contraction of airway smooth muscle and mucosal edema, the leukotrienes may also account for some of the other pathophysiologic features of asthma, such as increased mucus production and impaired mucociliary transport. This intense local event can then be followed by a more chronic one. The chemotactic factors elaborated (eosinophil and neutrophil chemotactic factors of anaphylaxis and leukotriene B_4) bring eosinophils, platelets, and polymorphonuclear leukocytes to the site of the reaction. These infiltrating cells as well as resident macrophages and the airway epithelium itself potentially are an additional source of mediators to enhance both the immediate and the cellular phase.

Like the mast cell in the early reaction, the eosinophil appears to play an important part in the infiltrative component. The granular proteins in this cell (major basic protein and eosinophilic cationic protein) are capable of destroying the airway epithelium, which then is sloughed into the bronchial lumen in the form of Creola bodies. Besides resulting in a loss of barrier and secretory function, such damage elicits the production of chemotactic cytokines, leading to further inflammation. In theory, it also can expose sensory nerve endings, thus initiating neurogenic inflammatory pathways. That, in turn, could convert a primary local event into a generalized reaction via a reflex mechanism.

T lymphocytes also appear to be important in the inflammatory response. These cells are present in increased numbers in asthmatic airways and produce cytokines that activate cell-mediated immunity, as well as humoral (IgE) immune responses. Furthermore, the T_H1 and T_H2 lymphocyte subtypes have functions that may influence the asthmatic response. The T_H1 cytokines interleukin (IL) 2 and interferon (IFN) γ can promote the growth and differentiation of B cells and the activation of macrophages, respectively. The T_H2 cytokine IL-4 and IL-5 stimulate B-cell growth and immunoglobulin secretion, and IL-5 promotes eosinophil proliferation, differentiation, and activation. It can also facilitate granule release from basophils.

The relative roles of each of these components in the production of heightened airway reactivity and clinical asthma has yet to be determined. It is unlikely that any one cell type or mediator accounts for every feature. For example, mast cell–derived mediators cannot explain the whole picture, for they have been found in the blood of individuals with mast cell–related diseases such as cold-induced and cholinergic-induced urticaria and in the airways of atopic nonasthmatics. Since these individuals had no lower respiratory illness or complaints, these alleged mediators of asthma would appear to need a unique background from which to exhibit their effects. Similarly, the inflammatory cells believed to be relevant to asthma are also found in the airways of atopic nonasthmatics, raising the possibility that they are merely nonspecific markers of atopy rather than specific indexes of asthma. Finally, therapeutic administration of IL-2 and granulocyte-macrophage colony stimulating factor to cancer patients results in eosinophilia with cell activation but not in asthma.

The stimuli that interact with airway responsiveness and incite acute episodes of asthma can be grouped into seven major categories:

allergenic, pharmacologic, environmental, occupational, infectious, exercise-related, and emotional.

Allergens Allergic asthma is dependent on an IgE response controlled by T and B lymphocytes and activated by the interaction of antigen with mast cell–bound IgE molecules. Most of the allergens that provoke asthma are airborne, and to induce a state of sensitivity they must be reasonably abundant for considerable periods of time. Once sensitization has occurred, however, the patient can exhibit exquisite responsivity, so that minute amounts of the offending agent can produce significant exacerbations of the disease. Immune mechanisms appear to be causally related to the development of asthma in 25 to 35 percent of all cases and to be contributory in perhaps another third. Higher prevalences have been suggested, but it is difficult to know how to interpret the data because of confounding factors. Allergic asthma is frequently seasonal, and it is most often observed in children and young adults. A nonseasonal form may result from allergy to feathers, animal danders, dust mites, molds, and other antigens that are present continuously in the environment. Exposure to antigen typically produces an immediate response in which airways obstruction develops in minutes and then resolves. In 30 to 50 percent of patients, a second wave of bronchoconstriction, the so-called late reaction, develops 6 to 10 h later. In a minority, only a late reaction occurs. It was formerly thought that the late reaction was essential to the development of the increase in airways reactivity that follows antigen exposure. Recent data show that not to be the case.

The mechanism by which an inhaled allergen provokes an acute episode of asthma depends in part on antigen-antibody interactions on the surface of pulmonary mast cells, with the subsequent generation and release of the mediators of immediate hypersensitivity. Current hypotheses hold that very small antigenic particles penetrate the lung's defenses and come in contact with mast cells that interdigitate with the epithelium at the luminal surface of the central airways. (No mechanism has yet been proposed that explains how antigen can contact the mast cells in the submucosa.) The subsequent elaboration of mediators and cytokines then produces the sequence outlined above.

Pharmacologic Stimuli The drugs most commonly associated with the induction of acute episodes of asthma are aspirin, coloring agents such as tartrazine, beta-adrenergic antagonists, and sulfiting agents. It is important to recognize drug-induced bronchial narrowing because its presence is often associated with great morbidity. Furthermore, death sometimes has followed the ingestion of aspirin (or other nonsteroidal anti-inflammatory agents) or beta-adrenergic antagonists. The typical aspirin-sensitive respiratory syndrome primarily affects adults, although the condition may be seen in childhood. This problem usually begins with perennial vasomotor rhinitis that is followed by a hyperplastic rhinosinusitis with nasal polyps. Progressive asthma then appears. On exposure to even very small quantities of aspirin, affected individuals typically develop ocular and nasal congestion and acute, often severe episodes of airways obstruction. The prevalence of aspirin sensitivity in asthmatic subjects varies from study to study, but many authorities feel that 10 percent is a reasonable figure. There is a great deal of cross reactivity between aspirin and other nonsteroidal anti-inflammatory compounds. Indomethacin, fenoprofen, naproxen, zomepirac sodium, ibuprofen, mefenamic acid, and phenylbutazone are particularly important in this regard. On the other hand, acetaminophen, sodium salicylate, choline salicylate, salicylamide, and propoxyphene are well tolerated. The exact frequency of cross reactivity to tartrazine and other dyes in aspirin-sensitive asthmatic subjects is also controversial; again, 10 percent is the commonly accepted figure. This peculiar complication of aspirin-sensitive asthma is particularly insidious, however, in that tartrazine and other potentially troublesome dyes are widely present in the environment and may be unknowingly ingested by sensitive patients.

Patients with aspirin sensitivity can be desensitized by daily administration of the drug. Following this form of therapy, cross tolerance also develops to other nonsteroidal anti-inflammatory agents. The mechanism by which aspirin and other such drugs produce bronchospasm has not yet been elucidated but may be related to aspirin-induced preferential generation of leukotrienes. Immediate hypersensitivity does not seem to be involved. The availability of effective inhibitors of leukotriene synthesis or receptor activity should aid materially in the treatment of this problem.

Beta-adrenergic antagonists regularly obstruct the airways in asthmatics as well as in others with heightened airway reactivity and should be avoided by such individuals. Even the selective $beta_1$ agents have this propensity, particularly at higher doses. In fact, the local use of $beta_1$ blockers in the eye for the treatment of glaucoma has been associated with worsening asthma.

Sulfiting agents, such as potassium metabisulfite, potassium and sodium bisulfite, sodium sulfite, and sulfur dioxide, which are widely used in the food and pharmaceutical industries as sanitizing and preserving agents, also can produce acute airways obstruction in sensitive individuals. Exposure usually follows ingestion of food or beverages containing these compounds, e.g., salads, fresh fruit, potatoes, shellfish, and wine. Exacerbation of asthma has been reported following the use of sulfite-containing topical ophthalmic solutions, intravenous glucocorticoids, and some inhalational bronchodilator solutions. The incidence and mechanism of action of this phenomenon are unknown. When suspected, the diagnosis can be confirmed by either oral or inhalational provocations.

Environment and Air Pollution (See Chap. 254) Environmental causes of asthma are usually related to climatic conditions that promote the concentration of atmospheric pollutants and antigens. These conditions tend to develop in heavily industrial or densely populated urban areas and are frequently associated with thermal inversions or other situations creating stagnant air masses. In these circumstances, although the general population can develop respiratory symptoms, patients with asthma and other respiratory diseases tend to be more severely affected. The air pollutants known to have this effect are ozone, nitrogen dioxide, and sulfur dioxide. The last needs to be present in high concentrations and produces its greatest effects during periods of high ventilation. In some regions of North America, seasonal concentrations of airborne antigens such as pollen, can rise high enough to result in epidemics of asthma admissions to hospitals and an increase in the death rate. These events may be ameliorated by treating patients prophylactically with mast cell–stabilizing drugs before the allergy season begins.

Occupational Factors (See Chap. 254) Occupation-related asthma is a significant health problem, and acute and chronic airways obstruction has been reported to follow exposure to a large number of compounds used in many types of industrial processes. Bronchoconstriction can result from working with or being exposured to *metal salts* (e.g., platinum, chrome, and nickel), *wood and vegetable dusts* (e.g., those of oak, western red cedar, grain, flour, castor bean, green coffee bean, mako, gum acacia, karay gum, and tragacanth), *pharmaceutical agents* (e.g., antibiotics, piperazine, and cimetidine), *industrial chemicals and plastics* (e.g., toluene diisocyanate, phthalic acid anhydride, trimellitic anhydride, persulfates, ethylenediamine, *p*-phenylenediamine, and various dyes), *biologic enzymes* (e.g., laundry detergents and pancreatic enzymes), and *animal and insect dusts, serums, and secretions*. It is important to recognize that exposure to sensitizing chemicals, particularly those used in paints, solvents, and plastics, also can occur during leisure or non-work-related activities.

There seem to be three underlying mechanisms for this airways obstruction: (1) In some cases, the offending agent results in the formation of a specific IgE, and the cause seems immunologic (the immunologic reaction can be immediate, late, or dual); (2) in other cases, the substance causes a direct liberation of bronchoconstrictor substances; and (3) in other cases, the substance causes direct or reflex stimulation of the airways of either latent or frank asthmatics. In the case of asthmatic symptoms caused by occupational exposures that do not produce an immediate and dual immunologic reaction, patients give a characteristic cyclic history. They are well when they arrive at work, and symptoms develop toward the end of the shift, progress after the work site is left, and then regress. Absence from work during weekends or vacations brings about remission. Frequently, there are similar symptoms in fellow employees.

Infections Respiratory infections are the most common of the stimuli that evoke acute exacerbations of asthma. Well-controlled investigations have demonstrated that respiratory viruses and not bacteria or allergy are the major etiologic factors. In young children, the most important infectious agents are respiratory syncytial virus and parainfluenza virus. In older children and adults, rhinovirus and influenza virus predominate as pathogens. Simple colonization of the tracheobronchial tree is insufficient to evoke acute episodes of bronchospasm, and attacks of asthma occur only when symptoms of an ongoing respiratory tract infection are, or have been, present. The mechanism by which viruses induce exacerbations of asthma may be related to the production of T cell–derived cytokines that potentiate the infiltration of inflammatory cells into already susceptible airways.

Exercise Exercise is one of the most common precipitants of acute episodes of asthma. This stimulus differs from other naturally occurring provocations, such as antigens or viral infections, in that it does not evoke any long-term sequelae, nor does it change airway reactivity. Exercise probably provokes bronchospasm to some extent in every asthmatic patient, and in some it is the only trigger that produces symptoms. When such patients are followed for sufficient periods, however, they often develop recurring episodes of airway obstruction independent of exercise; thus, the onset of this problem frequently is the first manifestation of the full-blown asthmatic syndrome. There is a significant interaction between the ventilation produced by the exercise, the temperature, and the water content of the inspired air and the magnitude of the postexertional obstruction. Thus, for the same inspired air conditions, running will produce a more severe attack of asthma than will walking. Conversely, for a given task, the inhalation of cold air will markedly enhance the response, while warm, humid air will blunt or abolish it. Consequently, activities such as ice hockey, cross-country skiing, and ice skating are more provocative than is swimming in an indoor, heated pool. The mechanism by which exercise produces obstruction may be related to a thermally produced hyperemia and engorgement of the microvasculature of the bronchial wall and does not appear to involve smooth-muscle contraction.

Emotional Stress Abundant objective data demonstrate that psychological factors can interact with the asthmatic diathesis to worsen or ameliorate the disease process. The pathways and nature of the interactions are complex but have been shown to be operational to some extent in almost half the patients studied. Changes in airway caliber seem to be mediated through modification of vagal efferent activity, but endorphins also may play a role. The most frequently studied variable has been that of suggestion, and the weight of current evidence indicates that it can be quite important in selected asthmatics. When psychically responsive individuals are given the appropriate suggestion, they can actually decrease or increase the pharmacologic effects of adrenergic and cholinergic stimuli on their airways. The extent to which psychological factors participate in the induction and/or continuation of any given acute exacerbation is not established but probably varies from patient to patient and in the same patient from episode to episode.

PATHOLOGY In a patient who has died of acute asthma, the most striking feature of the lungs at necropsy is their gross overdistention and failure to collapse when the pleural cavities are opened. When the lungs are cut, numerous gelatinous plugs of exudate are found in most of the bronchial branches down to the terminal bronchioles. Histologic examination shows hypertrophy of the bronchial smooth muscle, hyperplasia of mucosal and submucosal vessels, mucosal edema, denudation of the surface epithelium, pronounced thickening of the basement membrane, and eosinophilic infiltrates in the bronchial wall. In asthmatic patients who die from trauma and causes other than asthma itself, mucus casts, basement membrane thickening, and eosinophilic infiltrates are frequently observed. In both situations there is an absence of any of the well-recognized forms of destructive emphysema. In a small proportion of asthmatics who die, the eosinophilic infiltration is replaced by neutrophils, and mucus plugging is conspicuously absent. The reasons for these differences are not yet clear.

PATHOPHYSIOLOGY The pathophysiologic hallmark of asthma is a reduction in airway diameter brought about by contraction of smooth muscle, vascular congestion, edema of the bronchial wall, and thick, tenacious secretions. The net result is an increase in airway resistance, a decrease in forced expiratory volumes and flow rates, hyperinflation of the lungs and thorax, increased work of breathing, alterations in respiratory muscle function, changes in elastic recoil, abnormal distribution of both ventilation and pulmonary blood flow with mismatched ratios, and altered arterial blood gas concentrations. Thus, although asthma is considered to be primarily a disease of airways, virtually all aspects of pulmonary function are compromised during an acute attack. In addition, in very symptomatic patients there frequently is electrocardiographic evidence of right ventricular hypertrophy and pulmonary hypertension. When a patient presents for therapy, his or her forced vital capacity tends to be $\leq$50 percent of normal. The 1-s forced expiratory volume (FEV_1) averages 30 percent or less of predicted, while the maximum and minimum midexpiratory flow rates are reduced to 20 percent or less of expected. In keeping with the alterations in mechanics, the associated air trapping is substantial. In acutely ill patients, residual volume (RV) frequently approaches 400 percent of normal, while functional residual capacity doubles. The patient tends to report that the attack has ended clinically when the RV has fallen to 200 percent of its predicted value and the FEV_1 reaches 50 percent of the predicted level.

Hypoxia is a universal finding during acute exacerbations, but frank ventilatory failure is relatively uncommon, being observed in 10 to 15 percent of patients presenting for therapy. Most asthmatics have hypocapnia and a respiratory alkalosis. In acutely ill patients, the finding of a normal arterial carbon dioxide tension tends to be associated with quite severe levels of obstruction. Consequently, when found in a symptomatic individual, it should be viewed as representing impending respiratory failure, and the patient should be treated accordingly. Equally, the presence of metabolic acidosis in the setting of acute asthma signifies severe obstruction. Usually, there are no clinical counterparts to the derangements in blood gases. Cyanosis is a very late sign. Hence, a dangerous level of hypoxia can go undetected. Likewise, signs attributable to carbon dioxide retention, such as sweating, tachycardia, and wide pulse pressure, or to acidosis, such as tachypnea, tend not to be of great value in predicting the presence of hypercapnia or hydrogen ion excess in individual patients, because they are too frequently seen in anxious patients with more moderate disease. Trying to judge the state of an acutely ill patient's ventilatory status on clinical grounds alone can be extremely hazardous, and clinical indicators should not be relied on with any confidence. Therefore, in patients with suspected alveolar hypoventilation, arterial blood gas tensions must be measured.

CLINICAL FEATURES The symptoms of asthma consist of a triad of dyspnea, cough, and wheezing, the last often being regarded as the *sine qua non*. In its most typical form, asthma is an episodic disease, and all three symptoms coexist. At the onset of an attack, patients experience a sense of constriction in the chest, often with a nonproductive cough. Respiration becomes audibly harsh, wheezing in both phases of respiration becomes prominent, expiration becomes prolonged, and patients frequently have tachypnea, tachycardia, and mild systolic hypertension. The lungs rapidly become overinflated, and the anteroposterior diameter of the thorax increases. If the attack is severe or prolonged, there may be a loss of adventitial breath sounds, and wheezing becomes very high pitched. Further, the accessory muscles become visibly active, and a paradoxical pulse often develops. These two signs have been found to be extremely valuable in indicating the severity of the obstruction. In the presence of either, pulmonary function tends to be significantly more impaired than in their absence. It is important to note that the development of a paradoxical pulse depends on the generation of large negative intrathoracic pressures.

Thus, if the patient's breathing is shallow, this sign and/or the use of accessory muscles could be absent even though obstruction is quite severe. The other signs and symptoms of asthma only imperfectly reflect the physiologic alterations that are present. Indeed, if the disappearance of subjective complaints or even of wheezing is used as the end point at which therapy for an acute attack is terminated, an enormous reservoir of residual disease will be missed.

The end of an episode is frequently marked by a cough that produces thick, stringy mucus, which often takes the form of casts of the distal airways (Curschmann's spirals) and, when examined microscopically, often shows eosinophils and Charcot-Leyden crystals. In extreme situations, wheezing may lessen markedly or even disappear, cough may become extremely ineffective, and the patient may begin a gasping type of respiratory pattern. These findings imply extensive mucus plugging and impending suffocation. Ventilatory assistance by mechanical means may be required. Atelectasis due to inspissated secretions occasionally occurs with asthmatic attacks. Other complications, such as spontaneous pneumothorax and/or pneumomediastinum, are rare.

Less typically, a patient with asthma may complain of intermittent episodes of nonproductive cough or exertional dyspnea. Unlike other asthmatics, when these patients are examined during symptomatic periods, they tend to have normal breath sounds but may wheeze after repeated forced exhalations and/or may show ventilatory impairments when tested in the laboratory. In the absence of both these signs, a bronchoprovocation test may be required to make the diagnosis.

DIFFERENTIAL DIAGNOSIS The differentiation of asthma from other diseases associated with dyspnea and wheezing is usually not difficult, particularly if the patient is seen during an acute episode. The physical findings and symptoms listed above and the history of periodic attacks are quite characteristic. A personal or family history of allergic diseases such as eczema, rhinitis, or urticaria is valuable contributory evidence. An extremely common feature of asthma is nocturnal awakening with dyspnea and/or wheezing. In fact, this phenomenon is so prevalent that its absence raises doubt about the diagnosis. *Upper airway obstruction by tumor* or *laryngeal edema* can occasionally be confused with asthma. Typically, a patient with such a condition will present with stridor, and the harsh respiratory sounds can be localized to the area of the trachea. Diffuse wheezing throughout both lung fields is usually absent. However, differentiation can sometimes be difficult, and indirect laryngoscopy or bronchoscopy may be required. Asthma-like symptoms have been described in patients with glottic dysfunction. These individuals narrow their glottis during inspiration and expiration, producing episodic attacks of severe airway obstruction. Occasionally carbon dioxide retention develops. However, unlike asthma, the arterial oxygen tension is well preserved, and the alveolar-arterial gradient for oxygen narrows during the episode, instead of widening as with lower airway obstruction. To establish the diagnosis of glottic dysfunction, the glottis should be examined when the patient is symptomatic. Normal findings at such a time exclude the diagnosis; normal findings during asymptomatic periods do not.

Persistent wheezing localized to one area of the chest in association with paroxysms of coughing indicates *endobronchial disease* such as foreign-body aspiration, a neoplasm, or bronchial stenosis.

The signs and symptoms of *acute left ventricular failure* occasionally mimic asthma, but the findings of moist basilar rales, gallop rhythms, blood-tinged sputum, and other signs of heart failure (Chap. 233) allow the appropriate diagnosis to be reached.

Recurrent episodes of bronchospasm can occur with *carcinoid tumors* (Chap. 95), *recurrent pulmonary emboli* (Chap. 261), and *chronic bronchitis* (Chap. 258). In chronic bronchitis there are no true symptom-free periods, and one can usually obtain a history of chronic cough and sputum production as a background upon which acute attacks of wheezing are superimposed. Recurrent emboli can be very difficult to separate from asthma. Frequently, patients with this condition will present with episodes of breathlessness, particularly on exertion, and they sometimes wheeze. Pulmonary function studies may show evidence of peripheral airway obstruction (Chap. 250); when these changes are present, lung scans also may be abnormal. The therapeutic response to bronchodilators and to institution of anticoagulant therapy may be helpful, but pulmonary angiography may be necessary to establish the correct diagnosis.

Eosinophilic pneumonias (Chap. 253) are often associated with asthmatic symptoms, as are various chemical pneumonias and exposures to insecticides and cholinergic drugs. Bronchospasm occasionally is a manifestation of *systemic vasculitis* with pulmonary involvement.

DIAGNOSIS The diagnosis of asthma is established by demonstrating reversible airway obstruction. *Reversibility* is traditionally defined as a 15 percent or greater increase in FEV_1 following two puffs of a beta-adrenergic agonist. When the spirometry results are normal at presentation, the diagnosis can be made by showing heightened airway responsiveness to challenges with histamine, methacholine, or isocapnic hyperventilation of cold air. Once the diagnosis is confirmed, the course of the illness and the effectiveness of therapy can be followed by measuring peak expiratory flow rates (PEFRs) at home and/or the FEV_1 in the laboratory. Positive wheal-and-flare reactions to skin tests can be demonstrated to various allergens, but such findings do not necessarily correlate with the intrapulmonary events. Sputum and blood eosinophilia and measurement of serum IgE levels are also helpful but are not specific for asthma. Chest roentgenograms showing hyperinflation are also nondiagnostic.

Rx TREATMENT

Elimination of the causative agent(s) from the environment of an allergic asthmatic is the most successful means available for treating this condition (for details on avoidance, see Chap. 310). Desensitization or immunotherapy with extracts of the suspected allergens has enjoyed widespread favor, but controlled studies are limited and have not proved it to be highly effective.

Drug Treatment The available agents for treating asthma can be divided into two general categories: drugs that inhibit smooth muscle contraction (beta-adrenergic agonists, methylxanthines, and anticholinergics) and agents that prevent and/or reverse inflammation (glucocorticoids and mast cell–stabilizing agents). Inhibitors of mediator synthesis and mediator-receptor antagonists are currently undergoing clinical trials.

ADRENERGIC STIMULANTS The drugs in this category consist of the catecholamines, resorcinols, and saligenins. These agents are analogues and produce airway dilation through stimulation of beta-adrenergic receptors and activation of G proteins with the resultant formation of cyclic adenosine monophosphate (AMP). They also decrease release of mediators and improve mucociliary transport. The catecholamines in widespread clinical use are epinephrine, isoproterenol, isoetharine, rimiterol, and hexoprenaline. The last two are not available in the United States. As a group, these compounds are short-acting (30 to 90 min) and are effective only when administered by inhalational or parenteral routes. Epinephrine and isoproterenol are not $beta_2$-selective and have considerable chronotropic and inotropic cardiac effects. Epinephrine also has substantial alpha-stimulating effects. The usual dose is 0.3 to 0.5 mL of a 1:1000 solution administered subcutaneously. Isoproterenol is devoid of alpha activity and is the most potent agent of this group. It is usually administered in a 1:200 solution by inhalation. Isoetharine is the most $beta_2$-selective compound of this class, but it is a relatively weak bronchodilator. It is employed as an aerosol and supplied as a 1% solution. The pharmacologies of hexoprenaline and rimiterol are similar to that of isoetharine.

The commonly used resorcinols are metaproterenol, terbutaline, and fenoterol, and the most widely known saligenin is albuterol (salbutamol). With the exception of metaproterenol, these drugs are highly selective for the respiratory tract and virtually devoid of significant cardiac effects except at high doses. Their major side effect is tremor. They are active by all routes of administration, and because their chemical structures allow them to bypass the metabolic processes used to degrade the catecholamines, their effects are relatively long-lasting (4 to 6 h). Differences in potency and duration among agents can be eliminated by adjusting doses and/or administration schedules.

Inhalation is the preferred route of administration because it increases the bronchial selectivity of these drugs and allows maximal bronchodilation with fewer side effects. This is true not just in maintenance therapy but also during the treatment of severe acute obstruction. In the past it was fashionable to treat episodes of severe asthma with intravenous sympathomimetics such as isoproterenol. This approach no longer appears justifiable. Isoproterenol infusions clearly can induce myocardial damage, and even for the beta$_2$-selective agents such as terbutaline and albuterol, intravenous administration offers no advantages over the inhaled route.

Salmeterol, a very long-lasting (9 to 12 h) congener of albuterol, is now available in the United States. When given every 12 h, it is effective in providing sustained symptomatic relief. It is particularly helpful for conditions such as nocturnal and exercise-induced asthma. It is not recommended for the treatment of acute episodes because of its relatively slow onset of action (approximately 30 min), nor is it intended as a rescue drug for breakthrough symptoms. In addition, its long half life means that administration of extra doses can cause cumulative side effects.

METHYLXANTHINES Theophylline and its various salts are medium-potency bronchodilators that work through an undefined mechanism. It was formerly thought that these drugs increased cyclic AMP by the inhibition of phosphodiesterase; however, the available evidence does not support this concept. The therapeutic plasma concentrations of theophylline traditionally have been thought to lie between 10 and 20 μg/mL. Some sources, however, recommend a lower target range between 5 and 15 μg/ml to avoid toxicity. The dose required to achieve the desired level varies widely from patient to patient owing to differences in the metabolism of the drug. Theophylline clearance, and thus the dosage requirement, is decreased substantially in neonates and the elderly and those with acute and chronic hepatic dysfunction, cardiac decompensation, and cor pulmonale. Clearance is also decreased during febrile illnesses. Clearance is increased in children. In addition, a number of important drug interactions can alter theophylline metabolism. Clearance falls with the concurrent use of erythromycin and other macrolide antibiotics, the quinolone antibiotics, and troleandomycin, allopurinol, cimetidine, and propranolol. It rises with use of cigarettes, marijuana, phenobarbital, phenytoin, or any other drug that has the capability of inducing hepatic microsomal enzymes.

For maintenance therapy, long-acting theophylline compounds are available and are usually given twice per day or once daily. The dose is adjusted on the basis of the clinical response with the aid of serum theophylline measurements. Single-dose administration in the evening reduces nocturnal symptoms and helps keep the patient complaint-free during the day. Aminophylline and theophylline are available for intravenous use. The recommendations for intravenous therapy in children aged 9 to 16 and in young adult smokers not currently receiving theophylline products are a loading dose of 6 mg/kg followed by an infusion of 1.0 mg/kg per hour for the next 12 h and then 0.8 mg/kg per hour thereafter. In nonsmoking adults, older patients, and those with cor pulmonale, congestive heart failure, and liver disease, the loading dose remains the same, but the maintenance dose is reduced to between 0.1 and 0.5 mg/kg per hour. In patients already receiving theophylline, the loading dose is frequently withheld or, in extreme situations, reduced to 0.5 mg/kg.

The most common side effects of theophylline are nervousness, nausea, vomiting, anorexia, and headache. At plasma levels greater than 30 μg/mL there is a risk of seizures and cardiac arrhythmias.

ANTICHOLINERGICS Anticholinergic drugs such as atropine sulfate produce bronchodilation in patients with asthma, but their use is limited by systemic side effects. Nonabsorbable quaternary ammonium congeners (atropine methylnitrate and ipratropium bromide) have been found to be both effective and free of untoward effects. They may be of particular benefit for patients with coexistent heart disease, in whom use of methylxanthines and beta-adrenergic stimulants may be dangerous. There is some evidence that addition of anticholinergics may enhance the bronchodilation achieved by sympathomimetics, but the effect is not large. The major disadvantages of the anticholinergics are that they are slow to act (60 to 90 min may be required before peak bronchodilation is achieved) and they are only of modest potency.

GLUCOCORTICOIDS Glucocorticoids are not bronchodilators, and their major use in asthma is in reducing airway inflammation. Systemic or oral steroids are most beneficial in acute illness when severe airway obstruction is not resolving or is worsening despite intense optimal bronchodilator therapy, and in chronic disease when there has been failure of a previously optimal regimen with frequent recurrences of symptoms of increasing severity.

The correct dose to use in acute situations is a matter of debate. The available data indicate that very high doses do not offer any advantage over more conventional amounts. In the United States, a usual starting dose is 40 to 60 mg of methylprednisolone intravenously every 6 h. Since intravenous and oral administration produce the same effects, prednisone, 60 mg every 6 h, can be substituted. Clinical impressions suggest that smaller quantities may work as effectively, but there are no confirmatory data. In the United Kingdom and elsewhere, acute asthma both in and out of hospital is frequently treated with doses of prednisolone ranging from 30 to 40 mg given once daily. It should be emphasized that the effects of steroids in acute asthma are not immediate and may not be seen for 6 h or more after the initial administration. Consequently, it is mandatory to continue vigorous bronchodilator therapy during this interval. Irrespective of the regimen chosen, it is important to appreciate that rapid tapering of glucocorticoids frequently results in recurrent obstruction. Most authorities recommend reducing the dose by one-half every third to fifth day following an acute episode. In situations in which it appears that continued steroid therapy will be needed, an alternate-day schedule should be instituted to minimize side effects. This is particularly important in children, since continuous corticosteroid administration interrupts growth. Long-acting preparations such as dexamethasone should not be used in this approach, for they defeat the purpose of alternate-day schedules by causing prolonged suppression of the pituitary-adrenal axis.

Several inhaled steroids of high topical potency are available and greatly facilitate the withdrawal of oral agents. They are also useful in reducing airways reactivity and as an alternative to oral glucocorticoids in situations where asthma symptoms are escalating. Some guidelines recommend starting aerosolized steroids in any patient whose disease is not controlled by inhaled bronchodilators. If symptoms are not eliminated at the standard dose, it has been suggested that the dose be increased twofold or more. While this course of action diminishes the need for oral glucocorticoids, it carries the risk of greater side effects. In addition to thrush and dysphonia, the increased systemic absorption that accompanies larger doses of inhaled steroids has been reported to produce adrenal suppression, cataract formation, decreased growth in children, interference with bone metabolism, and purpura. Many of the currently available inhaled steroid preparations require 2 to 4 weeks to produce a beneficial effect. Consequently, it is advisable to start a course of oral glucocorticoids simultaneously with the inhaled drug to facilitate symptom resolution. As the oral drugs are withdrawn, the improvements can be maintained via the inhaled route.

MAST CELL–STABILIZING AGENTS Cromolyn sodium and nedocromil sodium do not influence airway tone. Their major therapeutic effect is to inhibit the degranulation of mast cells, thereby preventing the release of the chemical mediators of anaphylaxis.

Cromolyn and nedocromil, like the inhaled steroids, improve lung function and reduce symptoms and lower airway reactivity in asthmatics. They are most effective in atopic patients who have either seasonal disease or perennial airways stimulation. A therapeutic trial of two puffs four times daily for 4 to 6 weeks frequently is necessary before the beneficial effects of the drug appear. Unlike steroids, nedocromil and cromolyn, when given prophylactically, will block the acute obstructive effects of exposure to antigen, industrial chemicals, exercise, or cold air. With antigen, the late response is also abolished. Therefore, a patient who has intermittent exposure to either antigenic or nonantigenic stimuli that provoke acute episodes of asthma need not use these drugs continuously but instead can obtain protection by taking the drug only 15 to 20 min before contact with the precipitant.

MISCELLANEOUS AGENTS It has been suggested that steroid-dependent patients might benefit from the use of immunosuppressant agents such as methotrexate or gold salts. The effects of these agents on steroid dosage and disease activity are minor, and side effects can be considerable. Consequently, this form of treatment can only be viewed as experimental. Opiates, sedatives, and tranquilizers should be absolutely avoided in the acutely ill asthmatic because the risk of depressing alveolar ventilation is great, and respiratory arrest has been reported to occur shortly after their use. Admittedly, most individuals are anxious and frightened, but experience has shown that they can be calmed equally well by the physician's presence and reassurances. Beta-adrenergic blockers and parasympathetic agonists are contraindicated because they can cause marked deterioration in lung function.

Expectorants and mucolytic agents have enjoyed great vogue in the past, but they do not add significantly to the treatment of the acute or chronic phases of this disease. Mucolytic agents such as acetylcysteine may actually produce bronchospasm when administered to susceptible asthmatics. This effect can be overcome by aerosolizing them in solution with a beta-adrenergic agent. The use of intravenous fluids in the treatment of acute asthma also has been advocated. There is little evidence that this adjunct hastens recovery. Nonstandard bronchodilators, such as intravenous magnesium sulfate for the treatment of acute asthma attacks, are not yet warranted in clinical practice because of the controversy surrounding their efficacy.

SPECIAL INSTRUCTIONS The treatment of patients with asthma who have coexisting conditions such as heart disease or pregnancy does not differ materially from that outlined above. Therapy with inhaled beta$_2$-selective and anti-inflammatory agents is the mainstay. The lowest doses of adrenergics that produce the desired effects should be used.

FRAMEWORK FOR MANAGEMENT **Emergency Situations** The most effective treatment for acute episodes of asthma is administration of aerosolized beta$_2$ agonists. These drugs provide three to four times more relief than intravenous aminophylline. In emergency situations, they can be given every 20 min by hand-held nebulizer for three doses. Thereafter, the frequency can be reduced to every 2 h until the attack has subsided. Aminophylline can be added to the regimen after the first hour in an attempt to speed resolution. Recent studies in a large series of patients demonstrate that beta$_2$ agonists alone terminate attacks in approximately two-thirds of patients, and that another 5 to 10 percent benefit from methylxanthine in combination with a sympathomimetic. The remainder have a poor acute response to all forms of therapy.

Acute episodes of bronchial asthma are one of the most common respiratory emergencies seen in the practice of medicine, and it is essential that the physician recognize which episodes of airway obstruction are life-threatening and which patients demand what level of care. These distinctions can be made readily by assessing selected clinical parameters in combination with measures of expiratory flow and gas exchange. The presence of a paradoxical pulse, use of accessory muscles, and marked hyperinflation of the thorax signify severe airways obstruction, and failure of these signs to remit promptly after aggressive therapy mandates objective monitoring of the patient using measurements of arterial blood gases and the peak expiratory flow rate (PEFR) or FEV$_1$.

In general, there is a direct correlation between the severity of the obstruction with which the patient presents and the time it takes to resolve it. Those individuals with the most impairment typically require the most extensive therapy for resolution. If the PEFR or FEV$_1$ is equal to or less than 20 percent of predicted on presentation and does not double within an hour of receiving the preceding therapy, the patient is likely to require extensive treatment including glucocorticoids before the obstruction dissipates. This group represents approximately 20 percent of all the patients who present for acute care. They generally require 24 h or more of inpatient treatment before becoming asymptomatic. In such individuals, if the clinical signs of a paradoxical pulse and accessory muscle use are diminishing, and/or if PEFR is increasing, there is no need to change medications or doses; the patient need only be followed. However, if the PEFR falls by more than 20 percent of its previous value or if the magnitude of the pulsus paradoxicus is increasing, serial measures of arterial blood gases are required, as well as a reconsideration of the therapeutic modalities being employed. If the patient has hypocarbia, one can afford to continue the current approaches a while longer. On the other hand, if the Pa_{CO_2} is within the normal range or is elevated, the patient should be monitored in an intensive care setting, and therapy should be intensified to reverse or arrest the patient's respiratory failure.

Chronic Treatment The goal of chronic therapy is to achieve a stable, asymptomatic state with the best pulmonary function possible. A number of algorithms have been proposed to accomplish this task. The first step is to educate patients to function as partners in their management. The severity of the illness needs to be assessed and monitored with objective measures of lung function. Asthma triggers should be avoided or controlled, and plans should be made for both chronic management and treatment of exacerbations. Regular follow-up care is mandatory. With respect to pharmacologic interventions, in general, the simplest approach works best. Infrequent symptoms require only the use of an inhaled sympathomimetic on an "as needed" basis. When the disease worsens, as manifested by nocturnal awakenings and daytime symptoms, inhaled steroids and/or mast cell–stabilizing agents should be added. If symptoms do not abate, the dose of inhaled steroids can be increased. An upper limit has not yet been established, but side effects of glucocorticoid excess begin to appear more frequently when the dose exceeds 2.0 mg/d. Persistent asthma complaints can be treated with long-acting inhaled beta$_2$ agonists, sustained-release theophylline, and/or parasympatholytics. In patients with recurrent or perennial symptoms and unstable lung function, oral steroids in a single daily dose are added to the regimen. Once control is reached and sustained for several weeks, a step-down reduction in therapy should be undertaken, beginning with the most toxic drug, to find the minimum amount of medication required to keep the patient well. During this process, the PEFR should be monitored and medication adjustments should be based on objective changes in lung function as well as on the patient's symptoms.

PROGNOSIS AND CLINICAL COURSE The mortality rate from asthma is small. The most recent figures indicate fewer than 5000 deaths per year out of a population of approximately 10 million patients at risk. Death rates, however, appear to be rising in inner-city areas where there is limited availability of health care.

Information on the clinical course of asthma suggests a good prognosis for 50 to 80 percent of all patients, particularly those whose disease is mild and develops in childhood. The number of children who still have asthma 7 to 10 years after the initial diagnosis varies from 26 to 78 percent, averaging 46 percent; however, the percentage who continue to have severe disease is relatively low (6 to 19 percent).

Unlike other airway diseases such as chronic bronchitis, asthma is not progressive. Although there are reports of patients with asthma developing irreversible changes in lung function, these individuals frequently have comorbid stimuli such as cigarette smoking that could account for these findings. Even when untreated, asthmatics do not continuously move from mild to severe disease with time. Rather, their clinical course is characterized by exacerbations and remissions. Some studies suggest that spontaneous remissions occur in approximately 20 percent of those who develop the disease as adults and that 40 percent or so can be expected to experience improvement, with less frequent and severe attacks, as they grow older.

BIBLIOGRAPHY

American Thoracic Society: Guidelines for the evaluation of impairment/disability in patients with asthma. Am Rev Respir Dis 147:1056, 1993

American Thoracic Society: Progress of the interface of inflammation and asthma. Am J Respir Crit Care Med 152:385, 1995

Burr ML: Epidemiology of asthma. Monogr Allergy 31:80, 1993

McFadden ER Jr: Evolving concepts in the pathogenesis and management of asthma. Adv Intern Med 39:357, 1994

McFadden ER Jr, Gilbert IA: Exercise-induced asthma. N Engl J Med 330:1362, 1994

McFadden ER Jr, Hejal R: Asthma. Lancet 345:1215, 1995

McFadden ER Jr et al: Protocol therapy for acute asthma: Therapeutic benefits and cost savings. Am J Med 99:651, 1995

Sheffer AL, Taggart VS: The National Asthma Education Program. Expert panel report guidelines for the diagnosis and management of asthma. Med Care 31:MS20, 1993

Skorodin MS: Pharmacotherapy for asthma and chronic obstructive pulmonary disease. Current thinking, practices, and controversies. Arch Intern Med 153:814, 1993

Wardlaw AJ: The role of air pollution in asthma. Clin Exp Allergy 23:81, 1993

253

Gary W. Hunninghake, Hal B. Richerson

HYPERSENSITIVITY PNEUMONITIS AND EOSINOPHILIC PNEUMONIAS

HYPERSENSITIVITY PNEUMONITIS

Hypersensitivity pneumonitis (HP), or extrinsic allergic alveolitis, is an immunologically induced inflammation of the lung parenchyma, involving alveolar walls and terminal airways, secondary to repeated inhalation of a variety of organic or other agents by a susceptible host. In contrast to many of the other interstitial lung diseases, etiologic agents of this interstitial and alveolar filling disease have been identified. The prevalence of HP is unknown but varies with the environmental exposure and the specific antigen involved. The prevalence of farmer's lung among Wisconsin dairy farmers has been reported as 4.2 per 1000. The diagnosis of HP requires a constellation of clinical, radiographic, physiologic, pathologic, and immunologic criteria, each of which is rarely pathognomonic alone, and the preferred treatment is avoidance of the causative antigen when practical.

ETIOLOGY Agents implicated as causes of HP include those listed in Table 253-1. Many cases of HP occurring in various occupations involve exposure to similar agents, particularly the thermophilic actinomycetes. Common sources of causative antigens are "moldy" hay, silage, or grain; pet birds; and heating, cooling, and humidification systems. Simple chemicals, such as isocyanates, may also cause hypersensitivity pneumonitis.

PATHOGENESIS The finding that precipitating antibodies against extracts of moldy hay were demonstrable in most patients with farmer's lung led to the early conclusion that HP was an immune-complex–mediated reaction. Subsequent investigations of HP in human beings and animal models provided evidence for the importance of cell-mediated hypersensitivity. The very early (acute) reaction is characterized by an increase in polymorphonuclear leukocytes in the alveoli and small airways. This early lesion is followed by an influx of mononuclear cells into the lung and the formation of granulomas that appear to be the result of a classic delayed (T cell mediated) hypersensitivity reaction to repeated inhalation of antigen and adjuvant-active materials.

Bronchoalveolar lavage (Chap. 251) in patients with HP consistently demonstrates an increase in T lymphocytes in lavage fluid (a finding that is also observed in patients with other granulomatous lung disorders). Patients with recent or continual exposure to antigen may have an increase in polymorphonuclear leukocytes in lavage fluid. Increased numbers of mast cells have also been reported. In most patients examined during recovery from acute disease, the T lymphocytes in lavage fluid are predominantly the CD8+ T cell subset. In patients with very recent exposure to antigen, however, the numbers of CD4+ T cells may increase in lavage fluid. Similar findings may be present in similarly exposed, asymptomatic individuals. These observations suggest that there is an active modulation of granuloma formation in the lung by immunoregulatory T cells and associated cytokines in this disorder.

CLINICAL PRESENTATION The *clinical picture* is that of an interstitial pneumonitis, although it varies from patient to patient and seems related to the frequency and intensity of exposure to the causative antigen and perhaps other host factors. The presentation can be *acute, subacute*, or *chronic*. In the *acute form*, symptoms such as cough, fever, chills, malaise, and dyspnea may occur 6 to 8 h after exposure to the antigen and usually clear within a few days if there is no further exposure to antigen. The *subacute form* often appears insidiously over a period of weeks marked by cough and dyspnea and may progress to cyanosis and severe dyspnea requiring hospitalization. In some patients, a subacute form of the disease may persist after an acute presentation of the disorder, especially if there is continued exposure to antigen. In most patients with the acute or subacute form of HP, the symptoms, signs, and other manifestations of HP disappear within days, weeks, or months if the causative agent is no longer inhaled. Transformation to a chronic form of the disease may occur in patients with continued antigen exposure, but the frequency of such progression is uncertain. The *chronic form* may also present as a gradually progressive interstitial disease associated with cough and exertional dyspnea without a prior history consistent with acute or subacute manifestations. Such a gradual onset frequently occurs with low-dose exposure to the antigen.

DIAGNOSIS Following acute exposure to antigen, neutrophilia and lymphopenia are frequently present. Eosinophilia is not a feature. All forms of the disease may be associated with elevations in erythrocyte sedimentation rate, C-reactive protein, rheumatoid factor, and serum immunoglobulins. Antinuclear antibodies are rarely present.

Examination for *serum precipitins* against suspected antigens, such as those listed in Table 253-1, is an important part of the diagnostic workup and should be performed on any patient with interstitial lung disease, especially if a suggestive exposure history is elicited. If found, precipitins indicate sufficient exposure to the causative agent for generation of an immunologic response. The diagnosis of HP is not established solely by the presence of precipitins, however, as precipitins are found in sera of many individuals exposed to appropriate antigens who demonstrate no other evidence of HP. False-negative results may occur because of poor-quality antigens or an inappropriate choice of antigens. Extraction of antigens from the suspected source may at times be helpful.

No specific or distinctive *chest roentgenogram* occurs in HP. It can be normal even in symptomatic patients. The acute or subacute phase may be associated with poorly defined, patchy, or diffuse infiltrates or with discrete, nodular infiltrates. In the chronic phase, the chest x-ray usually shows a diffuse reticulonodular infiltrate. Honeycombing may eventually develop as the condition progresses. Abnormalities rarely seen in HP include pleural effusion or thickening, and hilar adenopathy. High-resolution chest computed tomography (CT) has been reported to show a characteristic constellation of abnormalities, including (1) global lung involvement with increased lung density, (2) prominence of medium-sized bronchial walls, (3) patchy air space opacification with reticular and nodular patterns and midzone prominence, and (4) absence of hilar lymph node enlargement. No pathognomonic CT features of HP have been described.

Pulmonary function studies in all forms of HP typically show a restrictive pattern with loss of lung volumes, impaired diffusion capacity, decreased compliance, and an exercise-induced hypoxemia. A resting hypoxemia may be found. Functional abnormalities may gradually increase in severity or may occur rapidly following acute or subacute exposure to antigen.

Bronchoalveolar lavage is used in some centers to aid in diagnostic evaluation, and the characteristic features of the lavage fluid are described above.

Lung biopsy may be indicated in patients without sufficient other criteria to make a definitive diagnosis. The initial biopsy procedure is usually a transbronchial biopsy. In some patients, an open-lung biopsy may be necessary, as this procedure will provide adequate material for pathologic studies whereas transbronchial biopsy may not. Although the histopathology is distinctive, it may not be pathognomonic of HP. When the biopsy is taken during the active phase of disease, typical findings include an interstitial alveolar infiltrate consisting of plasma cells, lymphocytes, and occasional eosinophils and neutrophils, usually with accompanying granulomas. Interstitial fibrosis may be present but most often is mild in earlier stages of the disease. Some degree of bronchiolitis is found in about half the cases, whereas vasculitis is not a feature of the disorder. The triad of mononuclear bronchiolitis; interstitial infiltrates of lymphocytes and plasma cells; and single, nonnecrotizing, and randomly scattered parenchymal granulomas without mural vascular involvement is consistent with but not specific for HP.

The lack of standardized, nonirritating antigens and of proven controlled protocols makes *skin testing* and *inhalational challenge* useful only for research purposes. Similarly, *in vitro tests of cell-mediated (delayed) hypersensitivity* have not consistently been shown to correlate with clinical HP and have no place in the routine diagnostic workup.

In summary, the diagnosis in most cases is established by (1) consistent history, physical findings, pulmonary function tests, and chest x-ray; (2) exposure to a recognized antigen; and (3) finding an antibody to that antigen. In a few circumstances, bronchoalveolar lavage and/or lung biopsy may be needed. Provocation tests are research procedures and are not indicated.

DIFFERENTIAL DIAGNOSIS Chronic HP may often be difficult to distinguish from a number of other interstitial lung disorders such as idiopathic pulmonary fibrosis, sarcoidosis, interstitial lung disease associated with a collagen vascular disorder, and drug-induced lung diseases. A negative history for use of relevant drugs and no evidence of a systemic disorder usually exclude the presence of drug-induced lung disease or a collagen vascular disorder. Bronchoalveolar lavage often shows predominance of neutrophils in idiopathic pulmonary fibrosis and a predominance of CD4+ lymphocytes in sarcoidosis. The diagnosis of sarcoidosis is also favored by hilar/paratracheal lymphadenopathy or evidence of multisystem involvement. In some patients, a lung biopsy may be required to differentiate chronic HP from other interstitial diseases.

Table 253-1

Selected Examples of Hypersensitivity Pneumonitis (HP)

Disease	Antigen	Source of Antigen
Bagassosis	Thermophilic actinomycetes*	"Moldy" bagasse (sugar cane)
Bird fancier's, breeder's, or handler's lung	Parakeet, budgerigar, pigeon, chicken, turkey proteins	Avian droppings or feathers
Cephalosporium HP	Contaminated basement (sewage)	*Cephalosporium*
Cheese washer's lung	*Penicillium casei*	Moldy cheese
Chemical worker's lung	Isocyanates	Polyurethane foam, varnishes, lacquer, foundry casting
Coffee worker's lung	Coffee bean dust	Coffee beans
Compost lung	*Aspergillus*	Compost
Detergent worker's disease	*Bacillus subtilis* enzymes	Detergent
Familial HP	*Bacillus subtilis*	Contaminated wood dust in walls
Farmer's lung	Thermophilic actinomycetes*	"Moldy" hay, grain, silage
Fish meal worker's lung	Fish meal dust	Fish meal
Furrier's lung	Animal fur dust	Animal pelts
Hot tub lung	*Cladosporium* sp.	Mold on ceiling
Humidifier or air-conditioner lung (ventilation pneumonitis)	*Aureobasidium pullulans* or other microorganisms	Contaminated water in humidification and forced-air air-conditioning systems
Japanese summer house HP	*Trichosporon cutaneum*	House dust? Bird droppings
Laboratory worker's HP	Male rat urine	Laboratory rat
Lycoperdonosis	*Lycoperdon* puffballs	Puffball spores
Malt worker's lung	*Aspergillus fumigatus* or *A. clavatus*	Moldy barley
Maple bark disease	*Cryptostroma corticale*	Maple bark
Miller's lung	*Sitophilus granarius* (wheat weevil)	Infested wheat flour
Mushroom worker's lung	Thermophilic actinomycetes,* other	Mushroom compost
Paulis HP	Paulis reagent	Laboratory reagent
Pituitary snuff taker's lung	Animal proteins	Heterologous pituitary snuff
Potato riddler's lung	Thermophilic actinomycetes,* *Aspergillus*	"Moldy" hay around potatoes
Sauna taker's lung	*Aureobasidium* sp., other	Contaminated sauna water
Sequoiosis	*Aureobasidium, Graphium* sp.	Redwood sawdust
Streptomyces albus HP	*Streptomyces albus*	Contaminated fertilizer
Suberosis	Cork dust mold	Cork dust
Tap water lung	Unknown	Contaminated tap water
Thatched roof disease	*Sacchoromonospora viridis*	Dried grasses and leaves
Tobacco worker's disease	*Aspergillus* sp.	Mold on tobacco
Winegrower's lung	*Botrytis cinerea*	Mold on grapes
Wood trimmer's disease	*Rhizopus* sp., *Mucor* sp.	Contaminated wood trimmings
Woodman's disease	*Penicillium* sp.	Oak and maple trees
Woodworker's lung	Wood dust; *Alternaria*	Oak, cedar, and mahogany dusts; pine and spruce pulp

* Thermophilic actinomycetes species include *Micropolyspora faeni*, *Thermoactinomyces vulgaris*, *T. saccharrii*, *T. viridis*, and *T. candidus*.

The lung disease associated with acute or subacute HP may clinically resemble other disorders that present with systemic symptoms and recurrent pulmonary infiltrates, including the allergic bronchopulmonary mycoses and other eosinophilic pneumonias. Eosinophilic pneumonia is often associated with asthma and is typified by peripheral eosinophilia; neither of these is a feature of HP. Allergic bronchopulmonary aspergillosis (ABPA) is the most common example of the allergic bronchopulmonary mycoses and is sometimes confused with HP because of the presence of precipitating antibodies to *Aspergillus fumigatus*. ABPA is an obstructive rather than a restrictive lung disease, however, and is associated with allergic (atopic) asthma.

The term *organic dust toxic syndrome* (ODTS) has been applied to a condition that is more common than HP and is often mistaken for it; it follows heavy exposure to organic dusts and is characterized by transient fever and muscle aches, with or without respiratory symptoms. Serum precipitins are absent, and the chest x-ray is usually normal. Studies have shown no immunologic basis for ODTS. Endotoxin may be involved in its pathogenesis.

Massive exposure to moldy silage may result in a syndrome termed *pulmonary mycotoxicosis*, or *atypical farmer's lung*, with fever, chills, and cough and the presence of pulmonary infiltrates within a few hours of exposure. No previous sensitization is required, and precipitins are absent to *Aspergillus*, the suspected causative agent.

℞ TREATMENT

Because effective treatment depends largely on avoiding the antigen, identification of the causative agent and its source is essential. This is usually possible if the physician takes a careful environmental and occupational history or, if necessary, visits the patient's environment.

The simplest way to avoid the incriminated agent is to remove the patient from the environment or the source of the agent from the patient's environment. This recommendation cannot be taken lightly when it completely changes the life-style or livelihood of the patient. In many cases, however, the source of exposure (birds, humidifiers) can easily be removed. If occupational exposure is involved, an initial attempt can be made at antigen avoidance maneuvers least disruptive to the patient's livelihood, which usually means avoiding areas associated with heavy exposure and wearing an appropriate mask. This will not suffice for small-molecular-weight agents such as isocyanates, which require more elaborate respiratory systems. Pollen masks, personal dust respirators, airstream helmets, and ventilated helmets with a supply of fresh air are increasingly efficient means of purifying inhaled air. If symptoms recur or physiologic abnormalities progress in spite of these measures, then more effective measures to avoid antigen exposure must be pursued.

Compromises with environmental control pertain primarily to the acute, recurrent, transient clinical form of HP and must be accompanied by careful follow-up. Subacute forms are ordinarily the result of a heavy, sustained exposure. The chronic form typically results from low-grade or recurrent exposure over many months to years, and the lung disease may already be partially irreversible. These patients are usually advised to avoid completely all possible contact with the offending agent, although follow-up studies of farmer's lung and bird fancier's lung have found resolution of the disease despite continued exposure in some patients.

Patients with the *acute*, recurrent form of HP usually recover without need for glucocorticoids. *Subacute* HP may be associated with severe symptoms and marked physiologic impairment and may continue to progress for several days despite hospitalization. Urgent establishment of the diagnosis and prompt institution of glucocorticoid treatment are indicated in such patients. Such therapy may also hasten recovery in patients with lesser involvement. Prednisone at a dosage of 1 mg/kg per day or its equivalent is continued for 7 to 14 days and then tapered over the ensuing 2 to 6 weeks at a rate that depends on the patient's clinical status.

Patients with *chronic* HP may gradually recover without therapy following environmental control. In many patients, however, a trial of prednisone may be useful to obtain maximal reversibility of the lung disease. Following initial prednisone therapy (1 mg/kg per day for 2 to 4 weeks), the drug is tapered to the lowest dosage that will maintain the functional status of the patient. Many patients will not require or benefit from long-term therapy if there is no further exposure to antigen. Available studies report no effect of glucocorticoid therapy on long-term prognosis of farmer's lung.

EOSINOPHILIC PNEUMONIAS

Eosinophilic pneumonias are composed of distinct individual syndromes characterized by eosinophilic pulmonary infiltrates and, commonly, peripheral blood eosinophilia. Since Loeffler's initial description of a transient, benign syndrome of migratory pulmonary infiltrates and peripheral blood eosinophilia of unknown cause, this group of disorders has been enlarged to include several diseases of both known and unknown etiology (Table 253-2). These diseases may be considered as putative hypersensitivity lung diseases but are not to be confused with HP (extrinsic allergic alveolitis), in which eosinophilia is not a feature.

When an eosinophilic pneumonia is associated with bronchial asthma, it is important to determine if the patient has extrinsic (allergic, atopic) asthma and has wheal-and-flare skin reactivity to *Aspergillus* or other relevant fungal antigens. If so, other criteria should be sought for diagnosis of allergic bronchopulmonary aspergillosis (ABPA) (Table 253-3) or other, rarer examples of allergic bronchopulmonary mycosis such as those caused by *Penicillium*, *Candida*, *Curvularia*, or *Helminthosporium* spp. *Aspergillus fumigatus* is the most common cause of ABPA, although other *Aspergillus* species have also been implicated. ABPA has been reported to complicate cystic fibrosis. The chest roentgenogram in ABPA may show transient, recurrent infiltrates or may suggest the presence of proximal bronchiectasis. High-resolution chest CT is a sensitive, noninvasive technique for the recognition of proximal bronchiectasis. The bronchial asthma of ABPA likely involves an IgE-mediated hypersensitivity, whereas the bronchiectasis associated with this disorder is thought to result from a deposition of immune complexes in proximal airways. Adequate treatment usually requires the long-term use of systemic glucocorticoids.

Tropical eosinophilia is usually caused by filarial infection; however, eosinophilic pneumonias also occur with other parasites such as *Ascaris*, *Ancyclostoma* sp., *Toxocara* sp., and *Strongyloides stercoralis*. Tropical eosinophilia due to *Wuchereria bancrofti* or *Wuchereria malayi* occurs most commonly in southern Asia, Africa, and South America, and is treated successfully with diethylcarbamazine.

Drug-induced eosinophilic pneumonias are exemplified by acute reactions to nitrofurantoin, which may begin 2 h to 10 days after nitrofurantoin is started, with symptoms of dry cough, fever, chills, and dyspnea; an eosinophilic pleural effusion accompanying patchy or diffuse pulmonary infiltrates may also occur. Other drugs associated with eosinophilic pneumonias include sulfonamides, penicillin, chlorpropamide, thiazides, tricyclic antidepressants, hydralazine, meph-

Table 253-2

Eosinophilic Pneumonias
ETIOLOGY KNOWN
Allergic bronchopulmonary mycoses
Parasitic infestations
Drug reactions
Eosinophilia-myalgia syndrome
IDIOPATHIC
Loeffler's syndrome
Acute eosinophilic pneumonia
Chronic eosinophilic pneumonia
Allergic granulomatosis of Churg and Strauss
Hypereosinophilic syndrome

Table 253-3

Diagnostic Features of Allergic Bronchopulmonary Aspergillosis (ABPA)

MAIN DIAGNOSTIC CRITERIA
Bronchial asthma
Pulmonary infiltrates
Peripheral eosinophilia (>1000/μL)
Immediate wheal-and-flare response to *Aspergillus fumigatus*
Serum precipitins to *A. fumigatus*
Elevated serum IgE
Central bronchiectasis
OTHER DIAGNOSTIC FEATURES
History of brownish plugs in sputum
Culture of *A. fumigatus* from sputum
Elevated IgE (and IgG) class antibodies specific for *A. fumigatus*

enesin, mecamylamine, nickel carbonyl vapor, gold salts, isoniazid, para-aminosalicylic acid, and others. Treatment consists of withdrawal of the incriminated drugs and the use of glucocorticoids, if necessary.

The eosinophilia-myalgia syndrome, caused by dietary supplements of L-tryptophan, is occasionally associated with pulmonary infiltrates.

The group of idiopathic eosinophilic pneumonias consists of diseases of varying severity. *Loeffler's syndrome* was originally reported as a benign, acute eosinophilic pneumonia of unknown cause characterized by migrating pulmonary infiltrates and minimal clinical manifestations. In some patients, these clinical characteristics may prove to be secondary to parasites or drugs. *Acute eosinophilic pneumonia* has been described recently as an idiopathic acute febrile illness of less than 7 days' duration with severe hypoxemia, pulmonary infiltrates, and no history of asthma. *Chronic eosinophilic pneumonia* presents with significant systemic symptoms including fever, chills, night sweats, cough, anorexia, and weight loss of several weeks' to months' duration. The chest x-ray classically shows peripheral infiltrates resembling a photographic negative of pulmonary edema. Some patients also have bronchial asthma of the intrinsic or nonallergic type. Dramatic clearing of symptoms and chest x-rays is often noted within 48 h after initiation of glucocorticoid therapy.

Allergic angiitis and granulomatosis of Churg and Strauss is a multisystem vasculitic disorder that frequently involves the skin, kidney, and nervous system in addition to the lung (Chap. 319). The disorder may occur at any age and favors persons with a history of bronchial asthma. The asthma often is progressive until the onset of fever and exaggerated eosinophilia, at which time the symptoms of asthma may ease. The illness may be fulminating and the prognosis grave unless treated aggressively with glucocorticoids and, at times, immunosuppressive therapy.

The *hypereosinophilic syndrome* is characterized by presence of over 1500 eosinophils per microliter of peripheral blood for 6 months or longer; lack of evidence for parasitic, allergic, or other known causes of eosinophilia; and signs or symptoms of multisystem organ dysfunction. Consistent features are blood and bone marrow eosinophilia with tissue infiltration by relatively mature eosinophils. The heart may be involved with tricuspid valve abnormalities or endomyocardial fibrosis and a restrictive, biventricular cardiomyopathy. Other organs affected typically include the lungs, liver, spleen, skin, and nervous system. Therapy of the disorder consists of glucocorticoids and/or hydroxyurea, plus therapy as needed for cardiac dysfunction, which is frequently responsible for much of the morbidity and mortality in this syndrome.

BIBLIOGRAPHY

HYPERSENSITIVITY PNEUMONITIS

DENIS M: Proinflammatory cytokines in hypersensitivity pneumonitis. Am J Respir Crit Care Med 151:164, 1995

GURNEY JW et al: Agricultural disorders of the lung. Radiographics 11:625, 1991

KOKKARINEN JI et al: Recovery of pulmonary function in farmer's lung. A five-year followup study. Am Rev Respir Dis 147:793, 1993

MARX JJ et al: Cohort studies of immunologic lung disease among Wisconsin dairy farmers. Am J Int Med 18:263, 1990

RICHERSON HB: Hypersensitivity pneumonitis, in *Organic Dusts: Exposure, Effects, and Prevention,* R Rylander, RR Jacobs (eds). Boca Raton, FL, CRC Press, 1994, pp 139–160

——— et al: Guidelines for the clinical evaluation of hypersensitivity pneumonitis. J Allergy Clin Immunol 84:839, 1989

ROSE C, KING TE: Controversies in hypersensitivity pneumonitis. Am Rev Respir Dis 145:1, 1992

SHARMA OP: Hypersensitivity pneumonitis. Dis-Mo 37:409, 1991

EOSINOPHILIC PNEUMONIA

BUCHEIT J et al: Acute eosinophilic pneumonia with respiratory failure: A new syndrome? Am Rev Respir Dis 145:716, 1992

FISESELMANN JF, RICHERSON HB: Respiratory diseases, in *Basic and Clinical Immunology,* 8th ed, DP Stites, AI Terr, TG Parslow (eds). Norwalk, CT, Appleton & Lange, 1994, pp 528–540

HAYAKAWA H et al: A clinical study of idiopathic eosinophilic pneumonia. Chest 105:1462, 1994

MROUEH S, SPOCK A: Allergic bronchopulmonary aspergillosis in patients with cystic fibrosis. Chest 105:32, 1994

PATTERSON R, GREENBERGER PA, ROBERTS ML (eds): *Allergic Bronchopulmonary Aspergillosis.* Providence, RI, OceanSide Pub, 1995

ROSENOW ECIII et al: Drug-induced pulmonary disease: An update. Chest 102:239, 1992

254 ENVIRONMENTAL LUNG DISEASES

Frank E. Speizer

This chapter provides perspectives on ways to assess pulmonary diseases for which environmental causes are suspected. This assessment is important because removal of the patient from a harmful environment is often the only intervention that might prevent further significant deterioration or lead to improvement in a patient's condition. Furthermore, the identification of an environment-associated disease in a single patient may lead to primary preventive strategies affecting other similarly exposed people who have not yet developed disease.

The exact magnitude of the problem is unknown, but there is no question that large numbers of people are at risk of developing serious respiratory disease as a result of occupational or environmental exposures. For example, recent estimates suggest that approximately 2.3 million workers in the United States have been exposed to crystalline silica or asbestos dust in mining and nonmining industries. Even if only 5 percent of these workers (a conservative estimate) are to suffer from respiratory disease as a result of their exposure, this figure represents more than 100,000 individuals.

Although industries are required to spend substantial amounts of capital in efforts to protect their workers, occupationally related respiratory diseases continue to occur. These diseases are often attributed to exposures in the past, at a time when we were not aware of the risk incurred and the need for worker protection to the degree that we are today.

HISTORY AND PHYSICAL EXAMINATION The patient's history is of paramount importance in assessing any potential occupational or environmental exposure and the physician must ask the patient to describe a suspected environmental exposure in detail.

Inquiry into specific work practices should include questions about specific contaminants involved, the availability and use of personal respiratory protection devices, the size and ventilation of workspaces, and whether coworkers have similar complaints. In addition, the patient must be questioned about alternative sources for potentially toxic exposures, including hobbies or other environmental exposures at home. Short-term exposures to potential toxic agents in the distant past also must be considered (see Chap. 390).

Many people are aware of the potential hazards in their workplaces, and many states require that employees be informed about potentially hazardous exposures. These requirements include the provision of specific educational materials (including Material Safety Data Sheets), personal protective equipment and instructions in its use, and information on environmental control procedures. Reminders posted in the workplace may warn workers about hazardous substances. Protective clothing, lockers, and shower facilities may be considered necessary parts of the job. However, even in these more progressive industries, the introduction of new processes, particularly when related to the use of new chemical compounds, may change exposure significantly, and often only the employee on the production line is aware of the change. For the physician who regularly sees patients from a particular industry, a visit to the work site can be very instructive. Alternatively, physicians can request inspections by appropriate federal and/or state authorities.

The physical examination of patients with environment-related lung diseases may help to determine the nature and severity of the pulmonary condition. Unfortunately, the pulmonary response to most injurious agents is the development of a limited number of nonspecific physical signs. These findings do not point to the specific causative agent, and other types of information must be used to arrive at an etiologic diagnosis.

PULMONARY FUNCTION TESTS AND CHEST RADIOGRAPHY Many mineral dusts produce characteristic alterations in the mechanics of breathing and lung volumes that clearly indicate a restrictive pattern (Chaps. 250 and 259). Exposures to a number of organic dusts or chemical agents capable of producing occupational asthma result in pronounced obstructive patterns of pulmonary dysfunction that may be reversible (Chap. 252). Measurement of change in forced expiratory volume (FEV_1) before and after a working shift can be used to detect an acute inflammatory or bronchoconstrictive response. An acute decrement of FEV_1 over the Monday work shift is a characteristic feature of cotton textile workers with byssinosis.

The chest radiograph is useful in detecting and monitoring the pulmonary response to mineral dusts. The International Labour Organization (ILO) International Classification of Radiographs of Pneumoconioses classifies chest radiographs according to the nature and size of opacities seen and the extent of involvement of the parenchyma. In general, opacities may be round or irregular, small ($<$10 mm in diameter) or large. They may be few in number, with visible normal lung markings, partially obscure normal markings, or totally obscure normal markings. Although useful for screening large numbers of workers, the ILO system lacks specificity and may over- or underestimate the functional impact of pneumoconiosis. With dusts causing rounded, regular opacities like those evident in coal worker's pneumoconiosis, the degree of involvement on the chest radiograph may be extensive, while pulmonary function may be only minimally impaired. In contrast, in pneumoconiosis causing linear, irregular opacities like those seen in asbestosis, the radiograph may lead to underestimation of the severity of the impairment. It is possible for a patient to have a history of exposure, a moderately reduced forced vital capacity (FVC), and a reduced diffusion capacity in asbestosis with a relatively normal chest radiograph. The radiographic findings of irregular or linear opacities are simply more difficult to separate from normal markings until relatively late in the disease. When shadows become large, the condition is termed *complicated pneumoconiosis*, sometimes called progressive massive fibrosis (PMF). For the individual patient with a history of exposure, conventional computed tomography (CT) and high-resolution computed tomography (HRCT) have improved the sensitivity of identifying diffuse parenchymal abnormalities of the lung. The procedures have been shown to provide earlier detection of silicosis and asbestosis.

Other diagnostic procedures of use in identifying environment-induced lung disease include evaluation of heavy metal concentrations in urine (arsenic in smelter workers, cadmium in battery plant workers); bacteriologic studies (tuberculosis in medical care personnel, anthrax in wool sorters); fungal studies (coccidioidomycosis in southwestern farm workers, histoplasmosis in poultry or pigeon handlers); and serologic studies (psittacosis in pet shop workers or owners of sick birds, Q fever in tanners or slaughterhouse workers). Ultimately, a lung biopsy may be required both for morphologic diagnosis of the underlying pulmonary disease and for attempted identification of the specific etiologic agent.

MEASUREMENT OF EXPOSURE If reliable environmental sampling data are available, this information should be used in assessing a patient's exposure. Since many of the chronic diseases result from exposure over many years, current environmental measurements should be combined with work histories to arrive at estimates of past exposure. Even in acute conditions, when monitoring of exposure may be possible, little may be known about the actual dose received by the lung. Most of the research on health effects of air pollutants (discussed later in this chapter) has relied on fixed-station monitoring of outdoor air, often at locations somewhat distant from the residences of the people being studied. In addition, most people spend less than 20 percent of their time outdoors. Therefore, outdoor measurements can be used only in a relative sense, and they cannot be relied on to estimate actual dose.

In situations where individual exposure to specific agents—either in a work setting or via ambient air pollutants—has been determined, transport of these agents through the airways may be an important factor affecting dose. Highly soluble gases such as sulfur dioxide are absorbed in the upper airway and presumably produce their effects by reflex response of sensitive neural fibrils in the trachea or larger airways. In contrast, nitrogen dioxide, which is less soluble, may reach the bronchioles and alveoli in sufficient quantities to result in an acute life-threatening disease in farmers exposed even briefly to the gas evolved from moldy hay in silos (silo-filler's disease).

Particle size and chemistry of air contaminants also must be considered. Particles above 10 to 15 μm in diameter, because of their settling velocities in air, do not penetrate beyond the upper airways. These larger particles are often referred to as "fugitive dusts" and include pollens, other windblown dusts, and dusts resulting from mechanical industrial processes. They have little or no role in chronic respiratory disease except perhaps as related to cancer (see below).

Particles below 10 μm in size are created by the burning of fossil fuels or high-temperature industrial processes resulting in condensation products from gases, fumes, or vapors. These particles are divided into two size fractions on the basis of their chemical characteristics. Particles of approximately 2.5 to 10 μm (coarse-mode fraction) contain crustal elements, such as silica, aluminum, and iron. These particles mostly deposit relatively high in the tracheobronchial tree. Particles of less than approximately 2.5 μm (fine-mode fraction or accumulation mode) contain sulfates, nitrates, and organic compounds. The fine-mode particles more often deposit in the terminal bronchioles and alveoli. The smallest particles, those less than 0.1 μm in size, remain in the airstream and deposit in the lung only on a random basis as they come into contact with the alveolar walls.

Besides the size characteristics of particles and the solubility of gases, the actual chemical composition, mechanical properties, and immunogenicity or infectivity of inhaled material determine in large part the nature of the diseases found among exposed persons.

OCCUPATIONAL EXPOSURES AND PULMONARY DISEASE

ASBESTOSIS Except in localized regions with single industrial exposures, such as coal-mining or granite-quarrying regions, the most frequent inorganic dust–related chronic pulmonary diseases are associated with industries using *asbestiform fibers*. *Asbestos* is a generic term for several different mineral silicates, including chrysolite, amosite, anthophyllite, and crocidolite. Besides workers involved in the mining, milling, and manufacturing of asbestos products, workers in the building trades, including pipe fitters and boilermakers, were exposed to asbestos, which was widely used in construction because of its exceptional thermal and electric insulation properties. In addition, asbestos was used in the manufacture of fire-smothering blankets and safety garments, as filler for plastic materials, in cement and floor tiles, and in friction materials, such as brake and clutch linings.

Exposure to asbestos is not limited to persons who directly handle the material. Cases of asbestos-related diseases have been encountered in individuals with only moderate exposure, such as the painter or electrician who works alongside the insulation worker in a shipyard or the housewife who does no more than shake out and wash her husband's work clothes. Community exposure has probably resulted from the use of asbestos-containing material sprayed on steel girders in many large buildings as a safety feature to prevent buckling in case of fire.

Asbestos was first used extensively in the 1940s. Starting in 1975 it was mostly replaced with synthetic mineral fibers, such as fiberglass or slag wool. However, asbestos is still used in the manufacture of brake linings and remains as pipe and boiler insulation in hundreds of thousands of workplaces and homes. Despite current regulations mandating adequate training for any worker potentially exposed to asbestos, exposure probably continues among inexperienced demolition workers. The major health effects from exposure to asbestos are pulmonary fibrosis (asbestosis) and cancers of the respiratory tract, the pleura, and (in rare cases) the peritoneum.

Asbestosis is a diffuse interstitial fibrosing disease of the lung that is directly related to the intensity and duration of exposure. Except for its association with a history of exposure to asbestos (generally in a work setting), asbestosis resembles the other forms of diffuse interstitial fibrosis (Chap. 259). Usually, moderate to severe exposure has taken place for at least 10 years before the disease becomes manifest.

Physiologic studies reveal a restrictive pattern with a decrease in lung volumes. Flow rates are commonly reduced less than would be predicted on the basis of the volume reduction. An early sign of severe disease may be a reduction in diffusing capacity.

Pulmonary fibrosis may occur following sufficient exposure to any of the asbestiform fiber types. The fibrotic lesions do not appear to relate to either shape or chemical composition of any fiber type. During phagocytosis of the asbestos fiber, the membrane of the macrophage is damaged and this damage results in the release of lysosomes containing enzymes that may act to damage the lung parenchyma. The clinical manifestations are typical of those physical findings in any patient with pulmonary fibrosis (Chap. 259).

Diagnosis The chest radiograph can be used to detect a number of manifestations of asbestos exposure as well as to identify specific lesions. Past exposure is specifically indicated by pleural plaques, which are characterized by either thickening or calcification along the parietal pleura, particularly along the lower lung fields, the diaphragm, and the cardiac border. Without additional manifestations, pleural plaques imply only exposure, not pulmonary impairment. Benign pleural effusions may occur, particularly in patients with asbestosis, but are not necessarily restricted to those with overt disease. The fluid is sterile but may be a serous or blood-stained exudate and may occur bilaterally. The effusion may be slowly progressive or may resolve spontaneously.

The radiographic diagnosis of asbestosis depends on the presence of irregular or linear opacities, usually first noted in the lower lung fields and spreading into the middle and upper lung fields as the disease progresses. An indistinct heart border or a "ground glass" appearance in the lung fields is seen in some cases. As the fibrotic changes in the parenchyma begin to coalesce, the patient develops obliteration of entire acinar units, with eventual formation of the classical honeycombed lung, which appears on chest radiographs as coarse infiltrates with small (about 7- to 10-μm) air spaces. In cases in which the x-ray changes are less obvious, HRCT may show distinct changes of subpleural curvilinear lines 5 to 10 cm in length that appear to be parallel to the pleural surface; these alterations increase the positive predictive value of radiographic evidence from approximately 85 percent to about 100 percent.

In general, newly diagnosed cases will have resulted from exposure levels that were present many years before and, in spite of the patients' having left the industry, are attributable to that former exposure. Since the patient may be eligible for compensation within a specific time frame after the diagnosis of an asbestos-related disease is made, the physician making the diagnosis should be certain to inform the patient promptly. On occasion, the physician may have reason to suspect ongoing exposure from a patient's current job description or actual monitoring data. In such cases, federal or state health authorities may need to be notified. Present-day occupational safety and health regulations, if followed properly, protect workers from exposure.

Casual, nonoccupational exposure to undisturbed sources of asbestos-containing materials—e.g., in walls of schools or other buildings—represents little if any hazard to people who inhabit or work in such buildings. Because the association of smoking and asbestos exposure increases the risk of developing lung cancer (see below), it is extremely important to advise patients with a history of exposure to asbestos to stop smoking. No specific therapy is available in the management of patients with asbestosis. The supportive care is the same as that given to any patient with diffuse interstitial fibrosis from any cause.

Lung cancer (Chap. 90), either squamous cell carcinoma or adenocarcinoma, is the most frequent cancer associated with asbestos exposure. The excess frequency of lung cancer in asbestos workers is associated with a minimum lapse of 15 to 19 years between first exposure and development of the disease. Persons with more exposure are at greater risk of disease. In addition, there appears to be a significant multiplicative effect that leads to a far greater risk of lung cancer in persons who are cigarette smokers and have asbestos exposure than would be expected from the additive risk of each factor. To date, efforts to consider these high-risk individuals for special surveillance studies, including sputum cytologic examinations and repeated chest x-rays as frequently as every 4 to 6 months, have resulted in neither significant early detection nor prolonged survival once the lung cancer is found.

Mesotheliomas (Chap. 262), both pleural and peritoneal, are also associated with asbestos exposure. In contrast to lung cancers, these tumors do not appear to be associated with smoking. Relatively short-term asbestos exposures of 1 to 2 years or less occurring some 20 to 25 years in the past have been associated with the development of mesotheliomas (an observation that emphasizes the importance of obtaining a complete environmental exposure history). The risk for this type of tumor peaks 30 to 35 years after initial exposure. Although approximately 50 percent of mesotheliomas metastasize, the tumor generally is locally invasive, and death usually results from local extension. Most patients present with effusions that may obscure the underlying pleural tumor. In contrast to the findings in effusion due to other causes, because of the restriction placed on the chest wall, no shift of mediastinal structures toward the opposite side of the chest will be seen. The major diagnostic problem is differentiation from peripherally spreading pulmonary adenocarcinoma or from adenocarcinoma metastasized to pleura from an extrathoracic primary site. Although a needle biopsy may be diagnostic, an open biopsy is often necessary, and even the latter procedure may not provide a definitive diagnosis of the origin of the tumor.

Since epidemiologic studies have shown that more than 80 percent of mesotheliomas may be associated with asbestos exposure, documented mesothelioma in a worker with occupational exposure to asbestos may be compensable in many parts of the United States.

SILICOSIS In spite of the technical adequacy of existing protective equipment, *free silica* (SiO_2), or crystalline quartz, is still a major occupational hazard. In the United States, estimates of potential numbers of exposed workers range between 1.2 and 3 million people. The major occupational exposures include mining, stonecutting, employment in abrasive industries, foundry work, packing of silica flour, and quarrying, particularly of granite. Most often, progressive pulmonary fibrosis (silicosis) occurs in a dose-response fashion after many years of exposure.

Workers exposed through sandblasting in confined spaces, tunneling through rock with high quartz content (15 to 25 percent), or the manufacture of abrasive soaps may develop acute silicosis with as little as 10 months' exposure. The disease may be rapidly fatal in less than 2 years, despite the discontinuation of exposure. A radiographic picture of profuse miliary infiltration or consolidation is characteristic of acute silicosis.

In long-term, less intense exposure, small rounded opacities in the upper lobes, with retraction and hilar adenopathy, classically appear on the radiograph after 15 to 20 years. Calcification of hilar nodes may occur in as many as 20 percent of cases and produces the characteristic "eggshell" pattern. These changes may be preceded by or associated with a reticular pattern of irregular densities that are uniformly present throughout the upper lung zones.

The nodular fibrosis may be progressive in the absence of further exposure, with coalescence and formation of nonsegmental conglomerates of irregular masses in excess of 1 cm in diameter. These masses become quite large and are characteristic of PMF. Significant functional impairment with both restrictive and obstructive components may be associated with this form of silicosis. In the late stages of the disease, ventilatory failure may develop. In more subtle cases, CT may be helpful both in identifying nodules, which are preferentially located in the posterior aspect of the upper lobes, as well as in identifying larger opacities and more coalescence than might be noted on regular chest x-rays. Patients with silicosis are at greater risk of acquiring *Mycobacterium tuberculosis* infections (silicotuberculosis) and atypical mycobacterial infections. Because the frequency with which tuberculosis has been found at autopsy in patients with PMF exceeds considerably the frequency of premorbid diagnosis, treatment for tuberculosis is indicated in any patient with silicosis and a positive tuberculin test.

Other less hazardous silicates include Fuller's earth, kaolin, mica, diatomaceous earths, silica gel, soapstone, carbonate dusts, and cement dusts. The production of fibrosis in workers exposed to these agents is believed to be related to either the free silica content of these dusts or, for substances that contain no free silica, to the potentially large dust loads to which these workers may be exposed.

Other silicates, including *talc dusts*, may be contaminated with asbestos and/or free silica. Accidental exposure to significant quantities of talc may result in an acute syndrome with cough, cyanosis, and labored breathing (acute talcosis). Severe progressive fibrosis with respiratory failure may ensue within a few years. Far more common is the fibrosis and/or pleural or lung cancer associated with chronic exposure in rubber workers who use commercial talc as a lubricant in tire molds. Pure talc does not produce fibrosis; thus it is difficult to sort out whether the effects are due to the contamination of commercial talc by asbestos or by free silica.

COAL WORKER'S PNEUMOCONIOSIS (CWP) *Coal dust* is associated with CWP, which has enormous social, economic, and medical significance in every nation in which coal mining is an important industry. Simple radiographically identified CWP is seen in 12 percent of all miners and in as many as 50 percent of anthracite miners with more than 20 years' work on the coal face. The prevalence of disease is lower in workers in bituminous coal mines. Since much western U.S. coal is bituminous, CWP is less prevalent in that region.

Much of the symptomatology associated with simple CWP appears to be similar and additive to the effects of cigarette smoking on the development of chronic bronchitis and obstructive lung disease (Chap. 258). In the early stages of simple CWP, radiographic abnormalities consist of small, irregular opacities (reticular pattern). With prolonged exposure, one sees small, rounded, regular opacities, 1 to 5 mm in diameter (nodular pattern). Calcification is generally not seen, although approximately 10 percent of older anthracite miners have calcified nodules.

Complicated CWP is manifested by the appearance on the chest radiograph of nodules ranging from 1 cm in diameter to the size of an entire lobe, generally confined to the upper half of the lungs. This condition, considered a form of PMF, is accompanied by a significant reduction in diffusing capacity and is associated with premature mortality. In contrast to patients with silicosis, underground miners with simple CWP develop PMF at a rate of only 5 to 15 percent, depending on the type of coal.

The mechanism whereby PMF occurs in CWP is not fully understood. Several hypotheses have been proposed, including (1) sufficient free silica is present in the dust, (2) normal clearance mechanisms are unable to clear the excessive dust loads, (3) an interplay occurs between an intrinsic immunologic mechanism and the dust and/or damaged lung tissue, and (4) atypical reactions to *M. tuberculosis* occur. As previously described, PMF in silicosis is associated with prolonged duration and high intensity of exposure to free silica. Heavy exposure to carbon particles free of silica occurs in carbon black, graphite, and charcoal workers. The prolonged exposure of these workers may result in sufficient accumulation of carbon in the lung to produce PMF. The mechanism appears to relate to a breakdown of the clearance capacity of the airways.

Caplan's syndrome, which includes seropositive rheumatoid arthritis with characteristic PMF, is consistent with an immunopathologic mechanism. The syndrome was first described in coal miners but subsequently has been found in patients with a variety of pneumoconioses.

BERYLLIOSIS Beryllium may produce an acute pneumonitis or, far more commonly, a chronic interstitial pneumonitis. Unless one inquires specifically about occupational exposures to beryllium in the manufacture of alloys, ceramics, high-technology electronics, and (before the 1950s) the production of fluorescent lights, one may miss entirely the etiologic relationship to an occupational exposure. Nonspecific pulmonary function tests may be normal or may indicate evidence of restrictive disease. Between 2 and 15 years of exposure, depending on its intensity, are required for the disease to become manifest. On open lung biopsy, granulomatous formation similar to that seen in sarcoidosis (Chap. 320) may make differentiation impossible unless tissue levels of beryllium are measured.

Rarely, other hard metals, including aluminum powders, chromium, cobalt, titanium dioxide, and tungsten, may produce an interstitial pneumonitis.

OTHER INORGANIC DUSTS Other dusts are considered *nuisance dusts* because their major impact seems to be reduction in visibility and irritation of eyes, ears, nasal passages, and other mucous membranes. If they penetrate to the lower airways, these dusts do not affect the architecture of the terminal bronchioles or acinar spaces nor do they destroy collagen. Generally, clinical effects are reversible. Pulmonary function tests are usually normal unless another disease process coexists. If the dusts are radiodense, macular collections may produce striking radiographic pictures that are so characteristic that patients with a history of significant exposure are easily diagnosed as having the condition that bears the name reflecting the nature of the dust. Examples of radiodense dusts include iron and iron oxides from welding or silver finishing (*siderosis*); tin oxide used in metallurgy, color stabilization, printing, and the manufacture of porcelain, glass, and fabric (*stannosis*); and barium sulfate used as a catalyst for organic reactions, drilling mud components, and electroplating (*baritosis*). Other metal dusts producing similar radiodense pictures include *cerium dioxide* and *antimony salts*.

Most of the inorganic dusts discussed thus far are associated with the production of either dust macules or interstitial fibrotic changes in the lung. Another set of dusts (see Table 254-1), along with some of the dusts previously discussed, is associated with chronic mucous hypersecretion (chronic bronchitis), with or without reduction of expiratory flow rates. These conditions may be caused by cigarette smoking, and any effort to attribute some component of the disease to occupational and environmental exposures must take cigarette smoking into account. Most studies suggest an additive effect of dust exposure and smoking. The pattern of the effect is similar to that of cigarette smoking, suggesting that small airway inflammation may be the initial site of pathologic response in those cases as-

Table 254-1

Selected Occupational Dusts Believed to be Associated with Mucous Hypersecretion and/or Obstructive Airway Disease and Other Respiratory Diseases*

Agent (Exposure)	Mucous Hypersecretion	Obstruction	Other Conditions†
INORGANIC DUSTS			
Antimony (storage batteries, solder, ceramics, glass, plastics)	X		P
Arsenic (manufacture of pesticides, pigments, glass, alloys)	X		C
Barium and compounds including BaO, $BaSO_4$, $BaCO_3$ (catalysts, drilling mud, electroplating)	X		P
Cadmium dust (electroplating, battery manufacture, welding, smelting, aluminum soldering)	X	X	P
Cement dust (construction trades, manufacture of cement blocks)	X	X	
Chromium and CrO_3, CrF_2 (corrosion inhibitor pigment, metallurgy, electroplating)	X		C
Coal dust (mining)	X		P
Coke oven emissions (retort house, coke ovens)	X	X	P, C
Graphite (steelmaking, lubricants, pencils, paints, stove polish)	X	X	P
Iron dust (steel and nonferrous foundry workers, welding)	X		P
Mica (insulation, roofing shingles, oil refining, rubber manufacturing)	X		P
Phosphorus, elemental chlorides, sulfides (manufacture of fireworks, agricultural chemicals, insecticides, pesticides)	X	X	
Rock dusts (miners, tunnelers, quarry workers)	X		P
Vanadium pentoxide (welding electrodes, additive to steel, by-product in ash from oil burning)	X	X	
ORGANIC DUSTS (see Chap. 253)			
Cotton dust, flax, hemp (manufacture of yarns for linen, rope, cotton; ginning, cottonseed crushing; waste fiber processing)	X	X	
Grain dusts (farmers, workers in grain elevators, barge and grain ship crew members)	X	X	
Moldy hay (farmers, other animal attendants)	X		HP

* The table excludes agents associated with asthma as the primary disease (see Chap. 252).

† Other conditions include hypersensitivity pneumonitis (HP), pneumoconiosis (P), and cancers (C).

NOTE: X indicates that mucous hypersecretion or obstruction is associated with exposure.

sociated with the development of obstructive lung disease. Cigarette smoke is usually the more noxious agent, and dust effects may be discernible only in nonsmokers.

ORGANIC DUSTS Some of the specific diseases associated with organic dusts are discussed in detail in the chapters on asthma (Chap. 252) and hypersensitivity pneumonitis (Chap. 253). Many of these diseases are named for the specific setting in which they are found, e.g., farmer's lung, malt worker's disease, or mushroom worker's disease. Occupational and other environmental exposures must be sought when these conditions are suspected. Often the temporal relation of symptoms to exposure furnishes the best evidence for the diagnosis. Three occupational groups are singled out for discussion because they represent the largest proportion of people affected by the diseases resulting from organic dusts.

Cotton Dust (Byssinosis) Estimates of the number of exposed persons in the United States vary, but probably over 800,000 persons are exposed occupationally to cotton, flax, or hemp in the production of yarns for cotton, linen, and rope making. Although this discussion focuses on cotton, the same syndrome—albeit somewhat less severe—has been reported in association with exposure to flax, hemp, and jute.

Exposure occurs throughout the manufacturing process but is most pronounced in those portions of the factory involved with the treatment of the cotton prior to spinning—i.e., blowing, mixing, and carding (straightening of fibers). Attempts to control dust levels by use of exhaust hoods, general increases in ventilation, and wetting procedures in some settings have been highly successful. However, respiratory protective equipment appears to be required during certain operations to prevent workers from being exposed to levels of dust that exceed the current U.S. cotton dust standard.

Byssinosis is characterized clinically as occasional (early stage) and then regular (late stage) chest tightness toward the end of the first day of the workweek ("Monday chest tightness"). In epidemiologic studies, depending on the level of exposure via the carding room air, up to 80 percent of employees may show a significant drop in their FEV_1 over the course of a Monday shift.

Initially the symptoms do not recur on subsequent days of the week. However, in 10 to 25 percent of workers, the disease may be progressive, with chest tightness recurring or persisting throughout the workweek. After more than 10 years of exposure, workers with recurrent symptoms are more likely to have an obstructive pattern on pulmonary function testing. These higher grades of impairment are seen in workers exposed both to high levels of dust and for greater durations. There is an additive effect of cotton dust exposure plus cigarette smoking. The highest grades of impairment are generally seen in smokers.

Treatment in the early stages of the disease is directed toward reversing the bronchospasm with bronchodilators; however, the chest tightness appears to relate, at least in part, to histamine release, and antihistamines have been shown to lessen the anticipated fall in FEV_1 the first day of the week. Clearly, reduction of dust exposure is of primary importance. All workers with persistent symptoms or significantly reduced levels of pulmonary function should be moved to areas of lower risk of exposure. Regular surveillance of pulmonary function in the industry has made it easier to identify affected persons. Persons with reduced pulmonary function, a personal history of respiratory allergy, and a history of continued cigarette smoking should be considered at increased risk of developing byssinosis in association with work in the cotton industry.

Grain Dust Although the exact number of workers at risk in the United States is not known, at least 500,000 people work in grain elevators, and over 2 million farmers are potentially exposed to grain dust. The presentation of disease in grain elevator employees or in workers in flour or feed mills is virtually identical to the characteristic findings in cigarette smokers, i.e., persistent cough, mucous hypersecretion, wheeze and dyspnea on exertion, and reduced FEV_1 and FEV_1/FVC ratio (Chap. 250).

Dust concentrations in grain elevators vary greatly but appear to be in excess of 10,000 μg/m³; approximately one-third of the particles, by weight, are in the respirable range. The effect of grain dust exposure is additive to that of cigarette smoking, with approximately 50 percent of workers who smoke having symptoms. Among nonsmoking grain elevator operators, approximately one-quarter have mucous hypersecretion, about five times the number that would be expected in unexposed nonsmokers. However, evidence of obstruction on pulmonary function studies is observed only in workers who smoke. It is not clear whether the reason is an enhancement of the cigarette smoking effect in exposed workers or a greater susceptibility of smokers to the effects of grain dust.

Farmer's Lung This condition results from exposure to moldy hay containing spores of thermophilic actinomycetes that produce a hypersensitivity pneumonitis (Chap. 253). There are few good population-based estimates of the frequency of occurrence of this condition in the United States. However, among farmers in Great Britain, the rate of disease ranges from approximately 10 to 50 per 1000. The prevalence of disease varies in association with rainfall, which determines the amount of fungal growth, and with differences in agricultural practices related to turning and stacking hay.

The patient with acute farmer's lung presents 4 to 8 h after exposure with fever, chills, malaise, cough, and dyspnea without wheezing. The history of exposure is obviously essential to distinguish this disease from influenza or pneumonia with similar symptoms. In the chronic form of the disease, the history of repeated attacks after similar exposure is important in differentiating this syndrome from other causes of patchy fibrosis (e.g., sarcoidosis).

A wide variety of other organic dusts are associated with the occurrence of hypersensitivity pneumonitis (Chap. 253). For those patients who present with hypersensitivity pneumonitis, specific and careful inquiry about occupations, hobbies, or other home environmental exposures will, in most cases, reveal the source of the etiologic agent.

ASSESSMENT OF DISABILITY Significant reduction of dust levels in coal mines has resulted from federal legislation, enacted in the United States in 1969, that requires that respirable dust levels in underground mines be reduced to less than 2000 μg/m³. This same legislation authorizes payment to coal miners (or their survivors) totally disabled by CWP. The criteria for disability from CWP remain unclear and arbitrary. It is critical that physicians involved in occupational lung disease claim cases be aware of detailed exposure histories of their patients, in terms of both occupational exposures and other environmental exposures (cigarette smoking). To assess disability properly may require input not only from physicians but also from experts in ergonomics and vocational rehabilitation, lawyers, and employer and employee representatives.

Most commonly, the patient presents with asthma, and it is the physician's task to decide whether the asthma is occupation-induced or work-aggravated asthma. The distinction is important not only because of the implications for disability compensation but also because the longer one is exposed to an inciting agent, the worse the prognosis for recovery from occupation-induced asthma. The clinical evaluation of such a patient requires adherence to a prescribed protocol that may include not only the components of the evaluation previously described but also rechallenge of the patient in a controlled setting or under a carefully monitored program in a work setting.

TOXIC CHEMICALS Exposure to toxic chemicals affecting the lung generally involves gases and vapors. A common accident is one in which the victim is trapped in a confined space where the chemicals have accumulated to toxic levels. In addition to the specific toxic effects of the chemical, the victim will often sustain considerable anoxia, which can play a dominant role in determining whether the individual survives.

Table 254-2 lists a variety of toxic agents that can produce acute and sometimes life-threatening reactions in the lung. All these agents in sufficient concentrations have been demonstrated, at least in animal studies, to affect the lower airways and disrupt alveolar architecture, either acutely or as a result of chronic exposure. Some of these agents may be generated acutely in the environment. For example, when plastics burn, a number of compounds, including hydrogen cyanide and hydrochloric acid, may be formed and released. → ***The effects and treatment of exposure to these toxic gases are discussed in Chap. 391.***

Firefighters and fire victims are at risk of *smoke inhalation*, a numerically important cause of acute cardiorespiratory failure. Smoke inhalation kills more fire victims than does thermal injury. Carbon monoxide poisoning with resulting significant hypoxemia can be life-threatening (Chap. 391). Firefighters may inappropriately use the "blackness" of the smoke to indicate the degree of incomplete combustion and thus of carbon monoxide elevation. The use of synthetic materials (plastic, polyurethanes), which, when burned, may release a variety of other toxic agents, must be considered when evaluating smoke inhalation victims. Exposed victims may suffer some degree of lower respiratory tract inflammation, similar to that seen with exposure to other irritant gases (e.g., chlorine). Severe cases may include pulmonary edema.

Firefighters and victims also may be exposed to large quantities of particulate smoke. Significant long-term effects are not clearly associated with this particulate exposure except as related to the production of irritating effects on the upper airways; however, increased airway responsiveness in firefighters with repeated episodes of smoke inhalation has been demonstrated.

Some agents used in the manufacture of synthetic materials such as plastics, polyurethanes, and other polymers have resulted in some workers' being sensitized to extremely low levels of *isocyanates, aromatic amines*, or *aldehydes*. Repeated exposure to these agents causes some workers to develop chronic cough and sputum production, asthma, or episodes of low-grade fever and malaise.

Exposure occurs by an unusual route in *polymer fume fever*. Polymers, notably fluorocarbons, which at normal temperatures produce no reaction, may be transmitted from a worker's hands to his or her cigarettes. As the cigarette burns, the polymer is volatilized, and the inhaled agent causes a characteristic syndrome of fever, chills, malaise, and occasionally mild wheezing. The same scenario applies when workers are exposed to heated polymers without cigarette use. The syndrome is obviously controlled by proper attention to hygiene in the workplace. A similar self-limited, influenza-like syndrome—*metal fume fever*—results from acute exposure to fumes or smoke of zinc, copper, magnesium, and other volatilized metals. The syndrome may begin several hours after work and resolves within 24 h, only to return on repeated exposure. A proper occupational history should make the diagnosis evident.

ENVIRONMENTAL RESPIRATORY CARCINOGENS Historically, it has been the astute clinician who has recognized a higher incidence of malignant tumors associated with certain environmental exposures. When these observations are linked to an occupational setting, they must be pursued by epidemiologic studies of relatively large groups of both current and former workers. Often the concentration and/or exact nature of the substances involved in the putative exposures cannot be determined. Rarely, the possibility that a substance can play an etiologic role in cancer is supported by observing that a few cases of a very rare tumor in a particular group represent "an epidemic." Examples are nasal sinus and lung cancer in nickel workers, angiosarcomas of the liver in vinyl chloride workers, and adenocarcinomas of the nose in woodworkers.

Only in those few cases in which animal studies have been carried out can one confirm that a given suspected agent is really a carcinogen. For example, bis(chloromethyl) ether (BCME) has been shown to produce tumors in animals and oat cell cancer of the lung in humans. In this particular case, BCME, used as a chemical intermediary in the manufacture of a number of organic compounds, was found to produce tumors in animals at about the same time as the substance was introduced into industry.

In addition to asbestos exposures, other occupational exposures associated with either proven or suspected respiratory carcinogens include those to acrylonitrile, arsenic compounds, beryllium (animal studies only), BCME, chromium, polycyclic hydrocarbons (through coke ovens), iron oxide, isopropyl oil (nasal sinuses), mustard gas, the various ores used to produce pure nickel, talc (possible asbestos contamination in both mining and milling), vinyl chloride, welding materials, wood used in woodworking (nasal cancer only), and uranium. The occurrence of excess cancers in uranium miners raises the possibility that a large number of workers are at risk by virtue of exposure to similar radiation hazards. This number includes not only workers involved in processing uranium but also workers exposed in underground mining operations where radon daughters may be emitted from rock formations.

GENERAL ENVIRONMENTAL EXPOSURES

AIR POLLUTION Dramatic and disastrous episodes of air pollution inversion have been documented in many industrialized centers in the world. Each of these episodes has been associated with excess acute mortality in the very old, the very young, and those with chronic cardiopulmonary diseases. The most dramatic event was the London fog of 1952, in which approximately 4000 excess deaths occurred over a 2-week period following 5 days of severe cold and dense fog. Similar episodes in the United States, although less dramatic in terms of total deaths, occurred in Donora, Pennsylvania, in 1948 and in New York City in the 1960s. In these episodes, which were generally associated with cold temperature and air stagnation, patients with underlying cardiopulmonary disease were most severely affected.

In addition to significant excess mortality during these episodes, a large number of people required medical care for cardiorespiratory complaints. Subsequent follow-up studies failed to implicate these

Table 254-2

Selected Common Toxic Chemical Agents Affecting the Lung

Agent(s)	Selected Exposures	Acute Effects from High or Accidental Exposure	Chronic Effects from Relatively Low Exposure
Acid fumes; H_2SO_4, HNO_3	Manufacture of fertilizers, chlorinated organic compounds, dyes, explosives, rubber products, metal etching, plastics	Mucous membrane irritation, followed by chemical pneumonitis 2–3 days later	Bronchitis and suggestion of mildly reduced pulmonary function in children with lifelong residential exposure to high levels; clinical significance unknown
Ammonia	Refrigeration; petroleum refining; manufacture of fertilizers, explosives, plastics, and other chemicals	Same as for acid fumes	Chronic bronchitis
Cyanides	Electroplating; extraction of gold or silver; manufacture of mirrors, fumigants, photo supplies	Increase in respiratory rate followed by respiratory arrest, lactic acidosis, pulmonary edema, death	No data
Diazomethane	Methylating agent for acid compounds; laboratory workers	Violent coughing, dyspnea, wheezing, pulmonary edema	No data
Formaldehyde	Manufacture of resins, leathers, rubber, metals, and woods; laboratory workers, embalmers; emission from urethane foam insulation	Same as for acid fumes	Cancers in one species; no data on humans
Halides (Cl, Br, F)	Bleaching in pulp, paper, textile industry; manufacture of chemical compounds; synthetic rubber, plastics, disinfectant, rocket fuel, gasoline	Mucous membrane irritation, pulmonary edema; possible reduced FVC 1–2 yrs after exposure	Dryness of mucous membrane, epistaxis, dental fluorosis, tracheobronchitis
Hydrogen sulfide	By-product of many industrial processes, oil, other petroleum processes and storage	Respiratory paralysis similar to cyanides	Conjunctival irritation, chronic bronchitis, recurrent pneumonitis
Isocyanates (TDI, HDI, MDI)	Production of polyurethane foams, plastics, adhesives, surface coatings	Mucous membrane irritation, dyspnea, cough, wheeze, pulmonary edema	Upper respiratory tract irritation, cough, asthma, allergic alveolitis
Nitrogen dioxide	Silage, metal etching, explosives, rocket fuels, welding, by-product of burning fossil fuels	Cough, dyspnea, pulmonary edema may be delayed 4–12 h; possible result from acute exposure: bronchiolitis obliterans in 2–6 wks	Emphysema in animals, ?chronic bronchitis
Ozone	Arc welding, flour bleaching, deodorizing, emissions from copying equipment, photochemical air pollutant	Mucous membrane irritant, pulmonary hemorrhage and edema, reduced pulmonary function transiently in children and adults exposed to summer haze	Chronic eye irritation
Phosgene	Organic compound, metallurgy, volatilization of chlorine-containing compounds	Delayed onset of bronchiolitis and pulmonary edema	Chronic bronchitis
Phthalic anhydride	Manufacture of resin esters, polyester resins, thermoactivated adhesives	Nasal irritation, cough	Asthma, chronic bronchitis
Sulfur dioxide	Manufacture of sulfuric acid, bleaches, coating of nonferrous metals, food processing, refrigerant, burning of fossil fuels, wood pulp industry	Mucous membrane irritant, epistaxis	?Chronic bronchitis

episodic disasters in the etiology of chronic respiratory disease in adults. On the other hand, many epidemiologic studies of both international and regional differences in the prevalences of chronic respiratory disease suggest that long-term exposures in polluted areas in the early to middle part of the twentieth century were associated with excess chronic respiratory disease.

In 1970, the U.S. government established air quality standards for several pollutants believed to be responsible for excess cardiorespiratory diseases. Primary standards regulated by the Environmental Protection Agency (EPA) designed to protect the public health with an adequate margin of safety exist for sulfur dioxide, particulates <10 μm in size, nitrogen dioxide, ozone, lead, and carbon monoxide. Standards for each of these pollutants are updated regularly through an extensive review process conducted by the EPA.

Pollutants are generated from both stationary sources (power plants and industrial complexes) and mobile sources (automobiles), and none of the pollutants occurs in isolation. Thus, except for the change in carboxyhemoglobin from carbon monoxide exposure, it becomes extremely difficult to relate any specific health effect to any single pollutant. Furthermore, pollutants may be changed by chemical reactions after being emitted. For example, reducing agents, such as sulfur dioxide and particulate matter from a power plant stack, may react in air to produce acid sulfates and aerosols, the precursors of acid rain, which can be transported long distances in the atmosphere. Oxidizing substances, such as oxides of nitrogen and oxidants from automobile exhaust, may react with sunlight to produce ozone. Although originally a problem confined to the southwestern part of the United States, in recent years, at least during the summertime, elevated ozone and acid aerosol levels have been documented throughout the United States. Both acute and chronic effects of these exposures are currently under investigation.

The symptoms and diseases associated with air pollution are the same as the nononcogenic conditions commonly associated with cigarette smoking. In addition, respiratory illness in early childhood has been associated with chronic exposure to only modestly elevated levels of SO_2 and respirable particles. Recent population-based studies comparing cities that have relatively high levels of particulate exposures with less polluted communities suggest excess morbidity and mortality from cardiorespiratory conditions in long-term residents of the former communities. This finding, in part, has led to greater emphasis on publicizing pollution alert levels. One can only advise individuals with significant cardiopulmonary impairment to stay indoors during periods when pollution exceeds current standards.

INDOOR EXPOSURE Because of increased concern about energy costs, efforts to become energy efficient have led to reduced air-exchange rates in indoor environments. The unintentional effect of these efforts has been to increase exposures to a variety of air contaminants heretofore not considered important.

Until relatively recently, little attention was given to the effects of *passive cigarette smoking*. Several studies have shown that the respirable particulate load in any household is directly proportional to the number of cigarette smokers living in the home. Increases in prevalence of respiratory illnesses and reduced levels of pulmonary function measured with simple spirometry have been found in children of smoking parents in a number of studies. Although a modest increase in the risk of lung cancer is found in the aggregate of studies, the long-term consequences in terms of nononcogenic respiratory diseases are unknown.

Radon gas is believed to be a risk factor for lung cancer. The main radon product (radon 222) is a gas that results from the decay series of uranium 238, with the immediate precursor being radium 226. The amount of radium in earth materials determines how much radon gas will be emitted. Outdoors, the concentrations are trivial. Indoors, levels are dependent on the ventilation rate and the size of the space into which the gas is emitted. Levels associated with excess lung cancer risk may be present in as many as 10 percent of the houses in the United States. When smokers reside in the household, the problem is potentially greater, since the molecular size of radon particles allows them to readily attach to smoke particles that are inhaled. Fortunately, technology is available for assessing and reducing the level of exposure.

Other indoor exposures associated with an increased risk of atopy and asthma include those to such specific recognized putative biologic agents as cockroach antigen, dust mites, and pet danders. Other indoor chemical agents include formaldehyde, perfumes, and latex particles. Of recent interest are the nonspecific responses associated with "tight-building syndrome," in which no particular agent has been implicated; the affected individuals suffer from a wide variety of complaints, including respiratory symptoms, that are relieved only by avoiding exposure in the building in question. The degree to which "smells" or other sensory stimuli are involved in the triggering of potentially incapacitating psychological or physical responses has yet to be determined, and the long-term consequences of such environmental exposures are as yet unknown.

PORTAL OF ENTRY The lung is a primary point of entry into the body for a number of toxic agents that affect other organ systems. For example, the lung is a route of entry for benzene (bone marrow), carbon disulfide (cardiovascular and nervous systems), cadmium (kidney), and metallic mercury (kidney, central nervous system). Thus, in any disease state of obscure origin, it is important to consider the possibility of inhaled environmental agents. Such consideration can sometimes furnish the clue needed to identify a specific external cause for a disorder that might otherwise be labeled "idiopathic."

BIBLIOGRAPHY

BALAAN MR et al: Clinical aspects of coal workers' pneumononiosis and silicosis. Occup Med 8:19, 1993

BECKLAKE MR et al: The relationship between acute and chronic airway responses to occupational exposures. Curr Pulmonol 9:25, 1988

BERRY G: Prediction of mesothelioma, lung cancer, and asbestosis in former Wittenoom asbestos workers. Br J Ind Med 48:793, 1991

CHAN-YEUNG M, MALO J-L: Occupational asthma. N Engl J Med 333: 107, 1995

COCHRANE AL, MOORE FA: A 20-year follow-up of men aged 55–64 including coal miners and foundry workers in Staveley. Br J Ind Med 37:226, 1980

Guidelines for the Use of International Labour Office Classification of Radiographs of Pneumoconiosis. Occupational Safety and Health Sciences 22 (Revised 1980). Geneva, ILO, 1980

LAPP NL, CASTRANOVA V: How silicosis and coal workers' pneumoconioses develop—a cellular assessment. Occup Med 8:35, 1993

LEONARD JF, TEMPLETON PA: Pulmonary imaging techniques in the diagnosis of occupational interstitial lung disease, in *Occupational Medicine: State of the Art Reviews*, vol 7, no 2, WS Beckett, R Bascon (eds). Philadelphia, Hanley and Belfus, 1992, pp 241–260

MULLOY KB et al: Use of chest radiographs in epidemiological investigations of pneumoconioses. Br J Ind Med 50:273, 1993

PARKES WR: *Occupational Lung Disorders*, 2d ed. London, Butterworth, 1982

ROGGLI VL et al: Asbestos fiber type in malignant mesothelioma: An analytical scanning electron microscopic study of 94 cases. Am J Ind Med 23:605, 1993

SAMET JM, SPENGLER JD: *Indoor Air Pollution: A Health Perspective*, Baltimore, The Johns Hopkins University, 1991, chaps 2 and 15

SCHENKER MB: Regulatory and policy issues, in *Occupational and Environmental Respiratory Disease*, P Harber et al: (eds). St Louis, Mosby Year Books, 1996, Chaps. 55–58

SHERSON D, LANDER F: Morbidity of pulmonary tuberculosis among silicotic and nonsilicotic foundry workers in Denmark. J Occup Med 32:110, 1990

255

Matthew E. Levison

PNEUMONIA, INCLUDING NECROTIZING PULMONARY INFECTIONS (LUNG ABSCESS)

Pneumonia is an infection of the pulmonary parenchyma. Various bacterial species, mycoplasmas, chlamydiae, rickettsiae, viruses, fungi, and parasites can cause pneumonia. Thus pneumonia is not a single disease but a group of specific infections, each with a different epidemiology, pathogenesis, clinical presentation, and clinical course. Identification of the etiologic microorganism is of primary importance, since this is the key to appropriate antimicrobial therapy. However, because of the serious nature of the infection, antimicrobial therapy generally needs to be started immediately, often before laboratory confirmation of the causative agent. The specific microbial etiology remains elusive in about one-third of cases—e.g., when no sputum is available for examination, blood cultures are sterile, and there is no pleural fluid. Serologic confirmation requires weeks because of the late formation of specific antibody.

Initial antimicrobial therapy is often empirical and is based on the setting in which the infection was acquired, the clinical presentation, patterns of abnormality on chest radiography, results of staining of sputum or other infected body fluids, and current patterns of susceptibility of the suspected pathogens to antimicrobial agents. After the etiologic agent is identified, specific antimicrobial therapy can be chosen.

DEFENSE MECHANISMS The lung is a complex structure composed of aggregates of units that are formed by the progressive branching of the airways. Approximately 80 percent of the cells lining the central airways are ciliated, pseudostratified, columnar epithelial cells; the percentage decreases in the peripheral airways. Each ciliated cell contains about 200 cilia that beat in coordinated waves about 1000 times per minute, with a fast forward stroke and a slower backward recovery. Ciliary motion is also coordinated between adjacent cells so that each wave is propagated toward the oropharynx. The cilia are covered by a liquid film that is about 5 to 10 μm thick and is composed of two layers. The outer, or gel, layer is viscous and traps deposited particles. The cilia beat in the less viscous inner, or sol, layer. During the forward stroke, the tips of the cilia just touch the viscous gel and propel it toward the oropharynx. During recovery, the cilia move entirely within the low-resistance sol layer. Ciliated cells are interspersed with mucus-secreting cells in the trachea and bronchi but not in the bronchioles.

The alveolar walls, from blood to air, consist of the endothelium that lines the network of anastomotic capillaries, the capillary basement membrane, the interstitial tissue, the alveolar basement membrane, the alveolar lining epithelial cells (either flattened type I pneumocytes that cover 95 percent of the alveolar surface or rounded, granular surfactant-producing type II pneumocytes), and epithelial lining fluid. The epithelial lining fluid contains surfactant, fibronectin, and immunoglobulin, which may opsonize or—in the presence of complement—lyse microbial pathogens deposited on the alveolar surface. Loosely attached to the lining cells or lying free within the lumen are the alveolar macrophages, lymphocytes, and a few polymorphonuclear leukocytes.

The lower respiratory tract is normally sterile, despite being adjacent to enormous numbers of microorganisms that reside in the oropharynx and being exposed to environmental microorganisms in inhaled air. This sterility is the result of efficient filtering and clearance mechanisms.

Infectious particles deposited on the squamous epithelium of distal nasal surfaces normally are removed by sneezing, while those deposited on the more proximal ciliated surfaces are swept posteriorly in the mucous lining into the nasopharynx, where they are swallowed or expectorated. Reflex closure of the glottis and cough protect the lower respiratory tract. Those particles deposited on the tracheobronchial surface are swept by ciliary motion toward the oropharynx. Infectious particles that bypass defenses in the airways and are deposited on the alveolar surface are cleared by phagocytic cells and humoral factors. Alveolar macrophages are the major phagocytes in the lower respiratory tract. Some phagocytosed microorganisms are killed by the phagocyte's oxygen-dependent systems, lysosomal enzymes, and cationic proteins. Other microorganisms can evade microbicidal mechanisms and persist within the macrophage. For example, *Mycobacterium tuberculosis* persists within the lysosome, while *Legionella* resides within intracellular inclusions that fail to fuse with lysosomes. Intracellular pathogens can then be transported to the ciliated surfaces and into the oropharynx or via the lymphatics to regional lymph nodes. The alveolar macrophages process and present microbial antigens to the lymphocyte and also secrete cytokines (e.g., tumor necrosis factor and interleukin 1) that modulate the immune process in T and B lymphocytes. Cytokines facilitate the generation of an inflammatory response, activate alveolar macrophages, and recruit additional phagocytes and other immunologic factors from plasma. The inflammatory exudate is responsible for many of the local signs of pulmonary consolidation and the systemic manifestations of pneumonia, such as fever, chills, myalgias, and malaise.

TRANSMISSION Microbial pathogens enter the lung by one of several routes.

Aspiration of Organisms That Colonize the Oropharynx Most pulmonary pathogens originate in the oropharyngeal flora. Aspiration of these pathogens is the most common mechanism for the production of pneumonia. At various times during the year, healthy individuals transiently carry common pulmonary pathogens in the nasopharynx; these pathogens include *Streptococcus pneumoniae*, *Streptococcus pyogenes*, *Mycoplasma pneumoniae*, *Haemophilus influenzae*, and *Moraxella catarrhalis*. The sources of anaerobic pulmonary pathogens, such as *Porphyromonas gingivalis*, *Prevotella melaninogenica*, *Fusobacterium nucleatum*, *Actinomyces* spp., spirochetes, and anaerobic streptococci, are the gingival crevice and dental plaque, which contain more than 10^{11} colony-forming units (CFU) of microorganisms per gram. The frequency of aerobic gram-negative bacillary colonization of the oropharyngeal mucosa, which is unusual in healthy persons (<2 percent), increases with hospitalization, worsening debility, severe underlying illness, alcoholism, diabetes, and advanced age. This change may be a consequence of increased salivary proteolytic activity, which destroys fibronectin, a glycoprotein coating the surface of the mucosa. Fibronectin is the receptor for the normal gram-positive flora of the oropharynx. Loss of fibronectin exposes the receptors for aerobic gram-negative bacilli on the epithelial cell surface. The source of aerobic gram-negative bacilli may be the patient's own stomach (which can become colonized with these organisms as the result of an increase in gastric pH with atrophic gastritis or after the use of H_2-blocking agents or antacids), contaminated respiratory equipment, hands of health care workers, or contaminated food and water. Nasogastric tubes can facilitate the transfer of gastric bacteria to the pharynx.

About 50 percent of healthy adults aspirate oropharyngeal secretions into the lower respiratory tract during sleep. Aspiration occurs more frequently and may be more pronounced in individuals with an impaired level of consciousness (e.g., alcoholics; drug abusers; and patients who have had seizures, strokes, or general anesthesia), neurologic dysfunction of the oropharynx, and swallowing disorders or mechanical impediments (e.g., nasogastric or endotracheal tubes). Pneumonia due to anaerobes is an especially likely outcome if the aspirated material is large in volume or contains virulent components of the anaerobic microbial flora or foreign bodies, such as aspirated food or necrotic tissue. Impairment of the cough reflex increases the risk of pneumonia, as does mucociliary or alveolar macrophage dysfunction.

Inhalation of Infectious Aerosols Deposition of inhaled particles within the respiratory tract is determined primarily by particle diameter. Particles that are more than 10 μm in diameter are deposited mostly in the nose and upper airways. Particles that are less than 3 to 5 μm in diameter (also called *airborne droplet nuclei*) and that contain one or perhaps two microorganisms fail to settle out by gravity but rather remain suspended in the atmosphere for long periods unless removed by ventilation or by filtration in the lungs of the individual breathing the contaminated air. These infectious aerosols are small enough to bypass host defenses in the upper respiratory tract and airways. More particles are deposited in small bronchioles and alveoli as particle size decreases below 5 μm. One inhaled particle of appropriate size may be sufficient to reach the alveolus and initiate infection. The etiologies of pneumonia typically acquired by inhalation of infectious aerosols include tuberculosis, influenza, legionellosis, psittacosis, histoplasmosis, and Q fever.

Hematogenous Dissemination from an Extrapulmonary Site Infection, usually with *Staphylococcus aureus*, disseminates hematogenously to the lungs in patients (such as intravenous drug abusers) who have either right- or left-sided bacterial endocarditis and in patients with intravenous catheter infections. *Fusobacterium* infections of the retropharyngeal tissues (Lemierre's syndrome—i.e., retropharyngeal abscess and jugular venous thrombophlebitis) also disseminate to the lungs.

Direct Inoculation and Contiguous Spread Two additional routes of transmission of bacteria to the lungs are direct inoculation as a result of either tracheal intubation or stab wounds of the chest and contiguous spread from an adjacent site of infection.

PATHOLOGY The pneumonic process may involve primarily the interstitium or the alveoli. Involvement of an entire lobe is called *lobar pneumonia*. When the process is restricted to alveoli contiguous to bronchi, it is called *bronchopneumonia*. Confluent bronchopneumonia may be indistinguishable from lobar pneumonia. Cavities develop when necrotic lung tissue is discharged into communicating airways, resulting in either necrotizing pneumonia (multiple small cavities, each <2 cm in diameter, in one or more bronchopulmonary segments or lobes) or lung abscess (one or more cavities >2 cm in diameter). The classification of pneumonia is best based upon the causative microorganism rather than upon these anatomic characteristics (the criteria used in the past).

EPIDEMIOLOGY The patient's living circumstances, occupation, travel history, pet or animal exposure history, and contacts with other ill individuals as well as the physician's knowledge of the epidemic curve of community outbreaks provide useful clues to the microbial etiology of a given case of pneumonia (see Table 255-1).

The relative frequency of various pulmonary pathogens varies with the setting in which the infection was acquired—e.g., community, nursing home, or hospital. In patients hospitalized with community-acquired pneumonia, the most frequent pathogens are *S. pneumoniae*, *H. influenzae*, *Chlamydia pneumoniae*, and *Legionella pneumophila*. *M. pneumoniae*, which usually causes mild illness, is common among outpatients with community-acquired pneumonia. In contrast, enteric aerobic gram-negative bacilli and *Pseudomonas aeruginosa*, uncommon causes of community-acquired pneumonia, are estimated to account for more than 50 percent of cases of hospital-acquired pneumonia, while *S. aureus* is responsible for more than 10 percent. The relative frequencies of pathogens in pneumonia acquired in nursing homes fall somewhere between those of community- and hospital-acquired pneumonia. Enteric aerobic gram-negative bacilli and *P. aeruginosa* are more common among nursing home residents than among patients who acquire pneumonia in noninstitutional settings.

The season of the year and the geographic location are other predictors of etiology. The frequency of influenza virus as a cause of both community-acquired and institutionally acquired pneumonia increases during the winter months. Moreover, influenza virus infection causes an increase in the frequency of secondary bacterial pneumonia due to *S. pneumoniae*, *S. aureus*, and *H. influenzae*. Outbreaks of influenza in a community tend to be explosive and widespread, with many secondary cases resulting from the short incubation period of several days and the high degree of communicability. Legionellosis also occurs in explosive outbreaks when large numbers of susceptible people are exposed to an infectious aerosol; however, no secondary cases occur because of the low level of communicability of *L. pneumophila*. *Mycoplasma* can cause outbreaks, usually in relatively closed populations such as those at military bases, at colleges, or in households; however, because of its long incubation period (2 to 3 weeks) and its relatively low degree of communicability, *Mycoplasma* infection moves through the community slowly, affecting another person as the first is recovering. In communities where infection with human immunodeficiency virus (HIV) type 1 is endemic, *Pneumocystis carinii* and *M. tuberculosis* are more prominent causes of community-acquired pneumonia. Histoplasmosis, blastomycosis, and coccidioidomycosis are causes of pneumonia that have specific geographic distributions, and *Chlamydia psittaci* produces illness in bird handlers.

AGE AND COMORBIDITY Age is an important predictor of the infecting agent in pneumonia. *Chlamydia trachomatis* and respiratory syncytial virus are common among infants under 6 months of age; *H. influenzae* among children between 6 months and 5 years of age; *M. pneumoniae* and *C. pneumoniae* among young adults; and *H. influenzae*, *L. pneumophila*, and *M. catarrhalis* among elderly persons with chronic lung disease.

Oral anaerobes, frequently in combination with aerobic bacterial components of the human flora (e.g., viridans streptococci), are causes of community-acquired pneumonia and anaerobic lung abscess in patients who are prone to aspiration. Edentulous persons, who have lower numbers of oral anaerobes, are less likely to develop pneumonia due to anaerobes. When the etiology of community-acquired pneumonia in unselected hospitalized patients has been studied by methods that entail strict anaerobic bacteriology and that avoid contamination of lower respiratory tract secretions by the oral flora, anaerobic bacteria have been found to account for as many as 20 to 30 percent of cases. In hospital-acquired pneumonia, anaerobes are the pathogens—with or without aerobic copathogens—in about one-third of cases. However, the aerobic copathogens in hospital-acquired pneumonia are frequently virulent microorganisms in their own right (e.g., enteric aerobic gram-negative bacilli, *P. aeruginosa*, and *S. aureus*).

The patient's underlying disease may be characterized by specific immunologic or inflammatory defects that predispose to pneumonia due to specific pathogens (see Table 255-2). For example, patients who have severe hypogammaglobulinemia (<2.0 g/L) are at risk of infection with encapsulated bacteria such as *S. pneumoniae* and *H. influenzae*. HIV-infected patients also may exhibit ineffective antibody formation, which predisposes to infection with these encapsulated bacteria. Severe neutropenia (<500 neutrophils/μL) increases the risk of infections due to *P. aeruginosa*, Enterobacteriaceae, *S. aureus*, and (if neutropenia is prolonged) *Aspergillus*. The risk is unusually high for infections due to *M. tuberculosis* among HIV-infected patients

Table 255-1

Microbial Pathogens That Cause Pneumonia

Community-Acquired	Hospital-Acquired	HIV Infection–Associated
Mycoplasma pneumoniae	Enteric aerobic gram-negative bacilli	*Pneumocystis carinii*
Streptococcus pneumoniae	*Pseudomonas aeruginosa*	*Mycobacterium tuberculosis*
Haemophilus influenzae	*Staphylococcus aureus*	*Streptococcus pneumoniae*
Chlamydia pneumoniae	Oral anaerobes	*Haemophilus influenzae*
Legionella pneumophila		
Oral anaerobes		
Moraxella catarrhalis		
Staphylococcus aureus		
Nocardia spp.		
Viruses*		
Fungi†		
Mycobacterium tuberculosis		
Chlamydia psittaci		

* Influenza virus, cytomegalovirus, respiratory syncytial virus, measles virus, and vari-a-zoster virus.

toplasma, *Coccidioides*, and *Blastomyces* spp.

with circulating CD4 lymphocyte counts <500/μL; for infections due to *P. carinii*, *Histoplasma capsulatum*, and *Cryptococcus neoformans* among those with CD4 counts <200/μL; and for infections due to *Mycobacterium avium-intracellulare* and cytomegalovirus among those with CD4 counts <50/μL. Long-term glucocorticoid therapy increases the risk of tuberculosis and nocardiosis.

CLINICAL MANIFESTATIONS **Community-Acquired Pneumonia** Community-acquired pneumonia has traditionally been thought to present as either of two syndromes: the typical presentation and the atypical presentation. Although recent data suggest that these two syndromes may be less distinct than was once thought, the characteristics of the clinical presentation may nevertheless have some diagnostic value.

The "typical" pneumonia syndrome is characterized by the sudden onset of fever, cough productive of purulent sputum, and in some cases pleuritic chest pain; signs of pulmonary consolidation (dullness, increased fremitus, egophony, bronchial breath sounds, and rales) may be found on physical examination in areas of radiographic abnormality. The typical pneumonia syndrome is usually caused by the most common bacterial pathogen in community-acquired pneumonia, *S. pneumoniae*, but can also be due to other bacterial pathogens, such as *H. influenzae* and mixed anaerobic and aerobic components of the oral flora.

The "atypical" pneumonia syndrome is characterized by a more gradual onset, a dry cough, a prominence of extrapulmonary symptoms (such as headache, myalgias, fatigue, sore throat, nausea, vomiting, and diarrhea), and abnormalities on chest radiographs despite minimal signs of pulmonary involvement (other than rales) on physical examination. Atypical pneumonia is classically produced by *M. pneumoniae* but can also be caused by *L. pneumophila*, *C. pneumoniae*, oral anaerobes, and *P. carinii* as well as by *S. pneumoniae* and the less frequently encountered pathogens *C. psittaci*, *Coxiella burnetii*, *Francisella tularensis*, *H. capsulatum*, and *Coccidioides immitis*. *Mycoplasma* pneumonia (see Chap. 180) may be complicated by erythema multiforme, hemolytic anemia, bullous myringitis, encephalitis, and transverse myelitis. *Legionella* pneumonia (see Chap. 153) is frequently associated with deterioration in mental status, renal and hepatic abnormalities, and marked hyponatremia; pneumonia due to *H. capsulatum* or *C. immitis* is often accompanied by erythema nodosum. In *C. pneumoniae* pneumonia (see Chap. 181), sore throat, hoarseness, and wheezing are relatively common. The atypical pneumonia syndrome in patients whose behavioral history places them at risk of HIV infection suggests *Pneumocystis* infection. These patients may have concurrent infections due to other opportunistic pathogens, such as pulmonary (and frequently extrapulmonary) tuberculosis, oral thrush due to *Candida albicans*, or extensive perineal ulcers due to herpes simplex virus.

Certain viruses also produce pneumonia that is usually characterized by an atypical presentation—i.e., chills, fever, dry nonproductive cough, and predominance of extrapulmonary symptoms. Primary viral pneumonia can be caused by influenza virus infection (usually as part of a community outbreak in winter), by respiratory syncytial virus infection (in children and immunosuppressed individuals), by measles or varicella-zoster virus infection (accompanied by the characteristic rash), and by cytomegalovirus infection (in patients immunocompromised by HIV infection or by therapy given in association with organ transplantation). In addition, influenza, measles, and varicella can predispose to secondary bacterial pneumonia as a result of the destruction of the mucociliary barrier of the airways. Secondary bacterial infection may either follow the viral infection without interruption or be separated from the viral infection by several days of transient relief of symptoms. Bacterial infection may be heralded by sudden worsening of the patient's clinical condition, with persisting or renewed chills, fever, and cough productive of purulent sputum, possibly accompanied by pleuritic chest pain.

Patients with hematogenous *S. aureus* pneumonia may present with fever and dyspnea only. In these cases the inflammatory response is initially confined to the pulmonary interstitium. Cough, sputum production, and signs of pulmonary consolidation develop only after the infection extends into the bronchi. These patients are usually gravely ill, with intravascular infection as well as pneumonia, and may have signs of endocarditis (see Chap. 126).

Nocardiosis (see Chap. 167) is frequently complicated by metastasis of lesions to the skin and central nervous system. Signs of pulmonary consolidation, cough, and sputum production may be lacking in patients who are unable to mount an inflammatory response, such as those with agranulocytosis. The major manifestations in these patients may be limited to fever, tachypnea, agitation, and altered mental status. Elderly or severely ill patients may fail to develop fever.

Tuberculosis also produces an atypical presentation that is characterized by fever, night sweats, cough, and shortness of breath and sometimes by pleuritic chest pain and blood-streaked sputum. Several weeks usually elapse before the patient seeks medical attention because of the gradual worsening of these symptoms, by which time he or she will have lost considerable weight.

Nosocomial Pneumonia Patients with nosocomial pneumonia often pose a diagnostic challenge. The differential diagnosis of acute respiratory disease in critically ill, hospitalized patients is diverse and includes noninfectious entities, such as congestive heart failure, acute respiratory distress syndrome, preexisting lung disease, atelectasis, and oxygen- or drug-related toxicities, that may be difficult to distinguish clinically or radiologically from pneumonia. The usual criteria for nosocomial pneumonia, which include new or progressive pulmonary infiltrates, purulent tracheobronchial secretions, fever, and leukocytosis, are frequently unreliable in these patients, who often have preexisting pulmonary disease, endotracheal tubes that irritate the tracheal mucosa and may elicit an inflammatory exudate in respiratory secretions, or multiple other problems likely to produce fever and leukocytosis. Patients with nosocomial pneumonia complicating an underlying illness associated with significant neutropenia often have no purulent respiratory tract secretions or pulmonary infiltrates, and patients with nosocomial pneumonia complicating uremia or cirrhosis often remain afebrile. In addition, the patients at greatest risk for nosocomial pneumonia are most likely to be heavily colonized with potential pulmonary pathogens in the oropharyngeal or tracheobronchial mucosa; thus the presence of these organisms in gram-stained preparations or cultures of respiratory tract secretions does not necessarily confirm the diagnosis of pneumonia.

Aspiration Pneumonia and Anaerobic Lung Abscess Although the aspiration of oral anaerobes can initially lead to an infiltrative process, it ultimately results in putrid sputum, tissue necrosis, and pulmonary cavities. In about three-quarters of cases, the clinical course of an abscess of anaerobic, polymicrobial etiology is indolent and mimics that of pulmonary tuberculosis, with cough, shortness of breath, chills, fever, night sweats, weight loss, pleuritic chest pain, and blood-streaked sputum lasting for several weeks or more. In other patients

Table 255-2

Pulmonary Pathogens Associated with Specific Defects in Host Defenses

Defect	Pathogens
Severe hypogammaglobulinemia	Encapsulated bacteria: *Streptococcus pneumoniae*, *Haemophilus influenzae*
Severe neutropenia	*Pseudomonas aeruginosa*, Enterobacteriaceae, *Staphylococcus aureus*, *Aspergillus*
Defective cell-mediated immunity	
CD4 lymphocyte count	
<500/μL	*Mycobacterium tuberculosis*
<200/μL	*Pneumocystis carinii*, *Histoplasma capsulatum*, *Cryptococcus neoformans*
<50/μL	*Mycobacterium avium-intracellulare*, cytomegalovirus
Long-term glucocorticoid therapy	*M. tuberculosis*, *Nocardia*

the disease may present more acutely. Patients with anaerobic abscesses are usually prone to aspiration of oropharyngeal contents and have periodontal disease. One genus of oral anaerobes, *Actinomyces,* produces a chronic fibrotic necrotizing process that crosses tissue planes and may involve the pleural space, ribs, vertebrae, and subcutaneous tissue, with eventual discharge of sulfur granules (macroscopic bacterial masses) through the skin (empyema necessitatis).

DIAGNOSIS **Radiography** Chest radiographs can confirm the presence and location of the pulmonary infiltrate; assess the extent of the pulmonary infection; detect pleural involvement, pulmonary cavitation, or hilar lymphadenopathy; and gauge the response to antimicrobial therapy. However, chest radiographs may be normal when the patient is unable to mount an inflammatory response (e.g., in agranulocytosis) or is in the early stage of an infiltrative process (e.g., in hematogenous *S. aureus* pneumonia or in *Pneumocystis* pneumonia associated with AIDS).

The anatomic localization of the inflammatory process, as visualized in chest radiographs, occasionally has diagnostic implications. Most pulmonary pathogens produce focal lesions. A multicentric distribution suggests hematogenous infection, in which case the remote location of the primary infection (e.g., endocarditis or thrombophlebitis) should be sought. Hematogenous pneumonia, which results from septic embolization in patients with thrombophlebitis or right-sided endocarditis and from bacteremia in patients with left-sided endocarditis, appears on the chest radiograph as multiple areas of pulmonary infiltration that subsequently may cavitate. A diffuse distribution suggests the involvement of *P. carinii*, cytomegalovirus, measles virus, or varicella-zoster virus (with pneumonia due to the last two pathogens diagnosed by the characteristic accompanying rash). Pleurisy and hilar nodal enlargement are unusual with *Pneumocystis* and cytomegalovirus pneumonia; their presence suggests another etiology. Diffuse lesions in immunocompromised patients also suggest legionellosis, tuberculosis, histoplasmosis, *Mycoplasma* infection, or disseminated strongyloidiasis.

Oral anaerobes, *S. aureus*, *S. pneumoniae* serotype III, aerobic gram-negative bacilli, *M. tuberculosis*, and fungi as well as certain noninfectious conditions can produce tissue necrosis and pulmonary cavities (Table 255-3). In contrast, *H. influenzae*, *M. pneumoniae*, viruses, and most other serotypes of *S. pneumoniae* almost never cause cavities. Apical disease, with or without cavities, suggests reactivation tuberculosis. Anaerobic abscesses are located in dependent, poorly ventilated, and poorly draining bronchopulmonary segments and characteristically have air-fluid levels unlike the well-ventilated, well-drained upper-lobe cavities caused by *M. tuberculosis*, an obligate aerobe. Air-fluid levels may also be present in cavities due to pulmonary necrosis of other infectious etiologies. *Mucor* and *Aspergillus* invade blood vessels and cause pleura-based, wedge-shaped areas of pulmonary infarction; these infarcts may subsequently cavitate.

In the patient with an uncomplicated course, chest radiographs need not be repeated before discharge, since the resolution of infiltrates

Table 255-3

Causes of Pulmonary Cavities

INFECTIOUS
Bacteria: Oral anaerobes (*Bacteroides* spp., fusobacteria, *Actinomyces* spp., anaerobic and microaerophilic cocci), enteric aerobic gram-negative bacilli, *Pseudomonas aeruginosa*, *Legionella* spp., *Staphylococcus aureus*, *Streptococcus pneumoniae* serotype III, *Mycobacterium tuberculosis*, *Nocardia* spp.
Fungi: *Histoplasma capsulatum*, *Coccidioides immitis*, *Blastomyces* spp.
NONINFECTIOUS
lasms, Wegener's granulomatosis, infarction, infected bullae and cysts

may take up to 6 weeks after initial presentation. However, patients who do not respond clinically, who have a pleural effusion on admission, who may have postobstructive pneumonia, or who are infected with certain pathogens (e.g., *S. aureus*, aerobic gram-negative bacilli, or oral anaerobes) need more intensive surveillance. At times, computed tomography may be especially helpful in distinguishing different processes—e.g., pleural effusion versus underlying pulmonary consolidation, hilar adenopathy versus pulmonary mass, and pulmonary abscess versus empyema with an air-fluid level.

Sputum Examination Examination of the sputum remains the mainstay of the evaluation of a patient with acute bacterial pneumonia. Unfortunately, expectorated material is frequently contaminated by potentially pathogenic bacteria that colonize the upper respiratory tract (and sometimes the lower respiratory tract) without actually causing disease. This contamination reduces the diagnostic specificity of any lower respiratory tract specimen. In addition, it has been estimated that the usual laboratory processing methods detect the pulmonary pathogen in fewer than 50 percent of expectorated sputum samples from patients with bacteremic *S. pneumoniae* pneumonia. This low sensitivity may be due to misidentification of the alpha-hemolytic colonies of *S. pneumoniae* as nonpathogenic alpha-hemolytic streptococci ("normal flora"), overgrowth of the cultures by hardier colonizing organisms, or loss of more fastidious organisms due to slow transport or improper processing. In addition, certain very common pulmonary pathogens, such as anaerobes, mycoplasmas, chlamydiae, *Pneumocystis*, mycobacteria, fungi, and legionellae, cannot be cultured by routine methods.

Since expectorated material is routinely contaminated by oral anaerobes, the diagnosis of anaerobic pulmonary infection is frequently tentative. Confirmation of such a diagnosis requires the culture of anaerobes from pulmonary secretions that are uncontaminated by oropharyngeal secretions, which in turn requires the collection of pulmonary secretions by special techniques, such as transtracheal aspiration, transthoracic lung puncture, and protected brush via bronchoscopy. These procedures are invasive and usually are not used unless the patient fails to respond to empirical therapy.

Gram's staining of sputum specimens, screened initially under low-power magnification (10× objective and 10× eyepiece) to determine the degree of contamination with squamous epithelial cells, is of utmost diagnostic importance. In patients with the typical pneumonia syndrome who produce purulent sputum, the sensitivity and specificity of Gram's staining of sputum minimally contaminated by upper respiratory tract secretions (>25 polymorphonuclear leukocytes and <10 epithelial cells per low-power field) in identifying the pathogen as *S. pneumoniae* are 62 and 85 percent, respectively. Gram's staining in this case is more specific and probably more sensitive than the accompanying sputum culture. The finding of mixed flora on Gram's staining of an uncontaminated sputum specimen suggests an anaerobic infection. Acid-fast staining of sputum should be undertaken when mycobacterial infection is suspected. Examination by an experienced pathologist of Giemsa-stained expectorated respiratory secretions from patients with AIDS has given satisfactory results in the diagnosis of *Pneumocystis* pneumonia. The sensitivity of sputum examination is enhanced by the use of monoclonal antibodies to *Pneumocystis* and is diminished by prior prophylactic use of inhaled pentamidine. Blastomycosis can be diagnosed by the examination of wet preparations of sputum. Sputum stained directly with fluorescent antibody can be examined for *Legionella*, but this test yields false-negative results relatively often. Thus sputum should also be cultured for *Legionella* on special media.

Expectorated sputum usually is easily collected from patients with a vigorous cough but may be scant in patients with an atypical syndrome, in the elderly, and in persons with altered mental status. If the patient is not producing sputum and can cooperate, respiratory secretions should be induced with ultrasonic nebulization of 3% saline. An attempt to obtain lower respiratory secretions by passage of a catheter through the nose or mouth rarely achieves the desired results in an alert patient and is discouraged; usually the catheter can be found coiled in the oropharynx.

In some cases that do not require the patient's hospitalization (see Table 255-4), an accurate microbial diagnosis may not be crucial, and empirical therapy can be started on the basis of clinical and epidemiologic evidence alone. This approach may also be appropriate for hospitalized patients who are not severely ill and who are unable to produce an induced sputum specimen. Use of invasive procedures to establish a microbial diagnosis carries risks that must be weighed against potential benefits. However, the decision to initiate empirical therapy without an evaluation of induced sputum should be undertaken with caution and, in the case of hospitalized patients, should always be accompanied by the culture of several blood samples. The ability to understand the cause of a poor response to empirical antimicrobial therapy (see Table 255-5) may be compromised by the lack of an initial sputum culture.

Invasive Procedures The sensitivities and specificities of the invasive procedures described below for obtaining pulmonary material vary with the type of immunocompromised patient, the type of pulmonary lesion, and the degree of prior exposure to therapeutic or prophylactic antimicrobial agents.

Transtracheal aspiration (TTA) Popular several decades ago, TTA is rarely performed today. Although the sensitivity of the procedure is high (approaching 90 percent), the specificity is low. The material obtained by TTA (from a catheter inserted through the cricothyroid cartilage and advanced toward the carina) is not contaminated by upper respiratory tract secretions but can contain organisms that colonize the tracheobronchial tree without necessarily causing pneumonia. Significant morbidity and even death have attended the use of TTA. Contraindicated in patients with a bleeding diathesis, TTA may cause infection at the puncture site and may lead to severe subcutaneous and mediastinal emphysema in patients who are coughing vigorously.

Percutaneous transthoracic lung puncture This procedure employs a skinny (small-gauge) needle that is advanced into the area of pulmonary consolidation with computed tomographic guidance. It requires that the patient cooperate, have good hemostasis, and be able to tolerate a possible associated pulmonary hemorrhage or pneumothorax. Patients on mechanical ventilation cannot undergo lung puncture because of the high incidence of complicating pneumothorax.

Fiberoptic bronchoscopy Fiberoptic bronchoscopy is safe and relatively well tolerated and has become the standard invasive procedure used to obtain lower respiratory tract secretions from seriously ill or immunocompromised patients with complex or progressive pneumonia. This technique provides a direct view of the lower airways. Specimens obtained by bronchoscopy should be subjected to Gram's, acid-fast, *Legionella* direct fluorescent antibody, and Gomori's methenamine silver staining and should be cultured for routine aerobic and anaerobic bacteria, *Legionella*, mycobacteria, and fungi. Samples are collected with a protected double-sheathed brush (PSB), by bronchoalveolar lavage (BAL), or by transbronchial biopsy (TBB) at the site of pulmonary consolidation. The PSB sample is usually contaminated by oropharyngeal flora; quantitative cultures of the 1 mL of sterile culture medium into which the brush is placed after withdrawal from the inner catheter must be performed to differentiate contamination (<1000 CFU/mL) from infection (≥1000 CFU/mL). The results of PSB are highly specific and highly sensitive, especially when the patient has not received antibiotics before culture. BAL is usually performed with 150 to 200 mL of sterile, nonbacteriostatic saline. When used to facilitate endoscopy, local anesthetic agents with antibacterial activity can lower the sensitivity of culture results. Quantitative bacteriologic evaluation of BAL fluid has given results similar to those obtained with the PSB technique. Gram's staining of the cytocentrifuged BAL fluid specimen can serve as an immediate guide in the selection of antimicrobial therapy to be administered while culture results are awaited.

Open-lung biopsy This procedure is most commonly needed when specimens obtained bronchoscopically from an immunocompromised patient with progressive pneumonia have been unrevealing. Limitations on the performance of an open-lung biopsy include hypoxemia and a bleeding diathesis, which may supervene while the physician is deciding whether to undertake this procedure. Results of an open-lung biopsy are considered diagnostic because of the large size of the tissue sample. The diagnostic yield of this procedure is greatest in focal lesions, whereas bronchoscopic evaluation is most useful in diffuse lesions.

Other Diagnostic Tests In the initial evaluation of a patient with pneumonia, at least two blood samples for culture should be obtained from different venipuncture sites; if empyema is a clinical consideration, diagnostic thoracentesis is indicated. Positive blood or pleural fluid culture is generally considered diagnostic of the etiology of pneumonia. However, bacteremia and empyema each occur in fewer than 10 to 30 percent of patients with pneumonia.

Serologic studies are sometimes helpful in defining the etiology of certain types of pneumonia, although serologic diagnosis, because it is often delayed by the need to demonstrate at least a fourfold rise in convalescent-phase antibody titer, is usually retrospective. A single IgM antibody titer of >1:16, a single IgG antibody titer of >1:128, or a fourfold or greater rise in the IgG titer obtained by indirect immunofluorescence is diagnostic of *M. pneumoniae* infection. A single IgM antibody titer of ≥1:20, a single IgG antibody titer of ≥1:128, or a fourfold or greater rise in the IgG titer obtained by micro-indirect immunofluorescence is diagnostic of *C. pneumoniae* infection. A single legionella antibody titer of ≥1:256 or a fourfold rise to a titer of ≥1:128 suggests acute legionellosis. A highly sensitive and specific urinary antigen test is available to detect *L. pneumophila* serogroup 1 in patients with pneumonia; this organism accounts for about 70 percent of cases of *L. pneumophila* infection.

DECISION TO HOSPITALIZE Use of hospital services is costly and at times poses a risk to the patient (e.g., the risk of nosocomial infections). Thus hospitalization must be justified by the patient's poor functional status or by an inadequate social-support system that would compromise care at home, poor prognostic factors, unstable vital signs, or the need for intensive nursing care or specialized diagnostic procedures. Guidelines for hospitalization are given in Table 255-4. Discharge from the hospital should be guided by similar considerations.

Table 255-4

Criteria for Hospitalization of Patients with Pneumonia

1. Elderly patient (>65 years of age)
2. Significant comorbidity (e.g., kidney, heart, or lung disease; diabetes mellitus; neoplasm; immunosuppression)
3. Leukopenia (<5000 white blood cells/μL) not attributable to a known condition
4. *Staphylococcus aureus*, gram-negative bacilli, or anaerobes as the suspected cause of pneumonia
5. Suppurative complications (e.g., empyema, arthritis, meningitis, endocarditis)
6. Failure of outpatient management
7. Inability to take oral medication
8. Tachypnea (>30/min); tachycardia (>140/min); hypotension (<90 mmHg systolic); hypoxemia (arterial P_{O_2}, <60 mmHg); acute alteration of mental status

Table 255-5

Factors Involved in Poor Response to Empirical Antimicrobial Therapy

Incorrect microbiologic diagnosis
Inappropriate antimicrobial agent or dosing regimen
Drug hypersensitivity or other adverse effect (e.g., *Clostridium difficile* colitis)
Infectious complication: empyema, metastatic spread, superinfection
Atelectasis, parapneumonic effusion, phlebitis
Poor host defenses (e.g., endobronchial obstruction, life-threatening comorbidity)

℞ TREATMENT

Community-Acquired Pneumonia: Outpatient Management Most cases of community-acquired pneumonia in otherwise-healthy adults do not require hospitalization. Since it is often impractical to make a microbial diagnosis in an office setting, the oral antimicrobial therapy administered is frequently empirical (see Table 255-6). The pathogen in such a situation is likely to be *M. pneumoniae*, *S. pneumoniae*, or *C. pneumoniae*. In older patients with underlying chronic respiratory disease, *L. pneumophila*, *H. influenzae*, or *M. catarrhalis* should also be considered. In patients at risk of aspiration, oral anaerobes may be involved. No oral regimen has a reliable spectrum encompassing all these pathogens (see Table 255-6). Whatever regimen is chosen, its antimicrobial activity should encompass *S. pneumoniae*, the most common cause of pneumonia. Increasing resistance among pneumococci to all available oral antimicrobial agents precludes the designation of any one agent as the clear drug of choice.

Strains of *S. pneumoniae* that have a minimal inhibitory concentration (MIC) of penicillin (as determined by the broth dilution method) of 0.1 to 1.0 μg/mL are considered to have intermediate-level resistance, while strains that have an MIC of >1.0 μg/mL are considered to have high-level resistance. The current, less time-consuming method to screen for penicillin resistance is the use of a 1-μg oxacillin disk in a disk diffusion assay. Penicillin resistance (i.e., an MIC of ≥0.1 μg/mL) is indicated by a zone of growth inhibition of ≤19 mm. A new method, the E-strip, which is as accurate as the MIC broth dilution technique and can be performed as rapidly as the oxacillin disk diffusion assay, may replace the oxacillin test in the future.

The resistance of *S. pneumoniae* to penicillin varies greatly with the source of the clinical sample tested (e.g., strains isolated from middle-ear fluid are most often resistant), the age of the patient (e.g., resistance is more frequent among children than among adults), the setting (e.g., resistance is more common in day-care centers and hospitals than in the community), the patient's socioeconomic status (the frequency of resistance is highest in samples from suburban and white patients), and the geographic region in which the specimen was collected. Caution must be exercised in the interpretation of surveys of antimicrobial resistance among pneumococci in the United States, which can be strongly affected by these types of sampling bias. In a national survey of clinical isolates from normally sterile body sites that was conducted by the Centers for Disease Control and Prevention (CDC) from October 1991 to September 1992, 6.6 percent of 544 isolates of *S. pneumoniae* were resistant to ≥0.1 μg of penicillin/mL and 1.3 percent were resistant to ≥2 μg/mL. However, in another national survey of the antimicrobial susceptibility of clinical isolates from respiratory tract sites in 1992 and 1993, 15 percent of 799 isolates (with a range of 4 to 50 percent in the various medical centers) displayed intermediate-level penicillin resistance, and an additional 7 percent (with a range of 0 to 33 percent) were highly penicillin-resistant.

Penicillin-resistant strains can be expected to exhibit decreased susceptibility to oral cephalosporins as well as to other antimicrobial agents. In the CDC survey, 5.9 percent of isolates were resistant to erythromycin (MIC, ≥1 μg/mL), but erythromycin resistance has been reported in 10 to 20 percent of pneumococcal isolates from some centers in the United States. Erythromycin-resistant strains are also resistant to other macrolides, such as clarithromycin and azithromycin. Fewer than 5 percent of strains were resistant to tetracycline in the CDC survey. Resistance to all of these antibiotics currently is much more common in many other parts of the world than in the United States. The potential for increased resistance in the United States in the future deserves close scrutiny; such an increase would require changes in antibiotic recommendations.

Neither trimethoprim-sulfamethoxazole nor the fluoroquinolones should be considered options for empirical therapy. The former drug is not active against more than 10 percent of strains of *S. pneumoniae*, and the latter agents exhibit—at best—borderline activity against pneumococci in vitro.

Penicillin, ampicillin, or amoxicillin (e.g., 500 mg of amoxicillin every 8 h for 7 to 10 days) remains the drug of choice for the treatment of suspected pneumococcal pneumonia in the United States and is recommended for the treatment of community-acquired pneumonia with a "typical" presentation in young adult outpatients without preexisting disease. Erythromycin (500 mg every 6 h) or doxycycline (100 mg every 12 h) is another option.

In older patients or adult outpatients with preexisting respiratory disease and a "typical" presentation of community-acquired pneumonia (among whom β-lactamase-producing pathogens such as *H. influenzae* and *M. catarrhalis* are common), either amoxicillin plus the β-lactamase inhibitor clavulanic acid or doxycycline can be used. Erythromycin displays poor activity against *H. influenzae*; two new oral antibiotics related to erythromycin, azithromycin (a single dose of 500 mg on the first day and 250 mg once daily for 4 more days) and clarithromycin (500 mg twice daily for 7 to 10 days), show equal or greater potency against many lower respiratory pathogens and may elicit gastrointestinal intolerance less frequently. Although more costly than erythromycin, these new macrolides may replace the older drug as therapy for community-acquired pneumonia in outpatients if pneumococcal resistance to macrolides does not become a widespread problem.

Doxycycline and erythromycin are active against *M. pneumoniae* and *C. pneumoniae* and can be used in young adults with an atypical presentation in whom mild pneumonia due to these pathogens is suspected. Ciprofloxacin is also active against these pathogens but is inadequately active against the pneumococcus to justify empirical use in this situation. Although erythromycin is the drug of choice for the treatment of legionellosis, doxycycline, trimethoprim-sulfamethoxazole, and ciprofloxacin have been used successfully for this indication (according to anecdotal reports). The duration of therapy for *Mycoplasma* and *Legionella* infection is 2 to 3 weeks;

Table 255-6

Empirical Oral Antimicrobial Therapy for Outpatient Management of Community-Acquired Pneumonia

	Value of Indicated Antimicrobial*						
Pathogen	**Penicillin G**	**Amoxicillin/ Clavulanate**	**Cefuroxime**	**Trimethoprim-Sulfamethoxazole**	**Doxycycline**	**Erythromycin**	**Ciprofloxacin**
Streptococcus pneumoniae	+†	+†	+†	±	+	+†	±
Haemophilus influenzae	−	+	+	+	+	±‡	+
Moraxella catarrhalis	−	+	+	+	+	+	+
Anaerobes	±	+	±	−	−	−	−
Mycoplasma pneumoniae	−	−	−	−	+	+	+
Chlamydia pneumoniae	−	−	−	−	+	+	+
Legionella pneumophila	−	−	−	±	±	+	±

* +, effective; −, ineffective; ±, sometimes effective.

tween 10 and 20 percent of strains have recently been reported to be resistant to β-lactams and macrolides in some locations in the United States.

ıe new macrolides azithromycin and clarithromycin are more active against *H. influenzae* than erythromycin and are equally or more active against other respiratory pathogens.

the longer duration is frequently recommended to prevent relapse. The optimal duration of therapy for *C. pneumoniae* infection is unknown but probably is 2 to 3 weeks.

Pneumonia due to anaerobes can be treated with clindamycin (300 mg every 6 h or 450 mg every 8 h for 7 to 10 days), with amoxicillin (500 mg every 8 h) plus metronidazole (500 mg every 6 h), or with amoxicillin/clavulanic acid (500 mg every 8 h or 875 mg every 12 h). Metronidazole exhibits poor activity against microaerophilic gram-positive cocci and must be supplemented by a β-lactam agent that compensates for this deficit in coverage.

Community-Acquired Pneumonia: Inpatient Management Patients who have community-acquired pneumonia and are ill enough to be hospitalized (Table 255-4) must undergo prompt microbiologic evaluation, receiving empirical therapy based on Gram's staining of sputum and knowledge of the current antimicrobial sensitivities of the pulmonary pathogens in the local geographic area (Tables 255-7 and 255-8). Parenteral antimicrobial therapy in the hospitalized patient is usually mandatory. A lack of sputum production, an atypical clinical presentation, the presence of diffuse radiographic infiltrates, a rapidly progressive downhill course, and a poor response to prior empirical therapy are some of the indications for the use of invasive procedures to detect the pulmonary pathogen, especially in the immunocompromised patient. Although broad-spectrum antibacterial therapy should be started during a full evaluation in severely ill patients with rapidly progressing illness, these empirical regimens cannot encompass all the possible pathogens without unnecessary toxicity and expense. Indeed, in immunocompromised patients (including those with neutropenia or HIV infection), the number of microbial and noninfectious causes of pulmonary disease is large and increasing. Since failure to provide specific treatment can prove rapidly fatal, a diagnosis should be sought aggressively so that optimal therapy can be started promptly.

Penicillin or ampicillin remains the drug of choice for infection due to penicillin-susceptible pneumococci. Studies suggest that high-dose intravenous penicillin G (e.g., 10 to 20 million units daily), ampicillin (2 g every 6 h), ceftriaxone (1 or 2 g every 24 h), or cefotaxime (1 to 2 g every 6 h) constitutes adequate therapy for pneumonia due to strains exhibiting intermediate resistance to penicillin (MIC, 0.1 to 1 μg/mL). The effectiveness of high-dose intravenous penicillin against pneumonia due to highly resistant pneumococcal strains is unknown, but MICs of cefotaxime and ceftriaxone for these strains are usually lower than those of penicillin or ampicillin and most other β-lactam antibiotics. Ceftriaxone or cefotaxime may be effective when the MIC of penicillin is ≥ 1 μg/mL and those of ceftriaxone and cefotaxime are ≤ 2 μg/mL. However, highly cephalosporin-resistant strains have become a problem in certain geographic areas. Since all penicillin-resistant strains are sensitive to vancomycin, initial empirical therapy should include this antibiotic (1 g intravenously every 12 h) when the patient with pneumococcal pneumonia is severely ill, has significant comorbidity, and lives in a region where highly penicillin- or cephalosporin-resistant strains have become common.

Table 255-8

Dosage of Antimicrobial Agents for the Treatment of Pneumonia in Hospitalized Patients*

Drug	Dosage
Ampicillin/sulbactam	3 g IV q6h
Aztreonam	2 g IV q8h
Cefazolin	1–2 g IV q8h
Cefotaxime, ceftizoxime	1–2 g q8–12h
Ceftazidime	2 g IV q8h
Ceftriaxone	1–2 g IV q12–24h
Cefuroxime	750 mg IV q8h
Ciprofloxacin	400 mg IV or 750 mg PO q12h
Clindamycin	600–900 mg IV q8h
Erythromycin	0.5–1.0 g IV q6h
Gentamicin (or tobramycin)	5 mg/kg/d in 3 equally divided doses IV q8h
Imipenem	500 mg IV q6h
Metronidazole	500 mg IV or PO q6h
Nafcillin	2 g IV q4h
Penicillin G	1–3 million units IV q4–6h
Ticarcillin/clavulanate	3.1 g IV q4h
Vancomycin	1 g IV q12h

* Dosage must be modified for patients with renal failure. Guidelines on the duration of therapy for each pathogen are given in the text of this chapter and of chapters on specific infecting agents.

If the result of Gram's staining of sputum is not interpretable or not available, either (1) a third-generation cephalosporin plus metronidazole or (2) ampicillin plus sulbactam is generally an adequate empirical regimen; when *Legionella* or *Chlamydia* is the likely pathogen, erythromycin should be added to the regimen. Therapy can be switched from intravenous to oral agents to complete a 7- to 10-day course if the patient's clinical condition improves rapidly and if antimicrobial agents that are readily absorbed after oral administration and that reach tissue levels above the MIC are available. The presence of *S. aureus* or aerobic gram-negative bacilli or the development of suppurative complications requires a more prolonged course of therapy. Legionellosis should be treated with 1 g of erythromycin intravenously every 6 h for 3 weeks to prevent relapses; rifampin should be added to the regimen if the patient is critically ill. Anaerobic lung abscess should be treated with the regimens suggested for aspiration pneumonia until a chest radiograph (with radiography performed at 2-week intervals) is clear or shows only a small stable scar. Therapy is prolonged for 6 weeks or more to prevent relapse, although shorter courses are probably sufficient for most patients. Surgery is rarely required for lung abscess; indications for surgery include massive hemoptysis and suspected neoplasm. Supportive measures include the administration of supplemental oxygen and intravenous fluids, assistance in clearing secretions, fiberoptic bronchoscopy, and (if necessary) ventilatory support. Caution should be exercised in bronchoscopic drainage of large, fluid-filled

Table 255-7

Empirical Antimicrobial Therapy for the Management of Hospitalized Patients with Community-Acquired Pneumonia

	Value of Indicated Antimicrobial*						
Pathogen	Penicillin G	First-Generation Cephalosporin	Third-Generation Cephalosporin	Metronidazole	Trimethoprim-Sulfamethoxazole	Erythromycin	Ampicillin/Sulbactam
Streptococcus pneumoniae	+†	+†	+	−	±	+†	+‡
Staphylococcus aureus	−	+	+	−	+	−	+
Haemophilus influenzae	−	−	+	−	+	±	+
Moraxella catarrhalis	−	+	+	−	+	+	+
Anaerobic gram-positive cocci	+	+	+	+	−	−	+
Anaerobic gram-negative bacilli	−	−	−	+	−	−	+
Chlamydia pneumoniae	−	−	−	−	−	+	−
Legionella pneumophila	−	−	−	−	±	+	−

* +, effective; −, ineffective; ±, sometimes effective.
† Between 10 and 20 percent of strains have recently been reported to be resistant to β-lactams and macrolides in some locations in the United States.
‡ Ampicillin/sulbactam does cover penicillin-resistant *S. pneumoniae*.

lung abscesses because of the potential for sudden massive spillage of large collections of pus into the airways.

Patients with risk factors for HIV infection and an atypical pneumonia syndrome should be evaluated for *Pneumocystis* infection because of its frequency as an index diagnosis in HIV infection and its potential severity. Tuberculosis and other causes of atypical pneumonia must be excluded as part of the evaluation of these patients. Empirical therapy can consist of either trimethoprim-sulfamethoxazole (15 to 20 mg/kg of trimethoprim, given daily in four divided doses intravenously or by mouth) or pentamidine (3 to 4 mg/kg daily, given intravenously), and treatment is continued for 3 weeks in confirmed cases of *Pneumocystis* infection. Although some data suggest that trimethoprim-sulfamethoxazole is more effective than pentamidine, further studies directly comparing the two agents are needed. The frequency and severity of the adverse effects of the two drugs are generally thought to be equivalent. The addition of glucocorticoids (prednisone, 40 mg twice daily, with subsequent tapering of the dose) early in the course of *Pneumocystis* pneumonia in patients with an arterial P_{O_2} of <70 mmHg decreases the need for mechanical ventilation and improves the patient's chances of survival and functional status. Prophylaxis for recurrent *Pneumocystis* pneumonia must be started at the end of therapy.

Institutionally Acquired Pneumonia Pneumonia acquired in institutions such as nursing homes or hospitals is frequently caused by enteric aerobic gram-negative bacilli, *P. aeruginosa*, or *S. aureus*, with or without oral anaerobes. Again, the selection of empirical antimicrobial therapy should be guided by Gram's staining of sputum (see Tables 255-8 and 255-9) and knowledge of the prevalent nosocomial pathogens and their current in vitro antimicrobial sensitivity patterns in the institution involved. An aggressive diagnostic approach is needed in some circumstances, especially for the immunocompromised patient (as outlined above).

S. aureus acquired in some institutions is frequently methicillin-resistant. Such strains are resistant to all β-lactam antibiotics and may also be resistant to clindamycin, erythromycin, and the fluoroquinolones. Only vancomycin is predictably active against these organisms, and this drug should be added to the empirical regimen when methicillin-resistant organisms may be involved in pneumonia.

When multiantibiotic resistance is a problem, pneumonia due to gram-negative bacilli in the institutionalized patient can be treated initially with a β-lactam active against *P. aeruginosa* (ceftazidime, piperacillin/tazobactam, ticarcillin/clavulanate, aztreonam, or imipenem) or a parenterally administered fluoroquinolone (ciprofloxacin or ofloxacin). Ticarcillin/clavulanate and piperacillin/tazobactam are preferred over other penicillins with activity against *P. aeruginosa* (e.g., ticarcillin or piperacillin alone), which are not sufficiently active against *Klebsiella pneumoniae*, a relatively common pathogen. However, if piperacillin/tazobactam is to be used for infection suspected to be due to *P. aeruginosa*, a higher dose (3.375 g every 4 h) than is recommended by the package insert is required; a lower dose contains less piperacillin than is needed to be effective against this organism. Ampicillin/sulbactam, the other parenterally administered β-lactam antibiotic/β-lactamase inhibitor combination, is not active against many nosocomial pathogens, such as *P. aeruginosa*, *Enterobacter* spp., and *Serratia* spp., and therefore is inappropriate as empirical therapy for nosocomial pneumonia.

In seriously ill patients, especially those infected with *P. aeruginosa*, use of a β-lactam/aminoglycoside combination for bactericidal synergy is prudent. Such combinations are also used to broaden the spectrum of antibacterial activity to cover the possibility of infection with resistant pathogens, to treat polymicrobial infection, and to prevent the emergence of antimicrobial resistance. Combinations of β-lactams or aminoglycosides with a fluoroquinolone are not expected to enhance the already-rapid bactericidal activity of the fluoroquinolone alone; nevertheless, they are expected to broaden the spectrum covered and perhaps prevent the emergence of resistance. A fluoroquinolone plus either a β-lactam or an aminoglycoside can be used in institutions where there is a relatively high expectation of infection with a fluoroquinolone-resistant nosocomial pathogen (e.g., *Acinetobacter calcoaceticus*) or with organisms in which resistance frequently emerges during therapy (e.g., *P. aeruginosa*).

Pneumonia due to possible coinfection with aerobic gram-negative bacilli and anaerobes, as reflected by a polymicrobial flora on Gram's staining of sputum, may usually be treated with any of the following regimens: (1) ceftazidime plus metronidazole or clindamycin, (2) aztreonam or a fluoroquinolone plus clindamycin, or (3) imipenem or ticarcillin/clavulanate. The regimens that include a β-lactam agent usually should also include an aminoglycoside (see Table 255-9).

The production of chromosomally encoded, inducible β-lactamases by some aerobic gram-negative bacilli, including *Serratia marcescens*, *Enterobacter cloacae*, *Citrobacter freundii*, *Morganella morganii*, *P. aeruginosa*, and *A. calcoaceticus*, has important implications for the treatment of nosocomial pneumonia in institutions where these organisms are common nosocomial pathogens. Antibiotic resistance in these pathogens has been attributed to two related mechanisms: inducible production of chromosomally encoded β-lactamases and selection of mutants that have lost a gene that controls expression of β-lactamase production. The control gene represses β-lactamase production in the absence of a β-lactam agent and allows β-lactamase production in the presence of a β-lactam agent. This group of organisms has a relatively high mutation rate for loss of this control gene, and the loss of the gene results in continuous production of large amounts of β-lactamase (stable derepression). The derepressed mutants are resistant to third-generation cephalosporins, aztreonam, and broad-spectrum penicillins. These chromosomally encoded, inducible β-lactamases are not inhibited by clavulanic acid or sulbactam.

Selection by the β-lactam antibiotic of the derepressed mutants present in the dense bacterial populations of infected pulmonary tissue at the initiation of antibiotic therapy apparently accounts for the emergence of resistance during therapy, which is especially problematic in severely compromised patients whose defective host defenses are unable to control the growth of a few resistant mutants. The only β-lactam agent that maintains activity against the dere-

Table 255-9

Empirical Antimicrobial Therapy, Based on Gram's Staining of Sputum, for Institutionally Acquired Pneumonia

Etiology	Regimen
Presumptive *Staphylococcus aureus*	Nafcillin or vancomycin*
Presumptive enteric aerobic gram-negative bacilli or *Pseudomonas aeruginosa*	1. Ceftazidime ± aminoglycoside 2. Ticarcillin/clavulanate ± aminoglycoside 3. Aztreonam ± aminoglycoside 4. Imipenem[†] ± aminoglycoside 5. Fluoroquinolone[†] ± aminoglycoside or β-lactam
Mixed flora	1. Ceftazidime + clindamycin (or metronidazole) ± aminoglycoside[‡] 2. Ticarcillin/clavulanate or piperacillin/tazobactam ± aminoglycoside[‡] 3. Aztreonam + clindamycin (or metronidazole[§]) ± aminoglycoside[‡] 4. Imipenem[†] ± aminoglycoside[‡] 5. Fluoroquinolone[†] + clindamycin (or metronidazole[‡,§]) ± aminoglycoside or β-lactam

* If methicillin-resistant *S. aureus* is known to exist in the institution, use vancomycin; otherwise, use an antistaphylococcal β-lactam such as nafcillin or cefazolin.

† Use when chromosomally encoded, inducible β-lactamase producers are endemic in the institution.

[illegible]d vancomycin if methicillin-resistant *S. aureus* is present in the institution.

[illegible]tronidazole must be combined with vancomycin or another antimicrobial that covers [illegible]croaerophilic and anaerobic gram-positive cocci.

pressed mutants is imipenem. Ciprofloxacin and aminoglycosides may also retain activity against these mutants. Trimethoprim-sulfamethoxazole may remain active against all of these gram-negative bacilli except *P. aeruginosa*, which is inherently resistant to this agent. Some clinicians have questioned the efficacy of aminoglycosides alone for the treatment of gram-negative bacillary pneumonia. The poor clinical efficacy of aminoglycosides has been attributed to the low levels attained in bronchial secretions and to a loss of antimicrobial activity due to the relative acidity of purulent secretions, the anaerobic conditions in infected lung, and (in the case of *P. aeruginosa*) the divalent cations calcium and magnesium. The nephrotoxicity and ototoxicity of aminoglycosides frequently lead to underdosing with these agents. These problems are compounded by unpredictable pharmacokinetics that necessitate measurement of serum levels of aminoglycosides. If multiantibiotic-resistant nosocomial organisms are likely to be pathogens in severely compromised patients, reliable empirical agents may be fluoroquinolones or imipenem—unless resistance to these drugs is also endemic in the institution. Up-to-date knowledge of the antimicrobial sensitivities of an institution's nosocomial pathogens and use of various preventive practices are mandatory.

Amantadine (200 mg/day for most adults and 100 mg/day for persons over 65 years of age) is effective for the prevention of influenza A virus infection in the unimmunized patient during an influenza A outbreak and for the treatment (for 5 to 7 days) of early influenza A virus infection. Ribavirin is effective for respiratory syncytial virus infection. Intravenous acyclovir (5 to 10 mg/kg every 8 h for 7 to 14 days) is appropriate for varicella pneumonia. Treatment of cytomegalovirus pneumonia has yielded unsatisfactory results, but intravenous immunoglobulin combined with ganciclovir may be effective in some instances.

PREVENTION The prevention of pneumonia involves either (1) decreasing the likelihood of encountering the pathogen or (2) strengthening the host's response once the pathogen is encountered. The former approach can include measures such as hand washing and glove use by persons who care for patients infected with contact-transmitted pathogens (e.g., aerobic gram-negative bacilli); use of face masks or negative-pressure isolation rooms for patients with pneumonia due to pathogens spread by the aerosol route (e.g., *M. tuberculosis*); prompt institution of effective chemotherapy for patients with contagious illnesses; and correction of conditions that facilitate aspiration. The latter approach includes the use of chemoprophylaxis or immunization for patients at risk. Chemoprophylaxis may be administered to patients who have encountered or are likely to encounter the pathogen before they become symptomatic (e.g., amantadine during a community outbreak of influenza A, isoniazid for tuberculosis, or trimethoprim-sulfamethoxazole for pneumocystosis) or to patients who are likely to have a recurrence following recovery from a symptomatic episode (e.g., trimethoprim-sulfamethoxazole for pneumocystosis in patients with HIV infection). Gastric acidity is a major factor that prevents colonization of the gastrointestinal tract by nosocomial gram-negative bacillary pathogens. To prevent stress ulceration, it is preferable to use sucralfate, which maintains gastric acidity, rather than H_2-blocking agents. Vaccines (see Chaps. 122, 141, and 152) are available for immunization against *S. pneumoniae*, *H. influenzae* type b, influenza viruses A and B, and measles virus. Influenza and pneumococcal vaccines are strongly recommended for individuals over 65 years of age and for persons of any age who are at risk of adverse consequences of influenza or pneumonia because of underlying conditions. Pneumococcal, haemophilus, and influenza vaccines are recommended for HIV-infected patients who are still capable of responding to a vaccine challenge. The currently available 23-valent pneumococcal vaccine covers 88 percent of the serotypes causing systemic disease as well as 8 percent of related serotypes. The increasing prevalence of multiantibiotic resistance among pneumococci makes pneumococcal immunization of high-risk individuals of utmost importance. Immune serum globulin is available for intravenous replacement therapy in those patients with congenital or acquired hypogammaglobulinemia.

The prevention of nosocomial pneumonia requires good infection control practices, judicious use of broad-spectrum antimicrobial agents, and maintenance of patients' gastric acidity.

BIBLIOGRAPHY

APPELBAUM PC: Antimicrobial resistance in *Streptococcus pneumoniae*: An overview. Clin Infect Dis 15:77, 1992

BARRY AL et al: In vitro activities of 12 orally administered antimicrobial agents against four species of bacterial respiratory pathogens from U.S. medical centers in 1992 and 1993. Antimicrob Agents Chemother 38:2419, 1994

BREIMAN RF et al: Emergence of drug-resistant pneumococcal infections in the United States. JAMA 271:1831, 1994

CRAVEN DE et al: Nosocomial pneumonia in the 1990s: Update of epidemiology and risk factors. Semin Respir Infect 5:157, 1990

FAIRCHOK MP et al: Carriage of penicillin-resistant pneumococci in a military population in Washington, DC: Risk factors and correlation with clinical isolates. Clin Infect Dis 22:966, 1996

FANG GD et al: New and emerging etiologies for community-acquired pneumonia with implications for therapy. Medicine 69:307, 1990

FINE MJ: Pneumonia in the elderly: The hospital admission and discharge decisions. Semin Respir Infect 65:303, 1990

HAHN DL et al: Association of *Chlamydia pneumoniae* (strain TWAR) infection with wheezing, asthmatic bronchitis and adult-onset asthma. JAMA 266:225, 1991

HOFFMAN J et al: The prevalence of drug-resistant *Streptococcus pneumoniae* in Atlanta. N Engl J Med 333:481, 1995

JACOBS MR: Treatment and diagnosis of infections caused by drug-resistant *Streptococcus pneumoniae*. Clin Infect Dis 15:119, 1992

LEVISON ME, BUSH L: Pharmacodynamics of antimicrobial agents. Bactericidal and postantibiotic effects. Infect Dis Clin North Am 3:415, 1989

——— et al: Clindamycin compared with penicillin for the treatment of anaerobic lung abscess. Ann Intern Med 98:466, 1983

LORBER B, SWENSON RM: Bacteriology of aspiration pneumonia, a prospective study of community and hospital acquired cases. Ann Intern Med 81:329, 1974

PALLARES R et al: Resistance to penicillin and cephalosporin and mortality from severe pneumococcal pneumonia in Barcelona, Spain. N Engl J Med 333:474, 1995

RIES K et al: Transtracheal aspiration in pulmonary infection. Arch Intern Med 133:453, 1974

RILEY RL: Airborne infection. Am J Med 57:466, 1974

SANDERS CC, SANDERS WE JR: Clinical significance of inducible beta-lactamase in gram-negative bacteria. Eur J Clin Microbiol 6:435, 1987

SHELHAMER JH et al: NIH Conference: Respiratory disease in the immunosuppressed patient. Ann Intern Med 117:415, 1992

STEINHOFF D et al: *Chlamydia pneumoniae* as a cause of community-acquired pneumonia in hospitalized patients in Berlin. Clin Infect Dis 22:958, 1996

THORNSBERRY C et al: Increased penicillin resistance in recent U.S. isolates of *Streptococcus pneumoniae*, in *Abstracts of the General Meeting of the American Society for Microbiology*. ASM, Washington, DC, 1992, abstract C-268

VERGHESE A, BERK SL: Bacterial pneumonia in the elderly. Medicine 62:271, 1982

WOODHEAD MA et al: Prospective study of the aetiology and outcome of pneumonia in the community. Lancet 1:671, 1987

256

Steven E. Weinberger

BRONCHIECTASIS

DEFINITION Bronchiectasis is an abnormal and permanent dilatation of bronchi. It may be either focal, involving airways supplying a limited region of pulmonary parenchyma, or diffuse, involving airways in a more widespread distribution. Although this definition is based on pathologic changes in the bronchi, diagnosis is often suggested by the clinical consequences of chronic or recurrent infection in the dilated airways and the associated secretions that pool within these airways.

PATHOLOGY The bronchial dilatation of bronchiectasis is associated with destructive and inflammatory changes in the walls of medium-sized airways, often at the level of segmental or subsegmental bronchi. The normal structural components of the wall, including cartilage, muscle, and elastic tissue, are destroyed and may be replaced by fibrous tissue. The dilated airways frequently contain pools of thick, purulent material, while more peripheral airways are often occluded by secretions or obliterated and replaced by fibrous tissue. Additional microscopic features include bronchial and peribronchial inflammation and fibrosis, ulceration of the bronchial wall, squamous metaplasia, and mucous gland hyperplasia. The parenchyma normally supplied by the affected airways is abnormal, containing varying combinations of fibrosis, emphysema, bronchopneumonia, and atelectasis. As a result of the inflammation, vascularity of the bronchial wall increases, with associated enlargement of the bronchial arteries and anastomoses between the bronchial and pulmonary arterial circulations.

Three different patterns of bronchiectasis were described by Reid in 1950. In *cylindrical bronchiectasis* the bronchi appear as uniformly dilated tubes that end abruptly at the point that smaller airways are obstructed by secretions. In *varicose bronchiectasis* the affected bronchi have an irregular or beaded pattern of dilatation resembling varicose veins. In *saccular (cystic) bronchiectasis* the bronchi have a ballooned appearance at the periphery, ending in blind sacs without recognizable bronchial structures distal to the sacs.

ETIOLOGY AND PATHOGENESIS Bronchiectasis is a consequence of inflammation and destruction of the structural components of the bronchial wall. Infection is the usual cause of the inflammation; microorganisms such as *Pseudomonas aeruginosa* and *Haemophilus influenzae* produce pigments, proteases, and other toxins that injure the respiratory epithelium and impair mucociliary clearance. The host inflammatory response induces epithelial injury, largely as a result of mediators released from neutrophils. As protection against infection is compromised, the dilated airways become more susceptible to colonization and growth of bacteria. Thus, a reinforcing cycle can result, with inflammation producing airway damage, impaired clearance of microorganisms, and further infection, which then completes the cycle by inciting more inflammation.

Infectious Causes A wide variety of infectious agents can initiate bronchiectasis. In the past, bronchiectasis during childhood was often a complication of measles or pertussis; these are now rare causes, as a result of effective immunization. At present, adenovirus and influenza virus are the main viruses that cause bronchiectasis in association with lower respiratory tract involvement. Although not as common as in the preantibiotic era, virulent bacterial infections, especially with potentially necrotizing organisms such as *Staphylococcus aureus*, *Klebsiella*, and anaerobes, remain important causes of bronchiectasis when antibiotic treatment of a pneumonia is not given or is significantly delayed. Bronchiectasis has been reported in patients with human immunodeficiency virus (HIV) infection, perhaps at least partly due to recurrent bacterial infection. Tuberculosis can produce bronchiectasis by a necrotizing effect on pulmonary parenchyma and airways and indirectly as a consequence of airway obstruction from bronchostenosis or extrinsic compression by lymph nodes. Nontuberculous mycobacteria are frequently associated with bronchiectasis, usually as secondary infections or colonizing organisms, though occasionally as primary pathogens. Mycoplasmal and necrotizing fungal infections are rare causes.

Impaired host defense mechanisms are often involved in the predisposition to recurrent infections. The major cause of localized impairment of host defenses is endobronchial obstruction. Bacteria and secretions cannot be cleared adequately from the obstructed airway, which develops recurrent or chronic infection. Although primary lung cancer is the most common cause of endobronchial obstruction, it is an infrequent cause of bronchiectasis, since either the involved area is removed surgically or the disease progresses before bronchiectasis becomes an important problem. Slowly growing endobronchial neoplasms such as carcinoid tumors are more commonly associated with bronchiectasis. Foreign body aspiration is another important cause of endobronchial obstruction, particularly in children. Airway obstruction can also result from bronchostenosis, from impacted secretions, or from extrinsic compression by enlarged lymph nodes.

Generalized impairment of pulmonary defense mechanisms occurs with immunoglobulin deficiency, primary ciliary disorders, or cystic fibrosis. Infections and bronchiectasis are therefore often more diffuse. With panhypogammaglobulinemia, the best described of the immunoglobulin disorders associated with recurrent infection and bronchiectasis, patients often also have a history of sinus or skin infections. Selective IgA deficiency can be associated with bronchiectasis, frequently with coexisting deficiency of IgG subclasses (especially IgG2 or IgG4).

The primary disorders associated with ciliary dysfunction are termed *primary ciliary dyskinesia*. Numerous defects are encompassed under this category, including structural abnormalities of the dynein arms, radial spokes, and microtubules. The cilia become dyskinetic, their coordinated, propulsive action is diminished, and bacterial clearance is impaired. The clinical effects include recurrent upper and lower respiratory tract infections, such as sinusitis, otitis media, and bronchiectasis. Because normal sperm motility also depends on proper ciliary function, males are generally infertile (see also Chap. 336). Approximately half of patients with primary ciliary dyskinesia fall into the subgroup of *Kartagener's syndrome*, in which situs inversus accompanies bronchiectasis and sinusitis. It has been hypothesized that ciliary motility is necessary for proper rotation of the viscera during embryogenesis, so that visceral rotation is random when normal ciliary motion is lost.

In cystic fibrosis (see Chap. 257), the tenacious secretions in the bronchi are associated with impaired bacterial clearance, resulting in colonization and recurrent infection with a variety of organisms, particularly mucoid strains of *P. aeruginosa* but also *S. aureus*, *H. influenzae*, *Escherichia coli*, and *P. cepacia*.

Noninfectious Causes Some cases of bronchiectasis are associated with exposure to a toxic substance that incites a severe inflammatory response. Examples include inhalation of a toxic gas such as ammonia or aspiration of acidic gastric contents, though the latter problem is often also complicated by aspiration of bacteria. An immune response in the airway may also trigger inflammation, destructive changes, and bronchial dilatation. This mechanism is presumably responsible at least in part for bronchiectasis with allergic bronchopulmonary aspergillosis (ABPA), which is due to an immune response to *Aspergillus* organisms that have colonized the airway (Chap. 253). Bronchiectasis accompanying ABPA often involves proximal airways and is associated with mucoid impaction. Bronchiectasis also occurs rarely in ulcerative colitis, rheumatoid arthritis, and Sjögren's syndrome, but it is not known whether an immune response triggers airway inflammation in these patients.

In α_1*-antitrypsin deficiency*, the usual respiratory complication is the early development of panacinar emphysema, but affected individuals may occasionally have bronchiectasis. In the *yellow nail syndrome*, which is due to hypoplastic lymphatics, the triad of lymphedema, pleural effusion, and yellow discoloration of the nails is accompanied by bronchiectasis in approximately 40 percent of patients.

CLINICAL MANIFESTATIONS Patients typically present with persistent or recurrent cough and purulent sputum production. Hemoptysis occurs in 50 to 70 percent of cases and can be due to bleeding from friable, inflamed airway mucosa. More significant, even massive bleeding is often a consequence of bleeding from hypertrophied bronchial arteries.

When a specific infectious episode initiates bronchiectasis, patients may describe a severe pneumonia followed by chronic cough and sputum production. Alternatively, patients without a dramatic initiating event often describe the insidious onset of symptoms. In some cases, patients are either asymptomatic or have a nonproductive cough, often associated with "dry" bronchiectasis in an upper lobe. Dyspnea or wheezing generally reflects either widespread bronchiectasis or underlying chronic obstructive pulmonary disease. With exacerbations of infection, the amount of sputum increases, the appearance becomes more purulent and often more bloody, and patients may become febrile. Such episodes may be due solely to exacerbations of the airway infection, but associated parenchymal infiltrates sometimes reflect an adjacent pneumonia.

Physical examination of the chest overlying an area of bronchiectasis is quite variable. Any combination of crackles, rhonchi, and wheezes may be heard, all of which reflect the damaged airways containing significant secretions. As with other types of chronic intrathoracic infection, clubbing may be present. Patients with severe, diffuse disease, particularly those with chronic hypoxemia, may have associated cor pulmonale and right ventricular failure. Amyloidosis can result from chronic infection and inflammation but is now seldom seen.

RADIOGRAPHIC AND LABORATORY FINDINGS Though the chest radiograph is important in the evaluation of suspected bronchiectasis, the findings are often nonspecific. At one extreme, the radiograph may be normal with mild disease. Alternatively, patients with saccular bronchiectasis may have prominent cystic spaces, either with or without air-liquid levels, corresponding to the dilated airways. These may be difficult to distinguish from enlarged airspaces due to bullous emphysema or from regions of honeycombing in patients with severe interstitial lung disease. Other findings are due to dilated airways with thickened walls, which result from peribronchial inflammation. Because of decreased aeration and atelectasis of the associated pulmonary parenchyma, these dilated airways are often crowded together in parallel. When seen longitudinally, the airways appear as "tram tracks"; when seen in cross-section, they produce "ring shadows." Because the dilated airways may be filled with secretions, the lumen may appear dense rather than radiolucent, producing an opaque tubular or branched tubular structure.

Bronchography, which involves coating the airways with a radiopaque, iodinated lipid dye instilled through a catheter or bronchoscope, can provide excellent visualization of bronchiectatic airways. However, this technique has now been replaced by computed tomography (CT), which also provides an excellent view of dilated airways as seen in cross-sectional images (Fig. 256-1). With the advent of high-resolution CT scanning, in which the images are 1.0 to 1.5 mm thick, the sensitivity for detecting bronchiectasis has improved even further.

Examination of sputum often reveals an abundance of neutrophils and colonization or infection with a variety of possible organisms. Although common bacterial pathogens such as *Streptococcus pneumoniae* and *H. influenzae* may be present, a number of other organisms are seen frequently. *P. aeruginosa* is particularly common and may be a clue to the presence of previously unsuspected bronchiectasis. Other organisms include *Staph. aureus*, anaerobes, and nontuberculous (atypical) mycobacteria. Appropriate staining and culturing of sputum often provides a guide to antibiotic therapy.

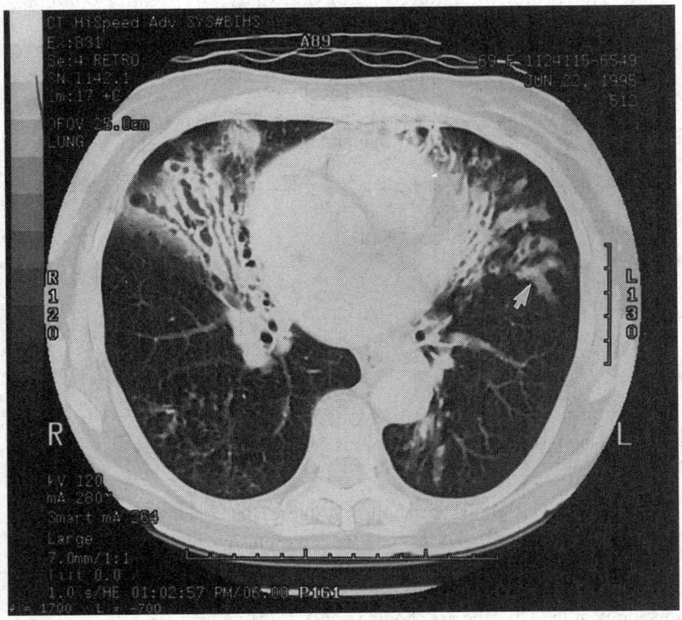

FIGURE 256-1 Chest CT section demonstrating extensive bronchiectasis, best seen in the right middle lobe and the lingula. The airways are dilated, crowded, and surrounded by poorly aerated pulmonary parenchyma. The arrow marks an opacity that represents a mucous plug in a dilated, branching airway.

Additional evaluation is aimed at diagnosing the cause for the bronchiectasis. When bronchiectasis is focal, fiberoptic bronchoscopy may reveal an underlying endobronchial obstruction. In other cases, upper lobe involvement may be suggestive of either tuberculosis or ABPA. With more widespread disease, measurement of sweat chloride levels for cystic fibrosis, structural or functional assessment of nasal or bronchial cilia or sperm for primary ciliary dyskinesia, and quantitative assessment of immunoglobulins may explain recurrent airway infection. In an asthmatic person with proximal bronchiectasis or other historical features to suggest ABPA, skin testing, serology, and sputum culture for *Aspergillus* are helpful in confirming the diagnosis.

Pulmonary function tests may demonstrate airflow obstruction as a consequence of diffuse bronchiectasis or associated chronic obstructive lung disease. Bronchial hyperreactivity, e.g., to methacholine challenge, and some reversibility of the airflow obstruction with inhaled bronchodilators are relatively common for reasons not well defined. Other laboratory evaluation is often relatively nonspecific. For example, as a result of chronic infection within the thorax, patients may develop the normocytic, normochromic anemia of chronic disease.

℞ TREATMENT

Therapy has four major goals: (1) elimination of an identifiable underlying problem; (2) improved clearance of tracheobronchial secretions; (3) control of infection, particularly during acute exacerbations; and (4) reversal of airflow obstruction. Appropriate treatment should be instituted when a treatable cause is found, for example, treatment of hypogammaglobulinemia with immunoglobulin replacement, tuberculosis with antituberculous agents, and ABPA with glucocorticoids.

Secretions are typically copious and thick and contribute to the symptoms. Chest physical therapy with vibration, percussion, and postural drainage frequently helps patients with copious secretions. Mucolytic agents to thin secretions and allow better clearance are controversial. Aerosolized recombinant DNase, which decreases viscosity of sputum by breaking down DNA released from neutrophils, has been shown to improve pulmonary function in cystic fibrosis, but similar benefits have not been found with bronchiectasis due to other etiologies.

Chronic or recurrent bacterial infections cause much of the morbidity of bronchiectasis. Antibiotics have an important role in management, but which antibiotic should be given and the frequency and duration of administration are not well established. For patients with infrequent exacerbations characterized by an increase in quantity and purulence of the sputum, antibiotics are commonly used only during acute episodes. Although choice of an antibiotic may be guided by Gram's stain and culture of sputum, empiric coverage (e.g., with ampicillin, amoxicillin, trimethoprim-sulfamethoxazole, or cefaclor) is often given initially. When *P. aeruginosa* is present, oral therapy with a quinolone or parenteral therapy with an aminoglycoside or third-generation cephalosporin may be appropriate. In patients with chronic purulent sputum despite short courses of antibiotics, more prolonged courses, e.g., with oral amoxicillin or inhaled aminoglycosides, or intermittent but regular courses of single or rotating antibiotics have been used.

Bronchodilators to improve obstruction and aid clearance of secretions are particularly useful in patients with airway hyperreactivity and reversible airflow obstruction. Although surgical therapy was common in the past, more effective antibiotic and supportive therapy has largely replaced surgery. However, when bronchiectasis is localized and the morbidity is substantial despite adequate medical therapy, surgical resection of the involved region of lung should be considered.

Complications present additional treatment issues. When massive hemoptysis, often originating from the hypertrophied bronchial circulation, does not resolve with conservative therapy, including rest and antibiotics, therapeutic options are either surgical resection or bronchial arterial embolization (Chap. 33). Although resection may be successful if disease is localized, embolization is preferable with widespread disease. In patients with extensive disease, chronic hypoxemia and cor pulmonale may indicate the need for long-term supplemental oxygen. For selected patients who are disabled despite maximal therapy, lung transplantation is a therapeutic option.

BIBLIOGRAPHY

BARKER AF: Bronchiectasis. Semin Thorac Cardiovasc Surg 7:112, 1995

COLE PJ: Inflammation: A two-edged sword—the model of bronchiectasis. Eur J Respir Dis 69(Suppl 147):6, 1986

GREENSTONE M et al: Primary ciliary dyskinesia: Cytological and clinical features. Q J Med 67:405, 1988

HOLMES AH et al: Bronchiectasis in HIV disease. Q J Med 85:875, 1992

KANG EY et al: Bronchiectasis: Comparison of preoperative thin-section CT and pathologic findings in resected specimens. Radiology 195:649, 1995

MCGUINNESS G et al: Bronchiectasis: CT evaluation. Am J Roentgenol 160:253, 1993

SHADICK NA et al: Bronchiectasis. A late feature of severe rheumatoid arthritis. Medicine 73:161, 1994

TRUCKSIS M, SWARTZ MN: Bronchiectasis: A current view. Curr Clin Top Infect Dis 11:170, 1991

257 CYSTIC FIBROSIS

Richard C. Boucher

Cystic fibrosis (CF) is a monogenetic disorder that presents as a multisystem disease. The first signs and symptoms typically occur in childhood, but nearly 4 percent of patients are diagnosed as adults. Due to improvements in therapy, approximately 34 percent of patients reach adulthood and nearly 10 percent live past the age of 30. The average life span for both male and female CF patients is similar, ~28 years. Thus, CF is no longer only a pediatric disease, and internists must be prepared to recognize and treat its many complications. This disease is characterized by chronic airway infection that ultimately leads to bronchiectasis and bronchiolectasis, exocrine pancreatic insufficiency and intestinal dysfunction, abnormal sweat gland function, and urogenital dysfunction.

PATHOGENESIS Genetic Basis CF is an autosomal recessive disease resulting from mutations in a gene located on chromosome 7. The prevalence of CF varies with the ethnic origin of a population. CF is detected in approximately 1 in 3000 live births in the Caucasian population of North America and northern Europe, 1 in 17,000 live births of African-Americans, and 1 in 90,000 live births of the Asian population of Hawaii. The most common mutation in the CF gene (~70 percent of CF chromosomes) is a 3-base-pair deletion that results in an absence of phenylalanine at amino acid position 508 (ΔF_{508}) of the CF gene protein product, known as the CF transmembrane regulator (CFTR). The large number (>400) of relatively uncommon (<2 percent) mutations identified in the CF gene makes it difficult to use DNA diagnostic technologies for identifying heterozygotes in populations at large, and no simple physiologic measurements allow heterozygote detection.

CFTR Protein The CFTR protein is a single polypeptide chain containing 1480 amino acids that appears to function both as a cyclic AMP–regulated Cl^- channel and, as its name implies, as a regulator of other ion channels. The fully processed form of CFTR is found in the plasma membrane in normal epithelia (Fig. 257-1). Biochemical studies indicate that the ΔF_{508} mutation leads to improper processing and intracellular degradation of the CFTR protein. Thus, absence of CFTR at appropriate cellular sites is often part of the pathophysiology of CF. However, other mutations in the CF gene produce CFTR proteins that are fully processed but are nonfunctional or only partially functional at the appropriate cellular sites.

Epithelial Dysfunction The epithelia affected by CF exhibit different functions in their native state; i.e., some are volume-absorbing (airways and intestinal epithelia), some are salt-absorbing but not volume-absorbing (sweat duct), whereas others are volume-secretory (pancreas). Given this diverse array of native activities, it should not be surprising that CF produces very different effects on patterns of electrolyte and water transport. However, the unifying concept is that all affected tissues express abnormal ion transport function.

ORGAN-SPECIFIC PATHOPHYSIOLOGY Lung The diagnostic biophysical hallmark of CF is the raised transepithelial electric potential difference (PD) detected in airway epithelia. The transepithelial PD reflects components of both the rate of active ion transport and the resistance to ion flow of the superficial epithelium. CF airway epithelia exhibit both raised transport rates (Na^+) and decreased ion permeability (Cl^-) (Fig. 257-2). The Cl^- transport defect reflects at least in part the absence of cyclic AMP–dependent kinase and protein kinase C–regulated Cl^- transport that is mediated by the Cl^- channel functions of CFTR. An important observation is that there is an alternative Cl^- channel expressed in airway epithelia. This "alternative" Cl^- channel ($Cl^-{}_a$) is different from CFTR and is regulated by intracellular Ca^{2+} levels or by extracellular triphosphate nucleotides, e.g., uridine–adenine triphosphate (UTP), and perhaps by CFTR itself. This channel can substitute for CFTR with regard to net Cl^- transport and may be a potential therapeutic target.

Raised Na^+ absorption is a feature of CF airway epithelia. Na^+ transport abnormalities are not a widespread feature of the CF epithelial phenotype and appear confined to volume-absorbing epithelia. Recent studies demonstrate that the increased Na^+ transport reflects the absence of CFTR's tonic inhibitory regulatory function on Na^+ channel activity. It appears that CFTR inhibits Na^+ channel activity as a part of its general function to act as a "switch" that coordinates the balance between Na^+ absorption and Cl^- secretion.

The central hypothesis of CF airways pathophysiology has been that the abnormal Na^+ and Cl^- transport rates produce secretions that are dehydrated and poorly cleared. The unique predisposition of CF airways to chronic infection by *Staphylococcus aureus* and *Pseudomo-*

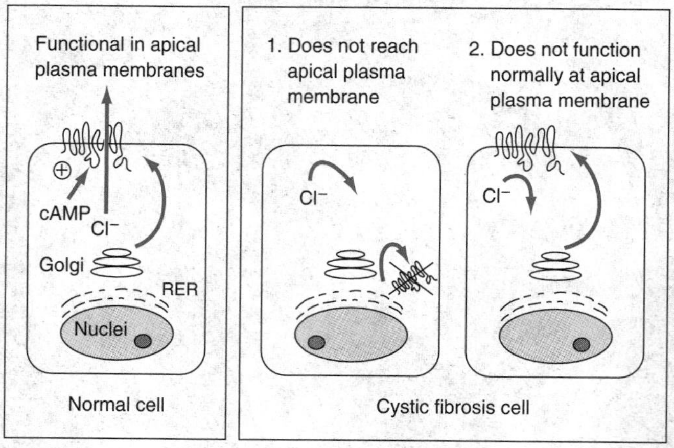

FIGURE 257-1 Cellular metabolism of the CFTR protein. In a normal cell (*left*), CFTR is synthesized in the rough endoplasmic reticulum (RER), glycosylated in the Golgi apparatus, and functions as a Cl^- channel and regulator of other ion channels when located in the plasma membrane. Two possible outcomes of mutations in the CF gene are shown (*right*). (1) If a mutation disturbs protein folding, e.g., the ΔF_{508} mutation, CFTR is degraded intracellularly so that no protein is transported to the plasma membrane. (2) With other mutations, the abnormal protein is processed and trafficks to the plasma membrane but functions abnormally at that site.

nas aeruginosa raises the issue that other as yet undefined abnormalities in airway surface liquid ionic composition also may contribute to the failure of lung defense.

Gastrointestinal Tract The gastrointestinal effects of CF are diverse. In the exocrine pancreas, the absence of the CFTR Cl^- channel in the apical membrane of pancreatic ductal epithelia limits the function of an apical membrane Cl^--HCO_3^- exchanger to secrete bicarbonate and Na^+ (by a passive process) into the duct. The failure to secrete $NaHCO_3$ and water leads to retention of enzymes in the pancreas and ultimately destruction of virtually all pancreatic tissue. The CF intestinal epithelium, because of the lack of Cl^- and water secretion, fails to flush the secreted mucins and other macromolecules from intestinal crypts. The diminished CFTR-mediated secretion of liquid may be exacerbated by excessive absorption of liquid, reflecting abnormalities of CFTR-mediated regulation of Na^+ absorption (both mediated by Na^+ channels and possibly other Na^+ transporters, e.g., Na^+-H^+ exchangers). Both dysfunctions lead to dessicated intralumenal contents and obstruction of both the small and large intestines. In the hepatobiliary system, defective hepatic ductal salt (Cl^-) and water secretion causes retention of biliary secretions and focal biliary cirrhosis and bile duct proliferation in approximately 25 to 30 percent of CF patients. The inability of the CF gallbladder epithelium to secrete salt and water can lead to both chronic cholecystitis and cholelithiasis.

Sweat Gland CF patients secrete nearly normal volumes of sweat in the sweat acinus. However, CF patients are not able to absorb NaCl from sweat as it moves through the sweat duct due to the inability to absorb Cl^- across the ductal epithelial cells.

DIAGNOSIS Because of the large number of CF mutations, DNA analysis is not used for primary diagnosis. The diagnosis of CF rests on a combination of clinical criteria and analyses of sweat Cl^- values. The values for the Na^+ and Cl^- concentration in sweat vary with age, but typically in adults a Cl^- concentration of >70 mmol/L discriminates between CF patients and patients with other lung disease. Between 1 and 2 percent of patients with the clinical syndrome of CF have normal sweat Cl^- values. In most of these patients, the nasal transepithelial PD is raised into the diagnostic range for CF and sweat acini do not secrete in response to injected beta-adrenergic agonists. A single mutation of the CFTR gene, 3849 + 10 kb C→T, is associated with approximately 50 percent of CF patients with normal sweat Cl^- values.

It is likely that DNA analyses will be performed increasingly in CF patients. Comprehensive genotype-phenotype relationships have not yet been established sufficiently for prognosis. A relationship between ΔF_{508} homozygosity or other mutations and pancreatic insufficiency has been established, but no predictive relationship holds for ΔF_{508} homozygosity and lung disease.

CLINICAL FEATURES Most CF patients present with signs and symptoms of the disease in childhood. Approximately 15 percent of patients present within the first 24 h of life with gastrointestinal obstruction, termed *meconium ileus*. Other common presentations within the first year or two of life include respiratory tract symptoms, most prominently cough and/or recurrent pulmonary infiltrates, and failure to thrive. A significant proportion of patients (~4 percent), however, are diagnosed after age 18.

Respiratory Tract Upper respiratory tract disease is almost universal in CF patients. Chronic sinusitis is common in childhood and leads to nasal obstruction and rhinorrhea. The occurrence of nasal polyps approaches 25 percent and often requires surgery.

In the lower respiratory tract, the first symptom of CF is cough. With time, the cough becomes persistent and produces viscous, purulent, often greenish-colored sputum. Inevitably, periods of clinical stability are interrupted by "exacerbations," defined by increased cough, weight loss, increased sputum volume, and decrements in pulmonary function. These exacerbations require aggressive therapy, including frequent postural drainage and oral antibiotics, and often intravenous antibiotics (see below), with the goal being recovery of lost lung function. Over the course of years, the exacerbations become more frequent and the recovery of lost lung function less complete, leading to respiratory failure.

CF patients exhibit a characteristic sputum microbiology. *Haemophilus influenzae* and *S. aureus* are often the first organisms recovered from samples of lung secretions in newly diagnosed CF patients. *P. aeruginosa* is typically cultured from lower respiratory tract secretions thereafter. After repetitive antibiotic exposure, *P. aeruginosa*, often in a mucoid form, is usually the predominant organism recovered from sputum and may be present as several strains with different antibiotic sensitivities. *Burkholderia* (formerly *Pseudomonas*) *cepacia* has been recovered from CF sputum and is pathogenic. Patient-to-patient spread of certain strains of this organism indicates that infection control in the hospital should be practiced. Other gram-negative rods recovered from CF sputum include *Xanthomonas zylosoxida* and *P. gladioli*, and occasionally, mucoid forms of *Proteus*, *Escherichia coli*, and *Klebsiella*. Up to 50 percent of CF patients have *Aspergillus fumigatus* in their sputum, and up to 10 percent of these patients exhibit the syndrome of allergic bronchopulmonary aspergillosis. *Mycobacterium tuberculosis* is rare in CF patients. However, 10 to 20 percent of adult CF patients have sputum cultures positive for nontuberculous mycobacteria, and in some patients these microorganisms are associated with disease.

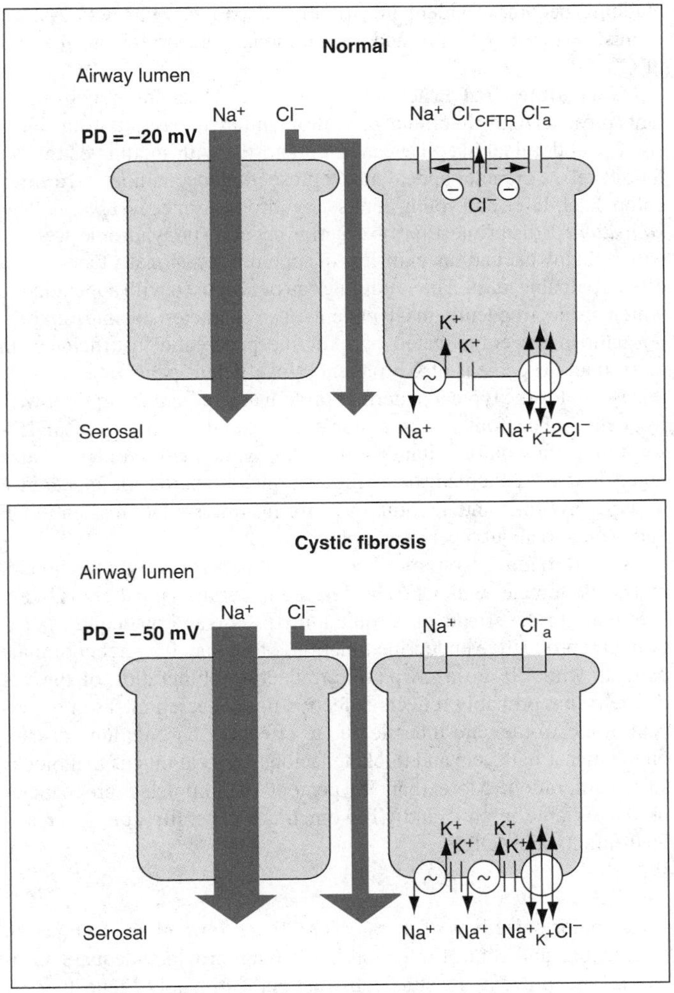

FIGURE 257-2 Comparison of ion transport properties of normal (*top*) and CF (*bottom*) airway epithelia. The vectors describe routes and magnitudes of Na^+ and Cl^- transport. The normal basal pattern for ion transport is absorption of Na^+ from the lumen via an amiloride-sensitive Na^+ channel. This process is accelerated in CF. The capacity to initiate cyclic cAMP–mediated Cl^- secretion is diminished in CF airway epithelia due to absence/dysfunction of the CFTR Cl^- channel. The accelerated Na^+ absorption in CF reflects the absence of CFTR inhibitory effects on Na^+ channels. Cl_a^-, alternative Cl^- channel; PD, potential difference; CFTR, cystic fibrosis transmembrane regulator.

The first lung function abnormalities observed in CF children, increased ratios of residual volume to total lung capacity, suggest that small airways disease is the first functional lung abnormality in CF. As the disease progresses, both reversible and irreversible changes in forced vital capacity (FVC) and forced expiratory volume (FEV_1) are noted. The reversible component reflects accumulation of intraluminal secretions and/or airway reactivity, which occurs in 40 to 60 percent of CF patients. The irreversible component reflects chronic destruction of the airway wall and bronchiolitis.

The earliest chest x-ray change in CF lungs is hyperinflation, reflecting small airways obstruction. Later, signs of luminal mucus impaction, bronchial cuffing, and finally, bronchiectasis, e.g., ring shadows, are noted. For reasons that are still unknown, the right upper lobe displays the earliest and most severe changes. Neither CT nor MRI scanning are routinely performed on CF patients.

CF pulmonary disease is associated with many intermittent complications. Pneumothorax is common (>10 percent of patients). The production of small amounts of blood in sputum is common in CF patients with advanced pulmonary disease and appears to be associated with lung infection. Massive hemoptysis is life-threatening and difficult to localize bronchoscopically. With advanced lung disease, digital clubbing becomes evident in virtually all patients with CF. As late events, respiratory failure and cor pulmonale are prominent features of CF.

Gastrointestinal Tract The syndrome of meconium ileus in infants presents with abdominal distention, failure to pass stool, and emesis. The abdominal flat plate can be diagnostic, with small intestinal air fluid levels, a granular appearance representing meconium, and a small colon. In children and young adults, a syndrome termed *meconium ileus equivalent* or distal intestinal obstruction occurs. The syndrome presents with right lower quadrant pain, loss of appetite, occasionally emesis, and often a palpable mass. The syndrome can be confused with appendicitis, which occurs frequently in CF patients. The characteristic intestinal abnormalities are complicated by exocrine pancreatic insufficiency in more than 90 percent of CF patients. Insufficient pancreatic enzyme release yields the typical pattern of protein and fat malabsorption, with frequent, bulky, foul-smelling stools. Signs and symptoms of malabsorption of fat-soluble vitamins, including vitamins E and K, are also noted. Because pancreatic beta cells are typically spared, the appearance of hyperglycemia and a requirement for insulin is a late finding in CF and occurs in about 5 percent of patients.

Genitourinary System Late onset of puberty is common in both males and females with CF. The delayed maturational pattern is likely secondary to the effects of chronic lung disease and inadequate nutrition on reproductive endocrine function. More than 95 percent of male patients with CF are azoospermic, reflecting obliteration of the vas deferens that probably reflects defective liquid secretion. Twenty percent of CF women are infertile due to effects of chronic lung disease on the menstrual cycle and thick, tenacious cervical mucus that blocks sperm migration. More than 90 percent of completed pregnancies produce viable infants, and CF women are generally able to breast-feed infants normally.

Rx TREATMENT

The major objectives of therapy for CF are to promote clearance of secretions and control infection in the lung, provide adequate nutrition, and prevent intestinal obstruction. Ultimately, gene therapy may be the treatment of choice.

Lung Disease At present, the principal technique for clearing pulmonary secretions is a combination of breathing exercises and chest percussion. It should be stressed that regular use of these maneuvers is effective in preserving lung function. More than 95 percent of CF patients die of complications resulting from lung infection. Antibiotics are the principal agents available for treating lung infection, and their use should be guided by sputum culture results. Early intervention with antibiotics is useful, and long courses of treatment are the rule. Because of increased total-body clearance and volume of distribution of antibiotics in CF patients, the required doses are higher for CF patients than for non-CF patients with similar chest infections.

Increased cough and mucus production are treated with antibiotics given by the oral route. Typical oral agents used to treat *Staphylococcus* include a semisynthetic penicillin or a cephalosporin. Oral ciprofloxacin may reduce pseudomonal bacterial counts and control symptoms. However, its clinical usefulness may be limited by rapid emergence of resistant organisms, and accordingly, courses should be intermittent (2 to 3 weeks) and not chronic. More severe exacerbations, or exacerbations associated with bacteria resistant to oral antibiotics, require intravenous antibiotics. Traditionally, intravenous therapy is given in the hospital, but outpatient intravenous antibiotic administration is gaining widespread acceptance. Usually, two drugs, often one of them an aminoglycoside, are used to treat *P. aeruginosa* to hinder emergence of resistant organisms. Drug dosage should be monitored so that levels for gentamicin or tobramycin peak at ranges of ~10 μg/mL and exhibit troughs of <2 μg/mL. Usually, a cephalosporin, e.g., ceftazadime, and/or a penicillin derivative is used as the second drug. Antibiotics directed at *Staphylococcus* and/or *H. influenzae* are added depending on the results of the culture. Aerosolization of antibiotics also may have an important role in treating CF lung infection. Large doses of aminoglycosides, e.g., 600 mg tobramycin twice daily, via aerosol are effective at delaying exacerbations. Aerosol administration also permits other drugs, e.g., colistin, to be utilized that are relatively ineffective by the intravenous route.

A number of pharmacologic agents for increasing mucus clearance are being tested. *N*-acetyl-cysteine, which solubilizes mucous glycoproteins, has not been shown to have clinically significant effects on mucus clearance and/or lung function. Recombinant human DNAse, however, degrades the concentrated DNA in CF sputum, decreases sputum viscosity, and increases airflow during short-term administration. Long-term (6 months) DNAse treatment also increases the time between pulmonary exacerbations, although mild adverse effects have been noted. Most patients receive a therapeutic trial of DNAse to test for efficacy, and a minority appear to demonstrate persistent objective benefits. Clinical trials of experimental drugs aimed at restoring salt and water content of secretions are underway. The combination of a sodium channel blocker (amiloride) to reduce excessive Na^+ absorption and UTP to initiate Cl^- secretion via non-CFTR-mediated Cl^- transport, although experimental, appears synergistic and promising.

Inhaled beta-adrenergic agonists can be useful to control airways constriction. They achieve a short-term increase in airflow, but long-term benefit has not been shown. Inhaled anticholinergics provide an alternative. Oral glucocorticoids are not first-line agents for controlling airways constriction and are of no use in improving the nonreversible component of lung function. Glucocorticoids may be useful for treating allergic bronchopulmonary aspergillosis.

The chronic damage to airway walls reflects to some degree the destructive activities of inflammatory enzymes generated in part by inflammatory cells. To date, specific therapies with antiproteases have not been successfully developed. However, a subset of adolescents with CF appears to benefit from long-term, high dose nonsteroidal (ibuprofen) therapy.

A number of pulmonary complications require acute interventions. Atelectasis is best treated with chest physiotherapy and antibiotic therapy. Pneumothoraces involving 10 percent or less of the lung can be observed without intervention. The use of chest tubes to expand collapsed, diseased lung often requires long periods of time, and sclerosing agents should be used with caution because of possible limitations for subsequent lung transplantation. Small-volume hemoptysis requires no specific therapy other than treatment of lung infection and assessment of coagulation and vitamin K status. If massive hemoptysis occurs, bronchial artery embolization can be successful. The most ominous complications of CF are respiratory failure and cor pulmonale. The most effective conventional therapy for these conditions is vigorous medical management of the lung disease and O_2 supplementation. Ultimately, the only effective treatment for respiratory failure in CF is lung transplantation. The 2-year survival for lung transplantation exceeds 60 percent, and deaths in transplant patients result principally from graft rejection, often involving obliterative bronchiolitis. The transplanted lungs do not develop a CF-specific phenotype.

Gastrointestinal Disease Maintenance of adequate nutrition is critical for the health of the CF patient. Most (>90 percent) of CF patients benefit from pancreatic enzyme replacement. Capsules generally contain between 4000 and 24,000 units of lipase. The dose of enzymes (typically no more than 2000 units/kg per meal) should be adjusted on the basis of weight gain, abdominal symptomatology, and character of stools. Replacement of fat-soluble vitamins, particularly vitamins E and K, is usually required. Hyperglycemia most often becomes manifest in the adult. Principles for treating other causes of nonketotic hyperglycemia should be employed.

For treatment of acute obstruction due to meconium ileus equivalent, megalodiatrizoate or other hypertonic radiocontrast materials delivered by enema to the terminal ileum are utilized. For control of symptoms, adjustment of pancreatic enzymes and the supplementation of intake by salt solutions containing osmotically active agents, e.g., propyleneglycol, are utilized. Persistent symptoms may indicate a diagnosis of gastrointestinal malignancy, which is increased in incidence in CF patients. Hepatic and gallbladder complications are treated as for non-CF patients. End-stage liver disease can be treated by transplantation, which has a 2-year survival rate exceeding 50 percent.

Psychosocial Factors CF imposes a tremendous burden on patients. Health insurance, career options, family planning, and life expectancy become major issues; thus, assisting patients with the psychosocial adjustments required by CF is critical.

BIBLIOGRAPHY

AITKEN ML, FIEL SB: Cystic fibrosis. Dis Mon 39:1, 1993

CHENG SH et al: Defective intracellular transport and processing of CFTR is the molecular basis of most cystic fibrosis. Cell 63:827, 1990

FITZSIMMONS SC: *CFF Patient Registry. 1994 Annual Report.* Bethesda, MD, Cystic Fibrosis Foundation, 1995

FUCHS HJ et al: Effect of aerosolized recombinant DNase on exacerbations of respiratory symptoms and on pulmonary function in patients with cystic fibrosis. The Pulmoenzyme Study Group. N Engl J Med 331:637, 1994

HARRIS A, ARGENT BE: The cystic fibrosis gene and its product CFTR. Semin Cell Biol 4:37, 1993

HIGHSMITH WE et al: A novel mutation in the cystic fibrosis gene in patients with pulmonary disease but normal sweat chloride concentrations. N Engl J Med 331:974, 1994

KONSTAN MW et al: Effect of high-dose ibuprofen in patients with cystic fibrosis. N Engl J Med 332:848, 1995

O'LOUGHLIN EV et al: Abnormal epithelial transport in cystic fibrosis jejunum. Am J Physiol 260:G758, 1991

RAMSEY BW et al: Efficacy of aerosolized tobramycin in patients with cystic fibrosis. N Engl J Med 328:1740, 1993

SFERRA TJ, COLLINS FS: The molecular biology of cystic fibrosis. Annu Rev Med 44:133, 1995

STUTTS MJ et al: CFTR as a cAMP-dependent regulator of sodium channels. Science 269:847, 1995

258

Eric G. Honig, Roland H. Ingram, Jr.

CHRONIC BRONCHITIS, EMPHYSEMA, AND AIRWAYS OBSTRUCTION

Chronic bronchitis and emphysema are two distinct processes, most often present in combination in patients with chronic airways obstruction. The diagnosis of chronic bronchitis is made by history, chronic airways obstruction is assessed physiologically, and emphysema can

be diagnosed with certainty in most instances by high resolution CT scans or by histologic examination of sections of whole lung fixed at inflation. Although the relationships among clinical characteristics, physiologic derangements, and morphologic changes have been studied for many years, uniform clinical criteria are still not available.

DEFINITIONS *Chronic bronchitis* is a condition associated with excessive tracheobronchial mucus production sufficient to cause cough with expectoration for at least 3 months of the year for more than 2 consecutive years. *Simple chronic bronchitis* describes a condition characterized by mucoid sputum production. *Chronic mucopurulent bronchitis* is characterized by persistent or recurrent purulence of sputum in the absence of localized suppurative diseases such as bronchiectasis. Since there may or may not be obstruction as assessed by the use of the forced expiratory vital capacity maneuver, *chronic bronchitis with obstruction* deserves a separate classification. There is a further subset of patients with chronic bronchitis and obstruction who experience severe dyspnea and wheezing in association with inhaled irritants or during acute respiratory infections. Such patients are said to have *chronic infective asthma* or *chronic asthmatic bronchitis*. Since there is considerable but not complete reversibility of airflow obstruction with bronchodilator treatment and abatement of inflammation, and since hyperresponsiveness of airways to nonspecific stimuli is seen in patients with chronic bronchitis with obstruction, confusion is possible between patients with this condition and those with asthma who may also have chronic airways obstruction (Chap. 252). The differentiation is based mainly on the history of the clinical illness. The patient with chronic bronchitis with obstruction has a long history of cough and sputum production with a later onset of wheezing, whereas the asthma patient with chronic obstruction gives a long history of wheezing with later onset of chronic productive cough.

Emphysema is defined as the permanent, abnormal distention of the air spaces distal to the terminal bronchiole with destruction of alveolar septa. *Chronic obstructive lung disease* is defined as a condition in which there is chronic obstruction to airflow due to chronic bronchitis and/or emphysema (see below). Although the degree of obstruction may be less when the patient is free from respiratory infection and may improve somewhat with bronchodilator drugs, significant obstruction is always present in patients with this condition.

PATHOLOGY Chronic bronchitis is associated with hypertrophy of the mucus-producing glands found in the submucosa of large cartilaginous airways. Quantitation of this anatomic change, known as the Reid index, is based on the ratio of the thickness of the submucosal glands to that of the bronchial wall. In persons without a history of chronic bronchitis, the mean ratio is 0.44 ± 0.09, whereas in those with such a history the mean ratio is 0.52 ± 0.08. Although a low index is rarely associated with symptoms and a high index is commonly associated with symptoms during life, there is a great deal of overlap. Therefore, many persons will have morphologic changes in large airways without having had chronic bronchitis.

In lungs from patients with chronic obstructive lung disease which have been studied at postmortem, the major site of airflow obstruction has been shown to be in the small airways. Goblet cell hyperplasia, mucosal and submucosal inflammatory cells, edema, peribronchial fibrosis, intraluminal mucus plugs, and increased smooth muscle are characteristic findings in small airways.

The alveolar epithelium is both the target and the initiator of inflammation in chronic bronchitis. Bronchitic inflammation differs from the predominantly eosinophilic inflammation of asthma because of the predominance of neutrophils and the peribronchiolar location of fibrotic changes. It is the consequence of the actions of interleukin 8 and a variety of other chemotactic and proinflammatory cytokines and of colony stimulating factors released by airway epithelial cells in response to toxic, infectious, or inflammatory stimuli. Injured epithelium may also release reduced amounts of regulatory products such as angiotensin-converting enzyme or neutral endopeptidase. As with asthma, the strength of these inflammatory reactions correlates with bronchial reactivity. Sputum production is stimulated by increased exocytosis from secretory cells, lipid mediators, and inflammatory cell products, especially macrophage mucus secretagogue. Mucin gene expression is amplified by tumor necrosis factor α, and secretory cell hyperplasia is encouraged by the neutrophil enzymes elastase and cathepsin G.

Emphysema is classified according to the pattern of involvement of the gas-exchanging units (acini) of the lung distal to the terminal bronchiole. With *centriacinar emphysema*, the distention and destruction are mainly limited to the respiratory bronchioles with relatively less change peripherally in the acinus. Because of the large functional reserve in the lung, many units must be involved in order for overall dysfunction to be detectable. The centrally destroyed regions of the acinus have a high ventilation/perfusion ratio because the capillaries are missing, yet ventilation continues. This results in a deficit of perfusion relative to ventilation, while the peripheral portions of the acinus have crowded and small alveoli with intact, perfused capillaries giving a low ventilation/perfusion ratio. This results in a deficit of ventilation relative to blood flow, giving a high alveolar-arterial P_{O_2} difference ($P_{A_{O_2}} - P_{a_{O_2}}$) (Chap. 250). During normal aging, airspaces enlarge and alveolar ducts increase in diameter. These changes are extremely common in lungs from persons above age 50 and may be misidentified as emphysema.

Panacinar emphysema involves both the central and peripheral portions of the acinus, which results, if the process is extensive, in a reduction of the alveolar-capillary gas exchange surface and loss of elastic recoil properties. When emphysema is severe, it may be difficult to distinguish between the two types, which most often coexist in the same lung.

CONTRIBUTIONS TO PATHOGENESIS

SMOKING Cigarette smoking is the most commonly identified correlate with both chronic bronchitis during life and extent of emphysema at postmortem. Experimental studies have shown that prolonged cigarette smoking impairs ciliary movement, inhibits function of alveolar macrophages, and leads to hypertrophy and hyperplasia of mucus-secreting glands; massive exposure in dogs can produce emphysematous changes. It is probable that smoke also inhibits antiproteases and causes polymorphonuclear leukocytes to release proteolytic enzymes acutely. Inhaled cigarette smoke can produce an acute increase in airways resistance due to vagally mediated smooth-muscle constriction, presumably by way of stimulating submucosal irritant receptors. Increased airways responsiveness is associated with more rapid progression in patients with chronic airways obstruction. Obstruction of small airways is the earliest demonstrable mechanical defect in young cigarette smokers, and the obstruction may disappear completely after cessation of smoking. Although smoking cessation does not result in complete reversal of more pronounced obstruction, there is a significant slowing of the decline in lung function in all smokers who give up cigarettes. In effect, it is never too late to quit smoking cigarettes.

Passive exposure to tobacco smoke correlates with respiratory symptoms such as cough, wheeze, and sputum production. Not only is cigarette smoking the most common single factor leading to chronic airways obstruction, it also adds to the effects of every other contributory factor to be discussed below.

AIR POLLUTION The incidence and mortality rates of both chronic bronchitis and emphysema may be higher in heavily industrialized urban areas. Exacerbations of bronchitis are clearly related to periods of heavy pollution with sulfur dioxide (SO_2) and particulate matter. While nitrogen dioxide (NO_2) can produce small-airways ob-ction (bronchiolitis) in experimental animals exposed to high con-ations, there are no data convincingly implicating NO_2, at even the st pollutant levels, in the pathogenesis or worsening of airways tion in humans (Chap. 254).

OCCUPATION Chronic bronchitis is more prevalent in workers who engage in occupations exposing them to either inorganic or organic dusts or to noxious gases. Epidemiologic surveys have succeeded in demonstrating an accelerated decline in lung function in many such workers—e.g., workers in plastics plants exposed to toluene diisocyanate, and carding room workers in cotton mills (Chap. 254)—suggesting that their occupational exposure contributes to their future disability.

INFECTION Morbidity, mortality, and frequency of acute respiratory illnesses are higher in patients with chronic bronchitis. Many attempts have been made to relate these illnesses to infection with viruses, mycoplasmas, and bacteria. However, only the rhinovirus is found more often during exacerbations; that is to say, pathogenic bacteria, mycoplasmas, and viruses other than rhinovirus are found just as often between as during exacerbations. Epidemiologic studies, however, implicate acute respiratory illness as one of the major factors associated with the etiology as well as the progression of chronic airways obstruction. Cigarette smokers may either transitorily develop or worsen small-airways obstruction in association with even mild viral respiratory infections. There is also some evidence that severe viral pneumonia early in life may lead to chronic obstruction, predominantly in small airways.

FAMILIAL AND GENETIC FACTORS Familial aggregation of chronic bronchitis has been well demonstrated. Children of smoking parents may experience more frequent and severe respiratory illnesses and have a higher prevalence of chronic respiratory symptoms. In addition, nonsmokers who remain in the presence of cigarette smokers (passive smokers) have increased blood levels of carbon monoxide, which indicate that they are significantly exposed to smoke. Another well-documented form of indoor air pollution relates to the use of natural gas for cooking. The role of such pollution, however, remains controversial. Thus a part of the familial aggregation may be related to home air pollution. However, some studies of monozygotic twins have suggested some genetic predisposition to the development of chronic bronchitis independent of personal or familial smoking habits and other indoor air pollution. The exact genetic mode of transmission, if it exists at all, is uncertain.

Alpha$_1$-Antitrypsin Deficiency The protease inhibitor α_1-antitrypsin (α1AT) is an acute-phase reactant, and normally the serum levels rise in association with many inflammatory reactions and with estrogen administration. Either deficient or absent serum levels of α1AT are found in some patients with the early onset of emphysema. By use of the techniques of acid starch gel and immunoelectrophoresis, genetic typing of the protease inhibitor types has been possible. Most members of the normal population have two M genes, designated as protease inhibitor type MM, and have serum α1AT levels in excess of 2.5 g/L. Several genes are associated with alterations in levels of serum α1AT, but the most common ones associated with emphysema are the Z and S genes. Individuals who are homozygous ZZ or SS have serum levels often near 0 but always less than 0.5 g/L and develop severe panacinar emphysema in the third and fourth decades of life. The panacinar process predominates at the lung bases. Progressive dyspnea with minimal cough characterizes the clinical presentation, although chronic bronchitis is prominent in smokers. Given that α_1-protease inhibitors can be chemically synthesized or biologically produced in significant quantities and can be shown with intravenous infusion to restore the protease-antiprotease balance in liquid lavaged from the lungs of ZZ patients, it has been suggested that replacement therapy with α1AT should be of value in preventing the development of emphysema in these patients. Since replacement therapy was available before efficacy had been assessed, a prospective, randomized trial has not been possible. Through a national registry, a natural history study is underway from which it might be possible to evaluate the effects of therapy if the treated and untreated groups turn out to be sufficiently comparable at entry.

The MZ and MS heterozygotes have intermediate levels of serum α1AT (i.e., between 0.5 and 2.5 g/L); hence the genetic expression is that of an autosomal codominant allele. It is a matter of some controversy whether the heterozygous state is associated with lung function abnormalities. The matter is of some importance, since the heterozygous state is common, with incidence estimates varying between 5 and 14 percent of the general population.

The precise way in which antitrypsin deficiency produces emphysema is unclear. In addition to inhibition of trypsin, $\alpha 1AT$ is an effective inhibitor of elastase and several other proteolytic enzymes. There is experimental evidence that the structural integrity of lung elastin depends on this antienzyme, which protects the lung from proteases released from leukocytes. It is tempting to speculate that recurrent inflammatory reactions related to infection and pollutants play some role in pathogenesis by calling forth leukocytes whose released proteases are uninhibited and are free to cause the damage.

The role of proteolytic enzymes in the induction of emphysema is not restricted to patients with $\alpha 1AT$ deficiency. Evidence is accumulating that proteolytic enzymes derived from neutrophilic leukocytes and alveolar macrophages can produce emphysema even in subjects with normal circulating levels of antiproteases. It is possible that local concentrations of proteolytic enzymes may exceed the inhibitory capacity of antiproteases, that some proteases present are not susceptible to the available antiproteases, or that some of the proteolytic enzymes may be physically inaccessible to the antiprotease activity. The ultimate clinical utility of exogenously produced protease inhibitors currently under development will undoubtedly depend on which of the protease-antiprotease interactions predominates in the production of emphysema. Reduction of endogenous elastase release from leukocytes in the lung has been achieved by colchicine (0.6 mg/d orally) in a randomized, placebo-controlled trial in ex-smokers with chronic airways obstruction. Current smokers showed no such reductions. An assessment of the clinical efficacy of this inexpensive and nontoxic form of therapy in ex-smokers must await a large, prospective clinical trial.

PATHOPHYSIOLOGY Although both chronic bronchitis and emphysema can exist without evidence of obstruction, by the time a patient begins to experience dyspnea as a result of these processes, obstruction is always demonstrable. Although chronic bronchitis and emphysema are usually combined, one process may dominate over the other, and to the extent that inflammatory airways disease, secretions, and bronchospasm are present, there are therapeutic possibilities with some hope for improvement. Both chronic bronchitis and emphysema result in airways narrowing. In addition to the primary airways processes of chronic bronchitis, loss of elastic recoil of the lung in emphysema accounts for a decrease in airways caliber through loss of radial traction on airways. Narrowing of airways is often associated with both an increase in airways resistance and a diminution in maximal expiratory flow rates.

There are occasions in which a normal or only slightly elevated airways resistance is accompanied by low maximal expiratory flow rates. Under such circumstances, an increase in the dynamic collapsibility of intrathoracic airways during forced exhalation is a possible explanation. Also in this context, the elastic recoil pressure of the lung must be considered in a slightly different way. In addition to providing radial support to airways during quiet breathing, the elastic recoil properties of the lung serve as a major determinant of maximal expiratory flow rates. The static recoil pressure of the lung is the difference between alveolar and intrapleural pressure. During forced exhalations, when alveolar and intrapleural pressures are high, there are points in the airway at which bronchial pressure equals pleural pressure. Flow does not increase with higher pleural pressure after these points become fixed, so that the effective driving pressure between alveoli and such points is the elastic recoil pressure of the lung (Fig. 258-1). Hence maximal expiratory flow rates represent a complex and dynamic interplay between airways caliber, elastic recoil pressures, and collapsibility of airways. As a direct consequence of the altered pressure-airflow relationships, the work of breathing is increased in bronchitis and emphysema. Since flow-resistive work is flow rate–dependent, there is a disproportionate increase in the work of breathing with increased ventilation.

The designated subdivisions of the lung volume outlined in Chap. 250 are abnormal to varying degrees in both bronchitis and emphysema. The residual volume (RV) and functional residual capacity (FRC) are almost always higher than normal. Since the normal FRC is the volume at which the inward recoil of the lung is balanced by the outward recoil of the chest wall, loss of elastic recoil of the lung results in a higher FRC. In addition, prolongation of expiration in association with obstruction would lead to a dynamic increase in FRC if inspiration is initiated before the respiratory system reaches its static balance point. Elevations of total lung capacity (TLC) are frequent. The exact cause is uncertain, but increases in TLC are often found in association with decreases in the elastic recoil of the lung. Although the vital capacity is frequently decreased, significant airways obstruction can be present with a normal to near-normal vital capacity.

Time constants for expiration are prolonged in all obstructive lung diseases because of increased airways resistance, increased lung compliance (e.g., emphysema), or a combination of both. When time constants are sufficiently prolonged, there may be insufficient time for expiration, even at normal respiratory rates, and the lungs may be unable to return to their mechanical equilibrium volume, FRC. The consequent progressive increase in lung volume moves tidal breathing to a higher, less compliant portion of the pressure-volume curve of the respiratory system and increases the work of breathing. The increased elastic recoil pressure associated with the higher end-tidal volume is

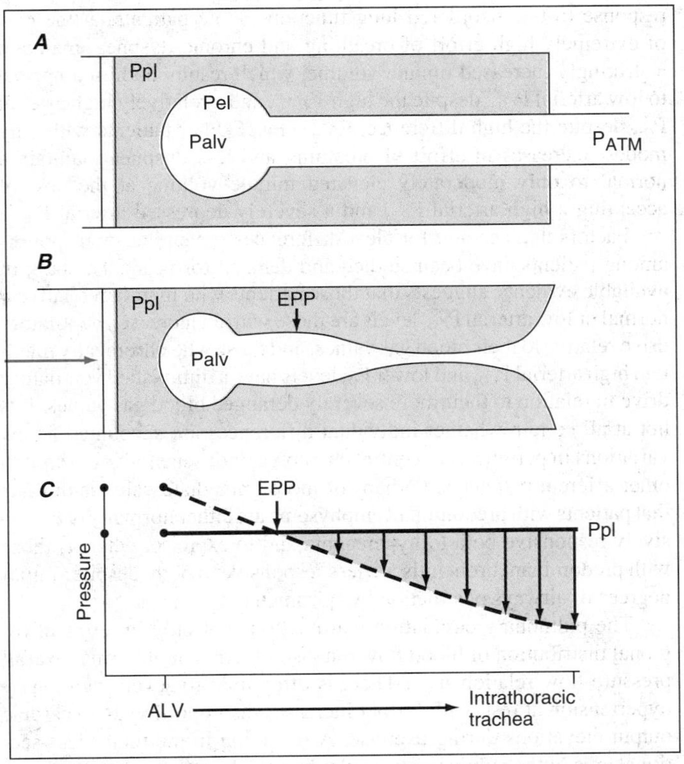

FIGURE 258-1 *A.* A schematic diagram of the lung and intrathoracic airways with no airflow. The alveolar pressure (Palv) is greater than pleural pressure (Ppl) by an amount equal to the elastic recoil pressure of the lung (Pel)—i.e., Palv is the algebraic sum of Ppl + Pel. With no airflow Palv equals atmospheric pressure (P_{ATM}), and for all of the intrathoracic airways, pressure outside is less than the pressure inside due to the Pel. *B.* The same schematic lung during forced exhalation when pleural pressure becomes quite positive (*arrow*). Palv is still greater than Ppl by an amount equal to Pel. However, there is a pressure drop along the airway associated with flow, and at some point Ppl equals local bronchial pressure (so-called equal pressure point, EPP). Mouthward from this point, Ppl exceeds local bronchial pressure and hence acts to compress the airways. *C.* Pressure within the airways from alveoli to the intrathoracic trachea is shown as a dashed line (---) and Ppl is shown as a constant (—). Therefore, the driving pressure from alveoli to EPP is equal to Pel, and a decrease in Pel (i.e., loss of elastic recoil) would mean a smaller driving pressure and smaller flow rates.

termed *intrinsic positive end-expiratory pressure (PEEP)*, or auto-PEEP (PEEPi), and represents an added threshold load that must be overcome to initiate the next inspiration. PEEPi is a common finding in patients with chronic airflow obstruction and contributes to their work of breathing and dyspnea. Hyperinflation contributes additionally to the discomfort associated with airflow obstruction by flattening the diaphragm and placing it at a mechanical disadvantage due to the length-tension relationship, the angle of diaphragmatic insertion with the lower ribs, and Laplace's law.

Maldistribution of inspired gas and blood flow is always present to some extent. When the mismatching is severe, impairment of gas exchange is reflected in abnormalities of arterial blood gases. There are regions of the lung with a deficit of perfusion in relation to ventilation that increase the wasted ventilation ratio (that is, V_d/V_t; Chap. 250). At a normal resting CO_2 production, the net effective alveolar ventilation, as reflected by the arterial P_{CO_2}, may be excessive, normal, or insufficient depending on the relationship of the overall minute volume to the wasted ventilation ratio. The net contribution of regions with perfusion in excess of ventilation can be assessed by either estimating or measuring the alveolar-arterial P_{O_2} difference (that is, $PA_{O_2} - Pa_{O_2}$; Chap. 250). In chronic bronchitis and emphysema, there are increases in both wasted ventilation and wasted blood flow.

The clinical manifestations depend, in large part, on the ventilatory response to the disordered lung function. Some patients, at the cost of extremely high effort of breathing and chronic dyspnea, maintain a strikingly increased minute volume, which results both in a normal to low arterial P_{CO_2}, despite the high V_d/V_t, and a relatively high arterial P_{O_2}, despite the high difference, $PA_{O_2} - Pa_{O_2}$. Other patients with only modest increases in effort of breathing and less dyspnea maintain a normal to only moderately elevated minute volume at the cost of accepting a high arterial P_{CO_2} and a severely depressed arterial P_{O_2}.

Factors that account for clear differences in ventilatory responses among patients have been studied and debated for years. The bulk of available evidence suggests that those patients who maintain relatively normal or low arterial P_{CO_2} levels are those with an increased ventilatory drive relative to their blood gas values, and those who chronically maintain high arterial P_{CO_2} and lower P_{O_2} levels have a diminished ventilatory drive in relation to their more severely deranged blood gas values. It is not at all certain whether individual differences are accounted for by variations in peripheral or central chemoreceptor sensitivity or through other afferent pathways. Perhaps of more immediate value is the fact that patients with predominant emphysema are either normally or excessively responsive both to hypercapnia and to exercise, whereas those with predominant bronchitis are less responsive to both, despite similar degrees of airways obstruction by spirometry.

The pulmonary circulation malfunctions not only in terms of regional distribution of blood flow but also in terms of abnormal overall pressure-flow relationships. There is often mild to severe pulmonary hypertension at rest, with further increases disproportionate to cardiac output elevations during exercise. A reduction in the total cross-sectional area of the pulmonary vascular bed can be attributed to anatomic changes and constriction of vascular smooth muscle in pulmonary arteries and arterioles as well as destruction of alveolar septa with loss of capillaries. Rarely does loss of capillaries alone lead to severe pulmonary hypertension with cor pulmonale, except as a near-terminal event (Chap. 238). Of more importance is the constriction of pulmonary vessels in response to alveolar hypoxia. The constriction is reversible upon increase in alveolar P_{O_2} with therapy. There is a synergism between hypoxia and acidosis that assumes importance during episodes of acute or chronic respiratory insufficiency. Chronic hypoxia leads not only to pulmonary vascular constriction but also to secondary erythrocytosis. The latter, although not proved to be a significant tributor to pulmonary hypertension, could add an unfavorable rheo- load. As discussed in Chap. 238, the chronic afterload on the entricle leads to hypertrophy and, in association with disordered ases, ultimately to failure.

CLINICAL-FUNCTIONAL CORRELATIONS Dyspnea and impairment of physical work capacity are characteristic only of severe to moderately severe airways obstruction. There is considerable variation among patients, and those with predominant emphysema have greater dyspnea and restriction of physical activity with lesser degrees of obstruction than those in whom chronic bronchitis predominates. The majority of patients have functionally mixed disease, usually experience exertional dyspnea when the forced expiratory volume in 1 s (FEV_1) falls below 50 percent of that predicted, and have dyspnea at rest when the FEV_1 is less than 25 percent of that predicted. In addition to dyspnea at rest, CO_2 retention and cor pulmonale frequently occur when the FEV_1 falls to 25 percent of that predicted. However, those with predominant bronchitis often have CO_2 retention and cor pulmonale with FEV_1 values above 25 percent of normal, in contrast to patients with predominant emphysema, whose FEV_1 usually falls well below that level before the onset of CO_2 retention and cor pulmonale. With a respiratory infection, small changes in the degree of obstruction can make a large difference in symptoms and gas exchange. Thus small therapeutic gains have rewarding results.

In general, the more severe the obstruction, the poorer the prognosis. Despite the general relationship, 20 to 30 percent of patients with severe obstruction and CO_2 retention will survive beyond 5 years.

CLINICAL SYNDROMES

The clinical presentation varies in severity from simple chronic bronchitis without disability to the severely disabled state with chronic respiratory failure. From a practical standpoint, it is well to consider that any symptom or any measurable abnormality may foreshadow the development of severe disabling disease; hence cessation of smoking and avoidance of environmental irritants and toxins are to be advised. However, the advice to modify behavior and life patterns is rarely taken, and most physicians are called on to categorize and treat patients with fully developed, chronic airways obstruction. Thus the approach taken here is to describe two polar opposite types of fully developed, chronic obstructive pulmonary disease with the realization that the majority of patients will have some features of both types. The salient features of each type are outlined in Table 258-1.

PREDOMINANT EMPHYSEMA These patients often give a long history of exertional dyspnea with minimal cough that is productive of only small amounts of mucoid sputum. Mucopurulent exacerba-

Table 258-1

Chronic Obstructive Lung Disease: Salient Features of the Two Types

	Predominant Emphysema	Predominant Bronchitis
Age at time of diagnosis, y	60±	50±
Dyspnea	Severe	Mild
Cough	After dyspnea starts	Before dyspnea starts
Sputum	Scanty, mucoid	Copious, purulent
Bronchial infections	Less frequent	More frequent
Respiratory insufficiency episodes	Often terminal	Repeated
Chest film	"Hyperinflation" ± bullous changes, small heart	Increased bronchovascular markings at bases, large heart
Chronic Pa_{CO_2}, mmHg	35–40	50–60
Chronic Pa_{O_2}, mmHg	65–75	45–60
Hematocrit, %	35–45	50–55
Pulmonary hypertension:		
Rest	None to mild	Moderate to severe
Exercise	Moderate	Worsens
Cor pulmonale	Rare, except terminally	Common
Elastic recoil	Severely decreased	Normal
Resistance	Normal to slight increase	High
Diffusing capacity	Decreased	Normal to slight decrease

tions in association with infections are not frequent. The body build is asthenic, with evidence of weight loss resulting from energy expenditure in excess of caloric intake. The patient appears distressed, with obvious use of accessory muscles of respiration which serve to lift the sternum in an anterosuperior direction with each inspiration. There is tachypnea with a relatively prolonged expiration through pursed lips, or expiration is begun with a grunting sound. While sitting, these patients often lean forward, extending the arms to brace themselves. The neck veins may be distended during expiration, yet they collapse briskly with inspiration. The lower intercostal spaces retract with each inspiration, and by palpation the lower lateral chest wall can be felt to move inward. The percussion note is hyperresonant, and by auscultation the breath sounds are diminished, with faint, high-pitched rhonchi heard toward the end of expiration. The cardiac impulse, if at all visible, is seen only in the xiphoid and subxiphoid regions, and cardiac dullness is either absent or severely reduced. By palpation there is frequently a sustained forward and downward right ventricular impulse in the subxiphoid region, and a presystolic gallop accentuated during inspiration is commonly heard.

The arterial P_{O_2} is often in the mid-70s (mmHg), and the P_{CO_2} is low to normal. Because of the maintained increase in minute volume and the maintenance of arterial P_{O_2} sufficient to nearly saturate hemoglobin, these patients have been referred to as "pink puffers." Their increased ventilatory drive probably accounts for their relatively preserved oxygenation and lack of hypercapnia; however, this increased drive with attendant increases in ventilation undoubtedly contributes to the severity of their dyspnea.

The TLC and RV are invariably increased, the vital capacity is low, and the maximal expiratory flow rates are diminished. The elastic recoil properties of the lung are severely impaired, and in direct proportion to this impairment, the capacity of the lung to transfer CO is lowered.

On radiographic examination the diaphragms are low and flattened, the bronchovascular shadows do not extend to the periphery of the lung, and the cardiac silhouette is lengthened and narrowed. These findings in association with a large retrosternal translucency on lateral chest radiographs are interpreted as hyperinflation, which correlates well with increases in TLC and loss of elastic recoil. Peripheral attenuation of bronchovascular markings and increased retrosternal lucency correlate best with subsequent postmortem demonstration of extensive and severe emphysema, predominantly of the panacinar type. Computed tomography (CT) has been shown to localize and quantitate emphysema. However, determining the localization of such regions most often is of little practical value, and the overall quantitative assessments from elastic recoil properties and CO transfer are just as good. Hence CT scans are not ordinarily employed for this purpose.

The patient with predominant emphysema is less prone to mucopurulent relapses than is the patient with predominant bronchitis, but such relapses frequently lead to severe respiratory failure and death. That is to say, right-sided heart failure and hypercapnic respiratory failure are often terminal events in those patients with predominant emphysema. In the absence of such relapses, the clinical course is characterized by severe and progressive dyspnea for which little can be done. The physician's role is to seek out and treat any factor that is possibly reversible and help the patient to avoid pollutants and infections.

PREDOMINANT BRONCHITIS The patient with predominant bronchitis usually has an impressive history of cough and sputum production for many years with an immodest history of cigarette smoking. Initially the cough is present only in the winter months, and the patient is apt to seek medical attention, if at all, only during the more severe of the frequent mucopurulent relapses. Over the years the cough progresses from hibernal to perennial, and mucopurulent relapses increase in frequency, duration, and severity. After beginning to experience exertional dyspnea, the patient often seeks medical help and will be found to have a severe degree of obstruction. Occasionally, such a patient will seek out a physician only after the onset of peripheral edema secondary to overt right ventricular failure. More rarely the initial medical contact is made by family members who present the physician with a deeply cyanotic, edematous, and stuporous patient with acute respiratory insufficiency.

The patient with predominant bronchitis is often overweight and cyanotic. There is usually no apparent distress at rest, the respiratory rate is normal or only slightly increased, and there is no apparent usage of accessory muscles. The chest percussion note is normally resonant, and by auscultation one can usually hear coarse rhonchi and wheezes that change in location and intensity after a deep and productive cough. There may be a sustained heave along the lower left sternal border which indicates right ventricular hypertrophy. In the presence of right ventricular failure, there are often an early diastolic gallop and occasionally a holosystolic murmur, both of which are accentuated by inspiration. The latter finding is indicative of functional tricuspid regurgitation, which is frequently accompanied by neck vein distention characterized by large v waves and brisk y descents. With right ventricular failure, the cyanosis deepens and peripheral edema becomes prominent. Clubbing of the digits is unusual.

With or without right ventricular failure, the minute volume is only slightly increased due to an overall diminution in ventilatory drive which modulates the level of dyspnea. However, failure to increase minute volume greatly in the face of significant proportions of wasted ventilation and blood flow results in severely deranged arterial blood gases, with arterial P_{CO_2} values that are chronically increased to the range of the high 40s to low 50s (mmHg). The lowered P_{O_2} produces desaturation of hemoglobin, serves to stimulate erythropoiesis, and results in hypoxic pulmonary vasoconstriction. Desaturation and erythrocytosis combine to produce the cyanosis, and hypoxic pulmonary vasoconstriction accentuates the right-sided heart failure. Because of cyanosis and edema secondary to heart failure, such patients have been referred to as "blue bloaters." It has been proposed, with some supporting data, that one of the pathophysiologic events in blue bloaters is the occurrence of repeated episodes of severe nocturnal oxygen desaturation in association with episodes of sleep apnea or periods of worsening hypoventilation. Such sleep-related ventilatory events worsen the degree of pulmonary hypertension and secondary erythrocytosis.

The TLC is often normal, and there is a moderate elevation of RV. The vital capacity is mildly diminished, and maximal expiratory flow rates are invariably low. The elastic recoil properties of the lung are normal or only slightly impaired, and the capacity of the lung to transfer CO is either normal or minimally decreased.

There are no roentgenographic features that are definitive for chronic bronchitis. The two findings most commonly encountered are thickened bronchial walls manifested by tubular or "tramline" shadows, and a generalized increase in bronchovascular markings. In the presence of chronic pulmonary hypertension, the main pulmonary arterial segments enlarge and the cardiac silhouette may become more prominent due to right atrial and right ventricular chamber enlargement.

Despite well-planned management (see below), the patient with predominant bronchitis may experience many episodes of respiratory failure from which recovery is frequent with proper therapy (see later). The ability to recover from such repeated episodes in these patients is in striking contrast to the frequently fatal outcome of such events in those with predominant emphysema. Ultimately, the lungs at postmortem exhibit severe bronchitic changes in both large and small airways and only moderate emphysema, predominantly of the centriacinar variety.

The preceding syndromes—predominant emphysema and predominant bronchitis—are described as polar ends of a continuous spectrum of clinical features. Most patients have some characteristics of each syndrome. Recognizing and understanding the pathophysiologic bases for these aids in the planning of appropriate management strategies for each patient.

℞ TREATMENT

Intelligent management must be based on as complete knowledge as possible of the degree of obstruction, the extent of disability, and the relative reversibility of the patient's illness. To the extent that obstructive processes in the airways are contributory, there is a chance for treatment to be effective. Since emphysema is an irreversible process, prevention of progression and avoidance of acute insults constitute the main approach. History, physical examination, and chest radiographs should be supplemented by tests of lung function performed during a symptomatically stable period. Ideally, complete spirometry, plethysmographic lung volumes, transfer of CO, arterial blood gases, and lung elastic recoil properties should be measured. Spirometry and lung volumes should be remeasured after the administration of bronchodilators in order to assess the degree of acutely reversible airways obstruction. Failure to respond to a single bronchodilator agent at one point in time does not rule out the possibility of improvement with more prolonged administration of one or more of these agents and should not preclude their use. In instances in which the degree of exertional dyspnea appears to be disproportionately greater than the degree of obstruction, measurements of blood gases, minute volume, CO_2 production, and O_2 consumption during exercise are indicated in order to determine whether impaired lung function is sufficient to account for the symptoms. After the initial assessment, the physician has some idea of the relative emphasis to be placed on patient education, rehabilitative and preventive measures, and direct therapeutic interventions in management of the patient and the illness.

Smoking and the Environment Cessation of smoking is the only certain means of influencing the progression of the chronic obstructive airways syndromes, and although such behavior modification is most effective at early stages of the disease processes, it is effective in slowing the rate of decline in lung function, even when such function is severely compromised. The physician should always ask the patient about smoking, urge the patient to stop smoking, help the patient set a date to stop, and provide close follow-up support for the patient's efforts. Smoking cessation produces sustained reductions in the rate of the decline of FEV_1 that are greater in magnitude and more persistent than those achieved with bronchodilator therapy alone. Nicotine replacement therapy has been shown to be an effective modality in helping patients to stop smoking, producing average increments in abstinence rates of 10 to 15 percent over behavioral and educational programs without pharmacologic intervention. Benefits are greater for nicotine patches than for nicotine gum and are most marked in patients who are highly dependent upon nicotine. Nonetheless, 6 to 12 month abstinence rates for smoking cessation programs remain 20 to 25 percent in most reports. The best results have been achieved with highly motivated patients in dedicated smoking cessation clinics.

In patients in whom occupational or environmental exposures are thought to play a significant role, change of occupation or relocation of dwelling is advisable. The validity of such advice should be considered carefully, since the impact on both the patient and the family is likely to be great. A simple environmental change is that of eliminating aerosol sprays such as deodorants, hair sprays, and insecticides from the household. Hair sprays have been shown to produce acute airways responses even in normal subjects. Other preventive measures include yearly vaccination against the common or expected influenza virus strains. Patients need be given pneumococcal polysaccharide vaccine only once in a lifetime due to prolonged effectiveness of the immune response. However, if an earlier vaccine was used that contained only 14 capsular antigen types, revaccination with the current 23-valent vaccine is probably advisable.

Respiratory Infections Infections cannot be totally avoided, and the patient should be made aware that increasing purulence, ˌiscosity, or volume of secretions signals the onset of an infection, ˌich should be treated early. The most common pathogenic bacteria ˌd are *Haemophilus influenzae*, *Streptococcus pneumoniae*, and ˌ*xella catarrhalis*. As mentioned above, however, the role of such bacteria is in question, since they are just as often isolated during periods of relative clinical quiescence. Nonetheless, an antibiotic effective against β-lactamase-producing organisms should be given for a 7- to 10-day course. It is practical to have the patient keep a 7- to 10-day supply of antibiotics at home and to begin treatment at the onset of symptoms. In Great Britain it is common practice to give continuous antibiotic therapy during winter months in order to prevent mucopurulent relapses. Although there is evidence that viruses are frequent causes of mucopurulent relapses, some clinical studies have shown that the standard antibiotic regimens decrease the duration and severity of infective episodes unrelated to culturable bacterial pathogens. The greatest benefits are seen in patients with more than four purulent exacerbations per year. Microscopic examination and culture of sputum are indicated if there are chills, fever, or chest pain or if purulence fails to respond to usually administered antibiotics.

Exercise and Nutrition Exercise programs, although not accompanied by measurable improvement in lung function, result in increased exercise tolerance and an improved sense of well-being. The improvement is usually task-specific, so most physicians advise walking in preference to the use of special apparatus, such as stationary bicycles. Arm exercise is poorly tolerated; the necessary muscles required for breathing are also recruited for the exercise task and hence are doing double duty.

If malnutrition (body weight less than 85 percent of ideal) is present, oral dietary supplements can result in improved muscle strength, less fatigability, and lessening of breathlessness. A carefully taken dietary history and elimination of other serious causes for low body weight and weight loss should precede the start of any major nutritional supplement effort. As with exercise programs, there is no direct and measurable effect on lung function from treating malnutrition, yet subjective relief and objective improvement in strength and exercise performance have been of great benefit in such patients.

Bronchodilator Drugs These are often quite helpful in alleviating symptoms, especially in patients who respond to them acutely in the laboratory. These drugs form three categories: the methylxanthines, sympathomimetics with strong $beta_2$-adrenergic-stimulating properties, and anticholinergics. The ethylene diamine salt of theophylline (aminophylline), the most commonly used methylxanthine, can be given orally or parenterally; in addition to bronchodilatation, it stimulates respiration and has cardiotonic and diuretic properties and may increase diaphragmatic contractility, especially in the setting of hypoxemia or muscle fatigue. Although it is a relatively weak bronchodilator and mechanical benefits are not consistently demonstrated, improved exercise performance and well-being are often seen. Oral theophylline preparations vary greatly in their intestinal release and rate of absorption. There is extreme variability in rates of absorption, degradation, and secretion among patients. Theophylline blood levels should be measured in those patients who, with standard doses, either fail to benefit or show signs of toxicity. Measurements at expected peak absorption and just before the subsequent dose will allow adjustment of dose. Blood levels between 10 and 15 mg/L should be maintained. Side effects such as insomnia and nervousness are frequent when levels are in the therapeutic range. Nausea, vomiting, tachyarrhythmias, and seizures are seen mainly when blood levels exceed 20 mg/L. Parenteral administration of theophylline is rarely indicated in the chronic obstructive syndromes, except during episodes of respiratory failure when agents cannot be given orally.

Selective $beta_2$-stimulating drugs such as albuterol, terbutaline, and metaproterenol can be given both orally and by aerosol with fewer cardiac side effects than are experienced with isoproterenol. Orally and parenterally administered $beta_2$ agonists are effective but are associated with greater tremulousness and cardiovascular side effects than result from inhaled agents. The latter can be most conveniently given in metered-dose inhalers at two to four puffs four to six times a day. Collecting chambers or spacers may improve the reliability of deposition of these agents. Anticholinergic agents such as atropine have been avoided in the past because of their tendency to desiccate secretions; however, ipratropium bromide, an anticholinergic agent in metered-dose inhaler form, is an effective bronchodilator in chronic bronchitic patients. It is considered by many to be the bronchodilator of choice for these patients.

Glucocorticoids The use of systemic glucocorticoids is based on very little scientific data from properly controlled clinical trials. Since these agents have time- and dose-related side effects that vary from deleterious to catastrophic, the almost invariable subjective benefit must be supported by objective measurements. There is little room for doubt in the minds of physicians that some patients respond well, even dramatically, to these agents in both objective and subjective terms. The real problem is how to select those patients most likely to benefit. Eosinophilia in the sputum, rather than in the blood, appears in some instances to identify this subgroup in advance. However, the best guidelines are, first, to try these agents only after maximal bronchodilator and bronchopulmonary drainage measures have been tried without success; second, to begin prednisone at 30 mg once per day; third, to confirm the objective change in terms of spirometry and gas exchange, stopping these agents if no objective benefit is seen; and fourth, to decrease to the smallest dose that will maintain the improved level of function. Though some objective benefit has been shown in patients with bronchial hyperresponsiveness, the role, if any, of inhaled glucocorticoid agents for these patients, in contrast to asthmatic patients, has not been established in the syndromes with chronic obstruction.

Hypoxia and Erythrocytosis When arterial hypoxia is persistent and severe (Pa_{O_2} of 55 to 60 mmHg) in association with cor pulmonale (see Chap. 238), erythrocytosis, and signs of right heart failure, continuous O_2 therapy is indicated. If the Pa_{O_2} is persistently <55 mmHg, with or without cor pulmonale, continuous O_2 supplementation also should be prescribed. The available data indicate that supplemental O_2 improves both exercise tolerance and neuropsychological function and alleviates pulmonary hypertension and right heart failure. In patients with severe hypoxemia, the need for hospitalization occurs less frequently and life span is lengthened by the use of supplemental O_2. Although long-term O_2 therapy has been shown to produce improvements in cognitive performance, quality of life, and exercise endurance, a survival benefit has not yet been demonstrated in those patients with less severe hypoxemia and who do not have cor pulmonale.

Since most patients with chronic airways obstruction, especially those with features of predominant bronchitis, can be shown to decrease their Pa_{O_2} values significantly during sleep, most prominently during the rapid eye movement phase, nocturnal O_2 administration has been suggested. While the rationale is clear and the results quite good, a cooperative clinical trial that compared nocturnal with continuous O_2 supplementation in severely hypoxic patients found that continuous O_2 administration was associated with a significantly lower mortality rate. Patients in both treatment groups experienced neuropsychological and hemodynamic benefits. Thus supplemental nocturnal O_2 is better than none, but continuous O_2 is better than nocturnal in such severely ill patients. Those patients not requiring continuous O_2 therapy may require supplementation during air travel. Even with modern pressurization, cabin altitudes may reach the equivalent of 8000 ft, at which the Pa_{O_2} may fall by 25 mmHg below that found at sea level. Hence O_2 supplementation during prolonged flights should be considered for patients with sea level Pa_{O_2} values in the mid-70s.

Secondary erythrocytosis with the hematocrit in excess of 50 percent is most easily viewed as a mechanism allowing greater O_2 delivery to compensate for the chronically lowered arterial P_{O_2}; hence improvement in oxygenation through improved lung function or by O_2 administration is the most physiologic means to reverse erythrocytosis. Since erythrocytosis results in elevation of blood viscosity at all shear rates, the proposal has been made that pulmonary vascular hypertension is aggravated by its presence. Although no study has demonstrated an objective improvement in hemodynamics, lung mechanics, or gas exchange at rest following phlebotomy, ventilatory and cardiovascular function during exercise improve. Some patients who complain of headaches and a sense of head fullness show a favorable subjective response to periodic phlebotomy when the hematocrit is in excess of 55 percent. In support of this subjective improvement is the demonstration that, following phlebotomy, cerebral blood flow, previously diminished, returns toward normal.

Other Measures *Bronchopulmonary drainage* should be maintained in patients with hypersecretion. If the coughing mechanism is ineffective or if paroxysms of coughing are exhausting, postural drainage is often a useful adjunct. Although liquefaction of secretions by means of orally administered expectorants or aerosol delivery of mucolytic agents is an appealing idea, it has never been shown by properly designed trials to be more effective than simple maintenance of total-body hydration.

Intermittent positive-pressure breathing devices were formerly advocated for home management. The various rationales included diminution in the work of breathing, promotion of bronchopulmonary drainage, and more efficient delivery of bronchodilator drugs. The first of the rationales has been shown to have no basis in fact, and the goals of the last two have been shown to be as well accomplished by postural drainage and use of less elaborate aerosol generators. In fact, metered-dose inhalers, when used properly, are as effective as any powered nebulizer system. Hence the use of intermittent positive-pressure breathing devices and compressor-driven aerosol generators for home management cannot be justified.

Despite employing all the aforementioned measures, some patients remain severely incapacitated. For these patients, *lung transplantation* can return them to both a functional and comfortable state (see Chap. 267). Criteria for transplanting such patients are being evolved in the several centers performing this procedure. Medical directors of such programs should be consulted if the possibility of a lung transplant is being considered.

Surgical bullectomy may provide symptomatic relief in patients with large emphysematous bullae that are expanded by the greater retractive force exerted by the normal parenchyma. Benefit is seen only in patients who have stopped smoking, and long-term effects have not been clearly established. Thoracoscopic laser bullectomy procedures have recently been described. A favorable risk:benefit profile remains to be established for this procedure. Lung volume–reduction surgery has recently been reintroduced with the aim of improving elastic recoil by resecting multiple regions of overdistended lung in patients with diffuse, nonhomogeneous emphysema. The procedure is currently experimental and should be applied only within the confines of a well-designed clinical trial.

There are two therapeutic interventions well short of lung transplantation that have been proposed repeatedly by a few investigators and that remain extremely controversial. It cannot be denied that some supporting data exist; the counterintuitive nature of the interventions and the absence of controlled trials preclude their wide acceptance. These are (1) bilateral carotid body resection, and (2) periodic use of negative-pressure ventilation. The initial rationale for bilateral carotid body resection was to relieve dyspnea by diminishing the ventilatory responsiveness to hypoxemia and hypercapnia, which would present its own set of dangers. Several studies have shown improved lung mechanics and exercise performance after the procedure. Use of negative-pressure ventilation for periods up to 8 h/d for 2 consecutive days has been shown to improve gas exchange, muscle strength, and ventilatory responsiveness for several subsequent days. Negative-pressure ventilation is most effective in patients with hypercapnia and when care is taken to ensure that sufficient mechanical support is provided to truly rest the respiratory muscles. Patients who are unable to synchronize upper airway motor output with the negative-pressure ventilator have been reported to experience obstructive sleep apnea as a complication of this form of therapy.

ACUTE RESPIRATORY FAILURE IN PATIENTS WITH CHRONIC BRONCHITIS, EMPHYSEMA, AND AIRWAYS OBSTRUCTION

DIAGNOSIS Although it may be strongly suspected on clinical grounds, the firm diagnosis of acute respiratory failure in chronic airways obstruction is based on measurements of arterial blood gas (Pa_{O_2}, Pa_{CO_2}) and pH values that must be interpreted in relation to the patient's chronic status. Since many patients have chronically lowered Pa_{O_2} levels and increased Pa_{CO_2} values, the diagnosis is based on the degree of change from the usual state of the individual patient. With regard to oxygenation, an acute decrease in Pa_{O_2} from a usual mid-70 range to the low 60s (mmHg) is just as indicative of acute respiratory failure as is an acute drop from a chronic mid-50 range to the mid-40s (mmHg). Thus a drop in Pa_{O_2} equal to or greater than 10 to 15 mmHg indicates acute failure.

Since renal compensation for chronic hypercapnia results in adjustment of arterial pH to near-normal values, the acuteness of the increase in Pa_{CO_2} can often be judged by the pH, unless there is a concomitant metabolic acidemia. As a practical guide, any level of hypercapnia associated with an arterial pH value less than 7.30 should be considered as acute respiratory failure.

PRECIPITATING FACTORS Increases in volume, viscosity, and/or purulence of secretions, presumably due to infection of the tracheobronchial tree, are the most common antecedents of acute respiratory failure in chronic obstructive lung disease. Increasing airways obstruction with airways inflammation and secretion, especially in association with a relatively blunted ventilatory drive, leads to worsening hypoxia and increasing CO_2 retention. Agitation, insomnia, and increasing dyspnea with impending respiratory failure are occasionally treated, mistakenly, with either sedatives or narcotics, and these, too, may precipitate frank respiratory failure. In fact, depressant drugs that impair ventilatory drive should be avoided at all times in patients with severe chronic obstructive lung disease. Major episodes of air pollution also can lead to respiratory failure, and the physicians responsible for patients with severe bronchitis and emphysema should be alert to these environmental events.

Pneumonia, thromboembolism, left ventricular failure, and pneumothorax occasionally precipitate acute respiratory failure and are extremely difficult to detect unless considered and specifically sought. As a minimum, chest radiographs, electrocardiograms, and sputum examinations should be obtained in addition to arterial blood gas measurements in all patients with respiratory failure.

℞ TREATMENT

The management of acute respiratory failure consists of two simultaneous processes: (1) maintaining acceptable levels of oxygenation and ventilation, and (2) treatment of infection, removal of secretions, and reversal of any airways constriction present.

Control of Hypoxemia These patients need O_2 when they are severely hypoxic, and while fears of respiratory depression due to the removal of the hypoxic respiratory stimulus are realistic, O_2 must be used, yet in the smallest concentration possible, to give a Pa_{O_2} in the mid-50 range while the patient's Pa_{CO_2}, pH, and clinical status are carefully monitored. It is best to begin with only modest increases in FI_{O_2} to approximately 0.24 (cf. air at 0.21), which can be accomplished using nasal prongs with O_2 flows at 1 to 2 L/min or, more precisely, with the use of a 0.24 Venturi mask. These latter masks, based on Bernoulli's principle, deliver a fixed concentration of O_2 irrespective of the O_2 flow rate by entraining air in direct proportion to O_2 flow rate. They are high-flow masks (oxygen plus air entrained from the room), each designed for a specific FI_{O_2} (0.24, 0.28, 0.35, 40). Even small increases in Pa_{O_2} when starting from low levels lt in significant increases in arterial oxygen content due to the e of the oxygen-hemoglobin saturation curve over this range . 106).

With improved oxygenation some patients will increase their Pa_{CO_2} values. The standard explanation has been that this increase is due to the removal of the hypoxic drive to ventilation leading to further hypoventilation. While this is the most important mechanism, recent data indicate that worsening ventilation-perfusion relationships (Chap. 250) occur with O_2 treatment. This is attributed to reversal of hypoxic pulmonary arterial constriction in the more initially hypoxic, less well ventilated regions, which in turn leads to decreased perfusion of initially less hypoxic, better ventilated regions. The result is an increase in the wasted ventilation ratio (V_d/V_t; Chap. 250) leading to a smaller effective alveolar ventilation. In either case, the FI_{O_2} should be increased as little as possible to achieve a Pa_{O_2} in the mid-50 range. Some increase in Pa_{CO_2} can be expected and should not cause alarm if the patient is alert. The majority of patients can be managed in this conservative way with excellent results. However, occasionally, large increases in Pa_{CO_2} occur and lead to stupor and coma. This can be explained by CO_2-induced cerebral vascular dilatation with increased intracranial pressure, including the development of papilledema, combined with the effect of hypercapnia and hypoxia on cerebral function. Patients most at risk for O_2-induced CO_2 retention are those presenting with Pa_{O_2} below 50 mmHg and H^+ concentration greater than 55 nM (pH ~ 7.26). It must be emphasized that if stupor and coma supervene, stopping the administration of O_2 is the worst possible course of action. When CO_2 narcosis is present, respirations are sufficiently depressed from the CO_2 itself that the patient will no longer respond to the rapidly worsening hypoxia, and fatal arrhythmias, generalized seizures, and death may ensue.

ENDOTRACHEAL INTUBATION AND MECHANICAL VENTILATION These become necessary for patients who fail to respond to conservative management and who have hypercapnia with evidence of obtundation. Before committing to mechanical ventilation, the patient's wishes and expectations should be explored as carefully as circumstances permit. Where uncertainty exists, however, intubation should proceed. Ventilation may be withdrawn if it is later determined to be inappropriate or against the patient's wishes.

Noninvasive ventilation may be attempted as an alternative to endotracheal intubation. In the absence of anxiety, poor cooperation, impaired swallowing, severe hypoxemia, hemodynamic instability, or acute abdominal distress, the majority of patients with chronic airflow obstruction and acute respiratory failure can be successfully managed by continuous positive airway pressure or volume-controlled ventilation applied by face mask.

In any ventilated patient, the ventilator should be set to produce blood gases that support life while avoiding hyperinflation and barotrauma. Tidal volumes and respiratory rates should be kept as low as possible, and moderate degrees of hypercapnia may be tolerated. Once mechanical ventilation has been instituted, the tidal volume and frequency should be set to gradually decrease the Pa_{CO_2} only down to the chronically elevated level rather than to attempt to decrease it to or below a normal value. Since such patients have renal compensation for their chronic hypercapnia, Pa_{CO_2} values at or below the normal level result in significant alkalemia, which in turn can lead to severe tachyarrhythmias and generalized seizures.

Control of Infection, Bronchoconstriction, and Secretions As mentioned above, maintaining oxygenation and ventilation serves to buy time while secretion removal, bronchial dilatation, and treatment of infection are instituted. Removal of secretions is accomplished by urging the patient to cough or by passing suction catheters into the trachea which, in addition to removing secretions that are present, stimulate cough that brings more secretions up to the region of the catheter tip. The advantage, if any, from the use of mucolytic agents in this process has yet to be demonstrated. However, $beta_2$-adrenergic bronchodilating agents have been shown to increase the rate of transport of particles by the mucociliary blanket; thus, in addition to bronchodilatation, such agents should improve the clearance of airway secretions. Postural drainage and chest percussion are other often-used adjuncts that have been shown, especially when secretions are voluminous, to improve tracheobronchial clearance, to increase sputum volume beyond that produced by cough, and to reduce airways obstruction.

Bronchodilatation with beta$_2$-adrenergic agonists and/or anticholinergics by inhalation has assumed a prominent role in treatment of acute respiratory failure in chronic airways obstruction. The utility of adding oral or intravenous theophylline is controversial, but in addition to bronchodilatation, theophylline may improve bronchopulmonary clearance and may help induce diuresis and hemodynamic improvement when there is cor pulmonale with heart failure. Unless there is clearly an acute pneumonia, the use of antibiotics is more controversial in the setting of acute respiratory failure than in mucopurulent relapses without failure. Nonetheless, broad-spectrum antibiotics, if no single agent is suspected or isolated, or erythromycin, if legionellae or mycoplasmas are suspected, should be added to the regimen.

Management of Complications Complications arising in the course of treatment for acute respiratory failure are cardiac arrhythmias (most often multifocal supraventricular tachycardias), left ventricular failure, pulmonary emboli, and gastrointestinal hemorrhage from stress ulceration. *Cardiac arrhythmias* resulting from rapid decreases in oxygenation or increases in pH due to overventilation can be readily avoided. However, when giving multiple drugs having cardiotonic properties, the question always arises as to whether the arrhythmias are drug–related. Keeping serum theophylline levels in the 10 to 15 mg/L range and using relatively selective beta agonists, such as terbutaline or albuterol by inhalation, can minimize these effects.

Left ventricular failure, usually attributable to coronary atherosclerosis with acute myocardial infarction, systemic hypertension, or aortic valvular disease, is difficult to detect in the presence of cor pulmonale. Fortunately, improving lung function and oxygenation most often reverse the pulmonary hypertension and right ventricular failure (Chap. 238) and induce a brisk diuresis. If signs of congestive failure persist or worsen after providing adequate oxygenation, consideration must be given to left ventricular failure; an assessment in such patients is best made through echocardiography or radioventriculography, since the usual physical and radiographic findings are obscured in such patients. Only in the presence of adequate gas exchange and only with either the firm demonstration, or strong clinical suspicion, of left ventricular failure should digitalis be used. Diuretic agents should also be reserved for left ventricular failure. They almost invariably produce hypokalemic, hypochloremic metabolic alkalemia that results in depression of ventilatory drive and interference with removal from mechanical ventilatory support.

Pulmonary emboli are suspected to be common in the setting of acute respiratory failure and are difficult to detect, and signs of cor pulmonale fluctuate in concert with the degree of lung dysfunction. Although ventilation-perfusion scans of low and intermediate probability are frequent and are not diagnostically useful, high-probability scans are still unreliable in the presence of chronic airflow obstruction. Noninvasive evaluation of the lower extremities may be helpful in this setting. Low-dose heparin prophylaxis should be used to prevent pulmonary emboli.

Gastrointestinal hemorrhage in patients with chronic airflow obstruction and acute respiratory failure may be especially severe. Awareness of this complication enhances the ability to detect it and act quickly. Antacids, coating agents such as sucralfate, and/or H_2 blockers have been used to diminish the frequency.

Weaning from Mechanical Ventilation For those patients who have required mechanical ventilatory support, the process of removal from that support is largely empirical. Weaning should not be attempted until the patient is responsive and gas exchange and lung mechanics have been improved. Data such as a ratio of respiratory frequency to tidal volume less than 105, maximal voluntary inspiratory mouth pressures greater than 20 cmH_2O, vital capacity greater than 10 mL/kg of body weight, and spontaneous tidal volume greater than 5 mL/kg of body weight are reassuring. However, these indices carry an accuracy of only 70 to 80 percent, and many patients can be successfully removed from such support with lesser values than these.

Failure to maintain gas exchange after removal of mechanical ventilatory support can usually be explained. First on the list is the continued administration or persistence of sedative and tranquilizing drugs that may have been prescribed earlier for agitation. These should be discontinued, and time allowed for their metabolism. Second is the possibility that the endotracheal tube is of small bore and imposes a resistive load. If so, it should be replaced by a larger one. Third is worsening airways obstruction and accumulation of secretions; continued bronchial dilatation and airway suctioning avoid these. Fourth is a metabolic alkalemia, with or without diuretic therapy, that should be treated with potassium chloride. Fifth is having maintained, while on mechanical ventilation, a Pa_{O_2} and Pa_{CO_2} that are too high and too low, respectively. This can be avoided by using an FI_{O_2} just sufficient to keep the Pa_{O_2} around 60 mmHg and using the assist mode with small enough tidal volumes to keep the Pa_{CO_2} at the expected chronic level (i.e., that associated with a normal or slightly low arterial pH) before discontinuing mechanical support. Sixth is poor nutrition, hypokalemia, hypophosphatemia, or neuromuscular disease, making the patient too weak to maintain breathing or resulting in fatigue of the respiratory muscles. Nutrition, of course, is a longer range problem that should be anticipated, while hypokalemia is often handled along with the metabolic alkalemia. Hypophosphatemia can be addressed by specific parenteral repletion or by enteral administration of skim milk.

Muscle fatigue, especially diaphragmatic, has received a great deal of attention. From a practical standpoint, paradoxical (inward) movement of the upper abdomen with inspiration is the key clinical finding. Experimental evidence suggests that therapeutic levels of aminophylline or beta$_2$ agonists, such as fenoterol, reverse the manifestations of fatigue, but the role of respiratory stimulants continues to be debated, and the data to be inconclusive. In those patients with severely blunted ventilatory drive and improving lung function, stimulants may be tried cautiously. If there is severe metabolic alkalemia, acetazolamide can be tried as a stimulant while chloride replacement is being carried out. Medroxyprogesterone, a central stimulant, or almitrine, a peripheral chemoreceptor stimulant, appear to be safe and, in some instances, effective. Hypothyroidism is a metabolic condition with neuromuscular consequences and is difficult to detect in this clinical setting. Thus any prolonged and difficult weaning process should lead to the assessment of thyroid function.

PROGNOSIS

On the average, data collected on large populations demonstrate a slow and relentless diminution in ventilatory function in patients with chronic airways obstruction. Although slow, the decrement in function with time far exceeds the rate of change seen with normal aging. In general, the likelihood of episodes of acute respiratory failure increases when the FEV_1 falls below 25 percent of predicted normal values. Although the in-hospital mortality rate over the past 20 years averages 10 percent for a single episode and the 5-year survival rate after the initial episode of respiratory failure averages only 15 to 20 percent, the clinical syndrome is extremely important in determining both the short- and long-range prognosis. Pulmonary arterial pressure is a significant determinant of prognosis in patients with chronic airflow obstruction. As noted above, those patients with predominant emphysema have a poorer prognosis after the onset of respiratory failure than do those with predominant bronchitis. In either case, long-term O_2 treatment in those with severe hypoxemia results in prolongation of life and improvement in the quality of life.

VARIANTS OF EMPHYSEMA AND OBSTRUCTIVE AIRWAYS DISEASE

In addition to the centriacinar and panacinar forms of emphysema described above, other structural patterns have been described but are functionally less important. Often there is overdistention and alveolar septal destruction in lung regions surrounding scar tissue (paracicatricial or scar emphysema) or along the borders of the acinus (paraseptal emphysema). The latter form, when it occurs at the visceral pleural surface, may predispose to episodes of spontaneous pneumothorax (Chap. 262). Infants rarely develop a check valve mechanism in a lobar bronchus, which leads to rapid and life-threatening overdistention (congenital lobar emphysema).

Unilateral emphysema may be an incidental radiographic finding (Macleod's or Swyer-James's syndromes). Since, in this condition, the airways are normal in number and structure but the alveoli are reduced in number, this form of unilateral emphysema has been attributed to disease occurring before the age of 8 years when alveoli are normally increasing in number. Overdistention and alveolar septal destruction are not present, and so this condition does not fit the definition of true emphysema. Most often the pulmonary artery on the affected side is hypoplastic. Although usually an incidental finding, the affected lung may become repeatedly infected so that surgical excision may be indicated.

BULLOUS EMPHYSEMA Confluent air spaces with diameters in excess of 1 cm are occasionally congenital but most often are found in association with generalized emphysema or progressive fibrotic processes. Gradual increases in size of such air spaces (or bullae) result from traction applied by regions with better elastic recoil properties, and such regions lose volume as the bullae become enlarged. If disability is severe, if the bulla is extremely large, and if either lobar gas sampling or ventilation and perfusion scans demonstrate that sufficient function remains in the nonbullous regions, surgical excision of the bulla may lead to functional improvement. Usually, however, improvement is relatively transitory because other emphysematous regions gradually enlarge into bullae after surgery.

MISCELLANEOUS DIFFUSE OBSTRUCTIVE SYNDROMES *Bronchiolitis obliterans* is a term applied to widespread inflammatory and fibrotic obstruction of small airways. Initially this syndrome was thought to be restricted to those persons who had suffered severe viral infections in childhood, particularly those due to parainfluenza virus. However, recently this syndrome has also been described in adult patients with rheumatoid arthritis. The response to bronchodilator treatment is poor, as would be expected from the histopathologic findings, and fatal respiratory failure often ensues within 2 years. There have been reports suggesting a relationship between penicillamine therapy and the development of bronchiolitis obliterans in patients with rheumatoid arthritis; however, it is clear that this syndrome can develop in patients who have never received penicillamine.

A syndrome with similar histopathology has been described in recipients of autologous bone marrow transplants. Although most often interstitial pneumonitis and fibrosis are sequelae, it has been documented that some patients develop a bronchiolitis obliterans picture. It appears that the development of this process occurs most often in the setting of a chronic graft-versus-host syndrome; however, it is clear that diffuse airways obstruction has developed without evidence of this syndrome in bone marrow recipients.

Cystic fibrosis in the adult with chronic airways obstruction is discussed elsewhere (Chap. 257).

BIBLIOGRAPHY

ANTHONISEN NR et al: Effects of smoking intervention and the use of an inhaled anticholinergic bronchodilator on the rate of decline of FEV_1. The Lung Health Study. JAMA 272:1497, 1994

COOPER JD et al: Bilateral pneumectomy (volume reduction) for chronic obstructive pulmonary disease. J Thorac Cardiovasc Surg 109:106, 1995

…USON GT, CHERNIACK RM: Management of chronic obstructive pulmo…ry disease. N Engl J Med 328:1017, 1993

… HM et al: Predisposing conditions to bacterial infection in chronic …uctive pulmonary disease. Am J Respir Crit Care Med 151:2073, 1995

LEUENBERGER P et al: Passive smoking exposure in adults and chronic respiratory symptoms (SAPALDIA study). Am J Respir Crit Care Med 150:1222, 1994

NINANE V et al: Intrinsic PEEP in patients with chronic obstructive pulmonary disease. Am Rev Respir Dis 148:1037, 1993

OSWALD-MAMMOSSER M et al: Prognostic factors in COPD patients receiving long-term oxygen therapy. Importance of pulmonary artery pressure. Chest 107:1193, 1995

RIES AL: Effects of pulmonary rehabilitation on physiologic and psychosocial outcomes in patients with chronic obstructive pulmonary disease. Ann Intern Med 122:823, 1995

SHELHAMER JH et al: Airway inflammation. Ann Intern Med 123:288, 1995

ST JOHN RC et al: Chronic obstructive pulmonary disease: Less common causes. An algorithm for the primary care physician. J Gen Intern Med 8:564, 1993

VAZ FRAGOSO CA, MILLER MA: Review of the clinical efficacy of theophylline in the treatment of chronic obstructive pulmonary disease. Am Rev Respir Dis 147:S40, 1993

259 INTERSTITIAL LUNG DISEASES

Herbert Y. Reynolds

The interstitial lung diseases (ILDs) represent a variety of conditions that involve the alveolar walls (septa), perialveolar tissue, and other contiguous supporting structures. The ILDs are nonmalignant and are not caused by any defined infectious agents. Although an acute phase of illness may occur, the onset is often insidious, and the disease is usually chronic in duration. The initial insult is injury to the epithelial surface causing inflammation in the air spaces and alveolar walls, creating an acute phase of intraluminal and mural alveolitis. If the disease is chronic and smoldering, inflammation will spread to adjacent portions of the interstitium and vasculature and eventually produce interstitial fibrosis. The resultant scarring and distortion of lung tissue leads to significant derangement of gas exchange and ventilatory function. Inflammation also can involve the conducting airways, and bronchiolitis obliterans associated with an organizing pneumonia is now part of the spectrum of an ILD.

Although diverse, this group of diseases has many features in common, including similarity of symptoms, comparable appearance of chest imaging studies, consistent alterations in pulmonary physiology, and typical histologic features. Lung pathology is usually confined to several general patterns, showing a mixture of alveolar inflammatory infiltrates and fibrotic/scarred areas with cystic, honeycomb spaces evident in advanced stages, often called *usual interstitial pneumonia*. Recently, diffuse, temporally uniform, single-time-appearing reactions have defied customary classifications and are considered as nonspecific interstitial pneumonia/fibrosis. However, ILDs have been difficult to classify because approximately 150 known individual diseases are characterized by some interstitial lung involvement, either as primary disease or as a significant part of a multiorgan process, as may occur in the collagen vascular diseases. The chest radiograph is of limited aid in classification because it can have a similar appearance in many of the ILDs as well as in other unrelated lung diseases; however, high-resolution computed tomography (HRCT) scanning of the chest has enhanced diagnostic accuracy. One useful approach for classification is to separate ILDs into two groups, those with known and unknown causes; each of these groups can be divided into subgroups according to the presence or absence of histologic evidence of granulomas in interstitial or vascular areas (Table 259-1). For each ILD there may be an acute phase, and there is usually a chronic one as well.

Among the ILDs of known cause, the largest group comprises occupational and environmental inhalant exposures; these include diseases due to inhalation of inorganic dusts (Chap. 254), organic dusts, and various irritative or noxious gases (Chap. 253). The number of ILDs of unknown cause is also very large. The major ones within this category are idiopathic pulmonary fibrosis (IPF), sarcoidosis, and the ILD often associated with collagen vascular disorders. ILD secondary to inorganic dust exposure usually can be recognized if the occupational history is pursued. For the myriad (see Table 259-1) of other diffuse ILDs, however, a precise diagnosis is obtained with difficulty, usually only after interpretation of an open-lung biopsy specimen; most of these diseases are relatively rare. The HRCT scan promises to improve diagnostic accuracy as further histologic-image correlations are perfected.

Although the initiating agent(s) or circumstances of the various ILDs may be multiple, and many are unknown, the immunopathogenic responses of lung tissue are limited, so the initial mechanisms of injury to the epithelial surface, the development of alveolitis, and the attempts at repair sometimes leading to fibrosis will have common features. IPF is discussed as the prototype ILD, since it is encountered relatively frequently and much of the recent research on mechanisms of inflammation and lung fibrosis has focused on this disease.

IDIOPATHIC PULMONARY FIBROSIS

Many patients who present with nonproductive cough, progressive dyspnea, a chest radiograph showing lower lung zone reticular or reticulonodular shadows, and pulmonary function tests showing a restrictive ventilatory pattern (Chap. 250) will be said to have IPF after the diagnostic evaluation is completed. This condition is also known as *cryptogenic fibrosing alveolitis*. Although the terms *idiopathic* and *cryptogenic* mean that the etiologic agent is unknown, this is not a nebulous "wastebasket" diagnosis or just a diagnosis of exclusion but rather a well-defined clinical entity.

IMMUNOPATHOGENESIS Several parts of the alveolar structure are affected in IPF, including the alveolar walls lined with type I squamous epithelial cells and type II pneumocytes and the interstitial supporting structure composed of mesenchymal cells (especially fibroblasts, myofibroblasts, occasional monocyte-macrophage cells, and lymphocytes), noncellular matrix of collagen, and various adhesive proteoglycans. The capillary endothelium also may be involved. The disease process does not affect the upper or conducting airways, but bronchiolitis of respiratory bronchioles may be present and alveolar units are always involved.

Normally, overlying or interspersed on the alveolar surface are a variety of immune cells, including alveolar macrophages, dendritic macrophages, lymphocytes, and inflammatory cells, such as polymorphonuclear leukocytes (PMNs) and eosinophils. The cellular content of normal bronchoalveolar lavage (BAL) fluid consists of approximately 80 percent alveolar macrophages, 10 percent lymphocytes (of which 70 percent are T lymphocytes), 1 to 5 percent B lymphocytes or plasma cells, 1 to 3 percent PMNs, and 1 percent eosinophils. In the lymphocyte population, the ratio of CD4 T helper and CD8 T suppressor/cytotoxic cells is about 1.5.

In the earliest, reversible forms of alveolar injury, "leakiness" of the alveolar type I cell layer and the adjacent capillary endothelial surface occurs, causing alveolar and interstitial edema and the formation of intraalveolar hyaline membranes. With persistence of the disease, increased alveolar-capillary permeability and desquamation of intraalveolar cells (alveolitis), mural inflammation, and interstitial fibrosis are present on biopsy. Histologically, the reaction can be patchy in distribution and various stages of development found. The presence and severity of the disease process are spotty in distribution; a continuum of inflammatory and fibrotic changes can be found throughout the affected lung. Fibrosis follows from an organization of inflammatory exudate within the airspaces in which fibroblasts beneath the type I epithelium proliferate and increase their production of fibronectin and collagen. Cicatrization can create cystic spaces.

Immunopathogenic mechanisms that interconnect the intraalveolar (luminal) and alveolar mural (septal) tissue with the interstitial space and capillary vascular areas are depicted in Fig. 259-1. Although the inciting agent or stimulus is unknown, it is likely an antigen that can initiate an immunoglobulin response. This is reflected by an increased ratio of IgG subclasses IgG1 and G3, an increased number of IgG-releasing cells, and perhaps the formation of immune complexes. Speculation continues that a microbial etiology, possibly viral, is probable for some cases of IPF.

This process is also reflected in the composition of cells and enzymes recovered in BAL fluid and in cellular components present in lung biopsy tissue. An increased number of macrophages, which are activated phagocytes capable of producing many cytokines that affect other lung cells, is a hallmark of the alveolitis. These macrophage cytokines or mediators can operate in two directions. First, through the production of chemokines, which include leukotriene B_4, interleukin (IL) 8, and tumor necrosis factor α, inflammatory cells such as PMNs and eosinophils are attracted into the alveoli. IPF lung macrophages express increased mRNA for IL-8, which roughly correlates with the percent of PMNs in BAL fluid. An increased percentage of PMNs (20 percent or more) and eosinophils (2 to 4 percent) in the profile of BAL cells is usual in IPF; eosinophil cationic protein is increased in BAL fluid. Lymphocytes are not usually increased, unless the IPF is part of a collagen vascular disease. Enzymes, such as collagenase, or oxidant radicals from inflammatory cells and histamine may cause local injury or alter the permeability of type I cells. Conversely, the antioxidant glutathione is deficient in the BAL fluid, further impairing neutralization of oxidants.

Second, macrophages are also capable of secreting substances that stimulate mesenchymal cells. For fibroblasts to replicate in the interstitium and in the alveolar walls, they must be primed to enter the G_1 phase of a growth cycle to proliferate. Several products from alveolar macrophages can participate in these steps. Platelet-derived growth factor B (PDGF-B) is a chemoattractant for mesenchymal cells

Table 259-1

Major Categories of Alveolar and Interstitial Inflammatory Lung Diseases

Known Cause	Unknown Cause
LUNG RESPONSE: ALVEOLITIS, INTERSTITIAL INFLAMMATION, AND FIBROSIS	
Asbestos	Idiopathic pulmonary fibrosis
Fumes, gases	Collagen vascular diseases
Drugs (antibiotics) and chemotherapy drugs	Systemic lupus erythematosus, rheumatoid arthritis, ankylosing spondylitis, systemic sclerosis, Sjögren's syndrome, polymyositis-dermatomyositis
Radiation	
Aspiration pneumonia	
Residual of adult respiratory distress syndrome	Pulmonary hemorrhage syndromes
	Goodpasture's syndrome, idiopathic pulmonary hemosiderosis
	Pulmonary alveolar proteinosis
	Lymphocytic infiltrative disorders (lymphocytic interstitial pneumonitis associated with collagen vascular diseases)
	Eosinophilic pneumonias
	Lymphangioleiomyomatosis
	Amyloidosis
	Inherited diseases
	Tuberous sclerosis, neurofibromatosis, Niemann-Pick disease, Gaucher's disease, Hermansky-Pudlak syndrome
	Gastrointestinal or liver diseases (Crohn's disease, primary biliary cirrhosis, chronic active hepatitis, ulcerative colitis)
	Graft vs. host disease (bone marrow transplantation)
LUNG RESPONSE: AS ABOVE BUT WITH GRANULOMA	
Hypersensitivity pneumonitis (organic dusts)	Sarcoidosis
Inorganic dusts: beryllium silica	Langerhans cell granulomatosis (eosinophilic granuloma)
	Granulomatous vasculitides
	Wegener's granulomatosis, allergic granulomatosis of Churg-Strauss, lymphomatoid granulomatosis
	Bronchocentric granulomatosis

and a stimulus for fibroblasts to change from resting cells to cells entering G_1. Although PDGF-B is not produced by normal monocytes or macrophages, alveolar macrophages obtained from patients with IPF make it abundantly. This is correlated with c-*sis*, a proto-oncogene that codes for the beta chain of PDGF-B, which is increased in IPF-derived macrophages. Interferon γ upregulates this gene activation. This mediator also acts as a chemoattractant and a growth factor for fibroblasts. Later in the fibroblast replication cycle, alveolar macrophage–derived insulin-like growth factors (IGF-1 and IGFBP-3) can accelerate proliferation. Transforming growth factor β, insulin, and other cellular or metabolic substances are needed in these growth-regulatory steps, also. Collagen peptides can be released locally, and N-terminal type III procollagen peptides have been found in BAL fluid. Surfactant protein A is reduced. Smooth-muscle cells also can proliferate. With continued activity of macrophages, fibrosis becomes more widespread and may involve the vasculature. Obliteration of functional alveolar structures occurs with scar tissue formation, and cystic areas develop from retraction of the terminal airways that once subtended the alveolar unit.

CLINICAL PRESENTATION **History** On average, patients are about 55 years old, although the range spans infancy to old age. Several family clusters have been reported, and it is possible that genetic factors may determine susceptibility to the disease. The first clinical manifestations of ILD or IPF are dyspnea, effort intolerance, and a dry cough without other obvious cause. A detailed work and environmental history is essential. For example, casual exposure to asbestos many years previously may provide a crucial clue to the etiology. Causes for hypersensitivity lung disease can be missed. Work-related compensation may influence complaints for some individuals.

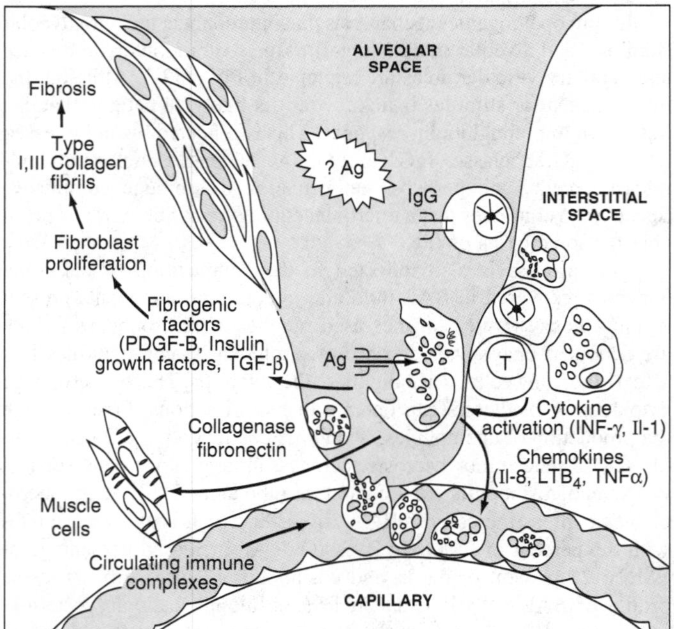

FIGURE 259-1 Immunologic mechanisms within the alveolar space, alveolar walls, and interstitium that can lead to inflammation and eventual fibrosis. The focus is the alveolar macrophage, which is activated, possibly by an immune complex and an as yet unidentified antigen (Ag). Through mediators, termed *chemokines*, the macrophage attracts PMNs and other cells from the circulation to the alveolar space, or it can initiate fibrogenesis with various mediators that can stimulate fibroblasts and muscle cells to proliferate. Interstitial fibrosis may result. Abbreviations: IL-8, interleukin 8; LTB_4, leukotriene B_4; TNF, tumor necrosis factor; INF-γ, interferon γ; IL-1, interleukin 1; TGF, transforming growth factor; PDGF-B, platelet-derived growth factor. *(After HY Reynolds, Chest 89:139, 1986.)*

Approximately one-third of patients can associate their awareness of dyspnea with the aftermath of a viral respiratory illness. Usually months or years elapse between the onset of exertional dyspnea and its progression perhaps to the point of breathlessness at rest. Dyspnea and frequent coughing are often accompanied by other constitutional symptoms such as fatigue, anorexia, weight loss, and arthralgias.

Physical Findings Initially, the physical examination may not be revealing, and auscultation of the chest may be normal. As the disease advances, dry crackles, or coarse crackles on inspiration, are usually heard at the lung bases. There may be tachypnea at rest, cyanosis, and clubbing of the fingers and toes, usually without hypertrophic osteoarthropathy. In later stages, cor pulmonale (Chap. 238) is evident, with findings of pulmonary hypertension, such as an accentuated pulmonic second sound or a right-sided lift, and eventually signs of right-sided heart failure. The right ventricular ejection fraction determined by radionuclide ventriculography is often depressed in the face of normal left ventricular performance.

LABORATORY AND DIAGNOSTIC TESTS **Imaging Studies** The chest radiograph usually reveals a pattern of diffuse reticular or reticulonodular markings, prominent in the lower lung zones. Several radiographic patterns on chest and HRCT scan can be seen that correlate roughly with the severity and duration of the disease. Early, a hazy "ground glass" appearance of the lower lung fields coincides with the stage of acute alveolitis. Later, curvilinear strands predominate and may coalesce into nodular infiltrates. With end-stage disease, the linear opacities are seen in all lung fields, the lung fields appear contracted, and ring-shaped opacities resulting from cystic and bronchiectatic changes are obvious, creating the *honey-combed* or *swiss cheese* appearance of the lung. HRCT patterns are helpful in monitoring disease activity also. Biopsy-proven forms of diffuse IPF occur occasionally in patients with normal chest radiographs (about 14 percent) despite significant exercise intolerance, abnormal pulmonary function tests (including a reduced diffusing capacity), and dry crackles. However, patients with biopsy-proven IPF may have no evidence of it on HRCT (found in only 3 of 25 patients, or 12 percent, in one study).

Laboratory Examination The erythrocyte sedimentation rate is usually elevated, circulating immune-complex titers and serum immunoglobulin levels may be increased, and cryoimmunoglobulins may be present. Serologic tests to screen for collagen vascular diseases are necessary to exclude these diagnoses. Although serum rheumatoid factor, antinuclear antibodies, depressed levels of complement, and other parameters of autoimmune diseases may be detected in approximately 10 percent of patients with IPF, the titers are generally quite low.

Lung Function Tests In patients with advanced disease, reductions in total lung capacity, vital capacity, and residual volume are found (Chap. 250). Usually, evidence of airway obstruction is minimal, and the FEV_1/FVC ratio is normal or increased. A restrictive ventilatory pattern is usually present, reflecting the stiff, noncompliant lungs characteristic of IPF and its common aftermath, fibrosis. There is usually resting arterial hypoxemia, but the carbon dioxide tension is normal or decreased. Blood pH is normal. The alveolar-arterial oxygen gradient during exercise is elevated, and exercise tolerance is reduced. The carbon monoxide diffusing capacity is usually reduced by 30 to 50 percent. Changes in these variables are useful in monitoring the course of the illness and in assessing the effectiveness of treatment. However, current or former cigarette smoking in IPF patients can alter lung function to misrepresent the extent of restriction and/or obstruction, if both emphysema and interstitial fibrosis are present. This has implications and raises caution for evaluating lung function in these patients.

Bronchoscopy Direct investigation of the airways by fiberoptic bronchoscopy is part of the evaluation, and four to six transbronchial biopsies are taken to obtain lung tissue for diagnosis. These provide a sufficient quantity of tissue for a definitive pathologic diagnosis in approximately one-fourth of all cases of IPF. In some diffuse granulomatous interstitial diseases, such as sarcoidosis (Chap. 320), transbronchial biopsy will yield a tissue diagnosis in about 80 percent of cases. Bronchoscopy also permits BAL, which gives useful information about cells and proteins in the airways that generally correlates with histologic changes in the interstitial and alveolar tissues. An analysis of BAL fluid and cells can reveal a number of changes in IPF.

Lung Biopsy The importance of an adequate sample of lung tissue to permit a full histologic evaluation, good microbial cultures, immunofluorescence and electron-microscopic studies, and analysis of inorganic substances cannot be overemphasized. Therefore, if a transbronchial biopsy does not yield sufficient tissue for a confident diagnosis, a thoracoscopic-guided or an open-lung biopsy should be considered. It is prudent to substantiate a tissue diagnosis before embarking on immunosuppressive therapy with its attendant complications.

DIAGNOSTIC APPROACH AND STAGING OF DISEASE ACTIVITY The importance of obtaining a thorough occupational and environmental history from the patient cannot be overemphasized. Also, a review of any prior chest films is usually helpful. Judging whether the lung disease is part of a multisystem process, related temporally to a new medication, or coincident with a change in neurologic status that would make aspiration and infection more likely are important in the differential diagnosis of ILD. Following the clinical examination, chest radiograph (or HRCT chest scan), pulmonary function tests [lung volumes, FEV_1/FVC, and diffusing capacity (Chap. 250)], and arterial blood gas determination measuring desaturation under exercising conditions, the functional disability from the lung disease can be estimated. However, a histologic analysis of lung tissue should be made before the disease is diagnosed definitively. Fiberoptic bronchoscopy is usually the first invasive procedure and is important for ruling out infection, malignancy, and other specific diseases. Although transbronchial biopsy has a lower diagnostic yield in IPF than in sarcoidosis and other granulomatous diseases, it is nevertheless a useful, low-risk procedure with a 20 to 30 percent success rate for obtaining an adequate sample for a confident pathologic diagnosis. BAL for cellular and protein analysis may be useful in judging the nature of alveolar inflammation and immunologic activity. However, the value of the periodic use of BAL analysis to monitor disease activity or its response to therapy has not been established. Use of gallium 67 lung scanning does not add more diagnostic accuracy or help with monitoring activity.

If the diagnosis is still in doubt after the bronchoscopy and related procedures, an imaged thorascopic or open-lung biopsy should be considered. The referring physician and the thoracic surgeon should cooperate in choosing the most representative areas of the lung for biopsy, and the proper microbial cultures and immunologic studies should be obtained.

Rx TREATMENT

Treatment is usually offered to patients with IPF, even to patients with advanced fibrotic disease. A trial of oral prednisone is begun in a dose of 1 mg/kg daily and continued for about 8 weeks. If lung disease shows objective improvement, the dose is tapered to a maintenance level of about 0.25 mg/kg for another 6 months or so. Should the disease not respond or be progressive, additional immunosuppression with cyclophosphamide should be considered. Cyclophosphamide is given at a dose of about 1.0 mg/kg daily (50 to 75 mg) with the patient continuing on a daily maintenance dose of oral prednisone (0.25 mg/kg). The dosages of cyclophosphamide may be increased as necessary by 50-mg increments at 7- to 10-day intervals. The objective is to reduce the white blood cell count to approximately half the normal baseline value, causing a distinct drop in the total blood lymphocyte count. However, a minimum count of 1000 PMNs/μL should be maintained. Alternatively, intravenous pulsed doses of cyclophosphamide given biweekly have been used with good success; 500 mg is given initially, and the dose can be increased in 100- to 200-mg increments to a total amount of 1.0 to 1.8 g and continued for a 12- to 18-month interval.

Use of high-dose, pulsed glucocorticoids does not offer special advantages over daily dosing. Azathioprine has been used in place of cyclophosphamide. Other agents such as penicillamine and cyclosporine have not been evaluated thoroughly. However, oral therapy with colchicine, which can inhibit macrophage-produced fibroblast growth factors, given in a dose of 0.6 mg daily has been found to improve or permit a stable condition to occur in some patients; more testing of this therapy is indicated.

Several other measures may help respiratory function. It is imperative that patients discontinue cigarette smoking. Since there is frequently a marked drop in Pa_{O_2} with exercise, supplemental oxygen therapy may be useful, sometimes using transtracheal catheter oxygen delivery, which can reduce oxygen requirements and help with the logistics of supplying high-flow therapy. As the pulmonary vascular bed is destroyed by progressive fibrosis, pulmonary hypertension and cor pulmonale can develop; right-sided congestive heart failure can be difficult to control. Judicious use of diuretics is advised. Adequate oxygenation is probably the best treatment for right-sided heart failure (Chap. 238). Some patients also may develop obstruction to airflow and wheezing and coughing, which may respond to bronchodilators. Severe coughing episodes may require a narcotic-containing antitussive medication. Infection may occur during immunosuppressive therapy and should be treated promptly and aggressively. Prophylactic use of pneumococcal and influenza vaccines is indicated. If refractory disease limited to the chest is present, the possibility of lung transplantation should be considered. Success with single-lung transplantation for ILD makes this therapy a reality for some patients. Selection criteria, contraindications, and availability of organs must be discussed candidly with patients so as not to create unrealistic expectations.

INDIVIDUAL FORMS OF ILD

ILD ASSOCIATED WITH COLLAGEN VASCULAR DISORDERS In these diseases, various pulmonary structures can be affected, especially the pleura, so that ILD is but one manifestation of intrathoracic involvement and is often a minor part of the multiorgan process. The same is true for fibrosis.

Systemic Lupus Erythematosus (See Chap. 312) About half of patients with systemic lupus erythematosus ultimately develop overt lung disease. Pleuritis, pleural effusion(s), and acute pneumonitis from pulmonary capillaritis causing alveolar hemorrhage are the most frequent forms of lung disease, while a chronic, progressive ILD is uncommon. It is important to exclude pulmonary infection. Although pleuropulmonary involvement may not be evident clinically, pulmonary function testing, particularly the diffusing capacity for carbon monoxide, reveals abnormalities in many patients. A lymphocytic alveolitis may occur, which usually indicates a better response to immunosuppressive therapy.

Rheumatoid Arthritis (See Chap. 313) A variety of pulmonary manifestations can occur, including pleural disease (pleural effusion and subpleural nodules), parenchymal nodular infiltrates associated with pneumoconiosis in miners (Caplan's syndrome), and diffuse interstitial fibrosis. The ILD can develop before joint disease becomes evident, particularly in men, and is accompanied by high titers of rheumatoid factor. Bronchiolitis obliterans with organizing pneumonia has been reported. Patients with rheumatoid arthritis who are receiving treatment with methotrexate or gold may develop ILD that represents a drug hypersensitivity, which must be differentiated from a preexisting or developing ILD associated with the underlying disease. Penicillamine therapy in patients with rheumatoid arthritis has been implicated as a cause of bronchiolitis obliterans.

Ankylosing Spondylitis (See Chap. 317) Bilateral upper lobe fibrosis, which can be complicated by fibrocavitary disease, may develop late in the course.

Systemic Sclerosis (See Chap. 314) Radiographic evidence of lung involvement develops in a majority of patients, but its severity or progression is variable. Because distal esophageal motor dysfunction is present in many patients, reflux with regurgitation and chronic aspiration is common. Mast cells and their mediators in BAL fluid may be important in the alveolitis that develops. In addition, cutaneous scleroderma can involve the anterior chest wall and abdomen, causing restrictive lung function.

Sjögren's Syndrome (See Chap. 316) General dryness and lack of airways secretions cause the major problems of hoarseness, cough, and bronchitis. Presence of an ILD in these patients may signify a lymphocytic infiltrate in lung tissue, which can behave as a low-grade lymphoma. As small terminal airways can be affected with bronchiolitis obliterans, lung hyperinflation on pulmonary function testing may be a clue (high residual volume to total lung capacity ratio).

Polymyositis and Dermatomyositis (See Chap. 315) Although ILD is reported to occur in only 5 to 10 percent of patients, its presence is more common in the subgroup of patients with an anti-Jo-1 antibody that is directed to histidyl tRNA synthetase. Weakness of respiratory muscles contributing to aspiration pneumonitis is a common occurrence.

SYNDROMES OF ILD WITH PULMONARY HEMORRHAGE Recurrent hemoptysis, dyspnea, and hypoxemia in the presence of a chest radiographic pattern of diffuse alveolar opacities should raise the possibility of alveolar hemorrhage. An association between vasculitis involving the kidney (lung-renal syndromes) or other organ systems should be investigated. Alveolar hemorrhage occurs rarely in all collagen vascular disorders, but it is described most often with systemic lupus erythematosus. It can occur with systemic necrotizing vasculitis and is described as an initial presentation of Wegener's granulomatosis; with Behçet's disease, in which aneurysm formation and rupture of small muscular arteries are manifestations of necrotizing vasculitis; in allergic Churg-Strauss granulomatosis; in Henoch-Schönlein purpura syndrome; and in essential (mixed) cryoimmunoglobulinemia. Serologic tests for antinuclear antibody, anti-glomerular basement membrane antibody, and complement to document a vasculitis and immunologic disorder are the first steps, but renal biopsy and possibly lung biopsy may be required for a definitive diagnosis. Some specific syndromes in this category will be discussed next.

Goodpasture's Syndrome (See Chap. 275) Pulmonary hemorrhage and glomerulonephritis are the features of this disease in which most patients have autoantibodies to renal glomerular and lung alveolar basement membranes.

Idiopathic Pulmonary Hemosiderosis Diffuse alveolar hemorrhage can occur in the absence of other organ involvement or an obvious immunologic cause and is therefore a diagnosis of exclusion after considering the many causes of alveolar bleeding associated with collagen vascular and vasculitic diseases. A lung biopsy is usually necessary to document the lack of inflammatory injury in the lung tissues and to exclude other diseases with confidence. Children and young adults are usually affected. The clinical course can be variable, ranging from recurrent and fulminant with development of progressive interstitial fibrosis to minimal disease that may remit without sequelae. Glucocorticoid treatment is useful for control of bleeding acutely but is not a predictable long-term remedy for keeping the disease suppressed and preventing recurrence.

PULMONARY ALVEOLAR PROTEINOSIS Similar clinical symptoms and the general appearance of the chest radiograph, showing diffuse alveolar consolidation and/or nodular shadows typically radiating from the hilar regions, place pulmonary alveolar proteinosis (PAP) in the ILD category. Histologically, the alveoli are filled with granular material that stains with periodic acid Schiff reagent, but they exhibit no inflammation and have relatively normal septal structure. Strictly speaking, then, PAP is an intraalveolar process that resembles, but is not, an ILD. Because the proteinaceous response can be associated with inhaled dust exposure (silica and aluminum), malignancy, and chronic infection, termed *secondary PAP*, these disorders should be differentiated from primary PAP by lung biopsy. The intraalveolar material is a combination of surfactant phospholipid produced by type II pneumocytes, lactate dehydrogenase, and other proteins and immunoglobulins found in alveolar lining fluid. The macrophages exhibit large phagolysosomes that have diminished microbial killing capacity in vitro, but lung infections with unusual organisms are not frequent. Whole-lung lavage(s) provides relief to many patients with dyspnea and progressive deterioration of arterial oxygenation and also may provide long-term benefit.

LYMPHOCYTIC INFILTRATIVE DISORDERS This group of disorders features lymphocyte and plasma cell infiltration of the lung parenchyma; the disorders either are benign or can behave as low-grade lymphomas. Within the spectrum of chronic interstitial pneumonias, a subset has been described with lung histology that shows diffuse interstitial infiltration with lymphocytes and plasma cells. In some of these patients, an autoimmune disease or dysproteinemia exists. However, lymphocytic interstitial pneumonia is probably not a distinct entity, belongs within the IPF group, and can be associated with Sjögren's syndrome. Lymphocytic interstitial pneumonia has been reported in patients, particularly children, with AIDS.

Included among these disorders is immunoblastic lymphadenopathy, also termed *angioimmunoblastic lymphadenopathy*, which usually is a fulminant lymphoma-like disease that may have an element of ILD in some cases. *Lymphomatoid granulomatosis* can be included, but its granulomatous response also places it with the granulomatous ILDs (see Table 259-1).

EOSINOPHILIC PNEUMONIAS (See Chap. 253) These pneumonias encompass a spectrum of diseases in which lung hypersensitivity plays a role and in which a specific cause may or may not be identified. For example, with extrinsic asthma and exposure to fungal antigens, allergic bronchopulmonary mycosis can develop; filarial and other parasitic infections can cause tropical pulmonary eosinophilia; many common drugs can induce eosinophilic pneumonia. Chronic eosinophilic pneumonia has features that make it difficult to distinguish from IPF and other forms of progressive ILD. This disease, which more commonly affects older females, has several radiologic characteristics that are helpful in diagnosis: (1) a peripheral pattern of dense lung infiltrates that appear to cross anatomic lobar boundaries with sparing of the central lung regions, (2) regression but reappearance of infiltrates in the same lung locations, and (3) extreme sensitivity of the infiltrates (and disease symptoms) to modest doses of oral glucocorticoids. The diagnosis can be established by lung biopsy, which shows an eosinophilic inflammatory process. Many other lung diseases have eosinophilia and eosinophils found in lung tissue or in respiratory secretions, including asthma, IPF (as mentioned), and forms of granulomatous vasculitis.

LYMPHANGIOLEIOMYOMATOSIS Immature smooth-muscle cells can proliferate in lung tissue around and throughout bronchial, vascular, and lymphatic structures, causing local obstruction or creating constricting lesions that develop into cysts. Lymphatics and lymph nodes in other organs are also usually affected. Because this disorder occurs predominantly in females of reproductive age, an association between estrogens and the disease is probable. Pulmonary symptoms consist of dyspnea, cough, and hemoptysis; a more overt presentation occurs with spontaneous pneumothorax, which can be recurrent, or with chylous effusion. In addition, the chest radiograph shows reticulonodular shadows and small cystlike areas or honeycombing throughout the lung fields. In contrast to most forms of ILD, lung volumes are normal or increased, as is also the case with Langerhans cell granulomatosis (see below). Therapy for progressive lung disease has not been particularly effective. Pneumothoraces and effusions may require chemical or surgical pleurodesis. Treatment with hormone manipulation, including oophorectomy or tamoxifen, has not been helpful, but medroxyprogesterone acetate injections (400 to 800 mg per month intramuscularly for 1 year) have improved dyspnea in some patients and could be considered. Lung transplantation may be considered for some patients.

AMYLOIDOSIS (See Chap. 309) As part of primary systemic amyloidosis or a plasma cell dyscrasia, an ILD may occur from amyloid deposits in alveolar septa and associated blood vessels, producing dyspnea, radiographic findings of diffuse reticulonodular shadows, and restrictive pulmonary function.

INHERITED DISORDERS ASSOCIATED WITH ILD Pulmonary infiltrates and respiratory symptoms typical of mild ILD can develop in related family members and in several inherited diseases. These include the phacomatoses tuberous sclerosis and neurofibromatosis and the lysosomal storage diseases (Chap. 346), such as Niemann-Pick disease and Gaucher's disease. The *Hermansky Pudlak syndrome* is an autosomal recessive disorder in which granulomatous colitis and ILD may occur. It is characterized by oculocutaneous albinism, bleeding diathesis from platelet dysfunction, and the accumulation of a chromolipid, lipofuscin material in cells of the reticuloendothelial system. The pulmonary fibrosis is similar to IPF, but the alveolar macrophages may contain cytoplasmic ceroid-like inclusions.

GASTROINTESTINAL AND LIVER DISEASE Rarely, inflammatory bowel disease and chronic hepatitis may be associated with a mild form of ILD. Crohn's disease, which has a number of similarities with sarcoidosis, also may be accompanied by asymptomatic lymphocytic alveolitis. For some patients with cirrhosis or end-stage liver disease, findings that can suggest an ILD include dyspnea, hypoxemia, digital clubbing, and basilar interstitial markings on chest radiograph, which may in fact be pulmonary vascular dilatations. The dyspnea often occurs in the upright position (platypnea).

GRAFT-VERSUS-HOST DISEASE (See Chap. 116) Some degree of graft-versus-host disease, manifested by variably progressive obstructive lung function and obliterative bronchoiolitis involving the terminal bronchioles, occurs in most patients receiving bone marrow transplantation and in between 20 and 50 percent of recipients of heart-lung or lung transplants. The syndrome occurs as an infection or part of an acute rejection episode, although there may be a more gradual, insidious onset of dry cough, mucositis, dyspnea, and airflow obstruction in the small airways, as demonstrated by pulmonary function testing. Chest radiographs reveal peribronchiolar infiltrates, and lung biopsy shows focal areas of interstitial infiltration with a mixture of lymphocytes and PMNs. The lesions are consistent with bronchiolitis; no vasculitis is present. Treatment includes increasing the doses of the immunosuppressive drugs together with bronchodilators and antibiotics. Infection, especially with a viral agent such as cytomegalovirus, is a common complication.

ILD WITH A GRANULOMATOUS RESPONSE IN LUNG TISSUE OR VASCULAR STRUCTURES Inhalation of organic dusts, which causes hypersensitivity pneumonitis, or of inorganic particles such as silica, which causes alveolitis and elicits a granulomatous inflammatory reaction leading to ILD, produces diseases of known etiology (see Table 259-1) that are discussed in Chaps. 253 and 254. Sarcoidosis (Chap. 320) is prominent among granulomatous diseases of *unknown cause* in which ILD is an important feature.

Langerhans Cell Granulomatosis (Eosinophilic Granuloma or Histiocytosis X) (See Chap. 61) This condition is being recognized with increasing frequency and may account for about 1 to 5 percent of ILD of unknown etiology. Previously, the proliferation of tissue macrophages (histiocytes) was thought to be characteristic of this disease that affects the lung, bones, and viscera. Now it is recognized that the precursor cell is the *dendritic cell*, which has potent stimulatory and accessory cell immune function, is normally found in the interstitium alveolar septal areas and in BAL fluid, and is distinctly different from a tissue macrophage. The dendritic cell can evolve into the Langerhans cell, characterized by a specific CD1a surface antigen that reacts with a monoclonal antibody identified as OKT_6. These cells have a low amount of autofluorescence and express L25, OK1a, RFD_1, and major histocompatibility complex class II antigens. Intracytoplasmic organelles that are called X bodies or Birbeck granules can be seen by electron microscopy. In Langerhans cell granulomatosis of the lung, 3 percent or more of the BAL cells may be so identified, which greatly exceeds the percentage found in other disorders. However, the Langerhans cells are not pathognomonic for this disease.

The pulmonary form of this disease occurs in young and middle-aged adults, usually males, and in those who use tobacco heavily; it may remain focal or involve one or several bony sites (long bones, spine, skull, or jaw). Occasionally, multifocal disease can affect the posterior pituitary gland, causing diabetes insipidus, a condition that is termed *Hand-Schüller-Christian disease*. In infants, *Letterer-Siwe disease* is a more fulminant visceral form of this disorder that mimics a malignant lymphoma. In adults, the presenting symptoms and signs do not distinguish this disease from other forms of ILD unless signs of a bone lesion exist. Chest radiographs will show diffuse micronodular shadows and cystic spaces, sparing the costophrenic angles and preserving lung volume, as occurs in lymphangioleiomyomatosis. Pulmonary function tests may disclose a combination of obstructive and restrictive defects. As the disease progresses, greater airway obstruction may develop, and the chest radiograph can resemble that in advanced chronic obstructive lung disease.

℞ TREATMENT

This involves a mandatory cessation of tobacco use, which may cause the pulmonary disease to stabilize or regress. Glucocorticoids usually are not helpful. Penicillamine has been used in an attempt to prevent fibrosis, with variable success. Local bone lesions may require irradiation treatment. For patients with increasing symptoms of airway obstruction, supportive therapy and bronchodilators may be tried, but their success has been modest. Lung transplantation should be considered for certain patients.

Granulomatous Vasculitis (See Chap. 319) Certain forms of vasculitis, accompanied by a granulomatous response, can involve the respiratory tract as part of a multiorgan process or can occasionally be localized to the respiratory tract, as occurs with a predominantly pulmonary form of Wegener's granulomatosis in which glomerulonephritis may not be prominent. It is very important to differentiate these conditions from lymphomatoid granulomatosis. Allergic angiitis and the granulomatosis of Churg and Strauss are forms of granulomatous vasculitis affecting many organs but especially the lungs; a history of asthma and the presence of eosinophilia are distinguishing features.

Lymphomatoid Granulomatosis (See Chaps. 61 and 319) This involves primarily the lungs and less frequently the skin, central and peripheral nervous systems, and kidneys with an infiltration of lymphocytoid, plasma-like cells and macrophages creating a necrotic granulomatous inflammatory reaction, especially in or near blood vessels. The disease can progress as a lymphoproliferative disorder and evolve into malignant lymphoma in as many as 50 percent of patients. Treatment of lymphomatoid granulomatosis with glucocorticoids and cyclophosphamide may induce a remission, and if this occurs, subsequent relapse and development of lymphoma are not likely.

BRONCHOCENTRIC GRANULOMATOSIS In contrast to the necrotizing granulomatous reaction in lung vessels, i.e., angiocentric vasculitis, granulomatous destruction of bronchioles occurs in this condition. There is usually associated parenchymal inflammation causing ILD. Eosinophils can be present if asthma and hypersensitivity to fungal antigens within the bronchi have occurred. In other cases without these associated conditions, hypersensitivity to other microbial antigens is postulated. Bronchocentric granulomatosis must be differentiated from hypersensitivity pneumonitis caused by inhalation of organic dusts. → ***For further discussion, see Chaps. 253 and 254.***

BIBLIOGRAPHY

BAUGHMAN RP, LOWER EE: Use of intermittent, intravenous cyclophosphamide for idiopathic pulmonary fibrosis. Chest 102:1090, 1992

EPLER GR et al: Bronchiolitis obliterans with organizing pneumonia. N Engl J Med 312:152, 1985

FUJIMOTO K et al: Eosinophil activation in patients with pulmonary fibrosis. Chest 108:48, 1995

HANSON D et al: Changes in pulmonary function test results after one year of therapy as predictors of survival in patients with idiopathic pulmonary fibrosis. Chest 108:305, 1995

HUNNINGHAKE GW, KALICA AR: Approaches to the treatment of pulmonary fibrosis. Am J Respir Crit Care Med 151:915, 1995

ORENS JB et al: The sensitivity of high-resolution CT in detecting idiopathic pulmonary fibrosis proved by open lung biopsy—a prospective study. Chest 108:109, 1995

PETERS SG et al: Colchicine in the treatment of pulmonary fibrosis. Chest 103:101, 1993
RAGHU G: Interstitial lung disease: A diagnostic approach (are CT scan and lung biopsy indicated in every patient?) Am J Respir Crit Care Med 151:909, 1995
REYNOLDS HY: Bronchoalveolar lavage. Am Rev Respir Dis 135:250, 1987
ALLEN JN, DAVIS WB: Eosinophilic lung diseases. Am J Respir Crit Care Med 150:1423, 1994
HELMERS R et al: Pulmonary manifestations associated with rheumatoid arthritis. Chest 100:235, 1991
HOFFMAN RM, ROGERS RM: Serum and lavage lactate dehydrogenase isoenzymes in pulmonary alveolar proteinosis. Am Rev Respir Dis 143:42, 1991
KITAICHI M et al: Pulmonary lymphangioleiomyomatosis: A report of 46 patients including a clinicopathologic study of prognostic factors. Am J Respir Crit Care Med 151:527, 1995
LAHDENSUO A, KORPELA M: Pulmonary findings in patients with primary Sjögren's syndrome. Chest 108:316, 1995
SCHWARZ MI et al: Pulmonary capillaritis and diffuse alveolar hemorrhage—a primary manifestation of polymyositis. Am J Respir Crit Care Med 151:2037, 1995
SOLER P et al: Pulmonary Langerhans' cell granulomatosis. Annu Rev Med 43:105, 1992
TROSHINSKY MB et al: Pulmonary function and gastroesophageal reflux in systemic sclerosis. Ann Intern Med 121:6, 1994

260

Stuart Rich

PRIMARY PULMONARY HYPERTENSION

Primary pulmonary hypertension is an uncommon disease characterized by increased pulmonary artery pressure and pulmonary vascular resistance without an obvious cause. The incidence has been estimated at approximately 2 cases per million. There is a female-to-male preponderance (1.7:1), with patients most commonly presenting in the third and fourth decades, although the age range is from infancy to greater than 60 years. Because the predominant symptom of primary pulmonary hypertension is dyspnea, which can have an insidious onset in an otherwise healthy person, the disease is typically diagnosed late in its course. By that time, the clinical and laboratory findings of severe pulmonary hypertension are usually present.

PATHOLOGY The histopathology of primary pulmonary hypertension is not pathognomonic for the disease but represents a pulmonary arteriopathy that is observed in pulmonary hypertension from a variety of causes. The most common patterns found are a plexogenic arteriopathy manifest by medial hypertrophy, concentric laminar intimal fibrosis, and plexiform lesions; and a thrombotic arteriopathy manifest by eccentric intimal fibrosis with medial hypertrophy, fibroelastic intimal pads in the arteries and arterioles, and scattered evidence of old recanalized thrombi appearing as fibrous webs. In most patients features of both patterns of vascular changes can be found.

The common pathogenetic denominator appears to be an undefined injury to the pulmonary vascular endothelium, which results in (1) an impaired ability to maintain a relaxed state of vasomotor tone, (2) intense medial hypertrophy and intimal proliferation that compromises the vascular lumen, and (3) a conversion to a procoagulant state within the pulmonary arteriolar bed that disposes to the development of in situ thrombosis. The types of vascular changes noted are likely determined by the nature of the injury to the pulmonary vascular endothelium and/or its duration, the patient's gender, and underlying genetic predisposition. The association of primary pulmonary hypertension with cirrhosis and portal hypertension, while statistically significant, remains unexplained.

Pulmonary venoocclusive disease is a rare and distinct pathologic entity, found in fewer than 10 percent of patients with primary pulmonary hypertension. Histologically, it is manifest by widespread intimal proliferation and fibrosis of the intrapulmonary veins and venules, occasionally extending to the arteriolar bed. The pulmonary venous obstruction explains the increased pulmonary capillary wedge pressure observed in patients with advanced disease. These patients may develop orthopnea that can mimic left ventricular failure.

Pulmonary capillary hemangiomatosis is also a very rare form of primary pulmonary hypertension. Histologically, it is characterized by infiltrating thin-walled blood vessels that are widespread throughout the pulmonary interstitium and walls of the pulmonary arteries and veins. These patients often have hemoptysis as a clinical feature.

ETIOLOGY The etiology of primary pulmonary hypertension remains unknown, although animal and human studies suggest an abnormality of the endothelial cell of the pulmonary arterial bed. In many individuals, a risk factor or "trigger" appears to influence pulmonary endothelial cell function, resulting in ineffective control of vasomotor tone, causing vasoconstriction, and platelet activation and thrombosis. Studies suggest that there is a release of growth factors and cytokines that act locally on the pulmonary arteriolar bed to induce vascular remodeling. Risk factors that have been linked to the development of unexplained pulmonary hypertension include essential hypertension, human immunodeficiency virus, portal hypertension, anorexigens, collagen vascular disease, and congenital shunts resulting in increased pulmonary blood flow.

A genetic basis for primary pulmonary hypertension appears likely. Familial primary pulmonary hypertension occurs in approximately 7 percent of cases, with the pattern of inheritance identified as autosomal dominant, with incomplete penetrance and genetic anticipation. The latter feature, which relates to offspring of subsequent generations manifesting the disease either at younger ages or by greater severity, is seen in other genetic diseases associated with a trinucleotide repeat expansion abnormality. The genetic basis of primary pulmonary hypertension may involve several genetic loci, with patients who present with sporadic disease possessing a genetic predisposition that becomes expressed following exposure to an external trigger or risk factor.

PATHOPHYSIOLOGY The underlying hemodynamic derangement in primary pulmonary hypertension is an increased resistance to pulmonary blood flow. Early in the disease there is a marked elevation in pulmonary artery pressure with relatively normal cardiac function. Over time the cardiac output becomes progressively reduced rather than the pulmonary artery pressure becoming progressively increased. Initially, the pulmonary arteries may respond to vasodilators, but as the disease progresses, the elevated pulmonary vascular resistance becomes fixed. The pulmonary capillary wedge pressure remains normal until the late stages, when it tends to rise in response to impaired diastolic filling of the left ventricle due to the altered configuration of the intraventricular septum. Eventually, as the right ventricle fails, the right atrial and right ventricular end-diastolic pressures rise in an attempt to compensate for the myocardial depression that has developed in response to chronic severe right ventricular pressure overload.

Pulmonary function is usually normal in primary pulmonary hypertension, although a mild restrictive pattern (see Chap. 250) is sometimes seen. Hypoxemia is common and is believed to be due to a mismatch between pulmonary ventilation and perfusion, magnified by a low cardiac output. Occasional patients with a patent foramen ovale may develop right-to-left shunting, which also can contribute to systemic arterial desaturation.

DIAGNOSIS A thorough diagnostic evaluation to look for all potential causes should be undertaken (see Fig. 260-1). The history usually reveals the gradual onset of shortness of breath with effort, progressing until the patient is dyspneic with minimal activity. The average duration from symptom onset until diagnosis is 2.5 years. Other common symptoms are fatigue, angina pectoris that likely represents right ventricular ischemia, syncope, near syncope, and peripheral edema.

The physical examination is characteristic. Increased jugular venous pressure, a reduced carotid pulse, and an easily palpable right ventricular lift are typical. Most patients have an increased pulmonic component of the second heart sound and right-sided third and fourth heart sounds. Tricuspid and pulmonic regurgitation and peripheral cyanosis and edema may be noted. Clubbing is not a feature.

The chest x-ray generally shows enlarged central pulmonary arteries and clear lung fields. The electrocardiogram usually reveals right axis deviation and right ventricular hypertrophy. The echocardiogram demonstrates right ventricular enlargement, a reduction in left ventricular cavity size, and abnormal septal configuration consistent with right ventricular pressure overload. Doppler studies have revealed a marked dependence on atrial systole for ventricular filling. Hypoxemia, hypocapnia, and an abnormal diffusing capacity for carbon monoxide are almost invariable findings. A mild restrictive pattern on pulmonary function is sometimes observed, but evidence of airways obstruction suggests a secondary etiology for the pulmonary hypertension. A perfusion lung scan may be normal or abnormal with multiple diffuse patchy filling defects of a nonsegmental nature and not suggestive of pulmonary thromboembolism. If the lung scan reveals perfusion defects of a segmental or subsegmental nature, a pulmonary angiogram must be done. Severe pulmonary hypertension in a patient with a high-probability lung scan should suggest a chronic process and *not* acute pulmonary embolism, since the nonconditioned right ventricle is unable to generate high systolic pressures acutely in the face of pulmonary thromboembolism. Chronic thromboembolic obstruction of the large pulmonary arteries (Chap. 261) can mimic primary pulmonary hypertension but can be amenable to treatment with surgical thromboendarterectomy.

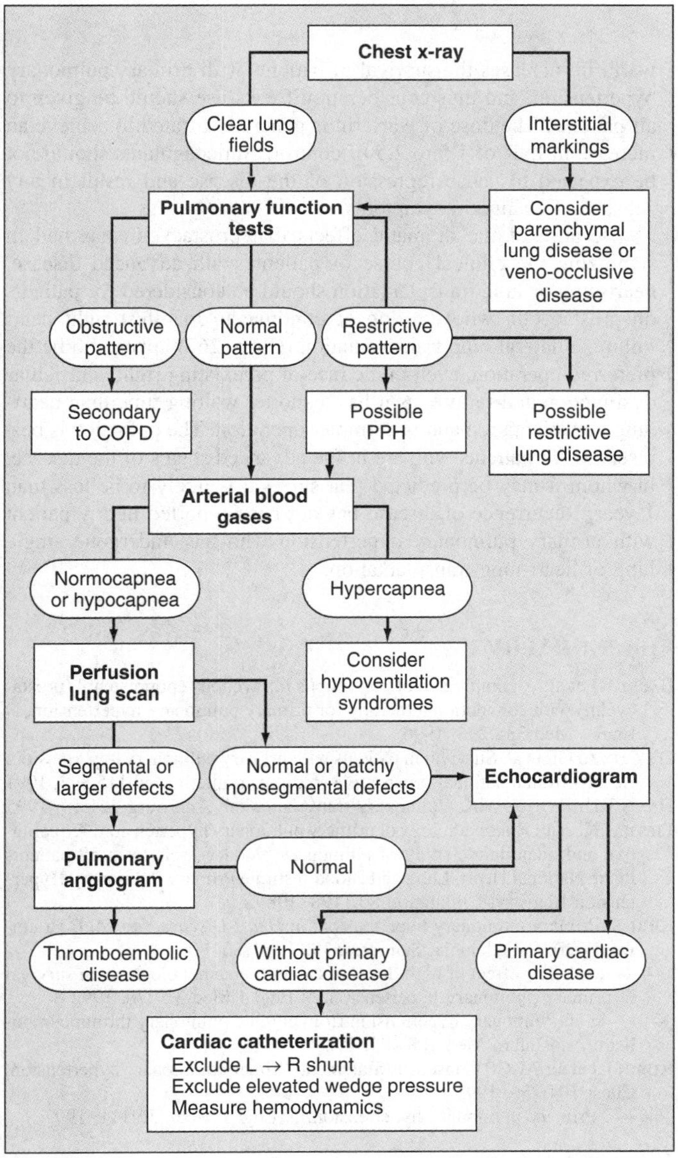

FIGURE 260-1 An algorithm for the workup of a patient with unexplained pulmonary hypertension. (*Adapted with permission from S Rich.*)

There is risk in performing pulmonary angiography in patients with primary pulmonary hypertension, and it is recommended that selective or subselective injections with small amounts of low-osmolar, nonionic contrast material be made following the pretreatment with 1 mg atropine to prevent vagally mediated bradycardia.

Cardiac catheterization is mandatory to characterize the disease and exclude an underlying cardiac shunt as the cause. The use of balloon-flotation catheters, especially those with removable guide-wires, can facilitate right heart catheterization. A right-to-left shunt might be attributable to a patent foramen ovale, but any left-to-right shunting implies the presence of a congenital defect. Although it may be difficult to obtain, the pulmonary capillary wedge pressure is normal. If it is increased, left heart catheterization also should be performed to exclude mitral stenosis or increased left ventricular end-diastolic pressures as the cause of the pulmonary hypertension. Although the diagnostic evaluation of these patients can be hazardous, experience from a national multicenter study revealed no mortality or serious morbidity in more than 300 patients whose evaluation included pulmonary angiography and cardiac catheterization. It is not necessary to perform an open lung biopsy in these patients to make an accurate diagnosis.

On occasion a patient may have marked elevations in pulmonary artery pressure and a relatively mild disease that is known to cause pulmonary hypertension. It would be a mistake to characterize these patients as having primary pulmonary hypertension on the belief that the pulmonary hypertension is out of proportion to the underlying associated condition. Since the pulmonary vascular bed has variable vasoreactivity, these cases probably reflect an exaggerated pulmonary vasoconstrictive response to the associated condition. Thus severe pulmonary hypertension can coexist with mild chronic obstructive pulmonary disease, small intracardiac shunts, mild mitral stenosis, and even ischemic heart disease. The distinction, however, is important because the treatment of pulmonary hypertension should always be focused toward the underlying cause.

NATURAL HISTORY The natural history of primary pulmonary hypertension is unknown because initially the disease is largely asymptomatic. Several older series have reported a mean survival of 2 to 3 years for patients from the time of diagnosis. Functional class is a strong predictor of survival, since patients who are functional classes II and III have a mean survival of 3.5 years compared with those who are functional class IV, in whom the mean survival is 6 months. The cause of death is usually right ventricular failure or sudden death; sudden death appears to be a late feature of the disease. Increased right atrial pressure above 15 mmHg and reduced cardiac index below 2 (L/min)/m^2 are hemodynamic predictors of a poor prognosis.

℞ TREATMENT

Because the pulmonary vascular resistance increases dramatically with exercise, patients should be cautioned against participating in activities that demand increased physical stress. The use of digoxin remains controversial, since no studies have documented a benefit or detriment. Diuretic therapy relieves dyspnea and peripheral edema and may be useful in reducing right ventricular volume overload in the presence of tricuspid regurgitation.

It is recommended that all patients in whom primary pulmonary hypertension is confirmed undergo acute drug testing with short-acting pulmonary vasodilators to determine the extent of pulmonary vasodilator reserve or reactivity (see Fig. 260-2). Intravenous adenosine, inhaled nitric oxide, and intravenous prostacyclin all appear to have similar effects in reducing pulmonary vascular resistance acutely with little effect on the systemic vascular bed. Adenosine is given as a constant infusion in doses of 50 (μg/kg)/min and increased every 2 min until side effects develop. Similarly, prostacyclin is given in doses of 2 (ng/kg)/min and increased every 30 min until side effects develop. Maximal physiologic effectiveness of the therapy is determined at the highest tolerated dose. Nitric oxide is generally administered via inhalation in 5 to 10 parts per million and increased every few minutes until no further effectiveness is obtained.

Patients who have substantial reductions in pulmonary vascular resistance from the short-acting vasodilators may be candidates to receive oral calcium channel blockers. These drugs must be administered under direct hemodynamic guidance in order to determine effectiveness and safety. Typically, patients will require high doses (e.g., nifedipine, 120 to 240 mg/d, or diltiazem, 540 to 900 mg/d,[1]). Patients who manifest significant reductions in mean pulmonary artery pressure and pulmonary vascular resistance should demonstrate improved symptoms, regression of right ventricular hypertrophy, and improved survival with chronic therapy. However, fewer than half the patients who are responsive to the short-acting vasodilators will respond to this regimen. It is unknown whether the response to calcium blockers depends on the histologic subtype, but the therapy appears to be more successful in patients who are diagnosed early and have less advanced disease.

Prostacyclin has recently been approved as a treatment of primary pulmonary hypertension for patients who are functional class III or IV and unresponsive to conventional therapy. Clinical trials have demonstrated that patients realize an improvement in symptoms and exercise tolerance and reduction in mortality. The drug can only be administered intravenously and requires placement of a permanent central venous catheter and continuous dose titration, as tolerance develops in all patients over a short period of time. The side effects of prostacyclin, which include flushing, jaw pain, and diarrhea, are generally tolerated by most patients. The major problems with this therapy have been infections related to the venous catheter, which requires close monitoring and diligence on behalf of the patient. Because of the complexity involved in managing patients on prostacyclin, it has been recommended that they be referred to centers with expertise in managing primary pulmonary hypertension for initiation of therapy.

None of the other classes of vasodilator drugs that have been investigated, including beta-adrenergic agonists, alpha-adrenergic blockers, smooth-muscle vasodilators, nitrates, and angiotensin-converting enzyme inhibitors, has shown similar sustained effectiveness.

The administration of vasodilators can have serious acute and chronic adverse effects. The most common response is a reduction in pulmonary vascular resistance, manifest by an increased cardiac output, without a reduction in the mean pulmonary artery pressure. This results in increased stroke work of the right ventricle, which can result in worsening of ventricular function and precipitate right ventricular failure over time. In addition, maintenance of adequate systemic blood pressure is crucial, since right ventricular coronary blood flow is already compromised due to the loss of the normal gradient for myocardial perfusion between the aorta and right ventricle. Vasodilator drugs can provoke acute right ventricular ischemia, and deaths have been reported. For these reasons, the pharmacologic evaluation of primary pulmonary hypertension should always be undertaken with direct monitoring of systemic and pulmonary arterial pressures and cardiac output.

Anticoagulant therapy also has been advocated based on the evidence that thrombosis in situ is common. One retrospective study and one prospective study have demonstrated that the anticoagulant

[1] These agents have not been approved for the treatment of primary pulmonary hypertension by the U.S. Food and Drug Administration.

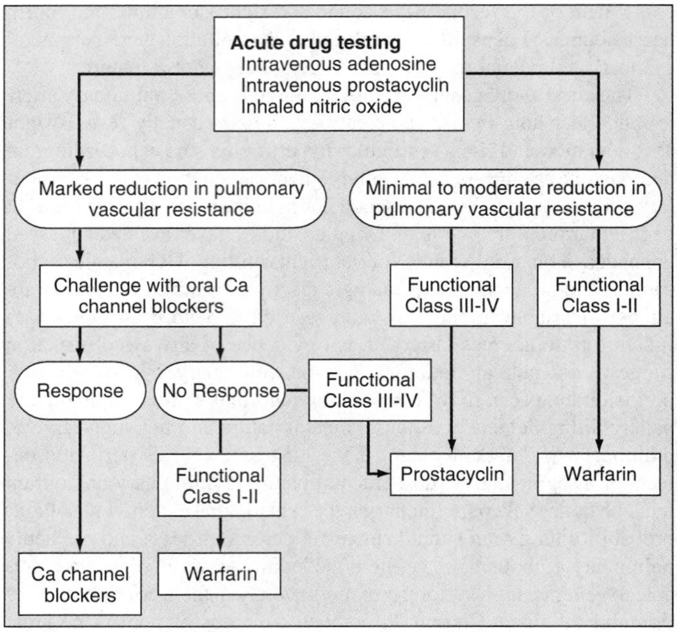

FIGURE 260-2 An algorithm for the evaluation and drug treatment of a patient with primary pulmonary hypertension.

warfarin increases the survival of patients with primary pulmonary hypertension, and thus consideration for its use should be given to all patients. The dose of warfarin is generally titrated to achieve an increase in INR of 1.5 to 2.5 of control. Anticoagulants should not be expected to cause regression of the disease and result in any substantial change in symptoms.

Because of the dramatic effects that prostacyclin has had in stabilizing the clinical course of patients with advanced disease, heart-lung or lung transplantation should be considered for patients on prostacyclin who develop or continue to manifest right heart failure. Bilateral lung transplantation (Chap. 267) appears to be the preferred operation, even in the face of preexisting right ventricular dysfunction and failure, as it has a shorter waiting time than heart-lung transplantation and is a simpler operation. The operation is best reserved for patients who are in the advanced stages of the disease, in whom it may be predicted that survival is likely to be less than 1 year. Recurrence of disease has not been reported in any patient with primary pulmonary hypertension who has undergone single lung or heart-lung transplantation.

BIBLIOGRAPHY

Barst RJ et al: A comparison of continuous intravenous epoprostenol (prostacyclin) with conventional therapy for primary pulmonary hypertension. N Engl J Med 334:296, 1996

D'Alonzo GE et al: Survival in patients with primary pulmonary hypertension: Results from a national prospective study. Ann Intern Med 115:343, 1991

Davis RD, Pasque MK: Pulmonary transplantation. Ann Surg 221:14, 1995

Pietra GG et al: Histopathology of primary pulmonary hypertension: A qualitative and quantitative study of pulmonary blood vessels from 58 patients in the National Heart, Lung and Blood Institute Primary Pulmonary Hypertension Registry. Circulation 80:1198, 1989

Rich S: Primary pulmonary hypertension, in *Heart Disease*, 5th ed, E Braunwald (ed). Philadelphia, Saunders, 1997 pp 780–806

——— et al: The effect of high doses of calcium-channel blockers on survival in primary pulmonary hypertension. N Engl J Med 327:76, 1992

——— et al: Pulmonary hypertension from chronic pulmonary thromboembolism. Ann Intern Med 108:425, 1988

Rubin LJ et al: ACCP Consensus Statement. Primary pulmonary hypertension. Chest 104:236, 1993

———: Primary pulmonary hypertension. N Engl J Med 336:111, 1997

261 PULMONARY THROMBOEMBOLISM

Samuel Z. Goldhaber

PATHOPHYSIOLOGY

Rudolf Virchow postulated more than a century ago that a triad of factors predisposed to venous thrombosis: (1) local trauma to the vessel wall, (2) hypercoagulability, and (3) stasis. We now believe that many patients who suffer pulmonary thromboembolism (PTE) have an underlying inherited predisposition that remains clinically silent until an acquired stressor occurs such as surgery, obesity, or pregnancy (Table 261-1).

FACTOR V LEIDEN The most frequent inherited predisposition to hypercoagulability is resistance to the endogenous anticoagulant protein, activated protein C. The phenotype of activated protein C resistance is associated with a single point mutation, designated *factor V Leiden*, in the factor V gene. This missense mutation—a single nucleotide substitution of adenine for guanine 1691—causes an amino acid substitution of glutamine for arginine at position 506.

The allelic frequency of this mutation is about 3 percent in healthy American male physicians participating in the Physicians' Health Study. However, the prevalence of the factor V mutation was three times higher among those physicians who subsequently developed venous thrombosis. Furthermore, after anticoagulation (for at least 3 months) was completed and discontinued, those participants with factor V Leiden had a much higher rate of recurrent venous thrombosis than those without. Factor V Leiden is more common than all other (identified) inherited hypercoagulable states combined, including deficiencies in protein C, protein S, antithrombin III, and disorders of plasminogen (Chap. 118).

EMBOLIZATION When venous thrombi become dislodged from their site of formation, they embolize to the pulmonary arterial circulation or, paradoxically, to the arterial circulation through a patent foramen ovale. About half of patients with pelvic vein thrombosis or proximal leg deep venous thrombosis (DVT) have PTE, which is usually asymptomatic. Isolated calf vein or upper extremity venous thromboses also pose a risk (albeit lower) of PTE. The small size of isolated calf vein thrombi does not necessarily render them benign; they can embolize through a patent foramen ovale and are the most common source of paradoxical embolism.

PHYSIOLOGY Pulmonary embolism can have the following effects:

1. *Increased pulmonary vascular resistance* due to vascular obstruction or neurohumoral agents including serotonin
2. *Impaired gas exchange* due to increased alveolar dead space from vascular obstruction and hypoxemia from alveolar hypoventilation in the nonobstructed lung, right-to-left shunting, and impaired carbon monoxide transfer due to loss of gas exchange surface
3. *Alveolar hyperventilation* due to reflex stimulation of irritant receptors
4. *Increased airway resistance* due to bronchoconstriction
5. *Decreased pulmonary compliance* due to lung edema, lung hemorrhage, and loss of surfactant.

Right Ventricular Dysfunction Progressive right heart failure is the usual immediate cause of death from PTE. As pulmonary vascular resistance increases, right ventricular wall tension rises and perpetuates further right ventricular dilatation and dysfunction. Consequently, the interventricular septum bulges into and compresses an intrinsically normal left ventricle. Increased right ventricular wall tension also compresses the right coronary artery and may precipitate myocardial ischemia and right ventricular infarction. Underfilling of the left ventricle may lead to a fall in left ventricular output and systemic arterial pressure, thereby provoking myocardial ischemia due to compromised coronary artery perfusion. Eventually, circulatory collapse and death may ensue.

Table 261-1

Stressors That May Precipitate Pulmonary Thromboembolism

Surgery, trauma
Obesity
Oral contraceptives, pregnancy, postpartum
Cancer (sometimes occult) or cancer chemotherapy
Immobilization (stroke or intensive care unit patients)
Indwelling central venous catheter

DIAGNOSIS

The clinical setting can be immensely helpful in suggesting the diagnosis of PTE (Table 261-1).

CLINICAL SYDNDROMES Patients with *massive PTE* present with systemic arterial hypotension and usually have anatomically widespread thromboembolism. Primary therapy with thrombolysis or embolectomy offers the greatest chance of survival. Those with *moderate to large PTE* have right ventricular hypokinesis on echocardiography but normal systemic arterial pressure. There is increasing evidence that such patients may benefit from primary therapy to prevent recurrent embolism. Patients with *small to moderate PTE* have both normal right heart function and normal systemic arterial pressure. They have a good prognosis with either adequate anticoagulation or an inferior vena caval filter. The presence of *pulmonary infarction* usually indicates a small PTE, but one that is exquisitely painful, because it lodges near the innervation of pleural nerves.

Nonthrombotic pulmonary embolism may be easily overlooked. Possible etiologies include fat embolism after blunt trauma and long bone fractures, tumor embolism, or air embolism. Intravenous drug users may inject themselves with a wide array of substances, such as hair, talc, or cotton. *Amniotic fluid embolism* occurs when fetal membranes leak or tear at the placental margin. The pulmonary edema seen in this syndrome is probably due primarily to alveolar capillary leakage.

PTE-DVT RELATIONSHIP When considering PTE, the interviewer should always ask about prior PTE or DVT and about a family history of venous thromboembolism. The presence of confirmed DVT is usually an adequate surrogate for PTE. Therefore, symptoms and signs of DVT (Chap. 248) should also be sought when investigating the possibility of PTE.

SYMPTOMS AND SIGNS Dyspnea is the most frequent symptom of PTE, and tachypnea is its most frequent sign. Whereas dyspnea, syncope, hypotension, or cyanosis indicate a massive PTE, pleuritic pain, cough, or hemoptysis often suggest a small embolism located distally near the pleura. On *physical examination*, young and previously healthy individuals may simply appear anxious but otherwise seem deceptively well, even with an anatomically large PTE. They need not have "classic" signs such as tachycardia, low-grade fever, neck vein distention, or an accentuated pulmonic component of the second heart sound. Sometimes, a paradoxical bradycardia occurs.

In older patients who complain of vague chest discomfort, the diagnosis of PTE may not be apparent unless signs of right heart failure are present. Unfortunately, because acute coronary ischemic syndromes are so common, one may overlook the possibility of life-threatening PTE and may inadvertently discharge these patients from the hospital after the exclusion of myocardial infarction with serial cardiac enzyme measurements and electrocardiograms.

DIFFERENTIAL DIAGNOSIS The differential diagnosis of PTE is broad (Table 261-2). Although PTE is known as "the great masquerader," quite often another illness simulates PTE. For example, when the proposed diagnosis of PTE is supposedly confirmed with a combination of dyspnea, chest pain, and an abnormal lung scan, the correct diagnosis of pneumonia might become apparent 12 h later when an infiltrate blossoms on chest x-ray, purulent sputum is first produced, and high fever and shaking chills develop.

Some patients have PTE and a coexisting illness such as pneumonia or heart failure. In such circumstances, clinical improvement will often fail to occur despite standard medical treatment of the concomitant illness. This situation can serve as a clinical clue to the possible coexistence of PTE.

NONIMAGING DIAGNOSTIC MODALITIES These are generally safer, less expensive, but also less specific than diagnostic modalities that employ imaging.

Blood Tests The quantitative *plasma* D-*dimer enzyme-linked immunosorbent assay (ELISA)* level is elevated (>500 ng/mL) in more than 90 percent of patients with PTE, reflecting plasmin's breakdown of fibrin and indicating endogenous (though clinically ineffective) thrombolysis. A qualitative latex agglutination D-dimer assay, which is more readily available and less expensive than an ELISA, can be obtained initially; if elevated, the ELISA will also be elevated. However, if the latex agglutination is normal, a D-dimer ELISA should be obtained, because the ELISA is much more sensitive than the latex agglutination D-dimer assay, which cannot be used to exclude PTE. The plasma D-dimer ELISA has a high negative predictive value and can be used to help exclude PTE. However, neither D-dimer assay is specific. Levels increase in patients with myocardial infarction, sepsis, or almost any systemic illness.

Data from the Prospective Investigation of Pulmonary Embolism Diagnosis (PIOPED) indicate that, contrary to classic teaching, *arterial blood gases* lack diagnostic utility for PTE. Among patients suspected of PTE, neither the room air arterial P_{O_2} nor calculation of the alveolar-arterial oxygen gradient can reliably differentiate or triage patients who actually have PTE at angiography.

Electrocardiogram Classic abnormalities include sinus tachycardia; new-onset atrial fibrillation or flutter; and an S wave in lead I, a Q wave in lead III, and an inverted T wave in lead III (Chap. 228). Often, the QRS axis is greater than 90°. T-wave inversion in leads V_1 to V_4 reflects right ventricular strain.

NONINVASIVE IMAGING MODALITIES **Chest Roentgenography** A normal or near-normal chest x-ray in a dyspneic patient suggests PTE. Well-established abnormalities include focal oligemia (Westermark's sign), a peripheral wedged-shaped density above the diaphragm (Hampton's hump), or an enlarged right descending pulmonary artery.

Venous Ultrasonography Ultrasonography of the deep venous system relies upon loss of vein compressibility as the primary criterion for DVT. About one-third of patients with PTE have no imaging evidence of DVT. In these situations, the clot may have already embolized to the lung or is in the pelvic veins, where ultrasonography is usually inadequate. Therefore, the workup for PTE should continue if there is high clinical suspicion, despite a normal ultrasound examination.

The reliability of venous ultrasonography is well established for proximal leg DVT among *symptomatic* outpatients. However, ultrasonography is notoriously insensitive for DVT screening among *asymptomatic* inpatients. Consequently, the use of ultrasonography to screen for DVT in postoperative orthopedic surgery or neurosurgery patients will underestimate the frequency of proximal leg vein thrombosis.

Table 261-2

Differential Diagnosis of Pulmonary Thromboembolism

Myocardial infarction, unstable angina
Pneumonia, bronchitis, COPD exacerbation
Congestive heart failure
Asthma
Pericarditis
Primary pulmonary hypertension
Rib fracture, pneumothorax
Costochondritis, "musculoskeletal pain," anxiety

NOTE: COPD, chronic obstructive pulmonary disease.

Lung Scanning (See also Chap. 251) Lung scanning is the principal imaging test for the diagnosis of PTE. Small particulate aggregates of albumin labeled with a gamma-emitting radionuclide are injected intravenously and are trapped in the pulmonary capillary bed. A perfusion scan defect indicates absent or decreased blood flow, possibly due to PTE. Ventilation scans, obtained with radiolabeled inhaled gases such as xenon or krypton, improve the specificity of the perfusion scan. Abnormal ventilation scans indicate abnormal nonventilated lung, thereby providing possible explanations for perfusion defects other than acute PTE. A high probability scan for PTE is defined as having two or more segmental perfusion defects in the presence of normal ventilation.

Lung scanning is particularly useful if the results are normal or near-normal, or if there is a high probability for PTE. The diagnosis of PTE is very unlikely in patients with normal and near-normal scans but, in contrast, is about 90 percent certain in patients with high-probability scans. Unfortunately, fewer than half of patients with angiographically confirmed PTE have a high-probability scan. Importantly, as many as 40 percent of patients with high clinical suspicion for PTE and "low-probability" scans do, in fact, have PTE at angiography.

Echocardiography This technique is useful for rapid triage of acutely ill patients who may have PTE. Bedside echocardiography can usually reliably differentiate among illnesses that have radically different treatment, including acute myocardial infarction, pericardial tamponade, dissection of the aorta, and PTE complicated by right heart failure. Detection of right ventricular dysfunction due to PTE helps to stratify the risk, delineate the prognosis, and plan optical management.

INVASIVE DIAGNOSTIC MODALITIES **Pulmonary Angiography** Selective pulmonary angiography is the most specific examination available for establishing the definitive diagnosis of PTE and can detect emboli as small as 1 to 2 mm. A definitive diagnosis of PTE depends upon visualization of an intraluminal filling defect in more than one projection. Secondary signs of PTE include abrupt occlusion ("cut-off") of vessels; segmental oligemia or avascularity; a prolonged arterial phase with slow filling; or tortuous, tapering peripheral vessels.

Pulmonary angiography can be carried out safely among properly selected patients at hospitals that perform at least several studies per month. In PIOPED, the procedure resulted in death in five patients (0.5 percent), two of whom had severe heart failure prior to the procedure. Angiography is most useful when the clinical likelihood of PTE differs substantially from the lung scan result or when the lung scan is of intermediate probability for PTE.

Contrast Phlebography This technique has been mostly replaced by ultrasonography. Venography is costly, uncomfortable, and occasionally results in contrast allergy or contrast-induced phlebitis. Contrast phlebography is worthwhile when there is a discrepancy between the clinical suspicion and the ultrasound result, or if it is clinically important to screen asymptomatic postoperative or trauma patients at high risk for DVT. Phlebography is also useful for diagnosing isolated calf vein thrombosis or recurrent DVT.

INTEGRATED DIAGNOSTIC APPROACH We advocate an integrated diagnostic approach to streamline the workup of PTE (Fig. 261-1). This strategy combines the clinical likelihood of PTE with the results of noninvasive testing to determine whether pulmonary angiography is warranted.

Rx TREATMENT

Risk Stratification Anticoagulation with heparin and warfarin constitutes secondary prevention of recurrent PTE rather than primary therapy. Primary therapy (Table 261-3) consists of clot dissolution with thrombolysis or removal of PTE by embolectomy and is reserved for patients at high risk of death from right heart failure and for those at risk of recurrent PTE despite adequate anticoagulation. The echocardiogram has a pivotal role in risk stratification. Patients with right ventricular dysfunction on echocardiography may be appropriate candidates for primary therapy of PTE, even if normal systemic arterial pressure is preserved (Fig. 261-2).

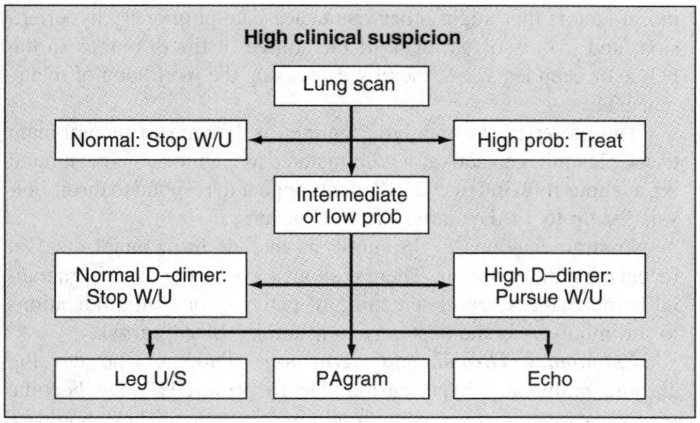

FIGURE 261-1 PTE diagnosis strategy. An integrated diagnostic approach. W/U, work up; U/S, ultrasound; PAgram, pulmonary arteriogram; ECHO, echocardiogram.

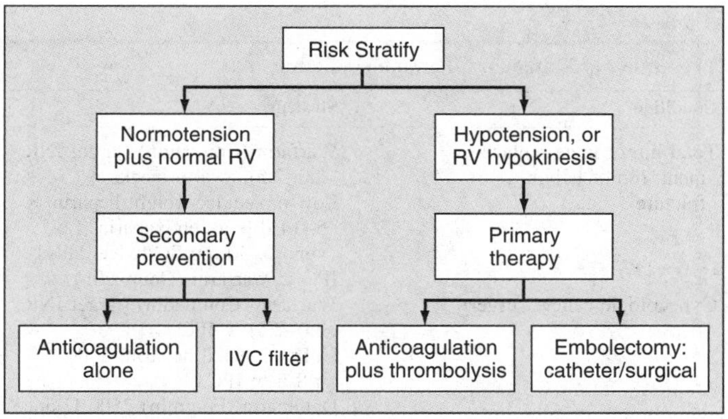

FIGURE 261-2 Acute PTE management: Risk stratification. RV, right ventricular; IVC, inferior vena cava.

When less than 30 percent of the lung scan is affected by PTE, then right ventricular function almost always remains normal. Such patients typically have good clinical outcomes with anticoagulation alone.

Adjunctive Therapy Important adjunctive measures include pain relief (especially with nonsteroidal anti-inflammatory agents), supplemental oxygenation, and psychological support. Dobutamine—a beta-adrenergic agonist with positive inotropic and pulmonary vasolidating effects—should be utilized to treat right heart failure and cardiogenic shock. In general, volume loading is ill advised because increased right ventricular dilatation can lead to even further reductions in left ventricular forward output.

Heparin Heparin binds to and accelerates the activity of antithrombin III, an enzyme that inhibits the coagulation factors thrombin (factor IIa), Xa, IXa, XIa, and XIIa. Heparin thus prevents additional thrombus formation and permits endogenous fibrinolytic mechanisms to lyse clot that has already formed. After 5 to 7 days of heparin, residual thrombus begins to stabilize in the endothelium of the vein or pulmonary artery. However, heparin does *not* directly dissolve thrombus that already exists.

DOSING Heparin administration can be instituted after major active bleeding has been excluded and after a rectal examination has been performed with testing for occult blood. The presence of occult blood does not preclude the use of heparin but indicates that the dose should be reduced. A typical bolus is 5000 to 10,000 units of unfractionated heparin followed by a continuous infusion of 1000 to 1500 units/h. An activated partial thromboplastin time that is at least twice the control value should provide a therapeutic level of heparin. Multiple nomograms (e.g., Raschke's) are available to assist in adjusting the infusion rate of heparin.

COMPLICATIONS The most important adverse effect of heparin is hemorrhage. For life-threatening or intracranial hemorrhage, protamine sulfate can be administered at the time heparin is discontinued.

Heparin-associated thrombocytopenia is usually of no clinical consequence. However, if the platelet count declines more than 50 percent from baseline, heparin should be discontinued. An ominous, immunologically mediated thrombocytopenia can promote platelet aggregation and destruction and may be associated with either thrombocytopenic bleeding or with life-threatening arterial ("white clot syndrome") and venous thrombosis.

Patients receiving prolonged heparin therapy may also develop osteopenia, osteoporosis, or pathologic bone fractures. Heparin-associated elevations in transaminase levels occur commonly but are rarely associated with clinical toxicity.

LOW-MOLECULAR-WEIGHT HEPARINS These fragments of unfractionated heparin exhibit less binding to plasma proteins and endothelial cells than does unfractionated heparin. They have a greater bioavailability, more predictable dose response, and longer half-life than unfractionated heparin. *Enoxaparin,* which has received Food and Drug Administration (FDA) approval for prophylaxis after total hip or knee replacement, has a lower rate of heparin-associated thrombocytopenia than does unfractionated heparin. *Dalteparin* has recently received FDA approval for once daily subcutaneous administration to prevent venous thromboembolism in patients undergoing general and pelvic surgery. Low-molecular-weight heparins have *not* received FDA approval for *treatment* of PTE or DVT.

Warfarin This is a vitamin K antagonist that prevents γ carboxylation activation of coagulation factors II, VII, IX, and X. The full effect of warfarin often requires 5 days, even if the prothrombin time, used for monitoring, becomes elevated more rapidly. When warfarin is initiated during an active thrombotic state, the levels of protein C and S decline, thus creating a thrombogenic potential. By overlapping heparin and warfarin for 5 days, the procoagulant effect of unopposed warfarin can be counteracted.

DOSING Warfarin is usually initiated in a dose of 7.5 to 10 mg. However, after several days, the dose usually needs to be reduced. Patients who are malnourished or who have received prolonged courses of antibiotics are probably deficient in vitamin K and should receive much smaller initial doses of warfarin, such as 2.5 mg. The prothrombin time should be reported according to the International Normalized Ratio (INR), not the prothrombin time ratio of the prothrombin time expressed in seconds (Chap. 119). The target INR should be approximately 3.0.

COMPLICATIONS As with heparin, bleeding is the most important and common complication associated with warfarin administration. Life-threatening bleeding can be treated with cryoprecipitate or fresh frozen plasma (usually 2 units) to achieve immediate hemostasis. For less serious bleeding, vitamin K may be administered, usually in an initial dose of 2.5 to 5 mg subcutaneously. This latter approach requires about 6 h to take effect and will help lower the INR toward the upper portion of the therapeutic range.

Warfarin induced skin necrosis is a rare complication that may be related to warfarin induced reduction of protein C. It is usually

Table 261-3

Primary Therapy for Pulmonary Thromboembolism

Classification	Specific Therapy
1. Medical	Thrombolysis (peripheral vein)
	Inotropic agents (e.g., dobutamine)
2. Catheter-based	Suction embolectomy
	Fragmentation and distal dispersion
	Mechanical pulverization
	Local, catheter-directed thrombolysis
	Balloon angioplasty (chronic)
3. Surgical	Embolectomy (acute)
	Thromboendarterectomy (chronic)

Table 261-4

Prevention of Pulmonary Thromboembolism

Condition	Strategy
Total hip or knee replacement; hip or pelvis fracture	Warfarin (Coumadin) (target INR 2.0–2.5) × 4–6 weeks
	Low-molecular-weight heparin × 5–14 d [e.g., enoxaparin (Lovenox), 30 mg SC twice daily]
	IPC ± warfarin (Coumadin)
Gynecologic cancer surgery	Warfarin (Coumadin) (target INR 2.0–2.5) ± IPC
	Unfractionated heparin, 5000 U q 8 h ± IPC
	Dalteparin (Fragmin) 2500 U once daily ± IPC
Urologic surgery	Warfarin (Coumadin) (target INR 2.0–2.5) ± IPC
Thoracic surgery	IPC *plus* unfractionated heparin, 5000 U q 8 h
High-risk general surgery (e.g., prior VTE, current cancer, or obesity)	IPC *or* graded-compression stockings *plus* unfractionated heparin, 5000 U q 8 h
	Dalteparin (Fragmin) 5000 U SC once daily
General, gynecologic, or urologic surgery (without prior VTE) for noncancerous conditions	Graded-compression stockings *plus* unfractionated heparin 5000 U q 12 h
	Dalteparin 2500 U SC once daily
	IPC alone
Neurosurgery, eye surgery, or other surgery when prophylactic anticoagulation is contraindicated	Graded-compression stockings ± IPC
Medical conditions	Graded-compression stockings ± heparin, 5000 U q 8–12 h
	IPC alone

NOTE: IPC, intermittent pneumatic compression; VTE, venous thromboembolism.

associated with administration of a high initial dose of warfarin during an acute thrombotic state in which heparin is withheld. During pregnancy, warfarin should be avoided if possible because of warfarin embryopathy, which is most common with exposure during the sixth through twelfth weeks of gestation. However, women can take warfarin postpartum and breast feed safely.

Duration of Anticoagulation After discontinuation of anticoagulation, the risk of recurrent PTE is surprisingly high. Schulman and colleagues found that after a 6-month course of anticoagulation, 14 percent of PTE patients suffered a recurrent venous thromboembolism within the ensuing 2 years. The recurrence rate was twice as high among patients who received only 6 weeks of anticoagulation. Patients with underlying cancer that is not cured or with massive obesity should probably be anticoagulated indefinitely. For other patients, it is reasonable to anticoagulate the first episode of isolated calf vein thrombosis for 3 months, proximal DVT for 6 months, and PTE for 1 year.

Inferior Vena Caval Filters When anticoagulation cannot be undertaken because of active bleeding, insertion of an inferior vena caval filter is usually necessary. Other indications include recurrent venous thrombosis despite adequate anticoagulation, prevention of recurrent PTE in patients with right heart failure who are not candidates for thrombolysis, or prophylaxis of extremely high risk patients. The Bird's Nest filter infrarenally or, if necessary, a Greenfield filter suprarenally are recommended.

Thrombolysis Thrombolytic therapy may rapidly reverse right heart failure and thus lead to a lower rate of death and recurrent PTE. Thrombolysis usually achieves the following: (1) dissolves much of the anatomically obstructing pulmonary arterial thrombus, (2) prevents the continued release of serotonin and other neurohumoral factors that might otherwise exacerbate pulmonary hypertension, and (3) dissolves much of the source of the thrombus in the pelvic or deep leg veins, thereby decreasing the likelihood of recurrent PTE.

The preferred thrombolytic regimen is 100 mg of recombinant tissue plasminogen activator administered as a continuous peripheral intravenous infusion over 2 h. Patients appear to respond to thrombolysis for up to 14 days after the PTE occurred.

Contraindications to thrombolysis include intracranial disease, recent surgery, or trauma. There is about a 1 percent risk of intracranial hemorrhage. Careful screening of patients for contraindications to thrombolysis is the best way to minimize bleeding risk.

Pulmonary Thromboendarterectomy Patients who develop chronic pulmonary hypertension due to prior PTE may become severely dyspneic at rest or with minimal extertion. They should be considered for pulmonary thromboendarterectomy which, if successful, can markedly reduce and at times even cure pulmonary hypertension.

Prevention Prevention of PTE is of paramount importance because it is both difficult to recognize and expensive to treat. Fortunately, effective mechanical and pharmacologic prophylaxis modalities are widely available and usually effective (Table 261-4).

BIBLIOGRAPHY

BERTINA RM et al: Mutation in blood coagulation factor V associated with resistance to activated protein C. Nature 369:64, 1994

BOUNAMEAUX H et al: Plasma measurement of D-dimer as diagnostic aid in suspected venous thromboembolism: An overview. Thromb Haemost 71:1, 1994

GOLDHABER SZ (ed): *Prevention of Venous Thromboembolism.* New York, Marcel Dekker, 1993

——— et al: Alteplase versus heparin in acute pulmonary embolism: Randomised trial assessing right-ventricular function and pulmonary perfusion. Lancet 341:507, 1993

——— (ed): Cardiopulmonary diseases and cardiac tumors, vol 3, in *Atlas of Heart Diseases,* E Braunwald (Series ed). Philadelphia, Current Medicine, 1995

———: Contemporary pulmonary embolism thrombolysis. Chest 107:45S, 1995

HIRSCH DR et al: A prospective study of deep venous thrombosis in medical intensive care unit patient. JAMA 274:335, 1995

LUALDI JC, GOLDHABER SZ: Right ventricular dysfunction after acute pulmonary embolism: Pathophysiologic factors, detection, and therapeutic implications. Am Heart J 130:1276, 1995

RASCHKE RA et al: The weight-based heparin dosing nomogram compared with a "standard care" nomogram: A randomized controlled trial. Ann Intern Med 119:874, 1993

RIDKER PM et al: Mutation in the gene coding for coagulation factor V and risks of future myocardial infarction, stroke, and venous thrombosis in apparently healthy men. N Engl J Med 332:912, 1995

SCHULMAN S et al: A comparison of six weeks with six months of oral anticoagulant therapy after a first episode of venous thromboembolism. N Engl J Med 332:1661, 1995

STEIN PD et al: Complications and validity of pulmonary angiography in acute pulmonary embolism. Circulation 85:462, 1992

——— et al: Arterial blood gas analysis in the assessment of suspected acute pulmonary embolism. Chest 109:78, 1996

262

Richard W. Light

DISORDERS OF THE PLEURA, MEDIASTINUM, AND DIAPHRAGM

DISORDERS OF THE PLEURA

PLEURAL EFFUSION The pleural space lies between the lung and chest wall and normally contains a very thin layer of fluid. This thin layer of liquid serves as a coupling system between the lung and chest wall. A pleural effusion is present when there is an excess quantity of fluid in the pleural space.

Etiology Pleural fluid accumulates when pleural fluid formation exceeds pleural fluid absorption. Normally, fluid enters the pleural space from the capillaries in the parietal pleura and is removed via the lymphatics situated in the parietal pleura. Fluid also can enter the pleural space from the interstitial spaces of the lung via the visceral pleura or from the peritoneal cavity via small holes in the diaphragm. The lymphatics have the capacity to absorb 20 times more fluid than is normally formed. Accordingly, a pleural effusion may develop when there is excess pleural fluid formation (from the parietal pleura, the interstitial spaces of the lung, or the peritoneal cavity) or when there is decreased fluid removal by the lymphatics.

Diagnostic Approach When a patient is found to have a pleural effusion, an effort should be made to determine the cause (Fig. 262-1). The first step is to determine whether the effusion is a transudate or an exudate. A *transudative* pleural effusion occurs when *systemic factors* that influence the formation and absorption of pleural fluid are altered. The leading causes of transudative pleural effusions in the United States are left ventricular failure, pulmonary embolism, and cirrhosis. An *exudative* pleural effusion occurs when *local factors* that influence the formation and absorption of pleural fluid are altered. The leading causes of exudative pleural effusions are bacterial pneumonia, malignancy, viral infection, and pulmonary embolism. The primary reason to make this differentiation is that additional diagnostic procedures are indicated with exudative effusions to define the cause of the local disease.

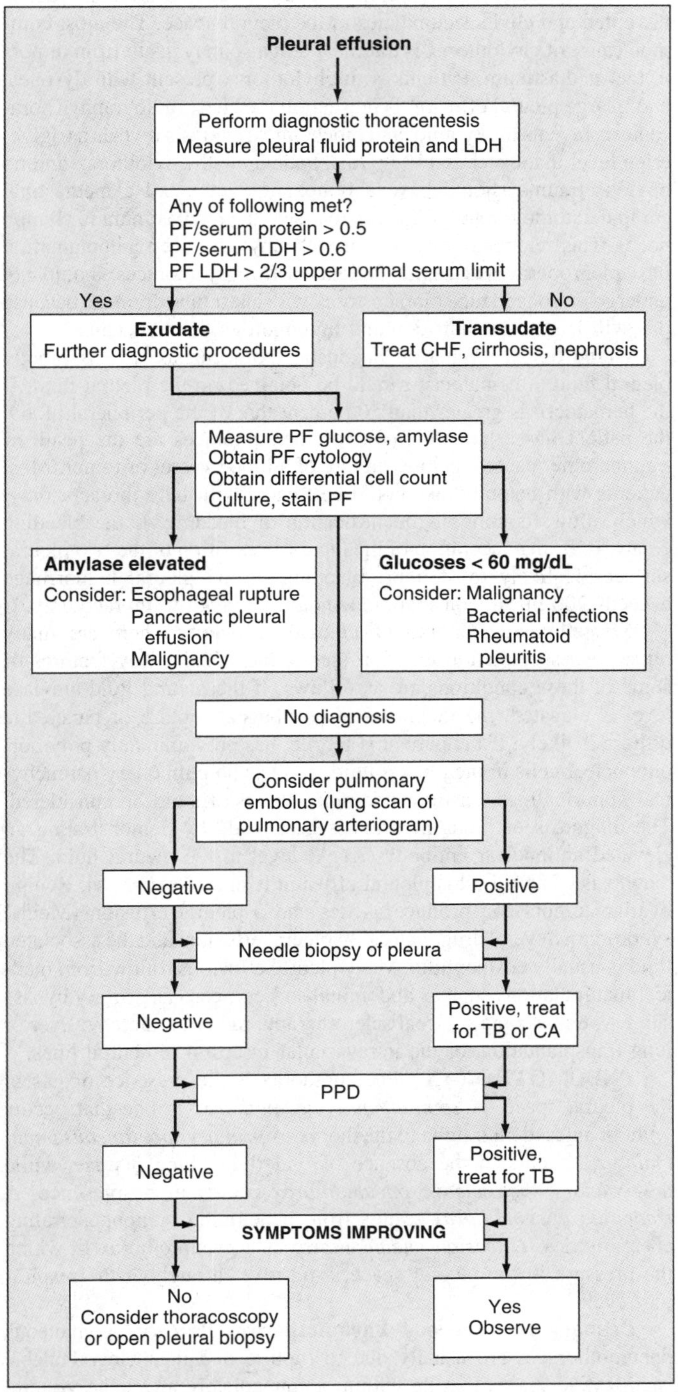

FIGURE 262-1 Approach to the diagnosis of pleural effusions; PF, pleural fluid.

Transudative and exudative pleural effusions are distinguished by measuring the lactate dehydrogenase (LDH) and protein levels in the pleural fluid. Exudative pleural effusions meet at least one of the following criteria, whereas transudative pleural effusions meet none.

1. Pleural fluid protein/serum protein >0.5
2. Pleural fluid LDH/serum LDH >0.6
3. Pleural fluid LDH more than two-thirds normal upper limit for serum

If a patient has an exudative pleural effusion, the following tests on the pleural fluid should be obtained: description of the fluid, glucose level, amylase level, differential cell count, microbiologic studies, and cytology.

Effusion due to Heart Failure The most common cause of pleural effusion is left ventricular failure. The effusion occurs because the increased amounts of fluid in the lung interstitial spaces exit in part across the visceral pleura. This overwhelms the capacity of the lymphatics in the parietal pleura to remove fluid. A diagnostic thoracentesis should be performed if the effusions are not bilateral and comparable in size, if the patient is febrile, or if the patient has pleuritic chest pain to verify that the patient has a transudative effusion. Otherwise the patient is best treated with diuretics. If the effusion persists despite diuretic therapy, a diagnostic thoracentesis should be performed. Diuretic therapy for a few days does not significantly change the biochemical characteristics of the pleural fluid.

Hepatic Hydrothorax Pleural effusions occur in approximately 5 percent of patients with cirrhosis and ascites. The predominant mechanism is the direct movement of peritoneal fluid through small holes in the diaphragm into the pleural space. The effusion is usually right-sided and frequently is large enough to produce severe dyspnea. If medical management does not control the ascites and the effusion, there are no good alternatives. Consideration can be given to inserting a peritoneal-venous shunt, thoracotomy with surgical repair of the leak, or tube thoracostomy with the injection of a sclerosing agent.

Parapneumonic Effusion Parapneumonic effusions are associated with bacterial pneumonia, lung abscess, or bronchiectasis and are probably the most common exudative pleural effusion in the United States. A *complicated parapneumonic effusion* requires tube thoracostomy for its resolution. *Empyema* refers to a grossly purulent effusion.

Patients with aerobic bacterial pneumonia and pleural effusion present with an acute febrile illness consisting of chest pain, sputum production, and leukocytosis. Patients with anaerobic infections present with a subacute illness with weight loss, a brisk leukocytosis, mild anemia, and a history of some factor that predisposes them to aspiration.

The possibility of a parapneumonic effusion should be considered whenever a patient with a bacterial pneumonia is initially evaluated. The presence of free pleural fluid can be demonstrated with a lateral decubitus radiograph. If the free fluid separates the lung from the chest wall by more than 10 mm on the decubitus radiograph, a diagnostic thoracentesis should be performed in order to determine whether or not a chest tube should be inserted. Any of the following is an indication for tube thoracostomy:

1. The presence of gross pus in the pleural space
2. Organisms visible on Gram stain of the pleural fluid
3. Pleural fluid glucose level of less than 50 mg/dL
4. Pleural fluid pH below 7.00 and 0.15 units lower than arterial pH

There should be no delay in its performance because a free-flowing parapneumonic effusion can become loculated within a matter of hours.

If the pleural fluid is loculated and is not adequately drained with one chest tube, either streptokinase, 250,000 units, or urokinase, 100,000 units, should be injected intrapleurally to dissolve the fibrin membranes that create the loculations. If the pleural drainage is inadequate after the intrapleural thrombolytic therapy, either thoracoscopy with breakdown of adhesions or thoracotomy with decortication should be performed.

Effusion Secondary to Malignancy Malignant pleural effusions secondary to metastatic disease are the second most common type of exudative pleural effusion. The three tumors that cause approximately 75 percent of all malignant pleural effusions are lung carcinoma, breast carcinoma, and lymphoma. Most patients complain of dyspnea, which is frequently out of proportion to the size of the effusion. The pleural fluid is an exudate, and its glucose level may be reduced if the tumor burden in the pleural space is high.

The diagnosis is usually made via cytology of the pleural fluid. If the initial cytologic examination is negative, then a needle biopsy of the pleura with repeat cytology is indicated. If there is still no diagnosis, thoracoscopy is likely to provide the diagnosis if the patient has malignancy. At the time of thoracoscopy, talc or some similar agent should be instilled into the pleural space to effect a pleurodesis.

Patients with a malignant pleural effusion are treated symptomatically for the most part, since the presence of the effusion indicates disseminated disease and most malignancies associated with pleural effusion are not curable with chemotherapy. The only symptom that can be attributed to the effusion itself is dyspnea. If the patient's lifestyle is compromised by dyspnea, and if the dyspnea is relieved with a therapeutic thoracentesis, then one of the following procedures should be performed: (1) tube thoracostomy with the instillation of a sclerosing agent such as talc, 5 g in a slurry, or doxycycline, 500 mg, (2) thoracoscopy with pleural abrasion or the insufflation of talc, or (3) insertion of a pleuroperitoneal shunt.

Mesothelioma Malignant mesotheliomas are primary tumors that arise from the mesothelial cells that line the pleural cavities. Most are related to asbestos exposure. Patients with mesothelioma present with chest pain and shortness of breath. The chest radiograph reveals a pleural effusion, generalized pleural thickening, and a shrunken hemithorax. Thoracoscopy or open pleural biopsy is usually necessary to establish the diagnosis. Various treatment modalities, including radical surgery, chemotherapy, and radiation therapy, have been tried, but none has been proven to be more effective than symptomatic therapy. It is recommended that chest pain be treated with opiates and that shortness of breath be treated with oxygen and/or opiates.

Effusion Secondary to Pulmonary Embolization The diagnosis most commonly overlooked in the differential diagnosis of a patient with an undiagnosed pleural effusion is pulmonary embolism. Dyspnea is the most common symptom. The pleural fluid can be either transudative or exudative. The diagnosis is suggested by lung scanning and/or pulmonary arteriography (see Chap. 261). Treatment of the patient with a pleural effusion secondary to pulmonary embolism is the same as for any patient with pulmonary emboli. If the pleural effusion increases in size after anticoagulation, the patient probably has recurrent emboli or another complication such as a hemothorax or a pleural infection.

Tuberculous Pleuritis (See Chap. 171) In many parts of the world, the most common cause of an exudative pleural effusion is tuberculosis, but this is relatively uncommon in the United States. Tuberculous pleural effusions are thought to be due primarily to a hypersensitivity reaction to tuberculous protein in the pleural space. Patients with tuberculous pleuritis present with fever, weight loss, dyspnea, and/or pleuritic chest pain. The pleural fluid is an exudate with predominantly small lymphocytes. The diagnosis is usually established by the demonstration of granulomas on needle biopsy of the pleura. Adequate treatment consists of isoniazide, 300 mg/d, plus rifampin, 600 mg/d, for 6 months. If the patient is suspected of having resistant organisms, ethambutol and pyrazinamide should also be included until the results of drug sensitivity tests are available.

Effusion Secondary to Viral Infection Viral infections are probably responsible for a sizable percentage of undiagnosed exudative pleural effusions. In many series, no diagnosis is established for approximately 20 percent of exudative effusions, and these effusions resolve spontaneously with no long-term residua. The importance of these effusions is that one should not be too aggressive in trying to establish a diagnosis for the undiagnosed effusion, particularly if the patient is improving clinically.

AIDS Pleural effusions are uncommon in such patients. The most common cause is Kaposi's sarcoma, followed by parapneumonic effusion. Other common causes are tuberculosis, cryptococcosis, and lymphoma. Pleural effusions are very uncommon with *Pneumocystis carinii* infection.

Chylothorax A chylothorax occurs when the thoracic duct is disrupted and chyle accumulates in the pleural space. The most common cause of chylothorax is trauma, but it also may result from tumors in the mediastinum. Patients with chylothorax present with dyspnea, and a large pleural effusion is present on the chest radiograph. Thoracentesis reveals milky fluid, and biochemical analysis reveals a triglyceride level that exceeds 110 mg/dL. Patients with chylothorax and no obvious trauma should have a lymphangiogram and a mediastinal computed tomographic (CT) scan to assess the mediastinum for lymph nodes. The treatment of choice for most chylothoraces is implantation of a pleuroperitoneal shunt. Patients with chylothoraces should not undergo prolonged tube thoracostomy with chest tube drainage because this will lead to malnutrition and immunologic incompetence.

Hemothorax When a diagnostic thoracentesis reveals bloody pleural fluid, a hematocrit should be obtained on the pleural fluid. If the hematocrit is greater than 50 percent that of the peripheral blood, the patient has a hemothorax. Most hemothoraces are the result of trauma; other causes include rupture of a blood vessel or tumor. Most patients with hemothorax should be treated with tube thoracostomy, which allows continuous quantification of bleeding. If the bleeding emanates from a laceration of the pleura, apposition of the two pleural surfaces is likely to stop the bleeding. If the pleural hemorrhage exceeds 200 mL/h, consideration should be given to thoracotomy.

Miscellaneous Causes of Pleural Effusion There are many other causes of pleural effusion (see Table 262-1). Key features of some of these conditions are as follows: If the pleural fluid amylase level is elevated, the diagnosis of esophageal rupture or pancreatic disease is likely. If the patient is febrile, has predominantly polymorphonuclear cells in the pleural fluid, and has no pulmonary parenchymal abnormalities, an intraabdominal abscess should be considered. The diagnosis of lupus pleuritis is best made by demonstrating an elevated antinuclear antibody (ANA) level in the pleural fluid. The diagnosis of an asbestos pleural effusion is one of exclusion. Benign ovarian tumors can produce ascites and a pleural effusion (Meigs' syndrome). Several drugs can cause pleural effusion, and the associated fluid is usually eosinophilic. Many pleural effusions follow from medical manipulations such as abdominal surgery, coronary artery bypass surgery, endoscopic variceal sclerotherapy, radiation therapy, liver or lung transplantation, or the intravascular insertion of central lines.

PNEUMOTHORAX Pneumothorax is the presence of gas in the pleural space. A *spontaneous pneumothorax* is one that occurs without antecedent trauma to the thorax. A *primary spontaneous pneumothorax* occurs in the absence of underlying lung disease, while a *secondary spontaneous pneumothorax* occurs in its presence. A *traumatic pneumothorax* results from penetrating or nonpenetrating chest injuries. A *tension pneumothorax* is a pneumothorax in which the pressure in the pleural space is positive throughout the respiratory cycle.

Primary Spontaneous Pneumothorax Primary spontaneous pneumothoraces are usually due to rupture of apical pleural blebs, small cystic spaces that lie within or immediately under the visceral pleura. Primary spontaneous pneumothoraces occur almost exclusively in smokers, which suggests that the patients indeed do have subclinical

Table 262-1

Differential Diagnoses of Pleural Effusions

TRANSUDATIVE PLEURAL EFFUSIONS	
1. Congestive heart failure	5. Superior vena cava obstruction
2. Cirrhosis	6. Myxedema
3. Nephrotic syndrome	7. Pulmonary emboli
4. Peritoneal dialysis	8. Urinothorax
EXUDATIVE PLEURAL EFFUSIONS	
1. Neoplastic diseases	6. Post-cardiac injury syndrome
a. Metastatic disease	7. Asbestos exposure
b. Mesothelioma	8. Sarcoidosis
2. Infectious diseases	9. Uremia
a. Bacterial infections	10. Meigs' syndrome
b. Tuberculosis	11. Yellow nail syndrome
c. Fungal infections	12. Drug-induced pleural disease
d. Viral infections	a. Nitrofurantoin
e. Parasitic infections	b. Dantrolene
3. Pulmonary embolization	c. Methysergide
4. Gastrointestinal disease	d. Bromocriptine
a. Esophageal perforation	e. Procarbazine
b. Pancreatic disease	f. Amiodarone
c. Intraabdominal abscesses	13. Trapped lung
d. Diaphragmatic hernia	14. Radiation therapy
e. After abdominal surgery	15. Electrical burns
f. Endoscopic variceal sclerotherapy	16. Hemothorax
g. After liver transplant	17. Iatrogenic injury
5. Collagen-vascular diseases	18. Ovarian hyperstimulation syndrome
a. Rheumatoid pleuritis	
b. Systemic lupus erythematosus	19. Pericardial disease
c. Drug-induced lupus	20. Chylothorax
d. Immunoblastic lymphadenopathy	
e. Sjögren's syndrome	
f. Wegener's granulomatosis	
g. Churg-Strauss syndrome	

lung disease. Approximately one-half of patients with an initial primary spontaneous pneumothorax will have a recurrence. The initial recommended treatment for primary spontaneous pneumothorax is simple aspiration. If the lung does not expand with aspiration, or if the patient has a recurrent pneumothorax, tube thoracostomy with instillation of a sclerosing agent such as doxycycline is indicated. Thoracoscopy or thoracotomy with pleural abrasion is almost 100 percent successful in preventing recurrences.

Secondary Spontaneous Pneumothorax Most secondary spontaneous pneumothoraces are due to chronic obstructive pulmonary disease, but pneumothoraces have been reported with virtually every lung disease. Pneumothorax in patients with lung disease is more life-threatening than it is in normal individuals because of the lack of pulmonary reserve in these patients. Nearly all patients with secondary spontaneous pneumothorax should be treated with tube thoracostomy and the instillation of a sclerosing agent such as doxycycline or talc. Patients with either primary or secondary spontaneous pneumothoraces who have a persistent air leak or an unexpanded lung after 5 days of tube thoracostomy should be subjected to thoracoscopy with bleb resection and pleural abrasion.

Traumatic Pneumothorax Traumatic pneumothoraces can result from both penetrating and nonpenetrating chest trauma. Traumatic pneumothoraces should be treated with tube thoracostomy. If a hemopneumothorax is present, one chest tube should be placed in the superior part of the hemithorax to evacuate the air, and another should be placed in the inferior part of the hemithorax to remove the blood. Iatrogenic pneumothorax is a type of traumatic pneumothorax which is becoming more common. The leading causes are transthoracic needle aspiration, thoracentesis, and the insertion of central intravenous catheters. The treatment differs according to the degree of distress and can be observation, supplemental oxygen, aspiration, or tube thoracostomy.

Tension Pneumothorax This condition usually occurs during mechanical ventilation or resuscitative efforts. The positive pleural pressure is life-threatening both because ventilation is severely compromised and because the positive pressure is transmitted to the mediastinum, which results in decreased venous return to the heart and reduced cardiac output.

Difficulty in ventilation during resuscitation or high peak inspiratory pressures during mechanical ventilation strongly suggest the diagnosis. The diagnosis is made by the finding of an enlarged hemithorax with no breath sounds and shift of the mediastinum to the contralateral side. Tension pneumothorax must be treated as a medical emergency. If the tension in the pleural space is not relieved, the patient is likely to die from inadequate cardiac output or marked hypoxemia. A large-bore needle should be inserted into the pleural space through the second anterior intercostal space. If large amounts of gas escape from the needle after insertion, the diagnosis is confirmed. The needle should be left in place until a thoracostomy tube can be inserted.

DISORDERS OF THE MEDIASTINUM

The mediastinum is the region between the pleural sacs. It is separated into three compartments. The *anterior mediastinum* extends from the sternum anteriorly to the pericardium and brachiocephalic vessels posteriorly. It contains the thymus gland, the anterior mediastinal lymph nodes, and the internal mammary arteries and veins. The *middle mediastinum* lies between the anterior and posterior mediastina and contains the heart; the ascending and transverse arches of the aorta; the venae cavae; the brachiocephalic arteries and veins; the phrenic nerves; the trachea, main bronchi, and their contiguous lymph nodes; and the pulmonary arteries and veins. The *posterior mediastinum* is bounded by the pericardium and trachea anteriorly and the vertebral column posteriorly. It contains the descending thoracic aorta, esophagus, thoracic duct, azygos and hemiazygos veins, and the posterior group of mediastinal lymph nodes.

MEDIASTINAL MASSES The first step in evaluating a mediastinal mass lesion is to place it in one of the three mediastinal compartments, since each has different characteristic lesions. The most common lesions in the anterior mediastinum are thymomas, lymphomas, teratomatous neoplasms, and thyroid masses. The most common masses in the middle mediastinum are vascular masses, lymph node enlargement from metastases or granulomatous disease, and pleuropericardial and bronchogenic cysts. In the posterior mediastinum, neurogenic tumors, meningoceles, meningomyeloceles, gastroenteric cysts, and esophageal diverticula are commonly found.

CT scanning is the most valuable imaging technique for evaluating mediastinal masses and is the only imaging technique that should be done. Barium studies of the gastrointestinal tract are indicated in many patients with posterior mediastinal lesions, since hernias, diverticula, and achalasia are readily diagnosed in this manner. An iodine 131 nuclear medicine scan can efficiently establish the diagnosis of intrathoracic goiter.

A definite diagnosis can be obtained with mediastinoscopy or anterior mediastinotomy in many patients with masses in the anterior or middle mediastinal compartments. A diagnosis can be established without thoracotomy via percutaneous fine-needle aspiration biopsy of mediastinal masses in any of the mediastinal compartments. In many cases the diagnosis can be established and the mediastinal mass removed with video-assisted thoracoscopy.

ACUTE MEDIASTINITIS Most cases of acute mediastinitis are either due to esophageal perforation or occur after median sternotomy for cardiac surgery. Patients with esophageal rupture are acutely ill with chest pain and dyspnea due to the mediastinal infection. The esophageal rupture can occur spontaneously or as a complication of esophagoscopy or the insertion of a Blakemore tube. Appropriate treatment is exploration of the mediastinum with primary repair of the esophageal tear and drainage of the pleural space and the mediastinum.

The incidence of mediastinitis following median sternotomy is 0.4 to 5.0 percent. Patients most commonly present with wound drainage. Other presentations include sepsis or a widened mediastinum. The diagnosis is usually established with mediastinal needle aspiration.

Treatment includes immediate drainage, debridement, and parenteral antibiotic therapy, but the mortality still exceeds 20 percent.

CHRONIC MEDIASTINITIS The spectrum of chronic mediastinitis ranges from granulomatous inflammation of the lymph nodes in the mediastinum to fibrosing mediastinitis. Most cases are due to tuberculosis or histoplasmosis, but sarcoidosis, silicosis, and other fungal diseases are at times causative. Patients with granulomatous mediastinitis are usually asymptomatic. Those with fibrosing mediastinitis usually have signs of compression of some mediastinal structure such as the superior vena cava or large airways, phrenic or recurrent laryngeal nerve paralysis, or obstruction of the pulmonary artery or proximal pulmonary veins. In most cases, mediastinal exploration is necessary to distinguish benign mediastinitis from malignant processes. Other than antituberculous therapy for tuberculous mediastinitis, no medical or surgical therapy has been demonstrated to be effective for mediastinal fibrosis.

PNEUMOMEDIASTINUM In this condition there is gas in the interstices of the mediastinum. The three main causes are (1) alveolar rupture with dissection of air into the mediastinum; (2) perforation or rupture of the esophagus, trachea, or main bronchi; and (3) dissection of air from the neck or the abdomen into the mediastinum. Typically, there is severe substernal chest pain with or without radiation into the neck and arms. The physical examination usually reveals subcutaneous emphysema in the suprasternal notch and *Hamman's sign*, which is a crunching or clicking noise synchronous with the heartbeat and best heard in the left lateral decubitus position. The diagnosis is confirmed with the chest radiograph. Usually no treatment is required, but the mediastinal air will be absorbed faster if the patient inspires high concentrations of oxygen. If mediastinal structures are compressed, the compression can be relieved with needle aspiration.

DISORDERS OF THE DIAPHRAGM

DIAPHRAGMATIC PARALYSIS The presence of bilateral diaphragmatic paralysis almost always causes severe morbidity in adults. The most common causes include high spinal cord injury, thoracic trauma (including cardiac surgery), multiple sclerosis, anterior horn disease, and muscular dystrophy. Most patients with severe diaphragmatic weakness present with hypercapnic respiratory failure, frequently complicated by cor pulmonale and right ventricular failure, atelectasis, and pneumonia.

The degree of diaphragmatic weakness is best quantitated by measuring transdiaphragmatic pressures. The treatment of choice is assisted ventilation for all or part of each day. This is best accomplished without tracheostomy using nasal intermittent positive airway pressure. If the nerve to the diaphragm is intact, diaphragmatic pacing may be a viable alternative. If the paralysis occurs during open heart surgery, recovery frequently occurs, but it may take 6 months or more.

Unilateral paralysis of the diaphragm is much more common than is bilateral paralysis. The most common cause is nerve invasion from malignancy, usually a bronchogenic carcinoma. If the patient does not have malignancy, then usually no cause for the paralysis is found. The diagnosis is suggested by finding an elevated hemidiaphragm on the chest roentgenogram. Confirmation is best established with the "sniff test." When a patient is observed with fluoroscopy while sniffing, the paralyzed diaphragm will move paradoxically upward due to the negative intrathoracic pressure. Patients with a unilateral paralyzed diaphragm are usually asymptomatic. Their vital capacity and total lung capacity are each reduced about 20 percent. If a patient has a mediastinal mass in conjunction with the diaphragmatic paralysis, further workup should be done. However, if the patient is asymptomatic with a normal chest radiograph, no invasive procedures are warranted.

BIBLIOGRAPHY

LIGHT RW: *Pleural Diseases*. Baltimore, Williams & Wilkins, 1995

———: Pleural diseases. Dis Mon 28:266, 1992

MULLER NL: Imaging of the pleura. Radiology 186:29, 1993

NAUNHEIM KS et al: Safety and efficacy of video-assisted thoracic surgical techniques for the treatment of spontaneous pneumothorax. J Thorac Cardiovasc Surg 109:1198, 1995

ROVIARO G et al: Videothoracoscopic excision of mediastinal masses: Indications and technique. Ann Thorac Surg 58:1679, 1994

WALKER-RENARD PB et al: Chemical pleurodesis for malignant pleural effusions. Ann Intern Med 120:56, 1994

WIENER-KRONISH JP, BROADDUS VC: Interrelationship of pleural and pulmonary interstitial liquid. Ann Rev Physiol 55:209, 1993

263

Eliot A. Phillipson

DISORDERS OF VENTILATION

HYPOVENTILATION

DEFINITION AND ETIOLOGY Alveolar hypoventilation exists by definition when arterial P_{CO_2} (Pa_{CO_2}) increases above the normal range of 37 to 43 mmHg, but in clinically important hypoventilation syndromes Pa_{CO_2} is generally in the range of 50 to 80 mmHg. Hypoventilation disorders can be acute or chronic. The acute disorders, which represent life-threatening emergencies, are discussed in Chap. 265; this chapter deals with chronic hypoventilation syndromes.

Chronic hypoventilation can result from numerous disease entities (Table 263-1), but in all cases the underlying mechanism involves a defect in either the metabolic respiratory control system, the respiratory neuromuscular system, or the ventilatory apparatus. Disorders associated with impaired respiratory drive, defects in the respiratory neuromuscular system, some chest wall disorders such as obesity, and upper airway obstruction produce an increase in Pa_{CO_2}, despite normal lungs,

Table 263-1

Chronic Hypoventilation Syndromes

Mechanism	Site of Defect	Disorder
Impaired respiratory drive	Peripheral and central chemoreceptors	Carotid body dysfunction, trauma Prolonged hypoxia Metabolic alkalosis
	Brainstem respiratory neurons	Bulbar poliomyelitis, encephalitis Brainstem infarction, hemorrhage, trauma Brainstem demyelination, degeneration Chronic drug administration Primary alveolar hypoventilation syndrome
Defective respiratory neuromuscular system	Spinal cord and peripheral nerves	High cervical trauma Poliomyelitis Motor neuron disease Peripheral neuropathy
	Respiratory muscles	Myasthenia gravis Muscular dystrophy Chronic myopathy
Impaired ventilatory apparatus	Chest wall	Kyphoscoliosis Fibrothorax Thoracoplasty Ankylosing spondylitis Obesity-hypoventilation
	Airways and lungs	Laryngeal and tracheal stenosis Obstructive sleep apnea Cystic fibrosis Chronic obstructive pulmonary disease

SOURCE: From Phillipson, with permission.

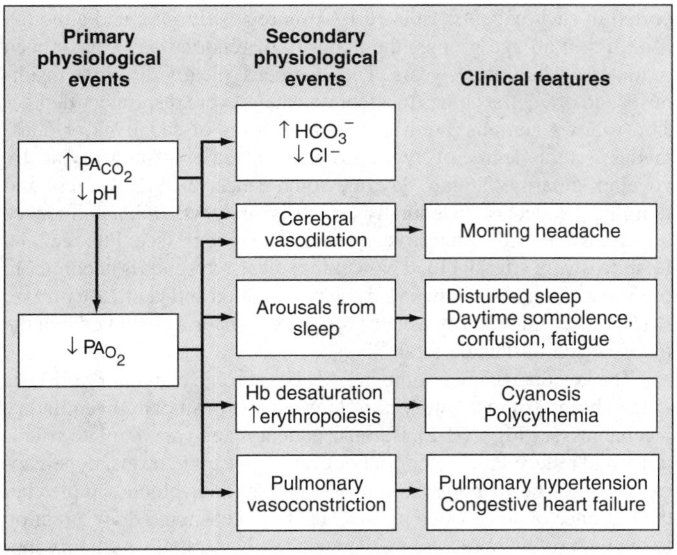

FIGURE 263-1 Physiologic and clinical features of alveolar hypoventilation. *(After Phillipson.)* Hb, hemoglobin; $P_{A_{CO_2}}$, alveolar P_{CO_2}; $P_{A_{O_2}}$, alveolar P_{O_2}.

because of a reduction in overall minute volume of ventilation and hence in alveolar ventilation. In contrast, most disorders of the chest wall and disorders of the lower airways and lungs may produce an increase in Pa_{CO_2}, despite a normal or even increased minute volume of ventilation, because of severe ventilation-perfusion mismatching that results in net alveolar hypoventilation.

Several hypoventilation syndromes involve combined disturbances in two elements of the respiratory system. For example, patients with chronic obstructive pulmonary disease may hypoventilate not simply because of impaired ventilatory mechanics but also because of a reduced central respiratory drive, which can be inherent or secondary to a coexisting metabolic alkalosis (related to diuretic and steroid therapy).

PHYSIOLOGIC AND CLINICAL FEATURES Regardless of cause, the hallmark of all alveolar hypoventilation syndromes is an increase in alveolar P_{CO_2} ($P_{A_{CO_2}}$) and therefore in Pa_{CO_2} (Fig. 263-1). The resulting respiratory acidosis eventually leads to a compensatory increase in plasma HCO_3^- concentration and a decrease in Cl^- concentration. The increase in $P_{A_{CO_2}}$ produces an obligatory decrease in $P_{A_{O_2}}$, resulting in hypoxemia. If severe, the hypoxemia manifests clinically as cyanosis and can stimulate erythropoiesis and induce secondary polycythemia. The combination of chronic hypoxemia and hypercapnia also may induce pulmonary vasoconstriction, leading eventually to pulmonary hypertension, right ventricular hypertrophy, and congestive heart failure. The disturbances in arterial blood gases are typically magnified during sleep because of a further reduction in central respiratory drive. The resulting increased nocturnal hypercapnia may cause cerebral vasodilation leading to morning headache; sleep quality also may be severely impaired, resulting in morning fatigue, daytime somnolence, mental confusion, and intellectual impairment. Other clinical features associated with hypoventilation syndromes are related to the specific underlying disease (see Table 263-1).

DIAGNOSIS Investigation of the patient with chronic hypoventilation involves several laboratory tests that will usually localize the disorder to either the metabolic respiratory control system, the neuromuscular system, or the ventilatory apparatus (Fig. 263-2). Defects in the control system impair responses to chemical stimuli, including ventilatory, occlusion pressure, and diaphragmatic electromyographic (EMG) responses. During sleep, hypoventilation is usually more marked, and central apneas and hypopneas are common. However, because the behavioral respiratory control system (which is anatomically distinct from the metabolic control system), the neuromuscular system, and the ventilatory apparatus are intact, such patients can usually hyperventilate voluntarily, generate normal inspiratory and expiratory muscle pressures (PI_{max}, PE_{max}, respectively) against an occluded airway, generate normal lung volumes and flow rates on routine spirometry, and have normal respiratory system resistance and compli-

Site of defect	Responses to CO_2, hypoxia: Ventil.	P.1	EMGdi	Sleep studies	Voluntary hyperventil.	PI_{max} PE_{max}	Volume flow rates	Resistance, compliance	(A-a) P_{O_2}
Metabolic control system (chemoreceptors, brainstem integrating neurons) ↓	↓	↓	↓	↑ Hypoventil, central apneas	N	N	N	N	N
Respiratory neuromuscular system (brainstem motoneurons, spinal cord, respiratory nerves and muscles) ↓	↓	↓	↓	↑ Hypoventil, central apneas	↓	↓	↓	N	N
Ventilatory apparatus (chest wall, lungs, airways)	↓	N	N	Variable	↓	N	Abnormal	Abnormal	↑

FIGURE 263-2 Pattern of laboratory test results in alveolar hypoventilation syndromes, based on the site of defect. Ventil, ventilation; P.1, mouth pressure generated after 0.1 s of inspiration against an occluded airway; EMGdi, diaphragmatic EMG; PI_{max}, PE_{max}, maximum inspiratory or expiratory pressure that can be generated against an occluded airway; (A − a) P_{O_2}, alveolar-arterial P_{O_2} difference; N, normal. Defects in the metabolic control system impair central respiratory drive in response to chemical stimuli (CO_2 or hypoxia); therefore responses of EMGdi, P.1, and minute volume of ventilation are reduced and hypoventilation during sleep is aggravated. In contrast, tests of voluntary respiratory control, muscle strength, lung mechanics, and gas exchange [(A − a)P_{O_2}] are normal. Defects in the respiratory neuromuscular system impair muscle strength; therefore all tests dependent on muscular activity (voluntary or in response to metabolic stimuli) are abnormal, but lung resistance, lung compliance, and gas exchange are normal. Defects in the ventilatory apparatus usually impair gas exchange. Because resistance and compliance are also impaired, all tests dependent on ventilation (whether voluntary or in response to chemical stimuli) are abnormal; in contrast, tests of muscle activity or strength that do not involve airflow (that is, P.1, EMGdi, PI_{max}, PE_{max}) are normal. *(After Phillipson.)*

ance and a normal alveolar-arterial P_{O_2} [$(A-a)P_{O_2}$] difference. Patients with defects in the respiratory neuromuscular system also have impaired responses to chemical stimuli but in addition are unable to hyperventilate voluntarily or to generate normal static respiratory muscle pressures, lung volumes, and flow rates. However, at least in the early stages of the disease, the resistance and compliance of the respiratory system and the alveolar-arterial oxygen difference are normal.

In contrast to patients with disorders of the respiratory control or neuromuscular systems, patients with disorders of the chest wall, lungs, and airways typically demonstrate abnormalities of respiratory system resistance and compliance and have a widened $(A-a)P_{O_2}$. Because of the impaired mechanics of breathing, routine spirometric tests are abnormal, as is the ventilatory response to chemical stimuli. However, because the neuromuscular system is intact, tests that are independent of resistance and compliance are usually normal, including tests of respiratory muscle strength and of respiratory control that do not involve airflow.

℞ TREATMENT

The management of chronic hypoventilation must be individualized to the patient's particular disorder, circumstances, and needs and should include measures directed toward the underlying disease. Coexistent metabolic alkalosis should be corrected, including elevations of HCO_3^- that are inappropriately high for the degree of chronic hypercapnia. Administration of supplemental oxygen is effective in attenuating hypoxemia, polycythemia, and pulmonary hypertension, but can aggravate CO_2 retention and the associated neurologic symptoms. For this reason, supplemental oxygen must be prescribed judiciously and the results monitored carefully. Pharmacologic agents that stimulate respiration (particularly progesterone) are of benefit in some patients, but generally, results are disappointing.

Most patients with chronic hypoventilation related to impairment of respiratory drive or neuromuscular disease eventually require mechanical ventilatory assistance for effective management. When hypoventilation is severe, treatment may be required on a 24-h basis, but in most patients ventilatory assistance only during sleep produces dramatic clinical improvement and lowering of daytime Pa_{CO_2}. In patients with reduced respiratory drive but intact respiratory lower motor neurons, phrenic nerves, and respiratory muscles, diaphragmatic pacing through an implanted phrenic electrode can be very effective. However, for patients with defects in the respiratory nerves and muscles, electrophrenic pacing is contraindicated. Such patients can usually be managed effectively with either intermittent negative-pressure ventilation in a cuirass or intermittent positive-pressure ventilation delivered through a tracheostomy or nose mask. For patients who require ventilatory assistance only during sleep, positive-pressure ventilation through a nose mask is the preferred method because it obviates a tracheostomy and avoids the problem of upper airway occlusion that can arise in a negative-pressure ventilator.

Hypoventilation related to restrictive disorders of the chest wall (see Table 263-1) also can be managed effectively with nocturnal intermittent positive-pressure ventilation through a nose mask or tracheostomy. Nocturnal ventilatory assistance also has been advocated for patients with hypercapnic chronic obstructive lung disease as a means of alleviating possible chronic respiratory muscle fatigue, but the efficacy of such an approach is variable and often disappointing.

HYPOVENTILATION SYNDROMES

PRIMARY ALVEOLAR HYPOVENTILATION Primary alveolar hypoventilation (PAH) is a disorder of unknown cause characterized by chronic hypercapnia and hypoxemia in the absence of identifiable neuromuscular disease or mechanical ventilatory impairment. The disorder is thought to arise from a defect in the metabolic respiratory control system, but few neuropathologic studies have been reported in such patients. Isolated PAH is relatively rare, and although it occurs in all age groups, the majority of reported cases have been in males aged 20 to 50 years. The disorder typically develops insidiously and often first comes to attention when severe respiratory depression follows administration of standard doses of sedatives or anesthetics. As the degree of hypoventilation increases, patients typically develop lethargy, fatigue, daytime somnolence, disturbed sleep, and morning headaches; eventually cyanosis, polycythemia, pulmonary hypertension, and congestive heart failure occur (see Fig. 263-1). Despite severe arterial blood gas derangements, dyspnea is uncommon, presumably because of impaired chemoreception and ventilatory drive. If left untreated, PAH is usually progressive over a period of months to years and ultimately fatal.

The key diagnostic finding in PAH is a chronic respiratory acidosis in the absence of respiratory muscle weakness or impaired ventilatory mechanics (see Fig. 263-2). Because patients can hyperventilate voluntarily and reduce Pa_{CO_2} to normal or even hypocapnic levels, hypercapnia may not be demonstrable in a single arterial blood sample, but the presence of an elevated plasma HCO_3^- level should draw attention to the underlying chronic disturbance. Despite normal ventilatory mechanics and respiratory muscle strength, ventilatory responses to chemical stimuli are reduced or absent (see Fig. 263-2), and breath-holding time may be markedly prolonged without any sensation of dyspnea.

Patients with PAH maintain rhythmic respiration when awake, although the level of ventilation is below normal. However, during sleep, when breathing is critically dependent on the metabolic control system, there is typically a further deterioration in ventilation with frequent episodes of central hypopnea or apnea, a disturbance that has been termed *Ondine's curse*.

PAH must be distinguished from other central hypoventilation syndromes that are secondary to underlying neurologic disease of the brainstem or chemoreceptors (see Table 263-1). This distinction requires a careful neurologic investigation for evidence of brainstem or autonomic disturbances. Unrecognized respiratory neuromuscular disorders, particularly those that produce diaphragmatic weakness, are often misdiagnosed as PAH. However, such disorders can usually be suspected on clinical grounds (see below) and can be confirmed by the finding of reduced voluntary hyperventilation, as well as PI_{max} and PE_{max}.

Some patients with PAH respond favorably to respiratory stimulant medications and to supplemental oxygen. However, the majority eventually require mechanical ventilatory assistance. Excellent long-term benefits can be achieved with diaphragmatic pacing by electrophrenic stimulation or with negative- or positive-pressure mechanical ventilation. The administration of such treatment only during sleep is sufficient in most patients.

RESPIRATORY NEUROMUSCULAR DISORDERS Several primary disorders of the spinal cord, peripheral respiratory nerves, and respiratory muscles produce a chronic hypoventilation syndrome (see Table 263-1). Hypoventilation usually develops gradually over a period of months to years and often first comes to attention when a relatively trivial increase in mechanical ventilatory load (such as mild airways obstruction) produces severe respiratory failure. In some of the disorders (such as motor neuron disease, myasthenia gravis, and muscular dystrophy), involvement of the respiratory nerves or muscles is usually a later feature of a more widespread disease. In other disorders, respiratory involvement can be an early or even isolated feature, and hence the underlying problem is often not suspected. Included in this category are the postpolio syndrome (a form of chronic respiratory insufficiency that develops 20 to 30 years following recovery from poliomyelitis), the myopathy associated with adult acid maltase deficiency, and idiopathic diaphragmatic paralysis.

Generally, respiratory neuromuscular disorders do not result in chronic hypoventilation unless there is significant weakness of the diaphragm. Distinguishing features of bilateral diaphragmatic weakness include orthopnea, paradoxical movement of the abdomen in the supine posture, and paradoxical diaphragmatic movement under fluoroscopy. However, the absence of these features does not exclude diaphragmatic weakness. Important laboratory features are a rapid deterioration of ventilation during a maximum voluntary ventilation maneuver and reduced PI_{max} and PE_{max} (see Fig. 263-2). More sophisticated investigations reveal reduced or absent transdiaphragmatic pressures, calculated from simultaneous measurement of esophageal and gastric pressures; reduced diaphragmatic EMG responses (recorded from an esophageal electrode) to transcutaneous phrenic nerve stimulation; and marked hypopnea and arterial oxygen desaturation during rapid eye movement sleep, when there is normally a physiologic inhibition of all nondiaphragmatic respiratory muscles and breathing becomes critically dependent on diaphragmatic activity.

The management of chronic alveolar hypoventilation due to respiratory neuromuscular disease involves treatment of the underlying disorder, where feasible, and mechanical ventilatory assistance as described for the primary alveolar hypoventilation syndrome. However, electrophrenic diaphragmatic pacing is contraindicated in these disorders, except for high cervical spinal cord lesions in which the phrenic lower motor neurons and nerves are intact.

OBESITY-HYPOVENTILATION SYNDROME Massive obesity represents a mechanical load to the respiratory system because the added weight on the rib cage and abdomen serves to reduce the compliance of the chest wall. As a result, the functional residual capacity (i.e., end-expiratory lung volume) is reduced, particularly in the recumbent posture. An important consequence of breathing at a low lung volume is that some airways, particularly those in the lung bases, may be closed throughout part or even all of each tidal breath, resulting in underventilation of the lung bases and widening of the $(A - a)P_{O_2}$. Nevertheless, in the majority of obese subjects, central respiratory drive is increased sufficiently to maintain a normal Pa_{CO_2}. However, a small proportion of obese subjects develop chronic hypercapnia, hypoxemia, and eventually polycythemia, pulmonary hypertension, and right-sided heart failure. Those patients who also develop daytime somnolence have been designated as having the *Pickwickian syndrome* (see Chap. 27). In many such patients, obstructive sleep apnea is a prominent feature, and even in those patients without sleep apnea, sleep-induced hypoventilation is an important element of the disorder and contributes to its progression. Most patients demonstrate a decrease in central respiratory drive, which may be inherent or acquired, and many have mild to moderate degrees of airflow obstruction, usually related to smoking. Based on these considerations, several therapeutic measures can be of considerable benefit, including weight loss, cessation of smoking, elimination of obstructive sleep apnea, and enhancement of respiratory drive by medications such as progesterone.

HYPERVENTILATION AND ITS SYNDROMES

DEFINITION AND ETIOLOGY Alveolar hyperventilation exists when Pa_{CO_2} decreases below the normal range of 37 to 43 mmHg. *Hyperventilation* is not synonymous with *hyperpnea*, which refers to an increased minute volume of ventilation without reference to Pa_{CO_2}. Although hyperventilation is frequently associated with dyspnea, patients who are hyperventilating do not necessarily complain of shortness of breath; and conversely, patients with dyspnea need not be hyperventilating.

Numerous disease entities can be associated with alveolar hyperventilation (Table 263-2), but in all cases the underlying mechanism involves an increase in respiratory drive that is mediated through either the behavioral or the metabolic respiratory control systems (Fig. 263-3). Thus hypoxemia drives ventilation by stimulating the peripheral chemoreceptors, and several pulmonary disorders and congestive heart failure drive ventilation by stimulating afferent vagal receptors in the lungs and airways. Low cardiac output and hypotension stimulate the peripheral chemoreceptors and inhibit the baroreceptors, both of which increase ventilation. Metabolic acidosis, a potent respiratory stimulant, excites both the peripheral and central chemoreceptors and increases the sensitivity of the peripheral chemoreceptors to coexistent hypoxemia. Hepatic failure also can produce hyperventilation, presumably as a result of metabolic stimuli acting on the peripheral and central chemoreceptors.

Table 263-2

Hyperventilation Syndromes

1. Hypoxemia
   a. High altitude
   b. Pulmonary disease
   c. Cardiac shunts
2. Pulmonary disorders
   a. Pneumonia
   b. Interstitial pneumonitis, fibrosis, edema
   c. Pulmonary emboli, vascular disease
   d. Bronchial asthma
   e. Pneumothorax
   f. Chest wall disorders
3. Cardiovascular disorders
   a. Congestive heart failure
   b. Hypotension
4. Metabolic disorders
   a. Acidosis (diabetic, renal, lactic)
   b. Hepatic failure
5. Neurologic and psychogenic disorders
   a. Psychogenic or anxiety hyperventilation
   b. Central nervous system infection, tumors
6. Drug-induced
   a. Salicylates
   b. Methylxanthine derivatives
   c. Beta-adrenergic agonists
   d. Progesterone
7. Miscellaneous
   a. Fever, sepsis
   b. Pain
   c. Pregnancy

Several neurologic and psychological disorders are thought to drive ventilation through the behavioral respiratory control system. Included in this category are psychogenic or anxiety hyperventilation and severe cerebrovascular insufficiency, which may interfere with the inhibitory influence normally exerted by cortical structures on the brainstem respiratory neurons. Rarely, disorders of the midbrain and hypothalamus induce hyperventilation, and it is conceivable that fever and sepsis also cause hyperventilation through effects on these structures. Several drugs cause hyperventilation by stimulating the central or peripheral chemoreceptors or by direct action on the brainstem respiratory neurons. Chronic hyperventilation is a normal feature of

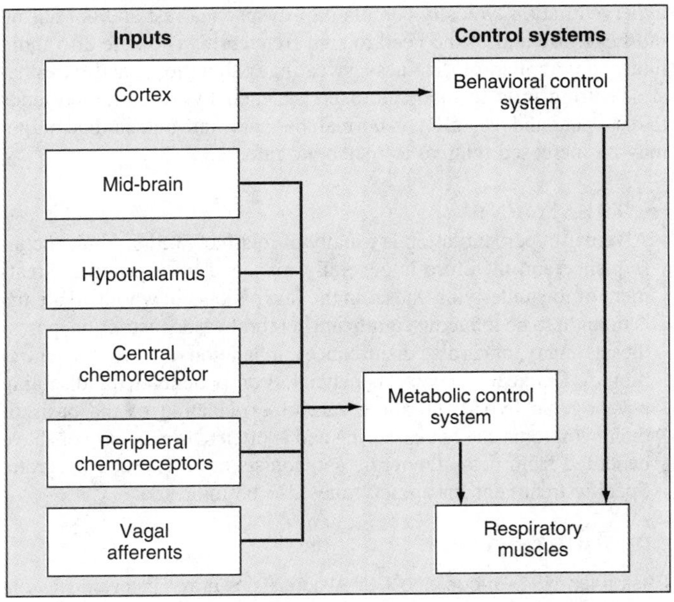

FIGURE 263-3 Schematic diagram of the mechanisms involved in alveolar hyperventilation. *(From Slutsky and Phillipson.)*

pregnancy and results from the effects of progesterone and other hormones acting on the respiratory neurons.

PHYSIOLOGIC AND CLINICAL FEATURES Because hyperventilation is associated with increased respiratory drive, muscle effort, and minute volume of ventilation, the most frequent symptom associated with hyperventilation is dyspnea. However, there is considerable discrepancy between the degree of hyperventilation, as measured by Pa_{CO_2}, and the degree of associated dyspnea. From a physiologic standpoint, hyperventilation is beneficial in patients who are hypoxemic, because the alveolar hypocapnia is associated with an increase in alveolar and arterial P_{O_2}. Conversely, hyperventilation can also be detrimental. In particular, the alkalemia associated with hypocapnia may produce neurologic symptoms, including dizziness, visual impairment, syncope, and seizure activity (secondary to cerebral vasoconstriction); parasthesias, carpopedal spasm, and tetany (secondary to decreased free serum calcium); and muscle weakness (secondary to hypophosphatemia). Severe alkalemia also can induce cardiac arrhythmias and evidence of myocardial ischemia. Patients with a primary respiratory alkalosis are also prone to periodic breathing and central sleep apnea (see Chap 264).

DIAGNOSIS In most patients with a hyperventilation syndrome, the cause is readily apparent on the basis of history, physical examination, and knowledge of coexisting medical disorders (see Table 263-2). In patients in whom the cause is not clinically apparent, investigation begins with arterial blood gas analysis, which establishes the presence of alveolar hyperventilation (decreased Pa_{CO_2}) and its severity. Equally important is the arterial pH, which generally allows the disorder to be classified as either a primary respiratory alkalosis (elevated pH) or a primary metabolic acidosis (decreased pH). Also of importance is the Pa_{O_2} and calculation of the $(A-a)P_{O_2}$, since a widened alveolar-arterial oxygen difference suggests a pulmonary disorder as the underlying cause. The finding of a reduced plasma HCO_3^- level establishes the chronic nature of the disorder and points toward an organic cause. Measurements of ventilation and arterial or transcutaneous P_{CO_2} during sleep are very useful in suspected psychogenic hyperventilation, since such patients do not maintain the hyperventilation during sleep.

The disorders that most frequently give rise to unexplained hyperventilation are pulmonary vascular disease (particularly chronic or recurrent thromboembolism) and psychogenic or anxiety hyperventilation. Hyperventilation due to pulmonary vascular disease is associated with exertional dyspnea, a widened $(A-a)P_{O_2}$ and maintenance of hyperventilation during exercise. In contrast, patients with psychogenic hyperventilation typically complain of dyspnea at rest and not during mild exercise and of the need to sigh frequently. They are also more likely to complain of dizziness, sweating, palpitations, and paresthesias. During mild to moderate exercise, their hyperventilation tends to disappear and $(A-a)P_{O_2}$ is normal, but heart rate and cardiac output may be increased relative to metabolic rate.

℞ TREATMENT

Alveolar hyperventilation is usually of relatively minor clinical consequence and therefore is generally managed by appropriate treatment of the underlying cause. In the few patients in whom alkalemia is thought to be inducing significant cerebral vasoconstriction, paresthesia, tetany, or cardiac disturbances, inhalation of a low concentration of CO_2 can be very beneficial. For patients with disabling psychogenic hyperventilation, careful explanation of the basis of their symptoms can be reassuring and is often sufficient. Others have benefited from beta-adrenergic antagonists or an exercise program. Specific treatment for anxiety may also be indicated.

BIBLIOGRAPHY

Cherniack NS, Longobardo GS: Abnormalities in respiratory rhythm, in *Handbook of Physiology*, section 3: *The Respiratory System*, vol 2, *Control of Breathing*, NS Cherniack, JG Widdicombe (eds). Bethesda, MD, Am Physiol Soc, 1986, pp 729–749

Fanburg BL, Sicilian L (eds): Respiratory dysfunction in neuromuscular disease. Clin Chest Med 15:(4)607, 1994

Meyer TJ, Hill NS: Noninvasive positive pressure ventilation to treat respiratory failure. Ann Intern Med 120:760, 1994

Phillipson EA: Hypoventilation syndromes, in *Textbook of Respiratory Medicine*, 2d ed, JF Murray, JA Nadel (eds). Philadelphia, Saunders, 1994, chap 83, pp 2291–2300

Slutsky AS, Phillipson EA: Hyperventilation syndromes, in *Textbook of Respiratory Medicine*, JF Murray, JA Nadel (eds). Philadelphia, Saunders, 1994, chap 85, pp 2325–2332

264 SLEEP APNEA

Eliot A. Phillipson

DEFINITION AND CLASSIFICATION *Sleep apnea* is defined as an intermittent cessation of airflow at the nose and mouth during sleep. By convention, apneas of at least 10 s duration have been considered important, but in most patients the apneas are 20 to 30 s in duration and may be as long as 2 to 3 min. *Sleep apnea syndrome* refers to a clinical disorder that arises from recurrent apneas during sleep. There is uncertainty as to the minimum number of apneas that should be considered clinically important, although by the time most patients come to attention they have at least 10 to 15 events per hour of sleep. The clinical importance of sleep apnea arises from the fact that it is one of the leading causes of excessive daytime sleepiness. Indeed, epidemiologic studies have established a prevalence of clinically important sleep apnea of at least 2 percent in middle-aged women and 4 percent in middle-aged men.

Sleep apneas have been classified into three types: central, obstructive, and mixed. In central sleep apnea (CSA) the neural drive to all the respiratory muscles is transiently abolished. In contrast, in obstructive sleep apnea (OSA) airflow ceases despite continuing respiratory drive because of occlusion of the oropharyngeal airway. Mixed apneas, which consist of a central apnea followed by an obstructive component, are a variant of OSA.

OBSTRUCTIVE SLEEP APNEA **Pathogenesis** The definitive event in OSA is occlusion of the upper airway usually at the level of the oropharynx (Fig. 264-1). The resulting apnea leads to progressive asphyxia until there is a brief arousal from sleep, whereupon airway patency is restored and airflow resumes. The patient then returns to sleep, and the sequence of events is repeated, often up to 400 to 500 times per night, resulting in marked fragmentation of sleep.

The immediate factor leading to collapse of the upper airway in OSA is the generation of a critical subatmospheric pressure during inspiration that exceeds the ability of the airway dilator and abductor muscles to maintain airway stability (see Fig. 264-1). Sleep plays a permissive but crucial role by reducing the activity of the muscles of the upper airways and the protective reflex response of the muscles to subatmospheric airway pressures. Alcohol is frequently an important cofactor because of its selective depressant influence on the upper airway muscles and on the arousal response that terminates each apnea. In most patients the patency of the airway is also compromised structurally and therefore predisposed to occlusion. In a minority of patients the structural compromise is due to obvious anatomic disturbances, such as adenotonsillar hypertrophy, retrognathia, and macroglossia. However, in the majority of patients the structural defect is simply a subtle reduction in airway size that can often be appreciated clinically as "pharyngeal crowding" and that can usually be demonstrated by imaging and acoustic reflection techniques. Obesity frequently contributes to the reduction in size of the upper airways, either by increasing fat deposition in the soft tissues of the pharynx or by compressing the pharynx by superficial fat masses in the neck. Snoring, a high-frequency vibration of the palatal and pharyngeal soft tissues that results from the decrease in size of the upper airway lumen, may aggravate the narrowing by producing edema of the soft tissues. More sophisticated studies also demonstrate a high airway compliance—

i.e., the airway is "floppy" and therefore prone to collapse. In some patients, a high upstream (i.e., nasal) resistance predisposes to collapse of the upper airway by increasing the subatmospheric pressure generated in the pharynx during inspiration as the strength of diaphragmatic contraction is increased to overcome airflow resistance in the nose.

Pathophysiologic and Clinical Features The narrowing of the upper airways during sleep, which predisposes to OSA, inevitably results in snoring. In most patients, snoring antedates the development of obstructive events by many years. However, the majority of snoring individuals do not have an OSA disorder. Although a few recent studies suggest that snoring per se may be associated with long-term health risks, definitive evidence in this regard is lacking. Hence, in the absence of other symptoms, snoring alone does not warrant an investigation for OSA but does call for preventive counselling, particularly with regard to weight gain and alcohol consumption.

The recurrent episodes of nocturnal asphyxia and of arousal from sleep that characterize OSA lead to a series of secondary physiologic events, which in turn give rise in some patients to the clinical complications of the syndrome (see Fig. 264-1). The most common manifestations are neuropsychiatric and behavioral disturbances that are thought to arise from the fragmentation of sleep and loss of slow-wave sleep induced by the recurrent arousal responses. Nocturnal cerebral hypoxia also may play an important role. The most pervasive manifestation is excessive daytime sleepiness. Initially, daytime sleepiness manifests under passive conditions, such as reading or watching television; but as the disorder progresses, sleepiness encroaches into all daily activities and can become disabling and dangerous. Several studies have demonstrated two to three times more motor vehicle accidents in patients with OSA compared with other drivers. Other related symptoms include intellectual impairment, memory loss, and personality disturbances. In men with OSA, impotence is a relatively frequent complaint.

The other major manifestations of OSA are cardiorespiratory in nature and are thought to arise from the recurrent episodes of nocturnal asphyxia (see Fig. 264-1). Many patients demonstrate a cyclical slowing of the heart during the apneas to 30 to 50 beats per minute, followed by a tachycardia of 90 to 120 beats per minute during the ventilatory phase. A small number of patients develop severe bradycardia with asystoles of 8- to 12-s duration or dangerous tachyarrhythmias, including unsustained ventricular tachycardia. The presence of such arrhythmias has led to the notion that OSA may result in sudden death during sleep, but firm corroborative data are lacking. Unlike in healthy subjects, in patients with OSA systemic blood pressure fails to decrease during sleep. In fact, blood pressure typically rises abruptly at the termination of each obstructive event. Furthermore, several epidemiologic studies have implicated OSA as a risk factor for the development of systemic hypertension, myocardial ischemia and infarction, stroke, and premature death. However, because these studies were cross-sectional or retrospective in design, the natural history of OSA remains largely undefined. OSA also markedly aggravates left ventricular failure in patients with underlying heart disease. This complication is probably due to the combined effects of increased left ventricular afterload during each obstructive event, secondary to increased negative intrathoracic pressure (see Fig. 264-1), recurrent nocturnal hypoxemia, and chronically elevated sympathoadrenal activity. Treatment of OSA in such patients often results in dramatic improvement in left ventricular function. Finally, a small proportion of patients with OSA (<10 percent) develop pulmonary hypertension, right ventricular failure, polycythemia, and chronic hypercapnia and hypoxemia. All such patients have evidence of sustained daytime hypoxemia in addition to the nocturnal ventilatory disturbance, usually as a result of reduced ventilatory drive and/or diffuse airways obstruction. Most of these patients are obese and sleepy and are therefore said to have the *Pickwickian syndrome*.

Diagnosis Although OSA occurs at any age, and is more prevalent in women than was previously thought, the typical patient is a male aged 30 to 60 years who presents with a history of snoring, excessive daytime sleepiness, nocturnal choking or gasping, witnessed apneas during sleep, moderate obesity, and often mild to moderate hypertension. The diagnosis can often be confirmed by direct observation of the patient during sleep. However, the definitive investigation for suspected OSA is polysomnography, a detailed overnight sleep study that includes recording of (1) electrographic variables (electroencephalogram, electrooculogram, and submental electromyogram) that

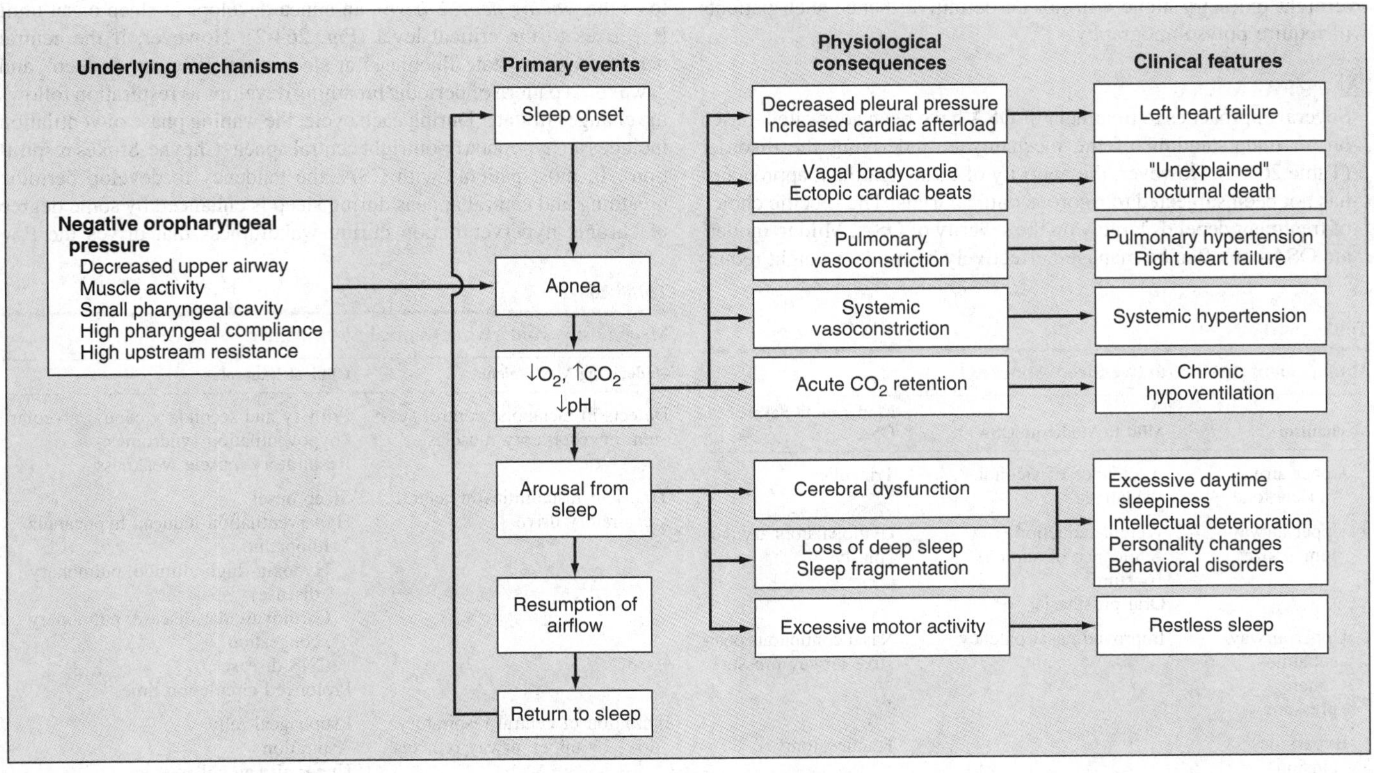

FIGURE 264-1 The primary sequence of events, underlying mechanisms, physiologic responses, and clinical features of obstructive sleep apnea. *(From EA Phillipson, Med Clin North Am 23:2314, 1982.)*

permit the identification of sleep and its various stages, (2) ventilatory variables that permit the identification of apneas and their classification as central or obstructive, (3) arterial O_2 saturation by ear or finger oximetry, and (4) heart rate. Continuous measurement of transcutaneous P_{CO_2} (which reflects arterial P_{CO_2}) can also be very useful, particularly in patients with central sleep apnea. The key diagnostic finding in OSA is episodes of airflow cessation at the nose and mouth despite evidence of continuing respiratory effort.

Because polysomnography is a time-consuming and expensive test, there is considerable interest in the role of simplified, unattended, ambulatory sleep monitoring for the investigation of OSA that would allow the patient to be studied at home, rather than in the sleep laboratory. The most useful test in this context is the recording of arterial O_2 saturation by oximetry. However, the reliability of overnight oximetry in the diagnosis of OSA is dependent on the pretest probability of the disorder. In patients with a high pretest probability (based on a history of daytime sleepiness, habitual snoring, nocturnal choking or gasping, and witnessed apneas during sleep), overnight oximetry can be used to *confirm* the diagnosis by demonstrating recurrent episodes of arterial O_2 desaturation (at a rate of at least 10 to 15 events per hour). Such findings obviate the need for full polysomnography and allow initiation of treatment with nasal continuous positive airway pressure (CPAP) during sleep (see "Treatment"). However, negative results in a patient with a high clinical probability of OSA do not exclude the diagnosis but mandate that the patient proceed to polysomnography to investigate the cause of the daytime sleepiness. In contrast, when the pretest probability of OSA is low (such as the patient with only occasional snoring, few witnessed apneas, and no daytime sleepiness), the absence of arterial O_2 desaturation can be used to *exclude* the diagnosis and thereby obviate the need for full polysomnography.

Studies suggest that overnight oximetry can obviate the need for polysomnography in about one-third of clinic patients referred for consideration of OSA, either by *confirming* the diagnosis in patients with a *high* pretest probability of the disorder, or by *excluding* the diagnosis in patients with a *low* pretest probability. In the remaining two-thirds of patients with an intermediate pretest probability of OSA, overnight oximetry alone will not be definitive; hence such patients will require polysomnography.

℞ TREATMENT

Several approaches to treatment of OSA have been advocated, based on an understanding of the mechanisms underlying the disorder (Table 264-1). However, the majority of these treatment approaches has not been subjected to rigorous clinical trials. The specific choice of treatment depends largely on the severity of OSA. Mild to moderate OSA can often be managed effectively by modest weight reduction, avoidance of alcohol, improvement of nasal patency, and avoidance of sleeping in the supine posture. Intraoral appliances, designed to keep the mandible and tongue forward, may also be effective. In some patients with more severe OSA, tricyclic medications, particularly protriptyline (20 to 30 mg at bedtime), have been beneficial. The role of nocturnal supplemental oxygen in managing OSA is uncertain but is generally not satisfactory. The most widely used treatments in moderate to severe OSA are uvulopalatopharyngoplasty and nasal CPAP during sleep. Uvulopalatopharyngoplasty is a surgical procedure designed to increase the pharyngeal lumen by resecting redundant soft tissue. When applied to unselected patients with OSA, it produces long-term benefits in only about 50 percent. More recent attempts to select patients based on the specific site of upper airway occlusion have yielded a higher success rate. Nasal CPAP, which prevents upper airway occlusion by splinting the pharyngeal airway with a positive pressure delivered through a nose mask, is currently the most successful long-term approach to treatment, being well tolerated and effective in over 80 percent of patients, provided that they have received proper training. For the few patients with severe OSA in whom all other treatment approaches fail, tracheostomy provides immediate relief.

CENTRAL SLEEP APNEA Pathogenesis The definitive event in CSA is transient abolition of central drive to the ventilatory muscles. The resulting apnea leads to a primary sequence of events similar to those of OSA (see Fig. 264-1). Several underlying mechanisms can result in cessation of respiratory drive during sleep (Table 264-2). First are defects in the metabolic respiratory control system and respiratory neuromuscular apparatus. Such defects usually produce a chronic alveolar hypoventilation syndrome (in addition to CSA) that becomes more severe during sleep when the stimulatory effect of wakefulness on breathing is abolished. In contrast are CSA disorders that arise from transient instabilities in an otherwise intact respiratory control system. Common to all these disorders is a P_{CO_2} level during sleep that falls transiently below the critical P_{CO_2} required for respiratory rhythm generation. The most frequent instability of this type occurs at sleep onset, because the P_{CO_2} level of wakefulness is often lower than that required for rhythm generation in sleep; hence with loss of the stimulatory effect of wakefulness on breathing (referred to as the *waking neural drive*), an apnea develops at sleep onset until P_{CO_2} rises to the critical level (Fig. 264-2). However, if the central nervous system state fluctuates at sleep onset between "asleep" and "awake," a pattern of periodic breathing develops as respiration follows the changes in state. During each cycle, the waning phase of ventilation includes an hypopnea or outright central apnea (Cheyne-Stokes respiration). In most patients with CSA, the tendency to develop periodic breathing and central apneas during sleep is enhanced by some degree of chronic hyperventilation during wakefulness that drives the P_{CO_2}

Table 264-1

Management of Obstructive Sleep Apnea (OSA)

Mechanism	Mild to Moderate OSA	Moderate to Severe OSA
↑ Upper airway muscle tone	Avoidance of alcohol, sedatives	Tricyclics
↑ Upper airway lumen size	Weight reduction Avoidance of supine posture Oral prosthesis	Uvulopalatopharyngoplasty
↓ Upper airway subatmospheric pressure	Improved nasal patency	Nasal continuous positive airway pressure
Bypass occlusion		Tracheostomy

SOURCE: Phillipson, with permission.

Table 264-2

Mechanisms Underlying Central Sleep Apnea

Underlying Mechanism	Clinical Example
Defects in metabolic control system or respiratory muscles	Primary and secondary central alveolar hypoventilation syndromes Respiratory muscle weakness
Transient instabilities in central respiratory drive	Sleep onset Hyperventilation-induced hypocapnia Idiopathic Hypoxia (high altitude, pulmonary disease) Cardiovascular disease, pulmonary congestion CNS disease Prolonged circulation time
Inhibition of central respiratory drive by upper airway reflexes	Esophageal reflux Aspiration Upper airway collapse

SOURCE: Phillipson, with permission.

level below the threshold required for rhythm generation during sleep. Such hyperventilation is frequently idiopathic in nature. Hypoxia, whether due to high altitude or to underlying cardiorespiratory disease, also enhances the tendency to periodic breathing and CSA for the same reasons. Hyperventilation due to central nervous system disease or to lung congestion secondary to heart failure produces periodic breathing and CSA by a similar mechanism. Circulatory slowing secondary to cardiac failure also may induce ventilatory instability by prolonging the time lag between changes in blood gas values by ventilation and the detection of those changes by the peripheral and central chemoreceptors (Chap. 233). Consequently, the ventilatory system overshoots the mark before reversing direction, resulting in periodic breathing that frequently includes central apneas.

Pathophysiologic and Clinical Features Many healthy individuals demonstrate a small number of central apneas during sleep, particularly at sleep onset and in rapid eye movement sleep. These apneas are not associated with any physiologic or clinical disturbances. In patients with clinically important CSA, the primary sequence of events that characterizes the disorder leads to prominent physiologic and clinical consequences (see Fig. 264-1). In those patients whose CSA is a component of an alveolar hypoventilation syndrome, daytime hypercapnia and hypoxemia are usually evident, and the clinical picture is dominated by a history of recurrent respiratory failure, polycythemia, pulmonary hypertension, and right-sided heart failure. Complaints of sleeping poorly, morning headache, and daytime fatigue and sleepiness are also prominent. In contrast, in patients whose CSA results from an instability in respiratory drive, the clinical picture is dominated by features related to sleep disturbance, including recurrent nocturnal awakenings, morning fatigue, and daytime sleepiness.

Diagnosis Initially, many patients with CSA are suspected clinically of having OSA because of a history of snoring, sleep disturbance, and daytime sleepiness. However, obesity and hypertension are less prominent in CSA than in OSA. Definitive diagnosis of CSA requires a polysomnographic study, with the *key observation being recurrent apneas that are not accompanied by respiratory effort*. Measurements of transcutaneous P_{CO_2} are particularly useful in CSA. Those patients with a defect in respiratory control or neuromuscular function typically demonstrate an elevated P_{CO_2} that tends to increase progressively during the night, particularly during rapid eye movement sleep. In contrast, patients with instabilities in the respiratory control system typically demonstrate a mild degree of hypocapnia, which is an integral pathogenetic feature of their disorder (see above).

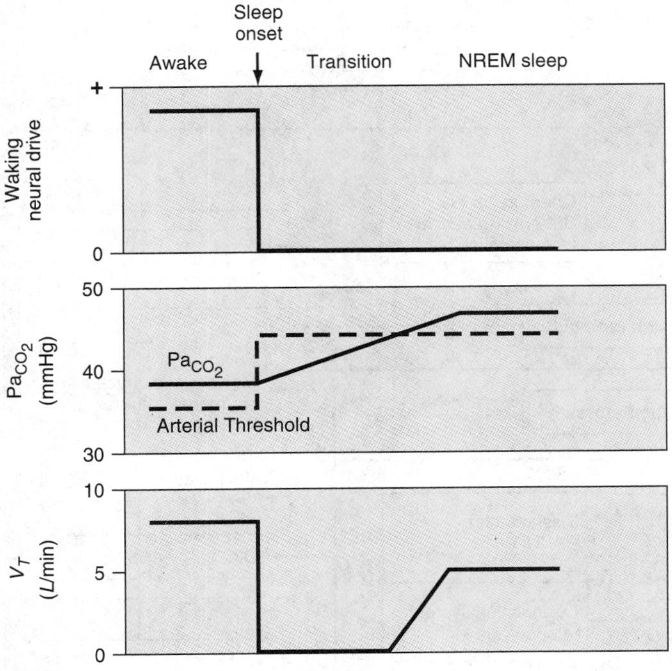

FIGURE 264-2 Schematic diagram of the mechanisms underlying central sleep apnea at sleep onset. With loss of the waking neural drive to breathing, the arterial threshold P_{CO_2} for rhythm generation increases above the Pa_{CO_2} present during wakefulness; hence tidal volume (V_T) falls to zero and apnea ensues until Pa_{CO_2} rises above the threshold for rhythm generation during sleep. NREM, non-rapid eye movement. *(From TD Bradley, EA Phillipson, Clin Chest Med 13:439, 1992.)*

TREATMENT

The management of patients whose CSA is a component of an alveolar hypoventilation syndrome is essentially the same as management of the underlying hypoventilation disorder (see Chap. 263). Management of patients whose CSA arises from an instability of respiratory drive is more problematic. Patients with hypoxemia usually respond favorably to nocturnal supplemental oxygen. Others have responded to acidification with acetazolamide, and recent reports indicate a good response to nasal CPAP (as for OSA). The mechanism by which CPAP abolishes central apneas probably involves a small increase in Pa_{CO_2} as a result of the added expiratory mechanical load. In patients whose CSA is secondary to congestive heart failure, CPAP is particularly effective in improving sleep quality and daytime cardiac function.

BIBLIOGRAPHY

Deegan PC, McNicholas WT: Pathophysiology of obstructive sleep apnoea. Eur Respir J 8:1161, 1995

National Commission on Sleep Disorders Research: *Wake up America: A National Sleep Alert.* Washington, DC, Government Printing Office, 1993

Naughton MT et al: Treatment of congestive heart failure and Cheyne-Stokes respiration during sleep by continuous positive airway pressure. Am J Respir Crit Care Med 151:92, 1995

Phillipson EA: Sleep disorders, in *Textbook of Respiratory Medicine,* 2d ed, JF Murray, JA Nadel (eds). Philadelphia, Saunders, 1994, chap 84, pp 2301–2324

———, Bradley TD (eds): Breathing disorders in sleep. Clin Chest Med 13:(3)383, 1992

Young T et al: The occurrence of sleep-disordered breathing among middle-aged adults. N Engl J Med 328:1230, 1993

265

Eric G. Honig, Roland H. Ingram, Jr.

ACUTE RESPIRATORY DISTRESS SYNDROME

The acute respiratory distress syndrome (ARDS; formerly known as the adult respiratory distress syndrome) is a condition characterized by acute hypoxemic respiratory failure due to pulmonary edema caused by increased permeability of the alveolar capillary barrier. ARDS represents the most serious manifestation of a spectrum of responses to acute lung injury (ALI); these responses occur as complications of a more widespread systemic response to acute inflammation or injury. Recent consensus groups have attempted to establish working definitions for ARDS and underlying systemic inflammatory states. ALI may be said to be present in the setting of severe hypoxemia of acute onset and bilateral diffuse opacities on a frontal chest radiograph when left atrial or pulmonary capillary hypertension have been excluded. ARDS is differentiated from ALI by the severity of the hypoxemia and is defined as a ratio of arterial P_{O_2} to inspired oxygen fraction (Pa_{O_2}/FI_{O_2}) ≤ 200 mmHg. ALI and ARDS should be viewed as the earliest and most recognizable manifestations of an infectious or inflammatory systemic disorder. The lung figures so prominently in systemic injury because it receives all of the cardiac output and because impairment of pulmonary function is readily apparent clinically.

ALI develops rapidly after a predisposing condition triggers a systemic inflammatory response, often within 90 min. Over half of all cases develop within 24 h of the underlying insult. ALI is most strongly associated with conditions that produce direct alveolar injury or indirect injury via the pulmonary capillary bed. These are listed in Table 265-1. The likelihood of ARDS varies with the precipitating causes, from a 13 percent risk associated with drug overdose to a 43 percent risk for patients with sepsis.

Table 265-1

Conditions That May Lead to the Acute Respiratory Distress Syndrome

Direct injury to alveolar epithelium	Indirect lung injury
Aspiration	Sepsis syndrome
Diffuse infection	Severe nonthoracic trauma
Near-drowning	Hypertransfusion
Toxic inhalation	Cardiopulmonary bypass
Airway contusion	

PATHOPHYSIOLOGY

ALI is the consequence of an unregulated overexpression of usual systemic inflammatory responses to infection and/or injury. Injury involves both the alveolar epithelium and the pulmonary capillary endothelium. The inciting event initiates a complex cascade of cellular and biochemical events outlined schematically in Fig. 265-1. These events may be thought of as occurring in three phases: *initiation*, in which the trigger event activates the cellular cascade; *amplification*, in which the effector cells are recruited and activated; and *injury*, i.e., expression of these events at the tissue level. Injury is produced by cellular events associated with neutrophils, macrophages, monocytes, and lymphocytes producing various cytokines, in turn producing cellular activation, chemotaxis, and adhesion. Activated cells produce a series of inflammatory mediators, including oxidants, proteases, kinins, growth factors, neuropeptides, activators of the complement cascade, intravascular coagulation, and fibrinolysis.

The pathophysiologic hallmark of ARDS is increased vascular permeability to proteins leaving the hydrostatic gradient unopposed so that even mild elevations in capillary pressures (due to increased intravenous liquid loads and cardiac dysfunction characteristic of sepsis) greatly increase interstitial and alveolar edema. This additive effect of permeability and hydrostatic factors is illustrated by the increased severity of disease involvement in dependent lung regions (Fig. 265-2). The increase in the ratio of lung tissue to gas in these lung zones causes alveolar closing pressures to exceed local transpulmonary pressures, leading to alveolar closure and collapse. The tendency to alveolar collapse is further exaggerated by the quantitative reduction in surfactant synthesis due to injury to type II pneumocytes as well as to further abnormalities in the size, composition, and metabolism of the remaining surfactant pool. Although these atelectatic regions of the lung contribute to a reduction in the compliance of the lung as a whole, significant regions of nondependent lung have relatively normal mechanical and gas-exchanging properties. The burden of ventilation and gas exchange is shifted to these uninvolved lung regions; by analogy, the respiratory function of the adult patient must be provided by a pair of baby-sized lungs.

Because of the decreased compliance, large inspiratory pressures must be generated by the respiratory muscles, so the work of breathing is elevated. The large mechanical load may lead to fatigue of the muscles of breathing with resulting diminution in tidal volumes and worsening gas exchange. Both hypoxemia and the stimulation of receptors in the stiff lung parenchyma cause an increase in respiratory frequency, decrease in tidal volume, and deterioration in gas exchange.

Airways resistance may be increased because minute volume must be handled by a decreased number of ventilating airways and because of airway narrowing from excess liquid and bronchospasm. Pulmonary vascular resistance and pulmonary arterial pressures are also elevated, initially because of neurohumoral factors and later due to obstruction, obliteration, and remodeling. Gas exchange is characterized by low ventilation-perfusion ratios and extensive shunt accompanied by an elevated dead space. Shunt is due to atelectasis, alveolar collapse,

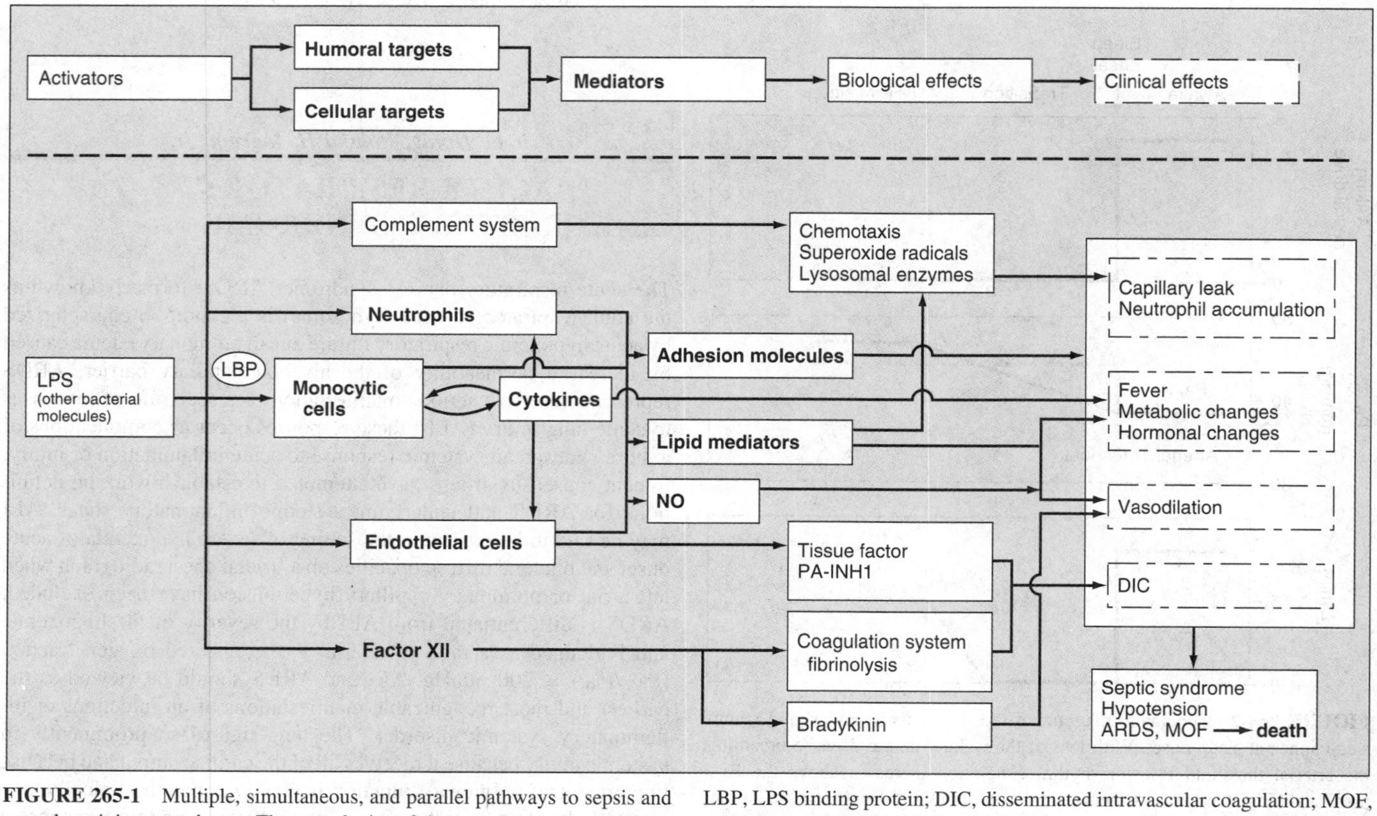

FIGURE 265-1 Multiple, simultaneous, and parallel pathways to sepsis and acute lung injury are shown. The complexity of the response and multiplicity of involved pathways present a formidable challenge to the design of effective pharmacotherapeutic approaches to sepsis and ARDS. LPS, lipopolysaccharide; LBP, LPS binding protein; DIC, disseminated intravascular coagulation; MOF, multiple organ failure. *[From MP Glauser et al, Clin Infect Dis 18(suppl 2):S205, 1994, with permission.]*

surfactant dysfunction, and attenuation of hypoxic vasoconstriction. Increase in dead space is caused by obstruction and obliteration of the pulmonary capillary bed.

PATHOLOGY Pathologic changes in ARDS evolve over three distinct phases, and the lesions correlate with these phases much better than the underlying cause of lung injury since the lung has a limited number of ways in which it reacts to a wide variety of injuries. Grossly, the lungs are heavy and edematous, with regions of hemorrhage, atelectasis, and consolidation.

The acute exudative phase, covering the first 3 days after lung injury, is characterized by the formation of hyaline membranes composed of fibrin and other matrix proteins in alveolar ducts and airspaces. Epithelial cell injury is represented by extensive necrosis of type I pneumocytes and a denuded basement membrane that allows free entry of liquid and macromolecules into the airspaces. Endothelial injury becomes manifest as cellular edema and a widening of intercellular junctions. Thromboemboli and in situ thrombi are found within the vasculature. Over the next week, the alveolar exudate is either resolved or undergoes organization, i.e., the proliferative phase. Cuboidal type II cells and squamous epithelium cover denuded alveolar basement membranes. Fibroblasts begin to enter the hyaline membranes and to produce collagen. After 3 to 4 weeks, changes characteristic of the fibrotic phase are seen. Microcystic airspaces enlarge to form cystic and honeycomb changes in dependent lung. Airspaces and alveolar ducts undergo fibrosis, while peripheral bronchi become dilated. Fibrocellular intimal proliferation occurs in small muscular arteries, veins, and pulmonary lymphatics. Extensive remodeling of the pulmonary capillary bed occurs, as well as muscularization of acinar blood vessels.

CLINICAL CHARACTERISTICS At the time of initial injury and for several hours thereafter, the patient may be free of respiratory symptoms or signs. The earliest sign often is an increase in respiratory frequency followed shortly by dyspnea. Arterial blood gas measurement in the earlier period will disclose a depressed P_{O_2} despite a decreased P_{CO_2}, so that the alveolar-arterial difference for oxygen (Chap. 250) is increased. At this early stage, administration of oxygen results in a significant increase in the Pa_{O_2}. The brisk rise in Pa_{O_2} indicates that ventilation-perfusion mismatching and, possibly, diffusion impairment account for the widened alveolar-arterial P_{O_2} difference [$(\text{A}-\text{a})P_{O_2}$] initially. Physical examination may be unremarkable, although a few fine inspiratory rales may be audible. Radiographically, the lung fields may be clear or demonstrate only minimal and scattered interstitial infiltrates. With progression, the patient becomes cyanotic and increasingly dyspneic and tachypneic. Rales become more prominent and easily heard throughout both lung fields, along with regions of tubular breath sounds; the chest radiograph demonstrates diffuse, extensive bilateral interstitial and alveolar infiltrates (Fig. 265-2). At this point, hypoxemia cannot be corrected simply by increasing the oxygen concentration of the inspired gas, and mechanical ventilatory support must be started. Right-to-left shunting of blood through collapsed or filled alveoli becomes the major mechanism for arterial hypoxemia at this more advanced stage. In contrast to ventilation-perfusion mismatching and diffusion impairment, with right-to-left shunts the $(\text{A}-\text{a})P_{O_2}$ remains high with breathing of pure oxygen. Positive end-expiratory pressure (PEEP) serves to increase lung volume, which in turn opens collapsed alveoli and decreases shunting. With further progression, and if mechanical ventilator and PEEP therapy are delayed, the combination of increasing tachypnea and decreasing tidal volumes results in alveolar hypoventilation, a rising P_{CO_2}, and worsening hypoxemia; these represent an ominous constellation of findings.

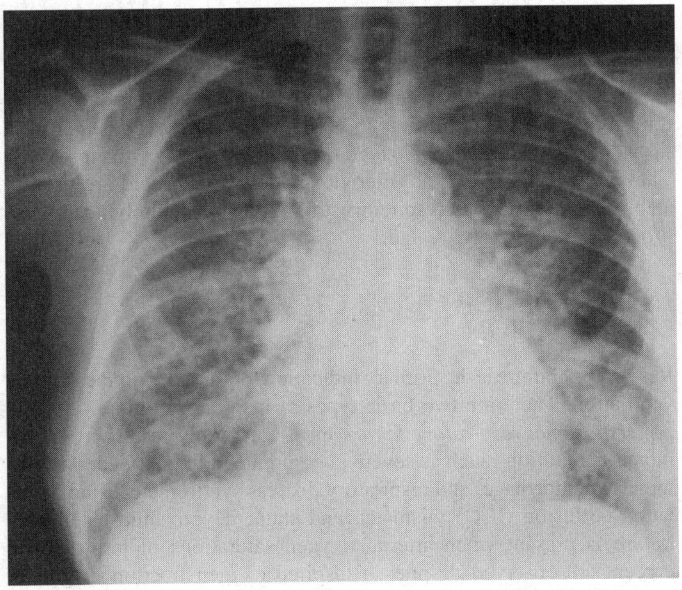

FIGURE 265-2 A standard posteroanterior chest radiograph from a patient with the acute respiratory distress syndrome secondary to a severe viral pneumonitis. Such a diffuse radiographic change is typical of all conditions listed in Table 265-1 when they are severe enough to cause acute hypoxemic respiratory failure. A similar radiographic picture is also seen in pulmonary edema due to left ventricular failure (Chap. 32). Often in such acutely ill patients, the radiograph must be taken with a portable unit and the film exposed from the anterior direction. Both the anteroposterior exposure and the failure to take a deep inspiration result in an apparent enlargement of the cardiac silhouette, which further obscures the reliable detection of left ventricular failure.

℞ TREATMENT

Supportive Management of Hypoxemia The simplest method and the lowest inspired fraction of oxygen (F_{IO_2}) should be used to achieve a Pa_{O_2} of 60 mmHg (O_2 saturation approximately 90%). Higher levels add little to oxygenation and introduce the risk of oxygen toxicity to the lung. The three main methods for delivering O_2, in order of increasing effectiveness, are soft nasal prongs, simple face masks, and face masks with inspiratory reservoir bags. It is reasonable to start with moderate flow rates (5 to 10 L/min of 100% O_2) and to monitor arterial blood gases, adjusting the flow rates and O_2 concentrations depending on results.

Mechanical Ventilatory Support In the presence of ARDS, adequate oxygenation is usually not maintained with these less invasive measures. Endotracheal intubation is needed, and mechanical ventilatory support with a volume-cycled ventilator should be instituted (see Chap. 266). The rationale behind mechanical ventilatory support in a patient who is hyperventilating is not to increase ventilation but to increase mean lung volume, thereby opening previously closed airways and improving oxygenation. The goal of ventilation for ARDS is to provide physiologic support for gas exchange while avoiding adverse mechanical consequences of the intervention. Because of the heterogeneous involvement of the lung in ARDS, setting tidal volumes to accomplish this goal for the lung as a whole carries the risk of overdistending or rupturing less affected alveoli and producing extraalveolar air (barotrauma). The latter is best avoided by limiting alveolar distending pressures through the use of relatively small tidal volumes (approximately 6 to 10 mL/kg of lean body weight) with a respiratory frequency set to deliver a minute volume that produces a pH above 7.25 to 7.30. Because of the small volume of aerated lung, high frequencies may be needed to provide an adequate minute volume. Alveolar inflation pressure, or peak inflation pressure, should be kept as low as possible consistent with sufficient ventilation and oxygenation. Inspired oxygen fraction (F_{IO_2}) is initially set at 1.0 and then decreased in steps to the lowest inspired fraction that will maintain a Pa_{O_2} of 60 mmHg.

If Pa_{O_2} cannot be maintained at 60 mmHg by an F_{IO_2} of 60% or less, PEEP may be added. PEEP improves oxygenation by elevating mean alveolar pressure, thereby recruiting atelectatic alveoli and preventing end-expiratory airway and alveolar closure. Because an adequate PEEP level for affected lung regions may overdistend uninvolved alveoli, PEEP should be added cautiously, starting at

5 cmH_2O and increasing in increments of 3 to 5 cmH_2O to a maximum of 15 cmH_2O. Because airway pressure is transmitted to the pleural space, cardiac output may be adversely affected. The optimal levels of PEEP are those associated with the greatest delivery of O_2 to the body; the latter is the product of cardiac output and arterial oxygen content.

It is desirable to minimize left atrial and left ventricular diastolic pressures. Small decrements in pulmonary capillary wedge pressure (PCWP) have been shown to produce significant decreases in extravascular lung water. However, caution must be exercised in reducing PCWP, since excessively vigorous diuresis, especially in the setting of PEEP, may reduce cardiac output and the perfusion of critical organs. During interventions that change intravascular volume, placement of a Swan-Ganz pulmonary arterial flotation catheter may be instructive in monitoring cardiac output and PCWP in order to assess the effects of therapeutic interventions. Mental status and urine output should also be followed closely. The development of a wide anion gap metabolic acidosis should alert the clinician to the possibility of lactic acidemia due to inadequate tissue perfusion. Insufficient intravascular volume can be identified by a decrease of arterial pressure with the addition of modest amounts of PEEP. For these patients, blood volume should be expanded as long as cardiac output increases in response to the infusion and PCWP does not rise above 12 mmHg. Where volume repletion is necessary, crystalloid solutions are preferable to colloids.

Recent reports have drawn attention to inhaled nitric oxide (NO) (5 to 80 parts per million) as a selective pulmonary vasodilator with therapeutic promise in ARDS (Chap. 71).

Mixed venous blood P_{O_2} values have long been considered to indicate the adequacy of oxygen delivery relative to demand. A low value (e.g., <20 mmHg) surely indicates that there is tissue hypoxemia, irrespective of measured cardiac output and Pa_{O_2}. However, a high value does not exclude serious tissue hypoxia, especially in gram-negative septicemia, in which systemic low-resistance shunts can develop and leave several capillary beds underperfused.

In situations where maximal PEEP with an FI_{O_2} of 1.0 does not supply sufficient oxygen, placing the patient in the prone position has been found to be helpful. Maintaining supranormal systemic oxygen transport does not improve, and may actually worsen, survival in ARDS.

Management of Sepsis Causing ARDS (See also Chap. 124) Therapy of the underlying infectious/inflammatory state should proceed along two lines: (1) identify and treat any infectious process, and (2) attempt to control the unregulated immune response that drives the acute lung injury. A localized source of sepsis must be drained quickly. Although the surgical mortality is high, failure to drain a purulent focus leads to an almost uniformly fatal outcome.

Glucocorticoids have shown no benefit in early ARDS, except in the settings of meningococcemia in children and *Pneumocystis carinii* pneumonia. Preliminary data suggest that glucocorticoids may be of some benefit in the fibroproliferative stage of late ARDS.

COMPLICATIONS Measures used in the management of ARDS have the potential to cause significant complications. Oxygen toxicity, due to prolonged use of FI_{O_2} above 50%, and excessive hydration may cause worsening of pulmonary infiltrates. High ventilator tidal volumes and pressures may lead to barotrauma. Prolonged mechanical ventilation predisposes to nosocomial pneumonia. ARDS and its underlying disorders may lead to the development of bronchopleural fistula or disseminated intravascular coagulation. Pulmonary fibrosis, irreversible pulmonary hypertension, or multiple organ failure suggest a poor prognosis when they are seen in ARDS.

PROGNOSIS Since the initial description of ARDS in the literature in 1967, mortality has ranged from 50 to 70 percent, although it may now be declining with optimal therapy. Age greater than 65 years, the number of associated organ system failures, sepsis, and severe gas exchange disturbances are negative prognostic factors, while patients with uncomplicated drug overdoses or aspiration have better outcomes. The majority of deaths in ARDS are due to nonrespiratory causes. Sepsis accounts for the majority of early deaths, and multiple organ failure is a prominent cause of late mortality.

In survivors with previously normal lung function, the long-term prognosis for recovery is excellent. Lung volumes and arterial blood gases have been shown to return to normal or near-normal levels within 6 months after respiratory failure. There are instances, however, when the fibrotic residua are sufficiently great that complete recovery is unlikely.

BIBLIOGRAPHY

Bernard GR et al: The American-European consensus conference on ARDS: Definitions, mechanisms, relevant outcomes, and clinical trial coordination. Am J Respir Crit Care Med 149:818, 1994

Hickling KG et al: Low mortality rate in ARDS using low-volume, pressure-limited ventilation with permissive hypercapnia: A prospective study. Crit Care Med 22:1568, 1994

Hudson LD et al: Clinical risks for development of the acute respiratory distress syndrome. Am J Respir Crit Care Med 151:293, 1995

Kollef MH, Schuster DP: The acute respiratory distress syndrome. N Engl J Med 332:27, 1995

Lewis JF, Jobe AH: Surfactant and the adult respiratory distress syndrome. Am Rev Respir Dis 147:218, 1993

McHugh LG et al: Recovery of function in survivors of the acute respiratory distress syndrome. Am J Respir Crit Care Med 150:90, 1994

Milberg JA et al: Improved survival of patients with acute respiratory distress syndrome (ARDS):1983–1993. JAMA 273:306, 1995

Mitchell JP et al: Improved outcome based on fluid management in critically ill patients requiring pulmonary artery catheterization. Am Rev Respir Dis 145:990, 1992

Rossaint R et al: Inhaled nitric oxide for the adult respiratory distress syndrome. N Engl J Med 328:399, 1993

266

Edward P. Ingenito, Jeffrey M. Drazen

MECHANICAL VENTILATORY SUPPORT

Ventilators are specially designed pumps that can support the ventilatory function of the respiratory system and improve oxygenation through application of high oxygen content gas and positive pressure. They are a mainstay of physiologic supportive care and are used to stabilize patients with respiratory failure as the underlying disease process is definitively treated.

INDICATIONS FOR MECHANICAL VENTILATION

Respiratory failure is the primary indication for initiation of mechanical ventilation. There are two basic types of respiratory failure.

Hypoxemic respiratory failure most commonly results from pulmonary conditions such as severe pneumonia, pulmonary edema, pulmonary hemorrhage, and respiratory distress syndrome causing ventilation-perfusion (V/Q) mismatch and shunt. Hypoxemic respiratory failure is present when arterial oxygen saturations of less than 90 percent are observed despite an inspired oxygen fraction of greater than 0.6. The goal of ventilator treatment in this setting is to provide adequate arterial oxygen saturation.

Hypercarbic respiratory failure results from disease states causing either a decrease in minute ventilation or an increase in physiologic dead space such that, despite adequate total minute ventilation, alveolar ventilation is inadequate to meet metabolic demands. Common clinical conditions associated with hypercarbic respiratory failure include neuromuscular diseases, such as myasthenia gravis, ascending polyradiculopathy, and myopathies, as well as diseases that cause respiratory muscle fatigue due to increased workload, such as asthma, chronic obstructive pulmonary disease, and restrictive lung disease. *Acute* hypercarbic respiratory failure is present when arterial P_{CO_2} values exceed 50 mmHg and the arterial pH is below 7.30 (Chap. 50). *Chronic* hypercarbic respiratory failure is characterized by arterial P_{CO_2} values of greater than 50 mmHg and an arterial pH above 7.30.

Mechanical ventilation generally should be instituted in acute hypercarbic respiratory failure. In contrast, the decision to institute mechanical ventilation when components of both acute and chronic hypercarbic respiratory failure are present depends on blood gas parameters and clinical evaluation. In particular, if a patient is not in respiratory distress and is not mentally impaired by CO_2 accumulation, it is not mandatory to initiate mechanical ventilation while other forms of treatment are being administered. The goal of ventilator treatment in hypercarbic respiratory failure is to normalize arterial pH through changes in carbon dioxide tensions. In patients with severe obstructive or restrictive lung disease, elevation in airway pressures may limit tidal volumes to the extent that normalization of pH is not possible, a situation known as *permissive hypercapnia*. Hypoxemic and hypercarbic respiratory failure may coexist in a given individual; in such cases, the indications for and goals of mechanical ventilation are similar to those in these two individual entities.

Accepted therapeutic applications of mechanical ventilation include controlled hyperventilation to reduce cerebral blood flow in patients with increased intracranial pressure or to improve pulmonary hemodynamics in patients with postoperative pulmonary hypertension. Mechanical ventilation also has been used to reduce the work of breathing in patients with congestive heart failure, especially in the presence of myocardial ischemia. Ventilator support is also frequently used in conjunction with endotracheal intubation to prevent aspiration of gastric contents in otherwise unstable patients during gastric lavage for suspected drug overdose or during upper gastrointestinal endoscopy. In the critically ill patient, intubation and mechanical ventilation are indicated before essential diagnostic or therapeutic studies if it appears that respiratory failure may occur during these maneuvers.

PHYSIOLOGIC ASPECTS OF MECHANICAL VENTILATION

Most modern mechanical ventilators function by providing warmed and humidified gas to the airway opening in conformance with various specific volume, pressure, and time patterns. The ventilator serves as the energy source for inspiration, replacing the muscles of the diaphragm and chest wall. Expiration is passive, driven by the recoil of the lungs and chest wall; at the completion of inspiration, internal ventilator circuitry vents the airway to atmospheric pressure or a specified level of positive end-expiratory pressure (PEEP).

PEEP helps maintain alveolar patency in the presence of destabilizing factors and therefore reverses hypoxemia and atelectasis by improving matching of ventilation and perfusion ($\dot{V}/Q$). PEEP levels between 0 and 5 cmH_2O are generally safe and effective; higher levels are recommended only in the management of significant refractory hypoxemia unresponsive to increments in inspired oxygen content up to an inspired oxygen content (F_{IO_2}) of 0.6.

ESTABLISHING AN AIRWAY A cuffed endotracheal tube must be inserted to allow positive-pressure ventilators to deliver conditioned gas, at pressures above atmospheric pressure, to the lungs in a controlled fashion. If neuromuscular paralysis is to be induced during intubation, the use of agents whose mechanism of action includes depolarization at the neuromuscular junction, such as succinylcholine chloride, should be avoided in patients with renal failure, tumor lysis syndrome, crush injuries, or medical conditions associated with elevated serum potassium levels because these agents may elevate the serum potassium to potentially lethal levels. Opiates and benzodiazepines can have a deleterious effect on hemodynamics in patients with depressed cardiac function or low systemic vascular resistance and should be used cautiously in this setting. Morphine can promote histamine release from tissue mast cells and may worsen bronchospasm in patients with asthma; fentanyl, sufentanil, and alfentanil are acceptable alternatives to morphine. Ketamine may increase systemic arterial pressure as well as intracranial pressure and has been associated with dramatic hallucinatory responses; it should be used with caution in patients with hypertensive crisis, increased intracranial pressures, or a history of psychiatric disorders.

VENTILATOR MODE This setting specifies the manner in which ventilator breaths are triggered, cycled, and limited; commonly used modes of mechanical ventilation are given in Table 266-1. The *trigger,* either an inspiratory effort or a time-based signal, defines what the ventilator senses to initiate an assisted cycle. *Cycle* refers to the factors that determine the end of inspiration. For example, in volume-cycled ventilation, inspiration ends when a specific tidal volume is delivered to the patient. Other types of cycling include pressure cycling, time cycling, and flow cycling. *Limiting factors* are operator-specified values, such as airway pressure, that are monitored by transducers internal to the ventilator circuit throughout the respiratory cycle; if the specified values are exceeded, inspiratory flow is immediately stopped and the ventilator circuit vented to atmospheric pressure or the specified PEEP.

Assist Control Mode Ventilation (ACMV) An inspiratory cycle is initiated either by the patient's inspiratory effort or, if no patient effort is detected within a specified time window, by a timer signal within the ventilator. Every breath delivered consists of the operator-specified tidal volume. Ventilatory rate is determined either by the patient or by the operator-specified backup rate, whichever is of higher frequency (Fig. 266-1*A*). ACMV is the recommended mode for initiation of mechanical ventilation because it ensures a backup minute ventilation in the absence of an intact respiratory drive and allows for synchronization of the ventilator cycle with the patient's inspiratory effort.

Problems can arise when ACMV is used in patients with tachypnea due to nonrespiratory or nonmetabolic factors such as anxiety, pain, or airway irritation. Respiratory alkalemia may develop and trigger myoclonus or seizures. Dynamic hyperinflation (so-called auto-PEEP) may occur if the patient's respiratory mechanics are such that inadequate time is available for complete exhalation between inspiratory cycles. Auto-PEEP can limit venous return, decrease cardiac output, and increase airway pressures, predisposing to barotrauma. ACMV is not effective for weaning patients from mechanical ventilation because it provides full ventilator assistance on each patient-initiated breath.

Synchronized Intermittent Mandatory Ventilation (SIMV) The major difference between SIMV and ACMV is that in the former the patient is allowed to breathe spontaneously, i.e., without ventilator assist, between delivered ventilator breaths. However, mandatory breaths are delivered in synchrony with the patient's inspiratory efforts at a frequency determined by the operator. If the patient fails to initiate a breath, the ventilator delivers a fixed-tidal-volume breath and resets the internal timer for the next inspiratory cycle (see Fig. 266-1*B*). SIMV differs from ACMV in that only the preset number of breaths is ventilator-assisted.

SIMV allows patients with an intact respiratory drive to exercise inspiratory muscles between assisted breaths. This characteristic makes SIMV a useful mode of ventilation for both supporting and weaning intubated patients. SIMV may be difficult to use in patients with tachypnea because they may attempt to exhale during the ventilator-programmed inspiratory cycle. When this occurs, the airway pressure may exceed the inspiratory pressure limit, the ventilator-assisted breath will be aborted, and minute volume may drop below that programmed by the operator. In this setting, if the tachypnea is in response to respiratory or metabolic acidosis, a change to ACMV will increase minute ventilation and help normalize the pH while the underlying process is further evaluated.

Continuous Positive Airway Pressure (CPAP) This is not a true support-mode of ventilation, since all ventilation occurs through the patient's spontaneous efforts. The ventilator provides fresh gas to the breathing circuit with each inspiration and charges the circuit to a constant, operator-specified pressure that can range from 0 to 20 cmH_2O (see Fig. 266-1*C*). CPAP is used to assess extubation potential in patients who have been effectively weaned and are requiring little ventilator support and in patients with intact respiratory system function who require an endotracheal tube for airway protection.

Pressure-Control Ventilation (PCV) This form of ventilation is time triggered, time cycled, and pressure limited. During the inspiratory phase, a given pressure is imposed at the airway opening, and the pressure remains at this user-specified level throughout inspiration (Fig. 266-2*A*). Since inspiratory airway pressure is specified by the operator, tidal volume and inspiratory flow rate are *dependent* rather than *independent* variables and are not user specified. PCV is the preferred mode of ventilation for patients with documented barotrauma, since airway pressures can be limited, and for postoperative thoracic surgical patients, in whom the shear forces across a fresh suture line should be limited. When using PCV, minute ventilation and tidal volume must be monitored; minute ventilation is altered through changes in rate or in the pressure-control value.

The major practical limitation of PCV is patient-ventilator asynchrony related to its time-cycled and time-triggered characteristics. Since PCV requires that the patient passively accept ventilator breaths, most patients require heavy sedation to be maintained on this ventilatory mode, which may be hazardous in the hemodynamically unstable patient.

Pressure-Support Ventilation (PSV) This form of ventilation is patient triggered, flow cycled, and pressure limited; it is specifically designed for use in the weaning process. During PSV, the inspiratory phase is terminated when inspiratory airflow falls below a certain level; in most ventilators this flow rate cannot be adjusted by the operator. When PSV is used, patients receive ventilator assist only when the ventilator detects an inspiratory effort (see Fig. 266-2*B*). PSV also can be used in combination with SIMV to ensure volume-cycled backup for patients whose respiratory drive is depressed either spontaneously or as a result of various therapeutic maneuvers.

PSV is well tolerated by most patients who are being weaned: PSV parameters can be set in such a way as to provide full or nearly full ventilatory support and can be withdrawn slowly over a period of days in a systematic fashion to gradually load the respiratory muscles.

Proportional Assist Ventilation (PAV) This recently developed mode of ventilation provides pressure assist at the airway opening in proportion to *patient effort* rather than at a preset designated pressure level or tidal volume. The level of ventilator support continuously varies throughout the respiratory cycle and from one cycle to the next as patient effort changes. This unique approach to ventilator support is thought to improve patient-ventilator synchrony by matching the level of support to inspiratory effort. It may, therefore, lower airways pressures and improve respiratory muscle conditioning.

Since PAV is strictly patient triggered, it cannot be used to support patients who lack an intact respiratory drive. It is currently being studied as an alternative to PSV for weaning patients from mechanical ventilation.

Table 266-1

Clinical Characteristics of Commonly Used Modes of Mechanical Ventilation

Independent Variables (Set by User)	Dependent Variables (Monitored by User)	Trigger/Cycle Limit	Advantages	Disadvantages	Initial Settings
ASSIST CONTROL MODE VENTILATION (ACMV)					
FI_{O_2} Tidal volume Ventilator rate Level of PEEP Inspiratory flow pattern Peak inspiratory flow Pressure limit	Peak airway pressure, Pa_{O_2}, Pa_{CO_2} Mean airway pressure I/E ratio	Patient/timer Pressure limit	Timer backup Patient-vent synchrony Patient controls minute ventilation	Not useful for weaning Potential for dangerous respiratory alkalosis	FI_{O_2} = 1.0* V_t = 10–15 mL/kg f = 12–15/min PEEP = 0–5 cmH_2O Inspiratory flow = 60 L/min
SYNCHRONIZED INTERMITTENT MANDATORY VENTILATION (SIMV)					
Same as for ACMV	Same as for ACMV	Same as for ACMV	Timer backup useful for weaning	Potential dysynchrony	Same as for ACMV
CONTINUOUS POSITIVE AIRWAY PRESSURE (CPAP)					
FI_{O_2} Level of CPAP	Tidal volume Rate, flow pattern Airway pressure Pa_{O_2}, Pa_{CO_2}, I/E ratio	No trigger Pressure limit	Allows assessment of spontaneous function Helps prevent atelectasis	No backup	FI_{O_2} = 0.5–1.0* CPAP = 5–15 cmH_2O
PRESSURE-CONTROL VENTILATION (PCV)					
FI_{O_2}	Tidal volume	Timer/patient	System pressures regulated	Requires heavy sedation	FI_{O_2} = 1.0* PC = 20–40 cmH_2O
Inspiratory pressure level	Flow rate, pattern	Timer/pressure limit	Useful for barotrauma treatment		
Ventilator rate Level of PEEP Pressure limit I/E ratio	Minute ventilation; Pa_{O_2}, Pa_{CO_2}		Timer backup	Not useful for weaning	PEEP = 5–10 cmH_2O f = 12–15/min I/E = 0.7/1–4/1
PRESSURE-SUPPORT VENTILATION (PSV)					
FI_{O_2}	Same as for PCV + I/E ratio	Inspiratory flow	Ensures synchrony	No timer backup	FI_{O_2} = 0.5–1.0* PS = 10–30 cmH_2O 5 cmH_2O usually the level used PEEP = 0–5 cmH_2O
Inspiratory pressure level PEEP Pressure limit		Pressure limit	Good for weaning		

* FI_{O_2} is usually set to 1.0 initially, unless there is a specific clinical indication to minimize FI_{O_2}, such as history of chemotherapy with bleomycin. Once adequate oxygenation is documented by blood gas analysis, FI_{O_2} should be decreased in decrements of 0.1 to 0.2 as tolerated, until the lowest FI_{O_2} required for an Sa_{O_2} of greater than 90 percent is achieved.

ABBREVIATIONS: f, frequency; I/E, inspiration/expiration.

EXTRACORPOREAL MEMBRANE OXYGENATION (ECMO) This nonconventional mode of ventilator support employs a large surface area membrane system connected in series with the patient's circulation to exchange CO_2 and O_2. The lung functions primarily as a passive conduit with gas exchange occurring by diffusion across the membrane. ECMO was first examined in 1970 as an alternative to positive-pressure ventilation in the management of patients with acute respiratory distress syndrome (ARDS). Initial studies failed to demonstrate an improvement in survival among patients treated with ECMO. Although several uncontrolled trials have since suggested that ECMO does improve outcome among ARDS patients, a 1993 study comparing survival among ARDS patients treated with ECMO and conventional ventilator therapy showed no mortality difference but increased morbidity and hospital costs among ECMO-treated patients. Presently, use of ECMO among patients with ARDS is not recommended.

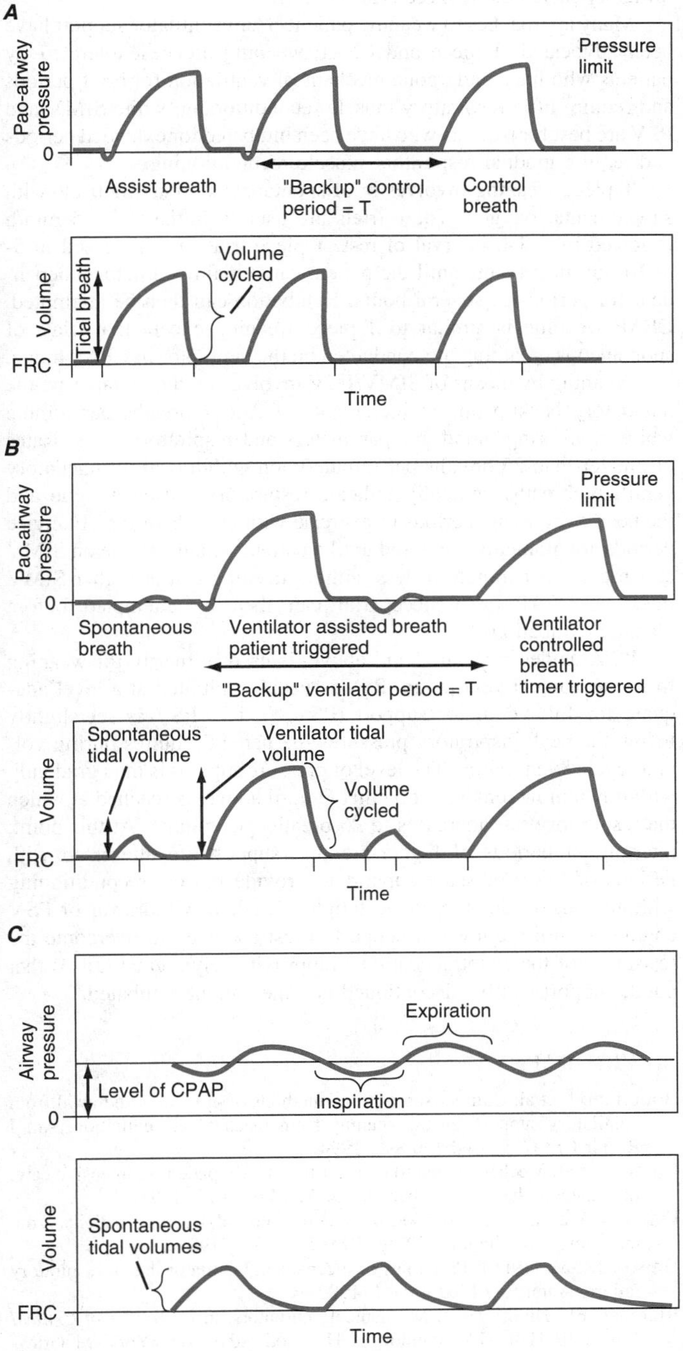

FIGURE 266-1 *A.* Airway pressure and lung volume versus time profile during ACMV. Assisted breaths are triggered by the patient's effort. Controlled breaths are triggered by the ventilator timer. Every breath, whether triggered by the patient or by the timer, is a complete volume-cycled breath, with airway pressure as a dependent variable. The pressure limit is set above the peak inspiratory pressure. *B.* Airway pressure and lung volume versus time profiles during SIMV. Spontaneous breaths occur between patient-triggered assisted breaths and timer-triggered breaths. The tidal volume of the spontaneous breaths is determined by the patient's effort and lung impedance. Assisted and controlled breaths are volume cycled. *C.* Airway pressure and lung volume versus time profiles during CPAP. Breathing is spontaneous, and no ventilator assist is provided. The spontaneous profile is superimposed on an elevated mean airway pressure that the user specifies.

COMPLICATIONS OF MECHANICAL VENTILATION

Endotracheal intubation and positive-pressure mechanical ventilation have direct and indirect effects on several organ systems, including the lung and upper airways, the cardiovascular system, and the gastrointestinal system. Pulmonary complications include barotrauma, nosocomial pneumonia, oxygen toxicity, tracheal stenosis, and deconditioning of respiratory muscles. *Barotrauma,* which occurs when high pressures (i.e., greater than 50 cmH_2O) disrupt lung tissue, is clinically

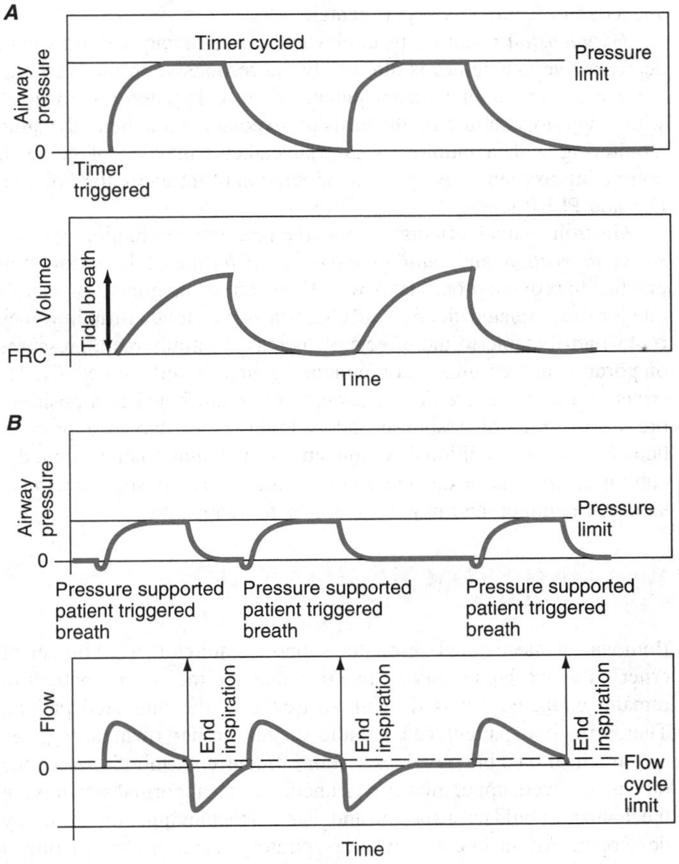

FIGURE 266-2 *A.* Airway pressure and lung volume versus time profiles during PCV. All breaths are timer triggered, timer cycled, and pressure limited. Peak airway pressure is set by the operator, and tidal volume is a dependent variable. The profiles shown here display the pressure limit as slightly higher than pressure-control level. This need not be the case, but it is appropriate to set the pressure limit only slightly above the pressure-control level when using this mode of ventilation for management of the patient with barotrauma. *B.* Airway pressure and airway flow versus time profiles during PSV. All breaths are patient triggered and flow cycled. Inspiration is cycled off when the inspiratory flow drops below a predetermined threshold internally set in the ventilator circuit. In the example shown, the pressure limit is slightly greater than the pressure-support level. Since each can be set independently, this need not be the case.

manifest by interstitial emphysema, pneumomediastinum, subcutaneous emphysema, or pneumothorax. Although the former conditions may resolve simply by reducing airway pressures, clinically significant pneumothorax, as indicated by hypoxemia, decreased lung compliance, and hemodynamic compromise, requires tube thoracostomy.

Patients intubated for longer than 72 h are at high risk for *nosocomial pneumonia* as a result of aspiration from the upper airways via small leaks around the endotracheal tube cuff; the most common organisms responsible for this condition are enteric gram-negative rods, *Staphylococcus aureus*, and anaerobic bacteria. Because the endotracheal tube and upper airways of patients on mechanical ventilation are commonly colonized with bacteria, the diagnosis of nosocomial pneumonia requires "protected brush" bronchoscopic sampling of airway secretions coupled with quantitative microbiologic techniques to differentiate colonization from infection.

Oxygen toxicity is a potential complication when an $F_{I_{O_2}}$ of 0.6 or greater is required for more than 72 h. The condition can be prevented in some cases through the use of PEEP to allow $F_{I_{O_2}}$ values below 0.6 to be used while primary therapy for the underlying condition is instituted. Although oxygen toxicity is thought to result from the effects of oxygen free radicals on the lung interstitium, the therapeutic use of antioxidants such as superoxide dismutase, catalase, selenium, and vitamin E remains experimental.

Hypotension resulting from elevated intrathoracic pressures with decreased venous return is almost always responsive to intravascular volume repletion. In patients judged to have hypotension together with respiratory failure on the basis of alveolar edema, hemodynamic monitoring with a pulmonary arterial catheter may be of value in optimizing oxygen delivery via manipulation of intravascular volume, $F_{I_{O_2}}$ and PEEP levels.

Gastrointestinal effects of positive-pressure ventilation include *stress ulceration* and *mild to moderate cholestasis*. It is common practice to provide prophylaxis with H_2-receptor antagonists or sucralfate for stress-related ulcers. Mild cholestasis (i.e., total bilirubin values ≤ 4.0) attributable to the effects of increased intrathoracic pressures on portal vein pressures is common and generally self-limited. Cholestasis of a more severe degree should not be attributed to a positive-pressure ventilation response and is more likely due to a primary hepatic process. Additional complications, including malnutrition, decubitus ulcers, muscle deconditioning, venous thrombosis, and depression, are common and require appropriate treatment.

WEANING FROM MECHANICAL VENTILATION

Removal of mechanical ventilator support requires that a number of criteria be met. Upper airway function must be intact for a patient to remain extubated but is difficult to assess in the intubated patient. Therefore, if a patient can breathe on his or her own through an endotracheal tube but develops stridor or recurrent aspiration once the tube is removed, upper airway dysfunction or an abnormal swallowing mechanism should be suspected and plans for achieving a stable airway developed. An intact cough when respiratory secretions are suctioned is a good indicator of a patient's ability to mobilize secretions. Respiratory drive and chest wall function are assessed by observation of respiratory rate, tidal volume, inspiratory pressure, and vital capacity. The weaning index, defined as the ratio of breathing frequency to tidal volume (breaths per minute per liter), has been shown to be both sensitive and specific for predicting the likelihood of successful extubation. When this ratio is less than 105 with the patient breathing without mechanical assistance through an endotracheal tube, successful extubation is likely. An inspiratory pressure of more than -30 cmH_2O and a vital capacity of greater than 10 mL/kg are considered indicators of acceptable chest wall and diaphragm function. Alveolar ventilation is generally adequate when systemic arterial P_{CO_2} is less than or equal to 45 mmHg, and arterial oxygen saturations greater than 90 percent can be achieved with an $F_{I_{O_2}}$ of less than 0.5 and a PEEP of 5 cmH_2O or less. Although many patients may not meet all criteria for weaning, the likelihood that a patient will tolerate extubation without difficulty increases as more criteria are met.

Many approaches to weaning patients from ventilator support have been advocated. T-piece and CPAP weaning are best tolerated by patients who have undergone mechanical ventilation for brief periods and require little respiratory muscle reconditioning, while SIMV and PSV are best for patients who have been intubated for extended periods and require gradual respiratory-muscle reconditioning.

T-piece weaning involves brief spontaneous breathing trials with supplemental oxygen. These trials are usually initiated for 5 min/h followed by a 1-h interval of rest. T-piece trials are increased in 5- to 10-min increments until the patient can remain ventilator independent for periods of several hours. Extubation can then be attempted. CPAP weaning is similar to T-piece weaning except that trials of spontaneous breathing are conducted on the ventilator in CPAP mode.

Weaning by means of SIMV/IMV involves gradually tapering the mandatory backup rate in increments of 2 to 4 breaths per minute while monitoring blood gas parameters and respiratory rates. Rates of greater than 25 breaths per minute upon withdrawal of mandatory ventilator breaths generally indicate respiratory muscle fatigue and the need to combine periods of exercise with periods of rest. Exercise periods are gradually increased until a patient remains stable on SIMV at 4 breaths per minute or less without needing rest at higher SIMV rates. A CPAP or T-piece trial can then be attempted before planned extubation.

PSV, as described in detail above, is used primarily for weaning from mechanical ventilation. PSV is usually initiated at a level adequate for full ventilator support (PSV_{max}); i.e., PSV is set slightly below the peak inspiratory pressures the patient requires during volume-cycled ventilation. The level of pressure support is then gradually withdrawn in increments of 5 cmH_2O until a level is reached at which the respiratory rate increases to 25 breaths per minute. At this point, intermittent periods of higher-pressure support are alternated with periods of lower-pressure support to provide muscle reconditioning without causing diaphragmatic fatigue. Gradual withdrawal of PSV continues until the level of support is just adequate to overcome the resistance of the endotracheal tube (approximately 5 cmH_2O). At that point, support can be discontinued and the patient extubated.

BIBLIOGRAPHY

Bouchard L et al: Comparison of three methods of gradual withdrawal from ventilatory support during weaning from mechanical ventilation. Am J Respir Crit Care Med 150:896, 1994

Cohn IL et al: Mechanical ventilation for the elderly patient in intensive care. Incremental changes and benefits. JAMA 269:1025, 1993

Esteban A et al: A comparison of four methods of weaning patients from mechanical ventilation. N Engl J Med 332:345, 1995

Hinson JR, Marini JJ: Principles of mechanical ventilator use in respiratory failure. Annu Rev Med 43:341, 1992

Ingenito EP, Drazen JM: Mechanical ventilators, in *Principles of Critical Care* , JB Hall, GA Schmidt, LDH Wood (eds). New York, McGraw-Hill, 1992, pp 142–154

Morris AH et al: Randomized clinical trial of pressure control inverse ratio ventilation and extracorporeal membrane oxygenation for adult respiratory distress syndrome. Am J Respir Crit Care Med 149:295, 1994

Ranieri VM et al: Physiologic effects of positive end expiratory pressure in patients with chronic obstructive pulmonary disease during acute ventilatory failure and controlled mechanical ventilation. Am Rev Respir Dis 147:5, 1993

Younes M: Proportional assist ventilation: A new approach to ventilatory support. Am Rev Respir Dis 145:114, 1992

267 *Janet R. Maurer*

LUNG TRANSPLANTATION

Lung transplantation for end-stage lung disease has been a therapeutic option since the 1980s. Several transplant options are available for carefully selected patients: unilateral lung transplant, bilateral lung transplant, heart-lung transplant, and living related lobar transplant. The first successful type of transplant was heart-lung, which was performed for a variety of indications in increasing numbers through 1989. Beginning in 1989, the numbers of both unilateral and bilateral lung transplants performed increased dramatically and greatly reduced the number of donor organs available for heart-lung procedures. By 1994, unilateral and bilateral lung transplants had plateaued, however, at around 500 and 400 per year respectively, and heart-lung procedures had dropped to approximately 100 per year. In late 1995, the Registry of the International Society for Heart and Lung Transplantation reported a cumulative total of 1708 heart-lung transplants. Unilateral and bilateral transplant recipients both have 1-year survivals of 67 percent and 3-year survivals of around 50 percent. Heart-lung recipient survivals are 56 percent at 1 year and less than 20 percent at 10 years. Among the unilateral transplant recipients, disease subcategories appear to affect early survival, with emphysema patients enjoying the best 1-year survival, approximately 75 percent, and pulmonary fibrosis patients experiencing the worst, at just over 60 percent. Data on survival of living related lobar recipients are not yet available.

INDICATIONS Emphysema, either smoking-induced or secondary to α_1-antitrypsin deficiency, has been the single largest indication for lung transplantation. This disease accounts for almost 60 percent of all single-lung transplants, more than 30 percent of all bilateral lung, and 9 percent of heart-lung transplants. Other major indications for single-lung transplantation include idiopathic pulmonary fibrosis, primary pulmonary hypertension, and a variety of other rarer diseases. Cystic fibrosis patients are the largest group of bilateral lung recipients, accounting for approximately 36 percent of the total, followed by emphysema patients and primary pulmonary hypertension patients. The major diagnoses among heart-lung recipients are primary and secondary pulmonary hypertension (60 percent of recipients) and cystic fibrosis (15 percent of recipients). With the widespread use of isolated unilateral and bilateral transplants, the indications for heart-lung transplant have become very circumscribed, so that most of these patients now have either concomitant left ventricular disease and end-stage lung disease or irreparable congenital heart disease with Eisenmenger's syndrome (Chap. 235). Patients receiving living related lobar donations have been either children or young adults, and most have suffered from cystic fibrosis. In the majority of living related donations, the recipient has received two lower lobes—one transplanted on the right, one on the left—taken from two separate donors.

Recipient Selection Because donor lungs are the scarcest of the common solid organs transplanted, patients with end-stage lung disease undergo extensive evaluation to select the best potential candidates. In general, good candidates have severe, progressive lung disease with a projected life span of less than 2 years. They must not be active smokers; the length of time of smoking abstinence required prior to consideration for transplant varies among programs but is usually at least 6 months. In addition, they should have no other systemic disease with significant end-organ damage that would impact on the post-transplant outcome. This includes significant coronary artery disease, renal insufficiency, hepatic disease, severe osteoporosis, or significant neurologic impairment. Other comorbid conditions such as previous malignancy, systemic illnesses, and chronic unresolved infections outside the lung may also preclude lung transplant. Considerations that are thought, though not proven, to enhance outcomes include ambulatory status, adequate nutrition, demonstrated motivation/compliance, and psychosocial stability.

In the early years of lung transplantation, patients with prior thoracic surgery were felt to have an unacceptably high risk of postoperative hemorrhage, and patients on glucocorticoids were felt to be at high risk of anastomotic healing complications. With improvements in surgical technique and refinements in early postoperative immunosuppressive management, potential candidates are now rarely rejected for either of these reasons provided the surgery has not been multiple or extensive and the glucocorticoid dose is less than 20 mg/d. Many programs use age cutoffs of between 55 and 65 years in selecting potential recipients. While these age limits are arbitrary, international registry data confirm that recipients older than age 60 have poorer survivals.

It is often difficult in the case of specific pulmonary diseases to determine when patients are within the transplant "window"—that is, have disease advanced enough to fit within the category of "end-stage" yet are not so ill that they will not survive the rigorous transplant operation or die during the long pretransplant waiting period. However, experience in evaluating patients and published longitudinal data has identified useful criteria for identifying appropriate candidates (Table 267-1). Emphysema patients and patients with Eisenmenger's physiology are the most difficult groups in which to predict life expectancy; patients with severe limitations even in activities of daily living may still have survivals at 3 to 5 years that are comparable to patients who have undergone transplantation. Thus, in many centers, the selection of emphysema candidates for transplantation involves not only projected survivals but also quality-of-life issues. Selecting patients with Eisenmenger's physiology is even more difficult. Survivals of patients waiting for at least a year for transplantation have been as good or better than the 1-year survival of similar transplanted patients. Clearly, this group of patients does not behave in the same way as primary pulmonary hypertensive patients, and more specific selection criteria are needed.

There are regional variations in waiting times for transplantation, and minor differences in the listing criteria for individual centers will reflect anticipated length of wait.

Selection of Transplant Procedure The only diseases that currently mandate a specific procedure are (1) irreparable congenital cardiac defects with Eisenmenger's syndrome, which requires heart-lung transplant; (2) advanced lung disease with concomitant left ventricular dysfunction, which requires heart-lung transplant; and (3) septic lung disease (e.g., cystic fibrosis), which requires bilateral lung transplant or bilobar related donor lung transplant to reduce the likelihood of lethal disseminated infection. In essentially all other diseases, single-lung transplantation can be performed with acceptable early and midterm results. Bilateral lung transplantation may be performed if there is anticipated difficulty in postoperative management, especially in pulmonary hypertension, significant bullous disease in emphysema, young age, surgeon preference, or as dictated by individual patient considerations. It is not yet known whether unilateral and

Table 267-1

Physiologic Guidelines for Determining Lung Transplant "Window"

Chronic obstructive pulmonary disease
Postbronchodilator $FEV_1 < 30$ percent predicted
Resting hypoxia ($Pa_{O_2} < 55$–60 mmHg) or hypercapnia
Significant secondary pulmonary hypertension
Severe limitation in activities of daily living
Cystic fibrosis
Postbronchodilator $FEV_1 < 30$ percent predicted
Resting hypoxia ($Pa_{O_2} < 55$ mmHg) or hypercapnia ($Pa_{CO_2} > 50$ mmHg)
Increasing numbers of exacerbations, complications
Idiopathic pulmonary fibrosis
Vital capacity or total lung capacity < 60 percent predicted
Resting hypoxia
Significant secondary pulmonary hypertension
Primary pulmonary hypertension
New York Heart Association functional class III or IV
Mean right atrial pressure > 10 mmHg
Mean pulmonary arterial pressure > 50 mmHg
Cardiac index < 2.5 $(L/min)/m^2$

bilateral lung transplant recipients will have similar long-term survivals and functional outcomes. However, most transplant physicians agree that maximizing the donor organ resource by performing unilateral transplants whenever possible is currently the optimum policy.

FUNCTIONAL OUTCOMES A variety of tests have been used to evaluate lung transplant outcomes including arterial blood gases, perfusion scans, pulmonary function studies, compliance measurements, and exercise studies. Arterial blood gases in both unilateral and bilateral lung recipients improve markedly by 3 months posttransplant. In both types of recipients, P_{CO_2} normalizes; in bilateral transplants, P_{O_2} also normalizes. Unilateral transplant recipients may continue to have mild hypoxemia but rarely require supplemental oxygen. Perfusion studies in unilateral transplant recipients have shown that by 3 months posttransplant the donor lung receives approximately 80 percent of the perfusion; this may be higher if the underlying diagnosis is pulmonary hypertension. Pulmonary function studies in patients receiving either one or two lungs reach their maximum values by between 3 and 12 months postoperatively. Unilateral lung recipients who had a preoperative diagnosis of pulmonary parenchymal disease reach 60 to 65 percent of the maximum predicted values of FVC and FEV_1. Bilateral lung recipients can reach normal predicted values but often have mild restriction. A moderate amount of restriction has been reported in heart-lung recipients, but this may reflect a policy of selecting relatively small donor lungs. Nongraded exercise tolerance (6-min walk test) is similar for all lung recipient groups and ranges between 600 and 700 m per 6 min. Bilateral lung transplant patients perform better on graded exercise studies (e.g., modified Bruce protocol) than do unilateral transplant patients, but both groups achieve only 40 to 60 percent of predicted maximums. The reason for this exercise limitation, particularly in bilateral recipients, is not clear. In most cases, the exercise limitation does not impact upon normal daily living, and patients report significant improvement in quality of life following lung transplantation.

POSTTRANSPLANT MANAGEMENT ISSUES **Acute Rejection** More than 75 percent of lung transplant recipients will experience at least one episode of acute rejection. Most episodes occur within the first 3 months, but acute rejection can occur up to several years posttransplant. Patients usually present primarily with dyspnea but can also have cough, fever, and malaise. Findings include rales, hypoxemia, deteriorating FVC and FEV_1, and, as the process advances, perihilar infiltrates on chest x-ray and leukocytosis. Often, however, if the patient presents early, the x-ray is unremarkable. The diagnosis is best made by transbronchial biopsy, which is sensitive and specific, and, especially in the early posttransplant period, it helps to rule out infections such as cytomegalovirus (CMV), which has a similar presentation. Most episodes respond to high-dose intravenous methylprednisolone. Up to 20 percent of asymptomatic patients will have at least one episode of acute rejection on surveillance transbronchial biopsy during the first 2 years posttransplant. It is not clear whether asymptomatic rejection requires therapy, since its impact on outcome is unknown. This uncertainty has led to varying practices among institutions concerning the use of surveillance bronchoscopy, which can be quite expensive.

Bronchiolitis Obliterans Bronchiolitis obliterans is the primary manifestation of chronic rejection in lung transplants. Some degree of bronchiolitis obliterans occurs in up to 50 percent of patients who survive at least 5 years and is the cause of death in more than one-fourth of long-term survivors. The only factors that clearly have been shown to predispose patients to the development of bronchiolitis obliterans are the number and severity of acute rejection episodes. The onset, usually at least 6 months posttransplant, is often subacute, with gradual onset of shortness of breath, viral-type symptoms, or malaise. It can be asymptomatic and detected incidentally by the insidious development of airflow obstruction on pulmonary function testing. Histology by transbronchial biopsy can confirm the diagnosis but is generally not very sensitive; therefore, a typical clinical picture with airflow obstruction in the absence of any other etiology is now considered sufficient to document *bronchiolitis obliterans syndrome*. Patients developing this syndrome may have a rapidly progressive loss of lung function, but more often they have a gradual progressive fall in FEV_1 over months or years or have a sudden drop in FEV_1 with subsequent stabilization.

Unfortunately treatment, which is with augmented immunosuppression, is rarely successful in reversing obstructive changes but may slow the loss of function for variable periods of time.

Infections Infections are second only to rejection as a cause of morbidity in the lung transplant population and are the most common cause of mortality, accounting for a third of all deaths occurring both during and after the first 3 postoperative months. Infections are more common in the lung transplant recipient than in any other solid-organ recipient. The transplanted lung may be uniquely vulnerable to infection because of impaired mucociliary clearance, loss of cough reflex, and other poorly defined local factors. In addition, the donor lungs are often colonized with organisms that are transmitted directly to the recipient. Some series have reported that at least 60 percent of lung recipients experience an infectious episode requiring treatment. Most of the infections are pulmonary, either pneumonia or bronchitis, and most are bacterial or viral, though recently fungal infections, especially with *Aspergillus*, have been increasingly reported. Bacterial infections are caused most often by gram-negative bacilli or staphylococcal organisms. CMV infection with pneumonitis, as with all solid-organ transplants, remains a significant threat, especially in the highest risk group in which the donor is CMV serology–positive and the recipient is CMV serology–negative. Elaborate systems of antimicrobial prophylaxis, employed now by most centers, along with the increased experience of transplant physicians appear to have been effective in reducing the morbidity from the viral, bacterial, and *Pneumocystis carinii* organisms. Antifungal prophylaxis is also often used since invasive fungal infections have a high mortality rate. The two particularly high-risk periods for infection are in the first 3 post-operative months and late after transplant if the patient develops bronchiolitis obliterans. In the early posttransplant period, it may be very difficult to distinguish infection from rejection, and bronchoscopy with transbronchial biopsies and appropriate cultures are often required to make a diagnosis.

Late after transplant, many patients with bronchiolitis obliterans have an increased risk of bacterial infection. These patients often develop bronchiectasis, become chronically colonized with *Pseudomonas* organisms, and experience repeated episodes of *Pseudomonas* bronchitis or pneumonia.

Airway Complications Careful examination of posttransplant airways in the first few postoperative weeks reveals many small dehiscences, but approximately 15 percent of lung transplant recipients experience airway stenosis requiring either dilation, laser resection, or stenting. Other airway problems include impairment of the mucociliary clearance and the development of bronchial hyperreactivity by many patients. These changes may be due to denervation, ischemia, and low-grade chronic airway inflammation.

Immunosuppressive Complications These are common in lung transplant recipients. Nephrotoxicity, hypertension, and hyperlipidemia occur in the majority of patients treated with current immunosuppressive regimens; however, fewer than 5 percent develop renal failure requiring dialysis or renal transplant. Neurotoxicity, including strokes, coma, severe headaches, and seizures, occurs in up to 20 percent of patients, as does osteoporosis with vertebral compressions or other fractures. Lymphoproliferative disorders occur within the first year in approximately 5 percent of lung transplant recipients; many of these appear to be related to infection with Epstein-Barr virus. Late after transplant, there is an increased incidence of many types of carcinoma and non-Hodgkin's lymphoma.

Recurrence of Underlying Disease Recently, several episodes of recurrence of the underlying disease have been reported in patients undergoing lung transplantation. Several transplant centers have reported the recurrence of sarcoidosis in transplanted lungs, usually as a histologic diagnosis and not clinically apparent. There have also been case reports of recurrent lymphangioleiomyomatosis, giant cell interstitial pneumonitis, and panbronchiolitis. Presumably, α_1-antitrypsin deficiency–related emphysema (Chap. 258) will recur in susceptible patients if they survive long enough, but this has not yet been reported; α_1-antitrypsin replacement therapy is not universally employed in these patients. It must be made clear to all lung transplant recipients that permanent abstinence from smoking is necessary. The abnormal electrical potentials characteristic of cystic fibrosis epithelium (Chap. 257) do not develop in the normal lungs transplanted into cystic fibrosis patients.

BIBLIOGRAPHY

American Thoracic Society: Lung transplantation. Report of the ATS workshop on lung transplantation. Am Rev Respir Dis 147:772, 1993

Grover FL, Zamora MR (eds): Lung transplantation. Semin Resp Crit Care Med 17(2):1996

Hosenpud JD et al: The Registry of the International Society for Heart and Lung Transplantation. Twelfth official report, 1995. J Heart Lung Transplant 14:805, 1995

Patterson GA (ed): Lung transplantation. Semin Thorac Cardiovasc Surg 4(2):1992

PART TEN

DISORDERS OF THE KIDNEY AND URINARY TRACT

268

Fredric L. Coe, Barry M. Brenner

APPROACH TO THE PATIENT WITH DISEASES OF THE KIDNEYS AND URINARY TRACT

Diseases of the kidneys and urinary tract frequently give rise to consistent arrays or clusters of clinical signs, symptoms, and laboratory findings called *syndromes*. Syndromes are useful diagnostically because each has fewer causes than the individual clinical signs and symptoms it contains. For example, any injured capillary bed from glomerulus to urethral meatus can cause hematuria, but only glomerular injury also can cause heavy albuminuria and erythrocyte casts (Chap. 47), and only a few of the diseases that injure the glomerular capillaries enough to cause hematuria and proteinuria also cause a rapid fall in glomerular filtration rate. Routine clinical evaluation is often sufficient to suggest that a particular syndrome may be present (Table 268-1), but additional laboratory measurements beyond the routine, as well as radiologic and/or urologic evaluation and sequential clinical observations, are usually required to establish the diagnosis. This chapter presents the general features of the syndromes, lists the clinical and laboratory data required for their recognition, and outlines the diseases that cause them. Succeeding chapters describe the diseases and their treatment in detail.

ACUTE AND RAPIDLY PROGRESSIVE RENAL FAILURE Whether the glomerular filtration rate (GFR) falls over days (acute renal failure; ARF) or weeks (rapidly progressive renal failure; RPRF) is a useful distinction, because the causes of these two syndromes are somewhat different (Table 268-1). For example, acute tubular necrosis, from sepsis, nephrotoxic materials, shock, or other cause (see Chap. 270), is the usual cause of ARF, whereas extracapillary proliferative (crescentic) glomerulonephritis, due to immunologic injury or to vasculitis, is an important cause of RPRF but not ARF (Chap. 274).

Proof for the existence of either syndrome requires serial determination of the GFR, blood urea nitrogen, or serum creatinine level. Anuria or oliguria (Chap. 47) strongly suggests ARF, since life cannot be sustained for long with such inadequate renal function. Symptoms and signs of uremia of recent onset suggest RPRF or ARF but also could result from chronic renal failure (CRF) that has only recently become life-threatening. Although edema, hypertension, and abnormalities of electrolytes and the urine sediment (Table 268-1) are frequent in both ARF and RPRF, they occur in other syndromes as well and are not specific.

Urinary obstruction, acute tubular necrosis, some forms of vasculitis, major renal vascular accidents, and endogenous and exogenous nephrotoxins are common causes of ARF. Vasculitis and crescentic glomerulonephritis are common causes of RPRF. Hemolytic-uremic syndrome, malignant nephrosclerosis, and essential mixed cryoimmunoglobulinemia occasionally present as RPRF. Idiopathic rapidly progressive glomerulonephritis—the prototype of a disease that produces RPRF—sometimes causes ARF. CRF may occur in some patients with diseases that typically cause ARF. Nevertheless, despite some variability of disease presentations, the finding of ARF or RPRF narrows the range of causes.

ACUTE NEPHRITIS A number of diseases involve the glomeruli and, to a generally lesser extent, the tubules in an acute but transient inflammatory process, manifested clinically by acute reduction in GFR and salt and water retention. This process is called *glomerulonephritis*. Expansion of the extracellular volume, if marked, causes hypertension, pulmonary vascular congestion, and facial and peripheral edema (Chap. 274). Since the causes of this syndrome all can damage the glomerular wall enough to permit red blood cells and plasma proteins to enter the urinary space and appear in the urine, gross or microscopic hematuria, red blood cell casts, and proteinuria are necessary for the diagnosis of acute glomerulonephritis, and their absence suggests other diagnoses. Acute glomerulonephritis is a transient inflammatory process, so its clinical and laboratory manifestations wax and wane over days to weeks. Many of the diseases that cause acute glomerulonephritis also cause ARF or RPRF. When acute glomerulonephritis is associated with RPRF, the term *rapidly progressive glomerulonephritis* is often applied as a clinical diagnosis, pending biopsy delineation of the precise disease process. Other diseases cause an acute but transitory inflammation of the tubules and interstitium (acute tubulointerstitial nephritis) but not of the glomerular capillaries. Hematuria, red blood cell casts, and reduction of GFR occur, as in acute glomerulonephritis, but proteinuria is less marked and, when present, consists mainly of low-molecular-weight proteins rather than albumin. Apart from the lesser proteinuria, tubulointerstitial nephritis may be manifested by increased urine leukocytes and especially urine eosinophils, as well as by peripheral blood eosinophilia.

Acute glomerulonephritis following infection with group A streptococci is the prototype of a disease that causes acute nephritis alone (Chap. 274). Immune complexes deposit in the subepithelial region of the glomerular capillary wall, between the basement membrane and the visceral epithelial cells that separate the membrane from the urinary space, and provoke an intense but transient inflammatory process. GFR falls but returns to normal within weeks to months in most patients. Deposition of immune complexes is also believed to be the cause of acute nephritis following other bacterial and viral infections and of lupus nephritis, membranoproliferative glomerulonephritis, Henoch-Schönlein purpura, and Berger's disease, i.e., IgA nephropathy. That the typical presentations of the last four diseases are chronic renal failure, nephrotic syndrome, and asymptomatic urinary abnormalities illustrates the weakness of relationships between pathogenesis and final clinical manifestations.

Renal biopsy is usually required for the evaluation of patients with acute nephritis, whether or not ARF or RPRF is also present. In patients with RPRF and glomerulonephritis (rapidly progressive glomerulonephritis), the usual histologic picture is that of proliferative glomerulonephritis, often with extracapillary crescent formation. However, this picture may also occur in patients without RPRF, and many other forms of histologic abnormality may be found in patients with acute glomerulonephritis. Thus, prediction of histopathology from clinical course is very uncertain. Prognosis and treatment are influenced strongly by the precise histologic and ultrastructural pattern, as well as the types of immune complexes and immunoglobulins deposited in the renal tissues. In patients with acute tubulointerstitial nephritis, inflammatory changes are prominent in the renal interstitium and evidence of tubule cell injury may be present, but glomerular abnormalities are often absent altogether.

CHRONIC RENAL FAILURE CRF results from progressive and irreversible destruction of nephrons, regardless of cause (Chap. 271). This diagnosis implies that the GFR is known to have been reduced for at least 3 to 6 months (see Table 268-1). Often a gradual decline in GFR occurs over a period of years. Proof of chronicity is also provided by the demonstration of bilateral reduction of kidney size by scout film, ultrasonography, intravenous pyelography, or tomography. Other findings of long-standing renal failure, such as renal osteodystrophy or symptoms of uremia, also help to establish this syndrome. Several laboratory abnormalities are often regarded as reliable indicators of chronicity of renal disease, such as anemia, hyperphosphatemia, or hypocalcemia, but these are not specific (Chap. 269).

In contrast, the finding of broad casts in the urinary sediment (Chap. 47) is specific for CRF, the wide diameters of these casts reflecting the compensatory dilatation and hypertrophy of surviving nephrons. Proteinuria is a frequent but nonspecific finding, as is hematuria. Chronic obstructive uropathy, polycystic and medullary cystic diseases, analgesic nephropathy, and the inactive end stage of any chronic tubulointerstitial nephropathy are conditions in which the urine often contains little or no protein, cells, or casts even though nephron destruction has progressed to chronic renal failure.

When ARF occurs in the presence of CRF, the acute component must be evaluated as if CRF were not present, because the acute component is potentially reversible. In most instances, depletion of extracellular fluid volume is the cause of acute deterioration of renal function, but urinary tract obstruction, drug-induced nephrotoxicity, or exacerbation of underlying renal disease also may be responsible (Chap. 271).

NEPHROTIC SYNDROME This diagnosis previously implied that a patient excretes more than 3.5 g protein per 1.73 m^2 surface area per 24 h; the proteinuria consists mainly of albumin; and that the patient has reduced serum albumin, edema, and hyperlipidemia (Table 268-1). Massive proteinuria alone has now come to define the syndrome, since this finding connotes serious renal disease whether or not the protein losses lead to hypoalbuminemia, lipid disturbances, or edema (Chap. 47). Provided the proteins in the urine are not paraproteins readily excreted by the normal kidney (e.g., immunoglobulin light chains in multiple myeloma), massive proteinuria is invariably a sign of injury to the glomeruli.

Common causes of the nephrotic syndrome include minimal change disease, idiopathic membranous glomerulopathy, focal and segmental glomerulosclerosis, and diabetic glomerulosclerosis (Chaps. 274 and 275). Because these diseases typically cause less inflammation than those that cause acute nephritis, the urine usually contains fewer cellular elements, and acute changes in GFR and urine volume are uncommon. Hematuria may occur in some forms of nephrotic syndrome, however, especially chronic membranoproliferative glomerulonephritis (Chap. 274). The presence of cellular or granular casts should suggest lupus nephritis (Chap. 275) or acute nephritis associated with massive proteinuria, such as essential mixed cryoimmunoglobulinemia, acute bacterial endocarditis, visceral sepsis, and Henoch-Schönlein purpura.

ASYMPTOMATIC URINARY ABNORMALITIES Mild microscopic hematuria, pyuria, and casts or less than 3.5 g protein per 1.73 m^2 surface area per 24 h may be present in the urine of a patient with no evidence of other nephrologic syndromes. By exclusion, these patients belong to the syndrome of asymptomatic urinary abnormalities. Isolated hematuria or proteinuria, or unexplained pyuria, are the most frequent abnormalities in this syndrome.

Isolated hematuria, without proteinuria or casts, may be the sole clue to the presence of neoplasm, stone, or infection (e.g., tuberculosis) in any part of the urinary tract (Chaps. 47, 96, 270, and 280). Isolated hematuria also may arise from renal papillae in analgesic and sickle cell nephropathies (Chaps. 276 and 277). Persistent isolated hematuria often requires intravenous pyelography, cystoscopy, and, occasionally,

Table 268-1

Initial Clinical and Laboratory Data Base for Defining Major Syndromes in Nephrology

Syndromes	Important Clues to Diagnosis	Findings that are Common	Location of Discussion of Diseases Causing Syndrome
Acute or rapidly progressive renal failure	Anuria Oliguria Documented recent decline in GFR	Hypertension, hematuria Proteinuria, pyuria Casts, edema	Chaps. 270, 274, 276, 277, 280
Acute nephritis	Hematuria, RBC casts Azotemia, oliguria Edema, hypertension	Proteinuria Pyuria Circulatory congestion	Chaps. 273, 274, 275
Chronic renal failure	Azotemia for >3 months Prolonged symptoms or signs of uremia Symptoms or signs of renal osteodystrophy Kidneys reduced in size bilaterally Broad casts in urinary sediment	Hematuria, proteinuria Casts, oliguria Polyuria, nocturia Edema, hypertension Electrolyte disorders	Chaps. 269, 271
Nephrotic syndrome	Proteinuria >3.5 g per 1.73 m^2 per 24 h Hypoalbuminemia Hyperlipidemia Lipiduria	Casts Edema	Chaps. 270, 275
Asymptomatic urinary abnormalities	Hematuria Proteinuria (below nephrotic range) Sterile pyuria, casts		Chap. 274
Urinary tract infection	Bacteriuria >10^5 colonies per milliliter Other infectious agent documented in urine Pyuria, leukocyte casts Frequency, urgency Bladder tenderness, flank tenderness	Hematuria Mild azotemia Mild proteinuria Fever	Chap. 131
Renal tubule defects	Electrolyte disorders Polyuria, nocturia Symptoms or signs of renal osteodystrophy Large kidneys Renal transport defects	Hematuria "Tubular" proteinuria Enuresis	Chaps. 276, 278
Hypertension	Systolic/diastolic hypertension	Proteinuria Casts Azotemia	Chaps. 38, 246, 277
Nephrolithiasis	Previous history of stone passage or removal Previous history of stone seen by x-ray Renal colic	Hematuria Pyuria Frequency, urgency	Chap. 279
Urinary tract obstruction	Azotemia, oliguria, anuria Polyuria, nocturia, urinary retention Slowing of urinary stream Large prostate, large kidneys Flank tenderness, full bladder after voiding	Hematuria Pyuria Enuresis, dysuria	Chap. 280

renal arteriography to identify the source of bleeding. *Nephronal hematuria*, in which casts contain red blood cells or hemoglobin pigment, indicates damage to the nephron (Chap. 47). It occurs without proteinuria, mainly in benign recurrent hematuria and Berger's disease (Chap. 274). *Nephronal hematuria and proteinuria* occur together in many renal diseases that may lead to chronic renal failure (Chap. 271). In general, the combination of nephronal hematuria and proteinuria suggests a worse prognosis than either alone.

Isolated proteinuria, without red blood cells or other formed elements in the urinary sediment, is characteristic of many renal diseases that manifest little or no inflammatory reaction within the glomeruli (e.g., diabetes mellitus, amyloidosis). Less than nephrotic-range proteinuria is common in mild forms of all the diseases that can cause overt nephrotic syndrome (Chaps. 274 and 275). "Tubular" proteinuria (Chap. 47) is the rule in cystinosis; in intoxication from cadmium, lead, or mercury; and in the peculiar Balkan nephropathy localized to a small region along the Danube River (Chap. 276).

Pyuria (leukocyturia) also may be a sole urinary abnormality and may reflect infection or inflammation of the lower urinary tract rather than parenchymal renal disease. Nevertheless, prominent pyuria can occur in any inflammatory disease of the kidneys, especially tubulointerstitial nephritis, lupus nephritis, pyelonephritis, and renal transplant rejection, but usually in association with mild proteinuria or hematuria. The finding of leukocyte casts (Chap. 47) establishes the kidney as the site of the inflammatory reaction.

Pyuria associated with urine that is sterile on *routine* bacteriologic culture presents a special problem. Causes of "sterile pyuria" include (1) recent bacterial urinary infection being treated with antibiotics, (2) glucocorticoid therapy, (3) acute febrile episodes, (4) cyclophosphamide administration, (5) pregnancy, (6) renal transplant rejection, (7) genitourinary trauma, (8) prostatitis and cystourethritis, and (9) all forms of tubulointerstitial nephritis. Leukocytes from vaginal secretions may contaminate the urine, so a midstream, clean-catch urine sample should be collected to substantiate a urinary origin. Pyuria associated with proteinuria, nephronal hematuria (Chap. 47), or casts usually signifies inflammatory disease of the renal glomeruli, tubules, interstitium, or microcirculation, and evaluation should focus not on the pyuria but on the nature of the renal disease.

Persistent sterile pyuria that cannot be ascribed to any of the foregoing causes has a narrow differential diagnosis. Unusual infections, such as tuberculosis, fungi, atypical mycobacteria, *Haemophilus influenzae*, anaerobic bacteria, fastidious bacteria that grow only on enriched media, and L forms, all must be sought. Intravenous pyelography may be needed to detect causes such as urinary tract calculi, papillary necrosis, and renal infiltration by lymphoma or myeloma cells. The latter is usually suspected because of other evidence of myeloma or lymphoma, for both rarely involve only the kidneys. If all tests are negative, cystoscopy may reveal cystitis or trigone inflammation.

URINARY TRACT INFECTION This syndrome is defined by the demonstration in urine of pathogenic organisms, either bacteria, tubercle bacilli, or fungi (Chap. 131). When urine is obtained for culture, the condition under which the urine is collected must minimize contamination from external surfaces. Women should void into a wide-mouthed sterile container after preliminary cleansing of the vulva with a moist, sterile gauze pledget. In men, midstream collection is usually adequate. Bacterial colony counts of 10^5 organisms per milliliter or greater in urine generally indicate urinary tract colonization and infection. Levels above 10^2 colonies per milliliter are sufficient to indicate infection in symptomatic patients (Table 268-1) and in urine samples obtained by suprapubic aspiration or bladder catheter. When the urinary tract is anatomically normal, *Escherichia coli* is the usual pathogen. After prolonged antibiotic treatment of persistent infections, particularly when urinary drainage is impaired or stones are present, *Klebsiella*, *Enterobacter*, and *Proteus* species predominate.

As discussed in Chap. 131, a positive urine culture need not imply that an organism is producing tissue inflammation or injury. In some patients, tissue effects may be trivial; in others, injury may occur even though symptoms or urinary abnormalities are not present at the time of evaluation. When bacteriuria is associated with tissue inflammation or injury, clinical manifestations usually depend on the site(s) involved. Dysuria, frequency, urgency, and suprapubic tenderness are common symptoms of bladder and urethral inflammation (Chap. 47 and Table 268-1). Prostatitis also leads to frequency, dysuria, and urgency, and the prostate may be boggy and tender on rectal examination. Flank pain, chills, fever, nausea and vomiting, hypotension from sepsis, and leukocyte casts all suggest true renal parenchymal infection, i.e., pyelonephritis; their absence, however, does not exclude pyelonephritis.

RENAL TUBULE DEFECTS This syndrome encompasses a large number of acquired and hereditary disorders, all of which tend to affect tubules more than glomeruli. Hereditary anatomic defects, including polycystic renal disease, medullary cystic disease, and medullary sponge kidney, are readily detected by ultrasonography or intravenous pyelography, which are usually performed because of hematuria, bacteriuria, flank pain, or unexplained azotemia (Chap. 278).

Defects in tubule transport functions, on the other hand, tend not to be associated with prominent renal anatomic defects and arise either as inherited traits (Chap. 278) or during the course of acquired renal disease (Chap. 276). In general, these functional defects impair secretion and/or reabsorption of electrolytes and organic solutes or limit urinary concentrating and diluting ability (see Table 268-1). Typical manifestations of such functional disturbances include polyuria and nocturia (Chap. 47), metabolic acidosis (Chap. 50), and various disorders of fluid and electrolyte balance (Chap. 49). Such defects are defined by direct physiologic measurements; their elucidation requires a sound understanding of normal renal physiology.

HYPERTENSION Hypertension implies that the average of a series of reliable blood pressure measurements exceeds 140 mmHg systolic or 90 mmHg diastolic (see Table 268-1). The pathogenetic mechanisms, clinical and laboratory manifestations, and therapeutic approaches are discussed in detail elsewhere (Chaps. 38 and 246). In addition, a number of renal complications of hypertension are reviewed in Chap. 277, as is the entity of renal artery stenosis, an infrequent but potentially curable cause of hypertension.

NEPHROLITHIASIS This syndrome is recognized with certainty when a stone is passed, visualized by x-ray, or removed at surgery or cystoscopy (see Table 268-1 and Chap. 279). Less certain, but suggestive, evidences of nephrolithiasis include renal colic; painful hematuria; or unexplained pyuria, dysuria, and urinary frequency (Chap. 47). Colic varies in its symptomatology but usually begins suddenly in one flank, radiates downward toward the groin, and is excruciatingly painful.

Most renal stones are composed of calcium, uric acid, cystine, or struvite (magnesium ammonium phosphate). All are radiopaque except for uric acid stones and are therefore visible by routine abdominal radiography. Uric acid stones appear as radiolucent filling defects and can be mistaken for tumor or blood clot.

URINARY TRACT OBSTRUCTION Documentation of the various structural or functional causes of urinary tract obstruction usually requires radiologic or surgical visualization. The most common initial evaluation at present is renal ultrasonography, although false-negative evaluations are not rare, especially when urine flow rate is low. The manifestations of obstruction, which initiate the search for its causes, are numerous (see Table 268-1) and are reviewed in Chap. 280. Anuria in an adult is almost always due to obstruction of bladder outflow. Less commonly, blockage of upper urinary drainage from both kidneys or from a solitary functioning kidney accounts for total or near-total cessation of urine flow. A large bladder after voiding is a sign of outflow obstruction, usually due to urethral stricture, tumor, stone, neurogenic causes, or prostatic hypertrophy. Nocturia, frequency and overflow incontinence, and slowing or hesitancy of micturition also suggest outflow obstruction (Chap. 47). Upper tract obstruction often produces few manifestations. When it is incomplete or unilateral, urine volume may be normal or even increased because of a loss of renal concentrating ability. Urinary stasis secondary to obstruction predisposes to recurrent urinary tract infection; chronic obstruction predisposes to progressive loss of renal function.

BIBLIOGRAPHY

Kasiske BL, Keane WF: Laboratory assessment of renal disease. Clearance, urinalysis, and renal biopsy, in *The Kidney,* 5th ed, BM Brenner (ed). Philadelphia, Saunders, 1996, p 1137

Rosenberg ME, Hostetter TH: Proteinuria, in *The Kidney,* DW Seldin, G Giebisch (eds). New York, Raven, 1992, p 3039

Tisher CC, Croker BP: Indications for and interpretation of the renal biopsy. Evaluation by light, electron and immunofluorescence microscopy, in *Diseases of the Kidney,* RW Schrier, CW Gottschalk (eds). Boston, Little, Brown, 1993, p 485

269

Barry M. Brenner, Harald S. Mackenzie

DISTURBANCES OF RENAL FUNCTION

Near constancy of the composition of the internal environment, including the volume, tonicity, and compartmental distribution of the body fluids, is essential to survival. With day-to-day variations in the intake of food and water, preservation of the internal environment requires the excretion of these substances in amounts that balance the quantities ingested. Although losses from intestines, lungs, and skin contribute to this excretory capacity, the greatest responsibility for solute and water excretion is borne by the kidneys.

The kidneys regulate the composition and volume of the plasma water. This, in turn, determines the composition and volume of the entire *extracellular* fluid compartment. Through the continuous exchange of water and solutes across all cell membranes, the kidneys influence the *intracellular* fluid compartment as well. These functions are served by a variety of physiologic mechanisms that enable individuals to excrete excesses of water and nonmetabolized solutes contained in the diet, as well as the nonvolatile end products of nitrogen metabolism, such as urea and creatinine. Conversely, when faced with deficits of water or solute, excretion of water or specific solute(s) is curtailed via appropriate mechanisms for renal conservation, reducing the likelihood of volume or solute depletion. The purpose of this chapter is to review the excretory functions of the kidney and to examine how these functions are affected by chronic renal disease.

EFFECTS OF NEPHRON LOSS ON RENAL EXCRETORY MECHANISMS

The volume of urine excreted (averaging 1.5 L/day or roughly 1 mL/min) represents the sum of two large, directionally opposite processes—namely, *ultrafiltration* of 180 L/day or more of plasma water (or 125 mL/min) and *reabsorption* of more than 99 percent of this filtrate by transport processes in the renal tubules. Renal blood flow accounts for about 20 percent of resting cardiac output, yet the kidneys comprise only about 1 percent of total body weight. This disproportionate allocation of cardiac output, greatly exceeding blood flow per gram of brain, heart or liver, is required for the process of ultrafiltration.

GLOMERULAR ULTRAFILTRATION Urine production begins at the glomerulus where an ultrafiltrate of plasma is formed. The rate of glomerular ultrafiltration (glomerular filtration rate, GFR) is governed chiefly by forces favoring filtration on the one hand (hydraulic pressure in the glomerular capillaries) and forces opposing filtration on the other (the sum of hydraulic pressure in Bowman's space and colloid osmotic pressure in the glomerular capillaries). The rate of glomerular plasma flow and the total surface area of the glomerular capillaries are also determinants of glomerular filtration rate. Decreased glomerular filtration rate can therefore be expected when (1) glomerular hydraulic pressure is reduced (as in circulatory shock); (2) tubule (hence Bowman's space) hydraulic pressure is elevated, as in urinary tract obstruction; (3) plasma colloid osmotic pressure rises to high levels (hemoconcentration due to severe volume depletion, myeloma, or other dysproteinemias); (4) renal, and hence glomerular, blood flow is reduced (severe hypovolemia, cardiac failure); (5) permeability is reduced (diffuse glomerular disease); or (6) filtration surface area is diminished, through focal or diffuse nephron loss in progressive renal failure.

The glomerular capillary wall is specially adapted to allow passage of extremely large volumes of water yet retain all but the smallest solute molecules. Molecules the size of inulin (approximately 5200 mol wt) pass freely across the glomerular filtration barrier, appearing at approximately the same concentration in Bowman's space as in plasma. The passage of solutes across the glomerular barrier decreases progressively with increasing molecular size such that, as the molecular weight of albumin is approached, most of the solute is retained in the plasma. Albumin, a polyanionic molecule in plasma, is further retarded at the glomerular filtration barrier by *electrostatic forces* imparted by negatively charged cell surface molecules on the epithelial foot processes that form the *filtration slits* and the *slit diaphragms*. With disruption of these structural and electrostatic barriers, as in many forms of glomerular injury (see Chaps. 273 to 275), large quantities of plasma proteins gain access to the glomerular filtrate.

Glomerular Adaptations to Nephron Loss With loss of nephron mass, the remaining healthy (or least injured) nephrons tend to hypertrophy and take on an increased functional burden so that the overall loss of function is offset. For example, a patient with a unilateral nephrectomy loses one half of the nephron mass, resulting in a 50 percent reduction in GFR at the time of surgery. However, the GFR in the remaining kidney begins to increase after 1 or 2 weeks, and within several months GFR may rise to 80 percent of the preoperative value. This indicates that the GFR of the individual remaining nephrons has increased above normal. Increases in single-nephron GFR may be achieved by renal hemodynamic adjustments (increased glomerular plasma flow and increased glomerular capillary hydraulic pressure), which augment the forces driving ultrafiltration, and by glomerular hypertrophy, which increases the maximum surface area available for filtration. These structural adaptations are evident from the enlargement of glomeruli (and tubules) seen on histologic sections from people with single kidneys. Similar structural changes are observed in kidneys damaged by chronic disease processes; foci of hypertrophied glomeruli and tubules are interspersed with areas of atrophic or scarred parenchyma. Although direct measurements of single-nephron GFR cannot be made in humans, it is reasonable to assume that focal nephron enlargement in chronically diseased kidneys generally signifies focally increased single-nephron GFR, and that these adaptations represent compensatory adjustments for the effects of nephron loss through disease.

Glomerulotubular Balance The close integration of glomerular and tubular functions (*glomerulotubular balance*) seen in chronic renal failure (CRF) supports the notion that progressive nephron obliteration is the usual mode of GFR reduction in CRF. Preservation of glomerulotubular balance until the terminal stages of CRF is fundamental to the *intact-nephron hypothesis*, which essentially states that as CRF advances, kidney function is supported by a diminishing pool of functioning (or hyperfunctioning) nephrons, rather than relatively constant numbers of nephrons, each with diminishing function. This concept has important implications for the mechanisms of disease progression in CRF. A considerable amount of evidence suggests that nephrons subjected to increased excretory burdens for prolonged periods actually sustain injury as a result of these adaptations: thus the cost of these compensatory adaptations to nephron loss may ultimately be relentless destruction of the remaining nephron pool.

The magnitude of the single-nephron *hyperfiltration* induced by loss of 50 percent of the total nephron mass usually has no serious adverse consequences, even when sustained over two to three decades. When more than 50 percent of the total nephron mass is lost, however, as in renal-sparing surgery for bilateral trauma or neoplasm or from a renal disease whose activity has abated, the remaining nephrons are forced to the limits of their compensatory capacity. While these adaptations achieve remarkable short-term success at offsetting the tendency for GFR to fall, over time, proteinuria and focal and segmental glomerulosclerosis develop, the more so where greater amounts of nephrons are lost or removed. As a result, a progressive decline in GFR ensues. Experimental study of the processes that advance glomerular injury show that the adverse long-term consequences of severe nephron deficits are invariably preceded by increases in glomerular capillary hydraulic pressure (glomerular capillary hypertension), glomerular hyperperfusion, and hypertrophy. Interventions directed against these adaptive responses can greatly ameliorate the subsequent development of renal failure. In particular, drugs (e.g., angiotensin-converting enzyme inhibitors) and other interventions (such as dietary protein restriction) that lower glomerular pressure can slow the rate of progression of experimental and human renal disease. Otherwise, more and more glomeruli cease to function through advancing glomerulosclerosis and disruption of tubule structure and function, leading eventually to total loss of GFR (i.e., end-stage renal disease). This *final common pathway* for chronic renal injury helps to explain the progressive nature of chronic renal failure resulting from many different kidney diseases.

Biologic Consequences of Sustained Reductions in GFR Although nephron loss can proceed, to some extent, without equivalent loss of GFR due to the compensatory mechanisms described above, determination of the total GFR of both kidneys remains the most reliable clinical index of overall excretory function. The effects of impaired GFR are to reduce the total rate of delivery of solute into the glomerular filtrate. When accompanied by comparably reduced rates of urinary excretion, *retention* and *accumulation* of the unexcreted solute occurs, resulting in increased concentrations of the substance in the plasma and other body fluids.

Figure 269-1 depicts the major types of response to impaired GFR. The degree of reduction in total GFR is plotted on the abscissa, expressed as a percentage of normal (100 percent). The renal handling of most solutes normally present in glomerular filtrate conforms to one of three patterns. Curve *A* describes the pattern with substances such as creatinine and urea that normally depend largely on glomerular filtration for urinary excretion; i.e., secretion contributes little to overall excretion. Therefore, as illustrated, gradual reductions in GFR are accompanied by progressive increases in plasma levels of creatinine, urea, and other substances normally excreted primarily by filtration.

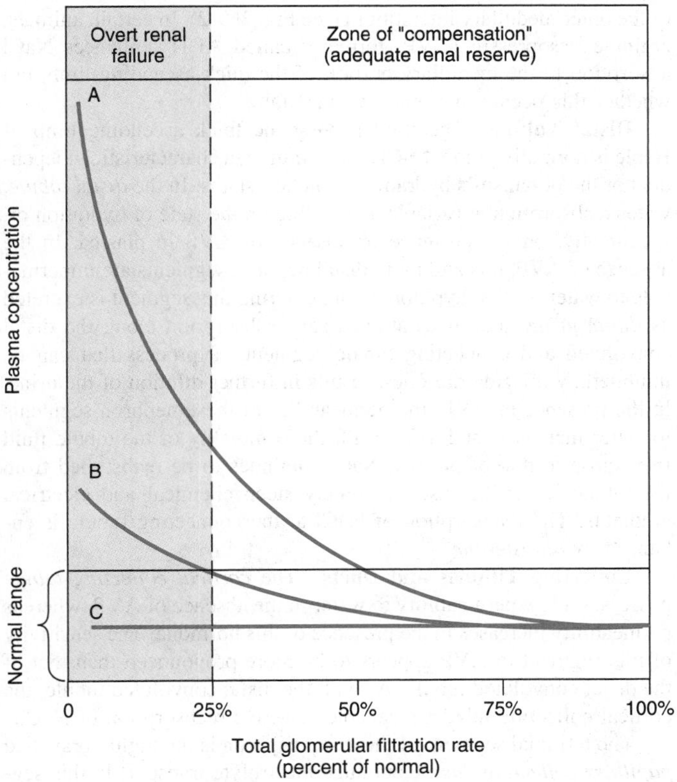

FIGURE 269-1 Representative patterns of adaptation for different types of solutes in body fluids in chronic renal failure. *(After NS Bricker et al, in Brenner, 1976.)*

The clinical course of CRF usually also approximates the pattern described by curve *A*. Patients with CRF usually pass from a long asymptomatic period of "compensation" to a more accelerated and clinically overt terminal phase. In other words, despite chronic injury leading to destruction of more than 50 percent of nephrons, plasma elevations of creatinine and urea may still lie within the normal limits for these substances. With further nephron loss and reduction in GFR, however, the limits of renal reserve are exceeded and continued accumulations of curve *A*–type solutes lead to abnormally elevated plasma concentrations (see Fig. 269-1). Because some of these retained solutes are thought to exert "toxic" effects on all organ systems, clinical manifestations of CRF may now become apparent. Consequently, in patients with substantial reductions in nephron mass but near-normal plasma creatinine, overt uremia may be precipitated by relatively modest additional decrements in GFR.

The accumulation of curve *A*–type solutes with chronic loss of renal function proceeds until external balance is restored, i.e., intake and/or production rates exactly match excretion rates. In the case of creatinine, for example, assuming a constant rate of creatinine production, a 50 percent reduction in GFR results in an approximate doubling of the plasma creatinine concentration. The latter restores the filtered load of creatinine (i.e., the product of GFR and plasma creatinine concentration) to normal, and the urinary excretion rate once again is equivalent to creatinine production. Since no alternative mechanisms exist for significantly augmenting creatinine excretion beyond this level, elimination of the retained creatinine is not possible and the plasma concentration remains twice normal. With further loss of GFR, elevations in plasma creatinine are compounded by loss of nephron excretory function and creatinine retained as the result of earlier nephron destruction (see Fig. 269-1). *In practice, so long as the net rates of acquisition and production (i.e., liver function and muscle mass) remain reasonably constant, the inverse relationship between plasma concentrations of solutes such as creatinine and urea and GFR is sufficiently reliable and predictable to serve as clinical indices of GFR.* However, where muscle mass is low or reduced by wasting, unremarkable plasma levels of creatinine may nevertheless belie substantial reductions in GFR.

In contrast to solutes of the curve *A* type, plasma levels of phosphate, urate, and potassium (K^+) and hydrogen (H^+) ions usually do not rise until the GFR falls to a small percentage of normal. With progressive renal failure this pattern of response (curve *B* in Fig. 269-1) reflects the participation of tubule transport mechanisms in the excretion of these substances. In other words, *as GFR declines, the tubules facilitate greater elimination of these substances, by enhancing secretion and/or by diminishing reabsorption, so that a greater fraction of the filtered load is excreted.* Plasma levels of curve *B*–type solutes, therefore, rise less than those of curve *A* because, with progressive reductions in GFR, *excretion rate per nephron* and therefore *fractional excretion* both increase. Eventually, however, with further loss of GFR, enhanced fractional excretion can no longer offset the reduction in net filtered load of these solutes and plasma levels rise (see Fig. 269-1). For urate, phosphate, and K^+, at least, increased fractional excretion serves to maintain normal plasma levels until GFR falls to less than one-fourth of normal.

Finally, for certain solutes, such as sodium chloride (NaCl), plasma concentrations remain normal throughout the course of CRF, despite unrestricted intake of these substances (curve *C* in Fig. 269-1). The compensatory mechanism required to achieve this represents a fundamental adaptation to chronic renal injury. To illustrate the magnitude of the adaptation involved, it is useful to compare the excretion of sodium (Na^+) in a normal individual (GFR of 125 mL/min) with that of a patient with advanced renal failure (GFR of 2 mL/min). Both individuals consume a diet containing 7 g/day of salt (120 mmol Na^+). With a normal serum Na^+ concentration of 140 mmol/L, external Na^+ balance is achieved by excreting approximately 0.5 percent of the filtered load. By contrast, for external balance to be maintained in the patient with CRF, fractional excretion of Na^+ must rise to 30 percent. In other words, *to maintain external Na^+ balance, the same amount of Na^+ must be excreted into the urine each day in the patient with CRF as in the normal individual.* Given the drastic reduction in GFR in CRF, external balance can only be maintained by large-magnitude adaptations in the reabsorptive processes in surviving tubules so that a progressively larger fraction of the filtered load escapes reabsorption and appears in the final urine. In short, *the rate of excretion of Na^+ per surviving nephron increases in inverse proportion to the composite GFR in surviving nephrons.*

ADAPTATIONS IN TUBULE TRANSPORT MECHANISMS IN RESPONSE TO NEPHRON LOSS

Despite progressive nephron loss, many mechanisms that regulate renal solute and water balance differ only quantitatively, and not qualitatively, from those that operate normally. Thus, glomerulotubular balance is maintained. The most important of these mechanisms are considered below.

TUBULAR TRANSPORT OF SODIUM CHLORIDE AND WATER Most of the filtered water and sodium salts are reabsorbed by the tubules, leaving small and variable amounts, equivalent on average to the quantities ingested, to reach the final urine. About two-thirds of the glomerular ultrafiltrate is reabsorbed in the *proximal tubule* with little change in the osmolality or Na^+ concentration of the unreabsorbed fraction (Fig. 269-2). In other words, fluid reabsorption in the proximal tubule is nearly *isosmotic* and is coupled to the active transport of Na^+. Since chloride (Cl^-) and bicarbonate (HCO_3^-) are the primary anions in the extracellular fluid, they constitute the main solutes that accompany Na^+ reabsorption in the renal tubules. In the earliest portion of the proximal tubule, bicarbonate is the principal anion that accompanies the reabsorption of Na^+. This process occurs via a Na^+/H^+ exchanger at the luminal brush border and is dependent on the activity of carbonic anhydrase. Glucose, amino acids, and other organic solutes (e.g., lactate) are also extensively reabsorbed in the proximal tubule by cotransport mechanisms that link the cellular entry of these organic molecules with Na^+. The coupling of water absorption (i.e., volume) with solute absorption appears to be dependent upon three processes. First, given the remarkably high water permeability of this segment, very small transepithelial osmolality differences, i.e., *luminal hypotonicity* of the order of 2 to 3 mosmol/L produced by solute absorption, could drive water absorption. Second, due to preferential absorption of HCO_3^- and organic solutes in the early portions of the proximal tubule, the concentrations of these substances decrease along the proximal tubule while that of chloride increases. Volume reabsorption would then occur if the diffusion of Na^+ and Cl^- down their respective electrochemical gradients across the proximal tubule epithelium occurred more easily than the back-diffusion of sodium bicarbonate into the lumen, creating an *effective osmotic pressure gradient.* Finally, *lateral interstitial space hypertonicity* produced by differences in the rates at which solutes are transported into the spaces or exit them by diffusion may also contribute to the coupling of water and solute reabsorption.

Reabsorption of Fluid from Proximal Convoluted Tubules This is sensitive to *Starling forces*, i.e., the hydraulic and colloid osmotic (or oncotic) pressures across the walls of the peritubular capillaries. Because the plasma proteins in glomerular capillaries are concentrated by ultrafiltration, oncotic pressure rises markedly along the glomerular capillary network. This step-up in oncotic pressure is transmitted largely unchanged to the first branches of the peritubular capillaries via the efferent arterioles. These resistance vessels cause a substantial drop in hydraulic pressure, however, so that when the plasma reaches the peritubular capillaries, oncotic pressure greatly exceeds hydraulic pressure. The Starling forces are therefore oriented in an *uptake* mode, in contrast to their configuration at the glomerulus where hydraulic pressure exceeds oncotic pressure, favoring *filtration.* The extent to which oncotic pressure exceeds hydraulic pressure in the peritubular capillary network modulates the overall rate of fluid absorption by the peritubular capillaries. Therefore, when peritubular capillary oncotic pressure falls, or hydraulic pressure rises, uptake of fluid by these capillaries is reduced. As a result, fluid is retained in the interstitial space, tending to increase hydraulic pressure, ultimately retarding the egress of fluid from the lateral intercellular channels. Without an adequate route of drainage, fluid in the intercellular channels leaks back into the lumen, thereby *diminishing net fluid reabsorption* from this tubule segment. The opposite occurs in states where peritubular oncotic pressure is increased (increased filtration fraction) or hydraulic pressure is decreased (enhanced efferent arteriolar tone). Under these circumstances, peritubular capillary uptake of reabsorbate is augmented, leading ultimately to *enhanced net fluid reabsorption* by the proximal tubule. Although physical factors appear to be the major determinants of fluid reabsorption in the proximal tubule, hormones (e.g., angiotensin II) may also modulate fluid reabsorption directly, by enhancing luminal Na^+ entry into proximal tubule cells via an apical Na^+/H^+ exchanger.

Thin Ascending Limb of Henle's Loop In contrast to the proximal tubule, active outward transport of Na has not been established for the *thin ascending limb of Henle's loop*. However, passive outward salt transport does occur, as indicated in Fig. 269-2. In the next nephron segment, the *medullary thick ascending limb of Henle*, the concentration of NaCl is reduced as fluid traverses this segment. Here Cl^- absorption occurs by an active process involving a furosemide-sensitive Na^+:K^+:$2Cl^-$ cotransport mechanism in the luminal membrane, with one-half of Na^+ absorption proceeding passively, driven by the lumen positive transepithelial voltage difference. Since the ascending limb of Henle is impermeable to water, net NaCl reabsorption generates hypotonic tubule fluid and gives rise to the high NaCl concentration of the outer medullary interstitium (see Fig. 269-2). In certain animals, arginine vasopressin (AVP; formerly called ADH) enhances NaCl absorption in the medullary portion of the thick ascending limb, but whether this occurs in humans is uncertain.

Distal Tubule The fluid leaving the thick ascending limb of Henle is normally of low NaCl concentration, a characteristic independent of the organism's hydration or dietary status. In the *distal tubule*, water reabsorption is variable, depending on the state of hydration or, specifically, on the presence or absence of AVP in plasma. In the absence of AVP, this and more distal nephron segments are impermeable to water, so that hypotonic fluid entering this segment is excreted as *dilute urine.* Indeed, continued salt reabsorption along the distal convoluted and connecting tubule segments, a process that can be inhibited by thiazide diuretics, results in further dilution of the urine. In the presence of AVP, the permeability of these nephron segments to water increases, and as a result, the osmolality of the tubule fluid rises close to that of plasma. NaCl continues to be reabsorbed from the tubule lumen against moderately steep chemical and electrical gradients. The reabsorption of NaCl at the connecting tubule is enhanced by *aldosterone.*

Collecting Tubules and Ducts The *cortical collecting tubule* possesses a low permeability to water in the absence of AVP, whereas permeability increases in the presence of this hormone. The sensitivity of this segment to AVP appears to be more pronounced than that of the distal convoluted tubule. As with the distal convoluted tubule, the cortical collecting tubule is capable of active reabsorption of NaCl.

The terminal segment of the distal nephron is the highly branched *papillary collecting duct.* Continued electrolyte transport in this segment results in the large ion concentration differences that normally exist between urine and plasma. As in the cortical collecting tubule, Na^+ transport appears to be active, since reabsorption proceeds against sizeable electrochemical gradients. The rate of Na^+ transport in this segment depends on the load of Na^+ delivered from more proximal segments and is also affected by aldosterone. The permeability to water is also increased markedly in the presence of AVP.

EFFECTS OF NEPHRON LOSS ON SODIUM CHLORIDE TRANSPORT IN SURVIVING NEPHRONS With progressive nephron loss, *maintenance of external balance for NaCl requires that fractional salt excretion increases as GFR decreases.* Several mechanisms contribute to this adaptive increase in fractional sodium excretion. With loss of functioning nephron units, peritubular capillary Starling forces are probably altered in directions that serve to reduce proximal tubule reabsorption of NaCl and water. For example, a rise in peritubular capillary hydraulic pressure, which tends to inhibit net proximal fluid reabsorption, might be anticipated with systemic hypertension, a common feature of chronic renal failure. Similarly, reductions in peritubular capillary oncotic pressures may be anticipated due to reductions in both filtration fraction and hypoalbuminemia.

Aldosterone, which normally exerts a potent influence on tubule transport, probably does not figure prominently in reducing fractional

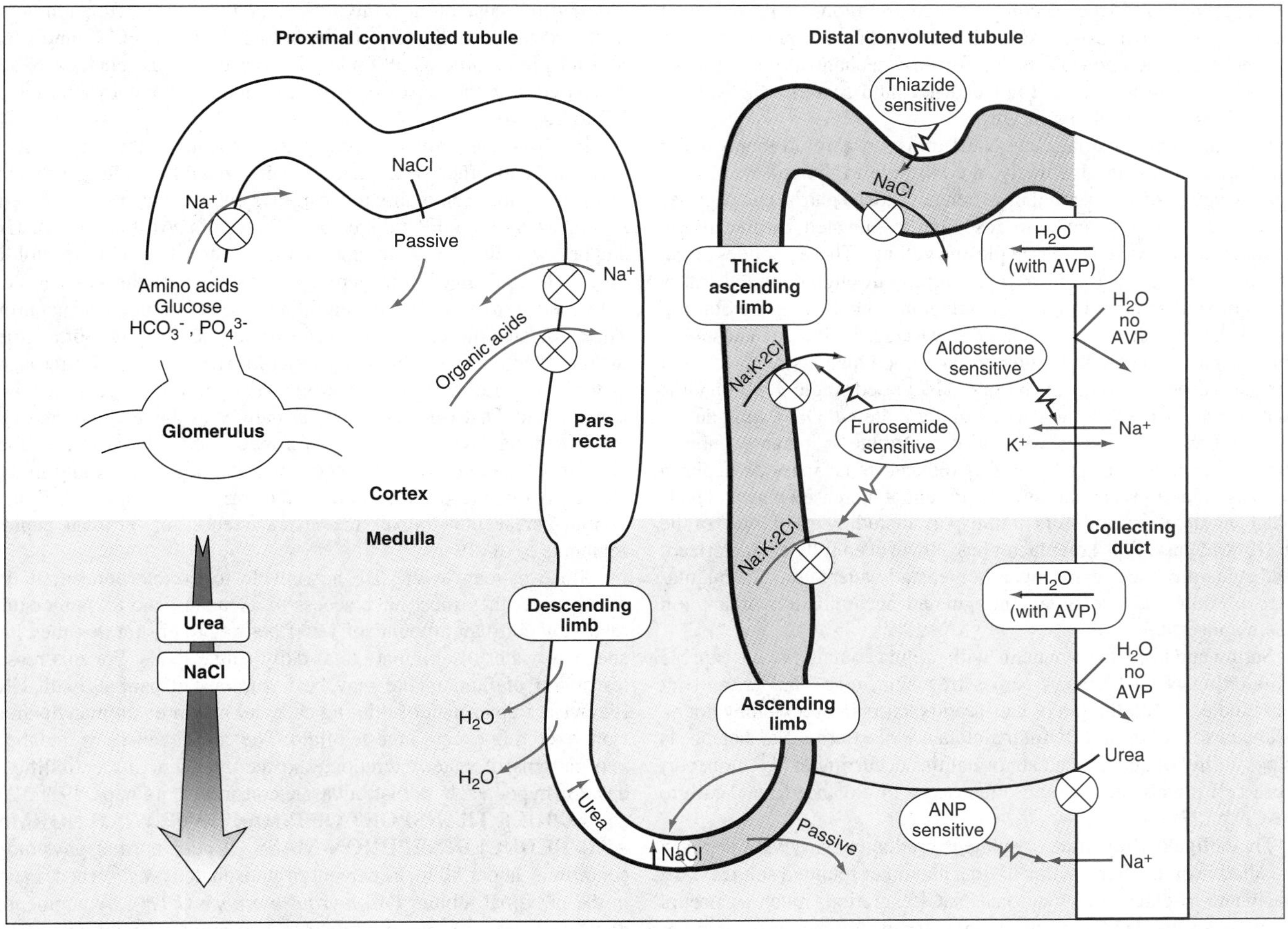

FIGURE 269-2 Transport functions of the various anatomic segments of the mammalian nephron. Fluid reabsorption across the proximal tubule is isosmotic and accounts for reabsorption of approximately two-thirds of the filtered Na^+ and H_2O. The major portions of the filtered HCO_3^-, amino acids, glucose, and phosphate are reabsorbed in the early proximal convoluted tubule. Reabsorption of glucose and amino acids is coupled to Na^+ transport and thereby generates a negative potential difference within the tubule lumen. At the same time, HCO_3^- is reabsorbed by a nonelectrogenic mechanism, via H^+ secretion. The active transport of these solutes results in transepithelial concentration and effective osmotic pressure gradients promoting H_2O flow across the proximal tubule, into the peritubular capillaries. The rise in tubule fluid Cl^- concentration is a necessary reciprocal consequence of the decreased luminal HCO_3^- concentration. The resultant high concentration of Cl^- becomes an important force for the outward passive transport of Cl^- down its concentration gradient, resulting in a lumen-positive potential difference in the late proximal convoluted tubule. The pars recta of the proximal tubule is capable of active electrogenic transport of Na^+ independent of organic solute transport. Under normal conditions, approximately one-third of the glomerular filtrate enters the descending limb of Henle's loop. Because the thin descending limb is incapable of active outward NaCl transport and is characterized by low permeability to Na^+ but high H_2O permeability, H_2O is abstracted passively as the fluid approaches the bend of Henle's loop. Hypertonic fluid with a greater NaCl concentration but lower urea concentration than the surrounding medullary interstitium thus enters the thin ascending limb of Henle, which is largely impermeable to H_2O and urea but highly permeable to NaCl. This permits passive outward diffusion of NaCl. Active Na:K:2Cl transport across the water-impermeable thick ascending limb of Henle allows for separation of solute and water. In consequence, tubule fluid becomes dilute and the medullary interstitium hypertonic.

Irrespective of the final osmolality of the urine, the fluid that enters the distal convoluted tubule is always hypoosmotic. This segment exhibits active Na^+ reabsorption. All but the terminal portion of the distal convoluted tubule is water-impermeable, even in the presence of AVP. Aldosterone exerts its effect in this segment by enhancing Na^+ reabsorption, which is variably coupled to K^+ and H^+ secretion. The cortical and papillary portions of the collecting duct are sites where AVP exerts its principal effect. The permeability of these segments to H_2O in the absence of AVP is very low but can be greatly enhanced in the presence of AVP. These segments are also characterized by active Na^+ reabsorption, which appears to depend on the presence of mineralocorticoid. In the absence of AVP, the collecting tubule is water-impermeable so that hypotonic tubule fluid courses through it. However, in the presence of AVP, water is avidly reabsorbed here, resulting in hypertonic final urine. Sites of action of furosemide and thiazide diuretics and of aldosterone and atrial natriuretic peptide (ANP) are shown.

Na^+ excretion, since aldosterone levels are seldom reduced in CRF. Furthermore, external Na^+ balance is preserved in bilaterally adrenalectomized dogs on fixed replacement doses of mineralocorticoid. Yet another factor contributing to the suppression of fractional NaCl reabsorption in CRF may relate to the retention of solutes as GFR declines. In addition to urea and creatinine, *organic acids* (including *hippurates*) also accumulate. These substances are normally excreted by both glomerular filtration and tubule secretion; the latter process involves a carrier-mediated organic transport system in proximal tubule cells. When GFR is reduced and plasma levels of these organic acids increase, sufficient fluid may accompany their secretion into the proximal tubule lumen (by osmosis) to diminish net fluid reabsorption and even favor net fluid secretion. Evidence for this mechanism derives from studies in which uremic sera induced net fluid secretion in isolated proximal tubules of rabbits in vitro.

Several factors that regulate NaCl transport across tubules under resting conditions are also likely to contribute to the enhanced fractional excretion of salt in renal insufficiency. Atrial natriuretic peptides are released from the heart in response to elevated cardiac filling pressures secondary to increased plasma volume. These peptides effect natriuresis by reducing net Na^+ reabsorption through complementary actions on Na^+ transport in the collecting duct and by altering Starling forces in the adjacent vasa recta. The vascular actions of natriuretic peptides may also extend to glomerular hemodynamics, with afferent arteriolar vasodilatation contributing to increased single-nephron GFR and hence an increase in the amount of Na^+ filtered. Other modulators of tubule transport processes may also contribute to increased single-nephron natriuresis in the setting of reduced renal mass or nephron loss. Vasodilator prostaglandins are present at increased plasma levels in CRF, as are other inhibitors of transport, including inhibitor(s) of the Na^+,K^+-ATPase. This latter factor has not yet been fully characterized; whether its presence represents a homeostatic adaptation for maintenance of fluid balance or an unregulated accumulation of a toxin remains uncertain.

Serum and urine from patients with uremia contain factors capable of inhibiting NaCl transport across frog skin, toad bladder, and rat renal tubule. Accumulation of natriuretic factors in uremia may not be without cost; the "trade-off" for maintenance of external Na^+ balance is the possibility of generalized abnormalities occurring in Na^+ transport across cell membranes, which often occur in advanced renal failure (see Chap. 271).

The obligatory high rate of solute excretion per surviving nephron (so-called osmotic diuresis due to urea and other retained solutes) also contributes to enhancing fractional NaCl excretion, much as occurs in normal individuals after the administration of mannitol or other nonreabsorbable solutes. Finally, certain forms of CRF are associated with unusually large losses of salt in the urine. These *salt-wasting nephropathies* include chronic pyelonephritis and other tubulointerstitial diseases (see Chap. 276) as well as polycystic and medullary cystic diseases. These disorders have in common greater destruction of medullary and tubulointerstitial, rather than cortical and glomerular, portions of the renal parenchyma. Preferential impairment of tubule reabsorptive function, rather than a primary reduction in glomerular filtration, may, therefore, underlie the salt-losing tendency in these disorders. Clinical derangements that alter renal handling of NaCl in CRF (including hypo- and hypervolemia, hypertension, etc.) are considered in Chap. 271.

EFFECTS OF NEPHRON LOSS ON WATER REABSORPTION IN SURVIVING NEPHRONS As with NaCl, there is a progressive increase in the fractional excretion of water with advancing renal insufficiency so that external water balance can be maintained even with a total GFR of 5 mL/min or less. The adaptations of water handling by the diseased kidney are of importance in the defects in urinary concentration and dilution and hence the polyuria and nocturia and tendency to develop water overload encountered in CRF (see Chap. 47). To appreciate the mechanisms involved, the responses of a normal and a uremic individual maintaining external water balance need to be considered. Assuming both individuals have the same dietary and fluid intakes, total solute and volume excretion in both should be identical as well. If the *obligatory solute load* to be excreted by each is 600 mmol/d (600 mosmol/d) and the urine osmolality is 300 mmol/kg water (300 mosmol/kg), a urine volume of 2 L/d will be required to excrete the total solute. If the GFR in normal and uremic individuals totals 180 and 4 L/d, respectively, urinary volume excretion of 2 L/d represents excretion of slightly more than 1 percent of the total glomerular filtrate in the normal subject compared with 50 percent in the uremic patient. Since the range of urine osmolalities that the diseased kidney can achieve [250 to 350 mmol/kg (250 to 350 mosmol/kg)] is narrower than in the normal kidney [40 to 1200 mmol/kg (40 to 1200 mosmol/kg)], the individual with normal function is able to excrete the obligatory daily solute load of 600 mmol (600 mosmol) in as little as 500 mL urine per day or as much as 15 L/d, compared with the narrower range in renal insufficiency, from about 1.7 to 2.4 L/d.

In CRF, the limited capacity to concentrate the urine usually correlates with other measures of impaired renal function. Isosthenuria (urine of similar osmolality to plasma) is therefore an almost universal finding when the GFR falls below 25 mL/min. At this level of GFR and below, urine osmolality does not rise even when supraphysiologic doses of AVP are administered, suggesting that the concentrating defect relates to impaired concentrating capacity in surviving nephrons. The associated increased fractional excretion per nephron of a variety of solutes produces an obligatory water loss (solute diuresis) at roughly isotonic proportions. Consequently, formation of a concentrated urine is prevented. Disease-induced abnormalities of the architecture of the renal medulla (loops of Henle, vasa recta), aberrations in medullary blood flow, and defective transport of NaCl in the ascending limb of Henle also contribute to this defect in urine concentration. Finally, uremia per se may impair the responsiveness of terminal nephron segments to AVP.

Since patients with CRF are unable to excrete concentrated or dilute urine, they must have access to adequate, and to some extent, relatively constant amounts of water per day to ensure that they have adequate water to eliminate total daily solute loads. For this reason, restriction of fluid intake may be hazardous in patients with CRF. Likewise, impairment of diluting capacity may prevent many patients from excreting excess ingested fluid. The consequences of the abnormal patterns of water excretion, and the attendant susceptibilities to develop hypo- and hypernatremia, are considered in Chaps. 49 and 271.

TUBULE TRANSPORT OF PHOSPHATE WITH NORMAL AND REDUCED NEPHRON MASS Under normal physiologic conditions, about 80 to 90 percent of phosphate is reabsorbed, mainly in the proximal tubule. *Parathyroid hormone* (*PTH*), by augmenting phosphate excretion via inhibition of this proximal reabsorptive process (Chap. 353), plays a key role in phosphate homeostasis. When dietary phosphate intake increases, a *transient* rise in plasma phosphate concentration is usually observed. This results in a similarly transient reduction in the plasma ionized calcium level (due largely to deposition of calcium phosphate in bone), which is sensed by a specific receptor on parathyroid cells, stimulating PTH secretion. By enhancing fractional phosphate excretion, PTH restores external phosphate balance and normophosphatemia. This enables plasma ionized calcium levels to return to normal, thereby removing the stimulus to PTH release and restoring the phosphate control system to the original steady state.

With advancing renal failure and constant dietary intake of phosphate, external phosphate balance is achieved by progressive reduction in fractional phosphate reabsorption. Enhanced PTH secretion is an important determinant of this phosphaturic response. With succeeding decrements in total GFR, the amount of phosphate filtered by surviving glomeruli is reduced, leading to transient phosphate retention and, therefore, a rise (albeit small) in plasma phosphate concentration. This leads to a small, reciprocal decline in plasma levels of ionized calcium and a corresponding increase in PTH secretion. Although the phosphaturic response of surviving tubules to this elevation in circulating PTH restores plasma phosphate and calcium to normal levels (at least in the "compensated" stage of CRF described by curve *B* in Fig. 269-1), the new steady-state conditions are only achieved at the cost of *persistently elevated plasma PTH levels.* With progressive reductions in GFR, the process is repeated but at ever-increasing cost in terms of elevated PTH levels.

Alterations in Vitamin D Metabolism These alterations also contribute to elevated PTH levels in CRF. The kidney is normally the major site of *conversion of vitamin D to its active metabolites.* As discussed in Chap. 353, vitamin D, synthesized in skin or acquired in the diet, undergoes initial hydroxylation in the liver to form 25-hydroxyvitamin D [25(OH)D]. The kidney is the site of a second important conversion to 1,25-hydroxyvitamin D [$1,25(OH_2)D$]. This active form of vitamin D acts directly on the parathyroid gland to suppress PTH secretion as well as to enhance intestinal absorption of calcium and phosphate resorption and promote resorption of these ions from bone. In addition, $1,25(OH)D_2$ probably opposes the phosphaturic actions of PTH in the renal tubule by augmenting, rather than diminishing, phosphate reabsorption. With advancing renal disease, nephron loss reduces the renal capacity for vitamin D hydroxylation; phosphate retention also impairs this reaction. Not only are the circulating levels of $1,25(OH)D_2$ diminished in uremia, but the receptors that mediate its action at the parathyroid gland are also diminished. These two effects remove inhibitory influences on PTH secretion, leading to increased plasma PTH levels. Reduction in circulating $1,25(OH)D_2$ levels, by suppressing intestinal calcium absorption, contributes to the development of the hypocalcemia and hyperparathyroidism of CRF (see Chap. 271).

Hyperparathyroidism in Chronic Renal Failure At least two additional processes are thought to contribute to hyperparathyroidism in CRF. One relates to resistance of bone to the calcemic effect of PTH in uremia. This resistance necessitates a higher level of PTH to demineralize bone and maintain the plasma calcium concentration. The other derives from the finding that reductions in renal mass impair the kidneys' capacity to degrade circulating PTH. Ultimately, however, phosphate conforms more to a curve *B*– rather than a curve *C*–type pattern in Fig. 269-1, and phosphate retention occurs when the GFR falls below about 25 mL/min, signifying that these latter forms of adaptation play limited roles.

Since PTH exerts major effects on bone as well as renal tubules, the external balance of phosphate in CRF is achieved at the expense of elevated PTH levels, which, in turn, account for many of the bone changes of renal osteodystrophy (i.e., *secondary hyperparathyroidism*; see Fig. 271-1). In support of this *trade-off hypothesis*, when dietary phosphate intake is reduced in proportion to the reduction in GFR in animals with CRF, external balance of phosphate no longer requires augmentation of fractional phosphate excretion in surviving nephrons. Accordingly, circulating levels of PTH no longer rise, and the bone changes of secondary hyperparathyroidism are diminished, if not prevented.

HYDROGEN AND BICARBONATE TRANSPORT WITH NORMAL AND REDUCED RENAL MASS As discussed in Chap. 50, the pH of extracellular fluid is normally maintained within a narrow range (7.36 to 7.44) despite day-to-day fluctuations in the quantity of acids added to the extracellular fluid from dietary and metabolic sources (approximately 1 mmol H^+ per kilogram of body weight per day). These acids consume buffers from both extracellular and intracellular fluid, of which HCO_3^- is the most important in the intracellular compartment. Such buffering minimizes changes in pH. Long-term effectiveness of the HCO_3^- buffer system, however, requires mechanisms for replenishment, otherwise unrelenting acquisition of nonvolatile acids from dietary and metabolic sources would ultimately exhaust buffering capacity, culminating in fatal acidosis. The kidneys normally function to prevent this eventuality by *regenerating* bicarbonate, thereby maintaining plasma concentrations of HCO_3^-. In addition, the kidneys also *reclaim* HCO_3^- in the glomerular ultrafiltrate. Reclamation of filtered HCO_3^- takes place largely in the proximal tubule and, under normal circumstances, is virtually complete below a critical plasma HCO_3^- concentration—the threshold concentration—which in humans is

normally about 26 mmol/L, identical to the concentration of HCO_3^- in plasma. As a consequence, HCO_3^- wastage is prevented. Alternatively, when plasma HCO_3^- rises above this threshold, reabsorption becomes less complete, allowing escape of excess HCO_3^- into the final urine, which restores the plasma HCO_3^- towards normal levels. Despite complete reabsorption of HCO_3^-, metabolic acidosis would still ensue if HCO_3^- consumed in buffering nonvolatile acids were not constantly regenerated.

The *reabsorption* of filtered HCO_3^- occurs by the following mechanism. Filtered bicarbonate combines with H^+ secreted from proximal tubule cells, probably via a Na^+/H^+ exchanger, to form carbonic acid (H_2CO_3). Dehydration of carbonic acid under the influence of *luminal carbonic anhydrase* yields CO_2, which is free to diffuse from lumen to peritubular blood. In the proximal tubule cell, the OH^- left behind by the H^+ secretion reacts with CO_2, under the influence of *intracellular carbonic anhydrase*, forming HCO_3^-. This ion is transported across the contraluminal proximal tubule cell membrane, via an electrogenic Na/HCO_3^- cotransporter, to reenter the extracellular HCO_3^- pool. The net result is *reclamation of a filtered bicarbonate ion.* Secreted H^+ is also free to react with nonbicarbonate buffers [e.g., phosphate or ammonia (NH_4^+)] in the tubule lumen, and hydrogen ions are excreted in these forms in the final urine. Again, the OH^- left behind in the proximal tubule cell from H^+ secretion reacts with CO_2, forming bicarbonate—also representing *regeneration of an* HCO_3^- *ion.*

Hydrogen ions in the urine are bound to filtered buffers (e.g., phosphate) in amounts equivalent to the amounts of alkali required to titrate the pH of the urine up to the pH of the blood (the so-called titratable acid). It is not usually possible to eliminate all the daily acid load in the form of titratable acid due to limits of urinary pH. Metabolism of glutamine by proximal tubule cells to yield ammonium (ammoniagenesis) serves as an additional mechanism for H^+ elimination and bicarbonate regeneration. Glutamine metabolism forms not only NH_4^+ (i.e., NH_3 plus H^+) but also HCO_3^-, which is transported across the proximal tubule (HCO_3^- regeneration). The NH_4^+ must be excreted in the urine for this process to be effective in bicarbonate regeneration. The excretion of ammonium involves secretion by proximal tubule cells (possibly by the Na^+/H^+ exchanger as $Na^+:NH_4^+$), generation of high medullary interstitial NH_4^+ concentration by an elaborate countercurrent multiplication/exchange system, and finally, secretion of the interstitial NH_4^+ by the collecting duct by a combination of H^+ secretion and passive NH_3 diffusion. *Ammoniagenesis* is responsive to the acid-base needs of the individual. When faced with an acute acid burden and an increased need for HCO_3^- regeneration, the rate of renal ammonia synthesis increases sharply.

The quantity of hydrogen ions excreted as titratable acid and NH_4^+ is equal to the quantity of HCO_3^- regenerated in tubule cells and added to plasma. Under steady-state conditions, the net quantity of acid excreted into the urine (the sum of titratable acid and NH_4^+ less HCO_3^-) must equal the quantity of acid gained by the extracellular fluid from all sources. Metabolic acidosis and alkalosis result when this delicate balance is perturbed, the former the result of insufficient net acid excretion, and the latter due to excessive acid excretion.

Progressive loss of renal function usually causes little or no change in arterial pH, plasma bicarbonate concentration, or arterial carbon dioxide tension (P_{CO_2}) until GFR falls below 30 percent of normal. Thereafter, all three tend to decline as *metabolic acidosis* ensues. In general, the metabolic acidosis of CRF is not due to overproduction of acids but is rather a reflection of nephron loss, which limits the amount of NH_3 (and therefore also HCO_3^-) that can be generated. Although surviving nephrons appear to be capable of generating supranormal amounts of NH_3 *per nephron*, the diminished nephron population causes overall production to be reduced to an extent that is insufficient to permit sufficient buffering of H^+ in urine. As a result, although patients with CRF may be able to acidify their urine normally (i.e., urine pH as low as 4.5), the defect in NH_3 production limits daily net acid excretion to 30 to 40 mmol, or one-half to two-thirds the quantity of nonvolatile acid added to the extracellular fluid in the same time period. Metabolic acidosis resulting from this daily positive balance of H^+ is seldom florid in CRF of mild to moderate severity. Relative stability of plasma bicarbonate (albeit at reduced levels of 14 to 18 mmol/L) is maintained at the expense of buffering by bone. Because it contains large reserves of alkaline salts (calcium phosphate and calcium bicarbonate), bone constitutes a major reserve of buffering capacity. Dissolution of these buffers contributes to the osteodystrophy of CRF (see Fig. 271-1).

Although the acidosis of CRF is due to loss of tubule mass, it nevertheless depends to a large part on the level of GFR. When GFR is reduced to only a moderate extent (i.e., to about 50 percent of normal), retention of anions, principally sulfates and phosphates, is not pronounced. Therefore, as the plasma HCO_3^- falls owing to dysfunction or loss of tubules, retention of Cl^- by the kidneys leads to a *hyperchloremic acidosis*. At this stage *the anion gap is normal*. With further reductions in GFR and more pronounced azotemia, however, the retention of phosphates, sulfates, and other *unmeasured* anions ensues and plasma Cl^- falls to normal levels despite the reduction in plasma HCO_3^- concentration. *A moderate to large anion gap therefore develops.*

TUBULE POTASSIUM TRANSPORT WITH NORMAL AND REDUCED NEPHRON MASS As with H^+, the concentration of K^+ in extracellular fluid is normally maintained within a relatively narrow range, 4 to 5 mmol/L. Ninety-five percent or more of total-body K^+ is in the intracellular compartment, where the intracellular concentration is approximately 160 mmol/L. Normal individuals maintain external K^+ balance by excreting amounts into the urine that equal the intake, less the relatively small losses in stool and sweat. K^+ is freely filtered at the glomerulus, although the amount excreted usually represents no more than about 20 percent of the quantity filtered. The great bulk of the K^+ filtered is reabsorbed in the early portions of the nephron, about two-thirds in the proximal tubule, and an additional 20 to 25 percent in the loop of Henle. A K^+ *secretory process* operates in the distal tubule and terminal nephron segments. This process is largely dependent on Na^+ reabsorption and the accompanying lumen-negative voltage creating an electrical gradient across the tubule wall, favoring K^+ secretion into the lumen of the distal tubule and collecting duct.

The ability to maintain external K^+ balance and normal plasma K^+ concentration until relatively late in the course of CRF is a consequence primarily of a progressive increase in fractional excretion of K^+. Greatly enhanced rates of K^+ secretion occur in distal portions of surviving tubules. The augmented secretion rate of aldosterone contributes to enhanced tubule secretion of K^+. In addition, both the increased distal tubule flow rates in residual functioning nephrons due to the osmotic diuresis and enhanced luminal electronegativity created by the increased presence of highly impermeable anions such as phosphate and sulfate enhance K^+ secretion. Aldosterone also stimulates net entry of K^+ into the lumen of the colon, a mechanism known to be enhanced in CRF. → ***More detailed discussions of abnormal K^+ homeostasis in acute and chronic forms of renal failure are given in Chaps. 270 and 271.***

BIBLIOGRAPHY

Brenner BM: Nephron adaptation to renal injury or ablation. Am J Physiol 249:F324, 1985

——— et al: Diverse biological actions of atrial natriuretic peptides. Physiol Rev 70:665, 1990

———: *The Kidney*, 5th ed. Philadelphia, Saunders, 1996

Feinfeld DA, Sherwood LM: Parathyroid hormone and $1,25(OH)_2D_3$ in chronic renal failure. Kidney Int 33:1049, 1988

Kaji D, Kahn T: Na^+-K^+ pump in chronic renal failure. Am J Physiol 252:F785, 1987

Warnock DG: Uremic acidosis. Kidney Int 34:278, 1988

270 ACUTE RENAL FAILURE

Hugh R. Brady, Barry M. Brenner

Acute renal failure (ARF) is a syndrome characterized by rapid decline in glomerular filtration rate (hours to weeks), retention of nitrogenous waste products, and perturbation of extracellular fluid volume and electrolyte and acid-base homeostasis. ARF complicates approximately 5 percent of hospital admissions and up to 30 percent of admissions to intensive care units. Oliguria (urine output <400 mL/d) is a frequent but not invariable clinical feature (~50 percent). ARF is usually asymptomatic and is diagnosed when biochemical screening of hospitalized patients reveals a recent increase in plasma urea and creatinine concentrations. It may complicate a wide range of diseases, which for purposes of diagnosis and management are conveniently divided into three categories: (1) diseases that cause renal hypoperfusion without compromising the integrity of renal parenchyma (*prerenal azotemia*, prerenal ARF) (~55 percent); (2) diseases that directly involve renal parenchyma (*renal azotemia*, intrinsic renal ARF) (~40 percent); and (3) diseases associated with urinary tract obstruction (*postrenal azotemia*, postrenal ARF) (~5 percent). Most ARF is reversible, the kidney being relatively unique among major organs in its ability to recover from almost complete loss of function. Nevertheless, ARF is associated with major in-hospital morbidity and mortality, in large part due to the serious nature of the illness that precipitated the ARF.

ETIOLOGY AND PATHOPHYSIOLOGY

PRERENAL AZOTEMIA (PRERENAL ARF) Prerenal azotemia is the most common form of ARF and represents a physiologic response to mild to moderate renal hypoperfusion. Prerenal azotemia is rapidly reversible upon restoration of renal blood flow and glomerular ultrafiltration pressure. Renal parenchymal tissue is not damaged; indeed, kidneys from individuals with prerenal azotemia function well when transplanted into recipients with normal cardiovascular function. More severe hypoperfusion may lead to ischemic injury of renal parenchyma and intrinsic renal azotemia. Thus, prerenal azotemia and ischemic ARF are part of a spectrum of manifestations of renal hypoperfusion. As shown in Table 270-1, prerenal azotemia can complicate any disease that induces hypovolemia, low cardiac output, systemic vasodilatation, or selective renal vasoconstriction.

Hypovolemia leads to a fall in mean systemic arterial pressure, which is detected as reduced stretch by arterial (e.g., carotid sinus) and cardiac baroreceptors. Activated baroreceptors trigger a coordinated series of neural and humoral responses designed to restore blood volume and arterial pressure. These include activation of the sympathetic nervous system and renin-angiotensin-aldosterone system and release of arginine vasopressin [AVP; formerly called antidiuretic hormone (ADH)]. Norepinephrine, angiotensin II, and AVP act in concert in an attempt to preserve cardiac and cerebral perfusion by stimulating vasoconstriction in relatively "nonessential" vascular beds such as the musculocutaneous and splanchnic circulations, inhibiting salt loss through sweat glands, stimulating thirst and salt appetite, and promoting renal salt and water retention. Glomerular perfusion, ultrafiltration pressure, and filtration rate are preserved during mild hypoperfusion through several compensatory mechanisms. Stretch receptors in afferent arterioles, in response to a reduction in perfusion pressure, trigger afferent arteriolar vasodilatation through a local myogenic reflex (autoregulation). Biosynthesis of vasodilator prostaglandins (e.g., prostacyclin, PGE_2) and possibly nitric oxide is also enhanced, and these compounds preferentially dilate afferent arterioles. In addition, angiotensin II induces preferential constriction of efferent arterioles. As a result, intraglomerular pressure is maintained, the fraction of plasma flowing through glomerular capillaries that is filtered is increased (filtration fraction), and glomerular filtration rate (GFR) is preserved. During states of more severe hypoperfusion, these compensatory responses are overwhelmed and GFR falls, leading to prerenal ARF.

Table 270-1

Classification and Major Causes of Acute Renal Failure

PRERENAL AZOTEMIA

I. Hypovolemia
   A. Hemorrhage, burns, dehydration
   B. Gastrointestinal fluid loss: vomiting, surgical drainage, diarrhea
   C. Renal fluid loss: diuretics, osmotic diuresis (e.g., diabetes mellitus), hypoadrenalism
   D. Sequestration in extravascular space: pancreatitis, peritonitis, trauma, burns, severe hypoalbuminemia
II. Low cardiac output
   A. Diseases of myocardium, valves, and pericardium, arrhythmias, tamponade
   B. Other: pulmonary hypertension, massive pulmonary embolus, positive pressure mechanical ventilation
III. Altered renal systemic vascular resistance ratio
   A. Systemic vasodilatation: sepsis, antihypertensives, afterload reducers, anesthesia, anaphylaxis
   B. Renal vasoconstriction: hypercalcemia, norepinephrine, epinephrine, cyclosporine, amphotericin B
   C. Cirrhosis with ascites (hepatorenal syndrome)
IV. Renal hypoperfusion with impairment of renal autoregulatory responses
   Cyclooxygenase inhibitors, angiotensin-converting enzyme inhibitors
V. Hyperviscosity syndrome (rare)
   Multiple myeloma, macroglobulinemia, polycythemia

INTRINSIC RENAL AZOTEMIA

I. Renovascular obstruction (bilateral or unilateral with one functioning kidney)
   A. Renal artery obstruction: atherosclerotic plaque, thrombosis, embolism, dissecting aneurysm, vasculitis
   B. Renal vein obstruction: thrombosis, compression
II. Disease of glomeruli or renal microvasculature
   A. Glomerulonephritis and vasculitis
   B. Hemolytic uremic syndrome, thrombotic thrombocytopenic purpura, disseminated intravascular coagulation, toxemia of pregnancy, accelerated hypertension, radiation nephritis, systemic lupus erythematosus, scleroderma
III. Acute tubular necrosis
   A. Ischemia: as for prerenal azotemia (hypovolemia, low cardiac output, renal vasoconstriction, systemic vasodilatation), obstetric complications (abruptio placentae, postpartum hemorrhage)
   B. Toxins
      1. Exogenous: radiocontrast, cyclosporine, antibiotics (e.g., aminoglycosides), chemotherapy (e.g., cisplatin), organic solvents (e.g., ethylene glycol), acetaminophen, illegal abortifacients
      2. Endogenous: rhabdomyolysis, hemolysis, uric acid, oxalate, plasma cell dyscrasia (e.g., myeloma)
IV. Interstitial nephritis
   A. Allergic: antibiotics (e.g., β-lactams, sulfonamides, trimethoprim, rifampicin), nonsteroidal anti-inflammatory agents, diuretics, captopril
   B. Infection: bacterial (e.g., acute pyelonephritis, leptospirosis), viral (e.g., cytomegalovirus), fungal (e.g., candidiasis)
   C. Infiltration: lymphoma, leukemia, sarcoidosis
   D. Idiopathic
V. Intratubular deposition and obstruction
   Myeloma proteins, uric acid, oxalate, acyclovir, methotrexate, sulphonamides
VI. Renal allograft rejection

POSTRENAL AZOTEMIA (OBSTRUCTION)

I. Ureteric
   Calculi, blood clot, sloughed papillae, cancer, external compression (e.g., retroperitoneal fibrosis)
II. Bladder neck
   Neurogenic bladder, prostatic hypertrophy, calculi, cancer, blood clot
III. Urethra
   Stricture, congenital valve, phimosis

Autoregulatory dilatation of afferent arterioles is maximal at mean systemic arterial blood pressures of ~80 mmHg, and hypotension below this level is associated with a precipitous decline in GFR. Lesser degrees of hypotension may provoke prerenal azotemia in the elderly and in patients with diseases affecting the integrity of afferent arterioles (e.g., hypertensive nephrosclerosis, diabetic vasculopathy). In addition, *drugs* that interfere with adaptive responses in the renal microcirculation may convert compensated renal hypoperfusion into overt prerenal azotemia or trigger progression of prerenal azotemia to ischemic ARF (see below). Pharmacologic inhibitors of either renal prostaglandin biosynthesis (*cyclooxygenase inhibitors*) or angiotensin-converting enzyme (ACE) activity (ACE inhibitors) are the major culprits and should be used judiciously in the setting of suspected renal hypoperfusion. *Nonsteroidal anti-inflammatory drugs*, which inhibit cyclooxygenases and prostaglandin biosynthesis, do not compromise GFR in healthy individuals but may precipitate prerenal azotemia in patients with volume depletion or in those with chronic renal insufficiency in whom GFR is maintained, in part, through prostaglandin-mediated hyperfiltration through the remaining functional nephrons. ACE inhibitors can also compromise GFR in subjects with renal hypoperfusion and should be used with special care in patients with bilateral renal artery stenosis or unilateral stenosis in a solitary functioning kidney. Glomerular perfusion and filtration may be exquisitely dependent on the actions of angiotensin II under the latter circumstances. Angiotensin II preserves glomerular filtration pressure distal to stenoses by elevating systemic arterial pressure and by triggering selective constriction of efferent arterioles. ACE inhibitors blunt these responses and precipitate ARF, usually reversible, in approximately ~30 percent of these patients.

Hepatorenal Syndrome This is a particularly aggressive form of ARF that frequently complicates hepatic failure due to advanced cirrhosis or other liver diseases, including malignancy, hepatic resection, and biliary obstruction. Intrarenal vasoconstriction and avid sodium retention are early sequelae of these diseases and may be detected before changes in systemic hemodynamics. Patients with advanced liver disease, portal hypertension, and ascites also have increased plasma volume but "effective" hypovolemia as a consequence of systemic vasodilatation and pooling of blood in the portal circulation. Azotemia typically develops slowly over weeks or months in parallel with deteriorating hepatic function but may accelerate dramatically following a variety of hemodynamic insults, including hemorrhage, paracentesis, and overzealous use of diuretics, vasodilators, or cyclooxygenase inhibitors. In full-blown hepatorenal syndrome, ARF progresses even after optimization of systemic hemodynamics and volume status and removal of nephrotoxins, probably as a result of ongoing intrarenal vasoconstriction, hypoperfusion, and ischemia triggered by a circulating or neural factor elaborated by the failing liver. Indeed, it must be remembered that patients with liver disease may develop other forms of ARF (e.g., sepsis, nephrotoxic medications), and a diagnosis of hepatorenal syndrome should be made only after exclusion of other possible reversible causes.

INTRINSIC RENAL AZOTEMIA (INTRINSIC RENAL ARF) Intrinsic renal azotemia can complicate many diverse diseases of the renal parenchyma. From a clinicopathologic viewpoint, it is useful to divide the causes of acute intrinsic renal azotemia into (1) diseases of large renal vessels, (2) diseases of the renal microcirculation and glomeruli, (3) ischemic and nephrotoxic ARF, and (4) tubulointerstitial diseases (Table 270-1). Most intrinsic renal azotemia is triggered by ischemia (ischemic ARF) or nephrotoxins (nephrotoxic ARF), insults that typically induce acute tubular necrosis (ATN). Accordingly, the terms ARF and ATN are usually used interchangeably in these settings. However, as many as 20 to 30 percent of patients with ischemic or nephrotoxic ARF do not have clinical (granular or tubular cell urinary casts) or morphologic evidence of tubular necrosis, underscoring the role of sublethal injury to tubular epithelium and injury to other renal cells (e.g., endothelial cells) in the pathophysiology of this syndrome.

Etiology and Pathophysiology of Ischemic ARF Prerenal azotemia and ischemic ARF are part of a spectrum of manifestations of renal hypoperfusion. Ischemic ARF differs from prerenal azotemia in that the hypoperfusion induces ischemic injury to renal cells, particularly tubular epithelium, and recovery typically takes 1 to 2 weeks after normalization of renal perfusion as it requires regeneration of tubular cells. In its most extreme form, ischemia leads to bilateral renal cortical necrosis and irreversible renal failure. Ischemic ARF occurs most frequently in patients undergoing major cardiovascular surgery or suffering severe trauma, hemorrhage, sepsis, and/or volume depletion (Table 270-1). Ischemic ARF can also complicate milder forms of true or "effective" hypovolemia if the latter occurs in the presence of other insults (e.g., nephrotoxins or sepsis) or in patients with compromised autoregulatory defense mechanisms or preexisting renal insufficiency.

The course of ischemic ARF is typically characterized by three phases: the initiation, maintenance, and recovery phases. The *initiation phase* (hours to days) is the initial period of renal hypoperfusion during which ischemic injury is evolving. GFR declines because (1) glomerular ultrafiltration pressure is reduced as a consequence of the fall in renal blood flow, (2) the flow of glomerular filtrate within tubules is obstructed by casts comprising epithelial cells and necrotic debris derived from ischemic tubule epithelium, and (3) there is backleak of glomerular filtrate through injured tubular epithelium (Fig. 270-1). Ischemic injury is most prominent in the terminal medullary portion of the proximal tubule (S_3 segment, pars recta) and the medullary portion of the thick ascending limb of the loop of Henle. Both segments have high rates of active (ATP-dependent) solute transport and oxygen consumption and are located in a zone of the kidney (the outer medulla) that is relatively ischemic, even under basal conditions, by virtue of the unique countercurrent arrangement of the medullary vasculature. Cellular ischemia results in a series of alterations in energetics, ion transport, and membrane integrity that ultimately lead to cell necrosis. These include depletion of ATP, inhibition of active sodium transport and transport of other solutes, impairment of cell volume regulation and cell swelling, cytoskeletal disruption and loss of cell polarity, accumulation of intracellular calcium, altered phospholipid metabolism, oxygen free radical formation, and peroxidation of membrane lipids. Importantly, renal injury can be limited by restoration of renal blood flow during this period.

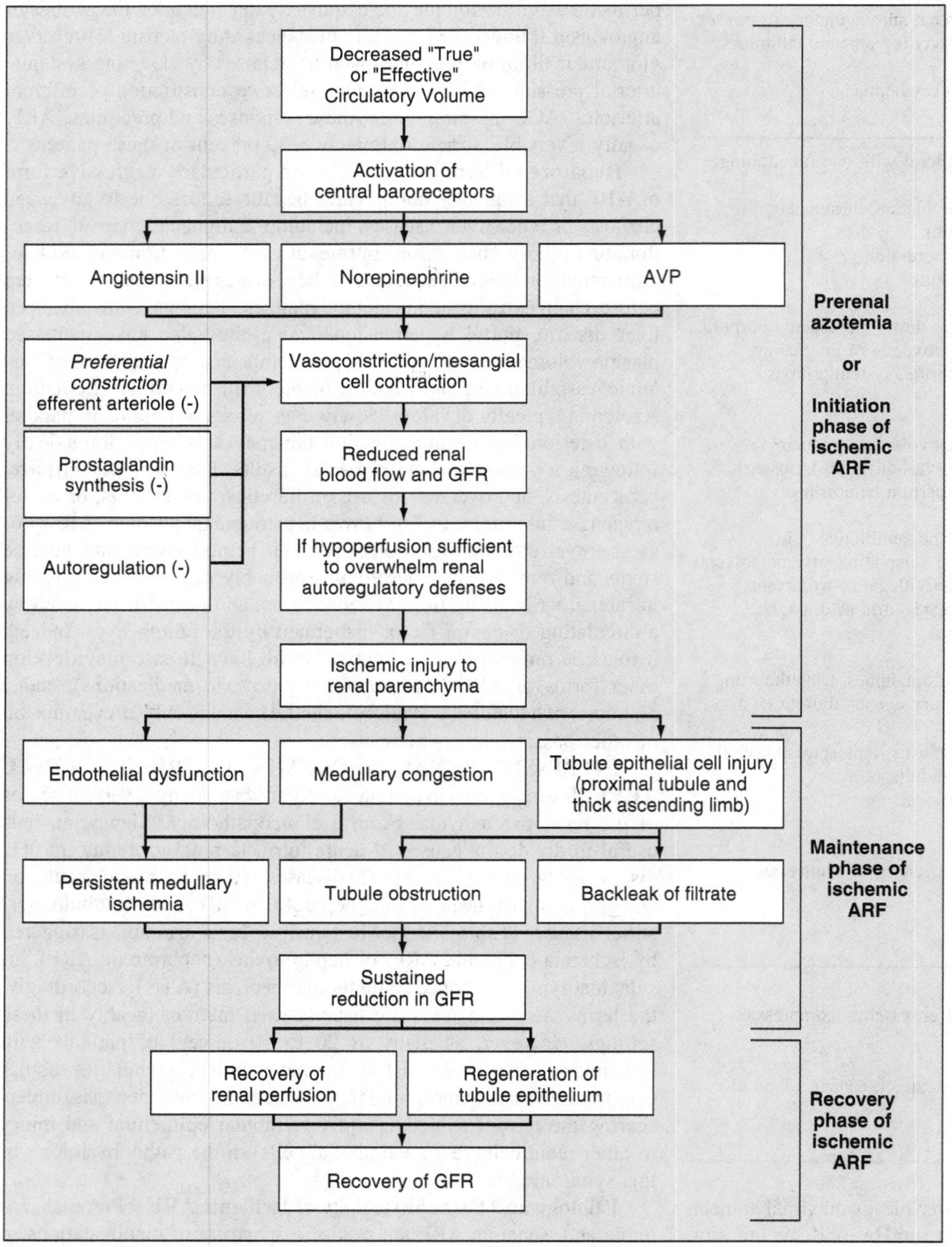

FIGURE 270-1 Overview of the pathophysiology of prerenal azotemia and ischemic ARF: A spectrum of manifestations of renal hypoperfusion (ARF, acute renal failure; AVP, arginine vasopressin; GFR, glomerular filtration rate.)

The initiation phase is followed by a *maintenance phase* (typically 1 to 2 weeks) during which epithelial cell injury is established, GFR stabilizes at its nadir (typically 5 to 10 mL/min), urine output is lowest, and uremic complications arise (see below). The reasons why the GFR remains low during this phase, despite correction of systemic hemodynamics, are still being defined. Putative mechanisms include persistent intrarenal vasoconstriction and medullary ischemia triggered by dysregulated release of vasoactive mediators from injured endothelial cells (e.g., decreased nitric oxide, increased endothelin), congestion of medullary blood vessels, and reperfusion injury induced by reactive oxygen species and other mediators derived from leukocytes or renal parenchymal cells (Fig. 270-1). In addition, epithelial cell injury per se may contribute to persistent intrarenal vasoconstriction by a process termed *tubuloglomerular feedback*. Specialized epithelial cells in the macula densa region of distal tubules detect increases in distal salt (probably chloride) delivery that occur as a consequence of impaired reabsorption by more proximal nephron segments. Macula densa cells in turn stimulate constriction of adjacent afferent arterioles by a poorly defined mechanism and further compromise glomerular perfusion and filtration, thereby contributing to a vicious cycle. A *recovery phase* is characterized by tubule cell regeneration and a gradual return of GFR to or towards premorbid levels. The recovery phase may be complicated by marked diuresis diuretic phase due to excretion of retained salt and water and other solutes, continued use of diuretics, and/or delayed recovery of epithelial cell function (solute and water reabsorption) relative to glomerular filtration (see below).

Etiology and Pathophysiology of Nephrotoxic ARF Acute intrinsic renal azotemia can complicate exposure to many structurally diverse pharmacologic agents (Table 270-1). With most nephrotoxins, the incidence of ARF is increased in the elderly and in patients with preexisting chronic renal insufficiency, true or "effective" hypovolemia, or concomitant exposure to other toxins.

Intrarenal vasoconstriction is a pivotal event in ARF triggered by *radiocontrast agents* (contrast nephropathy) and *cyclosporine*. In keeping with this pathophysiology, both agents induce ARF that shares features with prerenal azotemia: namely, an acute fall in renal blood flow and GFR, a relatively benign urine sediment, and a low fractional excretion of sodium (see below). Severe cases may show clinical or pathologic evidence of ATN. Contrast nephropathy classically presents as an acute (onset within 24 to 28 h) but reversible (peak 3 to 5 days, resolution within 1 week) rise in blood urea nitrogen and creatinine and is most common in individuals with preexisting chronic renal insufficiency, diabetes mellitus, congestive heart failure, hypovolemia, or multiple myeloma. The syndrome appears to be dose-related, and its incidence is only slightly reduced in high-risk individuals by use of more expensive low osmolality, nonionic contrast agents. Endothelin, a potent vasoconstrictor peptide released from endothelial cells, is an important mediator of intrarenal vasoconstriction and mesangial cell contraction in this setting. Endothelin has also been implicated as an important mediator of cyclosporine-induced ARF.

Direct toxicity to tubule epithelial cells and/or intratubular obstruction are major pathophysiologic events in ARF induced by many antibiotics and anticancer drugs. Frequent offenders are the antimicrobial agents, such as acyclovir, foscarnet, aminoglycosides, amphotericin B, and pentamidine, and chemotherapeutic agents, such as cisplatin and ifosfamide. ARF complicates 10 to 30 percent of courses of *aminoglycoside antibiotics*, even in the presence of therapeutic levels. *Amphotericin B* causes dose-related ARF through intrarenal vasoconstriction and direct toxicity to proximal tubule epithelium. Cisplatin, like the aminoglycosides, is accumulated by proximal tubule cells and typically provokes ARF after 7 to 10 days of exposure by inducing mitochondrial injury, inhibition of ATPase activity and solute transport, and free radical–mediated injury to cell membranes.

The most common endogenous nephrotoxins are calcium, myoglobin, hemoglobin, urate, oxalate, and myeloma light chains. Hypercalcemia can compromise GFR, predominantly by inducing intrarenal vasoconstriction. Calcium phosphate deposition within the kidney may also contribute. Both *rhabdomyolysis* and *hemolysis* can induce ARF, particularly in hypovolemic or acidotic individuals. Myoglobinuric ARF complicates approximately 30 percent of cases of rhabdomyolysis. Common causes of the latter include traumatic crush injury, muscle ischemia, seizures, excessive exercise, heat stroke or malignant hyperthermia, alcoholism, and infectious or metabolic disorders. ARF due to hemolysis is relatively rare and is observed following massive blood transfusion reactions. It has been postulated that myoglobin and hemoglobin or other compounds released from muscle or red blood cells cause ARF via toxic effects on tubule epithelial cells or by inducing intratubular cast formation. Hypovolemia or acidosis may contribute to the pathogenesis of ARF in this setting by promoting intranephronal cast formation. In addition, both hemoglobin and myoglobin are potent inhibitors of nitric oxide bioactivity and may trigger intrarenal vasoconstriction and ischemia in patients with borderline renal hypoperfusion. The formation of intratubular casts containing filtered immunoglobulin light chains and other proteins, including Tamm-Horsfall protein produced by thick ascending limb cells, is the major trigger for ARF in patients with *multiple myeloma* (myeloma-cast nephropathy). Light chains may also be directly toxic to tubule epithelial cells. Intratubular obstruction may also be an important cause of ARF in patients with severe *hyperuricosuria* or *hyperoxaluria*. Acute uric acid nephropathy typically complicates treatment of lymphoproliferative or myeloproliferative disorders but occasionally occurs in other forms of primary or secondary hyperuricemia if the urine is concentrated.

Pathology of Ischemic and Nephrotoxic ARF The classic pathologic features of ischemic ARF are patchy and focal necrosis of tubule epithelium with detachment from its basement membrane and occlusion of tubule lumens with casts composed of intact or degenerating epithelial cells, cellular debris, Tamm-Horsfall mucoprotein, and pigments. Leukocyte accumulation is frequently observed in vasa recta; however, the glomeruli and renal vasculature are characteristically normal. Necrosis is most severe in the straight portion (pars recta) of proximal tubules but may also be prominent in the medullary thick ascending limb of the loop of Henle.

In nephrotoxic ARF, morphologic changes tend to be most prominent in both the convoluted and straight portions of proximal tubules. Tubule cell necrosis is less pronounced than in ischemic ARF.

Other Causes of Acute Intrinsic Renal Azotemia Patients with advanced atherosclerosis can develop ARF after manipulation of the aorta or renal arteries at surgery or angiography, following trauma, or, rarely, spontaneously due to embolization of cholesterol crystals to the renal vasculature (atheroembolic ARF). Cholesterol crystals lodge in small- and medium-sized arteries and incite a giant cell and fibrotic reaction in the vessel wall with narrowing or obstruction of the vessel lumen. Atheroembolic ARF is frequently irreversible. A myriad of structurally diverse pharmacologic agents induce ARF by triggering allergic interstitial nephritis, a disease characterized by infiltration of the tubulointerstitium by granulocytes (typically but not invariably eosinophils), macrophages, and/or lymphocytes and by interstitial edema. The most common offenders are antibiotics (e.g., penicillins, cephalosporins, trimethoprim, sulfonamides, rifampicin) and nonsteroidal anti-inflammatory drugs (Table 270-1).

POSTRENAL AZOTEMIA (See also Chap. 280) Urinary tract obstruction accounts for fewer than 5 percent of cases of ARF. Since one kidney has sufficient clearance capacity to excrete nitrogenous waste products, ARF from obstruction requires either obstruction to urine flow between the external urethral meatus and bladder neck, bilateral ureteric obstruction, or unilateral ureteric obstruction in a patient with one functioning kidney or preexisting chronic renal insufficiency. Bladder neck obstruction represents the most common cause of postrenal azotemia and is usually due to prostatic disease (e.g., hypertrophy, neoplasia, or infection), neurogenic bladder, or therapy with anticholinergic drugs. Less common causes of acute lower urinary tract obstruction include blood clots, calculi, and urethritis with spasm. Ureteric obstruction may result from intraluminal obstruction (e.g., calculi, blood clots, sloughed renal papillae), infiltration of the ureteric wall (e.g., neoplasia), or external compression (e.g., retroperitoneal fibrosis, neoplasia or abscess, inadvertent surgical ligature). During the early stages of obstruction (hours to days), continued glomerular filtration leads to increased intraluminal pressure upstream to the site of obstruction. As a result there are gradual distention of proximal ureter, renal pelvis, and calyces and a fall in GFR. Acute obstruction is initially associated with modest increase in renal blood flow, but arteriolar vasoconstriction soon supervenes, leading to a further decline in glomerular filtration.

CLINICAL FEATURES AND DIFFERENTIAL DIAGNOSIS

Patients presenting with azotemia should be assessed initially to determine if the decline in GFR is acute or chronic. An acute process is easily established if a review of laboratory records reveals a recent rise in blood urea and creatinine levels, but previous measurements are not always available. Findings that suggest chronic renal failure (Chap. 271) include anemia, neuropathy, and radiologic evidence of renal osteodystrophy or small scarred kidneys. However, it should be noted that anemia may also complicate ARF (see below), and renal size may be normal or increased in several chronic renal diseases (e.g., diabetic nephropathy, amyloidosis, polycystic kidney disease). Once a diagnosis of ARF has been established, several issues should be addressed promptly: (1) the identification of the cause of ARF, (2) the elimination of the triggering insult (e.g., nephrotoxin) and/or institution of disease-specific therapies, and (3) the prevention and management of uremic complications.

CLINICAL ASSESSMENT Clinical clues to *prerenal azotemia* are symptoms of thirst and orthostatic dizziness and physical evidence of orthostatic hypotension and tachycardia, reduced jugular venous pressure, decreased skin turgor, dry mucous membranes, and reduced axillary sweating. Case records should be reviewed for documentation of a progressive fall in urine output and body weight and treatment with cyclooxygenase or ACE inhibitors. Careful clinical examination may reveal stigmata of chronic liver disease and portal hypertension, advanced cardiac failure, sepsis, or other causes of "effective" hypovolemia (Table 270-1).

Intrinsic renal azotemia due to ischemia is likely following prolonged or severe renal hypoperfusion complicating hypovolemic or septic shock or following major surgery. The likelihood of ischemic ARF is increased further if ARF persists despite normalization of systemic hemodynamics. Diagnosis of nephrotoxic ARF requires careful review of the clinical data and pharmacy, nursing, and radiology records for evidence of recent exposure to nephrotoxic medications or radiocontrast agents or to endogenous toxins (e.g., myoglobin, hemoglobin, uric acid, myeloma protein, or elevated levels of serum calcium).

Although ischemic and nephrotoxic ARF account for more than 90 percent of cases of intrinsic renal azotemia, other renal parenchymal diseases must be considered (Table 270-2). Flank pain may be a prominent symptom following occlusion of a renal artery or vein and with other parenchymal diseases distending the renal capsule (e.g., severe glomerulonephritis or pyelonephritis). Subcutaneous nodules, livido reticularis, bright orange retinal arteriolar plaques, and digital ischemia, despite palpable pedal pulses, are clues to atheroembolization. ARF in association with oliguria, edema, hypertension, and an "active" urine sediment (nephritic syndrome) suggests acute glomerulonephritis or vasculitis. Malignant hypertension is a likely cause of ARF in patients with severe hypertension and evidence of hypertensive injury to other organs (e.g., left ventricular hypertrophy and failure, hypertensive retinopathy and papilledema, neurologic dysfunction). Fever, arthralgias, and a pruritic erythematous rash following exposure to a new drug suggest allergic interstitial nephritis, although systemic features of hypersensitivity are frequently absent.

Acute postrenal azotemia presents with suprapubic and flank pain due to distention of the bladder and of the renal collecting system and capsule, respectively. Colicky flank pain radiating to the groin suggests acute ureteric obstruction. Prostatic disease is likely if there is a history of nocturia, frequency, and hesitancy and enlargement or induration of the prostate on rectal examination. Neurogenic bladder should be suspected in patients receiving anticholinergic medications or with physical evidence of autonomic dysfunction. Definitive diagnosis of postrenal azotemia hinges on judicious use of radiologic investigations and rapid improvement in renal function following relief of obstruction.

URINALYSIS Anuria suggests complete urinary tract obstruction but may complicate severe cases of prerenal or intrinsic renal azotemia. Wide fluctuations in urine output raise the possibility of intermittent obstruction, whereas patients with partial urinary tract obstruction can present with polyuria due to impairment of urine concentrating mechanisms.

In prerenal azotemia, the sediment is characteristically acellular and contains transparent hyaline casts ("bland," "benign," "inactive" urine sediment). Hyaline casts are formed in concentrated urine from normal constitutents of urine—principally Tamm-Horsfall protein, which is secreted by epithelial cells of the loop of Henle. Postrenal azotemia may also present with an inactive sediment, although hematuria and pyuria are common in patients with intraluminal obstruction or prostatic disease. Pigmented "muddy brown" granular casts and casts containing tubule epithelial cells are characteristic of tubule necrosis and suggest ischemic or nephrotoxic ARF. They are usually found in association with microscopic hematuria and mild "tubular" proteinuria (<1 g/d); the latter reflects impaired reabsorption and processing of filtered proteins by injured proximal tubules. Casts are absent, however, in 20 to 30 percent of patients with ischemic or nephrotoxic ARF and are not a requisite for diagnosis. In general, red blood cell casts indicate glomerular injury or, less often, acute tubulointerstitial nephritis. White cell casts and nonpigmented granular casts suggest interstitial nephritis, whereas broad granular casts are characteristic of chronic renal disease and probably reflect interstitial fibrosis and dilatation of tubules. Eosinophiluria (>5 percent of urine leukocytes) is a common finding (~90 percent) in antibiotic-induced allergic interstitial nephritis when studied using Hansel's stain; however, lymphocytes may predominate in allergic interstitial nephritis induced by nonsteroidal anti-inflammatory drugs. Eosinophiluria is also a feature of atheroembolic ARF. Occasional uric acid crystals (pleomorphic in shape) are common in the concentrated urine of prerenal azotemia but suggest acute urate nephropathy if seen in abundance. Oxalate (envelope-shaped) and hippurate (needle-shaped) crystals raise the possibility of ethylene glycol ingestion and toxicity.

Increased urine protein excretion, but <1 g/d, is common in ATN due to failure of injured proximal tubules to reabsorb filtered protein and excretion of cellular debris ("tubular proteinuria"). Proteinuria of >1 g/d suggests injury to the glomerular ultrafiltration barrier ("glomerular proteinuria") or excretion of myeloma light chains. The latter are not detected by conventional dipsticks (which detect albumin) and must be sought by other means (e.g., sulfosalicylic acid test, immunoelectrophoresis). Heavy proteinuria is also a frequent finding (~80 percent) in patients who develop combined allergic interstitial nephritis and minimal change glomerulopathy when treated with cyclooxygenase inhibitors. A similar syndrome can be triggered by ampicillin, rifampicin, or interferon α. Hemoglobinuria or myoglobinuria should be suspected if urine is strongly positive for heme by dipstick, but contains few red cells, and if the supernatant of centrifuged urine is positive for free heme. Bilirubinuria may provide a clue to the presence of hepatorenal syndrome.

RENAL FAILURE INDICES Analysis of urine and blood biochemistry is particularly useful for distinguishing prerenal azotemia from ischemic or nephrotoxic intrinsic renal azotemia (Table 270-3). The fractional excretion of sodium (FeNa) is most useful in this regard. The FeNa relates sodium clearance to creatinine clearance. Sodium is reabsorbed avidly from glomerular filtrate in patients with prerenal azotemia, in an attempt to restore intravascular volume, but not in patients with ARF, as a result of tubular epithelial cell injury. In contrast, creatinine is not reabsorbed in either setting. Consequently, patients with prerenal azotemia typically have a FeNa of <1.0 percent (frequently <0.1 percent, whereas the FeNa in patients with ischemic or nephrotoxic ARF is usually >1.0 percent. The *renal failure index* (Table 270-3) provides comparable information, since clinical variations in serum sodium concentration are relatively small. *Urine sodium concentration* is a less sensitive index for distinguishing prerenal azotemia from ischemic and nephrotoxic ARF as values overlap between groups. Similarly, indices of urinary concentrating ability such as urine specific gravity, urine osmolality, urine to plasma urea ratio, and blood urea to creatinine ratio are of limited value in differential diagnosis.

Many caveats apply when interpreting biochemical renal failure indices. FeNa may be >1.0 percent in prerenal azotemia if patients are receiving diuretics or have bicarbonaturia (accompanied by sodium to maintain electroneutrality), preexisting chronic renal failure complicated by salt wasting, or adrenal insufficiency. In contrast, the FeNa is <1.0 percent in approximately 15 percent of patients with nonoliguric ischemic or nephrotoxic ARF. The FeNa is often <1.0 percent in ARF due to urinary tract obstruction, glomerulonephritis, and vascular diseases.

LABORATORY FINDINGS Serial measurements of serum creatinine can provide useful pointers to the cause of ARF. Prerenal azotemia is typified by fluctuating levels that parallel changes in hemodynamic function. Creatinine rises rapidly (within 24 to 48 h) in patients with ARF following renal ischemia, atheroembolization, and radiocontrast exposure. Peak creatinine levels are observed after 3 to 5 days with contrast nephropathy and return to baseline after 5 to 7 days. In contrast, creatinine levels typically peak later (7 to 10 days) in ischemic ARF and atheroembolic disease. The initial rise in serum creatinine is characteristically delayed until the second week of therapy

Table 270-2

Useful Clinical Features, Urinary Findings, and Confirmatory Tests in the Differential Diagnosis of Major Causes of Acute Azotemia

Cause of Acute Renal Failure	Suggestive Clinical Features	Typical Urinalysis	Some Confirmatory Tests
I. Prerenal Azotemia	Evidence of true volume depletion (thirst, postural or absolute hypotension and tachycardia, low jugular venous pressure, dry mucous membranes/axillae, weight loss, fluid output > input) or decreased "effective" circulatory volume (e.g., heart failure, liver failure), treatment with NSAIDs or ACE inhibitors	Hyaline casts FeNa <1% U_{Na} <10 mmol/L SG >1.018	Occasionally requires invasive hemodynamic monitoring; rapid resolution of ARF upon restoration of renal perfusion
II. Intrinsic renal azotemia			
A. Diseases involving large renal vessels			
1. Renal artery thrombosis	History of atrial fibrillation or recent myocardial infarct; flank or abdominal pain	Mild proteinuria Occasionally red cells	Elevated LDH with normal transaminases, renal arteriogram
2. Atheroembolism	Age usually > 50 years, recent manipulation of aorta, retinal plaques, subcutaneous nodules, palpable purpura, livedo reticularis, vasculopathy, hypertension	Often normal, eosinophiluria, rarely casts	Eosinophilia, hypocomplementemia, skin biopsy, renal biopsy
3. Renal vein thrombosis	Evidence of nephrotic syndrome or pulmonary embolism, flank pain	Proteinuria, hematuria	Inferior vena cavagram and selective renal venogram
B. Diseases of small vessels and glomeruli			
1. Glomerulonephritis/vasculitis	Compatible clinical history (e.g., recent infection) sinusitis, lung hemorrhage, skin rash or ulcers, arthralgias, new cardiac murmur, history of hepatitis B or C infection	Red cell or granular casts, red cells, white cells, mild proteinuria	Low C3, ANCA, anti-GBM Ab, ANA, ASO, anti-DNAse, cryoglobulins, blood cultures, renal biopsy
2. Hemolytic-uremic syndrome/thrombotic thrombocytopenic purpura	Compatible clinical history (e.g., recent gastrointestinal infection, cyclosporine, anovulants), fever, pallor, ecchymoses, neurologic abnormalities	May be normal, red cells, mild proteinuria, rarely red cell/granular casts	Anemia, thrombocytopenia, schistocytes on blood smear, increased LDH, renal biopsy
3. Malignant hypertension	Severe hypertension with headaches, cardiac failure, retinopathy, neurologic dysfunction, papilledema	Red cells, red cell casts, proteinuria	LVH by echocardiography/ECG, resolution of ARF with control of blood pressure
C. ARF mediated by ischemia or toxins (ATN)			
1. Ischemia	Recent hemorrhage, hypotension (e.g., cardiac arrest), surgery	Muddy brown granular or tubular epithelial cell casts FeNa >1% U_{Na} >20 mmol/L SG <1.015	Clinical assessment and urinalysis usually sufficient for diagnosis
2. Exogenous toxins	Recent radiocontrast study, nephrotoxic antibiotics or anticancer agents often coexistent with volume depletion, sepsis, or chronic renal insufficiency	Muddy brown granular or tubular epithelial cell casts FeNa >1% U_{Na} >20 mmol/L SG <1.015	Clinical assessment and urinalysis usually sufficient for diagnosis
3. Endogenous toxins	History suggestive of rhabdomyolysis (seizures, coma, ethanol abuse, trauma)	Urine supernatant positive for heme	Hyperkalemia, hyperphosphatemia, hypocalcemia, increased circulating myoglobin, MM, CPK and uric acid
	History suggestive of hemolysis (blood transfusion)	Urine supernatant pink and positive for heme	Hyperkalemia, hyperphosphatemia, hypocalcemia, hyperuricemia, pink plasma positive for hemoglobin
	History suggestive of tumor lysis (recent chemotherapy), myeloma (bone pain), or ethylene glycol ingestion	Urate crystals, dipstick-negative proteinuria, oxalate crystals, respectively	Hyperuricemia, hyperkalemia, hyperphosphatemia (for tumor lysis); circulating or urinary monoclonal spike (for myeloma); toxicology screen, acidosis, osmolal gap (for ethylene glycol)
D. Acute diseases of the tubulointerstitium			
1. Allergic interstitial nephritis	Recent ingestion of drug, and fever, rash, or arthralgias	White cell casts, white cells (frequently eosinphiluria) red cells, rarely red cell casts, proteinuria (occasionally nephrotic)	Systemic eosinophilia, skin biopsy of rash (leukocytoclastic vasculitis), renal biopsy
2. Acute bilateral pyelonephritis	Flank pain and tenderness, toxic, febrile	Leukocytes, proteinuria, red cells, bacteria	Urine and blood cultures
III. Postrenal azotemia	Abdominal or flank pain, palpable bladder	Frequently normal, hematuria if stones, hemorrhage, malignancy, or prostatic hypertrophy	Plain film, renal ultrasound, IVP, retrograde or anterograde pyelography, CT scan

NOTE: NSAIDs, nonsteroidal anti-inflammatory drugs; U_{Na}, urine sodium concentration; SG, specific gravity; LDH, lactate dehydrogenase; C3, complement component; ANCA, antineutrophil cytoplasmic autoantibody; GBM Ab, glomerular basement membrane antibody; ANA, antinuclear antibody; ASO, antistreptolysin O; LVH, left ventricular hypertrophy; ECG, electrocardiogram; CPK, creatine phosphokinase; IVP, intravenous pyelogram; CT, computed tomography.

SOURCE: Adapted with permission from HR Brady et al in *The Kidney*, 5th ed, BM Brenner (ed). Philadelphia, Saunders, 1996

Table 270-3

Urine Diagnostic Indices in Differentiation of Prerenal versus Intrinsic Renal Azotemia

Diagnostic Index	Typical Findings: Prerenal Azotemia	Typical Findings: Intrinsic Renal Azotemia
Fractional excretion of sodium (%)* $\frac{U_{Na} \times P_{Cr}}{P_{Na} \times U_{Cr}} \times 100$	<1	>1
Urine sodium concentration (mmol/L)	<10	>20
Urine creatinine to plasma creatinine ratio	>40	>20
Urine urea nitrogen to plasma urea nitrogen ratio	>8	<3
Urine specific gravity	>1.018	<1.015
Urine osmolality (mosmol/kg H_2O)	>500	<300
Plasma BUN/creatinine ratio	>20	<10–15
Renal failure index* $\frac{U_{Na}}{U_{Cr}/P_{Cr}}$	<1	>1
Urinary sediment	Hyaline casts	Muddy brown granular casts

* Most sensitive indices

NOTE: U_{Na}, urine sodium concentration; P_{Cr}, plasma creatinine concentration; P_{Na}, plasma sodium concentration; U_{Cr}, urine creatinine concentration; BUN, blood urea nitrogen.

with many tubule epithelial cell toxins (e.g., aminoglycosides, cisplatin) and probably reflects the need for accumulation of these agents within cells before GFR falls.

Hyperkalemia, hyperphosphatemia, hypocalcemia, and elevations in serum uric acid and creatine kinase (MM isoenzyme) levels suggest a diagnosis of rhabdomyolysis. Hyperuricemia (>15 mg/dL) in association with hyperkalemia, hyperphosphatemia, and increased circulating levels of intracellular enzymes such as lactate dehydrogenase may indicate acute urate nephropathy and tumor lysis syndrome following cancer chemotherapy. A wide serum anion and osmolal gap (measured serum osmolality minus the serum osmolality calculated from serum sodium, glucose, and urea concentrations) indicate the presence of an unusual anion or osmole in the circulation and are clues to diagnosis of ethylene glycol or methanol ingestion. Severe anemia in the absence of hemorrhage raises the possibility of hemolysis, multiple myeloma, or thrombotic microangiopathy. Systemic eosinophilia suggests allergic interstitial nephritis but is also a feature of atheroembolic disease and polyarteritis nodosa.

RADIOLOGIC FINDINGS Imaging of the urinary tract by ultrasonography is useful to exclude obstructive uropathy. Computed tomography and magnetic resonance imaging are alternative imaging modalities. Whereas pelvicalyceal dilatation is usual with urinary tract obstruction (98 percent sensitivity), dilatation may be absent immediately following obstruction or in patients with ureteric encasement (e.g., retroperitoneal fibrosis, neoplasia). Retrograde or anterograde pyelography are more definitive investigations in complex cases and provide precise localization of the site of obstruction. Intravenous pyelography should be avoided as systemic radiocontrast may exacerbate ARF. A plain film of the abdomen, with tomography if necessary, is a valuable initial screening technique in patients with suspected nephrolithiasis. Doppler ultrasonography and magnetic resonance flow imaging appear promising for assessment of patency of renal arteries and veins in patients with suspected vascular obstruction; however, contrast angiography is usually required for definitive diagnosis.

RENAL BIOPSY Biopsy is reserved for patients in whom prerenal and postrenal failure have been excluded and the cause of intrinsic renal azotemia is unclear. Renal biopsy is particularly useful when clinical assessment and laboratory investigations suggest diagnoses other than ischemic or nephrotoxic injury that may respond to disease-specific therapy. Examples include glomerulonephritis, vasculitis, hemolytic-uremic syndrome, thrombotic thrombocytopenic purpura, and allergic interstitial nephritis.

COMPLICATIONS

ARF impairs renal excretion of sodium, potassium, and water and perturbs divalent cation homeostasis and urinary acidification mechanisms. As a result, ARF is frequently complicated by intravascular volume overload, hyponatremia, hyperkalemia, hyperphosphatemia, hypocalcemia, hypermagnesemia, and metabolic acidosis. In addition, patients are unable to excrete nitrogenous waste products and are prone to develop the uremic syndrome (Chap. 271). The speed of development and severity of these complications reflects the degree of renal impairment and catabolic state of the patient.

Expansion of extracellular fluid volume is an inevitable consequence of diminished salt and water excretion in oliguric or anuric individuals. Whereas milder forms are characterized by weight gain, bibasilar lung rales, raised jugular venous pressure, and dependent edema, continued volume expansion may precipitate life-threatening pulmonary edema. Hypervolemia may be particularly problematic in patients receiving multiple intravenous medications and enteral or parenteral nutrition. Excessive administration of free water either through ingestion or as hypotonic saline or isotonic dextrose solutions (dextrose being metabolized) can induce *hypoosmolality* and *hyponatremia*, which, if severe, lead to cerebral edema and neurologic abnormalities, including seizures.

Hyperkalemia is a frequent complication of ARF. Serum potassium typically rises by 0.5 mmol/L per day in oliguric and anuric patients due to impaired excretion of ingested or infused potassium and potassium released from injured tubular epithelium. Coexistent metabolic acidosis may exacerbate hyperkalemia by promoting potassium efflux from cells. Hyperkalemia may be particularly severe, even at the time of diagnosis, in patients with rhabdomyolysis, hemolysis, and tumor lysis syndrome. Mild hyperkalemia (<6.0 mmol/L) is usually asymptomatic. Higher levels are typically associated with electrocardiographic abnormalities (Chap. 228).

Metabolism of dietary protein yields between 50 and 100 mmol/d of fixed nonvolatile acids that are normally excreted by the kidneys. Consequently, ARF is typically complicated by *metabolic acidosis*, often with an increased serum anion gap (Chap. 50). Acidosis can be particularly severe when endogenous production of hydrogen ions is increased by other mechanisms (e.g., diabetic or fasting ketoacidosis; lactic acidosis complicating generalized tissue hypoperfusion, liver disease, or sepsis; metabolism of ethylene glycol or methanol).

Mild *hyperphosphatemia* is an almost invariable complication of ARF. Severe hyperphosphatemia may develop in highly catabolic patients or following rhabdomyolysis, hemolysis, or tumor lysis. Metastatic deposition of calcium phosphate can lead to *hypocalcemia*, particularly when the product of serum calcium (mg/dL) and phosphate (mg/dL) concentrations exceeds 70. Other factors that contribute to hypocalcemia include tissue resistance to the actions of parathyroid hormone and reduced levels of 1,25-dihydroxyvitamin D. Hypocalcemia is often asymptomatic but can cause perioral paresthesias, muscle cramps, seizures, hallucinations and confusion, and prolongation of the QT interval and nonspecific T-wave changes on electrocardiography (Chap. 354).

Anemia develops rapidly in ARF and is usually mild and multifactorial in origin. Contributing factors include impaired erythropoiesis, hemolysis, bleeding, hemodilution, and reduced red cell survival time. Prolongation of the *bleeding time* and *leukocytosis* are also common. Common contributors to the bleeding diathesis include mild thrombocytopenia, platelet dysfunction, and/or clotting factor abnormalities (e.g., factor VIII dysfunction), whereas leukocytosis usually reflects sepsis, a stress response, or other concurrent illness. *Infection* is a common and serious complication of ARF, occurring in 50 to 90 percent of cases and accounting for up to 75 percent of deaths. It is unclear whether patients with ARF have a clinically significant defect in host immune responses or whether the high incidence of infection reflects repeated breaches of mucocutaneous barriers (e.g., intravenous cannulae, mechanical ventilation, bladder catheterization). *Cardiac complications* of ARF include arrhythmias, myocardial infarction, and pulmonary embolism. Mild *gastrointestinal bleeding* is common (10 to 30 percent) and is usually due to stress ulceration of gastric or small intestinal mucosa.

Protracted periods of severe ARF are invariably associated with the development of the *uremic syndrome* (Chap. 271).

A vigorous diuresis can occur during the *recovery phase* of ARF (see above) and lead to intravascular volume depletion and delayed recovery of GFR by causing secondary prerenal azotemia. *Hypernatremia* can also complicate recovery if water losses via hypotonic urine are not replaced or if losses are inappropriately replaced by relatively hypertonic saline solutions. *Hypokalemia*, *hypomagnesemia*, *hypophosphatemia*, and *hypocalcemia* are less common metabolic complications during this period.

Rx TREATMENT

Prevention Because there are no specific therapies for treatment of ischemic or nephrotoxic ARF, prevention is of paramount importance. Many cases of ischemic ARF can be avoided by close attention to cardiovascular function and intravascular volume in high-risk patients. Indeed, aggressive restoration of intravascular volume has been shown to reduce the incidence of ARF dramatically after major surgery or trauma, burns, or cholera. The incidence of nephrotoxic ARF can be reduced by tailoring the dosage of potential nephrotoxins to body size and GFR; for example, reducing the dose or frequency of administration of drugs in patients with preexisting renal impairment. Adjusting drug dosage according to circulating drug levels also appears to limit renal injury in patients receiving aminoglycoside antibiotics or cyclosporine. Diuretics, cyclooxygenase inhibitors, ACE inhibitors, and other vasodilators should be used with caution in patients with suspected true or "effective" hypovolemia or renovascular disease as they may precipitate prerenal azotemia or convert the latter to ischemic ARF. Hypovolemia should be avoided in patients receiving nephrotoxic medications as renal hypoperfusion potentiates the toxicity of most nephrotoxins. Allopurinol and forced alkaline diuresis are useful in patients at high risk for acute urate nephropathy (e.g., cancer chemotherapy in hematologic malignancies) to limit uric acid generation and prevent precipitation of urate crystals in renal tubules. Forced alkaline diuresis may also prevent or attenuate ARF in patients receiving high-dose methotrexate or suffering from rhabdomyolysis. *N*-acetylcysteine limits acetaminophen-induced renal injury if given within 24 h of ingestion. Dimercaprol, a chelating agent, may prevent heavy metal nephrotoxicity. Ethanol inhibits ethylene glycol metabolism to oxalic acid and other toxic metabolites and is an important adjunct to hemodialysis in the emergency management of ethylene glycol intoxication. By inhibiting alcohol dehydrogenase, ethanol can also reduce the conversion of methanol to the highly toxic formic acid.

Specific Therapies By definition, *prerenal azotemia* is rapidly reversible upon correction of the primary hemodynamic abnormality, and *postrenal azotemia* resolves upon relief of obstruction. To date, there are no specific therapies for established intrinsic renal ARF due to ischemia or nephrotoxicity. Management of these disorders should focus on elimination of the causative hemodynamic abnormality or toxin, avoidance of additional insults, and prevention and treatment of complications. Specific treatment of other causes of intrinsic renal azotemia depends on the underlying pathology.

PRERENAL AZOTEMIA The composition of replacement fluids for treatment of prerenal azotemia due to hypovolemia must be tailored according to the composition of the lost fluid. Hypovolemia due to hemorrhage should be corrected with packed red blood cells in saline, whereas isotonic saline is usually appropriate replacement for plasma loss (e.g., burns, pancreatitis). Urinary and gastrointestinal fluids can vary greatly in composition but are usually hypotonic. Hypotonic solutions (e.g., 0.45 percent saline) are usually recommended as initial replacement in patients with prerenal azotemia due to increased urinary or gastrointestinal fluid losses, although isotonic saline may be more appropriate in severe cases. Subsequent therapy should be based on measurements of the volume and ionic content of excreted or drained fluids. Serum potassium and acid-base status should be monitored carefully, and potassium and bicarbonate supplemented as appropriate. Cardiac failure may require aggressive management with positive inotropes, preload and afterload reducing agents, antiarrhythmic drugs, and mechanical aids such as intraaortic balloon pumps. Invasive hemodynamic monitoring may be required to guide therapy for complicated conditions in patients in whom clinical assessment of cardiovascular function and intravascular volume proves unreliable.

Fluid management may be particularly difficult in patients with cirrhosis complicated by ascites. In this setting, it is important to distinguish between full-blown hepatorenal syndrome (Chap. 299), which carries a grave prognosis, and reversible ARF due to "true" or "effective" hypovolemia by overzealous use of diuretics or sepsis (e.g., spontaneous bacterial peritonitis). The contribution of hypovolemia to ARF can be definitively assessed only by administration of a fluid challenge. Fluids should be administered slowly and titrated against jugular venous pressure and, if necessary, central venous and pulmonary capillary wedge pressure, abdominal girth, and urine output. Patients with a reversible prerenal component typically have an increase in urine output and fall in serum creatinine, whereas patients with hepatorenal syndrome do not and may suffer increased ascites formation and pulmonary edema if not monitored closely. Large volumes of ascitic fluid can usually be drained by paracentesis without deterioration in renal function if intravenous albumin is administered simultaneously. Indeed, "large-volume paracentesis" may afford an increase in GFR, possibly by lowering intraabdominal pressure and improving flow in renal veins. Shunting of ascitic fluid from the peritoneum to a central vein (peritoneojugular shunt, LeVeen or Denver shunts) is an alternative approach in refractory cases. This maneuver can also improve GFR and sodium excretion transiently, probably because the increase in central blood volume stimulates release of atrial natriuretic peptides and inhibits secretion of aldosterone and norepinephrine.

ACUTE INTRINSIC RENAL AZOTEMIA Many different approaches have been tested for their ability to attenuate injury or hasten recovery in *ischemic* and *nephrotoxic ARF*. Whereas many of these are beneficial in experimental models of ischemic or nephrotoxic ARF, they have either failed to confer consistent benefit or have proved too toxic for use in humans.

Acute renal failure due to *other intrinsic renal diseases* such as acute glomerulonephritis or vasculitis may respond to glucocorticoids, alkylating agents, and/or plasmapheresis, depending on the primary pathology. Glucocorticoids also hasten remission in some cases of allergic interstitial nephritis. Aggressive control of systemic arterial pressure is of paramount importance in limiting renal injury in malignant hypertensive nephrosclerosis, toxemia of pregnancy, and other vascular diseases. Hypertension and ARF due to scleroderma may be exquisitely sensitive to treatment with ACE inhibitors.

POSTRENAL AZOTEMIA Management of postrenal azotemia requires close collaboration between nephrologist, urologist, and radiologist. Obstruction of the urethra or bladder neck are usually managed initially by transurethral or suprapubic placement of a bladder catheter, which provides temporary relief while the obstructing lesion is identified and treated definitively. Similarly, ureteric obstruction may be treated initially by percutaneous catheterization of the dilated renal pelvis or ureter. Indeed, obstructing lesions can often be removed percutaneously (e.g., calculus, sloughed papilla) or bypassed by insertion of a ureteric stent (e.g., carcinoma). Most patients experience an appropriate diuresis for several days following relief of obstruction. Approximately 5 percent of patients develop a transient salt-wasting syndrome that may require administration of intravenous saline to maintain blood pressure.

Supportive Measures (Table 270-4) Following correction of hypovelemia, salt and water intake are tailored to match losses. *Hypervolemia* can usually be managed by restriction of salt and water intake and diuretics. Indeed, there is, as yet, no proven rationale for administration of diuretics in ARF except to treat this complication. High doses of loop-blocking diuretics such as furosemide (up to 200 to 400 mg intravenously) or bumetanide (up to 10 mg intravenously) may promote diuresis in patients who fail to respond to conventional doses. Subpressor doses of dopamine (1 to 5 μg/kg per min) are claimed to promote salt and water excretion by increasing renal blood flow and GFR and by inhibiting tubule sodium reabsorption; however, its efficacy has not been definitively established. Ultrafiltration or dialysis is used to treat severe hypervolemia when conservative measures fail. *Hyponatremia* and *hypoosmolality* can usually be controlled by restriction of free water intake. Conversely, *hypernatremia* is treated by administration of water or intravenous hypotonic saline or isotonic dextrose–containing solutions.

The management of hyperkalemia is described in Chap. 49.

Metabolic acidosis is not treated unless serum bicarbonate concentration falls below 15 mmol/L or arterial pH falls below 7.2. More severe acidosis is corrected by oral or intravenous sodium bicarbonate. Initial rates of replacement are guided by estimates of bicarbonate deficit and adjusted thereafter according to serum levels (Chap. 50). Patients are monitored for complications of bicarbonate administration such as hypervolemia, metabolic alkalosis, hypocalcemia, and hypokalemia. From a practical point of view, most patients requiring sodium bicarbonate need emergency dialysis within days. *Hyperphosphatemia* is usually controlled by restriction of dietary phosphate and by oral aluminum hydroxide or calcium carbonate, which reduce gastrointestinal absorption of phosphate. *Hypocalcemia* does not usually require treatment unless severe, as may occur with rhabdomyolysis or pancreatitis or following administration of bicarbonate. *Hyperuricemia* is typically mild [<900 μmol/L (<15 mg/dL)] and does not require intervention.

The objective of *nutritional management* during the maintenance phase of ARF is to provide sufficient calories to avoid catabolism and starvation ketoacidosis, while minimizing production of nitrogenous waste. This is best achieved by restricting dietary protein to approximately 0.6 g/kg per day of protein of high biological value (i.e., rich in essential amino acids) and to provide most calories as carbohydrate (approximately 100 g daily). Nutritional management is easier in nonoliguric patients and following institution of dialysis. Vigorous parenteral hyperalimentation is claimed to improve prognosis; however, convincing benefit has yet to be demonstrated in controlled trials.

Anemia may necessitate blood transfusion or administration of recombinant human erythropoietin if severe or if recovery is delayed. Uremic bleeding usually responds to correction of anemia, administration of desmopressin or estrogens, or dialysis. Regular doses of antacids appear to reduce the incidence of *gastrointestinal hemorrhage* significantly and may be more effective in this regard than H_2 antagonists. Meticulous care of intravenous cannulae, bladder catheters, and other invasive devices is mandatory to avoid infections. Unfortunately, prophylactic antibiotics have not been shown to reduce the incidence of infection in these high-risk patients.

INDICATIONS AND MODALITIES OF DIALYSIS Dialysis replaces renal function until regeneration and repair restore renal function. Hemodialysis and peritoneal dialysis appear equally effective for management of ARF. Thus, the dialysis modality is chosen according to the needs of individual patients (e.g., peritoneal dialysis may be preferable if the patient is hemodynamically unstable, and hemodialysis after abdominal surgery involving the peritoneum), the expertise

Table 270-4

Management of Ischemic and Nephrotoxic Acute Renal Failure*

Management Issue	Therapy
REVERSE CAUSATIVE RENAL INSULT	
Ischemic ARF	Restore systemic hemodynamics and renal perfusion
Nephrotoxic ARF	Eliminate nephrotoxins
	Consider specific measures (e.g., forced alkaline diuresis, chelators: see text)
PREVENTION AND TREATMENT OF COMPLICATIONS	
Intravascular volume overload	Salt (1–2 g/d) and water (usually <1 L/d) restriction
	Diuretics (usually loop blockers ± thiazide)
	Ultrafiltration or dialysis
Hyponatremia	Restriction of enteral free water intake (<1 L/d)
	Avoid hypotonic intravenous solutions (including dextrose solutions)
Hyperkalemia	Restriction of dietary K^+ intake (usually <40 mmol/d)
	Eliminate K^+ supplements and K^+-sparing diuretics
	Potassium-binding ion-exchange resins (e.g., sodium polystyrene sulphonate)
	Glucose (50 mL of 50% dextrose) and insulin (10 units regular)
	Sodium bicarbonate (usually 50–100 mmol)
	Calcium gluconate (10 mL of 10% solution over 5 min)
	Dialysis (versus low K^+ dialysate)
Metabolic acidosis	Restriction of dietary protein (usually 0.6 g/kg per day of high biologic value)
	Sodium bicarbonate (maintain serum bicarbonate >15 mmol/L or arterial pH >7.2)
	Dialysis
Hyperphosphatemia	Restriction of dietary phosphate intake (usually <800 mg/d)
	Phosphate binding agents (calcium carbonate, aluminum hydroxide)
Hypocalcemia	Calcium carbonate (if symptomatic or if sodium bicarbonate to be administered)
	Calcium gluconate (10–20 mL of 10% solution)
Hypermagnesemia	Discontinue Mg^{2+}-containing antacids
Hyperuricemia	Treatment usually not necessary [if <900 μmol/L (<15 mg/dL)]
Nutrition	Restriction of dietary protein (~0.6 g/kg per day)
	Carbohydrate (~100 g/d)
	Enteral or parenteral nutrition (if recovery prolonged or patient very catabolic)
Indications for dialysis	Clinical evidence (symptoms or signs) of uremia
	Intractable intravascular volume overload
	Hyperkalemia or severe acidosis resistant to conservative measures
	?Prophylactic dialysis when urea >100–150 mg/dL or creatinine >8–10 mg/dL
PRESCRIBING OF MEDICATIONS	
Choice of agents	Avoid other nephrotoxins, ACE inhibitors, cyclooxygenase inhibitors, and radiocontrast unless absolute indication and no alternative agent
Drug dosing	Adjust doses and frequency of administration for degree of renal impairment

* These are general recommendations and must be tailored to needs of individual patients.

of the nephrologist, and the facilities of the institution. Absolute indications for dialysis include symptoms or signs of the uremic syndrome and management of refractory hypervolemia, hyperkalemia, or acidosis. Many nephrologists also initiate dialysis empirically for blood urea levels of >100 mg/dL, even in the absence of clinical uremia; however, this approach has yet to be validated in controlled clinical trials. Nor is it clear whether intensive dialysis prescribed to maintain blood urea and creatinine below a certain level is beneficial. The latter are important issues since unnecessary or intensive hemodialysis can exacerbate ATN and delay renal recovery by triggering hypotension and repeated renal hypoperfusion.

Continuous arteriovenous hemodiafiltration (CAVH) and continuous venovenous hemodiafiltration (CVVH) are alternative hemodialysis techniques for treatment of ARF. They are generally reserved for patients in whom intermittent hemodialysis fails to control hypervolemia or uremia and for those who do not tolerate intermittent hemodialysis and in whom peritoneal dialysis is not possible. CAVH requires both arterial and venous access. The patient's own blood pressure generates an ultrafiltrate of plasma across a porous biocompatible dialysis membrane. A physiologic crystalloid solution is passed along the other side of the membrane to achieve diffusive clearance. CVVH, in contrast, requires only a double-lumen venous catheter as a blood pump generates ultrafiltration pressure across the dialysis membrane. These newer techniques have not been compared to conventional intermittent hemodialysis in prospective, adequately controlled trials. Such evaluations are needed given that continuous hemodialysis techniques require immobilization in bed, systemic anticoagulation, arterial cannulation (in CAVH), and prolonged exposure of blood to synthetic, albeit relatively biocompatible, dialysis membranes.

OUTCOME AND LONG-TERM PROGNOSIS

The mortality rate among patients with ARF approximates 50 percent and has changed little over the past 30 years. It should be stressed, however, that patients usually die from sequelae of the primary illness that induced ARF and not from ARF itself. Indeed, the kidney is one of the few organs whose function can be replaced artificially (i.e., by dialysis) for protracted periods of time. In agreement with this interpretation, mortality rates vary greatly depending on the cause of ARF: ~15 percent in obstetric patients, ~30 percent in toxin-related ARF, and ~60 percent following trauma or major surgery. Oliguria (~400 mL/d) at time of presentation and a rise in serum creatinine of greater than 3 mg/dL are associated with a poor prognosis and probably reflect the severity of renal injury and of the primary illness. Mortality rates are higher in older debilitated patients and in those with multiple organ failure. Most patients who survive an episode of ARF recover sufficient renal function to live normal lives. However, 50 percent have subclinical impairment of renal function or residual scarring on renal biopsy. Approximately 5 percent of patients never recover function and require long-term renal replacement with dialysis or transplantation. An additional 5 percent suffer progressive decline in GFR, following an initial recovery phase, probably due to hemodynamic stress and sclerosis of remnant glomeruli (see Chap. 273).

BIBLIOGRAPHY

BRADY HR et al: Acute renal failure, in *The Kidney*, 5th ed., BM Brenner (ed). Philadelphia, Saunders, 1996, pp 1200–1252

BRENNER BM, LAZARUS JM (eds): *Acute Renal Failure*, 3d ed. New York, Churchill Livingstone, 1993

LIEBERTHAL W, LEVINSKY NG: Acute clinical renal failure, in *The Kidney, Physiology and Pathophysiology*, 2d ed, DW Seldin, G Giebisch (eds). New York, Raven Press, 1992, p 3181

WEINBERG J: Pathogenetic mechanisms of ischemic acute renal failure, in *The Principles and Practice of Nephrology*, 2d ed, HR Jacobsen, et al (eds). Philadelphia, BC Decker, 1991, p 544

OLSEN S, SOLEZ K: Acute tubular necrosis and toxic renal injury, in *Renal Pathology with Clinical and Functional Correlations*, 2d ed, CC Tisher, BM Brenner (eds). Philadelphia, Lippincott, 1994, pp 769–809

271

J. Michael Lazarus, Barry M. Brenner

CHRONIC RENAL FAILURE

In contrast to the capacity of the kidneys to regain function following acute renal injury (see Chap. 270), renal injury of a more prolonged nature often leads to progressive and irreversible destruction of nephron mass. Such reduction of renal mass, in turn, causes structural and functional hypertrophy of surviving nephrons. As discussed in Chap. 269, this compensatory hypertrophy is due to adaptive hyperfiltration mediated by increases in glomerular capillary pressures and flows. Eventually, these adaptations prove maladaptive, in that they predispose to sclerosis of the residual glomerular population.

Glomerulonephritis, in its several forms, was the most common initiating cause of chronic renal failure (CRF) in the past. Possibly because of more aggressive treatment of glomerulonephritis, diabetes mellitus and hypertensive renal disease are now the leading causes of CRF (Fig. 271-1). Irrespective of cause, the eventual impact of severe reduction in nephron mass is an alteration in function of virtually every organ system in the body. *Uremia* is the term generally applied to the clinical syndrome that results from profound loss of renal function. Although the cause(s) of the syndrome remain unknown, the term *uremia* was adopted originally because of the presumption that the abnormalities result from retention in the blood of urea and other end products of metabolism normally excreted in the urine. Uremia involves more than renal excretory failure alone, however. A host of metabolic and endocrine functions normally subserved by the kidney are also impaired, and the inexorable course to renal failure often is accompanied by anemia, malnutrition, impaired metabolism of carbohydrates, fats, and proteins, and defective utilization of energy. Therefore, *uremia* refers to the constellation of signs and symptoms associated with CRF, irrespective of cause.

The severity of signs and symptoms of uremia vary from patient to patient, depending, at least in part, on the magnitude of the reduction in functioning renal mass and the rapidity with which renal function is lost. As discussed in Chap. 269, in the relatively early stage of CRF—i.e., when total glomerular filtration rate (GFR) is reduced to about 35 to 50 percent of normal—overall renal function is sufficient to keep the patient symptom-free, although renal reserve is diminished. At this stage, the biosynthetic, excretory, and other regulatory functions of the kidney are generally well maintained. Blood urea nitrogen and serum creatinine levels may be within the normal range or are only

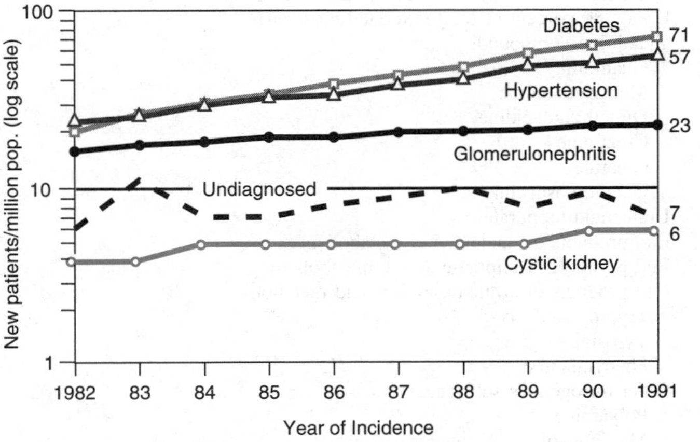

FIGURE 271-1 Incidence rates of treated end-stage renal disease (ESRD) per million population, by selected primary disease groups, 1982 through 1991. Rates are unadjusted. A semilog scale is used to show smaller rates. Rates do not include patients from Puerto Rico or U.S. Territories. Medicare patients only. *(From United States Renal Data System 1995 Annual Data Report. U.S. Department of Health and Human Services, Health Care Financing Administration.)*

slightly elevated and therefore serve as crude measures, at best, of the level of function (see Chap. 269). At a somewhat later stage in the course of CRF (GFR about 20 to 35 percent of normal), *azotemia* occurs, and initial manifestations of renal insufficiency usually appear. Although patients are still relatively asymptomatic, renal reserve is diminished sufficiently that sudden stress, such as intercurrent infection, urinary tract obstruction, dehydration, or administration of a nephrotoxic drug, may compromise renal function still further, inducing signs and symptoms of overt uremia. With further loss of nephron mass (GFR below approximately 20 percent of normal), the patient develops *overt renal failure*. Uremia may be viewed as the final stage in this inexorable process, when many or all of the untoward manifestations of CRF become evident clinically and biochemically.

PATHOPHYSIOLOGY AND BIOCHEMISTRY OF UREMIA

The finding that sera from patients with uremia exert toxic effects in a variety of biologic test systems has motivated an attempt to identify the responsible toxin(s). The most likely candidates as toxins in uremia are the byproducts of protein and amino acid metabolism. Unlike fats and carbohydrates, which are eventually metabolized to carbon dioxide and water—substances readily excreted even in uremic subjects via lungs and skin—the products of protein and amino acid metabolism depend primarily on the kidneys for excretion. A number of such products have been identified (Table 271-1). Nevertheless, the precise role of these substances in the pathogenesis of the uremic syndrome is unclear. As noted above, uremic symptoms correlate only in a rough and inconsistent way with concentrations of urea in blood. Although not the major cause of overt uremic toxicity, urea may contribute to some of the clinical abnormalities, including anorexia, malaise, vomiting, and headache. On the other hand, elevated levels of plasma *guanidinosuccinic acid*, by interfering with activation of platelet factor III by adenosine diphosphate (ADP), contribute to the impaired platelet function in CRF. *Creatinine* may cause adverse effects following conversion to metabolites such as sarcosine and methylguanidine. Nitrogenous compounds with a molecular mass of 500 to 12,000 daltons (so-called middle molecules) are also retained in CRF and similarly are believed to contribute to morbidity and mortality in uremic subjects. Decreased renal excretion is not the only reason why such middle-sized molecules, along with various cytokines and growth factors, accumulate in uremic plasma. The kidney normally catabolizes a number of circulating plasma proteins and polypeptides; with reduced renal mass, this capacity is impaired. Furthermore, plasma levels of many polypeptide hormones, including parathyroid hormone (PTH) insulin, glucagon, luteinizing hormone, and prolactin, rise with renal failure, often markedly, not only because of impaired renal catabolism but also because of enhanced glandular secretion. Of these, excessive PTH has been suggested to be an important uremic "toxin" because of its adverse effect of elevating cellular cytosolic calcium levels in several tissues and organs. The consequences of high circulating levels of PTH and other hormones in chronic renal failure are considered below.

Table 271-1

Uremic "Toxins"

By-products of protein and amino acid metabolism
- Urea—80 percent of total (excreted nitrogen)
- Guanidino compounds
  - Guanidine
  - Methylguanidine
  - Dimethylguanidine
  - Creatinine
  - Creatine
  - Guanidinosuccinic acid
- Urates and hippurates
- End-products of nucleic acid metabolism
- End-products of aliphatic amine metabolism
- End-products of aromatic amino acid metabolism
  - Tryptophan
  - Tyrosine
  - Phenylalanine
- Other nitrogenous substances
  - Polyamines
  - Myoinositol
  - Phenols
  - Benzoates
  - Indoles

Advanced glycation end-products
Inhibitors of ligand-protein binding
Glucuronoconjugates and aglycones
Inhibitors of somatomedin and insulin action

EFFECTS OF UREMIA ON CELLULAR FUNCTIONS Alterations in the composition of intracellular and extracellular fluids in CRF are believed to be a consequence, at least in part, of defective ion transport across cell membranes, with retained uremic toxins possibly mediating these alterations in transmembrane ion transport. The integrity of the volume and composition of cells throughout the body depends to a large extent on the active transport of Na^+ out of the cell, the resulting intracellular fluid being relatively low in Na^+ and high in K^+, whereas the reverse is true for extracellular fluid. Active Na^+ transport is metabolically costly, accounting for a major fraction of basal energy utilization and oxygen consumption. The consequences of this efflux of Na^+ from cells include (1) the generation of a resting electrical potential difference across the cell membrane, with the cell interior electronegative relative to the cell exterior, and (2) a mechanism for enhancing the influx of K^+ into cells. In animals, deliberate inhibition of this active efflux of Na^+ across cell membranes leads to alterations in body composition and cell functions similar to those seen in the erythrocytes, leukocytes, skeletal muscle, and other tissues of uremic subjects. These include increased and decreased intracellular concentrations of Na^+ and K^+, respectively, and reduction in magnitude of the transmembrane voltage. In addition to these abnormalities in Na^+ and K^+ flux, inhibition of Ca^{2+} flux has also been demonstrated in uremic patients. These alterations are largely reversed by efficient hemodialysis and, for erythrocytes at least, are recreated when cells from normal subjects are incubated in uremic serum. Whether the uremic "toxins" that account for these derangements in cellular function represent abnormally retained products of metabolism or substances whose production is increased as a homeostatic response to renal insufficiency remains unknown. Increased levels of parathyroid and natriuretic hormones, examples of both such derangements, are discussed in this context in Chap. 269.

EFFECTS OF UREMIA ON WHOLE-BODY COMPOSITION What is the impact of the above-described disturbances of active transcellular ion transport on the organism as a whole? From the pathophysiologic considerations discussed previously, CRF is likely to lead to abnormally high intracellular Na^+ concentrations and hence to osmotically induced overhydration of cells, whereas these same cells are relatively deficient in K^+. With the development of malaise, anorexia, nausea, vomiting, and diarrhea, patients with CRF may eventually develop protein-calorie malnutrition and negative nitrogen balance, often with profound losses of lean body mass and fat deposits. Owing to the concomitant tendency for salt and water retention due to impaired excretion, these losses often go unnoticed until the late stages of CRF. Because a large fraction of the increase in total body water in uremia is the result of expansion of intracellular volume, extracellular volume also expands. With initiation of intermittent hemodialysis or renal transplantation, there is often an immediate loss of body weight, due primarily to correction of this overhydration. With successful transplantation, the initial diuresis is followed by a period of weight gain due to restoration of lean body mass and fat deposits to preillness levels. For patients on chronic dialysis, the anabolic response is often less dramatic, even when therapy is regarded as optimal, and involves mainly reaccumulation of fat deposits. The failure of lean body mass to return to normal with chronic dialysis may reflect alterations in the catabolic rate but more likely results from insufficient intake of calories and protein, which, in adequately dialyzed patients, should be maintained at levels of 150 kJ/kg (35 kcal/kg) and 1.2 to 1.4 g/kg of body weight per day, respectively.

Deficits in intracellular K^+ concentration in CRF may result from inadequate intake (poor diet or overzealous K^+ restriction by the physician), excessive losses (vomiting, diarrhea, diuretics), reduction of Na^+- and K^+-stimulated ATPase, or a combination of these. In addition to promoting losses of K^+ into urine (which may be substantial if urine volume remains relatively normal in uremic subjects), the high levels of plasma aldosterone often seen in CRF also may augment the net secretion of K^+ into the colon, thereby contributing to K^+ losses in stool or diarrheal fluids. Despite deficits in intracellular K^+, serum K^+ is usually normal or high in CRF, owing to metabolic acidosis, which induces an efflux of K^+ from cells. Uremic patients are also relatively resistant to the action of insulin (see below), which normally enhances K^+ uptake by skeletal muscle (see also Chap. 49).

EFFECTS OF UREMIA ON METABOLISM **Hypothermia** In animals, injections of urine, urea, or other retained toxic metabolites can induce hypothermia, and basal heat production diminishes soon after nephrectomy. Since active Na^+ transport across cell membranes accounts for a major proportion of basal energy production, the inverse relationship between body temperature and degree of azotemia is believed to be due, in part, to inhibition of the Na^+ pump by some retained toxin(s). Dialysis usually returns body temperature to normal.

Carbohydrate Metabolism The ability to metabolize glucose is impaired in most patients with CRF, as evidenced by a slowing of the rate at which the blood glucose level declines to normal after administration of a glucose load. Fasting blood sugar levels are usually normal or only slightly elevated. Severe hyperglycemia and/or ketosis due to uremia alone are not seen, and, therefore, the glucose intolerance of CRF usually does not require specific therapy (hence the term *azotemic pseudodiabetes*). Because insulin is removed from the plasma largely by renal cells, which degrade it intracellularly, circulating insulin levels in plasma are slightly to moderately increased in most fasting uremic subjects, and levels in excess of normal are usually demonstrable after a glucose load. However, the response to intravenous insulin in patients with CRF is impaired, and the rate of utilization of glucose by peripheral tissues is diminished. The glucose intolerance of uremia results largely from this peripheral resistance to the action of insulin. Other factors that may contribute to glucose intolerance include intracellular deficits of K^+, metabolic acidosis, and increased levels of glucagon, catecholamines, growth hormone, and prolactin as well as of the myriad of potentially toxic metabolites that are retained in CRF. Patients with true insulin-dependent diabetes often show a decrease in insulin requirement with progressive azotemia, which is due to the reduced uptake and catabolism of insulin by the kidney as well as to decreased caloric intake.

Nitrogen and Lipid Metabolism The altered state of metabolism in uremic patients leads to abnormal amino acid profiles. In addition to the hypercatabolism seen in uremia, the capacity to eliminate nitrogenous end products of protein catabolism is reduced, so CRF may be regarded as a state of protein intolerance. As noted earlier, the retention of end products of increased nitrogen metabolism is a major cause of organ dysfunction, leading to the signs and symptoms of uremia.

Hypertriglyceridemia, decreased plasma levels of high-density lipoprotein cholesterol, and increased plasma levels of lipoprotein a antigen [Lp(a)] are common in uremia, whereas cholesterol levels in plasma are usually normal. Whether uremia accelerates triglyceride production by the liver and intestine is unknown. The enhancement of lipogenesis by insulin may contribute to increased triglyceride synthesis. In addition, the rate of removal of triglycerides from the circulation, which depends in large part on the enzyme lipoprotein lipase, is depressed in uremia, an effect not corrected appreciably by hemodialysis. The high incidence of premature atherosclerosis in patients on chronic dialysis (see "Cardiovascular and Pulmonary Abnormalities" below) may be related in part to these abnormalities in lipid metabolism.

Clinical Abnormalities in Uremia Chronic renal failure is associated with a constellation of signs and symptoms, which may or may not include reduced urine output but always include elevation in serum urea nitrogen and creatinine concentrations. As pointed out in Chap. 269, elevations of serum urea nitrogen and creatinine levels occur late in the course of renal failure. It can be difficult to differentiate acute from chronic renal failure. The usual hallmark of CRF is reduced kidney size as seen by ultrasound scanning or on an abdominal scout film or pyelogram. In the absence of small kidneys, renal biopsy may be necessary for diagnosis.

As noted earlier, CRF leads to disturbances in function of every organ system. The use of chronic dialysis reduces the incidence and severity of these disturbances, so that, where modern medicine is practiced, the overt and florid manifestations of uremia have largely disappeared. Unfortunately, as indicated in Table 271-2, even optimal dialysis therapy is not a panacea, because some disturbances resulting from impaired renal function fail to respond fully, while others continue to progress. Furthermore, as with many complex therapeutic modalities, dialysis may cause unique abnormalities not seen prior to initiation of therapy; these abnormalities should be viewed as complications of dialysis.

FLUID, ELECTROLYTE, AND ACID-BASE DISORDERS (See also Chaps. 49 and 50) **Sodium and Volume Homeostasis** In most patients with stable CRF, the total body contents of Na^+ and water are increased modestly, although expansion of the extracellular fluid (ECF) volume may not be apparent. With ingestion of excessive amounts of salt and water, however, control of excess volume becomes an important consideration. In general, excessive salt ingestion contributes to or aggravates congestive heart failure, hypertension, ascites, and edema. On the other hand, hyponatremia and weight gain are the consequence of excessive ingestion of water and in most patients are relatively mild or asymptomatic. In most predialysis patients, a daily intake of fluid equal in volume to the urine volume per day plus about 500 mL usually maintains the serum Na^+ concentration at normal levels. Patients on dialysis frequently demonstrate mild hyponatremia. Hypernatremia is relatively infrequent in CRF. In the edematous patient with CRF who is not on dialysis, diuretics and modest restriction of salt and water intake are the mainstays of therapy. In dialysis patients with volume expansion, management should include ultrafiltration and restriction of salt and water intake between dialyses. Patients with CRF have impaired renal mechanisms for conserving Na^+ and water (see Chap. 269). When an *extrarenal* cause for increased fluid loss is present (e.g., vomiting, diarrhea, fever), these patients are prone to volume depletion, leading to dry mucous membranes, dizziness, syncope, tachycardia, decreased filling of jugular veins, orthostatic hypotension, and eventual cardiovascular collapse. Depletion of extracellular fluid volume may result in deterioration of residual renal function and, in the previously stable and asymptomatic patient with mild CRF, signs and symptoms of overt uremia. Cautious fluid repletion usually restores extracellular and intravascular volumes to normal and often but not always restores renal function to prior levels.

Potassium Homeostasis Derangements in K^+ balance (see Chap. 49) are occasionally documented by laboratory analysis in patients with CRF but are rarely responsible for clinical symptoms unless the GFR is below 10 mL/min or unless an endogenous K^+ load (owing to hemolysis, trauma, infection) or an exogenous one (owing to administration of stored blood or K^+-containing medications) enters the system. Despite progression of renal failure, most patients maintain normal serum K^+ concentrations until the late stages of uremia. This ability to sustain K^+ balance in the face of advancing renal failure is due to adaptations in the renal distal tubules and colon, sites where aldosterone and other factors serve to enhance K^+ secretion.

Hyperkalemia Not surprisingly, oliguria or disruption of key adaptive mechanisms can lead to hyperkalemia and its potentially ominous effects on cardiac function. Antikaliuretic drugs such as spironolactone, triamterene, amiloride, trimethoprim, and pentamidine should be used with extreme caution in patients with CRF. Likewise, angiotensin converting enzyme inhibitors and beta blockers may cause or exacerbate hyperkalemia. In kidney transplant recipients, cyclosporine is another common cause of increased serum K^+. Hyperkalemia in CRF patients also may be induced by abrupt falls in blood pH, since acidosis is associated with efflux of K^+ from intracellular to extracellular fluids.

℞ TREATMENT

Correction of acidosis-induced hyperkalemia with sodium bicarbonate is the treatment of choice. This treatment is most often combined with the use of a loop diuretic, which not only enhances K^+ loss but also offsets the administered Na^+ load. Intravenous administration of insulin and dextrose, as well as administration of fludrocortisone and nebulized albuterol, are useful in lowering serum K^+ acutely, while the ion exchange resin sodium polystyrene sulfonate (Kayexalate) is the most effective agent in longer-term control of hyperkalemia. Oral administration of this agent may be accompanied by administration of a purgative, such as sorbitol, to expedite removal of the bound resin. However, sorbitol should not be used with rectal administration of sodium polystyrene sulfonate because of possible bowel dessication and perforation. When hyperkalemia persists in the absence of excessive K^+ intake, oliguria, or acute acidosis, the possibility of *hyporeninemic hypoaldosteronism* should be considered. Patients with this syndrome are often diabetic and have type 4 renal tubular acidosis (see Chap. 49).

Hypokalemia Hypokalemia is uncommon in most forms of CRF but may occur with poor dietary K^+ intake, usually in association with excessive diuretic therapy or gastrointestinal losses. When hypokalemia occurs as a result of primary K^+ wasting in urine, it may represent a solitary renal reabsorptive defect or, more commonly, may be associated with other solute transport abnormalities, as in Fanconi's syndrome, renal tubular acidosis, or other forms of hereditary or acquired tubulointerstitial diseases. The clinical consequences and management of hypokalemia and hyperkalemia are discussed more fully in Chap. 49.

Metabolic Acidosis With advancing renal failure, total daily acid excretion and buffer production fall below the level needed to maintain external balance of hydrogen ions. Metabolic acidosis is the inevitable result, and the mechanisms involved are considered in Chap. 50. In most patients with stable renal insufficiency, administration of 20 to 30 mmol/d of sodium bicarbonate or sodium citrate corrects the acidosis. In response to a sudden acid challenge (whether from an endogenous or an exogenous source), however, patients with CRF are susceptible to severe acidosis, which requires more substantial quantities of alkali for correction. Administration of Na^+ must be carried out with careful attention to volume status and the potential need for diuretic agents. Also, citrate enhances aluminum absorption in the large bowel, and citrate-containing antacids should be avoided if aluminum-containing drugs are also administered.

BONE, PHOSPHATE, AND CALCIUM ABNORMALITIES (Fig. 271-2) *Renal osteodystrophy* and *metabolic bone disease* are terms that encompass a number of skeletal abnormalities, including osteomalacia, osteitis fibrosa cystica, and, in children, impaired bone growth. Many experts also include adynamic or aplastic bone disease, aluminum-induced osteomalacia, and dialysis-related amyloid bone disease, all of which are consequences of long-term dialysis. Adynamic or aplastic bone disease is a recently described condition that is detected primarily on bone biopsy, which reveals a reduction in osteoid as well as fibrosis. Aluminum-induced osteomalacia also involves low bone turnover but is related to aluminum deposition at the osteoid front. Accumulation of β_2-microglobulin amyloid leads to dialysis-related amyloidosis (DRA), which consists of carpal tunnel syndrome, tenosynovitis of the hands, shoulder arthropathy, bone cysts, cervical spondyloarthropathy, and cervical pseudotumors.

Although clinical symptoms of bone disease are present before dialysis in less than 10 percent of patients with advanced renal failure, radiologic and histologic abnormalities are observed in about 35 and 90 percent, respectively, of these patients. Secondary hyperparathyroidism and osteitis fibrosa cystica are more common

Table 271-2

Clinical Abnormalities in Uremia*

Fluid and electrolyte disturbances	**Neuromuscular disturbances**	**Dermatologic disturbances**
Volume expansion and contraction (I)	Fatigue (I)†	Pallor (I)†
Hypernatremia and hyponatremia (I)	Sleep disorders (P)	Hyperpigmentation (I, P, or D)
Hyperkalemia and hypokalemia (I)	Headache (I or P)	Pruritus (P)
Metabolic acidosis (I)	Impaired mentation (I)†	Ecchymoses (I)
Hyperphosphatemia (I)	Lethargy (I)†	Uremic frost (I)
Hypocalcemia (I)	Asterixis (I)	**Gastrointestinal disturbances**
Endocrine-metabolic disturbances	Muscular irritability (I)	Anorexia (I)
Secondary hyperparathyroidism (I or P)	Peripheral neuropathy (I or P)	Nausea and vomiting (I)
Aluminum-induced osteomalacia (D)	Restless legs syndrome (I or P)	Uremic fetor (I)
Vitamin D–deficient osteomalacia (I)	Paralysis (I or P)	Gastroenteritis (I)
Carbohydrate intolerance (I)	Myoclonus (I)	Peptic ulcer (I or P)
Hyperuricemia (I or P)	Seizures (I or P)	Gastrointestinal bleeding (I, P, or D)
Hypertriglyceridemia (P)	Coma (I)	Hepatitis (D)
Increased Lp(a) level (P)	Muscle cramps (D)	Idiopathic ascites (D)
Decreased high-density lipoprotein level (P)	Dialysis disequilibrium syndrome (D)	Peritonitis (D)
Protein-calorie malnutrition (I or P)	Dialysis dementia (D)	**Hematologic and immunologic disturbances**
Impaired growth and development (P)	Myopathy (P or D)	Normocytic, normochromic anemia (I)†
Infertility and sexual dysfunction (P)	**Cardiovascular and pulmonary disturbances**	Microcytic (aluminum-induced) anemia (D)
Amenorrhea (P)	Arterial hypertension (I or P)	Lymphocytopenia (P)
Hypothermia (I)	Congestive heart failure or pulmonary edema (I)	Bleeding diathesis (I or D)†
Dialysis-induced β_2-microglobulin amyloidosis	Pericarditis (I)	Increased susceptibility to infection (I or P)
	Cardiomyopathy (I or P)	Splenomegaly and hypersplenism (P)
	Uremic lung (I)	Leukopenia (D)
	Accelerated atherosclerosis (P or D)	Hypocomplementemia (D)
	Hypotension and arrhythmias (D)	

* Virtually all abnormalities in this table are completely reversed in time by successful renal transplantation. The response of these abnormalities to hemodialysis or peritoneal dialysis therapy is more variable. (I) denotes an abnormality that usually improves with an optimal program of dialysis and related therapy; (P) denotes one that tends to persist or even progress, despite an optimal program; (D) denotes one that develops only after initiation of dialysis therapy.

† Improves with dialysis and erythropoietin therapy.

in children than in adults and are especially common in patients with slowly progressive renal insufficiency. Radiologic examination of uremic patients not yet on dialysis can reveal three types of lesions: (1) changes analogous to those of nutritional rickets, namely, widened osteoid seams at the growth margins of bones (so-called renal rickets); (2) the bone changes of secondary hyperparathyroidism (osteitis fibrosa cystica), characterized by osteoclastic bone resorption and subperiosteal erosions, especially of the terminal phalanges, long bones, and distal ends of the clavicles; and (3) osteosclerosis, often best evidenced by enhanced bone density in the upper and lower margins of vertebrae, producing the so-called rugger jersey spine. In patients being treated with dialysis, aluminum-induced osteomalacia and adynamic bone disease are generally not detected on x-ray films and are diagnosed principally by bone biopsy. DRA occurs only after many years of dialysis, particularly in the elderly, and is characterized on x-ray films by cysts in the carpal bones and femoral neck. Amyloid tumoral masses may be best appreciated by ultrasound examination or computed tomography.

With osteitis fibrosa cystica, vitamin D–deficient and aluminum-induced osteomalacia, and DRA, patients are prone to spontaneous fractures, which are slow to heal. The ribs are most commonly involved in the case of osteitis fibrosa cystica. The femoral neck is a frequent site of aluminum-induced osteomalacia and DRA and is also prone to pathologic fractures. Bone pain, even in the absence of fractures, is common in all of the above disorders. In osteitis fibrosa cystica, a proximal myopathy often coexists, giving rise to gait abnormalities and to impairment of ambulation. Similar myopathy may also occur with amyloid arthropathy due to disease. In CRF, there is a tendency to extraosseous or metastatic calcification when the calcium-phosphorus product is very high (>70). Medium-sized blood vessels, the subcutaneous, articular, and periarticular tissues, the myocardium, the eyes, and the lungs are common sites of metastatic calcification.

℞ TREATMENT

Secondary hyperparathyroidism is best treated by reducing the serum phosphate concentration through the use of a phosphate-restricted diet as well as oral phosphate-binding agents. Calcium carbonate and calcium acetate are the preferred phosphate-binding agents, but in some circumstances a combination of aluminum hydroxide and calcium carbonate is necessary. Aluminum levels should be monitored, and citrate antacids, which enhance aluminum absorption, should be avoided. Dialysate calcium, calcium carbonate, calcium acetate, aluminum hydroxide, and calcitriol must be properly balanced to maintain the serum phosphorus concentration at approximately 1.4 mmol/L (4.5 mg/dL) and the serum calcium at approximately 2.5 mmol/L (10 mg/dL) in an attempt to suppress parathyroid hypertrophy, thus avoiding or reversing osteitis fibrosa cystica, osteomalacia, and myopathy. It is particularly important to keep the calcium-phosphorus product in the normal range to avoid metastatic calcification.

The recently described disorder of adynamic bone disease is thought to be secondary to overzealous treatment of secondary hyperparathyroidism. Therefore, suppression of PTH levels to less than 120 pg/mL in uremic patients may not be desirable. The incidence of aluminum-induced osteomalacia has been greatly reduced with the recognition of aluminum as the principal culprit. Therapy for this disorder is continued avoidance of aluminum with possible use of a chelating agent such as desferoxamine along with high-flux dialysis. At present, there is no good therapy for DRA; local physical therapy, corticosteroid injections and nonsteroidal anti-inflammatory agents constitute current options.

Other Solutes Uric acid retention is a common feature of CRF but rarely leads to symptomatic gout. Hypophosphatemia is usually a consequence of overzealous oral administration of phosphate-binding gels. Because serum magnesium levels tend to rise in CRF, magnesium-containing antacids and cathartics should be avoided.

CARDIOVASCULAR AND PULMONARY ABNORMALITIES Fluid retention in uremia often results in congestive heart failure and/or pulmonary edema. A unique form of pulmonary congestion and edema may occur even in the absence of volume overload and is associated with normal or mildly elevated intracardiac and pulmonary capillary wedge pressures. This entity, characterized radiologically by peripheral vascular congestion giving rise to a "butterfly wing" distribution, is due to increased permeability of alveolar capillary membranes. This low-pressure pulmonary edema, as well as cardiopulmonary abnormalities associated with circulatory overload, usually respond promptly to vigorous dialysis.

Hypertension Hypertension is the most common complication of end-stage renal disease. When it is not found, the patient either has a salt-wasting form of renal disease (e.g., polycystic or medullary cystic disease, chronic tubulointerstitial disease, or papillary necrosis), is receiving antihypertensive therapy, or is volume-depleted, the last condition usually due to excessive gastrointestinal fluid losses or overzealous diuretic therapy. Since fluid overload is the major cause of hypertension in uremia, the normotensive state can usually be restored by aggressive ultrafiltration with dialysis. Nevertheless, because of hyperreninemia, some patients remain hypertensive despite rigorous salt and water restriction and ultrafiltration. Rarely, patients develop accelerated or malignant hypertension, manifested by markedly elevated systolic and diastolic pressures, extreme hyperreninemia, encephalopathy, seizures, retinal hemorrhages, and papilledema. Intravenous nitroprusside, labetolol, or enalaprilat, along with control of extracellular fluid volume, generally controls such hypertension. Subsequently, such patients usually require more than one oral antihypertensive drug. A high percentage of patients with CRF present with left ventricular hypertrophy or dilated cardiomyopathy. These changes are thought to be related to prolonged hypertension.

Pericarditis Retained metabolic toxins are thought to be the cause of uremic pericarditis. Once a common complication of CRF, pericarditis is now infrequent because of early initiation of dialysis.

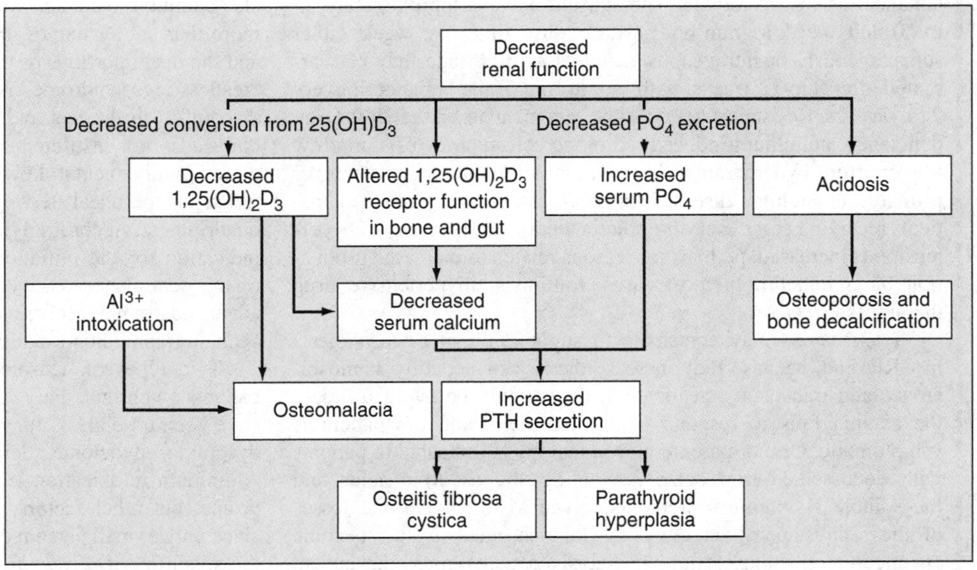

FIGURE 271-2 Flowchart for the development of bone, phosphate, and calcium abnormalities in CRF.

The rare occurrence of pericarditis in the well-dialyzed patient is due to viral infection, systemic disease, transmural myocardial infarction, or cardiac surgery. The clinical presentation of pericarditis in uremic subjects is similar to that seen in nonuremic subjects (Chap. 240), except that effusions are usually hemorrhagic. Treatment with intensive dialysis is recommended, and systemic anticoagulation should be avoided to minimize the occurrence of hemorrhagic tamponade. Pericardiocentesis with intrapericardial instillation of air or glucocorticoids is usually effective for pericardial tamponade. Pericardiectomy should be considered only if more conservative measures fail.

Chronically dialyzed patients have a high incidence of accelerated atherosclerosis, leading to coronary, cerebral, and peripheral vascular disease. Causes for these complications include hypertension, hyperlipidemia, glucose intolerance, chronic high cardiac output, and metastatic vascular and myocardial calcification.

HEMATOLOGIC ABNORMALITIES **Normochromic, Normocytic Anemia** This abnormality occurs regularly and contributes to the symptomatology in CRF. Erythropoiesis is depressed in CRF, owing to the effects of retained toxins on bone marrow, to diminished biosynthesis of erythropoietin by the diseased kidney or, much less often, to the presence of erythropoietin inhibitors. The administration of recombinant human erythropoietin results in a dramatic increase in hematocrit and hemoglobin concentration, suggesting that a reduced level of serum erythropoietin is perhaps the most important of these factors. Hemolysis is a minor component of uremic anemia and, when present, is due to an extracorpuscular effect, since survival of erythrocytes from normal subjects is reduced when these cells are transfused into uremic patients, and erythrocytes from patients with CRF have relatively normal survival times when experimentally transfused into normal individuals. Such hemolysis usually disappears with institution of dialysis. Gastrointestinal blood loss (due to gastrointestinal lesions and abnormal platelet function) may contribute to anemia. Blood loss is exaggerated in hemodialysis patients because of the need for heparin during dialysis and the retention of blood in the dialyzer and associated tubing.

℞ TREATMENT

Administration of recombinant human erythropoietin is the treatment of choice for anemia in patients with advanced renal insufficiency, both before and after initiation of dialysis. Treatment should be instituted if the hematocrit is less than 30 percent. The improvements in cardiovascular function, mental status, and energy level that occur with an increase in hematocrit to approximately 34 to 38 percent enhance the quality of life. The starting dose is approximately 25 to 50 units per kilogram body weight three times per week, either subcutaneously or intravenously. Increases in dosage may be warranted after 8 to 12 weeks, with monitoring of the hematocrit every 2 to 4 weeks. Resistance to erythropoietin mandates a search for iron deficiency, aluminum-induced red blood cell microcytosis, marrow fibrosis from hyperparathyroidism, chronic inflammatory states, or primary hematologic diseases. In approximately 30 percent of patients receiving chronic erythropoietin therapy, the severity of hypertension is increased, perhaps for reasons related to increased production of endothelin. In most cases, routine antihypertensive drug therapy is effective.

Transfusions may contribute to suppression of erythropoiesis in CRF, and, because they increase the risk of hepatitis, hemosiderosis, and transplant sensitization, they should be avoided unless the anemia fails to respond to erythropoietin and the patient is symptomatic. Oral or parenteral iron therapy is indicated in patients with documented iron deficiency. Folic and ascorbic acids and the soluble B vitamins should be given to offset chronic losses of these substances via dialysis. Hemochromatosis has become an uncommon complication in dialysis patients since the advent of erythropoietin therapy.

Abnormal Hemostasis Abnormal hemostasis is also common in CRF and is characterized by a tendency to abnormal bleeding and bruising. Bleeding from surgical wounds and spontaneous bleeding into the gastrointestinal tract, pericardial sac, or intracranial vault (in the form of subdural hematoma or intracerebral hemorrhage) are of the greatest concern. Prolongation of bleeding time, decreased activity of platelet factor 3, abnormal platelet aggregation and adhesiveness, and impaired prothrombin consumption contribute to the clotting defects. The abnormality in platelet factor 3 correlates with increased plasma levels of guanidinosuccinic acid and can be corrected by dialysis. Prolongation of the bleeding time is common even in well-dialyzed patients. Abnormal bleeding times and coagulopathy in patients with renal failure may be reversed with desmopressin, cryoprecipitate, conjugated estrogens, and blood transfusions, as well as by the use of erythropoietin.

Enhanced Susceptibility to Infection Changes in leukocyte formation and function in uremia lead to enhanced susceptibility to infection. Lymphocytopenia and atrophy of lymphoid structures occur, whereas neutrophil production is relatively unimpaired. Nevertheless, the function of all leukocyte cell types may be affected adversely by uremic serum. Alterations in monocyte, lymphocyte, and neutrophil function cause impairment of acute inflammatory responses, decreased delayed hypersensitivity, and altered late immune function. There is a tendency for uremic patients to have less fever in response to infection, perhaps because of the effects of uremia on the hypothalamic temperature control center.

Leukocyte function also may be impaired in patients with CRF because of coexisting acidosis, hyperglycemia, protein-calorie malnutrition, and serum and tissue hyperosmolarity (due to azotemia). In patients receiving hemodialysis, leukocyte function is disturbed because of the effects of the bioincompatibility of various dialysis membranes (see Chap. 272). Activation of cytokine and complement cascades likewise occurs when blood comes in contact with dialysis membranes. These substances in turn alter inflammatory and immune responses of the uremic patient. Mucosal barriers to infection also may be defective, and, in dialysis patients, vascular and peritoneal access devices are common portals of entry for pathogens, especially staphylococci. Glucocorticoids and immunosuppressive drugs used for various renal diseases further increase the risk of infection.

NEUROMUSCULAR ABNORMALITIES Subtle disturbances of central nervous system function, including inability to concentrate, drowsiness, and insomnia, are among the early symptoms of uremia. Mild behavioral changes, loss of memory, and errors in judgment soon follow and may be associated with neuromuscular irritability, including hiccups, cramps, and fasciculations and twitching of muscles. Asterixis, myoclonus, and chorea are common in terminal uremia, as are stupor, seizures, and coma. Peripheral neuropathy is also common in advanced CRF. Initially, sensory nerves are involved more than motor nerves, the lower extremities more than the upper, and the distal portions of the extremities more than the proximal. The "restless legs syndrome" is characterized by ill-defined sensations of discomfort in the feet and lower legs and frequent leg movement. If dialysis is not instituted soon after onset of sensory abnormalities, motor involvement follows, including loss of deep tendon reflexes, weakness, peroneal nerve palsy (foot drop), and, eventually, flaccid quadriplegia. Accordingly, evidence of peripheral neuropathy is a firm indication for the initiation of dialysis or for transplantation. Many of the central nervous system and neuromuscular complications of advanced uremia resolve with dialysis, although nonspecific electroencephalographic abnormalities may persist (Table 271-2).

Two types of neurologic disturbances appear to be unique to patients on chronic dialysis. *Dialysis dementia* is seen in patients who have been on dialysis for many years and is characterized by speech dyspraxia, myoclonus, dementia, and eventually seizures and death. Aluminum intoxication is probably a major contributor to this syndrome, but other factors, such as viral infections, may play a role since only a small percent of patients with aluminum exposure develop the syndrome. *Dialysis disequilibrium*, which occurs during the first few dialyses in association with rapid reduction of blood urea levels, consists of nausea, vomiting, drowsiness, headache, and even convulsions. It has been attributed to cerebral edema and increased intracranial pressure due to the rapid (dialysis-induced) changes in pH and osmolality between extracellular and intracellular fluids.

GASTROINTESTINAL ABNORMALITIES Anorexia, hiccups, nausea, and vomiting are common early manifestations of uremia. Protein restriction is useful in diminishing nausea and vomiting late in the course of renal failure. However, protein restriction should not be implemented in patients with early signs of protein-calorie malnutrition. *Uremic fetor*, a uriniferous odor to the breath, derives from the breakdown of urea in saliva to ammonia and is often associated with an unpleasant metallic taste sensation. Mucosal ulcerations leading to blood loss can occur at any level of the gastrointestinal tract in the very late stages of CRF. Peptic ulcer disease is common in uremic patients. Whether this high incidence is related to altered gastric acidity, enhanced colonization by *Helicobacter pylori*, or hypersecretion of gastrin is unknown. Patients with CRF, particularly those with polycystic kidney disease, have an increased incidence of diverticulosis. Pancreatitis and angiodysplasia of the large bowel with chronic bleeding have been noted more commonly in dialysis patients. Hepatitis B antigenemia was very common in the past, but it is much less so now because of the implementation of universal precautions, the use of hepatitis B vaccine, and the diminished need for blood transfusions resulting from the introduction of erythropoietin. A higher incidence of hepatitis C virus antibody has been noted in patients receiving chronic hemodialysis. This infection does not seem to cause significant liver disease in most patients, but it is a definite concern in patients who subsequently undergo transplantation and immunosuppression, in whom the incidence of active chronic hepatitis and cirrhosis is much higher.

ENDOCRINE-METABOLIC DISTURBANCES Disturbances in parathyroid function, glucose tolerance, and insulin metabolism, as well as the lipid, protein-calorie, and other nutritional abnormalities of uremia, have already been considered. The functioning of the pituitary, thyroid, and adrenal is relatively normal, often despite abnormalities in circulating thyroxine, growth hormone, aldosterone, and cortisol levels. In women, estrogen levels are low, and amenorrhea and inability to carry pregnancies to term are common manifestations of uremia. While menses frequently reappear after chronic dialysis is initiated, successful pregnancies are rare. In men with CRF, including those receiving chronic dialysis, impotence, oligospermia, and germinal cell dysplasia are common, as are reduced plasma testosterone levels. Like growth, sexual maturation is often impaired in adolescent children, even among those receiving chronic dialysis.

DERMATOLOGIC ABNORMALITIES The skin may show evidence of anemia (pallor), defective hemostasis (ecchymoses and hematomas), calcium deposition and secondary hyperparathyroidism (pruritus, excoriations), dehydration (poor skin turgor, dry mucous membranes), and the general cutaneous consequences of protein-calorie malnutrition. A sallow, yellow cast may reflect the combined influences of anemia and retention of a variety of pigmented metabolites, or *urochromes*. In advanced uremia, the concentration of urea in sweat may be so high that, after evaporation, a fine white powder can be found on the skin surface—so-called uremic (urea) frost. Although many of these cutaneous abnormalities improve with dialysis, *uremic pruritus* is usually resistant to dialysis as well as to most systemic and topical therapies. Hemochromatosis causes a slate gray to bronze discoloration of the skin and is now uncommon in dialysis patients because of reduced transfusion requirements.

CONSERVATIVE MANAGEMENT OF PROGRESSIVE RENAL FAILURE

Treatment directed to specific organ system abnormalities has been discussed in the preceding paragraphs. Principles of dialysis and transplant therapy are discussed in Chap. 272. Conservative (nondialytic, nontransplant) therapy must be instituted early to control symptoms, minimize complications, prevent long-term sequelae, and slow the progression of renal insufficiency. The level of renal function should be ascertained periodically, and any reversible component that is present should be corrected. Prerenal factors, such as volume depletion, decreased cardiac output, and renal artery stenosis, and postrenal components, such as urethral or ureteric obstruction, may exacerbate chronic renal insufficiency and must be identified and corrected. Hypertension, urinary tract infections, nephrolithiasis, structural abnormalities of the urinary tract, and the forms of glomerulonephritis that respond to immunosuppressive therapy also should be treated aggressively. Preventive measures include avoidance of nephrotoxic drugs and radiocontrast agents in patients with compromised renal function. In patients with slowly progressive renal failure, urine output is usually well maintained.

As noted earlier, blood urea nitrogen and serum creatinine levels correlate only roughly with symptoms and are poor measures of GFR (see Chap. 269). The creatinine clearance (the product of the volume of urine produced per minute multiplied by the ratio of the concentration of creatinine in urine to the concentration of creatinine in plasma) tends to overestimate the GFR, while the calculated urea clearance often underestimates the GFR. By averaging simultaneously determined creatinine and urea clearances, a reasonably accurate estimation of GFR can be obtained. More exact measures of GFR can be obtained by isotope clearance techniques, which involve the injection of radioisotope and the accurate collection of urine specimens at timed intervals over a 2- to 4-h period. Of these methods, the iothalamate clearance is the most useful clinically.

Restriction of dietary sodium intake is important in the management of hypertension. As renal insufficiency progresses, foods rich in phosphate and potassium should also be restricted. Debate continues as to the clinical usefulness of lowering the protein content of the diet. The strongest evidence suggests that this measure is most effective if initiated early in the course of renal failure. Reduction of dietary protein content reduces anorexia, nausea, and vomiting late in uremia. If initiated early (while the GFR is $>$ 40 to 50 mL/min), a low-protein diet (0.6 grams of protein per kilogram of body weight) may be effective in slowing the progression of renal disease.

The Modification of Diet in Renal Disease (MDRD) multicenter study sponsored by the U.S. National Institutes of Health/Health Care Financing Administration found that lowering the protein intake while the GFR was in the range of 25 to 55 mL/min was associated with a modest reduction in disease progression at 3 years of follow-up, especially in patients with proteinuria of $>$1 g per day. Because of the risk of malnutrition, aggressive reduction of dietary protein intake late in renal insufficiency should be discouraged if the patient's serum albumin concentration is below 3 g/dL or there is other evidence of malnutrition. The MDRD study demonstrated that the control of hypertension is as important as dietary protein restriction in slowing the progression of renal disease. The major finding of the MDRD study was that a decrease in blood pressure below a mean value of approximately 95 mmHg (i.e., 120/80) was effective in slowing progression of renal disease, again especially in patients with proteinuria of $>$1 g/d. Data from other studies, particularly in patients with early diabetic nephropathy, suggest a beneficial role for angiotensin converting enzyme (ACE) inhibitors in slowing progression of renal disease. Hyperkalemia and compromised renal function are complications of these drugs, especially in patients with bilateral renal artery stenosis (or unilateral stenosis in those with a solitary kidney). Combination therapy involving ACE inhibitors plus diuretics, alpha-adrenergic blockers, and/or beta-adrenergic blockers may be necessary to control hypertension as well as to delay progression to end-stage renal failure.

In more advanced uremia, it may be necessary to use sodium bicarbonate or calcium carbonate to correct metabolic acidosis and bicarbonate, dextrose-insulin combinations, or sodium-potassium exchange resins for treatment of hyperkalemia. Hypermagnesemia, hyperamylasemia, hypertriglyceridemia, and mild carbohydrate intolerance generally do not require or are not amenable to treatment.

Hyperuricemia should be treated with allopurinol (100 mg daily) only if gout develops. Treatment of anemia has been discussed above. Secondary hyperparathyroidism must be treated early to prevent bone disease. Vigorous use of phosphate-binding agents, calcium supplements, and vitamin D (dihydrotachysterol or calcitriol) to maintain the serum levels of calcium (9.5 to 10.5 mg/dL) and phosphorus (4.5 to 6.0 mg/dL) are often effective in suppressing parathyroid levels and preventing osteitis fibrosa and osteomalacia. However, the calcium-phosphorus product must be kept below 70 to avoid visceral, subcutaneous, joint and vascular calcifications.

Dietary restrictions of sodium, potassium, phosphate, and protein often prove unacceptable to patients. Consequently, when the complications of uremia worsen despite conservative management and malnutrition appears, dialysis and/or transplantation, along with an aggressive increase in calories and protein, should be instituted.

BIBLIOGRAPHY

ANDERSON S, BRENNER BM: Progressive renal disease: A disorder of adaptation. Q J Med 70:185, 1989

ATTMAN PO, ALAUPOVID P: Lipid abnormalities in chronic renal insufficiency. Kidney Int 39(Suppl 31):S16, 1991

CONVERSE RL JR et al: Sympathetic overactivity in patients with chronic renal failure. N Engl J Med 327:1912, 1992

ESCHBACH JW et al: Recombinant human erythropoietin in anemic patients with endstage renal disease: Results of phase III multicenter clinical trial. Ann Intern Med 111:992, 1989

FRASER CL, ARIEFF AF: Nervous system complications in uremia. Ann Intern Med 109:143, 1988

HAKIM RM, LAZARUS JM: Biochemical parameters in chronic renal failure. Am J Kidney Dis 11:238, 1988

KANG JY: The gastrointestinal tract in uremia. Digest Dis Sci 38:257, 1993

KLAHR S et al: The effects of dietary protein restriction and blood-pressure control on the progression of chronic renal disease. N Engl J Med 330:877, 1994

LEWIS EJ et al: The effect of angiotensin-converting-enzyme inhibition on diabetic nephropathy. N Engl J Med 329:1456, 1993

RITZ E, KOCH M: Morbidity and mortality due to hypertension in patients with renal failure. Am J Kidney Dis 21:113, 1993

ROSTAND SG et al: Cardiovascular complications in renal failure. J Am Soc Nephrol 2:1053, 1991

SHERRAD DJ et al: The spectrum of bone disease in end-stage renal failure—an evolving disorder. Kidney Int 43:436, 1993

272

Charles B. Carpenter, J. Michael Lazarus

DIALYSIS AND TRANSPLANTATION IN THE TREATMENT OF RENAL FAILURE

Over the past 30 years, dialysis and transplantation have prolonged the lives of thousands of patients with renal insufficiency. The approach to treatment in acute renal failure is different than in chronic renal failure because of the irreversible nature of the latter. Conservative medical management and dialysis are the mainstays of therapy for acute renal failure (Chap. 270). Obviously, transplantation is not a treatment for this group of patients.

The term *end-stage renal disease* (ESRD) is used by U.S. government agencies and has come to be synonymous with the late stages of chronic renal failure. Initially, patients with ESRD are managed with conservative therapy, but eventually they require hemodialysis, peritoneal dialysis, and/or transplantation. Because of limited success with each of these modalities, chronic renal failure should be approached with the concept of moving from one form of therapy to another as indicated by the degree of success and incidence of complications with each. Therapy for renal failure should *not* be initiated when the patient is totally asymptomatic; however, dialysis and/or transplant should be started sufficiently early to prevent serious complications, as noted in Chaps. 270 and 271. Early dialysis is appropriate in patients with acute renal failure in whom resumption of renal function can be expected and in patients with chronic renal failure who have a good immunologic match with a related donor and are to be transplanted without prior long-term dialysis. In the remainder of patients, the clinical judgment to move from conservative treatment to dialysis or transplantation is determined by the patient's quality of life and whether or not the benefits of treatment outweigh the risks.

The correlation of uremic symptoms with renal function varies from patient to patient depending on the cause of renal disease (earlier onset of symptoms in subjects with diabetes mellitus), muscle mass (large, muscular patients tolerate high levels of azotemia), diet, nutritional status, and coexisting conditions. Therefore, it is ill-advised to assign a certain "usual" level of blood urea nitrogen, serum creatinine, or glomerular filtration rate to the need to start dialysis. In the United States, the Health Care Financing Administration has assigned levels of creatinine and creatinine clearance to qualify for reimbursement from Medicare for patients receiving dialysis. The creatinine must be greater than or equal to 8.0 mg/dL (700 μmol/L) and the creatinine clearance must be less than or equal to 10 mL/min (0.17 mL/s). The recently introduced regulations will undoubtedly affect physician practice. Treatment with dietary protein restriction and aggressive control of hypertension, as described in Chap. 271, may prolong the time before the need for dialysis and/or transplantation but should be carried out only if complications of such therapy, specifically malnutrition, do not occur.

DIALYSIS AND/OR TRANSPLANTATION

Selection of patients to receive dialysis and/or transplantation is a matter of some debate. Because of the reversible nature of acute renal failure, all patients with this diagnosis should be supported with dialysis, at least for some period of time, to allow return of renal function (see Chap. 270). In patients with irreversible or chronic renal failure, criteria for selection for transplantation are generally more stringent than those for dialysis (see below) and are guided by the possibility of complications related to immunosuppressive therapy. Table 272-1 lists considerations in the selection of recipients for a human renal allograft. Transplantation should be undertaken only when conservative treatment has failed, when there are no reversible elements in the renal failure, and when the patient is too ill to be maintained comfortably with the usual methods of treatment. However, morbidity is less if transplantation is performed before the patient is critically ill. Transplantation should not be utilized in an attempt to salvage patients, particularly the elderly, from failure to thrive on dialysis.

The recipient should be free of life-threatening extrarenal complications such as cancer, severe coronary artery disease, and cerebrovascular disease. Provided that diffuse vascular involvement is not present,

Table 272-1

Contraindications to Kidney Transplantation
ABSOLUTE CONTRAINDICATIONS
Reversible renal involvement
Ability of conservative measures to maintain useful life
Advanced forms of major extrarenal complications (cerebrovascular or coronary disease, neoplasia)
Active infection
Active glomerulonephritis
Previous sensitization to donor tissue
RELATIVE CONTRAINDICATIONS
Age
Presence of vesical or urethral abnormalities
Iliofemoral occlusive disease
Psychiatric problems
Oxalosis

diabetes mellitus is not a contraindication. Oxalosis may recur in relatively short order in a transplanted kidney and is generally a contraindication for transplantation. Although advanced age may be a limiting factor, it is advanced "physiologic" rather than chronologic age that contraindicates transplantation. In general, patients reach a "physiologic" limit at approximately age 60 to 65 years, when the incidence of complications due to glucocorticoids becomes much higher. Although abnormalities of the bladder and urethra present additional hazards, successful renal allografts have been placed in patients with these abnormalities by prior constitution of an artificial bladder (i.e., ileal conduit) into which the donor ureter is placed. Patients with any disease process that may be aggravated by glucocorticoids, cyclosporine, azathioprine, or other immunosuppressive agents or any patient with coexisting medical conditions so severe that the risks of operation and drug therapy are high should not be offered transplantation.

Criteria for treatment with hemodialysis or peritoneal dialysis are more liberal because dialysis has less morbidity than transplantation in older patients with the aforementioned medical complications. Because of the cost of these programs, some have suggested that entry be restricted in patients of advanced age. Such decisions, based on moral, social, and economic issues, continue to be debated. In general, in the United States and some other countries, nearly all patients are accepted for dialysis if they or their families desire prolongation of life. The physician should inform the patient of the likelihood of success and review the complications and untoward effects. The patient and family should be given an estimate of prognosis and expected quality of life. In most areas of the world, the cost of medical care for chronic renal failure is borne by government. In the United States, the mechanism of coverage is by Medicare, with all patients eligible regardless of age.

PREPARATION FOR THERAPY OF END-STAGE RENAL DISEASE While conservative measures are being carried out in patients with chronic renal failure (Chap. 271), it is important to prepare them with an intensive educational program, explaining the likelihood and timing of complete renal failure and the various forms of therapy available. The more knowledgeable patients are concerning hemodialysis, peritoneal dialysis, and transplantation, the easier and more appropriate will be their decisions at a later time. With hemodialysis, the major method of obtaining blood for treatment is from an arteriovenous fistula. Since these devices often take months to develop, prophylactic placement of a fistula in a patient opting for hemodialysis is important in minimizing future complications of circulatory access. For those who select peritoneal dialysis [continuous ambulatory peritoneal dialysis (CAPD) or continuous cyclic peritoneal dialysis (CCPD)], placement of the peritoneal catheter does not require prior preparation, and catheter placement and peritoneal dialysis can be instituted when uremic signs and symptoms develop. In those who may perform home dialysis or undergo transplantation, early education of family members for selection and preparation as a home dialysis helper or a related donor for transplantation should occur before the onset of symptomatic renal failure.

In patients who have a good antigenic match with a willing donor, transplantation without intervening hemodialysis or peritoneal dialysis should be considered. Approximately 25 percent of patients receiving renal transplants at our institution do so without having had prior dialysis. In considering related-donor transplantation, the risk of unilateral nephrectomy in the donor, including development of proteinuria and hypertension, should be considered by the family. As discussed below, the success rate of cadaver-donor transplantation has improved sufficiently that this form of therapy should be considered both by the patient and by potential donors. Early referral of patients to ESRD programs will allow education of the patient and family and preparation for an appropriate therapy. In recent years, unrelated living donors have become acceptable in most programs.

DIALYSIS

HEMODIALYSIS Hemodialysis employs the process of diffusion across a semipermeable membrane to remove unwanted substances from the blood while adding desirable components. A constant flow of blood on one side of the membrane and a cleansing solution (dialysate) on the other allow removal of waste products by diffusive and convective transport. By altering the composition of the dialysate, the method of exposure of blood and dialysate (geometry of the dialyzer), the type and surface area of dialysis membrane, and the frequency and duration of exposure (the dialysis prescription), patients without renal function can be maintained in a relatively healthy state.

Hemodialysis equipment consists of three components—the blood delivery system, the composition and delivery system of the dialysate, and the dialyzer itself (Fig. 272-1). Blood is pumped to the dialyzer by a roller pump through lines with appropriate equipment to measure flow and pressures within the system; blood flow should be approximately 300 to 450 mL/min. Negative hydrostatic pressure on the dialysate side of the system can be manipulated to achieve desirable fluid removal, so-called ultrafiltration. Dialysis membranes have differing ultrafiltration coefficients (i.e., mL removed per mmHg/min), the selection of which, along with the hydrostatic pressure changes, determines fluid removal. The dialysate is delivered to the dialyzer from a storage tank or proportioning system that manufactures dialysate on-line. In most systems, dialysate passes once across the membrane, countercurrent to blood flow at a rate of 500 mL/min. The composition of the dialysate is similar to normal plasma water but may be altered depending on need. The dialysate potassium is varied most often; the concentration of calcium, chloride, and bicarbonate generally remain unchanged in each dialysis unit. Sodium concentration may be varied during the course of dialysis (sodium modeling) in order to optimize fluid removal.

The principal dialyzer in use in the United States is the hollow fiber or capillary dialyzer, in which membrane material is spun into fine capillaries, thousands of which are packed into bundles with blood flowing through the capillaries while dialysate is circulated on the outside of the fiber bundle. The type of membrane and surface area (size) are determinants of ultrafiltration and clearance and are important in the immunologic (i.e., biocompatible) response by the patient. Cuprophan (Cupra-ammonium cellophane) and cellulose acetate are "tighter" membranes with less diffusive and ultrafiltration capabilities and less biocompatibility. Polyacrylnitrile, polymethylmethacrylate, polysulphon, and certain newer cellulose derivatives are porous (high flux) and more biocompatible but are more expensive.

With current dialysis techniques, most patients require between 9 and 12 h of dialysis per week, equally divided into several sessions. The time depends on body size, residual renal function, dietary intake, complicating illnesses, and degree of anabolism or catabolism. The dialysis duration, frequency of treatments, type and size of dialyzer, dialysate composition, and blood or dialysate flow may all be altered to accomplish specific needs (see Fig. 272-2).

Urea kinetic modeling is a technique to measure the delivered dose of dialysis. This may be determined by use of a pre- and postdialysis urea sample [urea reduction ratio (URR)] or by determining the KT/V (K = clearance, T = dialysis time, and V = volume of distribution of the patient), which is a dimensionless measure of treatment. An acceptable URR is 65 percent, which is equivalent to a KT/V of approximately 1.0 to 1.2. The development of bicarbonate dialysis, sodium modeling, and high-flux or ultraefficient membranes has resulted in the ability to reduce dialysis time. It is mandatory, however, that such decreases in dialysis time be monitored by one of the above measures of adequacy. Reduction of dialysis time without documentation of adequacy of treatment is associated with an increased mortality and morbidity.

In addition to hemodialysis, a new method of treatment has been developed for patients with acute renal failure. Slow continuous ultrafiltration, continuous arteriovenous hemodialysis (CAVHD), or continuous venovenous hemodialysis (CVVHD) are techniques that employ high-efficiency dialyzers with continuous treatment utilizing very low blood and dialysate flow rates. These therapies are useful in

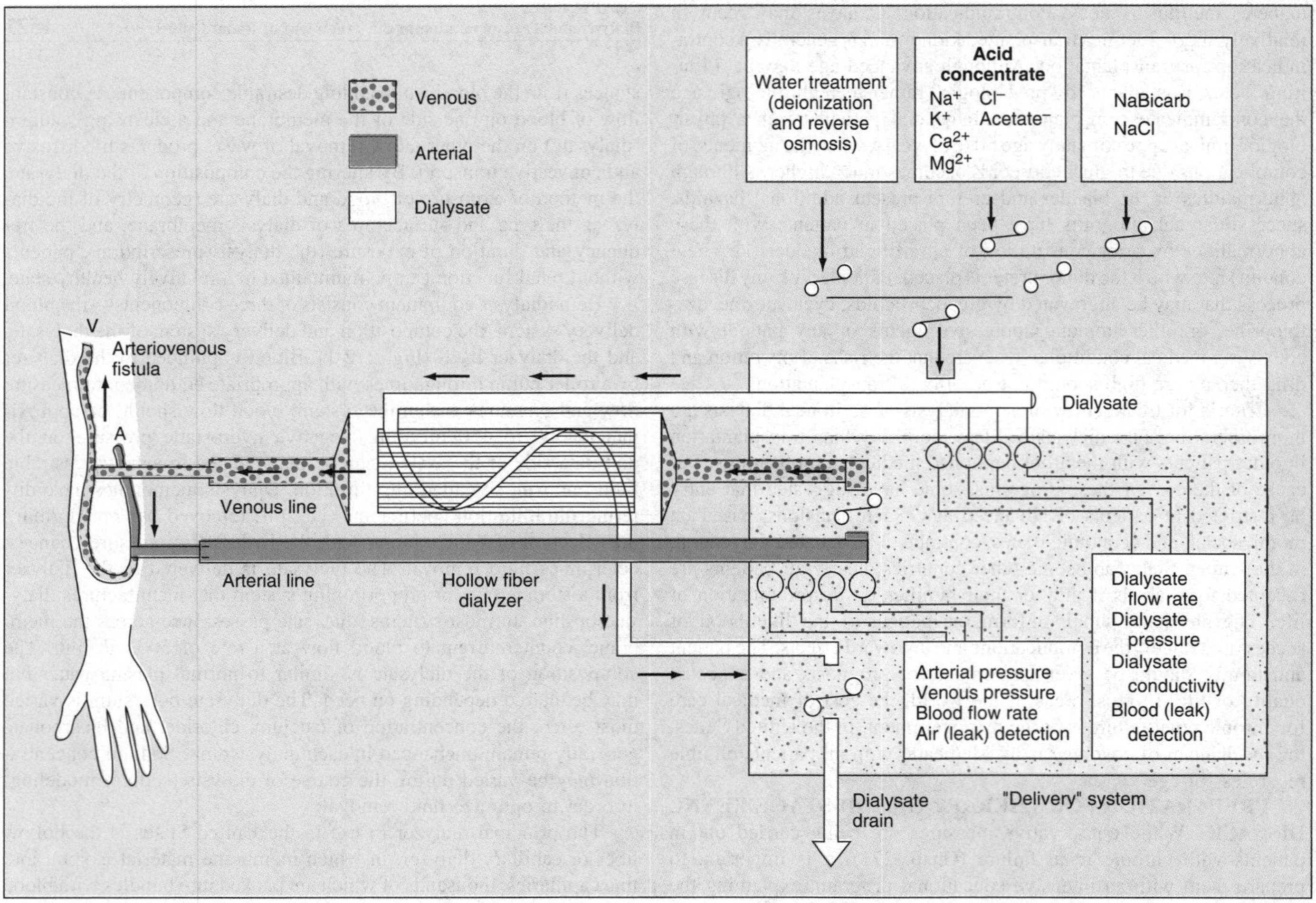

FIGURE 272-1 Schema for hemodialysis.

the unstable, acute renal failure patient and are often preferable to intermittent hemodialysis.

Complications of Hemodialysis Complications of chronic dialysis should be thought of as those related to unresolved uremia, direct complications of clearance and ultrafiltration, and complications created by long-term dialytic treatment. The persistent problems of uremia not corrected by dialysis are described in Chap. 271. Complications more directly related to the procedure include those related to access to the circulation or access to the peritoneal cavity, which are the Achilles' heel of dialysis treatment. Blood flows of 300 to 400 mL/min are necessary for hemodialysis. Blood from veins is inadequate,

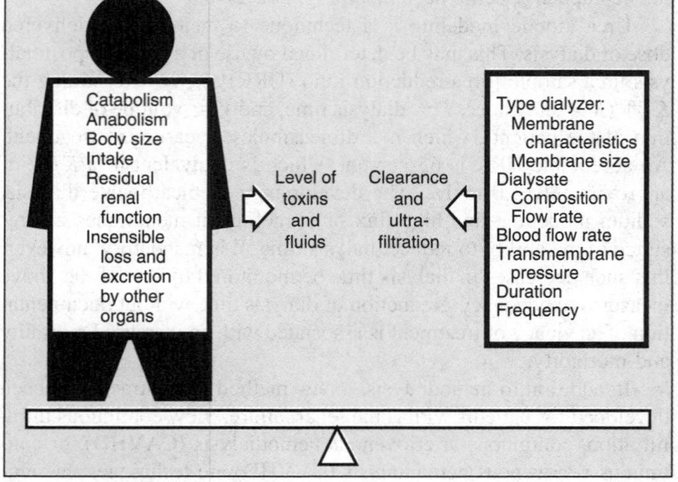

FIGURE 272-2 Factors in the development of the uremic syndrome and considerations in its treatment.

and repeated puncture of a large artery is not feasible. Therefore, by surgically anastamosing a superficial artery and nearby vein, a fistula is created. If a native vein is not available because of fibrosis and atrophy due to prior needling, phlebitis, or other injury, a prosthetic vascular graft (extended polytetrafluoroethylene), bridging an artery and a nearby vein, may be utilized. Repeated cannulation of arteriovenous fistulas or graft fistulas with 14- to 16-gauge needles permits blood flow sufficient to carry out hemodialysis. Some patients require placement of a semipermanent indwelling internal jugular catheter when a fistula cannot be developed or is slow to develop. Unfortunately, thrombosis, infection, and aneurysm formation commonly occur in arteriovenous fistulas, particularly in the prosthetic types, and are the leading causes of hospital admission in these patients. There is a high incidence of septicemia and septic embolization associated with fistula infections and semipermanent internal jugular catheters; the most common infecting agent is *Staphylococcus aureus*. Peritoneal dialysis is performed through the placement of an indwelling peritoneal catheter. On occasion, these catheters become nonfunctional, but the more common complication is peritonitis, generally related to contamination of the system during exchange of peritoneal fluid.

The rapid flux in osmolality with hemodialysis may cause a disequilibrium syndrome consisting of confusion, clouding of consciousness, and seizures. In addition, rapid changes in electrolytes (particularly potassium) may lead to arrhythmia during dialysis. Hypotension during hemodialysis is due to many factors—the size of the extracorporeal circulation, degree of ultrafiltration, change in serum osmolality, presence of autonomic neuropathy, concomitant use of antihypertensive agents, removal of catecholamines, or alterations in body temperature due to the dialysate temperature. Careful estimation of the extracellular fluid to be removed and use of isolated ultrafiltration and higher dialysate sodium are helpful in preventing hypotension. The occurrence of dialysis dementia (a condition of decreasing mental function with seizure activity and abnormal electroencephalogram), low-turnover osteomalacia, and microcytic anemia may be secondary to aluminum contamination of dialysate water or from high oral intake of aluminum hydroxide. These complications have nearly disappeared with awareness of the risk of aluminum exposure and its avoidance. An increased incidence of hepatitis B surface antigen (HBsAg) and hepatitis C virus (HCV) antigenemia are related to decreased immunology integrity and increased transfusions. Patients with chronic antigenemia are usually asymptomatic and have transient or mild derangement in liver function. The high rates of HCV infection and cytomegalovirus (CMV) infection do not have major impact on dialysis patients but do on patients who are subsequently transplanted. The use of recombinant human erythropoietin has reduced or eliminated the need for blood transfusion in hemodialysis patients (Chap. 271), thus reducing the risk of hepatitis and other bloodborne infections. In addition, the use of hepatitis vaccine has decreased the incidence of hepatitis B. Based on clinical experience and recommendations from the Centers for Disease Control and Prevention, only those patients with hepatitis B antigenemia need isolation. Strict compliance with universal precautions is absolutely essential in the dialysis unit, particularly because of patients with HCV and CMV and those who are positive for human immunodeficiency virus.

Mechanical and/or iatrogenic complications, such as hemolysis, air embolus, blood leaks, and contaminated dialysate, are less common with improved equipment. Membrane-induced adverse reactions may occur, as exemplified by complement-mediated leukopenia and hypoxemia. More prominent symptoms, such as back and chest pain, bronchospasm, and anaphylaxis, rarely occur from such reactions. Elaboration of cytokines, specifically interleukin (IL) 1, IL-6, and tumor necrosis factor, occur with exposure of blood to some dialysis membranes. Activation of the complement and cytokine systems likely plays a role in anorexia and hypercatabolism seen in hemodialysis patients. These cytokines also contribute, along with decreased excretion of β_2-microglobulin, to the development of dialysis-related amyloidosis—a syndrome consisting of carpal tunnel syndrome; destructive spondyloarthropathy; cervicooccipital pseudotumors; cyst formation in the femoral head and neck, carpal bones, and humoral head; scapulohumoral periarthritis; and increased visceral involvement with amyloidosis. Use of more biocompatible synthetic membranes (polycrilonitrile, polymethylmethacrylate, and polysulfone) rather than cellulosic-related membranes has been suggested to have a beneficial effect by reducing β_2-microglobulin production and increasing its removal. As mentioned earlier, these membranes are expensive. Reuse of such dialyzers, which occurs in approximately 70 to 75 percent of patients, makes their use feasible.

Heparin is necessary during the hemodialysis procedure to prevent clotting in the lines, but its use may lead to complications such as subdural hematoma and retroperitoneal, gastrointestinal, pericardial, and pleural hemorrhages. Recognition of the risks and modification of the dose of heparin reduce these complications.

The major cause of death in patients with ESRD receiving chronic hemodialysis or peritoneal dialysis is cardiovascular disease. Although this is not a direct complication of hemodialysis, it is probably related to inadequate treatment of hypertension, the persistence of hyperlipidemia in dialysis patients, and, in some cases, alterations in cardiovascular dynamics during the course of dialysis. In addition to aggressive removal of fluid, the appropriate use of antihypertensive agents may be necessary. One further major complication affecting morbidity and mortality in the dialysis population is malnutrition. Again, this is not directly related to the dialysis procedure except that the chronic exposure of the patient to dialysis may effect an increased catabolism and allow amino acid loss through the membrane. Recognition of amino acid loss, decreased protein and calorie intake, and hypercatabolism has led to the recommendation of more aggressive feeding of dialysis patients.

The potential for all of the above complications should cause the physician to evaluate the risk/benefit ratio of hemodialysis before proceeding with such treatment, particularly in the marginal patient. Advantages of hemodialysis are the relatively short treatment time and minimal interruption of life-style between treatments. It is more efficient than peritoneal dialysis, allowing rapid changes in abnormal serum values. Hemodialysis can be performed in the home, but the patient requires an assistant during treatment.

PERITONEAL DIALYSIS Peritoneal dialysis, like hemodialysis, may be performed in various settings and with several techniques. In patients with acute renal failure, intermittent peritoneal dialysis (IPD) has largely been replaced by CAVHD or CAVVHD. Chronic peritoneal dialysis was attempted in the late 1940s but was impractical until the development of a permanent peritoneal catheter—the Tenckhoff catheter. Use of this indwelling catheter and closed continuous-cycle dialysate delivery equipment led to treatment protocols with which patients were treated two to three times per week for a total of 30 to 40 h IPD to achieve clearances and fluid removal similar to those of hemodialysis. In 1978, the concept of continuous peritoneal lavage with prolonged dwell times led to the development of CAPD, which differs from IPD in that patients instill fluid into the peritoneal cavity, seal the catheter, continue in an ambulatory mode, and every 4 to 6 h empty the peritoneal cavity and replace the dialysate. This technique generally utilizes 2 L of dialysate and obviates the need for dialysis equipment. Modification of the technique using a cyclic dialysate delivery device to exchange dialysate during the night with dwelling of fluid during the waking hours (CCPD) is more acceptable to some patients.

IPD performed in a center is not a practical approach due to high costs. CCPD may be performed at home (usually overnight), while CAPD can be performed anywhere. As with hemodialysis, the composition of the dialysate can be modified for individual needs. The major difference in peritoneal dialysate formulas is in the amount of dextrose used as an osmotic agent (1.5, 2.5, or 4.25 g/dL). Advantages of peritoneal dialysis are avoidance of heparinization and vascular surgery and a slower clearance rate (helpful for some cardiovascular patients). It is more amenable to self-treatment. Disadvantages include the longer treatment time with continuous involvement by the patient. It should not be used in patients with pulmonary disease or extensive abdominal adhesions due to surgery. Inadequate clearance may occur in patients with scleroderma, vasculitis, malignant hypertension or peritoneal fibrosis or in heavy patients (>70 kg) with no residual renal function.

Determination of adequacy of treatment by CAPD or CCPD is performed by measuring the clearance of creatinine and urea in a 24-h dialysate collection. The most common complication is peritonitis, including catheter tunnel infections. Protein loss leading to malnutrition is another major complication, while hypertriglyceridemia, hypercholesterolemia, obesity, and inguinal and abdominal hernias are rare complications. The average peritonitis rate is approximately one episode every 10 to 12 months. Tunnel infections are much less frequent but usually require the catheter to be removed, whereas peritonitis can be treated with intravenous or intraparenteral antibiotics with the catheter remaining in place.

TREATMENT OPTIONS AND SETTINGS An acutely ill or medically complicated patient will likely undergo dialysis in a hospital dialysis unit or intensive care unit, while stable patients are generally dialyzed as outpatients in free-standing facilities or at home. Most centers attempt to have patients participate in their own care, so-called self-care dialysis. Home dialysis (either hemodialysis or peritoneal) is preferable for many because of self-reliance and freedom from hospital and center schedules. Patient motivation is the primary factor in the selection of home hemodialysis or peritoneal dialysis. Dialysis in the hospital setting is most expensive, while home dialysis with a nonpaid family assistant or alone (peritoneal dialysis only) is marginally less expensive than satellite dialysis. Despite the absence of equipment, peritoneal dialysis is nearly as expensive as home hemodialysis because of the cost of dialysate and of hospitalizations related to complications of peritoneal dialysis.

In 1995, the total Medicare budget for ESRD (inpatient and outpatient care including hemodialysis, peritoneal dialysis, and transplantation and all other related medical expenses) was estimated by the Health Care Financing Administration to be $9.5 billion. The cost of the ESRD program has grown to be substantially greater than anticipated at its initiation in 1973. This large expenditure reflects an increasing number of recipients treated, not an increasing cost per patient, which, in fact, has been significantly reduced over the past 30 years.

RESULTS The mean age for patients undergoing hemodialysis and peritoneal dialysis is approximately 64 years. Of new patients entering ESRD therapy, approximately 35 to 50 percent are physically and psychologically suitable for transplantation. Not all of these patients opt for transplantation. Only those patients with living related and unrelated donors or those fortunate enough to match a cadaver donor undergo prompt transplantation. These patients are usually younger and healthier than those patients left behind on hemodialysis. The age of patients on dialysis continues to rise, partly because of an increase in acceptance of patients with age-related nephrosclerosis but also because of the selection process favoring transplantation in younger patients.

Approximately 10 to 20 percent of patients with chronic renal failure are totally rehabilitated by dialysis, and another 30 to 40 percent of nondiabetic patients may be rehabilitated to a functional status even if they are not employed. Twenty percent of patients reach a level of function not considered rehabilitated but are able to care for themselves. The remainder (approximately 20 percent) are totally dependent on support from others. Diabetic patients, who have rehabilitation and survival rates lower than those of nondiabetic patients, make up much of the latter two groups. Mortality rates vary, depending on the age of the patient and the disease process(es) involved. Yearly gross mortality rates of patients in the ESRD program in the United States have increased from a low of 20 percent in 1982 to approximately 24 percent in 1991, which has persisted. This increase in mortality may be due to case-mix factors, i.e., acceptance in recent years of older patients with a higher incidence of comorbid conditions such as diabetes mellitus, nephrosclerosis, coronary artery disease, peripheral vascular disease, and pulmonary and hepatic disease. Others have suggested that treatment has become inadequate for financial reasons. In recent years, measurement of both quality and quantity of dialysis treatment has been implemented, leading to increased treatment intensity in many programs. It is anticipated that this will have a favorable effect on mortality and morbidity. In patients less than 50 years of age with no complicating medical illnesses, mortality with hemodialysis, peritoneal dialysis, and transplantation remains below 3 to 5 percent per year.

TRANSPLANTATION

Transplantation of the human kidney is frequently the most effective treatment of advanced chronic renal failure. Worldwide, tens of thousands of such procedures have been performed. When azathioprine and prednisone were initially used as immunosuppressive drugs, the results with properly matched familial donors were superior to those with organs from cadaveric donors, namely, 75 to 90 percent compared with 50 to 60 percent graft survival rates at 1 year. During the 1970s and 1980s, the success rate at the 1-year mark for cadaveric transplants rose progressively. By the time cyclosporine was introduced in the early 1980s, cadaveric donor grafts had a 70 percent 1-year survival and were at the 80 to 85 percent level in the mid 1990s. After the first year, graft survival curves show an exponential decline in numbers of functioning grafts from which a half-life ($t_{1/2}$) in years is calculated. Mortality rates are less than 5 percent in the first year and lower thereafter. Occasionally, acute irreversible rejection may occur after many months of good function, especially if the patient neglects to take the immunosuppressive drugs. Most grafts, however, succumb at varying rates to a chronic vascular and interstitial obliterative process termed *chronic rejection*, although its pathogenesis is incompletely understood. Second and even third transplants can be performed, and the overall results show a 10 to 20 percent reduction in expected survival compared with first transplants in those patients who rapidly rejected a prior transplant. Overall, transplantation returns the majority of patients to an improved life-style, as compared to patients on dialysis; however, careful prospective cohort studies have yet to be reported.

DONOR SELECTION Donors can be cadavers or volunteer living donors. The latter are usually family members selected to have at least partial compatibility for HLA antigens. Living volunteer donors should be normal on physical examination and of the same major ABO blood group, because crossing major blood group barriers prejudices survival of the allograft. It is possible, however, to transplant a kidney of a type O donor into an A, B, or AB recipient. Selective renal arteriography should be performed on donors to rule out the presence of multiple or abnormal renal arteries, because the surgical procedure is difficult and the ischemic time of the transplanted kidney long when vascular abnormalities exist. Cadaveric donors should be free of malignant neoplastic disease because of possible transmission to the recipient. Increased risk of graft failure exists when the donor is elderly or has renal failure and when the kidney has a prolonged period of ischemia and storage.

In the United States, there is a coordinated national system (United Network for Organ Sharing) of computerized information about and logistic support for the transportation of cadaver kidneys to suitable recipients. It is now possible to remove cadaver kidneys and to maintain them for over 48 h on cold pulsatile perfusion or simple flushing and cooling. This permits adequate time for typing, cross-matching, transportation, and selection problems to be solved.

TISSUE TYPING AND CLINICAL IMMUNOGENETICS Matching for antigens of the HLA major histocompatibility gene complex (Chap. 306) is the ideal criterion for selection of donors for renal allografts. Each mammalian species has a single chromosomal region that encodes the strong, or major, transplantation antigens, and this region on the human sixth chromosome is called *HLA*. HLA antigens have been classically defined by serologic techniques, but methods to define specific nucleotide sequences in genomic DNA are increasingly being used. Other antigens, called "minor," may nevertheless play crucial roles, especially the ABH(O) blood groups and endothelial antigens that are not shared with lymphocytes. Evidence for designation of HLA as the genetic region encoding major transplantation antigens comes from the success rate in living related donor renal and bone marrow transplantation, with superior results in HLA-identical sibling pairs. Nevertheless, 5 to 10 percent of HLA-identical renal allografts are rejected, often within the first weeks after transplantation. These failures represent states of prior sensitization to non-HLA antigens. Non-HLA antigens are relatively weak when initially encountered and are therefore suppressible by conventional immunosuppressive therapy. Once priming has occurred, however, secondary responses are much more refractory to treatment. ABO incompatibilities are hazardous because of the presence of natural anti-A and anti-B antibodies in recipients and the normal expression of A and B blood group substances on endothelium.

Living Donors When first-degree relatives are donors, graft survival rates at 1 year are slightly greater than those for cadaver grafts, with the exception of HLA-identical donors where 1-year results are approximately 95 percent. After the first year, the long-term survival rates as defined by the $t_{1/2}$ still favor the partially matched (one HLA haplotype) family donor over a randomly selected cadaver donor (Table 272-2). In addition, living donors provide the advantage of immediate availability. Waiting lists for cadaveric kidneys have grown faster than the available organ supply to the point where most new patients with end-stage renal disease wait for more than 3 years. In response to this increasing disparity between cadaver donor supply and patient demand, living unrelated volunteers, usually spouses or close friends, are being accepted as donors in increasing numbers. It is illegal in the United States to purchase organs for transplantation. The results of transplantation using living unrelated donors have been most satisfactory, with initial and long-term survival rates the same as for partial HLA-matched family donors and better than for partially matched cadaveric donors (Table 272-2).

Table 272-2

Effect of HLA-A, B, DR Mismatching on Kidney Graft Survival*

Donor Mismatches	Half-Life of Graft Survival, years	10-Year Graft Survival, %
Living related donor		
(HLA-identical sib = no mismatches)	24.0	74
Cadaver (no mismatches for 6 antigens)	20.3	65
Living related donor		
(1 haplotype = 3 mismatches)	12.0	54
Living unrelated donor		
(average 4 mismatches)	12.0	54
Cadaver (overall)	9.0	40
Cadaver (1 or 2 mismatches)	10.4	45
Cadaver (3 or 4 mismatches)	8.4	38
Cadaver (5 or 6 mismatches)	7.7	34

* HLA antigens are codominantly inherited: each person has two A, two B, and two DR antigens, for a total of six.

Concern has been expressed regarding the potential risk to a volunteer kidney donor of premature renal failure after several years of increased blood flow and hyperfiltration per nephron in the remaining kidney. There are a few reports of the development of hypertension, proteinuria, and even lesions of focal segmental sclerosis in donors under long-term follow-up. Difficulties in donors followed for 20 or more years are unusual, however, and it may be that having a single kidney becomes significant only when another condition, such as hypertension, is superimposed. It is also desirable to consider the risk of development of type 1 diabetes mellitus in a family member who is a potential donor to a diabetic renal failure patient. Anti-insulin and anti-islet antibodies should be measured, and glucose tolerance tests should be performed in such donors to rule out a prediabetic state.

HLA Matching and Cadaveric Donors The question of whether matching of HLA antigens in unrelated donor-recipient pairs would approximate the high initial success rates and slow rates of subsequent graft loss with HLA-identical sib pairs could not be answered until the late 1980s when reliable class II histocompatibility (DR) typing became widely available. Now that pooled data on tens of thousands of cadaveric renal transplants from all over the world are available, the HLA-matching effect can be clearly seen, especially in the long-term $t_{1/2}$ half-life survival figures. It is shown in Fig. 272-3 that there is an overall beneficial effect of HLA matching in first cadaveric grafts. When compared with HLA-identical transplants, where the 1-year graft survival rate is 95 percent and the subsequent half-life is 25 years, one-HLA-haplotype–matched family donor transplants have 1-year survival rates of 85 percent with a 12-year half-life (Table 272-2). With increasing numbers of mismatches for cadaveric donors, the half-life decreases from 20 to 7.7 years. The survival rates at the 10-year mark are projected to range from 65 (zero mismatches) to 34 percent (six mismatches). Many centers now report 1-year graft survival rates in the 85 to 90 percent range for all renal transplants, possibly the result of heavy initial immunosuppression, but the subsequent half-lives are similar to those above. There is controversy regarding the value of cadaveric organ-sharing rules that are based entirely upon the numbers of HLA mismatches. Avoidance of mismatching for six antigens (Table 272-2) is a top priority in the United States, however, and 20 percent of kidneys are transplanted on this basis. Table 272-2 also shows the interaction of HLA matching and graft ischemia on results; namely, kidneys from HLA-incompatible spousal donors do better than those from similarly mismatched cadaver donors, suggesting that the additional ischemic injury of organ storage is important. When such a cadaveric donor is HLA-compatible, however, ischemia and storage do not impede the matching benefit.

Presensitization A positive cross match of recipient serum with donor T lymphocytes representing anti-HLA class I is usually predictive of an acute vasculitic event termed *hyperacute rejection*. Patients with anti-HLA antibodies can be safely transplanted if careful cross matching is performed. Patients sustained by dialysis often show fluctuating antibody titers and specificity patterns. At the time of assignment of a cadaveric kidney, cross matches are performed with more than one highly reactive serum, and the previously analyzed antibody specificities are also taken into account. Techniques for cross matching are not universally standardized; however, at least two techniques are employed in most laboratories. The minimal criterion for the cross match is avoidance of hyperacute rejection mediated by recipient antibodies to donor HLA class I antigens. Sensitive tests, such as the use of flow cytometry, can be useful for avoidance of accelerated, and often untreatable, early graft rejection in patients receiving second or third transplants. Donor T lymphocytes, which express only class I antigens, are used as targets for detection of anti-class I (HLA-A and -B) antibodies. Anti-class II (HLA-DR) antibodies do not contraindicate transplantation, unless present in high titer. B lymphocytes, expressing both class I and class II antigens are used in these assays. Non-HLA antigens restricted in expression to endothelium and sometimes monocytes have been described, but clinical relevance is not well established.

Blood Transfusions Exposure to leukocyte HLA antigens during transfusions was a major cause of sensitization that limited transplantation access and increased the risk of early graft rejection. In the 1970s, attempts to avoid all blood exposure in dialysed patients paradoxically increased the risk of graft rejection. The beneficial "transfusion effect" was never fully explained, and it almost disappeared in the 1980s as overall management of patients improved with the use of cyclosporine and more effective means of rejection treatment. Currently, with the use of erythropoietin the need for transfusion is much reduced. It has been noted, however, that nontransfused patients do have more rejection activity. Ongoing studies with HLA-typed blood donors indicate that transfusions are beneficial only when they are not completely mismatched for HLA, and in particular when there is one DR and one B antigen matched with the recipient.

IMMUNOLOGY OF REJECTION Knowledge of the immunology of tissue transplantation stems largely from animal experimentation. However, enough evidence has accumulated in humans to indicate that the mechanisms are similar, and not qualitatively different from those found in other areas of immunology (Chap. 305). Early

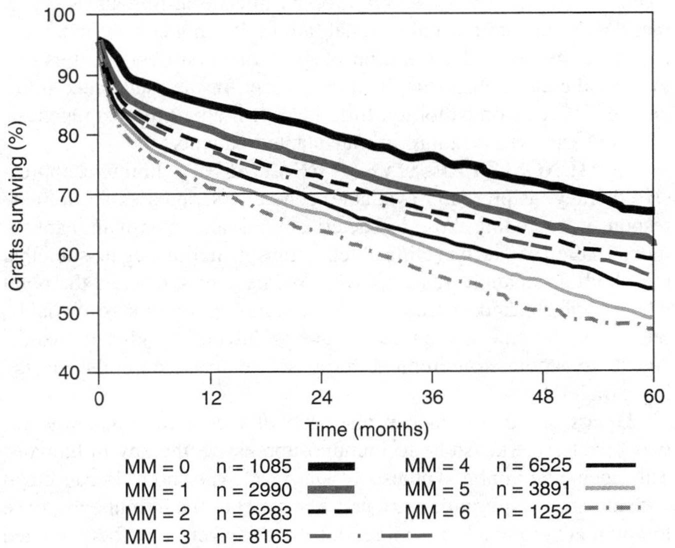

FIGURE 272-3 Survival of over 30,000 first cadaveric renal transplants over 5 years after transplantation. The transplants were performed in more than 200 centers around the world between 1982 and 1989. Cyclosporine was used in virtually all cases. The curves for each HLA matching grade are shown, according to the number of mismatches (MM) for HLA-A, -B, and -DR antigens. Since each individual has two genes for each locus, there is a potential for up to six mismatches. The overall effect of matching in this international Collaborative Transplant Study stratifies according to the mismatch grade (weighted regression, $p < 0.0001$) *(From Opelz.)*

rejection is associated with T lymphocytes having direct specificity against donor antigens. These may be cytotoxic cells (CD8+ or CD4+) or cells that mediate delayed hypersensitivity (CD4+); however, significant numbers of B lymphocytes, null cells, natural killer cells, and macrophages appear in the early infiltrate, and cells capable of mediating antibody-dependent cell-mediated cytotoxicity are also present (Fig. 272-4). Many of the B lymphocytes produce immunoglobulins. The spectrum of cellular and humoral response and graft injury is quite varied, depending on specific genetic differences between donor and recipient and states of presensitization. The greater the degree of presensitization, the more likely it is that one will find antibody-mediated vascular lesions. All the processes shown in Fig. 272-4 are possible, but their relative contribution varies from case to case. Monitoring of peripheral blood lymphocyte subsets utilizing monoclonal antibodies to functionally related surface molecules, such as CD4 (T helper cells) and CD8 (T suppressor/cytotoxic cells), has been related to the degree of rejection activity in some surveys. Since the principal role of the CD4 molecule is to promote interaction of T cells with class II HLA molecules on antigen-presenting cells, and similarly, CD8 interacts with class I HLA (see Chap. 305), it is not surprising that both types of T cells are usually present. Finally, the cytokine mediators of the cellular immune response [IL-1 to IL-4, IL-6, IL-10, IL-12, tumor necrosis factor (TNF), and interferon γ] are involved in the control and expression of the alloimmune rejection response. For example, T cell production of interferon γ causes increased expression of HLA antigens on endothelial cells. In normal immunobiology this effect may be to promote more efficient presentation of foreign antigen, while in transplantation it enhances the immunogenicity of the vascularized transplant. Also, IL-2, the major growth factor for expansion of effector T cells, is the product of a major subset of CD4 cells (Th1), while other CD4 cells (Th2) produce B cell growth factors, such as IL-4.

The failure of transplanted kidneys after several years of adequate function is said to be due to "chronic rejection." In such kidneys, the development of nephrosclerosis, with proliferation of the vascular intima of renal vessels, and intimal fibrosis, with marked decrease in the lumen of the vessels, takes place (Fig. 272-5). The result is renal ischemia, hypertension, tubular atrophy, interstitial fibrosis, and glomerular atrophy with eventual renal failure. It is not established, however, whether slow deterioration of graft function over years is due to the same mechanisms in all cases. Except for the established influence of HLA incompatibility, little is known about the pathogenesis of progressive renal failure in transplanted patients.

IMMUNOSUPPRESSIVE TREATMENT Immunosuppressive therapy, as presently available, generally suppresses all immune responses, including those to bacteria, fungi, and even malignant tumors. In the 1950s when clinical renal transplantation began, sublethal total-body irradiation was employed. We have now reached the point where sophisticated pharmacologic immunosuppression is available, but it still has the hazard of promoting infection and malignancy. Agents to suppress the immune response are discussed in the following paragraphs.

Drugs *Azathioprine*, an analogue of mercaptopurine, was for two decades the keystone to immunosuppressive therapy in humans. This agent can inhibit synthesis of DNA, RNA, or both. Because cell division and proliferation are a necessary part of the immune response to antigenic stimulation, suppression by this agent may be mediated by the inhibition of mitosis of immunologically competent lymphoid cells, interfering with synthesis of DNA. Alternatively, immunosuppression may be brought about by blocking the synthesis of RNA (possibly messenger RNA), inhibiting processing of antigens prior to lymphocyte stimulation. This drug has little effect in suppressing a secondary immune response, however. Therapy with azathioprine in doses of 1.5 to 2.0 mg/kg per day is generally added to cyclosporine as a means of decreasing the requirements for the latter. Because azathioprine is rapidly metabolized by the liver, its dosage need not

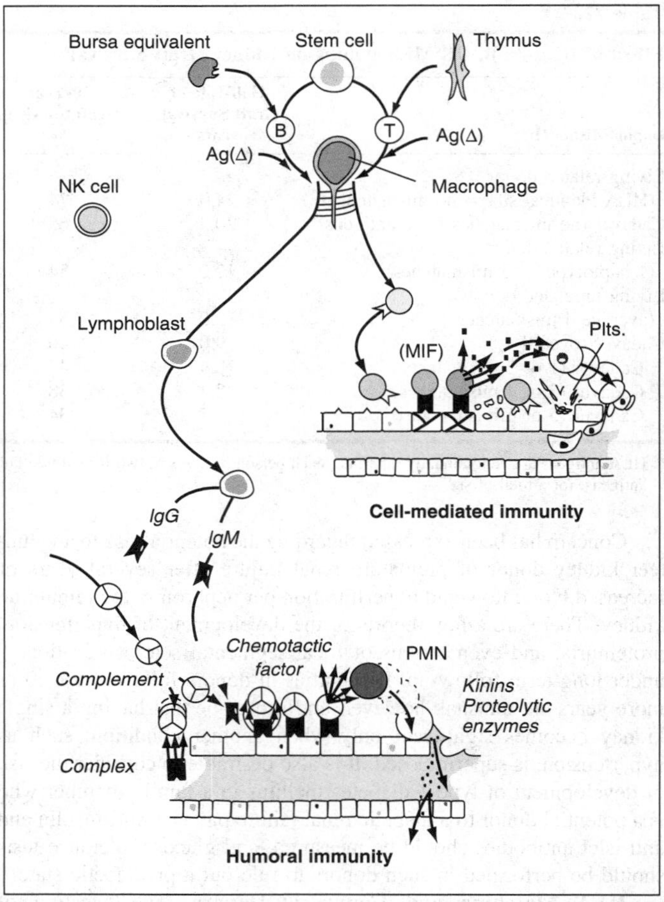

FIGURE 272-4 Overall scheme of the development of effector mechanisms in graft rejection. A set of bone marrow precursor stem cells is selected in the thymus gland to become mature thymus-derived (T) lymphocytes which are clonally determined to recognize non-self antigens (Δ) presented as fragments bound to self major histocompatibility molecules. These antigen-presenting structures are on the surfaces of macrophages, dendritic cells, and B lymphocytes. In transplantation, major histocompatibility antigens, such as HLA, may be recognized directly as the antigen-presenting molecules present in the grafted tissues or as fragments of donor HLA presented by recipient antigen-presenting cells. In avian species, but not in mammals, an anatomic site called the *bursa of Fabricius* provides the differentiating stimuli for maturation of B lymphocytes from bone marrow precursors. B lymphocytes with immunoglobulin receptors for a given antigen (Δ) proliferate and differentiate by a process of somatic mutation of immunoglobulin genes and selection by antigen for further growth. They begin to secrete IgM and, subsequently, IgG, IgE, and IgA. The response matures with help from T lymphocytes, which includes elaboration of the cytokines IL-4, IL-5, and IL-2. The proliferative phases of T and B lymphocyte response are illustrated by the lymphoblast.

Humoral immunity produces tissue injury following binding of immunoglobulins to tissue and, in particular, to the endothelium of a transplanted organ. Complement activation and chemotaxis of polymorphonuclear cells (PMN) are common in "hyperacute" rejection lesions when recipients have antidonor antibodies. Cell-mediated immunity is principally mediated by T lymphocytes bearing receptors for tissue antigens. These cells receive a major degree of help initially from macrophages that secrete the cytokines IL-6 and IL-1. Expanded populations of graft-specific T lymphocytes exert tissue damage by a delayed type hypersensitivity mechanism or by direct cytotoxic "killer" mechanisms. As noted in text, the T lymphocyte CD4 or CD8 phenotypes indicate whether the target antigens are HLA class II or class I, respectively.

The principal growth factor for T lymphocytes is an autocrine product, IL-2. Other T cell products include cytokines, such as interferon γ and tumor necrosis factor, which increase the pace of tissue injury. Activated macrophages can add nonspecifically to the inflammatory process. Natural killer cells (NK) play a minor role; however, they, along with other cells that bear receptors for the Fc portion of immunoglobulin, can provide cell-mediated target damage after fixation to IgG molecules previously bound to grafted cells (antibody-dependent cell-mediated cytotoxicity). Any of these mechanisms can result in vascular occlusion by platelet aggregation and thrombosis.

be varied directly in relation to renal function, even though renal failure results in retention of the metabolites of azathioprine. Some patients are unusually sensitive to this drug, particularly when renal function is compromised, and reduction in dosage is required because of leukopenia and occasionally thrombocytopenia. Excessive amounts of azathioprine also may cause jaundice, anemia, and alopecia. If it is essential to administer allopurinol concurrently, the azathioprine dose must be reduced, since inhibition of xanthine oxidase delays degradation. This combination is best avoided.

Mycophenolate mofetil is now used in place of azathioprine in many centers. It has a similar mode of action and a mild degree of gastrointestinal toxicity but produces minimal bone marrow suppression. Its advantage is its increased potency in preventing or reversing rejection.

Glucocorticoids are important adjuncts to immunosuppressive therapy. Of all the agents employed, prednisone has effects that are easiest to assess, and in large doses it is effective for the reversal of rejection. In general, 200 to 300 mg prednisone is given immediately prior to or at the time of transplantation, and the dosage is reduced to 30 mg within a week. The side effects of the glucocorticoids, particularly impairment of wound healing and predisposition to infection, make it desirable to taper the dose as rapidly as possible in the immediate postoperative period. Customarily, methylprednisolone, 0.5 to 1.0 g intravenously, is administered immediately upon diagnosis of beginning rejection and continued once daily for 3 days. When the drug is effective, the results are usually apparent within 96 h. Such "pulse" doses are not effective in chronic rejection. Most patients whose renal function is stable after 6 months or a year do not require large doses of prednisone; maintenance doses of 10 to 15 mg/d are the rule. Many patients tolerate an alternate-day course of steroids without an increased risk of rejection.

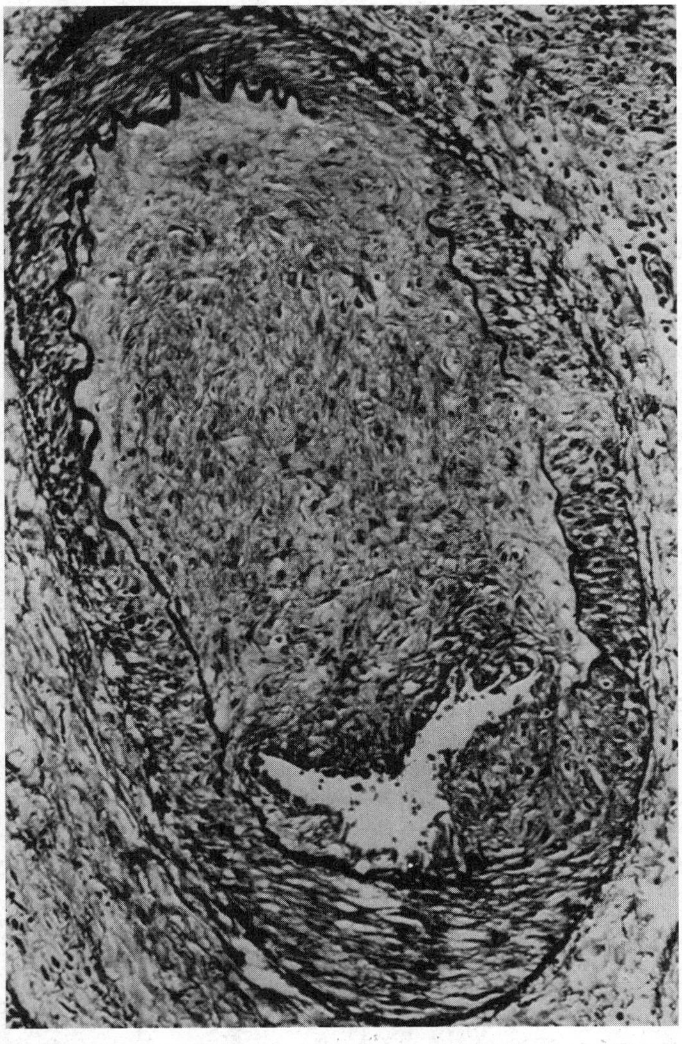

FIGURE 272-5 Biopsy of the renal cadaveric allograft illustrating obliterative endarteritis. Loss of the media is associated with intimal thickening. The elastic tissue shows dissolution of the elastica. The evidence for arteritis with subsequent thrombosis is typically the gaps in the elastica and media. The intimal thickening probably represents organization of a thrombus formed in response to the arteritis. *[From GJ Dammin, JP Merrill, in Structural Basis for Renal Disease, EL Becker (ed), New York, Hoeber-Harper, 1968.]*

A major effect of steroids is on the monocyte-macrophage system, preventing the release of IL-6 and IL-1. Lymphopenia after large doses of glucocorticoids is primarily due to sequestration of recirculating blood lymphocytes to lymphoid tissue.

Cyclosporine is a fungal peptide with potent immunosuppressive activity. It acts to block transcription of mRNA for IL-2 and other proinflammatory cytokines, thereby inhibiting T cell proliferation. Although it works alone, cyclosporine is more effective in conjunction with glucocorticoids. Since cyclosporine blocks production of IL-2 by T cells, its combination with steroids is expected to produce a double block in the macrophage → IL-6/IL-1 → T cell → IL-2 sequence. As noted, clinical results with tens of thousands of renal transplants have been impressive. Of its toxic effects (nephrotoxicity, hepatoxicity, hirsutism, tremor, gingival hyperplasia, diabetes), only nephrotoxicity presents a serious management problem and is further discussed below.

Tacrolimus (FK-506) is a fungal macrolide that has the same mode of action, and a similar side effect profile, as cyclosporine. De novo induction of diabetes mellitus is more common with tacrolimus. The drug is most useful in liver transplantation, for which it has received approval from the Food and Drug Administration, and may be tried as an alternative in renal patients whose rejections are poorly controlled by cyclosporine.

Sirolimus (previously called rapamycin) is another fungal macrolide, but has a different mode of action: namely, it inhibits T cell growth factor pathways, preventing the response to IL-2 and other cytokines. It shows some promise in clinical trials in combination with cyclosporine.

Antibodies to Lymphocytes When serum from animals made immune to host lymphocytes is injected into the recipient, a marked suppression of cellular immunity to the tissue graft results. The action on cell-mediated immunity is greater than on humoral immunity. A globulin fraction of serum [antilymphocyte globulin (ALG)] is the agent generally employed. For use in humans, peripheral human lymphocytes, thymocytes, or lymphocytes from spleens or thoracic duct fistulas have been injected into horses, rabbits, or goats to produce antilymphocyte serum, from which the globulin fraction is then separated. Although ALG or antithymocyte globulin (ATG) is unquestionably effective in prolonging grafts in animals, its efficacy in the transplantation of human tissue is less clear, since it varies from source to source. Heterologous antibody against defined T lymphocyte subsets, in the form of mouse antihuman monoclonal antibody, offers a more precise and standardized form of therapy. OKT3, at present, is the only such antibody in clinical use. It is directed to the CD3 molecules that form a portion of the T cell antigen-receptor complex; hence CD3 is expressed on all mature T cells. CD4 or CD8 molecules also form part of the fully activated cluster of molecules, and monoclonal antibodies to these offer the potential for more selective targeting of T cell subsets. Another approach to more selective therapy is to target the 55-kDa beta chain or the 70-kDa alpha chain of the IL-2 receptor, expressed only on T cells that have been recently activated. The problem with such mouse antibodies is the potential for developing human antimouse antibodies (HAMA), an event that limits the effective period of use. Clinical trials of genetically engineered "humanized" monoclonal antibodies are in progress. This approach offers the possibility of improved clearance and destruction of the targeted lymphocytes and reduced potential for development of HAMA.

CLINICAL COURSE AND MANAGEMENT OF THE RECIPIENT Bilateral nephrectomy at some point prior to transplantation is performed for a specific cause but not as a routine. Hypertension that is difficult to control or infection involving the end-stage kidneys are the two most common indications. Nephrectomized patients maintain a much lower hematocrit, but this is no longer considered a disadvantage because of the availability of recombinant erythropoietin. Nephrectomy per se does not appear to affect the survival of subsequent renal allografts.

Adequate hemodialysis should be performed within 48 h of surgery, and care should be taken that the serum potassium level is not markedly elevated so that intraoperative cardiac arrhythmias can be averted. The diuresis that commonly occurs postoperatively must be carefully monitored; in some instances it may be massive, reflecting the inability of ischemic tubules to regulate sodium and water excretion; with large diureses, massive potassium losses may occur. Most chronically uremic patients have some excess of extracellular fluid, and it is useful to maintain an expanded fluid volume in the immediate postoperative period. Acute tubular necrosis (ATN) may cause immediate oliguria or may follow an initial short period of graft function. ATN is most likely when cadaveric donors have been hypotensive or if the interval between cessation of blood flow and organ harvest (warm ischemic time) is more than a few minutes. Recovery usually occurs within 3 weeks, although periods as long as 6 weeks have been reported. Superimposition of rejection on ATN is common, and the differential diagnosis may be difficult without a graft biopsy. Cyclosporine therapy prolongs ATN, and some patients do not diurese until the dose is drastically reduced. Many centers avoid starting cyclosporine for the first several days, using ALG or a monoclonal antibody along with azathioprine and prednisone until renal function is established.

The Rejection Episode Early diagnosis of rejection allows prompt institution of therapy to preserve renal function and prevent irreversible damage. Clinical evidence of rejection is rarely characterized by fever, swelling, and tenderness over the allograft. Rejection may present only with a rise in serum creatinine, with or without a reduction in urine volume. The focus should be on ruling out other causes of functional deterioration.

Arteriography and radioactive iodohippurate sodium renograms of the transplanted kidney may be useful in ascertaining changes in the renal vasculature and in renal blood flow, even in the absence of urinary flow. Diagnostic ultrasound is the procedure of choice to rule out urinary obstruction or to confirm the presence of perirenal collections of urine, blood, or lymph. When renal function has been good initially, a rise in the serum creatinine level is the most sensitive and reliable indicator of possible rejection and may be the only sign.

Cyclosporine may cause deterioration in renal function in a manner similar to a rejection episode. In fact, rejection processes tend to be more indolent with cyclosporine, and the only way to make a diagnosis may be by renal biopsy. Cyclosporine has an afferent arteriolar constrictor effect on the kidney and, in addition, may produce permanent vascular and interstitial injury after sustained high-dose therapy. There is no universally accepted lesion(s) that makes a diagnosis of cyclosporine toxicity, although interstitial fibrosis, isometric tubular vacuolization, and thickening of arteriolar walls have been noted by some. Basically, if the biopsy does not reveal moderate and active cellular rejection activity, the serum creatinine will most likely respond to a reduction in cyclosporine dose. Blood levels of drug can be useful if very high or very low but do not correlate precisely with renal function. If rejection activity is present in the biopsy, appropriate therapy is indicated. The first rejection episode is usually treated with intravenous administration of methylprednisolone, 500 to 1000 mg daily for 3 days. Failure to respond is indication for antibody therapy, usually with OKT3.

OKT3 monoclonal antibody, given intravenously for 10 to 14 days, is effective in more than 90 percent of first rejections, and less so if methylprednisolone pulses have failed and in cases of severe recurrent rejection activity. A major problem with OKT3 is that severe systemic reactions may be produced during the first day or two of therapy. Chills, fever, hypotension, and headache are the direct result of the antibody effects on the targeted T cells, most likely related to the known potential of OKT3 to activate T cells nonspecifically. If the antibody is administered to overhydrated oliguric patients, pulmonary edema may be induced. These reactions are not characteristic of other monoclonal antibodies, such as those to the IL-2 receptor. Recurrent or rebound rejection activity may require additional therapy. In such circumstances, methylprednisolone may be effective even though it failed initially. Second courses of OKT3 may be given in spite of HAMA generated in response to the first course if the titers are low and the human antibodies are not directed to the combining-site region (idiotype) of the OKT3.

Management Problems The usual clinical manifestations of infection in the posttransplant period are blunted by immunosuppressive therapy. The major toxic effect of azathioprine is bone marrow suppression, while cyclosporine has no marrow effects. They both may predispose to unusual opportunistic infections, however. The signs and symptoms of infection may be masked and distorted, and fever without obvious cause is common. Only after days or weeks will it become apparent that it has a viral or fungal origin. Bacterial infections are most common during the first month after transplantation. The importance of blood cultures in such patients cannot be overemphasized, because systemic infection without obvious foci is frequent, although wound infections with or without urinary fistulas are most common. Particularly ominous are rapidly occurring pulmonary lesions, which may result in death within 5 days of onset. When these become apparent, immunosuppressive agents should be discontinued, except for maintenance doses of prednisone. Aggressive diagnostic procedures, including transbronchial and open lung biopsy, are frequently indicated. In the case of *Pneumocystis carinii* (Chap. 211) infection, trimethoprim-sulfamethoxazole is the treatment of choice; amphotericin B has been used effectively in systemic fungal infections. Prophylaxis against *P. carinii* with daily, or alternate day, low-dose trimethoprim-sulfamethoxazole is very effective. Involvement of the oropharynx with *Candida* (Chap. 207) may be treated with local nystatin. Small doses (a total of 300 mg) of amphotericin given over a period of 2 weeks may be effective in refractory oral candidiasis. *Aspergillus* (Chap. 208), *Nocardia* (Chap. 167), and CMV (Chap. 187) infections also occur.

CMV is a common and dangerous infection in transplant recipients. It does not generally appear until the end of the first posttransplant month. Active CMV infection is sometimes associated, or occasionally confused, with rejection episodes. Patients at highest risk for severe CMV disease are those without anti-CMV antibodies who receive a graft from a CMV antibody–positive donor (15 percent mortality). Serial intravenous administration of high-titer CMV immune globulin is effective in reducing this risk. Prophylactic use of ganciclovir is an effective alternative. Treatment of active CMV disease with ganciclovir is always indicated. Many patients immune to CMV can activate the virus after heavy immunosuppression, such as with OKT3. Concurrent treatment with ganciclovir during OKT3 administration appears to be effective for prophylaxis of CMV activation. The complications of glucocorticoid therapy are well known and include gastrointestinal bleeding, impairment of wound healing, osteoporosis, diabetes mellitus, cataract formation, and hemorrhagic pancreatitis. The treatment of unexplained jaundice in transplant patients should include cessation of azathioprine or cyclosporine if hepatitis or drug toxicity is suspected. It is surprising that cessation of azathioprine or cyclosporine therapy in such circumstances often does not result in rejection of a graft, at least for several weeks. Antiplatelet agents and anticoagulants, although effective in theory, have not been successful in the prevention of the chronic vascular lesion. Persistent elevation of serum creatinine levels above 220 μmol/L (2.5 mg/dL) in patients on cyclosporine is an indication for dose reduction, particularly if cyclosporine blood levels are elevated. Some centers convert patients from cyclosporine to azathioprine after 6 to 12 months, but some patients have rejection episodes, and some of those lose their grafts. The alternative to conversion is to use lower doses of cyclosporine indefinitely. The risk of long-term cumulative toxicity to the kidney now seems to be low.

In general, minimal or no rejection during the first 6 months after transplantation is a predictor of safety in reducing immunosuppression therapy over subsequent months to years.

Despite the potential teratogenic effects of immunosuppressive agents, both women and men have become parents after transplantation. The incidence of congenital abnormalities in the offspring is not increased.

Glomerular Lesions Glomerular lesions occur in 10 to 15 percent of allografts, even when the original disease was accidental removal of a solitary kidney. The pathogenesis is related to a chronic rejection process. In some cases the lesions resemble those of the original glomerular disease. In most instances, the recurrence of the original renal lesions represents no threat to the immediate prognosis, and a primary diagnosis of glomerulonephritis is rarely a contraindication to transplantation.

Malignancy The incidence of tumors in patients on immunosuppressive therapy is 5 to 6 percent, or approximately 100 times greater than that in the general population of the same age range. The most common lesions are cancer of the skin and lips and carcinoma in situ of the cervix, as well as lymphomas, such as non-Hodgkin's lymphomas. The risks are increased in proportion to the total immunosuppressive load administered and time elapsed since transplantation.

Other Complications *Hypercalcemia* after transplantation may indicate failure of hyperplastic parathyroid glands to regress. Aseptic necrosis of the head of the femur is probably due to preexisting hyperparathyroidism, with aggravation by glucocorticoid treatment. With improved management of calcium and phosphorus metabolism during chronic dialysis, the incidence of parathyroid-related complications has fallen dramatically.

Hypertension may be caused by (1) native kidneys; (2) rejection activity in the transplant; (3) renal artery stenosis, if an end-to-end anastomosis was constructed with an iliac artery branch; and (4) renal cyclosporine toxicity. The latter may improve with reduction in cyclosporine dose. Whereas angiotensin-converting enzyme inhibitors may be useful, calcium channel blockers are frequently more effective in cyclosporine-treated patients.

Chronic hepatitis, particularly when due to hepatitis B virus, can be a progressive, fatal disease over a decade or so. Patients who are persistently HBsAg-positive are at higher risk, according to some studies, but the presence of HCV is also a concern when one embarks on a course of immunosuppression in a transplant recipient.

Both chronic dialysis and renal transplant patients have a higher incidence of death from myocardial infarction and stroke than in the population at large, and this is particularly true in diabetic patients. Contributing factors are hypertension and hypertriglyceridemia. Increased low-density lipoprotein cholesterol and depressed high-density lipoprotein cholesterol concentrations may be exaggerated after transplantation and require treatment.

BIBLIOGRAPHY

Carpenter CB: Long-term failure of renal transplants: Adding insult to injury. Kidney Int 48(suppl 50):40, 1995

Daugirdas JT: Dialysis hypotension: A hemodynamic analysis. Kidney Int 39:233, 1991

Depner TA: Assessing adequacy of hemodialysis: Urea modeling. Kidney Int 45:1522, 1994

Institute of Medicine Special Report: The Medicare end-stage renal disease program. N Engl J Med 324:1143, 1991

Keane WF et al: Peritoneal dialysis–related peritonitis treatment recommendations, 1993 update. Perit Dial Int 13:14, 1993

McKay DB et al: Clinical aspects of renal transplantation, in *The Kidney*, 5th ed, B Brenner (ed). Philadelphia, Saunders, 1996, p 2602

Mehta RL: Therapeutic alternatives in renal replacement for critically ill patients in acute renal failure. Semin Nephrol 14:64, 1994

Opelz G: HLA matching should be utilized for improving kidney transplant success rates. Transplant Proc 23:46, 1991

Owen WF Jr et al: The urea reduction ratio and serum albumin concentration as predictors of mortality in patients undergoing hemodialysis. N Engl J Med 329:1001, 1993

Perkins DL, Carpenter CB: Immunobiology of transplantation, in *The Kidney*, 5th ed, B Brenner (ed). Philadelphia, Saunders, 1996, p 2576

Sprague SM, Popovtzer MM: Is β_2-microglobulin a mediator of bone disease? Kidney Int 47:1, 1995

Teehan B et al: Adequacy of continuous ambulatory peritoneal dialysis: Morbidity and mortality in chronic peritoneal dialysis. Am J Kidney Dis 24:990, 1994

Terasaki PI, Cecka JM (eds): *Clinical Transplants 1994*. Los Angeles, UCLA Tissue Typing Laboratory, 1995

273

Hugh R. Brady, Barry M. Brenner

PATHOGENETIC MECHANISMS OF GLOMERULAR INJURY

The glomerulus is a modified capillary network that delivers an ultrafiltrate of plasma to Bowman's space, the most proximal portion of the renal tubule. Approximately 1.6 million glomeruli are present in two mature kidneys (range 0.5 to 2.4 million) and collectively produce 120 to 180 L of ultrafiltrate daily. Glomerular filtration rate (GFR) is dependent on glomerular blood flow, ultrafiltration pressure, and surface area. These parameters are tightly regulated through changes in afferent and efferent arteriolar tone (for blood flow and ultrafiltration pressure) and mesangial cell contractility (for filtration surface area). Arteriolar tone and mesangial cell contractility are, in turn, modulated by neurohumoral factors, local myenteric reflexes, and endothelium-derived vasoactive substances, such as nitric oxide, prostacyclin, and endothelins. In health, glomerular endothelium is also antithrombotic and antiadhesive for leukocytes and platelets, thereby preventing inappropriate vascular thrombosis and inflammation during the filtration process. Filtration of most plasma proteins and all blood cells is normally prevented as a consequence of the physiochemical and electrostatic charge characteristics of the glomerular filtration barrier, the latter composed of fenestrated glomerular endothelium, basement membrane, and the foot processes and slit diaphragms of visceral epithelial cells (podocytes). Parietal epithelium facilitates glomerular filtration by maintaining the integrity of Bowman's space. In keeping with the physiologic functions of the glomerulus outlined above, virtually all glomerular injury results in impairment of glomerular filtration or the inappropriate appearance of plasma proteins and blood cells in the urine.

CLINICOPATHOLOGIC CORRELATES IN GLOMERULAR DISEASE

The major glomerulopathies are described in Chap. 274, and major morphologic patterns of glomerular disease and their clinical features are summarized in Table 273-1. These clinicopathologic entities can be induced by a variety of different pathogenetic mechanisms. Thus, prompt diagnosis, optimal management, and accurate prognostication is a three-step process that requires (1) recognition of the presenting clinical syndrome, (2) delineation of the underlying morphologic pattern of glomerular injury, and (3) elucidation of the specific renal-limited or systemic disease that triggered glomerular dysfunction.

NOMENCLATURE The terms *glomerulonephritis* and *glomerulopathy* are usually used interchangeably to denote glomerular injury, although some authorities reserve the former term for injury with evidence of inflammation such as leukocyte infiltration, antibody deposition, and complement activation. Glomerular diseases are classified as *primary* when the pathology is confined to the kidney and any systemic features are a direct consequence of glomerular dysfunction (e.g., pulmonary edema, hypertension, the uremic syndrome). Usually, but not always, the term primary is synonymous with *idiopathic*. Glomerular diseases are classified as *secondary* when part of a multisystem disorder. In general, *acute* refers to glomerular injury occurring

Table 273-1

Major Clinicopathologic Presentation of Glomerular Disease

Structural Pattern	Typical Clinical Presentation	Typical Pathology Findings	Most Common Etiologies*
Diffuse proliferative GN	Acute nephritic syndrome: Acute renal failure over days to weeks, hypertension, edema, oliguria, active urine sediment, subnephrotic proteinuria	Diffuse increase in cellularity of tufts of most glomeruli due to infiltration by neutrophils and monocytes, and proliferation of glomerular endothelial and mesangial cells.	Immune complex GN: idiopathic, postinfectious, SLE, SBE, cryoglobulinemia, Henoch-Schönlein purpura Pauci-immune GN and anti-GBM disease (crescentic GN common—see below)
Crescentic GN	Rapidly progressive glomerulonephritis (RPGN): Subacute renal failure over weeks to months, active urine sediment, variable amount of hypertension, edema, oliguria, and proteinuria	Majority of glomeruli contain areas of fibrinoid necrosis and crescents in Bowman's space, composed of proliferating parietal epithelial cells, infiltrating macrophages, and fibrin	Immune complex GN (as above) Pauci-immune GN: Wegener's granulomatosis, microscopic polyarteritis nodosa, renal-limited crescentic GN Anti-GBM disease (Goodpasture's syndrome if lung hemorrhage)
Focal proliferative GN	Mild to moderate glomerular inflammation: Active urine sediment and mild to moderate decline in GFR	Segmental areas of proliferation and necrosis in less than 50% of glomeruli, occasionally with crescent formation	Early and milder forms, or recovery phase of most diseases causing diffuse proliferative and crescentic GN IgA nephropathy/HSP
Mesangial proliferative GN	Chronic glomerular inflammation: Proteinuria, hematuria, hypertension, variable effect on GFR	Proliferation of mesangial cells and matrix	IgA nephropathy/HSP Early and milder forms, or recovery phases of most diseases causing diffuse proliferative and crescentic GN In association with minimal change glomerulopathy and FSGS
Membranoproliferative GN	Variable combination of nephritic and nephrotic features: Acute or subacute decline in GFR, active urine sediment, proteinuria often in nephrotic range	Diffuse proliferation of mesangial cells and infiltration of glomeruli by macrophages; increased mesangial matrix and thickening and reduplication of glomerular basement membrane	Immune complex GN (as for diffuse proliferative GN) In association with thrombotic microangiopathies (see below) In association with deposition diseases (see below) Postrenal or -marrow transplantation
Minimal change GN	Nephrotic syndrome: Proteinuria of >3–3.5 g/d, hypoalbuminemia, edema, hyperlipidemia, lipiduria, thrombotic diathesis, slow decline in GFR in 10–30%.	Light microscopy normal, but electron microscopy (EM) shows foot process effacement	Idiopathic In association with drug-induced interstitial nephritis, HIV infection, heroin, Hodgkin's and other lymphomas
Focal segmental glomerulosclerosis	Nephrotic syndrome: Proteinuria of >3–3.5 g/d, hypoalbuminemia, edema, hyperlipidemia, lipiduria, thrombotic diathesis, slow decline in GFR in 10–30%.	Segmental capillary collapse affecting <50% of glomeruli with entrapment of amorphous hyaline material. EM shows foot process effacement	Primary FSGS: idiopathic, HIV, heroin, lysosomal diseases, Charcot-Marie Tooth Secondary response to reduction in nephron number from any cause (hyperfiltration injury)
Nodular or global sclerosis	Proteinuria and chronic renal failure	Sclerosis of most glomeruli with interstitial fibrosis	Diabetic nephropathy Potential long-term consequence of most glomerulopathies listed above
Membranous GN	Nephrotic syndrome: Proteinuria of >3–3.5 g/d, hypoalbuminemia, edema, hyperlipidemia, lipiduria, thrombotic diathesis, slow decline in GFR in 10–30%	Diffuse thickening of the glomerular basement membrane with subepithelial projections ("spikes") around immune deposits	Idiopathic Infections (e.g., Hepatitis B & C, syphilis, schistasomiasis, malaria, leprosy) Drugs (e.g., gold, penicillamine, captopril) Autoimmune diseases (SLE, rheumatoid arthritis) Paraneoplastic
Deposition diseases	Combination of nephritic and nephrotic features: Renal failure over months to years, proteinuria, hematuria, and hypertension.	Mesangial expansion and thickening of glomerular capillary wall; variable cellular proliferation and crescent formation	Amyloid Cryoglobulinemia Light chain deposition disease Fibrillary/immunotactoid GN
Thrombotic microangiopathy	Acute or subacute renal failure: Variable degree of hypertension, edema and proteinuria, urine sediment usually contains red blood cells, but less activity than patients with nephritic syndrome or RPGN	Microthrombi in glomerular capillaries ± endothelial injury	Idiopathic In association with gastrointestinal infections, or drugs such as anovulants, mitomycin C Other diseases: SLE, scleroderma, toxemia, malignant hypertension
Nonimmune basement membrane abnormalities	Asymptomatic hematuria and variable renal failure	Alport's syndrome—mesangial hypercellularity with focal sclerosis and interstitial fibrosis; splintering of GBM on EM.	Alport's syndrome, Thin basement membrane disease, Nail patella syndrome, Lecithin–cholesterol acyltransferase deficiency

* Includes most common etiologies: For complete list, see Chap. 274.

NOTE: Diffuse, affecting ≥50% of glomeruli; focal, affecting <50% of glomeruli; global, affecting ≥50% of glomerular tuft; segmental, affecting <50% of glomerular tuft; GN, glomerulonephritis; FSGS, focal segmental glomerulosclerosis; HSP, Henoch-Schönlein purpura; SLE, systemic lupus erythematosus; HIV, human immunodeficiency virus; SBE, subacute bacterial endocarditis.

over days or weeks, *subacute* or *rapidly progressive* over weeks or a few months, and *chronic* over many months or years. Lesions are classified as *focal* or *diffuse* when they involve the minority (<50 percent) or majority (≥50 percent) of glomeruli, respectively. Lesions are termed *segmental* or *global* when they involve part of or almost all of the glomerular tuft, respectively. *Proliferative* is used to describe an increase in glomerular cell number, which can be due to infiltration by leukocytes or proliferation of resident glomerular cells. Proliferation of resident glomerular cells is classified as *intracapillary* or *endocapillary* when referring to endothelial or mesangial cells and *extracapillary* when referring to cells in Bowman's space. A *crescent* is a half-moon-shaped collection of cells in Bowman's space, usually composed of proliferating parietal epithelial cells and infiltrating monocytes. Because crescentic glomerulonephritis is often associated with renal failure that progresses rapidly over week to months, the clinical term *rapidly progressive glomerulonephritis* and pathologic term *crescentic glomerulonephritis* are often used interchangeably. The description *membranous* is applied to glomerulonephritis dominated by expansion of the glomerular basement membrane (GBM) by immune deposits. *Sclerosis* refers to an increase in the amount of homogeneous nonfibrillar extracellular material of the same ultrastructural appearance and chemical composition as GBM and mesangial matrix. This process is distinct from *fibrosis*, which involves deposition of collagens type I and III and is more commonly a consequence of healing of crescents or tubulointerstitial inflammation.

MAJOR CLINICOPATHOLOGIC ENTITIES Most glomerulopathies are still classified and named according to their morphologic features (Table 273-1). The major *inflammatory glomerulopathies* are focal proliferative glomerulonephritis (termed mesangial proliferative if the proliferating cells are predominantly mesangial cells), diffuse proliferative glomerulonephritis, and crescentic glomerulonephritis. These diseases typically present with a *nephritic-type* "active" urine sediment characterized by the presence of red blood cells, red blood cell casts, leukocytes, and *subnephrotic* proteinuria of <3 g/24 h. The severity of renal insufficiency varies in proportion to the degree of proliferation and necrosis.

The major morphologic patterns affecting the glomerular filtration barrier for proteins, namely the GBM and visceral epithelial cells, are membranous glomerulopathy, minimal change disease, and focal and segmental glomerulosclerosis. These entities typically present with *nephrotic-range* proteinuria of >3 g/24 h and the presence of few red blood cells, leukocytes, or cellular casts. As a consequence of the heavy proteinuria, nephrotic syndrome is associated with hypoalbuminemia, edema, hyperlipidemia, and lipiduria. Membranoproliferative glomerulonephritis, as the name suggests, is a hybrid lesion that presents with a combination of nephritic and nephrotic features.

The *glomerular deposition diseases* are a group of disorders characterized by prominent extravascular deposition of a paraprotein or fibrillar material. These diseases can also trigger nephritic-type and nephrotic-type responses (or a combination of both) and thus show marked clinical and morphologic overlap with the entities described above.

The *thrombotic microangiopathies* are a family of diseases in which the pathologic presentation is dominated by thrombi within the renal microvasculature, often leading to renal insufficiency.

MAJOR DETERMINANTS OF GLOMERULAR INJURY

Important determinants of the severity of glomerular injury include (1) the primary insult and the secondary mediator systems that it invokes, (2) the site of injury, and (3) the speed of onset, extent, and intensity of disease.

PRIMARY INSULT Glomeruli are susceptible to a variety of inflammatory, metabolic, hemodynamic, toxic, and infectious insults (Table 273-2). Most human glomerular disease is triggered by immune attack, diabetes mellitus, or hypertension. Diverse insults can induce similar clinicopathologic presentations, suggesting marked overlap among downstream molecular and cellular responses. For example, infections (e.g., streptococcal pharyngitis, bacterial endocarditis) and vasculitides (e.g., Henoch-Schönlein purpura, microscopic polyarteritis) can each trigger acute proliferative glomerulonephritis with the nephritic syndrome. Similarly, metabolic (e.g., diabetes mellitus) and deposition diseases (e.g., amyloid) can each induce glomerulosclerosis with nephrotic syndrome. An important corollary is that pharmacologic agents that inhibit common secondary mediator systems may prove effective in treating glomerular diseases of diverse etiologies (see below).

SITE OF INJURY The consequences of injury at different sites within the glomerulus can be predicted from the physiologic functions of the cells within the local milieu (Table 273-3). The major sequelae of injury to the *endothelium* and *subendothelial aspect of the GBM* are: (1) recruitment of leukocytes leading to inflammatory glomerulonephritis, (2) perturbed hemostasis leading to thrombotic microangiopathy, and (3) vasoconstriction and mesangial cell contraction leading to acute renal failure. It is usual for one of these phenotypes to dominate the presentation of specific diseases. *Mesangial* injury is usually immunologic in origin and, being more localized, induces less dramatic impairment of glomerular filtration. Patients typically present with

Table 273-2

Primary Mechanisms of Glomerular Injury

Mechanism of Injury	Some Renal Insults/Defects	Glomerular Disease
Immunologic*	Immunoglobulin†	Immune complex–mediated glomerulonephritis
	Cell-mediated injury†	Pauci-immune glomerulonephritis
	Cytokine (or other soluble factor)	Primary focal segmental glomerulosclerosis
	Persistent complement activation	Membranoproliferative glomerulonephritis (type II)
Metabolic*	Hyperglycemia†	Diabetic nephropathy
	Fabry's disease and sialidosis	Focal segmental glomerulosclerosis
Hemodynamic*	Systemic hypertension†	Hypertensive nephrosclerosis
	Intraglomerular hypertension†	Secondary focal segmental glomerulosclerosis
Toxic	*E. coli*–derived verotoxin	Thrombotic microangiopathy
	Therapeutic drugs (e.g., NSAIDs)	Minimal change disease
	Recreational drugs (heroin)	Focal segmental glomerulosclerosis
Deposition	Amyloid fibrils	Amyloid nephropathy
Infectious	Human immunodeficiency virus (HIV)	HIV nephropathy
	Subacute bacterial endocarditis	Immune complex glomerulonephritis
Inherited	Defect in gene for α5 chain of type IV collagen	Alport's syndrome
	Abnormally thin basement membrane	Thin basement membrane disease

* Most common categories.
† Most common insults within these categories.
NOTE: NSAIDs, nonsteroidal anti-inflammatory drugs.

asymptomatic abnormalities of the urinary sediment and mild renal insufficiency. Proteinuria dominates the clinical presentation of injury to *the subepithelial aspect of the GBM* and *visceral epithelial cells*. As with mesangial injury, GFR is often only mildly compromised in this setting. The classic pathologic manifestation of *parietal epithelial cell* injury is crescent formation. Crescents can be the dominant morphologic presentation of glomerular disease or complicate proliferative or membranous lesions.

SPEED OF ONSET, INTENSITY, AND EXTENT OF INJURY To illustrate the importance of the speed of onset, extent, and intensity of glomerular injury, it is instructive to compare acute postinfectious glomerulonephritis and IgA nephropathy, the latter being a more indolent disease of undetermined etiology. Postinfectious glomerulonephritis is characterized by rapid and extensive formation of immune complexes throughout the glomerular capillary wall, which often provokes acute renal failure with the classic hallmarks of acute inflammation: complement activation, leukocyte recruitment, lysosomal enzyme release, free radical generation, and perturbation of vascular tone and permeability. In contrast, IgA nephropathy is characterized by slow, but sustained, formation of immune complexes, largely confined to the mesangium; less dramatic activation of complement and other secondary mediator systems; and progressive renal insufficiency over 10 to 20 years.

IMMUNOLOGIC GLOMERULAR INJURY

Immune-mediated glomerulonephritis (see also Chaps. 274 and 275) accounts for a large fraction of acquired renal disease. The majority of cases are associated with the deposition of antibodies, often autoantibodies, within the glomerular tuft, indicating dysregulation of humoral immunity. Cellular immune mechanisms also contribute to the pathogenesis of antibody-mediated glomerulonephritis by modulating antibody production and through antibody-dependent cell cytotoxicity (see below). In addition, cellular immune mechanisms probably play a primary role in the pathophysiology of "pauci-immune" glomerulonephritides, notable for robust glomerular inflammation in the absence of immunoglobulin deposition.

ANTIBODY-MEDIATED INJURY (See Fig. 273-1) Most antibody-mediated glomerulonephritis in humans is initiated by reactivity of circulating antibodies with auto- or "planted" antigens. The major mechanisms of antibody deposition within the glomerulus are: (1) reactivity of circulating autoantibodies with intrinsic autoantigens that are components of normal glomerular parenchyma, (2) in situ formation of immune complexes through interaction of circulating antibodies and extrinsic antigens that have been planted within the glomerulus, and (3) intraglomerular trapping of immune complexes that have formed in the systemic circulation.

Generation of Nephritogenic Antibodies Exposure of the host to a foreign antigen (e.g., a prodromal infection) has been implicated as the trigger for the generation of nephritogenic autoantibodies in several forms of glomerulonephritis. Foreign antigens can provoke autoantibody formation through several mechanisms. First, a foreign

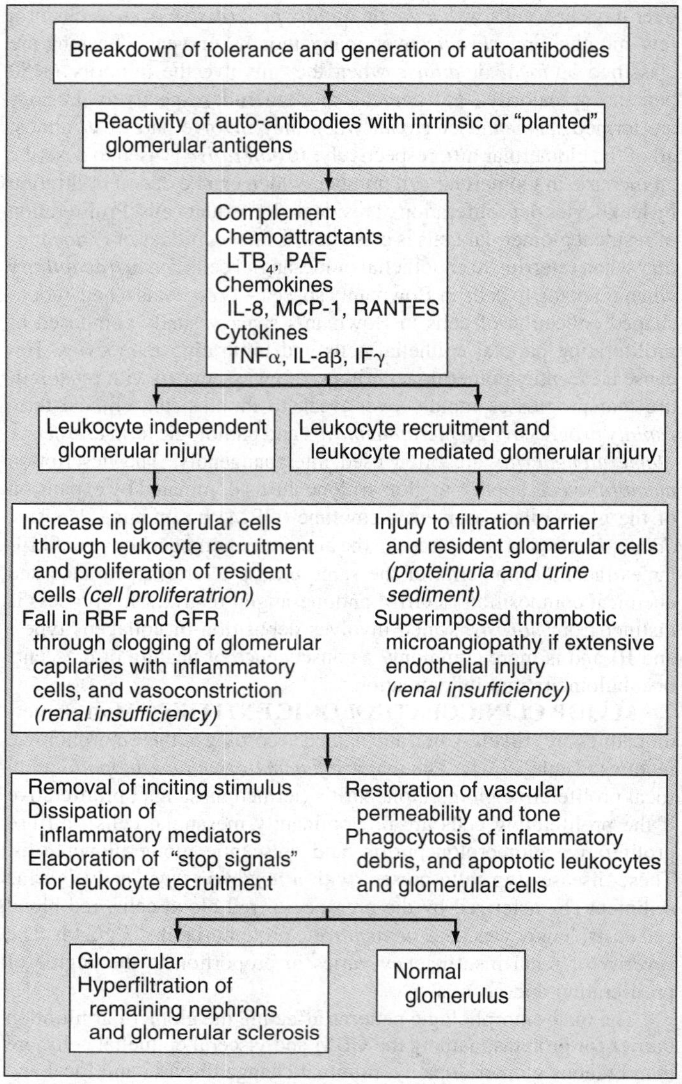

FIGURE 273-1 Mediator systems in acute immune complex–mediated glomerulonephritis: A paradigm of renal inflammation. Abbreviations: LTB_4, leukotriene B_4; PAF, platelet-activating factor; IL, interleukin; MCP-1, monocyte chemotactic peptide-1; TNFα, tumor necrosis factor alpha; Ifγ, interferon-gamma; RBF, renal blood flow; GFR, glomerular filtration rate.

antigen, whose structure resembles that of a host glomerular antigen, may stimulate the production of autoantibodies that cross-react with the intrinsic glomerular antigen ("molecular mimickry"). Second, the foreign antigen may trigger aberrant expression of major histocompatibility complex class II molecules on glomerular cells which present previously "invisible" autoantigens to T lymphocytes and thereby generate an autoimmune response. Third, the foreign antigen can trigger polyclonal activation of B lymphocytes, some of which generate nephritogenic antibodies. Alternatively, individuals may suffer a breakdown of immune tolerance through other mechanisms

Table 273-3

Correlation between Site of Glomerular Injury and Clinicopathologic Presentation

Target of Injury	Physiologic Role	Response to Injury	Representative Glomerular Disease
Endothelial cell	Maintains glomerular perfusion	Vasoconstriction	Acute renal failure
	Prevents leukocyte adhesion	Leukocyte infiltration	Focal or diffuse proliferative GN
	Prevents platelet aggregation and clotting	Intravascular microthrombi	Thrombotic microangiopathies
Mesangial cell	Controls glomerular filtration surface area	Proliferation/increased matrix	Mesangioproliferative GN/glomerulosclerosis
Basement membrane	Prevents filtration of plasma proteins	Proteinuria	Membranous nephropathy
Visceral epithelial cell	Prevents filtration of plasma proteins	Proteinuria	Minimal change disease and FSGS
Parietal epithelial cell	Maintains Bowman's space	Crescent formation	Crescentic GN

NOTE: GN, glomerulonephritis; FSGS, focal segmental glomerulosclerosis.

(e.g., genetically programmed). Autoreactive B cells are usually deleted in the thymus during development (clonal deletion) or rendered anergic in peripheral lymphoid tissue (clonal anergy). Similar tolerogenic mechanisms exist for deleting or anergizing autoreactive T helper cells that modulate immunoglobulin production by autoreactive B cells. Perturbation of either of these tolerogenic mechanisms could drive immunoglobulin production in some forms of autoimmune glomerulonephritis. Indeed, defective clonal deletion of autoreactive T cells has been demonstrated in experimental lupus nephritis due to defective synthesis of Fas, a cell-surface receptor that modulates T cell deletion through apoptosis (programmed cell death) within the thymus.

Deposition of Nephritogenic Antibodies within the Glomerulus Anti-GBM antibody disease (p. 1539) is the classic nephritis initiated by interaction of autoantibody with intrinsic glomerular antigen. Afflicted patients have a circulating antibody directed at a 28-kDa antigen (Goodpasture antigen) located in the noncollagenous NC1 domain of the α3 chain of type IV collagen. This type of collagen is preferentially expressed in glomerular and pulmonary alveolar basement membranes. Autoantibodies against mesangial cell antigens have been detected in the serum of patients with IgA nephropathy, the most common form of glomerulonephritis in humans; however, the pathogenicity of these autoantibodies has yet to be defined. Poststreptococcal glomerulonephritis and lupus nephritis are examples of glomerulonephritides that are probably initiated by interaction of circulating antibodies with planted antigens. Several streptococcal antigens have been isolated from immune deposits of kidneys with poststreptococcal glomerulonephritis, including a 46-kDa nephritis strain–associated antigen and a 46-kDa cytoplasmic protein endostreptosin. In addition, patients with poststreptococcal glomerulonephritis can have circulating antibodies against laminin, type IV collagen, and heparan sulphate proteoglycans, suggesting that molecular mimickry may also contribute. Similar findings have been reported in experimental and human lupus nephritis. Here, circulating anti-DNA antibodies induce immune complex glomerulonephritis by reacting with DNA bound to GBM or with planted DNA-histone complexes (nucleosomes). Cryoglobulinemia, due to chronic hepatitis C infection, is an example of glomerulonephritis initiated by trapping of immune complexes. These patients have circulating and intraglomerular immune complexes composed of hepatitis C antigens, polyclonal antihepatitis C IgG, and a second antibody, usually a monoclonal IgM, directed against the IgG. In support of the pathogenicity of circulating cryoglobulins, their injection into laboratory mice induces glomerulonephritis with many of the hallmarks of human disease.

Site of Antibody Deposition The site of antibody deposition within the glomerulus is a critical determinant of the clinicopathologic presentation. Among the factors that determine the site of deposition are the avidity, affinity, and quantity of the antibody; the size, charge, and site of the antigen; the size of the immune complexes; the efficiency of the clearance mechanisms for immune complexes; and local hemodynamic factors. Relatively anionic antigens are repelled by the GBM, which is negatively charged, and tend to be trapped in the subendothelial cell space and mesangium. In contrast, relatively cationic antigens tend to permeate the GBM and deposit within the GBM or in the subepithelial space. Acute deposition of antibody in the subendothelial cell space or mesangium typically triggers a nephritic-type response characterized by rapid recruitment of leukocytes and platelets, probably because inflammatory mediators generated at these sites are strategically positioned to activate endothelial and hematogenous cells. Inflammation is more severe when antibody is deposited in the subendothelial space, as compared with mesangium, at least in part because the mesangium abuts only 25 to 33 percent of the capillary wall. Antibody deposition in the subepithelial cell space typically induces a nephrotic-type response characterized by proteinuria without a pronounced inflammatory cell infiltrate, probably because the immune complexes are shielded from circulating inflammatory cells by the GBM and because the large fluid flux from blood to Bowman's space minimizes back-diffusion of inflammatory mediators towards the endothelium and vascular lumen.

Recruitment of Inflammatory Cells Leukocytes and platelets are important mediators of injury in most forms of acute and subacute glomerulonephritis. Immunoglobulin can provoke recruitment of leukocytes through several mechanisms. Many antibody subclasses activate the complement cascade, and complement proteins such as C3a, C5a, and C5b-9 (membrane attack complex) are potent stimuli for leukocyte recruitment. Complement-independent mechanisms also contribute. Leukocytes express Fc receptors that can directly engage the Fc portion of immunoglobulin. Resident glomerular macrophages, endothelial cells, and mesangial cells also express Fc receptors, engagement of which can trigger release of an array of inflammatory mediators that promotes directed locomotion of leukocytes (chemotaxis), binding of leukocytes to inflamed endothelium through cell surface leukocyte adhesion molecules, and diapedesis of leukocytes to the extravascular space.

The mechanisms of platelet recruitment in glomerulonephritis are less well defined. Potential mechanisms include direct binding of platelet Fc receptors with immunoglobulin, and interactions of platelets with endothelium, collagen, and other components of exposed GBM, and to products of the coagulation cascade such as fibrin.

Mediators of Glomerular Injury *Nephritic-type antibody-mediated glomerular injury* is a vivid example of host defense gone awry. In normal host defense, leukocytes engulf microorganisms into phagosomes, which then fuse with intracellular lysosomes. Microorganisms are destroyed within phagolysosomes through the actions of free radicals, proteolytic enzymes, and other toxic molecules. This process facilitates killing with relative protection and preservation of host tissue. When host defense is inappropriately activated in autoimmune diseases, the inciting antigens are often fixed to (planted antigens) or are a component of host tissue (autoantigen). As a result, phagocytosis is less efficient ("frustrated phagocytosis"), and there is release of toxic moieties into the parenchyma where they destroy host cells and matrix components. In addition, cytotoxic T lymphocytes and natural killer cells can damage resident glomerular cells by releasing toxic compounds, such as perforins, a process that is facilitated by binding of these cytotoxic cells to glomerular cells through HLA molecules, Fc portions of immunoglobulin (antibody-dependent cell cytotoxicity), and other immune recognition systems. Platelets promote nephritic injury by promoting leukocyte recruitment and intrarenal vasoconstriction and by triggering microthrombi formation.

Leukocytes play a lesser role in *nephrotic-type antibody-mediated glomerular injury* (Chap. 274). Membranous glomerulopathy is the prototypic entity and is initiated by the formation of subepithelial immune complexes; these provoke production of "spikes" of new basement membrane that eventually encircle and incorporate the immune complexes into the GBM. The antigenic targets in human membranous glomerulopathy have not been determined. The frequent association with infections, malignancies, and drugs suggests involvement of planted antigens or molecular mimickry (see above); however, many cases may represent a true loss of tolerance against autoantigens.

CELL PROLIFERATION AND ACCUMULATION OF EXTRACELLULAR MATRIX A hallmark of the nephritic-type proliferative glomerulopathies is an increase in glomerular cell number. Initially, this hypercellularity is due predominantly to infiltration of the glomerular tuft by leukocytes. Subsequently, resident glomerular cells proliferate in response to growth factors (e.g., epidermal growth factor, platelet-derived growth factor, thrombospondin) released into the local inflammatory milieu. The proliferating cells are typically mesangial in mesangioproliferative glomerulonephritis, and both endothelial and mesangial cells in diffuse proliferative glomerulonephritis. The visceral epithelial cell is, for the most part, a terminally differentiated cell that does not proliferate rapidly, even when injured.

Whereas acute antibody-mediated glomerulonephritis typically induces acute diffuse proliferative glomerulonephritis and acute renal failure over days to weeks (nephritic syndrome), subacute immune injury often induces the formation of glomerular crescents and renal failure over weeks or a few months (termed *rapidly progressive glomerulonephritis*). As discussed above, crescents are extracapillary proliferations of cells in Bowman's space, composed of infiltrating monocytes, proliferating parietal epithelial cells, and fibrin.

Sustained immune complex deposition over months to years can provoke a marked increase in basement membrane or mesangial matrix production. Mild to moderate accumulation of matrix usually manifests as proteinuria due to disruption of the glomerular filtration barrier; however, in its most severe form, matrix accumulation causes glomerulosclerosis and chronic renal insufficiency.

RESOLUTION, REPAIR, AND SCARRING Glomerular inflammation can resolve with complete recovery of renal function or with a variable amount of scarring and chronic renal insufficiency. Acute poststreptococcal glomerulonephritis (p. 1537), for example, usually resolves spontaneously and fully in children, whereas adults are frequently left with residual renal impairment. The resolution process requires cessation of further antibody production and immune complex formation, removal of deposited and circulating immune complexes, inhibition of further recruitment of inflammatory cells, dissipation of the gradients of inflammatory mediators, restoration of normal endothelial adhesiveness and permeability, normalization of vascular tone, and clearance of infiltrating inflammatory cells and proliferating resident glomerular cells (Fig. 273-1).

Unfortunately, the resolution phase of most inflammatory glomerulopathies in adults terminates in glomerular scarring. This is particularly true in patients with crescentic glomerulopathies who may be left with end-stage renal failure requiring dialysis or transplantation. Transforming growth factor β (TGFβ), a cytokine, stimulates production of extracellular matrix by most glomerular cells, inhibits synthesis of tissue proteases that normally degrade matrix proteins, and is a potent stimulus for scar formation immediately following glomerular injury.

Moderate-to-severe glomerulonephritis is usually associated with a variable degree of tubulointerstitial inflammation and scarring in addition to glomerular injury. Indeed, the severity of tubulointerstitial injury usually correlates closely with long-term impairment of renal function. The pathogenesis of tubulointerstitial inflammation in this setting is unclear. Potential mechanisms include primary involvement of the tubulointerstitium in autoimmune disease and induction of tubulointerstitial inflammation by mediators, generated by diseased glomeruli, which diffuse into the tubulointerstitium via blood, tubular fluid, or the interstitial space.

OTHER MECHANISMS OF ANTIBODY-MEDIATED INJURY Several other autoantibodies have been implicated as mediators of renal injury in patients with glomerulonephritis.

Antineutrophil Cytoplasmic Antibodies (ANCA) Immunoglobulin is not detected in the glomerulus in approximately 40 percent of patients with rapidly progressive glomerulonephritis ("pauci-immune crescentic glomerulonephritis"). The majority of these patients have Wegener's granulomatosis, microscopic polyangiitis nodosa, or renal-limited crescentic glomerulonephritis and have autoantibodies against neutrophil cytoplasmic antigens in their circulation. ANCA stimulate cytokine-primed human neutrophils to generate reactive oxygen species and injure endothelium in vitro. These findings raise the possibility that ANCA may be pathogenetic in vivo in the presence of circulating cytokines, as may occur following a prodromal infection.

Antiendothelial Cell Antibodies Circulating antibodies against endothelial antigens have been reported in several inflammatory vasculitides and glomerulonephritides. Their titers tend to correlate with disease activity, and some activate endothelial cells and increase their adhesiveness for leukocytes, suggesting a pathogenetic role.

C3 Nephritic Factor Some patients with membranoproliferative glomerulonephritis (p. 1543) have large deposits of electron-dense material within the GBM that does not stain for immunoglobulin (dense deposit disease; membranoproliferative glomerulonephritis type II). Intriguingly, most of these patients have a circulating IgG, termed the *C3 nephritic factor*, directed at C3bBb (C3 convertase) of the alternative pathway of complement.

CELL-MEDIATED INJURY Although cell-mediated injury is as yet less well defined than antibody-mediated glomerular injury, T cells have also been implicated as independent mediators of glomerular injury and as modulators of the production of nephritogenic antibodies. T cells may be particularly important as initiators of injury in pauci-immune glomerulonephritis. T cells interact, through their cell surface T cell receptor/CD3 complex, with antigens presented in the groove of major histocompatibility complex molecules of resident glomerular endothelial, mesangial, and epithelial cells, a process that is facilitated by cell-cell adhesion and costimulatory molecules. Cytokines and other mediators released by activated T cells are potent stimuli for further leukocyte recruitment, cytotoxicity, and fibrogenesis. CD4 T lymphocytes are important recruiters of macrophages and trigger clonal expansion of autoreactive B cells; they also promote glomerular cell injury by CD8 cytotoxic T lymphocytes and natural killer cells and through antibody-dependent cell cytotoxicity. Soluble factors derived from T cells have also been implicated in the pathogenesis of proteinuria in minimal change disease and primary focal segmental glomerulosclerosis. Their identity and molecular characterization remain to be determined.

NONIMMUNOLOGIC GLOMERULAR INJURY

METABOLIC Diabetic Nephropathy (See also Chaps. 275 and 334) Nephropathy complicates approximately 30 percent and 20 percent of cases of type 1 and type 2 diabetes mellitus, respectively, and is characterized clinically by proteinuria and progressive renal insufficiency. The typical glomerular lesion is glomerulosclerosis due to thickening of the GBM and expansion of the mesangium with extracellular matrix. Factors implicated as triggers for increased matrix production in diabetic glomerulosclerosis include glomerular hypertension; the direct effects of hyperglycemia on mesangial cells; advanced glycosylation end-products that result from nonenzymatic glycation of proteins; growth factors such as growth hormone, insulin-like growth factor 1, and angiotensin II; cytokines such as TGFβ; hyperlipidemia; and cell sorbitol accumulation and myoinositol deficiency secondary to activation of the aldose reductase polyol pathway. Complementary clinical and laboratory approaches suggest a central role for hemodynamic factors. The GFR increases by 20 to 30 percent within months of the development of hyperglycemia due, in large part, to extracellular fluid volume expansion and resulting afferent arteriolar dilatation and increased glomerular ultrafiltration pressure.

The mechanism by which diabetes mellitus induces glomerular hyperfiltration is still being defined but appears to involve atrial natriuretic peptide. In this framework, glycosuria triggers increased reabsorption of glucose coupled to sodium in the proximal tubule, thereby increasing total-body sodium and extracellular fluid volume. As a compensatory response, atrial natriuretic peptide is released from cardiac myocytes and induces natriuresis by triggering afferent arteriolar dilatation and thereby increasing intraglomerular pressure and GFR. Whereas this compensatory response is appropriate in the short term, sustained glomerular hypertension provokes thickening of the GBM, increased mesangial matrix production, and glomerulosclerosis and disruption of barrier function. In keeping with a central role for intra glomerular pressure in the pathogenesis of diabetic nephropathy, angiotensin-converting enzyme inhibitors, which lower intraglomerular pressure, dramatically slow the progression of diabetic nephropathy, even in normotensive patients. It is likely that hemodynamic and metabolic factors act in concert to generate the final glomerulosclerotic phenotype in genetically predisposed patients.

Other Metabolic Diseases Several rare inherited lysosomal enzyme defects induce focal segmental glomerulosclerosis, probably by allowing accumulation of toxic metabolites in renal cells. *Fabry's disease* (α-galactosidase deficiency; Chap. 346) and *sialidosis* (*N*-acetylneuraminic acid hydrolase deficiency; Chap. 346) are the major culprits in this regard. Both tend to induce focal segmental or global glomerulosclerosis by preferentially affecting visceral epithelial cells, probably because these are terminally differentiated cells with a very slow replication rate. *Partial lipodystrophy* (Chap. 352) is a rare metabolic disorder characterized by lipoatrophy affecting the arms, neck, and chest, often with redistribution of fat to the hips and legs. Approximately one-third of patients develop glomerular disease, usually type II membranoproliferative glomerulopathy (dense deposit disease; see Chap. 274).

HEMODYNAMIC GLOMERULAR INJURY High intraglomerular pressure is a major cause of glomerular injury in humans and can result from systemic hypertension or a local change in glomerular hemodynamics (glomerular hypertension).

Systemic Hypertension (See also Chap. 246) Although the kidneys have evolved sophisticated mechanisms for autoregulating glomerular blood flow and pressure, marked or sustained increments in systemic blood pressure can overwhelm these compensatory systems and perturb glomerular morphology and function. In its most dramatic form, namely malignant hypertension, hemodynamic stress causes massive fibrinoid necrosis of afferent arterioles and glomeruli, thrombotic microangiopathy, acute renal failure, and a nephritic urinary sediment. Chronic sustained hypertension typically leads to arteriolar vasoconstriction and sclerosis, which, in turn, cause secondary atrophy and sclerosis of glomeruli and the tubulointerstitium. A variety of molecular signals appear to couple elevations in intravascular pressure to myointimal proliferation and eventually sclerosis of the vessel wall. These include growth factors such as angiotensin II, epidermal growth factor, and platelet-derived growth factor; cytokines such as TGFβ; and activation of stretch activated ion channels and early response genes.

Glomerular Hypertension The pathophysiology of diabetic nephropathy, discussed above, illustrates the importance of intraglomerular pressure as a stimulus for mesangial matrix production and glomerulosclerosis. Glomerular hypertension is also a key factor in the pathogenesis of the progressive glomerulosclerosis and renal failure that complicate the adaptive response of remnant nephrons to increased workload following loss of the other nephrons from any cause (see below). Importantly, these changes in glomerular hemodynamics and pressure appear to precede the development of systemic hypertension and are independent risk factors for glomerular injury.

TOXIC GLOMERULOPATHIES The renal microvasculature is a relatively uncommon site for toxic injury, by comparison with the tubular interstitium; however, there are a few important exceptions. Verotoxin, derived from *Escherichia coli* during bouts of infective diarrhea, is directly toxic to renal endothelium and induces the hemolytic-uremic syndrome. In this setting, verotoxin interacts with a specific cell membrane receptor, perturbs the antithrombotic phenotype of endothelium, and triggers the development of thrombotic microangiopathy. Irradiation, mitomycin, and anovulants can induce a similar syndrome through ill-defined mechanisms. Nonsteroidal anti-inflammatory drugs, rifampin, ampicillin, and interferon α can induce an unusual combination of acute renal failure with nephrotic syndrome. The characteristic pathologic correlates of this syndrome are allergic interstitial nephritis and fusion of the foot processes of the visceral epithelial cells, the latter accounting for the marked proteinuria. How these structurally diverse agents induce epithelial cell injury is unclear.

DEPOSITION DISEASES The glomerular deposition diseases are a group of diverse conditions in which abnormal proteins are deposited in glomeruli where they provoke an inflammatory reaction and/or glomerulosclerosis. The major glomerular deposition diseases are cryoglobulinemia, amyloidosis, light and heavy chain deposition disease, and fibrillary/immunotactoid glomerulopathy. *Cryoglobulins* (Chap. 319) are immunoglobulins that precipitate in the cold and can be composed of either monoclonal immunoglobulin, usually generated by a lymphoproliferative malignancy (type I); a mixture of polyclonal immunoglobulin (usually IgG) and monoclonal immunoglobulin (usually IgM) directed to epitopes on polyclonal IgG (type II); or a mixture of polyclonal antibodies, one or more having anti-IgG activity (type III). As discussed above, cryoglobulins can induce nephritic-type and nephrotic-type injury depending on the rapidity, severity, and site of immunoglobulin deposition. *Glomerular amyloidosis* (Chaps. 275 and 309) is one of the five most common causes of nephrotic syndrome in adults and is characterized by extracellular deposition of amyloid fibrils composed, in part, of fragments of immunoglobulin light chains (AL amyloid) or serum amyloid A, the acute-phase reactant (AA amyloid). In light chain deposition diseases, intact immunoglobulin light chains, usually kappa, are deposited in a granular, rather than fibrillary, pattern. The composition of the deposits in *fibrillary/immunotactoid glomerulopathy* is still being defined and may also include immunoglobulin. These different types of deposits, in addition to directly disrupting glomerular architecture, provoke mesangial matrix production and glomerulosclerosis. Fibrillary/immunotactoid glomerulopathy can also present as acute or subacute glomerular inflammation. How these diverse deposits trigger glomerular matrix production and recruitment of inflammatory cells has yet to be determined.

INFECTIOUS CAUSES OF GLOMERULAR DISEASE Infectious organisms can induce glomerular disease through several different mechanisms: (1) by direct infection of renal cells, (2) by elaborating nephrotoxins such as *E. coli*–derived verotoxin, (3) by inciting intraglomerular deposition of immune complexes (e.g., postinfectious glomerulonephritis) or cryoglobulins (e.g., hepatitis B or C), and (4) by providing a chronic stimulus for amyloid fibril formation, as in AA amyloidosis. Direct infection of glomerular cells is a relatively rare mechanism of injury but has been implicated in the pathogenesis of nephropathy associated with human immunodeficiency virus. This entity is characterized histologically by focal segmental glomerulosclerosis, microcystic tubular dilatation, and interstitial fibrosis. Viral genome and p24 protein have been detected in glomerular and tubular cells in this disease, and infection of glomerular cells induces expression of TGFβ, a major stimulus for mesangial matrix production and sclerosis.

INHERITED GLOMERULAR DISEASES *Alport's syndrome* (hereditary nephritis; Chap. 275), the prototypical inherited glomerular disease, is usually transmitted as an X-linked dominant trait. Afflicted patients have a mutation in the COL4A5 gene that encodes the α5 chain of type IV collagen located on the X chromosome. As a result, the glomerular basement membrane is irregular with longitudinal layering, splitting, or thickening, and patients develop hematuria, progressive glomerulosclerosis, and renal failure. *Thin basement membrane disease* is another relatively common disorder of the GBM. In contrast to Alport's syndrome, this entity is usually inherited as an autosomal dominant or recessive trait and is benign. As the name suggests, the basement membrane is thin but otherwise ultrastructurally normal. Patients typically experience recurrent benign hematuria. The molecular basis for thin basement membrane disease has yet to be elucidated. Rarer hereditary glomerular diseases include *nail-patella syndrome* (osteoonychodysplasia), which is associated with a relatively benign mottling of the basement membrane with lucent rarefractions; *partial lipodystrophy*, which is associated with type II membranoproliferative glomerulonephritis (dense deposit disease); and *familial lecithin–cholesterol acyltransferase deficiency*, which is associated with distortion of the basement membrane by irregular rounded lucent zones, increased mesangial matrix production, and progressive sclerosis and renal insufficiency.

GLOMERULAR ADAPTATION TO NEPHRON LOSS

Nephron loss, from any cause, is followed by compensatory hyperfiltration in the remaining functional glomeruli. This adaptive response is appropriate in the short-term and maintains GFR. Over years, however, the hyperfiltering remnant nephrons develop focal and segmental glomerulosclerosis, and eventually global sclerosis, that manifests clinically as proteinuria, hypertension, and progressive renal insufficiency. Sustained glomerular capillary hypertension has been implicated as a major stimulus for glomerulosclerosis in this setting. Increased glomerular blood flow and ultrafiltration pressure are early findings in remnant nephrons in most experimental models in which the function of more than 50 percent of nephron mass has been lost through surgical ablation, immunologic or toxic injury, or other mechanisms. Sustained glomerular hypertension is thought to stimulate the accumulation of extracellular matrix by perturbing the function of visceral epithelial and mesangial cells, either directly or by increasing the flux of circulating macromolecules through the glomerular capillary wall. As with most forms of glomerulosclerosis, TGFβ may be an important regulator of matrix accumulation in remnant nephrons. Angiotensin II, platelet-derived growth factor, and endothelins are other potential modulators of this process. Maneuvers that lower intraglomerular pressure, such as low-protein diet or treatment with angiotensin-converting enzyme inhibitors, slow the development of glomerulosclerosis and renal failure. Glomerular hypertrophy, intracapillary microthrombi, recruited macrophages, and hyperlipidemia are other potential stimuli for glomerulosclerosis. Indeed, glomerular capillary hypertension and hypertrophy appear to be independent risk factors that could act synergistically to cause progressive renal insufficiency. Intriguingly, angiotensin II may trigger TGFβ production in remnant nephrons, suggesting that angiotensin-converting enzyme inhibitors may be renoprotective through complementary effects on glomerular hemodynamics and matrix production.

BIBLIOGRAPHY

ADLER SG et al: Secondary glomerular diseases, in *The Kidney*, 5th ed, BM Brenner (ed). Philadelphia, Saunders, 1996, pp 1498–1596

BRADY HR: Leukocyte adhesion molecules and kidney diseases. Kidney Int 45:1285, 1994

BRENNER BM: Hemodynamically mediated glomerular injury and the progressive nature of renal disease. Kidney Int 23:647, 1983

COTRAN R, RENNKE HG: Sites and the mechanisms of proteinuria. N Engl J Med 309:1050, 1983

COUSER WG: Mediation of glomerular injury. J Am Soc Nephrol 1:13, 1990

FALK RJ: ANCA-associated renal disease. Kidney Int 38:998, 1990

GLASSOCK RJ et al: Primary glomerular diseases, in *The Kidney*, 5th ed, BM Brenner (ed). Philadelphia, Saunders, 1996, pp 1392–1497

KELLY PT, HAPONIK EF: Goodpasture's syndrome: Molecular and clinical advances. Medicine (Baltimore) 73:171, 1994

MEYER TW et al: Nephron adaptation to renal injury, in *The Kidney*, 5th ed, BM Brenner (ed). Philadelphia, Saunders, 1995, pp 2011–2048

REES A: The immunogenetics of glomerulonephritis. Kidney Int 45:377, 1994

WILSON CB: Renal response to immunologic glomerular injury, in *The Kidney*, 5th ed, BM Brenner (ed). Philadelphia, Saunders, 1996, pp 1253–1391

274

Hugh R. Brady, Yvonne M. O'Meara, Barry M. Brenner

THE MAJOR GLOMERULOPATHIES

Glomerular injury can arise from diverse renal-limited and systemic diseases and is the major cause of end-stage renal disease (ESRD) requiring dialysis and transplantation. In this chapter, we describe the epidemiology, clinical presentations, pathology, and treatment of the major glomerulopathies. We focus on the *primary glomerulopathies*, glomerular diseases in which the pathologic process is confined to the kidney and in which systemic features are a direct consequence of impaired glomerular filtration (e.g., hypervolemia, hypertension, uremic syndrome). Considered here are the five major clinical presentations of glomerulopathy: acute nephritic syndrome, rapidly progressive glomerulonephritis (RPGN), nephrotic syndrome, asymptomatic abnormalities of the urinary sediment (hematuria, proteinuria), and chronic glomerulonephritis. Glomerulopathies associated with systemic diseases (*secondary glomerulopathies*) are discussed in Chap. 275. The nomenclature pertaining to the classification and clinicopathologic description of glomerular disease and the pathogenetic mechanisms of glomerular injury are reviewed in Chap. 273.

ACUTE NEPHRITIC SYNDROME AND RAPIDLY PROGRESSIVE GLOMERULONEPHRITIS

CLINICAL FEATURES AND CLINICOPATHOLOGIC CORRELATES The *acute nephritic syndrome* is the clinical correlate of acute glomerular inflammation. In its most dramatic form, the acute nephritic syndrome is characterized by sudden onset (i.e., over days to weeks) of *acute renal failure* and *oliguria* (<400 mL of urine per day). Renal blood flow and glomerular filtration rate (GFR) fall as a result of obstruction of the glomerular capillary lumen by infiltrating inflammatory cells and proliferating resident glomerular cells. Renal blood flow and GFR are further compromised by intrarenal vasoconstriction and mesangial cell contraction that result from local imbalances of vasoconstrictor (e.g., leukotrienes, platelet-activating factor, thromboxanes, endothelins) and vasodilator substances (e.g., nitric oxide, prostacyclin) within the renal microcirculation. *Extracellular fluid volume expansion*, *edema*, and *hypertension* develop because of impaired GFR and enhanced tubular reabsorption of salt and water. As a result of injury to the glomerular capillary wall, urinalysis typically reveals *red blood cell casts*, dysmorphic red blood cells, leukocytes, and subnephrotic proteinuria of <3.5 g per 24 h ("nephritic urinary sediment"). *Hematuria* is often macroscopic.

The classic pathologic correlate of the nephritic syndrome is *proliferative glomerulonephritis*. The proliferation of glomerular cells is due initially to infiltration of the glomerular tuft by neutrophils and monocytes and subsequently to proliferation of resident glomerular endothelial and mesangial cells (endocapillary proliferation). In its most severe form, the nephritic syndrome is associated with acute inflammation of most glomeruli, i.e., *acute diffuse proliferative glomerulonephritis*. When less vigorous, fewer than 50 percent of glomeruli may be involved, i.e., *focal proliferative glomerulonephritis*. In milder forms of nephritic injury, cellular proliferation may be confined to the mesangium, i.e., *mesangioproliferative glomerulonephritis*.

RPGN is the clinical correlate of more *subacute glomerular inflammation*. Patients develop renal failure over weeks to months in association with a nephritic urinary sediment, subnephrotic proteinuria and variable oliguria, hypervolemia, edema, and hypertension. The classic pathologic correlate of RPGN is crescent formation involving most glomeruli (*crescentic glomerulonephritis*), crescents being half-moon-shaped lesions in Bowman's space composed of proliferating parietal epithelial cells and infiltrating monocytes (*extracapillary proliferation*). In practice, the clinical term *rapidly progressive glomerulonephritis* and the pathologic term *crescentic glomerulonephritis* are often used interchangeably. In addition to classic crescentic glomerulonephritis, in which crescents dominate the glomerular pathology, crescents can also develop concomitantly with proliferative glomerulonephritis or as a complication of membranous glomerulopathy and other more indolent forms of glomerular inflammation.

The acute nephritic syndrome and RPGN are part of a spectrum of presentations of immunologically mediated proliferative glomerulonephritis. Studies of experimental models suggest that nephritic syndrome and diffuse proliferative glomerulonephritis represent an acute immune response to a sudden large antigen load, whereas RPGN and crescentic glomerulonephritis represent a more subacute immune response to a smaller antigen load in presensitized individuals. At the other end of the spectrum, chronic low-grade immune injury presents with slowly progressive renal insufficiency or asymptomatic hematuria in association with focal proliferative or mesangioproliferative glomerulonephritis. These more indolent forms of immune-mediated glomerulonephritis are discussed later in this chapter.

ETIOLOGY AND DIFFERENTIAL DIAGNOSIS Acute nephritic syndrome and RPGN can result from renal-limited *primary* glomerulopathy or *secondary* glomerulopathy complicating systemic disease. Figure 274-1 highlights the histopathologic and serologic features that help distinguish among the major causes of nephritic syndrome and RPGN. In general, rapid diagnosis and prompt treatment are critical to avoid the development of irreversible renal failure. Renal biopsy remains the "gold standard" for diagnosis. *Immunofluorescence* *microscopy* is particularly helpful and identifies three major patterns of deposition of immunoglobulin that define three broad diagnostic categories: (1) *granular* deposits of immunoglobulin, a hallmark of *immune-complex glomerulonephritis*; (2) *linear* deposition of immunoglobulin along the glomerular basement membrane (GBM), characteristic of *anti-GBM disease*; and (3) paucity or absence of immunoglobulin, typical of *pauci-immune glomerulonephritis* (Fig. 274-2). Most patients (>70 percent) with full-blown acute nephritic syndrome have immune-complex glomerulonephritis. Pauci-immune glomerulonephritis is less common in this setting (<30 percent) and anti-GBM disease is rare (<1 percent). Among patients with RPGN, immune-complex glomerulonephritis and pauci-immune glomerulonephritis are equally prevalent (~45 percent each), whereas anti-GBM disease again accounts for a minority of cases (<10 percent).

Three *serologic markers* often predict the immunofluorescence microscopy findings in nephritic syndrome and RPGN and may obviate the need for renal biopsy in classic cases. They are the serum C3 level and titers of anti-GBM antibody and antineutrophil cytoplasmic antibody (ANCA) (Fig. 274-1). As discussed in Chap. 273, the kidney is host to immune attack in immune-complex glomerulonephritis, most cases being initiated either by in situ formation of immune complexes or less commonly by glomerular trapping of circulating immune complexes. These patients typically have hypocomplementemia (low C3 and CH_{50} in 90 percent) and negative anti-GBM and ANCA serology. The glomerulus is the direct target of immune attack in anti-GBM disease, glomerular inflammation being initiated by an autoantibody directed at a 28-kDa autoantigen on the α3 chain of type IV collagen. Approximately 90 to 95 percent of patients with anti-GBM disease have circulating anti-GBM autoantibodies detectable by radioimmunoassay; serum complement levels are typically normal, and ANCA are usually not detected. The pathogenesis of pauci-immune glomerulonephritis is still being defined; however, most patients have circulating ANCA, implicating dysregulation of humoral immunity. The presence of mononuclear leukocytes in glomeruli and the paucity of glomerular immune deposits suggest that cellular mechanisms are also involved. Serum complement levels are typically normal, and anti-GBM titers are usually negative in ANCA-associated renal disease.

IMMUNE-COMPLEX GLOMERULONEPHRITIS Immune-complex glomerulonephritis may (1) be idiopathic, (2) represent a response to a known antigenic stimulus (e.g., postinfectious glomerulonephritis), or (3) form part of a multisystem immune-complex disorder (e.g., lupus nephritis, Henoch-Schönlein purpura, cryoglobulinemia, bacterial endocarditis; Fig. 274-1). Here, we focus on *postinfectious glomerulonephritis*, the best characterized *primary* immune-complex glomerulonephritis. The major *secondary* immune-complex glomerulonephritides are discussed in Chap. 275. Nephritic syndrome and RPGN occasionally complicate two other primary glomerulopathies, namely, membranoproliferative glomerulonephritis (MPGN) and IgA nephropathy when there is a florid proliferative component. Because nephrotic syndrome and asymptomatic hematuria are more common presentations of MPGN and IgA nephropathy, respectively, these glomerulopathies are discussed in later sections on nephrotic syndrome and asymptomatic urinary abnormalities.

POSTSTREPTOCOCCAL GLOMERULONEPHRITIS This is the prototypical postinfectious glomerulonephritis and a leading cause of acute nephritic syndrome. Most cases are sporadic, though the disease can occur as an epidemic. Glomerulonephritis develops, on average, 10 days after pharyngitis or 2 weeks after a skin infection (impetigo) with a nephritogenic strain of group A beta-hemolytic streptococcus. The known nephritic strains include M types 1, 2, 4, 12, 18, 25, 49, 55, 57, and 60. Immunity to these strains is type-specific and long-lasting, and repeated infection and nephritis are rare. Epidemic poststreptococcal glomerulonephritis is most commonly encountered in children of 2 to 6 years of age with pharyngitis during the winter months. This entity appears to be decreasing in frequency, possibly due to more widespread and prompt use of antibiotics. Poststreptococcal glomerulonephritis in association with cutaneous infections usually occurs in a setting of poor personal hygiene or streptococcal superinfection of another skin disease.

The classic clinical presentation of poststreptococcal glomerulonephritis is full-blown nephritic syndrome with oliguric acute renal failure; however, most patients have milder disease. Indeed, subclinical cases outnumber overt cases by four- to tenfold during epidemics.

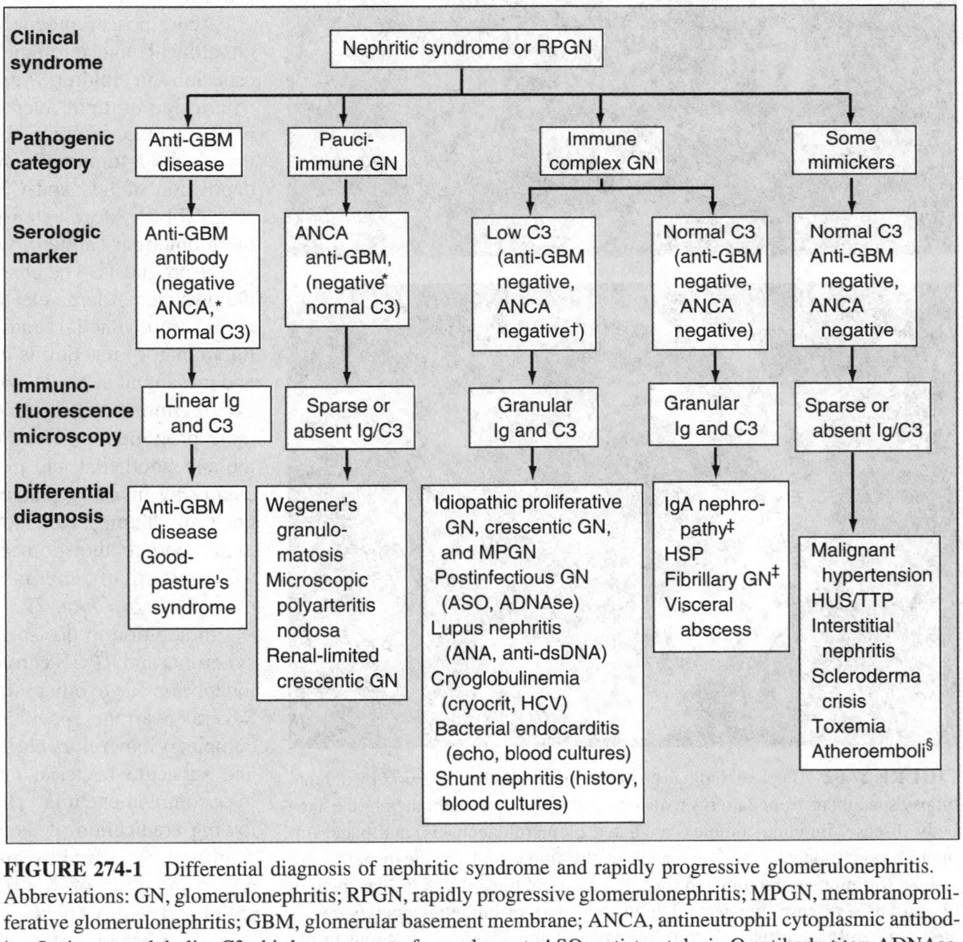

FIGURE 274-1 Differential diagnosis of nephritic syndrome and rapidly progressive glomerulonephritis. Abbreviations: GN, glomerulonephritis; RPGN, rapidly progressive glomerulonephritis; MPGN, membranoproliferative glomerulonephritis; GBM, glomerular basement membrane; ANCA, antineutrophil cytoplasmic antibodies; Ig, immunoglobulin; C3, third component of complement; ASO, antistreptolysin O antibody titer; ADNAse, anti-deoxyribonuclease antibody titer; ANA, antinuclear antibody; anti-dsDNA, anti-double-stranded DNA antibody; HCV, hepatitis C virus; echo, echocardiogram; HSP, Henoch-Schönlein purpura; HUS, hemolytic-uremic syndrome; TTP, thrombotic thrombocytopenic purpura.

*Approximately 20% of patients with anti-GBM disease have ANCA, which may portend a better prognosis.

†Nephritic syndrome and RPGN are unusual presentations of IgA nephropathy and fibrillary GN.

‡Atheroembolic renal disease may cause transient hypocomplementemia.

§ANCA occasionally detected in association with lupus nephritis.

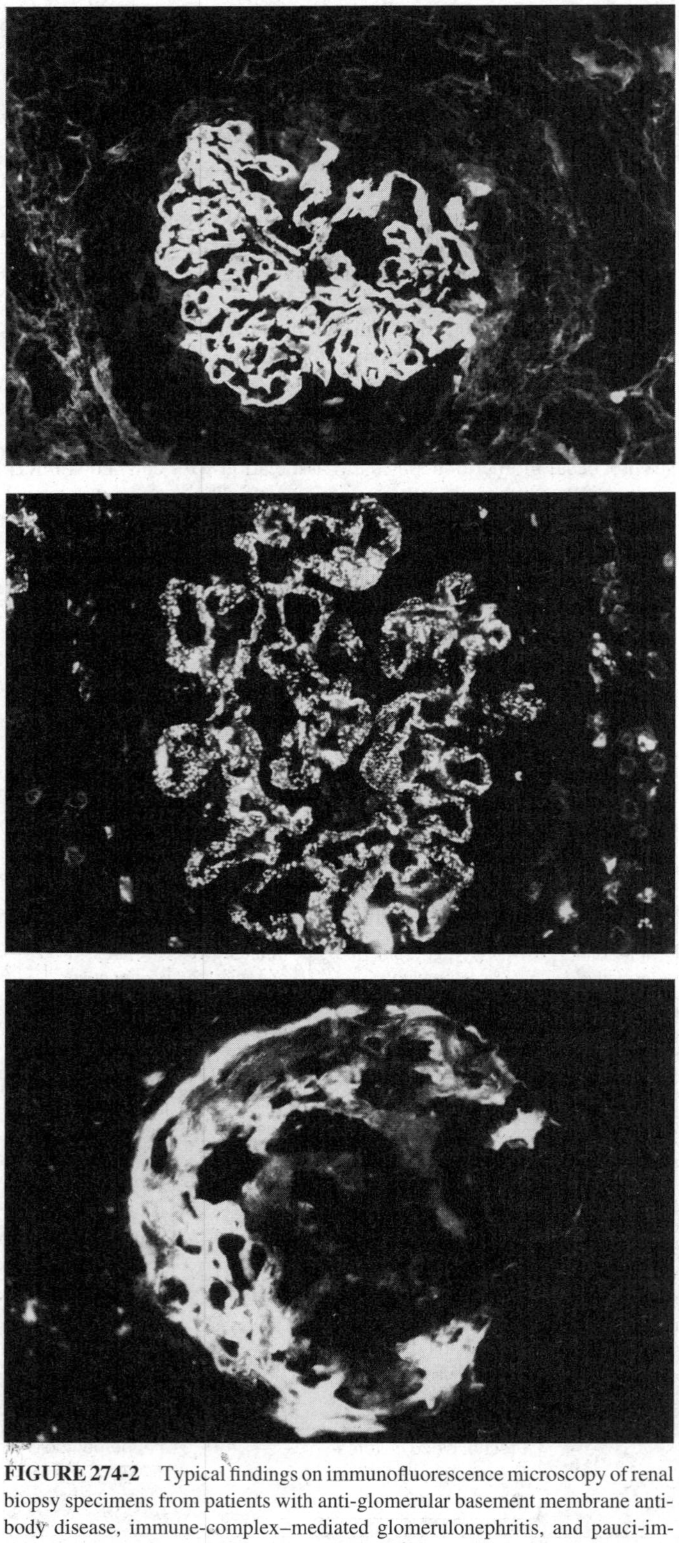

FIGURE 274-2 Typical findings on immunofluorescence microscopy of renal biopsy specimens from patients with anti-glomerular basement membrane antibody disease, immune-complex–mediated glomerulonephritis, and pauci-immune glomerulonephritis. Specimens in the upper and middle panels were stained for immunoglobulin and show the classical linear "ribbon-like" pattern of anti-GBM disease (*upper*) and granular pattern of immune-complex–mediated glomerulonephritis (*middle*). Immunoglobulin is sparse or absent in patients with pauci-immune glomerulonephritis; however, abundant fibrin is detected in crescents (*lower*). (*Micrographs courtesy of Dr. Helmut Rennke.*)

Patients with overt disease present with gross hematuria (red or "smoky" urine), headache, and generalized symptoms such as anorexia, nausea, vomiting, and malaise. Swelling of the renal capsule can cause flank or back pain. Physical examination reveals hypervolemia, edema, and hypertension. The urinary sediment is nephritic, with dysmorphic red blood cells, red cell casts, leukocytes, occasionally leukocyte casts, and proteinuria. Fewer than 5 percent of patients develop nephrotic-range proteinuria. The latter may only manifest as acute nephritis resolves and renal blood flow and GFR recover. Coexistent rheumatic fever is extremely rare.

The serum creatinine is typically elevated at presentation [88 to 177 μmol/L (1 to 2 mg/dL)]. Serum C3 levels and CH_{50} are depressed within 2 weeks in ~90 percent of cases. C4 levels are characteristically normal, indicating activation of the alternate pathway of complement. Complement levels usually return to normal within 6 to 8 weeks. Persistently depressed levels after this period should suggest another cause, such as the presence of a C3 nephritic factor (see "Membranoproliferative Glomerulonephritis"). The majority of patients (>75 percent) have transient hypergammaglobulinemia and mixed cryoglobulinemia. The antecedent streptococcal infection may still be evident or may have resolved either spontaneously or in response to antibiotic therapy. Most patients (>90 percent) have circulating antibodies against streptococcal exoenzymes such as antistreptolysin O (ASO), anti-deoxyribonuclease B (anti-DNAse B), antistreptokinase (ASKase), anti-nicotinyl adenine dinucleotidase (anti-NADase), and antihyaluronidase (AHase). ASO, anti-DNAse B, anti-NAD, and AHase are most useful after pharyngeal infection, whereas anti-DNAse B and AHase are more sensitive indices of streptococcal skin infection. Antibody titers tend to rise after 7 days, peak after 1 month, and return to normal levels after 3 to 4 months. These tests are relatively specific, with a false-positive rate of <5 percent. Early antibiotic therapy may prevent the development of an antibody response.

Acute poststreptococcal glomerulonephritis is usually diagnosed on clinical and serologic grounds, without resort to renal biopsy, especially in children with a typical antecedent history. The characteristic lesion on light microscopy is diffuse proliferative glomerulonephritis. Crescents are uncommon, and extraglomerular involvement is usually mild. Immunofluorescence microscopy reveals diffuse granular deposition of IgG and C3, giving rise to a "starry sky" appearance (Fig. 274-2). More extensive immunoglobulin deposition throughout the glomerular capillary wall ("garland pattern") is associated with a worse prognosis. The characteristic finding on electron microscopy is the presence of large electron-dense immune deposits in the subendothelial, subepithelial, and mesangial areas. It is likely that the acute inflammatory reaction is initiated, in large part, by the subendothelial and mesangial deposits, which activate complement and trigger leukocyte recruitment and glomerular injury. Subepithelial deposits may be more prominent on electron microscopy, however, probably because the subendothelial and mesangial deposits are scavenged more efficiently by invading phagocytes. Extensive subepithelial immune deposits, or "humps," tend to be associated with worse proteinuria, being juxtaposed to the glomerular filtration barrier for protein. → ***The pathogenesis of immune-complex glomerulonephritis is discussed extensively in Chap. 273.***

In addition to poststreptococcal glomerulonephritis, the nephritic syndrome and RPGN can complicate acute immune-complex glomerulonephritis due to other viral, bacterial, fungal, and parasitic infections. Several warrant specific mention. Diffuse proliferative immune-complex glomerulonephritis is a well-described complication of acute and subacute bacterial endocarditis and is usually associated with hypocomplementemia. The glomerular lesion typically resolves following eradication of the cardiac infection. *Shunt nephritis* is a syndrome characterized by immune-complex glomerulonephritis secondary to infection of ventriculoatrial shunts inserted for treatment of childhood hydrocephalus. The most common offending organism is coagulase-negative staphylococcus. Renal impairment is usually mild and associated with hypocomplementemia. Nephrotic syndrome complicates 30 percent of cases. Acute proliferative glomerulonephritis can also complicate *chronic suppurative infections* and *visceral abscesses*. Patients typically present with a fever of unknown origin and an active urine sediment. Although immune deposits containing IgG an C3 are detected on renal biopsy, serum complement levels are usually normal.

℞ TREATMENT

Treatment of poststreptococcal glomerulonephritis focuses on eliminating the streptococcal infection with antibiotics and providing supportive therapy until spontaneous resolution of glomerular inflammation occurs. Patients are usually confined to bed during the acute inflammatory phase. Diuretics and antihypertensive agents are employed to control extracellular fluid volume and blood pressure. Dialysis is rarely needed to control hypervolemia or the uremic syndrome. Poststreptococcal glomerulonephritis carries an excellent prognosis and rarely causes ESRD. Microscopic hematuria may persist for as long as 1 year after the acute episode but eventually resolves. Whereas complete recovery is the rule in children, adults may occasionally be left with residual renal impairment.

Antiglomerular Basement Membrane Disease Anti-GBM disease is an autoimmune disease in which autoantibodies directed against type IV collagen induce RPGN and crescentic glomerulonephritis. Acute nephritic syndrome is rare. Between 50 and 70 percent of patients have lung hemorrhage; the clinical complex of anti-GBM nephritis and lung hemorrhage is referred to as *Goodpasture's syndrome*. Anti-GBM disease is a rare disorder of unknown etiology with an annual incidence of 0.5 per million. There is a bimodal peak in incidence. Patients with Goodpasture's syndrome are typically young males (5 to 40 years; male-female ratio of 6:1). In contrast, patients presenting during the second peak in the sixth decade rarely suffer lung hemorrhage and have an almost equal sex distribution. The target antigen is a component of the noncollagenous domain (NCI) of the $\alpha3$ chain of type IV collagen, the $\alpha3$ chain being preferentially expressed in glomerular and pulmonary alveolar basement membrane. The trigger(s) for loss of self-tolerance to this Goodpasture antigen has not been well defined. A genetic predisposition is suggested by an association with HLA-DRw2 and occasional occurrence in identical twins. Patients with lung hemorrhage are more likely to be cigarette smokers and to have suffered a recent upper respiratory tract infection or exposure to volatile hydrocarbon solvents. These observations suggest that diverse insults to the alveolar basement membrane may render previously sequestered Goodpasture antigens available for interaction with circulating autoantibodies. It is not clear whether environmental factors also trigger the onset of nephritis. Binding of anti-GBM antibodies to the GBM induces activation of complement, leukocyte recruitment, necrotizing proliferative glomerulonephritis, disruption of the glomerular capillary wall, leakage of fibrin into Bowman's space, and crescent formation (see Chap. 273). A similar sequence of events in the lung leads to disruption of the alveolar capillary wall and pulmonary hemorrhage.

Anti-GBM disease commonly presents with hematuria, nephritic urinary sediment, subnephrotic proteinuria, and rapidly progressive renal failure over weeks, with or without pulmonary hemorrhage. When pulmonary hemorrhage occurs, it usually predates nephritis by weeks or months. Hemoptysis can vary from fluffy pulmonary infiltrates on chest x-ray and mild dyspnea on exertion to life-threatening pulmonary hemorrhage. Hypertension is unusual and occurs in fewer than 20 percent of cases.

The diagnostic serologic marker is circulating anti-GBM antibodies with a specificity for the NCI domain of the $\alpha3$ chain of type IV collagen (Fig. 274-1). Anti-GBM antibodies are detected in the serum of >90 percent of patients with anti-GBM nephritis by specific radioimmunoassay. If radioimmunoassay is not available, circulating anti-GBM antibodies can be detected in 60 to 80 percent of patients by indirect immunofluorescence, i.e., by incubating the patient's serum with stored sections of normal human kidneys. Complement levels are normal. About 20 percent of patients have low titers of ANCA, usually a perinuclear ANCA (see Chap. 275), the pathophysiologic significance of which is unclear. Occasional patients have a positive cytoplasmic ANCA, which may signal the presence of coexistent extraglomerular renal vasculitis. Patients with lung involvement frequently have microcytic, hypochromic, iron-deficiency anemia from alveolar hemorrhage, and abnormal bilateral hilar and basilar interstitial shadowing on chest x-ray that may be difficult to distinguish from pulmonary edema or infection. The diffusion capacity for carbon dioxide is a useful tool for distinguishing among the latter diagnoses, being increased in patients with lung hemorrhage due to uptake of carbon monoxide by alveolar blood, and reduced in patients with infection or pulmonary edema.

Renal biopsy is the gold standard for diagnosis of anti-GBM nephritis. The typical morphologic pattern on light microscopy is diffuse proliferative glomerulonephritis, with focal necrotizing lesions and crescents in >50 percent of glomeruli (crescentic glomerulonephritis). Immunofluorescence microscopy reveals linear ribbon-like deposition of IgG along the GBM (Fig. 274-2). C3 is present in the same distribution in 70 percent of patients. Prominent IgG deposition along the tubule basement membrane and tubulointerstitial inflammation is found occasionally. Electron microscopy reveals nonspecific inflammatory changes without immune deposits. Typical features on lung biopsy include alveolar hemorrhage, disruption of alveolar septa, hemosiderin-laden macrophages, and linear staining of IgG along the alveolar capillary basement membrane.

It should be noted that Goodpasture's syndrome is not the only cause of the pulmonary-renal syndrome (i.e., renal failure and lung hemorrhage). Other important causes of this clinical complex include severe cardiac failure complicated by pulmonary edema (often blood-tinged) and prerenal azotemia; renal failure from any cause complicated by hypervolemia and pulmonary edema; immune-complex–mediated vasculitides such as systemic lupus erythematosus (SLE), Henoch-Schönlein purpura, and cryoglobulinemia; pauci-immune vasculitides such as Wegener's granulomatosis and polyarteritis nodosa; infections such as Legionnaire's disease; and renal vein thrombosis with pulmonary embolism. In general, these disorders can be differentiated by astute analysis of the clinical, serologic, and histopathologic findings.

℞ TREATMENT

Prior to the introduction of immunosuppressive therapy, greater than 80 percent of patients with anti-GBM nephritis developed ESRD within 1 year, and many patients died from pulmonary hemorrhage or complications of uremia. With early and aggressive use of plasmapheresis, glucocorticoids, cyclophosphamide, and azathioprine, renal and patient survival have improved dramatically. In general, emergency plasmapheresis is performed daily or on alternate days until anti-GBM antibodies are not detected in the circulation (usually 1 to 2 weeks). Prednisone (1 mg/kg per day) is started simultaneously, in combination with either cyclophosphamide (2 to 3 mg/kg per day) or azathioprine (1 to 2 mg/kg per day) to suppress new synthesis of anti-GBM antibodies. The speed of initiation of therapy is a critical determinant of outcome. One-year renal survival approaches 90 percent if treatment is started before serum creatinine exceeds 442 μmol/L (5 mg/dL) and falls to about 10 percent if renal failure is more advanced. Patients who require dialysis at presentation rarely recover renal function. Serial anti-GBM titers are monitored to gauge response to therapy. Relapses are not unusual and are often heralded by rising antibody titers. In patients with ESRD, renal transplantation is a viable treatment option. Recurrence of anti-GBM nephritis in the allograft is extremely unusual provided that anti-GBM antibody titers have been consistently negative for 2 to 3 months prior to transplantation.

Pauci-Immune Glomerulonephritis The major pauci-immune glomerulonephritides are *idiopathic renal-limited crescentic glomerulonephritis*, *microscopic polyarteritis nodosa*, and *Wegener's granulomatosis* (Fig. 274-1). RPGN is a more common clinical presentation than acute nephritic syndrome, and the usual pathology is necrotizing glomerulonephritis with crescents affecting >50 percent of glomeruli (crescentic glomerulonephritis). The marked overlap of clinical features and glomerular histopathology, and the presence of circulating

ANCA in most patients, suggest that these entities are a spectrum of a single disease. Here, we focus on idiopathic renal-limited crescentic glomerulonephritis. The ANCA-associated glomerulopathies with extrarenal features, namely Wegener's granulomatosis and microscopic polyarteritis nodosa, are discussed in Chap. 275.

Idiopathic Renal-Limited Crescentic Glomerulonephritis This is more common in middle-aged and older patients and shows a slight male preponderance. Patients typically present with RPGN, nephritic syndrome being rare. ANCA, usually a perinuclear ANCA IgG with specificity for myeloperoxidase (see Chap. 275), are detected in 70 to 90 percent of patients (Fig. 274-1). The erythrocyte sedimentation rate and C-reactive protein levels may be elevated; however, C3 levels are typically normal, and circulating immune complexes, cryoglobulins, and anti-GBM antibodies are not detected. Most patients have crescents on light microscopy, often associated with necrotizing glomerulonephritis. Immune deposits are scanty or absent. Immunofluorescence microscopy reveals abundant fibrin deposits within crescents (Fig. 274-2). Most cases are treated aggressively with glucocorticoids, with or without cyclophosphamide or azathioprine (see Chap. 275).

NEPHROTIC SYNDROME

GENERAL FEATURES AND COMPLICATIONS The *nephrotic syndrome* is a clinical complex characterized by a number of renal and extrarenal features, the most prominent of which are proteinuria of >3.5 g per 1.73 m^2 per 24 h (in practice, >3.0 to 3.5 g per 24 h), hypoalbuminemia, edema, hyperlipidemia, lipiduria, and hypercoagulability. It should be stressed that the key component is *proteinuria*, which results from altered permeability of the glomerular filtration barrier for protein, namely the GBM and the podocytes and their slit diaphragms. The other components of the nephrotic syndrome and the ensuing metabolic complications are all secondary to urine protein loss and can occur with lesser degrees of proteinuria or may be absent even in patients with massive proteinuria.

In general, the greater the proteinuria, the lower the serum albumin level. *Hypoalbuminemia* is compounded further by increased renal catabolism and inadequate, albeit usually increased, hepatic synthesis of albumin. The pathophysiology of *edema* formation in nephrotic syndrome is poorly understood. The *underfilling hypothesis* postulates that hypoalbuminemia results in decreased intravascular oncotic pressure, leading to leakage of extracellular fluid from blood to the interstitium. Intravascular volume falls, thereby stimulating activation of the renin-angiotensin-aldosterone axis and the sympathetic nervous system and release of vasopressin (antidiuretic hormone), and suppressing atrial natriuretic peptide release. These neural and hormonal responses promote renal salt and water retention, thereby restoring intravascular volume and triggering further leakage of fluid to the interstitium. This hypothesis does not, however, explain the occurrence of edema in many patients in whom plasma volume is expanded and the renin-angiotensin-aldosterone axis is suppressed. The latter finding suggests that *primary renal salt and water retention* may also contribute to edema formation in some cases.

Hyperlipidemia is believed to be a consequence of increased hepatic lipoprotein synthesis that is triggered by reduced oncotic pressure and may be compounded by increased urine loss of proteins that regulate lipid homeostasis. Low-density lipoproteins and cholesterol are increased in the majority of patients, whereas very low density lipoproteins and triglycerides tend to rise in patients with severe disease. Although not proven conclusively, hyperlipidemia may accelerate atherosclerosis and progression of renal disease.

Hypercoagulability is probably multifactorial in origin and is caused, at least in part, by increased urinary loss of antithrombin III, altered levels and/or activity of proteins C and S, hyperfibrinogenemia due to increased hepatic synthesis, impaired fibrinolysis, and increased platelet aggregability. As a consequence of these perturbations, patients can develop spontaneous *peripheral arterial or venous thrombosis*, *renal vein thrombosis*, and *pulmonary embolism*. Clinical features that suggest acute renal vein thrombosis include sudden onset of flank or abdominal pain, gross hematuria, a left-sided varicocele (the left testicular vein drains into the renal vein), increased proteinuria, and an acute decline in GFR. Chronic renal vein thrombosis is usually asymptomatic. Renal vein thrombosis is particularly common (up to 40 percent) in patients with nephrotic syndrome due to membranous glomerulopathy, membranoproliferative glomerulonephritis, and amyloidosis.

Other metabolic complications of nephrotic syndrome include *protein malnutrition* and iron-resistant *microcytic hypochromic anemia* due to transferrin loss. *Hypocalcemia* and secondary hyperparathyroidism can occur as a consequence of vitamin D deficiency due to enhanced urinary excretion of cholecalciferol-binding protein, whereas loss of thyroxine-binding globulin can result in *depressed thyroxine levels*. An increased susceptibility to *infection* may reflect low levels of IgG that result from urinary loss and increased catabolism. In addition, patients are prone to unpredictable changes in the *pharmacokinetics* of therapeutic agents that are normally bound to plasma proteins.

ETIOLOGY AND DIFFERENTIAL DIAGNOSIS Proteinuria of greater than 150 mg per 24 h is abnormal and can result from a number of mechanisms. *Glomerular proteinuria* results from leakage of plasma proteins through a perturbed glomerular filtration barrier; *tubular proteinuria* results from failure of tubular reabsorption of low-molecular-weight plasma proteins that are normally filtered and then reabsorbed and metabolized by tubular epithelium; *overflow proteinuria* results from filtration of proteins, usually immunoglobulin light chains, that are present in excess in the circulation. Tubular proteinuria virtually never exceeds 2 g per 24 h and thus, by definition, never causes nephrotic syndrome. Overflow proteinuria should be suspected in patients with clinical or laboratory evidence of multiple myeloma or other lymphoproliferative malignancy. Suspicion is heightened when there is a discrepancy between proteinuria detected by dipsticks, which are sensitive to albumin but not light chains, and the sulfosalicylic acid precipitation method, which detects both.

Nephrotic syndrome can complicate any disease that perturbs the negative electrostatic charge or architecture of the GBM and the podocytes and their slit diaphragms. Six entities account for greater than 90 percent of cases of nephrotic syndrome in adults: minimal change disease (MCD), focal and segmental glomerulosclerosis (FSGS), membranous glomerulopathy, MPGN, diabetic nephropathy, and amyloidosis. Diabetic nephropathy and amyloidosis, being manifestations of systemic diseases, are discussed in Chap. 275. *Renal biopsy* is a valuable tool in adults with nephrotic syndrome for establishing a definitive diagnosis, guiding therapy, and estimating prognosis. Renal biopsy is not required in the majority of children with nephrotic syndrome as most cases are due to MCD and respond to empiric treatment with glucocorticoids.

MINIMAL CHANGE DISEASE This glomerulopathy accounts for about 80 percent of nephrotic syndrome in children of younger than 16 years and 20 percent in adults (Table 274-1). The peak incidence is between 6 and 8 years. Patients typically present

Table 274-1

Causes of Minimal Change Disease (Nil Disease, Lipoid Nephrosis)
Idiopathic (majority)
In association with systemic diseases or drugs
Drug-induced interstitial nephritis induced by NSAIDs, rifampin, interferon α
Hodgkin's disease and other lymphoproliferative malignancy
Human immunodeficiency virus infection
IgA nephropathy
Diabetes mellitus
Fabry's disease
Sialidosis
Heroin use
Iron dextran administration

with nephrotic syndrome and benign urinary sediment. Microscopic hematuria is present in 20 to 30 percent. Hypertension and renal insufficiency are very rare.

MCD (also called nil disease, lipoid nephrosis, or foot process disease) is so named because glomerular size and architecture are normal by light microscopy. Immunofluorescence studies are typically negative for immunoglobulin and C3. Mild mesangial hypercellularity and sparse deposits of C3 and IgM may be detected. Occasionally, mesangial proliferation is associated with scanty IgA deposits, similar to those found in IgA nephropathy. However, the natural history of this variant and response to therapy resemble classic MCD. Electron microscopy reveals characteristic *diffuse effacement of the foot processes of visceral epithelial cells* (Fig. 274-3). This morphologic finding is referred to as foot process fusion in the older literature.

The etiology of MCD is unknown and the vast majority of cases are idiopathic (Table 274-1). MCD occasionally develops after upper respiratory tract infection, immunizations, and atopic attacks. Patients with atopy and MCD have an increased incidence of HLA-B12, suggesting a genetic predisposition. MCD, often in association with interstitial nephritis, is a rare side effect of nonsteroidal anti-inflammatory drugs (NSAIDs), rifampin, and interferon α. Rare cases occur in association with inherited and acquired metabolic diseases such as Fabry's disease, sialidosis, and diabetes mellitus (see Chap. 275). The occasional association with lymphoproliferative malignancies (such as Hodgkin's lymphoma), the tendency for idiopathic MCD to remit during intercurrent viral infection such as measles, and the good response of idiopathic forms to immunosuppressive agents (see below) suggest an immune etiology. In children, the urine contains albumin principally and minimal amounts of higher molecular weight proteins such as IgG and α_2-macroglobulin. This *selective proteinuria* in conjunction with foot process effacement suggests injury to podocytes and loss of the fixed *negative charge* in the glomerular filtration barrier for protein. Proteinuria is typically nonselective in adults, suggesting more extensive perturbation of membrane permeability.

Rx TREATMENT

MCD is highly steroid-responsive and carries an excellent prognosis. Spontaneous remission occurs in 30 to 40 percent of childhood cases, but is less common in adults. Approximately 90 percent of children and 50 percent of adults enter remission following 8 weeks of high-dose oral glucocorticoids. In a typical regimen, children receive 60 mg of prednisone per m^2 of body surface area daily for 4 weeks, followed by 40 mg/m^2 on alternate days for an additional 4 weeks. Adults receive 1 to 1.5 mg/kg body weight per day for 4 weeks, followed by 1 mg/kg per day on alternate days for 4 weeks. Up to 90 percent of adults enter remission if therapy is extended for 20 to 24 weeks. Nephrotic syndrome relapses in over 50 percent of cases following withdrawal of glucocorticoids. Alkylating agents are reserved for the small number of patients who fail to achieve lasting remission. These include patients who relapse during or shortly after withdrawal of steroids (steroid-dependent) and those who relapse more than three times per year (frequently relapsing). In these settings, cyclophosphamide (2 to 3 mg/kg per day) or chlorambucil (0.1 to 0.2 mg/kg per day) is started after steroid-induced remission and continued for 8 to 12 weeks. Cytotoxic agents may also induce remission in occasional steroid-resistant cases. These benefits must be balanced against the risk of infertility, cystitis, alopecia, infection, and secondary malignancies, particularly in children and young adults. Azathioprine has not been proven to be a useful adjunct to steroid therapy. Cyclosporine induces remission in 60 to 80 percent of patients; it is an alternative to cytotoxic agents and an option in patients who are resistant to cytotoxic agents. Unfortunately, relapse is usual when cyclosporine is withdrawn, and long-term therapy carries the risk of nephrotoxicity and other side effects. Long-term renal and patient survival is excellent in MCD.

FOCAL AND SEGMENTAL GLOMERULOSCLEROSIS WITH HYALINOSIS The pathognomonic morphologic lesion in FSGS is sclerosis with hyalinosis involving portions (segmental) of

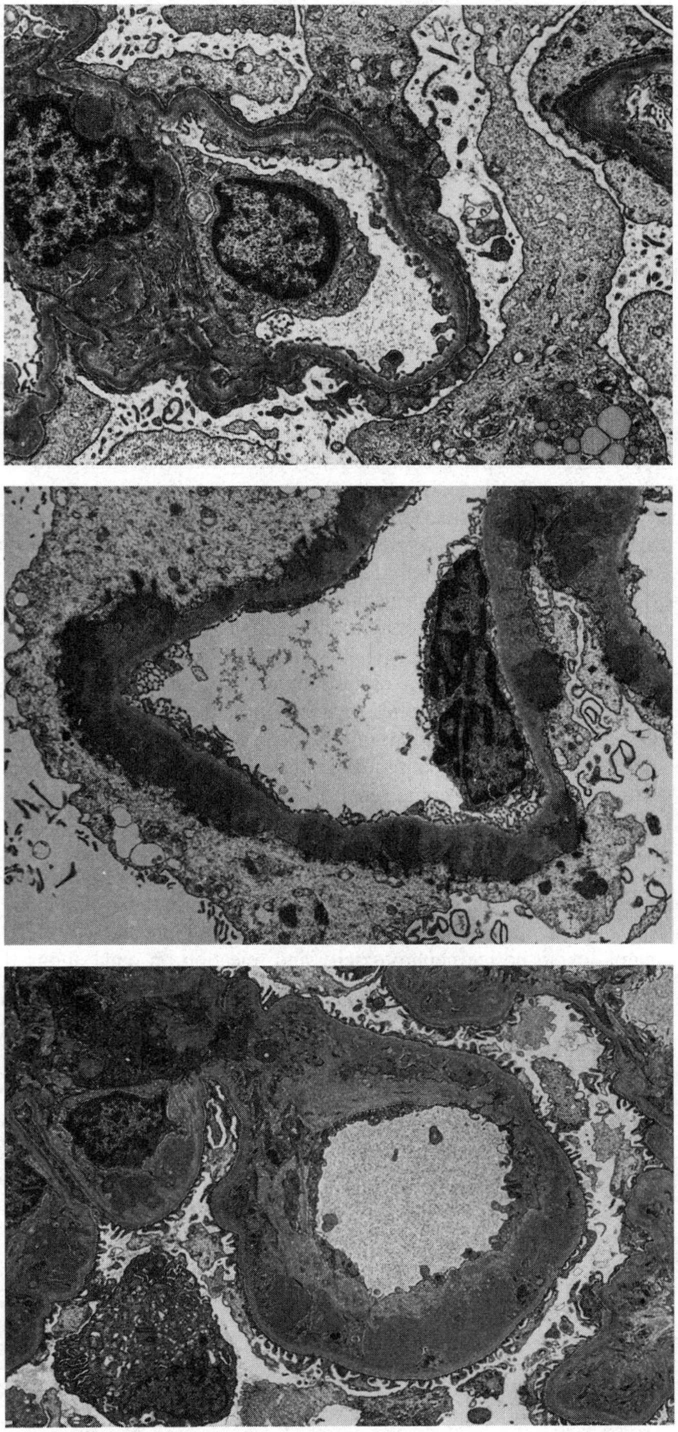

FIGURE 274-3 Typical findings on electron microscopy of renal biopsy specimens from patients with minimal change glomerulopathy, membranous glomerulopathy, and membranoproliferative glomerulonephritis. The pathognomonic feature of minimal change glomerulopathy (*upper*) is effacement of foot processes of visceral epithelial cells (podocytes), giving the impression of foot process fusion. Foot process effacement is also evident in focal and segmental glomerulosclerosis (not shown here); in addition, there is typically detachment of podocytes from basement membrane, areas of glomerular capillary collapse, deposits of hyaline material, and sclerosis. Membranous nephropathy (*middle*) is characterized by immune complexes in the subepithelial space. These electron-dense immune deposits stimulate production of new GBM, which eventually surrounds and incorporates the immune deposits into the GBM. The hallmarks of type I membranoproliferative glomerulonephritis (*lower panel*) are increased mesangial cellularity and matrix and thickening and reduplication of the GBM. The latter is initiated by formation of electron-dense immune complexes on the subendothelial aspect of the GBM, which are subsequently covered by a new layer of GBM, probably produced by regenerating endothelial cells. *(Micrographs courtesy of Dr. Helmut Rennke.)*

fewer than 50 percent (focal) of glomeruli on a tissue section. Idiopathic (primary) FSGS accounts for 10 to 15 percent of nephrotic syndrome in children and 15 to 25 percent in adults. FSGS can complicate a number of systemic diseases and sustained glomerular capillary hypertension following nephron loss from any cause (Table 274-2 and Chap. 273).

Idiopathic FSGS typically presents as nephrotic syndrome (~66 percent) or subnephrotic proteinuria (~33 percent) in association with hypertension, mild renal insufficiency, and an abnormal urine sediment that contains red blood cells and leukocytes. Proteinuria is nonselective in most cases.

Light microscopy of renal biopsy tissue reveals FSGS with entrapment of amorphous hyaline material, a process that shows a predilection for juxtamedullary glomeruli. The sclerotic scars contain areas of glomerular capillary collapse and hyaline material composed of collagen types I, III, and IV. Adhesions occur between areas of capillary collapse and Bowman's capsule. Immunofluorescence studies are usually negative. Electron microscopy reveals evidence of damage to visceral epithelial cells, including swelling and detachment of podocytes from the GBM, effacement of foot processes, transition to foam cells, and overt cell degeneration and necrosis.

The etiology of primary FSGS is unclear (Table 274-2). The overlap of clinical and morphologic features between MCD and FSGS has prompted some authorities to speculate that they are a spectrum of morphologic manifestations of a single pathogenetic process. FSGS is a potential long-term consequence of nephron loss from any cause. It can complicate congenital renal diseases such as congenital oligomeganephronia, in which both kidneys have a reduced complement of nephrons, and congenital unilateral agenesis. In addition, FSGS may develop following acquired loss of nephrons from extensive surgical ablation of renal mass, reflux nephropathy, glomerulonephritis, interstitial nephritis, sickle cell disease, and the combined effects of ischemia, cyclosporine nephrotoxicity and rejection on renal allograft function (Table 274-2). It appears that >50 percent of nephrons must be lost for development of secondary FSGS.

℞ TREATMENT

In contrast to MCD, spontaneous remission of primary FSGS is rare and renal prognosis is relatively poor. Proteinuria remits in only 20 to 40 percent of patients treated with glucocorticoids for 8 weeks. Uncontrolled studies suggest that up to 70 percent respond when steroid therapy is prolonged for 16 to 24 weeks. Cyclophosphamide and cyclosporine, when used at doses described above for MCD, induce partial or complete remission in 50 to 60 percent of steroid-responsive patients, but are generally ineffective in steroid-resistant cases. Poor prognostic factors at presentation include hypertension, abnormal renal function, black race, and persistent heavy proteinuria. Renal transplantation is complicated by recurrence of FSGS in the allograft in about 50 percent of cases and graft loss in about 10 percent. Factors associated with an increased risk of recurrence include a short time interval between the onset of the FSGS and ESRD, young age at onset, and possibly the presence of mesangial hypercellularity on renal biopsy.

MEMBRANOUS GLOMERULOPATHY This lesion is the most common cause of idiopathic nephrotic syndrome in adults (30 to 40 percent) and a rare cause in children (<5 percent). It has a peak incidence between the ages of 30 to 50 years and a male-female ratio of 2:1 (Table 274-3). Membranous glomerulopathy derives its name from the characteristic light-microscopic appearance on renal biopsy, namely diffuse thickening of the GBM, which is most apparent upon staining with periodic acid Schiff (PAS). Most patients (>80 percent) present with nephrotic syndrome, proteinuria usually being nonselective. Microscopic hematuria is present in up to 50 percent of cases, but red blood cells casts, macroscopic hematuria, and leukocytes are extremely rare. Hypertension is documented in only 10 to 30 percent of patients at the outset but is common later in patients with progressive renal failure. Serologic tests such as antinuclear antibody, ANCA, anti-GBM antibody, cryoglobulin titers, and complement levels are normal in the idiopathic form.

Light microscopy of renal biopsy sections reveals diffuse thickening of the GBM without evidence of inflammation or cellular proliferation. Silver staining demonstrates characteristic *spikes* along the GBM, which represent projections of new basement membrane engulfing subepithelial immune deposits. Immunofluorescence reveals granular deposition of IgG, C3, and the terminal components of complement (C_{5b-9}) along the glomerular capillary wall. Electron-microscopic appearances vary depending on the stage of disease. The earliest finding is the presence of subepithelial immune deposits (Fig. 274-3). As these deposits enlarge, spikes of new basement membrane extend out between the immune deposits and begin to engulf them. With time, the deposits are completely surrounded and incorporated into the basement membrane.

The pathogenesis of idiopathic human membranous glomerulopathy is incompletely understood. The presence of electron-dense immune deposits that contain IgG and C3 suggest an immune process. About one-third of adult membranous nephropathy occurs in association with systemic diseases such as SLE, infections such as hepatitis

Table 274-2

Etiology of Focal and Segmental Glomerulosclerosis

Idiopathic (majority)
In association with systemic diseases or drugs
- HIV infection
- Diabetes mellitus
- Fabry's disease
- Sialidosis
- Charcot-Marie-Tooth disease

As consequence of sustained glomerular capillary hypertension
- Congenital oligonephropathies
  - Unilateral renal agenesis
  - Oligomeganephronia
- Acquired nephron loss
  - Surgical resection
  - Reflux nephropathy
  - Glomerulonephritis or tubulointerstitial nephritis
- Other adaptive responses
  - Sickle cell nephropathy
  - Obesity with sleep apnea syndrome
  - Familial dysautonomia
- Miscellaneous
  - Heroin use

Table 274-3

Conditions Associated with Membranous Glomerulopathy

Idiopathic (majority)
In association with systemic diseases or drugs
- Infection
  - Hepatitis B and C, secondary and congenital syphilis, malaria, schistosomiasis, leprosy, hydatid disease, filariasis, enterococcal endocarditis
- Systemic autoimmune diseases
  - SLE, rheumatoid disease, Sjögren's syndrome, Hashimoto's disease, Graves' disease, mixed connective tissue disease, primary biliary cirrhosis, ankylosing spondylitis, dermatitis herpetiformis, bullous pemphigoid, myasthenia gravis
- Neoplasia
  - Carcinoma of the breast, lung, colon, stomach, and esophagus; melanoma; renal cell carcinoma; neuroblastoma; carotid body tumor
- Drugs
  - Gold, penicillamine, captopril, NSAIDs, probenecid, trimethadione, chlormethiazole, mercury
- Miscellaneous
  - Sarcoidosis, diabetes mellitus, sickle cell disease, Crohn's disease, Guillain-Barré syndrome, Weber-Christian disease, Fanconi's syndrome, α_1 antitrypsin deficiency, angiofollicular lymph node hyperplasia

B, malignancy, and drug therapy with gold and penicillamine (Table 274-3).

Nephrotic syndrome remits spontaneously and completely in up to 40 percent of patients with membranous glomerulopathy. The natural history of another 30 to 40 percent is characterized by repeated relapses and remissions. The final 10 to 20 percent suffer a slow progressive decline in GFR that typically culminates in ESRD after 10 to 15 years. Presenting features that predict a poor prognosis include male gender, older age, hypertension, severe proteinuria and hyperlipidemia, and impaired renal function. Controlled trials of glucocorticoids have failed to show consistent improvement in proteinuria or renal protection. Cyclophosphamide, chlorambucil, and cyclosporine have each been shown to reduce proteinuria and/or slow the decline in GFR in patients with progressive disease in small or uncontrolled studies. These observations need to be confirmed in controlled prospective studies. Transplantation is a successful treatment option for patients who reach ESRD.

MEMBRANOPROLIFERATIVE GLOMERULONEPHRITIS This morphologic entity, also known as mesangiocapillary glomerulonephritis, is characterized by thickening of the GBM and proliferative changes on light microscopy (Table 274-4). It is equally common in males and females and more common in whites. Two major types are identified. Both are characterized by a diffuse increase in mesangial cellularity and matrix and thickening and reduplication of the GBM such that the lobular pattern of the glomerular tuft is exaggerated. The hallmark of type I MPGN is the presence of subendothelial and mesangial deposits on electron microscopy that contain C3 and IgG or IgM; rarely, IgA deposits are demonstrated by immunofluorescence microscopy (Fig. 274-3). The hallmark of type II MPGN (dense deposit disease) is the presence of electron-dense deposits within the GBM and other renal basement membranes (shown by electron microscopy) that stain for C3 but little or no immunoglobulin.

Most patients with type I MPGN present with heavy proteinuria or nephrotic syndrome, active urinary sediment, and normal or mildly impaired GFR. C3 levels are usually depressed, and C1q and C4 levels are borderline or low. Type I MPGN is an immune-complex glomerulonephritis and can be associated with a variety of chronic infections (e.g., bacterial endocarditis, human immunodeficiency virus, hepatitis B and C), systemic immune-complex diseases (e.g., SLE, cryoglobulinemia) and malignancies (e.g., leukemias, lymphomas). Type I MPGN is a relatively benign disease, and 70 to 85 percent of patients survive without clinically significant impairment of GFR.

Table 274-4

Causes of Membranoproliferative (Mesangiocapillary) Glomerulonephritis

Idiopathic	
Type I	With subendothelial and mesangial immune deposits
Type II	With intramembranous dense deposits containing sparse or no Ig; associated with C3 nephritic factor
Type III	Features of type I MPGN and membranous nephropathy
In association with systemic diseases or drugs*	
Systemic immune-complex disease	SLE, mixed cryoglobulinemia, Sjögren's syndrome
Chronic infections	Hepatitis B and C, human immunodeficiency virus, bacterial endocarditis, ventriculoatrial shunts, visceral abscess
Malignancy	Leukemias, lymphomas
Liver disease	Chronic active hepatitis and cirrhosis (usually associated with hepatitis B or C)
Miscellaneous	Partial lipodystrophy, heroin use, sarcoidosis, inherited C2 deficiency, thrombotic microangiopathies

* Usual with morphologic features of idiopathic type 1 MPGN (see above).

There is no proven therapy for patients with progressive disease beyond eradicating the underlying infection, malignancy, or systemic disease, when possible.

Type II MPGN can also present with proteinuria and nephrotic syndrome; however, some patients present with nephritic syndrome, RPGN, or recurrent macroscopic hematuria. Type II MPGN is an autoimmune disease in which patients have an IgG autoantibody, termed *C3 nephritic factor*, that binds to C3 convertase, the enzyme that metabolizes C3, and renders it resistant to inactivation (see Chap. 273). Type II MPGN runs a variable course; the GFR remains stable in some patients and declines gradually to ESRD over 5 to 10 years in others. There is no effective therapy for this disease.

FIBRILLARY-IMMUNOTACTOID GLOMERULOPATHY This emerging clinicopathologic entity accounts for 1 percent of diagnoses in most large renal biopsy series. Virtually all patients present with proteinuria, and >50 percent have nephrotic syndrome. The majority of patients also have hematuria, hypertension, and renal insufficiency. The light-microscopic appearances vary from mesangial expansion and basement membrane thickening with PAS-positive material to proliferative and crescentic glomerulonephritis. On electron microscopy, this PAS-positive material is observed to be composed of randomly arranged (fibrillary glomerulopathy) or organized bundles (immunotactoid glomerulopathy) of microfibrils and microtubules, the compositon of which has yet to be defined. The etiology of fibrillary-immunotactoid glomerulopathy remains to be determined. Patients with the immunotactoid variant have an increased incidence of lymphoproliferative malignancy. There is no proven therapy for fibrillary-immunotactoid glomerulopathy, and many patients progress to ESRD over 1 to 10 years. Transplantation appears to be a viable option in the latter setting.

MESANGIAL PROLIFERATIVE GLOMERULONEPHRITIS In 5 to 10 percent of patients with idiopathic nephrotic syndrome, renal biopsy reveals a diffuse increase in glomerular cellularity, predominantly due to proliferation of mesangial and endothelial cells, and infiltration by monocytes. Findings on immunofluorescence microscopy vary and include deposits of IgA, IgG, IgM, and/or complement, or absence of immune reactants. It is likely that this morphologic entity is, in fact, a heterogeneous group of diseases that includes atypical forms of MCD and FSGS, and milder or resolving forms of the immune-complex and pauci-immune glomerulopathies described above under nephritic syndrome and RPGN. In keeping with the heterogeneity of this diagnosis, the prognosis is variable. In general, persistent nephrotic range proteinuria signals a poor prognosis, with many patients progressing to ESRD over 10 to 20 years despite immunosuppressive therapy.

℞ TREATMENT

Nephrotic Syndrome and Complications The treatment of nephrotic syndrome involves (1) specific treatment of the underlying morphologic entity and, when possible, causative disease (see above); (2) general measures to control proteinuria if remission is not achieved through immunosuppressive therapy and other specific measures; and (3) general measures to control nephrotic complications.

General measures may be warranted to control proteinuria in nephrotic syndrome if patients do not respond to immunosuppressive therapy and other specific measures and suffer progressive renal failure or severe nephrotic complications. Nonspecific measures that may reduce proteinuria include *dietary protein restriction*, *angiotensin-converting enzyme* (*ACE*) *inhibitors*, and *NSAIDs*. The first two of these measures aim to reduce proteinuria and slow the rate of progression of renal failure by lowering intraglomerular pressure and preventing the development of hemodynamically mediated focal segmental glomerulosclerosis. There is conclusive evidence that ACE inhibitors are renoprotective in human diabetic nephropathy (see Chap. 275) and that both ACE inhibitors and dietary protein restriction slow the development of secondary FSGS in experimental animals. Their role in the treatment of nephrotic syndrome in other settings is unproven. NSAIDs also reduce proteinuria in some patients with nephrotic syndrome, probably by altering glomerular hemodynamics or GBM permeability characteristics. This potential benefit must be balanced against the risk of inducing acute renal failure, hyperkalemia, salt and water retention, and other side effects.

Complications of nephrotic syndrome that may require treatment include edema, hyperlipidemia, thromboembolism, malnutrition, and vitamin D deficiency. Edema should be managed cautiously by moderate *salt restriction* usually 1 to 2 g/day, and the judicious use of *loop diuretics*. It is unwise to remove >1.0 kg of edema per day as more aggressive diuresis may precipitate intravascular volume depletion and prerenal azotemia. Administration of salt-poor albumin is not recommended as most is excreted within 24 to 48 h. Whereas many nephrologists advocate lowering low-density lipoproteins and cholesterol levels with *lipid-lowering drugs* to prevent accelerated atherosclerosis and slow the rate of decline of GFR, the value of such interventions in this setting has not been conclusively shown. *Anticoagulation* is indicated for patients with deep venous thrombosis, arterial thrombosis, and pulmonary embolism. Patients may be relatively resistant to heparin as a consequence of antithrombin III deficiency. Renal vein and vena caval angiography are probably indicated only when embolization occurs on anticoagulation and insertion of a caval filter is contemplated. There is no consensus regarding the optimal *diet* for patients with nephrotic syndrome. High-protein diets to prevent protein malnutrition are now in disfavor, since protein supplements have little, if any, effect on serum albumin levels and may hasten the progression of renal disease by increasing urinary protein excretion. The potential value of dietary protein restriction for reducing proteinuria and slowing the decline in GFR is discussed above. *Vitamin D* supplementation is advisable in patients with clinical or biochemical evidence of vitamin D deficiency.

ASYMPTOMATIC ABNORMALITIES OF THE URINARY SEDIMENT

HEMATURIA Most asymptomatic glomerular hematuria is due to *IgA nephropathy* (Berger's disease) or *thin basement membrane (TBM) disease* (benign hematuria). A rarer but more ominous cause of isolated hematuria is *Alport's syndrome*. The latter is the most common form of hereditary nephritis, is usually transmitted as an X-linked dominant trait, and is associated with sensorineural deafness, ophthalmologic abnormalities, and progressive renal insufficiency (see Chap. 275). TBM disease is sometimes familial but, in contrast to Alport's syndrome, is a benign disorder. Asymptomatic hematuria may also be the presenting feature of indolent forms of most other primary and secondary proliferative glomerulopathies (see Fig. 274-1). Glomerular hematuria must be distinguished from a variety of renal parenchymal and extrarenal causes of hematuria. It is particularly important to exclude malignancy of the kidney or urinary tract, particularly in older male patients (see Chap. 96). Other potential diagnoses include vascular, cystic, and tubulointerstitial diseases; papillary necrosis; hypercalciuria and hyperuricosuria; benign prostatic hypertrophy; and renal calculi. Important clues to the presence of glomerular hematuria are the presence of urinary red blood cell casts, dysmorphic urinary red blood cells, proteinuria of greater than 2.0 g per 24 h, and clinical or serologic evidence of nephritic syndrome, RPGN, or a compatible systemic disease.

IgA Nephropathy (Berger's Disease) IgA nephropathy is the most common glomerulopathy worldwide and accounts for 10 to 40 percent of glomerulonephritis in most series (Table 274-5). The disease is particularly common in southern Europe and Asia and appears to be more common in blacks than whites. Familial clustering has been reported but is rare. No consistent HLA association has emerged, although HLA-B35 appears to be more common in French patients. Most cases are idiopathic. The renal and serologic abnormalities in IgA nephropathy and Henoch-Schönlein purpura (see Chap. 275) are indistinguishable, and most authorities consider these to be a spectrum of a single disease. Less commonly, IgA nephropathy is found in association with systemic diseases, including chronic liver disease, Crohn's disease, gastrointestinal adenocarcinoma, chronic obstructive bronchiolitis, idiopathic interstitial pneumonia, dermatitis herpetiformis, mycosis fungoides, leprosy, ankylosing spondylitis, relapsing polychondritis, and Sjögren's syndrome. In many of these conditions, IgA is deposited in the glomerulus without inducing inflammation, and this may be a clinically insignificant consequence of perturbed IgA homeostasis.

Patients with IgA nephropathy typically present with gross hematuria, often 24 to 48 h after a pharyngeal or gastrointestinal infection, vaccination, or strenuous exercise. Other cases are diagnosed upon detection of microscopic hematuria during routine physical examinations. Hypertension (20 to 30 percent) and nephrotic syndrome (~10 percent) are unusual at presentation. Light microscopy of renal biopsy specimens typically shows mesangial expansion by increased matrix and cells. Diffuse proliferation, cellular crescents, interstitial inflammation, and areas of glomerulosclerosis may be evident in severe cases. The diagnostic finding, for which the disease is named, is mesangial deposition of IgA, detected by immunofluorescence microscopy. C3 is usually detected in the area of immune deposits, and IgG is observed in 50 percent of cases. Electron microscopy reveals electron-dense deposits in the mesangium and, in severe cases, these extend into the paramesangial subendothelial space. The pathogenesis of IgA nephropathy is incompletely understood.

℞ TREATMENT

There is no proven therapy for IgA nephropathy. A recent, relatively large randomized controlled trial suggested a benefit of fish oils in patients with progressive disease and heavy proteinuria; however, this experience has not been universal. Some authorities advocate a trial of high-dose immunosuppressive therapy in patients with severe nephrotic syndrome and those with nephritic syndrome or RPGN and evidence of active inflammation on renal biopsy.

IgA nephropathy typically smolders for decades, with patients often suffering exacerbations of hematuria and renal impairment during intercurrent infections. As many as 20 to 50 percent of patients develop ESRD within 20 years. Clinical predictors of a poor prognosis include older age, male sex, hypertension, nephrotic-range proteinuria, and renal insufficiency at presentation. Histologic features that predict an aggressive course include diffuse severe disease, extracapillary proliferation (crescents), extension of immune attack into the paramesangial subendothelial space, glomerulosclerosis, interstitial fibrosis, and arteriolar hyalinosis.

Thin Basement Membrane Disease (Benign Hematuria) This disorder can be heredofamilial or sporadic and is as common as IgA nephropathy in some series of asymptomatic hematuria. When familial,

Table 274-5

Diseases Associated with IgA Nephropathy

Idiopathic (majority)	
Renal-limited or as component of Henoch-Schönlein Purpura	
In association with systemic diseases or drugs*	
Liver	Chronic liver disease with involvement of biliary tree
Gastrointestinal	Celiac disease, Crohn's disease, adenocarcinoma
Respiratory	Idiopathic interstitial pneumonitis, obstructive bronchiolitis, adenocarcinoma
Skin	Dermatitis herpetiformis, mycosis fungoides, leprosy
Eyes	Episcleritis, anterior uveitis
Miscellaneous	Ankylosing spondylitis, relapsing polychondritis, Sjögren's syndrome, monoclonal IgA gammopathy, schistosomiasis

* Although prominent deposition of IgA has been reported with each of these conditions, significant glomerular inflammation and dysfunction is rare.

it is usually inherited as an autosomal dominant trait. TBM disease typically manifests in childhood as persistent hematuria. Intermittent hematuria and exacerbation of hematuria during upper respiratory tract infections have also been reported. The kidney is normal on light and immunofluorescence microscopy. The GBM is thin (usually <275 nm in children and <300 nm in adults) by comparison with normal subjects. TBM disease is almost always benign, and progressive renal impairment or proteinuria should prompt a search for an alternative diagnosis. The molecular basis for this disease has not been determined.

PROTEINURIA Between 0.5 and 10 percent of the population have isolated proteinuria, defined as proteinuria in the presence of an otherwise normal urinary sediment, a radiologically normal urinary tract, and the absence of known renal disease. The majority of these patients excrete <2 g of protein per day, and more than 80 percent have an excellent prognosis (*benign isolated proteinuria*). A minority (10 to 25 percent) are found to have persistent proteinuria (*persistent isolated proteinuria*), some of whom develop progressive renal insufficiency over 10 to 20 years.

Benign Isolated Proteinuria The major categories of benign isolated proteinuria are idiopathic transient proteinuria, functional proteinuria, intermittent proteinuria, and postural proteinuria. *Idiopathic transient proteinuria* is usually observed in young adults and refers to dipstick-positive proteinuria in an otherwise healthy individual that disappears spontaneously by the next clinic visit. *Functional proteinuria* refers to transient proteinuria during fever, exposure to cold, emotional stress, congestive cardiac failure, or obstructive sleep apnea. This phenomenon is presumed to be mediated through changes in glomerular ultrafiltration pressure and/or membrane permeability. Patients with *intermittent proteinuria* have proteinuria in approximately half of their urine samples in the absence of other renal or systemic abnormalities. *Postural proteinuria* is proteinuria (usually <2.0 g per 24 h) that is evident only in the upright position. This disorder affects 2 to 5 percent of adolescents and may be transient (~80 percent) or fixed (~20 percent). Fixed postural proteinuria resolves within 10 to 20 years in most cases. In each of these conditions, renal biopsy reveals either normal renal parenchyma or mild and nonspecific changes involving podocytes or the mesangium. All carry an excellent prognosis.

Persistent Isolated Proteinuria Isolated proteinuria detected on multiple ambulatory clinic visits in both the recumbent and upright position usually signals a structural renal lesion. Virtually all glomerulopathies that induce nephrotic syndrome (see above) can cause persistent isolated proteinuria. The most common lesion on renal biopsy is mild mesangial proliferative glomerulonephritis with or without focal and segmental glomerulosclerosis (30 to 70 percent), followed by focal or diffuse proliferative glomerulonephritis (~15 percent) and interstitial nephritis (~5 percent). Although this clinical entity carries a worse prognosis than benign isolated proteinuria, the prognosis is still relatively good, with only 20 to 40 percent of patients developing renal insufficiency after 20 years. Furthermore, progression to ESRD is extremely rare. It is wise to exclude monoclonal gammopathy by urinary electrophoresis in older patients.

CHRONIC GLOMERULONEPHRITIS

This syndrome is characterized by persistent proteinuria and/or hematuria and renal insufficiency that progresses slowly over years. Chronic glomerulonephritis usually comes to light (1) upon routine urinalysis, (2) when routine blood tests reveal unexplained anemia or elevated blood urea nitrogen and creatinine, (3) following discovery of bilateral small kidneys on abdominal imaging, (4) during evaluation for secondary causes of hypertension, or (5) during a clinical exacerbation of glomerulonephritis triggered by pharyngitis (synpharyngitic) or other infections. Chronic glomerulonephritis can be a manifestation of virtually all of the major glomerulopathies. Renal biopsy typically reveals a variable combination of proliferative, membranous, and sclerotic changes, depending on the causative glomerulopathy. Arteriosclerosis, induced by secondary hypertension, is a common finding in the renal vasculature. Tubulointerstitial inflammation and scarring are frequent

additional findings and portend a poor prognosis. Glomerular hypertension and hyperfiltration through remnant functioning nephrons can hasten progression to ESRD (see Chap. 273). Treatment is directed at lowering systemic and glomerular hypertension, usually with an ACE inhibitor, and controlling extracellular fluid volume, anemia, metabolic abnormalities, and the uremic syndrome through judicious use of diuretics, erythropoietin, and dietary modification (see "Chronic Renal Failure," Chap. 271). Some patients develop ESRD and require renal replacement therapy with dialysis or transplantation.

BIBLIOGRAPHY

Bernard DB, Salant DJ: Clinical approach to the patient with proteinuria and the nephrotic syndrome, in *The Principles and Practice of Nephrology*, 2d ed, HR Jacobsen, GE Striker, S Klahr (eds). St. Louis, Mosby, 1995, pp 110–121

Cotran R, Rennke HG: Sites and the mechanisms of proteinuria. N Engl J Med 309:1050, 1983

D'Amico G: Immunoglobulin A nephropathy, in *The Principles and Practice of Nephrology*, 2d ed, HR Jacobsen, GE Striker, S Klahr (eds). St. Louis, Mosby, 1995, pp 133–138

Falk RJ: ANCA-associated renal disease. Kidney Int 38:998, 1990

Glassock RJ et al: Primary glomerular diseases, in *The Kidney*, 5th ed, BM Brenner (ed). Philadelphia, Saunders, 1996, pp 1392–1497

Kelly PT, Haponik EF: Goodpasture's syndrome: Molecular and clinical advances. Medicine (Baltimore) 73:171, 1994

Meyer TW et al: Nephron adaptation to renal injury, in *The Kidney*, 5th ed, BM Brenner (ed). Philadelphia, Saunders, 1996, pp 2011–2048

275

Yvonne M. O'Meara, Hugh R. Brady, Barry M. Brenner

GLOMERULOPATHIES ASSOCIATED WITH MULTISYSTEM DISEASES

An array of multisystem diseases can cause glomerular injury, with glomerulopathy being either the dominant presenting feature or a relatively benign and clinically insignificant manifestation that is overshadowed by involvement of other organs. Glomerulopathies associated with multisystem diseases are often classified as *secondary* glomerulopathies to distinguish them from the *primary* glomerulopathies (Chap. 274) in which the pathology is limited to the kidneys. It should be emphasized, however, that most morphologic patterns of glomerular injury (Table 273-1) can manifest as a renal-limited process (i.e., primary) or as part of a systemic disease (i.e., secondary). It is best to approach glomerular disease by first identifying the presenting clinical syndrome (e.g., nephritic, nephrotic), then defining the pathologic features (e.g., proliferative, crescentic, membranous), and finally attempting to establish the specific disease that provoked glomerular injury [e.g., systemic lupus erythematosus (SLE), Henoch-Schönlein purpura].

In this chapter, we focus on the epidemiology, clinicopathologic features, and management of the major glomerulopathies associated with systemic diseases. The pathogenesis of glomerular injury is discussed in Chap. 273, and the overall place of the major glomerulopathies in the differential diagnosis of the major renal syndromes is described in Chap. 274.

DIABETIC NEPHROPATHY (See also Chaps. 273 and 334)

Diabetic nephropathy is the leading cause of end-stage renal disease (ESRD) in western societies and accounts for 30 to 35 percent of patients on renal replacement therapy in North America. Insulin-dependent diabetes mellitus (IDDM) and non-insulin-dependent diabetes mellitus (NIDDM) affect 0.5 and 4 percent of the population, respectively. Nephropathy complicates 30 percent of cases of IDDM and approximately 20 percent of cases of NIDDM. However, the majority of diabetic patients with ESRD have NIDDM because of the greater prevalence of NIDDM worldwide (90 percent of all diabetics). For reasons that are unclear, ESRD from diabetic nephropathy is more common in blacks with NIDDM than in whites (4:1 ratio), whereas the reverse is true for IDDM.

The clinical and morphologic features of diabetic nephropathy are similar in IDDM and NIDDM. Glomerular hypertension and hyperfiltration are the earliest renal abnormalities in experimental and human diabetes and are observed within days to weeks of diagnosis. Microalbuminuria, so named because the abnormal albumin excretion of 30 to 300 mg per 24 h is below the limits of detection of standard dipsticks, develops after approximately 5 years of sustained glomerular hypertension and hyperfiltration. Microalbuminuria is the first manifestation of injury to the glomerular filtration barrier and predicts the development of overt nephropathy. Dipstick-positive proteinuria, ultimately reaching nephrotic levels, typically develops 5 to 10 years after the onset of microalbuminuria (i.e., 10 to 15 years after the onset of diabetes) and is associated with hypertension and progressive loss of renal function. In addition, patients can display features of tubulointerstitial disease such as hyperkalemia and type IV renal tubular acidosis. ESRD typically develops 5 to 10 years after the development of overt nephropathy. Diabetic nephropathy is usually diagnosed on clinical grounds without a renal biopsy. Supportive clues are the presence of normal sized or enlarged kidneys, evidence of proliferative diabetic retinopathy, and a bland urinary sediment. Retinopathy is found in 90 and 60 percent of patients with IDDM and NIDDM, respectively, who develop nephropathy.

The earliest morphologic abnormalities in diabetic nephropathy are thickening of the glomerular basement membrane (GBM) and expansion of the mesangium due to accumulation of extracellular matrix. With time, matrix accumulation becomes diffuse and is evident as eosinophilic, periodic acid Schiff–positive glomerulosclerosis on renal biopsy. Prominent areas of nodular matrix expansion (nodular glomerulosclerosis, the classic Kimmelsteil-Wilson lesion) are often superimposed on this background. The glomeruli and kidneys are typically normal or increased in size, distinguishing diabetic nephropathy from most other forms of chronic renal insufficiency (renal amyloidosis and polycystic kidney disease being other important exceptions). Immunofluorescence microscopy may reveal deposition of IgG along the GBM in a linear pattern, but this does not appear to be immunopathogenetic as in anti-GBM disease. Immune deposits are not seen. The renal vasculature typically displays evidence of atherosclerosis, as a consequence of hyperlipidemia, and hypertensive arteriosclerosis.

℞ TREATMENT

Therapy is aimed at retarding the progression of nephropathy through control of blood sugar, systemic blood pressure, and glomerular capillary pressure. Glycemic control is achieved through regulation of diet and administration of oral hypoglycemic agents and insulin (see Chap. 334). Angiotensin-converting enzyme (ACE) inhibitors are the drugs of choice as they control both systemic hypertension and intraglomerular hypertension by inhibiting the actions of angiotensin II on the systemic vasculature and renal efferent arterioles. ACE inhibitors also attenuate the stimulatory effect of angiotensin II on glomerular cell growth and matrix production. Because ACE inhibitors have been shown conclusively to delay the time to ESRD by 50 percent in patients with IDDM in a large randomized controlled trial and to delay progression significantly in NIDDM, it is felt that all diabetic patients should receive an ACE inhibitor upon the development of microalbuminuria, even in the absence of systemic hypertension (Fig. 275-1).

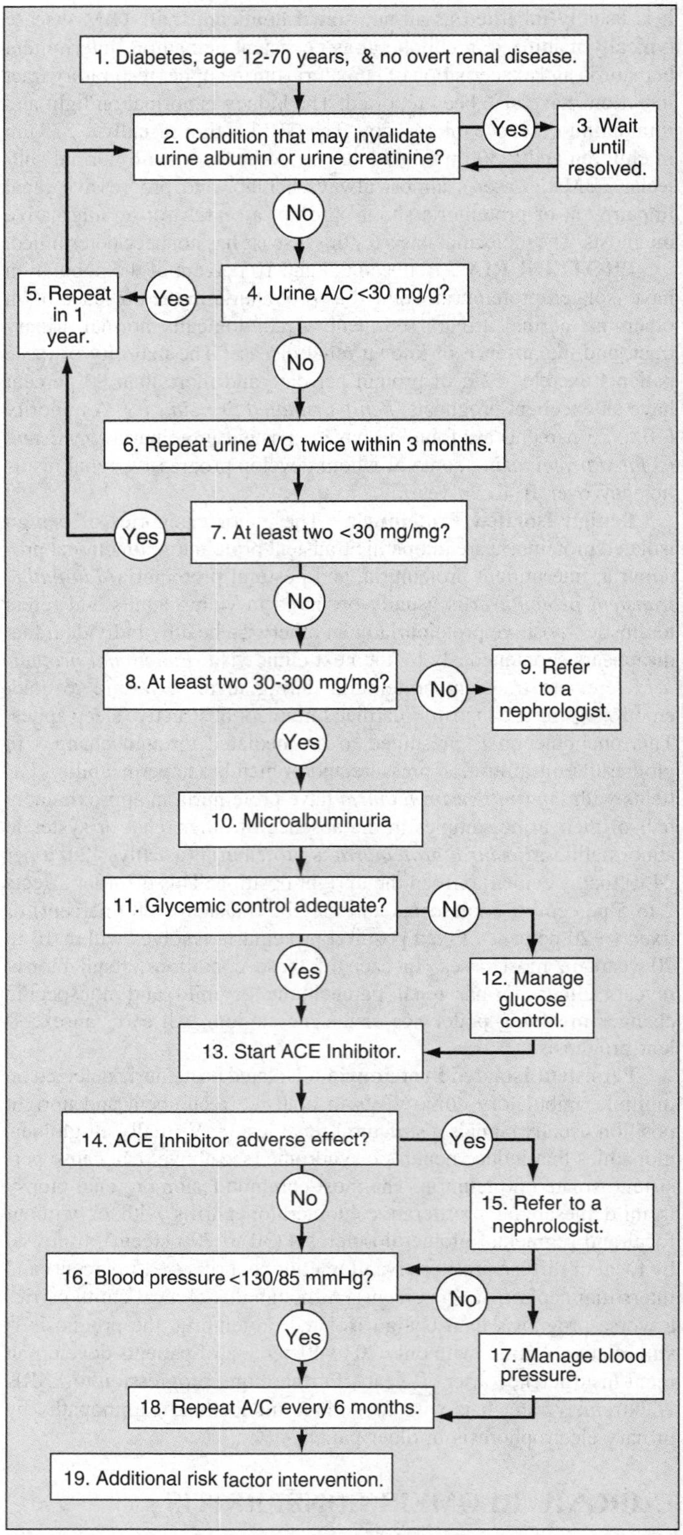

FIGURE 275-1 Algorithm for screening and management of microalbuminuria in patients with diabetes mellitus. A/C, albumin (in mg)/creatinine (in mg) in a spot urine sample. (*Reproduced with permission from Bennett et al.*)

Diabetic nephropathy is the most common cause of ESRD requiring renal replacement therapy, and diabetic patients have the highest annual mortality (20 to 30 percent) of any group on dialysis, in large part as a result of accelerated atherosclerosis. Survival of younger patients is comparable with either peritoneal dialysis or hemodialysis; however, older diabetics appear to have higher mortality on peritoneal dialysis. Transplantation is the preferred mode of renal replacement therapy in patients who are otherwise medically suitable.

The glomerulus is a frequent target of injury in a variety of immunologically mediated multisystem diseases, particularly systemic vasculitis and SLE. Systemic vasculitis is usually classified according to the size of the inflamed vessel (see Chap. 319). The major *large vessel* vasculitides are Takayasu's disease and giant cell arteritis. Glomerular injury is exceedingly rare in these diseases.

CLASSIC POLYARTERITIS NODOSA (See also Chap. 319) The typical glomerular lesion in classic polyarteritis nodosa (PAN) is ischemic collapse and obsolescence. Characteristic clinical and serologic features are hypertension, a bland urine sediment with subnephrotic proteinuria, slowly progressive renal insufficiency, normal serum complement levels, and absence of antineutrophil cytoplasmic antibodies (ANCA). Treatment with glucocorticoids and immunosupressive agents, such as cyclophosphamide, affords a 5-year patient survival of approximately 80 percent, as compared with 10 percent in untreated cases.

ANCA-ASSOCIATED SMALL-VESSEL VASCULITIS The ANCA-associated small-vessel vasculitides are Wegener's granulomatosis, the microscopic and Churg-Strauss variants of polyarteritis nodosa, and pauci-immune renal-limited glomerulonephritis. These diseases share a number of clinocopathologic and serologic features and may represent a spectrum of manifestations of a single disease. They are more common in whites and older patients (mean age 57 years) and show a slight male preponderance. Their incidence peaks in the winter months, and many patients have a viral-like prodrome, suggesting a pathogenetic role for an infective agent. Patients typically present with nonspecific constitutional symptoms and signs such as lethargy, malaise, anorexia, weight loss, fever, arthralgias, and myalgias. Nonspecific laboratory abnormalities include a rapid sedimentation rate, elevated C-reactive protein, leukocytosis, thrombocytosis, and normochromic, normocytic anemia. Serum complement levels are typically normal.

The majority of patients with these conditions have circulating ANCA. It is not clear whether ANCA are involved in the pathogenesis of vasculitis or merely represent an epiphenomenon of the vasculitic process, and there is debate whether serial ANCA titers are useful for monitoring disease activity and predicting relapse. Some ANCA activate cytokine-primed neutrophils in vitro and provoke them to injure endothelial cells, suggesting a pathogenetic role (see Chap. 273). It should be noted that ANCA are not entirely specific for vasculitis and are also found, albeit at low titers, in some cases (~20 percent) of anti-GBM disease and in patients with inflammatory bowel disease, primary biliary cirrhosis, and other autoimmune disorders.

Patients with ANCA-associated renal disease usually present with a nephritic urine sediment and moderate proteinuria. Renal dysfunction can vary from a mild decrement in glomerular filtration rate (GFR) to rapidly progressive glomerulonephritis (RPGN). Renal biopsy typically reveals focal, segmental, necrotizing glomerulonephritis with crescent formation. Immunofluorescence and electron microscopy are remarkable for the paucity or absence of immunoglobulin, complement, and immune deposits: so-called pauci-immune glomerulonephritis. These findings are in stark contrast to the prominent granular deposition of IgG and C3 in immune-complex glomerulonephritides such as Henoch-Schönlein purpura and lupus nephritis. ANCA-associated vasculitis is usually responsive to combined therapy with glucocorticoids and cyclophosphamide, and the 5-year patient survival usually exceeds 75 percent. The distinguishing features of individual ANCA-associated renal diseases are summarized below.

Wegener's Granulomatosis (See Chap. 319) Renal injury occurs in 80% of patients with Wegener's granulomatosis and varies from indolent smoldering inflammation to rapidly progressive renal failure. Cytoplasmic ANCA are detected at presentation in 80 percent of patients with renal disease and in a further 10 percent on follow-up. Renal biopsy typically reveals focal, segmental, necrotizing pauci-immune glomerulonephritis with crescent formation. In contrast to the lung, granulomas are rarely seen in the kidney.

℞ TREATMENT

Glucocorticoids and cyclophosphamide are the mainstay of treatment and dramatically ameliorate glomerular injury. Steroids are usually administered initially by pulse intravenous therapy on three consecutive days, followed by daily oral dosing of about 1 mg/kg body weight tapered to zero over 3 to 6 months. Cyclophosphamide is typically administered orally at a daily dose of 1 to 2 mg/kg or as monthly intravenous pulses of 1 g/m^2 of body surface area. Plasmapheresis may be a useful adjunct in patients with severe nephritis requiring dialysis. As many as 30% of patients relapse following treatment-induced remission. A persistently elevated or rising ANCA titer may predict relapse in individual patients; however, this relationship is not strong enough to justify treatment based on titers alone. Dialysis and renal transplantation afford excellent survival in patients with ESRD. Recurrence of Wegener's granulomatosis in the allograft is rare. ACE inhibitors may help to slow the progression to end-stage renal failure.

Microscopic Polyarteritis Nodosa (See Chap. 319) Microscopic PAN is a systemic disease characterized by leukocytoclastic vasculitis involving multiple organ systems including the lungs, skin, joints, and kidneys. Clinical renal disease ranges from a nephritic urinary sediment with mild impairment of GFR to RPGN. The usual histopathologic lesion is pauci-immune focal segmental necrotizing and crescentic glomerulonephritis. Circulating ANCA are detected in 70 to 80 percent of patients at presentation, cytoplasmic and perinuclear ANCA being equally prevalent. The treatment of microscopic PAN involves glucocorticoids and cyclophosphamide, as for Wegener's granulomatosis. Plasmapheresis may benefit patients with severe acute renal failure or massive pulmonary hemorrhage.

Churg-Strauss Syndrome (See Chap. 319) Clinical renal involvement in Churg-Strauss syndrome is relatively infrequent and usually limited to mild proteinuria and hematuria. Evolution to chronic renal failure is rare. Renal biopsy most frequently reveals extraglomerular pathology, with involvement of the renal vasculature and tubulointerstitium by granulomatous vasculitis. A minority of patients have focal segmental necrotizing glomerulonephritis.

Henoch-Schönlein Purpura (See Chap. 319) Nephritis is present in 80 percent of cases of Henoch-Schönlein purpura and manifests as a nephritic urine sediment and moderate proteinuria. Macroscopic hematuria and nephrotic-range proteinuria are uncommon. Light-microscopic appearances can vary from mild mesangial proliferation and expansion to diffuse proliferation with glomerular crescents. The glomerular lesion is identical to that found in IgA nephropathy (Berger's disease; see Chap. 274), suggesting that Henoch-Schönlein nephritis and IgA nephropathy are a spectrum of manifestations of a single disease. The *sine qua non* for diagnosis is the presence of mesangial IgA deposition on immunofluorescence microscopy. IgG and C3 are also detected. Electron microscopy reveals mesangial immune deposits. Immune complexes may also be seen in the peripheral glomerular capillary wall and paramesangial areas. Biopsy of involved skin reveals dermal IgA deposition and leukocytoclastic vasculitis. IgA deposition is also seen in areas of uninvolved skin.

℞ TREATMENT

Since there is no proven therapy for Henoch-Schönlein nephritis, treatment is supportive. Steroids and/or cytotoxic agents are often tried in patients with severe disease, but without compelling scientific evidence to support their use. The disease typically undergoes clinical exacerbations and remissions in the first year and then enters long-term remission. The prognosis is generally excellent; chronic renal failure and persistent hypertension occur in fewer than 10 percent of patients.

ESSENTIAL MIXED CRYOGLOBULINEMIA (See Chap. 319) Renal involvement is most common with the mixed cryoglobulinemias (types II and III), which are more common in females and usually begin in the sixth decade. Most patients present with a variable combination of leukocytoclastic vasculitis, skin ulcerations, arthralgias, fatigue, and Raynaud's phenomenon. Renal disease complicates 50 percent of cases and usually develops after 12 to 24 months. The typical clinical renal manifestations are nephrotic-range proteinuria, microscopic hematuria, and hypertension. Acute nephritic syndrome occurs in 20 to 30 percent, and oliguric acute renal failure in about 5 percent of patients with renal disease. The characteristic morphologic lesions are diffuse mesangial proliferative or membranoproliferative glomerulonephritis. The glomerular capillaries frequently contain eosinophilic hyaline "pseudothrombi" composed of precipitated immunoglobulins. Granular deposition of IgG, IgM, and C3 is usually prominent on immunofluorescence microscopy. Electron microscopy typically reveals subendothelial deposits containing microfibrils and microtubules that display a characteristic "thumbprint" appearance.

Circulating levels of C3, C4, and CH50 are depressed in about 80 percent of patients with renal involvement, and a transient antinuclear antibody (ANA) (speckled pattern) is sometimes detected. Abnormal liver function tests are found in about 15 percent of patients at presentation and in up to 50 percent subsequently. Many patients with "essential" mixed cryoglobulinemia (EMC) (i.e., idiopathic) are chronically infected with hepatitis C virus (HCV). In keeping with a pathogenetic role for this virus, HCV RNA has been isolated from the serum of patients with EMC, indicating active infection, and anti-HCV antibodies have been detected in both the serum and cryoprecipitates in association with viral antigens.

℞ TREATMENT

Traditionally, glucocorticoids, with or without cyclophosphamide, and plasmapheresis were the standard treatment for EMC. Recent reports indicate that interferon α controls viral replication and stabilizes renal function in most patients with EMC and HCV infection. Unfortunately, most patients relapse when interferon α is discontinued, a major problem given the prohibitive cost of the drug. In general, patient and renal survival are good in EMC, with 75 percent of patients being alive at 10 years.

SYSTEMIC LUPUS ERYTHEMATOSUS (See Chap. 312) Renal involvement is clinically evident in 40 to 85 percent of patients with SLE; it varies from isolated abnormalities of the urinary sediment to full-blown nephritic or nephrotic syndrome or chronic renal failure. Most glomerular injury is triggered by the formation of immune complexes within the glomerular capillary wall; however, thrombotic microangiopathy may be the dominant reason for renal dysfunction in a small subset of patients with the antiphospholipid antibody syndrome.

Immune Complex Mediated Lupus Nephritis The renal biopsy has proven very useful for identifying the different patterns of immune-complex glomerulonephritis in SLE, which are diverse, portend different prognoses, and do not necessarily correlate with the clinical findings. Indeed, clinically silent lupus nephritis is well described in which the urinalysis is virtually normal but renal biopsy demonstrates varying degrees of injury.

The World Health Organization categorizes lupus nephritis into six histologic classes. *Class I* consists of a normal biopsy on light microscopy with occasional mesangial deposits on immunofluorescence microscopy. Patients in this category usually do not have clinical renal disease. Patients with *class II* or mesangial lupus nephritis have prominent mesangial deposits of IgG, IgM, and C3 on immunofluorescence and electron microscopy. Mesangial lupus nephritis is designated as class IIA when the glomeruli are normal by light microscopy and class IIB when there is mesangial hypercellularity. Microscopic hematuria is common with this lesion, and 25 to 50 percent of patients have moderate proteinuria. Nephrotic syndrome is not seen, and renal survival is excellent (>90 percent at 5 years). *Class III* describes focal segmental proliferative lupus nephritis with necrosis or sclerosis affecting fewer than 50 percent of glomeruli. Up to one-third of patients have nephrotic syndrome, and glomerular filtration is impaired in 15 to 25 percent. In *class IV* or diffuse proliferative lupus nephritis, most glomeruli show cell proliferation, often with crescent formation. Other features on light microscopy include fibrinoid necrosis and "wire loops," which are caused by basement membrane thickening and mesangial interposition between basement membrane and endothelial cells. Deposits of IgG, IgM, IgA, and C3 are evident by immunofluorescence, and crescents stain positive for fibrin. Electron microscopy reveals numerous immune deposits in mesangial, subepithelial, and subendothelial locations. Tubuloreticular structures are frequently seen in endothelial cells. These are not specific for lupus nephritis and are also seen in human immunodeficiency virus (HIV)-associated nephropathy. Electron microscopy may also reveal curvilinear parallel arrays of microfibrils, measuring approximately 10 to 15 nm in diameter, with "thumbprinting," similar to those seen in cryoglobulinemia. Nephrotic syndrome and renal insufficiency are present in at least 50 percent of patients with class IV disease. Diffuse proliferative lupus nephritis is the most aggressive renal lesion in SLE, and as many as 30 percent of these patients progress to terminal renal failure. *Class V* is termed membranous lupus nephritis because of its similarity to idiopathic membranous glomerulopathy. Thickening of the GBM is evident by light microscopy. Electron microscopy reveals predominant subepithelial deposits in addition to subendothelial and mesangial deposits. Proliferative changes may also be evident, but the predominant pattern is that of membranous glomerulopathy. Most patients present with nephrotic syndrome (90 percent), but significant impairment of GFR is relatively unusual (10 percent). Tubulointerstitial changes such as active infiltration by inflammatory cells, tubular atrophy, and interstitial fibrosis are seen to varying degrees in lupus nephritis and are most severe in classes III and IV, especially in patients with long-standing disease. *Class VI* probably represents the end stages of proliferative lupus nephritis and is characterized by diffuse glomerulosclerosis and advanced tubulointerstitial disease. These patients are often hypertensive, may have nephrotic syndrome, and usually have impaired GFR.

Transformation from one class to another is relatively frequent. For example, class III often progresses to class IV spontaneously, and class IV can transform to class II or class V following treatment. Class II and class V lupus nephritis may predate other manifestations of lupus, whereas class III or IV usually occurs in patients who have systemic features of SLE. A semiquantitative analysis can be performed using a variety of features on renal biopsy, scored 0 to 3+, to derive indices of disease activity and chronicity. Features that suggest active inflammation include endocapillary proliferation, glomerular leukocyte infiltration, wire loop deposits, cellular crescents, and interstitial inflammation. In contrast, features that suggest chronicity include glomerulosclerosis, fibrous crescents, tubular atrophy, and interstitial fibrosis. In some, but not all, studies, these indices have been useful in predicting response to therapy and renal prognosis.

Patients with active lupus nephritis have a range of serologic abnormalities. Hypocomplementemia is present in 75 to 90 percent of patients and is most striking with diffuse proliferative glomerulonephritis. ANA are usually detected (95 to 99 percent), although not specific for SLE. ANA titers tend to fall with treatment, and ANA may not be detected during remissions. Anti-double-stranded DNA (dsDNA) antibodies are highly specific for SLE, and changes in their titers correlate with the activity of lupus nephritis. It should be noted that almost 100 percent of patients taking procainamide and 65 percent of patients taking hydralazine develop ANA; however, overt lupus, including nephritis, occurs in fewer than 10 percent of these patients, and anti-DNA antibodies are not usually detected. Other antibodies found in patients with SLE include anti-Sm (17 to 30 percent; highly specific, but not sensitive); anti-RNP, which frequently accompanies anti-Sm in low titer; anti-Ro (35 percent); anti-La (15 percent); and anti-histone antibodies (70 percent of SLE and 95 percent of drug-induced lupus).

℞ TREATMENT

The treatment of lupus nephritis is controversial and based largely on the class of injury and disease activity. Because there is relatively poor correlation between clinical features (urinalysis findings, serum creatinine) and histologic class, the renal biopsy findings are an important guide to therapy. Treatment is not indicated for class I and most cases of class II lupus nephritis, as these histologic patterns portend an excellent prognosis (100 percent and >90 percent 5-year survival, respectively). Extrarenal manifestations may warrant treatment with glucocorticoids, salicylates, or antimalarials. Glucocorticoids and cyclophosphamide are the mainstays of therapy for patients with proliferative nephritis (classes III and IV). High-dose steroids given as intravenous boluses (pulse therapy) are usually effective at rapidly controlling acute glomerular inflammation. Cyclophosphamide and azathioprine are important adjuncts to steroid therapy and appear to afford better long-term preservation of renal function than steroids alone. Intravenous pulse cyclophosphamide is as efficacious as oral therapy and appears to be less toxic. Most authorities advocate an initial regimen of monthly intravenous boluses of cyclophosphamide for 6 months. Subsequent therapy is tailored to disease activity and typically involves dosing every 3 to 6 months for a total treatment period of 18 to 24 months. The initial dose of cyclophosphamide is 0.5 g/m^2, and the dose is increased gradually to a maximum of 1 g/m^2 unless patients develop leukopenia or other side effects. Steroids are usually started simultaneously at 1 mg/kg per day and are tapered over the first 6 months to a maintenance dose of 5 to 10 mg/day for the duration of cyclophosphamide therapy. Five-year renal survivals of 60 to 90 percent have been obtained with this and similar regimens. A large randomized, prospective trial indicated that plasmapheresis does not offer additional benefit in patients with severe proliferative lupus nephritis. Plasmapheresis may have a role, albeit unproven, in patients with antiphospholipid syndrome and thrombotic microangiopathy (see below).

The management of membranous lupus nephritis is less well defined. As with idiopathic membranous glomerulopathy, the incidence of spontaneous remission approaches 50 percent in membranous lupus nephritis, and the course of the disease is generally indolent, with 70 to 90 percent renal survival at 5 years. Some authorities advocate steroids and ACE inhibitors at the time of diagnosis, whereas others reserve them for patients with progressive renal insufficiency or severe nephrotic syndrome. Useful parameters for monitoring the response to therapy and predicting relapse include the activity of the urine sediment, proteinuria, GFR, serum complement levels, and anti-dsDNA titers. Despite maximal immunosuppressive therapy, about 20 percent of patients with aggressive lupus nephritis develop ESRD requiring dialysis. SLE tends to become quiescent with advanced uremia, and patients rarely develop systemic flares once they commence dialysis. Recurrence of nephritis and systemic flares are also very uncommon following renal transplantation, and allograft survival rates are comparable to those in patients with other causes of ESRD.

Antiphospholipid Antibody Syndrome and Thrombotic Microangiopathy Patients with this syndrome can develop a variable degree of renal impairment due to thrombotic microangiopathy. The latter typically affects the interlobular arteries, arterioles, and glomerular capillaries and is characterized by intravascular microthrombi and swelling of endothelial cells. Decreased levels of tissue plasminogen activator and increased level of α_2-antiplasmin, both of which would tend to promote thrombosis, have been described in this syndrome.

RHEUMATOID ARTHRITIS (See Chap. 313) Although extra-articular manifestations are present in 35 percent of patients with rheumatoid arthritis, direct involvement of the kidney by rheumatoid disease is rare, and glomerular injury is usually secondary to AA amyloidosis or a side effect of drug therapy. AA amyloidosis complicates 10 to 20 percent of cases of rheumatoid arthritis, and renal involvement is evident clinically in 3 to 10 percent of these patients (nephrotic syndrome, renal insufficiency). Amyloidosis is more frequent in patients with rheumatoid arthritis of long duration (>10 years), with circulating rheumatoid factor, and with destructive arthropathy. Less frequent glomerular lesions include mesangial proliferative glomerulonephritis and basement membrane thickening by subepithelial immune deposits. Gold and penicillamine may cause nephrotic syndrome by inducing membranous glomerulopathy, whereas nonsteroidal anti-inflammatory drugs (NSAIDs) can trigger the nephrotic syndrome by inducing minimal change nephropathy, usually in association with acute interstitial nephritis (see below).

SJÖGREN'S SYNDROME (See Chap. 316) Tubulointerstitial injury is the most common form of renal involvement in Sjögren's syndrome and usually presents as either Fanconi's syndrome, distal renal tubular acidosis, or impairment of renal concentrating ability. Glomerulonephritis is relatively rare and should prompt a search for evidence of secondary causes. Membranous glomerulopathy and membranoproliferative glomerulonephritis (MPGN) are the most common lesions. Anecdotal reports describe successful therapy with glucocorticoids and cytotoxic agents.

POLYMYOSITIS AND DERMATOMYOSITIS (See Chap. 315) Occasional cases of focal mesangial proliferative glomerulonephritis with mesangial deposition of IgG and complement have been described in polymyositis/dermatomyositis. Membranous glomerulopathy has also been reported, particularly when polymyositis/dermatomyositis is associated with malignancy.

MIXED CONNECTIVE TISSUE DISEASE (See Chap. 314) Mixed connective tissue disease is a syndrome that includes features of SLE, scleroderma, and polymyositis and is associated with high titers of antiribonucleoprotein antibodies and negative antismooth muscle antibodies. Renal involvement occurs in fewer than 15 percent of patients and manifests as hematuria and subnephrotic proteinuria. The usual pathologic lesion is membranous or MPGN. The prognosis is usually excellent, and steroid therapy may be useful in rare patients with progressive renal disease.

GLOMERULAR DEPOSITION DISEASES

The glomerular deposition diseases are characterized by deposition of abnormal proteins, usually immunoglobulins or fragments thereof, within the glomerulus. They include amyloidosis, light and heavy chain deposition disease, cryoglobulinemia, and fibrillary/immunotactoid glomerulonephritis. Here, we focus on amyloidosis and light chain deposition disease (LCDD). Cryoglobulinemic nephropathy is described above in the discussion on systemic vasculitis. → ***Fibrillary and immunotactoid glomerulopathy are discussed in Chap. 274.***

AMYLOIDOSIS (See Chap. 309) Amyloidosis is classified according to the major component of its fibrils: for example, immunoglobulin light chains in AL amyloidosis, serum amyloid A in AA amyloidosis, β_2-microglobulin in dialysis-associated amyloidosis, and amyloid β protein in Alzheimer's disease and Down's syndrome. Amyloid deposits also contain a nonfibrillar component called the P component, a serum α_1 glycoprotein with a high affinity for the fibrillar components of all forms of amyloid. AL and AA amyloidosis frequently involve the kidneys, whereas involvement by other forms of amyloidosis is very rare.

There is substantial overlap in the renal clinicopathologic presentations of AL and AA amyloidosis. Glomeruli are involved in 75 to 90 percent of patients, usually in association with involvement of other organs. The clinical correlate of glomerular amyloid deposition is nephrotic-range proteinuria. In addition, over 50 percent of patients have impaired glomerular filtration at diagnosis. Hypertension is present in about 20 to 25 percent. Renal size is usually normal or slightly enlarged. A minority of patients present with renal failure due to amyloid deposition in the renal vasculature or with Fanconi's syndrome, nephrogenic diabetes insipidus, or renal tubular acidosis due to involvement of the tubulointerstitium. Rectal biopsy and abdominal fat pad biopsy reveal amyloid deposits in about 70 percent of patients and may obviate the need for renal biopsy.

Renal biopsy gives a very high yield if there is clinical evidence of renal involvement. The earliest pathologic changes are mesangial expansion by amorphous hyaline material and thickening of the GBM. Further amyloid deposition results in the development of large nodular eosinophilic masses. When stained with Congo red, these deposits show apple-green birefringence under polarized light. Immunofluorescence microscopy is usually only weakly positive for immunoglobulin light chains because amyloid fibrils are usually derived from the variable region of light chains. Electron microscopy reveals the characteristic nonbranching extracellular amyloid fibrils of 7.5 to 10 nm in diameter. Tubulointerstitial and vascular deposits of amyloid are also seen and may occasionally be more prominent than glomerular deposits.

℞ TREATMENT

Most patients with renal involvement by AL amyloidosis develop ESRD within 2 to 5 years. No treatment has been shown consistently to improve this prognosis; however, some success has been reported with a combination of melphalan and prednisone. Colchicine delays the onset of nephropathy in patients with familial Mediterranean fever but has not proved useful in patients with established disease or with other forms of amyloid. Remissions may be achieved in AA amyloidosis by eradication of the underlying cause. Renal replacement therapy is offered to patients who reach ESRD; however, 1-year survival on dialysis is low (~66 percent) by comparison with other causes of ESRD. Most patients die from extrarenal complications, particularly cardiovascular disease. Renal transplantation is a viable option in patients with AA amyloidosis whose primary disease has been eradicated. Transplantation is also an option for patients with AL amyloidosis, though a poor prognosis because of extrarenal organ involvement may preclude them as candidates. Here again, survival is lower by comparison with other causes of ESRD, most of the excess mortality being due to infectious and cardiovascular complications. Recurrence of amyloidosis in the allograft is common but rarely leads to graft loss.

LIGHT CHAIN DEPOSITION DISEASE (See Chap. 114) Renal involvement complicates 90 percent of cases of LCDD and is often the dominant feature. Nephrotic syndrome and renal impairment are the usual presenting features. Microscopic hematuria occurs in about 20 percent of cases. Defective hydrogen ion and potassium excretion and urinary concentration may be evident if light chains are deposited predominantly in the tubules. The most common pathologic lesion on renal biopsy is ribbon-like thickening of the tubular basement membrane due to light chain deposition. Mesangial expansion and nodular glomerulosclerosis are found in about 33 percent of patients. This light-microscopic appearance resembles that of idiopathic MPGN and diabetic nephropathy. Superimposed crescentic change is occasionally seen. Immunofluorescence studies are strongly positive for monoclonal light chains, in contrast to AL amyloid, because the constant region of the immunoglobulin is typically deposited. The tissue deposits in LCDD are granular rather than fibrillar on electron microscopy, appear more amorphous in character, do not stain with Congo red, and seem to have a greater affinity for basement membranes.

The prognosis of LCDD is poor when associated with multiple myeloma, and most patients progess rapidly to ESRD. Treatment with melphalan and prednisone has been reported to reduce proteinuria and stabilize renal function in uncontrolled studies. In the absence of myeloma, the prognosis is somewhat more variable, as several patients have undergone successful renal transplantation.

WALDENSTRÖM'S MACROGLOBULINEMIA (See Chap. 114) This disorder is characterized by monoclonal proliferation of an IgM-secreting clone of plasma cells. The circulating IgM paraprotein frequently gives rise to the hyperviscosity syndrome, which may compromise renal blood flow and GFR. Direct renal involvement is rare and, when present, involves deposition of large amorphous deposits of eosinophilic material in the glomerular capillaries. Renal amyloidosis can also occur.

DRUG-INDUCED GLOMERULAR DISEASE

A variety of drugs damage the glomerular filtration barrier and induce proteinuria and nephrotic syndrome. In contrast, drug-induced proliferative glomerulonephritis is rare. The more common drug-induced glomerulopathies are discussed here. Additional associations are included in Table 275-1 and Table 69-1.

NSAIDs have a variety of renal side effects, including hemodynamically mediated acute renal failure, salt and water retention, hyponatremia, hyperkalemia, papillary necrosis, acute interstitial nephritis, nephrotic syndrome, and ESRD. Nephrotic syndrome and acute renal failure frequently coexist due to a combination of acute interstitial nephritis and a glomerular lesion that is identical to that of minimal change disease. This entity occurs most commonly in patients on propionic acid derivatives such as fenoprofen, ibuprofen, and naproxen but can occur with other NSAIDS, ampicillin, rifampin, and interferon α. Withdrawal of the drug usually results in resolution of renal disease.

Gold therapy, administered by injection or orally, induces proteinuria in 5 to 25 percent of patients with rheumatoid arthritis. Proteinuria develops after 4 to 6 months of therapy, and up to 33 percent of patients develop full-blown nephrotic syndrome. Renal biopsy typically reveals membranous glomerulopathy, though minimal change disease or mesangial proliferative lesions have also been described. Progressive renal impairment is rare. Nephrotic syndrome is more common in patients who are HLA-B8/DR3 positive, suggesting a genetic susceptibility. Withdrawal of the drug leads to gradual resolution of the proteinuria.

Penicillamine also induces proteinuria in 5 to 30 percent of patients. As with gold, the underlying glomerular lesion is usually membranous glomerulopathy, and proteinuria gradually resolves following withdrawal of the drug.

Intravenous heroin use is associated with an increased incidence of focal and segmental glomerulosclerosis (heroin-associated nephropathy). It is not clear whether the nephrotoxin in this setting is heroin itself or a contaminant. Heroin-associated nepropathy occurs predominantly in blacks and is characterized by nephrotic syndrome, hyperten-

Table 275-1

Drug-Induced Glomerular Disease

Morphologic Lesion	Causative Agent
Minimal change diseases (usually with interstitial nephritis)	Nonsteroidal anti-inflammatory agents Recombinant interferon α Rifampin Ampicillin
Membranous nephropathy	Penicillamine Gold Mercury Trimethadione Captopril Chlormethiazole
Focal segmental glomerulosclerosis	Heroin
Pauci-immune necrotizing GN	Ciprofloxacin Hydralazine
Proliferative GN with vasculitis	Allopurinol Penicillin Sulfonamides Thiazides Intravenous amphetamines
RPGN	Rifampin Warfarin Carbimazole Amoxicillin Penicillamine

NOTE: GN, glomerulonephritis; RPGN, rapidly progressive glomerulonephritis.

sion, and a gradual progression to ESRD over a period of 3 to 5 years. The pathologic features are similar to those of idiopathic focal segmental glomerulosclerosis, though mesangial deposition of IgM and C3 may be more prominent. The incidence of this disease appears to be declining steadily. Potential reasons for the decline include increased purity of street heroin and a bias to attribute focal segmental glomerulosclerosis to HIV infection when both risk factors coexist. Intravenous *amphetamine* abuse is a rare cause of systemic necrotizing vasculitis.

HEREDITARY DISEASES WITH GLOMERULAR INVOLVEMENT

ALPORT'S SYNDROME (See Chap. 348) Alport's syndrome is the most common hereditary nephritis and is usually transmitted as an X-linked dominant trait. The genetic defect resides in the gene for the α5 chain of type IV collagen located on the long arm of the X chromosome, type IV collagen being a major structural component of the GBM. Numerous genetic mutations have been detected, ranging from major deletions to point mutations, and this genetic heterogeneity is reflected in the phenotypic variations of the disease. In the X-linked forms, males usually present with microscopic hematuria, proteinuria (nephrotic-range in 30 percent), and progressive renal insufficiency. Common extrarenal manifestations include sensorineural hearing loss (~60 percent) and bilateral anterior lenticonus (~15 to 30 percent). Platelet defects are described but are rare. Female carriers usually have mild disease and do not develop renal insufficiency. An autosomal recessive form also exists in which there are mutations in the gene for the α3 chain of type IV collagen, and males and females are equally affected.

Typical light-microscopic features on renal biopsy include mesangial hypercellularity, focal and segmental glomerulosclerosis, chronic tubulointerstitial fibrosis, atrophy, and accumulation of foam cells. Electron microscopy reveals thickening, fragmentation, and lamellation of the lamina densa of the GBM. Patchy thinning of the GBM may also be seen, especially early in the course of the disease and in female carriers.

Males with the disease tend to progress to ESRD and are suitable candidates for dialysis and transplantation. About 5 percent of transplant recipients develop anti-GMB disease in the renal allograft; their immune system recognizes normal GBM of the transplanted kidney as a foreign antigen. These patients can have antibodies against the α3 (Goodpasture antigen) or α5 chains of type IV collagen, probably because defective synthesis of the α5 chain results in defective incorporation or orientation of the α3 chain in the GBM.

SICKLE CELL DISEASE (See Chap. 107) Glomerular disease is common (15 to 30 percent) in homozygotes for sickle cell disease. Glomerular hyperfiltration and hypertrophy occur within the first 5 years of life. Approximately 15 to 30 percent of patients develop proteinuria in the first three decades, and 5 percent develop ESRD. The glomerular pathology is usually focal segmental glomerulosclerosis, probably due to sustained glomerular capillary hypertension, or MPGN. Predictors of chronic renal failure are worsening anemia, proteinuria, nephrotic syndrome, and hypertension. ACE inhibitors may slow the progression of renal disease by lowering systemic and glomerular capillary hypertension.

FABRY'S DISEASE (See Chap. 346) In patients with Fabry's disease, renal biopsy reveals accumulation of neutral glycosphingolipids with terminal α-galactosyl moieties in lysosomes of glomerular, tubular, vascular, and interstitial cells. Focal and global glomerulosclerosis are later features. Electron microscopy reveals stacked, concentric lamellar profiles known as "myeloid" bodies, which are characteristic. Renal disease manifests in the late teens to early twenties with lipiduria, proteinuria with minimal hematuria, nephrotic syndrome, hypertension, and progressive renal insufficiency. The most striking systemic manifestations are skin lesions (angiokeratomas), corneal and lens opacities, painful dysesthesias of the extremities, and arthropathy of the terminal interphalangeal joints. The diagnosis of Fabry's disease can often be made by careful physical examination, especially

if many of the typical clinical features are present. Measurement of urinary glycosphingolipids and estimation of peripheral leukocyte α-galactosidase levels help confirm the diagnosis. The renal lesion is progressive, and these patients often tolerate hemodynamic changes during dialysis poorly because of progressive vascular disease. Successful renal transplantation has been reported despite recurrence in the allograft.

NAIL-PATELLA SYNDROME The nail-patella syndrome is a rare hereditary disorder transmitted as an autosomal dominant trait. It is characterized by multiple osseous abnormalities, primarily affecting the elbows and knees, and nail dysplasia. About 50 percent of cases have clinically evident nephropathy. The light-microscopic features on renal biopsy include local GBM thickening, tubular atrophy, interstitial fibrosis, and varying degrees of glomerular sclerosis. Electron microscopy reveals irregular thickening of the GBM, with electrolucent areas giving it a "moth-eaten" appearance. Cross-striated fibrils with the periodicity of collagen can be identified in the mesangium and basement membrane. The disease usually manifests clinically as asymptomatic hematuria and proteinuria, occasionally in the nephrotic range, but may be silent. The renal lesion is usually benign, and progression to ESRD is rare ($<$10 percent).

LIPODYSTROPHY (See Chap. 352) MPGN type II (dense deposit disease) is the most frequent glomerular lesion (80 percent) in this condition, whereas MPGN type I affects the remainder (20 percent). The disease occurs mostly in females between the ages of 5 to 15 years, and the clinical presentation and course is similar to that of idiopathic MPGN, namely nephrotic-range proteinuria and progressive renal insufficiency. Low C3 levels are common in association with C3 nephritic factor (see Chap. 274).

LECITHIN-CHOLESTEROL ACYLTRANSFERASE DEFICIENCY (See Chap. 341) Renal manifestations of this disease include proteinuria, microscopic hematuria, and progressive renal insufficiency. Renal biopsy typically reveals focal and segmental glomerulosclerosis. Electron-microscopic findings include irregular rounded, lucent lacunae that contain solid or laminated dense structures in the GBM, mesangial matrix, and Bowman's capsular and renal tubular basement membranes. Endothelial cell detachment is also evident, and capillary lumens may be occluded by vacuolated foam cells. Recurrence of the disease has been documented in the renal allograft but without marked impairment of graft function.

GLOMERULAR LESIONS ASSOCIATED WITH INFECTIOUS DISEASES

VIRAL INFECTIONS Hepatitis B, hepatitis C, and HIV are strongly associated with glomerular disease (Table 275-2). Glomerular lesions associated with *hepatitis B virus* (HBV) infection include membranous glomerulopathy, MPGN, IgA nephropathy, essential mixed cryoglobulinemia, and polyarteritis nodosa. Membranous glomerulopathy is most common. In endemic areas, such as Asia and Africa, 80 to 100 percent of children and 30 to 45 percent of adults with membranous glomerulopathy have HBV surface antigenemia. HBV antigens have been identified in renal immune deposits, suggesting in situ immune complex formation following planting of HBV antigens or trapping of circulating immune complexes containing HBV antigens. Patients typically present with nephrotic syndrome and microscopic hematuria. Hypertension and renal impairment are rare. The most common associated hepatic lesion is chronic persistent or chronic active hepatitis. There is a male preponderance, and many patients are intravenous drug users or have other risk factor for acquisition of HBV. The asymptomatic carrier state of HBV is frequently associated with MPGN in endemic areas. Hypertension and azotemia are more common with this morphologic pattern than with membranous glomerulopathy. Children with HBV-associated membranous glomerulonephritis have a good prognosis, and almost two-thirds enter spontaneous remission within 3 years. ESRD is rare. In contrast, 30 percent of

Table 275-2

Glomerular Lesions Associated with Infectious Diseases

Morphologic Lesion	Common Disease or Inciting Organism
Diffuse proliferative glomerulonephritis (classic postinfectious glomerulonephritis)	Streptococcal pharyngitis
	Acute/subacute bacterial endocarditis
	Visceral sepsis
	Typhoid fever
	Syphilis
	Leptospirosis (*Mycobacterium leprae*)
	Toxoplasmosis
	Falciparum malaria
	Plasmodium falciparum
	Varicella, mumps, echovirus, coxsackievirus, measles
	Infectious mononucleosis
	Hepatitis B and C
Membranoproliferative glomerulonephritis	Subacute bacterial endocarditis
	Ventriculoatrial shunt infection
	Visceral sepsis
	Hepatitis C infection
	Hepatitis B infection
	P. falciparum
	Schistosomiasis
Mesangial proliferative glomerulonephritis	Recovery phase of postinfectious glomerulonephritis
Membranous nephropathy	Hepatitis C infection
	Hepatitis B infection
	Syphilis
	Filiariasis
	Hydatid disease
	Schistosomiasis
	Plasmodium malariae
	Leprosy
	Enterococcal endocarditis
Focal segmental glomerulosclerosis	HIV infection
	Schistosomiasis
Renal amyloidosis	Any chronic infection

adults develop progressive renal failure within 5 years, with 10 percent reaching ESRD. Steroids and cytotoxic agents are contraindicated as they may lead to increased viral replication and worsening of liver disease. Interferon α may reduce proteinuria and stabilize renal function in patients with progressive disease.

Hepatitis C infection (Chap. 295) should be considered in all patients with cryoglobulinemic proliferative glomerulonephritis, MPGN, and membranous glomerulopathy. These three clinicopathologic entities may represent a spectrum of morphologic manifestations of the same pathogenetic process, namely HCV-induced immune-complex disease. Up to 30 percent of patients with chronic HCV infection have an abnormal urinary sediment. HCV infection accounts for 10 to 20 percent of type I MPGN and is a major cause of essential mixed cryoglobulinemia. Renal biopsy reveals typical features of type I MPGN and IgG, IgM, C3, and/or cryoglobulin deposits. Most patients present with nephrotic syndrome and microscopic hematuria and may have red blood cell casts. Liver function tests are usually abnormal, and C3 levels are typically depressed. Anti-HCV antibodies are detected in most patients, and viral RNA has been documented in blood and cryoglobulins. A variety of treatments have been reported to be useful in HCV-induced renal disease including steroids, cytotoxic agents, and plasmapheresis; however, controlled trials to support their use are lacking. More recently, interferon α has been demonstrated to clear antigenemia, lower cryoglobulin levels, and stabilize renal disease. Unfortunately, relapse is usual once the drug is discontinued.

HIV infection (Chap. 308) has been associated with focal segmental glomerulosclerosis, acute diffuse proliferative glomerulonephritis, and mesangioproliferative glomerulonephritis, including IgA nephropathy, MPGN, and membranous glomerulopathy. The classic and most common HIV-associated glomerulopathy is focal segmental glomerulosclerosis, an entity that is termed *human immunodeficiency virus–associated nephropathy (HIVAN)*. The latter may be the first manifestation of infection in otherwise asymptomatic patients. HIVAN is more common in blacks than in other ethnic groups and is more frequent in intravenous drug abusers with HIV infection than in homosexuals. The disease has been described in all high-risk groups, however, including infants of HIV-positive mothers. Renal biopsy typically reveals glomerular collapse, severe tubulointerstitial inflammation, and microcystic dilatation of renal tubules. A number of characteristic abnormalities are noted on electron microscopy, including tubuloreticular inclusions in glomerular endothelial cells, tubular cells and infiltrating leukocytes, fibrillogranular degeneration of tubular nuclei, and the presence of complex nuclear bodies. The morphologic features distinguish HIVAN from idiopathic focal segmental glomerulosclerosis. The mechanisms of renal cell injury are still being defined. Viral DNA has been demonstrated in the renal epithelia of HIV-infected patients with and without nephropathy, suggesting that pathogenetic factors, other than infection of cells, are required for induction of disease. The typical clinical correlates of HIVAN are severe nephrotic syndrome and rapid progression to ESRD, occurring in weeks to months. Survival on dialysis is particularly poor for patients with clinical AIDS, though asymptomatic carriers have a better prognosis. There is no proven therapy for HIVAN. Anecdotal reports suggest a benefit of steroids, ACE inhibitors, and zidovudine (AZT) in reducing proteinuria, but there are no controlled trials to support their use.

BACTERIAL INFECTIONS (See Table 275-2) Immune-complex glomerulonephritis is a relatively frequent complication of infective *endocarditis* (Chap. 126). Other mechanisms of renal injury in bacterial endocarditis include embolic renal infarction, septic abscesses, acute tubular necrosis secondary to septicemia and drug therapy, disseminated intravascular coagulation, and antibiotic-induced acute interstitial nephritis. Patients typically present with microscopic hematuria, urinary red blood cell casts, pyuria and modest proteinuria (nephrotic range in 25 percent of patients), and mild, if any, renal failure. Rheumatoid factor is present in 10 to 70 percent, and circulating immune complexes in 90 percent. Serum complement levels are usually depressed. Renal biopsy reveals mild focal proliferative glomerulonephritis with mesangial and capillary wall deposition of IgG and C3 by immunofluorescence microscopy and subendothelial, mesangial, and subepithelial electron-dense deposits by electron microscopy. Occasional patients develop diffuse necrotizing glomerulonephritis with crescent formation and present with nephritic syndrome or RPGN. Endocarditis-associated glomerulonephritis typically has a good prognosis and resolves with eradication of the underlying infection.

Immune-complex glomerulonephritis complicates 1 to 4 percent of cases of *infected ventriculoatrial shunts*. Nephritis can manifest weeks to years after shunt insertion and usually presents with microscopic hematuria. Nephrotic syndrome occurs in 50 to 60 percent. The usual renal pathology is a membranoproliferative pattern, though diffuse proliferation can also occur. Immunofluorescence reveals IgM and C3 in the capillary wall and mesangial area, while subendothelial deposits and mesangial interposition are seen by electron microscopy. Up to one-third of patients may have residual renal impairment despite removal of the infected shunt and resolution of the infection.

Suppurative infections such as intrathoracic and intraabdominal abscesses, osteomyelitis, and dental abscesses have been associated with glomerulonephritis. The usual presentation is hematuria, urinary red blood cell casts, proteinuria, and acute renal failure. Oliguria and hypertension are common. Pathologic renal lesions include mesangial proliferative, membranoproliferative and diffuse proliferative glomerulonephritis with crescents. Immunofluorescence reveals mesangial and capillary wall deposition predominantly of C3, though IgG and IgM may also be seen.

Nephrotic syndrome complicates 0.3 percent of cases of secondary *syphilis* and 8 percent of congenital syphilis. The usual pathology is membranous glomerulopathy; however, mild mesangial and endocapillary proliferation can occur. IgG and IgM are evident in affected regions by immunofluorescence microscopy, and treponemal antigens have been identified in diseased glomeruli. C3 and C4 are typically depressed in congenital syphilis. The treatment consists of penicillin to eradicate the infection.

Leprosy most commonly causes AA amyloidosis; however, a syndrome resembling acute poststreptococcal glomerulonephritis has also been described.

PROTOZOAN AND PARASITIC INFECTIONS Transient proteinuria (50 percent of cases) and nephrotic syndrome (<1 percent of cases) are complications of infection with *Plasmodium falciparum*. Membranoproliferative glomerulonephritis is the usual pathologic lesion and may respond to eradication of infection. *Plasmodium malariae* has been associated with diffuse or focal proliferative glomerulonephritis, membranous glomerulopathy, and minimal change disease. Eradication of the malarial infection does not consistently induce remission of the nephrotic syndrome. *Schistosoma mansoni* causes nephrotic syndrome in 5 to 10 percent of cases. The usual pathology is MPGN or mesangial proliferative glomerulonephritis, though membranous glomerulonephritis and amyloidosis are occasionally seen. *Filiariasis* can trigger membranous glomerulonephritis (*Loa loa*) and occasionally induces proliferative glomerulonephritis (*Onchocerca volvulus*). *Congenital toxoplasmosis* infection occasionally induces immune-complex glomerulonephritis characterized by mesangial and subendothelial immune deposits that contain *Toxoplasma* antigens. Membranous glomerulopathy and proliferative glomerulonephritis occasionally complicate *hydatid disease* and *trichinosis*, respectively.

GLOMERULAR LESIONS ASSOCIATED WITH NEOPLASIA

Glomerulopathies associated with neoplasia include membranous glomerulopathy, minimal change disease, focal segmental glomerulosclerosis, immune-complex glomerulonephritis, fibrillary/immunotactoid glomerulonephritis, LCDD, and amyloidosis. Mild proteinuria is common in patients with *solid tumors*, but overt glomerulonephritis is rare. Patients with solid tumors of the lung, gastrointestinal tract, breast, kidney, and ovary have an increased incidence of nephrotic syndrome, frequently due to a membranous glomerulopathy. Estimates of the incidence of occult malignancy in patients presenting with membranous glomerulopathy range from 0.1 to 10 percent. Most authorities agree that an extensive search for malignancy is not indicated, unless there are other suggestive clinical features. As many as 35 percent of patients with renal cell carcinoma have mesangial deposition of IgG and C3 visible on immunofluorescence; however, morphologic abnormalities are detected in only 50 percent of these patients, and clinically significant glomerulopathy is rare. Glomerular amyloidosis has also been described in association with this tumor.

An array of glomerular disease has been reported in patients with lymphoproliferative malignancy. Nephrotic syndrome is a recognized complication of *Hodgkin's lymphoma*, 70 percent of cases being due to minimal change disease. The latter may occur concurrently with (40 to 45 percent), precede (10 to 15 percent), or follow (40 to 50 percent) diagnosis of the malignancy. It is postulated that a lymphokine or other mediator released by malignant T lymphocytes perturbs podocyte function and alters glomerular permeability in this setting. Nephrotic syndrome typically resolves with successful treatment and relapses with recurrence of disease. Less frequent associations with Hodgkin's lymphoma include focal segmental glomerulosclerosis, membranous glomerulopathy, MPGN, proliferative glomerulonephritis, and crescentic glomerulonephritis. Minimal change disease, membranous glomerulopathy, MPGN, and crescentic glomerulonephritis have also been reported in patients with *non-Hodgkin's lymphoma*. Glomerulopathy in the context of leukemia is rare. MPGN can complicate *chronic lymphatic leukemia* and related *B cell lymphomas*, particularly when associated with cryoglobulinemia. Other glomerular lesions associated with *paraproteinemia* include primary amyloid, LCDD, proliferative glomerulonephritis induced by cryoglobulinemia, and fibrillary/immunotactoid glomerulopathy. Here again, the renal lesion frequently improves or resolves with successful treatment of the underlying malignancy.

BIBLIOGRAPHY

Adler SG et al: Secondary glomerular diseases, in *The Kidney*, 5th ed, BM Brenner (ed). Philadelphia, Saunders, 1996, pp. 1498–1596

Balow J: Lupus nephritis. Ann Intern Med 79:106, 1987

Bennett PH et al: Screening and management of microalbuminuria in patients with diabetes mellitus: Recommendations to the Scientific Advisory Board of the National Kidney Foundation from an ad hoc committee of the Council on Diabetes Mellitus of the National Kidney Foundation. Am J Kidney Dis 25:107, 1995

Falk RJ: ANCA-associated renal disease. Kidney Int 38:998, 1990

Gregory MC, Atkin CL: Alport syndrome, in *Diseases of the Kidney*, 5th ed, RW Schrier, CW Gottschalk (eds). Boston, Little, Brown, 1992, pp 571–592

Humphreys MH: Human immunodeficiency virus–associated glomerulosclerosis. Kidney Int 48:311, 1995

Johnson R et al: Renal manifestations of hepatitis C virus infection. Kidney Int 46:1265, 1994

Parving HH et al: Diabetic nephropathy, in *The Kidney*, 5th ed, BM Brenner (ed). Philadelphia, Saunders, 1996, pp 1864–1892

Sealy FD et al: Acquired immunodeficiency syndrome and the kidney. Am J Kidney Dis 16:1, 1990

276

Barry M. Brenner, Elliott Levy, Thomas H. Hostetter

TUBULOINTERSTITIAL DISEASES OF THE KIDNEY

An etiologically diverse group of renal diseases can be distinguished from those considered in Chaps. 274 and 275 because the histologic and functional abnormalities involve the tubules and interstitium to a greater degree than the glomeruli and renal vasculature (see Table 276-1). Both clinically and histologically, these disorders can be divided into acute and chronic forms. The chronic group may be due to sustained insults by a factor or factors that initially cause acute disease or to a slower, progressive, cumulative insult without an identifiable acute episode. Morphologically, acute forms of these disorders are characterized by interstitial edema, often associated with cortical and medullary infiltration by polymorphonuclear leukocytes and patchy areas of tubule cell necrosis. In more chronic forms, interstitial fibrosis predominates, inflammatory cells are typically mononuclear, and abnormalities of the tubules tend to be more widespread, as evidenced by atrophy, luminal dilatation, and thickening of tubule basement membranes. Because of the nonspecific nature of the histology, particularly in chronic tubulointerstitial diseases, biopsy specimens rarely provide a specific diagnosis. The urine sediment is also unlikely to be diagnostic, except in allergic forms of acute tubulointerstitial disease, in which eosinophils may predominate in the urinary sediment.

Defects in renal function often accompany these alterations of tubule and interstitial structure (see Table 276-2). Proximal tubule dysfunction may be manifested as selective reabsorptive defects leading to hypokalemia, aminoaciduria, glycosuria, phosphaturia, uricosuria, or bicarbonaturia (proximal or type II renal tubular acidosis; see Chap. 278). In combination, these defects constitute the *Fanconi syndrome*. Protein excretion is usually modest, rarely exceeding 2 g/d.

Defects in urinary acidification and concentrating ability often represent the most troublesome of the tubule dysfunctions encountered in patients with tubulointerstitial disease. Hyperchloremic metabolic acidosis often develops at a relatively early stage in the course. Patients with this finding generally elaborate urine of maximal acidity (pH of 5.3 or less). In such patients the defect in acid excretion is usually caused by a reduced capacity to generate and excrete ammonia due to the reduction in renal mass. Preferential damage to the collecting ducts, as in amyloidosis or chronic obstructive uropathy, also may predispose to distal or type I renal tubular acidosis, characterized by high urine pH (>5.5) during spontaneous or NH_4Cl-induced metabolic

Table 276-1

Principal Causes of Tubulointerstitial Disease of the Kidney

TOXINS
Exogenous toxins
Analgesic nephropathy*
Lead nephropathy (see Chap. 397)
Miscellaneous nephrotoxins (e.g., antibiotics, cyclosporine, radiographic contrast media, heavy metals)*†
Metabolic toxins
Acute uric acid nephropathy (see Chap. 344)
Gouty nephropathy (see Chap. 344)*
Hypercalcemic nephropathy (see Chap. 354)
Hypokalemic nephropathy (see Chap. 49)
Miscellaneous metabolic toxins (e.g., hyperoxaluria, cystinosis, Fabry's disease, see Chap. 346)
NEOPLASIA
Lymphoma (see Chap. 113)
Leukemia (see Chap. 112)
Multiple myeloma (see Chap. 114)*
IMMUNE DISORDERS
Hypersensitivity nephropathy*†
Sjögren's syndrome (see Chap. 316)
Amyloidosis (see Chap. 309)
Transplant rejection (see Chap. 272)†
Tubulointerstitial abnormalities associated with glomerulonephritis (see Chaps. 274 and 275)
HIV–associated nephropathy (see Chap. 308)
VASCULAR DISORDERS (see Chaps. 270 and 277)
Arteriolar nephrosclerosis*
Atheroembolic disease
Sickle cell nephropathy
Acute tubular necrosis*†
HEREDITARY RENAL DISEASES
Hereditary nephritis (Alport's syndrome) (see Chaps. 275 and 348)
Medullary cystic disease (see Chap. 278)
Medullary sponge kidney (see Chap. 278)
Polycystic kidney disease (see Chap. 278)
INFECTIOUS INJURY (see Chap. 131)
Acute pyelonephritis*†
Chronic pyelonephritis
MISCELLANEOUS DISORDERS
Chronic urinary tract obstruction (see Chap. 280)*
Vesicoureteral reflux*
Radiation nephritis

* Common.
† Typically acute.

acidosis. Patients with tubulointerstitial diseases affecting medullary and papillary structures predominantly also may evidence concentrating defects, with resultant nocturia and polyuria. Analgesic nephropathy and sickle cell disease are prototypes of this form of injury.

TOXINS

Although the kidneys constitute less than 1 percent of total body mass, they receive approximately 20 percent of the cardiac output, and 90 percent or more of renal blood flow is distributed to the renal cortex. Exposure of tubules and interstitium of the renal cortex to circulating toxins is therefore greater than is that of most other tissues. Transport processes in renal tubules contribute further to the intrarenal accumulation of toxins, enhancing local concentrations of noxious agents. The urinary concentrating mechanism also can establish high levels of toxins within medullary and papillary portions of the kidney, predisposing these regions to chemical injury. Finally, the relatively acid pH of the fluid within most nephron segments may affect the ionization characteristics of potentially toxic compounds and thereby influence local concentration and solubility. Although these processes render the kidney vulnerable to toxic injury, the role of nephrotoxins in renal damage often goes unrecognized because the manifestations of such injury are usually nonspecific in nature and insidious in onset. Diagnosis largely depends on a history of exposure to a certain toxin. Particular attention should be paid to the occupational history, as well as to an assessment of exposure—current and remote—to drugs, especially antibiotics and analgesics. The recognition of a potential association between a patient's renal disease and exposure to a nephrotoxin is crucial, because, unlike many other forms of renal disease, progression of the functional and morphologic abnormalities associated with toxin-induced nephropathies may be prevented, and even reversed, by eliminating additional exposure.

Table 276-2

Transport Dysfunctions of Tubulointerstitial Disease

Defect	Cause(s)
Reduced GFR*	Obliteration of microvasculature and obstruction of tubules
Fanconi syndrome	Damage to proximal tubular reabsorption of glucose, amino acids, phosphate, and bicarbonate
Hyperchloremic acidosis*	1. Reduced ammonia production 2. Inability to acidify the collecting duct fluid (distal renal tubular acidosis) 3. Proximal bicarbonate wasting
Tubular or small-molecular-weight proteinuria*	Failure of proximal tubule protein reabsorption
Polyuria, isothenuria*	Damage to medullary tubules and vasculature
Hyperkalemia*	Potassium secretory defects including aldosterone resistance
Salt wasting	Distal tubular damage with impaired sodium reabsorption

* Common

EXOGENOUS TOXINS **Analgesic nephropathy** A distinct clinicopathologic syndrome has been described in heavy users of analgesic mixtures containing phenacetin in combination with aspirin, acetaminophen, or caffeine. These individuals have an approximately 20-fold increased risk of end-stage renal disease (ESRD). Analgesic nephropathy has been an important cause of chronic renal failure in Australia, Switzerland, Sweden, Belgium, and the southeastern United States.

Morphologically, analgesic nephropathy is characterized by papillary necrosis and tubulointerstitial inflammation. At an early stage, damage to the vascular supply of the inner medulla (vasa recta) leads to a local interstitial inflammatory reaction and, eventually, to papillary ischemia, necrosis, fibrosis, and calcification. The susceptibility of the renal papillae to damage by phenacetin is believed to be related to the establishment of a renal gradient for its acetaminophen metabolite, resulting in papillary tip concentrations tenfold higher than those in renal cortex. Hydration dissipates this gradient and may explain the protective effect of this maneuver in preventing phenacetin-induced papillary necrosis in animals. Aspirin in these analgesic compounds contributes to renal injury by uncoupling oxidative phosphorylation in renal mitochondria and by inhibiting the synthesis of renal prostaglandins, which are potent endogenous renal vasodilator hormones.

Analgesic nephropathy occurs some three to five times more commonly in women than in men. A direct relationship exists between the total amount of analgesic compounds ingested and the degree of renal impairment. The intake of 1.0 g phenacetin per day for 1 to 3 years or the total ingestion of 2 kg phenacetin in combination with other analgesics appears to represent minimum requirements for the development of analgesic nephropathy. In such patients, renal function usually declines gradually, in association with chronic necrosis of papillae and diffuse tubulointerstitial damage to the renal cortex. Occasionally, papillary necrosis may be associated with hematuria and even renal colic owing to obstruction of a ureter by necrotic tissue. More than half of patients with analgesic nephropathy have pyuria, which, if persistently associated with sterile urine, provides an important clue to the diagnosis. Nonetheless, active pyelonephritis may coexist in patients with analgesic nephropathy. Proteinuria, if present, is typically mild (less than 1 g/d). Patients with analgesic nephropathy are usually unable to generate maximally concentrated urine, reflecting the underlying medullary and papillary damage. An acquired form of distal renal tubular acidosis may contribute to the development of *nephrocalcinosis*. The occurrence of anemia out of proportion to the degree of azotemia also may provide a clue to the diagnosis of analgesic nephropathy. When analgesic nephropathy has progressed to renal insufficiency, the kidneys usually appear bilaterally shrunken on intravenous pyelography, and the calyces are deformed. A "ring sign" on the pyelogram is pathognomonic of papillary necrosis and represents the radiolucent sloughed papilla surrounded by the radiodense contrast material in the calyx. Renal sonography may reveal papillary calcifications surrounding the central sinus complex in a "garland" pattern. Transitional cell carcinoma may develop in the urinary pelvis or ureters as a late complication of analgesic abuse.

℞ TREATMENT

Every effort must be made to convince the patient who ingests excessive amounts of analgesic combinations to discontinue this hazardous practice. When renal damage is at an early stage, cessation of abuse usually arrests the progression of the nephrotoxic process; not infrequently, overall renal function improves with time. With continued abuse, however, progressive renal damage leads invariably to chronic renal failure.

Whether single-ingredient analgesics, used alone, cause renal disease is controversial. Recent reports have suggested a two- to threefold increase in the risk of ESRD among regular users of acetaminophen, and perhaps nonsteroidal antiinflammatory drugs (NSAIDs), but not among regular users of aspirin. Until conclusive evidence is available, physicians should consider screening regular users of acetaminophen and NSAIDs for evidence of renal disease. In patients with preexisting renal disease, the use of aspirin should be considered.

Lead Nephropathy (See also Chap. 397) Lead intoxication may produce a chronic tubulointerstitial renal disease. Children who repeatedly ingest lead-based paints may develop kidney disease as adults. Significant occupational exposure may occur in a diverse variety of workplaces where lead-containing metals or paints are heated to high temperatures, such as battery factories, smelters, salvage yards, and firing ranges. Alcohol, illegally distilled in an apparatus constructed from automobile radiators (so-called moonshine), is another cause of lead poisoning. Environmental lead exposure, particularly in industrial regions, may be great enough to produce changes in renal function.

Tubule transport processes enhance the accumulation of lead within renal cells, particularly in the proximal convoluted tubule, leading to cell degeneration, mitochondrial swelling, and eosinophilic intranuclear inclusion bodies rich in lead. In addition to tubule degeneration and atrophy, lead nephropathy is associated with ischemic changes in the glomeruli, fibrosis of the adventitia of small renal arterioles, and focal areas of cortical scarring. Eventually, the kidneys become atrophic. Urinary excretion of lead, porphyrin precursors such as δ-aminolevulinic acid and coproporphyrin, and urobilinogen, may be increased. Patients with chronic lead nephropathy are characteristically *hyperuricemic*, a consequence of enhanced reabsorption of filtered urate. Acute gouty arthritis (so-called saturnine gout) develops in about 50 percent of patients with lead nephropathy, in striking contrast to other forms of chronic renal failure in which de novo gout is rare (also see Chap. 344). Hypertension is also a complication. Therefore, in any patient with slowly progressive renal failure, atrophic kidneys, gout, and hypertension, the diagnosis of lead intoxication should be considered. Features of acute lead intoxication (abdominal colic, anemia, peripheral neuropathy, and encephalopathy) are usually absent.

The diagnosis may be suspected by finding elevated serum levels of lead. However, because blood levels may not be elevated even in the presence of a toxic total-body burden of lead, the quantitation of lead excretion following infusion of the chelating agent calcium disodium edetate is a more reliable indicator of serious lead exposure. Urinary excretion of more than 0.6 mg/d of lead is indicative of overt or potential toxicity.

℞ TREATMENT

Treatment includes removing the patient from the source of exposure and augmenting lead excretion with a chelating agent such as calcium disodium edetate.

Miscellaneous Nephrotoxins Use of *lithium salts* for manic-depressive illness has been associated with polyuria and polydipsia caused by tubulointerstitial disease. There are only rare reports of chronic renal insufficiency attributable to this agent. Renal function should be followed in patients taking this drug, and caution should be exercised if lithium is employed in patients with underlying renal disease.

The immunosuppressant *cyclosporine* causes both acute and chronic renal injury. The acute injury and the use of cyclosporine in transplantation are discussed in Chap. 272. The chronic injury results in an irreversible reduction in glomerular filtration rate (GFR), with mild proteinuria and arterial hypertension. Hyperkalemia is a relatively common complication and results in part from tubule resistance to aldosterone. Hypomagnesemia due to urinary magnesium wasting is less common but can cause hypocalcemia. The histologic changes in renal tissue include patchy interstitial fibrosis and tubular atrophy. In addition, the intrarenal vasculature often demonstrates hyalinosis, and focal segmental glomerular sclerosis can be present as well. Fibrosis may be the result of a cyclosporine-induced increase in renal collagen production. Vasoconstrictive mediators, such as angiotensin II, or vasoconstriction itself may also play a role in chronic cyclosporine toxicity. In patients receiving this drug for renal transplantation (see Chap. 272), chronic rejection and recurrence of the primary disease may coincide with chronic cyclosporine injury, and on clinical grounds, distinction among these may be difficult. Although most patients experience stable, albeit reduced, renal function, progressive renal injury can occur without a progressive reduction in GFR. Dose reduction appears to mitigate cyclosporine-associated renal fibrosis, but may increase the risk of rejection and graft loss. The optimal dosage of cyclosporine in renal transplantation remains controversial. Treatment of any associated arterial hypertension may lessen renal injury.

Many agents that commonly lead to acute renal failure are also capable of producing tubulointerstitial injury (see Chap. 270). These include antibiotics (e.g., aminoglycosides, amphotericin B), radiographic contrast agents, various hydrocarbons (e.g., carbon tetrachloride), and heavy metals (e.g., mercury, cadmium, and bismuth).

METABOLIC TOXINS Acute Uric Acid Nephropathy (See also Chap. 344) Acute overproduction of uric acid and extreme hyperuricemia often lead to a rapidly progressive renal insufficiency, so-called acute uric acid nephropathy. This tubulointerstitial disease is usually seen in patients given cytotoxic drugs for the treatment of lymphoproliferative or myeloproliferative disorders but also may occur in these patients before such treatment is begun. The pathologic changes are largely the result of deposition of uric acid crystals in the kidneys and their collecting systems, leading to partial or complete obstruction of collecting ducts, renal pelvis, or ureter. Since obstruction is often bilateral, patients typically show the clinical course of acute renal failure, characterized by oliguria and rapidly rising serum creatinine concentration. In the early phase uric acid crystals can be found in urine, usually in association with microscopic or gross hematuria. Peak serum uric acid levels vary but are almost always above 1200 μmol/L (20 mg/dL) and may even exceed 3500 μmol/L (60 mg/dL).

Prevention of hyperuricemia in patients at risk by treatment with allopurinol in doses of 200 to 800 mg/d prior to cytotoxic therapy reduces the danger of acute uric acid nephropathy. Once hyperuricemia develops, however, efforts should be directed to preventing deposition of uric acid within the urinary tract. Increasing urine volume with potent diuretics (furosemide or mannitol) effectively lowers intratubular uric acid concentrations, and alkalinization of the urine to pH 7 or greater with sodium bicarbonate and/or a carbonic anhydrase inhibitor (acetazolamide) enhances uric acid solubility. If these efforts, together with allopurinol therapy, are ineffective in preventing acute renal failure, dialysis should be instituted to lower the serum uric acid concentration as well as to treat the acute manifestations of uremia.

Gouty Nephropathy (See also Chap. 344) Patients with less severe but prolonged forms of hyperuricemia are predisposed to a more chronic tubulointerstitial disorder, often referred to as *gouty nephropathy*. The severity of renal involvement correlates with the duration and magnitude of the elevation of the serum uric acid concentration. Histologically, the distinctive feature of gouty nephropathy is the presence of crystalline deposits of uric acid and monosodium urate salts in kidney parenchyma. These deposits not only cause intrarenal obstruction but also incite an inflammatory response, leading to lymphocytic infiltration, foreign-body giant cell reaction, and eventual fibrosis, especially of medullary and papillary regions of the kidney. Bacteriuria and pyelonephritis occur in about one-fourth of cases, presumably as complications of intrarenal urinary stasis. Since patients with gout frequently suffer from hypertension and hyperlipidemia, degenerative changes of the renal arterioles may constitute a striking feature of the histologic abnormality, often out of proportion to other morphologic defects. Clinically, gouty nephropathy is an insidious cause of renal insufficiency. Early in its course, GFR may be near normal, often despite focal morphologic changes in medullary and cortical interstitium, proteinuria, and diminished urinary concentrating ability. Whether reducing serum uric acid levels with allopurinol exerts a beneficial effect on the kidney remains to be demonstrated. Although such undesirable consequences of hyperuricemia as gout and uric acid stones respond well to allopurinol, use of this drug in asymptomatic hyperuricemia has not been shown to improve renal function consistently. On the other hand, uricosuric agents such as probenecid, which may increase uric acid stone production, clearly have no role in the treatment of renal disease associated with hyperuricemia.

Hypercalcemic Nephropathy (See also Chap. 354) Chronic hypercalcemia, as occurs in primary hyperparathyroidism, sarcoidosis, multiple myeloma, vitamin D intoxication, or metastatic bone disease, can cause tubulointerstitial damage and progressive renal insufficiency. The earliest lesion is a focal degenerative change in renal epithelia, primarily in collecting ducts, distal convoluted tubules, and loops of Henle. Tubule cell necrosis leads to nephron obstruction and stasis of intrarenal urine, favoring local precipitation of calcium salts and infection. Dilatation and atrophy of tubules eventually occur, as do interstitial fibrosis, mononuclear leukocyte infiltration, and interstitial calcium deposition (nephrocalcinosis). Calcium deposition also may occur in glomeruli and the walls of renal arterioles.

Clinically, the most striking defect is an inability to concentrate the urine maximally, resulting in polyuria and nocturia. Defective transport of NaCl in the ascending limb of Henle's loop is responsible, at least in part, for this concentrating defect. Additionally, reduced collecting duct responsiveness to vasopressin may contribute. Reductions in GFR and renal blood flow also occur, both in acute severe hypercalcemia and with prolonged hypercalcemia of lesser severity. Distal renal tubular acidosis and sodium and potassium wasting also have been described in these chronic states. Eventually, uncontrolled hypercalcemia leads to severe tubulointerstitial damage and overt renal failure. Abdominal x-rays may demonstrate nephrocalcinosis as well as nephrolithiasis, the latter due to the hypercalciuria that often accompanies hypercalcemia.

℞ **TREATMENT**

This consists of reducing the serum calcium concentration toward normal and correcting the primary abnormality of calcium metabolism. The management of hypercalcemia is discussed in Chap. 354. Prognosis for recovery of renal function depends on the severity of the renal lesion at the time hypercalcemia is corrected. Renal dysfunction of acute hypercalcemia may be completely reversible. Gradual, progressive renal insufficiency related to chronic hypercalcemia, however, may not improve with correction of the calcium disorder. Nonetheless, every effort should be made to return serum calcium concentration to normal to minimize further loss of renal function.

Hypokalemic Nephropathy (See also Chap. 49) Disturbances of renal structure and function occur commonly in patients with moderate to severe potassium depletion of at least several weeks' duration. Histologically, renal epithelial cells are often seen to contain numerous vacuoles, most marked in proximal tubules. Glomeruli are reduced in size and may become sclerotic. Whether prolonged or recurrent potassium deficiency results in irreversible tubulointerstitial fibrosis, scarring, and atrophy is unresolved. Loss of urinary concentrating ability is the most commonly encountered functional defect and is due, at least in part, to defective operation of the countercurrent multiplier system. Elevated rates of intrarenal prostaglandin synthesis also may contribute to this concentrating defect. Nocturia, polyuria, and polydipsia are frequently encountered in patients with chronic potassium depletion. The polydipsia is probably due to both the impaired renal concentrating ability and a primary disorder of the thirst mechanism, which is believed to be a common feature of chronic potassium depletion. Patients with hypokalemic nephropathy may have an enhanced susceptibility to pyelonephritis. Urinalysis often reveals no abnormalities except for mild proteinuria. Serum creatinine and urea nitrogen concentrations usually remain within normal limits.

℞ **TREATMENT**

This should be directed at repleting body potassium stores and correcting the primary process responsible for potassium loss. With correction of body potassium, functional and histologic abnormalities of the kidneys usually disappear, although maximal urinary concentrating ability may not return to normal for several months.

Miscellaneous Metabolic Toxins Urinary oxalate, derived from the metabolism of glycine and, to a variable extent, from ingested oxalate, may deposit as insoluble intratubular calcium oxalate crystals and result in chronic tubulointerstitial damage in patients with hereditary or acquired forms of *hyperoxaluria*. *Cystinosis* and *Fabry's disease* are other hereditary depositional disorders affecting the renal tubules and interstitium (see Chaps. 275, 278, and 279).

RENAL PARENCHYMAL DISEASE ASSOCIATED WITH EXTRARENAL NEOPLASM

Except for the glomerulopathies associated with lymphomas and several solid tumors (see Chap. 275), the renal manifestations of primary extrarenal neoplastic processes are confined mainly to the interstitium and tubules. Although metastatic renal involvement by solid tumors is unusual, the kidneys are often invaded by neoplastic cells in various lymphomas and leukemias and in multiple myeloma. In postmortem studies of patients with *lymphoma*, renal involvement is found in approximately half. The involvement may be focal, in the form of multiple discrete nodules, or diffuse, with lymphomatous infiltration throughout the renal parenchyma. Diffuse infiltration is seen most commonly in lymphomas other than Hodgkin's disease. There may be flank pain related to massive renal infiltration, and x-rays may show enlargement of one or both kidneys. Renal insufficiency occurs in a minority of cases, and overt uremia is rare. Treatment of the primary disease may improve renal function in these cases.

The kidneys are also commonly involved in various forms of *leukemia*. At postmortem examination, bilateral renal involvement is present in approximately 50 percent of cases. As with lymphoma, uremia is rarely, if ever, a consequence of leukemic infiltration of the kidneys. The kidneys also can be involved in leukemias because of the associated high incidence of hyperuricemia, hypercalcemia, and lysozymuria. The myelogenous leukemias, particularly of the monocytic type, may be complicated by tubule defects involving potassium and magnesium wasting.

In contrast, infiltration of the kidneys with *myeloma* cells is infrequent (see also Chap. 114). When it occurs, the process is usually focal, so renal insufficiency from this cause is also uncommon. The more usual lesion is *myeloma kidney*, characterized histologically by atrophic tubules, many with eosinophilic intraluminal casts, and numerous multinucleated giant cells within tubule walls and in the interstitium. The frequent occurrence of myeloma kidney in patients with Bence Jones proteinuria has suggested a causal relation. Bence Jones proteins are thought to cause myeloma kidney through direct toxicity to renal tubule cells. In addition, Bence Jones proteins may precipitate within the distal nephron where the high concentrations of these proteins and the acid composition of the tubule fluid favor intraluminal cast formation and intrarenal obstruction. Occasionally, acute renal failure occurs after intravenous pyelography in patients with multiple myeloma and is believed to result from the further precipitation of Bence Jones proteins induced by dehydration prior to radiographic study. Dehydration of the patient with myeloma in preparation for intravenous pyelography should therefore be avoided. Multiple myeloma also may affect the kidneys indirectly. Hypercalcemia or hyperuricemia may lead to the nephropathies described above. Proximal tubule disorders are also seen occasionally, including type II proximal renal tubular acidosis and the Fanconi syndrome. Additionally, intrarenal deposits of *amyloid* (see below) may contribute to impaired excretory function.

IMMUNE DISORDERS

HYPERSENSITIVITY NEPHROPATHY An acute diffuse tubulointerstitial reaction may result from hypersensitivity to a number of drugs, including sulfonamides, many penicillins and cephalosporins, the fluoroquinolone antibiotics ciprofloxacin and norfloxacin, and the antituberculous drugs isoniazid and rifampin. Acute tubulointerstitial damage has also occurred after use of thiazide and loop diuretics, antiulcer medications (cimetidine, ranitidine, and omeprazole), and NSAIDs. Of note, the tubulointerstitial nephropathy that develops in some patients taking NSAIDs may be associated with nephrotic-range proteinuria and histologic evidence of minimal change glomerulopathy. Grossly, the kidneys are usually enlarged. Histologically, the glomeruli appear normal. The principal pathologic abnormalities are in the interstitium of the kidney, which reveals pronounced edema and infiltration with polymorphonuclear leukocytes, lymphocytes, plasma cells, and, in some cases, large numbers of eosinophils. If the process is severe, tubule cell necrosis and regeneration also may be apparent. Immunofluorescence studies either have been unrevealing or have demonstrated a linear pattern of immunoglobulin and complement deposition along tubule basement membranes. In a few cases of methicillin-induced acute tubulointerstitial disease, circulating anti-tubule basement membrane antibodies also have been found, suggesting that autoantibody formation may have been induced by the penicilloyl hapten of methicillin (by conjugation of hapten with tubule basement membrane proteins, thereby altering the native antigenicity of the basement membrane).

Most patients require several weeks of drug exposure before developing evidence of renal injury. Rare cases have occurred after only a few doses or after a year of more of use. Azotemia is usually present; a diagnostic triad of fever, skin rash, and peripheral blood eosinophilia is highly suggestive of acute tubulointerstitial nephritis but is often absent. Examination of the urine sediment reveals hematuria and often pyuria; occasionally, eosinophils may be present. Proteinuria is usually mild to moderate, except in cases of NSAID-induced tubulointerstitial nephritis with minimal change glomerulopathy. The clinical picture may be confused with acute glomerulonephritis, but when acute azotemia and hematuria are accompanied by eosinophilia, skin rash, and a history of drug exposure, a hypersensitivity reaction leading to acute tubulointerstitial nephritis should be regarded as the leading diagnostic possibility. Discontinuation of the drug usually results in complete reversal of the renal injury; rarely, renal damage may be irreversible. Glucocorticoids have been used, but their value has not been established.

SJÖGREN'S SYNDROME (See also Chap. 316) When the kidneys are involved in this disorder, the predominant histologic findings are those of chronic tubulointerstitial disease. Interstitial infiltrates are composed primarily of lymphocytes, causing the histology of the renal parenchyma in these patients to resemble that of the salivary and lacrimal glands. Renal functional defects include diminished urinary concentrating ability and distal (type I) renal tubular acidosis. Urinalysis may show pyuria (predominantly lymphocyturia) and mild proteinuria.

AMYLOIDOSIS (See also Chaps. 275 and 309) Glomerular pathology usually predominates and leads to heavy proteinuria and azotemia. However, tubule function also may be deranged, giving rise to a nephrogenic diabetes insipidus and to distal (type I) renal tubular acidosis. In several cases these functional abnormalities correlated with peritubular deposition of amyloid, particularly in areas surrounding vasa rectae, loops of Henle, and collecting ducts. Bilateral enlargement of the kidneys, especially in a patient with massive proteinuria and tubule dysfunction, should raise the possibility of amyloid renal disease.

HUMAN IMMUNODEFICIENCY VIRUS (HIV) INFECTION (See also Chap. 308) Chronic renal disease occurs in a small fraction of patients infected with HIV. This complication usually presents with nephrotic proteinuria and a rapid decline in renal function and may precede overt AIDS. Most patients have a characteristic renal lesion, HIV-associated nephropathy, comprising focal and segmental glomerulosclerosis with collapse of the glomerular tuft, tubular dilatation with cystic change, epithelial cell vacuolization, and a dense mononuclear cell infiltrate of the interstitium. A minority of patients have an immune-complex glomerulonephritis, with HIV-antigen-specific immune complexes. Uncertainty exists whether direct infection of renal cells by the virus or some indirect immune reaction is responsible for the renal disease. In addition to these HIV-specific renal diseases, a diverse array of mycobacterial, fungal, and viral diseases can affect the kidneys in HIV-infected individuals. Additional renal abnormalities may result from repeated exposure to nephrotoxic antibiotics. A thrombotic microangiopathy has also been reported. Black patients with HIV appear to be at particularly high risk for HIV-associated nephropathy. Once ESRD develops, survival depends primarily on the immunologic and functional status of the individual. The value of antiretroviral or steroid therapy in slowing the progression to ESRD has not been proved, whereas angiotensin-converting enzyme inhibitors appear to offer some benefit.

TUBULOINTERSTITIAL ABNORMALITIES ASSOCIATED WITH GLOMERULONEPHRITIS A number of primary glomerulopathies also may be associated with damage to tubules and interstitium. For example, in more than half of patients with the nephropathy of systemic lupus erythematosus, deposits of immune complexes can be identified in tubule basement membranes, usually accompanied by an interstitial mononuclear inflammatory reaction. Similarly, in many patients with glomerulonephritis associated with anti-glomerular basement membrane antibody, the same antibody is reactive against tubule basement membranes as well.

MISCELLANEOUS DISORDERS

VESICOURETERAL REFLUX (See also Chaps. 131 and 280) When the function of the ureterovesical junction is impaired, urine may reflux into the ureters due to the high intravesical pressure that develops during voiding. Clinically, reflux is often detected on the voiding and postvoiding films obtained during intravenous pyelography, although voiding cystourethrography may be required for definitive diagnosis. Bladder infection may ascend the urinary tract to the kidneys through incompetent ureterovesical sphincters. Not surprisingly, therefore, reflux is often discovered in patients with acute and/or chronic urinary tract infections. With more severe degrees of reflux, characterized by dilatation of ureters and renal pelves, progressive renal damage often appears, and although active infection also may be present, uncertainty exists as to the necessity of infection in producing the scarred kidney of reflux nephropathy. Substantial proteinuria is often present, and glomerular lesions similar to those of idiopathic focal glomerulosclerosis (Chap. 274) are often found in addition to the changes of chronic tubulointerstitial disease. Surgical correction of reflux is usually necessary only with the more severe degrees of reflux since renal damage correlates with the extent of reflux. Obviously, if extensive glomerulosclerosis already exists, urologic repair may no longer be warranted.

RADIATION NEPHRITIS Renal dysfunction can be expected to occur if 23 Gy (2300 rad) or more of x-ray irradiation is administered to both kidneys during a period of 5 weeks or less. Histologic examination of the kidneys reveals hyalinized glomeruli, atrophic tubules, extensive interstitial fibrosis, and hyalinization of the media of renal arterioles. Radiation-induced renal ischemia is believed to be the main pathogenic factor responsible for the tubulointerstitial damage, which may not become evident clinically for months after completion of radiation. The presentation of acute radiation nephritis includes rapidly progressive azotemia, moderate to malignant hypertension, anemia, and proteinuria that may reach the nephrotic range. More than 50 percent progress to chronic renal failure. A more insidious form is characterized by slower development of azotemia, anemia, and nephrotic syndrome. Malignant hypertension may follow unilateral renal irradiation and resolve with ipsilateral nephrectomy. Radiation nephritis has all but vanished because of heightened awareness of its pathogenesis by radiotherapists.

BIBLIOGRAPHY

Adler SG et al: Hypersensitivity phenomena and the kidney: Role of drugs and environmental agents. Am J Kidney Dis 5:75, 1985
Arant BS: Reflux nephropathy. Kidney 21:19, 1989
Bennet WM: Lead nephropathy. Kidney Int 28:218, 1985
———, Debroe ME: Analgesic nephropathy. A preventable renal disease. N Engl J Med 320, 1269, 1989
Kelly CJ, Neilson EG: Tubulointerstitial diseases, in *The Kidney*, 5th ed, BM Brenner (ed). Philadelphia, Saunders, 1996 pp 1655–1679
Boton R et al: Prevalence, pathogenesis, and treatment of renal dysfunction associated with chronic lithium therapy. Am J Kidney Dis 10:329, 1987
Cameron JS: Immunologically mediated interstitial nephritis: Primary and secondary. Adv Nephrol 18:207, 1989
Luke RG: New issues in therapy after renal transplantation. N Engl J Med 331:393, 1994
Myers BD et al: The long-term course of cyclosporine-associated chronic nephropathy. Kidney Int 33:590, 1988
Perneger TV et al: Risk of renal failure associated with the use of acetaminophen, aspirin, and nonsteroidal antiinflammatory drugs. N Engl J Med 331:1675, 1994
Rao TKS: Clinical features of human immunodeficiency virus associated nephropathy. Kidney Int 40(Suppl 35):S-13, 1991

277

Kamal F. Badr, Barry M. Brenner

VASCULAR INJURY TO THE KIDNEY

Adequate delivery of blood to the glomerular capillary network is crucial for glomerular filtration and overall salt and water balance. Thus, in addition to the threat to the viability of renal tissue, vascular injury to the kidney may compromise the maintenance of body fluid volume and composition. Involvement of the renal vessels by atherosclerotic, hypertensive, embolic, inflammatory, and hematologic disorders is usually a manifestation of generalized vascular pathology. The morphologic and clinical responses to these insults and the unique renal vasculopathy associated with the toxemias of pregnancy are considered in this chapter.

THROMBOEMBOLIC DISEASES OF THE RENAL ARTERIES Thrombosis of the major renal arteries or their branches is an important cause of deterioration of renal function, especially in the elderly. It is often difficult to diagnose and therefore requires a high index of suspicion. Thrombosis may occur as a result of intrinsic pathology in the renal vessels (posttraumatic, atherosclerotic, or inflammatory) or as a result of emboli originating in distant vessels, most commonly fat emboli, emboli originating in the left heart (mural thrombi following myocardial infarction, bacterial endocarditis, or aseptic vegetations), or "paradoxical" emboli passing from the right side of the circulation via a patent foramen ovale or atrial septal defect. Renal emboli are bilateral in 15 to 30 percent of cases.

The clinical presentation is variable, depending on the time course and the extent of the occlusive event. Acute thrombosis and infarction, such as follows embolization, may result in sudden onset of flank pain and tenderness, fever, hematuria, leukocytosis, nausea, and vomiting. If infarction occurs, renal enzymes may be elevated, namely aspartate aminotransferase (AST), lactic dehydrogenase (LDH; most reliable), and alkaline phosphatase, which rise and fall in the order listed. Urinary lactic dehydrogenase and alkaline phosphatase also may increase after infarction. Renal function deteriorates acutely, leading in bilateral thrombosis to acute oliguric renal failure. More gradual (i.e., atherosclerotic) occlusion of a single renal artery may go undetected. A spectrum of clinical presentations lies between these two extremes (Table 277-1). Hypertension usually follows renal infarction and results from renin release in the peri-infarction zone. Hypertension is usually transient but may be persistent. Diagnosis is established by renal arteriography.

℞ TREATMENT

Management of *acute* renal arterial thrombosis includes surgical intervention, anticoagulant therapy, conservative and supportive therapy, and control of hypertension. The choice of treatment depends mainly on (1) the condition of the patient, in particular the patient's ability to withstand major surgery, and (2) the extent of renovascular occlusion and amount of renal mass at risk of infarction. In general, supportive care and anticoagulant therapy are indicated in unilateral disease. In bilateral thrombosis, medical and surgical therapies yield comparable results. Twenty-five percent of patients die during the acute episode, usually from extrarenal complications. In *chronic* ischemic renal disease, surgical revascularization is more likely to preserve and improve renal function and to control the hypertension (see below).

ATHEROEMBOLIC DISEASE OF THE RENAL ARTERIES Atheroembolic disease typically results from multiple showers of cholesterol-containing microemboli dislodged from atheromatous plaques in large arteries. Such emboli occlude small (150- to 200-μm diameter) vessels in the kidneys and in other organs (retina, brain, pancreas, muscles, skin, and extremities). It usually occurs in an elderly individual with atherosclerotic disease elsewhere and usually follows aortic surgery or renal or coronary arteriography. Spontaneous atheroembolic disease has also been reported. Manifestations include deterioration of renal function (sudden or gradual), mild proteinuria, microscopic hematuria, and leukocyturia. Urine volume may remain normal or fall to oliguric levels depending on severity. Renal ischemia can induce or exacerbate preexisting hypertension.

Table 277-1

Clinical Presentations of Ischemic Renal Disease
Acute renal failure
Progressive azotemia in a patient with known renovascular hypertension (usually on medical therapy)
Unexplained progressive azotemia in an elderly patient with or without refractory hypertension
Hypertension and azotemia in a renal transplant patient

Antemortem diagnosis of atherosclerotic renal emboli is difficult. The demonstration of cholesterol emboli in the retina is helpful, but a firm diagnosis is established only by demonstration of cholesterol crystals in the smaller arteries and arterioles in renal biopsy or autopsy specimens. These also may be seen in asymptomatic skeletal muscle or skin. No specific treatment is available.

RENAL VEIN THROMBOSIS (RVT) Thrombosis of one or both main renal veins occurs in a variety of settings (Table 277-2). The pathogenesis is not always clear, particularly when it occurs in so-called hypercoagulable states such as may develop in pregnant women, users of oral contraceptives, subjects with nephrotic syndrome, or dehydrated infants. Nephrotic syndrome accompanying membranous glomerulopathy and certain carcinomas seems to predispose to the development of RVT, which occurs in 10 to 50 percent of patients with these disorders. RVT may exacerbate preexisting proteinuria but is infrequently the cause of the nephrotic syndrome.

The clinical manifestations depend on the severity and abruptness of its occurrence. Acute cases occur typically in children and are characterized by sudden loss of renal function, often accompanied by fever, chills, lumbar tenderness (with kidney enlargement), leukocytosis, and hematuria. Hemorrhagic infarction and renal rupture may lead to hypovolemic shock. In young adults RVT is usually suspected from an unexpected and relatively acute or subacute deterioration of renal function and/or exacerbation of proteinuria and hematuria in the appropriate clinical setting (underlying nephrotic syndrome, trauma, pregnancy, oral contraceptive use). In cases of gradual thrombosis, usually occurring in the elderly, the only manifestation may be recurrent pulmonary emboli or development of hypertension. A Fanconi-like syndrome and proximal renal tubular acidosis have been described.

The definitive diagnosis can only be established through selective renal venography with visualization of the occluding thrombus.

℞ TREATMENT

Treatment consists of anticoagulation, the main purpose of which is prevention of pulmonary embolization, although some authors have also claimed improvement in renal function and proteinuria. Encouraging reports have appeared concerning the use of streptokinase. Spontaneous recanalization with clinical improvement also has been observed. Anticoagulant therapy is more rewarding in the acute thrombosis seen in younger individuals. Nephrectomy is advocated in infants with life-threatening renal infarction. Thrombectomy is effective in some cases.

RENAL ARTERY STENOSIS / ISCHEMIC RENAL DISEASE Stenosis of the main renal artery and/or its major branches accounts for 2 to 5 percent of hypertension. The common cause in the middle-aged and elderly is an atheromatous plaque at the origin of the renal artery. In a large unselected autopsy series, stenosis producing > 50 percent renal artery diameter reduction was found in 18 percent of those between 65 and 74 years of age and in 42 percent of those older than 75 years. Bilateral involvement was found in half of the affected cases in both age groups. In younger women, stenosis is due to intrinsic structural abnormalities of the arterial wall caused by a heterogeneous group of lesions termed *fibromuscular dysplasia*.

Renal artery stenosis should be suspected when hypertension develops in a previously normotensive individual over 50 years of age or in the young (under 30 years) with suggestive features: symptoms of vascular insufficiency to other organs, high-pitched epigastric bruit on physical examination, symptoms of hypokalemia secondary to hyperaldosteronism (muscle weakness, tetany, polyuria), and metabolic alkalosis. If renovascular hypertension is suspected, a positive captopril test, which has a sensitivity and specificity of greater than 95 percent, constitutes an excellent screening procedure to assess the need for more invasive radiographic evaluation. The test relies on the exaggerated increase in plasma renin activity (PRA) following administration of captopril to patients with renovascular hypertension as compared with those with essential hypertension. It is considered positive when all the following criteria are satisfied: stimulated PRA of 12 (μg/L)/h, absolute increase in PRA of 10 (μg/L)/h or more, and increase in PRA of greater than 150 percent [or 400 percent if baseline PRA is less than 3 (μg/L)/h]. In the appropriate clinical setting, particularly in the presence of a positive captopril test, digital subtraction renal arteriography should be performed. This procedure obviates the need for cannulation of the arterial system and has a low incidence of false-positive (5 percent) and false-negative (10 percent) results. Since angiotensin I–converting enzyme (ACE) inhibitors magnify the impairment in renal blood flow and glomerular filtration rate (GFR) caused by functionally significant renal artery stenosis, use of these drugs in association with ^{99m}Tc-DTPA or ^{99m}MAG$_3$ renography greatly enhances the predictive value of radionuclide renography (>90 percent sensitivity and specificity). The most definitive diagnostic procedure is bilateral arteriography with repeated bilateral renal vein and systemic renin determinations. If renal vein renin measurements from the two kidneys differ by a factor of 1.5:1 or more (higher value from the affected kidney) in a patient with radiographic unilateral renal artery stenosis, the chance of cure of hypertension by surgical reconstruction is almost 90 percent, particularly if renal vein renin level from the unaffected kidney is equal to or less than systemic levels (suppressible). A ratio of less than 1.5:1, however, does not exclude the diagnosis of renovascular hypertension, particularly in the presence of bilateral disease. Two diagnostic modalities for the noninvasive evaluation of significant renal artery stenosis are duplex scanning (sensitivity 95 percent, specificity 90 percent) and magnetic resonance angiography (sensitivity 100 percent for lesions with ≥50 percent stenosis, specificity 92 percent).

℞ TREATMENT

The aims of treatment are control of the blood pressure and restoration of perfusion to the ischemic kidney. In general, it is now firmly established that interventional therapy (i.e., surgery or angioplasty) is superior to medical therapy, which, while controlling blood pressure, does little to salvage renal mass lost to ischemic injury. Success rates with percutaneous transluminal angioplasty in young patients with fibromuscular dysplasia are 50 percent cure and improvement in blood pressure control in another 30 percent. Angioplasty is best suited for noncalcified, segmental short lesions and is also useful in some elderly patients who are poor surgical risks. About half of elderly individuals with reduced renal function as a result of renal arterial stenosis improve following angioplasty or surgery, even when preintervention arteriography shows little evidence of cortical perfusion. Despite the risks associated with surgery, long-term follow-up studies demonstrate an advantage of surgery over angioplasty both with regard to the incidence of restenosis and to the preservation or improvement in GFR.

Renal artery stenosis, particularly if atherosclerotic, is a progressive disease that may lead to gradual and silent loss of renal functional tissue (ischemic renal disease). Progression of ipsilateral atherosclerotic narrowing can be expected in nearly 50 percent of individuals, resulting in complete occlusion in about 10 percent. Thus, these patients need careful follow-up of initially nonclinically significant narrowing (<70 percent) for the possibility of further occlusion or the development of contralateral disease (30 percent). Compensatory contralateral hypertrophy may maintain renal function until affected by superimposed pathologic processes, at which time azotemia supervenes. Ischemic renal disease is now recognized as a significant cause of end-stage renal dis-

Table 277-2

Conditions Associated with Renal Vein Thrombosis
Trauma
Extrinsic compression (lymph nodes, aortic aneurysm, tumor)
Invasion by renal cell carcinoma
Dehydration (infants)
Nephrotic syndrome
Pregnancy or oral contraceptives

ease in patients over 50 years of age (approximately 15 percent). Even if angioplasty or surgery fail to return blood pressure to normal, these procedures usually render medical therapy easier.

HEMOLYTIC UREMIC SYNDROME (HUS) AND THROMBOTIC THROMBOCYTOPENIC PURPURA (TTP) (See also Chap. 117) HUS and TTP, consumptive coagulopathies characterized by microangiopathic hemolytic anemia and thrombocytopenia, have a particular predilection for the kidney and the central nervous system, the latter especially in TTP. The kidneys of patients with HUS or TTP often exhibit a "flea-bitten" appearance, the result of multiple cortical hemorrhagic infarcts. The major sites of pathology are the small renal arteries and afferent arterioles, which are nearly occluded as a result of marked intimal hyperplasia (particularly in TTP) and fibrin deposits in the subintimal regions. When the vasoocclusive process is extensive, bilateral cortical necrosis may occur. In addition, arteriolar microaneurysms, glomerular infarction, or nonspecific focal changes may be seen. In keeping with the focal nature of the vascular lesions, patchy areas of interstitial edema, tubular necrosis, and, eventually, fibrosis occur. By immunofluorescence staining, complement components and immunoglobulins may be demonstrated in the arterioles, and fibrinogen deposits are present in arteries, arterioles, and glomerular capillary loops.

Several mechanisms have been implicated in the etiology of the intravascular coagulopathy seen in HUS and TTP, including induction of a generalized Shwartzman phenomenon by microorganisms or endotoxin, genetic predisposition, and deficiency of platelet antiaggregatory substance(s) (e.g., prostacyclin). Some patients improve following exchange transfusion or plasmapheresis, suggesting accumulation of an as yet unidentified toxin.

Renal failure is common in both HUS and TTP, usually manifested by azotemia, mild proteinuria, microscopic and/or gross hematuria, and cylindruria. Patients with HUS have more severe renal failure, often marked by oligoanuria and hypertension and commonly progressing to chronic renal failure. The prognosis in HUS is better in children than in adults. In TTP, the course of which may span days to months, renal failure is usually less severe.

Rx TREATMENT

In the management of TTP, high-dose glucocorticoids and plasma exchange often provide complete remission or cure. Plasma exchange should be initiated as early as possible, and the treatment cycles can be repeated if thrombocytopenia recurs. Splenectomy and antiplatelet therapy also have been used with varying degrees of success in TTP patients. The success of plasma exchange in adult HUS is less well established than in TTP.

ARTERIOLAR NEPHROSCLEROSIS (See also Chap. 242) Whether hypertension is "essential" or of known etiology, persistent exposure of the renal circulation to elevated intraluminal pressures results in development of intrinsic lesions of the renal arterioles (hyaline arteriolosclerosis) that eventually lead to loss of function (nephrosclerosis). Nephrosclerosis is divided into two distinct entities: "benign" and "malignant" (or accelerated).

Benign Arteriolar Nephrosclerosis Benign arteriolar nephrosclerosis is seen in patients who are hypertensive for an extended period of time (blood pressure more than 150/90 mmHg) but whose hypertension has not progressed to a malignant form (described below). Such patients, usually in the older age group, are often discovered to be hypertensive on routine physical examination or as a result of nonspecific symptomatology (e.g., headaches, weakness, palpitations).

Kidney size is normal to reduced, with loss of cortical mass leading to a fine granularity. Although the larger arteries may show atherosclerotic changes, the characteristic pathology is in the afferent arterioles, which have thickened walls due to deposition of homogeneous eosinophilic material (hyaline arteriolosclerosis). This material is composed of plasma proteins and fats that have been deposited in the arteriolar wall due to injury to the endothelium, probably secondary to the elevated intraluminal hydraulic pressure. Narrowing of vascular lumina results, with consequent ischemic injury to glomeruli and tubules.

Nephrosclerosis accompanying long-standing systemic arterial hypertension is only one manifestation of a generalized process affecting the cardiovascular system. Physical examination, therefore, may reveal changes in retinal vessels (arteriolar narrowing and/or flame-shaped hemorrhages), cardiac hypertrophy, and possibly signs of congestive heart failure. Renal disease may manifest as a mild to moderate elevation of serum creatinine concentration, microscopic hematuria, and/or mild proteinuria. In general, clinical evaluation does not reveal significant renal abnormalities. More specialized examination may disclose elevated urinary albumin excretion, tapering and loss of caliber of intrarenal vessels on arteriography, and an exaggerated natriuresis in response to a fluid challenge. Patients with benign nephrosclerosis maintain a near-normal GFR despite a reduction in renal blood flow.

Malignant Arteriolar Nephrosclerosis Patients with long-standing benign hypertension or patients not known to be hypertensive previously may develop malignant hypertension characterized by a sudden (accelerated) elevation of blood pressure (diastolic often above 130 mmHg) accompanied by papilledema, central nervous system manifestations, cardiac decompensation, and acute progressive deterioration of renal function. The absence of papilledema does not rule out the diagnosis in a patient with markedly elevated blood pressure and rapidly declining renal function. The kidneys are characterized by a flea-bitten appearance resulting from hemorrhages in surface capillaries. Histologically, two distinct vascular lesions can be seen. The first, affecting arterioles, is fibrinoid necrosis, i.e., infiltration of arteriolar walls with eosinophilic material including fibrin. There is thickening of vessel walls and, occasionally, an inflammatory infiltrate (necrotizing arteriolitis). The second lesion, involving the interlobular arteries, is a concentric hyperplastic proliferation of the cellular elements of the vascular wall with deposition of collagen to form a hyperplastic arteriolitis (onion-skin lesion). Fibrinoid necrosis occasionally extends into the glomeruli, which also may undergo proliferative changes or total necrosis. Most glomerular and tubular changes are secondary to ischemia and infarction. The sequence of events leading to the development of malignant hypertension is poorly defined. Two pathophysiologic alterations appear central in its initiation and/or perpetuation: (1) increased permeability of vessel walls to invasion by plasma components, particularly fibrin, which activates clotting mechanisms leading to a microangiopathic hemolytic anemia, thus perpetuating the vascular pathology; and (2) activation of the renin-angiotensin-aldosterone system at some point in the disease process, which contributes to the acceleration and maintenance of blood pressure elevation and, in turn, to vascular injury.

Malignant hypertension is most likely to develop in a previously hypertensive individual, usually in the third or fourth decade of life. There is a higher incidence among men, particularly black men. The presenting symptoms are usually neurologic (dizziness, headache, blurring of vision, altered states of consciousness, and focal or generalized seizures). Cardiac decompensation and renal failure appear thereafter. Renal abnormalities include a rapid rise in serum creatinine, hematuria (at times macroscopic), proteinuria, and red and white blood cell casts in the sediment. Nephrotic syndrome may be present. Elevated plasma aldosterone levels cause hypokalemic metabolic alkalosis in the early phase. Uremic acidosis and hyperkalemia eventually obscure these early findings. Hematologic indices of microangiopathic hemolytic anemia (i.e., schistocytes) are often seen.

Rx TREATMENT

Control of hypertension is the principal goal of therapy for both benign and malignant forms. The time of initiation of therapy, its effectiveness, and patient compliance are crucial factors in arresting the progression of benign nephrosclerosis. Untreated, most of these patients succumb to the extrarenal complications of hypertension. In contrast, malignant hypertension is a medical emergency; its natural course includes a death rate of 80 to 90 percent within 1 year of onset, almost always due to uremia. Supportive measures should be instituted to control the neurologic, cardiac, and other complications of acute renal failure, but the mainstay of therapy is prompt and aggressive reduction of blood pressure, which, if successful, can reverse all complications in the majority of patients. Presently, 5-year survival is 50 percent, and some patients have evidence of partial reversal of the vascular lesions and a return of renal function to near-normal levels.

SCLERODERMA (PROGRESSIVE SYSTEMIC SCLEROSIS) (See also Chap. 314) Renal vascular involvement in scleroderma is characterized by a distinctive lesion of the small arteries (diameters of 150 to 500 μm) consisting of intimal proliferation, medial thinning, and increased collagen deposition in the adventitial layer. Fibrinoid changes in the walls of afferent arterioles and microinfarcts may occur. Glomerular changes are generally nonspecific and secondary to ischemic damage. Tubules are often atrophic. As part of a generalized increase in vasomotor tone, a vasospastic (Raynaud-like) phenomenon at the level of the renal vasculature contributes to the renal insufficiency. Reduction in renal blood flow is the major mechanism underlying the deterioration in kidney function, being present in 80 percent of patients, even in the absence of other clinical abnormalities. As vascular narrowing progresses, hypertension, azotemia, and proteinuria eventually develop. Plasma renin rises in response to sustained renal ischemia. The resulting hypertension causes further renal injury and may play a role in the ultimate destruction of nephrons. As more and more nephrons are lost to the combined insults of ischemia and hypertension, development of azotemia heralds a particularly grim prognosis. Proteinuria, usually mild, is a consequence of ischemic and hypertensive glomerular injury.

Although the majority of patients with scleroderma present with extrarenal manifestations, renal involvement is eventually manifested in half of patients followed for up to 20 years. Renal involvement can present in one of two ways, depending on whether malignant hypertension is superimposed on the renal pathology: (1) *Persistent urinary abnormalities* with or without hypertension tend to follow an indolent course with mild proteinuria, occasional casts, cellular elements in the urinary sediment, and a propensity for development of hypertension. Azotemia is absent initially, but when it develops, dialysis is required within 1 year. (2) *Scleroderma renal crisis* is a rapid deterioration in renal function, usually accompanied by malignant hypertension, oliguria, fluid retention, microangiopathic hemolytic anemia, and central nervous system involvement. It may occur in patients with previously undemonstrable or slowly progressive renal disease. Untreated, it leads to chronic renal failure within days to months.

The prognosis of scleroderma renal disease is generally poor, particularly following the onset of azotemia. Aggressive antihypertensive therapy may be effective in delaying the progression of renal failure. In scleroderma renal crisis, prompt treatment with beta blockers, minoxidil, and particularly ACE inhibitors may reverse acute renal failure. The effect of these interventions on renal function over the long term is uncertain.

SICKLE CELL NEPHROPATHY (See also Chaps. 107 and 275) Sickle cell disease causes renal complications that arise mainly as a result of sickling of red blood cells in the microvasculature. The hypertonic and relatively hypoxic environment of the renal medulla, coupled with the slow blood flow in the vasa recta, favors the sickling of red blood cells, with resultant local infarction (papillary necrosis). Functional tubule defects in patients with sickle cell disease are likely the result of partial ischemic injury to the renal tubules.

In addition to the intrarenal microvascular pathology described above, young patients with sickle cell disease are characterized by renal hyperperfusion, glomerular hypertrophy, and hyperfiltration. Many of these individuals eventually develop a glomerulopathy leading to glomerular proteinuria (present in as many as 30 percent) and, in some, the nephrotic syndrome. Mild azotemia and hyperuricemia also can develop, but advanced renal failure and uremia are rare. Pathologic examination reveals the typical lesion of "hyperfiltration nephropathy," namely, focal segmental glomerular sclerosis. This has led to the suggestion that anemia-induced hyperfiltration in childhood is the principal cause of the adult glomerulopathy. Nephron loss secondary to ischemic injury also contributes to the development of azotemia in these patients.

In addition to the glomerulopathy described above, renal complications of sickle cell disease include the following: *Cortical infarcts* can cause loss of function, persistent hematuria, and perinephric hematomas. *Papillary infarcts*, demonstrated radiographically in 50 percent of patients with sickle trait, lead to an increased risk of bacterial infection in the scarred renal tissues and functional tubule abnormalities. Painless gross hematuria occurs with a higher frequency in sickle trait than in sickle cell disease and likely results from infarctive episodes in the renal medulla. *Functional tubule abnormalities* such as nephrogenic diabetes insipidus result from marked reduction in vasa recta blood flow, combined with ischemic tubule injury. This concentrating defect places these patients at increased risk of dehydration and, hence, sickling crises. The concentrating defect also occurs in individuals with sickle trait. Other tubule defects involve potassium and hydrogen ion excretion, occasionally leading to hyperkalemic metabolic acidosis and a defect in uric acid excretion which, combined with increased purine synthesis in the bone marrow, results in hyperuricemia.

Management of sickle nephropathy is not separate from that of overall patient management (see Chap. 107). In addition, however, the use of ACE inhibitors has been associated with improvement of the hyperfiltration glomerulopathy.

TOXEMIAS OF PREGNANCY (See also Chap. 7) Renal function is "reset" at a higher level during normal pregnancy. Renal plasma flow and GFR both increase by 30 to 50 percent. Therefore, serum creatinine levels above 70 μmol/L (0.8 mg/dL) or blood urea nitrogen (BUN) levels above 4.6 mmol/L (13 mg/dL) are abnormal in pregnant women and should be investigated. Systolic and diastolic blood pressures decrease by an average of 10 to 15 mmHg below pregravid values. A diastolic pressure above 75 mmHg during the second trimester or above 85 mmHg during the third trimester is therefore abnormal. Vasodilation in the uterine, renal, and cutaneous beds, vasodilator prostaglandin release from the uteroplacental unit, and a decrease in arteriolar sensitivity to angiotensin II all play a role in the decline of blood pressure during pregnancy.

Preeclampsia-Eclampsia The toxemia syndrome, usually occurring in the third trimester of primigravidas, includes hypertension, proteinuria, edema, consumptive coagulopathy, sodium retention, hyperreflexia (preeclampsia), and, if uncontrolled, convulsions (eclampsia). In pure preeclampsia (i.e., not superimposed on previously existing hypertensive or renal disease), the primary sites of pathology are the glomerular endothelial cells. These cells show marked swelling due to an increase in cytoplasmic volume with vacuolization (endotheliosis) and encroach on the vascular lumen, rendering the enlarged glomeruli ischemic. The glomerular basement membrane and the extraglomerular blood vessels are intact. The pathogenesis is unknown. Coagulation abnormalities, hormonal factors, uteroplacental ischemia, and immune mechanisms have all been implicated. Recent evidence suggests that increased microvascular reactivity is a result of endothelial cell change, which, in turn, alters the balance of endothelium-derived vasodilator/vasoconstrictor autacoids. These include reduced synthesis of nitric oxide and altered eicosanoid (thromboxane/prostacyclin) balance. Despite sodium retention, intravascular volume is contracted as compared with pregravid values. An increased sensitivity to angiotensin II is the basis for the "roll-over test" (an increase in diastolic blood pressure of 20 mmHg or more upon changing the patient's position from lateral recumbent to supine, presumably due to alterations in circulating angiotensin levels). In the supine position, the reduction in venous return due to compression by the gravid uterus increases circulating levels of angiotensin II. This results in a hypertensive response in preeclamptic patients, who are hyperresponsive to angiotensin II, but not in normal women, in whom pregnancy leads to a relative resistance to the pressor effects of this hormone.

A diagnosis of preeclampsia-related hypertension can be made when repeated measurements over a 4- to 6-h period show a blood pressure of 140/85 mmHg or more. The rise in blood pressure tends to be more severe at night. When preeclampsia occurs in a previously hypertensive patient, a rapid acceleration of the blood pressure elevation is accompanied by an increase in proteinuria, oliguria, edema, and coagulopathy. This is a life-threatening syndrome and tends to recur with future pregnancies. In addition to proteinuria, which correlates with the severity of the renal lesion, GFR and renal plasma flow are depressed. In view of the preexisting high levels, however, GFR in preeclamptic women often remains above nonpregnant levels. Uric acid clearance also falls, resulting in hyperuricemia. In the postpartum period, these patients are particularly susceptible to the development of "postpartum renal failure," which is thought to be a form of adult HUS.

℞ TREATMENT

This consists of bed rest in a quiet environment and control of neurologic manifestations and blood pressure, the former with magnesium sulfate and the latter usually with vasodilators such as hydralazine and methyldopa. Diuretics are avoided. The ultimate "treatment" is delivery, which should be induced if fetal maturity is adequate or if life-threatening coagulopathy or renal failure occur. The long-term prognosis is generally favorable.

Development of acute renal failure/preeclampsia in a pregnant woman should alert the physician to potential preexisting renal disease and/or hypertension. The latter is particularly likely if systolic blood pressure is greater than 200 mmHg. Hypertension and preexisting proteinuria tend to worsen in 50 percent of women during pregnancy. In addition, these abnormalities may be unmasked during pregnancy as the first manifestations of an underlying glomerulopathy. Conversely, patients with established underlying renal disease should be followed closely during pregnancy, with monthly measurements of 24-h urinary protein excretion and GFR. Sudden deterioration should raise suspicion of superimposed preeclampsia. There is no convincing evidence that pregnancy has an adverse effect on the long-term outcome of immunologic glomerular diseases or diabetic nephropathy. In all situations, control of blood pressure should be the primary therapeutic goal in view of its established beneficial effects on the progression of renal injury.

Bilateral Cortical Necrosis Acute bilateral cortical necrosis is associated with septic abortions, abruptio placentae, and preeclampsia. Coagulation in cortical vessels and arterioles leads to renal tissue necrosis. Anuria and renal failure ensue and may be irreversible. In other cases, renal function returns partially, but on long-term follow-up most patients slowly progress to uremia.

BIBLIOGRAPHY

BARRÉ P et al: Successful treatment with streptokinase of renal vein thrombosis associated with oral contraceptive use. Am J Nephrol 6:316, 1986

BAYLIS C: Nitric oxide and preeclampsia, in *Nitric Oxide and the Kidney: Physiology and Pathophysiology*, MS Goligorsky (ed). London, Chapman Hall, in press

BREYER JA, JACOBSON HR: Ischemic nephropathy. Curr Opin Nephrol Hypertens 2:216, 1993

EKNOYAN G, RIGGS SA: Renal involvement in patients with thrombotic thrombocytopenic purpura. Am J Nephrol 6:117, 1986

GUASCH A et al: Early detection and the course of glomerular injury in patients with sickle cell anemia. Kidney Int 49:786–791, 1996

HARDING MB et al: Renal artery stenosis: Prevalence and associated risk factors in patients undergoing routine cardiac catheterization. J Am Soc Nephrol 2:1608, 1992

KASHGARIAN M: Pathology of small blood vessels in hypertension. Am J Kidney Dis 5:A104, 1985

LLACH F: *Renal Vein Thrombosis*. New York, Futura, 1983

MANN SJ, PICKERING TG: Screening for renovascular hypertension. Ann Intern Med 118:906, 1993

McLEAN AG et al: Screening for renovascular disease with captopril-enhanced renography. Nephrol Dial Transplant 7:211, 1992

REDMAN CWG: Hypertension in pregnancy, in *Medical Disorders in Obstetric Practice*, M DeSwiet (ed). Oxford, Blackwell Scientific, 1995

RIMMER JM, GENNARI FJ: Atherosclerotic renovascular disease and progressive renal failure. Ann Intern Med 118:712, 1993

SYMPOSIUM ON ISCHEMIC RENAL DISEASE: Am J Kidney Dis 24:614, 1994

WILCOX CS: Use of angiotensin-converting enzyme inhibitors for diagnosing renovascular hypertension. Kidney Int 44:1379, 1993

WORKING GROUP ON RENOVASCULAR HYPERTENSION: Final Report: Detection, evaluation, and treatment of renovascular hypertension. Arch Intern Med 147:820, 1987

278

John R. Asplin, Fredric L. Coe

HEREDITARY TUBULAR DISORDERS

The hereditary renal tubular disorders and their morphologic and functional abnormalities, mode of inheritance, and associated abnormalities are summarized in Table 278-1. The individual disorders are discussed in detail below.

AUTOSOMAL DOMINANT POLYCYSTIC KIDNEY DISEASE

ETIOLOGY AND PATHOLOGY Autosomal dominant polycystic kidney disease (ADPKD) has a prevalence of 1:300 to 1:1000 and accounts for approximately 10 percent of end-stage renal disease (ESRD) in the United States. Ninety percent of cases are inherited as an autosomal dominant trait, and approximately 10 percent are spontaneous mutations. Three forms of ADPKD have been identified. ADPKD-1 accounts for 90 percent of cases, and the gene has been localized to the short arm of chromosome 16. The gene has recently been sequenced and found to encode a 4300-amino-acid protein; the function of the protein is unknown at this time. The gene for ADPKD-2 has been mapped to the short arm of chromosome 4. ADPKD-2 appears to have a later age of onset of symptoms and renal failure than ADPKD-1. A third form has been documented but has not been mapped to a gene at this point.

The kidneys are grossly enlarged, with multiple cysts studding the surface of the kidney. The cysts contain straw-colored fluid that may become hemorrhagic. The cysts are spherical, vary in size from a few millimeters to centimeters, and are distributed evenly throughout the cortex and medulla. Only 1 to 5 percent of nephrons will develop cysts. Hyperplastic polyps and renal adenomas are frequently found. The remaining renal parenchyma reveals varying degrees of tubular atrophy, interstitial fibrosis, and nephrosclerosis.

CLINICAL FEATURES The disease may present at any age but most frequently causes symptoms in the third or fourth decade. Patients may develop chronic flank pain from the mass effect of the enlarged kidneys. Acute pain indicates infection, urinary tract obstruction by clot or stone, or sudden hemorrhage into a cyst. Gross and microscopic hematuria are common, and impaired renal concentrating ability frequently leads to nocturia. Nephrolithiasis occurs in 15 to 20 percent of patients, calcium oxalate and uric acid stones being most common. Low urine pH, low urine citrate, and urinary stasis from distortion of the collecting system by cysts all play a role in stone formation. Hypertension is found in 20 to 30 percent of children and up to 75 percent of adults. It is secondary to intrarenal ischemia from distortion of the renal architecture, leading to activation of the renin-angiotensin system. Urinary tract infection is common and may involve the bladder or renal interstitium (pyelonephritis) or infect a cyst (pyocyst). Pyocysts can be difficult to diagnose but are more likely to be present if the patient has positive blood cultures, new renal pain, or failed to improve clinically after a standard course of antibiotic therapy.

Progressive decline in renal function is common, with approximately 50 percent of patients developing ESRD by age 60. However, there is considerable variation in age of onset of renal failure, even within the same family. Hypertension, recurrent infections, male sex, and early age of diagnosis are related to early onset renal failure. Renal failure usually progresses slowly; if a sudden decrement in kidney function occurs, ureteral obstruction from stone, clot, or compression by a cyst are likely causes. Patients usually have high hematocrits for their level of renal function, as erythropoietin production is high. Fluid overload is uncommon because of a tendency for renal salt wasting.

Extrarenal manifestations of this disease are frequent and underscore the systemic nature of the defect. Hepatic cysts occur in 50 to 70 percent of patients. Cysts are generally asymptomatic, and liver function is normal, though women may develop massive hepatic cystic disease on occasion. Cyst formation has also been observed in the spleen, pancreas, and ovaries. Intracranial aneurysms are present in 5 to 10 percent of asymptomatic patients, with potential for permanent neurologic injury or death from subarachnoid hemorrhage. Screening of all ADPKD patients for aneurysms is not recommended, but patients with a family history of subarachnoid hemorrhage should be studied noninvasively with magnetic resonance imaging angiography. Colonic diverticular disease is the most common extrarenal abnormality, and patients are more likely to develop perforation than the general population with colonic diverticula. Mitral valve prolapse is found in 25 percent of patients, and the prevalence of aortic and tricuspid valve insufficiency is increased.

Table 278-1

Renal Tubule Defects

Disease	Renal Morphologic Abnormalities	Renal Functional Abnormalities	Mode of Inheritance*	Associated Abnormalities
Autosomal dominant polycystic disease	Cortical and medullary cysts	Chronic renal failure, >20 yr	AD	Hepatic cysts, intracranial aneurysms, colonic diverticula
Autosomal recessive polycystic disease	Distal tubule and collecting duct cysts	Chronic renal failure, <20 yr	AR	Congenital hepatic fibrosis
Tuberous sclerosis	Renal cysts and angiomyolipomas	None	AD	Skin lesions, hamartomas of the central nervous system
Von Hippel–Lindau disease	Renal cysts, increased risk of renal cell cancer	None	AD	Hemangioblastoma of the retina and central nervous system
Medullary sponge kidney	Dilated collecting ducts	Nephrocalcinosis, hematuria	AD, S	None
Juvenile nephronophthisis	Medullary cysts, small kidneys	Chronic renal failure, <20 yr polyuria, salt wasting	AR	Hepatic fibrosis, retinal abnormalities
Medullary cystic disease	Medullary cysts, small kidneys	Chronic renal failure, >20 yr polyuria, salt wasting	AD	None
Liddle's syndrome	None	Hypokalemia, alkalosis, low aldosterone levels	AR	Hypertension
Bartter's syndrome	Juxtaglomerular apparatus hyperplasia	Hypokalemia, alkalosis, high aldosterone levels	AR, S	None
Congenital nephrogenic diabetes insipidus	None	Vasopressin renal concentrating defect	XL, AR	None
Renal tubular acidosis, type 1	Nephrocalcinosis	Impaired proton secretion in distal tubule, non-anion-gap metabolic acidosis	AD, AR, XL, S, ACQ	Rickets, osteomalacia, nephrolithiasis
Renal tubular acidosis, type 2	None	Reduced bicarbonate reabsorption, non-anion-gap metabolic acidosis	AR, AD, XL, ACQ	Fanconi syndrome, rickets
Renal tubular acidosis, type 4	Chronic renal insufficiency	Reduced proton and potassium secretion	ACQ	Renal insufficiency
X-linked hypophosphatemia	None	Reduced phosphate reabsorption	XL	Rickets, osteomalacia, normal serum $1,25(OH)_2D_3$
Vitamin D–dependent rickets, type 1	None	Defective renal $1,25(OH)_2D_3$ production	AR	Rickets, osteomalacia, low serum $1,25(OH)_2D_3$
Vitamin D–dependent rickets, type 2	None	Renal resistance to $1,25(OH)_2D_3$	AR, S	Rickets, osteomalacia, high serum $1,25(OH)_2D_3$
Oncogenic osteomalacia	None	Reduced phosphate reabsorption	ACQ	Osteomalacia, mesenchymal tumors
X-linked recessive nephrolithiasis	Interstitial fibrosis, medullary calcifications	Hypercalciuria, low-molecular-weight proteinuria	XL	Renal failure
Isolated hyperuricemia	None	Reduced urate reabsorption	AR	Variable hypercalciuria
Hartnup disorder	None	Reduced reabsorption of neutral amino acids	AR	Dermatitis, diarrhea, dementia
Cystinuria	Cystine stones	Reduced reabsorption of dibasic amino acids	AR	Short stature
Iminoglycinuria	None	Reduced reabsorption of proline, hydroxyproline, and glycine	AR	None
Fanconi syndrome	Swan neck deformity of proximal tubule	Reduced reabsorption of bicarbonate, glucose, phosphate, uric acid, and amino acids	AR	Rickets, osteomalacia, hypokalemia, metabolic acidosis

* AD, autosomal dominant; AR, autosomal recessive; XL, X-linked; ACQ, acquired; S, sporadic

DIAGNOSIS Ultrasound is the preferred technique for diagnosis of symptomatic patients and for screening asymptomatic family members. The ability to detect cysts increases with the subject's age: 80 to 90 percent of ADPKD patients over the age of 20 will have detectable cysts, and almost 100 percent over the age of 30 will have cysts. At least three to five cysts in each kidney is the standard diagnostic criteria for ADPKD. Computed tomography scan may be more sensitive than ultrasound in detection of small cysts. Genetic linkage analysis is now available for diagnosis of ADPKD-1 but is reserved for cases where radiographic imaging is negative and the need for definitive diagnosis critical, such as screening family members for potential kidney donation.

Rx TREATMENT

The goals of treatment are to slow the rate of progression of renal disease and minimize symptoms. Hypertension and renal infection should be treated aggressively to maintain renal function. Converting enzyme inhibitors are effective antihypertensive agents, though patients should be closely monitored as some develop renal insufficiency and hyperkalemia. Urinary infection is treated in a standard manner unless a pyocyst is suspected, in which case antibiotics that penetrate cysts should be used, such as trimethoprim-sulfamethoxazole, ciprofloxacin, and chloramphenicol. Chronic pain from cysts can be managed by cyst puncture and sclerosis with ethanol.

AUTOSOMAL RECESSIVE POLYCYSTIC KIDNEY DISEASE

ETIOLOGY AND PATHOLOGY Autosomal recessive polycystic kidney disease (ARPKD) is a rare genetic disease that has an incidence between 1:10,000 and 1:40,000. The gene for ARPKD has been localized to chromosome 6. In the past, ARPKD was considered to be a family of disorders, categorized as neonatal, infantile, and childhood forms depending on the age of onset and the relative degree of involvement of the kidneys and liver. However, variable clinical presentations within siblings in the same family, as well as the localization of the disease to chromosome 6 in multiple families, support the premise that this is a single genetic disease with variable phenotypic presentation.

At birth the kidneys are enlarged with a smooth external surface. The distal tubules and collecting ducts are dilated into elongated cysts that are arranged in a radial fashion. As the patient ages, the cysts may become more spherical and can be confused with ADPKD. Interstitial fibrosis is also seen as renal function deteriorates. Liver involvement includes proliferation and dilation of small intrahepatic bile ducts as well as periportal fibrosis.

CLINICAL FEATURES The majority of cases are diagnosed in the first year of life, presenting as bilateral abdominal masses. Death in the neonatal period is most commonly due to pulmonary hypoplasia. Hypertension and impaired urinary concentrating ability are common. The time course to ESRD is variable, though many children maintain adequate kidney function for years. Older children present with complications secondary to congenital hepatic fibrosis and generally have less severe kidney disease. Hepatosplenomegaly, portal hypertension, and esophageal varices are frequent complications of ARPKD.

DIAGNOSIS Ultrasound is the most common technique used to diagnose ARPKD, prenatally and in childhood. Ultrasound examination reveals enlarged kidneys with increased echogenicity. At times spherical cysts may be seen, potentially leading to an incorrect diagnosis of ADPKD. A thorough family history and imaging the kidneys of the parents aids in differentiation from other cystic diseases. The recent mapping of the gene should allow linkage studies to be used in diagnosis.

Rx TREATMENT

Aggressive treatment of hypertension and urinary tract infection are the major goals of therapy in order to maintain native renal function as long as possible. Dialysis and transplant are appropriate when kidney failure occurs. Hepatic fibrosis may lead to life-threatening variceal hemorrhage, requiring sclerotherapy or portocaval shunting.

TUBEROUS SCLEROSIS

Patients with this multisystem disease most commonly present with skin lesions and benign tumors of the central nervous system (Chap. 375). Renal involvement is common; angiomyolipomas are the most frequent abnormality and are usually bilateral. Renal cysts may be present as well and can give an appearance similar to that of ADPKD. Histologically, the cysts are unique—the cyst lining cells are large with an eosinophilic staining cytoplasm and they may form hyperplastic nodules that can fill the cyst space. The disease is inherited as an autosomal dominant trait, though spontaneous mutations do occur. Gene mutations have been identified on chromosomes 9 and 16. Tuberous sclerosis may be confused with ADPKD if the extrarenal manifestations are minimal.

VON HIPPEL–LINDAU DISEASE

This autosomal dominant disease is characterized by hemangioblastomas of the retina and the central nervous system (Chap. 375). Renal cysts occur in the majority of cases and are usually bilateral. Linkage studies have localized the gene to the short arm of chromosome 3 and it has been identified as a tumor-suppressor gene. Renal cell carcinoma may be found in up to 25 percent of patients and is frequently multifocal. Yearly screening of adults using computed tomography scans has been recommended in an attempt to diagnose renal cell cancers at an early stage.

MEDULLARY SPONGE KIDNEY (MSK)

ETIOLOGY AND PATHOLOGY MSK is a congenital disorder. Although some cases have apparent autosomal dominant inheritance, most are sporadic. It is found in 0.5 to 1 percent of all intravenous pyelograms. Males and females are affected equally. The pathologic lesion is cystic dilation of the inner medullary and papillary collecting ducts, with collecting diameters ranging from 1 to 5 mm. Bilateral renal involvement is present in 70 percent of cases, but not all papillae are equally affected. The dilated ducts are lined by cuboidal epithelium with areas of pseudostratified and stratified squamous epithelium. Calculi are frequently found in the dilated collecting ducts.

CLINICAL FEATURES Patients generally present in the third or fourth decade with kidney stones, infection, or recurrent hematuria. The disease is most commonly diagnosed by intravenous pyelogram, which shows linear striations radiating into the renal papillae or small cystic collections of contrast in the dilated ducts (Fig. 278-1). Approximately 60 percent of patients with MSK have stones, and 12 percent of all stone formers will have MSK. Hypercalciuria occurs with the same frequency in MSK as it does in random stone formers. Papillary nephrocalcinosis occurs more frequently in patients with MSK than in the random stone former. Proteinuria is minimal, if present at all, and renal function is normally preserved unless there is renal damage from recurrent infection or severe stone disease.

Rx TREATMENT

Asymptomatic patients require no specific therapy except to maintain high fluid intake to reduce the risk of nephrolithiasis. If stones are present, standard laboratory evaluation should be done and metabolic abnormalities treated as in any stone former (see Chap. 279). Infection should be treated aggressively, and instrumentation of the urinary tract should be minimized to avoid introducing infection.

JUVENILE NEPHRONOPHTHISIS/MEDULLARY CYSTIC DISEASE

ETIOLOGY AND PATHOLOGY Juvenile nephronophthisis (JN) and medullary cystic disease (MCD) have similar pathologic findings but differ in inheritance pattern and age of onset. JN is inherited as an autosomal recessive disease; linkage studies have shown 90 percent of the cases to map to a gene on the short arm of chromosome 2. MCD appears to be an autosomal dominant disease. In both conditions, the kidneys tend to be small, with cysts throughout the medulla; the cortex and papilla rarely have cysts. The cysts originate in the collecting ducts, distal convoluted tubules, and loops of Henle and range in size from 1 to 10 mm. Sclerotic glomeruli, tubule atrophy, and interstitial fibrosis are frequent findings on biopsy.

CLINICAL FEATURES Patients with JN present during childhood with symptoms of polyuria, growth retardation, anemia, and progressive renal insufficiency. Most patients develop ESRD prior to the age of 20; JN accounts for 2 to 10 percent of renal failure in children. Hepatic fibrosis, retinal abnormalities, and mental retardation have been reported in association with JN. MCD presents in the third or fourth decade, though some cases may be diagnosed in the elderly population. Presenting symptoms in MCD are the same as in JN except for growth retardation. In addition, MCD does not have extrarenal abnormalities. Severe salt wasting can be seen, though this is usually a transient phase that resolves as the disease progresses to ESRD. Other features of tubule damage are often found, including hyperkalemia and hyperchloremic metabolic acidosis. Proteinuria is mild, and hematuria is rare.

DIAGNOSIS The diagnosis is suggested by a family history of renal disease. The pattern of inheritance and age of onset aid in distinguishing JN/MCD from other inherited diseases. Radiographic studies show small kidneys, loss of the corticomedullary junction, and multiple cysts in the medulla. Computed tomography scan is more sensitive than ultrasound in making the diagnosis. Open renal biopsy, including medullary tissue, may be required for diagnosis in some cases.

Rx TREATMENT

Treatment is mainly supportive, as there is no specific therapy to prevent loss of renal function. Patients with salt wasting require a large oral intake of salt and water to maintain adequate extracellular volume. Alkali replacement and erythropoietin are required for acidosis and anemia, respectively. Renal transplantation has been performed in numerous patients, and the disease does not recur.

LIDDLE'S SYNDROME

Liddle's syndrome is a rare familial disease with a clinical presentation of hyperaldosteronism, consisting of hypertension, hypokalemia, and metabolic alkalosis. However, aldosterone levels are undetectable in these patients, and a nonaldosterone mineralocorticoid has not been isolated. Increased distal tubule sodium reabsorption, due to mutations in the β subunit of the amiloride-sensitive sodium channel, has been described in multiple families. Pharmacologic agents that block distal tubule sodium uptake, such as amiloride and triamterene, are effective in treating the hypertension and electrolyte abnormalities. As expected, spironolactone is ineffective, since the disease is not mediated via the aldosterone receptor.

BARTTER'S SYNDROME

CLINICAL FEATURES Hypokalemia secondary to renal potassium wasting, metabolic alkalosis, and normal to low blood pressure are the clinical features of Bartter's syndrome. Renin and aldosterone production are increased, and there is hyporesponsiveness to the pressor effects of angiotensin II infusion. Prostaglandin E_2, prostacyclin, kallikrein, and bradykinin production are frequently elevated. Hypomagnesemia with hypermagnesuria may be present. Most cases are diagnosed during childhood, with the presenting symptoms, such as polyuria and weakness, being attributable to hypokalemia. Inheritance is autosomal recessive, though sporadic cases do occur. Growth and developmental retardation may be associated with Bartter's syndrome. Although renal biopsy is rarely required for diagnosis, it reveals hyperplasia of the juxtaglomerular apparatus and prominence of medullary interstitial cells, with variable degrees of interstitial fibrosis.

PATHOGENESIS The pathogenesis of Bartter's syndrome is a matter of debate as the distinction between primary and secondary phenomena is difficult. Juxtaglomerular hyperplasia is most likely an epiphenomenon, as any form of chronic hyperreninemia will cause it. Resistance to the pressor effects of angiotensin II may be secondary to the high levels of vasodilatory prostaglandins. Inhibition of prostaglandin synthesis can reverse the vascular hyporesponsiveness. Prostaglandin overproduction has been implicated as the primary event, but variable clinical response to prostaglandin inhibitors suggests this is not the common etiology. Prostaglandin overproduction could be secondary to hypokalemia or volume depletion. Impaired chloride reabsorption in the thick ascending limb of the loop of Henle appears to be the most likely etiology. Inadequate chloride reabsorption would cause volume depletion and activate the renin-angiotensin system. Distal delivery of salt and water would be high in the presence of high aldosterone, promoting secretion of potassium and hydrogen ions. Hypokalemia and alkalosis would result. Prostaglandin synthesis would be increased by the volume contraction and hypokalemia. High aldosterone levels would increase production of kallikrein and bradykinin.

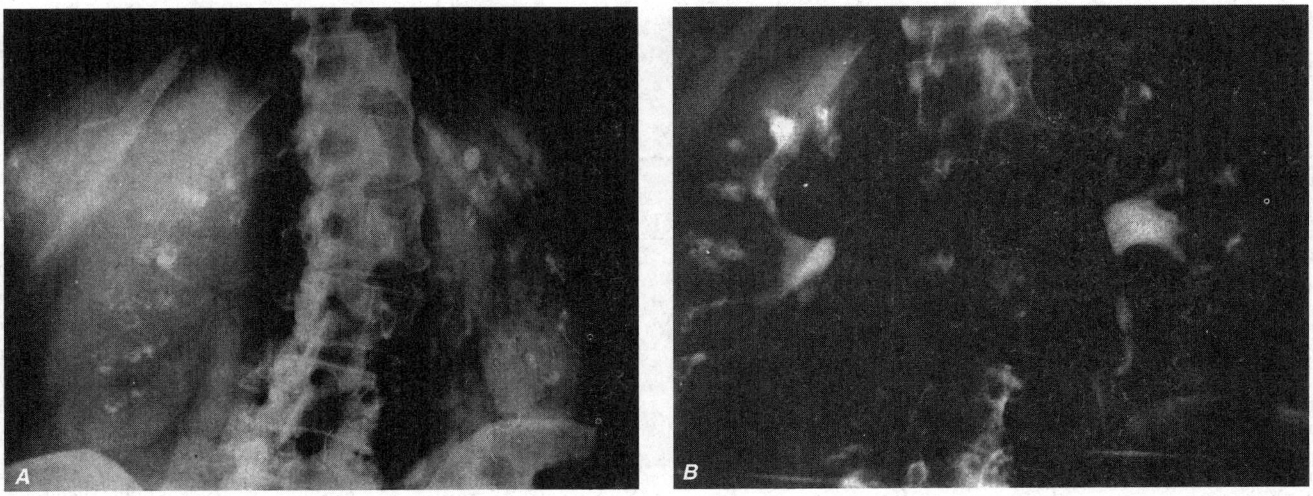

FIGURE 278-1 *A*. Radiographic appearance of medullary sponge kidney. Abdominal flat plate reveals multiple bilateral calcifications. *B*. Radiographic contrast material accumulates in the dilated and cystic terminal collecting ducts and obscures the calcifications.

However, Bartter's syndrome may be a disorder with a single phenotype caused by many physiologic abnormalities, further complicating investigation of its pathogenesis. Angiotensin II–receptor antagonists can produce some of the features of Bartter's syndrome in experimental studies. The gene for the angiotensin II receptor has been found to be abnormal in one of five Bartter's patients studied. Whether this will be a common finding in Bartter's syndrome remains to be seen.

DIAGNOSIS Most cases of Bartter's syndrome present during childhood. Symptoms such as weakness and cramps are secondary to the hypokalemia. Polyuria and nocturia are common due to the hypokalemia-induced nephrogenic diabetes insipidus (NDI). The disease is inherited as an autosomal recessive trait, though sporadic cases do occur. Differential diagnosis includes vomiting, surreptitious diuretic abuse, and magnesium deficiency. Chronic vomiting can be diagnosed by a low urine chloride concentration. Magnesium deficiency causes kaliuresis and alkalosis, simulating Bartter's syndrome. Serum and urine magnesium will be low in such cases. Diuretic abuse produces metabolic abnormalities indistinguishable from those of Bartter's syndrome. Urine should be screened for diuretics multiple times before the diagnosis of Bartter's syndrome is made in a patient without a family history of the disorder.

℞ **TREATMENT**

Dietary intake of sodium and potassium should be liberal. Potassium supplements are usually required. Magnesium supplements are needed in those patients with magnesuria. Spironolactone will reduce potassium wasting. Prostaglandin synthetase inhibitors are useful in some patients. Angiotensin-converting enzyme inhibitors have also been shown to be of use.

CONGENITAL NEPHROGENIC DIABETES INSIPIDUS

This rare genetic disorder is most commonly inherited as an X-linked disease, with full expression in males and variable penetrance in females. Vasopressin acts through two receptors; type 1 receptors are located in the vasculature, while type 2 receptors are found in the collecting ducts of the kidney. In NDI, only the actions requiring type 2 receptors are abnormal. Linkage analysis has localized the NDI gene to the long arm of the X chromosome in region 28 (Xq28), the same locus as the type 2 vasopressin receptor. Mutations in the gene that encodes the type 2 vasopressin receptor segregate with NDI, confirming it as the putative gene. Less frequently, NDI may be inherited as an autosomal recessive trait, in which mutations in the gene for the water channels in collecting duct cells (aquaporin 2) lead to abnormal cell routing of aquaporin 2.

Clinical presentation is that of persistent polyuria, dehydration, and hypotonic urine in the presence of hypernatremia. Vasopressin levels are appropriately elevated in the hypertonic state, but renal response is lacking. The onset of the disorder is in infancy. The recurrent hypernatremia may lead to seizures or mental retardation. Once old enough to satisfy their thirst, children will be clinically stable though in a chronic state of polyuria and polydypsia. Renal function is normal, and radiographic studies of the urinary system reveal dilated ureters and bladder secondary to the chronically high urine flow. Since the most common form of the disease is X-linked, most patients are male. Heterozygous females generally have mild concentrating defects, though a few have phenotypic expression similar to males due to skewed X-chromosome inactivation. In the autosomal recessive form, males and females are affected equally.

℞ **TREATMENT**

Treatment is aimed at maintaining adequate hydration. In the infant, low-solute feedings and high water intake are generally adequate. Addition of a thiazide diuretic reduces urine flow by inhibiting sodium reabsorption in the distal convoluted tubule. This lowers free water production and, by causing extracellular volume contraction, increases proximal salt and water reabsorption, reducing delivery to the distal nephron. Administration of vasopressin and its analogues has no role in the management of this disorder.

RENAL TUBULAR ACIDOSIS (RTA)

RTA is a disorder of renal acidification out of proportion to the reduction in glomerular filtration rate. RTA is characterized by hyperchloremic metabolic acidosis with a normal serum anion gap $[Na^+ - (Cl^- + HCO_3^-)]$. There are multiple forms of RTA, depending on which aspects of renal acid handling have been affected. Defective bicarbonate reabsorption in the proximal tubule, suppressed renal ammoniagenesis, and inadequate distal tublule proton secretion are the abnormalities that produce RTA. Three types of RTA exist (Table 278-2). Types 1 and 2 may be inherited or acquired. Type 4 is acquired and is associated with either hypoaldosteronism or tubular hyporesponsiveness to mineralocorticoids. Type 3 was formerly used to define distal RTA with bicarbonate wasting in children; however, the bicarbonaturia resolves with age and is not truly part of a pathologic process. The term *type 3 RTA* is no longer used.

TYPE 1 (DISTAL) RTA In this disorder the distal nephron does not lower urine pH normally, either because the collecting ducts permit excessive back-diffusion of hydrogen ions from lumen to blood or because there is inadequate transport of hydrogen ions. Excretion of titratable acid is low, as inadequate proton secretion prevents titration of urinary buffers such as phosphate. Urine ammonium excretion is inappropriately low for the level of acidosis, as the defect in acidification reduces the ion trapping required for ammonium excretion. Urinary concentration and potassium conservation also tend to be impaired.

Chronic acidosis lowers tubule reabsorption of calcium, causing renal hypercalciuria and mild secondary hyperparathyroidism. Buffering of bone by the daily metabolic acid load contributes to hypercalciuria. Urine citrate excretion is low, as acidosis and hypokalemia stimulate proximal tubule reabsorption of citrate. The hypercalciuria, alkaline urine, and low levels of urine citrate, which normally complexes about 40 percent of urine calcium, cause calcium phosphate stones and nephrocalcinosis. Growth in children is stunted because of rickets; this growth defect responds to amelioration of the acidosis with alkali. In the adult, osteomalacia occurs. In both children and adults, bone diseases may result, in part, from acidosis-induced loss of bone material and inadequate production of 1,25-dihydroxyvitamin D_3 $[1,25(OH)_2D_3]$. Since

Table 278-2

Comparison of Normal Anion-Gap Acidoses

Finding	Type 1 RTA	Type 2 RTA	Type 4 RTA	GI Bicarbonate Loss
Normal anion-gap acidosis	Yes	Yes	Yes	Yes
Minimum urine pH	>5.5	<5.5	<5.5	5 to 6
% filtered bicarbonate excreted	<10	>15	<10	<10
Serum potassium	Low	Low	High	Low
Fanconi syndrome	No	Yes	No	No
Stones/nephrocalcinosis	Yes	No	No	No
Daily acid excretion	Low	Normal	Low	High
Urine anion gap	Positive	Positive	Positive	Negative
Daily bicarbonate replacement needs	<4 mmol/kg	>4 mmol/kg	<4 mmol/kg	Variable

the kidney does not conserve potassium or concentrate the urine normally, polyuria and hypokalemia occur. With the stress of an intercurrent illness, acidosis and hypokalemia can be life-threatening.

Type 1 RTA can be familial, with autosomal dominant as the most common form of inheritance. X-linked, autosomal recessive, and sporadic cases have been reported. Other hereditary diseases that cause type 1 RTA include galactosemia, Ehler-Danlos syndrome, Fabry's disease, medullary sponge kidney, Wilson's disease, and hereditary elliptocytosis. The majority of cases of type 1 RTA are secondary to a systemic disorder such as Sjögren's syndrome, hypergammaglobulinemia, chronic active hepatitis, or lupus.

The diagnosis of type 1 RTA is suggested by a normal anion gap metabolic acidosis with a simultaneous urine pH greater than 5.5. Osteomalacia or rickets and calcium phosphate stones or nephrocalcinosis support the diagnosis, though they are not present in all cases. Bicarbonaturia is not present, which distinguishes this disorder from type 2 RTA. If acidosis is not severe and urine pH is equivocal, the oral ammonium chloride (NH_4Cl) loading test should be carried out: 0.1 g (1.9 mmol) NH_4Cl per kilogram of body weight is administered, and blood and urine pH are measured repeatedly over the next 6 h. Although systemic acidosis worsens, urine pH does not fall below 5.5. Urinary tract infection must not be present during this test because bacteria may possess urease, which hydrolyzes urea to ammonia and produces an alkaline urine.

Chronic diarrheal states cause normal anion gap acidosis and hypokalemia; urine pH may be above 5.5 if ammonium production is very high. The urine anion gap ($Na^+ + K^+ - Cl^-$) can be used to estimate renal ammonium production and distinguish RTA from gastrointestinal bicarbonate loss. Normally the urine anion gap is positive, as unmeasured anions exceeds unmeasured cations. If urine ammonium levels are high, urine chloride concentration increases to balance the charge. Unmeasured cation (predominantly ammonium) now exceeds unmeasured anion, and the urine anion gap is negative. During metabolic acidosis, a negative urine anion gap suggests an extrarenal cause of acidosis, whereas a positive urine anion gap suggests RTA. The urine anion gap cannot be used if there are large amounts of unmeasured anions, such as bicarbonate or ketones, in the urine.

Rx TREATMENT

Alkali supplements are the standard therapy. Enough alkali is prescribed to titrate the daily metabolic acid production, usually in the range of 0.5 to 2.0 mmol/kg body weight in four to six divided doses per day. Sodium bicarbonate and Shohl's solution (1 mmol sodium citrate and 1 mmol citric acid per mL) are common treatments. Potassium alkali salts can be used if hypokalemia is a persistent problem. Citrate requires less frequent dosing than bicarbonate salts as it is metabolized to bicarbonate after absorption. The dose of alkali should be raised until acidosis and hypercalciuria are both eliminated, and the patients should be followed by measurements of serum potassium, chloride, and CO_2 content approximately twice yearly. Requirements for alkali usually rise during intercurrent illnesses but are usually below 4 mmol/kg body weight per day. The relatives of patients with idiopathic type 1 RTA should be screened for this disorder, as timely treatment can prevent growth retardation in children. Incomplete RTA secondary to idiopathic hypercalciuria is best treated using thiazide diuretics in conjunction with potassium citrate (Chap. 279).

TYPE 2 (PROXIMAL) RTA Type 2 RTA usually occurs as part of a generalized disorder of proximal tubule function, presenting as hyperchloremic acidosis with other features of Fanconi syndrome. Bicarbonate reabsorption in the proximal tubule is defective. At normal concentrations of plasma bicarbonate, large amounts of bicarbonate are delivered to the distal tubule, overwhelming the absorptive capacity of the distal tubule and resulting in bicarbonaturia. As plasma bicarbonate levels fall, the lower filtered load of bicarbonate can be reabsorbed by the proximal tubule, resulting in normal distal delivery of bicarbonate. At this point the distal nephron can acidify the urine normally, resulting in normal excretion of daily metabolic acid production, albeit at a low serum bicarbonate level. Hypophosphatemia and low calcitriol levels are common and may lead to rickets or osteomalacia. Hypercalciuria occurs, but stone formation is unusual since urine citrate levels are normal or high because of reduced proximal tubule citrate reabsorption. Type 2 RTA may be inherited as autosomal dominant, autosomal recessive, or X-linked disorder. It may be acquired in association with other diseases (see "Fanconi Syndrome") or be secondary to drugs that inhibit carbonic anhydrase activity, such as acetazolamide.

Type 2 RTA may be distinguished from type 1 RTA by the ability to normally acidify urine during spontaneous or ammonium chloride–induced acidosis. Correction of acidosis with bicarbonate will result in bicarbonaturia in type 2 RTA but not type 1 RTA. Fractional excretion of bicarbonate is greater than 15 percent at normal or near-normal serum bicarbonate levels. In distal RTA it is less than 10 percent. It is unusual for serum bicarbonate levels to fall below 15 mmol/L in proximal RTA. The urine anion gap will be positive, as ammonium excretion is normal to handle daily acid production, but is not elevated as in nonrenal causes of acidosis.

Rx TREATMENT

Children should be treated to prevent growth retardation. Alkali must be given in large amounts daily, 5 to 15 mmol/kg body weight per day, because bicarbonate is rapidly excreted in the urine. A thiazide diuretic can be used in conjunction with a low-salt diet to reduce the amount of bicarbonate required. Potassium supplementation is often required.

TYPE 4 RTA In type 4 RTA, also called hyperkalemic distal RTA, distal tubule secretion of both potassium and hydrogen ions is abnormal, resulting in hyperchloremic acidosis with hyperkalemia. Type 4 RTA is an acquired disorder; a moderate degree of renal insufficiency is present in the majority of patients. Patients with type 4 RTA can be differentiated from patients with type 1 since they have an acid urine (pH < 5.5) during periods of acidosis (see Table 278-2) and hyperkalemia. They differ from type 2 patients by having a fractional excretion of bicarbonate less than 10 percent and a daily bicarbonate requirement of 1 to 3 mmol/kg body weight per day. Because potassium and hydrogen ion excretion are abnormal, such patients are considered to have generalized distal nephron dysfunction due to either insufficient aldosterone production or intrinsic renal disease causing aldosterone resistance. The resulting hyperkalemia reduces proximal tubule ammonia production, in addition to the inadequate proton secretion, leading to inadequate excretion of the daily metabolic proton load. These patients have an acid urine despite reduced proton secretion because there is inadequate ammonia to buffer protons in the distal tubule. If buffer delivery to the distal nephron is increased, urine pH will rise despite persistent acidosis.

Type 4 RTA due to inadequate aldosterone production has multiple etiologies. Hyporeninemic hypoaldosteronism is the most common cause of type 4 RTA. Plasma levels of renin and aldosterone are subnormal, even during extracellular volume depletion, and the most common causes of this are diabetic nephropathy and chronic tubulointerstitial nephropathies. Nonsteroidal anti-inflammatory drugs, angiotensin-converting enzyme inhibitors, and heparin can reduce aldosterone production and produce a type 4 RTA. Drug-induced type 4 RTA is usually seen in patients with preexisting renal insufficiency. Reduced aldosterone production may be due to adrenal disease, either occurring as an isolated defect or as part of a more generalized adrenal disorder (Chap. 332). Renin levels are normal to high in adrenal disorders.

Patients with tubular resistance to aldosterone present with the same clinical features as those with hyporeninemic hypoaldosteronism. A tubulointerstitial process damages the distal tubule, restricting potassium and hydrogen ion excretion, despite adequate aldosterone levels. Obstructive uropathy and sickle cell disease are the most common causes of acquired tubular resistance to aldosterone. Hyporeninemic hypoaldosteronism can be found in addition to tubular aldosterone resistance in many patients. Spironolactone, a competitive inhibitor of the aldosterone receptor, produces an aldosterone-resistant state. Amiloride and triamterene are diuretics that block sodium transport in the distal nephron, blunting the effect of aldosterone on the distal tubule.

Rx TREATMENT

This is aimed mainly at reducing serum potassium, as acidosis will usually improve once the hyperkalemic block of ammonium production is removed. All patients should be placed on a low-potassium diet. Any drug that suppresses aldosterone production or blocks aldosterone effect should be discontinued. Mineralocorticoid supplementation with fludrocortisone, 0.1 to 0.2 mg/d, will improve hyperkalemia and acidosis; however, the patients who also have a partial tubule resistance to mineralocorticoid will require a higher dose. Mineralocorticoid replacement may not be appropriate for patients with hypertension or a history of heart failure. In such situations, a loop diuretic with a liberal sodium intake can usually promote adequate potassium excretion. Exchange resins will reduce potassium levels but are usually not tolerated well enough to be used for long-term treatment.

IDIOPATHIC PSEUDOHYPOALDOSTERONISM This rare inherited disorder is transmitted as either an autosomal dominant or recessive trait. It is due to a defect in the high-affinity aldosterone receptor, resulting in hyperkalemia and metabolic acidosis unresponsive to mineralocorticoid supplementation. The disease presents during childhood and is usually complicated by salt wasting and volume depletion. Plasma renin and aldosterone levels are elevated. Treatment includes salt supplements, alkali, and potassium restriction.

VITAMIN D DISORDERS

X-LINKED HYPOPHOSPHATEMIC RICKETS (See also Chap. 355) This disorder, also called vitamin D–resistant rickets, is an X-linked dominant disorder characterized by hypophosphatemia with renal phosphate wasting, rickets, and short stature. Hypophosphatemia is present soon after birth; rachitic bowing of the legs develops when the child begins to walk. Children have growth retardation which is limited almost entirely to the lower extremities. Dentition is delayed, and skull abnormalities are common. Females generally have less severe disease than males. Presentation in adults ranges from disabling bone pain to no active symptoms, but generally some physical sign of childhood disease, such as short stature or bowed legs, is present. Overgrowth of bone at joints or sites of muscle attachment may reduce the mobility of the joint or cause nerve entrapment.

Hypophosphatemia secondary to reduced renal phosphate reabsorption is the hallmark of the disease. Intestinal phosphate absorption is low, worsening hypophosphatemia. Serum calcium levels are usually normal, with low intestinal absorption and renal excretion of calcium. Serum alkaline phosphatase and osteocalcin levels are elevated. Parathyroid hormone levels are normal, as would be expected with normal serum calcium. $1,25(OH)_2D_3$ levels are usually normal, though in the setting of hypophosphatemia $1,25(OH)_2D_3$ levels should be elevated. Inadequate 1α-hydroxylase activity appears to play some role in the disease. Linkage analysis has localized the gene to the Xp22.1 region of the X chromosome. A candidate gene has been identified and appears to be related to a family of endopeptidase genes.

Rx TREATMENT

The goal of therapy is to raise serum phosphorous to normal or near-normal levels to improve bone mineralization. Oral neutral phosphate, 1 to 4 g/d in four to six doses, combined with calcitriol is an effective therapy that improves growth rate, reduces bone pain, and leads to radiographically evident improvement of the bone disease. Patients should be closely monitored during therapy as they may develop nephrocalcinosis and renal insufficiency.

VITAMIN D–DEPENDENT RICKETS TYPE 1 This is an autosomal recessive disorder in which $1,25(OH)_2D_3$ levels are very low but 25-hydroxyvitamin D levels are normal. There appears to be a defect in renal 1α-hydroxylase activity, leading to a clinical syndrome of vitamin D deficiency. Symptoms usually appear before the age of 2, including rickets and growth retardation. Levels of serum calcium and phosphorous are low but that of alkaline phosphatase is elevated. Intestinal calcium absorption and urinary calcium excretion are low. Parathyroid hormone is elevated in response to the hypocalcemia, resulting in increased urinary phosphate losses.

Rx TREATMENT

Calcitriol (0.5 to 1 μg/d) leads to rapid correction of the biochemical abnormalities and resolution of the bone disease. Calcium and phosphorous supplementation are usually not required.

VITAMIN D–DEPENDENT RICKETS TYPE II (See also Chap. 355) End-organ resistance to $1,25(OH)_2D_3$ is the pathogenesis of this disorder. Serum calcium and phosphate levels are low, secondary hyperparathyroidism is present, and $1,25(OH)_2D_3$ levels are elevated. Inheritance is usually autosomal recessive, though sporadic cases have been reported. Most patients present during childhood with rickets, though some have a milder form of disease not recognized until adulthood. Alopecia is common and tends to be associated with the more severe childhood form of the disease. Multiple defects have been detected in $1,25(OH)_2D_3$ receptor interaction, including absent hormone binding to the receptor, decreased receptor affinity, deficient hormone-receptor localization, and abnormalities of the DNA-binding domain of the receptor. Pharmacologic doses of calcitriol (5 to 30 μg/d) along with mineral supplementation will improve the biochemical disorders and bone disease, though some patients have no response to massive doses of calcitriol.

ONCOGENIC OSTEOMALACIA This syndrome generally occurs in adults with highly vascular mesenchymal tumors. Patients present with bone pain and muscle weakness. Symptoms may be present for years before the correct diagnosis is made. Over 90 percent of the tumors are benign, and most are found in the extremities or maxillofacial region. Hypophosphatemia secondary to renal phosphate wasting and low levels of $1,25(OH)_2D_3$ are the major biochemical abnormalities. Serum calcium and parathyroid hormone levels are normal. It appears the tumor produces a humoral agent that reduces proximal tubule phosphate reabsorption and 1α-hydroxylase activity. Removal of the tumor leads to rapid resolution of the disease.

X-LINKED RECESSIVE NEPHROLITHIASIS

This disorder presents as calcium nephrolithiasis in male children and progresses to nephrocalcinosis and renal failure. Low-molecular-weight proteinuria and hypercalciuria are also prominent features of the disease. Kidney biopsy reveals tubular atrophy, interstitial fibrosis, and medullary calcifications. The gene has been mapped to the short arm of the X chromosome and encodes a voltage-gated chloride channel. Dent's disease has been mapped to the same gene and has a similar presentation, except for an increased incidence of rickets.

ISOLATED HYPOURICEMIA (See also Chap. 350)

This disorder is generally inherited as an autosomal recessive trait. Most commonly there is deficient urate reabsorption in the proximal tubule, though some patients have been demonstrated to oversecrete urate. Serum uric acid is usually below 120 μmol/L (2 mg/dL) and hyperuricosuria is common, possibly due to decreased intestinal urate excretion. Hypouricemia is usually an incidental finding, as patients with this disorder are asymptomatic except for an increased risk of nephrolithiasis. Other disorders associated with hypouricemia include Fanconi syndrome, Wilson's disease, Hodgkin's disease, and Hartnup disease. No treatment is required except for high fluid intake to prevent kidney stones. Alkali and allopurinol may be used to prevent stones if fluids alone are not sufficient. Hypercalciuria has been associated with isolated hypouricemia in some families.

SELECTED DISORDERS OF AMINO ACID TRANSPORT

HARTNUP DISEASE This disorder is characterized by reduced intestinal absorption and renal reabsorption of neutral amino acids. The defect involves an amino acid transporter on the brush border of the jejunum and the proximal tubule. Intestinal absorption of free amino acids is reduced, though the neutral amino acids can be absorbed when present in di- and tripeptides. Degradation of unabsorbed tryptophan by intestinal bacteria produces indolic acids that are absorbed and subsequently excreted at high levels in the urine of these patients. The disorder is inherited as an autosomal recessive trait, affecting males and females equally. Widespread screening of newborns has estimated an incidence of 1 in 24,000 live births.

The majority of subjects with this disorder are asymptomatic. Approximately 10 to 20 percent present with clinical symptoms similar to those seen in pellagra, including a photosensitive erythematous scaly rash, intermittent cerebral ataxia, delirium, and diarrhea. Short stature is noted in some patients. The symptoms are thought to be due to deficiency in the essential amino acid tryptophan and resultant inadequate synthesis of nicotinamide. Though the inheritance of the disorder is Mendelian autosomal recessive, the development of symptomatic disease appears to be multifactorial. Diet, environment, and polygenic traits controlling plasma amino acid levels all contribute to development of symptoms.

Clinically affected patients can be differentiated from patients with pellagra by dietary history and the presence of aminoaciduria. Diagnosis is made by the characteristic finding of large amounts of neutral amino acids in the urine. It can easily be distinguished from generalized aminoaciduria by the normal excretion of proline. There are no other renal tubule defects as in Fanconi syndrome. Heterozygotes have normal urinary amino acid excretion.

℞ TREATMENT

Symptomatic individuals should receive oral nicotinamide, 40 to 200 mg/d, and a high-protein diet to compensate for the poor amino acid absorption. Some patients who do not respond to nicotinamide may improve with tryptophan ethyl ester, which is lipid soluble and can be absorbed without an active transport system.

FANCONI SYNDROME Fanconi syndrome is a generalized defect in proximal tubule transport involving amino acids, glucose, phosphate, uric acid, sodium, potassium, bicarbonate, and proteins. Idiopathic Fanconi syndrome may be inherited as an autosomal dominant, autosomal recessive, or X-linked trait. Sporadic cases are also seen. A variety of inherited systemic disorders are also associated with Fanconi syndrome including Wilson's disease, galactosemia, tyrosinemia, cystinosis, fructose intolerance, and Lowe's oculocerebral syndrome. The syndrome may be acquired in multiple myeloma, amyloid, and heavy metal toxicity.

The patients may present with a wide array of laboratory abnormalities including proximal renal tubular acidosis, glucosuria with a normal serum glucose, hypophosphatemia, hypouricemia, hypokalemia, generalized aminoaciduria, and low-molecular-weight proteinuria. Some patients do not have abnormalities in all proximal tubule transporters and may present with only a few of the laboratory findings. Rickets and osteomalacia are common findings secondary to the hypophosphatemia; production of calcitriol may also be abnormal. Metabolic acidosis also contributes to the bone disease. Polyuria, salt wasting, and hypokalemia may be quite severe.

℞ TREATMENT

Treatment includes phosphate supplements and calcitriol to heal the bone lesions, alkali for the acidosis, and liberal intake of salt and water. Alkali in the form of potassium salts may be particularly useful in the patient with RTA and hypokalemia. Aminoaciduria, glucosuria, hypouricemia, and low-molecular-weight proteinuria do not require treatment.

BIBLIOGRAPHY

Buckalew VM Jr: Calcium nephrolithiasis and renal tubular acidosis, in *Disorders of Bone and Mineral Metabolism*, FL Coe, MJ Favus (eds). New York, Raven Press, 1992, p 729

Cantani A et al: Familial juvenile nephronophthisis: A review and differential diagnosis. Clin Pediatr 25:90, 1986

Clive DM: Bartter's syndrome: The unsolved puzzle. Am J Kidney Dis 25:813, 1995

Econs MJ, Drezner MK: Bone disease resulting from inherited disorders of renal tubule transport and vitamin D metabolism, in *Disorders of Bone and Mineral Metabolism*, FL Coe, MJ Favus (eds). New York, Raven Press, 1992, p 935

Gabow PA: Autosomal dominant polycystic kidney disease. N Engl J Med 329:332, 1993

Ginalski JM et al: Does medullary sponge kidney cause nephrolithiasis. AJR 155:299, 1990

Halperin ML et al: Urine ammonium: The key to the diagnosis of distal renal tubular acidosis. Nephron 50:1, 1988

International Polycystic Kidney Diseases Consortium: Polycystic kidney disease: The complete structure of the PKD1 gene and its protein. Cell 81:289, 1995

Lloyd SE et al: A common molecular basis for three inherited kidney stone diseases. Nature 379:445, 1996

Morris RC, Ives HE: Inherited disorders of the renal tubule, in *The Kidney*, 5th ed, BM Brenner (ed). Philadelphia, Saunders, 1996, p 1764

Schild L: A mutation in the epithelial sodium channel causing Liddle disease increases channel activity in the *Xenopus laevis* oocyte expression system. Proc Natl Acad Sci 92:5699, 1995

Scriver CR et al: The Hartnup phenotype: Mendelian transport disorder, multifactorial disease. Am J Hum Genet 40:401, 1987

Siris ES et al: Tumor-induced osteomalacia. Am J Med 82:307, 1987

Verge CF et al: Effects of therapy in X-linked hypophosphatemic rickets. N Engl J Med 325:1843, 1991

Welling LW, Grantham JJ: Cystic and developmental diseases of the kidney, in *The Kidney*, 5th ed, BM Brenner (ed). Philadelphia, Saunders, 1996, p 1828

Yoshida H et al: Angiotensin II type 1 receptor gene abnormality in a patient with Bartter's syndrome. Kidney Int 46:1505, 1994

279 NEPHROLITHIASIS

John R. Asplin, Fredric L. Coe, Murray J. Favus

TYPES OF STONES

Calcium salts, uric acid, cystine, and struvite ($MgNH_4PO_4$) are the basic constituents of most kidney stones in the western hemisphere. Calcium oxalate and calcium phosphate stones make up 75 to 85 percent of the total (Table 279-1) and may be admixed in the same stone. Calcium phosphate in stones is usually hydroxyapatite [$Ca_5(PO_4)_3OH$] or, less commonly, brushite ($CaHPO_4 \cdot H_2O$).

Calcium stones are more common in men; the average age of onset is the third decade. Approximately 60 percent of people who form a single calcium stone eventually form another within the next 10 years, and the intervals between successive stones shorten or remain constant. The average rate of new stone formation in patients who have had a previous stone is about one stone every 2 or 3 years. Calcium stone disease is frequently familial.

In the urine, calcium oxalate monohydrate crystals (whewellite) usually grow as biconcave ovals that resemble red blood cells in shape and size but may occur in a larger, "dumbbell" form. In polarized light the crystals appear bright against a dark background, with an intensity that is dependent on orientation, a property known as *birefringence.* Calcium oxalate dihydrate crystals (weddellite) are bipyramidal and only weakly birefringent. Apatite crystals do not exhibit birefringence and appear amorphous because the actual crystals are too small to be resolved by light microscopy. Brushite produces elongated lathlike (narrow, long, rectangular) crystals.

Uric acid stones (see Table 279-1) are radiolucent and are also more common in men. Half of patients with uric acid stones have gout; uric acid lithiasis is usually familial whether or not gout is present. In urine, uric acid crystals are red-orange in color because they absorb the pigment uricine. Anhydrous uric acid produces small crystals that appear amorphous by light microscopy. They are indistinguishable from apatite crystals, except for their birefringence. Uric acid dihydrate tends to form teardrop-shaped crystals as well as flat, square plates; both are strongly birefringent. Uric acid gravel appears like red dust, and the stones are also orange or red on some occasions. *Cystine stones* are uncommon (see Table 279-1), are lemon yellow, and sparkle; radiopacity is due to the sulfur content. Cystine crystals appear in the urine as flat, hexagonal plates.

Struvite stones are common (see Table 279-1) and potentially dangerous. These stones occur mainly in women or patients who require chronic bladder catheterization and result from urinary tract infection with urease-producing bacteria, usually *Proteus* species. The stones can grow to a large size and fill the renal pelvis and calyces to produce a "staghorn" appearance. They are radiopaque and have a variable internal density. In urine, struvite crystals are rectangular prisms said to resemble coffin lids.

MANIFESTATIONS OF STONES

As stones grow on the surfaces of the renal papillae or within the collecting system, they need not produce symptoms. Asymptomatic stones may be discovered during the course of radiographic studies undertaken for unrelated reasons. Stones rank, along with benign and malignant neoplasms, renal cysts, and genitourinary tuberculosis, among the common causes of isolated hematuria. Much of the time, however, stones break loose and enter the ureter or occlude the ureteropelvic junction, causing pain and obstruction.

STONE PASSAGE A stone can traverse the ureter without symptoms, but passage usually produces pain and bleeding. The pain begins gradually, usually in the flank, but increases over the next 20 to 60 min to become so severe that narcotic drugs may be needed for its control. The pain may remain in the flank or spread downward and anteriorly toward the ipsilateral loin, testis, or vulva. Pain that migrates downward indicates that the stone has passed to the lower third of the ureter, but if the pain does not migrate, the position of the stone cannot be predicted. A stone in the portion of the ureter within the bladder wall causes frequency, urgency, and dysuria that may be confused with urinary tract infection. Hematuria is usual with passage of a stone.

OTHER SYNDROMES Staghorn Calculi Struvite, cystine, and uric acid stones often grow too large to enter the ureter. They

Table 279-1

Major Causes of Renal Stones

Stone Type and Causes	Percent of all Stones*	Percent Occurrence of Specific Causes*	Ratio of Males to Females	Etiology	Diagnosis	Treatment
Calcium stones	75–85		2:1 to 3:1			
Idiopathic hypercalciuria		50–55	2:1	Hereditary (?)	Normocalcemia, unexplained hypercalciuria†	Thiazide diuretic agents
Hyperuricosuria		20	4:1	Diet	Urine uric acid >750 mg per 24 h (women), >800 mg per 24 h (men)	Allopurinol or diet
Primary hyperparathyroidism		5	3:10	Neoplasia	Unexplained hypercalcemia	Surgery
Distal renal tubular acidosis		Rare	1:1	Hereditary	Hyperchloremic acidosis, minimum urine pH >5.5	Alkali replacement
Intestinal hyperoxaluria		~1–2	1:1	Bowel surgery	Urine oxalate >50 mg per 24 h	Cholestyramine or oral calcium loading
Hereditary hyperoxaluria		Rare	1:1	Hereditary	Urine oxalate and glycolic or l-glyceric acid increased	Fluids and pyridoxine
Hypocitraturia		15–60	2:1 to 5:1	Hereditary (?), diet	Urine citrate <320 mg per 24 h	Alkali supplements
Idiopathic stone disease		20	2:1	Unknown	None of the above present	Oral phosphate, fluids
Uric acid stones	5–8					
Gout		~50	3:1 to 4:1	Hereditary	Clinical diagnosis	Alkali to raise urine pH
Idiopathic		~50	1:1	Hereditary (?)	Uric acid stones, no gout	Allopurinol if daily urine uric acid above 1000 mg
Dehydration		?	1:1	Intestinal, habit	History, intestinal fluid loss	Alkali, fluids, reversal of cause
Lesch-Nyhan syndrome		Rare	Males only	Hereditary	Reduced hypoxanthine-guanine phosphoribosyltransferase level	Allopurinol
Malignant tumors		Rare	1:1	Neoplasia	Clinical diagnosis	Allopurinol
Cystine stones	1		1:1	Hereditary	Stone type; elevated cystine excretion	Massive fluids, alkali, D-penicillamine if needed
Struvite stones	10–15		2:10	Infection	Stone type	Antimicrobial agents and judicious surgery

* Values are percent of patients who form a particular type of stone and who display each specific cause of stones.
† Urine calcium above 300 mg per 24 h (men), 250 mg per 24 h (women), or 4 mg/kg per 24 h either sex. Hyperthyroidism, Cushing syndrome, sarcoidosis, malignant tumors, immobilization, vitamin D intoxication, rapidly progressive bone disease, and Paget's disease all cause hypercalciuria and must be excluded in diagnosis of idiopathic hypercalciuria.

gradually fill the renal pelvis and may extend outward through the infundibula to the calyces themselves.

Nephrocalcinosis Calcium stones grow on the papillae. Most break loose and cause colic, but they may remain in place so that multiple papillary calcifications are found by x-ray, a condition termed *nephrocalcinosis*. Papillary nephrocalcinosis is common in hereditary distal renal tubular acidosis (RTA) and in other types of severe hypercalciuria. In medullary sponge kidney disease (see Chap. 278) calcification may occur in dilated distal collecting ducts.

Sludge Sufficient uric acid or cystine in the urine may plug both ureters with precipitate. Calcium oxalate crystals do not do this because less than 100 mg oxalate usually is excreted daily in the urine even in severe hyperoxaluric states, compared with 1000 mg uric acid in patients with hyperuricosuria and 400 to 800 mg cystine in patients with cystinuria. Calcium phosphate crystals can render the urine milky but do not plug the urinary tract.

INFECTION Although urinary tract infection is not a direct consequence of stone disease, it can occur after instrumentation and surgery of the urinary tract, which are frequent in the treatment of stone disease. Stone disease and urinary tract infection can enhance the seriousness of one another and interfere with treatment. Obstruction of an infected kidney by a stone may lead to sepsis and extensive damage of renal tissue, since it converts the urinary tract proximal to the obstruction into a closed, or partially closed, space that can become an abscess. Stones may harbor bacteria in the stone matrix, leading to recurrent urinary tract infection. On the other hand, infection due to bacteria that possess the enzyme urease can cause stones composed of struvite.

ACTIVITY OF STONE DISEASE *Active disease* means that new stones are forming or that preformed stones are growing. Sequential radiographs of the renal areas are needed to document the growth or appearance of new stones and to ensure that passed stones are actually newly formed, not preexistent ones.

PATHOGENESIS OF STONES

Urinary stones usually arise because of the breakdown of a delicate balance. The kidneys must conserve water, but they must excrete materials that have a low solubility. These two opposing requirements must be balanced during adaptation to diet, climate, and activity. The problem is mitigated to some extent by the fact that urine contains substances that inhibit crystallization of calcium salts and others that bind calcium in soluble complexes. These protective mechanisms are less than perfect. When the urine becomes supersaturated with insoluble materials, because excretion rates are excessive and/or because water conservation is extreme, crystals form and may grow and aggregate to form a stone.

SUPERSATURATION In a solution in equilibrium with crystals of calcium oxalate, the product of the chemical activities of the calcium and oxalate ions in the solution is termed the *equilibrium solubility product*. If crystals are removed, and if either calcium or oxalate ions are added to the solution, the activity product increases, but the solution may remain clear; no new crystals form. Such a solution is *metastably supersaturated.* If new calcium oxalate seed crystals are now added, they will grow in size. Ultimately, the activity product reaches a critical value at which a solid phase begins to develop spontaneously. This value is called the *upper limit of metastability*, or the *formation product*. Stone growth in the urinary tract requires a urine that, on average, is above the equilibrium solubility product. Persistence of a stone requires an average activity product at least equal to the solubility product. Excessive supersaturation is common in stone formation.

Calcium, oxalate, and phosphate form many stable soluble complexes among themselves and with other substances in urine, such as citrate. As a result, their free ion activities are below their chemical concentrations and can be measured only by indirect techniques. Reduction in ligands such as citrate can increase ion activity without changing total urinary calcium. Urine supersaturation can be increased by dehydration or by overexcretion of calcium, oxalate, phosphate, cystine, or uric acid. Urine pH is also important; phosphate and uric acid are weak acids that dissociate readily over the physiologic range of urine pH. Alkaline urine contains more urate and dibasic phosphate, favoring deposits of sodium hydrogen urate, brushite, and apatite. Below a urine pH of 5.5, uric acid crystals (pK 5.47) predominate, whereas phosphate crystals are rare. The solubility of calcium oxalate, on the other hand, is not influenced by changes in urine pH. Measurements of supersaturation in a pooled 24-h urine sample probably underestimate the risk of precipitation. Transient dehydration, variation of urine pH, and postprandial bursts of overexcretion may cause values considerably above average.

NUCLEATION **Homogeneous Nucleation** In urine that is supersaturated with respect to calcium oxalate, these two ions form clusters. Most small clusters eventually disperse because the internal forces that hold them together are too weak to overcome the random tendency of ions to move away. Clusters of over 100 ions can remain stable because attractive forces balance surface losses. Once they are stable, nuclei can grow at levels of supersaturation below that needed for their creation. The formation product marks the point at which stable nuclei become frequent enough to create a permanent solid phase.

Heterogeneous Nucleation If a supersaturated urine is seeded with preformed nuclei of a crystal that is similar in structure to calcium oxalate, calcium and oxalate ions in solution will bind to the crystal's surface as they would on a seed crystal of calcium oxalate itself. The organized growth of one crystal on the surface of another is called *epitaxial growth*, and the seeding of a supersaturated solution by foreign nuclei is called *heterogeneous nucleation.* Sodium hydrogen urate, uric acid, and hydroxyapatite crystals can serve as heterogeneous nuclei that permit calcium oxalate stones to form, even though urine calcium oxalate supersaturation never exceeds the metastable limit for homogeneous nucleation.

INHIBITORS OF CRYSTAL FORMATION Stable nuclei must grow and aggregate to produce a stone of clinical significance. Urine contains potent inhibitors of nucleation, growth, and aggregation for calcium oxalate and calcium phosphate but not for uric acid, cystine, or struvite. Inorganic pyrophosphate is a potent inhibitor that appears to affect calcium phosphate more than calcium oxalate crystals. Other urine components that appear to be glycoproteins inhibit all three processes of calcium oxalate stone formation. Slowing of crystal growth increases the apparent upper limit of metastability because the critical growth of ion clusters into stable nuclei is hindered. As a consequence of the presence of these inhibitors, crystal growth in urine is slow compared with growth in simple salt solutions, and the upper limit of metastability is higher. Citrate inhibits crystal growth and nucleation, though most of the stone inhibitory activity of citrate is due to lowering urine supersaturation via complexation of calcium.

EVALUATION AND TREATMENT OF PATIENTS WITH NEPHROLITHIASIS

Most patients with nephrolithiasis have remediable metabolic disorders that cause stones and can be detected by chemical analyses of serum and urine. A practical outpatient evaluation consists of two or three 24-h urine collections, each with a corresponding blood sample; measurements of serum and urine calcium, uric acid, electrolytes and creatinine and of urine pH, volume, oxalate, and citrate should be made. Since stone risks vary with diet, activity, and environment, at least one urine collection should be made on a weekend when the patient is at home and another on a work day. When possible, the composition of kidney stones should be determined because treatment depends on stone type (see Table 279-1). No matter what disorders are found, every patient should be counseled to avoid dehydration and to drink sufficient water so that they excrete at least 2 L of urine every day. Since treatment is prolonged, the use of medications must be justified by the activity and severity of stone disease and the importance of protection against new stones.

℞ TREATMENT

The management of stones already present in the kidneys or urinary tract requires a combined medical and surgical approach. The specific treatment depends on the location of the stone, the extent of obstruction, the function of the affected and unaffected kidney, the presence or absence of urinary tract infection, the progress of stone passage, and the risks of operation or anesthesia given the clinical state of the patient. In general, severe obstruction, infection, intractable pain, and serious bleeding are indications for removal of a stone.

In the past, stones were removed by operation or by passing a flexible basket retrograde up the ureter from the bladder during cystoscopy. There are now three alternatives. *Extracorporeal lithotripsy* causes the in situ fragmentation of stones in the kidney, renal pelvis, or proximal ureter by exposing them to shock waves. The kidney with the stone is centered at a focal point of parabolic reflectors, and high-intensity shock waves are created by high-voltage discharge. The waves are transmitted to the patient using water as a conduction medium, either by placing the patient in a water tank or by placing water-filled cushions between the patient and the shock-wave generators. The shock waves are focused by the reflectors so that they pass through the patient and fracture the stone as they pass. After multiple discharges, most stones are reduced to powder that moves through the ureter into the bladder. *Percutaneous ultrasonic lithotripsy* requires the passage of a rigid cystoscope-like instrument into the renal pelvis through a small incision in the flank. Stones can be disrupted by a small ultrasound transducer, and fragments can be removed directly. The last method is *laser lithotripsy via a ureteroscope* for removal of ureteral stones. These various forms of lithotripsy have largely replaced pyelolithotomy and ureterolithotomy.

CALCIUM STONES **Idiopathic Hypercalciuria** (See also Chap. 354) This condition appears to be hereditary, and its diagnosis is straightforward (see Table 279-1). In some patients, primary intestinal hyperabsorption of calcium causes transient postprandial hypercalcemia that suppresses secretion of parathyroid hormone. The renal tubules are deprived of the normal stimulus to reabsorb calcium at the same time that the filtered load of calcium is increased. In other patients, reabsorption of calcium by the renal tubules appears to be defective, and secondary hyperparathyroidism is evoked by urinary losses of calcium. Renal synthesis of 1,25-dihydroxyvitamin D is increased, enhancing intestinal absorption of calcium. In the past, the separation of "absorptive" and "renal" forms of hypercalciuria was used to guide treatment. However, these may not be distinct entities but the extremes of a continuum of behavior. Vitamin D overactivity, either through high vitamin D levels or excess vitamin D receptor, is a likely explanation for the hypercalciuria in many of these patients. Hypercalciuria contributes to stone formation by raising urine saturation with respect to calcium oxalate and calcium phosphate.

℞ TREATMENT

Thiazide diuretics lower urine calcium in idiopathic hypercalciuria and are effective in preventing the formation of stones. Two 3-year randomized trials have shown a 50 percent decrease in stone formation in the thiazide-treated group as compared to the placebo-treated controls. The drug effect requires slight contraction of the extracellular fluid volume, and massive use of NaCl reduces its therapeutic effect. Thiazide-induced hypokalemia should be aggressively treated since hypokalemia will reduce urine citrate, increasing urine calcium ion levels.

Hyperuricosuria About 20 percent of calcium oxalate stone formers are hyperuricosuric, primarily because of an excessive intake of purine from meat, fish, and poultry. The mechanism of stone formation probably is heterogeneous nucleation of calcium oxalate by crystals of sodium hydrogen urate or uric acid. A low-purine diet is desirable but difficult for many patients to achieve. The alternative is allopurinol, usually 100 mg bid.

Primary Hyperparathyroidism (See also Chap. 354) The diagnosis of this condition is established by documenting that hypercalcemia that cannot be otherwise explained is accompanied by inappropriately elevated serum concentrations of parathyroid hormone. Hypercalciuria, usually present, raises the urine supersaturation of calcium phosphate and/or calcium oxalate (see Table 279-1). Prompt diagnosis is important because parathyroidectomy should be carried out before renal damage or bone disease occurs.

Distal Renal Tubular Acidosis (See also Chap. 278) The defect in this condition seems to reside in the distal nephron, which cannot establish a normal pH gradient between urine and blood, leading to hyperchloremic acidosis. The diagnosis is suggested by a minimum urine pH in the presence of systemic acidosis above 5.5. If the diagnosis is in doubt because metabolic abnormalities are mild, oral challenge with NH_4Cl, 1.9 mmol/kg of body weight, will not lower urine pH below 5.5 in patients with distal RTA. Hypercalciuria, an alkaline urine, and a low urine citrate level cause supersaturation with respect to calcium phosphate. Calcium phosphate stones form, nephrocalcinosis is common, and osteomalacia or rickets may occur. Renal damage is frequent, and glomerular filtration rate falls gradually. Treatment with supplemental alkali reverses hypercalciuria and limits the production of new stones. The usual dose of sodium bicarbonate is 0.5 to 2.0 mmol/kg of body weight per day in four to six divided doses. An alternative is potassium citrate supplementation, given at the same dose per day but needing to be given only three to four times per day. In incomplete distal RTA, systemic acidosis is absent, but urine pH cannot be lowered below 5.5 after an exogenous acid load such as ammonium chloride. Incomplete RTA may develop in some patients who form calcium oxalate stones because of idiopathic hypercalciuria; the importance of the RTA in producing stones in this situation is uncertain, and thiazide treatment is a reasonable alternative. Some patients with incomplete RTA form calcium phosphate stones because of low urine citrate and an alkaline urine and are best treated with alkali as if RTA were complete.

Hyperoxaluria Overabsorption of dietary oxalate and consequent oxaluria, i.e., so-called intestinal oxaluria, is one consequence of fat malabsorption (Chap. 285). The latter can be caused by a variety of conditions, including bacterial overgrowth syndromes, chronic disease of the pancreas and biliary tract, jejunoileal bypass in treatment of obesity, or ileal resection for inflammatory bowel disease. With fat malabsorption, calcium in the bowel lumen is bound by fatty acids instead of oxalate, which is left free for absorption in the colon. Delivery of unabsorbed fatty acids and bile salts to the colon may injure the colonic mucosa and enhance oxalate absorption. Dietary excess of oxalate in patients with normal intestinal function is a common cause of mild elevation of urine oxalate, but seldom to the level of urine oxalate seen in patients with enteric hyperoxaluria. Hereditary hyperoxaluria states are rare causes of severe hyperoxaluria; patients usually present with recurrent calcium oxalate stones during childhood. Type I hereditary hyperoxaluria is inherited as an autosomal recessive trait and is due to a deficiency in the peroxisomal enzyme alanine:glyoxylate aminotransferase. Type II is due to a deficiency of D-glyceric dehydrogenase. Ethylene glycol intoxication and methoxyflurane also can cause oxalate overproduction and hyperoxaluria. Hyperoxaluria from any cause can produce tubulointerstitial nephropathy (Chap. 276) and lead to stone formation.

℞ TREATMENT

The oxalate-binding resin cholestyramine at a dose of 8 to 16 g/d, correction of fat malabsorption, and a low-fat diet are effective treatments for oxaluria secondary to intestinal overabsorption. Calcium lactate, 8 to 14 g/d, which precipitates oxalate in the gut lumen, is an alternative form of therapy. Treatment for hereditary hyperoxaluria includes a high fluid intake, neutral phosphate, and pyridoxine (25 to 200 mg/d). Citrate supplementation may also have some benefit. Even with aggressive therapy, irreversible renal failure secondary to recurrent stone formation often occurs. Segmental liver transplant, to correct the enzyme defect, combined with a kidney transplant have been successfully utilized in patients with hereditary hyperoxaluria.

Hypocitraturia Urine citrate prevents calcium stone formation by creating a soluble complex with calcium, effectively reducing free urine calcium. Hypocitraturia is found in 15 to 60 percent of stone formers, either as a single disorder or in combination with other metabolic abnormalities. It can be secondary to systemic disorders, such as RTA, chronic diarrheal illness, or hypokalemia, or it may be a primary disorder, in which case it is called *idiopathic hypocitraturia.*

TREATMENT

Treatment is with alkali, which increases urine citrate excretion; generally bicarbonate or citrate salts are used. Potassium salts are preferred as sodium loading increases urinary excretion of calcium, reducing the effectiveness of treatment. A recent randomized, placebo-controlled trial has demonstrated the effectiveness of potassium citrate in idiopathic hypocitraturia.

Idiopathic Calcium Lithiasis Some patients have no metabolic cause for stones despite a thorough metabolic evaluation (see Table 279-1). The best treatment appears to be high fluid intake so that the urine specific gravity remains at 1.005 or below throughout the day and night. Oral phosphate at a dose of 2 g phosphorus daily may lower urine calcium and increase urine pyrophosphate and thereby reduce the rate of recurrence. Orthophosphate causes mild nausea and diarrhea initially, but tolerance may improve with continued intake. Thiazide treatment to reduce calcium excretion and allopurinol to diminish uric acid output also may be helpful.

URIC ACID STONES These stones form because the urine becomes supersaturated with undissociated uric acid, uric acid that is protonated at its N-9 position. In gout, idiopathic uric acid lithiasis, and dehydration, the average pH is usually below 5.4 and often below 5.0. Undissociated uric acid therefore predominates and is soluble in urine only in concentrations of 100 mg/L. Concentrations above this level represent supersaturation that causes crystals and stones to form. Hyperuricosuria, when present, increases supersaturation, but urine of low pH can be supersaturated with undissociated uric acid even though the daily excretion rate is normal. Myeloproliferative syndromes, chemotherapy of malignant tumors, and the Lesch-Nyhan syndrome cause such massive production of uric acid and consequent hyperuricosuria that stones and uric acid sludge form even at a normal urine pH. Plugging of the renal collecting tubules by uric acid crystals can cause acute renal failure.

TREATMENT

The two goals of treatment are to raise urine pH and to lower excessive urine uric acid excretion to less than 1 g/d. Supplemental alkali, 1 to 3 mmol/kg of body weight per day, should be given in three or four evenly spaced, divided doses, one of which should be given at bedtime. The form of the alkali may be important. Potassium citrate may reduce the risk of calcium salts crystallizing when urine pH is increased, whereas sodium citrate or sodium bicarbonate may increase the risk. If the overnight urine pH is below 5.5, the evening dose of alkali may be raised or 250 mg acetazolamide added at bedtime. A low-purine diet should be instituted in those uric acid stone formers with hyperuricosuria. Patients who continue to form uric acid stones despite treatment with fluids, alkali, and a low-purine diet should have allopurinol added to their regimen. If hypercalciuria is also present, it should be specifically treated as alkali alone could lead to calcium phosphate stone formation.

CYSTINURIA AND CYSTINE STONES (See also Chap. 349) In this disorder, proximal tubular and jejunal transport of the dibasic amino acids cystine, lysine, arginine, and ornithine are defective, and excessive amounts are lost in the urine. Clinical disease is due solely to the insolubility of cystine, which forms stones.

Pathogenesis Cystinuria probably occurs because of defective transport of amino acids by the brush borders of renal tubule and intestinal epithelial cells. Cystine, lysine, arginine, and ornithine appear to share a common renal transport pathway, since infusion of lysine decreases tubular reabsorption of the other three. However, cystine is also transported by a separate transport mechanism, because cystinuria and dibasic aminoaciduria can occur independently. The intestinal defects are not similar in all patients who are homozygous for cystinuria, and the extent of aminoaciduria in individuals who are heterozygous carriers of the defect varies from family to family. Three types of inheritance have been described (see Chap. 349).

Diagnosis Cystine stones are formed only by patients with cystinuria, but 10 percent of stones in cystinuric patients do not contain cystine; therefore, every stone former should be screened for the disease. The sediment from a first morning urine specimen in many patients with homozygous cystinuria reveals typical flat, hexagonal platelike cystine crystals. Cystinuria also can be detected using the urine sodium nitroprusside test. The test is positive with 75 to 125 mg cystine per gram of creatinine, a concentration lower than that in the urine of patients with cystinuria but above the levels in normal urine. Because the test is sensitive, it is positive in many asymptomatic heterozygotes for cystinuria. A positive nitroprusside test or the finding of cystine crystals in the urine sediment should be evaluated by measurement of daily cystine excretion. Normal adults excrete 40 to 60 mg cystine per gram of creatinine, heterozygotes usually excrete less than 300 mg/g, and homozygotes almost always excrete above 250 mg/g.

TREATMENT

This consists of a high fluid intake, even at night. Daily urine volume should exceed 3 L. Raising urine pH with alkali is helpful, provided the urine pH exceeds 7.5. A low-salt diet (100 mmol/d) can reduce cystine excretion up to 40 percent. Because side effects are frequent, drugs such as penicillamine and tiopronin, which form the soluble disulfide cysteine-drug complexes, should be used only when fluid loading, salt reduction, and alkali therapy are ineffective. Captopril, which has a free sulfhydryl group to bind cysteine, has been used in a limited number of patients with some success. Low-methionine diets have not proved to be practical for clinical use, but patients should avoid protein gluttony.

STRUVITE STONES These stones are a result of urinary infection with bacteria, usually *Proteus* species, which possess urease, an enzyme that degrades urea to NH_3 and CO_2. The NH_3 hydrolyzes to NH_4^+ and raises urine pH to 8 or 9. The CO_2 hydrates to H_2CO_3 and then dissociates to CO_3^{2-} which precipitates with calcium as $CaCO_3$. The NH_4^+ precipitates PO_43^- and Mg^{2+} to form $MgNH_4PO_4$ (struvite). The result is a stone of calcium carbonate admixed with struvite. Struvite does not form in urine in the absence of infection, because NH_4^+ concentration is low in urine that is alkaline in response to physiologic stimuli. Chronic *Proteus* infection can occur because of impaired urinary drainage, urologic instrumentation or surgery, and especially with chronic antibiotic treatment, which can favor the dominance of *Proteus* in the urinary tract.

TREATMENT

Complete removal of the stone with subsequent sterilization of the urinary tract is the treatment of choice for patients who can tolerate the procedures. Open surgery is successful in debulking the stone and improving renal function if obstruction is present; however, there is recurrence of stone in 25 percent of the patients. Irrigation of the renal pelvis and calyces with hemiacidrin, a solution that dissolves struvite, can reduce recurrence after surgery. Newer procedures such as lithotripsy and percutaneous nephrolithotomy, alone or in combination, have largely replaced open surgery. Stone-free rates of 50 to 90 percent have been reported after these procedures.

Antimicrobial treatment is best reserved for dealing with acute infection and for maintenance of a sterile urine after surgery, in the hope of preventing recurrence or minimizing stone growth. Urine cultures and culture of stone fragments removed at surgery should guide the choice of antibiotic. Methenamine mandelate, which lowers urine pH and liberates formaldehyde, can be used for chronic suppression of infection when a stone is present. For patients who are not candidates for surgical removal of stone, acetohydroxamic acid, an inhibitor of urease, can be used. Though effective in treating the stones, acetohydroxamic acid has many side effects, such as headache, tremor, and thrombophlebitis, which limits its use. Lowering urine pH with chronic administration of NH_4Cl may retard stone growth but also may raise urine calcium level and promote the formation of calcium oxalate stones.

BIBLIOGRAPHY

BATAILLE P et al: Diet, vitamin D and vertebral mineral density in hypercalciuric calcium stone formers. Kidney Int 39:1193, 1991.

BARCELO P et al: Randomized double-blind study of potassium citrate in idiopathic hypocitraturic calcium nephrolithiasis. J Urol 150:1761, 1993

COE FL et al: The pathogenesis and treatment of kidney stones. N Engl J Med 327:1141, 1992

CONSENSUS CONFERENCE: Prevention and treatment of kidney stones. JAMA 260:977, 1988

GLEESON MJ, GRIFFITH DP: Struvite calculi. Br J Urol 71:503, 1993

LEMANN J JR: Pathogenesis or idiopathic hypercalciuria and nephrolithiasis, in *Disorders of Bone and Mineral Metabolism*, FL Coe, MJ Favus (eds). New York, Raven Press, 1992, p 685

LINGEMAN JE: Mechanisms of stone disruption and dissolution, in *Disorders of Bone and Mineral Metabolism*, FL Coe, MJ Favus (eds). New York, Raven Press, 1992, p 625

NEWMAN DM et al: Long-term follow-up of 1,900 ESWL treatments, in *Shock Wave Lithotripsy*, JE Lingeman, DM Newman (eds). New York, Plenum, 1988

RESNICK MI, PAK CYC: *Urolithiasis*. Philadelphia, Saunders, 1991

280

Julian L. Seifter, Barry M. Brenner

URINARY TRACT OBSTRUCTION

Obstruction to the flow of urine, with attendant stasis and elevation in urinary tract pressure, impairs renal and urinary conduit functions and is a common cause of acute and chronic renal failure. With early relief of obstruction, the defects in function usually disappear completely. However, chronic obstruction may produce permanent loss of renal mass (renal atrophy) and excretory capability, as well as enhanced susceptibility to local infection and stone formation. Early diagnosis and prompt therapy are therefore essential to minimize the otherwise devastating effects of obstruction on kidney structure and function.

ETIOLOGY Obstruction to urine flow can result from *intrinsic* or *extrinsic mechanical blockade* as well as from *functional defects* not associated with fixed occlusion of the urinary drainage system. Mechanical obstruction can occur at any level of the urinary tract, from the renal calyces to the external urethral meatus. Normal points of narrowing, such as the ureteropelvic and ureterovesical junctions, bladder neck, and urethral meatus, are common sites of obstruction. When blockage is above the level of the bladder, unilateral dilatation of the ureter (*hydroureter*) and renal pyelocalyceal system (*hydronephrosis*) occur; lesions at or below the level of the bladder cause bilateral involvement.

Common forms of obstruction are listed in Table 280-1. In childhood, *congenital malformations*, including marked narrowing of the ureteropelvic junction, anomalous (retrocaval) location of the ureter, and posterior urethral valves, predominate. The latter defect is the most common cause of bilateral hydronephrosis in boys. Children also may have bladder dysfunction secondary to congenital urethral stricture, urethral meatal stenosis, or bladder neck obstruction. In adults, urinary tract obstruction is due mainly to *acquired defects*. Pelvic tumors, calculi, and urethral stricture predominate. Ligation of, or injury to, the ureter during pelvic or colonic surgery can lead to hydronephrosis which, if unilateral, may remain relatively silent and undetected. *Schistosoma haematobium* and genitourinary tuberculosis are infectious causes of ureteral obstruction. Obstructive uropathy also may result from extrinsic neoplastic (carcinoma of cervix or colon, retroperitoneal lymphoma) or inflammatory disorders. One such inflammatory disorder is retroperitoneal fibrosis, a process of unknown cause seen most commonly in middle-aged men, which occasionally leads to bilateral ureteral obstruction. Retroperitoneal fibrosis must be distinguished from other retroperitoneal causes of ureteral obstruction, particularly lymphomas and pelvic neoplasms.

Functional impairment of urine flow usually results from disorders that involve both the ureter and bladder. Common functional lesions include neurogenic bladder, often with adynamic ureter, and vesicoureteral reflux. Reflux of urine from bladder to ureter(s) is more common in children than in adults and may result in severe unilateral or bilateral hydroureter and hydronephrosis. Abnormal insertion of the ureter into the bladder is the most common cause of vesicoureteral reflux in children. Reflux in the absence of urinary tract infection or bladder neck obstruction usually does not lead to renal parenchymal damage and often resolves spontaneously as the child matures. Surgical reinsertion of the ureter into the bladder is indicated if reflux is severe and unlikely to improve spontaneously, if renal function deteriorates, or if urinary tract infections recur despite chronic antimicrobial therapy. Hydronephrosis, usually more marked on the right than on the left, is common in pregnancy, due both to ureteral compression by the enlarged uterus and to functional effects of progesterone.

Table 280-1

Common Mechanical Causes of Urinary Tract Obstruction

Ureter	Bladder Outlet	Urethra
CONGENITAL		
Ureteropelvic junction narrowing or obstruction	Bladder neck obstruction	Posterior urethral valves
Ureterovesical junction narrowing or obstruction	Ureterocele	Anterior urethral valves
Ureterocele		Stricture
Retrocaval ureter		Meatal stenosis
		Phimosis
ACQUIRED INTRINSIC DEFECTS		
Calculi	Benign prostatic hyperplasia	Stricture
Inflammation	Cancer of prostate	Tumor
Trauma	Cancer of bladder	Calculi
Sloughed papillae	Calculi	Trauma
Tumor	Diabetic neuropathy	Phimosis
Blood clots	Spinal cord disease	
Uric acid crystals	Anticholinergic drugs and alpha-adrenergic antagonists	
ACQUIRED EXTRINSIC DEFECTS		
Pregnant uterus	Carcinoma of cervix, colon	Trauma
Retroperitoneal fibrosis	Trauma	
Aortic aneurysm		
Uterine leiomyomata		
Carcinoma of uterus, prostate, bladder, colon, rectum		
Lymphoma, pelvic inflammatory disease		
Accidental surgical ligation		

CLINICAL FEATURES The pathophysiology and clinical features of urinary tract obstruction are summarized in Table 280-2. *Pain* is the symptom that most commonly provokes the need for medical attention. The pain of urinary tract obstruction is due to distention of the collecting system or renal capsule. The severity of the pain is influenced more by the rate at which distention develops than by the degree of distention. Acute supravesical obstruction, as from a stone lodged in a ureter (Chap. 279), is associated with excruciatingly severe pain, usually called *renal colic*. This pain is relatively steady and continuous, with little fluctuation in intensity, and often radiates to the lower abdomen, testes, or labia. By contrast, more insidious causes of obstruction, such as chronic narrowing of the ureteropelvic junction, may produce little or no pain yet result in total destruction of the affected kidney. Flank pain that occurs only with micturition is pathognomonic of vesicoureteral reflux.

Azotemia develops in urinary tract obstruction when overall excretory function is impaired. This may occur in the setting of bladder outlet obstruction, bilateral renal pelvic or ureteric obstruction, or unilateral disease in a patient with a solitary functioning kidney. Complete bilateral obstruction should be suspected when acute renal failure is accompanied by anuria. Any patient with renal failure otherwise unexplained or with a history of nephrolithiasis, hematuria, diabetes mellitus, prostatic enlargement, pelvic surgery, trauma, or tumor should be evaluated for urinary tract obstruction.

In the acute setting, bilateral obstruction may result in sodium and water retention that may mimic prerenal azotemia. However, with more prolonged obstruction, symptoms of *polyuria* and *nocturia* commonly accompany partial urinary tract obstruction and result from impaired renal concentrating ability. This defect usually does not improve with administration of vasopressin and is therefore a form of acquired nephrogenic diabetes insipidus. Disturbances in sodium chloride transport in the ascending limb of Henle and, in azotemic patients, the osmotic (urea) diuresis per nephron lead to decreased medullary hypertonicity and hence a concentrating defect. Partial obstruction, therefore, may be associated with increased rather than decreased urine output. Indeed, wide fluctuations in urine output in a patient with azotemia should always raise the possibility of intermittent or partial urinary tract obstruction. If fluid intake is inadequate, severe dehydration and hypernatremia may develop. Hesitancy and straining to initiate the urinary stream, postvoid dribbling, urinary frequency, and (overflow) incontinence are common with obstruction at or below the level of the bladder (see Chap. 47).

In addition to loss of urinary concentrating ability and azotemia, partial bilateral urinary tract obstruction often results in other derangements of renal function, including *acquired distal renal tubular acidosis*, *hyperkalemia*, and *renal salt wasting*. These defects in tubule function are often accompanied by renal tubulointerstitial damage. Morphologic abnormalities appear early in the course of obstruction; initially the interstitium becomes edematous and infiltrated with mononuclear inflammatory cells. With continued obstruction, the interstitium becomes fibrotic; scarring and atrophy of the papillae and medulla occur and precede these processes in the cortex.

The possibility of urinary tract obstruction must always be considered in patients with urinary tract infections or urolithiasis. Urinary stasis encourages the growth of organisms as well as the formation of crystals, especially magnesium ammonium phosphate (struvite). *Hypertension* is frequent in acute and subacute unilateral obstruction and is usually a consequence of increased release of renin by the involved kidney. Chronic unilateral or bilateral hydronephrosis, in the presence of extracellular volume expansion or other renal disease, may result in significant hypertension. *Polycythemia*, an infrequent complication of obstructive uropathy, is probably secondary to increased erythropoietin production by the obstructed kidney.

DIAGNOSIS A history of difficulty in voiding, pain, infection, or changes in urinary volume is common. Evidence for distention of the kidney or urinary bladder often can be obtained by palpation and percussion of the abdomen. A careful rectal examination may reveal enlargement or nodularity of the prostate, abnormal rectal sphincter tone, or a rectal or pelvic mass. The penis should be inspected for evidence of meatal stenosis or phimosis. In the female, vaginal, uterine, and rectal lesions responsible for urinary tract obstruction are usually revealed by inspection and palpation.

Urinalysis and examination of the urine sediment may reveal hematuria, pyuria, and bacteriuria. Often, however, the urine sediment is normal, even when obstruction leads to marked azotemia and extensive structural damage. An abdominal scout film should be obtained to evaluate the possibility of nephrocalcinosis or a radiopaque stone at any level of the urinary collecting system. As indicated in Fig. 280-1, if urinary tract obstruction is suspected, a bladder catheter should be inserted. If diuresis does not follow, then abdominal ultrasonography should be performed to evaluate renal and bladder size, as well as pyelocalyceal contour. Ultrasonography is approximately 90 percent specific and sensitive for detection of hydronephrosis. False-positive results are associated with diuresis, renal cysts, or presence of an extrarenal pelvis, a normal congenital variant. Hydronephrosis may be absent on ultrasound when obstruction is associated with volume contraction, staghorn calculi, or retroperitoneal fibrosis.

In some cases, the intravenous urogram may define the site of obstruction. In the presence of obstruction, the appearance time of the nephrogram is often delayed. Eventually, however, the renal image becomes more dense than normal because of slow tubular fluid flow rate, which results in enhanced water reabsorption by the nephrons and greater concentration of contrast medium within tubules. The kidney involved by an acute obstructive process is usually slightly enlarged, and there is dilatation of the calyces, renal pelvis, and ureter above the obstruction. The ureter, however, is not tortuous, as is the case when the obstruction is chronic. In comparison with the nephrogram, the urogram may be extremely faint, especially if the dilated renal pelvis is voluminous, causing dilution of the contrast medium. The radiographic study should be continued until the site of obstruction is determined or the contrast medium is excreted. Radionuclide scans define less anatomic detail than intravenous urography and, like the urogram, are of limited value when renal function is poor. Nonetheless, such scans are sensitive for the detection of obstruc-

Table 280-2

Pathophysiology of Bilateral Ureteral Obstruction

Hemodynamic Effects	Tubule Effects	Clinical Features
ACUTE		
↑Renal blood flow ↓GFR ↓Medullary blood flow ↑Vasodilator prostaglandins	↑Ureteral and tubule pressures ↑Reabsorption of Na^+, urea, water	Pain (capsule distention) Azotemia Oliguria or anuria
CHRONIC		
↓Renal blood flow ↓↓GFR ↑Vasoconstrictor prostaglandins ↑Renin-angiotensin production	↓Medullary osmolarity ↓Concentrating ability Structural damage; parenchymal atrophy ↓Transport functions for Na^+, K^+, H^+	Azotemia Hypertension ADH-insensitive polyuria Natriuresis Hyperkalemic, hyperchloremic acidosis
RELEASE OF OBSTRUCTION		
Slow ↑ in GFR (variable)	↓Tubule pressure ↑Solute load per nephron (urea, NaCl) Natriuretic factors present	Postobstructive diuresis Potential for volume depletion and electrolyte imbalance due to losses of Na^+, K^+, PO_4^{2-}, Mg^{2+}, and water

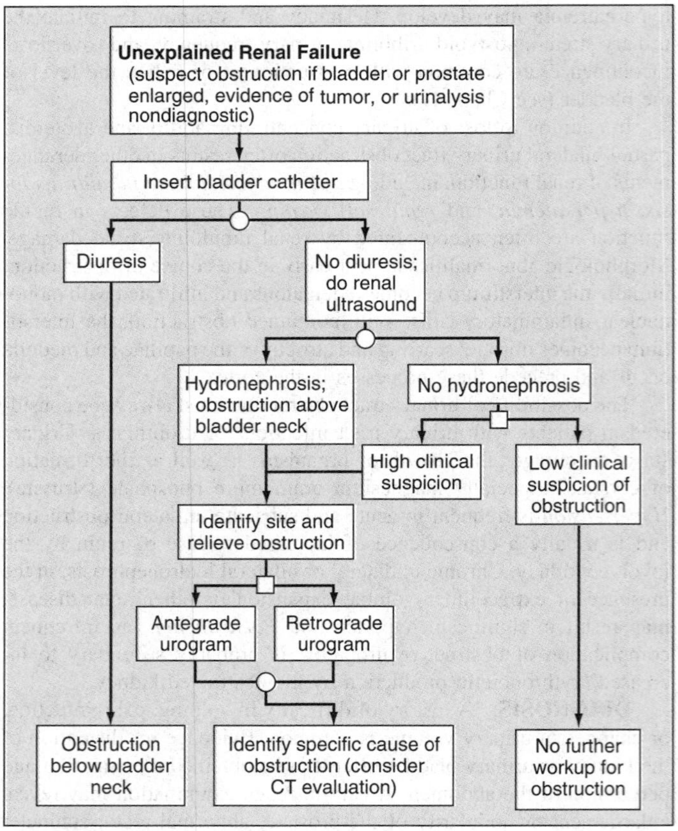

FIGURE 280-1 Diagnostic approach for urinary tract obstruction in unexplained renal failure. Circles represent diagnostic procedures, and squares indicate clinical decisions based on available data. CT, computed tomography.

tion and provide a substitute test in some patients at high risk for reaction to intravenous contrast.

To facilitate visualization of a suspected lesion in a ureter or renal pelvis, *retrograde* or *antegrade urography* should be attempted. These diagnostic studies may be preferable to the intravenous pyelogram in the azotemic patient, in whom poor excretory function precludes adequate visualization of the collecting system. Furthermore, intravenous urography carries the risk of contrast-induced renal failure in patients with renal insufficiency, diabetes mellitus, and multiple myeloma, particularly when performed under conditions of dehydration. The retrograde approach involves catheterization of the involved ureter under cystoscopic control, while the antegrade technique necessitates placement of a catheter into the renal pelvis via a needle inserted percutaneously under ultrasonic or fluoroscopic guidance. While the antegrade approach carries the added advantage of providing immediate decompression of a unilateral obstructing lesion, many urologists initially attempt the retrograde approach and resort to the antegrade method only when attempts at retrograde catheterization are unsuccessful or when cystoscopy or general anesthesia is contraindicated. Patients suspected of having intermittent ureteropelvic obstruction (whether functional or mechanical) should have radiologic evaluation while they are in pain, since a normal urogram is commonly seen during asymptomatic periods. Hydration often helps to provoke a symptomatic attack. Voiding cystourethrography is of great value in the diagnosis of vesicoureteral reflux and bladder neck and urethral obstructions. Patients with obstruction at or below the level of the bladder exhibit thickening, trabeculation, and diverticula of the bladder wall. Postvoiding films reveal residual urine. If these radiographic studies fail to provide adequate information for diagnosis, endoscopic visualization by the urologist often permits precise identification of lesions involving the urethra, prostate, bladder, and ureteral orifices.

Computed tomography is useful in the diagnosis of specific intraabdominal and retroperitoneal causes of obstruction but is less practical as an initial test to establish the presence of obstruction. Magnetic resonance imaging also may be useful in the identification of specific obstructive causes.

Rx TREATMENT

An individual with any form of urinary tract obstruction complicated by infection requires relief of obstruction as soon as possible to prevent development of generalized sepsis and progressive renal damage. On a temporary basis, depending on the site of obstruction, drainage is often satisfactorily achieved by nephrostomy, ureterostomy, or ureteral, urethral, or suprapubic catheterization. The patient with acute urinary tract infection and obstruction should be given appropriate antibiotics based on in vitro bacterial sensitivity and ability of the drug to concentrate in the kidney and urine. Treatment may be required for 3 to 4 weeks. Chronic or recurrent infections in an obstructed kidney with poor intrinsic function may necessitate nephrectomy. When infection is not present, immediate surgery often is not required, even in the presence of complete obstruction and anuria (because of the availability of dialysis), at least until acid-base, fluid and electrolyte, and cardiovascular status are restored to normal. Nevertheless, the site of obstruction should be ascertained as soon as feasible, in part because of the possibility that sepsis may occur and necessitate prompt urologic intervention. Elective relief of obstruction is usually recommended in patients with urinary retention, recurrent urinary tract infections, persistent pain, or progressive loss of renal function. Infrequently, mechanical obstruction can be alleviated by nonsurgical means, as with radiation therapy for retroperitoneal lymphoma. Likewise, functional obstruction secondary to neurogenic bladder may be decreased with the combination of frequent voiding and cholinergic drugs. → ***The approach to obstruction secondary to renal stones is discussed in Chap. 279.***

PROGNOSIS With relief of obstruction, the prognosis regarding return of renal function depends largely on whether irreversible renal damage has occurred. When obstruction is not relieved, the course will depend mainly on whether the obstruction is complete or incomplete, bilateral or unilateral, and whether urinary tract infection is also present. Complete obstruction with infection can lead to total destruction of the kidney within days. In dogs, relief of complete obstruction of 1 and 2 weeks' duration restores glomerular filtration rate to 60 and 30 percent of normal, respectively; after 8 weeks of obstruction, recovery does not occur. Nevertheless, in the absence of definitive evidence of irreversibility, every effort should be made to decompress in the hope of restoring renal function at least partially. A renal radionuclide scan, performed after a prolonged period of decompression, may be used to predict reversible renal function.

POSTOBSTRUCTIVE DIURESIS Relief of bilateral, but not unilateral, complete urinary tract obstruction commonly leads to a postobstructive diuresis, characterized by polyuria, which may be massive. The urine is usually hypotonic and may contain a large amount of sodium chloride. The natriuresis is due, at least in part, to the excretion of retained urea, which acts as a poorly reabsorbable solute and diminishes salt and water reabsorption in the tubules (osmotic diuresis). The increase in intratubular pressure very likely also contributes to the impairment in net sodium chloride reabsorption, especially in the terminal nephron segments. Natriuretic factors (other than urea) also may accumulate during uremia induced by obstruction and depress salt and water reabsorption when urine flow is reestablished. In the majority of patients this diuresis is physiologic, resulting in the *appropriate* excretion of the excesses of salt and water retained during the period of obstruction. When extracellular volume and composition return to normal, the diuresis usually abates spontaneously. Therefore, replacement of urinary losses should serve only to prevent hypovolemia, hypotension, or disturbances in serum electrolyte concentrations. Occasionally, iatrogenic expansion of extracellular volume, secondary to administration of excessive quantities of intravenous fluids, is responsible for, or sustains, the diuresis observed in the postobstructive period. Replacement of no more than two-thirds of urinary volume losses per day is usually effective in avoiding this complication. The loss of electrolyte-free water with urea may result in hypernatremia. Serum and urine sodium and osmolal concentrations should guide the use of appropriate intravenous replacement. Often replacement with 0.45% saline is required. In a rare patient, relief of obstruction may be followed by urinary salt and water losses severe enough to provoke profound dehydration and vascular collapse. In these patients, an intrinsic defect in tubule reabsorptive function is probably responsible for the marked diuresis. Appropriate therapy in such patients includes intravenous administration of large quantities of salt-containing solutions to replace sodium and volume deficits.

BIBLIOGRAPHY

Curhan GC, Zeidel ML: Urinary tract obstruction, in *The Kidney*, 5th ed, BM Brenner (ed). Philadelphia, Saunders, 1996, p 1936

Gillenwater JY: The pathophysiology of urinary obstruction, in *Campbell's Urology*, 6th ed, PC Walsh et al (eds). Philadelphia, Saunders, 1992, pp 499–532

Kaye AD, Pollack HM: Diagnostic imaging approach to the patient with obstructive uropathy. Semin Nephrol 2:55, 1982

Klahr S, Harris KPG: Obstructive uropathy, in *The Kidney: Physiology and Pathophysiology*, 2d ed, DW Seldin, G Giebisch (eds). New York, Raven Press, 1992, p 3327

Wilson DR: Renal function during and following obstruction. Annu Rev Med 28:329, 1977

PART ELEVEN

DISORDERS OF THE GASTROINTESTINAL SYSTEM

Section 1
DISORDERS OF THE ALIMENTARY TRACT

281

Kurt J. Isselbacher, Daniel K. Podolsky

APPROACH TO THE PATIENT WITH GASTROINTESTINAL DISEASE

BIOLOGIC CONSIDERATIONS The mucosal surface of the gastrointestinal (GI) tract is composed of a remarkably dynamic population of epithelial cells that are highly developed in their capacity for transmembrane absorption and secretion. These secretory and absorptive abilities facilitate the essential function of the digestive tract in digestion and nutrient uptake, which must be accomplished while maintaining the barrier between the host and potentially harmful pathogens and mutagens in the lumen. The latter is accomplished through both the physical integrity of the intact mucosal surface and the extensive population of resident immune cells.

The intestinal surface itself also contains the distinctive M cells that serve to sample the antigenic milieu of the lumen. They overlie lymphoid aggregates (Peyer's patches). The predominance of suppressor lymphocytes in the surface epithelial layer (intraepithelial lymphocytes) suggests that damping of the body's response to the enormous number of potentially antigenic substances in the lumen is necessary to prevent the constant and unrestrained activation of immune and inflammatory processes. Conversely, the presence of large numbers of helper lymphocytes as well as other cellular effectors of immune response in the lamina propria and submucosa attests to a large armamentarium ready to respond when surface defenses have been breached. No doubt the concentration of so many immune cells capable of attracting and activating inflammatory cells predisposes to the numerous inflammatory conditions to which the GI tract is subject.

The mucosal surface of the GI tract is also remarkable for the very rapid turnover of the epithelial cell population. It is likely that the epithelium turns over in its entirety every 24 to 72 h. This capacity may permit rapid restitution of a functional cell population following an acute insult and may reduce the risk of malignancy through the shedding of cells affected by the many mutagens in the luminal contents. Nevertheless, this proliferative potential creates the setting for neoplastic disorders, which are so common in the GI tract. Another fundamental feature of the GI mucosa is the spatial segregation of the proliferative compartment from the terminally differentiated cells. This is true throughout the GI tract but is most apparent in the small intestine, where a gradient of differentiation exists from the depths of the crypts of Lieberkühn to the villus tip. This organization has a strong effect on the histology and pathophysiology of many mucosal disorders, such as celiac sprue.

In view of the important secretory and absorptive activities of mucosal surface, diseases of the GI tract may result in clinical consequences owing to physical disruption of the mucosal layer (e.g., blood loss, fluid loss, pathogenic invasion) or to nutritional derangements caused by impaired digestion and nutrient absorption. In focal or localized disease processes the former effects predominate, whereas the latter may be especially prominent in disorders that affect extensive areas of the GI tract in a diffuse manner.

While the essential roles of the GI tract—the absorption of nutrients and the excretion of the products—are accomplished in large part at the luminal surface, these processes also depend on the deeper muscular layers for the coordinated propulsion of food through the lumen. The complexity of the local and distant neural and endocrine factors that contribute to the regulation of intestinal motility is only now becoming fully appreciated. Disruption of normal motility is quite common, with functional bowel complaints affecting as many as 15 percent of adults. Alterations in frequency of bowel movements, abdominal distention, abdominal pain, and nausea, individually or in varying combinations, may result from dysmotility. In addition, structural lesions may also indirectly lead to symptoms through their impact on motility involving some or all regions of the GI tract. These range from the *direct* effects of an obstructing lesion to the *indirect* actions of substances released by a primary mucosal disorder (e.g., inflammatory mediators such as arachidonic acid metabolites that also affect smooth-muscle activity).

Although valid unifying generalizations can be made about the GI tract in its entirety, the spectrum of diseases affecting this system and their clinical manifestations are significantly related to the constituent organ(s) involved (Table 281-1). Thus, esophageal disorders manifest themselves mainly through their relationship to swallowing; gastric disorders are dominated by features relating to acid secretion; and disease of the small and large intestine is evidenced mainly by disruption of nutrition and alterations of bowel movements. Similarly, diseases of the related ancillary organs, the exocrine pancreas and the hepatobiliary system, present characteristic clinical challenges. Finally, the GI tract may be affected by systemic disorders. These include vascular, inflammatory, infectious, and neoplastic conditions leading to focal or diffuse structural lesions. Metabolic and endocrine abnormalities as well as some drugs can disrupt normal bowel motility. Table 281-2 summarizes criteria that may be used to distinguish functional from organic or structural diseases of the GI tract.

CLINICAL CONSIDERATIONS **History** A thorough clinical history is essential in directing the clinician's attention to appropriate diagnostic considerations in the patient with GI symptoms. The most common complaints resulting from disorders involving the GI tract include pain and alterations in bowel habit, especially diarrhea or constipation. Of these complaints, *abdominal pain* is the most frequent and variable and may reflect a broad spectrum of problems, from the least threatening to the most urgent (see Chap. 14). In conjunction with an estimation of its intensity, an initial distinction should be made between pain of acute onset and more chronic discomfort. Pain of abrupt onset is often encountered in serious illness requiring urgent intervention, while a history of chronic discomfort is most often related to an indolent disorder. Dyspepsia, an ill-defined upper abdominal discomfort, is especially common. It is often accompanied in varying degrees by feelings of nausea, bloating, and distention. While it may be associated with peptic ulceration, non-ulcer dyspepsia (NUD) is common. A change in the pattern or character of pain may be equally important, possibly signifying the progression to a more critical stage of a problem (either recent or chronic) that was mild in onset. Ascertaining the location of the pain (upper or lower, localized or diffuse), its character (sharp, burning, cramping), and its relationship to meals will often provide significant insight into the most important diagnostic considerations. If eating produces the symptom, the clinician should determine whether the discomfort occurs while the patient is eating (as in esophageal disorders), shortly after the meal (as often occurs in biliary tract disease and abdominal angina), or 30 to 90 min later (as is typical of peptic disease). Pain that is not affected by eating suggests a process outside of the bowel lumen, such as abscess, peritonitis, pancreatitis, and some malignancies. Conversely, identification of factors that relieve the symptom is also helpful. For example, eating or antacid use typically gives relief in peptic ulcer disease or gastritis. A relationship of the discomfort to bowel movement, especially in association with an altered bowel habit, should focus attention on a disorder of the small or large bowel, such as inflammatory bowel disease.

Alterations in bowel habit can result from either disruption of normal intestinal motility or significant structural pathology. A thorough determination of the temporal evolution of the change and the nature of the alteration, in conjunction with other constitutional symptoms such as weight loss, fever, or anorexia, is important. A temporary variation in bowel habit in association with some life stress and in the absence of signs of systemic illness suggests the common "irritable bowel syndrome," especially when the alteration varies between diarrhea and constipation. Small, pellet-like stools are often described by the patient. Associated symptoms of dyspepsia (bloating, nausea, and "gas") are also common. This diagnosis can essentially be made on the basis of a thorough history and physical examination and very limited laboratory testing, to exclude structural disease. In contrast, the onset of worsening constipation in an adult with previously regular habits, especially when accompanied by systemic symptoms such as weight loss, suggests the possible presence of an underlying obstructing process, particularly malignancy. If diarrhea is present, one should determine the average number of stools, their consistency, their pattern, and the presence or absence of blood. Although *diarrhea* refers to an increased frequency of movements, patients will often use the term to describe loose or watery stools. The occurrence of nocturnal or true bloody diarrhea almost always reflects structural rather than functional bowel disease. A pungent stool odor or the presence of undigested meat in the movement are suggestive of pancreatic insufficiency. An alteration in color can be seen in cholestasis or steatorrhea (light-colored) or hemorrhage (melenic to maroon or bright red). Mucus in the movement is usually a sign of a functional bowel syndrome, while pus is more strongly suggestive of infectious or inflammatory disease. Less common but more dramatic are the symptoms of acute GI bleeding, including hematemesis, melena, and hematochezia, which usually lead to prompt efforts to find medical attention but should always be enquired after by the clinician.

In the evaluation of male patients, especially those with diarrhea, a tactful inquiry into sexual activity is essential. Homosexual males are at increased risk for a large variety of GI disorders, as well as AIDS, which may first manifest itself with GI symptoms. Such symptoms, especially diarrhea, are common in patients with AIDS. These patients are susceptible to a wide range of infections and neoplastic disorders of the GI tract, liver and biliary tract (see Chap. 308). Finally, careful attention must be given to a general medical history with an emphasis on present or past use of medications or nonprescription drugs. Thyroid and other metabolic disorders, especially those affecting calcium metabolism, can cause a variety of GI symptoms. Unless asked, patients may forget to mention that they take aspirin almost daily for headache, and this may account for occult blood found in the stool. The use of daily laxatives may explain chronic diarrhea.

Physical Examination, Endoscopy, and Radiology All of the cardinal methods of examination are helpful in evaluating the patient with GI symptoms. *Inspection* may disclose signs of cholestasis or nutritional deficiencies. Examination of the abdomen for an abnormal contour or inspection of the perianal region may reveal signs of a mass or a draining fistula. *Auscultation* is also important. A succussion splash may be elicited in the patients with symptoms of gastric outlet obstruction. The absence of bowel sounds or an alteration in pitch can lead to recognition of an evolving ileus or an obstructing process. A bruit may also be appreciated where there are symptoms of ischemic bowel disease. Careful *palpation* of the abdomen is especially important in detecting tenderness and masses, which in the appropriate clinical setting will lead to the recognition of cholecystitis, Crohn's disease, periappendiceal abscess, and many other disorders. Findings on abdominal palpation will often be complemented by *percussion*, which is essential to assessing liver and spleen size.

Elicitation of *rebound tenderness*, either direct or referred, after removal of the examining hand provides an important clue to localized or more generalized peritonitis, which is characteristic of many abdominal emergencies, including a perforated viscus, intraabdominal abscess, or tissue infarction. The clinician should be particularly alert to these signs in patients with severe pain of abrupt onset. Typically, the patient will remain immobile to avoid the accentuation of pain that may follow even slight movement and jarring of the abdomen. This contrasts with the sometimes frantic efforts to find a position of comfort in patients with severe pain deriving from visceral disease, e.g., pancreatitis or intestinal ischemia. In these disorders, the absence of findings on palpation of the abdomen may be in striking contrast to the evident distress of the patient. Only when the process progresses to tissue destruction (e.g., necrotizing pancreatitis or intestinal infarction) and secondary peritonitis will the abdominal examination prove remarkable, often in concert with striking signs of systemic illness, including hemodynamic instability. In addition to the examination of the abdomen, a carefully performed digital rectal examination is also essential. In the patient with complaints of incontinence, the integrity of the sphincter can be assessed. Most important, masses intrinsic to the rectum as well as abnormalities in the pelvis or the pouch of Douglas may only be detected by this examination, and the presence or absence of frank or occult blood in the stool is always important diagnostic information. Sigmoidoscopy should be viewed as a routine part of the physical examination in the patient with diarrhea or another alteration in bowel habit as well as when there is known or suspected blood loss from the lower bowel. Sigmoidoscopy, which can be performed with either a rigid or a flexible fiberoptic instrument, allows for direct inspection of the rectosigmoid mucosa, permitting the detection of cancers and polyps in this lower bowel segment that might well be missed by barium x-rays. Inflammatory changes of the mucosa can help identify patients with infectious dysentery or other forms of colitis, most notably ulcerative colitis. The findings of edema, granularity, and diffuse friability (easily induced mucosal bleeding) as well as superficial ulcerations are characteristic of the latter disorder. Fresh stool samples for microbiologic studies and superficial mucosal biopsies obtained at the time of sigmoidoscopy can also yield crucial diagnostic information.

Table 281-1

Distinguishing between Functional and Organic/Structural Disease of Gastrointestinal Tract

		Organic	
	Functional	**Neoplastic**	**Inflammatory**
Symptoms			
Weight loss	None	Common	Sometimes
Diarrhea	Daytime only	Nocturnal	Day and night
Blood loss	None	Frequent	Frequent
Fever	None	Rare	Frequent
Pain	Cramping, relieved by defecation	Minor to severe	May be localized; may be severe
Bowel habit (diarrhea or constipation)	Alternating diarrhea/constipation Pellet-like stools	Constipation (rarely diarrhea) Change in caliber	Diarrhea or normal
Laboratory tests			
Hematocrit	Normal	Often decreased	May be decreased
White blood cell count	Normal	Usually normal	Often elevated
Erythrocyte sedimentation rate	Normal	Usually increased	Usually increased

Definitive demonstration or exclusion of structural lesions of the GI tract, particularly the great majority of disorders that affect primarily the mucosal surface, often cannot be accomplished by physical examination alone. Many upper and lower GI tract disorders are accessible to inspection via fiberoptic instruments. As a result, endoscopy has supplanted conventional contrast x-ray studies for many clinical problems, both because of its heightened precision for diagnosis and the opportunity in many instances to accomplish meaningful therapeutic intervention. However, it should be emphasized that *no procedure should be considered routine* and used indiscriminately; there must be a rational basis for its use in the individual patient. These techniques are discussed in detail in Chap. 282. Upper GI endoscopy permits evaluation of the esophagus, stomach, duodenum, and, with specially designed instruments, proximal jejunum. When the clinical history warrants a diagnostic examination of the upper GI tract for a structural lesion, endoscopic examination is preferable to radiologic study in most patients when the choice is available. Side-viewing scopes permit inspection and cannulation of the ampulla of Vater, facilitating retrograde cholangiopancreatography. Evaluation of some patients will be further benefited by endoscopic ultrasound, which can delineate submucosal mass lesions and abnormalities in the pancreas. The colonoscope can be used to visualize the entire colon and often the terminal ileum, resulting in more accurate diagnosis of inflammatory bowel disease and mass lesions. Frequently, colonic polyps can be removed at the time of their initial identification.

Endoscopic techniques are relatively precise in defining many problems, but the limitations of these tools, as well as the continued advantages of x-ray studies in some situations, should be recognized. Endoscopic tools are not useful in assessing GI motility, which may be assessed more accurately by barium studies. In addition, some areas, notably the small intestine, remain relatively inaccessible to fiberoptic instruments. In hospitals where endoscopy is not feasible, the upper GI series and barium enema remain good diagnostic modalities to evaluate the upper and lower GI tract, especially when air-contrast techniques are employed. However, they should generally be avoided in patients with GI bleeding or suspected bowel obstruction. In addition the physician must exercise judgment in preparing the patient for these studies, recognizing that cathartics may markedly worsen the condition of a patient with obstructing lesions or colitis.

Although endoscopy has obviated the need for many conventional GI x-rays, other radiologic imaging modalities have assumed a crucial role in the approach to the patient with GI symptoms. These techniques include ultrasound (US), computed tomography (CT), and magnetic resonance imaging (MRI). Both US and CT are useful in the delineation of abdominal masses. CT, though more expensive, is often more effective in the evaluation of the lower abdomen, where inflammatory masses in patients with Crohn's disease or complications of diverticular disease may be accurately imaged. However, US is an effective and less expensive tool for the evaluation of the right upper quadrant, including the gall bladder and biliary tract. Imaging techniques are often complementary in the evaluation of pancreatic disease. In combination with Doppler analysis, US can be used to assess the patency and direction of blood flow in the portal vein in the patient with advanced liver disease. MRI may give exquisitely accurate information on the anatomic extent of invasive rectal cancers and blood flow in patients with vascular disorders, but the full range of its uses in GI disorders remains to be delineated. More sophisticated CT and MRI equipment can actually permit the performance of digital angiography without the invasive catheterization necessary in conventional visceral angiography.

DIAGNOSTIC APPROACHES **Abdominal Pain** Determination of the cause of abdominal pain remains an imposing clinical challenge. As noted above, disorders ranging from the acute and catastrophic to the chronic and indolent can cause abdominal pain. Further-

Table 281-2

Overview of Approach to Patients with Common Gastrointestinal Disorders

Site of Disorder	Common Symptoms	Possible Physical Signs	Potential Procedures or Laboratory Studies
Esophagus	Dysphagia Odynophagia Heartburn, chest pain Hematemesis/melena		Esophagoscopy Barium swallow Manometry Bernstein test
Stomach	Nausea and vomiting Epigastric pain Hematemesis/melena Early satiety	Distention Tenderness Succusion splash Mass	Gastroscopy Upper GI x-ray series Nasogastric aspiration Gastric emptying
Pancreas	Pain Weight loss Diarrhea Steatorrhea	Mass Jaundice	Kidney-ureter-bladder x-ray series Qualitative stool fat and muscle fiber US, CT, MRI, endoscopic retrograde cholangiopancreatography Pancreatic function tests
Small Intestine			
Duodenum	Pain Nausea/vomiting Hematemesis	Tenderness Altered bowel sounds Distention Mass	Duodenoscopy Small bowel follow-through, enteroclysis Kidney-ureter-bladder x-ray series D-Xylose absorption tests
Jejunum	Pain Diarrhea	Altered bowel sounds Distention Mass	CT Stool cultures, stool examination for ova and parasites Small bowel biopsy
Ileum	Pain Diarrhea	Altered bowel sounds Distention Mass	
Colon	Diarrhea Pain Blood	Tenderness Mass Distention	Sigmoidoscopy Colonoscopy Barium enema Stool culture, stool examination for ova and parasites *Clostridium difficile* toxin assay
Rectum	Pain Urgency Hematochezia Pruritus	Tenderness	Sigmoidoscopy Anoscopy
Nonspecific	Weight loss Fever Anorexia Nausea and vomiting		Complete blood count Erythrocyte sedimentation rate Fecal occult blood test

more, differential diagnostic considerations may encompass diseases extrinsic to the GI tract, such as disorders of the genitourinary tract (e.g., pelvic inflammatory disease) and the peritoneum. The history and physical examination are essential guides to a sensible diagnostic approach. The initial goal is to distinguish between an urgent problem requiring expeditious delineation and a nonacute disorder. In the former situation, initial clinical impressions based on the history and physical examination can be further refined through routine laboratory tests such as a complete blood count and differential as well as plain films of the abdomen. Particular features will dictate the appropriateness of urgent US or CT examination or the need to proceed promptly with surgery. In the patient with a long-standing and relatively stable problem, diagnostic evaluation can be more deliberate. The clinician may be able to reasonably establish a functional basis for the complaint on the strength of the history and physical examination alone. Radiologic contrast studies, other imaging modalities (e.g., US, CT), or endoscopic examination may be appropriate to exclude or identify certain of the gamut of disorders discussed above. If all these approaches do not determine the cause of the patient's symptoms, more unusual causes of abdominal pain may have to be excluded through specific urine or blood tests (e.g., porphyrins).

Problems of Swallowing The approach should be as follows:

1. *Thorough determination of the nature of dysphagia*. Is the difficulty primarily in swallowing liquids, solids, or both? The location of the difficulty from the patient's perspective and presence or absence of accompanying *odynophagia* are important to ascertain. These historical clues are complemented by careful visual and neurologic examination of the oropharynx when appropriate.
2. *Routine esophageal x-rays* in the upright and lateral or Trendelenburg position. The horizontal views are essential for demonstration of the swallowing mechanism, unaided by gravity, and of the esophagogastric junction. For details of the pharyngoesophageal area, cineradiography is necessary because of the rapidity with which the contrast medium passes through. Hiatus hernia is extremely common (in 15 to 35 percent of persons over 50) and often is asymptomatic unless spontaneous reflux of gastric contents can be demonstrated to occur repeatedly. Careful attention is usually needed to detect lower esophageal rings or webs, which may be visible as indentations in the barium column only from a limited angle.
3. *Esophagoscopy*. This procedure is desirable for lesions suggested by x-ray or, if the lesion is unsuspected, to biopsy masses or abnormal mucosa and to obtain washings for exfoliative cytologic study. The diagnoses of peptic esophagitis and Barrett's esophagus are made endoscopically. Endoscopy is the most sensitive technique for identifying esophageal or gastric varices, although they are seldom important in the absence of hemorrhage. Fiberoptic instruments with a US probe at the tip (endoscopic ultrasound) are increasingly useful diagnostic tools for particular problems of the esophagus (and other sites of the GI tract).
4. *Manometric studies* of the upper esophagus, particularly in conjunction with cineradiography. At present, this procedure offers the best means of differentiating among disorders originating in the central nervous system, primary pharyngeal muscular disease, and cricopharyngeal dystonia. Manometry of the lower esophagus is useful in the diagnosis of diffuse esophageal spasm, achalasia, and infiltrative diseases that can alter esophageal motility.

Peptic or Digestive Disorders The approaches to these disorders include the following.

1. *Insertion of a nasograstric tube*. This approach is used to establish whether significant gastric retention (more than 75 mL of gastric contents in the fasting state) exists and whether acid, bile, blood, or other materials are present. If pyloric obstruction or gastric atony is present, the tube is used to maintain suction while the patient's electrolyte and fluid balance is restored to normal; the stomach is kept as clean as possible so that reliable diagnostic investigation may be carried out.
2. *Upper gastrointestinal endoscopy*. This procedure is most helpful in assessing the mucosa in gastritis or, together with biopsy and brushings for cytology, in differentiating between peptic and neoplastic ulcerating lesions. It may identify a specific bleeding site in clinical situations where several potential bleeding sites could exist, as in the patient with portal hypertension. In addition, it may be possible to cauterize or otherwise intervene to control hemorrhage via the endoscope (e.g., by injections of vasoconstricting agents such as epinephrine). The frequent association of gastritis with *Helicobacter pylori* in patients with actual peptic ulceration, as well as in those with nonulcer dyspepsia, has been well documented. Although, at this time, *H. pylori* infection can be most reliably confirmed in the individual patient by endoscopy and biopsy, this approach may be superseded by other, less invasive modalities including breath and serologic tests. Endoscopy can detect a number of potential sources of upper GI bleeding that are often missed by x-ray studies (e.g., erosive gastritis, Mallory-Weiss tear). Gastroscopy is particularly helpful in inspecting the postoperative stomach, especially in detecting stomal ulceration or so-called alkaline reflux gastritis. The first and second portions of the duodenum can also be routinely examined, and important information about ulcers and other lesions can be obtained. Radiologic studies may be useful when endoscopy is not readily available or in the assessment of suspected motility disorders (e.g., gastroparesis). In addition, radiologic examination may be preferred when there are contraindications to safe endoscopy.
3. *Gastric acid secretory studies*. Although not routinely necessary, these studies are useful in the diagnosis of the Zollinger-Ellison syndrome or atrophic gastritis and for determination of completeness of vagotomy. They should not be performed for the routine diagnosis of uncomplicated duodenal ulcer; also, there is no convincing evidence that they are useful in determining the choice of surgery for peptic ulcer.

Obstructive and Vascular Disorders of the Small Intestine When intestinal problems present as obstructive syndromes, the plain x-ray film of the abdomen is the most important diagnostic adjunct to careful physical examination. Patterns of dilation of individual loops of intestine may be characteristic, as in volvulus or acute pancreatitis; erect and decubitus views will often show fluid levels in the affected segments. Motility disorders of the small intestine (temporary ileus or chronic intestinal pseudoobstruction) may also present with obstructive symptoms and similar x-ray findings but must be managed medically without surgical intervention. Air under the diaphragm is diagnostic of a perforated viscus; air in the portal vein usually results from intestinal necrosis secondary to mesenteric vascular occlusion. The diagnostic accuracy of the plain x-ray film in all types of intestinal obstruction is about 75 percent. In patients with symptoms of incomplete obstruction, the radiographic small-bowel series will often be diagnostic in defining the site and degree of obstruction. Infrequently, in this setting, all conventional x-ray studies are unremarkable. In such cases, the radiologist may perform a small bowel enteroclysis study by passing a special tube into the proximal jejunum; the rapid instillation of barium through the tube will distend the intestine and often reveal subtle lesions missed by other tests.

Vascular diseases of the small intestine are among the most difficult diseases to diagnose. In chronic mesenteric ischemia, radiographic, endoscopic, and laboratory tests are usually normal. Early in the course of acute mesenteric ischemia, the plain film of the abdomen may be unremarkable despite complaints of severe abdominal pain. In these settings, prompt mesenteric angiography is essential to confirm the diagnosis of vascular disease.

Inflammatory and Neoplastic Diseases of Small and Large Intestine Patients with these conditions are usually identified by history, physical examination, and careful examination of the stools for exudate and blood. Examination of fresh stool samples for common bacterial pathogens and parasites by laboratories skilled in these techniques is important in identifying or excluding infectious causes of diarrhea, particularly in the patient with colitis. Sigmoidoscopy is valuable in identifying mucosal and neoplastic lesions of the rectum and distal colon. The mucosal surface of the entire colon and terminal ileum can be examined directly and biopsied through the fiberoptic sigmoidoscope or colonoscope. The radiologic examination of the small intestine is highly reliable in identifying the prestenotic and stenotic lesions of Crohn's disease. In the colon, a single barium enema examination in a well-prepared patient has a diagnostic accuracy of 80 to 85 percent; the addition of air-contrast technique brings the accuracy up over 90 percent. None of these figures is meaningful if the patient is poorly prepared for the examination, however. Colonoscopy may be preferable because of its greater accuracy and the fact that it enables the operator to remove the vast majority of polyps that are encountered as well as to obtain preoperative tissue confirmation in the patient who probably has cancer.

Peroral biopsy of the small intestine (now most often accomplished during endoscopy) and forceps biopsy of the rectosigmoid are of considerable importance in revealing mucosal disease. Rectal biopsy is an excellent means of demonstrating amyloidosis, schistosomiasis, and amebiasis. Submucosal disease is not seen in these superficial biopsies. Hirschsprung's disease is diagnosed histologically by a deep surgical biopsy of the lower part of the rectum.

Malabsorption Syndromes Malabsorption may be suspected on the basis of history and physical examination and confirmed by examination of the stool. Radiologic examination is helpful to rule out local lesions and to suggest motor and secretory dysfunction, but it is rarely diagnostic unless an abnormal small bowel mucosa or fistulas between the intestine and stomach are demonstrated.

The tests useful in the diagnosis of malabsorption are discussed in Chap. 285. A simple screening test for excessive fat in the stools can be accomplished by the microscopic examination of a stool specimen stained with Sudan. Chemical analysis of 3-day stool collection for fat, with the patient on a standard diet, is used to establish the diagnosis of steatorrhea. The D-xylose absorption test is about 90 percent accurate in distinguishing mucosal disease from pancreatic insufficiency. Peroral biopsy of the small intestine via the endoscope or a specialized biopsy device is of value in the diagnosis of celiac disease, and it may show the less common infiltrations of the mucosa by amyloid or bacterial mucoproteins (Whipple's disease). Leakage of protein into the intestinal lumen may cause hypoproteinemia and can be demonstrated by the recovery in stools of the serum protein α_1-antitrypsin or intravenously administrated markers such as albumin labeled with iodine or chromium isotopes.

Pancreas The pancreas is difficult to study because of its anatomic location and relative inaccessibility. Calcification of the pancreas on a plain abdominal film is highly suggestive of chronic pancreatitis and may be associated with fat malabsorption. Pancreatic exocrine insufficiency can be demonstrated by intubation of the duodenum and collection of pancreatic juice after stimulation with secretin or a test meal, but a stool collection for qualitative determination of fat and muscle fiber content is usually sufficient as an initial diagnostic approach. Abdominal US and CT are the best radiographic means of searching for pancreatic enlargement (see Chaps. 303 and 304). Both techniques may also be used to guide needle biopsies of the pancreas and may provide sufficient diagnostic information to obviate the need for exploratory surgery. The pancreatic duct can be cannulated via the fiberoptic duodenoscope and visualized by the injection of radiographic dye. Visualization of the duct may be helpful in the diagnosis of pancreatic pseudocysts, carcinoma, or chronic pancreatitis.

BIBLIOGRAPHY

JOHNSON LR et al: *Physiology of the Gastrointestinal Tract*, 3d ed. New York, Raven, 1995

SLEISENGER MH, FORDTRAN JS: *Gastrointestinal Disease*, 5th ed. Philadelphia, Saunders, 1993

YAMADA T et al: *Textbook of Gastroenterology*, 2d ed. Philadelphia, Lippincott, 1995

282 GASTROINTESTINAL ENDOSCOPY*

Fred E. Silverstein

Endoscopes have revolutionized the examination of the gastrointestinal (GI) tract. Because of the flexibility of the instrument and the controllability of the instrument tip, the operator can steer the endoscope around multiple bends under visual control. A channel permits the passage of a variety of endoscopic tools, such as biopsy forceps, cytology brushes, wash tubes, injecting devices, and electrocautery probes and snares. The viewing window and the light at the instrument's distal end can be washed free of obscuring material. Fluid can be aspirated from hollow organs, and air can be insufflated as needed to improve visualization. The videoendoscope is a modification of the original fiberendoscope in which a charge-coupled device on the tip of the instrument transmits the image to a TV screen. This system is being used increasingly because it permits storage, analysis, and transmission of the endoscopic images. → ***The Color Atlas has plates of typical endoscopically visualized lesions.***

The usefulness of fiberendoscopy in diagnosing gastrointestinal disease is well established. Shallow lesions, such as erosions or healing ulcers, are missed by single-contrast x-ray examinations but not by endoscopy. The success of polypectomy via the colonoscope and of sphincterotomy via the duodenoscope have led to the development of other endoscopic therapeutic techniques, such as esophageal band ligation and endoscopic ultrasonography with fine needle aspiration; endoscopic approaches are now preferred to surgery in many situations.

Although esophagogastroduodenoscopy (EGD) is not a procedure for the occasional operator, it is widely available in both inpatient and outpatient settings. It is relatively easy to perform, but training and continued experience are necessary for optimal diagnostic accuracy and mastery of therapeutic techniques. The more complex procedures, such as colonoscopy and endoscopic retrograde cholangiopancreatography (ERCP), require special dexterity, a substantial investment of time for learning, and constant practice to maintain adequate skill; they are probably best performed by subspecialists. Complications are most frequent when the operator is inexperienced.

A history and physical examination should be done before any endoscopic procedure is undertaken. Special care is taken in patients with significant cardiac or pulmonary disease; blood clotting parameters should be checked in those with a history of excessive bleeding. Patients with prosthetic heart valves and those with a history of bacterial endocarditis or a significant right-to-left shunt should receive antibiotic prophylaxis. Contraindications to endoscopy in most situations include the inability of the patient to cooperate or give informed consent, an unstable cardiac or pulmonary condition, and an unstable neck prior to EGD. Intestinal perforation or full-thickness wall necrosis is also a contraindication to any endoscopic procedure.

Most endoscopists prefer to administer conscious sedation for endoscopic procedures other than flexible sigmoidoscopy and some screening upper endoscopies. After insertion of an intravenous catheter, a benzodiazepine such as diazepam or midazolam is titrated to light sedation. Supplementation with a narcotic such as meperidine also may be useful. Adequate monitoring of vital signs and oxygen saturation is important, as is the availability of oropharyngeal suction, resuscitation equipment, and antagonists to the sedative agents. Topical pharyngeal anesthesia with a gargle or spray of lidocaine or similar anesthetic is useful prior to upper endoscopic procedures.

Because of the risk of infection transmission, it is essential that every endoscope undergo meticulous cleaning and high-level disinfection or that the contaminated surfaces and tubing be replaced after each procedure.

* Dr. Michael Kimney contributed to this chapter in the 13th edition.

UPPER GASTROINTESTINAL ENDOSCOPY The tip of a forward-viewing endoscope is placed at the cricopharyngeal sphincter of the esophagus, and the patient is encouraged to swallow while gentle pressure is exerted. Small amounts of air are passed through the endoscope to visualize the esophageal lumen. The endoscope is then passed under direct vision into the stomach. The gastric body and antrum are carefully examined. The instrument tip is retroflexed in the stomach to view the gastric cardia, the fundus, and the whole lesser curvature. The pylorus is traversed, and the first and second portions of the duodenum are visualized. Visualized lesions can be recorded on photographs or videotape. Biopsies and brush cytologic examinations can be performed on suspicious areas.

EGD is a relatively safe procedure in experienced hands. Several large surveys suggest a risk of serious complications during diagnostic EGD of approximately 1 in 500 and a risk of death of approximately 1 in 10,000. The risks are higher in emergency procedures and in the elderly or seriously ill. In a survey of patients examined by endoscopy while experiencing upper GI bleeding, 1 in 200 had serious complications and 1 in 700 died from the procedure. The main causes of mortality were cardiopulmonary complications and perforations by the instrument. Endoscopy is preferred over x-ray examination in the urgent diagnosis of gastrointestinal illness in women who might be pregnant.

Gastroesophageal Reflux Disease (See Chap. 283) Esophageal pain may be confused with cardiac disease, or esophagitis may present as painless blood loss. Because esophagitis usually involves only the superficial mucosa, it cannot be diagnosed by routine single-contrast radiography. By endoscopy, friable mucosa, linear erosions, and ulcerations are clearly visible. Not every patient with heartburn requires esophagoscopy, but the procedure is indicated if the patient complains of dysphagia; if an x-ray shows a stricture, mass, or ulcer; if symptoms persist despite therapy; or if antireflux surgery is contemplated. Patients over age 40 with significant complaints of heartburn for over 10 years should be considered for endoscopy to detect Barrett's esophagus.

Barrett's esophagus is the progressive replacement of distal eroded squamous mucosa with metaplastic epithelium, which is more resistant to peptic digestion. This finding can be detected by visual inspection at endoscopy and confirmed by biopsy. Such epithelium is more prone to malignant transformation and, therefore, merits regular surveillance by esophagoscopy and biopsy every 12 to 24 months. Flow cytometry also may prove useful in the early detection of abnormal cell DNA populations (e.g., aneuploidy). If dysplasia is present, more frequent surveillance may be indicated to detect invasive carcinoma, or esophagectomy may be recommended, particularly if dysplasia is high-grade.

Esophagitis may progress to scarring and stricture formation. The endoscopic appearance of a benign stricture is characteristic but not diagnostic; a malignancy should be ruled out by biopsy and cytologic brushing; the whole length of the stricture should be sampled. Endoscopy may also facilitate dilatation of strictures (see below). Endoscopy is also indicated to biopsy the rim of an esophageal ulcer to rule out cancer.

The dilatation of a difficult stricture is best initiated by passing a flexible spring-tipped guidewire via the biopsy channel of the endoscope through the stricture under direct vision. The endoscope can then be withdrawn over the wire, which serves as a guide for passage of progressively larger polyvinyl dilators through the stricture under fluoroscopic control. An alternative technique uses balloon catheters passed via the endoscope channel or over a guidewire through the stricture. The balloon is inflated under endoscopic and/or fluoroscopic guidance to dilate the stricture.

Peptic Ulcer EDG is more accurate than upper GI x-ray examination for the detection of ulcers. It has been suggested that x-rays be abandoned entirely in favor of endoscopy for this purpose. Doing so makes sense when the source of acute upper GI bleeding is sought and urgent surgical intervention is being considered. However, in the workup of the patient with less pressing ulcer complaints, a double-contrast upper GI x-ray may still be used as the initial diagnostic test. Endoscopy may be indicated if the x-ray is equivocal or suggests that the ulcer may be malignant, if it is negative but the clinical picture suggests peptic ulceration, or if the patient is about to undergo surgery for ulcer. Patients with duodenal ulcers shown by x-ray or with classic ulcer deformities of the duodenal bulb do not require endoscopy for diagnosis if the presenting symptoms are characteristic and if the patient responds to antiulcer treatment. However, endoscopy also allows diagnosis of *Helicobacter pylori*, which is thought to cause most gastric and duodenal ulcers in patients not taking nonsteroidal antiinflammatory drugs. Screening endoscopy using small-diameter endoscopes without sedation is a reasonable alternative to contrast x-rays as the initial diagnostic test in a symptomatic patient.

Endoscopy is especially useful in visualizing postbulbar ulcers, giant duodenal ulcers, and stomal ulceration after partial gastrectomy, all of which can be missed by x-ray. Endoscopy is also of use in determining the cause of gastric outlet obstruction.

Cancer The endoscopic appearance of upper gastrointestinal cancer may seem obvious, especially if there is a mass growing into the lumen. On the other hand, malignant ulcers, infiltrative carcinomas, or small early carcinomas are frequently impossible to diagnose by their gross endoscopic appearance. Six to eight biopsy samples should be taken from the rim of a gastric ulcer to exclude malignancy. Experience and skill in choosing the biopsy sites improves the accuracy. A cytologic examination of lavage or brush specimens adds to the diagnostic accuracy in all areas of the upper gastrointestinal tract (see Chap. 92).

In patients with gastric ulcers, it has been standard practice to assess ulcer healing by endoscopy after 12 weeks of antiulcer therapy. Persistent ulcers should be biopsied if they were not biopsied at the time of the initial diagnosis or should be rebiopsied if they have not healed. Duodenal ulcers are rarely malignant and therefore do not need to be assessed for healing after therapy in most circumstances.

Primary gastric lymphoma can mimic benign gastric ulcer or adenocarcinoma on gastroscopy or x-ray. It can be diagnosed by biopsy or cytology, although the accuracy is not as high as in gastric adenocarcinoma. The diagnosis of lymphoma is aided by immunochemical staining of biopsy specimens.

If a polypoid lesion of the stomach is covered by mucosa that appears normal by gastroscopy, the likelihood of malignancy is small. Such lesions are often intramural subepithelial benign tumors such as leiomyomas or pancreatic rests. Biopsies are usually not diagnostic. These lesions can be evaluated by endoscopic ultrasonography, a technique that combines diagnostic ultrasound with endoscopy. Polyps covered by abnormal-appearing mucosa can be benign or malignant. Random biopsy can miss carcinoma within a polyp. If technically feasible, polyps should therefore be removed in their entirety by snare cautery for histologic examination. Polyps larger than 2 cm in diameter, are more likely to contain cancer (see Chap. 92). Large polyps may require surgical excision.

Ampullary carcinoma may be diagnosed by biopsy during duodenoscopy; a prior endoscopic sphincterotomy increases the diagnostic yield. Other primary duodenal malignancies are rare. Extensions from pancreatic or biliary tract cancer are difficult to diagnose because the tumor may not have extended into the mucosa and therefore may not be accessible for endoscopic biopsy or cytologic examination. In these secondary tumors, diagnosis must depend on some combination of ultrasonography (endoscopic and transabdominal), computed tomography, angiography, and ERCP with cytologic examination and/or biopsy of ductal strictures.

Upper GI Bleeding (See also Chap. 44) Endoscopy within the first 12 to 24 h of an upper GI hemorrhage is helpful in planning rational therapy by visualizing the bleeding source. Superficial lesions not visible by x-ray may be seen (esophagitis, a Mallory-Weiss tear, erosive gastritis, a stress ulcer, or telangiectasia). Moreover, lesions that are visible by x-ray may not be the source of bleeding. Endoscopy can determine the actual bleeding site and the degree of bleeding. For example, visualization of a spurting artery that is flooding the stomach indicates massive ongoing bleeding requiring prompt therapeutic intervention. Several studies have shown that the demonstration at endoscopy of any active bleeding whatsoever or of a nonbleeding 'visible' vessel (or "sentinel clot") in the ulcer base increases the likelihood of rebleeding. The diagnostic accuracy of emergency endoscopy in upper GI bleeding approaches 90 percent.

Every patient who is undergoing endoscopy for upper GI bleeding merits a complete endoscopic examination of the esophagus, stomach, and duodenum. Occasionally it is not possible to diagnose the exact lesion that is bleeding, but localizing the area of bleeding can be helpful; for example, bright red arterial blood may be seen pouring into the stomach from the duodenum when the esophagus and stomach show no signs of active bleeding.

There are three controversial areas relative to endoscopy and GI bleeding. First, *do all bleeders need endoscopy?* Endoscopy is indicated in all patients who may require surgery for continual bleeding or rebleeding, because the type of operation selected depends on the site and nature of the bleeding. Moreover, endoscopy provides critical information regarding the likelihood the bleeding will continue or recur. Finally, endoscopy permits therapeutic intervention. Second, *how early should endoscopy be performed in the acutely bleeding patient?* Most studies suggest that the diagnostic accuracy of EGD remains high for the first 12 to 24 h after the bleeding episode. All would agree that it is desirable to delay endoscopy if possible until vital signs have been stabilized after adequate blood replacement. Emergency endoscopy is critical in patients with continued massive bleeding or rebleeding requiring an immediate decision regarding surgery or other treatment. If the patient is exsanguinating, endoscopy can be performed after the induction of anesthesia and just before surgery. Thus, the patient's airway is protected by an endotracheal tube. Finally, *does endoscopy affect the clinical outcome?* Studies of the endoscopic treatment of bleeding lesions with heater probes, bipolar probes, and injection methods suggest that these methods are safe and reduce blood requirements, the need for surgery, and the risk of mortality in some patients.

Injection of various sclerosing solutions into or next to esophageal varices is an effective treatment for stopping active variceal bleeding. Rubber band ligation of varices at endoscopy has also been shown to stop bleeding and to obliterate varices with fewer sessions and less severe complications than occur with the use of sclerosing agents. Repeated injection sclerotherapy or band ligation may be performed to eradicate varices.

Percutaneous Endoscopic Gastrostomy (PEG) The placement of feeding or decompression gastrostomy tubes can be facilitated with the use of an endoscope. Under sedation, a suitable location for a gastrostomy is identified, a needle is introduced into the stomach percutaneously, and a snare is passed through the endoscope to capture a wire or suture placed through the needle. Using this wire, a feeding tube is advanced into the stomach. Feedings are generally begun the same or following day. Hospitalization time and morbidity and mortality rates are reduced compared to those for operative gastrostomy.

Patients with transfer dysphagia secondary to strokes and degenerative neurologic disorders benefit the most from percutaneous endoscopic gastrostomy. Other indications include dysphagia produced by head and neck neoplasms and the inability to eat secondary to diffuse cerebral injury. Patients with severe gastroparesis can be fed through a jejunal feeding tube placed through the gastrostomy and then directed through the pylorus. Simultaneous gastric decompression is possible through a separate lumen in the gastrostomy.

Palliation of Esophageal Carcinoma Patients with dysphagia caused by malignant esophageal strictures usually cannot be cured by esophagectomy. Surgical resection and radiation therapy are often chosen for palliation of dysphagia in this situation. The endoscopist also can help provide palliation in these patients when radiation therapy has failed or when surgical risks are too great.

Dilatation of malignant strictures is usually possible with polyvinyl dilators passed over an endoscopically placed guidewire. This procedure may improve the patient's swallowing initially, but more definitive therapy is usually needed. That can take the form of laser ablation or the placement of a prosthesis or stent. Tumor within the esophageal lumen can be destroyed by application of Nd:YAG laser energy using a laser waveguide placed through the biopsy channel of the endoscope. New approaches using photodynamic therapy are being evaluated. Alternatively, after stricture dilatation, large-caliber stents can be placed over a dilator. When the dilator is removed, the stent lumen is available for the passage of food. Stenting is especially useful in the palliation of malignant tracheoesophageal fistulas.

Other Indications Upper GI endoscopy is usually substituted for x-ray examination in the urgent diagnosis of GI illness in *pregnancy*. Patients with *dysphagia* merit esophagoscopy because the cause is frequently structural, the lesion can be missed by x-ray, and biopsy confirmation is possible during endoscopy. Dysphagia caused by esophageal dysmotility is best diagnosed by manometry or cineradiography. *Painful swallowing* (odynophagia), especially in immunosuppressed or diabetic patients, may merit esophagoscopy because biopsy and brushings of the involved esophageal wall may reveal monilial, herpetic, or cytomegalovirus infections. Soon after ingestion of a corrosive agent, if there is no indication of wall necrosis, limited and gentle upper endoscopy is useful in evaluating the severity of injury. Many impacted foreign bodies can be removed from the esophagus or stomach with a snare or forceps; sharp foreign bodies are usually best removed by pulling them into a rigid open-lumen tubular esophagoscope or into a protective overtube around a fiberoptic endoscope. Careful esophagoscopy after removal of an esophageal foreign body is important to determine whether there is an underlying lesion that caused the impaction (e.g., cancer, benign stricture, peptic esophagitis).

In the postoperative stomach, gastroscopy is especially useful in detecting carcinoma, recurrent ulceration, retrograde intussusception, and stomal stricture. Several studies have suggested that there is an increased risk of carcinoma developing in the gastric stump more than 20 years after a Billroth II gastrectomy, although the magnitude of the risk, if there is one, is controversial. The diagnosis of such postoperative carcinomas may require many biopsies of seemingly normal mucosa near the anastomosis.

A new endoscopic application is the combination of ultrasound with endoscopy. This can be achieved by attaching an ultrasound system to the endoscope or passing an ultrasound probe down the biopsy channel of the endoscope. High-resolution ultrasound applied endoscopically is an accurate tool in the staging of esophageal and gastric malignancies, the detection of pancreatic neoplasia, and the determination of vascular extension in pancreatic cancers. Endoscopic ultrasound can be used to evaluate masses and to guide endoscopic needle aspiration.

ENDOSCOPIC RETROGRADE CHOLANGIOPANCREATOGRAPHY ERCP involves placing a side-viewing instrument (duodenoscope) in the descending duodenum. The papilla of Vater is cannulated, x-ray contrast medium is injected, and the pancreatic ducts and hepatobiliary tree are visualized radiographically. Skilled operators can visualize 90 to 95 percent of pancreatic ducts and 90 percent of biliary ducts.

ERCP is performed on an x-ray table after sedation of the patient and induction of duodenal hypotonia with atropine or glucagon. The pancreatic duct is gently filled throughout its length with contrast material under constant fluoroscopic monitoring (Fig. 282-1*A*). Injection is continued until the first side branches are seen, and overfilling is avoided. Insertion of the cannula at a more acute cephalad angle makes it possible to visualize the common bile duct and the whole biliary tract including the gallbladder (Fig. 282-1*B*).

ERCP is a safe procedure when performed by an experienced operator. Asymptomatic amylase elevations occur in 40 to 75 percent of patients after pancreatography but are rarely of clinical significance. Pancreatitis occurs in approximately 1 to 7 percent of patients but is usually benign and self-limited. In a nationwide survey of complications, the morbidity rate was 3 percent and the mortality rate 0.2 percent. The main serious complication is retention of nonsterile con-

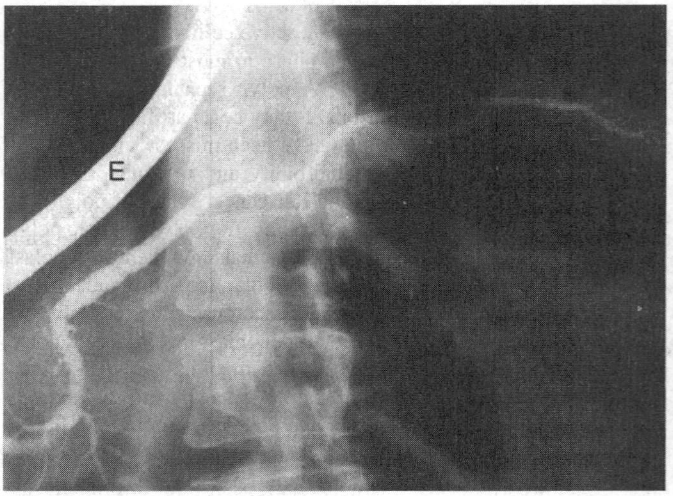

A

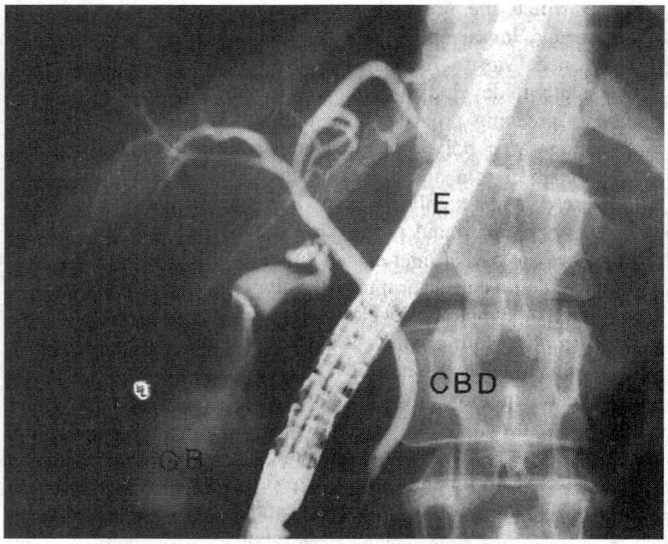

B

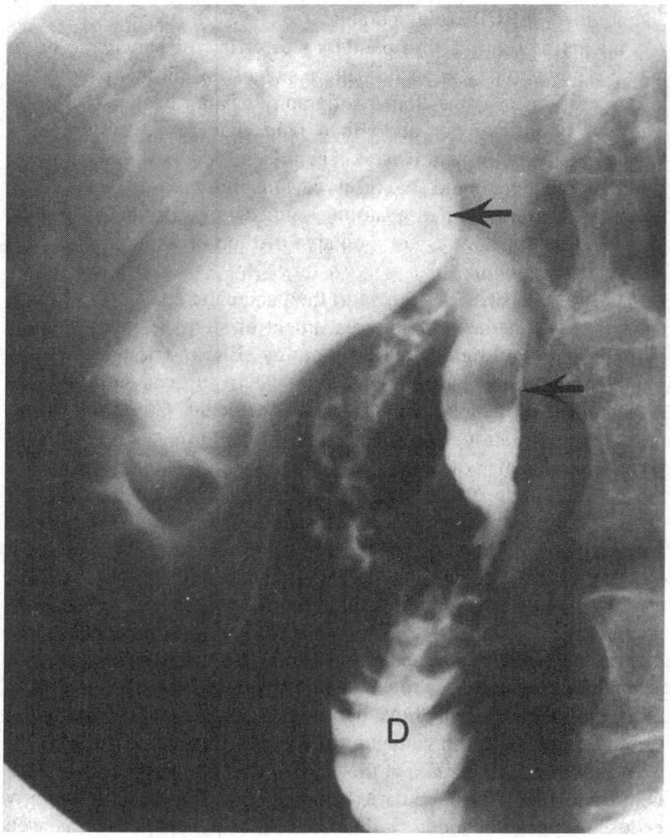

C

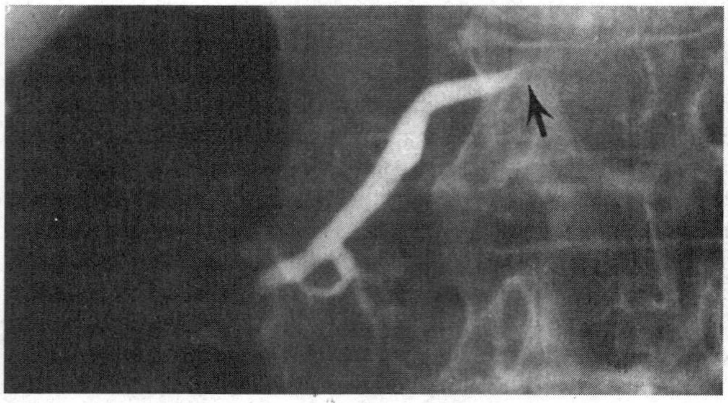

D

FIGURE 282-1 *A*. A tapering pancreatic duct of normal caliber is seen and may be compared to the endoscope (E) 1 cm in diameter. *B*. Normal cholangiogram. The diameter of the common bile duct (CBD) is normal. The intrahepatic ducts branch normally, and the gallbladder (GB) can be seen. The endoscope (E) is seen in the duodenum. *C*. Several stones (*arrows*) can be seen in an obstructed, dilated common duct. The gallbladder also contains several stones. Regurgitated contrast material is seen in the duodenum (D). *D*. The sharp cutoff (*arrow*) of the pancreatic duct is caused by a carcinoma of the body of the pancreas. *(Courtesy of Dr. Charles Rohrmann.)*

trast material proximal to an obstructed duct, causing cholangitis or pancreatic sepsis. If bile duct or pancreatic duct obstruction is first revealed by ERCP, the obstructed duct should be drained, if possible, either immediately by means of endoscopic techniques (papillotomy, stents, nasobiliary drains, etc.) or surgically within 36 h. Systemic antibiotics should be used immediately after filling an obstructed ductal system, especially if immediate endoscopic drainage cannot be accomplished.

Retrograde Cholangiography This procedure is especially useful in patients with persistent jaundice when the cause cannot be established by conventional diagnostic methods. The important differential diagnosis is between obstructive and nonobstructive jaundice. When the cause of jaundice is unclear, approximately 15 percent of patients thought to have nonobstructive jaundice prove to have extrahepatic biliary obstruction requiring endoscopic therapy or surgery; conversely, the same percentage of patients thought to have obstructive jaundice prove to have an open ductal system by ERCP.

Remediable causes of obstructive jaundice that can be diagnosed by retrograde cholangiography include common duct stones (Fig. 282-1*C*) and benign and malignant strictures. In jaundiced patients with suspected primary liver disease, such as primary biliary cirrhosis, ERCP can assure that no operable obstruction is being missed.

Most physicians first use ultrasound or computed tomography to see whether the biliary ducts are dilated and to seek the cause of the patient's jaundice (stones, a pancreatic mass, etc.). A radionuclide biliary scintigraphy scan can help to determine if the cystic duct and bile ducts are patent. Direct visualization is undertaken if the diagnosis is not established. Percutaneous transhepatic cholangiography (PTC) is often attempted first if an intrahepatic or proximal bile duct obstruction is suggested by imaging. ERCP is used first if distal obstruction is suspected. Advantages of the endoscopic approach are that the papilla and the pancreatic duct are seen (in addition to the biliary ducts) and that therapy can be performed with endoscopic sphincterotomy or drainage when appropriate. In the event of a technical failure or if the information provided by either ERCP or PTC is incomplete, the other technique is tried. This approach detects most lesions requiring surgical intervention.

ERCP or PTC also can be useful in patients with biliary pain, cholangitis, or impaired liver function after previous biliary surgery. Remediable postoperative lesions such as strictures can be discovered and sometimes treated endoscopically. Should endoscopic therapy fail, the precise anatomy of the lesion still has been outlined, so that reoperation is less difficult. Biliary manometry also can be performed in this setting to diagnose dysfunction of the sphincter of Oddi. A perfused catheter is placed into the sphincter via the endoscope, and pressures are recorded. A high basal sphincter pressure may predict a beneficial effect of sphincterotomy.

Retrograde Pancreatography Patients with recurrent or chronic pancreatitis may be candidates for retrograde pancreatography to seek a lesion that can be approached endoscopically or surgically, such as localized pancreatitis in the tail of the gland or ductal pathology amenable to endoscopic stenting or surgical drainage.

In patients with symptoms, signs, or laboratory findings suggesting pancreatic carcinoma, the pancreatogram may suggest malignancy by showing a narrowed, encased, or sharply "cut-off" pancreatic duct (Fig. 282-1*D*). Differentiation of pancreatic carcinoma from benign inflammatory disease on the basis of such ductal findings can be difficult. Cytologic examination of pancreatic duct brushings obtained during ERCP may prove helpful. Unfortunately, most patients with symptomatic pancreatic cancer diagnosed by ERCP are inoperable.

Patients presenting with painless steatorrhea of pancreatic origin may have a ductal pattern suggesting chronic pancreatitis or pancreatic carcinoma. Pancreatography has not been useful in the study of obscure upper abdominal pain. Pancreatic cysts can be better diagnosed by noninvasive techniques such as ultrasound, and pancreatography should be reserved for cases in which it is desirable to outline the anatomy immediately before surgery. Pancreatography alone is not a reliable method of screening for early pancreatic carcinoma.

Therapeutic ERCP Access to the pancreatic and biliary tree for the removal of stones and the placement of stents is made possible by endoscopic retrograde sphincterotomy (ERS). The pancreatic or biliary sphincter mechanism is cut using electrosurgical current passed through a wire attached to the ERCP catheter. Complications in the form of bleeding, perforation, pancreatitis, or cholangitis occur in 5 to 8 percent of patients, with a resulting mortality rate of 0.5 to 1 percent. The role of pancreatic sphincterotomy in the management of pancreatic stones and strictures is evolving; however, biliary sphincterotomy is an established therapy for several conditions.

Common bile duct stones in patients with prior cholecystectomy can be successfully removed from the bile duct after ERS 90 percent of the time. Small stones pass spontaneously or are pulled into the duodenum with a balloon catheter or after being captured by a basket. Stones larger than 1.5 cm in diameter may be difficult to extract without prior fragmentation by mechanical or other techniques. With the increasing use of laparoscopic cholecystectomy, endoscopic removal of common bile duct stones is being performed in this setting. Older patients with increased surgical risks can sometimes be managed with ERS and stone extraction alone; cholecystectomy can be delayed or avoided entirely. Urgent ERS is also indicated for acute cholangitis and has assumed an increasing role in the initial treatment of severe biliary pancreatitis, in which early endoscopic stone removal has been shown to improve outcome.

Patients with benign and malignant bile duct strictures may benefit from the endoscopic placement of biliary stents after ERS. Benign strictures frequently remain dilated following removal of stents that have been left in place for several months. In patients with either pancreatic carcinoma or cholangiocarcinoma and obstructive jaundice, palliation can be achieved by placement of a plastic or metal biliary stent. Plastic stents usually occlude after 3 to 6 months and must be exchanged if recurrent jaundice or cholangitis develops; wire-mesh metal stents are preferred in patients likely to survive at least 6 months. Strictures involving the hilum of the liver (see Chap. 302) are difficult to palliate endoscopically; stents sometimes must be placed into both sides of the liver. These patients may require additional percutaneous radiologic procedures to achieve adequate biliary drainage.

COLONOSCOPY The interior of the entire length of the colon from anus to cecum can be visualized by the experienced colonoscopist. This is one of the most significant diagnostic and therapeutic applications of endoscopy, because it can diagnose potentially curable colonic cancers that would be missed by other techniques, and it can be used for the removal of potentially precancerous adenomatous polyps.

Most initial colonoscopies are performed to investigate findings on an abnormal barium enema or to elucidate the cause of gastrointestinal bleeding. The ability to examine the whole colon is also useful in the management of some patients with inflammatory bowel disease and in patients with a strong family history of colonic polyps or cancer.

Patients are prepared for colonoscopy with laxatives and tap water enemas or by a total-gut lavage with a nonabsorbable electrolyte solution.

The main complications of colonoscopy are hemorrhage and perforation (morbidity rate, 0.5 to 1.3 percent; mortality rate, 0.02 percent). The complication rate for polypectomy is 1 to 2 percent. Diverticular or ischemic disease and prior irradiation make the procedure more difficult and hazardous. The risk of perforation is also increased in the patient with very active colitis; in most circumstances, colonoscopy should be avoided during the acute phase.

Polyps (See also Chap. 92) A polyp seen on barium enema merits colonoscopy for two reasons: It may be an artifact or a cancer, and a second polyp or cancer may have been missed. During colonoscopy, the polyp can usually be excised, with lower morbidity and mortality rates than with surgery. The best way to rule out cancer in a polyp is to remove the polyp completely for histologic examination. Hyperplastic polyps do not become malignant; colonic polyps that show benign neoplasia histologically may become malignant (tubular and villous adenomas). The risk that a neoplastic polyp is cancerous increases with its size. The risk is also higher in villous adenomas. Pedunculated polyps with moderately or well differentiated cancer confined to the mucosa and with an uninvolved stalk can be cured by removal with an electrocautery snare during colonoscopy. Thus, most colonoscopists will remove all polyps greater than 0.5 cm in diameter. Polyps smaller than 0.5 cm in diameter should be biopsied or removed, because more than 50 percent may be adenomatous, and the gross appearance of a polyp does not predict its histology. The wisdom of this course of action is suggested by several studies, including a sigmoidoscopic study in which the removal of all polyps reduced the expected incidence and invasiveness of subsequent cancers. Patients with adenomatous polyps are at increased risk of developing another polyp or cancer and therefore merit a regular screening program. The optimal frequency of follow-up examinations after polypectomy is not yet established. When a polyp is discovered, the entire colon should be examined for synchronous polyps or cancer. This examination should probably be repeated at 3- to 5-year intervals, and more frequently in patients with a history of colon cancer or multiple polyps. If stools are positive for occult blood or symptoms develop, immediate evaluation is indicated. In the average-risk patient without a known polyp, yearly digital examination and a stool test for occult blood are performed. Beginning at age 50, flexible sigmoidoscopy should be performed every 3 to 5 years.

Abnormal Findings on Barium Enema All filling defects on barium enema merit evaluation by colonoscopy. If the lesion is a pedunculated polyp, it can be removed for histologic examination; if its appearance suggests a cancer, it can be biopsied for histologic confirmation. When a polyp or a carcinoma is found, the remainder of the colon should be examined for additional polyps and synchronous carcinoma. A finding that is diagnosed as a mass by x-ray may be found on colonoscopy either not to exist or to represent a lesion such as a polyp rather than a cancer.

Narrowing Visualized by X-Ray Determining the cause of segmental narrowing may be difficult by x-ray but possible by colonoscopy, which can help in the differentiation of adenocarcinoma from inflammation secondary to ischemia, irradiation, diverticular disease, or Crohn's colitis. Even the most classic "apple-core" lesion seen on x-ray may be found on colonoscopy to be covered by normal mucosa, which suggests an extrinsic inflammatory lesion. In 10 to 30 percent of patients, narrowed segments seen on x-ray are not visualized during colonoscopy, probably because they were areas of temporary spasm.

Chronic Bleeding (X-Ray and Sigmoidoscopy Negative) Chronic bleeding is a common indication for colonoscopy. The x-ray is more likely to miss a lesion when a single-contrast technique is used rather than air contrast. The source of bleeding is found in approximately 40 percent of such patients and consists of such entities as an adenomatous polyp, an adenocarcinoma, and inflammatory bowel disease. If no bleeding site is found, it may be appropriate to search for an upper GI source with an upper GI x-ray or upper endoscopy, as well as to consider the possibiity of small intestinal bleeding.

Inflammatory Bowel Disease Colonoscopy may help in the initial diagnosis of this condition, especially in differentiating Crohn's colitis from ulcerative colitis. It also can aid the surgeon in assessing the activity and extent of the disease before surgery. Colonoscopy can help in the evaluation of radiographic abnormalities suggesting cancer, such as strictures, polyps, or masses. Colonoscopy is generally indicated in patients with ulcerative colitis of more than 10 years duration because of the increased risk of carcinoma; colonoscopy repeated at regular intervals helps to detect colonic dysplasia while the lesions are still curable. However, the benefit of such colonoscopic surveillance in terms of mortality and the optimal frequency of colonoscopy in such patients are still controversial. Nevertheless, if an expert gastrointestinal pathologist finds high-grade dysplasia in colonic biopsy samples from a patient with long-standing ulcerative colitis, most would consider it to be an indication for colectomy. Colonoscopy is contraindicated in patients with toxic megacolon, very active disease, or a possible intestinal perforation.

Other Indications The flexible sigmoidoscope has generally replaced the rigid 25-cm sigmoidoscope for routine screening because it can be passed to 40 to 60 cm with minimal preparation, less discomfort, and a higher diagnostic yield. After segmental colonic resection for carcinoma, colonoscopy may detect early mucosal recurrence and differentiate it from benign anastomotic strictures or bleeding suture granulomas. Colonoscopy is occasionally used during laparotomy to assist the surgeon in ruling out the presence of other lesions. The colonoscope can be advanced to the cecum rapidly with the surgeon's assistance, and additional polyps removed without colotomy. Colonoscopy is useful in the management of patients with lower GI bleeding (see Chap. 44). Bleeding polyps may be removed by snare electrocautery. Endoscopic hemostatic therapy may be useful in other bleeding lesions, such as colonic angiodysplasia.

Colonoscopy is usually not necessary for the diagnosis of familial polyposis because affected family members can be diagnosed by periodic flexible sigmoidoscopy. Carcinoma is a great threat in the familial polyposis syndromes that produce many adenomatous polyps (familial polyposis and Gardner's syndrome); in these conditions, polypectomy is useful for diagnosis, but colectomy is the only treatment that prevents development of carcinoma. These patients are also at risk of developing duodenal and periampullary adenomas and cancer and should probably undergo periodic surveillance with a side-viewing duodenoscope.

BIBLIOGRAPHY

HAGGITT RC et al: Prognostic factors in colorectal carcinomas arising in adenomas: Implications for lesions removed by endoscopic polypectomy. Gastroenterology 89:328, 1985

JENSEN DM, MACHICADO GA: Diagnosis and treatment of severe hematochezia: The role of urgent colonoscopy after purge. Gastroenterology 95:1569, 1988

LAI ECS et al: Endoscopic biliary drainage for severe acute cholangitis. N Engl J Med 326:1582, 1992

LAINE L: Multipolar electrocoagulation in the treatment of active upper gastrointestinal tract hemorrhage. N Engl J Med 316:1613, 1987

LIGHTDALE CJ et al: Localization of endocrine tumors of the pancreas with endoscopic ultrasonography. Cancer 68:1815, 1991

NIH CONSENSUS DEVELOPMENT CONFERENCE: Therapeutic endoscopy and bleeding ulcers. JAMA 262:1369, 1989

REID BJ et al: Flow cytometric and histologic progression to malignancy in Barrett's esophagus: Prospective endoscopic surveillance of a cohort. Gastroenterology 102:1212, 1992

SILVERSTEIN FE, TYTGAT GNJ: *Atlas of Gastrointestinal Endoscopy*, 3rd ed. London, Mosby-Wolfe, 1996

SPACH DH et al: Transmission of infection by gastrointestinal endoscopy and bronchoscopy. Ann Intern Med 118:117, 1993

STIEGMANN GV et al: Endoscopic sclerotherapy as compared with endoscopic ligation for bleeding esophageal varices. N Engl J Med 326:1527, 1992

TIO TL et al: Endosonography and computer tomography of esophageal carcinoma. Preoperative classification compared to the new TNM system. Gastroenterology 96:1478, 1989

283 DISEASES OF THE ESOPHAGUS

Raj K. Goyal

The two major functions of the esophagus are the transport of the food bolus from the mouth to the stomach and the prevention of retrograde flow of gastrointestinal contents. The transport function is achieved by peristaltic contractions (see Chap. 40). Retrograde flow is prevented by the two esophageal sphincters, which remain closed between swallows. The upper esophageal sphincter consists of the cricopharyngeus and inferior pharyngeal constrictor muscles, which are striated muscles and are innervated by excitatory somatic lower motor neurons. These muscles exhibit no myogenic tone and receive no inhibitory innervation. The upper sphincter remains closed owing to the elastic properties of its wall and to neurogenic tonic contraction of the sphincter muscles and is opened by inhibition of the sphincter muscles in concert with forward displacement of the larynx by the suprahyoid muscles. In contrast, the lower esophageal sphincter (LES) is composed of smooth muscle and is innervated by parallel sets of parasympathetic excitatory and inhibitory pathways. It remains closed because of its intrinsic myogenic tone, which is modulated by the excitatory and inhibitory nerves. It opens in response to the activity of the inhibitory nerves. The neuromuscular neurotransmitter of the excitatory nerves is acetylcholine, and those of the inhibitory nerves are vasoactive intestinal peptide (VIP) and nitric oxide. The function of the LES is supplemented by the striated muscle of diaphragmatic crura, which surrounds the sphincter and acts as external lower esophageal sphincter. A reflex decrease in the lower sphincter pressure occurs during belching and gastric distention. Fatty meals, smoking, and beverages with a high xanthine content (tea, coffee, cola) also cause a reduction in sphincter pressure. Many hormones and neurotransmitters can modify lower sphincter pressure. Muscarinic M_2 receptor agonists, alpha-adrenergic agonists, gastrin, substance P, and prostaglandin $F_{2\alpha}$ cause contraction; in contrast, nicotine, beta-adrenergic agonists, dopamine, cholecystokinin, secretin, VIP, calcitonin gene–related peptide (CGRP), adenosine, and nitric oxide donors such as nitrates cause relaxation of the sphincter.

SYMPTOMS

DYSPHAGIA → *See Chap. 40.*

ESOPHAGEAL PAIN *Heartburn*, or pyrosis, is characterized by burning retrosternal discomfort that may move up and down the chest like a wave. When severe, it may radiate to the sides of the chest, the neck, and the angles of the jaw. Heartburn is a characteristic symptom of reflux esophagitis and may be associated with regurgitation or a feeling of warm fluid climbing up the throat. It is aggravated by bending forward, straining, or lying recumbent and is worse after meals. It is relieved by an upright posture, by the swallowing of saliva or water, and, more reliably, by antacids. Heartburn appears to be produced by heightened mucosal sensitivity and can be reproduced by infusion of dilute (0.1 *N*) hydrochloric acid (Bernstein test) or neutral hyperosmolar solutions into the esophagus.

Odynophagia, or painful swallowing, is characteristic of nonreflux esophagitis, particularly monilial and herpes esophagitis. Odynophagia also may occur with peptic ulcer of the esophagus (Barrett's ulcer), carcinoma with periesophageal involvement, caustic damage of the esophagus, and esophageal perforation. Odynophagia is unusual in uncomplicated reflux esophagitis. Crampy chest pain associated with impaction of a food bolus should be distinguished from odynophagia.

Atypical chest pain other than heartburn and odynophagia occurs in reflux esophagitis or esophageal motility disorders such as diffuse esophageal spasm. The latter may occur spontaneously or during a meal. Chest pain due to periesophageal involvement caused by carcinoma or peptic ulcer may be constant and agonizing. Sometimes different types of esophageal pains exist together in the same patient, and frequently patients are not able to describe the pain accurately enough to allow its classification. Coronary artery disease should always be carefully excluded before the esophagus is considered as the cause of atypical chest pain. The most frequent esophageal cause of chest pain is reflux esophagitis. Some patients with atypical chest pain have nonspecific esophageal motor abnormalities of uncertain significance. Many of these patients have behavioral abnormalities, psychosomatic disorders, depression, anxiety, panic reactions, and other somatization disorders.

REGURGITATION *Regurgitation* is the effortless appearance of gastric or esophageal contents in the mouth. In distal esophageal obstruction and stasis, as in achalasia or the presence of a large diverticulum, the regurgitated material consists of tasteless mucoid fluid or undigested food. Regurgitation of sour or bitter-tasting material occurs in severe gastroesophageal reflux and is associated with incompetence of both the upper and lower esophageal sphincters. Regurgitation may result in laryngeal aspiration, with spells of coughing and choking that awaken the patient from sleep, and in aspiration pneumonia. Water brash is reflex salivary hypersecretion which occurs in response to peptic esophagitis; it should not be confused with regurgitation.

DIAGNOSTIC TESTS

RADIOLOGIC STUDIES Barium swallow with fluoroscopy and an esophagogram is the most widely used test for the diagnosis of esophageal disease and can be used to evaluate both structural and motor disorders. Since the oropharyngeal phase of swallowing lasts no more than a second, videofluoroscopy is necessary to permit detection and analysis of abnormalities of oral and pharyngeal function. The pharynx is examined to detect stasis of barium in the valleculae and piriform sinuses and regurgitation of barium into the nose and tracheobronchial tree. Spontaneous reflux of barium from the stomach into the esophagus should be sought in patients with suspected reflux esophagitis. Esophageal peristalsis is best studied in the recumbent position, because in the upright position the passage of most of the barium occurs by gravity alone. A double-contrast esophagogram, obtained by coating the esophageal mucosa with barium and distending the esophageal lumen with air using effervescent granules, is particularly useful in demonstrating mucosal ulcers and early cancers. A barium-soaked piece of bread or a 13-mm barium tablet is sometimes used to demonstrate an obstructive lesion. Figures 283-1 and 283-2 illustrate the radiographic appearance of some esophageal disorders.

ESOPHAGOSCOPY Fiberoptic esophagogastroduodenoscopy is described in Chap. 282. Esophagoscopy is the direct method of establishing the cause of mechanical dysphagia and of identifying mucosal lesions, such as superficial ulcers and esophagitis, which may not be identified by the usual barium swallow. If the lumen is markedly narrowed, it may be necessary to use a smaller-caliber endoscope, although on occasion a stricture must be dilated before the examination can be completed. Transendoscopic biopsies are useful in diagnosing carcinoma, reflux esophagitis, and other mucosal diseases. Obtaining cells by scraping the mucosa with a Teflon brush during endoscopy may enable the cytologist to detect carcinoma.

ESOPHAGEAL MOTILITY The study of esophageal motility entails simultaneous recording of pressures from different sites in the esophageal lumen using an assembly of pressure sensors that are positioned 5 cm apart. The upper and lower esophageal sphincters appear as zones of high pressure that relax on swallowing. The pharynx and esophageal body normally show peristaltic waves with each swallow.

Esophageal motility studies are very helpful in the diagnosis of achalasia, diffuse esophageal spasm and its variants, scleroderma, and other motor disorders of the esophagus (Fig. 283-3) but are of no value in the diagnosis of mechanical dysphagia. In patients with reflux

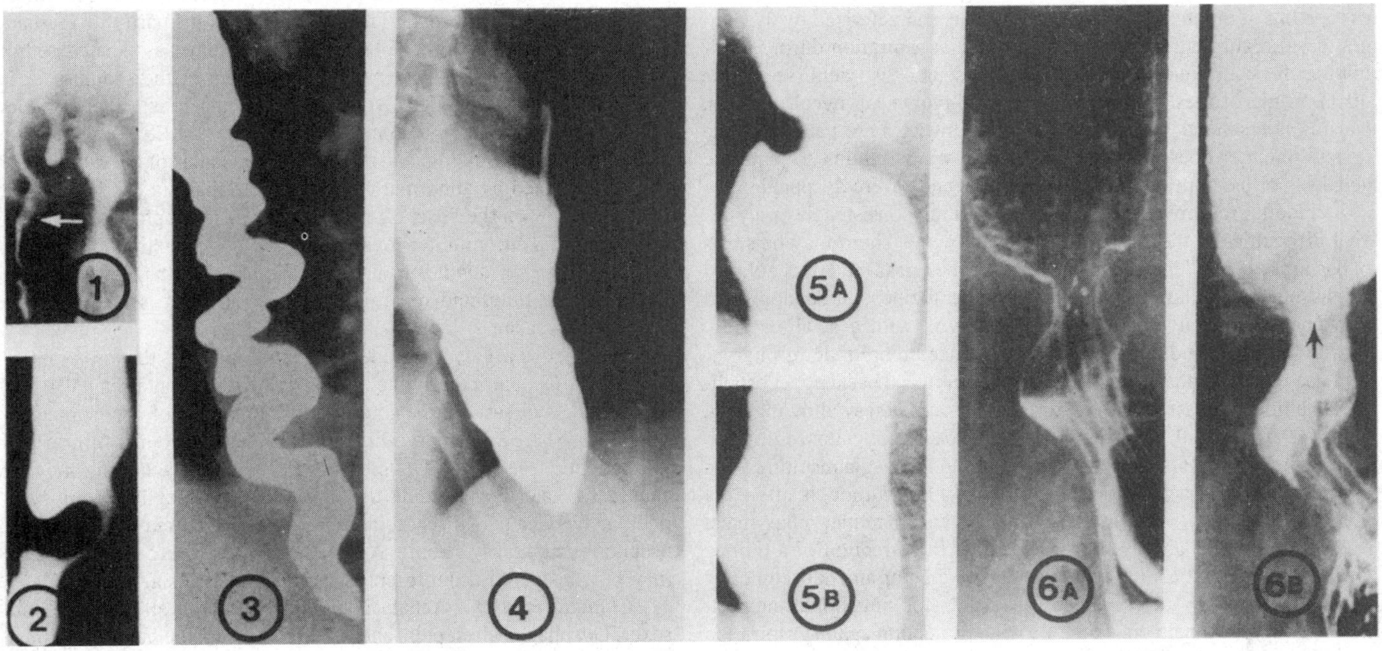

FIGURE 283-1 Radiographic appearance of some motor disorders of the pharynx and esophagus. *(1)* Pharyngeal paralysis with tracheal aspiration (*arrow*). *(2)* Cricopharyngeal achalasia. Note the prominent cricopharyngeus, which is recognized by its smoothness and location in the posterior wall. *(3)* Diffuse esophageal spasm. Note typical corkscrew appearance of the lower part of the esophagus. *(4)* Achalasia, showing a dilated esophageal body with an air-fluid level and a closed lower esophageal sphincter. *(5)* Muscular (contractile) lower esophageal ring. Note that the asymmetric contraction visible in *5A* has disappeared in *5B*, obtained during the same examination. *(6)* Scleroderma esophagus showing dilated esophagus with a stricture *(6A)* and reflux of barium from the stomach into the esophagus *(6B)*. *(Courtesy of Dr. Harvey Goldstein.)*

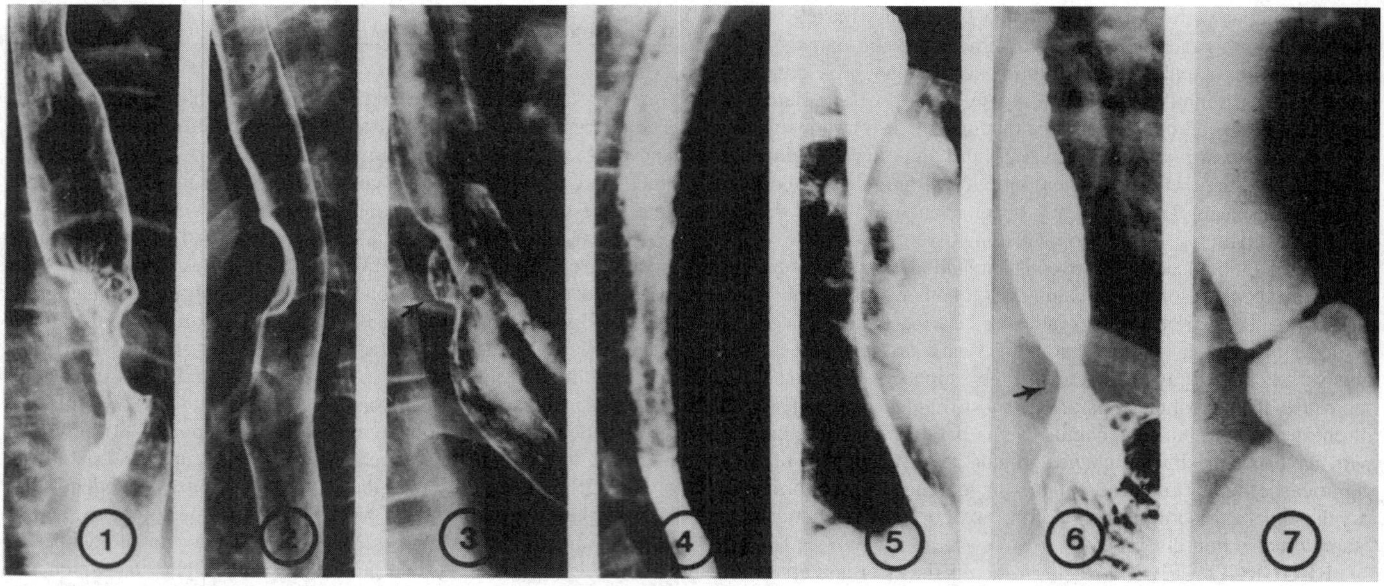

FIGURE 283-2 Selected structural lesions of the esophagus. *(1)* Carcinoma of the esophagus, with typical annular narrowing with overhanging margins and destruction of the mucosa. *(2)* Leiomyoma of the esophagus, with a smooth filling defect and right angles of origin from the esophageal wall. *(3)* Esophageal ulcer in columnar-cell-lined esophagus (Barrett's esophagus). *(4)* Monilial esophagitis, with irregular plaquelike filling defects. *(5)* Long stricture secondary to lye ingestion. *(6)* Peptic stricture, short and tubular, with associated hiatus hernia. *(7)* Lower esophageal mucosal (Schatzki) ring. A thin, weblike annular constriction at the esophagogastric junction is associated with a small hiatal hernia. *(Courtesy of Dr. Harvey Goldstein.)*

esophagitis, esophageal manometry is useful in quantitating lower esophageal competence and providing information on the status of the esophageal body motor activity. The information obtained by manometry is quantitative and cannot be obtained by barium swallow or endoscopy.

Special tests for the evaluation of reflux esophagitis are described later.

MOTOR DISORDERS

STRIATED MUSCLE Oropharyngeal Paralysis Paralysis of oral muscle leads to difficulty in initiating swallowing and to drooling of food out of mouth. Pharyngeal paralysis is characterized by dysphagia, nasal regurgitation, and tracheobronchial aspiration during swallowing. It occurs in a variety of neuromuscular disorders (see Table 40-1). Some of these disorders also may involve laryngeal muscles, causing hoarseness. When the suprahyoid muscles are paralyzed, the upper sphincter does not open with swallowing, leading to paralytic achalasia of the upper esophageal sphincter and severe dysphagia.

Videofluoroscopy using barium of various consistencies may reveal difficulties in the oral phase of swallowing. There may be stasis of barium in the valleculae and piriform sinuses, nasal and tracheobronchial aspiration, failure of the upper sphincter to open, and/or abnormal movement of the hyoid bone and the larynx with a swallow (Fig. 283-1). Motility studies demonstrate a reduced amplitude of pharyngeal and upper esophageal contractions and reduced basal upper esophageal sphincter pressure without further relaxation on swallowing (Fig. 283-3). Patients with myasthenia gravis and polymyositis respond to treatment for these diseases (see Chap. 381). Dysphagia resulting from a cerebrovascular accident improves with time, although often not completely. Treatment consists of maneuvers to reduce pharyngeal stasis and enhance airway protection under the direction of a trained swallow therapist. Feeding by a nasogastric tube or an endoscopically placed gastrostomy tube may be necessary for nutritional support; however, these maneuvers do not provide protection against aspiration of salivary secretions. Cricopharyngeal myotomy is sometimes performed, but its usefulness is unproven. Extensive operative procedures to prevent aspiration are rarely needed. Death is often due to pulmonary complications.

Cricopharyngeal Bar Failure of the cricopharyngeus to relax on swallowing leads to a contracted cricopharyngeus, which appears as a prominent bar on the posterior wall of the pharynx on barium swallow (Fig. 283-1). A transient cricopharyngeal bar is seen in up to 5 percent of subjects without dysphagia undergoing upper gastrointestinal studies; it can be produced in normal subjects during a Valsalva maneuver. A persistent cricopharyngeal bar may be caused by fibrosis in the cricopharyngeus. Some of these patients complain of food sticking in their throats. Cricopharyngeal myotomy may be helpful, but it is contraindicated in the presence of gastroesophageal reflux because, in such patients, it may lead to pharyngeal and pulmonary aspiration.

Globus Pharyngeus A sensation of a constant lump in the throat, but with no difficulty in swallowing, occurs especially in subjects with emotional disorders, particularly women. Results of barium studies and manometry are normal. Treatment consists primarily of reassurance. Some patients with globus pharyngeus have associated reflux esophagitis, and they may respond to treatment of the esophagitis.

SMOOTH MUSCLE Achalasia Achalasia is a motor disorder of the esophageal smooth muscle in which the LES does not relax properly with swallowing, and the normal peristalsis of the esophageal body is replaced by abnormal contractions. Achalasia can be divided into two types on the basis of the changes in the esophageal body. In *classic achalasia,* simultaneous small-amplitude contractions occur, while in *vigorous achalasia,* contractions are simultaneous in onset, large in amplitude, and repetitive, resembling those seen in diffuse esophageal spasm.

Pathophysiology The underlying abnormality is the loss of intramural neurons, particularly the inhibitory neurons containing VIP and nitric oxide synthase, in the smooth-muscle portion of the esophageal body and the LES. Primary idiopathic achalasia accounts for most of the patients seen in the United States. Secondary achalasia may be caused by gastric carcinoma that infiltrates the esophagus, by lymphoma, by Chagas' disease, and by neuropathic chronic intestinal pseudoobstruction syndrome. A hypertensive or hypercontracting LES may be considered to represent a variant of achalasia.

Clinical features Achalasia affects patients of all ages and both sexes. Dysphagia, chest pain, and regurgitation are the main symptoms. Dysphagia appears early, occurs with both liquids and solids, and is worsened by emotional stress and hurried eating. Various maneuvers designed to increase intraesophageal pressure, including the Valsalva maneuver, may aid the passage of the bolus into the stomach. Chest pain is more pronounced in vigorous achalasia than in classic achalasia. Regurgitation and pulmonary aspiration occur because of retention of large volumes of saliva and ingested food in the esophagus. The presence of gastroesophageal reflux argues against achalasia, and in patients with long-standing heartburn, cessation of heartburn and appearance of dysphagia suggest development of achalasia in a patient with reflux esophagitis. The overall course is usually chronic, with progressive dysphagia and weight loss over months to years. Achalasia associated with carcinoma is characterized by severe weight loss and a rapid downhill course if untreated.

Diagnosis A chest x-ray shows absence of the gastric air bubble and sometimes a tubular mediastinal mass beside the aorta. An air-fluid level in the mediastinum in the upright position represents retained food in the esophagus. Barium swallow shows esophageal dilation, and in advanced cases the esophagus may become sigmoid. On fluoroscopy, normal peristalsis is lost in the lower two-thirds of the esophagus. The terminal part of the esophagus shows a persistent beaklike narrowing representing the nonrelaxing LES (see Fig. 283-1). In patients with vigorous achalasia, there may be pronounced nonperistaltic contractions.

Manometry shows the basal lower esophageal sphincter pressure to be normal or elevated, and swallow-induced relaxation either does not occur or is reduced in degree, duration, and consistency. The esophageal body shows an elevated resting pressure. In response to swallows, primary peristaltic waves are replaced by simultaneous-onset contractions (Fig. 283-3). These contractions may be of poor amplitude (classic achalasia) or of large amplitude and long duration (vigorous achalasia). Administration of the cholinergic muscarinic agonist mecholyl causes a marked increase in baseline esophageal pressure, chest pain, and regurgitation of retained esophageal contents (Mecholyl test). Cholecystokinin (CCK), which normally causes a fall in the sphincter pressure, paradoxically causes contraction of the LES (the CCK test). This paradoxical response occurs because, in achalasia, the neurally transmitted inhibitory effect of CCK is absent owing to the loss of inhibitory neurons. Endoscopy is helpful in excluding the secondary causes of achalasia, particularly gastric carcinoma.

Rx TREATMENT

Medical treatment using soft foods, sedatives, and anticholinergic drugs is usually unsatisfactory. Nitroglycerin, 0.3 to 0.6 mg sublingually before meals and as needed for chest pain, is usually helpful. Isosorbide dinitrate, 2.5 to 5 mg sublingually or 10 to 20 mg orally before meals, can be used for longer-lasting relief of symptoms. Nitrates are associated with headache and postural hypotension. The calcium channel blocker nifedipine, 10 to 20 mg orally or sublingually before meals, is also effective. Injection of botulinum toxin in the LES during endoscopy has been reported to be effective. Botulinum toxin acts by blocking cholinergic excitatory nerves in the sphincter. A time-tested therapy involves balloon dilatation to reduce the basal LES pressure by tearing muscle fibers. In experienced hands, this technique is effective in about 85 percent of patients. Perforation and bleeding are potential complications. Heller's extramucosal myotomy of the lower sphincter, in which the circular muscle layer is incised, is equally effective. Reflux esophagitis and peptic stricture may follow successful treatment (more often with myotomy than with balloon dilatation). Laparoscopic myotomy of the sphincter also is successful.

Diffuse Esophageal Spasm and Related Motor Disorders Diffuse esophageal spasm is a motor disorder of the esophageal smooth muscle characterized by multiple spontaneous contractions and by swallow-induced contractions that are of simultaneous onset. The contractions may be of large amplitude, long duration, and repetitive occurrence. Variants show some but not all of these motor abnormalities.

Pathophysiology The pathogenesis of the various abnormalities of peristalsis in diffuse esophageal spasm is not known. Histopathologic studies show patchy neural degeneration localized to nerve processes, rather than the prominent degeneration of nerve cell bodies seen in achalasia.

Esophageal contractions that are peristaltic but of large amplitude constitute a condition (sometimes called "nutcracker" esophagus) that is diagnosed by manometry and is due to heightened excitatory activity. Cholinergic drugs cause large-amplitude contractions. Simultaneous contractions indicate loss of inhibitory nerve function; they frequently occur as a primary disease or in association with a variety of diseases as well as with emotional stress and aging. Collagen vascular disease, diabetic neuropathy, reflux esophagitis, irradiation esophagitis, esophageal obstruction, and anticholinergic drugs can cause simultaneous contractions. The relationship between reflux esophagitis and motor abnormalities is controversial. Overlapping features of diffuse esophageal spasm and achalasia occur in vigorous achalasia. The variant syndromes are more frequent in clinical practice than is classic diffuse esophageal spasm.

Clinical features The symptomatic patient with diffuse spasm or one of its variants presents with chest pain, dysphagia, or both. Chest pain is particularly marked in patients with esophageal contractions of large amplitude and long duration. Chest pain usually occurs at rest but may be brought on by swallowing or by emotional stress. The pain is retrosternal; it may radiate to the back, the sides of the chest,

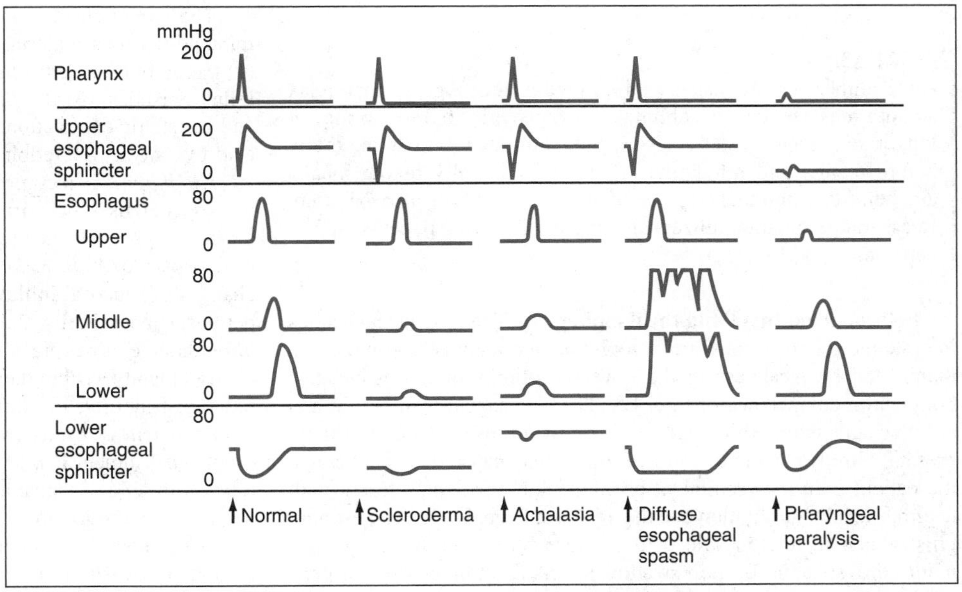

FIGURE 283-3 Motility patterns in selected esophageal and pharyngeal disorders. In normal subjects, the upper and lower esophageal sphincters (UES and LES) appear as zones of high pressure. With a swallow (indicated by ↑), pressure in the sphincters falls and a contraction wave starts in the pharynx and progresses down the esophagus. In scleroderma, the lower part of the esophagus (smooth muscle) shows a reduced amplitude of contractions, which may be peristaltic or simultaneous in onset, and hypotension of the lower sphincter. In achalasia, the lower part of the esophagus shows contractions that are reduced in amplitude and simultaneous in onset. In contrast to scleroderma, the lower esophageal sphincter in achalasia is hypertensive and fails to relax in response to a swallow. In diffuse esophageal spasm, the lower part of the esophagus shows simultaneous-onset, large-amplitude, prolonged, repetitive contractions. In pharyngeal paralysis, the smooth-muscle part of the esophagus is normal. The skeletal muscle part shows a reduced amplitude of contractions. The upper esophageal sphincter is hypotensive and may not relax normally on swallowing owing to associated weakness of the suprahyoid muscles.

both arms, or the sides of the jaw and may last from a few seconds to several minutes. It may be acute and severe, mimicking the pain of myocardial ischemia. Dysphagia for solids and liquids may occur with or without chest pain and is correlated particularly with simultaneous-onset contractions.

Diffuse esophageal spasm must be differentiated from other causes of chest pain, particularly ischemic heart disease with atypical angina. A complete cardiac workup should be done before an esophageal etiology is considered seriously. The presence of dysphagia in association with pain should point to the esophagus as the site of disease. Symptoms of esophageal spasm should be carefully distinguished from those of reflux esophagitis; the two conditions may coexist.

Diagnosis Barium swallow shows that normal sequential peristalsis below the aortic arch is replaced by uncoordinated simultaneous contractions that produce the appearance of curling or multiple ripples in the wall, sacculations, and pseudodiverticula—the "corkscrew" esophagus (Fig. 283-1). Sometimes an esophageal contraction obliterates the lumen, and barium is pushed away in both directions. The lower esophageal sphincter opens normally.

Manometry reveals the characteristic presence of prolonged, large-amplitude, repetitive contractions of simultaneous onset in the lower part of the esophagus (Fig. 283-3). Only one or two of these abnormalities may be present in variants of diffuse spasm. Because the disorder may be episodic, the results of manometry may be normal at the time of the study; therefore, several techniques are used in attempts to provoke esophageal spasm. Cold swallows produce chest pain but do not produce spasm on manometric studies. Solid boluses and pharmacologic agents, particularly edrophonium, induce both chest pain and motor abnormalities. However, there is a poor correlation between induction of pain and motility changes. Ergonovine can induce motor abnormalities but also may cause coronary artery spasm and therefore should not be used. Overall, the usefulness of pharmacologic provocative tests is limited.

℞ TREATMENT

Anticholinergics are usually of limited value. Agents that relax smooth muscle, such as sublingual nitroglycerin (0.3 to 0.6 mg) or longer-acting agents such as isosorbide dinitrate (10 to 30 mg orally before meals) and nifedipine (10 to 20 mg orally before meals) are helpful. Sublingual forms of these agents can also be used. Reassurance and tranquilizers are helpful in allaying patients' apprehension.

Scleroderma Involving the Esophagus The esophageal lesions in systemic sclerosis consist of atrophy of smooth muscle contraction, manifested by weakness in the lower two-thirds of the esophageal body and incompetence of the LES. The esophageal wall is thin and atrophic and may exhibit areas of patchy fibrosis. Patients usually present with dysphagia to solids. Liquids may cause dysphagia when the patient is in the recumbent position. Some patients present with heartburn and regurgitation due to gastroesophageal reflux and esophagitis, which in turn may lead to stricture formation and more pronounced dysphagia. Barium swallow shows dilation and loss of peristaltic contractions in the middle and distal portions of the esophagus. The LES is patulous, and gastroesophageal reflux may occur freely (Fig. 283-1). Mucosal changes due to esophageal ulceration may be detected, and esophageal stricture may be present. Motility studies show a marked reduction in the amplitude of smooth-muscle contractions, which may be peristaltic or nonperistaltic. The resting pressure of the LES is subnormal, but sphincter relaxation is normal (Fig. 283-3). Esophageal motor abnormalities are frequently found in patients with Raynaud's syndrome alone. Currently, there is no effective treatment for the motor difficulty. Reflux esophagitis and its complications should be treated aggressively, as described in the following section.

INFLAMMATORY DISORDERS

GASTROESOPHAGEAL REFLUX AND ESOPHAGITIS

Reflux esophagitis consists of esophageal mucosal damage caused by reflux of gastric or intestinal contents into the esophagus. Depending on the causative agent, it is referred to as *peptic*, *bile*, or *alkaline esophagitis*.

Pathophysiology Three considerations involved in the pathophysiology of reflux esophagitis are (1) the reflux episode, (2) the cumulative esophageal reflux, and (3) the pathogenesis of esophagitis.

Two conditions must be met for a *reflux episode* to occur: The gastrointestinal contents must be "ready" to reflux, and the antireflux mechanism at the lower end of the esophagus must be compromised. Gastrointestinal contents are most likely to reflux (1) when gastric volume is increased (after meals, in the presence of pyloric obstruction or gastric stasis syndrome, and in acid hypersecretory states), (2) when the gastric contents are located near the gastroesophageal junction (owing to recumbency, bending down, or the presence of a hiatus hernia), and (3) when gastric pressure is increased (owing to obesity, pregnancy, ascites, or tight binders or girdles).

The normal antireflux mechanisms consist of the LES and the anatomic configuration of the gastroesophageal junction. Reflux occurs only when the gradient of pressure between the LES and the stomach is lost. It can be caused by increased intragastric pressure or by a transient or sustained decrease in LES tone. The decrease in sphincter tone may be due to muscle weakness or to inappropriate sphincter relaxation mediated by inhibitory nerves. The secondary causes of LES incompetence include scleroderma-like diseases; a myopathic type of chronic intestinal pseudoobstruction syndrome; pregnancy; smoking; smooth-muscle relaxants (such as beta-adrenergic agents, aminophylline, nitrates, and calcium channel blockers); destruction of the sphincter by surgical resection, myotomy, or balloon dilatation; and esophagitis. Abnormal activity of the diaphragmatic crural muscle, which surrounds the esophageal hiatus in the diaphragm and changes the anatomic configuration of the esophagogastric junction—as occurs in hiatal hernia—also predisposes to gastroesophageal reflux.

The *cumulative esophageal reflux*—the amount and duration of refluxed noxious material remaining in the esophagus—depends on (1) the amount of refluxed material per episode, (2) the frequency of reflux episodes, (3) the rate of clearing of the esophagus by gravity and peristaltic contraction, and (4) the rate of neutralization of gastric acid by salivary secretion.

Esophagitis is a complication of reflux, and it develops when the mucosal defenses that normally counteract the effect of injurious agents on the esophageal mucosa succumb to the onslaught of the refluxed acid pepsin or bile. *Mild esophagitis* is manifested by microscopic changes of mucosal infiltration with granulocytes or eosinophils, hyperplasia of basal cells, and elongation of dermal pegs. It can occur with or without endoscopic abnormalities. *Erosive esophagitis* involves endoscopically visible damage to the mucosa in the form of marked redness, friability, bleeding, superficial linear ulcers, and exudates. *Peptic stricture* results from fibrosis that causes constriction of the esophageal lumen. Peptic strictures occur in about 10 percent of patients with reflux esophagitis. Short peptic strictures caused by spontaneous reflux are usually 1 to 3 cm long and are present in the distal esophagus near the squamocolumnar junction (see Fig. 283-2). Long, tubular peptic strictures can result from persistent vomiting or prolonged nasogastric intubation. Replacement of the squamous epithelium of the esophagus by columnar epithelium (*Barrett's esophagus*) also may result from reflux esophagitis. The columnar epithelium usually represents a specialized type of intestinal metaplasia, and the condition may be complicated further by a peptic ulcer or peptic stricture located in the upper part of the lower esophagus or in the midesophagus. Adenocarcinoma occurs in 2 to 5 percent of cases and is usually preceded by dysplasia of the columnar mucosa. Recently, a high prevalence of intestinal metaplasia localized to the gastroesophageal junction has been reported during upper endoscopic examination. This finding may explain the increased incidence of adenocarcinoma at the gastroesophageal junction.

Clinical Features Heartburn is the characteristic symptom and is produced by the contact of refluxed material with the inflamed esophageal mucosa. Angina-like or atypical chest pain occurs in some patients, while others experience no heartburn or chest pain. Dysphagia suggests development of a peptic stricture. Most patients with peptic stricture have a history of several years of heartburn preceding dysphagia. However, in one-third of patients, dysphagia is the presenting symptom. Rapidly progressive dysphagia and weight loss may indicate the development of adenocarcinoma in Barrett's esophagus. Bleeding occurs due to mucosal erosions or Barrett's ulcer. Reflux in the absence of esophagitis is usually asymptomatic. Severe reflux may reach the pharynx and mouth and result in laryngitis, morning hoarseness, and pulmonary aspiration. Recurrent pulmonary aspiration can cause aspiration pneumonia, pulmonary fibrosis, or chronic asthma.

Diagnosis The evaluation of reflux esophagitis is designed to assess the presence and severity of reflux, the nature of the refluxant, the presence and severity of esophagitis, and the pathophysiology of the reflux. A history is taken, and barium swallow, esophagoscopy, mucosal biopsy, esophageal motility testing, and a variety of special tests are performed.

The *presence of reflux* is suggested by the history. Spontaneous reflux from the stomach into the esophagus on barium examination suggests advanced reflux. Reflux of barium induced by stressful maneuvers is not very helpful, however, because of the high incidence of false-positive and false-negative results. A scintiscan using ^{99m}Tc-sulfur colloid has been used to quantitate gastroesophageal reflux. Several tests that involve the recording of the luminal pH of the esophagus with a small pH electrode have been proposed to detect and quantitate the reflux of gastric acid. In these tests, the pH electrode is swallowed, positioned in the stomach, gradually withdrawn across the LES, and then fixed at 5 cm above the sphincter. In the standard acid reflux test, a diagnosis of reflux can be made by failure of the pH to rise as the electrode enters the esophagus and by a decrease in esophageal pH with straining maneuvers. Quantitative information on acid reflux is obtained by ambulatory long-term (24-h) esophageal pH recording. The pH recordings are helpful only in the evaluation of acid reflux. The presence of bile or alkaline reflux is suggested by the occurrence of reflux symptoms in the absence of gastric acid and by the demonstration of bile in an aspirate of esophageal reflux fluid.

The *presence and complications of reflux esophagitis* are assessed by barium swallow, esophagoscopy, mucosal biopsy, and the Bernstein test. The results of barium swallow are usually normal in uncomplicated esophagitis but may reveal the complication of stricture or ulcer formation. A high esophageal peptic stricture, a deep ulcer, or adenocarcinoma suggest Barrett's esophagus. Uncomplicated Barrett's esophagus is not diagnosed reliably by barium studies. Esophagoscopy may reveal the presence of erosive esophagitis, distal peptic stricture, or a columnar-cell-lined lower esophagus with or without a proximally located peptic stricture, ulcer, or adenocarcinoma. Results of esophagoscopy may be normal in many patients with esophagitis; in such patients, mucosal biopsies and the Bernstein test are helpful. The mucosal biopsies should be performed at least 5 cm above the LES, because esophageal mucosal changes of chronic esophagitis are quite frequent in the most distal esophagus in otherwise normal subjects. Approximately 10 percent of biopsies yield a false-positive or false-negative result. Patients with Barrett's esophagus will show columnar mucosa lining the esophagus; the mucosa may be of a gastric fundic, cardiac, or specialized type. The Bernstein test consists of infusions of solutions of 0.1 *N* HCl and normal saline into the esophagus. It is useful in diagnosing reflux esophagitis that is not endoscopically obvious. In patients with reflux esophagitis, infusion of acid, but not of saline, reproduces the symptoms of heartburn. Infusion of acid in normal subjects usually produces no symptoms. Reflux esophagitis should be included in the differential diagnosis of chest pain, esophagitis, upper gastrointestinal bleeding, and dysphagia.

The *causative and predisposing factors* are assessed by the history and by studies of esophageal motility and esophageal clearance. Esophageal motility studies may provide useful quantitative information on the competence of the LES and on esophageal motor function. Barium swallow and scintiscans can be used to study esophageal clearance. An esophageal acid clearance test using a pH electrode quantifies the number of swallows necessary to clear the esophagus of 10 mL of instilled dilute 0.1 *N* HCl.

Full diagnostic evaluation is not necessary in every patient with reflux esophagitis. In transient and mild cases with a clear-cut history of reflux esophagitis, a therapeutic trial may be sufficient. In persistent cases and when the diagnosis is not clear, barium swallow, esophagoscopy, and esophageal motility with pH monitoring are indicated.

Patients with angina-like chest pain in whom coronary artery disease has been excluded may be investigated by the Bernstein test, 24-h ambulatory esophageal pH recording, and motility recording. Most of these patients are found to have reflux esophagitis, while a few have specific esophageal motor disorders. It also should be remembered that reflux esophagitis and nonspecific esophageal motility disorders frequently coexist with coronary artery disease.

℞ TREATMENT

The goals of treatment are to decrease gastroesophageal reflux, render the refluxate harmless, improve esophageal clearance, and protect the esophageal mucosa. These goals can be achieved by certain general measures and specific drug treatments. The management of uncomplicated cases generally includes weight reduction, sleeping with the head of the bed elevated by about 4 to 6 in with blocks, and elimination of factors that increase abdominal pressure. Patients should not smoke and should avoid consuming fatty foods, coffee, chocolate, alcohol, mint, orange juice, and certain medications (such as anticholinergic drugs, calcium channel blockers, and other smooth-muscle relaxants). They should also avoid ingesting of large quantities of fluids with meals. In mild cases, the use of H_2 receptor blocking agents (cimetidine, 300 mg; ranitidine, 150 mg; or famotidine, 20 mg) as needed may suffice.

In moderate to severe cases, the preceding measures are more strictly enforced. H_2 receptor blockers are used in higher doses (cimetidine, 300 mg qid; ranitidine, 150 mg bid; famotidine, 20 mg bid). If the patient does not respond fully, a prokinetic agent such as metoclopramide (10 mg) or cisapride (10 to 20 mg), taken 30 min before meals and at bedtime, is prescribed to raise sphincter pressure, hasten gastric emptying, and improve esophageal clearance. Metoclopramide may cause extrapyramidal central nervous system side effects. Inhibition of H^+,K^+-ATPase, the parietal cell pump that is responsible for acid secretion, with omeprazole (20 to 40 mg daily) is a most effective form of therapy that has been shown to heal erosive esophagitis. Reflux esophagitis requires prolonged therapy, for 3 to 6 months or longer if the disease recurs quickly. Patients with reflux esophagitis who have complications such as Barrett's esophagus (with or without a deep ulcer) should be treated vigorously. Patients who have an associated peptic stricture are treated with dilators to relieve dysphagia as well as with vigorous treatment for reflux. Patients who have specialized intestinal metaplasia must be monitored for the development of high-grade dysplasia and early adenocarcinoma, which must be treated if they occur. Monitoring consists of close follow-up with periodic endoscopic biopsies. Endoscopic surveillance is indicated every 1 to 2 years in patients without evidence of dysplasia; patients with dysplasia require more frequent surveillance. Suitable surgical candidates with high-grade dysplasia and early carcinoma are treated by esophagectomy and esophagogastric anastomosis.

Antireflux surgery, in which the gastric fundus is wrapped around the esophagus (fundoplication), increases the lower sphincter pressure and should be considered in patients with resistant and complicated reflux esophagitis that does not respond fully to medical therapy or in patients for whom long-term medical therapy is not desirable. Laproscopic fundoplication is used increasingly. In the ideal candidate for fundoplication, motility studies show persistently inadequate lower sphincter pressure but normal peristaltic contractions in the esophageal body.

Patients with alkaline esophagitis are treated with general antireflux measures and neutralization of bile salts with cholestyramine, aluminum hydroxide, or sucralfate. Sucralfate is particularly useful in these cases, as it also serves as a surface protector.

INFECTIOUS ESOPHAGITIS With the recent increase in the frequency of immunodeficiency states, infectious esophagitis has become increasingly important. Infectious esophagitis can be due to viral, bacterial, fungal, or parasitic organisms. In severely immunocompromised patients, multiple organisms may coexist.

Viral Esophagitis (See also Chap. 184) *Herpes simplex virus* (HSV) type 1 occasionally causes esophagitis in immunocompetent individuals, but either HSV type 1 or HSV type 2 may afflict patients who are immunosuppressed. These patients complain of an acute onset of chest pain, odynophagia, and dysphagia. Bleeding may occur in severe cases, and systemic manifestations such as nausea, vomiting, fever, chills, and mild leukocytosis may be present. Herpetic vesicles on the nose and lips sometimes provide a clue to the diagnosis. Barium swallow is inadequate to detect early lesions and cannot reliably distinguish HSV infection from other types of infections. Endoscopy shows vesicles and small, discrete, punched-out superficial ulcerations with or without a fibrinous exudate. In later stages, there is a diffuse erosive esophagitis caused by enlargement and coalescence of the ulcers. Mucosal cells from a biopsy sample taken at the edge of an ulcer or from a cytologic smear show ballooning degeneration, ground-glass changes in the nuclei with eosinophilic intranuclear inclusions (Cowdry type A), and giant cell formation on routine stains. Culture for HSV becomes positive within days and is helpful in diagnosis. For prophylaxis in a severely immunocompromised host, acyclovir, 800 mg orally twice daily or 250 mg per square meter of body surface every 12 h intravenously, is recommended. For treatment of esophagitis, intravenous therapy, 250 mg/m^2 every 8 h, is usually initiated. As swallowing improves, the therapy is changed to 200 to 400 mg orally five times daily. Symptoms usually resolve in 1 week, but large ulcerations may take longer to heal. Foscarnet (60 mg/kg intravenously every 8 h) may be useful if acyclovir resistance occurs. These patients also may have reflux esophagitis, which may worsen the symptoms and add to complications.

Varicella-zoster virus (VZV) (see also Chap. 185) sometimes produces esophagitis in children with chickenpox and adults with herpes zoster. Esophageal VZV also can be the source of disseminated VZV infection in the absence of skin involvement. In an immunocompromised host, VZV esophagitis causes vesicles and confluent ulcers and usually resolves spontaneously, but it may cause necrotizing esophagitis in a severely compromised host. On routine histologic examination of mucosal biopsy samples or cytology specimens, VZV is difficult to distinguish from HSV, but the distinction can be made immunohistologically or by culture. Acyclovir is effective in prevention and treatment of VZV esophagitis, but much higher doses are needed than for HSV.

Cytomegalovirus (CMV) infections occur only in immunocompromised patients. CMV is usually activated from a latent stage or may be acquired from blood product transfusions. CMV lesions initially appear as serpiginous ulcers in an otherwise normal mucosa. These may coalesce to form giant ulcers, particularly in the distal esophagus.

Patients present with painful swallowing, chest pain, hematemesis, nausea, and vomiting. Diagnosis requires endoscopy and biopsies of the center of the ulcer. Mucosal brushings are not useful. Routine histologic examination shows intranuclear and small intracytoplasmic inclusions in large fibroblasts and endothelial cells of blood vessels. Immunohistology with monoclonal antibodies to CMV and in situ hybridization of CMV DNA can be performed on centrifugation culture and are useful for early diagnosis. Ganciclovir (DHPG), 5 mg/kg every 12 h intravenously, is the treatment of choice. Foscarnet (60 mg/kg every 8 h intravenously) is used in resistant cases. Therapy is continued until healing, which may take weeks to months.

Human immunodeficiency virus (HIV) may be associated with a self-limited syndrome of acute esophageal ulceration associated with oral ulcers and a maculopapular skin rash, which occurs at the time of HIV seroconversion. Some patients with advanced disease have deep, persistent esophageal ulcers. They require treatment with oral steroids or thalidomide. Some ulcers respond to local steroid injection.

Bacterial Esophagitis *Bacterial esophagitis* is unusual, but esophagitis caused by *Lactobacillus* and beta-hemolytic streptococci has been described in the immunocompromised host. In profoundly granulocytopenic patients and in patients with cancer, bacterial esophagitis is often missed because it is commonly present with other organisms, including viruses and fungi, and because bacteria are difficult to identify on routine histologic examination. In patients with AIDS, infection with *Cryptosporidium* or *Pneumocystis carinii* may cause nonspecific inflammation, and *Mycobacterium tuberculosis* infection may cause deep ulcerations of the distal esophagus.

***Candida* Esophagitis** Many *Candida* species are normal commensals in the throat but become pathogenic and produce esophagitis in immunodeficiency states. Occasionally, monilial *Candida* esophagitis occurs in the absence of any predisposing factors. Patients may be asymptomatic or complain of odynophagia and dysphagia. Oral thrush or other evidence of mucocutaneous candidiasis may be absent. Rarely, *Candida* esophagitis is complicated by esophageal bleeding, perforation, and stricture or by systemic invasion. Results of barium swallow may be normal or may show multiple nodular filling defects of various sizes (Fig. 283-2). Large nodular defects may resemble clusters of grapes. Endoscopy shows small, yellow-white raised plaques with surrounding erythema in mild disease. In extensive disease, confluent linear and nodular plaques are seen. Diagnosis is made by demonstration of yeast or hyphal forms in plaque smears and exudate stained with Gram's, periodic acid–Schiff, or silver stains. Biopsy results usually are not positive. Culture is not useful in diagnosis but may be helpful in confirming the species and, if needed, the drug sensitivities of the yeast (see Chap. 209). In normal or minimally immunocompromised patients, nystatin or clotrimazole treatment is often successful. Nystatin is used as an oral suspension (100,000 units per milliliter) in doses of 10 to 20 mL every 6 h; clotrimazole is administered in the form of 10-mg tablets to be sucked five times a day. Ketoconazole (200 to 400 mg in a single daily oral dose) is an effective treatment; the higher dose is used in severely immunocompromised hosts. The bioavailability of ketoconazole is severely reduced at increased gastric pH; therefore, it should not be used concurrently with gastric acid suppression therapy or in achlorhydric subjects. Fluconazole (200 mg on the first day, followed by 100 mg daily) is the preferred treatment because its absorption is not affected by high gastric pH. Poorly responsive patients are treated with amphotericin, 10 to 15 mg as an intravenous infusion for 6 h daily to a total dose of 300 to 500 mg. Miconazole and amphotericin lozenges are currently not available in the United States. The treatment is for 7 to 10 days followed by nystatin, clotrimazole, ketoconazole, or fluconazole for as long as the host resistance remains low. In patients with AIDS and suspected *Candida* esophagitis, empirical treatment with fluconazole is often initiated.

OTHER TYPES OF ESOPHAGITIS *Radiation esophagitis* is a common occurrence during radiation treatment for lung, mediastinal, or esophageal carcinoma. The frequency and severity of esophagitis increase with the amount of radiation delivered to the area and with the subsequent use of certain chemotherapeutic agents, such as doxorubicin, bleomycin, cyclophosphamide, and cisplatin. Dysphagia and odynophagia may last several weeks to several months after the conclusion of therapy. The esophageal mucosa becomes erythematous, edematous, and friable. Superficial erosions coalesce to form larger superficial ulcers. Submucosal fibrosis and degenerative changes in the blood vessels, muscles, and myenteric neurons may be present. The treatment is relief of pain with viscous lidocaine during the acute phase; indomethacin treatment may lessen the radiation damage. Esophageal stricture may develop and require dilatation.

Corrosive esophagitis is caused by the ingestion of caustic agents, such as strong alkalies or acids. When severe, corrosive injury may lead to esophageal perforation, bleeding, and death. Steroids have not been shown to be useful in acute corrosive esophagitis. Healing is usually associated with stricture formation. Caustic strictures are usually long and rigid (Fig. 283-2) and generally require dilatation with dilators passed over a guidewire through the stricture. *Pill-induced esophagitis* is associated with the ingestion of certain pills and accounts for many cases of erosive esophagitis. Antibiotics such as doxycycline, tetracycline, and clindamycin account for over half the cases. Other commonly prescribed pills that cause esophageal injury include aspirin, potassium chloride, ferrous sulfate, quinidine, alprenolol, and various steroidal and nonsteroidal anti-inflammatory agents. Pill esophagitis can be prevented by having patients take pills in the upright position and wash them down with copious amounts of fluids.

Sclerotherapy for bleeding esophageal varices usually produces transient retrosternal chest pain and dysphagia; esophageal ulcer, stricture, hematoma, or perforation may occur. *Esophagitis associated with mucocutaneous and systemic diseases* is usually associated with blister and bulla formation, epithelial desquamation, and thin, weblike or dense esophageal strictures. Pemphigus vulgaris and bullous pemphigoid form intraepithelial and subepithelial bullae, respectively, and can be distinguished by specific immunohistology; they are both characterized by sloughing of epithelium or the presence of esophageal casts. Glucocorticoid treatment is usually effective. Dystrophic epidermolysis bullosa is an inherited disease that presents in childhood in which local trauma is associated with bulla formation and scarring. Cicatricial pemphigoid, Stevens-Johnson syndrome, and toxic epidermolysis bullosa can produce esophageal bullous lesions and strictures requiring gentle dilatation. Graft-versus-host disease occurs in patients who have received allogeneic bone marrow transplants and is associated with generalized desquamation and esophageal strictures. Behçet's disease and eosinophilic gastroenteritis may involve the esophagus and may respond to steroid therapy. Crohn's disease and an erosive lichen planus also can involve the esophagus, and Crohn's disease may cause inflammatory strictures, sinus tract, filiform polyps, and fistulas in the esophagus.

OTHER ESOPHAGEAL DISORDERS

DIVERTICULA Diverticula are outpouchings of the wall of the esophagus. A *Zenker's diverticulum* appears in the natural zone of weakness in the posterior hypopharyngeal wall and causes halitosis and regurgitation of saliva and food particles consumed several days previously. When it becomes large and filled with food, such a diverticulum can compress the esophagus and cause dysphagia or complete obstruction. Nasogastric intubation and endoscopy should be performed with utmost care in these patients, since they may cause perforation of the diverticulum. A *midesophageal diverticulum* may be caused by traction from old adhesions or by propulsion associated with esophageal motor abnormalities. An *epiphrenic diverticulum* may be associated with achalasia. Small or medium-sized diverticula and midesophageal and epiphrenic diverticula are usually asymptomatic. *Diffuse intramural diverticulosis* of the esophagus is due to dilation of the deep esophageal glands. This condition may lead to chronic candidiasis or to the development of a stricture high up in the esophagus. These patients may present with dysphagia. Symptomatic Zenker's diverticula are treated by cricopharyngeal myotomy with or without diverticulectomy. Very large symptomatic esophageal diverticula are removed surgically. When they are associated with motor abnormalities, distal myotomy is performed. Strictures associated with diffuse intramural diverticulosis are treated with rubber dilators.

WEBS AND RINGS Weblike constrictions of the esophagus are usually congenital or inflammatory in origin. Asymptomatic hypopharyngeal webs are demonstrated in up to 10 percent of normal individuals. When concentric, they cause intermittent dysphagia to solids. The combination of symptomatic hypopharyngeal webs and iron-deficiency anemia in middle-aged women constitutes *Plummer-Vinson syndrome*. The clinical importance of this syndrome is uncertain. Midesophageal webs are rare. A *lower esophageal mucosal ring* (Schatzki ring) is a thin, weblike constriction located at the squamocolumnar mucosal junction at or near the border of the LES (Fig. 283-2). It invariably produces dysphagia when the lumen diameter is less than 1.3 cm. Dysphagia to solids is the only symptom, and it is usually episodic. Asymptomatic rings may be present in about 10 percent of normal individuals. A lower esophageal ring is one of the common causes of dysphagia. Symptomatic webs and mucosal lower esophageal rings are easily treated by dilatation. A *lower esophageal muscular ring* (contractile ring) is located proximal to the site of mucosal rings and may represent an abnormal uppermost segment of the lower esophageal sphincter. These rings can be recognized by the fact that they are not constant in size and shape. They also may cause dysphagia and should be differentiated from peptic strictures, achalasia, and lower esophageal mucosal ring. They are treated by dilatation.

HIATAL HERNIA A *hiatal hernia* is a herniation of part of the stomach into the thoracic cavity through the esophageal hiatus in the diaphragm. A *sliding hiatal hernia* is one in which the gastroesophageal junction and fundus of the stomach slide upward. A sliding hernia may result from weakening of the anchors of the gastroesophageal junction to the diaphragm, from longitudinal contraction of the esophagus, or from increased intraabdominal pressure. Small sliding hernias can be demonstrated commonly during barium studies if intra-abdominal pressure is increased. Their incidence increases with age; in the sixth decade of life, the prevalence of such hernias is around 60 percent. It is unlikely that a small sliding hiatal hernia by itself produces any clinical symptoms, but it plays a role in the pathogenesis of reflux esophagitis. A *paraesophageal hernia* is one in which the esophagogastric junction remains fixed in its normal location and a pouch of stomach is herniated beside the gastroesophageal junction through the esophageal hiatus. A paraesophageal or mixed paraesophageal and sliding hernia may become incarcerated and strangulate. This situation leads to acute chest pain, dysphagia, and a mediastinal mass and requires prompt operative treatment. A herniated gastric pouch may cause dysphagia and may be the site of gastritis and ulceration causing chronic blood loss. A large paraesophageal hernia should be surgically repaired.

MECHANICAL TRAUMA *Esophageal rupture* may be caused by (1) iatrogenic damage from instrumentation of the esophagus or external trauma, (2) increased intraesophageal pressure associated with forceful vomiting or retching (*spontaneous rupture* or *Boerhaave's syndrome*), or (3) diseases of the esophagus such as corrosive esophagitis, esophageal ulcer, and neoplasm. The site of perforation depends on the cause. Instrumental perforation usually occurs in the pharynx or lower esophagus, often just above the diaphragm in the posterolateral wall. Esophageal perforation causes severe retrosternal chest pain, which may be worsened by swallowing and breathing. Free air enters the mediastinum and spreads to neighboring structures and causes palpable subcutaneous emphysema in the neck, mediastinal crackling sounds on auscultation, and pneumothorax. With time, secondary infection supervenes, and mediastinal abscess and pleuropulmonary suppurative complications may develop. Esophageal perforation associated with vomiting usually deposits gastric contents in the mediastinum and causes severe mediastinal complications. On the other hand, instrumental perforation may be clinically mild and free of severe complications. Spontaneous rupture of the esophagus may mimic myocardial infarction, pancreatitis, or rupture of an abdominal viscus. Symptoms of chest pain may be mild, particularly in the elderly. Mediastinal emphysema may develop late. An x-ray of the chest shows abnormalities in most patients, but computed tomography of the chest is more sensitive in detecting mediastinal air. Fluid from pleural effusions may have a high content of (salivary) amylase. The diagnosis is confirmed by swallow of radiopaque contrast material. Treatment includes esophageal and gastric suction and parenteral administration of broad-spectrum antibiotics. Surgical drainage and repair of the laceration should be performed as soon as possible. In patients with terminal carcinoma, surgical repair may not be feasible, and patients with minor instrumental perforation can be treated conservatively. Extensive corrosive damage may require esophageal diversion and subsequent excision of the damaged portion of the esophagus.

Mucosal Tear (Mallory-Weiss Syndrome) This tear is usually caused by vomiting, retching, or vigorous coughing. The tear usually involves the gastric mucosa just below the squamocolumnar mucosal junction. Patients present with upper gastrointestinal bleeding, which may be severe. In most patients bleeding ceases spontaneously; continued bleeding may respond to vasopressin therapy or angiographic embolization. Surgery is rarely needed.

Intramural Hematoma Emetogenic injury, particularly in patients with bleeding abnormalities, can cause bleeding between the mucosal and muscle layers of the esophagus. The patients develop sudden dysphagia. The diagnosis is made by barium swallow and computed tomography. Resolution is usually spontaneous.

FOREIGN BODIES Foreign bodies may lodge in the cervical esophagus just beyond the upper esophageal sphincter, near the aortic arch, or above the lower esophageal sphincter. Impaction of a bolus of food, particularly a piece of meat or bread, may occur when the esophageal lumen is narrowed due to stricture, carcinoma, or a lower esophageal ring. Acute impaction causes a complete inability to swallow and severe chest pain. Both foreign bodies and food boluses may be removed endoscopically. Use of a meat tenderizer to facilitate passage of an obstructed meat bolus is to be discouraged because of potential esophageal perforation and aspiration pneumonia.

For further discussion of cholinergic and anti-cholinergic agents and vasoconstrictors and vasodilators see Chaps. 7 and 32, in Goodman and Gilman's The Pharmacological Basis of Therapeutics, *9th ed, McGraw-Hill, New York, 1996.*

BIBLIOGRAPHY

ALLEN ML, DIMARINO AJ JR: Manometric diagnosis of diffuse esophageal spasm. Dig Dis Sci 41:1346, 1996

BOTT S et al: Medication-induced esophageal injury: Survey of the literature. Am J Gastroenterol 82:758, 1987

CONKLIN JL, CHRISTENSEN J: Neuromuscular control of the oropharynx and esophagus in health and disease. Annu Rev Med 45:13, 1994

DODDS WJ: The pathogenesis of gastroesophageal reflux disease. Am J Roentgenol 151:49, 1988

KLINKENBERG-KNOL EC et al: Long-term treatment with omeprazole for refractory reflux esophagitis: Efficacy and safety. Ann Intern Med 121:161, 1994

MITTAL RK et al: Transient lower esophageal sphincter relaxation. Gastroenterology 109:601, 1995

PASRICHA PH et al: Intrasphincteric botulinum toxin for treatment of achalasia. N Engl J Med 322:774, 1995

RICHTER JE et al: Esophageal chest pain: Current controversies in pathogenesis, diagnosis, and therapy. Ann Intern Med 110:66, 1989

RUBESIN SE: Oral and pharyngeal dysphagia. Gastroenterol Clin North Am 24:331, 1995

SINGARAM C et al: Nitrinergic and peptidergic innervation of the human esophagus. Gut 35:1690, 1994

SPECHLER SJ, GOYAL RK: Barrett's esophagus. N Engl J Med 315:362, 1986

——— et al: Prevalence of metaplasia at the gastroesophageal junction. Lancet 344:1533, 1994

SUTTON FM et al: Infectious esophagitis. Gastrointest Endosc Clin North Am 4:713, 1994

VAEZI MF et al: Role of acid and duodenogastric reflux in esophageal mucosal injury: A review of animal and human studies. Gastroenterology 108:1897, 1995

WEBB WA: Management of foreign bodies of the upper gastrointestinal tract: Update. Gastrointest Endosc 41:39, 1995

WILCOX CM et al: Esophageal ulceration in human immunodeficiency virus infection. Causes, response to therapy, and long-term outcome. Ann Intern Med 123:143, 1995

284

Lawrence S. Friedman, Walter L. Peterson

PEPTIC ULCER AND RELATED DISORDERS*

A peptic ulcer is a mucosal lesion of the stomach or duodenum in which acid and pepsin play major pathogenic roles. The major forms of peptic ulcer are duodenal ulcer (DU) and gastric ulcer (GU), both of which are chronic diseases often caused by the bacterium *Helicobacter pylori*. *H. pylori* is also an important risk factor for gastric cancer and certain types of gastric lymphoma. The term *peptic ulcer* also encompasses GUs and DUs associated with stress or the ingestion of drugs, most commonly aspirin and other nonsteroidal anti-inflammatory drugs (NSAIDs). Ulcer associated with the Zollinger-Ellison syndrome (ZES), caused by gastrin-secreting islet cell tumors (gastrinomas), is also considered a form of peptic ulcer.

Although our knowledge of the cause of peptic ulcer is incomplete, available information supports a central role for *H. pylori* and a necessary role for acid and pepsin. Whether an ulcer develops depends on the balance between aggressive factors (principally gastric acid and pepsin) and factors that participate in mucosal defense or resistance to ulceration. Peptic ulcer results when gastroduodenal mucosal defenses are unable to protect the epithelium from the corrosive effects of acid and pepsin.

In the past, ideas concerning the pathogenesis of peptic ulcer focused on the role of acid and pepsin, but recent observations suggest that many of the reported abnormalities of gastric acid secretion in patients with peptic ulcer may be a direct consequence of infection with *H. pylori*. Nevertheless, an understanding of basic gastric physiology remains central to a consideration of ulcer pathogenesis.

GASTRIC PHYSIOLOGY RELATED TO PEPTIC ULCER

Aggressive Factors: Acid and Pepsin The gastric mucosa has an extraordinary capacity to secrete acid. The parietal cells scattered along the course of the mucosal glands (oxyntic mucosa) of the body and fundus of the stomach secrete hydrochloric acid by a process involving oxidative phosphorylation (Fig. 284-1). The estimated concentration of HCl secreted by parietal cells is approximately 160 m*M*. Each secreted hydrogen ion (H^+) is accompanied by a chloride ion (Cl^-). For each hydrogen ion secreted into the gastric lumen, one bicarbonate ion (HCO_3^-) is released into the gastric venous circulation, accounting for the so-called alkaline tide; bicarbonate is released from carbonic acid generated from carbon dioxide by parietal cell carbonic anhydrase. The final step in hydrogen ion secretion is accomplished by an H^+,K^+-ATPase "proton pump" located in the apical microvillus membrane and tubovesicular apparatus of the parietal cell. This H^+,K^+-ATPase exchanges hydrogen for potassium across the microvillus membrane.

Multiple chemical, neural, and hormonal factors participate in the regulation of gastric acid secretion. Acid secretion is stimulated by gastrin and by postganglionic vagal fibers via muscarinic cholinergic receptors on parietal cells. Gastrin, the most potent known stimulant of gastric acid secretion, is contained in and released into the circulation from cytoplasmic secretory granules of gastrin cells (G cells), which are scattered singly or in small clusters among the epithelial lining cells of the middle and deeper portions of the pyloric glands of the antrum. Gastrin release is stimulated by the neuropeptide gastrin-releasing peptide and inhibited by somatostatin produced by D cells in the antrum. Gastrin in tissues and in the circulation exists in several molecular forms. The principal form of gastrin in gastric antral mucosa is heptadecapeptide gastrin (G-17), which contains 17 amino acid residues; the active site region is the C-terminal tetrapeptide amide (Trp-Met-Asp-Phe-NH_2). Gastrin II is the form in which the tyrosyl residue at position 12 is sulfated, while gastrin I is the nonsulfated form. Although G-17 accounts for more than 90 percent of the gastrin in antral mucosa, approximately two-thirds of the gastrin in serum is a larger species containing 34 amino acids (G-34). Although G-17 has a shorter half-life than G-34, circulating G-17 is approximately as potent as G-34 in stimulating gastric acid

* James McGuigan, M.D., was the author of this chapter in the 13th edition.

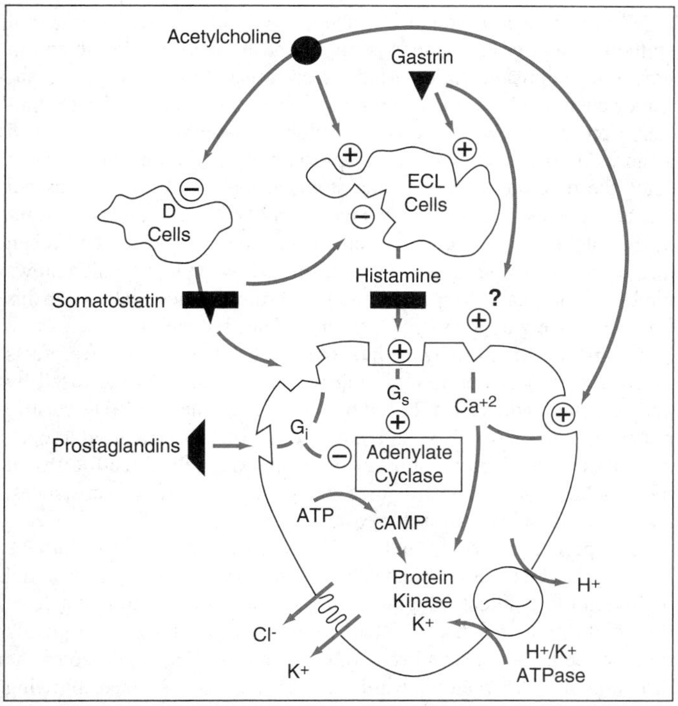

FIGURE 284-1 Biology of the parietal cell. G_i and G_s, inhibitory and stimulatory G protein subunits; ECL, enterochromaffin-like.

secretion. Gastrin is also present in duodenal mucosa, particularly in the most proximal duodenum (at approximately 10 percent of the antral concentration). The mucosal concentration of gastrin and the proportion of G-17 decrease progressively down the duodenum.

The effects of gastrin and vagal stimulation on gastric acid secretion are intimately interrelated. Vagal stimulation increases gastric acid secretion by cholinergic stimulation of parietal cell secretion, by enhancing release of gastrin from antral G cells (by both inhibition of the release of somatostatin by antral D cells and by direct stimulation of G cells), and by lowering the parietal cell threshold for response to circulating gastrin concentrations.

The gastric mucosa contains large amounts of histamine contained in cytoplasmic granules of mast cells and enterochromaffin-like (ECL) cells; the latter are epithelial endocrine cells distributed singly in the oxyntic glands, often in direct contact with parietal cells. Recognition of the role of histamine in acid secretion was fostered by discovery of H_2 receptor antagonists that competitively inhibit the action of histamine on H_2 receptors, which are located on gastric parietal, cardiac atrial, and uterine smooth-muscle cells. These drugs exert negligible effects on H_1 receptors, which are inhibited readily by conventional antihistamines (H_1 receptor antagonists). H_2 receptor antagonists (e.g., cimetidine, ranitidine, famotidine, and nizatidine) inhibit basal acid secretion as well as secretion in response to feeding, gastrin, histamine, hypoglycemia, or vagal stimulation. Histamine is the most important stimulant of gastric acid secretion and is released from ECL cells by the action of both gastrin and cholinergic activity.

The basolateral membranes of parietal cells contain receptors for histamine, gastrin, and acetylcholine that stimulate acid secretion and for prostaglandins and somatostatin that inhibit acid secretion (Fig. 284-1). The parietal cell histamine receptor is a membrane-spanning G protein-coupled receptor. Histamine stimulates gastric acid secretion by increasing parietal cell cyclic adenosine monophosphate (AMP), thereby activating cyclic AMP–dependent protein kinase(s). Gastrin stimulates gastric acid secretion by direct stimulation of parietal cells and by stimulation of histamine release from ECL cells. Gastrin and acetylcholine do not stimulate cyclic AMP production but, instead, stimulate acid secretion by increasing parietal cell cytosolic calcium. Prostaglandins and somatostatin act through inhibitory G proteins that decrease the generation of cyclic AMP; somatostatin also inhibits histamine release from ECL cells.

The major physiologic stimulus for gastric acid secretion is ingestion of food. Traditionally, regulation of gastric acid secretion has been classified into three phases: cephalic, gastric, and intestinal. This classification is of some value in analyzing factors that participate in regulation of gastric acid secretion. The cephalic phase encompasses the gastric acid secretory response to the sight, smell, taste, and anticipation of food; the gastric phase is induced by food in the stomach; and the intestinal phase occurs after entry of food into the lumen of the small intestine. The cephalic phase, which includes cortical and hypothalamic components, is mediated primarily by vagal activation, which increases gastric acid secretion principally by direct stimulation of ECL and parietal cells and to a lesser extent by promoting gastrin release. The gastric phase results from stimulation of chemical and mechanical receptors in the gastric wall by luminal contents. Mechanical distention of the stomach stimulates gastric acid secretion but results in little gastrin release; this mechanical effect is inhibited by atropine and appears to be mediated by vagal reflexes. Food (principally protein and the products of protein digestion) in the stomach promotes gastric acid secretion by increasing gastrin release. Food in the proximal small intestine stimulates the intestinal phase of gastric acid secretion by inducing the release of small amounts of gastrin and other peptides that stimulate gastric acid secretion and by a direct effect of absorbed amino acids on parietal cells. Basal or interdigestive gastric acid secretion can be considered to be a fourth phase of acid secretion. This phase is unrelated to feeding and reaches its peak around midnight and its lowest point about 7 A.M.; neural pathways are probably most important in its regulation.

Ingestion of both caffeine-containing and caffeine-free coffee stimulates gastric acid secretion by stimulating gastrin release. Ingestion of beer and wine also stimulate gastric acid secretion, presumably owing to the effects of amines and other congeners, because pure ethanol is a weak stimulant of acid secretion. Intravenous calcium stimulates gastric acid secretion and produces minimal increases in serum gastrin levels. Oral calcium has been reported to stimulate gastric acid secretion directly, i.e., without an increase in serum calcium or gastrin concentrations. Except in patients who harbor a gastrinoma, hypercalcemia is not usually associated with gastric acid hypersecretion or with an increase in serum gastrin.

Gastric acid secretion can be inhibited by acid in the stomach or duodenum, by hyperglycemia, or by hypertonic fluids or fat in the duodenum. Reduction of the intragastric pH to 3.0 produces partial inhibition of gastrin release; further reduction to pH 1.5 or below completely blocks release of gastrin in response to almost all stimuli. Somatostatin appears to play an important role in this acid-induced feedback inhibition of gastrin release. Somatostatin-containing antral mucosal endocrine cells (D cells) have cytoplasmic processes that extend to neighboring gastrin cells and to parietal cells. Somatostatin reduces gastric acid secretion by inhibiting gastrin release, by directly inhibiting parietal cell secretion, and by inhibiting the release of histamine by ECL cells. Acid in the duodenum decreases gastric acid secretion by the stomach, most likely by stimulating release into the circulation of intestinal peptides such as secretin that inhibit gastric acid secretion. Fat in the duodenum also inhibits gastric acid secretion; gastric inhibitory peptide (GIP) has been proposed as a candidate for this action. The mechanisms by which hyperglycemia or intraduodenal hyperosmolality inhibit gastric acid secretion are not known. Additional small intestinal mucosal peptides possessing the capacity to inhibit gastric acid secretion include vasoactive intestinal peptide (VIP), enteroglucagon, neurotensin, peptide YY, and urogastrone, but the extent to which these peptides contribute to the physiologic regulation of gastric acid secretion has not been defined.

The proteolytic effects of pepsins in concert with the corrosive properties of secreted gastric acid contribute to the tissue injury that produces peptic ulcer. Gastric acid catalyzes the cleavage of inactive pepsinogen molecules, converting them to proteolytically active pepsins, and also provides the low pH required for pepsin activity. Pepsins are maximally active at a pH of approximately 2.0, have substantially reduced activity above a pH of 4.0, and are irreversibly inactivated and denatured at neutral or alkaline pH. A variety of pepsinogens and their respective active pepsins are present in gastric juice. Pepsinogens (and their corresponding pepsins) have been classified by immunochemical techniques as either pepsinogen I or A (comprising pepsinogens 1 through 5) or pepsinogen II or C (comprising pepsinogens 6 and 7). Pepsinogen I is found in chief and mucous cells in the body and fundus of the stomach. Pepsinogen II is located in mucous cells in the body and fundus as well as in cells of the pyloric glands, cells of Brunner's glands of the duodenum, and mucous cells of the gastric cardiac glands. Both pepsinogen I and pepsinogen II are present in plasma, whereas only pepsinogen I is detected in urine. In general, there is a direct correlation between pepsinogen I serum concentrations and maximal gastric acid secretion. Most agents that stimulate gastric acid secretion also stimulate pepsinogen secretion; cholinergic action is particularly potent in promoting pepsinogen secretion. However, secretin inhibits gastric acid secretion but stimulates pepsinogen secretion.

In addition to secretion of hydrochloric acid, parietal cells also secrete intrinsic factor. Agents that stimulate gastric acid secretion also lead to secretion of intrinsic factor.

Measurement of Gastric Acid Secretion Gastric acid output is measured by collecting four consecutive 15-min samples to determine the 1-h basal acid output (BAO). Secretion volume and acid concentration (titrated with sodium hydroxide to pH 7.0 or calculated by formula from the pH of the aspirated gastric juice) are measured. Pentagastrin (which contains the biologically active C-terminal tetrapeptide amide portion of gastrin) is the preferred agent to stimulate maximal acid output (MAO) by the stomach. Following collection of basal acid secretion, gastric juice is collected for four additional consecutive 15-min periods after the subcutaneous injection of pentagastrin (6 μg/kg). The MAO is the amount of acid aspirated during the 1 h after pentagastrin administration. Peak acid output (PAO) is calculated by combining the two highest consecutive 15-min acid outputs following pentagastrin injection and multiplying by 2.

Measurement of basal and stimulated gastric acid secretion was used in the past in the clinical assessment of some patients with peptic ulcer and is still used as a research tool. The range of values for normal subjects is extremely broad and overlaps substantially with those for patients with DU, GU, and even ZES. Mean BAO in normal males without known ulcer disease is about 0.8 μmol/s (2 to 3 mEq/h). Mean MAO in normal males is about 6.4 μmol/s (23 mEq/h). In general, basal and stimulated acid outputs in females are approximately two-thirds to three-fourths those found in males. In patients with DU, the mean BAO averages 1 to 1.7 μmol/s (4 to 6 mEq/h) and the mean MAO is 8 to 11 μmol/s (30 to 40 mEq/h), again with wide variation. Patients with GU tend to have acid secretory rates that are normal or often slightly less than those for normal subjects. Whether variations in acid output from normal in patients with peptic ulcer reflect the effects of *H. pylori* infection is controversial, but the preponderance of evidence suggests that slight gastric acid hypersecretion persists in many patients with DU after eradication of *H. pylori* (see below).

Measurement of gastric acid output may be of value in selected clinical situations, particularly when ZES is suspected. Specifically, when hypergastrinemia is identified, measurement of gastric acid output will distinguish between clinical conditions characterized by gastric acid hypersecretion (e.g., ZES) and those that involve achlorhydria (e.g., atrophic gastritis associated with pernicious anemia).

Mucosal Defense The mechanisms by which the normal stomach and duodenum resist the corrosive effects of acid and pepsin (i.e., the mechanisms of mucosal resistance to injury or mucosal defense) have not been defined completely. However, a variety of factors have been identified that contribute to or compromise mucosal defense (Fig. 284-2).

Gastric mucus secreted by mucous cells of the gastric mucosal epithelium and gastric glands is important in mucosal defense and in preventing peptic ulceration. Mucus secretion is stimulated by mechanical or chemical irritation and by cholinergic stimulation. Gastric mucus is present in two phases: in a soluble phase in gastric juice and as an insoluble mucus gel layer, approximately 0.2 mm thick, which coats the mucosal surface of the stomach. Normally, the mucus gel is secreted constantly by gastric mucous epithelial cells and is continuously solubilized by pepsins secreted into the gastric lumen. When intact, the mucus gel serves as an unstirred water layer which slows ionic diffusion and is impermeable to macromolecules such as pepsins (molecular weight, 34,000). Pepsin molecules secreted into the gastric lumen are denied return by the intact mucus gel, which thereby protects mucosal cells from proteolytic injury. Gel thickness is increased by the E prostaglandins and reduced by aspirin and other NSAIDs. Gastric mucus glycoproteins also contain antigenic determinants used to classify AB(O) blood group substances. Approximately three-fourths of the population secrete gastric juice containing these AB(O) substances, and such individuals are referred to as secretors.

Nonparietal gastric epithelial cells secrete bicarbonate ions into the mucus gel, which help to create a microenvironment with a substantial hydrogen ion gradient, ranging from pH 1 to 2 in the luminal side of the gel layer to pH 6 to 7 in the zone in contact with the gastric mucosal cells. As an unstirred water layer, the mucus gel slows the diffusion of hydrogen ion toward the gastric mucosal surface, allowing buffering by bicarbonate within the gel. Gastric bicarbonate secretion is stimulated by calcium, certain prostaglandins of the E and F series, cholinergic agents, and dibutyryl cyclic guanosine monophosphate. It is inhibited by aspirin and NSAIDs, acetazolamide, alpha-adrenergic agents, and ethanol.

Normally, the luminal surfaces and intercellular tight junctions of the gastric epithelial cells create a gastric mucosal barrier that is almost completely impermeable to diffusion of hydrogen ions from the lumen. This barrier can be interrupted by bile acids, salicylates, ethanol, and weak organic acids, permitting hydrogen ions to diffuse into gastric tissue. The result may be cell injury, release of histamine from mast cells, further stimulation of acid secretion, damage to small blood vessels, mucosal hemorrhage, and erosion or ulceration. Interruption of the gastric mucosal barrier appears to contribute to the hemorrhagic erosive gastropathy associated with salicylate or ethanol ingestion and with other forms of gastric mucosal injury. Because of the high metabolic activity and substantial oxygen requirements of the gastric mucosa, maintenance of normal blood flow to the gastric mucosa is an essential component of mucosal resistance to injury. Decreased mucosal blood flow, accompanied by diffusion of luminal hydrogen

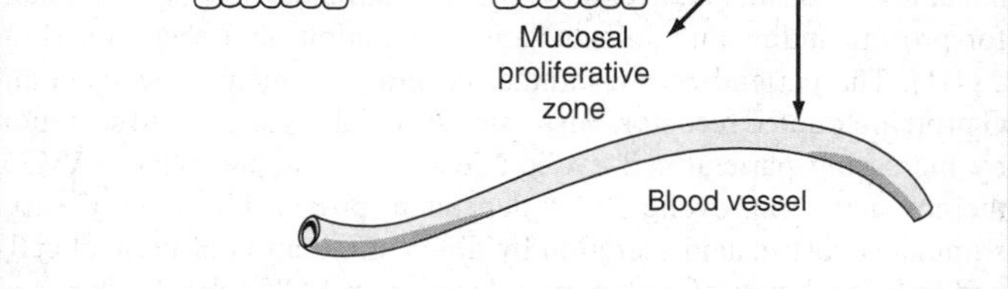

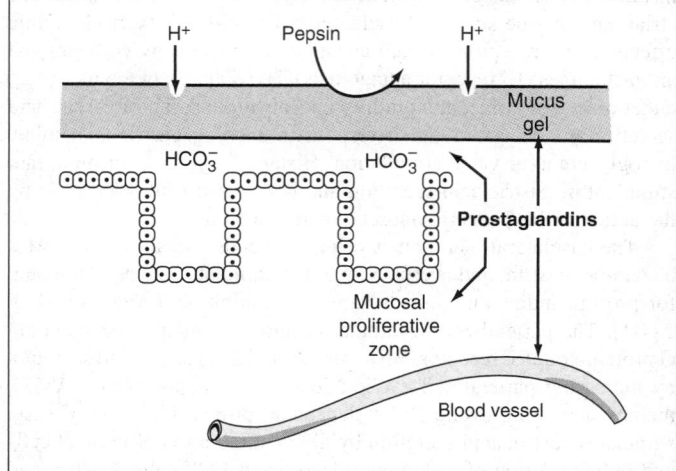

FIGURE 284-2 Gastric mucosal defense mechanisms. These include stimulation of secretion of mucus by gastric glands and of biocarbonate by gastric epithelial cells, epithelial cell renewal, and the gastric microcirculation, which provides nutrients to cells. Administration of prostaglandins enhances all of these mechanisms.

ions, is thought to be important in producing gastric mucosal damage.

Prostaglandins are abundant in the gastric mucosa. Administration to animals of various prostaglandins, particularly those of the E series, has been shown to prevent gastric mucosal injury caused by a wide variety of agents. Endogenous prostaglandins stimulate secretion of gastric mucus and gastric and duodenal mucosal bicarbonate. They participate in the maintenance of gastric mucosal blood flow and of the integrity of the gastric mucosal barrier and promote epithelial cell renewal in response to mucosal injury.

DUODENAL ULCER

DU is characteristically a chronic and recurrent disease. In contrast to erosions, which are superficial and limited to the mucosa, DUs are usually deep and sharply demarcated. They penetrate through the mucosa and submucosa, often into the muscularis propria. The ulcer floor contains no intact epithelium and usually consists of a zone of eosinophilic necrosis resting on a base of granulation tissue surrounded by variable amounts of fibrosis. The ulcer bed may be clear or may contain blood or a proteinaceous exudate with entrapped erythrocytes and acute and chronic inflammatory cells.

More than 95 percent of DUs occur in the first portion of the duodenum, and approximately 90 percent of those are located within 3 cm of the junction of the pyloric and duodenal mucosa. DUs are usually less than 1 cm in diameter; rarely, they are extremely large, 3 to 6 cm in diameter ("giant DUs"), and may be mistaken radiographically for the entire duodenal bulb.

The prevalence of DU is estimated to range from 6 to 15 percent of Western populations. During the past 40 years, the frequency of DU has been decreasing in the United States and England, especially in males. The reasons for this reduction are not known but are likely to relate to the changing epidemiology of *H. pylori* (see below). DUs now appear to be approximately as common in males as in females. Current estimates suggest that approximately 10 percent of the population has clinical evidence of DU at some time in their lives. The natural history of untreated DU consists of spontaneous healing and recurrence; at least 60 percent of healed DUs recur within 1 year, and 80 to 90 percent recur within 2 years.

ETIOLOGY AND PATHOGENESIS Peptic ulcer disease is thought to result from an imbalance between aggressive factors, especially gastric acid and pepsin, and protective factors, including gastric mucus, bicarbonate, and prostaglandins. Evidence that *H. pylori* plays a principal role in the pathogenesis of peptic ulcer disease is compelling. Indeed, infection with *H. pylori* is associated with a greatly increased risk of duodenal and gastric ulceration: from 95 to 100 percent of patients with DU and 75 to 85 percent of patients with GU (including virtually all cases not associated with NSAIDs) harbor the organism. Nested case-controlled studies in which IgG antibodies to *H. pylori* were measured in stored serum samples have demonstrated that preexisting *H. pylori* infection increases the risk of the subsequent development of either DU or GU; the level of antibody in serum correlates positively with the risk of DU and GU. On the other hand, only 15 to 20 percent of persons infected with *H. pylori* will develop an ulcer in their lifetimes, implying that additional pathogenic factors must be involved.

HELICOBACTER PYLORI *H. pylori* is a short (0.2 to 0.5 μm long), spiral-shaped, microaeropbilic gram-negative bacillus which invariably causes chronic active gastritis. With gastric colonization, *H. pylori* is found primarily in the deep portions of the mucus gel layer that coats the gastric mucosa and between the mucus gel layer and the apical surfaces of the gastric mucosal epithelial cells. *H. pylori* may adhere to the luminal surfaces of gastric epithelial cells but does not invade the gastric mucosa.

Pathophysiology *H. pylori* produces a variety of proteins that appear to mediate or facilitate its damaging effects on the gastric mucosa. Urease produced by *H. pylori* catalyzes the hydrolysis of urea to ammonia and carbon dioxide. Production of urease is required for gastric colonization by *H. pylori* and may protect *H. pylori* from

the effects of gastric acid, which normally prevents gastric colonization by other bacteria. Hydroxide ions generated by the equilibration of water with ammonia may contribute to gastric mucosal epithelial damage. *H. pylori* produces surface proteins that are chemotactic for human neutrophils and monocytes and secretes platelet-activating factor, which is also proinflammatory. *H. pylori* activates monocytes which express HLA-DR and interleukin 2 receptors on their cell surface and produce superoxides, interleukin 1, and tumor necrosis factor. The organism also produces proteases and phospholipases, which degrade the glycoprotein-lipid complex of the mucus gel layer. This activity reduces the thickness and viscosity of the mucus gel overlying the gastric mucosal epithelial cells, in spite of increased mucus synthesis and secretion. *H. pylori* produces an adhesin that facilitates its attachment to gastric epithelial cells. Different strains of *H. pylori* are thought to exist, and it has been proposed that only strains that have the cytotoxin-associated gene *cagA* and/or a 120-kDa vacuolating cytotoxin are associated with DU formation. In addition, there is some evidence that the likelihood of DU formation increases with increasing density of *H. pylori* (and hence urease activity) in the antrum.

Epidemiology In the United States, healthy persons under age 30 have prevalence rates of gastric colonization with *H. pylori* of approximately 10 percent. The prevalence of gastric colonization increases with age, with persons over age 60 having colonization rates that are approximately equal to their age. In contrast, in developing countries, *H. pylori* is generally acquired in childhood. Rates of *H. pylori* infection increase with deprived socioeconomic circumstances and also are increased in custodial institutions; they have been reported to be higher in black and Hispanic Americans. Transmission of *H. pylori* appears to be direct, from person to person; fecal-oral, oral-oral, and gastric-oral routes of transmission have been postulated. The risk of *H. pylori* infection is declining in developed countries, as is the risk of peptic ulcer. Most patients with gastric colonization by *H. pylori* never develop ulceration and remain asymptomatic.

Diagnosis *H. pylori* can be identified in gastric mucosal samples by histologic examination, culture, and detection of urease activity (Table 284-1). On stained tissue sections, *H. pylori* is positive for Giemsa and Warthin-Starry stains and faintly positive for hematoxylin. The organisms can be cultured successfully from biopsy samples but usually not from gastric secretions. *H. pylori* produces large amounts of urease. The rapid urease test of gastric biopsy material is a relatively simple and reliable method for presumptive identification of *H. pylori*. A positive test results from an increase in pH, with the phenol red indicator turning from light orange to red. The test is inexpensive, with a sensitivity of at least 90 percent and a specificity approaching 100 percent.

A urea breath test using ^{13}C or ^{14}C also has been developed for identifying *H. pylori* on the basis of urease production with release of labeled CO_2 (Fig. 284-3). This test has a sensitivity of 90 to 95 percent and a specificity of 98 to 99 percent.

Table 284-1

Diagnostic Tests for *Helicobacter pylori*

Test	Sensitivity (%)	Comments
Urease assay		
Breath	90–95	Simple; may be used to monitor therapy
Biopsy	90–98	Requires endoscopy
Histology	70–99	Requires endoscopy; may require special stains
Culture	70–95	Requires endoscopy; may be essential if antibiotic resistance emerges
Serology	95	Does not differentiate between active and remote infection; epidemiologic tool; titer decreases slowly after eradication

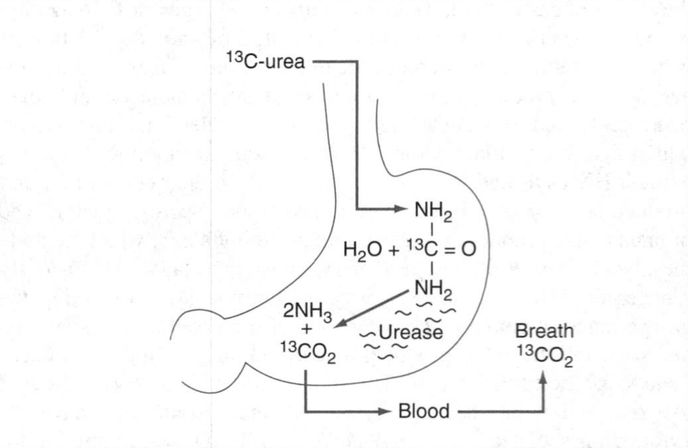

FIGURE 284-3 The urea breath test. Radiolabeled carbon dioxide is detectable in expired air after oral ingestion of radiolabeled urea in the presence of gastric urease produced by *H. pylori*.

Antibodies (IgG and IgA) to *H. pylori* have been identified in sera of individuals with *H. pylori* colonization. Serology is now used widely for routine detection of *H. pylori*. An enzyme-linked immunosorbent assay (ELISA) is the most commonly used serologic method, and a variety of diagnostic kits are available commercially. Compared with endoscopic detection of *H. pylori* infection, the ELISA has proved to be sensitive and specific and is particularly suited for epidemiologic studies. There is a high degree of correlation between the presence of serum antibodies and histologic evidence of gastritis.

Implications of Treatment The most compelling evidence for the role of *H. pylori* in the pathogenesis of peptic ulcer is that the 1-year relapse rate for DUs is less than 15 percent following therapy that successfully eradicates *H. pylori* but 70 to 80 percent after treatment only with H_2 receptor antagonists (see below) (Fig. 284-4). However, it should be emphasized that most persons with *H. pylori* infection never develop symptomatic DU or GU, suggesting that other factors have a role in the pathogenesis of peptic ulceration.

OTHER PATHOGENIC FACTORS It has long been observed that DU patients as a group secrete more acid than normal; however, most individual DU patients have acid secretory rates (BAO and MAO) within the normal range. In response to stimulation of gastric acid secretion, DU patients as a group also have comparable increases in gastric secretion of pepsin and in serum PGI levels. The variations in both groups are so large that most DU patients are in the normal range.

At initiation of infection by *H. pylori*, there may be a transient increase in gastric acid secretion. This phase is often followed by hypochlorhydria lasting for several months, after which rates of acid secretion return within a year to approximately their preinfection levels. Subsequently, *H. pylori* infection may be associated with an increase in basal and meal-stimulated serum gastrin levels, presumably owing to chronic antral inflammation. Somatostatin deficiency has been proposed as the mechanism responsible for enhanced gastrin release in patients with *H. pylori* infection, in whom gastric mucosal somatostatin levels are reduced and are correlated inversely with gastric luminal ammonia. An associated increase in gastric acid secretion (BAO and MAO in response to gastrin) in patients with DU has been attributed to an increase in parietal cell mass caused by the increased gastrin release, but a similar increase in gastric acid secretion is generally not observed in patients infected with *H. pylori* but without a DU, even though gastrin levels may be elevated. Therefore, increased gastric acid secretion in DU patients may be dependent on factors other than *H. pylori* infection. With eradication of *H. pylori*, the serum gastrin level and BAO slowly return to normal, but MAO in response to gastrin may remain mildly elevated.

The stomach tends to empty more rapidly in DU patients than in non-DU patients. This phenomenon, when coupled with relative gastric acid hypersecretion, may contribute to a greater rate of acid delivery to the first part of the duodenum in DU patients. In patients with DU and *H. pylori* infection, acidification of the proximal duodenum results in a smaller secretion of bicarbonate into the lumen by duodenal mucosal cells than in subjects not infected with *H. pylori*. Moreover, acidification of the proximal duodenum may lead to gastric metaplasia of the duodenal mucosa and subsequent colonization by *H. pylori*, which may in turn lead to ulcer formation.

A role for genetic factors in DU is suspected. DUs are approximately three times as common in first-degree relatives of DU patients than in the general population, although this finding may reflect a higher rate of *H. pylori* infection rather than genetic susceptibility. Patients with DUs have an increased frequency of blood group O and of the nonsecretor status [absence of secretion of AB(O) blood group antigens into the gastric juice], but these associations are weak. Moreover, the association with blood group O may relate to preferential binding of group O antigens to *H. pylori*. An increased incidence of HLA-B5 antigen has been reported in white male subjects with DU. Because the MAO in response to gastrin generally does not return to normal after eradication of *H. pylori* in patients with DU, despite return of serum gastrin elevations to normal, it is possible that at least some DU patients have an unusually large parietal cell mass (and hence MAO) on a genetic basis.

Cigarette smoking has been associated with an increased incidence of DU, a decreased response to DU therapy, and an increased mortality rate from DU. Although cigarette smoking does not increase gastric acid secretion, the increased incidence of DU among cigarette smokers may be due to inhibition of pancreatic bicarbonate secretion by nicotine or cigarette smoke, to accelerated emptying of gastric acid into the

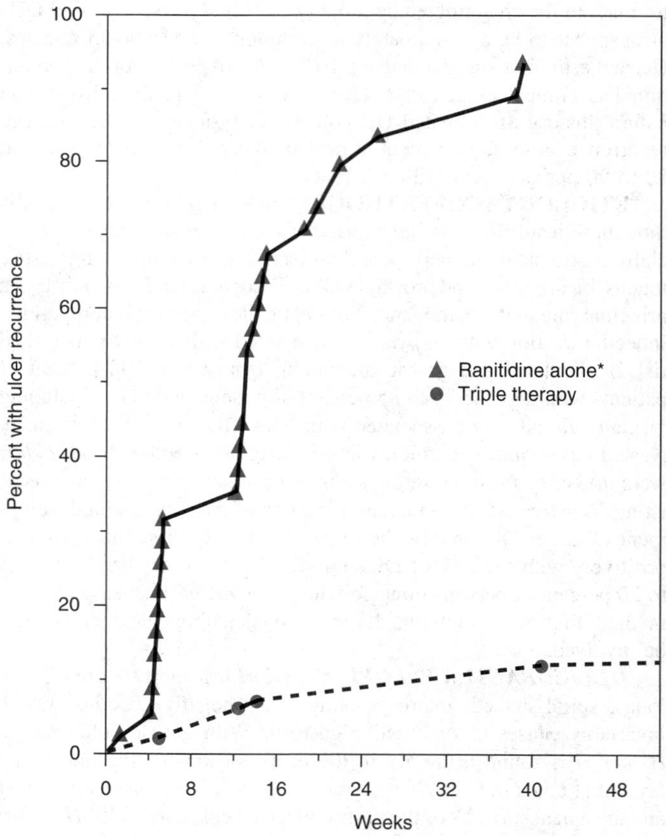

FIGURE 284-4 Lifetime recurrence of duodenal ulcers for the year after successful healing with an H-2 receptor antagonist alone or triple therapy plus an H-2 receptor antagonist. No maintenance therapy was given; the recurrence rate of ulcers in patients healed with an H-2 receptor antagonist alone was significantly greater ($p < 0.01$) than in those who received triple therapy plus a histamine-2 receptor antagonist. *(From DY Graham et al., 1992, with permission.)*

duodenum, or to a predisposition to (or association with) *H. pylori* infection.

The incidence of DU appears to be increased in patients with chronic renal failure, alcoholic cirrhosis, renal transplantation, hyperparathyroidism, systemic mastocytosis, and chronic obstructive pulmonary disease. Antibodies to herpes simplex have been reported to be present more often and in higher titers in sera of patients with DU than in normal subjects.

The importance of psychological factors in the pathogenesis of DU remains controversial. Contrary to earlier views, there is no typical DU personality. Chronic anxiety and psychological stress may, however, be factors in exacerbation of ulcer activity.

DU is uncommon before age 15, but GU may develop in children as young as age 5. It has been proposed that DU develops only in persons who acquire *H. pylori* infection at the end of childhood or later, because parietal cell mass is conserved after that point (see below).

CLINICAL FEATURES Epigastric pain is the most frequent DU symptom. The pain is often described as sharp, burning, or gnawing. However, it may be ill-defined, boring, or aching or may be perceived as abdominal pressure or fullness or as a hunger sensation. In approximately 10 percent of patients, the pain is located to the right of the epigastrium. The pain of DU characteristically occurs 90 min to 3 h after eating and frequently awakens the patient at night. It is usually relieved within a few minutes by food or antacids, presumably as a result of partial neutralization of gastric acid. However, ingestion of food leading to transient partial neutralization of gastric acid is followed by a rebound of gastrin release, resulting again in stimulation of acid secretion. With subsequent gastric emptying and increasing gastric acid secretion, the pH in the stomach and first portion of the duodenum becomes low enough to cause recurrent pain. Acid-induced pain in DU patients is believed to be due to acid stimulation of chemical receptors and/or alterations in gastric motility.

Episodes of pain may persist for periods of several days to weeks or months. Although symptoms tend to be recurrent and episodic, DUs often recur in the absence of pain. Periods of remission usually last from weeks to years and are almost always longer than the episodes of pain. However, in some patients the disease is more aggressive, with frequent and persistent symptoms or development of complications.

Changes in the character of ulcer pain may signal the development of complications. For example, ulcer pain that becomes constant, is no longer relieved by food or antacids, or radiates to the back or to either upper quadrant may herald penetration of the ulcer (often posteriorly into the pancreas). Pain associated with DU that is accentuated rather than relieved by food and/or is accompanied by vomiting often indicates gastric outlet obstruction. Abrupt, severe, or generalized abdominal pain is characteristic of free ulcer perforation into the peritoneal cavity. DU may cause acute gastrointestinal (GI) hemorrhage, with vomiting of blood or "coffee grounds" material or with the passage of black, tarry stools or even frankly red blood, if the bleeding is massive. Uncommonly, blood loss with DU is more subtle, with occult blood loss detected by stool examination or by variable degrees of anemia which may be accompanied by iron deficiency. Weight loss, in the absence of some degree of gastric outlet obstruction, is unusual in patients with DU.

It is important to emphasize that many patients with active DU have no ulcer symptoms. This situation leads to a significant underestimation of DU frequency in the population. Prospective studies using upper GI endoscopy suggest that approximately half of DU recurrences are without symptoms. Endoscopic studies also show a lack of good correlation among ulcer activity, symptom resolution, and ulcer healing. The absence of ulcer pain does not exclude DU as a potential cause for acute or chronic GI hemorrhage, gastric outlet obstruction, or ulcer perforation.

On physical examination, epigastric tenderness is the most frequent finding. The area of tenderness is usually in the midline, often midway between the umbilicus and the xiphoid process. In approximately 20 percent of patients, the tender area is to the right of the midline. Acute DU perforation into the peritoneal cavity often produces a rigid, boardlike abdomen, usually with generalized rebound tenderness. Auscultation of the abdomen initially may reveal hyperactive bowel sounds which, with clinical progression, may diminish or disappear. Patients with gastric outlet obstruction caused by a DU or a pyloric channel ulcer may have a succussion splash produced by retained fluid and air in the distended stomach.

The pyloric channel, which is 1 to 2 cm in length, is the narrowest portion of the gastric outlet. Because of their gastric acid secretory characteristics and clinical features, pyloric channel ulcers are classified with DU rather than with GU (Fig. 284-5). Ulcers in this location often produce symptoms similar to those of a DU; however, symptoms tend to be less responsive to food and antacids; food may accentuate rather than relieve ulcer pain and may produce vomiting due to partial gastric outlet obstruction. Surgery has been required more frequently for pyloric channel ulcers than for those in the duodenal bulb.

Nonulcer dyspepsia, also referred to as *essential* or *functional* dyspepsia, is a term used to describe a heterogeneous group of disorders characterized by persistent or recurrent upper abdominal pain or discomfort for which no underlying cause is detected. Although *H. pylori* is the primary cause of gastritis and an essential factor in the pathogenesis of peptic ulcer disease, it has not been proved to have a role in the pathogenesis of nonulcer dyspepsia. The prevalence of *H. pylori* infection in patients with nonulcer dyspepsia (50 percent) is no higher than that of the general population, and there is no convincing evidence that *H. pylori* accounts for the symptoms in these patients. Eradication of *H. pylori* infection with the subsequent resolution of histologic gastritis does not reliably lead to resolution of dyspepsia. Until and unless a clear association between *H. pylori* and nonulcer dyspepsia can be shown, there is no indication to treat such patients for *H. pylori*.

DIAGNOSIS Barium examination of the upper GI tract is of value in identifying DU and is still the most common initial method used to establish the diagnosis. Using conventional single-contrast barium techniques, 70 to 80 percent of DUs found at endoscopy can be identified by x-ray. With double-contrast barium examinations, the detection rate is about 90 percent. On x-ray, the typical DU appears as a discrete crater in the proximal portion of the duodenal bulb (Fig. 284-6). Marked deformity of the duodenal bulb, common in patients with chronic recurrent DU, may make radiographic identification of the ulcer difficult or impossible.

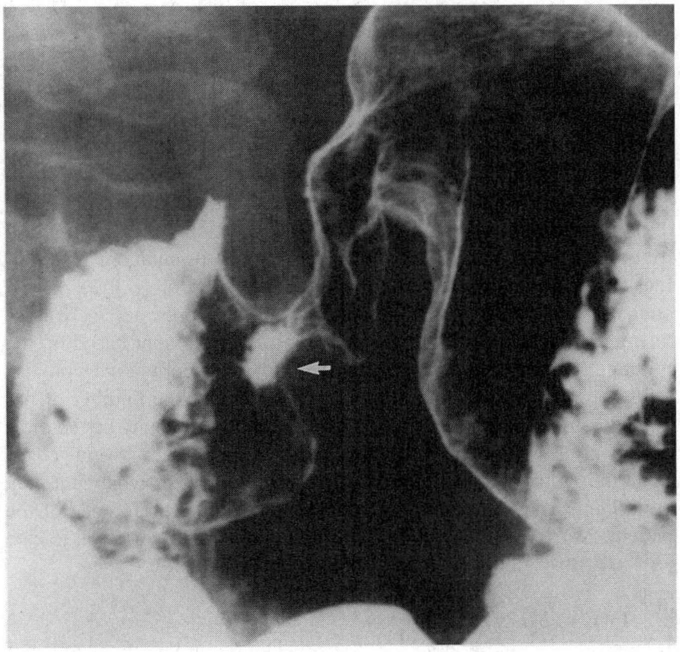

FIGURE 284-5 Barium radiograph of pyloric channel ulcer. *(Courtesy of Gary J. Whitman, M.D., Houston, TX)*

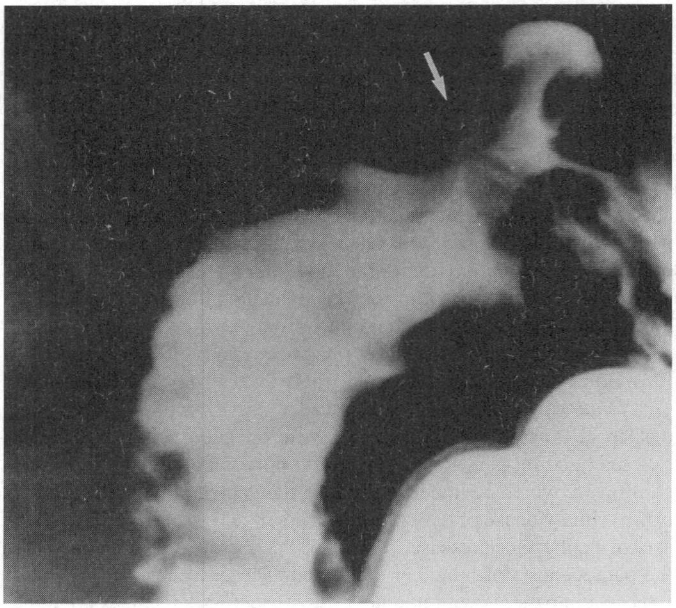

FIGURE 284-6 Barium radiograph of a DU. Note discrete ulcer in duodenal bulb (*arrow*). *(Courtesy of Gary J. Whitman, M.D., Houston, TX)*

Endoscopic examination of the upper GI tract is the most accurate means of diagnosing DU. Endoscopy is not required for this purpose when DU has been identified by barium radiographic examination. However, endoscopy may be of greatest value in (1) detecting DU suspected in the absence of a radiographically demonstrable ulcer, (2) evaluating patients with a radiographic deformity and uncertainty regarding ulcer activity, (3) identifying ulcers too small or too superficial to be recognized by x-ray, and (4) identifying (or excluding) an ulcer as the source of active GI hemorrhage. Endoscopy permits direct visualization and photographic documentation of the ulcer, including its size, shape, and location; permits mucosal biopsy of the antrum for detection of *H. pylori*; and may provide a reference base for assessment of ulcer healing.

In most patients with typical DUs, specific diagnostic testing for *H. pylori* may be unnecessary because the organism can be assumed to be present, as long as there is no recent history of NSAID use, symptoms or signs of a gastric hypersecretory state, or history of recent antibiotic therapy that might have eradicated *H. pylori*. Determination of the serum gastrin level is recommended only in patients for whom surgery is planned or in whom an underlying gastrinoma is suspected (see below). Patients with ulcer-like symptoms but no evidence of ulcer may be considered to have nonulcer dyspepsia.

Controversy exists as to the optimal approach to the patient presenting with chronic dyspepsia (see Chap. 41). Options include an initial trial of symptomatic treatment with an H_2 receptor antagonist, sucralfate, or omeprazole (see below), serologic testing for *H. pylori* and a course of therapy to eradicate the organism if it is present (see below), or immediate endoscopy followed by specific treatment based on the findings. Limited data suggest that early endoscopy gives precise guidance for diagnosis and treatment and reduces the number of patients treated inappropriately. While early endoscopy may be the most costly initial approach, its use may not lead to higher overall costs. In an individual case the approach to diagnosis and management may be influenced by other factors, such as the age and preference of the patient. Moreover, current practice is to limit treatment to eradicate *H. pylori* to patients with confirmed ulcers (see below).

Rx TREATMENT

Traditionally, the major objectives of DU therapy have been relief of pain, acceleration of ulcer healing, and prevention of ulcer recurrence and complications. Conclusions regarding the effectiveness of therapy were confused by the spontaneous healing of DU (a component of the natural history of the disease), and by imprecise methods used to assess ulcer activity. With the recognition that *H. pylori* plays a central role in the pathogenesis of DU, the objective of therapy now is eradication of *H. pylori* and cure of the disease.

There is general agreement that the only uniformly accepted indication for treating *H. pylori* infection is to prevent recurrent ulcer disease. Although eradication of *H. pylori* was originally reserved for recurrent or complicated ulcers that were unrelated to NSAIDs, a National Institutes of Health Consensus Development Conference Report has advocated routine eradication of *H. pylori* on first presentation of a peptic ulcer. Thus, patients with documented evidence of DU (by upper GI contrast radiography or endoscopy) should be treated for *H. pylori*, regardless of the severity of symptoms or the presence of other risk factors for ulcer disease, such as NSAID use. Treatment may be extended to patients who have a *history* of documented DU and evidence of *H. pylori* infection by serologic or breath test methods. While patients with complicated (e.g., bleeding) ulcers have generally been placed on long-term maintenance therapy with H_2 receptor antagonists to prevent recurrent complications (see below), data are emerging to suggest that maintenance therapy may not be necessary after eradication of *H. pylori*. Recent studies have suggested that rebleeding from recurrent DU is prevented by eradication of *H. pylori*. However, maintenance antisecretory therapy may be continued in patients for whom recurrent bleeding could be especially life-threatening.

Numerous drugs have been evaluated in the treatment of *H. pylori* infection, including bismuth compounds, amoxicillin, tetracycline, clarithromycin, metronidazole, omeprazole, and H_2 receptor antagonists, singly or in various combinations. *No single agent is optimally effective against the organism.* Although *H. pylori* is susceptible in vitro to most antibiotics, in vivo susceptibility cannot be assumed, because of the possibility of poor drug bioavailability, drug resistance, or patient noncompliance. Currently, therapy should consist of the most efficacious combination of agents, designed to maximize the eradication rate but minimize side effects and ensure patient compliance. The therapy of *H. pylori* infection is still evolving, and new drug regimens continue to be evaluated in an attempt to determine the best drug combinations, dosing regimens, and duration of treatment (Table 284-2).

Bismuth compounds have been used for the treatment of peptic ulcer disease for several centuries. The mechanism of action of bismuth is uncertain but may involve cytoprotective effects, including binding of the agent to the ulcer base and the stimulation of mucus and prostaglandin production. In addition, bismuth is thought to exert an antibacterial effect through inhibition of proteolytic, lipolytic, and urease enzyme activities. When used as monotherapy, bismuth compounds result in eradication of *H. pylori* in only 20 percent of patients, but when used in combination with antibiotics, they are associated with eradication in up to 95 percent of patients with documented *H. pylori* infection.

Currently, the most successful therapy for *H. pylori* infection is so-called triple therapy, which consists of a bismuth compound, metronidazole, and either amoxicillin or tetracycline. The most widely used and most effective regimen is a 2-week course of bismuth [usually a preparation such as bismuth subsalicylate (PeptoBismol)] at a dosage of two tablets qid together with metronidazole (250, 400, or 500 mg tid or qid) and tetracycline (500 mg qid); this regimen leads to eradication of *H. pylori* in about 90 percent of cases. Although tetracycline may be replaced with oral amoxicillin (500 mg qid), this change slightly increases the cost and slightly decreases the efficacy. Some studies suggest that a 1-week course of triple therapy may be as effective as a 2-week course.

Triple therapy for 2 weeks in combination with administration of an H_2 receptor antagonist for 6 weeks improves the ulcer healing rate slightly compared with use of an H_2 receptor antagonist alone and reduces the rate of ulcer recurrence to less than 15 percent at 1 year (compared to 60 to 100 percent after conventional antisecretory therapy). Although the requirement for gastric acid suppression in addition to therapy aimed at eradicating *H. pylori* has been questioned, the addition of omeprazole to a triple drug regimen appears to increase the rate of *H. pylori* eradication to about 98 percent. The precise role of gastric acid suppression as an essential component of the therapeutic regimen for *H. pylori* remains to be defined, but such therapy does contribute to the relief of symptoms in patients with DU.

Although triple therapy is the most effective and least expensive regimen, it has some drawbacks. Patient compliance is one of the important factors. A typical 2-week treatment requires that a patient ingest a total of approximately 200 tablets and take medication four times daily. Troublesome side effects occur in 20 to 30 percent of patients. Bismuth may cause darkening of the tongue and stool and lead to constipation. Amoxicillin may cause antibiotic-associated diarrhea, including pseudomembranous colitis, and may be associated with nausea, vomiting, skin rash, and allergic reactions. Tetracycline has been associated with skin rash and, rarely, anaphylaxis and hepatotoxicity. Potential adverse effects of long-term metronidazole use include paresthesias and, rarely, seizures, and those of short-term use include nausea, vomiting, diarrhea, and an altered taste sensation. In addition, patients must be cautioned to abstain from alcohol while taking metronidazole to avoid a disulfiram-like reaction.

Resistance to metronidazole is also a potentially significant problem in the treatment of *H. pylori* and has been found in about 30 percent of isolates from North America. The treatment of metronidazole-resistant strains of *H. pylori* with triple therapy does not necessarily result in failure of eradication. In fact, triple therapy has been reported to result in eradication of *H. pylori* in 91 percent of patients infected with a metronidazole-susceptible strain and 63 percent of those infected with a metronidazole-resistant strain.

Owing to the limitations of triple therapy, alternative regimens may be used. Dual therapy with amoxicillin (500 mg qid) and omeprazole (20 mg bid) for 2 weeks is associated with fewer side effects and improved compliance. However, this regimen may yield an eradication rate for *H. pylori* of only 36 to 60 percent, and the use of higher doses of omeprazole (40 mg bid or tid) and amoxicillin (750 mg tid) does not reliably increase the eradication rate.

Clarithromycin, a newer macrolide antimicrobial, may be used in place of metronidazole in a dose of 250 mg four times daily and, as part of a triple regimen, has resulted in a 90 percent eradication rate. Similar eradication rates have been achieved when clarithromycin is used in a dose of 500 mg three times daily in combination with omeprazole, 40 mg a day or 20 mg twice daily. Eradication rates of about 85 percent have been reported for a regimen of clarithromycin and the combination drug ranitidine bismuth citrate (RBC). There is much interest in simpler triple regimens of omeprazole (or lansoprazole), clarithromycin, and either metronidazole or amoxicillin given twice daily for 1 week (see Table 284-2). Combination therapy using clarithromycin is well-tolerated and may be especially useful in patients who are infected with metronidazole-resistant *H. pylori*, are allergic to penicillin, or have difficulty with compliance. However, resistance to clarithromycin may develop, and regimens that include omeprazole or clarithromycin are substantially more expensive than standard triple therapy.

Until now, confirmation that *H. pylori* has been eradicated has required repeat endoscopy with gastric mucosal biopsy and has generally been reserved for patients with complicated ulcer disease (e.g., bleeding). Serologic testing is unreliable for this purpose, because antibody levels generally decline slowly after successful therapy and often do not decline to zero. When eradication of *H. pylori* is demonstrated at least 1 month after the completion of treatment, subsequent reinfection is uncommon, with a frequency as low as 1 percent per year in Western countries. The availability of urea breath tests should make confirmation of *H. pylori* eradication simpler and less expensive.

Regardless of the treatment regimen used, it is becoming clear that eradication of *H. pylori* is the most cost-effective method of managing DU. In the past, drugs that neutralized or reduced secretion of gastric acid were the mainstays of DU therapy. With the advent

Table 284-2

Drugs Used in the Treatment of Peptic Ulcer

Drug and Mechanism	Dose	Side Effects
"Triple therapy": eradication of *H. pylori*	Bismuth subsalicylate 2 tabs qid, amoxicillin 500 mg qid or tetracycline 500 mg tid, plus metronidazole 250 mg tid. Treat for 2 weeks (combine with H_2 receptor antagonist or proton pump inhibitor)	Cumbersome; diarrhea, pseudomembranous colitis
"Dual therapy": eradication of *H. pylori* (plus proton pump inhibition)	Omeprazole 40 mg/d in the morning plus clarithromycin 500 mg tid. Treat for 2 weeks.	As for omeprazole and triple therapy, but frequency of side effects lower and cost greater
"New triple therapy": eradication of *H. pylori* (plus proton pump inhibition)	Omeprazole 20 mg bid plus either clarithromycin 250 mg bid and metronidazole 500 mg bid *or* clarithromycin 500 mg bid and amoxicillin 1 g bid. Treat for one week	Frequency of side effects lower than for standard triple therapy but cost greater
Ranitidine bismuth citrate plus antibiotic: eradication of *H. pylori*	Rantidine bismuth citrate 400 mg bid for 4 weeks plus clarithromycin 500 mg tid for first 2 weeks	Taste disturbance and diarrhea most common
Cimetidine: H_2 receptor blockade	300 mg qid or 400 mg bid or 800 mg at bedtime	Uncommon: antiandrogen (high doses), ↑ creatinine, ↓ hepatic drug metabolism, ↑ serum aminotransferase levels, rare blood dyscrasias
Ranitidine: H_2 receptor blockade	150 mg bid or 300 mg at bedtime	As for cimetidine but antiandrogen and drug metabolism effects are less frequent; rare cases of hepatitis
Famotidine: H_2 receptor blockade	40 mg at bedtime	As for ranitidine
Nizatidine: H_2 receptor blockade	300 mg at bedtime	Probably as for ranitidine
Misoprostol: raises prostaglandin levels (enhances mucosal defense, reduces gastric acid secretion)	200 μg qid for prevention of NSAID-induced ulcers	Diarrhea, uterine contraction (do not use in women of childbearing age)
Sucralfate: coats ulcers, binds pepsin	1 g 1 h before meals and at bedtime or 2 g bid	Constipation, binding to coadministered drugs
Omeprazole: inhibits H^+, K^+-ATPase (proton pump) on gastric parietal cell	20 mg/d in the morning	↓ Hepatic drug metabolism; prolonged use in high doses in rats causes gastric carcinoids
Lansoprazole: proton pump inhibitor	30 mg/d in the morning	As for omeprazole
Antacids: acid neutralization	140 mmol 1 h and 3 h after eating and at bedtime (e.g., 30 mL Maalox); lower doses (15 mL after eating and at bedtime) appear to be as effective	Diarrhea (Mg), constipation (Al), osteomalacia, milk-alkali syndrome (elevated serum Ca, P, BUN, creatinine, HCO_3; due to $CaCO_3$)

of therapy aimed at eradicating *H. pylori*, these drugs are now used in an adjunctive role or for symptomatic relief of DUs. In addition, they still form the mainstay of therapy for gastroesophageal reflux disease (see Chap. 283).

Antacids Although antacids have been used for decades to treat DU, only in the past 20 years has their effectiveness in accelerating DU healing been verified. They are now generally used on an as-needed basis for symptomatic relief in ulcer patients. The most widely used antacid preparations are mixtures of aluminum hydroxide and magnesium hydroxide that neutralize HCl. Complications of aluminum hydroxide treatment include constipation and systemic phosphate depletion, which can result in weakness, malaise, and anorexia in patients with phosphate-poor diets (e.g., dietary deficiency accompanying chronic alcoholism or other states of reduced dietary protein intake). Magnesium hydroxide may produce loose stools. This laxative effect and the constipating effects of aluminum hydroxide can be overcome by using antacids that contain these agents in combination. Ionic magnesium stimulates gastrin release, leading to increased gastric acid secretion ("acid rebound"). Magnesium trisilicate, which is included in various antacid mixtures, is a slow-acting weak antacid.

Calcium carbonate is a potent and inexpensive antacid that is converted to calcium chloride in the stomach. Approximately 10 percent of the ingested calcium is absorbed. Like magnesium hydroxide, calcium carbonate ingestion is associated with acid rebound. Chronic excessive calcium carbonate administration may be associated with the milk-alkali syndrome, producing elevations of serum calcium, urea nitrogen, creatinine, and bicarbonate levels and resulting in renal calcinosis and possibly progressive renal insufficiency. Sodium bicarbonate is a potent and rapidly acting antacid, but it has a tendency to induce systemic alkalosis.

H_2 Receptor Antagonists H_2 receptor antagonists are potent inhibitors of basal (unstimulated) and stimulated gastric acid secretion. H_2 receptor antagonists exhibit some structural similarities to histamine and to each other, with variations in ring structures and side chains (Fig. 284-7). Until recently, H_2 receptor antagonists were the preferred drugs in the treatment of peptic ulcer because of their safety and effectiveness in accelerating healing. Healing rates for treatment with H_2 receptor antagonists are similar to those for antacid treatment, but compliance appears to be better. Until recently, a daily maintenance dose of H_2 receptor antagonists (one-half the standard dose) was often used to reduce DU recurrence, with a reduction of 1-year recurrence rates by 50 to 70 percent after initial ulcer healing. H_2 receptor antagonists are now often used for 4 to 6 weeks in combination with triple therapy against *H. pylori*, as discussed above.

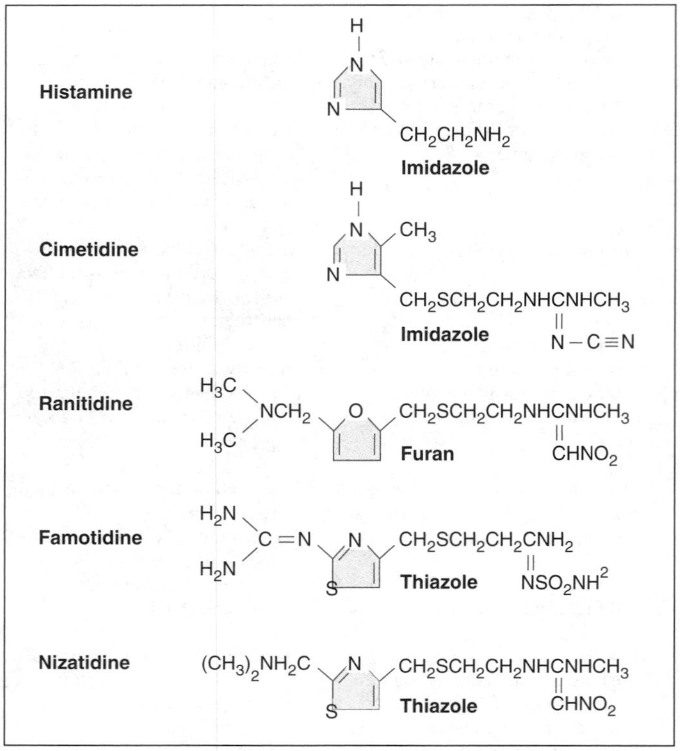

FIGURE 284-7 Chemical structures of H_2 receptor antagonists.

Cimetidine was the first H_2 receptor antagonist developed. At 300 mg, it inhibits basal acid secretion by more than 80 percent and meal-stimulated acid secretion by approximately 70 percent. It strikingly reduces acid secretory responses to histamine, caffeine, hypoglycemia, and gastrin. Initially, the oral dose of cimetidine recommended and used in treatment of DU was 300 mg four times daily, with meals and at bedtime. A dose of 400 mg twice daily (morning and bedtime) or 800 mg once daily (at bedtime) is also effective in the treatment of DU.

Few serious adverse effects have been experienced with cimetidine. Slight and reversible increases in serum aminotransferase and creatinine levels and brief increases in serum prolactin may occur after intravenous and oral use. Cimetidine has been shown to inhibit some cytochrome P450 hepatic microsomal enzyme systems and therefore may increase the blood level, duration of action, and pharmacologic effects of drugs metabolized by those systems. Tender gynecomastia due to the weak antiandrogenic effect of cimetidine has been reported in patients with ZES who required and were treated with extremely large doses for months to years. Although reversible confusional states have been attributed to cimetidine in a small number of severely ill patients with preexisting hepatic and/or renal functional impairment, a causative effect has not been proven.

Ranitidine is about six times as potent as cimetidine in inhibiting gastric acid secretion. Both drugs have similar half-lives, approximately 1.5 to 2 h. In the past, the recommended dose of ranitidine for treatment of DU was 150 mg twice a day, but 300 mg at bedtime is equally effective. Ranitidine may increase levels of serum asparate aminotransferase and alanine aminotransferase. There have been occasional reports of reversible hepatitis with ranitidine administration. This drug appears to have no antiandrogen properties and has a smaller inhibitory effect on cytochrome P450 mixed oxygenase enzyme systems than does cimetidine.

Famotidine and *nizatidine* are two other potent H_2 receptor antagonists. The recommended daily dose of famotidine in the treatment of DU is 40 mg once daily at bedtime, while that for nizatidine is 300 mg at bedtime. Associated blood dyscrasias have been noted rarely, and hepatotoxicity, similar to that with ranitidine and cimetidine, also has been reported.

Anticholinergic Agents Anticholinergic agents, such as atropine, were used in the past to block parietal cell muscarinic acetylcholine receptors and thereby decrease gastric acid secretion. However, they were not as effective as H_2 receptor antagonists and were associated with a variety of side effects, including dryness of the mouth, blurring of vision, cardiac arrhythmias, and urinary retention. *Pirenzepine*, a relatively selective anticholinergic agent, is more specific in inhibiting gastric acid secretion and has fewer side effects than other anticholinergic agents but is not available in the United States and is unlikely to find a role in ulcer treatment.

Coating Agents Several drugs that act neither by neutralization of gastric acid nor by inhibition of its secretion have been used in the treatment of DU. Among these is *sucralfate*, a complex polyaluminum hydroxide salt of sucrose sulfate (Fig. 284-8). Sucralfate becomes highly polar at acid pH and binds to the ulcer bed for up to 12 h, whereas relatively little of it binds to intact gastric or duodenal mucosa. It is believed that the adherence of sucralfate to granulation tissue impedes diffusion of H^+ to the base of the ulcer. In addition, sucralfate binds bile acids and pepsins and may therefore reduce their injurious effects. Sucralfate may increase the level of endogenous tissue prostaglandins and may bind epidermal growth factors and other growth factors and present them to the ulcer, thereby increasing mucosal defense. It is only minimally absorbed, with less than 5 percent appearing in the urine. Sucralfate is similar to antacids and H_2 receptor antagonists in its effectiveness in the treatment of DU and in prevention of DU recurrence. The recommended dose of sucralfate is 1 g 1 h before each meal and at bedtime.

Colloidal bismuth compounds also aid ulcer healing by forming (in an acid medium) a bismuth-protein coagulant which is believed to protect the ulcer from acid and pepsin digestion. Colloidal bismuth compounds have little acid-neutralizing effect and do not reduce gastric acid secretion. These compounds inhibit pepsin activity, bind to the gastric mucus gel layer, and may prevent diffusion of hydrogen ions. They stimulate gastric mucosal secretion of prostaglandins, bicarbonate, and glycoprotein mucus. As discussed above, the principal role of bismuth-containing compounds in the treatment of DU relates to their effects on *H. pylori*. Colloidal bismuth compounds are the only class of antiulcer drugs that eradicate *H. pylori* and cure the gastritis associated with its colonization (see below).

Prostaglandins A variety of prostaglandins, particularly those of the E series (PGE_1 and PGE_2), have been shown to be effective in clinical trials in the treatment of DU. They reduce basal and stimulated gastric acid secretion and appear to enhance mucosal resistance to tissue injury. In low doses, exogenous PGEs exert the following actions important in enhancing mucosal defense: they (1) stimulate gastric mucus secretion, (2) stimulate gastric and duodenal bicarbonate secretion, (3) maintain or increase gastric mucosal blood flow, (4) maintain the gastric mucosal barrier to diffusion of H^+, and (5) stimulate mucosal cell replacement. Because of side effects (diarrhea, uterine contraction) and the availability of other therapies, prostaglandins generally have not been used to treat DU. In the United States, misoprostol, a PGE_1 analogue, has been approved for use only for preventing ulcers caused by NSAIDs (see below).

Proton Pump Inhibitors The final step of hydrogen ion secretion by parietal cells is accomplished by H^+,K^+-ATPase, a proton pump that exchanges hydrogen for potassium. The H^+,K^+-ATPase is located in the apical membrane and tubulovesicular apparatus of parietal cells. The luminal surface of the transmembrane enzyme is exposed to the gastric luminal acid. Omeprazole and lansoprazole, specific inhibitors of this H^+,K^+-ATPase, are extraordinarily potent in decreasing gastric acid secretion (Fig. 284-9). These are substituted benzimidazoles that bind to the proton pump and irreversibly inactivate it. Both omeprazole and lansoprazole produce prolonged inhibition of all phases of gastric acid secretion, with acid secretory recovery requiring synthesis of new enzyme. The maximum effect of omeprazole occurs within 2 h; 50 percent of the maximum inhibition remains at 24 h; and inhibition persists for up to 72 h. With once-daily dosing, a plateau is reached after 4 days, and after discontinuation, gastric acid secretory activity returns gradually to normal over 3 to 5 days.

Omeprazole and lansoprazole are approved for treatment of DU, erosive esophagitis, and gastric acid hypersecretory states, including ZES. For DU, these drugs are used in conjunction with triple therapy or with antibiotics such as amoxicillin and/or clarithromycin, as discussed above. The standard dose of omeprazole is 20 mg daily and that for lansoprazole is 30 mg daily in the morning before breakfast for periods of 4 to 8 weeks. These drugs cause a small to moderate increase in serum gastrin because of their effect on gastric acidity. Serum gastrin levels return to normal within 2 weeks after drug discontinuance. Hypergastrinemia-induced hyperplasia of gastric mucosal ECL cells and carcinoid tumors, which were noted in rats receiving omeprazole, have not been documented in humans.

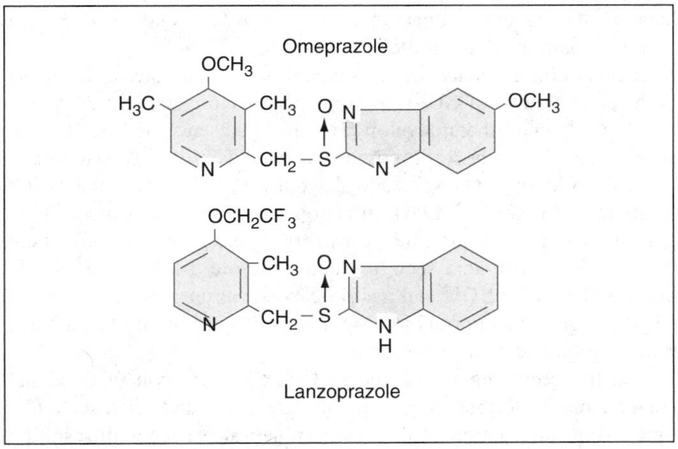

FIGURE 284-9 Chemical structures of omeprazole and lansoprazole.

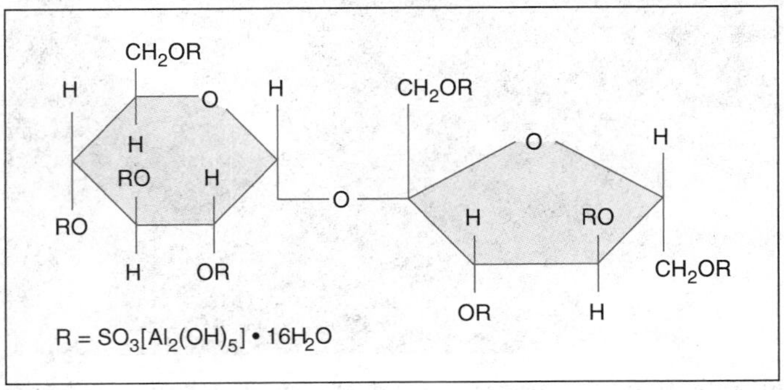

FIGURE 284-8 Chemical structure of sucralfate.

DIET In the past, many different diet programs were used for treatment of patients with DU. There is no evidence that bland diets reduce gastric acid secretion or promote healing, although they may relieve symptoms of DU. Similarly, soft diets or diets free of spices or fruit juices have not been proved beneficial. Although traditionally milk and cream were prescribed for ulcer patients, there is no evidence that they promote ulcer healing. They actually stimulate gastric acid secretion, contribute to the development of the milk-alkali syndrome, and probably accelerate atherogenesis. Many physicians recommend that patients with DU avoid coffee, with or without caffeine, and other caffeine-containing beverages because of their effects on gastric secretion. It also may be desirable to restrict alcohol intake in these patients. It is reasonable to suggest that patients avoid foods that exacerbate their symptoms.

GASTRIC ULCER

The incidence of GU peaks in the sixth decade, approximately 10 years later than for DU. Slightly more than half of GUs occur in males. The precise incidence of GU is not known, since many GUs are asymptomatic. Although DU is identified clinically more frequently than GU, most autopsy studies show an equal or greater proportion of GUs.

GUs are deep, penetrating beyond the mucosa of the stomach, and are similar histologically to DUs, but usually with more extensive gastritis surrounding the ulcer. Almost all benign GUs are found immediately distal to the junction of the antral mucosa and the acid-secreting mucosa of the body of the stomach. The location of this junction is variable. In general, antral mucosa extends approximately two-thirds of the way up the lesser curvature and one-third of the way up the greater curvature of the stomach.

Benign GUs are rare in the fundus of the stomach. Benign GUs are virtually always accompanied by antral gastritis as a result of *H. pylori* infection, with variable amounts of mucosal atrophy. When GU is associated with aspirin and other NSAIDs, gastritis is often absent.

ETIOLOGY AND PATHOGENESIS As for DU, acid and pepsin are important in the pathogenesis of GU. In contrast to DU patients, GU patients as a group have acid secretion rates that are normal or reduced compared with nonulcer subjects, although true achlorhydria (in response to pentagastrin stimulation) almost never occurs with benign GU. About 10 percent of patients with GUs also have a DU. Patients with both a DU and a GU tend to have acid secretory patterns that parallel those of DU.

Compelling evidence supports the primary importance of *H. pylori* in the pathogenesis of GU. Why some persons infected with *H. pylori* develop DU and others develop GU (in the absence of NSAID use) is not clear. It has been proposed that persons with GU, which can occur in children as young as age 5, acquire *H. pylori* infection earlier in life than do those with DU. Infection at a young age is more likely to result in chronic or atrophic gastritis (see below), with a subsequent decrease in gastric acid secretion and therefore a lower risk of DU but a higher risk of GU and gastric cancer. Serum gastrin levels are slightly higher than normal in a significant proportion of GU patients, reflecting gastric acid hyposecretion.

Gastric emptying is delayed in GU. Regurgitation of duodenal contents may contribute to gastric mucosal injury and subsequent GU by causing interruption of the gastric mucosal barrier with resulting diffusion of secreted hydrogen ions to the mucosa. NSAIDs are responsible for 15 to 25 percent of GUs, as is discussed below.

CLINICAL FEATURES As with DU, epigastric pain is the most common symptom, but the pattern is less characteristic. The pain may be precipitated or accentuated by food, and symptom relief with food or antacids is less consistent than with DU. Whereas in DU patients, nausea and vomiting almost always indicate gastric outlet obstruction, in patients with GU they may occur in the absence of mechanical obstruction. Weight loss may occur, due to anorexia or aversion to food developing from the discomfort produced by eating. GUs tend to heal but then recur, often in the same location.

Hemorrhage is a common complication of GU, occurring in approximately 25 percent of patients; gastric perforation is less common. The mortality rate with GU perforation is approximately three times that with DU perforation, owing partly to the greater average age of GU patients, the usually longer delay in diagnosis, and the greater soilage of the peritoneum with GU perforation. Gastric outlet obstruction may complicate GU in the distal antrum.

DIAGNOSIS While the history is of value in suggesting GU, it is not as characteristic as in DU. The two methods used for diagnosis are barium examination and endoscopy. GU usually can be identified by barium examination, although NSAID-associated GUs are frequently more superficial and are less often identified radiographically. Both benign GUs and malignant ulcers are more common on the lesser than on the greater curvature (Fig. 284-10). Radiation of gastric mucosal folds from the margin of the ulcer crater suggests a benign lesion. Large ulcers—i.e., those greater than 3 cm in diameter—are more often malignant than smaller ones. An ulcer within a mass, as defined radiographically, also suggests malignancy. From 1 to 8 percent of GUs that appear benign radiographically prove to be malignant (by endoscopic biopsy or at surgery). Because of false-positive and false-negative errors, radiographic appearance cannot be used as the sole criterion for judging the benign or malignant nature of an ulcer in the stomach.

Endoscopic visualization of the ulcer allows definition of its size, location, and, by biopsy, its histologic characteristics. To exclude malignancy at gastroscopy, a total of at least six biopsy samples are obtained from the inner margin of the ulcer. Brushings of the ulcer for cytology should be obtained prior to biopsy. The combination of radiographic, endoscopic, and histologic techniques makes it possible to distinguish malignant from benign ulcers with more than 97 percent confidence.

Gastric ulcer with pentagastrin-fast achlorhydria is rare. When it occurs, it almost always indicates gastric carcinoma. However, most patients with gastric carcinoma are capable of secreting gastric acid, although usually less than normal.

It is important in patients with GU to determine whether *H. pylori* is present, because the organism should be eradicated. Identification of *H. pylori* can be done by a rapid urease test on an antral mucosal biopsy specimen or histology preparation when endoscopy is the method used to diagnose the ulcer or by serology or urea breath testing (where available) when radiography is the method used. When GU is associated with *H. pylori* infection, treatment aimed at eradicating *H. pylori* is indicated, even if the GU occurs in the setting of NSAID use (see below).

℞ TREATMENT

On the basis of preliminary studies, it appears that GUs associated with *H. pylori* infection should be treated with triple therapy combined with an acid-suppressive agent, as for DU. In general, whatever the medical treatment modality selected, GUs tend to heal more slowly than DUs, and larger GUs take longer to heal than smaller ones. Although GU patients have normal or reduced gastric acid secretion, acid-inhibiting agents have been effective in promoting the acute healing of GUs, and GUs heal more rapidly with omeprazole than with H_2 receptor antagonists.

Since salicylates and other NSAIDs are associated with the development of GU, these agents should be discontinued if in use. Milk and cream, as well as bland or homogenized diets, have not been shown to be of value in treatment. In general, it is probably sufficient to recommend that patients consume a diet of their own choice. As in the case of DU, patients should be advised to avoid coffee (caffeine-containing or caffeine-free), other caffeine-containing beverages, and alcohol.

Carbenoxolone has been used in many countries (although it is not available in the United States) in GU treatment. This drug, a hydrolytic product of glycyrrhizic acid (derived from licorice), has been shown to decrease symptoms and increase the rate of GU healing. It does not decrease gastric acid secretion, but rather increases the life span of gastric mucosal epithelial cells as well as the secretion and viscosity of gastric mucus. Carbenoxolone possesses aldosterone-like effects, producing sodium and water retention. Its side effects and the availability of effective alternatives have led to its decreased use.

Benign GUs should heal completely within 2 to 3 months of the start of therapy. The failure of a GU to decrease satisfactorily in size and to heal with medical treatment has been taken as a sign of malignancy. Therefore, it may be reasonable, at least in selected cases, to monitor GU healing by a repeat gastroscopy after treatment, to check for healing of apparently benign GUs. If the ulcer is not healed, malignancy must be suspected, and exfoliative cytology samples and biopsy specimens of the ulcer should be obtained. Apparently complete healing with potent acid-suppressive therapy

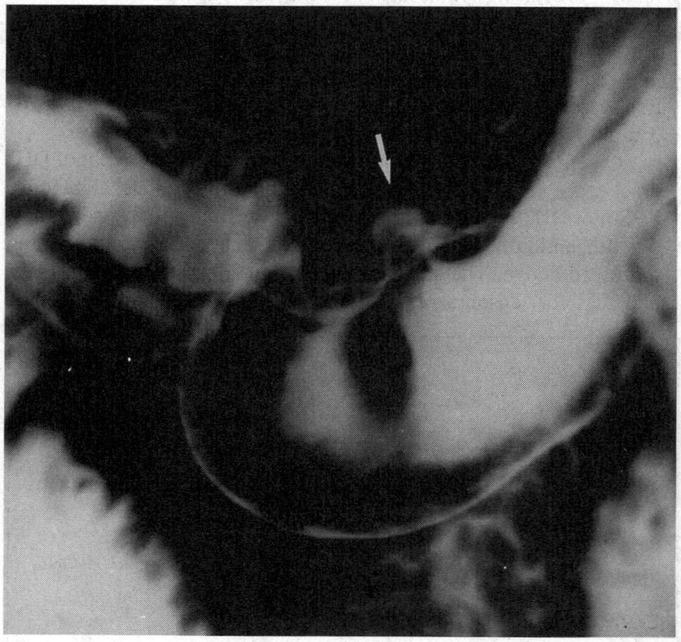

FIGURE 284-10 Barium radiograph of a benign GU. *(Courtesy of Gary J. Whitman, M.D., Houston, TX)*

does not guarantee the benign nature of a GU, since approximately 70 percent of ulcers that are eventually found to be malignant undergo significant (albeit usually incomplete) healing with such treatment.

COMPLICATIONS AND SURGERY FOR PEPTIC ULCER

Complications of ulcers include hemorrhage, obstruction, and perforation. Hemorrhage occurs in approximately 15 to 25 percent of patients with DUs; a recurrence of bleeding is estimated to occur in about 40 percent of patients with an initial hemorrhage if *H. pylori* eradication is not part of the treatment regimen or if maintenance therapy with an H_2 receptor antagonist is not prescribed. Hemorrhage related to an NSAID-associated ulcer occurs particularly frequently in the absence of prior peptic ulcer symptoms (approximately 50 percent of cases). In most patients, hemorrhage from a peptic ulcer is self-limited (see Chap. 44). In some cases, endoscopic intervention (use of a heater probe or bipolar electrocautery, laser photocoagulation, or injection of a vasoconstrictor or sclerosing agent) is needed to stop active bleeding or prevent recurrent bleeding in patients with ulcer characteristics, such as a *visible vessel*, that connote a high risk of rebleeding.

Free perforation into the peritoneal cavity occurs in approximately 2 to 3 percent of patients with DU. Of these patients, 5 to 10 percent will have had no recognizable prior ulcer symptoms. Simultaneous hemorrhage occurs in approximately 10 percent of patients with DU perforation; mortality is greatly increased in this group. DUs, especially those located posteriorly, may penetrate into adjacent structures, most often the pancreas, frequently resulting in modestly increased serum amylase levels. Less commonly, DUs penetrate into the liver, biliary tract, or colon.

Gastric outlet obstruction occurs in 2 to 4 percent of patients admitted to the hospital with duodenal or pyloric channel ulcers. Symptoms include abdominal bloating, nausea, vomiting, and weight loss. These patients usually have had ulcer symptoms for many years and, often, obstructive symptoms for several months.

℞ TREATMENT

For Duodenal Ulcer With the advent of curative therapy for ulcers associated with *H. pylori* infection as well as nonsurgical methods to arrest ulcer bleeding, the need for ulcer surgery has declined considerably. However, some patients will continue to need surgery for complicated ulcer disease, and there are many patients who have had ulcer surgery in the past. Therefore, there is a need for familiarity with the techniques and complications of ulcer surgery.

No single surgical procedure has been accepted universally as the most satisfactory DU operation. The most commonly performed surgical procedures are vagotomy with antrectomy, vagotomy with pyloroplasty, and proximal gastric vagotomy (also referred to as parietal cell or highly selective vagotomy) without a gastric drainage procedure (Table 284-3).

With truncal vagotomy and antrectomy, the vagal trunks are transected, the antrum is removed, and GI continuity is reestablished by anastomosis of the remaining stomach with the proximal duodenum (Billroth I anastomosis) or with a loop of jejunum (Billroth II anastomosis) (Fig. 284-11). Vagotomy with antrectomy has been an effective procedure with a low recurrence rate (approximately 1 percent), but morbidity and mortality rates have been slightly greater than with vagotomy with pyloroplasty and vary with patient selection and the skill of the surgeon.

Table 284-3

Principal Operations for Peptic Ulcer

Operation	Recurrence Rate, %	Complication Rate
Vagotomy + antrectomy (Billroth I or II)*	1	Highest
Vagotomy and pyloroplasty	10	Intermediate
Proximal gastric vagotomy	≥10	Lowest

* Billroth I, gastroduodenostomy; Billroth II, gastrojejunostomy.

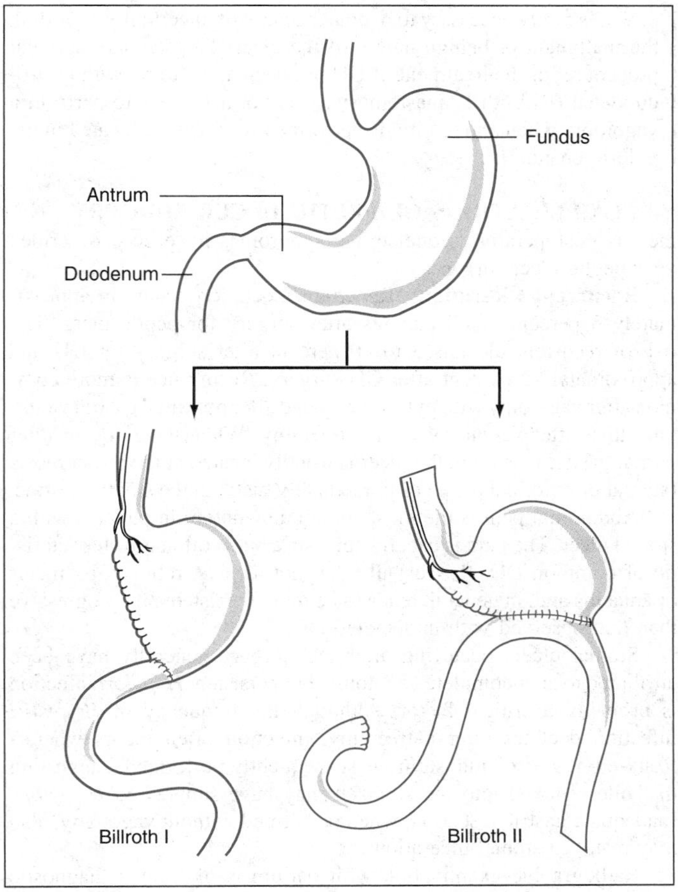

FIGURE 284-11 Diagram of Billroth I and II procedures.

With vagotomy and pyloroplasty, vagotomy is performed to inhibit vagal stimulation of gastric acid secretion, and a pyloroplasty is performed to facilitate gastric drainage after truncal or selective vagotomy. Three types of vagotomy have been used in the surgical treatment of duodenal or pyloric channel ulcer: truncal vagotomy, selective vagotomy, and proximal gastric vagotomy. Pyloroplasty with truncal vagotomy has been associated with a mortality rate of approximately 1 percent. Ulcer recurrence during the 5 years after surgery has been about 5 to 8 percent. With selective vagotomy, only the branches of the vagus that supply the stomach are transected, leaving intact the vagal innervation of other abdominal viscera. Selective vagotomy has been found by some surgeons to result in a more complete vagotomy, less ulcer recurrence, and fewer postvagotomy complications than truncal vagotomy. Proximal gastric vagotomy denervates only the acid-secreting portion of the stomach, sparing the branches of the vagus that innervate the antrum, which makes a gastric drainage procedure (e.g., pyloroplasty) unnecessary. Both immediate and late postoperative complications have been less common with proximal gastric vagotomy than with truncal vagotomy, and reductions in acid secretion are similar to those achieved with truncal or selective vagotomy. Mortality with proximal gastric vagotomy is less than 1 percent. With experience, recurrence has been comparable to that with vagotomy and pyloroplasty.

For Gastric Ulcer In the past, surgical treatment was required for GU patients who did not respond satisfactorily to medical therapy or who developed complications similar to those described for DU. With the current diagnostic accuracy of careful radiographic examination, endoscopy, biopsy of the ulcer margins, and exfoliative cytology, it is rarely necessary to operate because of uncertainty regarding the malignant or benign nature of the ulcer. The standard surgical procedure for the treatment of GU has been antrectomy with gastroduodenal (Billroth I) anastomosis. It is not necessary to perform a vagotomy when antrectomy is performed for GU (not located in the pyloric channel).

COMPLICATIONS OF PEPTIC ULCER SURGERY Numerous postoperative sequelae and syndromes have been described after peptic ulcer surgery.

Recurrent Ulceration Recurrent ulceration occurs in approximately 5 percent of all patients after surgery for peptic ulcer. The risk of recurrent ulcer is 3 to 10 percent after surgery for DU and approximately 2 percent after GU surgery. Recurrence is more common after vagotomy with pyloroplasty and after proximal gastric vagotomy than after vagotomy with antrectomy. When ulcers occur after partial gastric resection, the ulcer is usually located at the anastomosis (stomal or marginal ulcer) or immediately distal in the small intestine.

Abdominal pain is the most common symptom in patients with a stomal ulcer. The pain is usually epigastric but is often not characteristic of common DU. It is usually, but not always, relieved by meals or antacids and, in general, tends to be more persistent and progressive than that observed with unoperated DU.

Stomal ulcers occurring after DU surgery generally have been attributed to an incomplete vagotomy, but persistent *H. pylori* infection is probably a critical factor. Although the frequency of *H. pylori* infection declines after antrectomy, infection often recurs when a Roux-en-Y gastrojejunostomy is subsequently performed, suggesting that bile refluxed into the stomach may have suppressed *H. pylori.* Inadequate gastric resection, when performed without vagotomy, also may result in stomal ulceration.

Radiographic examination with barium is of limited diagnostic value and identifies only 50 to 60 percent of stomal ulcerations. Surgical deformity at the anastomotic site often may either mimic or conceal a stomal ulcer. When stomal ulceration is suspected, endoscopic examination is required to identify it. H_2 receptor antagonists and proton pump inhibitors have been reported to induce healing of stomal ulcers, although the long-term effectiveness of these agents in promoting healing of stomal ulcers and preventing their recurrence is uncertain. Transthoracic vagotomy may be effective when recurrent ulcer results from an incomplete vagotomy. Whether eradication of *H. pylori* should play a role in the treatment of stomal ulcers is uncertain.

Recurrent Ulcer due to Retained Antrum In a small number of patients who undergo antrectomy with gastrojejunostomy (Billroth II anastomosis), the antral resection is not complete, and residual distal antrum remains in continuity with the duodenum. These patients usually develop or continue to have gastric acid hypersecretion due to gastrin release by the residual antral mucosa, which is no longer in contact with gastric acid, the normal inhibitor of gastrin release. Fasting serum gastrin levels in these patients may be normal to moderately increased. Patients with retained antrum can be distinguished from those with gastrinoma by intravenous injection of secretin and measurements of serum gastrin levels. Gastrinoma patients exhibit substantial increases in serum gastrin (an increase of >200 ng/L), whereas those with retained antrum exhibit decreased, unchanged, or only slightly increased serum gastrin levels. The diagnosis of retained antrum may be suggested by a careful review of the original operative report or surgical pathology slides. In addition, endoscopy with biopsy of the anastomosis may disclose antral mucosa. These patients improve with removal of the remaining antrum.

Afferent Loop Syndromes Patients who have undergone partial gastric resection and gastrojejunostomy (Billroth II anastomosis) may experience abdominal bloating and pain 20 min to 1 h after eating, frequently followed by nausea and vomiting. The vomitus often contains large amounts of bile. Characteristically, the bloating and abdominal discomfort are relieved by vomiting. This type of afferent loop syndrome, which is uncommon, is believed to be caused by distention of an incompletely draining afferent intestinal loop by pancreatic and biliary secretions, which are stimulated by eating. Serum amylase levels may be mildly or moderately increased. Because of partial obstruction, it is often difficult to demonstrate the afferent loop by barium meal examination. Treatment is surgical correction of the incomplete afferent loop obstruction and, in some instances, revision to a gastroduodenal anastomosis.

A second form of afferent loop dysfunction is that due to stasis with bacterial overgrowth in the afferent loop. These patients may exhibit the same characteristics as those found with other forms of small intestinal bacterial overgrowth or blind loop syndromes (see Chap. 285), such as malabsorption, especially of fat and vitamin B_{12}. The syndrome can be corrected by surgical revision of the afferent loop.

Bile Reflux Gastropathy After peptic ulcer surgery, a small proportion of patients experience early satiety, abdominal discomfort, and vomiting, which is believed to be due to reflux of duodenal contents into the stomach. Endoscopic examination usually reveals regurgitated bile in the stomach and mucosal hyperemia, often involving the entire gastric remnant. Histologically, there is epithelial cell and foveolar injury with minimal inflammation. This entity has been referred to as alkaline reflux gastropathy, bile reflux gastropathy, duodenogastric reflux, and bilious vomiting. The substances in the refluxed intestinal contents that account for these symptoms have not been defined. Despite the term *bile reflux gastropathy*, there is no certainty that regurgitated bile is responsible for the syndrome. Administration of cholestyramine, intended to bind bile acids and facilitate their excretion, has not been proved of benefit in this disorder. In some cases, symptoms improve with administration of a gastric prokinetic agent such as cisapride, 10 to 20 mg before meals and at bedtime. Surgical diversion of duodenal contents from proximity to the stomach with a roux-en-Y anastomosis often alleviates bilious vomiting, particularly in patients in whom bile reflux is demonstrated by nuclear scanning after administration of ^{99m}Tc-HIDA; however, early satiety often does not improve with surgery.

Dumping Syndrome Following peptic ulcer surgery, some patients experience a spectrum of vasomotor symptoms after eating. These include palpitations, tachycardia, lightheadedness, diaphoresis, and, less frequently, postural hypotension. Abdominal discomfort and vomiting also may occur. This constellation of symptoms, called the *early dumping syndrome*, is usually experienced within 30 min after eating and is believed to result from rapid emptying of hyperosmolar gastric contents into the proximal small intestine, which leads to a shift of fluid into the gut lumen, intestinal distention, and contraction of plasma volume. Additional proposed mechanisms for these symptoms include stimulation of autonomic reflexes secondary to small intestinal distention and/or release of hormones from the gut and vasoactive substances into the circulation in response to the rapid entry of gastric contents into the duodenum or jejunum.

The *late dumping syndrome* is a symptom complex of dizziness, lightheadedness, palpitations, diaphoresis, confusion, and, in rare instances, syncope occurring 90 min to 3 h after eating. The symptoms can often be precipitated by meals rich in simple carbohydrates, especially sucrose, and appear to result from hypoglycemia due to excessive insulin release, which is stimulated by an abrupt increase in blood glucose secondary to rapid emptying of sugar-containing meals into the proximal small intestine.

Both forms of the dumping syndrome are treated by dietary measures, including limitation of simple sugar-continuing liquids and solids (sweets), elimination of liquids at mealtime, and the eating of frequent small meals. In severe cases, symptoms may improve with the somatostatin analogue octreotide (50 μg subcutaneously tid).

Postvagotomy Diarrhea Some patients experience diarrhea after peptic ulcer surgery, especially after truncal vagotomy. Diarrhea usually occurs within 2 h of eating. The mechanism of diarrhea is not clear but is thought to involve interruption of vagal fibers to the abdominal viscera. Loss of the pyloric regulatory emptying mechanism and rapid emptying of gastric contents into the small intestine, resulting in increased fluid volume within the intestinal lumen due to the osmotic action of the meal, also may contribute to the diarrhea.

Hematologic Complications Intrinsic factor secreted by gastric parietal cells is necessary for active absorption of vitamin B_{12} by the distal ileum (see Chap. 108). Although total gastrectomy invariably results in malabsorption of vitamin B_{12}, megaloblastic anemia due to vitamin B_{12} deficiency is rare after partial gastric resection; however, reduced serum vitamin B_{12} levels have been observed in about 14 percent of these patients. Gastritis in the remaining stomach is present in more than 60 percent of DU patients after vagotomy with antrectomy or vagotomy with pyloroplasty; it may progress to gastric atrophy and also may contribute to decreased vitamin B_{12} absorption. Because the stomach secretes approximately 100 times more intrinsic factor than is needed, peptic ulcer patients treated with partial gastric resection do not develop vitamin B_{12} deficiency as a result of the amount of stomach resected. Moreover, the resected portion of the stomach is almost always mainly antrum, which contains few parietal cells. Nevertheless, after peptic ulcer surgery, patients may develop decreased serum vitamin B_{12} levels as a result of reduced absorption of vitamin B_{12}. The precise mechanism of the malabsorption of vitamin B_{12} is not known but may in part involve hypochlorhydria and bacterial overgrowth.

Anemia may result from iron deficiency due to impaired absorption of dietary iron in patients with a Billroth II gastrojejunostomy. These patients have normal absorption of iron salts and respond favorably to oral iron preparations. Folate deficiency may result from either reduced dietary intake or impaired folate absorption. Except for anemia from blood loss caused by early recurrent ulcer, development of anemia after peptic ulcer surgery is gradual, usually occurring over several years.

Osteomalacia and Osteoporosis Osteoporosis and osteomalacia are common after partial or complete gastrectomy but are rare after vagotomy with pyloroplasty. Osteomalacia is extremely common after gastrojejunostomy or Billroth II anastomosis owing to malabsorption of calcium and vitamin D. The incidence of bone fractures in men following gastric resection has been estimated to be almost twice that of control subjects of similar age. Reduced bone density perceptible by x-ray requires years to develop. Patients may develop bone pain and pathologic fractures. Patients with osteomalacia usually have increased levels of serum alkaline phosphatase and may have reduced serum calcium concentrations. These patients should be treated with supplemental oral vitamin D and calcium. The frequency of osteoporosis and osteomalacia after partial or complete gastrectomy is sufficiently great to justify prophylactic treatment with vitamin D and calcium indefinitely after gastric resection, especially in females.

General Malabsorption (See also Chap. 285) Mild, chemically demonstrable steatorrhea is common after ulcer surgery. Weight loss is more common after partial gastric resection (approximately 60 percent of patients) than after vagotomy alone. The major cause of weight loss is reduced food intake. On a diet providing 100 g of fat per day, loss of stool fat seldom exceeds 15 g/d (normal, less than 7 g/d). The causes of maldigestion and malabsorption include rapid gastric emptying, a reduced dispersion of food in the stomach, reduced bile concentrations in the gut lumen, an increased rate of transit of the meal through the small intestine, and reduced or delayed pancreatic secretory responses to feeding. Steatorrhea and weight loss, sometimes accompanied by vitamin B_{12} malabsorption, also may develop as a result of bacterial overgrowth. Malabsorption after peptic ulcer surgery also may be due to preexisting conditions, including latent celiac sprue or chronic pancreatitis.

Carcinoma after Partial Gastrectomy Several studies have reported an increased incidence of adenocarcinoma of the stomach in DU patients 15 or more years after partial gastric resection for DU. This complication should be considered when abdominal symptoms (which may be similar to or distinct from those due to the original ulcer) appear many years after apparently successful ulcer surgery.

NONGASTRITIS EPITHELIAL CELL INJURY

STRESS-RELATED MUCOSAL INJURY Acute upper GI erosions and ulcers distinct from chronic peptic ulcer may occur in

patients with shock, massive burns, sepsis, and severe trauma (Table 284-4). These lesions, called *stress erosions* and *ulcers*, are frequently multiple and are most common in the acid-secreting portion of the stomach. They occur in about 80 to 90 percent of patients with massive injuries and burns (in the latter case, they are called *Curling's ulcers*). The most common clinical finding is painless GI hemorrhage. In critically ill patients in medical intensive care units, the principal risk factors for bleeding are the need for mechanical ventilation and the presence of coagulopathy. Blood loss is usually minimal but may be substantial and life-threatening. Usually, erosions develop about 24 h after trauma or shock. When massive hemorrhage occurs, it typically happens more than 2 or 3 days after the acute insult. The diagnosis is best established by upper GI endoscopy. Erosions are usually too superficial to be recognized by barium examination.

Many theories have been proposed to explain stress-associated acute mucosal ulceration, but mucosal ischemia and tissue injury from gastric acid appear to be the most important factors. Although there is usually no evidence of acid hypersecretion, the lesions cannot be produced in experimental animals in the absence of acid. It is believed that ischemia of the gastric mucosa, which has enormous oxygen requirements, is the most important element in producing stress erosions and ulceration.

Cushing's ulcers are acute ulcers of the upper GI tract associated with intracranial injury or an increase in intracranial pressure (e.g., due to a brain tumor or subdural hematoma). These ulcers may involve the stomach, proximal duodenum, or esophagus and frequently lead to hemorrhage or perforation. They do not differ histologically from acute stress ulceration; however, they are frequently associated with gastric acid hypersecretion. Treatment includes correction of increased intracranial pressure, when possible, and the usual measures for treatment of acute erosions and ulcerations, including vigorous therapy with antacids or H_2 receptor antagonists.

Management of acute stress ulcerations and erosions is principally preventive. With improvements in the hemodynamic management of critically ill patients in the past 20 years, the frequency of bleeding from stress ulcers in intensive care units has fallen from 20 to 30 percent to 1.5 to 14 percent. In fact, the need for routine therapy to prevent stress ulcer bleeding has been questioned. However, it is still standard practice to administer prophylactic therapy to high-risk patients, including patients in an intensive care unit who are being mechanically ventilated, who have coagulopathy or multiorgan failure, or who are severely burned. Standard preventive therapy consists of liquid antacids administered via a nasogastric tube hourly or as needed to maintain a gastric pH of at least 3.5 and/or intravenous administration of an H_2 receptor antagonist, either as bolus injections or by continuous infusion. Alternatively, sucralfate administered by nasogastric tube as a 1-g slurry every 6 h is equally effective in preventing stress ulcer bleeding, and, because it does not raise gastric pH, it may be associated with a lower risk of late-onset (4 or more days after initiation) pneumonia than antacids and H_2 receptor antagonists. When bleeding occurs and does not subside with medical therapy, endoscopic intervention and, in some cases, surgery, including pyloroplasty with vagotomy or total gastrectomy, may be necessary.

MUCOSAL INJURY INDUCED BY ASPIRIN AND OTHER NSAIDS Aspirin is associated with an increased incidence of GU and, to a lesser extent, DU and may cause hemorrhagic erosive gastro-

Table 284-4

Risk Factors for Stress-Related Mucosal Injury (Stress Erosions and Ulcers)

Mechanical ventilation
Coagulopathy
Sepsis and multiorgan failure
Burns (Curling's ulcers)
Central nervous system trauma (Cushing's ulcers)

pathy. Similar gastric mucosal injury is observed in patients ingesting other NSAIDs (e.g., indomethacin, ibuprofen, naproxen, tolmetin, sulindac, piroxicam, diflunisal, fenoprofen, and others). Several mechanisms by which salicylates and other NSAIDs induce ulcers and erosions have been proposed. NSAIDs are directly toxic to the gastric mucosa, and they deplete protective endogenous mucosal prostaglandins by inhibiting prostaglandin synthesis. They also may contribute to ulcer formation by interrupting the gastric mucosal barrier, permitting back-diffusion of hydrogen ions that may injure the gastric mucosa. They reduce gastric mucus secretion and gastric and duodenal bicarbonate secretion and may increase gastric acid secretion. Depletion of mucosal prostaglandins also impairs epithelial cell replacement after injury.

Gastric ulcers develop in 10 to 30 percent of patients receiving chronic NSAID treatment, while the prevalence of DU is 2 to 20 percent. Factors contributing to a high risk for ulcer are shown in Table 284-5. There is no convincing evidence that *H. pylori* infection, smoking, or caffeine or alcohol ingestion increase the risk of NSAID-induced ulcers. As yet, there is no conclusive evidence that any particular NSAID is associated with a lower or greater risk of gastroduodenal ulceration, but some observations suggest that newer NSAIDs, such as nabumetone, which selectively inhibit mucosal cyclooxygenase type 2, may be associated with a lower risk of ulceration than other NSAIDs. Glucocorticoids administered alone have not been proven to be ulcerogenic.

Most persons taking aspirin or NSAIDs experience some GI distress, but there is a poor correlation between symptoms and the development of chronic ulcers. In addition to causing GUs and DUs, NSAIDs have been implicated in occasional cases of small intestinal and colonic ulceration and strictures (which may be either broad or thin and diaphragm-like), as well as in exacerbations of Crohn's disease and ulcerative colitis.

Misoprostol, a PGE_1 analogue, in doses of 100 and 200 μg four times a day, reduces the risk of NSAID-associated GU by approximately 75 and 95 percent, respectively. Abdominal cramping and/or diarrhea may occur with abrupt initiation of the full dose. The drug causes uterine contraction and should not be used in women of childbearing age. NSAID-induced DUs can be prevented by H_2 receptor antagonists, and preliminary studies suggest that higher than standard doses (e.g., famotidine 40 mg orally bid) are also effective in preventing NSAID-induced GUs. These drugs and omeprazole are also effective in healing NSAID-induced ulcers, and omeprazole appears to accelerate the healing of such ulcers even if NSAID use is continued.

OTHER AGENTS THAT INDUCE MUCOSAL INJURY *Ethanol* damage to the gastric mucosa is associated with subepithelial hemorrhages with surrounding edema and only slight to moderate increases in mucosal inflammatory cells. Possible mechanisms for cell injury include the inherent lipophilic and lipolytic properties of ethanol, interruption of the gastric mucosal barrier, and direct damage to small mucosal blood vessels.

Ingestion of corrosive chemicals can cause severe damage to the gastric mucosa. Causative agents include strong acids (e.g., hydrochloric acid, sulfuric acid) and strong alkalis (e.g., sodium hydroxide). The esophagus is particularly susceptible to severe injury by alkalies (particularly lye), with a risk of necrosis and subsequent stricture formation. The stomach, especially the antrum, is more susceptible to acute injury from strong acid. Depending on the dose and concentration, these agents can cause injury ranging from mild inflammation to extensive tissue necrosis. Patients may describe burning of the mouth, throat, and retrosternal area. Epigastric pain and vomiting often signal gastric injury. Hemorrhage and/or perforation may occur. Treatment of strong acid ingestion includes dilution with water, followed by antacids and supportive therapy as required.

Table 284-5

Risk Factors for NSAID-Induced Mucosal Injury

Older age
Female sex
High NSAID doses
Protracted NSAID use
Combined use of NSAID and glucocorticoids
Severe intercurrent illness
Unproven: *H. pylori*, smoking, caffeine, alcohol

GASTRITIS

Gastritis, or inflammation of the gastric mucosa, is not a single disease but rather a group of disorders that all induce inflammatory changes in the gastric mucosa but that differ in their clinical features, histologic characteristics, and causative mechanisms. Several classifications of gastritis exist (Table 284-6). In general, these classifications have been based on (1) the acuteness or chronicity of the clinical manifestations, (2) histologic features, (3) anatomic distribution, or (4) proposed mechanism of pathogenesis. On the basis of clinical features, the two principal forms of gastritis are acute gastritis and chronic gastritis. Different types of chronic gastritis may be classified according to their presumed cause, their histologic features, and the anatomic distribution of the gastritis or associated mucosal atrophy.

ACUTE GASTRITIS ASSOCIATED WITH *H. PYLORI* The onset of *H. pylori* infection may result in acute gastritis associated with a transient increase in gastric acid secretion followed by hypochlorhydria for up to 1 year. Patients may have mild epigastric discomfort, although most remain asymptomatic. Several epidemics of acute gastritis have been attributed to *H. pylori*, but the endoscopic and histologic features have not been well characterized. Acute *H. pylori* gastritis is a precursor to chronic active gastritis (see below).

OTHER CAUSES OF INFECTIOUS GASTRITIS Infectious causes of gastritis, other than gastric *H. pylori* colonization, are unusual. *Phlegmonous gastritis*, a rare form of bacterial gastritis, is a life-threatening disease with extensive infiltration of the gastric wall, tissue necrosis, and manifestations of generalized sepsis. Responsible organisms include streptococci, staphylococci, *Proteus* species, and *Escherichia coli*. Treatment includes appropriate intravenous antibiotics and necessary supportive care with fluid and electrolyte replacement as required. Lack of response to therapy may necessitate gastrectomy.

Infectious gastritis may be found in immunocompromised patients, including patients with AIDS. Gastric erosions may be produced by herpes simplex virus. Typical intranuclear inclusions of cytomegalovirus, with positive cultures, may occur in disseminated cytomegalovirus infection.

Table 284-6

Classification of Gastritis

Acute gastritis
Acute *H. pylori* gastritis
Other acute infectious gastritides
Bacterial (other than *H. pylori*)
Helicobacter helmmanii
Phlegmonous
Mycobacterial
Syphilitic
Viral
Parasitic
Fungal
Chronic atrophic gastritis
Type A: Body-predominant, autoimmune
Type B: Antral-predominant, *H. pylori*–related, environmental
Type AB
Indeterminant type
Uncommon forms of gastritis
Lymphocytic gastritis
Eosinophilic gastritis
Crohn's disease
Sarcoidosis
Isolated granulomatous gastritis

CHRONIC GASTRITIS The inflammatory cell infiltrate in chronic gastritis consists mainly of lymphocytes and plasma cells. Polymorphonuclear leukocytes and eosinophils may be present in small numbers. Chronic gastritis is often patchy and irregular in distribution. It involves the superficial and glandular areas of the gastric mucosa initially and progresses to glandular destruction, which may be followed by gland metaplasia and a profound reduction in gland number (atrophy). Chronic gastritis has been classified descriptively on the basis of several characteristic histologic abnormalities.

Superficial gastritis appears to represent the initial stage in the development of chronic gastritis. Inflammatory changes are limited to the lamina propria of the superficial mucosa, with cellular infiltration and edema separating the gastric glands; the glands are preserved. There may be a decrease in the amount of mucus in glandular mucous cells and in the frequency of mitotic figures in cells of the glands.

Atrophic gastritis is the next stage in the development of chronic gastritis. The inflammatory infiltrate extends to the deep portions of the mucosa. There is progressive distortion and destruction of the glands, which become separated by the inflammatory process. In the more common form of chronic gastritis, the process begins in the antrum and extends proximally into the body and fundus of the stomach.

Gastric atrophy is the final stage of chronic gastritis. There is a profound loss of glandular structures, which are now separated widely by connective tissue, with a greatly reduced or absent inflammatory infiltrate. The mucosa becomes thin, and the underlying blood vessels may be evident on endoscopic examination.

There may be changes in the morphology of the gastric glandular elements as chronic gastritis progresses. *Intestinal metaplasia* is the conversion of gastric glands to a form resembling that of small intestinal mucosal glands containing goblet cells. Intestinal metaplasia may be patchy or extensive and is an important predisposing factor for gastric cancer (see Chap. 92); however, the magnitude of the risk is not sufficient to justify endoscopic surveillance for gastric cancer.

The two major forms of chronic gastritis traditionally have been called types A (body-predominant, autoimmune) and B (antral-predominant, related to *H. pylori* infection) on the basis of their distribution in the gastric mucosa coupled with implications regarding their pathogenesis, although the distinction is not always clear. In some cases, the designation *type AB gastritis* is used to reflect involvement of both body and antrum.

Type A Gastritis (Body-Predominant Gastritis, Autoimmune Chronic Atrophic Gastritis) Type A gastritis is the less common form of chronic gastritis. It characteristically involves the fundus and body of the stomach, with relative sparing of the antrum. This is the form of gastritis that may be associated with pernicious anemia (see Chap. 108). The frequent presence of antibodies to parietal cells and to intrinsic factor in sera of patients with type A gastritis and pernicious anemia has suggested an immune or autoimmune pathogenesis for this form of gastritis, although autoimmune features are often not present and it appears that a substantial number of cases may result from *H. pylori* infection (see below). Antibodies to parietal cells have been shown to be cytotoxic for gastric mucosal cells. Cell-mediated immune mechanisms also have been proposed to participate in gastric mucosal cell injury in pernicious anemia and related forms of type A gastritis. Antibodies to parietal cells have been found in sera of approximately 90 percent of patients with pernicious anemia and in more than half of other patients with type A gastritis. Relatives of patients with pernicious anemia have a higher than normal frequency of serum antibodies to parietal cells, atrophic gastritis, and reduced gastric acid secretion. In control populations, parietal cell antibodies may be found in up to 20 percent of individuals over age 60 and in approximately 20 percent of all patients with hypoparathyroidism, Addison's disease, and vitiligo. About 50 percent of patients with pernicious anemia have antibodies to thyroid antigens, and approximately 30 percent of patients with thyroid disease have circulating antibodies to parietal cells. Serum antibodies to intrinsic factor are more specific for type A gastritis than parietal cell antibodies and are present in about 40 percent of patients with pernicious anemia.

In patients with pernicious anemia, the gastric glands that contain parietal cells are invariably destroyed, accounting for their inability to secrete hydrochloric acid. Since, in humans, parietal cells also secrete intrinsic factor, type A atrophic gastritis also results in malabsorption of vitamin B_{12}, with resulting hematologic and/or neurologic consequences characteristic of pernicious anemia.

In general, the reduction in gastric acid secretion, which is complete in patients with pernicious anemia, is proportionate to the severity of parietal cell destruction and mucosal atrophy in the body and fundus of the stomach. Serum gastrin levels are usually elevated substantially in patients with pernicious anemia and are in approximately the same range as those of patients with ZES (gastrinoma). Since the antral mucosa is relatively spared, the antral gastrin-containing cells, deprived of the feedback control normally exerted by acid in the stomach, release gastrin continuously. As a result of pronounced hypergastrinemia, ECL-cell hyperplasia and carcinoid tumors of the stomach may develop in these patients. Carcinoids may regress following antrectomy to remove gastrin-producing cells. Serum gastrin levels are also often similarly elevated in patients with type A gastritis with achlorhydria or profound hypochlorhydria who do not have pernicious anemia.

Type B Gastritis (Antral-Predominant Gastritis, *H. pylori* Gastritis, Environmental Gastritis) Type B gastritis is the more common form of chronic gastritis. In younger patients, type B gastritis principally involves the antrum, whereas in older patients the entire stomach is affected. This transition is estimated to require about 15 to 20 years. The incidence of chronic gastritis, most of it type B gastritis, increases with age, reaching 78 percent in individuals over age 50 and virtually 100 percent after age 70.

Studies from various parts of the world have established that *H. pylori* is the agent responsible for type B gastritis and that eradication of *H. pylori* leads to resolution of the histologic findings. Gastric colonization with *H. pylori* is found in virtually all patients with chronic superficial gastritis, but fewer bacteria are demonstrable with progression to atrophic gastritis. In general, the degree of histologic abnormality correlates with the number of organisms identified histologically. Findings include a dense chronic inflammatory infiltrate of the lamina propria and invasion of the epithelial cell layer by polymorphonuclear leukocytes (Fig. 284-12). *H. pylori* are few in number or not demonstrated with severe gastric atrophy.

Patients with type B gastritis have fasting serum gastrin levels that are highly variable, not consistently elevated, and often in the normal range. A few patients with type B gastritis have serum antibodies to gastrin, leading some to propose an autoimmune mechanism for this form of gastritis. Alternatively, and probably more likely, these antibodies may represent responses to the inflammatory process rather than contributing factors.

Chronic *H. pylori* gastritis may lead to multifocal atrophic gastritis, gastric atrophy, and gastric metaplasia (Fig. 284-13). Moreover, treatment with acid-suppressive therapy (e.g., H_2 receptor antagonists or proton pump inhibitors) increases the rate of development of gastric atrophy, thereby possibly increasing the risk of gastric cancer. In addition, such therapy in patients infected with *H. pylori* may increase the activity of gastritis in the gastric body; this too may lead to atrophic gastritis and a predisposition to gastric cancer.

H. pylori appears to be an independent risk factor for the development of gastric cancer, although its effect may be indirect. The epidemiologic features of gastric carcinoma and *H. pylori* infection are similar, and socioeconomic conditions known to influence the risk of gastric cancer are also important determinants of *H. pylori* infection. Worldwide epidemiologic studies have shown a higher prevalence of *H. pylori* infection in patients with gastric cancer than in control subjects. Seropositivity for *H. pylori* is associated with a three- to sixfold increase in the risk of gastric cancer (as high as ninefold after adjustment for the inaccuracy of serological testing in the elderly), although no such association exists in patients with cancer located at the gastric cardia.

As for peptic ulcer, not all patients with gastric cancer are infected with *H. pylori*, and not all persons with *H. pylori* infection develop gastric cancer. In addition, gastric atrophy only sometimes progresses to gastric cancer. Therefore, the etiology of gastric cancer is most likely multifactorial, with *H. pylori* infection as one of several factors contributing to its development.

The mechanism by which *H. pylori* infection may initiate gastric carcinogenesis is not known. The organism alters the physical and chemical milieu of the gastric mucus, which may render the gastric mucosa less resistant to environmental or dietary carcinogens. *H. pylori* infection also causes a decrease in the gastric secretion of ascorbic acid, reduced levels of which may allow formation of carcinogenic *N*-nitroso compounds. In addition, the chronic inflammation produced by *H. pylori* infection may stimulate mucosal hyperproliferation in a manner similar to that observed in chronic ulcerative colitis. It remains to be determined if eradication of *H. pylori* will substantially reduce the risk of gastric cancer. Currently, eradication of *H. pylori* in asymptomatic persons to reduce gastric cancer risk is not recommended.

H. pylori may also be associated with gastric lymphoma. Whereas lymphoid tissue is not found in the normal stomach, gastric lymphoid tissue develops in response to local infection with *H. pylori*. Most primary gastric lymphomas are, in fact, derived from mucosa-associ-

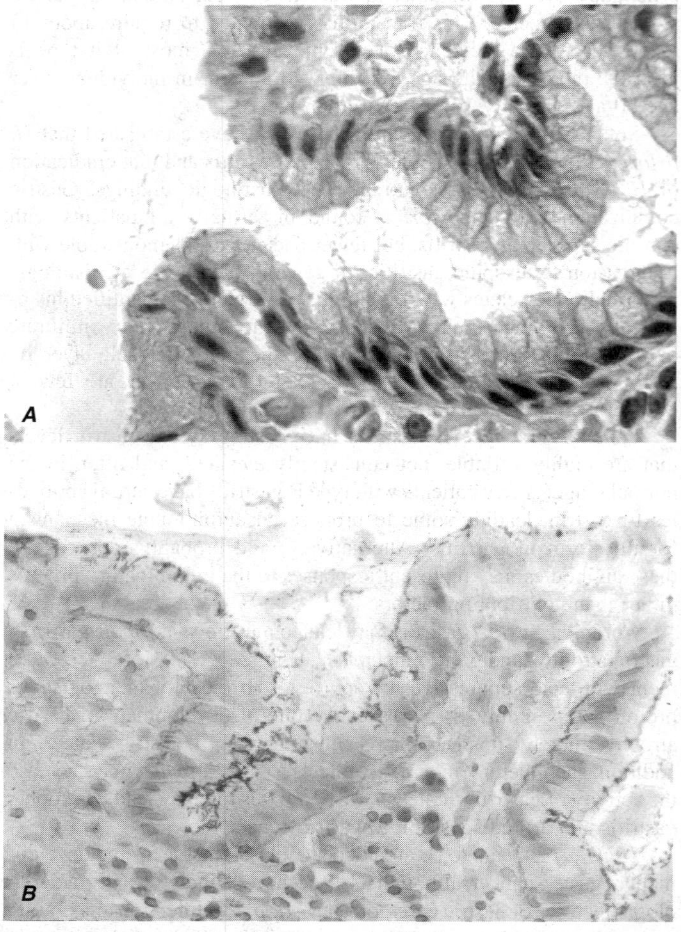

FIGURE 284-12 Chronic gastritis and *Helicobacter pylori* organisms. *A.* H&E stain of gastric mucosa showing surface foveolar cells, adherent mucus, and scattered bacillary forms within the mucus. *B.* Steiner silver stain of superficial gastric mucosa, showing abundant darkly staining microorganisms layered over the apical portion of the surface epithelium. Note that there is no tissue invasion. *[Courtesy of James M. Crawford, M.D., Ph.D. Reprinted with permission from JM Crawford, The oral cavity and gastrointestinal tract, in Basic Pathology, V Kumar, RS Cotran, and SL Robbins (eds.). Philadelphia, Saunders, 1997.]*

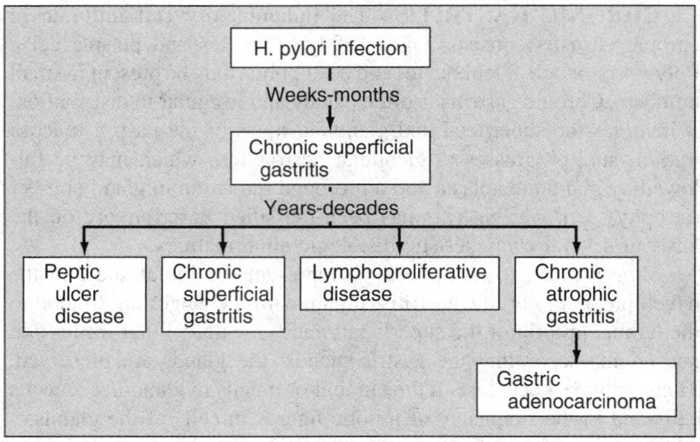

FIGURE 284-13 Possible long-term consequences of *H. pylori* infection.

ated lymphoid tissue (MALT). Epidemiologic studies in Europe have shown that regions with a high incidence of gastric lymphoma have higher rates of *H. pylori* infection than regions with a low incidence of gastric lymphoma. Moreover, patients with gastric lymphoma are more likely to have serologic evidence of *H. pylori* infection than matched controls. No association has been found between nongastric, non-Hodgkin's lymphoma and *H. pylori* infection.

The mechanism by which *H. pylori* infection leads to gastric lymphoma is unclear. Features of primary gastric B-cell lymphoma of MALT suggest that the tumor may be antigen-responsive; that is, the lymphoid follicles may result from chronic antigenic stimulation of the gastric mucosa by *H. pylori*. Given its close association with MALT lymphoma, *H. pylori* may initiate a malignant transformation by stimulating an immune response.

It has also been suggested that eradication of *H. pylori* from the gastric mucosa may result in the eventual loss of MALT, thereby removing the lymphoid precursor from which gastric lymphoma arises. Indeed, some studies have demonstrated that antibiotic treatment of *H. pylori* in patients with biopsy-proven low-grade B-cell MALT lymphoma results in eradication of the infection and regression of the lymphoma. It remains to be determined if prophylactic eradication of the infection will result in a substantially reduced risk of gastric lymphoma. Currently, the treatment of *H. pylori* in asymptomatic persons for the purpose of reducing the risk of gastric lymphoma is not recommended.

DIAGNOSIS Biopsy is the most reliable means of identifying and classifying gastritis as well as detecting *H. pylori*. However, caution must be exercised in the interpretation of a single gastric mucosal biopsy, because the patchy and irregular distribution of the gastritis may lead to substantial sampling error. Therefore, biopsy of several suspected areas is recommended when it is safe and possible.

℞ TREATMENT

In general, no specific treatment is required for type A or type B chronic gastritis with or without mucosal atrophy. However, pernicious anemia, a consequence of type A gastritis, requires lifelong regular parenteral vitamin B_{12} administration (see Chap. 108). In the absence of documented peptic ulcer or MALT lymphoma, eradication of *H. pylori* in patients with type B gastritis is generally not recommended.

OTHER TYPES OF GASTRITIS *Lymphocytic gastritis* is characterized histologically by intense lymphocytic infiltration of the gastric surface epithelium and the presence of superficial pits with a lymphocytosis of small mature T cells and plasmacytosis of the lamina propria. The cause is unknown, but some cases occur in patients with celiac sprue, and shared pathogenic mechanisms are suspected. Patients are usually asymptomatic, but endoscopy shows thickened gastric folds, often capped by small nodules with central depressions, an appearance often referred to as "varioliform gastritis." Lymphocytic gastritis has been treated with corticosteroids or sodium cromoglycate, with variable response. There is controversy as to whether lymphocytic gastritis may be caused by *H. pylori*.

Eosinophilic gastritis is characterized by extensive eosinophilic infiltration of the stomach wall, usually with circulating eosinophilia. It may occur as isolated involvement of the stomach or as a component of eosinophilic gastroenteritis. Biopsy reveals extensive eosinophilic infiltration, which may involve all layers of the stomach wall or may be limited to the mucosa, submucosa, or muscularis. The antrum is involved more often than the body or fundus. There may be prominent antral mucosal folds with edema and mucosal thickening, which uncommonly lead to gastric outlet obstruction. Epigastric pain, which may be accompanied by nausea and vomiting, is the most frequent symptom. Patients usually respond favorably to treatment with glucocorticoids.

A number of generalized diseases can involve the stomach, producing *granulomatous gastritis*. Crohn's disease may produce gastric ulceration, granulomatous infiltration, and/or scarring with stricture formation; associated small intestinal Crohn's disease is usually present. Infectious causes of granulomatous gastritis include histoplasmosis, candidiasis, syphilis, and tuberculosis. Multiple mucosal biopsies and cytology are usually required to establish the diagnosis of granulomatous gastritis and to exclude malignancy. If the diagnosis is not established by biopsy at endoscopy, surgical exploration may be required. Rarely, sarcoidosis, idiopathic granulomatous gastritis, and eosinophilic granulomas involve the stomach.

MÉNÉTRIER'S DISEASE

Ménétrier's disease is a clinical entity characterized by large, tortuous gastric mucosal folds, which may be localized or may involve the whole stomach. These mucosal folds are often most conspicuous in the gastric body and fundus. The mucosal thickening is due to massive foveolar hyperplasia (hyperplasia of surface and glandular mucous cells), which replaces most of the chief and parietal cells. The pits of the gastric glands elongate and may become extremely tortuous. The lamina propria may contain a mild chronic inflammatory infiltrate; however, technically Ménétrier's disease is not a form of gastritis.

The most common symptom is epigastric pain. Anorexia, nausea, vomiting, and weight loss are less frequent. Occult GI bleeding may occur, but overt bleeding is unusual and, when present, is due to superficial mucosal erosions. Uncommonly, GU or gastric carcinoma may develop. Patients often develop a protein-losing gastropathy resulting in hypoalbuminemia and edema. Gastric acid secretion is usually reduced or absent. Barium examination of the upper GI tract reveals the large gastric folds, which are readily confirmed by endoscopy. Deep mucosal biopsy (and cytology) is needed for diagnosis. The depth of these lesions and the disconcerting prominence of the folds may require a surgical full-thickness biopsy to exclude lymphoma or infiltrating carcinoma.

Anticholinergic agents and H_2 receptor antagonists have been reported to decrease protein loss in patients with Ménétrier's disease. Treatment includes a high-protein diet, when required, to replace protein losses. If ulcers are present, the treatment should be as for common GU. Severe disease with persistent and substantial protein loss may require total gastrectomy.

ZOLLINGER-ELLISON SYNDROME (GASTRINOMA)

Zollinger-Ellison syndrome (ZES) consists of ulcer disease of the upper GI tract, marked increases in gastric acid secretion, and non-beta islet cell tumors of the pancreas. These tumors are called gastrinomas because they contain gastrin, which circulates in large amounts, producing the pathophysiologic characteristics of ZES.

ETIOLOGY AND PATHOGENESIS In initial studies, gastrinomas were reported most often in the pancreas. They are most common in the head of the pancreas and may vary in size from 1 mm to more than 20 cm in diameter. One-half to two-thirds of patients have multiple gastrinomas. Recent studies suggest that, with careful searching, gastrinomas are found as frequently (or perhaps more frequently) in the wall of the duodenum as in the pancreas. Duodenal gastrinomas, approximately half of which are solitary, are usually found in the submucosa of the first or second part of the duodenum and are just as likely as pancreatic gastrinomas to be malignant. Rarely, gastrinomas are found in the stomach or in lymph nodes near to the pancreas, proximal duodenum, or spleen in the absence of demonstrated primary tumors. Approximately 90 percent of gastrinomas are found within an anatomic triangle ("the gastrinoma triangle") that is defined by the junction of the cystic and common bile ducts superiorly, the junction of the second and third portions of the duodenum inferiorly, and the junction of the pancreatic body and neck medially. In unusual instances, ZES has resulted from gastrinomas originating in remote organs, such as the parathyroids or ovaries.

About two-thirds of gastrinomas are histologically or biologically malignant; about one-third of all patients have metastatic disease on presentation. Malignant gastrinomas usually grow slowly; however, a small portion are rapidly invasive and may metastasize early and widely. Metastasis is most often to regional lymph nodes and the liver; other sites are peritoneal surfaces, spleen, bone, skin, and mediastinum. Gastrinomas have similarities by light microscopy to carcinoid tumors and may be mistaken for these tumors, especially when arising from the mucosa of the small intestine or stomach.

Pancreatic islet cell hyperplasia occurs in approximately 10 percent of patients with ZES. Islet hyperplasia accompanying recognized or unidentified gastrinoma appears to be a result, rather than a cause, of excess gastrin release, since gastrin is not present in the hyperplastic tissue.

In an estimated 20 to 60 percent of patients with ZES, the gastrinoma is a component of the multiple endocrine neoplasia type 1 (MEN 1) syndrome, an autosomal dominant disorder with a high degree of penetrance and great variability in expressivity (see Chap. 340). The MEN 1 locus is on chromosome 11 (11q11-q13). Patients with MEN 1 may have clinically recognized hyperplasia, adenomas, or carcinoma involving, in order of frequency, the parathyroid glands, pancreatic islets, and pituitary. Hyperparathyroidism has been reported in close to 90 percent of patients with MEN 1 syndrome, and gastrinoma has been reported in approximately half of them (see Chap. 340). However, a careful search would probably find involvement of all three organs in all patients with MEN 1, although frequently without overt clinical expression. Patients with MEN 1 usually present with multiple gastrinomas, which generally are smaller than sporadic gastrinomas. Gastrinomas with MEN 1 are located more frequently in the wall of the duodenum than in the pancreas. In fact, MEN 1 patients, including those with duodenal gastrinomas, usually have multiple pancreatic islet cell tumors, but most of these are not gastrinomas.

Most of the gastrin in gastrinomas is heptadecapeptide gastrin (G-17), with the remainder being mostly G-34. In contrast, approximately two-thirds of circulating gastrin in gastrinoma patients is G-34; most of the remainder is G-17. When examined carefully, almost all gastrin-secreting islet cell tumors contain multiple hormones, which are usually clinically silent. These may include adrenocorticotropic hormone (ACTH), glucagon, melanocyte-stimulating hormone, parathyroid hormone, growth hormone releasing factor (GRF), insulin, pancreatic polypeptide, and vasoactive intestinal peptide. Of these, ACTH is the most common; it is found in approximately one-third of gastrinomas. Cushing's syndrome with increased serum ACTH levels has been reported in 8 percent of patients with ZES. ACTH-releasing gastrinomas are often aggressively malignant. In contrast, ACTH may be released by pituitary tumors in patients with MEN 1, in whom symptoms of Cushing's syndrome are generally mild and gastrinomas are usually not metastatic. Approximately one-third of patients with gastrinomas have increases in serum concentrations of pancreatic polypeptide.

In patients with ZES, the parietal cell mass is substantially expanded (three to six times normal), owing to the trophic effects of circulating gastrin. Small, multicentric, noninvasive carcinoid tumors have been identified in the gastric mucosa of ZES patients. These tumors and associated focal areas of enterochromaffin-like (ECL) cell hyperplasia are believed to result from substantial and sustained hypergastrinemia and are more likely in patients with MEN 1 than in those with sporadic gastrinomas. Carcinoids and ECL hyperplasia also have been found in the gastric mucosa of patients with pernicious anemia and achlorhydria, who have increases in serum gastrin in the range of those found with gastrinoma.

CLINICAL FEATURES While the true incidence of ZES is not known, estimates are that it accounts for 0.1 to 1 percent of peptic ulcers. ZES may occur at any age, but initial manifestations occur most commonly between ages 30 and 60.

Most, if not all, patients with gastrinomas develop ulceration of the GI tract at some point in the course of their disease. Profound gastric acid hypersecretion is usually present. Especially early in the course of the disease, symptoms are usually similar to those of patients with typical peptic ulcer. However, ulcer symptoms may be more fulminant, progressive, and persistent and, in general, respond poorly to usual medical and surgical peptic ulcer treatments. The anatomic site of the ulcers in ZES is similar but not identical to that of common types of peptic ulcer. About 75 percent of ZES patients have ulcers in the first portion of the duodenum or in the stomach; these are usually single but may be multiple. When multiple ulcers occur, they are frequently located not only in the first portion of the duodenum, but also in the remainder of the duodenum and even the jejunum.

Diarrhea occurs in about 40 percent of patients owing to the outpouring of large amounts of hydrochloric acid into the proximal duodenum; it can be reduced or eliminated by aspiration of gastric juice. The excessive acid has been shown to reduce the pH of the contents of the proximal and distal jejunum to as low as 1 and 3.6, respectively. The large amounts of acid and pepsin may cause corrosive changes in the mucosa of the small intestine. Steatorrhea, which is less common than diarrhea, results from inactivation of pancreatic lipase by large concentrations of acid in the proximal small intestine and from decreases in luminal bile acids. The decrease in intraluminal bile acid concentration is caused by precipitation of the major bile acids at low pH, leading to impaired micelle formation, which, in turn, reduces intestinal absorption of fatty acids and monoglycerides (see Chap. 285). Vitamin B_{12} malabsorption not correctable by addition of intrinsic factor has been detected in some patients with ZES. Although gastric secretion of intrinsic factor appears normal, the reduced luminal pH prevents the activation of the pancreatic enzymes that are needed to split R proteins from vitamin B_{12} so that the vitamin can bind with intrinsic factor and undergo intestinal absorption (see Chap. 108).

DIAGNOSIS Gastrinoma should be suspected in patients with a compatible clinical history, especially in those with marked acid hypersecretion (Table 284-7). More than 90 percent of patients with ZES have a basal gastric acid output (BAO) that exceeds 4 μmol/s (15 mEq/h). In rare instances, the BAO may be greater than 40 μmol/s (150 mEq/h). However, there is substantial overlap in rates of gastric acid secretion among ZES patients, those with DU, and normal subjects. Patients with ZES often have a BAO that is greater than 60 percent of the output induced by maximal stimulation (the MAO). In most normal subjects and DU patients, the BAO is less than 60 percent of maximal secretion. However, exceptions are common, so the BAO/MAO ratio alone cannot be relied on to identify patients with gastrinoma.

Some radiographic and endoscopic features may suggest the diagnosis of ZES. Large mucosal folds may be demonstrated most prominently in the stomach but also in the duodenum and, in some instances, the jejunum. The lumen of the stomach and small intestine often contains large amounts of fluid. Radiographic and endoscopic features of most ulcers in these patients, except when they are distal in location, are similar to those of common peptic ulcer. *H. pylori* is usually absent.

The diagnosis of gastrinoma in a patient with clinical features consistent with ZES depends on the demonstration of increased serum gastrin levels by radioimmunoassay. Fasting serum gastrin levels in normal subjects and patients with typical DU average approximately 20 to 50 ng/L and usually do not exceed 150 ng/L. Patients with ZES almost always have fasting serum gastrin levels that are greater than 200 ng/L; levels may be as high as 450,000 ng/L. However, approximately half these patients have fasting serum gastrin levels less than 1000 ng/L (the approximate mean value for serum gastrin for patients with gastrinoma). Rarely, serum gastrin levels as measured by standard assays are normal in patients with ZES.

Several provocative tests have been used to evaluate patients with possible ZES, especially those who do not exhibit pronounced hypergastrinemia (i.e., serum gastrin of at least 1000 ng/L). These tests involve measurements of serum gastrin levels after intravenous secretin injection, calcium infusion, or ingestion of a standard test meal.

In the *secretin injection* test, secretin (Kabi secretin, 2 U/kg) is given intravenously over 30 to 60 s. Serum gastrin is measured in samples obtained immediately before injection of secretin, at 2 and 5 min after injection, and at 5-min intervals thereafter for a total of 30 min. In normal individuals and patients with common DU, secretin produces either no change or small reductions or increases in serum gastrin levels. However, in ZES patients, intravenous secretin induces substantial increases in serum gastrin; these levels increase promptly by at least 200 ng/L, usually at 5 min (and virtually always by 10 min), and then gradually decrease toward preinjection levels by 30 min.

In the *calcium infusion* test, serum gastrin measurements are obtained before and at 30-min intervals for 4 h after a 3-h constant-rate intravenous infusion of calcium gluconate (5 mg/kg per hour). In patients with ZES, serum gastrin concentrations usually increase above the basal serum gastrin level by more than 400 ng/L.

The third provocative test involves the *feeding of a standard meal*: gastrin is measured in serum samples obtained before the meal and at 15-min intervals thereafter for 90 min. This test has been used to attempt to distinguish between ZES patients and those with hypergastrinemia and gastric acid hypersecretion due to antral gastrin cell hypertrophy or hyperplasia (see below).

The secretin injection test is the most valuable provocative test in identifying patients with ZES. Positive serum gastrin response to intravenous secretin is found in more than 95 percent of ZES patients. Using the criteria suggested, substantial increases in serum gastrin following secretin injection occur only rarely in nongastrinoma patients. Because reduced gastric acid secretion (achlorhydria or profound hypochlorhydria) is the most common cause of hypergastrinemia, gastric acid secretion should be measured before using the secretin injection test (Table 284-8). Exaggerated release of gastrin in response to calcium infusion is found in more than 80 percent of ZES patients; however, this exaggerated response also occurs in some nongastrinoma patients with hypergastrinemia (e.g., with achlorhydria). Enhanced gastrin release with calcium infusion is rarely observed in ZES patients in the absence of the abnormally large gastrin release in response to secretin. Since the calcium infusion test does not add significantly to the sensitivity or specificity of the secretin injection

Table 284-7

Indications for Measuring Serum Gastrin Levels in Patients with Peptic Ulcer

Multiple ulcers or ulcers in unusual locations
Ulcers resistant to therapy or with frequent recurrences
Ulcers requiring surgery
Extensive family history of peptic ulcer disease
Postoperative ulcer recurrence
Severe esophagitis
Basal hyperchlorhydria
Unexplained diarrhea or steatorrhea
Hypercalcemia
Family history of pancreatic islet, pituitary, or parathyroid tumor
Prominent gastric or duodenal folds

Table 284-8

Causes of Hypergastrinemia

Hypochlorhydria or achlorhydria with or without pernicious anemia
Retained gastric antrum
Antral G-cell hyperplasia
Renal insufficiency
Massive small bowel resection
Gastric outlet obstruction
Pheochromocytoma

test, and since calcium infusion is potentially more hazardous, it is usually not necessary or recommended.

In a minority of DU patients (much less than 1 percent), gastric acid hypersecretion may be accompanied by increased serum gastrin levels due to hyperfunctioning and/or hyperplasia of antral gastrin cells (G cells). It is quite possible that this response is an effect, at least in part, of *H. pylori* infection. These patients can be distinguished from those with ZES by the secretin and meal stimulation tests. In patients with this antral gastrin cell abnormality, intravenous secretin does not produce the large increases in serum gastrin characteristic of ZES. On the other hand, serum gastrin concentrations may increase by greater than 200 percent after test meals in patients with gastrin cell hypertrophy or hyperplasia, suggesting that this response may be of value in distinguishing these patients from those with gastrinoma. More recently, however, other investigators have found similarly large amounts of gastrin released into the sera of patients with gastrinomas, suggesting that the meal-stimulated test is of limited value in distinguishing between patients with antral gastrin cell hyperplasia and those with ZES.

Gastrinomas are difficult to localize. In almost half of patients with clinical and laboratory evidence of ZES, the tumors cannot be identified at surgery. Selective arteriography identifies gastrinomas in about half of patients with clinical and biochemical evidence of ZES. Computed tomography (CT) localizes gastrinomas in 30 percent, and ultrasound in 20 percent, of ZES patients. Hepatic venous gastrin sampling after intra-arterial injection of secretin during arteriography appears to be useful in localizing duodenal gastrinomas. Magnetic resonance imaging is no better than CT in localizing primary tumors but is the most sensitive method of detecting hepatic metastases. Endoscopic retrograde pancreatography has not been helpful in the diagnosis or exclusion of pancreatic gastrinomas. A small number of duodenal wall gastrinomas have been identified and confirmed histologically by duodenoscopy and, more recently, by endoscopic ultrasonography, which shows great promise. Because gastrinomas express cell-surface receptors for somatostatin, nuclear scanning after intravenous injection of radiolabeled octreotide has proved useful for localizing small primary tumors and metastases.

℞ TREATMENT

In general, patients with ZES are resistant to the medical and surgical therapies that are effective in treating common peptic ulcer. In fact, partial gastric resection (with or without vagotomy) or pyloroplasty with vagotomy is frequently followed by prompt and often fulminant ulcer recurrence. In the past, many patients with gastrinoma underwent multiple surgical procedures, particularly in cases where the diagnosis was not established initially. The mortality rate was reported to be lowest in patients with ZES in whom gastrectomy was the initial gastric surgery. This report led to the conclusion that, when surgery was required in gastrinoma patients, total gastrectomy was the procedure of choice.

Development of effective drugs to reduce acid secretion and of more precise diagnostic techniques to locate gastrinomas have increased therapeutic options substantially. Management in these patients must be individualized, because patients with ZES are heterogeneous with respect to clinical manifestations and extent of disease. As with many other predominantly malignant tumors, the ideal treatment is removal of the gastrinoma.

H_2 receptor antagonists are effective in reducing gastric acid secretion, relieving symptoms, and inducing ulcer healing in patients with ZES. Improvement in clinical symptoms, a decrease in gastric acid output, and ulcer healing occur in 80 to 85 percent of patients. Daily doses four to eight times those used in the treatment of common DU may be required. H_2 receptor antagonist therapy must be continued indefinitely, since even temporary discontinuation is usually followed by ulcer recurrence. In approximately 25 percent of patients with ZES, ulcers fail to respond to treatment with H_2 receptor antagonists or recur during treatment. The dose of H_2 receptor antagonist required to maintain a satisfactory reduction in gastric acid secretion can be assessed by measuring the BAO during the hour immediately prior to the next anticipated dose of the drug; the goal is to reduce BAO to less than 2.8 μmol/s (10 mEq/h) at that time.

The parietal cell H^+,K^+-ATPase inhibitors omeprazole and lansoprazole are the most effective drugs and the agents of choice in reducing gastric acid secretion and healing ulcers in patients with ZES, including those with ulcers resistant to treatment with H_2 receptor antagonists. The usual initial daily recommended dose of omeprazole or lansoprazole is 60 mg in a single dose administered in the morning before breakfast. The dose is adjusted to maintain the BAO at less than 2.8 μmol/s (10 mEq/h) [or at less than 1.4 μmol/s (5 mEq/h) in patients who have had prior ulcer surgery] during the hour immediately before the next dose. Patients with esophagitis may require doses sufficient to reduce gastric hypersecretion to less than 0.25 μmol/s (1 mEq/h) to control symptoms. Twice-daily dosing is required in about one-third of patients. It may be possible to reduce the drug dose once symptoms are controlled.

Some patients with ZES in whom gastrinomas could not be identified or removed surgically have been treated with parietal cell vagotomy. In a few instances, this treatment has reduced the amount of H_2 receptor antagonist required or rendered the drug unnecessary.

In selecting the best therapy, the biologic behavior of the tumor and the clinical manifestations in each patient must be taken into consideration. Early studies indicated that morbidity and mortality in patients with ZES were due principally to complications of severe ulcer disease. However, with earlier diagnosis, more effective antiulcer treatment, and longer follow-up, more frequent consequences of the malignant properties of gastrinomas are being recognized. Approximately half of ZES patients in whom the gastrinoma has not been removed will die from malignant invasion by the tumor. Complete surgical resection of the tumors, when possible, is the optimal treatment. Exploratory surgery should include endoscopic transillumination of the duodenum and lateral duodenotomy with examination of the duodenum. The possible benefit of intraoperative ultrasonography remains to be determined. Complete surgical removal of gastrinoma, with cure, has been achieved in approximately 30 percent of patients with ZES.

Treatment with omeprazole or lansoprazole is indicated while the diagnosis is being established, while the location and extent of the tumor are being determined, and prior to anticipated surgery. At present, long-term treatment with omeprazole or lansoprazole is indicated for patients who are not suitable candidates for surgery, who refuse surgery, or in whom surgical removal of the tumor is not possible.

Patients with aggressively invasive gastrinoma have been treated with combinations of streptozotocin, 5-fluorouracil, and doxorubicin in attempts to reduce tumor bulk and associated symptoms. Response to chemotherapy is limited, with initial response rates of up to 65 percent and no complete responses. The efficacy of interferon and octreotide also appears limited. When metastatic or nonresectable gastrinoma is present, control of the ulcer disease may be achieved in most instances by treatment with omeprazole or lansoprazole or, rarely, when required, by total gastric resection. There is no convincing evidence that tumor progression is influenced by gastrectomy.

BIBLIOGRAPHY

PEPTIC ULCER AND *HELICOBACTER PYLORI*

El-Omar EM et al: *Helicobacter pylori* infection and abnormalities of acid secretion in patients with duodenal ulcer disease. Gastroenterology 109:681, 1995

Fendrick AM et al: Alternative management strategies for patients with suspected peptic ulcer disease. Ann Intern Med 123:260, 1995

Graham DY et al: Effect of treatment of *Helicobacter pylori* infection on the long-term recurrence of gastric or duodenal ulcer: a randomized, controlled study. Ann Intern Med 116:705, 1992

Hentschel E et al: Effect of ranitidine and amoxicillin plus metronidazole on the eradication of *Helicobacter pylori* and the recurrence of duodenal ulcer. N Engl J Med 328:308, 1993

McGowan CC et al: *Helicobacter pylori* and gastric acid: Biological and therapeutic implications. Gastroenterology 110:926, 1996

Modlin IM, Tang LH: The gastric enterochromaffin-like cell: An enigmatic cellular link. Gastroenterology 111:926, 1996

Soll AH: Medical treatment of peptic ulcer disease: Practice guidelines. JAMA 275:622, 1996

Talley TJ: A critique of therapeutic trials in *Helicobacter pylori*-positive functional dyspepsia. Gastroenterology 106:1174, 1994

Taylor JL et al: Pharmacoeconomic comparison of treatments for the eradication of *Helicobacter pylori.* Arch Intern Med 157:87, 1997

Walsh JH, Peterson WL: The treatment of *Helicobacter pylori* infection in the management of peptic ulcer disease. N Engl J Med 338:984, 1995

Wolfe MM, Soll AH: The physiology of gastric acid secretion. N Engl J Med 319:1707, 1988

STRESS ULCERS AND EROSIONS

Ben-Menachem T et al: Prophylaxis for stress-related gastric hemorrhage in the medical intensive care unit: A randomized, controlled single-blind study. Ann Intern Med 121:568, 1994

Peura DA, Johnson LF: Cimetidine for prevention and treatment of gastroduodenal lesions in patients in an intensive care unit. Ann Intern Med 103:173, 1985

Prod'hom G et al: Nosocomial pneumonia in mechanically ventilated patients receiving antacid, ranitidine, or sucralfate as prophylaxis for stress ulcer: A randomized controlled trial. Ann Intern Med 10:653, 1994

ASPIRIN AND NSAID-INDUCED MUCOSAL INJURY

Cryer B, Feldman M: Effects of nonsteroidal anti-inflammatory drugs on endogenous GI prostaglandins and therapeutic strategies for prevention and treatment of nonsteroidal anti-inflammatory drug-induced damage. Arch Intern Med 152:1145, 1992

Hollander G: GI complications of nonsteroidal anti-inflammatory drugs: Prophylactic and therapeutic strategies. Am J Med 96:274, 1994

Silverstein FE et al: Misoprostol reduces serious GI complications in patients with rheumatoid arthritis receiving nonsteroidal anti-inflammatory drugs: A randomized double-blind, placebo-controlled trial. Ann Intern Med 123:241, 1995

GASTRIC MUCOSAL DISEASE

Appleman HD: Gastritis: Terminology, etiology, and clinical correlations: Another biased view. Hum Pathol 25:1006, 1994

Kuipers EJ et al: Review article: The development of atrophic gastritis—*Helicobacter pylori* and the effects of acid suppressive therapy. Aliment Pharmacol Ther 9:331, 1995

Parsonnet J et al: *Helicobacter pylori* infection and the risk of gastric carcinoma. N Engl J Med 325:1127, 1991

——— et al: *Helicobacter pylori* infection and gastric lymphoma. N Engl J Med 330:1267, 1994

Wolfsen HC et al: Ménétrier's disease: A form of hypertrophic gastropathy or gastritis? Gastroenterology 104:1310, 1993

ZOLLINGER-ELLISON SYNDROME

Gibril F et al: Somatostatin receptor scintigraphy: Its sensitivity compared with that of other imaging methods in detecting primary and metastatic gastrinomas. Ann Intern Med 125:26, 1996

Jensen RT et al: Zollinger-Ellison syndrome: Advances in the treatment of gastric hypersecretion and the gastrinoma. JAMA 271:1429, 1994

Maton PN: Review article: The management of Zollinger-Ellison syndrome. Aliment Pharmacol Ther 7:467, 1993

Metz DC et al: Use of omeprazole in Zollinger-Ellison syndrome: A prospective nine-year study of efficacy and safety. Aliment Pharmacol Ther 7:597, 1993

Pipeleers-Marichal M et al: Gastrinomas in the duodenums of patients with multiple endocrine neoplasia type 1 and the Zollinger-Ellison syndrome. N Engl J Med 322:723, 1990

Pisegna JR et al: Effects of curative gastrinoma resection on gastric secretory function and antisecretory drug requirement in the Zollinger-Ellison syndrome. Gastroenterology 102:767, 1992

Termanini B et al: Value of somatostatin receptor scintigraphy: A prospective study in gastrinoma of its effects in clinical management. Gastroenterology 112:335, 1997

285

Norton J. Greenberger, Kurt J. Isselbacher

DISORDERS OF ABSORPTION

MECHANISMS OF ABSORPTION

Diseases of the small intestine are frequently accompanied by alterations in intestinal function, and clinically, this impaired function is seen as the malabsorption syndrome. To obtain a better appreciation of the derangements that occur in the many disorders of intestinal function, the processes of normal absorption will first be reviewed.

It is important to distinguish between digestion and absorption, since an increased loss of nutrients in the stool may reflect a derangement of either process. Digestion involves the breakdown or hydrolysis of nutrients to smaller molecules to prepare the ingested substances for absorption, or transport across the intestinal cell. It will be recalled that most of the digestive process is initiated in the stomach by acid and pepsin and is continued in the upper small intestine primarily by the action of pancreatic enzymes such as lipase, amylase, and trypsin. As a result of these digestive actions, carbohydrates are broken down to monosaccharides and disaccharides, proteins to peptides and amino acids, and fats to monoglycerides and fatty acids. In the adult, it is in this form that nutrients are largely transported across the epithelial surface of the intestinal cell.

ANATOMIC AND PHYSIOLOGIC FACTORS The intestine has an enormous surface area. This fact can be attributed in large part to the length of the intestine, which in the adult is more than 4 m, and to the foldings of the surface plicae. At the light-microscopic level, the villi of the small intestine provide additional surface area, which is further augmented by the presence of microvilli (approximately $2 \times 10^8/cm^2$) on the brush border region of epithelial cells.

Bowel motility is an important process which permits nutrients to remain in intimate contact with the intestinal cells and influences the continued movement of the nutrients into and along the absorbing channels, such as the lymphatics. Two types of motility aid in this process: the gross motility of the intestine itself and the motility of individual villi. The entrance of the nutrients into the general circulation is achieved via the capillaries into the portal system or via the lacteals into the intestinal lymphatics.

TYPES OF ABSORPTION (See also Chap. 42) Four mechanisms have been considered to be important in the transport of substances across the intestinal cell membrane, namely, active transport, passive diffusion, facilitated diffusion, and endocytosis.

Active transport involves the transport of a substance across the cell against an electric or chemical gradient; this process requires energy, is carrier-mediated, and is subject to competitive inhibition. *Passive diffusion* is the opposite of this process; energy is not required, transport is with (rather than against) the electric or chemical gradient, the process is not carrier-mediated, and it does not show properties of competitive inhibition. Thus, active transport may be viewed as "uphill" transport, whereas passive diffusion is equivalent to "downhill" transport. *Facilitated diffusion* is similar to passive diffusion except that it shows evidence of being carrier-mediated and frequently is subject to competitive inhibition.

Endocytosis is a process akin to phagocytosis. By this mechanism, nutrients (dissolved or particulate) are surrounded by the components of the outer plasma cell membrane as they enter the cell. In the intestinal tract, endocytosis occurs in the neonatal period and also to a limited extent in the adult. While quantitatively limited, it appears to account, at least in part, for uptake of antigens.

SITES OF ABSORPTION While many substances are absorbed throughout the length of the small intestine, certain nutrients tend to be absorbed more in one region than in others. The proximal intestine is a major area for the absorption of iron, calcium, water-soluble vitamins, and fat (monoglycerides and fatty acids). Sugars are absorbed in the proximal intestine as well as the midintestine. While amino acids are absorbed primarily in the middle of the small intestine, or jejunum, some absorption also occurs in the upper and lower areas. The distal small intestine is the *major* absorptive area for bile salts and vitamin B_{12}. As is emphasized below, this fact is of clinical significance in circumstances where there has been removal or disease of the ileum.

The colon is important for the absorption of water and electrolytes, a process that occurs predominantly in the cecum. Although the rectum is not a usual site for absorption of ingested nutrients, drugs introduced by rectum may be absorbed there. Thus, drugs introduced by this route, such as salicylates or steroids, may have systemic as well as local effects.

ABSORPTION OF SPECIFIC NUTRIENTS **Carbohydrate Absorption** Much of the carbohydrate we ingest is in the form of starch, a complex polysaccharide consisting of many hexose units. By the action of salivary and pancreatic amylase, starch is hydrolyzed to oligosaccharides and then to disaccharides (mostly maltose). While monosaccharides such as glucose are readily absorbed, disaccharides are not. Disaccharides are split enzymatically into their component sugars by brush border disaccharidases (or oligosaccharidases). The two types of disaccharidases are β-galactosidases (lactase) and α-glucosidases (sucrase, maltase). By the action of these enzymes, lactose is split into glucose and galactose, sucrose into glucose and fructose, and maltose into two molecules of glucose. The resulting monosaccharides are then transported through the cell into the portal circulation. Most disaccharides are hydrolyzed so rapidly by brush border enzymes that the capacity of the transport mechanism is exceeded, and some monosaccharides diffuse back into the intestinal lumen. Lactose, however, is hydrolyzed at a slower rate, and thus lactose hydrolysis is the rate-limiting step in lactose absorption.

Sugars such as glucose and galactose are absorbed by an active transport mechanism. Glucose (and galactose) enter the cell via the Na^+-dependent glucose transporter. Energy is required for the movement of glucose into the cell, and it comes largely from the Na^+,K^+-ATPase of the basolateral membrane (see below).

Protein and Amino Acid Absorption Dietary proteins undergo initial degradation in the stomach by pepsin. However, complete hydrolysis is largely achieved by the action of pancreatic trypsin and chymotrypsin, as well as by other endopeptidases and exopeptidases such as carboxypeptidase. These enzymatic processes yield oligopeptides, dipeptides, and amino acids. Just as there are disaccharidases on the surface of mucosal cells to digest disaccharides, so there are oligopeptidases to split small peptides. However, dipeptidases are located in the cytoplasm as well as on the microvilli. Dipeptides are absorbed more rapidly than amino acids, and presumably their uptake involves a separate mechanism. Thus, digestion of proteins to amino acids occurs in three locations: the intestinal lumen, the brush border, and the cytoplasm of mucosal cells. As indicated above, proteins also can be absorbed by the adult intestine. Although quantitatively limited, protein absorption can be immunologically significant.

Most naturally occurring amino acids are L-amino acids, and these are subject to a number of different transport processes. *Neutral* amino acids share a common carrier mechanism; thus, amino acids such as tryptophan and alanine show competitive inhibition. Among the *dibasic* amino acids that appear to have a distinct transport mechanism are arginine, ornithine, and lysine. The neutral amino acid cystine shares this mechanism. There is a separate transport system for *glycine* and the *imino acids* proline and hydroxyproline. There is also a transport system for *dicarboxylic* acids, such as glutamic and aspartic acids. Therefore, in genetic disorders such as cystinuria, there is impaired absorption not only of cystine but also of arginine, ornithine, and lysine. Similarly, in Hartnup disease, a defect in the transport of neutral amino acids (especially of tryptophan, phenylalanine, and histidine) is found. In these genetic disorders, uptake and absorption of dipeptides is normal (see Chap. 350).

Absorption of amino acids is rapid in the duodenum and jejunum but slow in the ileum. Sodium ions are necessary for the entry of these acids, and energy is needed for their concentration within the cell. Some amino acids have affinity for more than one mechanism. For example, glycine can be transported by both the neutral and the imino acid transport systems.

Fat Absorption (Fig. 285-1) Most of the ingested dietary fats are in the form of long-chain triglycerides. These contain both saturated fatty acids (such as palmitic and stearic) and unsaturated fatty acids (such as oleic and linoleic). The particle size of the fat is decreased largely by the churning action of the stomach. The entry of fat into the duodenum, plus the presence of acid, causes release of secretin and cholecystokinin, which in turn stimulate the flow of bile and pancreatic juice.

Role of pancreatic lipase The hydrolysis of triglycerides by pancreatic lipase is a complex process involving lipase, colipase, and bile salts. Pancreatic lipase binds to the oil-water interface of an emulsified triglyceride substrate. The detergent properties of bile salts permit pancreatic lipase to gain access to water-insoluble lipids. One of the important functions of bile salts is to clear the oil-water interface of dietary fat from proteins of exogenous and endogenous origin, thus making it available for pancreatic lipolysis. Colipase, a protein present in pancreatic juice, is also essential for the action of lipase; its function is to anchor the lipase close to the surface of the triglyceride droplet. All three components—i.e., pancreatic lipase, colipase, and bile salts—form a *ternary complex*, which generates lipolytic products that diffuse away from the complex and are absorbed. With colipase present, lipase remains at the interface and forms 2-monoglycerides and fatty acids, which are the major end products of triglyceride hydrolysis. Less than 5 percent of ingested fat remains in the form of diglycerides and triglycerides. Without colipase, bile acids would actually wash pancreatic lipase away from the interface, and the rate of hydrolysis of triglycerides would be reduced.

Role of bile salts (Fig. 285-2) Bile salts play an important role in the digestion and absorption of fat. They are synthesized from

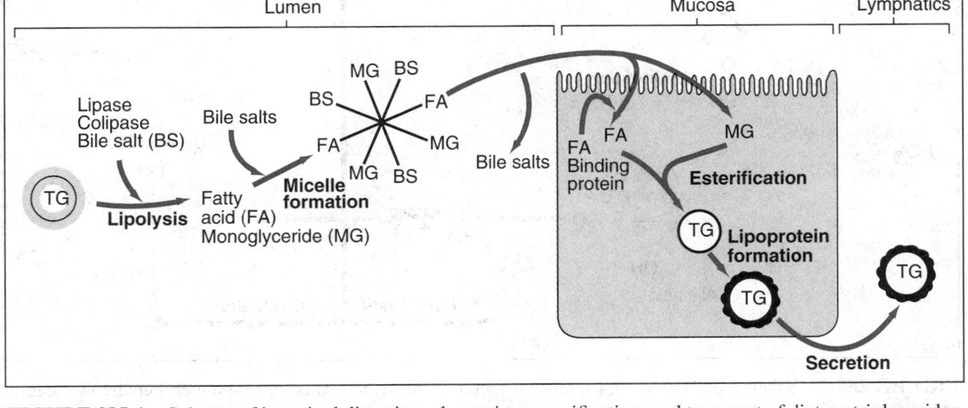

FIGURE 285-1 Scheme of intestinal digestion, absorption, esterification, and transport of dietary triglycerides. TG, triglycerides; FA, fatty acids; MG, monoglycerides; BS, bile salts.

cholesterol in the liver (in an amount of approximately 200 to 600 mg daily) and are excreted in the bile in the form of their glycine or taurine conjugates. In humans, the principal bile acids excreted are conjugates of cholic and chenodeoxycholic acid. Bile salts are good detergents, because they have both polar (hydrophilic) and nonpolar (hydrophobic) groups. During digestion, the concentration of conjugated bile salts in the lumen is in the range of 5 to 15 μmol/mL, and at these concentrations the bile salts aggregate to form *micelles*. Fatty acids and monoglycerides enter these micelles, forming mixed micelles. An emulsion of triglyceride is turbid; mixed micelles containing bile salts, fatty acids, and monoglycerides form clear solutions. The formation of *mixed micelles*, and hence the solubilization of fatty acids and monoglycerides, is much more effectively achieved with *conjugated bile salts* at the pH normally present in the intestinal lumen (see Fig. 285-2).

Most conjugated bile salts are absorbed in the ileum and, after entering the portal vein, are subject to an enterohepatic circulation. By this process, about 90 percent of the amount of conjugated bile salts reaching the ileum is reabsorbed. As a consequence, only about 200 to 600 mg of bile salts is excreted in the feces per day, even though the 3- to 4-g bile salt pool passes through the enterohepatic circulation many times each day, and, thus, 20 to 30 g of bile salts may enter the duodenum daily. When the enterohepatic circulation is intact, the size of the bile salt pool is determined largely by the rate of the enterohepatic circulation, i.e., the number of cycles occurring per day (see also Chap. 302). If the ileum is diseased or removed, absorption of bile salts is impaired, and a significant fecal loss of bile salts will occur. As a consequence of this bile salt depletion, the concentration of bile salts in the intestinal lumen also will decrease, leading to further impairment of fat absorption. A similar result will occur if bile salt reabsorption is prevented by chelating agents, such as cholestyramine (see "Regional Enteritis," below). Diarrhea per se may result in increased fecal excretion of bile salts. This effect has been demonstrated both in normal subjects in whom diarrhea has been induced and in patients with chronic idiopathic diarrhea.

Intramucosal aspects of fat absorption (Fig. 285-1) After triglycerides have been hydrolysed to fatty acids and monoglycerides and these products have interacted with bile salts to form mixed micelles, the lipids pass through an "unstirred" water layer covering the cell surface. The mixed micelles do not enter the cell; rather, the component fatty acids and monoglycerides are released from the micellar phase and then enter the cell by diffusion. In aqueous duodenal contents, large bile-salt mixed micelles saturated with products of lipolysis coexist with larger liquid crystal liposomes of the same lipids saturated with free fatty acids and mixed bile salts. These phases are interconvertible, and both may be important in fat digestion and absorption. Upon entry into the mucosal cell, fatty acids interact with specific fatty acid binding proteins. The subsequent fate of the intracellular lipid is strongly influenced by the fatty acid chain length. Fatty acids and monoglycerides derived from long-chain triglycerides (i.e., containing C_{16} to C_{18} fatty acids) are promptly *reesterified to triglycerides* by enzymes of the endoplasmic reticulum. These triglycerides then interact with specific apolipoproteins plus cholesterol and phospholipid to form chylomicrons and very low density lipoproteins. These initially accumulate in the Golgi region of the cell and then are secreted into the lacteals and the intestinal lymph. There are thus four major steps in the absorption of long-chain fatty acids and monoglycerides: (1) mucosal uptake and interaction with binding proteins, (2) reesterification to triglycerides, (3) lipoprotein formation, and (4) secretion into lymph.

By contrast, fatty acids derived from medium-chain triglycerides (i.e., those containing C_8 and C_{12} fatty acids) are *not reesterified* to any significant extent within the cell and are not incorporated into lipoproteins. Instead, they rapidly enter the portal venous system, where they are transported as fatty acids bound to albumin. The major aspects of fat absorption are summarized in Fig. 285-1.

Absorption of Cholesterol and Fat-Soluble Vitamins (A, D, E, K) In addition to contributing significantly to the total-body synthesis of cholesterol, the intestine also plays an active role in the absorption of cholesterol and its esters. Within the lumen, cholesterol esters from the bile and diet are hydrolyzed by a pancreatic esterase. There is also a separate cholesterol esterase in the intestinal microvilli which completes this hydrolysis. As a result, only free cholesterol enters the intestinal cell. However, just as in the case of long-chain fatty acids, much of the cholesterol is reesterified and is then secreted primarily into lymph.

The absorption mechanisms of the fat-soluble vitamins A, D, E, and K are not well understood. The intestine is able to convert β-carotene into vitamin A. The vitamin A thus formed or absorbed from the lumen is esterified in the mucosa primarily with palmitic acid, transported in the chylomicrons of the lymph, and stored as retinol palmitate in the liver. The other lipid-soluble vitamins also appear in lymph chylomicrons, but esterification with fatty acids does not appear to be necessary for their transport.

Water and Sodium Absorption (See also Chap. 42) The mechanisms responsible for fluid absorption differ in the jejunum, ileum, and colon. There are two pathways by which water and ions cross the intestinal mucosa: the paracellular and transcellular pathways. Individual intestinal mucosa cells are joined near their apex by a tight junction, and ions and water traverse this *paracellular* pathway during absorption and secretion. The tight-junction pathway contains water-filled channels or pores. Such intercellular spaces are closed in the resting state and dilated during absorption. Considerable evidence has accumulated indicating that pumps and carriers are involved in intestinal water and solute transport. For example, in the ileum, Na^+ enters in exchange for H^+, and Cl^- enters in exchange for HCO_3^-. Sodium entry into the cell also occurs coupled with glucose via the glucose-sodium carrier in the microvillus mem-

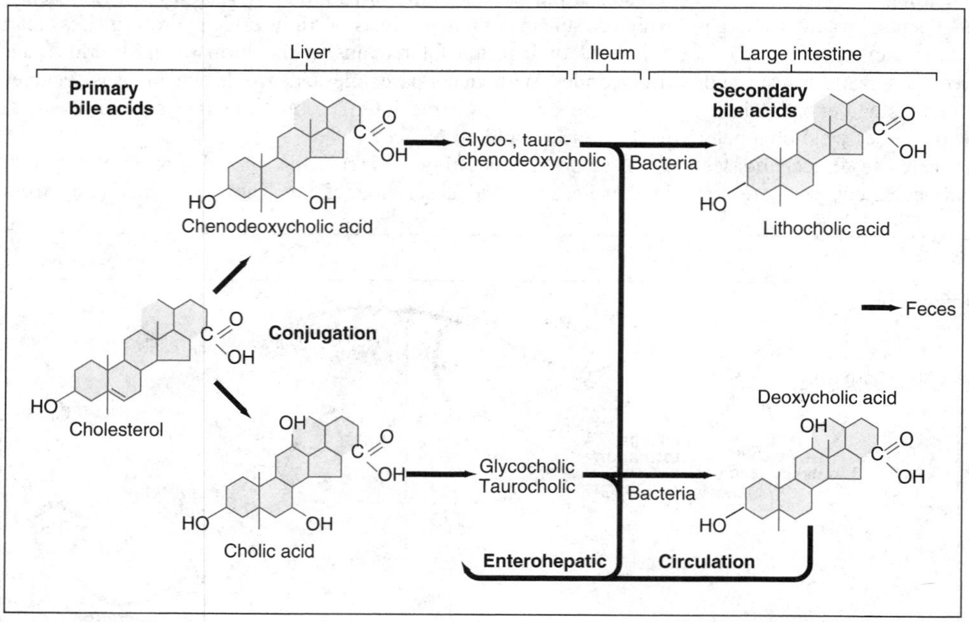

FIGURE 285-2 Scheme of hepatic and intestinal metabolism of bile salts and the enterohepatic circulation (from ileum to liver). Note that bacteria lead to the formation of secondary bile acids; of the latter, only deoxycholic acid is absorbed to any appreciable extent.

brane. Inside the cell, the Na^+ pump located in the basolateral membrane actively transports Na^+ out of the mucosal cell and into the intercellular space. *Transcellular* transport requires passage of ions through two membrane barriers, i.e., the apical brush border plasma membrane and the basolateral membrane. After Na^+ and Cl^- are transported across the brush border membrane into the cell, Na^+ is pumped across the basolateral membrane and Cl^- either follows passively or is also pumped into the intercellular space. The Na^+, K^+-ATPase is present in the basolateral but not in the brush border membrane and is the biochemical mediator of this pump. Bulk water movement obviously influences the movement of Na^+, K^+, and Cl^-. This "solvent drag" effect is explained by two mechanisms: (1) solutes may be caught in a moving stream of water and transported across a membrane, and (2) water movement results in increased concentration of solute on the side of the membrane from which water was transported, which causes solute to diffuse through the direction of flow. Diarrhea can be simply defined as impaired net absorption of water and electrolytes by the small intestine or colon. Some mechanisms producing diarrhea are listed in Table 285-1. The response to fasting is a practical way to distinguish secretory from osmotic diarrhea; stool volumes do not decrease with fasting in secretory diarrhea, whereas a reduction in stool volumes to under 300 g/d is characteristic of osmotic diarrhea. Steatorrheic stools are usually less than 700 g/d.

Calcium Absorption Calcium is actively transported by the small intestine, and this process is intimately linked to the active form of vitamin D_3, namely, 1,25-dihydroxycholecalciferol. The role of two other intestinal cell proteins, calcium-binding protein and calmodulin, in the absorption of calcium remains unclear. Recent studies indicate that calcium is absorbed to the same extent from various calcium salts (carbonate, citrate, gluconate, lactate, and acetate) and from milk in healthy subjects; an average of 32 percent of the ingested calcium was absorbed from the various sources.

Iron Absorption The formation of soluble iron complexes is important for maintaining intraluminal iron in an absorbable form. Gastric acid facilitates the chelation of inorganic iron with substances such as ascorbic acid, sugars, amino acids, and bile; these macromolecular complexes then remain soluble in the more alkaline duodenum and jejunum. In the average western diet, the iron intake averages 15 to 25 mg/d; iron absorption averages 0.5 to 1.0 mg/d in men and 1.0 to 2.0 mg/d in women during their reproductive years. Iron is actively transported by the small intestine, with the duodenum being the principal site of iron absorption. The transferrin receptor and also duodenal ferritin in small intestinal mucosal cells appear to have a regulatory/inhibitory role in iron absorption. The absorption of elemental iron in humans and animals involves at least two distinct steps: (1) mucosal uptake of iron from the lumen and (2) mucosal transfer of iron to the plasma. Much of the iron entering the mucosal cell is not transferred to the plasma but remains trapped in the cell and is excreted into the lumen when the cell is shed. The amount of iron lost by this mechanism seems to vary inversely with body iron stores. However, this mucosal regulatory mechanism can be overcome when pharmacologic doses of iron are ingested. Hemoglobin iron is also absorbed by human subjects in amounts that depend on body requirements for iron; the heme is split from globin in the lumen and absorbed as an intact metalloporphyrin. Organic iron in the form of hemoglobin is absorbed more effectively than iron from cereals and vegetables. The absorption of inorganic iron is increased by ascorbic acid. Similarly, the presence of anemia, liver injury, pregnancy, idiopathic hemochromatosis, or a portacaval shunt may result in increased iron absorption. Conversely, the prior ingestion of large doses of iron and the presence in the lumen of phosphates, carbonates, and phytates may lead to decreased absorption of inorganic iron. Impaired absorption of iron is frequent in disorders (such as celiac sprue) which involve the duodenal mucosa.

Water-Soluble Vitamins *Vitamin B_{12} absorption* is discussed in Chap. 108. In the case of *folic acid absorption*, it should be emphasized that folates exist in food conjugated with glutamyl peptides. These *polyglutamates* must be deconjugated (by folic deconjugase) to monoglutamates for absorption to occur. Certain drugs (such as oral contraceptives, sulfasalazine, diphenylhydantoin, trimethoprim, and pyrimethamine) inhibit the absorption of dietary folate and hence can cause folate deficiency. Sulfasalazine, for example, competitively inhibits three enzymes important in the intestinal metabolism of folate: dihydrofolate reductase, methylene tetrahydrofolate reductase, and serine transhydroxymethylase. Thiamine and riboflavin appear to be absorbed by passive diffusion.

TESTS USEFUL IN THE DIAGNOSIS OF MALABSORPTION Most of the tests useful in the diagnosis of malabsorption indicate the presence of abnormal absorptive or digestive function, and only a few tests may suggest a specific diagnosis. Accordingly, it is frequently necessary to employ a combination of tests to establish a diagnosis. To illustrate the use of various tests, the characteristic

Table 285-1

Some Mechanisms in the Production of Diarrhea

SECRETORY DIARRHEA
Secretory agents associated with adenylate cyclase system
Enterotoxin-producing bacteria (*Vibrio cholerae, Escherichia coli*)
Methylxanthines (caffeine, theophylline)
Prostaglandins
Vasoactive intestinal peptide (VIP)
Dihydroxy bile acids (affect colon primarily; effects seen after ileal resection)
Secretory agents *not associated* with adenylate cyclase system
Glucagon, secretin, cholecystokinin-pancreozymin, serotonin, calcitonin, gastric inhibitory polypeptide (GIP)
Some laxatives* (ricinoleic acid, bisacodyl, phenolphthalein, dioctyl sodium sulfosuccinate)
Bacterial enterotoxins (*Shigella, Staphylococcus aureus, Clostridium perfringens*)
Mucosal injury, altered cell permeability
Salmonella, Shigella, invasive *E. coli*, gastroenteritis viruses
Celiac sprue
Inflammatory bowel disease (ulcerative colitis, regional enteritis)
Neoplasms with or without hormone production
Gastrinoma (gastrin)
Carcinoid syndrome (serotonin, prostaglandins)
Medullary carcinoma of thyroid (calcitonin, prostaglandins)
Pancreatic cholera syndrome (VIP)
Villous adenoma
Medications
Diuretics
Theophylline
Colchicine
Prostaglandins (misoprostol)
Azodisalicylate
Congenital
Microvillus inclusion disease
Congenital chloridorrhea
OSMOTIC DIARRHEA
Impaired carbohydrate absorption
Disaccharidase deficiency (lactose or sucrose-isomaltose intolerance)
Glucose-galactose malabsorption
Nonabsorbable osmotically active agents (lactulose, sorbitol, mannitol, dietetic foods)
Laxative ingestion or abuse
Saline purgatives (magnesium phosphate, magnesium hydroxide–containing antacids)
Postoperative disorders
Vagotomy and pyloroplasty*
Gastrojejunostomy* (Billroth I and II)
MOTILITY DISORDERS
Laxative abuse*
Irritable bowel syndrome
Diverticular disease of the colon
Diabetic diarrhea with visceral neuropathy
Hyperthyroidism

* Multiple mechanisms involved in production of diarrhea.

findings in celiac sprue, an example of a primary malabsorptive disorder, and pancreatic insufficiency, an example of impaired digestion, are compared in Table 285-2.

Stool Fat The qualitative examination of the stool for undigested muscle fibers, neutral fat, and split fat is a simple and reliable screening test for steatorrhea. The finding of an increased number of muscle fibers indicates impaired intraluminal digestion. Properly performed, the qualitative microscopic examination of a stool specimen with the Sudan III stain is of value and correlates well with the quantitative determination of fecal fat. The latter remains the most reliable measurement of steatorrhea. Normal fecal fat excretion is less than 6 g for 24 h, representing a coefficient of fat absorption of >94 percent. It has been demonstrated that diarrhea itself can induce mild secondary steatorrhea. When the quantitative fecal fat test is used in patients with diarrhea, mild abnormalities (up to 14 g/d) are not specific for a primary defect in fat digestion or absorption, i.e., they may represent false-positive results.

Although not used frequently, oral [^{14}C]triolein can be used as an effective test for fat absorption. During the digestive process, the triolein is hydrolyzed, and the labeled glycerol is absorbed and metabolized by the liver. The $^{14}CO_2$ produced is exhaled and can then be measured hourly (for 6 h) in the expired air. Normally, more than 3.5 percent of the administered label [0.185 MBq (5 μCi)] appears in the breath per hour.

Xylose Absorption In the most commonly employed test of carbohydrate absorption, the patient ingests 25 g D-xylose. A 5-h urine xylose excretion of 26 mmol (4.0 g) or greater is considered normal. Low values may be obtained in patients with ascites, intestinal bacterial overgrowth, or renal insufficiency; after the administration of certain drugs (e.g., aspirin, indomethacin); and, most commonly, if the urine collection is incomplete. To prevent difficulties in interpreting the test, it is advisable to determine the blood xylose level 2 h after ingestion of xylose. A blood xylose level of 2 mmol/L (30 mg/dL) or greater indicates normal absorption of D-xylose. Abnormal D-xylose absorption is found most frequently in disorders affecting the mucosa of the proximal small intestine, such as celiac sprue and tropical sprue.

Gastrointestinal X-Ray Studies All patients with malabsorption should have radiographic examinations of the small intestine and, in many cases, of the esophagus, stomach, and colon as well. Occasionally, the latter two examinations may provide important clues to the presence of such disorders as celiac sprue, scleroderma, Zollinger-Ellison syndrome, regional enteritis, ulcerative colitis, and intestinal fistulas. Traditional radiographic findings suggesting a diagnosis of malabsorption include flocculation of barium in fluid-filled loops, which causes fragmentation and segmentation of the barium column. However, these patterns are no longer demonstrated reliably in small-bowel series because of the widespread use of barium products that contain a nonflocculating suspension of micropulverized barium sulfate. In celiac sprue, the most consistent abnormalities are thickened and nodular duodenal folds and dilation of the small bowel. However, these findings are nonspecific and may be found in several of the disorders listed in Table 285-3. Some representative examples of abnormal small-bowel radiographs are shown in Fig. 285-3.

Small-Intestinal Biopsy The most commonly used instrument for obtaining peroral biopsy specimens from the small intestine is the upper gastrointestinal endoscope, which has largely superseded the use of the Crosby, Carey, and Ross-Moore biopsy capsules. Examination of small bowel biopsy specimens is of considerable value in the differential diagnosis of malabsorptive disorders. Table 285-3 lists disorders associated with abnormalities in intestinal biopsies, and Fig. 285-4 depicts some illustrative lesions.

Schilling Test for Vitamin B_{12} Absorption The Schilling test is valuable in the differential diagnosis of malabsorption and is frequently carried out in three stages: (1) without intrinsic factor, (2) with intrinsic factor, and (3) after a course of treatment with antibiotics or anti-inflammatory drugs. Since vitamin B_{12} is absorbed primarily in the distal ileum, an abnormal response to a Schilling test may indicate a pathologic condition of the distal small bowel. In disorders affecting the terminal ileum, such as regional enteritis and lymphomas, the first- and second-stage Schilling tests are frequently abnormal. The ileal receptor site appears to be damaged in these disorders, and the impaired absorption of B_{12} is not corrected by the addition of intrinsic factor or the use of antibiotics. However, the Schilling test response may normalize after treatment with prednisone or sulfasalazine. The Schilling test also may be useful in establishing a diagnosis of intestinal bacterial overgrowth of the small bowel, as in disorders such as blind loop syndrome, scleroderma, and multiple small-bowel diverticula (see below). In the blind loop syndrome, for example, the bacteria can actually take up vitamin B_{12}, with resultant impaired absorption of B_{12}. Under these conditions, the first-stage Schilling test frequently gives an abnormal result, as does the second-stage test. After appropriate antibiotic treatment, the Schilling test response usually returns to normal. Vitamin B_{12} absorption is frequently abnormal in patients with exocrine pancreatic insufficiency (see Chap. 304).

Secretin and Other Pancreatic Tests The secretin test, secretin cholecystokinin test, intraduodenal perfusion with essential amino acids, and bentiromide test, which may be useful in establishing a diagnosis of pancreatic insufficiency, are discussed in detail in Chap. 303.

Serum Calcium, Albumin, Cholesterol, Magnesium, and Iron Abnormal serum calcium, albumin, cholesterol, magnesium, and iron values may be found in several malabsorptive disorders. The primary value of such findings is to suggest abnormal absorption. These tests are usually of limited value in the *differential diagnosis* of malabsorption, but an abnormal result may be helpful in supporting this diagnosis.

Serum Carotenes, Vitamin A, and Prothrombin Time Absorption of the fat-soluble vitamins A, D, K, and E is frequently impaired in patients with steatorrhea. Measurements of serum carotene and vitamin A levels are useful as screening tests for malabsorption. However, other tests not only are more sensitive but often give more specific information than the serum carotene and vitamin A levels. The blood prothrombin time is an important test, since patients with malabsorption may present with abnormal bleeding due to vitamin K deficiency. If the decreased prothrombin activity is due to malabsorption, it should be readily correctable with parenteral vitamin K.

Breath Tests The bile acid breath test utilizing [^{14}C]cholylglycine is a reasonably reliable screening test for bacterial overgrowth syndromes. Approximately two-thirds of patients with a positive small-bowel culture will have an abnormal bile acid breath test. However, in patients with suspected malabsorption of bile acids, the test is rather insensitive without the additional determination of fecal bile acid excretion. The excretion of breath hydrogen after ingestion of lactose is a sensitive, specific, and noninvasive test for detecting lactase deficiency. Lactulose and [^{14}C]xylose breath tests for bacterial overgrowth also have been found helpful.

PATHOPHYSIOLOGIC BASIS FOR SYMPTOMS AND SIGNS IN MALABSORPTIVE DISORDERS The common symptoms and signs found in malabsorptive disorders are listed in Table 285-4. The most frequent symptoms are those of malnutrition, weight loss, and diarrhea. However, in each of the clinical settings listed in Table 285-4, it is important to consider the cause of the malabsorption.

DISORDERS OF MALABSORPTION

See Table 285-5

INADEQUATE DIGESTION Liver and Biliary Tract Disease It is not generally appreciated that patients with acute or chronic liver disease may develop malabsorption owing to impaired intraluminal digestion. Steatorrhea has been described in acute viral hepatitis, chronic extrahepatic biliary tract obstruction, primary biliary cirrhosis, and postnecrotic and nutritional cirrhosis. Absorption of D-xylose and vitamin B_{12} is usually normal, and small-intestinal mucosal biopsy specimens are generally unremarkable. The steatorrhea associated with

Table 285-2

Tests Useful in the Diagnosis of Malabsorptive Disorders

		Typical Findings		
Test	Normal Values	Malabsorption (Celiac Sprue)	Maldigestion (Pancreatic Insufficiency)	Comment
Quantitative determination of stool fat	<6 g per 24 h: >95% coefficient of fat absorption	>6 g per 24 h	>6 g per 24 h	Best test for establishing presence of steatorrhea
Carbohydrate absorption				
D-Xylose absorption (25-g oral dose)	5-h urinary excretion >26 mmol (>4.5 g); peak blood level >2.0 mmol/L (>30 mg/dL)	↓	Normal	A good screening test for carbohydrate malabsorption
Small-intestine x-rays		Malabsorption pattern	Normal or minimal malabsorption pattern; occasionally pancreatic calcification	
Blood tests				
Serum calcium	2.2–2.7 mmol/L (9–11 mg/dL)	Frequently ↓	Usually normal	
Serum albumin	35–55 g/L (3.5–5.5 g/dL)	Frequently ↓	Usually normal	Decreased levels of both serum albumin and globulins should raise the question of protein-losing enteropathy
Serum cholesterol	3.90–6.45 mmol/L (150–250 mg/dL)	↓	Frequently ↓	Usually decreased in disorders associated with significant steatorrhea
Serum iron	14–24 μmol/L (80–150 μg/dL)	Frequently ↓	Normal	Low values may reflect decreased body iron stores
Serum magnesium	0.6–1.0 mmol/L (1.2–2.0 mEq/L)	Frequently ↓	Usually normal	
Serum zinc	12–20 μmol/L	Frequently ↓	Usually normal	Decreased levels common in malnutrition, cirrhosis, and malabsorption
Serum carotenes	>100 IU/dL	↓	Usually ↓	Fairly satisfactory screening tests for malabsorption
Serum vitamin A	>100 IU/dL	↓		
Prothrombin time	70–100%; 12–15 s	Frequently ↑	Frequently ↑ (prolonged)	
Small intestinal mucosal biopsy		Abnormal	Normal	A specific diagnosis can be established in a small number of disorders (see text)
Urine tests				
Vitamin B_{12} absorption	>8% urinary excretion in 48 h	Frequently ↓	Frequently ↓	Useful in determining whether vitamin B_{12} malabsorption is due to gastric or small-intestinal disorders or to pancreatic insufficiency
Urine 5-hydroxyindoleacetic acid (5-HIAA)	10–47 μmol per 24 h (2–9 mg per 24 h)	↑	Normal	Slightly increased level (12–16 mg per 24 h) characteristically found in celiac sprue
Breath tests				
Breath H_2 (after 50 g lactose)	Minimal breath H_2	May be ↑	Normal	Secondary to lactase deficiency (see text)
Breath H_2 (after 10 g lactulose)	Minimal breath H_2	May be normal or ↓	Normal	Early peak in bacterial overgrowth; can be used to determine intestinal transit time
Breath $^{14}CO_2$ (after [^{14}C]xylose)	Minute amounts $^{14}CO_2$	May be ↓	Usually normal	Increased in bacterial overgrowth
Glycocholic acid metabolism (oral glycine-1-[^{14}C]glycocholate)	<1% of dose excreted $^{14}CO_2$ in 4 h	Normal	Normal	Increased $^{14}CO_2$ excretion with bacterial overgrowth or bile acid malabsorption (due to ileal resection or inflammatory disease)
	<4% of dose excreted in stools	Normal	Normal	Increased fecal excretion of ^{14}C in bile acid malabsorption
[^{14}C]triolein absorption (breath test)	>3.5% of dose as breath $^{14}CO_2$ per hour	↓	↓	Correlates well with chemical stool fat; recently introduced test
Miscellaneous				
Bacteria (culture)	<10^3 organisms per milliliter	Normal	Normal	>10^5 organisms per milliliter indicates bacterial overgrowth
Secretin test	Volume >1.8 (mL/kg)/h Bicarbonate concentration >80 mmol/L	Normal	Abnormal	See discussion of pancreatic insufficiency in Chaps. 303 and 304
Bentiromide test	Urine excretion arylamines ≥50%	May be abnormal	Abnormal	See discussion of pancreatic disease in Chaps. 303 and 304

Table 285-3

Disorders Associated with Abnormalities in Small-Bowel Biopsy Specimens

BIOPSY HAS DIAGNOSTIC VALUE (DIFFUSE LESIONS)
Whipple's disease: Lamina propria infiltrated with macrophages containing PAS-positive glycoproteins
Abetalipoproteinemia: Villus structure normal; epithelial cells vacuolated due to excess fat
Agammaglobuinemia: Flattened or absent villi; increased lymphocyte infiltration; absence of plasma cells
Mycobacterium avium complex
BIOPSY MAY HAVE DIAGNOSTIC VALUE (PATCHY LESIONS)
Intestinal lymphoma: Infiltration of lamina propria and submucosa with malignant cells
Intestinal lymphangiectasia: Dilated lacteals and lymphatics in lamina propria; clubbed villi
Eosinophilic enteritis: Diffuse or patchy eosinophilic infiltration in lamina propria and mucosa
Amyloidosis: Presence of amyloid confirmed by special stains
Regional enteritis: Noncaseating granulomas
Parasitic infestations: Parasitic invasion of mucosa; adherence of trophozoites to mucosal surface, as in giardiasis
Systemic mastocytosis: Mast cell infiltration of lamina propria
BIOPSY IS ABNORMAL BUT NOT DIAGNOSTIC
Celiac sprue: Shortened or absent villi; hypertrophied crypts; damaged surface epithelium; mononuclear infiltrate
"Collagenous" sprue: Indistinguishable from celiac sprue; extensive subepithelial collagen deposition
Tropical sprue: Lesion similar to celiac sprue with shortened or absent villi; lymphocyte infiltration
Folate deficiency: Shortened villi; megalocytosis; decreased mitoses in crypts
Vitamin B_{12} deficiency: Similar to folate deficiency
Acute radiation enteritis: Similar to folate deficiency
Systemic scleroderma: Fibrosis around Brunner's glands
Bacterial overgrowth syndromes: Patchy damage to villi and increased lymphocyte infiltration

liver and biliary tract disease is thought to be due to impaired hepatic synthesis or excretion of conjugated bile salts, resulting in impaired formation of micellar lipid. In addition to steatorrhea, patients with liver disease may have impaired absorption of vitamin D and calcium, resulting in severe metabolic bone disease. This is particularly common in patients with primary biliary cirrhosis. Skeletal roentgenograms may show increased porosity of bone, cortical thinning, vertebral compression, and spontaneous pathologic fractures. Patients with alcohol-induced liver disease also may have exocrine pancreatic insufficiency. Accordingly, pancreatic function should be evaluated in patients with liver disease and malabsorption.

Postgastrectomy Malabsorption The presence of a malabsorption syndrome has been documented frequently in patients after subto-

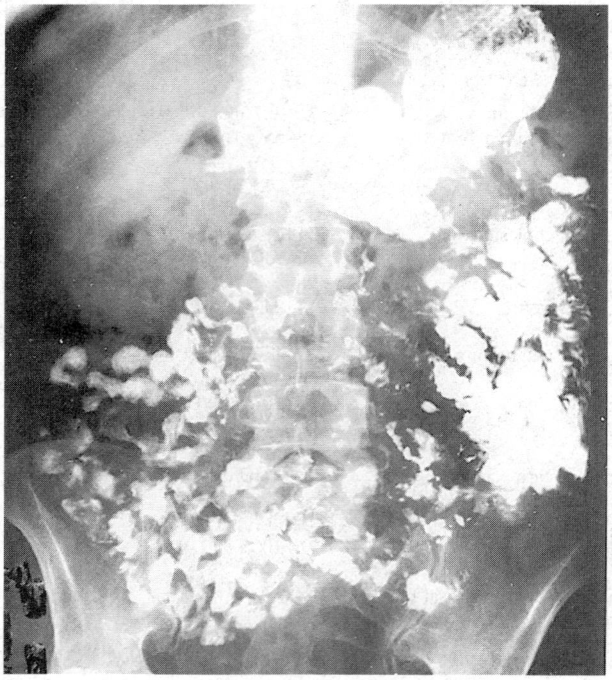

B

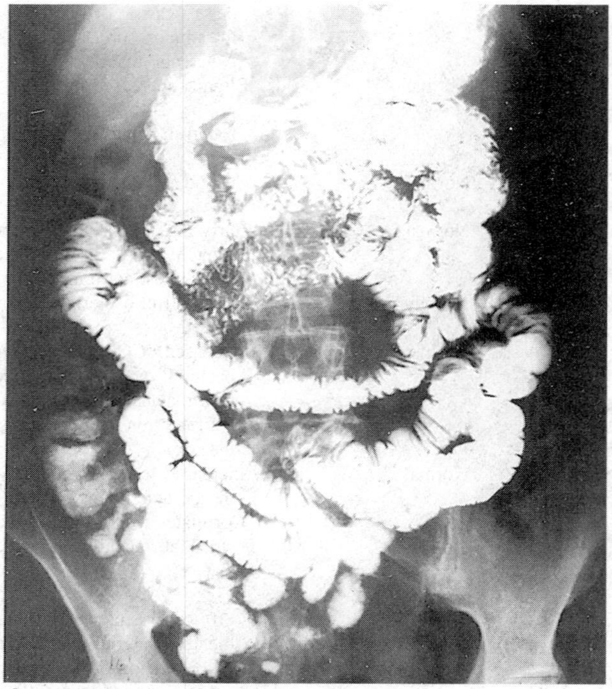

A

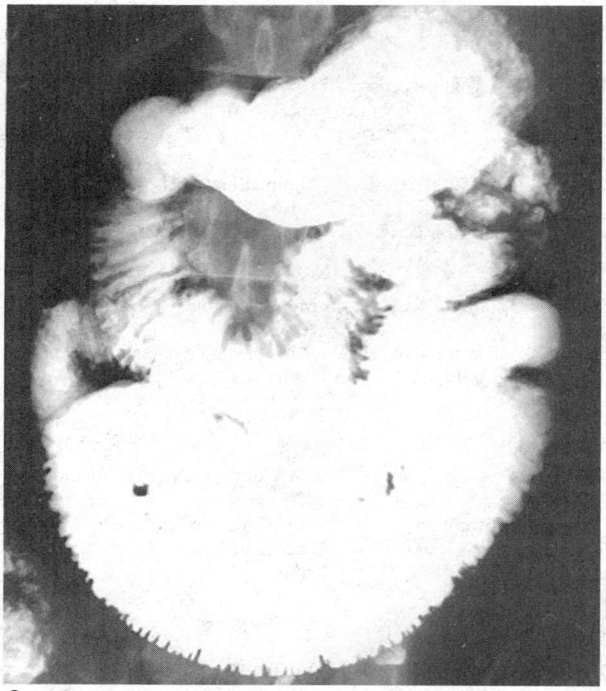

C

FIGURE 285-3 *A.* Radiograph of a normal small intestine showing good mucosal pattern. *B.* Intestinal radiograph of a patient with celiac sprue. Note dilation of small bowel, lack of mucosal markings, and segmentation and clumping of barium. *C.* Intestinal radiograph of patient with obstructed lymphatics due to Köhlmeier-Degos disease, with "accordion-pleated" pattern (lower edge).

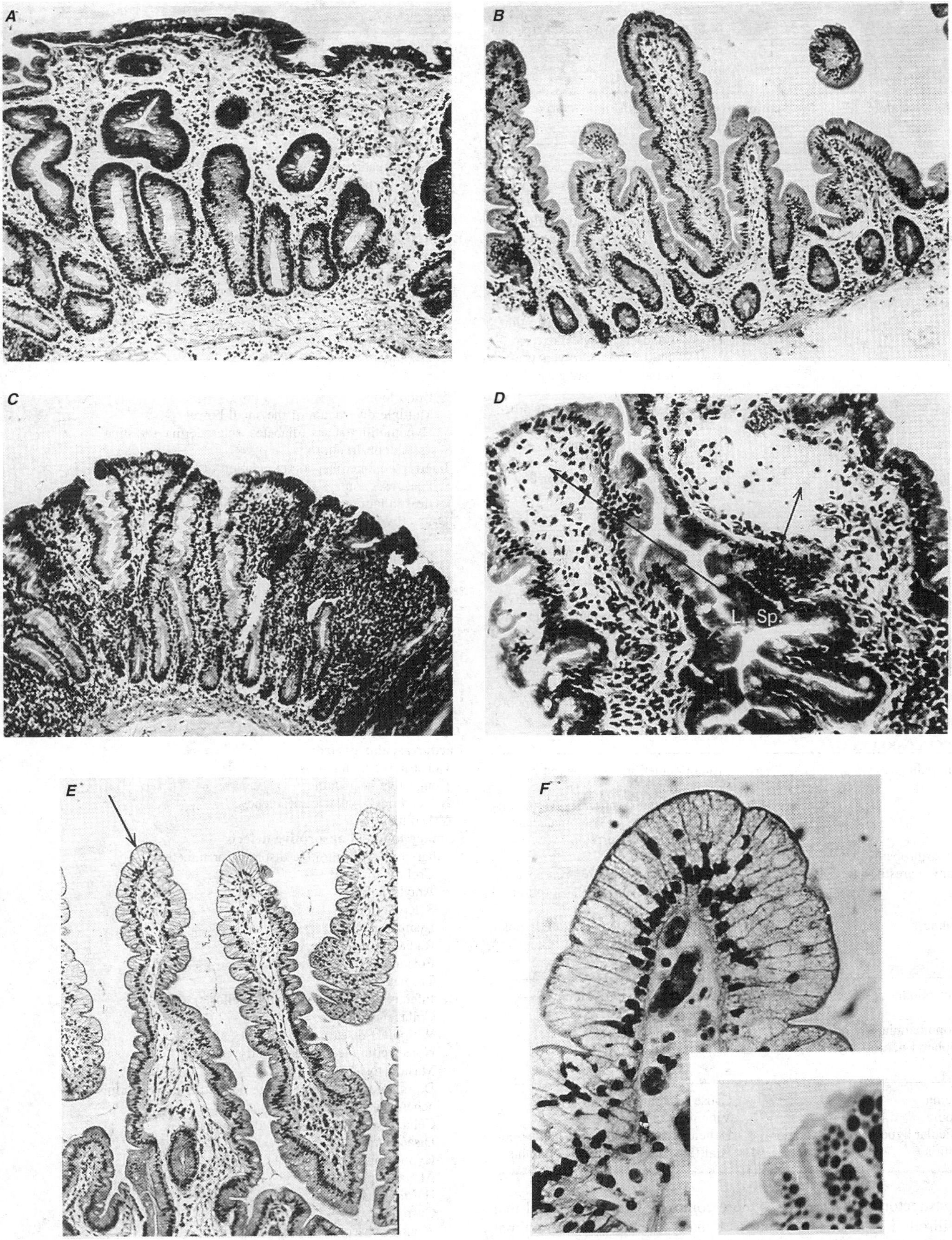

FIGURE 285-4 Typical peroral intestinal biopsy specimens. *A*. Jejunal mucosa of patient with celiac sprue. Note virtual absence of villi, elongated crypts (some cut in cross section), mononuclear infiltrate, and cuboidal instead of columnar epithelium on top of villi (300×). *B*. Biopsy specimen from the same patient as in *A*, after 9 months on a gluten-free diet. Note reappearance of villi with normal-appearing columnar cells and reduction in infiltrate and crypt height (300×). *C*. Biopsy specimen from patient with agammaglobulinemia. The features bear a striking resemblance to those of celiac sprue. There is a marked mononuclear infiltration, some of it in aggregates (200×). *D*. Close-up of villi of patient with protein-losing enteropathy. Note broadened and dilated tips, and lymphatic spaces (*arrows*). (450×). *E*. Intestinal biopsy specimen from patient with abetalipoproteinemia. The villus tips have a "lacy" appearance (*arrow*) due to retained fat (300×). *F*. High-power micrograph of villus in *E*. Vacuoles are filled with lipid (750×). Insert shows dark-staining (osmium) lipid droplets in mucosal cells (osmium counterstained with Giemsa; 800×).

Table 285-4

Pathophysiologic Basis for Symptoms and Signs in Malabsorptive Disorders

Symptom or Sign	Pathophysiology
GASTROINTESTINAL	
Generalized malnutrition and weight loss	Malabsorption of fat, carbohydrate, and protein → loss of calories, anorexia
Diarrhea	Impaired absorption or increased secretion of water and electrolytes; unabsorbed dihydroxy bile acids and fatty acids → decreased absorption of water and electrolytes; excess load of fluid and electrolytes presented to the colon may exceed its absorptive capacity
Flatus	Bacterial fermentation of unabsorbed carbohydrate
Glossitis, cheilosis, stomatitis	Deficiency of iron, vitamin B_{12}, folate, and other vitamins
Abdominal pain	Distention or inflammation of bowel, chronic pancreatitis
GENITOURINARY	
Nocturia	Delayed absorption of water, hypokalemia
Azotemia, hypotension	Fluid and electrolyte depletion
Amenorrhea, ↓ libido	Protein depletion and "caloric starvation" → secondary hypopituitarism
HEMATOPOIETIC	
Anemia	Impaired absorption of iron, vitamin B_{12}, folic acid, and pyridoxine
Hemorrhagic phenomena	Vitamin K malabsorption → hypoprothrombinemia
MUSCULOSKELETAL	
Bone pain	Protein depletion → impaired bone formation → osteoporosis Calcium malabsorption → demineralization of bone → osteomalacia Vitamin D malabsorption
Osteoarthropathy	Cause uncertain
Tetany, paresthesias	Calcium malabsorption → hypocalcemia; magnesium malabsorption → hypomagnesemia
Weakness	Anemia: electrolyte depletion (hypokalemia)
NERVOUS SYSTEM	
Night blindness	Impaired absorption vitamin A → vitamin A deficiency
Xerophthalmia	Vitamin A deficiency
Peripheral neuropathy	Vitamin B_{12}, thiamine deficiency
SKIN	
Eczema	Cause uncertain
Purpura	Vitamin K deficiency
Follicular hyperkeratosis and dermatitis	Deficiency of vitamin A, zinc, essential fatty acids, and other vitamins

tal gastrectomy. Steatorrhea is more common with a Billroth II than a Billroth I type of anastomosis. Usually the fat loss is minimal, ranging from 7 to 10 g per 24 h. Patients with gross steatorrhea usually have impaired intraluminal fat digestion due to several factors, as follows. (1) With a Billroth II anastomosis the duodenum is bypassed, and there is a decreased entry of stomach contents into the proximal duodenum (i.e., the afferent loop). This leads to a decreased stimulus for the release of *secretin* and *cholecystokinin* (CCK) from the duodenum and may result in a depressed pancreatic enzyme response. (2) There may be *inadequate mixing* of the pancreatic enzymes and bile

Table 285-5

Classification of the Malabsorption Syndromes

Inadequate digestion
- Postgastrectomy steatorrhea*
- Deficiency or inactivation of pancreatic lipase
  - Exocrine pancreatic insufficiency
    - Chronic pancreatitis
    - Pancreatic carcinoma
    - Cystic fibrosis
    - Pancreatic resection
  - Gastrinoma (Zollinger-Ellison syndrome)*

Reduced intestinal bile salt concentration (with impaired micelle formation)
- Liver disease
  - Parenchymal liver disease
  - Cholestasis (intrahepatic or extrahepatic)
- Abnormal bacterial proliferation in the small bowel
  - Afferent loop stasis
  - Strictures
  - Fistulas
  - Blind loops
  - Multiple diverticula of the small bowel
  - Hypomotility states (diabetes, scleroderma, intestinal pseudoobstruction)
- Interrupted enterohepatic circulation of bile sales
  - Ileal resection
  - Ileal inflammatory disease (Crohn's disease)
- Drugs (by sequestration or precipitation of bile salts)
  - Neomycin
  - Calcium carbonate
  - Cholestyramine

Inadequate absorptive surface
- Intestinal resection or bypass
  - Mesenteric vascular disease with massive intestinal resection
  - Regional enteritis with multiple bowel resections
  - Jejunoileal bypass
- Gastroileostomy (inadvertent)

Lymphatic obstruction
- Intestinal lymphangiectasia
- Lymphoma

Cardiovascular disorders
- Constrictive pericarditis
- Congestive heart failure
- Mesenteric vascular insufficiency
- Vasculitis

Primary mucosal absorptive defects
- Inflammatory, infiltrative disorders or infection
  - Crohn's disease*
  - Amyloidosis
  - Scleroderma*
  - Lymphoma*
  - Radiation enteritis
  - Eosinophilic enteritis
  - Tropical sprue
  - Infective enteritis (e.g., salmonellosis)
  - Collagenous sprue
  - Whipple's disease
  - Nonspecific ulcerative jejunitis
  - Mastocytosis
  - Dermatologic disorders (e.g., dermatitis herpetiformis)
- Biochemical or genetic abnormalities
  - Celiac sprue (gluten-induced enteropathy)
  - Disaccharidase deficiency
  - Hypogammaglobulinemia
  - Abetalipoproteinemia
  - Hartnup disease
  - Cystinuria
  - Monosaccharide malabsorption

Endocrine and metabolic disorders
- Diabetes mellitus*
- Hypoparathyrodism
- Adrenal insufficiency
- Hyperthyroidism
- Gastrinoma (Zollinger-Ellison syndrome)*
- Carcinoid syndrome

* Malabsorption caused by multiple defects.

salts secreted into the proximal duodenum with the gastric contents entering the jejunum. (3) There may be *stasis* of intestinal contents in the afferent loop, resulting in abnormal bacterial proliferation in the proximal small bowel. This in turn may lead to abnormalities in bile salt metabolism (see "Pathophysiology" under "Malabsorption Due to Bacterial Overgrowth of the Small Bowel," below). (4) The presence of maldigestion may lead to *protein depletion*, which in turn may produce further impairment in pancreatic function. (5) The *loss of the reservoir function of the stomach* may result in decreased intestinal transit time. Perhaps the most important factor is rapid gastric emptying, which results in low luminal concentrations of digestive secretions for the first 60 to 80 min after a meal. Such a disorder has been described in patients with subtotal gastrectomy and duodenostomy (Billroth I), gastrojejunostomy (Billroth II), and truncal vagotomy and pyloroplasty (V&P). That gastric emptying rates are somewhat slower in patients with V&P may account for the overall less severe nutritional deficiencies in such patients. In some patients, treatment with pancreatic enzymes leads to significant improvement. Specimens of duodenal or jejunal fluid should be obtained for culture of both aerobic and anaerobic organisms, and appropriate antibiotic therapy should be instituted if there is evidence of abnormal bacterial overgrowth (a colony count of $>10^5$/mL in jejunal fluid). Because the duodenum is the principal site of absorption of iron and calcium, in patients with a Billroth II anastomosis, impaired absorption of calcium and iron also may develop. Occult metabolic bone disease occurs frequently in this setting.

INADEQUATE ABSORPTIVE SURFACE (SHORT-BOWEL SYNDROME) Extensive intestinal resection often results in the short-bowel syndrome. The most common disorders resulting in this syndrome are (1) massive intestinal resection following a vascular insult to the small intestine, (2) regional enteritis with multiple bowel resections, and (3) a jejunoileal bypass for morbid obesity. In general, the absorption of nutrients will be influenced by the extent and site of small bowel resected, the presence of the ileocecal valve, and adaptation of the remaining small bowel. Resection of 40 to 50 percent of the small bowel is usually well tolerated, provided the proximal duodenum, the distal half of the ileum, and the ileocecal valve are spared. By contrast, resection of the ileum and the ileocecal valve alone may induce severe diarrhea and malabsorption, even though less than 30 percent of the small intestine is resected.

Several measures are important in the management of short-bowel syndrome: (1) The diet should contain at least 2500 kcal and consist primarily of carbohydrate and protein, with fat restricted to less than 40 g/d. A fat-restricted diet is effective in reducing diarrhea, presumably because there is decreased production of hydroxy fatty acids from long-chain fats. Such hydroxy fatty acids, in essence, are cathartics and increase net secretion of water and electrolytes by the colon as well as the small bowel. (2) It is often necessary to provide vitamin and mineral supplements, which usually include K^+, Cl^-, Mg^{2+}, Ca^{2+}, trace metals (Zn, Cd, Mn), iron, folate, vitamin B_{12}, other vitamins (A, D, E, K, B_1, B_2, B_6, biotin), and essential fatty acids. (3) Specific drugs (e.g., belladonna alkaloids, diphenoxylate, loperamide, and codeine) that decrease intestinal motility and prolong mucosal contact time are helpful in controlling diarrhea. These agents also decrease ileostomy outputs. (4) A bile salt–sequestering agent such as cholestyramine blunts the effects of bile salts, which stimulate net secretion of water and electrolytes by the colon. (5) Patients with short-bowel syndrome may have gastric acid hypersecretion, which is often transient and which results in dilution of pancreatic secretions as well as inactivation of pancreatic enzymes. Under these conditions, a histamine H_2 receptor antagonist or proton pump inhibitor is useful because it will suppress gastric acid secretion and decrease the volume of fluid entering the proximal small bowel, thus leading to an increased concentration of pancreatic enzymes. In addition, supplemental pancreatic enzyme therapy may be required. (6) A bypassed colon can be used to receive infusions of fluid and electrolytes, since a portion of the colon can still absorb 1000 to 1500 mL fluid per day. (7) Octreotide, a long-acting somatostatin analogue, reduces digestive secretions (biliary and pancreatic secretions and succus entericus) and thus may ameliorate diarrhea. Finally, (8) total parenteral nutrition is frequently required during the first 6 months after massive intestinal resection, until some degree of adaptation has occurred. Such patients also may require long-term parenteral hyperalimentation with a silicone rubber catheter in the superior vena cava; this can be done at home.

→ ***For a discussion of regional enteritis see Chap. 286.***

MALABSORPTION DUE TO BACTERIAL OVERGROWTH OF THE SMALL BOWEL The proximal small intestine is usually bacteriologically sterile because of three factors: (1) the acid milieu of the stomach, (2) intestinal peristalsis, which sweeps bacteria to the distal small bowel, and (3) secretion into the lumen of the intestine of immunoglobulins, which may serve as coproantibodies. When bacteria are isolated from the upper small bowel, they are frequently contaminants transported from the mouth and upper respiratory tract, and the colony count rarely exceeds 10^4 per milliliter of jejunal fluid. The major mechanism limiting the growth of bacteria in the small intestine is normal peristalsis. Any disorder leading to impaired intestinal motility may result in abnormal stasis of intestinal contents with ineffective mechanical cleansing of bacteria. This, in turn, may lead to abnormal bacterial proliferation and malabsorption. An intact ileocecal valve prevents reflux of colonic bacteria; loss of the ileocecal valve, as in the case of ileocecal resection, facilitates bacterial proliferation in the small bowel. Several malabsorptive disorders have been associated with bacterial overgrowth of the small bowel, and these are listed in Table 285-6.

Pathophysiology Bacterial overgrowth may result in changes in bile salt metabolism, leading directly and indirectly to steatorrhea. First, bacteria (especially anaerobic gram-positive bacteria) may lead to the intraluminal deconjugation of bile salts, with a consequent production of free bile acids. In contrast to conjugated bile salts, unconjugated bile salts may be absorbed in the proximal small bowel by nonionic diffusion, resulting in decreased intraluminal concentrations of bile salts in the jejunum. Second, the decreased bile salt concentrations, the increase of unconjugated bile salts, and the decrease of the conjugated salts all serve to contribute to impaired intraluminal micelle formation and hence fat malabsorption. In addition to these abnormalities, intestinal mucosal lesions have been demonstrated in patients with intestinal stasis. Such lesions are often patchy in distribu-

Table 285-6

Causes of Intestinal Bacterial Overgrowth (Intestinal Colonization)

Structural abnormalities producing stasis of intestinal contents
Multiple small-bowel diverticula
Strictures
Crohn's disease*
Radiation enteritis*
Occlusive vascular disease: vasculitis
Billroth II subtotal gastrectomy with afferent loop stasis*
Multiple laparotomies resulting in adhesions and partial small-bowel obstruction
Fistulas: Gastrocolic, gastroileal, jejunoileal, jejunocolic
Motor abnormalities resulting in intestinal hypomotility
Scleroderma*
Amyloidosis*
Diabetes mellitus*
Hypothyroidism
Vagotomy
Intestinal pseudoobstruction (see Table 285-7)
Miscellaneous
Hypogammaglobulinemia*
Nodular lymphoid hyperplasia
Pancreatic insufficiency
Gastric hypochlorhydria/achlorhydria
Subtotal gastrectomy
Pernicious anemia
Prolonged use of H_2 receptor antagonists, proton pump inhibitors

* No underlying disorder detected.

tion, and the histologic appearance ranges in severity from minimal changes in villous architecture to severe lesions with virtual absence of villi. The cause of these lesions is unclear; possible causes include damage caused by bacterial invasion, bacterial toxins, or metabolic products such as unconjugated bile salts. In this regard, certain bacteria such as *Bacteroides* elaborate proteases that solubilize brush border proteins and destroy disaccharidases such as sucrase and maltase. The impaired absorption of vitamin B_{12} is not related to the disturbed bile salt metabolism but appears to be due to uptake of vitamin B_{12} by microorganisms.

Many of the preceding abnormalities in bile salt metabolism may be reversed by appropriate antibiotic therapy. When such treatment is instituted, the level of unconjugated bile salts in the jejunal fluid decreases, the amount of micellar lipid phase increases, and steatorrhea diminishes or disappears. In addition, significant improvement in the absorption of vitamin B_{12} occurs with the use of broad-spectrum antibiotics such as tetracycline.

Clinical Manifestations Breath tests—i.e., tests with ^{14}C-labeled bile acid, [^{14}C]xylose, or lactulose—are useful screening tests for malabsorption syndromes due to abnormal bacterial overgrowth of the small intestine. The 2-h 50-g glucose breath hydrogen test reliably predicts the presence of bacterial overgrowth; a positive test is characterized by a rise in breath hydrogen of at least 12 parts per million (ppm) within 2 h of a 50-g glucose challenge *and* a high fasting breath hydrogen level of at least 15 ppm. A definitive diagnosis is established by demonstrating larger numbers of microorganisms (greater than 10^5/mL) and a polymicrobial flora in cultures of duodenal or jejunal fluid or in cultures of an unwashed mucosal biopsy specimen, especially when luminal secretions are scanty. Other clinical features include the following: (1) a moderate steatorrhea, usually in the range of 15 to 30 g fecal fat per 24 h, (2) macrocytic anemia with a megaloblastic bone marrow, (3) impaired absorption of vitamin B_{12} that is not corrected by intrinsic factor, and (4) correction of steatorrhea and impaired vitamin B_{12} absorption by antibiotic therapy. Absorption of D-xylose, peroral small-intestinal biopsy specimens, and results of other tests of absorptive function (see Table 285-2) may be normal in these patients. A single course or a series of intermittent courses (2 to 3 weeks per month) of therapy with antibiotics such as tetracycline, ciprofloxacin, clarithromycin, ampicillin, metronidazole, or trimethoprim-sulfamethoxazole is usually given. Finally, it should be noted that duodenal bacterial overgrowth occurs frequently after long-term treatment with omeprazole, and while it clearly causes impaired absorption of vitamin B_{12}, it is typically not associated with clinically significant fat or carbohydrate malabsorption.

Chronic Intestinal Pseudoobstruction (See also Chap. 288) Chronic intestinal pseudoobstruction is a heterogeneous syndrome with a variety of causes (Table 285-7). Primary or idiopathic intestinal pseudoobstruction is a chronic illness characterized by recurrent episodes of intestinal obstruction in which all known causes of mechanical obstruction and other illnesses known to produce intestinal pseudoobstruction have been excluded. In addition to abnormalities in small-bowel motility, derangements in esophageal, gastric, and colonic motility also have been described. The primary clinical manifestations are nausea and vomiting, abdominal pain, distention, constipation, diarrhea, and urinary tract symptoms. Patients typically exhibit a prolonged transit time for chyme along the gastrointestinal tract, especially the small bowel, where pressure-activity patterns are markedly disordered. Oral cisapride accelerates gastric emptying, normalizes intestinal transit, and improves propulsive small-bowel activity in patients with pseudoobstruction. Octreotide is also sometimes useful. Malabsorption secondary to stasis of intestinal contents with resultant abnormal bacterial proliferation in the small bowel is frequently a contributing factor.

Tropical Sprue Tropical sprue is a malabsorptive disorder of unknown cause affecting residents of or visitors to tropical regions. Both epidemic and endemic forms of the disease have been recognized. Tropical sprue may have its onset months or even years after a patient has returned from the tropics. The etiology of the disorder has not been elucidated, but it might well result from one or more of the following: (1) a nutritional deficiency, (2) a transmissible infectious microorganism, and (3) a toxin elaborated by a microorganism or contained in the diet. It is of interest that coliform organisms, shown to produce an enterotoxin causing fluid secretion, have been isolated from the jejunum of tropical sprue patients but not from other patients with bacterial overgrowth of the proximal small bowel. Anorexia, diarrhea, weight loss, symptoms of anemia, sequelae of nutritional deficiency (see Table 285-4), and abdominal distention are common findings. Patients are frequently deficient in iron as well as vitamin B_{12} and folate. Laboratory studies usually reveal anemia (megaloblastic in 60 percent of cases) and impaired absorption of fat, xylose, and vitamin B_{12}. Malabsorption of at least two nutrients is considered essential for the diagnosis. Jejunal biopsy classically reveals shortened and thickened villi, increased crypt depth, and increased infiltration of lymphocytes in the lamina propria and epithelium. Endoscopy may reveal scalloping of the valvulae conniventes and a mosaic-appearing mucosa (see Table 285-3). However, these biopsy findings are not specific, and the lesion may be patchy; in addition, interpretation is difficult because "control" biopsies from asymptomatic residents in the same tropical region are often considered abnormal when compared with normal biopsies from patients in temperate zones. Such histologic findings have been termed *tropical jejunitis*. Treatment with vitamin B_{12}, folate, and antibiotics have all been effective in inducing a remission. A short course (2 to 4 weeks) of combined therapy with a sulfonamide or tetracycline and folic acid is usually given. Occasional patients require more prolonged antibiotic therapy.

Scleroderma Although there are numerous reports of small-intestinal involvement in scleroderma, frank malabsorption has been reported in only one-third of patients. Malabsorption is due to three key factors: (1) impaired intestinal motility and jejunal pseudodiverticulosis leading to relative stasis of intestinal contents and hence bacterial overgrowth; (2) involvement of the intestinal wall by the disease; and (3) vascular ischemia. In some cases, abnormal bacterial proliferation in the upper small bowel can be documented, and in these patients antibiotic therapy with drugs such as ciprofloxacin, trimethoprim-sulfamethoxazole, and metronidazole may result in decreased steatorrhea, gain in weight, and increased absorption of vitamin B_{12}. In the intestinal wall there also may be extensive deposition of collagen, especially in the muscular mucosa, submucosa, and muscularis externa, with significant muscle atrophy. Studies of duodenal myoelectric activity in scleroderma revealed absence of migrating motor complexes in

Table 285-7

Causes of Chronic Intestinal Pseudoobstruction

Primary: Idiopathic
Visceral myopathy
Visceral neuropathy
Secondary
Collagen vascular disease
Scleroderma
Dermatomyositis/polymyositis
Systemic lupus erythematosus
Amyloidosis
Endocrine disorders
Hypothyroidism
Diabetes mellitus
Neurologic diseases
Chagas' disease
Paraneoplastic visceral neuropathy
Small cell lung carcinoma
Drugs
Chronic narcotic use (narcotic bowel syndrome)
Tricyclic antidepressants
Miscellaneous
Jejunal diverticulosis
Jejunoileal bypass

* See Chap. 288.

the basal state and decreased excitability of the bowel to mechanical stimuli, such as distention, and humoral stimuli, such as pentagastrin and secretin. This motor dysfunction is an important factor in the dilatation, atony, and stasis of intestinal contents in scleroderma. Therapy with prokinetic drugs such as octreotide, cisapride, and erythromycin may be beneficial.

Malabsorption in AIDS Diarrhea and weight loss occur frequently in patients with AIDS. These symptoms are often due to enteric infections or small-intestinal Kaposi's sarcoma. The jejunal mucosa is often abnormal in patients infected with human immunodeficiency virus (HIV), and such abnormalities can be masked by an opportunistic infection. However, such symptoms can be due to malabsorption, which has been well documented in patients with AIDS in whom identifiable enteric infections and intestinal involvement with Kaposi's sarcoma have been excluded. The presence of malabsorption in these patients has been documented by steatorrhea and abnormal D-xylose absorption tests. Serum zinc levels may be decreased. In addition, small-bowel biopsy specimens have revealed dense infiltration of mononuclear cells and histiocytes. Microorganisms also have been identified in the mucosa (see also Chap. 308).

DISORDERS ASSOCIATED WITH LYMPHATIC OBSTRUCTION **Whipple's Disease** This is a rare disorder characterized clinically by arthralgia, abdominal pain, diarrhea, progressive weight loss, dilated lacteals in the bowel wall, and impaired intestinal absorption. Wasting, low-grade fever, increased skin pigmentation, and peripheral lymphadenopathy are frequently present. In addition, heart failure, endocarditis, uveitis, and central nervous system manifestations, including confusion, memory loss, focal cranial nerve signs, nystagmus, and ophthalmoplegia, may be present. Laboratory examination usually reveals the presence of steatorrhea, impaired xylose absorption, abnormal small-bowel x-rays, hypoalbuminemia, and anemia. Hypoalbuminemia is due to excessive loss of serum albumin into the gastrointestinal tract as well as impaired synthesis of albumin.

The diagnosis is established by demonstrating the presence in the mucosa of macrophages containing large cytoplasmic granules that stain brilliant magenta with the periodic acid Schiff (PAS) reagent. Such macrophages also may be seen in other tissues, such as lymph nodes, spleen, or liver. The finding of PAS-positive macrophages in the lamina propria is not specific for Whipple's disease, but virtual replacement of most cellular elements in the lamina propria by these macrophages has been seen only in this disorder. In addition to the PAS-positive macrophages, jejunal biopsy specimens frequently show dilated lymphatics and some degree of blunting of the intestinal mucosal villi. Since many patients with Whipple's disease have bacteremia, testing of peripheral blood using the polymerase chain reaction is potentially useful in diagnosis.

Electron-microscopic studies have revealed the presence of rod-shaped structures (or bacilliform bodies) 0.3 by 1.5 to 2.5 μm in and adjacent to the macrophages in the lamina propria as well as in epithelial cells and polymorphonuclear leukocytes. The bacterium has not been cultured but has been identified as a gram-negative actinomycete with distinct morphologic characteristics and thus named *Tropheryma whippelii*. After treatment of the patient with antibiotics, the bacilliform bodies decrease or disappear together with a decrease in the number of PAS-positive macrophages. In addition, the reappearance of the bacteria often heralds the onset of a clinical relapse after antibiotics have been withdrawn. Positive blood tests for *T. whippelii* DNA have been reported in patients with AIDS.

Whipple's disease at one time was thought to be invariably fatal. However, it is now clear that therapy with antibiotics will usually induce a clinical remission. In a few cases there has been complete reversal of the histologic abnormalities in the jejunal mucosa, and some of these cases have been followed for more than 10 years. Patients with Whipple's disease should be treated with antibiotics such as trimethoprim-sulfamethoxazole for at least 1 year. Treatment with tetracycline alone or penicillin alone is not adequate initial therapy; relapse rates with these drugs are approximately 40 percent. The most important parameter for following the disease and predicting its course is the presence or absence of bacilli in sections of small-bowel biopsy specimens.

Intestinal Lymphoma Steatorrhea is a manifestation of *primary* intestinal lymphoma. The disease occurs predominantly in men, and the mean age of onset of symptoms is about 50 years. The diagnosis should be suspected in patients with malabsorption with the following findings: (1) a malabsorption syndrome in which clinical and biopsy features resemble those of celiac sprue but in which there is an incomplete response to a gluten-free diet, (2) the presence of *abdominal pain* and *fever*, and (3) signs and symptoms of intestinal obstruction. The usual stigmata of generalized lymphoma are frequently absent. Hepatomegaly, splenomegaly, palpable abdominal masses, and peripheral adenopathy are usually not found. Lymphangiography and computed tomography (CT) may reveal abnormal intraabdominal nodes. The diagnosis can be established by laparotomy and often may be made by thorough examination of multiple mucosal biopsy specimens obtained perorally. There may be a total absence of villi or lesser degrees of blunting and shortening of the villi. In contrast to celiac sprue, the lamina propria is usually massively infiltrated with lymphoid cells. Malignancy may be diagnosed by demonstrating lymphoid cells with the cytologic features of malignancy, the presence of reticulum cells outside germinal centers, and infiltration and destruction of crypts by pleomorphic lymphoid cells. Some patients elaborate or secrete a fragment of the heavy chain of IgA immunoglobulins (*α-chain disease*). The latter is probably a variant of intestinal lymphoma.

The mechanism of malabsorption in intestinal lymphoma may be related to several factors: (1) diffuse involvement of the small-intestinal mucosa, (2) involvement of the bowel wall with lymphatic obstruction, and (3) localized stenosis with stasis of intestinal contents and bacterial overgrowth. It should be emphasized that it is often difficult, by clinical and morphologic features alone, to distinguish Crohn's disease and celiac sprue from intestinal lymphoma. Indeed, there is evidence to suggest that lymphoma may develop as a late complication of celiac sprue.

The course of intestinal lymphoma has ranged from 4 months to 4 years from the onset of symptoms. Perforation, bleeding, and intestinal obstruction are common terminal complications. Multimodality treatment appears to be superior to therapy with either surgery or chemotherapy alone.

CARDIOVASCULAR DISORDERS Steatorrhea has been described in patients with chronic congestive heart failure, superior mesenteric artery insufficiency, and constrictive pericarditis. Abnormal dilated mucosal lymphatics and excessive enteric loss of protein have been demonstrated in patients with constrictive pericarditis. The mechanism of steatorrhea in patients with chronic heart failure remains uncertain. It might be due to congestion and edema of the mucosa, mucosal hypoxia, or abnormalities in pancreatic function. Although pronounced steatorrhea is uncommon in congestive heart failure, these patients are frequently anorectic, and a low fat intake could mask a latent steatorrhea. Steatorrhea is quite infrequent in patients with vasculitis and is thought to be due to segmental infarction of the small bowel in addition to intestinal ischemia.

DEFECTS IN MUCOSAL FUNCTION

INFLAMMATORY OR INFILTRATIVE DISORDERS **Regional Enteritis** The clinical features of regional enteritis are described in Chap. 286. Malabsorption in regional enteritis may result from several factors: (1) interruption of the enterohepatic circulation of bile salts by ileal disease or resection, (2) deconjugation of bile salts due to bacterial overgrowth, in turn related to strictures and/or fistulas, (3) active inflammatory bowel disease causing impaired mucosal cell function, (4) inadequate absorptive surface resulting from intestinal resection or fistulas, and (5) severe protein depletion producing impaired exocrine pancreatic function. Active ileal disease and/or ileal resection resulting in an interrupted enterohepatic circulation of and deficiency of conjugated bile salts appears to be the major factor responsible for steatorrhea as well as impaired absorption of vitamin B_{12}. Small-bowel absorptive function has been correlated with the extent of ileal disease or resection. When the length of dysfunctional ileum exceeds 90 to 100 cm, virtually all patients will have steatorrhea and vitamin B_{12} malabsorption. After intestinal resection, the functional capacity of the remaining small bowel will depend on the site and extent of resection as well as the presence of residual inflammatory disease. Massive intestinal resection usually results in impaired absorption of all food constituents. When the malabsorption is due to strictures and blind loops as a result of previous surgery, antibiotic therapy may be helpful, but surgical removal of these areas is usually necessary for long-term improvement. With diffuse inflammatory disease, a florid malabsorption syndrome may occur with steatorrhea, hypocalcemia, impaired vitamin B_{12} absorption, and hypoalbuminemia due to increased enteric protein loss. Treatment with sulfasalazine, glucocorticoids, and other immunosuppressive drugs may be beneficial (see Chap. 286).

After *ileal resection*, patients frequently have bothersome diarrhea. This appears to be due to *interruption of the enterohepatic circulation*, whereby increased amounts of bile salts reach the colon, where they interfere with water and electrolyte absorption and thus have a cathartic effect. The *bile salt–induced diarrhea* after ileal resection may respond to treatment with cholestyramine, an exchange resin that binds bile salts and causes them to lose their biochemical effect on the bowel. Patients with ileal resection of less than 100 cm and fecal fat excretion less than 20 g/d show the best symptomatic response to cholestyramine, usually at a dose of 4 g tid.

Chronic Nongranulomatous Ulcerative Jejunoileitis This disorder is characterized by abdominal pain, weight loss, fever, diarrhea, steatorrhea, hypoalbuminemia, and protein-losing enteropathy. Clinical features mimic those found in both regional enteritis and celiac sprue. Indeed, the intestinal lesion may be indistinguishable from celiac sprue. However, exclusion of gluten from the diet does not result in any benefit. Glucocorticoid treatment has resulted in transient improvement, but long-term effects are unpredictable.

Amyloidosis See Chap. 309

Radiation Injury to the Small Bowel Extensive morphologic damage of the small-intestinal mucosa often follows normal or excessive abdominal irradiation. These changes include a decrease in crypt mitoses, marked shortening of the villi, megalocytosis of epithelial cells, and inflammatory cell infiltration of the lamina propria. These may be associated with transient diarrhea and impaired intestinal absorption. However, restoration of normal intestinal architecture is usually complete within 2 weeks after cessation of therapy. Persistent diarrhea and malabsorption may develop shortly after x-ray therapy, or there may be a latent period of several years before the onset of diarrhea. Steatorrhea, ranging from 10 to 40 g/d, has been observed frequently, but impaired absorption of calcium, iron, D-xylose, or vitamin B_{12} is less common. In some patients, intestinal strictures due to vasculopathy and ischemia may develop following irradiation, and thus stasis of intestinal contents and abnormal bacterial proliferation may occur. In others, intestinal lymphangiectasia, presumably due to lymphatic obstruction, has been documented. Diarrhea and malabsorption may be refractory to all methods of management. Treatment with antibiotics, pancreatic enzymes, gluten-free diet, adrenal glucocorticoids, and opiates has met with but limited success.

Eosinophilic Enteritis Eosinophilic gastroenteritis is a disorder of the stomach, small bowel, and colon that is of unknown etiology and is characterized by peripheral blood eosinophilia and eosinophilic infiltration of the gut wall without evidence of vasculitis. The clinical manifestations, usually recurrent, are protean and relate to the site of gastrointestinal tract involvement. Three main patterns have been identified: (1) Predominant mucosal disease manifested by iron-deficiency anemia, hypoalbuminemia due to protein-losing enteropathy, and mild steatorrhea. Patients in this group often present with a malabsorption syndrome and a history of intolerance to specific foods. (2) Predominant muscle layer disease characterized by marked thickening and rigidity of the stomach and proximal small bowel with obstructive symptoms and radiologic features of pyloric narrowing and obstruction. (Because of this pattern, eosinophilic enteritis should be considered in the differential diagnosis of gastric outlet obstruction, diffuse small-bowel disease, and ileocolitis. Indeed, eosinophilic enteritis often mimics regional enteritis.) (3) Predominant subserosal disease in which the cardinal manifestation is ascites with marked eosinophilia in the ascitic fluid. Although this classification based on the tissue layer of major involvement is useful in understanding the principal manifestations, it should be emphasized that mixed clinical forms—e.g., ascites (serosal involvement) plus obstruction (muscular involvement)—also occur. Diarrhea occurs in 30 to 60 percent of patients regardless of whether eosinophils infiltrate the gut mucosal, muscular, or serosal layers. *Ancylostoma caninum*, the canine hookworm present in domestic pets throughout Northeastern Australia and possibly worldwide, has been identified as a cause of obscure abdominal pain with biopsy-proven eosinophilic enteritis. The diagnosis can be confirmed by serologic tests.

Previous reports have emphasized food allergy and mucosal features of this disease. However, food allergy is related to symptoms in less than 20 percent of patients. In such patients, fasting serum IgE levels are often elevated, and challenge with offending foods frequently evokes symptoms of abdominal pain and diarrhea in addition to a marked increase in serum IgE levels. In most patients with eosinophilic enteritis, however, immunologic studies, including measurement of serum immunoglobulins, serum complement, lymphocytes, and lymphocyte response to nonspecific mitogens, reveal no abnormalities. Thus both IgE-mediated and IgE-independent mechanisms may be operative in different patients with eosinophilic gastroenteritis. It seems clear that evidence of allergy or food sensitivity is often absent and is not required for the diagnosis of eosinophilic enteritis. In addition, even in patients with food allergies, elimination diets are frequently ineffective, and such patients may require prolonged glucocorticoid therapy to remain well. Ketotifen and cromolyn are also useful therapeutic adjuncts. However, surgical treatment for relief of obstructive symptoms and use of glucocorticoids are the mainstays of therapy.

Dermatitis and Malabsorption A malabsorption syndrome, usually mild, has been reported in patients with a variety of dermatologic disorders, including psoriasis, eczematoid dermatitis, and dermatitis herpetiformis. Proximal intestinal mucosal abnormalities are almost invariably found in patients with dermatitis herpetiformis. In one study, 21 of 22 patients had lesions ranging in severity from a completely "flat" to an almost normal intestinal mucosa. The mucosal lesions were often patchy in distribution. Clinical and laboratory evidence of significant malabsorption was infrequent, possibly owing to the limited length of small intestine involved in this skin disorder. While the skin lesions of dermatitis herpetiformis respond to sulfone, the gut lesions do not. By contrast, in some patients with blunted and flattened intestinal mucosal lesions and steatorrhea, there may be a striking improvement in villous architecture and regression of steatorrhea after withdrawal of gluten from the diet without improvement in the skin lesions. Further, in patients with dermatitis herpetiformis and a morphologically normal small-intestinal mucosa, administration of a high-gluten diet may result in blunted and flattened mucosal lesions indistinguishable from those of celiac sprue. As in the latter disease, an increased frequency of HLA-A1 and HLA-B8 is also seen. These observations raise the interesting question as to whether certain patients with dermatitis herpetiformis and a malabsorption syndrome have latent celiac sprue.

BIOCHEMICAL OR GENETIC ABNORMALITIES **Celiac Sprue** Celiac sprue is a disorder characterized by malabsorption, abnormal small-bowel structure, and intolerance to gluten, a protein found in wheat and wheat products. It has been appropriately referred to as *gluten-induced enteropathy*. Celiac disease in children and celiac sprue in adults are probably the same disorder with the same pathogenesis.

There are insufficient data to provide an accurate estimation of the incidence of celiac sprue in any population. This is largely because the severity of the disease varies greatly, and individuals may have typical mucosal change and yet have no overt symptoms. In most reported series, 70 percent of the cases are in women. The incidence in siblings appears to be many times higher than that in the general population, and it has been suggested that sprue may be inherited through a dominant gene with incomplete penetrance. Celiac sprue patients have an increased frequency of some serum histocompatibility antigens, particularly of the HLA-DR3 and HLA-DQw2 types. The HLA-DR3 phenotype has been found in 70 to 90 percent of sprue patients, as compared with 20 to 25 percent in normal subjects. The HLA antigens may be linked to immune response genes which may determine the immunologic recognition of certain substances (see Chap. 306). It has been suggested that such genetic factors may predispose to immunologic tolerance of dietary proteins such as the peptides in gluten or to the production of pathogenic antigluten antibodies, which could result in the binding of gluten to epithelial cells with subsequent tissue damage. The discordance for celiac sprue among HLA-identical siblings and some identical twins raises the question of whether an additional susceptibility gene (or genes) not yet identified is required for the development of celiac sprue.

Pathophysiology Gluten and the related substance gliadin are high-molecular-weight proteins found especially in wheat. The alcohol-soluble fraction of gluten consists of glutamine-rich gliadin polypeptides, which can be fractionated into γ, β, δ, and α subgroups; peptides from all four gliadin subgroups are toxic to celiac sprue patients and induce the intestinal lesion when administered to patients with sprue in remission. The exact mechanism for this effect is not clear, but two theories have been proposed, namely, a "toxic" and an immunologic theory. One possible mechanism is that patients with celiac sprue lack a specific mucosal peptidase, so that gluten or its larger glutamine-containing peptides are not effectively hydrolyzed to smaller peptides (i.e., dipeptides or amino acids). As a consequence, "toxic" peptides might accumulate in the mucosa. It has been demonstrated that patients with celiac sprue in remission will develop steatorrhea and typical mucosal changes when they are given gluten. Similar results will occur with the administration of peptide hydrolysates containing at least eight amino acids with a terminal glutamine residue. It has been shown that when gluten is instilled into the *ileum* of celiac sprue patients, histologic changes begin to occur within hours. This does not occur in the *upper jejunum*, suggesting that the effect is immediate and is local rather than systemic. After surface absorptive cells are damaged by noxious gluten fractions, they are sloughed rapidly from the mucosal surface into the gut lumen. To compensate for this loss, cell proliferation increases, crypts undergo hypertrophy, and cell migration accelerates to replace the damaged and sloughed epithelial cells. This accelerated epithelial cell renewal can be reversed by a gluten-free diet.

The intestinal mucosa of patients with celiac sprue shows many enzyme alterations, including decreased levels of disaccharidases, alkaline phosphatase, and peptide hydrolases, as well as impaired ability to digest gluten peptides. However, these abnormalities usually revert toward normal after successful treatment with a gluten-free diet. There is additional evidence supporting the concept of toxicity of gluten and gluten breakdown products in celiac sprue. First, gliadin, especially the A-gliadin moiety, is toxic to sprue mucosa maintained in organ culture, causing ultrastructural changes and depression of disaccharidase activity. Second, sprue mucosa hydrolyzes a specific fraction of a gliadin digest (fraction 9) in a defective manner, and fraction 9 is selectively toxic to sprue mucosa. Third, specific fractions of gluten fed to celiac sprue patients cause transient alterations in mucosal histology and depression of disaccharidase activity, but full recovery is observed in 72 h. The rapid onset of these changes and the prompt recovery are consistent with a direct toxic effect. Two key tetrapeptide sequences present in cereals are toxic to patients with celiac disease—namely, Pro-Ser-Gly-Gly and Gly-Gly-Gly-Pro. Despite intensive study, however, no persistent, specific, or selective peptidase or other enzyme deficiency has been demonstrated.

It also has been suggested that gluten or gluten metabolites may initiate an *immune reaction* in the intestinal mucosa. Alternatively, the interaction of T lymphocytes with crypt epithelium may be a primary event in the pathogenesis of the intestinal lesion. The presence of a mononuclear inflammatory cell infiltrate in the lamina propria of the mucosa, the beneficial effect of glucocorticoid drugs, the finding of abnormal antibodies to gliadin in the serum of celiac sprue patients, the synthesis of increased amounts of antigliadin antibody by sprue mucosa maintained in organ culture, and the elaboration of lymphokines such as migration inhibitory factor (MIF) by sprue mucosa incubated with gliadin have all been cited as evidence in support of this hypothesis.

A possible role for adenovirus serotype 12 (Ad12) in the pathogenesis of celiac sprue has been proposed on the basis of two observations: (1) There is amino acid sequence homology between a portion of A-gliadin and a viral-encoded protein (E16) produced by Ad12, and (2) patients with untreated celiac sprue have a much higher frequency of antibodies to Ad12 than treated celiac sprue patients and controls. Although other studies have not confirmed these results, these findings are in accord with the hypothesis that there must be *environmental* factors as well as a *genetic predisposition* to explain why only certain people develop celiac sprue. Despite intensive studies, there is not yet enough information to integrate the distinctive dietary, immunologic, and genetic features of celiac sprue into a clear understanding of the pathogenesis of the disease.

Jejunal biopsy specimens from patients with celiac sprue show a characteristic lesion. There is blunting and flattening of the mucosal surface, with villi either absent or broad and short. The crypts are elongated, and there is generally a dense infiltration of inflammatory cells in the lamina propria. The surface epithelium is altered with a sparse brush border, cuboidal rather than the normal columnar cells, and infiltration of inflammatory cells in the epithelial layer. These changes are usually most severe in the proximal small bowel, presumably because this area of the bowel is exposed to the highest gluten concentration. The typical morphologic changes illustrated in Fig. 285-4 are characteristic of celiac sprue but are not specific. Similar changes have been described in other conditions, including lymphoma, tropical sprue, and hypogammaglobulinemia associated with malabsorption. Many biochemical abnormalities have been demonstrated in mucosal biopsy specimens from celiac sprue patients. Impaired esterification of fatty acids to triglycerides, decreased uptake of amino acids, and decreased activity of intestinal disaccharidases (especially lactase) have been well documented. The latter observation may account for the high incidence of milk intolerance in untreated celiac sprue patients or those in relapse. However, the greater abundance of undifferentiated crypt cells may be important, since crypt cells normally have a lower capacity for nutrient uptake than do villus cells.

Since the mucosa is damaged and altered in patients with celiac sprue, there may be *decreased release of pancreatotropic hormones* (secretin and CCK). This effect results in decreased stimulation of the pancreas and abnormally low intraluminal levels of pancreatic enzymes in response to a meal. In addition, the gallbladder appears to be resistant to the action of CCK, resulting in absent or minimal contractions of the gallbladder, in turn leading to sequestration of bile salts in an inert gallbladder. These two defects may result in impaired intraluminal digestion of fat and protein, which will be superimposed on the defect in intestinal transport caused by a damaged mucosa.

Diarrhea is common in celiac sprue patients and is due to a number of factors, including *impaired absorption* of salt and water by duodenum and jejunum, net *secretion* of water and electrolytes by an abnormally permeable jejunal mucosa, and net colonic secretion of water and electrolytes induced by unabsorbed fatty acids and hydroxy fatty acids. However, the distal small intestine in celiac sprue has the ability to adapt to the damage and loss of absorptive capacity in the proximal small intestine. Indeed, increased ileal absorption of sodium, chloride, and water has been demonstrated in celiac sprue patients.

Clinical features Most patients with celiac sprue will have a typical malabsorption syndrome characterized by weight loss, abdominal distention and bloating, diarrhea, steatorrhea, and abnormal results on tests of absorptive function. The characteristic alterations in responses to these tests are outlined in Table 285-2. It should be emphasized, however, that some patients present with isolated abnormalities that initially do not suggest the diagnosis of celiac sprue. Thus a patient may be admitted for investigation of iron-deficiency anemia without apparent blood loss or of abnormal bleeding due to hypoprothrombinemia but may not have diarrhea or overt steatorrhea. Likewise, celiac sprue patients may present with puzzling metabolic bone disease without diarrhea or steatorrhea. Such patients usually complain of bone pain and tenderness and frequently are found to have extensive demineralization of bone, compression deformities, kyphoscoliosis, and Milkman's fractures. Emotional disturbances are common in these patients, and many individuals with a diagnosis of weight loss initially considered related to severe anxiety and depression are subsequently found to have celiac sprue. Neurologic manifestations of celiac sprue include cerebellar ataxia, sensory neuropathy, myopathy hyporeflexia, and seizures. In each of the preceding clinical settings, celiac sprue should be considered in the differential diagnosis. In addition to dermatitis herpetiformis, there are established associations between celiac sprue and diabetes mellitus, selective IgA deficiency, primary sclerosing cholangitis, primary biliary cirrhosis, ulcerative colitis, and lymphocytic or microscopic colitis (see Chaps. 286 and 298).

Three criteria should be met for a definite diagnosis of celiac sprue to be made: (1) evidence of malabsorption, (2) the finding of an abnormal small-bowel (jejunal) biopsy specimen showing blunting and flattening of the villi along with changes in the surface epithelium, and (3) clinical, biochemical, and histologic improvement after institution of a gluten-free diet.

In recent studies, distinctive endoscopic changes were found in 22 of 28 patients with microscopic changes characteristic of sprue on biopsy (6 of 9 with sprue in relapse and 16 of 19 with initial symptoms). The mucosa was atrophic and had a mottled appearance, with patchy areas of pale mucosa alternating with more edematous mucosa; the pale areas had a pronounced mosaic appearance. Importantly, the valvulae conniventes exhibited a lesion now recognized to be characteristic of sprue—a distinctive scalloped appearance. The duodenal folds should always be examined at upper gastointestinal endoscopy. If they are absent or reduced, duodenal biopsy is indicated. Abnormality of Kerkring's folds is a helpful sign of celiac disease, especially in patients with minimal or transient symptoms.

In equivocal cases, the patient can be challenged with 30 to 50 g gluten orally; if this challenge results promptly in increased diarrhea and steatorrhea, the diagnosis of gluten-induced enteropathy is established. It should be emphasized that tests of intestinal absorption may reveal abnormalities ranging from very minimal to severe. Abnormalities in absorption tests have been shown to correlate reasonably well with the length of small-bowel involvement and to a lesser extent with the severity of the proximal lesion. Antigliadin, antiendomysial, and antireticulin antibodies have been widely used in the diagnosis of celiac disease. Approximately 90 percent of patients with untreated clinically symptomatic celiac disease, and many patients with asymptomatic latent disease, have IgA and/or IgG antigliadin antibodies; titers frequently decrease after institution of a gluten-free diet. Elevated titers of antiendomysial antibodies are found in over 90 percent of patients with active celiac disease and also decrease with improvement following intitiation of a gluten-free diet. Antireticulin antibodies are less sensitive but more specific than antigliadin antibodies, which can be found in other disorders affecting the small-bowel mucosa, such as Crohn's disease. Combined determination of antigliadin, antiendomysial, and antireticulin antibodies offers optimal sensitivity and specificity for the detection of celiac disease. These antibodies are also useful in following the response to therapy and adherence to a gluten-free diet, and in screening for celiac disease among family members.

A possible variant of celiac sprue is *collagenous* sprue, in which small-bowel biopsy specimens characteristically reveal a blunted and flattened mucosa and large masses of eosinophilic hyaline material in the lamina propria. In one study of biopsy specimens from 145 patients with celiac sprue, 31 percent showed basement membrane thickening, which often was associated with collagen deposition, but dense collagen deposition was found in only 8 percent. Fatal, unremitting malabsorption developed in a third of the latter patients. These observations suggest that collagenous membrane thickening is a fairly frequent finding in jejunal biopsies of patients with sprue but that dense collagen deposits are unusual and may indicate a poor prognosis.

℞ TREATMENT

Despite the uncertainties concerned with the diagnosis of celiac sprue, approximately 80 percent improve after institution of a *gluten-free diet.* Symptomatic improvement usually occurs within a few weeks, but improvement in the response to tests of absorptive function and in small-bowel histologic characteristics may not occur for months. It has been demonstrated repeatedly that strict adherence to a gluten-free diet more consistently results in improvement than does suboptimal gluten restriction. Recent studies indicate that oats, when ingested in quantities of about 50 g/d, are safe for celiac sprue patients for a period of at least 6 to 12 months. Nevertheless, even with strict diet adherence, some patients show little improvement in intestinal histologic features. Patients with celiac sprue who are treated with glucocorticoids but continue to eat a normal gluten-containing diet have shown symptomatic improvement as well as improvement in intestinal histology and tests of intestinal absorptive function. The mechanism by which glucocorticoids protect the mucosa from the effects of gluten is not clear.

If a patient with celiac sprue does not respond to a gluten-free diet, other possibilities or complicating factors must be considered: (1) The diagnosis is incorrect; (2) the patient is not adhering strictly to the diet; (3) there may be another concurrent disease, such as pancreatic insufficiency; (4) the patient may have ulceration of the jejunum or ileum; (5) lactase deficiency may be present with resulting milk intolerance; (6) the patient may have collagenous sprue; (7) the patient may have developed intestinal lymphoma, a disease which appears to occur more frequently in patients with sprue than in the general population; and (8) the patient may have developed lymphocytic or microscopic colitis. Finally, it should be emphasized that a small number of patients show a markedly delayed response to a gluten-free diet, with significant improvement occurring only after 24 to 36 months of therapy. Approximately 50 percent of patients with refractory sprue respond to glucocorticoids; such patients also may require parenteral hyperalimentation or treatment with other immunosuppressive drugs such as 6-mercaptopurine.

Systemic Mastocytosis Some evidence of malabsorption occurs in 30 percent of patients with systemic mastocytosis. Malabsorption is usually not severe and is manifested primarily as minimal or moderate steatorrhea and impaired absorption of D-xylose and vitamin B_{12}. Small-bowel biopsy specimens typically show moderate blunting of villi and mast cell infiltration. Treatment with histamine H_1 and H_2 receptor antagonists and cromolyn provides relief of diarrhea in some patients.

Disaccharidase Deficiency Syndromes As indicated above, the hydrolysis of disaccharides occurs on or within the brush border (microvilli) of intestinal epithelial cells by specific disaccharidases. There are both primary (genetic or familial) and secondary (acquired) disaccharidase deficiencies.

Lactase deficiency in the adult Instances of isolated deficiency of mucosal lactase occur; they are associated with symptoms of lactose intolerance. Since lactose is the principal carbohydrate of milk, such individuals show milk intolerance, with symptoms of abdominal cramps, bloating or distention, and diarrhea. Similar symptoms will occur following the ingestion of lactose. When lactose is not hydrolyzed, it is not absorbed, and its osmotic effect in the lumen leads to shifts of fluid into the intestinal tract. The pH of the stool also will decrease because of the production of lactic acid and short-chain fatty acids from the fermentation of lactose by colonic bacteria. Although primary intestinal lactase deficiency seems to be hereditary, lactose or milk intolerance may not become clinically evident until puberty or late adolescence. There are significant racial differences in the incidence of this entity. It would appear that about 5 to 15 percent of the adult white population shows intestinal lactase deficiency, but in African Americans, Bantus, and Asians, the incidence is as high as 80 to 90 percent.

The diagnosis may be suspected when one obtains a history of gastrointestinal symptoms following milk ingestion. Bloating, cramps, and flatulence, but not diarrhea, are usually produced with ingestion of moderate amounts of lactose. The vast majority of lactose-intolerant persons are aware that they are milk-intolerant and avoid milk. These symptoms are not due to allergic reactions to the proteins in milk (i.e., milk allergy or hypersensitivity) and can be demonstrated by measurement of breath hydrogen after ingestion of 50 g lactose, which is a sensitive and specific test. The rationale for this test is that hydrogen is released from unabsorbed lactose by colonic bacteria, and breath hydrogen excretion subsequently rises. The test is noninvasive and is not influenced by gastric emptying or metabolic factors. Approximately 70 percent of patients with primary lactose intolerance will respond to a lactose-restricted diet, while the remaining 30 percent will not because of an underlying irritable bowel syndrome. When lactose intake is limited to less than 240 mL of milk per day, gastrointestinal symptoms are likely to be negligible in many patients who identify themselves as severely lactose intolerant. These findings suggest that a variety of abdominal complaints are frequently misattributed to lactose intolerance. The use of lactase-containing digestive aids may be unnecessary for milk intakes of <8 oz/d.

Acquired lactase deficiency is often seen in association with a variety of gastrointestinal diseases, in many of which there is histologic evidence of mucosal damage. These include celiac and tropical sprue, regional enteritis, viral and bacterial infections of the intestinal tract, giardiasis, abetalipoproteinemia, cystic fibrosis, and ulcerative colitis.

Deficiency of other disaccharidases Damage to the intestinal mucosa may produce decreased levels of other disaccharidases, such as sucrase-isomaltase, but usually these enzymes are not as depressed as lactase, and symptoms of specific intolerance, such as sucrose intolerance, are uncommon. There are instances of primary and apparently hereditary sucrose intolerance, but these always occur in association with sucrase-isomaltase deficiency. Sucrase-isomaltase deficiency, while not as common as lactase deficiency, is nonetheless an important cause of diarrhea, bloating, and cramping abdominal pain in children. Such patients are often unable to adhere to a low-sucrose diet. Thus, the observation that the symptoms of sucrose malabsorption can be ameliorated by the simple expedient of ingesting viable yeast cells is of considerable practical importance.

Hypogammaglobulinemia See Chap. 307

Abetalipoproteinemia See Chap. 341

Hartnup Disease, Cystinuria See Chap. 350

ENDOCRINE AND METABOLIC DISORDERS **Diabetes Mellitus** The occurrence of diarrhea and steatorrhea in patients with diabetes mellitus has been well documented. When steatorrhea accompanies diabetes, it may be due to the presence of (1) exocrine pancreatic insufficiency, (2) coexisting celiac sprue (6 percent of insulin-requiring diabetics have shown histologic evidence of celiac sprue), (3) abnormal bacterial proliferation in the proximal small bowel, or (4) severe and uncontrolled diabetes per se (e.g., so-called diabetic diarrhea). Patients falling into the first three categories will usually respond satisfactorily to treatment with pancreatic extracts, a gluten-free diet, and antibiotics, respectively. The pathogenesis of diarrhea and steatorrhea in patients in the fourth category remains poorly understood. They may have involvement of the autonomic nervous system with degenerative changes in the sympathetic and parasympathetic nerves and ganglia; in some, bacterial overgrowth may occur and contribute to the malabsorption.

The clinical features in patients with diarrhea and steatorrhea due to diabetes seem to be fairly uniform. Diabetes usually developed at a young age and is often severe and difficult to control. There is a distinct male predominance. Several signs of autonomic neuropathy are usually present, including postural hypotension, anhydrosis, impotence, and bladder irregularities. Peripheral vascular disease and peripheral neuropathy are also common. Gastrointestinal x-rays may show delayed gastric emptying and disordered transit through the small bowel. Small-bowel biopsy specimens appear normal. Tests of intestinal absorptive function give normal results except for showing the presence of steatorrhea and azotorrhea. There has been no consistent response to therapy with pancreatic extracts, a gluten-free diet, or glucocorticoids. When bacterial overgrowth is present, broad-spectrum antibiotics may be helpful. Persistent diarrhea may also result from ingestion of dietetic food containing large amounts of sorbitol, which often are erroneously labeled "sugarless." Clonidine has proved useful in patients with large-volume diarrhea not responding to dietary measures and anticholinergics.

Hypoparathyroidism Steatorrhea has been documented in several patients with idiopathic hypoparathyroidism. In addition to hypocalcemia, impaired absorption of D-xylose and vitamin B_{12}, decreased serum iron values, and abnormal small-intestinal roentgenograms have been demonstrated in some cases. In such patients the serum phosphorus level is elevated (owing to the hypoparathyroidism) rather than low (as in primary malabsorption). The cause of malabsorption in this disorder is unclear.

Adrenal Insufficiency Although there are few studies on fat excretion in adrenal insufficiency in human beings, malabsorption, especially of fat, appears to occur more frequently than has been generally appreciated. Patients with adrenal insufficiency have been found to have steatorrhea that is corrected by therapy with adrenal glucocorticoids.

Hyperthyroidism There are few detailed studies on intestinal absorptive function in patients with hyperthyroidism. Mild to moderate steatorrhea and hypoalbuminemia have been reported, but absorption of D-xylose and vitamin B_{12} is frequently normal. Steatorrhea usually remits after successful treatment of hyperthyroidism. Clinical studies suggest that steatorrhea in hyperthyroidism is not due to any defect of pancreatic, biliary, or small-intestinal mucosal function but is a result of hyperphagia with ingestion of unusually large amounts of fat occurring in association with rapid gastric emptying and intestinal transit.

Gastrinoma (Zollinger-Ellison Syndrome) The clinical features of gastrinomas are described in Chaps. 95 and 284. Malabsorption is frequently found in this disease. The acidification and dilution of intestinal contents caused by gastric acid hypersecretion leads to major disturbances in fat digestion and absorption. Impaired formation of micellar lipid due to inactivation of pancreatic lipase is probably the major factor in the production of steatorrhea. Other factors contributing to fat malabsorption include (1) precipitation of glycine-conjugated bile salts due to low intraluminal pH, (2) alteration of the intestinal mucosa with ulceration and metaplasia, and (3) impaired fatty acid esterification and chylomicron formation.

Carcinoid Syndrome (See also Chap. 95) Although diarrhea is common in the carcinoid syndrome, malabsorption with significant steatorrhea is unusual. In many cases of carcinoid syndrome with steatorrhea, there has been a prior intestinal resection (usually ileal), and in these cases the resection is the major cause of steatorrhea. However, direct involvement of the bowel wall and mesentery by the carcinoid tumor has been well documented. That abnormalities in serotonin metabolism also may be important is suggested from the decrease in the steatorrhea observed in some of these patients when treated with the antiserotonin drug methysergide. Although side effects may occur, for control of diarrhea and steatorrhea, patients may be given a trial of 8 to 12 mg methysergide per day.

PROTEIN-LOSING ENTEROPATHY The gastrointestinal tract plays a significant role in the metabolism and physiologic degradation of plasma proteins. While the exact magnitude of the normal gastrointestinal protein loss is unclear, studies with labeled albumin suggest that between 10 and 20 percent of the normal turnover of albumin may be accounted for by enteric protein loss. However, under certain pathologic conditions, excessive gastrointestinal protein loss may develop. Many disorders have been found to be associated with intestinal protein loss. Some of these are listed in Table 285-8.

Pathophysiology Several mechanisms have been proposed for the passage of plasma proteins across the gastrointestinal mucosa, both normally and in certain disease states. First, plasma proteins may pass into the gastrointestinal tract through an inflamed or ulcerated mucosa and account for the protein loss occasionally seen in Crohn's disease and ulcerative colitis. Second, plasma protein loss may occur as a result of disordered mucosal cell structure. For example, patients with celiac sprue have abnormal villous structure and surface epithelium, and these changes facilitate the diffusion of plasma protein between the cells. Third, in the presence of increased lymphatic pressure, there may be increased passage of plasma proteins into the lumen via the intercellular spaces of the mucosal epithelium. This might be expected to occur in disorders in which there is granulomatous or neoplastic involvement of lymphatics. Fourth, dilated lymph vessels in the mucosa may rupture through the surface epithelium, discharging their contents into the intestinal lumen. This is thought to be important in the pathogenesis of steatorrhea and hypoproteinemia in patients with idiopathic intestinal lymphangiectasia (see "Intestinal Lymphangiectasia," below).

In the past, the detection and quantitation of gastrointestinal protein loss primarily involved the use of intravenously administered radiolabeled macromolecules such as ^{125}I-labeled serum albumin, $^{51}CrCl_3$, ^{51}Cr-labeled albumin, and indium 111. Patients with excessive enteric protein loss may excrete from 2 to 40 percent of the injected radioactive label, versus 0.1 to 0.7 percent in normal subjects. False-positive results may be obtained if the stool specimen is contaminated with urine. However, tests with radiolabeled compounds have been superceded by a reliable and sensitive *nonisotopic* method to measure intestinal protein loss which involves the measurement of α_1-antitrypsin (AT). This serum enzyme, which has the same molecular weight as albumin (50,000), is resistant to proteolysis and, when leaked into the intestinal lumen, is not degraded. One can easily measure AT in serum and stool by radial immunodiffusion in order to measure the AT loss in stool (the normal loss is less than 2.6 mg per gram of stool) or intestinal clearance of AT (the normal value is less than 13 mL/d). Random fecal AT assays also can be used as a simple screening method for enteric protein loss.

Intestinal Lymphangiectasia *Pathophysiology* This disorder is characterized by increased enteric loss of protein, hypoproteinemia, edema, lymphocytopenia, malabsorption, and abnormal dilated lymphatic channels in the small intestine. The high incidence of chylous effusions and abnormal peripheral, retroperitoneal, and thoracic lymphatics indicates that intestinal lymphangiectasia is part of a generalized congenital disorder of the lymphatic system. It has been suggested that the hypoplastic visceral lymphatic channels result in obstruction to lymph flow, with the subsequent development of increased intestinal lymphatic pressure. This, in turn, may lead to dilated lymphatic vessels throughout the small-bowel wall and mesentery. Hypoproteinemia and steatorrhea are thought to be due to rupture of the dilated lymphatic vessels with discharge of lymph into the bowel lumen. In adults, approximately 1500 mL of lymph, containing 70 g fat and 50 g albumin, passes through the thoracic duct each day. The leakage of a small amount of this lymph might be expected to result in considerable loss of protein and fat into the intestinal lumen. In addition, absorption of dietary long-chain triglycerides stimulates lymph flow, and this may increase further the retrograde leakage of intestinal lymph into the lumen. Three lines of evidence support the concept of intestinal leakage of lymph in intestinal lymphangiectasia: (1) Chylous fluid has been recovered from the duodenum in these patients; (2) retrograde passage of contrast material from retroperitoneal lymphatics into the duodenum and jejunum has been documented; and (3) significant steatorrhea may persist in patients after institution of a completely fat-free diet, suggesting an increased enteric loss of endogenous fat present in lymph.

Table 285-8

Disorders Assocaited with Protein-Losing Enteropathy

Stomach	**Colon**
Gastric carcinoma	Colonic neoplasm
Ménétrier's disease	Ulcerative colitis
Atrophic gastritis	Granulomatous colitis
Postgastrectomy syndrome	Megacolon
Small intestine	**Heart**
Intestinal lymphangiectassia	Congestive heart failure
Celiac sprue	Constrictive pericarditis
Tropical sprue	Interatrial septal defect
Regional enteritis	Primary cardiomyopathy
Whipple's disease	**Miscellaneous**
Lymphoma	Esophageal carcinoma
Intestinal tuberculosis	Gastrocolic fistula
Acute infectious enteritis	Agammaglobulinemia
Scleroderma	Nephrosis
Jejunal diverticulosis	
Allergic gastroenteropathy	
Eosinophilic gastroenteritis	
Bacterial overgrowth	

Clinical features The disease affects primarily children and young adults. All patients have edema, which may be asymmetric because of hypoplastic peripheral lymphatics. Chylous effusions and diarrhea are common symptoms. The primary laboratory finding is hypoproteinemia with decreased serum levels of albumin, immunoglobulins IgG, IgA, and IgM, transferrin, and ceruloplasmin. Despite moderate to severe hypogammaglobulinemia, there does not appear to be an increased incidence of pyogenic bacterial infections. In addition, the circulating antibody response to challenge with *Brucella* and typhoid antigens is normal. Steatorrhea is usually mild, although in some instances fat loss may be as much as 40 g/d. Some patients have hypocalcemia and impaired absorption of vitamin B_{12}. Lymphocytopenia (due to the loss of lymphocytes in lymph) is common, with lymphocyte counts ranging from 400 to 1000/mL (normal: 1500 to 4000/mL). This deficiency is associated with abnormal delayed hypersensitivity, as evidenced by prolonged homograft survival and impaired cutaneous responsiveness to antigens such as mumps and monilia.

Small-bowel roentgenograms are frequently abnormal, showing changes of mucosal edema and a malabsorption pattern. Lymphangiograms may demonstrate hypoplastic peripheral and visceral lymphatics, with the absence of groups of retroperitoneal lymph nodes. Specimens of jejunal mucosa characteristically reveal dilated and telangiectatic lymphatic vessels in the lamina propria and submucosa. The villi may be club-shaped because of distortion from grossly dilated lymphatics (see Fig. 285-4). Such changes in the intestinal mucosa may be reversed after appropriate therapy. The diagnosis of intestinal lymphangiectasia is therefore established by (1) small-intestinal biopsy and (2) demonstration of increased enteric protein loss using radiolabeled macromolecules.

℞ TREATMENT

A low-fat diet, by decreasing lymph flow, usually results in significant improvement with decreased fecal fat excretion, decreased enteric protein loss, increased serum calcium and albumin levels, and an increased half-life of injected ^{125}I-labeled albumin. Similar results may be obtained by the substitution of medium-chain triglycerides for dietary long-chain triglycerides, since the former are transported as medium-chain fatty acids by the portal vein rather than via the lymph.

For further discussion of drugs affecting gastrointestinal function, see Chaps. 37 and 38, in Goodman and Gilman's The Pharmacological Basis of Therapeutics, *9th ed., McGraw-Hill, New York, 1996.*

BIBLIOGRAPHY

AMER MH, EL-AKKAD S: Gastrointestinal lymphoma in adults: Clinical features and management of 300 cases. Gastroenterology 106:840, 1994

ARRANZ E, FERGUSON A: Intestinal antibody pattern in celiac disease: Occurrence in patients with normal jejunal biopsy histology. Gastroenterology 104:1263, 1993

CHIN JS et al: Paraneoplastic visceral neuropathy as a cause of severe gastrointestinal motor dysfunction. Gastroenterology 95:1279, 1988

CORAZZA G et al: Gliadin immune reactivity is associated with overt and latent enteropathy in relatives of celiac patients. Gastroenterology 102:1517, 1992

FERGUSON A et al: Clinical and pathological spectrum of coeliac disease—active, silent, latent, potential. Gut 34:150, 1993

FINE KD, FORDTRAN JS: The effect of diarrhea on fecal fat excretion. Gastroenterology 102:1936, 1992

FINE KD: The prevalence of occult gastrointestinal bleeding in celiac sprue. N Engl J Med 334:1163, 1996

FRIED M et al: Duodenal bacterial overgrowth during treatment in outpatients with omeprazole. Gut 35:23, 1994

HAMMER HF et al: Carbohydrate malabsorption: Its measurement and its contribution to diarrhea. J Clin Invest 86:1936, 1990

JANATUINEN ER et al: A comparison of diets with and without oats in adults with celiac disease. N Engl J Med 333:1033, 1995

KAGNOFF M et al: Evidence for the role of human intestinal adenovirus in the pathogenesis of coeliac disease. Gut 28:5, 1987

KERLIN P, WONG L: Breath hydrogen testing in bacterial overgrowth of the small intestine. Gastroenterology 95:982, 1988

LADINSER B et al: Endomysium antibodies in coeliac disease. Gut 35:776, 1994

LOUGHRAN TP et al: T-cell intestinal lymphoma associated with celiac sprue. Ann Intern Med 104:44, 1986

MARCUARD SP et al: Omeprazole therapy causes malabsorption of cyanocobalamin (vitamin B-12). Ann Intern Med 120:211, 1994

RELMAN DA et al: Identification of the uncultured bacillus of Whipple's disease. N Engl J Med 327:293, 1992

SALTZMAN JR et al: Bacterial overgrowth without clinical malabsorption in elderly hypochlorhydric subjects. Gastroenterology 106:615, 1994

SUAREZ FL et al: A comparison of symptoms after the consumption of milk or lactose-hydrolyzed milk by people with self reported lactose intolerance. N Engl J Med 333:1, 1995

SCHILLER LR et al: Studies on the prevalence and significance of radiolabeled bile acid malabsorption in a group of patients with idiopathic chronic diarrhea. Gastroenterology 92:151, 1987

TRIER JS: Medical progress: Celiac sprue. N Engl J Med 325:1709, 1991

TRONCONE R et al: Gluten-sensitive enteropathy. Pediatr Clin North Am 43:355, 1996

VAN ELBURG RM et al: Intestinal permeability in patients with coeliac disease and relatives of patients with coeliac disease. Gut 34:354, 1993

286

Robert M. Glickman

INFLAMMATORY BOWEL DISEASE: Ulcerative Colitis and Crohn's Disease

DEFINITION *Inflammatory bowel disease* (IBD) is a general term for a group of chronic inflammatory disorders of unknown cause involving the gastrointestinal tract. Since these disorders have no pathognomonic features or specific diagnostic tests, in a strict sense they remain diagnoses of exclusion. Their features are sufficiently characteristic, however, to permit accurate diagnosis in most cases. Chronic IBD may be divided into two major groups, chronic nonspecific *ulcerative colitis* (UC) and *Crohn's disease* (CD). The original description of the latter disease by Crohn, Ginzberg, and Oppenheimer in 1932 localized it to segments of ileum. However, the same process may involve the buccal mucosa, esophagus, stomach, and duodenum, as well as the jejunum and ileum. Crohn's disease of the small bowel is also known as *regional enteritis*. A similar inflammatory picture may occur in the colon, either alone or with accompanying small intestinal involvement. In most instances, this form of colitis can be distinguished clinically and pathologically from ulcerative colitis and may be referred to as *Crohn's disease of the colon*. *Granulomatous colitis* is a less accurate term because only some cases exhibit granulomas. Clinically these disorders are characterized by recurrent inflammatory involvement of intestinal segments with diverse clinical manifestations, often resulting in a chronic, unpredictable course.

EPIDEMIOLOGY The epidemiology and etiology of UC and CD share many features and will be discussed together. These diseases are more common in whites than in blacks or Asians, and Jews have an incidence three to six times greater than that of non-Jews. The sexes are affected equally.

The incidence and prevalence of the two diseases differ slightly, UC being the more common. When analyzed in western Europe and the United States, UC (including ulcerative proctitis) has an incidence of approximately 6 to 8 cases per 100,000 population and an estimated prevalence of approximately 70 to 150 cases per 100,000 population. Estimates of the incidence of CD (colonic plus small bowel) are approximately 2 cases per 100,000 population; the prevalence is estimated at 20 to 40 per 100,000 population. Many believe the incidence of CD (especially colonic) to be increasing. In western Europe and North America, the incidence and prevalence of CD have been increasing five times faster than those of ulcerative colitis.

While the occurrence of both diseases peaks between the ages of 15 and 35, they have been reported from every decade of life. A familial incidence of IBD has been recorded, with estimates that 2 to 5 percent of persons with CD or UC will have one or more relatives affected. There is no specificity, however, for a given form of IBD within a given family. Such epidemiologic clustering of cases could be due to an effect of either genetic factors or common environmental influences on the development of these diseases (see below). It has been suggested that the pathogenesis of these disorders has both a probable hereditary basis and a strong environmental component.

ETIOLOGY AND PATHOGENESIS While the causes of UC and CD remain unknown, certain features of these diseases have suggested several areas of possible importance. These include familial or genetic, infectious, immunologic, and psychological factors.

As mentioned, the increased incidence of inflammatory bowel disease in whites and in Jews and the occurrence of familial clustering suggest a *genetic* predisposition to the development of the disease. An increased incidence of CD in monozygotic twins also is strong evidence for a genetic component. A search for genetic markers that might be of value in identifying susceptible individuals has not identified any single marker (i.e., a histocompatibility antigen) in patients with IBD.

The chronic inflammatory nature of these diseases has prompted a continuing search for an *infectious* cause. Despite numerous attempts, no bacterial, fungal, or viral agents has thus far been isolated. Preliminary reports of isolates of cell wall variants of *Pseudomonas* or of transmissible agents producing cytopathic effects in tissue culture have yet to be confirmed. As discussed below, many infectious agents can produce *acute* colitis or ileitis; however, there is no evidence that these agents are involved in *chronic* IBD.

The idea that an *immune* mechanism is involved is based on the reasoning that the extraintestinal manifestations that may accompany these disorders (e.g., arthritis and pericholangitis) may represent autoimmune phenomena and that therapeutic agents such as glucocorticoids, azathioprine, and cyclosporine may act via immunosuppressive mechanisms. Patients with IBD may have *humoral antibodies* to colon cells, to bacterial antigens such as *Escherichia coli*, to lipopolysaccharide, and to foreign proteins such as cow's milk protein. In general, the presence and titer of these antibodies do not correlate with disease activity. It is likely that these antigens gain access to immunocompetent cells as a consequence of epithelial damage. In addition, IBD has been described in association with agammaglobulinemia as well as IgA deficiency, casting further doubt on the pathogenetic role of humoral antibodies. *Immune complexes* also have been invoked to explain extraintestinal manifestations of IBD. While there are well-defined examples of tissue injury resulting from immune complexes, studies using specific detection techniques have failed to demonstrate an increased frequency of immune complexes in patients with IBD.

Abnormalities of *cell-mediated immunity* that have been reported in association with IBD include cutaneous anergy, diminished responsiveness to various mitogenic stimuli, and a decreased number of peripheral T cells. Since many of these changes may revert to normal when the disease is quiescent, they are probably secondary phenomena. Many abnormalities of cell-mediated immunity in the mucosa of patients with IBD also have been described. They include an increased concentration of mucosal IgG cells and changes in subsets of T cells, suggesting antigenic stimulation. Activation of mucosal immune cells results in a complex expression of cytokines, which may contribute to the mucosal inflammatory response. In addition, noncytokine inflammatory mediators, such as prostaglandin and thromboxane products, are present in elevated levels in the mucosa of patients with IBD and would further stimulate the inflammatory response. Animal models of IBD, including a transgenic rat model that expresses human HLA-B27, a mouse deficient in interleukin 2, and the spontaneous chronic colitis of the cotton-top tamarin, also may yield important insights into the pathogenesis of IBD. No immunologic alterations specific for either UC or CD have yet been found, however.

The *psychological* features of patients with IBD also have been stressed. It is not uncommon for these diseases to present initially or to flare up in association with major psychological stresses such as the loss of a family member. It has been suggested that patients with IBD have a characteristic personality that renders them susceptible to emotional stresses. While there is little evidence directly relating emotional factors to the etiology of IBD, there is little doubt that a chronic disease of unknown cause, affecting individuals in the prime of life, often results in anger, anxiety, and some degree of depression. These reactions are undoubtedly important factors in modifying the course of these diseases and the response to therapy.

PATHOLOGY In UC, there is an inflammatory reaction primarily involving the colonic mucosa. Grossly, the colon appears ulcerated, hyperemic, and usually hemorrhagic (Fig. 286-1). A striking feature of the inflammation is that it is *uniform* and *continuous*, with no intervening areas of normal mucosa. The rectum is usually involved (95 percent of cases), and the inflammation extends proximally in a continuous fashion for a variable distance. When the entire colon is involved, there may also be minimal involvement of a few centimeters of the terminal ileum, called "backwash ileitis." This involvement never leads to the thickening and narrowing characteristic of Crohn's disease. The surface mucosal cells as well as the crypt epithelium and submucosa are involved in an inflammatory reaction with neutrophilic infiltration (Fig. 286-2*A*). This reaction progresses to epithelial damage with loss of surface epithelial cells, resulting in multiple ulcerations. Infiltration of the crypts by neutrophils results in characteristic (but not specific) small crypt abscesses and eventual crypt destruction. There also may be loss of crypt epithelium, with a loss of goblet cells and submucosal edema. Repetitive cycles of inflammation lead to mild submucosal fibrosis. Regenerative activity is evidenced by crypts with irregular epithelium and often with a basal bifurcation. It is important to stress that, unlike Crohn's disease, deeper layers of the bowel, beneath the submucosa, usually are not involved. In severe UC, as seen with toxic megacolon, the bowel wall may become extremely thin and denuded of mucosa, with inflammation extending to the serosa, leading to dilation and subsequent perforation.

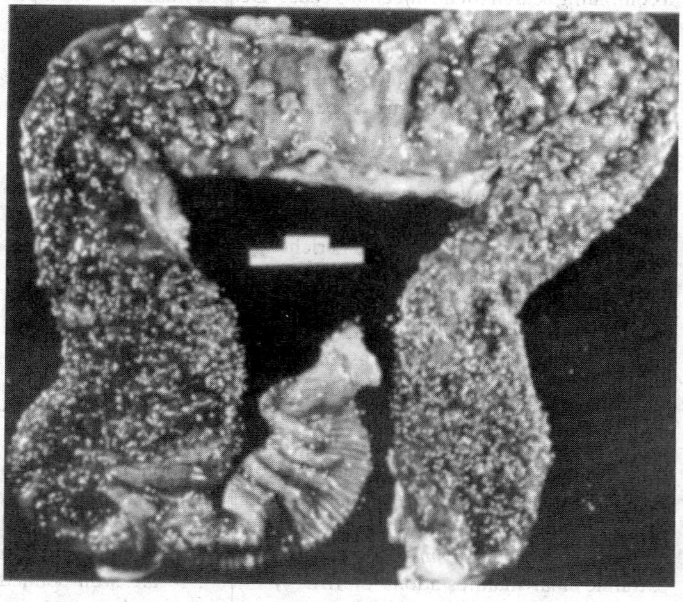

FIGURE 286-1 Ulcerative colitis. Resected colon with portion of terminal ileum. The specimen showed uniform inflammation, erythema, and hemorrhage and a normal terminal ileum.

Recurrent inflammation may lead to characteristic features of chronicity. Fibrosis and longitudinal retraction result in shortening of the colon. Loss of the normal haustral pattern leads radiologically to a smooth, "lead-pipe" appearance of the colon. Regenerating islands of mucosa surrounded by areas of ulceration and denuded mucosa appear as "polyps" protruding into the lumen. However, these protrusions are inflammatory rather than neoplastic and are therefore called *pseudopolyps* (Fig. 286-2*B*).

With long-standing UC, the surface epithelium may show features of *dysplasia*. Nuclear and cellular atypia are thought to represent premalignant changes occurring in the setting of long-standing UC. Marked dysplasia in colonic biopsy samples in the setting of long-standing colitis is associated with a significant risk of a carcinoma elsewhere in the colon and may influence the decision to advise colectomy.

Crohn's disease, in contrast to ulcerative colitis, is characterized by chronic inflammation extending through *all layers of the intestinal wall* and involving the mesentery as well as regional lymph nodes. Whether or not the small bowel or colon is involved, the basic pathologic process is the same for small bowel and colonic involvement.

The earliest pathologic changes in CD are poorly defined, since surgery is usually not undertaken electively early in the course of the disease. At laparotomy, the terminal ileum appears hyperemic and boggy, with mesentery and mesenteric lymph nodes swollen and reddened. At this stage, the bowel wall, although edematous, is usually pliable. While some patients with this initial presentation subsequently develop typical regional enteritis, a significant number recover completely. This acute form of ileitis will undoubtedly be shown to have diverse causes. Indeed, a significant number of patients with this presentation have been shown to be infected with *Yersinia enterocolitica*, an organism capable of producing a self-limited, acute inflammatory ileitis.

As the disease progresses, the gross appearance becomes characteristic. The bowel appears greatly thickened and leathery with a narrowed lumen (Fig. 286-3). This characteristic stenosis can occur in any portion of the intestine and may be associated with some degree of intestinal obstruction. The mesentery appears greatly thickened and fatty and often extends over the serosal surface of the bowel in characteristic finger-like projections. The appearance of the mucosa depends on the severity and stage of the disease, but it may be relatively normal, in sharp contrast to the mucosa in UC. In more advanced cases, the mucosa has a nodular, "cobblestone" look. This appearance is the result of submucosal thickening and mucosal ulceration, often linear in the long axis of the bowel at the base of mucosal folds. These ulcerations may penetrate into the submucosa and muscularis and coalesce to form intramural channels that become manifest as fistulas and fissures.

Other morphologic features also distinguish CD from UC. In CD, the disease is often *discontinuous*; severely involved segments of bowel are separated by "skip areas" of apparently normal bowel. In approximately 50 percent of cases of CD of the colon, the rectum is spared. In sharp contrast, in UC, the involvement is contiguous and the rectum almost always is involved. In addition, in CD, the transmural inflammatory process, involving serosa and mesentery, accounts for the characteristic fistula and abscess formation. As a result of serosal inflammation, adjacent loops of small intestine may become adherent

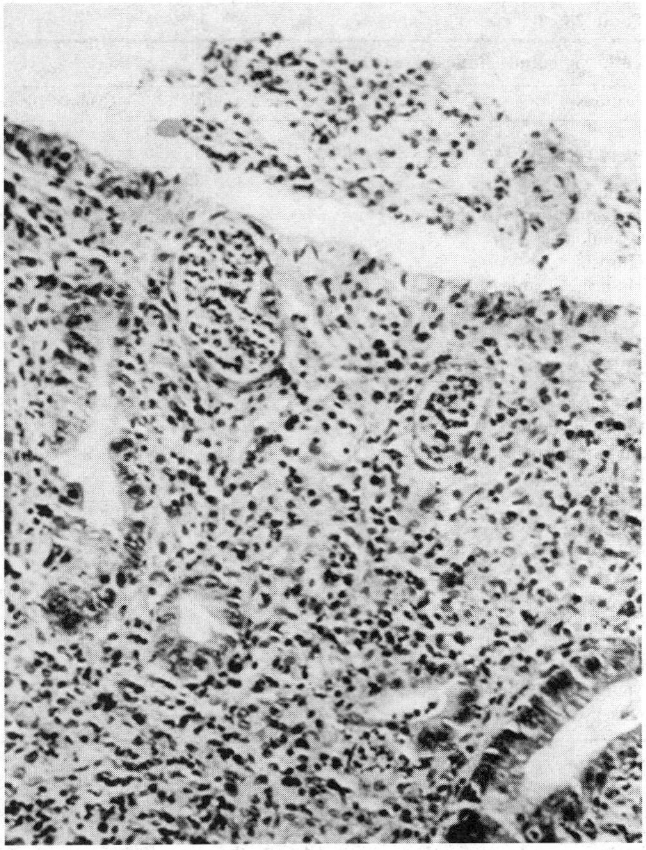

A

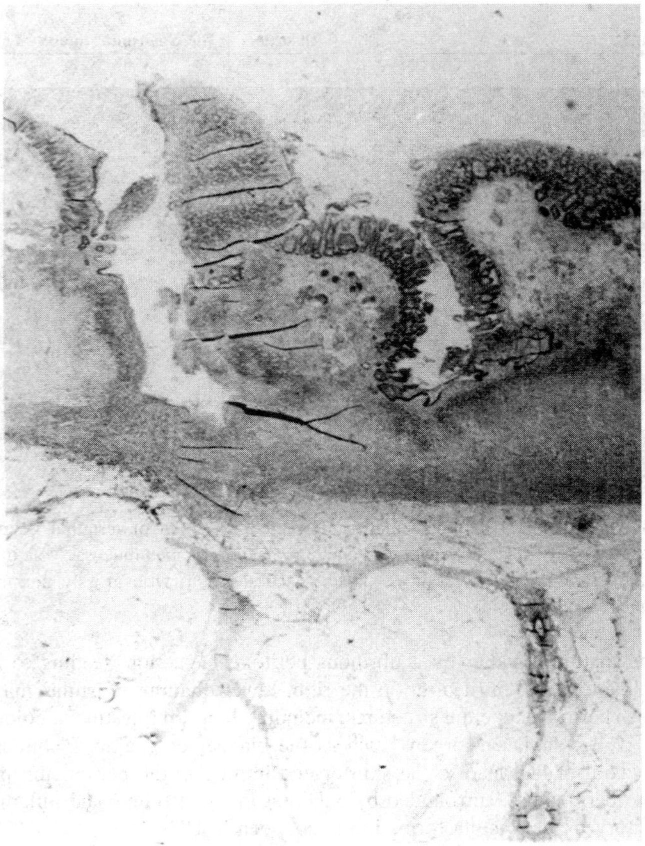

B

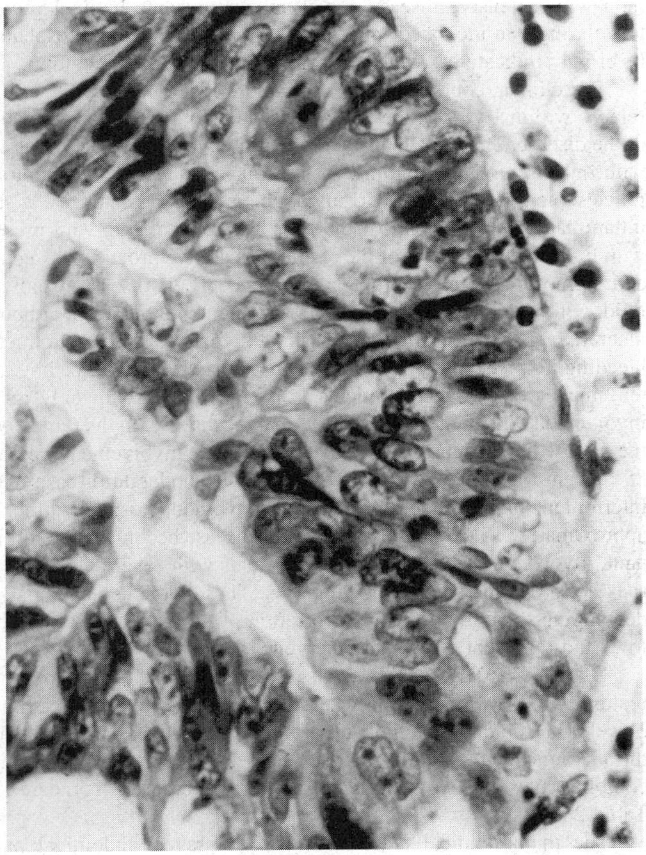

C

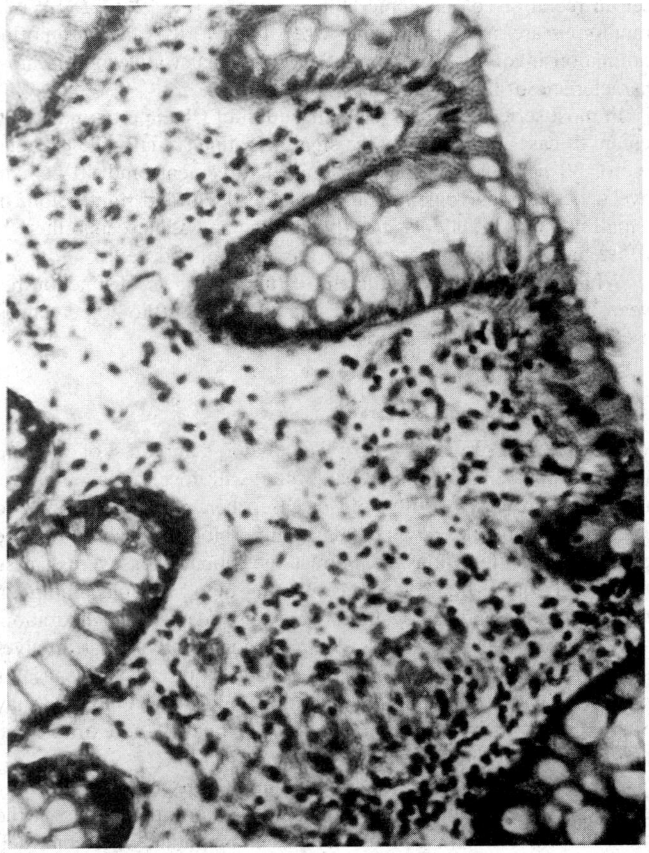

D

FIGURE 286-2 Colonic biopsy samples in inflammatory bowel disease. *A*. Ulcerative colitis. The surface mucosa is destroyed and the submucosa is diffusely infiltrated with polymorphonuclear leukocytes. Crypt abscesses are also present. *B*. Pseudopolyp. Regenerating island of mucosa with adjacent area of ulceration. *C*. Ulcerative colitis. Severe dysplasia occurring in long-standing chronic ulcerative colitis. Note atypical changes in the nuclei and marked palisading of nuclei of the crypt epithelium. *D*. Crohn's disease of the colon. Note the relatively intact mucosa with a solitary granuloma in the lamina propria.

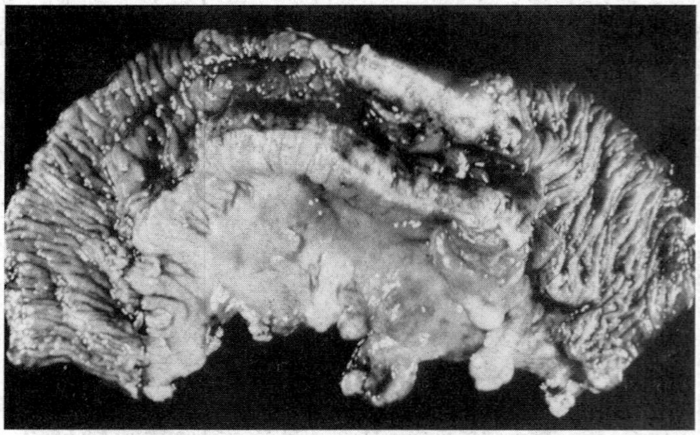

FIGURE 286-3 Regional enteritis. Resected specimen of terminal ileum demonstrates thickened bowel wall and chronically inflamed mucosa. Note the relatively sharp demarcation of the diseased segment, with grossly normal mucosa on either side.

and matted together by a fibrinous peritoneal reaction, leading to a palpable mass, most often in the right lower quadrant. Fistulas may form between adherent structures, including loops of intestine or colon as well as adjacent organs such as the bladder or vagina. Fistulous tracts also may lead to the skin or end blindly in the peritoneum or retroperitoneum, surrounded by adherent loops of bowel and inflammatory tissue. Fistula formation is not seen in UC.

Microscopically, granulomas are most helpful in distinguishing CD from other forms of IBD; they do not occur in UC. They may be seen in rectal or colonoscopic biopsy samples (Fig. 286-2*D*). While granulomas are a helpful finding when present, it is the chronic inflammation involving all layers of the intestinal wall which is most characteristic of CD.

In most series reporting the distribution of CD, approximately 30 percent of cases involve only the small intestine (usually the terminal ileum), 30 percent have only colonic involvement, and 40 percent have ileocolic involvement, usually of the ileum and right colon. In a small number of patients (mostly children and adolescents) there is diffuse and extensive ulceration of the jejunum and ileum.

While there often are sufficient features to permit distinction between UC and CD of the colon (Table 286-1), in 10 to 20 percent of cases this distinction is not possible.

Table 286-1

Pathologic and Clinical Features of IBD

Features	Ulcerative Colitis	Crohn's Disease
PATHOLOGIC FEATURES		
Segmental	0	+ +
Transmural involvement	+/−	+ +
Granulomas	0	+/+ + (50%)
Fibrosis	+	+ +
Fissuring, fistulas	+/−	+ +
Mesenteric fat, lymph node involvement	0	+ +
CLINICAL FEATURES		
Diarrhea	+ +	+ +
Rectal bleeding	+ +	+
Abdominal pain	+	+ +
Palpable mass	0	+ +
Fistulas	+/−	+ +
Strictures	+	+ +
Small bowel involvement	+/− ("backwash ileitis")	+ +
Rectal involvement	+ + (95%)	+/+ + (50%)
Extraintestinal disease	+ +	+ +
Toxic megacolon	+	+/−
Recurrence after colectomy	0	+
Malignancy (with long-standing disease)	+	+/−

NOTE: 0, never; +/−, rare; +, occasional; + +, frequent, common.

CLINICAL FEATURES

ULCERATIVE COLITIS The major symptoms of UC are bloody diarrhea and abdominal pain, often with fever and weight loss in more severe cases. With mild disease, there may be one or two semiformed stools per day, containing little blood, and there may be no systemic manifestations. In contrast, the patient with severe disease may have frequent liquid stools containing blood and pus, complain of severe cramps, and demonstrate symptoms and signs of dehydration, anemia, fever, and weight loss. With predominantly rectal involvement, constipation rather than diarrhea may be present, and tenesmus may be a major complaint. On occasion, intestinal symptoms may be overshadowed by fever, weight loss, or one of the extracolonic manifestations of the disease (see below).

The physical findings in UC are usually nonspecific; there may be some abdominal distention or tenderness along the course of the colon. In mild cases, the general physical examination will be normal. Extracolonic manifestations include arthritis, skin changes, or evidence of liver disease. Fever, tachycardia, and postural hypotension are usually associated with more severe disease. The laboratory findings are often nonspecific and usually reflect the degree and severity of bleeding and inflammation. There may be anemia, which reflects chronic disease as well as iron deficiency from chronic blood loss. Leukocytosis with a left shift and an elevated erythrocyte sedimentation rate are often seen in the severely ill, febrile patient. Electrolyte abnormalities, especially hypokalemia, reflect the degree of diarrhea. Hypoalbuminemia is common with extensive disease and usually represents luminal protein loss through an ulcerated mucosa. An elevated alkaline phosphatase level may indicate associated hepatobiliary disease (see below).

The clinical course of UC is variable. Most patients will suffer a relapse within 1 year of the first attack, reflecting the recurrent nature of the disease. There may, however, be prolonged periods of remission with only minimal symptoms. In general, the severity of symptoms reflects the extent of colonic involvement and the intensity of the inflammation. At one end of the spectrum are patients who present with limited involvement of the rectum (ulcerative proctitis) or rectum and sigmoid (ulcerative proctosigmoiditis). Their disease usually is mild, with minimal systemic or extracolonic manifestations, although ulcerative proctitis is sometimes difficult to treat, exhibiting protracted bleeding and tenesmus. The major symptoms are rectal bleeding and tenesmus. Most of these patients, especially those with only rectal involvement, do not develop more extensive disease. In the remainder, the disease may extend proximally with variable involvement. Perhaps 85 percent of patients with UC have mild to moderate disease of an intermittent nature and can be managed without hospitalization. In approximately 15 percent of patients, the disease becomes more fulminant, involves the entire colon, and presents with severe bloody diarrhea and systemic signs and symptoms. These patients are at risk of developing toxic dilation and perforation of the colon (described below) and represent a medical emergency.

CROHN'S DISEASE As discussed above, the basic pathologic features of CD are the same whether the disease involves the small bowel or the colon. The clinical presentation, however, largely reflects the anatomic location of the disease and to some degree predicts which complications may develop. The clinical features are compared in Table 286-1.

The major clinical features of CD are fever, abdominal pain, diarrhea (often without blood), and generalized fatigability. There may be associated weight loss. With *colonic involvement*, diarrhea and pain are the most frequent symptoms. Rectal bleeding is distinctly less common than with UC and reflects (1) sparing of the rectum in many patients and (2) the transmural nature of the disease, with only irregular mucosal involvement. There may be associated severe anorectal complications such as fistulas, fissures, and perirectal abscess. Such features may antedate the clinical onset of colitis and should always raise the suspicion of associated Crohn's disease. Recurrent perirectal inflammation may result in a thickened anal canal, and perianal fistulas or scarring may be present. Extensive colonic involvement may lead to dilation of the colon. However, since CD often results in a thickened colonic wall, this feature is less common with CD than with UC. Extracolonic manifestations (discussed below), particularly arthritis, are seen more commonly with colonic than with small-bowel CD.

Involvement of the *small bowel* may be accompanied by additional presenting signs and symptoms. Typically, the disease presents in a young adult with a history of fatigue, variable weight loss, right lower quadrant discomfort or pain, and diarrhea. Low-grade fever, anorexia, nausea, and vomiting also may be present. The abdominal pain may be steady and localized to the right lower quadrant or may assume a colicky or crampy pattern, reflecting various degrees of intestinal stenosis. The diarrhea is often moderate, usually without gross blood; if there is no rectal involvement, tenesmus is absent. Physical examination at this time often reveals right lower quadrant tenderness with an associated fullness or mass reflecting adherent loops of bowel. At this time the patient may have mild anemia, mild to moderate leukocytosis, and an elevated erythrocyte sedimentation rate.

Since acute ileitis may have an abrupt onset with fever, leukocytosis, and right lower quadrant pain, the clinical picture may be indistinguishable from that of acute appendicitis. Often the diagnosis can be made only at laparotomy, when the characteristic beefy red terminal ileum, boggy mesenteric fat, and succulent mesenteric lymph nodes indicate that appendicitis alone cannot be the culprit.

While the symptoms of diarrhea and abdominal pain will usually alert the clinician to the possibility of regional enteritis, other symptoms may dominate the clinical presentation. In children and the aged, fever of undetermined origin and unexplained weight loss may be prominent and initially may suggest an underlying malignancy. In some patients, the first manifestation of the disease is intestinal obstruction; in others, the disease presents with perianal sepsis or urinary tract infection resulting from an enterovesical fistula. Similarly, right ureteral obstruction and hydronephrosis may occur as a result of external compression of the ureter by a right lower quadrant inflammatory mass. On occasion, often in the setting of extensive small-bowel involvement, features of malabsorption may be prominent. These features, along with anorexia and the catabolic effects of the chronic inflammatory process, may combine to produce striking weight loss. The complications of the disease are often local, resulting from intestinal inflammation and involvement of adjacent structures.

Intestinal obstruction is a frequent complication, occurring in 20 to 30 percent of patients during the course of the disease. In the initial stages, the obstruction usually is due to acute inflammation and edema of the involved intestinal segment, which is usually the terminal ileum. However, as the disease progresses and fibrosis develops, obstruction may be due to a fixed narrowing of the bowel.

Fistula formation is a frequent complication of chronic regional enteritis as well as of CD of the colon. Fistulas may occur between contiguous segments of intestine; they also may burrow into the retroperitoneal spaces and present as cutaneous fistulas or indolent abscesses. In a significant number of patients, the first indication of the disease may be the presence of persistent rectal fissures, a perirectal abscess, or a rectal fistula. Although uncommon, pneumaturia should raise the suspicion of enterovesical fistula and is often associated with a persistent urinary tract infection.

Since CD is a transmural disease in which the bowel wall is greatly thickened, free *intestinal perforation* is uncommon. Rarely, however, it is the presenting feature, and the disease is first discovered at the time of laparotomy for a perforated viscus. The passage per rectum of bright red blood should alert one to the possible coexistence of rectal involvement (i.e., ileocolitis). CD can involve any portion of the gastrointestinal tract. Aphthous ulcers are the most common *oral* manifestation of CD. CD also may involve the *stomach* and *duodenum*, most often the antrum and/or the first and second portions of the

duodenum. Symptoms may include pain mimicking peptic ulcer disease. Later in the course of the disease, chronic scarring may produce gastric outlet or duodenal obstruction.

There are increasing reports of *small-bowel* and *colonic malignancy* developing in the setting of long-standing CD. The frequency of malignancy in this setting is low compared with the frequency of malignancy in UC, however (see below). The presence of extensive ileal disease, resulting in *bile salt malabsorption*, is associated with a decreased bile salt pool and increased bile lithogenicity (see Chap. 285). Up to 30 percent of patients with extensive ileal disease develop gallstones. Also, in the setting of ileal disease and an intact colon, there is increased colonic absorption of dietary oxalate, with resulting hyperoxaluria and the development of *urinary oxalate stones*. Dehydration due to diarrhea is an additional predisposing factor in renal stone formation.

DIAGNOSIS

The diagnosis of IBD should be entertained in all patients presenting with diarrhea or bloody diarrhea, persistent perianal sepsis, and abdominal pain. Atypical presentations also occur, such as fever of unexplained origin either in the absence of bowel symptoms or with extracolonic manifestations such as arthritis or liver disease that antedate or overshadow the bowel involvement. Since CD also may involve the small intestine, it should be considered in the differential diagnosis of all types of malabsorption syndromes, intermittent intestinal obstruction, and abdominal fistulas.

The results of laboratory tests usually are nonspecific and reflect the extent and severity of the inflammatory reaction. When CD involves the small bowel, laboratory features of malabsorption also may be present. There may be a variable degree of anemia, caused by occult blood loss or the effect of chronic inflammation on the bone marrow. Folate or vitamin B_{12} malabsorption also may contribute to the anemia. While the Schilling test may give abnormal results in patients with extensive ileal disease, frank macrocytic anemia due to vitamin B_{12} malabsorption alone is unusual, attesting to the efficiency of ileal absorption of the vitamin. When there is significant diarrhea, electrolyte abnormalities (hypokalemia, hypomagnesemia) may be prominent. Hypocalcemia may reflect extensive mucosal involvement and malabsorption of vitamin D. Hypoalbuminemia may result from amino acid malabsorption as well as from protein-losing enteropathy. A variable degree of steatorrhea may result from bile salt depletion and mucosal damage. Mild abnormalities of liver function markers (especially an increased level of serum alkaline phosphatase) may reflect the development of hepatosteatosis in a malnourished patient or a coexisting early sclerosing cholangitis. Significant jaundice is unusual.

Sigmoidoscopy and *radiologic studies* of the bowel are most important in establishing the diagnosis of IBD. Sigmoidoscopy must be performed in all patients presenting with chronic diarrhea and in all instances of rectal bleeding. While meticulous air-contrast barium enema examination of a perfectly prepared colon may disclose the earliest mucosal changes in either UC or CD (see below), a conventional barium enema examination is often "normal" in early disease. Direct visualization of the colonic mucosa combined with biopsy is the most sensitive way of determining whether rectal inflammation is present. This procedure can often be performed without prior enema preparation in a patient having active diarrhea. The goal of this initial sigmoidoscopy is to establish *whether* mucosal inflammation is present, not necessarily to determine its full *extent*. Thus, if changes are encountered within the first 8 to 10 cm, it is not necessary to pass the instrument to its full length, which may cause discomfort when the bowel is acutely inflamed. In UC, findings include a loss of mucosal vascularity, diffuse erythema, friability of the mucosa, and often an exudate consisting of mucus, blood, and pus. Mucosal friability and uniform involvement are characteristic. Once diseased mucosa is encountered (usually in the rectum), there are no areas of intervening normal mucosa before the proximal limit of the disease is reached. Ulcers are shallow and may be small or confluent, but ulceration invariably occurs in segments of active colitis. Full colonoscopic examination of the colon in UC is not indicated in the acutely ill patient. Rectal biopsy may corroborate mucosal inflammation. With more chronic disease, the mucosa may appear granular and pseudopolyps may be present.

Endoscopic examination of the colon is also of value in the diagnosis of colonic CD. The salient finding is ulcerations, which may be tiny, aphthous erosions or deep, longitudinal fissures. They usually occur in segments of otherwise normal mucosa. Since the mucosa is not uniformly involved, friability and diffuse granularity—hallmarks of UC—are not characteristic. Rather, a cobblestone appearance—that is, coarse irregularity of the mucosal surface, reflecting submucosal inflammation—is characteristic of CD. Pseudopolyps, edema, and strictures may be seen in CD as well as in UC. Colonic mucosal biopsy reveals granulomas in 30 to 50 percent of specimens taken from involved areas. Features such as crypt abscesses, infiltration with inflammatory cells, or ulcerations are nonspecific but compatible. Since skip areas and rectal sparing are characteristic of CD, colonoscopy may be better than sigmoidoscopy for the evaluation of CD. Colonoscopic examination is also indicated when CD appears only to involve the small bowel. Ileal biopsy may be feasible, and coexisting colonic involvement occurs in a significant number of cases. Perianal inflammatory lesions as well as areas of rectal disease seen at endoscopy often show granulomatous inflammation. In 5 to 15 percent of patients, rectal biopsy samples of seemingly uninvolved areas show microscopic evidence of granulomatous inflammation.

The *radiologic evaluation* of the bowel provides essential information in the diagnosis of IBD. In UC, barium enema may reveal the extent of the disease and help to define associated features such as stricture, pseudopolyposis, or carcinoma. The earliest features seen in UC are irritability and incomplete filling due to associated inflammation. Fine ulcerations may be seen at this time as serrations along the contour of the bowel, producing a hazy margin (Fig. 286-4). The ulcerations may become deeper and, with more fulminant disease, produce a grossly ragged and irregular contour. Polypoid defects appear as a result of edematous mucosa between ulcerations. The diffuse pattern of ulceration is best seen on the evacuation film or on air-contrast barium enema. In the chronic stage of the disease (Fig. 286-5), the characteristic features are shortening of the bowel, depression of the flexures, narrowing of the bowel lumen, and rigidity. The bowel has a symmetric, ahaustral, tubular appearance with a decreased mucosal pattern. Although strictures are uncommon, when they occur, they have a concentric lumen with fusiform tapering margins. Eccentricity should raise the suspicion of an associated carcinoma.

On barium enema examination, CD of the colon usually has features that distinguish it from UC. These features include rectal sparing, the presence of skip lesions, and small ulcerations occurring on small irregular nodules. Small ulcerations often extend to produce longitudinal ulcers (Fig. 286-6) and transverse fissures, which in reality are limited sinus tracts. These may extend into adjacent tissues to produce fistulas. Irregular thickening and fibrosis may lead to stricture formation, which may be multiple. In 10 to 15 percent of cases, the disease involves the entire colon uniformly, making differentiation from UC more difficult. Reflux of barium into the terminal ileum during barium enema may reveal characteristic ileal changes of regional enteritis.

The terminal ileum is the portion of the small intestine most often involved by CD, with features similar to those of colonic involvement. Careful x-ray examination of the small bowel may demonstrate loss of mucosal detail and rigidity of involved segments resulting from submucosal edema or stenosis. The submucosal inflammation may lead to the characteristic radiologic cobblestone appearance of the mucosa (Fig. 286-7), and fistulous tracts may be seen, especially in the ileocecal area (Fig. 286-8). Involvement of the stomach and duodenum usually appears radiologically as stiffening and infiltration of the mucosa and can mimic an infiltrative tumor. If such an appearance is due to regional enteritis, there is almost always coexisting involvement of the jejunum or ileum. In CD, computed tomography (CT) of the abdomen may be of value in the evaluation of thickened, separated bowel loops and may help distinguish thickened, matted loops (phlegmon) from intraabdominal abscess.

While barium studies often provide information on the pattern and extent of IBD, caution must be exercised in performing these studies

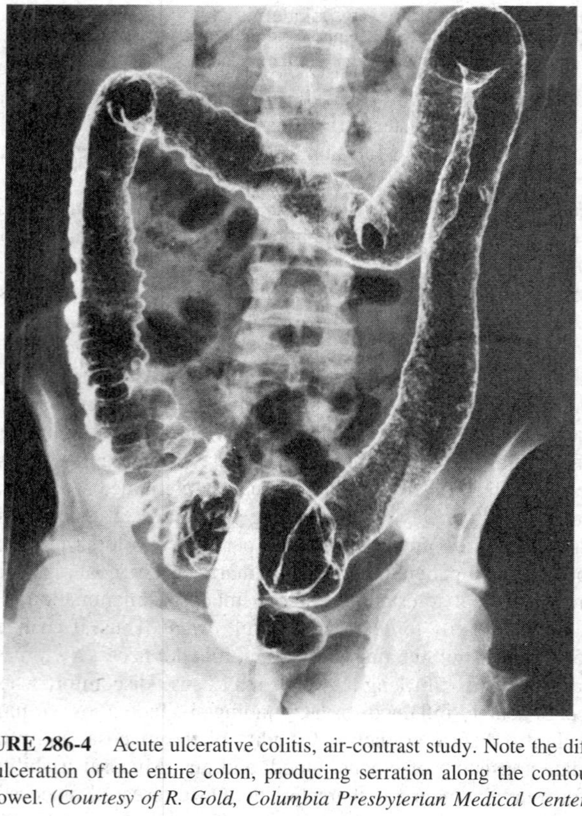

FIGURE 286-4 Acute ulcerative colitis, air-contrast study. Note the diffuse fine ulceration of the entire colon, producing serration along the contour of the bowel. *(Courtesy of R. Gold, Columbia Presbyterian Medical Center.)*

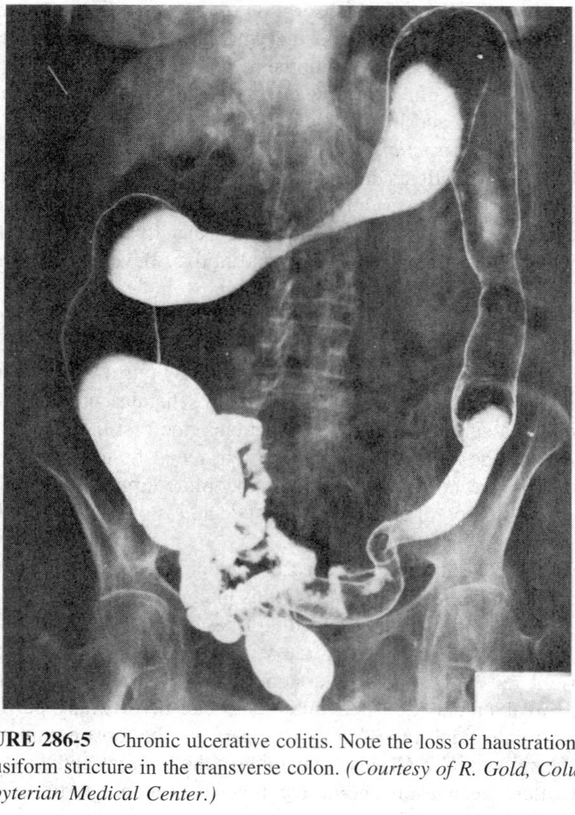

FIGURE 286-5 Chronic ulcerative colitis. Note the loss of haustrations and the fusiform stricture in the transverse colon. *(Courtesy of R. Gold, Columbia Presbyterian Medical Center.)*

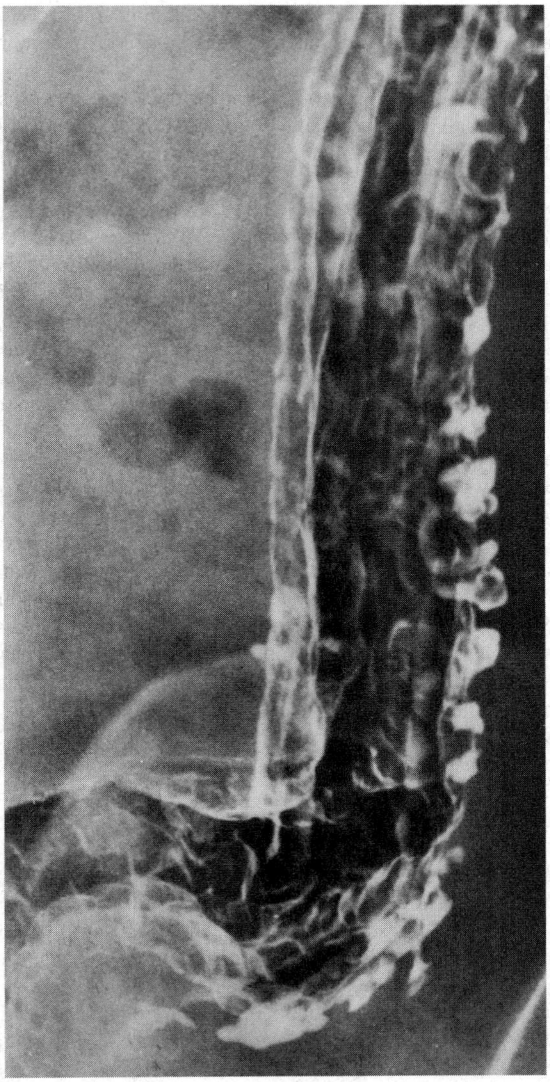

FIGURE 286-6 Crohn's colitis. Air-contrast study.

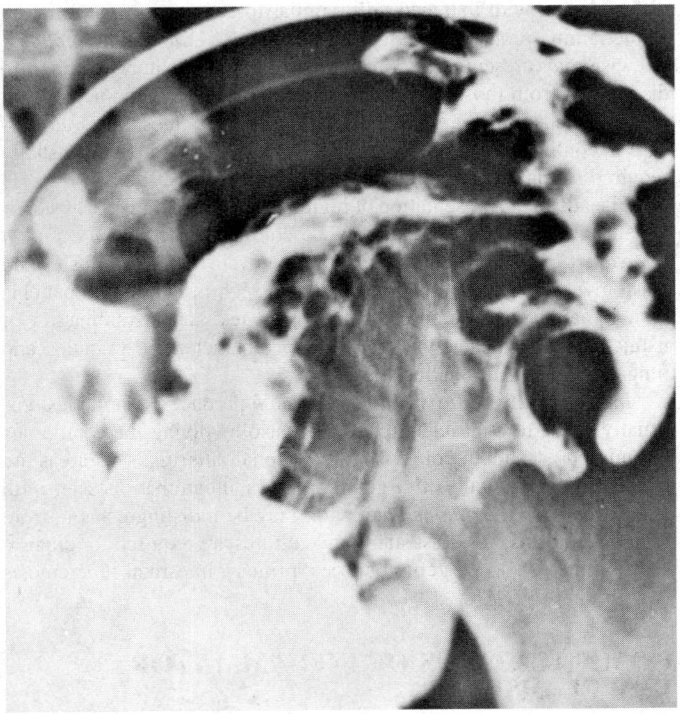

FIGURE 286-7 Crohn's ileocolitis. Note the nodularity and ulceration of the terminal ileum and the deformity of the cecum.

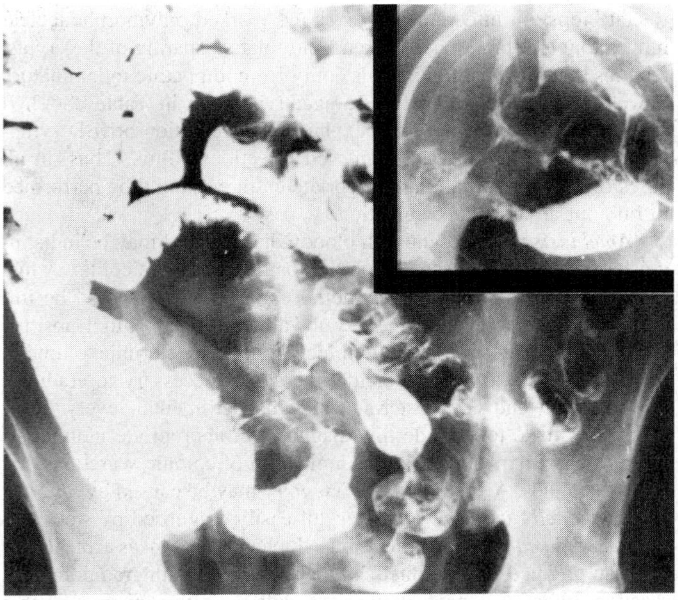

FIGURE 286-8 Regional enteritis. X-ray showing fistulas between loops of bowel. Insert is a compression film of this area; note fistulas between adjacent loops of bowel.

in acutely ill patients with severe colitis, as the procedure and the bowel cleansing that precedes it may cause a worsening of the disease and can precipitate toxic dilation of the colon.

Fiberoptic colonoscopy is a powerful tool in the diagnosis of colonic IBD. Areas beyond the reach of the sigmoidoscope can now be directly visualized and biopsied. Early in the course of colonic inflammation, endoscopic examination and biopsy are the most sensitive techniques for demonstrating mucosal involvement. Polypoid lesions, strictures, and unclear x-ray features can usually be defined fully. Periodic colonoscopic examination and biopsy are being used increasingly in cancer surveillance in patients with long-standing IBD (see below).

DIFFERENTIAL DIAGNOSIS

Many entities must be considered in the differential diagnosis of IBD. The focus of the differential diagnosis is determined largely by the presenting features of the disease. When *rectal bleeding* is the presenting complaint, a colonic source should be considered. While *hemorrhoids* are commonly found, they must be considered a tentative source of bleeding until sigmoidoscopy, colonoscopy, and/or barium enema examination have ruled out other colonic lesions. Colonic *neoplasms* (carcinoma, adenomatous polyps) also may present with rectal bleeding and can usually be diagnosed by barium enema with subsequent sigmoidoscopic or colonoscopic biopsy. It should be remembered that carcinoma may complicate long-standing colitis. Rectal bleeding from *colonic diverticula* or *arteriovenous malformations* usually presents no problem in differential diagnosis, since radiologic and endoscopic features of IBD are absent. *Radiation proctitis*, which may present as a localized area of colitis, is usually found in the setting of pelvic irradiation. The onset may be months to years after irradiation. Characteristic features on sigmoidoscopy include mucosal atrophy and telangiectasia along with friability and small ulcerations. A colitis sometimes indistinguishable from ulcerative colitis may occur in Behçet's syndrome and is associated with aphthous oral ulceration, uveitis, and urethritis.

Acute colitis may be caused by a variety of *infectious* agents (Chap. 128). Often presenting with bloody diarrhea, infectious colitis may be difficult to distinguish from IBD at initial presentation, and severe cases may present with colonic dilation mimicking toxic megacolon.

Rectal biopsy in infectious colitis shows marked polymorphonuclear infiltration with pronounced edema and relative sparing of the crypts, features that may distinguish this entity from idiopathic inflammatory bowel disease. A listing of these agents is given in Table 286-2. It should also be noted that an unexplained exacerbation of IBD symptoms may be due to a superimposed infectious colitis. Thus, in all cases of IBD exacerbation, appropriate cultures should be performed to rule out an associated infection.

Amebiasis may present with bloody diarrhea and may be indistinguishable by sigmoidoscopy from idiopathic ulcerative colitis. A history of recent foreign travel or homosexual exposure would be important. Serologic testing may be of value, although initial positive titers may indicate prior amebic infection at an indeterminate time in the past. Since specific amebicidal therapy is necessary to eradicate this infection and corticosteroids may be detrimental, every effort should be made to exclude this diagnosis in appropriate individuals via serologic titers and careful examination of colonic secretions and biopsy samples. Acute *bacillary dysentery* may be caused by *Shigella* and *Salmonella* or *Campylobacter*, all easily diagnosed by stool culture. *Yersinia enterocolitis* infection, which may present as acute ileitis, also can produce a self-limited colitis, sometimes with granulomatous reaction. Infectious agents may cause acute proctitis indistinguishable from idiopathic ulcerative proctitis. Such infections, often seen in homosexuals, may represent herpes simplex virus infection, *gonorrhea*, *lymphogranuloma venereum* (LGV), cytomegalovirus infection, *Isospora* infection, or *Treponema pallidum* infection, as well as *amebiasis*. In homosexual men, non-LGV strains of *Chlamydia* have been shown to produce a granulomatous proctitis closely resembling Crohn's disease of the rectum.

Pseudomembranous colitis (antibiotic-associated colitis) is caused by a necrolytic toxin elaborated by *Clostridium difficile*, which proliferates the bowel under certain circumstances (see Chap. 148). Most often the disease is a result of antibiotic therapy, which presumably upsets the normal ecologic balance of the bowel flora and permits *C. difficile* to proliferate. Almost every antibiotic has been implicated, although cases related to the use of vancomycin or aminoglycosides are rare. Most often diarrhea is profuse and watery, although bloody diarrhea occurs in 5 percent of cases. Characteristic multiple, discrete yellowish plaques are seen on sigmoidoscopy, which on biopsy show features of acute inflammation and ulceration with a pseudomembrane of fibrin and necrotic material. On occasion, lesions may be beyond the reach of the sigmoidoscope and require colonoscopy. Diagnosis is best made by detecting *C. difficile* toxin in the stool. Treatment is initially directed at eradicating *C. difficile* from the stool. Vancomycin (250 mg orally qid for 7 to 14 days) is the treatment of choice for more severely ill patients and should produce clinical improvement within 5 days. Since vancomycin therapy is expensive, alternative therapies have been proposed. The use of metronidazole (500 mg orally qid for 7 to 14 days) has been shown to be as effective as vancomycin. Bacitracin (20,000 units qid for 7 to 14 days) is also quite effective. With all forms of therapy, relapse rates of 15 to 30 percent have been observed, and a second course of therapy may be required to eradicate the organism.

Table 286-2

Microbiologic Causes of Colitis

Shigella infection
Salmonella infection
Amebiasis (infection with *Entamoeba histolytica*)
Yersinia enterocolitica infection
Campylobacter jejuni infection
Lymphogranuloma venereum (LGV)
"Non-LGV" *Chlamydia* infection
Neisseria gonorrhoeae infection
Pseudomembranous colitis (caused by *Clostridium difficile* toxin)
Tuberculosis (*Mycobacterium tuberculosis* infection)
Infection with enteropathogenic *Escherichia coli* O157:H7
Aeromonas hydrophila infection
Plesiomonas shigelloides infection

Occasionally, infectious colitis is superimposed on an unsuspected case of UC or CD. In this situation, once the acute infection has subsided, symptoms and inflammatory mucosal changes may persist, raising the possibility of associated idiopathic IBD. Similar considerations apply to the rare patient with IBD who develops associated *pseudomembranous colitis*. The finding of *C. difficile* toxin in the stool and subsequent treatment will serve to clarify this presentation.

Abdominal pain in association with rectal bleeding, especially in older patients, may be due to *ischemic colitis*; this condition may be most difficult to distinguish from IBD, especially CD. Because of an excellent collateral circulation, the rectum is usually spared. Radiologic features are often characteristic, showing submucosal edema or hemorrhage (thumb-printing) which typically resolves spontaneously over several weeks.

IBD may be difficult to distinguish from functional diarrhea early in the course of disease. The presence of constitutional symptoms such as fatigue, fever, weight loss, and nocturnal diarrhea, coupled with laboratory findings of anemia, an elevated erythrocyte sedimentation rate, or occult blood in the stool, should alert the clinician to the possibility of IBD. Similarly, the presence of leukocytes in a stained stool specimen points to an inflammatory basis for the diarrhea. In all cases, stool cultures and parasitologic examination of the stool are required to rule out enteric bacterial pathogens or amebiasis. In the *irritable bowel syndrome*, sigmoidoscopy, rectal biopsy, and barium enema examination all give normal results (see Chap. 287).

Once the diagnosis of idiopathic IBD has been established, it is usually possible to distinguish between UC and CD of the colon (see Table 286-1).

With small-intestinal involvement (regional enteritis), the differential diagnosis should include disorders presenting with intraabdominal abscesses, fistulas, intestinal obstruction, and malabsorption. The finding of associated colonic involvement in patients with ileal disease will often serve to distinguish CD from other ileal disorders. With diffuse involvement of the jejunum and ileum, regional enteritis must be distinguished from *nongranulomatous ulcerative jejunoileitis*. Abdominal pain and diarrhea are prominent features of the latter disorder, and weight loss, malabsorption, and hypoproteinemia tend to be more prominent than in regional enteritis. Small-bowel biopsy shows a more diffuse lesion with flattened villi (similar to celiac sprue), infiltration of the lamina propria, and mucosal ulceration. *Abdominal lymphoma* likewise may present with clinical and radiologic features difficult to distinguish from those of regional enteritis. Hepatosplenomegaly and peripheral adenopathy, when present, are helpful clues, but often disease is confined to the intestine. In such cases, laparotomy is usually required to make the definitive histologic diagnosis.

The advanced presentation of regional enteritis with areas of stenosis and draining fistulas also may be confused with *chronic fungal infection of the bowel*, including actinomycosis, aspergillosis, and blastomycosis. These infections often are seen in debilitated patients with impaired host defenses. Fungal skin tests and examination of fistula drainage and biopsy material for characteristic granules and fungi are helpful in making the diagnosis.

Intestinal tuberculosis characteristically produces stenotic lesions, usually in the terminal ileum and often also involving the contiguous cecum and ascending colon. Unlike regional enteritis, skip areas are unusual. Histologically, the granulomatous inflammation seen with *Mycobacterium tuberculosis* infection may be indistinguishable from regional enteritis; acid-fast stains and cultures are required for diagnosis. Fortunately, in western countries, primary intestinal tuberculosis is now rare.

COMPLICATIONS OF INFLAMMATORY BOWEL DISEASE

The complications of IBD may be classified as local or systemic, the former being direct consequences of inflammation or its extension

(Table 286-3). Local complications of IBD including fistulas, abscesses, and strictures are described above. In addition, perforation, toxic dilation, and the development of carcinoma may complicate both UC and CD.

PERFORATION Intestinal perforation can occur in severe UC because extensive ulceration may greatly thin the bowel wall. The clinical features are those of acute peritonitis, with signs of peritoneal inflammation and the demonstration of free air under the diaphragm on upright film of the abdomen. These signs are an indication for immediate colectomy.

Toxic dilation of the colon may occur in CD but is more common in UC. This complication can best be considered as a severe form of ulcerative colitis with the additional feature of colonic dilation. The dilation is thought to result from an effect of the severe inflammation on the neuromuscular tone of the bowel. Injudicious use of hypomotility agents (codeine, diphenoxylate, loperamide, paregoric, anticholinergic agents) to treat diarrhea in the setting of acute colitis can precipitate this complication. Similarly, cathartic preparation for a barium enema examination, as well as the examination and superimposed hypokalemia, may be contributing factors. Clinically, features of severe colitis are present, with high fever, tachycardia, volume depletion, electrolyte imbalance, and abdominal pain. On examination, the patient appears toxic, and colonic dilation may be evident. There is abdominal tenderness, and, if perforation has already occurred, peritoneal signs. Diarrhea may actually decrease markedly owing to colonic atony, creating the false impression that the colitis is clinically improved. Plain film of the abdomen will show colonic dilation with a colon diameter of more than 6 cm. There may be air in the wall of the colon, and irregular, ulcerated islands of mucosa may be silhouetted against the air shadow. While the transverse colon is the most common site of dilation, this effect is probably largely positional, since with the patient supine this is the highest portion of the colon. This presentation of colitis represents a true medical emergency and is associated with a mortality of greater than 30 percent if perforation has occurred. Appropriate therapy is discussed below.

CARCINOMA AND INFLAMMATORY BOWEL DISEASE Patients with chronic IBD have a higher incidence of carcinoma than the general population, especially patients who have extensive mucosal involvement (i.e., pancolitis) and those whose disease is of long duration. The cumulative risk of cancer begins to rise 10 years after the disease is diagnosed. While the incidence of cancer varies among patient populations, the overall incidence of cancer is estimated to be 0.5 to 1 percent per year after 10 years. For patients with pancolitis, the risk of cancer has been estimated to be 12 percent at 15 years, 23 percent at 20 years, and 42 percent at 24 years, although estimates in community-based practices have been lower (a 10 percent risk of colon cancer at 26 years). In children, the risk of cancer appears to rise more sharply after the first 10 years of disease, perhaps because of the higher incidence of pancolitis in children. Patients with ulcerative proctitis (disease limited to the rectum) have no increased risk of cancer. Rates of malignancy in patients with CD of the colon or small bowel are less well documented, but the incidence of both small- and large-bowel malignancy is higher than in the general population. However, it is lower than in patients with UC, perhaps because less mucosa usually is chronically involved with CD than with UC.

The development of colon carcinoma in the setting of IBD differs in important ways from that of carcinoma arising in a noncolitic population. Many of the earlier warning signs of a colonic neoplasm (rectal bleeding, a change in bowel habits) are difficult to interpret in the setting of colitis. In colitic patients, carcinomas are distributed more uniformly throughout the colon than in noncolitic patients; in the latter, most carcinomas are in the rectosigmoid region, within reach of the sigmoidoscope. In colitis patients, the tumors are more often multiple, flat, and infiltrating and appear to have a higher grade of malignancy. There is some evidence that these features may reflect the younger age at which they occur rather than the associated colitis. Further adding to the difficulty of diagnosis is the frequent occurrence of mucosal irregularities, ulcerations, and pseudopolyps, which make a small carcinoma difficult to diagnose radiologically or endoscopically.

Efforts have been made to devise effective screening procedures to detect carcinoma developing in the setting of IBD. Plasma levels of carcinoembryonic antigen may be elevated in UC, but this finding is nonspecific and therefore of limited value. Periodic barium enema examination and/or sigmoidoscopy or colonoscopy has been suggested, but interpretation of these studies is sometimes hampered by abnormalities related to the colitis itself. The addition of colonic mucosal biopsy may add a significant dimension. It was originally suggested that a generalized precancerous lesion may be present in high-risk patients with colitis who either harbor an occult malignancy or will develop cancer. Subsequent studies in patients who had long-standing colitis and subsequently underwent colectomy showed that if severe dysplasia was present, there was approximately a 50 percent chance that an associated malignancy also was present. Complicating these findings was the fact that dysplastic changes were found by rectal biopsies only 60 percent of the time, making colonoscopy with multiple biopsies desirable. In addition, in some patients who did not undergo colectomy, dysplasia was not a consistent finding on subsequent biopsies. In any event, it seems prudent to examine patients with colonic IBD of greater than 8 to 10 years' duration with colonoscopy and multiple mucosal biopsies at regular intervals. The optimal frequency for such examinations has not been established; recommendations vary from every 6 months to every 2 years. If severe dysplasia is found, confirmation at less than 6-month intervals seems prudent. While most authorities would not advise "prophylactic" colectomy in patients with long-standing colitis and mild or moderate dysplasia, the finding of severe dysplasia may well identify a subgroup who already harbor an occult carcinoma or are at high risk for carcinoma. There can be no uniform recommendation for this small group of patients, but many physicians will advise colectomy in this setting.

Table 286-3

Some Systemic Complications of Inflammatory Bowel Disease
Nutritional and metabolic complications
Weight loss, reduced muscle mass, growth retardation (children)
Electrolyte deficiency (K^+, Ca^{2+}, Mg^{2+})
Hypoalbuminemia (inadequate nutrition, protein-losing enteropathy)
Anemia (chronic disease, iron deficiency; rarely folate or vitamin B_{12} deficiency in Crohn's disease)
Bile salt deficiency with ileal disease (steatorrhea and fat-soluble vitamin deficiency; increased colonic oxalate absorption leading to renal stones; increased lithogenicity of bile leading to gallstones)
Musculoskeletal complications
Peripheral arthralgia, arthritis
Ankylosing spondylitis, sacroileitis
Granulomatous myositis (rare)
Hepatobiliary disease
Hepatosteatosis
Cholelithiasis
Pericholangitis, biliary cirrhosis (rare)
Sclerosing cholangitis
Bile duct carcinoma
Chronic active hepatitis and cirrhosis
Skin and mucous membrane complications
Erythema nodosum
Pyoderma gangrenosum
Aphthous stomatitis
Crohn's disease of buccal mucosa, gingiva, vagina
Ocular complications: iritis, uveitis, episcleritis
Venous thrombosis and thromboembolism (hypercoagulability, dehydration, stasis)

EXTRAINTESTINAL MANIFESTATIONS OF INFLAMMATORY BOWEL DISEASE

A variety of nonintestinal symptoms and signs may be associated with IBD and occur in both UC and CD (see Table 286-3). Because some of these manifestations may not coincide with or may overshadow the underlying bowel disease, they sometimes pose difficult diagnostic problems. Their cause is currently unknown.

Joint manifestations occur in 25 percent of patients with IBD. They range from arthralgia to an acute arthritis with painful, swollen joints. The nondeforming arthritis is mono- or polyarticular and often migratory. Knees, ankles, and wrists are most commonly involved, but any joint may be affected. Joint fluid, if aspirated, reveals findings of an acute arthritis without crystals or evidence of infection. Tests for markers of specific forms of arthritis (rheumatoid factor, antinuclear antibody, and lupus erythematosus factor) are negative. Typically, the severity of arthritis varies with the activity of the underlying bowel disease. Rarely, peripheral arthritis truly predates clinical bowel symptoms. Arthritis is more common in patients with colonic than with only small-bowel involvement (regional enteritis).

In contrast, the central arthritis or ankylosing spondylitis associated with IBD is unrelated to the activity of the underlying bowel disease. It may antedate the bowel disease by years and persist after surgical or medical remission of the disease has been achieved. Symptoms consist of low backache and stiffness with eventual limitation of motion. Sacroileitis may be present as well. X-rays usually reveal characteristic changes. In contrast to the peripheral arthritis, there is a strong association of HLA-B27 with ankylosing spondylitis, whether or not IBD is present.

Like the peripheral arthritis, *skin manifestations* are more common with colonic disease. They occur in about 15 percent of patients, and their severity correlates with activity of the bowel disease. *Erythema nodosum* may be seen and heals without scarring. *Pyoderma gangrenosum*, an ulcerating lesion often occurring on the trunk, is relatively painless and may heal with scarring. In rare patients, the lesion persists even after colectomy for UC. *Aphthous ulcers* resemble "canker sores" of the mouth, and in approximately 5 to 10 percent of patients they are present during periods of active disease and then resolve. Their cause is unknown, and they are treated symptomatically. *Ocular manifestations* such as episcleritis, recurrent iritis, and uveitis occur in approximately 5 percent of patients and may represent a severe manifestation of the disease. In general, their activity parallels the course of the bowel disease, and they may respond dramatically when colectomy is done for other indications.

Abnormalities of *liver function* are common in IBD. In the severely ill, malnourished patient, mild abnormalities of serum levels of aminotransferases and alkaline phosphatase are often seen and represent nonspecific focal hepatitis or fatty infiltration. Factors favoring hepatosteatosis in the severely ill patient are poor nutrition and, often, concomitant steroid therapy. The lesion is not progressive and resolves with disease remission. *Pericholangitis* is characterized histologically by portal tract inflammation, some bile ductular proliferation, and concentric fibrosis around bile ductules. Some workers think that this lesion represents the intrahepatic form of sclerosing cholangitis. Most often, the lesion is clinically insignificant, and its sole manifestation is an elevated serum alkaline phosphatase level. It is usually nonprogressive and requires no therapy. Rarely, there is apparent progression to cirrhosis of either the postnecrotic or biliary type. Uncommonly, patients with IBD develop *sclerosing cholangitis* (Chap. 302), a chronic inflammation of unknown cause involving the extrahepatic and intrahepatic bile ducts, which may produce various degrees of extrahepatic biliary obstruction. Corticosteroids and immunosuppressive therapy are not beneficial. The disease only sometimes reverses after colectomy and should not be the sole indication for colectomy. Cholangiocarcinoma, arising in the extrahepatic biliary tree, has an increased incidence in patients with chronic UC, especially patients with sclerosing cholangitis. Such patients will present with extrahepatic biliary obstruction, which must be distinguished from sclerosing cholangitis. Finally, *autoimmune chronic active hepatitis*, which may progress to *cirrhosis*, may be seen in IBD, although the exact relationship between these disorders is unknown. There is no clear evidence that colectomy influences the course of this form of liver disease.

Rx TREATMENT

Certain common principles govern the treatment of UC and CD. Initial treatment of all forms of uncomplicated IBD is primarily medical, and the principles of medical therapy are similar for the two types of disease. Surgery is reserved for (1) specific complications and (2) intractable disease. There are important differences between the treatment of UC and CD however: the response to drug therapy may differ, complications often differ, and the prognosis after surgical therapy is not the same.

Ulcerative Colitis MEDICAL THERAPY Once the diagnosis is established, the severity of the disease must be assessed. Mild UC, including ulcerative proctitis, can usually be treated on an ambulatory basis. It should be noted that the disease is occasionally severe, even though it is limited to the rectum. The disease can worsen rapidly, and the course of a given attack cannot be predicted at the outset. The aims of therapy are to control the inflammatory process and to replace nutritional losses. A degree of improvement usually follows intravenous correction of fluid and electrolyte disturbances. Blood transfusions may be required, especially when there is continued active bleeding. Agents to control diarrhea (diphenoxylate, loperamide, codeine, anticholinergics) should be used with extreme caution for fear of precipitating colonic dilation and toxic megacolon. The decision to institute specific nutritional replacement therapy is determined by the patient's nutritional status and by whether the clinical course is expected to be protracted. In the severely ill patient, even clear liquids taken orally may stimulate colonic activity, and it is often wise to give the patients nothing by mouth. In this setting, intravenous alimentation, either peripheral or central, has been used as interim nutritional replacement therapy (see Chap. 78). While there is no evidence that intravenous alimentation is effective as primary therapy, it is an important component of a treatment program. In less severely ill patients able to tolerate fluids by mouth, the use of elemental oral diets may be beneficial, providing supplemental nutrition with low fecal volume.

The principal drugs used in the therapy of ulcerative colitis are the anti-inflammatory agents *sulfasalazine* (Azulfidine) and *glucocorticoids*. Sulfasalazine consists of a sulfonamide (sulfapyridine) moiety chemically bound to a salicylate (5-aminosalicylate); it undergoes bacterial cleavage in the colon. The liberated sulfapyridine is efficiently absorbed and largely excreted in the urine; the liberated 5-aminosalicylate, believed to be the active component, remains largely in the colon and is excreted in the stool. The salicylate moiety is thought to exert its action through inhibition of prostaglandin synthesis. While most physicians are familiar with the use of sulfasalazine to prevent recurrences of UC, it is less well appreciated that this agent is effective in the therapy of acute UC of mild to moderate severity. Therapeutic doses of 4 to 6 g/d are required. The drug is usually started at a dose of 500 mg bid and then increased daily or every other day by 1 g until the therapeutic dose is achieved. Topical preparations of 5-aminosalicylate (mesalamine) given as an enema are effective in the control of distal proctocolitis. Some of the oral and rectal 5-aminosalicylic acid products and their uses are listed in Table 286-4.

In the severely ill patient who may not tolerate oral medication, and for whom more rapid therapy is often desired, initial therapy is begun with glucocorticoids. While adrenocorticotropic hormone is as effective as glucocorticoids when given in equivalent dosages and by comparable routes of administration, most physicians seldom use it. The choice is one of individual preference; oral prednisone (45 to 60 mg/d) is usually employed initially. In the severely ill patient, parenteral administration of corticosteroids (i.e., intravenous prednisolone, 45 to 60 mg/d) is preferable to avoid the uncertainty of oral absorption. Improvement is usually noted after 7 to 10 days of such therapy by a reduction in fever, a decrease in bloody diarrhea, and improvement in appetite.

After initial improvement, low-roughage oral feedings can be resumed. At this point, the dose of steroids can be tapered. While there is no specific tapering schedule, the guiding principle is that, once clinical remission is achieved, there is no evidence that chronic glucocorticoid administration improves the long-term outlook or helps to prevent recurrences. In practice, steroid therapy can be tapered and discontinued over a 2- to 3-month period after discharge. In some patients (10 to 15 percent), efforts to completely eliminate steroids may be associated with a flare-up of the disease, and low to moderate steroid doses (10 to 15 mg prednisone daily) may be required to suppress disease activity. This regimen should not be confused with prophylactic administration of steroids to patients in remission but rather represents treatment of incompletely responsive disease. Once the acutely ill patient is taking oral feedings, sulfasalazine should be added as described above in a daily dose of 2 g. Controlled trials have shown that this dose of sulfasalazine, when administered chronically to patients with UC, is effective in decreasing the frequency of relapses and should be continued chronically after glucocorticoids have been discontinued. Patients with glucose phosphate dehydrogenase deficiency and those exhibiting severe allergic reactions to the sulfa moiety of the drug unfortunately cannot be maintained on it. Patients who exhibit intolerance for the drug (headache, nausea) or allergic reactions can be treated with one of the oral preparations of 5-aminosalicylate listed in Table 286-4. Mesalamine enemas are effective topical therapy for distal UC and are necessary to maintain remission.

The use of immunosuppressive therapy with drugs such as azathioprine is less well established in UC. As a single agent in the therapy of acute UC, the drug is ineffective. However, it may be added to the regimen at a dose of 1.5 to 2.0 mg/kg when glucocorticoids fail or when the steroid dose needed to reduce inflammation is too high. It is desirable to monitor the blood count and observe the patient carefully for infection. Azathioprine also may have a limited role as a "steroid-sparing agent" in the patient with chronic UC who must be maintained on glucocorticoids to control disease activity. Cyclosporine (4 mg/kg per day), a potent immunosuppressive agent, is also beneficial in severely ill patients, producing marked improvement in patients who otherwise would require colectomy.

Toxic megacolon is a major complication of severe UC that requires rapid, intensive management, best carried out jointly by the internist or gastroenterologist and the surgeon. Once the diagnosis is established, prompt and vigorous use of intravenous fluids, electrolyte replacement therapy, and blood transfusions are indicated. Because of the fear of perforation and high likelihood that bacteremia and occult perforation have occurred, many physicians institute broad-spectrum antibiotic coverage after appropriate cultures have been obtained. The patient is given nothing by mouth and nasogastric suction is instituted. Full intravenous glucocorticoid therapy is also begun. Most workers favor an initial period of medical stabilization for the first 24 to 48 h. If significant objective improvement has not occurred, and if perforation seems imminent, emergency colectomy should be carried out. While some patients slowly improve under maximal medical therapy and thus avoid colectomy, this approach is risky, because mortality rates rise sharply if perforation occurs, approaching 50 percent in patients who subsequently undergo colectomy.

At the other end of the spectrum is the patient with mild UC limited to the rectum or rectosigmoid. Therapy is started with sulfasalazine, 0.5 to 1.0 g four times a day with meals. Alternatively, in the sulfa-allergic patient, 5-aminosalicylate enemas or oral 5-aminosalicylate preparations can be given. If rectal symptoms such as tenesmus are prominent, topical steroid enemas may produce marked improvement. The equivalent of 100 mg of hydrocortisone (20 mg of prednisone) in 60 to 100 mL of saline is used as a bedtime enema. On occasion, steroid foam preparations may be better tolerated in patients with severe tenesmus. Retention enemas have been shown to deliver medication as far as the descending colon, and absorption of steroid is slight (10 to 20 percent). If large doses of rectal steroids are required for control, it is preferable to use oral prednisone at a moderate dosage (20 mg/d).

PSYCHOTHERAPY The elements of trust and mutual understanding combined with the compassion and expertise of the physician are essential in the therapy of any chronic disease and are particularly important in the long-term management of patients with IBD. Often these patients are intelligent young adults, who frequently are resentful of a disease that affects them during their most productive years. However, through the vigorous participation of the physician, many patients are able to lead reasonably stable and productive lives. More formal psychiatric assistance may be required in chronically ill patients, in particular children or adolescents, and in the elderly, in whom severe depressive reactions are common. This is particularly true when colectomy is being advised and for the emotional adjustment that must be made after colectomy.

PREGNANCY AND ULCERATIVE COLITIS While many physicians are apprehensive about the management and prognosis of UC in the pregnant patient, the outcome for the patient and fetus is excellent. In general, the pregnancy is not threatened by coexisting colitis, with no increase in stillbirths or premature deliveries when compared with the general population. When patients with inactive colitis become pregnant, approximately 50 percent have an exacerbation of their disease, with some clustering of these flare-ups during the first trimester and in the postpartum period. The therapy of UC during pregnancy is largely the same as in the nonpregnant patient. Sulfasalazine is used to treat mild to moderate disease, since there is no evidence that the drug is harmful to the fetus or leads to fetal malformations. Women with inactive colitis who enter a pregnancy on maintenance sulfasalazine should be continued on the drug to protect the mother during the postpartum period from a relapse of disease. Both sulfasalazine and 5-aminosalicylate preparations may be taken during breast feeding. Corticosteroids should be used in the same dosage and for the same indications as in the nonpregnant patient. However, other immunosuppressive agents should not be

Table 286-4

5-Aminosalicylic Acid Products and Their Uses

Drug	Delivery Method	Dose	Use in Ulcerative Colitis	Use in Crohn's Disease
Sulfasalazine (Azulfidine)	Colonic bacterial azo reductases	2–4 g	Active colitis Maintenance	Active colonic disease
Olsalazine (Dipentum)	Colonic bacterial azo reductases	1 g	Active colitis Maintenance	Active colonic disease
Mesalamine (Asacol)	Eudragit-S Release at pH > 7	800–2400 mg	Active colitis Maintenance	Active colonic disease
Mesalamine (Pentasa)	Ethylcellulose microgranules Time-release	1500–4000 mg	Active colitis Maintenance	Active disease Maintenance
Mesalamine enemas (Rowasa)	Directly available	4 g	Active left-sided disease Maintenance	Distal colonic disease
Mesalamine suppositories (Rowasa)	Directly available	500 mg	Active proctitis Maintenance	Crohn's proctitis

SOURCE: Modified from Griffin and Miner.

used during pregnancy. Similar therapeutic approaches apply to the management of CD during pregnancy.

SURGICAL THERAPY Approximately 20 to 25 percent of patients with UC require colectomy during the course of their disease. A major indication for colectomy is failure to respond to intensive medical management. This group includes patients who do not improve after 7 to 10 days of optimal medical therapy, even if they do not show signs of colonic dilation. Fever, persistent bloody diarrhea, and severe fatigue may persist, and consideration should be given to semielective colectomy. Elective colectomy may be performed in patients whose disease remains chronically active and who require continuous glucocorticoid administration. Such patients are at risk of developing the complications of chronic steroid therapy. After colectomy, these patients often feel more energetic and usually gain weight to their preillness level. As discussed above, the patient with long-standing colitis is at high risk for colonic cancer. While most authorities do not advise "prophylactic" colectomy in patients with quiescent disease, the finding of marked dysplasia on colonoscopic biopsies performed as a part of a surveillance program should make the physician think seriously about advising colectomy.

The decision to advise colectomy in other than emergency circumstances is difficult for both patient and physician. Many patients have an understandable reluctance to undergo colectomy and have difficulty in viewing life with an ileostomy. In most metropolitan centers there are ileostomy groups who visit patients preoperatively and can provide answers to many practical questions. It is also desirable for the patient to be visited by a nurse familiar with stoma care to instruct the patient on the practical aspects of handling the ileostomy.

While total proctocolectomy with permanent ileostomy has been the standard surgical procedure for almost all patients undergoing colectomy, several alternative approaches are available. The *continent ileostomy* is an ileal loop reservoir fashioned under the skin with a nipple valve to prevent spilling of ileal contents. Ileal effluent collects in this reservoir, which must be emptied with a soft rubber catheter. Only a small stoma is externally visible, thus eliminating an external ileostomy appliance. Problems with leakage and frequent revisions have made this procedure less attractive. There is great enthusiasm for *ileal-rectal anastomosis* with an internal ileal pouch created to act as a reservoir. This often produces a highly satisfactory result, with continence and five to seven stools per day. Complications such as pouchitis or the need for surgical revision seem less frequent than with the continent ileostomy. Refinement in technique has permitted an *ileoanal anastomosis* with an internal pouch fashioned from small intestine anastomosed to the anal canal. When the procedure is performed by experienced surgeons, continence is excellent; however, nocturnal leakage occurs in about 20 percent of patients. Since some residual rectal mucosa may remain after these anastomotic procedures, surveillance proctoscopy for dysplasia should be performed.

Crohn's Disease The medical management of colonic CD is similar in most respects to that of UC. In a multicenter study (National Cooperative Crohn's Disease Study), sulfasalazine was shown to be effective in the therapy of active colonic disease. Glucocorticoids also were efficacious, but less so than with small-bowel involvement. The indications and dosages for these medications are similar to those for UC. Since, in CD, intraabdominal sepsis can result from fistula or abscess formation, glucocorticoids must be used with caution, and constant attention is required to detect sepsis, which can be masked by these agents. In general, the disease is less explosive in onset, and toxic dilation and perforation are less common than in UC. The principles of management are the same. Because of the indolent nature of the disease, the response to therapy is often less complete than in UC, and the disease tends to progress despite apparent clinical inactivity. It may be more difficult to achieve a clinical remission and to withdraw steroids completely. As in UC, controlled studies have shown no benefit to continuing steroids after remission, since the frequency of recurrence is not altered by prophylactic steroid therapy. Disappointingly, sulfasalazine has not decreased recurrence rates in CD.

While response to treatment of the initial attack of Crohn's colitis may be satisfactory, many patients continue to have persistently active disease. This may express itself as progressive weight loss, diarrhea, and deterioration of general health. Perianal disease with predominantly left-sided colonic involvement (fistula formation and perirectal abscesses) may be a recurrent problem. In one controlled study, *metronidazole* (20 mg/kg per day in divided doses) resulted in marked improvement in some patients with chronic perineal fistulas associated with CD. It is not clear whether the drug is active because of its antibacterial properties or through anothermechanism. It is possible that metronidazole may be of value in treating the perineal complications of CD before surgical therapy is attempted. In patients taking these doses of metronidazole on a chronic basis, peripheral sensory neuropathy is a significant side effect and may necessitate reducing the dose or discontinuing the drug if symptoms persist. The role of immunosuppressive therapy in the treatment of CD has become better established in recent years. The use of 6-mercaptopurine or azathioprine (1.5 to 2.0 mg/kg) has been shown to decrease disease activity, cause fistulas to close or become less active, and exert a steroid-sparing effect; it may decrease the relapse rate if used as maintenance therapy. Often, adding these drugs to a maximal program in a nonresponding patient produces beneficial results. However, a positive response may take 3 to 4 months to appear.

The management of CD of the small intestine (regional enteritis) is similar to that for colonic CD, and, as noted, many patients have both small- and large-bowel disease. Several additional considerations are pertinent, however. *Intestinal obstruction* is not uncommonly a presenting feature with ileal involvement. Initially, this problem may be secondary to acute inflammation and will respond to glucocorticoids. With recurrent involvement and the development of fibrosis, steroid therapy is less effective, and surgical decompression is required. *Nutritional problems* often are more severe with involvement of the small intestine than with colonic involvement alone. Added to the general catabolic nature of the disease may be loss of absorptive surface, either from progressive involvement or because of surgical resection. Refinements in the technique of parenteral alimentation have made it possible to provide a patient's total daily caloric intake intravenously for a period of weeks or even months (see Chap. 78). Parenteral alimentation has been employed with increasing frequency in severely ill patients as a means of "resting" the gastrointestinal tract and in preparing the malnourished patient for surgery. However, disease activity frequently recurs when oral feedings are resumed. On occasion, prolonged intravenous alimentation, administered at home, may be required when oral feedings are not effective or in children exhibiting severe growth failure associated with CD. Most often it is possible to design a dietary program of oral supplementation to nourish the patient adequately.

In patients with extensive small-bowel involvement and in those with a short bowel resulting from extensive intestinal resection, supplementation of electrolytes, minerals, and vitamins will be necessary. Extensive ileal disease or resection often results in diarrhea induced by impaired bile salt absorption; cholestyramine may be needed to control the diarrhea, and medium-chain triglycerides may need to be added to reduce fat malabsorption (see Chap. 285). In patients with stenotic segments of intestine, a low-residue (low-fiber) diet should be recommended. A lactose-free diet should be instituted if there is an associated lactase deficiency. Other dietary modifications have not been shown to have any beneficial effect on the primary disease process. Patients should be encouraged to eat a nutritious, appealing diet of their own choosing.

Surgical therapy in general should be reserved for the complications of CD rather than used as a primary form of therapy. More patients with CD than with UC require surgery in the chronic management of the disease. Approximately 70 percent of patients require at least one operation during the course of their disease. Although each case must be assessed individually, surgery may be required (1) for persistent or fixed bowel narrowing or obstruction, (2) for symptomatic fistula formation to the bladder, vagina, or skin, (3) for persistent anal fistulas or abscesses, and (4) for intraabdominal abscesses, toxic dilation of the colon, or perforation. In contrast to UC, where colectomy is curative, in CD surgical resection of the small or large intestine is followed by a high rate of recurrence. With resection of segments of small bowel or ileum and reanastomosis, a recurrence rate of 50 to 75 percent over a 5-year period is not unusual. The site of recurrence invariably is proximal to the created anastomosis. When total colectomy and ileostomy are performed for CD of the colon without significant small-intestinal involvement, recurrence rates are lower, varying from 10 to 30 percent. Despite these recurrences, most patients do not develop a short bowel syndrome, and most can expect significant improvement. Faced with the possibility of recurrent disease, many physicians are reluctant to advise surgery in CD, except for the clear-cut complications described above. Alternatively, surgery may be indicated for patients with persistently active disease that requires chronic maintenance therapy with unacceptably high levels of corticosteroids. While patients with Crohn's colitis without major small-bowel involvement also have a definite rate of recurrence, such recurrences often are not disabling. When extensive small-bowel disease is present, surgical therapy often is not feasible and should only be reserved for specific disease complications.

The therapy of CD in children presents special problems, since active disease may retard normal growth and development. In addition to conventional drug therapy, intensive nutritional therapy or the judicious use of surgery may be required.

PROGNOSIS

The overall prognosis of IBD has been improved by the use of glucocorticoids and sulfasalazine, as well as supportive measures such as intravenous alimentation. In *acute* UC, these therapeutic modalities can produce a remission in almost 90 percent of patients. The mortality rate from an initial acute attack is less than 5 percent. The prognosis is poorer and the mortality rate higher when there is total colonic involvement, when disease onset is after age 60, and when toxic megacolon develops.

The long-term prognosis of *chronic* UC is more difficult to assess owing to the variable and intermittent nature of the disease and improvements in therapy. Left-sided colitis and ulcerative proctitis have a very favorable prognosis and probably cause no increase in mortality rate; similarly, the long-term prognosis for extensive colitis has improved greatly. Previous studies suggested a poor prognosis for extensive colitis, with less than 50 percent of patients surviving 15 years after onset. However, more recent observations (longest follow-up, 11 years) show 10-year mortality rates of 5 and 10 percent for severe first attacks (excluding toxic megacolon). Approximately 75 percent of patients will experience relapses, and 20 to 25 percent will require colectomy. The problem of carcinoma developing in the setting of long-standing chronic UC is important in determining the long-term prognosis of UC. As discussed above, periodic colonoscopic surveillance with multiple biopsies to detect dysplastic changes is indicated to detect a high-risk group in whom to advise colectomy.

The prognosis for CD is not as favorable as for UC. An exception is *acute regional enteritis*, often discovered during laparotomy for suspected appendicitis; this condition has an excellent prognosis. More than two-thirds of such patients may show no subsequent evidence of regional enteritis, and this form of acute ileitis may well be due to *Yersinia* infection (see above). Surgical opinion favors a conservative approach in this situation, and in general operative resection is not advised.

In most patients with CD, the course is chronic and intermittent regardless of the site of involvement. The disease responds less well to medical therapy with time, and over two-thirds of patients develop complications requiring surgery at some point in their disease. In contrast to UC, where mortality appears greatest early in the disease, in CD the mortality rate increases with the duration of the disease and probably ranges from 5 to 10 percent. Most deaths are caused by peritonitis and sepsis. As indicated above, patients with CD often have recurrence and relapses after surgery. Nevertheless, therapy results in reasonably stable and productive lives for most CD patients.

BIBLIOGRAPHY

GENERAL

KIRSNER JB, SHORTER RG (eds): *Inflammatory Bowel Disease*, 4th ed. Philadelphia, Lea & Febiger, 1995

PODOLSKY DK: Inflammatory bowel disease. N Engl J Med 325:928, 1991

SLEISENGER MH, FORDTRAN JS (eds): *Gastrointestinal Diseases*, 5th ed. Philadelphia, Saunders, 1993

STENSON WF, MACDERMOTT RP: Inflammatory bowel disease, in *Textbook of Gastroenterology*, 2d ed, T Yamada et al (eds). Philadelphia, Lippincott, 1995

ETIOLOGY AND DIAGNOSTIC ASPECTS

BLASER MJ, RELLER LB: *Campylobacter* enteritis. N Engl J Med 305:1444, 1981

COLOMBEL JF et al: Clinical characteristics of Crohn's disease. Gastroenterology 111:604, 1996

GOLDBERG HI et al: Computed tomography in the evaluation of Crohn's disease. Am J Roentgenol 140:277, 1983

MACDERMOTT RP, STENSON WF: Alterations of the immune system in ulcerative colitis and Crohn's disease. Adv Immunol 42:285, 1988

SURAWICZ CM, BELIC L: Rectal biopsy helps to distinguish acute self limited colitis from idiopathic inflammatory bowel disease. Gastroenterology 86:104, 1984

THERAPY OF INFLAMMATORY BOWEL DISEASE

BOHR J et al: Collagenous colitis: A retrospective study of clinical presentation and treatment in 163 patients. Gut 39:846, 1996

COLLINS RH et al: Colon cancer in ulcerative colitis. Gastroenterology 94:1089, 1988

EKBOM A et al: Ulcerative colitis and colorectal cancer. N Engl J Med 323:1228, 1990

FARMER RG et al: Long-term follow-up of patients with Crohn's disease. Relationship between clinical pattern and prognosis. Gastroenterology 88:1818, 1985

GAGINELLA TS, WALSH RE: Sulfasalazine: Multiplicity of action. Dig Dis Sci 37:801, 1992

GIONCHETTI P, CAMPIERI M: Medical treatment of ulcerative colitis. Curr Opin Gastroenterol 12:352, 1996

GRIFFIN MG, MINER PB JR: Conventional drug therapy in inflammatory bowel disease. Gastroenterol Clin North Am 24:509, 1995

HANAUER SB: Drug therapy: Inflammatory bowel disease. N Engl J Med 334:841, 1996

LICHTIGER S et al: Cyclosporine in severe ulcerative colitis refractory to steroid therapy. N Engl J Med 330:1841, 1994

PEMBERTON JH et al: Ileal ulcerative colitis—anal anastomosis for chronic ulcerative colitis. Long-term results. Ann Surg 206:504, 1987

PEPPERCORN MA: Advances in drug therapy for inflammatory bowel disease. Ann Intern Med 112:50, 1990

PRESENT DH et al: 6-Mercaptopurine in the management of inflammatory bowel disease: short- and long-term toxicity. Ann Intern Med 111:641, 1989

PROVENCALE D et al: Prophylactic colectomy or surveillance for chronic ulcerative colitis. Gastroenterology 109:1188, 1995

RANSOHOFF DF et al: Ulcerative colitis and colon cancer: Problems in analyzing the diagnostic usefulness of mucosal dysplasia. Dis Colon Rectum 28:383, 1985

RIDDELL RH et al: Dysplasia in inflammatory bowel disease. Hum Pathol 14:931, 1983

SANDBORN WJ et al: Ulcerative colitis disease activity following treatment of associated primary sclerosing cholangitis with cyclosporine. Gut 34:242, 1993

SCHROEDER KW et al: Coated oral 5-aminosalicylate acid therapy for mild to moderately active ulcerative colitis. A randomized study. N Engl J Med 317:1625, 1987

SUGITA A et al: Colorectal cancer in ulcerative colitis: Influence of anatomical extent and age at onset in colitis-cancer interval. Gut 32:169, 1991

287

Richard B. Lynn, Lawrence S. Friedman

IRRITABLE BOWEL SYNDROME

The irritable bowel syndrome (IBS) is the most common gastrointestinal disease in clinical practice. Although not a life-threatening illness, it can cause great distress to patients and a feeling of frustration for physicians. IBS is characterized by abdominal pain and altered bowel habits, including diarrhea, constipation, or alternating diarrhea and constipation. Symptoms are typically intermittent but may be continuous and should be present for at least 3 months before a diagnosis of IBS is considered.

DEFINITION AND CLINICAL PRESENTATION Abdominal pain and altered bowel habits are nonspecific symptoms found in patients with a wide variety of illnesses (see Table 287-1). However, several characteristic symptoms, known as the *Manning criteria*, have been identified that, when present, increase the likelihood of IBS. The Manning criteria include abdominal pain or discomfort that is relieved by defecation or associated with a change in stool frequency or consistency, abdominal distention, the sensation of incomplete evacuation, and the passage of mucus. Diagnostic criteria for IBS that incorporate the Manning criteria have been established to standardize research and may be useful in clinical practice (Table 287-2). Patients presenting with abdominal pain in the absence of altered bowel habits or with altered bowel habits in the absence of abdominal pain may be considered to have IBS if no alternative explanation for the symptoms is found. However, patients with otherwise unexplained chronic constipation in the absence of abdominal pain are generally considered to have a distinct disorder (see Chap. 42).

In addition to altered bowel habits and abdominal pain, patients with IBS may have symptoms referable to the upper gastrointestinal (GI) tract, including noncardiac chest pain, heartburn, dysphagia, and globus sensation. Patients with IBS also may have a broad range of nongastrointestinal symptoms, such as fatigue, urologic dysfunction, and gynecologic complaints.

EPIDEMIOLOGY Estimates of the prevalence of IBS vary depending on the definition used and the population studied. Symptoms compatible with IBS are reported by 10 to 22 percent of the U.S. adult population, with a female predominance $> 2:1$ among patients presenting to a physician. However, fewer than half of adults with symptoms seek medical attention (see below). Symptoms typically begin in young adulthood, and the prevalence of IBS is similar in elderly and younger adults. IBS is a worldwide disorder with similar prevalence rates reported in a variety of industrialized and nonindustrialized countries. Until now, patients with symptoms of IBS have constituted fully 25 to 50 percent of outpatients referred to gastroenterologists, a reflection of the high prevalence and chronicity of IBS as well as the difficulty in treating the disorder.

ETIOLOGY AND PATHOGENESIS IBS is often considered a "functional" disorder because no structural, biochemical, or infectious etiology has been found. The fundamental disturbance is thought to relate to disordered motor or sensory function of the GI tract. Other functional disorders of the GI tract include noncardiac chest pain, nonulcer dyspepsia, and biliary dyskinesia. Similarities among these disorders and IBS suggest that they share underlying pathophysiologic mechanisms. Functional bowel disorders are often attributed erroneously to stress. Despite extensive investigation, however, there is no proof that emotional stress is the cause of IBS, but for many patients stress can lead to exacerbations of IBS.

IBS is probably a heterogeneous group of disorders. Numerous studies have reported motility or sensory abnormalities of the GI tract in some patients with IBS, but none of the findings is present in all patients nor accounts for the entire symptom complex. Some of these findings may characterize subgroups of patients with IBS. Studies describing motility and sensory abnormalities in IBS have generally been performed on patients either at rest or subjected to acute stimulation but not while experiencing the spontaneous painful episodes characteristic of IBS. Therefore, the relevance of the observed abnormalities to the pathophysiology of IBS remains uncertain.

IBS is often assumed to be caused by altered colonic motility because the characteristic symptoms are consistent with colonic dysfunction and the abdominal pain is frequently located in areas referable to the colon. Abnormal colonic motility has been reported in some patients, but these findings have not been convincingly linked with the pathogenesis of IBS. Similarly, continuous recording techniques have identified abnormalities of small intestinal motility, but their relevance to IBS is unclear. The most reproducible finding in IBS patients is altered visceral sensation. Balloon distention of the rectum, sigmoid colon, or small intestine causes abdominal pain in IBS patients at volumes usually not painful in control subjects. Little is understood, however, about either the mechanism of this abnormality in pain sensation or whether the fundamental defect resides in sensory recep-

Table 287-1

Some Conditions That May Present with Symptoms Similar to IBS

Intestinal malabsorption: Lactose intolerance
Infections: Giardiasis
Inflammatory bowel diseases: Crohn's disease, ulcerative colitis, collagenous colitis, lymphocytic colitis
Neoplasms: Colon cancer, villous adenoma, small-bowel tumors
Obstructing disorders: Fecal impaction, intermittent sigmoid volvulus, megacolon
Vascular insufficiency: Abdominal angina, ischemic colitis
Gynecologic disorders: Endometriosis
Psychiatric disorders: Depression, panic disorders, somatization, anxiety
Chronic idiopathic intestinal pseudoobstruction

Table 287-2

Evaluation of Patients with Symptoms of IBS

I. Diagnosite criteria for IBS
  A. At least 3 months of continuous or recurrent symptoms of
    1. Abdominal pain or discomfort that is
      a. Relieved with defecation
      b. Associated with a change in frequency of stool, or
      c. Associated with a change in consistency of stool, and
    2. Two or more of the following, at least on one-fourth of occasions or days:
      a. Altered stool frequency (>3 bowel movements daily or <3 bowel movements weekly)
      b. Altered stool consistency (lumpy/hard or loose/watery stool)
      c. Altered stool passage (straining, urgency, or feeling of incomplete evacuation),
      d. Passage of mucus,
      e. Bloating or feeling of abdominal distention
II. Essential history to exclude other causes
  A. Exclude symptoms not compatible with IBS only:
    1. Visible or occult blood in the stool
    2. Weight loss
    3. Fever
    4. Pain or diarrhea awakening the patient from sleep
  B. Obtain dietary history to exclude lactose intolerance or excessive use of sorbitol, fructose, or caffeine
  C. Review medications with possible GI side effects
  D. Consider depression or panic disorders
III. Physical examination: Should be unremarkable; if positive, further evaluation required
IV. Laboratory examination
  A. Complete blood count; erythrocyte sedimentation rate; chemistry panel
  B. Flexible sigmoidoscopy (patients >40 years old; all patients with diarrhea)
  C. If diarrhea is predominant symptom:
    1. Examine stool for ova and parasites, fecal leukocytes, excessive fat
    2. Thyroid function tests
    3. Mucosal biopsy of rectosigmoid for microscopic colitis

SOURCE: Adapted from Thompson et al, with permission.

tors and neurons in the bowel wall or in the central nervous system where pain sensation is processed and reaches awareness. Lower pain thresholds have been found at multiple locations in the gut in patients with IBS, suggesting that the disease involves a generalized disorder of visceral pain sensation.

PSYCHOSOCIAL FACTORS Psychosocial factors play an important role in IBS. Only 15 to 50 percent of adults with IBS symptoms seek medical attention. Compared to non-IBS controls and persons with symptoms of IBS who do not seek medical attention, patients with symptoms of IBS presenting to a physician have an increased frequency of psychiatric diagnoses, including personality disorders, anxiety, depression, hysteria, and somatization. Symptomatic patients not seeking medical attention are not psychologically different from healthy subjects. Therefore, while psychosocial factors do not cause the IBS symptoms, they can influence how symptomatic patients respond. While presenters report more severe GI distress, it is unclear whether they actually have more severe symptoms because their psychiatric disturbances affect pain sensation or whether they experience similar symptoms but report them as more severe.

The origin of psychosocial dysfunction in IBS patients probably varies. One hypothesis is that symptomatic IBS patients who seek medical attention have a learned illness behavior originating in childhood. In some cases, there may be a history of childhood sexual or physical abuse.

DIAGNOSTIC EVALUATION A diagnosis of IBS is based on a careful history to identify characteristic symptoms (e.g., Manning criteria), physical examination, selected laboratory tests, and, if necessary, further testing to exclude other disorders (see Table 287-2). In most cases, postponing designation of IBS as the likely diagnosis until all other possible etiologies of abdominal pain and altered bowel habits have been excluded by additional radiologic or endoscopic studies is unnecessary. Such an approach can lead to expensive, often invasive testing that increases the patient's anxiety and reinforces the unrealistic expectation that a demonstrable abnormality needs to be found. On the other hand, in persons with the recent onset of symptoms, particularly those over age 40, and those with previously stable IBS who have a change in symptoms, a thorough investigation of the GI tract may be indicated.

The history should include a detailed description of the abdominal pain, but it should be recognized that wide variations may be found in patients with IBS. Careful description of bowel frequency, consistency, and volume should be elicited. A complete list of medications should be reviewed, as many medications cause diarrhea or constipation (see Chap. 42). A careful dietary history is essential, including excessive use of caffeinated beverages or foods and beverages sweetened with fructose or sorbitol, which may cause diarrhea, bloating, or cramps. Consideration should be given to a 3-week trial of a lactose-free diet to exclude lactose intolerance. It is especially important to explore the psychosocial factors that may have influenced the patient to seek medical attention, including the specific events prompting the patient's initial visit. Panic disorders and depression often present with GI symptoms.

The physical examination in IBS patients is generally unremarkable. Abdominal tenderness, often in the left lower quadrant, may be elicited but is typically mild. A mass, an enlarged liver or spleen, or a positive fecal occult-blood test are not compatible with IBS alone and require further evaluation. In women, a pelvic examination should be performed to look for endometriosis.

Certain procedures may be needed to exclude other disorders. Flexible sigmoidoscopy is generally included in the evaluation of all patients over age 40 to exclude colonic neoplasms. In younger patients with IBS in whom diarrhea is the predominant symptom, flexible sigmoidoscopy is also indicated to exclude inflammatory bowel disease. If there is persistent diarrhea, sigmoidoscopic biopsies should be performed to exclude disorders such as collagenous or lymphocytic colitis. In many patients with suspected IBS, barium enema or colonoscopy may not be needed but should be considered if the patient is over age 40 or if there is a strong family history of colorectal neoplasms. Symptoms suggestive of upper GI or biliary tract disease may require additional evaluation.

Rx TREATMENT

The most important aspect of treatment is to establish a therapeutic physician-patient relationship. A beneficial outcome is most likely when the physician is nonjudgmental, establishes realistic expectations and consistent limits, encourages the patient's understanding of the illness, and involves the patient in treatment decisions. Discussion of the circumstances leading to the decision to seek medical attention may be particularly beneficial. The patient needs to be reassured of the benign nature of the illness and of the excellent long-term prognosis. It may be helpful to emphasize that although there is no cure for IBS, there are steps that both the physician and patient can take to improve the symptoms.

Initial recommendations generally focus on dietary modifications. These include avoidance of dairy products; foods, beverages, or medications containing fructose or sorbitol; excessive caffeine; or gas-forming foods such as legumes. Fiber supplements can often be recommended regardless of the presenting complaint but are particularly useful when constipation is the predominant symptom (see Table 287-3). Natural fiber, such as wheat bran, is inexpensive, but fiber supplements such as psyllium, polycarbophil, and methylcellulose may cause less bloating and discomfort. In fact, all fiber supplements can cause bloating and discomfort, but these symptoms often resolve within a few weeks. Although the efficacy of fiber supplements in IBS has never been proven, in part because of the high placebo response rate in controlled trials, a trial of fiber is generally safe and reasonable.

While most patients will improve with the simple measures outlined above, some with persistent symptoms may benefit from additional medications as shown in Table 287-3. While no medication has been proven effective in controlled trials, some patients may benefit from one or more of them. On the other hand, a trial-and-error approach using a series of medications should be avoided, as it may mislead the patient that a cure can be found.

Treatment should be directed to the predominant symptom. With diarrhea-predominant IBS, an antidiarrheal agent such as loperamide or diphenoxylate with atropine may be used. For symptoms of abdominal pain and bloating, an anticholinergic agent (e.g., belladonna)

Table 287-3

Drugs of Potential Benefit in IBS

Drug Type and Examples	Typical Starting Dose	Indications
Fiber supplements		Constipation-predominant IBS
Wheat bran	1/2 cup; 10–30 g/d	May be tried for any IBS symptom complex
Psyllium	1/2 to 1 tbsp qd to bid	
Antispasmodics (anticholinergics)		Pain-predominant IBS
Tincture of belladonna	5–10 drops PO tid	Prevention of postcibal abdominal pain
Dicyclomine	10–20 mg tid–qid	
Cimetropium bromide	50 mg tid	
Antidiarrheals		Diarrhea-predominant IBS
Diphenoxylate	2.5–5 mg qid	
Loperamide	2 mg bid	
Cholestyramine	1/2–1 pck qd to bid	
Tricyclic antidepressants		Pain-predominant IBS
Amitriptyline	10–25 mg qhs	
Desipramine	50 mg qhs	
Prokinetic agents		Constipation-predominant IBS
Cisapride	5–10 mg tid	
Domperidone	10–20 mg qid	
Benzodiazepine-type anxiolytics		Anxiety, use for brief periods

may be used as an antispasmodic. Newer anticholinergic agents (e.g., dicyclomine and cimetropium) appear to act more selectively on GI smooth muscle than older anticholinergic agents and therefore may have fewer side effects. Tricyclic antidepressants, which have proven effective in some chronic pain syndromes, may also benefit some patients with pain-predominant IBS; however, it is unclear whether a response to tricyclic antidepressants is due to their antidepressant or anticholinergic effects or to a direct effect on sensory pathways mediating pain perception. Anxiolytic agents may be used for brief periods when there are stress-related exacerbations of symptoms but should not be used on a long-term basis because of the risk of habituation, rebound effect on withdrawal, and drug interactions.

Other medications may be useful in selected cases. For example, cholestyramine may be helpful in some patients with apparent diarrhea-predominant IBS, in whom diarrhea is the result of bile salt malabsorption by the terminal ileum (see Chap. 42). Cisapride may improve constipation and abdominal pain in patients with constipation-predominant IBS. Other drugs being tried in the treatment of IBS include calcium channel blockers, gonadotropin-releasing hormone, serotonin-receptor antagonists, somatostatin agonists, and kappa opioid agonists. In refractory or severe cases, psychotherapy, hypnotherapy, and biofeedback may be helpful. In all cases, efforts should be directed toward firm and empathetic psychosocial support in the context of a sustained physician-patient relationship.

BIBLIOGRAPHY

Camilleri M, Prather CM: The irritable bowel syndrome: Mechanisms and a practical approach to management. Ann Intern Med 116:1001, 1992

Drossman DA et al: Psychosocial factors in the irritable bowel syndrome: A multivariate study of patients and nonpatients with irritable bowel syndrome. Gastroenterology 95:701, 1988

———: Sexual and physical abuse and gastrointestinal illness. Ann Intern Med 123:782, 1995

———, Thompson WG: The irritable bowel syndrome: Review and a graduated multicomponent treatment approach. Ann Intern Med 116:1009, 1992

Klein KB: Controlled treatment trials in the irritable bowel syndrome: A critique. Gastroenterology 95:232, 1988

Lynn RB, Friedman LS: Irritable bowel syndrome. N Engl J Med 329:1940, 1993

———, ———: Irritable bowel syndrome: managing the patient with abdominal pain and altered bowel habits. Med Clin North Am 79:373, 1995

Manning AP et al: Towards positive diagnosis of the irritable bowel. BMJ 2:653, 1978

Talley NJ et al: Psychological treatments for irritable bowel syndrome: A critique of controlled treatment trials. Am J Gastroenterol 91:277, 1996

Thompson WG et al: Functional bowel disorders and functional abdominal pain, in *The Functional Gastrointestinal Disorders*, DA Drossman et al (eds). Boston, Little, Brown, 1994

Whitehead WE et al: Symptoms of psychologic distress associated with irritable bowel syndrome: Comparison of community and medical clinic samples. Gastroenterology 95:709, 1988

288

Kurt J. Isselbacher, Alan Epstein

DIVERTICULAR, VASCULAR, AND OTHER DISORDERS OF THE INTESTINE AND PERITONEUM

DIVERTICULAR DISEASE

Diverticula may be either congenital or acquired and may affect either the small or large intestine. Congenital diverticula are herniations of the entire thickness of intestinal wall, while the more common acquired diverticula consist of herniations of the mucosa through the muscularis, generally at the site of a nutrient artery.

SMALL-INTESTINAL DIVERTICULA Diverticula may occur in any portion of the small intestine; however, with the exception of Meckel's diverticulum, the most common locations are in the duodenum and jejunum. Most often diverticula are asymptomatic and discovered incidentally on upper gastrointestinal x-rays. On occasion, however, they may cause symptoms either because of their anatomic proximity to other structures or rarely from inflammation or bleeding.

Duodenal diverticula arise singly from the medial surface of the second portion of the duodenum. In most patients, they cause no symptoms. Rarely, they may present as acute diverticulitis with abdominal pain, fever, gastrointestinal bleeding, or, most rarely, perforation. Periampullary diverticula are occasionally associated with cholangitis or pancreatitis. Jejunal diverticula, while less common, also may be the site of acute inflammation, bleeding, or perforation with resulting abscess or peritonitis.

Multiple jejunal diverticula may be associated with malabsorption related to bacterial overgrowth within the diverticula, similar to other situations where intestinal stasis (e.g., blind loops) permits bacterial proliferation. The consequences of bacterial proliferation with resultant mucosal damage, deconjugation of bile salts, and vitamin B_{12} malabsorption are discussed in Chap. 285.

Meckel's diverticulum, a persistent omphalomesenteric duct, is the most frequent congenital anomaly of the digestive tract, occurring in approximately 2 percent of autopsied adults. The diverticulum is wide-mouthed, about 5 cm long, and arises from the antimesenteric border of the ileum, usually within 100 cm of the ileocecal valve. The sac may be lined with normal ileal mucosa (approximately 50 percent) or contain gastric, duodenal, pancreatic, or colonic mucosa. While rarely symptomatic after age 5, Meckel's diverticulum may produce hemorrhage, inflammation, and obstruction in children and teenagers.

Hemorrhage occurs almost exclusively before age 10 and invariably results from peptic ulceration of ileal mucosa adjacent to a Meckel's diverticulum lined with gastric mucosa. The diagnosis may be established by isotope scanning of the abdomen after injection of technetium, which is taken up by the ectopic gastric mucosa in the diverticulum. False-negative and false-positive Meckel's scans are not uncommon; thus, other clinical and laboratory features must be assessed carefully before recommending surgery. In older children and young adults, inflammation of the diverticulum may mimic acute appendicitis. Mechanical obstruction also may occur if the diverticulum intussuscepts into the lumen of the bowel or twists on a fibrous remnant of the omphalomesenteric duct which extends from the diverticulum to the abdominal wall. The treatment of any of these complications of Meckel's diverticulum is surgical excision.

COLONIC DIVERTICULA Diverticula of the colon are herniations or saclike protrusions of the mucosa through the muscularis, at the point where a nutrient artery penetrates the muscularis. Diverticula occur most commonly in the sigmoid colon and decrease in frequency in the proximal colon. They increase with age, and the incidence ranges between 20 and 50 percent in western populations over age 50. The exact mechanism for their formation is unknown but may be related to an increase in intraluminal pressure. Thickening of the muscle coat of the colon in most patients with diverticula suggests that herniations of mucosa are caused by increased pressure produced by colonic muscle contractions. The rarity of colonic diverticula in underdeveloped nations has led to the speculation that diverticula result from the highly refined western diet, which is deficient in dietary fiber or roughage. It is proposed that such diets result in decreased fecal bulk, narrowing of the colon, and an increase in intraluminal pressure in order to move the smaller fecal mass. However, the role of dietary fiber in the etiology and treatment of diverticular disease remains to be determined.

Colonic diverticula are usually asymptomatic and are an incidental finding on barium enema or colonoscopy. The major complications of inflammation, both acute and chronic, and hemorrhage occur in only a small percentage of individuals with diverticulosis. Since diverticulosis is quite common in older patients, one must avoid the temptation of attributing pain or bleeding to the diverticula unless other conditions, especially colonic neoplasm, have been excluded.

DIVERTICULITIS Inflammation can occur in or around the diverticular sac. The cause of diverticulitis is probably mechanical, related to retention in the diverticula of undigested food residues and bacteria, which may form a hard mass called a *fecalith*. This compromises the blood supply to the thin-walled sac (made up solely of mucosa and serosa) and renders it susceptible to invasion by colonic bacteria. The inflammatory process may vary from a small intramural or pericolic abscess to generalized peritonitis. Some attacks are accompanied by minimal symptoms and seem to heal spontaneously. Studies of resected specimens indicate that most perforations of the diverticular sac are small and result in inflammation of the sac itself and the adjacent serosal surface. Diverticulitis occurs more often in men than in women and three times as often in the left as in the right colon. This suggests that diverticulitis may be related to the higher intraluminal pressures and the more solid fecal material in the sigmoid and descending colon.

Acute colonic diverticulitis is a disease of variable severity characterized by fever, left lower quadrant abdominal pain, and signs of peritoneal irritation—muscle spasm, guarding, rebound tenderness. Rectal examination may reveal a tender mass if the area of inflammation is close to the rectum. Although constipation may not have been noted prior to onset of the illness, the inflammation around the colon often results in some degree of acute constipation or obstipation. Rectal bleeding, usually microscopic, is noted in 25 percent of cases; it is rarely massive. Polymorphonuclear leukocytosis is common. Complications include free perforation, which results in acute peritonitis, sepsis, and shock, particularly in the elderly. The perforation may be walled off by adherent omentum or neighboring structures such as the bladder or small bowel. Abscess formation or fistulas then occur as the inflammatory mass burrows into other organs. Severe pericolitis may cause a fibrous stricture around the bowel, which can be associated with colonic obstruction and may mimic a neoplasm.

Diagnosis During the acute phase of diverticulitis, barium enema and sigmoidoscopy may be hazardous, since contrast material or air under pressure may lead to rupture of an inflamed diverticulum and convert a walled-off inflammatory lesion to a free perforation. These examinations are usually safe after adequate treatment and healing of the diverticulitis. The radiologic findings on barium enema suggestive of diverticulitis are leakage of barium from a diverticular sac, stricture formation, and the presence of a pericolic inflammatory mass. In many patients, the distortion caused by inflammation prevents a clear distinction between cancer and diverticulitis. In these cases, colonoscopy or surgical excision may be required for accurate diagnosis. Abdominal computed tomography scan may be useful in demonstrating the presence of a pericolic abscess.

℞ TREATMENT

Most patients with acute diverticulitis require bowel rest, intravenous fluids, and broad-spectrum antibiotics. Repeated attacks of diverticulitis in the same area generally require surgical resection. Severe attacks with acute peritoneal signs, suspected abscess, or perforation require intravenous antibiotics directed against gram-negative anaerobic bacteria, followed by surgical drainage or resection. The usual procedure is a diverting colostomy with resection of the involved colon; reanastomosis is then performed at a second operation.

PAINFUL DIVERTICULAR DISEASE WITHOUT DIVERTICULITIS Some patients with diverticulosis develop recurrent left lower quadrant colicky pain without clinical or pathologic evidence of acute diverticulitis. They often have bouts of alternating constipation and diarrhea, and the pain may be relieved by defecation or passage of flatus. These features suggest the coexistence of the irritable bowel syndrome (see below). Examination during a bout of pain reveals tenderness of the sigmoid colon, but signs of peritoneal inflammation such as rebound tenderness, muscle guarding, fever, and leukocytosis are absent. Barium enema shows typical diverticula without evidence of inflammation and stricture, plus a "sawtooth" irregularity of the lumen reflecting muscle hypertrophy and spasm. In some patients the pain is severe enough to warrant observation in a hospital and restriction of food, since feeding aggravates the pain by causing colonic contraction. Anticholinergics, which reduce sigmoid contractions, and mild sedation are usually all that is required. After recovery, the patient should be started on a high-residue diet or given a bulk laxative such as hemicellulose, unprocessed bran, or psyllium extract. Surgical excision is usually not indicated unless acute diverticulitis or its complications occur.

HEMORRHAGE FROM DIVERTICULA Massive hemorrhage from colonic diverticula is one of the most common causes of hematochezia in patients over age 60. This complication of diverticulosis is caused by erosion of a vessel by a fecalith within the diverticular sac. The bleeding is painless and not accompanied by signs or symptoms of diverticulitis. Most cases of mild or moderate hemorrhage stop spontaneously with bed rest and blood transfusion. Localization of bleeding can be obtained by bleeding scan or angiography. In patients with severe hemorrhage, mesenteric angiography can be both diagnostic in localizing the bleeding site and therapeutic, since vasoconstrictive drugs or artificial blood clot infused intraarterially can sometimes effectively control hemorrhage. Colonoscopy is also useful in evaluating acute hematochezia and the endoscopist may be able to cauterize angiodysplasias (see Chap. 44). The location of bleeding diverticula demonstrated at angiography on several series has been more commonly in the right colon, particularly the ascending colon, in contrast to the sigmoid colon, where diverticula are more numerous.

MOTILITY DISORDERS

Normal intestinal motility involves the delicate interplay of the gut motor system, neural influences of the autonomic and central nervous system, as well as hormonal factors, specifically gut neuropeptides. In addition, many drugs used in the treatment of disease (e.g., opioids, antibiotics) affect and influence intestinal motility directly or indirectly. The reader is referred to several excellent reviews cited in the bibliography, dealing with the complex mechanism involved in the regulation of intestinal motility.

Table 288-1 lists some of the common and unusual disorders of the enteric motor and neural system. Only some of the more clinically relevant and important ones are discussed below.

MEGACOLON Megacolon, or giant colon, is characterized by massive distention of the colon, usually accompanied by severe constipation or obstipation. This condition can be either congenital or acquired and is seen in all age groups. Acute toxic megacolon is a severe complication of ulcerative colitis (see Chap. 286).

Aganglionic Megacolon (Hirschsprung's Disease) This is a congenital disorder due to absence of enteric neurons (ganglions) in the distal colon and rectum. This aganglionic segment loses its neural inhibition and remains contracted. Hirschsprung's disease is a heterogeneous genetic disorder—some patients have an autosomal dominant form of the disease with mutations in the *RET* gene; many have an autosomal recessive form with a mutation in the endothelin-B receptor gene. These defects result in the gestational failure of neural crest cells to migrate to the distal colon. The disease becomes manifest in early infancy, occurring more frequently in males, and is often familial. These infants have massive abdominal distention, absent bowel movements, and impaired nutrition due to chronic obstruction of the colon. In some individuals with less severe symptoms, the disease may not be diagnosed until adolescence or early adulthood. The aganglionic and contracted segment of bowel is unable to relax to permit passage of stool, causing the normal proximal colon to become greatly dilated. On rectal examination, the ampulla is empty of feces and the anal sphincter is normal. Barium enema reveals a narrowed segment in the rectosigmoid, with massive dilatation above. Diagnosis is made by full-thickness surgical biopsy under anesthesia and demonstration of absent ganglion cells in the diseased segment. In most patients the aganglionic segment is in the rectosigmoid colon. The treatment of choice is a pull-through procedure in which normally innervated colon is anastomosed to the distal rectum just above the internal sphincter, thus bypassing the contracted aganglionic segment and restoring normal defecation.

Acquired Megacolon In Central and South America, infection with *Trypanosoma cruzi* (Chagas' disease) can result in destruction of the ganglion cells of the colon, producing a clinical picture similar to congenital megacolon, except that the onset is in adult life rather than childhood. A number of other diseases are associated with megacolon in adults. Patients with schizophrenia or depression, particularly institutionalized patients, may have obstipation and massive colonic dilatation. Severe neurologic disorders, including cerebral atrophy, spinal cord injury, and parkinsonism, also may cause megacolon. Myxedema, infiltrative diseases such as amyloidosis, and primary systemic sclerosis also can reduce colonic motility and produce marked colonic distention. Narcotic drugs, particularly morphine and codeine, can cause severe constipation, especially when administered to bedridden patients. Digital rectal examination of adults with acquired megacolon reveals a rectum distended with feces, as opposed to the empty rectum in aganglionic megacolon. Treatment is aimed at the underlying disease, as well as the careful use of enemas and cathartics.

INTESTINAL PSEUDOOBSTRUCTION Intestinal pseudoobstruction is an acute or chronic motility disorder characterized by distention or dilatation of the small and large intestine. Abdominal pain, nausea, and vomiting may lead to diagnostic confusion with mechanical obstruction, but as the name of this condition implies, the underlying cause is not obstruction but rather a severe dysmotility resulting in distention. Pseudoobstruction may be primary or secondary and acute or chronic. In primary or idiopathic pseudoobstruction, no other contributing condition can be identified, and the motility disorder is attributed to abnormalities of sympathetic innervation or of the muscle layers of the intestine. Secondary pseudoobstruction may result from primary systemic sclerosis, diabetes, amyloidosis, neurologic diseases, drugs, or sepsis.

Chronic or Intermittent Secondary Pseudoobstruction Numerous medical conditions can cause chronic dilatation of the large and small bowel. Some of these may involve the intestinal smooth muscle, such as primary systemic sclerosis, amyloidosis, or muscular dystrophy. Endocrine disorders, including myxedema and diabetes mellitus, may result in chronic distention, which in the diabetic patient results from autonomic visceral neuropathy. Chronic neurologic diseases, including Parkinson's disease and stroke, may be complicated by chronic pseudoobstruction; in these patients, drugs and relative immobility are contributing features. Finally, psychotic patients (especially those who are institutionalized) may suffer from prolonged megacolon.

The symptoms of chronic secondary pseudoobstruction are chronic or intermittent constipation, crampy abdominal pain, anorexia, and bloating. Gastric distention and disordered swallowing may be present. Abdominal x-rays reveal gaseous distention of the large and small

Table 288-1

Some Motility Disorders of the Enteric Nervous System

Disorder	Comment
Intestinal pseudo-obstruction	
Visceral neuropathy	Autosomal dominant disorder characterized by dilatation of jejunum and ileum and degeneration and loss of neurons.
Visceral neuropathy with basal ganglia calcifications	Autosomal recessive disorder with dilatation of duodenum and small bowel and mental retardation. Calcification of basal ganglia and degeneration of myenteric plexus.
Megacolon	
Hirschsprung's disease	Congenital disorder characterized by colonic dilatation proximal to an aganglionic, contracted distal colon and rectum. Caused by gestational failure of neural crest cells to migrate to distal colon. An autosomal dominant form is associated with mutations of the *RET* gene, and an autosomal recessive form with mutation of the endothelin, B–receptor gene.
Multiple endocrine neoplasia type 2A (MEN-2A)	Features similar to those of Hirschsprung's disease. Medullary thyroid cancer, parathyroid hyperplasia, and pheochromocytoma are characteristic. ? Mutation of *RET* gene.
Generalized, with hyperganglionosis	
MEN-2B (Sipple's syndrome)	Achalasia and pseudoobstruction reported with ganglioneuromatosis of myenteric and submucosal plexuses. Medullary thyroid cancer, pheochromocytoma, and mucosal neuromas are characteristic. Mutation of *RET* gene reported.
Neurofibromatosis(von Recklinghausen's disease)	Achalasia and megacolon reported, with neuronal dysplasia of the myenteric plexus. Central nervous system tumors, neurofibromas, pigmented iris, hamartomas, café au lait spots, and mental retardation are characteristic.
Generalized, with hypoganglionosis	
Chagas' disease	Achalasia, intestinal, and colonic pseudoobstruction; megaloureter; and myocarditis due to infection with *Trypanosoma cruzi*. Possible autoimmune response to parasitic antigen.
Paraneoplastic syndrome	Achalasia, gastroparesis, and intestinal pseudoobstruction reported in some patients with small-cell lung cancer and carcinoid tumors. Serum antibodies reactive to enteric neurons.
Cytomegalovirus infection	Esophageal dysmotility, delayed gastric emptying, achalasia, and pseudoobstruction reported, with intranuclear neuronal viral inclusions and loss of myenteric neurons.
Myotonic dystrophy	Autosomal dominant disorder with impaired esophageal and gastric transit and intestinal pseudoobstruction, selective loss of substance P– and enkephalin-containing enteric neurons and preservation of neurons containing neuropeptide Y or vasoactive intestinal polypeptide. Myotonia, weakness, cataracts, cardiac abnormalities, gonadal atrophy, and mental retardation are characteristic.
Generalized, other	
Parkinson's disease	Achalasia, pseudoobstruction, and megacolon reported in some patients, with Lewy bodies in the myenteric plexus of the esophagus and colon.
Diabetes mellitus	Gastroparesis and intestinal and colonic dysmotility, with generalized autonomic neuropathy. Myenteric plexus morphologically intact.
Amyloidosis	Achalasia, gastroparesis, and pseudoobstruction, with amyloid deposits in both smooth muscle and the myenteric plexus.
Fabry's disease	Impaired gastric emptying, jejunal and colonic diverticulosis, and malabsorption, with glycolipid deposition in neurons of the myenteric plexus and decreased numbers of enlarged ganglion cells. Cutaneous angiokeratoma, renal insufficiency, and cardiovascular and central nervous system damage are also seen.
Disorders caused by exogenous neural toxins	Intestinal and colonic pseudoobstruction, with increased argyrophilia of the myenteric plexus.

SOURCE: Modified from Goyal and Hirano, with permission.

bowel and occasionally of the stomach. Air-fluid levels are unusual and should raise the possibility of mechanical obstruction. Upper gastrointestinal series and barium enema do not reveal specific abnormalities of the intestine such as tumor, stricture, or volvulus. The presence of an autoimmune disorder or endocrinopathy may require confirmation by serologic or blood tests; biopsy may be needed as in amyloidosis or muscular dystrophy.

The treatment of chronic intestinal pseudoobstruction is made difficult by the complexity and chronicity of the underlying systemic disease. Patients with primary systemic sclerosis may respond to broad-spectrum antibiotics if intestinal bacterial overgrowth is suspected. Metoclopramide may benefit gastric dysmotility in the diabetic patient. Discontinuation of psychotropic or anti-Parkinson drugs occasionally may result in improvement. Cathartics and enemas may be required to relieve fecal impaction, and the regular use of stool softeners and a high-fiber diet may help prevent recurrences.

Idiopathic Intestinal Pseudoobstruction This term is used to describe the condition of patients with signs and symptoms of pseudoobstruction in whom no systemic disease can be identified. The typical patient has recurrent attacks of abdominal pain and distention with nausea and vomiting. The small intestine is primarily involved, and chronic constipation is much less frequent than in secondary pseudoobstruction. Steatorrhea secondary to bacterial overgrowth of the small intestine is common and may lead to chronic diarrhea and malnutrition. Many patients exhibit abnormalities of motility in the esophagus and urinary bladder, in addition to the small and large intestine. Neuromuscular defects have been described in patients with this syndrome, including abnormalities of the mesenteric plexus and myopathy of the intestinal and urinary bladder smooth muscle (so-called hollow visceral myopathy). Elevated prostaglandin E levels have been reported in some patients.

Management of idiopathic pseudoobstruction is unsatisfactory. Surgery to relieve "obstruction" is to be avoided, since the condition is often worsened by abdominal surgery. Medical therapy with metoclopramide and cholinergic agents has been unsuccessful. Nutritional support in the form of low-residue elemental diets or parenteral hyperalimentation may be helpful. Unfortunately, the lack of effective therapy and the progressive nature of the illness make the prognosis of idiopathic pseudoobstruction rather unfavorable. Death from malnutrition and steatorrhea are common. The long-term impact of total parenteral nutrition on this disease is not yet clear.

Acute Intestinal Pseudoobstruction This entity, sometimes referred to as *Ogilvie's syndrome*, is characterized by acute intestinal dilatation involving primarily the colon but occasionally also the small intestine. As in other forms of pseudoobstruction, the clinical features are difficult to distinguish from mechanical obstruction. The patient may complain of colicky lower abdominal pain and acute constipation. Examination reveals a distended, tympanitic abdomen, with reduced or absent bowel sounds. Localized tenderness over the distended colon is common, but diffuse abdominal tenderness, rigidity, or rebound tenderness are unusual. Abdominal films reveal massive dilatation of the colon and small intestine, occasionally with the presence of air-fluid levels. The cecum, being the most capacious part of the colon, is often massively dilated and tender. The onset of these symptoms usually occurs in patients who have recently undergone severe surgical or medical stress such as major surgery, myocardial infarction, sepsis, or respiratory failure. Patients with acute pseudoobstruction are frequently on respirators, have received narcotics or sedatives, and have metabolic and electrolyte disturbances. Ogilvie's syndrome may also be due to paraneoplastic obstruction.

Management of acute pseudoobstruction requires careful correction of fluid and electrolyte abnormalities, intubation of the stomach or small intestine for decompression, and avoidance of drugs that depress intestinal motility. Barium enema may be hazardous because of the risk of perforating the already dilated bowel. Decompressive colonoscopy is beneficial in some patients, and cecostomy may be required in some patients with massive cecal dilatation. The outcome depends in large part on the prognosis of the associated medical or surgical conditions. Patients who recover from the underlying medical or surgical conditions usually have a return of normal colonic function.

IRRITABLE BOWEL SYNDROME See Chap. 287

CHRONIC CONSTIPATION The mechanism of defecation is discussed in Chap. 42. Chronic constipation is widespread in western society, with approximately 10 percent of the population taking laxatives on a regular basis. Most cases of chronic constipation arise from habitual neglect of afferent impulses, failure to initiate defecation, and accumulation of large, dry fecal masses in the rectum. This voluntary suppression of the call to stool may arise during the period of toilet training in childhood or later in life because of a sense of social impropriety, unaccustomed surroundings, uncomfortable toilet facilities, or illnesses that require confinement to bed. Chronic constipation is much more common in women, with onset typically in late adolescence or early adulthood. As constant distention of the rectum with feces becomes chronic, the patient grows less aware of rectal fullness. Bowel movements become progressively more difficult, and painful hemorrhoids or anal fissures reinforce suppression of the urge to defecate. To avoid these problems, the patient begins the chronic use of laxatives or enemas, without which defecation becomes impossible.

℞ TREATMENT

The physician should make every attempt to educate the patient about the chain of events that has led to chronic constipation. Attempts should be made to alter patterns of many years' duration, and the patient must recognize the importance of responding to, rather than suppressing, the urge to defecate. It is helpful to initiate a routine whereby defecation is attempted at a given time each day. In most individuals the call to stool occurs in the morning after breakfast. Physical exercise such as a brisk walk just before attempts at defecation may be helpful. Patients are instructed to increase dietary bulk with foods rich in fiber, such as green vegetables and unprocessed cereal grains, or by the regular use of bulk laxatives, such as hemicellulose, psyllium extract, and powdered unprocessed bran. The success of such a regimen depends to some extent on the duration of symptoms. Elderly patients with long-standing constipation and reliance on enemas or laxatives are more resistant to these measures than younger patients whose bowel patterns are less established. Moreover, poor muscle tone, reduced physical activity, and increased incidence of other medical conditions make the problem more difficult in the older age group. Bedridden elderly patients often develop severe constipation and even fecal impaction unless preventive measures are taken. This applies not only to patients with previous constipation but also to those with regular bowel movements prior to their confining illness. Regular administration of stool softeners, bulk laxatives, or mild cathartics is necessary until full ambulation and a normal diet are resumed. The onset of fecal impaction in bedridden patients is heralded by a feeling of rectal distention, urgency of defecation, or tenesmus. Occasionally, the fecal impaction will result in low-grade chronic obstruction with dilatation and increased fluid content proximal to the impaction; "paradoxical diarrhea" may thus occur as fluid moves past the obstructing fecal mass. This situation will be aggravated if antidiarrheal drugs are given because the underlying constipation will be worsened. The appropriate maneuver is to disimpact the rectum manually or to administer gentle enemas if the impaction is beyond the reach of the finger.

DISORDERS OF THE MESENTERIC CIRCULATION

Ischemia of the intestine is the end result of interruption or reduction of its blood supply. However, the clinical manifestations of intestinal ischemia range from mild chronic symptoms to a catastrophic acute episode, depending on the vascular supply involved, the extent of the occlusion or ischemia, and the rapidity of the process. The clinician should be aware of the spectrum of clinical manifestations (Table 288-2). The gut derives its arterial blood supply from the celiac axis and the superior and inferior mesenteric arteries. The small intestine is supplied by the celiac and superior mesenteric arteries; the colon by branches of the superior and inferior mesenteric arteries. A rich network of anastomotic vessels and the possible development of collateral circulation determine the clinical picture of acute or chronic intestinal arterial insufficiency.

MESENTERIC ISCHEMIA AND INFARCTION Acute intestinal ischemia may be classified as occlusive or nonocclusive. *Occlusion* may result from an arterial thrombus or embolus of the celiac or superior mesenteric arteries or from venous occlusion in the same distribution. Arterial embolus occurs most commonly in patients with chronic or recurrent atrial fibrillation, artificial heart valves, or valvular heart disease; arterial thrombosis is usually associated with extensive atherosclerosis or low cardiac output. Venous occlusion is rare; it is occasionally seen in women taking oral contraceptives. Approximately one-half of patients with mesenteric ischemia have no definite occlusion of a major vessel, a condition referred to as *nonocclusive ischemia*. The exact cause of nonocclusive disease is obscure; systemic arterial hypotension, cardiac arrhythmias, prolonged heart failure, digitalis therapy, dehydration, and endotoxemia can be contributing factors.

The major clinical feature of acute mesenteric ischemia is severe abdominal pain, often colicky and periumbilical at the onset, later becoming diffuse and constant. Vomiting, anorexia, diarrhea, and constipation are also frequent but of little diagnostic help. Examination of the abdomen may reveal tenderness and distention. Bowel sounds are often normal even in the face of severe infarction. Some patients have a surprisingly normal abdominal examination in spite of severe pain. Mild gastrointestinal bleeding is often detected by examination of stool for occult blood; gross hemorrhage is unusual except in ischemic colitis (see below). A typical laboratory finding is a pronounced polymorphonuclear leukocytosis. Late in the course of the disease (24 to 72 h), gangrene of the bowel occurs with diffuse peritonitis, sepsis, and shock. Abdominal plain films in patients with mesenteric ischemia may reveal air-fluid levels and distention. Barium study of the small intestine reveals nonspecific dilatation, poor motility, and evidence of thick mucosal folds ("thumbprinting") (Fig. 288-1).

Acute mesenteric ischemia is a grave condition with a high morbidity and mortality. Patients suspected of having acute arterial embolus should undergo immediate celiac and mesenteric angiography to localize the embolus, followed by embolectomy. Restoration of normal circulation may allow complete recovery if performed before irreversible necrosis or gangrene has occurred. Unfortunately, infarction and transmural necrosis are frequently found at surgery, necessitating resection. Arterial or venous thrombosis is not generally amenable to surgical removal of the thrombus, and resection of the affected bowel is required. Similarly, patients with nonocclusive ischemia are not candidates for corrective vascular surgery (as major vessels are patent).

Table 288-2

Patterns of Intestinal Ischemia

Condition	Etiology	Clinical Features	Management
Mesenteric artery embolus	Arterial embolus associated with atrial fibrillation or rheumatic heart disease	Acute central abdominal pain, shock, peritonitis	Immediate angiography and embolectomy if possible
Abdominal angina	Atherosclerosis of celiac and superior mesenteric arteries	Chronic postprandial pain, weight loss	Angiography and surgery in selected cases
Ischemic colitis	Low-flow state	Acute lower abdominal pain, rectal bleeding	Sigmoidoscopy; surgery only for peritonitis

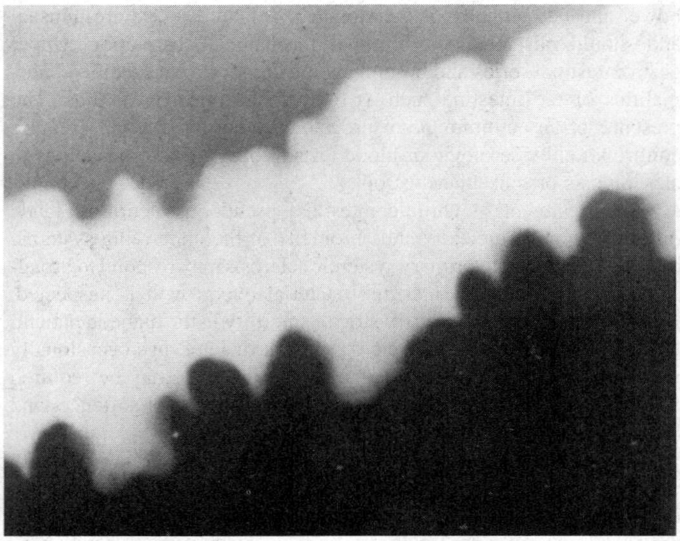

FIGURE 288-1 Barium enema showing "thumbprinting" or submucosal edema of the inferior margin of the transverse colon in a patient with acute ischemic colitis.

These individuals often have extensive necrosis of the small or large intestine because of the widespread nature of the ischemic event. The decision to operate when mesenteric ischemia is suspected is often difficult, because the typical patient is a poor surgical risk owing to advanced age, dehydration, sepsis, and other serious medical conditions.

Chronic arterial insufficiency may precede acute vascular insufficiency, producing so-called abdominal angina. As in angina pectoris, the pain of chronic mesenteric insufficiency occurs under conditions of increased demand for splanchnic blood flow. The patient complains of intermittent dull or cramping midabdominal pain 15 to 30 min after a meal, lasting for several hours postprandially. There may be significant weight loss due to decreased food intake; however. Chronic intestinal ischemia also may produce mucosal damage and malabsorption, which in turn aggravates the weight loss. Since abdominal angina may progress to bowel infarction, serious consideration should be given to performing arteriographic studies to confirm the diagnosis in those patients who are candidates for abdominal vascular surgery. The only definitive treatment is vascular surgery or balloon angioplasty to remove the thrombus or the construction of bypass arterial grafts to the ischemic bowel.

A number of systemic conditions are associated with *vasculitis* of the large and small arteries supplying the intestine. Most often these disorders can be recognized by the associated extraintestinal manifestations, as in polyarteritis nodosa, lupus erythematosus, dermatomyositis, Henoch-Schönlein purpura (allergic vasculitis), and rheumatoid vasculitis. When larger arteries are involved, as in polyarteritis nodosa, the picture of acute intestinal infarction is similar to that of embolic or atherosclerotic vascular occlusion. Often the involvement of smaller vessels leads to areas of intramural hemorrhage and edema resulting in abdominal pain, variable degrees of intestinal obstruction, and bleeding. Barium enema may show "thumbprinting" and "spiculation" due to localized edema, hemorrhage, and ulceration (see Fig. 288-1). In many instances, treatment of the underlying disorder may lead to regression of symptoms. If signs of an acute abdomen develop, surgical exploration is usually indicated.

Intramural small-intestinal hemorrhage may occur with vasculitis, trauma, or impaired coagulation, especially in patients receiving anticoagulants. The clinical and radiologic features resemble those seen with vasculitis and local mucosal hemorrhage.

ISCHEMIC COLITIS Ischemia of the colon most often affects the elderly because of the greater frequency of vascular disease in that group. Ischemic colitis is almost always a nonocclusive disease. Shunting of blood away from the mucosa may contribute to this condition, but the mechanism of ischemia is not known.

The clinical picture depends on the degree of ischemia and its rate of development. In *acute fulminant ischemic colitis*, the major manifestations are severe lower abdominal pain, rectal bleeding, and hypotension. Dilatation of the colon and physical signs of peritonitis are seen in severe cases. Abdominal films may reveal thumbprinting from submucosal hemorrhage and edema (Fig. 288-1). Barium enema is hazardous in the acute situation because of the risk of perforation. Sigmoidoscopy or colonoscopy may detect ulcerations, friability, and bulging folds from submucosal hemorrhage. Angiography is not helpful in the management of patients with presumed ischemic colitis because a remediable occlusive lesion is very rarely found. Surgical resection may be required in some patients with fulminant ischemic colitis to remove gangrenous bowel; others with lesser degrees of ischemia may respond to conservative medical management.

Subacute ischemic colitis is the most common clinical variant of ischemic colonic disease. It produces lesser degrees of pain and bleeding, often occurring over several days or weeks. The left colon may be involved, but the rectum is usually spared because of the collateral blood supply, a feature distinguishing it from acute ulcerative colitis. Barium enema reveals edema, cobblestoning, thumbprinting, and occasionally superficial ulceration. Angiography is not indicated because almost all cases are nonocclusive. Occasionally, *stricture formation* may follow a bout of ischemic colitis or may present de novo without a history of antecedent pain or bloody diarrhea. Most cases of nonocclusive ischemic colitis resolve in 2 to 4 weeks and do not recur. Surgery is not required except for obstruction secondary to postischemic stricture.

ANGIODYSPLASIA OF THE COLON These are vascular ectasias or arteriovenous malformations (AVMs) that occur in the right colon of many older individuals and may cause bleeding (see Chap. 44). Angiodysplasia is a degenerative lesion consisting of dilated, distorted, thin-walled vessels lined by vascular endothelium. It may result from partial obstruction of the submucosal venous plexus by the tension generated in the cecal wall during muscular contraction. Grossly, angiodysplasias look similar to spider angiomas of the skin and on colonoscopy appear as star-shaped branching vessels in the submucosa measuring from 2 mm to 1 cm in diameter. The lesions are usually multiple and are found primarily in the cecum and ascending colon, but in some patients they may be distributed from the stomach to rectum.

Cecal angiodysplasia is important because of the likelihood of bleeding, either massively or chronically. In patients over age 60, approximately one-quarter of colonic bleeding episodes are secondary to angiodysplasia. The diagnosis is easiest to establish by colonoscopy, which allows treatment by laser photocoagulation, electrocautery, or injection with sclerosant. Some patients with massive uncontrolled bleeding or multiple sites of angiodysplasia may require right hemicolectomy. Angiodysplasias also may respond to chronic estrogen-progesterone therapy.

ANORECTAL PROBLEMS

HEMORRHOIDS The internal hemorrhoidal plexus of veins is located in the submucosal space above the valves of Morgagni. The anal canal separates it from the external hemorrhoidal venous plexus, but the two spaces communicate under the anal canal, the submucosa of which is attached to underlying tissue to form the interhemorrhoidal depression. Whenever the internal hemorrhoidal plexus is enlarged, there is associated increase in supporting tissue mass, and the resultant venous swelling is called an *internal hemorrhoid*. When veins in the external hemorrhoidal plexus become enlarged or thrombosed, the resultant bluish mass is called an *external hemorrhoid*.

Both types of hemorrhoids are very common and are associated with increased hydrostatic pressure in the portal venous system, such as during pregnancy, straining at stool, or with cirrhosis. When internal hemorrhoids enlarge, pain is not a usual feature until the situation is complicated by thrombosis, infection, or erosion of the overlying mucosal surface. Most persons complain of bright red blood on the toilet tissue or coating the stool, with a feeling of vague anal discomfort.

The discomfort is increased when the hemorrhoid enlarges or prolapses through the anus: prolapse is often accompanied by edema and sphincteric spasm. Prolapse, if not treated, usually becomes chronic as the muscularis stays stretched, and the patient complains of constant soiling of underclothing with very little pain. Prolapsed hemorrhoids may be detected or thrombosed; the overlying mucous membrane may bleed profusely from the trauma of defecation.

External hemorrhoids, because they lie under the skin, are quite often painful, particularly if there is a sudden increase in their mass. These episodes result in a tender blue swelling at the anal verge due to thrombosis of a vein in the external plexus and need not be associated with enlargement of the internal veins. Since the thrombus usually lies at the level of the sphincteric muscles, anal spasm often occurs.

The diagnosis of internal and external hemorrhoids is made by inspection, digital examination, and direct vision through the anoscope and proctoscope. Since such lesions are very common, they must not be regarded as the cause of rectal bleeding or chronic hypochromic anemia until a thorough investigation has been made of the more proximal gastrointestinal tract. Acute blood loss can occasionally be attributed to internal hemorrhoids. Chronic anemia or occult blood in the stool in the presence of large but not definitely bleeding hemorrhoids requires a search for a polyp, cancer, or ulcer.

℞ TREATMENT

Most hemorrhoids respond to conservative therapy such as sitz baths or other forms of moist heat, suppositories, stool softeners, and bed rest. Internal hemorrhoids that remain permanently prolapsed are best treated surgically; milder degrees of prolapse or enlargement with pruritus ani or intermittent bleeding can be handled successfully by banding or injection of sclerosing solutions. External hemorrhoids that become acutely thrombosed are treated by incision, extraction of the clot, and compression of the incised area following clot removal. No surgical procedure should be carried out in the presence of acute inflammation of the anus, ulcerative proctitis, or ulcerative colitis. Proctoscopy or colonoscopy should always be performed before a patient is subjected to hemorrhoidectomy.

ANAL INFLAMMATION Perianal inflammatory lesions may be primary or may be associated with inflammatory bowel disease or diverticular disease, as mentioned above. *Anal fissures* are superficial erosions of the anal canal which usually heal rapidly with conservative therapy. *Anal ulcers* are more chronic and deep and give symptoms largely as the result of painful spasm of the external anal sphincter during and after defecation. Bleeding may occur with either fissure or ulcer; healing of the ulcer often is associated with a hypertrophied anal papilla and some degrees of anal contracture. *Fistula in ano*, a tract leading from the rectal lumen to the perianal skin, usually results from local crypt abscesses. The fistula is a chronically inflamed canal made up of fibrous tissue surrounding granulation tissue, the lumen of which may be difficult to demonstrate. *Perirectal abscesses* often represent the tracking down into the anal area of purulent material escaping from the rectosigmoid; diverticulitis, Crohn's disease, ulcerative colitis, or previous surgery may be the underlying cause. Fistulas between the rectum and vagina or the rectum and bladder represent serious complications of granulomatous, septic, or malignant disorders and require the patient to be hospitalized for definitive diagnostic and therapeutic procedures.

PERITONEAL AND MESENTERIC DISEASES

ACUTE PERITONITIS Peritonitis is a localized or generalized inflammatory process of the peritoneum that may appear in both acute and chronic forms. In the acute form, the motor activity of the intestine is decreased, and the intestinal lumen becomes distended with gas and fluid. Fluid accumulates as a result of failure to reabsorb the 7 or 8 L normally secreted daily into the lumen and absorbed from the distal small bowel and colon. Because of accumulation of fluid in the peritoneal cavity as well as decreased oral intake, rapid depletion of the plasma volume with impaired cardiac and renal function may occur.

Etiology *Bacterial peritonitis* may be due to entry of bacteria into the peritoneal cavity from a perforation in the gastrointestinal tract or from an external penetrating wound. *Chemical peritonitis* results from spillage of pancreatic enzymes, gastric acid, or bile as a result of injury or perforation of the intestine or biliary tract. *Sterile peritonitis* occurs in patients with systemic lupus erythematosus, porphyria, and familial Mediterranean fever (FMF) during attacks of their disease (see below).

The most common causes of bacterial peritonitis are appendicitis, perforations associated with diverticulitis, peptic ulcer, gangrenous gallbladder, and gangrenous obstruction of the small bowel from adhesive bands, incarcerated hernia, or volvulus. Any lesion leading to the escape of intestinal bacteria may be a source, including a perforating carcinoma, foreign body, and ulcerative colitis. The peritoneal cavity is remarkably resistant to contamination, and unless continuing contamination occurs, the peritonitis remains localized. Patients with alcoholic cirrhosis and ascites have an increased susceptibility to *spontaneous bacterial peritonitis*, usually from enteric pathogens. This complication occurs in the absence of recognizable perforation of a viscus and may be due to leakage of bacteria through the intestinal wall (see Chap. 299).

Clinical Features The cardinal manifestations of peritonitis are acute abdominal pain and tenderness. The location of the pain and tenderness depends on the underlying cause and whether the inflammation is localized or generalized. In *localized peritonitis*, as seen in uncomplicated appendicitis or diverticulitis, the physical findings are limited to the area of inflammation. With widespread peritoneal inflammation there is *generalized peritonitis* with diffuse abdominal tenderness and rebound. Rigidity of the abdominal wall is a common finding in peritonitis and may be localized or generalized.

Peristalsis may be present initially but usually disappears as the illness progresses and bowel sounds disappear. Hypotension, tachycardia, oliguria, and leukocytosis, with cell counts greater than 20,000 cells per microliter, are common, especially in generalized peritonitis. Plain abdominal films may reveal dilatation of the large and small bowel with edema of the small-bowel wall, as evidenced by the distance between adjacent loops of gas-filled small intestine. Diagnostic paracentesis is sometimes valuable in determining the nature of the exudate as well as whether bacteria can be demonstrated or cultured.

GONOCOCCAL PERITONITIS This usually involves an extension of gonococcal infection from a primary focus in the female reproductive tract. The signs of inflammation usually are limited to the pelvis, but there may be findings of a mild generalized peritonitis. Occasionally, the patient has right upper quadrant pain and tenderness caused by gonococcal perihepatitis involving the liver capsule and adjacent peritoneum (Fitz-Hugh–Curtis syndrome; see also Chap. 150).

STARCH PERITONITIS An acute granulomatous peritonitis can develop in some patients as a foreign-body reaction to cornstarch used to powder surgical gloves. The clinical picture is that of acute abdominal pain and fever 10 to 30 days after an abdominal operation. The diagnosis can be made by paracentesis and demonstration of starch granules in monocytes. However, most patients are reexplored because of the fear of abscess or bacterial peritonitis, with the finding of foreign-body granuloma studding the peritoneum.

PSEUDOMYXOMA PERITONEI This is a rare condition resulting from rupture of a mucocele of the appendix, a mucinous ovarian cyst, or mucin-secreting intestinal or ovarian adenocarcinoma. The abdomen becomes filled with masses of jelly-like mucus. Occasionally, with removal of the mucocele or the ovarian cyst and most of the myxomatous material, a cure may ensue. In other cases, however, the mucoid material recurs, leading to progressive wasting and eventual death. Colloid carcinoma arising from the stomach or colon with peritoneal implants may resemble pseudomyxoma at laparotomy. The course of this type of highly malignant tumor is one of rapid cachexia and early death. The diagnosis usually can be made by the appearance of many highly malignant cells in the peritoneal implants.

PNEUMATOSIS CYSTOIDES INTESTINALIS This is a condition in which multiple gas-filled blebs or cysts accumulate in the intestinal wall beneath the serosal surface of the bowel. The exact source of the gas has not been explained satisfactorily. In some instances, this disease is associated with specific ulceration of the intestinal mucosa, in particular peptic ulcer with outlet obstruction. Cysts in the wall of the small bowel are seen as an occasional complication of mesenteric vascular occlusion. In the large bowel, these cysts are usually benign, may be seen with a variety of other disorders, and usually disappear over time.

There are no specific physical findings secondary to the pneumatosis, and the diagnosis is made either by x-ray or at laparotomy. Occasionally, the subserosal cysts may rupture, resulting in pneumoperitoneum.

CHYLOUS ASCITES See Chap. 46

MESENTERIC LIPODYSTROPHY This is a rare disorder usually affecting middle-aged women and characterized pathologically by infiltration of the mesentery with lipid-laden macrophages and fibrous tissue. These patients present with ill-defined abdominal pain and occasionally an abdominal mass. The diagnosis is made at laparotomy by demonstration of thick fibrofatty masses at the root of the mesentery with retraction and distortion of the bowel loops.

FAMILIAL MEDITERRANEAN FEVER*

Familial Mediterranean fever (FMF, familial paroxysmal polyserositis) is an inherited disorder of unknown etiology, characterized by recurrent episodes of fever, peritonitis, and/or pleuritis. Arthritis, skin lesions, and amyloidosis are seen in some patients.

FMF occurs predominantly in patients of non-Ashkenazi (Sephardic) Jewish, Armenian, and Arabic ancestry. However, the disease has been seen in patients of Italian, Ashkenazi Jewish, and Anglo-Saxon descent as well as others.

The earliest studies of the genetics of FMF were done in Israel, where the disease appears to be inherited in an autosomal recessive manner. Consanguinity among the parents of FMF patients is as high as 20 percent, a figure that may be an underestimate. Approximately 60 percent of patients are male. The gene believed to cause FMF is located in the short arm of chromosome 16.

ETIOLOGY The cause of FMF is unknown. Fever and inflammation are such prominent signs that frequent attempts have been made to implicate infectious agents and/or their products. However, extensive studies have failed to implicate these or any other specific infectious agents. Others have suggested a deficiency in an inhibitor of C5a, thus implicating alterations in the immune system. The demonstration that FMF is inherited as an autosomal recessive disorder has led to the thesis that it is an inborn error of metabolism. However, no such error has been found.

PATHOLOGY Despite the striking clinical manifestations during an acute attack of FMF, no specific pathologic alterations have been found. At laparotomy, there is acute peritoneal inflammation with an exudate that contains a predominance of polymorphonuclear leukocytes. A disproportionately large number of male patients develop gallbladder disease with and without cholelithiasis. Pleural and joint inflammation are also nonspecific.

In the amyloidosis that accompanies FMF, amyloid is deposited in the intima and media of the arterioles, the subendothelial region of venules, the glomeruli, and the spleen. Aside from their vessels, the heart and liver are uninvolved.

MANIFESTATIONS The symptoms of FMF often begin between the ages of 5 and 15, although attacks sometimes commence during infancy and onset has occurred as late as age 50. The duration

* The late Sheldon M. Wolff was the previous author of this topic.

and frequency of attacks vary greatly in the same patient, and there is no set pattern to their occurrence. The usual acute episode lasts 24 to 48 h, but some may be prolonged for 7 to 10 days. The attacks range in frequency from twice weekly to once a year, but 2 to 4 weeks is the commonest interval. Spontaneous remissions lasting years have been seen. There may be a decrease in the severity and frequency of the attacks with age or with development of amyloidosis.

Fever Fever is a cardinal manifestation and is present during most attacks. Rarely, fever may be present without serositis. The temperature may be preceded by a chill and will peak in 12 to 24 h. Defervescence is often accompanied by diaphoresis. The fever ranges from 38.5 to 40°C but is quite variable.

Abdominal Pain Abdominal pain occurs in more than 95 percent of patients and may vary in severity in the same patient. Minor premonitory discomfort may precede an acute episode by 24 to 48 h. The pain usually starts in one quadrant and then spreads to involve the whole abdomen. The initial site is usually very tender. Tenderness may remain localized with referred pain in other areas, and there may be radiation to the back. There may be splinting of the chest and pain in one or both shoulders, typical of diaphragmatic irritation. Nausea and vomiting sometimes occur. The abdomen is usually distended and may become rigid, with decreased or absent bowel sounds. On x-ray, the wall of the small intestine may appear edematous, transit of barium is slowed, and fluid levels may be seen. An abdominal operation may precipitate an acute attack of FMF, which may be confused with other postoperative complications.

Chest Pain Most patients with abdominal attacks have referred chest pain at one time or another, and 75 percent also develop acute pleuritic pain with or without abdominal symptoms. In 30 percent, the attacks of pleuritis precede the onset of abdominal attacks by varying periods of time, and a small number of patients never develop abdominal attacks. Chest pain is usually unilateral and is associated with diminished breath sounds, a friction rub, or a transient pleural effusion.

Joint Pain In Israel, 75 percent of patients report at least one episode of acute arthritis. Arthritis can be distinct from abdominal or pleural attacks, can be acute or, rarely, chronic, and may involve one or several joints. Effusions are common, with large joints most frequently involved. Radiologic findings are nonspecific. Despite careful search, frank arthritis rarely has been seen in the United States. Some patients have a history of rheumatic fever–like illness in childhood, but in a large series of patients, including 30 from the Middle East, acute arthritis was not observed. Mild arthralgia is common during acute attacks but is nonspecific.

Skin Manifestations Skin involvement occurs in a third of patients. These lesions consist of painful, erythematous areas of swelling from 5 to 20 cm in diameter, usually located on the lower legs, the medial malleolus, or the dorsum of the foot. They may occur without abdominal or pleural pain and subside within 24 to 48 h.

Other Signs and Symptoms Involvement of other serosal membranes has been reported, but pericarditis and meningitis are rare. Hematuria, splenomegaly, and small white dots called *colloid bodies* in the ocular fundus are findings of questionable significance. Rarely migraine-like headaches accompany acute abdominal attacks, and some patients have become somewhat irrational or show extreme emotional lability during attacks. Whether these are primary manifestations of FMF or secondary effects of pain and fever is unclear.

Complications Depression and lack of motivation are common, and patients with FMF require considerable support. A striking number of patients have developed gallbladder disease.

Amyloidosis has been reported in Israel, North Africa, and elsewhere in the Middle East, but its occurrence is rare in the United States. These findings are even more striking because there are probably as many known FMF patients in the United States as in Israel. Thus, environmental or nutritional, as well as genetic, factors may play a role in the development of amyloidosis in FMF.

LABORATORY FINDINGS Polymorphonuclear leukocytosis ranging from 10,000 to 30,000 cells/μL is almost invariable during acute attacks. The erythrocyte sedimentation rate is elevated during

attacks but returns to normal between attacks. Plasma fibrinogen, serum haptoglobin, ceruloplasmin, and C-reactive protein increase during the episodes. Plasma lipids are normal, and there are no consistent abnormalities of hepatic or renal function. When amyloidosis is present, laboratory findings are typical of a nephrotic syndrome followed by renal insufficiency.

DIAGNOSIS When the typical acute attacks of FMF occur in an individual of appropriate ethnic background with a family history of FMF, the diagnosis is easy. When a patient is seen for the first time, a variety of other febrile illnesses must be excluded, such as acute appendicitis, pancreatitis, porphyria, cholecystitis, intestinal obstruction, and other major abdominal catastrophes.

Some inherited hyperlipidemias may mimic the clinical picture of FMF, but lipid analysis will eliminate them from consideration. The FMF patient is not immune to other diseases, and when an attack differs from the usual pattern or is more prolonged, consideration should be given to other diagnostic possibilities. The pleural form of the disease is sometimes difficult to differentiate from acute pulmonary infection or infarction, but the rapid disappearance of signs and symptoms resolves the problem. The erythema is sometimes difficult to differentiate from superficial thrombophlebitis or cellulitis.

The most difficult diagnostic problem in FMF is the patient who presents with fever alone. In this situation, an extensive diagnostic workup for fever of unknown origin may be required. Fortunately, such patients are rare, and all eventually develop serosal involvement. Until specific diagnostic tests for FMF are available, patients with recurrent fever but without signs of inflammation of one of the serosal membranes should not be categorized as having FMF.

PROGNOSIS Despite the severity of the symptoms during some acute attacks, most patients are remarkably free of debilitation between attacks and are able to lead fairly normal lives. The greatest hazard to patients is prolonged periods of hospitalization due to erroneous diagnoses or failure to understand the disease. In the United States, the prognosis of patients with FMF does not seem to be different from that of patients with other chronic nonfatal illnesses. Death usually results from causes unrelated to the underlying disease.

In the past, approximately 25 percent of FMF patients in Israel developed amyloidosis, and this complication usually led to death. However, the widespread use of colchicine has resulted in dramatically decreasing the incidence of amyloidosis.

℞ TREATMENT

Among the therapies tried have been antibiotics, hormones (including estrogens and glucocorticoids), antipyretic drugs, immunotherapy, psychotherapy, elimination and low-fat diets, chloroquine, and phenylbutazone. When carefully studied and followed up, none of these therapies proved effective.

During the past 25 years, the outlook of patients with FMF has been altered dramatically. In 1972, Goldfinger showed that the prophylactic use of colchicine dramatically reduced the number of attacks. Subsequently, controlled trials in the United States and Israel have shown that chronic administration of colchicine greatly reduces the number of acute attacks of FMF. It is recommended that 0.6 mg colchicine be taken by mouth three times a day. Patients often develop gastrointestinal side effects with this dose, however, in which case the dose should be reduced to 0.6 mg taken twice a day. Although an occasional patient will respond to 0.6 mg taken only once a day, this amount is less likely to be beneficial. Most FMF patients will respond favorably to colchicine prophylaxis.

BIBLIOGRAPHY

DISORDERS OF MOTILITY

Colemont LJ, Camilleri M: Chronic intestinal pseudo-obstruction: Diagnosis and treatment. Mayo Clin Proc 64:60, 1989

Drossman DA, Thompson WG: The irritable bowel syndrome: Review and a graduated multicomponent treatment approach. Ann Intern Med 116:1009, 1992

Goyal RK, Hirano I: Mechanisms of disease: The enteric nervous system. N Engl J Med 334:1106, 1996

Johnson LR (ed): *Physiology of the Gastrointestinal Tract*, 2d ed. New York, Raven Press, 1987

Kellow JE, Malcolm A: Motility. Curr Opin Gastroenterol 12:134, 1996

Lynn RB, Friedman LS: Irritable bowel syndrome. Managing the patient with abdominal pain and altered bowel habits. Med Clin North Am 79:373, 1995

Preston DM, Lennard-Jones JE: Severe chronic constipation of young women: Idiopathic slow transit constipation. Gut 27:41, 1986

DIVERTICULAR DISEASES

Brian JE, Stair JM: Non-colonic diverticular disease. Surg Gynecol Obstet 161:189, 1985

Stefansson T et al: Increased risk of left sided colon cancer in patients with diverticular disease. Gut 34:499, 1993

Thompson WG, Patel DG: Clinical picture of diverticular disease of the colon. Clin Gastroenterol 15:903, 1986

INTESTINAL ISCHEMIA AND ANGIODYSPLASIA

Clavin PA: Diagnosis and management of mesenteric infarction. Br J Surg 77:601, 1990

Kitchens CS: Evolution of our understanding of the pathophysiology of primary mesenteric venous thrombosis. Am J Surg 163:346, 1992

Naveau S et al: Long-term results of treatment of vascular malformation of the gastrointestinal tract by neodynium YAG laser photocoagulation. Dig Dis Sci 35:821, 1990

Sargeant IR et al: Laser ablation of upper gastrointestinal vascular ectasias: Long term results. Gut 34:470, 1993

Van Cutsem et al: Treatment of bleeding gastrointestinal vascular malformations with oestrogen-progesterone. Lancet I:953, 1990

PERITONEAL AND MESENTERIC DISEASES

Gortine SR: Treatment of benign anal disease with topical nitroglycerine. Dis Colon Rectum 38:453, 1995

Press OW et al: Evaluation and management of chylous ascites. Ann Intern Med 96:358, 1982

Schwartz SI et al: *Principles of Surgery*, 6th ed. New York, McGraw-Hill, 1994

Tito L et al: Spontaneous bacterial peritonitis. Hepatology 8:27, 1988

Yamada T et al (eds): *Textbook of Gastroenterology*, 2d ed. Philadelphia, Lippincott, 1995

FAMILIAL MEDITERRANEAN FEVER

Daniels M et al: Familial Mediterranean fever: High gene frequency among the Jewish populations in Israel. Am J Med Genet 55:311, 1995

Dinarello CA et al: Colchicine therapy for familial Mediterranean fever. A double-blind trial. N Engl J Med 291:934, 1974

Meyerhoff J: Familial Mediterranean fever: Report of a large family, review of the literature, and discussion of the frequency of amyloidosis. Medicine 59:66, 1980

Pras E et al: Mapping of a gene causing familial Mediterranean fever to the short arm of chromosome 16. N Engl J Med 326:1509, 1992

Zemer D et al: Colchicine in the prevention and treatment of the amyloidosis of familial Mediterranean fever. N Engl J Med 314:1001, 1986

289

William Silen

ACUTE INTESTINAL OBSTRUCTION

ETIOLOGY AND CLASSIFICATION Intestinal obstruction may be *mechanical* or *nonmechanical* (resulting from neuromuscular disturbances that produce either *adynamic* or *dynamic ileus*). The causes of mechanical obstruction of the lumen are conveniently divided into (1) lesions *extrinsic* to the intestine, e.g., adhesive bands, internal and external hernias; (2) lesions *intrinsic* to the wall of the intestine, e.g., diverticulitis, carcinoma, regional enteritis; and (3) obturation of the lumen, e.g., gallstone obstruction, intussusception. Clinically, however, it is most useful to consider whether the obstructive mechanism involves the small or large intestine, because the causes, symptoms, and treatments are different (see below). Adhesions and external hernias are the most common causes of obstruction of the small intestine, constituting 70 to 75 percent of cases of this type. Adhesions, however, almost never produce obstruction of the colon, whereas carcinoma, sigmoid diverticulitis, and volvulus, in that order, are the most common causes and together account for about 90 percent of the cases. Primary intestinal pseudoobstruction (see Chap. 288) is a chronic motility disorder that frequently mimics mechanical obstruction. Unnecessary operations in such patients should be avoided.

Adynamic ileus is probably the most common overall cause of obstruction. The development of this condition is mediated via the hormonal component of the sympathoadrenal system. Adynamic ileus may occur after any peritoneal insult, and its severity and duration will be dependent to some degree on the type of peritoneal injury. Hydrochloric acid, colonic contents, and pancreatic enzymes are among the most irritating substances, whereas blood and urine are less so. Adynamic ileus occurs to some degree after any abdominal operation. Retroperitoneal hematomas, particularly associated with vertebral fracture, commonly cause severe adynamic ileus, and the latter may occur with other retroperitoneal conditions, such as ureteral calculus or severe pyelonephritis. Thoracic diseases, including lower-lobe pneumonia, fractured ribs, and myocardial infarction, frequently produce adynamic ileus, as do electrolyte disturbances, particularly potassium depletion. Finally, intestinal ischemia, whether the result of vascular occlusion or intestinal distention itself, may perpetuate an adynamic ileus.

Spastic ileus or *dynamic ileus* is very uncommon and results from extreme and prolonged contraction of the intestine. It has been observed in heavy metal poisoning, uremia, porphyria, and extensive intestinal ulcerations.

PATHOPHYSIOLOGY Distention of the intestine is caused by the accumulation of gas and fluid proximal to and within the obstructed segment. Between 70 and 80 percent of intestinal gas consists of swallowed air, and because this is composed mainly of nitrogen, which is poorly absorbed from the intestinal lumen, removal of air by continuous gastric suction is a useful adjunct in the treatment of intestinal distention. The accumulation of fluid proximal to the obstructing mechanism results not only from ingested fluid, swallowed saliva, gastric juice, and biliary and pancreatic secretions but also from interference with normal sodium and water transport. During the first 12 to 24 h of obstruction, there is a marked depression of flux from lumen to blood of sodium and consequently water in the distended proximal intestine. After 24 h, there is movement of sodium and water into the lumen, contributing further to the distention and fluid losses. Intraluminal pressure rises from a normal of 2 to 4 cmH_2O to 8 to 10 cmH_2O. During peristalsis, when simple obstruction or a "closed loop" is present, pressures reach 30 to 60 cmH_2O. Closed-loop obstruction of the small intestine results when the lumen is occluded at two points by a single mechanism such as a hernial ring or adhesive band, thus producing a closed loop whose blood supply is often obstructed at the same time. Strangulation of the loop itself is thus common in association with marked distention proximal to the involved loop. A form of closed-loop obstruction is encountered when complete obstruction of the colon exists in the presence of a competent ileocecal valve (85 percent of individuals). Although the blood supply of the colon is not entrapped within the obstructing mechanism, distention of the cecum is extreme because of its greater diameter (Laplace's law), and impairment of the intramural blood supply is considerable with consequent gangrene of the cecal wall, usually anteriorly. Necrosis of the small intestine may occur by the same mechanism of interference with intramural blood flow when distention is extreme, but this sequence is uncommon in the small intestine. Once impairment of blood supply occurs, bacterial invasion supervenes, and peritonitis develops. The systemic effects of extreme distention include elevation of the diaphragm with restricted ventilation and subsequent atelectasis. Venous return via the inferior vena cava also may be impaired.

The loss of fluids and electrolytes may be extreme and, unless replacement is prompt, leads to hemoconcentration, hypovolemia, renal insufficiency, shock, and death. Vomiting, accumulation of fluids within the lumen by the mechanisms described above, and the sequestration of fluid into the edematous intestinal wall and peritoneal cavity as a result of impairment of venous return from the intestine all contribute to massive loss of fluid and electrolytes, especially potassium. As soon as significant impedance to venous return is present, the intestine becomes severely congested, and blood begins to seep into the intestinal lumen. Blood loss may reach significant levels when long segments of intestine are involved.

SYMPTOMS *Mechanical small-intestinal obstruction* is characterized by cramping midabdominal pain, which tends to be more severe the higher the obstruction. The pain occurs in paroxysms, and the patient is relatively comfortable in the intervals between the pains. Audible borborygmi are often noted by the patient simultaneously with the paroxysms of pain. The pain may become less severe as distention progresses, probably because motility is impaired in the edematous intestine. When strangulation is present, the pain is usually more localized and may be steady and severe without a colicky component, a fact that often causes delay in diagnosis of obstruction. Vomiting is almost invariable, and it is earlier and more profuse the higher the obstruction. The vomitus initially contains bile and mucus and remains as such if the obstruction is high in the intestine. With low ileal obstruction, the vomitus becomes feculent, i.e., orange-brown in color with a foul odor, which results from the overgrowth of bacteria proximal to the obstruction. Hiccups (singultus) are common. Obstipation and failure to pass gas by rectum are invariably present when the obstruction is complete, although some stool and gas may be passed spontaneously or after an enema shortly after onset of the complete obstruction. Diarrhea is occasionally observed in partial obstruction. Blood in the stool is rare but does occur in cases of intussusception. Other than some minor but inconsistent differences in pain patterns noted above, the symptoms of strangulating obstructions cannot be distinguished from those of nonstrangulating obstructions.

Mechanical colonic obstruction produces colicky abdominal pain similar in quality to that of small-intestinal obstruction but of much lower intensity. Complaints of pain are occasionally absent in stoic elderly patients. Vomiting occurs late, if at all, particularly if the ileocecal valve is competent. Paradoxically, feculent vomitus is very rare. A history of recent alterations in bowel habits and blood in the stool is common because carcinoma and diverticulitis are the most frequent causes. Constipation becomes progressive, and obstipation with failure to pass gas ensues. Acute symptoms may develop over a period of a week. Cecal volvulus more closely resembles obstruction of the small intestine clinically, whereas patients with sigmoid volvulus more typically have the picture of colonic obstruction in which marked distention predominates, with relatively less pain.

In *adynamic ileus*, colicky pain is absent, and only discomfort from distention is evident. Vomiting may be frequent but is rarely profuse. It usually consists of gastric contents and bile and is almost never feculent. Complete obstipation may or may not occur. Singultus (hiccups) is common.

PHYSICAL FINDINGS *Abdominal distention* is the hallmark of all forms of intestinal obstruction. It is least marked in cases of obstruction high in the small intestine and most marked in colonic obstruction. Early, especially in closed-loop strangulating small-bowel obstruction, distention may be barely perceptible or absent. Tenderness and rigidity are usually minimal; the temperature is rarely above 37.8°C (100°F) in nonstrangulating obstruction of the small and large intestine. Contrary to popular belief, the same is true of strangulating obstruction until very late, a fact that has often resulted in unfortunate delay in treatment. Signs and symptoms of shock also occur *very late* in strangulating obstruction. The appearance of shock, tenderness, rigidity, and fever often means that there has been contamination of the peritoneum with infected intestinal content. Hernial orifices should always be carefully examined for the presence of a mass. The presence of a palpable abdominal mass usually signifies a closed-loop strangulating small-bowel obstruction because the tense fluid-filled loop is the palpable lesion. Auscultation may reveal loud, high-pitched borborygmi coincident with the colicky pain, but this finding is often absent late in strangulating or nonstrangulating obstruction. A quiet abdomen does not eliminate the possibility of obstruction, nor does it necessarily establish the diagnosis of adynamic ileus.

LABORATORY AND X-RAY FINDINGS Leukocytosis, with shift to the left, usually occurs when strangulation is present, but a normal white blood cell count does not exclude strangulation. Elevation of the serum amylase level is encountered occasionally in all forms of intestinal obstruction, especially the strangulating variety.

The x-ray is extremely valuable but under certain circumstances also may be misleading. In nonstrangulating complete small-bowel obstruction, x-rays are almost completely reliable. Distention of fluid- and gas-filled loops of small intestine usually arranged in a "stepladder" pattern with air-fluid levels and an absence or paucity of colonic gas are pathognomonic (Fig. 289-1). These findings, however, are absent in slightly over half the cases of strangulating small-bowel obstruction, especially early in the disease. A general haze due to peritoneal fluid and sometimes a "coffee bean"–shaped mass are seen in strangulating obstruction. Occasionally, the films are normal, but when symptoms are consistent with obstruction of the small intestine, a normal film should suggest strangulation. Roentgenographic differentiation of partial mechanical small-bowel obstruction from adynamic ileus may be impossible because gas is present in both the small and large intestines; however, colonic distention is usually more prominent in adynamic ileus. A radiopaque dye given by mouth is useful in making this distinction.

Colonic obstruction with a competent ileocecal valve is easily recognized because distention with gas is mainly confined to the colon. Barium enema, sigmoidoscopy, or colonoscopy, depending on the suspected site of obstruction, is usually advisable to determine the nature of the lesion, except when concomitant perforation is suspected,

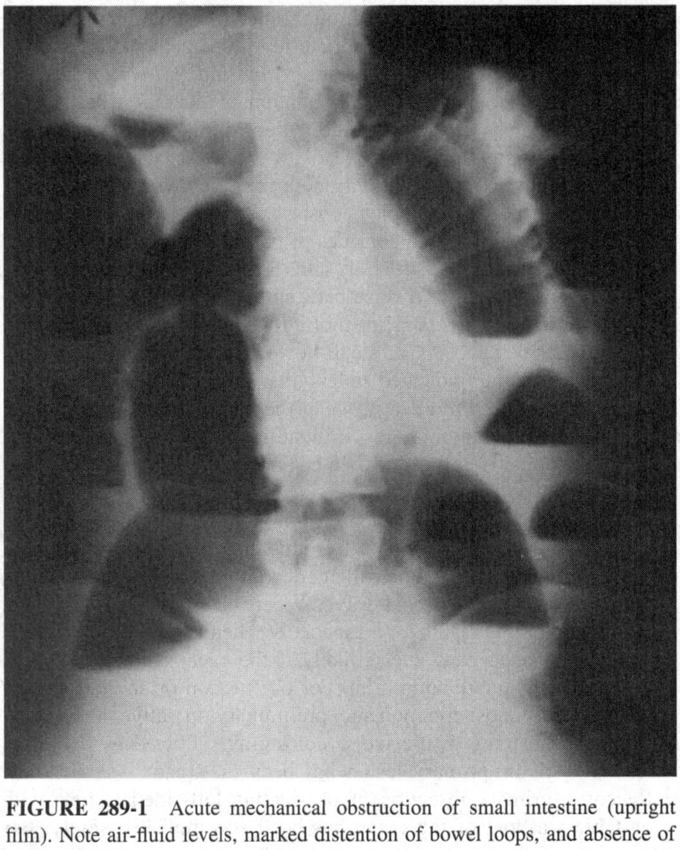

FIGURE 289-1 Acute mechanical obstruction of small intestine (upright film). Note air-fluid levels, marked distention of bowel loops, and absence of colonic gas.

a rare occurrence. Sigmoidoscopy may be therapeutic in cases of sigmoid volvulus. When the ileocecal valve is incompetent, the films resemble those of partial small-bowel obstruction or adynamic ileus, and barium enema or colonoscopy is necessary to establish the correct diagnosis. Barium given by mouth is perfectly safe when obstruction is in the small intestine, since the barium sulfate does not become inspissated in this location. *Barium should never be given by mouth to a patient with possible colonic obstruction* until that possibility has been excluded by barium enema.

℞ TREATMENT

Small-Intestinal Obstruction The overall mortality rate for obstruction of the small intestine is about 10 percent, even under the most optimal conditions. While the mortality rate for nonstrangulating obstruction is as low as 5 to 8 percent, that for strangulating obstruction has been reported to be between 20 and 75 percent. Well over half the deaths from small-bowel obstruction occur in those with strangulation; however, the latter constitute only one-fourth to one-third of the cases. Careful studies indicate that the clinical, laboratory, and x-ray findings are not reliable in distinguishing strangulating from nonstrangulating obstruction when obstruction is complete. Complete obstruction is suggested when there has been a total cessation in the passage of gas or stool per rectum and when gas is absent in the distal intestine by x-ray. Since strangulating small-bowel obstruction is always complete, operation should always be undertaken in such patients after suitable preparation. Prior to operation, fluid and electrolyte balance should be restored and decompression instituted by means of a nasogastric tube. Replacement of potassium is especially important because intake is nil and losses in vomitus are large. Six to eight hours of preparation may be necessary. During this period, broad-spectrum antibiotics are indicated if strangulation is felt to be likely, but operation should not be delayed unless there is unequivocal clinical and roentgenographic evidence of resolution of the obstruction during the period of preparation. Attempts to pass a long tube into the small intestine usually fail while putting the patient through uncomfortable, unproductive manipulations that delay appropriate fluid replacement and decompression. *There are probably few, if any, indications for the use of a long intestinal tube*. Procrastination of operation because of improvement in well-being of the patient during resuscitation and gastric decompression usually leads to unnecessary and hazardous delay in proper treatment. Purely nonoperative therapy is safe only in the presence of incomplete obstruction and is best utilized in patients with (1) repeated episodes of partial obstruction, (2) recent postoperative partial obstruction, and (3) partial obstruction following a recent episode of diffuse peritonitis.

Colonic Obstruction The mortality rate for colonic obstruction is about 20 percent. As in small-bowel obstruction, nonoperative treatment is contraindicated unless the obstruction is incomplete. Occasionally, but not always, when the obstruction is incomplete, nonoperative therapy may result in sufficient decompression that a definitive operative procedure can be undertaken at a later date. This usually can be accomplished by discontinuation of all oral intake and perhaps by nasogastric suction, although attempts to decompress a *completely* obstructed colon by intubation are almost invariably futile. A long intestinal tube will not decompress an obstructed colon with a competent ileocecal valve. When obstruction is complete, early operation is mandatory, especially when the ileocecal valve is competent; cecal gangrene is likely if the cecal diameter exceeds 10 cm on plain abdominal film. For obstruction on the left side of the colon, the most common site, preliminary operative decompression by cecostomy or transverse colostomy followed by definitive resection of the primary lesion has been the treatment of choice. Recently, primary resection of obstructing left-sided lesions with on-table washout of the colon has been accomplished safely. For a lesion of the right or transverse colon, primary resection and anastomosis can be performed safely because distention of the ileum with consequent discrepancy in size and hazard in suture are not present.

Adynamic Ileus This type of ileus usually responds to nonoperative continuous decompression and adequate treatment of the primary disease. The prognosis is usually good. Successful decompression of severe colonic ileus has been accomplished by colonoscopy, but this should be avoided if tenderness in the right lower quadrant suggests possible cecal gangrene. Rarely, adynamic colonic distention may become so great that cecostomy is required if cecal gangrene is feared. Spastic ileus usually responds to treatment of the primary disease.

BIBLIOGRAPHY

Bulkley GB et al: Intraoperative determination of small intestinal viability following ischemic injury: Prospective controlled trial of two adjuvant methods (Doppler and fluorescein) compared with standard clinical judgement. Ann Surg 193:628, 1981

Dubois A et al: Postoperative ileus: Physiopathology, etiology and treatment. Ann Surg 178:781, 1973

Eskelinen M et al: Contributions of history-taking, physical examination, and computer assistance to diagnosis of acute small-bowel obstruction. A prospective study of 1333 patients with acute abdominal pain. Scand J Gastroenterol 29:715, 1994

Hofsetter SR: Acute adhesive obstruction of the small intestine. Surg Gynecol Obstet 152:141, 1981

Jackson BR: The diagnosis of colonic obstruction. Dis Colon Rectum 25:603, 1982

Peschiera JL, Beerman SP: Intestinal dysfunction associated with acute thoracolumbar fractures. Orthop Rev 19:284, 1990

Silen W: *Cope's Early Diagnosis of the Acute Abdomen*, 18th ed. London, Oxford, 1991

290

William Silen

ACUTE APPENDICITIS

INCIDENCE AND EPIDEMIOLOGY The maximum incidence of acute appendicitis occurs in the second and third decades of life. While the disease may be encountered at any time of life, it is relatively rare at the extremes of age. Males and females are equally affected, except between puberty and age 25, when males predominate in a 3:2 ratio. Perforation is relatively much more common in infancy and in the aged, during which periods mortality rates are highest. The mortality rate has decreased steadily in Europe and the United States from 8.1 per 100,000 of the population in 1941 to less than 1 per 100,000 in 1970 and subsequently. The absolute incidence of the disease also decreased by about 40 percent between 1940 and 1960 but since then has remained unchanged. Although various factors such as changing dietary habits, altered intestinal flora, and better nutrition and intake of vitamins have been suggested to explain the reduced incidence, the exact reasons have not been elucidated. The overall incidence of appendicitis is much lower in underdeveloped countries, especially parts of Africa, and in lower socioeconomic groups.

PATHOGENESIS The primary pathogenetic hallmark has always been thought to be luminal obstruction. While obstruction can be identified in 30 to 40 percent of cases, recent studies have shown that ulceration of the mucosa is the initial event in the majority. The causation of the ulceration is unknown, although a viral etiology has been postulated. It has been suggested that infection with *Yersinia* organisms may cause the disease, since high complement fixation titers have been found in as many as 30 percent of cases of proven appendicitis 1 week after operation. Whether the inflammatory reaction attendant with ulceration is sufficient to obstruct the tiny appendiceal lumen even transiently is not clear. Obstruction, when present, is most commonly caused by a fecalith, which results from accumulation and inspissation of fecal matter around vegetable fibers. Enlarged lymphoid follicles associated with viral infections (e.g., measles), inspissated barium, worms (e.g., pinworms, *Ascaris*, and *Taenia*), and tumors (e.g., carcinoid or carcinoma) also may obstruct the lumen. Secretion of mucus distends the organ, which has a capacity of only 0.1 to 0.2 mL, and luminal pressures rise as high as 60 cmH_2O. Luminal bacteria multiply and invade the appendiceal wall as venous engorgement and subsequent arterial compromise result from the high intraluminal pressures. Finally, gangrene and perforation occur. If the process evolves slowly, adjacent organs such as the terminal ileum, cecum, and omentum may wall off the appendiceal area so that a localized abscess will develop, whereas rapid progression of vascular impairment may cause perforation with free access to the peritoneal cavity. Subsequent rupture of primary appendiceal abscesses may produce fistulas between the appendix and bladder, small intestine, sigmoid, or cecum. Occasionally, acute appendicitis may be the first manifestation of Crohn's disease. While chronic infection of the appendix with tuberculosis, amebiasis, and actinomycosis may occur, a useful clinical aphorism states that *chronic appendiceal inflammation is not usually the cause of prolonged abdominal pain of weeks' or months' duration.* In contrast, it is clear that recurrent acute appendicitis does occur, often with complete resolution of inflammation and symptoms between attacks. Recurrent acute appendicitis may become more frequent as antibiotics are dispensed more freely and if a long appendiceal stump becomes more prevalent as laparoscopic appendectomy is used more often.

CLINICAL MANIFESTATIONS The history and sequence of symptoms are among the most important diagnostic features of appendicitis. The initial symptom is almost invariably *abdominal pain* of the visceral type, resulting from appendiceal contractions or distention of the lumen. It is usually poorly localized in the periumbilical or epigastric region. There is often an accompanying urge to defecate or pass flatus, neither of which relieves the distress. This visceral pain is mild, often cramping, and rarely catastrophic in nature, usually lasting 4 to 6 h, but it may not be noted by stoic individuals or by some patients during sleep. As inflammation spreads to the parietal peritoneal surfaces, the pain becomes somatic, steady, and more severe, aggravated by motion or cough, and usually located in the *right lower quadrant. Anorexia* is so frequent that the presence of hunger should arouse suspicion of the diagnosis of acute appendicitis. *Nausea* and *vomiting* occur in 50 to 60 percent of cases, but vomiting is rarely profuse and protracted. The development of nausea and vomiting before the onset of pain is extremely rare. Change in bowel habit is of little diagnostic value, since any or no alteration may be observed, although the presence of diarrhea caused by an inflamed appendix in juxtaposition to the sigmoid may cause serious diagnostic difficulties. Urinary frequency and dysuria occur if the appendix lies adjacent to the bladder. The typical sequence of symptoms (poorly localized periumbilical pain followed by nausea and vomiting with subsequent shift of pain to the right lower quadrant) occurs in only 50 to 60 percent of patients, and some variations are considered below.

Physical findings vary with time after onset of the illness and according to the location of the appendix, which may be situated deep in the pelvic cul-de-sac; in the right lower quadrant in any relation to the peritoneum, cecum, and small intestine; in the right upper quadrant (especially during pregnancy); or even in the left lower quadrant. *The diagnosis cannot be established unless tenderness can be elicited.* While tenderness is sometimes absent in the early visceral stage of the disease, it ultimately always develops and is found in any location corresponding to the position of the appendix. Abdominal tenderness may be completely absent if a retrocecal or pelvic appendix is present, in which case the sole physical finding may be tenderness in the flank or on rectal or pelvic examination. Percussion, rebound tenderness, and referred rebound tenderness are often, but not invariably, present; they are most likely to be absent early in the illness. Flexion of the right hip and guarded movement by the patient are due to parietal peritoneal involvement. Hyperesthesia of the skin of the right lower quadrant and a positive psoas or obturator sign are often late findings and are rarely of diagnostic value. When the inflamed appendix is in close proximity to the anterior parietal peritoneum, muscular rigidity is present yet is often minimal early. The temperature is usually normal or slightly elevated [37.2 to 38°C (99 to 100.5°F)], but a temperature above 38.3°C (101°F) should always suggest the presence of perforation. Tachycardia is commensurate with the elevation of the temperature. Rigidity and tenderness become more marked as the disease progresses to perforation and localized or diffuse peritonitis. Distention is rare unless severe diffuse peritonitis has developed. The alleged disappearance of pain and tenderness just prior to perforation is extremely unusual. A mass may develop if localized perforation has occurred but usually will not be detectable before 3 days after onset of the disease. Earlier presence of a mass suggests carcinoma of the cecum or Crohn's disease. Perforation is rare before 24 h after onset of symptoms, but the rate may be as high as 80 percent after 48 h.

Laboratory examination does not establish the diagnosis because the latter is based primarily on clinical grounds. Although moderate leukocytosis of 10,000 to 18,000 cells/μL is frequent (with a concomitant shift to immature cells), the absence of leukocytosis does not eliminate the possibility of acute appendicitis. Leukocytosis of greater than 20,000 cells/μL should alert the clinician to the probability of perforation. Anemia and blood in the stool suggest a primary diagnosis of carcinoma of the cecum, especially in elderly individuals. The urine may contain a few white or red blood cells without bacteria if the appendix lies close to the right ureter or bladder.

Urinalysis is most useful, however, in excluding genitourinary conditions that may mimic acute appendicitis. X-rays are rarely of value except when an opaque fecalith (5 percent of patients) is observed in the right lower quadrant (especially in children) together with other clinical findings consistent with appendicitis. Consequently, there is no routine need to obtain films of the abdomen unless there is a possibility of other conditions such as intestinal obstruction or ureteral calculus. In some patients in whom symptoms are either recurrent or more prolonged, a careful barium enema or computed tomography scan may disclose an extrinsic defect on the medial wall of the cecum or a calcified fecalith. The diagnosis also may be established by the ultrasonic demonstration of an enlarged and thick-walled appendix, but if the appendix cannot be seen, the diagnosis cannot be excluded. Ultrasound is most useful to exclude ovarian cysts, ectopic pregnancy, or tuboovarian abscess.

While the typical historical sequence and physical findings are present in 50 to 60 percent of cases, it is obvious that a wide variety of atypical patterns of disease are encountered, especially at the age extremes and during pregnancy. The 70 to 80 percent incidence of perforation and generalized peritonitis in infants under 2 years of age is dramatic testimony to the importance of the history in the early detection of the disease. Any infant or child with diarrhea, vomiting, and abdominal pain is highly suspect. Fever is much more common in this age group, and abdominal distention is often the only physical finding. In the elderly, pain and tenderness are often obtunded, and thus the diagnosis is frequently delayed. A 30 percent incidence of perforation in patients over 70 attests to the importance of this delay. Elderly patients often present themselves initially with a slightly painful mass (a primary appendiceal abscess) or sometimes appear with adhesive intestinal obstruction 5 or 6 days after a previously undetected perforated appendix. Appendicitis occurs about once in every 1000 pregnancies and is the most common extrauterine condition requiring abdominal operation. The diagnosis may be missed or delayed because of the frequent occurrence of mild abdominal discomfort and nausea and vomiting during pregnancy. During the last trimester, when the mortality rate from appendicitis is highest, uterine displacement of the appendix to the right upper quadrant and laterally leads to confusion in diagnosis because pain and tenderness are similarly displaced.

DIFFERENTIAL DIAGNOSIS A listing of the differential diagnoses of acute appendicitis would produce an encyclopedic compendium of all conditions that cause abdominal pain, since appendicitis may simulate any of these diseases. Diagnostic accuracy is about 75 to 80 percent for experienced clinicians and must be based solely on the clinical criteria outlined above. It is probably better to err slightly in the direction of overdiagnosis, since delay is associated with perforation and increased morbidity and mortality. In unperforated appendicitis, the mortality rate is 0.1 percent, little more than that associated with general anesthesia; for perforated appendicitis, there is an overall mortality of 3 percent, a figure that increases to 15 percent in the elderly. In doubtful cases, 4 to 6 h of observation is always more beneficial than harmful, however. The most common conditions discovered at operation when acute appendicitis is erroneously diagnosed are, in rough order of frequency, mesenteric lymphadenitis, no organic disease, acute pelvic inflammatory disease, ruptured graafian follicle or corpus luteum cyst, and acute gastroenteritis. In addition, acute cholecystitis, perforated ulcer, acute pancreatitis, acute diverticulitis, strangulating intestinal obstruction, ureteral calculus, and pyelonephritis frequently present diagnostic difficulties.

It is useful to consider separately some of the more common and difficult diagnostic possibilities, especially in the female. Differentiation of *pelvic inflammatory disease* from acute appendicitis may be virtually impossible. Gram-negative intracellular diplococci on cervical smear are not pathognomonic unless *Neisseria gonorrhoeae* can be cultured. Pain on movement of the cervix is not specific and may occur in appendicitis if perforation has occurred or if the appendix lies adjacent to the uterus or adnexa. *Rupture of a graafian follicle* (mittelschmerz) occurs at midcycle with spill of blood and fluid to produce pain and tenderness more diffuse and usually of a less severe degree than in appendicitis. Fever and leukocytosis are usually absent. *Rupture of a corpus luteum cyst* is identical clinically to rupture of a graafian follicle but develops about the time of menstruation. The presence of an adnexal mass, evidence of blood loss, and a positive pregnancy test help differentiate *ruptured tubal pregnancy*, but a negative pregnancy test is present when tubal abortion has occurred. *Twisted ovarian cyst* and *endometriosis* occasionally are difficult to distinguish from appendicitis. In all these female conditions, ultrasonic examination of the pelvis and laparoscopy may be of great value.

Acute mesenteric lymphadenitis is the appellation usually given when enlarged, slightly reddened lymph nodes at the root of the mesentery and a normal appendix are encountered at operation in a patient who usually has right lower quadrant tenderness and a somewhat higher temperature than most patients with acute appendicitis. Whether this is a single, discrete entity is unclear, since the causative factor is not known. It has been recognized that some of these patients have infection with *Y. pseudotuberculosis* or *Y. enterocolytica*, in which case the diagnosis can be established by culture of the mesenteric nodes or by serologic titers (see Chap. 164). The diagnosis is essentially impossible clinically, although retrospectively there often appears to have been more diffuse pain and tenderness. Children seem to be affected more frequently than adults. Operation should be undertaken unless there is rapid resolution of all symptoms and findings. *Acute gastroenteritis* usually causes profuse watery diarrhea, often with nausea and vomiting, but without localized findings. Between cramps, the abdomen is completely relaxed. In *Salmonella* gastroenteritis, the abdominal findings are similar, although the pain may be more severe and more localized, and fever and chills are common. The occurrence of similar symptoms among other members of the family may be helpful. When the diagnosis of acute pelvic appendicitis with perforation has been missed, gastroenteritis is the most common previous working diagnosis. Persistent abdominal or rectal tenderness should eliminate the diagnosis of gastroenteritis. *Regional enteritis* (Crohn's disease) is usually associated with a more prolonged history, often with previous exacerbations regarded by the patient or physician as episodes of gastroenteritis unless the diagnosis has been established previously. *Meckel's diverticulitis* usually cannot be distinguished from acute appendicitis but is very rare.

℞ TREATMENT

Cathartics and enemas should be avoided if appendicitis is under consideration, and antibiotics should not be administered when the diagnosis is in question, since they will only mask the presence or development of perforation. The treatment is early operation and appendectomy as soon as the patient can be prepared. Appendectomy is increasingly accomplished laparoscopically, but there is no demonstrable value of this technique over open operation except where a diagnostic dilemma exists. Preparation rarely takes more than 1 to 2 h in early appendicitis but may require 6 to 8 h in cases of severe sepsis and dehydration associated with late perforation. The *only* circumstance in which operation is *not* indicated is the presence of a palpable mass 3 to 5 days after the onset of symptoms. Should operation be undertaken at that time, a phlegmon rather than a definitive abscess will be found, and complications from dissection of such a phlegmon are frequent. Such patients treated with broad-spectrum antibiotics, parenteral fluids, and rest usually show resolution of the mass and symptoms within 1 week. *Interval appendectomy* can and should be done safely 3 months later. Should the mass enlarge or the patient become more toxic, drainage of the abscess is necessary. The complications of subphrenic, pelvic, or other intra-abdominal abscesses usually follow perforation with generalized peritonitis and can be avoided by early diagnosis of the disease.

BIBLIOGRAPHY

Butler C: Surgical pathology of acute appendicitis. Hum Pathol 12:870, 1981

Sarfati MR et al: Impact of adjunctive testing on the diagnosis and clinical course of patients with acute appendicitis. Am J Surg 166:660, 1993

Tate JJ et al: Conventional versus laparoscopic surgery for acute appendicitis. Br J Surg 80:761, 1993

Wade DS et al: Accuracy of ultrasound in the diagnosis of acute appendicitis compared with the surgeon's clinical impression. Arch Surg 128:1039, 1993

SECTION 2
LIVER AND BILIARY TRACT DISEASE

291 APPROACH TO THE PATIENT WITH LIVER DISEASE

Kurt J. Isselbacher, Daniel K. Podolsky

BIOLOGIC CONSIDERATIONS An understanding of diseases of the liver and their clinical manifestations can be derived from a knowledge of fundamental normal hepatic structure and function. An appreciation of anatomic aspects of the liver and biliary tree from the gross level to that of the individual hepatocyte and other cellular constituents is needed to understand the spectrum of clinical manifestations of liver disease. The dual blood supply, unique to the liver and including the portal venous system, makes the liver an intermediate filter for most of the venous drainage of the abdominal viscera. This often leads to secondary hepatic involvement in a number of extrahepatic diseases and makes the liver a relatively common site of solid tumor metastases. Furthermore, an appreciation of the relevant anatomy, especially that of the portal venous system, is important in understanding clinically important manifestations of portal hypertension, a common complication of chronic liver disease when scarring and regeneration lead to distortion of the intrahepatic microvasculature. These anatomic considerations lead the clinician to look for evidence of splenic enlargement and hypersplenism, gastrointestinal bleeding, accumulation of ascites, and signs of portal-systemic encephalopathy. An understanding of the anatomy of the biliary tract from canaliculus to common bile duct is integral to understanding the basis and sequelae of obstructive jaundice. While inflammation of the gallbladder may lead to fever and pain, choledocholithiasis will cause biliary colic as well as jaundice. Diffuse processes affecting the intrahepatic ducts, such as primary sclerosing cholangitis, will lead to cholestasis and its attendant symptoms, while a focal process affecting a single branch of the biliary tree, such as a neoplasm, usually will not.

The structural organization at a level intermediate between the gross anatomic and the cellular also contributes to the clinical patterns seen with disorders of the liver. While various concepts have been offered, the most useful is that of the traditional liver lobule. Blood emanates from the portal venules at the periphery and passes through the hepatic sinusoids to the central vein. The portal venules, terminal bile ductules, and hepatic arterioles are arranged in a *triad*. Appreciation of this organization and the presence of concentric zones of function within the lobule explain distinct patterns of injury such as the centrilobular injury resulting from ischemia. These structural features no doubt also provide the basis for the relative preservation of hepatocellular function in many disorders that can lead to significant portal hypertension, such as schistosomiasis and biliary cirrhosis.

As important as the anatomic features are in understanding liver disease, many liver disorders and their manifestations can only be appreciated in the context of the functional complexity of the liver at the cellular level. As detailed in Chap. 293, the hepatocyte plays an important role in diverse general metabolic processes that may be deranged as a consequence of liver disease. In addition, this metabolic diversity leads to hepatic involvement in many inborn errors of metabolism, including a wide variety of storage diseases, and less well-understood disorders of iron metabolism (hemosiderosis and hemochromatosis) and copper homeostasis (Wilson's disease).

Some other functional aspects also should be emphasized. The hepatocyte modifies numerous endogenous (e.g., bilirubin) and exogenous (e.g., alcohol, acetaminophen) potentially toxic compounds through oxidation, reduction, and conjugation carried out by several enzymes of the endoplasmic reticulum. Conjugation of substrates generally facilitates their hepatic excretion, converting water-insoluble substances to water-soluble derivatives. It is therefore not surprising that parenchymal liver disease may lead to either conjugated or unconjugated hyperbilirubinemia and jaundice. Metabolic modifications may significantly alter the pharmacologic activity of drugs through formation of derivatives with either decreased or enhanced activity. These metabolic processes may create intermediates that are toxic to the liver itself. This explains the selective susceptibility of the liver to the toxicity of carbon tetrachloride, acetaminophen, and, most important, alcohol, which is converted initially to acetaldehyde.

Additional functions of the hepatocyte that may have significant clinical ramifications include the production of a variety of soluble proteins for secretion into the circulation and the presence of receptors specific for various circulating ligands. The latter is a property shared with the Kupffer cell, which fulfills much of its function as a constituent of the reticuloendothelial system by clearing a number of serum glycoproteins through asialoglycoprotein receptor–mediated endocytosis. There is evidence to suggest that some of the substances taken up by this endocytotic mechanism may subsequently pass to and through the hepatocyte to complete an enterohepatic circulation. Carcinoembryonic antigen (CEA) is a glycoprotein and tumor-associated marker that is handled in this manner, leading to artifactual elevations in hepatobiliary disease. In contrast to the Kupffer cell, the spectrum of ligands taken up by hepatocytes via specific receptors is much broader. In addition to ligands targeted for lysosomal degradation, the hepatocyte possesses receptors for ligands that are metabolically active after their uptake and dissociation from their receptors. These include transferrin-bound iron and, most important, low-density lipoprotein, which contributes to regulation of overall body cholesterol metabolism. Disruption of lysosomal degradation of specific ligands in hereditary storage disease leads to hepatomegaly and a variety of infiltrative disorders. Disruption of the nonlysosomal endocytotic pathway ligands can lead to systemic disorders. It is not clear whether specific receptors or other hepatocyte membrane components play a role in the relative or absolute tropism of infectious agents (particularly the hepatitis viruses) that account for a large proportion of both acute and chronic liver disease. However, the relative selectivity of the hepatitis viruses (A, B, C, E, and indirectly D) for the hepatocyte is essential in understanding the clinical features of the illnesses caused by these agents, which derive from the extent of hepatocyte destruction, largely due to immune destruction rather than direct cytopathic effects of the virus. At the same time, the hepatocyte may be infected by less strictly organotropic agents including other viruses (e.g., Epstein-Barr virus) and a wide variety of bacterial and parasitic organisms. The vascular supply of the liver leads to its frequent involvement in disseminated infections.

A final feature of hepatocyte cell biology that contributes to the expression of liver disease is the potential for proliferation and regeneration. Although few mitotic figures are seen in normal hepatic parenchyma, rapid regeneration involving both proliferation and cellular hypertrophy occurs following hepatic resection in experimental animals and humans. The capacity for hepatocellular regeneration is evident in the complete recovery that usually occurs following fulminant hepatitis (due either to viral or toxic agents) if the patient can be sustained through the period of acute injury. Architecturally disordered regeneration in concert with fibrosis is an essential factor in the development of cirrhosis and leads both to disruption of blood flow through the hepatic parenchyma and to uneven hepatocellular function due to distortion of normal lobular structure.

CLINICAL CONSIDERATIONS In approaching the patient with known or suspected liver disease, consideration of the patient's problem in the context of a few salient questions permits the clinician to focus on the most important diagnostic possibilities and the severity of the illness. Is the problem primarily hepatocellular or cholestatic? Was the onset of the illness abrupt or gradual? Has the problem led to clinically significant impairment of normal hepatocellular function, such as signs of altered mentation or coagulopathy? Are there signs or symptoms of portal hypertension? Important and reliable clues that address these questions often may be obtained from a careful history and physical examination.

Clinical History A number of historic features may distinguish cholestatic and hepatocellular disease processes. A history of marked right upper quadrant pain or previous indigestion suggests cholelithiasis, cholecystitis, or choledocholithiasis, whereas vague, nagging discomfort suggests hepatocellular or infiltrative disease with hepatomegaly causing pain due to acute distention of Glisson's capsule. Additional important symptoms that should be elicited include pruritus, jaundice, anorexia, weight loss, and fever. Complaints of easy bruising or mental confusion by the patient (or family) should be regarded as ominous signs of either fulminant acute or advanced chronic liver disease.

Family history is important with respect to jaundice, anemia, splenectomy, or cholecystectomy; a positive history may be helpful in diagnosing hemolytic anemia, congenital or familial hyperbilirubinemia, or gallstones. *Occupation* should be reviewed in detail, and *environmental factors* need to be examined. Note should be made of the use of any medications or exposure to known or putative toxins such as carbon tetrachloride, beryllium, or vinyl chloride. The patient should be asked about travel to other countries, especially to areas where hepatitis may be endemic. Careful questioning regarding alcohol intake is important in most cases. Since the alcoholic often denies or understates the amounts consumed, it may be desirable to check the validity of the history with relatives or close friends. History of concomitant use of acetaminophen and alcohol may be particularly important.

Contact with jaundiced patients (especially intimate or sexual relations) should be noted. If the patient has had any *injections*, hepatitis B or C infection may be the underlying disease. Injections include blood or plasma transfusions, tattooing, and dental treatment. Postoperative jaundice may be due to the anesthetic, especially after multiple uses of halothane, or to impaired hepatic excretory function resulting from relative hypoxemia of liver cells during the operative or postoperative period.

As suggested, the manner of the *onset of the illness* should be ascertained. The relatively abrupt onset of nausea, anorexia, and aversion to smoking followed by progressive jaundice suggests viral hepatitis. A gradual development of jaundice associated with pruritus suggests cholestasis. Intermittent right upper quadrant abdominal pain followed by cholestatic jaundice points to gallstone disease, while the gradual onset of painless jaundice with weight loss is suggestive of tumor, such as carcinoma of the head of the pancreas. Jaundice associated with fever and chills makes cholangitis and extrahepatic biliary obstruction likely possibilities. The awareness of progressive abdominal swelling, perhaps first noticed because of tightness of clothing, suggests ascites, which may be due to malignancy or an insidious first manifestation of cirrhosis. The patient with hepatitis generally feels ill, and dark urine and light stools occur before the appearance of scleral or skin icterus. In cholestatic hepatitis, the patient may feel relatively well and complain only of symptoms due to the obstruction, such as pruritus.

Physical Examination Jaundice is looked for in the sclera as well as the skin. Pallor indicative of anemia may be a reflection of hemolysis, cirrhosis, or neoplasm. Significant cachexia, especially of the extremities, may be associated with cancer or cirrhosis. In the cirrhotic patient, one should look for stigmata of alcohol abuse such as parotid and lacrimal gland enlargement and Dupuytren's contracture, as well as other features of cirrhosis, such as gynecomastia, testicular atrophy, and diminished axillary or pubic hair.

The *skin examination* may reveal ecchymoses due to prothrombin deficiency or purpura due to thrombocytopenia. *Palmar erythema* or *spider angiomas* may reflect acute or chronic liver disease. Spider angiomas are usually found above the umbilicus and especially on the face, neck, shoulders, forearms, and dorsum of the hands. The presence of a few spider angiomas is not abnormal in women, especially during pregnancy. However, their appearance in men is always abnormal and should be carefully searched for. In chronic cholestasis, *scratch marks*, *finger clubbing*, and *xanthoma* of the eyelids and extensor surfaces of the tendons of the wrists and ankles may be found. A *slate color* to the skin due to increased iron or bronze discoloration resulting from melanin deposition should suggest the presence of hemochromatosis.

Evaluation of the *mental state* and *neurologic function* is important. Slight deterioration of the intellect and minimal personality changes may suggest hepatocellular disease or the presence of portal-systemic venous shunts, but care must be taken to exclude other causes such as neurologic disease. The presence of flapping tremor of the hands (asterixis) may be found in association with portal-systemic encephalopathy or impending hepatic coma.

Abdominal examination may reveal ascites, which, together with dilated periumbilical veins, suggests cirrhosis and extensive portal collateral circulation. If additional features of liver disease are lacking, malignancy must be considered more seriously. A very large, nodular, and rock-hard liver suggests the presence of hepatoma or hepatic metastases. Careful percussion is necessary to evaluate the size of a nonpalpable liver. A small liver may indicate cirrhosis (especially postnecrotic); a small liver that diminishes in size suggests severe hepatitis or massive hepatic necrosis. In the alcoholic, fatty infiltration and cirrhosis often produce a uniform enlargement of the liver. The liver edge is tender in hepatitis, in congestive heart failure, and occasionally in malignant disease and with alcoholism (especially "alcoholic hepatitis").

A palpable, enlarged gallbladder (Courvoisier's sign) suggests extrahepatic biliary obstruction, often due to pancreatic cancer. A tender gallbladder and positive Murphy's sign suggest cholelithiasis or choledocholithiasis. A palpable spleen may indicate hepatitis or cirrhosis; significant splenomegaly may be a reflection of portal hypertension.

Table 291-1

Suggested Guidelines for Ordering Hepatobiliary Imaging Studies in Various Clinical Situations

Clinical Problem	Initial Imaging Study	Supplemental Imaging Studies (if Necessary)
Suspected gallbladder disease	US to detect stones or evidence of acute or chronic cholecystitis Nuclear medicine biliary scan for suspicion of acute cholecystitis	OCG to assess gallbladder function and number of stones CT if abscess suspected
Suspected bile duct abnormalities	US to detect dilatation, stones, or mass ERCP or THC to define ductal anatomy	CT to detect stones or cause of extrinsic compression
Jaundice	US to detect biliary obstruction, liver masses, or obvious hepatic parenchymal disease	CT if dilated ducts to detect obstructing lesion or if suspicion of a mass in the pancreas or porta hepatitis ERCP or THC to determine site and exact cause of dilated ducts
Hepatic parenchymal disease	US ^{99m}TC-labeled sulfur colloid scan MRI	Doppler, color Doppler, or MRI with flow sequences if a vascular abnormality is suspected and in some instances of portal hypertension
Screening for liver mass	US ^{99m}Tc-labeled sulfur colloid scan	MRI
Characterizing known liver mass		
Suspicion of malignancy	US- or CT-directed biopsy	CT portogram MRI Intraoperative US
Suspicion of benign lesion (hemangioma, regenerative nodule, focal nodular hyperplasia, adenoma)	MRI (after detection on US or CT) Nuclear medicine scan (e.g., ^{99m}TC-labeled red blood cell scan for suspected hemangioma)	Angiography US- or CT-directed biopsy
Suspicion of abscess	US or CT US- or CT-directed aspiration	Nuclear medicine abscess scan (gallium or ^{111}In-labeled white blood cell scan)

NOTE: US, ultrasound; OCG, oral cholecystogram; CT, computed tomography; THC, transhepatic cholangiography; ERCP, endoscopic retrograde cholangiopancreatography; MRI, magnetic resonance imaging; Tc, technetium; In, indium.

Table 291-2

Classification of Liver Disease

PARENCHYMAL

1. Hepatitis (viral, drug-induced, toxic, ischemic)
   a. Acute
   b. Chronic (persistent or active)
2. Cirrhosis
   a. Alcoholic (portal, nutritional, Lacnnec's cirrhosis)
   b. Postnecrotic
   c. Biliary
   d. Hemochromatosis
   e. Rare types (e.g., Wilson's disease, galactosemia, cystic fibrosis of pancreas, alpha$_1$-antitrypsin deficiency)
3. Infiltrations
   a. Glycogen
   b. Fat (neutral fat, cholesterol, gangliosides, cerebrosides)
   c. Amyloid
   d. Lymphoma, leukemia
   e. Granuloma (e.g., sarcoidosis, tuberculosis, idiopathic)
4. Space-occupying lesions
   a. Hepatocellular carcinoma, metastatic tumor
   b. Abscess (pyogenic, amoebic)
   c. Cysts (polycystic disease, *Echinococcus*)
   d. Gummas
5. Functional disorders associated with jaundice (hereditary or acquired)
   a. Gilbert's syndrome
   b. Crigler-Najjar syndrome
   c. Dubin-Johnson and Rotor syndromes
   d. Cholestasis of pregnancy and benign recurrent cholestasis

HEPATOBILIARY

1. Extrahepatic biliary obstruction (by stone, stricture, or tumor)
2. Cholangitis (septic, primary biliary cirrhosis, primary sclerosing cholangitis, drug, toxic)

VASCULAR

1. Chronic passive congestion and cardiac cirrhosis
2. Hepatic vein thrombosis (Budd-Chiari syndrome)
3. Portal vein thrombosis
4. Pylophlebitis
5. Arteriovenous malformations
6. Venocclusive disease

Abdominal auscultation may reveal the presence of a venous hum over dilated collateral veins radiating from the umbilicus, the so-called caput medusae. In advanced cirrhosis this venous hum is virtually diagnostic of significant portal hypertension. A bruit may sometimes be heard over large regenerating nodules in cirrhosis and occasionally over hepatomas and metastatic nodules in the liver. A friction rub occasionally may be heard over hepatomas and metastatic liver nodules.

Laboratory Evaluation Serum assays for biochemical markers of liver disease are an integral part of the proper evaluation of liver and biliary tract disease. In general, the serum bilirubin level is measured to confirm the presence and severity of jaundice and determine the extent of bilirubin conjugation. Aminotransferase (transaminase) elevations reflect the severity of active hepatocellular damage, though not necessarily the aggregate severity of liver injury (e.g., aminotransferase levels may actually decline with near-complete hepatic parenchymal destruction), while alkaline phosphatase elevations are found with cholestasis and hepatic infiltrates. Serum albumin level and the prothrombin time are used as indexes of hepatic synthetic function. → *These and other tests are reviewed in Chaps. 45 and 292.*

The further evaluation of patients with hepatobiliary disease should be individualized depending on the history, physical findings, and initial screening laboratory tests. Hepatocellular disease such as hepatitis is often sufficiently clear that only serologic tests are needed. Nonetheless, in many patients, computed tomography (CT), ultrasound, scintiscans, magnetic resonance imaging (MRI), or liver biopsy may be needed to determine the nature of the liver disease. When hepatic tumors are suspected, CT, ultrasound, MRI, or scintiscan may be performed followed by liver biopsy or laparoscopy for a more specific diagnosis. When biliary obstruction is suspected, the first examination is usually an ultrasound study to determine the size of the bile ducts, whether gallstones are present, or whether there is the suggestion of a mass in the head of the pancreas. Frequently, more information is needed, and thus a cholangiogram, performed through the endoscope (endoscopic retrograde cholangiopancreatography) or through percutaneous puncture under ultrasound or CT guidance, should be obtained. An overview of the utilization of imaging studies in the evaluation of patients with suspected hepatic and biliary disorders is provided in Table 291-1. More detailed consideration of imaging modalities is presented in the context of the discussion of specific conditions (Chaps. 302 and 304).

CLASSIFICATION OF LIVER DISEASE No single classification of the various types of liver disease is entirely satisfactory because in many instances the etiology and pathogenetic mechanism are obscure. As a consequence, one finds an abundance of labels and names applied to hepatic disorders. Some individuals use the term *hepatitis* to imply viral infection; others, simply to connote evidence of hepatic inflammation. The often used words *acute*, *subacute*, and *chronic* are ambiguous. *Chronicity* should refer to continuing or recurrent disease (i.e., duration). *Activity* should refer to evidence of the presence of perpetuation of liver cell injury; this is most readily identified by serum transaminase elevations and by the degree of hepatocellular necrosis on biopsy.

Because of the difficulties involved in defining the etiology of many types of liver disease, in most instances the process is best defined and described by an examination of the morphologic character of the lesion. Therefore, a *morphologic classification* of liver disease, as outlined in Table 291-2, appears at present more practical than one based on etiology.

BIBLIOGRAPHY

MILLWARD-SADLER GH et al: *Wright's Liver and Biliary Disease*, 3d ed. London, Saunders, 1992

SHERLOCK S, DOOLEY J: *Diseases of the Liver and Biliary System*, 9th ed., Oxford, Blackwell, 1993

ZAKIM D, BOYER TD: *Hepatology: A Textbook of Liver Disease*, 3d ed. Philadelphia, Saunders, 1996

292

Daniel K. Podolsky, Kurt J. Isselbacher

EVALUATION OF LIVER FUNCTION

The diversity of normal liver functions and the disruption of these functions by the spectrum of disorders that may affect the liver preclude the use of any single test as a reliable measure of overall liver function. Many disease processes may lead to severe impairment of some liver functions, while others remain entirely unaffected. Since no battery of tests is universally applicable, those most appropriate to a given clinical problem must be selected, their potential value and risks considered, and the results interpreted in relation to the clinical findings.

In assessing the severity and course of liver disease, the physician should be guided by several practical principles. The tests selected should (1) assess different parameters of liver function, (2) be used *serially* in order to evaluate the evolution or course of the disease, and (3) be interpreted within the total clinical context, with recognition that any single laboratory test may be fallible.

BLOOD TESTS OF LIVER FUNCTION

See Table 292-1

BILIRUBIN Bilirubin metabolism and its assessment are discussed in detail in Chaps. 45 and 294. Spectrophotometric determinations of serum bilirubin in the clinical laboratory measure two pigment

Table 292-1

Abnormalities Shown by Tests of Liver Function

	Type of Liver Disease	
Test	Obstructive	Parenchymal
AST and ALT (SGOT and SGPT)	↑	↑–↑↑↑
Alkaline phosphatase	↑↑↑	↑
Albumin	N	↓–↓↓↓
Prothrombin time	N–↑*	↑–↑↑↑
Bilirubin	N–↑↑↑	N–↑↑↑
γ-Glutamyl transpeptidase (GGT)	↑↑↑	N–↑↑↑
5′-Nucleotidase	↑–↑↑↑	N–↑

* Correctable with parenteral vitamin K if elevated.
NOTE: N, normal; ↑, elevated; ↓, decreased.

fractions: (1) the water-soluble conjugated fraction that gives a *direct reaction* with the diazo reagent and consists largely of conjugated bilirubin (as the mono- and diglucuronide) and (2) the lipid-soluble *indirect-reaction* fraction (total minus direct) that represents primarily unconjugated bilirubin. The serum of normal adults (when measured by the van den Bergh reaction) contains less than 4.2 μmol/L (0.25 mg/dL) direct-reacting bilirubin and 17 μmol/L (1 mg/dL) or less of total bilirubin. Studies with high-performance liquid chromatography suggest that even these levels may be artifactually high in normal persons (see Chap. 45).

Conjugated hyperbilirubinemia with elevated direct- and indirect-reacting material indicates impairment of secretion into the bile, while unconjugated hyperbilirubinemia reflects impaired conjugation. The latter is found in a limited number of processes, including such nonhepatic conditions as hemolytic anemia and ineffective erythropoiesis (increased pigment load) and a few hepatic disorders, principally Gilbert's syndrome or the relatively rare Crigler-Najjar syndrome. Although measurement of both the direct and total serum bilirubin will determine whether the patient has predominantly unconjugated or conjugated hyperbilirubinemia, this distinction is of limited usefulness, since the majority of hepatobiliary disorders lead to conjugated hyperbilirubinemia. In most instances, fractionation of serum bilirubin does not distinguish cholestasis due to parenchymal disease from that arising from biliary tract disease.

Bilirubin appears in the urine only after it is converted to a water-soluble form; generally this involves conjugation with polar glucuronide groups that enhance water solubility. Rapid assessment of bilirubinuria is possible using commercially available dipsticks and may be helpful as an initial screening measure. Bilirubinuria occurs with even minimal degrees of jaundice and may be detected before jaundice is clinically evident. Its usefulness is otherwise quite limited. Urobilinogen, a product of luminal bacterial metabolism of bilirubin, is reabsorbed from the bowel and secreted in the urine. Complete bile duct obstruction blocks excretion of bilirubin into the gut and results in disappearance of urobilinogen from the urine. Assessment of urobilinogen in a freshly collected 2-h urine specimen by the Watson method (normal values 0.2 to 1.2 units) may distinguish biliary tract obstruction from parenchymal dysfunction, but this test has been largely superseded by other methods.

SERUM ENZYME ASSAYS A number of serum enzymes have been used to distinguish and assess hepatocellular injury and biliary tract dysfunction or obstruction. All have inherent limitations in sensitivity and specificity, and none truly distinguishes these processes definitively. Elevations in enzyme activities also may be seen in association with nonhepatic disorders. Nevertheless, with proper and careful interpretation, a number of serum enzymes provide important clinical tools.

Aminotransferases (Transaminases) Assays of many serum enzymes have been proposed as indicators of hepatocellular damage. Of these, aspartate aminotransferase (AST, SGOT) and alanine aminotransferase (ALT, SGPT) activities have proven most useful. These enzymes catalyze the transfer of the γ-amino groups of aspartate and alanine, respectively, to the γ-keto group of ketoglutarate, leading to the formation of oxaloacetic acid and pyruvic acid. In contrast to ALT, which is found primarily in the liver, AST is present in many tissues, including heart, skeletal muscle, kidney, and brain, and is thus somewhat less specific as an indicator of liver function. The source of serum AST and ALT in the normal person [less than 0.58 μkat/L (35 U/L)] is unclear, and the mechanism responsible for clearance of these enzymes is uncertain. In the hepatocyte, ALT is found exclusively in the cytosol, while different isoenzymes of AST exist in mitochondria and the cytosol. Although elevated serum levels of AST or ALT may be observed in a variety of nonhepatic diseases, notably in myocardial infarction and skeletal muscle disorders, these disorders can usually be distinguished clinically from liver disease. Conversely, uremia may lead to spuriously low aminotransferase values.

Serum AST and ALT are elevated to some extent in nearly all liver disorders. Highest levels are found in association with conditions causing extensive hepatic necrosis, such as severe viral hepatitis, toxin-induced liver injury, or prolonged circulatory collapse. Lesser elevations are encountered in mild acute viral hepatitis as well as in both diffuse and focal chronic liver diseases (e.g., chronic active hepatitis, cirrhosis, and hepatic metastases). However, the absolute levels of aminotransferases correlate poorly with severity of liver injury or prognosis, and serial determinations are usually most helpful. Thus, in the patient with massive hepatic necrosis, there may be marked elevations in the early phase (i.e., 24 to 48 h), but by the time the patient is tested 3 to 5 days later, the levels may be in the range of 3.34 to 5.8 μkat/L (200 to 350 U/L). It is noteworthy that in severe alcoholic hepatitis one commonly finds only modest increases in these enzymes (generally less than 5.0 μkat/L). Minimal elevations of AST and ALT (less than 1.67 μkat/L) also may be found in association with biliary tract obstruction; higher levels suggest the development of cholangitis with resultant hepatic cell necrosis.

In general AST and ALT levels parallel each other, with a couple of exceptions. In alcoholic hepatitis the AST/ALT ratio may be greater than 2; this appears to result from a reduction in hepatic ALT content due to a deficiency in the cofactor pyridoxine-5-phosphate. An increase in the ratio of AST/ALT (>1) also can be seen occasionally in patients with the fatty liver associated with pregnancy, but is typically <1 in other causes of steatohepatitis.

Alkaline Phosphatase Human serum contains several forms of alkaline phosphatase, a plasma membrane–derived enzyme of uncertain physiologic function that hydrolyzes synthetic phosphate esters at pH 9. These activities arise from bone, intestine, liver, and placenta. A number of different assays have been developed that utilize different substrates.

In the absence of bone disease or pregnancy, elevated levels of alkaline phosphatase activity usually reflect impaired biliary tract function. The increased levels reflect increased synthesis of the enzyme by hepatocytes and biliary tract epithelium rather than regurgitation of enzyme due to obstruction. Bile acids may play a role both by inducing synthesis and by promoting solubilization of the membrane-associated enzyme activity.

Slight to moderate increases in alkaline phosphatase (one to two times normal) occur in many patients with parenchymal liver disorders such as hepatitis and cirrhosis; transient increases may occur in all types of liver disease. Occasionally very high levels of alkaline phosphatase may be found in association with some infiltrative disorders, e.g., mycobacterial infection. However, striking increases in alkaline phosphatase (10 times normal or more) occur more consistently with extrahepatic biliary tract (mechanical) obstruction or with intrahepatic (functional) cholestasis, as in drug-induced cholestasis or primary biliary cirrhosis. Conversely, it is unusual for the serum alkaline phosphatase to remain normal when there is obstructive jaundice, and a normal enzyme level argues strongly against the presence of cholestasis. The alkaline phosphatase is usually mildly elevated in metastatic or infiltrative liver disease (e.g., leukemia, lymphoma, and sarcoid). The enzyme may be elevated in the presence of incomplete biliary obstruction or when there is obstruction of only one hepatic duct, conditions in which the serum bilirubin is often normal or only slightly elevated. Serum alkaline phosphatase is also elevated in nonhepatic disorders, most notably in some bone disorders (e.g., Paget's disease, osteomalacia, and metastases to bone) and sometimes with malignancy. Occasionally, tumors produce an alkaline phosphatase that is identical or similar to the placental form (Regan isoenzyme).

Although one can usually make a reasonable assessment as to whether an elevation of the alkaline phosphatase is of hepatic or nonhepatic origin, several methods can distinguish the different isoenzymes, facilitating resolution of any uncertainty. In contrast to that derived from bone, the hepatic isozyme is stable to treatment with heat (56°C for 15 min) or urea. These enzymes also can be separated by electrophoresis, but this is usually impractical. Parallel determination of serum 5′-nucleotidase activity is also helpful; an increase of both 5′-nucleotidase and alkaline phosphatase is consistent with an hepatobiliary source of the enzyme elevation. Even after correction for age and sex (higher levels being found in the young and in older women), isolated elevations in alkaline phosphatase may occasionally be encountered in adults with no apparent disease.

5′-Nucleotidase This enzyme catalyzes the hydrolysis of phosphate from the 5′ position of the pentose component of the nucleotide. Although tissue distribution is widespread, elevations are generally associated with hepatobiliary disease. The principal value of the 5′-nucleotidase measurement is to confirm the hepatic origin of an elevated alkaline phosphatase level in children or pregnant women or in those settings where coincident bone disease may be present. However, 5′-nucleotidase levels do not always parallel alkaline phosphatase in liver disease, and lack of elevation does not exclude an hepatic source of elevated serum alkaline phosphatase.

γ-Glutamyltranspeptidase (GGT) GGT catalyzes the transfer of the γ-glutamyl group from peptides such as glutathione to other amino acids and may play a role in amino acid transport. It is found throughout the hepatobiliary system as well as in other tissues. In liver disease, GGT correlates with alkaline phosphatase levels and is the most sensitive indicator of biliary tract disease. However, elevations of GGT are nonspecific and may be associated with pancreatic, cardiac, renal, and pulmonary disorders as well as with diabetes and alcoholism. The overall lack of specificity of GGT has limited its clinical usefulness.

Other Enzymes Measurement of total serum lactic dehydrogenase (LDH) or its isoenzymes is usually not helpful in diagnosis of liver disease because of this enzyme's nearly ubiquitous body distribution. Moderate LDH elevations are common in acute viral hepatitis, cirrhosis, and metastatic carcinoma to the liver. Biliary tract disease also may produce slight elevations. Marked elevations of LDH in association with abnormal results of other tests of liver function may reflect a hematologic malignancy such as lymphoma. Elevation of serum ornithine carbamyl transferase, a urea cycle enzyme present only in liver and intestine, occurs primarily in liver disease, but its lack of association with any specific type of liver disease has limited its diagnostic usefulness.

SERUM PROTEINS Extensive liver injury may lead to *decreased* blood levels of albumin, prothrombin, fibrinogen, and other proteins synthesized exclusively by hepatocytes. In contrast to measurements of serum enzymes, serum protein levels reflect liver synthetic function rather than just cell injury. There are three important caveats in the interpretation of serum protein levels: (1) they are neither early nor sensitive indicators of liver disease (because of the extent of hepatic reserve and their half-life, see below), (2) they are of little value in the differential diagnosis of liver disease, and (3) decreases in their serum levels are not specific for liver disease.

Albumin and Globulin Albumin is quantitatively the most important serum protein synthesized by the liver; the normal serum value ranges from 35 to 55 g/L (see Chap. 293). Albumin has a fairly long half-life (14 to 20 days), with less than 5 percent turnover daily; it is therefore not a good indicator of acute or mild liver injury. Furthermore, there is a substantial reserve of hepatic albumin synthesis; thus adequate synthesis may continue until there is extensive hepatocellular injury. Serum levels are influenced by a variety of nonhepatic factors, most notably nutritional status, hormonal factors, and plasma oncotic pressure. Routes of degradation in health remain undefined, but nonhepatic conditions may lead to depressed serum albumin levels mainly due to excessive loss (e.g., nephrotic syndrome or protein-losing enteropathy) despite adequate synthetic function. Nonetheless, reduction in the serum albumin levels provides an excellent indication of the severity of chronic liver disease. In the patient with ascites, an increased volume of distribution as well as an absolute reduction in protein synthesis may contribute to hypoalbuminemia.

Serum globulins are a heterogeneous group of proteins whose production in a variety of tissues is influenced by a number of factors. Serum globulins (normal value ranges from 20 to 35 g/L) include alpha and beta globulins as well as serum immunoglobulins, the latter largely accounting for the gamma fraction. Serum globulins are often diffusely elevated in association with chronic liver disease and in other nonhepatic disorders. In cirrhosis, varying degrees of hyperglobulinemia may occur; this may reflect increased stimulation of the peripheral reticuloendothelial compartment due to shunting of antigens past the liver and impaired clearance by hepatic Kupffer cells. Although some have suggested that elevations in different globulin fractions as assessed by electrophoretic or other means may have a differential diagnostic value, this remains a largely unfulfilled promise. Similarly, the albumin/globulin ratio has no physiologic significance.

Clotting Factors The liver is the major site of synthesis of virtually all coagulation proteins (factors I, II, V, VII, IX, X, XII, and XIII). With the exception of factors V, XII, and XIII, production of functional proteins requires the presence of the cofactor vitamin K. Because most of these factors are normally present in excess concentrations, impaired coagulation is usually seen only in severe liver disease. Abnormalities of these factors can be most efficiently determined by the one-stage *prothrombin time*, which measures the rate of prothrombin conversion to thrombin in the presence of thromboplastin and calcium and requires the integrity of most of the vitamin K–dependent clotting factors (see Chap. 60). Factor VII is the rate-limiting factor in this pathway and thus has the greatest influence on the prothrombin levels. The prothrombin time is dependent on normal hepatic synthesis of clotting factors and sufficient intestinal uptake of vitamin K. Absorption of this fat-soluble vitamin itself requires adequate dietary intake and normal function of intestinal mucosa and biliary secretion. Severe acute or chronic parenchymal liver injury may lead to prolongation of the prothrombin time due to impaired synthesis of the clotting proteins. Because these proteins have a shorter half-life than that of albumin, the prothrombin time may be an earlier indicator than serum albumin level of severe liver injury. In both acute and chronic hepatocellular injury, an increase in the prothrombin time serves as an ominous prognostic sign. Because vitamin K is a fat-soluble vitamin, prolongation of the prothrombin time can result from vitamin K malabsorption, which may occur with cholestasis due to biliary tract disease or due to fat malabsorption (steatorrhea) of any cause (e.g., pancreatic insufficiency). Poor dietary intake, antibiotic therapy, and use of warfarin-type anticoagulants are additional causes of a prolonged prothrombin time, owing to deficiencies of active vitamin K. These processes can be distinguished from hepatic synthetic failure by demonstrating normalization of the prothrombin time (within 24 to 48 h) after parenteral injections of vitamin K. The *partial thromboplastin time*, which reflects the activities of fibrinogen, prothrombin, and factors V, VIII, IX, X, XI, and XII, also may be prolonged in severe liver disease. Clotting functions should be assessed in all patients with liver disease prior to any surgical procedure, including liver biopsy (see Chaps. 60 and 118). Of interest, hepatocellular carcinomas have been found to produce an abnormal form of prothrombin that has not been fully carboxylated by vitamin K–dependent mechanisms (des-γ-prothrombin).

BLOOD AMMONIA Ammonia is elevated in the blood of some patients with either acute or chronic liver disease. Although influenced by a number of factors (summarized in Chap. 293), elevations in blood ammonia reflect disruption of the pathways of urea synthesis by which the liver detoxifies amine groups. A markedly elevated blood ammonia usually reflects severe hepatocellular injury. Cirrhotic patients, especially those with endogenous or surgically created portal-systemic shunting, often have varying degrees of hyperammonemia and hepatic encephalopathy. However, there is only a rough correlation between blood ammonia levels and the degree of hepatic encephalopathy; some patients will function normally with a twofold elevation, while others will be stuporous at the same concentration. Ammonia levels may increase before the onset of coma; similarly, they may return to normal some 48 to 72 h before improvement of the neurologic status.

SERUM LIPIDS AND LIPOPROTEINS AND BILE ACIDS- Abnormalities in serum lipids and lipoproteins are sensitive but nonspecific indicators of liver diseases. Acute parenchymal liver disease is commonly associated with increased plasma triglycerides, decreased cholesterol esters, and abnormal lipoproteins. The absence of alpha and prebeta bands with a concomitant increase in the beta fraction is typical of acute viral hepatitis. Less marked but more persistent abnormalities are found in patients with chronic parenchymal disease, reflecting deficiencies in lecithin:cholesterol acyltransferase (LCAT) and hepatic triglyceride lipase. Either intra- or extrahepatic cholestasis may lead to an increase in unesterified cholesterol and in serum phospholipids.

Removal of bile acids from portal blood is impaired in liver disease because of parenchymal damage and portal-systemic shunts; there also may be reentry of bile acids into blood from injured hepatocytes or an obstructed biliary tract. Although there are a variety of techniques for measuring serum bile acids, these determinations are not yet of proven value for routine clinical use.

IMMUNOLOGIC AND OTHER TESTS

A number of immunologic derangements may be seen in liver disease. These are summarized in Table 292-2. Antimitochondrial antibodies (AMA) are found in 85 to 90 percent of patients with primary biliary cirrhosis. These antibodies appear to be directed against components of the pyruvate dehydrogenase complex and other related mitochondrial enzyme complexes. In this test, serum is incubated with rabbit hepatocytes. The presence of AMA can then be assessed after subsequent staining with a fluorescein-tagged second antibody. However, this marker is not entirely specific and is occasionally found in patients with autoimmune hepatitis and drug-induced hepatitis. Its primary value is in helping to distinguish primary biliary cirrhosis from extrahepatic biliary obstruction. In autoimmune hepatitis, the *lupus erythematosus–cell test* may be positive, and *antinuclear antibodies* (ANA) as well as *anti-smooth-muscle antibodies* (ASM) may be present (see Chap. 312). Patients with autoimmune hepatitis have clinical and histologic features similar to those of primary biliary cirrhosis but serologic tests resembling those of autoimmune hepatitis (negative AMA and positive ANA or ASM). Alpha fetoprotein is of value in the diagnosis of hepatocellular carcinoma (see Chap. 93). Measurements of serum α_1-antitrypsin and ceruloplasmin should be performed in infants with cirrhosis or hepatitis since they may reflect α_1-antitrypsin deficiency or Wilson's disease, respectively (see Chaps. 300 and 345).

Table 292-2

Immunologic Tests in Diagnosis of Hepatic Disorders

Test	Disease Association	Comment
Antimitochondrial antibody (AMA)	Primary biliary cirrhosis (90%); chronic active hepatitis (occasional)	Antibodies against component of pyruvate dehydrogenase and other 2-oxo-acid complexes
Antinuclear antibody (ANA)	Autoimmune hepatitis (10%)	
Anti-smooth-muscle antibody (ASM)	Autoimmune hepatitis	
Antineutrophil cytoplasmic antibody (ANCA)	Primary sclerosing cholangitis	Perinuclear pattern; antigen unknown but distinct from myeloperoxidase
Anti-liver/kidney microsomal antibody (anti-LKM)	Autoimmune hepatitis, type II	

Studies assessing iron stores are essential in the evaluation of those patients suspected of hemochromatosis on clinical grounds, those exhibiting compatible nonspecific abnormal liver function tests results (e.g., unexplained mild to moderate elevation of aminotransferase), or those with evidence of liver disease, early or advanced, of uncertain cause. Routine tests include iron, total serum iron-binding capacity (TIBC), and ferritin. Hemochromatosis is associated with elevated levels of both iron and TIBC and an increased ratio of iron/TIBC, consistent with a high degree of saturation of iron-binding capacity. While iron-binding saturations of >90% are typical, hemochromatosis should be suspected at levels about 50%, especially in women. Although high iron saturation may be seen in many chronic systemic illnesses, the overall levels of iron and TIBC will be diminished. Serum levels of ferritin, the intrahepatic ion storage protein, are typically markedly elevated in hemochromatosis. Somewhat less pronounced increases may be seen in other forms of liver injury, including alcoholic liver disease and other diseases (e.g., lymphoma). Particular confusion may arise in distinguishing secondary hemosiderosis, most commonly seen in alcoholics but also encountered in patients receiving numerous transfusions (e.g., sickle cell anemia), from primary hemochromatosis by these initial serum determinations. Diagnosis often ultimately requires percutaneous liver biopsy or other more specific tests. → ***For further discussion, see Chap. 342.***

OTHER DIAGNOSTIC PROCEDURES **Percutaneous Needle Biopsy of the Liver** Percutaneous needle biopsy is a safe, simple, and valuable method for the diagnostic evaluation of liver disease. *Diffuse parenchymal disorders* such as cirrhosis, hepatitis, and drug reactions may be diagnosed with remarkable accuracy. In *disseminated focal diseases* (such as granulomas or tumor infiltrates), serial sections may demonstrate characteristic lesions.

Biopsy is usually performed "blindly," under local anesthesia, by either a transpleural or subcostal approach. If the operator is skillful and patients are carefully selected, morbidity should be quite low and limited to occasional postbiopsy pain or vasovagal reactions.

Some of the most frequent indications for needle biopsy are (1) unexplained hepatomegaly or hepatosplenomegaly; (2) cholestasis of uncertain cause; (3) persistently abnormal liver function tests; (4) suspected systemic or infiltrative diseases such as sarcoidosis, miliary tuberculosis, or fever of unknown origin; and (5) suspected primary or metastatic liver tumor. Percutaneous liver biopsy may be performed either for diagnostic purposes or to evaluate the extent and severity of a known disease process. However, other new and improved noninvasive diagnostic methods have obviated the need for biopsy in many circumstances, and thus biopsy should be performed only when information from these other techniques is inadequate.

Needle biopsy should not be performed if (1) the patient is unable to cooperate; (2) clinical or laboratory evidence indicates impaired hemostasis (prothrombin time prolonged by 3 s or more over control, thrombocytopenia less than 80×10^9 platelets per liter, or partial thromboplastin time or bleeding time prolonged); (3) there is infection of the right pleural space or septic cholangitis; (4) tense ascites is present, with risk of continued leakage of ascitic fluid; (5) compatible blood is not available for transfusion in case of hemorrhage; (6) high-grade biliary obstruction is suspected and there is an increased risk of bile peritonitis; (7) there is a possible echinococchal cyst; or (8) a vascular lesion is suspected. In patients in whom a percutaneous biopsy cannot be performed safely due to impaired hemostasis or ascites, biopsy can sometimes be carried out by a transjugular approach, in which the tissue is obtained via the hepatic vein and any bleeding occurs directly into the vascular space. With the increasing use of computed tomography scanning and ultrasonography, it is possible to perform "directed" aspiration biopsies of isolated focal lesions with very thin needles. Aspirated material can be used for cytology (tumors) and culture (abscesses) but is often inadequate for assessment of liver architecture.

BIBLIOGRAPHY

Schiff L, Schiff ER: *Diseases of the Liver*, 7th ed. Philadelphia, Lippincott, 1993
Zakim D, Boyer TD: *Hepatology: A Textbook of Liver Disease*, 3d ed. Philadelphia, Saunders, 1996

293

Daniel K. Podolsky, Kurt J. Isselbacher

DERANGEMENTS OF HEPATIC METABOLISM

The liver plays a central role in the maintenance of metabolic homeostasis. It is therefore not surprising that the development of clinically important liver disease is accompanied by diverse manifestations of disordered metabolism. Although some functions are more sensitive than others, the liver has considerable reserve capacity, so minimal or even moderate cell injury may not be reflected by measurable metabolic changes. However, a variety of defects may be seen, depending on the nature and extent of the initial insult.

The biochemical functions in which the liver plays a major role include (1) the intermediate metabolism of amino acids and carbohydrates, (2) synthesis and degradation of proteins and glycoproteins, (3) metabolism and degradation of drugs and hormones, and (4) regulation of lipid and cholesterol metabolism. The derangements of these functions are discussed in connection with their occurrence in various forms of parenchymal liver disease. Alterations of bilirubin, bile salt, and porphyrin metabolism are discussed elsewhere (Chaps. 45, 285, and 343).

Metabolic derangements are most evident in the patient with advanced liver disease, and the manifestations are similar regardless of the initial etiologic insult. To a varying degree, similar abnormalities are observed in patients with severe chronic hepatitis, micronodular cirrhosis, and postnecrotic cirrhosis. Since the many functions of the liver may be affected to varying degrees in individual patients, no single test effectively measures the overall state of liver function. The proper evaluation of tests of liver function is discussed in Chap. 292.

CARBOHYDRATE METABOLISM The liver functions to maintain normal levels of blood sugar by a combination of glycogenesis, glycogenolysis, glycolysis, and gluconeogenesis. These pathways are regulated by a number of hormones, including insulin, glucagon, growth hormone, and certain catecholamines. Although it has been presumed that exquisite sensitivity of the hepatocytes to insulin is responsible for the uptake of an oral glucose load by the liver, there are also data that have challenged the importance of insulin-mediated glucose uptake by the hepatocyte. In the fasting state, the liver contributes to glucose homeostasis by glycogenolysis and gluconeogenesis in response to hypoinsulinemia and hyperglucagonemia. Maintenance of normal blood glucose levels through gluconeogenesis is ultimately related to catabolism of muscle protein, which provides the necessary amino acid precursors, especially alanine. In a complementary fashion, in the postprandial state, the liver directs alanine and branched-chain amino acids to the peripheral tissues, where they are then incorporated into muscle protein. These reciprocal pathways form a glucose-alanine shuttle, which is modulated by ambient changes in the hormones mentioned above. While it has been presumed that synthesis of glycogen and fatty acid in the postprandial state arises from direct conversion of glucose, there are data to suggest that, in fact, these pathways are *indirect*, with products deriving from three-carbon metabolites of glucose or other gluconeogenic compounds such as lactate, fructose, and alanine.

Abnormalities of glucose homeostasis are common in cirrhosis (Table 293-1). Most frequently, hyperglycemia and glucose intolerance are observed. Glucose intolerance is associated with normal or increased levels of plasma insulin (except in patients with hemochromatosis), suggesting that insulin resistance rather than insulin deficiency may be responsible. One of the factors that may play a role in the apparent insulin resistance is an absolute decrease in the liver's ability to metabolize a glucose load because of a decrease in functioning hepatocellular mass. There is also evidence that response to insulin is diminished due to both receptor and postreceptor defects in hepatocytes of patients with cirrhosis. In addition, both hyperinsulinemia and hyperglucagonemia may be present due to decreased hepatic clearance of this hormone resulting from portal-systemic shunting. In patients with hemochromatosis, however, insulin levels, may indeed be low due to pancreatic iron deposition and sometimes concomitant diabetes mellitus. Patients with cirrhosis also may have elevated serum lactate levels, reflecting the decreased capacity of the liver to utilize lactate for gluconeogenesis.

Hypoglycemia, although more common in acute fulminant hepatitis, also may be seen with end-stage cirrhosis. Because the capacity of the liver to store glycogen is limited (approximately 70 g) and glucose consumption continues at a constant rate (approximately 150 g/d), hepatic glycogen stores are depleted after 1 day of fasting. Hypoglycemia in end-stage cirrhosis may be due to decreased hepatic glycogen stores, diminished glucagon responsiveness, or decreased capacity to synthesize glycogen due to extensive parenchymal destruction.

AMINO ACID AND AMMONIA METABOLISM Through a variety of anabolic and catabolic processes, the liver is the major site of amino acid interconversion. Amino acids utilized for hepatic protein synthesis are derived from dietary protein, metabolic turnover of endogenous protein (primarily from muscle), and direct synthesis in the liver. Most of the amino acids entering the liver via the portal vein are catabolized to urea (except for the branched-chain amino acids leucine, isoleucine, and valine). Some of these amino acids are released into the general circulation as free amino acids and may play an important role in the glucose-alanine cycle mentioned above. In addition, amino acids are utilized for the synthesis of liver intracellular proteins, plasma proteins, and special compounds such as glutathione, glutamine, taurine, carnosine, and creatine. Disruption of normal amino acid metabolism may be reflected in altered plasma amino acid concentrations. In general, levels of aromatic amino acids normally metabolized by the liver (as well as methionine) are elevated, while those of

Table 293-1

Alteration of Glucose Metabolism in Cirrhosis

Factors Leading to Hyperglycemia
Decreased hepatic glucose uptake
Decreased hepatic glycogen synthesis
Hepatic resistance to insulin
Portal-systemic glucose shunting
Peripheral insulin resistance
Hormonal abnormalities (serum)
↑ Glucagon
↓ Cortisol
↑ Insulin (↓ in hemochromatosis)
Factors Leading to Hypoglycemia
Decreased gluconeogenesis
Decreased hepatic glycogen content
Hepatic resistance to glucagon
Poor oral intake
Hyperinsulinemia secondary to portal-systemic shunting

the branched-chain amino acids, largely utilized by skeletal muscle, tend to be normal or depressed. It was previously suggested that an alteration in the ratio of these two types of amino acids plays a role in the development of hepatic encephalopathy (see below), but there is not agreement on this concept.

Hepatic catabolism or degradation of amino acids involves two major reactions: transamination and oxidative deamination. In transamination, an amino group of an amino acid is transferred to a keto acid. This process is catalyzed by aminotransferases, which are found in very high amounts in liver but are also present in other tissues, such as kidney, muscle, heart, lung, and brain. Glutamic-oxaloacetic acid transaminase (aspartate aminotransferase, AST) has been studied most extensively, and increased levels are found in the serum secondary to various types of liver injury (e.g., acute viral and drug-induced hepatitis). As a result of transamination, amino acids can enter the citric acid cycle and then function in the intermediary metabolism of carbohydrates and lipids. Most of the nonessential amino acids are also synthesized in the liver by transamination. Oxidative deamination, which results in conversion of amino acids to keto acids (and ammonia), is catalyzed by L-amino acid oxidase with two exceptions: glycine oxidation is catalyzed by glycine oxidase, and glutamic oxidation is catalyzed by glutamic dehydrogenase. With severe liver damage (e.g., massive hepatic necrosis), utilization of amino acids is impaired, free amino acids in the bloodstream increase, and an "overflow" type of aminoaciduria may occur (unless renal function is also impaired).

Urea production is intimately related to the metabolic pathways outlined above, providing a means for disposal of ammonia, the toxic product of nitrogen metabolism. Disruption of this process is of particular clinical importance in the patient with severe acute and chronic liver disease. The fixation of amino acid–derived NH_3 in the form of urea is carried out via the Krebs-Henseleit cycle. The final step of this cycle, the formation of urea by arginase, is irreversible. In advanced liver disease, urea synthesis is often depressed, leading to an accumulation of NH_3, usually with a significant reduction in blood urea nitrogen, an ominous sign of liver failure. This finding may be obscured by superimposed renal impairment, which often develops in patients with severe hepatic failure. Urea is mostly excreted by the kidney, but approximately 25 percent will diffuse into the intestine, where it is converted to NH_3 by bacterial urease. The intestinal production of ammonia also occurs from the bacterial deamination of unabsorbed amino acids and of protein derived from the diet, exfoliated cells, or blood in the gastrointestinal tract.

Gut NH_3 is absorbed and transported to the liver via the portal vein, where it is again converted to urea. The kidney also produces varying amounts of NH_3, largely by the deamination of glutamine. The contributions of the gut and kidney to ammonia synthesis have important implications for the management of the hyperammonemic state frequently seen in patients with advanced liver disease, usually in association with portal-systemic shunting of blood.

While the exact chemical mediators of hepatic encephalopathy remain unknown and may include endogenous benzodiazepine compounds, elevated levels of blood NH_3 are generally associated with the development of encephalopathy, although approximately 10 percent of such patients have normal levels of blood ammonia (see Chap. 299). In addition, therapeutic measures that reduce serum NH_3 levels also usually lead to clinical improvement. The several mechanisms known to lead to increased blood NH_3 levels in patients with cirrhosis are illustrated in Fig. 293-1 and include the following:

1. If there is excessive nitrogenous material in the intestine (from bleeding or dietary protein), excessive amounts of NH_3 will be formed by bacterial deamination of amino acids. If intestinal motility is diminished, as manifest by constipation, bacterial production of ammonia will increase due to prolonged time for degradation of luminal protein and amino acids.
2. If renal function declines (as in the hepatorenal syndrome), blood urea nitrogen rises, leading to increased diffusion of urea into the intestinal lumen, where bacterial urease converts it to NH_3.
3. If hepatic function is significantly depressed, diminished urea synthesis may occur with a resultant decrease in the removal of NH_3.
4. If alkalosis (often due to central hyperventilation) and hypokalemia accompany hepatic decompensation, there may be a decrease in the renal availability of H^+ ions; as a result, the NH_3 produced from glutamine by the action of renal glutaminase is permitted to enter the renal vein (rather than being excreted as NH_4^+), leading to increased peripheral blood NH_3 levels. In addition, hypokalemia itself leads to increased renal NH_3 production.
5. If portal hypertension is present and anastomoses exist between the portal vein and systemic venous channels, these portal-systemic shunts will allow NH_3 from the gut to bypass hepatic detoxification, leading to elevated blood NH_3 levels. Thus, with portal-systemic shunting of blood, elevated NH_3 levels may develop with relatively modest hepatocellular dysfunction.

It is unclear what effects these same factors may have on other compounds that may play a role in the development of hepatic encephalopathy.

An additional factor important in determining whether a given NH_3 level in the blood will be detrimental to the central nervous system is the blood pH. The more alkaline the pH, the more toxic a given level of NH_3 is likely to be. At 37°C, the pK of NH_3 is 8.9; this is close enough to the pH of blood that minor changes in pH can affect the NH_4^+/NH_3 ratio. Because un-ionized NH_3 crosses membranes more readily than NH_4^+ ions, alkalosis favors the entry of ammonia into the brain (with subsequent changes in cell metabolism) by shifting the equilibrium of the following reaction to the right

$$NH_4^+ + OH^- \rightleftharpoons NH_3 + HOH$$

As a result, alkalosis not only increases peripheral blood NH_3 levels by renal mechanisms but also increases tissue levels by influencing the diffusion of NH_3 across membranes. Similarly, alterations in the pH of intestinal luminal contents also will affect the equilibrium between NH_4^+ and NH_3; a more alkaline lumen will shift the balance in favor of NH_3, permitting increased absorption. In theory, laxatives that cause relative acidification of luminal contents (e.g., lactulose) may be more effective than others as agents for the treatment of hepatic encephalopathy. However, this theoretical effect on the equilibrium

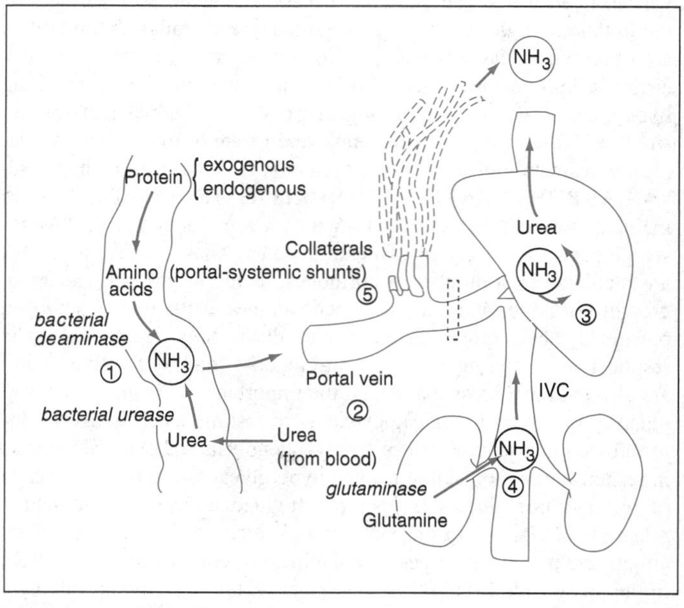

FIGURE 293-1 Major factors (steps 1 to 4) influencing the level of blood ammonia. In cirrhosis with portal hypertension, venous collaterals allow ammonia to bypass the liver (step 5), permitting the entry of ammonia into the systemic circulation (portal-systemic shunting).

between NH_4^+ and NH_3 has never been convincingly demonstrated for available laxatives.

PROTEIN SYNTHESIS AND DEGRADATION The liver is an important site of protein synthesis and degradation. Although the body muscle mass produces the greatest total amount of protein, the liver has the highest rate of synthesis per gram of tissue. The liver synthesizes not only the proteins it needs, but also produces numerous export proteins. Among the latter, albumin is the most important; *it is produced at a rate of approximately 12 g/d*, representing 25 percent of total hepatic protein synthesis and half of all exported protein. The average normal half-life of serum albumin is 17 to 20 days. The proportion of hepatocytes carrying out active albumin synthesis varies from 10 to 60 percent, depending on the body's requirements. Approximately 60 percent of albumin is found in the extravascular spaces, but plasma albumin is still the most abundant circulating protein.

Albumin contributes significantly to the plasma oncotic pressure. In addition, it is the principal binding and transport protein for numerous substances, including some hormones, fatty acids, trace metals, tryptophan, bilirubin, and other organic anions of both endogenous and exogenous origin. Despite the many important functions of albumin, rare individuals with congenital analbuminemia appear to have no major physiologic derangements other than the excessive accumulation of extravascular fluid. While many of the less hydrophobic ligands may be transported in the unbound form, this suggests that other serum proteins also may play a role in binding and transport.

Much has been learned about the mechanisms involved in the synthesis of secretory proteins, especially albumin. Polyribosomes bound to the rough endoplasmic reticulum (RER) of the hepatocyte are the principal site of translation of messenger RNA coding for export proteins; in contrast, proteins destined for intracellular use, such as ferritin, are synthesized on free rather than bound polyribosomes in the cytoplasm. Albumin, like secretory proteins produced by other organs, appears to be synthesized initially as a larger precursor, preproalbumin. This precursor molecule contains an additional 24 extra amino acid residues on the *N* terminus, referred to as a *signal peptide*, which undergoes two sequential cleavages (or "processing"). The "pre" portion of preproalbumin is cleaved within the RER even before protein synthesis is completed; the "pro" segment is removed within the lumen of the RER. The molecule is then transported to the Golgi apparatus prior to secretion. Once synthesis and processing are completed, albumin is transported from the Golgi vesicles to the hepatocyte surface by mechanisms that are unclear but almost certainly involve the microfilaments and microtubule apparatus of the cell. Although the hepatic lymph space of Disse provides a potential avenue for the newly released albumin, most secreted proteins such as albumin enter the plasma.

Albumin synthesis is subject to a number of regulatory influences. These include the rate of transcription of specific messenger RNAs and the availability of the substrate transfer RNA. At the translational level, the integrity of polyribosomes and their synthetic abilities are modified by factors affecting initiation, elongation, and release of peptides and proteins as well as by the availability of ATP, GTP, and magnesium ions. The rate of albumin synthesis is also influenced by the availability of amino acid precursors, especially tryptophan, the scarcest of the essential amino acids. Indeed, in patients with large carcinoid tumors, albumin synthesis may decrease precipitously when tryptophan is consumed by carcinoid cells in the production of 5-hydroxytryptophan (serotonin) (see Chap. 95). The rate of albumin synthesis is also affected by colloid oncotic pressure, with increased production occurring in response to falling oncotic pressure. Finally, influences of hormones such as insulin and glucagon on hepatic protein metabolism are closely integrated with the nutritional factors discussed above.

The liver also produces a wide variety of other secretory proteins, most of which have a synthetic pathway and processing procedure similar to that of albumin. The presence of a signal peptide such as the "prepro" segment of albumin, which is subsequently removed during protein maturation, appears to be a general mechanism for orienting proteins in the membranes of the endoplasmic reticulum and directing them for export rather than for intracellular use or degradation. Most proteins undergo even further modification in the form of sequential *glycosylation* in the RER and Golgi apparatus. The carbohydrate moieties of these glycoproteins appear to be important in determining their site of action and their rate of tissue uptake after secretion. Some of the clinically important secretory glycoproteins include ceruloplasmin, α_1-antitrypsin, and most other alpha and beta globulins. While the site of albumin catabolism is uncertain, the removal of terminal sialic acid residues after secretion and the resultant exposure of penultimate galactose or *N*-acetylglucosamine residues appears to result in receptor-mediated uptake of "aged" proteins by hepatocytes and Kupffer cells, followed by their subsequent degradation. Reduced amounts of the hepatic receptor for asialoglycoproteins appear to result in elevated serum concentrations of these glycoproteins in patients with severe and chronic liver disease.

One of the clinically most important derangements in protein metabolism is the development of *hypoalbuminemia*, which results largely from reduced synthetic activity. Decreased synthesis may be caused by a decrease in the number as well as the function of hepatocytes. A decrease in the dietary supply of amino acids also can contribute to deficient synthesis. To some extent the body attempts to compensate for decreased albumin synthesis by reducing the rate of degradation. Attempts to raise the serum albumin level by intravenous infusions are often futile because this compensatory mechanism can be blunted and the decrease in albumin degradation may not occur. The reduced degradation of albumin is not a general phenomenon in chronic liver disease because other proteins such as fibrinogen are degraded more rapidly than normal. In the patient with ascites, the degree of hypoalbuminemia is worsened by the loss of large amounts of the body's albumin into the ascitic fluid. When there is increased hepatic venous pressure (as in postsinusoidal or hepatic vein outflow block), there may be increased hepatic lymph production with extravasation into the peritoneal cavity. In contrast to intestinal lymph, the protein content of hepatic lymph appears to be relatively uninfluenced by ascitic oncotic pressure, most likely reflecting the lack of tight junctions between sinusoidal endothelial cells.

Other proteins produced by the liver include many of the blood-clotting factors: fibrinogen (factor I), prothrombin (factor II), and factors V, VII, IX, X, XII, and XIII, as well as inhibitors of both coagulation and fibrinolysis. Factors II, VII, IX, and X are vitamin K–responsive and are dependent on normal intestinal fat absorption. Vitamin K activates an enzyme system in liver endoplasmic reticulum which catalyzes the γ carboxylation of selected glutamyl residues in clotting factor precursors. The γ carboxylation enhances the Ca^{2+}- and phospholipid-binding capacity of prothrombin and permits its rapid conversion to thrombin in the presence of factors V and X (Chap. 118).

The liver is involved in the process of hemostasis by virtue of both anabolic and catabolic functions. As expected, severe liver disease leads to reduced synthesis of prothrombin, a vitamin K–dependent clotting factor. The presence of malnutrition, the use of broad-spectrum antibiotics, or concomitant impairment of fat absorption due to reduction in intestinal bile salt concentration (e.g., cholestasis) may accentuate hypoprothrombinemia by decreasing the amount of vitamin K that can be absorbed from the intestine. In these situations, prothrombin levels may be at least partially corrected by parenteral vitamin K administration. However, when the coagulopathy results from impaired hepatocellular function and not cholestasis or intestinal factors, exogenous vitamin K is unlikely to correct or improve prothrombin synthesis. The vitamin K–dependent clotting proteins have a substantially shorter serum half-life than albumin; therefore, hypoprothrombinemia usually precedes the development of hypoalbuminemia, especially in the patient with acute hepatocellular disease. In cirrhosis, coagulopathy may be further aggravated by the thrombocytopenia resulting from hypersplenism.

Since the liver is also the site of production of non-vitamin K–dependent clotting factors, severe liver disease injury may lead to decreased plasma concentrations of factor V. It is unusual for fibrinogen to be reduced significantly, unless there is an associated disseminated intravascular coagulation. For unclear reasons, the damaged liver may actually produce increased amounts of fibrinogen as well as other proteins, collectively designated *acute-phase reactants* (C-reactive proteins, haptoglobin, ceruloplasmin, and transferrin). The latter are produced both in response to liver injury and in association with systemic illnesses such as cancer, rheumatoid arthritis, bacterial infections, burns, and myocardial infarctions. Cytokines, including interleukins 1 and 6, appear to be major stimuli of hepatic synthesis of acute-phase reactants. However, while the diseased liver may produce normal or increased amounts of fibrinogen, the molecules themselves may be qualitatively abnormal (i.e., structurally and functionally), reflecting more subtle derangements in protein synthesis. These functionally abnormal fibrinogen molecules may contribute to the altered hemostasis frequently found in patients with chronic liver disease.

DETOXIFICATION MECHANISMS Water-soluble drugs and endogenous substances usually are excreted unchanged in the urine or bile. However, lipid-soluble compounds tend to accumulate in the body and affect cellular processes, unless they are converted to less active compounds or to more water-soluble metabolites that are more easily excreted. Hepatic blood flow, protein binding, and the intrinsic capacity of the liver to eliminate a drug are all primary determinants of hepatic drug clearance. The liver has an important role in the metabolism of many exogenous drugs and endogenous hormones by virtue of several enzyme systems involved in biochemical transformation, as well as the "first-pass effect" of blood flow from virtually the entire gastrointestinal tract through the liver via the portal circulation. The relative importance of these various factors differs depending on how well a drug is extracted by the liver. There are two major types of reactions. The first, *phase I reactions*, results in chemical modification of reactive groups by oxidation, reduction, hydroxylation, sulfoxidation, deamination, dealkylation, or methylation. Such modifications usually involve one of several enzymatic systems, including the mixed-function oxidases, cytochromes b_5 and P450 (microsomal), and the glutathione *S*-acyltransferases (cytoplasmic). These biochemical reactions usually lead to *inactivation* of drugs such as benzodiazepines. However, *activation* also may occur. For example, cortisone is activated to cortisol and prednisone to prednisolone (both products being more potent than the parent compounds); imipramine, a depressant, is converted to desmethylimipramine, an antidepressant. In the same manner, phase I reactions may even convert a nontoxic compound to a toxic one, as in the metabolism of isoniazid and acetaminophen. Similarly, some carcinogens may be activated by formation of highly reactive epoxide intermediates in the liver, while other carcinogens may be detoxified.

The enzymes responsible for phase I reactions, especially those involving the cytochrome P450 system, can be induced by drugs such as ethanol, barbiturates, haloperidol, and glutethimide. Conversely, hepatic microsomal enzymes may be inhibited by agents such as chloramphenicol, cimetidine, disulfiram, dextropropoxyphene, allopurinol, and, paradoxically, ethanol. The concomitant administration of two drugs metabolized by the same microsomal enzyme may result in modification, potentiation, or diminution of the pharmacologic efficacy of either or both drugs. Activity of phase I reactions also may change with aging.

Phase II reactions involve the conversion of substances to their glucuronide, sulfate, acetyl, taurine, or glycine derivatives, thereby converting lipophilic substances to water-soluble derivatives and permitting their excretion in bile or urine. Conjugation catalyzed by microsomal UDP (uridine diphosphate)-glucuronosyltransferases to form glucuronide derivatives is one of the most common phase II reactions. In general, the conjugates are more soluble than the parent compound and are pharmacologically inactive.

An awareness that there may be varying degrees of impairment in the hepatic uptake, detoxification, and excretion of certain drugs is important in the clinical management of patients with chronic liver disease. Portal-systemic shunting of blood may decrease the first-pass effect of drugs absorbed from the gut. In cirrhosis, altered intrahepatic hemodynamics due to a disordered liver architecture also may reduce the rates of hepatic drug clearance. Hypoalbuminemia will permit drugs usually bound to albumin to be present in increased concentrations of their unbound form in the circulation and extracellular spaces; this may result in their increased activity. Most important, a decrease in the amount of functional microsomal enzymes responsible for phase I and phase II reactions will result in slower rates of drug inactivation and elimination. Drugs for which there may be a decreased hepatic clearance include anticonvulsants (e.g., phenytoin, phenobarbital), anti-inflammatory agents (e.g., acetaminophen, phenylbutazone, glucocorticoids), minor tranquilizers, cardioactive drugs (e.g., lidocaine, quinidine, propranolol), and antibiotics (e.g., nafcillin, chloramphenicol, tetracyclines, clindamycin, trimethoprim, rifampin, pyrazinamide). This will lead to decreased dosage requirements and a narrowing of the range between therapeutic and toxic drug levels. Finally, the patient with chronic liver disease may demonstrate alterations in the pharmacologic effects of drugs in addition to or independent of changes in their pharmacokinetics, such as an increased central nervous system sensitivity to opiates and other sedatives.

The difficulties in safely administering pharmacologic agents to patients with both acute and chronic liver disease are underscored by the frequency with which administration of benzodiazepines precipitates hepatic coma. It may be very difficult clinically to determine whether agitation, confusion, and irrational behavior are due to early hepatic encephalopathy or are related to the concurrent use of benzodiazepines, opiates, barbiturates, and other depressants. It should be recognized that there is great variation of drug clearance in patients with liver disease; although data on average clearances may provide a reasonable estimate for initial dosages, subsequent adjustments in dose need to be individualized in order to attain the desired plasma drug concentration.

The mechanism by which some agents exert a hepatotoxic effect may involve the same metabolic pathways responsible for normal drug detoxification. The mechanism of acetaminophen toxicity is particularly illustrative. Acetaminophen is metabolized and detoxified by the hepatic mixed-function oxygenase system, but one of the intermediate products is a potent free radical (postulated metabolite *N*-acetylimidoquinone) that can inactivate many enzymes and proteins by binding irreversibly to their sulfhydryl groups. Normally, this interaction can be prevented by reduced glutathione. In the presence of excessive amounts of the acetaminophen free radical (e.g., from overdosage or underlying liver disease), the glutathione levels of the hepatocytes are readily exhausted, and the excess free radicals can lead to inactivation of cellular proteins and produce widespread hepatocellular necrosis. In the case of acetaminophen overdosage, the very early administration of sulfhydryl groups in the form of *N*-acetylcysteine can often prevent this drug-induced liver injury.

HORMONE METABOLISM In addition to its role in the metabolism of diverse pharmacologic agents, the liver is also responsible for inactivation or modification of several endogenous hormones; therefore, chronic liver disease may be accompanied by signs of apparent hormonal imbalance. Some hormones (e.g., insulin and glucagon) are inactivated in the liver by proteolysis or deamination. Thyroxine and triiodothyronine are metabolized in the liver by reactions involving deiodination. Steroid hormones, such as glucocorticoids and aldosterone, are first inactivated to their tetrahydro derivative (by reduction of the Δ^4 double bond and the 3-keto group), followed by conjugation, mostly with glucuronic acid. Testosterone is metabolized to the isomeric 17-ketosteroids androsterone and etiocholanolone and excreted in the urine mostly as sulfate conjugates. Estrogens, such as estradiol, may be converted to estriol and estrone and then conjugated with glucuronic acid or sulfate. Abnormalities in estrogen (and testosterone) metabolism are believed to be involved in the development of the spider angiomas, loss of axillary or pubic hair, and testicular atrophy frequently seen in patients with chronic liver disease. In addition, increased portal-systemic shunting of testosterone and androstenedione secondary to portal hypertension may lead to the development of gynecomastia in cirrhotic males due to increased peripheral conversion to estradiol and estrone, especially in patients with alcoholic cirrhosis. In patients with alcoholic liver disease, feminization also may be related to the direct toxic effects of alcohol on the gonadal-pituitary-hypothalamic axis, which lead to an overall reduction in serum testosterone. Similar effects are also seen in patients with hemochromatosis due to deposition of iron in these sites. However, gynecomastia is often lacking in the latter, apparently due to a coincident reduction in plasma concentration of androstenedione, a major precursor for estrogen synthesis.

Estrogens also act directly on the liver to impair hepatic secretory activity. Estradiol and related estrogens, such as those present in contraceptive pills, interfere with bile salt excretion and worsen the preexisting defect in secretion of conjugated bilirubin in patients with Dubin-Johnson syndrome; they also may elevate plasma alkaline phosphatase levels (see Chap. 292). Related steroids such as etiocholanolone and pregnanediol have been shown to stimulate δ-aminolevulinic acid (ALA) synthetase activity, leading to increased porphobilinogen excretion. Since these steroids exert their effects only in their unconjugated form, the increased hepatic levels of δ-aminolevulinic acid synthetase in patients with alcoholic cirrhosis may be secondary to the action of gonadal steroids. The liver also serves to remove some important circulating vasoactive substances, including epinephrine and bradykinin. Elevated levels of epinephrine, perhaps reflecting in part diminished hepatic uptake, may promote the hyperdynamic state that contributes to the development of ascites and the hepatorenal syndrome.

LIPID METABOLISM: FATTY ACIDS AND TRIGLYCERIDES Under normal conditions, most of the fatty acids taken up by the liver and esterified to triglyceride are derived from adipose tissue or the diet. Some fatty acids (especially saturated ones) are synthesized in the liver from acetate. The fatty acids may then be converted enzymatically to triglyceride, esterified with cholesterol, incorporated into phospholipids, or oxidized to CO_2 or ketone bodies. Most of the triglyceride is produced for export, but in order to be secreted it must be converted to lipoproteins by combining with relatively specific apoprotein moieties. This emphasizes the importance of protein synthesis for the release and secretion of triglyceride from the liver. The liver plays a major role in regulating lipoprotein levels by virtue of both its degradative and synthetic functions. Thus the liver is quantitatively the major site of low-density lipoprotein (LDL) catabolism, with dual high- and low-affinity receptor-mediated pathways playing a role. In addition, chylomicron remnants are removed and degraded by the liver, where their constituents have a number of metabolic effects. The liver is not only the primary site of very low density lipoprotein (VLDL) secretion but also accounts for a major portion of its subsequent degradation by mechanisms similar to that of chylomicron remnant degradation and the conversion to LDL. The liver also may play a role in high-density lipoprotein (HDL) catabolism. It is noteworthy that with the exception of cholestatic disease (see below), clinically significant alterations in lipoprotein and cholesterol metabolism are usually not found in patients with chronic liver disease.

Studies on the production of fatty liver have shown that, singly or in combination, one or more of the steps depicted in Fig. 293-2 may be involved. An increased influx of fatty acids mobilized from adipose tissue due to drugs (e.g., ethanol or glucocorticoids) or secondary to diabetic ketosis may lead to a fatty liver. Similarly, increased levels of fatty acids in the liver, either from enhanced fatty acid synthesis or from decreased fatty acid oxidation, may lead to increased triglyceride formation. In some instances (e.g., ethanol excess) there also may be increases in the carbohydrate backbone, α-glycerophosphate, involved in fatty acid esterification to triglyceride. Since release of triglyceride involves the formation of lipoproteins, lipid accumulation may occur because of decreased apoprotein synthesis. This appears to be the case in fatty livers seen in patients with protein-calorie malnutrition (kwashiorkor) and due to toxins such as carbon tetrachloride, phosphorus, or ethionine, as well as following excessive doses of antibiotics such as tetracycline that can inhibit protein synthesis. Finally, there may be impaired lipoprotein secretion from the liver. Different alterations disrupting hepatic fat metabolism may lead to different patterns of fat accumulation designated *macrovesicular* (most common) and *microvesicular*; these are reviewed in Chap. 300. Alcohol is perhaps the most common agent leading to hepatic steatosis, but the mechanism(s) whereby alcohol leads to increased liver triglyceride is not clear. Depending on factors such as dose or duration, alcohol ingestion may affect any of the seven steps shown in Fig. 293-2; however, the primary factor for the production of the alcohol-induced fatty liver remains to be determined. The alterations in the redox state due to excessive accumulation of NADH resulting from oxidation of alcohol also may contribute.

CHOLESTEROL Cholesterol and bile acid synthesis is carried out primarily by the liver. Cholesterol synthesis is subject to a number of metabolic controls, most of them mediated via the rate-limiting biosynthetic enzyme 3-hydroxy-3-methylglutaryl coenzyme A reductase (HMG-CoA reductase). Cholesterol exists either free or combined with fatty acids in the form of cholesterol esters; in the plasma, both are found primarily in association with β-lipoproteins. The plasma and liver also contain lecithin–cholesterol acyltransferase (LCAT), an enzyme involved in the conversion of free cholesterol to its esterified form. Since there is exchange of free cholesterol between tissues, changes in plasma cholesterol levels reflect changes in total body cholesterol. However, decreases in plasma cholesterol esters may reflect hepatic damage and impaired hepatic cholesterol esterification.

Severe liver injury often leads to a decrease in *total* serum cholesterol levels, including both free and esterified fractions. This may be due to decreased synthesis of cholesterol and cholesterol esters, decreased apoprotein synthesis, or both. In cholestasis (either intra- or extrahepatic), total serum cholesterol often increases strikingly. Disorders of cholestasis are associated with marked abnormalities of lipoprotein metabolism. In primary biliary cirrhosis there are pronounced elevations in serum free cholesterol and LDL; conversely, serum HDL is reduced and may disappear from the serum in patients with long-standing disease. Similar but less marked changes are seen in other cholestatic conditions.

The increase in serum free cholesterol (and phospholipid) and the concomitant decrease in esterified cholesterol in cholestasis may be related to a decrease in the hepatic production of LCAT. Reduced levels of LCAT are also correlated with the appearance of an abnormal

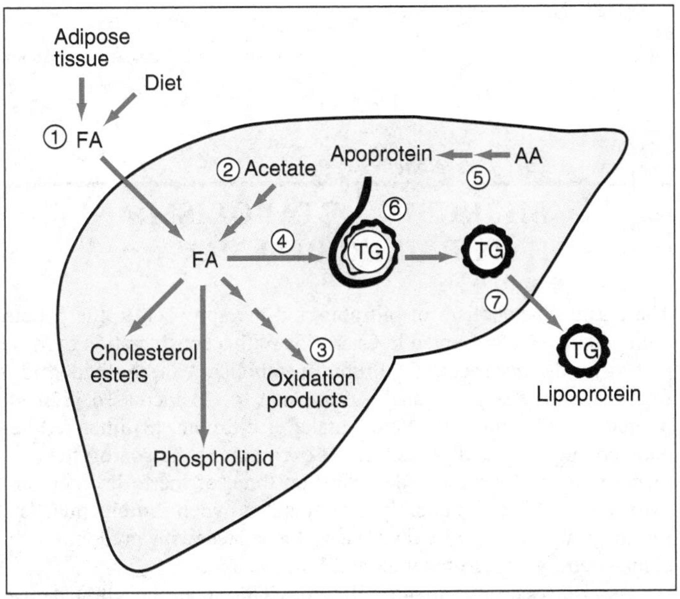

FIGURE 293-2 Factors in the uptake and esterification of fatty acids to triglyceride by the liver, including the formation and release of triglyceride as lipoprotein. The numbers refer to steps, which, if altered, may result in increased liver triglyceride (i.e., fatty liver).

LDL, referred to as *lipoprotein X* (LP-X). Although LP-X, which has a high content of free cholesterol and triglyceride, was originally thought to be a specific indicator of biliary tract obstruction, it is evident that it appears in any cholestatic condition. While the depressed hepatic production of LCAT may be responsible for altered lipid content and composition of lipoproteins, the factors leading to the overall increase in total serum cholesterol are not clear. In experimental animals, bile duct ligation results in a net increase in hepatic cholesterol synthesis and in "regurgitation" of bile salts, cholesterol, and LP-X into venous radicals. However, it is difficult to translate these experimental findings to the patient with primary biliary cirrhosis unless any insult to cells lining the biliary canaliculi and ductules can impair the delicate balance of lipid synthesis and removal.

The alterations in cholesterol and related substances resulting from liver disease may lead to significant changes in the composition of erythrocyte membranes. Such changes in composition lead to altered morphology with the development of spur and burr cell forms. The presence of these altered erythrocytes is usually an ominous sign of advanced liver disease.

BIBLIOGRAPHY

Arias IM et al: *The Liver: Biology and Pathophysiology*, 3d ed. New York, Raven, 1994

Cooper AD: Role of the liver in the degradation of lipoproteins. Gastroenterology 88:192, 1984

Flannery DB et al: Current status of hyperammonemic syndromes. Hepatology 2:495, 1982

Hoyumpa AM et al: Hepatic encephalopathy. Gastroenterology 77:803, 1979

Kleg HK et al: Conversion of androgens to estrogens in idiopathic hemochromatosis: Comparison with alcoholic liver disease. J Clin Endocrinol Metab 61:1, 1985

Owen OE et al: Hepatic, gut and renal substrate flux rates in patients with hepatic cirrhosis. J Clin Invest 68:240, 1981

Petrides A et al: Pathogenesis of glucose intolerance and diabetes mellitus in cirrhosis. Hepatology 19:616, 1994

Rothschild MA et al: Serum albumin. Hepatology 8:355, 1988

Schiff L, Schiff ER: *Diseases of the Liver*, 7th ed. Philadelphia, JB Lippincott, 1993

Smith AR et al: Alteration in plasma and CSF amino acids, amines and metabolites in hepatic coma. Ann Surg 187:343, 1978

Williams RC: Drug administration in hepatic disease. N Engl J Med 309:1616, 1983

Zakim D, Boyer TD: *Hepatology: A Textbook of Liver Disease*, 3d ed. Philadelphia, Saunders, 1996

294

Kurt J. Isselbacher

BILIRUBIN METABOLISM AND HYPERBILIRUBINEMIA

The normal metabolism of bilirubin and the approach to the patient with jaundice are presented in Chap. 45. With a consideration of these pathways, the disorders of bilirubin metabolism can be divided into four major categories, namely, those due to (1) increased pigment production, (2) reduced hepatic uptake of bilirubin, (3) impaired hepatic conjugation, and (4) decreased excretion of the conjugated pigment from the liver into bile. The first three of these disorders are associated with predominantly unconjugated hyperbilirubinemia. The fourth group, defective excretion, is associated with predominantly conjugated hyperbilirubinemia and bilirubinuria.

As discussed in Chap. 45, bilirubin UDP-glucuronosyltransferase (UGT) is essential for the normal excretion of bilirubin mono- or diglucuronide from liver to bile. There are two isoforms of UGT that are encoded by the UGT1 gene by the process of alternative splicing. Mutation in either the variable or common exons of this gene accounts for the hereditary unconjugated hyperbilirubinemic syndromes described below.

DISORDERS CAUSING PREDOMINANTLY UNCONJUGATED HYPERBILIRUBINEMIA

The plasma concentration of unconjugated bilirubin is determined by (1) the rate at which newly synthesized bilirubin enters the plasma (bilirubin turnover) and (2) the rate of removal of bilirubin by the liver (hepatic bilirubin clearance). Disturbances of the latter can result from derangements of hepatic bilirubin uptake, conjugation, or both. Measurements of these variables, although not routinely available, permit a classification of patients into those with *increased bilirubin turnover* (e.g., hemolysis), those with *decreased bilirubin clearance* (e.g., Gilbert's syndrome), and those in whom both mechanisms operate.

OVERPRODUCTION OF BILIRUBIN (INCREASED TURNOVER) Increased Destruction of Circulating Erythrocytes (Intravascular and Extravascular Hemolysis) In disorders associated with hemolysis, most commonly the hemolytic anemias, the rate of bilirubin production is increased and may even exceed the amount that can be removed by a normal liver. The resulting jaundice is primarily an unconjugated hyperbilirubinemia. There is often also a small increase in the serum conjugated bilirubin. If significant anemia or other adverse factors are present (e.g., fever, sepsis, hypoxemia, or vascular collapse), the ability of the liver to handle the pigment load will be compromised, and the degree of jaundice will be greater.

The clinical and diagnostic features of the various hemolytic anemias are described in Chap. 109. The presence of reticulocytosis, shortened red blood cell survival, and increased fecal urobilinogen, in the absence of clinical and laboratory evidence of liver disease, strongly suggest hemolysis and overproduction of bilirubin as the cause of the jaundice. It is obvious, however, that in some cases (e.g., cirrhosis, tumors, and sepsis), hemolysis *plus* deranged liver function may be present. In most cases of uncomplicated hemolytic states, the mean serum bilirubin level will be in the range of 51 to 68 μmol/L (3 to 4 mg/dL); rarely, higher levels may be seen.

Jaundice due to increased pigment production also may be seen as a consequence of *tissue infarction* (e.g., pulmonary infarcts) and large *collections of blood in tissues* (e.g., leakage from blood vessels after catheterization studies, rupture of an aortic aneurysm). If hypotension and hypoxemia also supervene, jaundice is usually more pronounced, and the resulting impairment of liver function also may lead to a significant increase in the serum conjugated bilirubin level (see "Postoperative Jaundice," below).

Except in early infancy, elevations of serum unconjugated bilirubin levels are not harmful per se, and the prognosis is that of the hemolytic process itself. However, in the neonatal state and infancy, unconjugated bilirubin levels above 340 μmol/L (20 mg/dL) may lead to *kernicterus* due to bilirubin deposition in the lipid-rich basal ganglia. Chronic overproduction of bilirubin may result in the formation of gallstones composed predominantly of bilirubin ("pigment stones"). In this situation, all the potential complications of calculus disease of the biliary tract (Chap. 302) may be superimposed on the chronic hemolytic state that produced it.

Increased Production of Bilirubin from Sources Other Than Circulating Erythrocytes About 15 to 20 percent of the circulating bilirubin is normally derived from sources other than the destruction of circulating red blood cells. This represents the so-called early-labeled fraction; it includes the synthesis of bilirubin from nonhemoglobin heme in the liver and from hemoglobin heme in the marrow.

In some conditions, jaundice results from an increased destruction of red blood cells or their precursors in the marrow—a process referred to as *ineffective erythropoiesis* (see Chap. 59). In patients with thalassemia, pernicious anemia, and congenital erythropoietic porphyria, such an increased rate of formation of the early-labeled bilirubin fraction has been demonstrated. It is possible that some cases of unexplained unconjugated hyperbilirubinemia may be caused by an increased hepatic production of bilirubin from nonhemoglobin heme, but this phenomenon has not been demonstrated clinically.

IMPAIRED HEPATIC UPTAKE OF BILIRUBIN **Drugs** Only a few drugs have been definitely shown to influence the uptake of bilirubin by the liver. Flavaspidic acid, used in the treatment of tapeworm infestation, may cause unconjugated hyperbilirubinemia during its administration. The jaundice readily subsides with cessation of the drug. Flavaspidic acid competes with bilirubin for binding to ligandin, leading thereby to unconjugated hyperbilirubinemia. The jaundice that may occur with novobiocin and some cholecystogrphic dyes is also apparently due to an interference in bilirubin uptake.

Gilbert's Syndrome Some cases of this syndrome of chronic unconjugated hyperbilirubinemia may be due to a defect in hepatic uptake. In most cases, however, a mild deficiency of bilirubin glucuronosyltransferase can be demonstrated. Hence this syndrome is best considered as a defect in bilirubin conjugation (see below).

IMPAIRED BILIRUBIN CONJUGATION (DECREASED ACTIVITY OF BILIRUBIN GLUCURONOSYLTRANSFERASE) **Neonatal Jaundice (Physiologic Jaundice of the Newborn)** Almost every infant exhibits some transient unconjugated hyperbilirubinemia between the second and fifth days of life. While during gestation the placenta serves to clear bilirubin from the fetus, after birth infants must detoxify the pigments themselves. However, at this stage the hepatic enzyme glucuronosyltransferase is still "immature." In addition, lack of intestinal bacteria prevents bilirubin conversion to urobilinogen, permitting unconjugated bilirubin to be absorbed. As a result, unconjugated bilirubinemia develops, usually not exceeding 86 μmol/L (5 mg/dL). The activity of glucuronosyltransferase increases within several days to 2 weeks after birth, and concomitantly, the serum bilirubin level returns to normal. In infants with a superimposed hemolytic process (e.g., erythroblastosis), the excessive pigment load leads to more pronounced jaundice, and bilirubin levels may exceed 340 μmol/L (20 mg/dL). It should be emphasized that neonatal jaundice is not present at the time of delivery; if jaundice is present at birth, other causes must be considered.

The cytoplasmic liver cell protein ligandin (glutathione-*S*-transferase B) binds bilirubin in the hepatocyte and may assist in the transfer of bilirubin to the endoplasmic reticulum for conjugation (Chap. 45).

An additional facet of the "immature" liver is a concomitant defect in the excretion of *conjugated* bilirubin. Rarely this defect persists beyond the time needed for the development of adequate glucuronide conjugation and may explain the occasional presence of conjugated hyperbilirubinemia in infants with erythroblastosis (*inspissated bile syndrome*).

When in the neonatal state unconjugated bilirubin levels approach or exceed 340 μmol/L (20 mg/dL), the infants may develop and die of kernicterus (bilirubin encephalopathy). This condition results from unconjugated bilirubin deposition in the lipid-rich basal ganglia. The current therapeutic approach involves *phototherapy*; intense illumination of these patients with strong white or blue light leads to the *photoisomerization* of bilirubin to water-soluble isomers that are rapidly excreted in the bile without the prior need for conjugation. Another novel approach involves decreasing bilirubin production from heme by inhibitors of heme oxygenase. Synthetic protoporphyrins, such as tin protoporphyrin, have been administered successfully to patients with neonatal hyperbilirubinemia with marked reduction in the serum bilirubin and with no major side effects.

Hereditary Glucuronosyltransferase Deficiency There are currently three syndromes that fall into this category. As indicated in Table 294-1, they reflect progressive decreases in the activity of glucuronosyltransferase and thus may be part of a spectrum, i.e., from minimal deficiency to complete absence of bilirubin glucuronosyltransferase.

Gilbert's syndrome Since the original report by Gilbert in 1907, there has been an increased recognition of this benign but chronic disorder characterized by mild, persistent, unconjugated hyperbilirubinemia. The patient usually does not manifest this disorder until after the second decade and is often unaware of the jaundice until it is detected by physical examination or routine laboratory testing. The total serum bilirubin level usually ranges and fluctuates from 21 to 51 μmol/L (1.2 to 3 mg/dL) and rarely exceeds 86 μmol/L (5 mg/dL). With the van den Bergh diazo reaction, less than 20 percent of bilirubin gives a direct reaction; however, studies using more accurate methods (such as high-pressure liquid chromatography) show that *the serum bilirubin in patients with Gilbert's syndrome is almost all unconjugated.* Typically, the jaundice fluctuates and is exacerbated following prolonged fasting (see below), surgery, fever or infection, and excessive exertion or alcohol ingestion. Liver function tests are normal, and the liver cells usually appear normal by light microscopy.

With the exception of hemolytic anemias, Gilbert's syndrome is probably the most common cause of mild unconjugated hyperbilirubinemia. On the basis of serum bilirubin levels, 3 to 10 percent of the general population are estimated to have Gilbert's syndrome. These patients have a partial deficiency of bilirubin glucuronosyltransferase; their hepatic glucuronidating activity is approximately 30 percent of normal.

Genetic data indicate that patients with Gilbert's syndrome have reduced expression of the UGT1 gene due to the presence of two extra nucleotides (TA) in the promotor region (the TATAA element) of the gene. This expanded nucleotide repeat interferes with the binding for the transcription factor IID resulting in reduced expresion of UGT1. Some patients also manifest decreased bilirubin uptake and increased hemolysis. Decreased glucuronosyltransferase alone or together with a decrease in bilirubin uptake appears to account for the observed *decrease in hepatic bilirubin clearance.* A decreased clearance and hepatic uptake of bile salts also have been shown.

Previously, Gilbert's syndrome was traditionally defined as mild, chronic, unconjugated hyperbilirubinemia occurring in the absence of hemolysis. However, with the use of radiobilirubin kinetics and erythrocyte half-life studies, at least two forms of Gilbert's syndrome have been described. One group includes patients with decreased bilirubin clearance and *no hemolysis.* A second group includes those who also have *evidence of hemolysis* (often occult) and hence increased bilirubin turnover. The simultaneous presence of both derangements appears to be a chance occurrence of two not uncommon disorders in the same patient and does not imply a causal relationship. There is additional evidence of the heterogeneity of patients with Gilbert's syndrome. Thus, some patients have an increase in hepatocyte lipofuscin and an increase in the smooth endoplasmic reticulum (SER); others show an increase in hepatic lysosomal enzymes.

A feature of Gilbert's syndrome that can be useful diagnostically is the increase in serum bilirubin following prolonged fasting or calorie deprivation. Patients with this disorder, when placed on 1260 kJ (300 kcal) per day for 2 days, will increase their serum bilirubin by 25 μmol/

Table 294-1

Hereditary Unconjugated Hyperbilirubinemias with Deficiency of Glucuronosyltransferase

Features	Mild (Gilbert's Syndrome)	Moderate (Crigler-Najjar Syndrome Type II)	Severe (Crigler-Najjar Syndrome Type I)
Inheritance	Unclear*	Dominant†	Recessive
Serum bilirubin, μmol/L (mg/dL)	17–102 (1–6)	102–340 (6–20)	340–770 (20–45)
Kernicterus	No	Rare	Yes
Conjugated bilirubin in bile	Yes (↑ monoconjugates)	Yes (↑↑ monoconjugates)	No
Response to phenobarbital	Yes	Yes	No
Bilirubin conjugation	↓‡	↓↓	Absent

* Many cases have no familial incidence.
† Variable expressivity.
‡ Other defects such as occult hemolysis and decreased bilirubin uptake may coexist.

L (1.5 mg/dL) or more, the major increase being in the unconjugated fraction. A decrease in glucuronosyltransferase activity is needed to obtain this effect. Patients with hemolysis do not show an increase in serum bilirubin with fasting. As a reflection of the mild decrease in glucuronosyltransferase in Gilbert's syndrome, (1) serum bilirubin levels will diminish when the enzyme activity is enhanced following phenobarbital administration, and (2) the bile shows a modest increase in monoconjugates of bilirubin (see Table 294-1).

In general, the diagnosis of this benign but not uncommon disorder is made by exclusion. The syndrome is suspected in a patient with low-grade unconjugated hyperbilirubinemia with (1) no systemic symptoms, (2) *no overt* or clinically recognizable hemolysis, (3) normal tests of routine liver function, and (4) a liver biopsy (although usually not necessary) that is normal by light microscopy.

Crigler-Najjar syndrome (types I and II) This disorder exists in two forms. Type I is the clinically *severe* form (originally described by Crigler and Najjar) and is due to *absence of glucuronosyltransferase activity* as a result of a mutation in one of the common 3′ regions of the UGT1 gene (or lack of function of one or more isoenzymes of the transferase). Type II has more *moderate* clinical findings due to *partial deficiency of glucuronosyltransferase* resulting from a mutation in the variable region (exon 1) of the UGT1 gene. The major differences of types I and II are summarized in Table 294-1.

Type I (Crigler-Najjar) is a rare disorder. Infants develop high unconjugated bilirubin levels in the serum [340 to 770 μmol/L (20 to 45 mg/dL)]. Absence of the enzyme can be demonstrated in the liver by enzymatic or molecular genetic techniques. Routine liver function tests are normal, as is liver histology. Because of the lack of glucuronosyltransferase activity, no conjugated bilirubin is formed by the liver; hence no bilirubin is secreted into the bile and liver, and the bile is colorless.

Phototherapy may temporarily and transiently reduce the unconjugated bilirubin level. Phenobarbital has no effect, since the enzyme defect is complete and no drug "induction" is therefore possible. Other options include plasmapheresis, orthotopic liver transplantation, and, perhaps in the future, gene therapy with insertion of the normal UGT gene. Affected infants usually die within the first year of life, although some patients have survived to the second or third decade of life. Death is usually from kernicterus. A strain of rats (Gunn rat) with the type I defect exists and is widely used as an animal model of the Crigler-Najjar syndrome (type I).

Type II patients with only a *partial deficiency* of glucuronosyltransferase have a less severe disorder. Serum unconjugated bilirubin levels are lower [103 to 340 μmol/L (6 to 20 mg/dL)], jaundice may not appear until adolescence, and neurologic complications are uncommon. The bile contains variable amounts of conjugated bilirubin with a significant increase in monoconjugates. Phenobarbital is effective in lowering the serum bilirubin level in type II patients. However, the disorder is relatively benign in those patients with bilirubin levels less than 308 to 340 μmol/L (18 to 20 mg/dL).

Acquired Deficiency of Glucuronosyltransferase (UGT) As with any enzyme, glucuronosyltransferase is susceptible to inhibition by a variety of agents, and because of the decreased activity of the enzyme in the neonatal state, such inhibition may be more evident at that time. Neonatal jaundice may be aggravated or prolonged in infants treated with *drugs* such as chloramphenicol or novobiocin or with *vitamin K.* In some breast-fed infants, jaundice has been ascribed to glucuronosyltransferase inhibitors in *breast milk*, including pregnane-3β,20α-diol and free fatty acids. When the infant is removed from the breast, the "breast-milk jaundice" subsides.

Hypothyroidism delays the normal "maturation" of glucuronosyltransferase. In cretins, neonatal jaundice may be prolonged for weeks or months. In fact, the presence of prolonged unconjugated hyperbilirubinemia after birth may be a clue to an underlying hypothyroidism.

In the infant, as well as in the adult, *liver cell damage* leads to impairment in glucuronide conjugation as a result of decreased transferase activity. However, since excretion is probably the rate-limiting step in bilirubin metabolism, and since this step appears to be interfered with to a greater extent than conjugation in parenchymal liver disease, the pigment that accumulates in the blood is predominantly conjugated bilirubin.

DISORDERS CAUSING COMBINED CONJUGATED AND UNCONJUGATED HYPERBILIRUBINEMIA

In jaundice due to primary liver disease, the plasma usually exhibits elevated levels of both conjugated and unconjugated bilirubin, and the *urine contains bilirubin.* The relative proportions of the two pigments are highly variable. In many familial hepatic abnormalities (described below) and in some forms of liver injury, the jaundice is largely due to increases in conjugated bilirubin. Such a serum pigment pattern is also seen with extrahepatic biliary obstruction. One *cannot differentiate* intrahepatic and extrahepatic causes of jaundice from either the levels or proportions of unconjugated and conjugated bilirubin in serum. Thus the main purpose of the initial fractionation of the serum bilirubin is to distinguish hepatic parenchymal and biliary obstructive disease from the disorders associated with predominantly unconjugated hyperbilirubinemia.

FAMILIAL DEFECTS IN HEPATIC EXCRETORY FUNCTION **Dubin-Johnson Syndrome** This relatively rare disorder, also called *chronic idiopathic jaundice*, is a benign, autosomally inherited hyperbilirubinemia characterized by the presence of a dark pigment in the centrilobular region of the liver cells. On direct visual inspection, the liver is black. Functionally, there exists a *defect in biliary excretion* of bilirubin, cholephilic dyes, and porphyrins. Using the diazo method for measuring bilirubin, the serum pigment in these patients typically is in the range of 51 to 257 μmol/L (3 to 15 mg/dL) and predominantly of the conjugated type. However, with the newer and more accurate method (alkaline methanolysis and high-pressure liquid chromatography), homozygous patients with the Dubin-Johnson syndrome have been shown to also have significant levels of serum *unconjugated bilirubin.* The latter finding may in part reflect pigment that, after conjugation by the liver, is deconjugated in the hepatobiliary system and refluxed back into the plasma. Moreover, the serum contains more diconjugated than monoconjugated bilirubin, just the reverse of what is seen in acquired hepatobiliary disease and Rotor syndrome. This reversed ratio is believed to be characteristic and diagnostic for homozygous patients.

Patients with Dubin-Johnson syndrome may be asymptomatic or have vague constitutional or gastrointestinal symptoms. Pruritus is absent, and serum bile acid levels are normal. The degree of jaundice is increased by intercurrent illness, oral contraceptives, and pregnancy. Not infrequently the liver is slightly enlarged; in about one-fourth of cases there is mild hepatic tenderness. Oral and intravenous cholangiography fail to visualize the biliary tract. There is typically and characteristically a late rise in the plasma sodium sulfobromophthalein (BSP) elimination curve at *90 min.* This is caused by the reflux from the liver of the conjugated dye and reflects the defect in the hepatic excretory transport maximum. It is noteworthy that there is no such secondary rise in plasma when dyes that are not conjugated by the liver are given, such as indocyanine green. When bile salts such as ursodeoxycholic acid are given, these patients show a decreased hepatic uptake and clearance. In the liver the striking feature is the presence of a *brown or black pigment in the hepatocytes.* Some findings suggest that this unique pigment is "melanin-like"; others indicate it to be a polymer of epinephrine metabolites.

These patients also show an abnormality in coproporphyrin excretion. Normal urine contains mostly coproporphyrin III and small amounts of coproporphyrin I; Dubin-Johnson patients show the opposite, i.e., they excrete predominantly coproporphyrin I. Heterozygotes show an intermediate excretory pattern.

There is impaired excretion of many metabolites, including conjugated bilirubin, BSP, and iodinated dyes. Excretion of bile acids, however, is normal. Oral contraceptive agents may accentuate hyperbilirubinemia or may produce jaundice for the first time. Features of cholestasis such as pruritus or steatorrhea are usually lacking, and specifically, serum alkaline phosphatase levels are *not* elevated. The overall prognosis of the disorder is excellent.

Rotor Syndrome This is similar in many respects to the Dubin-Johnson syndrome. However, *there is no pigment in the liver cells*, and the serum conjugated bilirubin has more monoconjugates than diglucuronide conjugates. The liver looks grossly normal. The gallbladder is usually visualized on cholecystography, and there is an increase in the *total* urinary coproporphyrins but *not* an increased percentage in excretion of coproporphyrin I. The BSP excretion pattern does *not* show a secondary rise at 90 min. The impairment in excretion that is typical of Dubin-Johnson syndrome is not present; instead, in most cases with Rotor syndrome there is impairment of *hepatic storage capacity*. This rare syndrome is inherited as an autosomal recessive trait and is genetically distinct from Dubin-Johnson syndrome.

Benign Recurrent Intrahepatic Cholestasis This is a relatively rare syndrome characterized by recurrent attacks of pruritus and jaundice. During an attack, the serum alkaline phosphatase and bile acid levels are markedly elevated, and liver biopsy shows the morphologic features of cholestasis. However, there is no mechanical biliary obstruction, with cholangiography revealing a patent biliary tree. Remissions are the rule, and at such times hepatic function tests and liver morphologic features are normal. The cause of the disorder is unknown; cirrhosis does not develop, and the disorder is benign. A congenital origin has been postulated on the basis of the early age of onset and familial incidence.

Recurrent Jaundice of Pregnancy This form of jaundice is also known as *intrahepatic cholestasis of pregnancy*. During a normal pregnancy, some derangements in liver function occur, especially during the last trimester. Usually these consist of slight increases in BSP retention and in serum alkaline phosphatase. This mild increase in alkaline phosphatase during pregnancy is normally of placental rather than of hepatic origin. With a normal pregnancy, elevations of serum bilirubin level either do not occur or are less than 34 μmol/L (2 mg/dL).

In a small number of pregnant women, intrahepatic cholestasis may appear. This usually occurs in the third trimester but may develop any time after the seventh week of gestation. The clinical features consist primarily of pruritus and jaundice. Serum bilirubin levels are usually less than 103 μmol/L (6 mg/dL). The serum alkaline phosphatase and cholesterol levels are elevated significantly, while other liver function tests are only mildly deranged. Histologically, the liver shows varying degrees of cholestasis but only a few parenchymal cell changes. The clinical and laboratory abnormalities subside promptly after delivery and are usually normal within 7 to 14 days.

This condition has been seen more frequently in Scandinavia and Europe than in the United States. Since steroid hormones and specifically estrogens can induce changes in hepatic excretory function in normal individuals (see Chap. 293), these patients probably have an increased susceptibility or sensitivity to the hepatic effects of estrogenic and progestational hormones. The intrahepatic cholestasis is usually termed *recurrent*, since the syndrome often (but not always) reappears in subsequent pregnancies. The process is benign and self-limited, and treatment is usually not needed, but cholestyramine administration will diminish the pruritus. This disorder must be distinguished from the many other causes of jaundice not unique to pregnancy, such as viral hepatitis. It also must be distinguished from the idiopathic *acute fatty liver of pregnancy* and the *tetracycline-induced fatty liver*. The latter two conditions are rare, occur in the last trimester, and have a high fatality rate; however, in these disorders there is evidence of diffuse parenchymal damage and not only cholestasis.

ACQUIRED DEFECTS OF HEPATIC EXCRETORY FUNCTION **Drug-Induced Cholestasis** A condition entirely analogous to the intrahepatic cholestasis of pregnancy may occur in some women following the use of oral contraceptive agents. In some, mild cholestatic jaundice may occur, liver function returns to normal when the drugs are withdrawn, and chronic liver disease does not result. It is relevant that one-third of the reported patients with jaundice due to oral contraceptives also have a history of recurrent intrahepatic cholestasis of pregnancy.

The nature of these changes produced by the natural and synthetic female sex hormones is very similar to those resulting from the administration of certain testosterone analogues, especially those with α substitutions at the 17 position of the steroid nucleus. These agents (such as methyltestosterone and norethandrolone), unlike the female hormones, have been implicated as a cause of chronic liver disease, especially biliary cirrhosis.

Because of these phenomena, synthetic steroid sex hormones should not be used in patients with liver disease. Conversely, in individuals using these agents, the appearance of jaundice or elevations in serum aminotransferase or alkaline phosphatase levels contraindicates their further use.

There are many drugs that may produce not only cholestasis but liver injury resembling acute hepatitis or cholestatic hepatitis. In contrast to the jaundice produced by the steroid hormones, the clinical features are those of fever, rash, arthralgia, and sometimes eosinophilia, with the liver showing a pronounced inflammatory reaction. These features suggest that such reactions are *allergic* or *toxic* in nature and therefore differ from the effects caused by the steroid hormones, which probably represent an exaggerated response by the liver to the normal action of these hormones. → *For further discussion, see Chap. 296.*

Postoperative Jaundice The occurrence of postoperative jaundice is a problem of increasing importance. It is perhaps seen more frequently now than in earlier years because patients are able to undergo more major surgical procedures (i.e., cardiac surgery, repair of ruptured aneurysms) and survive. In approaching this problem, the possible pathogenic mechanisms listed in Table 294-2 need to be considered. The patient may have *pigment overload*, especially from blood transfusions (with hemolysis of stored blood), from resorption of blood in extravascular spaces, and, less commonly, from hemolytic anemia. *Hepatocellular damage* and decreased liver cell function may occur due to concurrent use of hepatotoxic drugs (Chap. 296) or anesthetics such as halothane. Hepatocellular necrosis may follow profound shock; with lesser degrees of hypotension or hypoxemia, morphologic damage may be slight, but significant impairment of function may occur. Hence prior shock or hypotension plus pigment overload may produce significant jaundice. Extensive sepsis also can produce jaundice, often of a cholestatic type. Concurrent renal impairment due to hypotension and hypoxemia may enhance the degree of jaundice because the renal excretion of conjugated bilirubin is decreased. *Extrahepatic obstruction* due to surgical damage or stones needs to be considered and may be excluded by sonography.

A form of jaundice referred to as *benign postoperative intrahepatic cholestasis* may be seen. In the typical case, the patient has had major

Table 294-2

Conditions Causing or Contributing to Postoperative Jaundice

I. Increased pigment load
    A. Hemolytic anemia
    B. Transfusions (especially of stored blood)
    C. Resorption of hematomas, blood in extravascular spaces
II. Impaired hepatocellular function
    A. Hepatitis-like picture
        1. Anesthetic agents (e.g., halothane)
        2. Drugs
        3. Shock
        4. Infection with hepatitis viruses
    B. Cholestatic picture
        1. Hypotension, hypoxemia
        2. Drugs
        3. Sepsis
III. Extrahepatic obstruction
    A. Bile duct injury
    B. Choledocholithiasis

and prolonged surgery for a catastrophic event such as a ruptured aortic aneurysm complicated by hypotension and hypoxemia, extensive blood loss into tissues, and massive blood replacement. Jaundice may be noted on the second or third postoperative day, and the serum bilirubin, predominantly conjugated, may reach 340 to 680 μmol/L (20 to 40 mg/dL) by the eighth to tenth day. Serum alkaline phosphatase levels may be elevated three- to tenfold. Typically, the serum aspartate aminotransferase (AST, SGOT) is only mildly elevated. The liver morphology is striking in that necrosis is not seen, only cholestasis and erythrophagocytosis.

The cause of this type of postoperative cholestatic jaundice is uncertain. However, it probably reflects (1) increased pigment load, (2) decreased liver function due to hypoxemia and hypotension, and (3) decreased renal bilirubin excretion due to varying degrees of tubular necrosis as a result of shock. This diagnostic possibility must be considered in the postoperative patient with marked cholestatic jaundice. The course of the jaundice is self-limited and will subside if the other systemic complications do not predominate and lead to death.

Hepatitis and Cirrhosis These disorders constitute the *most common disorders associated with jaundice*. As has been stated previously, when the liver cell is damaged, as in viral hepatitis, there is often impairment in all three major hepatic phases of bilirubin metabolism, namely, uptake, conjugation, and excretion. Since the excretory step is the one which is rate-limiting and most readily affected by injury, significant amounts of conjugated bilirubin reenter the systemic circulation. There are also lesser increases in the serum unconjugated bilirubin. This phenomenon is probably a reflection of the impaired uptake and conjugation and is due in part to the shortened life span of red blood cells often found in liver disease. In most patients with hepatitis and cirrhosis, the total serum bilirubin levels tend not to exceed 860 μmol/L (50 mg/dL). (For a summary of laboratory features in icteric states, see Table 294-3.) → ***For detailed discussion, see Chaps. 295 to 298.***

EXTRAHEPATIC BILIARY OBSTRUCTION Anatomic or mechanical obstruction of the bile ducts is most commonly due to stones, tumors, or strictures. The clinical picture is quite similar to that of intrahepatic cholestasis, with pronounced elevations of the serum conjugated bilirubin and alkaline phosphatase levels. Usually, but not always, fever, pain, and chills may be present. In contrast to hepatitis and cirrhosis, the serum bilirubin level often tends to plateau and rarely exceeds levels of 600 μmol/L (35 mg/dL). The reason for this plateau is not clear but may be related to renal excretion of conjugated bilirubin or alternative pathways of bilirubin catabolism in obstructive jaundice.

Table 294-3

Laboratory Features in Icteric States

Bilirubin Disorder	Serum Bilirubin: Unconjugated	Serum Bilirubin: Conjugated	Urine Bilirubin	Comments
OVERPRODUCTION				
I. Hemolysis (intra- and extravascular)	↑	N	0	↑ Bilirubin turnover; serum bilirubin rarely exceeds 68 μmol/L (4 mg/dL)
II. Ineffective erythropoiesis	↑	N	0	Splenomegaly; normal RBC survival; normoblasts in marrow
DEFECTIVE HEPATIC UPTAKE				
I. Some drugs (e.g., flavaspidic acid, novobiocin)				
II. Gilbert's syndrome (some cases)	↑	N	0	Normal liver biopsy
DEFECTIVE CONJUGATION				
I. Neonatal jaundice	↑	Low	0	↓ Glucuronosyltransferase; ↓ conversion of bilirubin to urobilinogen
II. Gilbert's syndrome	↑	Low	0	↓ Glucuronosyltransferase and ↓ bilirubin uptake; some may have ↑ hemolysis; bile contains ↑ monoconjugates
III. Crigler,Najjar syndrome (types I and II)	↑	Low	0	Type I = absence of transferase Type II = deficiency of transferase; bile contains ↑↑ monoconjugates
DEFECTIVE EXCRETION				
I. Intrahepatic obstruction				
A. Familial syndromes				
1. Dubin-Johnson	↑	↑	+	Abnormal BSP curve, hepatic lipochrome pigment; ↑ urinary coproporphyrin type I
2. Rotor	↑	↑		No liver pigment; ↑ total urinary coproporphyrin
B. Drugs (e.g., chloramphenicol, methyltestosterone)	↑	↑	+	↑ Alkaline phosphatase but other function tests usually normal
C. Benign recurrent intrahepatic cholestasis	↑	↑	+	↑ Alkaline phosphatase
D. Recurrent jaundice of pregnancy (third trimester)	↑	↑	+	↑ Alkaline phosphatase; may be reproduced in afflicted subjects by estrogens or progesterone
II. Extrahepatic obstruction (tumors, stone, stricture of bile duct)				↑↑ Alkaline phosphatase (often > fourfold)
A. Partial	↑	↑	+	
B. Complete	↑	↑	+	
HEPATOCELLULAR DISEASE*				
I. Hepatitis	↑	↑	+	Conjugated/total serum bilirubin >50–70%; liver biopsy important for diagnosis
II. Cirrhosis: Same as hepatitis	↑	↑		

* Note that in hepatocellular disease there is generally an interference in all pathways of bilirubin metabolism (i.e., impaired uptake, conjugation, and excretion).

BIBLIOGRAPHY

BENIGN RECURRENT INTRAHEPATIC CHOLESTASIS

DEPAGTER AGF et al: Familial benign intrahepatic cholestasis. Gastroenterology 71:202, 1976

ENDO T et al: Bile acid metabolism in benign recurrent intrahepatic cholestasis. Gastroenterology 76:1002, 1979

DUBIN-JOHNSON AND ROTOR SYNDROMES

PAULUSMA CC et al: Congenital jaundice in rats with a mutation in a multidrug resistance-associated protein gene. Science 271:1126,1996

ROSENTHAL P et al: Homozygous Dubin-Johnson syndrome exhibits a characteristic serum bilirubin pattern. Hepatology 1:540, 1981

SWARTZ HM et al: On the nature and excretion of the hepatic pigment in the Dubin-Johnson syndrome. Gastroenterology 76:958, 1979

WOLPERT E et al: Abnormal sulfobromophthalein metabolism in Rotor's syndrome and obligate heterozygotes. N Engl J Med 206:1099, 1977

BILIRUBIN GLUCURONOSYL TRANSFERASE (UGT) DEFICIENCY STATES

AONO S et al: Analysis of genes for bilirubin UDP-glucuronosyltransferase in Gilbert's syndrome. Lancet 345:958, 1995

BOSMA PJ et al: The genetic basis of the reduced expression of UDP-glucuronosyltransferase 1 in Gilbert's syndrome. N Engl J Med 333:1171, 1995

BURCHELL B et al: Function and regulation of UDP-glucuronosyltransferase genes in health and liver disease. Hepatology 20:1622, 1994

CHOWDURY JR et al: Hereditary jaundice and disorders of bilirubin metabolism, in *The Metabolic and Molecular Bases of Inherited Disease*, 7th ed. CR Scriver et al (eds). New York, McGraw-Hill, 1995, pp 2161–2208

———, CHOWDURY NR: Unveiling the mysteries of inherited disorders of bilirubin glucuronidation. Gastroenterology 105:288, 1993

MONAGHAN G et al: Genetic variation in bilirubin UDP-glucuronosyltransferase gene promotor and Gilbert's syndrome. Lancet 347:578, 1996

RITTER JK et al: Identification of a genetic alteration in the code for bilirubin UDP-glucuronosyltransferase in the UGT1 gene complex of a Crigler-Najjar type I patient. J Clin Invest 90:150, 1992

SEPPEN J et al: Discrimination between Crigler-Najjar type I and II by expression of mutant bilirubin uridine diphosphate-glucuronosyltransferase. J Clin Invest 94:2385, 1994

SOEDA Y et al: Predicted homozygous missense mutation in Gilbert's syndrome. Lancet 346:1494, 1995

POSTOPERATIVE JAUNDICE

HOOTEGEM PV et al: Serum bilirubins in hepatobiliary disease: Comparison with other liver function tests and changes in the postobstructive period. Hepatology 5:112, 1985

LAMONT JT, ISSELBACHER KJ: Postoperative jaundice, in *Wright's Liver and Biliary Disease*, 3d ed, GH Millward-Sadler et al (eds). Philadelphia, Saunders, 1992, pp 1372–1380

295

Jules L. Dienstag, Kurt J. Isselbacher

ACUTE VIRAL HEPATITIS

Acute viral hepatitis is a systemic infection affecting the liver predominantly. Almost all cases of acute viral hepatitis are caused by one of five viral agents: hepatitis A virus (HAV), hepatitis B virus (HBV), hepatitis C virus (HCV), the HBV-associated delta agent or hepatitis D virus (HDV), and hepatitis E virus (HEV). A sixth agent, hepatitis G virus (HGV), has been discovered, but its role in acute viral hepatitis remains to be established. All these human hepatitis viruses are RNA viruses, except for hepatitis B, which is a DNA virus. Although these agents can be distinguished by their molecular and antigenic properties, all types of viral hepatitis produce clinically similar illnesses. These range from asymptomatic and inapparent to fulminant and fatal acute infections common to all types, on the one hand, and from subclinical persistent infections to rapidly progressive chronic liver disease with cirrhosis and even hepatocellular carcinoma, common to the blood-borne types (HBV, HCV, and HDV), on the other.

VIROLOGY AND ETIOLOGY **Hepatitis A** Hepatitis A virus is a nonenveloped 27-nm, heat-, acid-, and ether-resistant RNA virus in the hepatovirus genus of the picornavirus family (Fig. 295-1). Its virion contains four capsid polypeptides, designated VP1 to VP4, which are cleaved posttranslationally from the polyprotein product of a 7500-nucleotide genome. Inactivation of viral activity can be achieved by boiling for 1 min, by contact with formaldehyde and chlorine, or by ultraviolet irradiation. Despite nucleotide sequence variation of up to 20 percent among isolates of HAV, all strains of this virus are immunologically indistinguishable and belong to one serotype. Hepatitis A has an incubation period of approximately 4 weeks. Its replication is limited to the liver, but the virus is present in the liver, bile, stools, and blood during the late incubation period and acute preicteric phase of illness. Despite persistence of virus in the liver, viral shedding in feces, viremia, and infectivity diminish rapidly once jaundice becomes apparent. HAV is the only one of the human hepatitis viruses that can be cultivated in vitro.

Antibodies to HAV (anti-HAV) can be detected during acute illness when serum aminotransferase activity is elevated and fecal HAV shedding is still occurring. This early antibody response is predominantly of the IgM class and persists for several months, rarely for 6 to 12 months. During convalescence, however, anti-HAV of the IgG class becomes the predominant antibody (Fig. 295-2). Therefore, the diagnosis of hepatitis A is made during acute illness by demonstrating anti-HAV of the IgM class. Following acute illness, anti-HAV of the IgG class remains detectable indefinitely, and patients with serum anti-HAV are immune to reinfection. Indeed, neutralizing antibody activity parallels the appearance of anti-HAV, and the IgG anti-HAV present in immune globulin accounts for the protection it affords against HAV infection.

Hepatitis B Hepatitis B virus is a DNA virus with a remarkably compact genomic structure; despite its small, circular, 3200-base-pair size, HBV DNA codes for four sets of viral products and has a complex, multiparticle structure. HBV achieves its genomic economy by relying on an efficient strategy of encoding proteins from four overlapping genes: S, C, P, and X (Fig. 295-3), as detailed below. Once thought to be unique among viruses, HBV is now recognized as one of a family of animal viruses, hepadnaviruses (hepatotropic DNA viruses), and is classified as hepadnavirus type 1. Similar viruses infect certain species of woodchucks, ground and tree squirrels, and Pekin ducks, to mention the most carefully characterized. Like HBV, all have the same distinctive three morphologic forms, have counterparts to the envelope and nucleocapsid virus antigens of HBV, replicate within the liver but exist in extrahepatic sites, contain their own endogenous DNA polymerase, have partially double-stranded and partially single-stranded genomes, are associated with acute and chronic hepatitis and hepatocellular carcinoma, and rely on a replicative strategy unique among DNA viruses but typical of retroviruses. Instead of DNA replication directly from a DNA template, hepadnaviruses rely on reverse transcription (effected by the DNA polymerase) of minus-strand DNA from a "pregenomic" RNA intermediate. Then plus-strand DNA is transcribed from the minus-strand DNA template by the DNA-dependent DNA polymerase. Viral proteins are translated by the pregenomic RNA, and the proteins and genome are packaged into virions and secreted from the hepatocyte. Although HBV is difficult to cultivate in vitro in the conventional sense from clinical material, several cell lines have been transfected with HBV DNA. Such transfected cells support in vitro replication of the intact virus and its component proteins.

Three particulate forms of HBV (Table 295-1) can be demonstrated by electron microscopy (see Fig. 295-1). The most numerous are the 22-nm particles, which appear as spherical or long filamentous forms; these are antigenically indistinguishable from the outer surface or envelope protein of HBV and are thought to represent excess viral envelope protein. Outnumbered in serum by a factor of 100 or 1000 to 1 compared with the spheres and tubules are large, 42-nm, double-shelled spherical particles, which represent the intact hepatitis B virion. The envelope protein expressed on the outer surface of the virion and on the smaller spherical and tubular structures is referred to as *hepatitis B surface antigen* (HBsAg). The concentration of HBsAg and virus

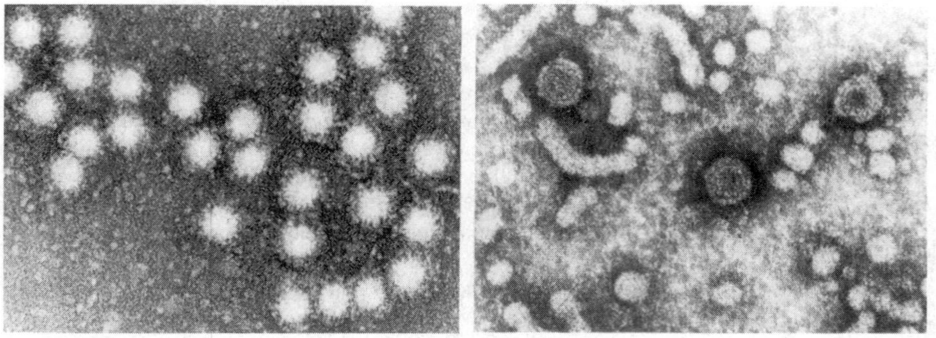

FIGURE 295-1 *A.* Electron micrograph of 27-nm hepatitis A virus particles purified from stool of a patient with acute hepatitis A virus infection and aggregated by hepatitis A antibody. *B.* Electron micrograph of concentrated serum from a patient with acute hepatitis B infection, demonstrating the 42-nm virions, tubular forms, and spherical 22-nm particles of hepatitis B surface antigen. 132,000×. (Hepatitis D resembles 42-nm virions of hepatitis B but is smaller, 35 to 37 nm; hepatitis E resembles hepatitis A virus but is slightly larger, 32 to 34 nm; hepatitis C has not been visualized definitively.)

particles in the blood may reach 500 μg/mL and 10 trillion particles per milliliter, respectively. The envelope protein, HBsAg, is the product of the S gene of HBV.

HBsAg consists primarily of two major polypeptides, one of 24,000 mol wt and its glycosylated counterpart of 28,000 mol wt. A number of different HBsAg subdeterminants have been identified. There is a common group-reactive antigen, *a*, shared by all HBsAg isolates. In addition, HBsAg may contain one of several subtype-specific antigens, namely, *d* or *y, w* or *r*, as well as other more recently characterized specificities. These HBsAg subtypes provide additional epidemiologic markers in evaluating the transmission of hepatitis B infection in that subtypes "breed true." For example, studies of hepatitis outbreaks have shown that index cases and their contacts have identical HBsAg subtypes. Clinical course and outcome, however, are independent of subtype.

Upstream of the S gene are the pre-S genes (Fig. 295-3), which code for pre-S gene products, including receptors on the HBV surface of polymerized human serum albumin and for hepatocyte membrane proteins. The pre-S region actually consists of both pre-S1 and pre-S2. Depending on where translation is initiated, three potential HBsAg gene products are synthesized. The protein product of the S gene is HBsAg (*major protein*), the product of the S region plus the adjacent pre-S2 region is the *middle protein*, and the product of the pre-S1 plus pre-S2 plus S regions is the *large protein*. Compared with the smaller spherical and tubular particles of HBV, complete 42-nm virions are enriched in the large protein. Both pre-S proteins and their respective antibodies can be detected during HBV infection, and the period of pre-S antigenemia appears to coincide with other markers of virus replication, as detailed below.

The intact 42-nm virion can be disrupted by mild detergents, and the 27-nm nucleocapsid core particle isolated. Nucleocapsid proteins are coded for by the C gene. The antigen expressed on the surface of the nucleocapsid core is referred to as *hepatitis B core antigen* (HBcAg), and its corresponding antibody is anti-HBc. A third HBV antigen is *hepatitis B e antigen* (HBeAg), a soluble, nonparticulate, nucleocapsid protein that is immunologically distinct from intact HBcAg but is a product of the same C gene. The C gene has two initiation codons, a precore and a core region (Fig. 295-3). If translation is initiated at the precore region, the protein product is HBeAg, which has a signal peptide that binds it to the smooth endoplasmic reticulum and leads to its secretion into the circulation. If translation begins with the core region, HBcAg is the protein product; it has no signal peptide, it is not secreted, but it assembles into nucleocapsid particles, which bind to and incorporate RNA and which, ultimately, contain HBV DNA. Also packaged within the nucleocapsid core is a DNA polymerase, which directs replication and repair of HBV DNA. In vitro, the polymerase can repair the single-stranded gap and render it double-stranded; it directs the synthesis of plus-strand DNA from a minus-strand template. When packaging within viral proteins is complete, synthesis of the incomplete plus strand stops; this accounts for the single-stranded gap and for differences in the size of the gap. HBcAg particles remain in the hepatocyte, where they are readily detectable by immunohistochemical staining, and are exported after encapsidation by an envelope of HBsAg. Therefore, naked core parti-

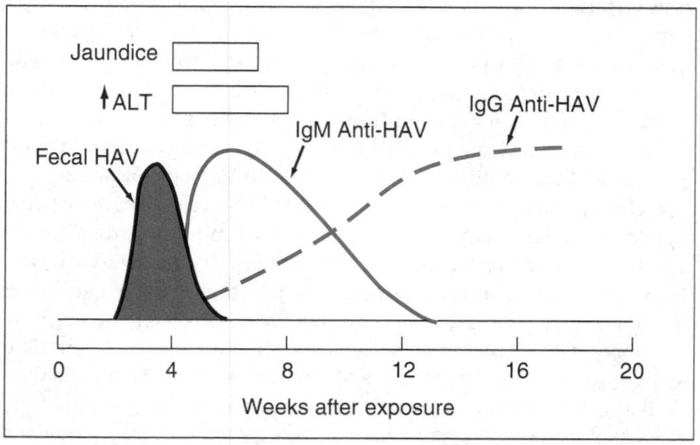

FIGURE 295-2 Scheme of typical clinical and laboratory features of viral hepatitis type A.

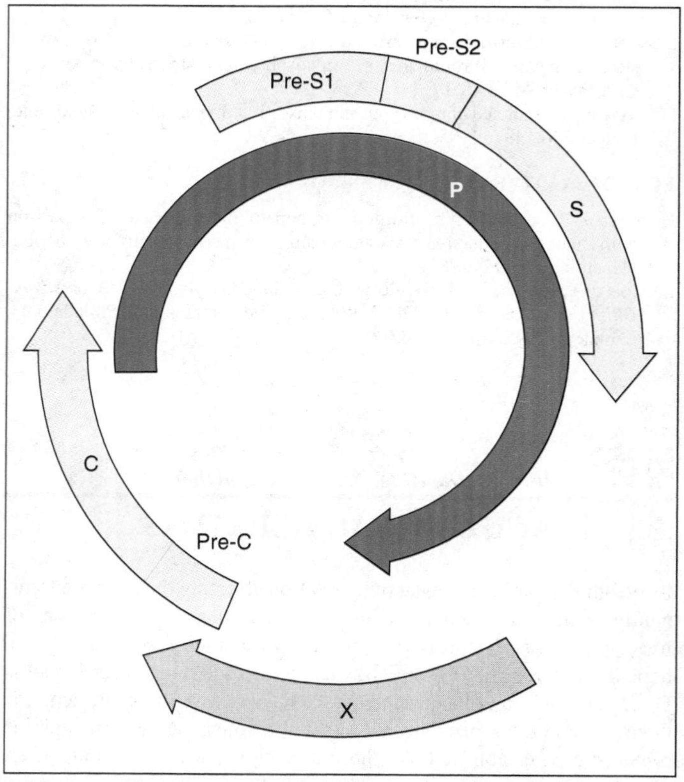

FIGURE 295-3 Its compact genomic structure, with overlapping genes, permits HBV to code for multiple proteins. The S gene codes for the "major" envelope protein, HBsAg. Pre-S1 and pre-S2, upstream of S, combine with S to code for two larger proteins, "middle" protein, the product of pre-S2 + S, and "large" protein, the product of pre-S1 + pre-S2 + S. The largest gene, P, codes for DNA polymerase. The C gene codes for two nucleocapsid proteins, HBeAg, a soluble, secreted protein (initiation from the pre-C region of the gene) and HBcAg, the intracellular core protein (initiation after pre-C). The X gene codes for HBxAg, which can transactivate the transcription of cellular and viral genes; its clinical relevance is not known.

Table 295-1

Nomenclature and features of hepatitis viruses

Hepatitis Type	Virus Particle	Morphology	Genome*	Classification	Antigen(s)	Antibodies	Remarks
HAV	27 nm	Icosahedral nonenveloped	7.5-kb RNA, linear, ss, +	Hepatovirus	HAV	anti-HAV	Early fecal shedding Diagnosis: IgM anti-HAV Previous infection: IgG anti-HAV
HBV	42 nm	Double-shelled virion (surface and core) spherical	3.2-kb DNA, circular, ss/ds	Hepadnavirus	HBsAg HBcAg HBeAg	anti-HBs anti-HBc anti-HBe	Bloodborne virus; carrier state Acute diagnosis: HBsAg, IgM anti-HBc Chronic diagnosis: IgG anti-HBc, HBsAg Markers of replication: HBeAg, HBV DNA Liver, lymphocytes, other organs.
	27 nm	Nucleocapsid core			HBcAg HBeAg	anti-HBc anti-HBe	Nucleocapsid contains DNA and DNA polymerase; present in hepatocyte nucleus; HBcAg does not circulate; HBeAg (soluble, nonparticulate) and HBV DNA circulate—correlate with infectivity and complete virions.
	22 nm	Spherical and filamentous; represents excess virus coat material			HBsAg	anti-HBs	HBsAg detectable in >95% of patients with acute hepatitis B; found in serum, body fluids, hepatocyte cytoplasm; anti-HBs appears following infection—protective antibody.
HCV	Approx. 30–60 nm	Enveloped	9.4-kb RNA, linear, ss, +	Flavivirus-like	HCV C100-3 C33c C22-3 NS5	anti-HCV	Bloodborne agent, formerly labeled non-A, non-B hepatitis Acute diagnosis: anti-HCV (C33c, C22-3, NS5), HCV RNA Chronic diagnosis: anti-HCV (C100-3, C33c, C22-3, NS5) and HCV RNA; cytoplasmic location in hepatocytes
HDV	35–37 nm	Enveloped hybrid particle with HBsAg coat and HDV core	1.7-kb RNA, circular, ss, −	Resembles viroids and plant satellite viruses	HBsAg HDV antigen	anti-HBs anti-HDV	Defective RNA virus, requires helper function of HBV (hepadnaviruses); HDV antigen present in hepatocyte nucleus Diagnosis: anti-HDV, HDV RNA; HBV/HDV coinfection—IgM anti-HBc and anti-HDV; HDV superinfection—IgG anti-HBc and anti-HDV.
HEV	32–34 nm	Nonenveloped icosahedral	7.6-kb RNA, linear, ss, +	Alphavirus-like	HEV antigen	anti-HEV	Agent of enterically transmitted hepatitis; rare in USA; occurs in Asia, Mediterranean countries, Central America Diagnosis: IgM/IgG anti-HEV (assays being developed); virus in stool, bile, hepatocyte cytoplasm
HGV	?	?	9.4-kb RNA, linear, ss, +	Flavivirus-like	?	?	Bloodborne agent, definitive role as pathogen inconclusive Diagnosis: HGV RNA, serologic assays being developed

* ss, single-stranded; ss/ds, partially single-stranded, partially double-stranded; −, minus-stranded; +, plus-stranded.

cles do not circulate in the serum. The secreted nucleocapsid protein, HBeAg, provides a convenient, readily detectable, qualitative marker of HBV replication and relative infectivity.

HBsAg-positive serum containing HBeAg is more likely to be highly infectious and to be associated with the presence of hepatitis B virions (and DNA polymerase and HBV DNA, see below) than HBeAg-negative or anti-HBe-positive serum. For example, HBsAg carrier mothers who are HBeAg-positive almost invariably (>90 percent) transmit hepatitis B infection to their offspring, while HBsAg carrier mothers with anti-HBe rarely (10 to 15 percent) infect their offspring.

Early during the course of acute hepatitis B, HBeAg appears transiently; its disappearance may be a harbinger of clinical improvement and resolution of infection. Persistence of HBeAg in serum beyond the first 3 months of acute infection may be predictive of the development of chronic infection, and the presence of HBeAg during chronic hepatitis B is associated with ongoing viral replication, infectivity, and inflammatory liver injury.

The third of the HBV genes is the largest, the P gene (Fig. 295-3), which codes for the DNA polymerase; as noted above, this enzyme has both DNA-dependent DNA polymerase and RNA-dependent reverse transcriptase activities. The fourth gene, X, codes for a small, nonparticulate protein that has been shown to be capable of transactivating the transcription of both viral and cellular genes (Fig. 295-3). Such transactivation may enhance the replication of HBV, leading to the clinical association observed between the expression of the product of the X gene, hepatitis B x antigen (HBxAg), and antibodies to it in patients with severe chronic hepatitis and hepatocellular carcinoma. The transactivating activity can enhance the transcription of other viruses besides HBV, such as human immunodeficiency virus (HIV). Therefore, HBV may be responsible for enhanced replication of other viruses. Cellular processes transactivated by X include the human interferon γ gene and class I major histocompatibility genes; potentially, these effects could contribute to enhanced susceptibility of HBV-infected hepatocytes to cytolytic T cells. The X gene and its protein product, however, are absent in nonmammalian hepadnaviruses; therefore, X is not essential for hepadnavirus replication.

After infection with HBV, the first virologic marker detectable in serum is HBsAg (Fig. 295-4). Circulating HBsAg precedes elevations of serum aminotransferase activity and clinical symptoms and remains

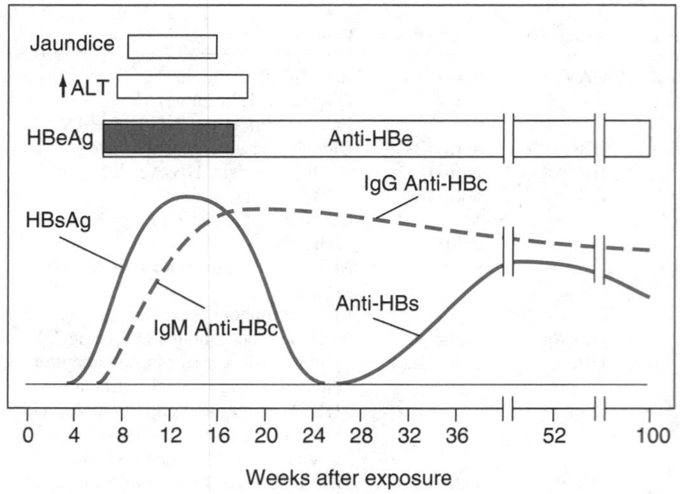

FIGURE 295-4 Scheme of typical clinical and laboratory features of acute viral hepatitis type B.

detectable during the entire icteric or symptomatic phase of acute hepatitis B and beyond. In typical cases, HBsAg becomes undetectable 1 to 2 months following the onset of jaundice and rarely persists beyond 6 months. After HBsAg disappears, antibody to HBsAg (anti-HBs) becomes detectable in serum and remains detectable indefinitely thereafter. Because HBcAg is sequestered within an HBsAg coat, HBcAg is not detectable routinely in the serum of patients with HBV infection. On the other hand, anti-HBc is readily demonstrable in serum, beginning within the first 1 to 2 weeks after the appearance of HBsAg and preceding detectable levels of anti-HBs by weeks to months. Because variability exists in the time of appearance of anti-HBs following HBV infection, occasionally a gap of several weeks or longer may separate the disappearance of HBsAg and the appearance of anti-HBs. During this "gap" or "window" period, anti-HBc may represent serologic evidence of current or recent HBV infection, and blood containing anti-HBc in the absence of HBsAg and anti-HBs has been implicated in the development of transfusion-associated hepatitis B. In part because the sensitivity of immunoassays for HBsAg and anti-HBs has increased, however, this window period is rarely encountered. In some persons, years after HBV infection, anti-HBc may persist in the circulation longer than anti-HBs. Therefore, isolated anti-HBc does not necessarily indicate active virus replication; most instances of isolated anti-HBc represent hepatitis B infection in the remote past. Rarely, however, isolated anti-HBc represents low-level hepatitis B viremia, with HBsAg below the detection threshold; occasionally, isolated anti-HBc represents a cross-reacting or false-positive immunologic specificity. Distinction between recent and remote HBV infection can be accomplished by determination of the immunoglobulin class of anti-HBc. Anti-HBc of the IgM class (IgM anti-HBc) predominates during the first 6 months approximately after acute infection, whereas IgG anti-HBc is the predominant class of anti-HBc beyond 6 months. Therefore, patients with current or recent acute hepatitis B, including those in the anti-HBc window, have IgM anti-HBc in their serum. In patients who have recovered from hepatitis B in the remote past as well as those with chronic HBV infection, anti-HBc is predominantly of the IgG class. Infrequently, in no more than 1 to 5 percent of patients with acute HBV infection, levels of HBsAg are too low to be detected; in such cases, the presence of IgM anti-HBc establishes the diagnosis of acute hepatitis B. When isolated anti-HBc occurs in the rare patient with chronic hepatitis B whose HBsAg level is below the sensitivity threshold of contemporary immunoassays (a low-level carrier), the anti-HBc is of the IgG class. Generally, in persons who have recovered from hepatitis B, anti-HBs and anti-HBc persist indefinitely.

The temporal association between the appearance of anti-HBs and resolution of HBV infection as well as the observation that persons with anti-HBs in serum are protected against reinfection with HBV suggest that *anti-HBs is the protective antibody*. Therefore, strategies for prevention of HBV infection are based on providing susceptible persons with circulating anti-HBs (see below). Occasionally, in 10 to 20 percent of patients with chronic hepatitis B, low-level, low-affinity anti-HBs can be detected. This antibody is directed against a subtype determinant different from that represented by the patient's HBsAg; its presence is thought to reflect the stimulation of a related clone of antibody-forming cells, but it has no clinical relevance and does not signal imminent clearance of hepatitis B.

The other readily detectable serologic marker of HBV infection, HBeAg, appears concurrently with or shortly after HBsAg. Its appearance coincides temporally with high levels of virus replication and reflects the presence of circulating intact virions, DNA polymerase, and HBV DNA. Pre-S1 and pre-S2 proteins are also expressed during periods of peak replication, but assays for these gene products are not routinely available. In self-limited HBV infections, HBeAg becomes undetectable shortly after peak elevations in aminotransferase activity, before the disappearance of HBsAg, and anti-HBe then becomes detectable, coinciding with a period of relatively lower infectivity (see Fig. 295-4). Because markers of HBV replication appear transiently during acute infection, testing for such markers is of little clinical utility in typical cases of acute HBV infection. In contrast, markers of HBV replication provide valuable information in patients with protracted infections. Departing from the pattern typical of acute HBV infections, in chronic HBV infection, HBsAg remains detectable beyond 6 months, anti-HBc is primarily of the IgG class, and anti-HBs is either undetectable or detectable at low levels (see "Laboratory Features," below) (Fig. 295-5). During early chronic HBV infection, HBV DNA can be detected both in serum and in hepatocyte nuclei, where it is present in free or episomal form. This *replicative stage* of HBV infection is the time of maximal infectivity and liver injury; HBeAg is a qualitative marker and HBV DNA a quantitative marker of this replicative phase, during which all three forms of HBV circulate, including intact virions. Over time, the replicative phase of chronic HBV infection gives way to a relatively *nonreplicative phase*. This occurs at a rate of approximately 10 percent per year and is accompanied by seroconversion from HBeAg-positive to anti-HBe-positive. In most cases, this seroconversion coincides with a transient, acute hepatitis–like elevation in aminotransferase activity, believed to reflect cell-mediated clearance of virus-infected hepatocytes. In the nonreplicative phase of chronic infection, when HBV DNA is demonstrable in hepatocyte nuclei, it tends to be integrated into the host genome. In this phase, only spherical and tubular forms of HBV, *not intact*

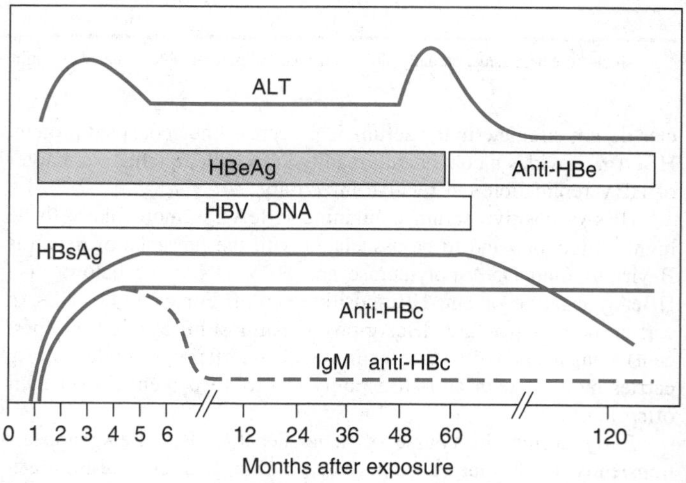

FIGURE 295-5 Scheme of typical laboratory features of chronic viral hepatitis type B. HBeAg and HBV DNA can be detected in serum during the *replicative phase* of chronic infection, which is associated with infectivity and liver injury. Seroconversion from the replicative phase to the *nonreplicative phase* occurs at a rate of approximately 10 to 15 percent per year and is heralded by an acute hepatitis–like elevation of ALT activity; during the nonreplicative phase, infectivity and liver injury are limited.

virions, circulate, and liver injury tends to subside. Most such patients would be characterized as asymptomatic HBV *carriers*. In reality, the designations *replicative* and *nonreplicative* are only relative; even in the so-called nonreplicative phase, HBV replication can be detected with highly sensitive amplification probes such as the polymerase chain reaction. Still, the distinctions are pathophysiologically and clinically meaningful. Occasionally, nonreplicative HBV infection converts back to replicative infection. Such spontaneous reactivations are accompanied by reexpression of HBeAg and HBV DNA as well as by exacerbations of liver injury.

Molecular variants of HBV have been recognized. Variation occurs throughout the HBV genome, and clinical isolates of HBV that do not express typical viral proteins have been attributed to mutations in individual or even multiple gene locations. For example, variants have been described that lack nucleocapsid proteins, envelope proteins, or both. Two categories of HBV have attracted the most attention. One of these was identified initially in Mediterranean countries among patients with an unusual serologic-clinical profile. They have severe chronic HBV infection and detectable HBV DNA but with anti-HBe instead of HBeAg. These patients were found to be infected with an HBV mutant that contained an alteration in the precore region rendering the virus incapable of encoding HBeAg. Although several potential mutation sites exist in the pre-C region, the region of the C gene necessary for the expression of HBeAg (see "Virology and Etiology," above), the most commonly encountered in such patients is a single base substitution, from G to A, which occurs in the second to last codon of the pre-C gene at nucleotide 1896. This substitution results in the replacement of the TGG tryptophan codon by a stop codon (TAG), which prevents the translation of HBeAg. Another mutation in the core promoter region prevents transcription of the coding region for HBeAg and yields an HBeAg-negative phenotype. Patients with such precore mutants that are unable to secrete HBeAg tend to have severe liver disease that progresses rapidly to cirrhosis and that does not respond readily to antiviral therapy. Both "wild-type" HBV and precore mutant HBV can coexist in the same patient, or mutant HBV may arise during wild-type HBV infection. In addition, clusters of fulminant hepatitis B in Israel and Japan have been attributed to common-source infection with a precore mutant. Fulminant hepatitis B in North America and western Europe, however, occurs in patients infected with wild-type HBV, in the absence of precore mutants, and both precore mutants and other mutations throughout the HBV genome occur commonly even in patients with typical, self-limited, milder forms of HBV infection. Therefore, additional investigation will be necessary to define the effect of precore mutants on the pathogenicity and natural history of HBV infection.

The second important category of HBV mutants consists of *escape mutants*, in which a single amino acid substitution, from glycine to arginine, occurs at position 145 of the immunodominant *a* determinant common to all subtypes of HBsAg. This change in HBsAg leads to a critical conformational change that results in a loss of neutralizing activity by anti-HBs. This specific HBV/*a* mutant has been observed in two situations, active and passive immunization, in which humoral immunologic pressure may favor evolutionary change ("escape") in the virus—in a small number of hepatitis B vaccine recipients who acquired HBV infection despite the prior appearance of neutralizing anti-HBs and in liver transplant recipients who underwent the procedure for hepatitis B and who were treated with a high-potency human monoclonal anti-HBs preparation. Although such mutants have not been appreciated frequently, their existence raises a concern that may complicate vaccination strategies and serologic diagnosis.

Hepatitis B antigens and HBV DNA have been identified in extrahepatic sites, including lymph nodes, bone marrow, circulating lymphocytes, spleen, and pancreas. Although the virus does not appear to be associated with tissue injury in any of these extrahepatic sites, its presence in these "remote" reservoirs has been invoked to explain the recurrence of HBV infection after orthotopic liver transplantation. A more complete understanding of the clinical relevance of extrahepatic HBV remains to be defined.

Hepatitis D The delta hepatitis agent, or HDV, is a defective RNA virus that coinfects with and requires the helper function of HBV (or other hepadnaviruses) for its replication and expression. Slightly smaller than HBV, delta is a formalin-sensitive, 35- to 37-nm virus with a hybrid structure. Its nucleocapsid expresses delta antigen, which bears no antigenic homology with any of the HBV antigens, and contains the virus genome. The delta core is "encapsidated" by an outer envelope of HBsAg, indistinguishable from that of HBV except in its relative compositions of major, middle, and large HBsAg component proteins. The genome is a small, 1700-nucleotide, circular, single-stranded RNA (minus strand) that is nonhomologous with HBV DNA (except for a small area of the polymerase gene) but that has features and the rolling circle model of replication common to genomes of plant satellite viruses or viroids. HDV RNA contains many areas of internal complementarity; therefore, it can fold on itself by internal base pairing to form an unusual, very stable, rodlike structure. HDV RNA replicates via RNA-directed RNA synthesis by transcription of genomic RNA to a complementary antigenomic (plus strand) RNA; the antigenomic RNA, in turn, serves as a template for subsequent genomic RNA synthesis. Between the genomic and antigenomic RNAs of HDV, there are coding regions for nine proteins. Delta antigen, which is a product of the antigenomic strand, exists in two forms, a small, 195-amino-acid species, which plays a role in facilitating HDV RNA replication, and a large, 214-amino-acid species, which appears to suppress replication but is required for assembly of the antigen into virions. Although complete hepatitis D virions and liver injury require the cooperative helper function of HBV, intracellular replication of HDV RNA can occur without HBV. Genomic heterogeneity among HDV isolates has been described; however, pathophysiologic and clinical consequences of this genetic diversity have not been recognized.

HDV can either infect a person simultaneously with HBV (*coinfection*) or superinfect a person already infected with HBV (*superinfection*); when HDV infection is transmitted from a donor with one HBsAg subtype to an HBsAg-positive recipient with a different subtype, the HDV agent assumes the HBsAg subtype of the recipient, rather than the donor. Because HDV relies absolutely on HBV, the duration of HDV infection is determined by the duration of (and cannot outlast) HBV infection. HDV antigen is expressed primarily in hepatocyte nuclei and is occasionally detectable in serum. During acute HDV infection, anti-HDV of the IgM class predominates, and 30 to 40 days may elapse after symptoms appear before anti-HDV can be detected. In self-limited infection, anti-HDV is low titer and transient, rarely remaining detectable beyond the clearance of HBsAg and HDV antigen. In chronic HDV infection, anti-HDV circulates in high titer, and both IgM and IgG anti-HDV can be detected. HDV antigen in the liver and HDV RNA in serum and liver can be detected during HDV replication.

Hepatitis C Hepatitis C virus, which, before its identification was labeled "non-A, non-B hepatitis," is a linear, single-stranded, positive-sense, 9500-nucleotide RNA virus, the genome of which is similar in organization to that of flaviviruses and pestiviruses; HCV constitutes its own genus in the family Flaviviridae. The HCV genome contains a single large open reading frame (gene) that codes for a virus polyprotein of approximately 3000 amino acids. The 5′ end of the genome consists of an untranslated region adjacent to the genes for structural proteins, the nucleocapsid core protein and two envelope glycoproteins, E1 and E2/NS1. The 5′ untranslated region and core gene are highly conserved among genotypes, but the envelope proteins are coded for by the hypervariable region, which varies from isolate to isolate and may allow the virus to evade host immunologic containment directed at accessible virus-envelop proteins. The 3′ end of the genome contains the genes for nonstructural (NS) proteins. The first reported HCV clone, 5-1-1, and the nucleotide sequence coding for C100-3, the recombinant virus protein used in the first immunoassay for antibodies to HCV, reside within the NS4 gene, and the RNA-dependent RNA polymerase, through which HCV replicates, is encoded by the NS5 region (Fig. 295-6). Because HCV does not replicate via a DNA

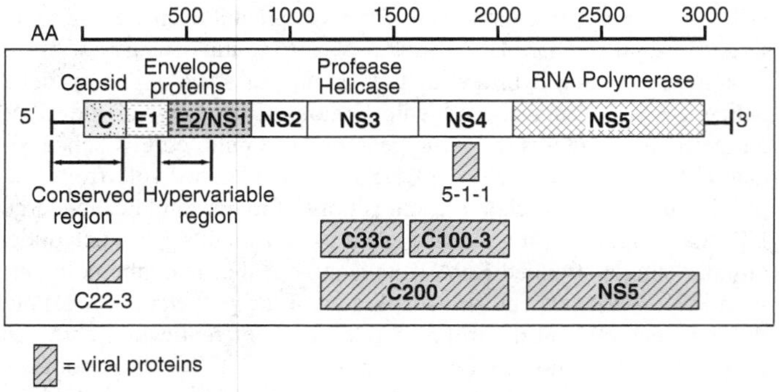

FIGURE 295-6 Organization of the hepatitis C virus genome and its associated proteins. Structural genes at the 5′ end include the nucleocapsid region, C, and the envelope regions, E1 and E2. The 5′ untranslated region and the C region are highly conserved among isolates, while the envelope domain E2/NS1 contains the hypervariable region. At the 3′ end are five nonstructural (NS) regions. Viral proteins included in the first-generation (C100-3), second-generation (C200, a fusion protein of C100-3 and C33c, and C22-3), and third-generation (C22-3, C200, or C33c and C100-3, and NS5) immunoassays and in the recombinant immunoblot assay (5-1-1, C100-3, C33c, C22-3, NS5) are presented below their corresponding genes (AA = amino acid).

intermediate, it does not integrate into the host genome. Because HCV tends to circulate in very low titer, visualization of virus particles has been difficult. Although in vitro HCV replication remains difficult to accomplish convincingly, the chimpanzee has proven to be an invaluable experimental animal model.

At least six distinct genotypes, as well as subtypes within genotypes, of HCV have been identified by nucleotide sequencing. Because divergence of HCV isolates within a genotype or subtype, and within the same host, may vary insufficiently to define a distinct genotype, these intragenotypic differences are referred to as *quasispecies*. The genotypic and quasispecies diversity of HCV, resulting from its high mutation rate, interferes with effective humoral immunity. Neutralizing antibodies to HCV have been demonstrated, but they tend to be short-lived, and HCV infection has not been shown to induce lasting immunity against reinfection with different virus isolates or even the same virus isolate. Thus, neither *heterologous* nor *homologous* immunity appears to develop after acute HCV infection. Some HCV genotypes are distributed worldwide, while others are more geographically confined. In addition, differences in pathogenicity and responsiveness to antiviral therapy have been reported among genotypes; however, the biological impact of genotype and quasispecies differences remains incompletely defined.

As noted above, the first assay detected antibodies to C100-3, a recombinant polypeptide derived from the NS4 region of the genome. In most patients with acute hepatitis C, antibody detected with this assay appears between 1 to 3 months after the onset of acute hepatitis but sometimes not for a year or longer. Second-generation assays incorporate recombinant proteins from the nucleocapsid core region, C22-3, and the NS3 region, C33c (expressed in combination with C100-3 as C200); these assays are more sensitive (by approximately 20 percent) and detect anti-HCV 30 to 90 days earlier, during the period of acute hepatitis. A third-generation immunoassay, which incorporates proteins from the NS5 region and replaces some recombinant proteins with synthetic peptides, may detect anti-HCV even earlier. Because nonspecificity has been encountered in clinical samples tested for anti-HCV, a supplementary recombinant immunoblot assay was introduced. Reactivity in an immunoassay is "confirmed" by incubation with a nitrocellulose strip that contains individual bands of recombinant or synthetic HCV proteins. This approach allows the demonstration of individual antibodies to nonstructural and structural viral proteins and identifies false-positive reactivity associated with nonviral specificities. It is useful to support the validity of anti-HCV-reactive samples, especially in patients with a low prior probability of true infection (e.g., blood donors) or in patients with confounding activity in serum (such as a rheumatoid factor) that may yield false-positive antibody reactivity. Still, detection of anti-HCV is insufficient to identify all persons infected with HCV. The most sensitive indicator is the presence of HCV RNA, which requires molecular amplification by polymerase chain reaction (PCR) (Fig. 295-7). An alternative method for detection of HCV RNA, more easily automated but one or two orders of magnitude less sensitive, is branched-chain complementary DNA hybridization. HCV RNA can be detected within a few days of exposure to HCV, well before the appearance of anti-HCV, and tends to persist for the duration of HCV infection; however, in patients with chronic HCV infection, occasionally, HCV RNA may be detectable only intermittently. Application of sensitive molecular probes for HCV RNA has revealed the presence of replicative HCV in peripheral blood lymphocytes of infected persons; however, as is the case for HBV in lymphocytes, the clinical relevance of HCV lymphocyte infection is not known.

Hepatitis E Previously labeled *epidemic* or *enterically transmitted non-A, non-B hepatitis*, HEV is an enterically transmitted virus that occurs primarily in India, Asia, Africa, and Central America. This agent, with epidemiologic features resembling those of hepatitis A, is a 32- to 34-nm, nonenveloped, HAV-like virus with a 7600-nucleotide, single-stranded, positive-sense RNA genome. HEV has three open reading frames (genes), the largest of which encodes nonstructural proteins involved in virus replication. A middle-sized gene encodes the nucleocapsid protein, and the smallest, whose function is not known, encodes protein specificities to which antibodies appear in human serum. All HEV isolates appear to belong to a single serotype, despite genomic heterogeneity of up to 25 percent. There is no genomic or antigenic homology, however, between HEV and HAV or other picornaviruses, and HEV, although resembling calciviruses, appears to be sufficiently distinct from any known agent to merit a new classification of its own within the alphavirus group. The virus has been detected in stool, bile, and liver from infected patients as well as from experimentally infected nonhuman primates. Studies in humans and experimental animals have shown that HEV is excreted in the stool during the late incubation period and that immune responses to viral antigens occur very early during the course of acute infection. Both IgM anti-HEV and IgG anti-HEV can be detected, but both fall rapidly after acute infection, reaching low levels within 9 to 12 months. Currently, serologic testing for HEV infection is not available routinely.

Hepatitis G A sixth hepatitis virus was discovered independently by two different groups, one calling it hepatitis G (HGV), the other calling it GB virus C (GBV-C; a viral agent isolated in the 1960s from a surgeon with viral hepatitis and transmitted in tamarins). This

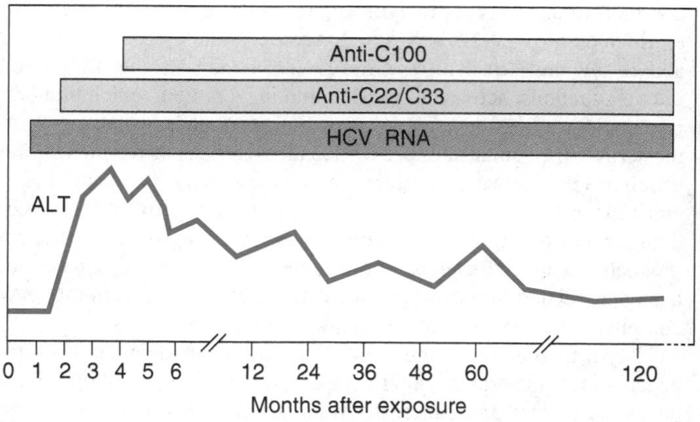

FIGURE 295-7 Scheme of typical laboratory features during acute hepatitis type C progressing to chronicity. HCV RNA is the first detectable event, preceding ALT elevation and the appearance of anti-HCV. The appearance of antibody to C100, detectable with first-generation assays, is delayed from 1 to 3 months after the appearance of antibody to C22 and C33, antibodies that are included in second-generation immunoassays. Anti-HCV detectable with second-generation assays appears during acute hepatitis C.

agent may contribute to cases of acute and chronic viral hepatitis unaccounted for by the other five hepatitis viruses. Like HCV, HGV is a bloodborne RNA virus with a flavivirus-like genomic structure. Its 2900-amino-acid polyprotein is encoded by a 9400 nucleotide genome, the 5′ end of which codes for structural (nucleocapsid and envelope) proteins and the 3′ end of which codes for nonstructural proteins with replicative function (helicase, protease, and RNA polymerase). HGV and GBV-C share almost complete nucleotide and amino acid sequence homology, and they are distantly related to HCV (approximate nucleotide homology of 25 percent), from which they diverged evolutionarily in the remote past. Infection with this agent, identified reliably by PCR amplification of RNA (much less reliably by antibody testing), occurs in approximately 1.5 percent of blood donors, is transmitted by blood transfusion, and can be detected in some patients with acute, chronic, and fulminant hepatitis. Data available to date, however, indicate that a sizable proportion of clinically apparent HGV infections occur in patients coinfected with hepatitis C, that HGV does not alter the severity of hepatitis C, and that most isolated instances of HGV infection are not associated with acute or chronic liver injury. Thus, although HGV may play a small role in viral hepatitis and may be transmitted by transfusion, its contribution to acute and chronic liver disease requires better definition.

PATHOGENESIS Under ordinary circumstances, none of the hepatitis viruses is known to be directly cytopathic to hepatocytes. Evidence suggests that the clinical manifestations and outcomes following acute liver injury associated with viral hepatitis are determined by the immunologic responses of the host. Among the viral hepatitides, the immunopathogenesis of hepatitis B has been studied most extensively. Certainly for this agent, the existence of asymptomatic hepatitis B carriers with normal liver histology and function suggests that the virus is not directly cytopathic. The facts that lymphoid cells are juxtaposed with necrotic hepatocytes in the livers of patients with liver injury and that patients with defects in cellular immune competence are more likely to remain chronically infected rather than to clear the virus are cited to support the role of cellular immune responses in the pathogenesis of hepatitis B–related liver injury. The model that has the most experimental support involves cytolytic T cells sensitized specifically to recognize host and hepatitis B viral antigens on the liver cell surface. Although HBsAg was initially thought to be the most likely viral target antigen on the hepatocyte surface, recent laboratory observations suggest that nucleocapsid proteins (HBcAg and possibly HBeAg), present on the cell membrane in minute quantities, are the viral target antigens that, with host antigens, invite cytolytic T cells to destroy HBV-infected hepatocytes. Still, this hypothesis is insufficient to explain differences in outcomes between those who recover after acute hepatitis and those who progress to chronic hepatitis or between those with mild and severe (fulminant) acute HBV infection. As convincing as are the cumulative data supporting nucleocapsid proteins as the target of cell-mediated immunologic injury, attention has been refocused on the envelope protein, HBsAg, by the demonstration that in transgenic mice with the gene for HBsAg inserted into their genomes, cytolytic T cells directed against HBsAg can be shown to destroy hepatocytes. Therefore, HBsAg cannot be dismissed as a potential immunologic target.

Moreover, debate continues over the relative importance of viral and host factors in the pathogenesis of HBV-associated liver injury and its outcome. As noted above, precore genetic mutants of HBV have been associated with the more severe outcomes of HBV infection (severe chronic and fulminant hepatitis), suggesting that, under certain circumstances, relative pathogenicity is a property of the virus, not the host. The fact that concomitant HDV and HBV infections are associated with more severe liver injury than HBV infection alone and the fact that cells transfected in vitro with the gene for HDV (delta) antigen express HDV antigen and then become necrotic in the absence of any immunologic influences are also consistent with a viral effect on pathogenicity. Similarly, in patients who undergo liver transplantation for end-stage chronic HBV infection, occasionally, rapidly progressive liver injury appears in the new liver. This clinical pattern is associated with an unusual histologic pattern in the new liver, *fibrosing cholestatic hepatitis*, which, ultrastructurally, appears to represent a choking of the cell with overwhelming quantities of HBsAg. This observation suggests that under the influence of the potent immunosuppressive agents required to prevent allograft rejection, HBV may have a direct cytopathic effect on liver cells, independent of the immune system.

Although the precise mechanism of liver injury in HBV infection remains elusive, studies of nucleocapsid proteins have shed light on the profound immunologic tolerance to HBV of babies born to mothers with highly replicative (HBeAg-positive), chronic HBV infection. In HBeAg-expressing transgenic mice, in utero exposure to HBeAg, which is sufficiently small to traverse the placenta, induces T cell tolerance to both nucleocapsid proteins. This, in turn, may explain why, when infection occurs so early in life, immunologic clearance does not occur, and protracted, lifelong infection ensues.

Immune complex–mediated tissue damage appears to play a pathogenetic role in the extrahepatic manifestations of acute hepatitis B. The occasional prodromal serum sickness–like syndrome observed in acute hepatitis B appears to be related to the deposition in tissue blood vessel walls of circulating immune complexes leading to activation of the complement system. The clinical consequences are urticarial rash, angioedema, fever, and arthritis. During the early prodrome of HBV infection in these patients, HBsAg in high titer in association with small amounts of anti-HBs leads to the formation of soluble, circulating immune complexes (in antigen excess). Complement components in the serum are depressed during the arthritic phase of the illness and are also detectable in the circulating immune complexes. In addition to complement components, these complexes contain HBsAg, anti-HBs, IgG, IgM, IgA, and fibrin. After the patient recovers from the serum sickness–like syndrome, these immune complexes disappear.

In patients with chronic hepatitis B, other types of immune-complex disease may be seen. Glomerulonephritis with the nephrotic syndrome is occasionally observed; HBsAg, immunoglobulin, and C3 deposition has been found in the glomerular basement membrane. While polyarteritis nodosa develops in considerably fewer than 1 percent of patients with HBV infection, 20 to 30 percent of patients with polyarteritis nodosa have HBsAg in serum. In these patients, the affected small and medium-sized arterioles have been shown to contain HBsAg, immunoglobulins, and complement components. Another extrahepatic manifestation of viral hepatitis, essential mixed cryoglobulinemia (EMC), was reported initially to be associated with hepatitis B. The disorder is characterized clinically by arthritis and cutaneous vasculitis (palpable purpura) and serologically by the presence of circulating cryoprecipitable immune complexes of more than one immunoglobulin class. Many patients with this syndrome have chronic liver disease, but the association with HBV infection has always been controversial. Recent reevaluation of patients with EMC suggests instead that a substantial proportion have chronic HCV infection. Their circulating immune complexes contain HCV RNA at a concentration that exceeds its serum concentration; this observation argues against secondary trapping of HCV in the immune complexes and favors a primary role for the virus in the pathogenesis of EMC.

PATHOLOGY The typical morphologic lesions of all types of viral hepatitis are similar and consist of panlobular infiltration with mononuclear cells, hepatic cell necrosis, hyperplasia of Kupffer cells, and variable degrees of cholestasis. Hepatic cell regeneration is present, as evidenced by numerous mitotic figures, multinucleated cells, and "rosette" or "pseudoacinar" formation. The mononuclear infiltration consists primarily of small lymphocytes, although plasma cells and eosinophils are occasionally seen. Liver cell damage consists of hepatic cell degeneration and necrosis, cell dropout, ballooning of cells, and acidophilic degeneration of hepatocytes (forming so-called Councilman-like bodies). Large hepatocytes with a ground glass appearance of the cytoplasm may be seen in chronic but not in acute HBV infection; these cells have been shown to contain HBsAg and can be identified histochemically with orcein or aldehyde fuchsin. In uncomplicated viral hepatitis, the reticulin framework is preserved.

In hepatitis C, the histologic lesion is often remarkable for a relative paucity of inflammation, a marked increase in activation of sinusoidal lining cells, lymphoid aggregates, the presence of fat, and, occasionally, bile duct lesions in which biliary epithelial cells appear to be piled up without interruption of the basement membrane. Occasionally, microvesicular steatosis occurs in hepatitis D. In hepatitis E, a common histologic feature is marked cholestasis. A cholestatic variant of slowly resolving acute hepatitis A also has been described.

A more severe histologic lesion, *bridging hepatic necrosis*, also termed *subacute* or *confluent necrosis*, is occasionally observed in some patients with acute hepatitis. "Bridging" between lobules results from large areas of hepatic cell dropout, with collapse of the reticulin framework. Characteristically, the bridge consists of condensed reticulum, inflammatory debris, and degenerating liver cells that span adjacent portal areas, portal to central veins, or central vein to central vein. This lesion had been thought to have prognostic significance; in many of the originally described patients with this lesion, a subacute course terminated in death within several weeks to months, or severe chronic hepatitis and postnecrotic cirrhosis developed. More recent investigations have failed to uphold the association between bridging necrosis and such a poor prognosis in patients with acute hepatitis. Although the frequency of bridging may be higher among hospitalized patients with severe acute hepatitis, and although cirrhosis, chronic hepatitis, and even death have been observed in this group, the frequency of bridging necrosis in uncomplicated acute viral hepatitis is probably on the order of 1 to 5 percent. Prospective studies have failed to demonstrate a difference in prognosis between patients with acute hepatitis who have bridging necrosis and those who do not. Therefore, although demonstration of this lesion in patients with chronic hepatitis has prognostic significance (see Chap. 297), its demonstration during acute hepatitis is less meaningful, and liver biopsies to identify this lesion are no longer undertaken routinely in patients with acute hepatitis. In *massive hepatic necrosis* (fulminant hepatitis, acute yellow atrophy), the striking feature at postmortem examination is the finding of a small, shrunken, and soft liver. Histologic examination reveals massive necrosis and dropout of liver cells of most lobules with extensive collapse and condensation of the reticulin framework.

Immunofluorescence and immunoperoxidase antibody studies have localized HBsAg to the cytoplasm and plasma membrane of infected liver cells. In contrast, HBcAg predominates in the nucleus, but occasionally, scant amounts are also seen in the cytoplasm and on the cell membrane. Electron-microscopic studies of liver biopsy material have demonstrated the presence of HBsAg particles in the cytoplasm and HBcAg particles in the nucleus of liver cells during hepatitis B infection. These morphologic observations suggest that DNA is synthesized and packaged within core particles in the nucleus, while the envelope is assembled in the cytoplasm, resulting in the formation of intact hepatitis B virus. HDV antigen is localized to the hepatocyte nucleus, while HAV, HCV, and HEV antigens are localized to the cytoplasm.

EPIDEMIOLOGY Prior to the availability of serologic tests for hepatitis viruses, all viral hepatitis cases were labeled either as "infectious" or "serum" hepatitis. Modes of transmission overlap, however, and *a clear distinction among the different types of viral hepatitis cannot be made solely on the basis of clinical or epidemiologic features* (Table 295-2). The most accurate means to distinguish the various types of viral hepatitis involves specific serologic testing.

Hepatitis A *This agent is transmitted almost exclusively by the fecal-oral route*. Person-to-person spread of HAV is enhanced by poor personal hygiene and overcrowding, and large outbreaks as well as sporadic cases have been traced to contaminated food, water, milk, and shellfish. Intrafamily and intrainstitutional spread are also com-

Table 295-2

Clinical and Epidemiologic Features of Viral Hepatitis

Feature	HAV	HBV	HCV	HDV	HEV
Incubation (days)	15–45, mean 30	30–180, mean 60–90	15–160, mean 50	30–180, mean 60–90	14–60, mean 40
Onset	Acute	Insidious or acute	Insidious	Insidious or acute	Acute
Age preference	Children, young adults	Young adults (sexual and percutaneous), babies, toddlers	Any age, but more common in adults	Any age (similar to HBV)	Young adults (20–40 years)
Transmission:					
Fecal-oral	+ + +	–	–	–	+ + +
Percutaneous	Unusual	+ + +	+ + +	+ + +	–
Perinatal	–	+ + +	±[a]	+	–
Sexual	±	+ +	±[a]	+ +	–
Clinical:					
Severity	Mild	Occasionally severe	Moderate	Occasionally severe	Mild
Fulminant	0.1%	0.1–1%	0.1%	5–20%[b]	1–2%[e]
Progression to chronicity	None	Occasional (1–10%) (90% of neonates)	Common (50–70% chronic hepatitis; 80–90% chronic infection)	Common[d]	None
Carrier	None	0.1–30%[c]	0.5–1.0%	Variable[f]	None
Cancer	None	+ (neonatal infection)	+	±	None
Prognosis	Excellent	Worse with age, debility	Moderate	Acute, good; Chronic, poor	Good
Prophylaxis	IG; Inactivated vaccine	HBIG; Recombinant vaccine	None	HBV vaccine (none for HBV carriers)	Unknown
Therapy	None	Interferon 40% effective	Interferon 50% response; sustained response <15%	Unknown	None

[a] Primarily with HIV coinfection and high-level viremia in index case; risk approximately 5 percent.
[b] Up to 5% in acute HBV/HDV coinfection; up to 20% in HDV superinfection of chronic HBV infection.
[c] Varies considerably throughout the world and in subpopulations within countries; see text.
[d] In acute HBV/HDV coinfection, the frequency of chronicity is the same as that for HBV; in HDV superinfection, chronicity is invariable.
[e] 10–20% in pregnant women.
[f] Common in Mediterranean countries, rare in North America and western Europe.

mon. Early epidemiologic observations suggested that there is a predilection for hepatitis A to occur in late fall and early winter. In temperate zones, epidemic waves have been recorded every 5 to 20 years as new segments of nonimmune population appeared; however, in developed countries, the incidence of type A hepatitis has been declining, presumably as a function of improved sanitation, and these cyclic patterns are no longer being observed. No HAV carrier state has been identified after acute type A hepatitis; perpetuation of the virus in nature depends presumably on nonepidemic, inapparent subclinical infection.

In the general population, anti-HAV, an excellent marker for previous HAV infection, increases in prevalence as a function of increasing age and of decreasing socioeconomic status. In the 1970s, serologic evidence of prior hepatitis A infection occurred in about 40 percent of urban populations in the United States, most of whom never recalled having had a symptomatic case of hepatitis. In subsequent decades, however, the prevalence of anti-HAV has been declining in the United States. In developing countries, exposure, infection, and subsequent immunity are almost universal in childhood. As the frequency of subclinical childhood infections declines in developed countries, a susceptible cohort of adults emerges. Hepatitis A tends to be more symptomatic in adults; therefore, paradoxically, as the frequency of HAV infection declines, the likelihood of clinically apparent, even severe, HAV illnesses increases in the susceptible adult population. Travel to endemic areas is a common source of infection for adults from nonendemic areas. More recently recognized epidemiologic foci of HAV infection include child-care centers, neonatal intensive care units, promiscuous homosexual men, and intravenous drug users. Although hepatitis A is rarely bloodborne, several outbreaks have been recognized in recipients of clotting factor concentrates.

Hepatitis B It has long been recognized that a major route of hepatitis B transmission is percutaneous, but the outmoded designation "serum hepatitis" is an inaccurate label for the epidemiologic spectrum of HBV infection recognized today. As detailed below, most of the hepatitis transmitted by blood transfusion is not caused by HBV; moreover, in approximately half of patients with acute type B hepatitis, there is no history of an identifiable percutaneous exposure. We now recognize that many cases of type B hepatitis result from less obvious modes of nonpercutaneous or covert percutaneous transmission. HBsAg has been identified in almost every body fluid from infected persons—saliva, tears, seminal fluid, cerebrospinal fluid, ascites, breast milk, synovial fluid, gastric juice, pleural fluid, and urine, and even rarely in feces. Although there is abundant evidence to suggest that feces are not infectious, at least some of these body fluids—most notably semen and saliva—have been shown to be infectious, albeit less so than serum, when administered percutaneously or nonpercutaneously to experimental animals. Among the nonpercutaneous modes of HBV transmission, oral ingestion has been documented as a potential route of exposure but one whose efficiency is quite low. On the other hand, the two nonpercutaneous routes considered to have the greatest impact are intimate (especially sexual) contact and perinatal transmission.

In sub-Saharan Africa, intimate contact among toddlers is considered instrumental in contributing to the maintenance of the high frequency of HBsAg in the population. Perinatal transmission occurs primarily in infants born to HBsAg carrier mothers or mothers with acute hepatitis B during the third trimester of pregnancy or during the early postpartum period. Perinatal transmission is uncommon in North America and western Europe but occurs with great frequency and is the most important mode of HBV perpetuation in the Far East and developing countries. Although the precise mode of perinatal transmission is unknown, and although approximately 10 percent of infections may be acquired in utero, epidemiologic evidence suggests that most infections occur approximately at the time of delivery and are not related to breast feeding. The likelihood of perinatal transmission of HBV correlates with the presence of HBeAg; 90 percent of HBeAg-positive mothers but only 10 to 15 percent of anti-HBe-positive mothers transmit HBV infection to their offspring. In most cases, acute infection in the neonate is clinically asymptomatic, but the child is very likely to become an HBsAg carrier.

The more than 200 million HBsAg carriers in the world constitute the main reservoir of hepatitis B in human beings. Serum HBsAg is infrequent (0.1 to 0.5 percent) in normal populations in the United States and western Europe; however, a prevalence of up to 5 to 20 percent has been found in the Far East and in some tropical countries and in persons with Down's syndrome, lepromatous leprosy, leukemia, Hodgkin's disease, polyarteritis nodosa, patients with chronic renal disease on hemodialysis, and needle-using drug addicts.

Other groups with high rates of HBV infection include spouses of acutely infected persons, sexually promiscuous persons (especially promiscuous homosexual men), health care workers exposed to blood, persons who require repeated transfusions especially with pooled blood product concentrates (e.g., hemophiliacs), residents and staff of custodial institutions for the mentally retarded, prisoners, and, to a lesser extent, family members of chronically infected patients. In volunteer blood donors, the prevalence of anti-HBs, a reflection of previous HBV infection, ranges from 5 to 10 percent, but the prevalence is higher in lower socioeconomic strata, older age groups, and persons—including those mentioned above—exposed to blood products.

Prevalence of infection, modes of transmission, and human behavior conspire to mold geographically different epidemiologic patterns of HBV infection. In the Far East and Africa, hepatitis B, a disease of the newborn and young children, is perpetuated by a cycle of maternal-neonatal spread. In North America and western Europe, hepatitis B is primarily a disease of adolescence and early adulthood, the time of life when intimate sexual contact as well as recreational and occupational percutaneous exposures tend to occur.

Hepatitis D Infection with HDV has a worldwide distribution, but two epidemiologic patterns exist. In Mediterranean countries (northern Africa, southern Europe, the Middle East), HDV infection is endemic among those with hepatitis B, and the disease is transmitted predominantly by nonpercutaneous means, especially close personal contact. In nonendemic areas, such as the United States and northern Europe, HDV infection is confined to persons exposed frequently to blood and blood products, primarily drug addicts and hemophiliacs. HDV infection can be introduced into a population through drug addicts or by migration of persons from endemic to nonendemic areas. Thus, patterns of population migration and human behavior facilitating percutaneous contact play important roles in the introduction and amplification of HDV infection. Occasionally, the migrating epidemiology of hepatitis D is expressed in explosive outbreaks of severe hepatitis, such as those which have occurred in remote South American villages as well as in urban centers in the United States. Ultimately, such outbreaks of hepatitis D—either of coinfections with acute hepatitis B or of superinfections in those already infected with HBV—may blur the distinctions between endemic and nonendemic areas.

Hepatitis C Routine screening of blood donors for HBsAg and the elimination of commercial blood sources in the early 1970s reduced the frequency of, but did not eliminate, transfusion-associated hepatitis. During the 1970s, the likelihood of acquiring hepatitis after transfusion of voluntarily donated, HBsAg-screened blood was approximately 10 percent per patient (up to 0.9 percent per unit transfused). Although hepatitis B accounted for up to 5 to 10 percent of these cases, the remaining 90 to 95 percent were classified, based on serologic exclusion, as "non-A, non-B" hepatitis. For patients requiring transfusion of pooled products, such as clotting factor concentrates, the risk was even higher, up to 20 to 30 percent, while for those receiving such products as albumin and immune globulin, because of prior treatment of these materials by heating to 60°C or cold ethanol fractionation, there was no risk of hepatitis.

During the 1980s, voluntary self-exclusion of blood donors with risk factors for AIDS and then the introduction of donor screening for anti-HIV reduced further the likelihood of transfusion-associated hepatitis to under 5 percent. During the late 1980s and early 1990s, the introduction first of "surrogate" screening tests for non-A, non-B hepatitis [alanine aminotransferase (ALT) and anti-HBc, both shown to identify blood donors with a higher likelihood of transmitting non-A, non-B hepatitis to recipients] and, subsequently, after the discovery of HCV, first-generation immunoassays for anti-HCV reduced the frequency of transfusion-associated hepatitis even further. A prospective analysis of transfusion-associated hepatitis conducted between 1986 and 1990 showed that the incidence of transfusion-associated hepatitis at one urban university hospital fell from a baseline of 3.8 percent per patient (0.45 percent per unit transfused) to 1.5 percent per patient (0.19 percent per unit) after the introduction of surrogate testing and to 0.6 percent per patient (0.03 percent per unit) after the introduction of first-generation anti-HCV assays. The introduction of second-generation anti-HCV assays has reduced the frequency of transfusion-associated hepatitis C to almost imperceptible levels.

In addition to being transmitted by transfusion, hepatitis C can be transmitted by other percutaneous routes, such as self-injection with intravenous drugs. In addition, this virus can be transmitted by occupational exposure to blood, and the likelihood of infection is increased in hemodialysis units. Although the frequency of transfusion-associated hepatitis C fell as a result of blood donor screening, the overall frequency of hepatitis C remained the same until the early 1990s, when the overall frequency fell in parallel with a reduction in the number of new cases in intravenous drug users. After the exclusion of anti-HCV-positive plasma units from the donor pool, rare, sporadic instances have occurred of hepatitis C among recipients of immune globulin preparations for intravenous (but not intramuscular) use.

Serologic evidence for HCV infection occurs in >90 percent of patients with transfusion-associated hepatitis, hemophiliacs, and intravenous drug users; 60 to 70 percent of patients with sporadic non-A, non-B hepatitis (in the absence of a known risk factor); 0.5 percent of volunteer blood donors; and 1.5 percent of the general population. The vast majority of asymptomatic blood donors found to have circulating, reproducible anti-HCV do not belong to high-risk groups. How they become infected remains a mystery. The potential exists that such infections of undefined source represent sexually transmitted infection or infection acquired by perinatal transmission. Although these routes of infection can occur (in some studies especially when the source of infection is also infected with HIV, in other studies primarily when the level of viremia in the source is very high), their efficiency is low; the risk of sexual (primarily in those with multiple sexual partners, rarely for monogamous couples) and perinatal transmission is only approximately 5 percent, insufficient to account for the large reservoir of epidemiologically unexplained cases. In all likelihood, the inefficiency of these less than direct routes of transmission is a reflection of the relatively low infectivity titer of HCV. Infections of household contacts are rare as well. Among patients with reported cases of acute hepatitis C, 40 percent have no readily identifiable risk factor, but they do have in common the fact that they tend to belong to lower socioeconomic groups.

The risk of HCV infection is increased in organ transplant recipients and in patients with AIDS; in all immunosuppressed groups, levels of anti-HCV may be undetectable, and a diagnosis may require testing for HCV RNA. Chronic hepatitis C occurs in as many as 20 percent of renal transplant recipients. In the early years after transplantation, the death rate in these patients with hepatitis is increased not as a result of liver failure but of severe infections outside the hepatobiliary tree. This effect has been attributed to the immunosuppressive impact of HCV infection on the host. Five to 10 years after transplantation, however, complications of chronic liver disease account for increased morbidity and mortality. The impact of HCV infection on liver transplant recipients is controversial, associated with severe liver disease in some series but with trivial morbidity in others.

Hepatitis E The enteric form of non-A, non-B hepatitis identified in India, Asia, Africa, and Central America resembles hepatitis A in its primarily enteric mode of spread. The commonly recognized cases occur after contamination of water supplies such as after monsoon flooding, but sporadic, isolated cases occur. An epidemiologic feature that distinguishes HEV from other enteric agents is the rarity of secondary person-to-person spread from infected persons to their close contacts. Infections arise in populations that are immune to HAV and favor young adults. It is not known if hepatitis E occurs outside of recognized endemic areas, for example, in the United States, but preliminary studies suggest that HEV does not account for any of the sporadic "non-A, non-B" cases in nonendemic areas. Cases imported from endemic areas have been found in the United States.

Hepatitis G Hepatitis G is a bloodborne agent whose modes of transmission have not been defined adequately but tend to parallel those of HCV infection. Evidence for infection occurs in approximately 1.5 percent of blood donors, but the frequency of infection is the same in blood donors with normal and with elevated ALT levels. Among sporadic, community-acquired cases of acute viral hepatitis unexplained by hepatitis viruses A through E, HGV accounts for only 10 to 15 percent, which represents less than 0.5 percent of all community-acquired cases.

CLINICAL AND LABORATORY FEATURES **Symptoms and Signs** Acute viral hepatitis occurs after an incubation period that varies according to the responsible agent. Generally, incubation periods for hepatitis A range from 15 to 45 days (mean 4 weeks), for hepatitis B and D from 30 to 180 days (mean 4 to 12 weeks), for hepatitis C from 15 to 160 days (mean 7 weeks), and for hepatitis E from 14 to 60 days (mean 5 to 6 weeks). The *prodromal symptoms* of acute viral hepatitis are systemic and quite variable. Constitutional symptoms of anorexia, nausea and vomiting, fatigue, malaise, arthralgias, myalgias, headache, photophobia, pharyngitis, cough, and coryza may precede the onset of jaundice by 1 to 2 weeks. The nausea, vomiting, and anorexia are frequently associated with alterations in olfaction and taste. A low-grade fever between 38 and 39°C (100 to 102°F) is more often present in hepatitis A and E than in hepatitis B or C, except when hepatitis B is heralded by a serum sickness–like syndrome; rarely, a fever of 39.5 to 40°C (103 to 104°F) may accompany the constitutional symptoms. Dark urine and clay-colored stools may be noticed by the patient from 1 to 5 days prior to the onset of clinical jaundice.

With the onset of *clinical jaundice*, the constitutional prodromal symptoms usually diminish, but in some patients mild weight loss (2.5 to 5 kg) is common and may continue during the entire icteric phase. The liver becomes enlarged and tender and may be associated with right upper quadrant pain and discomfort. Infrequently, patients present with a cholestatic picture, suggesting extrahepatic biliary obstruction. Splenomegaly and cervical adenopathy are present in 10 to 20 percent of patients with acute hepatitis. Rarely, a few spider angiomas appear during the icteric phase and disappear during convalescence. During the *recovery phase*, constitutional symptoms disappear, but usually some liver enlargement and abnormalities in liver biochemical tests are still evident. The duration of the posticteric phase is variable, ranging from 2 to 12 weeks, and usually is more prolonged in acute hepatitis B and C. Complete clinical and biochemical recovery is to be expected 1 to 2 months after all cases of hepatitis A and E and 3 to 4 months after the onset of jaundice in three-quarters of uncomplicated cases of hepatitis B and C. In the remainder, biochemical recovery may be delayed. A substantial proportion of patients with viral hepatitis never become icteric.

Infection with HDV can occur in the presence of acute or chronic HBV infection; the duration of HBV infection determines the duration of HDV infection. When acute HDV and HBV infection occur simultaneously, clinical and biochemical features may be indistinguishable from those of HBV infection alone, although occasionally they are more severe. As opposed to patients with *acute* HBV infection, patients with *chronic* HBV infection can support HDV replication indefinitely. This can happen when acute HDV infection occurs in the presence of a nonresolving acute HBV infection. More commonly, acute HDV infection becomes chronic when it is superimposed on an underlying chronic HBV infection. In such cases, the HDV superinfection appears as a clinical exacerbation or an episode resembling acute viral hepatitis in someone already chronically infected with HBV. Superinfection with HDV in a patient with chronic hepatitis B often leads to clinical deterioration (see below).

In addition to superinfections with other hepatitis agents, acute hepatitis-like clinical events in persons with chronic hepatitis B may accompany spontaneous HBeAg–to–anti-HBe seroconversion or spontaneous reactivation, i.e., reversion from nonreplicative to replicative infection. Such reactivations can occur as well in therapeutically immunosuppressed patients with chronic HBV infection when cytotoxic-immunosuppressive drugs are withdrawn; in these cases, restoration of immune competence is thought to allow resumption of previously checked cell-mediated cytolysis of HBV-infected hepatocytes. Occasionally, acute clinical exacerbations of chronic hepatitis B may represent the emergence of a precore mutant (see "Virology and Etiology," above).

Laboratory Features The serum aminotransferases AST and ALT (previously designated SGOT and SGPT) show a variable increase during the prodromal phase of acute viral hepatitis and precede the rise in bilirubin level (see Figs. 295-2 and 295-4). The acute level of these enzymes, however, does not correlate well with the degree of liver cell damage. Peak levels vary from 400 to 4000 IU or more; these levels are usually reached at the time the patient is clinically icteric and diminish progressively during the recovery phase of acute hepatitis. The diagnosis of anicteric hepatitis is difficult and requires a high index of suspicion; it is based on clinical features and on aminotransferase elevations, although mild increases in conjugated bilirubin also may be found.

Jaundice is usually visible in the sclera or skin when the serum bilirubin value exceeds 43 μmol/L (2.5 mg/dL). When jaundice appears, the serum bilirubin typically rises to levels ranging from 85 to 340 μmol/L (5 to 20 mg/dL). The serum bilirubin may continue to rise despite falling serum aminotransferase levels. In most instances, the total bilirubin is equally divided between the conjugated and unconjugated fractions. Bilirubin levels above 340 μmol/L (20 mg/dL) extending and persisting late into the course of viral hepatitis are more likely to be associated with severe disease. In certain patients with underlying hemolytic anemia, however, such as glucose-6-phosphate dehydrogenase deficiency and sickle cell anemia, a high serum bilirubin level is common, resulting from superimposed hemolysis. In such patients, bilirubin levels greater than 513 μmol/L (30 mg/dL) have been observed and are not necessarily associated with a poor prognosis.

Neutropenia and lymphopenia are transient and are followed by a relative lymphocytosis. Atypical lymphocytes (varying between 2 and 20 percent) are common during the acute phase. These atypical lymphocytes are indistinguishable from those seen in infectious mononucleosis. Measurement of the prothrombin time (PT) is important in patients with acute viral hepatitis, for a prolonged value may reflect a severe synthetic defect, signify extensive hepatocellular necrosis, and indicate a worse prognosis. Occasionally, a prolonged PT may occur with only mild increases in the serum bilirubin and aminotransferase levels. Prolonged nausea and vomiting, inadequate carbohydrate intake, and poor hepatic glycogen reserves may contribute to hypoglycemia noted occasionally in patients with severe viral hepatitis. Serum alkaline phosphatase may be normal or only mildly elevated, while a fall in serum albumin is uncommon in uncomplicated acute viral hepatitis. In some patients, mild and transient steatorrhea has been noted as well as slight microscopic hematuria and minimal proteinuria.

A diffuse but mild elevation of the gamma globulin fraction is common during acute viral hepatitis. Serum IgG and IgM are elevated in about one-third of patients during the acute phase of viral hepatitis, but serum IgM elevation is seen more characteristically during acute hepatitis A. During the acute phase of viral hepatitis, antibodies to smooth muscle and other cell constituents may be present, and low titers of rheumatoid factor, antinuclear antibody, and heterophil antibody also can be found occasionally. In hepatitis C and D, antibodies to liver-kidney microsomes (LKM) may occur; however, the species of LKM antibodies in the two types of hepatitis are different from each other as well as from the LKM antibody species characteristic of autoimmune chronic hepatitis type 2 (see Chap. 297). The autoantibodies in viral hepatitis are nonspecific and also can be associated with other viral and systemic diseases. In contrast, virus-specific antibodies, which appear during and after hepatitis virus infection, are serologic markers of diagnostic importance.

As described above, serologic tests are available with which to establish a diagnosis of hepatitis A, B, D, and C. Tests for fecal or serum HAV are not routinely available. Therefore, a diagnosis of type A hepatitis is based on detection of IgM anti-HAV during acute illness (see Fig. 295-2). Rheumatoid factor can give rise to false-positive results in this test.

A diagnosis of HBV infection can usually be made by detection of HBsAg in serum. Infrequently, levels of HBsAg are too low to be detected during acute HBV infection, even with the current generation of highly sensitive immunoassays. In such cases, the diagnosis can be established by the presence of IgM anti-HBc.

The titer of HBsAg bears little relation to the severity of clinical disease. Indeed, there may be an inverse correlation between the serum concentration of HBsAg and the degree of liver cell damage. For example, titers are highest in immunosuppressed patients, lower in chronic liver disease (but higher in mild chronic than in severe chronic hepatitis), and very low in acute fulminant hepatitis. These observations suggest that in hepatitis B the degree of liver cell damage and the clinical course are probably related to variations in the patient's immune response to HBV rather than to the amount of circulating HBsAg. In immunocompetent persons, however, there is a correlation between markers of HBV *replication* and liver injury (see below).

Another serologic marker that may be of value in patients with hepatitis B is HBeAg. Its principal clinical usefulness is as an indicator of relative infectivity. Because HBeAg is invariably present during early acute hepatitis B, HBeAg testing is indicated primarily during follow-up of chronic infection.

In patients with hepatitis B surface antigenemia of unknown duration, e.g., blood donors found to be HBsAg-positive and referred to a physician for evaluation, testing for IgM anti-HBc may be useful to distinguish between acute or recent infection (IgM anti-HBc-positive) and chronic HBV infection (IgM anti-HBc-negative, IgG anti-HBc-positive). A false-positive test for IgM anti-HBc may be encountered in patients with high-titer rheumatoid factor.

Anti-HBs is rarely detectable in the presence of HBsAg in patients with *acute* hepatitis B, but 10 to 20 percent of persons with *chronic* HBV infection may harbor low-level anti-HBs. This antibody is directed not against the common group determinant, *a*, but against the heterotypic subtype determinant (e.g., HBsAg of subtype *ad* with anti-HBs of subtype *y*). In most cases, this serologic pattern cannot be attributed to infection with two different HBV subtypes, and the presence of this antibody is not a harbinger of imminent HBsAg clearance. When such antibody is detected, its presence is of no recognized clinical significance (see "Virology and Etiology," above).

After immunization with hepatitis B vaccine, which consists of HBsAg alone, anti-HBs is the only serologic marker to appear. A summary of the commonly encountered serologic patterns of hepatitis B and their interpretations appears in Table 295-3. Tests for the detection of HBV DNA in liver and serum are now available. Like HBeAg, serum HBV DNA is an indicator of HBV replication, but tests for HBV DNA are more sensitive and quantitative. These markers are useful in following the course of HBV replication in patients with chronic hepatitis B receiving antiviral chemotherapy, e.g., with interferon (see Chap. 297). In immunocompetent persons, a general correlation does appear to exist between the level of HBV replication, as reflected by the level of HBV DNA in serum, and the degree of liver injury. High serum HBV DNA levels, increased expression of viral antigens, and necroinflammatory activity in the liver go hand in hand unless immunosuppression interferes with cytolytic T cell responses to virus-infected cells; reduction of HBV replication with antiviral drugs, such as interferon, tends to be accompanied by an improvement in liver histology.

In patients with hepatitis C, an episodic pattern of aminotransferase elevation is common. A specific serologic diagnosis of hepatitis C can be made by demonstrating the presence in serum of anti-HCV. When a second- or later-generation immunoassay (that detects antibodies to nonstructural and nucleocapsid proteins) is used, anti-HCV can be detected in acute hepatitis C during the initial phase of elevated aminotransferase activity. This antibody may never become detectable in 5 to 10 percent of patients with acute hepatitis C, and levels of anti-HCV may become undetectable after recovery from acute hepatitis C. In patients with chronic hepatitis C, anti-HCV is detectable in >90 percent of cases. Because nonspecificity can confound immunoassays for anti-HCV, a supplementary recombinant immunoblot assay should be done, especially in persons with a low prior probability of infection, to establish the specific viral proteins to which anti-HCV is directed (see "Virology and Etiology," above). Assays for HCV RNA are the most sensitive tests for HCV infection. HCV RNA can be detected even before acute elevation of aminotransferase activity and before the appearance of anti-HCV in patients with acute hepatitis C. In addition, HCV RNA remains detectable indefinitely, continuously in most but intermittently in some, in patients with chronic hepatitis C (even detectable in some persons with normal liver tests, i.e., asymptomatic carriers). Thus a diagnosis of hepatitis C can be supported by detection of anti-HCV and by exclusion of false-positive reactivity. In the small minority of patients with hepatitis C who lack anti-HCV, a diagnosis can be supported by detection of HCV RNA. If all these tests are negative and the patient has a well-characterized case of hepatitis following percutaneous exposure to blood or blood products, a diagnosis of hepatitis G or, perhaps, hepatitis caused by another agent as yet unidentified can be entertained. A proportion of patients with hepatitis C have isolated anti-HBc in their blood, a reflection of a common risk in certain populations to multiple bloodborne hepatitis agents. The anti-HBc in such cases is almost invariably of the IgG class and usually represents HBV infection in the remote past, rarely current HBV infection with low-level virus carriage.

The presence of HDV infection can be identified by demonstrating intrahepatic HDV antigen or, more practically, an anti-HDV seroconversion (a rise in titer of anti-HDV or de novo appearance of anti-HDV). Circulating HDV antigen, also diagnostic of acute infection, is detectable only briefly, if at all. Because anti-HDV is often undetectable once HBsAg disappears, retrospective serodiagnosis of acute self-limited, simultaneous HBV and HDV infection is difficult. Early diagnosis of acute infection may be hampered by a delay of up to 30 to 40 days in the appearance of anti-HDV.

When a patient presents with acute hepatitis and has HBsAg and anti-HDV in the serum, determination of the class of anti-HBc is helpful in establishing the relationship between infection with HBV and HDV. Although IgM anti-HBc does not distinguish *absolutely* between acute and chronic HBV infection, its presence is a reliable indicator of recent infection and its absence a reliable indicator of infection in the remote past. In simultaneous acute HBV and HDV infections, IgM anti-HBc will be detectable, while in acute HDV infection superimposed on chronic HBV infection, anti-HBc will be of the IgG class.

Tests for the presence of HDV RNA are useful for determining the presence of ongoing HDV replication and relative infectivity. Currently, probes for this marker are restricted to a limited number of research laboratories. Similarly, diagnostic tests for hepatitis E and G are confined to a small number of research laboratories.

Liver biopsy is rarely necessary or indicated in acute viral hepatitis, except when there is a question about the diagnosis or when there is clinical evidence suggesting a diagnosis of chronic hepatitis.

A diagnostic algorithm can be applied in the evaluation of cases of acute viral hepatitis. A patient with acute hepatitis should undergo four serologic tests, HBsAg, IgM anti-HAV, IgM anti-HBc, and anti-HCV (Table 295-4). The presence of HBsAg, with or without IgM anti-HBc, represents HBV infection. If IgM anti-HBc is present, the HBV infection is considered acute; if IgM anti-HBc is absent, the HBV infection is considered chronic. A diagnosis of acute hepatitis B can be made in the absence of HBsAg when IgM anti-HBc is detectable. A diagnosis of acute hepatitis A is based on the presence of IgM anti-HAV. If IgM anti-HAV coexists with HBsAg, a diagnosis of simultaneous HAV and HBV infections can be made; if IgM anti-HBc (with or without HBsAg) is detectable, the patient has simultaneous acute hepatitis A and B, and if IgM anti-HBc is undetectable, the patient has acute hepatitis A superimposed on chronic HBV infection. The presence of anti-HCV, if confirmable, supports a diagnosis of acute hepatitis C. Occasionally, repeat anti-HCV testing later during the illness is necessary to establish the diagnosis. Absence of all serologic markers is consistent with a diagnosis of "non-A, non-B, non-C" hepatitis, if the epidemiologic setting is appropriate.

In patients with chronic hepatitis, initial testing should consist of HBsAg and anti-HCV. Anti-HCV supports the diagnosis of chronic hepatitis C. If a

Table 295-4

Simplified Diagnostic Approach in Patients Presenting with Acute Hepatitis

Serologic Tests of Patient's Serum				
HBsAg	**IgM Anti-HAV**	**IgM Anti-HBc**	**Anti-HCV**	**Diagnostic Interpretation**
+	–	+	–	Acute hepatitis B
+	–	–	–	Chronic hepatitis B
+	+	–	–	Acute hepatitis A superimposed on chronic hepatitis B
+	+	+	–	Acute hepatitis A and B
–	+	–	–	Acute hepatitis A
–	+	+	–	Acute hepatitis A and B (HBsAg below detection threshold)
–	–	+	–	Acute hepatitis B (HBsAg below detection threshold)
–	–	–	+	Acute hepatitis C

Table 295-3

Commonly Encountered Serologic Patterns of Hepatitis B Infection

HBsAg	Anti-HBs	Anti-HBc	HBeAg	Anti-HBe	Interpretation
+	–	IgM	+	–	Acute HBV infection, high infectivity
+	–	IgG	+	–	Chronic HBV infection, high infectivity
+	–	IgG	–	+	Late-acute or chronic HBV infection, low infectivity
+	+	+	+/–	+/–	1. HBsAg of one subtype and heterotypic anti-HBs (common) 2. Process of seroconversion from HBsAg to anti-HBs (rare)
–	–	IgM	+/–	+/–	1. Acute HBV infection 2. Anti-HBc window
–	–	IgG	–	+/–	1. Low-level HBsAg carrier 2. Remote past infection
–	+	IgG	–	+/–	Recovery from HBV infection
–	+	–	–	–	1. Immunization with HBsAg (after vaccination) 2. Remote past infection (?) 3. False-positive

serologic diagnosis of chronic hepatitis B is made, testing for HBeAg and anti-HBe is indicated to evaluate relative infectivity. Testing for HBV DNA in such patients provides a more quantitative and sensitive test for the level of virus replication and, therefore, is very helpful during antiviral therapy (see Chap. 297). In patients with hepatitis B, testing for anti-HDV is useful under the following circumstances: severe and fulminant cases, severe chronic cases, cases of acute hepatitis-like exacerbations in patients with chronic hepatitis B, persons with frequent percutaneous exposures, and persons from areas where HDV infection is endemic.

PROGNOSIS Virtually all previously healthy patients with hepatitis A recover completely from their illness with no clinical sequelae. Similarly, in acute hepatitis B, 95 percent of patients have a favorable course and recover completely. There are, however, certain clinical and laboratory features that suggest a more complicated and protracted course. Patients of advanced age and with serious underlying medical disorders may have a prolonged course and are more likely to experience severe hepatitis. Initial presenting features such as ascites, peripheral edema, and symptoms of hepatic encephalopathy suggest a poorer prognosis. In addition, a prolonged PT, low serum albumin level, hypoglycemia, and very high serum bilirubin values suggest severe hepatocellular disease. Patients with these clinical and laboratory features deserve prompt hospital admission. The case-fatality rate in hepatitis A and B is very low (approximately 0.1 percent) but is increased by advanced age and underlying debilitating disorders. Among patients ill enough to be hospitalized for acute hepatitis B, the fatality rate is 1 percent. Hepatitis C occurring after transfusion is less severe during the acute phase than type B hepatitis and is more likely to be anicteric; fatalities are rare, but the precise case-fatality rate is not known. In outbreaks of waterborne hepatitis E in India and Asia, the case-fatality rate is 1 to 2 percent and up to 10 to 20 percent in pregnant women. Patients with simultaneous acute hepatitis B and hepatitis D do not necessarily experience a higher mortality rate than do patients with acute hepatitis B alone; however, in several recent outbreaks of acute simultaneous HBV and HDV infection among drug addicts, the case fatality rate has been approximately 5 percent. In the case of HDV superinfection of a person with chronic hepatitis B, the likelihood of fulminant hepatitis and death is increased substantially. Although the case-fatality rate for hepatitis D has not been defined adequately, in outbreaks of severe HDV superinfection in isolated populations with a high hepatitis B carrier rate, the mortality rate has been recorded in excess of 20 percent.

COMPLICATIONS AND SEQUELAE A small proportion of patients with hepatitis A experience *relapsing hepatitis* weeks to months after apparent recovery from acute hepatitis. Relapses are characterized by recurrence of symptoms, aminotransferase elevations, occasionally jaundice, and fecal excretion of HAV. Another unusual variant of acute hepatitis A is *cholestatic hepatitis*, characterized by protracted cholestatic jaundice and pruritus. Rarely, liver test abnormalities persist for many months, even up to a year. Even when these complications occur, hepatitis A remains self-limited and does not progress to chronic liver disease. During the prodromal phase of acute hepatitis B, a serum sickness–like syndrome characterized by arthralgia or arthritis, rash, angioedema, and rarely hematuria and proteinuria may develop in 5 to 10 percent of patients. This syndrome occurs prior to the onset of clinical jaundice, and these patients are often erroneously diagnosed as having rheumatoid arthritis or other rheumatologic diseases such as systemic lupus erythematosus. The diagnosis can be established by measuring serum aminotransferase levels, which are almost invariably elevated, and serum HBsAg. As noted above, EMC is an immune-complex disease that can complicate hepatitis C. Attention has been drawn as well to associations between hepatitis C and such cutaneous disorders as porphyria cutanea tarda and lichen planus. A mechanism for these associations is unknown.

The most feared complication of viral hepatitis is *fulminant hepatitis* (massive hepatic necrosis); fortunately, this is a rare event. This is primarily seen in hepatitis B and D, as well as hepatitis E, but rare fulminant cases of hepatitis A occur primarily in older adults and in persons with underlying chronic liver disease. Hepatitis B accounts for more than 50 percent of fulminant hepatitis cases, a sizable proportion of which are associated with HDV infection. Participation of HDV can be documented in approximately one-third of patients with acute fulminant hepatitis B and two-thirds of patients with fulminant hepatitis superimposed on chronic hepatitis B. Fulminant hepatitis is seen rarely in hepatitis C, but hepatitis E, as noted above, can be complicated by fatal fulminant hepatitis in 1 to 2 percent of all cases and in up to 20 percent of cases occurring in pregnant women. Patients usually present with signs and symptoms of encephalopathy that may evolve to deep coma. The liver is usually small and the PT excessively prolonged. The combination of rapidly shrinking liver size, rapidly rising bilirubin level, and marked prolongation of the PT, together with clinical signs of confusion, disorientation, somnolence, ascites, and edema, indicates that the patient has hepatic failure with encephalopathy. Cerebral edema is common; brainstem compression, gastrointestinal bleeding, sepsis, respiratory failure, cardiovascular collapse, and renal failure are terminal events. The mortality is exceedingly high (greater than 80 percent in patients with deep coma), but patients who survive may have a complete biochemical and histologic recovery. If a donor liver can be located on time, liver transplantation may be life-saving in patients with fulminant hepatitis.

It is particularly important to document the disappearance of HBsAg following apparent clinical recovery from acute hepatitis B. Before laboratory methods were available to distinguish between acute and acute hepatitis–like exacerbations (*spontaneous reactivations*) of chronic hepatitis B, observations suggested that approximately 10 percent of patients remained HBsAg-positive for longer than 6 months after the onset of clinically apparent acute hepatitis B. Half these persons were found to clear the antigen from their circulations during the next several years, but the other 5 percent remained chronically HBsAg-positive. More recent observations suggest that the true rate of chronic infection after clinically apparent acute hepatitis B is as low as 1 percent in normal, immunocompetent, young adults. Earlier, higher estimates may have been biased by inadvertent inclusion of acute exacerbations in chronically infected patients; these patients, chronically HBsAg-positive before exacerbation, were unlikely to seroconvert to HBsAg-negative thereafter. Whether the rate of chronicity is 10 or 1 percent, such patients have anti-HBc in serum; anti-HBs is either undetected or detected at low titer against the opposite subtype specificity of the antigen (see "Laboratory Features," above). These patients may (1) be asymptomatic carriers, (2) have low-grade, mild chronic hepatitis, or (3) have moderate to severe chronic hepatitis with or without cirrhosis. The likelihood of becoming an HBsAg carrier after acute HBV infection is especially high among neonates, persons with Down's syndrome, chronically hemodialyzed patients, and immunosuppressed patients, including persons with HIV infection.

Chronic hepatitis is an important late complication of acute hepatitis B occurring in a small proportion of acute cases but more common in those who present with chronic infection without having experienced an acute illness (see Chap. 297). Certain clinical and laboratory features suggest progression of acute hepatitis to chronic hepatitis: (1) lack of complete resolution of clinical symptoms of anorexia, weight loss, and fatigue and the persistence of hepatomegaly; (2) the presence of bridging or multilobular hepatic necrosis on liver biopsy during protracted, severe acute viral hepatitis; (3) failure of the serum aminotransferase, bilirubin, and globulin levels to return to normal within 6 to 12 months following the acute illness; and (4) the continued presence of HBsAg and HBeAg 6 months or more after acute hepatitis, suggesting chronic, replicative viral infection of the liver.

Although acute hepatitis D infection does not increase the likelihood of chronicity of simultaneous acute hepatitis B, hepatitis D has the potential for contributing to the severity of chronic hepatitis B. Hepatitis D superinfection can transform asymptomatic or mild chronic hepatitis B into severe, progressive chronic hepatitis and cirrhosis; it also can accelerate the course of chronic hepatitis B. Some HDV superinfections in patients with chronic hepatitis B lead to fulminant hepatitis. Although HDV and HBV infections are associated with severe liver disease, mild hepatitis and even asymptomatic carriage have been identified in some patients. After transfusion-associated acute hepatitis C, at least 50 percent of patients have abnormal biochemical liver tests for more than a year. In some experiences, the frequency of progression to chronicity after acute hepatitis C is as high as 70 percent. In most of these patients, liver histology is consistent with moderate to severe chronic hepatitis. Even among those who recover biochemically, the likelihood of retaining circulating HCV RNA is high. Thus, after acute HCV infection, the likelihood of remaining chronically *infected* approaches 85 to 90 percent. Although many patients with chronic hepatitis C have no symptoms, cirrhosis may develop in as many as 20 percent within 10 years of acute illness; in some series of cases, cirrhosis has been reported in as many as 50 percent of patients with chronic hepatitis C. Although chronic hepatitis C accounts for a quarter of cases of chronic liver disease and a quarter of patients undergoing liver transplantation for end-stage liver disease in the United States and Europe, in the majority of patients with chronic hepatitis C, morbidity and mortality are limited during the initial 20 years after the onset of infection. Progression of chronic hepatitis C may be influenced by hepatitis C genotype, level of hepatitis C viremia, age of acquisition, duration of infection, immunosuppression, as well as coexisting excessive alcohol use or other hepatitis virus infection. In contrast, neither HAV nor HEV causes chronic liver disease.

Rare complications of viral hepatitis include pancreatitis, myocarditis, atypical pneumonia, aplastic anemia, transverse myelitis, and peripheral neuropathy. *Carriers* of HBsAg, particularly those infected in infancy or early childhood, have an enhanced risk of hepatocellular carcinoma. The risk of hepatocellular carcinoma is increased as well in patients with chronic hepatitis C, almost exclusively in patients with cirrhosis, and almost always after at least a decade, usually after three decades of disease (see Chap. 93). In children, hepatitis B may present rarely with anicteric hepatitis, a nonpruritic papular rash of the face, buttocks, and limbs, and lymphadenopathy (papular acrodermatitis of childhood or Gianotti-Crosti syndrome).

DIFFERENTIAL DIAGNOSIS Viral diseases such as infectious mononucleosis; those due to cytomegalovirus, herpes simplex, and coxsackieviruses; and toxoplasmosis may share certain clinical features with viral hepatitis and cause elevation in serum aminotransferase and less commonly in serum bilirubin levels. Tests such as the differential heterophile and serologic tests for these agents may be helpful in the differential diagnosis if HBsAg, anti-HBc, IgM anti-HAV, and anti-HCV determinations are negative. Aminotransferase elevations can accompany almost any systemic viral infection; other rare causes of liver injury confused with viral hepatitis are infections with *Leptospira*, *Candida*, *Brucella*, *Mycobacteria*, and *Pneumocystis*. A complete drug history is particularly important, for many drugs and certain anesthetic agents can produce a picture of either acute hepatitis or cholestasis (see Chap. 296). Equally important is a past history of unexplained "repeated episodes" of acute hepatitis. This should alert the physician to the possibility that the underlying disorder is chronic hepatitis. Alcoholic hepatitis also must be considered, but usually the serum aminotransferase levels are not as markedly elevated and other stigmata of alcoholism may be present. The finding on liver biopsy of fatty infiltration, a neutrophilic inflammatory reaction, and "alcoholic hyaline" would be consistent with alcohol-induced rather than viral liver injury. Because acute hepatitis may present with right upper quadrant abdominal pain, nausea and vomiting, fever, and icterus, it is often confused with acute cholecystitis, common duct stone, or ascending cholangitis. Patients with acute viral hepatitis may tolerate surgery poorly; therefore, it is important to exclude this diagnosis, and in confusing cases, a percutaneous liver biopsy may be necessary prior to laparotomy. Viral hepatitis in the elderly is often misdiagnosed as obstructive jaundice resulting from a common duct stone or carcinoma of the pancreas. Because acute hepatitis in the elderly may be quite severe and the operative mortality high, a thorough evaluation including biochemical tests, radiographic studies of the biliary tree, and even liver biopsy may be necessary to exclude primary parenchymal liver disease. Another clinical constellation that may mimic acute hepatitis is right ventricular failure with passive hepatic congestion or hypoperfusion syndromes, such as those associated with shock, severe hypotension, and severe left ventricular failure. Also included in this general category is any disorder that interferes with venous return to the heart, such as right atrial myxoma, constrictive pericarditis, hepatic vein occlusion (Budd-Chiari syndrome), or venoocclusive disease. Clinical features are usually sufficient to distinguish between these vascular disorders and viral hepatitis. Acute fatty liver of pregnancy, cholestasis of pregnancy, eclampsia, and the HELLP syndrome (hemolysis, elevated liver tests, and low platelets) can be confused with viral hepatitis during pregnancy. Very rarely, malignancies metastatic to the liver can mimic acute or even fulminant viral hepatitis. Occasionally, genetic or metabolic liver disorders (e.g., Wilson's disease, α_1-antitrypsin deficiency) are confused with viral hepatitis.

℞ TREATMENT

Treatment of Acute Attack There is no specific treatment for *typical acute viral hepatitis*. Although hospitalization may be required for clinically severe illness, most patients do not require hospital care. Forced and prolonged bed rest is not essential for full recovery, but many patients will feel better with restricted physical activity. A high-calorie diet is desirable, and because many patients may experience nausea late in the day, the major caloric intake is best tolerated in the morning. Intravenous feeding is necessary in the acute stage if the patient has persistent vomiting and cannot maintain oral intake. Drugs capable of producing adverse reactions such as cholestasis and drugs metabolized by the liver should be avoided. If severe pruritus is present, the use of the bile salt–sequestering resin cholestyramine will usually alleviate this symptom. Glucocorticoid therapy has no value in acute viral hepatitis. Even in severe cases associated with *bridging necrosis*, controlled trials have failed to demonstrate the efficacy of steroids. In fact, such therapy may be hazardous.

Physical isolation of patients with hepatitis to a single room and bathroom is rarely necessary except in the case of fecal incontinence for hepatitis A and E or uncontrolled, voluminous bleeding for hepatitis types B (with or without concomitant hepatitis D) and hepatitis C. Because most patients hospitalized with hepatitis A excrete little if any HAV, the likelihood of HAV transmission from these patients during their hospitalization is low. Therefore, burdensome *enteric precautions are no longer recommended*. Although gloves should be worn when the bedpans or fecal material of patients with hepatitis A are handled, these precautions do not represent a departure from sensible procedure for all hospitalized patients. For patients with hepatitis types B and C, emphasis should be placed on blood precautions, i.e., avoiding direct, ungloved hand contact with blood and other body fluids. Enteric precautions are unnecessary. The importance of simple hygienic precautions, such as hand washing, cannot be overemphasized. Universal precautions that have been adopted for all patients apply to patients with viral hepatitis.

Hospitalized patients may be discharged when there is substantial symptomatic improvement, a significant downward trend in the serum aminotransferase and bilirubin values, and a return to normal of the PT. Mild aminotransferase elevations should not be considered contraindications to the gradual resumption of normal activity.

In *fulminant hepatitis*, the goal of therapy is to support the patient by maintenance of fluid balance, support of circulation and respiration, control of bleeding, correction of hypoglycemia, and treatment of other complications of the comatose state in anticipation of liver regeneration and repair. Protein intake should be restricted, and oral lactulose or neomycin administered. Glucocorticoid therapy has been shown in controlled trials to be ineffective. Likewise, exchange transfusion, plasmapheresis, human cross-circulation, porcine liver cross-perfusion, and hemoperfusion have not been proven to enhance survival. Meticulous intensive care is the one factor that does appear to improve survival. Orthotopic liver transplantation is resorted to with increasing frequency, with excellent results, in patients with fulminant hepatitis (see Chap. 301).

PROPHYLAXIS Because there is no therapy for acute viral hepatitis, and because antiviral therapy for chronic viral hepatitis is effective in only a proportion of patients (see Chap. 297), emphasis is placed on prevention through immunization. The prophylactic approach differs for each of the types of viral hepatitis. In the past, immunoprophylaxis relied exclusively on passive immunization with antibody-containing globulin preparations purified by cold ethanol fractionation from the plasma of hundreds of normal donors. Currently, for hepatitis A and B, active immunization with vaccines is available as well.

Hepatitis A Both passive immunization with immune globulin (IG) and active immunization with a killed vaccine are available. All preparations of IG contain anti-HAV. Although the titers may vary, all IG preparations have an antibody concentration sufficient to be protective. When administered before exposure or during the early incubation period, IG is effective in preventing clinically apparent type A hepatitis. In some cases, IG does not abort infection but, by attenuating it, renders it inapparent. As a result, long-lasting "passive-active" immunity occurs; however, this is now considered to be the exception rather than the rule. For postexposure prophylaxis of intimate contacts (household, institutional) of persons with hepatitis A, administration of 0.02 mL/kg is recommended as early after exposure as possible; it may be effective even when administered as late as 2 weeks after exposure. Prophylaxis is not necessary for casual contacts (office, factory, school, or hospital), for most elderly persons, who are very likely to be immune, or for those known to have anti-HAV in their serum. In day-care centers, recognition of hepatitis A cases in children or staff should provide a stimulus for immunoprophylaxis in the center and in the children's family members. By the time most common-source outbreaks of type A hepatitis are recognized, it is usually too late in the incubation period for IG to be effective; however, prophylaxis may limit the frequency of secondary cases. For travelers to tropical countries, developing countries, and other areas outside standard tourist routes, IG prophylaxis had been recommended, before a vaccine became available. When such travel lasted less than 3 months, 0.02 mL/kg was given; for longer travel or residence in these areas, a dose of 0.06 mL/kg every 4 to 6 months was recommended. The high-dose, repeated approach was recommended as well for certain primate handlers and laboratory personnel who work with HAV or fecal specimens. Administration of plasma-derived globulin is safe; it has not been associated with transmission of AIDS to recipients, and the AIDS virus (HIV) is inactivated by 25% alcohol, to which plasma is subjected during the cold ethanol fractionation process.

A formalin-inactivated vaccine made from a strain of HAV attenuated in tissue culture has been shown to be safe, immunogenic, and effective in preventing hepatitis A. It is approved for use in persons who are at least 2 years old and appears to provide adequate protection 4 weeks after a primary inoculation. If it can be given within 4 weeks of an expected exposure, such as by travel to an endemic area, hepatitis A vaccine is the preferred approach to *preexposure* immunoprophylaxis. If travel is more imminent, IG (0.02 mL/kg) should be administered at a different injection site, along with the first dose of vaccine. Because vaccination provides long-lasting protection (protective levels of anti-HAV should last 20 years after vaccination), persons whose risk will be sustained (e.g., frequent travelers or those remaining in endemic areas for prolonged periods) should be vaccinated, and vaccine should supplant the need for repeated IG injections. Other groups who are candidates for hepatitis A vaccination include military personnel, populations with cyclic outbreaks of hepatitis A (e.g., Alaskan natives), employees of day-care centers, primate handlers, laboratory workers exposed to hepatitis A or fecal specimens, and other populations whose recognized risk of hepatitis A is increased. For adults, a complete course of hepatitis A vaccine consists of two intramuscular injections (a 1-mL dose contains 1440 enzyme immunoassay units of viral antigen) given 6 to 12 months apart. For children, aged 2 to 18, three transmuscular injections (a 0.5-mL dose contains 360 enzyme immunoassay units) are recommended, the first two a month apart and the third 6 to 12 months after the first. The role of hepatitis A vaccine in *postexposure* prophylaxis remains to be demonstrated.

Hepatitis B Until 1982, prevention of hepatitis B was based on *passive* immunoprophylaxis either with standard IG, containing modest levels of anti-HBs, or hepatitis B immune globulin (HBIG), containing high-titer anti-HBs. The efficacy of standard IG has never been established and remains questionable; even the efficacy of HBIG, demonstrated in several clinical trials, has been challenged, and its contribution appears to be in reducing the frequency of clinical *illness*, not in preventing *infection*. The first vaccine for *active* immunization, introduced in 1982, was prepared from purified, noninfectious 22-nm spherical forms of HBsAg derived from the plasma of healthy HBsAg carriers. In 1987, the plasma-derived vaccine was supplanted by a genetically engineered vaccine derived from recombinant yeast. The latter vaccine consists of HBsAg particles that are nonglycosylated but are otherwise indistinguishable from natural HBsAg. Current recommendations can be divided into those for preexposure and postexposure prophylaxis.

For *preexposure* prophylaxis against hepatitis B in settings of frequent exposure (health workers exposed to blood, hemodialysis patients and staff, residents and staff of custodial institutions for the developmentally handicapped, intravenous drug abusers, inmates of long-term correctional facilities, promiscuous homosexual men as well as promiscuous heterosexuals, persons such as hemophiliacs who require long-term, high-volume therapy with blood derivatives, household and sexual contacts of HBsAg carriers, persons living in or traveling extensively in endemic areas, and unvaccinated children under the age of 11 who are Alaskan natives, Pacific Islanders, or residents in households of first-generation immigrants from endemic countries), three intramuscular (deltoid, not gluteal) injections of hepatitis B vaccine are recommended at 0, 1, and 6 months. Pregnancy is *not* a contraindication to vaccination. In areas of low HBV endemicity such as the United States, despite the availability of safe and effective hepatitis B vaccines, a strategy of vaccinating persons in high-risk groups has not been effective. The incidence of new hepatitis B cases continued to increase in the United States after introduction of vaccines; fewer than 10 percent of all targeted persons in high-risk groups have actually been vaccinated, and approximately 30 percent of persons with sporadic acute hepatitis B do not fall into any high-risk-group category. Therefore, to have an impact on the frequency of HBV infection in an area of low endemicity such as the United States, universal hepatitis B vaccination in childhood has been recommended. For unvaccinated children born after the implementation of universal infant vaccination, vaccination during early adolescence, at age 11 to 12 years, has been recommended.

There are two comparable recombinant hepatitis B vaccines available, one containing 10 μg of HBsAg (Recombivax-HB) and the other containing 20 μg of HBsAg (Engerix-B), and recommended doses for each injection vary between the two preparations. For Recombivax-HB, 2.5 μg is recommended for children <11 years of age of HBsAg-negative mothers, 5 μg for infants of HBsAg-positive mothers (see below) and for children and adolescents 11 to 19 years of age; 10 μg for immunocompetent adults; and 40 μg for dialysis patients and other immunosuppressed persons. For Engerix-B, 10 μg is recommended for children aged 10 and under, 20 μg for immunocompetent children older than 10 years of age and adults, and 40 μg for dialysis patients and other immunocompromised persons.

For unvaccinated persons sustaining an exposure to HBV, *postexposure* prophylaxis with a combination of HBIG (for rapid achievement of high-titer circulating anti-HBs) and hepatitis B vaccine (for achievement of long-lasting immunity as well as its apparent efficacy in attenuating clinical illness after exposure) is recommended. For *perinatal* exposure of infants born to HBsAg-positive mothers, a single dose of HBIG, 0.5 mL, should be administered intramuscularly in the thigh *immediately after birth*, followed by a complete course of three injections of recombinant hepatitis B vaccine (see doses above) to be started within the first 12 h of life. For those experiencing a direct percutaneous inoculation or transmucosal exposure to HBsAg-positive blood or body fluids (e.g., accidental *needle stick*, other mucosal penetration, or ingestion), a single intramuscular dose of HBIG, 0.06 mL/kg, administered as soon after exposure as possible, is followed by a complete course of hepatitis B vaccine to begin within the first week. For those exposed by *sexual* contact to a patient with acute hepatitis B, a single intramuscular dose of HBIG, 0.06 mL/kg, should be given within 14 days of exposure, to be followed by a complete course of hepatitis B vaccine. When both HBIG and hepatitis B vaccine are recommended, they may be given at the same time but at separate sites.

The precise duration of protection afforded by hepatitis B vaccine is unknown; however, approximately 80 to 90 percent of immunocompetent vaccinees retain protective levels of anti-HBs for at least 5 years. Thereafter and even after anti-HBs becomes undetectable, protection persists against clinical hepatitis B, hepatitis B surface antigenemia, and chronic HBV infection. Currently, *booster* immunizations are not recommended routinely, except in immunosuppressed persons who have lost detectable anti-HBs or immunocompetent persons who sustain percutaneous HBsAg-positive inoculations after losing detectable antibody. Specifically, for hemodialysis patients, annual anti-HBs testing is recommended after vaccination; booster doses are recommended when anti-HBs levels fall below 10 mIU/mL.

Hepatitis D Infection with hepatitis D can be prevented by vaccinating susceptible persons with hepatitis B vaccine. No product is available for immunoprophylaxis to prevent HDV superinfection in HBsAg carriers; for them, avoidance of percutaneous exposures and limitation of intimate contact with persons who have HDV infection are recommended.

Hepatitis C IG has been shown to be ineffective in preventing hepatitis C and is no longer recommended for postexposure prophylaxis in cases of perinatal, needle stick, or sexual exposure. Although a prototype vaccine that induces antibodies to HCV envelope protein has been developed, currently, hepatitis C vaccination is not feasible practically. Genotype and quasispecies viral heterogeneity, as well as rapid evasion of neutralizing antibodies by this rapidly mutating virus, conspire to render HCV a difficult target for immunoprophylaxis with a vaccine. Prevention of transfusion-associated hepatitis C has been accomplished by the following successively introduced measures: Exclusion of commercial blood donors and reliance on a volunteer blood supply; screening donor blood with surrogate markers such as ALT (no longer recommended) and anti-HBc, markers that identify segments of the blood donor population with an increased risk of bloodborne infections; exclusion of blood donors in high-risk groups for AIDS and the introduction of anti-HIV screening tests; and progressively sensitive serologic screening tests for anti-HCV. Chemical and heat treatment of blood products used for large-pool and concentrated blood derivates are being pursued.

Hepatitis E Whether IG prevents hepatitis E remains undetermined. Development of a vaccine is in progress.

BIBLIOGRAPHY

Advisory Committee on Immunization Practices: Licensure of inactivated hepatitis A vaccine and recommendations for use among international travelers. Morb Mort Week Rep 44:559, 1995

Alter HJ: To C or not to C: These are the questions. Blood 85:1681, 1995

Alter MJ et al: The epidemiology of viral hepatitis in the United States. Gastroenterol Clin North Am 23:437, 1994

———: Acute non-A-E hepatitis in the United States and the role of hepatitis G virus infection. N Engl J Med 336:741, 1997

Barrera JM et al: Persistent hepatitis C viremia after acute self-limiting posttransfusion hepatitis C. Hepatology 21:639, 1995

Centers for Disease Control: Update: Recommendations to prevent hepatitis B virus transmission—United States. Morb Mort Week Rep 44:574, 1995

Choo Q-L et al: Isolation of a cDNA clone derived from a blood-borne non-A, non-B viral hepatitis genome. Science 244:359, 1989

Cohen JI: Hepatitis A virus: Insights from molecular biology. Hepatology 9:889, 1989

Di Bisceglie AM et al: Long-term clinical and histologic follow-up of chronic posttransfusion hepatitis. Hepatology 14:969, 1991

Dienstag JL: Non-A, non-B hepatitis: I. Recognition, epidemiology, and clinical features. II. Experimental transmission, putative virus agents and markers, and prevention. Gastroenterology 85:439, 743, 1983

——— (ed): Viral hepatitis. Semin Liver Dis 11:73, 1991

Dobson S et al: Assessment of a universal, school-based hepatitis B vaccination program. JAMA 274:1209, 1995

Donahue JG et al: The declining risk of post-transfusion hepatitis C virus infection. N Engl J Med 327:369, 1992

Farci P et al: Lack of protective immunity against reinfection with hepatitis C virus. Science 258:135, 1992

Hoofnagle JH: Type D (delta) hepatitis. JAMA 261:1321, 1989

Houghton M et al: Molecular biology of the hepatitis C viruses: Implications for diagnosis, development and control of viral disease. Hepatology 14:381, 1991

Innis BL et al: Protection against hepatitis A by an inactivated vaccine. JAMA 271:1328, 1994

Krawczynski K: Hepatitis E. Hepatology 17:932, 1993

Lemon SM, Thomas DL: Vaccines to prevent viral hepatitis. N Engl J Med 336:196, 1997

Linnen J et al: Molecular cloning and disease association of hepatitis G virus: A transfusion-transmissible agent. Science 271:505, 1996

Margolis HS et al: Prevention of hepatitis B virus transmission by immunization: An economic analysis of current recommendations. JAMA 274:1201, 1995

Miller RH et al: Compact organization of the hepatitis B virus genome. Hepatology 9:322, 1989

Nishioka K et al (eds): *Viral Hepatitis and Liver Disease*. New York, Springer-Verlag, 1994

Nousbaum J-B et al: Hepatitis C virus type 1b (II) infection in France and Italy. Ann Intern Med 122:161, 1995

Okamoto H et al: Superinfection of chimpanzees carrying hepatitis C virus of genotype II/1b with that of genotype III/2a or I/1a. Hepatology 20:1131, 1994

Purcell RH: Hepatitis viruses: Changing patterns of human disease. Proc Natl Acad Sci USA 91:2401, 1994

Reyes GR et al: Isolation of a cDNA from the virus responsible for enterically transmitted non-A, non-B hepatitis. Science 247:1335, 1990

Sato S et al: Hepatitis B virus strains with mutations in the core promoter in patients with fulminant hepatitis. Ann Intern Med 122:241, 1995

Seeff LB: Natural history of viral hepatitis, type C. Semin Gastrointest Dis 6:20, 1995

———: Hepatitis C. Semin Liver Dis 15:1, 1995

Shakil AO et al: Volunteer blood donors with antibody to hepatitis C virus: Clinical, biochemical, virologic, and histologic features. Ann Intern Med 123:330, 1995

Sheth SG et al: Nonalcoholic steatohepatitis. Ann Intern Med 126:137, 1997

Simmonds P: Variability of hepatitis C virus. Hepatology 21:570, 1995

Simons JN et al: Isolation of novel virus-like sequences associated with human hepatitis. Nature 1:564, 1995

——— et al: Identification of two flavivirus-like genomes in the GB hepatitis agent. Proc Natl Acad Sci USA 92:3401, 1995

Takahashi M et al: Natural history of chronic hepatitis C. Am J Gastroenterol 88:240, 1993

Thomas DL et al: Sexual transmission of hepatitis C virus among patients attending sexually transmitted disease clinics in Baltimore—an analysis of 309 sex partnerships. J Infect Dis 171:768, 1994

Tong MJ et al: Clinical outcomes after transfusion-associated hepatitis C. N Engl J Med 332:1463, 1995

296

Jules L. Dienstag, Kurt J. Isselbacher

TOXIC AND DRUG-INDUCED HEPATITIS

Liver injury may follow the inhalation, ingestion, or parenteral administration of a number of pharmacologic and chemical agents. These include industrial toxins (e.g., carbon tetrachloride, trichloroethylene, and yellow phosphorus), the heat-stable toxic bicyclic octapeptides of certain species of *Amanita* and *Galerina* (hepatotoxic mushroom poisoning), and more commonly, pharmacologic agents used in medical therapy. It is essential that any patient presenting with jaundice or altered biochemical liver tests be questioned carefully about exposure to chemicals used in work or at home and drugs taken by prescription or bought "over the counter." In general, two major types of chemical hepatotoxicity have been recognized: (1) direct toxic type and (2) idiosyncratic type.

As shown in Table 296-1, direct toxic hepatitis occurs with predictable regularity in individuals exposed to the offending agent and is dose-dependent. The latent period between exposure and liver injury is usually short (often several hours), although clinical manifestations may be delayed for 24 to 48 h. Agents producing toxic hepatitis are generally systemic poisons or are converted in the liver to toxic metabolites. The direct hepatotoxins result in morphologic abnormalities that are reasonably characteristic and reproducible for each toxin. For example, carbon tetrachloride and trichloroethylene characteristically produce a centrilobular zonal necrosis, whereas yellow phosphorus poisoning typically results in periportal injury. The hepatotoxic octapeptides of *Amanita phalloides* usually produce massive hepatic necrosis. The lethal dose of the toxin is about 10 mg, the amount found in a single deathcap mushroom. Tetracycline, when administered in intravenous doses greater than 1.5 g daily, leads to microvesicular fat deposits in the liver. Liver injury, which is often only one facet of the toxicity produced by the direct hepatotoxins, may go unrecognized until jaundice appears.

In idiosyncratic drug reactions the occurrence of hepatitis is usually infrequent and unpredictable, the response is not dose-dependent, and it may occur at any time during or shortly after exposure to the drug. Extrahepatic manifestations of hypersensitivity, such as rash, arthralgias, fever, leukocytosis, and eosinophilia, occur in about one-quarter of patients with idiosyncratic hepatotoxic drug reactions; this observation and the unpredictability of idiosyncratic drug hepatotoxicity contributed to the hypothesis that this category of drug reactions is immunologically mediated. More recent evidence, however, suggests that, in most cases, even idiosyncratic reactions represent direct hepatotoxity but are caused by drug metabolites rather than by the intact compound. Even the prototype of idiosyncratic hepatoxicity reactions, halothane hepatitis, and isoniazid hepatotoxicity, associated frequently with hypersensitivity manifestations, are now recognized to be mediated by toxic metabolites that damage liver cells directly. Currently, most idiosyncratic reactions are thought to result from differences in metabolic reactivity to specific agents; host susceptibility is mediated by the kinetics of toxic metabolite generation, which differs among individuals. Occasionally, however, the clinical features of an allergic reaction (prominent tissue eosinophilia, autoantibodies, etc.) are difficult to ignore. In vitro models have been described in which lymphocyte cytotoxicity can be demonstrated against rabbit hepatocytes altered by incubation with the potential offending drug. Similarly, in selected cases, a drug or its metabolite has been shown to bind to a host cellular component forming a hapten; the immune response to this "neoantigen" is postulated to play a role in the pathogenesis of liver injury. Therefore, some authorities subdivide idiosyncratic drug hepatotoxicity into hypersensitivity (allergic) and "metabolic" categories. Several unusual exceptions notwithstanding, true drug allergy is difficult to support in most cases of idiosyncratic drug-induced liver injury.

Idiosyncratic reactions lead to a morphologic pattern that is more variable than those produced by direct toxins; a single agent is often capable of causing a variety of lesions, although certain patterns tend to predominate. Depending on the agent involved, idiosyncratic hepatitis may result in a clinical and morphologic picture indistinguishable from that of viral hepatitis (e.g., halothane) or may simulate extrahepatic bile duct obstruction clinically with morphologic evidence of cholestasis and minimal hepatocellular damage (e.g., chlorpromazine). Morphologic alterations also may include bridging hepatic necrosis (e.g., methyldopa), or, infrequently, hepatic granulomas (e.g., sulfonamides).

Not all adverse hepatic drug reactions can be classified as either toxic or idiosyncratic in type. For example, oral contraceptives, which combine estrogenic and progestational compounds, may result in impairment of hepatic tests and occasionally in jaundice. However, they do not produce necrosis or fatty change, manifestations of hypersensitivity are generally absent, and susceptibility to the development of oral contraceptive–induced cholestasis appears to be genetically determined.

Because drug-induced hepatitis is often a presumptive diagnosis and many other disorders produce a similar clinicopathologic picture, evidence of a causal relationship between the use of a drug and subsequent liver injury may be difficult to establish. The relationship is most convincing for the direct hepatotoxins, which lead to a high frequency of hepatic impairment after a short latent period. Idiosyncratic reactions may be reproduced, in some instances, when rechallenge, after an asymptomatic period, results in a recurrence of signs, symptoms, and morphologic and biochemical abnormalities. Rechallenge, however, is often ethically unfeasible, because severe reactions may occur.

℞ TREATMENT

Treatment of toxic and drug-induced hepatic disease is largely supportive, as in acute viral hepatitis, except in acetaminophen hepatotoxicity (see below). Withdrawal of the suspected agent is indicated at the first sign of an adverse reaction. In the case of the direct toxins, liver involvement should not divert attention from renal or other organ involvement, which also may threaten survival.

In Table 296-2, several classes of chemical agents are listed, together with examples of the pattern of liver injury produced by them. Certain drugs appear to be responsible for the development of chronic as well as acute hepatic injury. For example, oxyphenisatin, alpha methyldopa, and isoniazid have been associated with moderate to severe chronic hepatitis, and halothane and methotrexate have been implicated in the development of cirrhosis. A syndrome resembling primary biliary cirrhosis has been described following treatment with chlorpromazine, methyl testosterone, tolbutamide, and other drugs. Portal hypertension in the absence of cirrhosis may result from alterations in hepatic architecture produced by vitamin A or arsenic intoxication, industrial exposure to vinyl chloride, or administration of thorium dioxide. The latter three agents also have been associated with

Table 296-1

Some Features of Toxic and Drug-Induced Hepatic Injury

Features	Direct Toxic Effect		Idiosyncratic			Other
	(Carbon Tetrachloride, e.g.)	(Acetaminophen, e.g.)	(Halothane, e.g.)	(Isoniazid, e.g.)	(Chlorpromazine, e.g.)	(Oral Contraceptive Agents, e.g.)
Predictable and dose-related toxicity	+	+	0	0	0	+
Latent period	Short	Short	Variable	Variable	Variable	Variable
Arthralgia, fever, rash, eosinophilia	0	0	+	0	+	0
Liver morphology	Necrosis, fatty infiltration	Centrilobular necrosis	Similar to viral hepatitis	Similar to viral hepatitis	Cholestasis *with* portal inflammation	Cholestasis *without* portal inflammation, vascular lesions

Table 296-2

Principal Alterations of Hepatic Morphology Produced by Some Commonly Used Drugs and Chemicals*

Principal Morphologic Change	Class of Agent	Example
Cholestasis	Anabolic steroid	Methyl testosterone.
	Anti-inflammatory	Sulindac
	Antithyroid	Methimazole
	Antibiotic	Erythromycin estolate, nitrofurantoin, rifampin
	Oral contraceptive	Norethynodrel with mestranol
	Oral hypoglycemic	Chlorpropamide
	Tranquilizer	Chlorpromazine†
	Oncotherapeutic	Anabolic steroids, busulfan, tamoxifen
	Immunosuppressive	Cyclosporine
	Anticonvulsant	Carbamazine
	Calcium channel blocker	Nifedipine, verapamil
Fatty liver	Antibiotic	Tetracycline
	Anticonvulsant	Sodium valproate
	Antiarrhythmic	Amiodarone
	Antiviral	Dideoxynucleosides (e.g., zidovudine)
	Oncotherapeutic	Asparaginase, methotrexate
Hepatitis	Anesthetic	Halothane‡
	Anticonvulsant	Phenytoin, carbamazine
	Antihypertensive	Methyldopa,‡ captopril, enalapril
	Antibiotic	Isoniazid,‡ rifampin, nitrofurantoin
	Diuretic	Chlorothiazide
	Laxative	Oxyphenisatin‡
	Antidepressant	Iproniazid, amitriptyline, imipramine
	Anti-inflammatory	Ibuprofen, indomethacin, diclofenac, sulindac
	Antifungal	Ketoconazole, fluconazole, itraconazole
	Antiviral	Zidovudine, dideoxy inosine
	Calcium channel blocker	Nifedipine, verapamil, diltiazem
	Antiandrogen	Flutamide
Mixed hepatitis/ cholestatic	Immunosuppressive	Azathioprine
	Lipid-lowering	Nicotinic acid, lovastatin
Toxic (necrosis)	Hydrocarbon	Carbon tetrachloride
	Metal	Yellow phosphorus
	Mushroom	*Amanita phalloides*
	Analgesic	Acetaminophen
	Solvent	Dimethylformamide
Granulomas	Anti-inflammatory	Phenylbutazone
	Antibiotic	Sulfanomides
	Xanthine oxidase inhibitor	Allopurinol
	Antiarrhythmic	Quinidine
	Anticonvulsant	Carbamazine

* Several agents cause more than one type of liver lesion and appear under more than one category.
† Rarely associated with primary biliary cirrhosis–like lesion.
‡ Occasionally associated with chronic hepatitis or bridging hepatic necrosis or cirrhosis.

angiosarcoma of the liver. Oral contraceptives have been implicated in the development of hepatic adenoma and, rarely, hepatocellular carcinoma and occlusion of the hepatic vein (Budd-Chiari syndrome). Another unusual lesion, peliosis hepatis (blood cysts of the liver), has been observed in some patients treated with anabolic steroids. The existence of these hepatic disorders expands the spectrum of liver injury induced by chemical agents and emphasizes the need for a thorough drug history in all patients with liver dysfunction.

The following are the patterns of adverse hepatic reactions for some prototypic agents.

ACETAMINOPHEN HEPATOTOXICITY (DIRECT TOXIN) Acetaminophen has caused severe centrolobular hepatic necrosis when ingested in large amounts in suicide attempts or accidentally by children. A single dose of 10 to 15 g, occasionally less, may produce clinical evidence of liver injury. Fatal fulminant disease is usually (although not invariably) associated with ingestion of 25 g or more. Blood levels of acetaminophen correlate with the severity of hepatic injury (levels above 300 μg/mL 4 h after ingestion are predictive of the development of severe damage, while levels below 150 μg/mL suggest that hepatic injury is highly unlikely). Nausea, vomiting, diarrhea, abdominal pain, and shock are early manifestations occurring 4 to 12 h after ingestion. Then 24 to 48 h later, when these features are abating, hepatic injury becomes apparent. Maximal abnormalities and hepatic failure may not be evident until 4 to 6 days after ingestion, and aminotransferase levels approaching 10,000 units are not uncommon. Renal failure and myocardial injury may be present.

Acetaminophen hepatotoxicity is mediated by a toxic reactive metabolite formed from the parent compound by the cytochrome P450 mixed-function oxidase system of the hepatocyte. This metabolite is detoxified by binding to glutathione. When excessive amounts of the metabolite are formed, glutathione levels in the liver fall, and the metabolite is covalently bound to nucleophilic hepatocyte macromolecules. This process is believed to lead to hepatocyte necrosis; the precise sequence and mechanism are unknown. Hepatic injury may be potentiated by prior administration of alcohol or other drugs, by conditions that stimulate the mixed-function oxidase system, or by conditions such as starvation that reduce hepatic glutathione levels. Cimetidine, which inhibits P450 enzymes, has the potential to reduce generation of the toxic metabolite. In chronic alcoholics, the toxic dose of acetaminophen may be as low as 2 g.

℞ TREATMENT

Treatment of acetaminophen overdosage includes gastric lavage, supportive measures, and oral administration of activated charcoal or cholestyramine to prevent absorption of residual drug. Neither of these agents appears to be effective if given more than 30 min after acetaminophen ingestion; if they are used, the stomach lavage should be done before other agents are administered orally. In patients with high acetaminophen blood levels (>200 μg/mL measured at 4 h or >100 μg/mL at 8 h after ingestion), the administration of sulfhydryl compounds (e.g., cysteamine, cysteine, or *N*-acetylcysteine) appears to reduce the severity of hepatic necrosis. These agents appear to act by providing a reservoir of sulfhydryl groups to bind the toxic metabolites or by stimulating synthesis and repletion of hepatic glutathione. Therapy should be begun within 8 h of ingestion but may be effective even if given as late as 24 to 36 h after overdose. Later administration of sulfhydryl compounds is of uncertain value. Routine use of *N*-acetylcysteine has reduced substantially the occurrence of fatal acetaminophen hepatotoxicity. When given orally, *N*-acetylcysteine is diluted to yield a 5% solution. A loading dose of 140 mg/kg is given, followed by 70 mg/kg every 4 h for 15 to 20 doses. Treatment can be stopped when plasma acetominophen levels indicate that the risk of liver damage is low.

Survivors of acute acetaminophen overdose usually have no evidence of hepatic sequelae. In a few patients, prolonged or repeated administration of acetaminophen in therapeutic doses appears to have led to the development of chronic hepatitis and cirrhosis.

HALOTHANE HEPATOTOXICITY (IDIOSYNCRATIC REACTION) Administration of halothane, a nonexplosive fluorinated hydrocarbon anesthetic agent that is structurally similar to chloroform, results in severe hepatic necrosis in a small number of individuals, many of whom have previously been exposed to this agent. The failure to produce similar hepatic lesions reliably in animals, the rarity of hepatic impairment in human beings, and the delayed appearance of hepatic injury suggest that halothane is not a direct hepatotoxin but rather a sensitizing agent. However, manifestations of hypersensitivity are seen in fewer than 25 percent of cases. A genetic predisposition leading to an idiosyncratic metabolic reactivity has been postulated and appears to be the most likely mechanism of halothane hepatotoxicity. Adults (rather than children), obese people, and women appear to be particularly susceptible. Fever, moderate leukocytosis, and eosinophilia may occur in the first week following halothane administration. Jaundice usually is noted 7 to 10 days after exposure but may occur earlier in previously exposed patients. Nausea and vomiting may precede the onset of jaundice. Hepatomegaly is often mild, but liver tenderness is common. The serum aminotransferase levels are elevated. The pathologic changes at autopsy are indistinguishable from massive hepatic necrosis resulting from viral hepatitis. The case-fatality rate of halothane hepatitis is not known but may vary from 20 to 40 percent in cases with severe liver involvement. It is strongly suggested that patients in whom unexplained spiking fever, especially delayed fever, or jaundice develops after halothane anesthesia not receive this agent again. Because cross-reactions between halothane and methoxyfluorane have been reported, the latter agent should not be used after halothane reactions. Later-generation halogenated hydrocarbon anesthetics, which have supplanted halothane except in rare instances, are felt to be associated with a lower risk of hepatotoxicity.

METHYLDOPA HEPATOTOXICITY (TOXIC AND IDIOSYNCRATIC REACTION) Minor alterations in liver tests are reported in about 5 percent of patients treated with this antihypertensive agent. These trivial abnormalities typically resolve despite continued drug administration. In fewer than 1 percent of patients, acute liver injury resembling viral or chronic hepatitis or, rarely, a cholestatic reaction is seen 1 to 20 weeks after methyldopa is started. In 50 percent of cases the interval is shorter than 4 weeks. A prodrome of fever, anorexia, and malaise may be noted for a few days before the onset of jaundice. Rash, lymphadenopathy, arthralgia, and eosinophilia are rare. Serologic markers of autoimmunity are detected infrequently, and fewer than 5 percent of patients have a Coombs-positive hemolytic anemia. In about 15 percent of patients with methyldopa hepatotoxicity, the clinical, biochemical, and histologic features are those of moderate to severe chronic hepatitis, with or without bridging necrosis and macronodular cirrhosis. With discontinuation of the drug, the disorder usually resolves.

ISONIAZID HEPATOTOXICITY (TOXIC AND IDIOSYNCRATIC REACTION) In approximately 10 percent of adults treated with the antituberculosis agent isoniazid, elevated serum aminotransferase levels develop during the first few weeks of therapy; this appears to represent an adaptive response to a toxic metabolite of the drug. Whether or not isoniazid is continued, these values (usually below 200 units) return to normal in a few weeks. In about 1 percent of treated patients, an illness develops that is indistinguishable from viral hepatitis; approximately half of these cases occur within the first 2 months of treatment, while in the remainder, clinical disease may be delayed for many months. Liver biopsy reveals morphologic changes similar to those of viral hepatitis or bridging hepatic necrosis. The disease may be severe, with a case-fatality rate of 10 percent. Important liver injury appears to be age-related, increasing substantially after age 35; the highest frequency is in patients over age 50, the lowest under the age of 20. Isoniazid hepatotoxicity is enhanced by alcohol and rifampicin. Fever, rash, eosinophilia, and other manifestations of drug allergy are distinctly unusual. A reactive metabolite of acetylhydrazine, a metabolite of isoniazid, may be responsible for liver injury, and patients who are rapid acetylators would be more prone to such injury. A picture resembling chronic hepatitis has been observed in a few patients.

SODIUM VALPROATE HEPATOTOXICITY (TOXIC AND IDIOSYNCRATIC REACTION) Sodium valproate, an anticonvulsant useful in the treatment of petit mal and other seizure disorders, has been associated with the development of severe hepatic toxicity and, rarely, fatalities in both children and adults. Asymptomatic elevations of serum aminotransferase levels have been recognized in as many as 45 percent of treated patients. These "adaptive" changes, however, appear to have no clinical importance, for major hepatotoxicity is not seen in the majority of patients despite continuation of drug therapy. In those rare patients in whom jaundice, encephalopathy, and evidence of hepatic failure are found, examination of liver tissue reveals microvesicular fat and bridging hepatic necrosis, predominantly in the centrolobular zone. Bile duct injury also may be apparent. It seems likely that sodium valproate is not directly hepatotoxic but that its metabolite, 4-pentenoic acid, may be responsible for hepatic injury.

PHENYTOIN HEPATOTOXICITY (IDIOSYNCRATIC REACTION) Phenytoin, formerly diphenylhydantoin, a mainstay in the treatment of seizure disorders, has been associated in rare instances with the development of severe hepatitis-like liver injury leading to fulminant hepatic failure. In many patients the hepatitis is associated with striking fever, lymphadenopathy, rash (Stevens-Johnson syndrome or exfoliative dermatitis), leukocytosis, and eosinophilia, suggesting an immunologically mediated hypersensitivity mechanism. Despite these observations, there is also evidence that metabolic idiosyncrasy may be responsible for hepatic injury. In the liver, phenytoin is converted by the cytochrome P450 system to metabolites, which include the highly reactive electrophilic arene oxides. These metabolites are normally metabolized further by epoxide hydrolases. A defect (genetic or acquired) in epoxide hydrolase activity could permit covalent binding of arene oxides to hepatic macromolecules, thereby leading to hepatic injury. Regardless of the mechanism, hepatic injury is usually manifest within the first 2 months after beginning phenytoin therapy. With the exception of an abundance of eosinophils in the liver, the clinical, biochemical, and histologic picture resembles that of viral hepatitis. In rare instances, bile duct injury may be the salient feature of phenytoin hepatotoxicity, with striking features of intrahepatic cholestasis. Asymptomatic elevations of aminotransferase and alkaline phosphatase levels have been observed in a sizable proportion of patients receiving long-term phenytoin therapy. These liver changes are believed by some authorities to represent the potent hepatic enzyme–inducing properties of phenytoin and are accompanied histologically by swelling of hepatocytes in the absence of necroinflammatory activity or evidence of chronic liver disease.

CHLORPROMAZINE HEPATOTOXICITY (CHOLESTATIC IDIOSYNCRATIC REACTION) In about 1 percent of patients receiving chlorpromazine, intrahepatic cholestasis with jaundice develops after 1 to 4 weeks of treatment. In rare instances, jaundice has been reported after a single exposure. Anicteric reactions are frequent. The onset may be abrupt, with fever, rash, arthralgias, lymphadenopathy, nausea, vomiting, and epigastric or right upper quadrant pain. Pruritus may precede the appearance of jaundice, dark urine, and light stools. Eosinophilia with or without mild leukocytosis may be present, and conjugated hyperbilirubinemia, moderately elevated serum alkaline phosphatase, and mildly elevated serum aminotransferase levels (100 to 200 units) are noted. Liver biopsy reveals cholestasis, bile plugs in dilated bile canaliculi, and a dense portal infiltrate of polymorphonuclear, eosinophilic, and mononuclear leukocytes. Occasionally, scattered foci of hepatic parenchymal necrosis may be evident. Jaundice and pruritus usually subside within 4 to 8 weeks following cessation of therapy, without sequelae, and fatalities are rare. Cholestyramine may be of value in relieving severe pruritus. In a small number of patients, jaundice is prolonged for several months to years; rarely, a disorder resembling but distinct from primary biliary cirrhosis may develop.

AMIODARONE HEPATOTOXICITY (TOXIC AND IDIOSYNCRATIC REACTION) Therapy with this potent antiarrhythmic drug is accompanied in 15 to 50 percent of patients by modest elevation of serum aminotransferase levels that may remain stable or diminish despite continuation of the drug. Such abnormalities may appear days to many months after beginning therapy. A proportion of those with elevated aminotransferase levels have detectable hepatomegaly, and clinically important liver disease develops in fewer than 5 percent of patients. Features that represent a direct effect of the drug on the liver and that are common to the majority of long-term recipients are ultrastructural phospholipidosis, unaccompanied by clinical liver disease, and interference with hepatic mixed-function oxidase metabolism of other drugs. The relatively common elevations in aminotransferase levels are also considered a predictable, dose-dependent, direct hepatotoxic effect. On the other hand, in the rare patient with clinically apparent, symptomatic liver disease, liver injury resembling that seen in alcoholic liver disease is observed. The so-called pseudoalcoholic liver injury can range from steatosis, to alcoholic hepatitis–like neutrophilic infiltration and Mallory's hyaline, to cirrhosis. Electron-microscopic demonstration of phospholipid-laden lysosomal lamellar bodies can help to distinguish amiodarone hepatotoxicity from typical alcoholic hepatitis. This category of liver injury appears to be a metabolic idiosyncracy that allows hepatotoxic metabolites to be generated. Rarely, an acute idiosyncratic hepatocellular injury resembling viral hepatitis or cholestatic hepatitis occurs. Hepatic granulomas have occasionally been observed. Because amiodarone has a long half-life, liver injury may persist for months after the drug is stopped.

ERYTHROMYCIN HEPATOTOXICITY (CHOLESTATIC IDIOSYNCRATIC REACTION) The most important adverse effect associated with erythromycin is the infrequent occurrence of a cholestatic reaction. Although most of these reactions have been associated with erythromycin estolate, other erythromycins also may be responsible. The reaction usually begins during the first 2 or 3 weeks of therapy and includes nausea, vomiting, fever, right upper quadrant abdominal pain, jaundice, leukocytosis, and moderately elevated aminotransferase levels. The clinical picture can resemble acute cholecystitis or bacterial cholangitis. Liver biopsy reveals variable cholestasis; portal inflammation comprising lymphocytes, polymorphonuclear leukocytes, and eosinophils; and scattered foci of hepatocyte necrosis. Symptoms and laboratory findings usually subside within a few days of drug withdrawal, and evidence of chronic liver disease has not been found on follow-up. The precise mechanism remains ill-defined.

ORAL CONTRACEPTIVE HEPATOTOXICITY (CHOLESTATIC REACTION) The administration of oral contraceptive combinations of estrogenic and progestational steroids leads to intrahepatic cholestasis with pruritus and jaundice in a small number of patients weeks to months after taking these agents. Especially susceptible seem to be patients with recurrent idiopathic jaundice of pregnancy, severe pruritus of pregnancy, or a family history of these disorders. With the exception of liver biochemical tests, laboratory studies are normal, and extrahepatic manifestations of hypersensitivity are absent. Liver biopsy reveals cholestasis with bile plugs in dilated canaliculi and striking bilirubin staining of liver cells. In contrast to chlorpromazine-induced cholestasis, portal inflammation is absent. The lesion is reversible on withdrawal of the agent. The two steroid components appear to act synergistically on hepatic function, although the estrogen may be primarily responsible. Oral contraceptives are contraindicated in patients with a history of recurrent jaundice of pregnancy. Primarily benign, but rarely malignant, neoplasms of the liver, hepatic vein occlusion, and peripheral sinusoidal dilatation have also been associated with oral contraceptive therapy.

17,α-ALKYL-SUBSTITUTED ANABOLIC STEROIDS (CHOLESTATIC REACTION) In the majority of patients receiving these agents, used therapeutically mainly in the treatment of bone marrow failure but used surreptitiously and without medical indication by athletes to improve their performance, mild hepatic dysfunction develops. Impaired excretory function is the predominant defect, but the precise mechanism is uncertain. Jaundice, which appears to be dose-related, develops in only a minority of patients and may be the sole clinical manifestation of hepatotoxicity, although anorexia, nausea, and malaise may occur. Pruritus is not a prominent feature. Serum aminotransferase levels are usually under 100 units, and serum alkaline phosphatase levels are normal, mildly elevated, or, in fewer than 5 percent of patients, three or more times the upper limit of normal. Examination of liver tissue reveals cholestasis without inflammation or necrosis. Hepatic sinusoidal dilatation and peliosis hepatis have been found in a few patients. The cholestatic disorder is usually reversible on cessation of treatment, although fatalities have been linked to peliosis. An association with hepatic adenoma and hepatocellular carcinoma has been reported.

TRIMETHOPRIM-SULFAMETHOXAZOLE HEPATOTOXICITY (IDIOSYNCRATIC REACTION) This antibiotic combination is used routinely for urinary tract infections in immunocompetent persons and for prophylaxis against and therapy of *Pneumocystis carinii* pneumonia in immunosuppressed persons (transplant recipients, patients with AIDS). With its increasing use, its occasional hepatotoxicity is being recognized with growing frequency. Its likelihood is unpredictable, but when it occurs, trimethoprim-sulfamethoxazole hepatotoxicity follows a relatively uniform latency period of several weeks and is often accompanied by eosinophilia, rash, and other features of a hypersensitivity reaction. Biochemically and histologically, acute hepatocellular necrosis predominates, but cholestatic features are quite frequent. Occasionally, cholestasis without necrosis occurs, and very rarely, a severe cholangiolytic pattern of liver injury is observed. In most cases, liver injury is self-limited, but rare fatalities have been recorded. The hepatotoxicity is attributable to the sulfamethoxazole component of the drug and is similar in features to that seen with other sulfonamides; tissue eosinophilia and granulomas may be seen.

BIBLIOGRAPHY

Black M et al: Isoniazid-associated hepatitis in 114 patients. Gastroenterology 69:389, 1975

———: Acetaminophen hepatotoxicity. Ann Rev Med 35:577, 1984

Harrison PM et al: Improved outcome of paracetamol-induced fulminant hepatic failure by late administration of acetylcysteine. Lancet 335:1572, 1990

Kaplowitz N et al: Drug-induced hepatotoxicity. Ann Intern Med 104:826, 1986

——— (ed): Recent advances in drug metabolism and hepatotoxicity. Semin Liver Dis 10:233, 1990

Lee WM: Drug-induced hepatotoxicity. N Engl J Med 333:1118, 1995

Lewis JH et al: Amiodarone hepatotoxicity: Prevalence and clinicopathologic correlations among 104 patients. Hepatology 9:679, 1989

Ludwig J, Axelsen R: Drug effects on the liver: An updated tabular compilation of drugs and drug-related hepatic diseases. Dig Dis Sci 28:651, 1983

Morgan DJ, Smallwood RA: Drug-induced liver disease. Curr Opinion Gastroenterol 12:246, 1996

Rabinovitz M et al: Hepatotoxicity of nonsteroidal anti-inflammatory drugs. Am J Gastroenterol 87:1696, 1992

Seeff LB et al: Acetaminophen hepatotoxicity in alcoholics: A therapeutic misadventure. Ann Intern Med 104:399, 1986

Smilkstein MJ et al: Efficacy of *N*-acetylcysteine in the treatment of acetaminophen overdose. N Engl J Med 319:1557, 1988

Tarazi EM et al: Sulindac-associated hepatic injury: Analysis of 91 cases reported to the Food and Drug Administration. Gastroenterology 104:569, 1993

Whitcomb DC et al: Association of acetaminophen hepatotoxicity with fasting and ethanol use. JAMA 272:1845, 1994

Zimmerman HJ, Ishak KG: Valproate-induced hepatic injury: Analysis of 23 fatal cases. Hepatology 2:591, 1982

297 CHRONIC HEPATITIS

Jules L. Dienstag, Kurt J. Isselbacher

Chronic hepatitis represents a series of liver disorders of varying causes and severity in which hepatic inflammation and necrosis continue for at least 6 months. Milder forms are nonprogressive or only slowly progressive, while more severe forms may be associated with scarring and architectural organization, which, when advanced, lead ultimately to cirrhosis. Several categories of chronic hepatitis have been recognized. These include chronic viral hepatitis (see Chap. 295), drug-induced chronic hepatitis (see Chap. 296), and autoimmune chronic hepatitis. In many cases, clinical and laboratory features are insufficient to allow assignment into one of these three categories; these "idiopathic" cases are also believed to represent autoimmune chronic hepatitis. Finally, clinical and laboratory features of chronic hepatitis are observed occasionally in patients with such hereditary/metabolic disorders as Wilson's disease (copper overload) and even occasionally in patients with alcoholic liver injury (see Chap. 298). Although all types of chronic hepatitis share certain clinical, laboratory, and histopathologic features, chronic viral and chronic autoimmune hepatitis are sufficiently distinct to merit separate discussions.

CLASSIFICATION OF CHRONIC HEPATITIS Common to all forms of chronic hepatitis are histopathologic distinctions based on localization and extent of liver injury. These vary from the milder forms, previously labeled chronic persistent hepatitis and chronic lobular hepatitis, to the more severe form, formerly called chronic active hepatitis. When first defined, these designations were felt to have prognostic implications, which have been challenged by more recent observations. Compared to the time more than two decades ago when the histologic designations chronic persistent, chronic lobular, and chronic active hepatitis were adopted, much more information is currently available about the causes, natural history, pathogenesis, serologic features, and therapy of chronic hepatitis. Therefore, categorization of chronic hepatitis based primarily upon histopathologic features has been replaced by a more informative classification based upon a combination of clinical, serologic, and histologic variables. Classification of chronic hepatitis is based upon (1) its *cause*, (2) its histologic activity, or *grade*, and (3) its degree of progression, or *stage*. Thus, neither clinical features alone nor histologic features—requiring liver biopsy—alone are sufficient to characterize and distinguish among the several categories of chronic hepatitis.

Classification by Cause Clinical and serologic features allow the establishment of a diagnosis of *chronic viral hepatitis*, caused by hepatitis B, hepatitis B plus D, hepatitis C, or other viruses; *autoimmune hepatitis*, including several subcategories, types 1, 2, and 3, based on serologic distinctions; *drug-associated chronic hepatitis*; and a category of unknown cause, or *cryptogenic* chronic hepatitis (Table 297-1). These are addressed in more detail below.

Classification by Grade Grade, a histologic assessment of necroinflammatory activity, is based upon examination of the liver biopsy. An assessment of important histologic features includes the degree of *periportal necrosis* and the disruption of the limiting plate of periportal hepatocytes by inflammatory cells (so-called *piecemeal necrosis*); the degree of confluent necrosis that links, or forms bridges between vascular structures—between portal tract and portal tract or even more important bridges between portal tract and central vein—referred to as *bridging necrosis*; the degree of hepatocyte degeneration and focal necrosis within the lobule; and the degree of *portal inflammation*. Several scoring systems that take these histologic features into account have been devised, and the most popular is the numerical histologic activity index (HAI), based on the work of Knodell and Ishak (Table 297-2). Technically, the HAI, which is primarily a measure of *grade*, also includes an assessment of fibrosis, which is currently used to categorize *stage* of the disease, as described below. Such precise HAI scoring tends to be used more in measuring disease activity before and after therapy in clinical studies. In clinical practice, more qualitative grading suffices. Based on the presence and degree of these features of histologic activity, chronic hepatitis can be graded as mild, moderate, or severe.

Table 297-1

Clinical and Laboratory Features of Chronic Hepatitis

Type of Hepatitis	Diagnostic Test(s)	Autoantibodies	Therapy
Chronic hepatitis B	HBsAg, IgG anti-HBc, HBeAg, HBV DNA	Uncommon	Interferon α
Chronic hepatitis C	Anti-HCV (EIA and RIBA), HCV RNA	Anti-LKM1*	Interferon α
Chronic hepatitis D	Anti-HDV, HDV RNA, HBsAg, IgG anti-HBc	Anti-LKM3	Interferon α (?)
Other viral	?Anti-HGV, ?HGV RNA	?	?
Autoimmune hepatitis	ANA† (homogeneous), anti-LKM1(±), hyperglobulinemia	ANA, anti-LKM1, anti-SLA‡	Prednisone, azathioprine
Drug-associated	—	Uncommon	Withdraw drug
Cryptogenic	All negative	None	Prednisone (?), azathioprine (?)

* Antibodies to liver-kidney microsomes type 1 (autoimmune hepatitis type II and some cases of hepatitis C).
† Antinuclear antibody (autoimmune hepatitis type I).
‡ Antibodies to soluble liver antigen (autoimmune hepatitis type III).
NOTE: HBsAg, hepatitis B surface antigen; EIA, enzyme immunoassay; RIBA, recombinant immunoblot assay; HGV, hepatitis G virus.

Table 297-2

Histologic Activity Index (Knodell-Ishak Score) in Chronic Hepatitis

Histologic Feature	Severity	Score
1. Periportal necrosis, including piecemeal necrosis (PN), and/or bridging necrosis (BN)	None	0
	Mild PN	1
	Moderate PN	3
	Marked PN	4
	Moderate PN + BN	5
	Marked PN + BN	6
	Multilobular necrosis	10
2. Intralobular necrosis	None	0
	Mild	1
	Moderate	3
	Marked	4
3. Portal inflammation	None	0
	Mild	1
	Moderate	3
	Marked	4
4. Fibrosis	None	0
	Expanding portal tract	1
	Bridging fibrosis	3
	Cirrhosis	4
Maximum score		22

Classification by Stage The stage of chronic hepatitis, which reflects the level of progression of the disease, is based on the degree of fibrosis. When fibrosis is so extensive that fibrous septa surround parenchymal nodules and alter the normal architecture of the liver lobule, the histologic lesion is defined as cirrhosis. Staging is based on the degree of fibrosis as follows:

0 = no fibrosis
1 = mild fibrosis
2 = moderate fibrosis
3 = severe fibrosis, including bridging fibrosis
4 = cirrhosis

Reconciliation Between Histologic Classification and New Classification For historical purposes, and to provide the basis for navigating several decades worth of literature on chronic hepatitis, the histologic categories chronic persistent hepatitis, chronic lobular hepatitis, and chronic active hepatitis are worth reviewing and linking with their new-classification counterparts (Table 297-3).

In *chronic persistent hepatitis*, a mononuclear inflammatory infiltrate expands, but is localized to and contained within, portal tracts. The "limiting plate" of periportal hepatocytes is intact, and there is no extension of the necroinflammatory process into the liver lobule. A "cobblestone" arrangement of liver cells, indicative of hepatic regenerative activity, is a common feature, and although minimal periportal fibrosis may be present, *cirrhosis is absent.* As a general rule, patients with chronic persistent hepatitis are asymptomatic or have relatively

Table 297-3

Correlation Between Earlier and Contemporary Nomenclature of Chronic Hepatitis

	Contemporary Classification	
Old Classification	**Grade (Activity)**	**Stage (Fibrosis)**
Chronic persistent hepatitis	Minimal or mild	None or mild
Chronic lobular hepatitis	Mild or moderate	Mild
Chronic active hepatitis	Mild, moderate, or severe	Mild, moderate, or severe

mild constitutional symptoms (e.g., fatigue, anorexia, nausea); have normal physical findings, except perhaps for liver enlargement, without the usual stigmata of chronic liver disease (see below); and have modest elevations of aminotransferase activities. Progression to more severe lesions (chronic active hepatitis and cirrhosis) was felt to be very unlikely, especially in patients with autoimmune or idiopathic chronic persistent hepatitis; however, progressive disease occurs in patients with chronic persistent *viral* hepatitis and in those with chronic persistent hepatitis following spontaneous or therapeutic remission of autoimmune hepatitis. In the new nomenclature, chronic persistent hepatitis would be classified by *grade* as minimal or mild chronic hepatitis and by *stage* as absent or mild fibrosis.

In patients with *chronic lobular hepatitis*, in addition to portal inflammation, histologic examination of the liver reveals foci of necrosis and inflammation in the liver lobule. Morphologically, chronic lobular hepatitis resembles slowly resolving acute hepatitis. The limiting plate remains intact, periportal fibrosis is absent or limited, lobular architecture is preserved, and progression to chronic active hepatitis and cirrhosis was felt to be rare. Thus chronic lobular hepatitis can be considered a variant of chronic persistent hepatitis with a lobular component, and clinical/laboratory features are comparable. Occasionally, the clinical activity of chronic lobular hepatitis may increase spontaneously; elevation of aminotransferase activity may resemble that seen in acute hepatitis, and transient histologic deterioration can be documented. The same qualifications in prognostic import mentioned above for chronic persistent hepatitis apply to chronic lobular hepatitis. Chronic lobular hepatitis corresponds in the new nomenclature to a mild or moderate *grade* and a *stage* of absent or minimal fibrosis.

Chronic active hepatitis is characterized clinically by continuing hepatic necrosis, portal/periportal and, to a lesser extent, lobular inflammation, and fibrosis. Varying in severity from mild to severe, chronic active hepatitis was recognized to be a progressive disorder that can lead to cirrhosis, liver failure, and death. Morphologic characteristics of chronic active hepatitis include (1) a dense mononuclear infiltrate of the portal tracts, which are substantially expanded into the liver lobule (in the autoimmune type, plasma cells represent a component of the infiltrate); (2) destruction of the hepatocytes at the periphery of the lobule, with erosion of the limiting plate of hepatocytes surrounding the portal triads (piecemeal necrosis); (3) connective tissue septa surrounding portal tracts and extending from the portal zones into the lobule, isolating parenchymal cells into clusters and enveloping bile ducts; and (4) evidence of hepatocellular regeneration—"rosette" formation, thickened liver cell plates, and regenerative "pseudolobules." This process may be patchy, with individual liver lobules spared, or it may be diffuse. Histologic evidence of single-cell coagulative necrosis, Councilman or acidophilic bodies, appear in the periportal areas. Piecemeal necrosis is the minimal histologic requirement to establish a diagnosis of chronic active hepatitis, but this change is seen even in mild, relatively nonprogressive forms of chronic active hepatitis. A more severe lesion, *bridging hepatic necrosis* (originally termed *subacute hepatic necrosis*), characterizes a more severe and progressive form of chronic active hepatitis. Although bridging necrosis can be seen occasionally in patients with acute hepatitis, in whom it carries no prognostic importance, in chronic active hepatitis this lesion is associated with progression to cirrhosis. Bridging necrosis is characterized by hepatocellular dropout that spans lobules (i.e., between portal tracts—the periphery of the lobule—or between portal tracts and central veins—the centrizonal part of the lobule). Collapse of the reticulin network is a hallmark of bridging necrosis, and bridging fibrosis follows, leading ultimately to architectural reorganization by nodular regeneration, i.e., cirrhosis. A more extensive and ominous variant of bridging necrosis is multilobular collapse, in which bridging necrosis is widespread throughout the liver and which is associated clinically with rapid deterioration and even acute liver failure.

Although progression to cirrhosis is difficult to demonstrate in patients with chronic active hepatitis who have isolated piecemeal necrosis, in more severe forms of chronic active hepatitis, progression to cirrhosis is common. Among patients with chronic active hepatitis on liver biopsy, 20 to 50 percent also have cirrhosis, even early during the course of the disease. Generally, chronic active hepatitis is more severe clinically than chronic persistent and lobular hepatitis. Although a sizable proportion of patients with chronic active hepatitis are asymptomatic, the majority tend to have mild to severe constitutional symptoms, especially fatigue. Generally, physical findings associated with chronic liver disease and portal hypertension are more common, aminotransferase levels tend to be higher, and jaundice and hyperbilirubinemia are more frequent in this form of chronic hepatitis.

In the new nomenclature for chronic hepatitis, what used to be called chronic active hepatitis spans the entire spectrum of activity *grade* from minimal, to mild, to severe chronic hepatitis, based on the degree of periportal and piecemeal necrosis, on the degree of lobular inflammation and injury, and on the degree of portal inflammation. Similarly, *stage* in chronic active hepatitis can translate to mild, moderate, or severe fibrosis as well as to cirrhosis.

CHRONIC VIRAL HEPATITIS Both the enterically transmitted forms of viral hepatitis, hepatitis A and E, are self-limited and do not cause chronic hepatitis (rare reports notwithstanding in which acute hepatitis A serves as a trigger for the onset of autoimmune hepatitis in genetically susceptible patients). In contrast, the entire clinicopathologic spectrum of chronic hepatitis occurs in patients with chronic viral hepatitis B and C as well as in patients with chronic hepatitis D superimposed on chronic hepatitis B.

Chronic Hepatitis B The likelihood of chronicity after acute hepatitis B varies as a function of age. Infection at birth is associated with a clinically silent acute infection but a 90 percent chance of chronic infection, while infection in young adulthood in immunocompetent persons is associated typically with clinically apparent acute hepatitis but a risk of chronicity of only approximately 1 percent. Most cases of chronic hepatitis B among adults, however, occur in patients who never had a recognized episode of clinically apparent acute viral hepatitis. The degree of liver injury (grade) in patients with chronic hepatitis B is variable, ranging from none in asymptomatic carriers, to mild, to severe. Among adults with chronic hepatitis B, histologic features are of prognostic importance. In one long-term study of patients with chronic hepatitis B, investigators found a 5-year survival of 97 percent for patients with chronic persistent hepatitis (mild chronic hepatitis), of 86 percent for patients with chronic active hepatitis (moderate to severe chronic hepatitis), and of only 55 percent for patients with chronic active hepatitis and postnecrotic cirrhosis. On the other hand, more recent observations do not allow us to be so sanguine about the prognosis in patients with mild chronic hepatitis; among patients with what used to be labeled chronic persistent hepatitis followed for 1 to 13 years, progression to more severe chronic hepatitis and cirrhosis has been observed in more than a quarter of cases.

Probably more important to consider than histology alone in patients with chronic hepatitis B is the degree of hepatitis B virus (HBV) replication. As reviewed in Chap. 295, chronic hepatitis B can be divided into two phases based on the relative level of HBV replication. The relatively *replicative phase* is characterized by the presence in the serum of markers of HBV replication [hepatitis B e antigen (HBeAg) HBV DNA], by the presence in the liver of detectable intrahepatocyte nucleocapsid antigens [primarily hepatitis B core antigen (HBcAg)], by high infectivity, and by accompanying liver injury;

HBV DNA can be detected in the liver but is extrachromosomal. In contrast, the relatively *nonreplicative phase* is characterized by the absence of conventional markers of HBV replication (HBeAg and HBV DNA detectable by hybridization) but associated with anti-HBe, the absence of intrahepatocytic HBcAg, limited infectivity, and minimal liver injury; HBV DNA can be detected in the liver but is integrated into the host genome. Those in the replicative phase tend to have more severe chronic hepatitis, while those in the nonreplicative phase tend to have minimal or mild chronic hepatitis or to be asymptomatic hepatitis B carriers; however, distinctions in HBV replication and in histologic category do not always coincide. The likelihood of converting spontaneously from relatively replicative to nonreplicative chronic HBV infection is approximately 10 to 15 percent per year. As noted in Chap. 295, the conversion from replicative to nonreplicative chronic hepatitis B is associated with a transient elevation in aminotransferase activity resembling acute hepatitis; occasionally, spontaneous resumptions of replicative activity occur in nonreplicative infection; and occasionally, HBV variants occur in which serologic markers of replication (HBeAg) are absent, despite the presence of replicative infection. As reviewed in Chap. 93, chronic HBV infection, especially when acquired at birth or in early childhood, is associated with an increased risk of hepatocellular carcinoma. A discussion of the pathogenesis of liver injury in patients with chronic hepatitis B appears in Chap. 295.

The spectrum of *clinical features* of chronic hepatitis B is broad, ranging from asymptomatic infection to debilitating disease or even end-stage, fatal hepatic failure. As noted above, the onset of the disease tends to be insidious in most patients, with the exception of the very few in whom chronic disease follows failure of resolution of clinically apparent acute hepatitis B. The clinical and laboratory features associated with progression from acute to chronic hepatitis B are discussed in Chap. 295. *Fatigue* is a common symptom, and persistent or intermittent *jaundice* is a common feature in severe or advanced cases. Intermittent deepening of jaundice and recurrence of malaise and anorexia, as well as worsening fatigue, are reminiscent of acute hepatitis; such exacerbations may occur spontaneously, often coinciding with evidence of virologic reactivation, may lead to progressive liver injury, and, when superimposed on well-established cirrhosis, may cause hepatic decompensation. Complications of cirrhosis occur in end-stage chronic hepatitis and include ascites, edema, bleeding gastroesophageal varices, hepatic encephalopathy, coagulopathy, or hypersplenism. Occasionally, these complications bring the patient to initial clinical attention. Extrahepatic complications of chronic hepatitis B, similar to those seen during the prodromal phase of acute hepatitis B, are associated with deposition of circulating hepatitis B antigen–antibody immune complexes. As reviewed in Chap. 295, these include arthralgias and arthritis, which are common, and the more rare purpuric cutaneous lesions (leukocytoclastic vasculitis), immune-complex glomerulonephritis, and generalized vasculitis (polyarteritis nodosa).

Laboratory features of chronic hepatitis B do not distinguish adequately between histologically mild and severe hepatitis. Aminotransferase elevations tend to be modest for chronic hepatitis B but may fluctuate in the range of 100 to 1000 units. As is true for acute viral hepatitis B, alanine aminotransferase (ALT, or SGPT) tends to be more elevated than aspartate aminotransferase (AST, or SGOT); however, once cirrhosis is established, AST tends to exceed ALT. Levels of alkaline phosphatase activity tend to be normal or only marginally elevated. In severe cases, moderate elevations in serum bilirubin [51.3 to 171 μmol/L (3 to 10 mg/dL)] occur. Hypoalbuminemia and prolongation of the prothrombin time occur in severe or end-stage cases. Hyperglobulinemia and detectable circulating autoantibodies are distinctly absent in chronic hepatitis B (in contrast to autoimmune hepatitis). → *Viral markers of chronic HBV infection are discussed in Chap. 295.*

℞ TREATMENT

Management of chronic hepatitis B depends on the level of virus replication. Although progression to cirrhosis is more likely in severe chronic than in mild or moderate chronic hepatitis B, all forms of chronic viral hepatitis can be progressive. Randomized, prospective, controlled trials have established that patients with well-compensated chronic replicative hepatitis B, selected to have chronic hepatitis on liver biopsy and aminotransferase elevations, regardless of histologic features, respond to antiviral therapy with interferon α. A 4-month (16-week) course of subcutaneous injections, daily at a dose of 5 million units or three times a week at a dose of 10 million units, is associated with an approximately 40 percent seroconversion from replicative (HBeAg and HBV DNA detectable in serum) to nonreplicative (anti-HBe detectable) HBV infection, with a concomitant improvement in liver histologic features and an approximately 10 percent chance of losing detectable HBsAg. In most cases, successful interferon therapy and seroconversion is accompanied by an acute hepatitis–like elevation in aminotransferase activity, which is believed to represent an immunostimulatory effect of interferon on the interaction between the cellular immune system and virus-infected hepatocytes. Relapse after successful therapy is rare indeed (1 to 2 percent). The likelihood of responding to interferon is greater in patients with moderate to low levels of HBV DNA (<200 pg/mL) and in patients with substantial elevations of aminotransferase activities (e.g., >100 to 200 units). The likelihood of losing HBsAg *during therapy* is increased in patients with brief-duration disease (mean duration 1½ years); if patients are followed sufficiently long after successful interferon-induced loss of replicative markers, approximately 60 to 70 percent have been estimated to lose HBsAg, i.e., all serologic markers of infection, over a 5-year period. Immunosuppressed patients with chronic hepatitis B and children infected at birth do not appear to be responsive to interferon therapy. Indications for interferon therapy in patients with chronic hepatitis B are summarized in Table 297-4.

Complications of interferon therapy include systemic "flulike" symptoms, marrow suppression, emotional lability (irritability commonly, depression rarely), autoimmune reactions (especially autoimmune thyroiditis), and miscellaneous side effects such as alopecia, rashes, diarrhea, and numbness and tingling of the extremities. With the possible exception of autoimmune thyroiditis, all these side effects are reversible upon dose lowering or cessation of therapy.

In patients with chronic hepatitis B, long-term therapy with glucocorticoids is not only ineffective but also detrimental. Under certain circumstances, however, the predicted impact of glucocorticoids on HBV and the immune system can be exploited for the patient's benefit. Glucocorticoids increase HBV replication and expression in hepatocytes and depress the activity of cytolytic T cells. Theoretically, if steroids are administered for a brief time and then withdrawn, cytolytic T cells, suppressed while HBV replication was being steroid-induced, could resume their presteroid function and be capable of attacking and destroying the new crop of HBV antigen–expressing hepatocytes. Such appears to be the case; an acute hepatitis–like elevation of aminotransferase activity follows and may be accompanied by a dramatic drop in, or even a loss of, HBV replication. A preliminary 6-week period of glucocorticoid therapy (prednisone at doses of 60 mg for 2 weeks, 40 mg for 2 weeks, and 20 mg for 2 weeks), followed by its abrupt withdrawal, has been shown to be of benefit in conjunction with interferon therapy (5 million units subcutaneously daily for 4 months) in patients with chronic hepatitis B, primarily those with near-normal or only modest eleva-

Table 297-4

Characteristics of Patients with Chronic Hepatitis B Who Are Candidates for Interferon Therapy

Detectable markers of chronic, replicative hepatitis B (HBeAg and HBV DNA)
Elevated ALT activity
Immunocompetence
Acquisition of HBV infection in adulthood
Compensated liver disease
"Wild-type" chronic hepatitis B (not "pre-core" mutants)

tions in aminotransferase levels. This approach, however, has not attracted broad acceptance by clinicians and is used rarely.

No treatment is indicated or available for asymptomatic, nonreplicative hepatitis B carriers, and antiviral therapy should be withheld from patients with decompensated hepatitis B, in whom treatment may be associated with hepatic decompensation. Such patients should be referred to research centers involved in clinical trials. Several nucleoside analogues active against HBV are being evaluated in experimental trials. Famciclovir and ganciclovir have activity against hepatitis B, but the dideoxynucleoside lamivudine (3 thiacytidine), active against reverse transcriptase activity of human immunodeficiency virus and HBV, is a more potent inhibitor of HBV replication than these other antivirals and has shown promise in initial trials among patients with chronic replicative hepatitis B.

For patients with end-stage chronic hepatitis B, liver transplantation is the only potential lifesaving intervention. Reinfection of the new liver is almost universal; however, the likelihood of liver injury associated with hepatitis B in the new liver is variable. The majority of patients become high-level viremic carriers with minimal liver injury. Unfortunately, an unpredictable proportion experience severe hepatitis B–related liver injury, sometimes a fulminant-like hepatitis, sometimes a rapid recapitulation of the original severe chronic hepatitis B (see Chap. 301). Prevention of recurrent hepatitis B after liver transplantation has been achieved by *prophylaxis* with hepatitis B immune globulin and with nucleoside analogues; in addition, nucleoside analogues have been used successfully to *reverse* post-transplantation liver injury associated with recurrent hepatitis B (see Chap. 301).

Chronic Hepatitis D (Delta Hepatitis) The clinical and laboratory features of chronic hepatitis D virus (HDV) infection are summarized in Chap. 295. Chronic hepatitis D may follow acute coinfection with HBV but at a rate no higher than the rate of chronicity of hepatitis B. That is, although HDV coinfection can increase the severity of acute hepatitis B, HDV does not increase the likelihood of progression to chronic hepatitis B. However, when HDV superinfection occurs in a person who is already chronically infected with HBV, long-term HDV infection is the rule and a worsening of the liver disease the expected consequence. Except for severity, chronic hepatitis B plus D has similar clinical and laboratory features to those seen in chronic hepatitis B alone. Relatively severe chronic hepatitis, with or without cirrhosis, is the rule, and mild chronic hepatitis the exception. A distinguishing serologic feature of chronic hepatitis D is the presence in the circulation of antibodies to liver-kidney microsomes (anti-LKM); however, the anti-LKM seen in hepatitis D are designated anti-LKM3 and are distinct from anti-LKM1 seen in patients with autoimmune hepatitis and in a subset of patients with chronic hepatitis C (see below).

℞ TREATMENT

Management is not well defined. Glucocorticoids are ineffective and are not used. Preliminary experimental trials of interferon α suggested that conventional doses and durations of therapy lower levels of HDV RNA and aminotransferase activity only transiently during treatment but have no impact on the natural history of the disease. Although high-dose interferon α (9 million units) three times a week for 12 months may be associated with a sustained loss of HDV replication and clinical improvement in up to 50 percent of patients, ultimately recurrent HDV replication becomes universal after cessation of therapy. Antiviral therapy for chronic hepatitis D remains the subject of experimental trials. In patients with end-stage liver disease secondary to chronic hepatitis D, liver transplantation has been effective. If hepatitis D recurs in the new liver without the expression of hepatitis B (an unusual serologic profile in immunocompetent persons, but common in transplant patients), liver injury is limited. In fact, the outcome of transplantation for chronic hepatitis D is superior to that for chronic hepatitis B (see Chap. 301).

Chronic Hepatitis C Regardless of the epidemiologic mode of acquisition of hepatitis C virus (HCV) infection, chronic hepatitis follows acute hepatitis C in 50 to 70 percent of cases. Furthermore, in patients with chronic transfusion-associated hepatitis followed for 10 years, progression to cirrhosis occurs in about 20 percent. Such is the case even for patients with relatively clinically mild chronic hepatitis, including those without symptoms, with only modest elevations of aminotransferase activity, and with mild chronic hepatitis on liver biopsy. Even in cohorts of well-compensated patients with chronic hepatitis C (no complications of chronic liver disease and with normal hepatic synthetic function), the prevalence of cirrhosis may be as high as 50 percent. Many cases of hepatitis C are identified in asymptomatic patients who have no history of acute hepatitis C, e.g., those discovered while attempting to donate blood or as a result of routine laboratory screening tests. The source of HCV infection in most of these cases is not defined, although a long-forgotten percutaneous exposure in the remote past can be elicited in a substantial proportion. The natural history of chronic hepatitis C identified under these circumstances remains to be determined. Among asymptomatic persons with anti-HCV, even when aminotransferase levels are normal, between a third and a half have been reported to have chronic hepatitis on liver biopsy, although mild in most cases. In these asymptomatic persons with normal aminotransferase levels, the presence of detectable circulating HCV RNA appears to distinguish those with chronic hepatitis on biopsy from those with normal liver histology.

Despite this substantial rate of progression of chronic hepatitis C, and despite the fact that liver failure can result from end-stage chronic hepatitis C, the long-term prognosis for chronic hepatitis C in a majority of patients is relatively benign. Mortality over 10 to 20 years among patients with transfusion-associated chronic hepatitis C has been shown not to differ from mortality in a matched population of transfused patients in whom hepatitis C did not develop. Although death in the hepatitis group is more likely to result from liver failure, and although hepatic decompensation may occur in approximately 15 percent of such patients over the course of a decade, the majority (almost 60 percent) of patients remain asymptomatic and well compensated, with no clinical sequelae of chronic liver disease. Overall, then, chronic hepatitis C tends to be very slowly and insidiously progressive, if at all, in the vast majority of patients, while in approximately a quarter of cases, chronic hepatitis C will progress eventually to end-stage cirrhosis. The degree of progression of liver disease in chronic hepatitis C has been shown to be greater in patients with higher levels of HCV RNA and longer durations of infection; HCV-associated liver disease also tends to be worse in patients with certain genotypes (e.g., 1b). Among these variables, however, duration of infection appears to be the most important. In addition, severity of chronic hepatitis is greater and progression of chronic liver disease is more accelerated in patients who have chronic hepatitis C as well as other liver processes, including alcoholic liver disease, chronic hepatitis B, hemochromatosis, and α_1-antitrypsin deficiency. No other epidemiologic or clinical features of chronic hepatitis C (e.g., severity of acute hepatitis, level of aminotransferase activity, presence or absence of jaundice) are predictive of eventual outcome. Despite the relative benignity of chronic hepatitis C over time, cirrhosis following chronic hepatitis C has been associated with the late development, after several decades, of hepatocellular carcinoma (see Chap. 93).

Clinical features of chronic hepatitis C are similar to those described above for chronic hepatitis B. Generally, *fatigue* is the most common symptom; jaundice is rare. Immune-complex–mediated extrahepatic complications of chronic hepatitis C are less common than in chronic hepatitis B, with the exception of essential mixed cryoglobulinemia (see Chap. 295). This is the case, despite the fact that assays for immune-complex-like activity are often positive in patients with chronic hepatitis C. In addition, chronic hepatitis C has been associated with extrahepatic complications unrelated to immune-complex injury. These include Sjögren's syndrome, lichen planus, and porphyria cutanea tarda. *Laboratory features* of chronic hepatitis C are similar to those in patients with chronic hepatitis B, but aminotransferase levels tend to fluctuate more (the characteristic episodic pattern of aminotransferase activity) and to be lower, especially in patients with long-standing disease. An interesting and occasionally confusing finding in patients with chronic hepatitis C is the presence of autoantibodies. Rarely, patients with autoimmune hepatitis (see below) and hyperglobulinemia have false-positive enzyme immunoassays for anti-HCV. On the other hand, some patients with serologically confirmable chronic hepatitis C have circulating anti-LKM. These antibodies are anti-LKM1, as seen in patients with autoimmune hepatitis *type 2* (see below), and are directed against a 33-amino-acid sequence of P450 IID6. The occurrence of anti-LKM1 in some patients with chronic hepatitis C may result from the partial sequence homology between the epitope recognized by anti-LKM1 and two segments of the HCV polyprotein. In addition, the presence of this autoantibody in some patients with chronic hepatitis C suggests that autoimmunity may be playing a role in the pathogenesis of chronic hepatitis C. Histopathologic features of chronic hepatitis C, especially those that distinguish hepatitis C from hepatitis B, are described in Chap. 295.

℞ TREATMENT

In the management of chronic hepatitis C, glucocorticoids are ineffective. Based on the outcome of prospective, randomized, controlled clinical trials, interferon α has been approved for the treatment of chronic hepatitis C. Doses ranging from 2 to 5 million units three times a week have been shown to be effective in these trials, but the initial dose recommendation was 3 million units by subcutaneous injection three times a week for 6 months (24 weeks). This regimen is associated with a likelihood of biochemical response (return of ALT to normal or a 50 percent reduction of ALT to within 1.5 times the upper limit of normal) in approximately 50 percent of patients. Other regimens are being evaluated (see below). Unlike in hepatitis B, in chronic hepatitis C a successful response to interferon is not accompanied by an acute hepatitis–like elevation in aminotransferase activity; instead, ALT levels fall precipitously. Between 85 and 90 percent of responses occur within the first 3 months of therapy; responses thereafter are rare. In addition, histologic improvement in periportal and lobular inflammation has been demonstrated, primarily in biochemically responding patients but also in biochemical nonresponders. Clinical trials have demonstrated that, after 6 months of therapy, at least 50 percent of responding patients experience a biochemical relapse; based on this relapse rate, the likelihood of a sustained response would be 25 percent. In practice, however, the relapse rate can approach 90 percent, and the likelihood of a sustained response is probably no greater than 10 to 15 percent. Still, in a proportion of cases, all markers of HCV infection can be eradicated by interferon therapy, and durable responses have been documented many years after successful therapy. In those who relapse after responding, retreatment with interferon invariably leads to a subsequent response. A small proportion of patients, approximately 10 percent, experience biochemical "breakthrough" *during* interferon therapy. In general, they remain refractory to retreatment thereafter; some such breakthroughs are associated with interferon antibodies, while others may reflect mutations in the HCV genome that render HCV nonresponsive to interferon.

Levels of HCV RNA fall in tandem with ALT levels during interferon therapy, but loss of detectable HCV RNA does not preclude relapse. When a patient experiences an apparently sustained biochemical response after discontinuing interferon but continues to remain viremic, as reflected by the persistence of detectable HCV RNA, future biochemical relapse is likely. Patient variables that tend to correlate with *sustained* responsiveness to interferon include a low baseline level of HCV RNA and histologically mild hepatitis. Patients with cirrhosis can respond, but they are less likely to do so and especially unlikely to have a *sustained* response. In certain countries, patients with HCV genotype 1b are less likely to respond than patients with other genotypes, but in the United States, where most patients are infected with either genotypes 1a or 1b, genotype appears to have less of an impact on interferon responsiveness. Other variables reported to correlate with increased responsiveness include brief duration of infection, low HCV quasispecies diversity, immunocompetence, and low liver iron levels. High levels of HCV RNA, more histologically advanced liver disease, and high quasispecies diversity all go hand in hand with advanced duration of infection, which may be the single most important variable determining interferon responsiveness. The ironic fact, then, is that patients whose disease is *least* likely to progress are the ones *most* likely to respond to interferon and vice versa. Finally, among patients with genotype 1b, responsiveness to interferon is enhanced in those with amino-acid-substitution mutations in the nonstructural protein 5A gene.

Among the approaches to increasing the response rate and decreasing the relapse rate associated with interferon therapy are longer-duration, higher-dose, and/or higher-frequency therapy. In several European studies, durations of therapy of 12 to 18 months increased the frequency of sustained responses, but this effect has not been observed as conclusively in studies conducted in the United States. Other approaches that have been suggested but not yet supported by adequate clinical trials include the initiation of therapy with a higher dose followed by maintenance with a standard dose; reliance on alternative types of interferons; tapering therapy slowly rather than discontinuing therapy abruptly; and, because of the observation that a high liver iron level is associated with nonresponsiveness, the addition of phlebotomy to interferon therapy. Pending clinical trials to the contrary, none of these approaches can be recommended. Several small clinical trials have suggested that the nucleoside analogue ribavirin, which is ineffective when used alone, may increase the efficacy of interferon when given as combination therapy; large-scale, multicenter trials are underway to pursue this potential approach. Whether sustained, long-term (even indefinite) therapy will be necessary or effective in those who relapse remains to be determined. Similarly, the impact of short-term therapy on the long-term natural history of chronic hepatitis C continues to be studied.

Although a consensus exists that patients with symptomatic chronic hepatitis C should be treated with interferon, treatment of asymptomatic patients and those with mild chronic hepatitis remains controversial. Because progression to cirrhosis can occur in an unpredictable proportion of such cases, the potential benefit of therapy should not be dismissed out of hand in these patients. Additional study is needed. Currently, the treatment of asymptomatic hepatitis C "carriers" with normal aminotransferase levels or patients with decompensated cirrhosis secondary to chronic hepatitis C is not recommended. Interferon therapy has been advocated for patients with symptomatic essential mixed cryoglobulinemia, but results are mixed (Table 297-5). For those with decompensated, end-stage disease, liver transplantation is an option. Although the likelihood of reexpressing detectable anti-HCV after transplantation is low, the likelihood of reinfection of the new liver is almost universal. Nevertheless, and the occasional exception notwithstanding, most patients who undergo liver transplantation for chronic hepatitis C experience little, if any, morbidity, allograft loss, or mortality associated with recurrent hepatitis C infection during the early postoperative years (see Chap. 301).

AUTOIMMUNE HEPATITIS **Definition** Autoimmune hepatitis (formerly called autoimmune chronic active hepatitis) is a chronic disorder characterized by continuing hepatocellular necrosis and inflammation, usually with fibrosis, which tends to progress to cirrhosis and liver failure. When fulfilling criteria of severity, this type of chronic hepatitis may have a 6-month mortality of as high as 40 percent. The prominence of extrahepatic features of autoimmunity as well as seroimmunologic abnormalities in this disorder supports an autoimmune process in its pathogenesis, and this concept is reflected in the labels "lupoid," plasma cell, or autoimmune hepatitis. Because autoantibodies and other typical features of autoimmunity do not occur in all cases, however, a broader, more appropriate designation for this type of chronic hepatitis is "idiopathic" or cryptogenic. Cases in which

Table 297-5

Indications for Interferon Therapy in Patients with Chronic Hepatitis C

ACCEPTED INDICATIONS
Elevated ALT activity (≥1.5 times the upper limit of normal)
Chronic hepatitis of moderate severity on liver biopsy
Detectable HCV RNA
CONTROVERSIAL INDICATIONS
Histologically mild hepatitis
Near-normal ALT activity (<1.5 times the upper limit of normal)
History of relapse after an initial course of interferon
Hepatitis C–associated essential mixed cryoglobulinemia
FEATURES ASSOCIATED WITH REDUCED RESPONSIVENESS
Advanced histologic lesion (e.g., advanced cirrhosis)
Long-duration disease
High-level HCV RNA
Genotype 1b (especially so in Europe and Japan, less so in the United States)
High HCV RNA quasispecies diversity
ABSENCE OF BENEFIT
Decompensated liver disease
Normal aminotransferase activity
Failure to respond to a previous course of interferon

hepatotropic viruses, metabolic/genetic derangements, and hepatotoxic drugs have been excluded merit this designation and probably include a spectrum of heterogeneous liver disorders of unknown cause, a proportion of which have characteristic autoimmune features.

Immunopathogenesis The weight of evidence suggests that the progressive liver injury in patients with idiopathic/autoimmune hepatitis is the result of a cell-mediated immunologic attack directed against liver cells; in all likelihood, predisposition to autoimmunity is inherited, while the liver specificity of this injury is triggered by environmental (e.g., chemical or viral) factors. For example, patients have been described in whom apparently self-limited cases of acute hepatitis A or B led to autoimmune hepatitis, presumably because of genetic susceptibility or predisposition. Evidence to support an autoimmune pathogenesis in this type of hepatitis includes the following: (1) In the liver, the histopathologic lesions are composed predominantly of cytotoxic T cells and plasma cells; (2) circulating autoantibodies (nuclear, smooth muscle, thyroid, etc.; see below), rheumatoid factor, and hyperglobulinemia are common; (3) other autoimmune disorders—such as thyroiditis, rheumatoid arthritis, autoimmune hemolytic anemia, ulcerative colitis, proliferative glomerulonephritis, juvenile diabetes mellitus, and Sjögren's syndrome—occur with increased frequency in patients who have autoimmune hepatitis and in their relatives; (4) histocompatibility haplotypes associated with autoimmune diseases, such as HLA-B1, -B8, -DRw3, and -DRw4, are common in patients with autoimmune hepatitis; and (5) this type of chronic hepatitis is responsive to glucocorticoid/immunosuppressive therapy, effective in a variety of autoimmune disorders.

Cellular immune mechanisms appear to be important in the pathogenesis of autoimmune hepatitis. In vitro studies have suggested that in patients with this disorder, lymphocytes are capable of becoming sensitized to hepatocyte membrane proteins and of destroying liver cells. Abnormalities of immunoregulatory control over cytotoxic lymphocytes (impaired suppressor cell influences) may play a role as well. Studies of genetic predisposition to autoimmune hepatitis demonstrate that certain haplotypes are associated with the disorder, as enumerated above. The precise triggering factors, genetic influences, and cytotoxic and immunoregulatory mechanisms involved in this type of liver injury remain poorly defined.

Intriguing clues into the pathogenesis of autoimmune hepatitis come from the observation that circulating autoantibodies are prevalent in patients with this disorder. Among the autoantibodies described in these patients are antibodies to nuclei [so-called antinuclear antibodies (ANA), primarily in a homogeneous pattern] and smooth muscle (so-called anti-smooth-muscle antibodies, directed at actin), anti-LKM (see below), antibodies to "soluble liver antigen" (directed at cytokeratins), as well as antibodies to the liver-specific asialoglycoprotein receptor (or "hepatic lectin") and other hepatocyte membrane proteins. Although some of these provide helpful diagnostic markers, their involvement in the pathogenesis of autoimmune hepatitis has not been established.

Humoral immune mechanisms have been shown to play a role in the extrahepatic manifestations of autoimmune/idiopathic hepatitis. Arthralgias, arthritis, cutaneous vasculitis, and glomerulonephritis occurring in patients with autoimmune hepatitis appear to be mediated by the deposition in affected tissue vessels of circulating immune complexes, followed by complement activation, inflammation, and tissue injury. While specific viral antigen-antibody complexes can be identified in acute and chronic viral hepatitis, the nature of the immune complexes in autoimmune hepatitis has not been defined.

Many of the *clinical features* of autoimmune hepatitis are similar to those described for chronic viral hepatitis. The onset of disease may be insidious or abrupt; the disease may present initially like, and be confused with, acute viral hepatitis; and a history of recurrent bouts of what had been labeled acute hepatitis is not uncommon. A subset of patients with autoimmune hepatitis has distinct features. Such patients are predominantly young to middle-aged women with marked hyperglobulinemia and high-titer circulating ANA. This is the group with positive LE preparations (initially labeled "lupoid" hepatitis) in whom other autoimmune features are common. Fatigue, malaise, anorexia, amenorrhea, acne, arthralgias, and jaundice are common. Occasionally, arthritis, maculopapular eruptions (including cutaneous vasculitis), erythema nodosum, colitis, pleurisy, pericarditis, anemia, azotemia, and sicca syndrome (keratoconjunctivitis, xerostomia) occur. In some patients, complications of cirrhosis, such as ascites and edema (associated with hypoalbuminemia), encephalopathy, hypersplenism, coagulopathy, or variceal bleeding, may bring the patient to initial medical attention.

The course of autoimmune hepatitis may be variable. In those with mild disease or limited histologic lesions (e.g., piecemeal necrosis without bridging), progression to cirrhosis is limited. In those with severe symptomatic autoimmune hepatitis (aminotransferase levels >10 times normal, marked hyperglobulinemia, "aggressive" histologic lesions—bridging necrosis or multilobular collapse, cirrhosis), then 6-month mortality without therapy may be as high as 40 percent. Such severe disease accounts for only 20 percent of cases; the natural history of milder disease is variable, often accentuated by spontaneous remissions and exacerbations. Especially poor prognostic signs include multilobular collapse at the time of initial presentation and failure of the bilirubin to improve after 2 weeks of therapy. Death may result from hepatic failure, hepatic coma, other complications of cirrhosis (e.g., variceal hemorrhage), and intercurrent infection. In patients with established cirrhosis, hepatocellular carcinoma may be a late complication (see Chap. 93).

Laboratory features of autoimmune hepatitis are similar to those seen in chronic viral hepatitis. Liver biochemical tests are invariably abnormal but may not correlate with the clinical severity or histopathologic features in individual cases. Many patients with autoimmune hepatitis have normal serum bilirubin, alkaline phosphatase, and globulin levels with only minimal aminotransferase elevations. Serum AST and ALT levels are increased and fluctuate in the range of 100 to 1000 units. In severe cases, the serum bilirubin level is moderately elevated [51 to 171 μmol/L (3 to 10 mg/dL)]. Hypoalbuminemia occurs in patients with very active or advanced disease. Serum alkaline phosphatase levels may be moderately elevated or near normal. In a small proportion of patients, marked elevations of alkaline phosphatase activity occur; in such patients, clinical and laboratory features overlap with those of primary biliary cirrhosis (see Chap. 298). The prothrombin time is often prolonged, particularly late in the disease or during active phases.

Hypergammaglobulinemia (>2.5 g/dL) is common in autoimmune hepatitis. Rheumatoid factor is common as well. As noted above, circulating autoantibodies are also common. The most characteristic are ANA in a homogeneous staining pattern. Smooth-muscle antibodies are less specific, seen just as frequently in chronic viral hepatitis. Because of the high levels of globulins achieved in the circulation of some patients with autoimmune hepatitis, occasionally the globulins may bind nonspecifically in solid-phase binding immunoassays for viral antibodies. This has been recognized most commonly in tests for antibodies to hepatitis C virus, as noted above. In fact, studies of autoantibodies in autoimmune hepatitis have led to the recognition of new categories of autoimmune hepatitis. *Type I autoimmune hepatitis* is the classic syndrome occurring in young women, associated with marked hyperglobulinemia, lupoid features, and circulating ANA. *Type II autoimmune hepatitis*, often seen in children and more common in Mediterranean populations, is associated not with ANA but with anti-LKM. Actually, anti-LKM represent a heterogeneous group of antibodies. In type II autoimmune hepatitis, the antibody is anti-LKM1, directed against P450 IID6. This is the same anti-LKM seen in some patients with chronic hepatitis C. Anti-LKM2 is seen in drug-induced hepatitis, and anti-LKM3 is seen in patients with chronic hepatitis D. Type II autoimmune hepatitis has been subdivided by some authorities into two categories, one more typically autoimmune and the other associated with viral hepatitis type C. Autoimmune hepatitis type IIa is felt to be autoimmune, is more likely to occur in young women, is associated with hyperglobulinemia, is associated with high-titer anti-LKM1, responds to glucocorticoid therapy, and is seen commonly in western Europe and the United Kingdom. Type IIb autoimmune hepatitis is associated with hepatitis C virus infection, tends to occur in older men, is associated with normal globulin levels and low-titer anti-LKM1, responds to interferon, and occurs most commonly in Mediterranean countries. In addition, another type of autoimmune hepatitis has been recognized, *autoimmune hepatitis type III*. These patients, who lack ANA and anti-LKM1, have circulating antibodies to soluble liver antigen, which are directed at hepatocyte cytoplasmic cytokeratins 8 and 18. Most of these patients are women and have clinical features similar to those of patients with type I autoimmune hepatitis.

℞ TREATMENT

The mainstay of management in autoimmune or idiopathic (nonviral) hepatitis is glucocorticoid therapy. Several controlled clinical trials have documented that such therapy leads to symptomatic, clinical, biochemical, and histologic improvement as well as increased survival. A therapeutic response can be expected in up to 80 percent of patients. Unfortunately, therapy has not been shown to prevent ultimate progression to cirrhosis. Although some advocate the use of prednisolone, the hepatic metabolite of prednisone, prednisone is just as effective and is favored by most authorities. Therapy may be initiated at 20 mg/d, but a popular regimen in the United States relies on an initiation dose of 60 mg/d. This high dose is tapered successively over the course of a month down to a maintenance level of 20 mg/d. An alternative, but equally effective, approach is to begin with half the prednisone dose (30 mg/d) along with azathioprine (50 mg/d). With azathioprine maintained at 50 mg/d, the prednisone dose is tapered over the course of a month down to a maintenance level of 10 mg/d. The advantage of the combination approach is a reduction, over the span of an 18-month course of therapy, in serious, life-threatening complications of steroid therapy from 66 percent down to under 20 percent. Azathioprine alone, however, is not effective in achieving remission, nor is alternate-day glucocorticoid therapy. Although therapy has been shown to be effective for severe autoimmune hepatitis, therapy is not indicated for mild forms of chronic hepatitis (which used to be labeled chronic persistent hepatitis or chronic lobular hepatitis), and the efficacy of therapy in mild or asymptomatic autoimmune hepatitis (which used to be labeled mild chronic active hepatitis) has not been established.

Improvement of fatigue, anorexia, malaise, and jaundice tends to occur within days to several weeks; biochemical improvement occurs over the course of several weeks to months, with a fall in serum bilirubin and globulin levels and an increase in serum albumin. Serum aminotransferase levels usually drop promptly, but improvements in AST and ALT alone do not appear to be a reliable marker of recovery in individual patients; histologic improvement, characterized by a decrease in mononuclear infiltration and in hepatocellular necrosis may be delayed for 6 to 24 months. Still, if interpreted cautiously, aminotransferase levels are valuable indicators of relative disease activity, and many authorities do *not* advocate serial liver biopsies to assess therapeutic success or to guide decisions to alter or stop therapy. Therapy should continue for at least 12 to 18 months. After tapering and cessation of therapy, the likelihood of relapse is at least 50 percent, even if posttreatment histology has improved to show mild chronic hepatitis, and the majority of patients require therapy at maintenance doses indefinitely. Continuing azathioprine alone after cessation of prednisone therapy may reduce the frequency of relapse.

If medical therapy fails, or when chronic hepatitis progresses to cirrhosis and is associated with life-threatening complications of liver decompensation, liver transplantation is the only recourse (see Chap. 301). Recurrence of autoimmune hepatitis in the new liver has not been documented to occur.

DIFFERENTIAL DIAGNOSIS Early during the course of chronic hepatitis, the disease may resemble typical *acute viral hepatitis*. Without histologic assessment, severe chronic hepatitis cannot be readily distinguished based on clinical or biochemical criteria from mild chronic hepatitis. In adolescence, *Wilson's disease* may present with features of chronic hepatitis long before neurologic manifestations become apparent and before the formation of Kayser-Fleischer rings; in this age group, serum ceruloplasmin and serum and urinary copper determinations and measurement of liver copper levels will establish the correct diagnosis. *Postnecrotic* or *cryptogenic cirrhosis* and *primary biliary cirrhosis* share clinical features with autoimmune hepatitis; biochemical, serologic, and histologic assessments are usually sufficient to allow these entities to be distinguished from autoimmune hepatitis. Of course, the distinction between autoimmune ("idiopathic") and viral chronic hepatitis is not always straightforward, especially when viral antibodies occur in patients with autoimmune disease or when autoantibodies occur in patients with viral disease. Finally, the presence of extrahepatic features such as arthritis, cutaneous vasculitis, or pleuritis—not to mention the presence of circulating autoantibodies—may cause confusion with *rheumatologic disorders* such as rheumatoid arthritis and systemic lupus erythematosus. The existence of clinical and biochemical features of progressive necroinflammatory liver disease distinguishes chronic hepatitis from these other disorders, which are not associated with severe liver disease.

For further discussion of interferon and other antiviral agents, see Chap. 50, in Goodman and Gilman's The Pharmacological Basis of Therapeutics, *9th ed., McGraw-Hill, New York, 1996.*

BIBLIOGRAPHY

Alter HJ: The cloning and clinical implications of HGV and HGBV-C. N Engl J Med 334:1536, 1996

Brillanti S et al: A pilot study of combination therapy with ribavirin plus interferon alfa for interferon alfa-resistant chronic hepatitis C. Gastroenterology 107:812, 1994

Chemello L et al: Randomized trial comparing three different regimens of alpha-2a-interferon in chronic hepatitis C. Hepatology 22:700, 1995

Czaja AJ et al: Frequency and significance of antibodies to liver/kidney microsome type 1 in adults with chronic active hepatitis. Gastroenterology 103:1290, 1992

———: Autoimmune hepatitis: Evolving concepts and treatment strategies. Dig Dis Sci 40:435, 1995

———: The variant forms of antoimmune hepatitis. Ann Intern Med 125:588, 1996

Davis GL et al: Treatment of chronic hepatitis C with recombinant interferon alfa: A multicenter randomized, controlled trial. N Engl J Med 321: 1501, 1989

Desmet VJ et al: Classification of chronic hepatitis: Diagnosis, grading, and staging. Hepatology 19:1513, 1994

DIENSTAG JL et al: A preliminary trial of lamivudine for chronic hepatitis B infection. N Engl J Med 333:1657, 1995

ENOMOTO N et al: Mutations in the nonstructural protein 5A gene and response to interferon in patients with chronic hepatitis C virus 1b infection. N Engl J Med 334:77, 1996

FARCI P et al: Treatment of chronic hepatitis D with interferon alfa-2a. N Engl J Med 330:88, 1994

GARSON JA et al: Analysis of clinical and virological factors associated with response to alpha interferon therapy in chronic hepatitis C. J Med Virol 45:348, 1995

HOOFNAGLE JH, DIBISCEGLIE AM: The treatment of chronic viral hepatitis. N Engl J Med 336:347, 1997

———, JONES EA (GUEST EDS.): Interferon therapy of chronic viral hepatitis. Semin Liver Dis 9:231, 1989

———: Therapy of acute and chronic viral hepatitis. Adv Intern Med 39:241, 1994

ISHAK K et al: Histologic grading and staging of chronic hepatitis. J Hepatol 22:696, 1995

JOHNSON PJ et al: Azathioprine for long-term maintenance of remission in autoimmune hepatitis. N Engl J Med 333:958, 1995

KASAHARA A et al: Ability of prolonged interferon treatment to suppress relapse after cessation of therapy in patients with chronic hepatitis C: A multicenter randomized controlled trial. Hepatology 21:291, 1995

KATKOV WN, DIENSTAG JL: Prevention and therapy of viral hepatitis. Semin Liver Dis 11:165, 1991

KORENMAN J et al: Long-term remission of chronic hepatitis B after alpha-interferon therapy. Ann Intern Med 114:629, 1991

KRAWITT EL: Autoimmune hepatitis. N Engl J Med 334:897, 1996

MADDREY WC: Chronic hepatitis. Dis Mon 39:53, 1993

MASUKO K et al: Infection with hepatitis GB virus C in patients on maintenance dialysis. N Engl J Med 334:1485, 1996

NIEDERAU C et al: Long-term follow-up of HBeAg-positive patients treated with interferon alfa for chronic hepatitis B. N Engl J Med 334:1422, 1996

PERRILLO RP et al: A randomized, controlled trial of interferon alpha-2b alone and after prednisone withdrawal for the treatment of chronic hepatitis B. N Engl J Med 323:295, 1990

POYNARD T et al: A comparison of three interferon alfa-2b regimens for the long-term treatment of chronic non-A, non-B hepatitis. N Engl J Med 332:1457, 1995

REICHARD O et al: High sustained response rate and clearance of viremia in chronic hepatitis C after treatment with interferon-α2b for 60 weeks. Hepatology 19:280, 1994

——— et al: Two-year biochemical, virological, and histological follow-up in patients with chronic hepatitis C responding in a sustained fashion to interferon alfa-2b treatment. Hepatology 21:918, 1995

ROMEO R et al: Eradication of hepatitis C virus RNA after alpha-interferon therapy. Ann Intern Med 121:276, 1994

SHINDO M et al: Hepatic hepatitis C virus RNA as a predictor of a long-term response to interferon-α therapy. Ann Intern Med 122:586, 1995

TONG MJ et al: Clinical outcomes after transfusion-associated hepatitis C. N Engl J Med 332:1463, 1995

298

Daniel K. Podolsky, Kurt J. Isselbacher

CIRRHOSIS AND ALCOHOLIC LIVER DISEASE

Cirrhosis is a pathologically defined entity that is associated with a spectrum of characteristic clinical manifestations. The cardinal pathologic features reflect irreversible chronic injury of the hepatic parenchyma and include extensive fibrosis in association with the formation of regenerative nodules. These features result from hepatocyte necrosis, collapse of the supporting reticulin network with subsequent connective tissue deposition, distortion of the vascular bed, and nodular regeneration of remaining liver parenchyma. The pathologic process should be viewed as a final common pathway of many types of chronic liver injury. Clinical features of cirrhosis derive from the morphologic alterations and often reflect the severity of hepatic damage rather than the etiology of the underlying liver disease. Loss of functioning hepatocellular mass may lead to jaundice, edema, coagulopathy, and a variety of metabolic abnormalities; fibrosis and distorted vasculature lead to portal hypertension and its sequelae, including gastroesophageal varices and splenomegaly. Ascites and hepatic encephalopathy result from both hepatocellular insufficiency and portal hypertension.

Classification of the various types of cirrhosis based on either etiology or morphology alone is unsatisfactory. A single pathologic pattern may result from a variety of insults, while the same insult may produce several morphologic patterns. Nevertheless, most types of cirrhosis may be usefully classified by a mixture of etiologically and morphologically defined entities as follows: (1) alcoholic; (2) cryptogenic and postviral or postnecrotic; (3) biliary; (4) cardiac; (5) metabolic, inherited, and drug-related; and (6) miscellaneous. This chapter considers the various types of cirrhosis. → ***The major complications of cirrhosis are discussed in Chap. 299.***

ALCOHOLIC LIVER DISEASE AND CIRRHOSIS

Definition *Alcoholic cirrhosis*, historically referred to as *Laennec's cirrhosis*, is the most common type of cirrhosis encountered in North America and many parts of western Europe and South America. It is characterized by diffuse fine scarring, fairly uniform loss of liver cells, and small regenerative nodules, and therefore it is sometimes referred to as *micronodular cirrhosis*. However, micronodular cirrhosis also may result from other types of liver injury (e.g., following jejunoileal bypass), and thus alcoholic cirrhosis and micronodular cirrhosis are not necessarily synonymous. Conversely, alcoholic cirrhosis may progress to macronodular cirrhosis with time.

Alcoholic cirrhosis is only one of many consequences resulting from chronic alcohol ingestion, and it often accompanies other forms of alcohol-induced liver injury. The three principal alcohol-induced hepatic lesions are designated (1) *alcoholic fatty liver (steatosis)*, (2) *alcoholic hepatitis*, and (3) *alcoholic cirrhosis*. These morphologic categories are rarely found in a pure form, and features of each may be present to varying degrees in an individual patient.

Etiology Although chronic alcoholism is the most common cause of cirrhosis, the quantity and duration of drinking necessary to cause cirrhosis remain unclear. The typical alcoholic patient with cirrhosis has had a daily consumption of a pint or more of whiskey, several quarts of wine, or an equivalent amount of beer for at least 10 years. The amount and duration of ethanol ingestion, rather than the type of alcoholic beverage or the pattern of ingestion, appear to be the important determinants of liver injury. In general, the latent period preceding the development of cirrhosis is inversely related to the level of daily alcohol intake. Rates of ethanol metabolism are under genetic control, but no metabolic defect has been identified in cirrhotic patients or their families to suggest a unique "susceptibility" to ethanol or its toxic effects. Although malnutrition per se does not appear to lead to cirrhosis, it is possible that nutritional factors may augment the detrimental effects of chronic alcohol ingestion on the liver. The finding that only 10 to 15 percent of alcoholics develop cirrhosis suggests that other factors may affect the impact of alcohol on the liver. Women, on average, appear to develop alcohol-induced liver injury at lesser levels of consumption than men, suggesting that hormonal factors may play a role in susceptibility. Lower levels of alcohol dehydrogenase in gastric mucosa and resultant diminished rates of alcohol metabolism may also contribute to a greater predisposition to alcohol-related liver injury in women. The finding of increased concordance of alcoholic liver disease among monozygotic twins compared to dizygotic twins ingesting excessive amounts of alcohol suggests that genetic factors contribute, though no genetic alterations have yet been consistently identified. Other observations suggest that immune mechanisms may also play a significant role.

Alcoholic fatty liver occurs in most heavy drinkers but is reversible on cessation of alcohol consumption and is not thought to be an inevitable precursor of alcoholic hepatitis or cirrhosis. In contrast, alcoholic hepatitis, an inflammatory lesion characterized by infiltration of the liver with leukocytes, liver cell necrosis, and alcoholic hyaline, is thought to be the major precursor of cirrhosis. Subsequent healing accompanied by fibrosis distorts the normal lobular architecture. Indeed, *deposition of collagen in perivenular spaces* may be the earliest manifestation of the process that ultimately leads to cirrhosis.

Pathology and Pathogenesis *Alcoholic fatty liver* The liver is enlarged, yellow, greasy, and firm. Hepatocytes are distended by large macrovesicular cytoplasmic fat vacuoles that push the hepatocyte nucleus against the cell membrane. Accumulation of fat in the liver of the alcoholic results from the combination of impaired fatty acid oxidation, increased uptake and esterification of fatty acids to form triglycerides, and diminished lipoprotein biosynthesis and secretion.

Alcoholic hepatitis Morphologic features include hepatocyte degeneration and necrosis, often with ballooned cells, and an infiltrate of polymorphonuclear leukocytes and lymphocytes. The polymorphonuclear cells may encircle damaged hepatocytes that contain *Mallory bodies*, or *alcoholic hyaline*. These are clumps of perinuclear, deeply eosinophilic material believed to represent aggregated intermediate filaments. Mallory bodies are highly suggestive of, but *not specific* for, alcoholic hepatitis, since morphologically similar material is seen in association with morbid obesity, jejunoileal bypass surgery, poorly controlled diabetes mellitus, and a variety of other disorders, including Wilson's disease and Indian childhood cirrhosis. Deposition of collagen around the central vein and in perisinusoidal areas, often termed *central hyaline sclerosis*, is associated with an increased likelihood of progression to cirrhosis.

Alcoholic cirrhosis With continued alcohol intake and destruction of hepatocytes, fibroblasts (including myofibroblasts with contractile properties) appear at the site of injury and stimulate collagen formation. Weblike septa of connective tissue appear in periportal and pericentral zones and eventually connect portal triads and central veins. This fine connective tissue network surrounds small masses of remaining liver cells, which regenerate and form nodules. Although regeneration occurs within the small remnants of parenchyma, cell loss generally exceeds replacement. With continuing hepatocyte destruction and collagen deposition, the liver shrinks in size, acquires a nodular appearance, and becomes hard as "end-stage" cirrhosis develops. Although alcoholic cirrhosis is usually a progressive disease, appropriate therapy and strict avoidance of alcohol may arrest the disease at most stages and permit functional improvement.

Clinical Features *Signs and symptoms* Clinical manifestations of *alcoholic fatty liver* are often minimal or entirely absent, and the disorder may not be recognized unless another illness (frequently alcohol-related) brings the patient to medical attention. Hepatomegaly, at times accompanied by tenderness, may be the only finding. Jaundice, ascites, and edema are seen only with more serious liver injury.

The clinical severity of *alcoholic hepatitis* varies enormously, ranging from asymptomatic or mild illness to fatal hepatic insufficiency. Typically, the clinical features of alcoholic hepatitis resemble those of viral or toxic liver injury. Patients often experience anorexia, nausea and vomiting, malaise, weight loss, abdominal distress, and jaundice. Fever sometimes as high as 39.4°C (103°F) is seen in about half of cases. On physical examination, tender hepatomegaly is common, and splenomegaly is found in about one-third of patients. The patient may have cutaneous arterial "spider" angiomas and jaundice. More severe cases may be complicated by ascites, edema, bleeding, and encephalopathy. At the time of initial presentation, the central nervous system findings may be difficult to distinguish from manifestations of concurrent alcohol intoxication or withdrawal (see below).

Although jaundice, ascites, and encephalopathy may subside with abstinence, continued alcohol excess and poor dietary habits usually lead to repeated acute episodes of hepatic decompensation. Some patients die during these acute exacerbations, but most recover after several weeks or months. Even after complete abstinence, clinical recovery may be protracted, and histologic abnormalities can persist up to 6 months or longer. Cholestatic jaundice mimicking biliary tract obstruction also may develop in some cases of acute alcoholic hepatitis.

Alcoholic cirrhosis also may be clinically silent and many (10 to 40 percent) cases are discovered incidentally at laparotomy or autopsy. In many cases symptoms are insidious in onset, occurring usually after 10 or more years of excessive alcohol use and progressing slowly over subsequent weeks and months. Anorexia and malnutrition lead to weight loss and a reduction in skeletal muscle mass. The patient may experience easy bruising, increasing weakness, and fatigue. Eventually the clinical manifestations of hepatocellular dysfunction and portal hypertension ensue, including progressive jaundice, bleeding from gastroesophageal varices, ascites, and encephalopathy. The abrupt onset of one of these complications may be the first event prompting the patient to seek medical attention. In other cases, cirrhosis first becomes evident when the patient requires treatment of symptoms related to alcoholic hepatitis.

A firm, nodular liver may be an early sign of disease; the liver may be either enlarged, normal, or decreased in size. Other frequent findings include jaundice, palmar erythema, spider angiomas, parotid and lacrimal gland enlargement, clubbing of fingers, splenomegaly, muscle wasting, and ascites with or without peripheral edema. Men may have decreased body hair and/or gynecomastia and testicular atrophy, which, like the cutaneous findings, result from disturbances in hormonal metabolism, including increased peripheral formation of estrogren due to diminished hepatic clearance of the precursor androstenedione. Testicular atrophy may reflect hormonal abnormalities or the toxic effect of alcohol on the testes. In women, signs of virilization or menstrual irregularities may occasionally be encountered. Dupuytren's contractures resulting from fibrosis of the palmar fascia with resulting flexion contracture of the digits are associated with alcoholism but are not specifically related to cirrhosis.

Although the cirrhotic patient may stabilize if drinking is discontinued, over a period of years, the patient may become emaciated, weak, and chronically jaundiced. Ascites and other signs of portal hypertension may become increasingly prominent. Ultimately, most patients with advanced cirrhosis die in hepatic coma, commonly precipitated by hemorrhage from esophageal varices or intercurrent infection. Progressive renal dysfunction often complicates the terminal phase of the illness.

Laboratory findings Routine hematologic and biochemical blood tests are usually normal in patients with alcoholic fatty liver, except for minimal elevations of the serum AST (aspartate aminotransferase); occasionally alkaline phosphatase and bilirubin levels are also elevated. In more advanced alcoholic liver disease, abnormalities of laboratory tests are more common. Anemia may result from acute and chronic gastrointestinal blood loss, coexistent nutritional deficiency (notably of folic acid and vitamin B_{12}), hypersplenism, and a direct suppressive effect of alcohol on the bone marrow. Hemolytic anemia, presumably due to effects of hypercholesterolemia on erythrocyte membranes resulting in unusual spurlike projections (acanthocytosis), has been described in some alcoholics with cirrhosis. Leukocytosis is often present in severe alcoholic hepatitis; however, some patients with this disorder may have leukopenia and thrombocytopenia due to hypersplenism or an inhibitory effect of alcohol on the bone marrow. Mild or pronounced hyperbilirubinemia may be found, usually in association with varying elevations of serum alkaline phosphatase levels. Levels of serum AST are frequently elevated, but levels greater than 5 μkat (300 units) are unusual and should prompt one to look for other coincident or complicating factors. In contrast to viral hepatitis, the serum AST is usually disproportionately elevated relative to ALT (alanine aminotransferase), i.e., AST/ALT ratio >2. In nonalcoholic steatohepatitis, the ALT level is also typically greater than the AST level. This discrepancy in alcoholic hepatitis may result from the proportionally greater inhibition of ALT synthesis by ethanol, which may be partially reversed by pyridoxal phosphate.

The serum prothrombin time is frequently prolonged, reflecting reduced synthesis of clotting proteins, most notably the vitamin K–dependent factors (see "Coagulopathy" in Chap. 299). The serum albumin level is usually depressed, while serum globulins are increased. Hypoalbuminemia reflects in part overall impairment in hepatic protein synthesis, while hyperglobulinemia is thought to result from nonspecific stimulation of the reticuloendothelial system. Elevated blood ammonia levels in patients with hepatic encephalopathy reflect diminished hepatic clearance because of impaired liver function and shunting of portal venous blood around the cirrhotic liver into the systemic circulation (see Chaps. 293 and 299).

A variety of metabolic disturbances may be detected. Glucose intolerance due to endogenous insulin resistance may be present; however, clinical diabetes is uncommon. Central hyperventilation may lead to respiratory alkalosis in patients with cirrhosis. *Dietary deficiency* and *increased urinary losses* lead to hypomagnesemia and *hypophosphatemia*. In patients with ascites and dilutional hyponatremia, hypokalemia may occur from increased urinary potassium losses due in part to hyperaldosteronism. Prerenal azotemia is also observed in such patients.

Diagnosis *Alcoholic fatty liver* should be suspected in alcoholic patients with hepatomegaly and normal or minimally deranged liver function tests. Alcoholic fatty liver may be seen in combination with alcoholic hepatitis or established cirrhosis. *Alcoholic hepatitis* should be considered in an alcoholic who has been drinking heavily and demonstrates jaundice, fever, an enlarged, tender liver, or ascites. The clinical impression is often supported by the deranged results of tests of liver function and other laboratory abnormalities described above. Alcoholic hepatitis or fatty liver may be present in association with alcoholic cirrhosis.

Alcoholic cirrhosis should be strongly suspected in patients with a history of prolonged or excessive alcohol intake and physical signs of chronic liver disease. However, since only 10 to 15 percent of individuals with excessive alcohol intake develop cirrhosis, other causes and types of liver disease may have to be excluded. The clinical features and laboratory findings are usually sufficient to provide reasonable indication of the presence and extent of hepatic injury. Although a percutaneous needle biopsy of the liver is not usually necessary to confirm the typical findings of alcoholic hepatitis or cirrhosis, it may be helpful in distinguishing patients with less advanced liver disease from those with cirrhosis and in excluding other forms of liver injury such as viral hepatitis. Biopsy also may be helpful as a diagnostic tool in evaluating patients with clinical findings suggestive of alcoholic liver disease who deny alcohol intake. In patients with features of cholestasis, ultrasonography may be appropriate to exclude the presence of extrahepatic biliary obstruction. When the clinical status of an otherwise stable cirrhotic patient deteriorates without an obvious explanation, complicating conditions, such as infection, portal vein thrombosis, and hepatocellular carcinoma, should be sought.

Prognosis The patient with an alcoholic fatty liver and no complications has a good prognosis; rapid and complete resolution usually follows cessation of alcohol intake. In patients with alcoholic hepatitis, the presence of marked hyperbilirubinemia, rising serum creatinine, marked prolongation of the prothrombin time (>1.5 times control), ascites, and encephalopathy are associated with a poor short-term prognosis; the in-hospital mortality in these patients may exceed 50 percent. A discriminant function calculated as $4.6 \times$ [prothrombin time $-$ control time (seconds)] + serum bilirubin (μm/L)/17 can be used to distinguish between those with especially poor prognosis (value > 32). In milder cases, clinical recovery may be complete, but repeated bouts of alcoholic hepatitis usually lead to irreversible and progressive chronic liver injury. Abstinence from alcohol as well as early and appropriate medical care can decrease long-term morbidity and mortality and delay or prevent the appearance of further complications. Patients who have had a major complication of cirrhosis and who continue to drink have a 5-year survival of less than 50 percent. However, those patients who remain abstinent have a substantially better prognosis. In general, overall outlook in patients with advanced liver disease remains poor; most of these patients eventually die as a result of massive variceal hemorrhage and/or profound hepatic encephalopathy (see Chap. 299).

Rx TREATMENT

Alcoholic hepatitis and cirrhosis are serious illnesses that require long-term medical supervision and careful management. Therapy of the underlying liver disease is largely supportive. Specific treatment is directed at particular complications such as variceal bleeding and ascites (see Chap. 299). Some studies suggest that administration of prednisone or prednisolone in moderately large doses may be helpful in patients with severe alcoholic hepatitis and encephalopathy. However, the use of glucocorticoids in acute alcoholic hepatitis remains controversial and should probably be reserved for those with a discriminant function greater than 32, as described above. Maintenance therapy with colchicine (0.6 mg PO bid) has been shown to slow disease progression and increase longevity of the patient with alcoholic liver disease in one long-term study.

In the absence of signs of impending hepatic coma, the patient should be placed on a diet containing at least 1 g protein per kilogram of body weight and 8500 to 12,500 kJ (2000 to 3000 kcal) per day. Use of diets enriched in branched-chain amino acids has been advocated in patients predisposed to hepatic encephalopathy, but the value of these diets in patients with compensated cirrhosis is unproven. Daily multivitamin supplements should be prescribed, with the addition of large parenteral doses of thiamine in patients with Wernicke-Korsakoff disease (see Chap. 380). The patient should be made to realize that there is no medication that will protect the liver against the effects of further alcohol ingestion. Therefore, alcohol should be absolutely forbidden. An important component of the complete care of such patients is encouragement to become involved in an appropriate alcohol counseling program.

All medicines must be administered with caution in the patient with cirrhosis, especially those eliminated or modified through hepatic metabolism or biliary pathways. In particular, care must be taken to avoid overzealous use of drugs that may directly or indirectly precipitate complications of cirrhosis. For example, vigorous treatment of ascites with diuretics may result in electrolyte abnormalities or hypovolemia, which can lead to coma. Similarly, even modest doses of sedative can lead to deepening encephalopathy. Furthermore, patients may be sensitive to the toxic effects of acetaminophen, particularly in conjunction with alcohol, which can lead to excess concentrations of a toxic metabolite even at doses that are not generally toxic.

POSTNECROTIC CIRRHOSIS, POSTVIRAL CIRRHOSIS

Definition Postnecrotic cirrhosis represents the final common pathway of many types of advanced liver injury. *Coarsely nodular*, *posthepatitic*, and *multilobular cirrhosis* are terms synonymous with *postnecrotic cirrhosis*. The term *cryptogenic cirrhosis* has been used interchangeably with *postnecrotic cirrhosis*, but this designation should be reserved for those cases in which the etiology of cirrhosis is unknown (approximately 10 percent of all patients with cirrhosis).

Postnecrotic cirrhosis is characterized morphologically by (1) extensive confluent loss of liver cells, (2) stromal collapse and fibrosis resulting in broad bands of connective tissue containing the remains of many portal triads, and (3) irregular nodules of regenerating hepatocytes, varying in size from microscopic to several centimeters in diameter.

Etiology *Postnecrotic cirrhosis* is a morphologic term referring to a defined stage of advanced chronic liver injury of both specific and unknown (cryptogenic) causes. Epidemiologic and serologic evidence suggests that viral hepatitis (hepatitis B or hepatitis C) may be an antecedent factor in from one-fourth to three-fourths of cases of apparently cryptogenic postnecrotic cirrhosis. In areas where hepatitis B virus infection is endemic (e.g., Southeast Asia, sub-Saharan Africa), up to 15 percent of the population may acquire the infection in early childhood, and cirrhosis may ultimately develop in one-fourth of these chronic carriers. Although hepatitis B infection is much less prevalent in the United States, it is relatively common among certain high-risk groups (e.g., promiscuous homosexual men, intravenous drug abusers) and contributes to an increased incidence of cirrhosis. In the United States, hepatitis C accounts for many cases of cirrhosis following blood transfusions. Before hepatitis C screening of blood donors was introduced, hepatitis C occurred in 5 to 10 percent of blood recipients. In over 20 percent of those surviving 20 years or more, cirrhosis may ultimately develop. More than half of patients who would previously have been designated as having cryptogenic chronic liver disease have evidence of hepatitis C infection. Postnecrotic cirrhosis also may develop in patients with autoimmune hepatitis (see Chap. 297).

Other probable causes of postnecrotic cirrhosis, including drugs and toxins, are listed in Table 298-1. In some instances, advanced alcoholic liver disease and primary biliary cirrhosis may lead to postnecrotic cirrhosis.

Pathology The postnecrotic liver is typically shrunken in size, distorted in shape, and composed of nodules of liver cells separated by dense and broad bands of fibrosis. The microscopic picture is consistent with the gross impression: Nodules are highly variable in size, with large amounts of connective tissue separating the disorganized islands of regenerating parenchyma.

Clinical Features In patients with cirrhosis of known etiology in whom there is progression to a postnecrotic stage, the clinical manifestations are an extension of those resulting from the initial disease process. Usually clinical symptoms are related to portal hypertension and its sequelae, such as ascites, splenomegaly, hypersplenism, encephalopathy, and bleeding esophageal varices. The hematologic and liver function abnormalities resemble those seen with other types of cirrhosis. In a few patients with postnecrotic cirrhosis the diagnosis may be made incidentally at operation, at postmortem, or by a needle biopsy of the liver performed to investigate asymptomatic hepatosplenomegaly.

Table 298-1

Cirrhosis and/or Liver Disease Associated with Various Disorders

INFECTIOUS DISEASES
Brucellosis (Chap. 162)
Echinococcus (Chap. 225)
Schistosomiasis (Chap. 224)
Toxoplasmosis (Chap. 219)
Viral hepatitis [hepatitis B, C, D, E, G; cytomegalovirus (Chaps. 187, 295, and 297)]
INHERITED AND METABOLIC DISORDERS (see also Chap. 300)
Alpha$_1$-antitrypsin deficiency (Chap. 300)
Fanconi's syndrome (Chap. 346)
Galactosemia (Chap. 351)
Gaucher's disease (Chap. 346)
Glycogen storage disease (Chap. 347)
Hemochromatosis (Chap. 342)
Hereditary fructose intolerance (Chap. 351)
Hereditary tyrosinemia (Chap. 349)
Wilson's disease (Chap. 345)
DRUGS AND TOXINS (Chap. 296)
Arsenicals
Isoniazid
Methotrexate
Methyldopa
Oral contraceptives (Budd-Chiari)
Oxyphenisatin
Perhexilene maleate
Pyrrolidizine alkaloids (venoocclusive disease)
OTHER OR UNPROVEN CAUSES
Chronic inflammatory bowel disease (Chap. 286)
Cystic fibrosis (Chap. 257)
Diabetes mellitus (Chap. 334)
Graft-versus-host disease (Chap. 116)
Jejunoileal bypass (Chap. 43)
Sarcoidosis (Chap. 320)

Diagnosis and Prognosis Postnecrotic cirrhosis should be suspected in patients with signs and symptoms of cirrhosis or portal hypertension. Needle or operative liver biopsies confirm the diagnosis, although nonuniformity of the pathologic process may result in sampling errors. The diagnosis of cryptogenic cirrhosis is reserved for those patients in whom no known etiology can be demonstrated. About 75 percent of patients have progressive disease despite supportive therapy and die within 1 to 5 years from complications, including exsanguinating variceal hemorrhage, hepatic encephalopathy, or superimposed hepatocellular carcinoma.

℞ TREATMENT

Management is usually limited to treatment of the complications of portal hypertension, including control of ascites, avoidance of drugs or excessive protein intake that may induce hepatic coma, and prompt treatment of infections (see Chap. 299). In patients with asymptomatic cirrhosis, expectant management alone is appropriate. In those patients in whom postnecrotic cirrhosis has developed as a result of a treatable condition, therapy directed at the primary disorder may limit further progression (e.g., Wilson's disease, hemochromatosis).

BILIARY CIRRHOSIS

Biliary cirrhosis results from injury to or prolonged obstruction of either the intrahepatic or extrahepatic biliary system. It is associated with impaired biliary excretion, destruction of hepatic parenchyma, and progressive fibrosis. Primary biliary cirrhosis is characterized by chronic inflammation and fibrous obliteration of intrahepatic bile ductules. Secondary biliary cirrhosis is the result of long-standing obstruction of the larger extrahepatic ducts. Although primary and secondary biliary cirrhosis are separate pathophysiologic entities with respect to the initial insult, many clinical features are similar.

PRIMARY BILIARY CIRRHOSIS Etiology and Pathogenesis The cause of primary biliary cirrhosis (PBC) remains unknown. Several observations suggest that a disordered immune response may be involved. PBC is frequently associated with a variety of disorders presumed to be autoimmune in nature, such as the syndrome of calcinosis, Raynaud's phenomenon, esophageal dysmotility, sclerodactyly, telangiectasia (CREST); the sicca syndrome (dry eyes and dry mouth); autoimmune thyroiditis; and renal tubular acidosis.

Most important, a circulating IgG antimitochondrial antibody (AMA) is detected in more than 90 percent of patients with primary biliary cirrhosis and only rarely in other forms of liver disease. It has been demonstrated that these autoantibodies recognize three to five inner mitochondrial membrane proteins identified as enzymes of the pyruvate dehydrogenase complex (PDC), the branched chain α-keto-acid dehydrogenase complex (BCKDC), and the α-ketoglutarate dehydrogenase complex (KGDC). The major autoantigen in PBC (found in 90 percent of patients) has been identified as the 74-kDa E2 component of the PDC, dihydrolipoamide acetyltransferase. The antibodies are directed to a region essential for binding of a lipoic acid cofactor and inhibit the overall enzymatic activity of the PDC. Other AMA autoantibodies in PBC patients are directed to similar constituents of BCKDC and KGDC and also inhibit their enzymatic function. It remains unclear whether these properties have a direct pathogenetic role in the development of PBC. In addition to AMA, elevated serum levels of IgM and cryoproteins consisting of immune complexes capable of activating the alternative complement pathway are found in 80 to 90 percent of patients. Aberrant expression of major histocompatibility complex class II molecules has been found on biliary epithelium in association with PBC, suggesting that these cells may serve as antigen-presenting cells in this setting. Lymphocytes are prominent in the portal regions and surround damaged bile ducts. These histologic findings resemble those noted in graft-versus-host disease following liver and bone marrow transplantation and suggest that damage to bile ducts may be immunologically mediated, perhaps reflecting a defect in a suppressor cell population.

Pathology PBC is often divided into four stages based on morphologic findings. The earliest recognizable lesion (stage I), termed *chronic nonsuppurative destructive cholangitis*, is a necrotizing inflammatory process of the portal triads. It is characterized by destruction of medium and small bile ducts, a dense infiltrate of acute and chronic inflammatory cells, mild fibrosis, and occasionally, bile stasis. At times, periductal granulomas and lymph follicles are found adjacent to affected bile ducts. Subsequently, the inflammatory infiltrate becomes less prominent, the number of bile ducts is reduced, and smaller bile ductules proliferate (stage II). Progression over a period of months to years leads to a decrease in interlobular ducts, loss of liver cells, and expansion of periportal fibrosis into a network of connective tissue scars (stage III). Ultimately, cirrhosis, which may be micronodular or macronodular, develops (stage IV).

Clinical Features *Signs and symptoms* Many patients with PBC are asymptomatic, and the disease is initially detected on the basis of elevated serum alkaline phosphatase levels during routine screening. The majority of such patients remain asymptomatic for prolonged periods, although many may ultimately develop progressive liver injury.

Among patients with symptomatic disease, 90 percent are women aged 35 to 60. Often the earliest symptom is pruritus, which may be either generalized or limited initially to the palms and soles. In addition, fatigue is commonly a prominent early symptom. After several months or years, jaundice and gradual darkening of the exposed areas of the skin (melanosis) may ensue. Other early clinical manifestations of PBC reflect impaired bile excretion. These include steatorrhea and the malabsorption of lipid-soluble vitamins, often resulting in easy bruising (vitamin K deficiency); bone pain due to osteomalacia (vitamin D deficiency), which is typically present in conjunction with osteoporosis; occasionally night blindness (vitamin A deficiency); and dermatitis (possibly vitamin E and/or essential fatty acid deficiency). Protracted elevation of serum lipids, especially cholesterol, leads to subcutaneous lipid deposition around the eyes (xanthelasmas) and over joints and tendons (xanthomas). Over a period of months to years, the itching, jaundice, and hyperpigmentation slowly worsen. Eventually signs of hepatocellular failure and portal hypertension develop and ascites appears. Progression may be quite variable. Whereas a proportion of asymptomatic patients may show no signs of progression for a decade or longer, in others, death due to hepatic insufficiency may occur within 5 to 10 years after the first signs of the illness. Such decompensation is often precipitated by uncontrolled variceal hemorrhage or infection.

Physical examination may be entirely normal in the early phase of the disease, when patients are asymptomatic or pruritus is the sole complaint. Later, there may be jaundice of varying intensity, hyperpigmentation of the exposed skin areas, xanthelasmas and tendinous and planar xanthomas, moderate to striking hepatomegaly, splenomegaly, and clubbing of the fingers. Bone tenderness, signs of vertebral compression, ecchymoses, glossitis, and dermatitis may all be noted. Clinical evidence of the sicca syndrome can be found in as many as 75 percent of patients, and serologic evidence of autoimmune thyroid disease in 25 percent. Other conditions encountered with increased frequency include rheumatoid arthritis, CREST syndrome, scleroderma, pernicious anemia, and renal tubular acidosis. Bone disease is often a significant problem encountered over the course of the disease. While osteomalacia occurs due to diminished vitamin D absorption, accelerated osteoporosis in this patient population (the majority of whom are postmenopausal women) is even more common.

Laboratory findings PBC is increasingly diagnosed at a presymptomatic stage, prompted by the finding of a two- to fivefold elevation of the serum alkaline phosphatase during routine screening. Serum 5′-nucleotidase activity is also elevated. In this setting, serum bilirubin and aminotransferase levels are usually normal, but the diagnosis is supported by a positive antimitochondrial antibody test (titer $>$ 1:40). The latter is both *relatively* specific and sensitive; a positive test is found in over 90 percent of symptomatic patients. As the disease evolves, the serum bilirubin level rises progressively and may reach 510 μmol/L (30 mg/dL) or more in the final stages. Serum aminotransferase values rarely exceed 2.5 to 3.3 μkat (150 to 200 units). Hyperlipidemia is common, and a striking increase of the serum unesterified cholesterol is often noted. An abnormal serum lipoprotein (lipoprotein X) may be present in PBC but is not specific and appears in other cholestatic conditions. A deficiency of bile salts in the intestine leads to moderate steatorrhea and impaired absorption of the fat-soluble vitamins and hypoprothrombinemia. Patients with PBC have elevated liver copper levels, but this finding is not specific and is found in all disorders in which there is prolonged cholestasis.

Diagnosis PBC should be considered in middle-aged women with unexplained pruritus or an elevated serum alkaline phosphatase level and in whom there may be other clinical or laboratory features of protracted impairment of biliary excretion. Although a positive serum AMA determination provides important diagnostic evidence, false-positive results do occur, and therefore, liver biopsy should be performed to confirm the diagnosis. Rarely, the AMA test may be negative in patients with histologic features of PBC. Frequently, patients have antibodies to the E2 protein in tests using these specific antigens. In some cases with histologic features of PBC and a negative AMA, antinuclear or smooth muscle antibodies are present (as in autoimmune hepatitis), and the designation *autoimmune cholangitis* is applied. In most cases the biliary tract should be evaluated to exclude remediable extrahepatic biliary tract obstruction, especially in view of the frequent presence of coexisting cholelithiasis.

Rx TREATMENT

There is no specific therapy for PBC. Glucocorticoids are ineffective and may actually worsen the bone disease. D-Penicillamine has been tried because of its ability to chelate copper and because of its possible antifibrotic and immunomodulating activities. However, the drug appears to be ineffective and has a high incidence of unacceptable side effects. While some have suggested that azathioprine may be helpful in slowing the progression of disease, this has not been established. Colchicine has been shown to have some limited effectiveness in slowing the progression of disease in symptomatic patients and should be tried (0.6 mg PO bid) unless gastrointestinal intolerance is limiting. Treatment with either low-dose methotrexate or cyclosporine has been reported to halt or reverse progression of PBC, but definitive trials have not been reported and these drugs are not appropriate for routine use. Only ursodiol treatment (13 to 15 mg/kg per day) has been consistently observed to achieve both symptomatic improvement and "improvement" in serum biochemical markers in patients with clinically overt PBC. The mechanism of action of ursodeoxycholic acid in achieving this benefit remains obscure. This agent is generally well tolerated and safe and should be considered for use in PBC patients. However, it may have limited ability to prevent ultimate progression to advanced cirrhosis.

Treatment is generally directed toward the relief of symptoms. As noted, ursodiol may be helpful in controlling symptoms and improving the patient's sense of well-being. Although the mechanism of the protracted pruritus is not entirely clear, cholestyramine, an oral bile salt–sequestering resin, may be helpful in doses of 8 to 12 g/d to decrease both the pruritus and the hypercholesterolemia. Occasionally orthotopic liver transplantation has been performed for intractable pruritus. Rifampin, opiate antagonists, plasmapheresis, and ultraviolet light have all been tried for control of pruritus with varying results. Steatorrhea can be reduced by a low-fat diet and substituting medium-chain triglycerides for dietary long-chain triglycerides. Fat-soluble vitamins A and K should be given by parenteral injection at regular intervals to prevent or correct night blindness and hypoprothrombinemia, respectively. Zinc supplementation may be necessary if night blindness is refractory to vitamin A therapy. Osteomalacia and osteoporosis may be ameliorated by dietary calcium supplements in conjunction with oral vitamin D. In advanced disease, $25(OH)D_3$ or $1,25(OH_2)D_3$ may be preferred to vitamin D, since poor hepatic function may limit conversion of vitamin D to the active metabolites. Progression of PBC leads to the typical complications of advanced liver disease.

The management of ascites, variceal hemorrhage, and encephalopathy are described in Chap. 299. In recent years, it has become evident that orthotopic liver transplantation is a highly effective treatment for patients with advanced PBC. Stratified analysis of patients with a wide variety of risk levels utilizing a validated prognostic model has demonstrated enhanced survival for all. Thus, hepatic transplantation is the treatment of choice for advanced PBC.

SECONDARY BILIARY CIRRHOSIS **Etiology** Secondary biliary cirrhosis (SBC) results from prolonged partial or total obstruction of the common bile duct or its major branches. In adults, obstruction is most frequently caused by postoperative strictures or gallstones, usually with superimposed infectious cholangitis. Chronic pancreatitis may lead to biliary stricture and secondary cirrhosis. SBC also may develop in patients with pericholangitis or primary sclerosing cholangitis. Patients with malignant tumors of the common bile duct or pancreas rarely survive long enough to develop SBC. In children, congenital biliary atresia and cystic fibrosis are common causes of SBC. Choledochal cysts, if unrecognized, also may be a rare cause of SBC.

Pathology and Pathogenesis Unrelieved obstruction of the extrahepatic bile ducts leads to (1) bile stasis and focal areas of centrilobular necrosis followed by periportal necrosis, (2) proliferation and dilatation of the portal bile ducts and ductules, (3) sterile or infected cholangitis with accumulation of polymorphonuclear infiltrates around bile ducts, and (4) progressive expansion of portal tracts by edema and fibrosis. Extravasation of bile from ruptured interlobular bile ducts into areas of periportal necrosis leads to the formation of "bile lakes" surrounded by cholesterol-rich pseudoxanthomatous cells. As in other forms of cirrhosis, injury is accompanied by regeneration in residual parenchyma. These changes gradually lead to a finely nodular cirrhosis. In general, at least 3 to 12 months is required for biliary obstruction to result in cirrhosis. Relief of the obstruction is frequently accompanied by biochemical and morphologic improvement.

Clinical Features *Signs and symptoms* The signs and symptoms of SBC are similar to those of PBC. Jaundice and pruritus are usually the most prominent features. In addition, fever and/or right upper quadrant pain, reflecting bouts of cholangitis or biliary colic, are typical. The manifestations of portal hypertension are found only in advanced cases.

Laboratory tests Elevations in serum alkaline phosphatase and 5′-nucleotidase as well as conjugated hyperbilirubinemia are almost always present. There is a moderate increase in serum aminotransferases. When the disease is complicated by cholangitis, elevations in aminotransferase levels and leukocytosis are more pronounced. As in PBC, there are abnormalities in serum lipids (including the presence of lipoprotein X) and laboratory findings consistent with steatorrhea. However, the antimitochondrial antibody test is usually negative.

Diagnosis SBC should be considered in any patient with clinical and laboratory evidence of prolonged obstruction to bile flow, especially when there is a history of previous biliary tract surgery or gallstones, bouts of ascending cholangitis, or right upper quadrant pain. Cholangiography (either percutaneous or endoscopic) usually demonstrates the underlying pathologic process. Liver biopsy, although not always necessary from a clinical standpoint, can document the development of cirrhosis.

℞ TREATMENT

Relief of obstruction to bile flow, by either endoscopic or surgical means, is the most important step in the prevention and therapy of SBC. Effective decompression of the biliary tract results in a significant improvement in both symptoms and survival, even in patients with established cirrhosis. When obstruction cannot be relieved, as in sclerosing cholangitis, antibiotics may be helpful acutely in controlling superimposed infection or, when administered on a chronic basis, as prophylactic therapy in suppressing recurring episodes of ascending cholangitis. Without relief of obstruction, there is a steady progression to end-stage cirrhosis and its terminal manifestations.

CARDIAC CIRRHOSIS

Definition Prolonged, severe right-sided congestive heart failure may lead to chronic liver injury and cardiac cirrhosis. The characteristic pathologic features of fibrosis and regenerative nodules distinguish cardiac cirrhosis from both reversible passive congestion of the liver due to acute heart failure and acute hepatocellular necrosis ("ischemic hepatitis" or "shock liver") resulting from systemic hypotension and hypoperfusion of the liver.

Etiology and Pathology In right-sided heart failure, retrograde transmission of elevated venous pressure via the inferior vena cava and hepatic veins leads to congestion of the liver. Hepatic sinusoids become dilated and engorged with blood, and the liver becomes tensely swollen. With prolonged passive congestion and ischemia from poor perfusion secondary to reduced cardiac output, necrosis of centrilobular hepatocytes ensues and leads to fibrosis in these central areas. Ultimately, centrilobular fibrosis develops, with collagen extending outward in a characteristic stellate pattern from the central vein. Gross examination of the liver shows alternating red (congested) and pale (fibrotic) areas, a pattern often referred to as "nutmeg liver." Improvement in management of cardiac disorders, particularly advances in surgical treatment, has reduced the frequency of cardiac cirrhosis.

Clinical Features In acute passive congestion, the liver becomes enlarged and tender, and the patient may complain of severe right upper quadrant pain due to stretching of Glisson's capsule. A range of abnormalities of liver function tests may be found, though none is uniformly present. The serum bilirubin is usually only mildly increased and may be predominantly either conjugated or unconjugated. Mild to moderate elevation in alkaline phosphatase and prothrombin time prolongation are sometimes present. The AST level is also typically mildly elevated but may be transiently very high following a period of marked systemic hypotension (shock liver), when the clinical picture can mimic acute viral or drug-induced hepatitis. In cases of tricuspid insufficiency the liver may be pulsatile, but this finding disappears as cirrhosis develops. With prolonged right-sided heart failure the liver becomes enlarged, firm, and usually nontender. The signs and symptoms of heart failure usually overshadow the liver disease. Bleeding from esophageal varices is rare, but chronic encephalopathy may be prominent, with a waxing and waning course reflecting variations in the severity of right-sided heart failure. Ascites and peripheral edema, often primarily related to the underlying cardiac dysfunction, may be worsened by the superimposed liver disease.

Diagnosis The presence of a firm, enlarged liver with signs of chronic liver disease in a patient with valvular heart disease, constrictive pericarditis, or cor pulmonale of long duration (>10 years) should suggest cardiac cirrhosis. Liver biopsy can confirm the diagnosis but is usually contraindicated because of coagulopathy or ascites. Coexistent chronic heart and liver disease should also raise the possibility of hemochromatosis, amyloidosis, or other infiltrative diseases.

Budd-Chiari syndrome resulting from the occlusion of the hepatic veins or inferior vena cava may be confused with acute congestive hepatomegaly. In this condition the liver is grossly enlarged and tender, and severe intractable ascites is present. However, signs and symptoms of heart failure are notably absent. The most common cause is thrombosis of the hepatic veins, often in the setting of polycythemia rubra vera, myeloproliferative syndromes, paroxysmal nocturnal hemoglobinuria, oral contraceptive use, or other hypercoagulable states; it also may result from invasion of the inferior vena cava by tumor, such as renal cell or primary hepatocellular carcinoma. Idiopathic membranous obstruction of the inferior vena cava is the most common cause of this syndrome in Japan. Hepatic venography or liver biopsy showing centrilobular congestion and sinusoidal dilatation in the absence of right-sided heart failure establishes the diagnosis of Budd-Chiari syndrome. Venoocclusive disease affecting the sublobular branches of the hepatic veins and the hepatic venules may result from hepatic irradiation, treatment with certain antineoplastic agents, or ingestion

Table 298-2

Some Causes of Noncirrhotic Hepatic Fibrosis

Idiopathic portal hypertension (noncirrhotic portal fibrosis, Banti's syndrome); three variants:
- Intrahepatic phlebosclerosis and fibrosis
- Portal and splenic vein sclerosis
- Portal and splenic vein thrombosis

Schistosomiasis ("pipe-stem" fibrosis with presinusoidal portal hypertension)
Congenital hepatic fibrosis (may be associated with polycystic disease of liver and kidneys)

of pyrrolidizine alkaloids present in some herbal teas ("bush tea disease") and can mimic congestive hepatomegaly.

Rx TREATMENT

Prevention or treatment of cardiac cirrhosis depends on the diagnosis and therapy of the underlying cardiovascular disorder. Improvement in cardiac function frequently results in improvement of liver function and stabilization of the liver disease.

METABOLIC, HEREDITARY, DRUG-RELATED, AND OTHER TYPES OF CIRRHOSIS (See Table 298-1)

Cirrhosis or hepatitis may result from a wide variety of other processes encompassing the spectrum of etiologic factors listed in Table 298-2. Although some of these disorders have distinctive clinical or morphologic features, the manifestations of cirrhosis are largely independent of the underlying pathogenic mechanism.

NONCIRRHOTIC FIBROSIS OF THE LIVER

Several diseases, either congenital or acquired, may be associated with localized or generalized hepatic fibrosis. They are distinguished from cirrhosis by the absence of hepatocellular damage and the lack of nodular regenerative activity. The clinical manifestations in such cases are largely secondary to portal hypertension. The different types of these disorders are indicated in Table 298-2; with the exception of schistosomiasis, all these conditions are relatively rare.

BIBLIOGRAPHY

ALCOHOLIC AND POSTNECROTIC CIRRHOSIS

Arroyo V, Ginés P: Arteriolar vasodilation and the pathogenesis of the hyperdynamic circulation and renal sodium and water retention in cirrhosis. Gastroenterology 102:1077, 1992

Bacon BR et al: Nonalcoholic steatohepatitis: An expanded clinical entity. Gastroenterology 107:1103, 1994

Brown J et al: Seroprevalence of hepatitis C virus nucleocapsid antibodies in patients with cryptogenic chronic liver disease. Hepatology 15:175, 1992

Carithers RL et al: Methylprednisolone therapy in patients with severe alcoholic hepatitis: A randomized multicenter trial. Ann Intern Med 110:685, 1989

Jeffers LJ et al: Prevalence of antibodies to hepatitis C virus among patients with cryptogenic chronic hepatitis and cirrhosis. Hepatology 15:187, 1992

Lieber CS: Alcohol and the liver: 1994 update. Gastroenterology 106:1085, 1994

Ramond M-J et al: A randomized trial of prednisolone in patients with severe alcoholic hepatitis. N Engl J Med 326:507, 1992

Sheth SG et al: Nonalcoholic steatohepatitis. Ann Intern Med 126:137, 1997

BILIARY CIRROHOSIS

Christensen E et al: Updating prognosis in primary biliary cirrhosis using a time-dependent cox regression model. Gastroenterology 105:1865, 1993

Combes B et al: A randomized, double-blind, placebo-controlled trial of ursodeoxycholic acid in primary biliary cirrhosis. Hepatology 22:759, 1995

Fregeau DR et al: Antimitochondrial antibodies of primary biliary cirrhosis recognize dihydrolipoamide acyltransferase and inhibit enzyme function of the branched chain α-ketoacid dehydrogenase complex. J Immunol 142:3815, 1989

Kaplan MM: Medical progress: Primary biliary cirrhosis. N Engl J Med 335:1570, 1996

Locke III GR et al: Time course of histological progression in primary biliary cirrhosis. Hepatology 23:52, 1996

Markus BH et al: Efficacy of liver transplantation in patients with primary biliary cirrhosis. N Engl J Med 320:1709, 1989

Metcalf JV et al: Natural history of early primary biliary cirrhosis. Lancet 348:1399, 1996

Poupon RE et al: Ursodial for the long-term treatment of primary biliary cirrhosis. N Engl J Med 330:1342, 1994

Tsuneyama K et al: Abnormal expression of the E2 component of the pyruvate dehydrogenase complex on the luminal surface of biliary epithelium before major histocompatibility complex class II and BB1/BB7 expression. Hepatology 21:103, 1995

299 MAJOR COMPLICATIONS OF CIRRHOSIS

Daniel K. Podolsky, Kurt J. Isselbacher

The clinical course of patients with advanced cirrhosis is often complicated by a number of important sequelae that are independent of the etiology of the underlying liver disease. These include portal hypertension and its consequences (e.g., gastroesophageal varices and splenomegaly), ascites, hepatic encephalopathy, spontaneous bacterial peritonitis, hepatorenal syndrome, and hepatocellular carcinoma.

PORTAL HYPERTENSION Definition and Pathogenesis Normal pressure in the portal vein is low (10 to 15 cm saline) because vascular resistance in the hepatic sinusoids is minimal. Portal hypertension (>30 cm saline) most commonly results from increased resistance to portal blood flow. Because the portal venous system lacks valves, resistance at any level between the right side of the heart and splanchnic vessels results in retrograde transmission of an elevated pressure. Increased resistance can occur at three levels relative to the hepatic sinusoids: (1) presinusoidal, (2) sinusoidal, and (3) postsinusoidal. Obstruction in the *presinusoidal* venous compartment may be anatomically outside the liver (e.g., portal vein thrombosis) or within the liver itself but at a functional level proximal to the hepatic sinusoids so that the liver parenchyma is not exposed to the elevated venous pressure (e.g., schistosomiasis).

Postsinusoidal obstruction also may occur outside the liver at the level of the hepatic veins (e.g., Budd-Chiari syndrome), the inferior vena cava, or, less commonly, within the liver (e.g., venoocclusive disease in which the central hepatic venules are the primary site of injury). When cirrhosis is complicated by portal hypertension, the increased resistance is usually *sinusoidal.* While distinctions between pre-, post-, and sinusoidal processes are conceptually appealing, functional resistance to portal flow in a given patient may occur at more than one level. Portal hypertension also may arise from increased blood flow (e.g., massive splenomegaly or arteriovenous fistulas), but the low outflow resistance of the normal liver makes this a rare clinical problem.

Cirrhosis is the most common cause of portal hypertension in the United States. Clinically significant portal hypertension is present in greater than 60 percent of patients with cirrhosis. *Portal vein obstruction* is the second most common cause; it may be idiopathic or occur in association with cirrhosis, infection, pancreatitis, or abdominal trauma. Portal vein thrombosis may develop in a variety of hypercoagulable states including polycythemia vera, essential thrombocythemia, and deficiencies of protein C, protein S, or antithrombin III. Portal vein thrombosis may be idiopathic, though some of these patients may have a subtle myeloproliferative disorder. *Hepatic vein thrombosis* (Budd-Chiari syndrome) and hepatic venoocclusive disease are relatively infrequent causes of portal hypertension (see above). Portal vein occlusion may result in massive hematemesis from gastroesophageal varices, but ascites is usually found only when cirrhosis is present. Noncirrhotic portal fibrosis accounts for only a few cases of portal hypertension.

Clinical Features The major clinical manifestations of portal hypertension include hemorrhage from gastroesophageal varices, splenomegaly with hypersplenism, ascites, and acute and chronic hepatic encephalopathy. These are related, at least in part, to the development of portal-systemic collateral channels. The absence of valves in the portal venous system facilitates retrograde (hepatofugal) blood flow from the high-pressure portal venous system to the lower-pressure systemic venous circulation. Major sites of collateral flow involve the veins around the rectum (hemorrhoids), cardioesophageal junction (esophagogastric varices), retroperitoneal space, and the falciform ligament of the liver (periumbilical or abdominal wall collaterals). Abdominal wall collaterals appear as tortuous epigastric vessels that radiate from the umbilicus toward the xiphoid and rib margins (caput medusae).

Diagnosis In patients with known liver disease, the development of portal hypertension usually becomes evident by the appearance of splenomegaly, ascites, encephalopathy, and/or esophageal varices. Conversely, the finding of any of these features should lead one to evaluate the patient for the presence of underlying portal hypertension and liver disease. Varices are most reliably documented by fiberoptic esophagoscopy; their presence lends indirect support to the diagnosis of portal hypertension. Although rarely necessary, portal venous pressure may be measured directly by percutaneous transhepatic "skinny needle" catheterization or indirectly through transjugular cannulation of the hepatic veins. Both free and wedged hepatic vein pressure (WHVP) should be measured. While WHVP is elevated in sinusoidal and postsinusoidal portal hypertension, including cirrhosis, this measurement is usually normal in presinusoidal portal hypertension. In patients in whom additional information is necessary (e.g., preoperative evaluation before portal-systemic shunt surgery) or when percutaneous catheterization is not feasible, mesenteric and hepatic angiography may be helpful. Particular attention should be directed to the venous phase to assess the patency of the portal vein and the direction of portal blood flow.

Rx TREATMENT

Although treatment is usually directed toward a specific complication of portal hypertension, attempts are sometimes made to reduce the pressure in the portal venous system. Surgical decompression procedures have been used for many years to lower portal pressure in patients with bleeding esophageal varices (see below). However, portal-systemic shunt surgery does not result in improved survival rates in patients with cirrhosis. Decompression can now be accomplished without surgery through the percutaneous placement of a portal-systemic shunt, termed a transjugular intrahepatic portosystemic shunt (TIPS). Beta-adrenergic blockade with propranolol or nadolol reduces portal pressure through vasodilatory effects on both the splanchnic arterial bed and the portal venous system in combination with reduced cardiac output. Such therapy has been shown to be effective in preventing both a first variceal bleed and subsequent episodes after an initial bleed. Treatment of patients with clinically significant sequelae of portal hypertension, especially variceal bleeding, with doses of propranolol titrated to reduce the resting pulse by 25 percent is reasonable if no contraindications exist.

Vigorous treatment of patients with alcoholic hepatitis and cirrhosis, chronic active hepatitis, and other liver diseases may lead to a fall in portal pressure and to a reduction in variceal size. In general, however, portal hypertension due to cirrhosis is not reversible. In appropriately selected patients hepatic transplantation will be beneficial.

VARICEAL BLEEDING

Pathogenesis While vigorous hemorrhage may arise from any portal-systemic venous collaterals, bleeding is most common from varices in the region of the gastroesophageal junction. The factors contributing to bleeding from gastroesophageal varices are not entirely understood but include the degree of portal hypertension and the size of the varices.

Clinical Features and Diagnosis Variceal bleeding often occurs without obvious precipitating factors and usually presents with painless but massive hematemesis with or without melena. Associated signs range from mild postural tachycardia to profound shock, depending on the extent of blood loss and degree of hypovolemia. Because patients with varices may bleed from other gastrointestinal lesions (e.g., peptic ulcer, gastritis), exclusion of other bleeding sources is important even in patients with prior variceal hemorrhage. Fiberoptic endoscopy is the best approach to evaluate upper gastrointestinal hemorrhage in patients with known or suspected portal hypertension.

Rx TREATMENT

(See Fig. 299-1) Variceal bleeding is a life-threatening emergency. Prompt estimation and vigorous replacement of blood loss to maintain intravascular volume are essential and take precedence over diagnostic studies and more specific intervention to stop the bleeding. However, excessive fluid administration can increase portal pressure with resultant further bleeding and should therefore be avoided. Replacement of clotting factors with fresh frozen plasma is important in patients with coagulopathy. Patients are best managed in an intensive care unit and require close monitoring of central venous or pulmonary capillary wedge pressures, urine output, and mental status. Only when the patient is hemodynamically stable should attention be directed toward specific diagnostic studies (especially endoscopy) and other therapeutic modalities to prevent further or recurrent bleeding.

About half of all episodes of variceal hemorrhage cease without intervention, although the risk of rebleeding is very high. The medical management of acute variceal hemorrhage includes the use of vasoconstrictors (vasopressin or somatostatin), balloon tamponade, and endoscopic sclerosis of varices (sclerotherapy) or endoscopic ligation of varices and beta-adrenergic blockade (see Chap. 44). Intravenous infusion of *vasopressin* at a rate of 0.1 to 0.4 U/min results in generalized vasoconstriction leading to diminished blood flow in the portal venous system. Intravenous infusion of vasopressin is as effective as selective intraarterial administration. Control of bleeding can be achieved in up to 80 percent of cases, but bleeding recurs

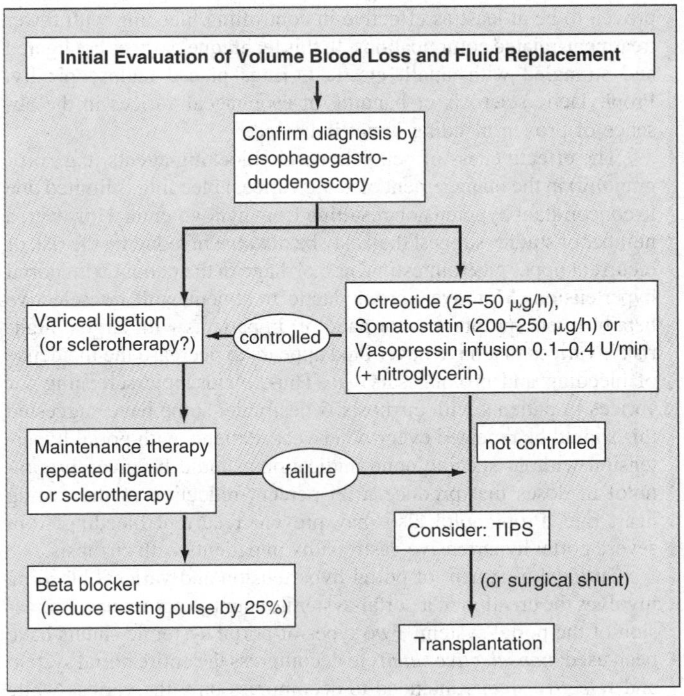

FIGURE 299-1 Approach to the patient with variceal bleeding. Use of a beta blocker is the only intervention demonstrated to offer prophylactic benefit in a patient who has never bled.

in more than half after the vasopressin is tapered and discontinued. Furthermore, a number of serious side effects, including cardiac and gastrointestinal tract ischemia, acute renal failure, and hyponatremia, may be associated with vasopressin therapy. Concurrent use of venodilators such as nitroglycerin as an intravenous infusion or isosorbide dinitrate sublingually may enhance the effectiveness of vasopressin and reduce complications. Somatostatin and its analogue, octreotide, are direct splanchnic vasoconstrictors. In some studies somatostatin, given as an initial 250-μg bolus followed by constant infusion (250 μg/h), has been found to be as effective as vasopressin. Octreotide at doses of 25 to 50 μg/h is also effective. These agents may be preferable to vasopressin, offering equivalent efficacy with fewer complications. If bleeding is too vigorous or endoscopy is not available, *balloon tamponade* of the bleeding varices may be accomplished with a triple-lumen (Sengstaken-Blakemore) or four-lumen (Minnesota) tube with esophageal and gastric balloons. Because of the high risk of aspiration, endotracheal intubation should be performed prior to placing one of these tubes. After the tube is introduced into the stomach, the gastric balloon is inflated and pulled back into the cardia of the stomach. If bleeding does not stop, the esophageal balloon is inflated for additional tamponade. Complications occur in 15 percent or more of patients and include aspiration pneumonitis as well as esophageal rupture.

Where available, *endoscopic intervention* should be employed as the first line of treatment to control bleeding acutely (see Chap. 44). Over the past 15 years, endoscopic sclerosis of varices has been extensively employed. In this procedure, the varices are injected with one of several sclerosing agents via a needle-tipped catheter passed through the endoscope. After endoscopic identification of varices as the presumed source of bleeding, sclerotherapy controls acute bleeding in up to 90 percent of cases. In addition, repeated sclerotherapy can be performed until obliteration of all varices is accomplished in an effort to prevent recurrent bleeding. While available data support the efficacy of sclerotherapy in controlling bleeding acutely, repeated sclerotherapy has not been documented to prolong survival. Mucosal ulceration resulting from injection of the caustic sclerosant may occur and result in further hemorrhage or stenosis. More recently, endoscopic ligation (rubber banding) of varices has proven to be at least as effective in controlling bleeding with fewer treatment-related complications. In this technique, varices are ligated and strangled with small, elastic O-rings placed endoscopically. Prophylactic sclerosis or banding of esophageal varices in the absence of proven bleeding is not indicated.

The effectiveness of beta-adrenergic blocking agents (e.g., propranolol) in the management of acute variceal bleeding is limited due to concomitant hypotension resulting from hypovolemia. However, a number of studies suggest they may be of value in reducing the risk of recurrent upper gastrointestinal hemorrhage in the patient with portal hypertension. Moreover, prophylactic treatment with nonselective beta blockers (propranolol or nadolol) in patients with large ("high-risk") varices that have never bled appears to decrease the incidence of bleeding and prolong survival. Thus, endoscopic screening for varices in patients with cirrhosis is desirable; some have suggested this should be repeated every other year. Patients with portal hypertension without specific contraindications should be given propranolol in doses that produce a 25 percent reduction in the resting heart rate. Propranolol also may prevent recurrent bleeding from severe portal hypertensive gastropathy in patients with cirrhosis.

Surgical treatment of portal hypertension and variceal bleeding involves the creation of a portal-systemic shunt to permit decompression of the portal system. Two types of portal systemic shunts have been used: *nonselective shunts* to decompress the entire portal system and *selective shunts* intended to decompress only the varices while maintaining blood flow to the liver itself. Nonselective shunts include end-to-side or side-to-side portacaval and proximal splenorenal anastomoses; selective shunts include the distal splenorenal shunt. Nonselective shunts are more likely to be complicated by encephalopathy than selective shunts. Emergency portal-systemic nonselective shunts may control acute hemorrhage, but such surgery is usually used only as a last resort because early operative mortality is greater than 30 percent. The role of portal-systemic shunt surgery after initial control of bleeding by nonoperative means is also uncertain. Surgically created shunts effectively reduce the risk of recurrent hemorrhage, but the overall mortality of patients undergoing such surgery is comparable to that of unoperated patients. Although patients who have undergone portal-system surgery succumb to recurrent bleeding less commonly than unoperated patients, this improvement is counterbalanced by increased morbidity from encephalopathy and death from progressive liver failure. Increasingly, therapeutic portal-systemic shunts have been reserved for patients who experience further bleeding despite serial endoscopic sclerotherapy or band ligation. Using TIPS, a technique developed to create a portal-systemic shunt by a percutaneous approach, an expandable metal stent is advanced to the hepatic veins under angiographic guidance and then through the substance of the liver to create a direct portacaval channel. This technique offers an alternative to surgery for refractory bleeding due to portal hypertension, but stents frequently undergo stenosis or occlude over a period of months, prompting the need for a second TIPS or an alternative approach. Encephalopathy may be encountered after TIPS just as in the surgical shunts. Procedures such as esophageal transection also have been advocated for the management of acute variceal bleeding, but their efficacy remains unproven. Even though recent trials found that esophageal transection was as effective as endoscopic sclerotherapy, transection is usually considered a last resort.

Portal Hypertensive Gastropathy Although variceal hemorrhage is the most commonly encountered bleeding complication of portal hypertension, many patients will develop a congestive gastropathy due to the venous hypertension. In this condition, identified by endoscopic examination, the mucosa appears engorged and friable. Indolent mucosal bleeding occurs rather than the brisk hemorrhage typical of a variceal source. Beta-adrenergic blockade with propranolol (reducing splanchnic arterial pressure as well as portal pressure) is sometimes effective in ameliorating this condition. H_2 receptor antagonists or other agents useful in the treatment of peptic disease are usually not helpful.

SPLENOMEGALY Definition and Pathogenesis Congestive splenomegaly is common in patients with severe portal hypertension. Rarely, massive splenomegaly from nonhepatic disease leads to portal hypertension due to increased blood flow in the splenic vein.

Clinical Features Although usually asymptomatic, splenomegaly may be massive and contribute to the thrombocytopenia or pancytopenia of cirrhosis. In the absence of cirrhosis, splenomegaly in association with variceal hemorrhage should suggest the possibility of splenic vein thrombosis.

TREATMENT

Splenomegaly usually requires no specific treatment, although massive enlargement of the spleen may occasionally necessitate splenectomy at the time of shunt surgery. However, it should be noted that splenectomy without an accompanying shunt may actually increase portal pressure. Splenectomy also may be indicated if splenomegaly is the cause rather than the result of portal hypertension. Thrombocytopenia alone is rarely severe enough to necessitate removal of the spleen.

ASCITES Definition Ascites is the accumulation of excess fluid within the peritoneal cavity. It is most frequently encountered in patients with cirrhosis and other forms of severe liver disease, but a number of other disorders may lead to either transudative or exudative ascites (see Chap. 46).

Pathogenesis The accumulation of ascitic fluid represents a state of total-body sodium and water excess, but the event that initiates this imbalance is unclear. Three theories have been proposed (see Fig.

299-1). The "underfilling" theory suggests that the primary abnormality is inappropriate sequestration of fluid within the splanchnic vascular bed due to portal hypertension and a consequent decrease in effective circulating blood volume. According to this theory, an apparent decrease in intravascular volume (underfilling) is sensed by the kidney, which responds by retaining salt and water. The "overflow" theory suggests that the primary abnormality is inappropriate renal retention of salt and water in the absence of volume depletion. A third theory, the peripheral arterial vasodilation hypothesis, has been proposed to account for the constellation of arterial hypotension and increased cardiac output in association with high levels of vasoconstrictor substances that are routinely found in patients with cirrhosis and ascites. Again, sodium retention is considered secondary to arterial vascular underfilling and the result of a disproportionate increase of the vascular compartment due to arteriolar vasodilation rather than from decreased intravascular volume. According to this theory, portal hypertension results in splanchnic arteriolar vasodilation, possibly mediated by nitric oxide, and leading to underfilling of the arterial vascular space and baroreceptor-mediated stimulation of renin-angiotensin, sympathetic output, and antidiuretic hormone release.

Regardless of the initiating event, a number of factors contribute to accumulation of fluid in the abdominal cavity (see Fig. 299-2). Elevated levels of serum epinephrine and norepinephrine have been well documented. *Increased central sympathetic outflow* is found in patients with cirrhosis and ascites but not in those with cirrhosis alone. Increased sympathetic output results in diminished natriuresis by activation of the renin-angiotensin system and diminished sensitivity to atrial natriuretic peptide. *Portal hypertension* plays an important role in the formation of ascites by raising hydrostatic pressure within the splanchnic capillary bed. *Hypoalbuminemia* and *reduced plasma oncotic pressure* also favor the extravasation of fluid from plasma to the peritoneal cavity, and thus ascites is infrequent in patients with cirrhosis unless both portal hypertension and hypoalbuminemia are present. *Hepatic lymph* may weep freely from the surface of the cirrhotic liver due to distortion and obstruction of hepatic sinusoids and lymphatics and contribute to ascites formation. In contrast to the contribution of transudative fluid from the portal vascular bed, hepatic lymph may weep into the peritoneal cavity even in the absence of marked hypoproteinemia because the endothelial lining of the hepatic sinusoids is discontinuous. This mechanism may account for the high protein concentration present in the ascitic fluid of some patients with the Budd-Chiari syndrome.

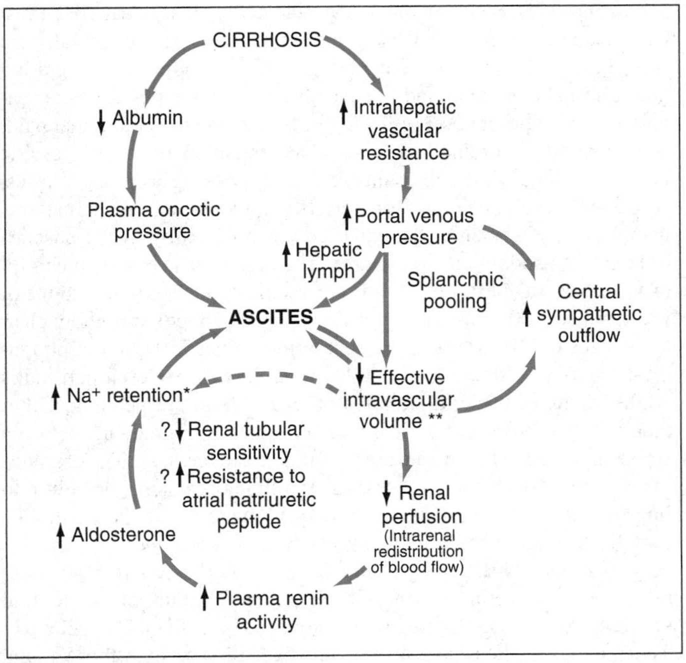

FIGURE 299-2 Multiple factors involved in development of ascites. Current concepts suggest that initiating factor may be primary sodium retention (*"overflow"), diminished effective intravascular volume (**"underfilling"), or arteriolar vasodilation.

Renal factors also play an important role in perpetuating ascites. Patients with ascites fail to excrete a water load in a normal fashion. They have increased renal sodium reabsorption by both proximal and distal tubules, the latter due largely to increased plasma renin activity and secondary hyperaldosteronism. Insensitivity to circulating atrial natriuretic peptide, often present in elevated concentrations in patients with cirrhosis and ascites, may be an important contributory factor in many patients. This insensitivity has been documented in those patients with the most severely impaired sodium excretion, who typically also exhibit low arterial pressure and marked overactivity of the renin-aldosterone axis. Renal vasoconstriction, perhaps resulting from increased serum prostaglandin or catecholamine levels, also may contribute to sodium retention. Recently a role for endothelin, a potent vasoconstrictor peptide, has been proposed. While elevated levels have been reported by some, this has not been observed by others.

As discussed in Chap. 46, ascites may arise in a number of clinical settings in addition to cirrhosis and portal hypertension. Although historically ascites was classified as either transudative or exudative, similar to the characterization of pleural fluids, this schema has limitations. Instead, the serum-ascites albumin gradient (SAAG) provides a better classification than total protein content or other parameters. Ascites resulting from cirrhosis typically has a high SAAG (>1.1 g/dL), reflecting indirectly the abnormally high hydrostatic pressure gradient between the portal bed and the ascitic compartment.

Clinical Features and Diagnosis Usually ascites is first noticed by the patient because of increasing abdominal girth. More pronounced accumulation of fluid may cause shortness of breath because of elevation of the diaphragm. When peritoneal fluid accumulation exceeds 500 mL, ascites may be demonstrated on physical examination by the presence of shifting dullness, a fluid wave, or bulging flanks. Ultrasound examination, preferably with a Doppler study, can detect smaller quantities of ascites and should be performed when physical examination is equivocal or when the cause of the recent onset of ascites is not clear (e.g., exclude Budd-Chiari syndrome or portal vein thrombosis).

℞ TREATMENT

(See Fig. 299-3) A thorough search should be made for precipitating factors in the patient with recent onset of or worsening ascites, e.g., excessive salt intake, medication noncompliance, superimposed infection, worsening liver disease, portal vein thrombosis, or development of hepatocellular carcinoma. When ascites develops in the setting of severe, acute liver disease, resolution of ascites is likely to follow improvement in liver function. More commonly, ascites develops in patients with stable or steadily worsening liver function. Paracentesis usually should be performed with a small-gauge needle at the time of initial evaluation or at the time of any clinical deterioration of a cirrhotic patient with ascites. A small amount of fluid (<200 mL) should be obtained and examined for evidence of infection, tumor, or other possible causes and complications of ascites. Therapeutic intervention is indicated both to prevent potential complications and to control progressive increase in ascites, which may become pronounced enough to cause physical discomfort. For the patient with a modest accumulation, therapy can be undertaken as an outpatient and should be gentle and incremental (see below). The goal is the loss of no more than 1.0 kg/d if both ascites and peripheral edema are present and no more than 0.5 kg/d in patients with ascites alone. In some patients, particularly those with a large accumulation of fluid, it may be desirable to hospitalize the patient so that daily weights and frequent serum electrolyte levels can be monitored and compliance ensured. Although abdominal girth measurements are frequently used as an index of fluid loss, they tend to be unreliable.

Strict bed rest is often recommended because of improved renal clearance in the supine position. However, salt restriction is the most important cornerstone of therapy. A diet containing 800 mg sodium

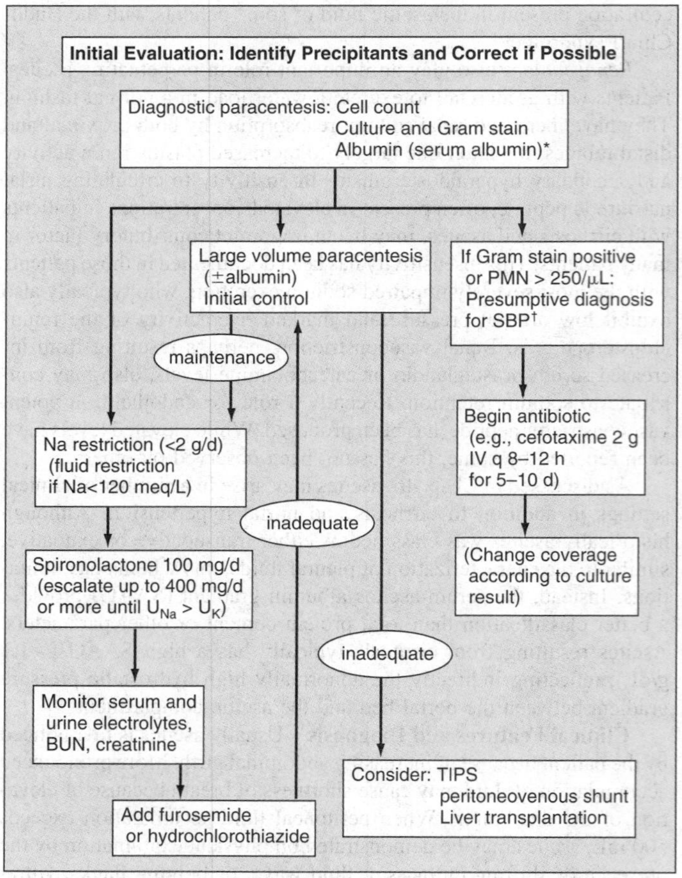

FIGURE 299-3 Approach to the patient with ascites [and spontaneous bacterial peritonitis (SBP)]. PMN, polymorphonuclear leukocytes; TIPS, transjugular intrahepatic portosystemic shunt. *Calculate SAAG [serum ascites albumin gradient = serum albumin − ascites albumin (g/dL)] to confirm high gradient (>1.1 g/dL) in portal hypertension. †If PMN > 250/μL but culture is negative = culture negative neutrocytic ascites; begin empiric antibiotic and retap at 48 h; if culture is positive but PMN < 250/μL normal = monomicrobial nonneutrocytic bacterascites; retap; treat if PMN > 250/μL; if polymicrobial infection, exclude secondary peritonitis.

(2 g NaCl) is often adequate to induce a negative sodium balance and permit diuresis. Response to salt restriction and bed rest alone is more likely to occur if the ascites is of recent onset, the underlying liver disease is reversible, a precipitating factor can be corrected, or the patient has a high urinary sodium excretion (~25 mmol/d) and normal renal function. Fluid restriction of approximately 1000 mL/d does little to enhance diuresis but may be necessary to correct hyponatremia. If sodium restriction alone fails to result in diuresis and weight loss, diuretics should be prescribed. Because of the role of hyperaldosteronism in sustaining salt retention, spironolactone or other distal tubule–acting diuretics (triamterene, amiloride) are the drugs of choice. These agents are also preferred because of their gentle action and specific potassium-sparing properties. Spironolactone is initially given in a dose of 25 mg four times a day and is increased as needed by 100 mg/d every several days to a maximum dose that should rarely exceed 400 mg/d. An indication of the minimum effective dose of spironolactone may be obtained by monitoring urinary electrolyte concentrations for a rise in sodium and fall in potassium levels, reflecting effective competitive inhibition of aldosterone. Conversely, the development of azotemia or hyperkalemia may be dose-limiting or even warrant a reduction in the amount of this medication. In some patients, diuresis cannot be initiated despite maximal doses of distal tubule–acting agents (e.g., 400 mg spironolactone) because of avid proximal tubular sodium absorption. More potent and proximally acting diuretics (furosemide, thiazide, or ethacrynic acid) may then be added cautiously to the regimen. Spironolactone plus furosemide, 20 or 80 mg/d, is usually sufficient to initiate a diuresis in most patients. However, such aggressive therapy must be used with great caution to avoid plasma volume depletion, azotemia, and hypokalemia, which may lead to encephalopathy.

In patients with pronounced ascites, particularly those requiring hospitalization, large-volume paracentesis has proven to be an effective and less costly approach to initial management than prolonged bed rest and conventional diuretic treatment. In this approach, ascitic fluid is removed by peritoneal cannula using strict aseptic techniques and monitoring hemodynamic and renal function. This can be safely accomplished in a single session. The need for concomitant albumin replacement by intravenous infusion remains controversial but may be prudent in the patient without peripheral edema, to avoid depleting the intravascular space and precipitating hypotension. Maintenance diuretic therapy in conjunction with sodium restriction may then be instituted to avoid recurrent ascites.

A minority of patients with advanced cirrhosis have "refractory ascites" or rapidly reaccumulate fluid after control by paracentesis. In some patients, a side-to-side *portacaval shunt* may result in improvement in ascites, although generally these patients are extremely poor surgical risks. In the past, intractable ascites has also been treated with the surgical implantation of a plastic *peritoneovenous shunt*, which has a pressure-sensitive, one-way valve allowing ascitic fluid to flow from the abdominal cavity to the superior vena cava. However, the usefulness of this technique is limited by a high rate of complications such as infection, disseminated intravascular coagulation, and thrombosis of the shunt. More recently, TIPS has been used effectively to control refractory ascites, although portal decompression, while mobilizing ascitic fluid, has precipitated severe hepatic encephalopathy in some patients.

SPONTANEOUS BACTERIAL PERITONITIS (SBP) Patients with ascites and cirrhosis may develop acute bacterial peritonitis without an obvious primary source of infection. Patients with very advanced liver disease are particularly susceptible to SBP. The ascitic fluid in these patients typically has especially low concentrations of albumin and other so-called opsonic proteins, which normally may provide some protection against bacteria. Although key steps in the pathogenesis of SBP remain to be elucidated, it is clear that most bacteria contributing to SBP derive from the bowel and eventually are spread to ascitic fluid by the hematogenous route after transmigration through the bowel wall and transversing the lymphatics. Typical features include abrupt onset of fever, chills, generalized abdominal pain, and rebound abdominal tenderness accompanied by cloudy ascitic fluid with a high white cell count and usually positive bacterial cultures. However, the clinical symptoms *may be minimal*, and some patients manifest only worsening jaundice or encephalopathy in the absence of localizing abdominal complaints. The diagnosis is based on careful examination of the ascitic fluid. An ascitic fluid leukocyte count of greater than 500 cells/μL (with a proportion of polymorphonuclear leukocytes of 50 percent or greater) or more than 250 polymorphonuclear leukocytes should suggest the possibility of bacterial peritonitis while results of bacterial cultures of ascitic fluid are pending. Other measurements such as fluid pH or determination of gradients between serum and fluid pH or lactate are generally not necessary. The presence of more than 10,000 leukocytes/μL, multiple organisms, or failure to improve after standard therapy for 48 h suggest that the peritonitis may be secondary to an infection elsewhere in the body.

A variant of SBP, designated *monomicrobial nonneutrocytic bacterascites*, is sometimes seen. In these patients, culture of ascitic fluid yields bacteria, but the neutrophil count is less than 250 cells/μL. These patients often have less severe liver disease than those found initially to have typical SBP. While many patients with this variant have cleared the bacterascites at the time of a subsequent paracentesis, nearly 40 percent will develop typical SBP; thus follow-up paracentesis is usually warranted in this setting.

℞ TREATMENT

Empirical therapy with cefotaxime or ampicillin and an aminoglycoside should be initiated when the diagnosis is first suspected because enteric gram-negative bacilli are found in the majority of cases; less frequently, the infection is caused by pneumococci and other gram-positive bacteria. Cefotaxime may be preferable due to the lower rate of renal toxicity. Specific antibiotic therapy can be selected once the specific organism is identified. Therapy is usually administered for 10 to 14 days, although one controlled study has suggested that a 5-day course of intravenous antibiotics may be as effective when repeat paracentesis at 48 h demonstrates a decline in the ascitic polymorphonuclear leukocytes count by more than 50 percent and negative cultures.

While appropriate antibiotic therapy is usually effective in the treatment of an episode of SBP, recurrent episodes are relatively common; as many as 70 percent of patients will experience at least one recurrence within a year of the first episode. The risk of recurrence likely reflects the predisposing role of the underlying advanced liver disease that contributed to the development of the first episode of SBP. Recent trials have demonstrated that prophylactic maintenance therapy with norfloxacin (400 mg/d) can reduce the frequency of recurrent SBP. This agent presumably causes elective decontamination of the intestine, eliminating many aerobic gram-negative bacilli. Trimethoprim-sulfamethoxazole given for 5 days a week has also proven effective. Antibiotics may be administered as infrequently as once a week (e.g., ciprofloxacin, 750 mg once weekly). While maintenance therapy reduces the frequency of SBP and need for hospitalization, it is unclear whether this is associated with prolonged survival.

HEPATORENAL SYNDROME **Definition and Pathogenesis** Hepatorenal syndrome is a serious complication in the patient with cirrhosis and ascites and is characterized by worsening azotemia with avid sodium retention and oliguria in the absence of identifiable specific causes of renal dysfunction. The exact basis for this syndrome is not clear, but altered renal hemodynamics appear to be involved. The kidneys are structurally intact; urinalysis and pyelography are usually normal. Renal biopsy, although rarely needed, is also normal, and in fact, kidneys from such patients have been used successfully for renal transplantation. There are indications that an imbalance in certain metabolites of arachidonic acid (prostaglandins and thromboxane) may play a pathogenetic role.

Clinical Features and Diagnosis Worsening azotemia, hyponatremia, progressive oliguria, and hypotension are the hallmarks of the hepatorenal syndrome. This syndrome, which is distinct from prerenal azotemia, may be precipitated by severe gastrointestinal bleeding, sepsis, or overly vigorous attempts at diuresis or paracentesis; it also may occur without an obvious cause. It is essential to exclude other causes of renal impairment often seen in these patients. These include prerenal azotemia or acute tubular necrosis due to hypovolemia (e.g., secondary to gastrointestinal bleeding or diuretic therapy) or an increased nitrogen load such as that seen as a result of bleeding. Drug nephrotoxicity is also often a consideration, particularly in the patient who has received agents such as aminoglycosides or contrast dye. The diagnosis is supported by the demonstration of avid urinary sodium retention. Typically, the urine sodium concentration is less than 5 mmol/L, a concentration lower than that generally found in uncomplicated prerenal azotemia. The urinary sediment is unremarkable.

℞ TREATMENT

Treatment is usually unsuccessful. Although some patients with hypotension and decreased plasma volume may respond to infusions of salt-poor albumin, volume expansion must be undertaken with caution to avoid precipitating variceal bleeding. Vasodilator therapy, including intravenous infusion of dopamine, is not effective.

HEPATIC ENCEPHALOPATHY **Definition** Hepatic (portal-systemic) encephalopathy is a complex neuropsychiatric syndrome characterized by disturbances in consciousness and behavior, personality changes, fluctuating neurologic signs, asterixis or "flapping tremor," and distinctive electroencephalographic changes. Encephalopathy may be *acute* and reversible or *chronic* and progressive. In severe cases, irreversible coma and death may occur. Acute episodes may recur with variable frequency.

Pathogenesis The specific cause of hepatic encephalopathy is unknown. The most important factors in the pathogenesis are severe hepatocellular dysfunction and/or intrahepatic and extrahepatic shunting of portal venous blood into the systemic circulation so that the liver is largely bypassed. As a result of these processes, various toxic substances absorbed from the intestine are not detoxified by the liver and lead to metabolic abnormalities in the central nervous system (CNS). Ammonia is the substance most often incriminated in the pathogenesis of encephalopathy. Many, but not all, patients with hepatic encephalopathy have elevated blood ammonia levels, and recovery from encephalopathy is often accompanied by declining blood ammonia levels. Other compounds and metabolites that may contribute to the development of encephalopathy include mercaptans (derived from intestinal metabolism of methionine), short-chain fatty acids, and phenol. Several observations suggest that excessive concentrations of gamma-aminobutyric acid (GABA), an inhibitory neurotransmitter, in the CNS are important in the reduced levels of consciousness seen in hepatic encephalopathy. Increased CNS GABA may reflect failure of the liver to extract precursor amino acids efficiently or to remove GABA produced in the intestine. False neurochemical transmitters (e.g., octopamine), resulting in part from alterations in plasma levels of aromatic and branched-chain amino acids, also may play a role. An increase in the permeability of the blood-brain barrier to some of these substances may be an additional factor involved in the pathogenesis of hepatic encephalopathy. There is also evidence to suggest that endogenous benzodiazepines may contribute to the development of hepatic encephalopathy. This evidence includes isolation of 1,4-benzodiazepines from brain tissue of patients with fulminant hepatic failure as well as the partial response observed in some patients and experimental animals after administration of flumazenil, a benzodiazepine antagonist. The benzodiazepine receptor is closely associated with the GABA receptor and may facilitate GABA neurotransmission. However, the inconsistent effect of flumazenil in patients with encephalopathy, as well as potential methodologic pitfalls in the measurement of endogenous benzodiazepines, precludes definitive attribution of a role to these substances in the pathogenesis of hepatic encephalopathy.

In the patient with otherwise stable cirrhosis, hepatic encephalopathy often follows a clearly identifiable precipitating event (see Table 299-1). Perhaps the most common predisposing factor is *gastrointestinal bleeding*, which leads to an increase in the production of ammonia

Table 299-1

Common Precipitants of Hepatic Encephalopathy

Increased Nitrogen Load
Gastrointestinal bleeding
Excess dietary protein
Azotemia
Constipation
Electrolyte and Metabolic Imbalance
Hypokalemia
Alkalosis
Hypoxia
Hyponatremia
Drugs
Narcotics, tranquilizers, sedatives
Diuretics (see "Electrolyte imbalance")
Miscellaneous
Infection
Surgery
Superimposed acute liver disease
Progressive liver disease

and other nitrogenous substances which are then absorbed. Similarly, *increased dietary protein* may precipitate encephalopathy as a result of increased production of nitrogenous substances by colonic bacteria. *Electrolyte disturbances*, particularly hypokalemic alkalosis secondary to overzealous use of diuretics, vigorous paracentesis, or vomiting, may precipitate hepatic encephalopathy. Systemic alkalosis causes an increase in the amount of nonionic ammonia (NH_3) relative to ammonium ions (NH_4^+). Only nonionic (uncharged) ammonia readily crosses the blood-brain barrier and accumulates in the central nervous system. Hypokalemia also directly stimulates renal ammonia production. Hypoxia, injudicious use of CNS-depressing drugs (e.g., barbiturates, benzodiazepines), and acute infection may trigger or aggravate hepatic encephalopathy, although the mechanisms involved are not clear. Other potential precipitating factors include superimposed acute viral hepatitis, alcoholic hepatitis, extrahepatic bile duct obstruction, surgery, and other coincidental medical complications.

Clinical Features and Diagnosis Hepatic encephalopathy has protean manifestations, and any neurologic abnormality, including focal deficits, may be encountered. In patients with acute encephalopathy, neurologic deficits are completely reversible upon correction of underlying precipitating factors and/or improvement in liver function, but in patients with chronic encephalopathy, the deficits may be irreversible and progressive. Cerebral edema is frequently present and contributes to the clinical picture and overall mortality in patients with both acute and chronic encephalopathy.

The diagnosis of hepatic encephalopathy should be considered when four major factors are present: (1) acute or chronic hepatocellular disease and/or extensive portal-systemic collateral shunts (the latter may be either spontaneous, e.g., secondary to portal hypertension, or surgically created, e.g., portacaval anastomosis); (2) disturbances of awareness and mentation, which may progress from forgetfulness and confusion to stupor and finally coma; (3) shifting combinations of neurologic signs, including asterixis, rigidity, hyperreflexia, extensor plantar signs, and rarely, seizures; and (4) a characteristic (but nonspecific) symmetric, high-voltage, slow-wave (2 to 5 per second) pattern on the electroencephalogram. Asterixis ("liver flap," "flapping tremor") is a nonrhythmic asymmetric lapse in voluntary sustained position of the extremities, head, and trunk. It is best demonstrated by having the patient extend the arms and dorsiflex the hands. Because elicitation of asterixis depends on sustained voluntary muscle contraction, it is not present in the comatose patient. Asterixis is nonspecific and also occurs in patients with other forms of metabolic brain disease. Disturbances of sleep with reversal of sleep/wake cycles are among the earliest signs of encephalopathy. Alterations in personality, mood disturbances, confusion, deterioration in self-care and handwriting, and daytime somnolence are additional clinical features of encephalopathy. *Fetor hepaticus*, a unique musty odor of the breath and urine believed to be due to mercaptans, may be noted in patients with varying stages of hepatic encephalopathy. Some patients may develop spastic paraparesis or *chronic progressive hepatocerebral degeneration*, the latter a clinical variant of hepatic encephalopathy characterized by a slow decline in intellectual function, tremor, cerebellar ataxia, choreoathetosis, and psychiatric symptoms.

Grading or classifying the stages of hepatic encephalopathy is often helpful in following the course of the illness and assessing response to therapy. One useful classification is shown in Table 299-2.

The diagnosis of hepatic encephalopathy is usually one of exclusion. There are no diagnostic liver function test abnormalities, although an elevated serum ammonia level in the appropriate clinical setting is highly suggestive of the diagnosis. Examination of the cerebrospinal fluid is unremarkable, and computed tomography of the brain shows no characteristic abnormalities. A number of conditions, particularly disorders related to acute and chronic alcoholism, can mimic the clinical features of hepatic encephalopathy. These include acute alcohol intoxication, sedative overdose, delirium tremens, Wernicke's encephalopathy, and Korsakoff's psychosis (see Chap. 379). Subdural hematoma, meningitis, and hypoglycemia or other metabolic encephalopathies also must be considered, especially in patients with alcoholic cirrhosis. In young patients with liver disease and neurologic abnormalities, Wilson's disease should be excluded.

Table 299-2

Clinical Stages of Hepatic Encephalopathy

Stage	Mental Status	Asterixis	EEG
I	Euphoria or depression, mild confusion, slurred speech, disordered sleep	+/−	Usually normal
II	Lethargy, moderate confusion	+	Abnormal
III	Marked confusion, incoherent speech, sleeping but arousable	+	Abnormal
IV	Coma; initially responsive to noxious stimuli, later unresponsive	−	Abnormal

Rx TREATMENT

(See Fig. 299-4) Early recognition and prompt treatment of hepatic encephalopathy are essential. Patients with acute, severe hepatic encephalopathy (stage IV) require the usual supportive measures for the comatose patient. Specific treatment of hepatic encephalopathy is aimed at (1) elimination or treatment of precipitating factors and (2) lowering of blood ammonia (and other toxin) levels by decreasing the absorption of protein and nitrogenous products from the intestine. In the setting of acute gastrointestinal bleeding, blood in the bowel should be promptly evacuated with laxatives (and enemas if necessary) in order to reduce the nitrogen load. Protein should be excluded from the diet, and constipation should be avoided. Ammonia absorption can be decreased by the administration of lactulose, a nonabsorbable disaccharide that acts as an osmotic laxative. Metabolism of lactulose by colonic bacteria also may result in an acid pH that favors conversion of ammonia to the poorly absorbed ammonium ion. In addition, lactulose may actually diminish ammonia production through its direct effects on bacterial metabolism. Acutely, lactulose syrup can be administered in a dose of 30 to 50 mL every hour until diarrhea occurs; thereafter the dose is adjusted (usually 15 to 30 mL three times daily) so that the patient has two to four soft stools daily.

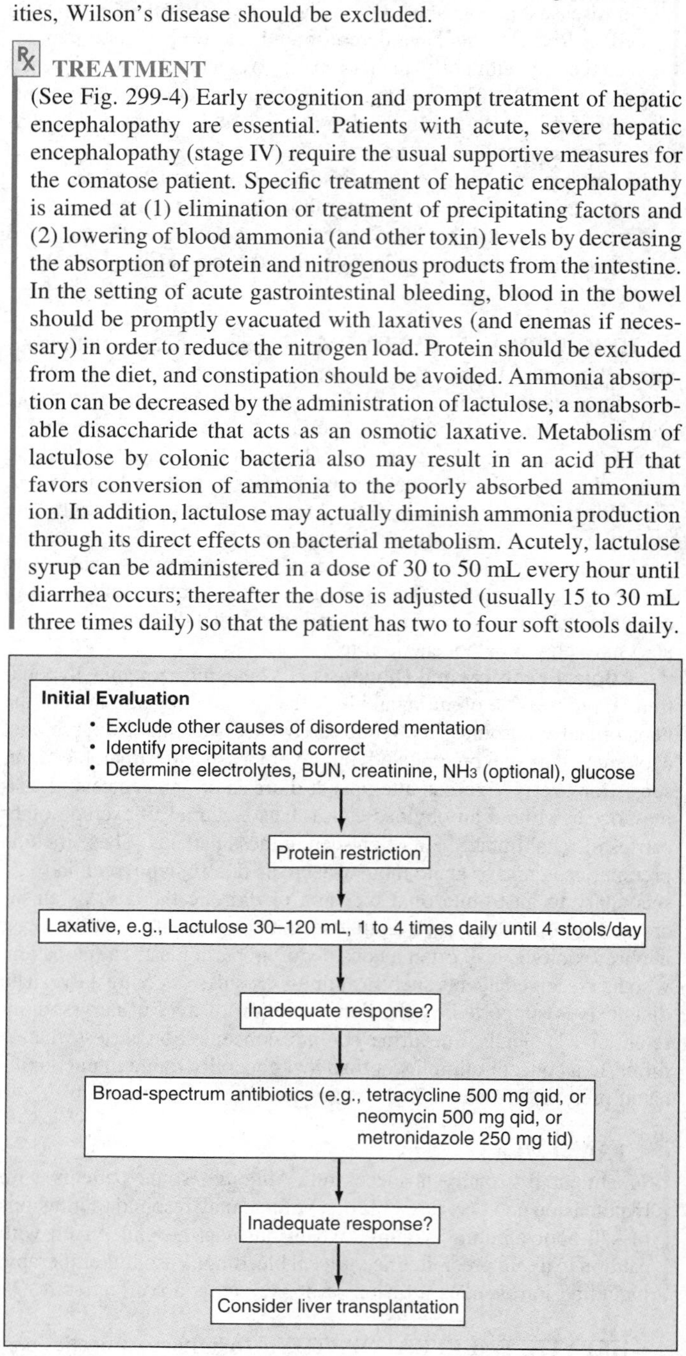

Initial Evaluation
• Exclude other causes of disordered mentation
• Identify precipitants and correct
• Determine electrolytes, BUN, creatinine, NH3 (optional), glucose
Protein restriction
Laxative, e.g., Lactulose 30–120 mL, 1 to 4 times daily until 4 stools/day
Inadequate response?
Broad-spectrum antibiotics (e.g., tetracycline 500 mg qid, or neomycin 500 mg qid, or metronidazole 250 mg tid)
Inadequate response?
Consider liver transplantation

FIGURE 299-4 Approach to the patient with hepatic encephalopathy.

Intestinal ammonia production by bacteria also can be decreased by oral administration of a "nonabsorbable" antibiotic such as neomycin (0.5 to 1.0 g every 6 h). However, despite poor absorption, neomycin may reach sufficient concentrations in the bloodstream to cause real toxicity. Equal benefits may be achieved with broad-spectrum antibiotics such as tetracycline, ampicillin, or metronidazole. The use of agents such as levodopa, bromocriptine, keto analogues of essential amino acids, and intravenous amino acid formulations rich in branched-chain amino acids in the treatment of acute hepatic encephalopathy remains of unproven benefit. Flumazenil, a short-acting benzodiazepine antagonist, may have a role in management of hepatic encephalopathy precipitated by use of benzodiazepines, if there is a need for urgent therapy. Hemoperfusion to remove toxic substances and therapy directed primarily toward coincident cerebral edema in acute encephalopathy are also of unproven value.

Chronic encephalopathy may be effectively controlled by administration of lactulose. Management of patients with chronic encephalopathy should include dietary protein restriction (usually to 60 g/d) in combination with low doses of lactulose or neomycin. Nephrotoxicity or ototoxicity may be limiting in prolonged usage of neomycin. There are suggestions that vegetable protein may be preferable to animal protein.

OTHER SEQUELAE OF CIRRHOSIS **Coagulopathy** Patients with cirrhosis often demonstrate a variety of abnormalities in both cellular and humoral clotting function. Thrombocytopenia may result from hypersplenism. In the alcoholic patient, there may be direct bone marrow suppression by ethanol. Diminished protein synthesis may lead to reduced production of fibrinogen (factor I), prothrombin (factor II), and factors V, VII, IX, and X. Reduction in levels of all factors except factor V may be worsened by the coincident malabsorption of the fat-soluble cofactor vitamin K due to cholestasis (see Chap. 285). Recent reports have documented the appearance of normal factor VIII levels following liver transplantation in patients with classical hemophilia, probably as a result of production by nonhepatocellular components of the donor organ.

Hepatocellular Carcinoma See Chap. 93.

HYPOXEMIA AND HEPATOPULMONARY SYNDROME

Definition and Pathogenesis Mild hypoxemia occurs in approximately one-third of patients with chronic liver disease. The hepatopulmonary syndrome is manifest by dyspnea, platypnea, and orthopnea. Hypoxemia results from right-to-left intrapulmonary shunts through dilatations in intrapulmonary vessels that can be detected by contrast-enhanced echocardiography.

℞ TREATMENT

No specific treatment is consistently effective, though large arteriovenous shunts may be embolized.

BIBLIOGRAPHY

HEPATIC ENCEPHALOPATHY

BASILE AS et al: Elevated brain concentrations of 1,4-benzodiazepines in fulminant hepatic failure. N Engl J Med 325:473, 1991

FRASER CL, ARIEFF AI: Hepatic encephalopathy. N Engl J Med 313:865, 1985

JALAN R et al: Review article: Pathogenesis and treatment of chronic hepatic encephalopathy. Aliment Pharmacol Ther 10:681, 1996

JONES EA et al: The neurobiology of hepatic encephalopathy. Hepatology 4:1235, 1984

MORGAN MY, HAWLEY KE: Lactitol vs. lactulose in the treatment of acute hepatic encephalopathy in cirrhotic patients: A double-blind randomized study. Hepatology 7:1278, 1987

SKOLNICK P: The γ-aminobutyric acid A ($GABA_A$)-benzodiazepine receptor complex, pp 534–536, in, Jones EA, moderator: The γ-aminobutyric A ($GABA_A$) receptor complex and hepatic encephalopathy: Some recent advances. Ann Intern Med 110:532, 1989

VARICEAL HEMORRHAGE

LAINE L et al: Endoscopic ligation compared with sclerotherapy for treatment of esophageal variceal bleeding: A meta-analysis. Ann Intern Med 123:280, 1995

——— et al: Endoscopic ligation compared with sclerotherapy for the treatment of bleeding esophageal varices. Ann Intern Med 119:1, 1993

LO G-H et al: A prospective, randomized trial of sclerotherapy versus ligation in the management of bleeding esophageal varices. Hepatology 22:466, 1995

PAGLIARO L et al: Prevention of first bleeding in cirrhosis: A meta-analysis of randomized trials of nonsurgical treatment. Ann Intern Med 117:59, 1992

PLANAS R et al: A prospective randomized trial comparing somatostatin and sclerotherapy in the treatment of acute variceal bleeding. Hepatology 20:370, 1994

STIEGMANN GV et al: Endoscopic sclerotherapy as compared with endoscopic ligation for bleeding esophageal varices. N Engl J Med 326:1527, 1992

SUNG JJY et al: Octreotide infusion or emergency sclerotherapy for variceal haemorrhage. Lancet 342:637, 1993

PORTAL HYPERTENSION AND ASCITES

D'AMICO G et al: The treatment of portal hypertension: A meta-analytic review. Hepatology 22:332, 1995

FLORAS JS et al: Increased sympathetic outflow in cirrhosis and ascites: Direct evidence from intraneural recordings. Ann Intern Med 114:373, 1991

GINÉS P et al: Comparison of paracentesis and diuretics in the treatment of cirrhotics with tense ascites: Results of a randomized study. Gastroenterology 93:234, 1987

——— et al: Paracentesis with intravenous infusion of albumin as compared with peritoneovenous shunting in cirrhosis with refractory ascites. N Engl J Med 325:829, 1991

——— et al: Incidence, predictive factors, and prognosis of the hepatorenal syndrome in cirrhosis with ascites. Gastroenterology 105:229, 1993

JAFFE D et al: Management of portal hypertension and its complications. Med Clin North Am 80:1021, 1996

OCHES A et al: The transjugular intrahepatic portosystemic stent-shunt procedure for refractory ascites. N Engl J Med 332:1192, 1995

PINTO PC et al: Large-volume paracentesis in nonedematous patients with tense ascites: Its effect on intravascular volume. Hepatology 8:207, 1988

PYNARD T et al: Beta-adrenergic-antagonist drugs in the prevention of gastrointestinal bleeding in patients with cirrhosis and esophageal varices. N Engl J Med 324:1532, 1991

RING EJ et al: Using transjugular intrahepatic portosystemic shunts to control variceal bleeding before liver transplantation. Ann Intern Med 116:304, 1992

STANLEY AJ et al: Long-term follow up of transjugular mitrahepatic portosystemic stent shunt (TIPSS) for the treatment of portal hypertension: Results in 130 patients. Gut 39:479, 1996

STIEGMANN GV et al: Endoscopic sclerotherapy as compared with endoscopic ligation for bleeding esophageal varices. N Engl J Med 326:1527, 1992

SPONTANEOUS BACTERIAL PERITONITIS

NAVASA M et al: Randomized, comparative study of oral ofloxacin versus intravenous cefotaxime in spontaneous bacterial peritonitis. Gastroenterology 111:1011, 1996

ROLACHON A et al: Ciprofloxacin and long-term prevention of spontaneous bacterial peritonitis: Results of a prospective controlled trial. Hepatology 22:1171, 1995

RUNYON BA et al: Short-course versus long-course antibiotic treatment of spontaneous bacterial peritonitis: A randomized controlled study of 100 patients. Gastroenterology 100:1737, 1991

300

Kurt J. Isselbacher, Daniel K. Podolsky

INFILTRATIVE AND METABOLIC DISEASES AFFECTING THE LIVER

Many disseminated, systemic, or metabolic diseases involve the liver in a diffuse manner by the infiltration of abnormal cells or the accumulation of chemical substances or metabolites. Chemical accumulation may be extracellular or intracellular and may involve hepatocytes, Kupffer cells, or other elements of the reticuloendothelial system. Although infiltrative diseases may vary widely in cause and extrahepatic manifestations, the findings in the liver may be quite similar.

Generalized enlargement and firmness of the liver, gradual and nonspecific deterioration of liver function, and, less often, signs of portal hypertension or ascites are typical features of this group of diseases. Differential diagnosis by clinical means may be difficult on occasion, but in patients in whom ancillary clinical findings do not establish the diagnosis, the diffusely infiltrated liver provides an excellent source of tissue for diagnostic purposes.

HEPATIC STEATOSIS (FATTY LIVER) AND STEATOHEPATITIS (See also Chap. 293)

Slight to moderate enlargement of the liver due to a diffuse accumulation of neutral fat (triglycerides) in hepatocytes is an important clinical and pathologic finding. Imaging techniques such as computed tomography (CT), ultrasound, and magnetic resonance imaging (MRI) may each yield alterations suggesting increased fat in the liver. As discussed in Chap. 293, several mechanisms can contribute to lipid accumulation in the liver. Fatty liver can be separated into two categories based on whether the fat droplets in the hepatocytes are macrovesicular or microvesicular (Table 300-1). In addition, fatty infiltration may be accompanied by necroinflammatory activity, a condition designated *steatohepatitis*.

MACROVESICULAR FATTY LIVER This is the most common type of fatty liver and is seen most frequently in alcoholism or alcoholic liver disease, diabetes mellitus, obesity, and prolonged parenteral nutrition. Hematoxylin and eosin–stained liver sections show hepatocytes with large, empty vacuoles with the nucleus "pushed" to the periphery of the cell. In general, fat in the liver is not damaging per se, and the fat will disappear with improvement or elimination of the predisposing condition.

Etiology The major causes of fatty liver with macrovesicular fat depend on the age, geographic location, and metabolic-nutritional status of the patient population. *Chronic alcoholism* is the most common cause of hepatic steatosis in this country and in other countries with a high alcohol intake. The severity of fatty involvement is roughly proportional to the duration and degree of alcoholic excess. *Protein malnutrition*, especially in infancy and early childhood, accounts for most cases of severe fatty liver in the tropical zones of Africa, South America, and Asia. The hepatic changes may be associated with other clinical and pathologic features of kwashiorkor. Patients with adult-onset *diabetes mellitus*, especially those who are overweight and are poorly controlled, often have fatty livers. *Obesity* is commonly associated with fatty infiltration of the liver; this recedes as weight reduction occurs. *Jejunoileal bypass* for surgical treatment of morbid obesity was sometimes associated with severe fatty liver and hepatic failure that could be fatal. In patients with Cushing's syndrome and in those receiving large doses of glucocorticoids, fatty infiltration of the liver may occur. In many *chronic illnesses*, especially those complicated by impaired nutrition or malabsorption, increased fat is found in liver cells. For example, patients with severe ulcerative colitis, chronic pancreatitis, or protracted heart failure frequently have moderate hepatic steatosis at the time of death. Patients maintained on prolonged *total parenteral nutrition* also may develop a fatty liver. In some cases, fatty infiltration and steatohepatitis may occur in the absence of an identifiable cause.

Table 300-1

Causes of Hepatic Steatosis

MACROVESICULAR (LARGE FAT DROPLETS IN HEPATOCYTES)
Alcohol, alcoholic liver disease*
Diabetes mellitus*
Obesity*
Protein-calorie malnutrition
Total parenteral nutrition*, jejunoileal bypass
Drugs*, e.g., methotrexate, aspirin, vitamin A, glucocorticoids, amiodarone, and synthetic estrogen
MICROVESICULAR (SMALL FAT DROPLETS IN HEPATOCYTES)
Reye's syndrome
Acute fatty liver of pregnancy
Jamaican vomiting sickness
Drugs, e.g., valproic acid, tetracycline

* May also be associated with necroinflmmatory activity

Acute fatty liver is caused by a number of hepatotoxins and is frequently accompanied by signs and symptoms of liver failure. Carbon tetrachloride intoxication, DDT poisoning, and ingestion of substances containing yellow phosphorus result in severe hepatic steatosis. Acute and prolonged alcohol ingestion also may be considered in this category and may be associated with a rapidly enlarging and fat-laden liver.

Clinical Features The signs and symptoms of hepatic steatosis are related to the degree of fat infiltration, the time course of its accumulation, and the underlying cause. The obese or diabetic patient with a chronic fatty liver is usually asymptomatic and has only mild tenderness over the enlarged liver. The liver function tests are normal or show mild elevations of alkaline phosphatase or aminotransferases. In contrast, the rapid accumulation of fat seen in the setting of hyperalimentation may lead to marked tenderness, presumably resulting from stretching of Glisson's capsule. Similarly, alcoholic patients with acute fatty liver following a bout of heavy drinking may have right upper quadrant pain and tenderness often with laboratory evidence of cholestasis. The clinical presentation of fatty liver from hepatotoxins is similar to that of fulminant hepatic failure arising from any cause, with evidence of hepatic encephalopathy, marked elevations of prothrombin time and aminotransferases, and variable degrees of jaundice. Although steatohepatitis is generally thought to have a benign clinical course with improvement following elimination of the associated precipitant, in some individuals it may result in significant fibrosis and even cirrhosis.

Diagnosis The findings of a firm, nontender, and generally enlarged liver with minimal hepatic dysfunction in a patient with chronic alcoholism, malnutrition, poorly controlled diabetes mellitus, or obesity should suggest hepatic steatosis. This can usually be detected by CT, MRI, or ultrasound. Modest elevations of aminotransferases are often found in association with hepatic steatohepatitis. A disproportional elevation in AST leading to an AST/ALT ratio greater than 2 is generally associated with alcoholic hepatitis; ratios below one are usually found in non-alcoholic steatohepatitis. When diagnostic uncertainty exists, needle biopsy of the liver will demonstrate the increased fat content and possibly the underlying primary disorder.

℞ TREATMENT

Adequate nutritional intake, removal of alcohol or offending toxins, and correction of any associated metabolic disorders usually result in recovery. There is no clinical rationale for the use of lipotropic agents such as choline. When indicated, attention should be directed to abstinence from alcohol, careful control of diabetes, weight loss, or correction of intestinal absorptive defects. In the alcoholic fatty liver there is gradual disappearance of fat from the liver after 4 to 8 weeks of adequate diet and abstinence from alcohol. Similarly, fatty infiltration usually resolves within 2 weeks after discontinuation of parenteral hyperalimentation.

MICROVESICULAR FATTY LIVER This is the less common form of fatty liver. On microscopic examination, the fat is present in many small vacuoles. Although the droplets consist of triglycerides in both the macrovesicular and microvesicular forms, the reason for this difference in morphologic appearance is not clear.

Acute fatty liver of pregnancy is a syndrome that occurs late in pregnancy and is often associated with jaundice and hepatic failure. In half the cases it is associated with preeclampsia. If diagnosed in time, the disease usually resolves with termination of the pregnancy.

Microvesicular fat accumulation also may be seen as a toxic reaction to *valproic acid* and with excessive doses of *tetracycline*. It is a typical finding in *Jamaican vomiting sickness*, which is caused by hypoglycin A present in unripened ackee fruit.

REYE'S SYNDROME (FATTY LIVER WITH ENCEPHALOPATHY) This acute illness is encountered exclusively in children below 15 years of age. It is characterized clinically by vomiting and signs of progressive central nervous system damage, signs of hepatic injury, and hypoglycemia. Morphologically, there is extensive fatty vacuolization of the liver and renal tubules. There is mitochondrial dysfunction with decreased activity of hepatic mitochondrial enzymes. The cause is unknown, although viral agents and drugs, especially salicylates, have been implicated. Increased aspirin use and much higher serum salicylate levels in children with this illness than in the general population have been described during outbreaks of Reye's syndrome. Recognition of this relationship and reduced aspirin use in this setting may account for the decreasing incidence of Reye's syndrome. However, this illness may occur in the absence of exposure to salicylates. In fatal cases, the liver is enlarged and yellow with striking diffuse fatty microvacuolization of cells. Peripheral zonal hepatic necrosis also has been present in some cases. Fatty changes of the renal tubular cells, cerebral edema, and neuronal degeneration of the brain are the major extrahepatic changes. Electron-microscopic studies show structural alterations of mitochondria in liver, brain, and muscle.

The onset usually follows an upper respiratory tract infection, especially influenza or chickenpox. Within 1 to 3 days, persistent vomiting occurs, together with stupor, which usually progresses rapidly to generalized convulsions and coma. The liver is enlarged, but *jaundice is characteristically absent or minimal.* Elevations in serum aminotransferases and prothrombin time, hypoglycemia, metabolic acidosis, and elevated serum ammonia levels are the major laboratory findings. The mortality rate in Reye's syndrome is approximately 50 percent. Therapy consists of infusions of glucose and fresh frozen plasma, as well as intravenous mannitol to reduce the cerebral edema. Chronic liver disease has not been reported in survivors.

STORAGE DISEASES

Lipid storage diseases include the hereditary disorders of Gaucher's and Niemann-Pick disease. Other rare diseases associated with increased fat in the liver include abetalipoproteinemia, Tangier disease, Fabry's disease, and types I and V hyperlipoproteinemia (see Chap. 341 for details). Hepatic enlargement caused by distention of liver cells with glycogen is present in some poorly controlled diabetics and frequently in juvenile diabetes. More often, however, hepatomegaly is due to fatty infiltration (see above). Ketoacidosis and vigorous insulin therapy may further enhance hepatic enlargement.

HEPATIC MINERAL ACCUMULATION

WILSON'S DISEASE This is a rare disorder, predominantly of young people, in which excess copper accumulates in the liver and other tissues. Deficiency of the plasma copper protein ceruloplasmin is a characteristic feature. The accumulation appears to result from impaired copper excretion due to a mutation in a gene that encodes a P-type ATPase copper transporter. Clinically, patients may present in teenage or early adult years with chronic hepatitis, cirrhosis or their complications. A small number of patients will present with fulminant hepatitis. Liver disease is often accompanied by softening and degeneration of the basal ganglia (hepatolenticular degeneration) due to copper deposition, which results in extrapyramidal neurologic and psychiatric symptoms. Pigmentation of the cornea (Kayser-Fleischer rings) is frequently present. Hemolytic anemia is also common, especially with fulminant disease. Liver biopsy may reveal findings ranging from fulminant hepatitis to macronodular cirrhosis in addition to excess copper levels. Typically, liver cells are ballooned and show increased glycogen with glycogen vacuolization in the nuclei. All patients under age 40 with unexplained chronic hepatitis or cirrhosis should be evaluated for possible Wilson's disease. Prompt diagnosis is important; treatment, which must be continued throughout life, can prevent progression of end-organ damage. → *For further discussion, see Chap. 345.*

HEMOCHROMATOSIS Hemochromatosis may be the most common genetic disorder of humans; it involves accumulation of abnormal amounts of iron due to inappropriate absorption from the intestine. The liver, as a primary site of iron storage, is affected most directly. There is diffuse deposition of excess iron in hepatocytes, in contrast to the characteristic accumulation of iron in the reticuloendothelial compartment typical of secondary iron overload and hemosiderosis. Excess hepatic iron commonly results in hepatomegaly. Although liver function is initially well preserved, if the disease is untreated, progressive impairment is followed by the development of cirrhosis. Prompt diagnosis can permit the institution of effective lifelong therapy to reduce the iron load and halt progression of the disease. → *For further discussion, see Chap. 342*

OTHER INFILTRATIVE DISEASES

HURLER'S SYNDROME This is an uncommon hereditary disease that is characterized by the widespread tissue deposition of mucopolysaccharide (chondroitin sulfate B and heparan sulfate) in many tissues. The liver is frequently enlarged and firm. Microscopically, Kupffer cells and other macrophages are enlarged and filled with metachromatic granular material. Cirrhosis may be a late complication. → *For further discussion, see Chap. 346*.

α_1-ANTITRYPSIN DEFICIENCY Patients with homozygous deficiency of serum α_1-antitrypsin (α_1AT) are prone to develop emphysema in adult life. The disease is suggested by the absence of alpha$_1$ globulin on serum electrophoresis (α_1AT makes up 90 percent of this fraction normally) and confirmed by direct measurement of α_1AT. The exact phenotype can then be determined by starch electrophoresis. Although there are approximately 75 recognized alleles, only PiZ and PiS are associated with clinical disease. The molecular bases of these altered products have been related to single nucleic acid substitutions, e.g., PiZ is caused by a G (guanine) to A (adenine) transposition, which results in a substitution of a glutamic acid for lysine at residue 292 in the α_1AT protein. Hepatocytes of some patients with this deficiency contain globules positive to the periodic acid Schiff reaction. Approximately 10 percent of children with homozygous deficiency (PiZZ phenotype) of α_1AT will develop significant liver disease, including neonatal hepatitis and progressive cirrhosis. It has been suggested that 15 to 20 percent of all chronic liver disease in infancy may be attributed to α_1AT deficiency. In adults, the most common manifestation of α_1AT deficiency is asymptomatic cirrhosis, which may progress from a micronodular to a macronodular state and may be complicated by the development of hepatocellular carcinoma. The occurrence of liver disease in these patients is not dependent on the development of lung disease. → *For further discussion, see Chap. 258*).

RETICULOENDOTHELIAL DISORDERS (See also Chaps. 61 and 113)

Moderate to massive hepatomegaly and splenomegaly occur frequently in the various types of *leukemia* and *lymphoma*. Jaundice, when present, is usually slight and results from hemolysis, although cholestasis may occasionally be associated with lymphoma as a paraneoplastic syndrome. Deep and protracted jaundice is distinctly rare and is caused by obstruction of the intrahepatic or extrahepatic bile ducts by tumor. Liver biopsy specimens reveal portal and sinusoidal infiltrates in most cases of leukemia, but the cellular pattern may be mixed and nonspecific. Liver biopsy is diagnostic in only 5 percent of patients with *Hodgkin's disease*. This percentage is increased in those with advanced disease or splenomegaly. Directed biopsy at laparoscopy or laparotomy is more likely to be positive than "blind" needle biopsy. Nonspecific histologic changes in the liver have been described in patients with lymphoma and may contribute to the abnormal liver function tests.

Myeloid metaplasia and other myeloproliferative disorders associated with extramedullary hematopoiesis produce hepatomegaly which may reach huge proportions, especially following splenectomy. Serum alkaline phosphatase elevations are often found. Ascites and portal hypertension, resulting from diffuse involvement of portal venules and lymphatics, are rare complications.

GRANULOMATOUS INFILTRATIONS

Perhaps as a result of the large population of mononuclear phagocytes, a number of systemic granulomatous diseases involve the liver, including sarcoidosis, miliary tuberculosis, histoplasmosis, brucellosis, schistosomiasis, berylliosis, and drug reactions (Table 300-2). In addition, isolated granulomas of no diagnostic importance may be found occasionally in patients with various forms of cirrhosis and hepatitis. The liver infiltrated by granulomas may be slightly enlarged and firm, but hepatic dysfunction is usually limited. Increases in serum alkaline phosphatase are common and may range from mild to marked. Occasionally mild serum elevations in aminotransferases are also present. In a few patients with sarcoidosis or brucellosis, portal hypertension may develop, and extensive postnecrotic scarring or postnecrotic cirrhosis may follow healing of the granulomatous lesions, as in schistosomiasis.

In AIDS, evidence of liver disease is quite common but is usually mild with minimal morbidity. In these patients, hepatic granulomatous disease is often present and may be caused by opportunistic infections, with *Mycobacterium avium-intracellulare* being the most frequent pathogen. Cytomegalovirus hepatitis and hepatic mycoses are less common. These patients are frequently being treated for *Pneumocystis carinii* infections with sulfonamides, which also may cause hepatic granulomatous disease. AIDS cholangiopathy has become a well recognized entity. It exhibits features similar to those found in primary sclerosing cholangitis and is typically associated with cryptosporidia, microsporidia, and/or cytomegalovirus infection in the biliary tract. Papillary stenosis is frequently present.

Needle biopsy of the liver often provides the first definite evidence of a systemic or disseminated granulomatous disease. In patients with sarcoidosis who have neither clinical nor laboratory evidence of hepatic involvement, needle biopsy is positive in about 80 percent of cases. In cases of suspected miliary tuberculosis, a portion of the biopsy should be cultured and stained for mycobacteria. The organism can be detected in the majority of cases, particularly when caseating granulomas are present. Serial sections of the biopsy specimen should be examined if granulomas are not apparent. Individual granulomas are rarely specific in their microscopic appearance, and final diagnosis usually requires other clinical, laboratory, or histologic data.

In approximately 20 percent of patients it is not possible to identify a cause for the granulomatous infiltration. When these infiltrates are accompanied by fever of unknown origin, the diagnosis of granulomatous hepatitis should be considered. This is an uncommon disorder of unknown cause and is diagnosed by exclusion. While granulomatous hepatitis invariably responds to moderate doses of glucocorticoids, relapses are frequent, and such therapy should never be undertaken unless tuberculous disease or other causes of granulomatous infiltration have been excluded. This may include an initial empiric trial of antituberculous therapy.

Table 300-2

Some Causes of Hepatic Granulomas

SYSTEMIC DISEASE	
Sarcoidosis	Crohn's disease
Hodgkin's and non-Hodgkin's lymphoma	Wegener's granulomatosis
Primary biliary cirrhosis	Granulomatous hepatitis, idiopathic
Berylliosis	
INFECTIONS	
Bacterial	Parasitic
Tuberculosis	Schistosomiasis
Mycobacterium avium intracellulare	Rickettsial
Brucellosis	Q fever
Leprosy	Spirochetes
Viral	Syphilis
Epstein-Barr virus	Drugs
Cytomegalovirus	Sulfonamides
Chicken pox	Isoniazid
	Allopurinol

AMYLOIDOSIS (See also Chap. 309)

Systemic amyloidosis, whether primary and idiopathic, familial, or secondary to chronic inflammatory or neoplastic diseases, often involves the liver. Grossly, the liver infiltrated with amyloid is enlarged and pale and rubbery in consistency. Microscopically, the birefringent amyloid deposits appear as homogeneous waxy material within the space of Disse, often being concentrated in the periportal areas and associated with atrophy of adjacent liver cell plates. Selective involvement of the walls of blood vessels, especially of the hepatic arterioles, may be a striking feature of primary amyloidosis. With this possible exception, however, the hepatic lesions are the same in all forms of amyloidosis and are present in 60 to 90 percent of cases.

An enlarged and firm liver is found in about 60 percent of patients, and ascites occurs in advanced stages of the disease in about 20 percent. Jaundice, portal hypertension, and other signs of chronic liver disease are usually absent. Liver function changes, although frequent, correlate poorly with the extent of liver infiltration. Hypoalbuminemia and elevated serum alkaline phosphatase are common. Hypoalbuminemia, however, may be related to the presence of nephrosis; the prothrombin time is usually normal. The diagnosis is established by biopsy of rectum, skin, liver, or other involved organs and demonstration of the characteristic Congo red–staining deposits by polarizing microscopy.

BIBLIOGRAPHY

Arias IM et al: *The Liver: Biology and Pathobiology*, 3d ed. New York, Raven Press, 1994

Crystal RG: Alpha 1-antitrypsin deficiency, emphysema and liver disease: Genetic basis and strategy for therapy. J Clin Invest 85:1343, 1990

Hurwitz ES et al: Public Health Service Study on Reye's syndrome and medications. N Engl J Med 313:842, 1985

Hutchison DC: Natural history of alpha 1-protease inhibitor deficiency. Am J Med 84:3, 1988

Lee WM: Drug-induced hepatotoxicity. N Engl J Med 333:1118, 1995

Minakami H et al: Pre-eclampsia: A microvesicular fat disease of the liver. Am J Obstet Gynecol 159:1043, 1988

Perlmutter DH: The cellular basis for liver injury in alpha 1-antitrypsin deficiency. Hepatology 13:172, 1991

Riley C et al: Acute fatty liver of pregnancy: A reassessment based on observations in nine patients. Ann Intern Med 106:703, 1987

Rustgi VK: Liver disease in pregnancy. Med Clin North Am 73:1041, 1989

Schiff L, Schiff ER: *Diseases of the Liver*, 7th ed. Philadelphia, Lippincott, 1993

Scriver CR et al (eds): *The Metabolic and Molecular Bases of Inherited Disease*, 7th ed. New York, McGraw-Hill, 1995

Sherlock S, Dooley J: *Diseases of the Liver and Biliary System*, 9th ed. Oxford, Blackwell, 1993

Sternlieb I: Perspectives on Wilson's disease. Hepatology 12:1234, 1990

Van Costa RN et al: Adult Reye's syndrome: A review with new evidence for a generalized defect in intramitochondrial enzyme processing. Neurology 41:1815, 1991

Zakim D, Boyer TD: *Hepatology: A Textbook of Liver Disease*, 3d ed. Philadelphia, Saunders, 1996

301 LIVER TRANSPLANTATION

Jules Dienstag

Liver transplantation, the replacement of the native, diseased liver by a normal organ (allograft) recovered from a brain-dead donor, has matured from an experimental procedure reserved for desperately ill patients to an accepted, lifesaving operation applied much earlier in the natural history of end-stage liver disease. The preferred and technically most advanced approach is *orthotopic transplantation*, in which the native organ is removed and the donor organ is inserted in the same anatomic location. Pioneered in the 1960s by Starzl at the University of Colorado and, later, at the University of Pittsburgh and by Calne in Cambridge, England, liver transplantation is now performed routinely by dozens of centers throughout North America and western Europe. Success and survival have improved from approximately 30 percent in the 1970s to >80 percent today. These improved prospects for prolonged survival, dating back to the early 1980s, resulted from refinements in operative technique (including the introduction of venovenous bypass to allow venous return from the extremities and visceral circulation during clamping of the inferior vena cava), improvements in organ procurement and preservation, advances in immunosuppressive therapy, and, perhaps most influentially, more enlightened patient selection and timing. Despite the perioperative morbidity and mortality, the technical and management challenges of the procedure, and its costs, liver transplantation has become the approach of choice for selected patients whose chronic or acute liver disease is progressive, life-threatening, and unresponsive to medical therapy. Based on the current level of success, the number of liver transplants has continued to grow each year; in 1995, 3700 patients received liver allografts in the United States. Still, the demand for new livers continues to outpace availability; in 1995, as many as 6000 patients in the United States were on a waiting list for a donor liver.

INDICATIONS Potential candidates for liver transplantation are children and adults who, in the absence of contraindications (see below), suffer from severe, irreversible liver disease for which alternative medical or surgical treatments have been exhausted or are unavailable. *Timing of the operation is of critical importance*. Indeed, improved timing and better patient selection are felt to have contributed more to the increased success of liver transplantation in the 1980s and beyond than all the impressive technical and immunologic advances combined. Although the disease should be advanced, and although opportunities for spontaneous or medically induced stabilization or recovery should be allowed, the procedure should be done sufficiently early to give the surgical procedure a fair chance for success. Ideally, transplantation should be considered in patients with end-stage liver disease who are experiencing or have experienced a life-threatening complication of hepatic decompensation, whose quality of life has deteriorated to unacceptable levels, or whose liver disease will result predictably in irreversible damage to the central nervous system (CNS). If this is done sufficiently early, the patient will not have developed any contraindications or extrahepatic systemic deterioration. Although patients with well-compensated cirrhosis can survive for many years, many patients with quasi-stable chronic liver disease have much more advanced disease than may be apparent. As discussed below, the better the status of the patient prior to transplantation, the higher will be the anticipated success rate of transplantation. The decision about *when* to transplant is complex and requires the combined judgment of an experienced team of hepatologists, transplant surgeons, anesthesiologists, and specialists in support services, not to mention the well-informed consent of the patient and the patient's family.

Transplantation in Children Indications for transplantation in children are listed in Table 301-1. The most common is *biliary atresia*. *Inherited or genetic disorders of metabolism* associated with liver failure constitute another major indication for transplantation in children and adolescents. In Crigler-Najjar disease type I and in certain hereditary disorders of the urea cycle and of amino acid or lactate-pyruvate metabolism, transplantation may be the only way to prevent impending deterioration of CNS function, despite the fact that the native liver is structurally normal. Combined heart and liver transplantation has yielded dramatic improvement in cardiac function and in cholesterol levels in children with homozygous familial hypercholesterolemia; combined liver and kidney transplantation has been successful in patients with hereditary oxalosis. In hemophiliacs with transfusion-associated hepatitis and liver failure, liver transplantation has been associated with recovery of normal factor VIII synthesis.

Transplantation in Adults Liver transplantation is indicated for end-stage *cirrhosis* of all causes (see Table 301-1). In sclerosing cholangitis and *Caroli's disease* (multiple cystic dilatations of the intrahepatic biliary tree), recurrent infections and sepsis associated with inflammatory and fibrotic obstruction of the biliary tree may be an indication for transplantation. Because prior biliary surgery complicates, and is a relative contraindication for, liver transplantation, surgical diversion of the biliary tree has been all but abandoned for patients with sclerosing cholangitis. In patients who undergo transplantation for *hepatic vein thrombosis (Budd-Chiari syndrome)*, postoperative anticoagulation is essential; underlying myeloproliferative disorders may have to be treated but are not a contraindication to liver transplantation. If a donor organ can be located quickly, before life-threatening complications—including cerebral edema—set in, patients with *fulminant hepatitis* are candidates for liver transplantation. More controversial as candidates for liver transplantation are patients with *alcoholic cirrhosis*, *chronic viral hepatitis*, and *primary hepatocellular malignancies*. Although all three of these categories are considered to be high risk, liver transplantation can be offered to carefully selected patients. Patients with alcoholic cirrhosis can be considered as candidates for transplantation if they meet strict criteria for abstinence and reform. Patients with chronic hepatitis C have done as well as any other subset of patients after transplantation, despite the fact that recurrent infection in the donor organ is the rule. In patients with chronic hepatitis B, in the absence of measures to prevent recurrent hepatitis B, survival after transplantation is reduced by approximately 10 to 20 percent; however, prophylactic use of hepatitis B immune globulin (HBIG) during and after transplantation increases the success of transplantation compared to that seen in patients with nonviral causes of liver decompensation. Issues of disease recurrence are discussed in more detail below. Patients with nonmetastatic primary hepatobiliary tumors—primary hepatocellular carcinoma, cholangiocarcinoma, hepatoblastoma, angiosarcoma, epithelioid hemangioendothelioma, and multiple or massive hepatic adenomata—have undergone liver transplantation; however, for hepatobiliary malignancies,

Table 301-1

Indications for Liver Transplantation

Children	Adults
Biliary atresia	Primary biliary cirrhosis
Neonatal hepatitis	Secondary biliary cirrhosis
Congenital hepatic fibrosis	Primary sclerosing cholangitis
Alagille's disease*	Caroli's disease‡
Byler's disease†	Cryptogenic cirrhosis
α_1-Antitrypsin deficiency	Chronic hepatitis with cirrhosis
Inherited disorders of metabolism	Hepatic vein thrombosis
Wilson's disease	Fulminant hepatitis
Tyrosinemia	Alcoholic cirrhosis
Glycogen storage diseases	Chronic viral hepatitis
Lysosomal storage diseases	Primary hepatocellular malignancies
Protoporphyria	Hepatic adenomas
Crigler-Najjar disease type I	
Familial hypercholesterolemia	
Hereditary oxalosis	
Hemophilia	

* Arteriohepatic dysplasia, with paucity of bile ducts, and congenital malformations, including pulmonary stenosis.
† Intrahepatic cholestasis, progressive liver failure, mental and growth retardation.
‡ Multiple cystic dilatations of the intrahepatic biliary tree.

overall survival is significantly lower than that for other categories of liver disease. To minimize the very high likelihood of recurrent tumor after transplantation, some centers are evaluating experimental adjuvant chemotherapy protocols. Some transplantation centers have reported excellent long-term, recurrence-free survival in patients with unresectable hepatocellular carcinoma for single tumors <5 cm in diameter or for three or fewer lesions all <3 cm. Because the likelihood of recurrent cholangiocarcinoma is almost universal, this tumor is no longer considered an indication for transplantation.

CONTRAINDICATIONS *Absolute contraindications* for transplantation include life-threatening systemic diseases, uncontrolled extrahepatic bacterial or fungal infections, preexisting advanced cardiovascular or pulmonary disease, multiple uncorrectable life-threatening congenital anomalies, metastatic malignancy, active drug or alcohol abuse, and human immunodeficiency virus (HIV) infection. Because carefully selected patients in their sixties and even seventies have undergone transplantation successfully, advanced age per se is no longer considered an absolute contraindication; however, in older patients, a more thorough preoperative evaluation should be undertaken to exclude ischemic cardiac disease. Advanced age (>60 years), however, may be considered a *relative contraindication*, that is, a factor to be taken into account with other relative contraindications. Other relative contraindications include highly replicative hepatitis B, portal vein thrombosis, preexisting renal disease not associated with liver disease, intrahepatic or biliary sepsis, severe hypoxemia resulting from right-to-left intrapulmonary shunts, previous extensive hepatobiliary surgery, and any uncontrolled serious psychiatric disorder. Any one of these relative contraindications is insufficient in and of itself to preclude transplantation. For example, the problem of portal vein thrombosis can be overcome by constructing a graft from the donor liver portal vein to the recipient's superior mesenteric vein.

TECHNICAL CONSIDERATIONS **Donor Selection** Donor livers for transplantation are procured primarily from victims of head trauma. Organs from brain-dead donors up to age 60 are acceptable if the following criteria are met: hemodynamic stability, adequate oxygenation, absence of bacterial or fungal infection, serologic exclusion of hepatitis B and C viruses and HIV, absence of abdominal trauma, and absence of hepatic dysfunction. Cardiovascular and respiratory functions are maintained artificially until the liver can be removed. Compatibility in ABO blood group and organ size between donor and recipient are important considerations in donor selection; however, ABO-incompatible or reduced-donor-organ transplants can be performed in emergency or marked donor-scarcity situations. Tissue typing for HLA matching is not required, and preformed cytotoxic HLA antibodies do not preclude liver transplantation. Following perfusion with cold electrolyte solution, the donor liver is removed and packed in ice. The use of University of Wisconsin (UW) solution, rich in lactobionate and raffinose, has permitted the extension of cold ischemic time up to 20 h; however, 12 h may be a more reasonable limit. Improved techniques for harvesting multiple organs from the same donor have increased the availability of donor livers, but the availability of donor livers is far outstripped by the demand. Currently, in the United States, all donor livers are distributed through a nationwide organ-sharing network (United Network of Organ Sharing) designed to allocate available organs based on regional considerations and recipient acuity. Recipients who require the highest level of care (intensive care) have the highest priority.

Surgical Technique Removal of the recipient's native liver is technically difficult, particularly in the presence of portal hypertension with its associated collateral circulation and extensive varices, and even more so in the presence of scarring from previous abdominal operations. The combination of portal hypertension and coagulopathy (elevated prothrombin time and thrombocytopenia) translates into large blood product transfusion requirements. After the portal vein and infrahepatic and suprahepatic inferior vena cavae are dissected, a pump-driven venovenous bypass system is applied to reroute blood from the portal vein and inferior vena cava, preventing congestion of visceral organs. After the hepatic artery and common bile duct are dissected, the native liver is removed and the donor organ inserted. During the anhepatic phase, coagulopathy, hypoglycemia, hypocalcemia, and hypothermia are encountered and must be managed by the anesthesiology team. Caval, portal vein, hepatic artery, and bile duct anastomoses are performed in succession, the last by end-to-end suturing of the donor and recipient common bile ducts or by choledochojejunostomy to a Roux en Y loop if the recipient common bile duct cannot be used for reconstruction (e.g., in sclerosing cholangitis). A typical transplant operation lasts 8 h, with a range of 6 to 18 h. Because of excessive bleeding, large volumes of blood, blood products, and volume expanders may be required during surgery.

POSTOPERATIVE COURSE AND MANAGEMENT **Immunosuppressive Therapy** The introduction in 1980 of cyclosporine as an immunosuppressive agent contributed substantially to the improvement in survival after liver transplantation. Cyclosporine inhibits early activation of T cells and is specific for T cell functions that result from the interaction of the T cell with its receptor and that involve the calcium-dependent signal transduction pathway; as a result, the activity of cyclosporine leads to inhibition of lymphokine gene activation, blocking interleukins 2, 3, and 4, tumor necrosis factor α, as well as other lymphokines. Cyclosporine also inhibits B cell functions. This process occurs without affecting rapidly dividing cells in the bone marrow, which may account for the reduced frequency of posttransplantation systemic infections. The most common and important side effect of cyclosporine therapy is nephrotoxicity. Cyclosporine causes dose-dependent renal tubular injury and direct renal artery vasospasm. Following renal function, therefore, is important in monitoring cyclosporine therapy, perhaps even a more reliable indicator than blood levels of the drug. Nephrotoxicity is reversible and can be managed by dose reduction. Other adverse effects of cyclosporine therapy include hypertension, hyperkalemia, tremor, hirsutism, glucose intolerance, and gum hyperplasia.

Tacrolimus (originally labeled FK 506) is a macrolide lactone antibiotic isolated from a Japanese soil fungus, *Streptomyces tsukubaensis*. It has the same mechanism of action as cyclosporine but is 10 to 100 times more potent. Initially applied as "rescue" therapy for patients in whom rejection occurred despite the use of cyclosporine, tacrolimus has been shown in two large, multicenter, randomized trials to be associated with a reduced frequency of acute rejection, refractory rejection, and chronic rejection. Although patient and graft survival are the same with these two drugs, the advantage of tacrolimus in minimizing episodes of rejection, reducing the need for additional glucocorticoid doses, and reducing the likelihood of bacterial and cytomegalovirus infection has simplified the management of patients undergoing liver transplantation. In addition, the oral absorption of tacrolimus is more predictable than that of cyclosporine, especially during the early postoperative period when T-tube drainage interferes with the enterohepatic circulation of cyclosporine. As a result, in most transplantation centers, tacrolimus has now supplanted cyclosporine for primary immunosuppression, and many centers rely on oral, rather than intravenous, administration from the outset. For transplantation centers that prefer cyclosporine, a new, better-absorbed, microemulsion preparation is now available.

Although tacrolimus is more potent than cyclosporine, it is also more toxic and more likely to be discontinued for adverse events. The toxicity of tacrolimus is similar to that of cyclosporine; nephrotoxicity and neurotoxicity are the most commonly encountered adverse effects, and neurotoxicity (tremor, seizures, hallucinations, psychoses, coma) is more likely and more severe in tacrolimus-treated patients. Both drugs can cause diabetes mellitus, but tacrolimus does not cause hirsutism or gingival hyperplasia. Because of overlapping toxicity between cyclosporine and tacrolimus, especially nephrotoxicity, and because tacrolimus reduces cyclosporine clearance, these two drugs should not be used together. Because 99 percent of tacrolimus is metabolized by the liver, hepatic dysfunction reduces its clearance; in primary graft nonfunction (when, for technical reasons or because of ischemic damage prior to its insertion, the allograft is defective and does not function normally from the outset) tacrolimus doses have to be reduced substantially, especially in children. Both cyclosporine and tacrolimus are metabolized by the cytochrome P450 IIIA system, and so drugs that induce cytochrome P450 (e.g., phenytoin, phenobarbital, carbamazepine, rifampin) reduce available levels of cyclosporine and tacrolimus; drugs that inhibit cytochrome P450 (e.g., erythromycin, fluconazole, ketoconazole, clotrimazole, itraconazole, verapamil, diltiazem, nicardipine, cimetidine, danazol, metoclopramide, bromocriptine) increase cyclosporine and tacrolimus blood levels. Like azathioprine, cyclosporine and tacrolimus appear to be associated with a risk of lymphoproliferative malignancies (see below), which may occur earlier after cyclosporine or tacrolimus than after azathioprine therapy. Because of these side effects, combinations of cyclosporine or tacrolimus with prednisone and azathioprine—all at reduced doses—are preferable regimens for immunosuppressive therapy.

In patients with pretransplant renal dysfunction or renal deterioration that occurs intraoperatively or immediately postoperatively, tacrolimus or cyclosporine therapy may not be practical; under these circumstances, induction or maintenance of immunosuppression with monoclonal antibodies to T cells, OKT3, may be appropriate. Therapy with OKT3 has been especially effective in reversing acute rejection in the posttransplant period and is the standard treatment for acute rejection that fails to respond to methylprednisolone boluses. Intravenous infusions of OKT3 may be complicated by transient fever, chills, and diarrhea. When this drug is used to induce immunosuppression initially or to provide "rescue" in those who reject despite "conventional" therapy, the incidence of bacterial, fungal, and especially cytomegalovirus infections is increased during and after such therapy. In some centers, ganciclovir antiviral therapy is initiated prophylactically as a routine along with OKT3. Another immunosuppressive drug that is likely to be used in the future for patients undergoing liver transplantation is mycophenolic acid, a nonnucleoside purine metabolism inhibitor derived as a fermentation product from several *Penicillium* species. Mycophenolate has been shown to be better than azathioprine, when used with other standard immunosuppressive drugs, in preventing rejection after renal transplantation and has been approved for use in renal transplantation. Rapamycin, an inhibitor of later events in T cell activation, is yet another drug undergoing experimental evaluation as an immunosuppressive agent.

The most important principle of immunosuppression is that the ideal approach strikes a balance between immunosuppression and immunologic competence. Given sufficient immunosuppression, acute liver allograft rejection is always reversible; however, if the cumulative dose of immunosuppressive therapy is too large, the patient will succumb to opportunistic infection. Therefore, immunosuppressive drugs must be used judiciously, with strict attention to the infectious consequences of such therapy.

Postoperative Complications Complications of liver transplantation can be divided into hepatic and nonhepatic categories. In addition, both immediately postoperative and late complications are encountered. Patients who undergo liver transplantation as a rule have been chronically ill for protracted periods and may be malnourished and wasted. The impact of such chronic illness and the multisystem failure that accompanies liver failure continues to require attention in the postoperative period. Because of the massive fluid losses and fluid shifts that occur during the operation, patients may remain fluid overloaded during the immediate postoperative period, straining cardiovascular reserve; this effect can be amplified in the face of transient renal dysfunction and pulmonary capillary vascular permeability. Continuous monitoring of cardiovascular and pulmonary function, measures to maintain the integrity of the intravascular compartment and to treat extravascular volume overload, and scrupulous attention to potential sources of and sites of infection are of paramount importance. Cardiovascular instability may result as well from the electrolyte imbalance that may accompany reperfusion of the donor liver. Pulmonary function may be compromised further by paralysis of the right hemidiaphragm associated with phrenic nerve injury. The hyperdynamic state with increased cardiac output that is characteristic of patients with liver failure reverses rapidly after successful liver transplantation.

Other immediate management issues include renal dysfunction; prerenal azotemia, acute kidney injury associated with hypoperfusion (acute tubular necrosis), and renal toxicity caused by antibiotics, tacrolimus, or cyclosporine are frequently encountered in the postoperative period, sometimes necessitating dialysis. Occasionally, postoperative intraperitoneal bleeding may be sufficient to increase intraabdominal pressure, which, in turn, may reduce renal blood flow—this effect is rapidly reversible when abdominal distention is relieved by exploratory laparotomy to identify and ligate the bleeding site and to remove intraperitoneal clot. Anemia also may result from acute upper gastrointestinal bleeding or from transient hemolytic anemia, which may be autoimmune, especially when blood group O livers are transplanted into blood group A or B recipients. This autoimmune hemolytic anemia is mediated by donor intrahepatic lymphocytes that recognize red blood cell A or B antigens on recipient erythrocytes. Transient in nature, this process resolves once the donor liver is repopulated by recipient bone marrow–derived lymphocytes; the hemolysis can be treated by transfusing blood group O red blood cells and/or by administering higher doses of glucocorticoids. Transient thrombocytopenia is encountered commonly as well. Aplastic anemia, a late occurrence, is rare but has been reported in almost 30 percent of patients who underwent liver transplantation for acute, severe hepatitis of unknown cause.

Bacterial, fungal, or viral infections are common and may be life-threatening postoperatively. Early after transplant surgery, common postoperative infections predominate—pneumonia, wound infections, infected intraabdominal collections, urinary tract infections, and intravenous line infections—rather than opportunistic infections; these infections may involve the biliary tree and liver as well. Beyond the first postoperative month, the toll of immunosuppression becomes evident, and opportunistic infections—cytomegalovirus, herpes viruses, fungal infections (*Aspergillus*, *Candida*, cryptococcal disease), mycobacterial infections, parasitic infections (*Pneumocystis*, *Toxoplasma*), bacterial infections (*Nocardia*, *Legionella*, and *Listeria*)—predominate. Rarely, early infections represent those transmitted with the donor liver, either infections present in the donor or infections acquired during procurement processing. De novo viral hepatitis infections acquired from the donor organ or from transfused blood products occur after typical incubation periods for these agents (well beyond the first month). Obviously, infections in an immunosuppressed host demand early recognition and prompt management; prophylactic antibiotic therapy is administered routinely in the immediate postoperative period. Use of sulfamethoxazole with trimethoprim reduces the incidence of postoperative *Pneumocystis carinii* pneumonia.

Neuropsychiatric complications include seizures (commonly associated with cyclosporine and tacrolimus toxicity), encephalopathy, depression, and difficult psychosocial adjustment. Rarely, diseases are transmitted by the allograft from the donor to the recipient. In addition to viral and bacterial infections, malignancies of donor origin have occurred. Lymphoproliferative malignancies, especially B cell lymphoma, are a recognized complication associated with immunosuppressive drugs such as azathioprine, tacrolimus, and cyclosporine (see above). Epstein-Barr virus has been shown to play a contributory role in some of these tumors, which may regress when immunosuppressive therapy is reduced.

Hepatic Complications Hepatic dysfunction after liver transplantation is similar to the hepatic complications encountered after major abdominal and cardiothoracic surgery; however, in addition, there may be complications such as primary graft failure, vascular compromise, failure or obstruction of the biliary anastomoses, and rejection. As in nontransplant surgery, postoperative jaundice may result from prehepatic, intrahepatic, and posthepatic sources. *Prehepatic* sources represent the massive hemoglobin pigment load from transfusions, hemolysis, hematomas, ecchymoses, and other collections of blood. *Early intrahepatic* liver injury includes effects of hepatotoxic drugs and anesthesia; hypoperfusion injury associated with hypotension, sepsis, and shock; and benign postoperative cholestasis. *Late intrahepatic* sources of liver injury include posttransfusion hepatitis and recurrent primary disease (see below). *Posthepatic* sources of hepatic dysfunction include biliary obstruction and reduced renal clearance of conjugated bilirubin. Hepatic complications unique to liver transplantation include primary graft failure associated with ischemic injury to the organ during harvesting; vascular compromise associated with thrombosis or stenosis of the portal vein or hepatic artery anastomoses; stenosis, obstruction, or leakage of the anastomosed common bile duct; and rejection.

Transplant Rejection Despite the use of immunosuppressive drugs, rejection of the transplanted liver still occurs in a majority of patients, beginning 1 to 2 weeks after surgery. Clinical signs suggesting rejection are fever, right upper quadrant pain, and reduced bile pigment and volume. Leukocytosis may occur, but the most reliable indicators are increases in serum bilirubin and aminotransferase levels. Because these tests lack specificity, distinguishing among rejection and biliary obstruction, primary graft nonfunction, vascular compromise, viral hepatitis, cytomegalovirus infection, drug hepatotoxicity, and recurrent primary disease may be difficult. Radiographic visualization of the biliary tree and/or percutaneous liver biopsy often help to establish the correct diagnosis. Morphologic features of acute rejection include portal infiltration, bile duct injury, and/or endothelial inflammation ("endothelialitis"); some of these findings are reminiscent of graft-versus-host disease and primary biliary cirrhosis. As soon as transplant rejection is suspected, treatment consists of intravenous methylprednisolone in repeated boluses; if this fails to abort rejection, many centers use antibodies to lymphocytes, such as OKT3, or polyclonal antilymphocyte globulin.

Chronic rejection is a relatively rare outcome that may follow repeated bouts of acute rejection or that occurs unrelated to preceding rejection episodes. Morphologically, chronic rejection is characterized by progressive cholestasis, focal parenchymal necrosis, mononuclear infiltration, vascular lesions (intimal fibrosis, subintimal foam cells, fibrinoid necrosis), and fibrosis. This process may be reflected as ductopenia—the vanishing bile duct syndrome. Some of the histologic hallmarks of chronic rejection may be so similar to those of chronic viral hepatitis that differentiation between the two may be difficult. Reversibility of chronic rejection is limited; in patients with therapy-resistant chronic rejection, retransplantation has yielded encouraging results.

OUTCOME Survival The survival rate for patients undergoing liver transplantation has improved steadily since 1983. One-year survival rates have increased from approximately 70 percent in the early 1980s to 80 to 90 percent in the mid-1990s. Currently, the 5-year survival rate approaches 60 percent. An important observation is the relation between clinical status before transplantation and outcome. For patients who undergo liver transplantation when their level of compensation is high (e.g., still working or only partially disabled), a 1-year survival rate of 85 percent is common. For those whose level of decompensation mandates continuous in-hospital care prior to transplantation, the 1-year survival rate is about 70 percent, while for those who are so decompensated that they require life support in an intensive care unit, the 1-year survival rate is approximately 50 percent. Indeed, the trend toward transplantation earlier in the natural history of end-stage liver disease is a major factor in the increased success of liver transplantation during the 1980s and 1990s. Another important distinction in survival has been drawn between high-risk and low-risk patient categories. For patients who do not fit any "high-risk" designations, 1-year and 5-year survival rates of 85 and 80 percent, respectively, have been recorded. In contrast, among patients in high-risk categories—cancer, fulminant hepatitis, hepatitis B, age >65, concurrent renal failure, respirator dependence, portal vein thrombosis, and history of a portacaval shunt or multiple right upper quadrant operations—survival statistics fall into the range of 60 percent at 1 year and 35 percent at 5 years. Survival after retransplantation for primary graft nonfunction is approximately 50 percent. Causes of failure of liver transplantation vary with time. Failures within the first 3 months result primarily from technical complications, postoperative infections, and hemorrhage. Transplant failures after the first 3 months are more likely to result from infection, rejection, or recurrent disease (such as malignancy or viral hepatitis).

Recurrence of Primary Disease The recurrence of autoimmune hepatitis or primary sclerosing cholangitis has not been reported. There have been reports of recurrent primary biliary cirrhosis after liver transplantation; however, the histologic features of primary biliary cirrhosis and acute rejection are virtually indistinguishable and occur as frequently in patients with primary biliary cirrhosis as in patients undergoing transplantation for other reasons. Hereditary disorders such as Wilson's disease and α_1-antitrypsin deficiency have not recurred after liver transplantation; however, recurrence of disordered iron metabolism has been observed in some patients with hemochromatosis. Hepatic vein thrombosis (Budd-Chiari syndrome) may recur; this can be minimized by treating underlying lymphoproliferative disorders and by anticoagulation. Cholangiocarcinoma recurs almost invariably; therefore, few centers now transplant such patients. In patients with hepatocellular carcinoma, tumor recurrence in the liver is common after approximately 1 year, although better success has been reported in patients with an unresectable isolated lesion <5 cm or with three or fewer lesions all <3 cm. Trials are underway to assess the benefit of adjuvant chemotherapy.

Hepatitis A can recur after transplantation for fulminant hepatitis A, but such acute reinfection has no serious clinical sequelae. In fulminant hepatitis B, recurrence is not the rule; however, in the absence of any prophylactic measures, hepatitis B usually recurs after transplantation for end-stage chronic hepatitis B. With sufficient immunosuppressive therapy to prevent allograft rejection, levels of hepatitis B viremia increase markedly, regardless of pretransplantation values. A majority of patients undergoing transplantation for chronic hepatitis B become carriers of hepatitis B virus (HBV) with high levels of virus replication but without liver injury; however, some patients experience a rapid recapitulation of severe injury—severe chronic hepatitis or even fulminant hepatitis—after transplantation. *Fibrosing cholestatic hepatitis* is a histologic feature linked to rapidly progressive liver injury in approximately 10 percent of patients who undergo liver transplantation for hepatitis B. These patients experience marked hyperbilirubinemia, substantial prolongation of the prothrombin time (both out of proportion to relatively modest elevations of aminotransferase activity), and rapidly progressive liver failure. This lesion has been suggested to represent a "choking off" of the hepatocyte by an overwhelming density of HBV proteins. Complications such as sepsis and pancreatitis also have been observed more frequently in patients undergoing liver transplantation for hepatitis B. Although the risk of recurrent hepatitis B is approximately 20 percent higher in patients with pretransplantation markers of HBV replication (hepatitis B e antigen and HBV DNA), recurrent hepatitis B occurs in at least 60 percent of patients whose replicative markers were undetectable prior to transplantation, probably because of the enhancing impact of immunosuppressive drugs on HBV replication. Most transplantation centers will not undertake liver transplantation in patients with hepatitis B unless immunoprophylaxis with HBIG is used. Neither preoperative hepatitis B vaccination, preoperative or postoperative interferon therapy, nor short-term (≤2 months) HBIG prophylaxis has been shown to be effective, but a retrospective analysis of data from several hundred patients followed for 3 years after transplantation has shown that long-term (≥6 months) prophylaxis with HBIG is associated with a lowering of the risk of HBV reinfection from approximately 75 percent to 35 percent and a reduction in mortality from approximately 50 percent to 20 percent. Passive immunoprophylaxis with HBIG is begun during the anhepatic stage of surgery, repeated daily for the first 6 postoperative days, then continued with infusions that are given either at regular intervals of 4 to 6 weeks or, alternatively, when anti-HBs levels fall below a threshold of 100 mIU/mL. In all likelihood, indefinite HBIG infusions will be required, and, occasionally "breakthrough" HBV infection occurs. This approach is very expensive, approximately $20,000 per year, and involves the intravenous administration of a globulin preparation designed for intramuscular injection. Although this approach is now practiced universally, it has not been approved officially by the U.S. Food and Drug Administration; clinical trials of HBIG preparations produced specifically for intravenous administration are in progress.

An alternative, promising but still experimental approach to the prophylaxis of patients with chronic hepatitis B undergoing liver transplantation is the use of nucleoside analogues such as famciclovir and lamivudine (see Ch. 297). Limited evidence available to date suggests that they have the potential to prevent recurrence of HBV infection when administered *prior* to transplantation, to treat hepatitis B that recurs *after* transplantation, including in patients who break through HBIG prophylaxis, and to reverse the course of otherwise fatal fibrosing cholestatic hepatitis. Clinical trials are underway to define the role of these antiviral agents in the management of patients undergoing liver transplantation for chronic hepatitis B.

Patients who undergo liver transplantation for chronic hepatitis B plus D have a better survival rate than patients undergoing transplantation for hepatitis B alone. Recurrence of hepatitis C virus (HCV) after liver transplantation can be documented in almost every patient, if sufficiently sensitive virus markers are used. Although acute and chronic liver injury occur after transplantation in patients with chronic hepatitis C, and although histologic analyses reveal moderate to severe HCV-associated hepatic injury in approximately half of all patients, HCV-induced liver injury is mild or absent in the other half of patients, and clinical consequences of recurrent hepatitis C are limited during the first 5 years after transplantation. About 5 to 10 percent of patients have sufficiently severe recurrent hepatitis C to merit antiviral therapy with interferon (which can *suppress* HCV-associated liver injury in approximately half of patients but rarely leads to *sustained* benefit), a small number succumb to HCV-associated liver injury, and a syndrome reminiscent of fibrosing cholestatic hepatitis (see above) has been observed rarely. Because patients with more episodes of rejection receive more immunosuppressive therapy, and because immunosuppressive therapy enhances HCV replication, patients with severe or multiple episodes of rejection are more likely to experience early recurrence of hepatitis C after transplantation. In addition, patients with HCV genotype 1b are more likely to have recurrent HCV-induced liver disease and to experience disease recurrence earlier after transplantation than patients with other genotypes. On the other hand, in the vast majority of patients, the impact of recurrent hepatitis C on graft and patient survival appears to be negligible, at least for the first 5 years after transplantation.

Patients who undergo liver transplantation for end-stage alcoholic cirrhosis are at risk of resorting to drinking again after transplantation, a potential source of recurrent alcoholic liver injury. Currently, alcoholic liver disease is one of the most common indications for liver transplantation, and most transplantation centers screen candidates carefully for predictors of continued abstinence. Recidivism is more likely in patients whose sobriety prior to transplantation was shorter than 6 months.

Posttransplantation Quality of Life Full rehabilitation is achieved in the majority of patients who survive the early postoperative months and escape chronic rejection or unmanageable infection. Psychosocial maladjustment interferes with medical compliance in a small number of patients, but most manage to adhere to immunosuppressive regimens, which must be continued indefinitely. In one study, 85 percent of patients who survived their transplants returned to gainful activities. In fact, some women have conceived and carried pregnancies to term after transplantation without demonstrable injury to their infants.

BIBLIOGRAPHY

Bismuth H (ed): Consensus conference on indications of liver transplantation. Hepatology 20(Suppl):1, 1994

Davies SE et al: Hepatic histological findings after transplantation for chronic hepatitis B virus infection, including a unique pattern of fibrosing cholestatic hepatitis. Hepatology 13:150, 1991

European FK506 Multicentre Liver Study Group: Randomised trial comparing tacrolimus (FK506) and cyclosporin in prevention of liver allograft rejection. Lancet 344:423, 1994

Féray C et al: Reinfection of liver graft by hepatitis C virus after liver transplantation. J Clin Invest 89:1361, 1992

———: Influence of the genotype of hepatitis C virus on the severity of recurrent liver disease after liver transplantation. Gastroenterology 108: 1088, 1995

Gane EJ et al: Long-term outcome of hepatitis C infection after liver transplantation. N Engl J Med 334:815, 1996

Keefe EB, Esquivel CO: Liver transplantation. Current Opinion in Gastroenterology 12:290, 1996

Lau JYN et al: High-level expression of hepatitis B viral antigens in fibrosing cholestatic hepatitis. Gastroenterology 102:956, 1992

Lucey MR et al: Selection for and outcome of liver transplantation in alcoholic liver disease. Gastroenterology 102:1736, 1992

Mazzaferro V et al: Liver transplantation for the treatment of small hepatocellular carcinoma in patients with cirrhosis. N Engl J Med 334:693, 1996

Osorio RW et al: Predicting recidivism after orthotopic liver transplantation for alcoholic liver disease. Hepatology 20:105, 1994

Samuel D et al: Liver transplantation in European patients with the hepatitis B surface antigen. N Engl J Med 329:1842, 1993

Starzl TE et al: Liver transplantation. N Engl J Med 321:1014, 1092, 1989

Todo S et al: Orthotopic liver transplantation for patients with hepatitis B virus–related liver disease. Hepatology 13:619, 1991

U.S. Multicenter FK506 Liver Study Group: A comparison of tacrolimus (FK506) and cyclosporine for immunosuppression in liver transplantation. N Engl J Med 331:1110, 1994

Wade JJ et al: Bacterial and fungal infections after liver transplantation: An analysis of 284 patients. Hepatology 21:1328, 1995

Wright TL: Liver transplantation for chronic hepatitis C viral infection. Gastroenterol Clin North Am 22:231, 1993

——— et al: Interferon-α therapy for hepatitis C infection after liver transplantation. Hepatology 20:773, 1994

Zetterman RK (guest ed): Long-term management of the liver transplant patient. Semin Liver Dis 15:123, 1995

302

Norton J. Greenberger, Kurt J. Isselbacher

DISEASES OF THE GALLBLADDER AND BILE DUCTS

PHYSIOLOGY OF BILE PRODUCTION AND FLOW **Bile Secretion and Composition** Bile formed in the hepatic lobules is secreted into a complex network of canaliculi, small bile ductules, and larger bile ducts that run with lymphatics and branches of the portal vein and hepatic artery in portal tracts situated between hepatic lobules. These interlobular bile ducts coalesce to form larger septal bile ducts that join to form the right and left hepatic ducts, which in turn unite to form the common hepatic duct. The common hepatic duct is joined by the cystic duct of the gallbladder to form the common bile duct (CBD), which enters the duodenum (often after joining the main pancreatic duct) through the ampulla of Vater.

Hepatic bile is a pigmented isotonic fluid with an electrolyte composition resembling blood plasma. The electrolyte composition of gallbladder bile differs from that of hepatic bile because most of the inorganic anions, chloride and bicarbonate, have been removed by reabsorption across the basement membrane.

Major components of bile by weight include water (82 percent), bile acids (12 percent), lecithin and other phospholipids (4 percent), and unesterified cholesterol (0.7 percent). Other constituents include conjugated bilirubin, proteins (IgA, by-products of hormones, and other proteins metabolized in the liver), electrolytes, mucus, and, often, drugs and their metabolic by-products.

The total daily basal secretion of hepatic bile is approximately 500 to 600 mL. The metabolic products of hepatocyte uptake and synthesis are secreted into the bile canaliculi, which are lined by microvillus membrane components associated with microfilaments of actin, microtubules, and other contractile elements. Within the hepatocyte, conjugation of many of the bile constituents may occur, while other components of bile, such as primary bile acids, lecithin, and some cholesterol, are synthesized de novo. Three mechanisms are important in regulating bile flow: (1) active transport of bile acids from hepatocytes into the canaliculi, (2) bile acid–independent ATPase-mediated transport of sodium, and (3) ductular secretion. The last is a secretin-mediated and cyclic AMP–dependent phenomenon that appears to result from the active transport of sodium and bicarbonate into the ductule, with resulting passive movement of water across the cell membrane.

The Bile Acids The primary bile acids, cholic and chenodeoxycholic acids, are synthesized from cholesterol in the liver, conjugated with glycine or taurine, and excreted into the bile. Secondary bile acids, including deoxycholate and lithocholate, are formed in the colon as bacterial metabolites of the primary bile acids. However, lithocholic acid is much less efficiently absorbed from the colon than deoxycholic acid. Other secondary bile acids, found in trace amounts, which include ursodeoxycholic acid [(UDCA) a stereoisomer of chenodeoxycholate (CDCA)] and a variety of other unusual or "aberrant" bile acids, may be produced in increased amounts in patients with chronic cholestatic syndromes. In normal bile, the ratio of glycine to taurine conjugates is about 3:1, while in patients with cholestasis, increased concentrations of sulfate and glucuronide conjugates of bile acids are often found.

Bile acids are detergents that in aqueous solutions and above a critical concentration of about 2 m*M* form molecular aggregates called *micelles*. Cholesterol alone is poorly soluble in aqueous environments, and its solubility in bile depends on both the lipid concentration and the relative molar percentages of bile acids and lecithin. Normal ratios of these constituents favor the formation of solubilizing *mixed micelles*, while abnormal ratios promote the precipitation of cholesterol crystals in bile.

In addition to facilitating the biliary excretion of cholesterol, bile acids are necessary for the normal intestinal absorption of dietary fats via a micellar transport mechanism (see Chap. 285). Bile acids also serve as a major physiologic driving force for hepatic bile flow and aid in water and electrolyte transport in the small bowel and colon.

Enterohepatic Circulation Bile acids are efficiently conserved under normal conditions. Conjugated and unconjugated bile acids are absorbed by *passive diffusion* along the entire gut. Quantitatively much more important for bile salt recirculation, however, is the *active transport* mechanism for conjugated bile acids in the distal ileum (see Chap. 285). The reabsorbed bile acids enter the portal bloodstream and are taken up rapidly by hepatocytes, reconjugated, and resecreted into bile (enterohepatic circulation).

The normal bile acid pool size is approximately 2 to 4 g. During digestion of a meal, the bile acid pool undergoes at least one or more enterohepatic cycles, depending on the size and composition of the meal. Normally, the bile acid pool circulates approximately 5 to 10 times daily. Intestinal absorption of the pool is about 95 percent efficient, so fecal loss of bile acids is in the range of 0.3 to 0.6 g/d. This fecal loss is compensated by an equal daily synthesis of bile acids by the liver, and thus the size of the bile salt pool is maintained. Bile acids returning to the liver suppress de novo hepatic synthesis of primary bile acids from cholesterol by inhibiting the rate-limiting enzyme 7α-hydroxylase. While the loss of bile salts in stool is usually matched by increased hepatic synthesis, the maximum rate of synthesis is approximately 5 g/d, which may be insufficient to replete the bile acid pool size when there is pronounced impairment of intestinal bile salt reabsorption.

Gallbladder and Sphincteric Functions In the fasting state, the sphincter of Oddi offers a high-pressure zone of resistance to bile flow from the common bile duct into the duodenum. This tonic contraction serves to (1) prevent reflux of duodenal contents into the pancreatic and bile ducts and (2) promote bile filling of the gallbladder. The major factor controlling the evacuation of the gallbladder is the peptide hormone cholecystokinin (CCK), which is released from the duodenal mucosa in response to the ingestion of fats and amino acids. CCK produces (1) powerful contraction of the gallbladder, (2) decreased resistance of the sphincter of Oddi, (3) increased hepatic secretion of bile, and thus (4) enhanced flow of biliary contents into the duodenum.

Hepatic bile is "concentrated" within the gallbladder by energy-dependent transmucosal absorption of water and electrolytes. Almost the entire bile acid pool may be sequestered in the gallbladder following an overnight fast for delivery into the duodenum with the first meal of the day. The normal capacity of the gallbladder is 30 to 75 mL of bile.

DISEASES OF THE GALLBLADDER

CONGENITAL ANOMALIES Anomalies of the biliary tract may be found in 10 to 20 percent of the population, including abnormalities in number, size, and shape (e.g., agenesis of the gallbladder, duplications, rudimentary or oversized "giant" gallbladders, and diverticula). Phrygian cap is a clinically innocuous entity in which a partial or complete septum (or fold) separates the fundus from the body. Anomalies of position or suspension are not uncommon and include left-sided gallbladder, intrahepatic gallbladder, retrodisplacement of the gallbladder, and "floating" gallbladder. The latter condition predisposes to acute torsion, volvulus, or herniation of the gallbladder.

GALLSTONES Pathogenesis Gallstones are quite prevalent in most western countries. In the United States, autopsy series have shown gallstones in at least 20 percent of women and in 8 percent of men over the age of 40. It is estimated that 16 to 20 million persons in the United States have gallstones and that approximately 1 million new cases of cholelithiasis develop each year.

Gallstones are crystalline structures formed by concretion or accretion of normal or abnormal bile constituents. These stones are divided into three major types; cholesterol and mixed stones account for 80 percent of the total, with pigment stones comprising the remaining 20 percent. Mixed and cholesterol gallstones usually contain more than 70 percent cholesterol monohydrate plus an admixture of calcium salts, bile acids and bile pigments, proteins, fatty acids, and phospholipids. Pigment stones are composed primarily of calcium bilirubinate; they contain less than 10 percent cholesterol.

Cholesterol and mixed stones and biliary sludge Cholesterol is relatively water insoluble and requires aqueous dispersion into either micelles or vesicles, both of which require the presence of a second lipid to "liquefy" the cholesterol. When the cholesterol content of bile exceeds the amount that can be solubilized by bile salt and bile salt–lecithin micelles, the excess is dispersed in larger lipid vesicles (Fig. 302-1). Vesicles are spherical particles composed of lecithin and cholesterol and contain only traces of bile salts. Vesicles and micelles are important cholesterol-solubilizing and -transport agents in bile supersaturated with cholesterol.

There are several important mechanisms in the formation of lithogenic (stone-forming) bile. The most important is increased biliary secretion of cholesterol. This may occur in association with obesity, high-caloric diets, or drugs (e.g., clofibrate) and may result from increased activity of hydroxymethylglutaryl–coenzyme A (HMG-CoA) reductase, the rate-limiting enzyme of hepatic cholesterol synthesis. In some patients, impaired hepatic conversion of cholesterol to bile acids also may occur, resulting in an increase of the lithogenic cholesterol/bile acid ratio. Lithogenic bile also results from decreased hepatic secretion of bile salts and phospholipids, which may follow impaired hepatic synthesis (e.g., rare inborn errors of metabolism such as cerebrotendinous xanthomatosis), or conditions affecting the enterohepatic circulation of these constituents (e.g., prolonged parenteral alimentation or ileal disease or resection). In addition, most patients with gallstones appear to have reduced activity of hepatic cholesterol 7α-hydroxylase, the rate-limiting enzyme for primary bile acid synthesis.

Thus an excess of biliary cholesterol in relation to bile acids and phospholipids may be due to hypersecretion of cholesterol, hyposecretion of bile acids, or both. While cholesterol saturation of bile is an important prerequisite for gallstone formation, it is not sufficient by itself to produce cholesterol precipitation in vivo. Most people with supersaturated bile do not develop stones because the time required for cholesterol crystals to nucleate and grow is longer than the time bile spends in the gallbladder. Two additional disturbances of bile acid metabolism that are likely to contribute to supersaturation of bile with cholesterol are (1) reduction of the bile acid pool and (2) enhanced conversion of cholic acid to deoxycholic acid, with replacement of the cholic acid pool by an expanded deoxycholic acid pool. The first disorder may be caused by more rapid loss of primary bile acid from the small intestine into the colon. The second disturbance may result from enhanced dehydroxylation of cholic acid and increased absorption of newly formed deoxycholic acid.

A second important abnormality is defective vesicle formation. Ordinarily, cholesterol and phospholipid are secreted into bile as unilamellar bilayered vesicles, which are unstable and are converted, along with bile acids, into other lipid aggregates such as micelles. During micellation of vesicles, more phospholipid than cholesterol is transferred to mixed micelles, leading to unstable cholesterol-rich vesicles that aggregate into larger multilamellar vesicles from which cholesterol crystals aggregate.

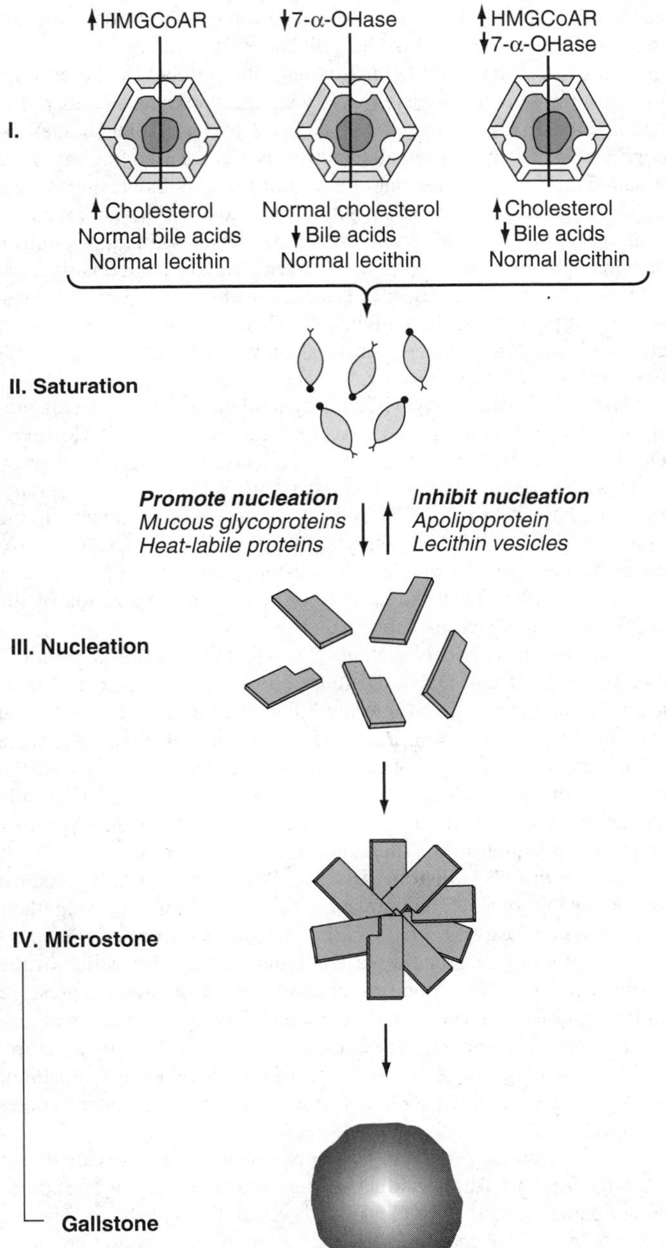

FIGURE 302-1 Scheme showing pathogenesis of gallstone formation. Conditions or factors that increase the ratio of cholesterol to bile acids and lecithin favor gallstone formation (HMG-CoAR, hydroxymethylglutaryl–coenzyme A reductase; 7-α-OHase, 7α-hydroxylase).

A third important mechanism is *nucleation* of cholesterol monohydrate crystals, which is greatly accelerated in human lithogenic bile; it is this feature rather than the degree of cholesterol supersaturation that distinguishes lithogenic from normal gallbladder bile. Accelerated nucleation of cholesterol monohydrate in bile may be due to either an *excess of pronucleating factors* or a *deficiency of antinucleating factors*. Nonmucin and mucin glycoproteins and lysine phosphatidylcholine appear to be pronucleating factors, while apolipoproteins AI and AII and other glycoproteins appear to be antinucleating factors. However, the characterization of additional pronucleating and antinucleating factors remains incomplete. Cholesterol monohydrate crystal nucleation and crystal growth probably occur within the mucin gel layer. Vesicle fusion leads to liquid crystals, which, in turn, nucleate into solid cholesterol monohydrate crystals. Continued growth of the crystals occurs by direct nucleation of cholesterol molecules from supersaturated unilamellar or multilamellar biliary vesicles.

A fourth important mechanism in cholesterol gallstone formation concerns *biliary sludge*. Biliary sludge is a thick mucous material that upon microscopic examination reveals lecithin-cholesterol crystals, cholesterol monohydrate crystals, calcium bilirubinate, and mucin thread or mucous gels. Biliary sludge typically forms a crescent-like layer in the most dependent portion of the gallbladder and is recognized by characteristic echoes on ultrasonography (see below). In vitro, cholesterol monohydrate crystals (>50 μm) mixed with mucus produce echoes that are indistinguishable from gallbladder sludge observed in patients. The presence of biliary sludge implies two abnormalities: (1) the normal balance between gallbladder mucin secretion and elimination has become deranged; and (2) nucleation from biliary solutes has occurred. That biliary sludge is a precursor form of gallstone disease is evident from several observations. In one study, 96 patients with gallbladder sludge were followed prospectively by serial ultrasound studies. In 17 patients (18 percent), biliary sludge disappeared and did not recur for at least 2 years. In 58 patients (60 percent), biliary sludge disappeared and reappeared. Importantly, gallstones developed in 14 patients, in 8 of whom the gallstones were "silent." In 12 patients, cholecystectomies were performed, 6 for gallstone-associated biliary pain and 3 in symptomatic patients with sludge but without gallstones who had prior attacks of pancreatitis; the latter did not recur after cholecystectomy. It should be emphasized that biliary sludge can develop with disorders that cause gallbladder hypomotility, i.e., surgery, burns, total parenteral nutrition, pregnancy, and oral contraceptives—all of which are associated with gallstone formation. Finally, biliary sludge can account for the observation that most cholesterol gallstones have a pigmented center.

Two other conditions are associated with cholesterol stone or biliary sludge formation: pregnancy and very low calorie diet. There appear to be two key changes during pregnancy that contribute to a "cholelithogenic state." First, the composition of the bile acid pool and the cholesterol-carrying capacity of bile change, with a resultant marked increase in cholesterol saturation during the third trimester. Second, ultrasonographic studies have demonstrated that gallbladder contraction in response to a standard meal is sluggish, resulting in impaired gallbladder emptying. That these changes are related to pregnancy per se is supported by several studies that show reversal of these abnormalities after delivery. During pregnancy, gallbladder sludge develops in 20 to 30 percent of women and gallstones in 5 to 12 percent. While biliary sludge is a common finding during pregnancy, it is usually asymptomatic and often resolves spontaneously after delivery. Gallstones that are less common and frequently associated with biliary colic may also disappear after delivery because of spontaneous dissolution related to bile becoming unsaturated with cholesterol post partum.

Ten to 20 percent of people having rapid weight reduction through very low calorie dieting develop gallstones. In a study involving close to 800 patients who completed a 16-week, 520-kcal/d diet, UDCA in a dosage of 600 mg/d proved highly effective in preventing gallstone formation; gallstones developed in only 2 percent of UDCA recipients compared to 28 percent of placebo-treated patients.

There is increasing evidence for the association between dietary cholesterol and gallstone formation. In patients with gallstones, an increase in dietary cholesterol further *increases* biliary cholesterol secretion and *decreases* bile acid synthesis and pool size, changes known to predispose to cholesterol gallstone formation. These changes do not occur in control (non-gallstone) patients on high-cholesterol diets. These findings help explain the presence of supersaturated bile in individuals predisposed to form gallstones.

To summarize, cholesterol gallstone disease occurs because of several defects, which include (1) bile supersaturation with cholesterol, (2) nucleation of cholesterol monohydrate with subsequent crystal retention and stone growth, and (3) abnormal gallbladder motor function with delayed emptying and stasis. Other important factors known to predispose to cholesterol stone formation are summarized in Table 302-1.

Pigment stones Gallstones composed largely of calcium bilirubinate are much more common in the orient than in western countries.

Table 302-1

Predisposing Factors for Cholesterol and Pigment Gallstone Formation

CHOLESTEROL AND MIXED STONES

1. Demography
   a. Northern Europe and North and South America greater than Asia, native Americans, probable familial, hereditary aspects
2. Obesity
   a. Normal bile acid pool and secretion but increased biliary secretion of cholesterol
3. Weight loss
   a. Mobilization of tissue cholesterol leads to increased biliary cholesterol secretion while enterohepatic secretion of bile salt is decreased
4. Female sex hormones
   a. Estrogens stimulate hepatic lipoprotein receptors, increase uptake of dietary cholesterol, increase biliary cholesterol secretion, and inhibit synthesis of chenodeoxycholic acid
   b. Natural estrogens, other estrogens, and oral contraceptives lead to decreased bile salt secretion and decreased conversion of cholesterol to cholesteryl esters
5. Ileal disease or resection
   a. Malabsorption of bile acids leads to decreased bile acid pool, decreased biliary secretion of bile salts, and decreased 7α-hydroxylase activity
6. Increasing age
   a. Increased biliary secretion of cholesterol, decreased size of bile acid pool, decreased biliary secretion of bile salts
7. Gallbladder hypomotility leading to stasis and formation of sludge/stools
   a. Prolonged parenteral nutrition
   b. Fasting
   c. Pregnancy
   d. Drugs such as octreotide
8. Clofibrate therapy
   a. Increased biliary secretion of cholesterol
9. Decreased bile acid secretion
   a. Primary biliary cirrhosis
   b. Chronic intrahepatic cholestasis
10. Miscellaneous
    a. High-calorie, high-fat diet
    b. Spinal cord injury

PIGMENT STONES

1. Demographic/genetic factors: Asia, rural setting
2. Chronic hemolysis
3. Alcoholic cirrhosis
4. Chronic biliary tract infection, parasite infestation
5. Increasing age

The presence of increased amounts of unconjugated, insoluble bilirubin in bile results in the precipitation of bilirubin, which may aggregate to form pigment stones or may fuse to form the nidus for growth of mixed cholesterol gallstones. In western countries, chronic hemolytic states (with increased conjugated bilirubin in bile) or alcoholic liver disease are associated with an increased incidence of pigment stones. Deconjugation of soluble bilirubin mono- and diglucuronide may be mediated by the enzyme β-glucuronidase, which is sometimes produced when bile is chronically infected by bacteria. Pigment stone formation is especially prominent in Asians and is often associated with infections in the biliary tree (see Table 302-1).

Diagnosis Procedures of potential use in the diagnosis of cholelithiasis and other diseases of the gallbladder are detailed in Table 302-2. The plain abdominal film may detect gallstones containing sufficient calcium to be radiopaque (10 to 15 percent of cholesterol and mixed stones and approximately 50 percent of pigment stones). Plain radiography also may be of use in the diagnosis of emphysematous cholecystitis, porcelain gallbladder, limey bile, and gallstone ileus.

Ultrasonography of the gallbladder is very accurate in the identification of cholelithiasis and has several advantages over oral cholecystography (see Fig. 302-2*A*). The gallbladder is easily visualized with the technique, and in fact, failure to image the gallbladder successfully in a fasting patient correlates well with the presence of underlying gallbladder disease. Stones as small as 2 mm in diameter may be confidently identified provided that firm criteria are used [e.g., acoustic "shadowing" of opacities that are within the gallbladder lumen and that change with the patient's position (by gravity)]. In major medical centers, the false-negative and false-positive rates for ultrasound in gallstone patients are about 2 to 4 percent. Biliary sludge is material of low echogenic activity that typically forms a layer in the most dependent position of the gallbladder. This layer shifts with postural changes but fails to produce acoustic shadowing; these two characteristics distinguish sludges from gallstones.

Oral cholecystography (OCG) is a useful procedure for the diagnosis of gallstones but has been largely replaced by ultrasound. However, OCG is still useful for the selection of patients for nonsurgical therapy of gallstone disease such as lithotripsy or bile acid dissolution therapy. In both these settings, OCG is used to assess the patency of the cystic duct and gallbladder emptying function. Further, OCG can also delineate the size and number of gallstones and determine whether they are calcified. Factors that may produce nonvisualization of the OCG are summarized in Table 302-2.

Radiopharmaceuticals such as ^{99m}Tc-labeled *N*-substituted iminodiacetic acids (HIDA, DIDA, DISIDA, etc.) are rapidly extracted from the blood and are excreted into the biliary tree in high concentration even in the presence of mild to moderate serum bilirubin elevations. Failure to image the gallbladder in the presence of biliary ductal visualization may indicate cystic duct obstruction, acute or chronic cholecystitis, or surgical absence of the organ. Such scans have their greatest application in the diagnosis of acute cholecystitis.

Symptoms of Gallstone Disease Gallstones usually produce symptoms by causing inflammation or obstruction following their migration into the cystic duct or CBD. The most specific and characteristic symptom of gallstone disease is biliary colic. Obstruction of the cystic duct or CBD by a stone produces increased intraluminal pressure and distention of the viscus that cannot be relieved by repetitive biliary contractions. The resultant visceral pain is characteristically a severe, steady ache or pressure in the epigastrium or right upper quadrant (RUQ) of the abdomen with frequent radiation to the interscapular area, right scapula, or shoulder.

Biliary colic begins quite suddenly and may persist with severe intensity for 1 to 4 h, subsiding gradually or rapidly. An episode of biliary pain is sometimes followed by a residual mild ache or soreness in the RUQ, which may persist for 24 h or so. Nausea and vomiting frequently accompany episodes of biliary colic, and mild elevations of serum bilirubin [not exceeding 85.5 μmol/L (5 mg/dL)] occur in 25 percent of patients. Persistence of a high serum bilirubin level suggests common duct stones. Fever or chills (rigors) with biliary colic usually imply an underlying complication, i.e., cholecystitis, pancreatitis, or cholangitis. Complaints of vague epigastric fullness, dyspepsia, eructation, or flatulence, especially following a fatty meal, should not be confused with biliary colic. Such symptoms are frequently elicited from patients with gallstone disease but are not specific for biliary calculi. Biliary colic may be precipitated by eating a fatty meal, by consumption of a large meal following a period of prolonged fasting, or by eating a normal meal.

Natural History Gallstone disease discovered in an asymptomatic patient or in a patient whose symptoms are not referable to cholelithiasis is a common clinical problem. The natural history of "silent" or asymptomatic gallstones has occasioned much debate. In contrast to previous reports, a study of predominantly male silent gallstone patients suggests that the cumulative risk for the development of symptoms or complications requiring surgery is relatively low—10 percent at 5 years, 15 percent at 10 years, and 18 percent at 15 years. Patients remaining asymptomatic for 15 years were found to be unlikely to develop symptoms during further follow-up, and most patients who did develop complications from their gallstones experienced *prior* warning symptoms. Similar conclusions apply to diabetics with silent gallstones. Decision analysis has suggested that (1) the cumulative risk of death due to gallstone disease while on expectant management is small, and (2) prophylactic cholecystectomy is not warranted.

Complications requiring cholecystectomy appear to be much more common in gallstone patients who have developed symptoms of biliary colic. Patients found to have gallstones at a young age are more likely to develop symptoms from cholelithiasis than are patients older than 60 years at the time of initial diagnosis. Patients with diabetes mellitus and gallstones may be somewhat more susceptible to septic complications, but the magnitude of risk of septic biliary complications in diabetic patients is incompletely defined. In addition, asymptomatic gallstone patients with nonvisualization of the gallbladder on OCG appear to have an increased tendency to develop symptoms and complications.

TREATMENT

Surgical Therapy Although the management of silent gallstones remains controversial, the risk of developing symptoms or complications requiring surgery is quite small (in the range of 1 to 2 percent per year) in most asymptomatic gallstone patients. Thus a recommendation for prophylactic cholecystectomy in a patient with gallstones should probably be based on assessment of three factors: (1) the presence of symptoms that are frequent enough or severe enough to interfere with the patient's general routine; (2) the presence of a prior complication of gallstone disease, i.e., history of acute cholecystitis, pancreatitis, gallstone fistula, etc.; or (3) the presence of an underlying condition predisposing the patient to increased risk of gallstone complications (e.g., calcified or porcelain gallbladder, cholesterolosis, adenomyomatosis, and/or a previous attack of acute cholecystitis regardless of current symptomatic status). Patients with very large gallstones (over 2 cm in diameter) and patients having gallstones in a congenitally anomalous gallbladder also might be considered for prophylactic cholecystectomy. Although age under 50 years is a worrisome factor in asymptomatic gallstone patients, few authorities would now recommend routine cholecystectomy in all young patients with silent stones. Laparoscopic cholecystectomy is a minimal-access approach for the removal

Table 302-2

Diagnostic Evaluation of the Gallbladder

Diagnostic Advantages	Diagnostic Limitations	Comment
PLAIN ABDOMINAL X-RAY		
Low cost Readily available	Relatively low yield ?Contraindicated in pregnancy	Pathognomonic findings in: Calcified gallstones Limey bile, porcelain GB Emphysematous cholecystitis Gallstone ileus
ORAL CHOLECYSTOGRAM		
Low cost Readily available Accurate identification of gallstones (90–95%) Identification of GB anomalies, hyperplastic cholecystoses Identification of chronic GB disease after nonvisualization on double dose	?Contraindicated in pregnancy ?Contraindicated with history of reaction to iodinated contrast Nonvisualization with: Serum bilirubin >34–68 μmol/L (2–4 mg/dL) Failure to ingest or absorb tablets Impaired hepatic excretion Very small stones may be undetected More time-consuming than GBUS	Largely replaced by GBUS A useful procedure in identification of gallstones if diagnostic limitations prevent GBUS
GALLBLADDER ULTRASOUND		
Rapid Accurate identification of gallstones (>95%) Simultaneous scanning of GB, liver, bile ducts, pancreas "Real-time" scanning allows assessment of GB volume, contractility Not limited by jaundice, pregnancy May detect very small stones	Bowel gas Massive obesity Ascites Recent barium study	Procedure of choice for detection of stones
RADIOISOTOPE SCANS (HIDA, DIDA, ETC.)		
Accurate identification of cystic duct obstruction Simultaneous assessment of bile ducts	?Contraindicated in pregnancy Serum bilirubin >103–205 μmol/L (6–12 mg/dL) Cholecystogram of low resolution	Indicated for confirmation of suspected acute cholecystitis; less sensitive and less specific in chronic cholecystitis; useful in diagnosis of acalculous cholecystopathy, especially if given with CCK to assess gallbladder emptying

NOTE: GB, gallbladder; GBUS, gallbladder ultrasound.

of the gallbladder together with its stones. Because of a markedly shortened hospital stay as well as decreased cost and a mortality rate of less than 1 percent, it is the procedure of choice for most patients referred for elective cholecystectomy; in only 4 to 5 percent of patients are surgeons compelled to convert to open cholecystectomy.

From several studies involving over 4000 patients undergoing laparoscopic cholecystectomy, the following key points emerge: (1) complications develop in about 4 percent of patients; (2) conversion to laparotomy occurs in 5 percent; (3) the death rate is remarkably low (i.e., <0.1 percent); and (4) bile duct injuries are unusual (i.e., 4 percent). Preoperative endoscopic retrograde cholangiopancreatography (ERCP) was carried out in about 5 percent, intraoperative cholangiography in about 30 percent, and postoperative ERCP in approximately 1.5 percent of patients. These data indicate why laparoscopic cholecystectomy has become the "gold standard" for treating symptomatic cholelithiasis.

Medical Therapy—Gallstone Dissolution UDCA and CDCA decrease HMG-CoA reductase activity, which in turn results in decreased hepatic cholesterol synthesis. UDCA administration also appears to produce a lamellar liquid crystalline phase in bile that allows a dispersion of cholesterol from stones by physiochemical means. UDCA also may retard cholesterol crystal nucleation. In carefully selected patients with a functioning gallbladder and with radiolucent stones <15 mm in diameter, complete dissolution can be achieved in 50 to 60 percent of patients within 2 years with UDCA at a dose of 10 to 13 mg/kg per day. The highest success rate (i.e., >70 percent) occurs in patients with small (<5 mm) floating radiolucent gallstones. Probably no more than 10 percent of patients with *symptomatic* cholelithiasis are candidates for such treatment. However, in addition to the vexing problem of recurrent stones (30 to 50 percent over 3 to 12 years of follow-up), there is also the factor of taking an expensive drug for an indefinite period of time. The advantages and success of laparoscopic cholecystectomy have largely reduced the role of gallstone dissolution to patients who either refuse or are not candidates for elective cholecystectomy. One role for UDCA is in the treatment of patients with recurrent calculous disease after cholecystectomy.

Gallbladder stones may be fragmented by extracorporeal shock waves generated by the use of electrohydraulic, piezoceramic, or electromagnetic devices. While such shock wave lithotripsy combined with medical litholytic therapy is safe and effective in carefully selected patients with gallbladder calculi, the procedure is employed infrequently for several reasons: (1) the rapid emergence of laparoscopic cholystectomy as the procedure of choice for symptomatic cholelithiasis and/or chronic cholecystitis, (2) recurrence of gallstones in 10 to 15 percent of patients within 2 years after lithotripsy combined with medical litholytic therapy, and (3) the considerable cost of taking UDCA or UDCA plus CDCA for an indefinite period.

ACUTE AND CHRONIC CHOLECYSTITIS **Acute Cholecystitis** Acute inflammation of the gallbladder wall usually follows obstruction of the cystic duct by a stone. Inflammatory response can be evoked by three factors: (1) *mechanical inflammation* produced by increased intraluminal pressure and distention with resulting ischemia of the gallbladder mucosa and wall, (2) *chemical inflammation* caused by the release of lysolecithin (due to the action of phospholipase on lecithin in bile) and other local tissue factors, and (3) *bacterial inflammation*, which may play a role in 50 to 85 percent of patients with acute cholecystitis. The organisms most frequently isolated by culture of gallbladder bile in these patients include *Escherichia coli*, *Klebsiella* species, group D *Streptococcus*, *Staphylococcus* species, and *Clostridium* species.

Acute cholecystitis often begins as an attack of biliary colic that progressively worsens. Approximately 60 to 70 percent of patients report having experienced prior attacks that resolved spontaneously. As the episode progresses, however, the pain of acute cholecystitis becomes more generalized in the right upper abdomen. As with biliary colic, the pain of cholecystitis may radiate to the interscapular area, right scapula, or shoulder. Peritoneal signs of inflammation such as increased pain with jarring or on deep respiration may be apparent. The patient is anorectic and often nauseated. Vomiting is relatively common and may produce symptoms and signs of vascular and extracellular volume depletion. Jaundice is unusual early in the course of acute cholecystitis but may occur when edematous inflammatory changes involve the bile ducts and surrounding lymph nodes.

A low-grade fever is characteristically present, but shaking chills or rigors are not uncommon. The RUQ of the abdomen is almost invariably tender to palpation. An enlarged, tense gallbladder is palpa-

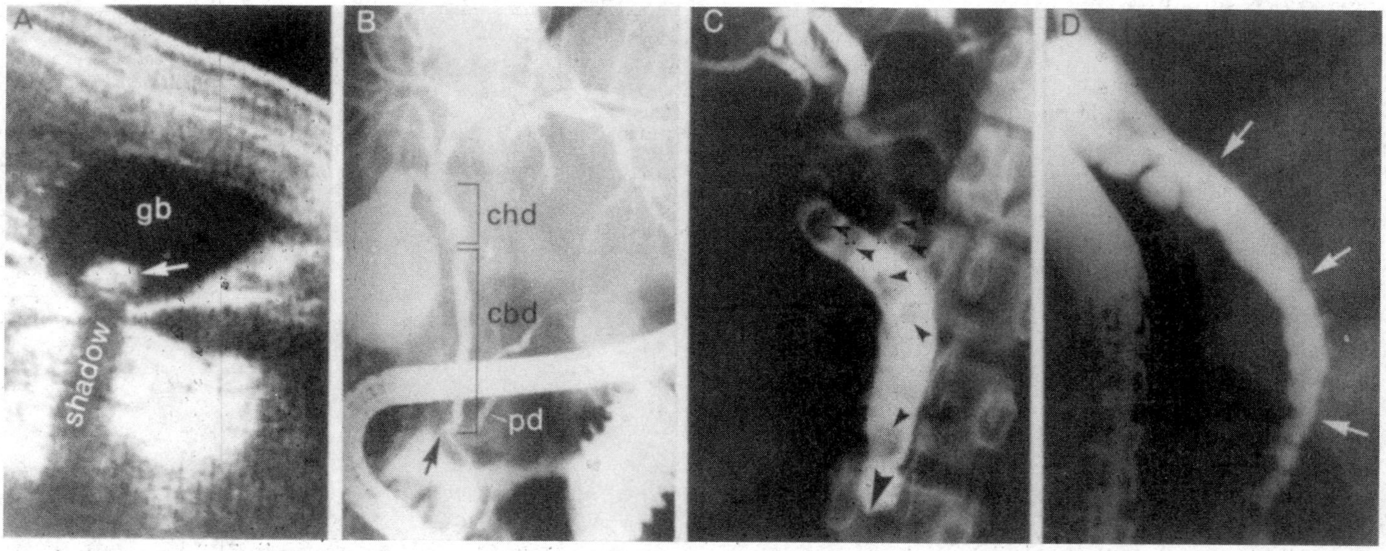

FIGURE 302-2 Examples of ultrasound and radiologic studies of the biliary tract. *A*. An ultrasound study showing a distended gallbladder containing a single large stone (*arrow*) which casts an acoustic shadow. *B*. Endoscopic retrograde cholangiopancreatogram (ERCP) showing normal biliary tract anatomy. In addition to the endoscope and large vertical gallbladder filled with contrast dye, the common hepatic duct (chd), common bile duct (cbd), and pancreatic duct (pd) are shown. The arrow points to the ampulla of Vater. *C*. Percutaneous transhepatic cholangiogram (PTHC) showing choledocholithiasis. The biliary tract is dilatated and contains multiple radiolucent calculi (*small arrows*). The dilatation is due to obstruction by a large stone in the distal portion of the duct (*large arrow*). *D*. ERCP showing sclerosing cholangitis. The common bile duct is to the right of the endoscope. Following retrograde cholangiography, the common bile duct shows thickening of the wall with a narrow, beaded lumen typical of sclerosing cholangitis.

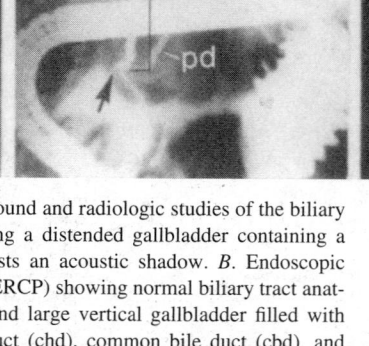

ble in one-quarter to one-half of patients. Deep inspiration or cough during subcostal palpation of the RUQ usually produces increased pain and inspiratory arrest (Murphy's sign). A light blow delivered to the right subcostal area may elicit a marked increase in pain. Localized rebound tenderness in the RUQ is common, as are abdominal distention and hypoactive bowel sounds from paralytic ileus, but generalized peritoneal signs and abdominal rigidity are usually lacking, absent perforation.

The diagnosis of acute cholecystitis is usually made on the basis of a characteristic history and physical examination. The triad of sudden onset of RUQ tenderness, fever, and leukocytosis is highly suggestive. Typically, leukocytosis in the range of 10,000 to 15,000 cells per microliter with a left shift on differential count is found. The serum bilirubin is mildly elevated [<85.5 μmol/L (5 mg/dL)] in 45 percent of patients, while 25 percent have modest elevations in serum aminotransferases (usually less than a fivefold elevation). The radionuclide (e.g., HIDA) biliary scan may be confirmatory if bile duct imaging is seen without visualization of the gallbladder. Ultrasound will demonstrate calculi in 90 to 95 percent of cases.

Approximately 75 percent of patients treated medically have remission of acute symptoms within 2 to 7 days following hospitalization. In 25 percent, however, a complication of acute cholecystitis will occur despite conservative treatment (see below). In this setting, prompt surgical intervention is required. Of the 75 percent of patients with acute cholecystitis who undergo remission of symptoms, approximately one-quarter will experience a recurrence of cholecystitis within 1 year, and 60 percent will have at least one recurrent bout within 6 years. In view of the natural history of the disease, acute cholecystitis is best treated by early surgery whenever possible.

Acalculous cholecystitis In 5 to 10 percent of patients with acute cholecystitis, calculi obstructing the cystic duct are not found at surgery. In over 50 percent of such cases an underlying explanation for acalculous inflammation is not found. An increased risk for the development of acalculous cholecystitis is especially associated with serious trauma or burns, with the postpartum period following prolonged labor, and with orthopedic and other nonbiliary major surgical operations in the postoperative period. Other precipitating factors include vasculitis, obstructing adenocarcinoma of the gallbladder, diabetes mellitus, torsion of the gallbladder, "unusual" bacterial infections of the gallbladder (e.g., *Leptospira*, *Streptococcus*, *Salmonella*, or *Vibrio cholerae*), and parasitic infestation of the gallbladder. Acalculous cholecystitis also may be seen with a variety of other systemic disease processes (sarcoidosis, cardiovascular disease, tuberculosis, syphilis, actinomycosis, etc.) and may possibly complicate periods of prolonged parenteral hyperalimentation.

Although the clinical manifestations of acalculous cholecystitis are indistinguishable from those of calculous cholecystitis, the setting of acute gallbladder inflammation complicating severe underlying illness is characteristic of acalculous disease. Ultrasound, computed tomography (CT) scanning, or radionuclide examinations demonstrating a large, tense, static gallbladder without stones and with evidence of poor emptying over a prolonged period may be diagnostically useful in some cases. The complication rate for acalculous cholecystitis exceeds that for calculous cholecystitis. Successful management of acute acalculous cholecystitis appears to depend primarily on early diagnosis and surgical intervention, with meticulous attention to postoperative care.

Acalculous cholecystopathy Disordered motility of the gallbladder can produce recurrent biliary pain in patients without gallstones. Infusion of an octapeptide of CCK can be used to measure the gallbladder ejection fraction during cholescintigraphy. In a representative study, CCK cholescintigraphy using ^{99m}Tc-diisopropyl iminodiacetic acid (DIDA) identified 21 patients with an abnormal gallbladder ejection fraction (<40 percent at 45 min); 10 of 11 patients who underwent surgery became asymptomatic, whereas all 10 who did not undergo surgery showed abnormalities, i.e., chronic cholecystitis, gallbladder muscle hypertrophy, and/or a markedly narrowed cystic duct. From this and other similar studies, the following criteria can be used to identify patients with acalculous cholecystopathy: (1) recurrent episodes of typical RUQ pain characteristic of biliary tract pain, (2) abnormal CCK cholescintigraphy demonstrating a gallbladder ejection fraction of less than 40 percent, (3) infusion of CCK reproduces the patient's pain, and (4) prior history of transient abnormalities in liver tests that accompanied episodes of RUQ pain. An additional clue would be the identification of a large gallbladder on ultrasound examination. Finally, it should be noted that sphincter of Oddi dysfunction also can give rise to recurrent RUQ pain and CCK-scintigraphic abnormalities.

Emphysematous cholecystitis So-called emphysematous cholecystitis is thought to begin with acute cholecystitis (calculous or acalculous) followed by ischemia or gangrene of the gallbladder wall and infection by gas-producing organisms. Bacteria most frequently cultured in this setting include anaerobes, such as *Clostridium welchii* or *Clostridium perfringens*, and aerobes, such as *E. coli*. This condition occurs most frequently in elderly men and in patients with diabetes mellitus. The clinical manifestations are essentially indistinguishable from those of nongaseous cholecystitis. The diagnosis is usually made on plain abdominal film by the finding of gas within the gallbladder lumen, dissecting within the gallbladder wall to form a gaseous ring, or in the pericholecystic tissues. The morbidity and mortality rates with emphysematous cholecystitis are considerable. Prompt surgical intervention coupled with appropriate antibiotics is mandatory.

Chronic Cholecystitis Chronic inflammation of the gallbladder wall is almost always associated with the presence of gallstones and is thought to result from repeated bouts of subacute or acute cholecystitis or from persistent mechanical irritation of the gallbladder wall. The presence of bacteria in the bile occurs in more than one-quarter of patients with chronic cholecystitis. Although the presence of infected bile in a patient with *chronic* cholecystitis undergoing elective cholecystectomy probably adds little to the operative risk, intraoperative Gram's staining and routine culturing of bile have been advocated to identify those patients whose gallbladder is colonized with *Clostridium* species. Appropriate antibiotics intra- and postoperatively are recommended in such patients because colonization with these organisms may be associated with devastating septic complications following surgery. Chronic cholecystitis may be asymptomatic for years, may progress to symptomatic gallbladder disease or to acute cholecystitis, or may present with complications (see below).

Complications of Cholecystitis *Empyema and hydrops* Empyema of the gallbladder usually results from progression of acute cholecystitis with persistent cystic duct obstruction to superinfection of the stagnant bile with a pus-forming bacterial organism. The clinical picture resembles that of cholangitis with high fever, severe RUQ pain, marked leukocytosis, and often, prostration. Empyema of the gallbladder carries a high risk of gram-negative sepsis and/or perforation. Emergency surgical intervention with proper antibiotic coverage is required as soon as the diagnosis is suspected.

Hydrops or mucocele of the gallbladder also may result from prolonged obstruction of the cystic duct, usually by a large solitary calculus. In this instance, the obstructed gallbladder lumen is progressively distended, over a period of time, by mucus (mucocele) or by a clear transudate (hydrops) produced by mucosal epithelial cells. A visible, easily palpable, nontender mass often extending from the RUQ into the right iliac fossa may be found on physical examination. The patient with hydrops of the gallbladder frequently remains asymptomatic, although chronic RUQ pain also may occur. Cholecystectomy is indicated, since empyema, perforation, or gangrene may complicate the condition.

Gangrene and perforation Gangrene of the gallbladder results from ischemia of the wall and patchy or complete tissue necrosis. Underlying conditions often include marked distention of the gallbladder, vasculitis, diabetes mellitus, empyema, or torsion resulting in arterial occlusion. Gangrene usually predisposes to perforation of the gallbladder, but perforation also may occur in chronic cholecystitis without premonitory warning symptoms. *Localized perforations* are usually contained by the omentum or by adhesions produced by recurrent inflammation of the gallbladder. Bacterial superinfection of the walled-off gallbladder contents results in abscess formation. Most patients are best treated with cholecystectomy, but some seriously ill patients may be managed with cholecystostomy and drainage of the abscess. *Free perforation* is less common but is associated with a mortality rate of approximately 30 percent. Such patients may experience a sudden transient relief of RUQ pain as the distended gallbladder decompresses; this is followed by signs of generalized peritonitis.

Fistula formation and gallstone ileus *Fistulization* into an adjacent organ adherent to the gallbladder wall may result from inflammation and adhesion formation. Fistulas into the duodenum are most common, followed in frequency by those involving the hepatic flexure of the colon, stomach or jejunum, abdominal wall, and renal pelvis. Clinically "silent" biliary-enteric fistulas occurring as a complication of chronic cholecystitis have been found in up to 5 percent of patients undergoing cholecystectomy. Asymptomatic cholecystoenteric fistulas may sometimes be diagnosed by finding gas in the biliary tree on plain abdominal films. Barium contrast studies or endoscopy of the upper gastrointestinal tract or colon may demonstrate the fistula, but oral cholecystography will almost never result in opacification of either the gallbladder or the fistulous tract. Treatment in the symptomatic patient usually consists of cholecystectomy, CBD exploration, and closure of the fistulous tract.

Gallstone ileus refers to mechanical intestinal obstruction resulting from the passage of a large gallstone into the bowel lumen. The stone customarily enters the duodenum through a cholecystoenteric fistula at that level. The site of obstruction by the impacted gallstone is usually at the ileocecal valve, provided that the more proximal small bowel is of normal caliber. The majority of patients do not give a history of either prior biliary tract symptoms or complaints suggestive of acute cholecystitis or fistulization. Large stones over 2.5 cm in diameter are thought to predispose to fistula formation by gradual erosion through the gallbladder fundus. Diagnostic confirmation may occasionally be found on the plain abdominal film (e.g., small-intestinal obstruction with gas in the biliary tree and a calcified, ectopic gallstone) or following an upper gastrointestinal series (cholecystoduodenal fistula with small bowel obstruction at the ileocecal valve). Laparotomy with stone extraction (or propulsion into the colon) remains the procedure of choice to relieve obstruction. Evacuation of large stones within the gallbladder should also be performed. In general, the gallbladder and its attachment to the intestines should be left alone.

Limey (milk of calcium) bile and porcelain gallbladder Calcium salts may be secreted into the lumen of the gallbladder in sufficient concentration to produce calcium precipitation and diffuse, hazy opacification of bile or a layering effect on plain abdominal roentgenography. This so-called limey bile or milk of calcium bile is usually clinically innocuous, but cholecystectomy is recommended because limey bile most often occurs in a hydropic gallbladder. In the entity called *porcelain gallbladder*, calcium salt deposition within the wall of a chronically inflamed gallbladder may be detected on the plain abdominal film. Cholecystectomy is advised in all patients with porcelain gallbladder because in a high percentage of cases this finding appears to be associated with the development of carcinoma of the gallbladder.

℞ TREATMENT

Medical Therapy Although surgical intervention remains the mainstay of therapy for acute cholecystitis and its complications, a period of in-hospital stabilization may be required before cholecystectomy. Oral intake is eliminated, nasogastric suction is initiated, and extracellular volume depletion and electrolyte abnormalities are repaired. Meperidine or pentazocine are usually employed for analgesia because they may produce less spasm of the sphincter of Oddi than drugs such as morphine. Intravenous antibiotic therapy is usually indicated in patients with severe acute cholecystitis even though bacterial superinfection of bile may not have occurred in the early stages of the inflammatory process. Postoperative complications of wound infection, abscess formation, or sepsis are reduced in antibiotic-treated patients. Effective single-agent antibiotics include ampicillin, cephalosporins, ureidopenicillins, or aminoglycosides, but in diabetic or debilitated patients and in those with signs of gram-negative sepsis, combination antibiotic treatment may be preferable (see also Chap. 138).

Surgical Therapy The optimal timing of surgical intervention in patients with acute cholecystitis depends on stabilization of the patient. The clear trend is toward earlier surgery, and this is due in part to requirements for shorter hospital stays. Urgent (emergency) cholecystectomy or cholecystostomy is probably appropriate in most patients in whom a complication of acute cholecystitis such as empyema, emphysematous cholecystitis, or perforation is suspected or confirmed. In uncomplicated cases of acute cholecystitis, up to 30 percent of patients fail to resolve their symptoms on appropriate medical therapy, and progression of the attack or a supervening complication leads to the performance of early operation (within 24 to 72 h). The technical complications of surgery are not increased in patients undergoing early as opposed to delayed cholecystectomy. Delayed surgical intervention is probably best reserved for (1) patients in whom the overall medical condition imposes an unacceptable risk for early surgery and (2) patients in whom the diagnosis of acute cholecystitis is in doubt. Early cholecystectomy is the treatment of choice for most patients with acute cholecystitis. Mortality figures for emergency cholecystectomy in most centers approach 3 percent, while the mortality risk for elective or early cholecystectomy approximates 0.5 percent in patients under age 60. Of course, the operative risks increase with age-related diseases of other organ systems and with the presence of long- or short-term complications of gallbladder disease. Seriously ill or debilitated patients with cholecystitis may be managed with cholecystostomy and tube drainage of the gallbladder. Elective cholecystectomy may then be done at a later date.

Postcholecystectomy Complications Early complications following cholecystectomy include atelectasis and other pulmonary disorders, abscess formation (often subphrenic), external or internal hemorrhage, biliary-enteric fistula, and bile leaks. Jaundice may indicate absorption of bile from an intraabdominal collection following a biliary leak or mechanical obstruction of the CBD by retained calculi, intraductal blood clots, or extrinsic compression. Routine performance of intraoperative cholangiography during cholecystectomy has helped to reduce the incidence of these early complications.

Overall, cholecystectomy is a very successful operation that provides total or near-total relief of preoperative symptoms in 75 to 90 percent of patients. The most common cause of persistent postcholecystectomy symptoms is an overlooked extrabiliary disorder (e.g., reflux esophagitis, peptic ulceration, postgastrectomy syndrome, pancreatitis, or irritable bowel syndrome). In a small percentage of patients, however, a disorder of the extrahepatic bile ducts may result in persistent symptomatology. These so-called postcholecystectomy syndromes may be due to (1) biliary strictures, (2) retained biliary calculi, (3) cystic duct stump syndrome, (4) stenosis or dyskinesia of the sphincter of Oddi, or (5) bile salt–induced diarrhea or gastritis.

Cystic duct stump syndrome In the absence of cholangiographically demonstrable retained stones, symptoms resembling biliary colic or cholecystitis in the postcholecystectomy patient have frequently been attributed to disease in a long (>1 cm) cystic duct remnant (cystic duct stump syndrome). Careful analysis, however, reveals that postcholecystectomy complaints are attributable to other causes in almost all patients in whom the symptom complex was originally thought to result from the existence of a long cystic duct stump. Accordingly, considerable care should be taken to investigate the possible role of other factors in the production of postcholecystectomy symptoms before attributing them to cystic duct stump syndrome.

Papillary dysfunction, papillary stenosis, spasm of the sphincter of Oddi, and biliary dyskinesia Symptoms of biliary colic accompanied by signs of recurrent, intermittent biliary obstruction may be produced by papillary stenosis, papillary dysfunction, spasm of the sphincter of Oddi, and biliary dyskinesia. Papillary stenosis is thought to result from acute or chronic inflammation of the papilla of Vater or from glandular hyperplasia of the papillary segment. Five criteria have been used to define papillary stenosis: (1) upper abdominal pain, usually RUQ or epigastric, (2) abnormal liver tests, (3) dilatation of the common bile duct upon ERCP examination, (4) delayed (>45 min) drainage of contrast material from the duct, and (5) increased basal pressure of the sphincter of Oddi, a finding that may be of only minor significance. A useful alternative to ERCP is hepatobiliary scintigraphy using ^{99m}Tc-DIDA, especially if ERCP and/or biliary manometry are either unavailable or not feasible. In patients with papillary stenosis, quantitative hepatobiliary scintigraphy has revealed delayed transit from the common bile duct to the bowel, ductal dilatation, and abnormal time-activity dynamics. This technique also can be used before and after sphincterotomy to document improvement in biliary emptying. Treatment consists of endoscopic or surgical sphincteroplasty to ensure wide patency of the distal portions of both the bile and pancreatic ducts. The greater the number of the preceding criteria present, the greater the likelihood that a patient does have a degree of papillary stenosis sufficient to justify correction. The factors usually considered as indications for sphincterotomy include (1) prolonged duration of symptoms, (2) lack of response to symptomatic treatment, (3) presence of severe disability, and (4) the patient's choice of sphincterotomy over surgery (given a clear understanding on his or her part of the risks involved in both procedures).

Criteria for diagnosing dyskinesia of the sphincter of Oddi are even more controversial than those for papillary stenosis. Proposed mechanisms include spasm of the sphincter, denervation sensitivity resulting in hypertonicity, and abnormalities of the sequencing or frequency rates of sphincteric contraction waves. When thorough evaluation has failed to demonstrate another cause for the pain, and when cholangiographic and manometric criteria suggest a diagnosis of biliary dyskinesia, medical treatment with nitrites or anticholinergics to attempt pharmacologic relaxation of the sphincter has been proposed. Endoscopic sphincterotomy or surgical sphincteroplasty may be indicated in patients who fail to respond to a 2- to 3-month trial of medical therapy, especially if basal sphincter of Oddi pressures are elevated.

Bile salt–induced catharsis and gastritis Postcholecystectomy patients may develop symptoms and signs of gastritis, which has been attributed to duodenogastric reflux of bile. However, firm data linking an increased incidence of bile gastritis with surgical removal of the gallbladder are lacking. Similarly, the occurrence of cholestyramine-responsive diarrhea in a small number of patients following cholecystectomy has been attributed to an alteration of the enterohepatic circulation of bile acids induced or unmasked by removal of the gallbladder.

THE HYPERPLASTIC CHOLECYSTOSES The term *hyperplastic cholecystoses* is used to denote a group of disorders of the gallbladder characterized by excessive proliferation of normal tissue components.

Adenomyomatosis is characterized by a benign proliferation of gallbladder surface epithelium with glandlike formations, extramural sinuses, transverse strictures, and/or fundal nodule ("adenoma" or "adenomyoma") formation. Outpouchings of mucosa termed *Rokitansky-Aschoff sinuses* may be seen on oral cholecystography in conjunction with hyperconcentration of contrast medium. Characteristic dimpled filling defects also may be seen.

Cholesterolosis is characterized by abnormal deposition of lipid, especially cholesterol esters, in the lamina propria of the gallbladder wall. In its diffuse form ("strawberry gallbladder"), the gallbladder mucosa is brick red and speckled with bright yellow flecks of lipid. The localized form shows solitary or multiple "cholesterol polyps" studding the gallbladder wall. Cholesterol stones of the gallbladder are found in nearly half the cases. Cholecystectomy is indicated in both adenomyomatosis and cholesterolosis when symptomatic or when cholelithiasis is present.

DISEASES OF THE BILE DUCTS

CONGENITAL ANOMALIES **Biliary Atresia and Hypoplasia** Atretic and hypoplastic lesions of the extrahepatic and major intrahepatic bile ducts are the most common biliary anomalies of clinical relevance encountered in infancy. The clinical picture is one of severe obstructive jaundice during the first month of life, with pale stools. The diagnosis is confirmed by surgical exploration with operative cholangiography. Approximately 10 percent of cases of biliary atresia are treatable with roux-en-Y choledochojejunostomy, with the Kasai procedure (hepatic portoenterostomy) being attempted in the remainder in an effort to restore some bile flow. Most patients, even those having successful biliary-enteric anastomoses, eventually develop chronic cholangitis, extensive hepatic fibrosis, and portal hypertension.

Choledochal Cysts Cystic dilatation may involve the free portion of the CBD, i.e., choledochal cyst, or may present as diverticulum formation in the intraduodenal segment. In the latter situation, chronic reflux of pancreatic juice into the biliary tree can produce inflammation and stenosis of the extrahepatic bile ducts leading to cholangitis or biliary obstruction. Because the process may be gradual, approximately 50 percent of patients present with onset of symptoms after age 10. The diagnosis may be made by ultrasound, abdominal CT, or cholangiography. Only one-third of patients show the classic triad of abdominal pain, jaundice, and an abdominal mass. Ultrasonographic detection of a cyst separate from the gallbladder should suggest the diagnosis of choledochal cyst, which can be confirmed by demonstrating the entrance of extrahepatic bile ducts into the cyst. Surgical treatment involves excision of the "cyst" and biliary-enteric anastomosis. Patients with choledochal cysts are at increased risk for the subsequent development of cholangiocarcinoma.

Congenital Biliary Ectasia Cystic dilatation of the intrahepatic bile ducts may involve either the major intrahepatic radicles (Caroli's disease), the inter- and intralobular ducts (congenital hepatic fibrosis), or both. In Caroli's disease, clinical manifestations include recurrent cholangitis, abscess formation in and around the affected ducts, and, sometimes, gallstone formation within portions of ectatic intrahepatic biliary radicles. The CT scan and cholangiographic patterns are usually diagnostic, and treatment with ongoing antibiotic therapy is usually undertaken in an effort to limit the frequency and severity of recurrent bouts of cholangitis. Progression to secondary biliary cirrhosis with portal hypertension, amyloidosis, extrahepatic biliary obstruction, cholangiocarcinoma, or recurrent episodes of sepsis with hepatic abscess formation is common.

CHOLEDOCHOLITHIASIS **Pathophysiology and Clinical Manifestations** Passage of gallstones into the CBD occurs in approximately 10 to 15 percent of patients with cholelithiasis. The incidence of common duct stones increases with increasing age of the patient so that up to 25 percent of elderly patients may have calculi in the common duct at the time of cholecystectomy. Undetected duct stones are left behind in approximately 1 to 5 percent of cholecystectomy patients. The overwhelming majority of bile duct stones are cholesterol or mixed stones formed in the gallbladder, which then migrate into the extrahepatic biliary tree through the cystic duct. Primary calculi arising de novo in the ducts are usually pigment stones developing in patients with (1) chronic hemolytic diseases, (2) hepatobiliary parasitism or chronic, recurrent cholangitis, (3) congenital anomalies of the bile ducts (especially Caroli's disease), or (4) dilated, sclerosed, or strictured ducts. Common duct stones may remain asymptomatic for years, may pass spontaneously into the duodenum, or (most often) may present with biliary colic or a complication.

Complications *Cholangitis* Cholangitis may be acute or chronic, and symptoms result from inflammation, which usually requires at least partial obstruction to the flow of bile. Bacteria are present on bile culture in approximately 75 percent of patients with acute cholangitis early in the symptomatic course. The characteristic presentation of acute cholangitis involves biliary colic, jaundice, and spiking fevers with chills (Charcot's triad). Blood cultures are frequently positive, and leukocytosis is typical. *Nonsuppurative* acute cholangitis is most common and may respond relatively rapidly to supportive measures and to treatment with antibiotics. In *suppurative* acute cholangitis, however, the presence of pus under pressure in a completely obstructed ductal system leads to symptoms of severe toxicity—mental confusion, bacteremia, and septic shock. Response to antibiotics alone in this setting is relatively poor, multiple hepatic abscesses are often present, and the mortality rate approaches 100 percent unless prompt surgical correction of the obstructing lesion and drainage of infected bile is carried out. Endoscopic management of bacterial cholangitis is as effective as surgical intervention. ERCP with endoscopic sphincterotomy is safe and the preferred initial procedure for both establishing a definitive diagnosis and providing effective therapy.

Obstructive jaundice Gradual obstruction of the CBD over a period of weeks or months usually leads to initial manifestations of jaundice or pruritus without associated symptoms of biliary colic or cholangitis. Painless jaundice may occur in patients with choledocholithiasis, but this manifestation is much more characteristic of biliary obstruction secondary to malignancy of the head of pancreas, bile ducts, or ampulla of Vater.

In patients whose obstruction is secondary to choledocholithiasis, associated chronic calculous cholecystitis is very common, and the gallbladder in this setting may be relatively indistensible. The absence of a palpable gallbladder in most patients with biliary obstruction from duct stones is the basis for *Courvoisier's law*, i.e., that the presence of a palpably enlarged gallbladder suggests that the biliary obstruction is secondary to an underlying malignancy rather than to calculous disease. Biliary obstruction causes progressive dilatation of the intrahepatic bile ducts as intrabiliary pressures rise. Hepatic bile flow is suppressed, and regurgitation of conjugated bilirubin into the bloodstream leads to jaundice accompanied by dark urine (bilirubinuria) and light-colored (acholic) stools.

CBD stones should be suspected in any patient with cholecystitis whose serum bilirubin level exceeds 85.5 μmol/L (5 mg/dL). The maximum bilirubin level is seldom over 256.5 μmol/L (15.0 mg/dL) in patients with choledocholithiasis unless concomitant hepatic disease or another factor leading to marked hyperbilirubinemia exists. Serum bilirubin levels of 342.0 μmol/L (20 mg/dL) or more should suggest the possibility of neoplastic obstruction. The serum alkaline phosphatase level is almost always elevated in biliary obstruction. A rise in alkaline phosphatase often precedes clinical jaundice and may be the only abnormality in routine liver function tests. There may be a two- to tenfold elevation of serum aminotransferases, especially in association with acute obstruction. Following relief of the obstructing process, serum aminotransferase elevations usually return rapidly to normal, while the serum bilirubin level may take 1 to 2 weeks to return to normal. The alkaline phosphatase level usually falls slowly, lagging behind the decrease in serum bilirubin.

Pancreatitis The most common associated entity discovered in patients with nonalcoholic acute pancreatitis is biliary tract disease. Biochemical evidence of pancreatic inflammation complicates acute cholecystitis in 15 percent of cases and choledocholithiasis in over 30 percent, and the common factor appears to be the passage of gallstones through the common duct. Coexisting pancreatitis should be suspected in patients with symptoms of cholecystitis who develop (1) back pain or pain to the left of the abdominal midline, (2) prolonged vomiting with paralytic ileus, or (3) a pleural effusion, especially on the left side. Surgical treatment of gallstone disease is usually associated with resolution of the pancreatitis.

Secondary biliary cirrhosis Secondary biliary cirrhosis may complicate prolonged or intermittent duct obstruction with or without recurrent cholangitis. Although this complication may be seen in patients with choledocholithiasis, it is more common in cases of prolonged obstruction from stricture or neoplasm. Once established, secondary biliary cirrhosis may be progressive even after correction of the obstructing process, and increasingly severe hepatic cirrhosis may lead to portal hypertension or to hepatic failure and death. Prolonged biliary obstruction also may be associated with clinically relevant deficiencies of the fat-soluble vitamins A, D, and K.

Diagnosis and Treatment The diagnosis of choledocholithiasis is usually made by cholangiography (Table 302-3), either preoperatively by ERCP or intraoperatively at the time of cholecystectomy. As many as 20 percent of patients undergoing cholecystectomy will prove to have CBD stones. With the advent of laparoscopic cholecystectomy, the management of CBD stones in the presence of gallstones is gradually being clarified. Preoperative ERCP with endoscopic papillotomy and stone extraction is the preferred approach. It not only provides stone clearance but also defines the anatomy of the biliary tree in relationship to the cystic duct. ERCP is indicated in gallstone patients who have any of the following risk factors: (1) a history of jaundice or pancreatitis, (2) abnormal tests of liver function, and (3) ultrasonographic evidence of a dilated CBD or stones in the duct. Alternatively, if routine cholangiography of the cystic duct reveals retained stones, postoperative ERCP can be carried out. The need for preoperative ERCP is expected to decrease further as laparoscopic techniques improve.

The widespread use of laparoscopic cholecystectomy and ERCP has decreased the incidence of complicated biliary tract disease and the need for choledocholithotomy and T-tube drainage of the bile ducts. Endoscopic sphincterotomy followed by spontaneous passage or stone extraction is a nonoperative alternative in the management of patients with common duct stones, especially in elderly or poor-risk patients.

TRAUMA, STRICTURES, AND HEMOBILIA Benign strictures of the extrahepatic bile ducts result from surgical trauma in approximately 95 percent of cases and occur in about 1 in 500 cholecystectomies. Strictures may present with bile leak or abscess formation in the immediate postoperative period or with biliary obstruction or cholangitis as long as 2 years or more following the inciting trauma. The diagnosis is established by percutaneous or endoscopic cholangiography. Endoscopic brushing of biliary strictures is an effective way to establish the nature of the lesion and is more accurate than bile cytology alone. When positive exfoliative cytology is obtained, the diagnosis of a neoplastic stricture is established. This procedure is especially important in patients with primary sclerosing cholangitis who are predisposed to the development of cholangiocarcinomas. Successful operative correction by a skillful surgeon with duct-to-bowel anastomosis is usually possible, although mortality rates from surgical complications, recurrent cholangitis, or secondary biliary cirrhosis are high.

Hemobilia may follow traumatic or operative injury to the liver or bile ducts, intraductal rupture of a hepatic abscess or aneurysm of the hepatic artery, biliary or hepatic tumor hemorrhage, or mechanical complications of choledocholithiasis or hepatobiliary parasitism. Diagnostic procedures such as liver biopsy, percutaneous transhepatic cholangiography (PTHC), and transhepatic biliary drainage catheter placement also may be complicated by hemobilia. Patients often present with a classic triad of biliary colic, obstructive jaundice, and melena or occult blood in the stools. The diagnosis is sometimes made by cholangiographic evidence of blood clot in the biliary tree, but selective angiographic verification may be required. Although minor episodes of hemobilia may resolve without operative intervention, surgical ligation of the bleeding vessel is frequently required.

EXTRINSIC COMPRESSION OF THE BILE DUCTS Partial or complete biliary obstruction may sometimes be produced by extrinsic compression of the ducts. The most common cause of this form of obstructive jaundice is carcinoma of the head of the pancreas. Biliary obstruction also may occur as a complication of either acute or chronic pancreatitis or involvement of lymph nodes in the porta hepatis by lymphoma or metastatic carcinoma. The latter should be distinguished from cholestasis resulting from massive replacement of the liver by tumor.

Table 302-3

Diagnostic Evaluation of the Bile Ducts

Diagnostic Advantages	Diagnostic Limitations	Contraindications	Complications	Comment
HEPATOBILIARY ULTRASOUND				
Rapid Simultaneous scanning of GB, liver, bile ducts, pancreas Accurate identification of dilated bile ducts Not limited by jaundice, pregnancy Guidance for fine-needle biopsy	Bowel gas Massive obesity Ascites Barium Partial bile duct obstruction Poor visualization of distal CBD	None	None	Initial procedure of choice in investigating possible biliary tract obstruction
COMPUTED TOMOGRAPHY				
Simultaneous scanning of GB, liver, bile ducts, pancreas Accurate identification of dilated bile ducts, masses Not limited by jaundice, gas, obesity, ascites High-resolution image Guidance for fine-needle biopsy	Extreme cachexia Movement artifact Ileus Partial bile duct obstruction High cost May not be readily available	Pregnancy	Reaction to iodinated contrast, if used	Indicated for evaluation of hepatic or pancreatic masses Procedure of choice in investigating possible biliary obstruction if diagnostic limitations prevent HBUS
MAGNETIC RESONANCE CHOLANGIOPANCREATOGRAPHY				
Useful modality for visualizing pancreatic and biliary ducts Can identify pancreatic duct dilatation or stricture, pancreatic duct stenosis, and pancreas divisum Has excellent sensitivity for bile duct dilatation, biliary stricture, and intraductal abnormalities	Cannot offer therapeutic intervention			
PERCUTANEOUS TRANSHEPATIC CHOLANGIOGRAM				
Extremely successful when bile ducts dilated Best visualization of proximal biliary tract Possible separate visualization of obstructed left ductal system Bile cytology/culture Percutaneous transhepatic drainage	Nondilated or sclerosed ducts	Pregnancy Uncorrectable coagulopathy Massive ascites ? Hepatic abscess	Bleeding Hemobilia Bile peritonitis Bacteremia, sepsis	Usually, initial cholangiogram of choice when bile ducts are dilated
ENDOSCOPIC RETROGRADE CHOLANGIOPANCREATOGRAM				
Simultaneous pancreatography Visualization/biopsy of ampulla and duodenum Best visualization of distal biliary tract Bile or pancreatic cytology Endoscopic sphincterotomy and stone removal Biliary manometry Not limited by ascites, coagulopathy, abscess	Gastroduodenal obstruction ? Roux en Y biliary-enteric anastomosis	Pregnancy ? Acute pancreatitis ? Severe cardiopulmonary disease	Pancreatitis Cholangitis, sepsis Infected pancreatic pseudocyst Perforation (rare) Hypoxemia, aspiration	Cholangiogram of choice in: Absence of dilated ducts ? Pancreatic, ampullary or gastroduodenal disease Prior biliary surgery PTHC contraindicated or failed Endoscopic sphincterotomy a treatment possibility

NOTE: GB, gallbladder; HBUS, hepatobiliary ultrasound. Intravenous cholangiography is an obsolete technique because 40 percent of common duct stones are missed and there is poor resolution even with tomography. There are few indications for its use, especially since other cholangiographic techniques are usually available.

HEPATOBILIARY PARASITISM Infestation of the biliary tract by adult helminths or their ova may produce a chronic, recurrent pyogenic cholangitis with or without multiple hepatic abscesses, ductal stones, or biliary obstruction. This condition is relatively rare but does occur in inhabitants of southern China and elsewhere in Southeast Asia. The organisms most commonly involved are trematodes or flukes, including *Clonorchis sinensis*, *Opisthorchis viverrini* or *Opisthorchis felineus*, and *Fasciola hepatica*. The biliary tract also may be involved by intraductal migration of adult *Ascaris lumbricoides* from the duodenum or by intrabiliary rupture of hydatid cysts of the liver produced by *Echinococcus* species. The diagnosis is made by cholangiography and the presence of characteristic ova on stool examination. When obstruction is present, the treatment of choice is laparotomy under antibiotic coverage, with common duct exploration and a biliary drainage procedure. It should be emphasized that in the Orient, one also sees cholangiohepatitis associated with pigment lithiasis, which may, in fact, be more common than cholangitis due to parasites.

SCLEROSING CHOLANGITIS Primary or idiopathic sclerosing cholangitis is a disorder characterized by a progressive, inflammatory, sclerosing, and obliterative process affecting the extrahepatic and, often, the intrahepatic bile ducts. The lesion may appear as an isolated entity or may occur in association with inflammatory bowel disease, especially ulcerative colitis, or with multifocal fibrosclerosis syndromes such as retroperitoneal, mediastinal, and/or periureteral fibrosis; Riedel's struma; or pseudotumor of the orbit. In patients with AIDS, cholangiopancreatography may demonstrate a broad range of biliary tract changes as well as pancreatic duct obstruction and occasionally pancreatitis (see Chap. 308). Further, biliary tract lesions in AIDS include infection and cholangiopancreatographic changes similar to primary sclerosing cholangitis. Changes noted include: (1) diffuse involvement of intrahepatic bile ducts alone, (2) involvement of both intra- and extrahepatic bile ducts, (3) ampullary stenosis, (4) stricture of the intrapancreatic portion of the common bile duct, and (5) pancreatic duct involvement. Associated infectious organisms include *Cryptosporidium*, *Mycobacterium avium-intracellulare*, cytomegalovirus, *Microsporidia*, and *Isospora*. In addition, acalculous cholecystitis occurs in up to 10 percent of patients. ERCP sphincterotomy, while not without risk, provides significant pain reduction in patients with AIDS-associated papillary stenosis. Secondary sclerosing cholangitis may occur as a long-term complication of choledocholithiasis, cholangiocarcinoma, operative or traumatic biliary injury, or contiguous inflammatory processes.

Patients with primary sclerosing cholangitis often present with signs and symptoms of chronic or intermittent biliary obstruction: jaundice, pruritus, RUQ abdominal pain, or acute cholangitis. Late in the course, complete biliary obstruction, secondary biliary cirrhosis, hepatic failure, or portal hypertension with bleeding varices may occur. The diagnosis is usually established by finding thickened ducts with narrow, beaded lumina on cholangiography (see Fig. 302-2*D*). The cholangiographic technique of choice in suspected cases is probably ERCP, since intrahepatic ductal involvement may make PTHC difficult. When a diagnosis of sclerosing cholangitis has been established, a search for associated diseases, especially for chronic inflammatory bowel disease, should be carried out.

℞ TREATMENT

Therapy with cholestyramine may help control symptoms of pruritus, and antibiotics are useful when cholangitis complicates the clinical picture. Vitamin D and calcium supplementation may help prevent the loss of bone mass frequently seen in patients with chronic cholestasis. Glucocorticoids, UDCA, methotrexate, and cyclosporine have not been shown to be efficacious. In cases where complete or high-grade biliary obstruction has occurred, balloon dilatation or surgical intervention may be appropriate. Efforts at biliary-enteric anastomosis or stent placement may, however, be complicated by recurrent cholangitis and further progression of the stenosing process. The role of colectomy in patients with sclerosing cholangitis complicating chronic ulcerative colitis is uncertain. The prognosis is unfavorable, with a mean survival of 4 to 10 years following the diagnosis, regardless of therapy. Four variables (age, serum bilirubin level, histologic stage, and splenomegaly) predict survival in patients with primary sclerosing cholangitis and serve as the basis for a risk score. Primary sclerosing cholangitis is one of the most common indications for liver transplantation. In one study, the mean follow-up time from the diagnosis of primary sclerosing cholangitis to the time of liver transplantation was 5.8 years.

BIBLIOGRAPHY

ABEI M et al: Isolation and characterization of a cholesterol crystallization promoter from human bile. Gastroenterology 104:539, 1993

BARKUN JS et al: Randomised controlled trial of laparoscopic versus mini cholecystectomy. Lancet 340:1116, 1992

CAREY MC et al: Whither biliary sludge? Gastroenterology 95:508, 1988

DICKSON ER: Primary sclerosing cholangitis: Refinement and validation of survival models. Gastroenterology 103:1893, 1992

EVERSON GT: Pregnancy and gallstones. Hepatology 17:160, 1993

GEENEN JE et al: The efficacy of endoscopic sphincterotomy after cholecystectomy in patients with sphincter-of-Oddi dysfunction. N Engl J Med 320:82, 1989

GRACIE WA, RANSOHOFF DF: The natural history of silent gallstones. The innocent gallstone is not a myth. N Engl J Med 307:798, 1982

JOHNSTON DE, KAPLAN MM: Medical progress: Pathogenesis and treatment of gallstones. N Engl J Med 328:412, 1993

LEE SP et al: Origin and fate of biliary sludge. Gastroenterology 94:170, 1988

MARINGHINI A et al: Gallstones, gallbladder cancer, and other gastrointestinal malignancies: An epidemiologic study in Rochester, Minnesota. Ann Intern Med 107:30, 1987

MEYERS WC: A prospective analysis of 1518 laparoscopic cholecystectomies. N Engl J Med 324:1073, 1991

PAUMGARTNER G et al: Gallstones: Pathogenesis. Lancet 338:1117, 1991

PODDA M et al: Efficacy and safety of a combination of dienodeoxycholic acid and ursodeoxycholic acid for gallstone dissolution. Gastroenterology 96:222, 1989

PORAYKO MK et al: Patients with asymptomatic primary sclerosing cholangitis frequently have progressive disease. Gastroenterology 98:1594, 1990

SHAFFER EA et al: Cholescintigraphic detection of functional obstruction of the sphincter of Oddi: Effect of papillotomy. Gastroenterology 90:728, 1986

SHIFFMAN M et al: Prophylaxis against gallstone formation with ursodeoxycholic acid in patients. Ann Intern Med 122:999, 1995

SOTO JA et al: Magnetic resonance cholangiography: Comparison with endoscopic retrograde cholangiopancreatography. Gastroenterology 110:598, 1996

WIESNER RH et al: Comparison of clinicopathologic features of primary sclerosing cholangitis and primary biliary cirrhosis. Gastroenterology 88:108, 1985

YAP L et al: Acalculous biliary pain: Cholecystectomy alleviates symptoms in patients with abnormal cholescintigraphy. Gastroenterology 101:786, 1991

303

Phillip P. Toskes, Norton J. Greenberger

APPROACH TO THE PATIENT WITH PANCREATIC DISEASE

GENERAL CONSIDERATIONS

Inflammatory disease of the pancreas may be acute or chronic. Although good data exist concerning the frequency of acute pancreatitis (about 5000 new cases per year in the United States, with a mortality rate of about 10 percent), the number of patients who suffer with recurrent acute pancreatitis or chronic pancreatitis is largely undefined. Only one prospective study on the incidence of chronic pancreatitis is available; it showed an incidence of 8.2 new cases per 100,000 per year and a prevalence of 26.4 cases per 100,000. These numbers probably underestimate considerably the true incidence and prevalence, since non-alcohol-induced pancreatitis was largely ignored. At autopsy, the prevalence of chronic pancreatitis ranges from 0.04 to 5 percent. The relative inaccessibility of the pancreas to direct examination and the nonspecificity of the abdominal pain associated with pancreatitis make the diagnosis of pancreatitis difficult and usually dependent on elevation of blood amylase levels. Many patients with chronic pancreatitis do not have elevated blood amylase levels. Some patients with chronic pancreatitis develop signs and symptoms of pancreatic exocrine insufficiency, and thus objective evidence for pancreatic disease can be demonstrated. However, there is a very large reservoir of pancreatic exocrine function. More than 90 percent of the pancreas must be damaged before maldigestion of fat and protein is manifested. Even the secretin stimulation test, which is the most sensitive method of assessing pancreatic exocrine function, is probably abnormal only when more than 60 percent of exocrine function has been lost. Noninvasive, indirect tests of pancreatic exocrine function (bentiromide, serum trypsinogen) are much more likely to give abnormal results in patients with obvious pancreatic disease, i.e., pancreatic calcification, steatorrhea, or diabetes mellitus, than in patients with occult disease. Thus, the number of patients who have subclinical exocrine dysfunction (less than 90 percent loss of function) is unknown.

The clinical manifestations of acute and chronic pancreatitis and pancreatic insufficiency are protean. Thus, patients may present with hypertriglyceridemia, vitamin B_{12} malabsorption, hypercalcemia, hypocalcemia, hyperglycemia, ascites, pleural effusions, and chronic abdominal pain with normal blood amylase levels. Indeed, if the clinician considers pancreatitis as a possible diagnosis only when presented with a patient having classic symptoms (i.e., severe, constant epigastric pain that radiates through to the back, along with an elevated blood amylase level), only a minority of patients with pancreatitis will be diagnosed correctly.

As emphasized in Chap. 304, the etiologies as well as the clinical manifestations of pancreatitis are quite varied. Although it is well appreciated that pancreatitis is frequently secondary to alcohol abuse and biliary tract disease, it can also be caused by drugs, trauma, and viral infections and is associated with metabolic and connective tissue disorders. In approximately 30 percent of patients with acute pancreatitis and 25 to 40 percent of patients with chronic pancreatitis, the etiology is obscure.

TESTS USEFUL IN THE DIAGNOSIS OF PANCREATIC DISEASE

Several tests have proved of value in the evaluation of pancreatic exocrine function. Examples of specific tests and their usefulness in the diagnosis of acute and chronic pancreatitis are summarized in Table 303-1. At most institutions, pancreatic function tests are performed if the diagnosis of pancreatic disease remains a possibility after noninvasive tests [ultrasound, computed tomography (CT)] and invasive tests [endoscopic retrograde cholangiopancreatography (ERCP)] have given normal or inconclusive results. In this regard, tests employing *direct* stimulation of the pancreas are the most sensitive.

PANCREATIC ENZYMES IN BODY FLUIDS The serum amylase level is widely used as a screening test for acute pancreatitis in the patient with acute abdominal pain or back pain. A value greater than 65 U/L should raise the question of acute pancreatitis. Levels greater than 130 U/L make the diagnosis more likely, and values greater than three times normal virtually clinch the diagnosis if gut perforation or infarction is excluded. In acute pancreatitis, the serum amylase is usually elevated within 24 h of onset and remains so for 1 to 3 days. Levels return to normal within 3 to 5 days unless there is extensive pancreatic necrosis, incomplete ductal obstruction, or pseudocyst formation. Approximately 85 percent of patients with acute pancreatitis will have an elevated serum amylase level. This index may be normal, however, if (1) there is a delay (of 2 to 5 days) before blood samples are obtained, (2) the underlying disorder is chronic pancreatitis rather than acute pancreatitis, or (3) hypertriglyceridemia is present. Patients with hypertriglyceridemia and proven pancreatitis have been found to have spuriously low levels of amylase and lipase activity.

The serum amylase is often elevated in other conditions (Table 303-2), in part because the enzyme is found in many organs in addition to the pancreas (salivary glands, liver, small intestine, kidney, fallopian tube) and can be produced by various tumors (carcinomas of the lung, esophagus, breast, and ovary). Isoenzymes of amylase fall into two general categories: those arising from the pancreas (P isoamylases) and those arising from nonpancreatic sources (S isoamylases). The measurement of serum isoamylases is of clinical importance. In normal serum, about 35 to 45 percent of the amylase is of pancreatic origin. For example, in patients with acute pancreatitis, the total serum amylase level returns to normal more rapidly than the level of pancreatic isoamylase. Thus, in patients seen after the first day, the pancreatic isoamylase level is a more sensitive indicator of pancreatitis than the total serum amylase level. In the past, elevations in serum amylase seen in certain conditions, such as the postoperative state, acute alcohol intoxication, and diabetic ketoacidosis, were assumed to indicate acute pancreatitis. However, the elevation of serum amylase in such conditions has been shown to be due to an elevation of the S isoamylase. Simple tests to distinguish pancreatic from nonpancreatic amylase are no longer readily available, and such tests are often not reliable when the total amylase is minimally to moderately elevated. An assay of serum trypsinogen (performed by several commercial laboratories) is quite helpful in this regard. Since this enzyme is secreted specifically by the pancreas, a normal serum trypsinogen level in a patient with minimal elevation of serum amylase essentially rules out acute pancreatitis. Urinary amylase measurements, including the amylase/creatinine clearance ratio, are no more sensitive or specific than blood amylase levels.

Elevation of ascitic fluid amylase occurs in acute pancreatitis as well as in (1) pancreatogenous ascites due to disruption of the main pancreatic duct of a leaking pseudocyst and (2) other abdominal disorders that simulate pancreatitis (e.g., intestinal obstruction, intestinal infarction, and perforated peptic ulcer). Elevation of pleural fluid amylase occurs in acute pancreatitis, chronic pancreatitis, carcinoma of the lung, and esophageal perforation.

Lipase may now be the single best enzyme to measure for the diagnosis of acute pancreatitis. Improvements in substrates and technology offer clinicians improved options, especially when a turbidometric assay is used. The newer lipase assays have colipase as a cofactor and are fully automated.

An assay for trypsinogen (or for trypsin-like immunoreactivity) has a theoretical advantage over amylase and lipase determinations

Table 303-1

Tests Useful in the Diagnosis of Acute and Chronic Pancreatitis and Pancreatic Tumors

Test	Principle	Comment
PANCREATIC ENZYMES IN BODY FLUIDS		
Amylase		
1. Serum	Pancreatic inflammation leads to increased enzyme levels	Simple; 20–40% false negatives and positives; reliable if test results are three times the upper limit of normal
2. Urine	Renal clearance of amylase is increased in acute pancreatitis	May be abnormal when serum levels normal; false negatives and positives
3. Amylase/creatinine clearance ratio (C_{am}/C_{cr})	Renal clearance of amylase greater than clearance of creatinine	No more sensitive than serum amylase; many false positives
4. Ascitic fluid	Disruption of gland or main pancreatic duct leads to increased amylase concentration	Can establish diagnosis of pancreatitis; false positives occur with intestinal obstruction and perforated ulcer
5. Pleural fluid	Exudative pleural effusion with pancreatitis	False positives occur with carcinoma of the lung and esophageal perforation
6. Isoenzymes	P isoamylases arise from the pancreas; S isoamylases are from other sources	More sensitive than total serum amylase in diagnosis of acute pancreatitis; useful in identifying nonpancreatic causes of hyperamylasemia
Serum lipase	Pancreatic inflammation leads to increased enzyme levels	New methods have greatly simplified determination; positive in 70–85% of cases.
Serum trypsin-like immunoreactivity (TLI)	Pancreatic inflammation leads to increased levels	*Elevated* in acute pancreatitis; *decreased* in chronic pancreatitis *with* steatorrhea; normal in chronic pancreatitis *without* steatorrhea and in steatorrhea with normal pancreatic function
Pancreatic polypeptide (PP)	PP confined almost totally to the pancreas; release stimulated by nutrients and hormones; such release parallels pancreatic enzyme secretion	Basal, meal-simulated, and hormone-stimulated (by secretin or CCK) PP levels *decreased* in chronic pancreatitis; a fasting PP level >125 pg/mL argues against chronic pancreatitis and pancreatic cancer
STUDIES PERTAINING TO PANCREATIC STRUCTURE		
Radiologic and radionuclide tests		
1. Plain film of the abdomen	Abnormal in acute and chronic pancreatitis	Simple; normal in >50% of cases of both acute and chronic pancreatitis
2. Upper gastrointestinal x-rays	Abnormally thickened duodenal folds; displacement of stomach or widening of duodenal loop suggests a pancreatic mass (inflammatory, neoplastic, cystic)	Simple; frequently normal; largely superseded by US and CT scanning
3. Ultrasonography (US)	Can provide information on edema, inflammation, calcification, pseudocysts, and mass lesions	Simple, noninvasive; sequential studies quite feasible; useful in diagnosis of pseudocyst
4. CT scan	Permits detailed visualization of pancreas and surrounding structures	Useful in the diagnosis of pancreatic calcification, dilated pancreatic ducts, and pancreatic tumors; may not be able to distinguish between inflammatory and neoplastic mass lesions
5. Selective angiography	Can identify pancreatic neoplasms (1) by sheathing of celiac or superior mesenteric branches by tumor or (2) by tumor staining; displacement of vessels by tumor	Indicated (1) in suspected islet cell tumors and (2) prior to pancreatic or duodenal resection; most reliable features reflect nonresectable pancreatic cancer
6. Endoscopic retrograde cholangiopancreatography (ERCP)	Cannulation of pancreatic and common bile duct permits visualization of pancreatic-biliary ductal system	Provides diagnostic data in 60–85% of cases; differentiation of chronic pancreatitis from pancreatic carcinoma may be difficult
Pancreatic biopsy with US or CT guidance	Percutaneous biopsy with skinny needle and localization of lesion by US	High diagnostic yield; laparotomy avoided; requires special technical skills
TESTS OF EXOCRINE PANCREATIC FUNCTION		
Direct stimulation of the pancreas with analysis of duodenal contents		
1. Secretin-pancreozymin (CCK) test	Secretin leads to increased output of pancreatic juice and HCO_3^-; CCK leads to increased output of pancreatic enzymes; pancreatic secretory response is related to the functional mass of pancreatic tissue	Sensitive enough to detect occult disease; involves duodenal intubation and fluoroscopy; poorly defined normal enzyme response; overlap in chronic pancreatitis; large secretory reserve capacity of the pancreas
Indirect stimulation of pancreas with measurement of pancreatic enzymes		
1. Lundh test meal	Test meal (fat, carbohydrate, and protein) causes increased release of CCK, which causes increased enzyme output; trypsin concentration measured	Useful in pancreatic exocrine insufficiency; false negatives with delayed gastric emptying; false positives in primary mucosal disease of the gut and choledocholithiasis; does not measure secretory capacity
2. Benzoyl-tyrosyl-*p*-aminobenzoic acid (Bz-Ty-PABA, bentiromide) test	Synthetic peptide (Bz-Ty-PABA) is specifically cleaved by chymotrypsin, liberating PABA, which is absorbed; PABA metabolite is excreted in the urine	Simple and reliable test of pancreatic exocrine function. Measurement of blood PABA level increases sensitivity.

(continued)

Table 303-1—*(Continued)*

Tests Useful in the Diagnosis of Acute and Chronic Pancreatitis and Pancreatic Tumors

Test	Principle	Comment
3. Pancreolauryl test	Fluorescein dilaurate is hydrolyzed by pancreatic elastase and absorbed; fluorescein is measured in urine	Sensitivity and specificity similar to those of Bentiromide test
Measurement of intraluminal digestion products		
1. Microscopic examination of stool for undigested meat fibers and fat	Lack of proteolytic and lipolytic enzymes causes decreased digestion of meat fibers and triglycerides	Simple, reliable; not sensitive enough to detect milder cases of pancreatic insufficiency
2. Quantitative stool fat determination	Lack of lipolytic enzymes brings about impaired fat digestion	Reliable, reference standard for defining severity of malabsorption; does not distinguish between maldigestion and malabsorption
3. Fecal nitrogen	Lack of proteolytic enzymes leads to impaired protein digestion, resulting in an increase in stool nitrogen	Does not distinguish between maldigestion and malabsorption; low sensitivity
Measurement of pancreatic enzymes in feces		
1. Chymotrypsin	Pancreatic secretion of proteolytic enzymes	May be useful in cystic fibrosis; tedious; 10% false-positive and false-negative results
Miscellaneous tests		
1. Dual-labeled Schilling test	Intrinsic factor [^{57}Co]cobalamin and Hog R protein [^{58}Co]cobalamin are given together. Since proteases are necessary to cleave R protein, the ratio of labeled cobalamin excreted in urine is an index of exocrine dysfunction.	Time-consuming and expensive

in that the pancreas is the only organ that contains this enzyme. The test appears to be useful in the diagnosis of both acute and chronic pancreatitis. Sensitivity and specificity are comparable to those of amylase and lipase determinations. Since trypsinogen is also excreted by the kidney, elevated serum values are found in renal failure, as is the case with serum amylase and lipase levels. *No single blood test is reliable for the diagnosis of acute pancreatitis in patients with renal failure.* Determinating whether a patient with renal failure and abdominal pain has pancreatitis remains a difficult clinical problem. A recent study found that serum amylase levels were elevated in patients with renal dysfunction only when creatinine clearance was less than 50 mL/min. In such patients, the serum amylase level was invariably less than 500 IU/L in the absence of objective evidence of acute pancreatitis. In that study, serum lipase and trypsin levels paralleled serum amylase values.

A recent study evaluated the sensitivity and specificity of five assays used to diagnose acute pancreatitis: two for amylase, one for lipase, one for trypsin-like immunoreactivity (TLI), and one for pancreatic isoamylase. The data obtained (1) show that, if the best cutoff level is used, all these assays have similar specificities and (2) suggest that total serum amylase is as good an indicator of acute pancreatitis as any of the alternatives. However, inherent in many such studies is the problem that the recognition and diagnosis of acute pancreatitis hinge on the finding of an elevated serum amylase level. The question arises as to whether any diagnostic test result can be proved superior to the total serum amylase level if hyperamylasemia is required for the diagnosis. In other studies, when "objective" confirmation of the clinical diagnosis of pancreatitis was required (ultrasonography, CT, laparotomy), the sensitivity of the serum amylase has been found to be as low as 68 percent. With these limitations in mind, the recommended screening tests for acute pancreatitis are *total serum amylase* and *serum lipase activities.* Serum amylase values greater than three times normal are highly specific.

Table 303-2

Causes of Hyperamylasemia and Hyperamylasuria

PANCREATIC DISEASE

- I. Pancreatitis
  - A. Acute
  - B. Chronic: ductal obstruction
  - C. Complications of pancreatitis
    - 1. Pancreatic pseudocyst
    - 2. Pancreatogenous ascites
    - 3. Pancreatic abscess
- II. Pancreatic trauma
- III. Pancreatic carcinoma

NONPANCREATIC DISORDERS

- I. Renal insufficiency
- II. Salivary gland lesions
  - A. Mumps
  - B. Calculus
  - C. Irradiation sialadenitis
  - D. Maxillofacial surgery
- III. "Tumor" hyperamylasemia
  - A. Carcinoma of the lung
  - B. Carcinoma of the esophagus
  - C. Breast carcinoma, ovarian carcinoma
- IV. Macroamylasemia
- V. Burns
- VI. Diabetic ketoacidosis
- VII. Pregnancy
- VIII. Renal transplantation
- IX. Cerebral trauma
- X. Drugs: morphine

OTHER ABDOMINAL DISORDERS

- I. Biliary tract disease: cholecystitis, choledocholithiasis
- II. Intraabdominal disease
  - A. Perforated or penetrating peptic ulcer
  - B. Intestinal obstruction or infarction
  - C. Ruptured ectopic pregnancy
  - D. Peritonitis
  - E. Aortic aneurysm
  - F. Chronic liver disease
  - G. Postoperative hyperamylasemia

STUDIES PERTAINING TO PANCREATIC STRUCTURE Radiologic Tests Plain films of the abdomen provide useful information in 30 to 50 percent of patients with acute pancreatitis. The most frequent abnormalities include (1) a localized ileus, usually involving the jejunum ("sentinel loop"), (2) a generalized ileus with air-fluid levels, (3) the "colon cutoff sign," which results from isolated distention of the transverse colon, (4) duodenal distention with air-fluid levels, and (5) a mass, which is frequently a pseudocyst. In chronic pancreatitis, an important radiographic finding is pancreatic calcification, which characteristically is localized adjacent to and superimposed on the second lumbar vertebra (see Fig. 304-3*A*).

Upper gastrointestinal x-rays may reveal displacement of the stomach by the retroperitoneal mass (see Fig. 304-2*A*) or widening and effacement of the duodenal C loop, which also suggest the presence of a pancreatic mass, which could be inflammatory, cystic, or neoplastic. However, the use of x-ray films has been largely superseded by ultrasound.

Ultrasonography can provide important information in patients with acute pancreatitis, chronic pancreatitis, pancreatic calcification, pseudocyst, and pancreatic carcinoma. Echographic appearances can indicate the presence of edema, inflammation, and calcification (not obvious on plain films of the abdomen), as well as pseudocysts, mass lesions, and gallstones (see Figs. 304-2*B* and 304-3*B*). In acute pancreatitis, the pancreas is characteristically enlarged. In pancreatic pseudocyst, the usual appearance is that of an echo-free, smooth, round fluid collection. Pancreatic carcinoma distorts the usual landmarks, and mass lesions greater than 3.0 cm are usually detected as localized, echo-free solid lesions. Ultrasound is often the initial investigation for most patients with suspected pancreatic disease. However, obesity, excess small- and large-bowel gas, and recently performed barium contrast examinations can interfere with ultrasound studies.

CT is the best imaging study for initial evaluation of a suspected chronic pancreatic disorder and for the complications of acute and chronic pancreatitis. It is especially useful in the detection of pancreatic tumors, fluid-containing lesions such as pseudocysts and abscesses, and calcium deposits (see Figs. 304-3*C* and 304-4*A*). Most lesions are characterized by (1) enlargement of the pancreatic outline, (2) distortion of the pancreatic contour, and/or (3) a fluid filling that has a different attenuation coefficient than normal pancreas. However, it is occasionally difficult to distinguish between inflammatory and neoplastic lesions. Oral water-soluble contrast agents may be used to opacify the stomach and duodenum during CT scans; this strategy permits more precise delineation of various organs as well as mass lesions. Dynamic CT (using rapid intravenous administration of contrast)is useful in estimating the degree of pancreatic necrosis and in predicting morbidity and mortality. Spiral (helical) CT provides clear images much more rapidly and essentially negates artifact caused by patient movement (Fig. 304-2*D*).

Selective catheterization of the celiac and superior mesenteric arteries combined with superselective catheterization of others arteries, such as the hepatic, splenic, and gastroduodenal arteries permits visualization of the pancreas and detection of pancreatic neoplasms and pseudocysts. Pancreatic neoplasms can be identified by the sheathing of blood vessels by a mass lesion (see Fig. 304-1*D*). Hormone-producing pancreatic tumors are especially likely to exhibit increased vascularity and tumor staining. Angiographic abnormalities are noted in many patients with pancreatic carcinoma but are uncommon in patients without pancreatic disease. Angiography complements ultrasonography and ERCP in the study of patients with a suspected pancreatic lesion and may be carried out if ERCP is either unsuccessful or nondiagnostic. The recently introduced technique of *magnetic resonance cholangiopancreatography* (MRCP) appears to be of value under these conditions.

ERCP may provide useful information on the status of the pancreatic ductal system and thus aid in the differential diagnosis of pancreatic disease (see Figs. 304-1*C*, 304-3*D*, and 304-4*B*). Pancreatic carcinoma is characterized by stenosis or obstruction of either the pancreatic duct or the common bile duct; both ductal systems are often abnormal. In chronic pancreatitis, ERCP abnormalities include (1) luminal narrowing, (2) irregularities in the ductal system with stenosis, dilation, sacculation, and ectasia, and (3) blockage of the pancreatic duct by calcium deposits. The presence of ductal stenosis and irregularity can make it difficult to distinguish chronic pancreatitis from carcinoma. It is important to be aware that ERCP changes interpreted as indicating chronic pancreatitis actually may be due to the effects of aging on the pancreatic duct or to the fact that the procedure was performed within several weeks of an attack of acute pancreatitis. Although aging may cause impressive ductal alterations, it does not affect the results of pancreatic function tests (i.e., the secretin test). Elevated serum and/or urine amylase levels following ERCP have been reported in 25 to 75 percent of patients, but clinical pancreatitis is uncommon. In a series of 300 patients, pancreatitis occurred in only 5 patients following ERCP. If no lesion is found in the biliary and/or pancreatic ducts in a patient with repeated attacks of acute pancreatitis, manometric studies of the sphincter of Oddi may be indicated. Such studies, however, do increase the risk of post-ERCP/manometry acute pancreatitis. Such pancreatitis appears to be more common in patients with a nondilated pancreatic duct.

Pancreatic Biopsy with Radiologic Guidance Percutaneous aspiration biopsy of a pancreatic mass often distinguishes a pancreatic inflammatory mass from a pancreatic neoplasm.

TESTS OF EXOCRINE PANCREATIC FUNCTION

Pancreatic function tests (Table 303-1) can be divided into the following:

1. *Direct stimulation of the pancreas* by intravenous infusion of secretin or secretin plus cholecystokinin (CCK) followed by collection and measurement of duodenal contents
2. *Indirect stimulation of the pancreas* using nutrients or amino acids, fatty acids, and synthetic peptides followed by assays of proteolytic, lipolytic, and amylolytic enzymes
3. Study of *intraluminal digestion products,* such as undigested meat fibers, stool fat, and fecal nitrogen
4. *Measurement of fecal pancreatic enzymes* such as chymotrypsin

The secretin test, used to detect diffuse pancreatic disease, is based on the physiologic principle that the pancreatic secretory response is directly related to the functional mass of pancreatic tissue. In the standard assay, secretin is given intravenously in a dose of 1 clinical unit (CU) per kilogram, as either a bolus or a continuous infusion. Obviously, the results will vary with the secretin preparation used, the dose, the mode of administration, and the completeness with which the duodenal contents are collected. Normal values for the standard secretin test are (1) volume output >2.0 mL/kg per hour, (2) bicarbonate (HCO_3^-) concentration >80 mmol/L, and (3) HCO_3^- output >10 mmol in 1 h. The most reproducible measurement, giving the highest level of discrimination between normal subjects and patients with chronic pancreatitis, appears to be the maximal bicarbonate concentration.

The *combined secretin-CCK test* permits measurement of pancreatic amylase, lipase, trypsin, and chymotrypsin. Although there is overlap in the distributions of enzyme output in normal subjects and patients with pancreatitis in response to this test, markedly low enzyme outputs suggest advanced damage and destruction of acinar cells. With frank exocrine pancreatic insufficiency, there is usually an overall reduction in both HCO_3^- concentration and output of several enzymes. However, with lesser degrees of pancreatic damage there may be a dissociation between HCO_3^- concentration and enzyme output. There also may be a dissociation between the results of the secretin test and those of tests of absorptive function. For example, patients with chronic pancreatitis often have abnormally low outputs of HCO_3^- after secretin but have normal fecal fat excretion. Thus the secretin test measures the secretory capacity of ductular epithelium, while fecal fat excretion indirectly reflects intraluminal lipolytic activity. Steatorrhea does not occur until intraluminal levels of lipase are markedly reduced, underscoring the fact that only small amounts of enzymes are necessary for intraluminal digestive activities. An abnormal secretin test result suggests only that chronic pancreatic damage is present; it will not consistently distinguish between chronic pancreatitis and pancreatic carcinoma.

Another test of exocrine pancreatic function, which indirectly reflects intraluminal chymotrypsin activity, has been evaluated in patients with pancreatic disease. This test (the *tripeptide hydrolysis* or *bentiromide test*) uses a synthetic peptide, *N*-benzoyl-L-tyrosyl-*p*-aminobenzoic acid (Bz-Ty-PABA), that is specifically cleaved by chymotrypsin to Bz-Ty and PABA. Normally, after oral administration, the peptide is hydrolyzed in the small intestine by chymotrypsin with the liberation of PABA, which is rapidly absorbed and excreted in the urine. Results in several hundred patients with chronic pancreatitis and other disorders indicate that PABA excretion is significantly lower in patients with chronic pancreatitis than in control subjects. Depending on the severity of pancreatic exocrine impairment, the overall sensitivity is 60 percent (range, 46 to 74 percent), and the specificity if coupled with a D-xylose test approximates 90 percent. Measurement of blood PABA levels increases sensitivity.

Measurement of *intraluminal digestion products*, i.e., undigested muscle fibers, stool fat, and fecal nitrogen, is discussed in Chap. 285. The amount of chymotrypsin in stool reflects the pancreatic output of this proteolytic enzyme. Decreased chymotrypsin activity in stool has been reported in patients with chronic pancreatitis and cystic fibrosis. However, normal values may occur in patients with pancreatic insufficiency, and false-positive results have been reported in up to 10 percent of normal individuals. → ***Tests useful in the diagnosis of exocrine pancreatic insufficiency and the differential diagnosis of malabsorption are also discussed in Chaps. 285 and 304***

Norton J. Greenberger, Phillip P. Toskes, Kurt J. Isselbacher

304 ACUTE AND CHRONIC PANCREATITIS

BIOCHEMISTRY AND PHYSIOLOGY OF PANCREATIC EXOCRINE SECRETION

GENERAL CONSIDERATIONS The pancreas secretes 1500 to 3000 mL of isosmotic alkaline (pH >8.0) fluid per day containing about 20 enzymes and zymogens. The pancreatic secretions provide the enzymes needed to effect the major digestive activity of the gastrointestinal tract and provide an optimal pH for the function of these enzymes.

REGULATION OF PANCREATIC SECRETION The exocrine pancreas is influenced by intimately interacting hormonal and neural systems. *Gastric acid* is the stimulus for the release of secretin, a peptide with 27 amino acids. Sensitive radioimmunoassay studies for secretin suggest that the pH threshold for its release from the duodenum and jejunum is 4.5. Secretin stimulates the secretion of pancreatic juice rich in *water and electrolytes*. Release of cholecystokinin (CCK) from the duodenum and jejunum is largely triggered by long-chain fatty acids, certain essential amino acids (tryptophan, phenylalanine, valine, methionine), and gastric acid itself. CCK evokes an *enzyme-rich secretion from the pancreas*. Gastrin, although it has the same terminal tetrapeptide as CCK, is a weak stimulus for pancreatic enzyme output. The *parasympathetic nervous system* (via the vagus nerve) exerts significant control over pancreatic secretion. Secretion evoked by secretin and CCK depends on permissive roles of vagal afferent and efferent pathways. This is particularly true for enzyme secretion, whereas water and bicarbonate secretion is heavily dependent on the hormonal effects of secretin and CCK. Also, vagal stimulation effects the release of vasoactive intestinal peptide (VIP), a secretin agonist. Bile salts also stimulate pancreatic secretion, thereby integrating the functions of the biliary tract, pancreas, and small intestine.

Somatostatin acts on multiple sites to induce inhibition of pancreatic secretion. The appropriate roles of other peptides, such as peptide YY, pancreastatin, gastrin-releasing peptide, pituitary adenylate cyclase–activating polypeptide, calcitonin gene–related peptide, and galanin are still being defined. Nitric oxide is an important neurotransmitter in the regulation of pancreatic exocrine secretion, although its mechanism of action has not been fully elucidated.

WATER AND ELECTROLYTE SECRETION Although sodium, potassium, chloride, calcium, zinc, phosphate, and sulfate are found in pancreatic secretions, *bicarbonate is the ion of primary physiologic importance*. In the acini and in the ducts, secretin causes the cells to add water and bicarbonate to the fluid. In the ducts, an exchange occurs between bicarbonate and chloride. There is a good correlation between the maximal bicarbonate output after stimulation with secretin and the pancreatic mass. The bicarbonate output of 120 to 300 mmol/d helps neutralize gastric acid and creates the appropriate pH for the activity of the pancreatic enzymes.

ENZYME SECRETION The pancreas secretes amylolytic, lipolytic, and proteolytic enzymes. *Amylolytic enzymes*, such as amylase, hydrolyze starch to oligosaccharides and to the disaccharide maltose. The *lipolytic enzymes* include lipase, phospholipase A, and cholesterol esterase. Bile salts *inhibit* lipase in isolation, but colipase, another constituent of pancreatic secretion, binds to lipase and prevents this inhibition. Bile salts *activate* phospholipase A and cholesterol esterase. *Proteolytic enzymes* include *endopeptidases* (trypsin, chymotrypsin), which act on internal peptide bonds of proteins and polypeptides; *exopeptidases* (carboxypeptidases, aminopeptidases), which act on the free carboxyl- and amino-terminal ends of peptides, respectively; and elastase. The proteolytic enzymes are secreted as inactive precursors (zymogens). Ribonucleases (deoxyribonucleases, ribonuclease) are also secreted. While parallel secretion of pancreatic enzymes usually occurs, nonparallel secretion can occur as a result of exocytosis from heterogeneous sources in the pancreas. *Enterokinase*, an enzyme found in the duodenal mucosa, cleaves the lysine-isoleucine bond of trypsinogen to form trypsin. Trypsin then activates the other proteolytic zymogens in a cascade phenomenon. All pancreatic enzymes have pH optima in the alkaline range.

AUTOPROTECTION OF THE PANCREAS Autodigestion of the pancreas is prevented by the packaging of proteases in precursor form and by the synthesis of protease inhibitors. These protease inhibitors are found in the acinar cell, the pancreatic secretions, and the alpha$_1$- and alpha$_2$-globulin fractions of plasma.

EXOCRINE-ENDOCRINE RELATIONSHIPS Insulin appears to be needed locally for secretin and CCK to promote exocrine secretion; thus, it acts in a permissive role for these two hormones.

ENTEROPANCREATIC AXIS AND FEEDBACK INHIBITION Pancreatic enzyme secretion is controlled, at least in part, by a negative feedback mechanism induced by the presence of active serine proteases in the duodenum. To illustrate, perfusion of the duodenal lumen with phenylalanine causes a prompt increase in plasma CCK levels as well as increased secretion of chymotrypsin. However, simultaneous perfusion with trypsin blunts both responses. Conversely, perfusion of the duodenal lumen with protease inhibitors actually leads to enzyme hypersecretion. It appears that serine proteases inhibit pancreatic secretion by acting on a CCK-releasing peptide in the lumen of the small intestine.

ACUTE PANCREATITIS

GENERAL CONSIDERATIONS Pancreatic inflammatory disease may be classified as (1) acute pancreatitis and (2) chronic pancreatitis. The pathologic spectrum of acute pancreatitis varies from *edematous pancreatitis*, which is usually a mild and self-limited disorder, to *necrotizing pancreatitis*, in which the degree of pancreatic necrosis correlates with the severity of the attack and its systemic manifestations. The term *hemorrhagic pancreatitis* is less meaningful in a clinical sense because variable amounts of interstitial hemorrhage can be found in pancreatitis as well as in other disorders such as pancreatic trauma, pancreatic carcinoma, and severe congestive heart failure.

The incidence of pancreatitis varies in different countries and depends on cause, e.g., alcohol, gallstones, metabolic factors, and drugs (Table 304-1). In the United States, for example, acute pancreatitis is related to alcohol ingestion more commonly than to gallstones; in England, the opposite obtains.

ETIOLOGY AND PATHOGENESIS There are many causes of acute pancreatitis (Table 304-1), but the mechanisms by which these conditions trigger pancreatic inflammation have not been identified. Alcoholic patients with pancreatitis may represent a special subset, since most alcoholics do not develop pancreatitis. The list of identifiable causes is growing, and it is likely that pancreatitis related to viral infections, drugs, and as yet undefined factors is more common than heretofore recognized.

Approximately 5 percent of cases of acute pancreatitis are drug-related (Table 304-1). Drugs cause pancreatitis either by a hypersensi-

Table 304-1

Causes of Acute Pancreatitis

- Alcohol ingestion (acute and chronic alcoholism)
- Biliary tract disease (gallstones)
- Postoperative state (after abdominal or nonabdominal operation)
- Endoscopic retrograde cholangiopancreatography (ERCP), especially manometric studies of sphincter of Oddi
- Trauma (especially blunt abdominal type)
- Metabolic causes
  - Hypertriglyceridemia
  - Apolipoprotein CII deficiency syndrome
  - Hypercalcemia (e.g., hyperparathyroidism), drug-induced
  - Renal failure
  - After renal transplantation*
  - Acute fatty liver of pregnancy†
- Hereditary pancreatitis
- Infections
  - Mumps
  - Viral hepatitis
  - Other viral infections (coxsackievirus, echovirus, cytomegalovirus)
  - Ascariasis
  - Infections with *Mycoplasma, Campylobacter, Mycobacterium avium* complex, other bacteria
- Drugs
  - Drugs for which association is definite
    - Azathioprine, 6-mercaptopurine
    - Sulfonamides
    - Thiazide diuretics
    - Furosemide
    - Estrogens (oral contraceptives)
    - Tetracycline
    - Valproic acid
    - Pentamidine
    - Dideoxyinosine (ddI)
  - Drugs for which association is probable
    - Acetaminophen
    - Nitrofurantoin
    - Methyldopa
    - Erythromycin
    - Salicylates
    - Metronidazole
    - Nonsteroidal anti-inflammatory drugs
    - Angiotensin-converting enzyme (ACE) inhibitors
- Vascular causes and vasculitis
  - Vascular
    - Ischemic-hypoperfusion state (after cardiac surgery)
    - Atherosclerotic emboli
  - Connective tissue disorders with vasculitis
    - Systemic lupus erythematosus
    - Necrotizing angiitis
    - Thrombotic thrombocytopenic purpura
- Penetrating peptic ulcer
- Obstruction of the ampulla of Vater
  - Regional enteritis
  - Duodenal diverticulum
- Pancreas divisum
- Causes to be considered in patients having recurrent bouts of acute pancreatitis without an obvious cause
  - Occult disease of the biliary tree or pancreatic ducts, especially occult gallstones (microlithiasis, sludge)
  - Drugs
  - Hypertriglyceridemia
  - Pancreas divisum
  - Pancreatic cancer
  - Sphincter of Oddi dysfunction
  - Cystic fibrosis
  - Truly idiopathic

* Pancreatitis occurs in 3 percent of renal transplant patients and is due to many factors, including surgery, hypercalcemia, drugs (glucocorticoids, azathioprine, L-asparaginase, diuretics), and viral infections.

† Pancreatitis also occurs in otherwise uncomplicated pregnancy and is most often associated with cholelithiasis.

tivity reaction or by the generation of a toxic metabolite, although in some cases it is not clear which of these mechanisms is operative.

Autodigestion is one pathogenetic theory, according to which pancreatitis results when proteolytic enzymes (e.g., trypsinogen, chymotrypsinogen, proelastase, and phospholipase A) are activated in the pancreas rather than in the intestinal lumen. A number of factors (e.g., endotoxins, exotoxins, viral infections, ischemia, anoxia, and direct trauma) are believed to activate these proenzymes. Activated proteolytic enzymes, especially trypsin, not only digest pancreatic and peripancreatic tissues but also can activate other enzymes, such as elastase and phospholipase. The active enzymes then digest cellular membranes and cause proteolysis, edema, interstitial hemorrhage, vascular damage, coagulation necrosis, fat necrosis, and parenchymal cell necrosis. Cellular injury and death result in the liberation of activated enzymes. In addition, activation and release of bradykinin peptides and vasoactive substances (e.g., histamine) are believed to produce vasodilation, increased vascular permeability, and edema. Thus, a cascade of events culminates in the development of acute necrotizing pancreatitis.

The autodigestion theory has largely eclipsed two older theories. First, according to the "common channel" theory, the existence of a common anatomic channel for pancreatic secretions and bile permits reflux of bile into the pancreatic duct, which results in activation of pancreatic enzymes. (Actually, a common channel with free communication between the common bile duct and the main pancreatic duct is infrequently encountered.) The second theory is that obstruction and hypersecretion are pivotal in the development of pancreatitis. Obstruction of the main pancreatic duct, however, produces pancreatic edema but generally not pancreatitis.

A recent hypothesis to explain the intrapancreatic activation of zymogens is that they become activated by *lysosomal hydrolases* in the pancreatic acinar cell itself. In two different types of experimental pancreatitis, it has been demonstrated that digestive enzymes and lysosomal hydrolases become admixed; as a result, the latter can activate the former in the acinar cell. In vitro, lysosomal enzymes such as cathepsin B can activate trypsinogen, and trypsin can activate the other protease precursors. It is still not clear, however, whether the human acinar cell can provide the pH (about 3.0) necessary for activation of trypsinogen by lysosomal hydrolases. It is now believed that ischemia/hypoperfusion can alone result in activation of trypsinogen and pancreatic injury.

CLINICAL FEATURES *Abdominal pain* is the major symptom of acute pancreatitis. Pain may vary from a mild and tolerable discomfort to severe, constant, and incapacitating distress. Characteristically, the pain, which is steady and boring in character, is located in the epigastrium and periumbilical region and often radiates to the back as well as to the chest, flanks, and lower abdomen. The pain is frequently more intense when the patient is supine, and patients often obtain relief by sitting with the trunk flexed and knees drawn up. Nausea, vomiting, and abdominal distention due to gastric and intestinal hypomotility and chemical peritonitis are also frequent complaints.

Physical examination frequently reveals a distressed and anxious patient. Low-grade fever, tachycardia, and hypotension are fairly common. Shock is not unusual and may result from (1) hypovolemia secondary to exudation of blood and plasma proteins into the retroperitoneal space (a "retroperitoneal burn"); (2) increased formation and release of kinin peptides, which cause vasodilation and increased vascular permeability; and (3) systemic effects of proteolytic and lipolytic enzymes released into the circulation. Jaundice occurs infrequently; when present, it usually is due to edema of the head of the pancreas with compression of the intrapancreatic portion of the common bile duct. Erythematous skin nodules due to subcutaneous fat necrosis may occur. In 10 to 20 percent of patients, there are pulmonary findings, including basilar rales, atelectasis, and pleural effusion, the latter most frequently left-sided. Abdominal tenderness and muscle rigidity are present to a variable degree, but, compared with the intense pain, these signs may be unimpressive. Bowel sounds are usually diminished or absent. A pancreatic pseudocyst may be palpable in the upper abdomen. A faint blue discoloration around the umbilicus

(Cullen's sign) may occur as the result of hemoperitoneum, and a blue-red-purple or green-brown discoloration of the flanks (Turner's sign) reflects tissue catabolism of hemoglobin. The latter two findings, which are uncommon, indicate the presence of a severe necrotizing pancreatitis.

LABORATORY DATA The diagnosis of acute pancreatitis is usually established by the detection of an increased level of serum amylase. Values threefold or more above normal virtually clinch the diagnosis if overt salivary gland disease and gut perforation or infarction are excluded. However, there appears to be no definite correlation between the severity of pancreatitis and the degree of serum amylase elevation. After 48 to 72 h, even with continuing evidence of pancreatitis, total serum amylase values tend to return to normal. However, pancreatic isoamylase and lipase levels may remain elevated for 7 to 14 days. It will be recalled that amylase elevations in serum and urine occur in many conditions other than pancreatitis (see Table 303-2). Importantly, patients with *acidemia* (arterial pH ≤7.32) may have spurious elevations in serum amylase. In one study, 12 of 33 acidemic patients had elevated serum amylase, but only 1 had an elevated lipase value; in 9, salivary-type amylase was the predominant serum isoamylase. This finding explains why patients with diabetic ketoacidosis may have marked elevations in serum amylase without any other evidence of acute pancreatitis. The urine amylase:creatinine clearance ratio (C_{am}/C_{cr}) is usually elevated in patients with severe pancreatitis; this ratio usually is not increased in patients with a normal level of serum amylase. Serum lipase activity increases in parallel with amylase activity, and measurement of both enzymes increases the diagnostic yield. An elevated serum lipase or trypsin value is usually diagnostic of acute pancreatitis; these tests are especially helpful in patients with nonpancreatic causes of hyperamylasemia (see Table 303-2). Markedly increased levels of peritoneal or pleural fluid amylase [>1500 nmol/L (>5000 U/dL)] are also helpful, if present, in establishing the diagnosis.

Leukocytosis (15,000 to 20,000 leukocytes per microliter) occurs frequently. More severe cases may show hemoconcentration with hematocrit values exceeding 50 percent because of loss of plasma into the retroperitoneal space and peritoneal cavity. *Hyperglycemia* is common and is due to multiple factors, including decreased insulin release, increased glucagon release, and an increased output of adrenal glucocorticoids and catecholamines. *Hypocalcemia* occurs in approximately 25 percent of cases, and its pathogenesis is incompletely understood. While earlier studies suggested that the response of the parathyroid gland to a decrease in serum calcium is impaired, subsequent observations have failed to confirm this idea. Intraperitoneal saponification of calcium by fatty acids in areas of fat necrosis occurs occasionally, with large amounts (up to 6.0 g) dissolved or suspended in ascitic fluid. Such "soap formation" also may be significant in patients with pancreatitis, mild hypocalcemia, and little or no obvious ascites. *Hyperbilirubinemia* [serum bilirubin >68 μmol/L (>4.0 mg/dL)] occurs in approximately 10 percent of patients. However, jaundice is transient, and serum bilirubin levels return to normal in 4 to 7 days. Serum alkaline phosphatase and aspartate aminotransferase (AST) levels are also transiently elevated and parallel serum bilirubin values. Markedly elevated serum lactic dehydrogenase (LDH) levels [>8.5 μmol/L (>500 U/dL)] suggest a poor prognosis. Serum albumin is decreased to ≤30 g/L (≤3.0 g/dL) in about 10 percent of cases; this sign is associated with more severe pancreatitis and a higher mortality rate (Table 304-2). *Hypertriglyceridemia* occurs in 15 to 20 percent of cases, and serum amylase levels in these patients are often spuriously normal (see Chap. 303). Most patients with hypertriglyceridemia and pancreatitis, when subsequently examined, show evidence of an underlying derangement in lipid metabolism which probably antedated the pancreatitis (see below). Approximately 25 percent of patients have *hypoxemia* (arterial $P_{O_2} \leq 60$ mmHg), which may herald the onset of adult respiratory distress syndrome. Finally, the electrocardiogram is occasionally abnormal in acute pancreatitis with ST-segment and T-wave abnormalities simulating myocardial ischemia.

Radiologic studies useful in the diagnosis of acute pancreatitis are discussed in Chap. 303 and listed in Table 303-1. Although one or more radiologic abnormalities are found in over 50 percent of patients, the findings are inconstant and nonspecific. The chief value of conventional x-rays [chest films; kidney, ureter, and bladder (KUB) studies] in acute pancreatitis is to help exclude other diagnoses, especially a perforated viscus. Upper gastrointestinal tract x-rays have been superseded by ultrasonography and computed tomography (CT). A CT scan may confirm the clinical impression of acute pancreatitis even in the face of normal serum amylase levels. Importantly, CT is quite helpful in indicating the severity of acute pancreatitis and the risk of morbidity and mortality (see below). Sonography and radionuclide scanning [*N-p*-isopropylacetanilide-iminodiacetic acid (PIPIDA) scan; hepatic 2,6-dimethyliminodiacetic acid (HIDA) scan] are useful in acute pancreatitis to evaluate the gallbladder and biliary tree.

DIAGNOSIS Any severe acute pain in the abdomen or back should suggest acute pancreatitis. The diagnosis is usually entertained when a patient with a possible predisposition to pancreatitis presents with severe and constant abdominal pain, nausea, emesis, fever, tachycardia, and abnormal findings on abdominal examination. Laboratory studies frequently reveal leukocytosis, an abnormal appearance on x-rays of the abdomen and chest, hypocalcemia, and hyperglycemia. The diagnosis is usually confirmed by the finding of an elevated level of serum amylase and/or lipase. Obviously, not all the above features have to be present for the diagnosis to be established.

The *differential diagnosis* should include the following disorders: (1) perforated viscus, especially peptic ulcer, (2) acute cholecystitis and biliary colic, (3) acute intestinal obstruction, (4) mesenteric vascular occlusion, (5) renal colic, (6) myocardial infarction, (7) dissecting aortic aneurysm, (8) connective tissue disorders with vasculitis, (9) pneumonia, and (10) diabetic ketoacidosis. A penetrating duodenal ulcer usually can be identified by upper gastrointestinal x-rays and/or endoscopy. A perforated duodenal ulcer is readily diagnosed by the presence of free intraperitoneal air. It may be difficult to differentiate acute cholecystitis from acute pancreatitis, since an elevated serum amylase may be found in both disorders. Pain of biliary tract origin is more right-sided and gradual in onset, and ileus is usually absent; sonography and radionuclide scanning are helpful in establishing the diagnosis of cholelithiasis and cholecystitis. Intestinal obstruction due to mechanical factors can be differentiated from pancreatitis by the history of colicky pain, findings on abdominal examination, and x-rays of the abdomen showing changes characteristic of mechanical

Table 304-2

Factors That Adversely Affect Survival in Acute Pancreatitis

Ranson/Imrie criteria
- At admission or diagnosis
  - Age >55 years
  - Leukocytosis >16,000/μL
  - Hyperglycemia >11 mmol/L (>200 mg/dL)
  - Serum LDH >400 IU/L
  - Serum AST >250 IU/L
- During initial 48 h
  - Fall in hematocrit by >10 percent
  - Fluid deficit of >4000 mL
  - Hypocalcemia [calcium concentration <1.9 mmol/L (<8.0 mg/dL)]
  - Hypoxemia (P_{O_2} <60 mmHg)
  - Increase in BUN to >1.8 mmol/L (>5 mg/dL) after IV fluid administration
  - Hypoalbuminemia [albumin level <32 g/L (<3.2 g/dL)]

Acute physiology and chronic health evaluation (APACHE II) score > 12

Hemorrhagic peritoneal fluid

Obesity

Key indicators of organ failure
- Hypotension (blood pressure <90 mmHg) or tachycardia >130 beats per minute
- P_{O_2} <60 mmHg
- Oliguria (<50 mL/h) or increasing blood urea nitrogen (BUN), creatinine
- Metabolic indicators: serum calcium <1.9 mmol/L (<8.0 mg/dL) or serum albumin <32 g/L (<3.2 g/dL)

obstruction. Acute mesenteric vascular occlusion is usually evident in elderly debilitated patients with brisk leukocytosis, abdominal distention, and bloody diarrhea, in whom paracentesis shows sanguineous fluid and arteriography shows vascular occlusion. Serum as well as peritoneal fluid amylase levels are increased, however, in patients with intestinal infarction. Systemic lupus erythematosus and polyarteritis nodosa may be confused with pancreatitis, especially since pancreatitis may develop as a complication of these diseases. Diabetic ketoacidosis is often accompanied by abdominal pain and elevated total serum amylase levels, thus closely mimicking acute pancreatitis. However, the serum lipase and pancreatic isoamylase levels are not elevated in diabetic ketoacidosis.

COURSE OF THE DISEASE AND COMPLICATIONS It is important to identify patients with acute pancreatitis who have an increased risk of dying. Ranson and Imrie have used multiple prognostic criteria and have demonstrated that there is an increased mortality rate when three or more risk factors are identifiable either at the time of admission to the hospital or during the initial 48 h of hospitalization (see Table 304-2). Recent studies indicate that obesity is a major risk factor for severe pancreatitis, presumably because the increased deposits of peripancreatic fat in such patients may predispose them to more extensive pancreatic and peripancreatic necrosis. The acute physiology and chronic health evaluation scoring system (APACHE II) uses the worst values of 12 physiologic measurements plus age and previous health status and provides a good description of illness severity for a wide range of common diseases; this score also correlates with outcome. Prospective studies have compared APACHE II with multiple prognostic criteria, i.e., Ranson and Imrie scores, in predicting the severity of acute pancreatitis. On admission, APACHE II identified approximately two-thirds of severe attacks, and after 48 h, the prognostic accuracy of APACHE II is comparable with that of Ranson and Imrie's scoring system. The drawbacks of APACHE II are (1) its complexity, (2) the requirement of a computer for scoring, and (3) standardization regarding peak values and cutoff scores. McMahon and colleagues have shown that the presence of a "toxic broth" or dark (hemorrhagic) fluid in abdominal pancreatitis is also an important prognostic indicator in acute pancreatitis. These multiple-factor scoring systems are difficult to use and have not been embraced consistently by clinicians. There is a great need for a reliable, simple biochemical test that consistently predicts outcome in patients with acute pancreatitis. Three candidate markers that show great promise are C-reactive protein, serum granulocyte elastase, and urinary trypsinogen activation peptide (TAP). The key indicators of a severe attack of acute pancreatitis are also listed in Table 304-2. Importantly, the presence of any one of these factors is associated with an increased risk of complications, and the presence of any two, with a 20 to 30 percent mortality rate. The high mortality rate of such severely ill patients is due in large part to infection and warrants intensive radiologic intervention and monitoring and/or a combination of radiologic and surgical means, as discussed in detail below.

The local and systemic complications of acute pancreatitis are listed in Table 304-3. Patients frequently develop an inflammatory mass in the first 2 to 3 weeks after pancreatitis. This may be due to pancreatic necrosis (with or without infection) or may represent an abscess or pseudocyst (see below). Systemic complications include pulmonary, cardiovascular, hematologic, renal, metabolic, and central nervous system abnormalities. Pancreatitis and hypertriglyceridemia constitute an association in which cause and effect remain incompletely understood. However, several reasonable conclusions can be drawn. First, hypertriglyceridemia can precede and apparently cause pancreatitis. Second, the vast majority (>80 percent) of patients with acute pancreatitis do not have hypertriglyceridemia. Third, almost all patients with pancreatitis and hypertriglyceridemia have preexisting abnormalities in lipoprotein metabolism. Fourth, many of the patients with this association have persistent hypertriglyceridemia after recovery from pancreatitis and are prone to recurrent episodes of pancreatitis. Fifth, any factor (e.g., drugs or alcohol) that causes an abrupt increase in serum triglycerides to levels greater than 11 mmol/L (1000 mg/dL) can precipitate a bout of pancreatitis that can be associated with significant complications and even become fulminant. To avert the risk of triggering pancreatitis, a fasting serum triglyceride measurement should be obtained before estrogen replacement therapy is begun in postmenopausal women. Fasting levels less than 300 mg/dL pose no risk, whereas levels greater than 750 mg/dL are associated with a high probability of developing pancreatitis. Finally, patients with a defi-

Table 304-3

Complications of Acute Pancreatitis

LOCAL

- Necrosis
  - Sterile
  - Infected
- Pancreatic fluid collections
  - Pancreatic abscess
  - Pancreatic pseudocyst
    - Pain
    - Rupture
    - Hemorrhage
    - Infection
    - Obstruction of gastrointestinal tract (stomach, duodenum, colon)
- Pancreatic ascites
  - Disruption of main pancreatic duct
  - Leaking pseudocyst
- Involvement of contiguous organs by necrotizing pancreatitis
  - Massive intraperitoneal hemorrhage
  - Thrombosis of blood vessels (splenic vein, portal vein)
  - Bowel infarction
- Obstructive jaundice

SYSTEMIC

- Pulmonary
  - Pleural effusion
  - Atelectasis
  - Mediastinal abscess
  - Pneumonitis
  - Adult respiratory distress syndrome
- Cardiovascular
  - Hypotension
    - Hypovolemia
    - Hypoalbuminemia
  - Sudden death
  - Nonspecific ST-T changes in electrocardiogram simulating myocardial infarction
  - Pericardial effusion
- Hematologic
  - Disseminated intravascular coagulation
- Gastrointestinal hemorrhage*
  - Peptic ulcer disease
  - Erosive gastritis
  - Hemorrhagic pancreatic necrosis with erosion into major blood vessels
  - Portal vein thrombosis, variceal hemorrhage
- Renal
  - Oliguria
  - Azotemia
  - Renal artery and/or renal vein thrombosis
  - Acute tubular necrosis
- Metabolic
  - Hyperglycemia
  - Hypertriglyceridemia
  - Hypocalcemia
  - Encephalopathy
  - Sudden blindness (Purtscher's retinopathy)
- Central nervous system
  - Psychosis
  - Fat emboli
- Fat necrosis
  - Subcutaneous tissues (erythematous nodules)
  - Bone
  - Miscellaneous (mediastinum, pleura, nervous system)

* Aggravated by coagulation abnormalities (disseminated intravascular coagulation).

ciency of apolipoprotein CII have an increased incidence of pancreatitis; apolipoprotein CII activates lipoprotein lipase, which is important in clearing chylomicrons from the bloodstream.

Purtscher's retinopathy, a relatively unusual complication, is manifested by a sudden and severe loss of vision in a patient with acute pancreatitis. It is characterized by a peculiar funduscopic appearance with cotton-wool spots and hemorrhages confined to an area limited by the optic disk and macula; it is believed to be due to occlusion of the posterior retinal artery with aggregated granulocytes.

The two most common causes of acute pancreatitis are alcoholism and biliary tract disease; other causes are listed in Table 304-1. However, after a conventional workup, a specific cause will not be identified in about 30 percent of patients. It is important to note that ultrasound examinations will fail to detect gallstones, especially microlithiasis and/or sludge, in 4 to 7 percent of patients. In one series of 31 patients diagnosed initially as having idiopathic acute pancreatitis, 23 were found to have occult gallstone disease. Thus, approximately two-thirds of patients with recurrent acute pancreatitis without an obvious cause actually have occult gallstone disease due to microlithiasis. Examination of duodenal aspirates in such cases often reveals cholesterol crystals, which confirm the diagnosis. Other diseases of the biliary tree and pancreatic ducts that can cause acute pancreatitis include choledochocele, ampullary tumors, pancreas divisum, and pancreatic duct stones, stricture, and tumor. Approximately 2 percent of patients with pancreatic carcinoma present with acute pancreatitis.

Pancreatitis in AIDS Patients The incidence of acute pancreatitis is increased in patients with AIDS for two reasons: (1) the high incidence of infections involving the pancreas, such as infections with cytomegalovirus, *Cryptosporidium*, and the *Mycobacterium avium* complex; and (2) the frequent use by AIDS patients of medications such as didanosine, pentamidine, and trimethoprim-sulfamethoxazole (see also Chap. 308).

℞ TREATMENT

In most patients (approximately 85 to 90 percent) with acute pancreatitis, the disease is self-limited and subsides spontaneously, usually within 3 to 7 days after treatment is instituted. Conventional measures include (1) analgesics for pain, (2) intravenous fluids and colloids to maintain normal intravascular volume, (3) no oral alimentation, and (4) nasogastric suction to decrease gastrin release from the stomach and prevent gastric contents from entering the duodenum. Recent controlled trials, however, have shown that nasogastric suction offers no clear-cut advantages in the treatment of mild to moderately severe acute pancreatitis. Its use, therefore, must be considered elective rather than mandatory.

It has been demonstrated that CCK-stimulated pancreatic secretion is almost abolished in four different experimental models of acute pancreatitis. This probably explains why drugs to block pancreatic secretion in acute pancreatitis have failed to have any therapeutic benefit. For this and other reasons, anticholinergic drugs are not indicated in acute pancreatitis. In addition to nasogastric suction and anticholinergic drugs, other therapies designed to "rest the pancreas" by inhibiting pancreatic secretion have not changed the course of the disease. Although antibiotics have been used in the treatment of acute pancreatitis, randomized, prospective trials have shown no benefit from their use in acute pancreatitis of mild to moderate severity. However, recent studies of antibiotic use in patients with extensive pancreatic necrosis have demonstrated a reduced mortality rate. Furthermore, because secondary infection of necrotic pancreatic tissue (abscess, pseudocyst) or obstructed biliary passages (ascending cholangitis, complicating choledocholithiasis) contributes to much of the late mortality from pancreatitis, appropriate *antibiotic therapy of established infection* is obviously quite important. Several other drugs have been evaluated by prospective, controlled trials and found *ineffective* in the treatment of acute pancreatitis. The list, by no means complete, includes glucagon, H_2 blockers, protease inhibitors such as aprotinin, glucocorticoids, calcitonin, somatostatin analogues such as octreotide, and nonsteroidal anti-inflammatory drugs (NSAIDs). However, prophylactic treatment with gabexate, a protease inhibitor, has reduced pancreatic damage related to endoscopic retrograde cholangiopancreatography (ERCP).

A CT scan, especially a contrast-enhanced dynamic CT (CECT) scan, provides valuable information on the severity and prognosis of acute pancreatitis (Fig. 304-1 and Table 304-4). In particular, CECT allows estimation of the presence and extent of pancreatic necrosis. Recent studies suggest that the likelihood of prolonged pancreatitis or a serious complication is negligible when the CT severity index is 1 or 2 and low with scores of 3 to 6. However, patients with scores of 7 to 10 had a 92 percent morbidity and 17

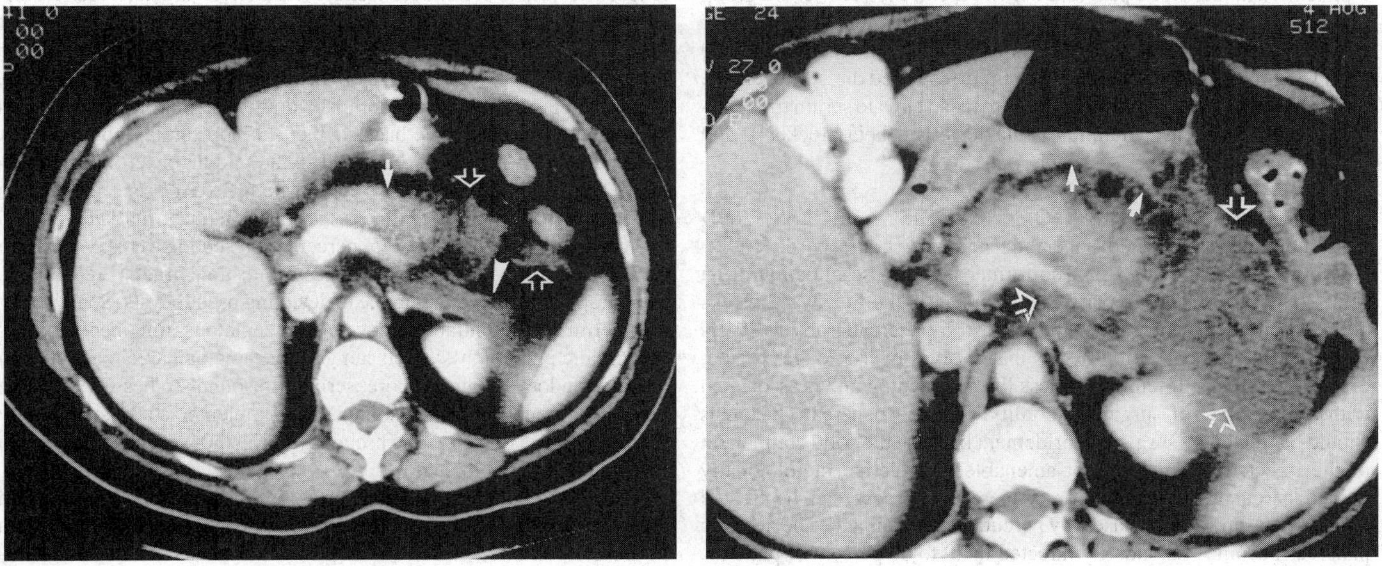

A *B*

FIGURE 304-1 Acute pancreatitis: CT evolution. *A*. Contrast-enhanced CT scan of the abdomen performed on admission of a patient with clinical evidence of acute pancreatitis. Note the mildly decreased density of the body of the pancreas to the left of the midline (*arrow*). There are a few linear strands in the peripancreatic fat, suggesting inflammation (*open arrows*). A small amount of fluid is seen in the anterior pararenal space (*arrowhead*). *B*. Nine days after admission, there is a marked worsening with severe inflammation of the pancreas evidenced by anterior displacement of the posterior gastric wall (*arrows*), increased inflammation of the peripancreatic fat, and increased pancreatic effusion in the anterior perirenal space and around the splenic vein (*open arrows*). *(Courtesy of Dr. PR Ros, University of Florida College of Medicine.)*

Table 304-4

Severity Index in Acute Pancreatitis

	Points
Grade of Acute Pancreatitis	
A. Normal pancreas	0
B. Pancreatic enlargement alone	1
C. Inflammation compared with pancreas and peripancreatic fat	2
D. One peripancreatic fluid collection	3
E. Two or more fluid collections	4
Degree of Pancreatic Necrosis	
A. No necrosis	0
B. Necrosis of one-third of pancreas	2
C. Necrosis of one-half of pancreas	4
D. Necrosis of more than one-half of pancreas	6

percent mortality. A CECT scan is indicated in patients with three or more of Ranson's signs, in all seriously ill patients, and in patients who show evidence of clinical deterioration. The patient with mild to moderate pancreatitis usually requires treatment with intravenous fluids, fasting, and possibly nasogastric suction for 2 to 4 days. A clear liquid diet is frequently started on the third to sixth day, and a regular diet by the fifth to seventh day. The patient with unremitting *fulminant pancreatitis* usually requires inordinate amounts of fluid and close attention to complications such as cardiovascular collapse, respiratory insufficiency, and pancreatic infection. The latter should be managed by a combination of radiologic and surgical means (see below). While earlier uncontrolled studies suggested that *peritoneal lavage* via a percutaneous dialysis catheter was helpful in severe pancreatitis, subsequent studies indicate that this treatment does not influence the outcome of such attacks. Laparotomy with adequate drainage and removal of necrotic tissue should be considered if conventional therapy does not halt the patient's deterioration. The use of parenteral nutrition makes it possible to give nutritional support to patients with severe, acute, or protracted pancreatitis who are unable to eat normally. Patients with severe gallstone-induced pancreatitis may improve dramatically if papillotomy is carried out within the first 36 to 72 h of the attack. Recent studies indicate that only those patients with gallstone pancreatitis who are in the very severe group should be considered for urgent ERCP. Finally, the treatment for patients with hypertriglyceridemia-associated pancreatitis include (1) weight loss to ideal weight, (2) a lipid-restricted diet, (3) exercise, (4) avoidance of alcohol and of drugs that can elevate serum triglycerides (i.e., estrogens, vitamin A, thiazides, and beta-blockers), and (5) control of diabetes.

INFECTED PANCREATIC NECROSIS, ABSCESS, AND PSEUDOCYST Infected pancreatic necrosis should be differentiated from pancreatic abscess. The former is a diffuse infection of an acutely inflamed, necrotic pancreas occurring in the first 1 to 2 weeks after the onset of pancreatitis. In contrast, a pancreatic abscess is an ill-defined, liquid collection of pus that evolves over a longer period, often 4 to 6 weeks. It tends to be less life-threatening and is associated with a lower rate of surgical mortality. Infected pancreatic necrosis should be treated by surgical debridement because the solid component of the infected pancreas is not amenable to effective radiologically guided percutaneous evacuation. Pancreatic abscess can be treated surgically or, in selected cases, by percutaneous drainage. The necrotic pancreas becomes secondarily infected in 40 to 60 percent of patients, most frequently with gram-negative bacteria of alimentary origin. Whether infection occurs depends on several factors, including the extent of pancreatic and peripancreatic necrosis, the degree of pancreatic ischemia and hypoperfusion, and the presence of organ or multiorgan failure.

The early diagnosis of pancreatic infection can be accomplished by CT-guided needle aspiration. In one study, 60 patients, representing 5 percent of all admissions for acute pancreatitis, were suspected of harboring a pancreatic infection on the basis of fever, leukocytosis, and an abnormal CT scan (phlegmon, pseudocyst, or extrapancreatic fluid collection). Importantly, 60 percent of these patients had a pancreatic infection, and 55 percent of these infections developed in the first 2 weeks. These findings suggest that only guided aspiration can reliably distinguish sterile from infected pancreatic necrosis. The following are guidelines for patients meeting the above selection criteria: (1) Pseudocysts and phlegmons should be aspirated promptly, because more than half may be infected; (2) extrapancreatic fluid collections need not be aspirated promptly, because most are sterile; (3) if a phlegmon is found initially to be sterile but fever and leukocytosis persist, several days of observation should be allowed to pass before reaspiration is considered, as clinical improvement frequently occurs; and (4) if fever and leukocytosis recur after an interval of well-being, reaspiration should be considered.

Severe pancreatitis with the presence of three or more risk factors, postoperative pancreatitis, early oral feeding, early laparotomy, and perhaps injudicious use of antibiotics predispose to the development of pancreatic abscess, which occurs in 3 to 4 percent of patients with acute pancreatitis. Pancreatic abscess also may develop because of a communication between a pseudocyst and the colon, inadequate surgical drainage of a pseudocyst, or needling of a pseudocyst. The characteristic signs of abscess are fever, leukocytosis, ileus, and rapid deterioration in a patient previously recovering from pancreatitis. Sometimes, however, the only manifestations are persistent fever and signs of continuing pancreatic inflammation. Drainage of pancreatic abscesses by percutaneous catheter techniques, using CT guidance, has been only moderately successful (resolution in 50 to 60 percent of patients). Accordingly, laparotomy with radical sump drainage and possibly resection of necrotic tissue is usually required, because the mortality rate for undrained pancreatic abscess approaches 100 percent. Multiple abscesses are common, and reoperation is frequently necessary.

Pseudocysts of the pancreas are collections of tissue, fluid, debris, pancreatic enzymes, and blood which develop over a period of 1 to 4 weeks after the onset of acute pancreatitis; they form in approximately 15 percent of patients with acute pancreatitis. In contrast to true cysts, pseudocysts do not have an epithelial lining, the walls consisting of necrotic tissue, granulation tissue, and fibrous tissue. Disruption of the pancreatic ductal system is common. However, the subsequent course of this disruption varies widely, ranging from spontaneous healing to continuous leakage of pancreatic juice, which results in tense ascites. Pseudocysts are preceded by pancreatitis in 90 percent of cases and by trauma in 10 percent. Approximately 85 percent are located in the body or tail of the pancreas and 15 percent in the head. Some patients have two or more pseudocysts. Abdominal pain, with or without radiation to the back, is the usual presenting complaint. A palpable, tender mass may be found in the middle or left upper abdomen. The serum amylase level is elevated in 75 percent of patients at some point during their illness and may fluctuate markedly.

On x-ray examination, 75 percent of pseudocysts can be seen to displace some portion of the gastrointestinal tract (Fig. 304-2). Sonography, however, is reliable in detecting pseudocysts. Sonography also permits differentiation between an edematous, inflamed pancreas (pancreatic phlegmon), which can give rise to a palpable mass, and an actual pseudocyst. Furthermore, serial ultrasound studies will indicate whether a pseudocyst has resolved. CT complements ultrasonography in the diagnosis of pancreatic pseudocyst (Fig. 304-2), especially when the pseudocyst is infected.

In studies using sonography, pseudocysts were seen to resolve in 25 to 40 percent of patients. Pseudocysts that are greater than 5 cm in diameter and that persist for longer than 6 weeks should be considered for drainage. Recent natural history studies have suggested that noninterventional, expectant management is the best course in selected patients with minimal symptoms and no evidence of active alcohol use in whom the pseudocyst appears mature by radiography and does not resemble a cystic neoplasm. A significant number of these pseudocysts will resolve spontaneously more than 6 weeks after their formation. Also, these studies demonstrate that large pseudocyst size is not an absolute indication for interventional therapy and that many peripancreatic fluid collections detected on CT in cases of acute pancreatitis resolve spontaneously. A pseudocyst that does not resolve spontaneously may lead to serious complications, such as (1) pain caused by expansion of the lesion and pressure on other viscera, (2) rupture, (3) hemorrhage, and (4) abscess. Rupture of a pancreatic pseudocyst is a particularly serious complication. Shock almost always supervenes, and mortality rates range from 14 percent if the rupture is not associated with hemorrhage to over 60 percent if hemorrhage has occurred. Rupture and hemorrhage are the prime causes of death from pancreatic pseudocyst. A triad of findings—an increase in the size of the mass, a localized bruit over the mass, and a sudden decrease in hemoglobin level and hematocrit without obvious external blood loss—should alert one to the possibility of hemorrhage from a pseudocyst. Thus, in patients who are stable and free of complications and in whom serial ultrasound studies show that the pseudocyst is shrinking, conservative therapy is indicated. Conversely, if the pseudocyst is expanding and is complicated by rupture, hemorrhage, or abscess, the patient should be operated on. Using ultrasound or CT guidance, sterile chronic pseudocysts can be treated safely with single or repeated needle aspiration or more prolonged catheter drainage with a success rate of 45 to 75 percent. The success rate of these techniques for infected pseudocysts is considerably less (40 to 50 percent). Patients who do not respond to drainage require surgical therapy for internal or external drainage of the cyst.

Pseudoaneurysms develop in up to 10 percent of patients with acute pancreatitis at sites reflecting the distribution of pseudocysts and fluid collections (Fig. 304-2*D*). The splenic artery is most frequently involved, followed by the inferior and superior pancreatic duodenal

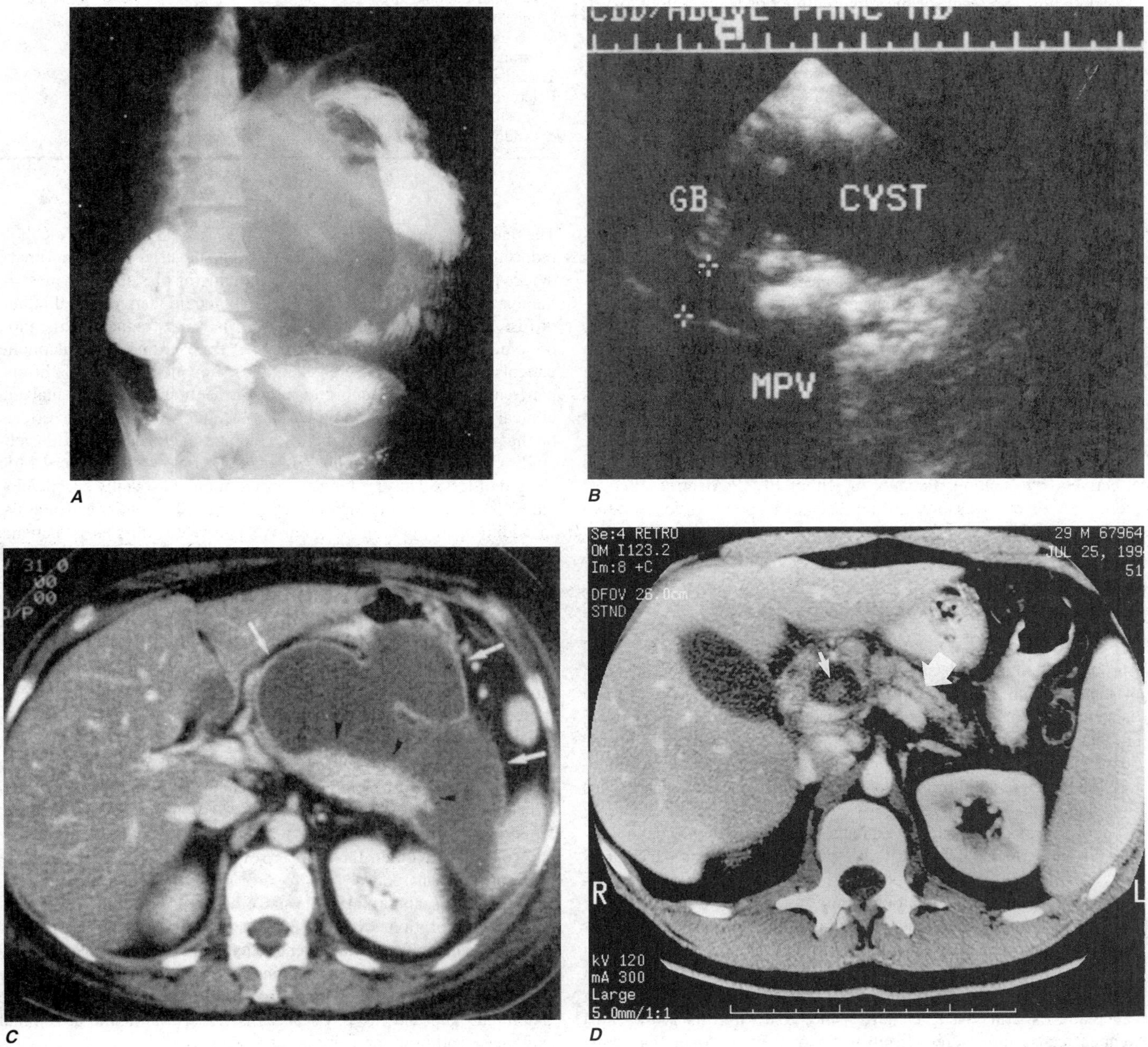

FIGURE 304-2 Pseudocyst of pancreas. *A*. Upper gastrointestinal x-ray showing displacement of stomach by pseudocyst. *B*. Sonogram showing pseudocyst (*cyst*). GB, gallbladder; MVP, portal vein. Behind the large pseudocyst is seen the calcified head of the pancreas. A dilated common bile duct (*asterisk*) is noted. *C*. CT scan showing pseudocyst. Note the large, lobulated fluid collection (*arrows*) surrounding the tail of the pancreas (*arrowheads*). Note also the dense, thin rim in the periphery representing the fibrous capsule of the pseudocyst. *D*. Spiral CT showing a pseudocyst (*small arrow*) with a pseudoaneurysm (light area in pseudocyst). Note the demonstration of the main pancreatic duct (*big arrow*), even though this duct is minimally dilated by ERCP. *(A, B courtesy of Dr. CE Forsmark, University of Florida College of Medicine; C, D courtesy of Dr. PR Ros, University of Florida College of Medicine.)*

arteries. This diagnosis should be suspected in patients with pancreatitis who develop upper gastrointestinal bleeding without an obvious cause or in whom thin-cut CT scanning reveals a contrast-enhanced lesion within or adjacent to a suspected pseudocyst. Arteriography is necessary to confirm the diagnosis.

PANCREATIC ASCITES AND PANCREATIC PLEURAL EFFUSIONS Pancreatic ascites is usually due to disruption of the main pancreatic duct, often by an internal fistula between the duct and the peritoneal cavity or a leaking pseudocyst (see also Chap. 43). This diagnosis is suggested in a patient with an elevated serum amylase level in whom the ascites fluid has both increased levels of albumin [>30 g/L (>3.0 g/dL)] and a markedly elevated level of amylase. The fluid in true pancreatic ascites usually has an amylase concentration of >20,000 U/L as a result of the ruptured duct or leaking pseudocyst. Lower amylase elevations may be found in the peritoneal fluid of patients with acute pancreatitis. In addition, ERCP will often demonstrate passage of contrast material from a major pancreatic duct or a pseudocyst into the peritoneal cavity. As many as 15 percent of patients with pseudocysts have concurrent pancreatic ascites. The differential diagnosis should include intraperitoneal carcinomatosis, tuberculous peritonitis, constrictive pericarditis, and Budd-Chiari syndrome.

If the pancreatic duct disruption is posterior, an internal fistula may develop between the pancreatic duct and the pleural space, producing a pleural effusion, which is usually left-sided and often massive. This complication often requires thoracentesis or chest tube drainage.

Treatment usually involves using nasogastric suction and parenteral alimentation to decrease pancreatic secretion. In addition, paracentesis is performed to keep the peritoneal cavity free of fluid and, it is hoped, to effect sealing of the leak. The long-acting somatostatin analogue octreotide, which inhibits pancreatic secretion, is useful in cases of pancreatic ascites and pleural effusion. If ascites continues to recur after 2 to 3 weeks of medical management, the patient should be operated on following pancreatography to define the anatomy of the abnormal duct. A disrupted main pancreatic duct can also be treated effectively by stenting. Patients in whom ERCP identifies two or more sites of extravasation are unlikely to respond to conservative management and/or stenting.

CHRONIC PANCREATITIS AND PANCREATIC EXOCRINE INSUFFICIENCY

GENERAL AND ETIOLOGIC CONSIDERATIONS Chronic inflammatory disease of the pancreas may present as episodes of acute inflammation in a previously injured pancreas or as chronic damage with persistent pain or malabsorption. The causes of relapsing chronic pancreatitis are similar to those of acute pancreatitis (Table 304-1), except that there is an appreciable incidence of cases of undetermined origin. In addition, the pancreatitis associated with gallstones is predominantly acute or relapsing-acute in nature. A cholecystectomy is almost always performed in patients after the first or second attack of gallstone-associated pancreatitis. Patients with chronic pancreatitis may present with persistent abdominal pain, with or without steatorrhea; some present with steatorrhea and no pain.

Patients with chronic pancreatitis in whom there is extensive destruction of the pancreas (less than 10 percent of exocrine function remaining) will have steatorrhea and azotorrhea. Among American adults, alcoholism is the most common cause of clinically apparent pancreatic exocrine insufficiency, while cystic fibrosis is the most frequent cause in children. In up to 25 percent of American adults with chronic pancreatitis, the cause is not known; that is, they have idiopathic chronic pancreatitis. In other parts of the world, severe protein-calorie malnutrition is a common cause. Table 304-5 lists other causes of pancreatic exocrine insufficiency, but they are relatively uncommon.

PATHOPHYSIOLOGY Unfortunately, the events that initiate an inflammatory process in the pancreas are still not well understood. The many hypotheses will not be reviewed here. In the case of alcohol-induced pancreatitis, however, it has been suggested that the primary defect may be the precipitation of protein (inspissated enzymes) in the ducts. The resulting ductal obstruction could lead to duct dilation, diffuse atrophy of the acinar cells, fibrosis, and eventual calcification of some of the protein plugs. However, the fact that some alcoholic patients with recurrent acute pancreatitis show no evidence of chronic pancreatitis does not support this hypothesis. In fact, experimental and clinical observations have shown that alcohol has direct toxic effects on the pancreas. While patients with alcohol-induced pancreatitis generally consume large amounts of alcohol, some consume very little (50 g/d or less). Thus prolonged consumption of "socially acceptable" amounts of alcohol is compatible with the development of pancreatitis. In addition, the finding of extensive pancreatic fibrosis in patients who died during their first attack of clinical acute alcohol-induced pancreatitis supports the concept that such patients already have chronic pancreatitis.

Table 304-5

Causes of Pancreatic Exocrine Insufficiency

Alcohol, chronic alcoholism
Idiopathic pancreatitis
Cystic fibrosis
Hypertriglyceridemia
Severe protein-calorie malnutrition with hypoalbuminemia
Tropical pancreatitis (Africa, Asia)
Pancreatic and duodenal neoplasms
Pancreatic resection
Gastric surgery
Subtotal gastrectomy with Billroth I anastomosis
Subtotal gastrectomy with Billroth II anastomosis
Truncal vagotomy and pyloroplasty
Gastrinoma (Zollinger-Ellison syndrome)
Hereditary pancreatitis
Traumatic pancreatitis
Abdominal radiotherapy
Hemochromatosis
Shwachman's syndrome (pancreatic insufficiency and bone marrow dysfunction)
Trypsinogen deficiency
Enterokinase deficiency
Isolated deficiencies of amylase, lipase, or proteases
α_1-Antitrypsin deficiency

CLINICAL FEATURES Patients with relapsing chronic pancreatitis may present with symptoms identical to those of acute pancreatitis, but pain may be continuous, intermittent, or absent. The pathogenesis of this pain is poorly understood. Although the classic description is of epigastric pain radiating through the back, the pain pattern is often atypical; the pain may be worst in the right or left upper quadrant of the back or may be diffuse throughout the upper abdomen; it may even be referred to the anterior chest or flank. Characteristically it is persistent, deep-seated, and unresponsive to antacids. It often is worsened by ingestion of alcohol or a heavy meal (especially one rich in fat). Often the pain is severe enough to necessitate the frequent use of narcotics.

Weight loss, abnormal stools, and other signs or symptoms suggestive of malabsorption (see Table 285-5) are common in chronic pancreatitis. However, clinically apparent deficiencies of fat-soluble vitamins are surprisingly rare. The physical findings in these patients are usually not impressive, so that there is a disparity between the severity of the abdominal pain and the physical signs (other than some abdominal tenderness and mild temperature elevation).

DIAGNOSTIC EVALUATION (See Chap. 303) In contrast to relapsing acute pancreatitis, the serum amylase and lipase levels are usually not elevated in chronic pancreatitis. Elevations of serum bilirubin and alkaline phosphatase levels may indicate cholestasis secondary to chronic inflammation around the common bile duct (Fig. 304-3). Many patients demonstrate impaired glucose tolerance, and some have an elevated fasting blood glucose level.

The classic triad of pancreatic calcification, steatorrhea, and diabetes mellitus usually establishes the diagnosis of chronic pancreatitis and exocrine pancreatic insufficiency but is found in less than one-third of chronic pancreatitis patients. Accordingly, it is often necessary to perform an intubation test such as the *secretin stimulation test*, which usually gives abnormal results when 60 percent or more of pancreatic exocrine function has been lost. Approximately 40 percent of patients with chronic pancreatitis have *cobalamin (vitamin B_{12}) malabsorption*, which can be corrected by the administration of oral pancreatic enzymes. There is usually a marked excretion of fecal fat (see Chap. 285), which can be reduced by the administration of oral pancreatic enzymes. The bentiromide test (Chap. 303) and the D-xylose urinary excretion test are useful in patients with "pancreatic steatorrhea," since the bentiromide test will be abnormal, and D-xylose excretion usually is normal. A decreased serum trypsinogen level strongly suggests pancreatic exocrine insufficiency.

The radiographic hallmark of chronic pancreatitis is the presence of scattered calcification throughout the pancreas (Fig. 304-3). Diffuse pancreatic calcification indicates that significant damage has occurred and obviates the need for a secretin test. While alcohol is by far the most common cause, pancreatic calcification also may be seen in cases of severe protein-calorie malnutrition, hereditary pancreatitis, posttraumatic pancreatitis, hyperparathyroidism, islet cell tumors, and idiopathic chronic pancreatitis. A large prospective study has shown convincingly that pancreatic calcification decreases or even disappears spontaneously in one-third of patients with severe chronic pancreatitis; this outcome may also follow ductal decompression. Pancreatic calcification is a dynamic process that is incompletely understood.

Sonography, CT, and ERCP greatly aid the diagnosis of pancreatic disease. In addition to excluding pseudocysts and pancreatic cancer, sonography and CT may show calcification or dilated ducts associated with chronic pancreatitis (Fig. 304-4). ERCP is the only major technique that provides a direct view of the pancreatic duct. In patients with alcohol-induced pancreatitis, ERCP may reveal a pseudocyst missed by sonography or CT.

COMPLICATIONS OF CHRONIC PANCREATITIS The complications of chronic pancreatitis are protean. *Cobalamin (vitamin B_{12}) malabsorption* occurs in 40 percent of patients with alcohol-induced chronic pancreatitis and in virtually all with cystic fibrosis. It is consistently corrected by the administration of pancreatic enzymes (containing proteases). It may be due to excessive binding of cobalamin by cobalamin-binding proteins other than intrinsic factor, which ordinarily are destroyed by pancreatic proteases and therefore do not

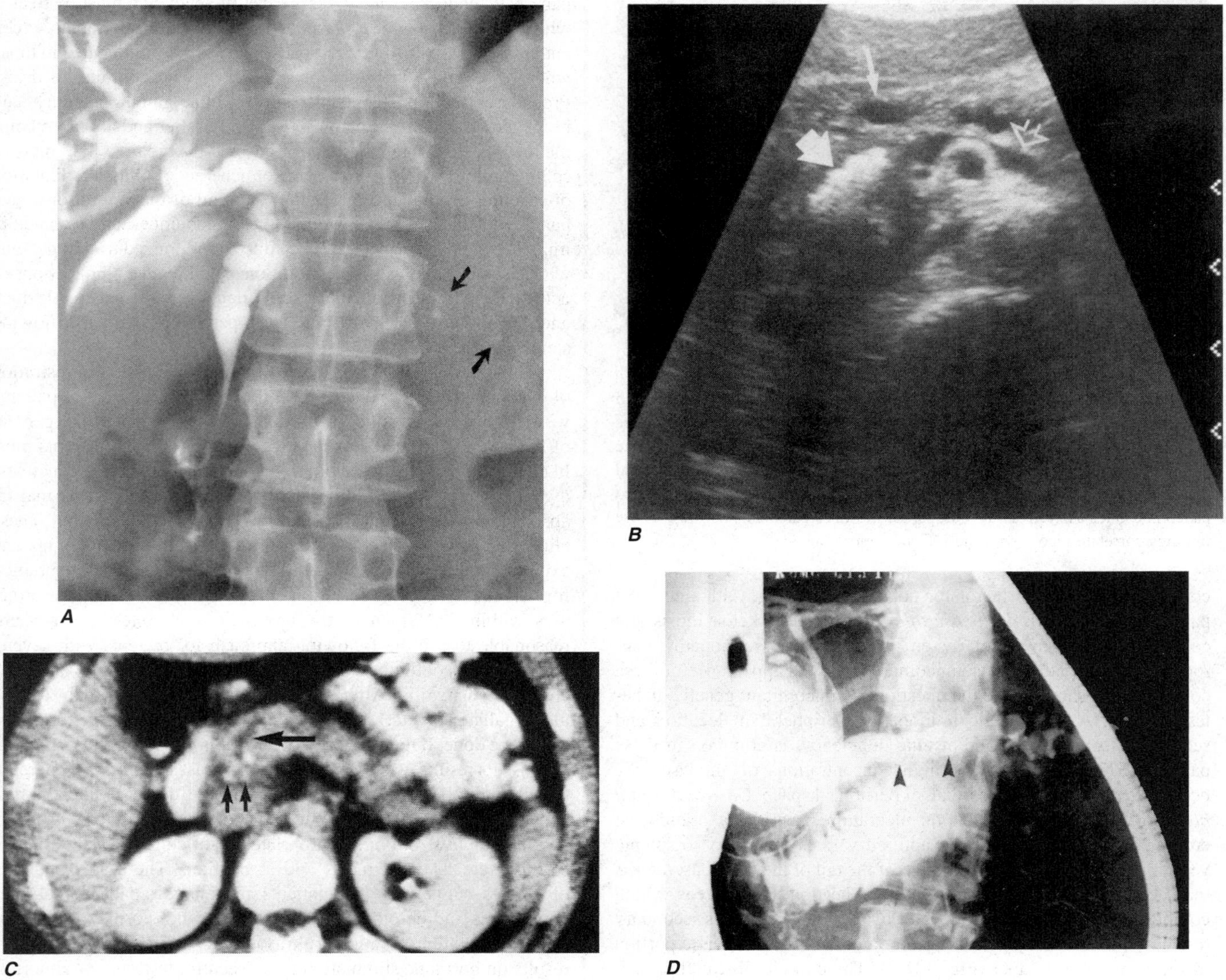

FIGURE 304-3 Radiologic abnormalities in chronic pancreatitis. *A*. Pancreatic calcification (*arrows*) and stenosis (tapering) of the intrahepatic portion of the common bile duct demonstrated by percutaneous transhepatic cholangiography. *B*. Pancreatic calcification (*large white arrow*) demonstrated by sonography. Note dilated pancreatic duct (*thin white arrow*) and splenic vein (*open arrow*). *C*. Pancreatic calcification (*vertical arrows*) and dilated pancreatic duct (*horizontal arrow*) demonstrated by CT scan. *D*. Endoscopic retrograde cholangiogram shows grossly dilated pancreatic ducts (*arrows*) in a patient with long-standing pancreatitis.

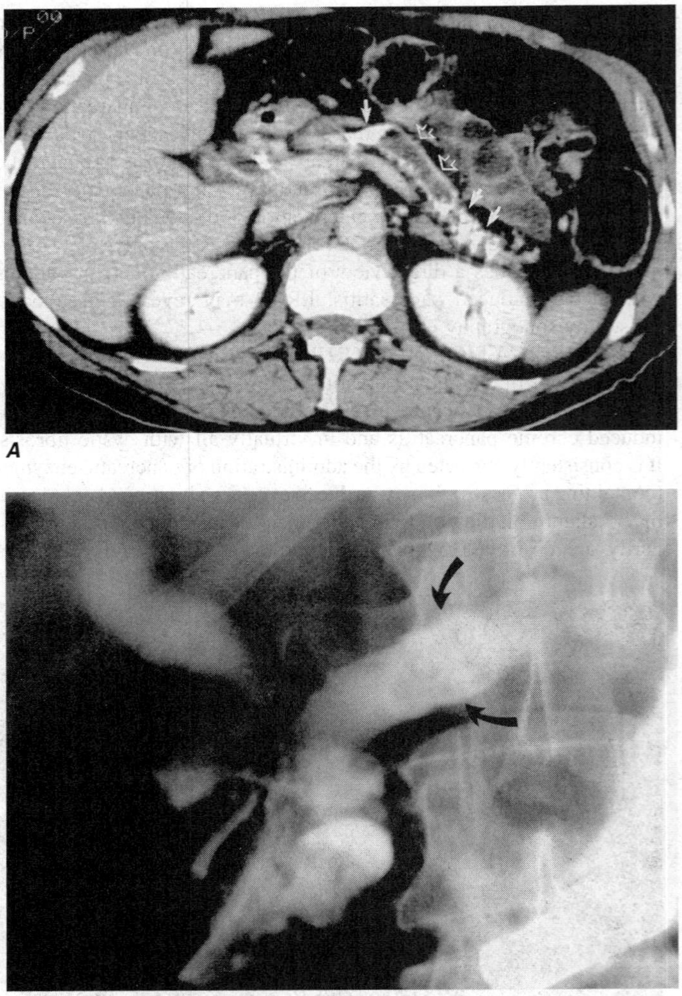

A

B

FIGURE 304-4 Chronic pancreatitis and pancreatic calculi: CT scan and ERCP appearance. *A*. In this contrast-enhanced CT scan of the abdomen, there is evidence of an atrophic pancreas with multiple calcifications (*arrows*). Note the markedly dilated pancreatic duct seen in this section through the body and tail (*open arrows*). *B*. ERCP in the same patient demonstrates the dilated pancreatic duct as well as an intrapancreatic duct calculus (*arrows*). These findings correlate nicely with the CT scan appearance.

compete with intrinsic factor for cobalamin binding. Although most patients show *impaired glucose tolerance*, diabetic ketoacidosis and coma are uncommon. Similarly, end-organ damage (retinopathy, neuropathy, nephropathy) is also uncommon, and the appearance of these complications should raise the question of concomitant genetic diabetes mellitus. A nondiabetic retinopathy, peripheral in location and secondary to vitamin A and/or zinc deficiency, is common in these patients. *Effusions* containing high concentrations of amylase may occur into the pleural, pericardial, or peritoneal space. *Gastrointestinal bleeding* may occur from peptic ulceration, gastritis, a pseudocyst eroding into the duodenum, or ruptured varices secondary to splenic vein thrombosis due to inflammation of the tail of the pancreas. *Icterus* may occur, caused either by edema of the head of the pancreas, which compresses the common bile duct, or by chronic cholestasis secondary to a chronic inflammatory reaction around the intrapancreatic portion of the common bile duct (Fig. 304-3). The chronic obstruction may lead to cholangitis and ultimately to biliary cirrhosis. *Subcutaneous fat necrosis* may appear as tender red nodules on the lower extremities. *Bone pain* may be secondary to intramedullary fat necrosis. Inflammation of the large and small joints of the upper and lower extremities may occur. The incidence of pancreatic carcinoma is increased in patients with chronic pancreatitis who have been followed for 2 or more years. Perhaps the most common and troublesome complication is addiction to narcotics.

℞ TREATMENT

Therapy for patients with chronic pancreatitis is directed toward two major problems—pain and malabsorption. Patients with intermittent attacks of pain are treated essentially like those with acute pancreatitis (see above). Patients with severe and persistent pain should avoid alcohol completely and avoid large meals rich in fat. Since the pain is often severe enough to require frequent use of narcotics (and hence addiction), a number of surgical procedures have been developed for pain relief. ERCP allows the surgeon to plan the operative approach. If there is a stricture of the pancreatic duct, a *local resection* may ameliorate the pain. Unfortunately, isolated localized strictures are not common. In most patients with alcohol-induced disease, the pancreas is diffusely involved, and surgically correctible localized ductal disease is rare. When there is primary ductal obstruction and dilation, ductal decompression may provide effective pain palliation. Short-term pain relief may be achieved in up to 80 percent of patients, while long-term pain relief occurs in approximately 50 percent. In some of these patients, however, pain relief can be achieved only by resecting 50 to 95 percent of the gland. Although pain relief is achieved in three-quarters of these patients, they tend to develop pancreatic endocrine and exocrine insufficiency and must be treated with pancreatic enzyme replacement therapy. It is important to screen patients carefully, for such radical surgery is contraindicated in those who are severely depressed or suicidal or who continue to drink. Procedures such as splanchnicectomy, celiac ganglionectomy, and nerve blocks usually bring only temporary relief and are not recommended. Endoscopic treatment of chronic pancreatitis may involve sphincterotomy of the minor or major pancreatic sphincter, dilatation of strictures, removal of calculi, or stenting of the ventral or dorsal pancreatic duct. While many of these techniques are technically impressive, none has been subjected to a randomized trial in patients with chronic pancreatitis. In addition, significant complications—acute pancreatitis, pancreatic abscess, damage to the pancreatic duct, and death—have occurred in up to 36 percent of patients following stent placement.

Three double-blind trials have demonstrated that administration of pancreatic enzymes decreases abdominal pain in selected patients with chronic pancreatitis. In these trials, approximately 75 percent of the patients evaluated experienced pain relief. The patients most likely to respond are those with mild to moderate exocrine pancreatic dysfunction, as evidenced by an abnormal secretin test, normal fat absorption, and minimal abnormalities on ERCP examination. These clinical observations seem to fit with data from human beings and experimental animals demonstrating a negative feedback regulation for pancreatic exocrine secretion controlled by the amount of proteases within the lumen of the proximal small intestine. It seems reasonable to use the following approach for patients with severe, persistent or continuous abdominal pain thought to be caused by chronic pancreatitis. After other causes of abdominal pain (peptic ulcer, gallstones, etc.) have been excluded, a pancreatic *sonogram* should be done. If no mass is found, a *secretin test* may be performed, because its results usually are abnormal in cases of chronic pancreatitis with pain. If the results are abnormal (i.e., decreased bicarbonate concentration or volume output), a 3- to 4-week *trial of pancreatic enzyme administration* is appropriate. Eight conventional tablets or capsules are taken at meals and at bedtime. There are a number of studies suggesting that patients may have small-duct chronic pancreatitis and chronic abdominal pain with a normal appearance on radiographic evaluations (ultrasound, CT, ERCP) but abnormal results on hormone stimulation tests (secretin test) and/or abnormal pancreatic histology. Such minimal-change chronic pancreatitis may respond well to pancreatic enzyme therapy (non-enteric-coated) for relief of abdominal pain. If no relief is obtained, and especially if the volume secreted during the secretin test is very low, ERCP should be performed. If a pseudocyst or a localized ductal obstruction is found, surgery should be considered. A patient who has dilated ducts may be a candidate for a surgical ductal decompression procedure. This procedure provides short-term relief in up to 80 percent of patients, although long-term results are closer to 50 percent. Some studies have shown octreotide to be effective in decreasing abdominal pain in patients with severe large-duct disease. If no surgically remediable lesion is found and severe pain continues despite abstinence from alcohol, subtotal pancreatic resection may be necessary.

The treatment of malabsorption rests on the use of pancreatic enzyme replacement therapy. Diarrhea and steatorrhea are usually improved by this treatment, although the steatorrhea may not be completely corrected. The major problem is delivering enough active enzyme into the duodenum. Steatorrhea could be abolished if 10 percent of the normal amount of lipase could be delivered to the duodenum at the proper time. This concentration of lipase cannot be achieved with the current preparations of pancreatic enzymes, even if the latter are given in large doses. The reason for these poor results may be that lipase is inactivated by gastric acid, that food empties from the stomach faster than do the pancreatic enzymes, and that batches of commercially available pancreatic extracts vary in enzyme activity.

For the usual patient, two or three enteric-coated capsules or eight conventional (non-enteric-coated) tablets of a potent enzyme preparation should be administered with meals. Some patients using conventional tablets require adjuvant therapy to improve enzyme replacement treatment. H_2 receptor antagonists, sodium bicarbonate, and proton pump inhibitors are effective adjuvants. Antacids containing calcium carbonate or magnesium hydroxide are not effective and may actually result in increased steatorrhea. Adjuvant therapy should not be given with enteric-coated microsphere preparations, because the resulting increase in gastric pH might cause these preparations to release their enzymes into the stomach rather than the small intestine. Several publications have reported colonic strictures in patients with cystic fibrosis receiving extraordinarily high doses of high-potency pancreatic enzyme preparations. Such lesions have not been reported in adults with chronic pancreatitis.

Supportive measures include diet restriction and pain medications. The diet should be moderate in fat (30 percent), high in protein (24 percent), and low in carbohydrate (40 percent). Restriction of long-chain triglyceride intake can help patients who do not respond satisfactorily to pancreatic enzyme therapy. Use of foods containing mainly medium-chain fatty acids, which do not require lipase for digestion, may be beneficial. Nonnarcotic analgesics should be emphasized. Patients taking narcotic drugs for pain relief often become addicted and continue to have pain.

Patients with severe exocrine pancreatic insufficiency secondary to alcohol who continue to drink have a high mortality rate (in one series, 50 percent of patients who were followed for 5 to 12 years died during this period) and significant morbidity (weight loss, lassitude, vitamin deficiency, and narcotic addiction). Chronic pancreatitis carries significant medical and social costs. A recent study found that pancreatitis led to retirement in 11 percent of patients with the disease, accounting for 45 percent of all retirements. In 87 percent of patients with chronic pancreatitis unable to maintain gainful employment, alcoholism was a contributing factor. Patients with chronic pancreatitis also use substantial medical resources. In 1987 in the United States, this diagnosis accounted for 122,000 recorded outpatient visits and 56,000 hospital admissions. Pain may abate if progressive severe exocrine insufficiency continues. Patients who abstain from alcohol and use vigorous replacement therapy for maldigestion-malabsorption do reasonably well.

HEREDITARY PANCREATITIS Hereditary pancreatitis is a rare disease that is similar to chronic pancreatitis except for an early age of onset and evidence of hereditary factors (involving an autosomal dominant gene with incomplete penetrance). These patients have recurring attacks of severe abdominal pain which may last from a few days to a few weeks. The serum amylase and lipase levels may be elevated during acute attacks but usually are normal. Patients frequently develop pancreatic calcification, diabetes mellitus, and steatorrhea, and, in addition, they have an increased incidence of pancreatic carcinoma. Such patients often require ductal decompression for pain relief. Abdominal complaints in relatives of patients with hereditary pancreatitis should raise the question of pancreatic disease.

PANCREATIC ENDOCRINE TUMORS

→ *Pancreatic endocrine tumors are summarized in Table 304-6 and are discussed in Chap. 95.*

OTHER CONDITIONS

ANNULAR PANCREAS When the ventral pancreatic anlage fails to migrate correctly to make contact with the dorsal anlage, the result may be a ring of pancreatic tissue encircling the duodenum. Such an annular pancreas may cause intestinal obstruction in the neonate or the adult. Symptoms of postprandial fullness, epigastric pain, nausea, and vomiting may be present for years before the diagnosis is entertained. The radiographic findings are symmetric dilation of the proximal duodenum with bulging of the recesses on either side of the annular band, effacement but not destruction of the duodenal mucosa, accentuation of the findings in the right anterior oblique position, and lack of change on repeated examinations. The differential diagnosis should include duodenal webs, tumors of the pancreas or duodenum, postbulbar peptic ulcer, regional enteritis, and adhesions. Patients with annular pancreas have an increased incidence of pancreatitis and peptic ulcer. Because of these and other potential complications, the treatment is surgical even if the condition has been present for years. Retrocolic duodenojejunostomy is the procedure of choice, although some surgeons advocate Billroth II gastrectomy, gastroenterostomy, and vagotomy.

PANCREAS DIVISUM Pancreas divisum occurs when the embryologic ventral and dorsal pancreatic anlagen fail to fuse, so that pancreatic drainage is accomplished mainly through the accessory papilla. Pancreas divisum is the most common congenital anatomic variant of the human pancreas. Current evidence indicates that this anomaly does not predispose to the development of pancreatitis in the great majority of patients who harbor it. However, the combination of pancreas divisum and a small accessory orifice could result in dorsal duct obstruction. The challenge is to identify this subset of patients with dorsal duct pathology. Cannulation of the dorsal duct by ERCP is not as easily done as is cannulation of the ventral duct. Patients with pancreatitis and pancreas divisum demonstrated by ERCP should be treated with conservative measures, including pancreatic enzyme therapy. In many of these patients, the pancreatitis is idiopathic and unrelated to the pancreas divisum and will respond well to pancreatic enzyme therapy. Endoscopic or surgical intervention is indicated only when the above methods fail. If marked dilation of the dorsal duct can be demonstrated, surgical ductal decompression should be performed. The appropriate therapy for patients without dilation of the dorsal duct is not yet defined. It should be stressed that the ERCP appearance of pancreas divisum—i.e., a small-caliber ventral duct with an arborizing pattern—may be mistaken as representing an obstructed main pancreatic duct secondary to a mass lesion.

MACROAMYLASEMIA In macroamylasemia, amylase circulates in the blood in a polymer form too large to be easily excreted by the kidney. Patients with this condition demonstrate an elevated serum amylase value, a low urinary amylase value, and a C_{am}/C_{cr} ratio of less than 1 percent. The presence of macroamylase can be documented by chromatography of the serum. The prevalence of macroamylasemia is 1.5 percent of the nonalcoholic general adult hospital population. Usually macroamylasemia is an incidental finding and is not related to disease of the pancreas or other organs. It is important

Table 304-6

Pancreatic Endocrine Tumors

Syndrome	Hormone(s) Produced	Primary Hormone Effects	Pathologic Features	Clinical Features
Zollinger-Ellison	Gastrin	Gastric acid hypersecretion with basal acid outputs usually >15 mmol/h (>15 mEq/h)	Delta cell islet tumors; 10% aberrant (duodenal); 60% malignant	Severe peptic ulcer disease often refractory to therapy; ectopic ulcers; diarrhea; multiple endocrine adenomas (parathyroid, pituitary, adrenal, thyroid)
Insulinoma	Insulin	Hypoglycemia with inappropriately increased serum insulin levels	Beta cell islet tumors; 80–90% benign	Hypoglycemic symptoms
Glucagonoma	Glucagon; pancreatic polypeptide	Hyperglucagonemia → glucose intolerance	Alpha cell islet tumors; 60% malignant	Slow-growing pancreatic tumor; hyperglycemia; bullous and ezcematoid dermatitis, weight loss; anemia; gastric and intestinal motor abnormalities
Somatostatinoma	Somatostatin; pancreatic polypeptide	Somatostatin inhibits insulin, gastrin, and pancreatic enzyme secretion; decreased bile flow	Delta cell islet tumor	Pancreatic tumor; diarrhea; steatorrhea; gallstones; diabetes mellitus; anemia
Pancreatic cholera	Vasoactive intestinal peptide ? Gastric inhibitory polypeptide ? Prostaglandin E ? Pancreatic peptide	Net secretion of salt and water by gut	? Delta cell tumor; >50% malignant	Pancreatic tumor with severe watery diarrhea; flushing; weight loss; hypokalemia; hypercalcemia; hypochlorhydria; hyperglycemia; inordinate fecal water and electrolyte losses
Carcinoid	Serotonin; prostaglandins	Altered gut motility; diarrhea	Enterochromaffin cells; non-beta-cell islet tumors	Carcinoid syndrome with flushing; wheezing; diarrhea; alcohol intolerance; hepatomegaly

to be aware of this fact, so that patients with macroamylasemia will not be needlessly evaluated and treated for pancreatic disease.

Macrolipasemia has now been documented in a few patients with cirrhosis or non-Hodgkin's lymphoma. In these patients, the pancreas appeared normal on ultrasound and CT examination. Lipase was shown to be complexed with immunoglobulin A. Thus, the possibility of *both* macroamylasemia and macrolipasemia should be considered in patients with elevated blood levels of these enzymes.

BIBLIOGRAPHY

Balthazar EJ et al: Acute pancreatitis: Value of CT in establishing prognosis. Radiology 174:331, 1990

Bozkurt T et al: Comparison of pancreatic morphology and exocrine functional impairment in patients with chronic pancreatitis. Gut 35:1132, 1994

Cavallini G et al: Gabexate for the prevention of pancreatic damage related to endoscopic retrograde cholangiopancreatography. N Engl J Med 335:919, 1996

Fan ST et al: Early treatment of acute biliary pancreatitis by endoscopic papillotomy. N Engl J Med 328:228, 1993

Fernandez del Castillo C et al: Acute pancreatitis. Lancet 342:475, 1993

Karimgani I et al: Prognostic factors in sterile pancreatic necrosis. Gastroenterology 103:1636, 1992

Lee SP et al: Biliary sludge as a cause of acute pancreatitis. N Engl J Med 326:589, 1992

Neoptolemos JP et al: Control trial of urgent endoscopic retrograde cholangiopancreatography and endoscopic sphincterotomy versus conservative treatment for acute pancreatitis due to gallstones. Lancet 2:979, 1988

Sainio V et al: Early antibiotic treatment in acute necrotizing pancreatitis. Lancet 346:663, 1995

Steer ML et al: Chronic pancreatitis. N Engl J Med 332:1482, 1995

Steinberg WM et al: Diagnostic assays in acute pancreatitis: A study of sensitivity and specificity. Ann Intern Med 102:576, 1985

———, Tenner S: Medical progress. Acute pancreatitis. N Engl J Med 330:1198, 1994

Whitcomb DC et al: Hereditary pancreatitis is caused by a mutation in the cationic trypsinogen gene. Nature Genetics 13:141, 1996

Wilson C et al: Prediction of outcome in acute pancreatitis: A comparative study of APACHE II, clinical assessment, and multiple screening systems. Br J Surg 77:1260, 1990

PART TWELVE

DISORDERS OF THE IMMUNE SYSTEM, CONNECTIVE TISSUE, AND JOINTS

SECTION 1
DISORDERS OF THE IMMUNE SYSTEM

305

Barton F. Haynes, Anthony S. Fauci

INTRODUCTION TO THE IMMUNE SYSTEM

Basic research in immunology has resulted in advances in a wide range of clinical disciplines, from allergy and rheumatology to neurology and cardiology. Monoclonal antibody technology has revolutionized the study of cell surface molecules of effector and regulatory immune cells and has provided specific reagents for essentially any target molecule. Advances in cell biology have resulted in the ability to expand and characterize isolated immune cell populations with specific functions in vitro. The ability to manipulate ("overexpress" or "knockout") genes in the living animal has created the opportunity to study the immune function of virtually any protein in vivo. The cloning and sequencing of genes for antigen receptors and their associated molecules on B cells and T cells, the delineation of the structures of major histocompatibility complex (MHC) class I and class II molecules (see Chap. 306), the identification of soluble mediators (cytokines) as cell-to-cell messengers in the immune system, and the elucidation of the molecular and biochemical mechanisms of signal transduction in immune competent cells have provided the information necessary to understand immune cell recognition and effector function. Thus, in recent years, breakthroughs in new technology have provided molecular explanations for specificity and diversity of the immune system, induction and maintenance of self-tolerance (self-antigen nonreactivity), and regulation of immune cell growth and differentiation.

The normal function of the immune system is essential for health, and dysfunction of the immune system leads to a wide diversity of diseases (Table 305-1). Deficiency of immune cell production or defective immune cell function can lead to a spectrum of immunodeficiency diseases (see Chap. 307). Overactivity of various components of the immune system leads to the development of allergic or autoimmune diseases. Leukemias and lymphomas are the result of malignant transformation in cells of the immune system (see Chaps. 112 and 113). With these new insights into immune system function have come new and specific modes of therapy for autoimmune, immunodeficiency, and malignant immune system diseases. The aim of this chapter is to provide the essentials of the cellular and molecular basis of immunity, with emphasis on those principles relevant to understanding at a basic level the protean clinical and laboratory manifestations of disordered immunity.

THE CD CLASSIFICATION OF HUMAN LYMPHOCYTE DIFFERENTIATION ANTIGENS The development of monoclonal antibody technology led to the discovery of a large number of new leukocyte surface molecules. In 1982, the First International Workshop on Leukocyte Differentiation Antigens was held to establish a nomenclature for cell surface molecules of human leukocytes. From this and subsequent leukocyte differentiation workshops has come the cluster of differentiation (CD) classification of leukocyte antigens (Table 305-2). The data presented in Table 305-2 establish a context to facilitate study of the extraordinarily complex series of events that transpire during normal and aberrant human immune system function.

CYTOKINES Cytokines are soluble proteins produced by a wide variety of hematopoietic and nonhematopoietic cell types. They are critical for normal immune system function, and their expression may be perturbed in disease states. They are involved in the regulation of the growth, development, and activation of immune system cells and the mediation of the inflammatory response. In general, cytokines are characterized by considerable redundancy in that different cytokines have similar functions. In addition, many cytokines are pleotropic in that they are capable of acting on many different cell types. This pleotropism results from the expression on multiple cell types of receptors for the same cytokine (see below), leading to the formation of "cytokine networks." The action of cytokines may be: (1) autocrine when the target cell is the same cell that secretes the cytokine, (2) paracrine when the target cell is nearby, and (3) endocrine when the cytokine is secreted into the circulation and acts distal to the source. A number of categorizations have been proposed for the grouping of cytokines according to functions. However, these are all imperfect because of the fact that a number of cytokines overlap these groupings. One empiric categorization divides the cytokines into the following three groups: (1) Immunoregulatory cytokines that are involved in the activation, growth, and differentiation of lymphocytes and monocytes, e.g., interleukin (IL)-2, IL-4, and transforming growth factor beta (TGFβ); (2) proinflammatory cytokines that are produced predominantly by mononuclear phagocytes in response to infectious agents, e.g., IL-1, tumor necrosis factor (TNF) alpha, and IL-6, and the chemokine family of inflammatory cytokines, within which are included IL-8, monocyte chemotactic protein (MCP)-1, MCP-2, MCP-3, macrophage inflammatory protein (MIP)-1α, MIP-1β, and regulation-upon-activation, normal T expressed and secreted (RANTES) (see also Chap. 62); and (3) cytokines that regulate immature leukocyte growth and differentiation, e.g., IL-3, IL-7, and granulocyte-macrophage colony stimulating factor (GM-CSF). In general, cytokines exert their effects by influencing gene activation that results in cellular activation, growth, differentiation, functional cell surface molecule expression, and cellular effector function. In this regard, cytokines can have dramatic effects on the regulation of immune responses and the pathogenesis of a variety of diseases. Indeed, T cells have been categorized on the basis of the pattern of cytokines that they secrete that results in either an allergic humoral immune response or a cell-mediated immune response (see below).

Cytokine receptors can be grouped into five general families based on similarities in their extracellular amino acid sequences and conserved structural domains (Fig. 305-1). The immunoglobulin (Ig) superfamily represents a large number of cell surface and secreted proteins. All members of the Ig superfamily must have at least one domain in their protein structure. The IL-1 receptors (type 1, type 2) are examples of cytokine receptors with extracellular Ig domains. The hallmark of the hematopoietic growth factor (type 1) receptor family is that the extracellular regions of each receptor contain two conserved motifs. One motif located at the N terminus is rich in cysteine residues. The other motif is located at the C terminus proximal to the transmembrane region and comprises five amino acid residues, tryptophan-serine-X-tryptophan-serine (WSXWS). Cytokine receptors expressing the WSXWS motif are also referred to as "type I family of cytokine receptors." This family can be further grouped on the basis of the number of receptor subunits they have and utilization of shared subunits. The shared common receptors often have a critical role in signal transduction. A number of cytokine receptors, i.e., IL-6, IL-11, IL-12, and leukemia inhibitory factor, are paired with gp130. There is also a common 150-kDa subunit shared by IL-3, IL-5, and GM-CSF receptors. The gamma chain (γ_c) of the IL-2 receptor is common to the IL-2, IL-4, IL-7, IL-9, and IL-15 receptors. Thus, the specific cytokine receptor is responsible for ligand-specific binding, while the subunits such as gp130, the 150-kDa subunit, and γ_c are important in

Table 305-1

Disorders of the Immune System

IMMUNODEFICIENCIES

- **Primary immunodeficiencies**
  - Combined immunodeficiencies
    - Severe combined immunodeficiency
      - X-linked
      - Autosomal recessive
    - Adenosine deaminase (ADA) deficiency
    - Purine nucleoside phosphorylase (PNP) deficiency
    - MHC class II deficiency
    - MHC class I deficiency (bare leukocyte syndrome)
    - Reticular dysgenesis
    - CD3γ or CD3ε deficiency
    - CD8 deficiency
  - Predominantly antibody deficiencies
    - X-linked agammaglobulinemia (Bruton)
    - Hyper-IgM syndrome
      - X-linked
      - Other
    - Ig heavy chain gene deletions
    - κ chain deficiency
    - IgA deficiency
    - Selective deficiency of IgG subclasses
    - Common variable immunodeficiency (CVID)
    - Antibody deficiency with normal Igs
    - Transient hypogammaglobulinemia of infancy
    - Secretory component deficiency
  - Other well-defined immunodeficiency syndromes
    - Wiskott-Aldrich syndrome
    - Ataxia-telangiectasia
    - DiGeorge anomaly
  - Syndromes associated with immunodeficiency
    - Chromosomal instability or defective repair
      - Bloom syndrome
      - Fanconi anaemia
      - ICF syndrome
      - Nijmegen breakage syndrome
      - Seckel syndrome
      - Xeroderma pigmentosa
    - Chromosomal defects
      - Down syndrome
      - Turner syndrome
      - Chromosome 18 rings and deletions
    - Skeletal abnormalities
      - Short-limbed skeletal dysplasia
      - Cartilage-hair hypoplasia
    - Immunodeficiency with generalized growth retardation
      - Schimke immunoosseous dysplasia
      - Immunodeficiency with absent thumbs
      - Dubowitz syndrome
      - Growth retardation, facial anomalies, and immunodeficiency
      - Progeria (Hutchinson-Gilford syndrome)
    - Immunodeficiency with dermatologic defects
      - Partial albinism
      - Dyskeratosis congenita
      - Netherton syndrome
      - Acrodermatitis enteropathica
      - Anhidrotic ectodermal dysplasia
      - Papillon-Lefèvre syndrome
    - Hereditary metabolic defects
      - Transcobalamin 2 deficiency
      - Methylmalonic acidaemia
      - Type I hereditary orotic aciduria
      - Biotin-dependent carboxylase deficiency
      - Mannosidosis
      - Glycogen storage disease, type 1b
      - Chédiak-Higashi syndrome
    - Hypercatabolism of immunoglobulin
      - Familial hypercatabolism
      - Intestinal lymphangiectasia
    - Other
      - Hyper-IgE syndrome
      - Chronic mucocutaneous candidiasis
      - Hereditary or congenital hypo- or asplenia
      - Ivermark syndrome
      - X-linked lymphoproliferative syndrome
- **Acquired immunodeficiencies**
  - Acquired immunodeficiency syndrome (AIDS)
  - Iatrogenic
  - Idiopathic CD4+ T lymphocytopenia

ALLERGIC DISEASES

- Generalized
  - Anaphylaxis
  - Serum sickness
  - Generalized drug reactions
  - Food allergy
  - Insect venom allergy
  - Mastocytosis
- Airways
  - Allergic rhinitis
  - Asthma
  - Hypersensitivity pneumonitis
- Skin
  - Urticaria
  - Angioedema
  - Eczema
  - Atopic dermatitis
  - Allergic contact dermatitis
  - Erythema multiforme and Stevens-Johnson syndrome
- Ocular allergy
  - Allergic conjunctivitis
  - Atopic keratoconjunctivitis
  - Venereal keratoconjunctivitis
  - Giant papillary conjunctivitis
  - Contact allergy

AUTOIMMUNITY

- **Organ specific**
  - Endocrine system
    - Thyroid gland
      - Hashimoto's thyroiditis
      - Graves' disease
      - Thyroiditis with hyperthyroidism
    - Type I autoimmune polyglandular syndrome
    - Type II autoimmune polyglandular syndrome
    - Insulin-dependent diabetes mellitus
    - Immune-mediated infertility
    - Autoimmune Addison's disease
  - Skin
    - Pemphigus vulgaris
    - Pemphigus foliaceus
    - Paraneoplastic pemphigus
    - Bullus pemphigoid
    - Dermatitis herpetiformis
    - Linear IgA disease
    - Epidermolysis bullosa acquisita
    - Autoimmune alopecia
    - Erythema nodosa
    - Pemphigoid gestationis
    - Cicatricial pemphigoid
    - Chronic bullous disease of childhood
  - Hematologic system
    - Autoimmune hemolytic anemia
    - Autoimmune thrombocytopenic purpura
      - Idiopathic
      - Drug-related
    - Autoimmune neutropenia
  - Neuromuscular system
    - Myasthenia gravis
    - Eaton-Lambert myasthenic syndrome
    - Stiff-man syndrome
    - Acute disseminated encephalomyelitis
    - Multiple sclerosis
    - Guillain-Barré syndrome
    - Chronic inflammatory demyelinating polyradiculoneuropathy
    - Multifocal motor neuropathy with conduction block
    - Chronic neuropathy with monoclonal gammopathy
  - Paraneoplastic neurologic disorders
    - Opsoclonus-myoclonus syndrome
    - Cerebellar degeneration
    - Encephalomyelitis
    - Retinopathy
  - Hepatobiliary system
    - Autoimmune chronic active hepatitis
    - Primary biliary sclerosis
    - Sclerosing cholangitis
  - Gastrointestinal tract
    - Gluten-sensitive enteropathy
    - Pernicious anemia
    - Inflammatory bowel disease
- **Organ nonspecific**
  - Connective tissue diseases
    - Systemic lupus erythematosus
    - Rheumatoid arthritis
    - Systemic sclerosis (scleroderma)
    - Ankylosing spondylitis
    - Reactive arthritides
    - Polymyositis/dermatomyositis
    - Sjögren's syndrome
    - Mixed connective tissue disease
    - Behçet's syndrome
    - Psoriasis
  - Vasculitic syndromes
    - Systemic necrotizing vasculitides
      - Classic polyarteritis nodosa
      - Allergic angiitis and granulomatosis (Churg-Strauss disease)
      - Polyangiitis overlap syndrome
    - Hypersensitivity vasculitis
    - Wegener's granulomatosis
    - Temporal arteritis
    - Takayasu's arteritis
    - Kawasaki's disease
    - Isolated vasculitis of the central nervous system
    - Thromboangiitis obliterans
    - Miscellaneous vasculitides
  - Sarcoidosis
  - Graft-versus-host disease
  - Cryopathies

(*continued*)

Table 305-1 *(continued)*

Disorders of the Immune System

NEOPLASMS

- T cell neoplasms
  - Adult T cell leukemia/lymphoma
  - Cutaneous T cell lymphoma
  - Non-Hodgkin's lymphoma
  - Acute lymphoblastic leukemia
  - Chronic lymphocytic leukemia (rare)
- B cell neoplasms
  - Chronic lymphocytic leukemia
  - Multiple myeloma
  - Burkitt's lymphoma
  - Hairy cell leukemia
  - Acute lymphoblastic leukemia
  - Non-Hodgkin's lymphoma
  - Waldenström's macroglobulinemia
  - Primary amyloidosis
  - Heavy chain diseases
    - Gamma (Franklin's disease)
    - Alpha (Seligmann's disease)
    - Mu
- Monocyte neoplasms
  - Acute monocytic leukemia
  - Hodgkin's disease
  - True histiocytic lymphoma
  - Histiocytosis X
    - Eosinophilic granuloma
    - Letterer-Siwe disease
    - Hand-Schüller-Christian disease
  - Malignant histiocytosis (histiocytic medullary reticulosis)
- Other
  - Large granular lymphocyte (LGL) leukemia

Table 305-2

CD Classification of Human Lymphocyte Surface Molecule

CD	Other Names	Molecular Mass, kDa	Chromosome Location	Molecular Structure	Tissue/Lineage	Function
CD1	T6	49	1q22-23	Ig superfamily associated with β2M	Cortical thymocytes, Langerhans cells, interdigitating cells	Antigen presentation to TCR$\gamma\delta$ cells
CD2	T11, LFA-3 receptor, E-rosette receptor	50	1p13	Ig superfamily	T lymphocytes	Binds LFA-3 (CD58) on RBC, monocytes, thymic epithelial cells; alternative pathway of T cell activation
CD3	T3, CD3 complex, Leu4	CD3γ—26 CD3δ—20 CD3ϵ—20 CD3ζ—16 CD3η—28	11q23 11q23 11q23 1q22 1q22	CD3γ,δ,ϵ Ig superfamily; CD3η, ζ; homologous to each other and with FcRϵ ζ chain comprise α family of signal transducers	CD3$\gamma,\delta,\epsilon,\zeta,\eta$, T lymphocytes, cytoplasmic CD3ϵ, NK cells	T cell–associated molecules; transduce signals from T cell receptors
CD4	T4, Leu3a	59	12pter-p12	Ig superfamily	T lymphocytes, monocytes, tissue macrophages, microglial cells, EBV-transformed B lymphocytes	Receptor for HIV env gp120; binds to MHC class II; associated with p56-lck tyrosine kinase
CD5	T1	67	11q13	Ig superfamily	T lymphocytes, B lymphocyte subset	Comitogenic for T lymphocytes; ligand for CD72
CD6	T12	100	?	Scavenger receptor type I superfamily	Subset of T and B lymphocytes	?
CD7	3A1, Leu9	40	17	Ig superfamily	T lymphocytes, NK cells; on subsets of T, B, and myeloid precursors	Comitogenic for T lymphocytes; Ca^{2+} inducible gene; signals T and NK cells through phosphoinositide-3-phosphate kinase
CD8	T8, Leu2a	CD8α—38 CD8β—38	2p12 2	CD8 α, β, Ig superfamily	T cell subset	Receptor for MHC class I; associated with p56-lck tyrosine kinase
CD9	p24	24	12p13	Type III transmembrane protein	Platelets, megakaryocytes, monocytes, pre B cells, activated T cells	Plays a signal transduction role in platelet activation and aggregation
CD10	J5, CALLA, neutral endopeptidase	100	3q21-27	Endopeptidase enzyme	B lymphoid progenitor cells	Peptide cleavage
CD11a	LFA-1α chain	180	16p13.1-11	α^L integrin	T, B, NK lymphocytes, monocytes	With β2 integrin, ligand for ICAM-1 (CD54), ICAM-2, and ICAM-3; mediates leukocyte adhesion and leukocyte-endothelial adherence

(continued)

CD Classification of Human Lymphocyte Surface Molecule

CD	Other Names	Molecular Mass, kDa	Chromosome Location	Molecular Structure	Tissue/Lineage	Function
CD11b	MAC-1, MO-1α chain, CR3	165	16p13.1-11	α^M integrin	NK cells, PMNs, monocytes	With β2 integrin, receptor for C3bi, fibrinogen, factor X
CD11c	gp150/95 α chain, CR4	150	16p13.1-11	α^X integrin	NK cells, PMNs, monocytes	With β2 integrin, mediates cell binding to C3bi
CD14	LeuM3, MO-2	55	5q31	Phosphoinositol-linked transmembrane glycoprotein	Monocytes	Endotoxin-binding protein
CD15	Sialyl Lewis X (sLe^x)	Carbohydrate	11q	Neu Acα 2–3 Gal β1–4 (Fucα1–3) GlcNac	Granulocytes; cryptic form of CD15 is on T cells [Cutaneous lymphocyte antigen (CLA)]	Ligand for ELAM-1 on endothelial cells; CLA mediates T cell homing to skin
CD16	Fc receptor for IgG (low affinity) FcRγIII	50–65	1q23	Ig superfamily, PI and TM forms	NK cells, PMN, macrophages	FcR for IgG
CD18	LFA-1β chain	95	21q22.3	β2 integrin	T, B, NK lymphocytes, monocytes	Ligand for ICAM-1, (CD54), ICAM-2, and ICAM-3; mediates leukocyte-endothelial interactions
CD19	B4	90	?	Ig superfamily	B lymphocytes	Regulates B cell activation
CD20	B1, Bp35	35–37	11q12-13.1	Calcium channel	B lymphocytes	Mediates B cell activation
CD21	B2	140	1q32	Complement regulatory protein family	B lymphocytes	C3d/EBV receptor, complement receptor 2 (CR2), ligand for CD23
CD22	Bgp135	135	19p13.1	Ig superfamily, homology with N-CAM, myelin-associated glycoprotein (MAG)	B lymphocytes	Comitogenic for B cell activation, interacts with CD45RO on T cells and CD75 on B cells
CD23	Low-affinity receptor for IgE FcϵRII	45–50	19	Homology with asialoglycoprotein receptor (lectin)	Activated B lymphocytes, subset of activated T lymphocytes, thymic epithelial cells, macrophages, eosinophils, platelets	FcϵRII, soluble CD23 activates immature T cells, ligand for CD21
CD25	TAC, IL-2 receptor α chain	55	10p15-14	Type I transmembrane protein	Activated T and B lymphocytes, monocytes	Low-affinity receptor for IL-2
CD26	Dipeptidylpeptidase IV, gp120	120	11pter-p11.2	Dipeptidylpeptidase IV enzyme	Activated T and B lymphocytes, monocytes	Serine exopeptidase; binds collagen
CD27		55	12p13	TNF receptor family	T cells	Involved in T cell activation; CD70 ligand
CD28	Tp44	44	2q33-34	Ig superfamily	T lymphocytes and activated B cells	Comitogenic for T lymphocytes, regulates T cell cytokine stability, Ligand for B7/BB1 (CD80) molecules
CD29	Integrin β1 chain; common β subset of VLA-1-6, GPIIa	130	10p11.2	β1 integrin	Panhematopoietic, many other cell types	Ligand for many extracellular matrix molecules; conserved cytoplasmic domain binds to cytoskeleton
CD30	Ki-1	105–120	1p36	TNF receptor family	Activated T and B cells	Involved in T cell activation
CD30 ligand		40	9q33	TNF receptor family	Activated T cells and monocytes	Activates or kills CD30+ cells
CD32	FcδRII, gp40	39, 48	1q23	Polymorphic transmembrane glycoproteins, two chains	Macrophages, PMNs, B cells, eosinophils	Fc receptor for aggregated IgG, ligation leads to cell activation

(*continued*)

Table 305-2 *(continued)*

CD Classification of Human Lymphocyte Surface Molecule

CD	Other Names	Molecular Mass, kDa	Chromosome Location	Molecular Structure	Tissue/Lineage	Function
CD34	MY10	105–120	1q32	Sialomucin with unique protein sequence	Pluripotent stem cells, other hematopoietic precursors, endothelial cells	Phosphorylated upon cell activation
CD35	CR1, C3b receptor	160–250	1q32	Type I transmembrane receptor	B cells, subset NK cells, PMNs, monocytes, RBC	Binds immune complexes; ? Binds complement-opsonized HIV
CD38	OKT10, T10	45	4	Single-chain glycoprotein	T and B cells, NK cells, and macrophages	Ligand for hyaluronate; modulates immune cell function via ADP-ribosylation of intracellular signal-transducing mediators
CD39	gp80	70–100	?	—	Activated B lymphocytes, T lymphocytes, and NK cells	Mediates homotypic adhesion of B cells
CD40	gp50	44–48	20	Homology with nerve growth factor receptor, fas(APO-1), and TNF receptor	B cells, follicular dendritic cells, macrophages	B cell activation, homotypic adhesion; binds to a TNF-like molecule, gp39, that is defective in X-linked hyper-IgM syndrome
CD40 ligand	gp39	39	Xq26	TNF receptor family	Activated CD4+ cells	Induces activation of CD40-expressing cells
CD43	Leukosialin, sialophorin, leukocyte sialoglycoprotein	95	16p11.2	Cell surface sialomucin	T, B, NK cells, monocytes	Involved in leukocyte activation, deficient in Wiskott-Aldrich syndrome, ligand for ICAM-1 (CD54)
CD44	Pgp-1, In(Lu)-related p80, Hermes, extracellular matrix receptor III	80–120	11p13	Cartilage link protein, core proteoglycan homology; multiple isoforms generated by alternative splicing	T, B, NK cells, monocytes, RBC	Transmembrane hyaluronate receptor, promotes leukocyte adhesion; comitogenic for T cells, mediates leukocyte-endothelial binding; promotes carcinoma metastasis
CD45	Leukocyte common antigen, T200	CD45RO—180 CD45RA—220 CD45RB—220, 205, 190	1q31-32 1q31-31 1q31-32	Multiple isoforms generated by alternative splicing	Leukocytes	Cytoplasmic domain is a tyrosine phosphatase, regulates lymphocyte activation, CD45RO in T cells is a ligand for CD22 on B cells
CD49a	VLA-1	210	5	α1 integrin, assembles with CD29 to form α1β1 integrin	Activated T cells, monocytes	Laminin and collagen receptor
CD49b	VLA-2α chain	170	5q23-31	α2 integrin, assembles with CD29, β1 integrin	Activated T cells, platelets	With β1 integrin (CD29), binds collagen types I, II, III, and IV
CD49c	VLA-3	125	17	α3 integrin, assembles with CD29, β1 integrin	B cells	Laminin, collagen, fibronectin receptor
CD49d	VLA-4α chain	150	2q31-32	α4 integrin, assembles with CD29, β1 integrin	T and B lymphocytes, monocytes	With β integrin (CD29), is the receptor for endothelial VCAM-1; mediates leukocyte-endothelial cell binding in Peyer's patches

(continued)

CD Classification of Human Lymphocyte Surface Molecule

CD	Other Names	Molecular Mass, kDa	Chromosome Location	Molecular Structure	Tissue/Lineage	Function
CD54	ICAM-1	40	19	Ig superfamily	Endothelial cells, activated lymphocytes	Ligand for LFA-1, rhinoviruses, falciparum malaria, CD43
CD55	Decay accelerating factor	70	1q32	Complement control protein superfamily	Hematopoietic and nonhematopoietic cells	Binds C3b, C3/C5 convertase
CD56	N-CAM, NKH-1	140	11q23-24	Ig superfamily, homology with N-CAM	NK cells, neuroectodermal cells	Mediates NK cell homotypic adhesion
CD57	HNK1, Leu7	110	?		NK cells, subset of T cells	?
CD58	LFA-3	40–65	1p13	Ig superfamily	Widespread, activated lymphocytes	Ligand for CD2
CD62E	ELAM; E-selectin; LECAM-2	140	1q12-qter	Selectin family; C-type lectin	Endothelium	Binds sialyl Lewis X; mediates neutrophil-endothelial interactions
CD62L	LAM-1, L-selectin, LECAM-1, Leu-8, MEL-14	75–80	1q23-25	Selectin family; C-type lectin	B, T, NK cells, monocytes	Binds CD34, GlyCAM, mediates leukocyte-endothelial interactions; leukocyte rolling
CD62P	P-selectin, PADGEM; LECAM-3	140	1q21-24	Selectin family; C-type lectin	Platelets, endothelium	Binds sialyl Lewis X; mediates platelet interaction with leukocytes and neutrophil-endothelial cell interactions
CD64	FcγRI, high-affinity receptor for IgG	72	1q	Ig superfamily	Monocytes, tissue macrophages	Binds monomeric IgG with high affinity, leads to cell activation
CD69	Activation inducer molecule, EA-1, gp34/28; Leu-23	28, 34	12p12.3-13.2	Homodimer; type II membrane protein related to NK cell activation protein family	Activated B, T, NK cells, monocytes	Ligand binding to CD69 triggers cytolytic activity of NK and TCR γδ T cells
CD70	Ki-24	75, 95, 170	19p13	Type II membrane protein	Activated T cells	CD27 ligand; involved in T cell activation
CD71	T9, transferrin receptor	95	3q26.2-qter	Heterodimer	Activated T and B lymphocytes, monocytes, proliferating cells of many types	Binds transferrin
CD72	Mouse Lyb2	39, 43	9p	Heterodimer	B cells	Ligand for CD5 molecule
CD73	Ecto-5′ nucleotidase L-VAP-2	69	6q14-21	Nucleotidase enzyme	Subsets of B and T lymphocytes	Regulates uptake of nucleotides; mediates binding of lymphocytes to endothelial cells
CD74	Invariant chain of MHC class II	33–43	5q31-33	Glycoprotein	MHC class II–positive cells	MHC class II–associated invariant chains prevents binding of endogenous peptide to class II; associates with CD44
CD79α, β	B cell receptor–associated molecules	α:32–33 β:37–39	?	Ig superfamily	B cells	Component of B cell antigen receptor involved in signal transduction
CD80	B7, BB1	60	3q13.3-21	Ig superfamily	Antigen-presenting cells, B cells, NK cells	Ligand for CTLA-4 and CD28; involved in co-stimulation of T cells

(*continued*)

Table 305-2 *(continued)*

CD Classification of Human Lymphocyte Surface Molecule

CD	Other Names	Molecular Mass, kDa	Chromosome Location	Molecular Structure	Tissue/Lineage	Function
CD81	TAPA-1	26	11p	Tetraspanning membrane protein	Lymphocytes	Associates with CD19 and CD21 to form B cell signal–transduction complex
CD83	HB15	43	6p23-21.3	Type I transmembrane protein	Activated B, T cells, bone marrow dendritic cells	Unknown
CD86	B7-2, FUN-1	80	3q13.3-21	Ig superfamily	Monocytes, activated B cells	Ligand for CD28 and CTLA-4
CD87	UPA-R	50–65	19q13.1-13.2	Glycoprotein	Granulocytes, monocytes-macrophages, activated T cells	Urokinase plasminogen activator receptor
CD89	FcαR	50–70	19q13.4	Ig superfamily	Leukocytes	Receptor for IgA
CD95	fas/APO-1	43	10q24.1	TNF receptor family	Wide variety of leukocytes, thymic epithelial cells	Binds fas ligand, induces programmed cell death (apoptosis)
CD98	4F2	80, 40	11q12-22	Glycoprotein heterodimer	Monocytes, activated T cells	Involved in T cell activation
CD99	E2, MIC2	32	Xp22.32-pter or Yp11.2-pter (pseudoautosomal)	Glycoprotein	T, B, NK cells, erythrocytes	Involved in T cell activation and adhesion
CD102	ICAM-2	55–65	17q23	Ig superfamily	Lymphocytes, monocytes, endothelial cells	Ligand for CD11a/CD18 (LFA-1)
CD115	M-CSF, c-fms	150	5q33.2-33.3	Ig superfamily, transmembrane tyrosine kinase receptor	Monocytes-macrophages	Receptor for M-CSF
CDw116	GM-CSFRα	70–85	Xp22.32; Yp11.3; pseudoautosomal	Hematopoietin receptor family	Granulocytes, endothelium	GM-CSF receptor α chain
CD117	SCFR, c-kit	145	4cen-q21	Ig superfamily	Hematopoietic progenitors	Tyrosine kinase that is receptor for stem cell factor (kit ligand)
CD119	IFN γR	90–100	6q23-24	Glycoprotein	Monocytes, B cells, endothelium	IFN γ receptor
CD120a,b	TNFRI(a) TNFRII(b)	55 75–85	12p13.2 1p36.3-36.2	TNF receptor family	Hematopoietic and nonhematopoietic cells	Binds both TNFα and TNFβ
CD121a	IL-1R type I	80	2q12	Ig superfamily	Thymocytes, T cells	Binds IL-1α and IL-1β
CD121b	IL-1R type II	60–70	2q12	Ig superfamily	Monocytes, B cells	Binds IL-1α and IL-1β
CD122	IL-2Rβ	75	2q12-22	Hematopoietin receptor family	NK cells, T and B cells	Binds IL-2
CD123	IL-3Rα	70	?	Hematopoietin receptor family	Stem cells, granulocytes, monocytes	Binds IL-3
CD124	Il-4R	130–150	16p12.1-11.2	Hematopoietin receptor family	T and B cells, hematopoietic precursors	Binds IL-4
CD125	IL-5R	55–60	?	Hematopoietin receptor family	Eosinophils, basophils	Binds IL-5
CD126	IL-6Rα	80	1	Hematopoietin receptor and Ig superfamilies	Activated B cells, granulocytes, monocytes	Binds IL-6
CD127	IL-7R	75	?	Hematopoietin receptor family	Lymphoid precursors, T cells, monocytes	Binds IL-7
CD128	IL-8R	58–67	2	Chemokine (rhodopsin) family	Neutrophils, basophils, T cell subset	Binds IL-8
CD130	IL-6Rβ, IL-11Rβ, OSMRβ, L1FRβ	130	?	Hematopoietin and Ig superfamilies	Activated B cells, monocytes, T cells, NK cells	Common β subunit of IL-6, IL-11, oncostatin M, and leukemia inhibitory factor receptors

NOTE: LFA, lymphocyte function-associated (glycoprotein); RBC, red blood cell; EBV, Epstein-Barr virus; ICAM, intercellular adhesion molecule; PMNs, polymorphonuclear leukocytes; ELAM, endothelial-leukocyte adhesion molecule; VCAM, vascular cell adhesion molecule; VLA, very late activation (antigen).

SOURCE: After Haynes and Denning; Janeway and Travers; and SF Schlossman et al (eds), *Leucocyte Typing V. White Cell Differentiation Antigens,* vols 1 and 2, Oxford, Oxford Univ Press, 1995, with permission.

signal transduction. The members of the interferon (IFN) (type II) receptor family include the receptors for IFN γ, and IFN α/β, which share a similar 210-amino-acid binding domain with conserved cysteine pairs at both the amino and carboxy termini. The receptors for the interferons consist of at least two distinct subunits. The members of the TNF (type III) receptor family share a common binding domain composed of repeated cysteine-rich regions. Members of this family include the p55 and p75 receptors for TNF (TNFR1 and TNFR2, respectively); CD40 antigen, which is an important B cell surface marker involved in isotype switching; fas/Apo-1, whose triggering induces apoptosis; CD27 and CD30, which are found on activated T cells and B cells; and nerve growth factor receptor. The common motif for the seven transmembrane helix family was originally found in receptors that are linked to GTP-binding proteins. This family includes receptors for chemokines, beta-adrenergic receptors, and retinal rhodopsin. It is important to note that two members of the chemokine receptor family, CXC chemokine receptor type 4 (CXCR4) and beta chemokine receptor type 5 (CCR5), have recently been found to serve as coreceptors during infection of CD4-expressing host cells for syncytium-inducing and non-syncytium-inducing HIV, respectively. Both cytokines and their receptors share similar structures and functions. For example, ligands for the TNF receptor family of receptors regulate and determine cell death (apoptosis) program activation and all ligate molecules of the same structural family. Similarly IL-3, IL-5, and GM-CSF are all produced by T helper (TH) 2 cells, and the receptors of these cytokines share common β chains. Thus, cytokines and their receptors may have diversified together during evolution.

Significant advances have been made in defining the signaling pathways through which cytokines exert their effects intracellularly. This is particularly true with regard to the diverse family of hematopoietin receptors. The Janus family of protein tyrosine kinases (JAK) is a critical element involved in signaling via the hematopoietin receptors. There are four known JAK kinases, JAK1, JAK2, JAK3, and Tyk2, which preferentially bind different receptor subunits. Cytokine binding to its receptor brings the subunits into apposition and allows a pair of JAKs to transphosphorylate and activate one another. The JAKs then phosphorylate the receptor on the tyrosine residues and allow signaling molecules to bind to the receptor, where these molecules in turn can become phosphorylated. These signaling molecules can bind the receptor because they have domains (SH2, or src homology 2 domains) that can bind phosphorylated tyrosine residues. There are a number of these important signaling molecules that bind the receptor, such as the adapter molecule SHC, which can couple the receptor to the activation of the mitogen-activated protein kinase pathway. In addition, a very important class of substrate of the JAKs is the signal transducers and activators of transcription (STAT) family of transcription factors. STATs have SH2 domains that enable them to bind to phosphorylated receptors, where they are then phosphorylated by the JAKs. It appears that different STATs have specificity for different receptor subunits. The STATs then dissociate from the receptor and translocate to the nucleus, bind to DNA motifs that they recognize, and regulate gene expression. The STATs preferentially bind DNA motifs that are slightly different from one another and thereby presumably control transcription of specific genes. The importance of this pathway is particularly relevant to lymphoid development. The receptors for IL-2, IL-4, IL-7, IL-9, and IL-15 all contain a common receptor subunit termed the *common γ subunit*, or γc. The gene for γc is on the X chromosome, and mutations of γc result in the disease X-linked severe combined immunodeficiency (SCID). Mutations of JAK3 itself also result in a disorder identical to X-SCID; however, since JAK3 is found on chromosome 19 and not on the X chromosome, JAK3 deficiency occurs in boys and girls (see Chap. 307). In this chapter the cytokines that affect various cell types are discussed in the context of each type of immune cell.

PHENOTYPE AND FUNCTION OF IMMUNE CELLS

The host defense system is divided into two major categories: immune and nonimmune. Immunity is characterized by an antigen-specific response to a foreign antigen or pathogen and generally takes several days or longer to materialize. A key feature of immunity is memory for the antigen such that subsequent exposure leads to more rapid and often a more vigorous response. Nonimmune host defense is not antigen-specific and is an immediate response system (beginning within minutes of an insult) without memory for the eliciting stimulus. This process is called inflammation. Neutrophils, eosinophils, basophils, natural killer (NK) cells, monocytes, and macrophages are the mediators of this immediate response system. They also play a role in the subsequent development of an immune response.

The dual limbs of the immune system consist of cellular and humoral immunity. The principal effector of cellular immunity is the thymus-derived (T) lymphocyte, and of humoral immunity is the bone marrow–derived or bursa-equivalent (B) lymphocyte. Both B and T lymphocytes derive from a common stem cell. Other key effector and regulator cells of the immune system are large granular lymphocytes (LGL), monocytes-macrophages, and dendritic/Langerhans cells (Fig. 305-2).

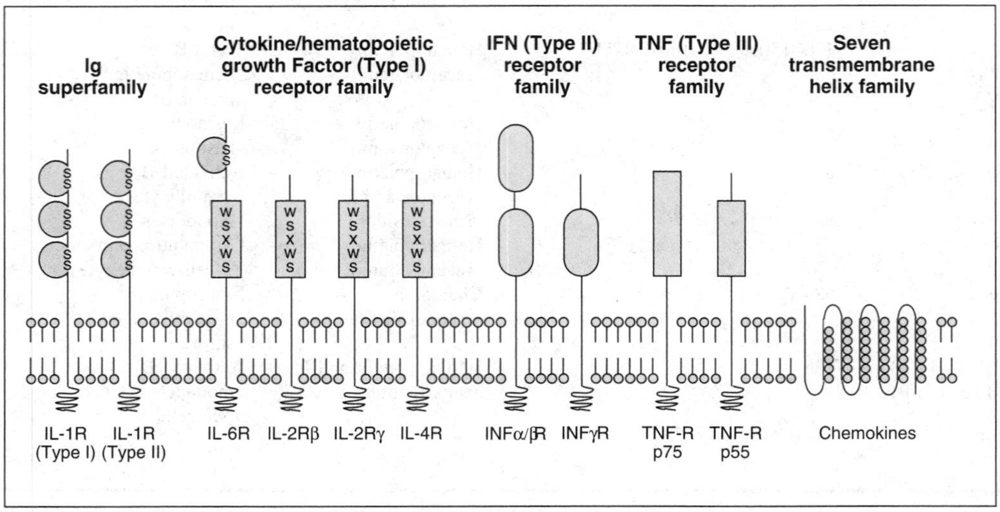

FIGURE 305-1 Cytokine family receptor members. Cytokine receptors have been segregated into several large families based on similarities in their extracellular amino acid sequences and conserved structural domains. There are five cytokine receptor family members. See text for details. *(After Abbas et al, with permission.)*

The proportion and distribution of immunocompetent cells in various tissues reflect cell traffic, homing patterns, and functional capabilities. Bone marrow is the major site of maturation of B cells, monocytes-macrophages, and granulocytes and contains pluripotent stem cells which, under the influence of various colony stimulating factors, are capable of giving rise to all hematopoietic cell types (Table 305-3). Granulocyte colony stimulating factor (G-CSF) stimulates the production of neutrophils and stem cell division; GM-CSF stimulates neutrophil, monocyte, eosinophil, and erythroid and megakaryocytoid cell growth and synergizes with IL-3, IL-11, and stem cell factor (SCF) for stem cell activation. Macrophage colony stimulating factor (M-CSF) drives monocyte differentiation; GM-CSF, IL-4, and TNFα drive dendritic/Langerhans cell differentiation; IL-3 drives neutrophil, monocyte, eosinophil, basophil, and erythroid and megakaryocytoid cell differentiation and promotes hematopoietic stem cell survival (see Chap. 105). T cell precursors also arise from hematopoietic stem cells but leave the yolk sac, fetal liver, or bone marrow while they are immature and home to the thymus for completion of maturation. Mature T lymphocytes, B lymphocytes, monocytes, and dendritic/Langerhans cells enter the circulation and home to peripheral lymphoid organs (lymph nodes, spleen) and the gut-associated lymphoid tissue (tonsil, Peyer's patches, and appendix) as well as the skin and mucous membranes and await activation by foreign antigen.

T CELLS T lymphocytes differ from other immune effector cell types in that the pool of effector T cells is established in the thymus early in life and is maintained throughout life by antigen-driven expansion of virgin peripheral T cells into "memory" T cells that reside primarily in peripheral lymphoid organs. Mature T lymphocytes constitute 70 to 80 percent of normal peripheral blood lymphocytes (only 2 percent of the total body lymphocytes are contained in peripheral blood), 90 percent of thoracic duct lymphocytes, 30 to 40 percent of lymph node cells, and 20 to 30 percent of spleen lymphoid cells. In lymph nodes, T cells occupy deep paracortical areas around B cell germinal centers, and in the spleen, they are located in periarteriolar areas of white pulp (see Chap. 61). T cells are the primary effectors of cell-mediated immunity, with subsets of T cells maturing into cytotoxic cells capable of lysis of virus-infected or foreign cells. T cells are also the primary regulatory cells of T and B lymphocyte and monocyte function by the production of cytokines and by direct cell contact. In addition, T cells regulate erythroid cell maturation in bone marrow.

Human T cells express cell surface proteins that mark stages of intrathymic T cell maturation or identify specific functional subpopulations of mature T cells. Many of these molecules mediate or participate in important T cell function (Table 305-2; Fig. 305-3).

A number of cytokines regulate the process of T cell proliferation and differentiation (Table 305-4). The earliest identifiable cells of T lineage are CD34+ pro-T cells (i.e., cells in which T cell receptor genes are neither rearranged nor expressed); they are found in fetal liver, yolk sac, and postnatal bone marrow. In the thymus, CD7lo+, CD34+ T cell precursors begin cytoplasmic (c) synthesis of components of the CD3 complex of T cell receptor–associated molecules (see Fig. 305-3). Within CD7+, CD2+, and cCD3+ T cell precursors, T cell receptor (TCR) gene rearrangement begins under the influence of IL-7 and eventuates in two T cell lineages, expressing either TCRαβ chains or TCRγδ chains (see Chap. 307). T cells expressing the TCRαβ

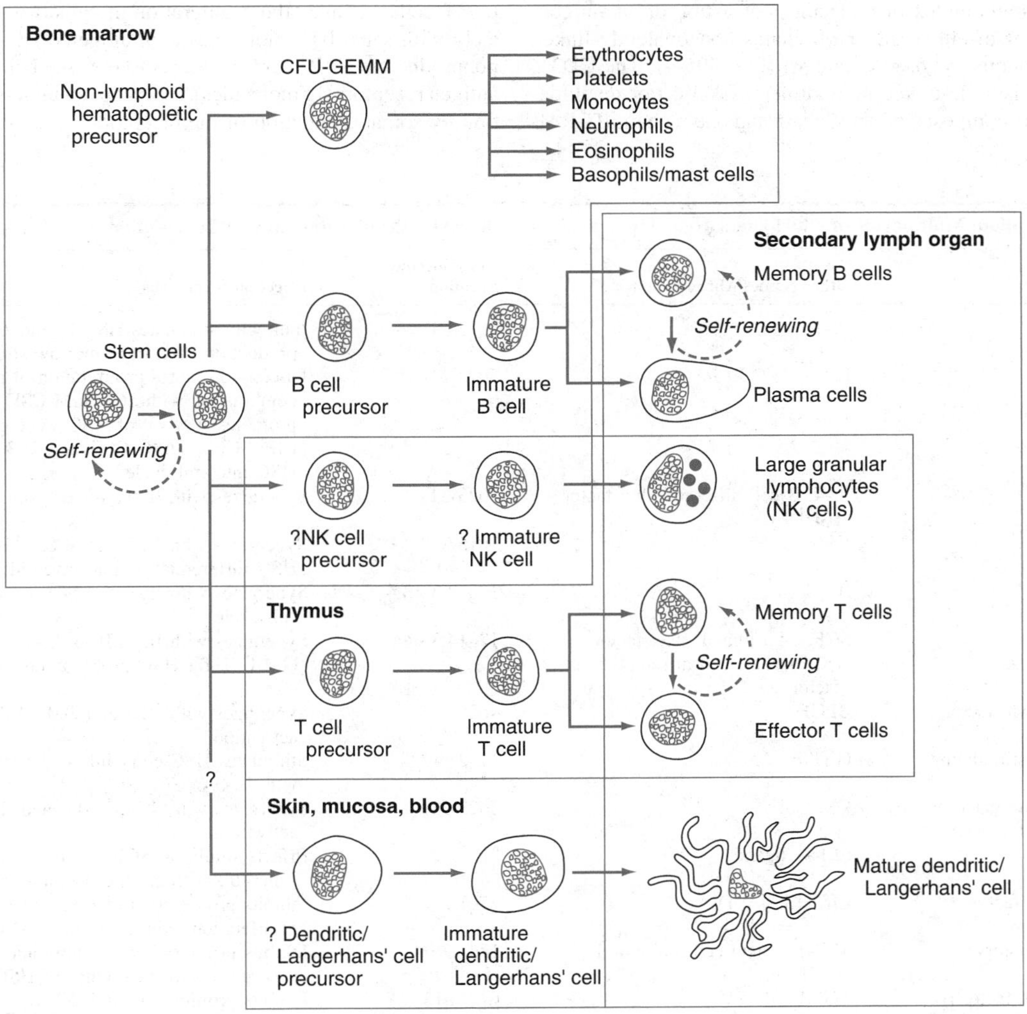

FIGURE 305-2 Hematopoietic stem cell differentiation in bone marrow, thymus, and secondary lymphoid organs. *(After Haynes and Denning, with permission.)*

chains comprise the majority of peripheral T cells in blood, lymph node, and spleen and terminally differentiate into either CD4+ or CD8+ cells. Cells expressing TCRγδ chains circulate as a minor population in blood; their functions, although not fully known, have been postulated as immune surveillance at epithelial surfaces and as cellular defenses against mycobacterial organisms and other intracellular bacteria. Immature cortical thymocytes express, in addition to CD1, both CD4 and CD8 (i.e., they are double positive); however, upon reaching functional maturity, T cell expression of CD1 ceases, and CD4 and CD8 are reciprocally expressed. Mature CD4+ TCRαβ+ cells induce B cell differentiation, induce CD8+ cytotoxic T cell proliferation, produce various cytokines, and regulate certain stages of erythropoiesis. A subset of CD4+ cells also functions as cytotoxic effector cells, recognizing foreign peptide antigen fragments that are physically associated with MHC class II molecules on antigen-presenting cells (APC). CD8+ TCRαβ+ cells function as cytotoxic effector T cells or as immunoregulatory cells that modulate B and T cell function; CD8+ T cells recognize foreign peptide antigen fragments associated with MHC class I molecules (see Chap. 306).

Elucidation of the stages of T cell development has found clinical relevance in the understanding of T cell malignancies. T cell acute lymphoblastic leukemia and lymphomas are malignancies of pro-T, pre-T, or immature T cells, while forms of cutaneous T cell lymphoma (mycosis fungoides, Sézary syndrome), peripheral T cell lymphomas, and the syndrome of adult T cell leukemia (associated with HTLV-I infection) share the phenotype of mature (usually CD4+) T cells.

Molecular Basis of T Cell Recognition of Antigen The T cell antigen receptor is a complex of molecules consisting of an antigen-binding heterodimer of either αβ or γδ chains noncovalently linked with five CD3 subunits (γ, δ, ϵ, ζ, and η) (Fig. 305-4). The CD3 ζ chains are either disulfide-linked homodimers (CD3-ζ_2) or disulfide-linked heterodimers composed of one ζ chain and one η chain. TCRαβ or TCRγδ molecules must be associated with CD3 molecules to be inserted into the T cell surface membrane, TCRα being paired with TCRβ and TCRγ being paired with TCRδ. Molecules of the CD3 complex mediate transduction of T cell activation signals via T cell receptors, while TCRα and β or γ and δ molecules combine to form the TCR antigen-binding site.

The α, β, γ, and δ T cell antigen receptor molecules have amino acid sequence homology and structural similarities to immunoglobulin heavy and light chains and are thus members, along with other important molecules of immune cells (e.g., MHC class I or II, CD2, CD4, CD8), of the *immunoglobulin gene superfamily* of molecules. The genes encoding the TCR molecules are encoded as clusters of gene segments that rearrange during the course of T cell maturation. This creates an efficient and compact mechanism for housing the diversity requirements of antigen receptor molecules. The TCRβ and δ chains contain four separate regions, namely, the V (variable), D (diversity), J (joining), and C (constant) regions, each encoded by a different gene segment; the TCRα and γ chains consist of V, J, and C regions. Thus, molecules of the T cell antigen receptor have constant (framework) and variable regions, and the gene segments encoding the α, β, γ, and δ chains of these molecules are selected in an antigen-independent fashion during T cell maturation in the thymus, culminating in synthesis of the completed molecule.

TCR diversity is created by the different V, (D), and J segments that are possible for each receptor chain, extensive junctional diversity due to large numbers of possible segments, "N-region diversification" due to the addition of nucleotides at the junction of rearranged gene segments, and the pairing of individual chains to form a TCR dimer. As T cells mature in the thymus, the repertoire of antigen-reactive T cells is modified by selection processes that eliminate many autoreactive T cells, enhance the proliferation of cells that function appropriately with self-MHC molecules and antigen, and allow T cells with nonproductive TCR rearrangements to die (see below). Unlike B cell antigen receptors (Ig molecules), TCRs do not undergo affinity maturation by somatic mutation of the receptor.

Table 305-3

Cytokines That Regulate Multipotent or Pluripotent Hematopoietic Stem Cell (HSC) Proliferation and Differentiation

Cytokine	Other Names/Abbreviation	Chromosome Location	Effect on Stem Cells
Interleukin 1α,β	IL-1αβ	2q13-21	Indirectly stimulates HSC by inducing IL-6 production from bone marrow stromal cells
Interleukin 3	IL-3	5q23-31	Directly promotes proliferation of progenitors in combination with SCF, GM-CSF, or M-CSF; promotes survival of HSC; synergizes with IL-11, LIF, SCF, IL-6, G-CSF, and flt-3 ligand for entry of HSC into cell cycle
Interleukin 4	IL-4, B cell differentiating factor (BCDF)	5q23-31	Synergizes with IL-11 for entry of HSC into cell cycle
Interleukin 6	IL-6	7p15	Synergizes with IL-3, GM-CSF, G-CSF, or SCF for HSC differentiation into myeloid lineages
Interleukin 11	IL-11	19q13.3-13.4	Synergizes with IL-3 and SCF for entry of HSC into cell cycle
Stem cell factor	SCF, c-kit ligand, steel factor (SLF), mast cell differentiating factor	12q14.3-qter	Synergizes with IL-3, IL-6, IL-11, G-CSF, and GM-CSF for HSC proliferation
Basic fibroblast growth factor	BFGF	4q25	Synergizes with IL-3 and GM-CSF for HSC activation
Granulocyte colony stimulating factor	G-CSF	17q21	Stimulates HSC entry into cell cycle and synergizes with IL-3 or SCF
Granulocyte/monocyte-macrophage colony stimulating factor	GM-CSF	5q23-31	Synergizes with SCF, IL-11, and IL-3 for HSC activation
Flt-3 ligand	FLK-2 ligand	?	Effects similar to SCF but, in contrast, does not synergize with erythropoietin (EPO)
Leukemia inhibitory factor	LIf, HILDA, DIA	22q12	Inhibits proliferation of HSC alone but enhances proliferation induced by IL-3, M-CSF, and SCF
Macrophage inflammatory protein 1α	MIP-1α, stem cell inhibitor 1 (SCI-1)	17q	Inhibits proliferation of embryonic stem cells but synergizes with SCF entry of HSC into cell cycle
Transforming growth factor β	TGFβ	β_1:19q13 β_2:1q41	Inhibits proliferation of HSC

SOURCE: After Haynes and Denning, with permission.

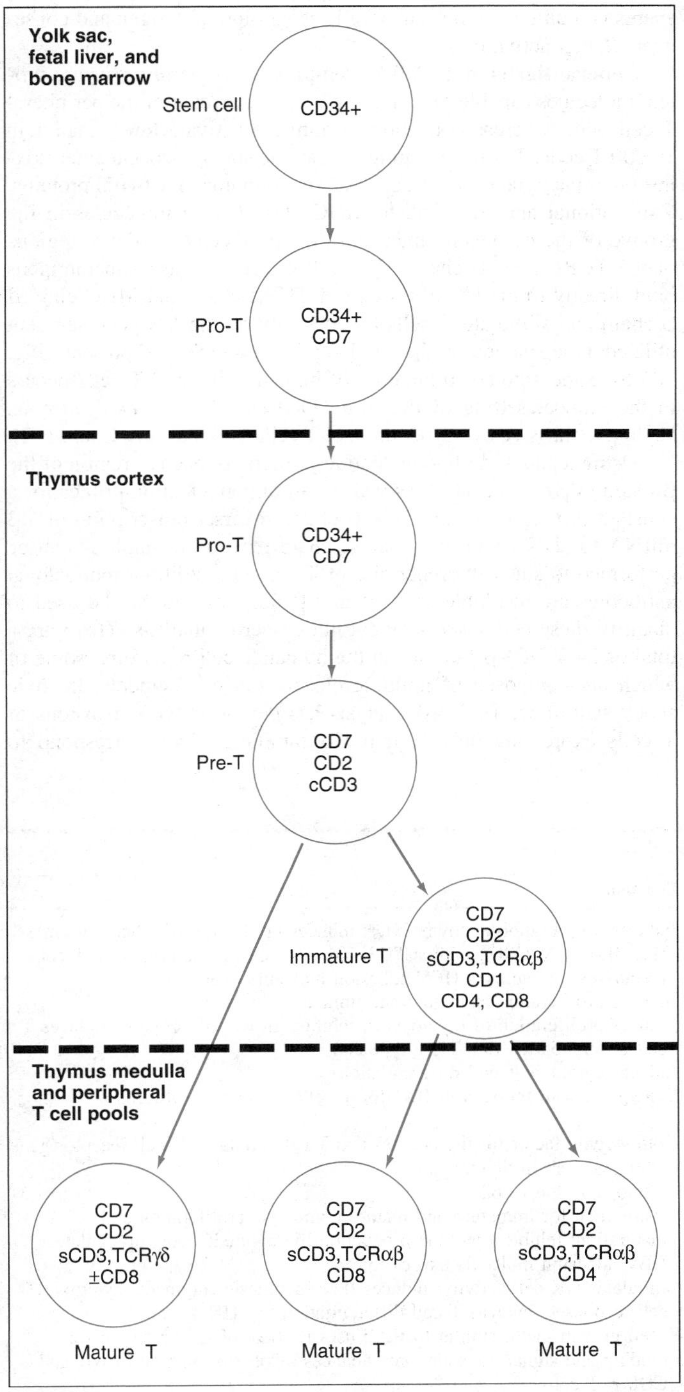

FIGURE 305-3 Human T cell maturation. sCD3, surface CD3 expression; cCD3, cytoplasmic CD3 expression.

T cells do not recognize native protein or carbohydrate antigens. Instead, T cells recognize only short (approximately 9 to 13 amino acids) peptide fragments derived from protein antigens taken up or produced in APC. Foreign antigens (such as mycobacteria pathogens) may be taken up by endocytosis into acidified intracellar vesicles and degraded into small peptides that associate with MHC class II molecules (exogenous antigen-presentation pathway). Other foreign antigens arise endogenously in the cytosol (such as from replicating viruses) and are broken down into small peptides that associate with MHC class I molecules (endogenous antigen-presenting pathway). Thus, APC proteolytically degrade foreign proteins and display peptide fragments embedded in the MHC class I or II antigen-recognition site on the MHC molecule surface (Fig. 305-5), where foreign peptide fragments are available to bind to TCRαβ or TCRγδ chains of reactive T cells. CD4 molecules act as an adhesive and, by direct binding to MHC class II (DR, DQ, or DP) molecules, stabilize the interaction of TCR with peptide antigen (see Fig. 305-4). Similarly, CD8 molecules also act as adhesives to stabilize the TCR-antigen interaction by direct CD8 molecule binding to MHC class I (A, B, or C) molecules.

Antigens that arise in the cytosol and are processed via the endogenous antigen-presentation pathway are cleaved into small peptides by a 28-subunit complex of proteases called the *proteasome*. From the proteasome, antigen peptide fragments are transported from the cytosol into the lumen of the endoplasmic reticulum by a heterodimeric complex termed *transporters associated with antigen processing*, or TAP proteins. There, MHC class I molecules in the endoplasmic reticulum membrane physically associate with processed cytosolic peptides. Following peptide association with class I molecules, peptide–class I complexes are exported to the Golgi apparatus, and then to the cell surface, for recognition by CD8+ T cells.

Antigens that are taken up from the extracellular space via endocytosis into intracellular acidified vesicles are degraded by vesicle proteases into peptide fragments. Intracellular vesicles containing MHC class II molecules fuse with peptide-containing vesicles, thus allowing peptide fragments to physically bind to MHC class II molecules. Peptide–MHC class II complexes are then transported to the cell surface for recognition by CD4+ T cells.

Whereas it is generally agreed that the TCRαβ receptor recognizes peptide antigens in MHC class I or class II molecules, recent data suggest that lipids in the cell wall of intracellular bacteria such as mycobacteria can be presented to TCRγδ T cells in the context of MHC-related CD1 molecules.

Just as foreign antigens are degraded and their peptide fragments presented in the context of MHC class I or class II molecules on APC, endogenous self-proteins are also degraded and self-peptide fragments are presented to T cells in the context of MHC class I or class II molecules on APC. In peripheral lymphoid organs, T cells are present that are capable of recognizing self-protein fragments but normally are *anergic*, i.e., nonresponsive to self-antigenic stimulation.

The immune repertoire of mature T cells is largely determined within the thymus during fetal and early postnatal development. In the thymus, the recognition of self-peptides on thymic epithelial cells and thymic macrophages and dendritic cells is thought to play an important role in shaping the T cell repertoire to recognize foreign antigen (*positive selection*) and in eliminating highly autoreactive T cells (*negative selection*). As immature cortical thymocytes begin to express surface TCR, autoreactive thymocytes are destroyed (negative selection), thymocytes with TCR capable of interacting with foreign antigen peptides in the context of self–MHC antigens are activated and develop to maturity (positive selection), and thymocytes with TCR that are incapable of binding to self–MHC antigens die of attrition (*no selection*). Mature thymocytes that are positively selected are either CD4+ helper T cells or MHC class II–restricted cytotoxic (killer) T cells, or they are CD8+ T cells destined to become MHC class I–restricted cytotoxic T cells. For T cells to be *MHC class I–* or *class II–restricted* means that T cells recognize antigen peptide fragments as immunogenic only when they are presented in the antigen-recognition site of a class I or class II MHC molecule, respectively.

Once engagement of mature T cell TCR by foreign peptide occurs in the context of self–MHC class I or class II molecules (see Fig. 305-4), binding of non-antigen-specific adhesion ligand pairs such as CD54-CD11/CD18 and -CD58/CD2 stabilizes MHC peptide–TCR binding and the expression of these adhesion molecules is upregulated (see Fig. 305-4).

Once TCR-MHC binding is stabilized, activation signals are transmitted through the cell to the nucleus that lead to the expression of gene products that are important in mediating the wide diversity of T cell functions. The TCR does not have intrinsic signaling activity but is linked to a variety of signaling pathways via tyrosine-based activation motifs expressed on the various CD3 chains that bind to enzymes that mediate signal transduction. Each of the pathways results in the activation of particular transcription factors that control the expression of cytokine and cytokine receptor genes. Thus, antigen-MHC binding to the TCR induces the activation of the src family kinases, fyn and lck (lck is associated with CD4 or CD8 co-stimulatory molecules); phosphorylation of CD3ζ chain; activation of the related tyrosine kinases ZAP-70 and syk; and downstream activation of the calcium-dependent calcineurin pathway, the ras pathway, and the protein kinase pathway. Each of these pathways leads to activation of specific families of transcription factors (including NF-AT, fos and jun, and rel/NF-κB) that form heteromultimers capable of inducing expression of IL-2, IL-2 receptor, IL-4, TNF, and other T cell mediators. The src family kinases require dephosphorylation of an inactivation site by CD45 phosphatase before they can be phosphorylated on an activation site. Furthermore, the activity through the receptor is downregulated by the csk kinase, which inactivates the src family kinases.

In addition to the signals delivered to the T cell from the TCR and CD4 and CD8 molecules, other co-stimulatory receptors [including CD2 activated by CD58, and CD28 activated by CD80 (B7/BB1)] also deliver important signals that affect the function of the T cell. The CD28 signal transduction pathway appears particularly important. CD28 signals through phosphoinositide-3-phosphate kinase; its downstream effects are not completely clear. However, if signal transduction through CD28 is blocked, the T cell becomes inactivated or anergic rather than activated. Thus, a concert of molecular and biochemical events is required for normal T cell recognition of antigen and consequent T cell activation.

Superantigens in T Cell Development *Superantigens* are protein molecules capable of activating up to 20 percent of the peripheral T cell pool, whereas conventional antigens activate fewer than 1 in 10,000 T cells. T cell superantigens include staphylococcal enterotoxins, other bacterial products, and certain nonhuman retroviral proteins. Conventional antigens bind to MHC class I or II molecules in the groove of the αβ heterodimer and bind to T cells via the V regions of the TCRα and -β chains (Fig. 305-5). In contrast, superantigens bind directly to the lateral portion of TCRβ chain and MHC class II β chain and stimulate T cells based solely on the Vβ gene segment utilized independent of the D, J, and Vα sequences present (Fig. 305-6). Superantigen stimulation of human peripheral T cells occurs in the clinical setting of the *staphylococcal toxic shock syndrome*, leading to massive overproduction of T cell cytokines (see Chap. 142).

Using a panel of oligonucleotide primers for each V region of the β chain (Vβ) of the TCR, as well as an oligonucleotide primer for a constant (C) region of the TCR β chain, reverse transcription of Vβ mRNA to cDNA with polymerase chain reaction technology can be performed to study the repertoire of T cells. In addition, monoclonal antibodies are available for certain Vβ families and can be used to quantify these cell subsets by cytofluorometric analysis. There are a total of 24 TCR Vβ families in the human T cell repertoire, some of which are composed of multiple closely related segments. In toxic shock syndrome, TCR Vβ analysis has demonstrated expansions of T cells expressing only certain Vβ families, which correspond to

Table 305-4

Roles of Cytokines in T Cell Proliferation and Differentiation

Cytokine	Source	Function
IL-1α,β	Macrophages, E cells, fibroblasts, endothelial cells, dendritic cells	Induces proliferation of thymocytes; induces production of other cytokines (i.e., IL-6, GM-CSF); with sCD23, induces TCRαβ maturation in T cell precursors; upregulates HEV adhesion molecule expression
IL-2	Activated T cells	Induces proliferation of mature and immature thymocytes
IL-4	T cells	Induces proliferation of thymocytes; inhibits growth of TE cells; induces T cell differentiation to a TH-2 type cell
IL-5	Activated T cells	Induces cytotoxic T cell differentiation
IL-6	Activated T and B cells, macrophages, fibroblasts, TE cells, endothelial cells	Synergizes with mitogen or IL-1 for T cell/thymocyte proliferation
IL-7	Fibroblasts, BM stromal cell line	Comitogenic factor for thymocytes and T cells; induces T cell receptor gene rearrangement in thymocytes
IL-8	Monocytes-macrophages	Chemotactic for T cells
IL-10	Fetal and postnatal thymocytes, B cells	Costimulant for immature and mature thymocyte proliferation and maturation; inhibits cytokine production by mature T cells; upregulates HEV adhesion molecule expression
IL-12	B cells, macrophages	Stimulates NK cell activity; induces IFNγ synthesis; augments cytotoxic T cell responses; induces T cell differentiation to TH-1 type cell
IL-15	Activated monocytes-macrophages; wide variety of tissues; not T cells	T cell growth factor similar to IL-2; uses β chain of IL-2 receptor for binding and signal transduction; enhances cytotoxic function of NK and CD8+ T cells
Soluble CD23 (FcεRII)	TE cells, B cells	With IL-1, induces TCRαβ maturation in T cell precursors
GM-CSF	Activated T cells, fibroblasts, endothelial cells, T cells	Promotes growth of early T cell leukemias; promotes proliferation of immature thymocytes
G-CSF	TE cells, macrophages, fibroblasts	?Mitogenic for immature thymocytes
M-CSF	TE cells, monocytes, fibroblasts, endothelial cells	Supports differentiation of progenitors committed to the monocyte-macrophage lineages; ?mitogenic for immature thymocytes
LIF	TE cells, activated cells	?Prevents multilineage differentiation of intrathymic stem cells prior to signal to become T cell precursors
IFNγ	Activated T cells, thymocytes	Upregulates expression of TE, fibroblast, and macrophage CD54 (ICAM-1) and MHC class II; antiproliferative effect on thymocytes via adenylate cyclase pathway; induced HEV adhesion molecule expression
TNFα	Macrophages, activated T and B cells, thymocytes	IL-1–like effects
TGFα	Activated macrophages, TE cells	Regulates production of other cytokines (IL-1 and IL-6) by TE cells; drives TE cell proliferation and/or differentiation via EGF receptor
TGFβ	?TE cells, T cells	Regulates expression of several oncogenes; suppresses lymphocyte responses to other cytokines; ?inhibits TE cell proliferation
EGF	?Monocytes-macrophages, ?fibroblasts, ?TE cells	Drives TE and other epithelial cell proliferation

NOTE: Unless otherwise stated, effect reported or postulated is in humans, TE; thymic epithelial; BM, bone marrow; EGF, epidermal growth factor; LIF, leukemia inhibitory factor; IFNγ, interferon γ; TNF, tumor necrosis factor; TGF, transforming growth factor; HEV, high endothelial venule; FcεRII, Fc receptor for IgE type II; IL, interleukin.

SOURCE: After BF Haynes et al, Semin Immunol 2:67, 1990.

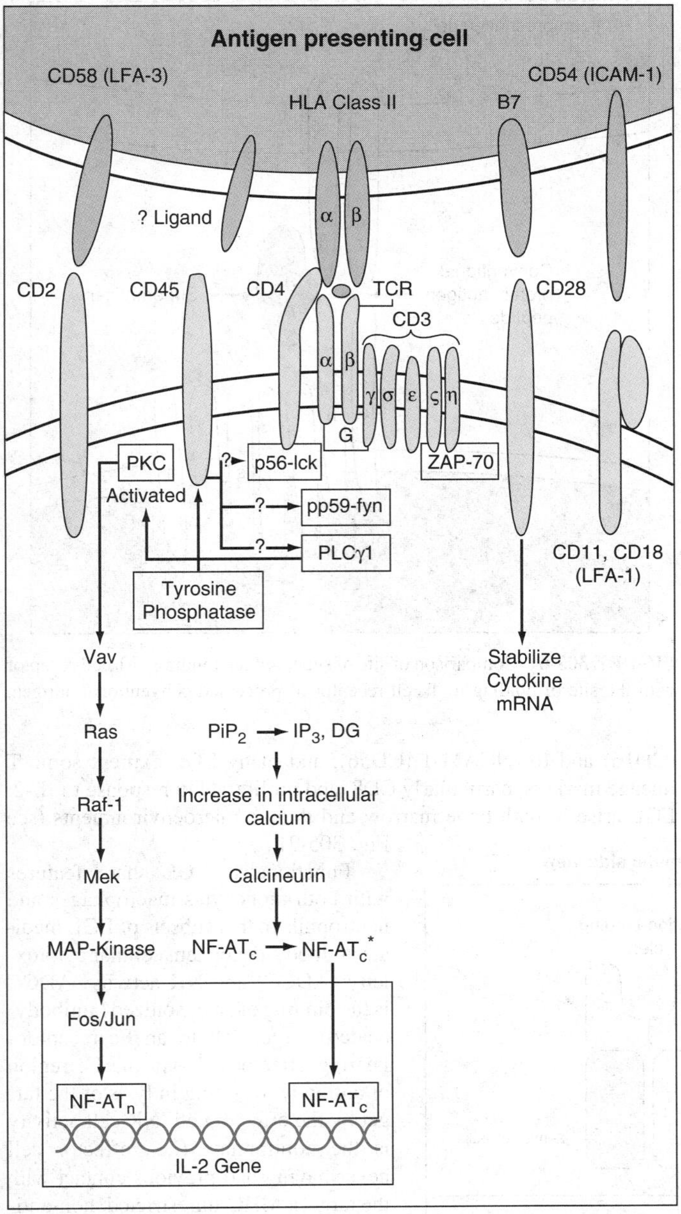

FIGURE 305-4 Molecules involved in human T cell recognition of antigen and in human T cell activation. The black circle at the tip of the αβ chains of MHC class II molecules represents a peptide fragment of "processed" protein antigen. See text for details of the activation and signal transduction process. The asterisk on $NF\text{-}AT_c$ represents the activated form of the molecule. *(After Robey and Allison; and Weiss and Littman, with permission.)*

those Vβ families capable of binding to (and being activated by) the staphylococcal enterotoxin superantigen of *Staphylococcus aureus*. The demonstration of selective expansions of certain Vβ subsets in diseases such as rheumatoid arthritis (see Chap. 313) and Kawasaki disease (see Chap. 319) has led to suggestions that various microbes might be the inducing stimuli of these diseases; however, the role of superantigens in such diseases remains speculative.

B CELLS Mature B cells comprise 10 to 15 percent of human peripheral blood lymphocytes, 50 percent of splenic lymphocytes, and approximately 10 percent of bone marrow lymphocytes. B cells express on their surface intramembrane immunoglobulin (Ig) molecules that function as B cell antigen receptors in a complex of Ig-associated α and β signaling molecules with intracellular signaling events similar to those in T cells (Fig. 305-7). Unlike T cells, which recognize only processed peptide fragments of conventional antigens embedded in the notches of MHC class I and class II antigens of APC, B cells are capable of recognizing and proliferating to whole and unprocessed native antigens via antigen binding to B cell surface Ig (sIg) receptors. B cells also express surface receptors for the Fc region of IgG molecules (CD32) as well as receptors for activated complement components (C3d or CD21, C3b or CD35). The primary function of B cells is to produce antibodies. B cells also serve as APC and are highly efficient at antigen processing. Their antigen-presenting function is enhanced by a variety of cytokines. Mature B cells are derived from bone marrow precursor cells that arise continuously throughout life (see Fig. 305-2).

B lymphocyte development can be separated into antigen-independent and antigen-dependent phases (see Chap. 307). Antigen-independent B cell development occurs in primary lymphoid organs, including fetal liver and bone marrow, and includes all stages of B cell maturation up to the sIg+ mature B cell. Antigen-dependent B cell maturation is driven by the interaction of antigen with B cell sIg, leading to memory B cell induction, Ig class switching, and plasma cell formation. Antigen-dependent stages of B cell maturation occur in secondary lymphoid organs, including lymph node, spleen, and gut Peyer's patches. In contrast to the T cell repertoire that is for the most part generated intrathymically before contact with foreign antigen, the repertoire of B cells expressing diverse antigen-reactive sites is modified by further alteration of Ig genes after stimulation by antigen—a process called *somatic mutation*—which occurs in lymph node germinal centers.

During B cell development, diversity of the antigen-binding variable region of Ig is generated by an ordered set of Ig gene rearrangements. Heavy chain rearrangements precede those for light chains. For the heavy chain, there is first a rearrangement of D segments to J segments, followed by a second rearrangement between a V gene segment and the newly formed D-J sequence; the C segment is aligned to the V-D-J complex to yield a functional Ig heavy chain gene (V-D-J-C). During later stages, a functional κ or λ light chain gene is generated by rearrangement of a V segment to a J segment, ultimately yielding an intact Ig molecule composed of heavy and light chains (see Chaps. 114 and 307).

The process of Ig gene rearrangement is regulated to result in a single antibody specificity produced by each B cell with each Ig molecule comprising one type of heavy chain and one type of light chain. Although each B cell contains two copies of Ig light and heavy chain genes, only one gene of each type in each B cell is productively rearranged and expressed, a process termed *allelic exclusion*.

There are approximately 300 V_κ genes and 5 J_κ genes, resulting in the pairing of V_κ and J_κ genes to create 1500 different light chain combinations. The number of distinct κ light chains that can be generated is increased by somatic mutations within the V_κ and J_κ genes, thus creating large numbers of possible specificities from a limited amount of germ-line genetic information. As noted above, in heavy chain Ig gene rearrangement, the VH domain is created by the joining of three types of germ-line genes called V_H, D_H, and J_H, thus allowing for even greater diversity in the variable region of heavy chains than for light chains (see Chap. 307).

The most immature B cell precursors (pro-B cells) express surface CD10 and CD34, lack B lineage–specific antigens CD19 and CD22, and also lack cytoplasmic Ig (cIg) and surface sIg (Fig. 305-8). The next stage in B cell development, the pre-B cell I, is marked by the acquisition of CD19 and CD22 B cell antigens. Ig genes undergo rearrangement in pre-pre-B cells, but Ig heavy chain protein is not expressed. The hallmark of the next maturation stage, the pre-B cell II, is expression of cμ heavy chain in association with expression of CD73 and CD21 surface proteins. Immature B cells have rearranged Ig light chain genes and express sIgM. As immature B cells develop into mature B cells, sIgD is expressed as well as sIgM and CD23. At this point, B lineage development in bone marrow is complete, and B cells exit into the peripheral circulation and migrate to secondary lymphoid organs.

A number of cytokines synergize to drive sequential stages of B cell maturation (Table 305-5). Bone marrow stromal cell– and T cell–

derived IL-3 and IL-7 drive the earliest stages of B cell differentiation. Low-molecular-weight B cell growth factor binds to high-affinity receptors expressed on all B cell precursors except pro-B cells and also triggers B cell differentiation. IL-1, -2, -4, -5, and -6 synergize to drive mature B cells to proliferate and differentiate into Ig-secreting cells. TGFβ can be an antagonistic cytokine for B cells in that it can block the synthesis of κ light chains.

Evidence exists that the murine B cell compartment contains three B cell subsets, each derived from a distinct cell lineage. B-1a B cells are produced early in fetal development, express the pan–T cell marker CD5, and produce high levels of autoantibodies. B-1b B cells have similar properties to B-1a cells except that B-1b cells are CD5 negative. Both B-1a and B-1b B cells are capable of self-replenishment in the adult and are found in the peritoneum of adult animals. In contrast, B-2 B cells are conventional B cells that are continuously generated in adult bone marrow, produce low levels of autoantibodies, and are the predominant B cell type in lymph nodes, Peyer's patches, and peripheral blood. B-1a, B-1b, and B-2 B cells each display unique V_HDJ_H repertoires that are formed at distinct stages of fetal or adult development, confirming their separate lineages. Some evidence suggests that similar B cells are present in humans, with elevated levels of CD5+ B cells found in autoimmune diseases such as rheumatoid arthritis (see Chap. 313).

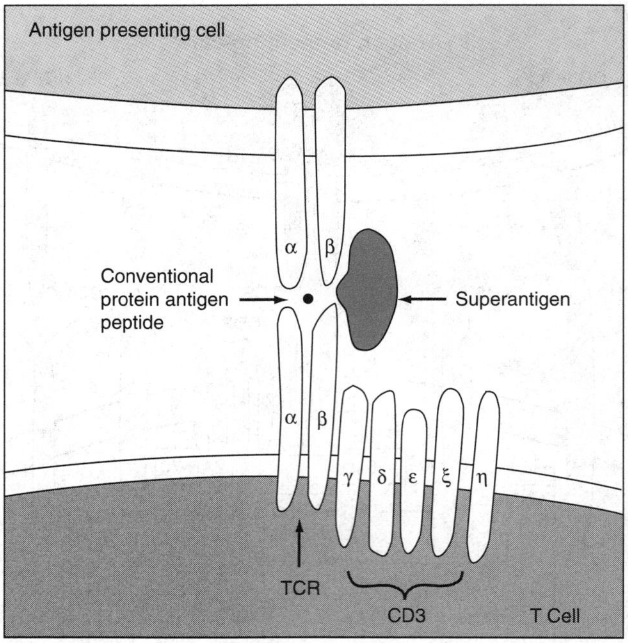

FIGURE 305-6 Comparison of site of superantigen binding to T cell receptor with the site of binding to T cell receptor of processed conventional antigen.

LARGE GRANULAR LYMPHOCYTES LGL constitute approximately 5 to 10 percent of peripheral blood lymphocytes. LGL are nonadherent, nonphagocytic cells with large azurophilic cytoplasmic granules. LGL express surface receptors for the Fc portion of IgG (CD16) and for NCAM-1 (CD56), and many LGL express some T lineage markers, particularly CD8, and proliferate in response to IL-2. LGL arise in both bone marrow and thymic microenvironments (see Fig. 305-2).

Functionally, LGL share features with both monocytes-macrophages and neutrophils in that subsets of LGL mediate antibody-dependent cellular cytotoxicity (ADCC) and NK activity. ADCC is the binding of an opsonized (antibody-coated) target cell to an Fc receptor–bearing effector cell via the Fc region of antibody, resulting in lysis of the target by the effector cell. NK cell activity is the nonimmune (i.e., effector cell never having had previous contact with the target), MHC-unrestricted, non-antibody-mediated killing of target cells, which are usually malignant cell types, transplanted foreign cells, or virus-infected cells. Thus, LGL that mediate NK activity may play an important role in immune surveillance and destruction of cells that spontaneously undergo malignant transformation in vivo. Subsets of NK cells may play a role in hematopoietic cell engraftment; some subsets stimulate bone marrow stem cells, and others stimulate engraftment. Lymphokine-activated killer (LAK) cells are NK lymphocytes that proliferate in vitro to high levels of IL-2 and develop the ability to kill tumor cells more efficiently than unstimulated NK cells. Rare patients with complete absence of NK cells have been described who lack both NK activity and CD56+, CD16+ lymphocytes but have normal T and B cell function. NK cell hyporesponsiveness is also observed in patients with the *Chédiak-Higashi syndrome*, an autosomal recessive disease associated with fusion of

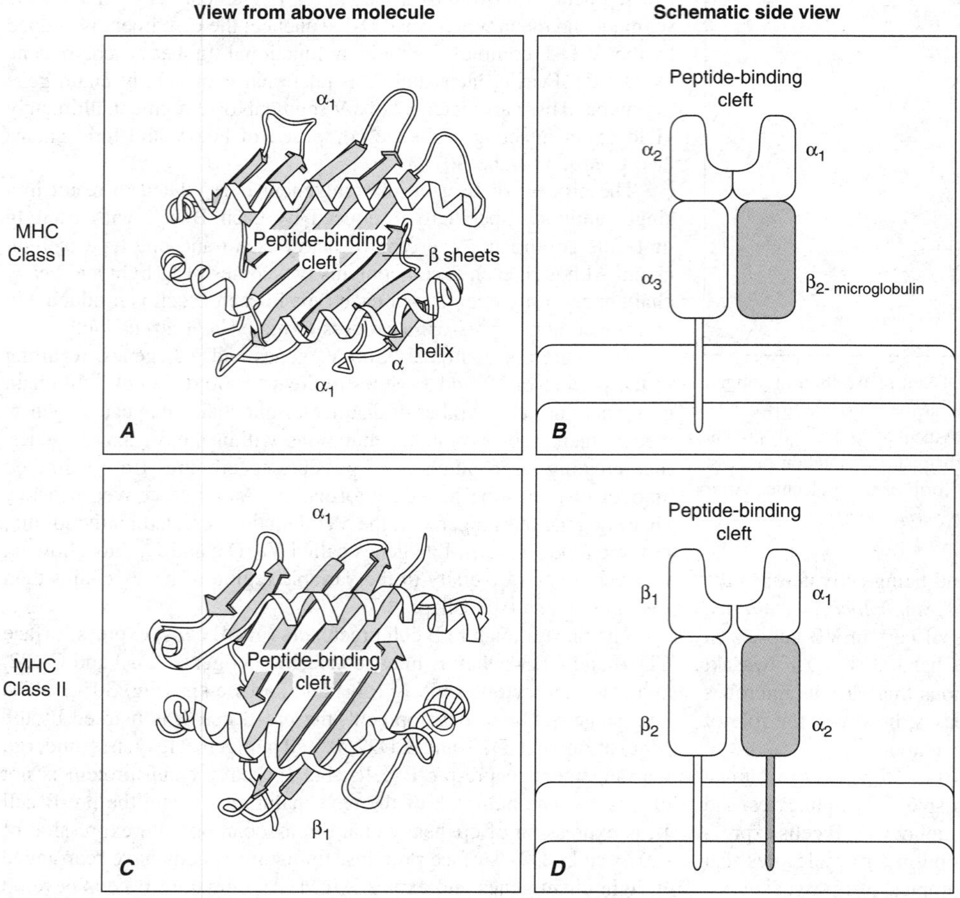

FIGURE 305-5 Structure of MHC class I and MHC class II molecules. *A* and *B*. Top and schematic side views of an MHC class I molecule. *C* and *D*. Top and schematic side views of an MHC class II molecule. Peptide-binding cleft is location of short peptide fragments derived from proteolytic cleavage of either foreign or self-proteins. Whereas the peptide-binding cleft comprises the α1, α2, and α3 domains of the class I α chain, the peptide-binding cleft of class II comprises the β1 and α1 domains of the class IIβ and α chains, respectively. *(From Janeway and Travers, with permission.)*

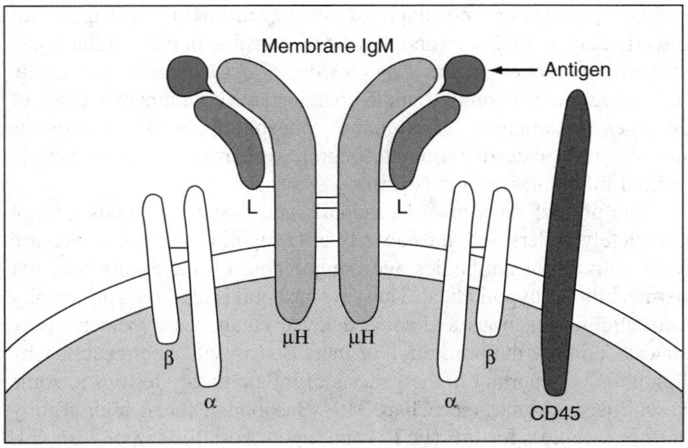

FIGURE 305-7 B cell antigen receptor for antigen-associated molecules. Immunoglobulin (Ig) associated α (CD79α) and β (CD79β) chains are disulfide-linked molecules that mediate the delivery of intracellular activation signals to B cells following interaction of membrane Ig with antigen. CD45 modulates the activation state of B cells by the tyrosine phosphatase activity of the cytoplasmic domain of CD45 molecules.

cytoplasmic granules and defective degranulation of neutrophil lysosomes. Recently, a series of studies has suggested that subsets of NK cells can specifically recognize normal allogeneic cells in a clonal fashion. Studies of allogeneic target cells suggest that the genetic locus controlling NK alloantigen lysis is different from conventional MHC products, is inherited as an autosomal recessive trait, and is located on chromosome 6 in the same region as MHC class I genes.

The ability of NK cells to kill target cells is inversely related to target cell expression of MHC class I molecules. Thus, NK cells kill target cells with low or negative levels of MHC class I expression and are prevented from killing target cells with high levels of class I expression. Some viruses and cancers downregulate host cell MHC class I molecule expression, thereby making infected or transformed cells unable to be targeted by CD8+ MHC class I–restricted cytotoxic T cells. One hypothesis is that NK cells evolved to fill a niche in the host immune response to viruses and tumors by providing a surveillance component of the immune system that could kill MHC class I–negative infected or malignant cells. Recently, the NK surface receptors that bind to MHC class I molecules and prevent NK cell killing of class I–expressing target cells have been cloned in humans and shown to be a group of molecules in the Ig gene superfamily.

MONOCYTES-MACROPHAGES Monocytes arise from precursor cells within bone marrow (see Fig. 305-2) and circulate with a half-life ranging from 1 to 3 days. Monocytes leave the peripheral circulation by marginating in capillaries and then migrating into a vast extravascular pool. Tissue macrophages arise by migration of monocytes from the circulation and by proliferation of macrophage precursors in tissue. Common locations of tissue macrophages (and some of their specialized names) are lymph node, spleen, bone marrow, perivascular connective tissue, serous cavities such as the peritoneum, pleura, skin connective tissue, lung (alveolar macrophage), liver (Kupffer cell), bone (osteoclast), central nervous system (microglia), and synovium (type A lining cell).

The monocyte-macrophage system plays a major role in the expression of immune reactivity by mediation of functions such as the presentation of antigen to T lymphocytes and the secretion of factors such as IL-1 and IL-6 that are central to antigen-specific activation of T and B lymphocytes. Although monocytes-macrophages were first thought to be the major APC of the immune system, it is now clear that dendritic/Langerhans cells are the most potent and effective APC in the body (see below). Monocytes-macrophages mediate effector functions such as destruction of antibody-coated bacteria, tumor cells, or even normal hematopoietic cells in certain types of autoimmune cytopenias. Activated macrophages also can mediate antigen-nonspecific lytic activity and eliminate cell types such as tumor cells in the absence of antibody. This activity is largely mediated by cytokines (i.e., TNF and IL-1). Monocytes-macrophages express lineage-specific molecules (e.g., CD14) as well as surface receptors for a number of molecules, including the Fc region of IgG (CD16, CD32, CD64), activated complement components (CD35) (see Table 305-2), and various cytokines (see Tables 305-3 to 305-5). Finally, macrophage secretory products are more diverse than those known for any other cell of the immune system. These secretory products allow the macrophage to exert both pro- and anti-inflammatory effects and to regulate other cell types. Among monocyte-macrophage–secreted products are hydrolytic enzymes, products of oxidative metabolism, TNFα, IL-1, -6, -12, -15, and a number of chemoattractant cytokines (chemokines) involved in the orchestration of an immune response in tissues.

DENDRITIC/LANGERHANS CELLS Dendritic/Langerhans cells are bone marrow–derived APC that are distinct from monocytes-macrophages. They lack the standard T, B, NK, and monocyte cell markers and have very little expression of C3 and Fc receptors; they express CD83 and other molecules that aid in their identification. They can be expanded in culture and their function enhanced by the cytokines GM-CSF, IL-1, IL-4, and TNFα. They are distinguished by an exceptional ability to present antigen, by expression of high levels of MHC class II and adhesion molecules, and dendritic morphology with multiple thin membrane projections (veils). Their antigen-processing capability has not been well studied. When present in the skin and beneath the mucosal surfaces, they are referred to as *Langerhans cells.* They are the dendritic cells of the blood and the spleen, the veiled cells of afferent lymphatics, and form part of the interdigitating cell network of the lymphoid organs. Dendritic cells are present in the blood in very small numbers, fewer than 0.1 percent of total blood leukocytes;

	Stem Cell	Pro-B	Pre-B I	Pre-B II (Large)	Pre-B II (Small)	Immature B	Mature B
	CD34	CD34	CD34	CD34	-	-	-
		CD10	CD10	CD10	CD10	-	-
			CD19	CD19	CD19	CD19	CD19
			CD40	CD40	CD40	CD40	CD40
				CD73	CD73	CD73	CD73
				CD22	CD22	CD22	CD22
				CD38	CD38	-	-
					CD21	CD21	CD21
							CD23
IL-7 Receptor	-	+	+	-	-	-	-
IL-3 Receptor	-	+	+	+	+	-	-
IL-4 Receptor	-	-	-	-	+	+	+
Immunoglobulin gene rearrangement	-	-	+	+	+	+	+
IgM Expression	-	-	-	-	cytoplasm	surface	surface
IgD Expression	-	-	-	-	-	-	surface

FIGURE 305-8 Antigen-independent human B lymphocyte maturation. *(After Haynes and Denning, with permission.)*

Table 305-5

Cytokines That Regulate Human B Cell Development

Cytokine	Source	Function
IL-7	T cells, bone marrow stromal cells	Drives pro-B and pre-pre-B cells to proliferate and differentiate
BCG-F (low-molecular-weight B cell growth factor)	Activated T cells	B cell precursor proliferation
IL-3	T cells, stromal cells	Induces B cell precursor proliferation
IL-1, IL-2, IL-4, IL-5, IL-6	T cells (IL-2, IL-4, IL-5), monocytes (IL-1, IL-6)	Drives mature B cells to proliferate and differentiate into Ig-secreting cells
TGFβ	T cells, ?thymic epithelial cells	Blocks synthesis of κ light chains

their presence in the blood suggests that these cells traffic among different organs.

FOLLICULAR DENDRITIC CELLS Follicular dendritic cells (FDC) are APC for B cells and are distinct from the dendritic/Langerhans cells, which are APC for T cells. They are located in the germinal centers or follicles of secondary lymphoid organs. The origin of FDC is unclear. Their main function is to trap and retain antigen in the germinal centers of lymphoid organs and present the antigen to B cells. Antigen is retained on their membranes in the form of antigen-antibody complexes that bind to the cell via the cellular receptor for C3. The FDC have extensive, thin, finger-like projections that surround the B cells in the germinal centers, allowing for maximal exposure of trapped antigen. FDC show very little evidence of endocytosis. The retention of antigen on the surface of the FDC membranes is felt to be critical for the selection and growth of high-affinity clones of B cells and for the maintenance of B cell memory. CD4+ T cells migrate into the germinal centers to provide immunologic help to the B cells. Of note, the human immunodeficiency virus (HIV) is trapped in large quantities on the processes of FDC in lymphoid organs, allowing the lymphoid tissue to serve as a reservoir of virus and a source of infection for CD4+ T cells migrating into the area to provide help to B cells in the initiation and propagation of an HIV-specific humoral response (see Chap. 308).

NEUTROPHILS, EOSINOPHILS, AND BASOPHILS Granulocytes are present in nearly all forms of inflammation and are nonspecific amplifiers and effectors of specific immune responses. Unchecked accumulation and activation of granulocytes can lead to host tissue damage, as seen in neutrophil- and eosinophil-mediated *systemic necrotizing vasculitis*. Granulocytes are derived from stem cells in bone marrow (see Fig. 305-2). Each type of granulocyte (neutrophil, eosinophil, or basophil) is derived from a different subclass of progenitor cell, which is stimulated to proliferate by colony stimulating factors. During terminal maturation of granulocytes, class-specific nuclear morphology and cytoplasmic granules appear that allow for histologic identification of granulocyte type.

Neutrophils express Fc receptors for IgG (CD16) and receptors for activated complement components (C3b or CD35) (see Table 305-2). Upon interaction of neutrophils with immune complexes, azurophilic granules (containing myeloperoxidase, lysozyme, elastase, and other enzymes) and specific granules (containing lactoferrin, lysozyme, collagenase, and other enzymes) are released, and microbicidal superoxide radicals (O_2) are generated at the neutrophil surface. The generation of superoxide leads to inflammation by direct injury to tissue and by alteration of macromolecules such as collagen and DNA.

Eosinophils express Fc receptors for IgG (CD32) and are potent cytotoxic effector cells for various parasitic organisms. Intracytoplasmic contents of eosinophils, such as major basic protein, eosinophil cationic protein, and eosinophil-derived neurotoxin, are capable of directly damaging tissues and may be responsible in part for the organ system dysfunction in the *hypereosinophilic syndromes* (see Chap. 62). Since the eosinophil granule contains anti-inflammatory types of enzymes (histaminase, arylsulfatase, phospholipase D), eosinophils may downregulate or terminate ongoing inflammatory responses in normal inflammation homeostasis.

The normal functions of basophils and tissue mast cells are not completely understood; the capacity of basophil mediators to increase local delivery of antibodies and complement by increasing vascular permeability is hypothetical. Thus, the basophil is identified principally with allergic reactions and some delayed cutaneous hypersensitivity states. Certainly the promotion of increased vascular permeability by basophils is important in the genesis of inflammatory lesions in some vasculitis syndromes (see Chap. 319). Basophils express high-affinity surface receptors for IgE (Fc RI) and, upon cross-linking of basophil-bound IgE by antigen, release histamine, eosinophil chemotactic factor of anaphylaxis, and neutral protease—all mediators of immediate (anaphylaxis) hypersensitivity responses (Table 305-6). In addition, basophils express surface receptors for activated complement components (C3a, C5a), through which mediator release can be directly effected. → ***For further discussion of tissue mast cells, see Chap. 310.***

HUMORAL MEDIATORS OF SPECIFIC IMMUNITY: IMMUNOGLOBULINS

Immunoglobulins are the products of differentiated B cells and mediate the humoral arm of the immune response. The primary functions of antibodies are to bind specifically to antigen and bring about the inactivation or removal of the offending toxin, microbe, parasite, or other foreign substance from the body. The structural basis of Ig molecule function and Ig gene organization has provided insight into the role of antibodies in normal protective immunity, pathologic immune-mediated damage by immune complexes, and autoantibody formation against host determinants.

All immunoglobulins have the basic structure of two heavy and two light chains (Fig. 305-9). Immunoglobulin isotype (i.e., G, M, A, D, E) is determined by the type of Ig heavy chain present. IgG and IgA isotypes can be divided further into subclasses (G1, G2, G3, G4, and A1, A2) based on specific antigenic determinants on Ig heavy chains. The characteristics of human immunoglobulins are outlined in Table 305-7. The four chains are covalently linked by disulfide bonds. Each chain is made up of a V region and C regions (also called *domains*), themselves made up of units of approximately 110 amino acids. Light chains have one variable (VL) and one constant (CL) unit; heavy chains have one variable unit (VH) and three or four constant (CH) units, depending on isotype. As the name suggests, the

Table 305-6

Mediators Released from Human Mast Cells and Basophils

Mediator	Actions
Histamine	Smooth-muscle contraction, increased vascular permeability
Slow reacting substance of anaphylaxis (SRSA) (leukotriene C_4, D_4, E_4)	Smooth-muscle contraction
Eosinophil chemotactic factor of anaphylaxis (ECF-A)	Chemotactic attraction of eosinophils
Platelet-activating factor	Activates platelets to secrete serotonin and other mediators; smooth-muscle contraction; induces vascular permeability
Neutrophil chemotactic factor (NCF)	Chemotactic attraction of neutrophils
Leukotactic activity (leukotriene B_4)	Chemotactic attraction of neutrophils
Heparin	Anticoagulant
Basophil kallikrein of anaphylaxis (BK-A)	Cleaves kininogen to form bradykinin

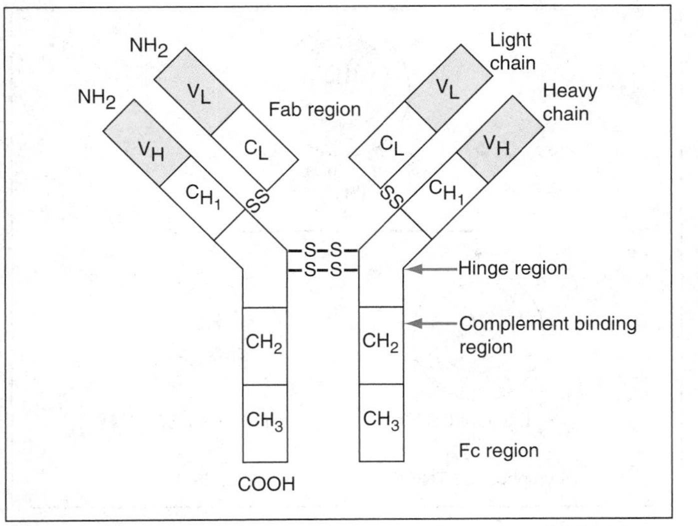

FIGURE 305-9 Schematic structure of the immunoglobulin G (IgG) molecule.

C regions of Ig molecules are made up of homologous sequences and share the same primary structure as all other Ig chains of the same isotype and subclass. Constant regions are involved in biologic functions of Ig molecules. The CH2 domain of IgG and the CH4 units of IgM are involved with the binding of the C1q portion of C1. The CH region at the carboxy-terminal end of the IgG molecule, the Fc region (see Fig. 305-9), binds to surface Fc receptors (CD16, CD32, CD64) of macrophages, LGL, B cells, neutrophils, and eosinophils.

Variable regions (VL and VH) constitute the antibody-binding (Fab) region of the molecule. Within the VL and VH regions are hypervariable regions (extreme sequence variability) that constitute the antigen-binding site unique to each Ig molecule. The idiotype is defined as the specific region of the Fab portion of the Ig molecule to which antigen binds. Antibodies against the idiotype portion of an antibody molecule are called *anti-idiotype antibodies*. The formation of such antibodies in vivo during a normal B cell antibody response may generate a negative (or "off") signal to B cells to terminate antibody production.

IgG comprises approximately 75 to 85 percent of total serum immunoglobulin. The four IgG subclasses are numbered in order of their level in serum, IgG1 being found in greatest amounts and IgG4 the least. IgG subclasses have clinical relevance in their varying ability to bind macrophage and neutrophil Fc receptors and to activate complement (see Table 305-7). Moreover, selective deficiencies of certain IgG subclasses give rise to clinical syndromes in which the patient is inordinately susceptible to bacterial infections. IgG antibodies are frequently the predominant antibody made after rechallenge of the host with antigen (secondary antibody response).

IgM antibodies normally circulate as a 950-kDa pentamer with 160-kDa bivalent monomers joined by a molecule called the *J chain*, a 15-kDa nonimmunoglobulin molecule that also effects polymerization of IgA molecules. IgM is the first immunoglobulin to appear in the immune response (primary antibody response) and is the initial type of antibody made by neonates. Membrane IgM in the monomeric form also functions as a major antigen receptor on the surface of mature B cells (see Fig. 305-7). IgM is an important component of immune complexes in autoimmune diseases. For instance, IgM antibodies against IgG molecules (rheumatoid factors) are present in high titers in *rheumatoid arthritis*, other collagen diseases, and some infectious diseases (*subacute bacterial endocarditis*). IgM antibody binds the C1 component of complement via the CH4 domain and thus is a potent activator of complement.

IgA comprises only 7 to 15 percent of total serum immunoglobulin but is the predominant class of immunoglobulin in secretions. IgA in secretions (tears, saliva, nasal secretions, gastrointestinal tract fluid, and human milk) is in the form of secretory IgA (sIgA), a polymer consisting of two IgA monomers, a joining molecule, again called the J chain, and a glycoprotein called the *secretory protein*. Of the two IgA subclasses, IgA1 is primarily found in serum, whereas IgA2 is more prevalent in secretions. IgA fixes complement via the alternative complement pathway and has potent antiviral activity in humans by

Table 305-7

Physical, Chemical, and Biologic Properties of Human Immunoglobulins

Property	IgG	IgA	IgM	IgD	IgE
Usual molecular form	Monomer	Monomer, dimer	Pentamer, hexamer	Monomer	Monomer
Other chains	None	J chain, SC	J chain	None	None
Subclasses	G1, G2, G3, G4	A1, A2	None	None	None
Heavy chain allotypes	Gm (≈30)	No A1, A2m (2)	None	None	None
Molecular mass, kDa	150	160, 400	950, 1150	175	190
Sedimentation constant, Sw20	6.6S	7S, 11S	19S	7S	8S
Carbohydrate content, %	3	7	10	9	13
Serum level in average adult, mg/mL	9.5–12.5	1.5–2.6	0.7–1.7	0.04	0.0003
Percentage of total serum Ig	75–85	7–15	5–10	0.3	0.019
Serum half-life, days	23	6	5	3	2.5
Synthesis rate, mg/kg per day	33	65	7	0.4	0.016
Antibody valence	2	2, 4	10, 12	2	2
Classical complement activation	+(G1, 2?, 3)	−	++	−	−
Alternate complement activation	+(G4)	+	−	+	−
Binding cells via Fc	Macrophages, neutrophils, large granular lymphocytes	Lymphocytes	Lymphocytes	None	Mast cells, basophils, B cells
Biologic properties	Placental transfer, secondary Ab for most antipathogen responses	Secretory immunoglobulin	Primary Ab responses	Marker for mature B cells	Allergy, antiparasite responses

SOURCE: After L Carayannopoulos and JD Capra, in Paul, with permission.

prevention of virus binding to respiratory and gastrointestinal epithelial cells.

IgD is found in minute quantities in serum (see Table 305-7) and along with IgM is a major receptor for antigen on the B cell surface. Present in serum in very low concentrations (see Table 305-7), IgE is the major class of immunoglobulin involved in arming mast cells and basophils by binding to these cells via the Fc region. Antigen cross-linking of IgE molecules on basophil and mast cell surfaces results in release of mediators of the immediate hypersensitivity response (see Table 305-6).

CELLULAR INTERACTIONS IN REGULATION OF THE NORMAL IMMUNE RESPONSE

The net result of activation of the humoral (B cell) and cellular (T cell) arms of the immune system by foreign antigen is the elimination of antigen directly by immune effector cells or in concert with specific antibody. In addition, a series of regulatory cells is activated that modulate T effector cell activation and B cell antibody production. Figure 305-10 is a simplified schematic diagram of the immune system outlining some of these cellular interactions.

T CELL–T CELL AND T CELL–B CELL INTERACTIONS The expression of immune cell function is the result of a complex series of immunoregulatory events that occur in phases. Both T and B lymphocytes mediate immune functions, and each of these cell types, when given appropriate signals, passes through stages, from activation and induction through proliferation, differentiation, and ultimately effector functions. The effector function expressed may be at the end point of a response, such as secretion of antibody by a differentiated plasma cell, or it might serve a regulatory function that modulates other functions, such as is seen with CD4+ inducer or CD8+ regulatory T lymphocytes, which modulate both differentiation of B cells and activation of CD8+ or CD4+ cytotoxic T cells.

CD4 inducer (or helper) T cells can be subdivided on the basis of cytokines produced (Fig. 305-11). Activated TH1-type inducer T cells secrete IL-2, IFNγ, and TNFβ, while activated TH2-type inducer T cells secrete IL-4, -5, -6, and -10. TH1 CD4+ T cells provide T cell help for generation of cytotoxic T cells and generally respond to

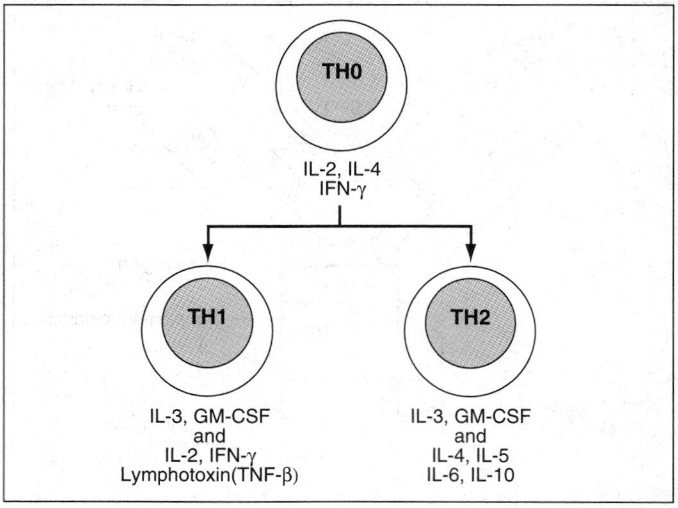

FIGURE 305-11 CD4+ T helper 1 (TH1) cells and TH2 T cells and their precursors (TH0 cells) secrete distinct but overlapping sets of cytokines. TH1 cells are frequently activated in immune and inflammatory reactions that involve CD8+ cytotoxic T cell induction and/or granuloma formation, while TH2 cells are frequently activated for certain types of antibody production and are activated in allergic diseases. *(From Janeway and Travers, with permission.)*

antigens that lead to delayed hypersensitivity types of immune responses (such as *Mycobacterium tuberculosis*). In contrast, TH2 cells regulate the intensity of immune responses by the secretion of a cytokine, IL-10, that inhibits the production of other cytokines (see Table 305-4). In addition, TH2 CD4+ T cells provide help to B cells for specific Ig production and respond to antigens that require high antibody levels for foreign antigen elimination (such as in certain parasite infections). Different cytokines can drive the immune response preferentially towards a TH1 or a TH2 response. For example, IL-12 induces T cell differentiation towards a TH1 type cell, whereas IL-4 drives differentiation towards a TH2 type cell.

As shown in Fig. 305-10, upon activation by APC, regulatory T cell subsets that produce IL-2, IL-3, IFNγ, and/or IL-4, -5, -6, and -10 are generated that exert positive and negative influences on effector T and B cells. For B cells, trophic effects are mediated by a variety of cytokines, particularly T cell–derived IL-3, -4, and -5, which act at sequential stages of B cell maturation, resulting in B cell proliferation, differentiation, and ultimately antibody secretion (see Table 305-5). For cytotoxic T cells, trophic factors include inducer T cell secretion of IL-2, IFNγ, IL-12, and IL-15 (see Table 305-4). In addition, B cells themselves are capable of serving as APC, processing and presenting antigens to T cells, and secreting TNFα and IL-6.

Although B cells recognize native antigen via B cell surface Ig receptors, B cells require T cell help to produce high-affinity antibody of multiple isotypes that will be the most effective antibody response in eliminating foreign antigen. This T cell dependence likely functions in the regulation of B cell responses and in protection against excessive autoantibody production. T cell–B cell interactions that lead to high-affinity antibody production require: (1) processing of native antigen by B cells and expressing peptide fragments on the B cell surface for presentation to TH cells, (2) the ligation of B cells both by the T

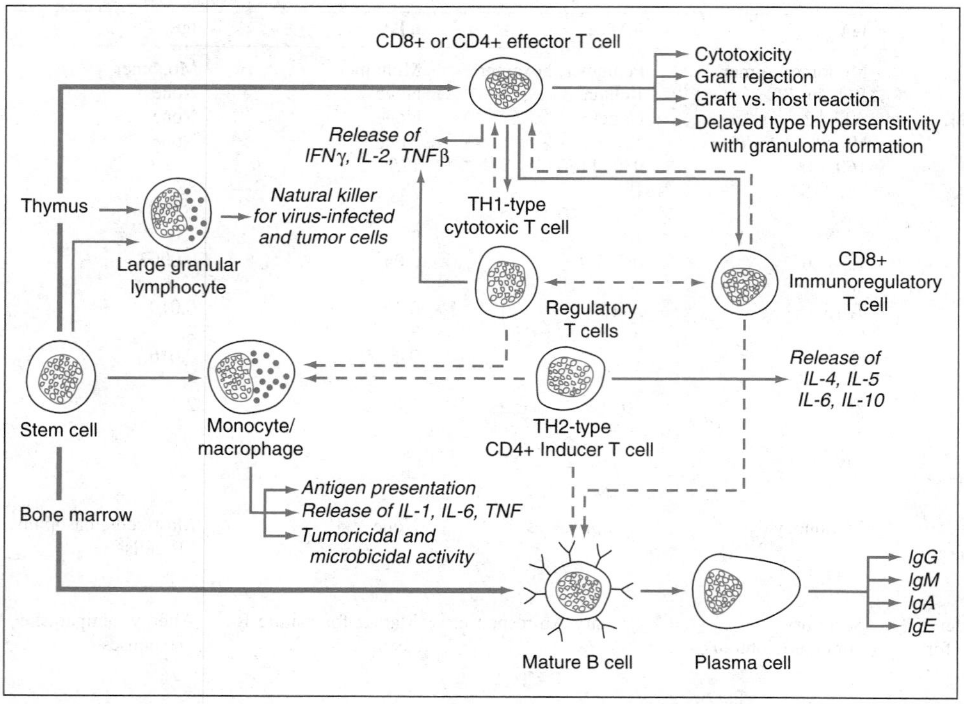

FIGURE 305-10 Schematic model of intercellular interactions of immune competent cells during the ontogeny and activation stages of immune responses.

cell receptor complex and the CD40 ligand, (3) induction of the process termed *antibody isotype switching* in antigen-specific B cell clones, and (4) induction of the process of *affinity maturation* of antibody in the germinal centers of B cell follicles of lymph node and spleen.

Naive B cells express cell-surface IgD and IgM, and initial contact of naive B cells with antigen is via B cell surface IgM binding to native antigen. T cell cytokines, released following TH cell contact with B cells or by a "bystander" effect, induce changes in Ig gene conformation that promote recombination of Ig genes. These events then result in the "switching" of expression of heavy chain exons in a triggered B cell, leading to IgG, IgA, or, in some cases, IgE antibody types secreted with the same V region antigen specificity as the original IgM antibody produced. Class switching may also occur by a posttranscriptional mechanism acting at the RNA level. The T cell cytokines that induce antibody isotype switching are IL-4, TGFβ, IL-5, and IFNγ. CD40 ligand expression by TH cells is critical for induction of antibody isotype switching, and patients with mutations in T cell CD40 ligand have B cells that are unable to undergo isotype switching, resulting in the immunodeficiency syndrome of *X-linked hyper-IgM syndrome* (see Chap. 307).

The gradual increase in the affinity of antibodies for antigen over time occurs in the germinal centers of lymph node and spleen and results from continued alteration of Ig V region genes, through a process of *somatic hypermutation*. Somatic hypermutation is a process whereby many mutations in V region genes occur, leading to a wide range of possibilities for changes in antibody specificity. Those changes that result in higher affinity antibodies are selected for continued usage by germinal center B cells by the firm binding of B cells to antigen on the surface of antigen-presenting FDC (see above), leading to B cell proliferation and clonal expansion.

ANTIGEN-PRESENTING CELL–T CELL INTERACTIONS The three cell types that are the primary presenters of antigen peptide fragments to T cells are dendritic/Langerhans cells, monocytes-macrophages, and B lymphocytes. Many of the activation and regulatory effects of these cell types occur via cytokines that regulate T and B cell maturation following direct APC–T cell contact (see Tables 305-3 to 305-5). APC are required for optimal activation of T cells by antigens or by mitogens (nonspecific activators of lymphocytes). Two signals are required to activate T cells by APC: signal 1, delivered to the T cell receptor/CD3 complex by antigen peptides embedded in MHC class I or class II clefts or grooves; and signal 2, delivered by an antigen-nonspecific co-stimulatory signal, mediated on APC by molecules, termed B7-1 (CD80) and B7-2 (CD86), that bind to the T cell molecule, CD28 (Fig. 305-4). Ligation of the T cell receptor/CD3 complex by MHC molecule/peptide complexes in the presence of co-stimulatory molecule ligation leads to T cell activation and clonal expansion of antigen-specific T cells; whereas, ligation of the T cell receptor in the absence of T cell CD28 ligation leads to T cell nonresponsiveness, termed *anergy*. Ingestion of foreign antigens such as bacteria by macrophage APC leads to induction of macrophage B7 molecule expression and the ability to activate bacteria-specific T cells, whereas presentation of host (self) peptides in APC MHC molecules does not lead to APC expression of B7, thus promoting the normal state of host T cell anergy to self-antigens. Upon contact with antigens or mitogens, APC secrete IL-1, IL-6, and TNFα, the effects of which are (1) the induction of receptors for IL-2 on T cells, and (2) the induction of T cell secretion of IL-2, IL-4, and other cytokines. These cytokines, in turn, activate other T cells in an antigen-nonspecific fashion, resulting in recruitment of effector and regulatory T cells that also have been induced to express IL-2, -4, and -7 receptors (see Fig. 305-10). Effector T cells mediate a variety of functions, including the killing of virus-infected cells, graft rejection, graft-versus-host reaction, delayed-type hypersensitivity, and the release of a wide spectrum of immunoregulatory cytokines (see Tables 305-3 to 305-5).

THE COMPLEMENT SYSTEM

The complement system is a cascading series of plasma enzymes, regulatory proteins, and proteins capable of cell lysis whose principal site of synthesis is the liver. There are two arms of the complement system (Fig. 305-12). Activation of the classic complement pathway via C1, C4, and C2 and activation of the alternative complement pathway via factor D, C3, and factor B both lead to cleavage and activation of C3. C3 is a protein whose activation fragments, when bound to target surfaces such as bacteria and other foreign antigens, are critical for opsonization (coating by antibody and complement) in preparation for phagocytosis.

The protein fragment C3b, split from C3, is necessary for activation of the terminal complement components C5–9. These form the membrane attack complex which, when inserted into cell membranes, brings about osmotic lysis of the cell.

C3b also joins with a cleavage product of factor B (called Bb) to form C3bBb, also known as the *alternative pathway C3 convertase*. Activation of the classic complement pathway results in cleavage of C4 and C2 with a resulting complex of fragments, C4b2a, also called the *classic pathway C3 convertase*. Both the classic pathway C3 convertase (C4b2a) and the alternative pathway C3 convertase (C3bBb) function to cleave C3 to form active C3b, thus driving activation of the C5–9 membrane attack complex. The fact that C3b can combine with Bb to form the alternative pathway C3 convertase gives rise to a potent positive feedback loop for production of C3b and thus continued activation of terminal complement components.

The classic complement pathway is activated by interaction of antigen and antibody to form immune complexes that bind C1q, a subunit of C1. Immunoglobulin isotypes that bind C1q and activate the classic pathway are IgM, IgG1, IgG2, and IgG3. In contrast, IgA1, IgA2, and IgD activate complement via the alternative pathway. Activation of the complement cascade via the classic pathway by IgG- or IgM-containing immune complexes is a rapid and efficient pathway to activation of terminal complement components. In contrast, activation of the alternative complement pathway via IgA-containing immune complexes or by bacterial endotoxin is a slower and less efficient pathway to terminal component activation. Thus the immunoglobulin isotype composition of immune complexes is a critical factor in determining complement activation and the efficiency of clearance of immune complexes by C3 receptor–bearing cells.

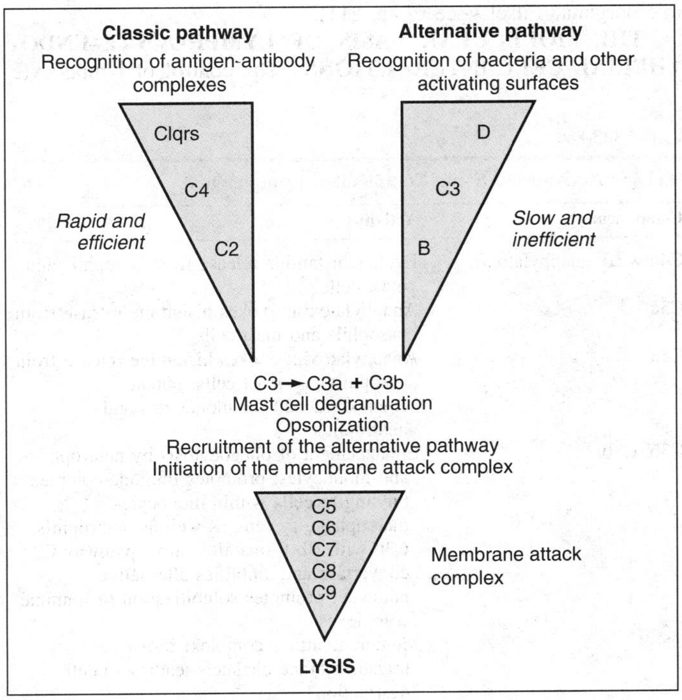

FIGURE 305-12 Components of the complement system. *(After Paul, with permission.)*

In addition to the role of complement in opsonization of bacteria and cell lysis, several complement fragments are potent mediators of immune cell activation. C3a and C5a bind to receptors on mast cells and basophils, resulting in release of histamine and other mediators of anaphylaxis. C5a is also a potent chemoattractant for neutrophils and monocytes-macrophages (Table 305-8).

MECHANISMS OF IMMUNE DAMAGE

Several responses by the host to foreign antigen culminate in the rapid and efficient elimination of nonself substances. In these scenarios, the classic weapons of the immune system (T cells, B cells, macrophages) interface with cells and soluble products that are mediators of inflammatory responses (neutrophils, eosinophils, basophils, kinin and coagulation systems, and complement cascade) (see Chaps. 62 and 310).

There are four general phases of host defenses: (1) migration of leukocytes to sites of antigen localization; (2) specific and nonspecific recognition of foreign antigens mediated by T and B lymphocytes, macrophages, and the alternative complement pathway; (3) amplification of the inflammatory response with recruitment of specific and nonspecific effector cells by complement components, lymphokines and monokines, kinins, arachidonic acid metabolites, and mast cell–basophil products; and (4) macrophage, neutrophil, and lymphocyte participation in antigen destruction with ultimate removal of antigen particles by phagocytosis (by macrophages or neutrophils) or by direct cytotoxic mechanisms (involving macrophages, neutrophils, and lymphocytes). Under normal circumstances, orderly progression of host defenses through these phases results in a well-controlled immune and inflammatory response that protects the host from the offending antigen. However, dysfunction of any of the host defense systems can damage host tissue and produce clinically apparent disease. Furthermore, for certain pathogens or antigens, the normal immune response itself might contribute substantially to the tissue damage. For example, the immune and inflammatory response in the brain to certain pathogens such as *M. tuberculosis* may be responsible for much of the morbidity of this disease in that organ system (see Chap. 171). In addition, the morbidity associated with certain pneumonias such as that caused by *Pneumocystis carinii* may be associated more with inflammatory infiltrates than with the tissue destructive effects of the microorganism itself (see Chap. 211).

THE MOLECULAR BASIS OF LYMPHOCYTE–ENDOTHELIAL CELL INTERACTIONS The control of lymphocyte circulatory patterns between the bloodstream and peripheral lymphoid organs operates at the level of lymphocyte–endothelial cell interactions to control the specificity of lymphocyte subset entry into organs. Similarly, lymphocyte–endothelial cell interactions regulate the entry of lymphocytes into inflamed tissue. Adhesion molecule expression on lymphocytes and endothelial cells regulates the retention and subsequent egress of lymphocytes within tissue sites of antigenic stimulation, delaying cell exit from tissue and preventing reentry into the circulating lymphocyte pool. All types of lymphocyte migration begin with lymphocyte attachment to specialized regions of vessels, termed *high endothelial venules* (HEV). An important concept for many of the adhesion molecules listed in Table 305-9 is that the molecules do not generally bind their ligand until a conformational change (ligand activation) occurs in the adhesion molecule that allows ligand binding. Induction of a conformation-dependent determinant on an adhesion molecule can be accomplished by cytokines or via ligation of other adhesion molecules on the cell.

Table 305-8

Biologic Activities of Some Complement Components

Component	Activity
C4a weak anaphylatoxin	Evokes histamine release from basophils and mast cells
C3a	Anaphylatoxin; evokes histamine release from basophils and mast cells
C5a	Anaphylatoxin; evokes histamine release from basophils and mast cells; potent chemoattractant for monocytes and neutrophils
C3b, C3bi	Enhancement of phagocytosis by neutrophils and monocytes; promotes immune-complex binding to cells within monocyte-macrophage system, as well as neutrophils; C3b with Bb forms alternative pathway C3 convertase and amplifies alternative pathway; promotes solubilization of immune complexes
C5–9	Membrane attack complex; forms transmembrane channels leading to cell destruction

SOURCE: After S Ruddy, in Kelley et al, with permission.

The first stage of lymphocyte–endothelial cell interactions, *attachment and rolling*, occurs when lymphocytes leave the stream of flowing blood cells in a postcapillary venule and roll along venule endothelial cells (Fig. 305-13). Lymphocyte rolling is mediated by the L-selectin molecule (LECAM-1, LAM-1) (see Table 305-9). Lymphocyte L-selectin ligands on HEV are sulfated oligosaccharides present on three different molecules: glycosylation-dependent cell adhesion molecule 1 (GlyCAM-1), CD34, and mucosal addressin cell adhesion molecule 1 (MAdCAM-1), leading to adhesion of lymphocytes to HEV. Lymphocyte rolling slows cell transit time through venules, allowing time for activation of adherent cells.

The second stage of lymphocyte–endothelial cell interactions, *adhesion triggering*, requires stimulation of lymphocytes by chemoattractants or by endothelial cell–derived cytokines. Cytokines thought to participate in adherent cell triggering include members of the IL-8–intercrine family, platelet-activation factor, leukotriene B_4, and C5a. Following activation by chemoattractants, lymphocytes shed L-selectin from the cell surface and upregulate cell CD11b/18 (MAC-1) or CD11a/18 (LFA-1) molecules (see Tables 305-2 and 305-9), resulting in firm attachment of lymphocytes to HEV.

Lymphocyte homing to peripheral lymph nodes involves adhesion of L-selectin to carbohydrate of peripheral node HEV, whereas homing of lymphocytes to intestine Peyer's patches primarily involves adhesion of the α4,β7 integrin to MAdCAM-1 oligosaccharides on Peyer's patch HEV. However, for migration to mucosal Peyer's patch lymphoid aggregates, naive lymphocytes primarily use L-selectin, whereas memory lymphocytes use α4,β7 integrin. α4, β1 (CD49d/CD29, VLA-4)–VCAM-1 interactions are important in the initial interaction of memory lymphocytes with HEV of multiple organs in sites of inflammation.

The third stage of leukocyte emigration in HEV, *sticking and arrest*, is sticking, of the lymphocyte and arrest at the site of sticking, mediated predominantly by ligation of αL,β2 integrin LFA-1 to the integrin ligands, ICAM-1 and ICAM-2 on HEV. While the first three stages of lymphocyte attachment to HEV takes only a few seconds, the fourth stage of lymphocyte emigration, *transendothelial migration*, takes approximately 10 min. Although the molecular mechanisms that control lymphocyte transendothelial migration are not fully characterized, the HEV CD44 molecule and molecules of the HEV glycocalyx (extracellular matrix) are thought to play important regulatory roles in this process (Fig. 305-13). Finally, expression of matrix metalloproteases capable of digesting the subendothelial basement membrane, rich in nonfibrillar collagen, appears to be required for the penetration of lymphoid cells into the extravascular sites.

Abnormal induction of HEV formation and use of the molecules discussed above have been implicated in the induction and maintenance of inflammation in a number of chronic inflammatory diseases. In animal models of insulin-dependent diabetes mellitus (IDDM), MAdCAM-1 and GlyCAM-1 have been shown to be highly expressed on HEV in inflamed pancreatic islets, and treatment of these animals with inhibitors of L-selectin and α4 integrin function blocked the development of IDDM (see Chap. 334). A similar role in human chronic inflammatory disease for abnormal induction of the adhesion

Table 305-9

Leukocyte–Endothelial Cell Adhesion Molecules

Molecule	Distribution	Ligand	Functions
SELECTIN FAMILY			
L-selectin (LECAM-1, LAM-1)	Leukocyte	Sulfated oligosaccharides on GlyCAM-1, MAdCAM-1, and CD34	Regulates leukocyte binding to inflamed endothelium; lymph node homing receptor
P-selectin (GMP-140)	Endothelial cells, alpha granules of platelets	Sialylated derivatives of Lewis X oligosaccharides	Involved in some initial PMN leukocyte–endothelial cell interactions
E-selectin (ELAM-1)	Endothelial cells	Sialylated derivatives of Lewis X oligosaccharides	Involved in some initial PMN leukocyte–endothelial cell interactions
INTEGRIN FAMILY			
$\alpha1\beta1$ (VLA-1, CD49a)	Activated T cells, monocytes, endothelial cells	Laminin, collagen	Activation-dependent adhesion receptor; marker for memory T cells
$\alpha2\beta1$ (VLA-2, CD49b)	Lymphocytes, endothelial cells, widespread	Collagen, laminin	Activation-dependent adhesion receptor
$\alpha3\beta1$ (VLA-3, CD49c)	Lymphocytes, endothelial cells, widespread	Fibronectin, collagen, laminin	Activation-dependent adhesion receptor
$\alpha4\beta1$ (VLA-4, CD49d)	Lymphocytes	VCAM-1, fibronectin fragment, vascular addressin	Involved in organ-specific homing in inflammation; activation upregulates adhesion
$\alpha4\beta7$	Lymphocytes	MAdCAM-1	Involved in organ-specific homing to Peyer's patches and to a variety of tissues in chronic diseases
$\alpha5\beta1$ (VLA-5, CD49c)	Lymphocytes, endothelial cells, widespread	Fibronectin	Activation-dependent adhesion receptor; marker for memory T cells
$\alpha6\beta1$ (VLA-6, CD49f)	Widespread	Laminin	Adhesion to endothelial cells
$\alpha L\beta2$ (LFA-1, CD11a)	Leukocytes	ICAM-1, ICAM-2, ICAM-3	Activation-dependent adhesion receptor
$\alpha M\beta2$ (MAC-1, CD11b)	Myeloid, NK cells	ICAM-1, C3bi, factor X	Activation-dependent adhesion receptor; mediates adhesion of myeloid cells to endothelial cells
$\alpha X\beta1$ (p150, 95, CD11c)	Myeloid cells, subset of lymphocyte	?	Activation-dependent adhesion receptor; mediates binding of myeloid cells to ligands derived from complement cascade
CD2	T cells, NK cells	CD58 (LFA-3)	Activation-dependent adhesion receptor; can transmit proliferation signal
CD54 (ICAM-1)	Activated lymphocytes, thymic epithelium, cytokine (IL-1, TNFα, IFNγ)–stimulated endothelial cells	LFA-1, rhinoviruses, *P. falciparum*	Upregulated expression on many tissues; mediates endothelial-leukocyte adherence
ICAM-2	Endothelial cells	LFA-1	Mediates leukocyte-endothelial adherence
ICAM-3	All resting leukocytes	LFA-1	Leukocyte-leukocyte interactions prior to leukocyte activation
CD58 (LFA-3)	Most tissue cell types	CD2	Upregulated expression in lymphoid tissues; involved in CTL–target cell interactions
VCAM-1 (InCAM-110)	TNFα– and IL-1–stimulated endothelial cells, follicular dendritic cells	VLA-4 ($\alpha4\beta1$)	Mediates homing of VLA-4+ leukocytes to Peyer's patches; mediates binding of B cells to germinal centers
CARTILAGE LINK PROTEIN FAMILY			
CD44 (Hermes, Pgpl, EcMRIII)	Leukocytes, widespread	Hyaluronan (hyaluronic acid)	Mediates leukocyte adhesion to extracellular matrix, probably by activation-dependent adhesion; binds to various cytokines; possibly involved in memory lymphocyte transendothelial migration

NOTE: ELAM, endothelial-leukocyte adhesion molecule; PMN, polymorphonuclear leukocytes; VLA, very late activation (antigen); VCAM, vascular cell adhesion molecule; LFA, lymphocyte function-associated (glycoprotein); ICAM, intercellular adhesion molecule; MAC, membrane attack complex.

SOURCE: From Haynes and Denning, with permission.

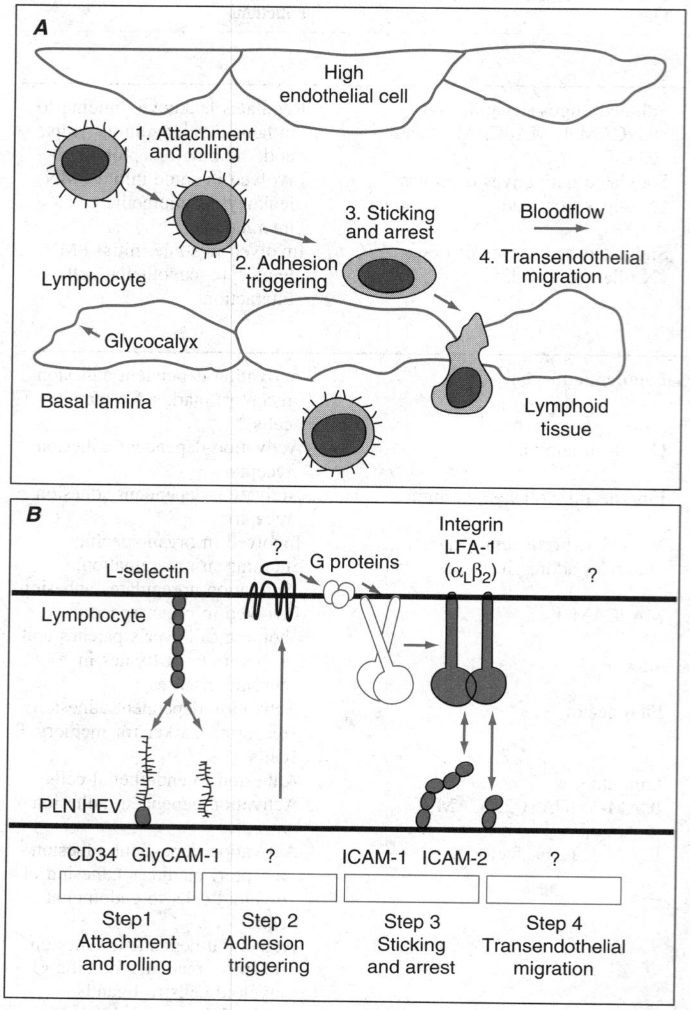

FIGURE 305-13 Lymphocyte emigration in high endothelial venules (HEV). *A*. Lymphocytes circulating in blood initiate contact with high endothelial cells via microvilli. This initial adhesion is transient and is often manifested in rolling of the interacting cells along the HEV endothelium (step 1: attachment and rolling). Activation of lymphocyte adhesiveness (step 2: adhesion triggering) results in firm attachment, which becomes stable to physiologic shear force (step 3: sticking and arrest). Lymphocytes then migrate through endothelial cell junctions and enter lymphoid tissue after crossing the HEV basal lamina (stage 4: transendothelial migration). The luminal surface of HEV is coated by a prominent glycocalyx, and this may play an important role in lymphocyte emigration (see text for details). *B*. The initial interaction of lymphocytes with HEV in peripheral lymph nodes (PLNs) is mediated by L-selectin, which recognizes the following HEV mucin-like counter-receptors: CD34 and glycosylation-dependent cell adhesion molecule 1 (GlyCAM-1). Activation of lymphocyte adhesiveness occurs via G protein–coupled receptors, but the local factors involved in physiologic activation of lymphocytes in HEV are not yet characterized. The integrin leukocyte function–associated molecule 1 (LFA-1) ($\alpha\beta$; CD11a/CD18) and its HEV counterreceptors intercellular adhesion molecule 1 (ICAM-1) and ICAM-2 play a major role in lymphocyte arrest in PLN HEV. The molecular mechanisms involved in lymphocyte transendothelial migration remain poorly characterized. *(After JP Girard, TA Springer. Immunology Today 16:449, 1995, with permission.)*

molecules of lymphocyte emigration has been suggested in rheumatoid arthritis (see Chap. 313), Hashimoto's thyroiditis (see Chap. 331), Graves' disease (see Chap. 331), multiple sclerosis (see Chap. 376), Crohn's disease (see Chap. 286), and ulcerative colitis (see Chap. 286). Cytokines that induce HEV expression of MAdCAM-1 and GlyCAM-1 are IFNγ, TNFα, IL-1, and IL-10.

IMMUNE-COMPLEX FORMATION Clearance of antigen by immune-complex formation between antigen and antibody is a highly effective mechanism of host defense. However, depending on the level of immune complexes formed and their physicochemical properties, immune complexes may or may not result in host and foreign cell damage. After antigen exposure, certain types of soluble antigen-antibody complexes freely circulate and, if not cleared by the reticuloendothelial system, can be deposited in blood vessel walls and in other tissues such as renal glomeruli. The precise mechanisms whereby immune complexes damage tissues, particularly blood vessels, are discussed in Chap. 319.

IgE-MEDIATED ALLERGIC REACTIONS—ANAPHYLAXIS T helper cells that drive antiallergen IgE responses are usually TH2-type inducer T cells that secrete IL-4, IL-5, IL-6, and IL-10. Mast cells and basophils have high-affinity receptors for the Fc portion of IgE (Fc RI), and cell-bound antiallergen IgE effectively "arms" basophils and mast cells. Mediator release is triggered by antigen (allergen) interaction with Fc receptor–bound IgE; the mediators released are responsible for the pathophysiologic changes of allergic diseases (see Table 305-6). Mediators released from mast cells and basophils can be divided into three broad functional types: (1) those that increase vascular permeability and contract smooth muscle (histamine, platelet-activating factor, SRS-A, BK-A); (2) those that are chemotactic for or activate other inflammatory cells (ECF-A, NCF, leukotriene B_4; and (3) those that modulate the release of other mediators (BK-A, platelet-activating factor) (see Chap. 310).

CYTOTOXIC REACTIONS OF ANTIBODY In this type of immunologic injury, complement-fixing (C1-binding) antibodies against normal or foreign cells or tissues (IgM, IgG1, IgG2, IgG3) bind complement via the classic pathway and initiate a sequence of events similar to that initiated by immune-complex deposition, resulting in cell lysis or tissue injury. Examples of antibody-mediated cytotoxic reactions include red cell lysis in *transfusion reactions*, *Goodpasture's syndrome* with anti-glomerular basement membrane antibody formation, and *pemphigus vulgaris* with antiepidermal antibodies inducing blistering skin disease.

CLASSIC DELAYED-TYPE HYPERSENSITIVITY REACTIONS Inflammatory reactions initiated by mononuclear leukocytes and not by antibody alone have been termed *delayed-type hypersensitivity reactions*. The term *delayed* has been used to contrast a secondary cellular response that appears 48 to 72 h after antigen exposure with an *immediate* hypersensitivity response generally seen within 12 h of antigen challenge and initiated by basophil mediator release or preformed antibody. For example, in an individual previously infected with *M. tuberculosis* organisms, intradermal placement of tuberculin purified-protein derivative as a skin test challenge results in an indurated area of skin at 48 to 72 h, indicating previous exposure to tuberculosis.

The cellular events that result in classic delayed-type hypersensitivity responses are centered around T cells (predominantly IFNγ, IL-2, and TNFβ-secreting TH1-type helper T cells) and macrophages. First, local immune and inflammatory responses at the site of foreign antigen upregulate endothelial cell adhesion molecule expression, promoting the accumulation of lymphocytes at the tissue site. In the general scheme outlined in Fig. 305-10, antigen is processed by dendritic/Langerhans cells or monocytes-macrophages and presented to small numbers of TH1 cells expressing a TCR specific for the antigen. IL-1 and IL-6 secreted by APC amplify the clonal expansion of antigen-specific T cells, and lymphokines (primarily IL-2, IFNγ, and TNFβ) are secreted that promote recruitment of diverse populations of T cells and macrophages to the site of the cellular inflammatory response. In particular, CD8+ cytotoxic T cells are induced to become active killer cells by IL-2. Once recruited, macrophages frequently undergo epithelioid cell transformation and form giant cells in response to IL-4 and IFNγ. This type of mononuclear cell infiltrate is termed *granulomatous inflammation*. Examples of diseases in which delayed-type hypersensitivity plays a major role are fungal infections (*histoplasmosis*) (see Chap. 203), mycobacterial infections (*tuberculosis, leprosy*) (see Chaps. 171 and 172), chlamydial infections (*lymphogranuloma venereum*) (see Chap. 181), helminth infections (*schistosomiasis*) (see Chap. 224), reactions to toxins (*berylliosis*) (see Chap. 254), and hypersensitivity reactions to organic dusts (*hypersensitivity pneu-*

monitis) (see Chap. 253). In addition, delayed-type hypersensitivity responses play important roles in tissue damage in autoimmune diseases such as *rheumatoid arthritis*, *temporal arteritis*, and *Wegener's granulomatosis* (see Chaps. 313 and 319).

AUTOIMMUNE DISEASE Autoimmune disease is characterized by production of either antibodies that react with host tissue or immune effector T cells that are autoreactive to endogenous self-peptides. Because most B cell responses in humans require helper T cells, a B cell autoantibody response generally implies disordered T cell immunoregulatory control. Exceptions to this rule are seen with T cell–independent and anti-idiotypic B cell responses. In some instances, autoantibodies may arise from normal T and B cell responses to foreign organisms or substances that contain antigens, particularly polysaccharides, that cross-react with similar self-antigens in body tissues. This phenomenon is called *molecular mimicry*. Examples of clinically relevant autoantibodies are antibodies against the acetylcholine receptor in *myasthenia gravis* (see Chap. 382) and anti-DNA, antierythrocyte, and antiplatelet antibodies in *systemic lupus erythematosus* (see Chap. 312).

As mentioned above in the description of immunoglobulins, the unique portion of the variable region of the immunoglobulin molecule where antigen binds is called the *idiotype*, and an antibody that reacts specifically with that region is called an *anti-idiotype antibody*. Anti-idiotype antibodies may arise during the course of the normal immune response. For example, anti-idiotypes against antitetanus antibodies develop during normal immunization of humans to tetanus toxoid and serve to deliver "off" signals to B cells secreting antitetanus antibodies. Antibodies may be an important component of the normal immunoregulatory network. Anti-idiotype antibodies also may be relevant to two types of autoimmunity: (1) dysfunction of the idiotype–anti-idiotype antibody system could lead to B cell hyperreactivity by failure to generate "off" signals for B cell differentiation, and (2) some antireceptor antibodies produced in autoimmune diseases (anti-insulin receptor antibodies in forms of type 1 diabetes mellitus and antithyrotropin receptor antibodies in autoimmune thyroid disease) may be anti-idiotype antibodies made against the antibody-combining site (idiotype) of an autoantibody. Despite these mechanistic considerations, the precise role, if any, of anti-idiotype antibodies in human disease remains speculative.

Genetic factors play a role in the genesis of many autoimmune diseases, as shown in studies of familial aggregation and high concordance for disease in monozygotic, but not dizygotic, twins. Based upon analogy to murine autoimmune disorders and on limited human data, polygenic inheritance (e.g., multiple independent genes) of autoimmune susceptibility is likely. It is possible that genetic factors operate via an influence on inherent B or T cell hyperreactivity via presentation of self- or foreign peptides that stimulate an inappropriate antiself response, or via abnormal downregulatory mechanisms. In this regard, many autoimmune disorders are associated with specific haplotypes (e.g., combinations of allelic genes) of the MHC, strongly suggesting that inherited differences in APC molecules or in APC–T cell interactions might influence susceptibility to autoimmunity. The strongest known association between an MHC molecule and an autoimmune disease is the class I molecule HLA-B27 and inflammatory spondyloarthropathy (ankylosing spondylitis) (see Chap. 317). In type 1 diabetes mellitus, a genome-wide search for disease genes has demonstrated that several genes contribute to diabetes, but that MHC-linked genes are the most important. Other genetic association studies have implicated the Ig heavy chain locus in some forms of autoimmunity.

Whereas organ-specific autoimmune diseases are likely the result of the combined effects of several factors that lead to inappropriate targeting of a particular organ or system to immune damage by induction of HEV adhesion molecules for memory and effector lymphocytes, generalized autoimmune diseases such as systemic lupus erythematosus (see Chap. 312) can be thought of as diseases in which there is episodic breakdown of immunologic tolerance to self-molecules. Recent studies have demonstrated that in a mouse model of autoimmunity (the MRL mouse), the cause of autoimmune disease is a defect in a cell surface molecule (fas/APO-1) on T cells that is required for the intrathymic death of autoreactive T lymphocytes. The defective fas/APO-1 molecule prevents negative selection of autoreactive T cells, leading to seeding of peripheral lymphoid organs with excessive numbers of autoreactive T cells. It is thought that rare serious multisystem lupus erythematosus–like syndromes in children may be the human homologues of murine MRL autoimmune disease. Instead of a defect in central (thymic) tolerance, adult acquired systemic lupus erythematosus is more likely to result from a generalized defect in maintenance of peripheral tolerance in which the peripheral immune system lacks the ability to maintain anergy to self-antigens. While the molecules involved in maintenance of peripheral tolerance/anergy to self-antigens are not fully known, recent data suggest that T cell CD28 and B cell B7/BB1 molecules are involved in regulating this process.

THE CELLULAR AND MOLECULAR CONTROL OF PROGRAMMED CELL DEATH (APOPTOSIS) The process of programmed cell death, or apoptosis, plays a crucial role in the tissue organization and modeling that occur during normal embryogenesis and development of many tissues. Induction of apoptosis leads to the removal of superfluous and damaged cells in many cell systems and is particularly critical to regulating normal responses to antigen in the immune system. In general, a wide variety of stimuli trigger cell surface receptors (e.g., TNF receptor family members or related proteins) or cytoplasmic receptors (e.g., ceramide, glucocorticosteroids) that activate groups of proteases such as IL-1β converting enzyme. These proteases either cleave molecules that lead to cell death themselves or activate other enzymes to cleave molecules that eventuate in cell death (Fig. 305-14). The end stages of this sequence of events lead to cell death characterized by degradation of cytoplasmic (actin) and nuclear cytoskeletal proteins as well as cleavage of DNA at regular intervals (nucleosomes), leading to nuclear disintegration seen on electron microscopy and "laddering" of DNA when analysed by agarose

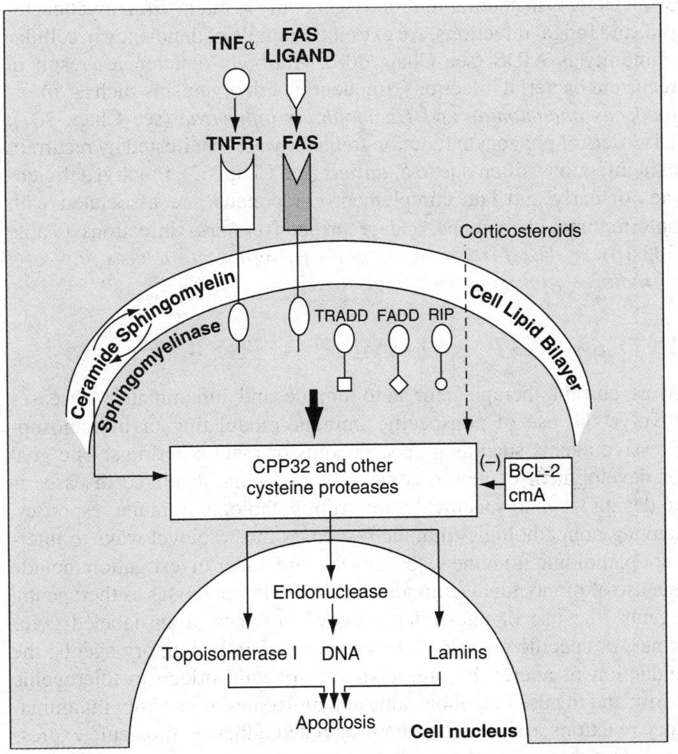

FIGURE 305-14 Pathways that regulate programmed cell death. Ceramide production via fas/APO-1 ligation or other stimuli, ligation of fas or TNFR1, and, for some cell types, stimulation with corticosteroids, can lead to triggering of cytosolic and nuclear proteases that degrade cytoskeletal proteins and DNA, leading to cell death. BCL-2 and crmA are two proteins that inhibit programmed cell death. TRADD, FADD, and RIP are cytoplasmic proteins thought to associate with either TNFR1 or fas via their cytoplasmic domains in the mediation of programmed cell death.

gel electrophoresis. The level of expression of certain cytosolic proteins, such as CrmA and Bcl-2, negatively regulates the process of apoptosis by inhibiting activation of cytosolic proteases that induce cell death. For example, T cells that are negatively selected in the thymus are induced to undergo apoptosis and have low levels of proteins such as Bcl-2, whereas medullary thymocytes that have been triggered to proliferate and survive thymocyte selection (positive selection) have high levels of Bcl-2.

Thus, in the immune system, apoptosis is a mechanism induced to remove autoreactive T cells from the thymus during negative selection, to remove autoreactive B and T cells from peripheral lymphoid organs upon immune cell contact with antigen or antigen-reactive T helper cells in spleen and lymph node, and to remove virus-infected or malignant cells after contact with antigen-specific CD8+ cytotoxic T lymphocytes. Induction of apoptosis is one of two principal mechanisms of target cell lysis by cytotoxic T lymphocytes, the other consisting of the release of cytotoxic perforin molecules.

CLINICAL EVALUATION OF IMMUNE FUNCTION

Clinical assessment of immunity requires investigation of the four major components of the immune system that participate in host defense and in pathogenesis of autoimmune diseases: (1) humoral immunity (B cells); (2) cell-mediated immunity (T cells, monocytes); (3) phagocytic cells of the reticuloendothelial system (macrophages), as well as polymorphonuclear leukocytes; and (4) complement. Clinical problems that require an evaluation of immunity include chronic infections, recurrent infection, unusual infecting agents, and certain autoimmune syndromes. The type of clinical syndrome under evaluation can provide information regarding possible immune defects (see Chap. 307). Defects in cellular immunity generally result in viral, mycobacterial, and fungal infections. An extreme example of deficiency in cellular immunity is AIDS (see Chap. 308). Antibody deficiencies result in recurrent bacterial infections, frequently with organisms such as *Streptococcus pneumoniae* and *Haemophilus influenzae* (see Chap. 307). Disorders of phagocyte function frequently are manifested by recurrent skin infections, often due to *S. aureus* (see Chap. 62). Finally, deficiencies of early and late complement components are associated with autoimmune phenomena and recurrent *Neisseria* infections (Table 305-10). → ***For further discussion of useful initial screening tests of immune function, see Chap. 307.***

INTERVENTIONAL IMMUNOTHERAPY

Most current therapies for autoimmune and inflammatory diseases involve the use of nonspecific immune-modulating or immunosuppressive agents such as glucocorticoids or cytotoxic drugs. The goal of development of new treatments for immune-mediated diseases is to design ways to specifically interrupt pathologic immune responses, leaving nonpathologic immune responses intact. Novel ways to interrupt pathologic immune responses that are under investigation include the use of monoclonal antibodies against T lymphocytes as therapeutic agents; the use of anti-inflammatory cytokines, toxin-labeled cytokines, or specific cytokine inhibitors as anti-inflammatory agents; the induction of anergy by administration of autoantigen in tolerogenic form; and the use of soluble adhesion molecules to interrupt inflammatory reactions associated with upregulated adhesion molecule expression. For some animal models of organ-specific autoimmune disease, the TCR types of pathogenic T cells have been found to be oligoclonal or monoclonal, raising hope that anti-TCR therapy (TCR peptides, inducing anti-TCR antibodies or anti-TCR regulatory T cells) may be feasible. However, to date, pathologic T cells in human autoimmune disease have remained difficult to define, and specific TCR-directed therapy of T cell–mediated autoimmune diseases remains only a theoretical possibility.

Table 305-10

Complement Deficiencies and Associated Diseases

Component	Associated Diseases
CLASSIC PATHWAY	
C1q, C1r, C1s, C4	Immune-complex syndromes,* pyogenic infections
C2	Immune-complex syndromes,* few with pyogenic infections
C1 inhibitor	Rare immune-complex disease, few with pyogenic infections
C3 AND ALTERNATIVE PATHWAY C3	
C3	Immune-complex syndromes,* pyogenic infections
D	Pyogenic infections
Properdin	*Neisseria* infections
I	Pyogenic infections
H	Hemolytic uremic syndrome
MEMBRANE ATTACK COMPLEX	
C5, C6, C7, C8	Recurrent *Neisseria* infections, immune-complex disease
C9	Rare *Neisseria* infections

* Immune-complex syndromes include systemic lupus erythematosus (SLE) and SLE-like syndromes, glomerulonephritis, and vasculitis syndromes.

SOURCE: After JA Schifferli and DK Peters, Lancet 88:957, 1983, with permission.

Immune-based therapy has been used with varying success to enhance host defense mechanisms as well as specific and nonspecific immune responses in a variety of host defense defects and immune deficiency diseases (see Chaps. 62, 307, 308). Of particular note has been the successful use of IFNγ in the treatment of the phagocytic cell defect in chronic granulomatous disease (see Chap. 62). Intermittent infusions of IL-2 in HIV-infected individuals in the early or intermediate stages of disease has resulted in substantial and sustained increases in CD4+ T cells. However, the long-term benefit of this therapeutic modality remains to be determined.

BIBLIOGRAPHY

ABBAS AK et al (eds): *Cellular and Molecular Immunology*, 2d ed. Philadelphia, Saunders, 1994

FINKEL TH et al: T-cell development and transmembrane signaling: Changing biological responses through an unchanging receptor. Immunol Today 12:79, 1991

GIRARD JP, SPRINGER TA: High endothelial venules (HEVs): Specialized endothelium for lymphocyte migration. Immunol Today 16:449, 1995

GLEICH GJ: Eosinophils, basophils and mast cells. J Allergy Clin Immunol 84:1024, 1989

HAYNES BF, DENNING SM: Lymphopoiesis, in *The Molecular Basis of Blood Diseases*, 2d ed, G Stamatoyannopoulos et al (eds). Philadelphia, Saunders, 1993, pp 425–462

HERMAN A et al: Superantigens: Mechanism of T-cell stimulation and the role in immune responses. Annu Rev Immunol 9:745, 1991

JANEWAY CA, TRAVERS P (eds): *Immunobiology. The Immune System in Health and Disease.* New York, Garland, 1994

KAYE PM: Costimulation and the regulation of anti-microbial immunity. Immunol Today 16:423, 1995

KELLEY WN et al (eds): *Textbook of Rheumatology*, 4th ed. Philadelphia, Saunders, 1993, chaps. 6, 7, 10, 13, 15, 16

MARTIN SJ, GREEN DR: Protease activation during apoptosis: Death by a thousand cuts. Cell 82:349, 1995

PAUL WE (ed): *Fundamental Immunology*, 2d ed. New York, Raven, 1989

RETH M et al: The B-cell antigen receptor complex. Immunol Today 12:196, 1991

ROBEY E, ALLISON JP: T-cell activation: Integration of signals from the antigen receptor and costimulatory molecules. Immunol Today 16:306, 1995

ROLINK A et al: B-cell development in mouse and man. The Immunologist 3:125, 1995

SPRINGER TA: Traffic signals for lymphocyte recirculation and leukocyte emigration: The multistep paradigm. Cell 76:301, 1994

WEISS A, LITTMAN DR: Signal transduction by lymphocyte antigen receptors. Cell 76:263, 1995

306 THE MAJOR HISTOCOMPATIBILITY GENE COMPLEX

Charles B. Carpenter

Antigenic differences between members of a species are called *alloantigens*, and when these play a determining role in the rejection of allogeneic tissue grafts, they are called *histocompatibility antigens*. Evolution has conserved a single closely linked region of histocompatibility genes, the products of which are prominently displayed on cell surfaces and provide a strong barrier to allotransplantation. The terms *major histocompatibility antigens* and *major histocompatibility gene complex* (MHC) refer to the gene products and genes of this chromosomal region. Their principal function is to bind peptide fragments of potentially pathogenic microbes and present them to T lymphocytes for recognition. Cell-surface antigen receptors on T lymphocytes [T cell receptors (TCR)] are virtually identical for each member of a clone, and they engage antigenic peptide fragments that have been previously bound to MHC molecules. Direct TCR binding to peptides in solution, or to antigenic determinants present on the surface of an intact protein molecule, does not occur. Much of the early evidence for MHC genetic control of the immune response came from work in animal models in which immune response genes were mapped within the mouse (H-2), rat (RT1), and guinea pig (GPLA) MHC. The response to a given antigenic determinant is now known to require the binding of the appropriate peptide fragment to an MHC molecule. In humans, the MHC is called HLA and is located on the short arm of chromosome 6. The individual letters of HLA have various unofficial meanings, and by international agreement HLA is the logo for the human MHC.

Several generalizations can be made about the MHC. *First*, three classes of gene products are encoded within the 4000-kilobase region of HLA. Class I molecules, expressed on virtually all cell surfaces, consist of one heavy and one light polypeptide chain and are the products of three reduplicated loci: HLA-A, HLA-B, and HLA-C. Class II molecules, restricted in expression to B lymphocytes, dendritic cells, monocytes, antigen-activated T lymphocytes, and to epithelial and endothelial cells that have been activated by interferon, consist of two noncovalently linked polypeptide chains (α and β) of unequal length. They are the products of several closely linked genes, collectively termed the *HLA-D region*. The class II heterodimers form a structure similar to that of class I. Class III molecules are the C4, C2, and Bf components of complement and share little structural similarity to classes I and II. *Second*, the expressed MHC genes in the thymus play a crucial role in the selection of the T cell receptor repertoire during maturation. Various self-peptide + MHC combinations promote survival or elimination of newly formed T cells. Clones with too high or too low an affinity to MHC are eliminated. Self versus nonself discrimination, based upon moderate affinity to self-peptide + MHC, is thereby imprinted on the T cell repertoire, providing the means for selective, also called restricted, recognition of peptides bound to self-peptide + MHC molecules. *Third*, genes for enzyme systems having no apparent relationship to immunity are located in the region of the MHC, as are genes of importance in skeletal growth and development. *Fourth*, genes for tumor necrosis factor (TNF) α and TNFβ, heat shock protein (Hsp_{70}), and peptide processing (LMP) and transport (TAP) lie also within the MHC (Fig. 306-1).

In contrast to the single linkage group for the MHC, many *minor* histocompatibility antigen genes are encoded throughout the genome. They represent weaker allotypic differences on molecules that serve functions apparently unrelated to the immune system, except that they can be a target for rejection of transplants. Whereas the MHC is a powerful stimulus to the immune system during a primary response, minor histocompatibility differences can be of clinical significance only after priming has occurred. Antibody responses to minor histocompatibility antigens are generally weak or absent, whereas cytotoxic CD8+ T cell responses, restricted to presentation of peptides derived from minor antigens by self-peptide + MHC molecules, are common.

LOCI OF THE HLA SYSTEM **Class I Antigens** HLA antigens of the class I type are defined serologically by human immune sera, principally from multiparous females, and to a limited extent by monoclonal antibodies. They are present in varying densities in most body tissues, including B cells, T cells, and platelets, but not in mature red blood cells. CD8+ T cells preferentially bind to MHC class I molecules via a CD8 binding site on class I. The number of serologically defined specificities is large, and the HLA system is the most polymorphic genetic system known in humans. Three clearly defined loci are recognized within the HLA complex for class I HLA antigens. Each class I antigen consists of an 11.5-kDa β_2-microglobulin subunit and a 44-kDa heavy chain that carries the antigenic specificities (Fig. 306-2). There are over 80 serologically defined A and B specificities, and 8 C-locus specificities are known. Antigens of the major complex are prefixed by HLA, but this may be omitted when the context is

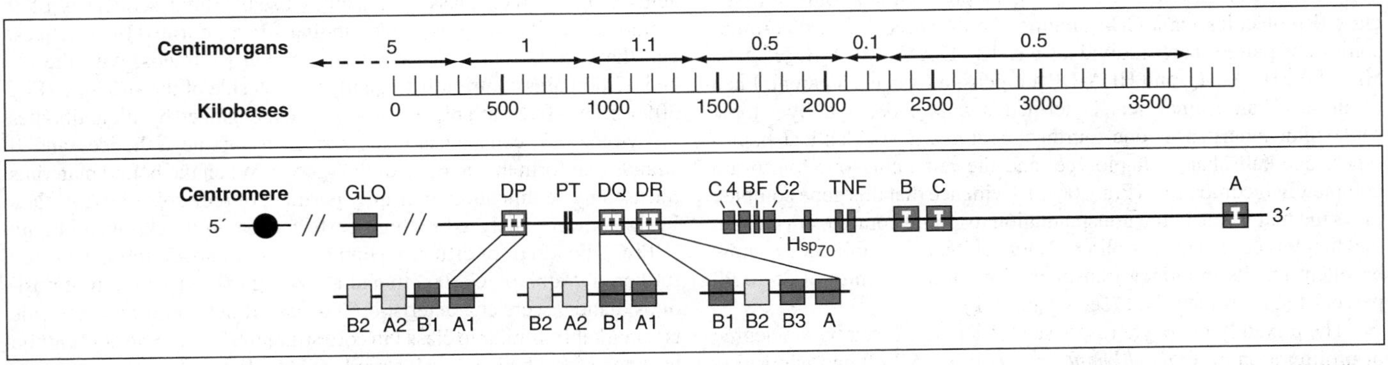

FIGURE 306-1 Schematic representation of human chromosome 6 showing the location of the HLA region in the 21 region of the short arm. The HLA-A, -B, and -C loci encode class I heavy chains (44 kDa), while the β_2-microglobulin light chain (11.5 kDa) of the class I molecule is encoded by genes of chromosome 15. HLA-D region (class II) is centromeric to the A, B, and C loci, with genes for closely linked complement components C4A, C4B, Bf, and C2 in the B–D region. Two genes for tumor necrosis factor (TNFα,β) also lie between HLA-B and the complement genes. The order of the complement genes is uncertain. Additional loci shown are P for the proteosome (LMP) and T for the peptide transporter (TAP) genes and the Hsp_{70} heat-shock protein gene. Each D region class II molecule is made up of an α and β chain (their genes are written as A and B). They appear on the cell surface in distinct heterodimers, DP, DQ, and DR. The numbers following A or B indicate that there are different genes for the chains of a given set; e.g., for DR, there are 9 β-chain genes (three are shown). The expressed molecule may be β1α(B1A) or β3α(B3A), for example. The β2 gene is not expressed (pseudogene). The antigens DR51, DR52, and DR53 are on the expressed B5, B3, and B4 chains, respectively, while the other DR antigens are on B1. DRA is not polymorphic, while the molecules bearing the DQ antigens have polymorphism in both A1 and B1 chains. DQA2 and DQB2 are pseudogenes. Polymorphism in DP is greater for B1 than for A1. The overall length of the HLA region is about 3 cM (3400 kilobases).

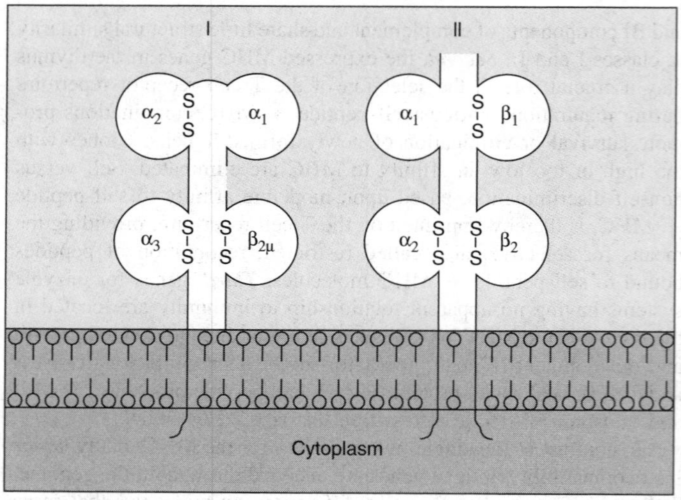

FIGURE 306-2 Schematic representation of class I and class II molecules on the cell surface. Class I molecules are composed of two polypeptide chains. The 44-kDa heavy chain passes through the plasma membrane. Its external portion consists of three domains (α_1, α_2, α_3) formed by disulfide bonding. The β_2-microglobulin ($\beta_{2\mu}$) light chain (11.5 kDa) encoded by chromosome 15 is noncovalently bound to the heavy chain. Amino acid sequence homology among class I molecules is 80 to 85 percent, falling to 50 percent or less in portions of α_1 and α_2 that represent the sites of alloantigenic polymorphism. Class II molecules consist of two noncovalently associated polypeptide chains, a 34-kDa α and a 29-kDa β. Each chain has two domains formed by disulfide bridging (the α_1 domains lack a sulfide bridge). (*From Carpenter and Strom.*)

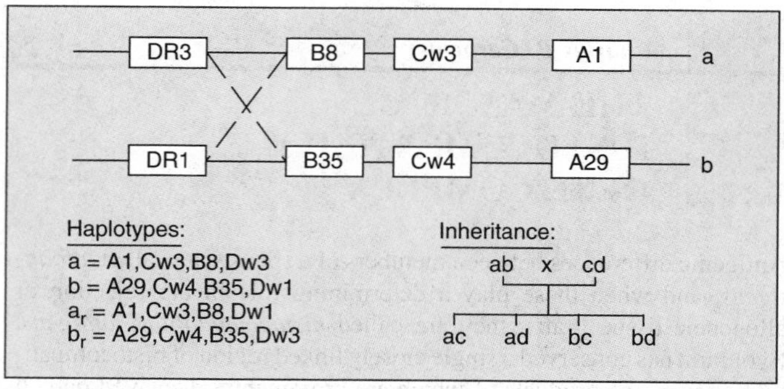

FIGURE 306-3 HLA region, chromosome 6: inheritance of HLA haplotypes. Each chromosomal segment of linked genes is termed a *haplotype*, and each individual inherits one haplotype from each parent. The A, B, C, and D antigens of haplotypes a and b are shown for this hypothetical individual in chromosomal order on the diagram and also below as they would be written in text. If individual ab were to marry cd, their offspring would be of four types only, as far as HLA is concerned. Occasionally (*dashed cross*) recombination occurs in the germ line (meiosis) of a parent, resulting in an altered haplotype. The frequency of recombinant children is a measure of the map distance (1 percent recombination frequency = 1 cM; see Fig. 306-1). (*From CB Carpenter, Kidney Int 14:283, 1978.*)

clear. The number following the locus designation is the name of the antigen (e.g., HLA-A2). HLA antigens of African, Asian, and Oceanic peoples include many of the antigens commonly found in people of western European ancestry. However, the distribution of HLA antigens is distinctive for certain racial groups and can serve as anthropologic markers in the study of migration patterns and diseases.

Class II Antigens The HLA-D region is separated from the class I loci on the short arm of chromosome 6 by 1000 kilobases (see Fig. 306-1). This region encodes a series of class II molecules, each consisting of a 29-kDa β chain and a 34-kDa α chain (see Fig. 306-2). Incompatibility for this region, particularly concerning the DR antigens, determines the in vitro proliferative response of lymphocytes to mismatched haplotypes. CD4+ T cells preferentially bind to MHC class II molecules via a CD4 binding site on class II. Since chromosomes are paired, each individual has 12 HLA-A, HLA-B, HLA-C, HLA-DR, HLA-DQ, and HLA-DP antigens, 6 from each parent. Each of these chromosomal sets is termed a *haplotype*, and by simple Mendelian inheritance, one-fourth of siblings have identical haplotypes, one-half share a haplotype, and the remaining one-fourth are completely incompatible (Fig. 306-3). Evidence that this gene complex plays the major role in the transplantation response comes from the fact that haplotype-matched sibling donor-recipient combinations show excellent results in kidney transplantation, in the vicinity of 85 to 90 percent long-term survival (see Chap. 272).

The mixed lymphocyte response (MLR) is assessed by the degree of proliferation of a *mixed lymphocyte culture* (MLC) and is positive even when HLA-A, HLA-B, and HLA-C antigens are identical (see Fig. 306-3). When parental recombination has occurred between HLA-B and -DR, for example, a new haplotype appears in the child, who will be identical for class I but different for class II (a versus a_r in Fig. 306-3). HLA-D antigens are defined by stimulation with reference lymphocytes that are homozygous for HLA-D and are inactivated by x-irradiation or mitomycin C to make the reaction unidirectional. There are over 35 such antigens recognized by homozygous typing cells.

Attempts to define HLA-D by serology first established a series of D-related (DR) antigens expressed on class II molecules of B lymphocytes, monocytes, and activated T lymphocytes. Macrophages, dendritic cells, and skin Langerhans cells are also class II–positive. There are 22 DR, 8 DQ, and 8 DP antigens recognized by serology. The class II gene map shown in Fig. 306-1 describes a minimal number of genes and molecular sets. Although a class II molecule may be composed of a DQα (DQA1 gene) from one parental haplotype and a DQβ (DQB1 gene) from the other parent (transcomplementation), α and β combinations among DP, DQ, and DR sets rarely, if ever, occur. DR, and to some extent DQ, molecules provide the stimuli for the primary MLR. A second round of MLR stimulation in culture (secondary MLR) is called the *primed lymphocyte test* (PLT) and occurs rapidly over 24 to 36 h instead of 6 to 7 days. DP alloantigens were discovered from their ability to provide PLT stimulation, although they do not contribute much to a primary MLR. DQ and DP molecules also can be identified serologically. While B lymphocytes and activated T lymphocytes express all three sets of class II molecules, DQ antigens are not expressed on 60 to 90 percent of monocytes, which are virtually all DP- and DR-positive.

Three-Dimensional Structure of HLA X-ray diffraction studies of crystallized HLA class I molecules show a groove or cleft on the surface facing away from the cell membrane with dimensions sufficient to bind a linearly extended peptide fragment 8 to 15 amino acids long. In fact, class I molecules usually bind sequences of 9 amino acids. The margins of the binding site are formed by α helices, and the base is floored by eight antiparallel β strands, with the $\alpha1$ and $\alpha2$ domains contributing equally to each side of the structure (Fig. 306-4). The HLA variable regions that are recognized by alloantibodies or cytotoxic T cells lie along the surfaces of the α helices and β strands that form the margins of the groove. When the bound materials released by acidification of affinity purified, or redissolved, HLA class I crystals were analyzed by high-performance liquid chromatography (HPLC), hundreds of different peptides were found. Of those analyzed further, a 9-amino-acid length and a binding consensus motif at positions 2 and 9 were characteristic. The class II heterodimeric molecule is remarkably similar to class I in core structure. The amino acid carbon backbone for α helices and β strands of class II is superimposable upon that of class I. Therefore, the overall size and shape of the binding grooves are the same, and the class II polymorphic regions are also arrayed along the margins of the α helices and β strands. The main difference is that the ends of the class II groove are more open, allowing peptides as long as 26 amino acids to bind.

Antigen Processing T lymphocyte receptors bind efficiently only to peptide fragments of proteins presented in the groove of a self-MHC molecule. Virtually all MHC molecules come to the surface of the cell with a peptide in place. These peptides may have originated from an intracellular or extracellular source. In the case of class I, the pathway is primarily one of selection of peptides generated from endogenous proteins within the cytosolic compartment (e.g., from intracellular viral infection); for class II, the pathway is primarily an exogenous one that processes endocytosed or pinocytosed proteins. Any cell that expresses MHC class II can serve as an antigen-presenting cell (APC) to CD4+ lymphocytes; in addition, the macrophage can also process exogenous proteins into the class I pathway for presentation to CD8+ lymphocytes, thereby providing a means for activating both CD4+ and CD8+ subsets to fragments of the same antigen.

Cytosolic proteins subject to proteolysis include normal cellular constituents, including self-peptide + MHC molecules, and foreign invaders such as viruses. Proteosome genes mapped to the class II region of the MHC (Fig. 306-1) encode cytosolic structures that cleave proteins into short peptides (8 to 9 amino acids); however, these particular genes (LMP2 and LMP7) do not account for all the immunogenic peptides formed in the cytosol. A heterodimeric channel encoded by TAP1 and TAP2 genes then transports peptides to the endoplasmic reticulum (ER) where binding to class I heavy chains and association with β_2-microglobulin complete the class I assembly before transport to the cell surface. The class II pathway utilizes proteases in acidic endocytic vesicles to produce random proteolysis of ingested proteins. The peptide-rich endosome then fuses with the ER where class II assembly occurs. The 13- to 26-amino-acid length of peptides eluted from class II molecules frequently consists of a nested set of sequences of various lengths, having a consensus binding region of 9 or so amino acids, and variably sized tails at either end of the groove. Eluted class II bound peptides also contain a high proportion of self-MHC fragments.

Understanding the precise topography of TCR binding to MHC + peptide awaits the full crystal structure of the α and β chains of the TCR; however, sequence analysis of TCR genes indicates three hypervariable regions (CDR) for each chain. A likely model is that the CDR-1 and CDR-2 regions of the TCR α chain bind to one of the MHC α helices, while the analogous CDRs of the TCR β chain bind to the other MHC α helix. Both CDR-3 regions would, by this model, contact the peptide. Alternatively, it may be possible that all contact points are to portions of the MHC α helices, the shape of which is modified by the peptide.

Molecular Genetics Each polypeptide chain of class I and class II molecules bears several polymorphic sites. The "private" antigen (e.g., B27 or B35) defined by alloantisera frequently depends upon more than one site on the face of the molecule. In the *cell-mediated lympholysis* (CML) test, the specificity of killer T cells (T_c), which arise during the proliferative events in MLR, is determined by testing on target cells from donors other than those providing the MLR stimulus. Antigen systems defined by this method show a close but imperfect correlation with class I private antigens. Cloning of cytotoxic cells has revealed the presence of a variety of polymorphic target determinants on HLA molecules, some of which are identifiable by alloantisera or monoclonal antibodies derived from immunization of mice with human cells. Some of these reagents can be used to identify private determinants of HLA, while others are directed to more "public" (sometimes called *supertypic*) determinants. The latter are epitopes found to be identical on molecules that have different private specificities. One such system of public HLA-B antigens has two alleles, Bw4 and Bw6. Most HLA-B private antigens are associated with either Bw4 or Bw6. HLA-B–bearing heavy chains carry additional sites that are common to B7, B27, B22, and B40, and others to B5, B15, B18, and B35. Other types of shared antigenic determinants exist, as exemplified by a monoclonal antibody that reacts with a site shared between HLA-A and HLA-B heavy chains. Increasingly, these complexities are more easily resolved by analysis of DNA sequences than by serology.

When genomic DNA for HLA is examined, typical exon-intron sequences of DNA have been found for class I and class II, exons having been identified for signal peptides (5′), each of the domains, a transmembrane hydrophobic segment, and a cytoplasmic segment (3′). cDNA probes are available for most of the HLA chains, and enzymatic digests have been used to study patterns of *restriction fragment length polymorphisms* (RFLP), many of which correlate with class II serologic and MLR patterns. There are 20 to 30 class I genes, however, making assessment of polymorphism by RFLP difficult. Many of these genes are not expressed (pseudogenes), while some could represent additional class I loci that are expressed only on activated T cells and are of uncertain function. Tissue typing by the detection of variable nucleotide sequences begins with the polymerase

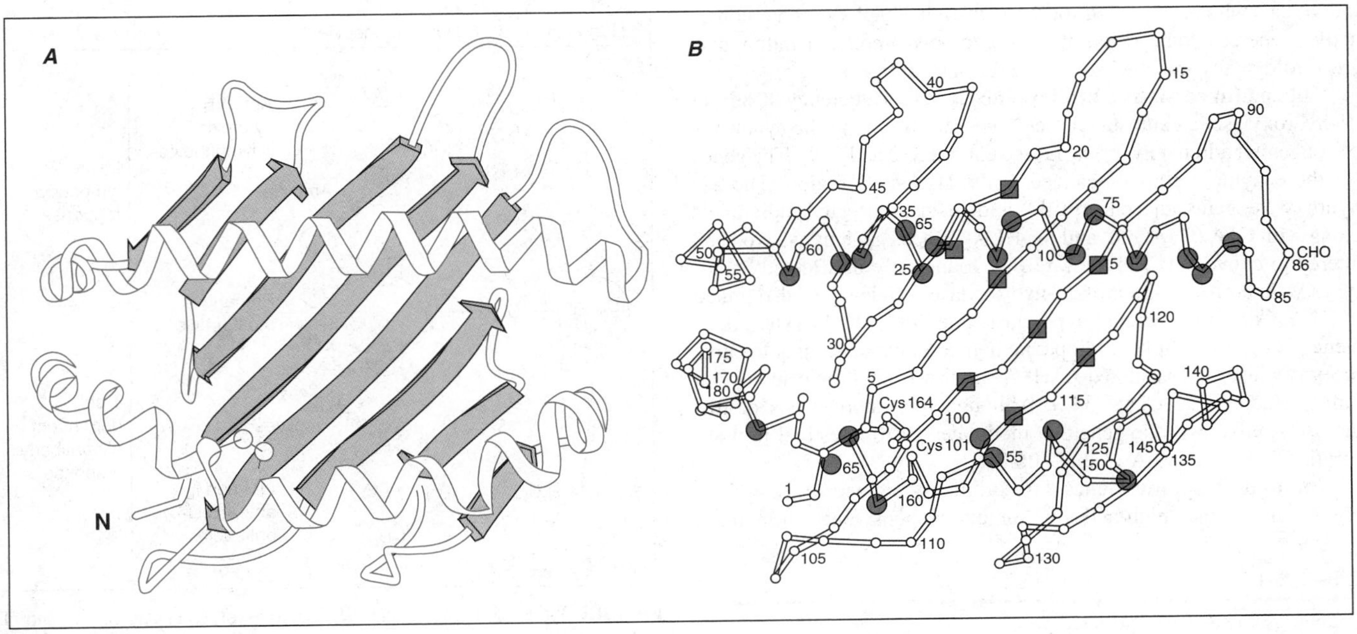

FIGURE 306-4 Structure of the HLA class I molecule as determined by x-ray crystallography. *A.* Shown is the face of the HLA-A2 molecule that points away from the cell surface. This ribbon diagram shows the groove that is formed by two α helices and is supported by a floor of eight β strands. N is the amino terminal of the α_1 domain; the two small circles represent a disulfide bond. *B.* Composite display of polymorphic sites from several human and mouse class I alleles using the HLA-A2 structure as the model. The symbols show a composite of the polymorphisms along the groove. Localization of variable amino acids and/or sites for alloantibody and/or cytotoxic T cell recognition is shown to be along the α helices (*circles*). Polymorphic sites exist also in the β strands (*squares*). The numbers indicate the amino acid sequence. (*After PJ Bjorkman et al.*)

chain reaction (PCR) technique to amplify specific segments of DNA, as defined by oligonucleotide primers, from genomic DNA obtained from a small sample of blood or tissue. The primers are usually locus-specific (e.g., the β1 chain of HLA-DR) or may be allele-specific (e.g., amplifying only genes having a particular polymorphic sequence). The products are then analyzed by hybridization with sequence-specific labeled probes or by RFLP analysis of the amplified DNA. The technique has already demonstrated ability to identify sequences in the human population in a more accurate fashion than with the established serologic technique. The official HLA nomenclature has been changed to reflect the definition of distinct sequences and to document the presence of polymorphisms not previously appreciated from the definitions of classical serology. To illustrate, HLA-DR1 is written as DRB1*0101. DRB1 indicates the β1 chain of the DR locus, and *0101 indicates that it is antigen 1, first variant. In similar fashion, DQA1*0302 indicates the α1 chain of the DQ locus, antigen 3, variant 2. Many recent observations of disease associations with HLA antigens use this more precise nomenclature in order to define the molecular basis for peptide binding, as well as to provide better genetic markers for ethnic and population diversity. Molecular typing for HLA-DR is proving to be of value in clinical typing for organ and bone marrow transplantation.

Complement (Class III) Structural genes for three complement components, C4, C2, and Bf (factor B), are present in the HLA-BD region (see Fig. 306-1). There are two loci for C4, coding for C4A and C4B, formerly recognized as the Rodgers and Chido red blood cell antigens, respectively. These antigens are, in fact, adsorbed plasma C4 molecules. Other complement components are not closely linked to HLA. No crossovers have been found between the C2, Bf, and C4 loci. They are all encoded within a 100-kilobase segment between HLA-B and HLA-DR. There are two alleles of C2, four of Bf, seven of C4A, and three of C4B, plus blanks (null genes) for each locus (QO). The extensive polymorphism of complement types (complotypes) makes them useful for genetic studies. The four most common extended haplotypes found in people of western European ancestry are shown in Table 306-1. Such identical extended haplotypes may be conserved from a common ancestor. MLRs between unrelated individuals who are matched for these extended haplotypes are nonreactive, whereas some reactivity is common if unrelated individuals are serologically matched for only HLA-DR antigens.

Other Linked Sixth-Chromosome Genes Deficiency of steroid 21-hydroxylase, an autosomal recessive trait, results in the syndrome of congenital adrenal hyperplasia (see Chaps. 332 and 339). The genes for the enzyme are also localized in the HLA-B-D region. The 21-hydroxylase gene adjacent to C4A is deleted in affected individuals along with C4A (C4AQO), and the HLA-B locus gene may have been altered to convert B13 to the rare B47 found only in affected haplotypes. A late-onset variant of 21-hydroxylase deficiency is also linked to HLA. Congenital adrenal hyperplasia due to 11β-hydroxylase deficiency is not HLA-linked. Idiopathic hemochromatosis, an autosomal recessive disorder, is linked to HLA, as has been shown in several family studies (see Chap. 342). Although the pathogenesis of this disease is unknown, the gene that modulates gastrointestinal iron absorption is near HLA-A (Table 306-2).

Immune-Response Genes As originally defined in the guinea pig and the mouse, high and low immune responsiveness to haptens or synthetic peptide motifs was shown to be determined by genes in the region of the MHC. It is now clear that these genes encode the class II molecules and that the ability to bind the relevant antigen is the major determinant of a strong T cell–dependent response initiated by CD4+ T cells. Class I genes are also important in the effector phases of a response, especially with regard to recognition by CD8+ T cells of foreign peptide bound to class I molecules. For example, human cell lines infected with the influenza virus are lysed by immune cytotoxic T cells (T_c) only if a class I (HLA-A or HLA-B) antigen is shared between the attacking and target cells. Class I and II molecules are said to be the *restriction elements* in immune responsiveness because they must be able to bind and present peptide fragments properly to T cells. In the allogeneic response, there is evidence that recognition may be of either the amino acid differences on the external face of the intact MHC molecule or of an MHC peptide fragment presented by a responder strain MHC molecule. In this special case, instead of restricting the response, the MHC antigenic differences become the stimulus. In transplantation, the induction and effector phases of a rejection response follow the general rules of CD4+ T_H (T helper cell) and CD8+ T_c interacting with MHC class II and I, respectively (Fig. 306-5). Although B lymphocytes can be directly activated via their surface immunoglobulin receptors, they also express high concen-

Table 306-1

Common Extended HLA Haplotypes

HLA-B	HLA-DR	Bf	C2	C4A	C4B
8	3	S	C	QO	1
7	2	S	C	3	1
57	7	S	C	6	1
44	7	F	C	3	1

Table 306-2

Linkage of Genetic Defects to HLA

	Gene Location	Common Haplotype Found
C2 deficiency	HLA-B-D	A25, B18, BfS, DR2
21-OH deficiency	HLA-B-D	A3, B47, BfF, DR7
21-OH deficiency (late onset)	HLA-B-D	B14, BfS, DR1
Idiopathic hemochromatosis	HLA-A	A3, B14
Paget's disease	HLA-A-D	
Spinocerebellar ataxia	HLA-A-D	
Hodgkin's disease	HLA-A-D	

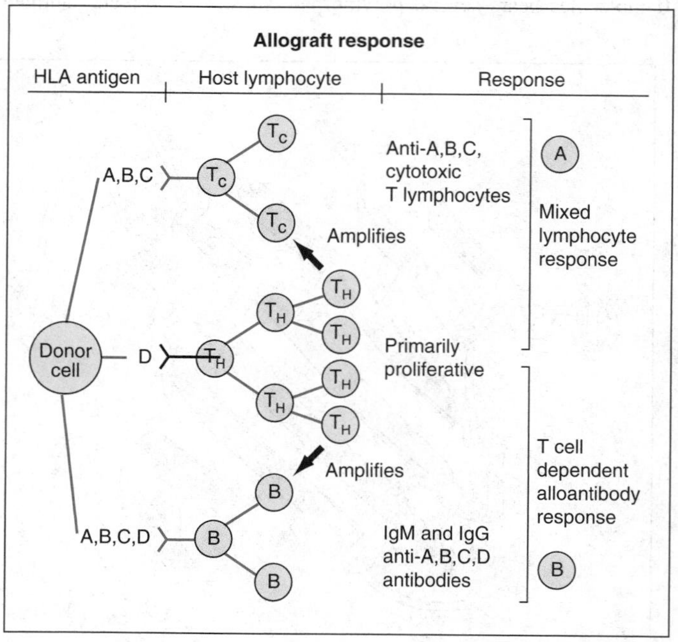

FIGURE 306-5 Schema of the relative roles of HLA-A, -B, -C, and -D antigens in initiation of the alloimmune response and in the development of effector cells and antibodies. Two main classes of T lymphocytes recognize antigens: T_c, the precursors to the cytotoxic "killer" cells, and T_H, the helper cells for amplification of the cytotoxic response. T_H also provide help to B lymphocytes for production of a fully mature IgG response. Note that T_c generally recognize class I antigens, while the T_H signal is provided by antigens of the HLA-D region (class II). (*From CB Carpenter, Kidney Int 14:283, 1978.*)

trations of class I and II molecules and can process antigens for presentation on the cell surface. It is the response of the T cell to such antigen presentation that provides the "help" required for a mature IgG secretory response by the B cells.

DISEASE ASSOCIATIONS Not all genes involved in regulating the immune response are in the MHC region. It is nevertheless a fact that most human inflammatory diseases thought to have some autoimmune basis are in some way promoted by genes of the HLA region. In most cases, these are *associations* of particular HLA antigens in populations of individuals with certain diseases. Since it is becoming apparent that the extensive polymorphism of the MHC is directly related to the ability of a given molecule to bind a particular peptide sequence, the critical biologic function of MHC polymorphism may be to ensure survival of the species in relation to the large numbers of microbiologic agents present in the environment. Self-tolerance that happens to crossreact with microbiologic agents would produce a high degree of susceptibility, resulting in lethal infection, whereas the polymorphism of the HLA system ensures that some individuals in segments of the human population will recognize offending agents as foreign and initiate the appropriate response. The value of the MHC for species survival is of such importance that there is need for local mechanisms, not entirely understood, to prevent allorecognition in the special case of pregnancy. The extent to which the MHC plays a role in immune surveillance against neoplasia and whether such a role contributes to survival in an evolutionary sense are not established.

Table 306-3 summarizes the most significant HLA and disease associations. Overall, the mechanisms in the induction of these diseases are not yet explained. It should be noted that such associations do not in themselves prove that variations in antigen presentation to T cells is necessarily at the root of autoimmunity. It also can be that HLA genes are markers for haplotypes in which mutations have occurred in other linked genes. A possible example of effects of linked genes is the recent observation that insulin-dependent diabetes is associated with a low density of MHC class I molecules on the patient's cells, explained by a defect in TAP peptide transporters. Since the genes for the latter map to the HLA class II region (Fig. 306-1), associations of diabetes with class II antigens could in part be on this basis.

Most striking is the increased frequency of HLA-B27 in certain rheumatic diseases, particularly ankylosing spondylitis, a condition

Table 306-3

HLA Antigens and Disease, Showing the Most Highly Associated Antigens

Disease	Antigen	Relative Risk*
RHEUMATIC		
Ankylosing spondylitis	B27	69.1
Reiter's syndrome	B27	37.0
Acute anterior uveitis	B27	8.2
Reactive arthritis (*Yersinia*, *Salmonella*, gonococcus)	B27	18.0
Psoriatic arthritis, central	B27	10.7
	B38	9.1
Psoriatic arthritis, peripheral	B27	2.0
	B38	6.5
Juvenile rheumatoid arthritis	B27	3.9
	DR8	3.6
Juvenile arthritis, pauciarticular	DR5	3.3
Rheumatoid arthritis	Dw4/DR4	3.8
Sjögren's syndrome	Dw3	5.7
Systemic lupus erythematosus		
Caucasian	DR3	2.6
Japanese	DR2	5.3
Chinese	DQ3	11.5
Systemic lupus erythematosus (hydralazine)	DR4	5.6
GASTROINTESTINAL		
Gluten-sensitive enteropathy	DR3	11.6
Chronic active hepatitis	DR3	6.8
Ulcerative colitis	B5	3.8
HEMATOLOGIC		
Idiopathic hemochromatosis	A3	6.7
	B14	2.7
	A3, B14	90.0
Pernicious anemia	DR5	5.4
Hodgkin's disease		
Caucasian	DP3	2.0
Japanese	DP4	0.2
SKIN		
Dermatitis herpetiformis	Dw3	17.3
Psoriasis vulgaris	Cw6	7.5
Psoriasis vulgaris (Japanese)	Cw6	8.5
Pemphigus vulgaris (Jews)	DR4	14.6
	A26	4.8
Behçet's disease		
Caucasian	B5	3.8
Japanese	B51	12.4
Chinese	B51	5.5
ENDOCRINE		
Type 1 diabetes mellitus	DR4	3.6
	DR3	4.8
	DR2	0.2
	BfF1	15.0
Hyperthyroidism (Graves')	B8	2.5
	DR3	3.7
Hyperthyroidism (Japanese)	B35	4.4
	A2	2.2
	DP5	4.4
	A2 + DP5	10.5
Adrenal insufficiency	Dw3	10.5
Subacute thyroiditis (de Quervain)	B35	13.7
Hashimoto's thyroiditis	DR5	3.2
Congenital adrenal hyperplasia	B47	15.4
NEUROLOGIC		
Myasthenia gravis	B8	2.7
	DR3	2.5
Multiple sclerosis	DR2	6.0
Manic-depressive disorder	B16	2.3
Narcolepsy	DR2	130.0
Schizophrenia	A28	2.3
RENAL		
Idiopathic membranous glomerulonephritis	DR3	5.7
Goodpasture's syndrome (anti-GBM)	DR2	15.9
Minimal change disease (steroid response)	B12	4.2
Polycystic kidney disease	B5	2.6
IgA nephropathy		
Caucasian	DR2	0.6
French, Japanese	DR4	3.1
Gold nephropathy	DR3	14.0
	DR4	0.3
INFECTIOUS		
Tuberculoid leprosy (Asians)	B8	6.8
Paralytic polio	B16	4.3
Low vs. high response to vaccinia virus	Cw3	12.7
IMMUNODEFICIENCY		
IgA deficiency (blood donors)	DR3	13.0

$$* \text{ Relative risk} = \frac{(\text{\% antigen-positive patients})(\text{\% antigen-negative controls})}{(\text{\% antigen-negative patients})(\text{\% antigen-positive controls})}.$$

with a strong familial tendency. B27 is present in about 7 percent of people of western European ancestry, while it appears in 80 to 90 percent of patients with ankylosing spondylitis. Expressed as a relative risk, the antigen B27 confers a susceptibility to the development of ankylosing spondylitis that is 69 times that in the general population. Similarly, acute anterior uveitis, Reiter's syndrome, and reactive arthritis to at least three bacterial infections (*Yersinia*, *Salmonella*, and gonococcus) show a high degree of association with B27. Although the ordinary form of juvenile rheumatoid arthritis (JRA) also shows a similar association with B27, the pauciarticular form of JRA with iritis is DR5-associated. The increased incidence of B27 in psoriatic arthritis is also significant for the central type (axial skeleton) of the disorder, while B38 is associated with both the central and peripheral types. Psoriasis is associated with Cw6. Patients with degenerative arthritis or gout show no alteration in antigen frequencies.

Most other disease associations are with HLA-D region antigens. The rheumatoid arthritis associations with DR4 involve 3 of the 22 DR4 variants (DRB1*0401, *0404, and *0405), as well as DRB1*0101 and DRB1*1402 in some ethnic groups. Such specificity adds weight to the argument for disease being the result of binding and presentation of particular peptides. Narcolepsy is virtually 100 percent associated with DR2 in both Japanese and Caucasians. Affected individuals need inherit only a single gene dose of DR2. Although there is no apparent autoimmune component to this condition, there is speculation that an abnormality in a neurotransmitter or its receptor may be influenced by the DR2 gene or another closely linked gene. Gluten-sensitive enteropathy (celiac disease, nontropical sprue) in children and adults is associated with DR3 (relative risk = 12). Recent DNA typing shows a higher relative risk of 52 with DQA1*0501 and DQB1*0201. The actual percentage of such patients having DR3 ranges from 63 to 96 percent compared with 22 to 27 percent of controls. The same antigen is also present in increased frequency in patients with chronic active hepatitis and in patients with dermatitis herpetiformis who also have gluten-sensitive enteropathy. Juvenile-onset insulin-dependent diabetes mellitus (type 1) is associated with DR4 and DR3 and is negatively associated with DR2. Resistance to type 1 diabetes is strongly associated with the inheritance of aspartate at position 57 of the β chain of HLA-DQ, in linkage disequilibrium with HLA-DR2. Other amino acids at position 57, especially when HLA-DR3 or -DR4 are on the same haplotype, are associated with an increased risk of disease. Recent studies show that not having aspartate at position 57 of DQB1 of both haplotypes confers a relative risk for type 1 diabetes of 7.4, whereas a single or double dose of aspartate at position 57, as with DQB1*0601 or *0602, provides protection (relative risk of 0.2). A rare allele of Bf (F1) is also found in 17 to 25 percent of patients with type 1 diabetes. Maturity-onset diabetes is not HLA-associated. Hyperthyroidism is an example of a disease in which racial differences display different HLA associations, in contrast with rheumatoid arthritis and type 1 diabetes, in which the DR4 associations are more universal. The common DR2 and DQ haplotype found in normal individuals (DRB1*1501, DQA1*0102, DQB1*0602) is also most commonly increased in multiple sclerosis. Renal diseases strongly HLA-DR–associated are Goodpasture's syndrome due to an autoantibody to glomerular basement membrane (DR2); idiopathic membranous glomerulonephritis (DR3 in Caucasians, DR2 in Japanese), which involves antibodies to an antigen of the glomerulus; and gold-induced nephritis (DR3). Studies of HLA associations with AIDS suggest that HLA-B35 is a risk factor for more rapid progression of the disease (see Chap. 308).

LINKAGE DISEQUILIBRIUM The most salient feature of population genetics of HLA antigens is the random distribution of HLA antigens within a given racial or ethnic group. The term *linkage disequilibrium* means that antigens of closely linked loci appear together more frequently than predicted by random association. In other words, nonrandom distribution of HLA antigens occasionally is found. The classic example is the frequency of the A-locus antigen HLA-A1 and the B-locus antigen HLA-B8 in people of western European ancestry. The coincidence of A1 and B8 should be the product of their individual gene frequencies ($0.17 \times 0.11 \cong 0.02$). The observed frequency of A1 and B8 is 0.08, four times that expected, an increase of 0.06. The latter value is termed Δ (delta) and is a measure of the disequilibrium. Other A- and B-locus haplotype disequilibria have been recognized and include (A3, B7), (A2, B12), (A29, B12), and (A11, B35). Furthermore, some D-region determinants are in linkage disequilibrium with B-locus antigens (e.g., DR3 and B8), as are some B- and C-locus antigens. Serologically defined HLA antigens can serve as markers for the genes of an entire haplotype within a family, but cannot predict other alleles within a population unless a linkage disequilibrium exists. Selective pressures during the course of evolution may have been the major factor in the survival of certain gene combinations in a haplotype. The conservation of certain extended haplotypes, mentioned above, supports this view.

On the other hand, the selection hypothesis is not necessary to explain linkage disequilibrium. When a population lacking certain antigens migrates into an area in which HLA antigens are in equilibrium, a Δ can develop within a few generations. For example, the increasing Δ value for A1, B8 found in populations from east to west, from India to western Europe, can be explained on the basis of migration and fusion. In smaller groups, consanguinity, founder effects, and gene drift may account for disequilibria. Finally, certain linkage disequilibria could occur as a result of nonrandom crossing over during gametic meiosis because of chromosomal segments that are either more or less likely to break. Unless there are selective pressures or restrictions in crossing over, linkage disequilibria disappear over a period of several generations.

LINKAGE VERSUS ASSOCIATION The diseases listed in Table 306-2 are examples of HLA linkage wherein the inherited conditions are marked within families by the relevant HLA haplotypes. For C2 deficiency, 21-hydroxylase deficiency, and idiopathic hemochromatosis, the mode of inheritance is recessive, with heterozygotes showing partial deficiencies. These genetic defects are also HLA-associated, with an excess of certain HLA alleles in affected unrelated individuals. Also, C2 deficiency is commonly linked to the HLA-A25, -B18, -BfS, Dw/DR2 haplotype, and idiopathic hemochromatosis exhibits both linkage and strong association with HLA-A3 and -B14. The high degree of linkage disequilibria in these HLA-linked diseases may result from mutations in a single founder, and a sufficient period of time may not have passed to bring the gene pool back into equilibrium. In this view, the HLA antigens are simple markers for the linked gene. Alternatively, expression of the defect may require interaction with specific HLA alleles. This latter hypothesis would require a higher mutation rate, with defective gene expression occurring only when linked with certain HLA genes.

HLA linkage can be demonstrated in the absence of association with a particular allele. Paget's disease and spinocerebellar ataxia are HLA-linked autosomal dominant traits, and Hodgkin's disease shows an HLA-linked recessive pattern of inheritance. As no HLA associations have been discerned for these disorders, it is suggested that there were multiple founders with mutations of as yet undefined genes in linkage with different HLA alleles.

CLINICAL APPLICATIONS The clinical value of HLA typing for diagnosis of disease is limited to B27 and ankylosing spondylitis, where nevertheless there are 10 percent false-positive and false-negative rates. HLA studies are also of value in genetic counseling and early recognition of disease in families with idiopathic hemochromatosis or congenital adrenal hyperplasia due to steroid 21-hydroxylase deficiency, particularly since HLA typing can be performed on cells obtained by amniocentesis. The high degree of polymorphism of the HLA system also makes it a powerful tool for paternity testing and other medicolegal applications. The implications for diseases such as type 1 diabetes mellitus and the other diseases showing HLA associations require further study of the components of the HLA system and their role in the pathogenesis of disease. Matching for HLA antigens in allogeneic transplantation shows the superiority of HLA identical sibs as donors and the immunodominance of HLA-A, -B, and -DR loci. Compatibility for these loci yields superior results in unrelated renal transplantation from cadaveric donors (see Chap. 272).

BIBLIOGRAPHY

BJORKMAN PJ et al: The foreign antigen binding site and T cell recognition regions of class I histocompatibility antigen. Nature 329:512, 1987

BODMER LG et al: Nomenclature for factors of the HLA system, 1995. Hum Immunol 43:149, 1995

BROWN JH et al: Three-dimensional structure of the human class II histocompatibility antigen HLA-DR1. Nature 364:33, 1993

CARPENTER CB, STROM TB: Immunobiology of renal transplantation, in *Contemporary Issues in Nephrology*, vol 19: *Renal Transplantation*, EL Milford et al (eds). New York, Churchill Livingstone, 1989

CHICZ RM et al: Specificity and promiscuity among naturally processed peptides bound to HLA-DR alleles. J Exp Med 178:27, 1993

GERMAIN RN: MHC-dependent antigen processing and peptide presentation: Providing ligands for T lymphocyte activation. Cell 76:287, 1994

ITESCU S et al: HLA-B35 is associated with accelerated progression to AIDS. J Acquir Immune Defic Syndr 5:37, 1992

POWIS SH et al: Alleles and haplotypes of the MHC-encoded ABC transporters TAP1 and TAP2. Immunogenetics 37:373, 1993

ROOPENIAN DC: What are minor histocompatibility loci? A new look at an old question. Immunol Today 13:7, 1992

SAYEGH MH et al: Mechanisms of T cell recognition of alloantigen: The role of peptides. Transplantation 57:1295, 1994

THOMSON G: HLA disease associations: Models for the study of complex human genetic disorders. Crit Rev Clin Lab Sci 32:183, 1995

WUCHERPFENNIG KW, STROMINGER JL: Selective binding of self peptides to disease-associated major histocompatibility complex (MHC) molecules: A mechanism for MHC-linked susceptibility to human autoimmune diseases. J Exp Med 181:1597, 1995

307

Max D. Cooper, Alexander R. Lawton III

PRIMARY IMMUNE DEFICIENCY DISEASES

Immunologic functions are mediated by developmentally independent, but functionally interacting, families of lymphocytes. The activities of B and T lymphocytes and their products in host defense are closely integrated with the functions of other cells of the reticuloendothelial system. Macrophages, dendritic cells, and the Langerhans' cells in the skin play an important role in the trapping and presentation of antigens to T and B cells to initiate the immune response. Macrophages also become effector cells, especially when activated by cytokine products of lymphocytes. The scavenger activity of polymorphonuclear leukocytes is directed and made specific by antibodies in concert with cytokines and the complement system. Natural killer (NK) cells, a population of granular lymphocytes, may spontaneously kill tumor and virus-infected cells, activities that are enhanced by the cytokine products of immune and inflammatory cells. Killing by NK cells also can be targeted by IgG antibodies for which NK cells have cell-surface receptors. The interaction of basophils and tissue mast cells with IgE antibodies in causation of immediate-type hypersensitivity is discussed in Chap. 310. Consideration of these interrelationships is an important part of the analysis of patients with suspected immune deficiency.

CLINICAL DISEASE FEATURES COMMON TO IMMUNE DEFICIENCY Immunodeficiency syndromes, whether congenital, spontaneously acquired, or iatrogenic, are characterized by unusual susceptibility to infection and not infrequently to autoimmune disease and lymphoreticular malignancies. The types of infection often provide the first clue to the nature of the immunologic defect.

Patients with *defects in humoral immunity* have recurrent or chronic sinopulmonary infection, meningitis, and bacteremia, most commonly caused by pyogenic bacteria such as *Haemophilus influenzae*, *Streptococcus pneumoniae*, and staphylococci. These and other pyogenic organisms also cause frequent infections in individuals who have either neutropenia or a deficiency of the pivotal third component of complement (C3). The tripartite collaboration of antibody, complement, and phagocytes in host defense against pyogenic organisms makes it important to assess all three systems in individuals with unusual susceptibility to bacterial infections.

Antibody-deficient patients in whom cell-mediated immunity is intact have an interesting response to viral infections. The clinical course of primary infection with viruses such as varicella zoster or rubeola, unless complicated by bacterial infection, does not differ significantly from that of the normal host. However, long-lasting immunity may not develop, and as a result, multiple bouts of chickenpox and measles may occur. Such observations suggest that intact T cells may be sufficient for control of established viral infections, while antibodies play an important role in limiting the initial dissemination of virus and in providing long-lasting protection. Exceptions to this generalization are becoming more widely recognized. Agammaglobulinemic patients fail to clear hepatitis B virus from their circulation and have a progressive, and often fatal, course. Poliomyelitis has occurred following live-virus vaccination in some patients. Chronic encephalitis, which may progress over a period of months to years, is a particular threat in congenitally agammaglobulinemic boys. Echoviruses and adenoviruses have been isolated from brain, spinal fluid, or other sites in such patients.

The occurrence of an unusually serious infection, for example, *H. influenzae* meningitis in an older child or adult, warrants consideration of humoral immune deficiency. Recurrent bacterial pneumonias also suggest this possibility. Chronic otitis media occurs frequently in patients with hypogammaglobulinemia and is significant because of its relative rarity in normal adults. Pansinusitis, although almost invariably present in immunoglobulin deficiency, is a less helpful finding because it is not rare in apparently normal people. Bacterial infections of the skin or urinary tract are less frequent problems in hypogammaglobulinemic patients.

Infestation with the intestinal parasite *Giardia lamblia* is a frequent cause of diarrhea in antibody-deficient patients.

Abnormalities of cell-mediated immunity predispose to disseminated virus infections, particularly with latent viruses such as herpes simplex (see Chap. 184), varicella zoster (see Chap. 185), and cytomegalovirus (see Chap. 187). In addition, patients so affected almost invariably develop mucocutaneous candidiasis and frequently acquire systemic fungal infections. Pneumonia caused by *Pneumocystis carinii* is also common (see Chap. 211).

T cell deficiency is always accompanied by some abnormality of antibody responses (see Fig. 307-1), although this may not be reflected by hypogammaglobulinemia. This explains in part why patients with primary T cell defects are also subject to overwhelming bacterial infection.

The most severe form of immune deficiency occurs in individuals, often infants, who lack both cell-mediated and humoral immune functions. Individuals with severe combined immunodeficiency (SCID) are susceptible to the whole range of infectious agents including organisms not ordinarily considered pathogenic. Multiple infections with viruses, bacteria, and fungi occur, often simultaneously. Because donor lymphocytes cannot be rejected by these recipients, blood transfusions can produce fatal graft-versus-host disease.

DIFFERENTIATION OF T AND B CELLS The functional deficits that occur in both congenital and acquired immunodeficiencies are usefully viewed as being caused by defects at various points along the differentiation pathways of immunocompetent cells. For this reason, certain features of the development and differentiation of T and B cells that are especially relevant to the analysis of immunodeficiency are briefly presented here; Chap. 305 provides a general account of their roles in cellular and humoral immunity.

A subpopulation of hematopoietic stem cells may become restricted to lymphoid differentiation prior to migration to the thymus, where T cells are generated, or to the fetal liver and adult bone marrow, where B cell development begins (see Fig. 307-1). A major function of these central lymphoid tissues is to generate the clonal diversity characteristic of the immune system. Each T or B lymphocyte expresses surface receptor molecules of a unique specificity for antigen. The receptors of B lymphocytes are immunoglobulin molecules that are formed by paired heavy and light chains of either κ or λ type. The heavy chain gene loci are on the long arm of chromosome 14; the 5′-3′ order of these is V_H (variable), D_H (diversity), and J_H (joining) minigene families followed by the C_H (constant region) genes, C_μ, C_δ, $C_{\gamma 3}$, $C_{\gamma 1}$, $C_{\alpha 1}$, $C_{\gamma 2}$, $C_{\gamma 4}$, C_ϵ, and $C_{\alpha 2}$. The κ gene family, consisting of V_κ, J_κ, and C_κ genes, is located on chromosome 2 and the homologous λ gene loci on chromosome 22.

The T cell receptors are related cell-surface molecules with antigen-binding specificity. The receptor on most T cells is composed of two polypeptide chains, called α and β. The β-chain family is located on chromosome 7 and consists of V_β, D_β, J_β, and C_β minigene loci. The α-chain family on chromosome 14 similarly consists of a series of V_α, D_α, J_α, and C_α genes. A smaller subpopulation of T cells express a T cell receptor composed of γ and δ polypeptide chains. The γ-chain gene family is located on chromosome 7, and the δ-chain family is located in the midst of the α gene locus on chromosome 14.

The genetic strategy for creating functional gene complexes encoding antigen receptors is similar for T and B cells. For example, a functional V region gene of the immunoglobulin heavy chain is formed by productive rearrangement of one each of the V_H, D_H, and J_H genes and deletion of the intervening DNA to generate a contiguous coding structure that is then transcribed together with the nearest C_H gene. Functional light chain genes are formed by a V-J rearrangement in either the κ or λ gene loci. The V_β gene is similarly composed of a rearranged set of V_β, D_H, and J_β genes forming a contiguous coding structure, which the T cell then transcribes along with the nearest C_β gene. Conserved flanking sequences serve as recombination signals for the V, D, and J gene segments in the T cell receptor (TCR) and immunoglobulin gene assembly processes. In both T and B cell precursors this DNA cutting and splicing operation involves the same recombinase proteins: the recombinase-activating gene (RAG) 1 and RAG-2, a DNA-dependent protein kinase, and at least two other proteins essential for DNA repair. Because there are many different V, D, and J genes, they can be put together in various combinations to encode a large number of receptor molecules having different antigen-binding specificities. Antibody and TCR variability are amplified further by nuclease nibbling around the DNA cuts needed to join the V, D, and J region segments and by addition of nonencoded nucleotides in the joins, a task that is performed by the nuclear enzyme, terminal deoxynucleotidyl transferase (TdT).

Generation of clonal diversity requires cellular proliferation, such that each of the different receptor specificities encoded in the genome

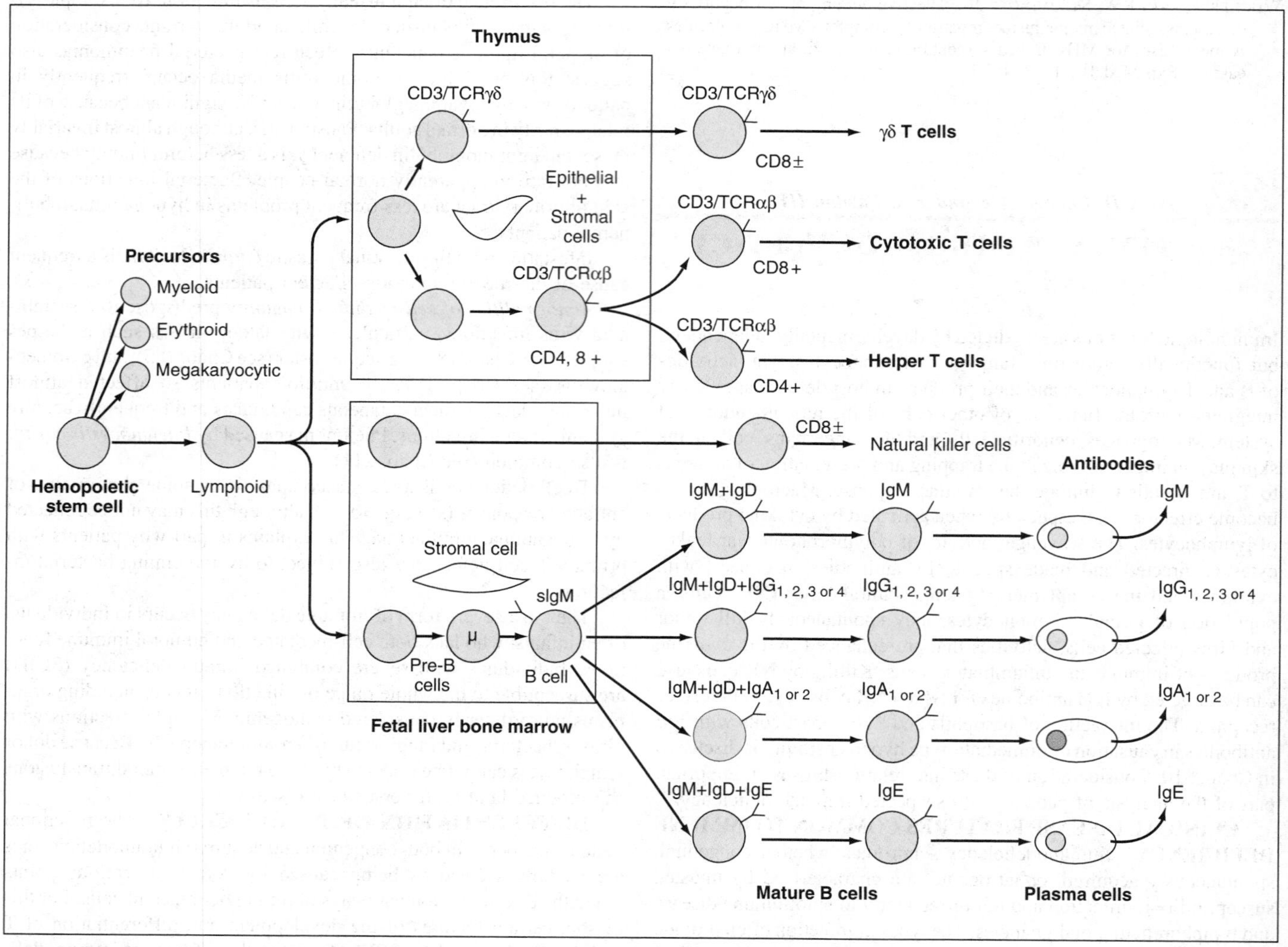

FIGURE 307-1 Hypothetical model outlining the differentiation of hemopoietic stem cells along T, B, and NK cell lineages. Failure to develop T and B cells may result from defective stem cells or from inborn metabolic errors affecting both cell types. Rarely, other hematopoietic cell lines are also absent. Absence of either T or B cells suggests malfunction of central lymphoid tissues, including the thymus and the fetal liver–bone marrow complex. B cell deficiency may result from failure to generate pre-B cells from their stem cell precursors or from failure of pre-B cells to give rise to their B lymphocyte progeny. Similarly, differentiation may be arrested at several levels within the T cell lineage; arrests at the thymocyte level and failure to develop the helper subset have been observed in immunodeficient patients. Agammaglobulinemia and deficiencies of some T cell functions may occur despite the presence of normal numbers of B or T cells in the circulation. Failure of B lymphocytes to differentiate to plasma cells can be due to intrinsic cellular abnormalities or to faulty T cell regulation.

comes to be uniquely expressed by individual cells. A clone consists of cells that express the identical antigen-binding receptors. Estimates for the total number of B cell clones usually vary between 10 and 100 million. T cell clonal diversity may be equally extensive. The initial step in clonal development is independent of antigen and reflects a genetically programmed sequence of differentiation analogous to that of primary erythropoiesis or myelopoiesis. This phase, termed *primary differentiation*, begins early in human fetal development and continues in adult life, albeit at reduced levels.

The most primitive morphologically identifiable cell in the B lineage is called a *pro-B cell*. These cells are marked by the cell surface CD19 antigen and nuclear TdT expression. Pro-B cells undergo productive $V_HD_HJ_H$ rearrangement to express cytoplasmic μ chains (the heavy chain of IgM) and become pre-B cells. Since light chain gene rearrangement usually occurs later, pre-B cells lack the characteristic membrane-bound immunoglobulin receptors that characterize B lymphocytes but they may express μ chain/surrogate light chain receptors encoded by the nonrearranged V pre-B and 14.1 genes in the λ light chain gene locus. Pre-B cells are generated in the fetal liver and in bone marrow throughout life, dividing in response to interleukin (IL)7 and other growth factors made by neighboring stromal cells. After undergoing a productive rearrangement of light chain VJ genes, pre-B cells become immature B lymphocytes that express surface IgM receptors. These B lymphocytes differ from their more mature counterparts in an important physiologic characteristic; they are highly susceptible to inactivation when their receptors bind antigen. Consequently, immature B cells encountering self-antigens may be eliminated or rendered anergic. The antigen receptors on B cells are multichain units. In order for membrane-bound immunoglobulins to reach the B cell surface, they require association with Ig-α and Ig-β chains, which serve as signal transduction elements for the antigen receptor complex. Antigen-mediated cross-linkage of the B cell receptors triggers the phosphorylation of tyrosines located in short conserved stretches of amino acids, called *immunomodulatory tyrosine activation motifs* in the cytoplasmic domains of the Ig-α and Ig-β chains. A cascade of enzymatic interactions is thus initiated that culminates in the binding of nuclear transcriptional factors to promoter regions of genes that determine the B cell's fate: death, survival, growth, or differentation. A pivotal enzyme in this B cell activation cascade is the *Syk* tyrosine kinase.

The developmental sequence for expression of diverse immunoglobulin classes by B lymphocytes begins with expression of IgM. The expression of IgD on immature IgM-bearing cells occurs after they leave the bone marrow. Lymphocytes committed to synthesis of IgG, IgA, and IgE are derived from the IgM- and IgD-bearing precursors via a genetic switch mechanism. Each of the heavy chain constant region genes except C_δ is preceded by a switch region composed of repetitive nucleotide sequences. The heavy chain class switch is accomplished by splicing of the switch region of μ with the switch region in front of the downstream heavy chain gene to be expressed next and deletion of the C_μ, C_δ, and other C_H genes in the intervening DNA. The switch process involves antigenic stimulation and the help of T cells. Class switching occurs within the germinal centers of peripheral lymphoid tissues, where pairs of B and T cells cooperate in an antigen response. Essential to this process is the signal-inducing interaction of the CD40 molecule on the B cell with the CD40 ligand that is transiently expressed on the antigen-activated T cell partner. The helper T cell also produces soluble factors that can direct the class switch. IL-4 and transforming growth factor β can promote IgE and IgA responses, for example. The germinal center B cells also undergo somatic mutations in the variable regions of their immunoglobulin genes, and those with the highest antigen affinity are selected for survival as memory B cells or for terminal differentiation into antibody-secreting plasma cells.

During their development T lineage cells also undergo sequential rearrangements of the minigene families encoding their antigen receptors. On entering the epithelial thymus, the precursor cells may follow one of two major pathways. The first involves rearrangement of V_γ and J_γ genes to express γ chains and rearrangement of V_δ, D_δ, and J_δ genes to express δ chains. These associate with the CD3 proteins to form the CD3/$\gamma\delta$ TCR complex of $\gamma\delta$ T cells. Pre-T cells beginning development along the second differentiation pathway in the thymus rearrange one each of the V_β, D_β, and J_β genes prior to the expression of a complete β chain together with a newly discovered pre-T chain. At a later differentiation stage, rearrangements of V_α and J_α genes occur in the α-chain family, and then the completed antigen receptor molecule of one α chain and one β chain is expressed together with the CD3 protein complex on the cell surface of an immature $\alpha\beta$ T cell. Initially, the $\alpha\beta$ T cells express both the CD4 and CD8 accessory molecules on their surface. As these cells mature under the influence of a selfantigen selection process, they either downregulate the CD8 molecule to become CD4+ T cells with helper cell potential or they cease to express the CD4 molecule to become CD8+ T cells with cytotoxic potential. The CD4+ $\alpha\beta$ T cells leaving the thymus have been selected to recognize peptide fragments presented in the groove of class II major histocompatibility complex (MHC) molecules of antigen presenting cells. The CD8+ $\alpha\beta$ T cells migrating from the thymus have been selected to recognize peptide fragments in the cleft of class I MHC molecules expressed by virtually all types of nucleated cells. The CD4 and CD8 molecules are called *accessory receptors* because they have binding affinity for class II or class I MHC molecules, respectively, and are coupled to tyrosine kinase molecules that are active in signal transduction. While the $\gamma\delta$ T cells express neither CD4 nor CD8 molecules during their intrathymic development, they may express CD8 molecules as mature T cells in the periphery. Expression of these and other cell surface molecules can be defined by specific monoclonal antibodies, thus providing a powerful tool for elucidating the developmental status of both T and B lymphocytes (see Fig. 307-1).

The $\alpha\beta$ T cells bearing the CD4 markers constitute approximately 70 percent of circulating T cells and function as helper cells that facilitate the effector functions of B cells, other T cells, NK cells, and macrophages. The $\alpha\beta$ T cells expressing CD8 molecules constitute 20 to 30 percent of circulating T cells, mediate cytotoxic reactions, and may suppress immune responses. The $\gamma\delta$ T cells constitute a minor population of T cells. They may serve a protective role along epithelial surfaces, where they predominate, and may modulate immune-based tissue damage. Developmental arrests or failure of function of one or more of these T cell subsets may result in immunodeficiency or autoimmune diseases.

The events designated *secondary differentiation* follow stimulation of specific clones of lymphocytes by antigen. These processes are synonymous with the immune response (see Chap. 305). Particularly important in consideration of immunodeficiencies are the collaborative interactions among macrophages, T cells, and B cells. While B lymphocytes may differentiate to become IgM-secreting plasma cells when stimulated by thymus-independent antigens, such as lipopolysaccharides, most antibody responses, particularly those of the IgG, IgA, and IgE classes, require intimate collaboration between T and B cells. Antigens bound to the antibody receptors on B cells are internalized, partially digested, and recycled to the cell surface, where they are presented on class II molecules to the T cell. The activated T cell in turn produces soluble factors that promote growth and differentiation of the B cell or inflammatory responses. These factors, which include interleukins IL-2, IL-4, IL-5, IL-6, IL-10, IL-12 and interferon γ (IFNγ), may be differentially produced by individual T cells. Depending on their initial activation stimulus, helper CD4 T cells may differentiate into different types of effector cells. The subset of helper T cells, designated TH1 cells, produces IL-2, IFNγ, tumor necrosis factor α, and other cytokines that regulate cell-mediated immunity, while the TH2 subset of cells typically produces IL-4, IL-5, IL-10, and other cytokines that regulate humoral immune responses. Antigen-presenting monocytes may produce IL-12 to bias the immune response toward TH1 effector cells, while IL-4 produced by a special subset of T cells or mast cells favors a TH2 effector cell response.

Differentiation of T or B cells may be arrested at either the primary or secondary stages. Reflecting the complex cellular interactions involved in immune responses and the pivotal role played by T lymphocytes, immune deficiencies primarily involving T cells are usually also associated with abnormal B cell function. Conversely, immunodeficiencies manifested primarily by inability to produce antibodies may be caused by T cell defects not associated with abnormal cell-mediated immunity.

EVALUATION OF IMMUNODEFICIENT PATIENTS A careful history and physical examination will usually indicate whether the major problem involves the antibody-complement-phagocyte system or cell-mediated immunity. A history of a normal response to smallpox vaccination or of contact dermatitis due to poison ivy suggests intact cellular immunity. Persistent mucocutaneous candidiasis suggests deficient cell-mediated immunity. Lymphopenia and the absence of palpable lymph nodes may be important findings. However, patients with profound immunodeficiency may have diffuse lymphoid hyperplasia. Most immunodeficiencies may be diagnosed by thoughtful use of tests available in local or regional clinical laboratories. More precise evaluation of immunologic functions and treatment may require referral to specialized centers. Table 307-1 presents a résumé of widely available laboratory investigations.

Humoral Immunity With rare exceptions, deficiency of humoral immunity is accompanied by diminished serum concentration of one or more classes of immunoglobulin. Normal values vary with age, and adult concentrations of IgM (1.0 g/L) are reached at about 1 year, of IgG (8.0 g/L) at 5 to 6 years, and of IgA (2.0 g/L) by puberty (see Chap. 305). Also, the wide range of values among normal adults creates difficulty in defining the lower limits of normal. Reasonable estimates for low normal values are 0.4 g/L for IgM, 5 g/L for IgG, and 0.5 g/L for IgA. In the presence of borderline hypogammaglobulinemia, assessing the patient's capacity to produce specific antibodies becomes particularly important. Isohemagglutinins, anti-streptolysin O, and "febrile agglutinins" are valuable standard assays, and measurements of pre- and postimmunization titers to tetanus toxoid, diphtheria toxoid, *H. influenzae* capsular polysaccharide, and *S. pneumoniae* serotypes provide a comprehensive assessment of humoral responsiveness.

Estimation of numbers of circulating B and T lymphocytes is of value in determining the pathogenesis of certain types of immune deficiency. B lymphocytes are identified by the presence of membrane-bound immunoglobulins, their associated α- and β-chain units, and other lineage-specific molecules on the B cell surface (Table 307-1), which can be identified and enumerated by specific monoclonal antibodies.

Since antibody deficiency may be mimicked clinically by deficiency of complement components, measurement of total hemolytic complement (CH_{50}) should be a part of the evaluation of host defense. Measurement of C3 alone is inadequate for screening, since deficiencies of both early and late complement components may predispose to bacterial infection (see Chap. 305).

Cellular Immunity T lymphocytes may be enumerated by their expression of the TCR/CD3 complex of surface molecules. The CD2 antigenic molecule is also expressed by almost all of the T cells and a few non-T lineage lymphocytes. The CD4 molecule serves as a marker for helper T cells, although macrophages also express this molecule in relatively low levels. Conversely, CD8αβ heterodimers are expressed by cytotoxic T cells. These cell-surface molecules are also expressed by some γδ T cells and by NK cells, although usually as CD8αα homodimeric molecules.

Normal levels of serum immunoglobulins and antibody responsiveness are reliable indices of intact helper T cell function. T lymphocyte function can be measured directly by delayed hypersensitivity skin testing using a variety of antigens to which the majority of older children and adults have been sensitized. A generally useful skin test antigen is a 1:5 dilution of tetanus toxoid injected intradermally, since almost all individuals will have been sensitized. Purified protein derivative (PPD), histoplasmin, mumps antigen, and extracts of *Candida* or *Trichophyton* also may be used.

T lymphocyte function may be estimated in vitro by the capacity of cells to proliferate in response to antigens to which the patient has been sensitized, to lymphocytes from an unrelated donor, to antibodies that cross-link the CD3/TCR complex, or to the T cell mitogens, which include phytohemagglutinin, concanavalin A, and pokeweed mitogen. The response is usually quantified by measurement of incorporation of radioactive thymidine into newly synthesized DNA. It is also possible to measure the production of cytokines (or interleukins) by activated T cells. The ability of T cells activated in mixed lymphocyte culture to lyse target cells can be measured. Finally, assays exist for detection of defects in T cell surface receptors and specific elements of the signal transduction pathways that they activate in T cell responses.

CLASSIFICATION *Primary immunodeficiencies* may be either congenital or acquired and are currently classified according to mode of inheritance and whether the defect involves T cells, B cells, or both (Table 307-2). The following discussion emphasizes three related concepts: (1) that immunodeficiencies are most logically viewed as defects of cellular differentiation, (2) that these defects may involve either primary development of T or B cells or the antigen-dependent phase of their differentiation, and (3) that defects of B cell differentiation may in some instances reflect faulty T-B collaboration.

Secondary immunodeficiencies are those not caused by intrinsic abnormalities in development or function of T and B cells. The best known of these is AIDS, which may follow infection with the human immunodeficiency virus (see Chap. 308). Other examples are immune deficiency associated with malnutrition, protein-losing enteropathy, and intestinal lymphangiectasia. Also considered secondary are immunodeficiencies resulting from hypercatabolic states such as occur in myotonic dystrophy, immunodeficiency associated with lymphoreticu-

Table 307-1

Laboratory Evaluation of Host Defense Status

INITIAL SCREENING ASSAYS*

Complete blood count with differential smear
Serum immunoglobulin levels: IgM, IgG, IgA, IgD, IgE

OTHER READILY AVAILABLE ASSAYS

Quantification of blood mononuclear cell populations by immunofluorescence assays employing monoclonal antibody markers†
- T cells: CD3, CD4, CD8, TCRαβ, TCRγδ
- B cells: CD19, CD20, CD21, Ig(μ, δ, γ, α, κ, λ), Ig-associated molecules (α, β)
- NK cells: CD16
- Monocytes: CD15
- Activation markers: HLA-DR, CD25, CD80 (B cells)

T cell functional evaluation
1. Delayed hypersensitivity skin tests (PPD, *Candida* histoplasmin, tetanus toxoid)
2. Proliferative response to mitogens (anti-CD3 antibody, phytohemagglutinin, concanavalin A) and allogeneic cells (mixed lymphocyte response)
3. Cytokine production

B cell functional evaluation
1. Natural or commonly acquired antibodies: isohemagglutinins; antibodies to common viruses (influenza, rubella, rubeola) and bacterial toxins (diphtheria, tetanus)
2. Response to immunization with protein (tetanus toxoid) and carbohydrate (pneumococcal vaccine, *H. influenzae B* vaccine) antigens
3. Quantitative IgG subclass determinations

Complement
1. CH_{50} assays (classic and alternative pathways)
2. C3, C4, and other components

Phagocyte function
1. Reduction of nitroblue tetrazolium
2. Chemotaxis assays
3. Bactericidal activity

* Together with a history and physical examination, these tests will identify more than 95 percent of patients with primary immunodeficiencies.

† The menu of monoclonal antibody markers may be expanded or contracted to focus on particular clinical questions.

Table 307-2

WHO Classification of Primary Immunodeficiencies

COMBINED IMMUNODEFICIENCIES
Severe combined immunodeficiency (SCID):
X-linked
Autosomal recessive ("Swiss-type agammaglobulinemia")
Adenosine deaminase (ADA) deficiency
Purine nucleoside phosphorylase (PNP) deficiency
MHC class II deficiency
Reticular dysgenesis
CD3γ or CD3ϵ deficiency
CD8 deficiency
PREDOMINANTLY ANTIBODY DEFICIENCIES
X-linked agammaglobulinemia
Hyper-IgM syndrome:
X-linked
Other
Ig heavy chain–gene deletions
κ-Chain deficiency
IgA deficiency
Selective deficiency of IgG subclasses (with or without IgA deficiency)
Common variable immunodeficiency (CVID)
Antibody deficiency with normal immunoglobulins
Transient hypogammaglobulinemia of infancy
OTHER WELL-DEFINED IMMUNODEFICIENCY SYNDROMES
Wiskott-Aldrich syndrome
Ataxia telangiectasia
DiGeorge anomaly
IMMUNODEFICIENCY ASSOCIATED WITH OR SECONDARY TO OTHER DISEASES
Chromosomal instability or defective repair
Bloom syndrome
Fanconi anaemia
ICF syndrome
Nijmegen breakage syndrome
Seckel syndrome
Xeroderma pigmentosa
Chromosomal defects
Down syndrome
Turner syndrome
Chromosome 18 rings and deletions
Skeletal abnormalities
Short-limbed skeletal dysplasia
Cartilage-hair hypoplasia
Immunodeficiency with generalized growth retardation
Schimke immunoosseous dysplasia
Immunodeficiency with absent thumbs
Dubowitz syndrome
Growth retardation, facial anomalies and immunodeficiency
Progeria (Hutchinson-Gilford syndrome)
Immunodeficiency with dermatologic defects
Partial albinism
Dyskeratosis congenita
Netherton syndrome
Acrodermatitis enteropathica
Anhidrotic ectodermal dysplasia
Papillon-Lefevre syndrome
Hereditary metabolic defects
Transcobalamin 2 deficiency
Methylmalonic acidaemia
Type 1 hereditary orotic aciduria
Biotin-dependent carboxylase deficiency
Mannosidosis
Glycogen storage disease, type 1b
Chédiak–Higashi syndrome
Hypercatabolism of immunoglobulin
Familial hypercatabolism
Intestinal lymphangiectasia
Other
Hyper-IgE syndrome
Chronic mucocutaneous candidiasis
Hereditary or congenital hypo- or asplenia
Ivermark syndrome

lar malignancy, and immunodeficiency resulting from treatment with x-rays, antilymphocyte serum, or cytotoxic drugs.

Incidence As a group, the primary immunodeficiencies are relatively common. The most frequent, isolated IgA deficiency, occurs in approximately 1 in 600 individuals in North America.

The more severe forms of primary immunodeficiency have their onset early in life and all too frequently result in death during childhood. Immunodeficiencies may become apparent at any age, however, and patients with congenital hypogammaglobulinemia may survive to middle age or beyond. In a referral center for patients with immunodeficiency diseases, approximately two-thirds of the immunodeficient patients will be adults.

Severe Combined Immunodeficiency The SCID syndrome is characterized by gross functional impairment of both humoral and cell-mediated immunity and by susceptibility to devastating fungal, bacterial, and viral infections. It is usually congenital, may be inherited either as an X-linked or autosomal recessive defect, or may occur sporadically. Affected infants rarely survive beyond 1 year without treatment.

The syndrome has been associated with a diversity of defects in development of immunocompetent cells, some of which are related to specific enzymatic abnormalities.

One form of SCID is characterized by severe lymphopenia and is inherited as an autosomal recessive disorder. The failure in both T and B cell development in some patients is due to *mutations in the RAG-1 or RAG-2 genes*, the combined activities of which are needed for V(D)J recombination. A function-loss *mutation in the DNA-dependent tyrosine kinase gene* is present in SCID mice and also may prove to be a cause for SCID in humans. Rarely, other hematopoietic cell lines fail to develop in a variant form of SCID called *reticular dysgenesia*. About half of patients with autosomal recessive SCID are deficient in an enzyme involved in purine metabolism, adenosine deaminase (ADA), due to deletions or point *mutations in the ADA gene*. Studies of the pathophysiologic relationship of ADA deficiency to abortive lymphoid differentiation suggest that intracellular accumulation of adenosine and deoxyadenosine nucleotides interferes with critical metabolic functions, including DNA synthesis. Improvement of both clinical status and immunologic function occurs in some patients treated with exogenous ADA conjugated to polyethylene glycol to prolong its half-life. The cellular defect in the lymphopenic forms of SCID logically rests with the precursor cells for both T and B lineages. The immunologic defects in all these types of SCID patients have been repaired following transplantation of bone marrow or fetal liver as a source of stem cells, indicating that the stromal microenvironments of the thymus and bone marrow of these patients are intact and capable of supporting T and B cell differentiation of normal stem cells.

SCID also may occur with an X-linked inheritance pattern. Aborted thymocyte differentiation and an absence of peripheral T cells and NK cells is seen in *X-linked SCID*. B lymphocytes are present in normal numbers but are functionally defective. The defective gene encodes a common γ chain of the receptors for IL-2, -4, -7, -9, and -15, thus disrupting the action of an important set of lymphokines. This developmental disorder can be repaired by transplantation of bone marrow stem cells from a histocompatible sibling. Transplants of haploidentical bone marrow, depleted of donor T cells to prevent graft-versus-host disease, also may correct the T cell deficit. However, antibody deficiency requiring immunoglobulin replacement therapy may persist for years unless the defective B cells are replaced by normal B cells of donor origin.

JAK3 protein kinase deficiency The same $T^{-}NK^{-}B^{+}$ SCID phenotype seen in X-linked SCID can be inherited as an autosomal recessive disease due to mutations in the gene for JAK3 protein kinase. This enzyme associates with the common γ chain of the receptors for IL-2, -4, -7, -9, and -15 as a key element in their signal transduction pathways.

℞ TREATMENT

Treatment of SCID patients should be performed in centers with a strong research interest in this problem. It is crucial that these patients be recognized early and not be given live viral vaccines or blood transfusions, which may cause fatal graft-versus-host disease.

T Cell Immunodeficiency Reflecting the diversity of T cell functions, abnormalities of T cell development may be responsible for a wide spectrum of immune deficiencies, including SCID, selective defects in cell-mediated immunity, and syndromes presenting as antibody deficiency. These defects may be acquired (see Chap. 308) as well as congenital.

DiGeorge's syndrome This classic example of isolated T cell deficiency results from maldevelopment of thymic epithelial elements derived from the third and fourth pharyngeal pouches. The gene defect has been mapped to chromosome 22q11. Defective development of organs dependent on cells of embryonic neural crest origin includes congenital cardiac defects, particularly those involving the great vessels; hypocalcemic tetany, due to failure of parathyroid development; and absence of a normal thymus. Facial abnormalities may include abnormal ears, shortened philtrum, micrognathia, and hypertelorism. Serum immunoglobulin concentrations are frequently normal, but antibody responses, particularly of IgG and IgA isotypes, are usually impaired. T cell levels are reduced, whereas B cell levels are normal. Affected individuals usually have a small, histologically normal thymus located near the base of the tongue or in the neck, allowing most patients to develop functional T cells in numbers that may or may not be adequate for host defense. Therapeutic intervention in the form of an epithelial thymic transplant is recommended only for the most severe cases of DiGeorge's syndrome.

T cell receptor deficiency Since the expression and function of antigenspecific TCR is dependent on their companion CD3γ, δ, ϵ, and ζ-η chains, defective genes for any of these receptor components can impair T cell development and function. Immunodeficiencies due to inherited CD3γ and CD3ϵ mutations have been identified. CD3γ mutations result in a selective deficit in CD8 T cells, whereas CD3ϵ mutations lead to a preferential reduction in CD4 T cells, thus implying differences in the signal transduction roles for each CD3 component.

MHC class II deficiency Because T cells are required for B cell responses to most antigens, any gene defect (or acquired disorder) that interferes with T cell development and cell-mediated immunity will also compromise antibody production and humoral immunity. MHC class II deficiency results in one such immunodeficiency in that the TCR must see protein antigens as peptide fragments held within the α helical grooves of class II and class I molecules encoded by the MHC. Antigen-presenting cells in individuals with this relatively rare disorder fail to express the class II molecules DP, DQ, and DR on their surface. Limited numbers of helper CD4 T cells are therefore generated in the thymus, and they fail to see antigen in the periphery. Affected individuals experience recurrent bronchopulmonary infections, chronic diarrhea, and severe viral infections that usually prove fatal before 4 years of age. The defect is caused by mutations in genes that encode essential transcriptional factors that bind to promoter elements for the MHC class II genes. In one subgroup of such patients the class II transactivator gene is mutated, whereas in other families mutations in genes encoding additional transcriptional factors for MHC class II genes are responsible for the defective development and function of CD4 T cells.

ZAP70 tyrosine kinase deficiency Recurrent and opportunistic infections begin within the first year of life in individuals with a deficiency in ZAP70 tyrosine kinase, a pivotal component in the TCR/CD3 signal transduction cascade. The rare inheritance of mutations in both alleles of the ZAP70 gene results in a selective deficiency of CD8 T cells and dysfunction of CD4 T cells, which are present in normal numbers. Severe immunodeficiency is the inevitable consequence.

Purine nucleoside phosphorylation deficiency Function-loss mutations of the purine nucleoside phosphorylase (PNP) gene are associated with an often severe and selective deficiency of T lymphocyte function. This enzyme functions in the same purine salvage pathway as ADA; toxic effects of the PNP deficiency may be related to intracellular accumulation of deoxyguanosine triphosphate.

Ataxia-telangiectasia Ataxia-telangiectasia (AT) is an autosomal recessive genetic disorder characterized by cerebellar ataxia, oculocutaneous telangiectasia, and immunodeficiency. The gene responsible is located in the q22–23 region on chromosome 11. The mutant AT gene has sequence similarity to the phosphatidyl-inositol-3 kinases that are involved in signal transduction. The AT gene belongs to a conserved family of genes that monitor DNA repair and coordinate DNA synthesis with cell division. The deleterious effects of the AT gene are widespread. Onset of truncal ataxia usually occurs in infancy and is progressive. Immunodeficiency may be clinically manifest by recurrent and chronic sinopulmonary infection leading to bronchiectasis, although not all patients have overt immunodeficiency. Ovarian agenesis is a frequent occurrence. Persistence of very high serum levels of oncofetal proteins, including alpha fetoprotein and carcinoembryonic antigen, may be of diagnostic value. Frequent causes of death are chronic pulmonary disease and malignancy. Lymphomas are most common, although carcinomas also have occurred.

The immunologic abnormalities seem to be related to maldevelopment of the thymus. The thymus is markedly hypoplastic and similar in appearance to an embryonic thymus. The peripheral T cell pool is frequently reduced in size, especially in lymphoid tissue compartments. Cutaneous anergy and delayed rejection of skin grafts are common. Although B lymphocyte development is normal, most patients are deficient in serum IgE and IgA, and a smaller number have reduced serum levels of IgG, particularly of the IgG2, IgG4 subclasses. IgM and IgD are usually normal.

The defect in DNA repair mechanisms in these patients renders their cells highly susceptible to radiation-induced chromosomal damage and results in a high incidence of malignancies.

Only symptomatic treatment is available. Unless a severe IgG deficiency is present, therapy with immunoglobulin is not indicated. Exposure to x-irradiation should be avoided in AT patients. AT is a rare disorder, one in 10,000 to 100,000 incidence, but 1 percent of the population is heterozygous for an AT mutation. The heterozygous state predisposes to enhanced cellular radiosensitivity and cancer, especially breast cancer in females.

Immunoglobulin deficiency syndromes *X-linked agammaglobulinemia* Males with this syndrome often begin to have recurrent bacterial infections late in the first year of life, when maternally derived immunoglobulins have disappeared. Affected individuals have very few immunoglobulin-bearing B lymphocytes in their circulation and lack primary and secondary lymphoid follicles. However, B cell progenitors are found in normal frequency in the bone marrow. This developmental block at the pre-B cell level contrasts with earlier and later arrests in B cell differentiation characterizing other immunodeficiencies (see below and Fig. 307-1). The defective Bruton's tyrosine kinase (Btk) gene responsible for X-linked agammaglobulinemia is located in the Xq 22 region. B cells from heterozygous female carriers utilize the X chromosome with the normal Btk gene exclusively, while T cells and myeloid cells express either X chromosome. *X-linked agammaglobulinemia with growth hormone deficiency* is a rare variant disorder caused by another gene defect that maps to the same region of the X chromosome.

Agammaglobulinemia is a misnomer, since most patients with this and other forms of severe panhypogammaglobulinemia synthesize some immunoglobulins. Within the same family, some affected males have had substantial levels of IgM, IgG, and IgA, while others have been nearly agammaglobulinemic. All of the Btk-deficient patients are very deficient in circulating B lymphocytes. This observation indicates that the few B lymphocytes that escape the block in differentiation are capable of plasma cell maturation and immunoglobulin synthesis.

However, antibody replacement therapy is needed in all these patients because of the limited number of B cell clones that are generated.

Sinopulmonary infections constitute the most frequent clinical problem. A form of arthritis with some of the features of rheumatoid disease occurs in some of these patients. *Mycoplasma* organisms are sometimes the cause of the arthritis. Chronic encephalitis of viral etiology can be a fatal complication. Some of these patients have an associated dermatomyositis. The frequency with which these complications occur is reduced by adequate treatment with intravenous immunoglobulin.

Transient hypogammaglobulinemia of infancy This diagnosis is reserved for those rare instances in which normal physiologic hypogammaglobulinemia of infancy is unusually prolonged and severe. IgG levels normally drop to 3.0 to 4.0 g/L between 3 and 6 months of age as maternally derived IgG is catabolized. The IgG levels subsequently rise, reflecting the infants' increased synthetic capacity. Periodic immunologic assessment is needed to differentiate transient hypogammaglobulinemia from other forms of antibody deficiency. Antibody replacement therapy is recommended only in the face of severe or recurrent infections.

Isolated deficiency of IgA This immunodeficiency occurs with a frequency of approximately 1 in 600 individuals of European origin. IgA deficiency is much less common in people of Asian and African origin. In Japan, for example, the incidence is approximately 1 in 18,500. While the precise genetic basis for this difference in incidence is unknown, IgA deficiency is frequently associated with certain MHC haplotypes in Caucasians.

With rare exceptions, IgA1 and IgA2 subclasses are both deficient in serum and in mucous secretions. While most individuals with isolated IgA deficiency appear healthy, others have an increased number of respiratory infections of varying severity, and a few have severe pulmonary disease such as bronchiectasis. Chronic diarrheal disease also occurs. The incidence of asthma and other atopic diseases among IgA-deficient patients is high, and conversely, the incidence of IgA deficiency among atopic children has been found to be 20 to 40 times that in the normal population. IgA deficiency is also significantly associated with autoimmune diseases such as rheumatoid arthritis (see Chap. 313) and systemic lupus erythematosus (see Chap. 312). Selective reductions in the IgG2 and IgG4 subclasses have been associated with the increased infections seen in some IgA-deficient individuals. Finally, IgA-deficient patients may develop significant levels of antibodies to IgA. These patients may have severe anaphylactic reactions when transfused with normal blood or blood products.

IgA deficiency is often familial. It also can occur in association with congenital intrauterine infections, such as toxoplasmosis, rubella, and cytomegalovirus infection, or following treatment with phenytoin, penicillamine, or other medications in genetically susceptible individuals.

The pathogenesis of IgA deficiency, whether genetic or induced by environmental insult, involves a block in terminal differentiation of B lymphocytes. The IgA-bearing lymphocytes in these patients also bear surface IgM. This immature phenotype, also prevalent in normal neonates, may reflect a primary defect in essential regulatory interactions between T and B cells.

Treatment of IgA deficiency is essentially symptomatic. IgA cannot be effectively replaced by exogenous immunoglobulin or plasma, and use of either can increase the risk of development of antibodies to IgA. IgA-deficient patients in need of transfusion should be screened for the presence of antibodies to IgA and ideally should be given blood only from IgA-deficient donors. Treatment with immunoglobulin may benefit the exceptional IgA-deficient person in whom IgG2 and IgG4 subclass deficiencies are associated with severe infections. The risk of anaphylactic reactions to contaminating IgA must always be considered in treating IgA-deficient patients.

IgG subclass deficiencies Selective deficiencies in one or more of the four IgG subclasses are seen in some patients with repeated infections. The IgG subclass deficiency may easily go undetected when the total serum IgG level is measured, because IgG2, IgG3, and IgG4 together account for only 30 to 40 percent of the IgG antibodies. Even a deficiency in IgG1 may be masked by increases in the remaining IgG isotypes. However, the availability of subclass-specific monoclonal antibodies allows precise measurement of IgG subclass levels.

Homozygous deletions of genes encoding the constant region of the different γ chains is the basis for the IgG subclass deficiency in some individuals. For example, deletion of the $C_{\alpha 1}$, $C_{\gamma 2}$, $C_{\gamma 4}$, and C_{ϵ} genes on both chromosomes 14 was responsible for one individual's inability to make IgA1, IgG2, IgG4, and IgE. Interestingly, individuals with this and other patterns of C_H-gene deletions may not have unusual infections.

Most of the IgG subclass–deficient individuals with repeated infections appear to have regulatory defects that prevent normal B cell differentiation. The defect may extend to other isotypes. IgA deficiency may accompany IgG2 and IgG4 subclass deficiencies (see "Isolated Deficiency of IgA," above), and an inability to produce IgM antibodies to polysaccharide antigens often reflects a broader defect in antibody responsiveness. While patients with IgG subclass deficiency may benefit from administration of immunoglobulin, a thorough immunologic assessment is needed to identify the relatively few who need this therapy.

Common variable immunodeficiency This diagnostic category includes a heterogeneous group of males and females, mostly adults, who have in common the clinical manifestations of deficient production of all major immunoglobulin classes. The majority of these panhypogammaglobulinemic patients have normal numbers of B lymphocytes that are clonally diverse but phenotypically immature. B lymphocytes in these patients are able to recognize antigens and can proliferate in response but fail to differentiate to become plasma cells. This abortive differentiation pattern leads to the frequent occurrence of nodular lymphoid hyperplasia, including splenomegaly and intestinal lymphoid hyperplasia. Several types of defects in B lymphocyte differentiation have been suggested. An intrinsic abnormality of B lymphocytes may prevent their differentiation into immunoglobulin-secreting plasma cells even when provided with differentiation factors from normal T cells. Alternatively, the defective B cell response may reflect a deficiency of helper T cell function which may be associated with reduced numbers of CD4+ T cells. Other possible causes include a deficiency in complement components, such as C4A, which facilitate antigen-mediated triggering of B cells.

Common variable immunodeficiency and IgA deficiency may represent polar ends of a clinical spectrum due to the same underlying gene defect in a large subset of these patients. The two disorders feature similar B cell differentiation arrests, differing only in the numbers of immunoglobulin classes involved. Both disorders occur frequently within the same family, and the same MHC haplotypes are associated with both immunodeficiency patterns. The data suggest an underlying susceptibility gene in both disorders.

It is important to consider the diagnosis of common variable immunodeficiency in adults with chronic pulmonary infections, some of whom will present with unexplained bronchiectasis. Intestinal diseases, including chronic giardiasis, intestinal malabsorption, and atrophic gastritis with pernicious anemia, are common in this group of patients. Patients with common variable immunodeficiency also may present with signs and symptoms highly suggestive of lymphoid malignancy, including fever, weight loss, splenomegaly, generalized lymphadenopathy, and lymphocytosis. Routine histologic examination of lymphoid tissues usually reveals germinal center hyperplasia which may be difficult to distinguish from nodular lymphoma (see Chap. 113). Demonstration of a normal distribution of immunoglobulin isotypes and light chain classes on circulating and tissue B lymphocytes can serve to distinguish these patients from those having a monoclonal B cell malignancy with secondary hypogammaglobulinemia. The monthly administration of intravenous immunoglobulin in adequate doses (see below) is an essential part of the prevention and treatment of all these complications.

X-linked immunodeficiency with increased levels of IgM In this syndrome, IgG and IgA levels are very low, while IgD levels may be high. The normal development of B lymphocytes bearing IgM and IgD and the absence of IgG and IgA B lymphocytes indicate a defect in isotype switching. The defective gene in most of these patients encodes a transmembrane molecule on activated T cells that is the ligand for the CD40 molecule on B cells. Gene mutations that preclude normal expression of this CD40 ligand prevent normal T and B cell cooperation, germinal center formation, and isotype switching. The clinical patterns of infection are similar to but more severe than those occurring with other hypogammaglobulinemic states. Probably because of a subtle defect in T cell responsiveness, pneumonia caused by *P. carinii*, severe enteritis due to cryptosporidial infection, and fungal infections sometimes occur. Neutropenia in affected males also can increase their vulnerability to infections. Adequate antibody replacement by immunoglobulin administration may reverse the neutropenia and reduce the frequency of infections requiring antibiotic therapy. Bone marrow transplantation can be curative, but this treatment presently is reserved for exceptional circumstances.

Isolated deficiency of IgM This syndrome has been reported rarely in the United States but was detected frequently in a British population. Approximately 60 percent of these patients had severe recurrent infections, often with bacteremia. Pneumococcal pneumonia and meningococcal meningitis have been noted in IgM-deficient patients. Other associated conditions included gastrointestinal disease, atopy, splenomegaly, and development of malignancy. The condition was frequently familial and was four times more common in males than in females. The number of circulating B lymphocytes has varied from very low to normal.

Miscellaneous Immunodeficiency Syndromes Infection with *Candida albicans* is the almost universal accompaniment of severe deficiencies in cell-mediated immunity. *Chronic mucocutaneous candidiasis* is different because superficial candidiasis is usually the only major manifestation of immunodeficiency in this syndrome. These patients rarely develop systemic infection with *Candida* or other fungal agents and are not unusually susceptible to virus or bacterial disease. The syndrome is often congenital and may be associated with single or multiple endocrinopathies as well as iron deficiency. Treatment of associated conditions may lead to improvement or even cure of *Candida* infection.

No uniformity of immunologic defects has been identified in these patients, although defects of antibody formation have been detected occasionally. Humoral immunity, including ability to make specific anti-*Candida* antibodies, is usually normal. Many patients are anergic, some to a variety of antigens and some only to *Candida*; anergy in some patients has been related to inability of their lymphocytes to produce the cytokine called *migration inhibition factor*.

Results of treatment with antifungal agents, such as amphotericin B, have been variable. In some patients, intensive treatment with amphotericin B coupled with surgical removal of infected nails has led to sustained improvement. Oral antifungal agents, such as fluconazole and itraconazole, also may be effective.

Immunodeficiency with thymoma The association of hypogammaglobulinemia with spindle cell thymoma usually occurs relatively late in adult life. Bacterial infections and severe diarrhea often reflect the antibody deficiency, whereas fungal and viral infections are infrequent complications. T cell numbers and cell-mediated immunity are usually intact, but these patients are very deficient in circulating B lymphocytes and pre-B cells in the bone marrow. They also frequently have eosinopenia and may develop erythroid aplasia. Complete bone marrow failure has occurred in a few immunodeficient patients with thymoma. The relationship between the thymoma and apparent abnormalities of hematopoietic stem cells remains conjectural.

Wiskott-Aldrich syndrome This is an X-linked genetic disease characterized by eczema, thrombocytopenia, and repeated infections. The platelets are small and have a shortened half-life. Affected male infants often present with bleeding, and most do not survive childhood, dying of complications of bleeding, infection, or lymphoreticular malignancy. The immunologic defects are well characterized phenotypically but are poorly understood. Serum concentrations of IgM are usually decreased, while IgA and IgG are normal and IgE is frequently increased. Synthetic rates for all three classes may be elevated, indicating a significant element of hypercatabolism. The number and class distribution of B lymphocytes are usually normal. Functionally, these boys are consistently unable to make antibodies to polysaccharide antigens normally; responses to protein antigens are often impaired late in the course of the disease. While most patients acquire T cell deficiencies, serial appraisal suggests that the T cell defects are secondary. Affected boys frequently become anergic, and their T cells do not respond normally to challenge with ubiquitous antigens. Mutations in the WASP gene on the short arm of the X chromosome are responsible for this disease. The WASP protein may serve an important role in transduction of cellular signals.

Transplantation of histocompatible bone marrow from a sibling donor has corrected both hematologic and immunologic abnormalities in several patients. In patients lacking a suitable donor, intravenous immunoglobulin infusions or splenectomy may improve platelet counts and reduce the risk of serious hemorrhage. Because of the increased risk of pneumococcal bacteremia, splenectomized patients should probably receive prophylactic penicillin.

X-linked lymphoproliferative syndrome This is an X-linked recessive disease in which there appears to be a selective impairment in immune elimination of Epstein-Barr virus (EBV). Infectious mononucleosis in affected males may have a fulminant and fatal outcome, may be associated with development of B cell malignancies, or may result in acquired hypogammaglobulinemia, aplastic anemia, or agranulocytosis. Antibodies to EBV can be detected in some patients but are often absent in the face of infection. Generation of cytotoxic T cells appears to be the primary mechanism of control of EBV infection in normal persons, and NK cells also may play a role in eliminating EBV-infected B cells. The gene defect has been mapped to the Xq 25 region, and the mutant gene responsible for the X-linked lymphoproliferative syndrome should be identified soon. Bone marrow transplantation from an HLA-matched donor may be curative, especially in younger children with this syndrome. Intravenous immunoglobulins should be administered to affected males who develop hypogammaglobulinemia.

Hyper-IgE syndrome The hyper IgE syndrome (see Chap. 62) is characterized by recurrent abscesses involving skin, lungs, and other organs and very high IgE levels. Staphylococcal infection is common to all patients, but most have infections with other pyogenic organisms as well. Males and females of all races are affected in an inheritance pattern suggesting an autosomal dominant defect with variable penetrance. A specific immunologic defect has not been identified. Abnormal neutrophil chemotaxis is an inconsistent finding, and diminished antibody responses to secondary immunization have been noted in some patients. Prophylaxis with penicillinase-resistant penicillins or cephalosporins is highly recommended to prevent staphylococcal infections. Pneumatocoeles, a frequent complication of penumonias, may require surgical excision.

Metabolic Abnormalities Associated with Immunodeficiency The relation of deficiencies of the purine salvage enzymes adenosine deaminase and purine nucleoside phosphorylase to immunodeficiency was discussed earlier. The syndrome of *acrodermatitis enteropathica* includes severe desquamating skin lesions, intractable diarrhea, bizarre neurologic symptoms, variable combined immunodeficiency, and an often fatal outcome. This disease is apparently caused by an inborn error of metabolism resulting in malabsorption of dietary zinc and can be treated effectively by parenteral or large oral doses of zinc. Zinc deficiency might in part account for the immunodeficiency that accompanies severe malnutrition. Inherited *deficiency of transcobalamin II*, the serum carrier molecule responsible for transport of vitamin B_{12} to tissues, is associated with failure of immunoglobulin production as well as megaloblastic anemia, leukopenia, thrombocytopenia, and severe malabsorption. All abnormalities of this rare disorder are reversed by administration of vitamin B_{12}.

℞ TREATMENT

Immunodeficiency diseases involving severe abnormalities of T cell function, with or without hypogammaglobulinemia, are often treatable with bone marrow transplants (see Fig. 307-1). Histocompatible marrow from a sibling donor is preferred, but haploidentical marrow may be used after removal of T cells. This therapy is complex and is best done by experienced research teams.

Replacement therapy with human immunoglobulin currently should be used in patients who have recurrent bacterial infections and are deficient in IgG. Maintenance of serum IgG levels above 5.0 g/L is sufficient to prevent most systemic infections and, together with antibiotic therapy, enhances reversal of chronic sinopulmonary infection. These serum levels usually can be achieved by intravenous administration of IgG, 400 mg/kg, at monthly intervals. In patients with mild to moderate IgG deficiency (3.0 to 4.0 g/L), the decision to treat should be based on clinical symptoms and response to antigenic challenge.

Immunoglobulin treatment is of no value in patients with deficiencies of immunoglobulins other than IgG, and this treatment is not benign. Some patients develop symptoms of diaphoresis, tachycardia, flank pain, and hypotension during or immediately following immunoglobulin administration. This reaction may be mediated by aggregates of IgG or other biologically active substances, but it also may occur as a consequence of antibodies produced by the patient against donor immunoglobulins, particularly IgA (see Chap. 115).

Therapy with exogenous IgG may not suffice to eliminate the chronic sinopulmonary inflammation and its progression to pulmonary fibrosis and bronchiectasis. Therefore, maintenance of good pulmonary toilet with regular postural drainage can be an especially important part of immunodeficient patient management. The principles of antibiotic therapy are not different in these than in other patients, except that the index of suspicion of bacterial infection should remain very high.

The availability of purified INFγ and other biologically active cytokines may prove to be valuable in the therapy of certain immunologic disorders. Gene replacement has been partially successful so far only in SCID patients with ADA deficiency. However, gene therapy holds great promise for treatment of a variety of genetic defects of the immune system, provided that the difficult problem of gene replacement in hemopoietic stem cells can be solved.

BIBLIOGRAPHY

Alarcon R et al: Familial defect in the surface expression of the T cell receptor-CD3 complex. N Engl J Med 319:1203, 1988

Blaese MR et al: T lymphocyte-directed gene therapy for ADA$^-$ SCID: Initial trial results after 4 years. Science 270:475, 1995

Buckley RH, Shiff RI: The use of intravenous immune globulin in immunodeficiency diseases. N Engl J Med 325:110, 1991

Elder ME et al: Human SCID due to a defect in ZAP70, a T cell tyrosine kinase. Science 264:4596, 1994

Fischer A, Arnaiz-Villena A: Immunodeficiencies of genetic origin. Immunol Today 16:510, 1995

Hollenbauh D et al: The role of CD40 and its ligand in the regulation of the immune response. Immunol Rev 138:23, 1994

Mach B: MHC class II regulation: Lessons from a disease. N Engl J Med 332:120, 1995

Paul WE: *Fundamental Immunology*, 3d ed. New York, Raven Press, 1993

Rosen FS et al: Primary immunodeficiency diseases. N Engl J Med 333:341, 1995

——— et al: Primary immunodeficiency diseases. Report of a WHO Scientific Group. Clin Exp Immunol 99(Suppl 1):1, 1995

Savitsky K et al: A single ataxia telangiectasia gene with a product similar to PI-3 kinase. Science 268:1749, 1995

Sideras P, Smith CIE: Molecular and cellular aspects of X-linked agammaglobulinemia. Adv Immunol 59:135, 1995

308

Anthony S. Fauci, H. Clifford Lane

HUMAN IMMUNODEFICIENCY VIRUS (HIV) DISEASE: AIDS AND RELATED DISORDERS

The acquired immune deficiency syndrome (AIDS) was first recognized in the United States in the summer of 1981, when the Centers for Disease Control and Prevention (CDC) reported the unexplained occurrence of *Pneumocystis carinii* pneumonia in five previously healthy homosexual men in Los Angeles and of Kaposi's sarcoma in 26 previously healthy homosexual men in New York and Los Angeles. Within months, the disease became recognized in male and female injection drug users (IDUs) and soon thereafter, in recipients of blood transfusions and in hemophiliacs. Because of the disproportionate number of cases of AIDS among Haitians in the United States early in the epidemic, this group was incorrectly designated as a "risk" group. Studies among Haitians in the United States and in Haiti soon revealed that the disease among Haitians was following a pattern of homosexual as well as heterosexual transmission; the latter was virtually identical to the predominant mode of transmissibility that was being recognized in developing countries in sub-Saharan Africa and elsewhere in the world (see below). As the epidemiologic pattern of the disease unfolded, it became clear that a microbe transmissible by sexual contact and blood or blood products was the most likely etiologic agent of the epidemic.

In 1983, human immunodeficiency virus (HIV) was isolated from a patient with lymphadenopathy, and by 1984 it was demonstrated clearly to be the causative agent of AIDS. The virus, which belongs to the lentivirus subfamily of the large family of retroviruses (Retroviridae) (see Chap. 192) was formerly called *lymphadenopathy associated virus* (LAV), *human T lymphotropic virus* (HTLV) *type III*, and *AIDS-associated retrovirus* (ARV). In 1985, a sensitive enzyme-linked immunosorbent assay (ELISA) was developed, which has led to an appreciation of the scope of HIV infection among cohorts of individuals in the United States who admit to practicing high-risk behavior (see below) as well as among selected populations that had been screened, such as blood donors, military recruits and active-duty military personnel, Job Corps applicants, and patients in selected sentinel hospitals. In addition, seroprevalance studies revealed the enormity of the global pandemic, particularly in developing countries (see below). Such surveillance approaches, when combined with monitoring of CD4+ T cell counts as a parameter of immunosuppression, led to the realization that there is a broad spectrum of HIV disease, ranging from asymptomatic infection and clinical latency to advanced clinical disease, the latter constituting AIDS.

During the early years of the AIDS epidemic in the 1980s, the care of HIV-infected individuals in the United States was, with few exceptions, confined to relatively restricted groups of physicians and hospitals, located predominantly in urban areas, particularly on the northeastern and western seaboards. Today, it is clear that virtually every practicing physician in the country and worldwide will be required to have some degree of familiarity with the workup, diagnosis, management, and specific treatment of HIV-infected individuals. HIV-infected patients are presenting in increasing numbers to family practice physicians, internists, obstetricians/gynecologists, pediatricians, and surgeons, with clinical problems that may be directly or indirectly related, or totally unrelated, to their HIV infection.

The staggering worldwide growth of the HIV pandemic is matched by an explosion of information in the areas of HIV virology, the pathogenesis (both immunologic and virologic) and treatment of HIV disease, the treatment and prophylaxis of the opportunistic diseases associated with HIV infection, and vaccine development. The information flow related to HIV disease is much greater than that for any other infectious or immunologic disease, or in fact for any other single disease in any subspecialty. It becomes almost impossible for the health care generalist to stay abreast of the literature. The purpose of this chapter is to present the most current information available on the scope of the epidemic; on its pathogenesis, treatment, and prevention; and on prospects for vaccine development. Above all, the aim is to provide a solid scientific basis and practical guidelines for a state-of-the-art approach to the HIV-infected patient.

DEFINITION AIDS was originally defined for surveillance purposes by the CDC (prior to the identification of HIV as the etiologic agent) as the presence of a reliably diagnosed "opportunistic" disease that is at least moderately predictive of an underlying defect in cell-mediated immunity in the absence of known causes of underlying immune defects, such as iatrogenic immunosuppression or malignant neoplasms. With the identification of HIV as the etiologic agent of AIDS and with the availability of sensitive and specific diagnostic tests for HIV infection, the case definition of AIDS has undergone several revisions. The latest revision took place in 1993; this revised CDC classification system for HIV-infected adolescents and adults categorizes persons on the basis of clinical conditions associated with HIV infection and CD4+ T lymphocyte counts. The system is based on three ranges of CD4+ T lymphocyte counts and three clinical categories and is represented by a matrix of nine mutually exclusive categories (Tables 308-1 and 308-2). Using this system, any HIV-infected individual with a CD4+ T cell count of <200/μL has AIDS by definition, regardless of the presence of symptoms or opportunistic diseases (Table 308-1). The clinical conditions in clinical category C now include pulmonary tuberculosis, recurrent pneumonia, and invasive cervical cancer (Table 308-2). Once individuals have had a clinical condition in category B, their disease cannot again be classified as category A, even if the condition resolves; the same holds true for category C in relation to category B.

While the definition of AIDS is complex and comprehensive, the clinician should not focus on whether AIDS is present but should view HIV disease as a spectrum ranging from primary infection, with or without the acute syndrome, to the asymptomatic stage, to advanced disease (see below). The definition of AIDS was established not for the practical care of patients but for surveillance purposes.

ETIOLOGIC AGENT

The etiologic agent of AIDS is HIV, which belongs to the family of human retroviruses and the subfamily of lentiviruses. Nononcogenic lentiviruses cause disease in other animal species, including sheep, horses, goats, cattle, cats, and monkeys. The four recognized human retroviruses belong to two distinct groups: the human T lymphotropic viruses, HTLV-I and HTLV-II, which are transforming retroviruses; and the human immunodeficiency viruses, HIV-1 and HIV-2, which are cytopathic viruses. The reader is referred to Chap. 192 for a detailed description of the biology of the human retroviruses. The most common cause of HIV disease throughout the world, and certainly in the United States, is HIV-1. HIV-1 comprises several subtypes with different geographic distributions (see below). HIV-2 was first identified in 1986 in West African patients and was originally confined to West Africa. However, a number of cases have been identified in Europe, South America, Canada, and the United States. HIV-2 is more closely related phylogenetically to the simian immunodeficiency virus (SIV) found in sooty mangabeys than it is to HIV-1. HIV-1 is more closely related to an SIV isolated from chimpanzees in 1990. The taxonomic relationship among primate lentiviruses is shown in Fig. 308-1.

Table 308-1

1993 Revised Classification System for HIV Infection and Expanded AIDS Surveillance Case Definition for Adolescents and Adults*

	Clinical Categories		
CD4+ T Cell Categories	A Asymptomatic, Acute (Primary) HIV or PGL†	B Symptomatic, Not A or C Conditions	C AIDS-Indicator Conditions
>500/μL	A1	B1	C1
200–499/μL	A2	B2	C2
<200/μL	A3	B3	C3

* The shaded areas indicate the expanded AIDS surveillance case definition.
† PGL, progressive generalized lymphadenopathy.
SOURCE: Morb Mort Week Rep 42(No. RR-17), December 18, 1992.

Table 308-2

Clinical Categories of HIV Infection

Category A: Consists of one or more of the conditions listed below in an adolescent or adult (>13 years) with documented HIV infection. Conditions listed in categories B and C must not have occurred.
- Asymptomatic HIV infection
- Persistent generalized lymphadenopathy
- Acute (primary) HIV infection with accompanying illness or history of acute HIV infection

Category B: Consists of symptomatic conditions in an HIV-infected adolescent or adult that are not included among conditions listed in clinical category C and that meet at least one of the following criteria: (1) The conditions are attributed to HIV infection or are indicative of a defect in cell-mediated immunity; or (2) the conditions are considered by physicians to have a clinical course or to require management that is complicated by HIV infection. Examples include, but are not limited to, the following:
- Bacillary angiomatosis
- Candidiasis, oropharyngeal (thrush)
- Candidiasis, vulvovaginal; persistent, frequent, or poorly responsive to therapy
- Cervical dysplasia (moderate or severe)/cervical carcinoma in situ
- Constitutional symptoms, such as fever (38.5°C) or diarrhea lasting >1 month
- Hairy leukoplakia, oral
- Herpes zoster (shingles), involving at least two distinct episodes or more than one dermatome
- Idiopathic thrombocytopenic purpura
- Listeriosis
- Pelvic inflammatory disease, particularly if complicated by tuboovarian abscess
- Peripheral neuropathy

Category C: Conditions listed in the AIDS surveillance case definition.
- Candidiasis of bronchi, trachea, or lungs
- Candidiasis, esophageal
- Cervical cancer, invasive*
- Coccidioidomycosis, disseminated or extrapulmonary
- Cryptococcosis, extrapulmonary
- Cryptosporidiosis, chronic intestinal (>1 month's duration)
- Cytomegalovirus disease (other than liver, spleen, or nodes)
- Cytomegalovirus retinitis (with loss of vision)
- Encephalopathy, HIV-related
- Herpes simplex: chronic ulcer(s) (>1 month's duration); or bronchitis, pneumonia, or esophagitis
- Histoplasmosis, disseminated or extrapulmonary
- Isosporiasis, chronic intestinal (>1 month's duration)
- Kaposi's sarcoma
- Lymphoma, Burkitt's (or equivalent term)
- Lymphoma, primary, of brain
- *Mycobacterium avium* complex or *M. kansasii*, disseminated or extrapulmonary
- *Mycobacterium tuberculosis*, any site (pulmonary* or extrapulmonary)
- *Mycobacterium*, other species or unidentified species, disseminated or extrapulmonary
- *Pneumocystis carinii* pneumonia
- Pneumonia, recurrent*
- Progressive multifocal leukoencephalopathy
- *Salmonella* septicemia, recurrent
- Toxoplasmosis of brain
- Wasting syndrome due to HIV

* Added in the 1993 expansion of the AIDS surveillance case definition.
SOURCE: Morb Mort Week Rep 42(No. RR-17), December 18, 1992.

MORPHOLOGY OF HIV Electron microscopy shows that the HIV virion is an icosahedral structure (Fig. 308-2*A*) containing numerous external spikes formed by the two major envelope proteins, the external gp120 and the transmembrane gp41. The virion buds from

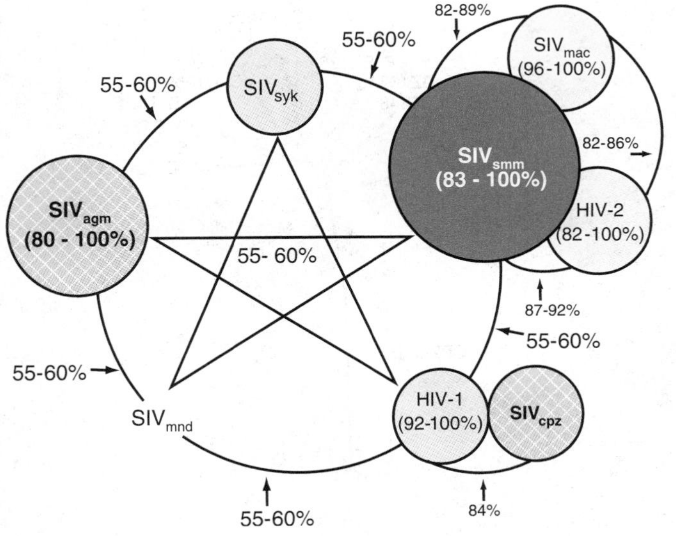

FIGURE 308-1 Five groups of primate lentiviruses. Five discrete groups of primate lentiviruses have been identified thus far on the basis of genetic sequence analysis. Members of each group share the same genomic organization and are more closely related to each other than to members of different groups. The percentages refer to the approximate amino acid identities in the relatively conserved *pol* gene. *(Adapted from RC Desrosiers, Nature 345:288, 1990; also from Desrosiers and Fauci.)*

the surface of the infected cell and incorporates a variety of host proteins, including major histocompatibility complex (MHC) class I and II antigens (see Chap. 306), into its lipid bilayer. The structure of HIV-1 is schematically diagrammed in Fig. 308-2*B* (see also Chap. 192).

LIFE CYCLE OF HIV HIV is an RNA virus whose hallmark is the reverse transcription of its genomic RNA to DNA by the enzyme *reverse transcriptase*. The life cycle of HIV begins with the high-affinity binding of the gp120 protein via a portion of its V1 region near the N terminus to its receptor on the host cell surface, the CD4 molecule (Fig. 308-3). The CD4 molecule is a 55-kDa protein found predominantly on a subset of T lymphocytes that are responsible for helper or inducer function in the immune system (see Chap. 305). It is also expressed on the surface of monocytes/macrophages and dendritic/Langerhans cells. It has recently been demonstrated that the coreceptor that must be present together with the CD4 molecule for fusion and entry of T cell–tropic strains of HIV-1 is a molecule termed CXCR4, while the coreceptor for macrophage-tropic strains of HIV-1 is the β-chemokine receptor CCR5. Both receptors belong to the family of seven-transmembrane-domain G protein–coupled cellular receptors (see below for details). Following binding, fusion with the host cell membrane occurs via the gp41 molecule, and the HIV genomic RNA is uncoated and internalized into the target cell. The reverse transcriptase enzyme, which is contained in the infecting virion, then catalyzes the reverse transcription of the genomic RNA into double-stranded DNA. The DNA translocates to the nucleus, where it is integrated randomly into the host cell chromosomes through the action of another virally encoded enzyme, *integrase*. This provirus may remain transcriptionally inactive (latent), or it may manifest varying levels of gene expression, up to active production of virus.

Cellular activation plays an important role in the life cycle of HIV and is critical to the pathogenesis of HIV disease (see below). Following initial binding and internalization of virions into the target cell, incompletely reverse-transcribed DNA intermediates are labile in quiescent cells and will not integrate efficiently into the host cell genome unless cellular activation occurs shortly after infection. Furthermore, activation of the host cell is required for the initiation of transcription of the integrated proviral DNA into either genomic RNA or mRNA. In this regard, activation of HIV expression from the latent state depends on the interaction of a number of cellular and viral factors. Following transcription, HIV mRNA is translated into proteins that undergo modification through glycosylation, myristylation, phosphorylation, and cleavage. The viral core is formed by the assembly of HIV proteins, enzymes, and genomic RNA at the plasma membrane of the cells. Budding of the progeny virion occurs through the host cell membrane, where the core acquires its external envelope (see Chap. 192). Each point in the life cycle of HIV is a real or potential target for therapeutic intervention (see below). Thus far, the reverse transcriptase and protease enzymes have proven to be susceptible to pharmacologic disruption (see below).

HIV GENOME Figure 308-4 schematically illustrates the arrangement of the HIV genome. Like other retroviruses, HIV-1 has genes that encode the structural proteins of the virus: *gag* encodes the proteins that form the core of the virion (including p24 antigen); *pol* encodes the enzymes responsible for reverse transcription and integration; and *env* encodes the envelope glycoproteins. However, HIV-1 is more complex than other retroviruses, particularly those of the nonprimate group, in that it also contains at least six other genes (*tat*, *rev*, *nef*, *vif*, *vpr*, and *vpu*), which code for proteins involved in the regulation of gene expression (see Chap. 192). Flanking these genes are the long terminal repeats (LTRs), which contain regulatory elements involved in gene expression (see below), such as the polyadenylation signal sequence, the TATA promotor sequence, the NF-κB and SP1 enhancer binding sites, the transactivating response (TAR) sequences, where the *tat* protein binds, and the negative regulatory element (NRE), whose deletion increases the level of gene expression (Fig. 308-4). The major difference between the genomes of HIV-1 and HIV-2 is the fact that HIV-2 lacks the *vpu* gene and has a *vpx* gene not contained in HIV-1.

MOLECULAR HETEROGENEITY OF HIV-1 Molecular analysis of various HIV isolates reveals sequence variation over many parts of the viral genome. For example, in different isolates, the degree of difference in the coding sequences of the viral envelope protein ranges from a few percent (very close) to 50 percent. These changes

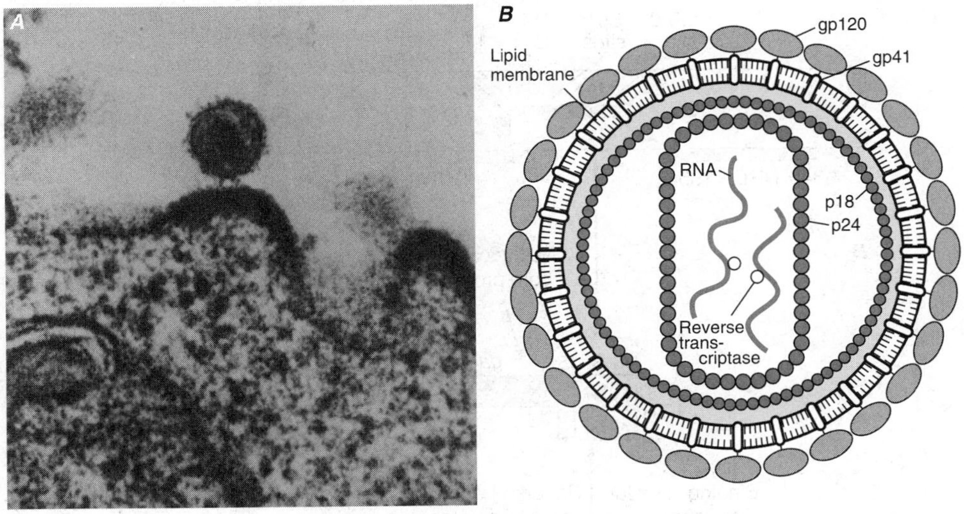

FIGURE 308-2 *A.* Electron micrograph of HIV. Figure illustrates a typical virion following budding from the surface of a CD4+ T lymphocyte, together with two additional incomplete virions in the process of budding from the cell membrane. *B.* Structure of HIV-1, including the gp120 outer membrane, gp41 transmembrane components of the envelope, genomic RNA, enzyme reverse transcriptase, p18(17) inner membrane, and p24 core protein. *[Adapted from RC Gallo. The human immunodeficiency virus (HIV), Sci Am, January 1987.]*

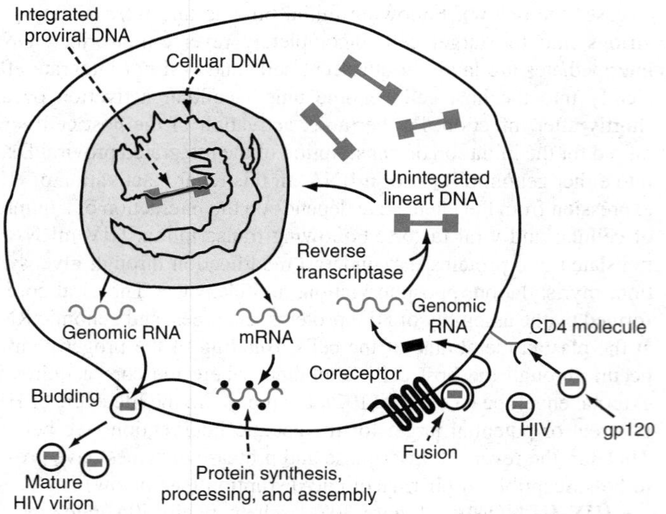

FIGURE 308-3 The life cycle of HIV. See text for description. *(From AS Fauci, Science 239:617, 1988.)*

tend to cluster in hypervariable regions. One such region, called V3, is a target for neutralizing antibodies and contains recognition sites for T cell responses (see below). Variability in this region is likely due to selective pressure from the host immune system. The extraordinary variability of HIV-1 is in marked contrast to the relative genetic stability of HTLV-I and -II.

There are two groups of HIV-1: group M (major), which is responsible for most of the infections in the world, and group O (outlier), a relatively rare viral form found at this time in Cameroon, Gabon, and France (see Chap. 192). The M group comprises at least eight sequence subtypes, or clades, designated A through H, which are distinguished by the fact that, at this time, they differ from each other by 30 percent in their *env* coding sequences and by 14 percent in their *gag* coding sequences. Curiously, the O-group viral sequences display subtype distances among each other of the same magnitude. As a result of the evolutionary process underlying these sequence differences, phylogenetic tree analyses produce starlike configurations suggestive of radiation from single ancestral viruses, one for the M group and one for the O group (Fig. 308-5).

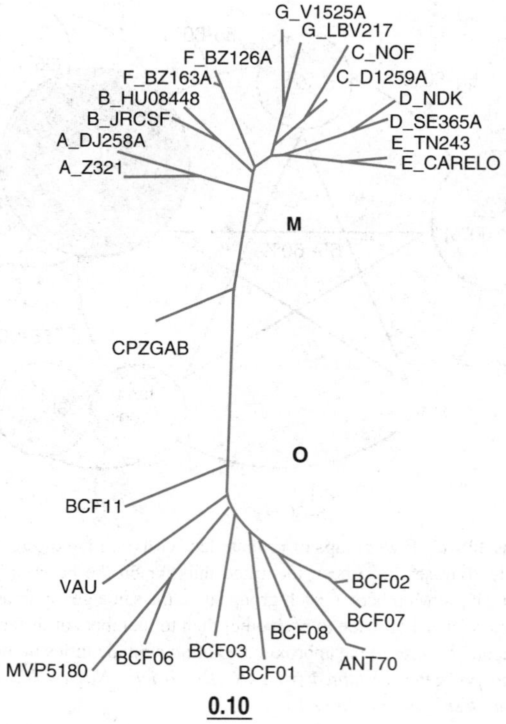

FIGURE 308-5 A phylogenetic tree constructed from HIV-1 M (major) and O (outlier) viral envelope sequences. Within the M group, subtypes A through G are represented (H is not shown); subtype B viruses predominate in the United States at this time. HIV-1 viruses are related to immunodeficiency viruses found in chimpanzees in the wild (CPZGAB). The M- and recently discovered O-group viruses each display a star-like configuration suggestive of two separate introductions of viruses into the human population. The scale-bar at the bottom indicates a 10 percent difference at the nucleotide level. *(Courtesy of Bette Korber and Gerald Myers, Los Alamos National Laboratory, Los Alamos, NM.)*

The global patterns of HIV-1 variation likely result from accidents of viral trafficking. Subtype B viruses, which now differ by up to 17 percent in their *env* coding sequences, are uniformly seen in the United States. It is thought that, purely by chance, this viral subtype was seeded into the United States in the late 1970s, thereby establishing

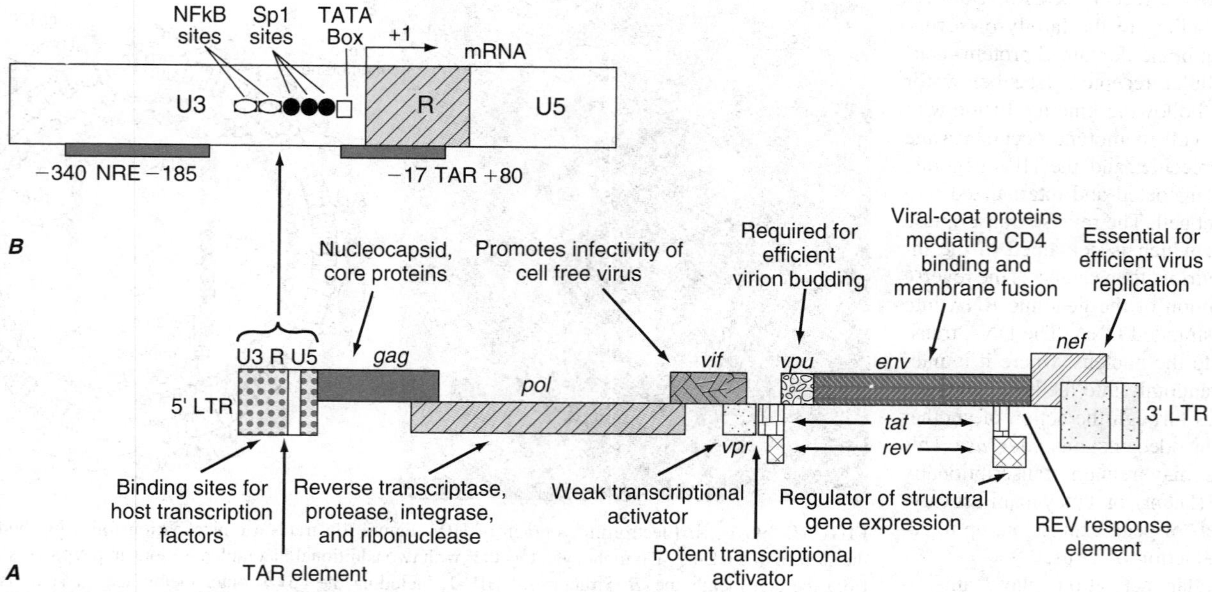

FIGURE 308-4 *A.* The genome of HIV. *B.* The long terminal repeat of HIV. *(A adapted from WC Greene, N Engl J Med 324:308, 1991; B from ZF Rosenberg, AS Fauci, Immunol Today 11:176, 1990.)*

an overwhelming founder effect. Subtype A viruses (of the M group) appear to be the most common form worldwide; many countries have cocirculating viral subtypes that are giving rise to recombinant forms. Figure 308-6 schematically diagrams the worldwide distribution of HIV-1 subtypes by region. The predominant subtype in Europe and the Americas is subtype B. In Africa, more than 75 percent of strains recovered to date have been of subtypes A, C, and D. In Asia, HIV-1 isolates of subtypes E, C, and B are found. Subtype E accounts for most infections in Southeast Asia, while subtype C is prevalent in India (see "HIV Infections and AIDS Worldwide," below). Sequence analyses of HIV-1 isolates from infected individuals indicate that recombination among viruses of different clades likely occurs as a result of infection of an individual with viruses of more than one clade, particularly in geographic areas where clades overlap.

TRANSMISSION

HIV is transmitted by both homosexual and heterosexual contact; by blood and blood products; and by infected mothers to infants either intrapartum, perinatally, or via breast milk. After more than 15 years of scrutiny, there is no evidence that HIV is transmitted by casual contact or that the virus can be spread by insects, such as by a mosquito bite.

SEXUAL TRANSMISSION HIV infection is predominantly a sexually transmitted disease worldwide. Although approximately one-half of reported cases of AIDS in the United States are still among homosexual men, heterosexual transmission is clearly the most common mode of infection worldwide, particularly in developing countries. Furthermore, the yearly incidence of new cases of AIDS contracted through heterosexual transmission is steadily increasing in the United States, mainly among minorities, particularly women minorities (see below).

HIV has been demonstrated in seminal fluid both within infected mononuclear cells and in the cell-free state. The virus appears to concentrate in the seminal fluid, particularly in situations where there are increased numbers of lymphocytes and monocytes in the fluid, as in genital inflammatory states such as urethritis and epididymitis, conditions closely associated with other sexually transmitted diseases (see below). The virus has also been demonstrated in cervical smears and vaginal fluid. There is a strong association of transmission of HIV with receptive anal intercourse, likely owing to the fact that only a thin and fragile rectal mucosal membrane separates the deposited semen from potentially susceptible cells in and beneath the mucosa, as well as the fact that trauma may be associated with anal intercourse. Anal douching and sexual practices such as insertion of hard objects or a clenched fist into the rectum ("fisting") traumatizes the rectal mucosa, thereby increasing the likelihood of infection during receptive anal intercourse. It is likely that anal intercourse provides at least two modalities of infection: direct inoculation into blood in cases of traumatic tears in the mucosa, and infection of susceptible target cells, such as Langerhans cells, in the mucosal layer in the absence of trauma (see below). Although the vaginal mucosa is several layers thicker than the rectal mucosa and less likely to be traumatized during intercourse, it is clear that the virus can be transmitted to either partner through vaginal intercourse. In the United States, there is approximately a 20-fold greater chance of transmission of HIV from a man to a woman than from a woman to a man through vaginal intercourse. This difference may be due in part to the prolonged exposure to infected seminal fluid of the vaginal and cervical mucosa, as well as the endometrium (when semen enters through the cervical os). By comparison, the penis and urethral orifice are exposed relatively briefly to infected vaginal fluid. Bidirectional heterosexual transmission appears to occur much more readily in Thailand than in the United States. The predominant strain of HIV-1 in Thailand is clade E, and the predominant strain in the United States is clade B (see above and below). Clade E has been observed to infect Langerhans cells, which reside in and beneath the mucosal surfaces of the vagina and other genital tract organs, more readily than does HIV clade B. It has been hypothesized that these differences account at least in part for the observed differences in transmission rates, but this hypothesis requires further investigation.

There is a close association between genital ulcerations and transmission, from the standpoints of both susceptibility to infection and infectivity. Infections with microorganisms such as *Treponema pallidum* (see Chap. 174), *Haemophilus ducreyi* (see Chap. 152), and herpes simplex virus (see Chap. 184) are important causes of genital ulcerations linked to transmission of HIV. Furthermore, there have been reports of associations of cervical ectopy as well as cervical erosions resulting from infection due to *Chlamydia trachomatis* (see Chap. 181) and *Neisseria gonorrhoeae* (see Chap. 150) with transmission of HIV infection. In a randomized trial, empirical treatment of genital ulcer disease was associated with a decrease in the risk of HIV infection. Finally, lack of circumcision has been reported to be associated with a higher risk of HIV infection in certain cohorts. This difference may be due to the higher risk of genital ulcerative disease in uncircumcised men as well as to other factors, such as microtrauma and a hospitable environment for the virus in the folds of the prepuce. Thus, in certain cases, all of these phenomena can be considered as *cofactors* for HIV transmission.

Oral sex appears to be a much less efficient mode of transmission of HIV than receptive anal intercourse. In this regard, there is a misperception by some people that oral sex, particularly among homosexual men, can be proposed as a form of "safe sex" and a substitute

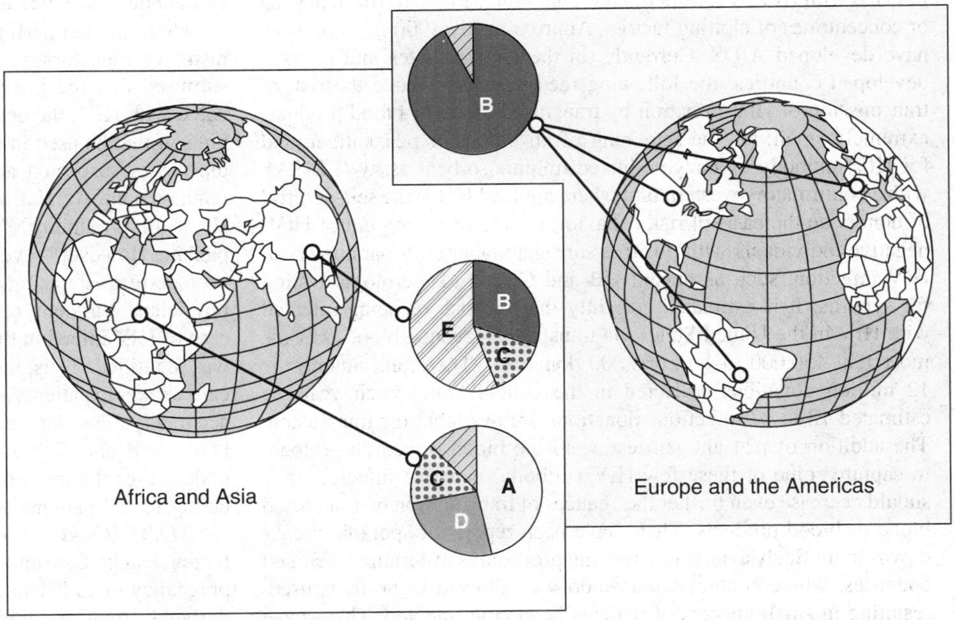

FIGURE 308-6 Geographic distribution of HIV-1 subtypes. The prevalence of HIV-1 genetic subtypes varies by geographic region. The proportions of subtypes in a particular region are indicated by the pie chart. The cross-hatched portion of the charts indicates the proportion of all other subtypes combined. Systematic evaluations of HIV-1 subtypes are needed to confirm and extend these initial observations. *(Courtesy of Dr. Francine E. McCutchan and Dr. Mika O. Salminen of The Henry Jackson Foundation for the Advancement of Military Medicine and of Col. Donald S. Burke of the Walter Reed Army Institute of Research.)*

for receptive anal intercourse. This is a dangerous approach, as there have been reports of documented HIV transmission resulting solely from receptive fellatio and insertive cunnilingus. There are probably many more cases that go unreported because of the frequent practice of both oral sex and receptive anal intercourse by the same person. In this regard, studies in the SIV model have clearly demonstrated the ease with which SIV infection can be transmitted by deposition of virus in the oral cavity. The association of alcohol consumption and crack cocaine use with unsafe sexual behavior, both homosexual and heterosexual, leads to an increased risk of sexual transmission of HIV.

TRANSMISSION BY BLOOD AND BLOOD PRODUCTS HIV can be transmitted by blood and blood products, both among individuals who share contaminated paraphernalia (needles and syringes) for injection drug use and in those who receive transfusions of blood and blood products. Among IDUs, HIV infection occurs through parenteral exposure to infected blood via contaminated drug paraphernalia. The risk of infection increases with the duration of injection drug use, the frequency of needle sharing, participation in the "shooting gallery" drug culture, where several individuals share the same paraphernalia, and the use of injection drugs in a geographic location with a high prevalence of HIV infection, such as inner city areas.

From the late 1970s until the spring of 1985, when mandatory testing of donated blood for HIV-1 was initiated, it has been estimated that over 10,000 individuals in the United States were infected through transfusions of blood or blood products (see Chap. 115). Approximately 7250 individuals who survived the illness for which the transfusion was administered have developed AIDS. It is estimated that 90 to 100 percent of individuals who were transfused with HIV-infected blood became infected. Transfusions of whole blood, packed red blood cells, platelets, leukocytes, and plasma are all capable of transmitting HIV infection. In contrast, hyperimmune gamma globulin, hepatitis B immune globulin, plasma-derived hepatitis B vaccine, and Rh_0 immune globulin have not been associated with transmission of HIV infection. The procedures involved in processing these products either inactivate or remove the virus.

In addition to the above, several thousand hemophiliacs were infected with HIV by receipt of HIV-contaminated fresh frozen plasma or concentrates of clotting factors. Approximately 4000 hemophiliacs have developed AIDS. Currently, in the United States and in most developed countries, the following measures have made the risk of transmission of HIV infection by transfused blood or blood products extremely small: (1) the screening of all blood for p24 antigen and for HIV antibody by enzyme-linked immunosorbent assay (ELISA), with a confirmatory western blot where applicable; (2) the self-deferral of donors on the basis of risk behavior; (3) the screening out of HIV-negative individuals with positive surrogate laboratory parameters of HIV infection, such as hepatitis B and C; and (4) serologic testing for syphilis. It is estimated currently that the risk of being infected with HIV in the United States via transfused screened blood is at the most 1 in 450,000 to 1 in 660,000 donations. Therefore, among the 12 million donations collected in the United States each year, an estimated 18 to 27 infectious donations are available for transfusion. The addition of p24 antigen testing to the blood screening protocol to capture some of these few HIV antibody–negative infected units should decrease even further the chances of transmission by transfused blood or blood products. There have been reports of sporadic breakdowns in routinely available screening procedures in certain developed countries, where contaminated blood was allowed to be transfused, resulting in small clusters of patients becoming infected. There have been no reported cases of transmission of HIV-2 in the United States via donated blood, and, currently, donated blood is screened for both HIV-1 and HIV-2 antibodies. The chance of infection of a hemophiliac via clotting factor concentrates has essentially been eliminated because of the added layer of safety resulting from heat treatment of the concentrates.

Prior to the screening of donors, a small number of cases of transmission of HIV via semen used in artificial insemination and tissues used in organ transplantation were well documented. At present, donors of such tissues are screened for HIV infection prior to transplantation.

OCCUPATIONAL TRANSMISSION OF HIV: HEALTH CARE AND LABORATORY WORKERS There is a small, but definite, occupational risk of HIV transmission among health care workers, laboratory personnel, and potentially others who work with HIV-infected specimens, particularly when sharp objects are used. It is estimated that 250,000 to 1 million health care workers are stuck with needles or other sharp medical instruments in the United States each year. Large, multiinstitutional studies have indicated that the risk of HIV transmission following skin puncture from a needle or a sharp object that was contaminated with blood from a person with documented HIV infection is approximately 0.3 percent (see "HIV and the Health Care Worker" below). The risk of hepatitis B infection following a similar type of exposure is 20 to 30 percent (see Chap. 295). An increased risk for HIV infection following percutaneous exposures to HIV-infected blood is associated with exposures involving a relatively large quantity of blood, as in the case of a device visibly contaminated with the patient's blood, a procedure that involves a needle placed directly in a vein or artery, or a deep injury. In addition, the risk increases for exposures to blood from patients with advanced-stage disease, probably owing to the higher titer of HIV in the blood as well as to other factors, such as the presence of more virulent strains of virus.

There have been reports of health care workers who became infected through the exposure of mucous membranes or abraded skin to HIV-infected material; however, the risk associated with mucocutaneous exposure has been difficult to quantify, because transmission by this route is rare. The risk that has been estimated by pooling data from several studies is 0.1 percent (95 percent confidence interval, 0.01 to 0.5 percent). Factors that might be associated with mucocutaneous transmission of HIV include exposure to an unusually large volume of blood, prolonged contact, and a potential portal of entry. The use of antiretroviral drugs after the exposure may be protective for occupationally exposed health care workers. Transmission of HIV through intact skin has not been documented (see "HIV and the Health Care Worker" below).

In 1990, the CDC reported that an HIV-infected dentist in Florida, by then deceased, had transmitted HIV infection to five of his patients on whom he had performed invasive dental procedures. The mechanisms of transmission were never fully delineated, although it was surmised that the infections occurred through instruments contaminated with HIV; the dentist supposedly used the same instruments on himself that he used in his practice, and a breakdown in sterile procedures was suspected although never proven. To this day, this case remains controversial, and for a time it caused considerable concern about the possibility of spread of HIV from health care provider to patient. However, several epidemiologic studies have subsequently been performed tracing thousands of patients of HIV-infected dentists, physicians, surgeons, obstetricians, and gynecologists, and not a single case of HIV infection that could be linked to the health care providers was identified. Thus, the risk of transmission from an infected health care worker to patients is extremely low; in fact, too low to be measured accurately. The very occurrence of transmission of HIV as well as hepatitis B and C to and from health care workers in the workplace underscores the importance of the use of universal precautions when caring for all patients (see below and Chap. 138).

MATERNAL-FETAL/INFANT TRANSMISSION HIV infection can be transmitted from an infected mother to her fetus during pregnancy or to her infant during delivery. This is an extremely important form of transmission of HIV infection in developing countries, where the proportion of infected women to infected men is approximately 1:1. In the United States, approximately 1600 newborns per year are infected with HIV from their mother. Virologic analysis of aborted fetuses indicate that HIV can be transmitted to the fetus during pregnancy, as early as the first and second trimester. However, maternal transmissions to the fetus occur most commonly in the perinatal period.

This conclusion is based on a number of considerations, including the time frame of identification of infection by the sequential appearance of classes of antibodies to HIV (i.e., the appearance of HIV-specific IgA antibody within 3 to 6 months after birth); a positive viral culture; the appearance of p24 antigenemia weeks to months after delivery, but not at the time of delivery; a polymerase chain reaction (PCR) assay of infant blood following delivery that is negative at birth and positive several months later; the demonstration that the firstborn twin of an infected mother is more commonly infected than is the second twin; and the evidence that cesarean section results in decreased transmission to the infant.

The rate of transmission of HIV from untreated mother to infant/fetus in the United States is approximately 25 percent. Studies in a variety of countries indicate a wide range of transmission rates, with a low of 12.9 percent in a European collaborative study to a high of approximately 45 to 48 percent in Nairobi, Kenya, and other cities in developing countries. These differences may relate to the adequacy of prenatal care as well as to the stage of HIV disease and the general health of the mother during pregnancy. Higher rates of transmission have been associated with advanced-stage disease, a low CD4+ T cell count, high levels of viremia, and vitamin A deficiency in the mother, as well as with chorioamniitis and funisitis. In addition, prolonged labor, a long interval between membrane rupture and delivery, and factors that increase the exposure of the infant to the mother's blood, including fetal-scalp electrodes, episiotomy, and severe cervical and vaginal lacerations, may contribute to transmission to the infant. With regard to levels of viremia, one report indicated that when the level of plasma viral RNA in the mother is less than 100,000 copies per milliliter, there is only a 3 percent likelihood that the infection will be passed to the infant. Finally, it has been speculated that if the mother experiences acute primary HIV infection during pregnancy, there is a higher rate of transmission to the fetus, owing to the high levels of viremia that follow primary infection (see below). Zidovudine treatment of HIV-infected pregnant women from the beginning of the second trimester through delivery and of the infant for 6 weeks following birth has dramatically decreased the rate of intrapartum and perinatal transmission of HIV infection from 22.6 percent in the untreated group to 7.6 percent in the zidovudine-treated group. It is expected that the rate of transmission will decrease even further as more potent combinations of drugs are used in HIV-infected pregnant women (see below and Table 308-26).

Postnatal transmission of HIV from mother to infant has been clearly documented, strongly implicating colostrum and breast milk as the vehicles of infection; virus can be isolated from both fluids. In rare cases, mothers have been infected by transfusions following delivery and have transmitted the infection to their infants, with the only risk factor being breast feeding. This is an important modality of transmission of HIV infection in developing countries, particularly where mothers continue to breast-feed for longer than is usual in developed countries. A meta-analysis of several prospective studies indicated that the risk attributable to breast feeding was 7 to 22 percent. Women with low CD4+ T cell counts, especially those with vitamin A deficiency, may be at increased risk of transmitting HIV to their infants through breast milk. Certainly, in developed countries breast feeding by an infected mother should be avoided. However, there is disagreement regarding recommendations for breast feeding in certain developing countries, where breast milk is the only source of adequate nutrition as well as immunity against potentially serious infections for the infant.

TRANSMISSION BY OTHER BODY FLUIDS There is no convincing evidence that saliva can transmit HIV infection, either through kissing or through other exposures, such as occupationally to health care workers. Although HIV can be isolated from saliva, this has been achieved in only a small percentage of infected individuals. Furthermore, a protein contained in saliva, called secretory leukocyte protease inhibitor, has been demonstrated to possess anti-HIV-1 activity in vitro. There have been outlier cases of suspected transmission by saliva, but these have probably been blood-to-blood transmissions. One case was reported of a 91-year-old man who was bitten during a robbery attempt by an HIV-infected person. He seroconverted, and there was no question that the source of the infection was the human bite. However, the individual who bit him had bleeding gums, and it was thought that the infection was actually transmitted via blood. In addition, a most unusual form of HIV transmission from infected children to mothers in the former Soviet Union has been identified. In those cases, the children (infected through transfusion) were said to have bleeding sores in the mouth, and the mothers were said to have lacerations and abrasions on and around the nipples of the breast resulting from trauma from the children's teeth. Breast feeding had been continued until the children were older than is usual in other developed countries.

Although virus can be identified, if not isolated, from virtually any body fluid, there is no evidence that HIV transmission can occur as a result of exposure to tears, sweat, and urine. However, there have been isolated cases of transmission of HIV infection by body fluids that may or may not have been contaminated with blood. For example, there is a documented case of a mother who very likely contracted HIV infection from her child who had a colostomy. The mother regularly rendered colostomy care, often without wearing gloves, and was exposed to potentially infected material from the colostomy as well as from blood and nasal secretions. Without question, bodily wastes of patients should be handled according to universal precautions (see below).

EPIDEMIOLOGY

HIV INFECTION AND AIDS WORLDWIDE HIV infection/AIDS is pandemic, with cases reported from virtually every country. The current estimate of the number of cases of HIV infection among adults worldwide is approximately 32.2 million, and among children it is approximately 1.2 million; the global distribution of these cases is illustrated in Fig. 308-7. The World Health Organization (WHO) estimates that approximately 10.7 million adults and 3.2 million children infected with HIV have died since the beginning of the epidemic. The global projections for the total number of HIV-infected individuals by the year 2000 range from 40 to 100 million. The HIV epidemic has occurred in "waves" in different regions of the world, each wave having somewhat different characteristics depending on the demographics of the country and region in question and the timing of the introduction of HIV into the population. Of note is the fact that different subtypes or clades of HIV-1 are prevalent in different regions of the world (see above and Fig. 308-6). The potential relevance of these differences relate in part to the development of vaccines. It is unlikely that a single vaccine will be applicable to all regions of the world, because of the substantial variations among viral subtypes throughout the world. In addition, it is likely that there will be gradual introduction of diverse HIV-1 genetic subtypes into the western hemisphere. In this regard, HIV-1 subtypes A, D, and E have been detected in United States and South American servicemen who had been deployed in southeast Asia and sub-Saharan Africa.

Figure 308-8 illustrates the beginnings, real and projected peaks, plateaus, and declines of the epidemic in different regions of the world. Although the epidemic was first recognized in the United States and shortly thereafter in western Europe, it very likely began in sub-Saharan Africa (see above and Chap. 192). The number of new cases of AIDS per year has already peaked and has begun to decline in North America and western Europe (Fig. 308-8). However, the demographics of the epidemic in the United States and western Europe are shifting with regard to the target populations (see below). Sub-Saharan Africa has been particularly devastated by the epidemic, with the prevalance of infection in many cities in the double digits. Indeed, in certain sub-Saharan African countries such as Zimbabwe, available seroprevalence data indicate that more than 25 percent of the adult population may be infected, with much higher prevalences in large trading centers. The epidemic is projected to peak in sub-Saharan Africa by the year 2000; however, it is possible that the epidemic will continue to accelerate there beyond the year 2000. Although the epidemic in Asian countries, particularly India and Thailand, has lagged somewhat behind that in Africa, the number of new cases in this region is accelerating rapidly, and the magnitude of the epidemic is projected to exceed that of sub-Saharan Africa as we enter the twenty-first century.

The actual reported cases of AIDS worldwide are a gross underestimate of the true prevalence, mainly because of the incomplete reporting mechanisms in certain developing countries. The reported cumulative cases of AIDS as of June 1998 are shown in Table 308-3.

The major mode of transmission of HIV worldwide is unquestionably heterosexual sex; this is particularly true in developing countries, where the numbers of infected men and women are approximately equal. Countries such as those in sub-Saharan Africa with a predominantly heterosexual mode of transmission have been termed by WHO as *pattern II* countries. In contrast, pattern I countries are those in which the vast majority of cases are among men who have sex with men or among IDUs. Originally, the United States and Canada, most countries in South America, western Europe, Scandinavia, Australia, and New Zealand were clearly pattern I countries. However, in most of these countries, including the United States, the pattern is gradually shifting, with a growing proportion of new cases among heterosexuals (see below). Pattern III countries are those in which there are relatively few cases of HIV infection/AIDS, and most of the infected individuals have had contact with individuals from pattern I or II countries. A striking index of the spread of the epidemic is the fact that, just a few years ago, India and Thailand, along with other Asian countries, countries in eastern Europe, North Africa, and the Middle East, and certain countries in the Pacific were considered pattern III countries. Both India and Thailand have rapidly evolved into pattern II countries. If educational and behavior-modification programs fail in other pattern III countries, there is no doubt that many of them will evolve to patterns I or II.

Apart from the tragic situation in certain countries in sub-Saharan Africa (see above), the potential for explosive spread of the epidemic can be illustrated dramatically by the situation in Thailand. A single HIV-positive person was identified in Thailand among 101 male prostitutes in Bangkok in 1985, and it was expected that gay men would experience the first wave of rapid transmission. From 1985 through 1987, serosurveys among IDUs in Thailand revealed a prevalence of 0 to 1 percent, and similar surveys conducted among female prostitutes from 1985 through 1989 reported prevalance rates of less than 1 percent. There was very little appreciation of the potential of the epidemic to emerge into the general population, and it was anticipated that it would remain confined largely to men who have sex with men and possibly to IDUs. However, a remarkable pattern began to emerge in 1988. There was an extraordinary explosion of HIV prevalence among IDUs, from 1 percent at the beginning of 1988 to 32 to 43 percent by August–September of 1988. Thus, unexpectedly, the first wave of HIV infection spread rapidly among IDUs. This was followed by successive waves of transmission, first to female commercial sex workers, then to their non-IDU male clients, and ultimately into the low-risk wives and girlfriends of these men in the general population. At present in Thailand, more than 70 percent of reported cases of AIDS are attributable to heterosexual transmission, and the major risk factor for infection is a history of sexual intercourse with commercial sex workers. The prevalence of HIV infection among military recruits bears witness to the growing rate of HIV infection among young men in Thailand, which is boosted by the frequent use of female commercial sex workers by young men in that country. Young men aged 19 to 23 are conscripted by lottery into the Royal Thai Army and Air Force and undergo mandatory HIV testing. Serosurveys of conscripts indicate that in the northern provinces of Thailand, including Chiang Mai, the overall prevalence of HIV infection has reached as high as 18 percent. Fortunately, an aggressive public health campaign to promote the use of condoms is showing signs of decreasing this accelerated spread of HIV in Thailand (see "Prevention" below). Such explosive patterns are being seen in other Asian countries, particularly developing countries such as India. It is projected that this region will equal and surpass sub-Saharan Africa as the most severely afflicted region in the remainder of the twentieth century and into the twenty-first century.

AIDS IN THE UNITED STATES AIDS has had and will continue to have an extraordinary public health impact in the United States. Despite recent declines in AIDS-related deaths, AIDS is the fifth leading cause of death among Americans aged 25 to 44 years (Fig. 308-9). As of June 30, 1998, more than 665,357 cumulative cases of AIDS had been reported in adults and adolescents in the United States (Table 308-4); approximately 60 percent of these patients have died so far. When one looks at the totality of data collected from the beginning of the epidemic, approximately one-half of cases are among men who have had sex with men. Given the large numbers of such individuals who are HIV-infected but do not yet have advanced HIV disease, it is clear that large numbers of new cases of AIDS will continue to emerge in this group. Although there have been progressively smaller annual increases in cases of AIDS among men who have sex with men, male-to-male sexual contact continues to represent the most frequently reported mode of HIV transmission among persons with AIDS. However, over the past few years, the numbers of newly reported cases of AIDS among other groups, including IDUs and heterosexuals (particularly women) from certain large cities such as New York City, have surpassed the numbers of newly reported cases among men who have had sex with men. The proportion of new cases of AIDS per year attributed to heterosexual contact has increased dramatically over the past 10 years in the United States. In the mid-1980s, this proportion was less than 2 percent; in 1998 it was approximately 23 percent (Fig. 308-10). The relationship between geographic areas of the country and the demography of HIV infection and AIDS compellingly links geography, injection

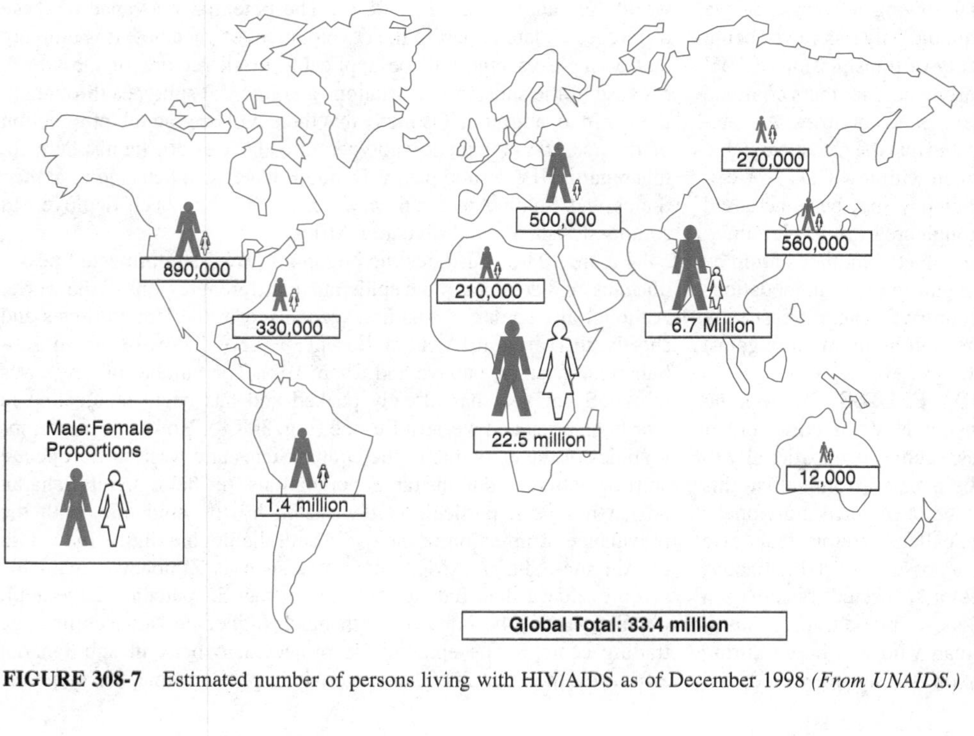

FIGURE 308-7 Estimated number of persons living with HIV/AIDS as of December 1998 *(From UNAIDS.)*

drug use, and heterosexual transmission, particularly among women, with consequent spread to children intrapartum or perinatally (see above). The rates of reported AIDS cases per 100,000 population in the United States by state from July 1997 through June 1998 are shown in Fig. 308-11. Most cases of transmission by injection drug use and heterosexual contact are reported from the northeast and southeast regions of the country, particularly among minorities. HIV infection and AIDS have disproportionately affected minority populations in the United States. African-Americans and Hispanics constitute only 12 and 9 percent of the population, respectively, yet they account for 36 and 18 percent, respectively, of adult/adolescent AIDS cases and for 58 and 23 percent, respectively, of AIDS cases in children.

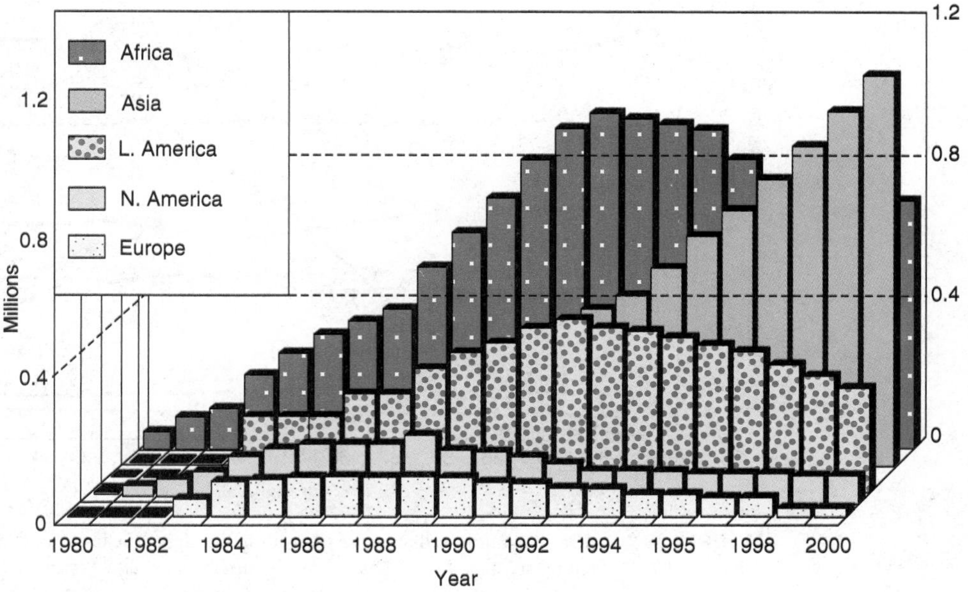

FIGURE 308-8 Estimated/projected annual adult HIV infections *(From WHO.)*

As of June 30, 1998, 8,280 cases of AIDS in children less than 13 years old had been reported, and more than 50 percent of these children have died (Table 308-5). Approximately 90 percent of these children were born to HIV-infected mothers, and, in approximately 60 percent of those cases, the mother was either an IDU or the heterosexual partner of an IDU. Forty-three percent of women with AIDS have become infected through injection drug use, compared to 22 percent of men with AIDS; 39 percent of women have become infected by heterosexual contact, compared to 4 percent of men with AIDS (Table 308-4). Only 1 percent of AIDS cases are among hemophiliacs, and 1 percent are among recipients of blood transfusions, blood products, or transplanted tissue. The relative contribution of the latter groups will gradually decrease, even though individuals infected previously through this mode of transmission will continue to develop AIDS. The risk of additional infections via this mode of transmission in the United States is extremely small (see above).

Since 1995, the incidence of AIDS has declined each year. This trend likely reflects both reduced infection rates since the mid-1980s, the availability of potent antiretroviral therapies and more widespread use of prophylactic therapies, which delay the onset of AIDS (see below). Also, the demography of newly infected individuals has changed considerably since the mid-1980s (see below).

HIV PREVALENCE IN THE UNITED STATES Using "back-calculation" mathematical modeling based on the national AIDS database compiled by the CDC and the distribution of the incubation period from initial infection with HIV to diagnosis with AIDS, it is estimated that between 630,000 and 897,000 adults and adolescents in the United States were living with HIV infection as of January, 1993, including 107,000 to 150,000 women. This estimate results in an overall nationwide prevalence of HIV infection of approximately 0.3 to 0.4 percent. The estimated incidence of HIV infection has declined among white males, especially those older than 30 years. In contrast, HIV incidence appears to have remained relatively constant among women and minorities (Fig. 308-12). As of January 1993, prevalence was highest among young adults in their late twenties and thirties and among minorities. An estimated 3 percent of black men and 1 percent of black women in their thirties were living with HIV infection as of that date. The estimated prevalence of HIV infection in the United States among different groups is shown in Table 308-6. The number of new infections per year is estimated to be approximately 40,000.

The seroprevalence rates differ greatly among groups practicing high-risk behaviors, and seroprevalence studies have given insight into the variability of HIV prevalence among diverse cohorts and the risk factors associated with seroconversion. There is a great deal of variability in seroprevalence and seroconversion rates related to geography, race, economic status, age, sex and, of course, behavior. Rates of seroconversion and seroprevalence have remained stable among certain groups and have increased or decreased among others over the past few years.

The routine and periodic nature of HIV-1 testing in the United States Army has allowed the direct measurement of the incidence of new infections among soldiers. Between November 1985 and October 1993, 978 HIV-1 seroconversions were noted among 1,061,768 soldiers with over 3.6 million person-years of follow-up. The seroconversion rate was 0.27 per 1000 person-years. A significant decreasing trend in seroconversion rates was seen over the period of analysis. The rate of new infections declined significantly from the first interval, 1985–1987 (0.43 per 1000 person-years), to the second interval, 1987–1988 (0.28 per 1000 person-years), but stabilized at approximately 0.22 per 1000 person-years after 1988. The latter figure represents approximately 100 to 150 new infections among soldiers annually. Subgroup analysis revealed that being young, male, of a minority race/ethnicity, and unmarried were strongly associated with HIV-1 seroconversion.

An important source of information regarding seroprevalence in various communities is the screening of patients who visit hospital emergency departments. A typical example of trends in inner-city HIV prevalence that is similar to results from a number of comparable studies is seen with data from the Johns Hopkins Hospital Department of Emergency Medicine. Of 1606 patients screened in 1992, 183 (11.4 percent) were HIV-positive, compared with 6.0 percent from an identical study conducted in 1988. The seroprevalence rose over this interval from 10.0 to 17.0 percent in black males, from 3.8 to 8.5 percent in black females, from 5.5 to 9.8 percent in white males, and from

Table 308-3

Cumulative Worldwide Cases of AIDS Reported to the World Health Organization as of June 1998

Country/Region	Cases
Africa	686,256
Americas	889,465
Canada	15,528
Caribbean/Bahamas	20,826
Central America	15,913
Mexico	35,119
South America	161,011
United States of America	641,068
Asia	101,429
Europe	207,890
Oceania	8744
TOTAL	1,893,784

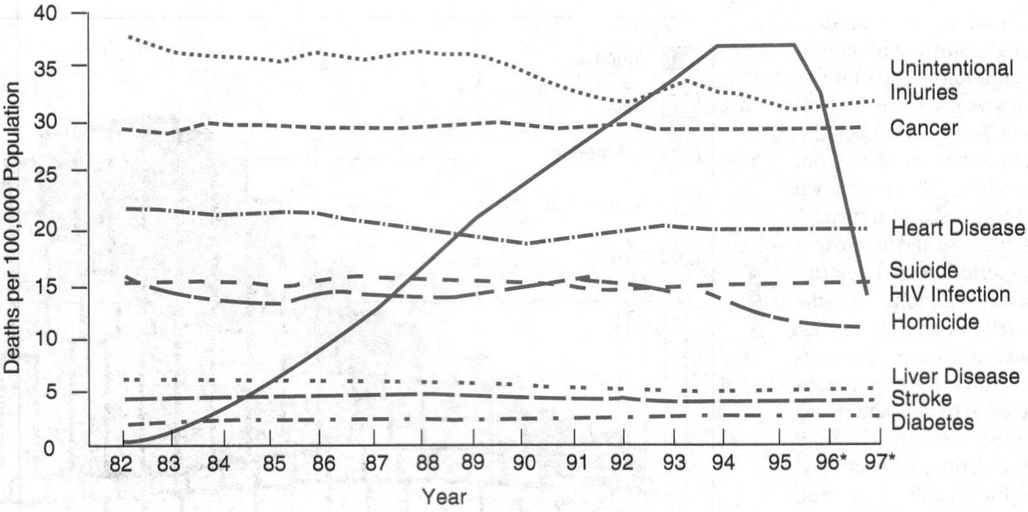

FIGURE 308-9 AIDS is the fifth leading cause of death in the United States among individuals 25 to 44 years old, 1982 to 1997. *, Preliminary data. *(From Centers for Disease Control and Prevention, 1998.)*

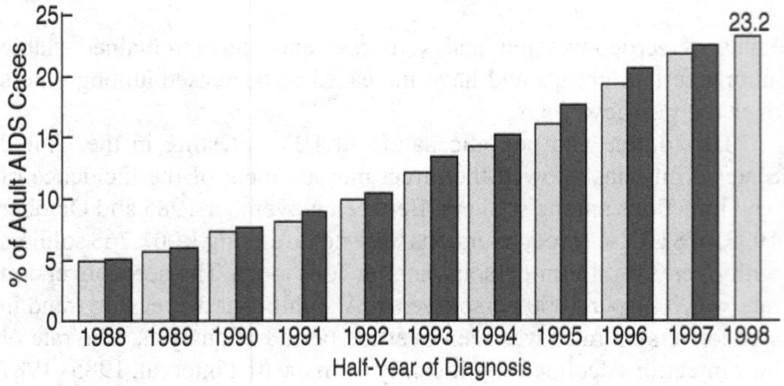

FIGURE 308-10 Percentage of AIDS cases attributed to heterosexual transmission, by year of diagnosis, in the United States from January 1988 to June 1998. *(From CDC.)*

1.6 to 1.9 percent in white females. Seroprevalence rates among patients whose only risk was heterosexual contact increased more than fourfold.

Other studies indicate high rates of seroprevalence among homeless people, inmates of prisons, and teenagers. In a cross-sectional study of inner-city shelters and free-meal programs in San Francisco, HIV seroprevalence was 8.5 percent. Of note, the prevalence of *Mycobacterium tuberculosis* infection was 32 percent, and 19 percent of the HIV-seropositive subjects had positive tuberculin skin tests (see below). Voluntary testing programs for HIV infection among prison inmates reveal a range of results depending on geographic location, from less than 1.0 percent in Oregon to 8.5 percent in Maryland. In anonymous, cross-sectional serosurveys of HIV infection among teenagers conducted in 130 clinics in 24 cities, the median clinic-specific prevalence was 0.2 percent in 22 adolescent medicine clinics, 0.3 percent in 33 correctional facilities, 0.5 percent in 70 sexually transmitted disease (STD) clinics, and 1.1 percent in 5 homeless youth centers. Rates were highest among young men who have sex with men; however, most teenagers practicing risk behaviors reported heterosexual activity as their only potential risk of exposure to HIV.

The seroprevalence and incidence rates among men who have sex with men has evolved dramatically since the beginning of the AIDS epidemic. The rate of new infection among homosexual men attending STD clinics in San Francisco in 1982 and 1983 was approximately 19 percent per year, and the prevalence of infection among this cohort was estimated at greater than 50 percent. By the mid and late 1980s, the seroconversion rate had dropped to less than 1 percent per year, likely owing to a combination of a saturation effect and significant behavioral modification. However, in the early 1990s, a disturbing upward trend in the annual rate of new infection was noted among young homosexual men who were "coming out." As a group, young homosexual men have not witnessed firsthand the devastation of the epidemic to the degree that their older counterparts have and are

Table 308-4

Adult/Adolescent AIDS Cases by Exposure Category and Race/Ethnicity in the United States Reported through June 30, 1998

Exposure Category	White, not Hispanic, No. (%)	Black, not Hispanic, No. (%)	Hispanic, No. (%)	Asian/Pacific Islander, No. (%)	Native American/ Alaskan Native, No. (%)	Total,* No. (%)
Men who have sex with men	204,339 (69)	67,346 (29)	41,862 (36)	3,114 (66)	884 (49)	317,862 (49)
Injection drug use (female and heterosexual male)	34,602 (12)	88,468 (37)	44,072 (38)	313 (7)	368 (20)	168,008 (26)
Men who have sex with men and inject drugs	21,803 (7)	13,337 (6)	6,532 (6)	147 (3)	257 (14)	42,093 (6)
Hemophilia or coagulation disorder	3,652 (1)	587 (0)	439 (0)	69 (1)	28 (2)	4,781 (1)
Heterosexual contact	13,637 (5)	33,681 (14)	14,695 (12)	379 (8)	147 (8)	62,599 (9)
Transfusions with blood or blood products	4,843 (2)	2,164 (1)	1,078 (1)	194 (4)	21 (1)	8,331 (1)
Risk not reported or identified	12,095 (4)	30,526 (13)	9,894 (7)	525 (11)	116 (6)	53,422 (8)
Total	294,971	236,109	118,572	4,741	1,821	657,076
% of total adult/adolescent AIDS cases	(45)	(36)	(18)	(<1)	(<1)	(100)

* Includes 862 persons whose race/ethnicity is unknown.

SOURCE: Centers for Disease Control and Prevention, *HIV/AIDS Surveillance Report* 10(No.1):1–40,1998.

engaging in a greater degree of high-risk behavior. A survey was conducted among 425 young (17 to 22 years) homosexual and bisexual men in public venues in San Francisco and Berkeley, California, including street corners, sidewalks, dance clubs, bars, and parks. HIV seroprevalence was 9.4 percent and was significantly higher among African-Americans (21.2 percent) than among other racial/ethnic groups. Approximately one-third of the participants reported unprotected anal intercourse, and 11.8 percent reported injection drug use in the previous 6 months. Of the HIV-infected men, 70 percent did not know that they were HIV seropositive.

During the earlier years of the epidemic, the HIV seroprevalence among IDUs in treatment programs in several metropolitan areas ranged from 0 to greater than 50 percent. The rates varied considerably with geographic location, with the highest rates observed on the eastern seaboard and much lower rates in the West and Southwest. To determine the trends in HIV seroprevalence and risk behavior among IDUs in New York City, comparisons were made between two surveys of IDUs at the same hospital-based drug abuse detoxification program. One survey was conducted among 141 IDUs in 1984, and the other among 974 IDUs from 1990 through 1992. The HIV seroprevalence remained stable over this period at slightly more than 50 percent. The estimated seroconversion rate among the new IDUs in the study was 6.6 per 100 person-years at risk. While still high, this rate was approximately half that of the rate of 13 per 100 person-years at risk estimated for IDUs seen at the same detoxification program from 1978 through 1983 and for whom historically collected serum samples were available for HIV testing. Large-scale decreases in risk behaviors were observed; for example, the use of potentially contaminated syringes declined from 51 percent to 7 percent of injections. Additional risk reduction was associated with the use of the underground syringe exchanges. In other studies, HIV prevalence rates among female prostitutes also varied greatly, from 0 to approximately 50 percent, with the rates directly reflecting the degree of injection drug use among the groups surveyed as well as the prevalence of HIV in the IDUs in that geographic location at the time of the survey.

Further information regarding changes in trends of HIV seroprevalence was obtained by annual studies of patients attending sentinel clinics for STDs in 40 metropolitan areas throughout the United States from 1988 through 1992. From 1988 to 1992, 552,665 specimens were tested in 80 STD clinics. The overall HIV prevalence was 33 percent (range among metropolitan areas, 5 to 52 percent) among homosexual and bisexual men; 3 percent (range, 0.3 to 11 percent) among heterosexual men; 2 percent (range, 0.1 to 11 percent) among women, and 10 percent (range, 0.5 to 45 percent) among heterosexual IDUs. HIV seroprevalence decreased among all homosexual and bisexual men, but especially among white homosexual and bisexual men, for whom it fell from 32 percent in 1989 to 22 percent in 1992. Among heterosexual men and women, HIV seroprevalence decreased among whites and, to a lesser degree, Hispanics, but it remained essentially stable among African-Americans over time. Among heterosexual IDUs, seroprevalence was also unchanged. This study clearly demonstrates a shift in the HIV epidemic in the United States, with an increasing burden of infection among heterosexuals and IDUs, particularly in minority populations (see above).

Thus, HIV infection and AIDS is widespread in the United States, and, although the epidemic on the whole is plateauing, it is spreading rapidly among certain populations, stabilizing in others, and decreasing in others. Similar to other STDs, HIV infection will not spread homogeneously throughout the population of the United States. However, it is clear that anyone who practices high-risk behavior is at risk for HIV infection. In addition, the alarming increase in infections and

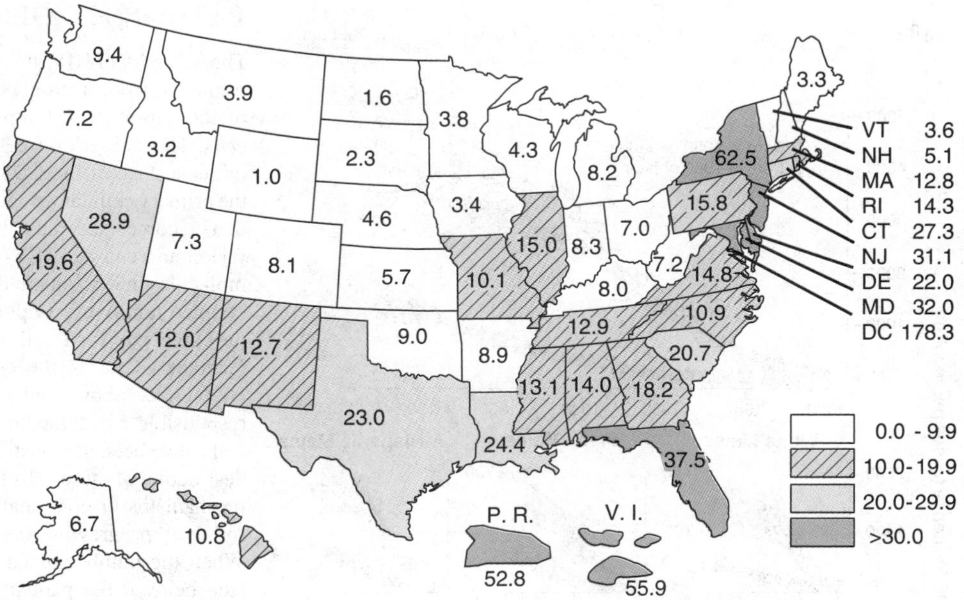

FIGURE 308-11 Annual rates of AIDS cases in the United States per 100,000 population by state (July 1997 through June 1998). *(From CDC HIV/AIDS Surveillance Report, 1998.)*

Table 308-5

Pediatric (<13 Years) AIDS Cases by Exposure Category and Race/Ethnicity in the United States Reported through June 30, 1998

Exposure Category	White, not Hispanic, No. (%)	Black, not Hispanic, No. (%)	Hispanic, No. (%)	Asian/Pacific Islander, No. (%)	Native American/ Alaskan Native, No. (%)	Total,* No. (%)
Hemophilia/coagulation disorder	158 (11)	35 (1)	37 (2)	3 (7)	1 (4)	234 (3)
Mother with/at risk for AIDS/HIV infection	1,097 (75)	4,587 (95)	1,758 (92)	30 (67)	26 (96)	7,512 (91)
IV drug related	*675*	*2,475*	*1,182*	*8*	*19*	*4,366*
Sex with bisexual male	*65*	*59*	*38*	*2*	—	*164*
Sex with person with hemophilia	*17*	*5*	*7*	—	—	*29*
Receipt of transfusion of blood, blood components, or tissue	*43*	*78*	*33*	*1*	—	*155*
Other	*297*	*1,970*	*498*	*19*	*7*	*2,798*
Receipt of transfusion of blood, blood components, or tissue	184 (13)	89 (2)	92 (5)	10 (22)	—	375 (5)
Risk not reported or identified	24 (2)	107 (2)	25 (1)	2 (4)	—	159 (2)
Pediatric subtotal	1,463	4,818	1,912	45	27	8,280
% of total pediatric AIDS cases	(18)	(58)	(23)	(<1)	(<1)	(100)

* Includes 15 children whose race/ethnicity is unknown.

SOURCE: Centers for Disease Control and Prevention, *HIV/AIDS Surveillance Report* 10(1): 1–40, 1998.

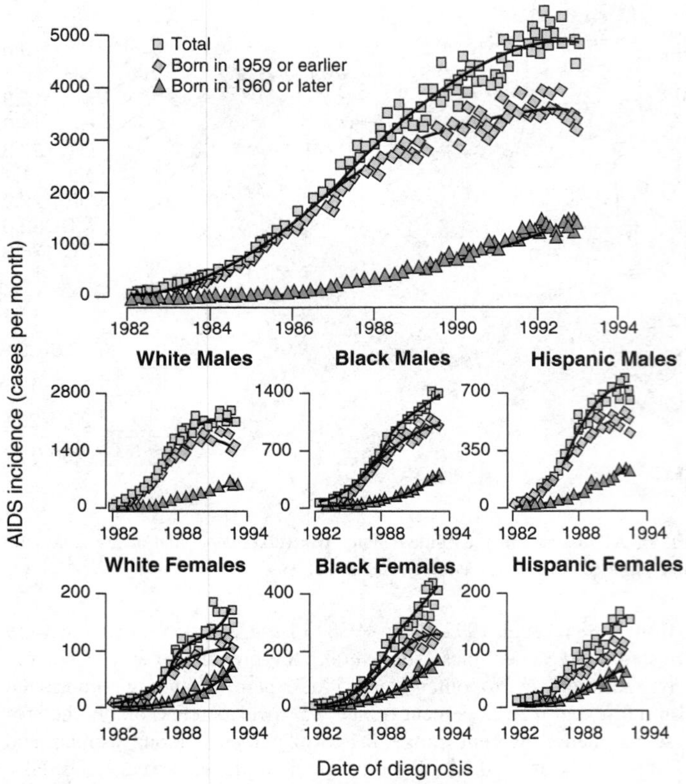

FIGURE 308-12 Monthly incidence of AIDS in the United States from 1982 through January, 1993. *A.* Monthly AIDS incidence for the total U.S. population (squares) and for individuals born in 1959 or earlier (diamonds) and in 1960 or later (triangles). *B.* Monthly AIDS incidence for white, black, and Hispanic men and women. Locally weighted regression smoothing with a bandwidth of 40 percent of the time axis was used to highlight trends in incidence (solid curves). The date axes mark 1 January of the years indicated. *(From Rosenberg.)*

AIDS cases among heterosexuals, particularly sexual partners of IDUs, women, infants born of infected women, and adolescents, as well as spread in certain inner city areas, particularly among underserved minority populations with inadequate access to health care, testifies to the fact that the epidemic of HIV infection in the United States is a public health problem of major proportions.

Table 308-6

Prevalence of HIV-1 Infection in the United States as of January 1, 1993, Estimated by Back-Calculation from AIDS Incidence Data*

Group	Alive with HIV-1 Infection†	HIV-1 Positive, Ages 18 to 59 y‡
MALES		
White	255 (248–370)	0.49 (0.48–0.70)
Black	184 (176–236)	2.29 (2.20–2.91)
Hispanic	97 (91–131)	1.44 (1.37–1.87)
Total	536 (523–747)	0.78 (0.77–1.04)
FEMALES		
White	25 (23–34)	0.05 (0.04–0.06)
Black	67 (63–82)	0.74 (0.69–0.90)
Hispanic	24 (21–32)	0.34 (0.31–0.45)
Total	116 (107–150)	0.16 (0.15–0.20)
Grand Total	652 (630–897)	0.47 (0.46–0.62)

* Plausible ranges, given in parentheses, reflect some uncertainty about the incubation distribution.
† Data given in thousands.
‡ Prevalence (%)

SOURCE: From Rosenberg.

PATHOPHYSIOLOGY AND PATHOGENESIS

The hallmark of HIV disease is a profound immunodeficiency resulting primarily from a progressive quantitative and qualitative deficiency of the subset of T lymphocytes referred to as *helper* or *inducer T cells*. This subset of T cells is defined phenotypically by the presence on its surface of the CD4 molecule (see Chap. 305), which serves as the primary cellular receptor for HIV. It has recently been demonstrated that a coreceptor must be present together with CD4 for efficient fusion and entry of HIV-1 into its target cells. These coreceptors are molecules that belong to the seven-transmembrane-domain G protein–coupled family of receptors. The molecule termed *fusin* or CXCR4 is the coreceptor for T cell–tropic strains of HIV-1, and the β-chemokine receptor CCR5 is the coreceptor for macrophage-tropic strains of HIV-1 (see above and below). Although a number of mechanisms responsible for cytopathicity and immune dysfunction of CD4+ T cells have been demonstrated in vitro, particularly direct infection and destruction of these cells by HIV (see below), it remains unclear which mechanisms or combination of mechanisms is primarily responsible for their progressive depletion and functional impairment in vivo. When the number of CD4+ T cells declines below a certain level (see below), the patient is at high risk of developing a variety of opportunistic diseases, particularly the infections and neoplasms that are AIDS-defining illnesses. Some features of AIDS, such as Kaposi's sarcoma and neurologic abnormalities, cannot be explained completely by the immunosuppressive effects of HIV, since these complications may occur prior to the development of severe immunologic impairment.

The combination of viral pathogenic and immunopathogenic events that occur during the course of HIV disease from the moment of initial (primary) infection through the development of advanced-stage disease is complex and varied. It is important to appreciate that the pathogenic mechanisms of HIV disease are multifactorial and multiphasic and are different at different stages of the disease. Therefore, it is essential to consider the typical clinical course of an HIV-infected individual in order to more fully appreciate these pathogenic events (Fig. 308-13).

PRIMARY HIV INFECTION, INITIAL VIREMIA, AND DISSEMINATION OF VIRUS The events associated with primary HIV infection are likely critical to the determination of the subsequent course of HIV disease. In particular, the phenomenon of dissemination of virus to lymphoid organs is a major factor in the establishment of a chronic and persisent infection (see below). The initial infection of susceptible cells may vary somewhat with the route of infection. Virus that enters directly into the bloodstream via infected blood or blood products (i.e., transfusions, use of contaminated needles for injecting drugs, sharp-object injuries, maternal-to-fetal transmission either intrapartum or perinatally, or, in certain cases, sexual intercourse where there is enough trauma to cause bleeding) is likely cleared from the circulation to the spleen and other lymphoid organs, where it replicates

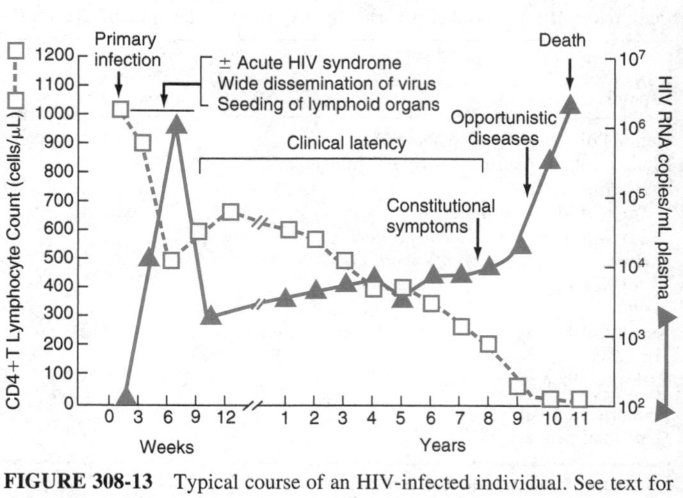

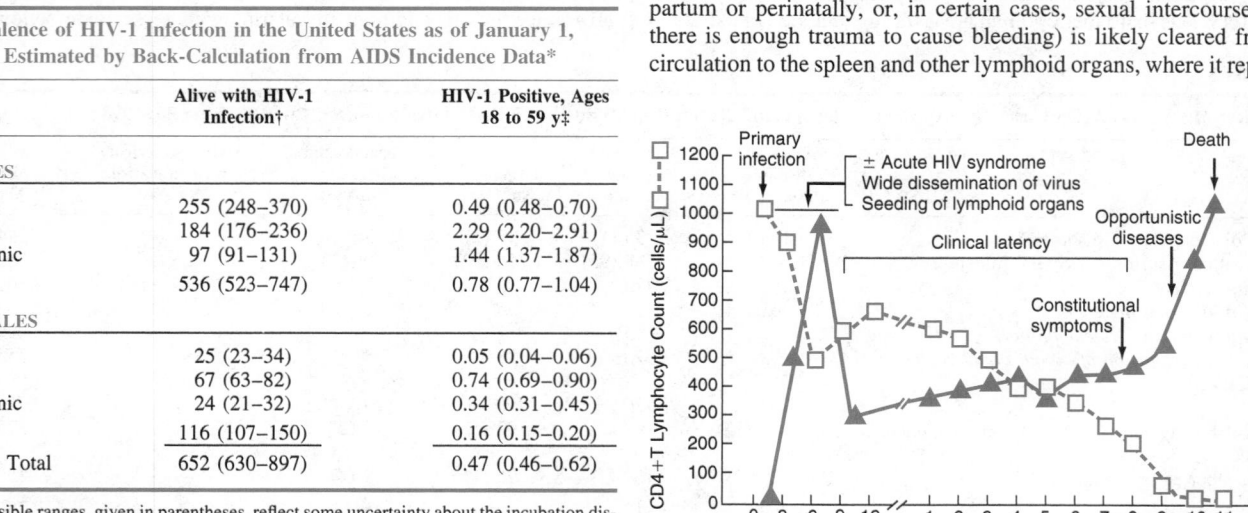

FIGURE 308-13 Typical course of an HIV-infected individual. See text for detailed description. *(From Fauci et al.)*

to a critical level and then leads to a burst of viremia that disseminates virus throughout the body. It is uncertain which cell in the blood or lymphoid tissue is the first actually to become infected. Certainly, CD4+ T cells and cells of monocyte lineage are the major ultimate targets of infection. Recent data indicate that dendritic cells are efficient transporters or presenters of HIV to CD4+ T cells, which is consistent with their role as extremely efficient antigen-presenting cells in the course of the normal immune response to antigen (see Chap. 305). The likely scenario in infection contracted via blood exposure is that free virus or virus-infected cells are cleared by the reticuloendothelial system and come into contact with susceptible target cells in these tissues, or that blood dendritic cells carry virus to tissues, particularly lymph nodes, where they put the virus in contact with susceptible CD4+ T cells. This is somewhat different from the role of follicular dendritic cells that reside in the germinal centers of lymphoid tissue and serve as traps or filters for the virus (see below). Dendritic cells have been reported to express low levels of CD4. However, there are conflicting reports as to whether blood dendritic cells themselves can actually become infected with HIV. Certain studies have shown that dendritic cells form conjugates with several CD4+ T cells and that active virus replication takes place within the conjugates. Data from the SIV-macaque model indicate that mucosal dendritic cells, known as Langerhans cells, become infected following mucosal exposure to the virus, as might occur when infected seminal fluid comes into contact with mucosal surfaces of the urogenital tract, the upper gastrointestinal tract, or the rectum. This mechanism likely operates when the virus enters "locally" (as opposed to directly into the blood), as via the vagina, rectum, or urethra during intercourse, or via the upper gastrointestinal tract from swallowed infected semen, vaginal fluid, or breast milk. The common denominator of local infection is the drainage of Langerhans cells to the regional lymph nodes; these cells either are themselves infected or carry virus to the lymphoid tissue. CD4+ T cells in the regional lymph nodes become infected after contact with the Langerhans cells, and virus replication intensifies prior to the initiation of an HIV-specific immune response (see below), leading to a burst of viremia (Fig. 308-13), which then leads to rapid dissemination of virus to other lymphoid organs, the brain, and other tissues. It is well documented that individuals who experience the "acute HIV syndrome" following primary infection have high levels of viremia which last for several weeks (see below). The acute mononucleosis-like symptoms are well correlated with the presence of viremia. It is highly likely that most patients develop some degree of viremia, which contributes to virus dissemination, even though they remain asymptomatic or do not recall experiencing symptoms. Many patients who have progressed to AIDS and who clearly have had wide dissemination of virus do not report having experienced such an acute viral syndrome. Careful examination of lymph nodes from more than one site in patients with established HIV infection who did not report symptoms that could have been related to primary infection strongly indicate that wide dissemination to lymphoid tissue occurs in most patients. A more detailed description of the role of lymphoid tissue in the immunopathogenesis of HIV disease is given below. It is unclear whether a high level of initial plasma viremia is associated with a poor prognosis. However, the set point of the level of steady state plasma viremia after approximately 1 year does seem to correlate with the rapidity of disease progression (see below).

ESTABLISHMENT OF CHRONIC AND PERSISTENT INFECTION HIV infection is relatively unique among human viral infections in that, despite the robust cellular and humoral immune responses that are mounted following primary infection (see below), the virus is, with very few exceptions, not cleared completely from the body. Rather, a chronic infection develops that persists with varying degrees of virus replication for a median of approximately 10 years before the patient becomes clinically ill (see below). It is this establishment of a chronic infection that is the hallmark of HIV disease. Throughout the often protracted course of chronic infection, virus replication can almost invariably be detected, if not by measurable plasma viremia, then by demonstration of virus replication in lymphoid tissue. In the vast majority of human viral infections, if the host survives, the virus is completely cleared from the body and a state of immunity against subsequent infection develops. HIV infection very rarely kills the host during primary infection. Certain viruses, such as herpes simplex virus (see Chap. 184), are not completely cleared from the body after infection but instead enter a latent state; in these cases, clinical latency is accompanied by microbiologic latency. This is not the case with HIV infection, in which some degree of virus replication invariably occurs during the period of clinical latency (see below). Chronicity associated with persistent virus replication can be seen in certain cases of hepatitis B and C infections (see Chap. 297); however, in these infections the immune system is not a target. As mentioned above, HIV usually does not abruptly kill the host; rather it generally succeeds in escaping from a rather vigorous immune response and establishing a state of chronic infection with persistently active virus replication.

HIV uses a number of mechanisms to evade elimination by the immune system. HIV has an extraordinary ability to mutate, but this mechanism probably acts mainly after the establishment of chronic infection and contributes to the maintenance of chronicity. Since the transmitted virus and the virus that initially becomes established as a chronic infection are relatively homogeneous, the initial escape from immune system control likely involves other mechanisms. Molecular analysis of clonotypes has demonstrated that clones of CD8+ cytolytic T lymphocytes (CTLs) that expand greatly during primary HIV infection and likely represent the high-affinity clones that would be expected to be most efficient in eliminating virus-infected cells disappear after their initial burst of expansion. The disappearance of these HIV-specific cells cannot be explained by mutations in the viral epitope to which they are directed, since virus sequencing studies indicate that the initial viral epitope is still present when the clones are no longer detected. Furthermore, other, less expanded clones of CD8+ T cells that recognize the same viral epitope persist and likely account for the partial control of virus replication. It is thought that the initially expanded clones are deleted owing to the overwhelming exposure to viral antigens during the initial burst of viremia, similar to the exhaustion of CD8+ CTLs that has been reported in the murine model of lymphocytic choriomeningitis virus (LCMV) infection. To compound this phenomenon, virus replication and thus saturation of antigen-presenting cells with viral antigen take place in the lymphoid tissue (see below), which is also the site of generation of HIV-specific CTLs.

Another important mechanism of HIV escape is related to the fact that, during primary HIV infection and the transition to established chronic infection, both activated HIV-specific CTLs and CTL precursors are preferentially and paradoxically segregated in the peripheral blood, where very little active virus replication takes place, rather than in the lymphoid tissue, which is the main site of virus replication and spreading and the major source of plasma viremia. Finally, the escape of HIV from elimination during primary infection allows the formation of a large pool of latently infected cells that cannot be eliminated by virus-specific CTLs. Thus, despite a potent immune response and the marked downregulation of virus replication following primary HIV infection, HIV succeeds in establishing a state of chronic infection with a variable degree of persistent virus replication. In most cases, during this period the patient makes the clinical transition from acute primary infection to a relatively prolonged state of clinical latency (see below).

Viral Dynamics It was originally thought that very little virus replication occurred during clinical latency. However, studies of lymphoid tissue using PCR analysis for HIV RNA and in situ hybridization for individual virus-expressing cells clearly demonstrated that HIV replication occurs throughout the course of HIV infection, even during clinical latency, when it is very difficult to culture virus from unfractionated peripheral blood mononuclear cells. The availability of sensitive PCR techniques led to the demonstration that plasma viremia is present at all stages of HIV disease. Subsequently, the dynamics of viral production and turnover were quantified using mathematical modeling in the setting of the administration of reverse transcriptase and protease inhibitors to HIV-infected individuals in clinical studies.

Treatment with these drugs resulted in a precipitous decline in the level of plasma viremia, which typically fell by 99 percent within 2 weeks. The number of CD4+ T cells in the blood increased concurrently, which implies that the killing of CD4+ T cells is linked directly to the levels of replicating virus. However, a contribution by redistribution of cells into the peripheral blood from other body compartments following the decrease in viremia has not been completely ruled out. It was determined on the basis of the emergence of resistant mutants during therapy that 99 percent of the circulating virus originated from recently infected cells. It was also determined that the half-life of a circulating virion was approximately 6 h and that of productively infected cells was 1.6 days. Given the relatively steady level of plasma viremia and of infected cells, it appears that extremely large amounts of virus (approximately 10^{10} virions) are produced and cleared from the circulation each day. In addition, data suggest that the minimum duration of the HIV-1 life cycle in vivo averages 1.2 days; the average generation time (the time from release of a virion until it infects another cell and causes the release of a new generation of viral particles) is estimated to be 2.6 days. Other studies have demonstrated that the decrease in plasma viremia that results from antiretroviral therapy correlates closely with a decrease in virus replication in lymph nodes, further confirming that lymphoid tissue is the main site of HIV replication and the main source of plasma viremia.

The level of steady-state viremia, called the viral *set point*, at approximately 1 year has important prognostic implications for the progression of HIV disease. It has been demonstrated that HIV-infected individuals who have a low set point at 6 months to 1 year progress to AIDS much more slowly than individuals whose set point is very high at that time. Levels of viremia generally increase as disease progresses. Measurement of the level of viremia is playing an increasingly important role in the guiding of therapeutic decisions in HIV-infected individuals (see below).

Immunopathogenic Events during Clinical Latency With few exceptions, the level of CD4+ T cells in blood decreases gradually and progressively in HIV-infected individuals. The slope of this decline, together with the level of plasma viremia (see above), predicts well the pattern of the clinical course and the development of advanced disease. Most patients are entirely asymptomatic while this progressive decline is taking place (see below), which led to the term *clinical latency*. However, clinical latency does not mean disease latency, since progression is generally relentless during this period. Furthermore, clinical latency should not be confused with microbiologic latency since, as mentioned above, although there are cells that are latently infected with virus, there is virtually always some degree of virus replication, even during the early stages of HIV disease.

ADVANCED HIV DISEASE After a variable period, usually measured in years, the CD4+ T cell count falls below a critical level (less than 200 cells per microliter), and the patient becomes highly susceptible to opportunistic disease. For this reason, the CDC case definition of AIDS was modified to include all HIV-infected individuals with CD4+ T cell counts below this level (see Table 308-1). Patients may experience constitutional signs and symptoms, or they may develop an opportunistic disease abruptly without any prior symptoms, although the latter scenario is unusual. The depletion of CD4+ T cells continues to be progressive and unrelenting in this phase. It is not uncommon for CD4+ T cell counts to drop as low as 10/μL or even to zero, yet the patients may survive for months or even for more than 1 year. This situation has become increasingly common as patients are treated more aggressively and are given prophylaxis against the common life-threatening opportunistic infections (see below). Ultimately, patients who progress to this severest form of immunosuppression usually succumb to opportunistic infections or neoplasms (see below).

LONG-TERM SURVIVORS AND LONG-TERM NONPROGRESSORS The median time from primary HIV infection to the development of AIDS is approximately 10 years. The definitions of *long-term survivor* and *long-term nonprogressor* continue to evolve as more data are collected from prospective cohort studies. Predictions from one study estimate that approximately 13 percent of homosexual/bisexual men who were infected at an early age may remain free of clinical AIDS for longer than 20 years. Currently, individuals are considered to be long-term survivors if they remain alive for 10 to 15 years after initial infection. In most such individuals the disease has progressed, in that they have significant immunodeficiency and many have experienced opportunistic diseases. Some of these individuals have CD4+ T cell counts that have decreased to 200/μL or lower but have remained stable at that level for years. The mechanisms of this stabilization are not entirely clear but may relate to the beneficial effects of antiretroviral therapy and prophylaxis against opportunistic infections. In addition, a number of viral and/or host determinants likely contribute to the long-term survival of these individuals. In some individuals, the virus may either have been less virulent initially or have mutated to a less virulent form. Quantitative and qualitative aspects of the HIV-specific immune response, as well as unrecognized genetic factors, may also contribute to the long-term survival of these individuals.

Less than 5 percent of HIV-infected individuals are characterized as *long-term nonprogressors*. While all long-term nonprogressors are long-term survivors the reverse is not true. Although different sets of empirical criteria have been proposed for the definition of long-term nonprogression, there is a common denominator. Individuals who have been infected with HIV for a long period (approximately 10 or more years), whose CD4+ T cell counts are in the normal range and have remained stable over years, and who have not received antiretroviral therapy are considered to be long-term nonprogressors. These patients are characterized by a low viral burden (low number of HIV-infected cells), low levels of plasma viremia, generally normal immune function according to commonly measured parameters (skin tests, in vitro lymphocyte responses to various mitogens and antigens), and normal-appearing lymphoid tissue architecture as determined on lymph node biopsy. In general, long-term nonprogressors manifest robust HIV-specific immune responses, both humoral (neutralizing antibodies) and cell-mediated (HIV-specific CTLs). Although viremia is consistently low in these patients, many have persistent viremia by the most sensitive PCR assays. No qualitative abnormalities in the virus could be detected in most of these patients. However, a small subset of patients do have defective virus; in particular, in one of five long-term nonprogressors, the virus had a defect in the *nef* gene. In another report, a blood donor in Australia who was HIV-infected and a group of six individuals who were infected by blood or blood products from that donor remain free of HIV-related disease and have normal and stable CD4+ T cell counts 10 to 14 years after infection. Sequence analysis of viruses isolated from the donor and recipients revealed similar deletions in the *nef* gene and the region of overlap of *nef* and the U3 region of the HIV LTR (see Fig. 308-4). The precise role of host factors in long-term nonprogression remains unclear. There is no obvious and consistent genetic determinant for nonprogression. However, recent studies indicate that the frequency of individuals heterozygous for a defect in the gene for CCR-5 (see below), which is the receptor for macrophage-tropic strains of HIV-1 (see above), may be increased among long-term nonprogressors, suggesting that heterozygosity for the genetic defect may provide some degree of protection. Although long-term nonprogressors have robust HIV-specific immune responses as well as competent CD8+ T cell suppressors of HIV replication, it is unclear whether these factors are directly responsible for the state of nonprogression. A substantial proportion of HIV-infected individuals manifest comparable immune responses early in the course of their disease and still experience disease progression. Long-term nonprogressors likely represent a heterogeneous group. The lack of disease progression may be explained in some by a defect in the virus, in others by any of a variety of host factors, including recognized and as yet unrecognized genetic factors, and in others by a combination of both.

ROLE OF LYMPHOID ORGANS IN HIV PATHOGENESIS The lymph nodes are the major anatomic sites for the establishment and propagation of HIV infection (see above). For practical reasons, most studies on the pathogenesis of HIV infection have focused on peripheral-blood mononuclear cells. However, lymphocytes in the peripheral blood represent only approximately 2 percent of the total body lymphocyte pool and so may not always accurately reflect the status of the entire immune system; most of the body's lymphocytes reside in lymphoid organs, such as the lymph nodes, spleen, and gut-associated lymphoid tissue. Furthermore, virus replication occurs mainly in lymphoid tissue and not in blood; the level of plasma viremia reflects virus production in lymphoid tissue. Finally, since HIV disease is an infectious disease of the immune system, it is critical to appreciate the pathogenic events that occur in the lymphoid tissue in HIV infection.

Certain patients experience progressive generalized lymphadenopathy (see below) early in the course of the infection; others experience varying degrees of transient lymphadenopathy. Lymphadenopathy reflects the cellular activation and immune response to the virus in the lymphoid tissue, which is generally characterized by follicular or germinal-center hyperplasia. Lymph node involvement is a common denominator of virtually all patients with HIV infection, even those without easily detectable lymphadenopathy. It has been suggested that progressive generalized lymphadenopathy represents an exaggerated immune response to HIV and carries a more favorable prognosis; however, long-term follow-up of such patients has not borne out this hope.

Simultaneous examination of lymph node and peripheral blood in the same patients during various stages of HIV disease, including the early asymptomatic stage (when CD4+ T cell counts generally are greater than 500/μL), the intermediate stage (when counts are usually 200 to 500/μL) and the advanced stage (when counts are <200/μL) has led to substantial insight into the pathogenesis of HIV disease. Using a combination of PCR techniques for HIV DNA and RNA in tissue and RNA in plasma, in situ hybridization for HIV RNA, and light and electron microscopy, the following picture has emerged. In most patients, early in the course of infection prior to significant immunodeficiency (CD4+ T cell counts >500/μL), plasma viremia generally is low, the viral burden (number of infected cells) in the peripheral blood is extremely low, and expression of HIV in these cells is minimal or undetectable. Remarkably, at this time copious amounts of extracellular virions are trapped on the processes of the follicular dendritic cells (FDCs) in the germinal centers of the lymph nodes (Fig. 308-14*A*). In situ hybridization reveals expression of virus in individual cells of the paracortical area and, to a lesser extent, the germinal center (Fig. 308-14*B*). The number of cells expressing virus is very low early in the course of disease and increases as disease progresses. Examination of lymph nodes during primary HIV infection in humans (see above) and SIV infection in macaques indicates that during the transition from primary infection to established chronic infection, germinal centers form and virus is trapped. This trapping, together with the generation of a vigorous HIV-specific immune response, likely contributes to the rapid decrease in plasma viremia seen in most patients following the initial burst of viremia associated with primary infection. A considerable amount of virus can be trapped during the period of high viremia associated with primary infection. The persistence of trapped virus after chronic infection has been established likely reflects a steady state whereby trapped virus turns over and is replaced by fresh virions, which are produced persistently, albeit usually at low levels during the early, clinically latent stage of disease.

During early-stage HIV disease, the architecture of the germinal centers is generally preserved and may even be hyperplastic owing to in situ proliferation of cells (mostly B lymphocytes) and recruitment to the lymph nodes of a number of cell types (B cells, CD4+ and CD8+ T cells). Electron microscopy demonstrates a fine network of FDCs with many long, finger-like processes that envelop virtually every lymphocyte in the germinal center (Fig. 308-14*C*). Extracellular virions can be seen attached to the processes, yet the FDCs appear to be relatively healthy. The trapping of antigen is a physiologically normal function for the FDCs, which present antigen to B cells and contribute to the generation of B cell memory. However, in the case of HIV, the trapped virions serve as a persistent source of cellular activation, resulting in the secretion of proinflammatory cytokines such as interleukin (IL) 1β, tumor necrosis factor (TNF)-α, and IL-6, which can upregulate virus replication in infected cells (see below). Furthermore, although trapped virus is coated by neutralizing antibodies, it has been demonstrated that these virions remain infectious for CD4+ T cells while attached to the processes of the FDCs. CD4+ T cells that migrate into the germinal center to provide help to B cells in the generation of an HIV-specific immune response thus are susceptible to infection by these trapped virions. Thus, in HIV infection, a normal physiologic function of the immune system, which contributes to the clearance of virus as well as to the generation of a specific immune response, can also have deleterious consequences. It is difficult to demonstrate infection of the FDCs at this point, or even in advanced disease; however, rare examples of virus budding off FDCs have been reported.

As the disease progresses, the architecture of the germinal centers begins to show disruption, and the trapping efficiency of the lymph node diminishes. Electron microscopy reveals swollen organelles, and the FDCs begin to undergo cell death. The mechanisms of FDC death remain unclear; there is no indication by electron microscopy of copious virus replication or budding of virions off the cell in great quantities. At this stage, the level of plasma viremia generally increases. In addition, both the relative number of infected cells in the blood and the expression of virus from these cells increases, approaching the levels in the lymph nodes. As the disease progresses to an advanced stage, there is complete disruption of the architecture of the germinal centers, accompanied by dissolution of the FDC network and massive dropout of FDCs (Fig. 308-14*D*). The trapping function of the lymph nodes is completely lost, and virus freely spills out into the circulation. Simultaneous PCR analysis of lymph node and peripheral blood mononuclear cells indicates that the relative number of infected cells in the blood and their expression of virus begins to equal the levels in the lymph nodes at this stage. Advanced disease is accompanied by high levels of plasma viremia, which represent a true increase in virus replication, due in part to a further diminution of immune control of virus replication (see below) as well as to the loss of the mechanical trapping function of the lymph nodes. At this point, the lymph nodes are "burnt out." This destruction of lymphoid tissue compounds the immunodeficiency of HIV disease and contributes to the inability to mount adequate immune responses against opportunistic pathogens. The events from primary infection to the ultimate destruction of the immune system are illustrated in Fig. 308-15.

ROLE OF CELLULAR ACTIVATION IN HIV PATHOGENESIS The immune system is normally in a state of homeostasis, awaiting perturbation by foreign antigenic stimuli. Activation of the immune system is an essential component of an appropriate immune response to a foreign antigen. Once the immune response deals with and clears the antigen, the system returns to relative quiescence (see Chap. 305). In HIV infection, however, the immune system is chronically activated owing to the chronicity of infection and the persistence of virus replication (see above). This activated state is reflected by hyperactivation of B cells leading to hypergammaglobulinemia; spontaneous lymphocyte proliferation; activation of monocytes; expression of activation markers on CD4+ and CD8+ T cells; lymph node hyperplasia, particularly early in the course of disease (see above); increased secretion of proinflammatory cytokines (see below); elevated levels of neopterin, β_2-microglobulin, acid-labile interferon, and soluble IL-2 receptors; and autoimmune phenomena (see below).

Persistent immune activation may have several deleterious consequences. From a virologic standpoint, although quiescent CD4+ T cells can be infected with HIV, reverse transcription, integration, and virus spread are much more efficient in activated cells. Furthermore, cellular activation induces expression of virus in cells latently infected with HIV. From an immunologic standpoint, chronic exposure of the immune system to a particular antigen over an extended period may ultimately lead to an inability to sustain an adequate immune response to the antigen. Furthermore, the ability of the immune system to respond to a broad spectrum of antigens may be compromised if immune-competent cells are maintained in a state of chronic activation. In addition, activation of the immune system may favor the elimination of cells via programmed cell death (apoptosis) (see below) as well as the secretion of certain cytokines that can induce HIV expression (see below).

Role of Apoptosis *Apoptosis* is a form of programmed cell death that is a normal mechanism for the elimination of effete cells in organogenesis as well as in the cellular proliferation that occurs during a normal immune response (see Chap. 305). Apoptosis is strictly dependent on cellular activation. It has been hypothesized that, in HIV infection, sequential activation signals delivered to CD4+ T cells induce apoptosis. Cross-linking of the CD4 molecule by gp120 or gp120/anti-gp120 complexes delivers the first of two signals required for apoptosis. The second signal supposedly leading to cell death is delivered via the T cell receptor by a conventional antigen or a superantigen (see below and Chap. 305). By this hypothesis, direct infection of CD4+ T cells is not required for apoptosis to occur, although it has been demonstrated that alterations in tyrosine kinase activity of HIV-infected cells may induce the cell to undergo apoptosis. A number of studies, including those examining lymphoid tissue, have demonstrated that the rate of apoptosis is elevated in HIV infection and that apoptosis is seen in CD8+ T cells and B cells as well as in CD4+ T cells. Furthermore, the intensity of apoptosis correlates with the general state of activation of the immune system and not with the stage of disease or with viral burden. It is likely that apoptosis of immune-competent cells contributes to the immune abnormalities in HIV disease; however, this is probably a nonspecific mechanism that merely reflects the aberrant state of immune activation.

Superantigens and HIV Pathogenesis It has been hypothesized that *superantigens*, either retrovirally coded or related to other microorganisms, may contribute to the pathogenesis of HIV disease. Conventional antigens bind in the groove of the MHC molecule of the antigen-presenting cell (see Chap. 305) and interact with the variable (V) components of the T cell receptor α and β chains to activate the T cell. Thus, any conventional antigenic peptide can stimulate only a very small fraction ($<1/100{,}000$) of total T cells. In contrast, certain microbial antigens are capable of binding to and activating entire subsets of T cells, not through true antigen-receptor binding, but by binding to another site on the V region of the β chain of the T cell receptor. There are 24 families or subsets of T cells that can be

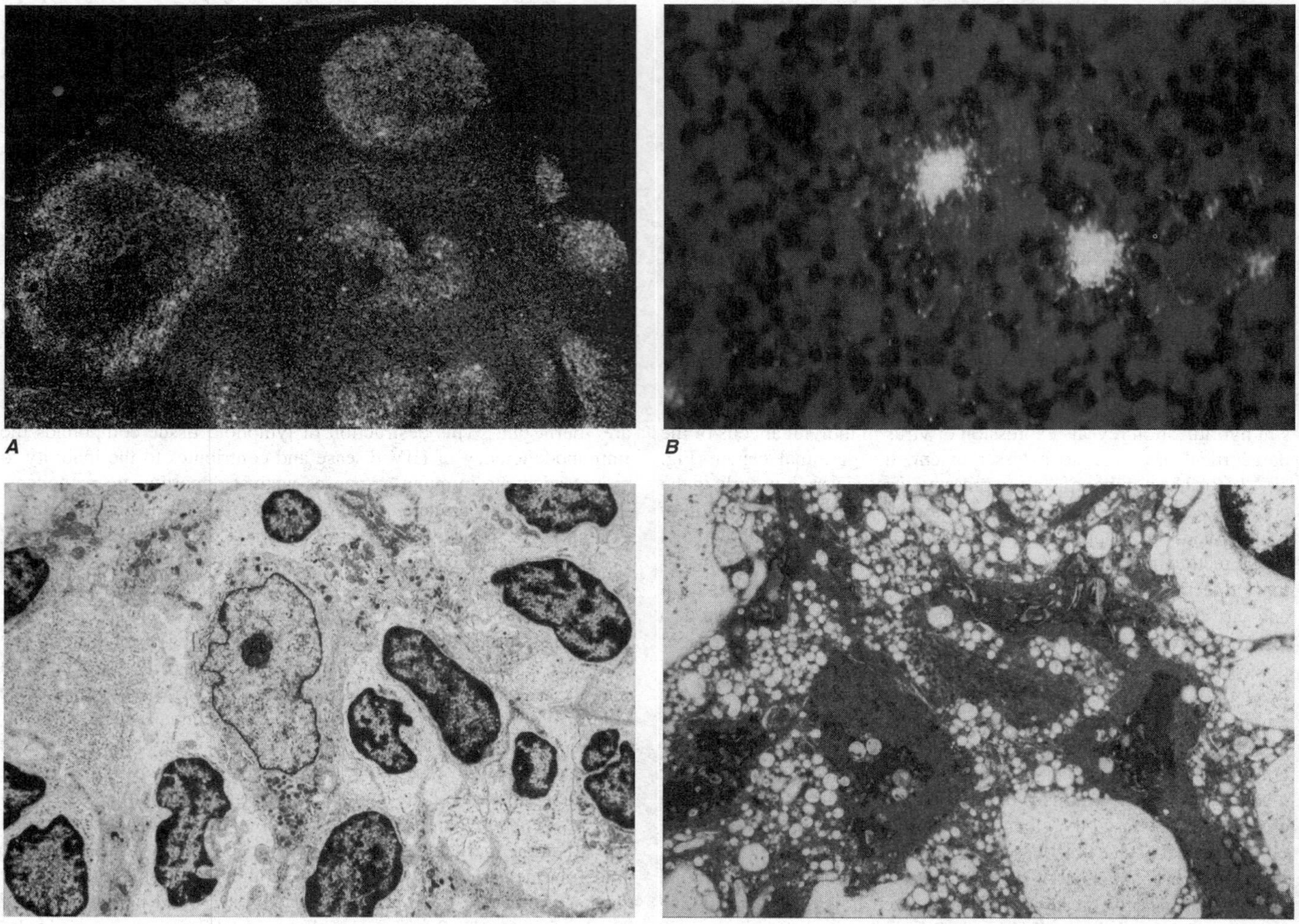

FIGURE 308-14 HIV in the lymph nodes of HIV-infected individuals. *A.* Cervical lymph node from an asymptomatic individual with very low levels of plasma viremia. In situ hybridization using a molecular probe for HIV RNA reveals copious virus demarcating the numerous germinal centers (bright areas) of the node. The virus was extracellular and bound to the processes of the follicular dendritic cells which form a matrix within the confines of the germinal centers. Original ×25. *B.* Individual cells infected with HIV. Two cells in the paracortical area of the lymph node are shown expressing HIV RNA by in situ hybridization using a radiolabeled molecular probe. Original ×250. *C.* Follicular dendritic cells in cervical node of an asymptomatic HIV-infected individual. Electron microscopy reveals a follicular dendritic cell with a prominant nucleolus surrounded by several lymphocytes within the germinal center of the node. Higher magnification of several fields indicates that multiple processes of the follicular dendritic cells are in contact with several lymphocytes. Original ×1920. *D.* Dissolution of follicular dendritic cells in the germinal center of a cervical lymph node from a patient with advanced HIV disease. Widespread death of follicular dendritic cells is associated with a loss of ability of the lymph node to trap virus late in the course of HIV disease. Original ×3744. *(A and B courtesy of Dr. Cecil Fox; C and D courtesy of Dr. Jan Orenstein. Adapted from G Pantaleo et al, N Engl J Med 328:327, 1993.)*

identified on the basis of their Vβ usage. Binding of a superantigen to all members of a particular Vβ subset of T cells (1 to 10 percent of all T cells) can induce massive stimulation of T cells and/or, depending on the original state of activation of the T cell, can result in deletion or anergy of T cells bearing the specific Vβs. There is no convincing evidence that HIV codes for a superantigen, nor is there any convincing evidence supporting the concept of true deletion of Vβ subsets by a superantigen mechanism in HIV disease. However, if superantigens associated with other microorganisms play any role in HIV disease, this role probably is related to the fact that superantigens can activate large numbers of CD4+ T cells and render them more susceptible to efficient virus infection (see above).

Autoimmune Phenomena The autoimmune phenomena that are common in HIV-infected individuals reflect, at least in part, chronic immune system activation. Although these phenomena usually occur in the absence of autoimmune disease, a wide spectrum of clinical manifestations that may be associated with autoimmunity have been described (see below). Autoimmune phenomena include antibodies to lymphocytes and, less commonly, to platelets and neutrophils. Antiplatelet antibodies have some clinical relevance, in that they may contribute to the thrombocytopenia of HIV disease (see below). Antibodies to nuclear and cytoplasmic components of cells have been reported, as have antibodies to cardiolipin, CD4 molecules, CD43 molecules, and IL-2. In addition, autoantibodies to a range of serum proteins, including albumin, immunoglobulin, and thyroglobulin, have been reported. There is antigenic cross-reactivity between HIV viral proteins (gp120 and gp41) and MHC class II determinants, and anti-MHC class II antibodies have been reported in HIV infection. These antibodies could potentially lead to the elimination of MHC class II-bearing cells via antibody-dependent cellular cytotoxicity (ADCC) (see Chap. 305). In addition, regions of homology exist between HIV envelope glycoproteins and IL-2 as well as MHC class I molecules.

Cofactors Contributing to HIV Pathogenesis Both endogenous and exogenous factors can contribute to HIV pathogenesis by a number of mechanisms; paramount among these is the upregulation of virus expression, a process intimately connected with cellular activation. The main endogenous factors that regulate HIV expression are cytokines (see below). Among exogenous factors, other microbes likely have important effects on HIV replication and HIV pathogenesis. They can thus be considered real or potential *cofactors* in the pathogenesis of HIV disease. Coinfection or simultaneous cotransfection of cells with HIV and other heterologous viruses or viral genes has demonstrated that certain viruses, such as herpes simplex virus type 1, cytomegalovirus, human herpesvirus 6, Epstein-Barr virus, hepatitis B virus, adenovirus, pseudorabies virus, and HTLV-I can upregulate HIV expression. Other microbes, such as *Mycoplasma* have been reported to contribute to the induction of HIV expression. *Mycobacterium tuberculosis* is a common opportunistic infection in HIV-infected individuals (see below and Chap. 171). In addition to the fact that HIV-infected individuals are more likely to develop active tuberculosis after exposure, it has been demonstrated that active tuberculosis can accelerate the course of HIV infection. It has also been shown that levels of plasma viremia are greatly elevated in HIV-infected individuals with active tuberculosis, compared to pretuberculosis levels and levels of viremia after successful treatment of the active tuberculosis. In vitro studies demonstrated that virus replication was markedly enhanced in lymphocytes of HIV-infected individuals who were skin test–positive for purified protein derivative (PPD) when PPD antigen was added to culture, resulting in cellular activation. Confirmatory evidence that antigen-induced activation was a major contributor to the accelerated viremia in HIV-infected individuals with active tuberculosis was provided by studies in which HIV-infected individuals were immunized with common recall antigens such as tetanus toxoid, influenza, or pneumococcal polysaccharide. Under these circumstances, a transient elevation of plasma viremia accompanied the cellular activation induced by the immunization.

THE CYTOKINE NETWORK IN HIV PATHOGENESIS The immune system is homeostatically regulated by a complex network of immunoregulatory cytokines, which are pleiotropic and

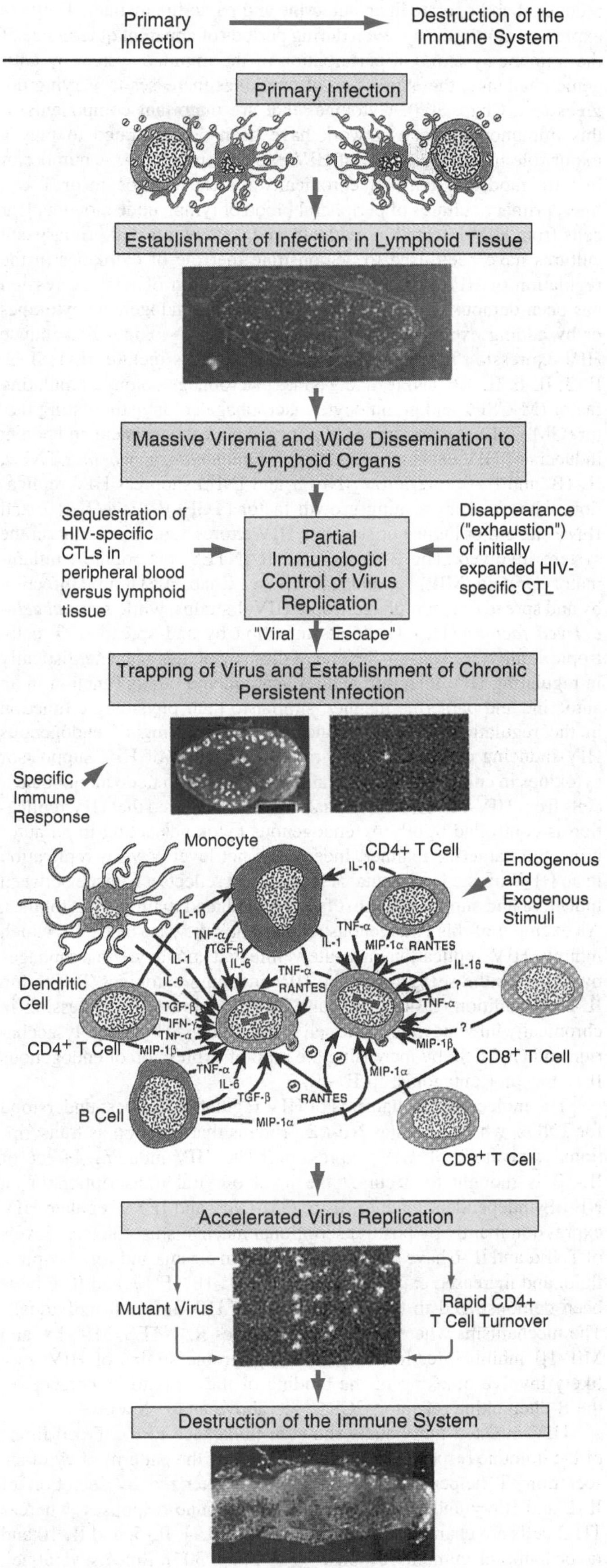

FIGURE 308-15 Events that transpire from primary HIV infection through the establishment of chronic persistent infection to the ultimate destruction of the immune system. See text for details.

redundant and operate in an autocrine and paracrine manner. They are expressed continuously, even during periods of apparent quiescence of the immune system. On perturbation of the immune system by antigenic challenge, the expression of cytokines increases to varying degrees (see Chap. 305). Cytokines that are important components of this immunoregulatory network have been demonstrated to play a major role in the regulation of HIV expression in vitro. A number of in vitro model systems of chronically infected monocyte or T cell lines, primary cultures of peripheral blood or lymph node mononuclear cells from HIV-infected individuals, and acutely infected primary cell cultures have been used to demonstrate the role of cytokines in the regulation of HIV expression. Potent modulation of HIV expression has been demonstrated either by manipulating endogenous cytokines or by adding exogenous cytokines to culture. Cytokines that induce HIV expression in one or more of these systems include IL-1, IL-2, IL-3, IL-6, IL-12, TNFα, and TNFβ, macrophage colony stimulating factor (M-CSF), and granulocyte-macrophage colony stimulating factor (GM-CSF). Among these cytokines, the most consistent and potent inducers of HIV expression are the *proinflammatory cytokines* TNFα, IL-1β, and IL-6. Interferon (INF) α and INFβ suppress HIV replication, whereas transforming growth factor (TGF)-β, IL-4, IL-10, and IFNγ can either induce or suppress HIV expression, depending on the system involved. The *β-chemokines* RANTES, macrophage inflammatory protein (MIP) 1α, and MIP-1β (see Chap. 305) inhibit infection by and spread of macrophage-tropic HIV-1 strains, while *stromal cell–derived factor* (SDF) 1 inhibits infection by and spread of T cell–tropic strains (see below). Several of these cytokines act synergistically in regulating HIV infection and replication, and others function in an autocrine and paracrine manner, similar to their physiologic function in the regulation of the immune system. Blocking of endogenous HIV-inducing cytokines or addition of inhibitors of HIV suppressor cytokines in cultures of peripheral blood and lymph node mononuclear cells from HIV-infected individuals has demonstrated that HIV replication is controlled tightly by endogenous cytokines acting in an autocrine and paracrine manner. Indeed, the net level of virus replication in an HIV-infected individual at least in part reflects a balance between inductive and suppressive host factors, mediated mainly by cytokines. An example of this endogenous regulation is the case of IL-10, which inhibits HIV replication in acutely infected monocyte/macrophages by blocking the secretion of the HIV-inducing cytokines TNFα and IL-6. In addition, IL-4, IL-13, and TGFβ inhibit HIV expression in chronically infected monocytic cell lines stimulated by lipopolysaccharide and GM-CSF by increasing the ratio of expression of endogenous IL-1 receptor antagonist to IL-1β.

The molecular mechanisms of HIV regulation are best understood for TNFα, which activates NF-κB proteins that function as transcriptional activators of HIV expression. The HIV-inducing effect of IL-1β is thought to occur at the level of viral transcription in an NF-κB-independent manner. IL-6, GM-CSF, and IFNγ regulate HIV expression mainly by posttranscriptional mechanisms. Elevated levels of TNFα and IL-6 have been demonstrated in plasma and cerebrospinal fluid, and increased expression of TNFα, IL-1β, IFNγ, and IL-6 have been demonstrated in the lymph nodes of HIV-infected individuals. The mechanisms whereby the β-chemokines RANTES, MIP-1α, and MIP-1β inhibit infection of macrophage-tropic strains of HIV very likely involve blocking of the binding of the virus to its coreceptor, the β-chemokine receptor CCR5 (see above and below).

HIV-infected individuals show an imbalance in the T cell limbs of the immune response, which are defined by the patterns of cytokine secretion. T helper (TH)-1 cells are characterized by secretion of IL-2 and IFNγ and favor cell-mediated immune responses, whereas TH-2 cells are characterized by secretion of IL-4, IL-5, and IL-10 and favor humoral immune responses (see Chap. 305). Since several cell types in addition to CD4+ T cells secrete these cytokines, it is more accurate to refer to immune responses that reflect one or the other cytokine pattern as *TH-1* or *TH-2 type responses*. HIV-infected individuals show a decrease in TH-1 type responses relative to TH-2 type cytokine patterns. It has also been demonstrated that in vitro apoptosis can be inhibited in T cells from HIV-infected donors by antibodies to IL-4 and IL-10 and enhanced by antibodies to IL-12. Although it has been proposed that a clear-cut switch from a TH-1 type to a TH-2 type of cytokine pattern is a critical step in the pathogenesis of HIV disease, no sharp dichotomy between these two types of cytokine patterns that is directly related to progression of disease has been corroborated.

CELLULAR TARGETS OF HIV Although the CD4+ T lymphocytes and CD4+ cells of monocyte lineage are the principal targets of HIV, virtually any cell that expresses the CD4 molecule together with coreceptor molecules (see above and below) can potentially be infected with HIV. Circulating dendritic cells have been reported to express low levels of CD4, and there have been conflicting reports on whether these cells can be infected with HIV. Epidermal Langerhans cells express CD4 and have been infected by HIV in vivo. In vitro, HIV has been reported also to infect a wide range of cells and cell lines that express low levels of CD4, no detectable CD4, or only CD4 mRNA; among these are follicular dendritic cells; megakaryocytes; eosinophils; astrocytes; oligodendrocytes; microglial cells; CD8+ T cells; B cells; natural killer cells; renal epithelial cells; cervical cells; rectal and bowel mucosal cells such as enterochromaffin, goblet, and columnar epithelial cells; trophoblastic cells; and cells from a variety of organs, such as liver, lung, heart, salivary gland, eye, prostate, testis, and adrenal gland. Since the only cells that have been shown unequivocally to be infected with HIV and to support replication of the virus are CD4+ T lymphocytes and cells of monocyte/macrophage lineage, the relevance of the in vitro infection of these other cell types is unclear and is questionable at present.

Of potentially important clinical relevance is the demonstration that thymic precursor cells, which were assumed to be negative for CD3, CD4, and CD8 molecules, actually do express low levels of CD4 and can be infected with HIV in vitro. In addition, human thymic epithelial cells transplanted into an immunodeficient mouse can be infected with HIV by direct inoculation of virus into the thymus. Since these cells may play a role in the normal replenishment of CD4+ T cells, it is possible that their infection and depletion contributes, at least in part, to the inability of the CD4+ T cell pool to replenish itself in infected individuals, including those in whom antiretroviral therapy has at least temporarily suppressed viral replication (see below). In addition, CD34+ monocyte precursor cells have been shown to be infected in vivo in patients with advanced HIV disease. It is likely that these cells express low levels of CD4, and therefore it is not essential to invoke CD4-independent mechanisms to explain the infection.

DETERMINANTS OF CELL TROPISM OF HIV The ability of HIV to infect different cell types varies from isolate to isolate. Many primary isolates of HIV replicate well in both primary T lymphocytes and monocytes, but not in transformed T cell lines. These isolates are often called *monocyte-tropic* or *macrophage-tropic* viruses, despite the fact that they actually can infect both primary T cells and monocytes. Isolates that replicate well only in primary macrophages, and not in lymphocytes, have been only rarely identified. Other isolates, particularly those that have been passaged in vitro in lymphoid cells (T cell line–adapted strains), infect primary T lymphocytes but not monocyte/macrophages; these isolates are referred to as *T cell–tropic* viruses. The viral determinant of cellular tropism maps to the gp120 subunit of the HIV-1 envelope protein, particularly the third variable region (V3 loop) of gp120 (see below). Early in the course of disease, macrophage-tropic viruses predominate in blood, whereas over time and as disease progresses, T cell–tropic viruses predominate. Similarly, viruses isolated from patients early in disease have been characterized as non-syncytia-inducing (NSI) in in vitro assays, while viruses isolated late in the course of disease are typically syncytia-inducing (SI) (see below). Thus, the term *macrophage-tropic* is often used synonymously with *NSI*, and the term *T cell–tropic* with *SI*. The transition from macrophage-tropic/NSI to T cell–tropic/SI virus in an infected individual (which may involve the transient appearance of dual-tropic viruses) is associated with the onset of a more rapid decline in CD4+ T cells. Transmitting viruses are usually macrophage-tropic. However, since most of these studies were done in homosexual men who were infected via receptive anal intercourse, this bias may be influenced somewhat by the route of transmission. Macrophage-tropic viruses are more efficient in infecting monocyte/macrophages and microglial cells of the brain. The *galactosyl ceramide* molecule can serve as an alternative receptor for HIV in CD4-negative neuronal and epithelial cells (see "Neuropathogenesis" below). The *env* gene is primarily responsible for the differences in the ability of different isolates to infect particular cell types, i.e., lymphocytes versus monocytes and primary mononuclear cells versus propagated cell lines. The V3 region of the viral envelope protein is a major determinant of cell tropism, and V3 appears to play a role in envelope protein–mediated fusion of viral and target cell membranes. Sequences within the envelope protein but outside of V3 can also influence the tropism of virus for different cells; however, the mechanisms involved have not been elucidated.

In mid-1996, it was demonstrated that cellular tropism actually reflects the presence of coreceptors specific for macrophage-tropic versus T cell-tropic strains of HIV-1. These coreceptors belong to the seven-transmembrane-domain G protein–coupled family of receptors. The coreceptor for T cell–tropic viruses is *fusin* or CXCR4, which is required for entry and fusion of these strains of virus. Its natural ligand is *stromal cell–derived factor* (SDF)-1. This ligand, as well as antibodies to fusin, can effectively block entry and infection of target cells by T cell–tropic viruses. The main coreceptor for macrophage-tropic viruses is the β chemokine receptor *CCR5*. This receptor binds all three of the β-chemokines (RANTES, MIP-1α, and MIP-1β) that have been shown to inhibit infection with macrophage-tropic strains of HIV-1. However, there is a great deal of redundancy among the β-chemokine receptors, and other members of this family, particularly CCR2b and CCR3, can support infection of dual-tropic strains of HIV-1. The mechanisms of inhibition of entry of macrophage-tropic and T cell–tropic strains of HIV-1 into their target cells by the β-chemokines and SDF-1, respectively, are not entirely clear. However, certain experiments indicate that at least for the β-chemokines, the mechanism involves a receptor blockade and not inhibition of signal transduction (Fig. 308-16). Given the already determined complexity in the interaction between HIV and its human host, it is highly likely that other coreceptors for HIV-1 entry will be identified.

T CELL ABNORMALITIES The range of T cell abnormalities in advanced HIV infection is broad. The defects are both quantitative and qualitative and involve virtually every limb of the immune system (see below), indicating the critical dependence of the integrity of the immune system on the inducer/helper function of CD4+ T cells. Virtually all of the immune defects in advanced HIV disease can ultimately be explained by the quantitative depletion of CD4+ T cells. However, T cell dysfunction (see below) can be demonstrated in patients early in the course of infection, even when the CD4+ T cell count is in the low-normal range. The degree and spectrum of dysfunctions increase as the disease progresses. One of the first abnormalities to be detected is a defect in response to remote recall antigens, such as tetanus toxoid and influenza, at a time when mononuclear cells can still respond normally to mitogenic stimulation. Defects in responses to soluble antigens are followed in time by the loss of T cell proliferative responses to alloantigens, and subsequently to mitogens. Essentially every T cell function has been reported to be abnormal at some stage of HIV infection. These abnormalities include defective T cell cloning and colony-forming efficiencies, impaired expression of IL-2 receptors, defective IL-2 production, decreased IFNγ production in response to antigens, and decreased help to B cells to produce immunoglobulins.

The level of CD8+ T cells varies throughout the course of disease. Following the resolution of acute primary infection, CD8+ T cells generally rebound to higher than normal levels, and they may remain that way throughout the clinically latent stage of disease. This CD8+ T lymphocytosis may in part reflect the expansion of clones of HIV-specific CD8+ CTLs. In addition, homeostatic mechanisms responsible for maintaining the total T cell count in the normal range in the face of CD4+ T cell destruction would replace lost CD4+ T cells with CD4+ T cells as well as with CD8+ T cells, thus leading to a CD8+ T lymphocytosis, at least prior to the advanced stage of disease (see below). However, during the late stages of HIV infection, there is a significant reduction in the numbers of CD8+ T cells. HIV-specific CD8+ CTLs have been demonstrated in HIV-infected individuals early in the course of disease (see below). As the disease progresses, this functional capability decreases and may be lost entirely. The cause of this loss of cytolytic activity is unclear. However, it has been demonstrated that, as disease progresses, CD8+ T cells assume an abnormal phenotype characterized by expression of activation markers such as HLA-DR with an absence of expression of the IL-2 receptor (CD25) and a loss of clonogenic potential. It has been reported that the phenotype of CD8+ T cells in HIV-infected individuals may be of prognostic significance. Those individuals whose CD8+ T cells developed a phenotype of HLA-DR+/CD38− following seroconversion had stabilization of their CD4+ T cell counts, whereas those whose CD8+ T cells developed a phenotype of HLA-DR+/CD38+ had a more aggressive course and a poorer prognosis. In addition to the defects in HIV-specific CTLs, functional defects in other MHC-restricted CTLs, such as those directed against influenza and cytomegalovirus, have been demonstrated. Since the integrity of CD8+ T cell function depends in part on adequate inductive signals from CD4+ T cells, the defect in CD8+ CTLs is likely compounded by the quantitative loss of CD4+ T cells.

Mechanisms of CD4+ T Lymphocyte Depletion and Dysfunction It is difficult to explain completely the profound immunodeficiency noted in HIV-infected individuals solely on the basis of direct infection and quantitative depletion of CD4+ T cells. This is particu-

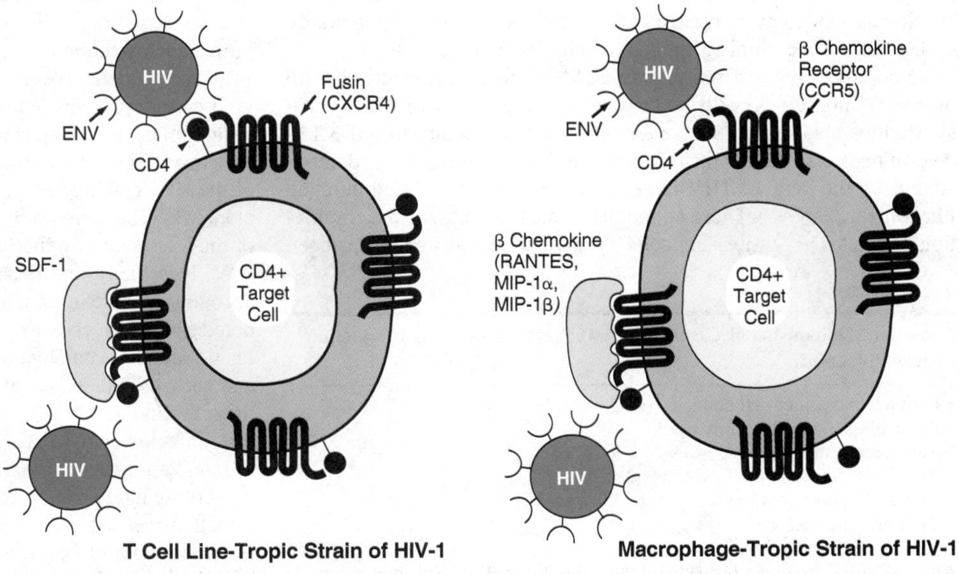

FIGURE 308-16 Model for the role of coreceptors fusin and CCR5 in the efficient binding and entry of T cell–tropic and macrophage-tropic strains of HIV-1, respectively, into CD4+ target cells. Blocking of this initial event in the virus life cycle can be accomplished by inhibition of binding to the coreceptor by the ligand for the receptor in question. The ligand for fusin is stromal cell–derived factor (SDF-1); the ligands for the β chemokine receptor CCR5 are RANTES, MIP-1α, and MIP-1β.

larly apparent during the early stages of HIV disease, when CD4+ T cell numbers may be only marginally decreased. Certainly, at the stage of advanced disease when the CD4+ T cell count is in the range of 0 to 50/μL, quantitative depletion alone can explain the immune defects. However, it is likely that CD4+ T cell dysfunction results from a combination of depletion of cells due to direct infection and a number of virus-related but indirect effects on the cell (Table 308-7).

Single-cell killing and the formation of syncytia between infected and uninfected cells have been demonstrated clearly in vitro, although the precise mechanisms of cell death in vivo have not been determined. Cytopathicity in an infected cell in vitro may result from a number of mechanisms, including copious budding of virions from the cell surface with resulting disruption of the integrity of the cell membrane; interference with cellular RNA processing or the accumulation of high levels of heterodisperse RNA molecules; disruption of cellular protein synthesis owing to high levels of viral RNA; accumulation of high levels of unintegrated viral DNA in the cell cytoplasm; induction of aberrant patterns of protein tyrosine phosphorylation; and the interaction between HIV gp120 and CD4 intracellularly. Strain differences in single-cell killing are determined largely by gp120 sequences, which supports the importance of the viral envelope in this process. *Syncytia formation* involves fusion of the cell membrane of an infected cell with the cell membranes of variable numbers of uninfected CD4+ cells. Although cell fusion has not been shown to be an important pathogenic process in vivo, a direct relationship between the presence of syncytia and the degree of cytopathic effect has been demonstrated in vitro, and a correlation has been reported between the presence of virus isolates that readily induce syncytia in vitro and a more aggressive clinical course in the patient. Efficient syncytia formation depends on the leukocyte adhesion molecule LFA-1 (see Chap. 305) on human CD4+ T cells acutely infected with HIV in vitro.

Humoral and cellular immune responses to HIV may contribute to protective immunity by eliminating virus and virus-infected cells (see below). However, since the main targets of HIV infection are immune-competent cells, these responses may contribute to immune-cell depletion and immunologic dysfunction by eliminating both infected cells and "innocent bystander" cells. Soluble viral proteins, particularly gp120, can bind with high affinity to the CD4 molecules on uninfected T cells and monocytes; in addition, virus and/or viral protein can bind to dendritic cells or follicular dendritic cells. HIV-specific antibody can recognize these bound molecules and potentially collaborate in the elimination of the cells by ADCC.

Nonpolymorphic determinants of MHC class I products share a degree of homology with gp120 and gp41 proteins of HIV. Such similarities may lead to the generation of autoantibodies to self-MHC determinants. In fact, anti-HLA-DR antibodies have been demonstrated in the sera of HIV-infected individuals (see "Autoimmune Phenomena," above). These antibodies could contribute to the elimination of HLA-DR–expressing cells by ADCC; in addition, it has been suggested that these antibodies may inhibit certain T cell functions that involve HLA-DR molecules.

It has been proposed that attempts by the immune system to maintain T cell homeostasis contribute to the progressive decline in numbers of CD4+ T cells. The theory of "blind" T cell homeostasis states that when CD4+ or CD8+ T cells are depleted selectively, the immune system is programmed to restore the total number of T cells blindly, without regard for which subset is depleted (see below). In HIV-infected individuals who experience a selective decrease in CD4+ T cells, both CD4+ and CD8+ T cells are produced to restore homeostasis. Thus, CD4+ T cells are further decreased relative to CD8+ T cells as the total number of T cells is maintained. This theory, if correct, can only apply to the early stages of HIV disease, since both CD4+ and CD8+ T cells decline as disease progresses to the advanced stages.

After gp120/anti-gp120 complexes bind to cell-surface CD4 molecules and cause cross-linking of these molecules, CD4+ T cells may become refractory to further stimulation in vitro via the CD3 molecule. Cross-linking of CD4 by gp120 and/or gp120/anti-gp120 complexes may result in cellular signal-transduction abnormalities, inhibition of IL-2 production and IL-2 receptor expression, steric interference with the MHC class II-CD4–mediated cell adhesion that is necessary for the induction of antigen-specific responses, and even inappropriate activation of the cell (see above). Inappropriate and sustained cellular activation play critical roles in the phenomenon of apoptosis, which may be an important mechanism of death of uninfected cells in HIV infection. In addition, putative superantigens associated with other microbes may contribute to this heightened state of cellular activation, and hence may contribute to immune dysfunction (see "Role of Cellular Activation in HIV Pathogenesis," above).

Finally, the inexorable decline in CD4+ T cell counts that occurs in most HIV-infected individuals may result in part from the inability of the immune system to regenerate the CD4+ T cell pool rapidly enough to compensate for both HIV-mediated destruction of cells and natural attrition of cells. At least two major mechanisms may contribute to the failure of the CD4+ T cell pool to adequately reconstitute itself over the course of HIV infection. The first is the destruction of lymphoid precursor cells, including thymic and bone marrow progenitor cells (see above); the other is the gradual disruption of the lymphoid tissue microenvironment, which is essential for efficient regeneration of immune-competent cells (see above).

B CELL ABNORMALITIES B cells from HIV-infected individuals manifest abnormal activation, which is reflected by spontaneous proliferation and immunoglobulin secretion and by increased spontaneous secretion of TNFα and IL-6. The enhanced spontaneous in vitro transformation of B cells with Epstein-Barr virus (EBV) is probably due to defective T cell immune surveillance and has as its in vivo counterpart an increase in the incidence of EBV-related B cell lymphomas. Untransformed B cells cannot be infected with HIV. However, HIV or its products can activate B cells directly; portions of the HIV gp41 envelope protein have been reported to induce polyclonal B cell activation. In addition, it has been reported that products of the VH_3 genes on the surface of B cells can serve as a receptor for HIV. It is likely that in vivo activation of B cells by virus products accounts at least in part for the spontaneous activation of these cells noted ex vivo. In vivo, this activated state manifests itself by hypergammaglobulinemia and by the presence of circulating immune complexes and autoantibodies (see above). The B cells are also defective in that they respond poorly to in vitro stimulation with antigens and mitogens. HIV-infected individuals respond poorly to primary and secondary immunizations with protein and polysaccharide antigens. These B cell defects are likely responsible in part for the increase in certain bacterial infections seen in advanced HIV disease in adults, as well as for the important role of bacterial infections in the morbidity and mortality of HIV-infected children, who cannot mount an adequate humoral response to common bacterial pathogens. The absolute number of circulating B cells may be depressed in primary HIV infection; however, this phenomenon is usually transient and likely reflects in part a redistribution of cells out of the circulation and into the lymphoid

Table 308-7

Potential Mechanisms of CD4+ T Lymphocyte Dysfunction/Depletion in HIV Infection

HIV-mediated direct cytopathicity (single-cell killing)
HIV-mediated syncytia formation
Virus-specific immune responses
HIV-specific cytolytic T lymphocytes
Antibody-dependent cellular cytotoxicity (ADCC)
Natural killer cells
Autoimmune mechanisms
Anergy caused by inappropriate cell signaling via gp120/CD4 interaction
Superantigen-mediated perturbation of T cell subsets
Programmed cell death (apoptosis)
Defect in CD4+ T cell regeneration

SOURCE: Adapted from G Pantaleo et al., N Engl J Med 328:327, 1993.

tissue. In certain patients, the number of circulating B cells decreases in advanced-stage disease.

MONOCYTE/MACROPHAGE ABNORMALITIES Circulating monocytes are generally normal in number in HIV-infected individuals. Monocytes express the CD4 molecule and coreceptor for HIV on their surface and thus are targets of HIV infection. Of note is the fact that the degree of cytopathicity of HIV for cells of the monocyte lineage is low, and HIV can replicate extensively in cells of the monocyte lineage with little cytopathic effect. Hence, monocyte-lineage cells can serve as reservoirs of HIV infection and may play a role in the dissemination of HIV in the body. In vivo infection of circulating monocytes is difficult to demonstrate; however, infection of tissue macrophages and macrophage-lineage cells in the brain (infiltrating macrophages or resident microglial cells) and lung (pulmonary alveolar macrophages) can be demonstrated easily. Infection of monocyte precursors in the bone marrow may directly or indirectly be responsible for certain of the hematologic abnormalities in HIV-infected individuals. A number of abnormalities of circulating monocytes have been reported in HIV-infected individuals, including defects in chemotaxis, secretion of IL-1, antigen presentation and induction of T cell responses, Fc receptor function, C3 receptor–mediated clearance, oxidative burst responses, and certain cytotoxic functions. The mechanisms of the monocyte defects are uncertain, but almost certainly they cannot be explained by direct infection with HIV. Exposure of monocytes to gp120 as well as to certain cytokines can cause abnormal activation, and this may play a role in cellular dysfunction (see above).

ABNORMALITIES OF DENDRITIC AND LANGERHANS CELLS There has been considerable disagreement regarding the HIV infectibility and hence the depletion as well as the dysfunction of circulating dendritic cells. Certain groups have reported infection and cellular dysfunction, particularly a decreased ability to present antigen to T cells, and other groups have found little if any HIV infection or functional abnormalities. There is more agreement regarding the ability of skin and mucous membrane Langerhans cells to be infected (see above). These latter cells likely play an important role in the initiation and propagation of HIV infection. The discrepancies in reported depletions and functional abnormalities in these cell types likely reflect the existence of different subsets of cells as well as the differences in isolation techniques and culture systems employed by various groups.

ABNORMALITIES OF NATURAL KILLER CELLS The presumed role of natural killer (NK) cells is to provide immunosurveillance against virus-infected cells, certain tumor cells, and allogeneic cells (see Chap. 305). Functional abnormalities in NK cells have been observed throughout the course of HIV disease, and the severity of these abnormalities increases as disease progresses. Most studies report that NK cells are normal in number and phenotype in HIV-infected individuals; however, a numerical decrease in the CD16+/CD56+ subpopulation of NK cells has been reported. The abnormality in NK cell function is thought to result from a defect in post-binding lysis. However, the lytic machinery does not appear to be impaired, since NK cells from HIV-infected individuals mediate ADCC normally. The addition of either IL-2 or IL-12 to cultures improves the defective in vitro NK cell function of HIV-infected individuals. The in vivo mechanisms for defective NK cell activity is unknown; however, it may be related to the lack of normal inductive signals from CD4+ T cells.

GENETIC FACTORS IN HIV PATHOGENESIS Several reports have described MHC alleles and other host factors that may influence the pathogenesis and course of HIV disease. These include associations with certain HIV-related manifestations, such as Kaposi's sarcoma and diffuse lymphadenopathy, or with the type of clinical course, such as long-term survival or rapid progression (Table 308-8). A number of mechanisms have been proposed whereby MHC-encoded molecules might predispose an individual either to rapid progression or to nonprogression to AIDS. These proposed mechanisms include the ability to present certain immunodominant HIV T helper or CTL epitopes, leading to a relatively protective immune response against HIV and hence to slow progression of disease. In contrast, certain MHC class I or class II alleles might predispose an individual to an immunopathogenic response against viral epitopes in certain tissues, such as the central nervous system or lungs, or against certain HIV-infected cell types, such as macrophages or dendritic cells/Langerhans cells. In addition, certain rare MHC class I and class II alleles might facilitate rapid recognition of HIV-infected cells from the infecting partner in primary HIV infection and promote rejection of these cells by alloreactive responses. Similarly, common MHC alleles could lead to less effective removal of HIV-infected allogeneic cells. Other data have indicated that transporter associated with antigen-presenting (TAP) genes play a role in determining the outcome of HIV infection. HLA profiles that reflect certain combinations of MHC-encoded TAP and class I and class II genes are strongly associated with different rates of progression to AIDS.

The most compelling data regarding the role of host genetic factors in the pathogenesis of HIV infection were reported in 1996. Rare individuals had been reported who had had repetitive sexual exposure to HIV in high-risk situations but who had remained uninfected. The peripheral blood mononuclear cells of two such individuals were found to be highly resistant to infection in vitro with macrophage-tropic strains of HIV-1, but they were readily infected with T cell–tropic strains. Genetic analysis revealed that these two individuals inherited a homozygous defect in the gene that codes for CCR5, the cellular coreceptor for macrophage-tropic strains of HIV-1. The defective

Table 308-8

Genetic Factors Implicated in the Pathogenesis of HIV Disease

Factor	Association
MAJOR HISTOCOMPATIBILITY LOCI-ENCODED GENES	
B35, C4, DR1, DQ1	Kaposi's sarcoma
DR1	Kaposi's sarcoma
DR2, DR5	Kaposi's sarcoma
DR5	Kaposi's sarcoma
Aw23, Bw49	Kaposi's sarcoma
B62	Fever, skin rash in primary HIV infection
Aw19	HIV seropositivity in individuals multiply exposed to HIV
A1, A24, C7, B8, DR3	Rapid progression to AIDS
DR4, DQB1*0302	Rapid progression to AIDS
DR3, DQ1	Rapid progression to AIDS
B35	Rapid progression to AIDS
TAP2.1	Promotes HIV progression to AIDS
DR5	Thrombocytopenia and lymphadenopathy in HIV infection
DR5, DR6	Diffuse infiltrative CD8+ lymphocytosis with Sjögren-like syndrome in HIV infection
Bw4	Slow decline in CD4+ T cell count
B13, B27, B51, B57, DQB1*0302,0303	Protects from progression to AIDS
A26, B38, TAP1.4, TAP2.3	Ability to clear HIV infection in transiently infected seronegative individuals
A28, Bw70, Aw69, B18	Protection from HIV infection
A32, B4, C2	Long-term survival in HIV infection
A11, A32, B13, C2, DQA1*0301, DQB1*0302, DRB1*0400, DRB4*0101	Long-term survival in HIV infection
OTHER GENES	
p53 tumor suppressor gene	Controls HIV replicative patterns and determinant of viral latency
CCR-5 gene	Homozygous defect results in resistance to infection; heterozygous defect appears to result in partial protection against disease progression

SOURCES: Haynes et al; Liu et al; Samson et al.

CCR5 allele contained a 32-base-pair deletion corresponding to the second extracellular loop of the receptor. The encoded protein was severely truncated, and the receptor was nonfunctional, explaining the refractoriness to infection with macrophage-tropic strains of HIV-1. Population studies revealed that approximately 1 percent of the Caucasian population of western European ancestry possessed the homozygous defect. Twenty percent of this group had the heterozygous defect. Of note, cohort studies of hundreds of DNA samples originating from western and central Africa and Japan did not reveal a single mutant allele, suggesting that the allele is either absent or extremely rare in Africa and Japan. In a cohort of 1400 HIV-1–infected Caucasian individuals, no subject homozygous for the mutation was found, strongly supporting the concept that the homozygous defect confers protection against infection. This finding is particularly compelling in light of the fact that transmitting viruses are strongly biased towards macrophage-tropic strains of HIV-1 (see above). Furthermore, there was a higher frequency of individuals heterozygous for the genetic defect among HIV-infected patients who were long-term nonprogressors compared to HIV-infected individuals who progressed more rapidly.

NEUROPATHOGENESIS HIV-infected individuals can experience a variety of neurologic abnormalities due either to opportunistic infections and neoplasms (see below) or to direct effects of HIV or its products. With regard to the latter, HIV has been demonstrated in the brain and cerebrospinal fluid of infected individuals with and without neuropsychiatric abnormalities. The main cell types that are infected in the brain in vivo are those of the monocyte/macrophage lineage, including monocytes that have migrated to the brain from the peripheral blood as well as resident microglial cells. HIV entry into brain is felt to be due, at least in part, to the ability of virus-infected and immune-activated macrophages to induce adhesion molecules such as E-selectin and vascular cell adhesion molecule-1 (VCAM-1) on brain endothelium. Other studies have demonstrated that HIV gp120 enhances the expression of intercellular adhesion molecule-1 (ICAM-1) in glial cells, and this effect may facilitate entry of HIV-infected cells into the central nervous system and may promote syncytia formation. Virus isolates from the brain are preferentially monocytotropic as opposed to T cell–tropic (see above); in addition, distinct HIV envelope sequences are associated with the clinical expression of the AIDS dementia complex (see below). Although there have been reports of infrequent HIV infection of neuronal cells and astrocytes, there is no convincing evidence that brain cells other than those of monocyte/macrophage lineage can be infected in vivo. Nonetheless, it has been demonstrated that galactosyl ceramide may be an essential component of the HIV gp120 receptor on neural cells, and antibodies to galactosyl ceramide inhibit entry of HIV into neural cell lines in vitro.

HIV-infected individuals may manifest white matter lesions as well as neuronal loss. Given the relative absence of evidence of HIV infection of neurons either in vivo or in vitro, it is unlikely that direct infection of these cells accounts for their loss. Rather, the HIV-mediated effects on brain tissue are thought to be due to a combination of direct effects, either toxic or function-inhibitory, of gp120 on neuronal cells and effects of a variety of neurotoxins released from infiltrating monocytes, resident microglial cells, and astrocytes. Neurotoxins can be released from monocytes as a consequence of infection and/or immune activation. Monocyte-derived neurotoxic factors have been reported to kill neurons via the *N*–methyl-D-aspartate (NMDA) receptor. In addition, HIV gp120 shed by virus-infected monocytes could cause neurotoxicity by antagonizing the function of vasoactive intestinal peptide (VIP), by elevating intracellular calcium levels, and by decreasing nerve growth factor levels in the cerebral cortex. A variety of monocyte-derived cytokines can contribute directly or indirectly to the neurotoxic effects in HIV infection; these include TNFα, IL-1, IL-6, TGFβ, INFγ, platelet-activating factor, and endothelin. In addition, infection and/or activation of monocyte-lineage cells can result in increased production of eicosanoids, nitric oxide, and quinolinic acid, which may contribute to neurotoxicity. Astrocytes may play diverse roles in HIV neuropathogenesis. Reactive gliosis or astrocytosis has been demonstrated in the brains of HIV-infected individuals, and TNFα and IL-6 have been shown to induce astrocyte proliferation. In addition, astrocyte-derived IL-6 can induce HIV expression in infected cells in vitro. Furthermore, it has been suggested that astrocytes may downregulate macrophage-produced neurotoxins. The likelihood that HIV or its products are involved in neuropathogenesis is supported by the observation that neuropsychiatric abnormalities may undergo remarkable and rapid improvement upon the initiation of antiretroviral therapy, particularly in HIV-infected children.

PATHOGENESIS OF KAPOSI'S SARCOMA Kaposi's sarcoma is an opportunistic disease in HIV-infected individuals. Unlike opportunistic infections, its occurrence is not strictly related to the level of depression of CD4+ T cell counts (see below). Kaposi's sarcoma does not result from a neoplastic transformation of cells in the classic sense, and so is not truly a sarcoma. It is a manifestation of excessive proliferation of spindle cells that are believed to be of vascular origin and have features in common with endothelial and smooth muscle cells. The initiation and/or propagation of Kaposi's sarcoma is mediated, at least in part, by cytokines. A number of factors, including TNFα, IL-1β, IL-6, GM-CSF, basic fibroblast growth factor, and oncostatin M, function in an autocrine and paracrine manner to sustain the growth and chemotaxis of the Kaposi's sarcoma spindle cells. In addition, the HIV-1 Tat protein has been shown to act synergistically with basic fibroblast growth factor in the induction of lesions resembling Kaposi's sarcoma lesions in mice. Glucocorticoids have been shown to have a stimulatory effect, and human chorionic gonadotrophin an inhibitory effect, on Kaposi's sarcoma spindle cells, suggesting that modulation of the balance of autocrine factors may have therapeutic potential in Kaposi's sarcoma.

The identification of Kaposi's sarcoma in HIV-seronegative homosexual men at high risk for HIV infection, as well as the disproportionate occurrence of Kaposi's sarcoma among HIV-infected homosexual men compared to other HIV-infected groups, has led to the suggestion that Kaposi's sarcoma is caused by a sexually transmitted agent other than HIV. In 1994, a molecular procedure called representational difference analysis succeeded in identifying unique herpesvirus sequences in more than 90 percent of Kaposi's sarcoma tissues obtained from HIV-infected individuals. The sequences showed similarities to herpesvirus saimiri of squirrel monkeys and to EBV. The virus is referred to as *Kaposi's sarcoma–associated herpesvirus* or *human herpesvirus (HHV)-8*. PCR analysis indicated that these same sequences were present not only in HIV-associated Kaposi's sarcoma, but also in classic Kaposi's sarcoma and the Kaposi's sarcoma that occurs in HIV-negative homosexual men (see above). In addition, the sequences were identified in AIDS-related, body cavity–based B cell lymphomas. HHV-8 has been detected in the blood of more than 50 percent of individuals with Kaposi's sarcoma of the skin. In addition, detection of HHV-8 in the blood is felt to be strongly predictive of later development of Kaposi's sarcoma. In 1996, the successful propagation of HHV-8 in culture made possible the performance of seroepidemiologic studies that strongly indicated that HHV-8 has a specific etiologic role in Kaposi's sarcoma. It is likely that the combination of immune activation, cytokine secretion, and HHV-8 act synergistically in the ultimate expression of this disease.

IMMUNE RESPONSE TO HIV

As detailed above and below, following the initial burst of viremia during primary infection, HIV-infected individuals generally mount a robust immune response that usually substantially curtails the levels of plasma viremia and almost certainly contributes to slowing the progression of infection and to delaying the ultimate development of clinically apparent disease for a median of 10 years. This immune response contains elements of both humoral and cell-mediated immunity (Table 308-9) and is directed against multiple antigenic determinants of the HIV virion, as well as against viral proteins produced in infected cells. Paradoxically, those CD4+ cellular elements of the immune system with T cell receptors specific for HIV are theoretically

Table 308-9

Elements of the Immune Response to HIV

Humoral immunity
- Binding antibodies
- Neutralizing antibodies
  - Type specific
  - Group specific
- Antibodies participating in ADCC
  - Protective
  - Pathogenic (bystander killing)
- Enhancing antibodies

Cell-mediated immunity
- Helper CD4+ T lymphocytes
- Class I MHC–restricted cytotoxic CD8+ T lymphocytes
- CD8+ T cell–mediated inhibition (noncytolytic)
- Antibody-dependent cellular cytotoxicity
- Natural killer cells

those CD4+ T cells most likely to bind to infected cells and themselves be infected and destroyed. Thus, relatively early in the course of HIV infection, it is likely that the cellular components of host defense that are most important for the control of HIV infection are preferentially infected and destroyed.

Although a great deal of investigation has been directed toward attempting to delineate and understand the individual elements of this immune response, it remains unclear which of these phenomena are most important in delaying progression of infection and which, if any, may actually be playing a role in the pathogenesis of HIV disease.

HUMORAL IMMUNE RESPONSE Antibodies to HIV usually appear within 2 weeks and almost invariably within 8 weeks of the onset of primary infection (Fig. 308-17). Detection of these antibodies forms the basis of most diagnostic screening tests for HIV infection. It should be noted that the appearance of HIV-binding antibodies detected by ELISA and western blot assays (see below) occurs prior to the appearance of neutralizing antibodies. The latter generally appear following the downregulation of plasma viremia, which is more closely associated with the appearance of HIV-specific CD8+ CTLs (see below). Despite earlier claims to the contrary, there is currently no evidence to suggest that, apart from extremely rare exceptions, the period between initial infection and development of an antibody response is any longer than 3 months. The first antibodies detected are those directed against the structural or *gag* proteins of HIV, p24 and p17, and the *gag* precursor p55. The development of antibodies to p24 is associated with a decrease in the serum levels of free p24 antigen. Antibodies to the *gag* proteins are followed by the appearance of antibodies to the envelope proteins (gp160, gp120, p88, and gp41) and to the products of the *pol* gene (p31, p51, and p66). In addition, one may see antibodies to low-molecular-weight proteins from HIV-

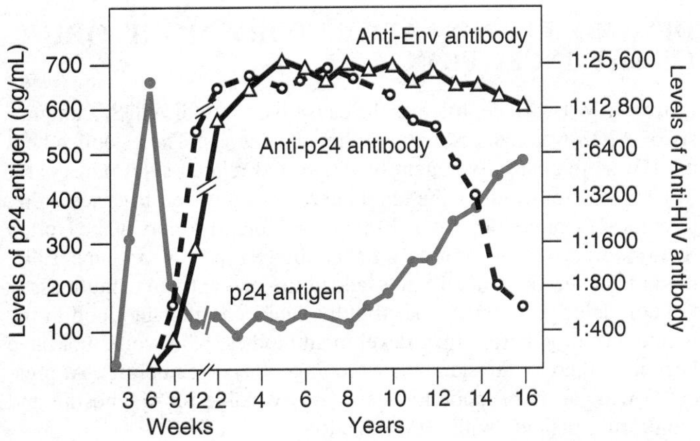

FIGURE 308-17 Relationship between antigenemia and the development of antibodies to HIV. Antibodies to HIV proteins are generally seen 6 to 12 weeks following infection and 3 to 6 weeks after the development of plasma viremia. Late in the course of illness, antibody levels to p24 decline, generally in association with a rising titer of p24 antigen.

infected cells corresponding to antibodies to the regulatory proteins produced by the HIV genes *vpr*, *vpu*, *vif*, *rev*, *tat*, and *nef*.

While antibodies are produced to multiple antigens of HIV, their precise functional significance is unclear. The best studied have been the antibodies directed toward the envelope proteins of the virus. As noted above, the envelope of HIV consists of an outer envelope glycoprotein, with a molecular weight of 120 kDa, and a transmembrane glycoprotein, with a molecular weight of 41 kDa. These are initially synthesized as a 160-kDa precursor. Most of the antienvelope antibodies are directed toward either an epitope in the gp41 region comprising amino acids 579 through 613, or towards a hypervariable region of the gp120 molecule known as the V3 loop region, comprising amino acids 303 through 338. This V3 region is a major site for the development of mutations that lead to variants of HIV that are not as well recognized by the immune system.

Antibodies directed toward the envelope proteins of HIV have been characterized both as being protective and as possibly contributing to the pathogenesis of HIV disease. Among the protective antibodies are those that function to neutralize HIV directly and prevent the infection of additional cells, as well as those that participate in ADCC. Neutralizing antibodies appear to be of two forms, type-specific and group-specific. Type-specific neutralizing antibodies are generally directed to the V3 loop region. These antibodies only neutralize viruses of a given strain and are present in low titer in most infected individuals. Group-specific antibodies, on the other hand, are capable of neutralizing a wide variety of HIV isolates. At least two forms of group-specific antibodies have been identified, those binding to amino acids 423 to 437 of gp120 and those binding to amino acids 728 to 745 of gp41. The other major class of protective antibodies are those that participate in ADCC. ADCC is actually a form of cell-mediated immunity (see Chap. 305) in which NK cells that bear Fc receptors and are armed with specific anti-HIV antibodies (which bind via their Fc portion to the cellular Fc receptors) bind to and destroy cells expressing HIV antigens (Fig. 308-18). Antibodies to both gp120 and gp41 have been shown to participate in ADCC-mediated killing of HIV-infected cells. The levels of antienvelope antibodies capable of mediating ADCC are highest in the earlier stages of HIV infection. ADCC-mediated killing can be augmented in vitro by IL-2.

In addition to playing a role in host defense, HIV-specific antibodies also have been implicated in the pathogenesis of the disease. In vitro, antibodies directed to gp41, when present in low titer, have been shown to be capable of facilitating infection of cells through an Fc receptor–mediated mechanism known as antibody enhancement. The same regions of the envelope protein of HIV that give rise to antibodies capable of mediating ADCC also elicit the production of antibodies that can facilitate infection of uninfected cells in vitro. In addition, it has been postulated that anti-gp120 antibodies that participate in the ADCC killing of HIV-infected cells might also kill uninfected CD4+ T cells if the uninfected cells had bound free gp120 from the circulation, a phenomenon referred to as *bystander killing* (Fig. 308-18).

CELLULAR IMMUNE RESPONSE Given the fact that T cell–mediated immunity is known to play a major role in host defense against most viral infections (see Chap. 305), it is generally thought to be an important component of the host immune response to HIV. T cell immunity can be divided into two major categories, mediated respectively by the helper/inducer or CD4+ T cells and the cytotoxic/immunoregulatory or CD8+ T cells.

It has been very difficult to demonstrate directly the presence of HIV-specific CD4+ T cells in HIV-infected patients. This difficulty may be related to the fact that these cells, with their high affinity for binding to HIV-infected cells, may be among the first to be infected and destroyed during HIV infection. Nonetheless, through the use of computer modeling, several regions of the HIV-1 envelope molecule have been identified that are structurally analogous to other known T cell epitopes by virtue of having structures known as *amphipathic helices*. Peptides from these envelope regions have been used to dem-

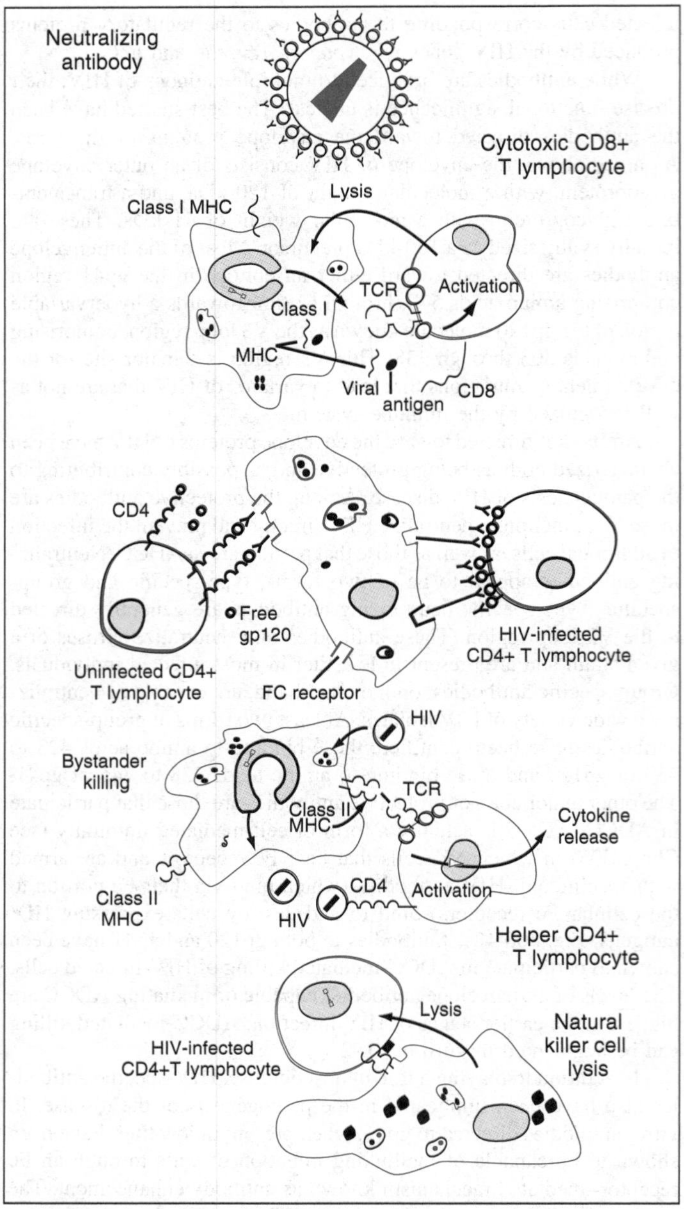

FIGURE 308-18 Schematic representation of the different immunologic effector mechanisms felt to be active in the setting of HIV infection. Detailed descriptions are given in the text.

onstrate the presence of CD4+ T cells specific for these regions in the peripheral blood of HIV-infected individuals. Other studies have demonstrated that peripheral blood T cells of some healthy, HIV-negative individuals also react to the envelope proteins of HIV.

Classic, MHC class I–restricted, HIV-specific CD8+ CTLs have been identified in the peripheral blood of patients within weeks of HIV infection. These CD8+ T lymphocytes, through their HIV-specific antigen receptors, bind to and cause the lytic destruction of target cells bearing identical MHC class I molecules associated with HIV antigens (Fig. 308-18). Two types of CD8+ CTL activity can be demonstrated in the peripheral blood and lymph node mononuclear cells of HIV-infected individuals. The first type directly lyses appropriate target cells in culture without in vitro stimulation (spontaneous CTL activity). The other type of CTL activity reflects the precursor frequency of CTLs (CTL_p); this type of CTL activity can be demonstrated by stimulation of CD8+ T cells in vitro with a mitogen such as phytohemagglutinin or anti-CD3 antibody. Following primary HIV infection, the qualitative nature of the HIV-specific CTL responses is an important predictor of eventual outcome. Patients who mount a broad CD8+ CTL response, involving several CD8+ T cell clonotypes none of which exhibits more than minor expansion, generally have a more favorable clinical course than patients who mount a more restricted CTL response, characterized by major expansions of a very restricted repertoire of CD8+ T cell clonotypes (see above). Longitudinal studies have demonstrated that the gradual loss of CD4+ T lymphocytes is paralleled by a loss of HIV-specific CD8+ CTL activity, which reinforces the concept that the CD4+ T lymphocyte is an important element in maintaining antigen-specific CTL responses. Multiple HIV antigens can elicit HIV-specific CTL responses. Class I–restricted CTLs directed against products of at least six HIV genes—*gag*, *env*, *pol*, *tat*, *rev*, and *nef*—have been identified. CD4+ CTLs, which are class II MHC–restricted, have also been identified in HIV-infected individuals and in uninfected individuals following vaccination with HIV proteins. The pathophysiologic significance of these CD4+ CTLs is unclear at present.

At least three other forms of cell-mediated immunity to HIV have been described. These are CD8+ T cell–mediated suppression of HIV replication, ADCC, and NK cell activity. *CD8+ T cell–mediated suppression of HIV replication* refers to the ability of CD8+ T cells from an HIV-infected patient to inhibit the replication of HIV in tissue culture in a noncytolytic manner. There is no requirement for HLA compatibility between the CD8+ T cells and the infected CD4+ T cells. In most culture systems that have been employed, the CD8+ T cells must be derived from an HIV-infected individual to suppress HIV replication. However, in certain systems, CD8+ T cells from uninfected individuals can also have this effect. It has been demonstrated that this effector mechanism is mediated by a soluble factor(s). CD8+ T cells, as well as monocytes, CD4+ T cells, and B cells, secrete the β-chemokines RANTES, MIP-1α, and MIP-1β (see above). These chemokines are potent suppressors of HIV replication and operate at least in part via blockade of the coreceptor (CCR5) for macrophage-tropic strains of HIV on peripheral blood mononuclear cells (see above). It is clear that other CD8+ T cell–derived soluble factors besides the β-chemokines suppress HIV replication; one of the mechanisms of suppression of HIV replication by these factors has been reported to be the inhibition of HIV transcription. The identity of these factors remain unknown.

ADCC, as described above in relation to humoral immunity, involves the killing of HIV-expressing cells by NK cells armed with specific antibody directed against HIV antigens. Finally, NK cells alone have been shown to be capable of killing HIV-infected target cells in tissue culture. This primitive cytotoxic mechanism of host defense is geared toward nonspecific surveillance for neoplastic transformation and viral infection through recognition of altered class I MHC molecules. Both NK and ADCC activity can be enhanced by IL-2.

DIAGNOSIS AND LABORATORY MONITORING OF HIV INFECTION

Before HIV-1 was identified as the causative agent of AIDS, a diagnosis of AIDS was made solely on clinical grounds. The establishment of HIV as the causative agent of AIDS and related syndromes early in 1984 was followed by the rapid development of sensitive screening tests for HIV infection, and by March 1985, blood donors in the United States were screened routinely for antibodies to HIV. In June 1996, blood banks in the United States added the p24 antigen capture assay to help identify the rare infected individuals who donate blood in the window of time before they develop antibodies, who would not have been identified by the standard screening assays (see below). At present, a wide array of laboratory tests are available for diagnosing and monitoring patients with HIV infection.

DIAGNOSIS OF HIV INFECTION The diagnosis of HIV infection depends on the demonstration of antibodies to HIV and/or the direct detection of HIV or one of its components. As noted above, antibodies to HIV generally appear in the circulation 4 to 8 weeks after infection.

The standard screening test for HIV is the *enzyme-linked immunosorbent assay* (ELISA). This solid-phase assay is an extremely good screening test, with a sensitivity of over 99.5 percent. Most diagnostic laboratories use a commercial ELISA kit that contains antigens from both HIV-1 and HIV-2 and that will detect either. These kits use both natural and recombinant antigens and are continuously updated to increase their sensitivity to newly discovered species, such as group O viruses (see Fig. 308-5). ELISA tests are generally scored as positive (highly reactive), negative (nonreactive), or indeterminate (partially reactive). While the ELISA is extremely sensitive, it is not optimal with regard to specificity. In fact, in studies of low-risk individuals, such as volunteer blood donors, only 13 percent of ELISA-positive individuals actually had HIV infection. Among the factors associated with false-positive ELISA tests are antibodies to class II antigens, autoantibodies, hepatic disease, and recent influenza vaccination. For these reasons, anyone suspected of having HIV infection on the basis of an inconclusive or positive ELISA result must have the result confirmed with a more specific assay.

The most commonly used confirmatory test is the *western blot* (Fig. 308-19). It takes advantage of the fact that multiple HIV antigens having different, well-characterized molecular weights elicit the production of specific antibodies. These antigens can be separated on the basis of molecular weight, and antibodies to each component can be detected as discrete bands on the western blot. A negative western blot is one in which no bands are present at molecular weights corresponding to HIV gene products. In a patient with a positive or indeterminate ELISA and a negative western blot, one can conclude with certainty that the ELISA reactivity was a false positive. On the other hand, a western blot demonstrating antibodies to products of all three of the major genes of HIV (*gag*, *pol*, and *env*) is conclusive evidence of infection with HIV. In fact, according to most experts, as well as the criteria established by the Association of State and Territorial Public Health Laboratory Directors and adopted by the CDC, a western blot can be considered positive for HIV-1 if it contains bands to at least two of the following gene products: p24, gp41, and gp120/160. By definition, western blot patterns of reactivity that do not fall into the positive or negative categories are considered "indeterminate." There are two possible explanations for an indeterminate western blot result. The most likely explanation is that the patient being tested has antibodies that cross-react with one of the proteins of HIV. The most common patterns of cross reactivity are antibodies that react with p24 and/or p55. The least likely explanation for an indeterminate western blot is that the individual is infected with HIV and is in the process of mounting a classic antibody response. In either instance, the western blot should be repeated in 1 month to confirm whether or not the indeterminate pattern is a pattern in evolution. In addition, one may attempt to confirm a diagnosis of HIV infection with the p24 antigen capture assay or one of the tests for HIV RNA (discussed below). While the western blot is an excellent confirmatory test for HIV infection in patients with a positive or indeterminate ELISA, it is a poor screening test. Among individuals with a negative ELISA and PCR for HIV, 20 to 30 percent may show one or more bands on western blot. While these bands are usually faint and represent cross reactivity, their presence creates a situation in which other diagnostic modalities (such as DNA PCR, RNA PCR, the bDNA assay, or p24 antigen capture) must be employed to ensure that the bands do not indicate early HIV infection.

A guideline for the use of these serologic tests in attempting to make a diagnosis of HIV infection is depicted in Fig. 308-20. In a patient in whom HIV infection is suspected, the appropriate initial test is the ELISA. If the result is negative, unless there is strong reason to suspect early HIV infection (as in a patient exposed within the previous 3 months), the diagnosis is ruled out and retesting should be performed only as clinically indicated. If the ELISA is indeterminate or positive, the test should be repeated. If the repeat is negative on two occasions, one can assume that the initial positive reading was due to a technical error in the performance of the assay and that the patient is negative. If the repeat is indeterminate or positive, one should proceed to the western blot. If the western blot is positive, the diagnosis is HIV infection. If the western blot is negative, the ELISA can be assumed to have been false positive, and the diagnosis of HIV infection is ruled out. If the western blot is indeterminate, it should be repeated in 1 month; in addition, one may proceed to a p24 antigen capture assay, HIV RNA assay, or HIV DNA PCR. If the p24 and HIV RNA assays are negative and there is no progression in the western blot, a diagnosis of HIV is ruled out. If either the p24 or HIV RNA assay is positive and/or the western blot shows progression, a tentative diagnosis of HIV infection can be made and later confirmed with a follow-up western blot demonstrating a positive pattern.

As mentioned earlier a variety of laboratory tests are available for the direct detection of HIV or its components (Table 308-10). These tests may be of considerable help in making a diagnosis of HIV infection when the western blot results are indeterminate. In addition, several of these can be used to assess the antiviral activity of therapies for HIV. The easiest to perform of these is the *p24 antigen capture assay*. This is an ELISA-type assay in which the solid phase consists of antibodies to the p24 antigen of HIV. It detects the viral protein p24 in the blood of HIV-infected individuals, where it exists either as free antigen or complexed to anti-p24 antibodies. Overall, approxi-

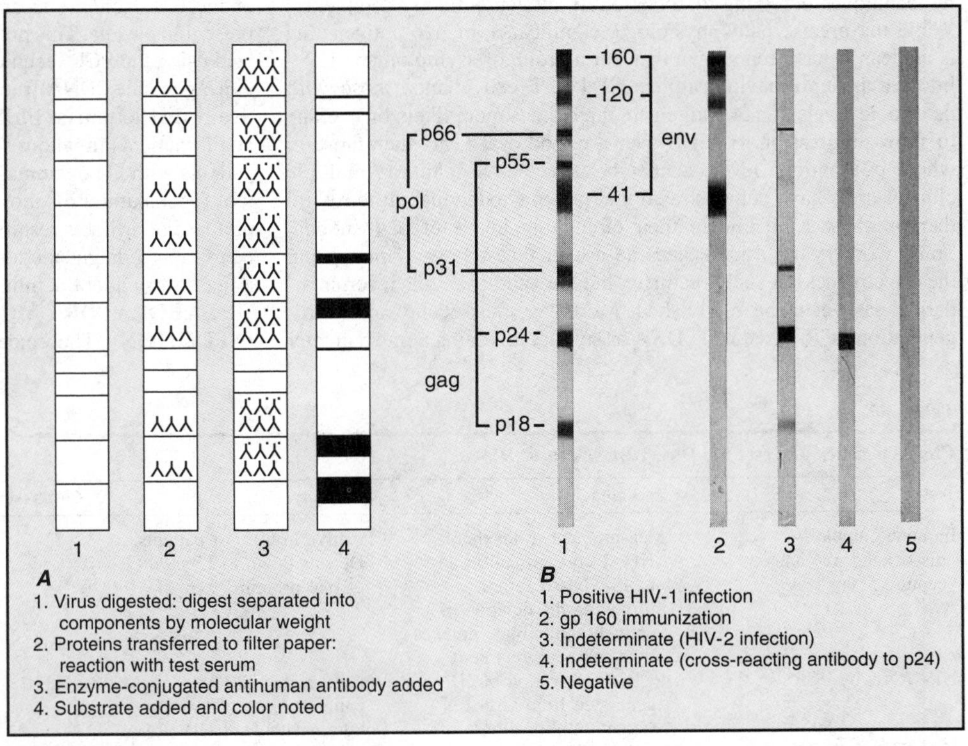

FIGURE 308-19 *A.* Schematic representation of how a western blot is performed. *B.* Examples of patterns of western blot reactivity. In each instance the western blot strip contains antigens to HIV-1. The sera from the patient immunized to the HIV-1 envelope only contains antibodies to the HIV-1 envelope proteins. The sera from the patient with HIV-2 infection cross-reacts with both reverse transcriptase and *gag* gene products of HIV-1.

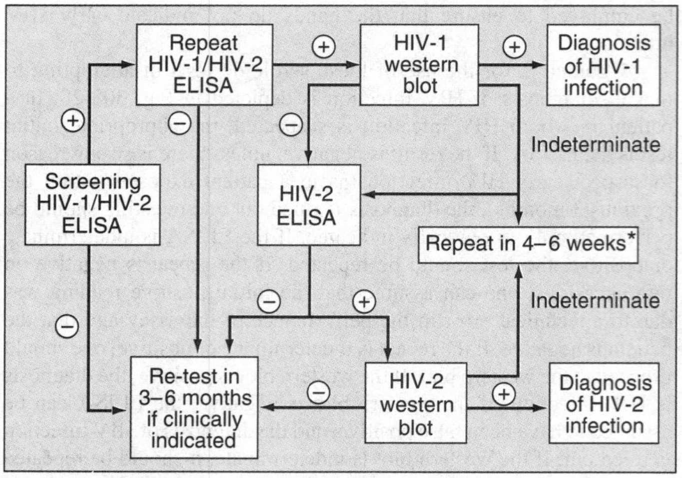

FIGURE 308-20 Algorithm for the use of serologic tests in the diagnosis of HIV-1 or HIV-2 infection. * Stable indeterminate western blot 4–6 weeks makes HIV infection unlikely. However, it should be repeated twice at 3-month intervals to rule out HIV infection. Alternatively, one may test for HIV-1 p24 antigen on HIV RNA.

mately 30 percent of individuals with HIV infection have detectable levels of free p24 antigen. This percentage increases to about 50 percent when samples are treated with a weak acid to dissociate antigen-antibody complexes prior to assay. Throughout the course of HIV infection, an equilibrium appears to exist between p24 antigen and anti-p24 antibodies. During the first few weeks of infection, before an immune response develops, there is a brisk rise in p24 antigen levels. After the development of anti-p24 antibodies, these levels decline. Late in the course of infection, when circulating levels of free virus are high, p24 antigen levels also increase, particularly when detected by techniques involving dissociation of antigen-antibody complexes. While the precise pathophysiologic significance of p24 antigenemia is unclear, it has been shown that, for a group of asymptomatic HIV-infected patients having similar CD4+ T cell counts, those with detectable levels of p24 antigen are three times more likely on average to show progression to AIDS over a period of 3 years than those in whom p24 antigen levels cannot be detected. In addition, multiple clinical trials have demonstrated that patients receiving antiretroviral therapy show a decline in their circulating levels of p24 antigen. Some workers have advocated the use of this assay for monitoring the effectiveness of such treatment, but the validity of this recommendation has yet to be established. Moreover, the second- and third-generation PCR-based and bDNA assays are assuming a much greater role in the decisions to initiate and/or modify antiretroviral therapy (see below). At present, the p24 antigen capture assay seems to be most useful as a screening test for HIV infection in patients suspected of having the acute HIV syndrome, as high levels of p24 antigen are present prior to the development of antibodies. It is currently used along with the HIV ELISA to screen blood donors in the United States for evidence of HIV infection.

The *polymerase chain reaction* is a diagnostic technique that has gained acceptance in many areas of clinical microbiology. Although the extreme sensitivity of this technique leads in many cases to false-positive results, in a well-controlled setting PCR has been of extraordinary value in furthering our understanding of the pathogenesis of HIV disease and has provided a gold standard for the diagnosis of HIV infection. This is particularly true for the diagnosis of HIV infection in at-risk neonates. Two forms of PCR are used in the study of HIV infection, DNA PCR and RNA PCR. The DNA PCR can be used for making a diagnosis of HIV infection by amplifying proviral DNA. In performing a DNA PCR test for HIV, peripheral blood mononuclear cells are lysed, and the DNA region of interest is amplified using primer pairs from relatively constant regions of the HIV genome. Primer pairs from both the *gag* and LTR regions are usually employed. The amplified DNA is then characterized using nucleic acid hybridization techniques. With the proper controls to check for contamination and success of amplification, it is possible to determine whether or not HIV proviral DNA is present at a frequency of one copy per 10,000 to 100,000 cells. Studies of this type have clearly documented that the interval between HIV infection and antibody positivity is on the order of 1 to 3 months. In addition to being a diagnostic tool, DNA PCR is also useful for amplifying defined areas of proviral DNA for sequence analysis and has become an important technique for studies of sequence diversity and microbial resistance to antiretroviral agents. While RNA PCR has been used most frequently for monitoring changes in the level of the HIV genome present in plasma, it can also be used for making an early diagnosis of HIV infection. In this technique, following DNAase treatment, a cDNA copy is made of all RNA species present in plasma. Insofar as HIV is an RNA virus (see above and Chap. 192), this will result in the production of DNA copies of the HIV genome in amounts proportional to the amount of HIV present in plasma. This proviral cDNA is then amplified and characterized using the PCR technique, employing primer pairs that can distinguish genomic cDNA from messenger cDNA. In patients with a positive or indeterminate ELISA test and an indeterminate western blot, and in patients in whom serologic testing may be unreliable (such as patients with hypogammaglobulinemia), PCR is a valuable diagnostic tool for making a diagnosis of HIV infection. Given its cost and the problem of artifacts resulting from contamination, however, it should be used as a diagnostic tool only when standard serologic testing has failed to provide a definitive result.

LABORATORY MONITORING OF PATIENTS WITH HIV INFECTION The epidemic of HIV infection and AIDS has provided the clinician with new challenges in the integration of clinical and laboratory data. The close relationship between clinical manifestations of HIV infection and CD4+ T cell count has made measurement of the latter quantity a routine part of the evaluation of HIV-infected individuals. Coupled with knowledge of the levels of HIV RNA in serum or plasma (see below), CD4+ T cell counts make a powerful set of tools for determining prognosis and monitoring response to therapy. While the CD4+ T cell count provides information on the current immunologic status of the patient, the HIV RNA level predicts what will happen to that CD4+ T cell count in the near future and hence predicts the clinical prognosis for the

Table 308-10

Characteristics of Tests for Direct Detection of HIV

Test	Technique	Sensitivity	Cost/Test
Immune complex–dissociated p24 antigen capture assay	Measurement of levels of HIV-1 core protein in an ELISA-based format following dissociation of antigen-antibody complexes by weak acid treatment	Positive in 50% of patients. Detects down to 15 pg/mL of p24 protein	$1–2
HIV RNA by PCR	PCR amplification of cDNA generated from viral RNA (target amplification)	Positive in >98% of patients. Detects down to 40 copies/mL of HIV RNA	$150
HIV RNA by bDNA	Measurement of levels of particle-associated HIV RNA in a nucleic acid capture assay employing signal amplification	Positive in 90% of patients. Detects down to 500 copies/mL of HIV RNA	$150

patient. Other tests, such as the p24 antigen capture assay (described above) and measurement of serum levels of neopterin and β_2-microglobulin, may also provide information of value to the clinician (see below).

The direct cultivation of HIV from plasma or peripheral blood mononuclear cells is a technique employed in many research laboratories and has proven very useful for generating HIV isolates for studies of antiviral resistance and analysis of genomic drift. Most of the techniques employed involve cocultivation of patient material with an indicator cell line capable of supporting HIV replication, most commonly peripheral blood mononuclear cells that have been activated with phytohemagglutinin. Cultures generally need to be maintained for up to 28 days, during which time they are periodically observed for the formation of syncytia or giant cells, and supernatants are sampled for the presence of either HIV p24 (using the antigen capture assays mentioned above) or reverse transcriptase. There is no role at present for HIV culture in the diagnosis or routine management of patients with HIV infection; however, such tests may be used more commonly as attempts are made to tailor antiretroviral therapy to the sensitivities of patient-derived viral isolates.

The CD4+ T cell count is the laboratory test generally accepted as an indicator of the immunologic competence of the patient with HIV infection. This measurement, which is the product of the percent of CD4+ T cells (determined by flow cytometry) and the total lymphocyte count [determined by the white blood cell count (WBC) and the differential count] has been shown to correlate very well with clinical progression. Patients with CD4+ T cell counts below 200/μL are at high risk of infection with *Pneumocystis carinii*, while patients with CD4+ T cell counts below 100/μL are at high risk of infection with cytomegalovirus and the *Mycobacterium avium-intracellulare* complex (Fig. 308-21). Patients with an initial diagnosis of HIV infection should have CD4+ T cell measurements performed approximately every 6 months, and more frequently if a declining trend is noted. At a minimum, antiretroviral therapy is generally indicated when the CD4+ T cell count falls below 500/μL, and a declining CD4+ T cell count may provide an indication for changing therapy (see below). Once the CD4+ T cell count is below 200/μL, patients should be placed on a regimen for *P. carinii* pneumonia (PCP) prophylaxis. All effective forms of antiretroviral therapy to date have been associated with at least a transient increase in either CD4+ T cell count or CD4 percent (see below).

Direct Measurements of HIV RNA Facilitated by techniques for the precise quantitation of small amounts of nucleic acids, the measurement of serum or plasma levels of HIV RNA has become the most commonly used approach for the direct detection of HIV. Two basic techniques are used: the reverse transcriptase PCR (RT-PCR) assay and the branched DNA (bDNA) assay. The RT-PCR assay involves the PCR amplification of cDNA generated from viral RNA. The bDNA assay involves the use of a solid-phase nucleic acid capture system and signal amplification through successive nucleic acid hybridizations to detect small quantities of HIV RNA. Both assays generate data in the form of number of copies of HIV RNA per milliliter of serum or plasma. The RT-PCR assay can detect as few as 40 copies of HIV RNA per milliliter and is positive in >98 percent of patients. The bDNA assay can detect as few as 500 copies of HIV RNA per milliliter and is positive in >90 percent of patients. Measurements of levels of HIV RNA over time have been of great value in delineating the relationship between levels of virus and rates of disease progression (Fig. 308-22), the rates of viral turnover, the relationship between immune system activation and viral replication, and the time to development of antiviral drug resistance. While the p24 antigen capture assays reflect changes in total viral burden over an extended period, the HIV RNA assays allow an evaluation of the changes in viral burden that occur over a matter of hours. Measurements of HIV RNA levels should be made approximately every 6 months and more frequently in the setting of changes in antiretroviral therapy. While precise guidelines have yet to be established, a level of HIV RNA of >20,000 copies per milliliter is felt by many experts to be an indication for antiretroviral therapy, regardless of the CD4+ T cell count. All effective forms of antiretroviral therapy to date have been associated with a drop in levels of HIV RNA.

β_2-Microglobulin Levels β_2-Microglobulin is an 11-kDa protein that is expressed on the surface of most nucleated cells. It forms a heterodimer with class I MHC molecules and exhibits amino acid homology with the constant region of immunoglobulin. Free β_2-microglobulin can be measured in both serum and urine. Levels of β_2-microglobulin are elevated in a variety of conditions characterized by lymphocyte activation and/or lymphocyte destruction; among these are lymphoproliferative syndromes, autoimmune diseases, and viral infections, including HIV infection. In addition, β_2-microglobulin is excreted by the renal tubules, and levels may be elevated in patients with renal disease. Levels of β_2-microglobulin correlate with the degree of progression of HIV disease. The highest levels are seen in patients with AIDS; the lowest levels in patients with asymptomatic HIV infection. The β_2-microglobulin level has a predictive value for progression to AIDS that is independent of its inverse relationship to CD4+ T cell counts. In one large study, the level of serum β_2-microglobulin was the single most important predictor of development of AIDS. In another study, 34 percent of patients with a β_2-microglobulin level of >3.8 μg/mL went on to develop AIDS over a 3-year period, compared to only 7 percent of patients with a β_2-microglobulin level of <2.9 μg/mL. Levels of β_2-microglobulin have been shown to decrease in a dose-dependent fashion in patients treated with zidovudine (AZT).

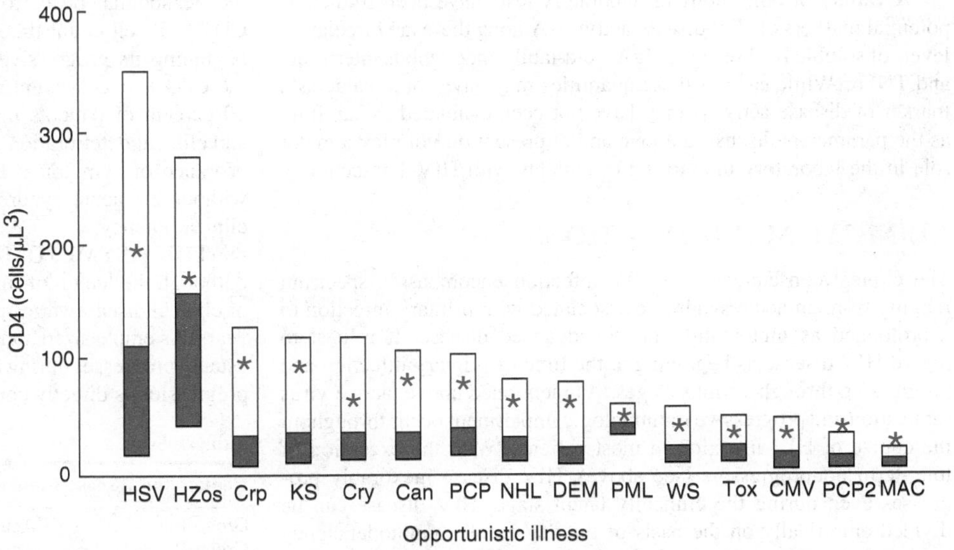

FIGURE 308-21 Relationship between CD4+ T cell counts and the development of opportunistic diseases. Boxplot of the median (line inside the box), first quartile (bottom of the box), third quartile (top of the box), and mean (asterisk) CD4+ lymphocyte count at the time of the development of opportunistic disease. Can, candidal esophagitis; CMV, cytomegalovirus infection; Crp, cryptosporidiosis; Cry, cryptococcal meningitis; DEM, AIDS dementia complex; HSV, herpes simplex virus infection; HZos, herpes zoster; KS, Kaposi's sarcoma; MAC, *Mycobacterium avium* complex bacteremia; NHL, non-Hodgkin's lymphoma; PCP, primary *Pneumocystis carinii* pneumonia; PCP2, secondary *Pneumocystis carinii* pneumonia; PML, progressive multifocal leukoencephalopathy; Tox, *Toxoplasma gondii* encephalitis; WS, wasting syndrome. *(From Moore & Chaisson.)*

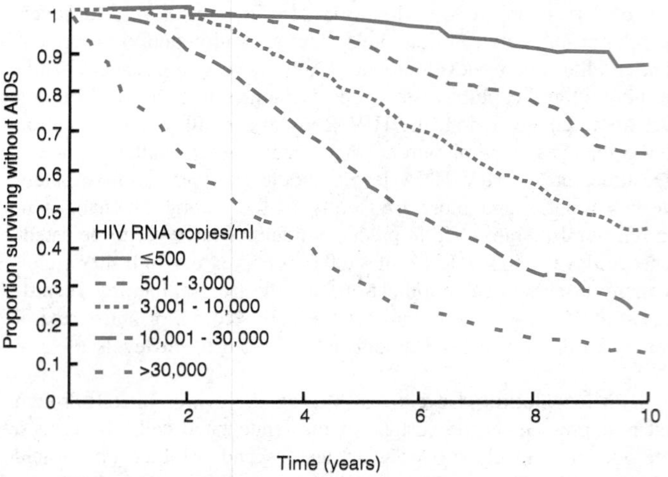

FIGURE 308-22 Relationship between levels of virus and rates of disease progression. Kaplan-Meier curves for AIDS-free survival stratified by baseline HIV-1 RNA categories (molecules per milliliter). *(From Mellors.)*

Neopterin Levels *Neopterin* (6-D-erythrotrihydroxypropylpterin) is a low-molecular-weight compound derived from an intermediate product of the de novo biosynthesis of tetrahydrobiopterin from guanosine triphosphate (GTP). It is produced by activated monocytes, and increased levels have been observed in patients with HIV infection. Elevated levels have also been reported in patients with other viral infections, autoimmune diseases, and atypical phenylketonuria, and in patients receiving immunostimulant therapy. As in the case of β_2-microglobulin, serum or urine levels of neopterin are highest in patients with advanced HIV disease and, in asymptomatic patients, higher levels are associated with an increased risk of progression to AIDS that is independent of CD4+ T cell count. Neopterin levels appear to measure a parameter linked to the same factor(s) that result in elevations in the level of β_2-microglobulin. The predictive value of these two parameters together does not exceed that provided by either one alone.

A variety of other nonviral laboratory tests have been studied as potential markers of HIV disease activity. Among these are circulating levels of soluble IL-2 receptor, IgA, acid-labile endogenous interferon, and TNFα. While each of these quantities may have some value as a marker of disease activity, they have not been evaluated as carefully as the parameters discussed above and at present do not play a major role in the laboratory monitoring of patients with HIV-1 infection.

CLINICAL MANIFESTATIONS

The clinical consequences of HIV infection encompass a spectrum ranging from an acute syndrome associated with primary infection to a prolonged asymptomatic state to advanced disease. It is best to regard HIV disease as beginning at the time of primary infection and progressing through various stages. As mentioned above, active virus replication and progressive immunologic impairment occur throughout the course of HIV infection in most patients. With the exception of long-term nonprogressors (see above), HIV disease inexorably progresses even during the clinically latent stage. HIV disease can be divided empirically on the basis of the degree of immunodeficiency into an early stage (CD4+ T cell count >500/μL), an intermediate stage (CD4+ T cell count 200 to 500/μL), and an advanced stage (CD4+ T cell count <200/μL). Most AIDS-defining opportunistic infections and true malignancies occur in the advanced stage of disease, while neurologic disease and Kaposi's sarcoma (see above) are not as strictly related to the degree of immunodeficiency. The two major classification systems for staging HIV disease are the CDC system (Table 308-11) and the Walter Reed Medical Center System (Table 308-12); these are to be distinguished from the case definition for AIDS, which is used for surveillance purposes (Table 308-1). Each classification system has advantages and disadvantages; the CDC system relies more on clinical condition, and the Walter Reed system more on markers of immunologic status, such as the CD4+ T cell count and the presence or absence of delayed cutaneous hypersensitivity. For the purposes of describing the clinical syndromes seen in patients with HIV disease, this chapter devotes sections to the acute syndrome, the asymptomatic stage, early symptomatic disease, neurologic disease, secondary infections, neoplasms, and organ-specific syndromes.

THE ACUTE HIV SYNDROME It is estimated that 50 to 70 percent of individuals with HIV infection experience an acute clinical syndrome approximately 3 to 6 weeks after primary infection (Fig. 308-23). Varying degrees of clinical severity have been reported, and it has been suggested that symptomatic seroconversion leading to the seeking of medical attention indicates an increased risk for an accelerated course of disease. The typical clinical findings are listed in Table 308-13; they occur along with a burst of plasma viremia and p24 antigenemia. The syndrome is typical of an acute viral syndrome and has been likened to acute infectious mononucleosis. Symptoms usually persist for 1 to several weeks and gradually subside as an immune response to HIV develops and the levels of plasma viremia decrease. Opportunistic infections have been reported during this stage of infection, reflecting the immunodeficiency that results from reduced numbers of CD4+ T cells and likely also from functional suppression of CD4+ T cells owing to cross-linking of the CD4 molecule on the cell surface (see "Mechanisms of CD4+ T Lymphocyte Depletion and Dysfunction," above) as a result of the extremely high levels of plasma viremia. A number of immunologic abnormalities accompany the acute HIV syndrome, including multiphasic perturbations of the numbers of circulating lymphocyte subsets. Total lymphocyte and T cell subsets (CD4+ and CD8+) are initially reduced. An inversion of the CD4+/CD8+ T cell ratio occurs later because of a rise in the number of CD8+ T cells. In fact, there may be a selective and transient expansion of CD8+ T cell subsets, as determined by T cell receptor analysis (see above). The total circulating CD8+ T cell count may remain elevated or return to normal; however, CD4+ T cell levels usually remain somewhat depressed, although there may be a slight rebound towards normal. Lymphadenopathy occurs in approximately 70 percent of individuals with primary HIV infection. Most patients recover spontaneously from this syndrome and have a mildly depressed CD4+ T cell count that remains stable for a variable period before beginning its progressive decline (see below); in some individuals, the CD4+ T cell count returns to the normal range. Approximately 10 percent of patients manifest a fulminant course of immunologic and clinical deterioration after primary infection, even after the disappearance of symptoms. In most patients, primary infection with or without the acute syndrome is followed by a prolonged period of clinical latency.

THE ASYMPTOMATIC STAGE—CLINICAL LATENCY Although the length of time from initial infection to the development of clinical disease varies greatly, the median time is approximately 10 years. As emphasized above, HIV disease with active virus replication usually progresses during this asymptomatic period. The rate of disease progression is directly correlated with HIV RNA levels. Patients with

Table 308-11

Centers for Disease Control Classification System for HIV Disease

Group I	Acute HIV syndrome
Group II	Asymptomatic infection
Group III	Persistent generalized lymphadenopathy
Group IV	Other diseases
Subgroup A	Constitutional disease
Subgroup B	Neurologic disease
Subgroup C	Secondary infectious diseases
Subgroup D	Secondary neoplasms
Subgroup E	Other conditions

SOURCE: Modified from the Centers for Disease Control and Prevention, USPHS, 1986 and 1987.

Table 308-12

Walter Reed Staging Classification of HIV Infection

Stage	HIV Antibody	Chronic Lymphadenopathy	CD4+ Cell Count, Cells/μL	DTH Skin Testing	Thrush	Opportunistic Infections
WR0	−	−	>400	Normal (reactive to ≥2 skin test antigens)	−	−
WR1	+	−	>400	Normal	−	−
WR2	+	+	>400	Normal	−	−
WR3	+	+/−	<400	Normal	−	−
WR4	+	+/−	<400	Partial defect (reactive to 1 skin test antigen)	−	−
WR5	+	+/−	<400	Anergy and/or thrush (reactive to 0 skin test antigens)		−
WR6	+	+/−	<400	Normal, partial defect or anergy	+/−	+

NOTE: [shaded box], absolute criteria to be fulfilled for stage assignment; +, present; −, absent; DTH, delayed-type hypersensitivity.

SOURCE: Modified from Redfield et al.

high levels of HIV RNA progress to symptomatic disease faster than do patients with low levels of HIV RNA (Fig. 308-22). Some patients, called long-term nonprogressors (see above), show little if any decline in CD4+ T cell counts over an extended period. These patients generally have extremely low levels of HIV RNA. Certain other patients remain entirely asymptomatic despite the fact that their CD4+ T cell counts fall extremely low. In these patients, the appearance of an opportunistic disease may be the first manifestation of HIV infection. Some patients, otherwise asymptomatic, develop persistent generalized lymphadenopathy during this time (Table 308-11) (see below). With few exceptions, CD4+ T cell counts fall progressively during this asymptomatic period at an average rate of approximately 50 cells/μL per year. When the CD4+ cell count falls below about 200/μL, the resulting state of immunodeficiency is severe enough to place the patient at high risk for opportunistic infections and neoplasms, and hence for clinically apparent disease.

EARLY SYMPTOMATIC DISEASE As noted above, viral replication continues during the period of clinical latency, and the immunologic function of the HIV-infected individual usually declines progressively. At some point, usually after the CD4+ T cell count has fallen below 500/μL, patients begin to develop signs and symptoms of clinical illness (Table 308-14). Many of these problems can be traced to minor opportunistic infections, not sufficiently indicative of a defect in cell-mediated immunity to be considered AIDS-defining illnesses, while some of them appear to be direct effects of long-standing HIV infection. This stage of HIV infection has been given a variety of names in the past, among them *pre-AIDS* and *AIDS-related complex* (ARC); however, these terms are rarely used today. The clinical findings at this stage of disease (described below), while indicative of a decline in immune function, are generally less predictive of the patient's overall status than are the data obtained from serial measurements of CD4+ T cell counts.

Generalized Lymphadenopathy This condition, defined as the presence of enlarged lymph nodes (>1 cm) in two or more extrainguinal sites for more than 3 months without an obvious cause, is often the earliest symptom of HIV infection after primary infection. It is due to marked follicular hyperplasia in response to HIV infection, and the nodes are generally discrete and freely movable. This feature of HIV disease, which may be seen at any point in the spectrum of immune dysfunction, is not associated with an increased likelihood of developing AIDS. Paradoxically, a loss in lymphadenopathy or a decrease in lymph node size may be a prognostic marker of disease progression. In the early and intermediate stages of HIV infection (CD4+ T cell counts >200/μL), the main differential diagnosis is an adenopathic form of Kaposi's sarcoma. Late in the course of disease, differential diagnosis expands to include lymphoma, mycobacterial infection, toxoplasmosis, systemic fungal infection, and bacillary angiomatosis. Lymph node biopsy is not indicated in patients with early-stage disease unless there are signs and symptoms of systemic illness, such as fever and weight loss, or unless the nodes begin to enlarge, become fixed, or coalesce.

Oral Lesions Oral lesions, including thrush, hairy leukoplakia, and aphthous ulcers, are particularly common during this phase of HIV infection. Thrush, due to *Candida* infection, and oral hairy leukoplakia, presumed due to Epstein-Barr virus, are usually indicative of fairly advanced immunologic decline, generally occurring in patients with fewer than 300 CD4+ T cells per microliter. In one study, 59 percent of patients with oral candidiasis went on to develop AIDS in the next year. Thrush appears as a white, cheesy exudate, often on an erythematous mucosa (**see Plate ID-42**). While most commonly seen on the soft palate, early lesions are often found along the gingival border. The diagnosis is made by direct examination of a scraping for pseudohyphal elements. Culturing is of no value, as most patients with HIV infection have a positive throat culture for *Candida* even in the absence of thrush. Oral hairy leukoplakia presents as a filamentous white lesion, generally along the lateral borders of the tongue **(see**

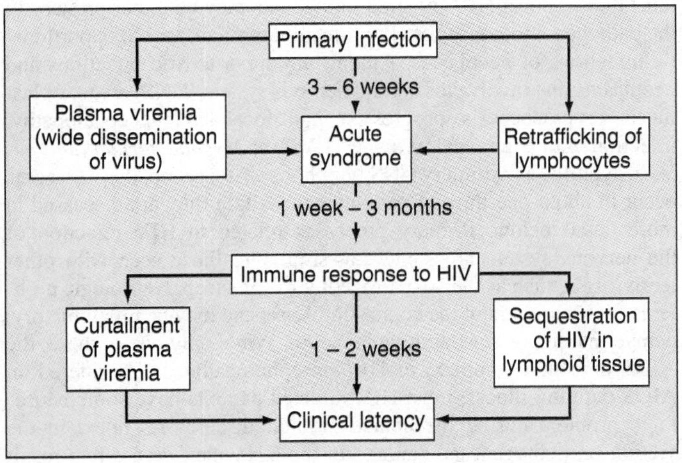

FIGURE 308-23 The acute HIV syndrome. See text for detailed description. *(From G Pantaleo et al, N Engl J Med 328:327, 1993.)*

Table 308-13

Clinical Findings in the Acute HIV Syndrome

General	Neurologic
Fever	Meningitis
Pharyngitis	Encephalitis
Lymphadenopathy	Peripheral neuropathy
Headache/retroorbital pain	Myelopathy
Arthralgias/myalgias	Dermatologic
Lethargy/malaise	Erythematous maculopapular rash
Anorexia/weight loss	Mucocutaneous ulceration
Nausea/vomiting/diarrhea	

SOURCE: From Tyndal and Cooper.

Table 308-14

Clinical Characteristics of Early Symptomatic Disease

Generalized lymphadenopathy
Thrush
Oral hairy leukoplakia
Shingles
Thrombocytopenia
Molluscum contagiosum
Recurrent herpes simplex
Condyloma acuminata
Aphthous ulcers

Plate ID-41). While usually more a sign of HIV-induced immunodeficiency than a clinical problem, severe cases have responded to therapy with acyclovir. Aphthous ulcers of the posterior oropharynx are also seen with regularity in patients with HIV infection. These lesions are of unknown etiology and can be quite painful and interfere with swallowing. Topical anesthetics provide immediate symptomatic relief of short duration. The fact that thalidomide is an effective treatment for this condition suggests that the pathogenesis may involve the action of tissue-destructive cytokines.

Reactivation Herpes Zoster (Shingles) This condition (**see Plate ID-37**) is seen in 10 to 20 percent of patients with HIV infection. This reactivation syndrome of varicella-zoster virus indicates a modest decline in immune function and is often the first clinical indication of immunodeficiency. In one series, patients who developed shingles did so an average of 5 years after HIV infection. In a cohort of patients with HIV infection, AIDS developed in 1 percent per month of the cohort after a diagnosis of localized zoster. In that study, AIDS was more likely to develop in patients with severe pain, extensive disease, or disease involving cranial or cervical dermatomes. In patients who developed shingles and oral hairy leukoplakia or thrush, shingles preceded the oral lesions by approximately 1 year. The clinical manifestations of reactivation zoster in HIV-infected patients, although indicative of immunologic compromise, are not as severe as those seen in other immunodeficient conditions. Thus, while lesions may extend over several dermatomes and frank cutaneous dissemination may be seen, visceral involvement has not been reported. In contrast to patients without a known underlying immunodeficiency state, patients with HIV infection tend to have recurrences of zoster, with a relapse rate of approximately 20 percent.

Thrombocytopenia Thrombocytopenia also may be an early consequence of HIV infection. Approximately 3 percent of patients with HIV infection and CD4+ T cell counts above 400/μL have platelet counts under 150,000/μL. For patients with CD4+ T cell counts below 400/μL, this incidence increases to 10 percent. Thrombocytopenia is rarely a serious clinical problem in these patients. Most such patients retain platelet counts above 50,000/μL, and the condition can be managed conservatively. As in other forms of thrombocytopenia, bleeding is rare unless the count falls below 10,000/μL, and bleeding of the gums, extremity petechiae, and easy bruisability are common presenting features. Bone marrow examination, which should be done to rule out other causes of thrombocytopenia, including drug toxicity, lymphoma, fungal infection, and mycobacterial infection, generally reveals a normal or increased number of megakaryocytes. In this regard, the idiopathic thrombocytopenia seen in patients with HIV infection is very similar to the thrombocytopenia seen in patients with idiopathic thrombocytopenic purpura (see Chap. 117). Immune complexes containing anti-gp120 antibodies and anti-anti-gp120 antibodies have been noted in the circulation and on the surface of platelets in patients with HIV infection. Patients with HIV infection also have been noted to have a platelet-specific antibody directed toward a 25-kDa component of the surface of the platelet. Because these data point to an immunologic basis for the thrombocytopenia seen in patients with AIDS, most of the therapeutic interventions that have been employed have been immune-based. Both high-dose intravenous immunoglobulin (IVIG) and glucocorticoids can induce a transient increase in platelet count, but they do not generally provide a long-term solution. It has been suggested that the thrombocytopenia in patients with HIV infection may be due to a direct effect of HIV on megakaryocytes, as evidenced by a decrease in platelet production. Consistent with this idea is the fact that the most effective medical approach to this problem has been the use of antiretroviral agents. Even in patients without thrombocytopenia, therapy with zidovudine has been associated with a significant increase in platelet count. Approximately 70 percent of patients with HIV-associated thrombocytopenia show a satisfactory response to zidovudine. Before combination antiretroviral therapy became the preferred treatment for HIV infection (see below), zidovudine alone was considered the treatment of choice for HIV-associated thrombocytopenia. Now, a combination of antiretroviral drugs that includes zidovudine is the treatment of choice. For patients with platelet counts below 20,000/μL, the approach should be initial treatment with IVIG or glucocorticoids for an immediate response, coupled with combination antiretroviral therapy for a more lasting response. Splenectomy is an option in patients refractory to medical management. Most patients with HIV-associated thrombocytopenia will respond to this surgical treatment. Because of the risk of serious infections with encapsulated organisms, physicians should ensure that all patients with HIV infection, especially those about to undergo splenectomy, are immunized with pneumococcal polysaccharide. It should be noted that, in addition to causing an increase in the platelet count, removal of the spleen will result in an increase in the peripheral blood lymphocyte count, making CD4+ T cell counts unreliable. In this situation, one should rely on the CD4 percent for making diagnostic decisions with respect to the likelihood of opportunistic infections. In patients with early HIV infection, thrombocytopenia has also been reported as a consequence of classic thrombotic thrombocytopenic purpura (see Chap. 117). This clinical syndrome, consisting of fever, thrombocytopenia, hemolytic anemia, and neurologic and renal dysfunction, is a rare complication of early HIV infection. As in other settings, the appropriate management is the use of salicylates and plasma exchange.

Miscellaneous Clinical Conditions Other conditions frequently seen in patients with early-stage HIV infection include molluscum contagiosum, basal cell carcinomas of the skin, headache, condyloma acuminata, and recurrent bouts of oral or genital herpes simplex. In the past, unexplained fever, weight loss, and diarrhea were included under the general heading of ARC. Many of these cases are now being diagnosed as specific opportunistic infections. In addition, this syndrome has been classified as an AIDS-defining illness in patients in whom no other diagnosis can be found; it is discussed below in the section "Generalized Wasting."

NEUROLOGIC DISEASE Clinical disease of the nervous system accounts for a significant degree of morbidity in a high percentage of patients with HIV infection (Table 308-15). The neurologic problems that occur in HIV-infected individuals may be either primary to the pathogenic processes of HIV infection or secondary to opportunistic infections or neoplasms. Among the opportunistic infections and neoplasms that involve the central nervous system (CNS) are toxoplasmosis, cryptococcosis, progressive multifocal leukoencephalopathy, infection with cytomegalovirus, HTLV-I, or *Mycobacterium tuberculosis*, syphilis, and primary CNS lymphoma. As a group, these diseases occur in about one-third of patients with AIDS; they are discussed in more detail below. Primary processes related to HIV infection of the nervous system are somewhat similar to those seen with other lentiviruses, such as the Visna-Maedi virus of sheep. Neurologic problems occur throughout the course of disease and may be inflammatory, demyelinating, or degenerative in nature. While only one of these, the AIDS dementia complex, or HIV encephalopathy, is considered an AIDS-defining illness, most HIV-infected patients have some neurologic problem during the course of their disease. As noted in the section on pathogenesis, damage to the CNS may be a direct result of viral infection of CNS macrophages or glial cells or may be secondary to the release of neurotoxins and potentially toxic cytokines such

Table 308-15

Neurologic Diseases in Patients with HIV Infection

- Opportunistic infections
  - Toxoplasmosis
  - Cryptococcosis
  - Progressive multifocal leukoencephalopathy
  - Cytomegalovirus
  - Syphilis
  - Mycobacterium tuberculosis
  - HTLV-I infection
- Neoplasms
  - Primary CNS lymphoma
  - Kaposi's sarcoma
- Result of HIV-1 infection
  - Aseptic meningitis
  - AIDS dementia complex (HIV encephalopathy)
  - Myelopathy
    - Vacuolar myelopathy
    - Pure sensory ataxia
    - Paresthesia/dysesthesia
  - Peripheral neuropathy
    - Acute demyelinating polyneuropathy
    - Mononeuritis multiplex
    - Distal symmetric polyneuropathy
  - Myopathy

as IL-1β, TNFα, IL-6, and TGFβ. Virtually all patients with HIV infection have some degree of involvement of the nervous system with HIV. This is evidenced by the fact that cerebrospinal fluid (CSF) findings are abnormal in approximately 90 percent of patients, even during the asymptomatic stage of HIV infection. Included among these abnormalities are pleocytosis (50 to 65 percent of patients), isolation of virus (approximately 50 percent), elevated CSF protein level (35 percent), and evidence of intrathecal synthesis of anti-HIV antibodies (89 percent). It should be pointed out, however, that evidence of infection of the CNS with HIV does not imply impairment of cognitive function, and, while neurologic problems related to HIV infection can be seen at all stages of disease, the mere presence of HIV infection in the CNS does not mean that the patient has a clinically relevant neurologic problem. The neurologic function of an HIV-infected individual should be considered normal unless clinical signs and symptoms suggest otherwise.

Aseptic Meningitis Aseptic meningitis may be seen in any but the very late stages of HIV infection. In the setting of acute primary infection (see above) patients may experience a syndrome of headache, photophobia, and, in some instances, frank encephalitis. CSF findings include a lymphocytic pleocytosis, elevated protein level, and normal glucose level. Cranial nerve involvement may be seen, predominantly cranial nerve VII, occasionally V, and/or VIII. This syndrome usually resolves spontaneously within 2 to 4 weeks; however, in some patients, signs and symptoms persist chronically. Such episodes may occur any time in the course of HIV infection; however, they become increasingly rare following the development of AIDS. This fact suggests that aseptic meningitis in the context of HIV infection is an immune-mediated disease.

HIV Encephalopathy HIV encephalopathy, also called *HIV-associated dementia* or *AIDS dementia complex*, consists of a constellation of signs and symptoms of CNS disease that generally occurs late in the course of HIV infection (Table 308-16). A major feature of this entity is the development of dementia, which is defined as a decline in cognitive ability from a previous level. It may present as impaired ability to concentrate, increased forgetfulness, difficulty reading, or increased difficulty performing complex tasks. Initially these symptoms may be indistinguishable from findings of situational depression or fatigue. In addition to dementia, patients with HIV encephalopathy also may have motor and behavioral abnormalities. Among the motor problems are unsteady gait, poor balance, tremor, and difficulty with rapid alternating movements. Increased tone and deep tendon reflexes may be found in patients with spinal cord involvement (see below). Late stages may be complicated by bowel and/or bladder incontinence. Behavioral problems include apathy and lack of initiative, with progression to a vegetative state in some instances. Some patients develop a state of agitation or mild mania. These changes usually occur without significant changes in level of alertness, in contrast to the findings in patients with dementia due to toxic/metabolic encephalopathies.

HIV encephalopathy is the initial AIDS-defining illness in approximately 3 percent of patients with HIV infection and thus only rarely precedes clinical evidence of immunodeficiency. Clinically significant HIV encephalopathy eventually develops in approximately one-fourth of patients with HIV infection. As immunologic function declines, the risk and severity of HIV encephalopathy increase. Autopsy series suggest that 80 to 90 percent of patients with HIV infection have histologic evidence of CNS involvement. Several classification schemes have been developed for grading HIV encephalopathy. The most commonly used clinical staging system is outlined in Table 308-16.

The precise cause of HIV encephalopathy remains unclear, although the condition is thought to be a result of direct effects of HIV on the CNS. HIV has been found in the brains of patients with HIV encephalopathy by Southern blot, in situ hybridization, PCR, and electron microscopy. Multinucleated giant cells, macrophages, and microglial cells appear to be the main cell types harboring virus in the CNS. Histologically, the major changes are seen in the subcortical areas of the brain and thus fall in the general category of subcortical dementia. In this regard, HIV encephalopathy is similar to the dementia seen in patients with Parkinson's disease (see Chap. 368) and Huntington's chorea (see Chap. 367) and distinct from that seen in patients with Alzheimer's disease (see Chap. 367). Among the histopathologic changes are pallor and gliosis, multinucleated giant cell encephalitis, and vacuolar myelopathy. Less commonly, diffuse or focal spongiform changes in the white matter occur.

There are no specific criteria for a diagnosis of HIV encephalopathy, and this syndrome thus must be distinguished from a number of other diseases that affect the CNS of HIV-infected patients (Table 308-17). The diagnosis of dementia depends on demonstrating a de-

Table 308-16

Clinical Staging of HIV Encephalopathy (AIDS Dementia Complex)

Stage	Definition
Stage 0 (normal)	Normal mental and motor function
Stage 0.5 (equivocal/ subclinical)	Absent, minimal, or equivocal symptoms without impairment of work or capacity to perform activities of daily living. Mild signs (snout response, slowed ocular or extremity movements) may be present. Gait and strength are normal.
Stage 1 (mild)	Able to perform all but the more demanding aspects of work or activities of daily living but with unequivocal evidence (signs or symptoms that may include performance on neuropsychological testing) of functional, intellectual, or motor impairment. Can walk without assistance.
Stage 2 (moderate)	Able to perform basic activities of self-care but cannot work or maintain the more demanding aspects of daily life. Ambulatory, but may require a single prop.
Stage 3 (severe)	Major intellectual incapacity (cannot follow news or personal events, cannot sustain complex conversation, considerable slowing of all output) or motor disability (cannot walk unassisted, usually with slowing and clumsiness of arms as well).
Stage 4 (end-stage)	Nearly vegetative. Intellectual and social comprehension and output are at a rudimentary level. Nearly or absolutely mute. Paraparetic or paraplegic with urinary and fecal incontinence.

SOURCE: Adapted from JJ Sidtis, RW Price, Neurology 40:197, 1990.

Table 308-17

Characterization of the Most Common Central Nervous System Diseases in Patients with HIV Infection

Disease	Approximate Incidence, %	Clinical Features	Characteristic CSF Findings	Characteristic Radiologic Findings
HIV encephalopathy (AIDS dementia complex)	25	Personality changes, dementia, unsteady gait, seizures	Nonspecific increases in cells and protein	Cortical atrophy, ventricular dilation, bright spots on T2-weighted MRI
Toxoplasmosis	15	Fever, headache, focal neurologic deficits, seizures, + antibodies in 95%	Nonspecific	Single or multiple ring-enhancing lesions in multiple locations
Cryptococcal meningitis	6–12	Fever, nausea, vomiting, confusion, headache	Elevated protein, low glucose, positive cryptococcal antigen or culture	Nonspecific
Progressive multifocal leukoencephalopathy	4	Multiple focal deficits without changes in level of consciousness	Nonspecific	Multiple white matter lesions on T2-weighted MRI images
Neurosyphilis	1	Meningitis, neuroretinitis, deafness, focal neurologic deficits	Positive VDRL, elevated protein, increase in cells	Nonspecific
Lymphoma	1	Seizure, focal neurologic deficits, headache	Nonspecific in primary CNS lymphoma; malignant cells in systemic lymphoma	Single or few ring-enhancing lesions
Tuberculous meningitis	1	Fever, headache, confusion, meningitis, cough	Elevated protein, low glucose, pleocytosis, positive smear/culture for acid-fast bacilli (AFB)	Mass lesions in approximately 50%, abnormal chest x-ray

cline in cognitive function. This can be accomplished objectively with the use of the Mini-Mental Status Examination (Table 308-18) in patients for whom prior scores are available. For this reason, it is advisable for all patients with a diagnosis of HIV infection to have a baseline Mini-Mental Status Examination. Imaging studies of the CNS, by either computed tomography (CT) or magnetic resonance imaging (MRI), often demonstrate evidence of cerebral atrophy (Fig. 308-24). MRI may also reveal small areas of increased density on T2-weighted images.

Table 308-18

The Folstein Mini-Mental Status Examination

Question	Scoring	Maximum Score
1. Where are you (state, county, city, hospital, clinic)?	1 point for each	5
2. What are the (day, date, month, season, year, time)?	1 point for each	5
3. "Say these three words after me: (yellow, apple, Ohio)."	1 point for each	3
4. Ask patient to begin with 100 and count backwards by 7's. Or, if patient refuses, ask to spell "world" backwards.	Stop after 5, score no. correct Or 1 point for each correct letter	5
5. Recall the three words given in question no. 3.	1 point for each	3
6. Ask the patient to name "watch" then "pencil".	1 point for each	2
7. Ask the patient to repeat "No ifs, ands, or buts."	1 point if correct	1
8. Three-stage command: Take this paper in your right hand, fold it in half, and put it on the door.	1 point for each correct	3
9. Ask the patient to read silently and obey the command (print in block letters): CLOSE YOUR EYES.	1 point if correct	1
10. Ask the patient to write a sentence.	1 point if contains a subject and verb and makes sense (ignore spelling and grammar)	1
11. Draw a clock with numbers and hands showing the time to be 8:20	2 points if correct	2
12. Have the patient copy this design: 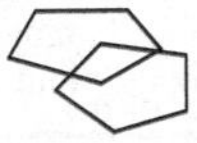	1 point if all sides and angles are preserved and if intersecting sides form a quadrangle	1

While a lumbar puncture is an important element of the evaluation of patients with HIV infection and neurologic abnormalities, it is generally most helpful in the diagnosis of opportunistic infections. In HIV encephalopathy, patients may have an increase in CSF cells and protein level; however, these findings are nonspecific, and the diagnosis is truly one that can be made only after opportunistic pathogens and neoplasms have been ruled out. While HIV can often be isolated from the CSF of these patients, this finding is not specific for HIV encephalopathy and, in fact, there appears to be no correlation between the presence of HIV in the CSF and the presence of HIV encephalopathy. Elevated levels of β_2-microglobulin, neopterin, and quinolinic acid (a metabolite of tryptophan reported to cause CNS injury) have been noted in the CSF of patients with AIDS dementia complex. These findings suggest that these factors as well as inflammatory cytokines may be involved in the pathogenesis of this syndrome; however, at this time definitive evidence is still lacking.

While there is no specific treatment for HIV encephalopathy, multiple reports suggest that treatment with antiretroviral agents may be of benefit. Improvement in neuropsychiatric test scores have been noted for both adult and pediatric patients treated with either zidovudine or didanosine. In fact, the rapid symptomatic improvement in cognitive function noted with the initiation of antiretroviral therapy suggests that at least some component of this problem is quickly reversible, again supporting at least a partial role of soluble mediators in the pathogenesis. It should also be noted that these patients have an increased sensitivity to the side effects of neuroleptic drugs. The use of these drugs for symptomatic treatment is associated with an increased risk of extrapyramidal

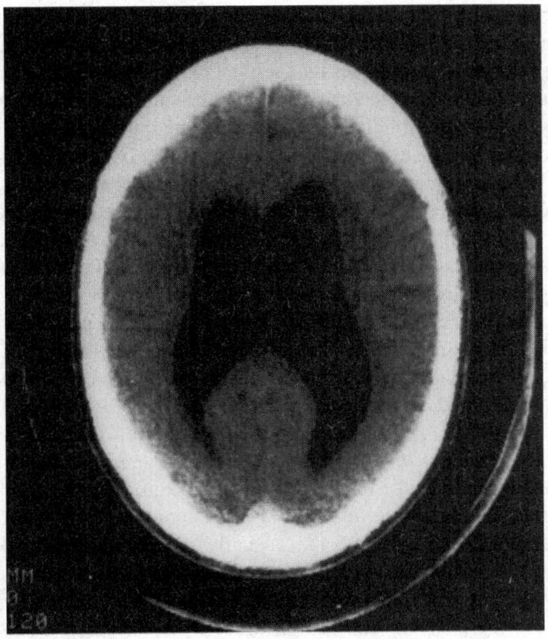

FIGURE 308-24 Computed tomogram of the central nervous system of a patient with AIDS dementia complex. CT demonstrates cortical thinning and dilation of the ventricles.

side effects, so patients with HIV encephalopathy who receive these agents must be monitored carefully.

Seizures Seizures are a relatively frequent complication of HIV infection and may be a consequence of opportunistic infections, neoplasms, or HIV encephalopathy (Table 308-19). The seizure threshold is often lower than normal in these patients owing to the frequent presence of electrolyte abnormalities. Seizures are seen in 15 to 40 percent of patients with cerebral toxoplasmosis, 15 to 35 percent of patients with primary CNS lymphoma, 8 percent of patients with cryptococcal meningitis, and 7 to 50 percent of patients with HIV encephalopathy. Seizures may also be seen in patients with CNS tuberculosis, aseptic meningitis, and progressive multifocal leukoencephalopathy. Seizures may be the presenting clinical symptom of HIV disease. In one study of 100 patients with HIV infection presenting with a first seizure, cerebral mass lesions were the most common cause, responsible for 32 of the 100 new-onset seizures. Of these 32 cases, 28 were due to toxoplasmosis and 4 to lymphoma. HIV encephalopathy accounted for an additional 24 new-onset seizures. Cryptococcal meningitis was the third most common diagnosis, responsible for 13 of the 100 seizures. In 23 cases, no cause could be found; it is possible that these cases represent a subcategory of HIV encephalopathy. Of these 23 cases, 16 (70 percent) had two or more seizures, suggesting that anticonvulsant therapy is indicated in all patients with HIV infection and seizures unless a rapidly correctable cause is found. While phenytoin remains the initial treatment of choice, hypersensitivity reactions to this drug have been reported in over 10 percent of patients with AIDS, and therefore the use of phenobarbital or valproic acid must be considered as alternatives.

Table 308-19

Causes of Seizures in Patients with HIV Infection

Disease	Overall Contribution to First Seizure, %	Fraction of Patients Who Have Seizures, %
AIDS dementia complex	24–47	7–50
Cerebral toxoplasmosis	28	15–40
Cryptococcal meningitis	13	8
Primary central nervous system lymphoma	4	15–30
Progressive multifocal leukoencephalopathy	1	

SOURCE: From Holtzman et al.

Spinal Cord Disease Spinal cord disease, or myelopathy, is present in approximately 20 percent of patients with AIDS, often as part of HIV encephalopathy. In fact, 90 percent of the patients with HIV-associated myelopathy have some evidence of dementia, suggesting that similar pathologic processes may be responsible for both conditions. Three main types of spinal cord disease are seen in patients with AIDS. The first of these is a vacuolar myelopathy, as discussed above under HIV encephalopathy. This condition is pathologically similar to subacute combined degeneration of the cord such as occurs with pernicious anemia. Although vitamin B_{12} deficiency is common in patients with AIDS, it does not appear to be responsible for the cord disease seen in these patients, given that there is no response to treatment with parenteral vitamin B_{12}. Vacuolar myelopathy is characterized by a subacute onset and often presents with gait disturbances, predominantly ataxia and spasticity; it may progress to include bladder and bowel dysfunction. Physical findings include evidence of increased deep tendon reflexes and extensor plantar responses. The second form of spinal cord disease involves the dorsal columns and presents as a pure sensory ataxia. The third form is also sensory in nature and presents with paresthesias and dysesthesias of the lower extremities. In contrast to the cognitive problems seen in patients with HIV encephalopathy, these spinal cord syndromes do not generally respond to therapy with antiretroviral drugs, and therapy is mainly supportive. One exception is a polyradiculopathy associated with cytomegalovirus (CMV). This entity is generally seen late in the course of HIV infection and is fulminant in onset, with lower extremity and sacral paresthesias, difficulty in walking, areflexia, ascending sensory loss, and urinary retention. CSF examination reveals a predominantly neutrophilic pleocytosis. Therapy with ganciclovir or foscarnet can lead to rapid improvement. Other diseases involving the spinal cord in patients with HIV infection include HTLV-I-associated myelopathy (HAM) (see Chap. 192), neurosyphilis (see Chap. 174), herpesvirus infections (varicella-zoster, simplex, and CMV) (see Chaps. 184 and 185), tuberculosis (see Chap. 171), and lymphoma (see Chap. 113).

Peripheral Neuropathies Peripheral neuropathies are common in patients with HIV infection; they occur at all stages of illness and take a variety of forms. Early in the course of HIV infection, an acute inflammatory demyelinating polyneuropathy resembling Guillain-Barré syndrome may occur (see Chap. 376). Patients commonly present with progressive weakness, areflexia, and minimal sensory changes. CSF examination reveals a pleocytosis, and peripheral nerve biopsy demonstrates a perivascular infiltrate suggesting an autoimmune etiology. Although generally a self-limited disease, in severe cases plasma exchange, intravenous immunoglobulin, or systemic glucocorticoids have been tried with variable degrees of success. Because of the immunosuppressive effects of glucocorticoids, they should be reserved for severe cases refractory to other measures. Another autoimmune peripheral neuropathy seen in patients with AIDS is mononeuritis multiplex (see Chap. 319). This necrotizing arteritis of peripheral nerves generally occurs in patients with a moderate degree of immunodeficiency and may be managed as outlined above. The most common peripheral neuropathy in patients with HIV infection is a distal sensory polyneuropathy, generally seen in patients with advanced HIV infection. Although it is present clinically in 30 to 40 percent of patients, two-thirds of patients with AIDS may be shown by electrophysiologic studies to have some evidence of peripheral nerve disease. This polyneuropathy, which is felt to be due to HIV-mediated axonal degeneration, most often presents as symmetric bilateral painful burning sensations in the feet and lower extremities. Antiretroviral agents have been of little benefit in the management of this problem and in fact may be the causative agent in some instances. Dideoxynucleoside-associated peripheral neuropathy may be a painful complication of didanosine, zalcitabine, or stavudine therapy, is most commonly seen at higher doses, and usually resolves following discontinuation of therapy. It is discussed in more detail below in relation to antiretroviral agents. Other entities in the differential diagnosis include diabetes mellitus, vitamin B_{12} deficiency, and side effects from flagyl or dapsone. For distal sensory polyneuropathy of unknown cause that fails to resolve following the discontinuation of dideoxynucleosides, therapy is symptomatic, involving the use of tricyclics and analgesics. Nerve growth factor is being investigated as a possible agent in this setting.

Myopathy Myopathy may also complicate the course of HIV infection. Among the causes of myopathy in the setting of HIV infection are HIV itself, zidovudine, and the generalized wasting syndrome. HIV-associated myopathy may range in severity from an asymptomatic elevation in creatine kinase to a subacute syndrome characterized by proximal muscle weakness and myalgias. Quite pronounced elevations in creatine kinase may occur in asymptomatic patients, particularly after exercise. The clinical significance of this finding is unclear. A variety of both inflammatory and noninflammatory pathologic processes have been noted in patients with more severe myopathy, including myofiber necrosis with inflammatory cells, nemaline rod bodies, cytoplasmic bodies, and mitochondrial abnormalities. Profound muscle wasting may be seen after prolonged zidovudine therapy. This toxic side effect of the drug appears to be related to its ability to interfere with the function of mitochondrial polymerases and is reversible following discontinuation of treatment. Histologically, red ragged fibers are a characteristic feature.

OPPORTUNISTIC INFECTIONS

Opportunistic infections are late complications of HIV infection, for the most part occurring in patients with less than 200 CD4+ T cells per microliter. While the causative agents characteristically are opportunistic organisms, such as *Pneumocystis carinii, Mycobacterium avium* complex, CMV, and other organisms that do not ordinarily cause disease in the absence of a compromised immune system, they also include common bacterial and mycobacterial pathogens. Opportunistic infections are the leading cause of morbidity and mortality in patients with HIV infection. Approximately 80 percent of AIDS patients die as a direct result of an infection other than HIV, with bacterial infections heading the list. The clinical spectrum of diseases caused by opportunistic infections is constantly changing as patients live longer and as new and better approaches to treatment and prophylaxis are developed.

PROTOZOAL INFECTIONS Pneumocystis carinii Infection (See Chap. 211) *P. carinii* is one of the most common causes of infection in patients with HIV infection; however, with the development of effective prophylactic regimens, the incidence of *P. carinii* infection and its relative contribution to morbidity and mortality have been decreasing. *P. carinii pneumonia* (PCP) is the initial AIDS-defining illness in close to 20 percent of patients, and approximately 50 percent of patients with HIV infection experience at least one bout of PCP during the course of their disease. As a result of increased awareness, improved diagnosis, and better treatment, the probability of death from a single episode of PCP has decreased from as high as 50 percent to 2 percent. Because of the AIDS epidemic, PCP has become a growing cause of community-acquired pneumonia. While the mode of transmission is unclear, infections with PCP probably represent reactivation of latent infection or failure of host defense mechanisms to suppress a ubiquitous microorganism. In the hospital setting, person-to-person spread of infection has been suggested anecdotally, and some feel it is prudent not to place a patient at risk for PCP (for example, an HIV-infected patient with fewer than 200 CD4+ T cells/μL) in the same room with someone suffering from an acute episode of PCP. Data are insufficient to make this a recommendation as standard practice. The risk of infection with *P. carinii* increases as the CD4+ T cell count declines. Among HIV-infected patients, PCP is most commonly seen among those who have experienced a previous bout of PCP and those who have fewer than 200 CD4+ T cells per microliter. In the absence of PCP prophylaxis, following a primary bout of PCP, 31 percent of HIV-infected individuals experience a second bout within 6 months, and 66 percent within 12 months. For patients with more than 200 CD4+ T cells per microliter, the attack rate for PCP is approximately 0.5 percent over a 6-month period. In contrast, for patients with less than 200 CD4+ T cells per microliter, the attack rate is 8 percent over 6 months and 18 percent over 12 months. For this reason, it is recommended that all patients with HIV infection who have either experienced a previous bout of PCP or have a CD4+ T cell count of <200/μL (or a CD4 percentage of less than 15), receive some form of PCP prophylaxis (discussed below). Owing to the implementation of these guidelines, the incidence of primary PCP for patients with HIV infection and CD4+ T cell counts of <300/μL has dropped to 8.9 cases per 100 person-years, and the incidence of secondary PCP has dropped to 5.1 cases per 100 person-years. Primary PCP is now occurring at a median CD4+ T cell count of 36/μL, while secondary PCP is occurring at a median CD4+ T cell count of 10/μL.

As suggested by its name, the most common manifestation of infection with *P. carinii* is pneumonia. Patients generally present with fever and a cough that is usually nonproductive or productive of only scant amounts of white sputum. They may complain of a characteristic retrosternal chest pain, which is usually worse on inspiration and described as either sharp or burning. In more severe cases, patients usually note dyspnea on exertion, fatigue, and weight loss. In stark contrast to PCP in the non-HIV setting, which is often a fulminant disease with patients usually presenting within 5 days of the onset of symptoms, HIV-associated PCP may have an indolent course characterized by weeks of vague symptoms prior to presentation or diagnosis. PCP should be included in the differential diagnosis of fever, pulmonary symptoms, or unexplained weight loss in any patient with HIV infection and fewer than 200 CD4+ T cells per microliter. Findings on physical examination are minimal, and the usual findings for pneumonia may not be present. Breath sounds are usually clear but may be slightly diminished. While occasional rhonchi or wheezes may be heard, especially in patients with some other underlying pulmonary disease, findings of consolidation are usually absent. While chest x-ray may reveal a variety of patterns, the most common finding is either a normal film, if the disease is suspected early, or a faint bilateral interstitial infiltrate. The classic finding of a dense, perihilar infiltrate described in patients with non-HIV-associated PCP is rarely seen in patients with AIDS. In patients with PCP who have been receiving aerosolized pentamidine for prophylaxis, one may see a chest x-ray pattern with upper lobe cavitary disease, reminiscent of tuberculosis. Other less common findings on chest film include lobar infiltrates and pleural effusions.

PCP is complicated by pneumothorax in approximately 2 percent of cases. Pneumothorax is more common in patients with prior episodes of PCP and in patients who have received aerosolized pentamidine for prophylaxis, presumably owing to the tendency of these patients to have apical cavitary disease. The mortality for patients with PCP-associated pneumothorax is approximately 10 percent, and aggressive medical (sclerotherapy) and/or surgical intervention may be required.

The laboratory evaluation is usually of little help in the differential diagnosis of PCP. A mild leukocytosis is common; however, given the fact that HIV-infected patients generally have leukopenia with baseline WBC values in the range of 1500 to 3000 cells/μL, a WBC on the order of 4000 to 6000/μL may represent an elevation. The serum lactate dehydrogenase (LDH) level is often elevated, and arterial blood gases may indicate hypoxemia, with a decline in Pa_{O_2} and an increase in the arterial-alveolar (a-A) gradient. Arterial blood gas measurements not only aid in making the diagnosis of PCP but also provide important information for staging the severity of the disease and directing treatment (see below and Chap. 211).

A definitive diagnosis of PCP requires demonstration of the trophozoite or cyst form of the organisms in samples obtained from induced sputum, bronchoalveolar lavage, transbronchial biopsy, or open lung biopsy (see Chap. 211). The diagnosis may be somewhat more difficult to make in patients who have been receiving aerosolized pentamidine for PCP prophylaxis, as the burden of organisms may be reduced. In this setting, the diagnostic yield from induced sputum decreases from 92 percent to 64 percent, while the yield from bronchoalveolar lavage

Table 308-20

Extrapulmonary Manifestations of *Pneumocystis carinii* Infection in Patients with HIV Infection

Acute otitis
Retinitis
Visceral cystic calcifications
Necrotizing vasculitis
Intestinal obstruction
Lymphadenopathy
Bone marrow involvement
Ascites
Thyroiditis

drops from 95 percent to 80 percent. More recently, PCR has been used in an attempt to identify specific DNA sequences for *P. carinii* in clinical specimens. This technique may provide somewhat better sensitivity than that obtained through histologic staining. The differential diagnosis of PCP in patients with HIV infection includes CMV pneumonia, fungal pneumonia, nonspecific interstitial pneumonitis, tuberculosis, and Kaposi's sarcoma (see below).

In addition to pneumonia, a number of other clinical problems have been reported in the HIV-infected patients as a result of infection with *P. carinii*. Many of these reports involve patients receiving aerosolized pentamidine as prophylaxis for PCP. This form of prophylaxis, while quite effective in preventing PCP, is ineffective in preventing disease outside the lung and has largely been replaced by oral systemic prophylaxis. *P. carinii* appears to be capable of hematogenous spread and of seeding a variety of organ systems as well as causing a primary infection of the ear (Table 308-20). "Extrapulmonary" manifestations of *P. carinii* infection occur in approximately 2.5 to 5.0 percent of patients with HIV infection.

Otic involvement with *P. carinii* is most commonly seen as a primary infection, i.e., in patients with no evidence of pulmonary disease. It usually presents as a unilateral polypoid mass that involves the external auditory canal. It may also involve the middle ear and may extend to the mastoid, resulting in radiographic abnormalities on plain films of the skull. Patients often complain of ear pain and decreased hearing. Perforation of the tympanic membrane has been reported in over half of the cases. In contrast, most of the other extrapulmonary forms of pneumocystosis are seen in patients with a history of PCP. Most common in this group are ophthalmic lesions of the choroid, which are usually noted on routine examination or in the context of evaluation for CMV retinitis. Multiple, bilateral lesions 0.5 to 2 disc diameters in size that appear as slightly elevated yellow-white plaques are generally seen. They are usually asymptomatic and are often confused with the cotton-wool spots of the retina associated with HIV infection. *P. carinii* has also been reported to cause a necrotizing vasculitis that resembles Buerger's disease, bone marrow hypoplasia, and intestinal obstruction. Other organs that have been involved include lymph nodes, spleen, liver, kidney, pancreas, pericardium, heart, thyroid, and adrenals. The presence of infection in either liver, kidney, or spleen may be asymptomatic and may be associated with cystic lesions that appear calcified on CT or ultrasound.

℞ TREATMENT

A variety of therapeutic options are available for the patient with PCP or disseminated pneumocystis (Table 308-21) (see Chap. 211). The gold standard for therapy at present is trimethoprim/sulfamethoxazole, which is available in both intravenous and oral forms and is effective in approximately 90 percent of patients. The major disadvantage of this therapy is the relatively high incidence of side effects. In contrast to the non-HIV population, in which there is a 10 percent incidence of side effects, the HIV-infected population has a 50 to 65 percent incidence of side effects, including rash, fever, leukopenia, thrombocytopenia, and hepatitis. Although therapy need not be discontinued when these occur, it is important to remain vigilant for more serious hypersensitivity reactions, such as Stevens-Johnson syndrome. In addition, it may be advisable to withhold other myelotoxic drugs, such as zidovudine and ganciclovir, during therapy with trimethoprim/sulfamethoxazole. In patients with mild disease, side effects may be minimized by slightly reducing dosage. Ideally, treatment with trimethoprim/sulfamethoxazole or the other agents mentioned below should be continued for 21 days. In contrast to many other infections, in which one expects to see stabilization, if not improvement, within 24 to 48 h of the initiation of appropriate antimicrobial therapy, AIDS patients with PCP often do not begin to improve until the end of the first week. In fact, during the first 5 days of treatment, particularly in moderate to severe cases, the patient's condition often worsens, presumably owing to the inflammatory response resulting from the death of large numbers of organisms in the lung. This inflammatory response and its adverse clinical consequences can be markedly reduced by the adjunct use of glucocorticoids. Glucocorticoids are indicated for use in the treatment of any patient with HIV infection and PCP in whom the Pa_{O_2} is under 70 mmHg or in whom the a-A gradient is over 35 mmHg. In this setting, several clinical trials have shown clear benefit from glucocorticoids, with approximately a 50 percent decrease in mortality (from 40 to 20 percent) and a 50 percent decrease in the number of patients requiring mechanical ventilatory support. The only significant side effect has been an increased incidence of thrush. Adjunct glucocorticoid therapy should be started as soon as possible after the diagnosis is made, preferably no later than 36 to 72 h. In fact, glucocorticoids added later in the course of disease have not been shown to confer any clinical benefit and have been associated with an increased risk of other opportunistic infections. The recommended length of glucocorticoid therapy is 21 days (Table 308-21), although some prefer to stop the drug 48 to 72 h prior to stopping antimicrobial therapy, to make it possible to assess the baseline status when the patient is still receiving antimicrobials but no longer receiving glucocorticoids.

Several options are available in patients unable to tolerate trimethoprim/sulfamethoxazole. Pentamidine isethionate is also licensed for treatment of PCP; this drug must be administered parenterally. The development of sterile abscesses following intramuscular administration makes intravenous administration the route of choice. In addition, it has been proposed that, for mild cases, the drug may be administered as an aerosol. Although some therapeutic successes have been noted with this route of administration, it is ineffective for extrapulmonary disease, and aerosolized pentamidine should be reserved for prophylaxis of PCP in the rare patient unable to tolerate systemic prophylaxis (see below). When given by the intravenous route, pentamidine must be administered slowly to prevent cardiovascular effects. Although comparable in efficacy to trimethoprim/sulfamethoxazole therapy, pentamidine therapy is associated with a greater number of serious side effects, including nephrotoxicity (which often necessitates reducing the dose by 20 to 50 percent), pancreatitis (necessitating discontinuation), thrombocytopenia, and dysregulation of glucose metabolism resulting in either hyper- or hypoglycemia. The latter side effect is seen in 14 percent of patients receiving pentamidine and is probably secondary to pancreatic injury during therapy. Fatal hypoglycemia as well as the development of insulin-requiring diabetes mellitus have occurred. These disorders of glucose metabolism are more common in patients who develop renal damage during therapy, generally occur late in the course of therapy, and are more common in patients receiving total doses above 4 g and in patients who have received pentamidine in the past. Pentamidine-associated hypoglycemia has been reported as late as 2 weeks following the discontinuation of drug; thus, patients must be alerted to watch for this side effect.

Among the alternatives to trimethoprim/sulfamethoxazole and intravenous pentamidine are trimethoprim/dapsone (oral only), clindamycin/primaquine (oral and parenteral), atovaquone (oral only), trimetrexate/leucovorin (oral and parenteral), and eflornithine (DFMO, oral and parenteral). The combination of trimethoprim and

Table 308-21

Manifestations and Treatment of Secondary Infections in Patients with HIV Disease

Infecting Agent	Manifestations	Treatment	Prophylaxis	Drug Toxicities	Comment
Pneumocystis carinii			TMP/SMX 1 DS tablet daily, or 3×/wk, or	Rash, fever, neutropenia	Begin once CD4+ T cell count <200/μL or CD4% <15
			Aerosolized pentamidine 300 mg/month, or	Bronchospasm	
			Dapsone 50 mg/d PO + Pyrimethamine 50 mg/wk PO + Folinic acid 25 mg/wk PO	Methemoglobinemia, neutropenia	Contraindicated in patients with G6PD deficiency
	Mild to moderate pneumonia [$Pa_{O_2} \geq$ 70 mmHg and (A-a)$dO_2 \leq$ 35 mmHg]	TMP/SMX 15–20 mg/kg/d PO		Rash, fever, neutropenia	Treat for 21 d if possible; no less than 14 d
		TMP 20 mg/kg/d PO qd + Dapsone 100 mg PO qd		Methemoglobinemia, *C. difficile* colitis	Contraindicated in patients with G6PD deficiency
		Clindamycin 600 mg PO q6h + Primaquine 15 mg PO qd		Rash, neutropenia, nephritis, pancreatitis, hypoglycemia, diabetes	Contraindicated in patients with G6PD deficiency
		IV Pentamidine 3–4 mg/kg/d			
		Atovaquone, 750 mg, PO, tid for 21 d			
		Aerosolized pentamidine 300 mg/d		Bronchospasm	Provides no systemic effects. Not recommended but an option for multidrug-allergic patient with mild pneumonia
	Severe pneumonia [Pa_{O_2} < 70 mmHg or (A-a)dO_2 > 35 mmHg]	TMP/SMX 15–20 mg/kg/d IV initially (total course 14–21 d)		Rash, fever, leukopenia, thrombocytopenia, hepatitis, nephritis, pancreatitis, hypoglycemia, diabetes, *C. difficile* colitis	Prednisone, 40 mg bid for 2 d, then 40 mg/d for 5 d, then 20 mg/d to the end of therapy (21 d total) added to specific antimicrobial ASAP and no later than 36 h after diagnosis
		Pentamidine 3–4 mg/kg/d IV for 14–21 d			
		Clindamycin 900 mg IV q8h then 450 mg PO q6h +			
		Primaquine 30 mg PO qd for total of 14–21 d		Rash, neutropenia	Contraindicated in patients with G6PD deficiency
		Trimetrexate 45 mg/m² IV (over 60–90 min) qd × 21 d + Leucovorin, 20 mg/m² IV q6h × 24 d		Rash, neutropenia	For patients intolerant of other regimens. Less effective than standard therapy. Bone marrow–suppressive effects blunted by use of leucovorin
		Eflornithine (DFMO) 100 mg/kg IV q6h for 14 d followed by 75 mg/kg PO q6h for 4–6 wk		Thrombocytopenia	Call 1-800-TRIALSA for information
	Disseminated disease	Any of the systemic therapies outlined above			
Toxoplasma gondii			TMP/SMX 1 DS tablet qd	Rash, fever, neutropenia	Alternative is dapsone, 50 mg, PO qd + pyrimethamine, 50 mg, PO weekly + folinic acid, 25 mg, PO weekly
	Encephalitis, brain abscess, chorioretinitis, myocarditis	Sulfadiazine 1–2 g PO q6h + Pyrimethamine 25–100 mg qd + Folinic acid 10–20 mg PO qd		Crystalluria, rash	Treatment is generally for life. Leucovorin to minimize bone marrow suppression
		Clindamycin initially 200–400 mg IV q6h +		Rash, fever, neutropenia *C. difficile* colitis	

(*continued*)

Table 308-21—*(continued)*

Manifestations and Treatment of Secondary Infections in Patients with HIV Disease

Infecting Agent	Manifestations	Treatment	Prophylaxis	Drug Toxicities	Comment
Toxoplasma gondii—(continued)		Pyrimethamine 25–100 mg qd + Folinic acid 10–20 mg qd followed by Clindamycin 300–900 mg PO q8h + Pyrimethamine 25–100 mg qd		Rash, fever, neutropenia	Leucovorin to minimize bone marrow suppression
		Atovaquone 250 mg PO tid + Pyrimethamine 25–100 mg qd + Folinic acid 10–20 mg qd		Rash, fever, neutropenia	Leucovorin to minimize bone marrow suppression
		Macrolides (clarithromycin or azithromycin) + Pyrimethamine			Early results disappointing
Isospora belli	Diarrhea	TMP/SMX 1 DS tablet PO qid for 10 d then bid for 3 weeks		Rash, fever, neutropenia	TMP/SMX 1 DS tablet PO 3×/week for maintenance
Cryptosporidia Microsporidia	Diarrhea	No known specific therapy; supportive measures include parenteral nutrition			NTZ; bovine colostrum in trials
Mycobacterium avium complex			Clarithromycin 500 mg PO bid or Azithromycin 1200 mg weekly or Rifabutin 300 mg PO qd		Begin prophylaxis once CD4+ T cell count <100/μL or <50/μL. Treatment is generally for life. Macrolides + rifabutin may be more effective; however, more toxic and costly
	Disseminated disease that may involve lung, bone marrow, liver	Ethambutol 15 mg/kg qd + Rifabutin 600 mg/qd + Clarithromycin 100 mg PO bid		Hepatitis, neuropathy (peripheral/optic)	
Mycobacterium tuberculosis	Asymptomatic, PPD test positive	Isoniazid 15 mg/kg up to 900 mg PO twice a wk or 300 mg PO daily for 1 y + Pyridoxine 50 mg/d		Hepatitis	
	Active disease	Isoniazid, 300 mg PO qd × 1 y +		Hepatitis	Treat with 3 drugs for 2 mo. If isolate is sensitive to isoniazid and rifampin, then switch to those 2 drugs. Treat a minimum of 9 mo and at least 6 mo after third negative culture. Quinolones may also be considered as a fifth drug
		Rifampin 600 mg PO qd × 1 y +		Hepatitis	
		Pyrazinamide 30 mg/kg/d in 2 doses		Hepatitis	
	Active disease in a setting where there is a possibility of multidrug resistance	Add ethambutol 15–25 mg/kg/d and		Neuropathy (peripheral/optic)	
		Streptomycin or Amikacin		Nephrotoxicity, hearing loss	
Candida albicans	Thrush, vaginitis	Clotrimazole troches, Nystatin prn	Fluconazole 200 mg PO qd (optional)	Hepatotoxicity	Primary prophylaxis generally not indicated. Treatment is generally prn
		Fluconazole 200 mg PO qd for 7–14 d		Hepatotoxicity	
		Amphotericin B 0.25 mg/kg/d IV for 7–10 d		Nephrotoxicity, fever/chills	
Cryptococcus neoformans	Meningitis, brain abscess, pneumonia, disseminated disease	Amphotericin B 0.3 mg/kg/d IV +	Fluconazole 200 mg PO qd (optional)	Hepatotoxicity	Begin prophylaxis if CD4+ T cell count <50/μL (optional; depending on risk). Approximately 50% will need to have flucytosine held during therapy due to neutropenia. An alternative is amphotericin B alone at a dose of 0.8 mg/kg/d
		Flucytosine 150 mg/kg/d PO for 6 wk		Nephrotoxicity, fever/chills, bone marrow suppression	
		followed by Fluconazole 100–200 mg PO qd indefinitely		Hepatotoxicity	

(continued)

Table 308-21—*(continued)*

Manifestations and Treatment of Secondary Infections in Patients with HIV Disease

Infecting Agent	Manifestations	Treatment	Prophylaxis	Drug Toxicities	Comment
Histoplasma capsulatum	Disseminated disease, pneumonia	Amphotericin B 0.6–1 mg/kg/d to a total 1 g then Itraconazole 200 mg qd indefinitely		Nephrotoxicity, fever/chills	
Bartonella henselae, (quintana)	Nodular skin lesions, peliosis hepatitis, trench fever	Erythromycin 500 g PO or IV qd for 2 months			
Penicillium marneffei	Disseminated disease, umbilicated skin lesions	Amphotericin B, 0.6–1 mg/kg/d to a total of 1 g then Itraconazole 200 mg qd indefinitely		Nephrotoxicity, fever, chills, hepatitis	
Cytomegalovirus	Retinitis, esophagitis, colitis, and pneumonia		Ganciclovir 1.0 g PO tid with food (optional)	Neutropenia	Expensive, marginal efficacy. Neutropenia may be ameliorated by colony-stimulating factors
		Ganciclovir 5 mg/kg q12h for 14 d followed by 5 mg/kg qd IV indefinitely			Retinitis may also be treated with ocular implant Oral ganciclovir, 1 g PO tid with food may be used for maintenance
		Foscarnet 90 mg/kg q12h for 14 d followed by 90–120 mg/kg qd IV indefinitely		Interstitial nephritis, seizure, hypocalcemia	Should be preceded by saline infusion to minimize nephrotoxicity
Herpes simplex virus	Recurrent perioral, perirectal, or genital ulcers	Acyclovir 200–400 mg PO 5id as needed			Foscarnet 60 mg/kg q8h × 14 d for patients with acyclovir-resistant herpes simplex or zoster
	Esophagitis; acute retinal necrosis	Acyclovir 5 mg/kg IV q8h for 10–14 d			
Varicella-zoster virus	Cutaneous (local or disseminated); retinal necrosis	Acyclovir 800 mg PO 5id or 10 mg/kg IV q8h for 10–14 d or longer			Famciclovir 500 mg PO q8h × 7 d is an alternative
Treponema pallidum	Early syphilis	Benzathine penicillin G 2.4 million units IM weekly for 3 wk			Approximately 20% relapse, need re-treatment. Immunologic abnormalities may cause inaccurate serology
	Late or neurosyphilis	Aqueous penicillin G 12–24 million units IV daily for 10–14 d Procaine penicillin G 2.4 million units IM daily for 10–14 d + Probenicid 500 mg PO qid Ceftriaxone 1–2 g IM or IV qd 10–14 d			

ABBREVIATIONS: DS, double-strength; NTZ, nitazoxanide; TMP/SMX, trimethaprim/sulfamethoxazole.

dapsone has been shown to be similar in efficacy to trimethoprim/sulfamethoxazole and to be associated with fewer toxicities. Some clinicians choose this combination as first-line treatment in patients with mild disease. One side effect of dapsone therapy is the development of methemoglobinemia, and its use is contraindicated in patients with glucose-6-phosphate dehydrogenase (G6PD) deficiency. Dapsone as a single agent is not effective. Similarly, while neither clindamycin alone nor primaquine alone is effective for the treatment of pneumocystosis, when they are used in combination, response rates are as high as 86 percent. The main side effects are rash and methemoglobinemia. Atovaquone is a hydroxynapthoquinone that interferes with electron transport in mitochondria and, as such, interferes with pyrimidine synthesis in protozoa. In a series of clinical trials, this drug has been shown to have activity against *P. carinii.* The incidence of side effects is lower than for trimethroprim/sulfamethoxazole, but overall response rates also are somewhat lower, and relapses are more common, so this agent must be considered second-line therapy. Trimetrexate, an inhibitor of dihydrofolate reductase, is another agent shown to be effective in the treatment of patients with PCP. This drug, whose side effect of bone marrow suppression can be greatly minimized by the concomitant use of folinic acid (leucovorin), is associated with response rates of approximately 70 percent. While not appropriate as initial therapy, trimetrexate may be of use in patients unable to tolerate or failing other forms of treatment. Eflornithine is an irreversible inhibitor of decarboxylase and thus interferes with the synthesis of polyamines. Its main side effect is thrombocytopenia. As in the case of trimetrexate, this drug has been shown to have some efficacy as a salvage treatment; however, the overall response rates to this agent are lower than for trimethoprim/sulfamethoxazole, which suggests that it not be used for initial therapy.

Once infection with *P. carinii* is diagnosed or suspected, appropriate systemic therapy is initiated with one of the agents or combinations discussed above. For patients with moderate to severe disease, glucocorticoids are included as part of the treatment regimen, and specific antimicrobial therapy should be administered parenterally (see above). After 7 to 14 days of therapy, clear-cut clinical improvement should be seen. If it is not, a change in therapy must be considered, with the general practice being to switch treatment regimens rather than add new drugs. If the situation is worsening, one should consider a repeat bronchoscopy to confirm the diagnosis and to rule out the possibility of a second infection. For patients who develop respiratory failure, intubation and mechanical ventilation remain an option; given the current range of therapeutic options available for treatment, such patients have been successfully treated and extubated.

Prophylaxis *Pneumocystis* prophylaxis is one of the cornerstones in the management of the HIV-infected patient. Prophylaxis is indicated for any HIV-infected individual who has experienced a previous bout of PCP, any patient who has fewer than 200 CD4+ T cells per microliter or a CD4 percentage of 15 or lower, any patient with unexplained fever (>100°F) for ≥2 weeks, and any patient with a history of oropharyngeal candidiasis. As in treatment, the preferred medication for prophylaxis is trimethoprim/sulfamethoxazole, which is given as a single double-strength tablet from three times a week to twice a day. The most common regimen is a single double-strength tablet daily. In studies of the twice-a-day regimen, no cases of PCP occurred in the treatment group, whereas 16 cases occurred in the untreated control group. In addition, in this study, which had a minimum follow-up of 24 months, the median survival in the treatment group was 22.9 months, compared to 12.6 months for the control group. In trials comparing a once-a-day regimen of trimethoprim/sulfamethoxazole to aerosolized pentamidine at a dose of 300 mg every 4 weeks, 1-year and 18-month recurrence rates of 4.5 percent and 11.4 percent, respectively, were found for the trimethoprim/sulfamethoxazole group, compared to 18.5 percent and 27.6 percent, respectively, for the aerosolized pentamidine group. These data, coupled with the increased incidence of pneumothorax and disseminated pneumocystosis seen with aerosolized pentamidine, point to systemic therapy with trimethoprim/sulfamethoxazole as the preferred regimen of prophylaxis. Unfortunately, however, some patients are unable to tolerate trimethoprim/sulfamethoxazole, and there is a great need for alternative regimens. Many such regimens, most of them variations on the treatment themes outlined above, have been proposed. A study of dapsone was stopped when it was observed that there was a higher incidence of death due to bacterial infections in the dapsone group than in the trimethoprim/sulfamethoxazole group. This result may have been due to the broad-spectrum antibacterial activity of the combination regimen or to some adverse effect of dapsone on neutrophil function. The combination of dapsone, pyrimethamine, and leucovorin has been recommended by some as a systemic alternative for those unable to tolerate trimethoprim/sulfamethoxazole. This regimen also provides protection against toxoplasmosis but not against most bacterial infections. Aerosolized pentamidine, 300 mg every 4 weeks delivered by a Respirgard II or equivalent nebulizer, remains an option for patients unable to tolerate systemic therapy.

Toxoplasmosis (See Chap. 219) *Toxoplasma gondii*, the etiologic agent of toxoplasmosis, is the most common cause of secondary CNS infection in patients with AIDS, accounting for 38 percent of all such infections. It accounts for 50 to 60 percent of all mass lesions in the CNS of patients with HIV infection and is responsible for 28 percent of first seizures. Overall, toxoplasmosis is seen in approximately 15 percent of patients with AIDS and is most common in patients from the Caribbean and from France. Toxoplasmosis is generally a late complication of HIV infection and usually occurs in patients with less than 100 CD4+ T cells per microliter. It is the initial AIDS-defining condition in 2 percent of AIDS patients in the United States. It is thought to represent a reactivation syndrome and is 10 times more common in patients with antibodies to the organisms, an indicator of prior infection, than in patients who are seronegative. However, owing to the abnormalities of B cell function seen in patients with HIV infection, serologic testing cannot be used to rule out a diagnosis of toxoplasmosis, and approximately 5 percent of cases occur in HIV-infected patients who are seronegative for *T. gondii*. Approximately 30 percent of AIDS patients with antibodies to *T. gondii* go on to develop CNS infection at some time during the course of their disease. Patients diagnosed with HIV infection should be screened for IgG antibody to *Toxoplasma* as part of their initial workup. Those who are seronegative should be counseled about ways to avoid infection, including avoiding the consumption of undercooked meat and careful hand washing after contact with soil or changing the cat litter box.

Primary infection with *T. gondii* is usually asymptomatic and occurs early in life, although some experience a chorioretinitis such as is seen following congenital infection. While primary infection in an immunocompromised host may result in a disseminated lethal infection involving lung, myocardium, and brain, this syndrome is rarely seen in patients with HIV infection. The most common clinical presentation in patients with HIV infection is one of fever, headache, and focal neurologic deficits, with the latter occurring in approximately 90 percent of patients. Patients may present with seizure, hemiparesis, or aphasia as a manifestation of focal neurologic defects or with a picture more related to accompanying cerebral edema and consisting of confusion, dementia, lethargy, and progression to coma. The latter manifestations are obviously similar to problems encountered in patients with HIV encephalopathy. In this clinical setting, the diagnosis is suspected on the basis of radiologic findings. MRI or double-dose contrast CT are the preferred techniques; MRI is clearly the most sensitive. Findings generally include multiple lesions in multiple locations, although in some cases only a single lesion is seen. Pathologically, these lesions generally exhibit inflammation and central necrosis and, as a result, show ring enhancement on contrast CT or MRI (Fig. 308-25). There is usually evidence of surrounding edema. The definitive diagnostic procedure is a brain biopsy. However, given the morbidity frequently associated with this procedure, it is usually more appropriate in the patient in whom one suspects toxoplasmosis (multiple ring-enhancing lesions on CT, seropositivity) to initiate specific therapy (see below) and proceed to biopsy only if there is no therapeutic response by 2 to 4 weeks. In a seronegative patient, the likelihood that a mass lesion of the CNS is due to *Toxoplasma* is less than 10 percent. In this setting, one may choose to be more aggressive and perform a biopsy sooner.

In addition to the classic presentation as a CNS mass lesion, *T. gondii* has been reported to cause a variety of other clinical problems in HIV-infected patients, including a CNS presentation more characteristic of herpes simplex, with a negative CT scan, chorioretinitis, pneumonia, peritonitis with ascites, gastrointestinal tract involvement, cystitis, and orchitis.

Rx TREATMENT

The standard treatment is combination therapy with pyrimethamine and sulfadiazine (Table 308-21). This regimen has a response rate of approximately 90 percent; however, since the relapse rate is over 50 percent at 6 months, the requirement for therapy is generally lifelong. Leukopenia, the main side effect of this combination, may be ameliorated by the concomitant use of folinic acid (leucovorin). If the patient is receiving other myelosuppressive agents, such as

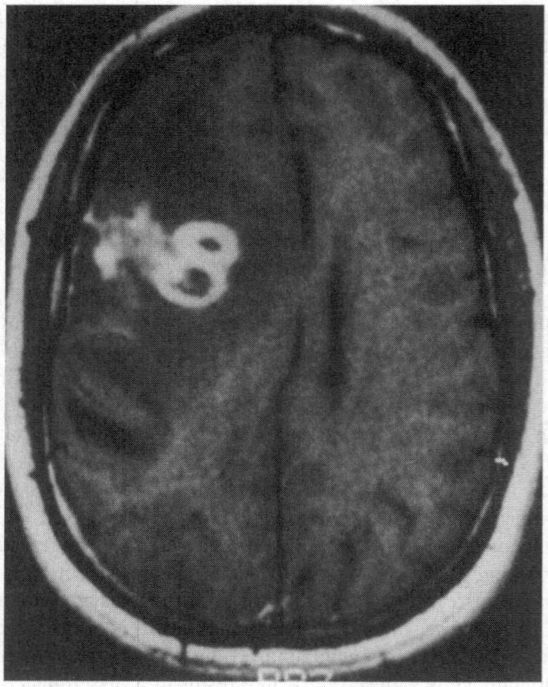

FIGURE 308-25 Contrast-enhanced MRI scan of the brain of a patient with CNS toxoplasmosis. Several ring-enhancing lesions can be seen in the temporoparietal area.

zidovudine or ganciclovir, the dosages of these medications may have to be modified. Other complications of therapy include fever, rash, thrombocytopenia, and renal failure due to sulfadiazine crystalluria. Crystalluria can be managed by administering fluids and alkalinizing the urine without discontinuing the medications. Overall, 45 to 70 percent of patients will develop side effects of treatment, and approximately 33 percent of patients will require a change in therapy. Treatment with clindamycin in combination with pyrimethamine is almost as good as treatment with sulfadiazine in combination with pyrimethamine and is an alternative for sulfa-allergic patients. Other treatment options include atovaquone plus pyrimethamine and azithromycin plus rifabutin plus pyrimethamine. Atovaquone has activity against a wide range of protozoa. Both as a single agent and in combination with pyrimethamine, it has been shown to be a viable alternative for treatment of toxoplasmosis in patients who have failed or developed adverse reactions to standard therapy. In patients for whom the sulfa component of treatment appears to cause side effects, the use of pyrimethamine alone as a maintenance regimen has been advocated. Although not as effective as the combination, it does appear to provide some protection from relapse. While animal model data suggest that the macrolide antibiotics clarithromycin and azithromycin might be of benefit for treatment of toxoplasmosis, clinical trial results thus far have been disappointing. Anecdotal reports suggest that the combination of a macrolide with rifabutin and pyrimethamine may have some activity. Glucocorticoids are recommended for the management of patients with cerebral edema.

Prophylaxis Given the frequency of toxoplasmosis in the HIV-infected population (overall incidence approximately 15 percent), there is a great need to develop effective prophylaxis. Unfortunately, aside from atovaquone, most of the agents and combinations of agents with therapeutic activity have severe enough side effects to make them dubious choices for primary prophylaxis. Fortunately, patients receiving trimethoprim/sulfamethoxazole or dapsone and pyrimethamine for prophylaxis of PCP have a decreased incidence of toxoplasmosis, which again underscores the potential importance of these particular regimens for antimicrobial prophylaxis.

Protozoal Diarrhea Cryptosporidia, microsporidia, and *Isospora belli* (see Chap. 220) are the most common opportunistic protozoa that infect the gastrointestinal tract and cause diarrhea in HIV-infected patients. *Cryptosporidium* is a well-known cause of diarrhea in animals and may cause a self-limited diarrheal infection in the immunocompetent host. It is spread through fecal-oral contact, and nosocomial outbreaks have been reported. In HIV-infected individuals, cryptosporidial infection may present in a variety of ways, ranging from a self-limited or intermittent diarrheal illness in patients in the early stages of HIV disease to a severe, life-threatening diarrhea in severely immunodeficient individuals. In patients with CD4+ T cell counts of $<300/\mu L$, the incidence of cryptosporidiosis is approximately 1 percent per year. Patients generally give a history of several months of intermittent diarrhea evolving to a several-month history of persistent diarrhea with copious watery stools, often up to several liters per day. In 75 percent of cases, diarrhea is accompanied by crampy abdominal pain; approximately 25 percent of patients have nausea and/or vomiting. This intestinal infection may be complicated by lactose intolerance and malabsorption. In addition to involving the intestinal tract, cryptosporidia may cause biliary tract disease in the HIV-infected population, which may present as cholecystitis with or without accompanying cholangitis. Radiographic studies of the biliary tree reveal thickening of the gallbladder wall with luminal abnormalities accompanying bile duct dilation and stricture. Cryptosporidia have also been noted in pulmonary specimens; however, the clinical significance of this finding is unclear. The diagnosis of cryptosporidial diarrhea is made by stool examination. The diarrhea is noninflammatory, and the characteristic finding is the presence of oocysts that stain with acid-fast dyes. Use of a sucrose flotation technique followed by procedures to concentrate the cysts and to separate them from other particles in the specimen may enhance detection. Organisms may be seen adhering to the brush border of intestinal epithelium on electron microscopy of small bowel biopsy specimens. Therapy is purely symptomatic at present. Patients can minimize their risk of developing cryptosporidiosis by avoiding contact with human and animal feces and by not drinking water from lakes or rivers.

Microsporidia are small, unicellular, obligate intracellular parasites that reside in the cytoplasm of enteric cells (see Chap. 220). The main species causing disease in humans is *Enterocytozoon bieneusi*. The clinical manifestations are similar to those described for *Cryptosporidium* and include abdominal pain and diarrhea. The small size of the organism may make it difficult to detect; however, with the use of chromotrope-based stains, organisms can be identified in stool samples by light microscopy. Definitive diagnosis generally depends on electron microscopic examination of a stool specimen, intestinal aspirate, or intestinal biopsy specimen. In contrast to cryptosporidia, microsporidia have been noted in a variety of extraintestinal locations, including the eye, muscle, and liver, and have been associated with conjunctivitis and hepatitis. As in the case of cryptosporidia, no effective therapy is known, and treatment is purely symptomatic.

Isospora belli is a coccidian parasite (see Chap. 220) most commonly found as a cause of diarrhea in patients from the Caribbean and Africa. Its cysts appear in the stool as large, acid-fast structures that can be differentiated from those of cryptosporidia on the basis of size, shape, and number of sporocysts. The clinical syndromes caused by these organisms appear to be identical to those caused by cryptosporidia; however, one important difference is that this infection can be treated with trimethoprim/sulfamethoxazole. While relapses are common, a three-times-a-week regimen, similar to that used to provide prophylaxis against PCP, appears adequate to prevent recurrence.

Entamoeba histolytica (see Chap. 215) and *Giardia lamblia* (see Chap. 220), although not strictly opportunistic pathogens in that they can also cause disease in immunocompetent individuals, are more common in patients with HIV infection. These treatable protozoal infections should be carefully looked for in any patient with HIV infection and persistent diarrhea. Other strains of Entamoeba and *Blastocystis hominis* are also seen with increased frequency in homosexual men with HIV infection; however, they are felt to be of little if any clinical significance.

Miscellaneous Protozoal Infections Miscellaneous protozoal infections are being reported with increased frequency as the AIDS epidemic spreads through the world. Visceral leishmaniasis (see Chap. 217) is recognized with increasing frequency in patients who live in or travel to endemic areas. The clinical presentation is one of hepatosplenomegaly, fever, and hematologic abnormalities. Lymphadenopathy and other constitutional symptoms may be present. Organisms can be isolated from cultures of bone marrow aspirates, while histologic stains are often negative and antibody titers are of little help in diagnosis. Patients usually respond well initially to standard therapy, although, as with most infections in HIV-infected individuals, eradication of the organisms is difficult and relapses are common. Among other protozoal infections that have been reported are severe and recurrent babesiosis (Chap. 179), Chagas' disease (Chap. 218) presenting as a CNS mass lesion, and meningoencephalitis due to *Acanthamoeba* or *Naegleria* (Chap. 215). No significant changes have been noted in the clinical manifestations of malaria in HIV-infected patients. Infections with *Cyclospora* species have been reported in HIV-infected individuals. Although infections in the general population have been linked to contaminated water, in 1996 outbreaks of infection with *Cyclospora cayetanensis* have been reported in association with the consumption of contaminated fruit, particularly strawberries and raspberries. Signs and symptoms include prolonged watery diarrhea, nausea, vomiting, crampy abdominal pain, and fever; these may be particularly severe and prolonged in HIV-infected individuals.

BACTERIAL INFECTIONS Bacterial infections are the leading cause of death in patients with HIV infection. While bacterial infections are often the terminal event in AIDS patients with multiple other problems, they also account for a substantial proportion of opportunistic infections earlier in the course of HIV disease. In the United States, disseminated mycobacterial infection, particularly due to the *Mycobacterium avium* complex (MAC), is the most common opportunistic bacterial infection. It is diagnosed antemortem in approximately 40 percent of HIV-infected patients and is seen at autopsy in 80 percent of patients. MAC accounts for 95 percent of the atypical mycobacterial infections seen in patients with AIDS in the United States; however, infections with at least 12 different mycobacteria, including *Mycobacterium bovis* and representatives of all four Runyon groups, have been reported. Infections with MAC, which consists of *M. avium* and *Mycobacterium intracellulare*, are seen mainly in patients in the United States and are rare in Africa. It has been suggested that prior infection with *M. tuberculosis* decreases the risk of MAC infection.

Infections with Atypical Mycobacteria MAC infection probably represents an acute infection with organisms that are ubiquitous in the environment in both soil and water. The presumed portals of entry are the gastrointestinal and respiratory tract. MAC infection is a late complication of HIV infection, occurring in patients with CD4+ T cell counts of $<100/\mu L$. Prior to the introduction of prophylactic regimens for MAC infections, the median CD4+ T cell count for patients with MAC was approximately $50/\mu L$. Now, with more widespread MAC prophylaxis, the CD4+ T cell count at the time of diagnosis is approximately $10/\mu L$. HIV-infected patients presenting with MAC infection have been reported to have a median survival of approximately 6 to 10 months. This fact likely reflects the late stage of their HIV infection. While a variety of clinical syndromes have been attributed to MAC infections, the most common presentation is fever, weight loss, and night sweats, presumably due to disseminated disease. At least 85 percent of HIV-infected patients with MAC infection are mycobacteremic, and enormous numbers of organisms can often be demonstrated on bone marrow biopsy. Liver involvement is common, and MAC infection should be suspected in any HIV-infected individual with a low CD4+ T cell count, unexplained fever, and an elevated alkaline phosphatase level. The chest x-ray is abnormal in approximately 25 percent of patients; the most common radiographic pattern is a bilateral lower lobe interstitial infiltrate, suggestive of miliary spread. In addition, alveolar or nodular infiltrates and hilar and/or mediastinal adenopathy occur. Endobronchial lesions have also been reported. Other clinical findings include lymphadenopathy, abdominal pain, and diarrhea. The diagnosis is suggested by the demonstration of long, slender acid-fast bacilli in biopsy specimens of bone marrow, lymph node, or liver or in stool specimens and is confirmed by culture of blood or involved tissue. The finding of two consecutive sputum samples positive for MAC is highly suggestive of pulmonary infection. Cultures generally turn positive within 2 weeks. In earlier studies, treatment with various combination regimens, which usually included ethambutol, clofazimine, and rifabutin, with or without an aminoglycoside, were shown to have little effect on mycobacteremia and to increase only marginally the median survival of patients with MAC infection (from 6 months to 8 months). The availability of the newer macrolide antibiotics (clarithromycin and azithromycin) changed this scenario considerably. Treatment with clarithromycin and ethambutol is thought by many to be the treatment of choice of MAC infection in patients with HIV infection. Some elect to add a third agent, either rifabutin, rifampin, clofazimine, ciprofloxacin, or amikacin, to the combination of ethambutol and a macrolide. At present, the data supporting the value of the third agent, particularly given the increased cost and complexity of such regimens, are weak. As with all of the potentially life-threatening infections seen in patients with AIDS, prophylactic regimens should be employed when available. In this regard, the use of rifabutin in patients with advanced HIV infection has been shown to delay the onset of bacteremia and death. Rifabutin has commonly been used as a prophylactic agent for patients with less than 75 to 100 CD4+ T cells per microliter. More recently, better results have been obtained with clarithromycin or azithromycin prophylaxis in patients with CD4+ T cell counts of less than $75/\mu L$, and many experts now recommend single-agent macrolide prophylaxis in preference to rifabutin.

A number of other atypical mycobacteria cause infections in patients with HIV infection. Infection with *Mycobacterium kansasii* generally presents as a pulmonary infection, with 20 to 30 percent of patients showing evidence of disseminated disease. Patients usually present with fever, cough, and night sweats. Chest x-ray reveals upper lobe cavitation in approximately half of these patients, while a lower lobe interstitial pattern consistent with hematogenous spread may be seen in other patients. Organisms are usually identified easily in pulmonary secretions; evidence of disease is found in over 75 percent of patients with a positive culture. It is particularly important to diagnose correctly *M. kansasii* infection, since it is relatively easy to treat with a combination regimen of isoniazid, rifampin, and ethambutol. *Mycobacterium fortuitum*, *Mycobacterium chelonae*, *Mycobacterium marinum*, *Mycobacterium scrofulaceum*, and *Mycobacterium haemophilum* all cause cutaneous lesions in patients with HIV infection; *M. haemophilum* also causes disseminated disease and septic arthritis. *Mycobacterium gordonae*, generally a nonpathogen in humans, and *Mycobacterium xenopi*, a colonizer of water storage tanks, may cause disseminated disease. Therapy of the latter organisms is extremely difficult.

Tuberculosis *M. tuberculosis*, once thought to be on its way to extinction in the United States, experienced a resurgence associated with the HIV epidemic (see Chap. 171). A 20-year decline in the number of new cases of tuberculosis in the United States ended in 1986, and the number of new cases per year increased for several years before reaching a new plateau. Approximately 5 percent of AIDS patients have active tuberculosis. While the prevalence and incidence of infection with *M. tuberculosis* in a given risk group, as determined by purified protein derivative (PPD) skin testing, appear not to be affected strongly by HIV status, HIV infection increases the risk of developing active tuberculosis by a factor of 15 to 30. For the patient with HIV infection and a positive PPD skin test, the rate of reactivation is 7 to 10 percent per year. Tuberculosis is a particularly important problem in patients with HIV infection. HIV disease progresses more rapidly in patients with tuberculosis; the level of plasma viremia increases during active tuberculosis; and successful treatment of tuberculosis causes plasma viremia to fall back to baseline levels. Although most cases of tuberculosis in the HIV-infected population are thought to represent reactivation, acute infection and reinfection are being seen increasingly often, especially in the context of outbreaks of multidrug resistant (MDR) tuberculosis. Active tuberculosis appears to be most common in patients 25 to 44 years of age, in African-Americans and Hispanics, in patients in New York City and Miami, and in patients in developing countries; in these demographic groups, 20 to 70 percent of the new cases of active tuberculosis are in patients with HIV infection. Given the fact that, in contrast to HIV infection, infection with *M. tuberculosis* can be spread via respiratory droplets and close, nonsexual contact, this epidemic of tuberculosis probably represents the greatest health risk to the general public and the health care profession associated with the HIV epidemic. In contrast to infection with MAC, active tuberculosis often develops relatively early in the course of HIV infection and may be among the earliest clinical signs of HIV infection. In one study, the median CD4+ T cell count at presentation of tuberculosis was 326/μL. The clinical manifestations of tuberculosis in HIV-infected patients are quite varied and generally show different patterns as a function of the CD4+ T cell count. In patients with relatively high CD4+ T cell counts, a typical pattern of pulmonary reactivation occurs in which patients present with fever, cough, dyspnea on exertion, weight loss, night sweats, and a chest x-ray revealing cavitary apical disease of the upper lobes. Disseminated disease is more common in patients with low CD4+ T cell counts. The chest x-ray in patients with disseminated disease may reveal diffuse or lower lobe bilateral reticulonodular infiltrates consistent with miliary spread, pleural effusions, and hilar and/or mediastinal adenopathy. Infection may be present in bone, brain, meninges, gastrointestinal tract, lymph nodes (particularly cervical nodes), and viscera. Abscesses of the liver and prostate have been reported. Approximately 60 to 80 percent of patients have pulmonary disease, and 30 to 40 percent have extrapulmonary disease.

Respiratory isolation and a negative-pressure room should be used for patients in whom a diagnosis of pulmonary tuberculosis is being considered. This approach is critical to limit nosocomial and community spread of infection. A definitive diagnosis is made by culture of the organisms from an involved site. Blood cultures are positive in 15 percent of cases. However, given the importance of making an early diagnosis and initiating treatment, especially with the emergence of MDR tuberculosis (see below), a presumptive diagnosis should be made based on a positive acid-fast stain or positive PCR and consistent clinical presentation while culture results are awaited. In such patients, treatment as indicated below should be initiated. PPD skin testing in HIV-infected individuals poses a particular problem. A positive PPD test in an HIV-infected person is defined as an area of induration ≥5 mm in diameter. While this test can be used to support the diagnosis and identify candidates for isoniazid prophylaxis, up to 50 percent of patients with HIV infection and active tuberculosis are anergic, and thus a negative skin test does not rule out a diagnosis. This fact underscores the importance of the anergy panel in evaluating a patient for tuberculosis. Some experts recommend that any anergic patient with HIV infection who is at high risk for tuberculosis should be given a 1-year course of isoniazid.

℞ TREATMENT

Standard therapy for tuberculosis is generally as successful in the HIV-infected patient as in the HIV-negative patient. Tuberculosis is one of the totally curable conditions seen in patients with HIV infection. Given the potential for the occurrence of MDR tuberculosis, a standard course of action for the HIV-infected patient with active tuberculosis is to initiate therapy with four drugs for 4 months followed by two drugs (four drugs if the isolate turns out to be resistant) for an additional 4 months and for no less than 6 months after a third negative culture. Given the plethora of gastrointestinal problems in patients with HIV infection, malabsorption should be considered in any patient in whom a tuberculosis infection fails to clear despite appropriate therapy. To ensure the best possible treatment outcome, daily therapy should be observed directly by a health care professional.

A major emerging problem is the increasing identification of strains of *M. tuberculosis* resistant to two or more first-line drugs, usually isoniazid and rifampin, so-called MDR tuberculosis (see Chap. 171). Of the first 87 reported cases of MDR tuberculosis, 83 occurred in HIV-infected patients. Owing to delays in obtaining results of antimicrobial sensitivity testing, patients often received inadequate treatment regimens, and the initial mortality from MDR tuberculosis was as high as 72 to 89 percent. Up to 20 percent of cases of tuberculosis in some series were due to resistant strains. Owing to more aggressive treatment strategies, particularly ones employing directly observed therapy, the incidence of MDR tuberculosis is decreasing.

Prevention Effective prevention of active tuberculosis can be a reality if the health care profession is aggressive in looking for evidence of latent tuberculosis by making sure that all patients at risk for tuberculosis and all patients with HIV infection receive a PPD skin test. The therapeutic approach to an HIV-infected patient with a positive PPD result or to an anergic HIV-infected patient at risk for tuberculosis is discussed above.

Infections with Bacteria Other than Mycobacteria Nonmycobacterial bacteria account for a high number of infections in patients with AIDS and are the leading cause of death in this patient population. Bacterial infections most frequently present clinically as respiratory tract infections, sepsis, and/or gastroenteritis. In addition, syphilis and bacillary angiomatosis may present with atypical features. Patients with HIV infection appear to be particularly prone to infections with encapsulated organisms, perhaps as a consequence of altered B cell activation and/or defects in neutrophil function that may be secondary to disease or drugs. *Streptococcus pneumoniae* (see Chap. 141) and *Haemophilus influenzae* (see Chap. 152) are among the most common bacterial causes of infection seen in patients with HIV infection. These two organisms are responsible for most cases of bacterial pneumonia in patients with AIDS and contribute to the increased incidence of sinusitis that has been reported in this patient population. Patients with HIV infection have a sixfold increase in the incidence of pneumococcal pneumonia and a 100-fold increase in the incidence of pneumococcal bacteremia. For these reasons, all patients with HIV infections should receive immunization with pneumococcal polysaccharide. *Staphylococcus aureus* infections (see Chap. 142) are seen with increased frequency in the setting of HIV infection and account for approximately one-third of all episodes of bacteremia in HIV-infected individuals. HIV-infected individuals also have about twice the rate of carriage of staphylococcal organisms as the general population. Staphylococcal infections are usually responsible for catheter-related sepsis, with the risk increasing as the CD4+ T cell count declines. Pyomyositis is another complication of staphylococcal infection and is seen with increased frequency in HIV-infected patients. This disease, which was formerly rare in the United States, is generally seen in association with muscle injury; it has been postulated that the myopathy of HIV infection may be a predisposing factor.

Infections with enteric pathogens such as *Salmonella*, *Shigella*, and *Campylobacter* are more common in homosexual men and are often more severe and more apt to relapse in patients with HIV infection. These patients have approximately a 20-fold increased risk of infection with *Salmonella typhimurium* (see Chap. 158). They may present with a variety of nonspecific symptoms, including fever, anorexia, fatigue, and malaise of several weeks' duration. Diarrhea is common but may be absent. Diagnosis is made by culture of blood and stool. Although treatment generally is not indicated for *Salmonella* gastroenteritis in the general population, among HIV-infected patients this disease often follows a protracted course and has a high rate of recurrence, and long-term therapy is usually prescribed for *Salmonella* infection in this setting. The greatest success has been reported with oral ciprofloxacin. HIV-infected patients also have an increased incidence of infection with *Salmonella typhi* in areas of the world where typhoid is a problem (see Chap. 158).

Shigella infections (see Chap. 159) cause particularly severe gastrointestinal disease in HIV-infected individuals, characterized by diarrhea and fever. *Shigella flexneri* is the most common species isolated, and up to 50 percent of patients with HIV infection and shigellosis are bacteremic, in contrast to otherwise healthy hosts, in whom bacteremia is rare.

Campylobacter infections (see Chap. 160) occur at an increased frequency in HIV-infected patients. While *Campylobacter fetus* and *Campylobacter jejuni* are the strains most frequently isolated, infections with many other strains have been reported. Patients usually present with crampy abdominal pain, fever, and bloody diarrhea; infection may also present as proctitis. Stool examination reveals the presence of fecal leukocytes. Systemic infection can occur, with up to 10 percent of infected patients exhibiting bacteremia. As in the case of the other enteric pathogens, infections with *Campylobacter* species are often persistent or recurrent, and prolonged therapy is usually required. Most strains are sensitive to erythromycin; however, resistant strains have been reported.

Infections with *Treponema pallidum*, the etiologic agent of syphilis, play an important role in the HIV epidemic (see Chap. 174). In HIV-negative individuals, genital syphilitic ulcers rank with the ulcers of chancroid as major predisposing factors for heterosexual transmission of HIV (see above). While most HIV-infected individuals with syphilis have a typical presentation, a variety of formerly rare clinical problems may be encountered. Among them are lues maligna, an ulcerating lesion of the skin due to a necrotizing vasculitis; unexplained fever; nephrotic syndrome; and neurosyphilis. The most common presentation is that of condyloma lata, a form of secondary syphilis. Neurosyphilis may be asymptomatic or may present as acute meningitis, neuroretinitis, deafness, or stroke. In one series, 44 percent of all cases of neurosyphilis occurred in patients with HIV infection; the rate of neurosyphilis in this population may be as high as 1.5 percent. The incidence is particularly high in users of crack cocaine. Given the immunologic abnormalities seen in patients with HIV infection, diagnosis of syphilis through standard serologic testing may be challenging. On the one hand, a significant number of patients have a false positive Venereal Disease Research Laboratories (VDRL) test due to polyclonal B cell activation. On the other hand, the development of a positive VDRL result may be delayed in patients with new infections, and the anti-fluorescent treponema antibody (anti-FTA) test may be negative owing to immunodeficiency. Dark-field examination of appropriate specimens should be performed in any patient in whom syphilis is suspected, even if the patient has a negative VDRL test. Similarly, given that the diagnosis of neurosyphilis may be difficult to make, any patient with a positive serum VDRL test, neurologic findings, and abnormal findings on spinal fluid examination, whether or not the CSF VDRL test is positive, should be considered to have possible neurosyphilis. In the HIV-infected patient with syphilis, standard treatment may be inadequate; treatment may need to be repeated in patients who fail to respond or show evidence of relapse. In these patients, it is necessary to have a high index of suspicion for neurosyphilis and to treat accordingly with high-dose intravenous penicillin if this diagnosis is suspected.

Infections with species of the small, gram-negative rickettsia-like organism *Bartonella* (see Chap. 165) are seen with increased frequency among HIV-infected patients. Among the clinical manifestations of *Bartonella* infection are bacillary angiomatosis, cat-scratch disease, and trench fever. Bacillary angiomatosis is usually due to infection with *Bartonella henselae*. It is characterized by a vascular proliferation that leads to a variety of skin lesions, which have been confused with Kaposi's sarcoma. In contrast to the lesions of Kaposi's sarcoma, the lesions of bacillary angiomatosis generally blanch and are painful, and they are often associated with systemic symptoms. Infection can also extend to the lymph nodes, liver (peliosis hepatis), spleen, bone, heart, nervous system, respiratory tract, and gastrointestinal tract. This infection is usually seen in relatively advanced HIV infection, with an average CD4+ T cell count of 60/μL. Cat-scratch disease generally begins with a papule at the site of inoculation. This is followed several weeks later by the development of regional adenopathy and malaise. Infection with *Bartonella quintana* is transmitted by lice and has been associated with case reports of trench fever, endocarditis, adenopathy, and bacillary angiomatosis.

FUNGAL INFECTIONS Candidiasis *Candida* infections are the most common fungal infections in patients with HIV infection; virtually all patients experience some type of *Candida* infection over the course of their illness (see Chap. 207). *Candida* infections often occur early in the course of HIV disease and may mark the onset of clinically apparent immunodeficiency. Although they are a significant cause of morbidity, *Candida* infections are generally easy to control and usually involve only the mucosal surfaces. Invasive disease is extremely rare and occurs predominantly as a consequence of iatrogenic measures, such as use of indwelling catheters or broad-spectrum antibiotics and/or drug-induced neutropenia.

Superficial infection of the oral cavity with *Candida* (thrush) generally presents as a white, cheesy exudate on the posterior oropharynx **(see Plate ID-42)**. Early lesions also may be detected along the gingival-labial margins. The exudate is easy to scrape, and branching pseudohyphae are readily detectable on wet-mount KOH preparations. In women with HIV infection, vaginal yeast infections are an early sign of immunodeficiency.

Later in the course of HIV infection, generally in association with CD4+ T cell counts below 100/μL, *Candida* infections of the esophagus, trachea, bronchi, or lungs may occur. These infections are thought to indicate a serious defect in cell-mediated immunity and are among the AIDS-defining conditions (Table 308-2). The most common of these is esophagitis. While generally a late manifestation of HIV infection, *Candida* esophagitis has also been reported during the acute syndrome associated with primary HIV infection. Esophagitis generally presents as odynophagia and retrosternal pain or burning. Oral thrush is often present as well, although it may be absent in patients who have been receiving topical oral medications. A definitive diagnosis is made through upper gastrointestinal endoscopy and observation of characteristic white plaques shown by wet mount to contain pseudohyphae. However, a high index of suspicion based on history and/or a barium swallow demonstrating a grossly irregular mucosa (Fig. 308-26) is sufficient to justify an empirical trial of antifungal therapy. If improvement does not occur after 4 to 6 days of therapy, upper gastrointestinal endoscopy should be performed to eliminate the other possible causes of esophagitis, namely CMV infection, herpes simplex, Kaposi's sarcoma, and lymphoma.

℞ TREATMENT

Oral and vaginal *Candida* infections can be treated with topical nystatin or clotrimazole troches; the frequency of administration should match the severity of disease. In severe cases, many clinicians find it more convenient to use systemic therapy with either ketoconazole or fluconazole, both of which are effective in most cases. Although fluconazole is more expensive, somewhat better results have been achieved with it, which may, at least in part, reflect the poor absorption of ketoconazole in patients with high gastric pH. A short course of intravenous therapy with amphotericin B followed by oral therapy with fluconazole may be indicated in particularly severe cases of *Candida* infection.

Cryptococcosis *Cryptococcus neoformans* is the leading cause of meningitis in patients with AIDS (see Chap. 206). This ubiquitous yeast-like fungus, which has a polysaccharide capsule, causes serious, life-threatening infection in 6 to 12 percent of patients with AIDS. It is the initial AIDS-defining condition in 2 percent of patients, generally occurring in patients with fairly advanced disease in whom CD4+ T cell counts are below 100/μL. The median survival of a patient with HIV infection following a diagnosis of cryptococcal infection is 9 months. Cryptococcal meningitis is particularly common in patients with AIDS in Africa, occurring in approximately 20 percent of individuals; it was the illness that first suggested that a new epidemic of

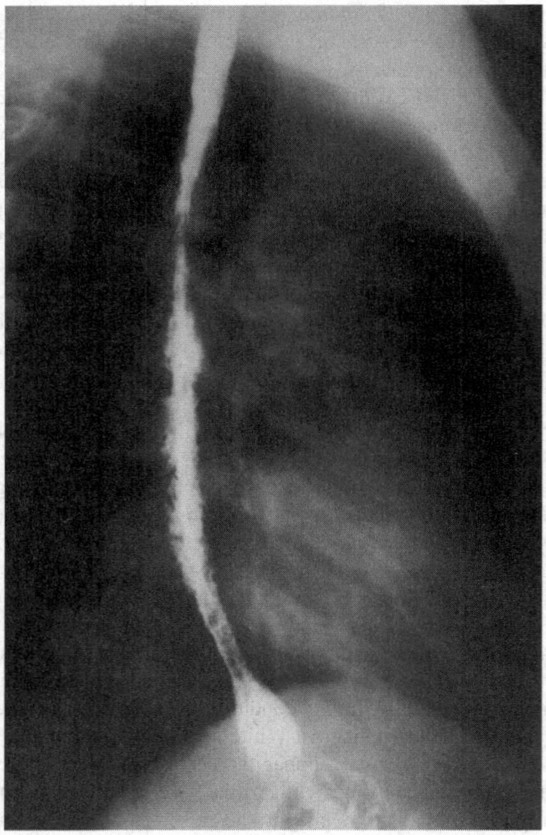

FIGURE 308-26 Barium swallow of a patient with *Candida* esophagitis. The flow of barium along the mucosal surface is grossly irregular.

immunodeficiency was occurring in Africa. Although the organism is thought to invade via the respiratory route, the most common sites of infection are the brain and meninges. CNS infection is seen in 67 to 85 percent of AIDS patients with cryptococcal disease; most patients present with a picture of subacute meningoencephalitis. In addition to meningitis, patients may develop cryptococcomas, which appear on MRI as multiple ring-enhancing lesions. Patients with CNS cryptococcal disease often experience symptoms for weeks to months prior to diagnosis; as with many AIDS-associated opportunistic infections, a high index of suspicion is essential to making an early diagnosis. Among the common symptoms are fever (in virtually 100 percent of patients), nausea and vomiting (40 percent), and altered mental status, headache, and meningeal signs (25 percent). The incidence of seizures and focal neurologic defects is low. Pulmonary disease occurs in 40 percent of patients, 90 percent of whom also have CNS infection. Patients with pulmonary disease present with fever, cough, dyspnea, and, in some cases, hemoptysis. A focal or diffuse interstitial infiltrate is seen on chest x-ray in over 90 percent of patients with pulmonary disease. Chest x-ray may also reveal lobar disease, cavitary disease, pleural effusions, and hilar or mediastinal adenopathy. Over half of patients are fungemic. In patients with fungemia, fever, malaise, and fatigue are common. While most patients with cryptococcal disease present with CNS infection, 4 to 10 percent present with pulmonary disease in the absence of other manifestations, and 4 to 8 percent present with fungemia as the only manifestation of infection. Uncommon manifestations of cryptoccocal infection in patients with HIV infection include skin lesions resembling molluscum contagiosum, lymphadenopathy, palatal and glossal ulcers, arthritis, gastroenteritis, myocarditis, and prostatitis. The prostate gland may serve as a reservoir for smoldering infection.

A presumptive diagnosis of cryptococcal infection can be made by the identification of organisms in spinal fluid with India ink examination, by the detection of cryptococcal antigen in blood or spinal fluid, or by histologic evidence of cryptococcal infection in a biopsy specimen. A definitive diagnosis is made by culturing organisms from spinal fluid, blood, bone marrow, sputum, or tissue. A positive culture for *Cryptococcus neoformans*, regardless of site, should be considered significant and an indication for treatment. Cryptococcal antigen is present in the CSF of virtually all patients with cryptococcal meningitis, although in 15 percent of these patients, all other findings are normal. In cryptococcal meningitis, the CSF WBC exceeds 20/μL in less than 50 percent of patients, the protein level is elevated in 35 to 70 percent, and the glucose level is low in about 50 percent. In patients with CNS cryptococcomas, both CSF antigen and culture may be negative, and biopsy may be required to make the diagnosis.

℞ TREATMENT

Therapy should be initiated immediately in any patient with evidence of cryptococcal infection, either by antigen or culture. Standard therapy in the HIV-infected patient consists of 6 weeks of amphotericin B at a daily dose of 0.3 to 0.5 mg/kg in combination with 150 mg/kg of flucytosine. In approximately 50 percent of patients the flucytosine will have to be omitted for at least part of the course of therapy owing to neutropenia. Given that over 50 percent of patients will relapse with this therapy alone, it is recommended that at the termination of amphotericin therapy, patients be placed on fluconazole, 100 to 200 mg daily, indefinitely. Many physicians choose to treat all patients with HIV infection with fluconazole, 100 to 200 mg daily, once the CD4+ T cell count falls below 100/μL as prophylaxis against both candidal and cryptococcal infections.

Histoplasmosis Histoplasmosis is an opportunistic infection that is seen most frequently in patients in the Mississippi and Ohio River valleys, Puerto Rico, the Dominican Republic, and South America; all of these are areas in which infection with *Histoplasma encapsulatum* is endemic (see Chap. 203). Because of this limited geographic distribution, the percentage of AIDS cases in the United States with histoplasmosis is only approximately 0.5 percent. In endemic areas, however, the incidence is much higher. The organism exists in the mycelial phase in soil, and large numbers of organisms are found in soil that contains droppings from birds or bats. The organism exists in the yeast phase at body temperature. Histoplasmosis is generally a late manifestation of HIV infection; however, it may be the initial AIDS-defining condition. The median CD4+ T cell count for patients with histoplasmosis was 33/μL in one study. While disease due to *H. encapsulatum* may present as a primary infection of the lung, disseminated disease, presumably due to reactivation, is the most common presentation in HIV-infected patients. These patients usually present with a 4- to 8-week history of fever and weight loss. Hepatosplenomegaly and lymphadenopathy are each seen in about 25 percent of patients. CNS disease, either meningitis or a mass lesion, is seen in 15 percent of patients. Bone marrow involvement is common, with thrombocytopenia, neutropenia, and anemia occurring in 33 percent of patients. Approximately 7 percent of patients have mucocutaneous lesions, consisting of a maculopapular rash and skin or oral ulcers. Although respiratory symptoms are usually minimal, with cough and dyspnea seen in 10 to 30 percent of patients, the chest x-ray is abnormal in about 50 percent of patients, revealing either a diffuse interstitial infiltrate or diffuse small nodules. The diagnosis is made by culturing the organisms from blood, bone marrow, or tissue. Fungal polysaccharide antigen may be detectable and quantifiable in the blood and can be used to follow the course of therapy; however, this test is not readily available commercially. Treatment consists of an initial course of amphotericin B, 0.6 mg/kg daily to a total dose of 1 g, followed by an indefinite maintenance regimen of either amphotericin, 1 mg/kg biweekly, or oral itraconazole.

***Penicillium marneffei* Infection** Following the spread of HIV infection to southeast Asia, disseminated infection with *Penicillium marneffei* was recognized as a complication of HIV infection. Clinical features include fever, generalized lymphadenopathy, hepatosplenomegaly, anemia, thrombocytopenia, and papular skin lesions with central umbilication. Treatment is with amphotericin B followed by itraconazole.

Coccidioidomycosis *Coccidioides immitis* is a mold that resides in the soil and causes a mainly pulmonary infection in both immunologically intact hosts and patients with HIV infection (see Chap. 204). As in the case of histoplasmosis, infection with *C. immitis* is limited to certain geographic areas; it is endemic in the southwest United States. In these endemic areas, the annual rate of infection is approximately 3 percent, and most of the disease seen in patients with HIV infection is thought to be a result of reactivation. Although coccidioidal infection may develop relatively early in the course of HIV infection, most patients with this condition have CD4+ T cell counts below 250/μL. Patients generally present with fever, weight loss, cough, and fairly extensive abnormalities on chest x-ray. Diffuse reticulonodular infiltrates are the most common finding on chest x-ray, although nodules, cavities, pleural effusions, and hilar adenopathy also occur. While pulmonary disease is the most common manifestation of infection, seen in almost 70 percent of patients, 12 percent develop meningitis; 9 percent, lymphadenopathy; 9 percent, hepatic involvement; and 5 percent, cutaneous disease. Abdominal infection and peritonitis have also been reported. Diagnosis is made by culture. While serologic testing is usually helpful in the immunocompetent host, serologies are negative in 25 percent of HIV-infected individuals with coccidioidal infection. Treatment is with amphotericin B, 1 mg/kg daily to a total dose of 1 g, followed by indefinite maintenance with either fluconazole or itraconazole.

Aspergillosis Invasive aspergillosis (see Chap. 208) is not an AIDS-defining illness and is generally not seen in patients with AIDS in the absence of neutropenia or administration of glucocorticoids. It does have an unusual presentation in the respiratory tract of patients with AIDS, where it gives the appearance of a pseudomembranous tracheobronchitis. As in other settings, treatment is with amphotericin B.

VIRAL INFECTIONS **Herpesvirus Infections** Human herpesvirus infections present substantial problems throughout the course of HIV infection. In addition to causing clinical disease in their own right, mainly in the form of reactivation syndromes, these DNA viruses are also thought to act as cofactors, enhancing the replication of HIV. Among the members of this group that are particularly disabling of patients with HIV infection are CMV (see Chap. 187), herpes simplex viruses (see Chap. 184), varicella-zoster viruses (see Chap. 185), Epstein-Barr virus (see Chap. 186) and HHV-8 (see above).

Cytomegalovirus infections CMV causes an acute infection, generally early in life, after which it exists in a latent state (see Chap. 187). Over 95 percent of patients with HIV infection are seropositive for CMV, and at autopsy 90 percent of patients have some evidence of reactivated CMV disease. Clinical manifestations of CMV generally occur late in the course of HIV infection, for the most part in patients with less than 50 CD4+ T cells per microliter; however, evidence of active CMV replication, such as excretion of CMV in throat washings or urine, can be detected quite early in the course of HIV disease. Retinitis, esophagitis, and colitis are the most common manifestations of CMV infection in patients with AIDS.

Among the most devastating manifestations of CMV is retinitis, occurring in 25 to 30 percent of patients. CMV retinitis usually presents as a painless, progressive loss of vision; patients may complain of "floaters." The disease is usually bilateral, affecting one eye more than the other, and the diagnosis is made purely on clinical grounds by an experienced ophthalmologist. The characteristic retinal appearance is that of perivascular hemorrhage and exudate **(see Plate III-1)**. CMV infection of the retina results in a necrotic inflammatory process, and the visual loss that develops is irreversible. As a consequence of retinal atrophy in areas of prior inflammation, CMV retinitis may be complicated by rhegmatogenous retinal detachment.

CMV esophagitis presents with substernal chest pain and odynophagia. Diagnosis usually requires endoscopy, which characteristically reveals a single large, shallow ulcer in the distal esophagus. Biopsy reveals characteristic intranuclear and intracytoplasmic inclusion bodies. While CMV may also involve the stomach and small intestine, the most frequent gastrointestinal manifestation of CMV infection is colitis, which is seen in 5 to 10 percent of all patients with AIDS and presents as diarrhea, abdominal pain, weight loss, and anorexia. The diarrhea is usually nonbloody and, as in the case of esophagitis, diagnosis is usually achieved through endoscopy and biopsy; characteristically, multiple mucosal ulcerations are seen. Barium enema examination is of little value and, in fact, may appear normal. Patients with CMV colitis may experience abdominal perforation and become bacteremic as a result. One consequence of CMV involvement of the gastrointestinal tract may be diffuse, generalized wasting.

Other manifestations of CMV disease are much less common in the HIV-infected patient. While histologic evidence of hepatitis is seen in 33 to 50 percent of patients who have CMV disease elsewhere in the body, clinical hepatitis is rare outside the setting of primary infection, which is almost exclusively seen in children. Approximately 33 percent of patients show some biochemical evidence of biliary tract disease, and CMV may cause a syndrome of papillary stenosis and sclerosing cholangitis. In patients with CMV-associated papillary stenosis, dilation of the extrahepatic common bile duct is usually demonstrated on ultrasound.

While the rate of pulmonary infection with CMV, as evidenced by positive cultures of pulmonary secretions, is quite high, the incidence of actual pulmonary disease due to CMV is quite low. In contrast to other manifestations of CMV infection in AIDS patients, CMV pneumonia responds quite poorly to therapy, as is the case in individuals without HIV infection.

CMV can cause an ascending myelitis and subacute polyneuropathy, which may respond to treatment. Other manifestations of CMV infection include adrenalitis, epididymitis, cervicitis, and pancreatitis.

The diagnosis of clinically significant CMV infection can be difficult. Given the fact that most patients with advanced HIV infection excrete CMV, positive throat, urine, blood, and/or tissue cultures are quite common and of little diagnostic significance. Aside from CMV retinitis, where the diagnosis is made on clinical grounds, a diagnosis of CMV infection requires the histologic demonstration of large intranuclear bodies and cytoplasmic inclusions in the suspect tissue, in the absence of other possible pathologic processes.

Rx TREATMENT

Three drugs—ganciclovir, foscarnet, and cidofovir—are currently licensed for systemic treatment of CMV infection, and formulations of ganciclovir and cidofovir are available for use as ocular implants. Initial response rates of retinitis to treatment with ganciclovir or foscarnet are approximately 80 to 90 percent; however, relapse rates are extremely high, and patients must receive long-term maintenance therapy. Of the two drugs, ganciclovir is somewhat easier to administer for initial therapy; it is given as a short infusion twice a day for 14 days. However, it is associated with a high incidence of bone marrow suppression and usually cannot be given in combination with zidovudine or trimethoprim/sulfamethoxazole. Foscarnet therapy is associated with a high incidence of renal and electrolyte disorders and, for initial therapy, foscarnet must be given as three 2-h infusions daily for 14 days. Maintenance therapy for both drugs consists of a single daily infusion. While both drugs were shown to have similar efficacy in a randomized controlled trial, patients without renal insufficiency treated with foscarnet had a slightly longer survival than patients treated with ganciclovir. The reason for this finding is unclear; however, it may be related to the fact that, in addition to being a potent anti-CMV agent, foscarnet also has activity against HIV. Hence, some clinicians recommend that patients with CMV retinitis be treated with an initial course of the more convenient drug, ganciclovir, followed by maintenance with foscarnet. Strains of CMV that are resistant to ganciclovir have been identified; foscarnet or cidofovir are clearly the agents of choice in this situation. Cidofovir was licensed for treating AIDS-related CMV retinitis based on two studies involving a total of 148 patients. One study showed that cidofovir was capable of delaying the progression of CMV retinitis.

The other demonstrated that cidofovir was effective in patients with relapsing CMV retinitis who had received other CMV therapy previously. While cidofovir may not be as potent as ganciclovir or foscarnet, it is clearly easier to administer. It is given once weekly for the first 2 weeks of treatment and once every 2 weeks thereafter. The major side effects include leukopenia, weakness, nausea, diarrhea, and decreased intraocular pressure. Another convenient way to treat CMV retinitis is to use intraocular implants that slowly release ganciclovir into the intraocular fluid. Although this approach is associated with an increased incidence of retinal detachments, it avoids the need for intravenous infusions. For the small percentage of HIV-infected individuals who are antibody-negative for CMV and who require blood products, such products should be obtained from CMV-negative donors if at all possible. The use of oral ganciclovir in the context of a medical center–based controlled clinical trial as a form of CMV prophylaxis has been associated with a delay in the development of CMV disease, and oral ganciclovir is licensed for this indication. A similar study taking place in a community-based setting failed to show any value for this form of prophylaxis.

Herpes simplex virus infections Infection with herpes simplex virus (HSV) in HIV-infected individuals is associated with recurrent orolabial, genital, and perianal lesions (see Chap. 184). As HIV disease progresses and the CD4+ T cell count declines, these infections become more frequent and severe. Lesions often appear beefy red, are exquisitely painful, and have a tendency to occur high in the gluteal cleft (Fig. 308-27). Perirectal HSV may be associated with proctitis and anal fissures. HSV should be high on the differential diagnosis in any HIV-infected patient with a poorly healing, painful perirectal lesion. As in the case of CMV, HSV may cause esophagitis. HSV esophagitis often occurs together with active orolabial lesions. In contrast to CMV, where esophagitis is usually associated with a single, large ulcer, HSV esophagitis generally occurs as multiple small ulcers.

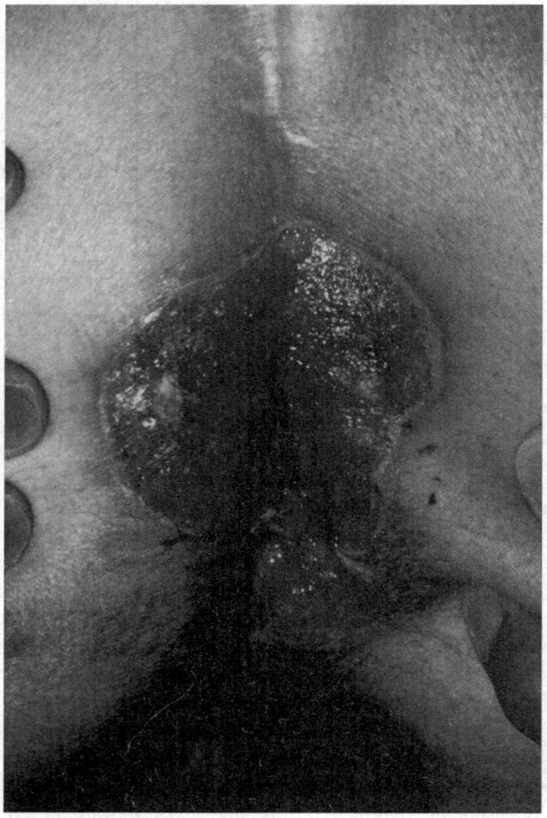

FIGURE 308-27 Severe, erosive perirectal herpes simplex in a patient with AIDS.

Recurrent *herpetic whitlow* is another problem in patients with HIV infection. It may present with painful vesicles or extensive cutaneous erosion and is a more severe version of the form seen in the immunologically intact host. Both HSV and varicella-zoster virus (see below) rarely cause a widespread, bilateral necrotizing retinitis referred to as the *acute retinal necrosis syndrome*. This syndrome, in contrast to CMV retinitis, is associated with pain, keratitis, and iritis. It is often associated with orolabial HSV or trigeminal zoster. Ophthalmologic examination reveals widespread pale gray peripheral lesions; this condition is often complicated by retinal detachment. Herpetic encephalitis is extremely rare in HIV-infected patients, despite its association with other immunocompromised conditions.

℞ TREATMENT

The treatment for severe or recurrent HSV infection is acyclovir. For most cases, 200 mg is given orally five times per day for 10 to 14 days; for more severe cases, the drug is given intravenously at higher doses. A more convenient alternative is famciclovir, 500 mg orally every 8 h for 7 days. Valacyclovir is licensed as a treatment for recurrent herpes simplex in the immunocompetent host; however, it has been associated with fatal cases of thrombotic thrombocytopenic purpura and should be avoided in immunocompromised patients, including patients with HIV infection. The development of microbial resistance to acyclovir due to alterations in the viral thymidine kinase enzyme is becoming an increasing problem in the HIV-infected population. These resistant strains are also resistant to ganciclovir; however, they are usually sensitive to foscarnet. The possibility of acyclovir resistance should be considered in patients with herpetic lesions refractory to acyclovir therapy.

Varicella-zoster virus infections Varicella-zoster virus (VZV), the etiologic agent of chickenpox, assumes a latent form in dorsal root ganglia following primary infection (see Chap. 185). Later in life, reactivation is associated with shingles; the appearance of shingles in any patient under 50 years of age should be an indication for workup of an underlying immunodeficiency, particularly HIV. Shingles is an early manifestation of HIV-induced immunodeficiency and, in one African study, 91 percent of patients developing shingles had underlying HIV infection. VZV infection in a patient with HIV infection is almost exclusively confined to the skin, although the skin eruptions may be extensive, over several dermatomes, and extremely painful (**see Plate ID-37**). A recurrence rate of 23 percent was noted in one report. A disseminated cutaneous form of zoster that very much resembles a mild form of chickenpox may be seen in patients with advanced HIV disease. As noted above, a small number of patients may develop the acute retinal necrosis syndrome, often in association with trigeminal shingles. Progression to visceral involvement is extremely rare as a reactivation syndrome in an HIV-infected patient, in contrast to many other severe immunodeficiency states. Hence, patients need not be hospitalized nor placed in strict isolation. Primary infection, on the other hand, can be lethal and should be treated aggressively with acyclovir and hyperimmune globulin. While treatment of shingles is not required, it can often result in a reduction in the time to resolution of lesions, and most physicians choose to treat it with high-dose oral or intravenous acyclovir or oral famciclovir. Acyclovir-resistant strains exist and characteristically produce hyperkeratotic lesions; under these circumstances, foscarnet is a useful alternative.

Epstein-Barr virus infections EBV, one of the causative agents of infectious mononucleosis, is also a very common infection in patients with HIV infection (see Chap. 186). Many patients with HIV actively shed EBV throughout the course of their illness. Aside from the association with lymphoma (discussed below), EBV is thought to play a causative role in *oral hairy leukoplakia*. This condition presents as white, frondlike lesions on the lateral aspect of the tongue and sometimes on the adjacent buccal mucosa (**see Plate ID-41**). These lesions are sometimes confused with candidiasis; however, they are quite distinct and, in contrast to *Candida* lesions, cannot be removed by scraping. The EBV genome has been demonstrated in these lesions by in situ hybridization. This observation, coupled with the fact that these lesions have been reported to regress following therapy with high-dose oral acyclovir, support the concept that EBV plays a causative role in this condition. Despite this therapeutic option, these lesions are rarely of sufficient clinical consequence to require therapy; they have a relatively high spontaneous remission rate (25 to 50 percent) and are more important for what they represent, namely, the presence of immunodeficiency.

Other human herpesvirus infections Human herpesvirus-8 (HHV-8) has been recognized in association with the lesions of Kaposi's sarcoma. It has also been associated with body cavity lymphoma in HIV-infected individuals. There is no specific therapy for HHV-8 infection at present (see "Pathogenesis of Kaposi's Sarcoma," above, for further details).

Human herpesvirus-6 is the first known human T-lymphotropic herpesvirus. It is the causative agent of exanthem subitum in infants. HHV-6 has been shown in some in vitro studies to act as a cofactor leading to an enhancement of HIV replication, and it is felt by some to accelerate the course of HIV disease. While antibodies to HHV-6 are present in 80 to 100 percent of individuals regardless of HIV status, HHV-6 replication is increased in patients with HIV infection, as evidenced by an increase in the fraction of patients harboring HHV-6 proviral DNA in peripheral blood (21 percent, versus 3 percent in HIV-negative individuals). HHV-6 is found in the retinal tissues of approximately 50 percent of HIV-infected individuals in whom it was sought, and it has been suggested that it may play a role in the subsequent development of CMV retinitis.

JC Virus Infection JC virus, a human papovavirus that is the etiologic agent of *progressive multifocal leukoencephalopathy* (PML), is an important opportunistic pathogen in patients with AIDS (see Chap. 379). While approximately 70 percent of the general adult population have antibodies to JC virus, indicative of prior infection, fewer than 10 percent of healthy adults show any evidence of ongoing viral replication. In contrast, close to 33 percent of HIV-infected individuals have evidence of active replication of JC virus. PML, the only known clinical manifestation of JC virus infection, is seen in 4 percent of HIV-infected individuals and is a late manifestation of AIDS. PML is a demyelinating disease; it begins as small foci in subcortical white matter, and the lesions eventually coalesce. The cerebral hemispheres, cerebellum, and brainstem may all be involved. Histologically, swollen oligodendritic nuclei with inclusions due to the nucleocapsid proteins of JC are seen. Death of the oligodendrocyte leads to demyelination without inflammation. Patients have a protracted clinical course, often developing multifocal neurologic deficits without changes in mental status. Patients with PML may exhibit ataxia, hemiparesis, visual field defects, aphasia, and sensory defects. The diagnosis is usually made by MRI, which reveals multiple white matter lesions on T2-weighted images. The clinical picture is generally much more impressive than the findings on MRI. Death usually occurs within 3 to 6 months of the onset of symptoms. Intrathecal administration of cytosine arabinoside has been reported to lead to improvement in some cases; however, no consistently effective therapy is currently available.

Human Papillomavirus Infection Evidence of infection with human papillomavirus is approximately twice as common in HIV-infected individuals (81 percent of patients in one series) as in the general population. The association of this virus with epidermal dysplasia suggests that both anal and cervical carcinomas will be seen in the HIV-infected population with increased frequency as survival is prolonged through the use of better antiretroviral regimens (see below).

Infection with Hepatitis Viruses Over 95 percent of HIV-infected individuals have evidence of infection with hepatitis B virus; coinfection with hepatitis C and/or D viruses is also quite common. HIV infection has several effects on hepatitis virus infection. It is associated with approximately a threefold increase in the development of persistent hepatitis B surface antigenemia. However, patients infected with both hepatitis B virus and HIV have decreased evidence of inflammatory liver disease, presumably owing to the effects of HIV on the immune system. Hepatitis D is a defective RNA virus that requires concomitant infection with hepatitis B in order to replicate, and thus infection is only seen together with hepatitis B infection. Hepatitis D infection is more common in patients with HIV infection, is associated with higher levels of hepatitis B virus replication, and seems to be associated with slightly worse hepatic disease, as evidenced by slightly higher levels of hepatic transaminases. Patients with HIV infection respond more poorly to treatment of hepatitis B with interferon-α than do HIV-negative individuals.

NEOPLASTIC DISEASES

A variety of neoplastic and premalignant diseases occur with increased frequency in HIV-infected individuals. Among them are Kaposi's sarcoma, lymphoma, and intraepithelial dysplasia of the cervix and anus. These diseases are significant contributors to the morbidity and mortality of patients with HIV infection. The clinical manifestations of these complications, as well as their epidemiologic profiles, have undergone considerable change as new approaches to treatment develop and as the epidemic involves different demographic groups.

KAPOSI'S SARCOMA Kaposi's sarcoma is a multicentric neoplasm consisting of multiple vascular nodules appearing in the skin, mucous membranes, and viscera. The course ranges from indolent, with only minor skin or lymph node involvement, to fulminant, with extensive cutaneous and visceral involvement. In the initial period of the AIDS epidemic, Kaposi's sarcoma was a prominent clinical feature of the first cases of AIDS, occurring in 79 percent of the patients diagnosed in 1981. By 1989 it was seen in only 25 percent of cases, and by 1992 this number had decreased to 9 percent. Part of this decrease is a reflection of the fact that AIDS-related Kaposi's sarcoma, in contrast to classic or endemic forms, occurs predominantly in homosexual men, with 96 percent of all cases occurring in that risk group. As the percentage of AIDS cases in other risk groups increases, the percentage of cases complicated by Kaposi's sarcoma decreases. This, however, is only a partial explanation for the observed decreased incidence of Kaposi's sarcoma in patients with AIDS. A growing body of epidemiologic and virologic data points to the high likelihood that a sexually transmitted cofactor plays an important role in the development of Kaposi's sarcoma. HHV-8 has been strongly implicated as this viral cofactor (see above). In this regard, Kaposi's sarcoma is four times more common in women who have had sexual contact with bisexual men than in other women, has been seen in homosexual men without evidence of HIV infection, and is more common among homosexual men in New York and Los Angeles than among homosexual men in the central states. As safer sex practices are employed, especially in the homosexual community, the risk of transmission of this cofactor and thus the risk of Kaposi's sarcoma has decreased. Kaposi's sarcoma can be an early manifestation of HIV infection, at times occurring in patients with normal CD4+ T cell counts. Thus, the rate of new cases of Kaposi's sarcoma may be influenced as much by the rate of new HIV infections as by the total number of HIV infections. As the rate of new HIV infections among homosexual men decreased, so did the incidence of new cases of Kaposi's sarcoma. However, as secondary opportunistic infections are better controlled, Kaposi's sarcoma is now appearing as a late complication of HIV infection. In these more advanced patients, Kaposi's sarcoma may be either quite indolent or aggressive. Overall, patients with Kaposi's sarcoma are more likely to die from causes other than those directly related to their tumor.

From a pathophysiologic perspective, Kaposi's sarcoma seems to be more a consequence of disordered cytokine regulation of cell growth than a true cancer (see above). Generally speaking, the tumor respects tissue planes and is rarely invasive.

Clinically, Kaposi's sarcoma may present in a variety of ways and may be seen at any stage of HIV infection, even in the presence of a normal CD4+ T cell count. The initial lesion may be a small, raised reddish-purple nodule on the skin, a discoloration on the oral mucosa, or a swollen lymph node (**see Plate IB-22**). Lesions often appear in sun-exposed areas, particularly the tip of the nose, and have a propensity to occur in areas of trauma (Koebner phenomenon). Because of the vascular nature of the tumors and the presence of extravasated red blood cells in the lesions, their color ranges from reddish to purple to brown and often take the appearance of a bruise, with yellowish discoloration and tattooing. Lesions range in size from a few millimeters to several centimeters in diameter and may be either discrete or confluent. Kaposi's sarcoma lesions most commonly appear as raised macules; however, they also can be papular, particularly in patients with higher CD4+ T cell counts. Confluent lesions may give rise to surrounding lymphedema and may be quite disfiguring when they involve the face and disabling when they involve the lower extremities or the surfaces of joints. Apart from the skin, the lymph nodes, gastrointestinal tract, and lung are the organ systems most commonly affected by Kaposi's sarcoma; however, lesions have been reported in virtually every organ, including the heart and the CNS. In contrast to most malignancies, in which lymph node involvement implies metastatic spread and a poor prognosis, lymph node involvement may be seen very early in Kaposi's sarcoma and is of no special clinical significance. In fact, some patients may present with disease limited to the lymph nodes. These are generally patients with relatively intact immune function and thus with the best prognosis. Pulmonary involvement generally presents as shortness of breath. Eighty percent of patients with pulmonary Kaposi's sarcoma have cutaneous lesions. The chest x-ray characteristically shows bilateral lower lobe infiltrates that obscure the margins of the mediastinum and diaphragm (Fig. 308-28). Pleural effusions are seen in 70 percent of cases of pulmonary Kaposi's sarcoma, a fact that is often helpful in the differential diagnosis. Gastrointestinal involvement is seen in 50 percent of patients and usually takes one of two forms. The first is submucosal involvement, which may lead to bleeding that can be severe. These patients sometimes also develop symptoms of gastrointestinal obstruction if lesions become large. The second gastrointestinal manifestation is biliary tract involvement. Kaposi's sarcoma lesions may infiltrate the gallbladder and biliary tree, leading to a clinical picture of obstructive jaundice similar to that seen with sclerosing cholangitis.

Several systems have been proposed for staging the extent of Kaposi's sarcoma. Given the unique nature of this disorder, standard oncologic staging systems have not been useful. An excellent staging system has been developed by the National Institute of Allergy and Infectious Diseases AIDS Clinical Trials Group; it distinguishes patients on the basis of tumor extent, immunologic function, and presence or absence of systemic disease (Table 308-22).

A diagnosis of Kaposi's sarcoma is based on biopsy of a suspicious lesion. Histologically one sees a proliferation of spindle cells and endothelial cells, extravasation of red blood cells, hemosiderin-laden macrophages, and, in early cases, an inflammatory cell infiltrate. Included in the differential diagnoses are lymphoma (oral lesions), bacillary angiomatosis, and cutaneous mycobacterial infections.

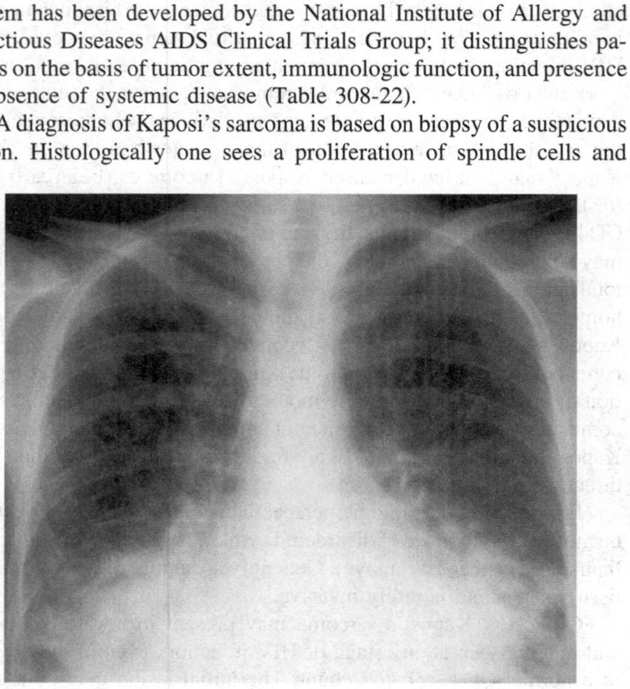

FIGURE 308-28 Chest x-ray of a patient with AIDS and pulmonary Kaposi's sarcoma. The characteristic findings include dense bilateral lower lobe infiltrates obscuring the heart borders and a pleural effusion.

℞ TREATMENT

Management of Kaposi's sarcoma (Table 308-23) should be carried out in consultation with an expert, since definitive therapeutic guidelines do not exist. In some cases, lesions remain quite indolent, and many of these patients can be managed with no specific treatment. Given the fact that less than 10 percent of AIDS patients with Kaposi's sarcoma die as a consequence of their malignancy and that death from opportunistic infections is much more common, whenever possible one should avoid treatment regimens that may further suppress the immune system and render the patients more susceptible to opportunistic infections. Furthermore, treatment is palliative and is not associated with improved survival.

Treatment is indicated under two main circumstances. The first is when a single lesion or a limited number of lesions are causing significant discomfort or cosmetic problems, such as with prominent facial lesions, lesions overlying a joint, or lesions in the posterior oropharynx that interfere with swallowing. Under these circumstances, treatment with localized irradiation, intralesional vinblastine, or cryotherapy may be indicated. It should be noted that patients with HIV infection are particularly sensitive to the side effects of radiation therapy. This is especially true with respect to the development of radiation-induced mucositis; doses of radiation directed at mucosal surfaces, particularly in the head and neck region, should be adjusted accordingly. The use of single-agent systemic chemotherapy should be considered in patients with a large number of lesions. Response rates varying from 26 to 80 percent have been seen with etoposide, vinblastine, doxorubicin, bleomycin, or IFNα. The single most important determinant of response appears to be the CD4+ T cell count. It is ironic that the patients most likely to respond to therapy are those who need it the least and who generally should not be treated aggressively for fear of further compromising immune function. This relationship between response rate and baseline CD4+ T cell count is particularly true for IFNα, where the response rate for patients with CD4+ T cell counts of $>600/\mu L$ is approximately 80 percent, while the response rate for patients with counts of $<150/\mu L$ is less than 10 percent. In contrast to the other single therapy agents, IFNα provides an added advantage of having antiretroviral activity; thus, it may be an appropriate first choice for single-agent systemic therapy for the early patient with disseminated disease. Combination chemotherapy offers the best overall response rate for patients with life-threatening disease, with close to 90 percent of all patients responding to a low-dose combination regimen of doxorubicin, bleomycin, and vinblastine. Liposome-encapulsated doxorubicin offers the potential for enhanced tumor uptake of this agent and thus lesser systemic side effects. As noted above, Kaposi's sarcoma is a radiation-sensitive tumor, and for patients with severe pulmonary involvement, one may also consider radiation therapy.

LYMPHOMAS Lymphomas occur with an increased frequency in patients with congenital or acquired T cell immunodeficiencies (see Chap. 307). AIDS is no exception; at least 6 percent of all patients develop lymphoma at some time during the course of their illness, which represents a 120-fold increase in incidence compared to the general population. Lymphoma occurs in all risk groups, with the highest incidence in patients with hemophilia and the lowest in patients from the Caribbean or Africa with heterosexually acquired infection. Lymphoma is a late manifestation of HIV infection, generally occurring in patients with less than 200 CD4+ T cells per microliter. As HIV disease progresses, the risk of lymphoma increases. In contrast to Kaposi's sarcoma, which occurs at a relatively constant rate (2.4 percent per year) throughout the course of illness, the attack rate for lymphoma rises exponentially with increasing duration of HIV infection and decreasing level of immunologic function. At 3 years after infection, the risk of lymphoma is 0.8 percent per year; by 8 years after infection, it is 2.6 percent per year. As people with HIV infection live longer because of improved antiretroviral therapy and more aggressive treatment and prophylaxis of opportunistic infections, the incidence of lymphomas may increase.

Three main categories of lymphoma are seen in patients with HIV infection: grade III or IV immunoblastic lymphoma, Burkitt's lymphoma, and primary CNS lymphoma (see Chap. 113). Approximately 90 percent of these lymphomas are B cell in phenotype, and half contain Epstein-Barr virus DNA. These tumors may be either monoclonal or oligoclonal in origin and are probably in some way related to the pronounced polyclonal B cell activation seen in patients with AIDS (see "Pathophysiology and Pathogenesis," above). Body cavity lymphomas have been associated with HHV-8.

Immunoblastic lymphomas account for approximately 60 percent of the cases of lymphoma in patients with AIDS. These are generally high-grade and would have been classified as diffuse histiocytic lymphomas in earlier classification schemes. This tumor is more common in older patients, increasing in incidence from 0 percent in HIV-infected individuals less than 1 year old to over 3 percent in those over 50 years old.

Small noncleaved cell lymphoma (Burkitt's lymphoma) accounts for approximately 20 percent of the cases of lymphoma in patients with AIDS. They are most frequent in patients 10 to 19 years old and usually demonstrate characteristic *c-myc* translocations from chromosome 8 to chromosomes 14 or 22. Burkitt's lymphoma is not commonly seen in the setting of immunodeficiency other than that due to HIV, and the incidence of this tumor in the setting of HIV infection is over 1000-fold higher than that in the general population. In contrast to African Burkitt's lymphoma, where 97 percent of cases contain an Epstein-Barr virus genome, only 50 percent of HIV-associated Burkitt's lymphomas are Epstein-Barr positive.

Primary CNS lymphoma accounts for approximately 20 percent of the cases of lymphoma in patients with HIV infection. In contrast to HIV-associated Burkitt's lymphoma, primary CNS lymphomas are usually positive for Epstein-Barr virus; in one study, the incidence of positivity was 100 percent, and the lymphomas did not appear to have a predilection for any particular age group. The median CD4+ T cell count at time of diagnosis of primary CNS lymphoma in AIDS patients is approximately 40/μL. CNS lymphoma generally presents at a later stage of HIV infection than does systemic lymphoma, and this fact may explain at least in part the poorer prognosis for this subset of patients (see below).

Table 308-22

National Institute of Allergy and Infectious Diseases AIDS Clinical Trials Group TIS Staging System for Kaposi's Sarcoma

Parameter	Good Risk (stage 0): All of the Following	Poor Risk (stage 1): Any of the Following
Tumor (T)	Confined to skin and/or lymph nodes and/or minimal oral disease	Tumor-associated edema or ulceration Extensive oral lesions Gastrointestinal lesions Nonnodal visceral lesions
Immune system (I)	CD4+ T cell count ≥200/μL	CD4+ T cell count <200/μL
Systemic illness (S)	No B symptoms* Karnofsky performance status >70 No history of opportunistic infection, neurologic disease, lymphoma, or thrush	B symptoms* present Karnofsky performance status <70 History of opportunistic infection, neurologic disease, lymphoma, or thrush

* Defined as unexplained fever, night sweats. >10% involuntary weight loss, or diarrhea persisting for more than 2 weeks.

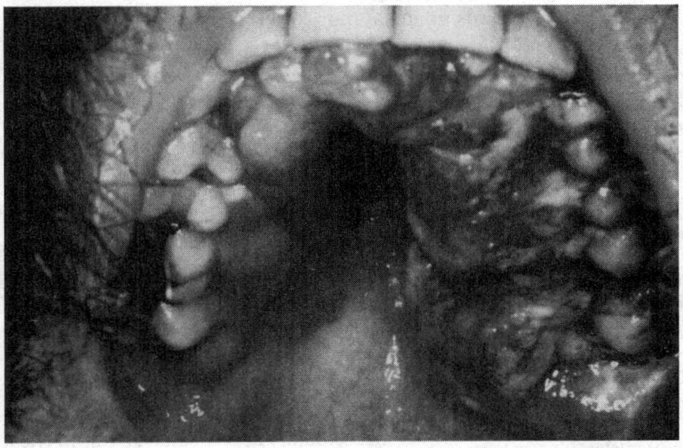

FIGURE 308-29 Diffuse histiocytic lymphoma involving the hard palate of a patient with AIDS.

The clinical presentation of lymphoma in patients with HIV infection is quite varied, ranging from focal seizures to rapidly growing mass lesions in the oral mucosa (Fig. 308-29) to persistent unexplained fever. At least 80 percent of patients present with extranodal disease, and a similar percentage have B-type symptoms of fever, night sweats, or weight loss. Virtually any site in the body may be involved. The most common extranodal site is the CNS, which is involved in approximately one-third of all patients with lymphoma; approximately 60 percent of these cases are primary CNS lymphoma. Primary CNS lymphoma generally presents with focal neurologic deficits, including cranial nerve findings, headaches, and/or seizures. MRI or CT generally reveals a limited number (one to three) of 3- to 5-cm lesions. The lesions often show ring-enhancement on contrast administration and may occur in any location. The main disease to be considered in the differential diagnosis is cerebral toxoplasmosis, although cerebral Chagas' disease may manifest a similar clinical picture. The prognosis is poor; the median survival following diagnosis is 2 to 3 months.

In addition to the 20 percent of all lymphomas in HIV-infected individuals that are primary CNS lymphomas, CNS disease is also seen in HIV-infected patients with systemic lymphoma; approximately 20 percent of patients with systemic lymphoma have CNS disease in the form of leptomeningeal involvement. This fact underscores the importance of a lumbar puncture in the staging evaluation of patients with systemic lymphoma.

Another common extranodal site of lymphoma in HIV-infected patients is the gastrointestinal tract, with involvement noted in 25 percent of patients. Any site in the gastrointestinal tract may be involved, and patients may complain of difficulty swallowing or abdominal pain. The diagnosis is usually suspected on the basis of CT or MRI of the abdomen. Bone marrow involvement occurs in approximately 20 percent of patients and may be associated with pancytopenia. Liver and lung involvement are each seen in approximately 10 percent of patients. Pulmonary disease may present as either a mass lesion, multiple nodules, or an interstitial infiltrate.

Table 308-23

Management of AIDS-Associated Kaposi's Sarcoma

- Observation
- Single or limited number of lesions
  - Radiation
  - Intralesional vinblastine
  - Cryotherapy
- Extensive, non-life-threatening disease
  - Single-agent chemotherapy (etoposide, vinblastine, adriamycin, or bleomycin)
  - Interferon-α (if CD4+ T cell >150/μL)
- Life-threatening disease
  - Combination chemotherapy with low-dose doxorubicin, bleomycin, and vinblastine (ABV)
  - Radiation treatment

TREATMENT Both conventional and unconventional approaches have been employed in an effort to treat HIV-related lymphomas. Initial attempts using standard intensive therapeutic regimens have largely been abandoned due to low response rates (20 to 30 percent) and a high incidence of fatal opportunistic infections. The median survival for patients treated with intensive regimens is approximately 4 to 6 months. These figures mainly reflect results in patients with fairly advanced HIV infection and low CD4+ T cell counts. Patients with higher CD4+ T cell counts do better with intensive chemotherapy, and in these earlier-stage patients, response rates as high as 72 percent and disease-free intervals exceeding 15 months have been reported. Clinical trials are under way comparing standard chemotherapeutic approaches with low-dose modified regimens. The median survival for patients with HIV-related systemic lymphoma is 10 months. Treatment of primary CNS lymphoma is almost uniformly unsuccessful. Palliative measures, such as radiation therapy and/or glucocorticoids, aimed at reducing the size of the lesion(s) and the accompanying edema may provide some symptomatic relief. The prognosis is poor for patients with primary CNS lymphoma; median survival is 2 to 4 months.

INTRAEPITHELIAL DYSPLASIA OF THE CERVIX OR ANUS This condition has been recognized increasingly as a complication of long-standing HIV infection. This human papillomavirus–associated condition correlates with the subsequent development of intraepithelial neoplasia and eventually invasive cancer. In two separate studies, HIV-infected men without anorectal symptoms were studied for evidence of dysplasia, and Papanicolaou smears were found to be abnormal in about 40 percent. These changes were persistent at 1 year follow-up, raising the possibility of a subsequent transition to a more malignant condition. While the incidence of an abnormal Papanicolaou smear of the cervix is approximately 5 percent in otherwise healthy women, the incidence of abnormal cervical smears in women with HIV infection is 60 percent. Based on this finding, invasive cervical carcinoma was added to the list of AIDS-defining conditions. Thus far, however, only small increases in the incidence of cervical or anal cancer have been seen as a consequence of HIV infection. However, given these findings, as patients with HIV infection live longer through the use of improved treatment strategies, it is likely that such conditions will begin to appear more frequently. For these reasons, all patients with HIV infection should have periodic pelvic examinations and/or rectal examinations with Papanicolaou smears to look for evidence of cellular dysplasia.

OTHER NEOPLASTIC CONDITIONS A variety of other neoplastic conditions have been described in patients with HIV infection. While none of these other conditions have been reported to occur at a higher rate than that seen in the general population, these cancers may be more fulminant and difficult to treat in HIV-infected patients. In this regard, Hodgkin's disease in the setting of HIV infection often presents as extensive disease, with mixed cellular or lymphocyte depletion pathologic types. In contrast to the excellent results and high cure rates for Hodgkin's disease in the general population, patients with advanced HIV infection and Hodgkin's disease have a median survival of only 12 to 15 months. As the epidemic of HIV infection continues, additional neoplastic complications are to be expected.

ORGAN-SPECIFIC SYNDROMES

Virtually every organ in the body is vulnerable to disease either as a direct consequence of HIV infection or secondary to other infectious or neoplastic conditions. While most of these diseases are due to opportunistic infections or neoplasms (see above), there are also a variety of clinical problems for which no specific pathogens are clearly identified.

PULMONARY DISEASE Pulmonary disease is seen in virtually every patient with HIV infection. Its evaluation is one of the most critical components in management, given the importance of early diagnosis and initiation of specific therapy. The most common manifestation of pulmonary disease is pneumonia. The two most common causes of pneumonia are bacterial infections and *P. carinii* infection. Other major causes of pneumonia include nonspecific interstitial pneumonitis, Kaposi's sarcoma, mycobacterial infections, and fungal infections. Although there are some distinguishing clinical and radiographic characteristics (Table 308-24), in most cases an accurate diagnosis is based on histologic or microbiologic identification of the causative organisms. Specimens for examination are derived from induced sputum, bronchoalveolar lavage, transbronchial biopsy, percutaneous aspiration, or open lung biopsy. In most of the conditions seen in HIV-infected patients, the chest x-ray reveals bilateral diffuse interstitial infiltrates. In patients with mycobacterial or fungal infections, hilar or mediastinal adenopathy may also be seen. *Aspergillus* may cause a pseudomembranous tracheobronchitis. In Kaposi's sarcoma, the infiltrates are dense and often obliterate the borders of the heart and diaphragm; there is usually an accompanying pleural effusion. Upper lobe cavitary disease is suggestive of reactivation tuberculosis or PCP in a patient receiving aerosolized pentamidine. The presence of a pneumothorax is most consistent with the latter condition. With the exception of bacterial pneumonias, sputum production is usually scant. Hemoptysis may be seen in the setting of cryptococcal pneumonia, tuberculosis, or Kaposi's sarcoma.

Two forms of *idiopathic interstitial pneumonia* have been described in patients with HIV infection: *lymphoid interstitial pneumonitis* (LIP) and *nonspecific interstitial pneumonitis* (NIP). LIP, a common finding in HIV-infected children, is rare in adults, occurring in approximately 1 percent of patients. This disorder is characterized by a benign lymphocytic infiltrate of the lung and is felt to be part of the systemic polyclonal activation of lymphocytes seen in the context of HIV and EBV infections. Transbronchial biopsy is diagnostic in 50 percent of cases; an open lung biopsy is required for diagnosis in the remainder. This condition is generally self-limited, and no specific treatment is necessary. Severe cases have been managed with a brief course of glucocorticoids. NIP is seen in up to half of all patients with AIDS and in some series is responsible for up to one-third of all pulmonary disease. Interstitial infiltrates with lymphocytes and plasma cells in a perivascular and peribronchial distribution are seen on histologic examination. Symptoms include fever and nonproductive cough, occasionally accompanied by mild chest discomfort. Chest x-ray, which is normal in 50 percent of cases, may reveal a faint

Table 308-24

Characteristics of Pneumonia in Patients with HIV Infection

Etiology	Sputum	Chest X-Ray
Pneumocystis carinii	Scant	Normal/interstitial infiltrate
Pneumocystis carinii in setting of aerosolized pentamidine	Scant	Upper lobe cavitary lesions; pneumothorax
Bacterial	Neutrophils, organisms	Consolidation
Atypical mycobacteria	Scant	Interstitial infiltrate; hilar adenopathy
Reactivation *Mycobacterium tuberculosis*	White blood cells, organisms, occasional hemoptysis	Cavitary or miliary infiltrates; hilar adenopathy
Nonspecific interstitial pneumonitis (NIP)	Scant	Normal/interstitial infiltrate
Kaposi's sarcoma	Scant, occasional hemoptysis	Dense, bilateral lower lobe infiltrates; pleural effusions

interstitial pattern. Like LIP, this is a self-limited process for which no therapy is indicated.

In addition to pneumonia, *sinusitis* is a common respiratory tract complication of HIV infection and is seen at all stages of disease. More severe cases are seen in patients with lower CD4+ T cell counts. Sinusitis presents as fever, nasal congestion, and headache; the diagnosis is best made by CT or MRI. The maxillary sinuses are most commonly involved; however, disease is also frequently seen in the ethmoid, sphenoid, and frontal sinuses. Although over 80 percent of patients show clinical improvement regardless of whether or not antibiotics are given, radiographic improvement is quicker and more pronounced in patients who have received antimicrobial therapy. It is postulated that this high incidence of sinusitis results from the increased frequency of infections with encapsulated organisms such as *Haemophilus influenzae* and *Streptococcus pneumoniae*, although this relationship has not been formally proven.

GASTROINTESTINAL DISEASE Gastrointestinal disease is a common feature of HIV infection and is most frequently due to a secondary infection. The oral mucosa, in addition to being involved with thrush, oral hairy leukoplakia, and Kaposi's sarcoma, may also be affected by large, shallow, painful aphthous ulcers. These lesions, which may be painful enough to result in a decrease in oral intake, are of unknown cause; however, they have been associated with dideoxynucleoside therapy in some instances. Brief courses of thalidomide have resulted in clearance of persistent aphthous ulcers. Esophagitis (Fig. 308-26) generally presents with odynophagia and retrosternal pain and may be due to *Candida*, CMV, or HSV. In addition, the esophagus may be involved with Kaposi's sarcoma and lymphoma. The esophageal mucosa, like the oral mucosa, may have large, painful ulcers of unclear etiology. These lesions are somewhat similar in appearance to the ulcers of CMV esophagitis but do not respond to antiviral therapy and can pose a significant problem with regard to nutrition. They may respond to therapy with thalidomide. Achlorhydria is a common problem in patients with HIV infection; however, gastric problems are otherwise rare. Kaposi's sarcoma as well as lymphoma may involve the stomach. Infections of the small and large intestine are among the most significant gastrointestinal problems in the HIV-infected patients. They usually present with diarrhea, abdominal pain, occasionally fever, and, in severe cases, weight loss. In addition to specific secondary infections, patients with HIV infection may also experience a chronic diarrheal syndrome for which no etiologic agent other than HIV can be identified and which is generally referred to as *AIDS* or *HIV enteropathy*. This is a clinical condition resembling chronic gastroenteritis with diarrhea of more than 1 month's duration for which no cause can be found. This condition is most likely a direct result of HIV infection in the gastrointestinal tract. Histologic examination of the small bowel in these patients reveals low-grade mucosal atrophy with a decrease in mitotic figures suggesting a hyporegenerative state. Patients often have decreased or absent small bowel lactase and malabsorption with accompanying weight loss.

In working up a patient with HIV infection and gastrointestinal problems, a set of stool examinations, including culture, examination for ova and parasites, and examination for *Clostridium difficile* toxin should form the initial part of the evaluation. Approximately 50 percent of the time, this workup will demonstrate infection with pathogenic bacteria, such as *Salmonella*, *Shigella*, or *Campylobacter*; mycobacteria (both atypical mycobacteria and *M. tuberculosis*); protozoa such as *Giardia*, *Entamoeba histolytica*, cryptosporidia, or *Isospora*; or *Clostridium difficile*. If these stool examinations are negative, additional evaluation, including upper and/or lower endoscopy with biopsy, establishes a diagnosis of microsporidial or mycobacterial infection of the small intestine or of CMV colitis in over half of patients. In patients for whom this diagnostic evaluation is nonrevealing, and if diarrhea has persisted for over 1 month, a presumptive diagnosis of HIV enteropathy can be made. An algorithm for the evaluation of diarrhea in patients with HIV infection is given in Fig. 308-30.

Rectal lesions are common in HIV-infected patients, particularly the perirectal ulcers and erosions due to the reactivation of HSV (Fig. 308-27). These may appear quite atypical, without vesicles, and respond well to treatment with acyclovir. Other rectal lesions more commonly seen in HIV-infected patients include condyloma acuminatum, Kaposi's sarcoma, and intraepithelial neoplasia.

Several different forms of hepatobiliary disease occur in patients with HIV infection. Biliary tract disease in the form of papillary stenosis or sclerosing cholangitis has been reported in the context of cryptosporidiosis, CMV infection, and Kaposi's sarcoma. Hepatic disease may take the form of hepatocellular injury due to hepatitis viruses, granulomatous hepatitis due to mycobacterial or fungal infections, or hepatic masses secondary to tuberculous abscess or peliosis hepatis. Fatty infiltration has also been reported; in some patients it may be related to nucleoside therapy. Asymptomatic hyperbilirubinemia may be seen as a consequence of indinavir therapy.

Pancreatic injury is most commonly due to drug toxicity, notably that secondary to pentamidine or dideoxynucleosides. While up to 50 percent of patients with HIV infection have biochemical evidence of pancreatic injury, and there is often evidence of pancreatic infection with CMV and/or MAC at autopsy, fewer than 5 percent of patients show any clinical evidence of pancreatitis that is not linked to a drug toxicity.

HEMATOLOGIC PROBLEMS Hematologic problems are common throughout the course of HIV infection and may be direct results of HIV, manifestations of secondary infections and neoplasms, or side effects of therapy (Table 308-25). Bone marrow suppression may be associated with disseminated mycobacterial infections, fungal infections, and lymphoma. Direct histologic examination and culture of bone marrow in patients with HIV infection and unexplained hematologic abnormalities are often diagnostic. A significant percentage of bone marrow aspirates have been reported to contain lymphoid aggregates, the precise significance of which is unknown.

Anemia is the most common hematologic abnormality in HIV-infected individuals, being present in 18 percent of asymptomatic seropositive individuals, 50 percent of patients with early symptoms, and 75 percent of patients with AIDS. While generally mild, anemia can be quite severe and may require chronic blood transfusions. Among the specific reversible causes of anemia in HIV-infected individuals are drug toxicity, systemic fungal and mycobacterial infections, nutritional deficiencies, and parvovirus B19 infections.

Zidovudine is a major contributor to the anemia seen in patients with advanced HIV infection. This nucleoside analogue (discussed

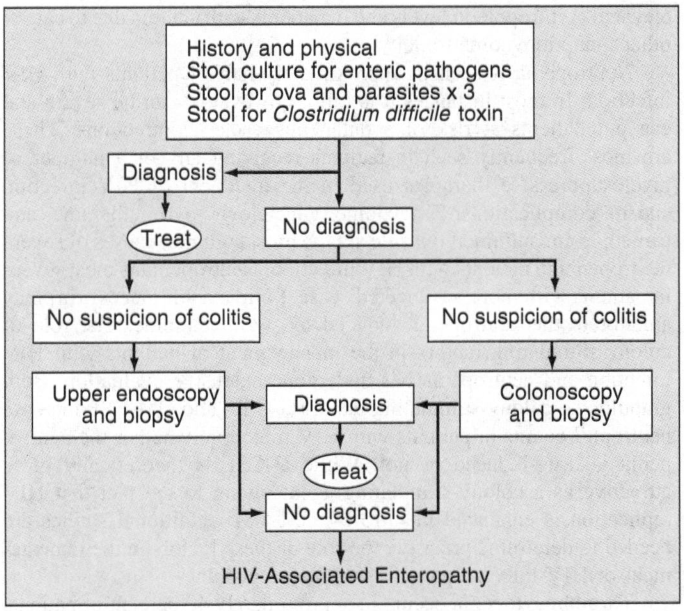

FIGURE 308-30 Algorithm for the evaluation of diarrhea in a patient with HIV infection. HIV-associated enteropathy is a diagnosis of exclusion and can be made only after other, generally treatable, forms of diarrheal illness have been ruled out.

Table 308-25

Causes of Bone Marrow Suppression in Patients with HIV Infection

HIV infection	Medications:
Mycobacterial infections	Zidovudine
Fungal infections	Dapsone
B19 parvovirus infection	Trimethoprim/sulfamethoxazole
Lymphoma	Pyrimethamine
	5-Flucytosine
	Ganciclovir
	Interferon-α
	Trimetrexate
	Foscarnet

below) has a somewhat selective ability to block erythroid maturation, an effect that precedes effects on other marrow elements. A characteristic feature of zidovudine therapy is an elevated mean corpuscular volume (MCV). Another drug with selective effects on the erythroid series is dapsone. This agent can cause a serious hemolytic anemia in patients who are G6PD-deficient and can create a functional anemia in others through induction of methemoglobinemia.

Folate levels are usually normal in HIV-infected individuals; however, vitamin B_{12} levels may be depressed in patients with AIDS, presumably as a consequence of long-standing achlorhydria and malabsorption. Replacement therapy with vitamin B_{12} seems to have a minimal effect on HIV-associated anemia. True autoimmune hemolytic anemia is rare, although approximately 20 percent of patients with HIV infection have a positive direct antiglobulin test, presumably as a consequence of polyclonal B cell activation.

In addition to the more common secondary infections described above, patients with HIV infection have been reported to develop anemia secondary to infection with parvovirus B19. It is important to be aware of this cause of anemia, as it responds to treatment with intravenous immunoglobulin.

Baseline erythropoietin levels in patients with HIV infection and anemia are generally less than expected, given the degree of anemia. The exception is zidovudine-associated anemia, in which levels may be quite high. In patients with zidovudine-associated anemia and low erythropoietin levels, treatment with erythropoietin at a dose of 100 μg/kg three times a week may result in an increase in hemoglobin levels. Erythropoietin seems to be of less benefit in patients with elevated erythropoietin levels and in patients with anemia due to causes other than zidovudine toxicity.

Neutropenia is seen in approximately half of patients with HIV infection. In most instances it is mild; however, it can be severe and can put patients at risk of spontaneous bacterial infections. These are most frequently seen in patients receiving any of a number of myelosuppressive therapies used in the treatment of HIV infection and its complications. Zidovudine, ganciclovir, pyrimethamine, and trimethoprim/sulfamethoxazole are the most common causes of severe neutropenia in patients with HIV infection. Neutropenia is most severe in patients with more advanced disease. Folinic acid (leucovorin) may ameliorate the neutropenia induced by pyrimethamine. The role of colony-stimulating factors in the management of patients with HIV infection and neutropenia has undergone extensive evaluation. Both granulocyte colony-stimulating factor (G-CSF) and GM-CSF increase neutrophil counts in patients with HIV infection, whether the neutropenia is drug-induced or not. While G-CSF is theoretically more attractive as a colony-stimulating agent owing to the fact that HIV replication is enhanced in vitro by GM-CSF, additional studies are needed to determine precisely the role of these factors in the management of HIV-infected patients with neutropenia.

Thrombocytopenia occurs in approximately 40 percent of patients with HIV infection and, in contrast to neutropenia and anemia, is often an early, primary manifestation of HIV infection. The thrombocytopenia seen as a direct result of HIV infection resembles that of idiopathic thrombocytopenic purpura (see Chap. 117) and responds not only to conventional strategies but, in a large number of cases, to therapy with antiretroviral agents. Thrombocytopenia may also be seen as a side effect of medications; however, it is rarely dose limiting. Other causes of thrombocytopenia in patients with HIV infection include bone marrow involvement by lymphoma, mycobacterial infection, and fungal infections.

LYMPHADENOPATHY Lymphadenopathy is also a common finding in patients with HIV infection, ranging from the generalized follicular hyperplasia seen early in disease (see above) to involvement secondary to opportunistic infections and neoplasms. Lymph node biopsy is not indicated in the lymphadenopathy seen early in disease unless it is associated with rapid enlargement, unusual consistency, or coalescence of nodes. While Kaposi's sarcoma may present in a lymphadenopathic form early in disease, there are no data to suggest that early treatment is indicated. In contrast, new-onset lymphadenopathy in the setting of more advanced HIV infection (CD4+ T cell counts under 200/μL) may be the first sign of a secondary infection or neoplasm and should be examined both histologically and microbiologically. Among the secondary infections commonly associated with lymphadenopathy are mycobacterial infections, fungal infections, and bacillary angiomatosis. In addition to Kaposi's sarcoma, lymphoma may also present as lymphadenopathy.

RENAL DISEASE Renal disease may be associated with HIV infection (see Chaps. 275 and 276). Although renal disease is often drug-induced, a significant portion of patients with AIDS (up to 10 percent in some series) develop renal disease as a direct consequence of HIV infection; this is designated *AIDS-* or *HIV-associated nephropathy*. Secondary infections rarely result in significant renal impairment; however, one may see nephrocalcinosis as a result of infection with mycobacteria or *P. carinii*.

Among the drugs commonly associated with renal damage in patients with AIDS are pentamidine, amphotericin, and foscarnet. In addition, trimethoprim/sulfamethoxazole may compete for tubular secretion with creatinine and cause an increase in the serum creatinine level. Sulfadiazine may crystallize in the kidney and result in an easily reversible form of renal shutdown, while the protease inhibitor indinavir can lead to renal calculi.

HIV-associated nephropathy closely resembles the heroin-associated nephropathy seen in IDUs and initially was thought to be that condition in patients with HIV infection; however, it is now recognized as a true direct complication of HIV infection. HIV-associated nephropathy can be an early manifestation of HIV infection and is also seen in children. The severity of renal disease and the propensity to develop end-stage renal failure appear to be a function of race and are much more of a problem among African Americans than whites, perhaps more so than any other manifestation of HIV infection. Given that in most series over 50 percent of patients with HIV-associated nephropathy were IDUs, it was originally thought that this racial predilection merely reflected the disproportionate number of African Americans in the IDU group rather than being a true race-related phenomenon. However, the incidence by race of HIV-associated end-stage renal failure in non-IDU homosexual men suggests that race does play a major role and that end-stage renal failure occurs disproportionately among African Americans.

The prototypic lesion of HIV-associated nephropathy is a focal segmental glomerulosclerosis, which is seen in approximately 80 percent of patients with this complication. Patients present with heavy proteinuria without edema or hypertension. Ultrasound examination usually reveals enlarged, hyperechogenic kidneys; a definitive diagnosis is obtained through renal biopsy. Progression to end-stage renal failure usually occurs within 1 year. The remainder of patients (approximately 20 percent) with HIV-associated nephropathy present with a mesangial hyperplasia with minimal glomerulosclerosis. It is believed that this may be the precursor lesion to focal segmental glomerulosclerosis.

There is no successful treatment for HIV-associated nephropathy. Antiretroviral therapy seems to have little overall beneficial effect on it, although temporary improvement following initiation of zidovudine therapy has been noted by some investigators. In patients in whom renal disease is detected relatively early, at the stage of mesangial hyperplasia with minimal glomerulosclerosis, it has been proposed that a short course of glucocorticoids may be of value. While this seems a reasonable therapeutic option, it must be carried out with awareness of the potential negative effects of long-term glucocorticoid use in patients with HIV infection.

DERMATOLOGIC PROBLEMS Dermatologic problems are common in patients with HIV infection (see Chap. 57). From the macular, roseola-like rash seen with the acute seroconversion syndrome to extensive end-stage Kaposi's sarcoma, cutaneous manifestations can be seen throughout the entire course of HIV infection. While many of these manifestations are covered elsewhere in this chapter under their respective causes and in the section "Early Symptomatic Disease," some additional ones occur (see Chaps. 55, 56, and 58). Among these are seborrheic dermatitis, eosinophilic pustular folliculitis, and several minor cutaneous infections.

Seborrheic dermatitis occurs in 3 percent of the general population, but it is seen in up to 50 percent of patients with HIV infection and is among the most common noninfectious manifestations of HIV infection. Seborrheic dermatitis increases in prevalence and severity as the CD4+ T cell count declines. In HIV-infected patients, seborrheic dermatitis may be aggravated by concomitant infection with *Pityrosporon*, a yeast-like fungus; use of topical antifungal agents has been recommended in cases refractory to standard topical treatment.

Eosinophilic pustular folliculitis is a rare dermatologic condition that is seen with increased frequency in patients with HIV infection. It presents as multiple urticarial perifollicular papules that may coalesce into plaque-like lesions. Skin biopsy reveals an eosinophilic infiltrate of the hair follicle, which in certain cases has been associated with the presence of a mite. Patients typically have an elevated IgE level and may respond to treatment with topical anthelmintics. There is at least one report of a patient with AIDS developing a severe form of Norwegian scabies with hyperkeratotic, psoriaform skin lesions.

Both psoriasis and ichthyosis, although they are not reported to be increased in frequency, may be particularly severe when they occur in patients with HIV infection. Preexisting psoriasis may become guttate in appearance and more refractory to treatment.

As mentioned above, a variety of secondary infections in HIV-infected patients can present with cutaneous manifestations. Among them are HSV infection, which can cause severe erosive orolabial, genital, and perirectal ulcers (Fig. 308-27) or whitlow lesions, and VZV infection, which can cause either shingles or a forme fruste of chickenpox secondary to cutaneous dissemination. Similarly, molluscum contagiosum and condyloma acuminatum may be significantly more serious in HIV-infected individuals. Atypical mycobacterial infections may present as erythematous cutaneous nodules, as may certain fungal infections and *Bartonella* infections. Extrapulmonary pneumocystosis may result in necrotizing vasculitis.

The skin of patients with HIV infection is often a target organ for drug reactions (see Chap. 56). Although most skin reactions are mild and not necessarily an indication to discontinue treatment, patients may have particularly severe cutaneous eruptions, including erythroderma and Stevens-Johnson syndrome, as a reaction to drugs, particularly sulfa drugs. Similarly, patients with HIV infection are often very photosensitive and burn easily following exposure to sunlight or as a side effect of radiation therapy (see Chap. 58).

HIV infection and treatment may be accompanied by cosmetic changes of the skin that are not of great clinical importance but nonetheless are troubling to patients. Both yellowing of the nails and straightening of the hair, particularly in African-American patients, have been reported as a consequence of HIV infection. Zidovudine therapy has been associated with elongation of the eyelashes and the development of a bluish discoloration to the nails, again more commonly among African Americans. Therapy with clofazimine may cause a yellow-orange discoloration of the skin.

HEART DISEASE While heart disease is a relatively common postmortem finding in HIV-infected patients (25 to 75 percent in autopsy series), it is rarely a clinical problem. The most common clinically significant finding is a dilated cardiomyopathy associated with congestive heart failure (see Chap. 239); this generally occurs as a late complication of HIV infection and, histologically, most closely resembles a myocarditis. HIV has been detected in cardiac tissue, and there is debate over whether it plays a direct role in this condition. Patients present with the classic findings of congestive heart failure, i.e., edema and shortness of breath. Treatment is no different than for any other patient with congestive heart failure, although one must be certain that drug toxicity is not the cause. Both IFNα and nucleoside analogues have been reported to cause a cardiomyopathy in patients with HIV infection that reverses once therapy is discontinued. Similarly, Kaposi's sarcoma, cryptococcosis, and toxoplasmosis can involve the myocardium, resulting in cardiomyopathy. In one series, most patients with a treatable myocarditis were found to have myocarditis associated with toxoplasmosis. Most of these patients also had evidence of CNS toxoplasmosis. Thus, an MRI or double-dose contrast CT scan of the brain should be included in the workup of any patient with advanced HIV infection and an unexplained cardiomyopathy.

A variety of other cardiovascular problems have been found in the setting of HIV infection. Pericardial disease may be due to Kaposi's sarcoma, mycobacterial infections, cryptococcal disease, or lymphoma. Tamponade and death have occurred in association with pericardial Kaposi's sarcoma, presumably owing to acute hemorrhage. Clinically significant ischemic heart disease is not seen to an increased degree in HIV-infected individuals, even though a high percentage of patients have hypertriglyceridemia, and coronary artery disease has been a relatively frequent finding at autopsy. Nonbacterial thrombotic endocarditis has been reported and should be considered in patients with unexplained embolic phenomena. Intravenous pentamidine, when given rapidly, can result in hypotension as a consequence of cardiovascular collapse.

IMMUNOLOGIC AND RHEUMATOLOGIC DISORDERS Disorders of these types are common in patients with HIV infection and range from excessive immediate hypersensitivity-type reactions (see Chap. 310) to an increase in the incidence of reactive arthritis (see Chap. 317) to conditions characterized by a diffuse infiltrative lymphocytosis. These phenomena occur in an apparent paradox to the profound immunodeficiency that characterizes this infection. Drug allergies are the most significant allergic reactions occurring in HIV-infected patients and seem to become more common as the disease progresses; they occur in 65 percent of patients who receive therapy with trimethoprim/sulfamethoxazole for PCP. In general, these drug reactions are characterized by an erythematous, morbilliform eruption that is pruritic, tends to coalesce, and is often associated with fever. Nonetheless, approximately 33 percent of patients can be maintained successfully on the offending therapy, and thus these reactions are not an immediate indication to stop the drug. Anaphylaxis is extremely rare in patients with HIV infection, and patients who have a cutaneous eruption during a single course of therapy can still be considered candidates for future treatment or prophylaxis with the same agent. In addition, desensitization regimens are moderately successful in HIV-infected patients. While the mechanisms underlying these allergic-type phenomena remain unknown, patients with HIV infection have been noted to have elevated IgE levels that increase as the CD4+ T cell count declines, and there are numerous examples of patients with multiple drug reactions, suggesting some common pathway. It is anticipated that allergic drug reactions will become an increasingly difficult aspect of managing patients with HIV infection, especially with the expanding need for multidrug regimens for the treatment of HIV infection itself and the treatment of tuberculosis, as well as for prophylaxis for opportunistic infections.

HIV infection shares many similarities with a variety of autoimmune diseases, including a substantial polyclonal B cell activation that is associated with a high incidence of antiphospholipid antibodies, such as anticardiolipin antibodies, VDRL antibodies, and lupus-like anticoagulants. In addition, HIV-infected individuals have an increased incidence of positive antinuclear antibodies. However, there is no evidence that HIV-infected individuals have an increase in two of the more common autoimmune diseases, namely systemic lupus erythematosus and rheumatoid arthritis. In fact, it has been observed that these diseases may be somewhat ameliorated by the concomitant presence of HIV infection, suggesting that an intact CD4+ T cell limb of the immune response plays an integral part in their pathogenesis. Similarly, there are anecdotal reports of patients with common variable immunodeficiency (see Chap. 307), characterized by hypogammaglobulinemia, who have had a normalization of Ig levels following the development of HIV infection, suggesting a possible role for overactive CD4+ T cell immunity in certain forms of that disease. The one autoimmune disease that may occur with an increased frequency in patients with HIV infection is a variant of primary Sjögren's syndrome (see Chap. 316). Patients with HIV infection may develop a syndrome consisting of parotid gland enlargement, dry eyes, and dry mouth that is characterized by lymphocytic infiltrates of the salivary gland and lung. In contrast to Sjögren's syndrome, in which these infiltrates are composed predominantly of CD4+ T cells, in patients with HIV infection the infiltrates are composed predominantly of CD8+ T cells. In addition, while patients with Sjögren's syndrome are mainly women who have autoantibodies to Ro and La and who frequently have HLA-DR3 or -B8, HIV-infected individuals with this syndrome are usually African-American men who do not have anti-Ro or anti-La and who most often have HLA-DR5. In at least one case, the syndrome improved following zidovudine therapy. The term *diffuse infiltrative lymphocytosis syndrome* (DILS) has been proposed to describe this entity and to distinguish it from Sjögren's syndrome.

Approximately 33 percent of HIV-infected individuals experience arthralgias; furthermore, 5 to 10 percent are diagnosed as having some form of reactive arthritis, such as Reiter's syndrome or psoriatic arthritis. These syndromes occur with increasing frequency as the competency of the immune system declines; this effect may be related to an increase in the number of infections with organisms that may trigger a reactive arthritis. These arthritides generally respond adequately to standard treatment (see Chap. 317); however, therapy with methotrexate has been associated with an increase in the incidence of opportunistic infections and should be used with caution and only in severe cases.

HIV-infected individuals also experience a variety of joint problems with no obvious cause, which are referred to generically as *HIV-* or *AIDS-associated arthropathy*. This syndrome is characterized by subacute obligoarticular arthritis developing over a period of 1 to 6 weeks and lasting 6 weeks to 6 months. It generally involves the large joints, predominantly knees and ankles, and is nonerosive with only a mild inflammatory response. X-rays of the joint are nonrevealing. Nonsteroidal anti-inflammatory drugs are marginally helpful; however, relief has been noted with the use of intraarticular steroids. A second form of arthritis also thought to be secondary to HIV infection is called "painful articular syndrome." This condition, described in as many as 10 percent of a cohort of AIDS patients, presents as acute, severe, sharp pain in the joint. It affects mainly the knees, elbows, and shoulders, lasts 2 to 24 h, and may be severe enough to require narcotic analgesics. The cause of this arthropathy is unclear; however, it is thought to result from a direct effect of HIV on the joint. This is a reasonable assumption, given the fact that other lentiviruses, in particular the caprine arthritis-encephalitis virus, are capable of causing arthritis.

A variety of other immunologic or rheumatologic diseases have been reported in HIV-infected individuals, either de novo or in association with opportunistic infections or drugs. Using the criteria of widespread musculoskeletal pain of at least 3 months' duration and the presence of at least 11 of 18 possible tender points by digital palpation, 11 percent of an HIV-infected cohort consisting of 55 percent IDUs could be diagnosed as having fibromyalgia (see Chap. 326). While the incidence of frank arthritis was less in this population than in other studied populations that consisted predominantly of homosexual men, these data support the concept that there are musculoskeletal problems that occur as a direct result of HIV infection. In addition, there have been reports of leukocytoclastic vasculitis in the setting of zidovudine therapy (see Chap. 319). CNS angiitis (see Chap. 319) and polymyositis (see Chap. 315) have also been reported in HIV-infected individuals. Septic arthritis is surprisingly rare, especially given the increased incidence of staphylococcal bacteremias seen in this population. When septic arthritis has been reported, it has usually been due to systemic fungal infections with *Sporothrix schenckii*, *Cryptococcus neoformans*, or *Histoplasma capsulatum*, or systemic mycobacterial infection with *Mycobacterium haemophilum*.

OPHTHALMIC PROBLEMS Ophthalmic problems are seen in over 50 percent of HIV-infected individuals, generally as a late manifestation of disease. The most common abnormal findings on funduscopic examination are cotton-wool spots—hard white spots that appear on the surface of the retina and often have an irregular edge. They represent areas of retinal ischemia secondary to microvascular disease. At times they are associated with small areas of hemorrhage and thus are difficult to distinguish from CMV retinitis. In contrast to CMV retinitis, however, these spots are not associated with visual loss and tend to remain stable or improve over time.

Apart from cotton-wool spots, the most common disease of the eye in HIV-infected individuals is CMV retinitis. This is almost invariably a late manifestation of HIV disease, occurring in patients with less than 50 CD4+ T cells per microliter. CMV causes a progressive necrotizing retinitis that results in permanent visual loss. Funduscopically one sees perivascular hemorrhage and exudate that is usually bilateral and progressive over time **(see Plate III-1)**. Retinal detachment may occur in areas of retinal scarring secondary to burned-out infection. Treatment is detailed above and at present is limited to either ganciclovir, foscarnet, or cidofovir.

Several other secondary infections may cause ocular problems in HIV-infected patients. Among them are *Pneumocystis carinii* infection, toxoplasmosis, and herpesvirus infections. *P. carinii* causes a severe choroiditis that is most commonly seen in the absence of pulmonary disease. Lesions appear as slightly raised yellow-white plaques and may be confused with cotton-wool spots. Toxoplasma retinitis is usually an accompaniment of CNS toxoplasmosis. It may be very difficult to distinguish from CMV retinitis and should be considered in anyone with a diagnosis of CMV retinitis who is not responding well to initial therapy. In contrast, infections of the retina caused by HSV and VZV, referred to as *acute retinal necrosis syndrome*, are quite distinct, causing a painful inflammation of the eye that may be associated with keratitis or iritis. Funduscopic examination reveals multiple, usually bilateral pale gray lesions. This entity is often seen in association with trigeminal zoster or orolabial herpes simplex and is associated with an increased risk of retinal detachment.

ENDOCRINE AND METABOLIC ABNORMALITIES Disorders of these types are frequently seen in HIV-infected individuals. The most common abnormality is hyponatremia, seen in up to 30 percent of patients. This is usually related to the syndrome of inappropriate antidiuretic hormone (vasopressin) secretion (SIADH) as a consequence of increased free water intake and decreased free water excretion (see Chap. 49). SIADH is generally seen in the context of pulmonary or CNS disease. A second cause of hyponatremia is adrenal insufficiency; the presence of a low serum sodium level combined with a high serum potassium level should alert one to this possibility. Although most HIV-infected individuals studied at autopsy had involvement of the adrenal gland, less than 10 percent had prior evidence of adrenal insufficiency. CMV is the most common cause of adrenal gland disease in HIV infection. Other causes include mycobacterial infections, Kaposi's sarcoma, cryptococcal disease, histoplasmosis, and ketoconazole toxicity.

Hypogonadism Hypogonadism is seen in approximately 50 percent of HIV-infected individuals and is generally a complication of the underlying illness. Testicular dysfunction may also be induced by ganciclovir therapy. In several surveys, 67 percent of patients with HIV infection reported decreased libido and 33 percent complained of impotence. Twenty-five percent of women with HIV infection in African studies were amenorrheic. Thyroid function is generally normal, despite histologic evidence of thyroid gland involvement with several pathologic processes, including Kaposi's sarcoma and infection with CMV, *Cryptococcus neoformans*, or *Pneumocystis carinii*.

PANCREATITIS As noted above, pancreatitis leading to abnormalities of glucose metabolism may be seen in HIV-infected individuals; however, this is most often due to complications of therapy with either pentamidine or dideoxynucleosides.

GENERALIZED WASTING Generalized wasting, defined as involuntary weight loss of greater than 10 percent associated with intermittent or constant fever and chronic diarrhea or fatigue lasting more than 30 days in the absence of a defined cause other than HIV infection, is an AIDS-defining condition (Table 308-11). It is the initial AIDS-defining illness in 9 percent of patients with AIDS in the United States and, thus, is currently the leading initial clinical indication of AIDS. A constant feature of this syndrome is major muscle wasting with scattered myofiber degeneration and occasional evidence of myositis. Glucocorticoids may be of some benefit; however, this approach must be carefully weighed against the risk of compounding the immunodeficiency of HIV infection. While similar findings may be seen with CMV disease or MAC bacteremia in the setting of advanced HIV infection, the generalized wasting syndrome appears to be a true direct effect of HIV. Androgenic steroids, growth hormone, and total parental nutrition have been used as therapeutic interventions with variable success.

IDIOPATHIC CD4+ T LYMPHOCYTOPENIA

A syndrome was recognized in 1992 that was characterized by an absolute CD4+ T cell count of less than 300/μL or less than 20 percent of total T cells on more than one occasion, no evidence of HIV-1, HIV-2, HTLV-I, or HTLV-II on testing, and the absence of any defined immunodeficiency or therapy associated with decreased levels of CD4+ T cells. By mid-1993, approximately 100 patients had been described. After extensive multicenter investigations, a series of reports were published in early 1993 which together allowed a number of conclusions. Idiopathic CD4+ lymphocytopenia (ICL) is a very rare syndrome, as determined by studies of blood donors and cohorts of HIV-seronegative homosexual men. Cases were clearly identified as early as 1983, and cases remarkably similar to ICL had been identified decades ago. The definition of ICL based on CD4+ T cell counts coincided with the ready availability of testing for CD4+ T cells in patients suspected of being immunosuppressed. Although, as a result of immunosuppression, certain patients with ICL develop some of the opportunistic diseases, particularly cryptococcosis, seen in HIV-infected patients, the syndrome is demographically, clinically, and immunologically unlike HIV infection and AIDS. Less than half of the ICL patients had risk factors for HIV infection, and there were wide geographic and age distributions. The fact that a significant proportion of patients did have risk factors probably reflects a selection bias, in that physicians who take care of HIV-infected patients are more likely to monitor CD4+ T cells. Approximately one-third of the patients are women, compared to 14 percent of women among HIV-infected individuals in the United States. Many patients with ICL remained clinically stable, and their condition did not progressively deteriorate as is common with seriously immunodeficient HIV-infected patients. Certain patients with ICL even experienced spontaneous reversal of the CD4+ T lymphocytopenia. Immunologic abnormalities in ICL are somewhat different from those of HIV infection. ICL patients often also have decreases in CD8+ T cells and in B cells. Furthermore, immunoglobulin levels were either normal or, more commonly, decreased in patients with ICL, compared to the usual hypergammaglobulinemia of HIV-infected individuals. Finally, virologic studies revealed no evidence of HIV-1, HIV-2, HTLV-I, or HTLV-II or of any other mononuclear cell–tropic virus. Furthermore, there was no epidemiologic evidence to suggest that a transmissible microbe was involved. The cases of ICL were widely dispersed, with no clustering. Close contacts and sexual partners who were studied were clinically well and were serologically, immunologically, and virologically negative for HIV. ICL is a heterogeneous syndrome, and it is highly likely that there is no common cause; however, there may be common causes among subgroups of patients that are currently unrecognized.

Patients who present with laboratory data consistent with ICL should be worked up for underlying diseases that could be responsible for the immunosuppression. If no underlying cause is detected, no specific therapy should be initiated. However, if opportunistic diseases occur, they should be treated appropriately (see above). Depending on the level of the CD4+ T cell count, patients should receive prophylaxis for the commonly encountered opportunistic infections.

TREATMENT OF HIV INFECTION AND ITS COMPLICATIONS

GENERAL PRINCIPLES OF PATIENT MANAGEMENT The treatment of patients with HIV infection requires not only a comprehensive knowledge of the possible disease processes but also the ability to deal with the problems of a chronic, life-threatening illness. Specific antiretroviral therapy and antimicrobial treatment and prophylaxis are critical measures in prolonging an acceptable quality of life; however, counseling and education are also of paramount importance in providing patients with optimal overall care. Patients must be educated about the potential transmission of their infection, including frank discussions concerning sexual practices and sharing of intravenous needles. The treating physician must not only be aware of the latest medications available for HIV infection and its complications but must also educate patients concerning the natural history of their illness and listen to and be sensitive to their fears and concerns. As with other diseases, therapeutic decisions should be made in consultation with the patient when possible and with the patient's proxy if the patient is incapable of making decisions. In this regard, it is recommended that all patients with HIV infection, and in particular those with less than 200 CD4+ T cells per microliter, designate a trusted individual with durable power of attorney to make medical decisions on their behalf, if necessary.

No matter how well prepared a person feels for adversity, the discovery of a diagnosis of HIV infection is a devastating event. For this reason it is recommended that anyone about to undergo testing have "pretest counseling" to prepare them at least partially should the results be positive. Following a diagnosis of HIV infection, the physician should be prepared to activate support systems immediately for the newly diagnosed patient; these should include an experienced social worker or nurse who can spend time talking to the person and ensuring that he or she is emotionally stable. Most communities have HIV crisis centers that can be of great help in these difficult situations.

Following a diagnosis of HIV infection, there are several examinations and laboratory studies that should be performed to help determine the extent of disease and provide baseline standards for future reference. In addition to routine chemistry, hematology screening panels, and chest x-ray, one should also obtain a CD4+ T cell count, two separate plasma HIV RNA levels, a VDRL test, and an anti-*Toxoplasma* antibody titer. A PPD skin test should be done and a Mini-Mental Status Examination performed and recorded (Table 308-18). In addition, patients should be counseled with regard to sexual practices and needle sharing, and counseling should be offered to those whom the patient knows or suspects may also be infected. Once these baseline activities are performed, short-term and long-term medical management strategies should be based on the most recent information and modified as new information becomes available.

ANTIRETROVIRAL THERAPY The cornerstone of medical management of HIV infection is antiretroviral therapy. Suppression of HIV replication is an important component in prolonging life as well as in improving the quality of life of patients with HIV infection. Many questions currently lack definitive answers, including when antiretroviral therapy should be started, what is the best regimen to start with, when therapy should be changed, and what it should be changed to. Nonetheless, the physician and patient must come to a mutually agreeable plan based on the best available data. At present an extensive clinical trials network, involving both clinical investigators and patient advocates, is in place, attempting to develop improved approaches to therapy. Consortia comprising representatives of academia, industry, and the governments of the United States and other nations are involved in the process of drug development and clinical trials. As a result, new therapies and new therapeutic strategies are continually emerging; in addition, new drugs are often available through expanded access programs prior to official licensure. For these reasons, management of patients with HIV infection is best accomplished primarily by or with significant input from someone who is an expert in the field.

Nucleoside Analogues *Zidovudine* Zidovudine (AZT; 3′-azido-2′,3′-dideoxythymidine) was the first drug approved for the treatment of HIV infection and is the prototype drug for the class of compounds referred to as nucleoside analogues (Table 308-26). These compounds, in which the hydroxyl group in the 3′ position of the ribose moiety is substituted with a hydrogen or other chemical group, act as DNA chain terminators owing to their inability to form a 3′-5′ phosphodiester linkage with another nucleoside. They bind much more avidly to the active site of the RNA-dependent DNA polymerase of HIV (reverse transcriptase) than to the active site of mammalian cell DNA polymerases. This fact may, at least in part, explain their selective effect on HIV replication. Zidovudine also has a relatively high avidity for the DNA polymerase γ of human mitochondria, which may contribute to the development of the myopathy sometimes observed in patients receiving zidovudine. The active form of zidovudine is the triphosphate, and the rate of phosphorylation, a thymidine kinase–dependent pathway, may be different in different cells. This may explain why zidovudine is more effective at inhibiting HIV replication in some cells than others. Zidovudine is well absorbed orally, with a serum half-life of approximately 1 h. Hence, the earliest dosing regimens employed an every-4-h (five times daily) schedule. Given that the intracellular half-life may be much longer than the plasma half-life (as is also true for didanosine; see below), the rationale for this dosing schedule is unsubstantiated, and a variety of more convenient schedules involving twice- or thrice-daily dosing are often employed, particularly when zidovudine is given as part of a combination regimen.

The clinical efficacy of zidovudine was clearly established in a phase II, placebo-controlled trial in which 282 patients who had either experienced a single bout of PCP or had a variety of AIDS-associated symptoms were randomized to receive either placebo or zidovudine at a dose of 200 mg every 4 h. The trial was stopped prematurely when it became clear that there were far fewer deaths and far fewer new opportunistic infections among the patients receiving zidovudine. In addition to this clinical benefit, patients treated with zidovudine had increases in lymphocyte counts, including CD4+ T cell counts, declines in circulating levels of p24 antigen, and weight gain. In subsequent trials, a beneficial effect was also noted in patients with neurologic disease. Considerable controversy arose regarding the use of zidovudine as monotherapy in asymptomatic HIV-infected individuals with CD4+ T cell counts greater than 200/μL. Initial studies indicated that elevations of CD4+ T cell counts resulted from this approach. At that time, the CD4+ T cell count was thought to be an adequate surrogate marker for monitoring antiretroviral therapy. However, subsequent studies demonstrated that this approach offered no clinical benefit over waiting until there was clear evidence of disease progression. Thus, these studies called into question the relevancy of CD4+ T cell counts as surrogate markers for monitoring therapy. In addition, it became clear that zidovudine monotherapy was not associated with a clear-cut clinical benefit in asymptomatic HIV-infected individuals with CD4+ T cell counts greater than 200/μL. More recent data have demonstrated that combination regimens of nucleosides are more effective than zidovudine monotherapy, and, at present, zidovudine is most appropriately used as part of combination antiretroviral therapy for patients with HIV infection and less than 500 CD4+ T cells per microliter and as monotherapy for the prevention of maternal-fetal transmission of HIV infection. These recommendations are based on the U.S. Food and Drug Administration (FDA) approval and licensure process, which in turn is based solely on the results of controlled clinical trials. Only such trials can indicate whether antiretroviral therapy should be started earlier than the point at which CD4+ T cell counts reach 500/μL. It should be pointed out that plasma levels of HIV RNA are assuming increasing importance in the decision as to when to initiate and/or modify antiretroviral therapy (see below).

A great deal of effort has been directed toward defining the optimal dose of zidovudine. While the earliest clinical trials employing doses of 1200 mg/d showed benefit, there was also substantial toxicity. Subsequent trials have demonstrated that doses as low as 400 to 600 mg/d are as effective as higher-dose regimens and significantly less toxic. At present, the dose usually employed is 200 mg three times a day in combination with other antiretroviral agents. The use of zidovudine monotherapy is currently restricted to the prevention of maternal-fetal transmission of HIV. Given the considerable advantage of combination regimens over monotherapy in other clinical settings, it is highly likely that combination regimens will also prove more effective in the prevention of maternal-fetal transmission and that recommendations for therapy in this setting will change accordingly.

While many patients experience fatigue, malaise, nausea, and headache on initiation of zidovudine therapy, these side effects often subside over time. The major toxicities of zidovudine involve the bone marrow. Patients often develop a macrocytic anemia which, when associated with low serum erythropoietin levels, may be ameliorated somewhat by injections of recombinant erythropoietin beginning at a dose of 100 μg/kg three times a week. Although zidovudine-induced anemia is macrocytic, there is no evidence that deficiencies in vitamin B_{12} or folate play a role; exogenous administration of these vitamins is of no benefit. In addition to anemia, patients receiving zidovudine, especially patients with advanced disease, may experience neutropenia and in some cases thrombocytopenia. Other common toxicities of zidovudine include a proximal myopathy characterized by weakness, muscle wasting, and in some patients an elevation in creatine kinase, which is felt to be secondary to mitochondrial dysfunction. This mechanism of action has also been postulated to play a role in some forms of zidovudine-associated cardiomyopathy, as well as in some cases of lactic acidosis associated with fatty infiltration of the liver. A bluish discoloration of the nails, which is particularly noticeable in black patients, has been observed. An increased incidence of tumors of the vaginal epithelium has been found in rodents treated with extremely high doses of zidovudine. In addition, in transplacental carcinogenicity studies, an increase in solid tumors occurred in adult mice whose mothers were treated with high doses of zidovudine during pregnancy. However, no increases in cancers in HIV-infected patients have thus far been attributed to zidovudine therapy. Given these potential side effects, it is recommended that patients starting therapy with zidovudine be monitored for toxicity at least every other week for the first month and then monthly.

Considerable concern has been raised over the existence of strains of HIV that are resistant to zidovudine. These have usually been identified in patients receiving zidovudine for periods of 6 months or longer; however, they have also been reported in isolates obtained at the time of seroconversion. Resistance emerges more rapidly in late-stage patients, in whom there is presumably a greater degree of viral replication and thus more chance for mutation. This resistance is secondary to mutations in the HIV reverse transcriptase; at least five different mutations have been identified that are associated with zidovudine resistance (codons Met41→Leu; Asp67→Asn; Lys70→Arg; Thr215→Tyr; and Phe/Lys219→Gln). While zidovudine resistance is not associated with resistance to either didanosine or zalcitabine, patients treated with zidovudine monotherapy are often less responsive to subsequent therapy with nucleoside analogues. The emergence of zidovudine-resistant strains of HIV certainly contributes to the limited long-term usefulness of this drug as monotherapy and provides a strong rationale for the use of combination regimens.

Didanosine Didanosine (ddI; 2′,3′-dideoxyinosine) was the second drug licensed for the treatment of HIV infection. In a series of open trials, didanosine therapy resulted in increases in CD4+ T cell counts and declines in p24 antigen levels. Licensure was based on the demonstration in a controlled, randomized trial that patients who had received zidovudine for a minimum of 16 weeks and were switched to didanosine experienced increases in CD4+ T cell counts and fewer

Table 308-26 Antiretroviral Drugs Used in the Treatment of HIV Infection

Drug	Status	Indication	Dose as Monotherapy	Dose in Combination	Supporting Data	Toxicity
REVERSE TRANSCRIPTASE INHIBITORS						
Zidovudine (AZT, azidothymidine, Retrovir, 3′azido-3′-deoxythymidine)	Licensed	Treatment of HIV infection when antiretroviral therapy is indicated	Not indicated	200 mg q8h	19 vs 1 death in original placebo-controlled trial in 281 patients with AIDS or ARC Decreased progression to AIDS in patients with CD4+ T cell counts <500/μL, n = 2051	Anemia, granulocytopenia, myopathy, lactic acidosis, hepatomegaly with steatosis, headache, nausea
		Prevention of maternal-fetal HIV transmission	*Mother:* 100 mg 5id until the start of labor, then 2 mg/kg over 1 h IV, followed by 1 mg/kg/h IV until clamping of umbilical cord; *Infant:* 2 mg/kg PO q6h beginning within 12 h birth, or 1.5 mg/kg IV over 30 min q6h		In pregnant women with CD4+ T cell count ≥200/μL, AZT PO beginning at weeks 14–34 of gestation plus IV drug during labor and delivery plus PO AZT to infant for 6 wk decreased transmission of HIV by 67.5% (from 25.5% to 8.3%), n = 363	
Didanosine (ddI, dideoxyinosine, Videx, 2′,3′-dideoxyinosine)	Licensed	For treatment of HIV infection when antiretroviral therapy is warranted	Not indicated	Requires 2 tablets to achieve adequate buffering of stomach acid; should be administered on an empty stomach ≥60 kg: 200 mg bid <60 kg: 125 mg bid	Clinically superior to AZT as monotherapy in 913 patients with prior AZT therapy. Clinically superior to AZT and comparable to AZT + ddI and AZT + ddC in 1067 AZT-naive patients with CD4+ T cell counts of 200–500/μL	Pancreatitis, peripheral neuropathy, abnormalities on liver function tests
Zalcitabine (ddC, HIVID, 2′3′-dideoxycytidine)	Licensed	In combination with AZT for treatment of patients with limited prior exposure to AZT	Not indicated	0.75 mg tid	Clinically inferior to AZT monotherapy as initial treatment. Clinically as good as ddI in advanced patients intolerant to AZT. In combination with AZT, was clinically superior to AZT alone in patient with AIDS or CD4+ T cell count <350/μL	Peripheral neuropathy, pancreatitis, lactic acidosis, hepatomegaly with steatosis, oral ulcers
Stavudine (d4T, Zerit, 2′3′-didehydro-3′-dideoxythymidine)	Licensed	Treatment of HIV-infected patients who have received prolonged prior AZT therapy	Not indicated	≥60 kg: 40 mg bid <60 kg: 30 mg bid	Superior to AZT with respect to changes in CD4+ T cell counts in 359 patients who had received ≥24 wk of AZT	Peripheral neuropathy, pancreatitis
Lamivudine (Epivir, 2′3′-dideoxy-3′-thiacytidine, 3TC)	Licensed	In combination with AZT for the treatment of HIV infection when treatment is indicated	Not indicated	150 mg bid	Lamivudine + AZT superior to AZT alone with regard to virologic and immunologic parameters. 54% decrease in progression to AIDS/death compared to AZT alone	Minimal toxicity

(continued)

Drug	Status	Indication	Dose as Monotherapy	Dose in Combination	Supporting Data	Toxicity
Abacavir (1592-U89; Ziagen)	Licensed	For treatment of HIV infection in combination with other antiretroviral agents	Not indicated	300 mg bid	Abacavir + AZT + 3TC equivalent to indinavir + AZT + 3TC with regard to viral load suppression and CD4 + T cell increase at 24 weeks	Hypersensitivity reaction, rash, nausea, vomiting, malaise, headache, diarrhea, loss of appetite
Delavirdine (Rescriptor)	Licensed	For use in combination with appropriate antiretroviral agents when treatment is warranted	Not indicated	400 mg tid	Increase in CD4+ T cell counts, decrease in HIV RNA when used in combination with nucleosides	Skin rash, abnormalities in liver function tests
Nevirapine (Viramune)	Licensed	In combination with nucleoside analogues for treatment of progressive HIV infection	Not indicated	200 mg qd x 14 days then 200 mg bid	Increases in CD4+ T cell count, decrease in HIV RNA when used in combination with nucleosides	Skin rash, abnormalities in liver function tests
Efavirenz (DMP-266; Sustiva)	Licensed	For treatment of HIV infection in combination with other antiretroviral agents	Not indicated	600 mg qHS	Efavirenz + AZT + 3TC comparable to indinavir + AZT + 3TC with regard to viral load suppression and CD4 cell increases at 24 weeks	Rash, CNS symptoms, abnormalities in liver function tests
Adefovir (Preveon)	Expanded access (1-800-445-3235)					
PROTEASE INHIBITORS						
Saquinavir mesylate (Invirase, hard gel capsule)	Licensed	In combination with other antiretroviral agents when therapy is warranted	Not indicated	600 mg q8h	Increases in CD4+ T cell counts, reduction in HIV RNA most pronounced in combination therapy with ddC. 50% reduction in first AIDS-defining event or death in combination with ddC compared to either agent alone.	Nausea
(Fortovase, soft gel capsule)	Licensed	For use in combination with other antiretroviral agents when treatment is warranted	Not indicated	1200 mg tid	Reducation in mortality rate and AIDS-defining events for patients who received hard gel formulation in combination with ddc	Diarrhea, nausea, abdominal pain, headaches
Ritonavir (Norvir)	Licensed	In combination with nucleoside analogues for treatment of HIV infection when treatment is warranted	Not indicated	600 mg bid	Reduction in the cumulative incidence of clinical progression or death from 34% to 17% in patients with CD4+ T cell count <100/μL treated for a median of 6 months	Nausea, abdominal pain, may alter levels of many other drugs, including saquinavir
Indinavir sulfate (Crixivan)	Licensed	For treatment of HIV infection when antiretroviral treatment is warranted	Not indicated	800 mg q8h 1000 mg q8h with nevirapine 400–600 mg q8h with delavirdine	Increase in CD4+ T cell count by 100/μL and 2-log decrease in HIV RNA levels when given in combination with AZT and lamivudine	Nephrolithiasis, indirect hyperbilirubinemia
Nelfinavir mesylate (Viracept)	Licensed	For treatment of HIV infection when antiretroviral therapy is warranted	Not indicated	750 mg tid	2.0-log decline in HIV RNA when given in combination with stavudine	Diarrhea, loose stools
Amprenavir (141-W94; agenerase)	Licensed	For treatment of HIV infection in combination with other antiretroviral agents	Not indicated	1200 mg bid	Amprenavir + AZT + 3TC superior to AZT + 3TC with regard to viral load suppression in treatment-naive patients	Rash, Stevens-Johnson syndrome, nausea, vomiting, diarrhea, paresthesia, mood alteration

new opportunistic infections compared to patients remaining on zidovudine. Two randomized trials comparing zidovudine to didanosine as initial therapy yielded different results. In the first study, zidovudine was found to be superior to didanosine as initial therapy. In the second study, involving a larger number of patients, didanosine was found to be superior to zidovudine with respect to survival and to development of AIDS-defining illnesses (Table 308-26). At present, didanosine is an FDA-approved agent for any patient with HIV infection who has received prolonged zidovudine therapy or as initial therapy in patients with less than 500 CD4+ T cells/μL. While this is the licensed indication, the more common practice is to initiate therapy with didanosine as part of a combination regimen. As is the case with most antiretroviral drugs, strains of HIV that are resistant to didanosine emerge in patients receiving the drug. At least some of these isolates, occurring in patients who had originally developed zidovudine-resistant isolates as a consequence of prior zidovudine therapy, have regained some degree of sensitivity to zidovudine. Strains of HIV that are resistant to didanosine are generally also resistant to zalcitabine.

The standard dose of didanosine is 200 mg twice a day for patients over 60 kg and 125 mg twice a day for patients under 60 kg. Didanosine is best absorbed on an empty stomach at a neutral pH. For this reason, the current formulations of didanosine contain a buffer, and each dose must be administered in no less than two tablets. Thus, a patient who requires 100 mg twice a day should take two 50 mg tablets twice a day rather than one 100 mg tablet twice a day.

The toxicity profile of didanosine is quite different from that of zidovudine. The most frequent toxicity is a painful sensory peripheral neuropathy, which occurs in approximately 30 percent of patients receiving more than 200 mg twice a day; it generally resolves with discontinuation of drug and may not recur when the drug is resumed at a reduced dose. The other major toxicity is pancreatitis; it was reported to occur in 9 percent of patients in early clinical trials, although the frequency was somewhat less in later studies using lower doses. Pancreatitis can be fatal, and for this reason all patients receiving didanosine should be monitored carefully. Didanosine should be discontinued if a patient experiences abdominal pain consistent with pancreatitis or if an elevated serum level of amylase and/or lipase is found and ultrasound examination shows an edematous pancreas. Such patients should not be treated again with didanosine, and, in general, didanosine is contraindicated for patients with a prior history of pancreatitis, regardless of etiology. Didanosine has minimal effects on the bone marrow and can be given in combination with bone marrow–toxic drugs such as zidovudine, ganciclovir, and trimethoprim/sulfamethoxazole.

Zalcitabine Zalcitabine (ddC; 2′,3′-dideoxycytidine) was the third drug licensed for the treatment of HIV infection. It is officially licensed as monotherapy for patients who are intolerant of zidovudine or whose disease progresses while they are receiving zidovudine, and as part of a combination regimen with zidovudine as initial therapy for patients with CD4+ T cell counts of less than 500/μL (Table 308-26). The latter indication reflects the results of the first clinical trials designed to assess the efficacy of zalcitabine in the initial therapy of HIV infection. A direct comparison of zalcitabine to zidovudine was stopped prematurely when it was noted that significantly more deaths were occurring in the zalcitabine-treated group (59 vs. 33). In a separate trial, however, the combination of zalcitabine and zidovudine was shown to cause greater and more sustained elevations in CD4+ T cell counts than zidovudine alone. Based on these results, zalcitabine (0.75 mg/kg three times a day) was licensed as part of a combination regimen with zidovudine (200 mg three times a day) for patients with advanced HIV infection. Subsequent trials in the United States and Europe (Table 308-26) have demonstrated the clinical superiority of this combination over zidovudine alone. As for didanosine, the major toxicity of zalcitabine is a reversible peripheral neuropathy. While cases of pancreatitis have been reported in patients receiving zalcitabine, it has not been observed to the same degree as with didanosine. Nonetheless, zalcitabine is also contraindicated in patients with a prior history of pancreatitis. The zidovudine/zalcitabine combination regimen is an option for the initial treatment of HIV infection. As in the case of other nucleoside analogues, the development of resistant strains of HIV is a common problem. Among the mutations in reverse transcriptase associated with resistance to zalcitabine are Lys65→Arg or Asn; Leu74→Val; Thr69→Asp; Val75→Thr; Met184→Val; and Tyr215→Cys. These mutations may also result in resistance to other nucleosides, including zidovudine, didanosine, stavudine, and lamivudine.

Stavudine Stavudine (d4T; 2′,3′-didehydro-3′-deoxythymidine) was the fourth nucleoside analogue licensed for the treatment of HIV infection. This agent is currently indicated for treatment of adults with advanced HIV disease who are intolerant of approved therapies with known clinical benefit or whose disease has progressed while they were receiving other therapies (Table 308-26). In preclinical studies, stavudine had an activity profile comparable to that of zidovudine. It demonstrates cross-resistance to ddI by mechanisms that have not yet been elucidated in vitro. Its activity is additive to that of ddI and in some situations antagonistic to that of zidovudine. For this reason, one should avoid the use of this agent in combination with zidovudine until definitive clinical data are available. Thus far, clinical trials have demonstrated that stavudine therapy is associated with increases in CD4+ T cell counts, declines in p24 antigen levels, and an improved sense of well-being. In a study of 359 zidovudine-experienced patients randomized to remain on zidovudine or switch to stavudine, the CD4+ T cell count in the patients who switched to stavudine increased by 22/μL, while in those remaining on zidovudine, it decreased by 22/μL. In contrast to zidovudine, stavudine appears to have minimal myelosuppressive toxicity. Peripheral neuropathy and elevations in the serum level of glutamic pyruvic transaminase have been the primary toxicities observed to date.

Lamivudine Lamivudine (3TC; 2′,3′-dideoxy-3′-thiacytidine) is the fifth of the nucleoside analogues to be licensed in the United States. This cytidine analogue is licensed for use only in combination with zidovudine in situations where zidovudine is indicated. However, it is often used as part of other combinations (Table 308-26). The broad language incorporated into the licensure of lamivudine reflects the increasing complexity of the field of antiretroviral therapy and acknowledges the fact that it will be impossible to test formally every monotherapy and combination regimen in every potential therapeutic setting. The combination of zidovudine and lamivudine in vitro is the most potent combination of nucleosides studied to date and is felt by many experts to be the preferred nucleoside combination. This potency may be due in part to the fact that strains of HIV that are resistant to lamivudine (Met184→Val) have an increased sensitivity to zidovudine, so that the development of dual resistance is more difficult. Another potential advantage of the combination regimen is the fact that some lamivudine-resistant mutants of the HIV reverse transcriptase are less able to generate errors in reverse transcription, thus potentially slowing the mutation rate of the virus. Licensure of this agent was based on laboratory data. Patients receiving the combination of zidovudine and lamivudine had increases in CD4+ T cell counts that were in the range of 40 to 70/μL greater than that seen with monotherapy. It is the opinion of many experts in the field that this is the most potent combination of nucleosides and should be considered first-line therapy either alone or together with a protease inhibitor (see below) as initial antiretroviral therapy. However, clinical data are not yet available to support this approach. Although the main toxicities of lamivudine are peripheral neuropathy and pancreatitis, it is among the best tolerated of the nucleoside analogues.

Nonnucleoside Reverse Transcriptase Inhibitors The nonnucleoside reverse transcriptase inhibitors interfere with the function of the viral enzyme reverse transcriptase by binding to regions outside the active site and causing conformational changes in the enzyme that render it inactive. Although these agents are potent in the nanomolar range, they are also very selective for the reverse transcriptase of HIV-1, have no activity against HIV-2, and, when used as monotherapy, are associated with the rapid emergence of drug-resistant mutants (Table 308-26). Two members of this class, *nevirapine* and *delavirdine*, are currently available for use. Nevirapine is licensed for use in combination with nucleoside analogues for the treatment of HIV-infected adults who have experienced clinical and/or immunologic deterioration. Delavirdine is licensed for use in combination with appropriate anti-HIV medications to treat patients with HIV infection when treatment is warranted. The main toxicities of these drugs are a maculopapular rash that generally resolves without the need for discontinuation of therapy and elevations in hepatic enzyme levels. In order to decrease the incidence of rash associated with nevirapine, it is recommended that it be given at a starting dose of 200 mg once a day for 2 weeks, followed by the full dose of 200 mg twice daily. When administered as part of combination regimens with nucleoside analogues, these agents lead to increases in CD4+ T cell counts and decreases in viral burden that are slightly greater and longer-lasting than those observed with nucleosides alone. These agents may play a valuable role in future multidrug combinations involving nucleosides and protease inhibitors.

Protease Inhibitors The licensure of four separate HIV-1 protease inhibitors (saquinavir, ritonavir, indinavir, and nelfinavir) heralded a major change in the options available for antiretroviral therapy of HIV infection. Unlike reverse transcriptase inhibitors, which interfere with cellular DNA polymerases as well as inhibiting the reverse transcriptase of HIV-1, the HIV protease inhibitors are exquisitely selective for the protease enzyme of HIV-1. These compounds are active in the nanomolar range and, thus far, are considerably less toxic than the reverse transcriptase inhibitors. Unfortunately, as in the case of the nonnucleoside reverse transcriptase inhibitors, this potency is accompanied by the rapid emergence of resistant isolates when these drugs are used alone. Thus, these compounds should be used in combination with other antiretroviral drugs.

Saquinavir Saquinavir was the first of the protease inhibitor compounds to be licensed (Table 308-26). In patients who had discontinued or were unable to take zidovudine, treatment with the combination of saquinavir and zalcitabine resulted in greater increases in CD4+ T cell counts and more pronounced decreases in plasma levels of HIV RNA than were seen with either agent alone. Subsequent clinical data revealed that at approximately 500 days of follow-up, there was a 50 percent decrease in the risk of either a first AIDS-defining event or death (rates of 15 percent, 27 percent, and 24 percent for saquinavir plus zalcitabine, zalcitabine alone, and saquinavir alone, respectively). Saquinavir is licensed to be given in combination with nucleoside analogues for the treatment of advanced HIV disease. Genotypic and/or phenotypic resistance to saquinavir has been observed in approximately 45 percent of patients. Viral resistance to the protease inhibitors is quite complex. Among the mutations in the HIV-1 protease codons associated with resistance to saquinavir are Leu90→Met and Gly48→Val. Of note is the fact that strains of HIV that are resistant to saquinavir are generally not resistant to either indinavir or ritonavir, suggesting that combination therapy with different protease inhibitors may be of considerable value. This possibility must be approached with caution, however, since saquinavir is metabolized by the cytochrome P450 system, and ritonavir therapy results in an inhibition of cytochrome P450 action. Thus, when both drugs are administered together, there is the potential for unpredictable increases in saquinavir levels. Of the first three protease inhibitors licensed for use in patients with HIV infection, saquinavir is among the better tolerated; however, it appears to be the least potent (Fig. 308-31).

Ritonavir Ritonavir is licensed for the treatment of HIV infection when treatment is warranted, either as monotherapy or in combination with nucleoside analogues. It was the first protease inhibitor for which clinical efficacy was demonstrated (Table 308-26). In a study of 1090 patients with CD4+ T cell counts less than 100/μL who were randomized to receive either placebo or ritonavir in addition to any other licensed medications, patients receiving ritonavir had a reduction in the cumulative incidence of clinical progression or death from 34 percent to 17 percent. Mortality decreased from 10.1 percent to 5.8 percent. Resistance to ritonavir has been associated with a variety of amino acid substitutions. Among them, a Val82→Phe substitution appears to be necessary but not sufficient for the development of phenotypic resistance. Other common mutations that have been described are Ile84→Val, Ala71→Val, and Met46→Ile. Strains of HIV-1 that are resistant to ritonavir are resistant to indinavir. The main side effects of ritonavir are nausea, diarrhea, abdominal pain, and circumoral paresthesias; these can be reduced somewhat by initiating therapy at 300 mg bid and then rapidly escalating the dose over 5 days to the full dose of 600 mg bid. Ritonavir has a high affinity for several isoforms of cytochrome P450, and thus it can produce large increases in the plasma concentrations of drugs metabolized by this pathway. Among the agents affected in this manner are saquinavir, macrolide antibiotics, R-warfarin, ondansetron, rifampin, most calcium channel blockers, glucocorticoids, and some of the chemotherapeutic agents used to treat Kaposi's sarcoma. In addition, ritonavir may increase the activity of glucuronyltransferases, thus decreasing the levels of drugs metabolized by this pathway. Overall, great care must be taken when prescribing additional drugs to patients taking ritonavir. Ritonavir is more potent than saquinavir, but it is generally the most poorly tolerated of these drugs because of the gastrointestinal side effects.

Indinavir Indinavir was the third protease inhibitor licensed for the treatment of HIV-1 infection. It is indicated for the treatment of HIV infection in adults in whom antiretroviral therapy is warranted (Table 308-26). As in the case of saquinavir, this indication is based on laboratory data demonstrating substantial increases in CD4+ T cell counts and reductions in plasma levels of HIV RNA during therapy. The strongest results were observed in treatment regimens that included zidovudine and lamivudine. Resistance to indinavir has been associated with over 10 different amino acid substitutions. Isolates of HIV-1 that are resistant to indinavir show cross-resistance to ritonavir and variable degrees of cross-resistance to saquinavir. The main side effects of indinavir are nephrolithiasis (seen in 4 percent of patients) and asymptomatic indirect hyperbilirubinemia (seen in 10 percent of patients). Indinavir is metabolized mainly by the liver, and the dose should be lowered in patients with cirrhosis. It shares metabolic pathways with terfenadine, astemizole, cisapride, triazolam, and midazolam. For this reason, these drugs should not be administered to patients taking indinavir, to avoid the potential for cardiac arrhythmias or prolonged sedation. Similarly, levels of indinavir are decreased during concurrent therapy with rifabutin and increased during concurrent therapy with ketoconazole. Dosages should be modified when these circumstances arise. Acidic conditions in the stomach favor the absorption of indinavir but decrease the availability of didanosine. Both are best absorbed on an empty stomach. Thus, when these drugs are prescribed together, they should be administered at different times. Compared to saquinavir and ritonavir, indinavir is both well tolerated and quite potent.

Nelfinavir Nelfinavir (Viracept) was approved early in March 1997 for the treatment of adult or pediatric HIV infection when antiretroviral therapy is warranted. This approval was based upon analysis of surrogate markers. In approximately 300 patients who had not previously received antiretroviral therapy, the combination of zidovudine, lamivudine, and nelfinavir (750 mg three times a day) resulted in an average decrease of at least 98 percent in viral load and a CD4 cell increase of 150 cells/μL. At present, no clinical data are available. Mild diarrhea, seen in approximately 20 percent of patients, is the main side effect.

℞ TREATMENT

Choice of Antiretroviral Treatment Strategy The large number of available antiretroviral agents coupled with a relative paucity of clinical end point studies make the subject of antiretroviral therapy one of the more controversial in the management of HIV-infected individuals. The relative merits of different therapeutic strategies should be discussed with the patient throughout the course of the illness, and new findings should be incorporated as they are reported. It is clear from our knowledge of the pathogenesis of HIV infection that there is a sufficient rationale for attempting to suppress viral replication from the time of initial infection. Indeed, the limited data on the treatment of patients with the acute seroconversion syndrome suggest that immediate intervention is of value in delaying the progression of disease. Unfortunately, at present, it is unclear whether currently available drugs are either potent enough or safe enough to be used over an indefinite period in multidrug combinations. The obvious hope is that virus replication will be suppressed to a low enough level and for long enough that the residual or regenerated immune system would be able to protect the patient from opportunistic diseases indefinitely. The best approach for this goal is unclear at present. For this reason, a variety of antiretroviral treatment strategies are currently employed. In an attempt to provide a range of potential approaches to therapy of the HIV-infected individual, we present a conservative approach, an aggressive approach, and our current approach (Table 308-27). The reader should bear in mind that the field of HIV therapeutics is evolving so rapidly that new drugs and new information on the use of currently available drugs may call for substantial modifications of the recommendations given. Nonetheless, the principles delineated will likely remain constant.

A *conservative approach*, which uses only strategies that have been shown to be of clinical benefit, would generally involve withholding antiretroviral therapy until the CD4+ T cell count falls below 500/μL. A choice would then be made among the proven options of didanosine monotherapy, zidovudine plus didanosine, zidovudine plus zalcitabine, and zidovudine plus lamivudine. The chosen regimen would be used until the disease demonstrated progression, as defined by a fall in the CD4+ T cell count below 200/μL. Therapy would then be changed. While a wide array of choices for the new regimen are available, the most prudent would seem to be one containing one or two new nucleosides and a protease inhibitor.

An *aggressive approach* would involve using combination therapy from the time of diagnosis of HIV infection. If the therapeutic decision were based on surrogate marker data, one option would be to use a combination of zidovudine, lamivudine, and indinavir. The patient would be monitored carefully for changes in CD4+ T cell count and plasma levels of HIV RNA. Evidence of increased disease activity, defined as a 0.5 log increase in plasma levels of HIV RNA or a 25 percent decrease in the CD4+ T cell count, would indicate that it was time for a change in therapy. Options would include the use of other nucleosides in combination with saquinavir; a combination of nucleosides, saquinavir, and ritonavir; and possibly the addition of a nonnucleoside reverse transcriptase inhibitor.

The *current approach of the authors* falls between these two options and is influenced by the fact that the median time from infection to clinical disease is 10 years and that some patients, particularly those with low levels of plasma viremia (Fig. 308-22), may do extremely well without therapy for extended periods of time. For the asymptomatic patient with a stable CD4+ T cell count of more than 500/μL and plasma viremia less than 20,000 copies of HIV RNA per milliliter, we would not treat but would perform repeat evaluations every 6 months. If the plasma levels of HIV RNA are greater than 20,000 copies per milliliter or the CD4+ T cell count is less than 500/μL, or if the patient is symptomatic, or if there is indication of progressive disease, therapy with two nucleosides and a protease inhibitor would be initiated. The goal of therapy, once begun, is to decrease plasma viremia as low as possible for as long as possible. We would then monitor the patient every 3 to 4 months. Therapy would be modified to replace the current regimen with two new nucleosides or one new nucleoside and a nonnucleoside in combination with one or two different protease inhibitors if the plasma HIV level rose above the baseline by 0.5 log or the CD4+ T cell count fell by more than 25 percent. The same holds true for a new patient whose care we assume and who is already receiving antiretroviral therapy. In the rare setting of diagnosing a patient with the acute retroviral syndrome, we would treat with two nucleosides and a protease inhibitor. This regimen should be continued for at least 1 year; many experts would continue treatment indefinitely. Definitive recommendations await the results of clinical trials. In any event, the patient should be evaluated every 3 to 4 months following initiation of therapy, and changes in therapy instituted where appropriate as indicated above.

Experimental Antiretroviral Agents In addition to the licensed drugs discussed above, a large number of experimental agents are being evaluated as possible therapies for HIV infection. Therapeutic strategies are being directed at virtually every step of the viral life cycle (Fig. 308-3). In addition, as more is learned about the role of the immune system in controlling viral replication, additional strategies, generically called *immune-based therapies*, are being developed as a complement to antiviral therapy. Among the antiviral agents in early clinical trials are additional nucleoside analogues, nucleotide analogues, additional protease inhibitors, integrase inhibitors, and antisense nucleic acids. Among the immune-based therapies being tested are IFNα, bone marrow transplantation with adoptive

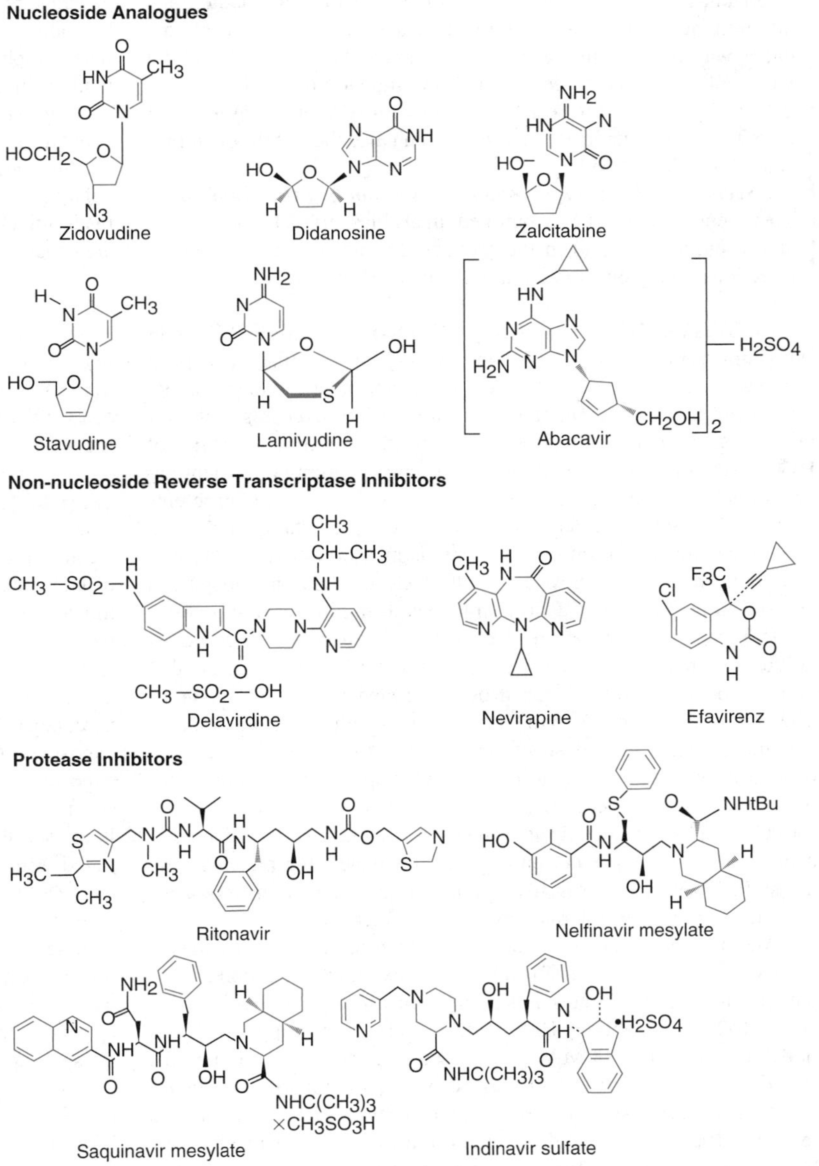

FIGURE 308-31 Molecular structures of antiretroviral agents.

Table 308-27

Different Antiviral Treatment Strategies*

	Aggressive	Conservative
When to start	Time of diagnosis	CD4+ T cell count <500/μL
What to start with	AZT plus lamivudine plus protease inhibitor	Didanosine AZT plus zalcitabine AZT plus didanosine AZT plus lamivudine
When to change	0.5-log increase in HIV RNA or 10% decrease in CD4+ T cell count	CD4+ T cell count <200/μL
What to change to	Two new nucleosides (or a new nucleoside and a nonnucleoside) plus a new protease inhibitor	Two new nucleosides plus a protease inhibitor

* See text for current approach of the authors.

transfer of lymphocytes, thymic implants, active immunotherapy with subunit envelope vaccines or autologous cells genetically engineered to express viral proteins, passive immunotherapy with inactivated anti-HIV antisera or HIV-specific monoclonal antibodies, and intermittent administration of IL-2. In addition, clinical trials are under way that use the techniques of molecular biology to inhibit HIV replication and spread through the infusion of CD4+ T cells genetically modified to resist infection with HIV or the infusion of CD8+ T cells genetically modified to enhance their ability to eliminate HIV-infected cells.

Secondary Infections, Kaposi's Sarcoma, and Lymphomas Treatment guidelines are outlined in Tables 308-21 and 308-23 and discussed in detail in the sections dealing with the secondary infections and neoplastic complications of HIV infection.

PROPHYLAXIS AGAINST SECONDARY INFECTIONS The improvements in survival and quality of life that have been achieved in patients with HIV infection are due not only to the introduction of antiretroviral compounds but also to improved regimens for preventing secondary infections. As a result, the clinical profile of HIV-infected patients is continually evolving as immunodeficient patients live longer and are at less risk of formerly inevitable problems such as PCP. Some secondary infections occur predictably only when the competence of the immune system, as measured by the CD4+ T cell count, has fallen below a certain level, and this knowledge can be used to help devise effective strategies to minimize these risks.

PCP rarely occurs before the CD4+ T cell count drops below 200/μL or the CD4 percentage declines below 15 percent. At that point, patients should be started on a regimen of PCP prophylaxis. The preferred regimen, for patients who can tolerate it, is trimethoprim/sulfamethoxazole at a dose of one double-strength tablet daily. A benefit of this regimen is that it also provides protection against toxoplasmosis as well as certain bacterial infections. Alternative strategies for PCP prophylaxis include dapsone/pyrimethamine and clindamycin/primaquine. These are currently being evaluated for patients who are sulfa intolerant. Aerosolized pentamidine remains an option for individuals unable to tolerate any systemic therapy.

Another opportunistic infection for which primary prophylaxis is clearly indicated is MAC. This infection is extremely common among patients in the United States; it is rarely seen with CD4+ T cell counts above 100/μL. Rifabutin, 100 mg/d, was effective in a clinical trial in delaying the onset of MAC bacteremia by an average of 6 months. Based on these data, rifabutin has been licensed for use as primary prophylaxis for MAC infection in patients with HIV infection and less than 100 CD4+ T cells per microliter. Even better results have been seen with the macrolides clarithyomycin and azithromycin. The median survival for patients receiving clarithromycin prophylaxis was >700 days, compared to 573 days for those receiving rifabutin. In a separate study, patients receiving azithromycin prophylaxis had an overall mortality of 10.5 percent, compared to 31 percent for those taking rifabutin. Of interest is the recent observation that patients with prior tuberculosis seem to have a decreased incidence of MAC. This finding raises the idea that it may be possible to develop a prophylactic vaccine for this complication.

Given the resurgence of tuberculosis in the HIV-infected population, any patient with HIV infection and at least 5 mm of induration upon PPD skin testing should receive a 1-year course of isoniazid. In addition, any patient with HIV infection who is anergic and at high risk of tuberculosis should be given 1 year of isoniazid therapy. These measures could be quite effective not only in helping the patient but also in curtailing the spread of tuberculosis in the community. All patients with tuberculosis should be treated with directly observed therapy to increase the chance of eradicating the infection and minimizing the risk of spread.

Patients with HIV infection are at increased risk for infection with encapsulated bacteria, particularly *H. influenzae* and *S. pneumoniae*. For this reason, these patients, and especially those in whom splenectomy is being considered, should be given the pneumococcal polysaccharide vaccine and possibly also the *H. influenzae* type b vaccine.

While no generally accepted guidelines exist, many physicians recommend primary prophylaxis against cryptococcal and candidal infections with fluconazole; clinical trials of a candidate cryptococcal vaccine are under way. In addition, clinical trials are being conducted to evaluate the role of intermittent clindamycin/pyrimethamine as primary prophylaxis for toxoplasmosis in patients unable to tolerate trimethoprim/sulfamethoxazole. Patients who are seronegative for *Toxoplasma gondii* should be encouraged to avoid ingestion of partially cooked meat and to use care when handling cat litter.

Secondary prophylaxis—the prevention of second or subsequent episodes of a given infection—is indicated for virtually every opportunistic infection experienced by patients with AIDS. These infections are usually impossible to eradicate and, with the exception of tuberculosis, life-long therapy or secondary prophylaxis is the rule (see Table 308-21). It is obvious that as the number of medications given to a patient increases, so do the chances of untoward drug reactions and interactions. Thus, patients must be monitored carefully for such reactions. However, the judicious use of prophylactic regimens clearly can yield a significant improvement in the quality and duration of life for the HIV-infected patient with advanced immunodeficiency.

HIV AND THE HEALTH CARE WORKER

Health care workers, especially those who deal with large numbers of HIV-infected patients, have a small but definite risk of becoming infected with HIV as a result of professional activities. By 1997, there were a total of 52 well-documented seroconversions in health care workers that occurred as a direct result of exposure to contaminated blood or bloody body fluids. Forty-five of these infections were due to percutaneous exposures, five were associated with mucous membrane exposures, one involved both percutaneous and mucous membrane exposures, and in one the route of exposure was unknown. Forty-seven of these accidents involved blood, one involved bloody pleural fluid, one involved an unspecified fluid, and three involved concentrated virus stocks. In addition, another 111 HIV-infected heath care workers have been identified with no identifiable risk for HIV infection other than possible occupational exposure. Taken together, the data from several large studies suggest that the risk of HIV infection following a percutaneous injury with an HIV-contaminated hollow-bore needle (in contrast to a solid-bore needle, i.e., a suture needle) is approximately 0.3 percent. A seroprevalence survey of 3420 orthopedic surgeons, 75 percent of whom practiced in an area with a relatively high prevalence of HIV infection and 39 percent of whom reported percutaneous exposure to patient blood, usually through an accident involving a suture needle, failed to reveal any cases of possible occupational infection, suggesting that the risk of infection with a suture needle may be considerably less than that with a blood-drawing needle.

Most cases of health care worker seroconversion occur as a result of needle-stick injuries. When one considers the circumstances that result in needle-stick injuries, it is immediately obvious that adhering to the standard guidelines for dealing with sharp objects would result in a significant decrease in this type of accident. In one study, 27 percent of needle-stick injuries resulted from improper disposal of the needle (over half of these were due to recapping the needle), 23 percent occurred during attempts to start an intravenous line, 22 percent occurred during blood drawing, 16 percent were associated with an intramuscular or subcutaneous injection, and 12 percent were associated with giving an intravenous infusion.

There is debate concerning the best management for a percutaneous injury with a needle contaminated with blood from an HIV-infected patient. The wound should be cleansed immediately and antiseptic applied. While there are multiple anecdotes of heath care workers who have seroconverted despite immediately beginning zidovudine prophylaxis, a case-control study among health care workers revealed that zidovudine postexposure prophylaxis was associated with a 79 percent decrease in the risk for HIV seroconversion after percutaneous exposure to HIV-infected blood. Based on this finding, a United States Public Health Service working group recommended that chemoprophylaxis be given after occupational exposure. While the precise regimen remains a topic of debate and will undoubtedly evolve, the authors currently recommend a combination of zidovudine, lamivudine, and indinavir. The side effects in this setting are considerable. In one study, 70 percent of health care workers taking zidovudine for postexposure prophylaxis reported one or more side effects, particularly nausea, malaise, and headache. The ultimate decision must be individualized and reached after careful discussion between the injured health care worker and the physician. Since antiretroviral prophylaxis, if it is going to be given, should probably be started as soon as possible after the injury, health care workers at potential risk should think beforehand about what they want to do. Given the prevalence of zidovudine resistance in the community, many experts advocate the use of combination therapy under such circumstances. Even if postexposure treatment fails to prevent primary infection, it almost certainly will decrease the initial burst of viremia (see above), which may have a significant long-term benefit.

Health care workers can minimize their risk of occupational HIV infection by following the CDC guidelines of July 1991, which include adherence to universal precautions; refraining from direct patient care if one has exudative lesions or weeping dermatitis; and disinfecting and sterilizing reusable devices employed in invasive procedures. The premise of universal precautions is that every specimen should be handled as if it came from someone infected with a bloodborne pathogen. All samples should be double-bagged, gloves should be worn when drawing blood, and spills should be immediately disinfected with bleach.

In attempting to put this small but definite risk to the health care worker in perspective, it is important to point out that approximately 200 health care workers die each year as a result of occupationally acquired hepatitis B infection. The tragedy in this instance is that these infections and deaths due to hepatitis B could be greatly decreased by more extended use of the hepatitis B vaccine. The risk of hepatitis B infection following a needle-stick injury from a hepatitis antigen–positive patient is much higher than the risk of HIV infection (see "Transmission," above). There are multiple examples of needle-stick injuries where the patient was positive for both hepatitis B and HIV and the health care worker became infected only with hepatitis B. For these reasons, it is advisable, given the high prevalence of hepatitis B infection in HIV-infected individuals, that all health care workers dealing with HIV-infected patients be immunized with the hepatitis B vaccine.

Tuberculosis is another infection common to HIV-infected patients that can be transmitted to the health care worker. For this reason, all health care workers should know their PPD status, have it checked yearly, and receive one year of isoniazid treatment if their skin test converts to positive. In addition, all patients in whom a diagnosis of tuberculosis is being entertained should be placed immediately in respiratory isolation, pending results of the diagnostic evaluation. The emergence of drug-resistant organisms has made tuberculosis an increasing problem for health care workers. This is particularly true for the health care worker with preexisting HIV infection.

One of the most charged issues ever to come between health care workers and patients is that of transmission of infection from HIV-infected health care workers to their patients. By the end of 1992, the well-publicized case of the Florida dentist (see above) was the only known or suspected case of such transmission, despite extensive investigation, including the testing of over 8000 patients who had received care from HIV-infected dentists or surgeons. This puts the risk of acquiring HIV infection from a doctor or dentist during an exposure-prone procedure at less than 1/1,000,000. That is one-half the risk that a given unit of screened blood is HIV-positive and 1/100th the risk of dying from general anesthesia. Thus, this level of risk seems acceptable and is within the scope of other risks taken by patients in the context of receiving health care. Theoretically, the same universal precautions that are used to protect the health care worker from the HIV-infected patient will also protect the patient from the HIV-infected health care worker.

VACCINES

Given the fact that human behavior, especially human sexual behavior, is extremely difficult to change, the best hope for preventing the spread of HIV infection rests with the development of a safe and effective vaccine. This task is extremely problematic for a number of reasons, including the high mutability of the virus, the fact that the infection can be transmitted by cell-free or cell-associated virus, and the likely need for the development of effective mucosal immunity. The fact that some HIV-infected individuals are long-term nonprogressors (see above), as well as the fact that a number of individuals have been exposed to HIV multiple times but remain uninfected, suggest that there are protective elements of an HIV-specific immune response. In addition, studies using animal models have been encouraging and suggest that an HIV vaccine is possible. It should be pointed out that while the ideal goal of an HIV vaccine is to prevent infection, a vaccine given to an uninfected individual that significantly alters the course of disease or the infectivity of the individual, should that person become infected, could have an impact not only on the individual in question, but on the spread of infection in the community.

Preclinical work in the area of vaccine development has been greatly facilitated by the use of animal models of lentivirus infections. Perhaps the most useful model to date has been the simian immunodeficiency virus (SIV) infection of rhesus monkeys. SIV, a lentivirus that is closely related to HIV-2 and differs from HIV-1 in lacking a *vpu* gene and having a *vpx* gene, causes an acute infection that leads to immunodeficiency, secondary infections, and death when administered to susceptible animals. Studies by several groups have clearly demonstrated that infection can be prevented by prior immunization of animals with either inactivated virus, recombinant vaccinia virus expressing the SIV envelope protein followed by a booster immunization with recombinant protein, or attenuated virus lacking an intact *nef* gene. Even in studies using antigens that did not confer protection from infection, the progression of disease following infection appeared to be decreased. Of note is the fact that in those studies that demonstrated protection it was not always obvious what components of the immune response conferred the protection. In fact, in certain studies of inactivated virus vaccines it was shown that the protective elements of the immune response were not directed toward genetic components of the virus at all but toward components of the cells used in growing up the viral stocks, which were incorporated into the viral envelope as the particles budded from the infected cells. These data suggest that antibodies to certain cell-surface proteins that participate in SIV binding may provide excellent protection against infection, a hypothesis that has been supported in studies of CD4-immunized monkeys. While the protection studies carried out with envelope-expressing recombinant vaccinia virus and recombinant envelope boosting point to an immune response to the envelope as potentially protective, there is still much to be learned about the correlates of immunity involved in protection against infection and/or disease.

The most suitable animal model for HIV infection is the chimpanzee. However, chimpanzees are expensive, they are an endangered species, and although they can be infected with HIV, they rarely develop disease over 10 years of observation. Thus, unless a candidate vaccine prevents infection in this model, its impact on disease progression is difficult to assess. Most recently, however, immunization of chimps either with whole inactivated virus followed by protein or peptide boosting or with recombinant envelope proteins has been shown to confer protection against infection with HIV-1. These data from animal models suggest the feasibility of inducing at least partial protection against HIV infection in humans by vaccination.

While clear signals from the preclinical animal studies are awaited, clinical trials of candidate vaccines have begun in humans. Both recombinant envelope proteins and recombinant viruses expressing a number of HIV proteins have been demonstrated to be safe and immunogenic in healthy uninfected volunteers. Certain of these vaccines are also being tested as forms of active immunotherapy in patients who are already infected. Different vaccine strategies lead to different immune responses. Live-virus vaccines and DNA vaccines are strategies in which the viral antigens are synthesized within the human cell. These types of vaccines tend to promote cytotoxic T cell responses. Recombinant proteins or killed-virus vaccines tend to promote antibody responses. A combination of these strategies tends to promote both. At present, one can state with a fair degree of certainty that humans can safely be immunized to several of the antigens of HIV. One or more of these vaccines candidates will be tested in vaccine efficacy trials. It is clear, however, that it will take several years of clinical trials to establish the efficacy or lack thereof of a candidate vaccine for HIV.

PREVENTION

Education, counseling, and behavior modification are the cornerstones of an HIV prevention strategy. Widespread voluntary testing of individuals who have practiced or are practicing high-risk behavior, together with counseling of infected individuals, is recommended. Information gathered from such an approach should serve as the basis for behavior-modification programs, both for infected individuals who may be unaware of their HIV status and who could infect others and for uninfected individuals practicing high-risk behavior. The practice of safe sex is the most effective way for sexually active uninfected individuals to avoid contracting HIV infection and for infected individuals to avoid spreading infection. Abstinence from sexual relations is the only absolute way to prevent sexual transmission of HIV infection. However, this may not be feasible, and there are a number of relatively safe practices that can markedly decrease the chances of transmission of HIV infection. Partners engaged in monogamous sexual relationships who wish to be assured of safety should both be tested for HIV antibody. If both are negative, it must be understood that any divergence from monogamy puts both partners at risk; open discussion of the importance of honesty in such relationships should be encouraged. When the HIV status of either partner is not known, or when one partner is positive, there are a number of options. Use of condoms, preferably together with the HIV-inhibiting spermicide nonoxynol-9, can markedly decrease the chance of HIV transmission. It should be remembered that condoms are not 100 percent effective in preventing transmission of HIV infection, and there is an approximately 10 percent failure rate of condoms used for contraceptive purposes. Most condom failures result from breakage or improper usage, such as not wearing the condom for the entire period of intercourse. Latex condoms are preferable, since virus has been shown to leak through natural skin condoms. Petroleum-based gels should never be used for lubrication of the condom, since they increase the likelihood of condom rupture. Mutual masturbation is considered safe provided there is no oral or open-cut exposure to or ingestion of semen, vaginal secretions, or other potentially infected body fluids. There has been a tendency among homosexual men to practice fellatio as a "minimal risk" activity compared to receptive anal intercourse. It should be emphasized that receptive oral fellatio is definitely not safe sex, and there has been clear-cut documentation of transmission of HIV where receptive fellatio was the only sexual act performed (see "Transmission," above). Topical microbicides for vaginal use are being pursued actively as a means by which women could avoid infection when the male partner cannot be relied on to use a condom. Kissing is considered safe, although there is a theoretical possibility of transmission via virus in saliva. The low concentration of virus in saliva of infected individuals, as well as the presence in saliva of HIV-inhibitory proteins (see above), lessens any risk of transmission by kissing.

The most effective way to prevent transmission of HIV infection among IDUs is to stop the use of injecting drugs. Unfortunately, that is extremely difficult to accomplish unless the addict enters a treatment program. For those who will not or cannot participate in a drug treatment program and who will continue to inject drugs, the avoidance of sharing of needles and other paraphernalia ("works") is the next best way to avoid transmission of infection. The cultural and social factors that contribute to the sharing of paraphernalia are complex and difficult to overcome. In addition, needles and syringes may be in short supply. Under these circumstances, paraphernalia should be cleaned after each usage with a virucidal solution, such as undiluted sodium hypochlorite (household bleach). Data from a number of studies have indicated that programs that provide sterile needles to addicts in exchange for used needles have resulted in a decrease in HIV transmission without increasing the use of injection drugs. It is important for IDUs to be tested for HIV infection and counseled, to avoid transmission to their sexual partners. Secondary and tertiary spread of HIV infection by the heterosexual route within settings of a high level of injection drug use has increased greatly in the United States (see above).

Transmission of HIV via transfused blood or blood products has been decreased dramatically by a combination of screening of all blood donors for HIV infection by assays for both HIV antibody and p24 antigen and self-deferral of individuals at risk for HIV infection. In addition, clotting factor concentrates are heat-treated, essentially eliminating the risk to hemophiliacs who require these products. Autologous transfusions are preferable to transfusions from another individual. However, logistic constraints as well as the unpredictability of the need for most transfusions limit the feasibility of this approach. At present the risk of becoming HIV-infected from a contaminated blood transfusion is approximately 2 in 1 million.

HIV can be transmitted via breast milk and colostrum. The avoidance of breast feeding may not be practical in developing countries, where nutritional concerns override the risk of HIV transmission. However, it is becoming appreciated that transmission by breast milk accounts for a considerable proportion of infections in infants in developing countries who were born of HIV-infected mothers and who were fortunate enough not to have been infected intrapartum or peripartum. Therefore, even in developing countries, breast feeding from an infected mother should be avoided if at all possible. In developed countries such as the United States, where bottled formula and milk are readily accessible, breast feeding is absolutely contraindicated when a mother is HIV positive.

BIBLIOGRAPHY

Alkhatib G et al: CC CKR5: A RANTES, MIP-1α, MIP-1β receptor as a fusion cofactor for macrophage-tropic HIV-1. Science 272:1955, 1996

Bleul CC et al: The lymphocyte chemoattractant SDF-1 is a ligand for LESTR/fusin and blocks HIV-1 entry. Nature 382:829, 1996

Brodine SK et al: Detection of diverse HIV-1 genetic subtypes in the USA. Lancet 346:1198, 1995

Cao Y et al: Virologic and immunologic characterization of long-term survivors of human immunodeficiency virus type-1 infection. N Engl J Med 332:201, 1995

Carpenter CJ et al: Antiretroviral therapy for HIV infection in 1996. Recommendations of an international panel. JAMA 276:146, 1996

CENTERS FOR DISEASE CONTROL AND PREVENTION: Update: Trends in AIDS diagnosis and reporting under the expanded surveillance definition for adolescents and adults—United States, 1993. Morb Mort Week Rep 43:826, 1994

———: Update: Trends in AIDS among men who have sex with men—United States, 1989–1994. Morb Mort Week Rep 44:401, 1995

———: Update: Mortality attributable to HIV infection among persons aged 25–44 years. Morb Mort Week Rep 45:121, 1996

———: Provisional recommendations for chemoprophylaxis after occupational exposure to human immunodeficiency virus. Morb Mort Week Rep 45:468, 1996

CESARMAN E et al: Kaposi's sarcoma-associated herpesvirus-like DNA sequences in AIDS-related body-cavity-based lymphomas. N Engl J Med 332:1186, 1995

CHANG Y et al: Identification of herpes-like DNA sequences in AIDS-associated Kaposi's sarcoma. Science 266:1865, 1994

CHOE H et al: The β-chemokine receptors CCR3 and CCR5 facilitate infection by primary HIV-1 isolates. Cell 85:1135, 1996

CLARK SJ, SHAW GM: The acute retroviral syndrome and the pathogenesis of HIV-1 infection. Semin Immunol 5:149, 1993

CLERICI M, SHEARER GM: The Th-1-Th-2 hypothesis of HIV infection: New insights. Immunol Today 15:575, 1994

COCCHI F et al: Identification of RANTES, MIP-1α, and MIP-1β as the major HIV-suppressive factors produced by CD8+ T cells. Science 270:1811, 1995

COLLIER AC et al: Treatment for human immunodeficiency virus infection with saquinavir, zidovudine, and zalcitabine. N Engl J Med 334:1011, 1996

CONNOR EM et al: Reduction of maternal-infant transmission of human immunodeficiency virus type 1 with zidovudine treatment. N Engl J Med 331:1173, 1994

D'AQUILA RT et al: Nevirapine, zidovudine and didanosine compared with zidovudine and didanosine in patients with HIV-1 infection. A randomized, double-blind, placebo controlled trial. Ann Intern Med 124:1019, 1996

DEACON NJ et al: Genomic structure of an attenuated quasi species of HIV-1 from a blood transfusion donor and recipients. Science 270:988, 1995

DEEKS SG et al: HIV-1 protease inhibitors. A review for clinicians. JAMA 277:145, 1997

DENG HK et al: Identification of a major co-receptor for primary isolates of HIV-1. Nature 381:661, 1996

DESROSIERS RC, FAUCI AS: Retroviral pathogenesis, Part II, in *Retroviruses*, H Varmus et al (eds). Cold Spring Harbor, NY, Cold Spring Harbor Laboratory Press, 1996

DICKOVER RE et al: Identification of levels of maternal HIV-1 RNA associated with risk of perinatal transmission. Effect of maternal zidovudine treatment on viral load. JAMA 275:599, 1996

DORANZ BJ et al: A dual-tropic primary HIV-1 isolate that uses fusin and the β-chemokine receptors CKR5, CKR3, and CKR-2b as fusion cofactors. Cell 85:1149, 1996

DRAGIC T et al: HIV-1 entry into CD4+ cells is mediated by the chemokine receptor CC-CKR-5. Nature 381:667, 1996

EMERY S, LANE HC: Immune-based therapies in HIV infection: Recent developments. AIDS 10(Suppl A):S159, 1996

ENSOLI B et al: Synergy between basic fibroblast growth factor and HIV-1 Tat protein in induction of Kaposi's sarcoma. Nature 371:674, 1994

ERON JJ et al: Treatment with lamivudine, zidovudine, or both in HIV-positive patients with 200 to 500 CD4+ cells per cubic millimeter. N Engl J Med 333:1662, 1995

EUROPEAN COLLABORATIVE STUDY: Caesarean section and risk of vertical transmission of HIV-1 infection. Lancet 343:1464, 1994

FANG G et al: Maternal plasma human immunodeficiency virus type 1 RNA level: A determinant and project threshold for mother-to-child transmission. Proc Natl Acad Sci USA 92:12100, 1995

FAUCI AS: CD4+ T lymphocytopenia without HIV infection—no lights, no camera, just facts. N Engl J Med 328:429, 1993

———: Multifactorial nature of human immunodeficiency virus disease: Implications for therapy. Science 262:1011, 1993

———: An HIV vaccine: Breaking the paradigms. Proc Assoc Am Physicians 108:6, 1996

———: Host factors and the pathogenesis of HIV-induced disease. Nature 384:529, 1996

——— et al: Immunopathogenic mechanisms of HIV infection. Ann Intern Med 124:654, 1996

FONG IW et al: The natural history of progressive multifocal leukoencephalopathy in patients with AIDS. Clin Infect Dis 20:1305, 1995

GALLANT JE et al: Prophylaxis for opportunistic infections in patients with HIV infection. Ann Intern Med 120:932, 1994

GERBERDING JL: Management of occupational exposures to blood-borne viruses. N Engl J Med 332:444, 1995

HAYNES BF et al: Toward an understanding of the correlates of protective immunity to HIV infection. Science 271:324, 1996

HO DD et al: Rapid turnover of plasma virions and CD4 lymphocytes in HIV infection. Nature 373:123, 1995

HOLTZMAN DM et al: New-onset seizures associated with human immunodeficiency virus infection: Causation and clinical features in 100 cases. Am J Med 87:173, 1989

JACOBSEN H et al: In vivo resistance to human immunodeficiency virus type 1 proteinase inhibitor: Mutations, kinetics and frequencies. J Infect Dis 173:1379, 1996

KAPLAN JE et al: USPHS/IDSA guidelines for the prevention of opportunistic infections in persons infected with human immunodeficiency virus. Clin Infect Dis 21(Suppl 1):1, 1995

——— et al: 14-year followup of HIV-infected homosexual men with lymphadenopathy syndrome. J Acquired Immune Defic Syndr Hum Retrovirol 11:206, 1996

KASLOW RA et al: Influence of combinations of human major histocompatibility complex genes on the course of HIV-1 infection. Nature Med 2:405, 1996

KELEN GD et al: Trends in human immunodeficiency virus (HIV) infection among a patient population of an inner-city emergency department: Implications for emergency department-based screening programs for HIV infection. Clin Infect Dis 21:867, 1995

KINLOCH-DE LOES S et al: A controlled trial of zidovudine in primary human immunodeficiency virus infection. N Engl J Med 333:408, 1995

KIRCHHOFF F et al: Brief report: Absence of intact *nef* sequences in a long-term survivor with nonprogressive HIV-1 infection. N Engl J Med 332:228, 1995

KORBER BTM et al: Mutational trends in V3 loop protein sequences observed in different genetic lineages of human immunodeficiency virus type 1. J Virol 68:6730, 1994

KOVACS JA et al: Controlled trial of interleukin-2 infusions in patients infected with the human immunodeficiency virus. N Engl J Med 335:1350, 1996

KROWN SE et al: Kaposi's sarcoma in the acquired immunodeficiency syndrome: A proposal for a uniform evaluation, response and staging criteria. J Clin Oncol 7:1201, 1989

KUHN L et al: Cesarean deliveries and maternal-infant HIV transmission: Results from a prospective study in South Africa. J Acquired Immune Defic Syndr Hum Retrovirol 11:478, 1996

LACKRITZ EM et al: Estimated risk of HIV transmission by screened blood in the United States. N Engl J Med 333:1721, 1995

LANE HC et al: Recent advances in the management of AIDS-related opportunistic infections. Ann Intern Med 120:945, 1994

LEVY JA: Pathogenesis of human immunodeficiency virus infection. Microbiol Rev 57:183, 1993

LIU R et al: Homozygous defect in HIV-1 coreceptor accounts for resistance of some multiply-exposed individuals to HIV-1 infection. Cell 86:367, 1996

LUSSO P, GALLO RC: Human herpesvirus 6 in AIDS. Immunol Today 2:67, 1995

MANNHEIMER SB, SOAVE R: Protozoal infections in patients with AIDS. Cryptosporidiosis, isosporiasis, cyclosporiasis, and microsporidiosis. Infect Dis Clin North Am 8:483, 1994

MELLORS JW et al: Prognosis in HIV-1 infection predicted by the quantity of virus in plasma. Science 272:1167, 1996

MOORE PS, CHANG Y: Detection of herpesvirus-like DNA sequences in Kaposi's sarcoma in patients with and those without HIV infection. N Engl J Med 332:1181, 1995

MOORE RD, CHAISSON RE: Natural history of opportunistic diseases in an HIV-infected urban clinical cohort. Ann Intern Med 124:633, 1996

NDUATI RW et al: Human immunodeficiency virus type 1-infected cells in breast milk: Association with immunosuppression and vitamin A deficiency. J Infect Dis 172:1461, 1995

OBERLIN E et al: The CXC chemokine receptor SDF-1 is the ligand for LESTR/fusin and prevents infection by T-cell-line-adapted HIV-1. Nature 382:833, 1996

O'BRIEN WA et al: Changes in plasma HIV-1 RNA and CD4+ lymphocyte count and the risk of progression to AIDS. N Engl J Med 334:426, 1996

PANTALEO G et al: Studies in subjects with long-term nonprogressive human immunodeficiency virus infection. N Engl J Med 332:209, 1995

———, FAUCI AS: New concepts in the pathogenesis of HIV infection. Annu Rev Immunol 13:487, 1995

——— et al: HIV infection is active and progressive in lymphoid tissue during the clinically latent stage of disease. Nature 362:355, 1993

PECKHAM C, GIBB D: Mother-to-child transmission of the human immunodeficiency virus. N Engl J Med 333:298, 1995

PERELSON AS et al: HIV-1 dynamics in vivo: Virion clearance rate, infected cell life-span, and viral generation time. Science 271:1582, 1996

PIATAK M et al: High levels of HIV-1 in plasma during all stages of infection determined by competitive PCR. Science 259:1749, 1993

PRICE RW: Neurological complications of HIV infection. Lancet 348:445, 1996

REDFIELD RR et al: The Walter Reed staging classification for HTLV-III/LAV infection. N Engl J Med 314:131, 1986
ROBERTSON DL et al: Recombination in HIV-1. Nature 374:124, 1995
ROSENBERG PS: Scope of the AIDS epidemic in the United States. Science 270:1372, 1995
SAMSON M et al: Resistance to HIV-1 infection in Caucasian individuals bearing mutant alleles of the CCR-5 chemokine receptor gene. Nature 382:722, 1996
SCHACKER T et al: Clinical and epidemiologic features of primary HIV infection. Ann Intern Med 125:257, 1996
SMITH KJ et al: Cutaneous findings in HIV-1 positive patients: a 42-month prospective study. J Am Acad Dermatol 31:746, 1994
SPARANO JA: Treatment of AIDS-related lymphomas. Curr Opin Oncol 7:442, 1995
SPECTOR SA et al: Oral ganciclovir for the prevention of cytomegalovirus disease in persons with AIDS. N Engl J Med 334:1491, 1996
SOCA ACTG: Mortality in patients with the acquired immunodeficiency syndrome treated with either foscarnet or ganciclovir for cytomegalovirus retinitis. N Engl J Med 326:213, 1992
SOTO-RAMIREZ LE et al: HIV-1 Langerhans' cell tropism associated with heterosexual transmission of HIV. Science 271:1291, 1996
SPIRA AI et al: Cellular targets of infection and route of viral dissemination after an intravaginal inoculation of simian immunodeficiency virus into rhesus macaques. J Exp Med 183:215, 1996
STANLEY SK, FAUCI AS: T cell homeostasis in HIV infection: Part of the solution or part of the problem? J Acquired Immune Defic Syndr Hum Retrovirol 6:142, 1993
TINDALL B, COOPER DA: Primary HIV infection. Host responses and intervention strategies. AIDS 5:1, 1991
WALKER CM et al: CD8+ lymphocytes can control HIV infection in vitro by suppressing virus replication. Science 234:1563, 1986
WEI X et al: Viral dynamics in human immunodeficiency virus type 1 infection. Nature 373:117, 1995
WHALEN C et al: Accelerated course of human immunodeficiency virus infection after tuberculosis. Am J Respir Crit Care Med 151:129, 1995
ZINKERNAGEL RM et al: Immunology taught by viruses. Science 271:173, 1996

309

Jean D. Sipe, Alan S. Cohen

AMYLOIDOSIS

DEFINITION AND CLASSIFICATION *Amyloidosis* results from the deposition of insoluble, fibrous amyloid proteins, nearly always in the extracellular spaces of organs and tissues. Named by Virchow in 1854 on the basis of color after staining with iodine and sulfuric acid, all amyloid proteins share a unique fibrillar ultrastructure. Depending upon the biochemical nature of the amyloid precursor protein, amyloid fibrils can be deposited locally or may involve virtually every organ system of the body. Amyloid fibril deposition may have no apparent clinical consequences or may lead to severe pathophysiologic changes. Often the disease falls between these two extremes. Regardless of etiology, the clinical diagnosis of amyloidosis is usually not made until the disease is far advanced.

There are multiple clinically and biochemically distinct forms of amyloid that share a unique morphology and secondary structure; some are systemic and others are localized or organ-limited (Table 309-1). Although the fibril precursors differ in their amino acid sequences, the polypeptide backbones of these protein precursors assume an identical secondary structure, the β-pleated sheet conformation, and similar fibrillar morphologies that render them resistant to proteolysis. All amyloid deposits contain an identical nonfibrillar component, the pentraxin or serum amyloid P (SAP). The amyloidoses are classified according to the biochemical nature of the fibril-forming protein. *Systemic amyloidoses* include biochemically distinct forms that are neoplastic, inflammatory, genetic, or iatrogenic in origin, while *localized* or *organ-limited amyloidoses* are associated with aging and diabetes and occur in isolated organs, often endocrine, without evidence of systemic involvement.

Despite their biochemical and clinical differences, the various amyloidoses share common features. These include the presence of an amyloidogenic precursor in appropriate concentration; the appropriate genetic background of the host; abnormalities in proteolysis of fibril precursors and nascent amyloid fibrils; and alterations in extracellular matrix constituents such as glycosaminoglycans, together with the presence of amyloid-enhancing factor (AEF). The most recent guidelines for nomenclature and classification of amyloid and amyloidosis were recommended in 1990 by the Nomenclature Committee of the International Society for Amyloidosis. Amyloid deposits should be classified using the capital letter A as the first letter of designation followed by the protein designation without any open space; for example, AL for amyloidosis involving immunoglobulin light chains (Table 309-1).

ETIOLOGY AND PATHOGENESIS **Light Chain Amyloidosis (AL)** The most common form of systemic amyloidosis seen in current clinical practice is AL (primary idiopathic amyloidosis, or that associated with multiple myeloma) resulting from fibril formation by monoclonal antibody light chains in primary amyloidosis and in some cases of multiple myeloma (see Chap. 114). Less than 20 percent of patients with AL have myeloma. The rest have other monoclonal gammopathies, light chain disease, or even agammablobulinemia (producing light chains, but not intact immunoglobulin). About 15 to 20 percent of patients with myeloma have amyloidosis. A monoclonal population of bone marrow plasma cells is present and consistently produces either small lambda or kappa fragments or immunoglobulins that are processed (cleaved) in an abnormal fashion by macrophage enzymes to produce the partially degraded light chains responsible for AL amyloidosis. Lambda chain class predominates over kappa in AL by a 2:1 ratio, whereas in multiple myeloma and normal immunoglobulin synthesis, the reverse is true. Indeed, almost all lambda VI family chains have been associated with amyloid. The primary structure of each amyloid-forming light chain is unique, reflecting the features of the B cell clone that produced it. In patients with multiple myeloma, light chains can be deposited as casts in kidney tubules or as punctate deposits on basement membranes. Also, nonfibrillar amyloid deposition diseases have been described; thus there are three forms of human light chain–associated renal and systemic diseases: AL amyloidosis, cast nephropathy, and light chain deposition disease. Rarely, heavy chain amyloid deposition has been reported.

Amyloid A Amyloidosis (AA) AA amyloidosis (secondary, reactive, or acquired amyloidosis) occurs most frequently as a complication of chronic inflammatory disease. Effective treatment of the underlying inflammatory condition has reduced incidence in developed countries. In the past in the United States, tuberculosis (see Chap. 171), osteomyelitis (see Chap. 132), and leprosy (see Chap. 172) were the most common precipitating diseases, and they remain so in developing countries. Familial deposition of the AA protein occurs in some groups of patients with familial Mediterranean fever (FMF) (see Chap. 288). However colchicine treatment has been very effective in reducing the incidence of AA amyloidosis in association with FMF. During inflammation, proinflammatory cytokines such as interleukin (IL) 1, IL-6, and tumor necrosis factor stimulate the synthesis in liver of serum amyloid A (apoSAA), a transient, injury-specific component of high-density lipoprotein (HDL). Thus, effective treatment of the underlying inflammatory disorder blocks the stimulus for precursor synthesis. SAA, the final protein product, is a chemokine, a chemoattractant cytokine that amplifies an inflammatory response.

Heredofamilial Amyloidoses Until the advent of biochemical studies, there was no generally accepted nosology for the heredofamilial amyloid syndromes. Some researchers emphasized the site of predominant organ involvement, classifying the disease as neuropathic, nephropathic, or cardiopathic amyloidosis, while others stressed the genetic aspects. With one exception, the amyloidosis of FMF, which is inherited as an autosomal recessive disorder and is an AA type of amyloid, the mode of inheritance of the heredofamilial amyloidoses is autosomal dominant. FMF is a disorder subdivided into phenotype I, with irregularly occurring fever and abdominal, chest, or joint pain, preceding or accompanying renal amyloid; and phenotype II, in which renal amyloidosis is the first or only manifestation of the disease (see

Chap. 288). Colchicine treatment prevents attacks of FMF and appears to prevent subsequent deposition of amyloid either by blocking precursor apoSAA production or by blocking AEF formation.

The heredofamilial amyloidoses primarily involve the nervous system. Familial amyloid polyneuropathies (FAP) are dominant hereditary diseases affecting kinships originating in Portugal, Japan, Sweden, Finland, Greece, Italy, and elsewhere. FAP can be subclassified based on clinical symptoms and the biochemical nature of the fibrils; in nearly all cases the fibrils are variants of transthyretin (TTR), apolipoprotein AI, gelsolin, cystatin C, and rarely the α chain of fibrinogen A or lysozyme. FAP are autosomal dominant conditions in which the mutant proteins, although present from birth, result in a delayed onset of disease symptoms, usually after three to seven decades of life. The FAP prototype is the lower limb neuropathy first described in Portugal, which has a poor prognosis and is characterized by progressively severe neuropathy, including marked autonomic nervous system involvement. In some of these individuals, bilateral "scalloped" pupils are pathognomonic of the disease.

ATTR The most frequently occurring form of FAP involves TTR, a 14-kDa protein originally described as prealbumin, that transports thyroxine and retinol-binding protein in the blood. The first mutation to be identified in Portuguese families and in families of Swedish origin was a single amino acid substitution, methionine for valine at position 30. To date, more than 50 TTR variants have been defined. Variant TTR gene carriers exhibit clinically heterogeneous amyloidoses according to the position and nature of the amino acid substitution. Substitution of proline for leucine at position 55 results in an early onset and rapidly progressing disease, whereas substitution of methionine for threonine at position 119 appears to protect against amyloid fibril formation. In Denmark, patients with a methionine substitution for leucine at position 111 have a severe cardiopathy. Nonpathogenic TTR mutants such as the substitution of serine for glycine at position 6 also exist, and several are associated with changes in association with retinol-binding protein.

AApoAI An autosomal dominant form of hereditary amyloidosis results from deposition of an apolipoprotein AI variant in which arginine is substituted for glycine at position 26 or for tryptophan at position 50 or for leucine at position 60. Gene carriers exhibit low levels of HDL and exhibit peripheral neuropathy that is clinically similar to the type of familial amyloidosis that is caused by variants of TTR. Another kindred carrying the same mutation presents clinically with renal failure but without neurologic symptoms.

AGel Two mutations at position 187, within the actin-binding domain of gelsolin, are associated with a unique form of hereditary systemic amyloidosis. Gelsolin is a calcium-binding protein that binds to and fragments actin filaments. The disease has been reported primarily in Finland but also in patients of Japanese and Dutch backgrounds. Fibrils of gelsolin fragments are deposited in blood vessels and basement membranes, leading to clinical manifestations of lattice corneal dystrophy and cranial neuropathy, followed by peripheral neuropathy, dystrophic skin changes, and involvement of other organs.

ALys Hereditary nonneuropathic systemic amyloidosis has been described in English families in which lysozyme is the major fibril protein. Two mutations have been described: one in which threonine is substituted for isoleucine at position 56, and the second in which histidine is substituted for aspartic acid at position 67.

AFib Hereditary nonneuropathic renal amyloidosis has been described in families with mutations in the fibrinogen A α chains.

Aβ_2M Deposition of β_2-microglobulin as amyloid fibrils in the musculoskeletal system can occur in the presence of renal problems that require long-term hemodialysis usually with cuprophane membranes. β_2-microglobulin contains a significant amount of β-pleated sheet structure and is thought to form amyloid fibrils because of high local concentrations of the precursor protein.

Localized or Organ-Limited Amyloidoses Depending upon the biochemical nature of the amyloid fibril protein, instead of systemic deposition involving the cardiovascular and gastrointestinal systems along with lymph nodes, spleen, liver, kidneys, and adrenals, amyloid deposition may be limited to a single organ such as the pancreas, brain, or heart.

Polypeptide hormone–derived amyloidosis Polypeptide hormone–derived amyloid deposits are common in polypeptide hormone–producing tissues and tumors. Calcitonin is deposited in the hereditary amyloid syndrome, medullary carcinoma of the thyroid (ACal) (see Chap. 331). Also AANF (atrial natriuretic factor–derived) amyloid deposits are found in the sarcolemma of ~80 percent of persons over 80 years of age. AIAPP (islet amyloid polypeptide–derived, or amylin) is deposited as amyloid fibrils in >90 percent of individuals with type 2 diabetes (see Chap. 334), in endocrine tumors (see Chap. 95), and in insulinoma (see Chap. 95). It is produced in β cells of the pancreas and stored and released together with insulin. Human insulin does not naturally form amyloid fibrils, although fibrils of porcine insulin, AIns, are sometimes found as subcutaneous nodules at sites of insulin injection in diabetic individuals.

Amyloidosis associated with Alzheimer's disease Alzheimer's disease (AD) is characterized by three lesions in the brain, i.e., senile or neuritic plaques, neurofibrillary tangles, and vascular lesions (see

Table 309-1

Abbreviated Classification of Amyloid

Amyloid Protein	Protein Precursor	Clinical Syndrome
AA	apoSAA	Reactive (secondary) Familial Mediterranean fever Muckle-Wells syndrome
AL	Igλ, Igκ	Idiopathic (primary) Multiple myeloma Local nodular
AH	γ1 heavy chain	Macroglobulinemia
Aβ_2M	β_2 microglobulin	Chronic hemodialysis arthropathy
Aβ	β-protein precursor	Alzheimer's disease Down's syndrome Hereditary cerebral angiopathy with bleeding (Dutch)
$APrP^{Sc}$	Prion protein	Creutzfeldt-Jakob disease Gerstmann-Straussler syndrome Kuru
AIAPP	Amyloid insulin polypeptide	Diabetes mellitus type 2 Insulinoma
AANF	Atrial natriuretic factor	Senile cardiac amyloid
ATTR	Transthyretin	FAP; multiple point mutations Senile systemic cardiac
AGel	Gelsolin	FAP-Finnish
AApoA1	Apolipoprotein A1	FAP-Iowa (Irish)
ACys	Cystatin C	Hereditary cerebral angiopathy with bleeding (Iceland)
AFibA	Fibrinogen A α	Nonneuropathic hereditary amyloid with renal disease
ALys	Lysozyme	Nonneuropathic hereditary amyloid with renal disease

Chap. 367). A novel protein, β-amyloid protein (Aβ), is the major fibril protein in the amyloid deposits of the cerebrovascular walls and the cores of neuritic plaques of AD patients and also in individuals with Down's syndrome (see Chap. 66). The intracellular neurofibrillary tangles are composed of paired helical filaments arranged in a twisted conformation and have as their major component an abnormally phosphorylated τ-protein, a microtubule-associated protein that, in spite of its intracellular localization, is sometimes considered to be amyloid in nature, i.e., APHF. Aβ varies in length from 39 to 43 amino acids and is derived from a large transmembrane glycoprotein called amyloid β-precursor protein (AβPP). Mutations in AβPP are associated with familial AD and also with a different type of amyloidosis, hereditary cerebral hemorrhage with amyloidosis (Dutch type).

Scrapie-associated prion proteins Prions are a unique class of infectious proteins associated with a group of neurodegenerative diseases, the transmissible spongiform encephalopathies. In humans, these diseases include kuru, Creutzfeldt-Jakob disease, Gerstmann-Straussler-Scheinker syndrome, and fatal familial insomnia (see Chap. 379); in animals, scrapie and bovine spongiform encephalopathy (mad cow disease). PrP^{Sc} is a pathogenic, transmissible spongiform encephalopathy-specific form of the host-encoded prion protein (PrP); PrP^{Sc} differs from PrP in that it contains a high amount of β-pleated sheet structure and is insoluble and resistant to proteolytic enzymes. PrP^{Sc} deposits either consist of or can be readily converted to amyloid fibrils. APrP is similar to Aβ and ATTR in that both familial and sporadic forms occur. It has been suggested that the earlier onset familial forms of amyloidosis are due to accelerated fibril formation from mutant precursors, whereas in sporadic cases, amyloid fibrils are formed more slowly from normal precursor molecules. The mutant PrP molecules are nearer the threshold for transition to the amyloidogenic PrP^{Sc} than are the normal. The transition from normal to amyloidogenic PrP^{Sc} is irreversible but very slow. The disease progresses because, once formed, amyloidogenic PrP^{Sc} can seed the conversion of normal molecules into an amyloidogenic form.

CLINICAL MANIFESTATIONS The clinical manifestations of amyloidosis are varied and depend entirely on the biochemical nature of the fibril protein and thus the area of the body that is involved (Table 309-2). The diagnosis of amyloidosis is usually not made until after the point of irreversible organ damage. Proteinuria is often the first symptom associated with systemic amyloidosis, particularly of the AA and AL type; peripheral neuropathies are associated with FAP, and dementia and cognitive dysfunction with amyloid deposits in brain. Organ enlargement, especially of the liver, kidney, spleen, and heart, may be prominent; however, this does not occur in FAP, AD, or PrP.

Table 309-2

Clinical Presentation of Systemic Amyloidosis

Disease	Symptoms
AL (primary)	Monoclonal immunoglobulin in urine or serum plus any of the following: Unexplained nephrotic syndrome Hepatomegaly Carpal tunnel syndrome Macroglossia Malabsorption or unexplained diarrhea or constipation Peripheral neuropathy Cardiomyopathy
AA (secondary)	Chronic infection (osteomyelitis, tuberculosis) or chronic inflammation (rheumatoid arthritis, granulomatous ileitis) plus development of any of the following: Proteinuria Hepatomegaly Unexplained gastrointestinal disease
Hereditary amyloidosis	Family history of neuropathy plus any of the following: Early sensorimotor disassociation Vitreous opacities Renal disease Autonomic nervous system symptoms Cardiovascular disease Gastrointestinal disease

Kidney Renal involvement may consist of mild proteinuria or frank nephrosis. In some cases, the urinary sediment may show a few red blood cells. The renal lesion is usually not reversible and in time leads to progressive azotemia and death. The prognosis does not appear to be related to the degree of the proteinuria; when azotemia finally develops, the prognosis is grave. Treatment by peritoneal or hemodialysis or kidney transplantation improves the prognosis considerably. Hypertension is rare, except in long-standing amyloidosis. Renal tubular acidosis or renal vein thrombosis may occur. Localized accumulation of amyloid may be noted in the ureter, bladder, or other parts of the genitourinary tract.

Heart With respect to systemic amyloidoses, cardiac amyloidosis is common in primary (AL) and heredofamilial amyloidosis and very rare in the secondary (AA) form. With respect to localized amyloidosis, cardiac amyloidosis of the TTR type is common after 80 years of age; also atrial natriuretic factor may be present in the atria. In systemic amyloidosis, cardiac manifestations consist primarily of congestive failure and cardiomegaly (with or without murmurs) and a variety of arrhythmias and are comparable in AL and FAP, the predominant forms with cardiomyopathy (see Chap. 239). Although these manifestations predominantly reflect diffuse myocardial amyloid, the endocardium, valves, and pericardium may also be involved. Pericarditis with effusion is rare, although the differential diagnosis of constrictive pericarditis versus restrictive cardiomyopathy frequently arises. Echocardiography has demonstrated symmetric thickening of the left ventricular wall; hypokinesia and decreased systolic contraction and thickening of the interventricular septum and left ventricular posterior wall; and left ventricular cavities of small to normal size. Two-dimensional echocardiography produces the characteristic findings of thickened right and left ventricles, a normal left ventricular cavity, and, especially, a diffuse hyperrefractile "granular sparkling" appearance. Hearts that are heavily infiltrated with amyloid may or may not show an enlarged silhouette. Fluoroscopy usually shows decreased mobility of the ventricular wall; angiographic studies usually demonstrate thickened ventricular wall, decreased ventricular mobility, and absence of rapid ventricular filling in early diastole. Cardiac amyloidosis can present as intractable heart failure. Electrocardiographic abnormalities include a low-voltage QRS complex and abnormalities in atrioventricular and intraventricular conduction, often resulting in varying degrees of heart block. Owing to their propensity to develop conduction defects and arrhythmias, patients with cardiac amyloidosis appear to be especially sensitive to digitalis, and this drug should be used with caution.

Liver While hepatic involvement is common except in heredofamilial amyloidosis of the TTR type, liver function abnormalities are minimal and occur late in the disease. Portal hypertension occurs but is uncommon. Intrahepatic cholestasis has been noted in about 5 percent of patients with AL (primary) amyloidosis. Hepatomegaly is common, and AL hepatic amyloid is usually accompanied by the nephrotic syndrome and congestive heart failure. Prognosis is poor, and one group of 80 patients with proven severe AL hepatic amyloid had a median survival of 9 months. Amyloidosis of the spleen characteristically is not associated with leukopenia and anemia.

Skin Involvement of the skin is one of the most characteristic manifestations of primary (AL) amyloidosis (see Chap. 57). Other forms of amyloidosis such as lichen amyloidosis are thought to involve forms of keratin. In AL amyloidosis, the lesions may consist of slightly raised, waxy papules or plaques that usually are clustered in the folds of the axillae, anal, or inguinal regions, the face and neck, or mucosal areas such as ear or tongue. Periorbital ecchymoses ("black eye" or "raccoon syndrome") have been reported. The lesions are seldom pruritic. Involvement of the skin or mucosa may not be apparent clinically but may induce bleeding into the skin, leading to purpura.

Cutaneous involvement can also be seen on biopsy in secondary amyloidosis; in one series it was found in 42 percent of such patients, in 55 percent of a group of patients with primary disease, and in all 11 patients with hereditary amyloid neuropathy.

Gastrointestinal Tract Gastrointestinal symptoms are common in all systemic types of amyloidosis. They may result from direct involvement of the gastrointestinal tract at any level or from infiltration of the autonomic nervous system with amyloid. The symptoms include those of obstruction, ulceration, malabsorption, hemorrhage, protein loss, and diarrhea (see Chap. 285). Infiltration of the tongue occasionally leads to macroglossia. When not enlarged, the tongue may become stiffened and firm to palpation. Infiltration of the tongue is characteristic of primary amyloidosis (AL) or amyloidosis accompanying multiple myeloma. Gastrointestinal bleeding may occur from any of a number of sites, notably the esophagus, stomach, or large intestine, and may be severe. Amyloid infiltration of the esophagus may lead to an incompetent or nonrelaxing lower esophageal sphincter, nonspecific motility disorders of the esophageal body, or rarely achalasia. Small-bowel lesions may lead to clinical and x-ray changes of obstruction. A malabsorption syndrome is common. Amyloidosis (AA or secondary) may also develop in association with other entities involving the gastrointestinal tract, especially tuberculosis (see Chap. 171), granulomatous enteritis (see Chap. 286), lymphoma (see Chap. 113), and Whipple's disease (see Chap. 285); differentiation of these conditions, which give rise to secondary amyloidosis, from diffuse primary amyloidosis of the small bowel may be difficult. Similarly, amyloidosis of the stomach may closely mimic gastric carcinoma, with obstruction, achlorhydria, and the radiologic appearance of tumor masses.

Nervous System Neurologic manifestations may include peripheral neuropathy, postural hypotension, inability to sweat, Adies's pupil, hoarseness, and sphincter incompetence. These manifestations are especially prominent in the heredofamilial amyloidoses. The cranial nerves are generally spared, except in the Finnish hereditary amyloidosis. Carpal tunnel syndrome may be caused by several amyloidoses, especially primary (AL) and chronic hemodialysis ($A\beta_2M$) amyloid. Peripheral neuropathy is frequent in the former type. Aβ amyloid occurs in the central nervous system as a component of senile plaques and in blood vessels ("congophilic angiopathy"). The protein concentration in the cerebrospinal fluid may be increased. Infiltrates of the cornea or vitreous body may be present in hereditary amyloid syndromes. Certain of these syndromes (advanced FAP) are characterized by a bilateral scalloping appearance of the pupil.

Endocrine Amyloid may infiltrate the thyroid or other endocrine glands but rarely causes endocrine dysfunction. Local amyloid deposits almost invariably accompany medullary carcinoma of the thyroid. Amyloid is often found in the adrenal gland, pituitary gland, and pancreas. Little if any clinical dysfunction is present unless there is massive replacement of the gland by amyloid.

Joints and Muscles Amyloid can directly, although rarely, involve articular structures by its presence in the synovial membrane and synovial fluid or in the articular cartilage. In these cases it is almost always of the AL type and associated with multiple myeloma. Amyloid arthritis can mimic a number of the rheumatic diseases because it can present as a symmetric arthritis of small joints with nodules, morning stiffness, and fatigue (see Chap. 321). The synovial fluid usually has a low white blood cell count, a good to fair mucin clot, a predominance of mononuclear cells, and no crystals. Studies of surgical specimens suggest a significant incidence of amyloid in cartilage, capsule, and synovium in osteoarthritis (see Chap. 322). Amyloid infiltration of muscle may lead to a pseudomyopathy. Shoulder muscle infiltration can produce the "shoulder pad" sign. Amyloid is found in muscle inclusion body disease, where Aβ and/or PrP have been identified.

Respiratory System The nasal sinuses, larynx, and trachea may be involved by accumulation of AL amyloid, which blocks the ducts, in the case of the sinuses, or the air passages. Amyloidosis of the lung involves the bronchi and alveolar septa diffusely. The lower respiratory tract is affected most frequently in primary (AL) amyloidosis and in the disease associated with dysproteinemia. Pulmonary symptoms

attributable to amyloid are present in about 30 percent of cases. In secondary (AA) amyloidosis, pulmonary disease is a frequent histopathologic accompaniment but seldom gives rise to clinically significant symptoms. Amyloid also may be localized in the bronchi or pulmonary parenchyma and may resemble a neoplasm. In these cases, local excision should be attempted and, when successful, may be followed by prolonged remissions.

Hematopoietic System Hematologic changes may include fibrinogenopenia, increased fibrinolysis, and selective deficiency of clotting factors. Deficient factor X seems to be due to nonspecific calcium-dependent binding to the polyanionic amyloid fibrils. Splenectomy in the patient with such a factor X deficiency can relieve the deficiency and the associated bleeding disorder, since factor X has been shown to bind to the large masses of splenic amyloid. Endothelial damage together with the clotting abnormalities lead to a propensity toward abnormal bleeding.

DIAGNOSIS Amyloid fibrils are identified in biopsy or necropsy tissue sections (Table 309-3). The systemic amyloidoses offer a choice of biopsy sites; abdominal fat aspirates or renal or rectal biopsies are often performed. Microscopically, amyloid deposits stain pink with the hematoxylin-eosin stain and show metachromasia with crystal violet. The Congo red stain imparts a unique green birefringence when stained tissue sections are viewed using the polarizing microscope. This is the single most widely used and useful procedure for establishing the presence of systemic amyloid. Fluorescent dyes such as thioflavin are sensitive screening stains for amyloid deposits in brain and other tissues; however, specificity should be confirmed. After amyloid has been identified by staining, it can be chemically classified by protein studies and by immunohistochemistry. In the case of FAP, the presence of mutant TTR (or gelsolin, apoAI, etc.) establishes the specific diagnosis of the disease. In order to establish the relationship of immunoglobulin-related amyloid to multiple myeloma, electrophoretic and immunoelectrophoretic studies on serum and urine should be performed when the biopsy reveals amyloid deposition. Most of these patients will have only relatively small paraprotein components, and only a few will have frank multiple myeloma.

PROGNOSIS Generalized amyloidosis is usually a slowly progressive disease that leads to death in several years, but in some instances, prognosis is improving. The average survival in most large series of AL amyloid is ~12 months and in FAP is ~7 to 15 years. A number of individuals with amyloid have been followed 5 to 10 years and longer. The course of amyloidosis is difficult to document, because dating the time of origin of the disease is rarely possible. When amyloidosis develops in patients with rheumatoid arthritis, it seldom becomes evident when the arthritis is less than 2 years in

Table 309-3

Diagnosis of Amyloidosis

BIOPSY	APPROPRIATE STAIN
Common sites	Congo red, viewed by polarization microscopy
Subcutaneous abdominal fat aspirate	Thioflavin (less specific)
Rectum	Potassium permanganate pretreatment, then Congo red stain
Skin	Other:
Gingiva	Cotton dyes (comparable with Congo red)
Occasional sites	Crystal violet (less sensitive)
Small intestine	**PROTEIN OR DNA STUDIES**
Muscle	Mutant protein identification
Nerve	Immunocytochemistry: immunofluorescent or immunoperoxidase stains with specific antisera
Rare sites	
Kidney	
Liver	
Bone marrow	
Synovium	
Spleen	

duration. When amyloidosis develops in patients with multiple myeloma, manifestations leading to initial hospitalization are more apt to be related to amyloid disease than to myeloma. In these cases, prognosis is very poor, and life expectancy is usually less than 6 months.

℞ TREATMENT

Rational therapy should be directed at (1) reducing precursor production, (2) inhibiting the synthesis and extracellular deposition of amyloid fibrils, and (3) promoting lysis or mobilization of existing amyloid deposits. There are new specific therapies for the various amyloidoses. In certain of the heredofamilial amyloidoses, genetic counseling is an important aspect of treatment, and the removal of the site of synthesis of the mutant protein by liver transplantation has proven remarkably successful. Liver transplantation has been carried out since 1990 for FAP patients in Sweden, the United States, Portugal, Spain, and other countries. It appears that disease progression is halted and that there is some improvement in autonomic nervous system function.

While instances have been reported of remission of amyloidosis accompanying treatable infections or inflammation, often these reports are not substantiated by biopsy proof of resorption. In one series, the mean survival of patients with renal amyloid from the time of biopsy was 29 months, but in a few cases, there was presumptive evidence of regression of the renal amyloid. The utilization of chronic hemodialysis and of kidney transplantation has clearly improved the prognosis of renal amyloid.

In the case of AL amyloid, the fact that immunoglobulin light chain is made by plasma cells has lead to the use of alkylating agents. However, these agents are toxic and not very effective. Recent trials have indicated that a prednisone/melphalan/colchicine program prolongs life. Hematopoietic stem cell transplantation appears promising. A novel anthracycline, iododoxorubicin, has been shown to bind to AL amyloid (similar to Congo red) in vivo and promote amyloid resorption. Only a small number of patients have received this experimental agent, but the majority have had objective improvement. Cardiac transplantation in selected cases of AL or FAP amyloidosis has its advocates.

Patients with severe renal amyloidosis and azotemia have been treated by dialysis or kidney transplantation with very good outcomes. This has significantly improved the prognosis in patients whose major manifestations are renal.

Colchicine has been shown to be effective in preventing acute attacks in patients with FMF (see Chap. 288). It has been determined from inhibition of AA amyloid deposition in the mouse model that colchicine inhibits formation of AEF. One large study has shown colchicine to be effective in prolonging life in primary (AL) amyloidosis using a life-table survivorship analysis, and it putatively reverses AA renal amyloid lesions.

The major causes of death are heart disease and renal failure. Sudden death, presumably due to arrhythmias, is common. Occasionally, gastrointestinal hemorrhage, respiratory failure, intractable heart failure, and superimposed infections are the terminal events.

BIBLIOGRAPHY

BENSON MD: Inherited amyloidosis. J Med Genet 28:73, 1991

COHEN AS: Amyloidosis. Bull Rheum Dis 40:1, 1991

———, JONES LA: Advances in amyloidosis. Curr Opin Rheumatol 5:62, 1993

———, SIPE JD: Amyloidosis; in *Clinical Immunology*, RR Rich et al (eds). St. Louis, Mosby Year Book, 1995, pp 1264–1272

GLENNER GG, MURPHY MA: Amyloidosis of the nervous system. J Neurol Soc 94:1, 1989

HUSBY G et al: The 1990 guidelines for nomenclature and classification of amyloid and amyloidosis, in *Amyloid and Amyloidosis*, JB Natvig et al (eds). Dordrecht, Netherlands, Kluwer, 1990, pp 813–816

——— et al: Serum amyloid A (SAA): Biochemistry, genetics and the pathogenesis of AA amyloidosis. Amyloid Int J Exp Clin Invest 1:119, 1994

LEWIS WD, SKINNER M: Liver transplantation for familial amyloidotic polyneuropathy: A potentially curative treatment. Amyloid Int J Exp Clin Invest 1:143, 1994

PRUSINER SB, DEARMOND SJ: Prion protein amyloid and neurodegeneration. Amyloid Int J Exp Clin Invest 2:39, 1995

SIPE JD: Amyloidosis. Crit Rev Clin Lab Sci 31:325, 1994

ZEMER D et al: Colchicine in the prevention and treatment of the amyloidosis of familial Mediterranean fever. N Engl J Med 314:1001, 1986

SECTION 2

DISORDERS OF IMMUNE-MEDIATED INJURY

310 *K. Frank Austen*

DISEASES OF IMMEDIATE TYPE HYPERSENSITIVITY

The term *atopic allergy* implies a familial tendency to manifest such conditions as asthma, rhinitis, urticaria, and eczematous dermatitis (atopic dermatitis) alone or in combination. However, individuals without an atopic background also may develop hypersensitivity reactions, particularly urticaria and anaphylaxis, associated with the same class of antibody, IgE, found in atopic individuals. The designation *diseases of immediate type hypersensitivity* presents a more suitable framework than the broad term *allergy* or the restrictive definition of atopy.

The fixation of IgE to human mast cells and basophils, a process termed *sensitization*, prepares these cells for subsequent antigen-specific activation. The high-affinity receptor for IgE, designated FcϵRI, is composed of one α, one β, and two disulfide-linked γ chains, which together cross the plasma membrane seven times. The α chain is solely responsible for IgE binding, and the β and γ chains are responsible for signal transduction that results from the aggregation of the tetrameric receptors by polymeric antigen.

Aggregation causes activation of an Src family–related tyrosine kinase, termed *Lyn*, which is constitutively associated with the β chain and which phosphorylates a particular motif [antigen recognition activation motif (ARAM)] in the γ chain. The phosphorylation of this motif in the γ chain induces an interaction with certain SH2 domains of a ZAP70/Syk family tyrosine kinase. The subsequent activation of Syk leads to phorphorylation and activation of phospholipase Cγ-1. This polyphosphatidyl inositol–selective phospholipase C elaborates 1,2-diacylglycerols (1,2-DAG) and inositol-1,4,5-*tris*-phosphate (IP_3), which in turn activate protein kinase C and mobilize intracellular calcium ions, respectively. These events may be augmented by the formation of calcium ion channels and attenuated by the activation of adenylate cyclase with formation of cyclic 3′,5′-adenosine monophosphate (cyclic AMP) and activation of cyclic AMP–dependent protein kinase. The calcium ion–dependent activation of phospholipases cleaves membrane phospholipids to generate lysophospholipids, which, like 1,2-DAG, are fusogenic and may facilitate the fusion of the secretory granule perigranular membrane with the cell membrane, a step that releases the membrane-free granule containing the preformed or primary mediators of mast cell effects.

The secretory granule of the human mast cell has a crystalline structure, unlike mast cells of lower species, and IgE-dependent cell activation can be characterized morphologically by solubilization and swelling of the granule contents within the first minute of receptor perturbation; this reaction is followed by the ordering of intermediate filaments about the swollen granule, movement toward the cell surface, and fusion of the perigranular membrane with that of other granules and with the plasmalemma to form extracellular channels for mediator release while maintaining cell viability.

In addition to exocytosis, aggregation of FcεRI initiates two other pathways for generation of bioactive products, namely, lipid mediators and cytokines. The biochemical steps involved in expression of such cytokines as tumor necrosis factor α (TNFα), interleukin (IL)-6, IL-4, IL-5, granulocyte-macrophage colony-stimulating factor (GM-CSF), and others have not been defined for mast cells in a manner comparable to T cells. Nonetheless, inhibition studies of cytokine production (IL-1β, TNFα, and IL-6) in mouse mast cells with cyclosporine or FK506 reveal binding to the ligand-specific immunophilin and attenuation of the calcium ion- and calmodulin-dependent serine/threonine phosphatase, calcineurin.

Lipid mediator generation (Fig. 310-1) involves translocation of calcium ion–dependent cytosolic phospholipase A_2 to the perinuclear membrane, with subsequent release of arachidonic acid for metabolic processing by the distinct prostanoid and leukotriene pathways. The constitutive prostaglandin endoperoxide synthase (PGHS-1/cyclooxygenase-1) or the de novo inducible PGHS-2 convert released arachidonic acid to the sequential intermediates prostaglandin (PG) G_2 and PGH_2. The glutathione-dependent hematopoietic PGD_2 synthase then converts PGH_2 to PGD_2, the predominant mast cell prostanoid.

For processing by the leukotriene pathway, the released arachidonic acid is translocated to an integral perinuclear membrane protein, the 5-lipoxygenase activating protein (FLAP). The calcium ion–dependent activation of 5-lipoxygenase involves translocation to the perinuclear membrane, which allows conversion of the arachidonic acid to the sequential intermediates, 5-hydroperoxyeicosatetraenoic acid and leukotriene (LT) A_4. LTA_4 is conjugated with reduced glutathione by

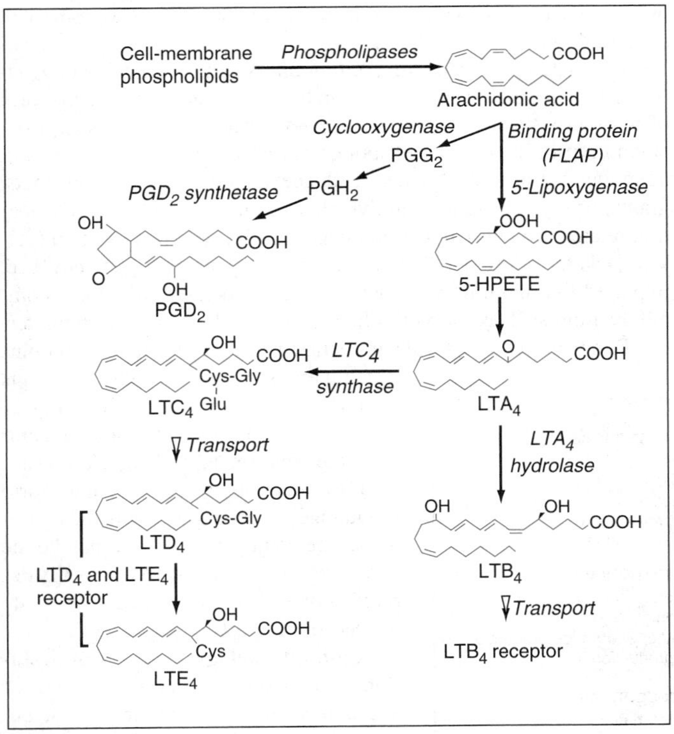

FIGURE 310-1 Pathways for biosynthesis and release of membrane-derived lipid mediators from mast cells. In the 5-lipoxygenase pathway leukotriene A_4 (LTA_4) is the intermediate from which the terminal-pathway enzymes generate the distinct final products, leukotriene C_4 (LTC_4) and leukotriene B_4 (LTB_4), which leave the cell by separate saturable transport systems. Gamma glutamyl transpeptidase and a dipeptidase then cleave glutamic acid and glycine from LTC_4 to form LTD_4 and LTE_4, respectively, for which there appears to be a common receptor. The only mast cell product of the cyclooxygenase system is PGD_2.

LTC_4 synthase, an integral membrane protein with significant homology to FLAP. Intracellular LTC_4 is released by a carrier-specific export step for extracellular conversion to the receptor-active cysteinyl leukotrienes LTD_4 and LTE_4 by sequential removal of glumatic acid and glycine. A cytosolic LTA_4 hydrolase converts some LTA_4 to the dihydroxy leukotriene LTB_4, which then undergoes specific export for extracellular receptor–mediated actions. The lysophospholipid formed during release of arachidonic acid from 1-*O*-alkyl-2-acyl-*sn*-glyceryl-3-phosphorylcholine can be acetylated in the second position to form platelet-activating factor (PAF).

Unlike other cells of bone marrow origin, mast cells do not mature in the marrow and do not circulate in a recognized mature form. In tissue they appear as mature populations with tissue-related phenotypes. It is thus assumed that unrecognized mast cell progenitors enter the tissue and undergo regulated proliferation, differentiation, and maturation. Based on the immunodetection of secretory granule neutral proteases, mast cells in the lung parenchyma and intestinal mucosa selectively express tryptase; those in the intestinal and airway submucosa, skin, lymph nodes, and breast parenchyma express tryptase, chymase, and carboxypeptidase A (CPA); and occasional mast cells in intestinal submucosa express chymase and CPA but not tryptase. The secretory granules of mast cells selectively positive for tryptase in lung and intestinal mucosa exhibit closed scrolls with a periodicity suggestive of a crystalline structure by electron microscopy; whereas the secretory granules of mast cells with mutiple proteases residing in skin, lymph nodes, breast parenchyma, and submucosa of airways and intestine are scroll-poor with an amorphous or latticelike appearance. These phenotypic distinctions are accompanied by differences in their T cell dependence; for example, intestinal mucosal but not submucosal mast cells are absent in patients with inborn or acquired cellular immunodeficiency.

Mast cells are distributed at cutaneous and mucosal surfaces and in deeper tissues about venules, are an expansile population during T cell stimulation, and could regulate the entry of foreign substances by their rapid response capability (Fig. 310-2). Upon stimulus-specific activation in vitro, histamine and selected secretory granule–associated acid hydrolases are solubilized, whereas the neutral proteases, which are cationic, remain largely complexed to the anionic proteoglycans, heparin and chrondroitin sulfate E. It is speculated that the macromolecular complex serves to deliver the neutral proteases so that the endo- and exoproteases can function in concert at the substrate site to clear damaged tissue and facilitate repair. Histamine and the various lipid mediators (PGD_2, LTD_4/E_4, PAF) alter venular permeability, thereby allowing influx of plasma proteins such as complement and immunoglobulins, whereas LTB_4 mediates leukocyte–endothelial cell adhesion with subsequent directed migration (chemotaxis). The accumulation of leukocytes and opsonins would facilitate defense of the microenvironment. The cysteinyl leukotrienes constrict both vascular and nonvascular smooth muscle and are much more potent than histamine in constricting human airway smooth muscle when administered by aerosol.

The cellular component of the inflammatory response elicited by preformed secretory granule–associated and membrane-derived lipid mediators would be augmented and sustained by the addition of cytokines of mast cell or T cell origin to the microenvironment. Activation of human skin mast cells in situ elicits TNFα production and augmented venular permeability and would provide endothelial cell responses favoring leukocyte adhesion. Activation of purified human lung mast cells in vitro results in substantial production of IL-5 and lesser quantities of IL-4. Biopsies of patients with bronchial asthma reveal that mast cells are immunohistochemically positive for IL-4 and IL-5, but that the predominant localization of IL-4, IL-5, and GM-CSF is to T cells, defined as TH2 by this profile. It is speculated that IL-4 modulates the T cell phenotype to the TH2 subtype, and that IL-5 or GM-CSF converts infiltrating eosinophils to an activated, autoaggressive phenotype with augmented capacity for cytotoxicity and generation of O_2^- and the cysteinyl leukotrienes.

The view of immediate and late, or cellular, phases of allergic inflammation is supported by the response of the skin, nose, or lung of allergic humans to local allergen challenge; greater quantities of allergen are needed to elicit the cellular phase. In the immediate phase of a local challenge, there is pruritus and watery discharge from the nose, bronchospasm and mucous secretion in the lungs, and a wheal-and-flare response with pruritus in the skin. The reduced nasal patency, pulmonary function, or evident erythema with swelling at the skin site in a late-phase response at 6 to 8 h are associated with biopsy findings of infiltrating and activated TH2 type T cells, eosinophils, and even some basophils and neutrophils. This allergic inflammation proceeding from early mast cell activation to late cellular infiltration is believed to promote end-organ hyperresponsivity, as would be characteristic of perennial rhinitis or bronchial asthma; for attenuation, it requires introduction of an anti-inflammatory agent such as a glucocorticoid. The particular cytokines responsible for eosinophil and T cell adhesion with subsequent directed migration are not yet defined, although numerous candidates are identified.

Consideration of the mechanism of immediate type hypersensitivity diseases in the human has focused largely on the IgE-dependent recognition of otherwise nontoxic substances. Support for this thesis has come from the finding that clinical atopic allergy is sometimes associated with elevated total levels of IgE and in some instances with an immune response that is specifically linked to the histocompatibility locus. IgE distribution in normal families is consistent with the dominant inheritance of the low-IgE phenotype. As a result of the action of a single IgE regulator gene, the majority of family members would have elevated IgE levels as a possible basis for their atopic state. The association between HLA histocompatibility type and the immediate hypersensitivity response has been noted in persons of the low-IgE phenotype who were studied with highly purified allergens, generally of small size. Such presumptive evidence of immune-response (Ir) genes by linkage disequilibrium, i.e., the association of the hypersensitivity response with a particular histocompatibility haplotype, represents an additional element in the polygenic atopic allergic state. It is also likely that diseases of immediate type hypersensitivity may occur because of deficient intracellular controls of mediator generation or release, or both, or that the extracellular controls directed against mediator inactivation may be impaired.

The induction of allergic disease requires sensitization of a predisposed individual to specific allergen. This sensitization can occur anytime in life, although the greatest propensity for the development of allergic disease appears to occur in childhood and early adolescence. Exposure of a susceptible individual to an allergen results in processing of the allergen by antigen-presenting cells, including macrophage-like cells located throughout the body at surfaces that contact the outside environment, such as the nose, lungs, eyes, skin, and intestine. These antigen-presenting cells process the allergen protein and present it in the context of select cell surface proteins to CD4+ T cells, which, in turn, become activated specifically by the peptide epitope resulting from processing of the allergen. T cells can potentially induce several responses to an allergen, including those typical of contact dermatitis, known as the TH1 type response; responses consistent with immediate hypersensitivity responses, known as TH2; or anergic, or nonresponses, known as TH0. These varying forms of T cell responsivity are associated with discrete cytokine products; interferon γ production is associated with TH1 responses, and IL-4, -5, and -6 and GM-CSF generation with TH2 responses. The TH2 response is associated with activation of specific B cells that transform into plasma cells that produce allergen-specific IgE. Release into the serum of allergen-specific IgE by plasma cells results in sensitization of IgE Fc receptor–bearing cells including mast cells and basophils, which subsequently are capable of becoming activated upon exposure to the specific allergen. In certain diseases, including those associated with atopy, the monocyte and eosinophil populations can express the high-affinity receptor, FcεRI, and respond to its aggregation.

ANAPHYLAXIS Definition The life-threatening anaphylactic response of a sensitized human appears within minutes after administration of specific antigen and is manifested by respiratory distress often followed by vascular collapse or by shock without antecedent respiratory difficulty. Cutaneous manifestations exemplified by pruritus and urticaria with or without angioedema are characteristic of such systemic anaphylactic reactions. Gastrointestinal manifestations include nausea, vomiting, crampy abdominal pain, and diarrhea.

Predisposing Factors and Etiology There is no convincing evidence that age, sex, race, occupation, or geographic location predisposes a human to anaphylaxis except through exposure to some immunogen. According to most studies, atopy does not predispose individuals to anaphylaxis from penicillin therapy or venom of a stinging insect.

The materials capable of eliciting the systemic anaphylactic reaction in humans include the following: heterologous proteins in the form of hormones (insulin, vasopressin, parathormone), enzymes (trypsin, chymotrypsin, penicillinase), pollen extracts (ragweed, grass, trees), nonpollen extracts (dust mites, cat dander), food (eggs, seafoods, nuts, grains, beans), antiserum (antilymphocyte gamma globulin), occupation-related proteins (rubber products), and Hymenoptera venom (yellow jacket, yellow and baldfaced hornets, paper wasp, honey bee, imported fire ants); polysaccharides such as dextran; and most commonly drugs such as antibiotics (penicillins, cephalosporins, amphotericin B, nitrofurantoin), local anesthetics (procaine, lidocaine), vitamins (thiamine, folic acid), diagnostic agents (sodium dehydrocholate, sulfobromophthalein), and occupation-related chemicals (ethylene oxide), which are considered to function as haptens that form immunogenic conjugates with host proteins. The conjugating hapten may be the parent compound, a nonenzymatically derived storage product, or a metabolite formed in the host.

Pathophysiology and Manifestations Individuals differ in the time of appearance of symptoms and signs, but the hallmark of the anaphylactic reaction is the onset of some manifestation within seconds to minutes after introduction of the antigen, generally by injection or less commonly by ingestion. There may be upper or lower airway obstruction or both. Laryngeal edema may be experienced as a "lump" in the throat, hoarseness, or stridor, while bronchial obstruction is associ-

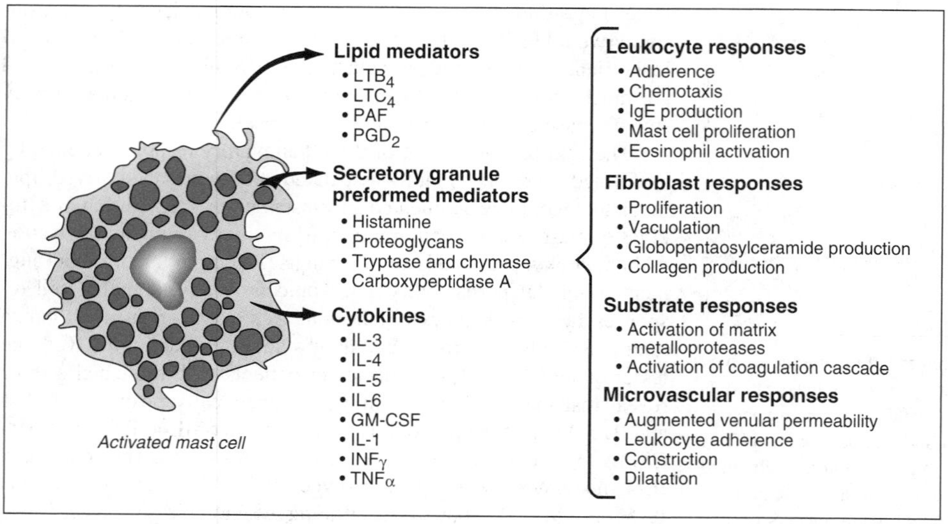

FIGURE 310-2 Bioactive mediators of three categories generated by IgE-dependent activation of murine mast cells can elicit common but sequential target cell effects leading to acute and sustained inflammatory responses.

ated with a feeling of tightness in the chest and/or audible wheezing. A characteristic feature is the eruption of well-circumscribed, discrete cutaneous wheals with erythematous, raised, serpiginous borders and blanched centers. These urticarial eruptions are intensely pruritic and may be localized or disseminated. They may coalesce to form giant hives, and they seldom persist beyond 48 h. A localized, nonpitting, deeper edematous cutaneous process, angioedema, also may be present. It may be asymptomatic or cause a burning or stinging sensation.

In fatal cases with clinical bronchial obstruction, the lungs show marked hyperinflation on gross and microscopic examination. The microscopic findings in the bronchi, however, are limited to luminal secretions, peribronchial congestion, submucosal edema, and eosinophilic infiltration, and the acute emphysema is attributed to intractable bronchospasm that subsides with death. The angioedema resulting in death by mechanical obstruction occurs in the epiglottis and larynx, but the process is also evident in the hypopharynx and to some extent in the trachea; on microscopic examination there is wide separation of the collagen fibers and the glandular elements; vascular congestion and eosinophilic infiltration are also present. Patients dying of vascular collapse without antecedent hypoxia from respiratory insufficiency have visceral congestion with a presumptive loss of intravascular blood volume. The associated electrocardiographic abnormalities, with or without infarction, noted in some patients may reflect a primary cardiac event or be secondary to a critical reduction in blood volume.

The angioedematous and urticarial manifestations of the anaphylactic syndrome have been attributed to release of endogenous histamine. A role for the cysteinyl leukotrienes in altering pulmonary mechanics by causing marked bronchiolar constriction seems likely. Vascular collapse without respiratory distress in response to experimental challenge with the sting of a hymenopteran was associated not only with marked and prolonged elevations in blood histamine but also with evidence of intravascular coagulation and kinin generation. Based on the findings that patients with systemic mastocytosis and episodic hypotension proceeding to vascular collapse excrete large amounts of PGD_2 in addition to histamine and are controlled by administration of a nonsteroidal agent but not by antihistamines alone, it may be that PGD_2 is also of importance in the hypotensive anaphylactic reactions. The cysteinyl leukotrienes may be involved in the pathobiologic process in patients with myocardial ischemia without or with infarction.

Diagnosis The diagnosis of an anaphylactic reaction depends largely on an accurate history revealing the onset of the appropriate symptoms and signs within minutes after the responsible material is encountered. When only a portion of the full syndrome is present, such as isolated urticaria, sudden bronchospasm in a patient with asthma, or vascular collapse after intravenous administration of an agent, it is difficult to exclude a nonimmunologic, toxicologic, or idiosyncratic response. Intravenous administration of a chemical mast cell–degranulating agent, including opiate derivatives and radiographic contrast media, may elicit generalized urticaria, angioedema, and a sensation of retrosternal oppression with or without clinically detectable bronchoconstriction or hypotension. Furthermore, nonsteroidal anti-inflammatory agents such as indomethacin, aminopyrine, mefenamic acid, and aspirin may precipitate a life-threatening episode of obstruction of upper or lower airways in patients with asthma that is clinically reminiscent of anaphylaxis but is not associated with a detectable IgE response. This syndrome, which is commonly associated with nasal polyposis, may reflect a unique reactivity to an imbalance in the ratio of prostaglandin to leukotriene biosynthesis when cyclooxygenase is inhibited.

The presence of specific IgE in the heart blood of patients dying of systemic anaphylaxis has been demonstrated at postmortem by passive transfer of the serum intradermally into a normal recipient, followed in 24 h by antigen challenge into the same site, with subsequent development of a wheal and flare, the Prausnitz-Küstner reaction. In order to avoid the hazards of transferring hepatitis or other infections to a recipient, it is preferable to employ a less sensitive monkey recipient or a human leukocyte suspension enriched with basophils for subsequent antigen challenge. Furthermore, radioimmunoassays have demonstrated specific IgE antibodies in patients with anaphylactic reactions, but such approaches require purified antigens. Elevations of tryptase levels in serum implicate mast cell activation in an adverse systemic reaction and are particularly informative with episodes of hypotension during general anesthesia or when there has been a fatal outcome. In the transfusion anaphylactic reaction that occurs in patients with IgA deficiency, the responsible specificity resides in IgG or IgE anti-IgA; the mechanism of the reaction mediated by IgG anti-IgA is presumed to be complement activation with secondary mast cell participation.

Rx TREATMENT

Early recognition of an anaphylactic reaction is mandatory, since death occurs within minutes to hours after the first symptoms. Mild symptoms such as pruritus and urticaria can be controlled by administration of 0.2 to 0.5 mL of 1:1000 epinephrine subcutaneously, with repeated doses as required at 20-min intervals for a severe reaction. If the antigenic material was injected into an extremity, the rate of absorption may be reduced by prompt application of a tourniquet proximal to the reaction site, administration of 0.2 mL of 1:1000 epinephrine into the site, and removal without compression of an insect stinger, if present. An intravenous infusion should be initiated to provide a route for administration of 2.5 mL epinephrine, diluted 1:10,000, at 5- to 10-min intervals, volume expanders such as normal saline, and vasopressor agents such as dopamine if intractable hypotension occurs. Replacement of intravascular volume due to postcapillary venular leakage may require several liters of saline. Epinephrine provides both alpha- and beta-adrenergic effects, resulting in vasoconstriction, bronchial smooth-muscle relaxation, and attenuation of enhanced venular permeability. Beta blockers are relatively contraindicated in persons at risk for anaphylactic reactions, especially those sensitive to Hymenoptera venom or those undergoing immunotherapy for respiratory system allergy. When epinephrine fails to control the anaphylactic reaction, hypoxia due to airway obstruction or related to a cardiac arrhythmia, or both, must be considered. Oxygen via a nasal catheter or intermittent positive-pressure breathing of oxygen with 0.5 mL isoproterenol diluted 1:200 in saline may be helpful, but either endotracheal intubation or a tracheostomy is mandatory for oxygen delivery if progressive hypoxia develops. Ancillary agents such as the antihistamine diphenhydramine, 50 to 100 mg intramuscularly or intravenously, and aminophylline, 0.25 to 0.5 g intravenously, are appropriate for urticaria-angioedema and bronchospasm, respectively. Intravenous glucocorticoids are not effective for the acute event but may alleviate later recurrence of bronchospasm, hypotension, or urticaria.

Prevention Prevention of anaphylaxis must take into account the sensitivity of the recipient, the dose and character of the diagnostic or therapeutic agent, and the effect of the route of administration on the rate of absorption. If there is a definite history of a past anaphylactic reaction, even though mild, it is advisable to select another agent or procedure. A knowledge of cross-reactivity among agents is critical since, for example, cephalosporins share a common β-lactam ring with the penicillins. A skin test should be performed before the administration of certain materials that are likely to elicit anaphylactic reactions, such as allergenic extracts, or when the nature of the past adverse reaction is unknown. A scratch test should precede an intradermal test in very sensitive patients. With regard to penicillin, two-thirds of patients with a positive reaction history and positive skin tests to benzylpenicilloyl-polylysine (BPL) and/or the minor determinant mixture (MDM) of benzylpenicillin products experience allergic reactions with treatment, and these are almost uniformly of the anaphylactic type in those patients with minor determinant reactivity. Even patients without a history of previous clinical reactions have a 2 to 6 percent incidence of positive skin tests to the two test materials, and about 3 per 1000 with a negative history experience anaphylaxis with therapy, with a mortality of about 1 per 100,000. Skin testing for antibiotics should be performed only on patients with a positive clinical history consistent with an immediate hypersensitivity reaction and in imminent need of the antibiotic in question; skin testing is of no value for non-IgE-mediated eruptions. Desensitization with most antibiotics can proceed by the intravenous, subcutaneous, or oral route. Typically, graded quantities of the antibiotic are given by the selected route using double doses until a therapeutic dosage is achieved. Due to the risk of systemic anaphylaxis during the course of desensitization, such a procedure should be performed only in a setting in which resuscitation equipment is at hand and an intravenous line is in place. It is critical to give the therapeutic agent at regular intervals to prevent the reestablishment of a sensitized cell pool of large size.

A different form of protection involves the development of blocking antibody of the IgG class, which is protective against Hymenoptera venom–induced anaphylaxis by interacting with antigen so that less reaches the sensitized tissue mast cells; to be effective, this immunotherapy requires the use of specific or cross-reacting Hymenoptera venom.

Because sensitization can be transient, the maximal risk for systemic anaphylactic reactions in persons with Hymenoptera sensitivity occurs in association with a currently positive skin test. Although there is only low-grade cross-reactivity between honey bee and yellow jacket venoms, there is a high degree of cross-reactivity between yellow jacket venom and the rest of the vespid venoms (yellow or baldfaced hornets and wasps). Prevention involves modification of outdoor activities to exclude bare feet, wearing perfumed toiletries, eating in certain areas, clipping hedges or grass, and hauling away trash or fallen fruit. As with each anaphylactic sensitivity, the individual should wear an informational bracelet and have immediate access to an unexpired epinephrine kit. The limitations of lifestyle and the psychological duress can be addressed by venom immunotherapy to achieve a venom-specific IgG titer above 3.0 μg/mL of serum. Although it has been recommended that venom therapy be continued indefinitely or until the skin and specific serum IgE tests are unremarkable, there is evidence that 5 years of treatment induces a state of resistance to sting reactions that is independent of serum levels of specific IgG or IgE. This contrasts with the definite relation of sting immunity to specific IgG earlier in the treatment regime. For children with a systemic reaction limited to skin, the likelihood of progression to more serious respiratory or vascular manifestations is low, and thus immunotherapy is not recommended.

URTICARIA AND ANGIOEDEMA Definition Urticaria and angioedema may appear separately or together as cutaneous manifestations of localized nonpitting edema; a similar process may occur at mucosal surfaces of the upper respiratory or gastrointestinal tract. *Urticaria* involves only the superficial portion of the dermis, presenting as well-circumscribed wheals with erythematous raised serpiginous borders with blanched centers that may coalesce to become giant wheals. *Angioedema* is a well-demarcated localized edema involving the deeper layers of the skin, including the subcutaneous tissue. Recurrent episodes of urticaria and/or angioedema of less than 6 weeks' duration are considered acute, whereas attacks persisting beyond this period are designated chronic.

Predisposing Factors and Etiology The occurrence of urticaria and angioedema is probably more frequent than usually described because of the evanescent, self-limited nature of such eruptions, which seldom require medical attention when limited to the skin. Although persons in any age group may experience acute or chronic urticaria and/or angioedema, these lesions increase in frequency after adolescence, with the highest incidence occurring in persons in the third decade of life; indeed, one survey of college students indicated that 15 to 20 percent had experienced a pruritic wheal reaction.

The classification of urticaria-angioedema presented in Table 310-1 focuses on the different mechanisms for eliciting clinical disease. Only the IgE-dependent and the IgG-mediated reactions in IgA-deficient persons should be considered immediate hypersensitivity. However, the other mechanisms are important for differential diagnosis, and most cases of chronic urticaria are idiopathic. The appearance of urticaria and angioedema in atopic persons in the absence of a specific exposure is attributed to the atopic diathesis and implies an IgE-dependent mechanism. Urticaria and/or angioedema occurring during the appropriate season in patients with seasonal respiratory allergy or as a result of exposure to animals or molds is attributed to inhalation or physical contact with pollens, animal dander, and mold spores, respectively. However, urticaria and angioedema secondary to inhalation are relatively uncommon compared to urticaria and angioedema elicited by ingestion of fresh fruits, shellfish, fish, milk products, chocolate, legumes including peanuts, and various drugs that may elicit not only the anaphylactic syndrome with prominent gastrointestinal complaints but also chronic urticaria.

Additional etiologies include physical stimuli such as cold, heat, solar rays, exercise, and mechanical irritation. The physical urticarias can be distinguished by the precipitating event and other aspects of the clinical presentation. *Dermographism*, which occurs in 1 to 4 percent of the population, is defined by the appearance of a linear wheal at the site of a brisk stroke with a firm object or by any configuration appropriate to the eliciting event. Dermographism has a prevalence that peaks in the second to third decades. It is not influenced by an atopic diathesis and has a duration generally of less than 5 years. *Pressure urticaria*, which often accompanies dermographism or chronic idiopathic urticaria, presents in response to a sustained stimulus such as a shoulder strap or belt, running (feet), or manual labor (hands). *Cholinergic urticaria* is distinctive in that the pruritic wheals are of small size (1 to 2 mm) and are surrounded by a large area of erythema; attacks are precipitated by fever, a hot bath or shower, or exercise and are presumptively attributed to a rise in core body temperature. *Exercise-related anaphylaxis* begins with erythema and pruritic urticaria but progresses to angioedema of the face, oropharynx, larynx, or intestine or to vascular collapse; it is distinguished from cholinergic urticaria by presenting with wheals of conventional size and by not occurring with fever or a hot bath. *Cold urticaria*, either acquired or hereditary, is local at the exposed site (ice cube) or exposed body areas (ambient temperature) but can progress to vascular collapse with immersion in cold water (swimming). *Solar urticaria* is subdivided into three groups by the response to specific portions of the light spectrum. *Vibratory angioedema* may occur after years of occupational exposure or can be idiopathic; it may be accompanied by cholinergic urticaria. Other rare forms of physical allergy, always defined by stimulus-specific elicitation, include *local heat urticaria*, *aquagenic urticaria* from contact with water of any temperature, and *contact urticaria* from direct interaction with some chemical substance.

Angioedema without urticaria occurs with $C\overline{1}$ inhibitor ($C\overline{1}INH$) deficiency that may be inborn as an autosomal dominant characteristic or may be acquired. The urticaria and angioedema associated with

Table 310-1

Classification of Urticaria with Angioedema

1. IgE-dependent
   a. Specific antigen sensitivity (pollens, foods, drugs, fungi, molds, Hymenoptera venom, helminths)
   b. Physical: dermographism, cold, solar, cholinergic, vibratory, exercise-related
2. Complement-mediated
   a. Hereditary angioedema: type 1, type 2
   b. Acquired angioedema: type 1, type 2
   c. Necrotizing vasculitis
   d. Serum sickness
   e. Reactions to blood products
3. Nonimmunologic
   a. Direct mast cell–releasing agents: opiates, antibiotics, curare, D-tubocurarine, radiocontrast media
   b. Agents that presumably alter arachidonic acid metabolism: aspirin and nonsteroidal anti-inflammatory agents, azo dyes, and benzoates
4. Idiopathic

classical serum sickness or with idiopathic cutaneous necrotizing angiitis are believed to be an immune-complex disease when hypocomplementemia is a concomitant. The idiosyncratic drug reactions to mast cell granule–releasing agents and to nonsteroidal anti-inflammatory drugs may be systemic, resembling anaphylaxis, or limited to cutaneous sites.

Pathophysiology and Manifestations Urticarial eruptions are distinctly pruritic, involve any area of the body from the scalp to the soles of the feet, and appear in crops of 24- to 72-h duration, with old lesions fading as new ones appear. The most common sites are the extremities, external genitalia, and face, particularly the region of the eyes and lips. Although self-limited in duration, angioedema of the upper respiratory tract may be life-threatening due to laryngeal obstruction, while gastrointestinal involvement may present with abdominal colic, with or without nausea and vomiting, and may precipitate unnecessary surgical intervention. No residual discoloration occurs with either urticaria or angioedema unless there is an underlying process leading to superimposed extravasation of erythrocytes.

The pathology of urticaria and angioedema is usually characterized by massive edema of the dermis in urticaria and of the subcutaneous tissue as well as the dermis in angioedema. Collagen bundles in affected areas are widely separated, and the venules are sometimes dilated. The perivenular infiltrate may consist of lymphocytes, eosinophils, and neutrophils that are present in varying combination and number throughout the dermis.

Perhaps the best-studied example of IgE- and mast cell–mediated urticaria and angioedema is *cold urticaria*. Cryoglobulins may be recognized, but not in the majority of patients. Immersion of an extremity in an ice bath precipitates angioedema of the distal portion with urticaria at the air interface within minutes of the challenge. Histologic studies reveal marked mast cell degranulation with associated edema of the dermis and subcutaneous tissues. The venous effluent of the cold-challenged and angioedematous extremity reveals a marked rise in plasma content of histamine, whereas the venous effluent of the contralateral normal extremity contains none of this mediator. Elevated levels of histamine have been found in the plasma content of venous effluent and in the fluid of suction blisters at experimentally induced lesional sites in patients with dermographism, pressure urticaria, vibratory angioedema, light urticaria, and heat urticaria. By ultrastructural analysis, the pattern of mast cell degranulation in cold urticaria resembles an IgE-mediated response with solubilization of granule contents, fusion of the perigranular and cell membranes, and discharge of granule contents, whereas in a dermographic lesion there is an additional superimposed zonal (piecemeal) degranulation. Elevations of plasma histamine levels with biopsy-proven mast cell degranulation have also been demonstrated with systemic attacks of *cholinergic urticaria* and *exercise-related anaphylaxis* precipitated experimentally by exercise on a treadmill while wearing a wet suit; however, only in cholinergic urticaria is there a concomitant decrease in pulmonary function.

Diagnosis The rapid onset and self-limited nature of urticarial and angioedematous eruptions are distinguishing features. Additional characteristics are the occurrence of the urticarial crops in various stages of evolution and the asymmetric distribution of the angioedema. Urticaria and/or angioedema involving IgE-dependent mechanisms are often appreciated by historical considerations implicating specific allergens or physical stimuli, by seasonal incidence, and by exposure to certain environments. Direct reproduction of the lesion with physical stimuli is particularly valuable because it so often establishes the cause of the lesion. The diagnosis of an environmental allergen based on the clinical history can be confirmed by skin testing or assay for allergen-specific IgE in serum. IgE-mediated urticaria and/or angioedema may or may not be associated with an elevation of total IgE or with peripheral eosinophilia. Fever, leukocytosis, and an elevated sedimentation rate are absent.

The classification of urticarial and angioedematous states noted in Table 310-1 in terms of possible mechanisms necessarily includes some differential diagnostic points. Hypocomplementemia is not observed in IgE-mediated mast cell disease and may reflect either an acquired abnormality generally attributed to the formation of immune complexes or a genetic deficiency of C$\overline{1}$INH. Chronic recurrent urticaria, generally in females, associated with arthralgias, an elevated sedimentation rate, and normo- or hypocomplementemia suggests an underlying cutaneous necrotizing angiitis. Vasculitic urticaria typically persists longer than 72 h, whereas conventional urticaria often has a duration of less than 24 to 48 h. Confirmation depends on a biopsy that reveals cellular infiltration, nuclear debris, and fibrinoid necrosis of the venules. The same pathobiologic process accounts for the urticaria in association with such diseases as systemic lupus erythematosus or viral hepatitis with or without an associated arteritis. Serum sickness per se or a similar clinical entity due to drugs includes not only urticaria but also pyrexia, lymphadenopathy, myalgia, and arthralgia or arthritis. Urticarial reactions to blood products or intravenous administration of immunoglobulin are defined by the event and generally are not progressive unless the recipient is IgA-deficient in the former case or the reagent is aggregated in the latter.

Hereditary angioedema is an autosomal dominant disease due to a deficiency of antigenic and/or functional C$\overline{1}$INH. The diagnosis is suggested not only by family history but also by the lack of pruritus and of urticarial lesions, the prominence of recurrent gastrointestinal attacks of colic, and episodes of laryngeal edema. Laboratory diagnosis depends on demonstrating a deficiency of C$\overline{1}$INH antigen (type 1) in most kindreds, but some kindreds have an antigenically intact nonfunctional protein (type 2) and require a functional assay to establish the diagnosis. The natural substrates of uninhibited C$\overline{1}$, C4 and C2, are chronically depleted but fall further during attacks due to the activation of additional C1. Because the C$\overline{1}$INH protein also regulates the Hageman factor–initiated activation of kallikrein and of plasmin, the vasoactive peptides responsible for the angioedema are likely some combination of bradykinin and a plasmin-derived fragment of C$\overline{1}$-cleaved C2. An acquired form of C$\overline{1}$INH deficiency, associated with lymphoproliferative disorders, has the same clinical manifestations but differs in the lack of a familial element; in the reduction of C1/C$\overline{1}$ as well as C$\overline{1}$INH, C4, and C2; and in the presence of an anti-idiotypic antibody to the monoclonal immunoglobulin expressed on the B cells. In a second acquired form of C$\overline{1}$INH deficiency with angioedema due to the appearance of IgG anti-C$\overline{1}$INH, B cell malignancy has not been prominent.

Urticaria and angioedema must be differentiated from contact sensitivity, a vesicular eruption that progresses to chronic thickening of the skin with continued allergenic exposure. They must also be differentiated from atopic dermatitis, a condition that may present as erythema, edema, papules, vesiculation, and oozing proceeding to a subacute and chronic stage in which vesiculation is less marked or absent and scaling, fissuring, and lichenification predominate in a distribution that characteristically involves the flexor surfaces. In cutaneous mastocytosis, the reddish brown macules and papules, characteristic of urticaria pigmentosa, urticate with pruritus upon trauma; and in systemic mastocytosis, without or with urticaria pigmentosa, there is an episodic systemic flushing with or without urticaria but no angioedema.

℞ TREATMENT

Identification of the etiologic factor(s) and their elimination provide the most satisfactory therapeutic program; this approach is feasible to varying degrees with IgE-mediated reactions to allergens or physical stimuli. For most forms of urticaria, H_1 antihistamines such as chlorpheniramine or diphenhydramine, and including the nonsedating class represented by astemizole, are effective in attenuating both urtication and pruritus. Cyproheptadine and especially hydroxyzine have proven effective when H_1 antihistamines have been inadequate. Doxepin, a dibenzoxepin tricyclic compound with both H_1 and H_2 receptor antagonist activity, is yet another alternative. Topical glucocorticoids are of no value in the management of urticaria and/or angioedema. Systemic glucocorticoids are generally avoided in idiopathic, allergen-induced, or physical urticarias due to their long-term toxicity. However, systemic glucocorticoids are useful in the management of patients with pressure urticaria, with vasculitic urticaria (especially with eosinophil prominence), or with idiopathic angioedema with or without urticaria. With persistent vasculitic urticaria, hydroxychloroquine or colchicine may be added to the regimen after hydroxyzine and before or along with systemic glucocorticoids.

The therapy of inborn C$\bar{1}$INH deficiency has been simplified by the finding that attenuated androgens correct the biochemical defect and afford prophylactic protection. Since the affected individuals are heterozygous, with the depletion of C$\bar{1}$INH being due to deficient synthesis and consequent excessive utilization of the limited amount available, the efficacy of the attenuated androgens is attributed to production by the normal gene of an amount of functional C$\bar{1}$INH sufficient to control the spontaneous activation of C1 to C$\bar{1}$. Since the use of such agents for children and pregnant women is not yet accepted, the antifibrinolytic agent ϵ-aminocaproic acid may be used occasionally to control spontaneous attacks or for preoperative prophylaxis in some patients. Infusion of isolated C$\bar{1}$INH protein appears useful in prophylaxis but is not widely available.

SYSTEMIC MASTOCYTOSIS **Definition** *Systemic mastocytosis* is defined by mast cell hyperplasia that in most instances is indolent and nonneoplastic. Since human mast cells originate from pluripotent bone marrow cells (CD34+), circulate as nonmetachromatically staining, c-*kit*-positive mononuclear cells, and undergo tissue-specific proliferation and maturation, the hyperplasia is generally recognized only in bone marrow and in the normal peripheral distribution sites of the cells, such as skin, gastrointestinal mucosa, liver, and spleen. Mastocytosis occurs at any age and has a slight preponderance in males. The prevalence of systemic mastocytosis is not known, and a familial occurrence has not been established.

Classification, Pathophysiology, and Clinical Manifestations A recent consensus classification for systemic mastocytosis recognizes four forms (Table 310-2). The form designated as *indolent* accounts for the majority of patients and is not known to alter life expectancy. When a patient is classified as having indolent systemic mastocytosis, the concomitant clinical findings must be carefully noted, since they define the complications and directions for management. In systemic mastocytosis *associated with hematologic disorders*, the prognosis is determined by the nature of that disorder, which can range from dysmyelopoiesis to leukemia. In *aggressive* systemic mastocytosis, mast cell proliferation in parenchymal organs such as liver, spleen, and lymph nodes is marked and in a subset of patients is associated with prominent eosinophilia; the prognosis is poor. *Mast cell leukemia* is the rarest form of the disease and is invariably fatal at present. In types II and IV systemic mastocytosis there is a point mutation of the c-*kit* tyrosine kinase in the leukocytes and mast cells, respectively. In types I and III there is excessive production of the c-*kit* ligand (stem cell factor) in the microenvironment of the mast cells, and this may be autocrine in type III. The clinical manifestations of systemic mastocytosis, distinct from a leukemic complication, are due to tissue occupancy by the mast cell mass, the tissue response to that mass, and the release of bioactive substances acting at both local and distal sites.

Table 310-2

Classification of Systemic Mastocytosis

Type	Description
I	*Indolent* with cutaneous manifestations, vascular collapse, ulcer disease, malabsorption, skeletal disease, hepatosplenomegaly, or lymphadenopathy
II	*Concomitant hematologic disorder*, either myelodysplastic or myeloproliferative
III	*Aggressive* per se or lymphadenopathic mastocytosis with eosinophilia
IV	*Mastocytic leukemia*

The pharmacologically induced manifestations are pruritus, flushing, palpitations and vascular collapse, gastric distress, lower abdominal crampy pain, and recurrent headache. The increase in cell burden is evidenced by the small, reddish brown macules or papules, termed *urticaria pigmentosa*, at skin sites, but it also contributes to bone pain and malabsorption. The mast cell–mediated fibrotic changes are limited to liver, spleen, and bone marrow and presumably relate to the functional characteristics of mast cells developing at those sites, as opposed to those at sites without fibrosis, such as the gastrointestinal tissue or skin. Immunofluorescent analysis of bone marrow and skin lesions in indolent mastocytosis and of spleen and skin in aggressive systemic mastocytosis has revealed only one mast cell phenotype, namely, scroll-poor cells expressing tryptase, chymase, and carboxypeptidase A.

The cutaneous lesions of urticaria pigmentosa respond to trauma with urtication and erythema (Darier's sign). The apparent incidence of these lesions is 90 percent or greater in patients with indolent systemic mastocytosis. Approximately 1 percent of patients with indolent mastocytosis have skin lesions that appear as tan-brown macules with striking patchy erythema and associated telangiectasia (telangiectasia macularis eruptive perstans). In the upper gastrointestinal tract, histamine-mediated hypersecretion is the most common problem, with resultant gastritis and peptic ulcer. In the lower intestinal tract, the occurrence of diarrhea and abdominal pain is attributed to increased motility due to mast cell mediators, and this can be aggravated by malabsorption with secondary nutritional insufficiency and osteomalacia. The periportal fibrosis associated with mast cell infiltration and a prominence of eosinophils may lead to portal hypertension and ascites. In some patients, flushing and recurrent vascular collapse are markedly aggravated by an idiosyncratic response to a minimal dosage of nonsteroidal anti-inflammatory agents. The neuropsychiatric disturbances are clinically most evident as impaired recent memory and "migraine-like" headaches. Patients in every category of systemic mastocytosis may experience exacerbation of a specific clinical sign or symptom with alcohol ingestion, use of mast cell–interactive narcotics, or ingestion of nonsteroidal anti-inflammatory agents.

Diagnosis Although the diagnosis is generally suspected on the basis of the clinical history and physical findings, the contention can be strengthened by certain laboratory procedures and established only by a tissue diagnosis. A 24-h urine collection for measurement of histamine, histamine metabolites, or metabolites of PGD_2 is currently the most common noninvasive approach. A convenient alternative, but with a lesser incidence of positivity, is to measure blood levels of histamine or the mast cell–derived neutral protease tryptase. Additional studies directed by the presentation include a bone scan or skeletal survey; contrast studies of the upper gastrointestinal tract with small-bowel follow-through, computed tomography (CT) scan, or endoscopy; and a neuropsychiatric evaluation, including an EEG. The tissue diagnosis is straightforward if there are lesions of urticaria pigmentosa, but the diagnosis of systemic mastocytosis requires involvement of other organs and is most frequently established by bone marrow biopsy and aspiration. The bone marrow lesions consist of focal and paratrabecular aggregates of mast cells, often mixed with eosinophils, lymphocytes, and, on occasion, plasma cells, histiocytes, and fibroblasts.

The differential diagnosis requires the exclusion of other flushing disorders. The 24-h urine assessment of 5-hydroxy-indoleacetic acid and metanephrines should exclude a carcinoid tumor or a pheochromocytoma. Most patients with recurrent anaphylaxis, including the idiopathic group, present with angioedema, which is not a manifestation of systemic mastocytosis.

℞ TREATMENT

The management of systemic mastocytosis uses a stepwise and symptom-sign–directed approach that includes an H_1 antihistamine for flushing and pruritus, an H_2 antihistamine or proton pump inhibitor for gastric acid hypersecretion, oral cromolyn sodium for diarrhea and abdominal pain, and a nonsteroidal anti-inflammatory agent for severe flushing associated with vascular collapse despite use of H_1 and H_2 antihistamines to block biosynthesis of PGD_2. Systemic glucocorticoids appear to alleviate the malabsorption. Headaches are generally managed with the medications customarily utilized for migraine disease. Ketotifen has been used to alleviate flushing in patients intolerant to nonsteroidal anti-inflammatory agents and in patients with bone pain or intractable headaches. The efficacy of α interferon in aggressive systemic mastocytosis is controversial, and this may relate to the difficulty in achieving the necessary dosage in some patients due to the attendant side effects. Chemotherapy is not appropriate for patients with indolent mastocytosis and apparently does not prolong survival in patients with mast cell leukemia. It is appropriate for leukemia of other cell types and for the aggressive form of systemic mastocytosis.

ALLERGIC RHINITIS **Definition** Allergic rhinitis is characterized by sneezing; rhinorrhea; obstruction of the nasal passages; conjunctival, nasal, and pharyngeal itching; and lacrimation, all occurring in a temporal relationship to allergen exposure. Although commonly seasonal due to elicitation by airborne pollens, it can be perennial in an environment of chronic exposure. The incidence of allergic rhinitis in North America is about 7 percent, with the peak occurring in childhood and adolescence.

Predisposing Factors and Etiology Allergic rhinitis generally presents in atopic individuals, i.e., in persons with a family history of a similar or related symptom complex and a personal history of collateral allergy expressed as eczematous dermatitis, urticaria, and/or asthma (see Chap. 252). Symptoms generally appear before the fourth decade of life and tend to diminish gradually with aging, although complete spontaneous remissions are uncommon. A relatively small number of weeds that depend on wind rather than insects for cross-pollination, as well as certain grasses and trees, produce sufficient quantities of pollen suitable for wide distribution by air currents to elicit seasonal allergic rhinitis. The dates of pollination of these species generally vary little from year to year in a particular locale but may be quite different in another climate. In the temperate areas of North America, trees typically pollinate from March through May, grasses in June and early July, and ragweed from mid-August to early October. Molds, which are widespread in nature because they occur in soil or decaying organic matter, may propagate spores in a pattern dependent on climatic conditions. Perennial allergic rhinitis occurs in response to allergens that are present throughout the year such as in desquamating epithelium in animal dander or cockroach dander, the processed materials or chemicals utilized in an industrial setting, or the dust accumulating at work or at home. Dust has a diverse allergen content including *Dermatophagoides farinae* and *D. pteronyssinus*, which may be present alone or together in house dust. Dust mites are scavengers of flecks of human skin and coat the digestate with mite-specific protein for subsequent excretion as part of a fecal ball. Dust mites are perennially present in warm, humid climates, but their presence diminishes in the winter in colder climates due to lack of indoor humidity. Some patients with perennial rhinitis are sensitive only to house dust. In up to two-thirds of patients with perennial rhinitis, no clear-cut allergen can be demonstrated. The ability of allergens to cause rhinitis rather than lower respiratory symptoms may be attributed to their size, 10 to 100 μm, and retention within the nose.

Pathophysiology and Manifestations Episodic rhinorrhea, sneezing, and obstruction of the nasal passages with lacrimation and pruritus of the conjunctiva, nasal mucosa, and oropharynx are the hallmarks of allergic rhinitis. The nasal mucosa is pale and boggy, but the nares are not reddened or excoriated. The conjunctiva may be congested and edematous; the pharynx is generally unremarkable but may appear injected. Swelling of the turbinates and mucous membranes with obstruction of the sinus ostia and eustachian tubes precipitates secondary infections of the sinuses and middle ear, respectively, commonly in perennial but rarely in seasonal disease. Nasal polyps often arise concurrently with edema and/or infection within the sinuses and increase obstructive symptoms.

The nose presents a large mucosal surface area through the folds of the turbinates and serves to adjust the temperature and moisture content of inhaled air and to filter out particulate materials. The convoluted nasal passages readily filter out particles above 10 μm in size by impingement in a mucous blanket at bends in their course; ciliary action then moves the entrapped particles toward the pharynx. Entrapment of pollen and digestion of the outer coat by mucosal enzymes such as lysozymes release protein allergens generally of 10,000 to 40,000 molecular weight. Although the initial interaction occurs between the allergen and intraepithelial mast cells sensitized with specific IgE, the bulk of the mast cells are located beneath the mucosal surface and are recruited secondarily. During the symptomatic season when the mucosa are already swollen and hyperemic, there is enhanced adverse reactivity to the seasonal pollen as well as to antigenically unrelated pollens for which there is underlying hypersensitivity. This priming effect is attributed to improved penetration of the allergens to the deeper perivenular mast cells. Biopsy specimens of nasal mucosa during an episodic allergic reaction show profound submucosal edema with infiltration predominantly by eosinophils, although some neutrophil polymorphonuclear leukocytes are present. Polyps, a feature in perennial rhinitis, are mucosal protrusions containing chiefly edema fluid with variable degrees of eosinophilic infiltration.

The mucosal surface fluid contains not only IgA that is present preferentially because of its secretory piece but also IgE, which apparently arrives by diffusion from plasma cells distributed in proximity to mucosal surfaces. IgE fixes to mucosal and submucosal mast cells, and the intensity of the clinical response to inhaled allergens is quantitatively related to the naturally occurring or experimentally defined pollen dose. Specific IgE is distributed not only to tissue mast cells but also to circulating basophilic leukocytes; patients with more severe clinical disease have basophils that release histamine in response to lesser concentrations of allergen in vitro than do cells from patients with milder disease. Human nasal polyps from ragweed-sensitive patients release histamine, eosinophilotactic factor(s), and leukotrienes upon challenge with ragweed allergen in vitro. In sensitive individuals, the introduction of allergen into the nose is associated with sneezing, "stuffiness," and discharge, and the fluid contains histamine, PGD_2, and leukotrienes. Thus the mast cells of nasal polyp tissue, and of the nasal mucosa and submucosa, generate and release mediators through IgE-dependent reactions that are capable of producing tissue edema and eosinophilic infiltration.

Diagnosis The diagnosis of seasonal allergic rhinitis depends largely on an accurate history of occurrence coincident with the pollination of the offending weeds, grasses, or trees. The continuous character of perennial allergic rhinitis due to contamination of the home or place of work makes historical analysis difficult, but there may be a variability in symptoms that can be related to exposure to animal dander, dust mite allergens, cockroach dander, or work-related allergens such as latex. Patients with perennial rhinitis commonly develop the problem in adult life, are more often women than men, and manifest nasal polyps and thickening of the sinus membranes demonstrated by radiography. The term *vasomotor rhinitis* designates a condition of enhanced reactivity of the nasopharynx in which a symptom complex resembling perennial allergic rhinitis occurs with nonspecific stimuli and in the absence of any established allergic basis. Other entities to be excluded are structural abnormalities of the nasopharynx; exposure to irritants; upper respiratory infection; pregnancy with prominent nasal mucosal edema; prolonged topical use of alpha-adrenergic agents in the form of nose drops (rhinitis medicamentosa); and the use of certain therapeutic agents such as rauwolfia, beta-adrenergic antagonists, or estrogens. Nasal polyps may be present independently of ostomeatal sinus obstruction on an allergic basis, especially in individuals with sensitivity to nonsteroidal anti-inflammatory agents, rhinosinusitis, and bronchial asthma.

The nasal secretions of allergic patients are rich in eosinophils, and peripheral eosinophilia with elevations in relation to clinical exacerbations is a common feature. Local or systemic neutrophilia implies infection. Total serum IgE is frequently elevated, but the demonstration of immunologic specificity for IgE is critical to an etiologic diagnosis.

A skin test by the epicutaneous route (scratch or prick) with the allergens of interest provides a rapid and reliable approach to identifying allergen-specific IgE that has sensitized cutaneous mast cells. An intradermal test may follow if indicated by history when the epicutaneous test is negative, but it is less reliable due to the reactivity by this route of some asymptomatic individuals at the test dose. Skin testing by scratch or prick for food allergens is controversial but does seem to have predictive value for the absence of specific IgE sensitivity; false-positive results may occur due to the histamine content of the allergen preparation, and false-negative results due to denaturation of the epitopes of importance. A double-blind, placebo-controlled challenge may document a food allergy, but such a procedure does bear the risk of an anaphylactic reaction. An elimination diet is safer but is tedious and less definitive. Food allergy is uncommon as a significant cause of allergic rhinitis.

Newer methodology for detecting total IgE, including the development of enzyme-linked immunosorbent assays (ELISA) employing anti-IgE bound to either a solid-phase or a liquid-phase paramagnetic particle, provides rapid and cost effective determinations. More important for patient management are the measurements of specific anti-IgE in serum by its binding to a solid-phase allergen and quantitation by subsequent uptake of radiolabeled anti-IgE. The radioallergosorbent technique (RAST) correlates with the bioassay of specific IgE by skin test, which is mast cell–dependent, and by histamine release from peripheral blood leukocytes, which is basophil-dependent. As compared to the skin test, the assay of specific IgE in serum is less sensitive, which is of concern for assessing patients with an equivocal clinical history. However, the serum assay has high specificity, with false-positive results being of much less concern than false-negative ones. Furthermore, ELISA utilizing reactions that generate visible light or fluorescence have replaced the radioimmunoassays, and newer chemiluminescent tracers provide additional sensitivity for detection of minute quantities of allergen-specific IgE.

Prevention Avoidance of exposure to the offending allergen is the most effective means of controlling allergic diseases; removal of pets from the home to avoid animal danders, utilization of air filtration devices to minimize the concentrations of airborne pollens, elimination of cockroach dander by chemical destruction of the pest and careful food storage, travel to nonpollinating areas during the critical periods, and even a change of domicile to eliminate a mold spore problem may be necessary. Control of dust mites by allergen avoidance includes use of plastic-lined and covers for mattresses, pillows, and comforters, elimination of carpets and drapes, and avoidance of humidification steps.

℞ TREATMENT

Management with pharmacologic agents represents the standard approach to seasonal or perennial allergic rhinitis. Antihistamines of the H_1 class are effective for nasopharyngeal itching, sneezing, and watery rhinorrhea and for such ocular manifestations as itching, tearing, and erythema, but they are not efficacious for the nasal congestion. The older antihistamines are sedating, and their anticholinergic (muscarinic) effects include visual disturbance, urinary retention, and even arrhythmias. Because the newer H_1 antihistaminics such as terfenadine or astemizole are less lipophilic, their ability to cross the blood-brain barrier is reduced, and thus their sedating and anticholinergic side effects are minimized. Because life-threatening ventricular arrhythmias with some fatalities have occurred due to inhibition of the metabolism of terfenadine or astemizole by the interactions of macrolide antibiotics such as erythromycin and clarithromycin or broad-spectrum antifungal agents of the ketoconazole class, these nonsedating H_1 antihistamines are contraindicated in combinations with such drugs or with concomitant medical illnesses impairing hepatic function or predisposing to an arrhythmia. Alpha-adrenergic agents such as phenylephrine or oximetazoline are generally used topically to alleviate nasal congestion and obstruction, but the duration of efficacy is limited because of rebound rhinitis and such systemic responses as insomnia, irritability, and hypertension. The latter are more frequent with use of oral alpha-adrenergic agonists. Nonetheless, oral alpha-adrenergic agonists are useful in enhancing the efficacy of antihistamines in relieving nasal congestion and may diminish their sedating effects. Cromolyn sodium, a liquid nasal metered-dose spray, is essentially without side effects and is the only intervention of a prophylactic nature; thus it is used to attenuate episodic allergen activation of nasal mast cells. To be efficacious, cromolyn sodium must be administered on a continuous basis during seasonal allergen exposure, generally four times daily, or immediately prior to a discrete exposure such as animal dander. The clinical efficacy of cromolyn sodium and that of nonsedating antihistamines are roughly equivalent. Intranasal high-potency glucocorticoids are the most potent drugs available for the relief of established rhinitis, seasonal or perennial, and even vasomotor rhinitis; they provide efficacy with substantially reduced side effects as compared with this same class of agent administered orally. Their most frequent side effect is local irritation, with *Candida* overgrowth being a rare occurrence. The topical-to-systemic activity of flunisolide or budesonide is significantly greater than for beclomethasone or triamcinolone with much less systemic absorption. Topical high-potency glucocorticoids exhibit superior efficacy as compared to antihistamines throughout the pollen seasons, especially when there is high pollen exposure. Thus, for patients who do not benefit adequately from a full dosage of nonsedating H_1 antihistamine and a maintenance dosage of cromolyn sodium, an alpha-adrenergic agent for short-term relief should be replaced by high-potency topical glucocorticoids. For systemic symptoms not related to the nasopharynx, such as allergic conjunctivitis, treatment may be local or by addition of an oral antihistamine.

Immunotherapy, often termed *hyposensitization*, consists of repeated subcutaneous injections of gradually increasing concentrations of the allergen(s) considered to be specifically responsible for the symptom complex. Controlled studies of ragweed, grass, dust mite, and cat dander allergens administered for treatment of allergic rhinitis have demonstrated at least partial relief of symptoms and signs. The duration of such immunotherapy is 3 to 5 years, with discontinuation being based upon minimal symptoms over two consecutive seasons of exposure. Clinical benefit appears related to the administration of a high dose of allergen at weekly or biweekly intervals. Patients should remain at the treatment site for at least 20 min after allergen administration so that any anaphylactic consequence can be managed. Local reactions with erythema and induration are not uncommon and may persist for 1 to 3 days. Immunotherapy is contraindicated in patients with significant cardiovascular disease or unstable asthma and should be conducted with particular caution in any patient requiring beta-adrenergic blocking therapy because of the difficulty in managing an anaphylactic complication. The immunologic characteristics of a response include a rise in antibodies of the IgG class, a small increase in specific IgE early in the treatment course followed by a plateau or decline, and a decline in the percentage of histamine released from peripheral blood basophilic leukocytes challenged with a fixed concentration of the allergen. The antibodies of the IgG class might well reduce or neutralize the quantity of allergen available for interaction with the tissue mast cells but, more important, could modify the seasonal booster response in specific IgE synthesis. None of the individual parameters of the response to immunotherapy correlates well with the assessments of clinical efficacy, suggesting that benefit is derived from a complex of effects that likely includes a reduction in T cell cytokine production. Immunotherapy should be reserved for clearly documented seasonal or perennial rhinitis, clinically related to defined allergen exposure with confirmation by the presence of allergen-specific IgE, which has failed management by allergen avoidance and pharmacotherapy due to lack of efficacy or side effects. A sequence for the management of allergic or perennial rhinitis based upon an allergen-specific diagnosis and stepwise management as required for symptom control would include the following: (1)

identification of the offending allergen(s) by history with confirmation of the presence of allergen-specific IgE by skin test (epicutaneous) and/or serum assay; (2) avoidance of the offending allergen; (3) for mild symptoms, prophylactic management with topical cromolyn sodium or treatment with a single bedtime dose of chlorpheniramine (if the latter is associated with undue side effects, substitute astemizole or terfenadine providing that there is no contraindication due to a concomitant medication or disease; (4) for prominent symptoms, utilization of topical beclomethasone with replacement by budesonide or flunisolide as needed for a satisfactory clinical outcome; and (5) for management failures despite avoidance and pharmacotherapy, progression to immunotherapy.

BIBLIOGRAPHY

Austen KF, Metcalfe DD: Anaphylactic syndrome, in *Immunological Diseases*, 5th ed, M Frank et al (eds). Boston, Little, Brown, 1995

Craig SS et al: Ultrastructural analysis of human T and TC mast cells identified by immunoelectron microscopy. Lab Invest 58:682, 1988

Gordon JR et al: Mast cells as a source of multifunctional cytokines. Immunol Today 11:458, 1990

Lewis RA et al: Leukotrienes and other products of the 5-lipoxygenase pathway: Biochemistry and relation to pathobiology in human diseases. N Engl J Med 323:645, 1990

McNeil HP, Austen KF: Biology of the mast cell, in *Immunological Diseases*, 5th ed, M Frank et al (eds). Boston, Little, Brown, 1995

Metcalfe DD, Austen KF: Mastocytosis, in *Immunological Diseases*, 5th ed, M Frank et al (eds). Boston, Little, Brown, 1995

Naclerio RM: Allergic rhinitis. N Engl J Med 325:860, 1991

Ravetch JV, Kinet J-P: Fc receptors. Annu Rev Immunol 9:457, 1991

Soter NA: Urticaria and angioedema, in *Dermatology In General Medicine*, 4th ed, TB Fitzpatrick et al (eds). New York, McGraw-Hill, 1993

Valentine MD: Insect venom allergy, in *Immunological Diseases*, 5th ed, M Frank et al (eds). Boston, Little, Brown, 1995

311

Kim B. Yancey, Thomas J. Lawley

IMMUNOLOGICALLY MEDIATED SKIN DISEASES

A number of immunologically mediated skin diseases and the cutaneous manifestations of immunologically mediated systemic disorders are now recognized as distinct entities with relatively consistent clinical, histologic, and immunopathologic findings. Many of these disorders are due to autoimmune mechanisms. Clinically, they are characterized by morbidity (pain, pruritus, disfigurement) and in some instances by mortality (largely due to loss of epidermal barrier function and/or secondary infection). The major features of the more common immunologically mediated skin diseases are summarized in this chapter (see Table 311-1).

PEMPHIGUS VULGARIS Pemphigus vulgaris (PV) is a blistering skin disease seen predominantly in elderly patients. Patients with PV have an increased incidence of the HLA-DR4 and -DRw6 serologically defined haplotypes. This disorder is characterized by the loss of cohesion between epidermal cells (a process termed *acantholysis*) with the resultant formation of intraepidermal blisters. Clinical lesions of PV typically consist of flaccid blisters on either normal-appearing or erythematous skin. These blisters rupture easily, leaving denuded areas that may crust and enlarge peripherally. Substantial portions of the body surface may be denuded in severe cases. Manual pressure to the skin of these patients may elicit the separation of the epidermis (Nikolsky's sign). This finding, while characteristic of PV, is not specific to this disorder and is also seen in toxic epidermal necrolysis, Stevens-Johnson syndrome, and a few other skin diseases. Lesions in PV typically present on the scalp, face, neck, axilla, trunk, and oral cavity. In half or more of patients, lesions begin in the mouth; approximately 90 percent of patients have oromucosal involvement at some time during the course of their disease. Involvement of other mucosal surfaces (e.g., pharyngeal, laryngeal, esophageal, conjunctival, vulval, or rectal) can occur in severe disease. Pruritus may be a feature of early pemphigus lesions; extensive denudation may be associated with severe pain. Lesions usually heal without scarring, except at sites complicated by secondary infection or mechanically induced dermal wounds. Nonetheless, postinflammatory hyperpigmentation is usually present at sites of healed lesions for some time.

Biopsies of early lesions demonstrate intraepidermal vesicle formation secondary to loss of cohesion between epidermal cells (i.e., acantholytic blisters). Blister cavities contain acantholytic epidermal cells, which appear as round homogeneous cells containing hyperchromatic nuclei. Basal keratinocytes remain attached to the epidermal basement membrane, hence blister formation is within the suprabasal portion of the epidermis. Lesional skin may contain focal collections of intraepidermal eosinophils within blister cavities; dermal alterations are slight, usually limited to an eosinophil-predominant leukocytic infiltrate. Direct immunofluorescence microscopy of lesional or normal skin shows deposits of IgG on the surface of keratinocytes; in contrast, deposits of complement are typically found in lesional but not normal skin. Keratinocyte IgG deposits are derived from a circulating autoantibody directed against cell surface antigens. Circulating autoantibodies can be demonstrated in 80 to 90 percent of PV patients by indirect immunofluorescence microscopy; monkey esophagus is the optimal substrate for demonstration of these autoantibodies. In PV, autoantibodies are directed against a 130-kDa desmosomal cadherin molecule (desmoglein 3) that forms a complex with plakoglobin, an 85-kDa protein found in both desmosomal and adherens junctions. Anti-desmoglein 3 autoantibodies in patients with PV are responsible for dysadhesion of epidermal cells. The titer of circulating autoantibody (determined by indirect immunofluorescence microscopy) correlates roughly with disease activity. These immunopathologic findings aid the diagnosis of PV and its differentiation from other blistering skin diseases.

PV can be life-threatening. Prior to the availability of glucocorticoids, the mortality ranged from 60 to 90 percent. The current mortality is approximately 5 to 15 percent. Common causes of morbidity and mortality are infection and complications of treatment with glucocorticoids. Bad prognostic factors include advanced age, widespread involvement, and the requirement for high doses of glucocorticoids (with or without other immunosuppressive agents) for control of disease. The course of PV in individual patients is variable and difficult to predict. Some patients achieve remission after variable periods (40 percent of patients in some series), but others may require long-term treatment or succumb to complications of their disease or its treatment. The mainstay of treatment is systemic glucocorticoids. Patients with moderate to severe disease are usually started on prednisone 60 to 80 mg/d. If new lesions continue to appear after 1 to 2 weeks of treatment, the dose should be increased. Many regimens have combined an immunosuppressive agent with systemic glucocorticoids for control of PV. The two most frequently used are either azathioprine (1 mg/kg per day) or cyclophosphamide (1 mg/kg per day). It is important to bring severe or progressive disease under control quickly to lessen the severity and/or duration of this disorder.

PEMPHIGUS FOLIACEUS Pemphigus foliaceus (PF) is distinguished from PV by several features. In PF, acantholytic blisters are located high within the epidermis, usually just beneath the stratum corneum. Hence PF is a more superficial blistering disease than PV. The distribution of lesions in the two disorders is much the same, except that in PF mucous membrane lesions are rare. Patients with PF rarely demonstrate intact blisters but rather exhibit shallow erosions associated with erythema, scale, and crust formation. Mild cases of PF resemble severe seborrheic dermatitis; severe PF may cause extensive exfoliation. Sun exposure (ultraviolet irradiation) may be an aggravating factor. A blistering skin disease endemic to south central Brazil known as fogo selvagem or Brazilian pemphigus is clinically, histologically, and immunopathologically indistinguishable from PF.

Patients with PF have immunopathologic features in common with PV. Specifically, direct immunofluorescence microscopy of normal, perilesional skin demonstrates IgG on the surface of keratinocytes. As in PV, patients with PF frequently have circulating IgG autoantibodies against keratinocyte cell surface antigens. Guinea pig esophagus is the optimal substrate for indirect immunofluorescence microscopy studies of sera from patients with PF. In PF, autoantibodies are directed against desmoglein 1, a 160-kDa desmosomal cadherin that (like PV antigen) is complexed to plakoglobin.

Although pemphigus has been associated with several autoimmune diseases, its association with thymoma and/or myasthenia gravis is particularly notable. To date, more than 30 cases of thymoma and/or myasthenia gravis have been reported in association with pemphigus, usually with PF. Patients also may develop pemphigus as a consequence of drug exposure. The most frequently implicated agent is penicillamine; other offenders include captopril, rifampin, piroxicam, penicillin, and phenobarbital. Drug-induced pemphigus usually resembles PF rather than PV; autoantibodies in these patients have the same antigenic specificity as they do in other pemphigus patients. In most patients, lesions resolve following discontinuation of the drug; however, some patients require treatment with systemic glucocorticoids and/or immunosuppressive agents.

PF is generally a far less severe disease than PV and carries a better prognosis. Localized disease can be treated conservatively with topical or intralesional glucocorticoids; more active cases can usually be controlled with systemic glucocorticoids.

PARANEOPLASTIC PEMPHIGUS Paraneoplastic pemphigus is a recently described autoimmune acantholytic mucocutaneous disease associated with an occult or confirmed neoplasm. Patients with paraneoplastic pemphigus typically show painful mucosal erosive lesions in association with pruritic papulosquamous eruptions that often progress to blisters. Palm and sole involvement is common in these patients and raises the possibility that prior reports of neoplasia-associated erythema multiforme actually may have represented unrecognized cases of paraneoplastic pemphigus. Biopsies of lesional skin from these patients show varying combinations of acantholysis, keratinocyte necrosis, and vacuolar-interface dermatitis. Direct immunofluorescence microscopy of patient skin shows deposits of IgG and complement on the surface of keratinocytes as well as similar immunoreactants in the epidermal basement membrane zone. Patients with paraneoplastic pemphigus have IgG autoantibodies that react with the surface of tissues containing desmosomes (i.e., complex and simple epithelia as well as myocardium). These autoantibodies immunoprecipitate a unique complex of four polypeptides (250, 230, 210, and 190 kDa) from keratinocyte cell extracts. In sodium dodecyl sulfate–polyacrylamide gel electrophoresis, the 250- and 210-kDa antigens comigrate with the desmosomal plaque–associated proteins desmoplakins I and II, respectively, whereas the 230-kDa antigen comigrates with bullous pemphigoid antigen (see below); the identity of the other antigen in this complex has not yet been conclusively determined. Interestingly, passive transfer of patient immunoglobulin to neonatal mice produces keratinocyte detachment, indicating that autoantibodies from patients with paraneoplastic pemphigus are pathogenic mediators of tissue damage. Paraneoplastic pemphigus is generally treatment-resistant, although patients may improve (or even remit) following resection of underlying benign neoplasms. The predominant neoplasms associated with this disorder are non-Hodgkin's lymphoma, chronic lymphocytic leukemia, Castleman's disease, thymoma, and spindle cell neoplasms.

BULLOUS PEMPHIGOID Bullous pemphigoid (BP) is a subepidermal blistering skin disease usually seen in the elderly. Lesions typically consist of tense blisters on either normal-appearing or erythematous skin. The lesions are usually distributed over the lower abdomen, groin, and flexor surface of the extremities; oral mucosal lesions are found in 10 to 40 percent of patients. Pruritus may be nonexistent or severe. As lesions evolve, tense blisters tend to rupture and be replaced by flaccid lesions or erosions with or without surmounting crust. Nontraumatized blisters heal without scarring. There is no ethnic or HLA association. Despite isolated reports, several studies have shown that patients with BP do not have an increased incidence of malignancy in comparison with appropriately age- and sex-matched controls.

While biopsies of early lesional skin demonstrate subepidermal blisters, the histologic features depend on the character of the particular lesion. Lesions on normal-appearing skin generally show a sparse perivascular leukocytic infiltrate with some eosinophils. Biopsies of inflammatory lesions typically show an eosinophil-rich, leukocytic infiltrate within the papillary dermis at sites of vesicle formation and in perivascular areas. In addition to eosinophils, these cell-rich lesions also contain mononuclear cells and neutrophils. It is not always possible to distinguish BP from other subepidermal blistering skin diseases by routine histologic techniques.

Immunopathologic studies have broadened our understanding of this disease and aided its diagnosis. Direct immunofluorescence microscopy of normal-appearing perilesional skin shows linear deposits of IgG and/or C3 in the epidermal basement membrane. The sera of approximately 70 percent of these patients contain circulating IgG autoantibodies that bind the epidermal basement membrane of normal human skin in indirect immunofluorescence microscopy. An even higher percentage of patients shows reactivity to the epidermal side of 1 M NaCl split skin

Table 311-1

Immunologically Mediated Blistering Skin Diseases

Disease	Clinical	Histology	Immunopathology
Pemphigus vulgaris	Flaccid blisters, denuded skin, oromucosal lesions	Blister formed in suprabasal layer of epidermis	Cell surface deposits of IgG on keratinocytes
Pemphigus foliaceus	Crusts and shallow erosions on scalp, central face, neck, upper chest, and back	Blister formed in superficial layers of epidermis	Cell surface deposits of IgG on keratinocytes
Bullous pemphigoid	Large tense blisters on flexor surfaces, oromucosal lesions	Blister formed in subepidermal region, usually eosinophil-rich	Linear band of IgG and/or C3 at BMZ*
Dermatitis herpetiformis	Extremely itchy small papules and vesicles on elbows, knees, buttocks, and posterior nuchal area	Subepidermal blister with neutrophils in dermal papillae	Granular deposits of IgA in dermal papillae
Linear IgA disease	Extremely itchy small papules and vesicles on extensor surfaces, occasionally larger arciform blisters	Subepidermal blister with neutrophils in dermal papillae	Linear band of IgA at BMZ
Epidermolysis bullosa acquisita	Blisters, scarring, and milia on dorsum of hands, elbows, knees; oromucosal lesions	Blister is subepidermal and can be inflammatory or not	Linear band of IgG and/or C3 at BMZ
Cicatricial pemphigoid	Erosive and/or blistering lesions of mucous membranes and possibly the skin; scarring at some sites	Blister is subepithelial and may or may not be associated with a mononuclear cell–rich infiltrate	Linear band of IgG, IgA, and/or C3 at BMZ

* BMZ, basement membrane zone of epidermis.

[an alternative immunofluorescence microscopy test substrate that is commonly used to distinguish circulating IgG anti-basement membrane autoantibodies in patients with BP from those in patients with similar, yet different, subepidermal blistering diseases (e.g., epidermolysis bullosa acquisita, see below)]. No correlation exists between the titer of these autoantibodies and disease activity. In BP, circulating autoantibodies recognize 230- and (in approximately 50 percent of BP patients) 180-kDa hemidesmosome-associated proteins in basal keratinocytes. Autoantibodies are thought to develop against these antigens, deposit in situ, and activate complement that subsequently produces dermal mast cell degranulation and granulocyte-rich leukocytic infiltrates that cause tissue damage and blister formation.

BP is generally benign, but it may persist for months to years, with exacerbations or remissions. Although extensive involvement may result in widespread erosions and compromise cutaneous integrity, the mortality rate is low even in the absence of treatment. Nonetheless, deaths may occur in elderly and/or debilitated patients. The mainstay of treatment is systemic glucocorticoids. Patients with local or minimal disease can sometimes be controlled with topical glucocorticoids alone; patients with more extensive lesions generally respond to systemic glucocorticoids either alone or in combination with immunosuppressive agents. Patients will usually respond to prednisone, 40 to 60 mg/d. In some instances, azathioprine (1 mg/kg per day) or cyclophosphamide (1 mg/kg per day) are necessary adjuncts.

PEMPHIGOID GESTATIONIS Pemphigoid gestationis (PG), also known as herpes gestationis, is a rare, nonviral, subepidermal blistering disease of pregnancy and the puerperium. PG may begin during any trimester of pregnancy or present shortly after delivery. Lesions are usually distributed over the abdomen, trunk, and extremities; mucous membrane lesions are rare. Skin lesions in these patients may be quite polymorphic and consist of erythematous urticarial papules and plaques, vesiculopapules, and/or frank bullae. Lesions are almost always very pruritic. Severe exacerbations of PG frequently occur after delivery, typically within 24 to 48 h. PG tends to recur in subsequent pregnancies, often beginning earlier during such gestations. Brief flare-ups of disease may occur with resumption of menses and may develop in patients later exposed to oral contraceptives. Occasionally, infants of affected mothers demonstrate transient skin lesions.

Biopsies of early lesional skin show teardrop-shaped subepidermal vesicles forming in dermal papillae in association with an eosinophil-rich leukocytic infiltrate. Differentiation of PG from other subepidermal bullous diseases by light microscopy is often difficult. However, direct immunofluorescence microscopy of normal perilesional skin from PG patients reveals the immunopathologic hallmark of this disorder—linear deposits of C3 in the epidermal basement membrane zone. These deposits develop as a consequence of complement activation produced by a low titer IgG anti-basement membrane zone autoantibody. Recent studies have shown that the majority of PG sera contain autoantibodies that recognize the same 180-kDa hemidesmosome-associated protein that is targeted by autoantibodies in roughly 50 percent of patients with BP—a subepidermal bullous disease that resembles PG morphologically, histologically, and immunopathologically.

The goals of therapy in patients with PG are to prevent the development of new lesions, relieve intense pruritus, and care for erosions at sites of blister formation. Most patients require treatment with moderate doses of daily glucocorticoids (i.e., 20 to 40 mg of prednisone) at some point in their course. Mild cases (or brief flare-ups) may be controlled by vigorous use of potent topical glucocorticoids. Although PG was once thought to be associated with an increased risk of fetal morbidity and mortality, the best evidence now suggests that these infants may only be at increased risk of being slightly premature or "small for dates." Current evidence suggests that there is no difference in the incidence of uncomplicated live births in PG patients treated with systemic glucocorticoids and in those managed more conservatively. If systemic glucocorticoids are administered, newborns are at risk for development of reversible adrenal insufficiency.

DERMATITIS HERPETIFORMIS Dermatitis herpetiformis (DH) is an intensely pruritic, chronic papulovesicular skin disease characterized by lesions symmetrically distributed over extensor surfaces (i.e., elbows, knees, buttocks, back, scalp, and posterior neck). The primary lesion in this disorder is a papule, papulovesicle, or urticarial plaque. Because pruritus is prominent, patients may present with excoriations and crusted papules but no observable primary lesions. Patients sometimes report that their pruritus has a distinctive burning or stinging component; the onset of such local symptoms reliably heralds the development of distinct clinical lesions 12 to 24 h later. Almost all DH patients have an associated, usually subclinical, gluten-sensitive enteropathy (see also Chap. 285), and more than 90 percent express the HLA-B8/DRw3 and HLA-DQw2 haplotypes. DH may present at any age, including childhood; onset in the second to fourth decades is most common. The disease is typically chronic.

Biopsy of early lesional skin reveals neutrophil-rich infiltrates within dermal papillae. Neutrophils, fibrin, edema, and microvesicle formation at these sites are characteristic of early disease. Older lesions may demonstrate nonspecific features of a subepidermal bulla or an excoriated papule. Because the clinical and histologic features of this disease can be variable and resemble other subepidermal blistering disorders, the diagnosis can be confirmed by direct immunofluorescence microscopy of normal-appearing perilesional skin. Such studies demonstrate granular deposits of IgA (with or without complement components) in the papillary dermis and along the epidermal basement membrane zone. IgA deposits in the skin are unaffected by control of disease with medication; however, these immunoreactants may diminish in intensity or disappear in patients maintained for long periods on a strict gluten-free diet (see below). Patients with granular deposits of IgA in their epidermal basement membrane zone typically do not have circulating IgA anti-basement membrane autoantibodies and should be distinguished from individuals with linear IgA deposits at this site (see below).

Although most DH patients do not report overt gastrointestinal symptoms or laboratory evidence of malabsorption, biopsies of small bowel usually reveal blunting of intestinal villi and a lymphocytic infiltrate in the lamina propria. As is true for patients with celiac disease, this gastrointestinal abnormality can be reversed by a gluten-free diet. Moreover, if maintained, this diet alone may control the skin disease and eventuate in clearance of IgA deposits from these patients' epidermal basement membrane zone. Subsequent gluten exposure in the latter patients alters the morphology of their small bowel, elicits a flare-up of their skin disease, and is associated with the reappearance of IgA in their epidermal basement membrane zone. Patients with DH also have an increased incidence of thyroid abnormalities, achlorhydria, atrophic gastritis, and antigastric parietal cell antibodies. These associations likely relate to the high frequency of the HLA-B8/DRw3 haplotype in these patients, since this marker is commonly linked to autoimmune disorders. The mainstay of treatment of DH is dapsone. Patients respond rapidly (24 to 48 h) to dapsone but require careful pretreatment evaluation and close follow-up to ensure that complications are avoided or controlled. All patients on more than 100 mg/d dapsone will have some hemolysis and methemoglobinemia. These are expected pharmacologic side effects of dapsone. It is important to employ the lowest possible maintenance dose of dapsone to control symptoms and lesions. Gluten restriction can control DH and lessen dapsone requirements; this diet must rigidly exclude gluten to be of maximal benefit. Moreover, many months of dietary restriction may be necessary before a beneficial result is achieved. Good dietary counselling by a trained dietitian is essential.

LINEAR IgA DISEASE Linear IgA disease, once considered a variant form of dermatitis herpetiformis, is actually a separate and distinct entity. Clinically, these patients may resemble typical cases of DH, bullous pemphigoid, or other subepidermal blistering diseases. Lesions typically consist of papulovesicles, bullae, and/or urticarial plaques, predominantly on extensor (as seen in "classic" DH), central, or flexural sites. Oral mucosal involvement does occur in some patients. Severe pruritus resembles that in patients with DH. Patients with linear IgA disease do not have an increased frequency of the HLA-B8/DRw3 haplotype or an associated enteropathy and hence are not candidates for a gluten-free diet.

The histologic alterations in early lesions may be virtually indistinguishable from those in DH. However, direct immunofluorescence microscopy of normal-appearing perilesional skin reveals linear deposits of IgA (and often C3) in the epidermal basement membrane zone. Many patients with linear IgA disease demonstrate circulating IgA autoantibodies against a 97-kDa protein in normal epidermal basement membrane. These patients generally respond to treatment with dapsone, 50 to 200 mg/d.

EPIDERMOLYSIS BULLOSA ACQUISITA (EBA) EBA is a rare, noninherited, polymorphic, subepidermal blistering disease. (The inherited form is discussed in Chap. 348.) Patients with classic or noninflammatory EBA have blisters on noninflamed skin, atrophic scars, milia, nail dystrophy, and oral lesions. Because lesions generally occur at sites exposed to minor trauma, classic EBA is considered to be a mechanobullous disease. Other patients with EBA have widespread inflammatory, scarring, bullous lesions and oromucosal involvement that resembles severe BP. Interestingly, some patients present with an inflammatory bullous skin disease that subsequently evolves into the classic noninflammatory form of this disorder. In general, EBA is chronic; associations with multiple myeloma, amyloidosis, inflammatory bowel disease, and diabetes mellitus have been reported. The HLA-DR2 haplotype is found with increased frequency in these patients.

The histology of lesional skin varies depending on the type or character of the lesion being studied. Noninflammatory bullae show subepidermal blisters with a sparse leukocytic infiltrate and resemble those in patients with porphyria cutanea tarda. Inflammatory vesiculobullous lesions consist of a subepidermal blister and neutrophil-rich leukocytic infiltrates in the superficial dermis. EBA patients have continuous deposits of IgG (and frequently C3 as well as other complement components) in a linear pattern within the epidermal basement membrane zone. Ultrastructurally, these immunoreactants are found in the sublamina densa region in association with anchoring fibrils, wheat stack–like structures that extend from the lamina densa into the underlying papillary dermis. Approximately 25 to 50 percent of EBA patients have circulating IgG autoantibodies directed against type VII collagen—the collagen species found in anchoring fibrils. Such IgG anti-basement membrane autoantibodies bind the dermal side of 1 M NaCl split skin (in contrast to IgG anti-basement membrane autoantibodies in patients with BP that bind either epidermal or both sides of this indirect immunofluorescence microscopy test substrate).

Treatment of EBA is generally unsatisfactory. Some patients with inflammatory EBA may respond to systemic glucocorticoids, either alone or in combination with immunosuppressive agents. Other patients (especially those with neutrophil-rich inflammatory lesions) may respond to dapsone. The chronic, noninflammatory form of this disease is largely resistant to treatment.

CICATRICIAL PEMPHIGOID Cicatricial pemphigoid (CP) is a rare, acquired, subepithelial blistering disease characterized by erosive lesions of mucous membranes and skin that result in scarring of at least some sites of involvement. Immunopathologically, perilesional mucosa and skin of patients with CP demonstrate in situ deposits of immunoreactants in epithelial basement membranes. Common sites of involvement include the oral mucosa (especially the gingiva) and conjunctiva; other sites that may be affected include the nasopharyngeal, laryngeal, esophageal, genital, and rectal mucosa. Skin lesions (present in about one-third of patients) tend to predominate on the scalp, face, and upper trunk and generally consist of a few scattered erosions or tense blisters on an erythematous or urticarial base. Less commonly, skin lesions present as a few blisters that occur repeatedly on the same sites on the head or neck; such lesions eventually scar and may not be associated with mucosal involvement. CP is typically a chronic and progressive disorder. Serious complications may arise as a consequence of ocular, laryngeal, or esophageal lesions. Erosive conjunctivitis may result in shortened fornices, symblephara, ankyloblepharon, entropion, corneal opacities, and (in severe cases) blindness. Similarly, erosive lesions of the larynx may cause hoarseness, pain, and tissue loss that if unrecognized and untreated may eventuate in complete destruction of the airway. Esophageal lesions may result in stenosis and/or strictures that may place patients at risk for aspiration.

Biopsies of lesional tissue generally demonstrate subepithelial vesiculobullae and a mononuclear leukocytic infiltrate. Neutrophils and eosinophils may be seen in biopsies of early lesions; older lesions may demonstrate a scant leukocytic infiltrate and fibrosis. Direct immunofluorescence microscopy of perilesional tissue typically demonstrates deposits of IgG, IgA, and/or C3 in these patients' epithelial basement membranes. Because many of these patients show no evidence of circulating anti-basement membrane autoantibodies, testing of perilesional skin is important diagnostically. Although CP was once thought to be a single nosologic entity, it is now largely regarded as a disease phenotype that may develop as a consequence of an autoimmune reaction against a variety of different molecules in epithelial basement membranes (e.g., bullous pemphigoid antigens, laminin 5, or other antigens yet to be completely defined). Treatment of CP is largely dependent upon sites of involvement. Due to potentially severe complications, ocular, laryngeal, and/or esophageal involvement require aggressive systemic treatment with dapsone, prednisone, or the latter in combination with another immunosuppressive agent (e.g., azathioprine or cyclophosphamide). Less threatening forms of the disease may be managed with topical or intralesional glucocorticoids.

AUTOIMMUNE SYSTEMIC DISEASES WITH PROMINENT CUTANEOUS FEATURES

DERMATOMYOSITIS The cutaneous manifestations of dermatomyositis (see Chap. 315) are often distinctive but at times may resemble those of systemic lupus erythematosus (SLE) (see Chap. 312), scleroderma (see Chap. 314), or other overlapping connective tissue diseases (see Chap. 314). The extent and severity of cutaneous disease may or may not correlate with the extent and severity of the myositis. Patients with severe muscle involvement may have relatively minor skin changes, whereas patients with marked skin involvement may have mild muscle disease. The cutaneous manifestations of dermatomyositis are similar whether the disease appears in childhood or old age, except that calcification of subcutaneous tissue is a common late sequela in childhood dermatomyositis.

The cutaneous signs of dermatomyositis may precede or follow the development of myositis by weeks to years. Cases lacking muscle involvement (i.e., dermatomyositis sine myositis) also have been reported. The most common manifestation is a purple-red discoloration of the upper eyelids, sometimes associated with scaling ("heliotrope" erythema) and periorbital edema. Erythema on the cheeks and nose in a "butterfly" distribution may resemble the eruption in SLE. Erythematous or violaceous scaling patches are common on the upper anterior chest, posterior neck, scalp, and the extensor surfaces of the arms, legs, and hands. Erythema and scaling may be particularly prominent over the elbows, knees, and the dorsal interphalangeal joints. Approximately one-third of patients have violaceous, flat-topped papules over the dorsal interphalangeal joints that are pathognomonic of dermatomyositis (Gottron's sign or Gottron's papules). These lesions can be contrasted with the erythema and scaling on the dorsum of the fingers in some patients with SLE which spares the skin over the interphalangeal joints. Periungual telangiectasia may be prominent, and a lacy or reticulated erythema may be associated with fine scaling on the extensor surfaces of the thighs and upper arms. Other patients, particularly those with long-standing disease, develop areas of hypopigmentation, hyperpigmentation, mild atrophy, and telangiectasia known as *poikiloderma vasculare atrophicans*. Poikiloderma is rare in both SLE and scleroderma and thus can serve as a clinical sign that distinguishes dermatomyositis from these two diseases. However, cutaneous changes may be similar in scleroderma and dermatomyositis and may include thickening and binding down of the skin of the hands (sclerodactyly) as well as Raynaud's phenomenon. However, the presence of severe muscle disease, Gottron's papules, heliotrope erythema, and poikiloderma serve to distinguish these patients as having dermatomyositis. Skin biopsy of erythematous, scaling lesions of dermatomyositis may reveal only mild nonspecific inflammation but sometimes may show changes indistinguishable from those found in SLE, including epidermal atrophy, hydropic degeneration of basal keratinocytes, edema of the upper dermis, and a mild mononuclear cell infiltrate. Direct immunofluorescence microscopy of lesional skin is usually negative. Treatment should be directed at the systemic disease. In the few instances where adjunctive cutaneous therapy is desirable, topical glucocorticoids are sometimes useful. These patients should avoid exposure to ultraviolet irradiation and use photoprotective measures such as sunscreens.

LUPUS ERYTHEMATOSUS The cutaneous manifestations of lupus erythematosus (LE) (see Chap. 312) can be divided into acute, subacute, and chronic (i.e., discoid LE) types. *Acute cutaneous LE* is characterized by erythema of the nose and malar eminences in a "butterfly" distribution. The erythema is often sudden in onset, accompanied by edema and fine scale, and correlated with systemic involvement. Patients may have widespread involvement of the face as well as erythema and scaling of the extensor surfaces of the extremities and upper chest. These acute lesions, while sometimes evanescent, usually last for days and are often associated with exacerbations of systemic disease. Skin biopsy of acute lesions may show only a sparse dermal infiltrate of mononuclear cells and dermal edema. In some instances, cellular infiltrates around blood vessels and hair follicles are notable, as is hydropic degeneration of basal cells of the epidermis. Direct immunofluorescence microscopy of lesional skin frequently reveals deposits of immunoglobulin(s) and complement in the epidermal basement membrane zone. Treatment is aimed at control of systemic disease; photoprotection in this, as well as in other forms of LE, is very important.

Subacute cutaneous lupus erythematosus (SCLE) is characterized by a widespread photosensitive, nonscarring eruption. About half of these patients have SLE in which severe renal and central nervous system involvement is uncommon. SCLE may present as a papulosquamous eruption that resembles psoriasis or annular lesions that resemble those seen in erythema multiforme. In the papulosquamous form, discrete erythematous papules arise on the back, chest, shoulders, extensor surfaces of the arms, and the dorsum of the hands but are uncommon on the face, flexor surfaces of the arms, and below the waist. The slightly scaling papules tend to merge into large plaques, some with a reticulate appearance. The annular form involves the same areas and also begins as an erythematous papule but tends to develop oval, circular, or polycyclic lesions. The lesions of SCLE are more widespread but have less tendency for scarring than do lesions of discoid LE. Skin biopsy reveals a dense mononuclear cell infiltrate around hair follicles and blood vessels in the superficial dermis, combined with hydropic degeneration of basal cells in the epidermis. Direct immunofluorescence microscopy of lesional skin reveals deposits of immunoglobulin(s) in the epidermal basement membrane zone in about half these cases. Most SCLE patients have anti-Ro antibodies. Local therapy is usually unsuccessful, and most patients require treatment with aminoquinoline antimalarials. Low-dose therapy with oral glucocorticoids is sometimes necessary; photoprotective measures against both ultraviolet B and A wavelengths are very important.

Discoid lupus erythematosus (DLE) is characterized by discrete lesions, most often on the face, scalp, or external ears. The lesions are erythematous papules or plaques with a thick, adherent scale that occludes hair follicles (follicular plugging). When the scale is removed, its underside will show small excrescences that correlate with the openings of hair follicles and is termed a "carpet tack" appearance. This finding is relatively specific for DLE. Long-standing lesions develop central atrophy, scarring, and hypopigmentation but frequently have erythematous, sometimes raised borders at the periphery. These lesions persist for years and tend to expand slowly. Only 5 to 10 percent of patients with DLE meet the American Rheumatism Association criteria for SLE. However, typical discoid lesions are frequently seen in patients with SLE. Biopsy of DLE lesions shows hyperkeratosis, follicular plugging, and atrophy of the epidermis. The dermal-epidermal junction reveals hydropic degeneration of basal keratinocytes, and a mononuclear cell infiltrate surrounds hair follicles and blood vessels. Direct immunofluorescence microscopy demonstrates immunoglobulin(s) and complement deposits at the basement membrane zone in about 90 percent of cases. Treatment is focused on control of local cutaneous disease and consists mainly of photoprotection and topical or intralesional glucocorticoids. If local therapy is ineffective, use of aminoquinoline antimalarials may be indicated.

SCLERODERMA AND MORPHEA The skin changes of scleroderma (see Chap. 314) usually begin on the hands, feet, and face, with episodes of recurrent nonpitting edema. Sclerosis of the skin begins distally on the fingers (sclerodactyly) and spreads proximally, usually accompanied by resorption of bone of the fingertips, which may have punched out ulcers, stellate scars, or areas of hemorrhage. The fingers may actually shrink in size and become sausage-shaped, and since the fingernails are usually unaffected, the nails may curve over the end of the fingertips. Periungual telangiectasias are usually present, but periungual erythema is rare. In advanced cases, the extremities show contractures and calcinosis cutis. Face involvement includes a smooth, unwrinkled brow, taut skin over the nose, shrinkage of tissue around the mouth, and perioral radial furrowing. Matlike telangiectasias are often present, particularly on the face and hands. Involved skin feels indurated, smooth, and bound to underlying structures; hyperpigmentation and hypopigmentation are also often present. Raynaud's phenomenon, i.e., cold-induced blanching, cyanosis, and reactive hyperemia, is present in almost all patients with scleroderma and can precede development of scleroderma by many years. The combination of calcinosis cutis, Raynaud's phenomenon, esophageal dysmotility, sclerodactyly, and telangiectasia has been termed the *CREST syndrome*. Anticentromere antibodies have been reported in a very high percentage of patients with the CREST syndrome but in only a small minority of patients with scleroderma. Skin biopsy reveals thickening of the dermis and homogenization of collagen bundles. Direct immunofluorescence microscopy of lesional skin is usually negative.

Morphea, which has been called *localized scleroderma*, is characterized by localized thickening and sclerosis of skin, usually affecting young adults or children. Morphea begins as erythematous or flesh-colored plaques that become sclerotic, develop central hypopigmentation, and demonstrate an erythematous border. In most cases, patients have one or a few lesions, and the disease is termed *localized morphea*. In some patients, widespread cutaneous lesions may occur, without systemic involvement. This form is called *generalized morphea*. Most patients with morphea do not have autoantibodies. Skin biopsy of morphea is indistinguishable from that of scleroderma. Linear scleroderma is a limited form of disease that presents in a linear, bandlike distribution and tends to involve deep as well as superficial layers of skin. Scleroderma and morphea are usually quite resistant to therapy with medications. For this reason, physical therapy to prevent joint contractures and to maintain function is employed and is often helpful.

Diffuse fasciitis with eosinophilia is a clinical entity that can sometimes be confused with scleroderma. There is usually the sudden onset of swelling, induration, and erythema of the extremities frequently following significant physical exertion. The proximal portions of extremities (arms, forearms, thighs, legs) are more often involved than are the hands and feet. While the skin is indurated, it is usually not bound down as in scleroderma. These skin findings are accompanied by peripheral blood eosinophilia, increased erythrocyte sedimentation rate, and sometimes hypergammaglobulinemia. Deep biopsy of affected areas of skin reveals inflammation and thickening of the deep fascia overlying muscle. An inflammatory infiltrate composed of eosinophils and mononuclear cells is usually found. Patients with eosinophilic fasciitis appear to be at increased risk to develop bone marrow failure or other hematologic abnormalities. While the ultimate course of eosinophilic fasciitis is uncertain, many patients respond favorably to treatment with prednisone in doses ranging from 40 to 60 mg/d.

The *eosinophilia-myalgia syndrome*, a disorder reported in epidemic numbers in 1989 and linked to ingestion of tryptophan manufactured by a single company in Japan, is a multisystem disorder characterized by debilitating myalgias and absolute eosinophilia in association with varying combinations of arthralgias, pulmonary symptoms, and peripheral edema. In a later phase (i.e., 3 to 6 months after initial symptoms), these patients often develop localized sclerodermatous skin changes, weight loss, and/or neuropathy (see Chap. 314). The precise cause of this syndrome, which may resemble other sclerotic skin conditions, is unknown. However, the clustering of cases suggests that an impurity or contaminant in a manufactured tryptophan preparation is likely.

BIBLIOGRAPHY

ANHALT GJ et al: Paraneoplastic pemphigus: An autoimmune mucocutaneous disease associated with neoplasia. N Engl J Med 323:1729, 1990

BRAVERMAN IM: Connective tissue diseases, in *Skin Signs of Systemic Disease*. Philadelphia, Saunders, 1981

FINE JD: Management of acquired bullous skin disease. N Engl J Med 333:1475, 1995

GAMMON WR et al: Epidermolysis bullosa acquisita—A pemphigoid-like disease. J Am Acad Dermatol 11:820, 1984

HALL RP: Dermatitis herpetiformis. J Invest Dermatol 99:873, 1992

KATZ SI et al: Dermatitis herpetiformis: The skin and the gut. Ann Intern Med 93:857, 1980

KORMAN N: Pemphigus. J Am Acad Dermatol 18:1219, 1988

SHORNICK JK: Herpes gestationis. J Am Acad Dermatol 17:539, 1987

SHULMAN LE: Diffuse fasciitis with eosinophilia: A new syndrome. Arthritis Rheum 20(Suppl):205, 1977

STANLEY JR: Cell adhesion molecules as targets of autoantibodies in pemphigus and pemphigoid, bullous diseases due to defective epidermal cell adhesion. Adv Immunol 53:291, 1992

YANCEY KB: Adhesion molecules. II: Interactions of keratinocytes with epidermal basement membrane. J Invest Dermatol 104:1008, 1995

312

Bevra Hannahs Hahn

SYSTEMIC LUPUS ERYTHEMATOSUS

DEFINITION AND PREVALENCE Systemic lupus erythematosus (SLE) is a disease of unknown etiology in which tissues and cells are damaged by pathogenic autoantibodies and immune complexes. Ninety percent of cases are in women, usually of child-bearing age, but children, men, and the elderly can be affected. In the United States, the prevalence of SLE in urban areas varies from 15 to 50 per 100,000 population; it is more common in blacks than in whites. Hispanic and Asian populations are also susceptible.

PATHOGENESIS AND ETIOLOGY SLE results from tissue damage caused by pathogenic subsets of autoantibodies and immune complexes. The abnormal immune responses include (1) polyclonal and antigen-specific T and B lymphocyte hyperactivity, and (2) inadequate regulation of that hyperactivity. These abnormal immune responses probably depend upon interactions between susceptibility genes and environment. Evidence for genetic predisposition includes increased concordance for disease in monozygotic (24 to 58 percent) compared with dizygotic (0 to 6 percent) twins, a 10 to 15 percent frequency of patients with more than one affected family member, and correlations of certain genes [especially major histocompatibility complex (MHC) class II and class III] with disease and with selected autoantibodies. C4AQO, a defective class III allele that fails to encode a functional C4A protein, is the most common genetic marker associated with SLE in many ethnic groups (found in 40 to 50 percent of patients compared with 15 percent of healthy controls). Most individuals with homozygous deficiencies of early complement components develop SLE or lupus-like diseases. Certain extended haplotypes, such as B8.DR3.DQw2.C4AQO, predispose to SLE in some populations. Single-gene associations occur between HLA class II (especially DQ_{beta}) and autoantibodies that define clinical subsets of lupus. For example, high titers of IgG anti-DNA are associated with lupus nephritis and with DQB1*0201, *0602, and *0302 inherited with either DR2 or DR3. Antibodies to Ro/La (SS-A/SS-B) are associated with the dermatitis of subacute cutaneous lupus and with certain DQA and DQB genes inherited with DR3 (occasionally DR2). The lupus anticoagulant, correlated clinically with clotting, is associated with DQB*0301, *0302, *0303, and *0602 inherited with DR4 or DR7. The DQA or DQB susceptibility genes in each group share amino acid sequences that may determine the ability to make a particular autoantibody. Family studies suggest that genes unlinked to HLA also confer susceptibility, and that females are more likely than males to express the autoimmune manifestations of their genotypes. The more susceptibility genes one has, the higher is the relative risk for SLE; for most individuals at least three or four different genes are probably required.

Environmental factors that cause flares of SLE are largely unknown, with the exception of ultraviolet (UV)-B (and sometimes UV-A) light. As many as 70 percent of patients are photosensitive. Other factors, such as ingested alfalfa sprouts, and chemicals, such as hydrazines, have been implicated. Searches for viral/retroviral disease inducers have been inconclusive. Although some drugs can induce lupus-like disease, there are notable clinical and autoantibody differences between drug-induced and spontaneous lupus. Femaleness is clearly a susceptibility factor, since the prevalence in women of child-bearing years is seven to nine times higher than in men, whereas the female:male ratio is 3:1 in pre- and postmenopausal years. Metabolism of estrogenic and androgenic hormones may be abnormal in lupus patients. Sex hormones also influence immune tolerance.

Abnormal immune responses permit sustained production of pathogenic subsets of autoantibodies and immune complexes. No immunoglobulin genes have been identified that exclusively encode harmful autoantibodies, although certain V-region genes (especially V_H) seem to be preferentially used, and there is probably clonal selection of B cells secreting high-avidity antibodies to autoantigens. In most murine lupus models, T cell help is critical to development of full-blown disease; cells of CD4+CD8−, CD4−CD8+, and CD4−CD8− phenotypes all help autoantibody production in murine and human SLE. The abnormalities that permit hyperactivated self-reactive B and T cells to dominate immune repertoires in murine and human SLE are multiple and include defects in tolerance, apoptosis, idiotypic networks, immune complex clearance, generation of regulatory cells, and production of autoantibodies that can affect quantities and functions of living cells. The structure of antigens that stimulate autoantibodies is under investigation. Some are clearly derived from self (nucleosomes, ribonucleoprotein, erythrocyte and lymphocyte surface antigens); others may be from the external environment and mimic self (e.g., components of vesicular stomatitis virus mimic peptides in Sm antigen). Some autoantibodies induce disease by direct reaction with their antigens, such as those directed against surface antigens on erythrocytes or platelets. Others may attach to cell membranes [such as glomerular basement membrane (GBM)] via cationic charge, or because they cross-react with tissue constituents (e.g., some anti-DNA antibodies react with laminin in GBM). If these antibodies when complexed with antigen can fix complement, tissue damage occurs. Alteration of cell function after antibodies bind to membranes also occurs independent of complement activation. Autoantibodies characteristic of SLE are listed in Table 312-1.

In summary, some individuals are genetically predisposed to SLE. Under the influence of multiple genes, often triggered by environmental challenges and highly influenced by sex, they may develop a number of different clinical syndromes that fulfill diagnostic criteria for SLE. The etiology of these syndromes is complex and probably differs between patients.

CLINICAL MANIFESTATIONS At onset, SLE may involve only one organ system (additional manifestations occur later) or may be multisystemic. Clinical manifestations are listed in Table 312-2;

those that fulfill American Rheumatism Association (currently the American College of Rheumatology) criteria for a diagnosis of SLE are listed in Table 312-3. Autoantibodies are detectable at disease onset. Severity varies from mild and intermittent to persistent and fulminant. Most patients experience exacerbations interspersed with periods of relative quiescence. True remissions with no symptoms and requiring no therapy occur in up to 20 percent. Systemic symptoms are usually prominent and include fatigue, malaise, fever, anorexia, and weight loss.

Musculoskeletal Manifestations Almost all patients experience arthralgias and myalgias; most develop intermittent arthritis. Pain is often out of proportion to physical findings of symmetric fusiform swelling in joints [most frequently proximal interphalangeal (PIP) and metacarpophalangeal (MCP) joints of the hands, wrists, and knees], diffuse puffiness of hands and feet, and tenosynovitis. Joint deformities are unusual, with 10 percent of patients developing swan-neck deformities of fingers and ulnar drift at MCP joints. Erosions are rare; subcutaneous nodules occur. Myopathy can be inflammatory (during periods of active disease), or secondary to treatment (hypokalemia, glucocorticoid myopathy, hydroxychloroquine myopathy). Ischemic necrosis of bone is a common cause of hip, knee, or shoulder pain in patients receiving glucocorticoids.

Cutaneous Manifestations The malar ("butterfly") rash is a fixed erythematous rash, flat or raised, over the cheeks and bridge of the nose, often involving the chin and ears. It is photosensitive. Scarring is absent; telangiectases may develop. A more diffuse maculopapular rash, predominant in sun-exposed areas, is also common and usually indicates disease flare. Loss of scalp hair is usually patchy but can be extensive; hair often regrows in SLE lesions but not in lesions of discoid lupus erythematosus (DLE). DLE occurs in about 20 percent of patients with SLE and can be disfiguring, since the lesions have central atrophy and scarring, with permanent loss of appendages. DLE lesions are circular and characterized by an erythematous raised rim, scaliness, follicular plugging, and telangiectasia. They occur over the scalp, ears, face, and sun-exposed areas of the arms, back, and chest. Only 5 percent of patients with DLE subsequently develop SLE. Less frequent SLE skin lesions include urticaria, bullae, erythema multiforme, lichen planus–like lesions, and panniculitis ("lupus profundus").

Patients with subacute cutaneous lupus erythematosus (SCLE) are a distinct subset with recurring extensive dermatitis. Arthritis and fatigue are frequent; central nervous system and renal involvement are not. Some patients are antinuclear antibody (ANA)–negative. Most have antibodies to Ro (SS-A) or to single-stranded (ss) DNA and are HLA-DR3, -DQw1, or -DQw2. Skin lesions are photosensitive and may be annular or papulosquamous psoriasiform lesions over the arms, trunk, and face; they become hypopigmented but do not scar.

Patients with SLE, DLE, or SCLE can develop vasculitic skin lesions. These include purpura, subcutaneous nodules, nail fold infarcts, ulcers, vasculitic urticaria, panniculitis, and gangrene of digits. Shallow, slightly painful ulcers in the mouth and nose are frequent in patients with SLE.

Renal Manifestations Most patients with SLE have immunoglobulins deposited in glomeruli, but only one-half have clinical nephritis, defined by proteinuria. Early in the disease most are asymptomatic, although some develop the edema of nephrotic syndrome. Urinalysis shows hematuria, cylindruria, and proteinuria. Most patients with mesangial or mild focal proliferative nephritis (see discussion under "Pathology" below) maintain good renal function. Patients with diffuse proliferative nephritis develop renal failure if untreated. Because severe nephritis requires aggressive immunosuppression with high-dose glucocorticoids and cytotoxic drugs and mild lesions do not, renal biopsy may provide information that affects therapy. Patients with rapidly deteriorating renal function and active urine sediment require prompt, aggressive therapy; biopsy is not necessary unless they fail to respond. However, patients with a slow rise in serum creatinine to levels >265 μmol/L (>3 mg/dL) may show a high

Table 312-1

Autoantibodies in Patients with SLE

	Incidence, %	Antigen Detected	Clinical Importance
Antinuclear antibodies	98	Multiple nuclear	Human cell substrates are more sensitive than murine. Repeatedly negative tests make SLE unlikely.
Anti-DNA	70	DNA (ds)	Anti-dsDNA is relatively disease-specific; anti-ssDNA is not. High titers are associated with nephritis and clinical activity.
Anti-Sm	30	Protein complexed to 6 species of small nuclear RNA	Specific for SLE.
Anti-RNP	40	Protein complexed to U1RNA	High titer in syndromes with features of polymyositis, lupus, scleroderma, and mixed connective tissue disease. If present in SLE without anti-DNA, risk for nephritis is low.
Anti-Ro (SS-A)	30	Protein complexed to y_1–y_5 RNA	Associated with Sjögren's syndrome, subacute cutaneous lupus, inherited C′ deficiencies, ANA-negative lupus, lupus in the elderly, neonatal lupus, congenital heart block. Can cause nephritis.
Anti-La (SS-B)	10	Phosphoprotein	Always associated with anti-Ro. Risk for nephritis is low if present. Associated with Sjögren's syndrome.
Antihistone	70	Histones	More frequent in drug-induced LE (95%) than in spontaneous SLE.
Antiphospholipid	50	Phospholipids	Three types—lupus anticoagulant (LA), anticardiolipin (aCL), and false-positive test for syphilis (BFP). The LA and aCL (particular high-titer IgG) are associated with clotting, fetal loss, thrombocytopenia, and valvular heart disease.
Antierythrocyte	60	Erythrocyte	A small proportion of these patients develop overt hemolysis.
Antiplatelet		Platelet surface	Associated with thrombocytopenia.
Antilymphocyte	70	Lymphocyte surface	Probably associated with leukopenia and abnormal T cell function.
Antineuronal	60	Neuronal and lymphocyte surface	In some series, high titers of IgG correlate with diffuse CNS lupus.
Antiribosomal P	20	Ribosomal P protein	In some series, antibody in serum correlates with psychosis or depression due to CNS SLE.

Table 312-2

Clinical Manifestations of SLE

		Percent of Patients Positive during Course of Disease
Systemic		95
Fatigue, malaise, fever, anorexia, nausea, weight loss		
Musculoskeletal		95
Arthralgias/myalgias	95	
Nonerosive polyarthritis	60	
Hand deformities	10	
Myopathy/myositis	40/5	
Ischemic necrosis of bone	15	
Cutaneous		80
Malar rash	50	
Discoid rash	15	
Photosensitivity	70	
Oral ulcers	40	
Other rashes—maculopapular, urticarial, bullous, subacute cutaneous lupus	40	
Alopecia	40	
Vasculitis	20	
Panniculitis	5	
Hematologic		85
Anemia (of chronic disease)	70	
Hemolytic anemia	10	
Leukopenia (<4000/mm³)	65	
Lymphopenia (<1500/mm³)	50	
Thrombocytopenia (<100,000/mm³)	15	
Circulating anticoagulant	10–20	
Splenomegaly	15	
Lymphadenopathy	20	
Neurologic		60
Cognitive dysfunction	50	
Organic brain syndromes	35	
Psychosis	10	
Seizures	20	
Headache	25	
Other CNS (see text)	15	
Peripheral neuropathy	15	
Cardiopulmonary		60
Pleurisy	50	
Pericarditis	30	
Myocarditis	10	
Endocarditis (Libman-Sachs)	10	
Pleural effusions	30	
Lupus pneumonitis	10	
Interstitial fibrosis	5	
Pulmonary hypertension	<5	
ARDS/hemorrhage	<5	
Renal		50
Proteinuria >500 mg/24 h	50	
Cellular casts	50	
Nephrotic syndrome	25	
Renal failure	5–10	
Gastrointestinal		45
Nonspecific (anorexia, nausea, mild pain, diarrhea)	30	
Vasculitis with bleeding or perforation	5	
Ascites	<5	
Abnormal liver enzymes	40	
Thrombosis		15
Venous	10	
Arterial	5	
Fetal loss		30 (of pregnancies)
Ocular		15
Retinal vasculitis	5	
Conjunctivitis/episcleritis	10	
Sicca syndrome	15	

Table 312-3

The 1982 Criteria for Classification of Systemic Lupus Erythematosus

1. Malar rash	Fixed erythema, flat or raised, over the malar eminences
2. Discoid rash	Erythematous raised patches with adherent keratotic scaling and follicular plugging; atrophic scarring may occur
3. Photosensitivity	
4. Oral ulcers	Includes oral and nasopharyngeal, observed by physician
5. Arthritis	Nonerosive arthritis involving two or more peripheral joints, characterized by tenderness, swelling, or effusion
6. Serositis	Pleuritis or pericarditis documented by ECG or rub or evidence of pericardial effusion
7. Renal disorder	Proteinuria greater than 0.5 g/d or greater than 3+, or cellular casts
8. Neurologic disorder	Seizures without other cause or psychosis without other cause
9. Hematologic disorder	Hemolytic anemia or leukopenia (less than 4000/μL) or lymphopenia (less than 1500/μL) or thrombocytopenia (less than 100,000/μL) in the absence of offending drugs
10. Immunologic disorder	Positive LE cell preparation or anti-dsDNA or anti-Sm antibodies or false-positive VDRL
11. Antinuclear antibodies	An abnormal titer of ANAs by immunofluorescence or an equivalent assay at any point in time in the absence of drugs known to induce ANAs

If four of these criteria are present at any time during the course of disease, a diagnosis of systemic lupus can be made with 98 percent specificity and 97 percent sensitivity.

SOURCE: Criteria published by EM Tan et al, Arthritis Rheum 25:1271, 1982

proportion of sclerotic glomeruli on biopsy; they are unlikely to respond to immunosuppressive therapies and are candidates for dialysis or transplantation. Patients with persistently abnormal urinalyses, high titers of anti-dsDNA, and/or hypocomplementemia are at risk for severe nephritis; kidney biopsy may guide therapy.

Nervous System Any region of the brain can be involved in SLE, as can the meninges, spinal cord, and cranial and peripheral nerves. Central nervous system (CNS) events may be single or multiple and often occur when SLE is active in other organ systems. Mild cognitive dysfunction is the most frequent manifestation. Headaches are common and may be migrainelike or nonspecific. Seizures of any type may occur. Less frequent manifestations include psychosis, organic brain syndromes, focal infarcts, extrapyramidal disorders, cerebellar dysfunction, hypothalamic dysfunction with inappropriate antidiuretic hormone (ADH) secretion, pseudotumor cerebri, subarachnoid hemorrhage, aseptic meningitis, transverse myelitis, optic neuritis, cranial nerve palsies, and peripheral sensorimotor neuropathy. Depression and anxiety, usually related to being chronically ill and not to active SLE, are frequent.

Laboratory diagnosis of CNS lupus can be difficult. Abnormal electroencephalograms occur in about 70 percent of patients and usually show diffuse slowing or focal abnormalities. Cerebrospinal fluid (CSF) shows elevated protein levels in 50 percent and increased mononuclear cells in 30 percent of patients; oligoclonal bands, increased Ig synthesis, and antineuronal antibodies may be found. Lumbar puncture should be performed whenever CNS symptoms could result from infection, especially in immunosuppressed patients. Computed tomography (CT) scans and angiograms are most likely to be positive when focal neurologic deficits are present and are less helpful in cases with diffuse manifestations. Magnetic resonance imaging is the most sensitive radiographic technique to detect changes of SLE; changes are often nonspecific. Laboratory measures of disease activity often do not correlate with neurologic manifestations. Neurologic problems (with the exception of deficits resulting from large infarcts) usually improve with immunosuppressive therapy and/or time; recurrences are seen in approximately one-third of patients.

Vascular System Thrombosis in vessels of any size can be a major problem. Although vasculitis may underly thrombosis, there is increasing evidence that antibodies against phospholipids (lupus anticoagulant, anticardiolipin) are associated with clotting without inflammation. In addition, degenerative vascular changes after years of exposure of blood vessels to circulating immune complexes and hyperlipidemia from glucocorticoid therapy predispose to degenerative coronary artery disease in lupus patients. Therefore, anticoagulation is more appropriate than immunosuppression in some patients.

Hematologic Manifestation Anemia of chronic disease occurs in most patients when lupus is active. Hemolysis occurs in a small proportion of those with positive Coombs' tests; it is usually responsive to high-dose glucocorticoids; resistant cases may respond to splenectomy. Leukopenia (usually lymphopenia) is common but is rarely associated with recurrent infections and does not require treatment. Mild thrombocytopenia is common; severe thrombocytopenia with bleeding and purpura occurs in 5 percent of patients and should be treated with high-dose glucocorticoids. Short-term improvement can be achieved by administration of intravenous gamma globulin. If the platelet count fails to reach acceptable levels in 2 weeks, addition of cytotoxic drugs and/or splenectomy should be considered.

The lupus anticoagulant (LA) belongs to a family of antiphospholipid antibodies. It is recognized by prolongation of the partial thromboplastin time and failure of added normal plasma to correct the prolongation. More sensitive tests include the Russell viper venom time and the rabbit brain neutral phospholipid test. Antibodies to cardiolipin (aCL) are detected in enzyme-linked immunosorbent assays (ELISA). Clinical manifestations of LA and aCL include thrombocytopenia, recurrent venous or arterial clotting, recurrent fetal loss, and valvular heart disease. If the LA is associated with hypoprothrombinemia or thrombocytopenia, bleeding may occur. Less commonly, antibodies to clotting factors (VIII, IX) arise; they cause bleeding. Bleeding syndromes usually respond to glucocorticoids; clotting syndromes do not.

Cardiopulmonary System Pericarditis is the most frequent manifestation of cardiac lupus; effusions can occur and occasionally lead to tamponade; constrictive pericarditis is rare. Myocarditis can cause arrhythmias, sudden death, and/or heart failure. Valvular insufficiency (usually aortic or mitral) is an uncommon sequel of Libman Sachs endocarditis and may be a source of cerebral emboli; this syndrome is probably associated with antiphospholipid antibodies. Myocardial infarcts usually result from degenerative disease, although they can result from vasculitis.

Pleurisy and pleural effusions are common manifestations of SLE. Lupus pneumonitis causes fever, dyspnea, and cough; x-rays show fleeting infiltrates and/or areas of platelike atelectasis; this syndrome responds to glucocorticoids. However, *the most common cause of pulmonary infiltrates in patients with SLE is infection.* Interstitial pneumonitis leading to fibrosis occurs occasionally; the inflammatory phase may respond to treatment; the fibrosis does not. Pulmonary hypertension is an uncommon, grave manifestation of SLE. Infrequent pulmonary manifestations with high mortality include adult respiratory distress syndrome and massive intraalveolar hemorrhage.

Gastrointestinal System Common gastrointestinal (GI) symptoms include nausea, diarrhea, and vague discomfort. Symptoms may result from lupus peritonitis and may herald a flare of SLE. Vasculitis of the intestine is the most dangerous manifestation, presenting with acute crampy abdominal pain, vomiting, and diarrhea. Intestinal perforation can occur and usually requires immediate surgery. Patients with pseudoobstruction have abdominal pain; x-rays show dilated loops of small bowel which may be edematous; surgery should be avoided unless frank obstruction is present. Glucocorticoid therapy is useful for all these GI syndromes. Some patients have GI motility disorders similar to those in scleroderma; they are not benefited by steroids. Acute pancreatitis occurs and can be severe, resulting from active SLE or from therapy with glucocorticoids or azathioprine. Elevated amylase levels may reflect pancreatitis, salivary gland inflammation, or macroamylasemia. Elevated serum transaminase levels are common in patients with active SLE but are not associated with significant hepatic damage; they return to normal as the disease is treated.

Ocular Manifestation Retinal vasculitis is a serious manifestation; blindness can develop over a few days, and aggressive immunosuppression should be instituted. Examination shows areas of sheathed, narrow retinal arterioles and cytoid bodies (white exudates) adjacent to vessels. Other ocular abnormalities include conjunctivitis, episcleritis, optic neuritis, and the sicca syndrome.

PATHOLOGY Cutaneous Lesions Lesions of acute SLE, DLE, and SCLE show similar histopathology, with degeneration of the basal layer of the epidermis, disruption of the dermal-epidermal junction (DEJ), and mononuclear infiltrates around vessels and appendages in the upper dermis. In DLE, follicular plugging and hyperkeratosis are prominent. Deposits of Ig and C′ are seen in the DEJ in 80 to 100 percent of lesional and 50 percent of nonlesional skin in active SLE; the proportions are lower during remissions. Only 50 percent of SCLE lesions are positive for Ig and C′ deposits. Ig deposition in the DEJ is not specific for SLE. Vasculitic skin lesions usually show leukocytoclastic angiitis.

Renal Lesions Glomerulonephritis (GN) is caused by deposition of circulating immune complexes or in situ complex formation in mesangium and GBM. Renal biopsy should be considered when results would affect therapy. Information regarding location of immune deposits, histologic pattern of renal damage, and activity and chronicity of lesions are all useful in predicting prognosis and selecting appropriate treatment. In mild GN unlikely to lead to renal failure, Ig deposits are confined to the mesangium, and histology shows no changes or mesangial proliferation. If Ig and C′ are deposited outside the mesangium in capillary GBM, prognosis worsens. Histologic changes that should be treated with aggressive immunosuppression include focal proliferative, membranoproliferative, and diffuse proliferative GN (see Chap. 275). Progression from focal to diffuse lesions can occur. Membranous changes without proliferation are uncommon but have a better prognosis than proliferative GN. Activity and chronicity scores indicate severity and reversibility of lesions. *Reversible "active" lesions* associated with high risk of progression to renal failure are glomerular necrosis, cellular epithelial crescents, hyaline thrombi, interstitial inflammatory infiltrates, and necrotizing vasculitis. *Irreversible changes unlikely to respond to immunosuppression* and highly associated with renal failure include glomerular sclerosis, fibrous crescents, interstitial fibrosis, and tubular atrophy. In patients with high chronicity scores, treatment of lupus should be determined by extrarenal disease.

LABORATORY MANIFESTATIONS The presence of characteristic antibodies (Table 312-1) confirms the diagnosis of SLE. ANAs are the best screening test. If the test substrate contains human nuclei (WIL-2 or HEP-2 cells), more than 95 percent of lupus patients will be positive. A positive ANA test is not specific for SLE; ANA occur in some normal individuals (usually in low titer); the frequency increases with aging. Other autoimmune diseases, viral infections, chronic inflammatory processes, and several drugs induce ANA. Therefore, a positive ANA test supports the diagnosis of SLE but is not specific; a negative ANA test makes the diagnosis unlikely but not impossible. Antibodies to double-stranded DNA (dsDNA) and to Sm are relatively specific for SLE; other autoantibodies listed in Table 312-1 are not. However, determining the complete autoantibody profile of each patient helps predict clinical subsets. High serum levels of ANA and anti-dsDNA and low levels of complement usually reflect disease activity, especially in patients with nephritis. Total functional hemolytic complement (CH_{50}) levels are the most sensitive measure of complement activation but are also most subject to laboratory error. Quantitative levels of C3 and C4 are widely available. Very low levels of CH_{50} with normal levels of C3 suggest inherited deficiency of a complement component, which is highly associated with SLE and with ANA negativity.

Hematologic abnormalities include anemia (usually normochromic normocytic but occasionally hemolytic), leukopenia, lymphopenia, and thrombocytopenia. The Westergren erythrocyte sedimentation rate correlates with disease activity in some patients.

Urinalysis should be performed and serum creatinine levels should be measured periodically in patients with SLE. With active nephritis, the urinalysis usually shows proteinuria, hematuria, and cellular or granular casts. Urinary protein excretion measured over 24 h increases during periods of activity. (See the discussion under "Pathology" for a description of renal biopsy.)

PREGNANCY Fertility rates are normal in patients with SLE, but spontaneous abortion and stillbirths are frequent (10 to 30 percent), especially in women with LA and/or aCL. Treatment of women with prior fetal loss and antiphospholipid antibodies is controversial. Options are no intervention, daily low-dose aspirin until the last month, low-dose aspirin plus daily high-dose glucocorticoids, and twice daily subcutaneous heparin in full anticoagulating doses; there are data to support each approach.

Pregnancy has varied effects on SLE activity. Disease flares in a small proportion, especially during the 6 weeks postpartum. If severe renal or cardiac disease is absent and SLE activity is controlled, most patients complete pregnancy safely and deliver normal infants. Glucocorticoids (except dexamethasone and betamethasone) are inactivated by placental enzymes and do not cause fetal abnormalities in humans; they should be used to suppress disease activity. Neonatal lupus, caused by transmission of maternal anti-Ro across the placenta, consists of transient skin rash and (rarely) permanent heart block. Transient thrombocytopenia from maternal antiplatelet antibodies also occurs.

DIFFERENTIAL DIAGNOSIS The American Rheumatism Association published diagnostic criteria for SLE (Table 312-3). Any four of the manifestations listed establish a diagnosis of SLE. Early disease confined to a few systems is more difficult to classify; it may take several years for a patient to fulfill criteria. Disorders with which SLE can be confused include rheumatoid arthritis; various forms of dermatitis; neurologic disorders such as epilepsy, multiple sclerosis, and psychiatric disorders; and hematologic diseases such as idiopathic thrombocytopenic purpura. Many autoimmune disorders have overlapping features so that exact classification may be difficult. Mixed connective tissue disease has features of SLE, rheumatoid arthritis, polymyositis, and scleroderma, accompanied by high titers of anti-RNP antibodies (Chap 314); patients have a low incidence of nephritis and CNS disease and a high incidence of pulmonary manifestations and evolution into scleroderma. The possibility of drug-induced lupus should always be considered. Figure 312-1 presents an algorithm for diagnosis of SLE.

DRUG-INDUCED LUPUS Several drugs can cause a syndrome resembling SLE, including procainamide, hydralazine, isoniazid, chlorpromazine, D-penicillamine, practolol, methyldopa, quinidine, interferon α, and possibly hydantoin, ethosuximide, and oral contraceptives. The syndrome is rare with all but procainamide, the most frequent offender, and hydralazine. There is genetic predisposition to drug-induced lupus, partly determined by drug acetylation rates. Procainamide induces ANA in 50 to 75 percent of individuals within a few months; hydralazine induces ANA in 25 to 30 percent. Between 10 and 20 percent of ANA-positive individuals develop lupuslike symptoms. Most common are systemic complaints and arthralgias; polyarthritis and pleuropericarditis occur in 25 to 50 percent. Renal and CNS diseases are rare. All patients have ANA and most have antibodies to histones. Antibodies to dsDNA and hypocomplementemia are rare—a helpful point in distinguishing drug-induced from idiopathic lupus. Anemia, leukopenia, LA, aCL, thrombocytopenia, cryoglobulins, rheumatoid factors, and false-positive VDRL, and positive direct Coombs' tests can occur. The initial therapeutic approach is withdrawal of the offending drug; most patients improve in a few weeks. If symptoms are severe, a short course (2 to 10 weeks) of glucocorticoids is indicated. Symptoms rarely persist more than 6 months; ANA may persist for years. Most lupus-inducing drugs can be used safely in patients with idiopathic SLE.

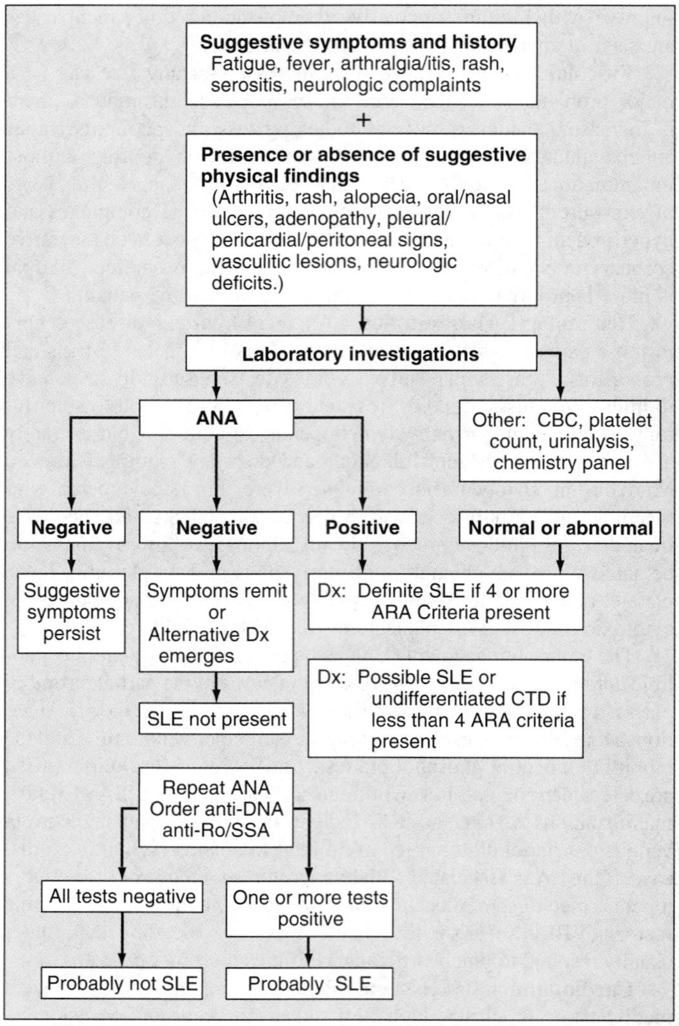

FIGURE 312-1 Algorithm for the diagnosis of SLE. ANA, antinuclear antibody; ARA, American Rheumatism Association; CTD, connective tissue disease; CBC, complete blood count; *, ANA titer ≥ 1 : 80.

PROGNOSIS Survival in patients with SLE is 90 to 95 percent at 2 years, 82 to 90 percent at 5 years, 71 to 80 percent at 10 years, and 63 to 75 percent at 20 years. The following factors have been associated with poor prognosis (approximately 50 percent mortality in 10 years) in multiple studies: high serum creatinine levels (>1.4 mg/dL), hypertension, nephrotic syndrome (24-h urine protein excretion >2.6 g), anemia, hypoalbuminemia and hypocomplementemia at the time of diagnosis, and low socioeconomic status. Other factors associated with a poor prognosis in some but not all studies include thrombocytopenia, serious CNS involvement, antibodies to phospholipids, and non-Caucasian race. Disability in SLE patients is common. However, aproximately 20 percent of patients experience disease remissions (with a mean duration of 5 years), regardless of the severity of disease at diagnosis. Some 50 percent in remission remain in remission for decades, and the likelihood of remission increases with each decade after diagnosis. Infections and renal failure are the leading causes of death in the first decade of disease. Thromboembolic events are frequent causes of death in the second decade.

℞ TREATMENT

There is no cure for SLE. Complete remissions are rare. Therefore, patient and physician should plan (1) to control acute, severe flares, and (2) to develop maintenance strategies in which symptoms are suppressed to an acceptable level, usually at the cost of some drug side effects. Approximately 25 percent of SLE patients have mild disease with no life-threatening manifestations, although pain and fatigue may be disabling. These patients should be managed without glucocorticoids. Arthralgias, arthritis, myalgias, fever, and mild serositis may improve on nonsteroidal anti-inflammatory drugs (NSAIDs) including salicylates. However, NSAID toxicities such as elevated serum transaminases, aseptic meningitis, and renal impairment are especially frequent in SLE. The dermatitides of SLE, fatigue, and lupus arthritis may respond to antimalarials. Doses of 400 mg hydroxychloroquine daily may improve skin lesions in a few weeks. Side effects are uncommon and include retinal toxicity, rash, myopathy, and neuropathy. Regular ophthalmologic examinations should be performed at least annually, since retinal toxicity is related to cumulative dose. Other therapies for rash include sunscreens (an SPF rating ≥15 is recommended), topical or intralesional glucocorticoids, quinacrine, retinoids, and dapsone. Recent studies suggest that daily oral doses of dihydroepiandrosterone (DHEA) may lower disease activity in patients with mild SLE. Systemic glucocorticoids should be reserved for patients with disabling disease unresponsive to these conservative measures.

Life-threatening, severely disabling manifestations of SLE that are responsive to immunosuppression should be treated with high doses of *glucocorticoids* (1 to 2 mg/kg per day). When disease is active, glucocorticoids should be given in divided doses every 8 to 12 h. After the disease is controlled, therapy should be consolidated to one morning dose; thereafter the daily dose should be tapered as rapidly as clinical disease permits. Ideally, patients should be slowly converted to alternate-day therapy with a single morning dose of short-acting glucocorticoid (prednisone, prednisolone, methylprednisolone) to minimize side effects. However, the disease may flare on the day off steroids, in which case the lowest single daily dose that suppresses disease should be used. Acutely ill lupus patients, including those with proliferative GN, can be treated with 3 to 5 days of 1000 mg intravenous "pulses" of methylprednisolone, followed by maintenance daily or alternate-day glucocorticoids. Disease flares are probably controlled more rapidly by this approach, but it is unclear whether long-term outcome is changed.

Undesirable effects of chronic glucocorticoid therapy include cushingoid habitus, weight gain, hypertension, infection, capillary fragility, acne, hirsutism, accelerated osteoporosis, ischemic necrosis of bone, cataracts, glaucoma, diabetes mellitus, myopathy, hypokalemia, irregular menses, irritability, insomnia, and psychosis. Prednisone doses of 15 mg daily (or less) given before noon usually do not suppress the hypothalamic-pituitary axis. Some side effects can be minimized; hyperglycemia, hypertension, edema, and hypokalemia should be treated; infections should be identified and treated early; immunizations with influenza and pneumococcal vaccines are safe and should be given if disease is stable. To minimize osteoporosis, supplemental calcium (1000 mg daily) should be added in most patients; in those with 24-h urinary calcium excretion <120 mg, vitamin D, 50,000 units one to three times weekly, can be added (monitor for hypercalcemia). Estrogen replacement therapy (ERT) should be considered at menopause. There is debate regarding the ability of oral contraceptives or ERT to cause flares of SLE in some patients; these therapies should be withheld from patients with a history of thrombosis. Calcitonin and bisphosphonates are also useful in preventing and treating osteoporosis.

The use of *cytotoxic agents* (azathioprine, chlorambucil, cyclophosphamide) in SLE is probably beneficial in controlling active disease, reducing the rate of disease flares, and reducing steroid requirements. Patients with lupus nephritis have significantly less renal failure if treated with combinations of glucocorticoids plus cyclophosphamide; azathioprine as the second drug is less beneficial but is also effective. However, overall survival is not different, probably because renal failure usually leads to dialysis or transplantation rather than to death. Undesirable side effects of cytotoxic drugs include bone marrow suppression, increased infection with opportunistic organisms such as herpes zoster, irreversible ovarian failure, hepatotoxicity (azathioprine), bladder toxicity (cyclophosphamide), alopecia, and increased risk for malignancy. Azathioprine is the least toxic; recommended doses are 2 to 3 mg/kg per day orally. Cyclophosphamide is the most effective and the most toxic. Intravenous pulse doses (10 to 15 mg/kg) once every 4 weeks have less

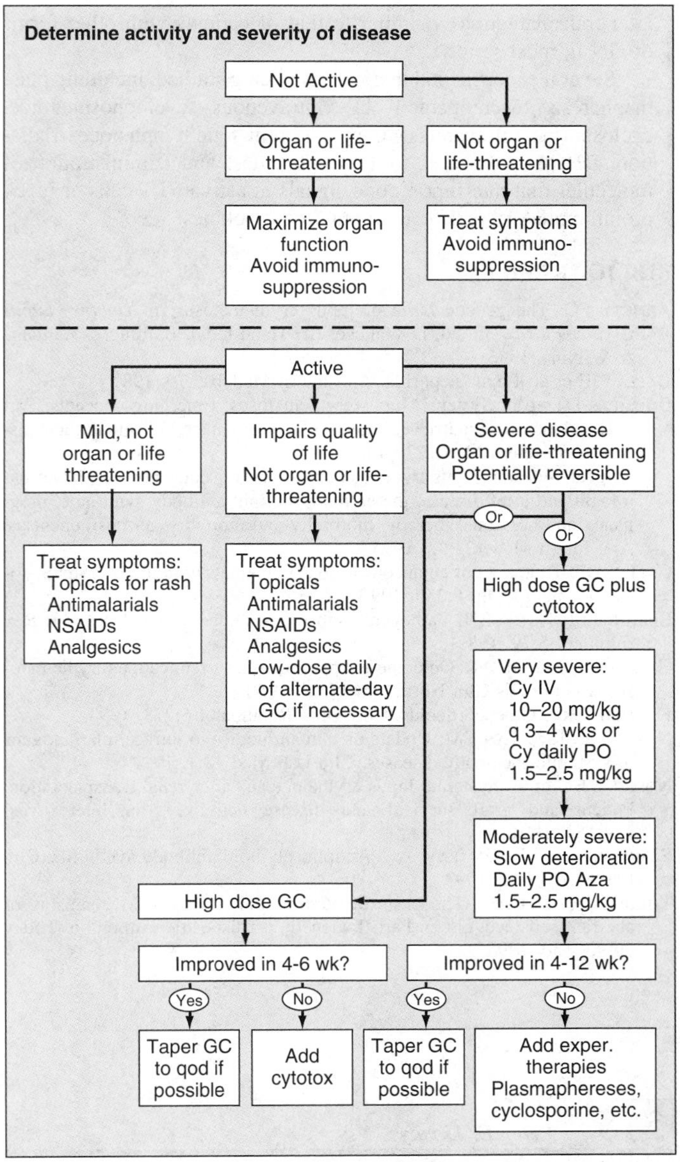

FIGURE 312-2 Algorithm for the treatment of SLE. GC, glucocorticoids; high-dose GC, methylprednisolone 1000 mg, IV, qd × 3, then 1 to 2 mg/kg prednisone per day orally, or 1 to 2 mg/kg prednisone per day orally; cytotox, cytotoxic drugs such as cyclophosphamide (Cy) and azathioprine (Aza); qod, alternate day therapy.

urinary bladder toxicity than daily oral doses, but bone marrow suppression can be severe. Cyclophosphamide can also be used in daily oral doses (1.5 to 2.5 mg/kg per day of each). After disease activity has been controlled for a few months, tapering of cytotoxic agents and attempts to discontinue them are appropriate. Figure 312-2 presents an algorithm for treatment of SLE.

Some manifestations of SLE do not respond to immunosuppression, including clotting disorders, some behavioral abnormalities, and end-stage GN. Anticoagulation is the therapy of choice for prevention of clotting; chronic warfarin therapy in relatively high doses (maintaining INR at 2.5 to 3.0) is effective in preventing venous and arterial clotting in patients with antiphospholipid syndromes; the effects of aspirin and heparin on arterial thrombosis are unclear. Psychoactive drugs should be used when appropriate. "Pure" membranous GN may not respond to immunosuppression; several weeks of therapy can be tried but should be abandoned if improvement is not obvious. The survival of lupus patients on dialysis or after transplantation is similar to that of patients with other forms of GN in most series.

Several experimental therapies are being studied, including plasmapheresis accompanied by intravenous cyclophosphamide, cyclosporine, intravenous gamma globulin, total lymph node irradiation, DHEA, antibodies to T lymphocytes, and administration of molecules that interrupt second signals in activated T cells or block proinflammatory or B cell stimulating cytokines.

BIBLIOGRAPHY

Arnett FC: The genetic basis of lupus erythematosus, in *Dubois' Lupus Erythematosus*, 5th ed, D Wallace, BH Hahn (eds). Baltimore, Williams & Wilkins, 1996

Balow JE et al: Lupus nephritis. Ann Intern Med 106:79, 1987

Boumpas DT et al: Systemic lupus erythematosus: Emerging concepts. Part 1: Renal, neuropychiatric, cardiovascular, pulmonary and hematologic disease. Ann Intern Med 122:940, 1995

——— et al: Systemic lupus erythematosus: Emerging concepts. Part 2: Dermatologic and joint disease, the antiphospholipid antibody syndrome, pregnancy and hormonal therapy, morbidity and mortality, and pathogenesis. Ann Intern Med 123:42, 1995

Callen JP: Treatment of cutaneous lesions in patients with lupus erythematosus. Dermatol Clin 8:355, 1990

Ebling FM, Hahn BH: Pathogenic subsets of antibodies to DNA. Int Rev Immunol 5:79, 1989

Ginzler E, Schorn AK: Outcome and prognosis in systemic lupus erythematosus. Rheum Dis Clin North Am 14:67, 1988

Kimberly RP: Glucocorticoids. Curr Opin Rheumatol 6:273, 1994

Nakamura RM, Tan EM: Update on autoantibodies to intracellular antigens in systemic rheumatic diseases. Clin Lab Med 12:1, 1992

Nossent HC et al: Systemic lupus erythematosus after renal transplantation: Patient and graft survival and disease activity. Ann Intern Med 114:183, 1991

Sammaritano LR, Gharavi AE: Antiphospholipid antibody syndrome. Clin Lab Med 12:41, 1992

Theofilopoulos AN: The basis of autoimmunity: Part I. Mechanisms of aberrant self-recognition. Part II. Genetic predisposition. Immunol Today 16:90, 150, 1995

313

Peter E. Lipsky

RHEUMATOID ARTHRITIS

Rheumatoid arthritis (RA) is a chronic multisystem disease of unknown cause. Although there are a variety of systemic manifestations, the characteristic feature of RA is persistent inflammatory synovitis, usually involving peripheral joints in a symmetric distribution. The potential of the synovial inflammation to cause cartilage destruction and bone erosions and subsequent changes in joint integrity is the hallmark of the disease. Despite its destructive potential, the course of RA can be quite variable. Some patients may experience only a mild oligoarticular illness of brief duration with minimal joint damage, whereas others will have a relentless progressive polyarthritis with marked functional impairment.

EPIDEMIOLOGY AND GENETICS The prevalence of RA is approximately 0.8 percent of the population (range 0.3 to 2.1 percent); women are affected approximately three times more often than men. The prevalence increases with age, and sex differences diminish in the older age group. RA is seen throughout the world and affects all races. However, the incidence and severity seem to be less in rural sub-Saharan Africa and in Caribbean blacks. The onset is most frequent during the fourth and fifth decades of life, with 80 percent of all patients developing the disease between the ages of 35 and 50. The incidence of RA is more than six times as great in 60- to 64-year-old women compared to 18- to 29-year-old women.

Family studies indicate a genetic predisposition. For example, severe RA is found at approximately four times the expected rate in first-degree relatives of individuals with disease associated with the presence of the autoantibody, rheumatoid factor; approximately 10 percent of patients with RA will have an affected first-degree relative. Moreover, monozygotic twins are at least four times more likely to be concordant for RA than dizygotic twins, who have a similar risk of developing RA as nontwin siblings. Approximately only 15 to 20 percent of monozygotic twins are concordant for RA, however, implying that factors other than genetics play an important etiopathogenic role. One of the major genetic factors in the etiology of RA is the class II major histocompatibility complex (MHC) gene product HLA-DR4. As many as 70 percent of patients with classic or definite RA express HLA-DR4 compared with 28 percent of control individuals. An association with HLA-DR4 has been noted in many populations, including North American and European whites, Chippewa Indians, Japanese, and native populations in India, Mexico, South America, and southern China. In a number of groups, including Israeli Jews, Asian Indians, and Yakima Indians of North America, however, there is no association between the development of RA and HLA-DR4. In these individuals, there is an association between RA and HLA-DR1 in the former two groups and HLA-Dw16 in the latter. Molecular analysis of HLA-DR antigens has provided insight into these apparently disparate findings. The HLA-DR molecule is composed of two chains, a nonpolymorphic α chain and a highly polymorphic β chain. Allelic variations in the HLA-DR molecule reflect differences in the amino acids of the β chain, with the major amino acid changes occurring in the three hypervariable regions of the molecule. Each of the HLA-DR molecules that is associated with RA has the same or a very similar sequence of amino acids in the third hypervariable region of the β chain of the molecule (Table 313-1). Thus the β chains of the HLA-DR molecules associated with RA, including HLA-Dw4 (DRβ1*0401), HLA-Dw14 (DRβ1*0404), HLA-Dw15 (DRβ1*0405), HLA-DR1 (DRβ1*0101), and HLA-Dw16 (DRβ1*1402), contain the same amino acids at positions 67 through 74, with the exception of a single change of one basic amino acid for another (arginine → lysine) in position 71 of HLA-Dw4. All other HLA-DR β chains have amino acid changes in this region that alter either their charge or hydrophobicity. These results indicate that a particular amino acid sequence in the third hypervariable region of the HLA-DR molecule is a major genetic element conveying susceptibility to RA, regardless of whether it occurs in HLA-DR4, HLA-Dw16, or HLA-DR1. It has been estimated that the risk of developing RA in a person with HLA-Dw4 (DRβ1*0401) or HLA-Dw14 (DRβ1*0404) is 1 in 35 and 1 in 20, respectively, whereas the presence of both alleles puts persons at an even greater risk. The lack of association of HLA-DR4 and RA in certain populations is explained by the major member of the DR4 family found in that population. HLA-DR4 is a family of closely related, serologically defined molecules, including HLA-Dw4, -Dw10, -Dw13, and -Dw15. Different members of the HLA-DR family of molecules are found to predominate in different ethnic groups. Thus, in HLA-DR4–positive North American

Table 313-1

Amino Acid Sequence of the Third Hypervariable Region of the β Chains of HLA-DR Alleles Associated with Rheumatoid Arthritis

		Amino Acid*								Associated with
HLA-DR	β Chain	67	68	69	70	71	72	73	74	Rheumatoid Arthritis
DR4/Dw4	β1*0401	L	L	E	Q	K	R	A	A	+
DR4/Dw14	β1*0404	—	—	—	—	R	—	—	—	+
DR4/Dw15	β1*0405	—	—	—	—	R	—	—	—	+
DR1	β1*0101	—	—	—	—	R	—	—	—	+
Dw16	β1*1402	—	—	—	—	R	—	—	—	+
DR4/Dw10	β1*0402	I	—	—	D	E	—	—	—	—
DR4/Dw13	β1*0403	—	—	—	—	R	—	—	E	—

* Single-letter amino acid code.

whites, HLA-Dw4 and -Dw14 are the most frequent, whereas HLA-Dw15 is most frequent in Japanese and southern Chinese. Each of these is associated with RA. By contrast, HLA-Dw10, which is not associated with RA and contains nonconservative amino acid changes in positions 70 and 71 of the β chain, is most common in Israeli Jews. Therefore, HLA-DR4 is not associated with RA in this population. In certain groups of patients, there does not appear to be a clear association between HLA-DR4–related epitopes and RA. Thus, nearly 75 percent of African-American RA patients do not have this genetic element. Moreover, there is an association with HLA-DR10 (DRβ1*1001) in Spanish and Italian patients.

Additional genes in the HLA-D complex also may convey altered susceptibility to RA. Certain HLA-DR alleles, including HLA-DR5 (DRβ1*1101), HLA-DR2 (DRβ1*1501), HLA-DR3 (DRβ1*0301), and HLA-DR7 (DRβ1*0701) may protect against the development of RA in that they tend to be found at lower frequency in RA patients than in controls. Moreover, the HLA-DQ alleles, DQβ1*0301, DQβ1*0302, and DQβ1*0501, that are frequently linked to HLA-DR4 or -DR1 have also been associated with RA. Disease manifestations have also been associated with HLA phenotype. Thus, early aggressive disease and extraarticular manifestations are more frequent in patients with DRβ1*0401 or DRβ1*0404, and more slowly progressive disease with DRβ1*0101. The presence of both DRβ1*0401 and DRβ1*0404 appears to increase the risk for both aggressive articular and extraarticular disease. It has been estimated that HLA genes contribute only a portion of the genetic susceptibility to RA. Thus genes outside the HLA complex also contribute. These include genes controlling the expression of the antigen receptor on T cells and both immunoglobulin heavy and light chains.

Genetic risk factors do not fully account for the incidence of RA, suggesting that environmental factors also play a role in the etiology of the disease. This is emphasized by epidemiologic studies in Africa that have indicated that climate and urbanization have a major impact on the incidence and severity of RA in groups of similar genetic background.

Besides an association between the development of RA and genes of the MHC, there appears to be a genetic predisposition for the development of certain toxic reactions induced by drugs used to treat RA. For example, the presence of the HLA-DR3 (DRβ1*0301) allele is highly associated with the development of side effects to gold therapy, including proteinuria, thrombocytopenia, and perhaps skin rash. Similarly, the presence of this allele appears to predispose to the development of proteinuria following therapy with D-penicillamine. In general, no association has been noted between HLA type and the response to therapy.

ETIOLOGY The cause of RA remains unknown. It has been suggested that RA might be a manifestation of the response to an infectious agent in a genetically susceptible host. Because of the worldwide distribution of RA, it has been hypothesized that if an infectious agent is involved, the organism must be ubiquitous. A number of possible causative agents have been suggested, including *Mycoplasma*, Epstein-Barr virus, cytomegalovirus, parvovirus, and rubella virus, but convincing evidence that these or other infectious agents cause RA has not emerged. The process by which an infectious agent might cause chronic inflammatory arthritis with a characteristic distribution also remains a matter of controversy. One possibility is that there is persistent infection of articular structures or retention of microbial products in the synovial tissues which generates a chronic inflammatory response. Alternatively, the microorganism or response to the microorganism might induce an immune response to components of the joint by altering its integrity and revealing antigenic peptides. In this regard, reactivity to type II collagen and heat shock proteins has been demonstrated. Another possibility is that the infecting microorganism might prime the host to cross-reactive determinants expressed within the joint as a result of "molecular mimicry." Recent evidence of similarity between products of certain gram-negative bacteria and the HLA-DR molecule itself has supported this possibility. Finally, products of infecting microorganisms might induce the disease. Recent work has focused on the possible role of "superantigens" produced

by a number of microorganisms, including staphylococci, streptococci and *M. arthritidis*. Superantigens are proteins with the capacity to bind to HLA-DR molecules and particular V_β segments of the heterodimeric T cell receptor and stimulate specific T cells expressing the V_β gene products (see Chap. 305). The role of superantigens in the etiology of RA remains speculative.

PATHOLOGY AND PATHOGENESIS Microvascular injury and an increase in the number of synovial lining cells appear to be the earliest lesions in rheumatoid synovitis. The nature of the insult causing this response is not known. Subsequently, an increased number of synovial lining cells is seen along with perivascular infiltration with mononuclear cells. As the process continues, the synovium becomes edematous and protrudes into the joint cavity as villous projections.

Light-microscopic examination discloses a characteristic constellation of features which include hyperplasia and hypertrophy of the synovial lining cells; focal or segmental vascular changes, including microvascular injury, thrombosis, and neovascularization; edema; and infiltration with mononuclear cells, often collected into aggregates around small blood vessels. The endothelial cells of the rheumatoid synovium have the appearance of high endothelial venules (HEV) of lymphoid organs and have been altered by cytokine exposure to facilitate entry of cells into tissue. Rheumatoid synovial endothelial cells express increased amounts of various adhesion molecules involved in this process. Although this pathologic picture is typical of RA, it also can be seen in a variety of other chronic inflammatory arthritides. The mononuclear cell collections are variable in composition and size. The predominant infiltrating cell is the T lymphocyte. CD4+ T cells predominate over CD8+ T cells and are frequently found in close proximity to HLA-DR+ macrophages and dendritic cells. An increased number of a separate population of T cells expressing the γδ form of the T cell receptor also has been found in the synovium, although they remain a minor population there and their role in RA has not been delineated. The major population of T cells in the rheumatoid synovium is composed of CD4+ memory T cells that form the majority of cells aggregated around postcapillary venules. Scattered throughout the tissue are CD8+ T cells. Both populations express the early activation antigen, CD69. Besides the accumulation of T cells, rheumatoid synovitis is also characterized by the infiltration of large numbers of B cells that differentiate locally into antibody-producing plasma cells. These cells produce both polyclonal immunoglobulin and the autoantibody rheumatoid factor that results in the local formation of immune complexes. Finally, the synovial fibroblasts in RA manifest evidence of activation in that they produce a number of enzymes such as collagenase and cathepsins that can degrade components of the articular matrix. These activated fibroblasts are particularly prominent in the lining layer and at the interface with bone and cartilage. Osteoclasts are also prominent at sites of bone erosion.

The rheumatoid synovium is characterized by the presence of a number of secreted products of activated lymphocytes, macrophages, and fibroblasts. The local production of these cytokines and chemokines appears to account for many of the pathologic and clinical manifestations of RA. These effector molecules include those that are derived from T lymphocytes such as interleukin (IL) 2, interferon γ (IFNγ), IL-6, IL-10, granulocyte-macrophage colony stimulating factor (GM-CSF), tumor necrosis factor α (TNFα), and transforming growth factor β (TGFβ); those originating from activated macrophages, including IL-1, TNFα, IL-6, IL-8, IL-10, GM-CSF, macrophage CSF, platelet-derived growth factor, insulin-like growth factor, and TGFβ; as well as those secreted by other cell types in the synovium, such as fibroblasts and endothelial cells, including IL-1, IL-6, IL-8, GM-CSF, and macrophage CSF. The activity of these chemokines and cytokines appears to account for many of the features of rheumatoid synovitis, including the synovial tissue inflammation, synovial fluid inflammation, synovial proliferation, and cartilage and bone damage, as well as the systemic manifestations of RA. In addition to the production of effector molecules that propagate the inflammatory process, local factors are produced that tend to slow the inflammation, including specific inhibitors of cytokine action and additional cytokines, such as TGFβ, which inhibits many of the features of rheumatoid synovitis including T cell activation and proliferation, B cell differentiation, and migration of cells into the inflammatory site.

These findings have suggested that the propagation of RA is an immunologically mediated event, although the original initiating stimulus has not been characterized. One view is that the inflammatory process in the tissue is driven by the CD4+ T cells infiltrating the synovium. Evidence for this includes (1) the predominance of CD4+ T cells in the synovium; (2) the increase in soluble IL-2 receptors, a product of activated T cells, in blood and synovial fluid of patients with active RA; and (3) amelioration of the disease by removal of T cells by thoracic duct drainage or peripheral lymphapheresis or suppression of their function by drugs, such as cyclosporine. In addition, the association of RA with certain HLA-DR alleles, whose only known functions are to shape the repertoire of CD4+ T cells during ontogeny in the thymus and bind and present antigenic peptides to CD4+ T cells in the periphery, strongly implies a role for CD4+ T cells in the pathogenesis of the disease. Finally, patients with established RA who become infected with the human immunodeficiency virus (HIV) also have been noted to improve, although this has not been a uniform finding. T lymphocytes produce a number of cytokines, including IFNγ and GM-CSF, that can lead to activation of macrophages and also increased expression of HLA molecules. Moreover, T lymphocytes produce a variety of cytokines that promote B cell proliferation and differentiation into antibody-forming cells and therefore also may promote local B cell stimulation. The resultant production of immunoglobulin and rheumatoid factor can lead to immune-complex formation with consequent complement activation and exacerbation of the inflammatory process by the production of the anaphylatoxins, C3a and C5a, and the chemotactic factor C5a. The tissue inflammation is reminiscent of delayed type hypersensitivity reactions occurring in response to soluble antigens or microorganisms, although it has become clear that the number of T cells producing cytokines such as IFNγ is less than is found in typical delayed type hypersensitivity reactions. It remains unclear whether the persistent T cell activity represents a response to a persistent exogenous antigen or to altered autoantigens such as collagen, immunoglobulin, or one of the heat shock proteins. Alternatively, it could represent persistent responsiveness to activated autologous cells such as might occur as a result of Epstein-Barr virus infection or persistent response to a foreign antigen or superantigen in the synovial tissue. Finally, rheumatoid inflammation could reflect persistent stimulation of T cells by synovial-derived antigens that cross-react with determinants introduced during antecedent exposure to foreign antigens or infectious microorganisms.

Overriding the chronic inflammation in the synovial tissue is an acute inflammatory process in the synovial fluid. The exudative synovial fluid contains more polymorphonuclear leukocytes than mononuclear cells. A number of mechanisms play a role in stimulating the exudation of synovial fluid. Locally produced immune complexes can activate complement and generate anaphylatoxins and chemotactic factors. Local production by mononuclear phagocytes of factors such as IL-1, TNFα, and leukotriene B_4, as well as products of complement activation, can stimulate the endothelial cells of postcapillary venules to become more efficient at binding circulating cells, whereas TNFα, IL-8, C5a, and leukotriene B_4 stimulate the migration of polymorphonuclear leukocytes into the synovial site. In addition, vasoactive mediators such as histamine produced by the mast cells that infiltrate the rheumatoid synovium also may facilitate the exudation of inflammatory cells into the synovial fluid. Finally, the vasodilatory effects of locally produced prostaglandin E_2 also may facilitate entry of inflammatory cells into the inflammatory site. Once in the synovial fluid, the polymorphonuclear leukocytes can ingest immune complexes, with the resultant production of reactive oxygen metabolites and other inflammatory mediators, further adding to the inflammatory milieu. Locally produced cytokines and chemokines such as TNFα, IL-8, and GM-CSF can additionally stimulate polymorphonuclear leukocytes. The production of large amounts of cyclooxygenase and lipoxygenase pathway products of arachidonic acid metabolism by cells in the synovial fluid and tissue further accentuates the signs and symptoms of inflammation.

The precise mechanism by which bone and cartilage destruction occurs has not been completely resolved. Although the synovial fluid contains a number of enzymes potentially able to degrade cartilage, the majority of destruction occurs in juxtaposition to the inflamed synovium, or pannus, that spreads to cover the articular cartilage. This vascular granulation tissue is composed of proliferating fibroblasts, small blood vessels, and a variable number of mononuclear cells and produces a large amount of degradative enzymes, including collagenase and stromelysin, that may facilitate tissue damage. The cytokines IL-1 and TNFα play an important role by stimulating the cells of the pannus to produce collagenase and other neutral proteases. These same two cytokines also activate chondrocytes in situ, stimulating them to produce proteolytic enzymes that can degrade cartilage locally. Finally, these two cytokines may contribute to the local demineralization of bone by activating osteoclasts. Prostaglandin E_2 produced by fibroblasts and macrophages also may contribute to bone demineralization. The common final pathway of bone erosion is likely to involve the activation of osteoclasts that are present in large numbers at these sites. Systemic manifestations of RA can be accounted for by release of inflammatory effector molecules from the synovium. These include IL-1, TNFα, and IL-6, which account for many of the manifestations of active RA, including malaise, fatigue, and elevated levels of serum acute phase reactants. The importance of TNFα in producing these manifestations is emphasized by the prompt amelioration of symptoms following administration of a monoclonal antibody to TNFα to patients with RA. In addition, immune complexes produced within the synovium and entering the circulation may account for other features of the disease, such as systemic vasculitis.

As shown in Fig. 313-1, the pathology of RA evolves over the duration of this chronic disease. The earliest event appears to be a nonspecific inflammatory response initiated by an unknown stimulus. Subsequently, an initial, and perhaps specific, response of CD4+ T cells is induced that amplifies and perpetuates the inflammation. The presence of activated T cells can induce polyclonal B cell stimulation and the local production of rheumatoid factor. As tissue damage occurs, additional autoantigens are revealed and the nature of the T cell response broadens as additional clones of CD4+ T cells are recruited to the inflammatory site. Finally, as a result of persistent exposure to the inflammatory milieu, the function of synovial fibroblasts is altered and they may acquire destructive potential that no longer requires stimulation from T cells or macrophages. Important features of this model include the following: (1) the pathologic events vary with time in this chronic disease; (2) the time required to progress from one

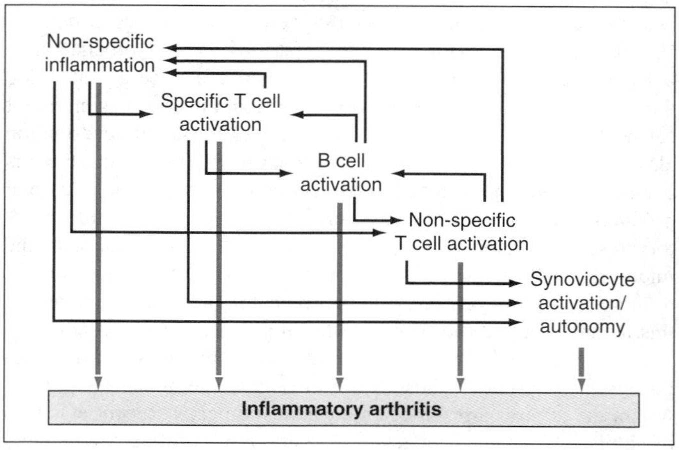

FIGURE 313-1 The progression of rheumatoid synovitis. This figure depicts the evolution of the pathogenic mechanisms and ultimate pathologic changes involved in the development of rheumatoid synovitis.

step to the next may vary in different patients; (3) once established, the major pathogenic events operative in an individual patient may vary at different times. These considerations have important implications with regard to appropriate treatment.

CLINICAL MANIFESTATIONS **Onset** Characteristically, RA is a chronic polyarthritis. In approximately two-thirds of patients, it begins insidiously with fatigue, anorexia, generalized weakness, and vague musculoskeletal symptoms until the appearance of synovitis becomes apparent. This prodrome may persist for weeks or months and defy diagnosis. Specific symptoms usually appear gradually as several joints, especially those of the hands, wrists, knees, and feet, become affected in a symmetric fashion. In approximately 10 percent of individuals, the onset is more acute, with a rapid development of polyarthritis, often accompanied by constitutional symptoms, including fever, lymphadenopathy, and splenomegaly. In approximately one-third of patients, symptoms may initially be confined to one or a few joints. Although the pattern of joint involvement may remain asymmetric in a few patients, a symmetric pattern is more typical.

Signs and Symptoms of Articular Disease Pain, swelling, and tenderness may initially be poorly localized to the joints. Pain in affected joints, aggravated by movement, is the most common manifestation of established RA. It corresponds in pattern to the joint involvement but does not always correlate with the degree of apparent inflammation. Generalized stiffness is frequent and is usually greatest after periods of inactivity. Morning stiffness of greater than 1-h duration is an almost invariable feature of inflammatory arthritis and may serve to distinguish it from various noninflammatory joint disorders. Recent evidence suggests, however, that the presence of morning stiffness may not reliably distinguish between chronic inflammatory and noninflammatory arthritides, as it is also found frequently in the latter. The majority of patients will experience constitutional symptoms such as weakness, easy fatigability, anorexia, and weight loss. Although fever to 40°C occurs on occasion, temperature elevation in excess of 38°C is unusual and suggests the presence of an intercurrent problem such as infection.

Clinically, synovial inflammation causes swelling, tenderness, and limitation of motion. Warmth is usually evident on examination, especially of large joints such as the knee, but erythema is infrequent. Pain originates predominantly from the joint capsule, which is abundantly supplied with pain fibers and is markedly sensitive to stretching or distention. Joint swelling results from accumulation of synovial fluid, hypertrophy of the synovium, and thickening of the joint capsule. Initially, motion is limited by pain. The inflamed joint is usually held in flexion to maximize joint volume and minimize distention of the capsule. Later, fibrous or bony ankylosis or soft tissue contractures lead to fixed deformities.

Although inflammation can affect any diarthrodial joint, RA most often causes symmetric arthritis with characteristic involvement of certain specific joints such as the proximal interphalangeal and metacarpophalangeal joints. The distal interphalangeal joints are rarely involved. Synovitis of the wrist joints is a nearly uniform feature of RA and may lead to limitation of motion, deformity, and median nerve entrapment (carpal tunnel syndrome). Synovitis of the elbow joint often leads to flexion contractures that may develop early in the disease. The knee joint is commonly involved with synovial hypertrophy, chronic effusion, and frequently ligamentous laxity. Pain and swelling behind the knee may be caused by extension of inflamed synovium into the popliteal space (Baker's cyst). Arthritis in the forefoot, ankles, and subtalar joints can produce severe pain with ambulation as well as a number of deformities. Axial involvement is usually limited to the upper cervical spine. Involvement of the lumbar spine is not seen, and lower back pain cannot be ascribed to rheumatoid inflammation. On occasion, inflammation from the synovial joints and bursae of the upper cervical spine leads to atlantoaxial subluxation. This usually presents as pain in the occiput but on rare occasions may lead to compression of the spinal cord.

With persistent inflammation, a variety of characteristic deformities develop. These can be attributed to a number of pathologic events, including laxity of supporting soft tissue structures; destruction or weakening of ligaments, tendons, and the joint capsule; cartilage destruction; muscle imbalance; and unopposed physical forces associated with the use of affected joints. Characteristic deformities of the hand include (1) radial deviation at the wrist with ulnar deviation of the digits often with palmar subluxation of the proximal phalanges ("Z" deformity), (2) hyperextension of the proximal interphalangeal joints, with compensatory flexion of the distal interphalangeal joints (swan-neck deformity), (3) flexion deformity of the proximal interphalangeal joints and extension of the distal interphalangeal joints (boutonnière deformity), and (4) hyperextension of the first interphalangeal joint and flexion of the first metacarpophalangeal joint with a consequent loss of thumb mobility and pinch. Typical deformities also may develop in the feet, including eversion at the hindfoot (subtalar joint), plantar subluxation of the metatarsal heads, widening of the forefoot, hallux valgus, and lateral deviation and dorsal subluxation of the toes.

Extraarticular Manifestations RA is a systemic disease with a variety of extraarticular manifestations. Although these occur frequently, not all of them have clinical significance. However, on occasion, they may be the major evidence of disease activity and source of morbidity and require management per se. As a rule, these manifestations occur in individuals with high titers of autoantibodies to the Fc component of immunoglobulin G (rheumatoid factors).

Rheumatoid nodules develop in 20 to 30 percent of persons with RA. They are usually found on periarticular structures, extensor surfaces, or other areas subjected to mechanical pressure, but they can develop elsewhere, including the pleura and meninges. Common locations include the olecranon bursa, the proximal ulna, the Achilles tendon, and the occiput. Nodules vary in size and consistency and are rarely symptomatic, but on occasion they break down as a result of trauma or become infected. They are found almost invariably in individuals with circulating rheumatoid factor. Histologically, rheumatoid nodules consist of a central zone of necrotic material including collagen fibrils, noncollagenous filaments, and cellular debris; a midzone of palisading macrophages that express HLA-DR antigens; and an outer zone of granulation tissue. Examination of early nodules has suggested that the initial event may be a focal vasculitis.

Clinical weakness and atrophy of skeletal muscle are common. Muscle atrophy may be evident within weeks of the onset of RA and usually is most apparent in musculature approximating affected joints. Muscle biopsy may show type II fiber atrophy and muscle fiber necrosis with or without a mononuclear cell infiltrate.

Rheumatoid vasculitis (see Chap. 319), which can affect nearly any organ system, is seen in patients with severe RA and high titers of circulating rheumatoid factor. Rheumatoid vasculitis is very uncommon in African Americans. In its most aggressive form, rheumatoid vasculitis can cause polyneuropathy and mononeuritis multiplex, cutaneous ulceration and dermal necrosis, digital gangrene, and visceral infarction. While such widespread vasculitis is very rare, more limited forms are not uncommon, especially in white patients with high titers of rheumatoid factor. Neurovascular disease presenting either as a mild distal sensory neuropathy or as mononeuritis multiplex may be the only sign of vasculitis. Cutaneous vasculitis usually presents as crops of small brown spots in the nail beds, nail folds, and digital pulp. Larger ischemic ulcers, especially in the lower extremity, also may develop. Myocardial infarction secondary to rheumatoid vasculitis has been reported, as has vasculitic involvement of lungs, bowel, liver, spleen, pancreas, lymph nodes, and testes. Renal vasculitis is rare.

Pleuropulmonary manifestations, which are more commonly observed in men, include pleural disease, interstitial fibrosis, pleuropulmonary nodules, pneumonitis, and arteritis. Evidence of pleuritis is found commonly at autopsy, but symptomatic disease during life is infrequent. Typically, the pleural fluid contains very low levels of glucose in the absence of infection. Pleural fluid complement is also low compared with the serum level when these are related to the total protein concentration. Pulmonary fibrosis can produce impairment of the diffusing capacity of the lung. Pulmonary nodules may appear singly or in clusters. When they appear in individuals with pneumoconiosis, a diffuse nodular fibrotic process (Caplan's syndrome) may develop. On occasion, pulmonary nodules may cavitate and produce a pneumothorax or bronchopleural fistula. Rarely, pulmonary hypertension secondary to obliteration of the pulmonary vasculature occurs. In addition to pleuropulmonary disease, upper airway obstruction from cricoarytenoid arthritis or laryngeal nodules may develop.

Clinically apparent heart disease attributed to the rheumatoid process is rare, but evidence of asymptomatic pericarditis is found at autopsy in 50 percent of cases. Pericardial fluid has a low glucose level and is frequently associated with the occurrence of pleural effusion. Although pericarditis is usually asymptomatic, on rare occasions death has occurred from tamponade. Chronic constrictive pericarditis also may occur.

RA tends to spare the central nervous system directly, although vasculitis can cause peripheral neuropathy. *Neurologic manifestations* also may result from atlantoaxial or midcervical spine subluxations. Nerve entrapment secondary to proliferative synovitis or joint deformities may produce neuropathies of median, ulnar, radial (interosseous branch), or anterior tibial nerves.

The rheumatoid process involves the *eye* in fewer than 1 percent of patients. Affected individuals usually have long-standing disease and nodules. The two principal manifestations are episcleritis, which is usually mild and transient, and scleritis, which involves the deeper layers of the eye and is a more serious inflammatory condition. Histologically, the lesion is similar to a rheumatoid nodule and may result in thinning and perforation of the globe (scleromalacia perforans). Fifteen to twenty percent of persons with RA may develop Sjögren's syndrome with attendant keratoconjunctivitis sicca.

Felty's syndrome consists of chronic RA, splenomegaly, neutropenia, and on occasion anemia and thrombocytopenia. It is most common in individuals with long-standing disease. These patients frequently have high titers of rheumatoid factor, subcutaneous nodules, and other manifestations of systemic rheumatoid disease. Felty's syndrome is very uncommon in African Americans. It may develop after joint inflammation has regressed. Circulating immune complexes are often present, and evidence of complement consumption may be seen. The leukopenia is a selective neutropenia with polymorphonuclear leukocyte counts of less than 1500 cells per microliter and sometimes less than 1000 cells per microliter. Bone marrow examination usually reveals moderate hypercellularity with a paucity of mature neutrophils. However, the bone marrow may be normal, hyperactive, or hypoactive; maturation arrest may be seen. Hypersplenism has been proposed as one of the causes of leukopenia, but splenomegaly is not invariably found and splenectomy does not always correct the abnormality. Excessive margination of granulocytes caused by antibodies to these cells, complement activation, or binding of immune complexes may contribute to granulocytopenia. Patients with Felty's syndrome have increased frequency of infections usually associated with neutropenia. The cause of the increased susceptibility to infection is related to the defective function of polymorphonuclear leukocytes as well as the decreased number of cells.

Osteoporosis secondary to rheumatoid involvement is common and may be aggravated by glucocorticoid therapy. Glucocorticoid treatment may cause significant loss of bone mass, especially early in the course of therapy, even when low doses are employed. Osteopenia involves both juxtaarticular bone and long bones distant from involved joints. RA is associated with a modest decrease in mean bone mass and a moderate increase in the risk of fracture. Bone mass appears to be adversely affected by functional impairment and active inflammation, especially early in the course of the disease.

RA in the Elderly The incidence of RA continues to increase past age 60. It has been suggested that elderly onset RA might have a poorer prognosis, as manifested by more persistent disease activity, more frequent radiographically evident deterioration, more frequent systemic involvement, and more rapid functional decline. Aggressive disease is largely restricted to those patients with high titers of rheumatoid factor. By contrast, elderly patients who develop RA without elevated titers of rheumatoid factor (seronegative disease) generally have less severe, often self-limited disease.

LABORATORY FINDINGS No tests are specific for diagnosing RA. However, rheumatoid factors, which are autoantibodies reactive with the Fc portion of IgG, are found in more than two-thirds of adults with the disease. Widely utilized tests largely detect IgM rheumatoid factors. The presence of rheumatoid factor is not specific for RA. Rheumatoid factor is found in 5 percent of healthy persons. The frequency of rheumatoid factor in the general population increases with age, and 10 to 20 percent of individuals over 65 years old have a positive test. In addition, a number of conditions besides RA are associated with the presence of rheumatoid factor. These include systemic lupus erythematosus, Sjögren's syndrome, chronic liver disease, sarcoidosis, interstitial pulmonary fibrosis, infectious mononucleosis, hepatitis B, tuberculosis, leprosy, syphilis, subacute bacterial endocarditis, visceral leishmaniasis, schistosomiasis, and malaria. In addition, rheumatoid factor may appear transiently in normal individuals after vaccination or transfusion and also may be found in relatives of individuals with RA.

The presence of rheumatoid factor does not establish the diagnosis of RA but can be of prognostic significance because patients with high titers tend to have more severe and progressive disease with extraarticular manifestations. Rheumatoid factor is uniformly found in patients with nodules or vasculitis. The predictive value of the presence of rheumatoid factor in determining a diagnosis of RA is poor. Thus fewer than one-third of unselected patients with a positive test for rheumatoid factor will be found to have RA. The test is not useful as a screening procedure but can be employed to confirm a diagnosis in individuals with a suggestive clinical presentation and, if present in high titer, to designate patients at risk for severe systemic disease.

Normochromic, normocytic anemia is frequently present in active RA. It is thought to reflect ineffective erythropoiesis; large stores of iron are found in the bone marrow. In general, anemia and thrombocytosis correlate with disease activity. The white blood cell count is usually normal, but a mild leukocytosis may be present. Leukopenia also may exist without the full-blown picture of Felty's syndrome. Eosinophilia, when present, usually reflects severe systemic disease.

The erythrocyte sedimentation rate is increased in nearly all patients with active RA. The levels of a variety of other acute phase reactants including ceruloplasmin and C-reactive protein are also elevated, and generally such elevations correlate with disease activity and the likelihood of progressive joint damage.

Synovial fluid analysis confirms the presence of inflammatory arthritis, although none of the findings is specific. The fluid is usually turbid, with reduced viscosity, increased protein content, and a slightly decreased or normal glucose concentration. The white cell count varies between 5 and 50,000 cells per microliter; polymorphonuclear leukocytes predominate. A synovial fluid white blood cell count of more than 2000 cells per microliter with more than 75 percent polymorphonuclear leukocytes is highly characteristic of inflammatory arthritis, although not diagnostic of RA. Total hemolytic complement, C3, and C4 are markedly diminished in synovial fluid relative to total protein concentration as a result of activation of the classic complement pathway by locally produced immune complexes.

RADIOGRAPHIC EVALUATION Early in the disease, roentgenograms of the affected joints are usually not helpful in establishing a diagnosis. They reveal only that which is apparent from physical examination, namely, evidence of soft tissue swelling and joint effusion. As the disease progresses, abnormalities become more pronounced, but none of the radiographic findings is diagnostic of RA. The diagnosis, however, is supported by a characteristic pattern of abnormalities, including the tendency toward symmetric involvement. Juxtaarticular osteopenia may become apparent within weeks of onset. Loss of articular cartilage and bone erosions develop after months of sustained activity. The primary value of radiography is to determine the extent of cartilage destruction and bone erosion produced by the disease, particularly when one is monitoring the impact of therapy with disease-modifying drugs or surgical intervention. Other means of imaging bones and joints, including ^{99m}Tc bisphosphonate bone scanning and magnetic resonance imaging, may be capable of detecting early inflammatory changes that are not apparent from standard radiography but are rarely necessary in the routine evaluation of patients with RA.

CLINICAL COURSE AND PROGNOSIS The course of RA is quite variable and difficult to predict in an individual patient. Most patients experience persistent but fluctuating disease activity, accompanied by a variable degree of joint abnormalities and functional impairment. After 10 to 12 years, fewer than 20 percent of patients will have no evidence of disability or joint abnormalities. A number of features are correlated with a greater likelihood of developing joint abnormalities or disability. These include the presence of more than 20 inflamed joints, a markedly elevated erythrocyte sedimentation rate, radiographic evidence of bone erosions, the presence of rheumatoid nodules, high titers of serum rheumatoid factor, the presence of functional disability, persistent inflammation, advanced age at onset, the presence of comorbid conditions, low socioeconomic status or educational level, or the presence of HLA-DRβ1*0401 or -DRβ*0404. The presence of one or more of these implies the presence of more aggressive disease with a greater likelihood of developing progressive joint abnormalities and disability. Patients who lack these features have more indolent disease with a slower progression to joint abnormalities and disability. The pattern of disease onset does not appear to predict the development of disabilities. Approximately 15 percent of patients with RA will have a short-lived inflammatory process that remits without major disability. These individuals tend to lack the aforementioned features associated with more aggressive disease.

Several features of patients with RA appear to have prognostic significance. Remissions of disease activity are most likely to occur during the first year. White females tend to have more persistent synovitis and more progressively erosive disease than males. Persons who present with high titers of rheumatoid factor, C-reactive protein, and haptoglobin also have a worse prognosis, as do individuals with subcutaneous nodules or radiographic evidence of erosions at the time of initial evaluation. Although sustained disease activity of more than 1 year's duration portends a poor outcome, the rate of progression of joint abnormalities is not constant; the greatest progression takes place during the first 6 years of disease and at a much slower rate thereafter. Indeed, the rate of progression of joint damage is greater during the first year of observation compared with the second and third years. Within 3 years of disease, as many as 70 percent of patients will have some radiographic evidence of damage to joints; more than 50 percent of these persons will have had evidence of erosions in the first year of disease. Foot joints are affected more frequently than hand joints. Despite the decrease in the rate of progressive joint damage with time, functional disability, which develops early in the course of the disease, continues to worsen at the same rate, although the most rapid rate of functional loss occurs within the first 2 years of disease.

The median life expectancy of persons with RA is shortened by 3 to 7 years. Of the 2.5-fold increase in mortality rate, RA itself is a contributing feature in 15 to 30 percent. The increased mortality rate seems to be limited to patients with more severe articular disease and can be attributed largely to infection and gastrointestinal bleeding. Drug therapy also may play a role in the increased mortality rate seen in these individuals. Factors correlated with early death include disability, disease duration or severity, glucocorticoid use, age at onset, and low socioeconomic or educational status.

DIAGNOSIS The mean delay from disease onset to diagnosis is 9 months. This is often related to the nonspecific nature of initial symptoms. The diagnosis of RA is easily made in persons with typical established disease. In a majority of patients, the disease assumes its characteristic clinical features within 1 to 2 years of onset. The typical picture of bilateral symmetric inflammatory polyarthritis involving small and large joints in both the upper and lower extremities with sparing of the axial skeleton except the cervical spine suggests the diagnosis. Constitutional features indicative of the inflammatory nature of the disease, such as morning stiffness, support the diagnosis. Demonstration of subcutaneous nodules is a helpful diagnostic feature.

Table 313-2

The 1987 Revised Criteria for the Classification of Rheumatoid Arthritis

1. Guidelines for classification
   a. Four of seven criteria are required to classify a patient as having rheumatoid arthritis.
   b. Patients with two or more clinical diagnoses are not excluded.
2. Criteria*
   a. Morning stiffness: Stiffness in and around the joints lasting 1 h before maximal improvement.
   b. Arthritis of three or more joint areas: At least three joint areas, observed by a physician simultaneously, have soft tissue swelling or joint effusions, not just bony overgrowth. The 14 possible joint areas involved are right or left proximal interphalangeal, metacarpophalangeal, wrist, elbow, knee, ankle, and metatarsophalangeal joints.
   c. Arthritis of hand joints: Arthritis of wrist, metacarpophalangeal joint, or proximal interphalangeal joint.
   d. Symmetric arthritis: Simultaneous involvement of the same joint areas on both sides of the body.
   e. Rheumatoid nodules: Subcutaneous nodules over bony prominences, extensor surfaces, or juxtaarticular regions observed by a physician.
   f. Serum rheumatoid factor: Demonstration of abnormal amounts of serum rheumatoid factor by any method for which the result has been positive in less than 5 percent of normal control subjects.
   g. Radiographic changes: Typical changes of RA on posteroanterior hand and wrist radiographs which must include erosions or unequivocal bony decalcification localized in or most marked adjacent to the involved joints.

* Criteria a–d must be present for at least 6 weeks. Criteria b–e must be observed by a physician.

SOURCE: Arnett et al.

Additionally, the presence of rheumatoid factor, inflammatory synovial fluid with increased numbers of polymorphonuclear leukocytes, and radiographic findings of juxtaarticular bone demineralization and erosions of the affected joints substantiate the diagnosis.

The diagnosis is somewhat more difficult early in the course when only constitutional symptoms or intermittent arthralgias or arthritis in an asymmetric distribution may be present. A period of observation may be necessary before the diagnosis can be established. A definitive diagnosis of RA depends predominantly on characteristic clinical features and the exclusion of other inflammatory processes. The isolated finding of a positive test for rheumatoid factor or an elevated erythrocyte sedimentation rate, especially in an older person with joint pains, should not itself be used as evidence of RA.

In 1987, the American College of Rheumatology developed revised criteria for the classification of rheumatoid arthritis (Table 313-2). These criteria demonstrate a sensitivity of 91 to 94 percent and a specificity of 89 percent when used to classify patients with RA compared with control subjects with rheumatic diseases other than RA. Although these criteria were developed as a means of disease classification for epidemiologic purposes, they are useful as guidelines for establishing the diagnosis. Failure to meet these criteria, however, especially during the early stages of the disease, does not exclude the diagnosis.

℞ TREATMENT

General Principles The goals of therapy of RA are (1) relief of pain, (2) reduction of inflammation, (3) protection of articular structures, (4) maintenance of function, and (5) control of systemic involvement. Since the etiology of RA is unknown, the pathogenesis is speculative, and the mechanisms of action of many of the therapeutic agents employed are uncertain, therapy remain empirical. None of the therapeutic interventions is curative, and therefore all must be viewed as palliative, aimed at relieving the signs and symptoms of the disease. The various therapies employed are directed at nonspecific suppression of the inflammatory or immunologic process in the hope of ameliorating symptoms and preventing progressive damage to articular structures.

Management of patients with RA involves an interdisciplinary approach, which attempts to deal with the various problems that these individuals encounter with functional as well as psychosocial interactions. A variety of physical therapy modalities may be useful in decreasing the symptoms of RA. Rest ameliorates symptoms and can be an important component of the total therapeutic program. In addition, splinting to reduce unwanted motion of inflamed joints may be useful. Exercise directed at maintaining muscle strength and joint mobility without exacerbating joint inflammation is also an important aspect of the therapeutic regimen. A variety of orthotic and assistive devices can be helpful in supporting and aligning deformed joints to reduce pain and improve function. Patient and family education is an important component of the therapeutic plan to help those involved become aware of the potential impact of the disease and make appropriate accommodations in life-style to maximize satisfaction and minimize stress on joints.

Medical management of RA involves four general approaches. The first is the use of aspirin and other nonsteroidal anti-inflammatory drugs (NSAIDs) and simple analgesics to control the symptoms and signs of the local inflammatory process. These agents are rapidly effective at mitigating signs and symptoms, but they appear to exert minimal effect on the progression of the disease. The second line of therapy involves use of low-dose oral glucocorticoids. Although these agents have been widely used to suppress signs and symptoms of inflammation, recent evidence suggests that low-dose oral glucocorticoids may also retard the development and progression of bone erosions. The third line of agents includes a variety of agents that have been classified as the disease-modifying or slow-acting antirheumatic drugs. These agents appear to have the capacity to decrease elevated levels of acute phase reactants in treated patients and, therefore, are thought to modify the destructive capacity of the disease. Other agents are the immunosuppressive and cytotoxic drugs that have been shown to ameliorate the disease process in some patients. The fourth approach involves the use of intraarticular glucocorticoids that can provide transient relief when systemic medical therapy has failed to resolve inflammation. A final approach that can be entertained when standard therapy has failed to control disease activity involves the use of a variety of investigational therapies, including combinations of disease-modifying antirheumatic drugs (DMARDs) and other more experimental agents. Recently, substituting omega-3 fatty acids such as eicosapentaenoic acid found in certain fish oils for dietary omega-6 essential fatty acids found in meat also has been shown to provide symptomatic improvement in patients with RA. A variety of nontraditional approaches also have been claimed to be effective in treating RA, including diets, plant and animal extracts, vaccines, hormones, and topical preparations of various sorts. Many of these are costly, and none has been shown to be effective. However, belief in their efficacy ensures their continued use by some patients.

Nonsteroidal Anti-Inflammatory Drugs Besides aspirin, there are now several additional NSAIDs available to treat RA. As a result of the capacity of these agents to block the activity of the enzyme cyclooxygenase and therefore the production of prostaglandins, prostacyclin, and thromboxanes, they have analgesic, anti-inflammatory, and antipyretic properties. In addition, the agents may exert other anti-inflammatory effects. These agents are all associated with a wide spectrum of toxic side effects. Some, such as gastric irritation, azotemia, platelet dysfunction, and exacerbation of allergic rhinitis and asthma, are related to the inhibition of cyclooxygenase activity, while a variety of others, such as rash, liver function abnormalities, and bone marrow depression, may not be. Elderly patients on diuretics may be at higher risk for certain toxic effects. None of the NSAIDs has been shown to be more effective than aspirin in the treatment of RA. However, these nonaspirin drugs are associated with a lower incidence of gastrointestinal intolerance. None of the newer NSAIDs appears to show significant therapeutic advantages over the other available agents. In addition, there is no consistent advantage of any of these newer agents over the others with respect to the incidence or severity of toxic manifestations. Recent evidence indicates that two separate enzymes, cyclooxygenase 1 and 2, are responsible for the initial metabolism of arachidonic acid into various inflammatory mediators. The former is constitutively present in many cells and tissues, including the stomach and the platelet, whereas the latter is specifically induced in response to inflammatory stimuli. Inhibition of cyclooxygenase 2 accounts for the anti-inflammatory effects of NSAIDs, and suppression of cyclooxygenase 1 induces much of the mechanism-based toxicity. As the currently available NSAIDs inhibit both enzymes, therapeutic benefit and toxicity are intertwined. Newer, specific cyclooxygenase 2 inhibitors are being developed that promise therapeutic benefit with less toxicity.

DISEASE-MODIFYING ANTIRHEUMATIC DRUGS Clinical experience has delineated a number of agents that appear to have the capacity to alter the course of RA. This group of agents includes gold compounds, D-penicillamine, the antimalarials, and sulfasalazine. Despite having no chemical or pharmacologic similarities, in practice these agents share a number of characteristics. They exert minimal direct nonspecific anti-inflammatory or analgesic effects, and therefore NSAIDs must be continued during their administration, except in a few cases when true remissions are induced with them. The appearance of benefit from DMARD therapy is usually delayed for weeks or months. As many as two-thirds of patients develop some clinical improvement as a result of therapy with any of these agents, although the induction of true remissions is unusual. In addition to clinical improvement, there is frequently an improvement in serologic evidence of disease activity, and titers of rheumatoid factor and C-reactive protein and the erythrocyte sedimentation rate frequently decline. Despite this, there is minimal evidence that DMARDs actually retard the development of bone erosions or facilitate their healing.

Each of these drugs is associated with considerable toxicity, and therefore careful patient monitoring is necessary. Which DMARD should be the drug of first choice remains controversial, and trials have failed to demonstrate a consistent advantage of one over the other. Toxicity of the various agents thus becomes important in determining the drug of first choice. Failure to respond or development of toxicity to one agent does not preclude responsiveness to another. For example, a similar percentage of RA patients who have failed to respond to gold will respond to D-pencillamine when it is given as the second disease-modifying drug.

No characteristic features of patients have emerged that predict responsiveness to a DMARD. Moreover, the indications for the initiation of therapy with one of these agents are not well defined, although recently the trend has been to begin DMARD therapy early in the course of the disease.

The folic acid antagonist methotrexate, given in an intermittent low dose (7.5 to 20 mg once weekly), is currently a frequently utilized DMARD. Most rheumatologists recommend use of methotrexate as the initial DMARD, especially in individuals with evidence of aggressive RA. Recent trials have documented the efficacy of methotrexate and have indicated that its onset of action is more rapid than other DMARDs, and patients tend to remain on therapy with methotrexate longer than they remain on other DMARDs because of better clinical responses and less toxicity. Long-term trials have indicated that methotrexate does not induce remission but rather suppresses symptoms while it is being administered. Maximal improvement is observed after 6 months of therapy, with little additional improvement thereafter. Major toxicity includes gastrointestinal upset, oral ulceration, and liver function abnormalities that appear to be dose-related and reversible and hepatic fibrosis that can be quite insidious, requiring liver biopsy for detection in its early stages. Drug-induced pneumonitis also has been reported. Liver biopsy is recommended for individuals with persistent or repetitive liver function abnormalities. Concurrent administration of folic acid or folinic acid may diminish the frequency of some side effects.

GLUCOCORTICOID THERAPY Systemic glucocorticoid therapy can provide effective symptomatic therapy in patients with RA. Low-dose (less than 7.5 mg/d) prednisone has been advocated as useful additive therapy to control symptoms. Moreover, recent evidence suggests that low-dose glucocorticoid therapy may retard the progression of bone erosions. Monthly pulses with high-dose glucocorticoids may be useful in some patients and may hasten the response when therapy with a DMARD is initiated.

IMMUNOSUPPRESSIVE THERAPY The immunosuppressive drugs azathioprine and cyclophosphamide have been shown to be effective in the treatment of RA and to exert therapeutic effects similar to those of the DMARDs. However, these agents appear to be no more effective than the DMARDs. Moreover, they cause a variety of toxic side effects, and cyclophosphamide appears to predispose the patient to the development of malignant neoplasms. Therefore, these drugs have been reserved for patients who have clearly failed therapy with DMARDs. On occasion, extraarticular disease such as rheumatoid vasculitis may require cytotoxic immunosuppressive therapy.

Recent trials have suggested that cyclosporine also may be effective in the treatment of RA. Although high-dose therapy may induce rapid improvement, it is associated with frequent renal and gastrointestinal toxicity. Lower doses of cyclosporine (<5 mg/kg per day), however, appear to cause slower but nonetheless significant improvement in disease activity with fewer toxic side effects that are reversed upon lowering the dose. In addition, concomitant use of methotrexate and cyclosporine may afford additional benefit. Currently, cyclosporine has not been approved for use in RA.

SURGERY Surgery plays a role in the management of patients with severely damaged joints. Although arthroplasties and total joint replacements can be done on a number of joints, the most successful procedures are carried out on hips, knees, and shoulders. Realistic goals of these procedures are relief of pain and reduction of disability. Reconstructive hand surgery may lead to cosmetic improvement and some functional benefit. Open or arthroscopic synovectomy may be useful in some patients with persistent monarthritis, especially of the knee. Although synovectomy may offer short-term relief of symptoms, it does not appear to retard bone destruction or alter the natural history of the disease. In addition, early tenosynovectomy of the wrist may prevent tendon rupture.

APPROACH TO THE PATIENT WITH RA An approach to the medical management of patients with rheumatoid arthritis is depicted in Fig. 313-2. The principles underlying care of these patients reflect the variability of the disease, the frequent persistent nature of the inflammation and its potential to cause disability, the relationship between sustained inflammation and bone erosions, and the need to reevaluate the patient frequently for symptomatic response to therapy, progression of disability and joint damage, and side effects of treatment. At the onset of disease it is difficult to predict the natural history of an individual patient's illness. Therefore, the usual approach is to attempt to alleviate the patient's symptoms with NSAIDs. Some patients may have mild disease that requires no additional therapy.

At some time during most patients' course, the possibility of initiating DMARD therapy and/or low-dose oral glucocorticoids is entertained. With aggressive disease this might occur sooner, often within 1 to 3 months of diagnosis, whereas in patients with more indolent disease, smoldering activity may not require such therapy for many years. The development of bone erosions or radiographic evidence of cartilage loss is clear-cut evidence of the destructive potential of the inflammatory process and indicates the need for DMARD therapy. The other indications as outlined above, including persistent pain, joint swelling, or functional impairment, are much more subjective, however. The decision to begin use of a DMARD and/or low-dose oral glucocorticoids requires experience and clinical judgment as well as the ability to assess joint swelling and functional activity and the patient's pain tolerance and expectation of therapy accurately. In this setting, the fully informed patient must play an active role in the decision to begin DMARD and/or low-dose oral glucocorticoid therapy, after careful review of the therapeutic and toxic potential of the various drugs.

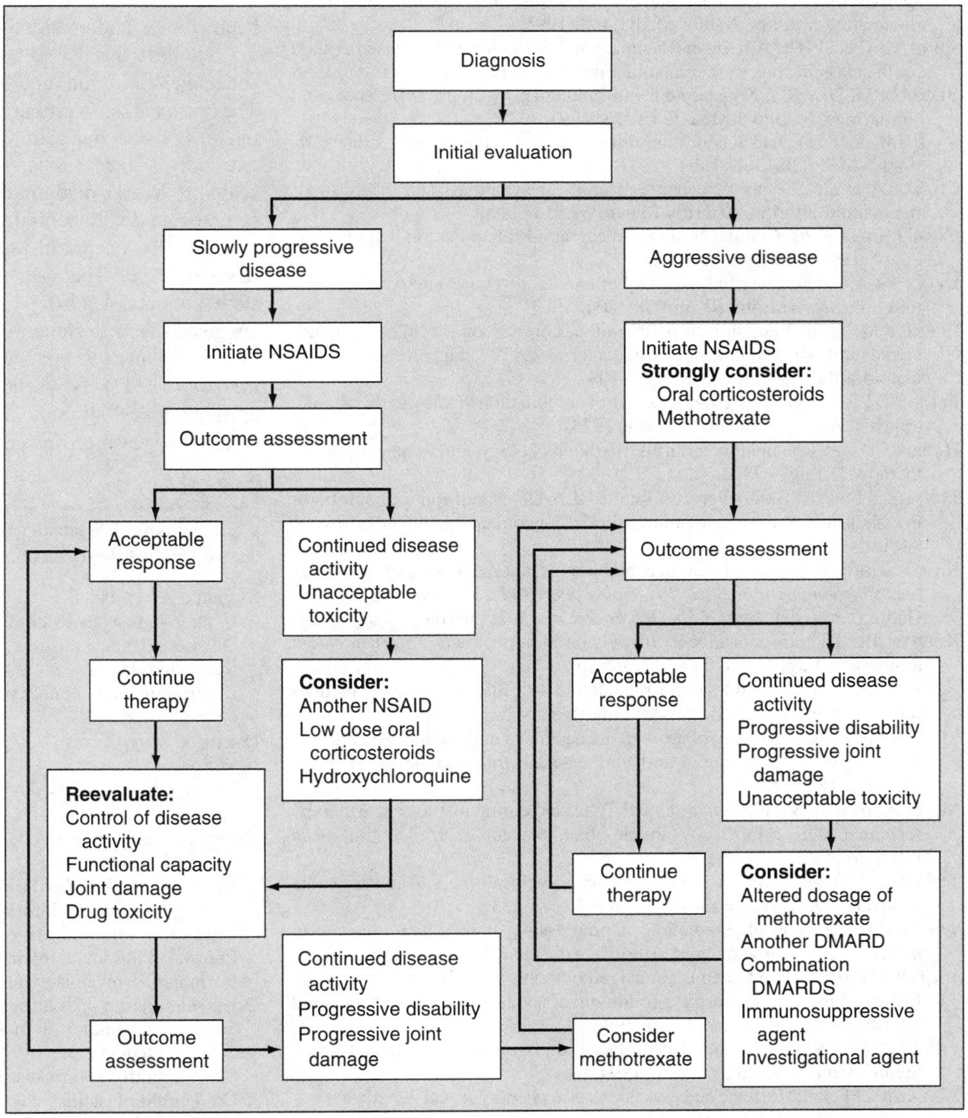

FIGURE 313-2 Algorithm for the medical management of rheumatoid arthritis. (*Courtesy of the University of Texas Southwestern Medical Center, Office of Continuing Education.*)

If a patient responds to a DMARD, therapy is continued with careful monitoring to avoid toxicity. All DMARDs provide a suppressive effect and therefore require prolonged administration. Even with successful therapy, local injection of glucocorticoids may be necessary to diminish inflammation that may persist in a limited number of joints. In addition, NSAIDs may be necessary to mitigate symptoms. Even after inflammation has totally resolved, symptoms from loss of cartilage and supervening degenerative joint disease or deformities may require additional treatment. Surgery also may be necessary to relieve pain or diminish the functional impairment secondary to deformity. Only when patients have persistent inflammatory disease or severe extraarticular manifestations is the use of cytotoxic immunosuppressive drugs or experimental procedures justified. Recently an alternative approach to treat patients with RA has been suggested. This involves the initiation of therapy with multiple agents early in the course of disease in an attempt to control inflammation, followed by maintenance on one or more agents as necessary to control disease activity. The effectiveness of this therapeutic alternative has not been proven.

BIBLIOGRAPHY

Albani S et al: Positive selection in autoimmunity: Abnormal immune responses to a bacterial dnaJ antigenic determinant in patients with early rheumatoid arthritis. Nature Med 1:448, 1995

Arnett FC et al: The American Rheumatism Association 1987 revised criteria for the classification of rheumatoid arthritis. Arthritis Rheum 31:315, 1988

Brooks PM, Day RO: Nonsteroidal anti-inflammatory drugs: Differences and similarities. N Engl J Med 324:1716, 1991

Cash JM, Klippel JH: Second-line drug therapy for rheumatoid arthritis. N Engl J Med 330:1368, 1994

Chan KA et al: The lag time between onset of symptoms and diagnosis of rheumatoid arthritis. Arthritis Rheum 37:814, 1994

Cush J, Lipsky PE: Cellular basis for rheumatoid inflammation. Clin Orthop 265:9, 1991

Deodhar AA et al: Longitudinal study of hand bone densitometry in rheumatoid arthritis. Arthritis Rheum 38:1204, 1995

Elliott MJ et al: Randomized double-blind comparison of chimeric monoclonal antibody to tumour necrosis factor α (cA2) versus placebo in rheumatoid arthritis. Lancet 344:1105, 1994

Felson DT et al: The efficacy and toxicity of combination therapy in rheumatoid arthritis. Arthritis Rheum 37:1487, 1994

Harris ED Jr: Rheumatoid arthritis: Pathophysiology and implications for therapy. N Engl J Med 322:1277, 1990

Jawaheer D et al: "Homozygosity" for the HLA-DR shared epitope contributes the highest risk for rheumatoid arthritis concordance in identical twins. Arthritis Rheum 37:681, 1994

Kavanaugh AF, Lipsky PE: Gold, penicillamine, antimalarials and sulfasalazine, on *Inflammation: Basic Principles and Clinical Correlates*, 2d ed, JI Gallin et al (eds). New York, Raven Press, 1992, pp 1083–1101

Kirwan JR: The effect of glucocorticoids on joint destruction in rheumatoid arthritis. N Engl J Med 333:142, 1995

Kremer JM et al: Methotrexate for rheumatoid arthritis: Suggested guidelines for monitoring liver toxicity. Arthritis Rheum 37:316, 1994

McDaniel DO et al: Most African-American patients with rheumatoid arthritis do not have the rheumatoid antigenic determinant (Epitope). Ann Intern Med 123:181, 1995

Morgan SL et al: Supplementation with folic acid during methotrexate therapy for rheumatoid arthritis: A double-blind, placebo-controlled trial. Ann Intern Med 121:833, 1994

Tugwell P et al: Combination therapy with cyclosporine and methotrexate in severe rheumatoid arthritis. N Engl J Med 333:137, 1995

van der Heide A et al: Prediction of progression of radiologic damage in newly diagnosed rheumatoid arthritis. Arthritis Rheum 38:1466, 1995

Van Der Heijde DMFM et al: Biannual radiographic assessments of hands and feet in a three-year prospective follow-up of patients with early rheumatoid arthritis. Arthritis Rheum 35:26, 1992

van Schaardenburg D, Breedveld FC: Elderly-onset rheumatoid arthritis. Semin Arthritis Rheum 23:367, 1994

Weyand CM et al: Correlation between disease phenotype and genetic heterogeneity in rheumatoid arthritis. J Clin Invest 95:2120, 1995

Zvaifler NJ, Firestein GS: Pannus and pannocytes: Alternative models of joint destruction in rheumatoid arthritis. Arthritis Rheum 37:783, 1994

314

Bruce C. Gilliland

SYSTEMIC SCLEROSIS (SCLERODERMA)

DEFINITION Systemic sclerosis (SSc) is a multisystem disorder of unknown cause characterized by fibrosis of the skin, blood vessels, and visceral organs, including the gastrointestinal tract, lungs, heart, and kidneys (Table 314-1). The degree and rate of skin and internal organ involvement vary among patients. Two subsets, however, can be identified, even though there is some overlap (Table 314-2). One subset is referred to as *diffuse cutaneous scleroderma* and is characterized by the rapid development of symmetric skin thickening of proximal and distal extremity, face, and trunk. These patients are at greater risk for developing kidney and other visceral disease early in their course. The other subset is *limited cutaneous scleroderma*, which is defined by symmetric skin thickening limited to distal extremities and face. This subset frequently has features of the *CREST syndrome*, an acronym standing for calcinosis, Raynaud's phenomenon, esophageal dysmotility, sclerodactyly, and telangiectasia. The prognosis in limited cutaneous scleroderma is better except for the occasional patient who, after many years, develops pulmonary arterial hypertension or biliary cirrhosis. Systemic sclerosis of visceral organs also may occur in the absence of any skin involvement, which is referred to as *systemic sclerosis sine scleroderma*. Survival is determined by the severity of visceral disease, especially involving the heart, lungs, and/or kidneys.

Scleroderma also can occur in a localized form limited to the skin, subcutaneous tissue, and muscle and without systemic involvement. The two localized forms are morphea, which occurs as single or multiple plaques of skin induration, and linear scleroderma, which involves an extremity or face. Linear scleroderma of one side of the forehead and scalp produces a disfiguration referred to as *en coup de sabre* and may be associated with hemiatrophy of the same side of the face.

SSc also occurs in association with features of other connective tissue diseases. The term overlap syndrome has been used to describe such patients. Undifferentiated connective tissue disease has been suggested as a designation for patients who do not have diagnostic criteria for any one connective tissue disease. *Mixed connective tissue disease* (MCTD) is a syndrome involving features of systemic lupus erythematosus, systemic sclerosis, polymyositis, and rheumatoid arthritis and very high titers of circulating antibody to nuclear ribonucleo-

Table 314-1

Classification of Scleroderma/Systemic Sclerosis and Scleroderma-Like Disorders

Systemic sclerosis
Limited cutaneous disease
Diffuse cutaneous disease
Sine scleroderma
Undifferentiated connective tissue disease
Overlap syndromes
Localized scleroderma
Morphea
Linear scleroderma
En coup de sabre
Chemically induced scleroderma-like disorders
Toxic-oil syndrome
Vinyl chloride–induced disease
Bleomycin-induced fibrosis
Pentazocine-induced fibrosis
Epoxy- and aromatic hydrocarbons–induced fibrosis
Eosinophilia-myalgia syndrome
Other scleroderma-like disorders
Sclerederma adultorum of Buschke
Scleromyxedema
Chronic graft-vs.-host disease
Eosinophilic fasciitis
Digital sclerosis in diabetes
Primary amyloidosis and amyloidosis associated with multiple myeloma

protein antigen, will be discussed later in the chapter. *Eosinophilic fasciitis* and the *eosinophilia-myalgia syndrome* associated with L-tryptophan ingestion are scleroderma-like illnesses and will also be discussed in this chapter.

EPIDEMIOLOGY SSc has a worldwide distribution and affects all races. The onset of disease is unusual in childhood and young men. The incidence increases with age, peaking in the third to fifth decade. Women overall are affected approximately three times as often as men, and even more often during the childbearing years (as high as 15:1). SSc is more frequent and severe in young black women. The annual incidence has been estimated to be 14.1 cases per million population based on a 20-year study performed in Allegheny County, Pennsylvania. The prevalence of SSc has been reported between 19 and 75 per 100,000 persons. An exceptionally high prevalence of SSc was recently reported in the Choctaw Native Americans in Oklahoma. The prevalence was 472 per 100,000 persons, which is the highest found to date in any ethnic group. Both incidence and prevalence may be underestimated because patients with early and atypical disease may be overlooked in surveys. The role of heredity has not been clarified. Several examples of familial SSc have been reported, and the finding of other connective tissue diseases and autoantibodies in relatives of involved patients suggests a hereditary predisposition. However, an increased incidence of antinuclear antibodies in spouses of SSc patients suggests an environmental role. Immunogenetic studies have not shown strong associations between the major histocompatibility complex and susceptibility to SSc. Some studies have shown an association of SSc with HLA-DR1, -DR2, -DR3, and -DR5. C4A null alleles and HLA-DQA2 have been reported by some investigators to be markers for disease susceptibility. A more consistent relationship has been found between certain HLA types and the occurrence of specific autoantibodies in SSc patients. Anticentromere antibodies have been shown to be associated with HLA-DR1, -DR4, and -DR5, and antitopoisomerase antibodies with HLA-DR5. Both autoantibodies appear to be more closely associated with HLA-DQB1 alleles.

Several environmental factors have been associated with the development of SSc and scleroderma-like illnesses. SSc appears to be more common in coal and gold miners, especially in those with more extensive exposure, suggesting that silica dust may be a predisposing factor. Workers exposed to polyvinyl chloride may develop Raynaud's phenomenon, acroosteolysis, scleroderma-like skin lesions, and nail fold capillary abnormalities similar to those observed in SSc. These workers also may develop hepatic fibrosis and angiosarcoma. The development of scleroderma has been associated with exposure to vinyl chloride, epoxy resins, and aromatic hydrocarbons such as benzine and toluene. In 1981, in Spain, a multisystem disease resembling scleroderma occurred following the ingestion of adulterated cooking oil (rapeseed oil). Approximately 20,000 people were affected. The patients initially develop interstitial pneumonitis, eosinophilia, arthralgias, arthritis, and myositis, followed subsequently by joint contractures, skin thickening, Raynaud's phenomenon, pulmonary hypertension, sicca syndrome, and resorption of the distal fingertips. Extensive sclerosis of the dermis and subcutaneous tissue has been noted in patients receiving pentazocine, a nonnarcotic analgesic agent. Bleomycin, an anticancer agent, produces fibrotic skin nodules, linear hyperpigmentation, alopecia, gangrene of fingers, and pulmonary fibrosis affecting mainly the lower lobes. Scleroderma and other connective tissue diseases have been reported in women who have had silicone breast implants. At present, the evidence is not conclusive that women with these implants carry an increased risk for developing scleroderma or other connective tissue diseases. Localized fibrosis, however, can occur around the implant. The development of a scleroderma-like illness has been associated with the ingestion of products containing L-tryptophan and is referred to as the *eosinophilia-myalgia syndrome* (see below and Chap. 315).

Table 314-2

Subsets of Systemic Sclerosis

	Diffuse	Limited*
Skin involvement	Distal and proximal extremities, face, trunk	Distal to elbows, face
Raynaud's phenomenon	Onset within 1 year or at time of skin changes	May precede skin disease by years
Organ involvement	Pulmonary (interstitial fibrosis); renal (renovascular hypertensive crisis); gastrointestinal; cardiac	Gastrointestinal; pulmonary arterial hypertension after 10–15 years of disease in fewer than 10% of patients; biliary cirrhosis
Nail fold capillaries	Dilatation and dropout	Dilatation without significant dropout
Antinuclear antibodies	Antitopoisomerase 1	Anticentromere

* Also referred to as CREST (calcinosis, Raynaud's, esophageal dysmotility, sclerodactyly, telangiectasia).

PATHOGENESIS The outstanding feature of SSc is overproduction and accumulation of collagen and other extracellular matrix proteins in skin and other organs. While the pathogenesis of SSc remains to be further elucidated, the disease process involves immunologic mechanisms, vascular damage, and activation of fibroblasts.

An early event in SSc that precedes fibrosis is vascular damage involving small arteries, arterioles, and capillaries in the skin, gastrointestinal tract, kidneys, heart, and lungs. Raynaud's phenomenon, the initial symptom of SSc in the majority of patients, is a clinical expression of the abnormal regulation of blood flow resulting from vascular injury. Injury to endothelial cells and basal lamina occurs early and is followed by thickening of the intima, narrowing of the lumen, and eventual obliteration of the vessel. As vascular damage progresses, the microvascular bed in the skin and other sites is diminished, producing a state of chronic ischemia. Vascular damage can be observed in the nail folds by wide-field microscopy, which shows drop-out of capillaries with dilatation and tortuosity of remaining ones. In the skin, remaining capillaries may proliferate and dilate to become visible telangiectasia.

Several mechanisms for endothelial injury in SSc patients have been proposed. In the sera of some patients an endothelial cytotoxic factor secreted by activated T cells has been found that degrades type IV collagen. This factor, termed granzyme A, is a serine proteinase and may be responsible for disruption of the basal lamina. The sera of some patients mediate antibody-dependent cellular cytotoxicity directed against human endothelial cells. Circulating antiendothelial antibodies, present in some patients, may be yet another mechanism for cell injury. Tumor necrosis factor also can induce endothelial injury as well as stimulate fibrosis. Vasoconstriction in SSc also contributes to endothelial damage through a mechanism of reperfusion injury resulting in fibrosis and vascular occlusion. Factors regulating vascular tone favor vasoconstriction. Endothelin 1, a vasoconstricting factor released from endothelial cells on cold exposure, is increased in SSc patients. Endothelin 1 has also been shown to stimulate fibroblasts and smooth-muscle cells. Its vasoconstriction action is normally opposed by endothelium-derived relaxation factor (EDRF, nitric oxide), also secreted by endothelial cells. The normal compensatory increase in EDRF was not seen in some patients with SSc, suggesting impairment of its synthesis. A deficiency of vasodilatory neuropeptides resulting from sensory system nerve damage may also contribute to a state favoring vasoconstriction.

Endothelial cell damage is reflected by elevated levels of factor VIII/von Willebrand factor in the sera of many but not all patients with SSc. The binding of von Willebrand factor to subendothelium mediates platelet activation with release of factors that alter vascular permeability, leading to edema. Activated platelets also release platelet-derived growth factor (PDGF), which is chemotactic and mitogenic for both smooth-muscle cells and fibroblasts, and transforming growth factor β (TGFβ), which stimulates fibroblast collagen synthesis. These and other cytokines stimulate intimal fibrosis and with their passage through the injured endothelium also could account for adventitial and perivascular fibrosis. Endothelial damage along with a deficiency of tissue plasminogen activator factor enhances intravascular coagulation and, when extensive, can lead to microangiopathic hemolytic anemia observed in those patients at risk for developing acute renal failure.

Existing evidence indicates that cell-mediated immunity plays an important role in the development of fibrosis. Perivascular and diffuse mononuclear infiltrates consisting predominantly of T cells and monocytes are found in macroscopically normal appearing skin adjacent to areas of skin fibrosis. The T cells in these infiltrates are mostly helper T cells (CD4). Elevated levels of circulating interleukin (IL) 2, IL-2 receptors, CD4 antigens, and adenine deaminase are found in SSc patients, indicating activation of helper T cells. In early SSc, elevated levels of circulating IL-2 and IL-2 receptors have been shown to be associated with disease progression. IL-4 and IL-6 have also been detected in the sera of SSc patients. IL-4 is produced by activated T cells and mast cells and stimulates fibroblast proliferation and collagen synthesis (see Chap. 305). It also enhances T cell adhesion to endothelial cells. IL-6 is produced by several cells including fibroblasts, T and B cells, and endothelial cells. One of its roles is induction of IL-2 and IL-2R, which are involved in immune activation in SSc. The CD4+/CD8+ T cell ratio is increased in peripheral blood of SSc patients due usually to an increased number of CD4+ T cells and a decreased number of CD8+ T cells. Laminin and type IV collagen, components of the endothelial basement membrane, induce in vitro transformation of lymphocytes from SSc patients, suggesting that the target of cell-mediated immunity might be endothelium. T cell interaction with endothelial cells is mediated by a group of molecules known as selectins (E-selectin and P-selectin) and adhesion molecules including intercellular adhesion molecule 1 (ICAM-1), and vascular cell adhesion molecule 1 (VCAM-1) (see Chap. 305). Correlation has been shown between serum, skin, and endothelial expression of ICAM-1, VCAM-1, and P-selectin and disease activity in early SSc. Increased levels of circulating IL-1 and tumor necrosis factor in SSc patients indicate in vivo activation of monocytes. These two cytokines have been shown to stimulate fibroblasts. Additional support for involvement of cell-mediated immunity in the pathogenesis of SSc is the appearance of scleroderma-like lesions in patients with graft-versus-host disease (GVHD) after bone marrow transplantation and in a murine model of chronic GVHD, conditions known to be associated with activated T cells. Mast cells also may be involved in the development of fibrosis. Increased numbers of mast cells are found in the dermis in both involved and uninvolved skin. Mast cell degranulation has been noted in skin that subsequently became fibrosed. Interaction with T cells may be one mechanism for mast cell degranulation resulting in release of products that stimulate fibroblast collagen synthesis. Release of histamine from mast cells also may contribute to edema observed in early disease.

Humoral immune abnormalities are also present in patients with SSc. Antinuclear antibodies are found in approximately 95 percent of patients (see "Laboratory Findings," below), and antibodies to type IV collagen and laminin may be present. The role of these antibodies in the pathogenesis of SSc is not presently understood.

Regulatory mechanisms control fibroblast growth and synthesis of collagen, fibronectin, and glycosaminoglycans. Compared with fibroblasts from normal persons, the fibroblasts from SSc appear to have aberrant regulation of growth. When fibroblasts from affected SSc skin are removed and cultured in vitro, they continue to produce excessive quantities of collagen. The collagen is biochemically normal, and the proportion of type I to type III is the same as in normal skin. Fibroblasts from SSc patients appear to be in a state of permanent activation most likely as a result of stimulation by cytokines. These activated cells are thought to represent an expanded subpopulation of fibroblasts that inherently express increased matrix genes. Studies have revealed a subpopulation of SSc fibroblasts that produces two to three times more collagen than other cells from the same tissue. Fibroblasts expressing elevated levels of messenger RNA for types I and III collagen have been demonstrated by in situ hybridization, particularly around dermal blood vessels in affected SSc skin. A small number of fibroblasts expressed increased levels of mRNA for type VI and type VII collagen. Type VII collagen is normally found at the dermal-epidermal basement membrane zone and is the major component of anchoring fibrils that act to stabilize the attachment of the basement membrane to the underlying dermis. In SSc patients, type VII collagen is found throughout the dermis and may account for the indurated, tightly bound skin in this disease. PDGF receptors are expressed on SSc fibroblasts not only from affected areas but also from macroscopically normal appearing skin. Fibroblasts from normal persons lack expression of these receptors. TGFβ has been shown to upregulate the expression of these receptors in SSc fibroblasts but not in normal cells and, in conjunction with PDGF, stimulates SSc fibroblast proliferation. Macrophages and fibroblasts are capable of secreting PDGF and TGFβ, and activated T cells release TGFβ.

Fibroblasts may activate T cells to release cytokines that stimulate fibrosis. Fibroblasts in SSc patients have been shown to have increased expression of an adhesion molecule, ICAM-1, which binds to specific integrins on T cells. This binding allows interaction between T cell antigen receptor and class II molecules and antigen on fibroblasts resulting in T cell activation and cytokine release. T cells also may be activated by their interaction with extracellular matrix molecules including collagen, fibronectin, and laminin.

Chromosomal abnormalities have been noted in greater than 90 percent of SSc patients. These acquired abnormalities include chromatid breaks, acentric fragments, and ring chromosomes and are found in approximately 30 percent of mitotic cells. A chromosomal breakage factor has been found in the serum of SSc patients and their first-degree relatives. The significance of these chromosomal abnormalities is unknown.

PATHOLOGY **Skin** In the skin, a thin epidermis overlies compact bundles of collagen that lie parallel to the epidermis. Finger-like projections of collagen extend from the dermis into the subcutaneous tissue and bind the skin to the underlying tissue. Dermal appendages are atrophied, and rete pegs are lost. In early stages of disease, increased numbers of T cells, monocytes, plasma cells, and mast cells are found, particularly in the lower dermis of involved skin.

Gastrointestinal Tract In the lower two-thirds of the esophagus, the histologic findings consist of a thin mucosa and increased collagen in the lamina propria, submucosa, and serosa. The degree of fibrosis is less than in the skin. Atrophy of the muscularis in the esophagus and throughout the involved portions of the gastrointestinal tract is more prominent than the amount of fibrotic replacement of muscle. Ulceration of the mucosa is often present and may be due to either SSc or superimposed peptic esophagitis. Striated muscles in the upper third of the esophagus are relatively spared. Similar changes may be found throughout the gastrointestinal tract, especially in the second and third portions of the duodenum, in the jejunum, and in the large intestine. Atrophy of the muscularis of the large intestine may lead to the development of large-mouth diverticula. In the later stages of the disease, the involved portions of the gastrointestinal tract become dilated. Infiltration of lymphocytes and plasma cells in the lamina propria is also present.

Lung With pulmonary involvement, diffuse interstitial fibrosis, thickening of the alveolar membrane, and peribronchial fibrosis are observed. Bronchiolar epithelial proliferation accompanies the pulmonary fibrosis. Rupture of septa produces small cysts and areas of bullous emphysema. Small pulmonary arteries and arterioles show intimal thickening, fragmentation of the elastica, and muscular hypertrophy; this may occur without interstitial pulmonary fibrosis and produce pulmonary hypertension.

Musculoskeletal System The synovium in patients with arthritis is similar to that seen in early rheumatoid arthritis and shows edema with infiltration of lymphocytes and plasma cells. A characteristic finding is a thick layer of fibrin overlying and within the synovium. Later in the disease the synovium may become fibrotic. Fibrinous deposits appear on the surfaces of tendon sheaths and in the overlying fascia and may lead to audible creaking over moving tendons.

Histologic features of primary myopathy consist of interstitial and perivascular lymphocytic infiltrations, degeneration of muscle fibers, and interstitial fibrosis. Arterioles may be thickened, and capillaries may be decreased in number. Pathologic and electrophysiologic findings of polymyositis in proximal muscles are present in the few patients who are considered to have the overlap syndrome of SSc and polymyositis.

Heart Cardiac involvement consists of degeneration of myocardial fibers and irregular areas of interstitial fibrosis that are most prominent around blood vessels. Fibrosis also involves the conduction system, leading to atrioventricular conduction defects and arrhythmias. The wall of smaller coronary arteries may be thickened. Fibrinous pericarditis and pericardial effusions are found in some patients.

Kidney Renal involvement is found in over half the patients and consists of intimal hyperplasia of the interlobular arteries; fibrinoid necrosis of the afferent arterioles, including the glomerular tuft; and thickening of the glomerular basement membrane. Small cortical infarctions and glomerulosclerosis may be present. The renal pathologic change is often indistinguishable from that observed in malignant hypertension. Renal vascular lesions, however, may be present in the absence of hypertension. Immunofluorescence studies of kidney have shown IgM, complement components, and fibrinogen in the walls of affected vessels. Angiographic renal studies in patients with SSc may show constriction of the intralobular arteries, a finding that simulates the vasospasm of the digital arteries observed in Raynaud's phenomenon. Cold-induced Raynaud's phenomenon has been shown to decrease renal blood flow.

Other Organs Primary liver involvement is not common. Primary biliary cirrhosis occurs in some patients, particularly in those with the limited cutaneous form of SSc. Fibrosis of the thyroid gland may develop in the presence or absence of autoimmune thyroiditis.

Thickening of the periodontal membrane with replacement of the lamina dura is demonstrated radiographically as widening of the periodontal space and rarely causes loosening of the teeth.

CLINICAL MANIFESTATIONS (See Table 314-3) **Raynaud's phenomenon** Systemic sclerosis usually begins insidiously; the first symptoms are frequently Raynaud's phenomenon and puffy fingers. Ninety-five percent of patients will experience Raynaud's phenomenon, which is defined as episodic vasoconstriction of small arteries and arterioles of fingers, toes, and sometimes the tip of the nose and earlobes. Episodes are brought on by cold exposure, vibration, or emotional stress. Patients experience pallor and/or cyanosis followed by rubor on rewarming. Pallor and/or cyanosis is usually associated with coldness and numbness of fingers and/or toes, and rubor with pain and tingling. Not all patients appreciate the three color phases. A history of digit pallor appears to be the most reliable symptom for the presence of Raynaud's phenomenon. Raynaud's phenomenon may precede skin changes by several months or even years in those patients who subsequently develop the limited cutaneous form of SSc. In diffuse cutaneous SSc, skin changes are seen typically within a year of the onset of Raynaud's phenomenon. After 2 or more years of Raynaud's phenomenon, few patients who have this as their only symptom will subsequently develop SSc.

Table 314-3

Clinical Features of Systemic Sclerosis

Clinical Feature	Percent of Patients with Clinical Feature during Course of Disease: Limited*	Diffuse*
Raynaud's phenomenon	95–100	90–95
Skin thickening	98†	100
Subcutaneous calcinosis	50	10
Telangiectasia	85	40
Arthralgias/arthritis	40	70
Myopathy	5	50
Esophageal dysmotility	80	80
Pulmonary fibrosis	35	40
Isolated pulmonary arterial hypertension	<10	<1
Congestive heart failure	<1	30
Renal crisis	<1	15

* Limited cutaneous and diffuse cutaneous subsets of SSc
† 2% or fewer of patients have SSc sine scleroderma

Skin Features In early disease, fingers and hands are swollen. Swelling also may involve forearms, feet, lower legs, and face. However, lower extremities are relatively spared. This edematous phase may last for a few weeks, months, or even longer. The edema may be pitting or nonpitting and accompanied by erythema. The skin changes begin distally in the extremities and advance proximally. The skin gradually becomes firm, thickened, and eventually tightly bound to underlying subcutaneous tissue (indurative phase). In patients with diffuse cutaneous scleroderma, skin changes will become generalized, involving initially the extremities, followed by the face and trunk over a period of time, varying from months to a few years. In some patients, the skin changes may develop gradually over several years. Rapid progression of these changes over a 2- to 3-year period is associated with a greater risk of visceral disease, particularly of the lungs, heart, or kidneys. Also in diffuse cutaneous SSc, the skin changes usually peak in 3 to 5 years and then slowly improve. On the other hand, patients with limited cutaneous scleroderma will usually have a more gradual progression of skin changes, which are restricted to fingers or distal extremity and face and may continue to worsen. In both subsets of SSc, skin thickening is usually greater in the distal extremity. After many years of disease, the skin may soften and return to normal thickness or become thin and atrophic.

In the extremities, the taut skin over fingers gradually limits full extension, and flexion contractures develop. Ulcers may appear on the volar pads of the fingertips and over bony prominences such as elbows, malleoli, and the extensor surface of the proximal interphalangeal joints of the hands. These ulcers may become secondarily infected. The volar pads of the fingertips develop pitting scars and lose soft tissue. In some instances, resorption of the terminal phalanges occurs. Skin over the extremities, face, and trunk may become darkly pigmented, even without exposure to the sun. Pigmentation of the skin may occur over superficial blood vessels and tendons. Areas of hypopigmentation may also develop. The skin loses hair, oil, and sweat glands and so becomes dry and coarse. Vaginal dryness occurs and may cause dyspareunia.

In some patients, particularly those with the limited cutaneous form of disease, calcific deposits develop in intracutaneous and subcutaneous tissue. The sites commonly involved are periarticular tissue, digital pads, olecranon and prepatellar bursae, and skin along the extensor surface of the forearms. The overlying skin may break down, with drainage of calcific material. Involvement of the face results in loss of skin wrinkles and facial expression, as well as microstomia, which may make eating and dental hygiene difficult. The nose takes on a pinched or beaklike appearance. Wrinkles appear around the mouth perpendicular to the lips. Small telangiectatic mats may appear on the fingers, face, lips, tongue, and buccal mucosa after several years. They are seen more frequently in patients with limited cutaneous SSc but also are observed in patients with long-standing diffuse cutaneous SSc. The capillary beds of nail folds of the fingers may show enlargement of capillaries with little or no capillary loss, usually indicative of limited cutaneous scleroderma. In diffuse cutaneous scleroderma, there is disorganization of the capillary beds with dilated capillaries interspersed with areas where capillaries have disappeared. These capillary changes, which are observed by wide-angle microscopy or with an ophthalmoscope used as a magnifier, are not found in patients who have only Raynaud's phenomenon.

Musculoskeletal Features More than half the patients with SSc complain of pain, swelling, and stiffness of the fingers and knees. A symmetric polyarthritis resembling rheumatoid arthritis may be seen. In more advanced stages of the disease, leathery crepitation can be palpated over moving joints, especially the knee. Extensive fibrotic thickening of the tendon sheaths in the wrist can produce a carpal tunnel syndrome. Muscle weakness usually is present in patients with severe skin involvement and, in most cases, is due to disuse atrophy. There is a distinctive histologic myopathy that accompanies SSc that is not associated with muscle enzyme abnormalities. A few patients develop a myositis characterized by proximal muscle weakness and muscle enzyme elevations that are identical to polymyositis (overlap syndrome). In addition to terminal phalanges, resorption of bone may involve ribs, clavicle, and angle of mandible.

Gastrointestinal Features The majority of patients from both subsets of SSc have gastrointestinal involvement. Symptoms attributable to esophageal involvement are present in more than 50 percent of patients and include epigastric fullness, burning pain in the epigastric or retrosternal regions, and regurgitation of gastric contents. These symptoms, most noticeable when the patient is lying flat or bending over, are due to the reduced tone of the gastroesophageal sphincter and to dilatation of the distal esophagus. Peptic esophagitis frequently occurs and may lead to strictures and narrowing of the lower esophagus. However, it seldom results in bleeding. Barrett's metaplasia may develop, but transition to adenocarcinoma is uncommon. Dysphagia, particularly of solid foods, may occur independent of other esophageal symptoms and is caused by loss of esophageal motility due to neuromuscular dysfunction. Manometry or cineradiography reveals decreased amplitude or disappearance of peristaltic waves in the lower two-thirds of the esophagus. Raynaud's phenomenon in the absence of a connective tissue disease is also associated with esophageal dysmotility. Later in the course of the illness, dilatation and atony of the lower portion of the esophagus as well as reflux are seen. With gastric involvement, barium studies show dilatation, atony, and delayed gastric emptying.

Hypomotility of the small intestine produces symptoms of bloating and abdominal pain and may suggest an intestinal obstruction or paralytic ileus (pseudoobstruction). Malabsorption syndrome with weight loss, diarrhea, and anemia is due to bacterial overgrowth in the atonic intestine or possibly to obliteration of lymphatics by fibrosis. Roentgenographic features of the second and third portions of the duodenum and of the jejunum include dilatation, loss of the usual feathery pattern, and delayed disappearance of barium. Pneumatosis intestinalis occasionally occurs and appears as radiolucent cysts or linear streaks within the wall of the small intestine. Benign pneumoperitoneum may result from the rupture of these cysts. Involvement of the large intestine may cause chronic constipation and fecal impaction with episodes of bowel obstruction. A segment of atonic bowel may act as a fulcrum for intussuception to occur. Barium studies of the large intestine may show dilatation, atony, and large-mouth diverticula. Laxity of the anal sphincter may cause incontinence or rarely anal prolapse. Some patients may have gastrointestinal features of SSc with little or no cutaneous or other organ involvement, referred to as SSC sine scleroderma. Telangiectasia may develop in the stomach and intestine and can be the source of gastrointestinal bleeding.

Pulmonary Features Pulmonary involvement occurs in at least two-thirds of SSc patients and is now the leading cause of death in SSc, replacing renal disease, which usually can be treated effectively. The most common symptom is exertional dyspnea, often accompanied by a dry, nonproductive cough. Symptoms may occur in the absence of pulmonary fibrosis, and patients with pulmonary fibrosis can be relatively asymptomatic. Bilateral basilar rales may be present. Restriction of chest movement caused by extensive skin involvement of the thorax rarely occurs. Aspiration pneumonia may result from gastric reflux due to lower esophageal atony. Superimposed bacterial or viral pneumonia can be a serious complication in patients with pulmonary fibrosis. There is an increased frequency of alveolar cell and bronchogenic carcinoma in patients with pulmonary fibrosis. Pulmonary function tests are frequently abnormal and show a reduction in vital capacity and decreased lung compliance. Impairment of gas exchange is reflected by a low diffusing capacity and low P_{O_2} with exercise. These abnormalities may be present even when the chest radiograph is normal. Chest film may show a pattern of linear densities, mottling, and honeycombing involving most prominently the lower two-thirds of the lung. Early pulmonary disease can be detected by high-resolution computed tomography (HRCT) and bronchoalveolar lavage (BAL). The recovery by BAL of increased number of cells, mostly alveolar macrophages accompanied by neutrophils and eosinophils, is evidence for alveolitis. Treatment of alveolitis with drugs such as cyclophosphamide conceivably may be more effective when alveolitis is detected early, although this is not proven. A controlled study of the effect of cyclophosphamide in diffuse cutaneous SSc patients with early active alveolitis is under consideration. In the absence of significant interstitial fibrosis, a severe form of pulmonary arterial hypertension develops after many years of disease in patients with limited cutaneous scleroderma. Fewer than 10 percent of patients will develop this complication, which is caused by narrowing and obliteration of pulmonary arteries and arterioles by intimal fibrosis and medial hypertrophy. Pulmonary hypertension is manifested by progressive worsening of dyspnea and eventually by the appearance of right-sided heart failure. Electrocardiographic evidence of pulmonary hypertension is usually present. The prognosis is extremely poor with the development of pulmonary hypertension; the mean duration of survival is approximately 2 years.

Cardiac Features Primary cardiac involvement in SSc includes pericarditis with or without effusions, heart failure, and varying degrees of heart block or arrhythmias. The majority of patients with diffuse cutaneous SSc have cardiac abnormalities. Cardiomyopathy attributable to myocardial fibrosis appears in fewer than 10 percent of patients and involves primarily those patients with diffuse cutaneous scleroderma. Radionuclide studies have shown abnormalities of left ventricular function due to myocardial fibrosis. Cold-induced vasospasm of the hands produces defects in myocardial thallium perfusion. The characteristic pathologic feature of contraction band necrosis results from cardiac muscle damage caused by intermittent vasospasm of coronary vessels. Patients may experience angina pectoris even though coronary angiograms are normal. Patients also can develop left ventricular failure secondary to systemic hypertension or cor pulmonale secondary to pulmonary arterial hypertension.

Renal Features Renal failure was the leading cause of death in SSc until the advent of effective treatment. Significant renal disease occurs mostly in those patients with diffuse cutaneous scleroderma. A high risk of renal crisis is present in those patients who have rapidly progressive widespread skin thickening in their first 2 to 3 years of disease. Renal crisis is characterized by malignant hypertension, which can rapidly progress to renal failure. These patients manifest hypertensive encephalopathy, severe headache, retinopathy, seizures, and left ventricular failure. Hematuria and proteinuria are followed by oliguria and renal failure. The mechanism for the hypertensive crisis is activation of the renin-angiotensin system. Before the advent of effective antihypertensive drugs, the majority of these patients died within 6 months. A small number of patients may develop renal crises in the absence of hypertension. Renal failure also can develop insidiously later in the course of disease in the setting of mild to moderate hypertension and proteinuria. In these patients or those with clinically unrecognized renal disease, reduction of renal plasma flow secondary to heart failure or volume depletion resulting from overdiuresis may precipitate renal crisis. An indicator of impending renal failure is microangiopathic anemia, which may occur in a normotensive patient. The presence of a chronic pericardial effusion may also herald subsequent renal failure.

Other Features Symptoms of dry eyes and/or dry mouth are frequently present in patients with SSc. Lip biopsy may show lymphocytic infiltration of minor salivary glands characteristic of Sjögren's syndrome or intraglandular or periglandular fibrosis secondary to SSc. Antibodies to SS-A (Ro) and/or SS-B (La) are found in those patients with lip biopsies consistent with Sjögren's syndrome and not in those with salivary gland fibrosis.

Hypothyroidism occurs in a significant number of patients and may be associated with high levels of antithyroid antibodies. Fibrosis of the thyroid gland may be present but also occurs in the absence of autoimmune thyroiditis. Other manifestations of SSc include trigeminal neuralgia and male impotence secondary to decreased penile tumescence. These men have normal serum levels of testosterone and gonadotropins. Pathogenesis of this abnormality has been considered to be vascular and/or autonomic nervous system abnormalities. Biliary cirrhosis is occasionally observed in patients with limited cutaneous SSc.

LABORATORY FINDINGS The erythrocyte sedimentation rate may be elevated. Hypoproliferative anemia related to chronic inflammation is the most common cause of anemia in SSc. Anemia also may be caused by iron deficiency secondary to gastrointestinal bleeding. Bacterial overgrowth due to atony of the small bowel may lead to vitamin B_{12} and/or folic acid–deficiency anemia. Microangiopathic hemolytic anemia is most often associated with renal involvement and is caused by the presence of intravascular fibrin in renal arterioles. Hypergammaglobulinemia, consisting mostly of IgG, is found in approximately half the patients. Rheumatoid factor, in low titer, is present in 25 percent of patients. Antinuclear antibodies detected by using a cultured human laryngeal carcinoma cell line (HEp-2) substrate are present in 95 percent of patients (Table 314-4). Antinuclear antibodies that have a high specificity for SSc are antitopoisomerase 1 (Scl-70), antinucleolar, and anticentromere. Antitopoisomerase 1, originally called anti-Scl-70, recognizes the nuclear enzyme DNA topoisomerase 1. These antibodies are found in about 20 percent of all SSc patients and in approximately 40 percent of those with diffuse cutaneous SSc. They are associated with diffuse cutaneous involvement, interstitial pulmonary disease, and other visceral organ involvement. A very high frequency of these antibodies has been reported in Choctaw Native Americans in association with diffuse cutaneous SSc. They are seldom present in other disorders or in conjunction with anticentromere antibodies. Anticentromere antibodies react with protein antigens located in the kinetochore region of chromosomes and are present in 60 to 80 percent of patients with limited cutaneous scleroderma or CREST syndrome. Anticentromere antibodies are found in only about 10 percent of patients with diffuse cutaneous scleroderma and rarely in other connective tissue diseases. They are found occasionally in patients with only Raynaud's phenomenon and may indicate subsequent development of limited cutaneous disease. Antinucleolar antibodies are relatively specific for SSc and are present in approximately 20 to 30 percent of patients. Several antinucleolar antibodies have been associated with SSc: Anti-RNA polymerases I, II, and III are found in patients with diffuse cutaneous SSc who have a higher prevalence of renal and cardiac involvement. Anti-Th ribonucleoprotein (RNP) has been found in patients with limited cutaneous SSc, and anti-PM-Scl, formerly referred to as anti-PM1, may be found in a subset of patients with overlapping features of limited cutaneous SSc and polymyositis. *Anti-U_3 RNP (anti-fibrillarin) is also highly specific for SSc and may be associated with skeletal muscle disease, bowel involvement, and pulmonary arterial hypertension.* Anti-U_1 RNP is found in approximately 5 to 10 percent of SSc patients and 95 to 100 percent of those patients with the overlap syndrome of MCTD. The titers in MCTD are usually high (see below). Anti-SS-A and/or anti-SS-B are present in those patients with overlap syndrome of SSc and Sjögren's syndrome.

Table 314-4

Autoantibodies in Systemic Sclerosis

Autoantibody	Clinical Association	Percent*
Antitopoisomerase 1	Diffuse cutaneous SSc	40
Anticentromere	Limited cutaneous SSc	60–80
Anti-RNA polymerase I, II, III	Diffuse cutaneous SSc	5–40
Anti-Th RNP	Limited cutaneous SSc	14
Anti-U_1 RNP	Limited cutaneous SSc	5–10
	Mixed connective tissue disease	95–100
Anti-PM/Scl	Overlap (SSc, polymyositis)	25

* Approximate percentages for the predominant clinical association.

DIAGNOSIS The diagnosis of SSc presents no difficulty in the presence of Raynaud's phenomenon, with typical skin lesions and visceral involvement. Although Raynaud's phenomenon may be the first symptom of SSc, most patients with Raynaud's phenomenon alone do not develop a connective tissue disease. Other causes of Raynaud's phenomenon include thoracic outlet (scalenus anticus and cervical rib) syndromes, shoulder-hand syndrome, trauma (jackhammer or vibratory machine operators), previous cold injury, vinyl chloride exposure, and circulating cryoglobulins or cold agglutinins. Linear scleroderma and morphea are localized forms of scleroderma that can usually be distinguished clinically. In early disease, SSc may initially be confused with rheumatoid arthritis, systemic lupus erythematosus, or polymyositis when articular or muscle involvement is prominent. SSc without cutaneous involvement should be considered in patients with unexplained pulmonary fibrosis, pulmonary hypertension, cardiomyopathies, heart block, dysphagia, or malabsorption syndrome. Several conditions have scleroderma-like features but lack the visceral involvement. Scleredema (scleredema adultorum of Buschke) occurs predominantly in children and is characterized by painless edematous induration involving the face, scalp, neck, trunk, and proximal portions of the extremities. Involvement of the hands and feet usually does not occur. Scleredema may be associated with previous streptococcal infection and is usually self-limited, resolving in 6 to 12 months. Histology reveals accumulation of mucopolysaccharides in the dermis and skeletal muscle. A rare entity, scleromyxedema is manifested by yellowish or pale red papules in association with diffuse skin thickening that may involve the face and hands. Acid mucopolysaccharide deposits are found in the dermis. Monoclonal IgG may be detected in some of these patients. Patients with insulin-dependent diabetes mellitus may develop digital sclerosis and contractures. Primary amyloidosis and amyloidosis associated with multiple myeloma may involve the skin of the extremities and face diffusely to give the appearance of scleroderma. Biopsy will clearly differentiate these entities.

COURSE AND PROGNOSIS The course of SSc is quite variable. Until the disease differentiates into recognizable subsets, prognosis in early disease is difficult to predict. Patients with limited cutaneous scleroderma, especially those with anticentromere antibodies, have a good prognosis, with the notable exception of those few patients, fewer than 10 percent, who after 10 to 20 years or longer develop pulmonary arterial hypertension. Malabsorption syndrome and primary biliary cirrhosis are the causes of morbidity and mortality in some patients with limited cutaneous disease. On the other hand, the prognosis is generally worse in patients with diffuse cutaneous disease, particularly when the onset occurs at an older age. In addition, males have a worse prognosis. Renal and other visceral organ disease may develop early in the course of those patients with rapidly progressive generalized skin thickening. Death occurs most often from cardiac, renal, or pulmonary involvement. With the advent of effective therapy for renal crisis along with renal dialysis for those patients with renal failure, the 10-year cumulative survival rate has increased to approximately 65 percent. In patients with diffuse cutaneous disease, the 10-year cumulative survival rate is approximately 55 percent, and in limited cutaneous disease is 75 percent.

Skin may spontaneously soften after years of disease. Softening occurs in the reverse order of original skin involvement, beginning with the trunk and followed by the proximal and then the distal extremities. Sclerodactyly and flexion contractures may persist. Skin thickness may eventually approach normal; however, the skin may be atrophic.

℞ TREATMENT

Even though SSc cannot be cured, treatment of involved organ systems can relieve symptoms and improve function. The doctor-patient relationship is extremely important in caring for patients with this chronic debilitating illness. Once the diagnosis of SSc has been made, the patient and family should be instructed about this disorder. The patient will need repeated explanations and reassurances throughout his or her illness. Depending on the severity of illness, the patient will require monitoring of blood pressure, blood counts, urinalysis, and monitoring of renal and pulmonary function on a regular basis.

Effectiveness of drug therapy in SSc is difficult to evaluate because of the variable course and severity of the disease. Many drugs have been used in the treatment of SSc without any consistent or prolonged benefit. In uncontrolled studies, D-penicillamine has been reported to reduce skin thickening and prevent development of significant organ involvement. This drug interferes with inter- and intramolecular cross-linking of collagen and is also immunosuppressive. Its immunosuppressive activity also may lead to decreased collagen production. Penicillamine is better tolerated when started at a low dose, usually 250 mg/d, and then increased at 1- to 3-month intervals up to 1.5 g/d as tolerated. Although a few patients can tolerate higher doses, most patients are maintained on a dose between 0.5 and 1 g/d. For optimal absorption, it is important to give this drug 1 h before or 2 h after a meal. This drug can be quite toxic; its more serious complications include glomerulonephritis with nephrotic syndrome, aplastic anemia, leukopenia, thrombocytopenia, and myasthenia gravis. Other side effects are fever, rash, anorexia, nausea, and loss of taste. Patients should have monthly complete blood counts (including platelet count) and urinalyses. Azathioprine and other immunosuppressives also have been used in SSc and should be reserved for those patients with rapidly progressive and life-threatening disease. Control studies are lacking. Trials of treatment with recombinant interferon γ, 5-fluorouracil, and *extracorporeal photochemotherapy* have shown improvement in some disease parameters. No therapy, however, has been clearly demonstrated in a controlled, prospective study to suppress or reverse the disease process of SSc.

Antiplatelet therapy may play a role in the treatment of SSc, since the biologic products of platelets affect blood vessels. Low doses of aspirin block the formation of thromboxane A_2, a powerful vasoconstrictor and platelet aggregator. In addition, dipyridamole, 200 to 400 mg in divided daily doses, also decreases platelet adhesion to damaged vessel walls. While these drugs have a reasonable therapeutic rationale, a 2-year double-blind study did not show any benefit from their use. Reports of beneficial effects of colchicine or chlorambucil have not been documented in controlled studies.

Glucocorticoids are indicated in those patients with inflammatory myositis or pericarditis. The initial dose is 40 to 60 mg/d and is tapered based on clinical improvement. They should not be used for the indolent primary form of muscle disease of SSc. Prednisone in the range of 20 to 40 mg/d may decrease edema associated with the edematous phase of early skin involvement. Glucocorticoids are not otherwise indicated in the long-term treatment of SSc. High doses of glucocorticoids may play a role in precipitating acute renal failure. However, this association remains unclear.

The management of Raynaud's phenomenon is directed at control of vasospasm. Patients should be advised to dress warmly and wear mittens and socks, not to smoke, to remove causes of external stress, and to avoid drugs such as amphetamine and ergotamine. Beta blocking drugs may make Raynaud's phenomenon worse. Warmth of the central body induces peripheral vasodilatation. Drugs that block sympathetic vasoconstriction, such as reserpine, α-methyldopa, phenoxybenzamine, and prazosin, may be useful in the treatment of Raynaud's phenomenon, but their side effects often curtail extended use. The calcium channel blockers nifedipine and diltiazem can be effective in alleviating Raynaud's phenomenon, but side effects of light-headedness and palpitations may limit their use. The sustained-release form of nifedipine is better tolerated; the dose is 30 mg/d up to 60 or 90 mg/d as required to control symptoms. Ketanserin, an oral serotonin antagonist, also has been shown to be effective. Studies with iloprost, a prostacyclin analogue, have shown a decrease in frequency and severity of Raynaud's phenomenon and healing of digital ulcers in some patients. Iloprost is still not available in the United States for general use. Pentoxifylline may also improve perfusion by increasing the deformability of the red cell plasma membranes. Techniques of biofeedback also have been used with variable success for teaching patients to control the temperature of their hands. Stellate ganglion blockage may be useful in temporarily alleviating severe ischemic pain in the fingers. Surgical sympathectomy usually provides only temporary improvement, and it, along with other forms of therapy, does not prevent progression of the vascular lesion. The response to any therapy for Raynaud's phenomenon is limited by the degree of existing structural narrowing of digital arteries. Gangrene of distal digits may occur and require surgical amputation.

Numerous drugs have been claimed to soften the hidebound skin, but documentation in controlled studies is lacking. These drugs include D-penicillamine, colchicine, *p*-aminobenzoic acid, and vitamin E. Dryness of the skin may be reduced by avoiding frequent use of detergent soaps and by regularly applying hydrophilic ointments and bath oils. Regular exercise helps to maintain flexibility of extremities and pliability of skin. Massaging the skin several times a day also may be beneficial. Fingertip ulcerations can be protected by applying a guard or cage over the end of the finger. The use of an occlusive dressing, such as the hydrocolloid duoDERM or other membranes, over a noninfected ulcer may promote healing and protect the finger. Skin ulcers should be kept clean by soaking or by surgical or chemical debridement. Sympatholytic drugs or local nitroglycerine paste applied to or adjacent to the ulcer may be beneficial in promoting healing. Infected ulcers can usually be treated with topical antibiotics but may require systemic antibiotics, especially when there is a question of underlying osteomyelitis. The development of calcinosis cannot be prevented, nor can deposits be dissolved. Warfarin has been reported to reduce calcinosis in a few patients.

Patients with reflux esophagitis are treated with small, frequent meals, antacids between meals, and elevation of the head of the bed. Patients should be advised not to lie down for a few hours after a meal and to avoid coffee, tea, and chocolate, which reduce the pressure of the lower esophageal sphincter. Cimetidine, ranitidine or other newer H_2 blockers may be beneficial. Omeprazole, a gastric acid (proton) pump inhibitor, has been effective in treating erosive esophagitis in some patients. Metoclopramide and cisapride increase gastrointestinal motility but do not significantly improve esophageal motility. They both increase lower esophageal sphincter tone and can be of help in some patients. Nifedipine and, to a lesser extent, diltiazem reduce lower esophageal sphincter tone resulting in esophageal reflux. Patients with dysphagia should be instructed to chew their food thoroughly and wash it down with fluids. Malabsorption syndrome due to duodenal hypomotility and bacterial overgrowth may improve with intermittent use of appropriate antibiotics. Patients with severe debilitating malabsorption may benefit from parenteral hyperalimentation. Stool softeners and mild laxatives are usually adequate for treating constipation caused by hypomotility of the colon.

Articular symptoms are treated with nonsteroidal anti-inflammatory agents. Low-dose prednisone (10 mg/d or less) may improve symptoms in those not responding to these agents. Physical therapy may help to reduce the loss of joint mobility that occurs in SSc.

In patients with diffuse cutaneous SSc, the early recognition of alveolitis as previously described (see "Pulmonary Features") may allow treatment that might slow or prevent the development of pulmonary fibrosis. Cyclophosphamide has been reported in uncontrolled studies to be beneficial, and a controlled study is presently under consideration by the American College of Rheumatology. The role of glucocorticoids in preventing progression of interstitial lung disease is not clear but may be of benefit in early disease. Pulmonary fibrosis is not reversible, and therefore treatment is directed at symptoms or complications. Pulmonary infection requires prompt treatment with antibiotics. Hypoxia necessitates giving low concentrations of oxygen. Patients should receive polyvalent pneumoccal vaccine (Pneumovax) and yearly influenza immunizations.

For patients with limited cutaneous SSc who develop isolated pulmonary arterial hypertension, the treatment is inadequate. A calcium channel blocker such as nifedipine lowers pulmonary arterial resistance and improves cardiac function, but in most patients this is only for a short period of time. Few patients survive more than 5 years. Heart-lung or single-lung transplantation may be a therapeutic option in those patients without other significant systemic involvement. Recognition of early signs of renal hypertensive crisis is important in order to preserve renal function and prevent hypertensive encephalopathy. Renal involvement is often accompanied by hypertension and mild to moderate proteinuria. An occasional patient may be normotensive. Antihypertensive agents are often effective in lowering blood pressure and stabilizing or reversing renal failure. These drugs include propranolol, clonidine, and minoxidil. Particularly effective are the angiotensin-converting enzyme inhibitors, which include captopril, enalapril, and lisinopril. Dialysis may be required in patients with progressive renal failure. Some patients, however, have a slow return of renal function after several months and may no longer require dialysis. Patients are usually not candidates for kidney transplantation because of the other systemic manifestations of SSc.

Patients with cardiac failure require careful monitoring of digitalis and diuretic administration. Noninflammatory pericardial effusions also may improve with diuretics. Care should be taken to avoid overdiuresis, which may lead to decreased renal blood flow, decreased cardiac output, and renal failure.

MIXED CONNECTIVE TISSUE DISEASE MCTD is an overlap syndrome characterized by combinations of clinical features of systemic lupus erythematosus (SLE) (see Chap. 312), SSc, polymyositis (see Chap. 315), and rheumatoid arthrisis (see Chap. 313) and the presence of very high titers of circulating autoantibodies to nuclear RNP antigen. This antibody in high titer, now referred to as *anti-U_1* RNP, has been a justification for considering MCTD as a distinct clinical entity. MCTD has been challenged as a distinct disorder by those who consider it as a subset of SLE or scleroderma. Others prefer to classify MCTD as an undifferentiated connective tissue disease. MCTD occurs worldwide and in all races. The peak onset of disease is in the second and third decades, but MCTD is seen in children and the elderly. Women are predominantly affected. The pathogenic mechanisms in MCTD reflect the disorders making up this syndrome.

Clinical Features The presenting symptoms of MCTD are most often Raynaud's phenomenon, puffy hands, arthralgias, myalgias, and fatigue. Occasionally, patients may present with the acute onset of high fever, polymyositis, arthritis, and neurologic features such as trigeminal neuralgia and aseptic meningitis. The various features of the connective tissue disorders making up MCTD develop over months and years.

The fingers as well as the entire hand may be puffy, followed later by sclerodactyly. Sclerodermal changes are usually limited to the distal extremities and sometimes the face but spare the trunk. Telangiectasia and calcinosis may develop. Some patients have mucocutaneous features of SLE including a classic malar rash, photosensitivity, discoid lesions, alopecia, and painful oral ulcerations. An erythematous rash over the knuckles, elbows, and knees and heliotropic eyelids, typical of dermatomyositis, are uncommon.

Joint pain, stiffness, and swelling involving the peripheral joints occur frequently. Deformities of the hands similar to those of rheumatoid arthritis may develop but usually without bony erosions. A destructive polyarthritis is occasionally observed. Myalgias are a frequent symptom. Some patients develop typical symptoms of polymyositis with proximal muscle weakness, abnormal electromyographic findings, elevated levels of muscle enzymes, and inflammatory changes on muscle biopsy.

Approximately 85 percent of patients have pulmonary involvement, which is often asymptomatic. Diffusing capacity for carbon monoxide may be the only abnormality. Pleurisy commonly occurs but is seldom associated with large pleural effusions. Some patients develop interstitial lung disease. Pulmonary arterial hypertension is the most common cause of death in MCTD.

Approximately 25 percent of patients develop renal disease. Membranous glomerulonephritis is most common and usually mild but can cause nephrotic syndrome. Diffuse proliferative glomerulonephritis is unusual in MCTD, perhaps because of the protective role played by the high titers of anti-U_1 RNP. Renal crisis secondary to malignant renovasculature hypertension, as occurs in scleroderma, is seen in a few patients.

Gastrointestinal involvement is seen in approximately 70 percent of patients. The most common manifestations are esophageal dysmotility, lower esophageal sphincter laxity, and gastroesophageal reflux. Bowel manifestations mimic those of scleroderma bowel disease.

Pericarditis occurs in 30 percent of patients. Other cardiac features include myocarditis, arrhythmia, conduction disturbances, and mitral valve prolapse. Other clinical features of MCTD include trigeminal neuropathy, peripheral neuropathy, aseptic meningitis, lymphadenopathy, and Sjögren's syndrome. The majority of patients have developed, or will develop within 5 years of presentation, diagnostic clinical criteria for one of the overlapping connective tissue diseases, most often SLE or SSc.

Laboratory Findings Anemia of chronic inflammation is seen in the majority of patients. A positive direct Coombs' test is found in about 60 percent of patients, but hemolytic anemia is unusual. Leukopenia, thrombocytopenia, or both are present in some patients. Hypergammaglobulinemia is common, and rheumatoid factor is present in 50 percent of patients.

All patients, by definition of MCTD, have antibodies to U_1 RNP. The specificity of this antibody is to the 70-kDa protein complexed to small nuclear RNA. The anti-U_1 RNP antibodies are associated with HLA-DR4 but not with -DR2 and -DR3 as found in SLE. Molecular mimicry has been demonstrated between U_1 RNP and retroviral antigens by some laboratories.

Rx TREATMENT

The treatment of MCTD is essentially the same as would be indicated for the respective connective tissue diseases defining this syndrome. More than half the patients have a favorable course. The 10-year survival rate overall is approximately 80 percent but varies depending on the connective tissue disease that may eventually develop.

EOSINOPHILIC FASCIITIS Eosinophilic fasciitis is a scleroderma-like syndrome of unknown cause characterized by inflammation followed later by sclerosis of the dermis, subcutis, and deep fascia. The disease affects adults and often occurs after strenuous physical activity. Patients do not have Raynaud's phenomenon or internal organ involvement. Several immunologic abnormalities have been associated with eosinophilic fasciitis and include aplastic anemia, myelodysplastic syndrome, and thrombocytopenia. Patients usually have the abrupt onset of symmetric tenderness and swelling of the extremities which is rapidly followed by induration of the skin and subcutaneous tissue. The skin takes on a cobblestone or puckered appearance. Carpal tunnel syndrome appears early in the course, and flexion contractures develop later. A low-grade myositis is often present, but creatinine kinase levels are usually normal. A marked eosinophilia is found in the early stage of disease and subsequently decreases. Increased levels of polyclonal IgG and immune complexes are often present in the serum. A full-thickness biopsy consisting of skin, fascia, and superficial muscle shows perivascular infiltration of histiocytes, eosinophils, lymphocytes, and plasma cells. Biopsies later in the course show sclerosis. Spontaneous improvement and occasionally complete remission may occur after 2 to 5 years of disease. Some patients have persistent disease, while others are left with flexion contractures. Administration of glucocorticoids may provide symptomatic improvement and will decrease the eosinophilia. Improvement has been reported with the use of the H_2 blocker cimetidine.

EOSINOPHILIA-MYALGIA SYNDROME In 1989, reports of patients with scleroderma-like skin changes, myalgias, and eosinophilia dramatically increased. Most, but not all, of these cases were associated with ingestion of L-tryptophan manufactured by a single Japanese company. Batches of L-tryptophan implicated in eosinophilia-myalgia syndrome (EMS) were found to contain trace amounts of a contaminant identified as a dimer of L-tryptophan that appeared in 1988 after changes were made in the method of manufacturing this drug. It is not clear whether this chemical contaminant is the etiologic agent or whether another unidentified substance is responsible. *L-Tryptophan products were taken off the market in 1990.* The onset of EMS can be either abrupt or insidious. In the early phases of the disease, clinical manifestations include low-grade fever, fatigue, dyspnea, cough, arthralgias/arthritis, evanescent erythematous rashes, muscle cramping, and severe myalgias. Pulmonary infiltrates may be present. Over the next 2 to 3 months, scleroderma-like skin changes appear. Some patients develop a peripheral neuropathy which may persist. An ascending polyneuropathy may lead to paralysis and respiratory failure requiring ventilatory assistance. Cognitive dysfunction with impairment of memory and concentration has been recognized in this syndrome. Myocarditis and cardiac arrhythmias occur in some patients, and a few patients develop pulmonary hypertension. Approximately a third of patients have features of eosinophilic fasciitis. EMS most closely resembles toxic oil syndrome; however, Raynaud's phenomenon does not occur, and there is a lower prevalence of pulmonary hypertension and thromboembolic disease. The peripheral eosinophil count is greater than 1000 cells per cubic millimeter in most patients. The histologic findings on biopsy of skin, fascia, and superficial muscle are similar to that found in eosinophilic fasciitis. The clinical features of EMS may persist after L-tryptophan has been discontinued. EMS may run a chronic course, and response to therapy has been variable. Treatment has included glucocorticoids, antimalarial drugs, immunosuppressive drugs, and plasmapheresis. Prednisone was beneficial during the acute inflammatory phase of the disease in the majority of patients and resulted in resolution of pulmonary infiltrates, peripheral edema, and eosinophilia. In the later phase of the illness, no treatment was found to be of particular value. The pathogenesis of this disease is not known. A follow-up of patients 2 years after their onset of illness showed that most symptoms and physical findings had resolved or improved except for cognitive dysfunction, which became worse in approximately one-third of the patients, and peripheral neuropathy, which remained unchanged (see also Chap. 315).

BIBLIOGRAPHY

ARNETT FC: HLA and autoimmunity in scleroderma (systemic sclerosis). Int Rev Immunol 12:107, 1995

BENNETT RM: Mixed connective tissue disease and other overlap syndromes, in *Textbook of Rheumatology*, 4th ed, WN Kelley et al (eds). Philadelphia, Saunders, 1993, p 1057

BLACK CM: The aetiopathogenesis of systemic sclerosis: Thick skin—thin hypotheses. J R Coll of Physicians Lond 29:119, 1995

CARPENTIER PH, MARICQ HR: Microvasculature in systemic sclerosis. Rheum Dis Clin North Am 16:75, 1990

HERTZMAN PA et al: The eosinophilia-myalgia syndrome: status of 205 patients and results of treatment 2 years after onset. Ann Intern Med 122:851, 1995

KAHALEH B, MATUCCI-CERINIC M: Raynaud's phenomenon and scleroderma. Dysregulated neuroendothelial control of vascular tone. Arthritis Rheum 38:1, 1995

LAKHANPAL S et al: Eosinophilic fasciitis: Clinical spectrum and therapeutic response in 52 cases. Semin Arthritis Rheum 17:221, 1988

LEGERTON CW III et al: Systemic sclerosis (scleroderma). Clinical management of its major complications. Rheum Dis Clin North Am 21:203, 1995

LEROY ED et al: Scleroderma (systemic sclerosis): Classification, subset and pathogenesis. J Rheumatol 15:202, 1988

MEDSGER TA JR: Systemic sclerosis (scleroderma), localized forms of scleroderma, and calcinosis, in *Arthritis and Allied Conditions*, 12th ed, DJ McCarty, WJ Koopman (eds). Philadelphia, Lea & Febiger, 1993, p 1253

POSTLETHWAITE AE: Role of T cells and cytokines in effecting fibrosis. Int Rev Immunol 12:247, 1995

SEIBOLD J: Scleroderma, in *Textbook of Rheumatology*, 4th ed, WN Kelley et al (eds). Philadelphia, Saunders, 1993, p 1113

SHARP GC, SINGSEN BH: Mixed connective tissue disease, in *Arthritis and Allied Conditions*, 12th ed, DJ McCarty, WJ Koopman (eds), Philadelphia, Lea & Febiger, 1993, p 1213

STEEN VD: Renal involvement in systemic sclerosis. Clin Dermatol 12:253, 1994

——— et al: Therapy for severe interstitial lung disease in systemic sclerosis. A retrospective study. Arthritis Rheum 37:1290, 1994

VARGA J, BASHEY RI: Regulation of connective tissue synthesis in systemic sclerosis. Int Rev Immunol 12:187, 1995

V'AZQUEZ AD, ROTHFIELD NF: Autoantibodies in systemic sclerosis. Int Rev Immunol 12:145, 1995

315

Rup Tandan

DERMATOMYOSITIS AND POLYMYOSITIS*

Dermatomyositis and polymyositis are conditions of presumed autoimmune etiology in which the skeletal muscle is damaged by a nonsuppurative inflammatory process dominated by lymphocytic infiltration. The term *polymyositis* is applied when the condition spares the skin, and the term *dermatomyositis* when polymyositis is associated with a characteristic skin rash. One-third of cases are associated with various connective tissue disorders, such as rheumatoid arthritis, lupus erythematosus, mixed connective tissue disorder, and progressive systemic sclerosis, and one-tenth with a malignancy. *Inclusion body myositis* is a distinct clinicopathologic entity characterized by the presence of vacuolated inclusions containing tubulofilaments in muscle.

ETIOLOGY The precise cause of these diseases is unknown, but interplay between host genetic factors, viral infection of muscle, and autoimmune mechanisms is probably contributory. Familial occurrence of these diseases, and the increased frequency of HLA-DR3 and -DRw52 antigens in patients, suggest an underlying genetic and immunologic predisposition. Experimental viral myositis can be induced in animals by coxsackievirus. A mild inflammatory myopathy can occur with influenza and coxsackieviruses in humans. However, the several electron-microscopic observations of virus-like particles in muscle fibers in dermatomyositis or polymyositis have not been confirmed by virus isolation or demonstration of rising viral antibody titers, and the disease has not been passed into animals by injection of extracts of skeletal muscles. Nevertheless, the presence of serum antibodies to several cytoplasmic ribonucleoproteins involved in translation [especially histidyl tRNA synthetase or Jo-1 and signal recognition particle (SRP)] may result from an immune response to an altered virus that serves as an immunogen in polymyositis. These antibodies probably represent a cross-reactive phenomenon.

A lymphocyte-mediated disease resembling polymyositis has been reported in laboratory animals injected with muscle antigens together with Freund's adjuvant (experimental allergic myositis). Immunohistochemical and muscle co-culture studies indicate that muscle fiber necrosis in polymyositis and inclusion body myositis probably derive from activation of CD8+ T lymphocytes, accompanied by CD4+ T lymphocytes and macrophages present in the inflammatory infiltrates. In dermatomyositis, deposition of immunoglobulins and the $C_{5b\text{-}9}$ complement membrane attack complex has been demonstrated on intramuscular blood vessels even in unaffected or minimally involved regions of muscle, suggesting that humorally mediated blood vessel damage initiates the angiopathy that precedes muscle destruction. The final pathway for muscle fiber damage in dermatomyositis may be T cell–dependent stimulation of B cells, with resultant antibody-mediated cytotoxicity. In inclusion body myositis, the accumulation of amyloid, paired helical filaments, and several other proteins typically seen at autopsy in brain specimens of patients with Alzheimer's disease suggest some overlap of pathogenic mechanisms in these disorders.

* The author acknowledges the contribution of Walter G. Bradley to this chapter in previous editions.

CLASSIFICATION A widely used classification of the dermatomyositis-polymyositis group is shown in Table 315-1. Other diseases uncommonly associated with polymyositis are sarcoidosis, giant cell myositis with thymoma, and myositis in systemic infections due to viruses, toxoplasma, or parasites. A focal infective myositis due to streptococcal or staphylococcal infection is mostly seen in the tropics. Focal nodular myositis is a variant of polymyositis in which focal areas of myositis cause hot, often painful, multifocal muscle masses.

INCIDENCE Current estimates of the annual incidence of the inflammatory myopathies are approximately five cases per million population. These estimates are probably low, however; the true incidence may be as high as two to three per hundred thousand.

CLINICAL MANIFESTATIONS **Group I: Primary Idiopathic Polymyositis** This group comprises about one-third of all cases of inflammatory myopathy. It is usually insidiously progressive over weeks, months, or even years. Rarely the disease is acute, producing severe muscle weakness in a matter of days or even rhabdomyolysis. The disease may develop at any age. Affected females outnumber males 2:1.

Patients first become aware of weakness of the proximal limb muscles, especially the hips and thighs, and find difficulty in arising from the squatting or kneeling position and in climbing or descending stairs. When shoulder girdle muscles are involved, placing an object on a high shelf or combing the hair becomes difficult. Occasionally the disease is more restricted, affecting only the neck, the shoulder, or the quadriceps muscles. Aching pain in the buttocks, thighs, and calves is experienced in about 10 percent of the cases, and tenderness on palpation in another 20 percent. In the majority of patients the disorder is painless. Early symptoms of dysphagia and weakness of flexor muscles of the neck in a patient with a chronic myopathy suggest the diagnosis of polymyositis.

When the patient is first seen, there may be weakness of the muscles of the trunk, the pectoral and pelvic girdles, the upper arms and thighs, the neck, and the pharynx. Ocular muscles are almost never affected except in a rare association with myasthenia gravis. The distal muscles are spared in about 75 percent of cases. Muscle atrophy, contractures, and diminished tendon reflexes are rare in early myositis and never as pronounced as in muscular dystrophies and denervating conditions. When the reflexes are disproportionately reduced, carcinoma with polymyositis and polyneuropathy or the Lambert-Eaton syndrome should be considered. Occasionally, the reflexes may be paradoxically brisk in dermatomyositis-polymyositis, perhaps due to irritation of muscle spindle receptors by the inflammation.

At presentation about 25 percent of patients have dysphagia, about 5 percent have significant respiratory impairment, and 5 percent are unable to walk. Dysphagia is due to involvement of striated muscles of the pharynx and upper esophagus. At some time in the course of the disease, cardiac abnormalities are observed in about 30 percent of cases; these include electrocardiogram (ECG) changes, arrhythmias, and heart failure secondary to myocarditis. About half of the fatal cases have pathologic evidence of cardiac disease with necrosis of myocardial fibers, usually with only modest inflammatory reaction. The frequency of myocardial infarction may be increased in those treated for long periods with glucocorticoids. In a few cases there is dyspnea due to lymphocytic pneumonitis, obliterating bronchiolitis, pulmonary edema, or pulmonary fibrosis. Arthralgia, Raynaud's phenomenon, and, rarely, low-grade fever may also be present.

Table 315-1

Classification of Polymyositis-Dermatomyositis

Group I	Primary idiopathic polymyositis
Group II	Primary idiopathic dermatomyositis
Group III	Dermatomyositis (or polymyositis) associated with neoplasia
Group IV	Childhood dermatomyositis (or polymyositis) associated with vasculitis
Group V	Polymyositis (or dermatomyositis) with associated collagen vascular disease

SOURCE: Classification suggested by Bohan et al.

Group II: Primary Idiopathic Dermatomyositis This group comprises just over one-third of all cases of myositis. The skin changes may precede or follow the muscle syndrome and include a localized or diffuse erythema, maculopapular eruption, scaling eczematoid dermatitis, or, rarely, an exfoliative dermatitis. The classic lilac-colored (heliotrope) rash is on the eyelids, bridge of the nose, cheeks (butterfly distribution), forehead, chest, elbows, knees and knuckles, and around the nail beds. Itching may be troublesome in some cases. The skin lesions may be subtle and easily overlooked. Periorbital edema is frequent, particularly in acute cases. The skin lesions may occasionally ulcerate. Subcutaneous calcification may occur, especially in children.

The typical rash and myositis allow a diagnosis of dermatomyositis, and such cases may be placed in this category (group II, Table 315-1) if idiopathic and into groups III, IV, and V if there are other features, namely malignancy, vasculitis in children, and an established collagen vascular disease. There should be concern about an underlying malignancy in patients over the age of 40 with dermatomyositis.

Group III: Polymyositis or Dermatomyositis with Neoplasia This syndrome, which comprises about 8 percent of all cases of myositis, is categorized separately, although muscle and skin changes are indistinguishable from those in the other groups. Malignancy, however, is uncommon in myositis seen in children and in association with a connective tissue disorder. The malignancy may antedate or postdate the onset of the myositis by up to 2 years. The incidence of neoplasia is higher in patients over the age of 40 and is particularly high in patients over age 60; therefore, in such patients a thorough history and clinical examination (including breast, gynecologic, and rectal) should be supplemented by complete blood count, biochemical profile, serum protein electrophoresis and immunofixation, screening for carcinoembryonic antigen, urine analysis for blood and cytology, stool samples for occult blood, chest x-ray, sputum for cytology, and bone scan seeking clues for an underlying malignancy. This relatively inexpensive search uncovers most malignancies; undirected radiologic screening procedures are costly and unhelpful in improving the yield. The most common malignancies are lung, ovary, breast, gastrointestinal tract, and lymphoproliferative disorders. The myositis is a paraneoplastic syndrome, the cause of which may lie in an altered immune status, cross-reactive antigens between tumor and muscle, or an occult viral infection of the muscle.

Group IV: Childhood Polymyositis and Dermatomyositis Associated with Vasculitis This group comprises about 8 to 20 percent of all cases of myositis in various series. Inflammatory myopathy in childhood is frequently associated with skin involvement and clinical or histologic evidence of vasculitis in skin, muscles, gastrointestinal tract, and other organs. Degeneration and loss of capillaries in a perifascicular distribution occur in the skeletal muscles; often necrotizing lesions of the skin, and ischemic infarction of kidneys, gastrointestinal tract, and rarely brain may be seen. Consequently, some authors have reported mortality rates of up to one-third in childhood dermatomyositis, though most have found that the prognosis is better than in adult dermatomyositis-polymyositis. Based upon current data, it is unclear whether or not all cases of childhood myositis should be included in group IV. Subcutaneous calcification is frequently present in childhood dermatomyositis.

Group V: Polymyositis or Dermatomyositis with an Associated Connective Tissue Disorder This "overlap group" of myositis comprises about one-fifth of all cases that occur in association with several connective tissue diseases. Progressive systemic sclerosis, rheumatoid arthritis, mixed connective tissue disease (the rheumatologic overlap disorder), and lupus erythematosus are the most common associated conditions; polyarteritis nodosa and rheumatic fever are more rarely associated. Criteria for placement in the "overlap group" combine the demonstration of the appropriate clinical and laboratory abnormalities required for the diagnosis of the connective tissue disorder together with clinical and laboratory evidence of myositis. The diagnosis of myositis is often difficult in patients with a connective tissue disorder producing arthritis with secondary (disuse) muscle weakness with type II fiber atrophy. Moreover, perivascular inflammatory foci are common in muscle in connective tissue disorders. Demonstration of increased serum creatine kinase (CK), electromyography (EMG), and muscle biopsy are often required to make this diagnosis. Though patients in this overlap group usually respond to glucocorticoid therapy, the prognosis for recovery of function is poorer than in pure dermatomyositis-polymyositis. Dysphagia in group V patients with progressive systemic sclerosis is often due to involvement of the smooth muscle of the distal third of the esophagus.

Other Disorders Associated with Myositis *Sarcoidosis and polymyositis* The skeletal muscle contains noncaseating granulomas with Langhans-type multinuclear giant cells in at least one-quarter of patients with sarcoidosis (Chap. 320). Symptomatic polymyositis is, however, uncommon. Regenerating multinuclear myoblasts resemble Langhans' giant cells, which has led to the misdiagnosis in many of the cases reported in the literature of "sarcoid myositis." Giant cell or granulomatous polymyositis and myocarditis, sometimes associated with myasthenia gravis, have been recorded in patients with thymomas.

Focal nodular myositis A syndrome of acutely developing and painful focal inflammatory nodules, sometimes occurring sequentially in different muscles, has been termed *focal nodular myositis*. The pathologic appearance and response to therapy are similar to those in generalized polymyositis. The differential diagnosis includes, when single, a muscle tumor (sarcoma or rhabdomyosarcoma) or proliferative fasciitis and myositis and, when multiple, muscle infarcts such as can occur in polyarteritis nodosa.

Infectious polymyositis Rare cases of polymyositis have been found to result from infection with known pathogens such as toxoplasma (Chap. 219), viruses (Chap. 195), and spirochetes (Lyme disease). Antibody screening will suggest the diagnosis in such cases. Trichinosis may be confused with idiopathic polymyositis, particularly if the history of raw or undercooked pork ingestion is not obtained (see Chap. 221). The symptoms of trichinosis are variable and depend upon the parasitic load. Low-grade fever, muscle pain of variable degree, conjunctival and periorbital edema, and fatigue are frequent. Weakness is generally mild. Heavy infestation is often associated with central nervous system symptoms of delirium, coma, or focal neurologic deficits. Myocardial involvement is common, manifested by tachycardia and ECG changes. The diagnosis is made by the history of ingestion of undercooked pork, marked eosinophilia, a positive skin test to *Trichina* antigen, and the appearance of serum antibodies to *Trichina* during the course of the disease. Occasionally the diagnosis is not recognized until a muscle is biopsied. Pyomyositis, a suppurative inflammation of muscle due to staphylococci or streptococci, is mainly seen in the tropics but has recently been reported in patients with AIDS. The presentation is that of a diffuse abscess of the muscle.

Myopathy in infection caused by human immunodeficiency virus (HIV) Polymyositis occurs in AIDS (see Chap. 308). It may be the presenting manifestation of the disorder or be due to therapy with zidovudine (AZT), which inhibits DNA polymerase gamma and presumably mitochondrial DNA replication. Weight loss greater than 10 percent of baseline body weight with associated chronic diarrhea or weakness characterizes the HIV wasting syndrome; a myopathy, among other causes, may underlie this entity. Raised serum CK, EMG evidence of myopathy, and muscle fiber necrosis with or without inflammatory infiltrates occur in AIDS myopathy. Rhabdomyolysis can occur in HIV-infected patients, possibly related to the use of drugs (such as didanosine or sulfonamides), or, in late cases, as part of opportunistic infection in muscle (such as *Staphylococcus aureus*), toxemia, or severe electrolyte disturbances. HIV antigens are present in macrophages associated with muscle inflammatory infiltrates but are absent in muscle fibers. The inflammatory myopathy associated with early HIV infection usually responds to glucocorticoids. AZT myopathy is dose related and usually improves after discontinuation of the drug or reduction of the dose. Structural and functional mitochondrial abnormalities are usually associated with AZT myopathy.

Polymyositis also occurs in patients displaying the spectrum of diseases associated with human T lymphotropic virus type I infection, especially in the Caribbean islands and Japan. Almost all such patients show other neurologic features, such as a myelopathy or neuropathy. Response to glucocorticoids is usually poor.

Inclusion Body Myositis The clinical features of this typically sporadic, but rarely familial, disorder are similar to those of chronic idiopathic polymyositis, except that onset is at an older age, focal and distal muscle involvement are more frequent, and disease duration is longer. Early and prominent involvement of finger or forearm flexors and leg extensors is characteristic. Muscle biopsy shows interstitial and occasional perivascular inflammatory infiltrates, necrosis, and regeneration of muscle fibers, but in addition there are "rimmed vacuoles" in the fibers that stain positively with Congo-red, like amyloid. Inflammation is rarely seen in the familial disorder. Electron microscopy reveals paramyxovirus-like 15- to 18-nm filaments in the nuclei and sarcoplasm. Immunohistochemistry reveals abnormal accumulation of beta-amyloid protein, α_1-antichymotrypsin, phosphorylated tau, apolipoprotein E, and ubiquitin within vacuolated muscle fibers. The nature of the inflammatory infiltrate and the mechanism of muscle fiber damage are probably similar to that in polymyositis. Immunocytochemical and in situ hybridization studies suggest that a previously reported etiologic link with the mumps virus seems unlikely. This disorder usually responds poorly to glucocorticoids and immunosuppressive therapy; however, some patients may improve following treatment with intravenous immunoglobulin. Prognosis is for a chronically progressive disorder with loss of ambulation about 5 to 10 years after presentation.

Eosinophilic Myositis This rare disease probably represents one manifestation of the spectrum of hypereosinophilic syndrome. There are a number of subtypes. Subacute onset of muscle pain and proximal weakness, elevated serum CK, myopathic features on EMG, and histologic appearance of a myositis with an eosinophilic inflammatory infiltrate are characteristic. Some patients may respond to glucocorticoids, methotrexate, or leukapheresis.

Eosinophilia-myalgia syndrome A syndrome that is more common in women has been associated with ingestion of the essential amino acid L-tryptophan. Fever, rash, arthralgia, cough, dyspnea, and edema are commonly accompanied by eosinophilia (more than 1000 cells per microliter), peripheral neuropathy, and myositis with endomysial, perimysial, and fascial infiltration of lymphocytes and eosinophils. 1,1′-Ethylidenebis (tryptophan), a contaminating by-product of the manufacture of some batches of L-tryptophan, has been incriminated. Immune-mediated muscle damage by cytotoxic T cells alone or with accompanying macrophages has been reported.

Eosinophilic fasciitis This disorder is characterized by painful swelling and thickening of the skin in the extremities, limitation of movement due to contractures, and mild muscle weakness. Raised sedimentation rate, peripheral eosinophilia, hypergammaglobulinemia, and mildly elevated CK are seen. The EMG may show myopathic features. Histologically there is marked thickening and infiltration of the deep fascia with mononuclear cells and eosinophils, some involvement of the epimysium and perimysium, and variable muscle degeneration. Most patients respond to treatment with glucocorticoids.

Relapsing eosinophilic perimyositis This disease is characterized by recurrent painful and tender areas in the neck or lower extremities, but without muscle weakness. An elevated sedimentation rate and peripheral eosinophilia are frequent, serum CK is sometimes raised, and histologically there is eosinophilic infiltration of the perimysium. Response to glucocorticoids is usually good.

LABORATORY FINDINGS In all forms of polymyositis there may be elevated serum levels of the enzymes present in skeletal muscle, such as CK, aldolase, serum glutamic oxaloacetic transaminase, lactic acid dehydrogenase, and serum glutamic pyruvate transaminase. The degree of elevation decreases from the first to the last in this series of enzymes, and the pattern is the reverse of that seen in liver disease. The erythrocyte sedimentation rate is elevated in about two-thirds of cases. Tests for circulating rheumatoid factor are positive in less than one-half and for antinuclear antibodies in about three-quarters of the cases. Most other hematologic indexes are normal. Several autoantibodies seem to be associated with clinically distinct groups of patients. Anti-Jo-1 antibodies are more common in polymyositis, especially in patients with interstitial lung disease, and anti-nRNP antibodies are often associated with polymyositis seen in lupus erythematosus. Other antibodies seen in patients with dermatomyositis and polymyositis in association with connective tissue diseases include anti-Scl-70 (progressive systemic sclerosis), anti-Sm (lupus erythematosus), anti-Ro and anti-La (Sjögren's syndrome and lupus erythematosus), and anti-ENA (mixed connective tissue disease). Myoglobin can be found in the urine when muscle destruction is acute and extensive; rarely, acute polymyositis causes the full syndrome of rhabdomyolysis and myoglobinuria. In about 40 percent of cases EMG reveals a markedly increased insertional activity (muscle irritability), together with the typical myopathic triad of motor unit action potentials, which are of low amplitude, are polyphasic, and have an abnormally early recruitment. In a further 40 percent of the patients only myopathic changes are present. The ECG is abnormal in about 5 to 10 percent of the cases at presentation. Since the pathologic process in myositis is patchy, greater diagnostic yield is accomplished by obtaining a biopsy from two clinically affected muscles and by skip serial sectioning of all specimens. Magnetic resonance imaging may serve to identify sites of muscle involvement. Muscles recently used for EMG or intramuscular injection must be avoided as these procedures can produce inflammatory changes and muscle fiber damage, leading to false-positive results. In about two-thirds of cases, the biopsies will demonstrate the typical pathologic changes of myositis, but despite following the above recommendations, about 10 percent of cases have normal muscle biopsy.

Skeletal Muscle Pathology The principal changes in muscle consist of infiltrates of inflammatory cells (lymphocytes, macrophages, plasma cells, and rare eosinophils and neutrophils) and destruction of muscle fibers with a phagocytic reaction. Perivascular (usually perivenular) inflammatory cell infiltration is the hallmark of polymyositis. Interstitial inflammatory cell infiltration is also a prominent feature of the disease, but lesser degrees of it may be seen in other conditions as a secondary reaction (e.g., in facioscapulohumeral and Becker's muscular dystrophy). Evidence of muscle fiber degeneration and regeneration is almost invariably present. Many of the residual muscle fibers are small, with increased numbers of sarcolemmal nuclei. Either the degeneration of muscle fibers or the infiltration of inflammatory cells may predominate in any given biopsy specimen. Blood vessel changes and perifascicular atrophy are more prominent in childhood dermatomyositis than in adult dermatomyositis and polymyositis. Capillary loss due to endothelial cell necrosis occurs particularly in the periphery of fascicles and may explain the perifascicular atrophy. Other features include reduplication of capillary basement membrane and the presence of tubular inclusions within endothelial cells. Type II muscle fiber atrophy and muscle infarcts also may be found. Vasculitis is also seen in polymyositis or dermatomyositis associated with connective tissue disorders.

DIAGNOSIS Patients with dermatomyositis who have the characteristic skin rash, muscle weakness, EMG changes, and elevation of serum CK may not require a muscle biopsy to confirm the diagnosis. In the case of idiopathic polymyositis, however, a firm diagnosis must be based on the presence of a typical clinical picture, a typical EMG, elevation of serum CK, and a diagnostic muscle biopsy. All four of these criteria are required to be certain of the diagnosis, since inflammatory changes may occasionally occur in other myopathies (e.g., facioscapulohumeral muscular dystrophy) and in other connective tissue disorders without clear muscle weakness. However, in fewer than one-third of cases of polymyositis are *all* these criteria satisfied. It may be particularly difficult to obtain a diagnostic muscle biopsy because of the patchy nature of the disease. Thus, a therapeutic trial of glucocorticoids should be given when full investigation of a patient with significant disability leaves a diagnosis of "possible polymyositis," usually because of a nondiagnostic muscle biopsy.

DIFFERENTIAL DIAGNOSIS The clinical picture of skin rash and proximal or diffuse muscle weakness has few causes other than dermatomyositis. However, proximal muscle weakness without skin involvement can be due to many conditions other than polymyositis and necessitates detailed investigation to establish the correct diagnosis.

Subacute or Chronic Progressive Muscle Weakness This may be due to denervating conditions such as the spinal muscular atrophies or amyotrophic lateral sclerosis (Chap. 370). Upper motor neuron signs in the latter in addition to the muscle weakness aid in the diagnosis. The muscular dystrophies, such as those of Duchenne and Becker and the limb-girdle and facioscapulohumeral types, may appear similar to polymyositis (Chap. 383). However, the muscular dystrophies usually develop more slowly (over years rather than weeks or months); rarely present after the age of 30; usually spare the pharyngeal, posterior neck, and deltoid muscles until late in the course; and may selectively involve other muscles, such as the biceps and brachioradialis, early in the course. Nevertheless, in rare patients it may be difficult, even with a muscle biopsy, to distinguish chronic polymyositis from a rapidly advancing muscular dystrophy. This is particularly true of facioscapulohumeral muscular dystrophy, where interstitial inflammatory cell infiltration is commonly found early in the disease. Such doubtful cases should always be given an adequate trial of glucocorticoid therapy. Myotonic dystrophy produces a characteristic facies with ptosis, facial myopathy, temporalis muscle wasting, and grip myotonia (Chap. 383). Some metabolic myopathies, including glycogen storage disease due to carnitine and carnitine palmityltransferase deficiency, produce exertional cramps, rhabdomyolysis, and muscle weakness; diagnosis rests upon biochemical studies of the muscle biopsy (Chap. 383). Glycogen storage disease due to acid maltase deficiency also requires muscle biopsy for diagnosis. The endocrine myopathies such as those due to hypercorticosteroidism, hyper- and hypothyroidism, and hyper- and hypoparathyroidism require the appropriate laboratory investigations for diagnosis. Muscle wasting in patients with an underlying neoplasm may be true polymyositis, but it can be due to a protein-wasting state (cachexia), a paraneoplastic neuropathy, or type II fiber atrophy.

Muscle Weakness with Marked Exercise-Induced Fatigue Fatigue without much muscle wasting may be due to neuromuscular junction disorders including myasthenia gravis or the Lambert-Eaton syndrome. Repetitive nerve stimulation and single-fiber EMG studies aid in the diagnosis of these conditions (Chap. 382).

Acute Muscle Weakness This may be caused by an acute neuropathy such as that due to the Guillain-Barré syndrome or a neurotoxin. When combined with painful muscle cramps, rhabdomyolysis, and myoglobinuria, it may be due to metabolic disorders including some of the glycogen storage diseases such as myophosphorylase deficiency (McArdle's disease), carnitine palmityltransferase deficiency, and myoadenylate deaminase deficiency. Acute viral infections may cause a similar syndrome. Chronic alcoholics may develop a painful myopathy with myoglobinuria after a bout of heavy drinking or may present with a painless acute hypokalemic myopathy, which is completely reversible, or may show an asymptomatic elevation of serum CK and myoglobin. Acute muscle weakness with myoglobinuria may occur in prolonged severe hypokalemia due to potassium loss or with hypophosphatemia and hypomagnesemia, often seen in chronic alcoholics and in patients on nasogastric suction receiving parenteral hyperalimentation. An acute necrotizing myopathy with myoglobinuria can rarely accompany hyper- and hyponatremia.

Drug-Induced Myopathies Rhabdomyolysis and myoglobinuria have been associated with intake of amphotericin B, ϵ-aminocaproic acid, fenfluramine, heroin, and phencyclidine. A predominantly hypokalemic myopathy may result from prolonged use of diuretics, carbenoxolone, and azathioprine. Penicillamine has been reported to produce a myositis. The use of clofibrate, cimetidine, chloroquine, colchicine, carbimazole, cyclosporine, emetine, gemfibrozil, growth hormone, ketoconazole, leuprolide, lovastatin, phenytoin, provastatin, tretinoin, and, recently, AZT has been associated with a myopathy. Toxic myopathies usually have a different pathology from polymyositis and require a careful drug history for diagnosis. In other cases investigation reveals no etiology, and these may be due to a true acute autoimmune polymyositis or to an as yet undiscovered metabolic defect.

Pain on Movement and Muscle Tenderness Patients with muscle pain and little or no weakness may be thought to be neurotic or hysterical. A number of conditions including *polymyalgia rheumatica* (Chap. 319) and arthritic disorders of adjacent joints enter into the differential diagnosis of polymyositis. The muscle biopsy either is normal or discloses type II fiber atrophy, but in polymyalgia rheumatica the temporal artery biopsy may show giant cell arteritis (Chap. 319). *Fibrositis* and *fibromyalgia* are syndromes that frequently enter into the differential diagnosis of polymyositis. Patients complain of focal or diffuse muscle tenderness, aching, and weakness, which is sometimes poorly separated from joint pain. In other patients there may be minor signs of a collagen vascular disorder, such as an increased erythrocyte sedimentation rate, antinuclear antibody, or rheumatoid factor, and occasionally there is slight elevation of the serum CK. The muscle biopsy occasionally shows a few interstitial inflammatory cells. Where there is a focal "trigger point," biopsy may show inflammatory infiltration of the connective tissue. Rarely does this syndrome develop into frank polymyositis, and the prognosis is therefore more benign than that of polymyositis (see below). Many such patients show some response to nonsteroidal anti-inflammatory agents, though most continue to have indolent complaints. *Chronic fatigue syndrome*, which may follow a viral infection, can present with debilitating fatigue, fever, sore throat, painful lymphadenopathy, myalgia, arthralgia, sleep disorder, and headache (Chap. 384). The presence of other cognitive and behavioral features, such as impaired memory and concentration, depression, and irritability, and a normal muscle biopsy usually help in the diagnosis.

℞ TREATMENT

(See Fig. 315-1) Glucocorticoids in high dosage is the accepted treatment for severe dermatomyositis-polymyositis, though there is no controlled trial to prove its effectiveness. Prednisone is generally started at a dose of 1 to 2 mg/kg body weight per day (60 to 100 mg/d for adults). Improvement may begin within 1 to 4 weeks, though in some patients treatment may need to be continued for 3 months before improvement occurs. When improvement is noted, the daily dose may be reduced by 5 mg every 4 weeks. Repeated manual muscle testing and serum CK determinations should be performed to ensure that the myositis does not relapse. At about 40 mg/d, the schedule is changed gradually to 80 mg every other day in order to reduce the incidence of glucocorticoid side effects. There is some evidence that the use of alternate-day glucocorticoids from the outset may be effective, particularly in patients with milder disease. Adults with acute to subacute dermatomyositis-polymyositis tend to improve more rapidly than those with chronic polymyositis; children also respond in most cases. If the dose is reduced too rapidly, or to too low a level, relapse will occur, necessitating return to high dosage. Prednisone therapy may have to be continued for several years, but an attempt should be made every year to withdraw the therapy from patients who are clinically stable in order to determine if the disease is still active.

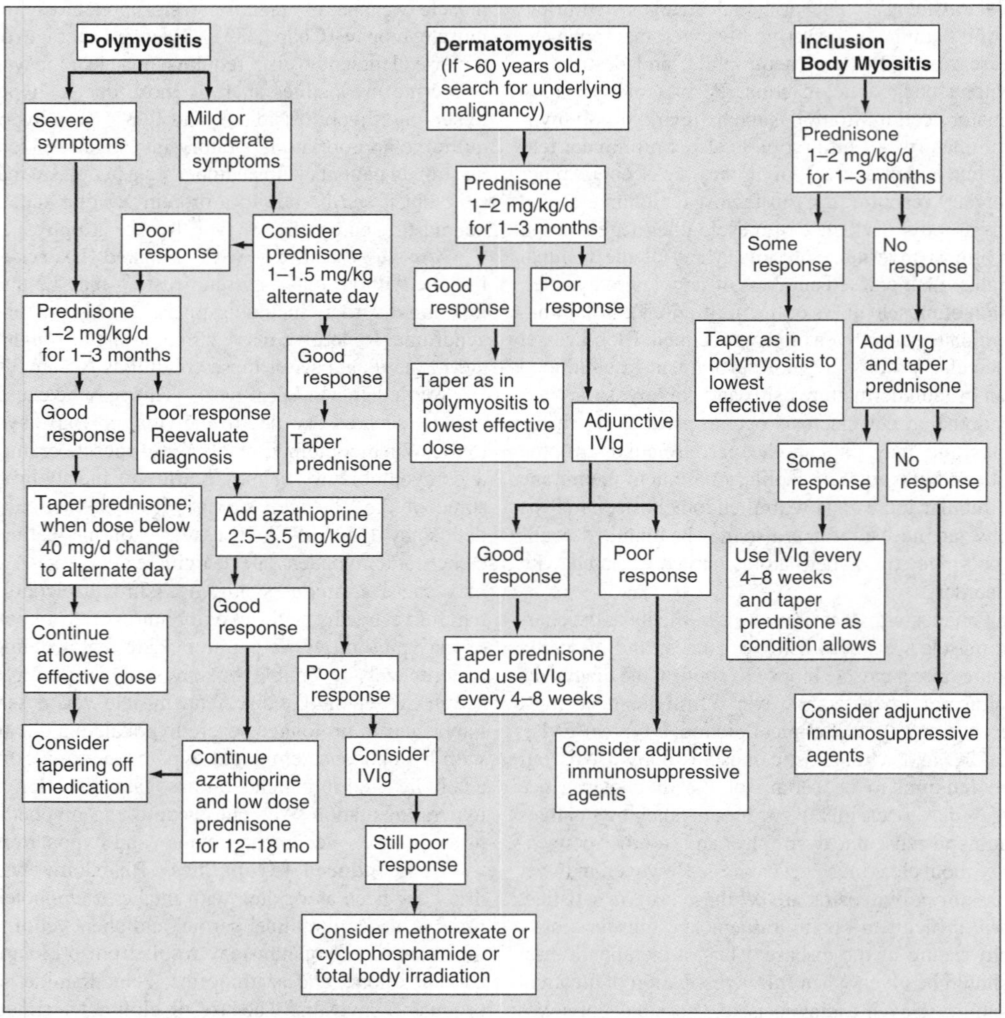

FIGURE 315-1 Algorithm for the treatment of polymyositis, dermatomyositis, and inclusion body myositis.

Cytotoxic drugs should be tried when the response to glucocorticoids is inadequate after 1 to 3 months or when relapses are frequent. The combined use of glucocorticoids and a cytotoxic drug usually allows a lower dose of glucocorticoids to be used. Azathioprine (2.5 to 3.5 mg/kg body weight per day in divided doses) is the most commonly used cytotoxic drug in this disease; preliminary studies have shown a benefit of azathioprine as adjunctive therapy in glucocorticoid-treated patients. The aim of therapy with azathioprine is to lower the total lymphocyte count to about 750/μL, while maintaining the hemoglobin level above 12 g/dL, the total white cell count above 3000/μL, and the platelet count about 125,000/μL. Periodic blood counts are required to monitor the cytotoxic drug therapy. Uncontrolled studies have shown some benefit with methotrexate, cyclophosphamide, and cyclosporine. Methotrexate is effective at doses that do not produce lymphopenia (usual dose about 0.5 mg/kg body weight per week achieved by slowly increasing from a starting dose of 10 mg). In a small controlled study, high-dose intravenous immunoglobulin (IVIg) therapy (0.4 g/kg daily for 5 consecutive days) produced improvement in patients with steroid-resistant dermatomyositis and probably should be used in severe or refractory cases. Anecdotal reports have suggested that IVIg may also be effective in polymyositis resistant to other forms of therapy. Total-body irradiation has been successfully used in some patients with disease refractory to glucocorticoids and immunosuppressants, but long-term follow-up and controlled studies are lacking for this potentially dangerous therapy. A controlled trial of plasma exchange and leukapheresis in a small number of patients with dermatomyositis-polymyositis resistant to glucocorticoids showed no benefit over sham pheresis. Bed rest has been recommended in the acute phase of the disease but is harmful in the long term. Physiotherapy and rehabilitative devices are important in the long-term treatment of patients with dermatomyositis-polymyositis.

Patients older than age 40, particularly those with dermatomyositis, should be followed closely for the possibility of malignant disease. If a malignant lesion is found, it should be treated, since the muscle weakness may disappear if the neoplasm is eradicated. However, a response to glucocorticoids can usually be obtained even in patients with dermatomyositis-polymyositis associated with a malignancy.

Monitoring serum CK levels during reduction of immunosuppressive therapy is useful, since a rise in level generally indicates an incipient clinical relapse. CK levels are not used to monitor initial response to prednisone, because prednisone reduces CK levels independent of any effects on the disease process.

Side effects of high-dose daily glucocorticoid therapy (see Chap. 332) are relatively common in patients treated for polymyositis and may limit therapy. However, these can be minimized by appropriate use of alternate-day therapy and judicious use of calcium supplements, vitamin D, and H_2-receptor blockers. When patients who have been stable on a static dose of prednisone develop increasing muscle weakness, this may be due to either a relapse of the myositis or to glucocorticoid myopathy. An EMG, serum CK measurement, and, rarely, muscle biopsy may help in differentiating these two conditions if the changes of myositis are present. Often, however, the only way to distinguish between these two conditions is to reduce the dose of prednisone slowly; if glucocorticoid myopathy is the cause of the weakness, it will improve as the dose is reduced; if a relapse of the myositis is responsible, the weakness will increase with reduction in the dose.

Side effects of cytotoxic drugs include marrow suppression, alopecia, gastrointestinal tract disorders, damage to the testes and ovaries, infections, and potential for malignancy.

PROGNOSIS The overall mortality rate of individuals with dermatomyositis-polymyositis is about four times that of the general population; death is usually due to pulmonary, renal, and cardiac complications. Females, blacks, and those severely affected at presentation or treated after long delays have a worse prognosis. Unfavorable outcome is also seen in patients with significant dysphagia, associated cancer or connective tissue diseases, and serum antibodies to Jo-1 and SRP. Evidence from several series suggests that patients seen at tertiary referral centers may have less favorable outcome when compared with patients seen at smaller community hospitals, probably because they represent a population with more severe disease that is less responsive to therapy. Nevertheless, the 5-year survival rate is about 75 percent overall, and is higher yet in children. Most patients improve with therapy. Many make a full functional recovery, though some weakness of the shoulders and hips, usually not disabling, remains at the conclusion of treatment. Relapse may occur at any time. Glucocorticoids should not be discontinued too soon, for the relapse that may follow is often more difficult to treat than the original presentation. About one-half of the patients with this disease recover and can discontinue therapy within 5 years after the onset of the symptoms; about 20 percent still have active disease requiring continued therapy. The remaining 30 percent have inactive disease but residual muscle weakness.

BIBLIOGRAPHY

Bohan A et al: A computer-assisted analysis of 153 patients with polymyositis and dermatomyositis. Medicine 56:255, 1977

Callen JP: Relationship of cancer to inflammatory muscle diseases. Dermatomyositis, polymyositis, and inclusion body myositis. Rheum Dis Clin North Am 20(4):943, 1994

Carpenter S, Karpati G: *Pathology of Skeletal Muscle*. New York, Churchill Livingstone, 1984, pp 515–592

Chariot P et al: Acute rhabdomyolysis in patients infected by human immunodeficiency virus. Neurology 44:1692, 1994

Cherin P, Herson S: Indications for intravenous gammaglobulin therapy in inflammatory myopathies. J Neurol Neurosurg Psychiatry 57:50, 1994

Dalakas MC: How to diagnose and treat the inflammatory myopathies. Semin Neurol 14:137, 1994

——— et al: A controlled trial of high dose intravenous immune globulin infusions as treatment for dermatomyositis. N Engl J Med 329:1993

DeVere R, Bradley WG: Polymyositis: Its presentation, mortality, and morbidity. Brain 98:637, 1975

Engel AG et al: The polymyositis and dermatomyositis syndromes, in *Myology*, 2d ed, AG Engel, C Franzini-Armstrong (eds). New York, McGraw-Hill, 1994, pp 1335–1383

Garlepp MJ, Mastaglia FL: Inclusion body myositis. J Neurol Neurosurg Psychiatry 60:251, 1996

Griggs RC et al: Inclusion body myositis and myopathies. Ann Neurol 38:705, 1995

Hohlfeld R, Engel AG: The immunobiology of muscle. Immunol Today 15:269, 1994

Joffe MM et al: Drug therapy of the idiopathic inflammatory myopathies: Predictors of response to prednisone, azathioprine, and methotrexate and a comparison of their efficacy. Am J Med 94:379, 1993

Martin RW et al: The clinical spectrum of the eosinophilia-myalgia syndrome associated with L-tryptophan ingestion. Ann Intern Med 113:124, 1990

McKenzie R, Straus SE: Chronic fatigue syndrome. Adv Intern Med 40:119, 1995

Sigurgeirsson B et al: Risk of cancer in patients with dermatomyositis or polymyositis: A population-based study. N Engl J Med 326:363, 1992

Targoff IN: Immune manifestations of inflammatory muscle disease. Rheum Dis Clin North Am 20(4):857, 1994

316

Haralampos M. Moutsopoulos

SJÖGREN'S SYNDROME

DEFINITION Sjögren's syndrome is a chronic, slowly progressive autoimmune disease characterized by lymphocytic infiltration of the exocrine glands resulting in xerostomia and dry eyes. Approximately one-third of patients present with systemic manifestations. A small but significant number of the patients may develop malignant lymphoma. The disease can be seen alone (primary Sjögren's syndrome) or in association with other autoimmune rheumatic diseases (secondary Sjögren's syndrome) (Table 316-1).

INCIDENCE AND PREVALENCE The disease affects predominantly middle-aged women (female-to-male ratio 9:1), although it can be seen in all ages, including childhood. The prevalence of primary Sjögren's syndrome is approximately 0.5 to 1.0 percent. In addition to the primary syndrome, 30 percent of patients with autoimmune rheumatic diseases suffer from secondary Sjögren's syndrome.

PATHOGENESIS Sjögren's syndrome is characterized by lymphocytic infiltration of the exocrine glands and B lymphocyte hyperreactivity, as illustrated by circulating autoantibodies. The latter is accompanied by an oligomonoclonal B cell process, which is characterized by serum and urine monoclonal light chains and cryoprecipitable monoclonal immunoglobulins.

Sera of patients with Sjögren's syndrome often contain a number of autoantibodies directed against non-organ-specific antigens such as immunoglobulins (rheumatoid factors) and extractable nuclear and cytoplasmic antigens (Ro/SS-A, La/SS-B). Ro/SS-A autoantigen consists of three polypeptide chains (52, 54, and 60 kDa) in conjunction with RNAs, whereas the 48-kDa La/SS-B protein is bound to RNA III polymerase transcripts. The presence of autoantibodies to Ro/SS-A and La/SS-B antigens in Sjögren's syndrome is associated with earlier disease onset, longer disease duration, salivary gland enlargement, severity of lymphocytic infiltration of minor salivary glands, and certain extraglandular manifestations such as lymphadenopathy, purpura, and vasculitis.

Phenotypic and functional studies have shown that the predominant cell infiltrating the affected exocrine glands is the helper/inducer T cell with characteristics of memory cells. Both B and T infiltrating lymphocytes are activated, as illustrated by production of immunoglobulins with autoantibody activity, spontaneous release of interleukin 2, as well as expression on the T cell surface of activation markers such as class II HLA molecules and lymphocyte function–associated antigen 1. Macrophages and natural killer cells are rarely detected in infiltrates, while epithelial cells of the affected glands inappropriately express class II molecules and possess messages for *c-myc* protooncogene and proinflammatory cytokines. All these phenomena suggest that the epithelial cell of the exocrine glands in Sjögren's syndrome may act as an antigen-presenting cell, and recent studies indicate that a retrovirus may be the initiator of the autoimmune process.

Immunogenetic studies have demonstrated that HLA-B8, -DR3, and -DRw52 are prevalent in primary Sjögren's syndrome patients as compared with the normal control population. Molecular analysis of HLA class II genes has revealed that Sjögren's syndrome patients, regardless of their ethnic origin, are highly associated with HLA DQA_1*0501 allele.

CLINICAL MANIFESTATIONS The majority of the patients with Sjögren's syndrome have symptoms related to diminished lacrimal and salivary gland function. In most patients, the primary syndrome runs a slow and benign course. The initial manifestations can be mucosal dryness or nonspecific, and 8 to 10 years elapse from the initial symptoms to full-blown development of the disease.

The principal oral symptom of Sjögren's syndrome is dryness (xerostomia). This is described as difficulty in swallowing dry food, inability to speak continuously, a burning sensation, increase in dental caries, and problems in wearing complete dentures. Physical examination shows a dry, erythematous, sticky oral mucosa. There is atrophy of the filiform papillae on the dorsum of the tongue, and saliva from the major glands is either not expressible or is cloudy. Enlargement of the parotid or other major salivary glands occurs in two-thirds of patients with primary Sjögren's syndrome but is uncommon in those with the secondary syndrome. Diagnostic tests include sialometry, sialography, and scintigraphy. The labial minor salivary gland biopsy permits histopathologic confirmation of the focal lymphocytic infiltrates.

Ocular involvement is the other major manifestation of Sjögren's syndrome. Patients usually complain of dry eyes, with a sandy or gritty feeling under the eyelids. Other symptoms include burning, accumulation of thick strands at the inner canthi, decreased tearing, redness, itching, eye fatigue, and increased photosensitivity. These symptoms are attributed to the destruction of corneal and bulbar conjunctival epithelium, defined as keratoconjunctivitis sicca. Diagnostic evaluation of keratoconjunctivitis sicca includes measurement of tear flow by Schirmer's I test and tear composition as assessed by the tear breakup time or tear lysozyme content. Slit-lamp examination of the cornea and conjunctiva after rose Bengal staining reveals punctate corneal ulcerations and attached filaments of corneal epithelium.

Involvement of other exocrine glands occurs less frequently and includes a decrease in mucous gland secretions of the upper and lower respiratory tree, resulting in dry nose, throat, and trachea (xerotrachea), and diminished secretion of the exocrine glands of the gastrointestinal tract, leading to esophageal mucosal atrophy, atrophic gastritis, and subclinical pancreatitis. Dyspareunia due to dryness of the external genitalia and dry skin also may occur.

Extraglandular (systemic) manifestations are seen in one-third of patients with Sjögren's syndrome (Table 316-2), while they are very rare in patients with Sjögren's syndrome associated with rheumatoid arthritis. These patients complain more often of easy fatigability, low-grade fever, myalgias, and arthralgias. Most patients with primary Sjögren's syndrome experience at least one episode of nonerosive arthritis during the course of their disease. Manifestations of pulmonary involvement are frequent but rarely important clinically, with subclinical diffuse interstitial lung disease being the most common. Renal involvement includes interstitial nephritis, clinically manifested by hypostenuria and renal tubular dysfunction with or without acidosis and Fanconi's syndrome. Untreated acidosis may lead to nephrocalcinosis. Glomerulonephritis is a rare finding that occurs in patients with systemic vasculitis, cryoglobulinemia, or systemic lupus erythematosus overlapping with Sjögren's syndrome. Vasculitis affects small and medium-sized vessels. The most common clinical features are purpura, recurrent urticaria, skin ulcerations, glomerulonephritis, and mononeuritis multiplex.

It has been suggested that primary Sjögren's syndrome with vasculitis also may present with multifocal, recurrent, and progressive nervous system disease, such as hemiparesis, transverse myelopathy, hemisensory deficits, seizures, and movement disorders. Aseptic meningitis and multiple sclerosis also have been reported in these patients.

Table 316-1

Association of Sjögren's Syndrome with Other Autoimmune Diseases

Rheumatoid arthritis
Systemic lupus erythematosus
Scleroderma
Mixed connective tissue disease
Primary biliary cirrhosis
Vasculitis
Chronic active hepatitis

Table 316-2

Incidence of Extraglandular Manifestations in Primary Sjögren's Syndrome

Clinical Manifestation	Percent
Arthralgias/arthritis	60
Raynaud's phenomenon	37
Lymphadenopathy	14
Lung involvement	14
Vasculitis	11
Kidney involvement	9
Liver involvement	6
Lymphoma	6
Splenomegaly	3
Peripheral neuropathy	2
Myositis	1

Table 316-3

Diagnostic Criteria for Sjögren's Syndrome*

Criteria	Definitions
1. Ocular symptoms	Dry eyes every day for more than 3 months, recurrent sensation of sand or gravel in the eyes, or use of tear substitutes more than three times a day
2. Oral symptoms	Daily feeling of dry mouth for more than 3 months, recurrent or persistently swollen salivary glands, or use of liquids to aid in swallowing dry food
3. Ocular signs	Positive Schirmer's I test (<5 mm in 5 min), or a rose Bengal score of ≥4 according to van Bijsterveld's scoring system
4. Histopathology	Focus score 1 in a minor salivary gland biopsy
5. Salivary gland involvement	Positive result in one of the following tests: salivary scintigraphy, parotid sialography, salivary flow (≤1.5 mL in 15 min)
6. Autoantibodies	Antibodies to Ro(SS-A) or La(SS-B), antinuclear antibodies, or rheumatoid factor

* Probable Sjögren's syndrome: three items are present.
Definite Sjögren's syndrome: four or more items are present.

Table 316-4

Differential Diagnosis of Sicca Symptoms

Xerostomia	Dry Eye	Bilateral Parotid Gland Enlargement
Viral infections	Inflammation	Viral infections
Drugs	Stevens-Johnson syndrome	Mumps
Psychotherapeutic	Pemphigoid	Influenza
Parasympatholytic	Chronic conjunctivitis	Epstein-Barr
Antihypertensives	Chronic blepharitis	Coxsackievirus A
Psychogenic	Sjögren's syndrome	Cytomegalovirus
Irradiation	Toxicity	HIV
Diabetes mellitus	Burns	Sarcoidosis
Trauma	Drugs	Amyloidosis
Sjögren's syndrome	Neurologic conditions	Sjögren's syndrome
	Impaired lacrimal gland function	Metabolic
	Impaired eyelid function	Diabetes mellitus
	Miscellaneous	Hyperlipoproteinemias
	Trauma	Chronic pancreatitis
	Hypovitaminosis A	Hepatic cirrhosis
	Blink abnormality	Endocrine
	Lid scarring	Acromegaly
	Anesthetic cornea	Gonadal hypofunction
	Epithelial irregularity	

Lymphoma and Waldenström's macroglobulinemia are well-known manifestations of Sjögren's syndrome. Most lymphomas are of B cell origin. Pseudolymphoma or frank lymphoma should always be suspected when persistent major salivary gland enlargement, lymphadenopathy, lung nodules, or hilar or mediastinal lymphadenopathy is observed. Parenchymal organs, such as lungs and gastrointestinal

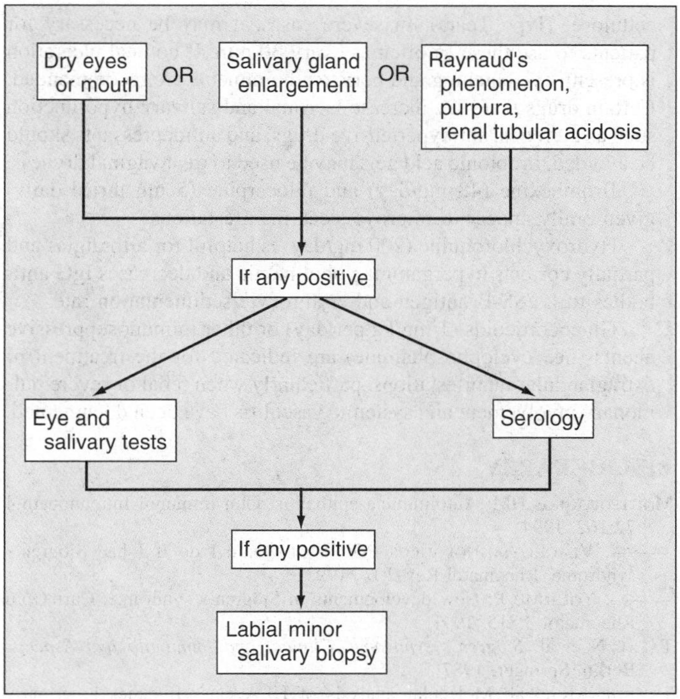

FIGURE 316-1 Algorithm for the diagnosis of Sjögren's syndrome.

tract, can be affected. Lymphomas may appear in Sjögren's syndrome patients after several years of an apparently benign course and are observed more often in patients with systemic disease.

Routine laboratory tests reveal mild normochromic, normocytic anemia. An elevated erythrocyte sedimentation rate is found in approximately 70 percent of patients.

DIAGNOSIS AND DIFFERENTIAL DIAGNOSIS A European multicenter study has developed diagnostic criteria of Sjögren's syndrome (Table 316-3), which have been validated and present high specificity and sensitivity. A diagnostic algorithm is depicted in Fig. 316-1.

The differential diagnosis of Sjögren's syndrome includes other conditions that may cause dry mouth or eyes or parotid salivary gland enlargement (Table 316-4). Human immunodeficiency virus (HIV) infection (see Chap. 308) and sarcoidosis (see Chap. 320) appear to produce a clinical picture indistinguishable from Sjögren's syndrome (Table 316-5).

℞ TREATMENT

Sjögren's syndrome remains fundamentally an incurable disease. Hence treatment of Sjögren's syndrome is aimed at symptomatic relief and limiting the damaging local effects of chronic xerostomia and keratoconjunctivitis sicca by substitution of the missing secretions.

The sicca complex is treated with fluid replacement supplied as often as necessary. To replace deficient tears, there are several readily available ophthalmic preparations (Tearisol; Liquifilm; 0.5% methyl-

Table 316-5

Differential Diagnosis of Sjögren's Syndrome with HIV Infection

HIV Infection and Sicca Syndrome	Sjögren's Syndrome	Sarcoidosis
Predominant in young males	Predominant in middle-aged women	Invariable
Lack of autoantibodies to Ro/SS-A and/or La/SS-B	Presence of autoantibodies	Lack of autoantibodies to Ro/SS-A and/or La/SS-B
Lymphoid infiltrates of salivary glands by CD8+ lymphocytes	Lymphoid infiltrates of salivary glands by CD4+ lymphocytes	Granulomas in salivary glands
Association with HLA-DR5	Association with HLA-DR3 and -DRw52	Unknown
Positive serologic tests for HIV	Negative serologic tests for HIV	Negative serologic tests for HIV

cellulose; Hypo Tears). In severe cases, it may be necessary for patients to use these as often as every 30 min. If corneal ulceration is present, eye patching and boric acid ointments are recommended. Certain drugs that may increase lacrimal and salivary hypofunction such as diuretics, antihypertensive drugs, and antidepressants should be avoided. Propionic acid gels may be used to treat vaginal dryness.

Bromhexine (48 mg/day) and pilocarpine (5 mg thrice daily) given orally appear to improve sicca manifestations.

Hydroxychloroquine (200 mg/day) is helpful for arthralgias and partially corrects hypergammaglobulinemia and decreases IgG antibodies to La/SS-B antigen and erythrocyte sedimentation rate.

Glucocorticoids (1 mg/kg per day) or other immunosuppressive agents (i.e., cyclophosphamide) are indicated for the treatment of extraglandular manifestations, particularly when renal or severe pulmonary involvement and systemic vasculitis have been documented.

BIBLIOGRAPHY

Moutsopoulos HM: Autoimmune epithelitis. Clin Immunol Immunopathol 72:162, 1994

———, Vlachoyiannopoulos PG: What would I do if I had Sjögren's syndrome. Rheumatol Rev 2:17, 1993

———, Youinou P: New developments in Sjögren's syndrome. Curr Opin Rheumatol 3:815, 1991

Talal N et al: *Sjögren's syndrome. Clinical and Immunological Aspects.* Berlin, Springer, 1987

Tambur AR et al: Molecular analysis of HLA class II genes in primary Sjögren's syndrome: A study of Israeli and Greek non-Jewish patients. Hum Immunol 36:235, 1993

Tzioufas AG, Moutsopoulos HM: Sjögren's syndrome, in *Connective Tissue Diseases*. JJF Belch, RB Zurier (eds). London, Chapman and Hall, 1995

Vitali C et al: Preliminary criteria for the classification of Sjögren's syndrome: Results of a prospective concerted action supported by the European Community. Arthritis Rheum 36:340, 1992

317

Joel D. Taurog, Peter E. Lipsky

ANKYLOSING SPONDYLITIS, REACTIVE ARTHRITIS, AND UNDIFFERENTIATED SPONDYLOARTHROPATHY

The spondyloarthropathies are a group of disorders that share certain clinical features and an association with the HLA-B27 allele. These disorders include ankylosing spondylitis, Reiter's syndrome, reactive arthritis, psoriatic arthritis and spondylitis, enteropathic arthritis and spondylitis, juvenile-onset spondyloarthropathy, and undifferentiated spondyloarthropathy. The similarity in clinical manifestations and in genetic predisposition suggests that these disorders share pathogenic mechanisms. Specific definitions and diagnostic criteria for the individual conditions will be provided in subsequent sections of this chapter.

ANKYLOSING SPONDYLITIS

Ankylosing spondylitis (AS) is an inflammatory disorder of unknown cause that primarily affects the axial skeleton; peripheral joints and extraarticular structures also may be involved. The disease usually begins in the second or third decade; the prevalence in men is approximately three times that in women. It is considered the prototype of the spondyloarthropathies. Older names include *Marie-Strümpell disease* or *Bechterew's disease*.

EPIDEMIOLOGY AS shows a striking correlation with the histocompatibility antigen HLA-B27 and occurs worldwide roughly in proportion to the prevalence of this antigen (see Chap. 306). In North American Caucasians, the general prevalence of B27 is 7 percent, whereas over 90 percent of patients with AS have inherited this antigen. The association with B27 is independent of disease severity.

In population surveys, 1 to 2 percent of adults inheriting B27 have been found to have AS. In contrast, in families of patients with AS, the prevalence is 10 to 20 percent among adult first-degree relatives inheriting B27. The concordance rate in identical twins is estimated to be 50 percent. These findings indicate that both genetic and environmental factors play a role in the pathogenesis of the disease and that the genetic factors probably include allelic genes in addition to B27. AS is strongly associated with inflammatory bowel disease (IBD), including both ulcerative colitis and Chrohn's disease. IBD is a risk factor for AS independent of HLA–B27, although 50 to 75 percent of patients with both AS and IBD are B27 positive. → *See also Chap. 286.*

PATHOLOGY Sacroiliitis is usually one of the earliest manifestations of AS. The early lesion consists of subchondral granulation tissue containing lymphocytes, plasma cells, mast cells, macrophages, and chondrocytes. Usually, the thinner iliac cartilage is eroded before the thicker sacral cartilage. The irregularly eroded, sclerotic margins of the joint are gradually replaced by fibrocartilage regeneration and then by ossification. Ultimately, the joint may be totally obliterated. This progression is evident radiographically (see below).

In the spine, the initial lesion consists of inflammatory granulation tissue at the junction of the annulus fibrosus of the disk cartilage and the margin of vertebral bone. The outer annular fibers are eroded and eventually replaced by bone, forming the beginning of a bony excrescence called a *syndesmophyte*, which then grows by continued enchondral ossification, ultimately bridging the adjacent vertebral bodies. Ascending progression of this process leads to the "bamboo spine" observed radiographically. Other lesions in the spine include diffuse osteoporosis, erosion of vertebral bodies at the disk margin, "squaring" of vertebrae, and inflammation and destruction of the disk-bone border. Inflammatory arthritis of the apophyseal joints is common, with erosion of cartilage by pannus, often followed by bony ankylosis.

Peripheral arthritis in AS can show synovial hyperplasia, lymphoid infiltration, and pannus formation, but the process lacks the exuberant synovial villi, fibrin deposits, ulcers, and plaques of plasma cells seen in rheumatoid arthritis (see Chap. 313). Central cartilaginous erosions caused by proliferation of subchondral granulation tissue are common in AS but rare in rheumatoid arthritis.

The enthesis, the site of tendinous or ligamentous attachment to bone, is another common site of pathology in AS, especially at sites localized around the spine and pelvis. Enthesitis is characterized by erosive, inflammatory lesions that may eventually undergo ossification.

Acute anterior uveitis (iritis) occurs in approximately 20 percent of patients with AS. Few cases have been studied histologically, none at an early stage. After recurrent attacks, the iris shows nonspecific inflammatory changes, scarring, increased vascularity, and pigment-laden macrophages.

Aortic insufficiency develops in a small percentage of cases. There is thickening of the aortic valve cusps and the aorta near the sinuses of Valsalva, with dense adventitial scar tissue and intimal fibrous proliferation. The scar tissue can extend into the ventricular septum with resultant heart block.

Microscopic inflammatory lesions of the colon and ileocecal valve have been found in 25 to 50 percent of patients with AS, even in those lacking any clinical evidence of inflammatory bowel disease. IgA nephropathy has been reported with increased frequency.

PATHOGENESIS The pathogenesis of AS is incompletely understood. A number of features of the disease implicate immune-mediated mechanisms, including elevated serum levels of IgA and acute phase reactants, inflammatory histology, and close association with HLA-B27. No specific event or exogenous agent that triggers the onset of disease has been identified, although overlapping features with reactive arthritis and inflammatory bowel disease suggest that enteric bacteria may play a role. Elevated serum titers of antibodies to certain enteric bacteria, particularly *Klebsiella pneumoniae*, are common in AS patients. Furthermore, antigenic interrelatedness between B27 and certain enteric bacteria has been documented, but it is not yet known whether these factors contribute to the pathogenesis of AS. Evidence that B27 plays a direct role is provided by the finding that rats transgenic for B27 spontaneously develop spondylitis, along with colitis, peripheral arthritis, and other lesions characteristic of the spondyloarthropathies (see below).

CLINICAL MANIFESTATIONS The symptoms of the disease are usually first noticed in late adolescence or early adulthood; onset after age 40 is unusual. The initial symptom is usually dull pain, insidious in onset, felt deep in the lower lumbar or gluteal region, accompanied by low-back morning stiffness of up to a few hours' duration that improves with activity and returns following periods of inactivity. Within a few months of onset, the pain usually has become persistent and bilateral. Nocturnal exacerbation of pain that forces the patient to rise and move around may be frequent.

In some patients bony tenderness may accompany back pain or stiffness, while in others it may be the predominant complaint. Common sites include the costosternal junctions, spinous processes, iliac crests, greater trochanters, ischial tuberosities, tibial tubercles, and heels. Occasionally, bony chest pain is the presenting complaint. Arthritis in the hips and shoulders ("root" joints) occurs in 25 to 35 percent of patients, in many cases early in the disease course. Arthritis of peripheral joints other than the hips and shoulders, usually asymmetric, occurs in up to 30 percent of patients and can occur at any stage of the disease. Neck pain and stiffness from involvement of the cervical spine are usually relatively late manifestations. Occasional patients present with predominantly constitutional symptoms such as fatigue, anorexia, fever, weight loss, or night sweats.

AS often has a juvenile onset in developing countries. In these individuals, peripheral arthritis and enthesitis usually predominate, with axial symptoms supervening in late adolescence.

The most common extraarticular manifestation is acute anterior uveitis, which can antedate the spondylitis. Attacks are typically unilateral and tend to recur, causing pain, photophobia, and increased lacrimation. Aortic insufficiency, sometimes producing symptoms of congestive heart failure, occurs in a few percent of patients, occasionally early in the course of the spinal disease. Up to half the patients have inflammation in the colon or ileum. This is usually asymptomatic, but in 5 to 10 percent of patients with AS, frank IBD will develop.

Initially, physical findings mirror the inflammatory process. The most specific findings involve loss of spinal mobility, with limitation of anterior and lateral flexion and extension of the lumbar spine and of chest expansion. Limitation of motion is usually out of proportion to the degree of bony ankylosis, reflecting muscle spasm secondary to pain and inflammation. Pain in the sacroiliac joints may be elicited either with direct pressure or with maneuvers that stress the joints, but these techniques are unreliable in discriminating inflammatory sacroiliitis. In addition, there is commonly tenderness upon palpation at the sites of symptomatic bony tenderness and paraspinous muscle spasm.

The Schober test is a useful measure of flexion of the lumbar spine. The patient stands erect, with heels together, and marks are made directly over the spine 5 cm below and 10 cm above the lumbosacral junction (identified by a horizontal line between the posterosuperior iliac spines.) The patient then bends forward maximally, and the distance between the two marks is measured. The distance between the two marks increases 5 cm or more in the case of normal mobility and less than 4 cm in the case of decreased mobility. Chest expansion is measured as the difference between maximal inspiration and maximal forced expiration in the fourth intercostal space in males or just below the breasts in females. Normal chest expansion is 5 cm or greater.

Limitation or pain with motion of the hips or shoulders is usually present if either of these joints is involved. Careful examination is also necessary to detect inflammatory disease of peripheral joints. It should be emphasized that early in the course of mild cases, symptoms may be subtle and nonspecific, and the physical examination may be completely normal.

The course of the disease is extremely variable, ranging from the individual with mild stiffness and radiographically equivocal sacroiliitis to the patient with a totally fused spine and severe bilateral hip arthritis, possibly accompanied by severe peripheral arthritis and extraarticular manifestations. Pain tends to be persistent early in the disease and then to become intermittent, with alternating exacerbations and quiescent periods. In a typical severe untreated case with progression of the spondylitis to syndesmophyte formation, the patient's posture undergoes characteristic changes. The lumbar lordosis is obliterated with accompanying atrophy of the buttocks. The thoracic kyphosis is accentuated. If the cervical spine is involved, there may be a forward stoop of the neck. Hip involvement with ankylosis may lead to flexion contractures, compensated by flexion at the knees. The progression of the disease may be followed by measuring the patient's height, chest expansion, Schober test, and occiput-to-wall distance when the patient stands erect with the heels and back flat against the wall. Occasional individuals are encountered with advanced physical findings suggestive of long-standing AS who report having never had significant symptoms.

Onset of the disease in adolescence correlates both with a worse prognosis and more frequent and severe hip involvement. The disease in women tends to progress less frequently to total spinal ankylosis, although there is some evidence for an increased prevalence of isolated cervical ankylosis and peripheral arthritis in women. In industrialized countries, peripheral arthritis (distal to hips and shoulders) occurs overall in about 25 percent of patients, usually as a late manifestation, whereas in developing countries, the prevalence is much higher, with onset typically early in the disease course.

The most serious complication of the spinal disease is spinal fracture, which can occur with even minor trauma to the rigid, osteoporotic spine. The cervical spine is most commonly involved, and this can lead to quadriplegia. Cauda equina syndrome and slowly progressive upper pulmonary lobe fibrosis are rare complications of long-standing AS. The prevalence of aortic insufficiency and of cardiac conduction disturbances, including third-degree heart block, increases with prolonged disease. Prostatitis has been reported to have an increased prevalence in men with AS. Amyloidosis is only rarely associated (see Chap. 309).

Despite the persistence of the disease, most patients with AS remain gainfully employed. Only in uncommon instances does the disease appear to shorten life, these being largely the result of spinal trauma, complications of therapy such as upper gastrointestinal hemorrhage, aortic insufficiency, respiratory failure, or amyloid nephropathy.

LABORATORY FINDINGS No laboratory test is diagnostic of AS. In most ethnic groups, the HLA-B27 gene is present in approximately 90 percent of patients with AS. Most patients with active disease have an elevated erythrocyte sedimentation rate and an elevated level of C-reactive protein. A mild normochromic, normocytic anemia may be present. Patients with severe disease may show an elevated alkaline phosphatase level. Elevated serum IgA levels are common. Rheumatoid factor and antinuclear antibodies are uniformly absent unless caused by a coexistent disease unrelated to AS. Synovial fluid from inflamed peripheral joints in AS is not distinctly different from that of other inflammatory joint diseases. In cases with restriction of chest wall motion, decreased vital capacity and increased functional residual capacity are common, but airflow measurements are normal and ventilatory function is usually well maintained.

RADIOGRAPHIC FINDINGS Radiographically demonstrable sacroiliitis is usually present in AS. The earliest changes in the sacroiliac joints demonstrable by standard radiography are blurring of the cortical margins of the subchondral bone, followed by erosions and sclerosis. Progression of the erosions leads to "pseudowidening" of the joint space; as fibrous and then bony ankylosis supervene, the joints may become obliterated radiographically. The changes and progression of the lesions are usually symmetric.

In mild cases, years may elapse before unequivocal sacroiliac abnormalities are evident on plain radiographs. Computed tomography (CT) and magnetic resonance imaging can detect abnormalities reliably at an earlier stage than plain radiography, but the role of these techniques in routine diagnosis is not yet settled.

Roentgenographic abnormalities generally appear in the sacroiliac joints before appearing elsewhere in the spine. In the lumbar spine, progression of the disease leads to straightening, caused by loss of lordosis, and reactive sclerosis, caused by osteitis of the anterior corners of the vertebral bodies with subsequent erosion, leading to "squaring" of the vertebral bodies. Progressive ossification of the superficial layers of the annulus fibrosus leads to eventual formation of marginal syndesmophytes, visible on plain films as bony bridges connecting successive vertebral bodies anteriorly and laterally.

DIAGNOSIS The diagnosis of early AS before the development of irreversible deformity can be difficult to establish. Currently, modified New York criteria (1984) are widely used for diagnosis. These consist of the following: (1) a history of inflammatory back pain (see below); (2) limitation of motion of the lumbar spine in both the sagittal and frontal planes; (3) limited chest expansion, relative to standard values for age and sex; and (4) definite radiographic sacroiliitis. Under these criteria, the presence of radiographic sacroiliitis plus any one of the other three criteria is sufficient for a diagnosis of definite AS.

Several studies have identified a sizable population of B27-positive individuals with symptoms suggestive of AS who lack definite radiographic sacroiliitis. Over time, most of these patients eventually develop radiographic changes. This indicates that diagnostic criteria based on plain radiographic findings may often be too insensitive for the diagnosis of early AS. The presence of B27 is neither necessary nor sufficient for the diagnosis, but the B27 test can be helpful in patients who have not yet developed radiographic sacroiliitis.

AS must be differentiated from numerous other causes of low-back pain, some of which are far more common than AS. The inflammatory back pain of AS is usually distinguished by the following five features: (1) age of onset below 40, (2) insidious onset, (3) duration greater than 3 months before medical attention is sought, (4) morning stiffness, and (5) improvement with exercise or activity. The most common causes of back pain other than AS are primarily mechanical or degenerative rather than inflammatory and do not show these features. Less common metabolic, infectious, and malignant causes of back pain also must be differentiated from AS.

Marked calcification and ossification of paraspinous ligaments occur in *diffuse idiopathic skeletal hyperostosis* (DISH). Although DISH is often categorized as a variant of osteoarthritis, diarthrodial joints are not involved. Ligamentous calcification and ossification are usually most prominent in the anterior spinal ligament and give the appearance of "flowing wax" on the anterior bodies of the vertebrae. However, a radiolucency may be seen between the newly deposited bone and the vertebral body, differentiating DISH from the marginal osteophytes in spondylosis. Intervertebral disk spaces are preserved, and sacroiliac and apophyseal joints appear normal, helping to differentiate DISH from spondylosis and from AS, respectively.

DISH occurs in the middle-aged and the elderly and is more common in men than in women. Patients are frequently asymptomatic but may have stiffness. Radiographic changes are generally much more severe than might be predicted from the mild symptoms caused by DISH.

℞ TREATMENT

There is no definitive treatment for AS. The principal goal of management is the conscientious participation by the patient in an exercise program designed to maintain functional posture and to preserve range of motion. There is evidence that exercise increases mobility and improves function. Most patients require anti-inflammatory agents to achieve sufficient symptomatic relief to be able to remain functional and carry out the exercise program. It is not known whether drug treatment alone can alter the progression of the disease.

Several nonsteroidal anti-inflammatory drugs (NSAIDs) have proved effective in reducing the pain and stiffness of AS and are commonly used. Indomethacin is particularly effective as a 75-mg slow-release preparation taken once or twice daily. Although phenylbutazone, at doses of 200 to 400 mg/d, has been considered by several authorities to be the most effective agent in AS, because of its greater potential for serious side effects such as aplastic anemia and agranulocytosis, its use in the United States is confined to patients with very severe disease whose symptoms do not respond at all to other agents. Recent controlled trials suggest that sulfasalazine,[1] in doses of 2 to 3 g/d, is useful in reducing peripheral joint symptoms as well as reversing laboratory evidence of inflammation. Some studies have not shown it to benefit axial arthritis, and its effect on natural progression of the disease is unproven. The peripheral arthritis also may respond to the folic acid antagonist methotrexate.[1] No therapeutic role for gold, penicillamine, immunosuppressive drugs, or systemic glucocorticoids has been documented in AS. Occasionally, intralesional or intraarticular glucocorticoid injections may be beneficial in patients with persistent enthesopathy or synovitis unresponsive to anti-inflammatory agents. Recent studies have suggested that symptomatic benefit can be achieved from CT-guided glucocorticoid injections into the sacroiliac joints.

The most common indication for surgery in patients with AS is severe hip joint arthritis, the pain and stiffness of which are often dramatically relieved by total hip arthroplasty. A small number of patients may benefit from surgical correction of extreme flexion deformities of the spine or of atlantoaxial subluxation.

Attacks of iritis are usually effectively managed with local glucocorticoid administration in conjunction with mydriatic agents. Coexistent cardiac disease may require pacemaker implantation or aortic valve replacement.

REACTIVE ARTHRITIS AND UNDIFFERENTIATED SPONDYLOARTHROPATHY

Reactive arthritis (ReA) refers to acute nonpurulent arthritis complicating an infection elsewhere in the body. In recent years, the term has been used primarily to refer to spondyloarthropathies following enteric or urogenital infections and occurring predominantly in individuals with the histocompatibility antigen HLA-B27. Included in this category is the constellation of clinical findings formerly commonly called *Reiter's syndrome*. Other forms of reactive arthritis not associated with B27 and showing a different spectrum of clinical features, such as rheumatic fever, are discussed elsewhere (see Chap. 236).

HISTORICAL BACKGROUND The association of acute arthritis with episodes of diarrhea or urethritis has been recognized for centuries. A large number of cases during World Wars I and II focused attention on the triad of arthritis, urethritis, and conjunctivitis, which became known as Reiter's syndrome, often occurring with additional mucocutaneous lesions.

The identification of bacterial species capable of triggering the clinical syndrome and the finding that up to three-fourths of the patients possess the B27 antigen have led to the unifying concept of ReA as a clinical syndrome triggered by specific etiologic agents in a genetically susceptible host. A similar spectrum of clinical manifestations can be triggered by enteric infection with any of several *Shigella*, *Salmonella*, *Yersinia*, and *Campylobacter* species, by genital infection with *Chlamydia trachomatis*, and possibly by other agents as well. Although Reiter's syndrome can be said to represent one part of the spectrum of the clinical manifestations of ReA, particularly that induced by *Shigella* or *Chlamydia*, the term is now largely of historical interest only. Since most patients with spondyloarthropathy do not have the classic features of Reiter's syndrome, it has become customary to employ the term *reactive arthritis*, regardless of whether or not there is evidence for a triggering infection. For the purposes of this chapter, the use of ReA will be restricted to those cases of spondyloarthropathy in which there is at least presumptive evidence for a related antecedent infection. Patients with clinical features of ReA who lack both evidence of an antecedent infection and the classic findings of Reiter's syndrome

[1] Azathioprine, methotrexate, and sulfasalazine have not been approved for this purpose by the Food and Drug Administration at the time of publication.

will be considered to have *undifferentiated spondyloarthropathy*, which is discussed at the end of this chapter.

EPIDEMIOLOGY Like AS, ReA occurs predominantly in individuals who have inherited the B27 gene; in most series, 60 to 85 percent of patients are B27 positive. In epidemics of arthritogenic bacterial infection, e.g., *S. flexneri*, it has been estimated that ReA develops in ~20 percent of exposed B27-positive individuals. In families with multiple cases of AS or ReA, the two conditions have been said to "breed true," i.e., to be uncommonly found together within an individual family. Whether this is caused by genetic or environmental factors is not known. The disease is most common in individuals 18 to 40 years of age, but it can occur both in children over 5 years of age and in older adults.

The sex ratio in ReA following enteric infection is nearly 1:1, whereas venereally acquired ReA is predominantly a male disease. The overall prevalence and incidence of ReA are difficult to assess because of the variable prevalence of the triggering infections and genetic susceptibility factors in different populations. For example, in Olmsted County, MN, the incidence was estimated as 3.5 cases per 100,000 population per year. In contrast, in a population with a high rate of genitourinary and/or gastrointestinal infections such as urban homosexual and bisexual men, the prevalence may approach 1 per 1000.

A particularly severe form of peripheral spondyloarthropathy has been described in patients with AIDS (see Chap. 308). Most of these patients are HLA-B27 positive, but human immunodeficiency virus (HIV) infection per se is not an independent risk factor for spondyloarthropathy.

PATHOLOGY Synovial histology is similar to that of other inflammatory arthropathies. Enthesitis is a common clinical finding in ReA; the histology of this lesion resembles that of AS. Microscopic histopathologic evidence of inflammation has occasionally been noted in the colon and ileum of patients with postvenereal ReA, but much less commonly than in postenteric ReA. The skin lesions of keratoderma blenorrhagica, which is associated mainly with venereally acquired ReA, are histologically indistinguishable from psoriatic lesions.

ETIOLOGY AND PATHOGENESIS The first bacterial infection noted to be causally related to ReA was *S. flexneri*. An outbreak of shigellosis among Finnish troops in 1944 resulted in numerous cases of ReA. Of the four species *S. sonnei*, *S. boydii*, *S. flexneri*, and *S. dysenteriae*, *S. flexneri* has most often been implicated in cases of ReA, both sporadic and epidemic. *S. sonnei*, although responsible for the majority of cases of shigellosis in the United States, has only rarely been implicated in cases of ReA.

Other bacteria that have been definitively identified as triggers of ReA include several *Salmonella* species, *Y. enterocolitica*, *C. jejuni*, and *C. trachomatis*. There is suggestive evidence implicating several other microorganisms, including *Y. pseudotuberculosis*, *Clostridium difficile*, *Neisseria gonorrhoeae*, and *Ureaplasma urealyticum*. *Chlamydia pneumoniae*, a respiratory pathogen, has also recently been implicated in triggering ReA. There are also numerous isolated reports of acute arthritis preceded by other bacterial, viral, or parasitic infections, but whether the microorganisms involved are actual triggers of ReA remains to be determined.

It has not been determined whether ReA occurs by the same pathogenic mechanism following infection with each of these microorganisms, nor has the mechanism been fully elucidated in the case of any one of the known bacterial triggers. Most, if not all, of the triggering organisms share a capacity to attack mucosal surfaces, to invade host cells, and survive intracellularly. Antigens from *Chlamydia*, *Yersinia*, *Salmonella*, and *Shigella* have been shown to be present in the synovium of patients with ReA for long periods following the acute attack. In the case of *C. trachomatis*, synovial persistence of microbial DNA and RNA suggests the presence of viable organisms, despite uniform failure to culture the organism from these specimens. It is thus conceivable that the disorder may be a form of chronic infection, rather than solely "reactive." T cells that specifically respond to antigens of the inciting organism are typically found in inflamed synovium but not in peripheral blood of patients with ReA. These T cells are predominantly CD4+, but CD8+ B27-restricted bacteria-specific cytolitic T cells have also been isolated in *Yersinia*- and *C. trachomatis*-induced ReA. The antibody response to *Yersinia*, *Salmonella*, and, in some studies, *C. trachomatis* tends to be more prolonged in patients developing ReA triggered by infection with these organisms than in individuals with uncomplicated infection. The role of these various immune responses in disease pathogenesis is not yet known.

The role of HLA-B27 in ReA remains to be determined. Transgenic rats with high expression of B27 spontaneously develop a multiple organ system inflammatory disease affecting the gut, peripheral and axial joints, male genital tract, and skin that resembles these human conditions clinically and histologically. When raised in a germ-free environment, the B27 rats do not develop gut or joint inflammation, but the skin and genital lesions are not prevented. These findings suggest that bacteria are necessary, and normal gut bacteria are sufficient, to induce B27-related joint inflammation. In both the rat and human diseases, it remains to be determined whether the primary process is an autoimmune response against host tissues or an immune response against antigens of the triggering organism that have disseminated to the target tissues, and the specific role of B27 itself remains to be determined.

CLINICAL FEATURES The clinical manifestations of ReA constitute a spectrum that ranges from an isolated, transient monarthritis to severe multisystem disease. In the majority of cases, a careful history will elicit some evidence of an antecedent infection 1 to 4 weeks before the onset of symptoms of the reactive disease. However, in a sizable minority, no clinical or laboratory evidence of an antecedent infection can be found. In many cases of presumed venereally acquired reactive disease, there is a history of a recent new sexual partner, even in the absence of laboratory evidence of infection.

Constitutional symptoms are common, including fatigue, malaise, fever, and weight loss. The musculoskeletal symptoms are usually acute in onset. Arthritis is usually asymmetric and additive, with involvement of new joints occurring over a period of a few days to 1 to 2 weeks. The joints of the lower extremities, especially the knee, ankle, and subtalar, metatarsophalangeal, and toe interphalangeal joints, are the most common sites of involvement, but the wrist and fingers can be involved as well. The arthritis is usually quite painful, and tense joint effusions are not uncommon, especially in the knee. Dactylitis, or "sausage digit," a diffuse swelling of a solitary finger or toe, is a distinctive feature of both ReA and psoriatic arthritis (see Chap. 325). Tendinitis and fasciitis are particularly characteristic lesions, producing pain at multiple insertion sites, especially the Achilles insertion, the plantar fascia, and sites along the axial skeleton. Spinal and low-back pain are quite common and may be caused by insertional inflammation, muscle spasm, acute sacroiliitis, or, presumably, arthritis in intervertebral articulations.

Urogenital lesions may occur throughout the course of the disease. In males, urethritis may be marked or relatively asymptomatic and may be either an accompaniment of the triggering infection or a result of the reactive phase of the disease. Prostatitis is also common. Similarly, in females, cervicitis or salpingitis may be caused either by the infectious trigger or by the sterile reactive process.

Ocular disease is common, ranging from transient, asymptomatic conjunctivitis to an aggressive anterior uveitis that occasionally proves refractory to treatment and may result in blindness.

Mucocutaneous lesions are frequent. Oral ulcers tend to be superficial, transient, and often asymptomatic. The characteristic skin lesions, *keratoderma blenorrhagica*, consist of vesicles that become hyperkeratotic, ultimately forming a crust before disappearing. They are most common on the palms and soles but may occur elsewhere as well. In patients with HIV infection, these lesions are often extremely severe and extensive, to the point of dominating the clinical picture (see Chap. 308). Lesions on the glans penis, termed *circinate balanitis*, are common; these consist of vesicles that quickly rupture to form painless superficial erosions, which in circumcised individuals can form crusts similar to those of keratoderma blenorrhagica. Nail changes are common and consist of onycholysis, distal yellowish discoloration, and/or heaped-up hyperkeratosis.

Less frequent or rare manifestations of ReA include cardiac conduction defects, aortic insufficiency, central or peripheral nervous system lesions, and pleuropulmonary infiltrates.

Long-term follow-up studies suggest that some joint symptoms persist in 30 to 60 percent of patients with ReA. Recurrences of the acute syndrome are common, and as many as 25 percent of patients either become unable to work or are forced to change occupations because of persistent joint symptoms. Chronic heel pain is often a particularly distressing symptom. Some aspects of ankylosing spondylitis are also common sequelae (see below). In some but not all studies, HLA-B27-positive patients have shown a worse outcome than B27-negative patients. The extent to which the long-term prognosis varies with different inciting agents is not known. However, patients with *Yersinia*-induced arthritis appear to have less chronic disease than those whose initial episode follows epidemic shigellosis.

LABORATORY AND RADIOGRAPHIC FINDINGS The erythrocyte sedimentation rate is elevated during the acute phase of the disease. Mild anemia may be present, and acute phase reactants tend to be increased. Synovial fluid is nonspecifically inflammatory, showing an elevated white cell count with a predominance of neutrophils. In most ethnic groups, 50 to 75 percent of the patients are B27 positive, although some recent studies of ReA following *Salmonella* epidemics have shown a B27 prevalence of 30 percent or less. It is unusual for the triggering infection to persist at the site of primary mucosal infection through the time of onset of the reactive disease, but it may occasionally be possible to culture the organism, e.g., in the case of *Yersinia*- or *Chlamydia*-induced disease. Serologic evidence of a recent infection may be present, such as a marked elevation of antibodies to *Yersinia*, *Salmonella*, or *Chlamydia*.

In early or mild disease, radiographic changes may be absent or confined to juxtaarticular osteoporosis. With long-standing persistent disease, marginal erosions and loss of joint space can be seen in affected joints. Periostitis with reactive new bone formation is characteristic of the disease, as it is with all the spondyloarthropathies. Spurs at the insertion of the plantar fascia are common.

Sacroiliitis and spondylitis may be seen as late sequelae. The sacroiliitis is more commonly asymmetric than in AS, and the spondylitis, rather than ascending symmetrically from the lower lumbar segments, can begin anywhere along the lumbar spine. The syndesmophytes may be coarse and nonmarginal, arising from the middle of a vertebral body, a pattern rarely seen in primary AS. Progression to spinal fusion as a sequela of ReA is uncommon.

DIAGNOSIS ReA is a clinical diagnosis, there being no definitively diagnostic laboratory test or radiographic finding. The diagnosis should be entertained in any patient with an acute inflammatory, asymmetric, additive arthritis or tendinitis. The evaluation of such a patient should include careful questioning regarding possible antecedent triggering events such as an episode of diarrhea or dysuria. On physical examination, careful attention must be paid to the distribution of the joint and tendon involvement and to possible sites of extraarticular involvement, such as the eyes, mucous membranes, skin, nails, and genitalia. Synovial fluid aspiration and analysis may be helpful in excluding septic or crystal-induced arthritis.

Although typing for B27 is not needed to secure the diagnosis in clear-cut cases, it may have prognostic significance in terms of severity, chronicity, and the propensity for spondylitis and uveitis. Furthermore, it can be helpful diagnostically in atypical cases, a positive test increasing and a negative test decreasing the probability of ReA.

It is particularly important to differentiate ReA from disseminated gonococcal disease, both of which can be venereally acquired and associated with urethritis (see Chap. 150). Gonococcal arthritis and tenosynovitis tend to involve both upper and lower extremities equally, whereas in ReA lower extremity symptoms usually predominate. Back pain is common in ReA but is not a feature of gonococcal disease, whereas the vesicular skin lesions characteristic of disseminated gonococcal disease are not found in ReA. A positive gonococcal culture from the urethra or cervix does not exclude a diagnosis of ReA; however, culturing gonococci from blood, skin lesion, or synovium establishes the diagnosis of disseminated gonococcal disease. Occasionally, the only definitive way to distinguish the two is through a therapeutic trial of antibiotics.

ReA shares many features in common with psoriatic arthropathy, including the asymmetry of the arthritis, a propensity for "sausage digits" and nail involvement, an association with uveitis, and skin lesions of similar histology (see Chap. 325). However, psoriatic arthritis is usually gradual in onset, the arthritis tends to affect primarily the upper extremities, and there is less associated periarthritis. Psoriatic arthritis is not associated with mouth ulcers or urethritis, or, usually, with bowel symptoms. Although psoriatic arthropathy shows some distinctive radiographic features that are not found in ReA, these occur only late in the disease and are of little help diagnostically. Only psoriatic spondylitis, not the peripheral arthritis, is associated with B27, about 50 percent of patients being positive. Occasional patients, usually B27 positive, following what appears to be a typical episode of ReA, will develop typical psoriasis and persistent arthritis such that the two entities become indistinguishable.

Undifferentiated spondyloarthropathy, or simply "spondyloarthropathy," is diagnosed in patients who lack evidence of an antecedent infection that might trigger ReA and who do not meet criteria for AS but who show clinical features of these disorders.

℞ TREATMENT

Most patients with ReA are benefitted to some degree by NSAIDs, although rarely are symptoms of the acute arthritis completely ameliorated, and some patients fail to respond at all. Indomethacin, 75 to 150 mg/d in divided doses, is the initial treatment of choice. Other NSAIDs may be tried, with phenylbutazone, 100 mg tid or qid, being the NSAID of last resort, to be used only in severe, refractory cases because of its potentially serious side effects.

It is unclear whether antibiotics have a role in the therapy of ReA. One controlled study suggested that prolonged administration of a long-acting tetracycline may accelerate recovery from *Chlamydia*-induced ReA, but subsequent results have been less encouraging, and therapy for other bacterial triggers of ReA has shown little or no benefit. However, there is evidence that prompt, appropriate antibiotic treatment of acute chlamydial urethritis may prevent subsequent reactive arthritis.

Two recent multicenter trials have suggested that sulfasalazine, up to 3 g/d in divided doses, may be beneficial to patients with persistent ReA.[1] Patients with debilitating symptoms refractory to NSAID and sulfasalazine therapy may respond to immunosuppressive agents such as azathioprine, 1 to 2 mg/kg per day, or to methotrexate, 7.5 to 15 mg per week. Systemic glucocorticoids are not generally used but in rare instances may be helpful in mobilizing a severely affected bedridden patient. Antimalarials, gold, and penicillamine are not useful in the treatment of ReA.

Tendinitis and other enthesitic lesions occasionally may benefit from intralesional glucocorticoids. Uveitis may require aggressive treatment with glucocorticoids to prevent serious sequelae. Skin lesions ordinarily require only symptomatic treatment. In patients with HIV infection and ReA, many of whom have severe skin lesions, the skin lesions in particular appear to respond to systemic treatment with zidovudine (see Chap. 308). Cardiac complications are managed conventionally; management of neurologic complications is symptomatic.

Patients need to be educated about the nature of the disease and the factors that predispose to its recurrence. Comprehensive management includes counseling of patients in the avoidance of sexually transmitted disease and exposure to enteropathogens, as well as appropriate use of physical therapy, vocational counseling, and continued surveillance for long-term complications such as ankylosing spondylitis.

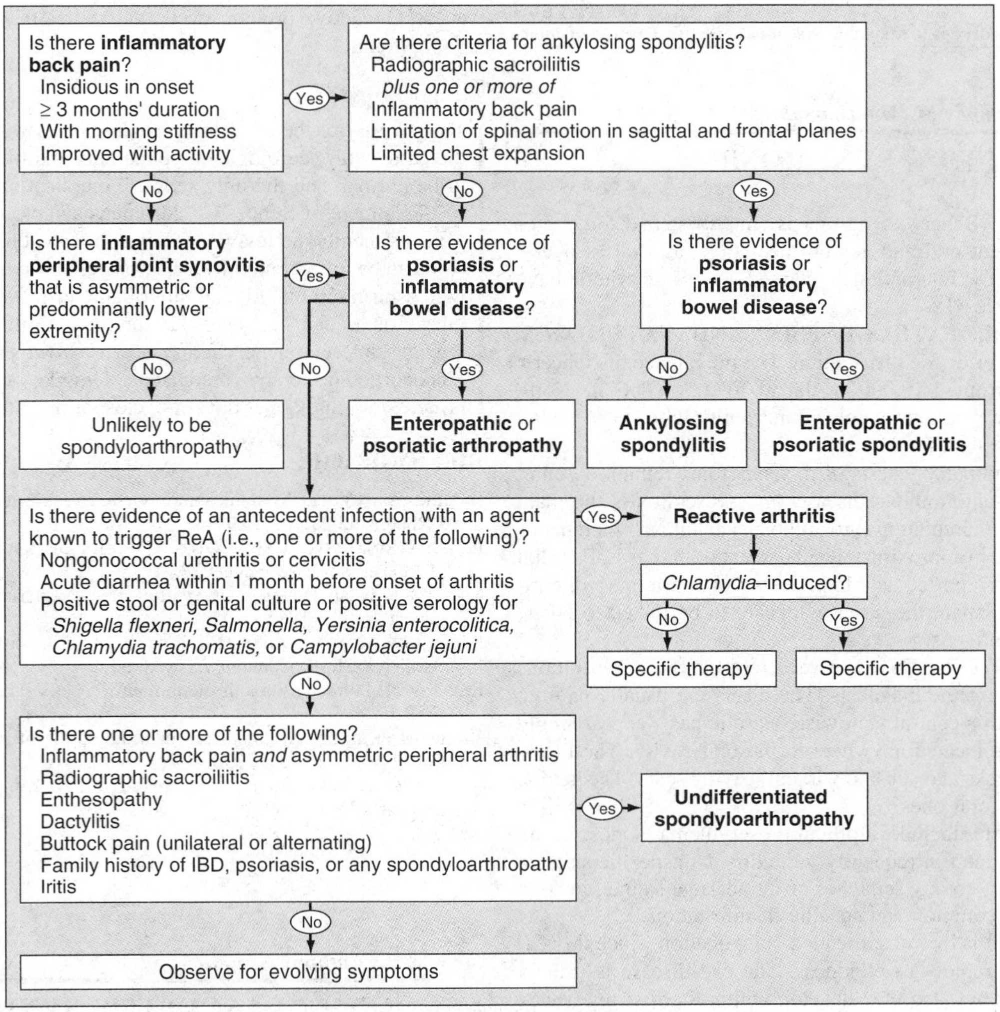

FIGURE 317-1 Algorithm for diagnosis of the spondyloarthropathies.

UNDIFFERENTIATED AND JUVENILE-ONSET SPONDYLOARTHROPATHY

It is not uncommon for clinicians to encounter patients, usually young adults, who do not have inflammatory bowel disease or psoriasis, lack evidence of an antecedent triggering infection, and do not have the classic triad of Reiter's syndrome or meet criteria for ankylosing spondylitis, who nonetheless present with some features of one or more of the spondyloarthropathies discussed above. For example, a patient may present with inflammatory synovitis of one knee, Achilles tendinitis, and dactylitis of one digit ("sausage digit"). It is now common to consider such patients as having *undifferentiated spondyloarthropathy*, or simply *spondyloarthropathy*. Other terms for this condition have included *seronegative oligoarthritis*, *undifferentiated oligoarthritis*, and the now-outmoded *incomplete Reiter's syndrome*. It is likely that some, perhaps most, of these patients have ReA in which the triggering infection remains undetected. In some other cases, the patient subsequently develops inflammatory bowel disease or psoriasis or the process eventually meets criteria for ankylosing spondylitis. Approximately half the patients with undifferentiated spondyloarthropathy are HLA-B27 positive, and thus the absence of B27 is not useful in establishing or excluding the diagnosis.

In *juvenile-onset spondyloarthropathy*, which begins most commonly in boys between ages 7 and 16, an asymmetric, predominantly lower extremity oligoarthritis and enthesitis without extraarticular features is the typical mode of presentation. The prevalence of B27 in this condition, which has been termed the *SEA syndrome* (seronegative, enthesopathy, arthropathy), is approximately 80 percent. Many of these patients go on to develop typical ankylosing spondylitis in late adolescence or adulthood.

Management of undifferentiated spondyloarthropathy is similar to that of the other spondyloarthropathies, with NSAIDs and physical therapy forming the mainstays of treatment. Textbooks of pediatrics should be consulted for information on management of juvenile-onset spondyloarthropathy. An algorithm for the diagnosis of the spondyloarthropathies in adults is presented in Fig. 317-1.

BIBLIOGRAPHY

Calin A and Taurog JD (eds): *The Spondyloarthritides.* Oxford, Oxford University Press, 1997

Dougados M et al: Sulfasalazine in the treatment of spondylarthrapathy. A randomized, multicenter, double-blind, placebo-controlled study. Arthritis Rheum 38:618, 1995

Gall V: Exercise in the spondyloarthropathies. Arthritis Care Res 7:214, 1994

Leirisalo-Repo M: Are antibiotics of any use in reactive arthritis? APMIS 101:575, 1993

Mielants H et al: The evolution of spondyloarthropathy in relation to gut histology. J Rheumatol 22:2266, 1995

Nanagara R et al: Alteration of *Chlamydia trachomatis* biologic behavior in synovial membranes: Suppression of surface antigen production in reactive arthritis and Reiter's syndrome. Arthritis Rheum 38:1410, 1995

Taurog JD et al: The germfree state prevents development of gut and joint inflammatory disease in HLA-B27 transgenic rats. J Exp Med 180:2359, 1994

318 BEHÇET'S SYNDROME

Haralampos M. Moutsopoulos

DEFINITION Behçet's syndrome is a multisystem disorder presenting with recurrent oral and genital ulcerations as well as ocular involvement. Recently, internationally agreed diagnostic criteria have been proposed (Table 318-1).

PREVALENCE, PATHOGENESIS, AND PATHOLOGY The disease has a worldwide distribution. The prevalence of Behçet's syndrome ranges from 1:10,000 in Japan to 1:500,000 in North America and Europe. It affects mainly young adults, with males having more severe disease than females.

The etiology and pathogenesis of this syndrome remain obscure; it is considered an autoimmune disease since vasculitis is the main pathologic lesion and circulating autoantibodies to human oral mucous membrane are found in approximately 50 percent of the cases. Familial occurrence has been reported, and in patients from eastern Mediterranean countries and Japan, the disease appears to be linked to HLA-B5 and -DR5 alloantigens.

CLINICAL FEATURES The recurrent aphthous ulcerations are a *sine qua non* for the diagnosis. The ulcers are usually painful, shallow or deep with a central yellowish necrotic base, appear singly or in crops, and are located anywhere in the oral cavity. The ulcers persist for 1 to 2 weeks and subside without leaving scars. The genital ulcers resemble the oral ones.

Skin involvement includes folliculitis, erythema nodosum, an acne-like exanthem, and infrequently vasculitis. Nonspecific skin inflammatory reactivity to any scratches or intradermal saline injection (pathergy test) is a common and specific manifestation.

Eye involvement is the most dreaded complication, since it occasionally progresses rapidly to blindness. The eye disease is usually present at the onset but also may develop within the first few years. In addition to iritis, posterior uveitis, retinal vessel occlusions, and optic neuritis can be seen in some cases of the syndrome. Hypopyon uveitis, which is considered the hallmark of Behçet's syndrome, is in fact a rare manifestation.

The arthritis of Behçet's syndrome is not deforming and affects the knees and ankles.

Superficial or deep peripheral vein thrombosis is seen in one-fourth of the patients. Pulmonary emboli are a rare complication. The superior vena cava is obstructed occasionally, producing a dramatic clinical picture. Arterial involvement occurs infrequently and presents with aortitis or peripheral arterial aneurysm and arterial thrombosis. Pulmonary artery vasculitis presenting with dyspnea, cough, chest pain, hemoptysis, and infiltrates on chest roentgenograms has been reported recently in 5 percent of patients.

Central nervous system involvement is found more frequently in northern Europe and the United States. The most common lesions are benign intracranial hypertension, a multiple sclerosis–like picture, pyramidal involvement, and psychiatric disturbances.

Gastrointestinal involvement is reported in patients from Japan and includes mucosal ulcerations of the gut.

Laboratory findings are mainly nonspecific indices of inflammation such as leukocytosis and elevated erythrocyte sedimentation rate as well as C-reactive protein levels; antibodies to human oral mucosa are also found.

Table 318-1

Diagnostic Criteria of Behçet's Disease

Recurrent oral ulceration plus 2 of the following:
- Recurrent genital ulceration
- Eye lesions
- Skin lesions
- Pathergy test

℞ TREATMENT

The severity of the syndrome usually abates with time. Apart from the cases with neurologic complications, the life expectancy seems to be normal, and the only serious complication is blindness.

Treatment of Behçet's syndrome is symptomatic and empirical. Mucous membrane involvement may respond to topical glucocorticoids in the form of mouthwash or paste. Thrombophlebitis is treated with aspirin, 500 mg/d, and dipyridamole, 150 mg/d. Colchicine or interferon α can be beneficial for the arthritis of the syndrome. Uveitis and central nervous system involvement require systemic glucocorticoid therapy (prednisone, 1 mg/kg per day) and azathioprine, 2 to 3 mg/kg per day, or cyclosporine, 5 to 10 mg/kg per day.

BIBLIOGRAPHY

Hamurgudan V et al: Systemic interferon α2b treatment in Behçet's syndrome. J Rheumatol 21:1098, 1994

International Study Group for Behçet's Disease: Criteria of diagnosis of Behçet's disease. Lancet 335:1078, 1990

Masuda K et al: Double masked trial of cyclosporin in Behçet's disease. Lancet 1:1093, 1989

Papiris SA, Moutsopoulos HM: Rare rheumatic disorders: Behçet's disease. Baillieres Clin Rheumatol 7:173, 1993

Raz I et al: Pulmonary manifestations in Behçet's syndrome. Chest 95:585, 1989

Yazici H et al: A controlled trial of azathioprine in Behçet's syndrome. N Engl J Med 322:281, 1990

———: Behçet's syndrome, in *Rheumatology*. JH Klippel, PA Dieppe (eds). London, Mosby, 1995

319 THE VASCULITIS SYNDROMES

Anthony S. Fauci

DEFINITION *Vasculitis* is a clinicopathologic process characterized by inflammation of and damage to blood vessels. The vessel lumen is usually compromised, and this is associated with ischemia of the tissues supplied by the involved vessel. A broad and heterogeneous group of syndromes may result from this process, since any type, size, and location of blood vessel may be involved. Vasculitis and its consequences may be the primary or sole manifestation of a disease; alternatively, vasculitis may be a secondary component of another primary disease. Vasculitis may be confined to a single organ such as the skin, or it may simultaneously involve several organ systems.

PATHOPHYSIOLOGY AND PATHOGENESIS Generally, most of the vasculitic syndromes are assumed to be mediated at least in part by immunopathogenic mechanisms (see Table 319-1). However, evidence to this effect is for the most part indirect and may reflect epiphenomena as opposed to true causality. Vasculitis is generally considered within the broader category of *immune complex diseases* that include serum sickness and certain of the connective tissue diseases of which systemic lupus erythematosus (see Chap. 312) is the prototype. Although deposition of immune complexes in vessel walls is the most widely accepted pathogenic mechanism of vasculitis, the causal role of immune complexes has not been clearly established in most of the vasculitic syndromes. Circulating immune complexes need not result in deposition of the complexes in blood vessels with ensuing vasculitis, and many patients with active vasculitis do not have demonstrable circulating or deposited immune complexes. The actual antigen contained in the immune complex has only rarely been identified in vasculitic syndromes. In this regard, hepatitis B antigen has been identified in both the circulating and deposited immune complexes in a subset of patients with systemic vasculitis, most notably within the polyarteritis nodosa group (see below). Essential mixed cryoglobulinemia has been associated with hepatitis C virus infection; hepatitis

C virions and hepatitis C virus antigen-antibody complexes have been identified in the cryoprecipitates of these patients. In addition, an association between persistent parvovirus B19 infection and certain vasculitides including Wegener's granulomatosis, polyarteritis nodosa, and Kawasaki's disease has been reported; however, the pathogenic mechanisms related to this association are unclear.

The mechanisms of tissue damage in immune-complex–mediated vasculitis resemble those described for serum sickness. In this model, antigen-antibody complexes are formed in antigen excess and are deposited in vessel walls whose permeability has been increased by vasoactive amines such as histamine, bradykinin, and leukotrienes released from platelets or from mast cells as a result of IgE-triggered mechanisms. The deposition of complexes results in activation of complement components, particularly C5a, which is strongly chemotactic for neutrophils. These cells then infiltrate the vessel wall, phagocytose the immune complexes, and release their intracytoplasmic enzymes, which damage the vessel wall. As the process becomes subacute or chronic, mononuclear cells infiltrate the vessel wall. The common denominator of the resulting syndrome is compromise of the vessel lumen with ischemic changes in the tissues supplied by the involved vessel.

In addition to the classic immune-complex–mediated mechanisms of vasculitis, other immunopathogenic mechanisms may be involved in damage to vessels. The most prominent of these are delayed hypersensitivity and cell-mediated immune injury as reflected in the histopathologic feature of granulomatous vasculitis. However, immune complexes themselves may induce granulomatous responses. Vascular endothelial cells can express HLA class II molecules following activation by cytokines such as interferon γ (IFNγ). This allows these cells to participate in immunologic reactions such as interaction with CD4+ T lymphocytes in a manner similar to antigen-presenting macrophages. Endothelial cells can secrete interleukin (IL)-1 which may activate T lymphocytes and initiate or propagate in situ immunologic processes within the blood vessel. In addition, IL-1 and tumor necrosis factor α (TNFα) are potent inducers of endothelial-leukocyte adhesion molecule 1 (ELAM-1) and vascular cell adhesion molecule 1 (VCAM-1), which may enhance the adhesion of leukocytes to endothelial cells in the blood vessel wall. Other mechanisms such as direct cellular cytotoxicity or antibody directed against vessel components or antibody-dependent cellular cytotoxicity have been suggested in certain types of vessel damage. However, there is no convincing evidence to support their causal contribution to the pathogenesis of any of the recognized vasculitic syndromes.

Antineutrophil Cytoplasmic Antibodies (ANCA) ANCA are antibodies directed against certain proteins in the cytoplasm of neutrophils. They are present in a high percentage of patients with systemic vasculitis, particularly Wegener's granulomatosis, as well as in patients with necrotizing and crescentic glomerulonephritis. They are important for the diagnosis and classification of Wegener's granulomatosis and other systemic vasculitides (see sections on individual diseases). There are two major categories of ANCA based on different targets for the antibodies. The terminology of cytoplasmic (c) ANCA refers to the diffuse, granular cytoplasmic staining pattern observed by immunofluorescence microscopy when serum antibodies bind to indicator neutrophils. Proteinase-3, the 29-kDa neutral serine proteinase present in neutrophil azurophilic granules is the major c-ANCA antigen. More than 90 percent of patients with typical Wegener's granulomatosis and active glomerulonephritis have a positive c-ANCA titer. The terminology of perinuclear (p) ANCA refers to the more localized perinuclear or nuclear staining pattern of the indicator neutrophils. The major target for p-ANCA is the enzyme myeloperoxidase; elastase is infrequently the target of p-ANCA. p-ANCA have been reported to occur in variable percentages of patients with polyarteritis nodosa, Churg-Strauss syndrome, polyangiitis overlap syndrome, crescentic glomerulonephritis, and Goodpasture's syndrome, as well as in some patients with characteristics of Wegener's granulomatosis.

It is unclear why patients with these vasculitis syndromes develop ANCA, whereas ANCA are rare in other inflammatory diseases. However, once ANCA are present, there are a number of in vitro observations that suggest feasible mechanisms whereby these antibodies can contribute to the pathogenesis of the vasculitis syndromes. When neutrophils are in the resting state, proteinase-3 exists in the azurophilic granules of the cytoplasm, apparently inaccessible to serum antibodies. However, when neutrophils are primed by TNFα or IL-1, proteinase-3 translocates to the cell membrane where it can interact with extracellular ANCA. The neutrophils then degranulate and produce reactive oxygen species that can cause tissue damage. Endothelial cells also translocate their cytoplasmic proteinase-3 to the cell membrane upon priming with TNFα, IL-1, or INFγ thus rendering them susceptible to interaction with ANCA and leading possibly to tissue damage due to complement-mediated cytotoxicity or antibody-dependent cellular cytotoxicity. Despite the attractiveness of these in vitro data, there is no conclusive evidence that ANCA are directly involved in the pathogenesis of the vasculitis syndromes, and they may represent merely an epiphenomenon; in fact, a number of clinical and laboratory observations argue against a primary pathogenic linkage. Patients may have vasculitis in the absence of ANCA; the absolute height of the antibody titers does not correlate well with disease activity; and patients with vasculitis, particularly Wegener's granulomatosis, in remission may continue to have high c-ANCA titers for years. Thus, their role in the pathogenesis of systemic vasculitis remains an open question.

It is unknown why certain individuals develop vasculitis in response to certain antigenic stimuli, whereas others do not. However, it is likely that a number of factors are involved in the ultimate expression of a vasculitic syndrome. These include the genetic predisposition and the regulatory mechanisms associated with immune response to certain antigens. When immune complexes are involved in the pathogenic process, the ability of the reticuloendothelial system to clear circulating complexes from the blood, the size and physicochemical properties of immune complexes, the relative degree of turbulence of blood flow, the intravascular hydrostatic pressure in different vessels, and the preexisting integrity of the vessel endothelium likely explain why only certain types of immune complexes cause vasculitis and why the vasculitic process is selective for only certain vessels in individual patients.

CLASSIFICATION OF VASCULITIC SYNDROMES A major feature of the vasculitic syndromes as a group is the fact that there is a great deal of heterogeneity at the same time as there is considerable overlap among them. This has led to both difficulty and confusion with regard to the categorization of these diseases. The classification scheme listed in Table 319-2 takes into account this heterogeneity and overlap and will serve as a matrix to emphasize the fact that certain syndromes are predominantly systemic in nature and

Table 319-1

Potential Pathogenic Mechanisms of Blood Vessel Damage in the Vasculitis Syndromes

IMMUNOPATHOGENIC MECHANISMS
In situ formation or deposition of immune complexes in blood vessel wall
Antineutrophil cytoplasmic antibody (ANCA)–mediated blood vessel damage
Direct antibody-mediated damage via antibodies directed at endothelial cells or other tissue components
Antibody-dependent cellular cytotoxicity directed against blood vessel tissue
Cytotoxic T lymphocytes directed at blood vessel components
Granuloma formation in blood vessel wall or adjacent to blood vessel
Cytokine (i.e., IL-1, TNFα)-induced mechanisms: expression of adhesion molecules for leukocytes on endothelial cells; induction of cytokine secretion by endothelial cells; procoagulant effects; prime neutrophils for ANCA-induced degranulation
NONIMMUNOPATHOGENIC MECHANISMS
Infiltration of blood vessel wall or surrounding tissue by microbial agents
Direct invasion of blood vessel wall by neoplastic cells
Unidentified mechanisms

almost invariably lead to irreversible organ system dysfunction and even death if untreated, while others are usually localized to the skin and rarely result in irreversible dysfunction of vital organs. The distinguishing and overlapping features of the diseases listed in Table 319-2, which justify this classification scheme, will be discussed below.

Approach to the Patient

Given the heterogeneous nature of the vasculitis syndromes, workup of a patient with suspected vasculitis should follow a series of progressive steps that establish the diagnosis of vasculitis, determine where possible the category of the vasculitis syndrome (Table 319-2), and determine the pattern and extent of disease activity. This information should then be utilized to determine the choice of therapeutic options (Fig. 319-1). This approach is of considerable importance since several of the vasculitis syndromes require aggressive therapy with glucocorticoids and immunosuppressive agents, while other syndromes usually resolve spontaneously and require symptomatic treatment only. Vasculitis is often suspected on clinical and laboratory grounds (see individual syndromes below). Depending on the individual category of vasculitis, measurement of ANCA titers may be helpful in this regard. However, a diagnosis of a vasculitis syndrome should not be made nor should treatment be initiated on the basis of a positive ANCA titer alone. The definitive diagnosis of vasculitis is made upon biopsy of involved tissue. The yield of "blind" biopsies of organs with no subjective or objective evidence of involvement is very low and should be avoided. When syndromes such as classic polyarteritis nodosa, Takayasu's arteritis, or the polyangiitis overlap syndrome are suspected, angiogram of organs with suspected involvement should be performed. However, angiograms should not be routinely performed when patients present with localized cutaneous vasculitis with no clinical indication of visceral involvement.

The constellation of clinical, laboratory, biopsy, and radiographic findings usually allows proper categorization to a specific syndrome, and therapy where appropriate should be initiated according to this information (see individual syndromes below). If an offending antigen that precipitates the vasculitis is recognized, the antigen should be removed where possible. If the syndrome resolves, no further action should be taken. If disease activity continues, treatment should be initiated. If the vasculitis is associated with an underlying disease such as an infection, neoplasm, or connective tissue disease, the underlying disease should be treated. If the syndrome resolves, no further action should be taken. If the syndrome does not resolve or if there is no recognizable underlying disease and the vasculitis persists, treatment should be initiated according to the category of the vasculitis syndrome. Treatment options will be considered under the individual syndromes, and general principles of therapy will be considered at the end of the chapter.

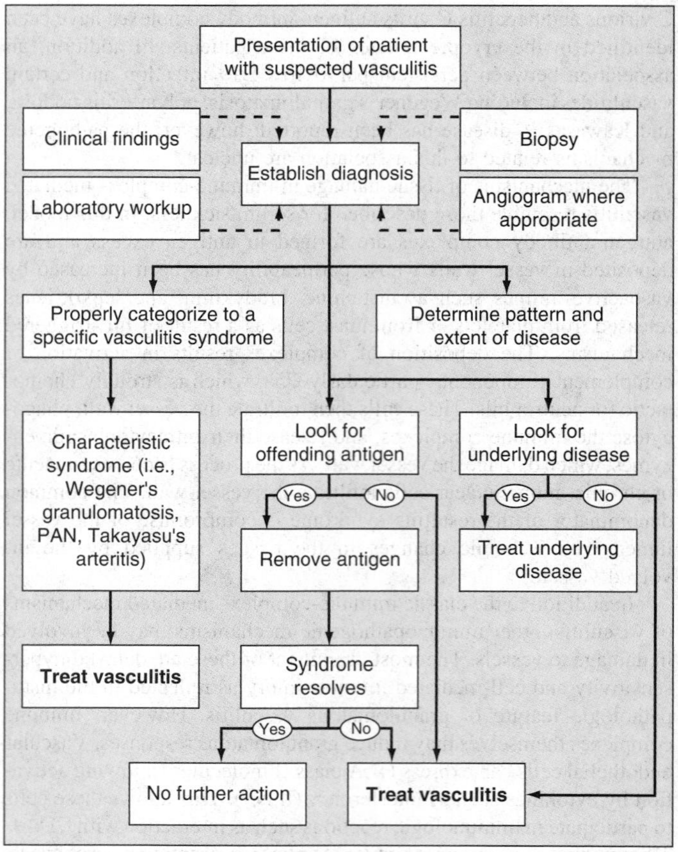

FIGURE 319-1 Algorithm for the approach to a patient with suspected diagnosis of vasculitis.

Table 319-2

Classification of the Vasculitis Syndromes

I. Systemic necrotizing vasculitis
  A. Polyarteritis nodosa (PAN)
    1. Classic PAN
    2. Microscopic polyangiitis
  B. Allergic angiitis and granulomatosis of Churg-Strauss
  C. Polyangiitis overlap syndrome
II. Wegener's granulomatosis
III. Temporal arteritis
IV. Takayasu's arteritis
V. Henoch-Schönlein purpura
VI. Predominantly cutaneous vasculitis (hypersensitivity vasculitis)
  A. Exogenous stimuli proven or suspected
    1. Drug-induced vasculitis
    2. Serum sickness and serum sickness–like reactions
    3. Vasculitis associated with infectious diseases
  B. Endogenous antigens likely involved
    1. Vasculitis associated with neoplasms (particularly lymphoid malignancies)
    2. Vasculitis associated with connective tissue diseases
    3. Vasculitis associated with other underlying diseases
    4. Vasculitis associated with congenital deficiencies of the complement system
VII. Other vasculitic syndromes
  A. Kawasaki disease
  B. Isolated central nervous system vasculitis
  C. Thromboangiitis obliterans (Buerger's disease)
  D. Behçet's syndrome
  E. Miscellaneous vasculitides

SYSTEMIC NECROTIZING VASCULITIS

POLYARTERITIS NODOSA Definition *Classic polyarteritis nodosa* (PAN) was described in 1866 by Kussmaul and Maier. It is a multisystem, necrotizing vasculitis of small and medium-sized muscular arteries in which involvement of the renal and visceral arteries is characteristic. Classic PAN does not involve pulmonary arteries, although bronchial vessels may be involved; granulomas, significant eosinophilia, and an allergic diathesis are not part of the classic syndrome. The term *microscopic polyangiitis* (microscopic polyarteritis) was introduced into the literature by Davson in 1948. The Chapel Hill Consensus Conference on the Nomenclature of Systemic Vasculitis held in 1992 officially adopted the term to connote a necrotizing vasculitis with few or no immune complexes (pauci-immune) affecting small vessels (capillaries, venules, or arterioles). Since necrotizing arteritis involving small and medium-sized arteries may also be present, it shares features with classic PAN except that glomerulonephritis is very common in microscopic polyangiitis, and pulmonary capillaritis often occurs.

Incidence and Prevalence It is difficult to establish an accurate incidence of this disease because of the fact that many reports of PAN actually have included both classic PAN and microscopic polyangiitis as well as other related vasculitides. Both diseases are uncommon, but classic PAN is felt to be more uncommon than microscopic polyangiitis. The mean age at onset in reports of PAN is 48 years, and the male-to-female ratio is 1.6:1.

Pathophysiology and Pathogenesis The vascular lesion in classic PAN is a necrotizing inflammation of small and medium-sized muscular arteries. The lesions are segmental and tend to involve bifurcations and branchings of arteries. They may spread circumferentially to involve adjacent veins. However, involvement of venules is not seen in classic PAN and, if present, suggests microscopic polyangiitis or the polyangiitis overlap syndrome (see below). In the acute stages of disease, polymorphonuclear neutrophils infiltrate all layers of the vessel wall and perivascular areas, which results in intimal proliferation and degeneration of the vessel wall. Mononuclear cells infiltrate the area as the lesions progress to the subacute and chronic stages. Fibrinoid necrosis of the vessels ensues with compromise of the lumen, thrombosis, infarction of the tissues supplied by the involved vessel, and, in some cases, hemorrhage. As the lesions heal, there is collagen deposition, which may lead to further occlusion of the vessel lumen. Aneurysmal dilatations up to 1 cm in size along the involved arteries are characteristic of classic PAN. Granulomas and substantial eosinophilia with eosinophilic tissue infiltrations are not characteristically found and suggest allergic angiitis and granulomatosis (see below).

Multiple organ systems are involved, and the clinicopathologic findings reflect the degree and location of vessel involvement and the resulting ischemic changes. As mentioned above, pulmonary arteries are not involved in classic PAN, and bronchial artery involvement is uncommon, whereas pulmonary capillaritis occurs frequently in microscopic polyangiitis. The pathology in the kidney in classic PAN is predominantly that of arteritis without glomerulonephritis. In contrast, glomerulonephritis is very common in microscopic polyangiitis. In patients with significant hypertension, typical pathologic features of glomerulosclerosis may be seen alone or superimposed on lesions of glomerulonephritis. In addition, pathologic sequelae of hypertension may be found elsewhere in the body.

The presence of hepatitis B antigenemia in approximately 20 to 30 percent of patients with systemic vasculitis, particularly of the classic PAN type, together with the isolation of circulating immune complexes composed of hepatitis B antigen and immunoglobulin, and the demonstration by immunofluorescence of hepatitis B antigen, IgM, and complement in the blood vessel walls, strongly suggest the role of immunologic phenomena in the pathogenesis of this disease. Hepatitis C infection has been reported in approximately 5 percent of patients with PAN; however, its pathogenic role in the vasculitis is unclear at present. Hairy cell leukemia can be associated with classic PAN; the pathogenic mechanisms of this association are unclear.

Clinical and Laboratory Manifestations Nonspecific signs and symptoms are the hallmarks of classic PAN. Fever, weight loss, and malaise are present in over one-half of cases. Patients usually present with vague symptoms such as weakness, malaise, headache, abdominal pain, and myalgias. Specific complaints related to the vascular involvement within a particular organ system also may dominate the presenting clinical picture as well as the entire course of the illness (Table 319-3). In classic PAN, renal involvement most commonly manifests as ischemic changes in the glomeruli, whereas in microscopic polyangiitis glomerulonephritis is the predominant renal lesion. Hypertension may be related to both the renal polyarteritis and the glomerulitis and may dominate the clinical picture. Classic PAN may involve any organ system; the clinical manifestations related to specific organ system involvement are listed in Table 319-3.

There are no diagnostic serologic tests for classic PAN. In over 75 percent of patients, the leukocyte count is elevated with a predominance of neutrophils. Eosinophilia is seen only rarely and, when present at high levels, suggests the diagnosis of allergic angiitis and granulomatosis. The anemia of chronic disease may be seen, and an elevated erythrocyte sedimentation rate (ESR) is almost always present. Other common laboratory findings reflect the particular organ involved. Hypergammaglobulinemia may be present, and up to 30 percent of patients have a positive test for hepatitis B surface antigen. Positive ANCA titers (usually of the p-ANCA type) are found in variable percentages of patients with classic PAN. Microscopic polyangiitis is strongly associated with ANCA that are usually of the p-ANCA type, but c-ANCA have also been reported. In contrast, the ANCA in Wegener's granulomatosis (see below) are almost always of the c-ANCA type, which can be helpful in distinguishing Wegener's granulomatosis from microscopic polyangiitis when both present with a pulmonary-renal syndrome. Arteriograms may demonstrate characteristic abnormalities such as aneurysms in the small and medium-sized muscular arteries of the kidneys and abdominal viscera.

Diagnosis The diagnosis of classic PAN is based on the demonstration of characteristic findings of vasculitis on biopsy material of involved organs. In the absence of easily accessible tissue for biopsy, the angiographic demonstration of involved vessels, particularly in the form of aneurysms of small and medium-sized arteries in the renal, hepatic, and visceral vasculature, is sufficient to make the diagnosis. Aneurysms of vessels are not pathognomonic of classic PAN; furthermore, aneurysms need not always be present, and angiographic findings may be limited to stenotic segments and obliteration of vessels. Biopsy of symptomatic organs such as nodular skin lesions, painful testes, and muscle groups provides the highest diagnostic yields, while blind biopsy of asymptomatic organs is frequently negative. The presence of small vessel vasculitis, particularly in the setting of glomerulonephritis and pulmonary capillaritis distinguishes microscopic polyangiitis from classic PAN.

Prognosis The prognosis of untreated classic PAN as well as that of microscopic polyangiitis is extremely poor. The usual clinical course is characterized either by fulminant deterioration or by relentless progression associated with intermittent acute flare-ups. Death usually results from renal failure; from gastrointestinal complications, particularly bowel infarcts and perforation; and from cardiovascular causes. Intractable hypertension often compounds dysfunction in other organ systems, such as the kidneys, heart, and central nervous system, leading to additional late morbidity and mortality. The 5-year survival rate of untreated patients has been reported to be 13 percent, while glucocorticoid treatment may increase this figure to over 40 percent.

Rx TREATMENT

Extremely favorable therapeutic results have been reported in classic PAN with the combination of prednisone, 1 mg/kg per day, and cyclophosphamide, 2 mg/kg per day (see "Wegener's Granulomatosis" for a detailed description of this therapeutic regimen). This regimen has been reported to result in up to a 90 percent long-term remission rate even following the discontinuation of therapy. In

Table 319-3

Clinical Manifestations Related to Organ System Involvement in Classic PAN

Organ System	Percent Incidence	Clinical Manifestations
Renal	60	Renal failure, hypertension
Musculoskeletal	64	Arthritis, arthralgia, myalgia
Peripheral nervous system	51	Peripheral neuropathy, mononeuritis multiplex
Gastrointestinal tract	44	Abdominal pain, nausea and vomiting, bleeding, bowel infarction and perforation, cholecystitis, hepatic infarction, pancreatic infarction
Skin	43	Rash, purpura, nodules, cutaneous infarcts, livedo reticularis, Raynaud's phenomenon
Cardiac	36	Congestive heart failure, myocardial infarction, pericarditis
Genitourinary	25	Testicular, ovarian, or epididymal pain
Central nervous system	23	Cerebral vascular accident, altered mental status, seizure

SOURCE: From Cupps and Fauci, p 29.

addition, long-term remissions have been reported in PAN associated with hepatitis B virus antigenemia using the antiviral agent vidarabine in combination with plasma exchange with and without glucocorticoids. Favorable results have also been reported in the treatment of PAN related to hepatitis B virus with IFNα and plasma exchange. Careful attention to the treatment of hypertension can lessen the acute and late morbidity and mortality associated with renal, cardiac, and central nervous system complications of PAN. The treatment regimen for microscopic polyangiitis is similar to that for classic PAN, particularly if glomerulonephritis is present.

ALLERGIC ANGIITIS AND GRANULOMATOSIS (CHURG-STRAUSS DISEASE) **Definition** *Allergic angiitis and granulomatosis* was described in 1951 by Churg and Strauss and is a disease characterized by granulomatous vasculitis of multiple organ systems, particularly the lung. It is similar in many respects to classic PAN, except that the former has a high frequency of lung involvement, vasculitis of blood vessels of various types or sizes (including veins and venules), intra- and extravascular granuloma formation together with eosinophilic tissue infiltration, and a strong association with severe asthma and peripheral eosinophilia.

Incidence and Prevalence Allergic angiitis and granulomatosis is an uncommon disease whose exact incidence, similar to classic PAN, is difficult to determine due to the grouping of multiple types of vasculitic syndromes in many reported series. The disease can occur at any age with the possible exception of infants. The mean age of onset is 44 years, with a male-to-female ratio of 1.3:1.

Pathophysiology and Pathogenesis The vasculitis that is characteristic of allergic angiitis and granulomatosis is similar to that of classic PAN (see above) with certain notable exceptions. In addition to small and medium-sized muscular arteries, capillaries, veins, and venules can be involved in the former disease. The characteristic histopathologic features of allergic angiitis and granulomatosis are granulomatous reactions that may be present in the tissues or even within the walls of the vessels themselves. These are usually associated with infiltration of the tissues with eosinophils. This process can occur in any organ in the body; however, in sharp contrast to classic PAN, lung involvement is predominant, with skin, cardiovascular system, kidney, peripheral nervous system, and gastrointestinal tract also commonly involved. Although the precise pathogenesis of this disease is uncertain, its strong association with asthma, its clinicopathologic manifestations which strongly suggest hypersensitivity phenomena, and its close similarity to classic PAN point to aberrant immunologic phenomena.

Clinical and Laboratory Manifestations Patients with allergic angiitis and granulomatosis exhibit nonspecific manifestations such as fever, malaise, anorexia, and weight loss similar to patients with classic PAN. In contrast to the latter disease, the pulmonary findings in allergic angiitis and granulomatosis clearly dominate the clinical picture with severe asthmatic attacks and the presence of pulmonary infiltrates. Clinically recognizable heart disease occurs in approximately one-third of patients. Heart involvement is seen at autopsy in 62 percent of cases and is the cause of death in 23 percent of patients. Skin lesions occur in approximately 70 percent of patients and include purpura in addition to cutaneous and subcutaneous nodules. Apart from the characteristic pulmonary findings, the multisystem involvement in this disease is quite similar to that of classic PAN (see above); an important exception is the fact that the renal disease in allergic angiitis and granulomatosis is less common and generally less severe than that of classic PAN.

The characteristic laboratory finding in virtually all patients with allergic angiitis and granulomatosis is a striking eosinophilia which reaches levels greater than 1000 cells/μL in more than 80 percent of patients. The other laboratory findings are similar to those of classic PAN and reflect the organ systems involved. Allergic angiitis and granulomatosis is associated with p-ANCA.

Diagnosis Similar to classic PAN, the diagnosis of allergic angiitis and granulomatosis is made by biopsy, demonstrating vasculitis in a patient with the characteristic clinical manifestations. The biopsy findings are distinctive in the latter disease in that granulomatous vasculitis with eosinophilic tissue involvement together with peripheral eosinophilia are typical. Furthermore, pulmonary involvement is extremely common and is usually manifested by severe asthma associated with pulmonary infiltrates that may be fleeting in nature.

Prognosis The prognosis of untreated allergic angiitis and granulomatosis is poor, with a reported 5-year survival of 25 percent. Unlike classic PAN, the cause of death is more likely to be related to pulmonary and cardiac disease as opposed to renal or gastrointestinal involvement.

Rx TREATMENT

Glucocorticoid therapy has been reported to increase the 5-year survival to more than 50 percent. In certain patients, the disease may be quite mild and may remit spontaneously or with short courses of glucocorticoids. In glucocorticoid failures or in patients who present with fulminant multisystem disease, the treatment of choice is a combined regimen of cyclophosphamide and alternate-day prednisone, which has resulted in a high rate of complete remission similar to the experience with classic PAN (see above).

POLYANGIITIS OVERLAP SYNDROME Many patients with systemic vasculitis manifest clinicopathologic characteristics that do not fit precisely into any classification but that have overlapping features of classic PAN, allergic angiitis and granulomatosis, Wegener's granulomatosis, Takayasu's arteritis, and the hypersensitivity group of vasculitides. This subgroup has been referred to as the *polyangiitis overlap syndrome* and is part of the major grouping of systemic necrotizing vasculitis. This entity has been designated with a distinct classification in order to avoid confusion in attempting to fit such overlap syndromes into one or other of the more classic vasculitic syndromes. This subgroup is truly a systemic vasculitis with the same potential for resulting in irreversible organ system dysfunction as the other systemic necrotizing vasculitides. The diagnostic and therapeutic considerations as well as the prognosis for this subgroup are the same as those for classic PAN and allergic angiitis and granulomatosis.

WEGENER'S GRANULOMATOSIS

DEFINITION *Wegener's granulomatosis* is a distinct clinicopathologic entity characterized by granulomatous vasculitis of the upper and lower respiratory tracts together with glomerulonephritis. In addition, variable degrees of disseminated vasculitis involving both small arteries and veins may occur.

INCIDENCE AND PREVALENCE Wegener's granulomatosis is an uncommon disease whose true incidence is difficult to determine. It is extremely rare in blacks compared with whites; the male-to-female ratio is 1:1. The disease can be seen at any age; approximately 15 percent of patients are less than 19 years of age, and only rarely does the disease occur before adolescence; the mean age of onset is approximately 40 years.

PATHOPHYSIOLOGY AND PATHOGENESIS The histopathologic hallmarks of Wegener's granulomatosis are necrotizing vasculitis of small arteries and veins together with granuloma formation which may be either intravascular or extravascular (Fig. 319-2). Lung involvement typically appears as multiple, bilateral, nodular cavitary infiltrates (Fig. 319-3), which on biopsy almost invariably reveal the typical necrotizing granulomatous vasculitis. Endobronchial disease, either in its active form or as a result of fibrous scarring, may lead to obstruction with atelectasis. Upper airway lesions, particularly those in the sinuses and nasopharynx, typically reveal inflammation, necrosis, and granuloma formation with or without vasculitis.

In its earliest form, renal involvement is characterized by a focal and segmental glomerulitis that may evolve into a rapidly progressive crescentic glomerulonephritis. Granuloma formation is only rarely seen on renal biopsy. In addition to the classic triad of upper and

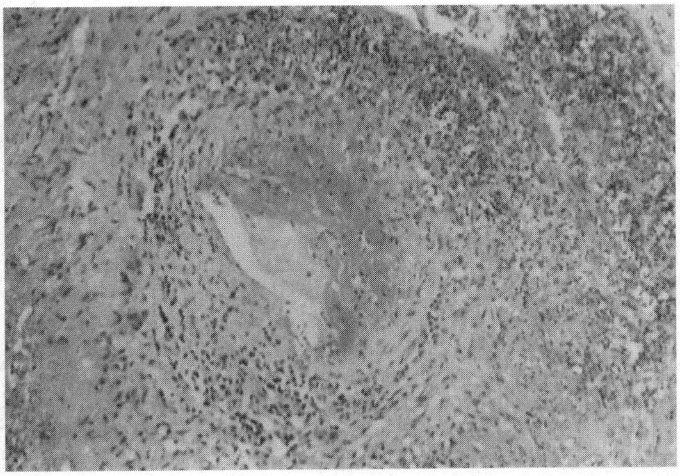

FIGURE 319-2 Lung biopsy in a patient with Wegener's granulomatosis. Biopsy revealed necrotizing vasculitis of medium-sized artery in the lung. Compromise of the vessel lumen, fibrinoid necrosis of the vessel wall, and mononuclear cell infiltration of vessel wall with early granuloma formation are seen.

lower respiratory tracts and kidney disease, virtually any organ can be involved with vasculitis, granuloma, or both.

The immunopathogenesis of this disease is unclear, although the involvement of upper airways and lungs suggests an aberrant hypersensitivity response to an exogenous or even endogenous antigen that enters through or resides in the upper airway. Chronic nasal carriage of *Staphylococcus aureus* has been reported to be associated with a higher relapse rate of Wegener's granulomatosis; however, there is no evidence for a role of this organism in the pathogenesis of the disease.

Although circulating and deposited immune complexes have been demonstrated in certain patients with Wegener's granulomatosis, there is no convincing evidence that immune complexes play a causal pathogenic role in this disease. The presence of granulomas with copious, well-defined multinucleated giant cells, particularly in involved pulmonary tissue, suggests delayed hypersensitivity and/or foreign-body reactions. However, direct evidence for either of these mechanisms is lacking.

A high percentage of patients with Wegener's granulomatosis develop ANCA; c-ANCA are the predominant ANCA in this disease. As with the other categories of vasculitis, there is no clear evidence that ANCA play a primary role in the pathogenesis of Wegener's granulomatosis.

The bronchoalveolar lavage fluid of patients with active Wegener's granulomatosis contains a high percentage of neutrophils compared with that of other granulomatous lung diseases such as sarcoidosis, in which increased numbers of lymphocytes are noted (see Chap. 320). The pathogenic significance of this difference is unclear.

CLINICAL AND LABORATORY MANIFESTATIONS A typical patient presents with severe upper respiratory tract findings such as paranasal sinus pain and drainage and purulent or bloody nasal discharge with or without nasal mucosal ulceration (Table 319-4). Nasal septal perforation may follow, leading to saddle nose deformity. Serous otitis media may occur as a result of eustachian tube blockage.

Pulmonary involvement may be manifested as asymptomatic infiltrates or may be clinically expressed as cough, hemoptysis, dyspnea, and chest discomfort. It is present in 85 to 90 percent of patients. Subglottic stenosis resulting from active disease or scarring occurs in approximately 16 percent of patients and may result in severe airway obstruction.

Eye involvement (52 percent of patients) may range from a mild conjunctivitis to dacryocystitis, episcleritis, scleritis, granulomatous sclerouveitis, ciliary vessel vasculitis, and retroorbital mass lesions leading to proptosis.

Skin lesions (46 percent of patients) appear as papules, vesicles, palpable purpura, ulcers, or subcutaneous nodules; biopsy reveals vasculitis, granuloma, or both. Cardiac involvement (8 percent of patients) manifests as pericarditis, coronary vasculitis, or, rarely, cardiomyopathy. Nervous system manifestations (23 percent of patients) include

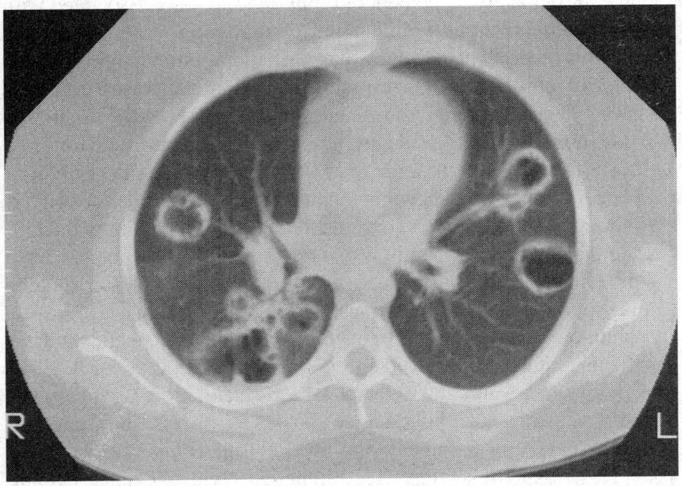

FIGURE 319-3 Computed tomography scan of a patient with Wegener's granulomatosis. The patient developed multiple, bilateral, and cavitary infiltrates.

Table 319-4

Wegener's Granulomatosis: Frequency of Clinical Manifestations in 158 Patients Studied at the National Institutes of Health

Manifestation	Percent at Disease Onset	Percent Throughout Course of Disease
Kidney		
Glomerulonephritis	18	77
Ear/nose/throat	73	92
Sinusitis	51	85
Nasal disease	36	68
Otitis media	25	44
Hearing loss	14	42
Subglottic stenosis	1	16
Ear pain	9	14
Oral lesions	3	10
Lung	45	85
Pulmonary infiltrates	25	66
Pulmonary nodules	24	58
Hemoptysis	12	30
Pleuritis	10	28
Eyes		
Conjunctivitis	5	18
Dacryocystitis	1	18
Scleritis	6	16
Proptosis	2	15
Eye pain	3	11
Visual loss	0	8
Retinal lesions	0	4
Corneal lesions	0	1
Iritis	0	2
Other*		
Arthralgias/arthritis	32	67
Fever	23	50
Cough	19	46
Skin abnormalities	13	46
Weight loss (greater than 10 percent body weight)	15	35
Peripheral neuropathy	1	15
Central nervous system disease	1	8
Pericarditis	2	6
Hyperthyroidism	1	3

* Fewer than 1 percent had parotid, pulmonary artery, breast, or lower genitourinary (urethra, cervix, vagina, testicular) involvement.

SOURCE: Hoffman et al., 1992.

cranial neuritis, mononeuritis multiplex, or, rarely, cerebral vasculitis and/or granuloma.

Renal disease (77 percent of patients) generally dominates the clinical picture and, if left untreated, accounts directly or indirectly for most of the mortality in this disease. Although it may smolder in some cases as a mild glomerulitis with proteinuria, hematuria, and red blood cell casts, it is clear that once clinically detectable renal functional impairment occurs, rapidly progressive renal failure usually ensues unless appropriate treatment is instituted.

While the disease is active, most patients have nonspecific symptoms and signs such as malaise, weakness, arthralgias, anorexia, and weight loss. Fever may indicate activity of the underlying disease but more often reflects secondary infection, usually of the upper airway.

Characteristic laboratory findings include a markedly elevated ESR, mild anemia and leukocytosis, mild hypergammaglobulinemia (particularly of the IgA class), and mildly elevated rheumatoid factor. Thrombocytosis may be seen as an acute-phase reactant; hypocomplementemia is not seen despite the presence of circulating immune complexes in some patients. In typical Wegener's granulomatosis with granulomatous vasculitis of the respiratory tract and glomerulonephritis, approximately 90 percent of patients have a positive c-ANCA. However, in the absence of renal disease, the sensitivity drops to approximately 70 percent.

DIAGNOSIS The diagnosis of Wegener's granulomatosis is a clinicopathologic one made by the demonstration of necrotizing granulomatous vasculitis on biopsy of appropriate tissue in a patient with the clinical findings of upper and lower respiratory tract disease together with evidence of glomerulonephritis. Pulmonary tissue, preferably obtained by open thoracotomy, offers the highest diagnostic yield, almost invariably revealing granulomatous vasculitis. Biopsy of upper airway tissue usually reveals granulomatous inflammation with necrosis but may not show vasculitis. Renal biopsy confirms the presence of glomerulonephritis.

The specificity of a positive c-ANCA titer for Wegener's granulomatosis is very high, especially if active glomerulonephritis is present. However, the presence of c-ANCA should be adjunctive and should not substitute for a tissue diagnosis. False-positive ANCA titers have been reported in certain infectious and neoplastic diseases. Furthermore, in evaluating patients for relapse, the ANCA titer can be misleading. Many patients who achieve remission continue to have elevated titers for years. In addition, over 40 percent of patients who were in remission and had a fourfold increase in c-ANCA titer did not have a relapse of disease.

In its typical presentation, the classic clinicopathologic complex of Wegener's granulomatosis usually provides ready differentiation from other disorders. However, if all the typical features are not present at once, it needs to be differentiated from the other vasculitides, particularly allergic angiitis and granulomatosis, Goodpasture's syndrome (see Chap. 275), tumors of the upper airway or lung, and infectious diseases such as mucocutaneous leishmaniasis (see Chap. 217) and rhinoscleroma (see Chap. 30) as well as noninfectious granulomatous diseases.

Of particular note is the differentiation from *midline granuloma* and *upper airway neoplasms*, which are part of the spectrum of *midline destructive diseases*. These diseases lead to extreme tissue destruction and mutilation localized to the midline upper airway structures including the sinuses; erosion through the skin of the face commonly occurs, a feature that is extremely rare in Wegener's granulomatosis. Although blood vessels may be involved in the intense inflammatory reaction and necrosis, primary vasculitis is seen rarely. When systemic involvement occurs, it usually declares itself as a neoplastic process. In this regard, it is likely that midline granuloma is part of the spectrum of *angiocentric immunoproliferative lesions* (AIL). The latter are considered to represent a spectrum of postthymic T cell proliferative lesions and should be treated as such (see Chap. 113). The term *idiopathic* has been applied to midline granuloma when extensive diagnostic workup including multiple biopsies has failed to reveal anything other than inflammation and necrosis. Under these circumstances, it is possible that the tumor cells were masked by the intensive inflammatory response. Such cases have responded to local irradiation with 50 Gy (5000 rad). Upper airway lesions should never be irradiated in Wegener's granulomatosis.

Wegener's granulomatosis must also be differentiated from *lymphomatoid granulomatosis*, the latter also being a part of the spectrum of AIL. Lymphomatoid granulomatosis is characterized by lung, skin, central nervous system, and kidney involvement in which atypical lymphocytoid and plasmacytoid cells infiltrate tissue in an angioinvasive manner. In this regard, it clearly differs from Wegener's granulomatosis in that it is not an inflammatory vasculitis in the classic sense but an infiltration of vessels with atypical mononuclear cells; granuloma may be present in involved tissues. Approximately 50 percent of patients develop a true malignant lymphoma. The presence of c-ANCA proves extremely helpful in the differentiation from all the preceding diseases.

℞ TREATMENT

Wegener's granulomatosis was formerly universally fatal, usually within a few months after the onset of clinically apparent renal disease. Glucocorticoids alone led to some symptomatic improvement, with little effect on the ultimate course of the disease. It has been well established that the treatment of choice in this disease is cyclophosphamide given in doses of 2 mg/kg per day orally. The leukocyte count should be monitored closely during therapy, and the dosage should be adjusted in order to maintain the count above 3000/μL, which generally maintains the neutrophil count at approximately 1500/μL. With this approach, clinical remission can usually be induced and maintained without causing severe leukopenia with its associated risk of infection. Cyclophosphamide should be continued for 1 year following the induction of complete remission and gradually tapered and discontinued thereafter.

At the initiation of therapy, glucocorticoids should be administered together with cyclophosphamide. This can be given as prednisone, 1 mg/kg per day initially (for the first month of therapy) as a daily regimen, with gradual conversion to an alternate-day schedule followed by tapering and discontinuation after approximately 6 months.

Using the above regimen, the prognosis of this disease is excellent; marked improvement is seen in more than 90 percent of patients, and complete remissions are achieved in 75 percent of patients. A number of patients who developed irreversible renal failure but who achieved subsequent remission on appropriate therapy have undergone successful renal transplantation.

Despite the dramatic remissions induced by the therapeutic regimen described above, long-term follow-up of patients has revealed that approximately 50 percent of remissions are later associated with one or more relapses. Reinduction of remission is almost always achieved; however, a high percentage of patients ultimately have some degree of morbidity from irreversible features of their disease, such as varying degrees of renal insufficiency, hearing loss, tracheal stenosis, saddle nose deformity, and chronically impaired sinus function.

Certain types of morbidity are related to toxic side effects of treatment. Since the preceding therapeutic regimen calls for conversion to alternate-day glucocorticoid therapy within 3 months and ultimate discontinuation within 6 to 12 months, glucocorticoid-related side effects such as diabetes mellitus, cataracts, life-threatening infectious disease complications, serious osteoporosis, and severe cushingoid features are infrequently encountered except in those patients requiring prolonged courses of daily glucocorticoids. However, cyclophosphamide-related toxicities are more frequent and severe. Cystitis to varying degrees occurs in 43 percent of patients, bladder cancer in 5 percent, and myelodysplasia in 2 percent.

Despite its life-saving effects in patients with Wegener's granulomatosis, cyclophosphamide cannot be tolerated by certain patients, such as those who develop severe neutropenia at low doses of drug or those who develop severe cystitis or bladder cancer. In these patients, alternative treatment regimens should be initiated. In one study, weekly methotrexate was shown to be an acceptable alternative therapy for selected patients with Wegener's granulomatosis who did not have immediately life-threatening disease or had developed serious cyclophosphamide-associated toxicity. Patients in this category were given oral prednisone as described above, and methotrexate was administered orally starting at a dosage of 0.3 mg/kg, with a maximum of 15 mg/week. If the treatment was well tolerated after 1 to 2 weeks, the dosage was increased by 2.5 mg weekly up to a dosage of 20 to 25 mg/week and maintained at that level. Remissions were achieved in 30 of 42 patients (71 percent). Eleven patients relapsed; eight of these were treated with a second course of methotrexate and prednisone and six of eight achieved a second remission. Toxicities of methotrexate included elevated transaminase levels (24 percent), leukopenia (7 percent), opportunistic infection (9.5 percent), methotrexate pneumonitis (7 percent), and stomatitis (2 percent). Azathioprine, in doses of 1 to 2 mg/kg per day, has proven effective in some patients, particularly in maintaining remission in those in whom remission was induced by cyclophosphamide. The drug should be administered together with the glucocorticoid regimen described above. Anecdotal reports have indicated therapeutic success with less frequent and severe toxic side effects using intermittent boluses of intravenous cyclophosphamide (1 g/m^2 per month) in place of daily drug administered orally. However, we have found that although 6 months of such a regimen induced improvement in approximately 90 percent of patients with remissions in 50 percent, 72 percent of patients were unable to maintain remission despite further treatment over 6 to 24 months. Although certain reports have indicated that trimethoprim-sulfamethoxazole may be of benefit in the treatment of Wegener's granulomatosis, there are no firm data to substantiate this, particularly in patients with serious renal and pulmonary disease.

TEMPORAL ARTERITIS

DEFINITION *Temporal arteritis*, also referred to as *cranial* or *giant cell arteritis*, is an inflammation of medium- and large-sized arteries. It characteristically involves one or more branches of the carotid artery, particularly the temporal artery, hence the name. However, it is a systemic disease that can involve arteries in multiple locations.

INCIDENCE AND PREVALENCE The incidence of temporal arteritis varies widely in different studies and in different geographic regions. A high incidence has been found in Scandanavia and in regions of the United States with large Scandanavian populations, compared to a lower incidence in southern Europe. The annual incidence rates in individuals 50 years of age and older range from 0.49 to 23.3 per 100,000 population. It occurs almost exclusively in individuals older than 55 years; however, well-documented cases have occurred in patients 40 years old or younger. It is more common in women than in men and is rare in blacks. Familial aggregation has been reported, as has an association with HLA-DR4. In addition, genetic linkage studies have demonstrated an association of temporal arteritis with alleles at the HLA-DRB1 locus, particularly HLA-DRB1*04 variants. The disease is closely associated with *polymyalgia rheumatica*, which is more common than temporal arteritis. In Olmsted County, Minnesota, the annual incidence of polymyalgia rheumatica in individuals 50 years of age and older is 52.5 per 100,000 population.

PATHOPHYSIOLOGY AND PATHOGENESIS Although the temporal artery is most frequently involved in this disease, patients often have a systemic vasculitis of multiple medium- and large-sized arteries, which may go undetected. Histopathologically, the disease is a panarteritis with inflammatory mononuclear cell infiltrates within the vessel wall with frequent giant cell formation. There is proliferation of the intima and fragmentation of the internal elastic lamina. Pathophysiologic findings in organs result from the ischemia related to the involved vessels. Distinct cytokine patterns as well as T lymphocytes expressing specific antigen receptors have been described suggesting the involvement of immunopathogenic mechanisms in temporal arteritis. IL-6 and IL-1β expression has been detected in a majority of circulating monocytes of patients with temporal arteritis and polymyalgia rheumatica. T cells recruited to vasculitic lesions in patients with temporal arteritis produce predominantly IL-2 and IFNγ, and the latter has been suggested to be involved in the progression to overt arteritis. Sequence analysis of the T cell receptor of tissue-infiltrating T cells in lesions of temporal arteritis indicates restricted clonal expansion, suggesting that an antigen residing in the arterial wall is recognized by a small fraction of T cells.

CLINICAL AND LABORATORY MANIFESTATIONS The disease is characterized clinically by the classic complex of fever, anemia, high ESR, and headaches in an elderly patient. Other manifestations include malaise, fatigue, anorexia, weight loss, sweats, and arthralgias. The polymyalgia rheumatica syndrome is characterized by stiffness, aching, and pain in the muscles of the neck, shoulders, lower back, hips, and thighs.

In patients with involvement of the temporal artery, headache is the predominant symptom and may be associated with a tender, thickened, or nodular artery, which may pulsate early in the disease but become occluded later. Scalp pain and claudication of the jaw and tongue may occur. A well-recognized and dreaded complication of temporal arteritis, particularly in untreated patients, is ocular involvement due primarily to ischemic optic neuritis, which may lead to serious visual symptoms, even sudden blindness in some patients. However, most patients have complaints relating to the head or eyes for months before objective eye involvement. Attention to such symptoms with institution of appropriate therapy (see below) will usually avoid this complication. Claudication of the extremities, strokes, myocardial infarctions, aortic aneurysms and dissections, and infarctions of visceral organs have been reported.

Characteristic laboratory findings in addition to the elevated ESR include a normochromic or slightly hypochromic anemia. Liver function abnormalities are common, particularly increased alkaline phosphatase levels. Increased levels of IgG and complement have been reported. Levels of enzymes indicative of muscle damage such as serum creatine kinase are not elevated.

DIAGNOSIS The diagnosis of temporal arteritis and its associated clinicopathologic syndrome often can be made clinically by the demonstration of the classic picture of fever, anemia, and high ESR with or without symptoms of polymyalgia rheumatica in an elderly patient. The diagnosis is confirmed by biopsy of the temporal artery. Since involvement of the vessel may be segmental, the diagnosis may be missed on routine biopsy; serial sectioning of biopsy specimens is recommended. When the temporal arteries appear clinically normal, but temporal arteritis is strongly suspected, a biopsy segment of a few centimeters may be required to establish the diagnosis. A temporal artery biopsy should be obtained as quickly as possible in the setting of ocular signs and symptoms, and under these circumstances therapy should not be delayed pending a biopsy. In this regard, it has been reported that temporal artery biopsies may show vasculitis even after more than 14 days of glucocorticoid therapy. A dramatic clinical response to a trial of glucocorticoid therapy can confirm the diagnosis.

℞ TREATMENT

Temporal arteritis and its associated symptoms are exquisitely sensitive to glucocorticoid therapy. Treatment should begin with prednisone, 40 to 60 mg per day for approximately 1 month, followed by a gradual tapering to a maintenance dose of 7.5 to 10 mg per day. In order to lessen glucocorticoid side effects in elderly individuals, conversion to alternate-day therapy may be attempted, but only after the disease has been put into remission with daily therapy. When ocular signs and symptoms occur, it is important that therapy be initiated or adjusted to control them. Because of the possibility of relapse, therapy should be continued for at least 1 to 2 years. The ESR can serve as a useful indicator of inflammatory disease activity in monitoring and tapering therapy and can be used to judge the pace of the tapering schedule. However, minor increases in the ESR can occur as glucocorticoids are being tapered and do not necessarily reflect an exacerbation of arteritis, particularly if the patient remains symptom free. Under these circumstances, the tapering should continue with caution. If one attempts to maintain a normal ESR throughout the tapering period, glucocorticoid toxicity will almost surely occur. The prognosis is generally good, and most patients achieve complete remission that is often maintained after withdrawal of therapy.

TAKAYASU'S ARTERITIS

DEFINITION *Takayasu's arteritis* is an inflammatory and stenotic disease of medium- and large-sized arteries characterized by a strong predilection for the aortic arch and its branches. For this reason, it is often referred to as the *aortic arch syndrome*.

INCIDENCE AND PREVALENCE Takayasu's arteritis is an uncommon disease, much less common than temporal arteritis. It is most prevalent in adolescent girls and young women. Although it is more common in the Orient, it is neither racially nor geographically restricted. An association of the disease has been described with HLA-DR2, MB1 in Japan and HLA-DR4, MB3 in the United States.

PATHOPHYSIOLOGY AND PATHOGENESIS The disease involves medium- and large-sized arteries, with a strong predilection for the aortic arch and its branches; the pulmonary artery also may be involved. The most commonly affected arteries seen by angiography are listed in Table 319-5. The involvement of the major branches of the aorta is much more marked at their origin than distally. The disease is a panarteritis with inflammatory mononuclear cell infiltrates and occasionally giant cells. There is marked intimal proliferation and fibrosis, scarring and vascularization of the media, and disruption and degeneration of the elastic lamina. Narrowing of the lumen occurs with or without thrombosis. The vasa vasorum are frequently involved. Pathologic changes in various organs reflect the compromise of blood flow through the involved vessels.

Immunopathogenic mechanisms, the precise nature of which is uncertain, are suspected in this disease. As with several of the vasculitis syndromes, circulating immune complexes have been demonstrated, but their pathogenic significance is unclear.

CLINICAL AND LABORATORY MANIFESTATIONS Takayasu's arteritis is a systemic disease with generalized as well as local symptoms. The generalized symptoms include malaise, fever, night sweats, arthralgias, anorexia, and weight loss which may occur months before vessel involvement is apparent. These symptoms may merge into those related to pain over the involved vessels, followed by symptoms of ischemia in organs supplied by the compromised vessels. Pulses are commonly absent in the involved vessels, particularly the subclavian artery. The frequency of arteriographic abnormalities and the potentially associated clinical manifestations are listed in Table 319-5.

The clinical course may be fulminant, may progress gradually, or may stabilize. Complications are related to the distribution of the involved vessels. Death usually occurs from congestive heart failure or cerebrovascular accidents.

Characteristic laboratory findings include an elevated ESR, mild anemia, and elevated immunoglobulin levels.

DIAGNOSIS The diagnosis of Takayasu's arteritis should be suspected strongly in a young woman who develops a decrease or absence of peripheral pulses, discrepancies in blood pressure, and arterial bruits. The diagnosis is confirmed by the characteristic pattern on arteriography, which includes irregular vessel walls, stenosis, poststenotic dilatation, aneurysm formation, occlusion, and evidence of increased collateral circulation. Complete aortic arteriography should be obtained unless this is renally contraindicated in order to fully delineate the distribution and degree of arterial disease. Histopathologic demonstration of inflamed vessels adds confirmatory data; however, tissue is rarely readily available for examination.

℞ TREATMENT

The course of the disease is variable, and spontaneous remissions may occur. Reported mortality statistics range from less than 10 percent to 75 percent. Although glucocorticoid therapy in doses of 40 to 60 mg prednisone per day alleviates symptoms, there are no convincing studies that indicate that they alone increase survival. The combination of glucocorticoid therapy for acute signs and symptoms and an aggressive surgical and/or angioplastic approach to stenosed vessels has markedly improved survival and decreased morbidity by lessening the risk of stroke, correcting hypertension due to renal artery stenosis, and improving blood flow to ischemic viscera and limbs. Unless it is urgently required, surgical correction of stenosed arteries should be undertaken only when the vascular inflammatory process is well controlled with medical therapy. Most recent mortality figures using this therapeutic approach are less than 10 percent. In individuals who are refractory to glucocorticoids, methotrexate in doses up to 25 mg per week has yielded encouraging results; however, long-term studies will be needed to confirm this.

Table 319-5

Frequency of Arteriographic Abnormalities and Potential Clinical Manifestations of Arterial Involvement in Takayasu's Arteritis

Artery	Percent of Arteriographic Abnormalities	Potential Clinical Manifestations
Subclavian	93	Arm claudication, Raynaud's phenomenon
Common carotid	58	Visual changes, syncope, transient ischemic attacks, stroke
Abdominal aorta*	47	Abdominal pain, nausea, vomiting
Renal	38	Hypertension, renal failure
Aortic arch or root	35	Aortic insufficiency, congestive heart failure
Vertebral	35	Visual changes, dizziness
Coeliac axis*	18	Abdominal pain, nausea, vomiting
Superior mesenteric*	18	Abdominal pain, nausea, vomiting
Iliac	17	Leg claudication
Pulmonary	10–40	Atypical chest pain, dyspnea
Coronary	<10	Chest pain, myocardial infarction

* Arteriographic lesions at these locations are usually asymptomatic but may potentially cause these symptoms.

SOURCE: G. Kerr et al., 1994.

HENOCH-SCHÖNLEIN PURPURA

DEFINITION *Henoch-Schönlein purpura,* also referred to as *anaphylactoid purpura* is a distinct systemic vasculitis syndrome that is characterized by palpable purpura (most commonly distributed over the buttocks and lower extremities), arthralgias, gastrointestinal signs and symptoms, and glomerulonephritis. It is a small vessel vasculitis.

INCIDENCE AND PREVALENCE Henoch-Schönlein purpura is usually seen in children; most patients range in age from 4 to 7 years; however, the disease may also be seen in infants and adults. It is not a rare disease; in one series it accounted for between 5 and 24 admissions per year at a pediatric hospital. The male to female ratio is 1.5:1. A seasonal variation with a peak incidence in spring has been noted.

PATHOPHYSIOLOGY AND PATHOGENESIS The presumptive pathogenic mechanism for Henoch-Schönlein purpura is immune-complex deposition. A number of inciting antigens have been suggested including upper respiratory tract infections, various drugs, foods, insect bites, and immunizations. IgA is the antibody class most often seen in the immune complexes and has been demonstrated in the renal biopsies of these patients.

CLINICAL AND LABORATORY MANIFESTATIONS In pediatric patients, presenting symptoms related to the skin, gut, and joints are present in 50 percent of cases. In adults, presenting symptoms related to the skin are seen in over 70 percent of patients, while initial complaints related to the gut or the joints are noted in fewer than 20 percent of cases. The typical palpable purpura is seen in virtually all patients; most patients develop polyarthralgias in the absence of frank arthritis. Gastrointestinal involvement, which is seen in almost 70 percent of pediatric patients, is characterized by colicky abdominal pain usually associated with nausea, vomiting, diarrhea, or constipation and is frequently accompanied by the passage of blood and mucus per rectum; bowel intussusception may occur rarely. The renal involvement is usually characterized by mild glomerulonephritis leading to proteinuria and microscopic hematuria, with red blood cell casts in the majority of patients (see also Chap. 275); it usually resolves spontaneously without therapy. Rarely, a progressive glomerulonephritis will develop. Renal failure is the most common cause of death in the rare patient who dies of Henoch-Schönlein purpura. Although certain studies have found that renal disease is more severe in adults, this has not been a consistent finding. However, the course of renal disease in adults may be more insidious and thus requires close follow-up. Myocardial involvement can occur in adults but is rare in children.

Routine laboratory studies generally show a mild leukocytosis, a normal platelet count, and occasionally eosinophilia. Serum complement components are normal, and IgA levels are elevated in about one-half of patients.

℞ TREATMENT

The prognosis of Henoch-Schönlein purpura is excellent. Most patients recover completely, and some do not require therapy. Treatment is similar for adults and children. When glucocorticoid therapy is required, prednisone in doses of 1 mg/kg per day and tapered according to clinical response has been shown to be useful in decreasing tissue edema, arthralgias, and abdominal discomfort; however, it has not proven beneficial in the treatment of skin or renal disease and does not appear to shorten the duration of active disease or lessen the chance of recurrence. Patients with rapidly progressive glomerulonephritis have been anecdotally reported to benefit from intensive plasma exchange combined with immunosuppressive drugs.

PREDOMINANTLY CUTANEOUS VASCULITIS

DEFINITION The term *predominantly cutaneous vasculitis* has been used in the literature interchangeably with the terms *hypersensitivity vasculitis* and *cutaneous leukocytoclastic vasculitis*. Due to the heterogeneity of this group of disorders, none of these terms is totally adequate. The common denominator of this group of diseases is the involvement of small vessels of the skin. The syndrome is presumed to be associated with an aberrant hypersensitivity reaction to an antigen such as an infectious agent, a drug, or other foreign or endogenous substances. In most instances, however, an antigen is never identified and the disease remains idiopathic. The Chapel Hill Consensus Conference on Nomenclature of Systemic Vasculitis does not use the term *hypersensitivity vasculitis*. Indeed, this is easily a misleading term since most of the other groups of vasculitis syndromes are probably also associated with some form of hypersensitivity or aberrant immunologic reaction to as yet unidentified antigens. The term *cutaneous leukocytoclastic vasculitis* is a better term; however, not all of these vasculitides are truly leukocytoclastic in nature. We have elected to use the term *"predominantly" cutaneous vasculitis* since skin involvement generally dominates the clinical picture, but the skin is not always the exclusive organ involved. Indeed, any organ system can be involved with this type of vasculitis; however, the extracutaneous involvement is usually much less severe than that of the systemic necrotizing vasculitides.

INCIDENCE AND PREVALENCE Although the exact incidence of this group of vasculitis syndromes is uncertain, it is clearly more common than the systemic necrotizing vasculitis group. The disease can occur at any age and in both sexes; however, different subgroups have a higher incidence in certain age groups, and some are more common in males than females, or vice versa.

PATHOPHYSIOLOGY AND PATHOGENESIS The typical histopathologic feature of the predominantly cutaneous vasculitides is the presence of vasculitis of small vessels. Postcapillary venules are the most commonly involved vessels; capillaries and arterioles may be involved less frequently. This vasculitis is characterized by a *leukocytoclasis*, a term that refers to the nuclear debris remaining from the neutrophils that have infiltrated in and around the vessels during the acute stages. In the subacute or chronic stages, mononuclear cells predominate; in certain subgroups, eosinophilic infiltration is seen. Erythrocytes often extravasate from the involved vessels, leading to palpable purpura.

Immune-complex deposition is generally considered to be the immunopathogenic mechanism of this type of vasculitis; however, formal proof that this is the case has not been established for all subgroups (see above). The predominantly cutaneous vasculitides can be broken down empirically into two major categories depending on the type of putative antigen involved in the hypersensitivity reaction. In the originally described group, the antigen was foreign to the host, i.e., a drug, microbe, or foreign protein. In this regard, essential mixed cryoglobulinemia has been associated with hepatitis C virus infection. In the second category, the antigen is felt to be endogenous to the host. Examples of these are the "self" proteins such as DNA or immunoglobulin, which form immune complexes with their respective antibodies and lead to vasculitic complications in systemic lupus erythematosus and rheumatoid arthritis, respectively; other examples are the recognized and putative tumor antigens that form immune complexes with antibody and lead to vasculitis associated with certain neoplasms. Certain lymphoid malignancies also may secrete cytokines that contribute to the pathogenic process (see Table 319-1).

CLINICAL AND LABORATORY MANIFESTATIONS The hallmark of this broad group of vasculitides is the predominance of skin involvement. Skin lesions may appear typically as palpable purpura; however, other cutaneous manifestations of the vasculitis may occur, including macules, papules, vesicles, bullae, subcutaneous nodules, ulcers, and recurrent or chronic urticaria. Despite the fact that skin lesions predominate, other organ systems may be involved to varying degrees, and the extent to which this occurs may define a relatively distinct subgroup. Even in patients with isolated cutaneous involvement, the disease may be characterized by systemic signs and symptoms such as fever, malaise, myalgia, and anorexia. The skin lesions may be pruritic or even quite painful, with a burning or stinging sensation. Lesions most commonly occur in the lower extremities in ambulatory patients or in the sacral area in bedridden patients due to the effects of hydrostatic forces on the postcapillary venules. Edema may accompany certain lesions, and hyperpigmentation often occurs in areas of recurrent or chronic lesions.

There are no specific laboratory tests diagnostic of this category of vasculitis. A mild leukocytosis with or without eosinophilia is characteristic, as is an elevated ESR. Cryoglobulins and rheumatoid factor may be seen in certain cases, and serum complement levels follow no definite pattern. Laboratory abnormalities related to specific organ dysfunction reflect the involvement of these organs in the particular syndrome in question.

Drug-Induced Vasculitis Cutaneous drug reactions take a number of forms, and vasculitis is only one of these (see Chaps. 56 and 57). Vasculitis associated with drug reactions usually presents as palpable purpura that may be generalized or limited to the lower extremities or other dependent areas; however, urticarial lesions, ulcers, and hemorrhagic blisters may also occur (see Chap. 56). Signs and symptoms may be limited to the skin, although systemic manifestations such as fever, malaise, and polyarthralgias may occur. Although the skin is the predominant organ involved, systemic vasculitis may result from drug reactions. Drugs that have been implicated in vasculitis include allopurinol, thiazides, gold sulfonamides, phenytoin, and penicillin.

Serum Sickness and Serum Sickness–Like Reactions These reactions are characterized by the occurrence of fever, urticaria, polyarthralgias, and lymphadenopathy 7 to 10 days after primary exposure and 2 to 4 days after secondary exposure to a heterologous protein (classic serum sickness) or a nonprotein drug such as penicillin or sulfa (serum sickness–like reaction). Most of the manifestations are not due to a vasculitis; however, occasional patients will have typical cutaneous venulitis that may progress rarely to a systemic vasculitis.

Vasculitis Associated with Other Underlying Primary Diseases A number of diseases have vasculitis as a secondary manifestation of the underlying primary process. Foremost among these are the connective tissue diseases, particularly *systemic lupus erythematosus* (Chap. 312), *rheumatoid arthritis* (Chap. 313), and *Sjögren's syndrome* (Chap. 316). The most common form of vasculitis in these conditions is the small vessel venulitis isolated to the skin and clinically indistinguishable from the predominantly cutaneous vasculitides noted in response to an exogenous antigen. However, certain patients may develop a fulminant systemic necrotizing vasculitis indistinguishable from the PAN group.

Cryoglobulinemia may be seen in a number of the diverse vasculitic syndromes. *Essential mixed cryoglobulinemia* (see Chap. 275) may present as a typical predominantly cutaneous vasculitis. However, typically, it is associated with glomerulonephritis, arthralgias, hepatosplenomegaly, and lymphadenopathy in addition to skin involvement.

Vasculitis can be associated with certain *malignancies*, particularly lymphoid or reticuloendothelial neoplasms. Leukocytoclastic venulitis confined to the skin is the most common finding; however, widespread systemic vasculitis may occur. Of particular note is the association of *hairy cell leukemia* (Chap. 113) with classic PAN.

A leukocytoclastic vasculitis predominantly involving the skin with occasional involvement of other organ systems may be a minor component of many other diseases. These include *subacute bacterial endocarditis, Epstein-Barr virus infection, human immunodeficiency virus infection, chronic active hepatitis, ulcerative colitis, congenital deficiencies of various complement components, retroperitoneal fibrosis*, and *primary biliary cirrhosis*. Association of predominantly cutaneous vasculitis with α_1-*antitrypsin deficiency, intestinal bypass surgery*, and *relapsing polychondritis* has been reported.

DIAGNOSIS The diagnosis of this category of vasculitis is made by the demonstration of vasculitis on biopsy. Given the predominance of cutaneous involvement, biopsy material is generally readily available. An important principle in the diagnostic approach to patients with presumed isolated cutaneous vasculitis is to search for an etiology of the vasculitis—be it an exogenous agent such as a drug or an infection or an endogenous condition such as an underlying disease (Fig. 319-1). In addition, a careful physical and laboratory examination should be performed to rule out the possibility of systemic disease. This should start with the least invasive diagnostic approach and proceed to the more invasive only if clinically indicated.

℞ TREATMENT

Most cases of predominantly cutaneous vasculitis resolve spontaneously, and others remit and relapse before finally remitting completely. In those patients in whom persistent cutaneous disease evolves or in whom extracutaneous organ system involvement occurs, a variety of therapeutic regimens have been tried with variable results. In general, the treatment of this type of vasculitis has not been satisfactory. This is in contrast to the systemic necrotizing vasculitis group and Wegener's granulomatosis (see above), which generally are much more serious diseases than predominantly cutaneous vasculitis but usually respond dramatically to the combination of prednisone and cyclophosphamide. Fortunately, since the disease is generally limited to the skin, this lack of consistent response to therapy usually does not lead to a life-threatening situation. When an antigenic stimulus is recognized as the precipitating factor in the vasculitis, it should be removed; if this is a microbe, appropriate antimicrobial therapy should be instituted. If the vasculitis is associated with another underlying disease, treatment of the latter often results in resolution of the former. In situations where disease is apparently self-limited, no therapy, except possibly symptomatic therapy, is indicated. When disease persists or results in progressive organ system dysfunction, as may occur with the vasculitis that may be associated with certain connective tissue diseases, treatment according to the regimen for systemic necrotizing vasculitis should be initiated. Glucocorticoid therapy should be instituted, usually as prednisone, 1 mg/kg per day, in a regimen aimed at rapid tapering where possible, either directly to discontinuation or by conversion to an alternate-day regimen followed by ultimate discontinuation. In cases that prove refractory to glucocorticoids in which irreversible organ system dysfunction is likely, a trial of a cytotoxic agent such as cyclophosphamide in the regimen described above for systemic vasculitis is warranted. Patients with chronic vasculitis isolated to cutaneous venules rarely respond dramatically to any therapeutic regimen, and cytotoxic agents should be used only as a last resort in these patients. Plasmapheresis has been used with some success in fulminant cases. Dapsone has been tried in a number of patients with isolated cutaneous vasculitis with rare anecdotal reports of success. However, this drug has been consistently beneficial as therapy for cutaneous vasculitis only in patients with erythema elevatum diutinum (see below).

KAWASAKI DISEASE

Kawasaki disease (mucocutaneous lymph node syndrome) is an acute, febrile, multisystem disease of children. It is characterized by unresponsiveness to antibiotics, nonsuppurative cervical adenitis, and changes in the skin and mucous membranes such as edema, congested conjunctivae, erythema of the oral cavity, lips, and palms, and desquamation of the skin of the fingertips. Although the disease is generally benign and self-limited, it is associated with coronary artery aneurysms in approximately 25 percent of cases, with an overall case fatality rate of 0.5 to 2.8 percent. These complications usually occur between the third and fourth weeks of illness during the convalescent stage. Vasculitis of the coronary arteries is seen in almost all the fatal cases that have been autopsied. There is typical intimal proliferation and infiltration of the vessel wall with mononuclear cells. Beadlike aneurysms and thromboses may be seen along the artery. Most investigators agree that many of the cases of PAN formerly reported in children were actually arteritic complications of unrecognized Kawasaki disease. Other manifestations include pericarditis, myocarditis, myocardial ischemia and infarction, and cardiomegaly.

It is likely that immune-mediated injury to blood vessel endothelium is involved in the pathogenesis of this disease. Patients with Kawasaki disease have been demonstrated to have evidence of increased immune activation characterized by increased activated helper T cells and monocytes, elevated serum-soluble IL-2 receptor levels, elevated levels of spontaneous IL-1 production by peripheral blood mononuclear cells, anti-endothelial cell antibodies, and increased cytokine-inducible activation antigens on their vascular endothelium. A strong association has been reported between a novel form of *S. aureus* that releases toxic shock syndrome toxin 1 and Kawasaki disease, suggesting that this was the causative organism and was acting as a superantigen similar to the superantigen effect in toxic shock syndrome. However, analysis of the T cell receptor repertoire of patients with Kawasaki disease suggests that the T cell response is driven by a conventional antigen and not a superantigen.

Apart from the up to 2.8 percent of patients who develop fatal complications, the prognosis of this disease for uneventful recovery is excellent. High-dose intravenous gamma globulin (2 g/kg as a single infusion over 10 h) together with aspirin (100 mg/kg per day for 14 days followed by 3 to 5 mg/kg per day for several weeks) have been shown to be effective in reducing the prevalence of coronary artery abnormalities when administered early in the course of the disease.

ISOLATED VASCULITIS OF THE CENTRAL NERVOUS SYSTEM

Isolated vasculitis of the central nervous system is an uncommon clinicopathologic entity characterized by vasculitis restricted to the vessels of the central nervous system without other apparent systemic vasculitis. Although the arteriole is most commonly affected, vessels of any size can be involved. The inflammatory process is usually composed of mononuclear cell infiltrates with or without granuloma formation. Cases have been associated with cytomegalovirus, syphilis, pyogenic bacterial, and varicella-zoster infections, as well as with Hodgkin's disease and amphetamine abuse; however, in most cases no underlying disease process has been identified.

Patients may present with severe headaches, altered mental function, and focal neurologic defects. Systemic symptoms are generally absent. Devastating neurologic abnormalities may occur depending on the extent of vessel involvement. The diagnosis is generally made by demonstration of characteristic vessel abnormalities on arteriography and confirmed by biopsy of the brain parenchyma and leptomeninges. In the absence of a brain biopsy, care should be taken not to misinterpret angiographic abnormalities that might actually be vessel spasm related to another cause with true primary vasculitis. The prognosis of this disease is poor; however, in certain patients the disease may remit spontaneously, and some reports indicate that glucocorticoid therapy alone or together with cyclophosphamide in steroid-resistant patients administered as described above for the systemic vasculitides has induced sustained clinical remissions in a small number of patients.

THROMBOANGIITIS OBLITERANS (BUERGER'S DISEASE)

Thromboangiitis obliterans is an inflammatory occlusive peripheral vascular disease of unknown etiology that affects arteries and veins. Thrombosis of the vessels is likely the primary event, and so this disease is not a classic vasculitis. However, it is considered among the vasculitides because of the intense inflammatory response within the thrombus and the fact that there is often a vasculitis of the vasa vasorum in the arterial wall. → ***The disease is discussed in detail in Chap. 248.***

BEHÇET'S SYNDROME

Behçet's syndrome is a clinicopathologic entity characterized by recurrent episodes of oral and genital ulcers, iritis, and cutaneous lesions. The underlying pathologic process is a leukocytoclastic venulitis, although vessels of any size and in any organ can be involved. → ***This disorder is described in detail in Chap. 318.***

MISCELLANEOUS VASCULITIDES

A variety of disorders, many of which are uncommon, are characterized by varying degrees of inflammatory responses involving blood vessels. *Cogan's syndrome* is a disease characterized by nonsyphilitic interstitial keratitis together with vestibuloauditory symptoms. It may be associated with a systemic vasculitis involving vessels of different sizes as well as the aortic valve.

Erythema elevatum diutinum is a rare chronic skin disorder of unknown etiology characterized by persistent red, purple, and yellowish papules, plaques, and nodules usually distributed symmetrically over the extensor surface of the limbs; on biopsy, they demonstrate a leukocytoclastic venulitis together with a marked dermal inflammatory infiltrate. An association with streptococcal infections has been reported. The disease responds dramatically to dapsone therapy.

Certain *infections* may directly trigger an inflammatory vasculitic process. For example, rickettsias can invade and proliferate in the endothelial cells of small blood vessels causing a vasculitis (see Chap. 179). In addition, the inflammatory response around blood vessels associated with certain systemic fungal diseases such as histoplasmosis (see Chap. 203) may mimic a primary vasculitic process.

℞ TREATMENT

Once a diagnosis of vasculitis has been established, a decision regarding therapeutic strategy must be made (Fig. 319-1). The vasculitis syndromes represent a wide spectrum of diseases with varying degrees of severity. Some require immediate and aggressive therapy with glucocorticoids and immunosuppressive agents, while others should be treated conservatively and symptomatically, usually with nonsteroidal anti-inflammatory drugs. Since the potential toxic side effects of certain therapeutic regimens may be substantial, the risk-versus-benefit ratio of any therapeutic approach should be weighed carefully. Specific therapeutic regimens are discussed above for the individual vasculitis syndromes; however, certain general principles regarding therapy should be considered. On the one hand, glucocorticoids and/or immunosuppressive therapy should be instituted immediately in diseases where irreversible organ system dysfunction and high morbidity and mortality have been clearly established. Wegener's granulomatosis is the prototype of a severe systemic vasculitis requiring such a therapeutic approach (see above). On the other hand, when feasible, aggressive therapy should be avoided for vasculitic manifestations that rarely result in irreversible organ system dysfunction and that usually do not respond to such therapy. For example, isolated cutaneous vasculitis usually resolves with symptomatic treatment, and prolonged courses of glucocorticoids uncommonly result in clinical benefit. Immunosuppressive agents have not proven to be beneficial in isolated cutaneous vasculitis, and their toxic side effects generally outweigh any potential beneficial effects. Glucocorticoids should be initiated in those systemic vasculitides that cannot be specifically categorized or for which there is no established standard therapy; immunosuppressive therapy should be added in these diseases only if an adequate response does not result or if remission can only be achieved and maintained with an unacceptably toxic regimen of glucocorticoids. When remission is achieved, one should continually attempt to taper glucocorticoids to an alternate-day regimen and discontinue when possible. When using immunosuppressive regimens, one should taper and discontinue the drug as soon as is feasible upon induction of remission (see below).

When glucocorticoids are used, prednisone is generally the formulation of choice and is administered as 1 mg/kg per day orally, first in divided doses and then converted to a single daily dose. After clinical improvement is noted (usually within a month), the regimen is gradually converted to an alternate-day schedule, followed by tapering and discontinuation after approximately 6 months or as the clinical response dictates. When an immunosuppressive agent is required, cyclophosphamide is the drug of choice and its efficacy has been clearly established in Wegener's granulomatosis and the severe systemic vasculitides (see above). It should be given in doses of 2 mg/kg per day orally. It is recommended that the drug be taken as a single dose in the morning together with large amounts of fluid. Dose adjustments should be based on the leukocyte count, which should be maintained above 3000/μL. Leukocyte counts at any given time will reflect the dosage of cyclophosphamide taken the previous week. Of note, neutropenia may become more pronounced as glucocorticoids are tapered. The regimen that has proven successful in Wegener's granulomatosis (see above) and that should be followed for the other severe systemic vasculitides has called for continuation of cyclophosphamide for approximately 1 year following the induction of complete remission, with gradual tapering (by 25-mg decrements of the daily dose) over several months until discontinuation. No other drug has proven to be as effective as cyclophosphamide for severe life-threatening vasculitis. However, immediate and long-range toxic side effects may be severe. Alternative immunosuppressive regimens may be instituted where indicated in those patients who cannot tolerate cyclophosphamide due to unacceptable side effects or who do not wish to take cyclophosphamide because of the potential side effects, particularly infertility or sterility in individuals of child-bearing age. Methotrexate has been shown to be an acceptable alternative to cyclophosphamide when the latter drug cannot be used. Methotrexate is administered initially at a dosage of 0.3 mg/kg, not to exceed 15 mg per week. If the treatment is well tolerated after 1 to 2 weeks, the dosage should be increased by 2.5 mg weekly up to a dosage of 20 to 25 mg/week and maintained at that level. Azathioprine at a

Table 319-6

Major Toxic Side Effects of Drugs Commonly Used in the Treatment of Systemic Vasculitis

GLUCOCORTICOIDS	
Osteoporosis	
Cataracts	Growth suppression in children
Glaucoma	Hypertension
Diabetes mellitus	Avascular necrosis of bone
Electrolyte abnormalities	Myopathy
Metabolic abnormalities	Alterations in mood
Suppression of inflammatory and immune responses leading to opportunistic infections	Psychosis
	Pseudotumor cerebri
	Peptic ulcer diathesis
Cushingoid features	Pancreatitis
CYCLOPHOSPHAMIDE	
Bone marrow suppression	Hypogammaglobulinemia
Cystitis	Pulmonary fibrosis
Bladder carcinoma	Myelodysplasia
Gonadal suppression	Oncogenesis
Gastrointestinal intolerance	
METHOTREXATE	
Gastrointestinal intolerance	Pneumonitis
Stomatitis	Teratogenicity
Neutropenia	Opportunistic infections
Hepatotoxicity (may lead to fibrosis or cirrhosis)	

dosage of 2 mg/kg per day orally has also been employed as an alternative to cyclophosphamide in severe systemic vasculitis with less favorable results. In unusual cases in which none of the above regimens have resulted in remission of the vasculitis, certain experimental approaches have been used, such as plasmapheresis together with immunosuppressive drugs, with anecdotal reports of limited success. In addition, other immunosuppressive agents such as cyclosporine have been employed with minimal success.

Physicians should be thoroughly aware of the toxic side effects of therapeutic agents employed (Table 319-6). Side effects of glucocorticoid therapy are markedly decreased in frequency and duration in patients on alternate-day regimens compared to daily regimens. When cyclophosphamide is administered chronically in doses of 2 mg/kg per day for substantial periods of time (one to several years), the incidence of cystitis as defined by nonglomerular hematuria is approximately 40 percent and the incidence of bladder cancer is 5 percent. Significant alopecia is unusual in the chronically administered, low-dose regimen. When patients are receiving low-dose cyclophosphamide, the white blood count (WBC) is maintained above 3000/μL, and the patient is not receiving daily glucocorticoids, the incidence of life-threatening opportunistic infections is very low. However, the WBC is not an accurate predictor of risk of opportunistic infections in patients receiving methotrexate; infections with *Pneumocystis carinii* and certain fungi can be seen in the face of WBC that are within normal limits.

Finally, it should be emphasized that each patient is unique and requires individual decision-making. The above outline should serve as a framework to guide therapeutic approaches; however, flexibility should be practiced in order to provide maximal therapeutic efficacy with minimal toxic side effects in each patient.

BIBLIOGRAPHY

CUPPS TR, FAUCI AS: *The Vasculitides*. Philadelphia, Saunders, 1981

——— et al: Isolated angiitis of the central nervous system. Prospective diagnostic and therapeutic experience. Am J Med 74:97, 1983

FAUCI AS et al: Wegener's granulomatosis: Prospective clinical and therapeutic experience with 85 patients for 21 years. Ann Intern Med 98:76, 1983

GIORDANO JM et al: Experience with surgical treatment of Takayasu's disease. Surgery 109:252, 1991

GUILLEVIN L et al: Treatment of polyarteritis nodosa related to hepatitis B virus with interferon-alpha and plasma exchanges. Ann Rheum Dis 53:334, 1994

HAYNES BF: Vasculitis: Pathogenic mechanisms of vessel damage, in *Inflammation: Basic Principles and Clinical Correlates*, JI Gallin et al (eds). New York, Raven Press, 1992, pp 921–941

HOFFMAN GS et al: Wegener's granulomatosis: An analysis of 158 patients. Ann Intern Med 116:488, 1992

HUNDER GG: Giant cell (temporal arteritis). Rheum Dis Clin North Am 16:399, 1990

JENNETTE JC et al: Nomenclature of systemic vasculitis. Proposal of an international consensus conference. Arthritis Rheum 37:187, 1994

KALLENBERG CGM et al: ANCA—pathophysiology revisited. Clin Exp Immunol 100:1, 1995

KERR G et al: Limited prognostic value of changes in antineutrophil cytoplasmic antibody titer in patients with Wegener's granulomatosis. Arthritis Rheum 36:365, 1993

——— et al: Takayasu arteritis. Ann Intern Med 120:919, 1994

NEWBURGER JW et al: A single intravenous infusion of gamma globulin as compared with four infusions in the treatment of acute Kawasaki disease. N Engl J Med 324:1633, 1991

NILES JL: Value of tests for antineutrophil cytoplasmic autoantibodies in the diagnosis and treatment of vasculitis. Curr Opin Rheumatol 5:18, 1993

PIETRA BA et al: TCR Vβ family repertoire and T cell activation markers in Kawasaki disease. J Immunol 153:1881, 1994

SNELLER MC et al: An analysis of forty-two Wegener's granulomatosis patients treated with methotrexate and prednisone. Arthritis Rheum 38:608, 1995

SOMER T, FINEGOLD SM: Vasculitis associated with infections, immunization, and antimicrobial drugs. Clin Infect Dis 20:1010, 1995

WEYLAND CM et al: Distinct vascular lesions in giant cell arteritis share identical T cell clonotypes. J Exp Med 179:951, 1994

——— et al: Tissue cytokine patterns in patients with polymyalgia rheumatica and giant cell arteritis. Ann Intern Med 121:484, 1994

320 SARCOIDOSIS

Ronald G. Crystal

DEFINITION Sarcoidosis is a chronic, multisystem disorder of unknown cause characterized in affected organs by an accumulation of T lymphocytes and mononuclear phagocytes, noncaseating epithelioid granulomas, and derangements of the normal tissue architecture. Although there are usually skin anergy and depressed cellular immune processes in the blood, sarcoidosis is characterized at the sites of disease by exaggerated T helper lymphocyte immune processes. All parts of the body can be affected, but the organ most frequently affected is the lung. Involvement of the skin, eye, and lymph nodes is also common. The disease is often acute or subacute and self-limiting, but in many individuals it is chronic, waxing and waning over many years.

ETIOLOGY The cause of sarcoidosis is unknown. A variety of infectious and noninfectious agents have been implicated, but there is no proof that any specific agent is responsible. However, all available evidence is consistent with the concept that the disease results from an exaggerated cellular immune response (acquired, inherited, or both) to a limited class of persistent antigens or self-antigens.

INCIDENCE AND PREVALENCE Sarcoidosis is a relatively common disease affecting individuals of both sexes and almost all ages, races, and geographic locations. Females appear to be slightly more susceptible than males. Cases of sarcoid have been described in all of the major races, and the disease is found throughout the world. It has been suggested that sarcoid is more common in certain geographic areas such as the southeastern part of the United States, but when case-matched controls have been used, these geographic differences are less convincing. There is a remarkable diversity of the prevalence of sarcoidosis among certain ethnic and racial groups, with a range of <1 to 64 per 100,000 worldwide. The prevalence of sarcoidosis is from 10 to 40 per 100,000 in the United States and Europe. In the United States, the majority of patients are black, with a ratio of blacks to whites ranging from 10:1 to 17:1. In Europe, however, the disease affects mostly whites. Furthermore, while the prevalence per 100,000 in Sweden is 64, in France it is 10, in Poland 3, yet for Irish females living in London it is 200. In contrast, the disease is very rare among Inuit, Canadian Indians, New Zealand Maoris, and Southeast Asians.

Most patients present with sarcoidosis between the ages of 20 and 40, but it can occur in children and in the elderly. Several hundred kindred groups with familial sarcoidosis have been described, and the disease has been observed in twins, more commonly in monozygotic than in dizygotic pairs. There also have been several instances of husband-wife pairs identified, and geographic foci of sarcoid among unrelated individuals living closely within a community, arguing for some environmental factors in the pathogenesis of the disease. Although the disease is believed to result from exaggerated cellular immune responses to a limited class of antigens, no clear patterns in any HLA locus have emerged. Unlike many diseases in which the lung is involved, sarcoidosis favors nonsmokers.

PATHOPHYSIOLOGY AND IMMUNOPATHOGENESIS

The first manifestation of the disease is an accumulation of mononuclear inflammatory cells, mostly T helper lymphocytes and mononuclear phagocytes, in affected organs. This inflammatory process is followed by the formation of granulomas, aggregates of macrophages and their progeny, epithelioid cells, and multinucleated giant cells. The typical sarcoid granuloma is a compact structure composed of an aggregate of mononuclear phagocytes surrounded by a rim of T helper-inducer lymphocytes and, to a far lesser extent, B lymphocytes. The overall structure is relatively discrete and is interspersed with fine collagen fibrils, presumably remnants of the underlying connective tissue matrix. The giant cells within the granuloma can be of the Langhans' or foreign-body variety and often contain inclusions such as Schaumann bodies (conchlike structures), asteroid bodies (stellate-like structures), and residual bodies (refractile calcium-containing inclusions).

Together the accumulated T cells, mononuclear phagocytes, and granulomas represent the active disease. Other than the fact that they take up space and thus their bulk modifies the local architecture, there is no evidence that the mononuclear inflammatory cells dispersed in the tissue or in the granuloma injure the affected organ by releasing mediators that damage the normal parenchymal cells or the extracellular matrix. Rather, organ dysfunction in sarcoid results mostly from the accumulated inflammatory cells distorting the architecture of the affected tissue; if a sufficient number of structures vital to the function of the tissue are involved, the disease becomes clinically apparent in that organ. Thus, while autopsy series show that, to some extent, sarcoidosis involves most organs in the majority of patients, the disease manifests clinically only in organs where it affects function (such as the lung and eye) or in organs where it is readily observed (such as the skin or, by x-ray, the hilar nodes). For example, in the lung, the inflammatory cells and granulomas distort the walls of the alveoli, bronchi, and blood vessels (Fig. 320-1*A*), thus altering the intimate relationships between air and blood necessary for normal gas exchange. When a sufficient amount of pulmonary tissue is involved, it is sensed by the individual as dyspnea. In contrast, most individuals with sarcoidosis have granulomatous mononuclear cell inflammation in the liver but usually do not have symptoms or functional derangements referable to that organ, likely because the disease process does not modify the local structures sufficiently to affect function.

If the disease is suppressed, either spontaneously or with therapy, the mononuclear inflammation is reduced in intensity and the number of granulomas is reduced. The granulomas resolve either by dispersion of the cells or by centripetal proliferation of fibroblasts from the periphery of the granuloma inward, to form a small scar. In chronic cases, the mononuclear cell inflammation persists for years. If the intensity of the inflammation is sufficiently high for a sufficiently long period, the derangements to the affected tissues result in extensive damage, the development of fibrosis, and permanent loss of organ function.

All available evidence suggests that active sarcoidosis results from an exaggerated cellular immune response to a variety of antigens or self-antigens, in which the process of T lymphocyte triggering, proliferation, and activation is skewed in the direction of helper-inducer T lymphocyte processes (Fig. 320-1*B*). The result is an exaggerated helper-inducer T cell response and thus the accumulation of large numbers of activated T cells in the affected organs. Since the activated helper-inducer T lymphocyte releases mediators that attract and activate mononuclear phagocytes, it is likely that the process of granuloma formation is a secondary phenomenon that is a consequence of the exaggerated helper-inducer T cell process. In this context, the current hypotheses of the cause of sarcoidosis, not mutually exclusive, include the following: (1) The disease is caused by a class of persistent antigens, nonself or self, that trigger only the helper-inducer T cell arm of the immune response; (2) the disease results from an inadequate suppressor arm of the immune response, such that helper-inducer T cell processes cannot be shut down in a normal fashion; or (3) the disease results from inherited (and/or acquired) differences in immune response genes, such that the response to a variety of antigens is an exaggerated, helper-inducer T cell process.

Independent of the inciting agent(s) or the reason why there is an exaggerated helper-inducer T cell response, there is a general understanding of the processes responsible for the maintenance of the inflammation and the development of the granuloma. The T helper-inducer lymphocytes accumulate at the sites of disease, at least in part, because they proliferate in these sites at an exaggerated rate. This T cell proliferation is maintained by the spontaneous release of interleukin (IL) 2, the T cell growth factor, by activated T helper-inducer cells in the local milieu. In this regard, sarcoidosis is a remarkable example of compartmentalization of the immune system and a dramatic illustration of why disease activity of sarcoidosis cannot be assessed by evaluating the immune system only in the blood. Whereas the T helper-inducer cells in the involved organs are releasing IL-2 and proliferating at an enhanced rate, the T cells in other sites, such as blood, are quiescent. Furthermore, while there is a marked enhancement of the number of T helper-inducer cells at the sites of disease, the numbers of T helper-inducer cells in the blood are normal or slightly reduced. In the involved organs, the ratio of helper-inducer to suppressor-cytotoxic T cells may be as high as 10:1 compared to the ratio of 2:1 found in normal tissues or in the blood of affected individuals.

In addition to driving other T helper-inducer cells in the affected organs to proliferate, the T helper-inducer cells at the sites of disease are activated and release mediators that both recruit and activate mononuclear phagocytes. The activated T helper-inducer cells accomplish this by releasing a variety of mediators (lymphokines) including proteins capable of recruiting blood monocytes to the local milieu of the activated T cells and interferon γ, a protein that, among its many actions, activates mononuclear phagocytes. Together with other cytokines released locally, these mediators recruit blood monocytes to the affected organs and activate them, providing the building blocks for the formation of the granuloma.

In addition to these exaggerated cellular immune processes, active sarcoid is also characterized by hyperglobulinemia. Included among the immunoglobulins are antibodies against a variety of infectious agents as well as IgM anti-T cell antibodies. However, there is no evidence that any of these antibodies plays a role in the pathogenesis of the disease, and they are thought to result from the nonspecific polyclonal stimulation of B cells by the activated T cells at the site of disease.

If the damage in the affected organs is sufficiently extensive that the remaining parenchymal cells cannot reestablish the normal tissue architecture, the usual result is fibrosis, the proliferation of mesenchymal cells, and deposition of their connective tissue products. There is convincing evidence that the fibroblast proliferation is directed by tissue macrophages spontaneously releasing growth signals for fibroblasts, including platelet-derived growth factor, fibronectin, and insulin-like growth factor 1. It is not known, however, why this fibrotic process occurs only in a relatively small proportion of individuals with sarcoidosis.

CLINICAL MANIFESTATIONS Sarcoidosis is a systemic disease, and thus the clinical manifestations may be generalized or focused on one or more organs. However, because the lung is almost always involved, most patients have symptoms referable to the respiratory system. Independent of the site, the clinical manifestations of the disease relate directly to the exaggerated helper-inducer T cell–mononuclear phagocyte granulomatous inflammatory process itself or to the sequelae resulting from the permanent damage caused by this process.

Sarcoidosis is occasionally discovered in a completely asymptomatic individual, but more commonly it presents abruptly over 1 to 2 weeks or the affected individual develops symptoms insidiously over several months. Independent of the mode of presentation, about 75 percent of all cases present when the individual is less than 40 years of age.

The asymptomatic form is usually detected by a routine examination, such as a chest film. In the United States, this represents about 10 to 20 percent of all cases, but in countries where chest films are mandatory in preemployment screening programs, the proportion of asymptomatic patients is higher.

So-called acute or subacute sarcoidosis develops abruptly over a period of a few weeks and represents 20 to 40 percent of all cases. These individuals usually have constitutional symptoms such as fever, fatigue, malaise, anorexia, or weight loss. These symptoms are usually mild, but in approximately 25 percent of the acute cases the constitutional complaints are extensive. Many patients have respiratory symptoms, including cough, dyspnea, a vague retrosternal chest discomfort and/or polyarthritis. Two syndromes have been identified in the acute group. Löfgren's syndrome, frequent in Scandinavian, Irish, and Puerto Rican females, includes the complex of erythema nodosum and x-ray findings of bilateral hilar adenopathy, often accompanied by joint symptoms, including arthritis at the ankles, knees, wrists, or elbows. The Heerfordt-Waldenström syndrome describes individuals with fever, parotid enlargement, anterior uveitis, and facial nerve palsy.

The insidious form of sarcoidosis develops over months and is associated usually with respiratory complaints without constitutional symptoms. In the United States, 40 to 70 percent of all sarcoid patients are in this category. About 10 percent of these individuals have symptoms referable to organs other than the lung. It is the individuals who present with the insidious form of sarcoidosis who most commonly go on to develop chronic sarcoidosis, with permanent damage to the lung and other organs.

Despite the fact that sarcoidosis is a systemic disease and some evidence of inflammation can be detected in most organs in the majority of patients, sarcoidosis is important clinically because of the pulmonary abnormalities and, to a lesser extent, lymph node, skin, and eye involvement. Far less commonly, other organs are involved significantly.

Lung Of individuals with sarcoidosis, 90 percent have an abnormal chest x-ray at some time during their course (Fig. 320-2*A*). Overall, approximately 50 percent develop permanent pulmonary abnormalities, and 5 to 15 percent have progressive fibrosis of the lung parenchyma. Sarcoidosis of the lung is primarily an interstitial lung disease (see Chap. 259) in which the inflammatory process involves the alveoli, small bronchi, and small blood vessels. These individuals typically have symptoms of dyspnea, particularly with exercise, and a dry cough. In acute and subacute cases, physical examination usually reveals dry rales. Hemoptysis is rare, as is production of sputum. Occasionally, the large airways are involved to a degree sufficient to cause dysfunc-

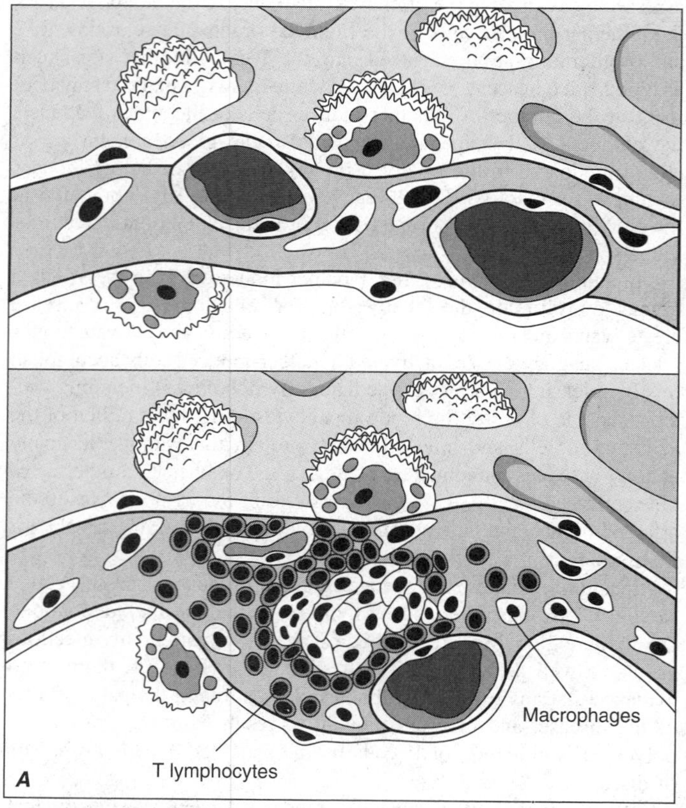

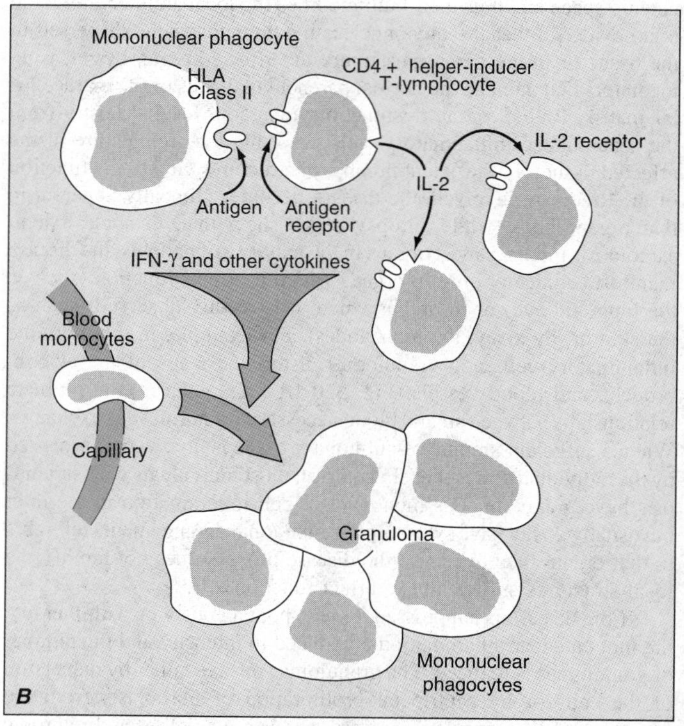

FIGURE 320-1 Pathogenesis of sarcoidosis. *A.* Histologic abnormalities. Normal alveoli (*left*) and alveoli in active sarcoidosis (*right*). The latter are distorted by the accumulated T helper-inducer lymphocytes, alveolar macrophages, and macrophages aggregated into granulomas. There is mild damage to alveolar epithelial and endothelial cells. *B.* The exaggerated processes of T helper-inducer lymphocytes in affected organs result in the accumulation of these cells along with macrophages and macrophages aggregated into granulomas. The trigger for the T helper-inducer cells is unknown. It may be a limited class of antigens or self-antigens presented in the context of class II HLA surface molecules by mononuclear phagocytes to the T helper-inducer lymphocyte. The antigen class II HLA complex is identified by the T cell antigen receptor, and the T cell is activated. Consequent to this process the immune response is exaggerated and skewed to produce activated T helper-inducer cells that release interleukin 2, which drives the accumulation of more T helper cells. The activated T helper-inducer cells also release interferon γ (INF-γ). Together with cytokines such as macrophage inflammatory protein 1α and granulocyte-macrophage colony stimulating factor released in the local milieu, there is recruitment and activation of blood monocytes and subsequent granuloma formation.

tion. Distal atelectasis can result from endobronchial sarcoidosis or from external compression from enlarged intrathoracic nodes. Rarely, wheezing is heard, incorrectly suggesting asthma. Large-vessel pulmonary granulomatous arteritis is common, but it rarely causes major problems. If it dominates the pulmonary lesions, it is sometimes called *necrotizing sarcoidal granulomatosis*. The pleura is involved in 1 to 5 percent of cases, almost always manifesting as a unilateral pleural effusion with characteristics of an exudate containing lymphocytes. The effusions usually clear within a few weeks, but chronic pleural thickening can result. Pneumothorax is very rare.

Lymph Nodes Lymphadenopathy is very common in sarcoidosis. Intrathoracic nodes are enlarged in 75 to 90 percent of all patients; usually this involves the hilar nodes, but the paratracheal nodes are commonly involved (Fig. 320-2*A*). Less frequently, there is enlargement of subcarinal, anterior mediastinal, or posterior mediastinal nodes. Peripheral lymphadenopathy is very common, particularly involving the cervical, axillary, epitrochlear, and inguinal nodes. The nodes in the retroperitoneal area and in the mesenteric chain also can enlarge. All these nodes are nonadherent, with a firm, rubbery texture. Palpation causes no pain. Unlike nodes in tuberculosis, the nodes do not ulcerate. The lymphadenopathy rarely causes a problem for the affected individual; however, if it is massive, it can be disfiguring and can impinge on other organs and lead to functional impairment.

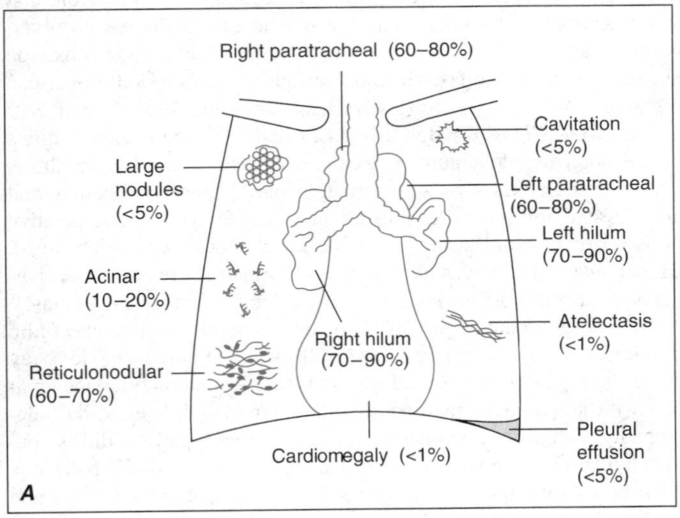

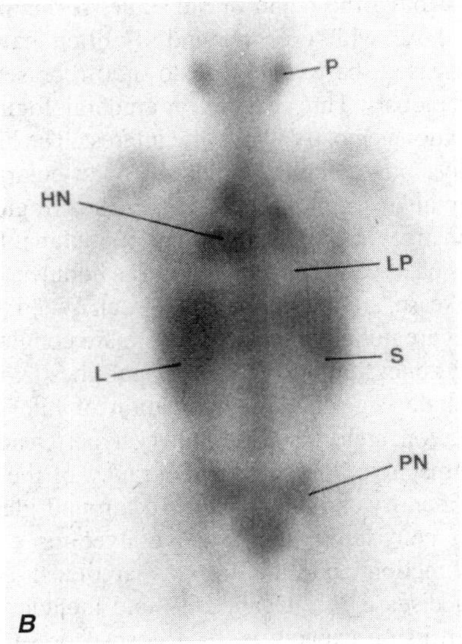

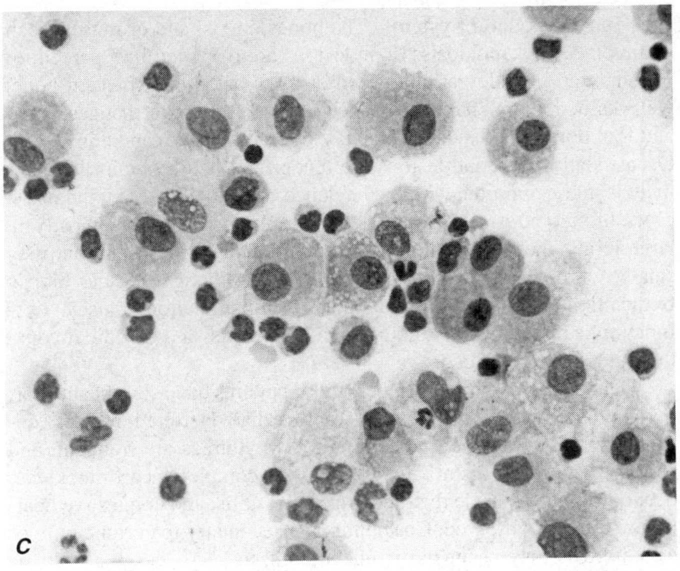

FIGURE 320-2 Common laboratory findings of sarcoidosis. *A*. Schematic view of the abnormal findings on the chest x-ray. Shown are changes observed with the average frequency of occurrence. *B*. Typical gallium 67 scan of an individual with active sarcoidosis. The isotope has accumulated in the lung parenchyma (LP), liver (L), spleen (S), parotid (P), hilar nodes (HN), and pelvic nodes (PN). *C*. Cells recovered by bronchoalveolar lavage of an individual with active pulmonary sarcoidosis. The lavage analysis reflects the inflammation in the tissue. Shown are alveolar macrophages (*large cells*) and lymphocytes (*small cells*). The cell population is dominated by lymphocytes, in contrast to normal individuals, in whom lymphocytes represent <20 percent of the cell population.

Skin Sarcoidosis involves the skin in about 25 percent of cases. The most common lesions are erythema nodosum, plaques, maculopapular eruptions, subcutaneous nodules, and lupus pernio. Erythema nodosum, comprising bilateral, tender red nodules on the anterior surface of the legs, is not specific for sarcoidosis but is common, particularly in acute sarcoidosis, in combination with systemic symptoms and polyarthralgias. Treatment is not required, since the lesions resolve spontaneously in 2 to 4 weeks. Erythema nodosum is much more common among sarcoid patients in Europe than in the United States. Skin plaques associated with sarcoid are purple, indolent lesions, often raised, and usually occur on the face, buttocks, and extremities. The maculopapular eruptions occur on the face around the eyes and nose, on the back, and on the extremities. These are elevated lesions less than 1 cm in diameter with a flat, waxy top. Subcutaneous nodules are most common on the trunk and extremities. Lupus pernio is characterized by indurated blue-purple, swollen, shiny lesions on the nose, cheeks, lips, ears, fingers, and knees. The lesions on the tip of the nose cause a bulbous appearance, sometimes associated with varicosities. The nasal mucosa is usually involved, and underlying bone can be destroyed. Sarcoidosis also can involve old surgical scars and tattoos. Although it may be disfiguring, cutaneous sarcoidosis rarely causes major problems. Clubbing of the fingers is occasionally observed in sarcoidosis, usually in association with extensive pulmonary fibrosis.

Eye Eye involvement occurs in approximately 25 percent of patients with sarcoidosis, and it can cause blindness. The usual lesions involve the uveal tract, iris, ciliary body, and choroid. Of those cases with eye involvement, approximately 75 percent have anterior uveitis and 25 to 35 percent have posterior uveitis. There is blurred vision, tearing, and photophobia. The uveitis can develop rapidly and may clear spontaneously over a 6- to 12-month period. It also can develop insidiously and be chronic. Conjunctival involvement is also common, usually with small, yellow nodules. When the lacrimal gland is involved, a keratoconjunctivitis sicca syndrome, with dry, sore eyes, can result.

Upper Respiratory Tract The nasal mucosa is involved in up to 20 percent of patients, usually presenting with nasal stuffiness. Any of the structures of the mouth can be involved, particularly the tonsils. Sarcoidosis involves the larynx in about 5 percent of cases. The epiglottis and areas around the true vocal cords are usually involved, but the cords themselves are not. These individuals are usually hoarse, and they have dyspnea, wheezing, and stridor; complete obstruction can occur.

Bone Marrow and Spleen Sarcoidosis of the marrow is reported in 15 to 40 percent of cases, but it rarely causes hematologic abnormalities other than a mild anemia, neutropenia, eosinophilia, and occasionally, thrombocytopenia. Although splenomegaly occurs in only 5 to 10 percent of patients, celiac angiography or splenic biopsy reveals involvement in 50 to 60 percent of cases. The presentation and complications of splenomegaly in sarcoidosis are similar to those of splenomegaly in general.

Liver Although liver biopsy reveals liver involvement in 60 to 90 percent of cases, liver dysfunction is usually not important clinically. Sarcoidosis involves generally the periportal areas. Approximately 20 to 30 percent have hepatomegaly and/or biochemical evidence of liver involvement. Usually these changes reflect a cholestatic pattern and include an elevated alkaline phosphatase level; the bilirubin and aminotransferase levels are only mildly elevated, and jaundice is rare. Rarely, portal hypertension can occur, as can intrahepatic cholestasis with cirrhosis.

Kidney Clinically apparent primary renal involvement in sarcoidosis is rare, although tubular, glomerular, and renal artery diseases have been reported. More commonly, but still in only 1 to 2 percent of all cases, there is a disorder of calcium metabolism with hypercalciuria, with or without hypercalcemia. If chronic, nephrocalcinosis and nephrolithiasis can result. It is believed that the calcium abnormalities are associated with enhanced calcium absorption in the gut, which is related to an abnormally high level of circulating 1,25-dihydroxyvitamin D produced by mononuclear phagocytes in the granulomas.

Nervous System All components of the nervous system can be involved in sarcoidosis. Neurologic findings are observed in about 5 percent of patients. Seventh nerve involvement with unilateral facial paralysis is most common. It occurs suddenly and is usually transient. Other common manifestations of neurosarcoid include optic nerve dysfunction, papilledema, palate dysfunction, hearing abnormalities, hypothalamic and pituitary abnormalities, chronic meningitis, and occasionally, space-occupying lesions. Psychiatric disturbances have been described, and seizures can occur. Rarely, multiple lesions occur that mimic multiple sclerosis, spinal cord abnormalities, and peripheral neuropathy.

Musculoskeletal System The bones, joints, and/or muscles can be involved in sarcoidosis. Bone lesions are observed in 5 percent of patients and include variable-sized cysts in areas of expanded bone; well-defined, round, punched-out lesions; or lattice-like changes. Hand and foot bones are the common sites, but most bones can be involved. Occasionally, the bone lesions are tender and painful. Joint involvement is more common, with an incidence of 25 to 50 percent in known cases of sarcoidosis. Arthralgias and frank arthritis occur mostly in large joints; they can be migratory and are usually transient, but they can be chronic and result in deformities. Although muscle biopsy frequently demonstrates granulomatous inflammation, muscle dysfunction is rare. However, nodules, polymyositis, and chronic myopathy have been described.

Heart Approximately 5 percent of patients have significant heart involvement, with clinical evidence of cardiac dysfunction. Left ventricular wall involvement is common. Arrhythmias are frequent, and serious conduction disturbances, including complete heart block, can occur. Papillary muscle dysfunction, pericarditis, and congestive heart failure are also observed. Cor pulmonale secondary to chronic pulmonary fibrosis may occur but is uncommon.

Endocrine and Reproductive System The hypothalamic-pituitary axis is the part of the endocrine system most commonly involved; this usually presents as diabetes insipidus. Anterior pituitary dysfunction is also seen, manifesting as a deficiency in one or more pituitary hormones. Complete hypopituitarism is rare. Much less frequently, sarcoidosis can cause primary dysfunction of other endocrine glands. Adrenal cortical involvement resulting in Addison's syndrome has been described. Involvement of the reproductive organs occurs, but infertility is rare. Pregnancy is not affected by sarcoidosis, and patients with sarcoidosis who become pregnant usually improve during pregnancy. However, the disease may flare post partum; presumably this variation results from fluctuations in endogenous glucocorticoid production.

Exocrine Glands Parotid enlargement is a classic feature of sarcoidosis, but clinically apparent parotid involvement occurs in fewer than 10 percent of patients. Bilateral involvement is the rule. The gland is usually nontender, firm, and smooth. Xerostomia can occur; other exocrine glands are affected only rarely.

Gastrointestinal Tract Although sarcoidosis involvement of the gastrointestinal tract is found occasionally at autopsy, it rarely has clinical importance. Occasionally, patients have esophageal or gastric symptoms.

COMPLICATIONS The respiratory tract abnormalities cause most of the morbidity and mortality associated with sarcoidosis. The major problems are those characteristic of interstitial lung disease (see Chap. 259), particularly dyspnea and insufficient oxygen delivery to vital organs. Respiratory failure with carbon dioxide retention is rare. In some patients, lung destruction results in formation of bullae that may harbor mycetomas, which are usually aspergillomas; erosion into the parenchyma can result in massive bleeding. The most common complications apart from the lung are associated with the eye; however, with therapy, blindness is rare. Complications of other organs include a gamut of abnormalities. The most serious are CNS lesions or cardiac involvement leading to congestive heart failure or sudden death.

LABORATORY ABNORMALITIES Common abnormalities in the blood include lymphocytopenia, an occasional mild eosinophilia, an increased erythrocyte sedimentation rate, hyperglobulinemia, and an elevated level of angiotensin-converting enzyme. False-positive tests for rheumatoid factor or antinuclear antibodies can be observed. Hypercalcemia is rare. Other serum abnormalities relate to involvement of specific organs such as liver, kidney, or endocrine glands.

Because the lung is involved so commonly, the routine chest film is almost always abnormal (Fig. 320-2*A*). The three classic x-ray patterns of pulmonary sarcoidosis are type I—bilateral hilar adenopathy with no parenchymal abnormalities; type II—bilateral hilar adenopathy with diffuse parenchymal changes; and type III—diffuse parenchymal changes without hilar adenopathy. The type III pattern is sometimes split into two categories, with films that show fibrosis and upper lobe retraction classified separately. Although patients with type I x-rays tend to have the acute or subacute, reversible form of the disease while those with types II and III often have the chronic, progressive disease, these patterns do not represent consecutive "stages" of sarcoidosis. Thus, except for epidemiologic purposes, this x-ray categorization is mostly of historic interest. The hilar adenopathy is almost always bilateral, but unilateral node enlargement can be seen. Nodes are also common in the paratracheal region. The diffuse parenchymal changes are typically reticulonodular infiltrates, but an acinar pattern is observed occasionally. Large nodules, similar to those of metastatic disease, are unusual but can occur. When there is massive fibrosis, the hila are pulled upward and there are conglomerate masses in the midlung zones. Some of the unusual chest x-ray findings in sarcoidosis include "egg shell" calcification of hilar nodes, pleural effusions, cavitation, atelectasis, pulmonary hypertension, pneumothorax, and cardiomegaly. Computed tomography of the chest is rarely helpful but can identify early fibrosis, and a "ground-glass" appearance is thought to be consistent with an active alveolitis.

The lung function abnormalities of sarcoidosis are typical for interstitial lung disease (see Chap. 259) and include decreased lung volumes and diffusing capacity with a normal or supernormal ratio of the forced expiratory volume in 1 s to the forced vital capacity. Occasionally there is evidence of airflow limitation. There is usually mild hypoxemia and a mild, compensated hypocarbia.

The gallium 67 lung scan is usually abnormal, showing a pattern of diffuse uptake. If present, enlarged nodes are detected in these scans, as is inflammation in a variety of extrathoracic sites that usually have no clinical importance (Fig. 320-2*B*). Bronchoalveolar lavage typically demonstrates an increased proportion of lymphocytes, most of which are activated helper-inducer T lymphocytes (Fig. 320-2*C*). The remainder of the cells are mostly alveolar macrophages. In patients with significant fibrosis, a small number of neutrophils are also found. Eosinophils are rare.

The other laboratory features of sarcoidosis depend on the specific organ involved.

DIAGNOSIS For a typical case, the diagnosis of sarcoidosis is made by a combination of clinical, radiographic, and histologic findings (Fig. 320-3*A*). In a young adult with constitutional complaints, respiratory symptoms, erythema nodosum, blurred vision, and bilateral hilar adenopathy, the diagnosis is almost always sarcoidosis. Commonly, however, the findings are more subtle. Furthermore, because sarcoidosis can occur in almost any place in the body, like tuberculosis or syphilis, it can be confused with many other disorders. In this context, the differential diagnosis of sarcoidosis must cover a wide range. However, it is confused most commonly with neoplastic diseases such as lymphoma or with disorders characterized also by a mononuclear cell granulomatous inflammatory process, such as the mycobacterial and fungal disorders.

The presence of skin anergy is typical but not diagnostic of sarcoidosis. Individuals with sarcoidosis who develop active tuberculosis react strongly to skin tests with purified protein derivative. The Kveim-Siltzbach skin test, the intradermal injection of a heat-treated suspension of a sarcoidosis spleen extract which is biopsied 4 to 6 weeks later, yields sarcoidosis-like lesions in 70 to 80 percent of individuals with sarcoidosis, with fewer than 5 percent false-positive results. However, the material is not widely available, and with the use of the transbronchial biopsy to obtain lung parenchyma for diagnostic purposes, the Kveim-Siltzbach test is not in general use.

No blood findings are diagnostic of the disease. Angiotensin-converting enzyme is elevated in the serum in approximately two-thirds of patients with sarcoidosis. Approximately 5 percent of all positive tests are not sarcoidosis and are seen in a variety of disorders, including asbestosis, silicosis, berylliosis, fungal infection, granulomatous hepatitis, hypersensitivity pneumonitis, leprosy, lymphoma, and tuberculosis. An elevated 24-h urine calcium level is consistent with the diagnosis but is not specific.

The chest x-ray cannot be used as the sole criterion for the diagnosis of sarcoidosis. While the finding of bilateral hilar adenopathy is the hallmark of this disease, a similar pattern is occasionally observed in lymphoma, tuberculosis, coccidioidomycosis, brucellosis, and bronchogenic carcinoma.

The pattern of the gallium 67 scan is not diagnostic for sarcoidosis, nor is the finding of an increased proportion of lymphocytes among the cells recovered by bronchoalveolar lavage. However, the typical patterns of these tests (Fig. 320-2*B* and *C*) put the diagnosis in the general category of granulomatous lung disorders.

Whether or not the presentation is "classic," biopsy evidence of a mononuclear cell granulomatous inflammatory process is mandatory in order to make a definitive diagnosis of sarcoidosis. Because the lung is involved so frequently, it is the most common site to be biopsied, usually through a fiberoptic bronchoscope. Less common, but acceptable, sites for biopsy are the hilar nodes (by mediastinoscopy), the skin, conjunctiva, or lip. Rarely, the spleen, intraabdominal nodes, muscle, parotid or other salivary glands, upper respiratory tract, or the heart is biopsied for diagnostic purposes. At any of these sites, the findings must include the typical noncaseating granulomas. However, although histologic evidence is mandatory for a definitive diagnosis of sarcoidosis, the histologic findings are not sufficiently specific to make the diagnosis by themselves, since noncaseating granulomas are found in a number of other diseases, including infections and malignancy. Furthermore, although the liver or scalene nodes often reveal "positive" biopsies in cases of sarcoidosis, noncaseating granulomas from other causes are so frequent in these sites that they are not considered acceptable sites for establishing the diagnosis. Thus the definitive diagnosis of sarcoidosis is based on the biopsy in the context of the history, physical examination, blood tests, x-ray, lung function, and, if available, gallium 67 scan and bronchoalveolar lavage. Patients with human immunodeficiency virus (HIV) infection commonly have lymphocytopenia, chest x-ray abnormalities, positive gallium 67 chest scans, and increased proportions of lavage lymphocytes (early in the course of the disease), and they can have lung granulomas; thus, serologic testing for HIV infection should always be done in individuals suspected of having sarcoidosis.

PROGNOSIS Overall, the prognosis in sarcoidosis is good. Most individuals who present with the acute disease are left with no significant sequelae. Approximately half of all patients have some permanent organ dysfunction, but for most this is mild, stable, and progresses rarely. In approximately 15 to 20 percent of cases, the disease remains active or recurs intermittently. Death is attributable directly to the disease in about 10 percent of all those affected.

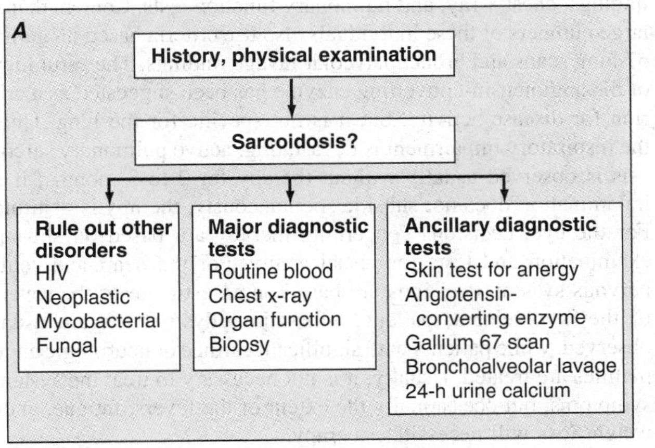

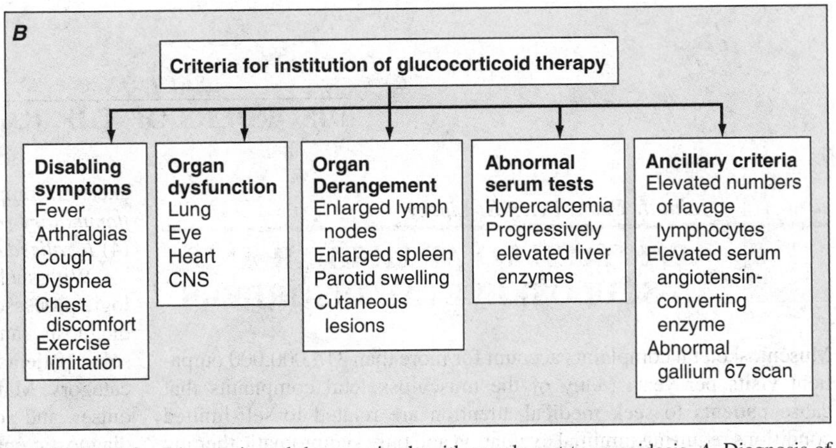

FIGURE 320-3 Diagnostic and therapeutic algorithms relevant to sarcoidosis. *A*. Diagnosis of sarcoidosis. If the history and physical examination suggest sarcoidosis, the diagnosis is made by a combination of history, physical examination, and diagnostic test. No tests are definitive for sarcoidosis; the diagnosis is made by a combination of findings. The major diagnostic tests carry the most weight, with biopsy and histologic assessment of the relevant organ the most important. Assessment of function of the organ systems that appear to be affected help with diagnosis and decisions about therapy. *B*. Therapy of sarcoidosis. Once the definitive diagnosis is made, the decision to not treat or to institute treatment with glucocorticoids is based on the presence or absence of disabling symptoms, organ dysfunction, organ derangement, and results of various tests of disease activity. Any organ can be threatened by sarcoidosis, but lung, eye, heart, and central nervous system are at greatest risk. The disease can wax and wane, and periodic assessments at 3- to 6-month intervals are used to reevaluate decisions regarding therapy.

Rx TREATMENT

The therapy of choice for sarcoidosis is glucocorticoids (Fig. 320-3*B*), A variety of other drugs have been tried, including indomethacin, oxyphenbutazone, chloroquine, methotrexate, *p*-aminobenzoate, allopurinol, levamisole, and cyclophosphamide, but there is no evidence, apart from anecdotal, uncontrolled reports, to support their efficacy. Cyclosporine is ineffective for the pulmonary manifestations of the disease; anecdotal reports suggest that it may be useful in extrathoracic sarcoid not responding to glucocorticoids.

The major problem in treating sarcoidosis is in deciding when to treat. Because the disease clears spontaneously in about 50 percent of patients, and because the permanent organ derangements often do not improve with glucocorticoids, there is controversy among clinicians as to the criteria for treatment. However, there is no question that glucocorticoids suppress effectively the activated T helper-inducer cell processes occurring at the sites of disease. Thus the major problem in making decisions concerning therapy in sarcoidosis is to determine the extent and activity of the inflammatory process in the organs at greatest risk, such as the lung, eye, heart, and central nervous system.

For the lung, this is based on a combination of history, physical findings, chest x-ray, and pulmonary function tests. Centers that see large numbers of these individuals also use criteria based on gallium 67 lung scans and bronchoalveolar lavage findings. The serum level of the angiotensin-converting enzyme has been suggested as a criterion for disease activity, but it is not specific for the lung. Unless the respiratory impairment is devastating, active pulmonary sarcoidosis is observed usually without therapy for 2 to 3 months; if the inflammation does not subside spontaneously, therapy is instituted. For the eye, decisions concerning therapy are based on slit-lamp examination and tests for visual acuity. For the heart and central nervous system, decisions are based on an estimate of the severity of the involvement; patients with minor dysfunction are usually observed, while patients with significant cardiac or neurologic abnormalities are treated. Usually, it is not necessary to treat the systemic symptoms, but occasionally the extent of the fevers, fatigue, and/or weight loss will necessitate therapy.

The usual therapy for sarcoidosis is prednisone, 1 mg/kg, for 4 to 6 weeks, followed by a slow taper over 2 to 3 months. This is repeated if the disease again becomes active. Alternate-day therapy is used by some clinicians, but there is no evidence that it is as effective. High-dose bolus intravenous glucocorticoids are used occasionally but are probably not as effective as oral therapy. There is no evidence that inhaled glucocorticoids are efficacious. Mild ocular disease responds usually to local therapy, but suppression of the uveitis often requires systemic glucocorticoids.

BIBLIOGRAPHY

CONSENSUS CONFERENCE: Activity of sarcoidosis. Third WASOG Meeting. Eur Respir J 7:624, 1994

CRYSTAL RG: Interstitial lung disease of unknown etiology: Disorders characterized by chronic inflammation of the lower respiratory tract. N Engl J Med 310:154, 235, 1984

DU BOIS RM: Corticosteroids in sarcoidosis: Friend or foe? Eur Respir J 7:1203, 1994

——— et al: Granulomatous processes, in *The Lung: Scientific Foundations*, 2d ed, RG Crystal et al (eds). Philadelphia, Lippincott-Raven, 1996, pp 2395–2409

FANBURG BL, PITT EA: Sarcoidosis, in *Textbook of Respiratory Medicine*, JF Murray, JA Nadel (eds). Philadelphia, Saunders, 1988, pp 1486–1500

JAMES DG (ed): *Sarcoidosis and Other Granulomatous Disorders*. New York, Marcel Dekker, 1994

MOLLER DR et al: Bias toward use of a specific T-cell receptor β-chain variable region in a subgroup of individuals with sarcoidosis. J Clin Invest 82:1183, 1988

NAGAI S, IZUMI T: Pulmonary sarcoidosis: Population differences and pathophysiology. South Med J 88:1001, 1995

PINKSTON P et al: Spontaneous release of interleukin-2 by lung T-lymphocytes in active pulmonary sarcoidosis. N Engl J Med 208:793, 1983

ROBINSON BWS et al: Gamma interferon is spontaneously released by alveolar macrophages and lung T-lymphocytes in patients with pulmonary sarcoidosis. J Clin Invest 75:1488, 1985

ROBINSON DS et al: Granulomatous processes, in *The Lung: Scientific Foundations*, 2d ed, RG Crystal et al (eds). Philadelphia, Lippincott-Raven, 1996, pp 2395–2410

SALTINI C et al: Spontaneous release of interleukin-2 by lung T-lymphocytes in active pulmonary sarcoidosis is primarily from the Leu3 + DR + T-cell subset. J Clin Invest 77:1962, 1986

SHARMA OP: Pulmonary sarcoidosis and corticosteroids. Am Rev Resp Dis 147:1598, 1993

VENET A et al: Enhanced alveolar macrophage-mediated antigen-induced T-lymphocyte proliferation in sarcoidosis. J Clin Invest 75:293, 1985

SECTION 3

DISORDERS OF THE JOINTS

321

John J. Cush, Peter E. Lipsky

APPROACH TO ARTICULAR AND MUSCULOSKELETAL DISORDERS

Musculoskeletal complaints account for more than 315,000,000 outpatient visits per year. Many of the musculoskeletal complaints that cause patients to seek medical attention are related to self-limited conditions requiring minimal evaluation and only symptomatic therapy and reassurance. However, some patients with similar symptoms have a more serious condition that requires further evaluation or additional laboratory testing to confirm the suspected diagnosis or determine the extent and nature of the pathologic process. The initial goal of the clinician is to formulate a differential diagnosis that leads to accurate diagnosis and timely therapy while avoiding excessive diagnostic testing and unnecessary treatment (Table 321-1).

Individuals with musculoskeletal complaints should be evaluated in a uniform, logical manner by means of a thorough history, a comprehensive physical examination, and if appropriate, laboratory testing. The goals of the initial encounter are to determine whether the musculoskeletal complaint is (1) *articular* or *nonarticular* in origin, (2) *inflammatory* or *noninflammatory* in nature, (3) *acute* or *chronic*, and (4) *localized*, *widespread*, or *systemic*.

With such an approach and an understanding of the pathophysiologic processes that underlie musculoskeletal complaints, an adequate diagnosis can be made in the vast majority of individuals. However, some patients will not fit immediately into an established diagnostic category. Many musculoskeletal disorders resemble each other at the outset, and some take months to evolve into a readily recognizable diagnostic entity. This consideration should temper the desire always to establish a definitive diagnosis at the first encounter.

ARTICULAR VERSUS NONARTICULAR SITE OF ORIGIN The musculoskeletal evaluation must discriminate the anatomic site(s) of origin of the patient's complaint. For example, ankle pain can result from a variety of pathologic conditions involving disparate anatomic structures, including gonococcal arthritis, calcaneal fracture, Achilles tendinitis, cellulitis, and peripheral neuropathy. Articular structures include the synovium, synovial fluid, articular cartilage, intraarticular ligaments, joint capsule, and juxtaarticular bone. Nonarticular (or periarticular) structures, such as supportive extraarticular ligaments, tendons, bursae, muscle, fascia, bone, nerve, and overlying skin, may be involved in the pathologic process. Pain from these structures may mimic true articular pain because of their proximity to the joint. Distinguishing between articular and nonarticular disease requires a careful and detailed examination. Articular disorders may be characterized by pain and limited range of motion on active and passive movement, swelling caused by synovial proliferation or effusion or bony enlargement, crepitation, instability, locking, or deformity. By contrast, nonarticular disorders tend to be painful on active but not passive range of motion, demonstrate point or focal tenderness in regions distinct from articular structures, and have physical findings remote from the joint capsule. Moreover, nonarticular disorders seldom demonstrate crepitus, instability, or deformity.

INFLAMMATORY VERSUS NONINFLAMMATORY DISORDERS In the course of a musculoskeletal evaluation, the examiner should elicit symptoms and signs that will narrow or establish the diagnosis. A primary objective is to identify the nature of the underlying pathologic process. Musculoskeletal disorders are generally classified as inflammatory or noninflammatory. Inflammatory disorders may be infectious (infection with *Neisseria gonorrhoea* or *Mycobacterium tuberculosis*), crystal-induced (gout, pseudogout), immune-related [rheumatoid arthritis (RA), systemic lupus erythematosus (SLE)], reactive (rheumatic fever, Reiter's syndrome), or idiopathic. Inflammatory disorders may be identified by the presence of some or all of the four cardinal signs of inflammation (erythema, warmth, pain, and swelling), by systemic symptoms (prolonged morning stiffness, fatigue, fever, weight loss), or by laboratory evidence of inflammation (elevated erythrocyte sedimentation rate or C-reactive protein level or thrombocytosis). Articular stiffness is common in chronic musculoskeletal disorders. However, the chronology and magnitude of stiffness may be diagnostically important. Morning stiffness related to inflammatory disorders (such as RA) is precipitated by prolonged rest, often lasts several hours, and may improve with activity and anti-inflammatory medications. By contrast, intermittent stiffness associated with noninflammatory conditions, such as osteoarthritis, is precipitated by brief periods of rest, usually lasts less than 60 min, and is exacerbated by activity. Noninflammatory disorders may be related to trauma (rotator cuff tear), ineffective repair (osteoarthritis), cellular overgrowth (pigmented villonodular synovitis), or pain amplification (fibromyalgia). They are often characterized by pain without swelling or warmth, the absence of inflammatory or systemic features, little or no morning stiffness, and normal laboratory findings.

Identification of the nature of the underlying process and the site of the complaint will enable the examiner to narrow the diagnostic considerations and to assess the need for immediate diagnostic or therapeutic intervention or for continued observation. Figure 321-1 presents a logical approach to the evaluation of patients with musculoskeletal complaints.

CLINICAL HISTORY Additional historic features may be helpful in establishing the nature and extent of the pathologic process and may provide important clues to the diagnosis. Aspects of the patient profile, including age, sex, race, and family history, can provide important information. Certain diagnoses are more frequent in specific age groups. SLE, rheumatic fever, and Reiter's syndrome are more common in the young, whereas fibromyalgia is most common in middle age, and osteoarthritis and polymyalgia rheumatica in old age. Some diseases are more common in a particular gender or race. Gout and the spondyloarthropathies (e.g., ankylosing spondylitis, Reiter's syndrome) are more common in men, whereas rheumatoid arthritis and fibromyalgia are more common in women. Polymyalgia rheumatica, giant cell arteritis, and Wegener's granulomatosis preferentially affect whites, whereas sarcoidosis and systemic lupus erythematosus are more common in blacks. *Familial aggregation* occurs in some disorders, such as ankylosing spondylitis, gout, RA, and Heberden's nodes of osteoarthritis.

The chronology of the complaint (*onset*, *evolution*, and *duration*) is an important diagnostic feature. The onset of disorders such as septic arthritis and gout tends to be abrupt, whereas osteoarthritis, rheumatoid arthritis, and fibromyalgia may develop more indolently In terms of evolution, disorders are classified as chronic (e.g., osteoarthritis), intermittent (e.g., gout), migratory (e.g., rheumatic fever, gonococcal or viral arthritis), or additive (e.g., RA, Reiter's syndrome). Musculoskeletal disorders typically are called *acute* if they last less than 6 weeks and *chronic* if they last longer. Acute arthropathies tend to be infectious, crystal-induced, or reactive. Noninflammatory and immune-related arthritides, such as osteoarthritis and RA, respectively, are often chronic. The duration of the patient's complaints may alter the diagnostic considerations. For example, the musculoskeletal signs and symptoms of hepatitis B virus infection may be identical with those of early RA at the onset but rarely persist beyond 3 weeks.

The *number and distribution* of involved articulations should be noted. Articular disorders are classified as *monarticular* (one joint involved), *oligoarticular* or *pauciarticular* (two to three joints involved), or *polyarticular* (more than three joints involved). Nonarticular disorders can be classified as either *focal* or *widespread*. Complaints secondary to trauma and gout are typically focal or monarticular, whereas polymyositis, RA, and fibromyalgia are more diffuse or polyarticular. Joint involvement tends to be symmetric in RA but is often asymmetric in the spondyloarthropathies and in gout. The upper extremities are frequently involved in rheumatoid arthritis, whereas lower extremity arthritis is characteristic of Reiter's syndrome and gout at their onset. Involvement of the axial skeleton is common in osteoarthritis and ankylosing spondylitis but infrequent in RA, with the notable exception of the cervical spine.

The clinical history should also identify *precipitating events*, such as trauma, drug administration, or antecedent or intercurrent illnesses, that may have contributed to the patient's complaint. Last, a thorough *rheumatic review of systems* may disclose associated features outside the musculoskeletal system and provide useful diagnostic information. A variety of musculoskeletal disorders may be associated with systemic features such as fever (SLE, infection), rash (SLE, Reiter's syndrome, dermatomyositis), myalgias, weakness (polymyositis, polymyalgia rheumatica), and morning stiffness (inflammatory arthritis). In addition, some conditions are associated with involvement of other organ systems, including the eyes (Behçet's disease, sarcoidosis, Reiter's syndrome), gastrointestinal tract (scleroderma, inflammatory bowel disease), genitourinary tract (Reiter's syndrome, gonococcemia), and nervous system (Lyme disease, vasculitis).

PHYSICAL EXAMINATION The goal of the physical examination is to ascertain the structures involved, the nature of the underlying pathology, the extent and functional consequences of the process, and the presence of systemic or extraarticular manifestations (Table 321-2). A knowledge of topographic anatomy is necessary to identify the primary site(s) of involvement and differentiate articular from nonarticular disorders. The musculoskeletal examination depends largely on careful inspection, palpation, and a variety of specific physical maneuvers to elicit diagnostic signs. Although most articulations of the appendicular skeleton can be examined in this manner, adequate inspection and palpation are not possible for many axial (e.g., zygapophyseal) and inaccessible (e.g., sacroiliac or hip) joints. For such

Table 321-1

Evaluation of Patients with Musculoskeletal Complaints

Goals
Accurate diagnosis
Timely provision of therapy
Avoidance of unnecessary diagnostic testing
Approach
Anatomic localization of complaint (articular vs. nonarticular)
Determination of the nature of the pathologic process (inflammatory vs. noninflammatory)
Determination of the extent of involvement (monarticular, polyarticular, focal, widespread)
Determination of chronology (acute vs. chronic)
Formulation of a differential diagnosis

joints, there is a greater reliance on specific maneuvers and imaging for assessment.

Examination of involved and uninvolved joints will determine whether *warmth*, *erythema*, or *swelling* is present. The examination should distinguish true articular swelling caused by synovial effusion or synovial proliferation from nonarticular or periarticular involvement, which usually extends beyond the normal joint margins or the full extent of the synovial space. Synovial effusion can be distinguished from synovial hypertrophy or bony hypertrophy by palpation or specific maneuvers. For example, small to moderate knee effusions may be identified by the "bulge sign" or "ballottement of the patella." Bursal effusions (e.g., effusions of the olecranon or prepatellar bursa) overlie bony prominences and are fluctuant with sharply defined borders. Joint *stability* can be assessed by palpation and by the application of manual stress. Subluxation or dislocation, which may be secondary to traumatic, mechanical, or inflammatory causes, can be assessed by inspection and palpation. Joint *volume* can be assessed by palpation. Distention of the articular capsule usually causes pain. The patient will attempt to minimize the pain by keeping the joint in the position of least intraarticular pressure and greatest volume, usually partial flexion. Clinically, joint distention may be detected as obvious swelling, voluntary or fixed flexion deformities, or diminished range of motion—especially on extension, which decreases joint volume. Active and passive *range of motion* should be assessed in all planes, with contralateral comparison. Serial evaluations of joint motion may be made using a goniometer to quantify the arc of movement. Each joint should be passively manipulated through its full range of motion (including, as appropriate, flexion, extension, rotation, abduction, adduction, inversion, eversion, supination, pronation, and medial or lateral deviation or bending). Limitation of motion is frequently caused by effusion, pain, deformity, or contracture. *Contractures* may reflect antecedent synovial inflammation or trauma. Joint *crepitus* may be felt during palpation or maneuvers and may be prominent in osteoarthritis. Joint *deformity* usually indicates a long-standing or aggressive pathologic process. Deformities may result from ligamentous destruction, soft tissue contracture, bony enlargement, ankylosis, erosive disease, or subluxation. Examination of the musculature will permit assessment of strength and reveal atrophy, pain, or spasm. The examiner should look carefully for nonarticular or periarticular involvement, especially when articular complaints are not supported by objective findings referable to the joint capsule. The identification of musculoskeletal pain of soft tissue origin (nonarticular pain) will prevent unwarranted and often expensive additional evaluations. Specific maneuvers may reveal nonarticular abnormalities, such as a carpal tunnel syndrome (which can be identified by Tinel's or Phalen's sign). Other examples of soft tissue abnormalities include olecranon bursitis, epicondylitis (tennis elbow), enthesitis (e.g., Achilles tendinitis), and trigger points associated with fibromyalgia.

LABORATORY INVESTIGATIONS The vast majority of musculoskeletal disorders can be diagnosed easily by a complete history and physical examination. An additional objective of the initial encounter is to determine whether additional investigations or immediate therapy are required. A number of features indicate the need for additional evaluation. *Monarticular* conditions require additional evaluation, as do *traumatic* or *inflammatory* conditions and conditions accompanied by *neurologic changes* or *systemic manifestations* of serious disease. Finally, individuals with *chronic* symptoms (lasting more than 6 weeks), especially when there has been a lack of response to symptomatic measures, are candidates for additional evaluation. The extent and nature of the

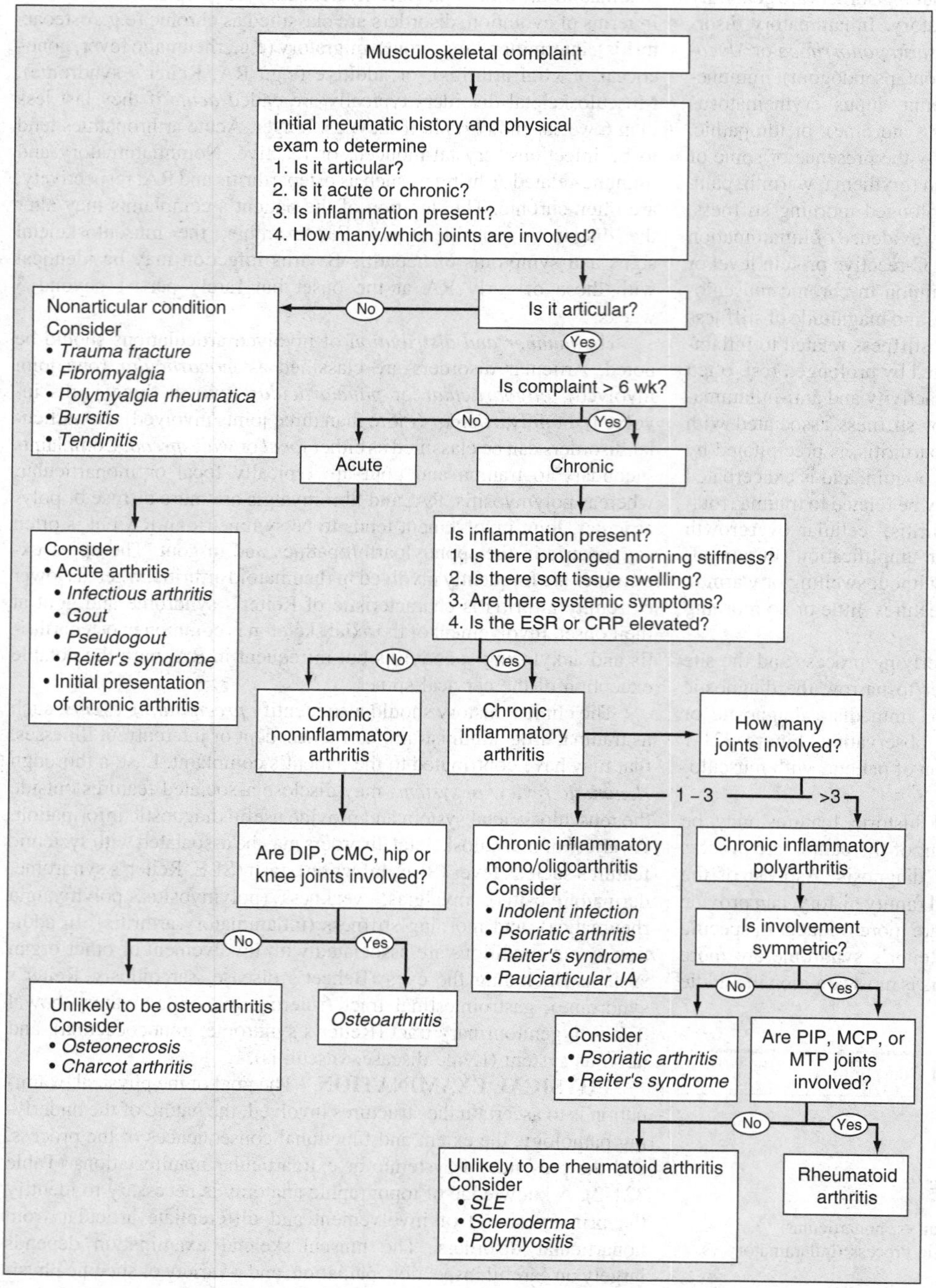

FIGURE 321-1 Algorithm for the diagnosis of musculoskeletal complaints. An approach to formulating a differential diagnosis (shown in italics). (ESR, erythrocyte sedimentation rate; CRP, C-reactive protein; DIP, distal interphalangeal; CMC, carpometacarpal; PIP, proximal interphalangeal; MCP, metacarpophalangeal; MTP, metatarsophalangeal; PMR, polymyalgia rheumatica; SLE, systemic lupus erythematosus; JA, juvenile arthritis.)

Table 321-2

Glossary of Musculoskeletal Terms

Subluxation	Alteration of joint alignment such that articulating surfaces incompletely approximate each other
Dislocation	Abnormal displacement of articulating surfaces such that the surfaces are not in contact
Range of motion	For diarthrodial joints, the arc of measurable movement through which the joint moves in a single plane
Contracture	Loss of full movement resulting from a fixed resistance due either to tonic spasm of muscle (reversible) or to fibrosis of periarticular structures (permanent)
Deformity	Abnormal shape or size of a structure; may result from bony hypertrophy, malalignment of articulating structures, or damage to periarticular supportive structures
Enthesitis	Inflammation of the entheses (tendinous or ligamentous insertions on bone)
Epicondylitis	Infection or inflammation involving an epicondyle

additional investigation should be dictated by the clinical features and suspected pathologic process. Broad batteries of diagnostic tests and radiographic procedures are rarely useful or cost-effective.

Besides a complete blood count, including a white blood cell and differential count, the routine evaluation should include determination of an acute-phase indicator, such as the erythrocyte sedimentation rate (ESR) or C-reactive protein (CRP), which can be useful in discriminating inflammatory from noninflammatory musculoskeletal disorders. Both tests are inexpensive and easily performed; the resulting values may be elevated with infections, inflammatory arthritis, autoimmune disorders, neoplasia, pregnancy, and advanced age. Serum uric acid determinations are only useful when gout has been diagnosed and therapy contemplated.

Serologic tests for rheumatoid factor, antinuclear antibodies, complement levels, Lyme disease antibodies, or antistreptolysin O (ASO) titer should be carried out only when there is substantive clinical evidence suggesting a relevant diagnosis, as these tests have poor predictive value when used in a screening fashion. They should not be performed arbitrarily in patients with minimal or nonspecific musculoskeletal complaints. IgM rheumatoid factor (autoantibodies against the Fc portion of IgG) is found in 80 percent of patients with RA and may also be seen in low titers in patients with chronic infections (tuberculosis, leprosy), other autoimmune diseases (SLE, Sjögren's syndrome), or chronic pulmonary, hepatic, or renal diseases. Antinuclear antibodies (ANAs) are found in nearly all patients with SLE and may also be seen in patients with other autoimmune diseases (polymyositis, scleroderma), drug-induced lupus (resulting from hydralazine, procainamide, or quinidine administration), or chronic hepatic or renal disorders. The interpretation of a positive ANA determination may depend on the titer and on the pattern observed by immunofluorescence microscopy. Diffuse and speckled patterns are the least specific, whereas a peripheral, or rim, pattern is highly specific and is suggestive of autoantibodies against double-stranded (native) DNA. This pattern is seen only in patients with SLE.

Aspiration and analysis of synovial fluid is always indicated in acute monarthritis or when an infectious or crystal-induced arthropathy is suspected. Synovial fluid analysis may be crucial in distinguishing between noninflammatory and inflammatory processes. This distinction can be made on the basis of the appearance, viscosity, and cell count of the synovial fluid. Tests for synovial fluid glucose, protein, lactate dehydrogenase, lactic acid, or autoantibodies are not recommended, as they are insensitive or have little discriminatory value. Noninflammatory synovial fluid is clear, viscous, and amber-colored, with a white blood cell count of $<2000/\mu L$ and a predominance of mononuclear cells. The viscosity of synovial fluid is assessed by expressing fluid from the syringe one drop at a time. Normally there is a stringing effect, with a long tail behind each drop. Effusions due to osteoarthritis or trauma usually have this typical viscosity. Inflammatory fluid is turbid and yellow, with an increased white cell count (2000 to 50,000 cells per microliter) and a predominance of polymorphonuclear leukocytes. Inflammatory fluid has a reduced viscosity, with little or no tail following each drop of synovial fluid. Such effusions are found in RA, gout, other inflammatory arthritides, and septic arthritis. Infectious fluid is turbid and opaque, with a white cell count usually $>50,000/\mu L$, a predominance of polymorphonuclear leukocytes (>75%), and low viscosity. Such effusions are typical of septic arthritis, but they occur rarely with sterile inflammatory arthritides such as RA or gout. In addition, hemorrhagic synovial fluid may be seen with hemarthrosis or trauma. An algorithm for synovial fluid aspiration and analysis is shown in Fig. 321-2. Synovial fluid should be analyzed immediately for appearance, viscosity, and cell count. Cellularity and the presence of crystals may be assessed by light or polarizing microscopy, respectively. Monosodium urate crystals, seen in gouty effusions, are long, needle-shaped, negatively birefringent, and usually intracellular, whereas calcium pyrophosphate dihydrate crystals, found in chondrocalcinosis and pseudogout, are usually short, rhomboid-shaped, and positively birefringent. Whenever infection is

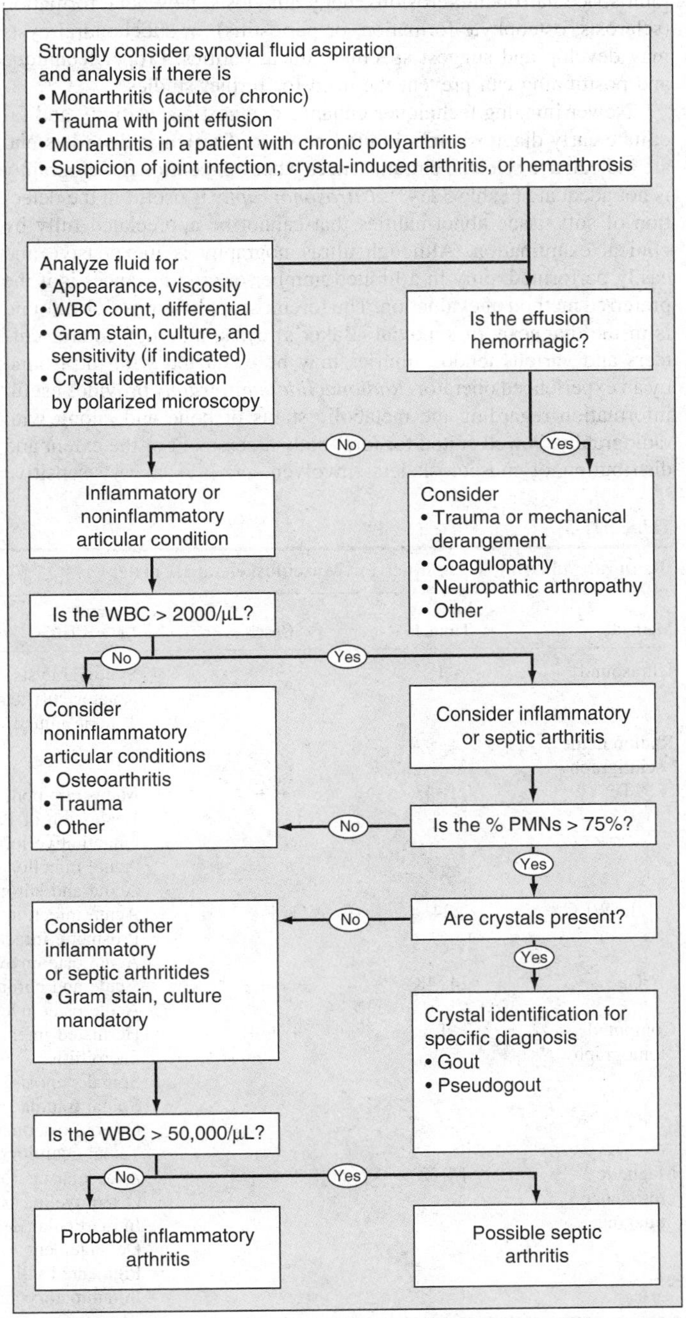

FIGURE 321-2 Algorithmic approach to the use and interpretation of synovial fluid aspiration and analysis.

suspected, synovial fluid should be Gram stained and cultured appropriately. If gonococcal arthritis is suspected, immediate plating of the fluid on appropriate culture medium is indicated. Synovial fluid from chronic monarthritis patients should also be cultured for *M. tuberculosis* and fungi. Last, it should be noted that crystal-induced arthritis and infection occasionally occur together in the same joint.

DIAGNOSTIC IMAGING IN JOINT DISEASES Conventional radiography has been a valuable tool in the diagnosis and staging of articular disorders. Plain x-rays are most appropriate when there is a history of trauma, suspected chronic infection, progressive disability, or monarticular involvement; when therapeutic alterations are considered; or when a baseline assessment is desired for what appears to be a chronic process. However, in most inflammatory disorders, early radiography is rarely helpful in establishing a diagnosis and may only reveal soft tissue swelling or juxtaarticular demineralization. As the disease progresses, calcification (of soft tissues, cartilage, or bone), joint space narrowing, erosions, bony ankylosis, new bone formation (sclerosis, osteophyte formation, or periostitis), or subchondral cysts may develop and suggest specific clinical entities. Proper technique and positioning can prevent the need for further studies.

Newer imaging techniques enhance diagnostic sensitivity and facilitate early diagnosis in a limited number of articular disorders and are indicated in selected circumstances when conventional radiography is not adequate (Table 321-3). *Ultrasonography* is useful in the detection of soft tissue abnormalities that cannot be appreciated fully by clinical examination. Although ultrasonography is inexpensive and easily performed, only in a limited number of circumstances is it the preferred method of evaluation. The foremost application of ultrasound is in the diagnosis of synovial (Baker's) cysts, although rotator cuff tears and various tendon injuries may be evaluated with ultrasound by an experienced operator. *Radionuclide scintigraphy* provides useful information regarding the metabolic status of bone and, along with radiography, is well suited for total-body assessment of the extent and distribution of musculoskeletal involvement. It is a very sensitive but poorly specific means of detecting inflammatory or metabolic alterations in bone or periarticular soft tissue structures. The limited tissue resolution of scintigraphy may obscure the distinction between bony and periarticular processes and may necessitate the use of additional imaging modalities. Scintigraphy, using ^{99m}Tc, ^{67}Ga, or white blood cells (WBCs) labeled with ^{111}In, has been applied to a variety of articular disorders with variable success (Table 321-2). [^{99m}Tc]pertechnetate or [^{99m}Tc]diphosphonate scintigraphy may be useful in identifying infection, neoplasia, inflammation, increased blood flow, bone remodeling, heterotopic bone formation, or avascular necrosis (Fig. 321-3). However, the poor specificity of ^{99m}Tc scanning has limited its use to investigational and serial assessments of joint or bone involvement, assessment of inflammatory or infectious processes, and surveys for bone metastases. ^{67}Ga binds to serum and cellular transferrin and lactoferrin and is preferentially taken up by neutrophils, macrophages, bacteria, and tumor tissue (e.g., lymphoma tissue) and is useful in the identification of infection and malignancies. Scanning with ^{111}In-labeled WBCs has been used to detect both infectious and inflammatory arthritis. Although both have been used with success, ^{111}In-labeled WBC scanning is superior to ^{67}Ga in the early diagnosis of osteomyelitis and infected prosthetic joints. Prior treatment with antibiotics may reduce the diagnostic sensitivity of both ^{67}Ga and ^{111}In-labeled WBC scintigraphy.

Computed tomography (CT) provides rapid reconstruction of sagittal, coronal, and axial images and thus of the spatial relationships among anatomic structures. It has proved most useful in the assessment of the axial skeleton because of its ability to visualize in the axial plane. Articulations that are difficult to visualize by conventional radiography, such as the zygapophyseal, sacroiliac, sternoclavicular, and hip joints, can be evaluated effectively using CT. CT has been demonstrated to be useful in the diagnosis of low back pain syndromes, sacroiliitis, osteoid osteoma, tarsal coalition, osteomyelitis, intraarticular osteochondral fragments, and advanced osteonecrosis.

Magnetic resonance imaging (MRI) has significantly advanced the ability to image musculoskeletal structures. MRI can provide multiplanar images with fine anatomic detail and contrast resolution (Fig. 321-4). Other advantages are the absence of ionizing radiation and adverse effects and the superior ability to visualize bone marrow and soft tissue periarticular structures. However, the high cost and long procedural time of MRI limit its use in the evaluation of musculoskeletal disorders. MRI should be used only when it will provide necessary information that cannot be obtained by less expensive and noninvasive means.

MRI can image fascia, vessels, nerve, muscle, cartilage, ligaments, tendons, pannus, synovial effusions, cortical bone, and bone marrow. Visualization of particular structures can be enhanced by altering the pulse sequence to produce either T1-weighted or T2-weighted spin echo, gradient echo, or inversion recovery (including STIR) images (Fig. 321-5). Because of its sensitivity to changes in marrow fat, MRI is a sensitive although nonspecific means of detecting osteonecrosis and osteomyelitis. Because of its greater ability to resolve soft tissue contrasts, MRI is more sensitive than arthrography or CT for the diagnosis of soft tissue injuries (e.g., meniscal and rotator cuff tears), intraarticular derangements, and spinal cord damage following injury, subluxation, or synovitis of the vertebrae.

Table 321-3

Diagnostic Imaging Techniques for Musculoskeletal Disorders

Method	Imaging Time, h	Cost*	Current Indications
Ultrasound†	<1	+	Synovial cysts Rotator cuff tears Tendon injury
Radionuclide scintigraphy			
^{99m}Tc	1–4	++	Metastatic bone survey Evaluation of Paget's disease Quantitative joint assessment Acute infection Acute and chronic osteomyelitis
^{111}In-WBC	24	+++	Acute infection Prosthetic infection Acute osteomyelitis
^{67}Ga	24–48	++++	Acute and chronic infection Acute osteomyelitis
Computed tomography	<1	+++	Herniated intervertebral disk Sacroiliitis Spinal stenosis Spinal trauma Osteoid osteoma Tarsal coalition
Magnetic resonance imaging	1/2–2	+++++	Avascular necrosis Osteomyelitis Intraarticular derangement and soft tissue injury Derangements of axial skeleton and spinal cord Pigmented villonodular synovitis Inflammatory and metabolic muscle pathology

* Relative cost for imaging study.
† Results depend on operator.

RHEUMATOLOGIC EVALUATION OF THE ELDERLY Muscu-

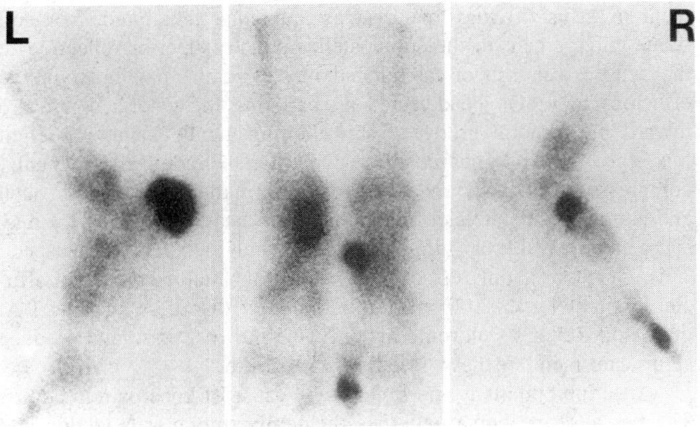

FIGURE 321-3 [^{99m}Tc]diphosphonate scintigraphy of the feet of a 33-year-old black male with Reiter's syndrome, manifested by sacroiliitis, urethritis, uveitis, asymmetric oligoarthritis, and enthesitis. This bone scan demonstrates increased uptake indicative of enthesitis involving the insertions of the left Achilles tendon, plantar aponeurosis, and right tibialis posterior tendon as well as arthritis of the right first interphalangeal joint.

loskeletal disorders in elderly patients are often not diagnosed because the signs and symptoms may be insidious or chronic in these patients. In addition, the nature of the problem is often obscured by the presence of multiple interacting factors, including other medical conditions and therapies. These difficulties are compounded by the diminished reliability of laboratory testing in the elderly, which is secondary to the wider range of nonpathologic variability. For example, erythrocyte sedimentation rates may be misleadingly high and titers of rheumatoid factor or antinuclear antibodies misleadingly low. Although nearly all rheumatic disorders can afflict the elderly, certain diseases and drug-induced disorders are more common in this age group. The elderly should be approached in the same manner as other patients with musculoskeletal complaints, but with additional inquiries to exclude common geriatric musculoskeletal disorders. An emphasis on identifying the rheumatic consequences of intercurrent medical conditions and therapies is extremely important. Drug-induced lupus erythematosus, polymyalgia rheumatica, gout, and chronic salicylate toxicity are all more common in the elderly than in other individuals. The physical examination should put an emphasis on coexisting diseases that may influence the diagnosis and choice of treatment.

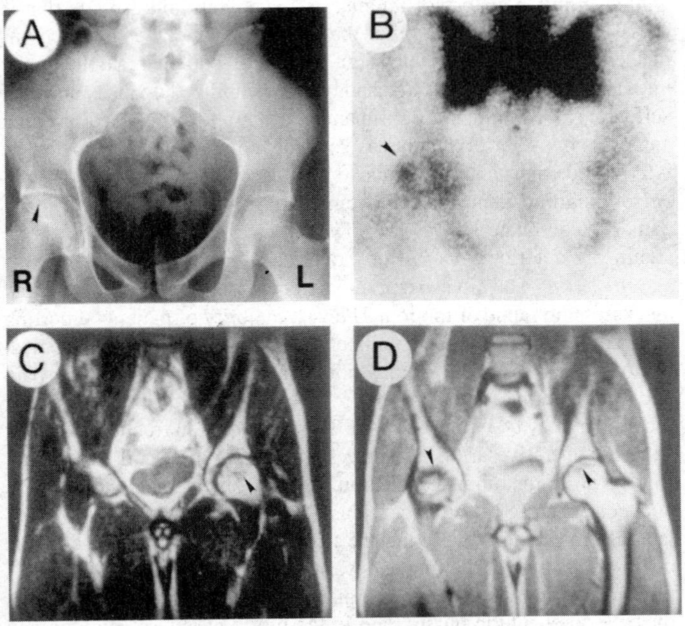

FIGURE 321-4 Superior sensitivity of magnetic resonance imaging in the diagnosis of osteonecrosis of the femoral head. A 25-year-old white man taking high-dose glucocorticoids for idiopathic thrombocytopenic purpura developed bilateral hip pain. Conventional x-ray films (*A*) demonstrated abnormalities only in the right hip consistent with stage II osteonecrosis (*arrow*). A bone scan (*B*) revealed increased uptake in the right hip only (*arrow*). MRI using spin-echo proton density images (*C* and *D*) demonstrated low-density signals from both femoral heads (*arrows*), indicative of bilateral osteonecrosis.

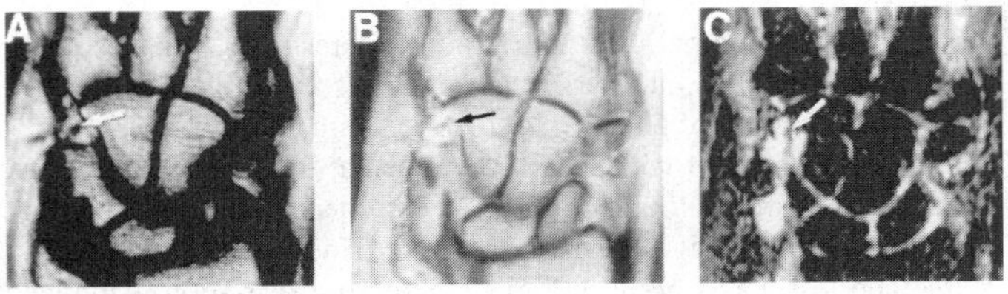

FIGURE 321-5 Coronal magnetic resonance images of the wrist in a 54-year-old woman with rheumatoid arthritis. *A*. T1-weighted image demonstrates an erosion of the triquetrum (*arrow*). *B*. Gadopentetate dimeglumine enhanced T1-weighted image demonstrates enhancement of the same erosion (*arrow*), indicating the presence of vascularized pannus. *C*. Inversion-recovery (STIR) image demonstrates a fluid-dense, high-intensity signal near the triquetrum (*arrow*) and in the intercarpal spaces, suggesting widespread intercarpal inflammation.

Approach to the Patient

With Regional Rheumatic Complaints Although all patients should be evaluated in a logical and thorough manner, many cases of focal musculoskeletal complaints are caused by commonly encountered disorders that exhibit a predictable pattern of onset, evolution, and localization and that often can be diagnosed immediately on the basis of limited historical information and selected maneuvers or tests. Although nearly every joint can be approached in this manner, the evaluation of four commonly involved anatomic regions—the hand, shoulder, hip, and knee—are reviewed here.

HAND PAIN Focal or unilateral hand pain may result from trauma, overuse, infection, or a reactive or crystal-induced arthritis. By contrast, bilateral hand complaints suggest osteoarthritis or a systemic or inflammatory/immune etiology. Patterns of joint involvement are highly suggestive of certain disorders. The distribution of affected joints in the hand may provide important diagnostic information. Thus, osteoarthritis (or degenerative arthritis) may manifest as distal interphalangeal (DIP) and proximal interphalangeal (PIP) joint pain with bony hypertrophy sufficient to produce Heberden's and Bouchard's nodes, respectively. Pain, with or without bony swelling, involving the base of the thumb (first carpometacarpal joint) is also highly suggestive of osteoarthritis. By contrast, RA tends to involve the proximal interphalangeal, metacarpophalangeal, intercarpal, and carpometacarpal joints (wrist) with pain, prolonged stiffness, and palpable synovial tissue hypertrophy. Psoriatic arthritis may also involve the DIP and PIP joints and the carpus with inflammatory pain, stiffness, and synovitis. Moreover, the diagnosis of psoriatic arthritis can be suggested by nail pitting or onycholysis. Soft tissue swelling may also be noted over the dorsum of the hand and wrist and may suggest an inflammatory extensor tendon tenosynovitis, possibly caused by gonococcal infection, gout, or inflammatory arthritis. The diagnosis of tenosynovitis may be suggested by local warmth and edema and is confirmed when pain is induced by maintaining the wrist in a fixed, neutral position and flexing the digits distal to the metacarpophalangeal joints to stretch the extensor tendon sheaths.

Focal wrist pain localized to the radial aspect may be caused by DeQuervain's tenosynovitis resulting from inflammation of the tendon sheath(s) involving the abductor pollicis longus or extensor pollicis brevis. This condition commonly results from overuse or develops after pregnancy and may be diagnosed with Finkelstein's test. A positive result in Finkelstein's test is present when local wrist pain is induced after the thumb is flexed across the palm and placed inside a clenched fist and the examiner passively deviates the hand towards the ulnar side. Carpal tunnel syndrome is another common disorder of the upper extremity and results from compression of the median nerve within the carpal tunnel to produce paresthesias in the thumb and the second, third, and radial half of the fourth fingers as well as, sometimes, atrophy of thenar musculature. Carpal tunnel syndrome is commonly associated with pregnancy, edema, trauma, osteoarthritis, inflammatory arthritis, and infiltrative disorders (e.g., amyloidosis). The diagnosis is suggested by a positive Tinel's or Phalen's sign. With each test, paresthesia in a median nerve distribution is induced or increased by either "thumping" the volar aspect of the wrist (Tinel's sign) or pressing the extensor surfaces of the two flexed wrists against each another (Phalen's sign).

SHOULDER PAIN During the evaluation of shoulder disorders, the examiner should carefully note any history of trauma, infection, inflammatory disease, occupational hazards, or previous cervical disease. In addition, the patient should be questioned as to the activities or movement(s) that elicit shoulder pain. Shoulder pain frequently is referred from the cervical spine, but it may also be referred from intrathoracic lesions (e.g., a Pancoast tumor) or from gallbladder, hepatic, or diaphragmatic disease. The shoulder should be put through its full range of motion both actively and passively (with examiner assistance): forward flexion, extension, abduction, adduction, and rotation. Manual inspection of the periarticular structures will often provide important diagnostic information. The examiner should apply direct manual pressure over the subacromial bursa, which lies lateral to and immediately beneath the acromion. Subacromial bursitis is a frequent cause of shoulder pain. Anterior to the subacromial bursa, the bicipital tendon traverses the bicipital groove. This tendon is best identified by palpating it in its groove as the patient rotates the humerus internally and externally. Direct pressure over the tendon may reveal pain indicative of bicipital tendinitis. Palpation of the acromioclavicular joint may disclose local pain, bony hypertrophy, or synovial swelling. Whereas osteoarthritis and RA commonly affect the acromioclavicular joint, osteoarthritis seldom involves the glenohumeral joint, unless there is a traumatic or occupational cause. The glenohumeral joint is best palpated anteriorly by placing the thumb over the humeral head (just medial and inferior to the coracoid process) and having the patient rotate the humerus internally and externally. Pain localized to this region is indicative of glenohumeral pathology. Synovial effusion or tissue is seldom palpable, but if present may suggest infection, RA, or an acute tear of the rotator cuff.

Rotator cuff tendinitis or tear is a very common cause of shoulder pain. The rotator cuff is formed by the tendons of the supraspinatus, infraspinatus, teres minor, and subscapularis muscles. Rotator cuff tendinitis is suggested by pain on active abduction (but not passive abduction), pain over the lateral deltoid muscle, night pain, and evidence of the impingement sign. This maneuver is performed by the examiner raising the patient's arm into forced flexion while stabilizing the scapula and preventing it from rotating. A positive sign is present if pain develops before 180° of forward flexion. A complete tear of the rotator cuff, which often results from trauma, may manifest in the same manner but is less common than tendinitis. The diagnosis is suggested by the drop arm test, in which the patient is asked to maintain the arm outstretched as it is passively abducted. If the patient is unable to hold the arm up once 90° of abduction is reached, the test is positive. Tendinitis or tear of the rotator cuff can be confirmed by MRI (tendinitis and tear) or arthrography (tear only).

KNEE PAIN A careful history should delineate the chronology of the knee complaint and whether there are predisposing conditions, trauma, or medications that might underlie the complaint. Observation of the patient's gait is also important. The knee should be carefully inspected in the upright (weight-bearing) and prone positions for swelling, erythema, contusion, laceration, and malalignment. The most common form of malalignment in the knee is genu varum (bow-legs) and genu valgum (knock-knees). Bony swelling of the knee joint commonly results from hypertrophic osseous changes seen with disorders such as osteoarthritis and neuropathic arthropathy. Swelling caused by hypertrophy of intrasynovial structures (synovial enlargement or effusion) may manifest as a fluctuant, ballotable, or soft tissue enlargement in the suprapatellar pouch (superior reflection of the synovial cavity) or lateral and medial to the patella. Synovial effusions may also be detected by balloting the patella downward toward the femoral groove or by eliciting a bulge sign. To elicit this sign, the examiner positions the knee extended and manually compresses or milks synovial fluid down from the suprapatellar pouch and lateral to the patellae. Manual pressure lateral to the patella may cause an observable shift in synovial fluid (bulge) to the medial aspect. This maneuver is only effective for detecting small to moderate effusions (smaller than 100 mL). Inflammatory disorders such as RA, gout, and Reiter's syndrome may involve the knee joint and produce significant pain, stiffness, swelling, or warmth.

Anserine bursitis is an often missed cause of knee pain in adults. The pes anserine bursa underlies the semimembranosus tendon and may become inflamed and painful owing to trauma, overuse, or inflammation. Anserine bursitis manifests primarily as point tenderness inferior and medial to the patella and overlying the medial tibial plateau. Swelling and erythema may not be present. Other forms of bursitis may also present as knee pain. The prepatellar bursa is superficial and is located over the inferior portion of the patella. The infrapatellar bursa is deeper and lies beneath the patellar ligament before its insertion on the tibial tubercle.

Internal derangement of the knee may result from trauma or degenerative processes. Damage to the meniscal cartilage (medial or lateral) frequently presents as chronic or intermittent knee pain. Such an injury should be suspected when there is a history of trauma or athletic activity and when the patient relates symptoms of locking, clicking, or "giving way" of the joint. Pain may be detected during direct palpation over the medial or lateral joint line. The diagnosis may also be suggested by ipsilateral joint-line pain when the knee is stressed laterally or medially. A positive McMurray test may indicate a meniscal tear. To perform this test, the knee is first flexed at 90°, and the leg is then extended while simultaneously the lower extremity is torqued medially or laterally. A painful click during inward rotation may indicate a lateral meniscus tear, and pain during outward rotation may indicate a tear in the medical meniscus. Finally, damage to the cruciate ligaments should be suspected if there is pain of acute onset, possibly with swelling, a history of trauma, or a synovial fluid aspirate that is grossly bloody. Examination of the cruciate ligaments is best accomplished by eliciting a drawer sign. With the patient recumbent, the knee should be partially flexed and the foot stabilized on the examining surface. The examiner should manually attempt to displace the tibia anteriorly or posteriorly with respect to the femur. If anterior movement is detected, then anterior cruciate ligament damage is likely. Conversely, significant posterior movement may indicate posterior cruciate damage. Contralateral comparison will assist the examiner in detecting significant anterior or posterior movement.

HIP PAIN The hip is best evaluated by observing the patient's gait and assessing range of motion. The vast majority of patients reporting "hip pain" localize their pain unilaterally to the posterior or gluteal musculature. Such pain may or may not be associated with low back pain and tends to radiate down the posterolateral aspect of the thigh. Range of movement may be limited by pain. This presentation frequently results from degenerative arthritis of the lumbosacral spine and commonly follows a dermatomal distribution with involvement of nerve roots between L2 and S1. Some individuals instead localize their "hip pain" laterally to the area overlying the trochanteric bursa. Because of the depth of this bursa, swelling and warmth are usually absent. Diagnosis of trochanteric bursitis can be confirmed by inducing point tenderness over the trochanteric bursa. Pain in the hip joint is less common and tends to be located anteriorly, over the inguinal ligament; it may radiate medially to the groin or along the anteromedial thigh. Uncommonly, iliopsoas bursitis may mimic true hip joint pain. Diagnosis of iliopsoas bursitis may be suggested by a history of trauma or inflammatory arthritis. Pain associated with an iliopsoas bursitis tends to worsen with hyperextension of the hip, and many patients prefer to flex and externally rotate the hip to reduce the pain from a distended bursa.

BIBLIOGRAPHY

BROWER AC: Imaging techniques and modalities, in *Arthritis in Black and White*, AC Brower (ed). Philadelphia, Saunders, 1988, p 1

GALL EP: Evaluation of the patient. A: History and physical examination, in *Primer on the Rheumatic Diseases*, 10th ed, HR Schumacher et al (eds). Atlanta, Arthritis Foundation, 1993, pp 60–64

HASSELBACHER P: Arthrocentesis, synovial fluid analysis and synovial biopsy, in *Primer on the Rheumatic Diseases*, 10th ed, HR Schumacher et al (eds). Atlanta, Arthritis Foundation, 1993, pp 67–72

LICHTENSTEIN MJ, PINCUS T: How useful are combinations of blood tests in "rheumatic panels" in diagnosis of rheumatic disease? J Gen Intern Med 3:435, 1988

SCHUMACHER HR JR: Arthritis of recent onset. A guide to evaluation and initial therapy for primary care physicians. Postgrad Med 97:52, 1995

SHMERLING RH, LIANG MH: Laboratory evaluation of rheumatic diseases, in *Primer on the Rheumatic Diseases*, 10th ed, HR Schumacher et al (eds). Atlanta, Arthritis Foundation, 1993, pp 64–66

——— et al: Synovial fluid tests: What should be ordered? JAMA 264:1009, 1990

WERNICK R: Avoiding laboratory test misinterpretation. Geriatrics 44:61, 1989

322 OSTEOARTHRITIS

Kenneth D. Brandt

Osteoarthritis (OA), also erroneously called degenerative joint disease, represents failure of a diarthrodial (movable, synovial-lined) joint. In idiopathic (primary) OA, the most common form of the disease, no predisposing factor is apparent. Secondary OA is pathologically indistinguishable from idiopathic OA but is attributable to an underlying cause (Table 322-1).

EPIDEMIOLOGY AND RISK FACTORS OA is the most common joint disease of humans. Among the elderly, knee OA is the leading cause of chronic disability in developed countries; some 100,000 people in the United States are unable to walk independently from bed to bathroom because of OA of the knee or hip.

Under the age of 55 years, the joint distribution of OA in men and women is similar; in older individuals, hip OA is more common in men, while OA of interphalangeal joints and the thumb base is more common in women. Similarly, radiographic evidence of knee OA and, especially *symptomatic* knee OA, is more common in women than in men (Table 322-2).

Racial differences exist in both the prevalence of OA and the pattern of joint involvement. The Chinese in Hong Kong have a lower incidence of hip OA than whites; OA is more frequent in native Americans than in whites. Interphalangeal joint OA and, especially, hip OA are much less common in South African blacks than in whites in the same population. Whether these differences are genetic or are due to differences in joint usage related to life-style or occupation is unknown.

In other cases, the relation of heredity to OA is less ambiguous. Thus, the mother and sister of a woman with distal interphalangeal joint OA (Heberden's nodes) are, respectively, twice and thrice as likely to exhibit OA in these joints as the mother and sister of an unaffected woman. Point mutations in the cDNA coding for articular cartilage collagen have been identified in families with chondrodysplasia and polyarticular secondary OA.

Age is the most powerful risk factor for OA. In a radiographic survey of women less than 45 years old, only 2 percent had OA; between the ages of 45 to 64 years, however, the prevalence was 30 percent, and for those older than 65 years it was 68 percent. In males, the figures were similar but somewhat lower in the older age groups.

Major trauma and repetitive joint use are also important risk factors for OA. In both humans and animal models, anterior cruciate ligament insufficiency and meniscus damage (and also meniscectomy) lead to knee OA. Although damage to the articular cartilage may occur at the time of injury or subsequently, with use of the affected joint, even normal cartilage will degenerate if the joint is unstable. A person with a trimalleolar fracture will almost certainly develop ankle OA.

The pattern of joint involvement in OA is influenced by prior vocational or avocational overload. Thus, ankle OA is common in

Supported in part by grant AR 20582 from the National Institute of Arthritis and Musculoskeletal and Skin Diseases.

Table 322-1

Classification of OA

I. **Idiopathic**
  A. Localized OA
    1. Hands: Heberden's and Bouchard's nodes (nodal), erosive interphalangeal arthritis (nonnodal), carpal–1st metacarpal
    2. Feet: hallux valgus, hallux rigidus, contracted toes (hammer/cock-up toes), talonavicular
    3. Knee:
      a. Medial compartment
      b. Lateral compartment
      c. Patellofemoral compartment
    4. Hip:
      a. Eccentric (superior)
      b. Concentric (axial, medial)
      c. Diffuse (coxae senilis)
    5. Spine:
      a. Apophyseal joints
      b. Intervertebral joints (disks)
      c. Spondylosis (osteophytes)
      d. Ligamentous (hyperostosis, Forestier's disease, diffuse idiopathic skeletal hyperostosis
    6. Other single sites, e.g., glenohumoral, acromioclavicular, tibiotalar, sacroiliac, temporomandibular
  B. Generalized OA includes 3 or more of the areas listed above (Kellgren-Moore)

II. **Secondary**
  A. Trauma
    1. Acute
    2. Chronic (occupational, sports)
  B. Congenital or developmental
    1. Localized diseases: Legg-Calvé-Perthes, congenital hip dislocation, slipped epiphysis
    2. Mechanical factors: unequal lower extremity length, valgus/varus deformity, hypermobility syndromes
    3. Bone dysplasias: epiphyseal dysplasia, spondyloapophyseal dysplasia, osteonychondystrophy
  C. Metabolic
    1. Ochronosis (alkaptonuria)
    2. Hemochromatosis
    3. Wilson's disease
    4. Gaucher's disease
  D. Endocrine
    1. Acromegaly
    2. Hyperparathyroidism
    3. Diabetes mellitus
    4. Obesity
    5. Hypothyroidism
  E. Calcium deposition diseases
    1. Calcium pyrophosphate dihydrate deposition
    2. Apatite arthropathy
  F. Other bone and joint diseases
    1. Localized: fracture, avascular necrosis, infection, gout
    2. Diffuse: rheumatoid (inflammatory) arthritis, Paget's disease, osteopetrosis, osteochondritis
  G. Neuropathic (Charcot joints)
  H. Endemic
    1. Kashin-Beck
    2. Mseleni
  I. Miscellaneous
    1. Frostbite
    2. Caisson disease
    3. Hemoglobinopathies

SOURCE: HJ Mankin et al: Workshop on etiopathogenesis of osteoarthritis. *J Rheumatol* 13:1127, 1986.

ballet dancers, elbow OA in baseball pitchers, and metacarpophalangeal joint OA in prize fighters, although OA is not very common at any of these sites in the general population.

Given the growing participation of the population of this country in sports, it is important to note that there are no convincing data to support an association between specific athletic activities and arthritis if major trauma is excluded. Neither long distance running nor jogging has been shown to cause OA. This apparent lack of association may, however, be due to the lack of good long-term studies, the difficulty of retrospective assessment of activities, and selection bias, i.e., early discontinuation of the activity by those incurring joint damage. In contrast, vocational activities, such as those performed by jackhammer operators, cotton mill and shipyard workers, and coal miners may lead to OA in the joints exposed to repetitive occupational use. Men whose jobs required knee bending and at least medium physical demands had a higher rate of radiographic evidence of knee OA, and more severe radiographic changes, than men whose jobs required neither.

Obesity is a risk factor for knee OA and hand OA. For those in the highest quintile for body mass index at baseline examination, the relative risk for developing knee OA in the ensuing 36 years was 1.5 for men and 2.1 for women. For *severe* knee OA, the relative risk rose to 1.9 for men and 3.2 for women, suggesting that obesity plays an even larger role in the etiology of the most serious cases of knee OA. Furthermore, obese subjects who have not yet developed OA can reduce their risk: A weight loss of only 5 kg was found to be associated with a 50 percent reduction in the odds of developing symptomatic knee OA.

The correlation between the pathologic severity of OA and symptoms is poor. Many individuals with radiographic changes of advanced OA have no symptoms. The risk factors for *pain and disability* in affected individuals are poorly understood. Disability in subjects with knee OA is more strongly associated with quadriceps muscle weakness than with either joint pain or radiographic severity of the disease. For the same degree of pathologic severity, women are more likely to be symptomatic than men, those on welfare more likely than those who are working, and those who are divorced more likely than those who are married. For individuals with OA who had poor social support, periodic telephone calls from a trained lay interviewer were as effective as a nonsteroidal anti-inflammatory drug (NSAID) in reducing joint pain, emphasizing the importance of psychosocial factors as determinants of pain.

PATHOLOGY The most striking changes in OA are usually seen in load-bearing areas of the articular cartilage. In the early stages the cartilage is thicker than normal, but with progression of OA, the joint surface thins, the cartilage softens, the integrity of the surface is breached, and vertical clefts develop (fibrillation) (Fig. 322-1). Deep cartilage ulcers, extending to bone, may appear. Areas of fibrocartilaginous repair may develop, but the repair tissue is inferior to pristine hyaline articular cartilage in its ability to withstand mechanical stress. All of the cartilage is metabolically active, and the chondrocytes replicate, forming clusters (clones). Later, however, the cartilage becomes hypocellular.

Remodeling and hypertrophy of bone are also major features of OA. Appositional bone growth occurs in the subchondral region, leading to the bony "sclerosis" seen radiographically. The abraded bone under a cartilage ulcer may take on the appearance of ivory (eburnation). Growth of cartilage and bone at the joint margins leads to osteophytes (spurs), which alter the contour of the joint and may restrict movement. A patchy chronic synovitis and thickening of the joint capsule may further restrict movement. Periarticular muscle wasting is common and may play a major role in symptoms and, as indicated above, in disability.

Table 322-2

Risk Factors for OA

Age	Repetitive stress, e.g., vocational*
Female sex	Obesity*
Race	Congenital/developmental defects*
Genetic factors	Prior inflammatory joint disease
Major joint trauma*	Metabolic/endocrine disorders

* Potentially modifiable

SOURCE: Adapted from M Hochberg: J Rheum 18:1438, 1991.

PATHOGENESIS The main load on articular cartilage—the major target tissue in OA—is produced by contraction of the muscles that stabilize or move the joint. Although cartilage is an excellent shock absorber in terms of its bulk properties, at most sites it is only 1 to 2 mm thick—too thin to serve as the sole shock-absorbing structure in the joint. Additional protective mechanisms are provided by subchondral bone and periarticular muscles.

Articular cartilage serves two essential functions in the joint, both of which are mechanical. First, it provides a remarkably smooth bearing surface, so that, with joint movement, the bones glide effortlessly over each other. With synovial fluid as lubricant, the coefficient of friction for cartilage rubbed against cartilage, even under physiologic loading, is 15 times lower than that of two ice cubes passed across each other! Second, articular cartilage prevents concentration of stresses, so the bones do not shatter when the joint is loaded.

OA develops in either of two settings: (1) the biomaterial properties of the articular cartilage and subchondral bone are normal, but excessive loading of the joint causes the tissues to fail, or (2) the applied load is reasonable, but the material properties of the cartilage or bone are inferior.

Although articular cartilage is highly resistant to wear under conditions of repeated oscillation, repetitive impact loading soon leads to joint failure. This fact accounts for the high prevalence of OA at specific sites related to vocational or avocational overloading. In general, the earliest changes occur at the sites in the joint that are subject to the greatest compressive loads. More than 80 percent of all cases of "idiopathic" OA of the hip may be due to subtle congenital or developmental defects, such as congenital subluxation/dislocation, acetabular dysplasia, Legg-Calvé-Perthes disease, or slipped capital femoral epiphysis, which increase joint congruity and concentrate the dynamic load. Notably, institution in the 1940s of screening of newborns and infants for congenital hip disease has been accompanied by a marked decrease in the prevalence of hip OA in adults in Brittany.

Clinical conditions that reduce the ability of the cartilage or subchondral bone to deform are associated with development of OA. In ochronosis, for example, accumulation of homogentisic acid polymers leads to stiffening of the cartilage; in osteopetrosis, stiffness of the subchondral trabeculae occurs. In both conditions, severe generalized OA is usually apparent by the age of 40. If the subchondral bone is stiffened experimentally, repetitive impact loading soon leads to breakdown of the overlying cartilage. Conversely, osteoporosis, in which the bone is abnormally soft, may protect against OA.

The Extracellular Matrix of Normal Articular Cartilage Articular cartilage is composed of two major macromolecular species: proteoglycans (PGs), which are responsible for the compressive stiffness of the tissue and its ability to withstand load, and collagen, which provides tensile strength and resistance to shear. Although lysomal proteases (cathepsins) have been demonstrated within the cells and matrix of normal articular cartilage, their low pH optimum makes it likely that the proteoglycanase activity of these enzymes will be confined to an intracellular site or the immediate pericellular area. However, cartilage also contains a family of matrix metalloproteinases (MMPs), including stromelysin, collagenase, and gelatinase, which can degrade all the components of the extracellular matrix at neutral pH. Each is secreted by the chondrocyte as a latent proenzyme that must be activated by proteolytic cleavage of its N-terminal sequence. The level of MMP activity in the cartilage at any given time represents the balance between activation of the proenzyme and inhibition of the active enzyme by tissue inhibitors.

The turnover of normal cartilage is effected through a degradative cascade, for which many investigators consider the driving force to be interleukin (IL) 1, a cytokine produced by mononuclear cells (including synovial lining cells) and synthesized by chondrocytes. IL-1 stimulates the synthesis and secretion of the latent MMPs and of tissue plasminogen activator. Plasminogen, the substrate for the latter enzyme, may be synthesized by the chondrocyte or may enter the cartilage from the synovial fluid. Both plasminogen and stromelysin may play a role in activation of the latent MMPs. In addition to its catabolic effect on cartilage, at concentrations even lower than those needed to stimulate cartilage degradation, IL-1 suppresses PG synthesis by the chondrocyte, inhibiting matrix repair (see below).

The balance of the system lies with at least two inhibitors, tissue inhibitor of metalloproteinase (TIMP) and plasminogen activator inhibitor-1 (PAI-1), which are synthesized by the chondrocyte and limit the degradative activity of MMPs and plasminogen activator, respectively. If TIMP or PAI-1 is destroyed or is present in concentrations that are insufficient relative to those of active enzymes, stromelysin and plasmin are free to act on matrix substrates. Stromelysin can degrade the protein core of the PG and activate latent collagenase. Conversion of latent stromelysin to an active, highly destructive protease by plasmin provides a second mechanism for matrix degradation.

Polypeptide mediators, e.g., insulin-like growth factor-1 (IGF-1) and transforming growth factor β (TGF-β), stimulate biosynthesis of PGs. They regulate matrix metabolism in normal cartilage and may play a role in matrix repair in OA. Notably, these growth factors modulate catabolic as well as anabolic pathways of chondrocyte metabolism; by down-regulating chondrocyte receptors for IL-1, they may decrease PG degradation.

In addition to its responsiveness to cytokines and a variety of other biologic mediators, chondrocyte metabolism in normal cartilage can be modulated directly by mechanical loading. Whereas static loading and prolonged cyclic loading inhibit synthesis of PGs and protein, loads of relatively brief duration may stimulate matrix biosynthesis.

Pathophysiology of Cartilage Changes in OA Most investigators feel that the primary changes in OA begin in the cartilage. A change in the arrangement and size of the collagen fibers is apparent. The biochemical data are consistent with the presence of a defect in the collagen network of the cartilage, perhaps due to disruption of the "glue" that binds adjacent fibers together in the matrix. This is among the earliest matrix changes observed and appears to be irreversible.

Although "wear" may be a factor in the loss of cartilage, strong evidence supports the concept that lysosomal enzymes and MMPs account for much of the loss of cartilage matrix in OA. Whether their synthesis and secretion are stimulated by IL-1 or by other factors (e.g., mechanical stimuli), MMPs, plasmin, and cathepsins all appear to be involved in the breakdown of articular cartilage in OA. TIMP and PAI-1 may work to stabilize the system, at least temporarily, while growth factors, such as IGF-1, TGF-β, and basic fibroblast growth factor (FGF), are implicated in repair processes that may heal the lesion or, at least, stabilize the process. A stoichiometric imbalance exists between the levels of active enzyme and the level of TIMP, which may be only modestly increased.

The chondrocytes in OA cartilage undergo active cell division and are very active metabolically, producing increased quantities of DNA, RNA, collagen, PG, and noncollagenous proteins. (For this reason, it is inaccurate to call OA a "degenerative" joint disease). Prior to cartilage loss and PG depletion, this marked biosynthetic activity may lead to an increase in PG concentration, which may be associated with thickening of the cartilage and a stage of homeostasis referred to as "compensated" OA. These mechanisms may maintain the joint in a reasonably functional state for years. The repair tissue, however, often does not hold up as well under mechanical stresses as normal hyaline cartilage, and eventually, at least in some cases, the rate of PG synthesis falls off and "end-stage" OA develops, with full-thickness loss of cartilage.

Table 322-3

Causes of Joint Pain in Patients with OA

Source	Mechanism
Synovium	Inflammation
Subchondral bone	Medullary hypertension, microfractures
Osteophyte	Stretching of periosteal nerve endings
Ligaments	Stretch
Capsule	Inflammation, distention
Muscle	Spasm

CLINICAL FEATURES The joint pain of OA is often described as a deep ache and is localized to the involved joint. Typically, the pain of OA is aggravated by joint use and relieved by rest, but, as the disease progresses, it may become persistent. Nocturnal pain, interfering with sleep, is seen particularly in advanced OA of the hip and may be enervating. Stiffness of the involved joint on arising in the morning or after a period of inactivity (e.g., an automobile ride) may be prominent but usually lasts less than 20 min. Systemic manifestations are not a feature of primary OA.

Because articular cartilage is aneural, the joint pain in OA must arise from other structures (Table 322-3). In some patients it may be due to stretching of nerve endings in the periosteum covering osteophytes. In others it may arise from microfractures in subchondral bone or from medullary hypertension caused by distortion of blood flow by thickened subchondral trabeculae. Joint instability, leading to stretching of the joint capsule, and muscle spasm also may be sources of pain.

In some patients with OA, joint pain may be due to synovitis. In advanced OA, histologic evidence of synovial inflammation may be as marked as that in the synovium of a patient with rheumatoid arthritis. Synovitis in OA may be due to phagocytosis of shards of cartilage and bone from the abraded joint surface (wear particles), to release from the cartilage of soluble matrix macromolecules, or to crystals of calcium pyrophosphate or hydroxyapatite. In other cases, immune complexes, containing antigens derived from cartilage matrix, may be sequestered in collagenous tissue of the joint, leading to low-grade

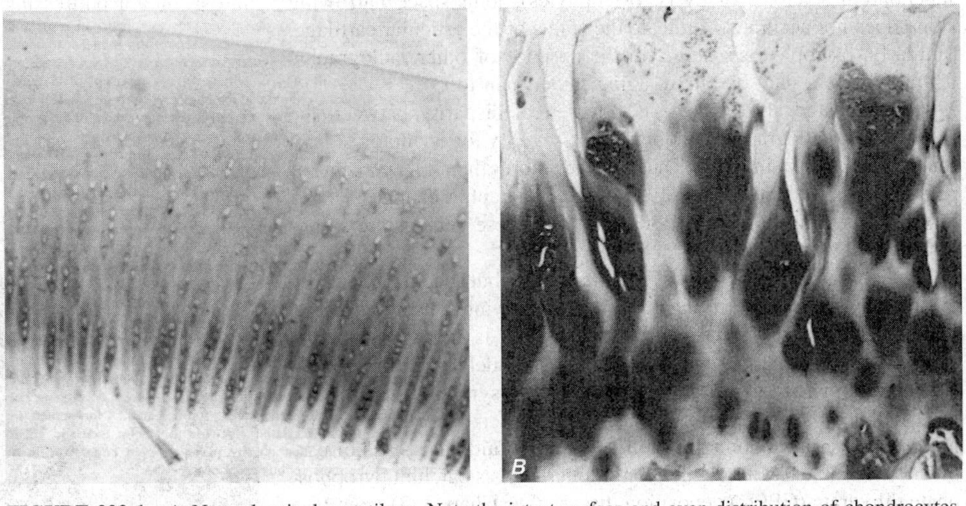

FIGURE 322-1 *A.* Normal articular cartilage. Note the intact surface and even distribution of chondrocytes. Mitotic figures are not present in normal adult articular cartilage. *B.* Osteoarthritic cartilage. Note the disruption of surface integrity, with vertical fissures (fibrillation) and irregular distribution of cells. Many of the chondrocytes have replicated and exist in clusters. Stained with safranin-O, which binds to the sulfated glycosaminoglycan chains of proteoglycans. Note patchy areas of diminished staining (pale extracellular matrix) due to proteoglycan depletion.

chronic synovitis. In contrast, in the earlier stages of OA, even in the patient with chronic joint pain, synovial inflammation may be absent, suggesting that the joint pain is due to one of the other factors mentioned above.

Physical examination of the OA joint may reveal localized tenderness and bony or soft tissue swelling. Bony crepitus (the sensation of bone rubbing against bone, evoked by joint movement) is characteristic. Synovial effusions, if present, are usually not large. Palpation may reveal some warmth over the joint. Periarticular muscle atrophy may be due to disuse or to reflex inhibition of muscle contraction. In the advanced stages of OA, there may be gross deformity, bony hypertrophy, subluxation, and marked loss of joint motion. The notion that OA is inexorably progressive, however, is incorrect. In many patients the disease stabilizes; in some, regression of joint pain and even of radiographic changes occurs.

Although the diagnosis of OA is often straightforward because of the high prevalence of radiographic changes of OA in asymptomatic individuals, it is important to ensure that joint pain in a patient with radiographic evidence of OA is not due to some other cause, such as soft tissue rheumatism (e.g., anserine bursitis at the knee, trochanteric bursitis at the hip), radiculopathy, referral of pain from another joint (e.g., 25 percent of patients with hip disease have pain referred to the knee, for example), entrapment neuropathy, vascular disease (claudication), or some other type of arthritis (e.g., crystal-induced synovitis, septic arthritis). These are all common pitfalls in the diagnosis of OA. It is usually not difficult to differentiate OA from a systemic rheumatic disease, such as rheumatoid arthritis, because, in the latter diseases, joint involvement is usually symmetric and polyarticular, with arthritis in wrists and metacarpophalangeal joints (which are generally not involved in OA), and there are also constitutional features such as prolonged morning stiffness, fatigue, and, occasionally, weight loss or fever (see Chap. 313).

LABORATORY AND RADIOGRAPHIC FINDINGS The diagnosis of OA is usually based on clinical and radiographic features. In the early stages, the radiograph may be normal, but joint space narrowing becomes evident as articular cartilage is lost. Other characteristic radiographic findings include subchondral bone sclerosis, subchondral cysts, and osteophytosis. A change in the contour of the joint due to bony remodeling and subluxation may be seen. Although tibiofemoral joint space narrowing has been considered to be a radiographic surrogate for articular cartilage thinning, in patients with early OA who do not have radiographic evidence of bony changes (e.g., subchondral sclerosis or cysts, osteophytes), joint space narrowing alone does not accurately indicate the status of the articular cartilage. Similarly, osteophytosis alone, in the absence of other radiographic features of OA, may be due to aging rather than to OA.

As indicated above, there is often great disparity between the severity of radiographic findings, the severity of symptoms, and functional ability in OA. Thus, while more than 90 percent of persons over the age of 40 have some radiographic changes of OA in weight-bearing joints, only 30 percent of these persons are symptomatic.

No laboratory studies are diagnostic for OA, but specific laboratory testing may help in identifying one of the underlying causes of secondary OA (Table 322-1). Because primary OA is not systemic, the erythrocyte sedimentation rate, serum chemistry determinations, blood counts, and urinalysis are normal. Analysis of synovial fluid reveals mild leukocytosis (<2000 white blood cells per microliter), with a predominance of mononuclear cells. Synovial fluid analysis is of particular value in excluding other conditions, such as calcium pyrophosphate dihydrate (CPPD) deposition disease (see Chap. 323), gout (see Chap. 344), or septic arthritis (see Chap. 324).

Prior to the appearance of radiographic changes, the ability to clinically diagnose OA without an invasive procedure (e.g., arthroscopy) is limited. Approaches such as magnetic resonance imaging (MRI) and ultrasonography have not been sufficiently validated, and their limits of resolution and cost do not justify their routine clinical use for diagnosis of OA or monitoring of disease progression.

OA AT SPECIFIC JOINT SITES **Interphalangeal Joints** Heberden's nodes, bony enlargements of the distal interphalangeal joints, are the most common form of idiopathic OA (Fig. 322-2). A similar process at the proximal interphalangeal joints leads to Bouchard's nodes. Often, Heberden's nodes develop gradually, with little or no discomfort. However, they may present acutely with pain, redness, and swelling, sometimes triggered by minor trauma. Gelatinous dorsal cysts filled with hyaluronic acid may develop at the insertion of the digital extensor tendon into the base of the distal phalanx.

Erosive OA In erosive OA distal and/or proximal interphalangeal joints of the hands are most prominently affected. Erosive OA tends to be more destructive than typical nodal OA. Radiographic evidence of collapse of the subchondral plate is characteristic, and bony ankylosis may occur. Joint deformity and functional impairment may be severe. Pain and tenderness are commonly episodic. The synovium is much more extensively infiltrated with mononuclear cells than in other forms of OA.

Generalized OA Generalized OA is characterized by involvement of three or more joints or groups of joints (distal interphalangeal and proximal interphalangeal joints are counted as one group each). Heberden's and Bouchard's nodes are prominent. Symptoms may be episodic, with "flare-ups" of inflammation marked by soft tissue swelling, redness, and warmth. The erythrocyte sedimentation rate may be elevated, but serum rheumatoid factor tests are negative.

Thumb Base The second most frequent area of involvement in OA is the thumb base. Swelling, tenderness, and crepitus on movement of the joint are typical. Osteophytes may lead to a "squared" appearance of the thumb base (Fig. 322-3). In contrast to Heberden's nodes, which usually do not interfere significantly with function, thumb base OA frequently causes loss of motion and strength. Pain with pinch leads to adduction of the thumb and contracture of the first web space, often resulting in compensatory hyperextension of the first metacarpophalangeal joint and swan-neck deformity of the thumb.

The Hip Congenital or developmental defects (e.g., acetabular dysplasia, Legg-Calvé-Perthes disease, slipped capital epiphysis) may be implicated in as many as 80 percent of cases of hip OA. Twenty percent of patients will develop bilateral involvement. Pain from hip OA is generally referred to the inguinal area but may be referred to the buttock or proximal thigh. Less commonly, hip OA presents as knee pain. Pain can be evoked by putting the involved hip through its range of motion. Flexion may be painless initially, but internal rotation will exacerbate pain. Loss of internal rotation occurs early, followed by loss of extension, adduction, and flexion due to capsular fibrosis and/or buttressing osteophytes.

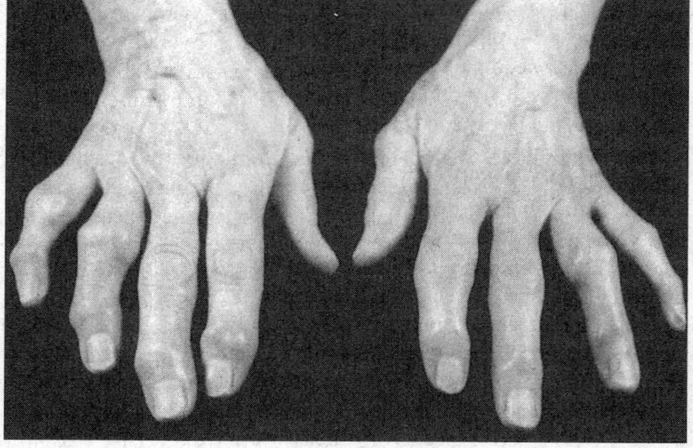

FIGURE 322-2 Nodal osteoarthritis. Note bony enlargement of distal and proximal interphalangeal joints (Heberden's nodes and Bouchard's nodes, respectively). *(Reprinted from the Clinical Slide Collection on the Rheumatic Diseases, © 1991, 1995. Used by permission of the American College of Rheumatology.)*

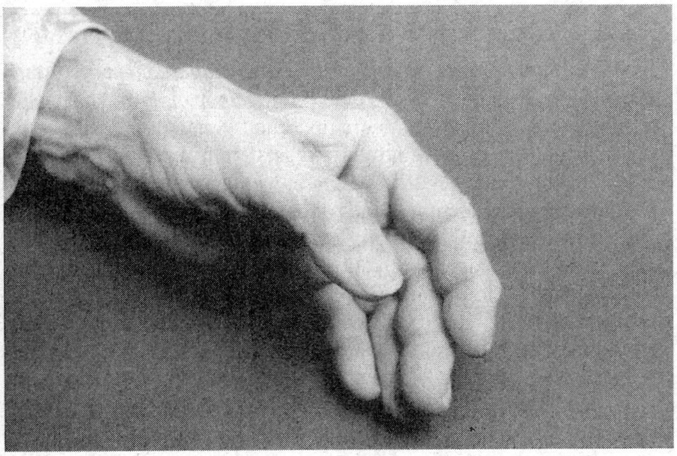

FIGURE 322-3 Osteoarthritis of the first carpometacarpal joint. Note the squared appearance of the thumb base, due to bony enlargement and remodeling of the joint.

The Knee OA of the knee may involve the medial or lateral femorotibial compartment and/or the patellofemoral compartment. Palpation may reveal bony hypertrophy (osteophytes) and tenderness. Effusions, if present, are generally small. Joint movement commonly elicits bony crepitus. OA in the medial compartment may result in a varus (bow-leg) deformity; in the lateral compartment it may produce a valgus (knock-knee) deformity. A positive "shrug" sign (pain when the patella is compressed manually against the femur during quadriceps contraction) may be a sign of patellofemoral OA.

Chondromalacia patellae, which also is characterized by anterior knee pain and a positive shrug sign, is a syndrome of patellofemoral pain, often bilateral, in teenagers and young adults. It is more common in females than in males. It may be caused by a variety of factors (e.g., abnormal quadriceps angle, patella alta, trauma). Although exploration of the knee may reveal softening and fibrillation of cartilage on the posterior aspect of the patella, this change is usually not progressive; chondromalacia patellae is usually not a precursor of OA. In most cases, analgesics or NSAIDs and physical therapy are effective; in some, pain may be relieved by surgical correction of patellar malalignment.

The Spine Degenerative disease of the spine can involve the apophyseal joint, intervertebral disks, and/or paraspinous ligaments. *Spondylosis* refers to degenerative *disk* disease. The diagnosis of spinal OA should be reserved for cases showing involvement of the apophyseal joints (true diarthrodial joints). Symptoms of spinal OA include localized pain and stiffness. Nerve root compression by an osteophyte blocking a neural foramen, prolapse of a degenerated disk, or subluxation of an apophyseal joint may cause radicular pain and motor weakness.

Marked calcification and ossification of paraspinous ligaments occur in diffuse idiopathic skeletal hyperostosis (DISH). Although DISH is often categorized as a variant of OA, diarthrodial joints are not involved. Ligamentous calcification and ossification in the anterior spinal ligaments give the appearance of "flowing wax" on the anterior vertebral bodies. However, a radiolucency may be seen between the newly deposited bone and the vertebral body, differentiating DISH from the marginal osteophytes in spondylosis. Intervertebral disk spaces are preserved, and sacroiliac and apophyseal joints appear normal, helping to differentiate DISH from spondylosis and from ankylosing spondylitis, respectively. DISH occurs in the middle-aged and elderly and is more common in men than in women. Patients are frequently asymptomatic but may have musculoskeletal stiffness. The radiographic changes are generally much more severe than might be predicted from the mild symptoms.

℞ TREATMENT

Treatment of OA is aimed at reducing pain, maintaining mobility, and minimizing disability. The vigor of the therapeutic intervention should be dictated by the severity of the condition in the individual patient. For those with only mild disease, reassurance, instruction in joint protection, and an occasional analgesic may be all that is required; for those with more severe OA, especially of the knee or hip, a comprehensive program comprising a spectrum of nonpharmacologic measures supplemented by an analgesic and/or anti-inflammatory drug is appropriate.

Nonpharmacologic measures *REDUCTION OF JOINT LOADING* OA may be caused or aggravated by poor body mechanics. Correction of poor posture and a support for excessive lumbar lordosis can be helpful. Excessive loading of the involved joint should be avoided. Patients with OA of the knee or hip should avoid prolonged standing, kneeling, and squatting. Obese patients should be counseled to lose weight. In patients with medial-compartment knee OA, a wedged insole may decrease joint pain.

Rest periods during the day may be of benefit, but complete immobilization of the painful joint is rarely indicated. In patients with unilateral OA of the hip or knee, a cane, held in the contralateral hand, may reduce joint pain by reducing the joint contact force. Bilateral disease may necessitate use of crutches or a walker.

PHYSICAL THERAPY Application of heat to the OA joint may reduce pain and stiffness. A variety of modalities are available; often, the least expensive and most convenient is a hot shower or bath. Occasionally, better analgesia may be obtained with ice than with heat.

Disuse of the OA joint because of pain will lead to muscle atrophy. Reflex inhibition of muscle contraction may have a similar effect. Because periarticular muscles play a major role in protecting the articular cartilage from stress, strengthening them is important. Exercises should be designed to maintain range of motion as well as to strengthen muscles surrounding the joint. In subjects with knee OA, strengthening of the periarticular muscles may result, within weeks, in a decrease in joint pain as great as that seen with NSAIDs.

Drug therapy of OA Therapy for OA today is palliative; no pharmacologic agent has been shown to prevent, delay the progression of, or reverse the pathologic changes of OA in humans.

Although NSAIDs often decrease joint pain and improve mobility in OA, the magnitude of this improvement is generally modest—on average, about 30 percent reduction in pain and 15 percent improvement in function. Patients with OA may obtain symptomatic benefit from an NSAID even when evidence of synovitis is lacking, consistent with the fact that these drugs have analgesic effects independent of their anti-inflammatory actions. In a double-blinded, controlled trial in patients with symptomatic knee OA, an anti-inflammatory dose of ibuprofen was no more effective than a low (i.e., essentially analgesic) dose of ibuprofen or than acetaminophen, a drug with essentially no anti-inflammatory effect. Other studies confirm that an analgesic dose of ibuprofen may be as effective as anti-inflammatory doses of other NSAIDs, including the potent agent phenylbutazone, in symptomatic treatment of patients with knee OA. Furthermore, even in the presence of clinical signs of inflammation (synovial swelling, tenderness), relief of joint pain by acetaminophen may be superior to that achieved with an NSAID. Nonetheless, if simple analgesics are inadequate, it is reasonable to cautiously prescribe an NSAID for a patient with OA. Although some NSAIDs have been claimed to have a "chondroprotective" effect, adequately controlled clinical trials of these claims in humans with OA are lacking.

Furthermore, concern is growing with respect to the appropriateness of NSAID administration in OA because of the side effects of these agents, especially those related to the gastrointestinal tract. The segment of the population at greatest risk for OA, i.e., the elderly, appears also to be at greater risk than younger individuals for gastrointestinal symptoms, ulceration, hemorrhage, and death as a result of NSAID use. The annual rate of hospitalization for peptic ulcer disease among elderly current NSAID users was 16 per 1000—four times greater than that for subjects not taking an NSAID.

Among people aged 65 and older, as many as 30 percent of all hospitalizations and deaths related to peptic ulcer disease have been attributed to NSAID use.

Systemic glucocorticoids have no place in the treatment of OA. However, intra- or periarticular injection of a depot glucocorticoid preparation may provide marked symptomatic relief for weeks to months. Because studies in animal models have suggested that glucocorticoids may produce cartilage damage, and frequent injections of large amounts of steroids have been associated with joint breakdown in humans, the injection should generally not be repeated in a given joint more often than every 4 to 6 months.

Capsaicin cream, which depletes local sensory nerve endings of substance P, a neuropeptide mediator of pain, may reduce joint pain and tenderness when applied topically by patients with hand or knee OA, even when used as monotherapy, i.e., without NSAIDs or systemic analgesics.

A rational approach to the nonsurgical management of OA It is being increasingly recognized that nonpharmacologic management is as important—and often more important—than drug treatment in the management of OA and that drugs should serve an *adjunctive* role in the management of this disease. Nonpharmacologic measures may comprise instruction of the patient in principles of joint protection; thermal modalities; exercises to strengthen periarticular muscles; weight reduction if the patient is obese; avoidance of excessive loading of the arthritic hip or knee joint by use of shoes with well-cushioned soles and a cane or walker, when appropriate; and prescription of orthotics for the patient with varus or valgus knee deformity. Medial taping of the patella may reduce knee pain in patients with patellofemoral OA. In patients with knee OA, if the above measures are ineffective, tidal irrigation of the painful joint warrants consideration. A health education program designed to assist the

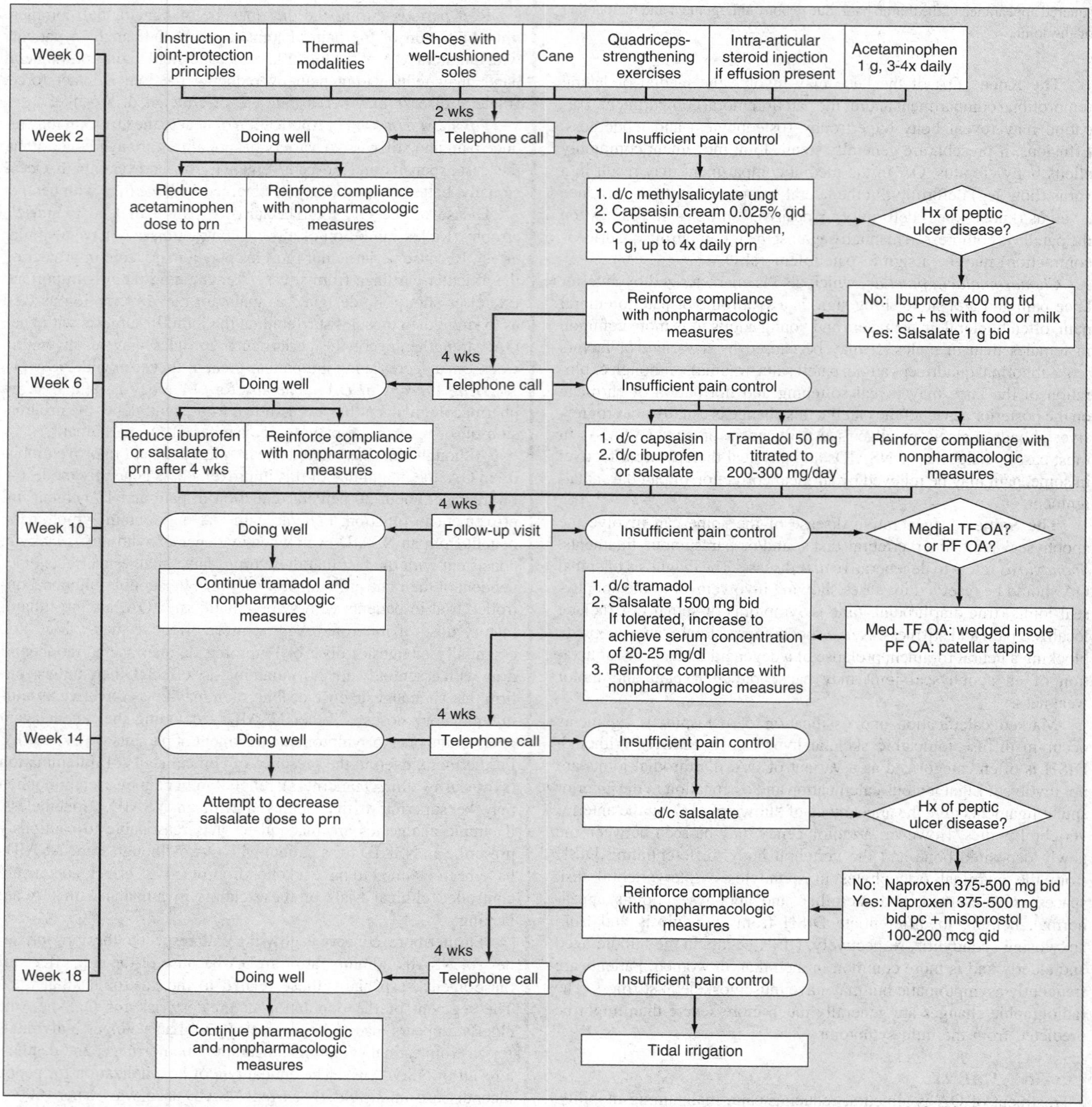

FIGURE 322-4 Algorithm for management of a newly diagnosed patient with knee OA. *(Modified from Brandt, 1996.)*

patient with self-management can reduce pain and decrease health care costs; the benefits may persist for years.

Figure 322-4 provides an algorithm which might be applied to treatment of a newly diagnosed patient with knee OA. The progressive levels of treatment are associated with increasing cost, decreasing convenience for the patient, and increasing risk of side effects. The scheme should not be interpreted dogmatically as a fixed progression of steps; rather, treatment of OA must be individualized. The treatment program should be flexible. For example, in some patients it may be reasonable to institute patellar taping or prescribe a wedged insole on the initial visit, or an intraarticular steroid injection on a later visit.

Because the symptomatic relief afforded by NSAIDs is often no greater than that achieved by a simple analgesic, because the side effects of NSAIDs are more frequent and more severe than those of acetaminophen, and because prescription NSAIDs cost considerably more than acetaminophen, when an analgesic drug is required for treatment of OA pain it is reasonable to prescribe acetaminophen initially, up to 4000 mg/d, as an adjunct to the nonpharmacologic measures mentioned above. If this regimen does not control joint symptoms in a reasonable period of time, a *low dose* or an NSAID (e.g., ibuprofen, 1200 mg/d; naproxen, 500 mg/d) may be substituted for, or added to, the acetaminophen. Should this modification be insufficient, tramadol, a weak opioid for which the risk of tolerance and addiction appear to be minimal, may be prescribed. If the above approach is not satisfactory, an antiinflammatory dose of an NSAID should be used.

Because the risk of an NSAID-associated gastrointestinal catastrophe (e.g., perforation, hemorrhage) is dose-dependent, the lowest effective dose should be employed. Salsalate and other nonacetylated salicylates, which have only a minimal effect on prostaglandin synthase, are as effective as other NSAIDs as have a lower rate of serious gastrointestinal side effects. When NSAIDs are required, they may be prescribed on an "as needed" basis, rather than in a fixed daily dose; pain control has been shown to be comparable and the risk of toxicity will be reduced. Once treatment with an NSAID or simple analgesic is initiated, the need for continuation of that treatment requires ongoing assessment. For many patients with OA, it will be possible eventually to reduce the dose of drug or to use the agent only intermittently, during exacerbations of joint pain.

Orthopedic surgery Joint replacement surgery should be reserved for patients with advanced OA in whom aggressive medical management has failed. In such cases it may be remarkably effective in relieving pain and increasing mobility. Osteotomy, which is surgically more conservative, can eliminate concentrations of peak dynamic loading and may provide effective pain relief in patients with hip or knee OA. It is of greatest benefit when the disease is only moderately advanced. Arthroscopic removal of loose cartilage fragments can prevent locking and relieve pain. Lavage of the OA knee with large quantities of saline or Ringer's lactate to flush out fibrin, cartilage shards, and other debris may provide months of comfort for the patient whose joint pain has been refractory to analgesics, NSAIDs, and intraarticular steroid injections. However, invasive procedures such as this are accompanied by a large placebo effect, and studies that include a sham lavage control group have not yet been reported.

Chondroplasty (abrasion arthroplasty) also has gained some popularity as treatment for OA, but well-controlled studies of its efficacy are lacking, and the fibrocartilage that resurfaces the abraded bone is inferior to normal hyaline cartilage in its ability to withstand mechanical loads. Notably, in patients who had undergone tibial osteotomy for medial compartment knee OA, knee pain and function were not related to the degree of cartilage regeneration seen at arthroscopy two years later.

BIBLIOGRAPHY

ANDERSON JJ, FELSON DT: Factors associated with osteoarthritis of the knee in the first national health and nutrition examination survey (HANES I). Evidence for an association with overweight, race, and physical demands of work. Am J Epidemiol 128:179, 1988

BRADLEY JD et al: Comparison of an anti-inflammatory dose of ibuprofen, an analgesic dose of ibuprofen, and acetaminophen in the treatment of patients with osteoarthritis of the knee. N Engl J Med 325:87, 1991

BRANDT KD: Management of osteoarthritis, in *Textbook of Rheumatology,* 5th ed, WN Kelley et al (eds). Philadelphia, Saunders, 1995

———: Nonsurgical management of osteoarthritis with an emphasis on nonpharmacologic measures. Arch Fam Med 4:1057, 1995

———: *Diagnosis and Nonsurgical Management of Osteoarthritis.* Caddo, OK, Professional Communications, Inc., 1996

———, FLUSSER D: Osteoarthritis, in *Prognosis in the Rheumatic Diseases,* N Bellamy (ed). Kluwer Academic Publishers, Lancaster, UK, 1991, pp 11–35

———, MANKIN HJ: Pathogenesis of osteoarthritis, in *Textbook of Rheumatology,* 4th ed, WN Kelley et al (eds). Philadelphia, Saunders, 1993

———, RADIN E: The physiology of articular stress: Osteoarthrosis. Hosp Pract 22: 103, 1987

GRIFFIN MR et al: Practical management of osteoarthritis: Integration of pharmacologic and nonpharmacologic measures. Arch Fam Med 4:1049, 1995

HOCHBERG MC et al: Guidelines for the medical management of osteoarthritis: Part I. Arthritis Rheum 38:1535, 1995

——— et al: Guidelines for the medical management of osteoarthritis: Part II. Arthritis Rheum 38:1541, 1995

MANKIN HJ: Clinical feature of osteoarthritis, in *Textbook of Rheumatology,* 3d ed, WN Kelley et al (eds). Philadelphia, Saunders, 1989, pp 1480–1500

——— et al: Workshop on etiopathogenesis of osteoarthritis. J Rheumatol 13:1127, 1986

323

Antonio J. Reginato, Gary S. Hoffman

ARTHRITIS DUE TO DEPOSITION OF CALCIUM CRYSTALS

"GOUT" CRYSTALLOGRAPHY AND ARTHRITIS The use of polarizing microscopy during synovial fluid analysis, and the application of other research tools such as electron microscopy, energy-dispersive elemental analysis, and x-ray diffraction have established the role of different microcrystals, including monosodium urate (MSU), calcium pyrophosphate dihydrate (CPPD), calcium hydroxyapatite (HA), and calcium oxalate (CaOx), in inducing arthritis (See Chap. 344). Each of these crystals may cause acute or chronic arthritis or periarthritis. In spite of differences in crystal morphology, chemistry, and physical properties, the clinical events that result from deposition and release of MSU, CPPD, HA, and CaOx may be indistinguishable. Prior to the use of crystallographic techniques in rheumatology, much of what was considered to be MSU gouty arthritis in fact was not. Simkin has suggested that the generic term *gout* be used to describe the whole group of crystal-induced arthritides (MSU gout, CPPD gout, HA gout, and CaOx gout). This concept further emphasizes the identical clinical presentations of these entities and the need to perform synovial fluid analysis to distinguish the type of crystal involved. In the setting of acute articular or periarticular inflammation, aspiration and analysis of effusions are most important to assess the possibility of infection and to identify the type of crystals present. Polarization microscopy alone can identify most typical crystals and allow diagnosis. HA, however, is an exception. Because these crystals are not birefringent and are extremely small, alizarin red S stain may be used as screening test, and more sophisticated techniques are required to confirm the presence of these crystals. Apart from the identification of specific microcrystalline materials or organisms, synovial fluid characteristics are nonspecific, and synovial fluid can be inflammatory or noninflammatory. The presence of crystals does not exclude the existence of an associated acute or, more rarely, chronic infection.

CPPD DEPOSITION DISEASE **Pathogenesis** The deposition of CPPD crystals in articular cartilage, synovium, and periarticular ligaments and tendons is most common in the elderly, affecting 10 to

15 percent of persons 65 to 75 years old and 30 to 60 percent of those more than 85 years old. In most cases this process is asymptomatic, and the cause of CPPD deposition is uncertain. Because over 80 percent of patients are more than 60 years old and 70 percent have preexisting joint damage from other conditions, it is likely that physical and chemical changes in aging cartilage favor crystal nucleation. Examples of such chemical alterations include the following. (1) There is an increased production of inorganic pyrophosphate and decreased levels of pyrophosphatases in cartilage extracts from patients with CPPD arthritis. The increase in pyrophosphate production appears to be related to enhanced activity of ATP pyrophosphohydrolase and 5′-nucleotidase, which catalyze the reaction of ATP to adenosine and pyrophosphate. This pyrophosphate could combine with calcium to form CPPD crystals in matrix vesicles. (2) There is a diminution in the levels of cartilage glycoproteins that normally inhibit and regulate crystal nucleation. These deficiencies may lead to increased crystal deposition. (3) In vitro studies have demonstrated that transforming growth factor β1 and epidermal growth factor both stimulate the production of pyrophosphate by articular cartilage and thus may contribute to the deposition of CPPD crystals. The release of CPPD crystals into the joint space is followed by the phagocytosis of these crystals by neutrophils, which respond by releasing inflammatory substances. In addition, neutrophils release a glycopeptide that is chemotactic for other neutrophils, thus augmenting the inflammatory events. The same substance is present in MSU gout. The production of this glycopeptide can be suppressed by colchicine.

A minority of patients with CPPD arthropathy have metabolic abnormalities or hereditary CPPD disease (Table 323-1). These associations suggest that a variety of different metabolic products may enhance CPPD deposition. Included among these conditions are hyperparathyroidism, hemochromatosis, gout, hypophosphatasia, hypomagnesemia, and ochronosis. Hemochromatosis and hyperparathyroidism are good examples. Ferrous ions and hypercalcemia may either directly alter cartilage or inhibit inorganic pyrophosphatases, leading to enhanced susceptibility to CPPD deposition. The presence of CPPD arthritis in individuals less than 50 years old should lead to consideration of these metabolic disorders and inherited forms of disease, including those identified in a variety of ethnic groups (Table 323-1). Genomic DNA studies performed on three different kindreds have shown a possible location of the genetic defects on chromosomes 5p and 8q. Identification of these genes will help elucidate the pathogenesis of both the familial and the more common sporadic form of the disease. Investigation should include inquiry for evidence of familial aggregation and evaluation of serum calcium, phosphorus, alkaline phosphatase, magnesium, serum ferritin, and transferritin saturation.

Clinical Manifestations CPPD arthropathy may be asymptomatic, acute, subacute, or chronic or cause acute synovitis superimposed on chronically involved joints. Acute CPPD arthritis was originally termed *pseudogout* by McCarty and coworkers because of its striking similarity to MSU gout. He and others have since recognized that the clinical sequelae of CPPD deposition include (1) induction or enhancement of peculiar forms of osteoarthritis, (2) induction of severe resorptive disease that may radiographically mimic neuropathic arthritis, (3) production of symmetric proliferative synovitis, clinically similar to rheumatoid arthritis and frequently seen in familial forms with early onset, (4) intervertebral disk and ligament calcification with restriction of spine mobility, mimicking ankylosing spondylitis (also seen in hereditary forms), and (5) rarely spinal stenosis (most commonly seen in the elderly).

Table 323-1

Conditions Associated with CPPD Disease

Aging
Disease-associated:
Primary hyperparathyroidism
Hemochromatosis
Hypophosphatasia
Hypomagnesemia
Chronic tophaceous gout
Post-meniscectomy
Epiphyseal dysplasias
Hereditary: Slovakian-Hungarian, Chilean-Spanish, French, Swedish, Dutch, Canadian, Mexican-American, Italian-American, German-American, Japanese, Tunisian, Jewish, English

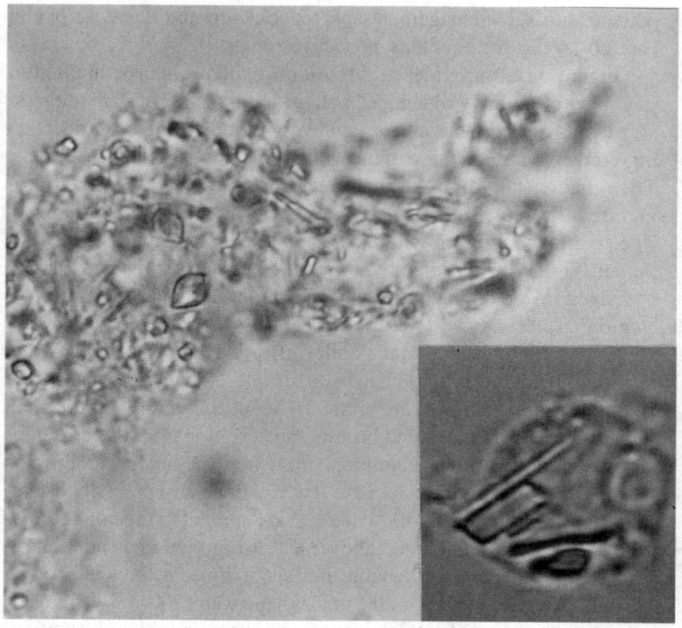

FIGURE 323-1 Intracellular and extracellular calcium pyrophosphate dihydrate crystals, as seen in a fresh preparation of synovial fluid, illustrate rectangular, rod-shaped, and rhomboid weakly birefringent crystals (compensated polarized light microscopy; 400×).

The knee is the joint most frequently affected in CPPD arthropathy. Other sites include the wrist, shoulder, ankle, elbow, and hands. Rarely, the temporomandibular joint and ligamentum flavum of the spinal canal are involved. Clinical and radiographic evidence indicates that CPPD deposition is polyarticular in at least two-thirds of patients. When acute synovitis occurs, diagnosis is made by identification of rod-shaped or rhomboid crystals with weak positive birefringence (Fig. 323-1) in synovial fluid. When the clinical picture resembles that of slowly progressive osteoarthritis, diagnosis may be more difficult. Joint distribution may provide important clues suggesting CPPD disease. For example, primary osteoarthritis rarely involves a metacarpophalangeal, wrist, elbow, shoulder, or ankle joint. If radiographs reveal punctate and/or linear radiodense deposits in fibrocartilaginous joint menisci or articular hyaline cartilage (chondrocalcinosis), the diagnostic certainty of CPPD is further enhanced. *Definitive diagnosis* requires demonstration of typical crystals in synovial fluid or articular tissue. In the absence of joint effusion or indications to obtain a synovial biopsy, chondrocalcinosis is presumptive of CPPD deposition. One exception is chondrocalcinosis due to CaOx in some patients with chronic renal failure.

Acute attacks of CPPD arthritis may be precipitated by trauma, such as physical injury to an extremity, joint surgery, a sprain, or even a long walk. Rapid diminution of serum calcium concentration, as may occur in severe medical illness or after surgery (especially parathyroidectomy), also can lead to pseudogout. How transient calcium disequilibrium may facilitate CPPD release is unclear.

In as many as 50 percent of cases, CPPD gout is associated with low-grade fever and, on occasion, temperatures as high as 40°C. Whether or not radiographic proof of chondrocalcinosis is evident in the involved joint(s), synovial analysis with microbial stains and cultures is essential to rule out the possibility of infection. In fact, infection in a joint with any microcrystalline deposition process can lead to crystal shedding and subsequent synovitis from both crystals and microorganisms. Synovial fluid in acute CPPD gout has inflammatory qualities. The white blood cell (WBC) count can range from several thousand cells to 100,000 cells/μL, the mean being about 24,000 cells/μL and the predominant cell being the neutrophil. Polarization microscopy usually reveals crystals with weak positive birefringence in the extracellular fluid and in neutrophils.

℞ TREATMENT

Untreated acute attacks may last a few days to as long as a month. *Treatment* by joint aspiration (to decrease intraarticular pressure) and nonsteroidal anti-inflammatory agents or intraarticular glucocorticoid injection may result in return to prior status in 10 days or less. For patients with frequent recurrent attacks of CPPD gout, daily prophylactic treatment with low doses of colchicine may be helpful in decreasing the frequency of the attacks. Severe polyarticular attacks usually require short courses of corticosteroids. Unfortunately, there is no effective way to remove CPPD deposits from cartilage and synovium. Uncontrolled studies suggest that radioactive synovectomy (with yttrium 90) or the administration of antimalarial agents may be helpful in controlling persistent synovitis. Patients with progressive destructive large joint arthropathy usually require joint replacement. There is no subsequent increased risk of soft tissue heterotopic calcification around the prosthesis.

CALCIUM HA DEPOSITION DISEASE **Pathogenesis** HA is the primary mineral of bone and teeth. Abnormal accumulation can occur in areas of tissue damage (dystrophic calcification), in hypercalcemic or hyperparathyroid states (metastatic calcification), and in certain conditions of unknown cause (Table 323-2). In chronic renal failure, hyperphosphatemia enhances HA deposition both in and around joints.

HA may be released from exposed bone and cause the acute synovitis occasionally seen in chronic stable osteoarthritis (e.g., "hot" Heberden's nodes). HA deposition is also an important factor in an extremely destructive chronic arthropathy of the elderly that occurs most often in knees and shoulders (Milwaukee shoulder). Joint destruction is associated with attenuation or rupture of supporting structures, leading to instability and deformity. Progression tends to be indolent, and synovial fluid WBC counts are usually less than 1000 cells/μL. Symptoms range from minimal to severe pain and disability that may lead to joint replacement surgery. Whether severely affected patients merely represent an extreme synovial tissue response to the HA crystals that are so common in osteoarthritis is uncertain. Observations that favor the idea that articular HA deposition and joint destruction constitute a unique entity rather than just a sequel of osteoarthritis include the following. (1) Primary osteoarthritis of the shoulders is infrequent. (2) High levels of activated collagenase and neutral protease, as well as fragments of collagen, have been found in the noninflammatory synovial fluids of patients with severe HA arthropathy; the concentration of these enzymes exceeded those found in rheumatoid arthritis and uncomplicated osteoarthritis. (3) Synovial membrane tissue cultures exposed to HA (or CPPD) crystals markedly increased release of these enzymes, underscoring the destructive potential of abnormally stimulated synovial lining cells.

Clinical Manifestations Periarticular and articular deposits may coexist and be associated with acute and/or chronic damage to the joint capsule, tendons, bursa, or articular surfaces. The most common sites of HA deposition include those in and/or around the knees, shoulders, hips, and fingers. Clinical manifestations include asymptomatic radiographic abnormalities, acute synovitis or tendinitis, and chronic destructive arthropathy. Most patients with HA arthropathy are elderly. Although the true incidence of HA arthritis is not known, 30 to 50 percent of patients with osteoarthritis have HA microcrystals in their synovial fluid. Such crystals can frequently be identified in clinically stable osteoarthritic joints, but they are more likely to come to attention in persons experiencing acute or subacute worsening of joint pain and swelling. The synovial fluid WBC count in HA arthritis is usually low (<2000 cells/μL) but may at times have as many as 50,000 cells/μL. Most synovial fluid analyses reveal a predominance of mononuclear cells. Occasionally, neutrophils may dominate.

Diagnosis Radiographic findings in HA arthropathy are not diagnostic. Intra- and/or periarticular calcifications with or without erosive, destructive, or hypertrophic changes may be present. X-ray films also may be normal.

Definitive diagnosis of HA arthropathy depends on identification of crystals from synovial fluid or tissue (Fig. 323-2). Individual crystals are very small, nonbirefringent, and can only be seen by electron microscopy. Clumps of crystals may appear as 1- to 20-μm shiny intra- or extracellular globules that stain purplish with Wright's stain and bright red with alizarin red S. Absolute identification depends on electron microscopy with energy-dispersive elemental analysis, x-ray diffraction, or infrared spectroscopy.

Table 323-2

Conditions Associated with HA Deposition Disease

Aging
Osteoarthritis
Hemorrhagic shoulder effusions in the elderly (Milwaukee shoulder)
Destructive arthropathy
Tendinitis, bursitis
Tumoral calcinosis (sporadic cases)
Disease-associated
Hyperparathyroidism
Milk alkali syndrome
Renal failure/long-term dialysis
Connective tissue diseases (e.g., progressive systemic sclerosis, CREST syndrome, idiopathic myositis)
Heterotopic calcification following neurologic catastrophes (e.g., stroke, spinal cord injury)
Hereditary
Bursitis, arthritis
Tumoral calcinosis

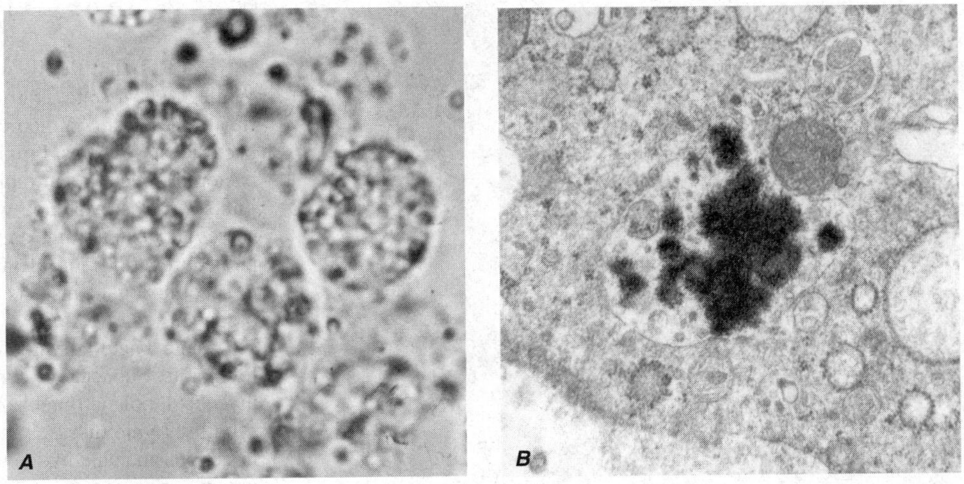

FIGURE 323-2 *A.* Cytoplasmic round inclusions inside synovial fluid cells represent aggregates of apatite crystals (fresh preparation, ordinary light microscopy; 288×). *B.* An electron micrograph demonstrates a cluster of dark apatite crystals within a synovial fluid mononuclear cell (21,600×).

℞ TREATMENT

Treatment of HA arthritis is nonspecific. Acute attacks of synovitis may be self-limiting, resolving in from days to several weeks. Aspiration of effusions and the use of either nonsteroidal anti-inflammatory agents or oral colchicine for 2 weeks or of intraarticular injection of glucocorticoid salts appear to shorten the duration and intensity of symptoms. In patients with underlying severe destructive articular changes, response to medical therapy is usually less rewarding.

CaOx DEPOSITION DISEASE **Pathogenesis** *Primary oxalosis* is a rare hereditary metabolic disorder (Chap. 349). Enhanced production of oxalic acid may result from at least two different enzyme defects, leading to hyperoxalemia and deposition of calcium oxalate crystals in tissues. Nephrocalcinosis, renal failure, and death usually occur before age 20. Acute and/or chronic CaOx arthritis and periarthritis may complicate primary oxalosis during later years of illness.

Secondary oxalosis is more common than the primary disorder. It is one of the many metabolic abnormalities that complicate end-stage renal disease (ESRD). In ESRD, calcium oxalate deposits have long been recognized in visceral organs, blood vessels, bones, and even cartilage. However, it was not until 1982 that such deposits were demonstrated to be one of the causes of arthritis in chronic renal failure. Thus far, reported patients have been dependent on long-term hemodialysis or peritoneal dialysis (see also Chap. 272), and many had received vitamin C (ascorbic acid) supplements. Ascorbic acid is metabolized to oxalate, which is inadequately cleared in uremia and by dialysis. Such supplements are now usually avoided in dialysis programs because of the risk of enhancing hyperoxalosis and its sequelae.

Clinical Manifestations and Diagnosis As was noted for the other calcium salts, CaOx aggregates can be found in bone, articular cartilage, synovium, and periarticular tissues. From these sites, crystals may be shed, causing acute synovitis. Persistent aggregates of CaOx may, like HA and CPPD, stimulate synovial proliferation and enzyme release, resulting in progressive articular destruction. Deposits have been documented in fingers, wrists, elbows, knees, ankles, and feet. Any articular site could potentially be involved.

Each of the known microcrystalline arthropathies may be a complication of ESRD, and rare patients have more than one type of crystal present in a joint effusion. The advent of crystallographic techniques has made it clear that most arthritic problems in ESRD are not, as was once believed, due to MSU gout. Clinical features of acute CaOx arthritis may not be distinguishable from those due to sodium urate, CPPD, or HA. Radiographs may reveal chondrocalcinosis, a feature of either CPPD or CaOx deposition. CaOx-induced synovial effusions are usually noninflammatory, with less than 2000 leukocytes/μL. Neutrophils or mononuclear cells have predominated. In most instances, crystals are extracellular, although CaOx has been identified in neutrophils. Synovial membranes show modest signs of inflammation. CaOx crystals have a variable shape and variable birefringence to polarized light. The most easily recognized forms are bipyramidal and have strong positive birefringence (Fig. 323-3).

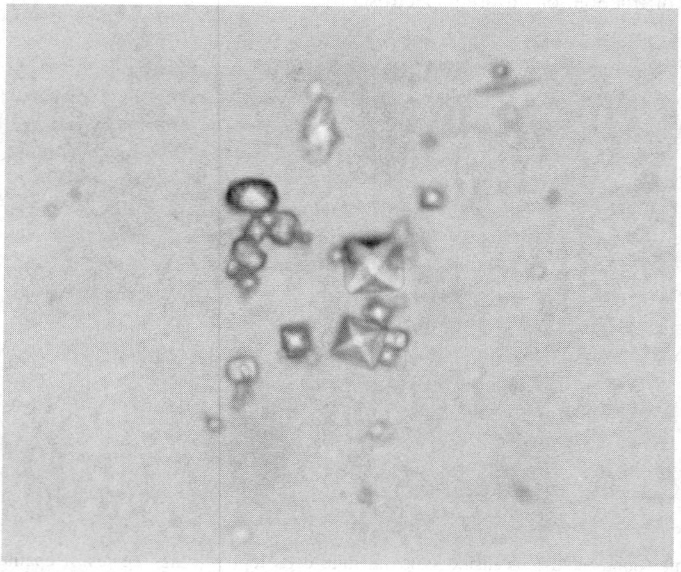

FIGURE 323-3 Bipyramidal and small polymorphic calcium oxalate crystals (ordinary light microscopy; 400×).

℞ TREATMENT

Treatment of CaOx arthropathy with nonsteroidal anti-inflammatory agents, colchicine, intraarticular glucocorticoids, and/or an increased frequency of dialysis has produced only slight improvement. In primary oxalosis, liver transplantation has induced a significant reduction in crystal deposits (see Chap. 349).

BIBLIOGRAPHY

ALVARELLOS A, SPILBERG I: Colchicine prophylaxis in pseudogout. J Rheumatol 13:804, 1986

BETH A et al: Articular cartilage vesicles generate calcium pyrophosphate dihydrate-like crystals in vitro. Arthritis Rheum 35:231, 1992

DIEPPE PA et al: Apatite deposition disease: A new arthropathy. Lancet 1:266, 1976

BALDWIN CT et al: Linkage of early onset osteoarthritis and chondrocalcinosis to human chromosome 8q. Am J Hum Genet 56:692, 1995

DOHERTY M et al: Inorganic pyrophosphate in metabolic diseases predisposing to calcium pyrophosphate dihydrate crystal deposition. Arthritis Rheum 34:1297, 1991

HOFFMAN GS et al: Calcium oxalate microcrystalline-associated arthritis in end-stage renal disease. Ann Intern Med 97:36, 1982

HUGHES A et al: Localisation of a gene for chondrocalcinosis to chromosome 5p. Hum Mol Genet 4:1225, 1995

MCCARTHY DJ: Crystals and arthritis. Dis Month 40:255, 1994

REGINATO AJ et al: Familial calcium pyrophosphate crystal deposition disease or calcium pyrophosphate gout. Rev Rheum [Engl Ed] 62:376, 1995

REGINATO AJ, SCHUMACHER HR: Apatite crystals in joint fluid; clinical relevance and search for a simple and accurate diagnostic test. Rheumatol Rev 3, 1994

ROSENTHAL AK, RYAN LM: Treatment of refractory crystal-associated arthritis. Rheum Dis Clin North Am 21:151, 1995

SIMKIN PA: Oxalate crystals and the taxonomy of gout. JAMA 260:1285, 1988

324

Scott J. Thaler, James H. Maguire

INFECTIOUS ARTHRITIS

INTRODUCTION AND APPROACH TO THE PATIENT While *Staphylococcus aureus*, *Neisseria gonorrhoeae*, and other bacteria are the most common causes of infectious arthritis, various mycobacteria, spirochetes, fungi, and viruses also infect joints. Since acute bacterial infection can rapidly destroy articular cartilage, all inflamed joints must be evaluated without delay to exclude noninfectious processes and to determine appropriate antimicrobial therapy and drainage procedures. For more detailed information on infectious arthritis due to specific organisms, the reader is referred to the chapters on those organisms.

Acute bacterial infection typically involves a single joint or a few joints. Subacute or chronic monarthritis or oligoarthritis suggests mycobacterial or fungal infection; episodic inflammation is seen in syphilis, Lyme disease, and the reactive arthritis that follows enteric infections and chlamydial urethritis (Table 324-1). Acute polyarticular inflammation occurs as an immunologic reaction during the course of endocarditis, rheumatic fever, disseminated neisserial infection, and acute hepatitis B. Bacteria and viruses occasionally infect multiple joints, the former most commonly in persons with rheumatoid arthritis.

Aspiration of synovial fluid, an essential element in the evaluation of potentially infected joints, can be performed without difficulty in most cases by the insertion of a large-bore needle into the site of maximal fluctuation or tenderness or by the route of easiest access. Ultrasonography or fluoroscopy may be used to guide aspiration of difficult-to-localize effusions of the hip and, occasionally, the shoulder and other joints. Normal synovial fluid contains fewer than 180 cells (predominantly mononuclear cells) per microliter. Synovial cell counts averaging 100,000/μL (range, 25,000 to 250,000/μL), with more than 90 percent neutrophils, are characteristic of acute bacterial infections. Crystal-induced, rheumatoid, and other noninfectious inflammatory arthritides are usually associated with fewer than 30,000 to 50,000 cells/μL; cell counts of 10,000 to 30,000/μL, with 50 to 70 percent neutrophils and the remainder lymphocytes, are common in mycobacterial and fungal infections. Definitive diagnosis of an infectious process relies on identification of the pathogen in stained smears of synovial fluid, isolation of the pathogen from cultures of synovial fluid and blood, or detection of microbial nucleic acids and proteins by polymerase chain reaction (PCR)–based assays and immunologic techniques.

ACUTE BACTERIAL ARTHRITIS **Pathogenesis** Bacteria enter the joint from the bloodstream, from a contiguous site of infection in bone or soft tissue, or by direct inoculation during surgery, injection, or trauma. In hematogenous infection, bacteria escape from synovial capillaries, which have no limiting basement membrane, and within hours provoke neutrophilic infiltration of the synovium. Neutrophils and bacteria enter the lumen of the joint; later, bacteria adhere to articular cartilage. Degradation of cartilage begins within 48 h as a result of increased intraarticular pressure, release of proteases and cytokines from chondrocytes, and invasion of the cartilage by bacteria and inflammatory cells. Histologic studies reveal bacteria lining the synovium and cartilage as well as abscesses extending into the synovium, cartilage, and—in severe cases—subchondral bone. Synovial proliferation results in the formation of a pannus over the cartilage, and thrombosis of inflamed synovial vessels develops. Bacterial factors that appear important in the pathogenesis of infective arthritis include collagen receptors in *S. aureus* that permit adherence to cartilage and endotoxins that promote chondrocyte-mediated breakdown of cartilage.

Microbiology The hematogenous route of infection is the most common route in all age groups. In infants, group B streptococci, gram-negative enteric bacilli, and *S. aureus* are the usual pathogens. Since the advent of the *Haemophilus influenzae* vaccine, *S. aureus* and *Streptococcus pyogenes* (group A *Streptococcus*) have predominated in children less than 5 years of age. Among young adults and adolescents, *N. gonorrhoeae* is the most commonly implicated organism. *S. aureus* accounts for most nongonococcal isolates in adults of all ages; gram-negative bacilli, pneumococci, and group B and other streptococci are involved in up to one-third of cases in older adults, especially those with underlying comorbid illnesses.

Infections following surgical procedures or penetrating injuries are due most often to *S. aureus* and occasionally to other gram-positive bacteria or gram-negative bacilli. Infections with coagulase-negative staphylococci are unusual except after the implantation of prosthetic joints or arthroscopy. Anaerobic organisms, often in association with aerobic or facultative bacteria, are found after human bites and when decubitus ulcers or intraabdominal abscesses spread into adjacent joints. Polymicrobial infections complicate traumatic injuries with extensive contamination. Cat bites or scratches may introduce *Pasteurella multocida* into joints.

Nongonococcal Bacterial Arthritis *Epidemiology* Although hematogenous infections with virulent organisms such as *S. aureus*, *H. influenzae*, and pyogenic streptococci occur in healthy persons, there is an underlying host predisposition in many cases of septic arthritis. Patients with rheumatoid arthritis have the highest incidence of infective arthritis, most often secondary to *S. aureus*, because of chronically inflamed joints, glucocorticoid therapy, and frequent breakdown of rheumatoid nodules, vasculitic ulcers, and skin overlying deformed joints. Diabetes mellitus, glucocorticoid therapy, hemodialysis, and malignancy all carry an increased risk of infection with *S. aureus* and gram-negative bacilli. Pneumococcal infections complicate alcoholism, deficiencies of humoral immunity, and hemoglobinopathies. Intravenous drug users acquire staphylococcal and streptococcal infections from their own flora and acquire pseudomonal and other gram-negative infections from drugs and injection paraphernalia.

Clinical manifestations Ninety percent of patients present with involvement of a single joint: most commonly the knee, less frequently the hip, and still less often the shoulder, wrist, or elbow. Small joints of the hands and feet are more likely to be affected after direct inoculation or a bite. Among intravenous drug users, infections of the spine, sacroiliac joints, or sternoclavicular joints are more common than infections of the appendicular skeleton. Polyarticular infection is most common among patients with rheumatoid arthritis and may resemble a flare of the underlying disease.

The usual presentation consists of moderate to severe pain that is uniform around the joint, effusion, muscle spasm, and decreased range of motion. Fever in the range of 38.3 to 38.9°C (101 to 102°F) and sometimes higher is common but may be lacking, especially in persons with rheumatoid arthritis, renal or hepatic insufficiency, or conditions requiring immunosuppressive therapy. The inflamed, swollen joint is usually evident on examination except in the case of a deeply situated joint, such as the hip or the sacroiliac joint. Cellulitis, bursitis, and acute osteomyelitis, which may produce a similar clinical picture, should be distinguished from septic arthritis by their greater range of motion and less-than-circumferential swelling. A focus of extraarticular infection, such as a boil or pneumonia, should be sought. Peripheral-blood leukocytosis and a left shift are common findings.

Plain radiographs show evidence of soft tissue swelling, joint-space widening, and displacement of tissue planes by the distended capsule. Narrowing of the joint space and bony erosions indicate

Table 324-1

Differential Diagnosis of Arthritis Syndromes

Acute Monarticular Arthritis	Chronic Monarticular Arthritis	Polyarticular Arthritis
Staphylococcus aureus	*Mycobacterium tuberculosis*	*Neisseria meningitidis*
Streptococcus pneumoniae	Nontuberculous mycobacteria	*Neisseria gonorrhoeae*
β-Hemolytic streptococci	*Borrelia burgdorferi*	Nongonococcal bacterial arthritis
Gram-negative bacilli	*Treponema pallidum*	Bacterial endocarditis
Neisseria gonorrhoeae	*Candida* species	*Candida* species
Candida species	*Sporothrix schenckii*	Poncet's disease (tuberculous rheumatism)
Crystal-induced arthritis	*Coccidioides immitis*	Hepatitis B virus
Fracture	*Blastomyces dermatitidis*	Parvovirus B19
Hemarthrosis	*Aspergillus* species	Human immunodeficiency virus
Foreign body	*Cryptococcus neoformans*	Human T lymphotropic virus type I
Osteoarthritis	*Nocardia* species	Rubella virus
Ischemic necrosis	*Brucella* species	Sickle cell disease flare
Monarticular rheumatoid arthritis	Legg-Calvé-Perthes disease	Reactive arthritis
	Osteoarthritis	Serum sickness
		Acute rheumatic fever
		Inflammatory bowel disease
		Systemic lupus erythematosus
		Rheumatoid arthritis/Still's disease
		Other vasculitides
		Sarcoidosis

advanced infection and a poor prognosis. Ultrasound is useful for detecting effusions in the hip, and computed tomography or magnetic resonance imaging can demonstrate infections of the sacroiliac joint and the spine very well.

Laboratory findings Specimens of peripheral blood and synovial fluid should be obtained before antibiotics are administered. Blood cultures are positive in up to 50 percent of *S. aureus* infections but are less frequently positive in infections due to other organisms. The synovial fluid is turbid, serosanguineous, or frankly purulent. Gram-stained smears confirm the presence of large numbers of neutrophils. Levels of total protein and lactate dehydrogenase in synovial fluid are elevated, and the glucose level is depressed; however, measurement of these levels is not necessary to make the diagnosis. The synovial fluid should be examined for crystals, because gout and pseudogout can resemble septic arthritis clinically, and infection and crystal-induced disease occasionally occur together. Organisms are seen on synovial fluid smears in nearly three-quarters of infections with *S. aureus* and streptococci and in 30 to 50 percent of infections due to gram-negative and other bacteria. Cultures of synovial fluid are positive in more than 90 percent of cases. Inoculation of synovial fluid into bottles containing liquid media for blood cultures increases the yield of culture.

℞ TREATMENT

Prompt administration of systemic antibiotics and drainage of the involved joint can prevent destruction of cartilage, postinfectious degenerative arthritis, joint instability, or deformity. Once cultures of blood and synovial fluid have been obtained, empirical antibiotics should be given that are directed against bacteria visualized on smears or against the pathogens that are likely, given the patient's age and risk factors. Initial therapy should consist of the intravenous administration of bactericidal agents; direct instillation of antibiotics into the joint is not necessary to achieve adequate levels in synovial fluid and tissue. An intravenous combination of a third-generation cephalosporin such as cefotaxime (1 g every 8 h) or ceftriaxone (1 to 2 g every 24 h) and either oxacillin or nafcillin (2 g every 4 h) will provide adequate coverage for most infections in adults. Intravenous vancomycin (1 g every 12 h) should be given if methicillin-resistant *S. aureus* is a possible pathogen in a hospitalized patient. In addition, an aminoglycoside should be given to intravenous drug users or other patients in whom *Pseudomonas aeruginosa* may be the responsible agent.

Definitive therapy is based on the identity and antibiotic susceptibility of the bacteria isolated in culture. Infections due to staphylococci are treated with oxacillin, nafcillin, or vancomycin for 4 weeks. Pneumococcal and streptococcal infections due to penicillin-susceptible organisms respond to 2 weeks of therapy with penicillin G (2 million units intravenously every 4 h); infections caused by *H. influenzae* and by strains of *S. pneumoniae* that are resistant to penicillin are treated with cefotaxime or ceftriaxone for 2 weeks. Most enteric gram-negative infections can be cured in 3 to 4 weeks by a second- or third-generation cephalosporin given intravenously. *P. aeruginosa* infection should be treated with at least 3 weeks of combination therapy with an aminoglycoside plus either an extended-spectrum penicillin such as mezlocillin (3 g intravenously every 4 h) or an antipseudomonal cephalosporin such as ceftazidime (1 g intravenously every 8 h). If tolerated, this regimen is continued for an additional 2 to 3 weeks; alternatively, a fluoroquinolone such as ciprofloxacin (750 mg orally twice daily) is substituted for the aminoglycoside.

Timely drainage of pus and necrotic debris from the infected joint is required for a favorable outcome. Needle aspiration of readily accessible joints such as the knee may be adequate if loculations or particulate matter in the joint does not prevent its thorough decompression. Arthroscopic drainage and lavage may be employed initially or within several days if repeated needle aspiration fails to relieve symptoms, decrease the volume of the effusion and the synovial white cell count, and clear bacteria from smears and cultures. In some cases, arthrotomy is necessary to remove loculations and debride infected synovium, cartilage, or bone. Septic arthritis of the hip is best managed with arthrotomy, particularly in young children, in whom infection threatens the viability of the femoral head. Septic joints do not require immobilization except for pain control before symptoms are alleviated by treatment. Weight bearing should be avoided until signs of inflammation have subsided, but frequent passive motion of the joint is indicated to maintain full mobility.

Gonococcal Arthritis *Epidemiology* Gonococcal arthritis, accounting for 70 percent of episodes of infectious arthritis in persons under 40 years of age, results from bacteremia arising from gonococcal infection or, more frequently, from asymptomatic gonococcal mucosal colonization of the urethra, cervix, or pharynx. Women are at greatest risk during menses and overall are two to three times more likely than men to develop disseminated gonococcal infection and arthritis. Persons with complement deficiencies, especially of the terminal components, are prone to recurrent episodes of gonococcemia. Strains of gonococci that are most likely to cause disseminated infection include those that produce transparent colonies in culture, have the type IA outer-membrane protein, or are of the AUH-auxotroph type.

Clinical manifestations and laboratory findings The most common manifestation of disseminated gonococcal infection is a syndrome of fever, chills, rash, and articular symptoms. Small numbers of papules that progress to hemorrhagic pustules develop on the trunk and the extensor surfaces of the distal extremities. Migratory arthritis and tenosynovitis of the knees, hands, wrists, feet, and ankles are prominent. The cutaneous lesions and articular findings are believed to be the consequence of an immune reaction to circulating gonococci and immune-complex deposition in tissues. Thus, cultures of synovial fluid are consistently negative, and blood cultures are positive in fewer than 45 percent of patients. Synovial fluid may be difficult to obtain from inflamed joints and usually contains only 10,000 to 20,000 leukocytes/μL.

True gonococcal septic arthritis is less common than the disseminated gonococcal infection syndrome and always follows disseminated infection, which is unrecognized in one-third of patients. A single joint, such as the hip, knee, ankle, or wrist, is usually involved. Synovial fluid that contains more than 50,000 leukocytes/μL can be obtained with ease; the gonococcus is only occasionally evident in gram-stained smears, and cultures of synovial fluid are positive in fewer than 40 percent of cases. Blood cultures are almost always negative.

Because it is difficult to isolate gonococci from synovial fluid and blood, specimens for culture should be obtained from potentially infected mucosal sites. Cultures and gram-stained smears of skin lesions occasionally are positive. All specimens for culture should be plated onto Thayer-Martin agar directly or in special transport media at the bedside and transferred promptly to the microbiology laboratory in an atmosphere of 5% CO_2, as generated in a candle jar. PCR-based assays are extremely sensitive in detecting gonococcal DNA in synovial fluid. A dramatic alleviation of symptoms within 12 to 24 h after the initiation of appropriate antibiotic therapy supports a clinical diagnosis of the disseminated gonococcal infection syndrome if cultures are negative.

℞ TREATMENT

Initial treatment consists of ceftriaxone (1 g intravenously or intramuscularly every 24 h) to cover possible penicillin-resistant organisms. Once local and systemic signs are clearly resolving, the 7-day course of therapy can be completed with an oral agent such as cefixime (400 mg twice daily) or ciprofloxacin (500 mg twice daily) or, if penicillin-susceptible organisms are isolated, amoxicillin (500 mg three times daily). Suppurative arthritis usually responds to needle aspiration of involved joints and 7 to 10 days of antibiotic treatment. Arthroscopic lavage or arthrotomy is rarely required.

It is noteworthy that arthritis symptoms similar to those seen in disseminated gonococcal infections occur in meningococcemia. A dermatitis-arthritis syndrome, purulent monarthritis, and reactive polyarthritis have been described. All respond to treatment with intravenous penicillin.

SPIROCHETAL ARTHRITIS **Lyme Disease** Lyme disease due to infection with the spirochete *Borrelia burgdorferi* causes arthritis in up to 70 percent of persons who are not treated. Intermittent arthralgias and myalgias, but not arthritis, occur within days or weeks of inoculation of the spirochete by the *Ixodes* tick. Later, there are three patterns of joint disease: (1) Fifty percent of untreated persons experience intermittent episodes of monarthritis or oligoarthritis involving the knee and/or other large joints. The symptoms wax and wane without treatment over months, and each year 10 to 20 percent of patients report loss of joint symptoms. (2) Twenty percent of untreated persons develop a pattern of waxing and waning arthralgias. (3) Ten percent of patients develop chronic inflammatory synovitis resulting in erosive lesions and destruction of the joint.

Rx TREATMENT

Lyme arthritis generally responds well to therapy. A regimen of oral doxycycline, oral amoxicillin plus probenecid, or parenteral ceftriaxone for a period of 3 to 4 weeks is recommended. Patients who do not respond to such a regimen are unlikely to benefit from additional therapy. Failure of therapy is associated with host features such as the HLA-DR4 genotype or persistent reactivity to OspA (outer surface protein A). New techniques using PCR amplification of spirochetal DNA may be useful in the monitoring of patients in whom conventional therapy fails. Patients who have negative results of synovial-fluid PCR and who fail to respond to initial therapy are highly unlikely to benefit from additional antimicrobial therapy.

Syphilitic Arthritis Articular manifestations occur in different stages of syphilis. In early congenital syphilis, periarticular swelling and immobilization of the involved limbs (Parrot's pseudoparalysis) complicate osteochondritis of long bones. Clutton's joint, a late manifestation of congenital syphilis that typically develops between the ages of 8 and 15, is caused by chronic painless synovitis with effusions of large joints, particularly the knees and elbows. Secondary syphilis may be associated with arthralgias; symmetric arthritis of the knees and ankles and occasionally of the shoulders and wrists; and sacroiliitis. The arthritis follows a subacute to chronic course with a mixed mononuclear and neutrophilic synovial-fluid pleocytosis (typical cell counts, 5,000 to 15,000/μL). Immunologic mechanisms may contribute to the arthritis, and symptoms usually improve rapidly with penicillin therapy. In tertiary syphilis, Charcot's joint is a result of sensory loss due to tabes dorsalis. Penicillin is not helpful in this setting.

MYCOBACTERIAL ARTHRITIS Tuberculous arthritis accounts for about 1 percent of all cases of tuberculosis and for 10 percent of extrapulmonary cases. The most common presentation is chronic granulomatous monarthritis. An unusual syndrome, Poncet's disease, is a reactive symmetric form of polyarthritis that affects persons with visceral or disseminated tuberculosis. No mycobacteria are found in the joints, and symptoms resolve with antituberculous therapy.

Unlike tuberculous osteomyelitis, which typically involves the thoracic and lumbar spine (50 percent of cases), tuberculous arthritis primarily involves the large weight-bearing joints, in particular the hips, knees, and ankles, and only occasionally involves smaller non-weight-bearing joints. Progressive monarticular swelling and pain develop over months to years, and systemic symptoms are seen in only half of all cases. Coexistent active pulmonary tuberculosis is unusual.

Aspiration of the involved joint yields fluid with an average cell count of 20,000/μL, with approximately 50 percent neutrophils. Acid-fast staining of the fluid yields positive results in fewer than one-third of cases, and cultures are positive in 80 percent. Culture of synovial tissue taken at biopsy is positive in about 90 percent of cases and shows granulomatous inflammation in most. Radiographs reveal peripheral erosions at the points of synovial attachment, periarticular osteopenia, and eventually joint-space narrowing. Therapy for tuberculous arthritis is the same as that for tuberculous pulmonary disease, requiring the administration of multiple agents for 6 to 9 months. Therapy is more prolonged in immunosuppressed individuals, such as those infected with human immunodeficiency virus (HIV).

Various atypical mycobacteria found in water and soil may cause chronic indolent arthritis. Such disease results from trauma and direct inoculation associated with farming, gardening, or aquatic activities. Smaller joints, such as the digits, wrists, and knees, are usually involved. Involvement of tendon sheaths and bursae is typical. The mycobacterial species involved include *M. marinum*, *M. avium-intracellulare*, *M. terrae*, *M. kansasii*, *M. fortuitum*, and *M. chelonae*. In persons who have HIV infection or are receiving immunosuppressive therapy, hematogenous spread to the joints has been reported for *M. kansasii*, *M. avium-intracellulare*, and *M. haemophilum*. Diagnosis usually requires biopsy and culture, and therapy is based on antimicrobial susceptibility patterns.

FUNGAL ARTHRITIS Fungi are an unusual cause of chronic monarticular arthritis. Granulomatous articular infection with the endemic dimorphic fungi *Coccidioides immitis*, *Blastomyces dermatitidis*, and (less commonly) *Histoplasma capsulatum* results from hematogenous seeding or direct extension from bony lesions in persons with disseminated disease. Joint involvement is an unusual complication of sporotrichosis (infection with *Sporothrix schenckii*) among gardeners and other persons who work with soil or sphagnum moss. Articular sporotrichosis is six times more common among men than among women, and alcoholics and other debilitated hosts are at risk for polyarticular infection.

Candida infection involving a single joint, usually the knee, hip, or shoulder, results from surgical procedures, intraarticular injections, or (among critically ill patients with debilitating illnesses such as diabetes mellitus or hepatic or renal insufficiency and patients receiving immunosuppressive therapy) hematogenous spread. *Candida* infections in intravenous drug users typically involve the spine, sacroiliac joints, or other fibrocartilaginous joints. Unusual cases of arthritis due to *Aspergillus* species, *Cryptococcus neoformans*, *Pseudallescheria boydii*, and the dematiaceous fungi have also resulted from direct inoculation or disseminated hematogenous infection in immunocompromised persons.

The synovial fluid in fungal arthritis usually contains 10,000 to 40,000 cells/μL, with about 70 percent neutrophils. Stained specimens and cultures of synovial tissue often confirm the diagnosis of fungal arthritis when studies of synovial fluid give negative results. Treatment consists of drainage and lavage of the joint and systemic administration of amphotericin B, fluconazole, or itraconazole (the exact drug depending on the species involved). The doses and duration of therapy are the same as for disseminated disease. Intraarticular instillation of amphotericin B has been used in addition to intravenous therapy.

VIRAL ARTHRITIS Viruses produce arthritis by infecting synovial tissue during systemic infection or by provoking an immunologic reaction that involves joints. As many as 50 percent of women report persistent arthralgias and 10 percent frank arthritis within 3 days of the rash that follows natural infection with *rubella virus* and within 2 to 6 weeks after receipt of live virus vaccine. Episodes of symmetric inflammation of fingers, wrists, and knees uncommonly recur for longer than a year, but a syndrome of chronic fatigue, low-grade fever, headaches, and myalgias can persist for months or years. Intravenous immunoglobulin has been helpful in selected cases. Self-limited monarticular or migratory polyarthritis may develop within 2 weeks of the parotitis of *mumps*; this sequela is more common in men than in women. Approximately 10 percent of children and 60 percent of women develop arthritis after infection with *parvovirus B19*. In adults, arthropathy sometimes occurs without fever or rash. Pain and stiffness, with less prominent swelling (primarily of the hands but also of the knees, wrists, and ankles), usually resolve within weeks, although a small proportion of women develop chronic arthropathy.

About 2 weeks before the onset of jaundice, up to 10 percent of persons with acute *hepatitis B* develop an immune complex–mediated, serum sickness–like reaction with maculopapular rash, urticaria, fever, and arthralgias. Less common developments include symmetric arthritis involving the hands, wrists, elbows, or ankles and morning stiffness that resembles a flare of rheumatoid arthritis. Symptoms resolve at the time jaundice develops. Painful arthritis involving larger joints often accompanies the fever and rash of several arthropod-borne viral infections, including those caused by *chikungunya, O'nyong-nyong, Ross River, Mayaro*, and *Barmah Forest* viruses. Symmetric arthritis involving the hands and wrists may occur during the convalescent phase of infection with *lymphocytic choriomeningitis virus*. Patients infected with an *enterovirus* frequently report arthralgias, and *echovirus* has been isolated from patients with acute polyarthritis.

Several arthritis syndromes are associated with *HIV* infection. Reiter's syndrome with persistent, painful, lower-extremity oligoarthritis often follows an episode of urethritis in HIV-infected persons. HIV-associated Reiter's syndrome appears to be extremely common among persons with the HLA-B27 haplotype, but sacroiliac joint disease is unusual. Up to one-third of HIV-infected persons with psoriasis develop psoriatic arthritis. Painless monarthropathy and persistent symmetric polyarthropathy occasionally complicate HIV infection. Chronic persistent oligoarthritis of the shoulders, wrists, hands, and knees occurs in women infected with human T-lymphotropic virus type I. Synovial thickening, destruction of articular cartilage, and leukemic-appearing atypical lymphocytes in synovial fluid are characteristic, but progression to T cell leukemia is unusual.

PARASITIC ARTHRITIS Arthritis due to parasitic infection is rare. The guinea worm *Dracunculus medinensis* may cause destructive joint lesions in the lower extremities as migrating gravid female worms invade joints or cause ulcers in adjacent soft tissues that become secondarily infected. Hydatid cysts infect bones in 1 to 2 percent of cases of infection with *Echinococcus granulosus*. The expanding destructive cystic lesions may spread to and destroy adjacent joints, particularly the hip and pelvis. In rare cases, chronic synovitis has been associated with the presence of schistosomal eggs in synovial biopsies. Monarticular arthritis in children with lymphatic *filariasis* appears to respond to therapy with diethylcarbamazine despite the absence of microfilariae in synovial fluid. Reactive arthritis has been attributed to *hookworm*, *Strongyloides*, *Cryptosporidium*, and *Giardia* infection in case reports, but confirmation is required.

REACTIVE ARTHRITIS OR REITER'S SYNDROME A syndrome of reactive arthritis associated with rash, urethritis, conjunctivitis, uveitis, and oral ulcers develops several weeks after approximately 1 percent of cases of nongonococcal urethritis and 2 percent of enteric infections, particularly with those due to *Yersinia enterocolitica*, *Shigella flexneri*, *Campylobacter jejuni*, and *Salmonella* species. Studies have identified microbial DNA or antigen in synovial fluid or blood in some cases, but the pathogenesis of this condition is poorly understood.

Reactive arthritis is most common among young men (except after *Yersinia* infection) and has been linked to the HLA-B27 locus as a potential genetic predisposing factor. Patients report painful, asymmetric oligoarthritis affecting mainly the knees, ankles, and feet. Low-back pain is common, and radiographic evidence of sacroiliitis is found in patients with long-standing disease. Most patients recover within 6 months, but prolonged recurrent disease is more common in cases following nongonococcal urethritis. Anti-inflammatory agents help to relieve symptoms, but the role of prolonged antibiotic therapy in eliminating microbial antigen from the synovium is controversial.

INFECTIONS IN PROSTHETIC JOINTS Infection complicates 1 to 4 percent of total joint replacements. The majority of infections are acquired intraoperatively or immediately postoperatively as a result of wound breakdown or infection; less commonly, these joint infections develop later after joint replacement and are the result of hematogenous spread or direct inoculation. The presentation may be acute, with fever, pain, and local signs of inflammation, especially in infections due to *S. aureus*, pyogenic streptococci, and enteric bacilli. Alternatively, infection may persist for months or years without causing constitutional symptoms when less virulent organisms, such as coagulase-negative staphylococci or diphtheroids, are involved. Such indolent infections are usually acquired during joint implantation and are discovered during evaluation of chronic unexplained pain or after a radiograph shows loosening of the prosthesis; the erythrocyte sedimentation rate is usually elevated in such cases.

The diagnosis is best made by needle aspiration of the joint; accidental introduction of organisms during aspiration must be meticulously avoided. Synovial fluid pleocytosis with a predominance of polymorphonuclear leukocytes is highly suggestive of infection, since other inflammatory processes uncommonly affect prosthetic joints. Culture and Gram's stain usually yield the responsible pathogen. Use of special media for unusual pathogens such as fungi, atypical mycobacteria, and *Mycoplasma* may be necessary if routine and anaerobic cultures are negative.

℞ TREATMENT

Treatment includes surgery and high doses of parenteral antibiotics, which are given for 4 to 6 weeks because bone is usually involved. In most cases, the prosthesis must be replaced to cure the infection. Implantation of a new prosthesis is best delayed for several weeks or months because relapses of infection occur most commonly within this time frame. In some cases, reimplantation is not possible, and the patient must manage without a joint, with a fused joint, or even with amputation. Cure of infection without removal of the prosthesis is occasionally possible in cases that are due to streptococci or pneumococci and that lack radiologic evidence of loosening of the prosthesis. In these cases, antibiotic therapy must be initiated within several days of the onset of infection, and the joint should be drained vigorously either by open arthrotomy or arthroscopically.

Prevention To avoid the disastrous consequences of infection, candidates for joint replacement should be selected with care. Rates of infection are particularly high among patients with rheumatoid arthritis, persons who have undergone previous surgery on the joint, and persons with medical conditions requiring immunosuppressive therapy. Perioperative antibiotic prophylaxis, usually with cefazolin, and measures to decrease intraoperative contamination, such as laminar flow, have lowered the rates of perioperative infection to <1 percent in many centers. After implantation, measures should be taken to prevent and rapidly treat extraarticular infections that might give rise to hematogenous spread to the prosthesis. The effectiveness of prophylactic antibiotics for the prevention of hematogenous infection following dental procedures has not been demonstrated; in fact, viridans streptococci and other components of the oral flora are extremely unusual causes of prosthetic joint infection.

BIBLIOGRAPHY

Baker DG, Schumacher HR: Acute monoarthritis. N Engl J Med 329:1013, 1993

Brower AC: Septic arthritis. Radiol Clin North Am 34:293, 1996

Calabrese LH: Human immunodeficiency virus (HIV) infection and arthritis. Rheum Dis Clin North Am 19:477, 1993

Cuckler JM et al: Diagnosis and management of the infected total joint arthroplasty. Orthop Clin North Am 22:523, 1991

Cunningham R et al: Clinical and molecular aspects of the pathogenesis of *Staphylococcus aureus* bone and joint infections. J Med Microbiol 44:157, 1996

Eustace SJ et al: Lyme arthropathy. Radiol Clin North Am 34:454, 1996

Evans J: Lyme disease. Curr Opin Rheumatol 7:322, 1995

Gardner GC, Weisman MH: Pyarthrosis in patients with rheumatoid arthritis: A report of 13 cases and a review of the literature from the past 40 years. Am J Med 88:503, 1990

Goldenberg DL: Bacterial arthritis. Curr Opin Rheumatol 7:310, 1995

———, Reed JI: Bacterial arthritis. N Engl J Med 312:764, 1985

Hughes RA, Keat AC: Reiter's syndrome and reactive arthritis: A current view. Semin Arthritis Rheum 24:190, 1994

Keat A: Reiter's syndrome and reactive arthritis in perspective. N Engl J Med 309:1606, 1983

Liebling MR et al: Identification of *Neisseria gonorrhoeae* in synovial fluid using the polymerase chain reaction. Arthritis Rheum 37:702, 1994

Meier JL, Beekmann SE: Mycobacterial and fungal infections of bones and joints. Curr Opin Rheumatol 7:329, 1995

Mitchell LA et al: Chronic rubella vaccine-associated arthropathy. Arch Intern Med 153:2268, 1993

MURADALI D et al: Multifocal osteoarticular tuberculosis: Report of four cases and review of management. Clin Infect Dis 17:204, 1993
PINALS RS: Polyarthritis and fever. N Engl J Med 330:769, 1994
PURVIS RS et al: Sporotrichosis presenting as arthritis and subcutaneous nodules. J Am Acad Dermatol 28:879, 1993
REGINATO AJ: Syphilitic arthritis and osteitis. Rheum Dis Clin North Am 19:379, 1993
SHMERLING R et al: Synovial fluid tests: What should be ordered? JAMA 264:1009, 1990
SILVEIRA LH et al: *Candida* arthritis. Rheum Dis Clin North Am 19:427, 1993
TSUKAYAMA DT et al: Infection after total hip arthroplasty. A study of the treatment of one hundred and six infections. J Bone Joint Surg [Am] 78A:512, 1996
WISE CM et al: Gonococcal arthritis in an era of increasing penicillin resistance. Arch Intern Med 154:2690, 1994

325

Peter H. Schur

PSORIATIC ARTHRITIS AND ARTHRITIS ASSOCIATED WITH GASTROINTESTINAL DISEASE

PSORIATIC ARTHRITIS

Psoriatic arthritis (PsA) is a chronic inflammatory arthritis that affects 5 to 42 percent of people with psoriasis.

ETIOLOGY AND PATHOGENESIS To date, the cause and pathogenesis of PsA are unknown. Indirect evidence has suggested that infections, trauma, increased cellular immunity (e.g., to streptococci), decreased suppressor cell activation, immune complexes, complement activation, adhesion molecules, dendritic cells, keratinocytes, and abnormal fibroblast and polymorphonuclear leukocyte (PMN) function may each play a role. Polyarthritis has developed in patients with psoriasis and hepatitis treated with interferon α. Most studies have observed an increased frequency of HLA-B17, CW6, DQ2, and/or B27 in patients with psoriatic spondylitis, while B27, BW62, B38, B39, and DR7a have been noted in association with peripheral arthritis in different studies. Fulminant disease should make one suspect human immunodeficiency virus (HIV) disease (see Chap. 308).

CLINICAL MANIFESTATIONS Three major types of psoriatic arthritis are generally recognized: asymmetric inflammatory arthritis, symmetric arthritis, and psoriatic spondylitis. A mean of 47 percent of patients (range, 16 to 70 percent) have an asymmetric inflammatory arthritis. Disease appears equally in men and women. Psoriasis tends to precede the arthritis by years, although many patients complain of morning stiffness. The proximal interphalangeal (PIP) and distal interphalangeal (DIP) joints are commonly involved [with characteristic sausage-shaped digits (dactylitis)], while knees, hips, ankles, temporomandibular joints, and wrists are less frequently involved. Most patients have onychodystrophy (onycholysis, ridging and pitting of nails), the course of which does not parallel that of the synovitis. The prognosis is good, with only one-fourth of the patients developing progressive destructive disease; one-third develop inflammatory ocular complications (conjunctivitis, iritis, episcleritis).

A mean of 25 percent of patients (range, 15 to 39 percent) develop symmetric arthritis resembling rheumatoid arthritis (see Chap. 313). This disease occurs twice as frequently in women. Psoriasis and inflammatory arthritis usually develop simultaneously; most patients experience morning stiffness. The DIP, PIP, metacarpophalangeal (MCP), metatarsophalangeal (MTP), sternoclavicular, and, in particular, large peripheral joints are involved. Practically all patients have onychodystrophy, which helps distinguish them from patients with rheumatoid arthritis. Over half of the patients in this group go on to develop destructive arthritis, including arthritis mutilans. Eye complications are uncommon. Subcutaneous nodules are not present, but one-fourth of patients have rheumatoid factors. Unilateral upper limb edema has been described.

A mean of 23 percent of the patients (range 5 to 40 percent) have psoriatic "spondylitis," with or without peripheral joint involvement. Psoriasis tends to precede the arthritis by a few years, and low back pain with morning stiffness is common. Psoriatic spondylitis is more common in men. About half the patients in this group have spondylitis and the other half have sacroiliitis. The back disease is usually slowly progressive, with little clinical deterioration as compared with ankylosing spondylitis; the peripheral disease also tends not to be destructive except for the occasional patient with arthritis mutilans. Enthesopathy, i.e., inflammation of tendons and ligamentous attachments to bone, is characteristic, viz., of the tendo Achillis, or of the plantar fascia causing heel pain. Many patients have onychodystrophy, but few have inflammatory ocular complications. Gut inflammation occurs in 30 percent (no gut inflammation was noted in patients with only peripheral arthritis).

Some authors have described additional subsets of psoriatic arthritis: predominant DIP joint involvement, arthritis mutilans, juvenile psoriatic arthritis, and SAPHO (synovitis, acne, pustulosis, hyperostosis, osteomyelitis).

The pathology of PsA is similar to that seen in rheumatoid arthritis: synoviocytic hyperplasia, early PMN infiltration and later mononuclear cell infiltration, cartilage erosion, and pannus formation. However, in PsA, the synovium is more vascular and there are fewer macrophages and less expression of endothelial cell leukocyte adhesion molecule-1 (ELAM-1). Skin lesions have more CD45RO+ cells in psoriasis. Fibrosis of the joint capsule and marrow is prominent in many patients.

LABORATORY FINDINGS There are a few laboratory abnormalities. Elevated erythrocyte sedimentation rates, C-reactive proteins, and complement levels reflect inflammation. Rheumatoid factors are uncommon and are more likely to be observed in those with symmetric arthritis. Immunoglobulin levels, especially IgA levels, may be elevated (IgA antibodies to cytokeratins and antienterobacteria antibodies are elevated). Uric acid levels may be elevated; sodium urate crystals in joint fluids suggest gout.

Radiologic investigation reveals findings similar to those of rheumatoid arthritis: soft tissue swelling, loss of the cartilage space, erosions, bony ankylosis of fingers, subluxations, and subchondral cysts; there is less demineralization, however. However, more unique and suggestive of psoriatic arthritis are erosions at DIP joints, expansion of the base of the terminal phalanx, tapering of the proximal phalanx and cuplike erosions of and bony proliferation of the distal terminal phalanx ("pencil-in-cup" appearance), proliferation of bone near osseous erosions, terminal phalangeal osteolysis, bone proliferation and periostitis (especially of phalanges), and telescoping of one bone into its neighbor, leading to the "opera-glass" deformity. The axial skeleton shows asymmetric or unilateral sacroiliitis, often asymptomatic paravertebral ossification, including cervical involvement, and large asymmetric nonmarginal syndesmophytes. Echocardiographic abnormalities resemble those of ankylosing spondilitis.

DIAGNOSIS The diagnosis of psoriatic arthritis should be considered in individuals with arthritis and psoriasis. Psoriasis should be distinguished from seborrheic dermatitis and eczema. Psoriatic lesions may be quite small peripherally and often are hidden in the scalp, umbilicus, and gluteal folds. Fungal infection of nails can be distinguished from psoriasis, for the latter will demonstrate pitting and onycholysis. Furthermore, onychodystrophy is uncommon (20 percent of cases) in uncomplicated psoriasis. It is often difficult to distinguish Reiter's syndrome (see Chap. 317) from psoriatic arthritis, since both manifest dactylitis. Reiter's syndrome usually presents in younger individuals, especially males, is less frequently progressive or destructive and is more likely to be associated with characteristic skin lesions (keratoderma blenorrhagica), urethritis, and conjunctivitis. Gout can be distinguished by the presence of intraarticular sodium urate crystals (see Chap. 344). Psoriasis in association with Heberden's nodes or Bouchard's nodes of the DIP and PIP joints, respectively, rather suggests osteoarthritis (see Chap. 322). Psoriatic arthritis differs from rheumatoid arthritis by the relative lack of rheumatoid factors; the tendency to asymmetry, dactylitis, iritis, enthesopathy, and onychodystrophy; the high frequency of HLA-B27, especially in patients with axial skeletal involvement; and characteristic radiologic features.

Rx TREATMENT

The treatment of psoriatic arthritis begins with patient education and physical and occupational therapy to maintain muscle strength and joint and muscle function. Orthotics and occasional intraarticular glucocorticoids for isolated acutely and severely inflamed joints may be added as needed (Fig. 325-1). The mainstay, however, is the use of nonsteroidal anti-inflammatory drugs (NSAIDs), which reduce inflammation and alleviate pain for most patients. For patients with more severe involvement, a disease-modifying antirheumatic drug should be used. While hydroxychloroquine is often successful in producing either amelioration or remission, it carries a significant risk of exacerbation of psoriasis and exfoliation. For more severe cases, especially with extensive skin involvement, 5 to 25 mg methotrexate per week is recommended. Most patients respond well with respect to both skin lesions and arthritis. Patients who are resistant to oral therapy may respond to intravenous therapy. Folic acid (1 mg/d) is recommended to prevent hematologic complications. Renal and liver function tests and a complete blood count should be performed frequently, and any abnormalities should suggest modification of the dosage. Liver biopsies are recommended after a total of 1.5 g methotrexate have been given and then every 2 years to identify the rare patient with fibrosis and cirrhosis, which necessitate withdrawal of the drug. Increased serum levels of the N-terminal propeptide of type III procollagen may predict liver fibrogenesis. However, patients are advised to avoid nephrotoxic and hepatotoxic (e.g., ethanol) drugs. Patients with HIV infection may have worsening of their disease when treated with methotrexate. Sulfasalazine (3 to 4 g/d), intramuscular gold, cyclosporine (2 to 5 mg/kg per day), etretinate (0.5 mg/kg per day), 6-mercaptopurine, and azathioprine have also proved successful. The arthritis may also respond to heliotherapy.

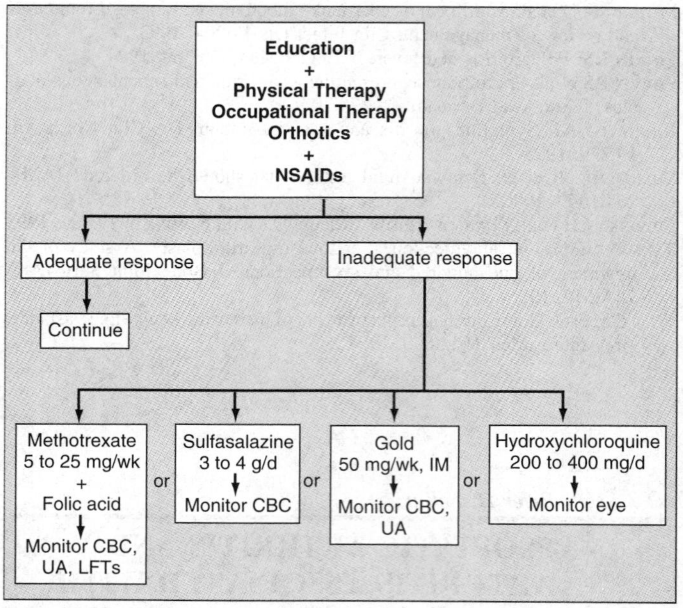

FIGURE 325-1 Algorithm for the treatment of psoriatic arthritis. See text for detailed description. NSAID, non-steroidal anti-inflammatory drugs; CBC, complete blood count; UA, urinalysis; LFTs, liver function tests.

ARTHRITIS ASSOCIATED WITH GASTROINTESTINAL DISEASE

INFLAMMATORY BOWEL DISEASE Peripheral arthritis occurs in 9 to 22 percent of patients with inflammatory bowel disease (IBD) (e.g., ulcerative colitis or Crohn's disease; see Chap. 286), and arthralgia is more common. Arthritis is somewhat more likely to occur in patients with large-bowel disease and in those patients with complications such as abscesses, pseudomembranous polyposis, perianal disease, massive hemorrhage, erythema nodosum, stomatitis, uveitis, and pyoderma gangrenosum. Males and females are affected equally. The arthritis tends to be acute, is associated with a flare-up of the bowel disease, occurs early in the course of the bowel disease, is self-limiting (90 percent of cases resolve within 6 months), and does not result in destruction. Most patients have a symmetric, migratory polyarthritis affecting primarily large joints of the lower extremity. Rheumatoid factors are not present. There is some association with HLA-BW62. Synovial fluids have 5000 to 12,000 white blood cells per microliter, mostly PMNs. Radiographs demonstrate soft tissue swelling and effusions without erosions or destruction. Pathologic examination of synovial biopsy specimens reveals only nonspecific inflammation. The peripheral arthritis responds to successful treatment of the bowel disease, such as colectomy (for ulcerative colitis), or administration of glucocorticoids, methotrexate, or sulfasalazine. NSAIDs relieve pain and inflammation but should be used with caution because of possible gastrointestinal side effects.

Spondylitis occurs in 1.1 to 43 percent of patients with IBD (while IBD develops in 5 percent of patients with ankylosing spondylitis). Spondylitis often precedes IBD; their clinical courses are unrelated. Males are affected more frequently. Patients typically complain of stiffness in the back and/or buttocks in the morning or after rest. The stiffness and associated pain are often relieved by exercise. Gastrointestinal infection/inflammation is thought to play a role in exacerbation of spondylitis. Physical examination reveals limitation of spinal flexion and reduced chest expansion. Some patients may have peripheral arthritis, especially of the hips and/or shoulders. Iritis is a frequent complication. Radiographs of the back show the typical findings of ankylosing spondylitis and bilateral sacroiliitis. HLA-B27 is found in 53 to 75 percent of these patients. Treatment includes physical therapy, NSAIDs, glucocorticoids for the bowel disease, and sulfasalazine. NSAIDs should be used with caution lest they exacerbate the IBD. The axial disease progresses slowly in a manner akin to that of ankylosing spondylitis.

Asymptomatic sacroiliitis detected by radiography occurs in 4 to 25 percent of patients with IBD. By contrast, 52 percent of patients with IBD have abnormalities on technetium pyrophosphate bone scans of the sacroiliac joint. There is no increased frequency of HLA-B27 in these patients. This "disease" does not necessarily progress to spondylitis.

Other complications of chronic IBD include (1) finger clubbing (observed in 4 to 13 percent of patients with Crohn's disease, especially those with small-bowel involvement), which may regress after surgery; (2) development of amyloid, especially in association with Crohn's disease; and (3) osteoporosis resulting from inactivity, malabsorption, and/or treatment with glucocorticoids. Osteomalacia can result from malabsorption. In this setting, with acutely increased back pain, one should suspect compression fracture.

INTESTINAL BYPASS ARTHRITIS Intestinal bypass surgery was developed for the treatment of obesity in 1952; 11 years later arthritis was recognized as a postoperative complication. Polyarthralgia and sometimes arthritis occur weeks, even years, after surgery in 8 to 36 percent of patients. Tenosynovitis is common, with episodes sometimes lasting for days and even months; it tends to affect the knee, wrist, ankle, shoulder, and finger joints and cause pain in the neck and back. This syndrome occurs more often after jejunocolic than after jejunoileal surgery and more often in females than in males. There is often an associated urticarial, vesicular, pustular, macular, or nodular eruption. Raynaud's symptoms appear in one-third of patients. X-rays generally show no joint damage, except marginal erosions in patients with persistent arthritis. Synovial fluids generally have white blood cell counts of 500 to 27,000 cells/μL, mostly PMNs. Synovial biopsy specimens show chronic synovitis with lymphocytes but without lymphoid follicles. Tests for rheumatoid factors, antinuclear antibodies, and HLA-B27 are usually negative, while immune complexes (and cryoglobulins) are often present. They contain bacterial antigens, the corresponding antibodies, IgA secretory component, and various complement components. These observations suggest that the syndrome has the following pathogenesis: Bacteria proliferate in intestinal blind loops; bacterial antigens are absorbed; and antibodies to these antigens develop and combine with them to form immune complexes, which deposit in synovial tissue to cause arthritis. NSAIDs and glucocorticoids can relieve the joint symptoms, but more lasting results can be achieved by tetracycline therapy to decrease the bacterial load; even better is reanastomosis of the bowel or resection of the blind loop.

WHIPPLE'S DISEASE (INTESTINAL LIPODYSTROPHY) Whipple's disease is rare and occurs mostly in middle-aged Caucasian males, who develop arthritis, prolonged diarrhea, malabsorption, and weight loss. Up to 90 percent of patients with the disease develop arthritis, usually prior to other symptoms. Knees and ankles and, to a lesser extent, fingers, hips, shoulders, elbows, and wrists are involved. The arthritis is acute in onset, migratory, usually lasts just a few days, and is rarely chronic or a cause of permanent joint damage. Associated symptoms may include fever (54 percent), edema, serositis (pleurisy, pericarditis, endocarditis), pneumonia, hypotension, lymphadenopathy (54 percent), hyperpigmentation (54 percent), subcutaneous nodules, clubbing, and uveitis. Central nervous system involvement may develop (43 percent), with loss of memory, confusion, depression, headache, diplopia, and papilledema, and may be appreciated by abnormalities in magnetic resonance images of the brain. Laboratory abnormalities include anemia (75 percent), low serum levels of carotene (95 percent), and albumin (93 percent). The presence of HLA-B27 (8 to 30 percent) occurs in those patients with axial arthritis. Synovial fluids have been reported to contain 450 to 36,000 white blood cells per microliter (30 to 95 percent neutrophils) or a mild monocytosis. Joint x-rays rarely show erosions but may show a sacroiliitis in the occasional patients who have axial skeletal symptoms; abdominal computed tomographic scans may reveal lymphadenopathy. The lamina propria and/or foamy macrophages in small intestine contain PAS-staining bacterial remnants, presumably of *Tropheryma whippelii* or related bacteria. Diagnosis is often established by polymerase chain reaction (PCR) of the 165 ribosomal gene sequences of these bacteria. These inclusion-containing foamy macrophages also have been detected in the synovium, lymph nodes, and other tissues. The syndrome responds best to long-term therapy with trimethoprim-sulfamethoxazole. However, CNS relapse may develop, which has been treated with cefixime.

REACTIVE ARTHRITIS A Reiter's-like syndrome of arthritis can develop 2 to 3 weeks following diarrhea caused by *Shigella*, *Salmonella*, *Yersinia*, *Chlamydia trachomatis*, or *Campylobacter* organisms. → ***This condition is described in Chap. 317.***

BIBLIOGRAPHY

BRUCKLE W et al: Treatment of psoriatic arthritis with auranofin and gold sodium thiomalate. Clin Rheumatol 13:209, 1994

DOUGADOS M et al: Sulfasalazine in the treatment of spondylarthropathy. A randomized multicenter, double-blind, placebo-controlled study. Arthritis Rheum 38:618, 1995

ESPINOZA LR et al: Psoriatic arthritis: Clinical response and side effects to methotrexate therapy. J Rheumatol 19:872, 1992

GLADMAN DD: Natural history of psoriatic arthritis. Baillieres Clin Rheumatol 8:379, 1994

———, FAREWELL VT: The role of HLA antigens as indicators of disease progression in psoriatic arthritis. Multivariate relative risk model. Arthritis Rheum 38:845, 1995

——— et al: Clinical and radiological progression in psoriatic arthritis. J Rheumatol 17:809, 1990

GOUPILLE P et al: Treatment of psoriatic arthritis. Semin Arthritis Rheum 21:355, 1992

HELLIWELL P et al: A re-evaluation of the osteoarticular manifestations of psoriasis. Br J Rheumatol 30:339, 1991

KAHN MF, CHAMOT AM: SAPHO syndrome. Rheum Dis Clin North Am 18:225, 1992

LEIRISALO-REPO M, REPO H: Gut and spondyloarthropathies. Rheum Dis Clin North Am 18:23, 1992

MAHRLE G et al: Low-dose short-term cyclosporine versus etretinate in psoriasis: Improvement of skin, nail, and joint involvement. J Am Acad Dermatol 32:78, 1995

PANAYI GS: Immunology of psoriasis and psoriatic arthritis. Baillieres Clin Rheumatol 8:419, 1994

PORTER GG: Psoriatic arthritis. Plain radiology and other imaging techniques. Baillieres Clin Rheumatol 8:465, 1994

SNELLMAN E et al: Effect of heliotherapy on skin and joint symptoms in psoriasis. A 6-month follow-up study. Br J Dermatol 128:172, 1993

TROUGHTON PR, MORGAN AW: Laboratory findings and pathology of psoriatic arthritis. Baillieres Clin Rheumatol 8:439, 1994

VEALE D et al: Classification of clinical subsets in psoriatic arthritis. Br J Rheumatol 33:133, 1994

WHITING-O'KEEFE QE et al: Methotrexate and histologic hepatic abnormalities: A meta-analysis. Am J Med 90:711, 1991

326

Bruce C. Gilliland

RELAPSING POLYCHONDRITIS AND OTHER ARTHRITIDES

RELAPSING POLYCHONDRITIS

Relapsing polychondritis is an episodic and often progressive inflammatory disorder of unknown cause affecting predominantly the cartilage of the ears, nose, and tracheobronchial tree, as well as internal structures of the eyes and ears. Other manifestations include polyarthritis, vasculitis, cardiac abnormalities, skin lesions, and glomerulonephritis. It is most common between the ages of 40 to 60 years but may affect children and the elderly. Relapsing polychondritis is an uncommon disorder which has been found in all races. Both sexes are equally affected, and no familial tendency is apparent. Approximately 30 percent of patients with relapsing polychondritis will have another rheumatologic disorder, the most frequent being systemic vasculitis, followed by rheumatoid arthritis, systemic lupus erythematosus, or Sjögren's syndrome. A significantly higher frequency of HLA-DR4 has been found in patients with relapsing polychondritis than in normal individuals. A predominant subtype of HLA-DR4 was not found, as has been the experience in patients with rheumatoid arthritis who are HLA-DR4 positive.

PATHOLOGY AND PATHOPHYSIOLOGY The earliest abnormality of cartilage noted histologically is a focal or diffuse loss of basophilic staining indicating depletion of proteoglycan from the cartilage matrix. Inflammatory infiltrates are found adjacent to involved cartilage and consist predominantly of mononuclear cells and occasional plasma cells. In acute disease, polymorphonuclear white cells also may be present. Destruction of cartilage begins at the outer edges and advances centrally. There is lacunar breakdown and loss of chondrocytes. Degenerating cartilage is replaced by granulation tissue and later by fibrosis and focal areas of calcification. Small loci of cartilage regeneration may be present. Immunofluorescence studies have shown immunoglobulins and complement at sites of involvement. Fine granular material observed in the degenerating cartilage matrix by electron microscopy has been interpreted to be enzymes or immunoglobulins.

Immunologic mechanisms play a role in the pathogenesis of relapsing polychondritis. Immunoglobulin and complement deposits are found at sites of inflammation. In addition, antibodies to type II collagen and immune complexes are detected in the sera of some patients. The possibility that an immune response to type II collagen may be important in the pathogenesis is supported experimentally by the occurrence of auricular chondritis in rats immunized with type II collagen. Antibodies to type II collagen are found in the sera of these animals, and immune deposits are detected at sites of ear inflammation. Cell-mediated immunity also may be operative in causing tissue injury, since lymphocyte transformation can be demonstrated when lymphocytes of patients are exposed to cartilage extracts. Humoral and cellular immune responses to type IX and type XI collagen have been demonstrated in some patients.

Dissolution of cartilage matrix can be induced by the intravenous injection of crude papain, a proteolytic enzyme, into young rabbits, which results in collapse of their normally rigid ears within 4 h. Reconstitution of the matrix occurs in about 7 days. In relapsing polychondritis, loss of cartilage matrix also most likely results from action of proteolytic enzymes released from chondrocytes, polymorphonuclear white cells, and monocytes that have been activated by inflammatory mediators.

CLINICAL MANIFESTATIONS Auricular chondritis is the most frequent presenting manifestation of relapsing polychondritis in 40 percent of patients and eventually affects about 85 percent of patients (Table 326-1). Usually both ears are involved. Patients experience the sudden onset of pain, tenderness, and swelling of the cartilaginous portion of the ear. Earlobes are spared because they do not contain cartilage. The overlying skin has a beefy red or violaceous color. Prolonged or recurrent episodes result in a flabby or droopy ear. Swelling may close off the eustachian tube (causing otitis media) or the external auditory meatus, either of which can impair hearing. Inflammation of the internal auditory artery or its cochlear branch produces hearing loss, vertigo, ataxia, nausea, and vomiting. The cartilage of the nose becomes inflamed during the first or subsequent attacks. Approximately 50 percent of patients will eventually have nose involvement. Patients may experience nasal stuffiness, rhinorrhea, and epistaxis. The bridge of the nose becomes red, swollen, and tender and may collapse, producing a saddle deformity. In some patients, the saddle deformity develops insidiously without overt inflammation. Saddle nose is observed more frequently in younger patients, especially in women.

Arthritis is the presenting manifestation in relapsing polychondritis in approximately one-third of patients and may be present for several months before other features appear. Eventually, more than half the patients will have arthritis. The arthritis usually is asymmetric and oligo- or polyarticular, and involves both large and small peripheral joints. An episode of arthritis lasts from a few days to several weeks and resolves spontaneously without residual joint deformity. Attacks of arthritis may not be temporally related to other manifestations of relapsing polychondritis. The joints are warm, tender, and swollen. Joint fluid has been reported to be noninflammatory. In addition to peripheral joints, inflammation may involve the costochondral, sternomanubrial, and sternoclavicular cartilages. Destruction of these cartilages may result in a pectus excavatum deformity or even a flail anterior chest wall. Relapsing polychondritis may occur in patients with preexisting rheumatoid arthritis, Reiter's syndrome, psoriatic arthritis, or ankylosing spondylitis. Myelodysplastic syndrome has been reported in several patients with relapsing polychondritis.

Eye manifestations occur in more than half of patients and include conjunctivitis, episcleritis, scleritis, iritis, and keratitis. Ulceration and perforation of the cornea may occur and cause blindness. Other manifestations include eyelid and periorbital edema, proptosis, cataracts, optic neuritis, extraocular muscle palsies, retinal vasculitis, and retinal vein occlusion.

Table 326-1

Clinical Manifestations of Relapsing Polychondritis

Clinical Feature	Frequency, % Presenting	Frequency, % Cumulative
Auricular chondritis	40	85
Hearing loss	10	30
Nasal chondritis	25	55
Saddle nose deformity	20	30
Ocular deformities	20	50
Respiratory disease	25	50
Arthritis	35	50
Aortic regurgitation	—	5
Vasculitis	3	10

SOURCE: Modified from Isaak et al.

Laryngotracheal involvement occurs in approximately 50 percent of patients. Symptoms include hoarseness, a nonproductive cough, and tenderness over the larynx and proximal trachea. Mucosal edema, strictures, and/or collapse of laryngeal or tracheal cartilage may cause stridor and life-threatening airway obstruction necessitating tracheostomy. Collapse of cartilage in bronchi leads to pneumonia and, when extensive, to respiratory insufficiency.

Aortic regurgitation occurs in about 5 percent of patients and is due to progressive dilation of the aortic ring or to destruction of the valve cusps. Mitral and other heart valves are less often affected. Other cardiac manifestations include pericarditis, myocarditis, and conduction abnormalities. Aneurysms of the proximal, thoracic, or abdominal aorta may occur and occasionally rupture.

Systemic vasculitis may occur in association with relapsing polychondritis. Vasculitides include leukocytoclastic vasculitis, polyarteritis, temporal arteritis, and Takayasu's arteritis (see Chap. 319). Neurologic abnormalities usually occur as a result of underlying vasculitis, manifesting as seizures, strokes, ataxia, and peripheral and cranial nerve neuropathies. Cranial nerves VI and VII are most often involved. Approximately 25 percent of patients have skin lesions, none of which are characteristic for relapsing polychondritis. These include purpura, erythema nodosum, erythema multiforme, angioedema/urticaria, livedo reticularis, and panniculitis. Segmental necrotizing glomerulonephritis with crescent formation has been noted in some patients in the absence of systemic vasculitis.

The course of disease is highly variable, with episodes lasting from a few days to several weeks and then subsiding spontaneously. In other patients, the disease has a chronic, smoldering course. In one study, the 5-year estimated survival rate was 74 percent and the 10-year survival rate 55 percent. In contrast to earlier series, only about half the deaths could be attributed to relapsing polychondritis or complications of treatment. Pulmonary complications accounted for only 10 percent of all fatalities. In general, patients with more widespread disease have a worse prognosis.

LABORATORY FINDINGS Mild leukocytosis and normocytic, normochromic anemia are often present. The erythrocyte sedimentation rate is usually elevated. Rheumatoid factor and antinuclear antibody tests are occasionally positive in low titers. Antibodies to type II collagen are present in most patients, but they are not specific. Circulating immune complexes may be detected, especially in patients with early active disease. Elevated levels of gamma globulin may be present. Antineutrophil cytoplasmic antibodies (ANCA), either cytoplasmic (C-ANCA) or perinuclear (P-ANCA), are found in some patients with active disease. The upper and lower airways can be evaluated by imaging techniques such as linear tomography, laryngotracheography, and computed tomography, and by bronchoscopy. Bronchography is performed to demonstrate bronchial narrowing. Intrathoracic airway obstruction also can be evaluated by inspiratory-expiratory flow studies. The chest film may show narrowing of the main bronchi, widening of the ascending or descending aorta due to an aneurysm, and cardiomegaly when aortic insufficiency is present. Radiographs may show calcification at previous sites of cartilage damage involving ear, nose, larynx, or trachea.

DIAGNOSIS Diagnosis is based on recognition of the typical clinical features. Biopsies of the involved cartilage from the ear, nose, or respiratory tract will confirm the diagnosis but are only necessary when clinical features are not typical. Patients with Wegener's granulomatosis may have a saddle nose and pulmonary involvement but can be distinguished by the absence of auricular involvement and the presence of granulomatous lesions in the tracheobronchial tree. Patients with Cogan's syndrome have interstitial keratitis and vestibular and auditory abnormalities, but this syndrome does not involve the respiratory tract or ears. Reiter's syndrome may initially resemble relapsing polychondritis because of oligoarticular arthritis and eye involvement, but it is distinguished in time by the appearance of urethritis and typical mucocutaneous lesions and the absence of nose or ear cartilage involvement. Rheumatoid arthritis may initially suggest relapsing polychondritis because of arthritis and eye inflammation. The arthritis in rheumatoid arthritis, however, is erosive and symmetric. In addition, rheumatoid factor titers are usually high compared with those in relapsing polychondritis. Bacterial infection of the pinna may be mistaken for relapsing polychondritis but differs by usually involving only one ear, including the earlobe. Auricular cartilage also may be damaged by trauma or frostbite.

Relapsing polychondritis may develop in patients with a variety of autoimmune disorders, including systemic lupus erythematosus, rheumatoid arthritis, Sjögren's syndrome, and vasculitis. In most cases, these disorders antedate the appearance of polychondritis, usually by months or years. It is likely that these patients have an immunologic abnormality that predisposes them to development of this group of autoimmune disorders.

℞ TREATMENT

In patients with active chondritis or associated vasculitis, prednisone, 40 to 60 mg/d, is often effective in suppressing disease activity; it is tapered gradually once disease is controlled. In some patients, prednisone can be stopped, while in others low doses in the range of 10 to 15 mg/d are required for continued suppression of disease. Immunosuppressive drugs such as cyclophosphamide or azathioprine should be reserved for patients who fail to respond to prednisone or who require high doses for control of disease activity. Dapsone and cyclosporine have been reported to be beneficial in a few patients. Patients with significant ocular inflammation often require intraocular steroids as well as high doses of prednisone. Heart valve replacement or repair of an aortic aneurysm may be necessary. In patients with obstructive subglottic disease, tracheostomy is required. Stents may be necessary in patients with tracheobronchial collapse.

OTHER ARTHRITIDES

NEUROPATHIC JOINT DISEASE Neuropathic joint disease (Charcot's joint) is a severe form of osteoarthritis associated with loss of pain sensation, proprioception, or both. In addition, normal muscular reflexes that modulate joint movement are decreased. Without these protective mechanisms, joints are subjected to repeated trauma, resulting in progressive cartilage damage. The distribution of joint involvement depends on the underlying neurologic disorder (Table 326-2). In tabes dorsalis, knees, hips, and ankles are most commonly affected; in syringomyelia, the glenohumeral joint, elbow, and wrist; and in diabetes mellitus, the tarsal and tarsometatarsal joints. Resorption of metatarsals and phalanges is also seen in diabetic patients. In children, neuropathic joint disease is caused by congenital indifference to pain or meningomyelocele. Neuropathic joint disease is also observed in patients with amyloidosis and leprosy or following frequent repeated intraarticular glucocorticoid injections. The mechanism of injury in the latter situation is thought to be an analgesic effect of steroids leading to overuse of a previously damaged joint, which results in accelerated cartilage deterioration.

Neuropathic joint disease usually begins in a single joint and then progresses to involve other joints, depending on the underlying neurologic disorder. The involved joint progressively becomes enlarged from bony overgrowth and synovial effusion. Loose bodies may be palpated in the joint cavity. Joint instability, subluxation, and crepitus occur as the disease progresses. Charcot's joints may develop rapidly, and a totally disorganized joint with multiple bony fragments may evolve in a patient within weeks or months. The amount of pain experienced by the patient is less than would be anticipated based on the degree of joint involvement. Patients may experience sudden joint pain from intraarticular fractures of osteophytes or condyles. Initially, radiographs show early features of osteoarthritis followed subsequently by marked destructive and hypertrophic changes. Large, bizarre-shaped osteophytes and intraarticular bone fragments are observed. The radiographic findings of the diabetic Charcot's foot may be difficult to distinguish from those of osteomyelitis. Osteomyelitis is often suspected when the diabetic patient has an infected cutaneous ulcer on the foot. The Charcot's joint radiographically shows osteopenia, sharp cortical margins, and severe disruption and disorganization of the midtarsal and tarsometatarsal joints. In osteomyelitis, the bone margins are indistinct. The synovial fluid from a neuropathic joint is usually noninflammatory, may be bloody or xanthochromic, and may contain fragments of synovium, cartilage, and/or bone.

Table 326-2

Disorders Associated with Neuropathic Joint Disease

Diabetes mellitus	Amyloidosis
Tabes dorsalis	Leprosy
Meningomyelocele	Congenital indifference to pain
Syringomyelia	

℞ TREATMENT

The primary focus of treatment is to provide stabilization of the joint. Treatment of the underlying disorder, even if successful, usually does not alter the joint disease. Braces and splints are helpful. Their use requires close surveillance, since patients may be unable to appreciate pressure from a poorly adjusted brace. In the diabetic patient, early recognition and treatment of a Charcot's foot by prohibiting weight bearing of the foot for at least 8 weeks may possibly prevent severe disease from developing. Fusion of a very unstable joint may improve function, but nonunion is frequent, especially when immobilization of the joint is inadequate.

HYPERTROPHIC OSTEOARTHROPATHY AND CLUBBING Hypertrophic osteoarthropathy (HOA) is characterized by clubbing of digits and, in more advanced stages, by periosteal new bone formation and synovial effusions. HOA occurs in primary and familial forms and begins usually in childhood. The secondary form of HOA is associated with intrathoracic malignancies, suppurative lung disease, congenital heart disease, and a variety of other disorders and is more common in adults. Clubbing is almost always a feature of HOA but can occur as an isolated manifestation (Fig. 326-1). The presence of clubbing in isolation is generally considered to represent either an early stage or an element in the spectrum of HOA. The presence of only clubbing in a patient usually has the same clinical significance as HOA.

Pathology and Pathophysiology In HOA, the bone changes in the distal extremities begin as a low-grade inflammatory process in the periosteum followed by new bone formation. At this stage, a radiolucent area may be observed between the new periosteal bone and subjacent cortex. As the process progresses, multiple layers of new bone are deposited, which become contiguous with the cortex

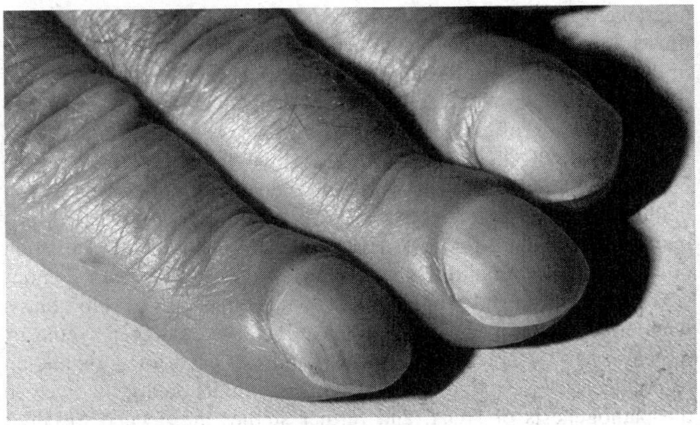

FIGURE 326-1 Clubbing of fingers. *(Reprinted from the Clinical Slide Collection on the Rheumatic Diseases, Copyright 1991, 1995. Used by permission of the American College of Rheumatology.)*

and result in cortical thickening. The outer portion of bone is laminated in appearance, with an irregular surface. Initially, the process of periosteal new bone formation involves the proximal and distal diaphyses of the tibia, fibula, radius, and ulna and, less frequently, the femur, humerus, metacarpals, metatarsals, and phalanges. Occasionally, scapulae, clavicula, ribs, and pelvic bones are also affected. In long-standing disease, these changes extend to involve metaphyses and musculotendinous insertions. The adjacent interosseous membranes may become ossified. The distribution of the bone manifestations is usually bilateral and symmetric. The soft tissue overlying the distal third of the arms and legs may be thickened. Mononuclear cell infiltration may be present in the adjacent soft tissue. Proliferation of connective tissue occurs in the nail bed and volar pad of digits, giving the distal phalanges a clubbed appearance. Small blood vessels in the clubbed digits are dilated and have thickened walls. In addition, the number of arteriovenous anastomoses is increased. The synovium of involved joints shows edema, varying degrees of synovial cell proliferation, thickening of the subsynovium, vascular congestion, vascular obliteration with thrombi, and small numbers of lymphocyte infiltrates.

Several theories have been suggested for the pathogenesis of HOA. Most have either been disproved or have not explained the development in all clinical disorders associated with HOA. Previously proposed neurogenic and humoral theories are no longer considered likely explanations for HOA. The neurogenic theory was based on the observation that vagotomy resulted in symptomatic improvement in a small number of patients with lung tumors and HOA. It was postulated that vagal stimuli from the tumor site led via a neural reflex to efferent nerve impulses to the distal extremities, resulting in HOA. This theory, however, did not explain HOA in conditions where vagal stimulation did not occur, as in cyanotic congenital heart disease or arterial aneurysms. The humoral theory postulated that soluble substances that normally are inactivated or removed during passage through the lung reached the systemic circulation in an active form and stimulated the changes of HOA. Substances proposed included prostaglandins, ferritin, bradykinin, estrogen, and growth hormone. These substances seemed unlikely candidates, since their blood levels in HOA patients overlapped those in individuals without HOA. Furthermore, these substances did not explain the development of localized HOA associated with arterial aneurysms or infected arterial grafts.

Recent studies have suggested a role for platelets in the development of HOA. It has been observed that megakaryocytes and large platelet particles, present in venous circulation, were fragmented in their passage through normal lung. In patients with cyanotic congenital heart disease and in other disorders associated with right-to-left shunts, these large platelet particles may bypass the lung and reach the distal extremities, where they can interact with endothelial cells. Platelet clumps have been demonstrated to form on an infected heart valve in bacterial endocarditis, in the wall of arterial aneurysms, and on infected arterial grafts. These platelet particles may also reach the distal extremities and interact with endothelial cells. Platelet-endothelial activation in the distal portion of extremities would then result in the release of platelet-derived growth factor (PDGF) and other factors leading to the proliferation of connective tissue and periosteum. Stimulation of fibroblasts by PDGF and transforming growth factor β (TGFβ) results in cell growth and collagen synthesis. Elevated plasma levels of von Willebrand factor antigen have been found in patients with both primary and secondary forms of HOA indicating endothelial activation or damage. Abnormalities of collagen synthesis have been demonstrated in the involved skin of patients with primary HOA. Fibroblasts from affected skin were shown to have increased collagen synthesis, increased α1 (I) procollagen mRNA, and evidence for upregulation of collagen transcription. Other factors are undoubtedly involved in the pathogenesis of HOA, and further studies are needed to better understand this disorder.

Clinical Manifestations Primary HOA, also referred to as *pachydermoperiostitis* or *Touraine-Solente-Golé syndrome*, usually begins insidiously at puberty. In a smaller number of patients, the onset is in the first year of life. The disorder is inherited as an autosomal dominant trait with variable expression and is nine times more common in boys than in girls. Approximately one-third of patients have a family history of primary HOA.

Primary HOA is characterized by clubbing, periostosis, and unusual skin features. A small number of patients with this syndrome do not express clubbing. The skin changes and periostitis are prominent features of this syndrome. The skin becomes thickened and coarse. Deep nasolabial folds develop, and the forehead may become furrowed. Patients may have heavy-appearing eyelids and ptosis. The skin is often greasy, and there may be excessive sweating of the hands and feet. Patients also may experience seborrhea and folliculitis. In a few patients, the skin over the scalp becomes very thick and corrugated, a feature that has been descriptively termed *cutis verticis gyrata*. The distal extremities, particularly the legs, become thickened owing to proliferation of new bone and soft tissue; when the process is extensive, the ankles resemble elephant feet. The periostosis is usually not painful, as it may be in secondary HOA. Clubbing of the fingers may be extensive, producing large, bulbous deformities and clumsiness. Clubbing also affects the toes. Patients may experience articular and periarticular pain, especially in the ankles and knees, and joint motion may be mildly restricted owing to periarticular bone overgrowth. Noninflammatory effusions occur in the wrists, knees, and ankles. Synovial hypertrophy is not found. Associated abnormalities observed in patients with primary HOA include hypertrophic gastropathy, bone marrow failure, female escutcheon, and cranial suture defects. In patients with primary HOA, the symptoms disappear when adulthood is reached.

HOA secondary to an underlying disease occurs more frequently than primary HOA. It accompanies a variety of disorders and may precede clinical features of the associated disorder by months. Clubbing is more frequent than the full syndrome of HOA in patients with associated illnesses. Because clubbing evolves over months and is usually asymptomatic, it is often recognized first by the physician and not the patient. Patients may experience a burning sensation in their fingertips. Clubbing is characterized by widening of the fingertips, enlargement of the distal volar pad, convexity of the nail contour, and the loss of the normal 15° angle between the proximal nail and cuticle. The thickness of the digit at the base of the nail is greater than the thickness at the distal interphalangeal joint. The base of the nail feels spongy when compressed, and the nail can be easily rocked on its bed. Marked periungual erythema is usually present. When clubbing is advanced, the finger may have a drumstick appearance. Periosteal involvement in the distal extremities may produce a burning or deep-seated aching pain. The pain can be quite incapacitating and is aggravated by dependency and relieved by elevation of the affected limbs. The overlying soft tissue may be swollen, and the skin slightly erythematous. Pressure applied over the distal forearms and legs may be quite painful.

Patients may also experience joint pain, most often in the ankles, wrists, and knees. Joint effusions may be present; usually they are small and noninflammatory. The small joints of the hands are rarely affected. Severe joint or bone pain may be the presenting symptom of an underlying lung malignancy and may precede the appearance of clubbing. In addition, the progression of HOA tends to be more rapid when associated with malignancies, most notably bronchogenic carcinoma. Unlike primary HOA, excessive sweating and oiliness of the skin and thickening of the facial skin are uncommon in secondary HOA.

HOA occurs in 5 to 10 percent of patients with intrathoracic malignancies, the most common being bronchogenic carcinoma and pleural tumors (Table 326-3). Lung metastases infrequently cause HOA. HOA is also seen in patients with intrathoracic infections, including lung abscesses, empyema, bronchiectasis, chronic obstructive lung disease, and, uncommonly, pulmonary tuberculosis. HOA also may accompany chronic interstitial pneumonitis, sarcoidosis, and cystic fibrosis. In the latter, clubbing is more common than the full syndrome of HOA. Other causes of clubbing include congenital heart

Table 326-3

Disorders Associated with Hypertrophic Osteoarthropathy

Pulmonary	
	Bronchogenic carcinoma and other neoplasms
	Lung abscesses, empyema, bronchiectasis
	Chronic interstitial pneumonitis
	Cystic fibrosis
	Chronic obstructive lung disease
	Sarcoidosis
Gastrointestinal	
	Inflammatory bowel disease
	Sprue
	Neoplasms: esophagus, liver, bowel
Cardiovascular	
	Cyanotic congenital heart disease
	Subacute bacterial endocarditis
	Infected arterial grafts*
	Aortic aneurysm*
	Aneurysm of major extremity artery*
	Patent ductus arteriosus
	Arteriovenous fistula of major extremity vessel*
Thyroid (thyroid acropachy)	
	Hyperthyroidism (Graves' disease)

* Unilateral involvement

disease with right-to-left shunts, bacterial endocarditis, Crohn's disease, ulcerative colitis, sprue, and neoplasms of the esophagus, liver, and small and large bowel. In patients with congenital heart disease with right-to-left shunts, clubbing alone occurs more often than the full syndrome of HOA.

Unilateral clubbing has been found in association with aneurysms of the aorta or the subclavian or innominate artery and with arteriovenous fistulas of brachial vessels. Clubbing of the toes but not fingers has been associated with an infected abdominal aortic aneurysm and patent ductus arteriosus. Clubbing of a single digit may follow trauma and has been reported in tophaceous gout and sarcoidosis. While clubbing occurs more commonly than the full syndrome in most diseases, periostosis in the absence of clubbing has been observed in the affected limb of patients with infected arterial grafts.

Hyperthyroidism (Graves' disease), treated or untreated, occasionally is associated with clubbing and periostitis of the bones of the hands and feet. This condition is referred to as *thyroid acropachy*. Periostitis is asymptomatic and occurs in the midshaft and diaphyseal portion of the metacarpal and phalangeal bones. The long bones of the extremities are seldom affected. Elevated levels of long-acting thyroid stimulator (LATS) are found in the serum of these patients.

Laboratory Findings The laboratory abnormalities reflect the underlying disorder. The synovial fluid of involved joints has fewer than 500 white cells per microliter, and the cells are predominantly mononuclear. Radiographs show a faint radiolucent line beneath the new periosteal bone along the shaft of long bones at their distal end. These changes are observed most frequently at the ankles, wrists, and knees. The ends of the distal phalanges may show osseous resorption. Radionuclide studies show pericortical linear uptake along the cortical margins of long bones that may be present before any radiographic changes.

Rx TREATMENT

The treatment of hypertrophic osteoarthropathy is to identify the associated disorder and treat it appropriately. The symptoms and signs of hypertrophic osteoarthropathy may disappear completely with removal or effective chemotherapy of a tumor or with antibiotic therapy and drainage of a chronic pulmonary infection. Vagotomy or percutaneous block of the vagus nerve leads to symptomatic relief in some patients. Aspirin, other nonsteroidal anti-inflammatory drugs, or analgesics may help control symptoms of hypertrophic osteoarthropathy.

FIBROMYALGIA Fibromyalgia is a commonly encountered disorder characterized by widespread musculoskeletal pain, stiffness, paresthesia, nonrestorative sleep, and easy fatigability along with multiple tender points which are widely and symmetrically distributed. Fibromyalgia affects predominantly women. This disorder is found in most countries, in most ethnic groups, and in all types of climates. The prevalence of fibromyalgia in the general population of a community in the United States using the 1990 American College of Rheumatology classification criteria was reported recently to be 3.4 percent in women and 0.5 percent in men. Contrary to some previous reports, fibromyalgia was not found to be present mainly in young women but, rather, to be most prevalent in women aged 50 and older. The prevalence increased with age, being 7.4 percent in women between the ages of 70 and 79 years. Although not common, fibromyalgia also occurs in children. The reported prevalence of fibromyalgia in some rheumatology clinics has been as high as 20 percent. Several causative mechanisms for fibromyalgia have been postulated. Disturbed sleep has been implicated as a factor in the pathogenesis. Nonrestorative sleep or awakening unrefreshed has been observed in most patients with fibromyalgia. Sleep electroencephalographic studies in patients with fibromyalgia have shown disruption of normal stage 4 sleep [non–rapid eye movement (NREM) sleep] by many repeated alpha-wave intrusions. The idea that stage 4 sleep deprivation has a role in causing this disorder was supported by the observation that symptoms of fibromyalgia developed in normal subjects whose stage 4 sleep was disrupted artificially by induced alpha-wave intrusions. This sleep disturbance, however, has been demonstrated in healthy individuals, in emotionally distressed individuals, and in patients with sleep apnea, fever, osteoarthritis, or rheumatoid arthritis. Low levels of serotonin metabolites have been reported in the cerebrospinal fluid of patients with fibromyalgia, suggesting that a deficiency of serotonin, a neurotransmitter that regulates pain and NREM sleep, might also be involved in the pathogenesis of fibromyalgia. Drugs that affect serotonin metabolism have not had a dramatic effect on fibromyalgia, however. Since patients experience pain from muscle and musculotendinous sites, many studies have been done to examine muscle, both structurally and physiologically. Inflammation or diagnostic muscle abnormalities have not been found. Evidence indicates deconditioning of muscles, and patients experience a greater degree of postexertional pain than do unaffected persons. Fibromyalgia patients as a group have been reported by some investigators to have lower levels of somatomedin C than normal individuals. Since somatomedin C is the major mediator of the anabolic function of growth hormone and is important for muscle repair and strength, low levels of somatomedin C therefore might retard the healing process in muscles of fibromyalgia patients and account for the extended periods of pain following exertion. The low levels of somatomedin C in these patients may result from lack of exercise or a disturbance in stage 4 sleep, both of which stimulate production of growth hormone. The observation of low somatomedin C levels therefore may indicate a mechanism connecting sleep abnormality and muscle pain. The level of the neurotransmitter substance P has been reported to be increased in the cerebrospinal fluid of fibromyalgia patients and may play a role in spreading muscle pain. Many patients with fibromyalgia have psychological abnormalities; there has been disagreement as to whether some of these abnormalities represent reactions to the chronic pain or whether the symptoms of fibromyalgia are a reflection of psychiatric disturbance. Many patients fit a psychiatric diagnosis, the most common being depression, anxiety, somatization, and hypochondriases. Studies have also shown a high prevalence of sexual and physical abuse and eating disorders. However, fibromyalgia also occurs in patients without significant psychiatric problems. Patients with fibromyalgia may have a lower pain threshold than usual, although not all investigators in the field agree on this point. A better understanding of fibromyalgia awaits further studies.

Symptoms are generalized aching and stiffness of the trunk, hip, and shoulder girdles. Other patients complain of generalized muscle aching and weakness. Patients may complain of low back pain, which may radiate into the buttocks and legs. Others complain of pain and tightness in the neck and across the upper posterior shoulders. Patients complain of muscle pain after even mild exertion. Some degree of pain is always present. The pain has been described as a burning or gnawing pain or as soreness, stiffness, or aching. While pain may begin in one region, such as the shoulders, neck, or lower back, it eventually becomes widespread. Patients may complain of joint pain and perceive that their joints are swollen; however, joint examination yields normal findings. Stiffness is usually present on arising in the morning; usually it improves during the day, but in some patients it lasts all day. Patients may complain of numbness of their hands and feet. They also may feel colder overall than others in the home, and some may experience Raynaud's-like phenomena or actual Raynaud's phenomenon. Patients complain of feeling fatigued and exhausted and wake up tired. They also awaken frequently at night and have trouble falling back to sleep. Symptoms are made worse by stress or anxiety, cold, damp weather, and overexertion. Patients often feel better during warmer weather and vacations.

The characteristic feature on physical examination is the demonstration of specific tender points, which are exclusively more tender or painful than adjacent areas. The American College of Rheumatology (ACR) Criteria for Fibromyalgia defines 18 tender points (Fig. 326-2). These points of tenderness are remarkably constant in location. Approximately 4 kg of force (4 kg·f/cm^2) should be used in digital palpation of these tender points. Some workers recommend that the tender site be palpated using a rolling motion, which may be more effective in eliciting the tenderness. The tender sites can also be examined using a dolorimeter, which is a spring-loaded pressure gauge. Digital palpation appears to be as effective and accurate for the diagnosis of fibromyalgia as dolorimetry. The amount of pressure applied by the examiner introduces variability in the interpretation, however. If too much pressure is applied, the pain will be produced even in normal subjects. Likewise, tenderness will not be appreciated if too little pressure is applied or the

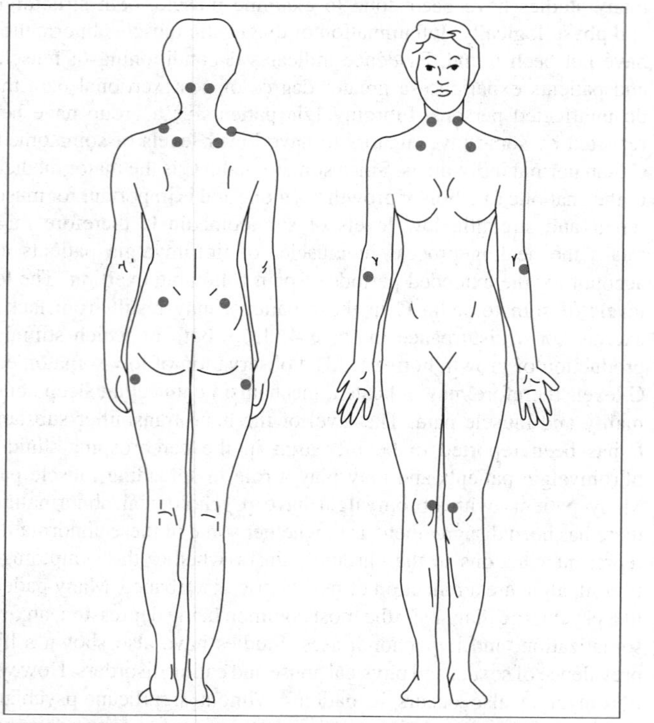

FIGURE 326-2 Tender points in fibromyalgia. Suboccipital muscle insertion at base of skull; anterior aspect of intertransverse process spaces at C5–7; midpoint of upper border of trapezius muscle; above scapular spine near medial border of scapula; second costochondral junction; lateral epicondyle; upper outer quadrant of buttocks; posterior aspect of trochanteric prominence; medial fat pad of knee (all bilateral). *(From the brochure "Fibromyalgia," Arthritis Information, Advise and Guidance, Disease Series. Used by permission of the Arthritis Foundation.)*

site is missed on palpation. Some investigators have quantitated their response, but the number of tender points sites is more diagnostic. Some patients are tender all over and not just at the specific tender point sites. These patients are still more tender over the specific tender point sites, however. Sites where there usually is no tenderness and which can be used as controls are the dorsum of the third digit between the proximal interphalangeal and distal interphalangeal joints, the medial third of the clavicle, the medial malleolus, and the forehead. If tenderness at these sites is also present, the diagnosis of fibromyalgia should be questioned, and possible psychiatric disorders investigated. Whether such patients can be diagnosed as also having fibromyalgia is debatable.

Skinfold tenderness may be present, particularly over the upper scapular region. Subcutaneous nodules may be felt at sites of tenderness. Nodules in similar locations are present in normal persons but are not tender.

Fibromyalgia may be triggered by emotional stress, medical illness, surgery, hypothyroidism, and trauma. It has appeared in some patients with human immunodeficiency virus (HIV) infection, parvovirus B19 infection, or Lyme disease. In the latter situation, fibromyalgia persisted despite adequate antibiotic treatment for Lyme disease. Disorders commonly associated with fibromyalgia include irritable bowel syndrome, irritable bladder, headaches (including migraine headaches), dysmenorrhea, premenstrual syndrome, restless legs syndrome, temporomandibular joint pain, and sicca syndrome.

The course of fibromyalgia is variable. Symptoms wax and wane in some patients, while in others pain and fatigue are persistent regardless of therapy. Studies from tertiary medical centers indicate a poor prognosis for most patients. The prognosis may be better in community-treated patients. In a community-based study reported after 2 years of treatment, 24 percent of patients were in remission, and 47 percent no longer fulfilled the ACR criteria for fibromyalgia.

Fibromyalgia is diagnosed by a history of widespread pain and the demonstration of at least 11 of the 18 tender point sites on digital palpation (Fig. 326-2). The ACR criteria are useful for standardizing the diagnosis; however, not all patients with fibromyalgia meet these criteria (Table 326-4). Some patients have fewer tender sites and more regional pain and may be considered to have probable fibromyalgia.

Table 326-4

The American College of Rheumatology 1990 Criteria for the Classification of Fibromyalgia*

A. History of widespread pain. Pain is considered widespread when all of the following are present:
   1. Pain in the left side of the body
   2. Pain in the right side of the body
   3. Pain above the waist
   4. Pain below the waist
   5. Axial skeletal pain (cervical spine or anterior chest or thoracic spine or low back)

B. Pain on digital palpation in at least 11 of the following 18 tender point sites (see Fig. 326-2):
   1. Occiput: bilateral, at the suboccipital muscle insertion
   2. Low cervical: bilateral, at the anterior aspect of the intertransverse spaces at C5–7
   3. Trapezius: bilateral, at the midpoint of the upper border
   4. Supraspinatus: bilateral, at the origin, above the scapular spine near the medial border
   5. Second rib: bilateral, at the second costochondral junction, just lateral to the junction on the upper surface
   6. Lateral epicondyle: bilateral, 2 cm distal to the epicondyle
   7. Gluteal: bilateral, in the upper outer quadrant of the buttock in the anterior fold of muscle
   8. Greater trochanter: bilateral, posterior to the trochanteric prominence
   9. Knee: bilateral, at the medial fat pad proximal to the joint line

Digital palpation should be performed with an approximate force of 4 kg. For a tender point to be considered positive, the subject must state that the palpation was painful. "Tender" is not to be considered painful.

* For purposes of classification, patients will be said to have fibromyalgia if both criteria are satisfied. Widespread pain must have been present for at least three months. The presence of a second clinical disorder does not exclude the diagnosis of fibromyalgia.

SOURCE: Modified from F Wolfe et al: Arthritis Rheum 33:171, 1990.

Results of joint and muscle examinations are normal in fibromyalgia patients, and there are no laboratory abnormalities. Fibromyalgia may occur in patients with rheumatoid arthritis, other connective tissue diseases, or other medical illness. A distinction is no longer made between primary and secondary fibromyalgia (concomitant with other disease), as the signs and symptoms are similar. Fibromyalgia and chronic fatigue syndrome have many similarities (see Chap. 384). Both are associated with fatigue, abnormal sleep, musculoskeletal pain, and psychiatric conditions such as less severe forms of depression and anxiety. Patients with chronic fatigue syndrome, however, are more likely to have symptoms suggesting a viral illness. These include mild fever, sore throat, and pain in the axillary and anterior and posterior cervical lymph nodes. The onset of chronic fatigue syndrome is usually sudden; patients are usually able to date the onset. Patients also have impaired memory and concentration. While many patients with chronic fatigue syndrome have tender points, the diagnosis does not require their presence. Polymyalgia rheumatica is distinguished from fibromyalgia in an elderly patient by the presence of more proximal muscle stiffness and pain and an elevated erythrocyte sedimentation rate. Patients should be evaluated for hypothyroidism, which may have symptoms similar to fibromyalgia or may accompany fibromyalgia.

The diagnosis of fibromyalgia has taken on a more complex significance in regard to labor and industry issues. This has become a significant issue since it has been reported that 10 to 25 percent of patients are not able to work in any capacity, while others require modification of their work. Disability evaluation in fibromyalgia is controversial. The diagnosis of fibromyalgia is not accepted by all. It is hard to evaluate patients' perceptions of their inability to function. The determination of tender points can also be subjective, on the part of both the physician and the patient, particularly when issues of compensation are pending. Patients also encounter difficulty in having their illness recognized as a disability. Physicians have been placed in the inappropriate role of assessing the patient's disability. Physicians are not in a position to quantitate disability at the workplace; that is better done by a work evaluation specialist. Better instruments are clearly needed for measuring disability, particularly in patients with fibromyalgia.

Patients should be informed that they have a condition that is not crippling, deforming, or degenerative, and that treatment is available. Salicylates or other nonsteroidal anti-inflammatory drugs only partially improve symptoms. Glucocorticoids have been of little benefit and should not be used in these patients. Opiate analgesics should be avoided. Local measures such as heat, massage, injection of tender sites with steroids or lidocaine, and acupuncture provide only temporary relief of symptoms. Other therapies that may help to varying degrees including biofeedback, hypnotherapy, and stress management and relaxation response training. The use of tricyclics such as amitriptyline (10 to 25 mg) and doxepin (10 to 25 mg) or a pharmacologically similar drug, cyclobenzaprine (10 to 20 mg), 1 to 2 h before bedtime will give the patient restorative sleep, resulting in clinical improvement. Higher doses of these medications may be necessary. Depression and anxiety should be treated with appropriate drugs and, when indicated, with psychiatric counseling. Alprazolam can be used for anxiety, while trazodone, sertraline, or fluoxetine can be used as antidepressants. Patients also may benefit by regular aerobic exercises. Exercise should be of a low-impact type and begun at a low level. Eventually, the patient should be exercising 20 to 30 min 3 to 4 days a week. Regular stretching exercises are also very important. Life stresses should be identified and discussed with the patient, and the patient should be provided with help on how to cope with these stresses. Patients may benefit from a multidisciplinary team approach involving a mental health professional, a physical therapist, and a physical medicine and rehabilitation specialist. Group therapy may be beneficial. Patients should be well educated about their disorder and taught the importance of self help. There are patient support groups in many communities. While treatment of fibromyalgia is effective in some patients, others continue to have chronic disease, which is relieved only partially if at all.

MYOFASCIAL PAIN SYNDROME Myofascial pain syndrome is characterized by localized musculoskeletal pain and tenderness in association with trigger points. The pain is deep and aching and may be accompanied by a burning sensation. Myofascial pain may follow trauma, overuse, or prolonged static contraction of a muscle or muscle group, which may occur when reading or writing at a desk or working at a computer. In addition, this syndrome may be associated with underlying osteoarthritis of the neck or low back. Trigger points are a diagnostic feature of this syndrome. Pain is referred from trigger points to defined areas distant from the original tender points. Palpation of the trigger point reproduces or accentuates the pain. The trigger points are usually located in the center of a muscle belly, but they can occur at other sites, such as costosternal junctions, the xyphoid process, ligamentous and tendinous insertions, fascia, and fatty areas. Trigger point sites in muscle have been described as feeling indurated and taut, and palpation may cause the muscle to twitch. These findings, however, have been shown not to be unique for myofascial pain syndrome, since in a controlled study they were also present in fibromyalgia patients and normal subjects. Myofascial pain most often involves the posterior neck, low back, shoulders, and chest. Chronic pain in the muscles of the posterior neck may involve referral of pain from the trigger point in the erector neck muscle or upper trapezius to the head, leading to persistent headaches which may last for days. Trigger points in the paraspinal muscles of the low back may refer pain to the buttock. Pain may be referred down the leg from a trigger point in the gluteus medius and can mimic sciatica. A trigger point in the infraspinatus muscle may produce local and referred pain over the lateral deltoid and down the outside of the arm into the hand. Injection of a local anesthetic such as 1% lidocaine into the trigger point site often results in pain relief. Another useful technique is first to spray from the trigger point toward the area of referred pain with an agent such as ethyl chloride and then to stretch the muscle. This maneuver may need to be repeated several times. Massage and application of ultrasound to the affected area may also be beneficial. Patients should be instructed in methods to prevent muscle stresses related to work and recreation. Posture and resting positions are important in preventing muscle tension. The prognosis in most patients is good. In some patients, myofascial pain syndrome may evolve into fibromyalgia. Patients at risk for developing fibromyalgia are thought to be those with anxiety, depression, nonrestorative sleep, and fatigue.

PSYCHOGENIC RHEUMATISM Patients may experience severe joint pain involving a few to several joints without physical findings of arthritis. These patients are often convinced that they have rheumatoid arthritis, systemic lupus erythematosus, or another connective tissue disease. This disorder is recognized by the inconsistencies, exaggerations, and emotional lability of the patient during the history and physical examination. Results of laboratory studies are normal. Organic disease needs to be excluded, which necessitates seeing the patient at regular intervals. This condition also needs to be distinguished from fibromyalgia. Anti-inflammatory or other drugs are not helpful.

REFLEX SYMPATHETIC DYSTROPHY SYNDROME The reflex sympathetic dystrophy syndrome (RSDS) is characterized by pain and swelling, usually of a distal extremity, accompanied by vasomotor instability, trophic skin changes, and the rapid development of bony demineralization. RSDS occasionally involves an isolated site such as a knee, hip, or one or two digits of a foot or hand. The contralateral side is affected clinically in approximately 25 percent of patients and may be involved in virtually all patients with RSOS, as shown by scintigraphic studies. A precipitating event can be identified in at least two-thirds of cases. These events include trauma, such as fractures and crush injuries; myocardial infarction; strokes; peripheral nerve injury; and use of certain drugs, including barbiturates, antituberculous drugs, and, more recently, cyclosporine administered to patients undergoing renal transplantation. The pathogenesis of RSDS is poorly understood and is thought to involve abnormal activity of the sympathetic nervous system following a precipitating event.

RSDS evolves through three clinical phases. The first phase is characterized by an intense burning pain and swelling of a distal extremity. The involved extremity is warm, edematous, and very tender, especially around joints. Sweating and hair growth are increased. Light touch causes pain, which may continue after the stimulus is removed. Passive or active motion of joints is very painful, and the joints are stiff. In the first phase, especially when both sides are involved, the clinical findings may suggest early rheumatoid arthritis. Redness and swelling over a distal extremity such as an ankle or wrist may also mimic inflammatory arthritis, or even an infectious arthritis. In 3 to 6 months, the skin gradually becomes thin, shiny, and cool. This is the second phase of the disease. The clinical features of the first and second phases often overlap. In another 3 to 6 months (third phase), the skin becomes atrophic and dry, and irreversible flexion contractures, palmar fibromatosis, and Dupuytren's contractures develop, resulting in a claw-like hand deformity. Similar changes occur in the feet. When RSDS occurs in the upper extremity, motion of the shoulder on the affected side may be painful and restricted, a condition referred to as *shoulder-hand syndrome* (see "Adhesive Capsulitis," below). → ***Reflex sympathetic dystrophy syndrome, including its treatment, is covered in greater detail in Chap. 371.***

TIETZE'S SYNDROME AND COSTOCHONDRITIS Tietze's syndrome is manifested by painful swelling of one or more costochondral articulations. The age of onset is usually before 40, and both sexes are affected equally. In most patients only one joint is involved, usually the second or third costochondral joint. The onset of anterior chest pain may be sudden or gradual. The pain may radiate to the arms or shoulder and is aggravated by sneezing, coughing, deep inspirations, or twisting motions of the chest. The term *costochondritis* is often used interchangeably with *Tietze's syndrome*, but some workers restrict the former term to pain of the costochondral articulations without swelling. Costochondritis is observed in patients over age 40, tends to affect the third, fourth, and fifth costochondral joints, and occurs more often in women. Both syndromes may mimic cardiac or upper abdominal causes of pain. Rheumatoid arthritis, ankylosing spondylitis, and Reiter's syndrome may involve costochondral joints but are distinguished easily by their other clinical features. Other skeletal causes of anterior chest wall pain are xiphoidalgia and the slipping rib syndrome, which usually involves the tenth rib. Malignancies such as breast cancer, prostate cancer, plasma cell cytoma, and sarcoma can invade the ribs, thoracic spine, or chest wall and produce symptoms suggesting Tietze's syndrome. They should be easily distinguishable by radiographs and biopsy. Analgesics, anti-inflammatory drugs, and local steroid injections usually relieve symptoms.

MUSCULOSKELETAL DISORDERS ASSOCIATED WITH HYPERLIPIDEMIA Musculoskeletal manifestations may be the first indication of a hereditary disorder of lipoprotein metabolism. Patients with type II hyperlipoproteinemia may have recurrent migratory polyarthritis involving knees and other large peripheral joints and, to a lesser degree, peripheral small joints. In a few patients, the arthritis is monarticular. Fever may accompany the arthritis. Pain ranges from moderate to very severe to incapacitating. The involved joints can be warm, erythematous, swollen, and tender. Arthritis usually has a sudden onset, lasts from a few days to 2 weeks, and does not cause joint damage. Several attacks occur a year. Synovial fluid from involved joints is not inflammatory and contains few white cells and no crystals. Joint involvement may actually represent inflammatory periarthritis or peritendinitis and not intraarticular disease. The recurrent, transient nature of the arthritis may suggest rheumatic fever, especially since patients with lipoproteinemia have an elevated erythrocyte sedimentation rate, a falsely elevated antistreptolysin O titer, and, in some cases, aortic valvular disease secondary to atherosclerosis. Patients heterozygous for type II hyperlipoproteinemia may also experience Achilles tendinitis, which can be very painful. Attacks of tendinitis come on gradually and last only a few days. Fever is not present. Patients may be asymptomatic between attacks. During an attack the Achilles tendon is warm, erythematous, swollen, and tender to palpation. Achilles tendinitis and other joint manifestations often precede the appearance of xanthomas and may be the first clinical indication of hyperlipoproteinemia. Patients with type II hyperlipoproteinemia also have tendinous xanthomas in the Achilles, patellar, and extensor tendons of the hands and feet. Xanthomas have also been reported in the peroneal tendon, the plantar aponeurosis, and the periosteum overlying the distal tibia. These xanthomas are located within tendon fibers. They appear in childhood in homozygous patients and after the age of 30 in heterozygous patients. Tuberous xanthomas appear only in patients homozygous for type II hyperlipoproteinemia. They are soft subcutaneous masses located over the extensor surfaces of the elbows, knees, and hands, as well as on the buttocks. Patients with type IV hyperlipoproteinemia also may have a mild inflammatory arthritis affecting large and small peripheral joints, usually in an asymmetric pattern with only a few joints involved at a time. The onset of arthritis is usually in middle age. Arthritis may be persistent or recurrent with episodes lasting a few days to weeks. Joint pain is severe in some patients. Patients may experience morning stiffness. Joint tenderness and periarticular hyperesthesia may also be present. Joint fluid is noninflammatory and without crystals. Radiographs may show juxtaarticular osteopenia and cystic lesions. Large bone cysts have been noted in a few patients. The pathogenesis of arthritis in both types of hyperlipoproteinemia is not well understood. Salicylates, other nonsteroidal anti-inflammatory drugs (NSAIDs), or analgesics usually provide relief of symptoms. Xanthomas and bone cysts are also observed in other hyperlipoproteinemias. Tendinous and tuberous xanthomas are seen in type III disorder. Also in type III disorder, lipids are deposited in the palms to form plane xanthomas. Eruptive xanthomas are found over the knees, shoulders, back, and buttocks in types I, IV, and V disorders. Large cystic lesions in both proximal femurs were reported in a patient with type V disorder.

ARTHROPATHY OF ACROMEGALY Acromegaly is the result of excessive production of growth hormone by an adenoma in the anterior pituitary gland (see Chap. 328). Middle-aged persons are most often affected. The excessive secretion of growth hormone along with insulin-like growth factor I stimulates proliferation of cartilage, periarticular connective tissue, and bone, resulting in several musculoskeletal abnormalities, including osteoarthritis, back pain, muscle weakness, and carpal tunnel syndrome.

An arthropathy resembling osteoarthritis is a common feature, affecting most often the knees, shoulders, hips, and hands. Single or multiple joints may be affected. The overgrowth of cartilage initially produces widening of the joint space. The newly synthesized cartilage is not developed in an organized manner, making it susceptible to fissuring, ulceration, and destruction. Ligamental laxity of the joint resulting from the growth of connective tissue also contributes to the development of osteoarthritis. With breakdown and loss of cartilage, the joint space narrows, and subchondral sclerosis and osteophytes appear on radiographs. Joint examination reveals marked crepitus and hypermobility. Joint fluid is noninflammatory. Calcium pyrophosphate dehydrate crystals are found in the cartilage in some cases of acromegaly arthropathy and, when shed into the joint, can produce attacks of pseudogout. Chondrocalcinosis may also be observed radiographically. Approximately half of the patients with acromegaly experience back pain, which is predominantly lumbosacral. Hypermobility of the spine may be a contributing factor in back pain. Radiograph of the spine shows normal or increased intervertebral disk spaces, hypertrophic anterior osteophytes, and ligamental calcification. These changes are similar to those observed in patients with diffuse idiopathic skeletal hyperostosis. Dorsal kyphosis in conjunction with elongation of the ribs contributes to the development of the barrel chest seen in acromegalic patients. The hands and feet become enlarged owing to soft tissue proliferation. The fingers are thickened and have spade-like distal tufts. One-third of patients have a thickened heel pad. Approximately 25 percent of patients have Raynaud's phenomenon.

Carpal tunnel syndrome occurs in about half of patients. The median nerve is compressed by the excessive growth of connective tissue in the carpal tunnel. The median nerve also becomes enlarged. Patients with acromegaly also develop proximal muscle weakness, which is thought to be caused by the effect of growth hormone on muscle. Results of muscle enzyme assays and electromyography are normal. Muscle biopsy specimens show muscle fibers of varying size and no inflammatory changes.

ARTHROPATHY OF HEMOCHROMATOSIS Hemochromatosis is a disorder of iron storage. Excessive amounts of iron are absorbed from the intestine, leading to iron deposition in parenchymal cells, which results in tissue damage and impairment of organ function (see Chap. 342). Symptoms of hemochromatosis usually begin between the ages of 40 and 60 but can occur earlier. Arthritis, which occurs in 20 to 40 percent of patients, usually begins after the age of 50 years and may be the first clinical feature of hemochromatosis. The arthropathy is an inflammatory osteoarthritis-like disorder affecting the small joints of the hands, followed later by larger joints such as knees, ankles, shoulders, and hips. The second and third metacarpophalangeal joints of both hands are often the first joints affected; they can provide an important clue to the possibility of hemochromatosis. Patients experience stiffness and pain. Morning stiffness usually lasts less than half an hour. The affected joints are enlarged and mildly tender. Synovial tissue is not appreciatively increased. Radiographs show irregular narrowing of the joint space, subchondral sclerosis, and subchondral cysts. There is juxtaarticular proliferation of bone, with frequent hook-like osteophytes. The synovial fluid is noninflammatory. The synovium shows mild to moderate proliferation of lining cells, fibrosis, and a low number of inflammatory cells, which are mononuclear. In approximately half of patients, there is evidence of calcium pyrophosphate deposition disease. Iron can be demonstrated in the lining cells of the synovium and also in chondrocytes.

Iron may damage the articular cartilage in several ways. Promotion by iron of superoxide-dependent lipid peroxidation may play a role in joint damage. In animal models, ferric iron has been shown to interfere with collagen formation. Iron has also been shown to increase the release of lysosomal enzymes from cells in the synovial membrane. Iron may also play a role in the development of chondrocalcinosis. Iron inhibits synovial tissue pyrophosphatase in vitro and, therefore, may inhibit pyrophosphatase in vivo, resulting in chondrocalcinosis. Iron in synovial cells may also inhibit the clearance of calcium pyrophosphate from the joint.

℞ TREATMENT

The treatment of hemochromatosis is repeated phlebotomy. Unfortunately, this treatment has little effect on the arthritis, which, along with chondrocalcinosis, usually continues to progress. Treatment of the arthritis consists of administration of acetaminophen and NSAIDs. Placement of a hip or knee prosthesis has been successful in advanced disease.

HEMOPHILIC ARTHROPATHY Hemophilia is a sex-linked recessive genetic disorder characterized by the absence or deficiency of factor VIII (hemophilia A, or classic hemophilia) or factor IX (hemophilia B, or Christmas disease) (see Chap. 118). Hemophilia A is by far the more common type, constituting 85 percent of cases. Spontaneous hemarthrosis is a common problem with both types of hemophilia and can lead to a chronic deforming arthritis. The frequency and severity of hemarthrosis are related to the degree of clotting factor deficiency. Hemarthrosis is not common in other inherited disorders of coagulation, such as von Willebrand's disease or factor V deficiency.

Hemarthrosis becomes evident after 1 year of age, when the child begins to walk and run. In order of frequency, the joints most commonly affected are the knees, ankles, elbows, shoulders, and hips. Small joints of the hands and feet are occasionally involved.

In the initial stage of arthropathy, hemarthrosis produces a warm, tensely swollen, and painful joint. The patient holds the affected joint in flexion and guards against any movement. Blood in the joint remains liquid because of the absence of intrinsic clotting factor and the absence of tissue thromboplastin in the synovium. The blood in the joint space is resorbed over a period of a week or longer, depending on the size of the hemarthrosis. Joint function usually returns to normal or baseline in about 2 weeks.

Recurrent hemarthrosis leads to the development of a chronic arthritis. The involved joints remain swollen, and flexion deformities develop. In the later stages of arthropathy, joint motion is restricted and function is severely limited. Joint ankylosis, subluxation, or laxity are features of end-stage disease.

Bleeding into muscle and soft tissue also causes musculoskeletal disorders. When bleeding into the iliopsoas muscle occurs, the hip is held in flexion because of the pain, resulting in a hip flexion contracture. Rotation of the hip is preserved, which distinguishes this problem from intraarticular hemorrhage. Expansion of the hematoma may place pressure on the femoral nerve, resulting in a femoral neuropathy. Another problem is shortening of the heel cord secondary to bleeding into the gastrocnemius. Hemorrhage into a closed compartment space, such as the volar compartment in the forearm, can result in muscle necrosis and flexion deformities of the wrist and fingers. When bleeding involves periosteum or bone, a pseudotumor forms. These occur distal to the elbows or knees in children and improve with treatment of the hemophilia. Surgical removal is indicated if the pseudotumor continues to enlarge. In adults, they occur in the femur and pelvis and are usually refractory to treatment. When bleeding occurs in muscle, cysts may develop over the muscle. Needle aspiration of a cyst is contraindicated because it can induce bleeding.

Septic arthritis can occur in hemophilia and is difficult at times to distinguish from acute hemarthrosis. Whenever there is suspicion of an infected joint, the joint should be aspirated immediately, the fluid cultured, and the patient started on a broad-spectrum antibiotic. The patient should be infused with the deficient clotting factor before the joint is tapped.

Radiographs of joints reflect the stage of disease. In early stages there is only capsule distention; later, juxtaarticular osteopenia, marginal erosions, and subchondral cysts develop. In late disease, the joint space is narrowed and there is bony overgrowth. The changes are similar to those observed in osteoarthritis. Unique features of hemophilic arthropathy are widening of the femoral intercondylar notch, enlargement of the proximal radius, and squaring of the distal end of the patella.

Recurrent hemarthrosis produces synovial hyperplasia and hypertrophy. A pannus covers the cartilage. Cartilage is damaged by collagenase and other degradative enzymes released by mononuclear cells in the overlying synovium. Hemosiderin is found in synovial lining cells, the subsynovium, and chondrocytes and may also play a role in cartilage destruction.

℞ TREATMENT

The treatment of hemarthrosis consists in the immediate infusion of factor VIII or IX at the first sign of joint or muscle hemorrhage. The patient is placed at bed rest, with the involved joint in as much extension as the patient can tolerate. Analgesic NSAIDs and local icing may help with the pain. NSAIDs can be given safely for short periods even though they have a stabilizing effect on platelets. Studies have shown no significant abnormalities in platelet function or bleeding time in hemophiliacs receiving ibuprofen. Synovectomy, open or arthroscopic, may be indicated in patients with chronic synovial proliferation and recurrent hemarthrosis. Hypertrophied synovium is very vascular and subject to bleeding. Both types of synovectomy reduce the number of hemarthroses and slow the roentgenographic progression of hemophilic arthropathy. Open surgical synovectomy, however, is associated with some loss of range of motion. Radiosynovectomy with either yttrium 90 silicate or phosphorus 31 colloid has also been effective and may be a useful alternative when surgical synovectomy is not practical. Total joint replacement is indicated for severe joint destruction and incapacitating pain. Because of the young age of hemophilic patients, total-joint prostheses may need to be replaced more than once during their lives.

ARTHROPATHIES ASSOCIATED WITH HEMOGLOBINOPATHIES **Sickle Cell Disease** Sickle cell disease (see Chap.

Table 326-5

Musculoskeletal Abnormalities in Sickle Cell Disease

Sickle cell dactylitis
Joint effusions in sickle cell crises
Osteomyelitis
Infarction of bone
Infarction of bone marrow
Avascular necrosis
Bone changes secondary to marrow hyperplasia
Septic arthritis
Gouty arthritis

107) is associated with several musculoskeletal abnormalities (Table 326-5). Children under the age of 5 may develop diffuse swelling, tenderness, and warmth of the hands and feet lasting from 1 to 3 weeks. The condition referred to as *sickle cell dactylitis* or *hand-foot syndrome* has also been observed in sickle cell disease and sickle cell thalassemia. Dactylitis is believed to result from infarction of the bone marrow and cortical bone leading to periostitis and soft tissue swelling. Radiographs show periosteal elevation, subperiosteal new bone formation, and areas of radiolucency and increased density involving the metacarpals, metatarsals, and proximal phalanges. These bone changes disappear after several months. The syndrome leaves little or no residual damage. Because hematopoiesis ceases in the small bones of hands and feet with age, the syndrome is rarely seen after age 4 or 5 and does not occur in adults.

Sickle cell crisis is often associated with periarticular pain and joint effusions. The joint and periarticular area are warm and tender. Knees and elbows are most often affected, but other joints can be involved. Joint effusions are noninflammatory, with fewer than 1000 white cells/μL; mononuclear cells predominate. There have been a few reports of sterile inflammatory effusion with high cell counts consisting of mostly polymorphonuclear white cells. Synovial biopsies have shown mild lining cell proliferation and microvascular thrombosis. Scintigraphic studies have shown decreased marrow uptake adjacent to the involved joint. The joint effusion and periarticular pain are considered to be the result of ischemia and infarction of the synovium and adjacent bone and marrow. The treatment is that for sickle cell crisis (see Chap. 107).

Patients with sickle cell disease may also develop osteomyelitis, which commonly involves the long tubular bones (see Chap. 132). These patients are particularly susceptible to bacterial infections, especially *Salmonella* infections, which are found in more than half of cases (see Chap. 158). Radiographs of the involved site show periosteal elevation initially, followed by disruption of the cortex. Treatment of the infection results in healing of the bone lesion. Sickle cell disease is also associated with bone infarction resulting from thrombosis secondary to the sickling of red cells. Bone infarction also occurs in hemoglobin S-C disease and sickle cell thalassemia (see Chap. 107). The bone pain in sickle cell crisis is due to bone and bone marrow infarction. In children, infarction of the epiphyseal growth plate interferes with normal growth of the affected extremity. Radiographically, infarction of the bone cortex results in periosteal elevation and irregular thickening of the bone cortex. Infarction in the bone marrow leads to lysis, fibrosis, and new bone formation.

Avascular necrosis of the head of the femur is seen in about 5 percent of patients. It also occurs in the humeral head and less commonly in the distal femur, tibial condyles, distal radius, vertebral bodies, and other juxtaarticular sites. The mechanism for avascular necrosis is most likely the same as for bone infarction. Subchondral hemorrhage may play a role in the deterioration of articular cartilage. Irregularity of the femoral head or of other bone surfaces affected by avascular necrosis eventually results in degenerative joint disease. Radiograph of the affected joint may show patchy radiolucency and density followed by flattening of the bone. Magnetic resonance imaging is a sensitive technique for detecting early avascular necrosis as well as bone infarction elsewhere. Total hip replacement and placement of prostheses in other joints may improve function and relieve pain in those patients with severe joint destruction.

Septic arthritis is occasionally encountered in sickle cell disease (see Chap. 324). Multiple joints may be infected. Joint infection may result from spread of contiguous osteomyelitis. Microorganisms identified include staphylococcus, *Streptococcus*, *Escherichia coli*, and *Salmonella*. The latter is not seen as frequently in septic arthritis as it is in osteomyelitis. Acute gouty arthritis is uncommon in sickle cell disease, even though 40 percent of patients are hyperuremic. Hyperuricemia is due to overproduction of uric acid secondary to increased red cell turnover. Attacks may be polyarticular.

The bone marrow hyperplasia in sickle cell disease results in widening of the medullary cavities, thinning of the cortices, coarse trabeculations and central cupping of the vertebral bodies. These changes are also seen to a lesser degree in hemoglobin S-C disease and sickle cell thalassemia. In normal individuals, red marrow is located mostly in the axial skeletal, but in sickle cell disease, red marrow is found in the bones of the extremities and even in the tarsal and carpal bones. Vertebral compression may lead to dorsal kyphosis, and softening of the bone in the acetabulum may result in protrusio acetabuli.

Thalassemia β-Thalassemia is a congenital disorder of hemoglobin synthesis characterized by impaired production of β chains (see Chap. 107). Bone and joint abnormalities occur in β-thalassemia, being most common in the major and intermedia groups. In one study, approximately 50 percent of patients with β-thalassemia had evidence of symmetric ankle arthropathy, characterized by a dull aching pain aggravated by weight bearing. The onset was most often in the second or third decade of life. The degree of ankle pain in these patients varied. Some patients experienced self-limited ankle pain, which occurred only after strenuous physical activity and lasted several days to weeks. Other patients had chronic ankle pain which became worse with walking. Symptoms eventually abated in a few patients. Compression of the ankle, calcaneus, or forefoot was painful in some patients. Synovial fluid from two patients was noninflammatory. Radiographs of ankle showed osteopenia, widened medullary spaces, thin cortices, and coarse trabeculations. These findings were largely the result of bone marrow expansion. The joint space was preserved. Specimens of bone from three patients revealed osteomalacia, osteopenia, and microfractures. Increased osteoblasts as well as increased foci of bone resorption were present on the bone surface. Iron staining was found in the bone trabeculae, in osteoid, and in the cement line. Synovium showed hyperplasia of lining cells which contained deposits of hemosiderin. This arthropathy was considered to be related to the underlying bone pathology. The role of iron overload or abnormal bone metabolism in the pathogenesis of this arthropathy is not known. This arthropathy was treated with analgesics and splints. Patients were also transfused to decrease hematopoiesis and marrow expansion.

Patients with β-thalassemia major and intermedia also have involvement of other joints, including the knees, hips, and shoulders. Acquired hemochromatosis with arthropathy has been described in a patient with thalassemia. Gouty arthritis and septic arthritis can occur. Avascular necrosis is not a feature of thalassemia because there is no sickling of red cells leading to thrombosis and infarction.

β-Thalassemia minor (trait) is also associated with joint manifestations. Chronic seronegative oligoarthritis affecting predominantly ankles, wrists, and elbows has been described. These patients had mild persistent synovitis without large effusions. Joint erosions were not seen. Recurrent episodes of an acute asymmetric arthritis also have been reported; episodes last less than a week and may affect knees, ankles, shoulders, elbows, wrists, and metacarpal phalangeal joints. The mechanism for this arthropathy is unknown. Treatment with nonsteroidal drugs was not particularly effective.

PERIARTICULAR DISORDERS **Bursitis** Bursitis is inflammation of a bursa, which is a thin-walled sac lined with synovial tissue. The function of the bursa is to facilitate movement of tendons and muscles over bony prominences. Excessive frictional forces, trauma, systemic disease (e.g., rheumatoid arthritis, gout), or infection may cause bursitis. Subacromial bursitis (subdeltoid bursitis) is the most common form of bursitis. Another form is trochanteric bursitis, which involves the bursa around the insertion of the gluteus medius onto the greater trochanter of the femur. Patients experience pain over the lateral aspect of the hip and upper thigh and have tenderness over the posterior aspect of the greater trochanter. External rotation and resisted abduction of the hip elicit pain. Olecranon bursitis occurs over the posterior elbow, and when the area is acutely inflamed, infection should be excluded by aspirating and culturing fluid from the bursa. Achilles bursitis involves the bursa located above the insertion of the tendon to the calcaneus and results from overuse and wearing tight shoes. Retrocalcaneal bursitis involves the bursa that is located between the calcaneus and posterior surface of the Achilles tendon. The pain is experienced at the back of the heel, and swelling appears on the medial and/or lateral side of the tendon. It occurs in association with spondyloarthropathies, rheumatoid arthritis, gout, and trauma. Ischial bursitis (weaver's bottom) affects the bursa separating the gluteus medius from the ischial tuberosity and develops from prolonged sitting on hard surfaces. Iliopsoas bursitis affects the bursa that lies between the iliopsoas muscle and hip joint and is lateral to the femoral vessels. Pain is experienced over this area and is made worse by hip extension and flexion. Bursitis results from trauma or overuse but can also be seen in patients with rheumatoid arthritis. Anserine bursitis is an inflammation of the sartorius bursa located over the medial side of the tibia just below the knee and is manifested by pain on climbing stairs. Tenderness is present over the insertion of the conjoint tendon of the sartorius, gracilis, and semitendinosus. Prepatellar bursitis (housemaid's knee) occurs in the bursa situated between the patella and overlying skin and is caused by kneeling on hard surfaces. Treatment of bursitis consists of prevention of the aggravating situation, rest of the involved part, administration of a NSAID, and local steroid injection.

Rotator Cuff Tendinitis and Impingement Syndrome Tendinitis of the rotator cuff is the major cause of a painful shoulder and is currently thought to be caused by impingement on the tendon(s). Of the tendons forming the rotator cuff, the supraspinatus tendon is the most often affected, probably because of its repeated confinement between the humeral head and the undersurface of the anterior third of the acromion and coracoacromial ligament above as well as the reduction in its blood supply that occurs with abduction of the arm (Fig. 326-3). The tendon of the infraspinatus or the long head of the biceps is less commonly involved. The process begins with edema and hemorrhage of the rotator cuff, which evolves to fibrotic thickening and eventually to rotator cuff degeneration with tendon tears and bone spurs. Subacromial bursitis also accompanies this syndrome. Symptoms usually appear after injury or overuse, especially with activities involving elevation of the arm with some degree of forward flexion. Impingement syndrome occurs in persons participating in baseball, tennis, swimming, or occupations that require repeated elevation of the arm. Those over age 40 are particularly susceptible. Patients complain of a dull aching in the shoulder, which may interfere with sleep. Severe pain is experienced when the arm is actively abducted into an overhead position. The arc between 60 and 120° is especially painful. Tenderness is present over the lateral aspect of the humeral head just below the acromion. Nonsteroidal anti-inflammatory drugs, local steroid injection, and physical therapy may relieve symptoms.

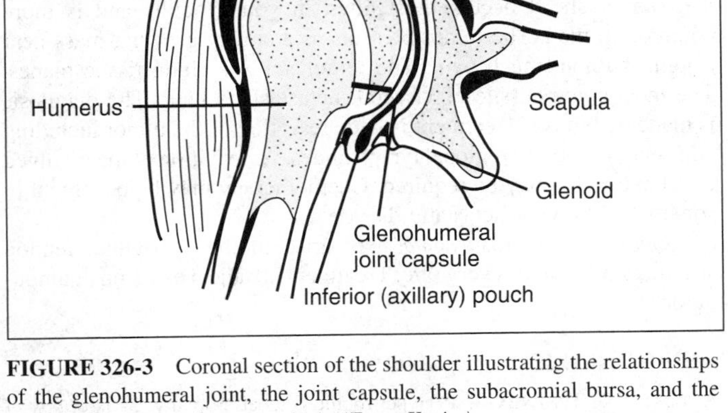

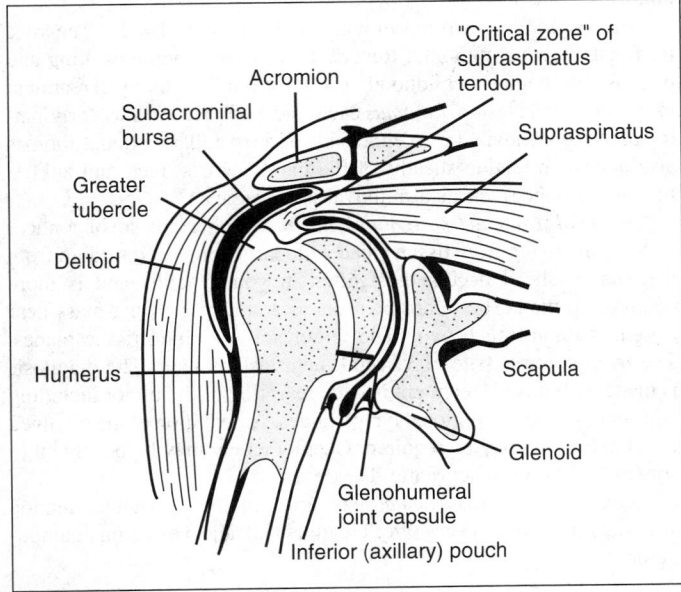

FIGURE 326-3 Coronal section of the shoulder illustrating the relationships of the glenohumeral joint, the joint capsule, the subacromial bursa, and the rotator cuff (supraspinatus tendon). *(From Kozin.)*

Patients may tear the supraspinatus tendon acutely by falling on an outstretched arm or lifting a heavy object. Symptoms are pain, along with weakness of abduction and external rotation of the shoulder. Atrophy of the supraspinatus muscles develops. The diagnosis is established by arthrogram or ultrasound. Surgical repair may be necessary in patients who fail to respond to conservative measures. In patients with moderate to severe tears and functional loss, surgery is indicated.

Calcific Tendinitis This condition is characterized by deposition of calcium salts, primarily hydroxyapatite, within a tendon. The exact mechanism of calcification is not known but may be initiated by ischemia or degeneration of the tendon. The supraspinatus tendon is most often affected because it is frequently impinged on and has a reduced blood supply when the arm is abducted. The condition usually develops after age 40. Calcification within the tendon may evoke acute inflammation, producing sudden and severe pain in the shoulder. However, it may be asymptomatic or not related to the patient's symptoms.

Bicipital Tendinitis and Rupture Bicipital tendinitis, or tenosynovitis, is produced by friction on the tendon of the long head of the biceps as it passes through the bicipital groove. When the inflammation is acute, patients experience anterior shoulder pain which radiates down the biceps into the forearm. Abduction and external rotation of the arm are painful and limited. The bicipital groove is very tender to palpation. Pain may be elicited along the course of the tendon by resisting supination of the forearm with the elbow at 90° (Yergason's supination sign). Acute rupture of the tendon may occur with vigorous exercise of the arm and is often painful. In a young patient, it should be repaired surgically. Rupture of the tendon in an older person may be associated with little or no pain and is recognized by the presence of persistent swelling of the biceps ("Popeye" muscle) produced by the retraction of the long head of the biceps. Surgery is usually not necessary in this setting.

Adhesive Capsulitis Often referred to as "frozen shoulder," adhesive capsulitis is characterized by pain and restricted movement of the shoulder, usually in the absence of intrinsic shoulder disease. Adhesive capsulitis, however, may follow bursitis or tendinitis of the shoulder or be associated with systemic disorders such as chronic pulmonary disease, myocardial infarction, and diabetes mellitus. Prolonged immobility of the arm contributes to the development of adhesive capsulitis, and reflex sympathetic dystrophy is thought to be a pathogenic factor. The capsule of the shoulder is thickened, and a mild chronic inflammatory infiltrate and fibrosis may be present.

Adhesive capsulitis occurs more commonly in women after age 50. Pain and stiffness usually develop gradually over several months to a year but progress rapidly in some patients. Pain may interfere with sleep. The shoulder is tender to palpation, and both active and passive movement are restricted. Radiographs of the shoulder show osteopenia. The diagnosis is confirmed by arthrography, in that only a limited amount of contrast material, usually less than 15 mL, can be injected under pressure into the shoulder joint.

In most patients, the condition improves spontaneously 12 to 18 months after onset, but some have permanent restriction of movement.

Early mobilization of the arm following an injury to the shoulder may prevent the development of this disease. Slow but forceful injection of contrast material into the joint may lyse adhesions and stretch the capsule, resulting in improvement of shoulder motion. Manipulation under anesthesia may be helpful in some patients. Once the disease is established, therapy may have little effect on its natural course. Local injections of glucocorticoids, nonsteroidal anti-inflammatory drugs and physical therapy may provide relief of symptoms.

Lateral Epicondylitis (Tennis Elbow) Lateral epicondylitis, or tennis elbow, is a painful condition involving the soft tissue over the lateral aspect of the elbow. The pain originates at or near the site of attachment of the common extensors to the lateral epicondyle and may radiate into the forearm and dorsum of the wrist. This painful condition is thought to be caused by small tears of the extensor aponeurosis resulting from repeated resisted contractions of the extensor muscles. The pain usually appears after work or recreational activities involving repeated motions of wrist extension and supination against resistance. Most patients with this disorder injure themselves in activities other than tennis, such as pulling weeds, carrying suitcases or briefcases, or using a screwdriver. The injury in tennis usually occurs when hitting a backhand with the elbow flexed. Shaking hands and opening doors can reproduce the pain. Striking the lateral elbow against a solid object may also induce pain.

The treatment is usually rest along with administration of a nonsteroidal anti-inflammatory drug. Ultrasound, icing, and friction massage may also help relieve pain. When pain is severe, the elbow is placed in a sling or splinted at 90° of flexion. When the pain is acute and well localized, injection of a steroid using a small-gauge needle may be effective. Following injection, the patient should be advised to rest the arm for at least 1 month and avoid activities that would aggravate the elbow. Once symptoms have subsided, the patient should begin rehabilitation to strengthen and increase flexibility of the extensor muscles before resuming physical activity involving the arm. A forearm band placed 2.5 to 5.0 cm (1 to 2 in) below the elbow may help to reduce tension on the extensor muscles at their attachment to the lateral epicondyle. The patient should be advised to restrict activities requiring forcible extension and supination of the wrist. Improvement may take several months. The patient may continue to experience mild pain but, with care, usually can avoid the return of debilitating pain. In an occasional patient, surgical release of the extensor aponeurosis may be necessary.

Medial Epicondylitis Medial epicondylitis is an overuse syndrome resulting in pain over the medial side of the elbow with radiation into the forearm. The cause of this syndrome is considered to be repetitive resisted motions of wrist flexion and pronation, which lead to microtears and granulation tissue at the origin of the pronator teres and forearm flexors, particularly the flexor carpi radialis. This overuse syndrome is usually seen in patients older than 35 years and is much less common than lateral epicondylitis. It occurs most often in work-related repetitive activities but also occurs with recreational activities such as swinging a golf club (golfer's elbow) or throwing a baseball. On physical examination, there is tenderness just distal to the medial epicondyle over the origin of the forearm flexors. Pain can be reproduced by resisting wrist flexion and pronation with the elbow extended. Radiographs are usually normal. The differential diagnosis of patients with medial elbow symptoms include tears of the pronator teres, acute medial collateral ligament tear, and medial collateral ligament instability. Ulnar neuritis has been found in 25 to 50 percent of patients with medial epicondylitis and is associated with tenderness over the ulnar nerve at the elbow as well as hypesthesia and paresthesias on the ulnar side of the hand.

The initial treatment of medial epicondylitis is conservative, involving rest, nonsteroidal anti-inflammatory drugs, friction massage, ultrasound, and icing. Some patients may require splinting. Injections of glucocorticoids at the painful site may also be effective. Patients should be instructed to rest at least 1 month. Also, patients should be started on physical therapy once the pain has subsided. In patients with chronic debilitating medial epicondylitis that remains unresponsive after at least a year of treatment, surgical release of the flexor muscle at its origin may be necessary and is often successful.

TUMORS OF JOINTS Primary tumors and tumor-like disorders of synovium are uncommon but should be considered in the differential diagnosis of monarticular joint disease. In addition, metastases to bone and primary bone tumors adjacent to a joint may produce joint symptoms.

Pigmented villonodular synovitis is characterized by exuberant proliferation of synovial cells, usually involving a single joint. It occurs most often in young adults and affects both sexes equally. The cause of this disorder is unknown.

The synovium has a brownish color and numerous large, finger-like villi which fuse to form pedunculated nodules. There is marked hyperplasia of synovial cells in the stroma of the villi. Hemosiderin granules and lipids are found in the cytoplasm of macrophages and in the interstitial tissue. Multinucleated giant cells may be present. The proliferative synovium grows into the subsynovial tissue and invades adjacent cartilage and bone.

The clinical picture of pigmented villonodular synovitis is characterized by the insidious onset of swelling and pain in one joint, most commonly the knee. Other joints affected include the hips, ankles, calcaneocuboid joints, elbows, and small joints of the fingers or toes. The disease also may involve the common flexor sheath of the hand. Symptoms may be mild and intermittent and may be present for years before the patient seeks medical attention. Radiographs may show joint space narrowing, erosions, and subchondral cysts. The joint fluid contains blood and is dark red or almost black in color. Lipid-containing macrophages may be present in the fluid. The joint fluid may be clear if hemorrhages have not occurred.

The treatment of pigmented villonodular synovitis is complete synovectomy. With incomplete synovectomy, the villonodular synovitis recurs, and the rate of tissue growth may be faster than originally. Irradiation of the involved joint has been successful in some patients.

Synovial chondromatosis is a disorder characterized by multiple focal metaplastic growths of normal-appearing cartilage in the synovium or tendon sheath. Segments of cartilage break loose and continue to grow as loose bodies. When calcification and ossification of loose bodies occur, the disorder is referred to as *synovial osteochondromatosis*. The disorder is usually monarticular and affects young to middle-aged individuals. The knee is most often involved, followed by hip, elbow, and shoulder. Symptoms are pain, swelling, and decreased motion of the joint. Radiographs may show several rounded calcifications within the joint cavity. Treatment is synovectomy; however, the tumor may recur.

Hemangiomas occur in synovium and in tendon sheaths. The knee is affected most commonly. Recurrent episodes of joint swelling and pain usually begin in childhood. The joint fluid is bloody. Treatment is excision of the lesion. *Lipomas* occur most often in the knee, originating in the subsynovial fat on either side of the patellar tendon. Lipomas also appear in tendon sheaths of the hands, wrists, feet, and ankles. In some instances, surgical removal is necessary.

Synovial sarcoma (malignant synovioma) is a neoplasm of connective origin arising from tissue adjacent to large joints and seldom from the joint itself. It occurs most often in young adults and is more common in men. The tumor presents as a slowly growing mass near a joint, without much pain. The tumor spreads along tissue planes. The most common site of visceral metastasis is lung. The diagnosis is made by biopsy. Treatment is wide resection of the tumor including adjacent muscle and regional lymph nodes. Amputation of the involved distal extremity may be required. Chemotherapy may be beneficial in some patients with metastatic disease.

Synovial chondrosarcoma may arise in the synovium, tendon sheath, or bursa and is very rare. Treatment is radical excision or amputation.

BIBLIOGRAPHY

ALTMAN RD, TENENBAUM J: Hypertrophic osteoarthropathy, in *Textbook of Rheumatology*, 5th ed, WN Kelley et al (eds). Philadelphia, Saunders, 1997

ARMAN MI et al: Brief report. Frequency and features of rheumatic findings in thalassaemia minor: A blind controlled study. Br J Rheumatol 31:197, 1992

BENNETT RM: The fibromyalgia syndrome, in *Textbook of Rheumatology*, 5th ed, WN Kelley et al (eds). Philadelphia, Saunders, 1997

BERKOVITCH M et al: Arthropathy in thalassaemia patients receiving deferiprone. Lancet 343:1471, 1994

CARELESS DJ, COHEN MG: Rheumatic manifestations of hyperlipidemia and antihyperlipidemia drug therapy. Semin Arthritis Rheum 23:90, 1993

CRONIN ME: Rheumatic aspects of endocrinopathies, in *Arthritis and Allied Conditions,* 13th ed, WJ Koopman (ed). Baltimore, Williams & Wilkins, 1997

ELLMAN MH: Neuropathic joint disease (Charcot joints), in *Arthritis and Allied Conditions*, 13th ed, WJ Koopman (ed). Baltimore, Williams & Wilkins, 1997

GOLDENBERG DL: Fibromyalgia: Why such controversy? Ann Rheum Dis 54:3, 1995

HECK LW JR: Arthritis associated with hematologic disorders, storage diseases, disorders of lipid metabolism, and dysproteinemias, in *Arthritis and Allied Conditions*, 13th ed, WJ Koopman (ed). Baltimore, Williams & Wilkins, 1997

HOCHBERG ME: Relapsing Polychondritis, in *Textbook of Rheumatology*, 5th ed, WN Kelley et al (eds). Philadelphia, Saunders, 1997

ISAAK BL et al: Ocular and systemic findings in relapsing polychondritis. Ophthalmology 93:681, 1986

KOZIN F: Painful shoulder and the reflex sympathetic dystrophy syndrome, in *Arthritis and Allied Conditions*, 13th ed, WJ Koopman (ed). Baltimore, Williams & Wilkins, 1997

LAMBERT RE, MCGUIRE JL: Iron storage disease, in *Textbook of Rheumatology*, 5th ed, WN Kelley et al (eds). Philadelphia, Saunders, 1997

LANG B et al: Susceptibility to relapsing polychondritis is associated with HLA-DR4. Arthritis Rheum 36:660, 1993

LINTNER SA et al: Sports medicine, in *Textbook of Rheumatology*, 5th ed, WN Kelley et al (eds). Philadelphia, Saunders, 1997

MARTINEZ-LAVIN M: Hypertrophic osteoarthropathy, in *Rheumatology*, JF Klippel, PA Dieppe (eds). St. Louis, Mosby, 1993, pp 40.1–40.4

MATSEN FA III, ARNTZ CT: Subacromial impingement, in *The Shoulder*, L Reines (ed). Philadelphia, Saunders, 1990

MICHET CJ: Relapsing polychondritis, in *Arthritis and Allied Conditions,* 13th ed, WJ Koopman (ed). Baltimore, Williams & Wilkins, 1997

NEER CS II: Impingement lesions. Clin Orthop 173:70, 1983

ROSENBERG EA, SCHILLER AC: Tumors and tumor-like lesions of joints and related structures, in *Textbook of Rheumatology*, 5th ed, WN Kelley et al (eds). Philadelphia, Saunders, 1997

SCHUMACHER RH JR: Hemoglobinopathies and arthritis, in *Textbook of Rheumatology*, 5th ed, WN Kelley et al (eds). Philadelphia, Saunders, 1997

UPCHURCH KS, BRETTLER DB: Hemophilic arthropathy, in *Textbook of Rheumatology*, 5th ed, WN Kelley et al (eds). Philadelphia, Saunders, 1997

WILKE WS: Treatment of "resistant" fibromyalgia. Rheum Dis Clin North Am 21:247, 1995

WOLFE F: When to diagnose fibromyalgia. Rheum Dis Clin North Am 20:485, 1994

——— et al: The prevalence and characteristics of fibromyalgia in the general population. Arthritis Rheum 38:19, 1995

PART THIRTEEN

ENDOCRINOLOGY AND METABOLISM

SECTION 1

ENDOCRINOLOGY

327

Jean D. Wilson

APPROACH TO THE PATIENT WITH ENDOCRINE AND METABOLIC DISORDERS

Communication between cells is mediated by the endocrine, nervous, and immune systems, which constitute an interlocking network. Not only do neurotransmitters such as norepinephrine circulate in blood as hormones, but neural impulses have major effects on the release of chemical mediators such as testosterone and insulin. Likewise, the immune system is subject to neural and hormonal modulation, and cytokine formation by lymphocytes can influence endocrine function. The interlocking nature of this relationship is most apparent in the hypothalamus, where a neuroendocrine-immunologic system evolved to integrate and coordinate the metabolic activities of higher organisms. Endocrinology deals largely with the chemical mediators that are secreted into the bloodstream, but in fact the functions of the three systems interlap at every level.

The term *hormone* originally referred to substances that are synthesized in a limited number of tissues and secreted into the circulation to act as chemical effectors in other tissues. However, the capacity to form such chemical mediators is not limited to so-called endocrine organs. Some hormones, such as angiotensins II and III, are formed in the bloodstream itself. Others, such as testosterone in women and dihydrotestosterone and estradiol in men, are both secreted from the gonads and formed in extraglandular tissues from circulating precursors (prohormones). Still other hormones circulate only in restricted compartments, such as the hypothalamic-pituitary portal system, and do not reach the systemic circulation in appreciable quantities. Finally, hormones such as insulin and dihydrotestosterone have *autocrine* actions in the cells of origin, *paracrine* actions in cells in the same tissues in which they are formed, *juxtacrine* actions on adjacent cells, and *endocrine* actions at distal sites. Other chemical mediators, such as müllerian-inhibiting hormone, appear to exert paracrine actions exclusively.

BIOCHEMISTRY

SYNTHESIS The approximately 150 known chemical mediators fall into three major categories—peptides or peptide derivatives, steroids, and amines. In the case of peptide hormones, genes code for messenger RNA, which is then translated into protein precursors. These proteins undergo posttranslational cleavage (preproparathyroid hormone → proparathyroid hormone → parathyroid hormone) and/or processing (thyroglobulin → thyroxine → triiodothyronine) to form the active hormone recognized by the target tissues. The distinct feature of peptide hormones is that one or a few structural genes code for the amino acid sequence of the peptide, and other genes are responsible for the alteration of the peptide to its final form. In the case of peptide hormones with subunits, the different subunits may be derived either from a single precursor (insulin) or from separate precursors [luteinizing hormone (LH)]. Furthermore, the same peptide hormone (somatostatin) can be formed from different prohormones encoded by distinct genes; individual prohormones such as proopiomelanocortin can be metabolized to different hormones in different cells, depending on the complement of processing enzymes in the cell in question; and the initial RNA transcripts of the calcitonin gene can be alternatively spliced in different tissues to form messenger RNA for either calcitonin or calcitonin gene–related peptide. Peptide hormones may also be formed ectopically in malignancies of nonendocrine origin, such as carcinoma of the lung, and in small amounts in normal nonendocrine tissues (see Chap. 102).

In the case of steroid hormones, the precursor—cholesterol (for most steroid hormones) or 7-dehydrocholesterol (for vitamin D metabolites)—undergoes a series of enzymatic transformations to form the final products. At least six enzymes, and consequently a minimum of six genes, are required to transform cholesterol to estradiol. Because of the number of enzymes required, the formation of steroid hormones is unusual in nonendocrine malignancies. However, many tissues—malignant and nonmalignant—that cannot synthesize steroid hormones from cholesterol contain enzymes that convert circulating steroids to other hormones; examples are the conversion of androgens to estrogens by trophoblastic tumors and by normal adipocytes and the conversion of progesterone to deoxycorticosterone by the kidney.

Amine hormones are formed by a process similar to that involved in steroid hormone synthesis except that the precursors are amino acids. For example, tyrosine is the precursor for epinephrine and norepinephrine (see Chap. 70).

STORAGE Most endocrine organs have a limited capacity to store the hormones they synthesize. For example, the normal adult testes contain only about one-fifteenth the quantity of testosterone secreted each day, and the testicular pool turns over several times to provide the normal daily output of hormone. Even when tissues have special storage organelles for hormones, the amount of hormone stored is usually limited: The insulin granules in the pancreatic beta cell ordinarily contain amounts of insulin sufficient only for short-term, reserve needs. (In contrast, nerve endings may contain a several-day supply of norepinephrine.) The limited storage capacity for hormones in tissues is due to the unsuitability of these compounds for incorporation into any of the three main storage compartments of the body (lipids, glycogen, or protein). For example, most steroid hormones are too polar to be stored in large quantities in lipid compartments, and peptide and amine hormones are unsuitable for incorporation into proteins. As a consequence, the body pools of most hormones tend to be small. The major exceptions to this rule occur when hormone precursors can be stored either as protein or in neutral lipid compartments; the normal thyroid gland contains the equivalent of a 2-week supply of thyroid hormones in the form of the protein thyroglobulin, and the precursor and intermediate forms of vitamin D can be stored in considerable quantity in hepatic lipid.

RELEASE Release of hormones into the blood stream can involve conversion of insoluble to soluble derivatives (proteolysis of thyroglobulin to thyroid hormones), exocytosis of storage granules (insulin, glucagon, prolactin, growth hormone), or passive diffusion of newly synthesized molecules such as steroid hormones down activity gradients into plasma.

Because of the limited capacity for storage, most hormones are released into plasma at a pace reflecting their rates of formation, and most trophic hormones enhance both the synthesis and release of their target hormones. Even when peptide hormones are stored in granules, release of the stored material is followed by an enhanced rate of synthesis (as, for instance, the two-phase release of insulin induced by glucose infusion). For some hormones, diurnal, sleep-related, developmental, and neural factors influence hormone release, and in most of these instances, synthesis and release are also tightly linked.

Hormone release may be periodic or rhythmic, the cycle varying in frequency from minutes to hours (*ultradian*) to daily (*circadian*) to months or years (*infradian*). The release of hormones such as LH and follicle-stimulating hormone (FSH) is *pulsatile*, with bursts of secretion occurring in a repetitive pattern; the release of adrenocorticotropic hormone (ACTH) (and of cortisol) varies over a 24-h cycle; and thyroid hormone release can vary on longer cycles. Whether this intermittent release is a function of alterations in synthetic rates, changes in blood flow, or other mechanisms is uncertain, but most such cycles are under neurogenic control. In some instances the physiologic significance of pulsatile release is not fully understood, but changes in frequency or amplitude of the release pattern on occasion have profound effects on hormone function; i.e., the pulsatile administration of luteinizing hormone–releasing hormone (LHRH) stimulates the release of LH by the pituitary, whereas the constant infusion of the same amount of hormone per unit time has the opposite effect. Furthermore, changes in frequency or amplitude of hormone release are characteristic of some disease states; the diurnal rhythm of cortisol release is lost in the early phase of Cushing's disease, and pulsatile release of LHRH is blunted in anorexia nervosa. Understanding the rhythms by which hormones are released is essential for interpreting plasma hormone levels.

TRANSPORT Hormones are transported via lymph, blood, and extracellular fluids to sites of cellular action and ultimately of metabolic inactivation and degradation. The plasma is probably a passive diluent for most peptide and amine hormones, and this feature explains the short half-lives (3 to 7 min) of most nonglycosylated peptide hormones. [Glycoprotein hormones such as human chorionic gonadotropin (hCG) have longer half-lives.] The more insoluble a hormone in water, the more important the role of transport proteins; for example, thyroid and steroid hormones are transported largely in protein-bound form. However, no transport protein is the sole carrier of its hormone; for example, testosterone can be transported both by a specific binding protein [testosterone-binding globulin (TeBG); also called sex hormone–binding globulin (SHBG)] and by albumin; thyroxine can be transported both by prealbumin and by thyroxine-binding globulin (TBG). Protein-bound hormone (HP) cannot enter most cellular compartments and serves as a reservoir from which free hormone (H) is liberated for diffusion into intracellular compartments:

$$H + P \rightleftarrows HP$$

Distribution of bound and free hormone in plasma is determined by the amount of hormone, the amount of binding protein(s), and the binding affinity of hormone for the proteins. The relation between free and bound hormone is complex. First, the free (dialyzable) fraction in vitro is usually an underestimate of the actual free fraction in vivo, because hormone bound to weakly binding proteins, such as albumin (in contrast to that bound to high-affinity binding proteins), dissociates rapidly as the free fraction diffuses from the capillary; consequently, the albumin-bound hormone approximates the free fraction in some capillary beds. In tissues, such as liver, that clear hormone-transport protein complexes, free hormone levels have less impact on hormone uptake by the tissue.

Second, the distribution of hormones between plasma and tissue is a function of the balance between tissue binding proteins and plasma binding proteins. Therefore, free hormone levels may not reflect the amounts of hormone within cells.

Third, only the free hormone interacts with receptors in target cells and participates in the regulatory feedback control of hormone synthesis. As a consequence, changes in the amount of transport protein cannot cause endocrine pathology in the steady state, provided the remainder of the endocrine feedback loop is intact. For example, profound elevations or decreases in TBG (because of either genetic or other factors) are both compatible with a euthyroid state. To illustrate, an increase in TBG would lower the level of free (dialyzable) hormone and lower the amount bound to albumin; as a consequence, secretion of thyroid-stimulating hormone (TSH) would increase, and the output of thyroxine by the thyroid would increase *until* TBG again became saturated and the level of free hormone returned to the normal range, at which time TSH levels and the rate of thyroid hormone secretion also would return to normal. Likewise, a decrease in TBG would temporarily increase the level of free hormone, and TSH secretion and thyroxine output would fall until the free level returns to normal.

To summarize, a change in the level of a transport protein can cause profound alterations in total hormone levels but does not cause either hormone excess or deficiency of the hormone, provided the regulatory feedback mechanisms that control hormone synthesis are intact. However, alterations in the level of transport protein can cause endocrine pathology when hormone formation is not regulated by feedback control mechanisms or when feedback control mechanisms are deranged. For example, testosterone production in women is not regulated by testosterone levels, and alterations in TeBG levels in women can change the steady-state levels of free testosterone. Likewise, changes in TBG levels in a hypothyroid patient receiving a fixed dose of levothyroxine can cause alterations in free thyroxine levels.

DEGRADATION AND TURNOVER The plasma level (PL) of any hormone is dependent on the secretion rate (SR) of the hormone and the rates of metabolism and excretion, the so-called metabolic clearance rate (MCR):

$$PL = SR/MCR \quad \text{or} \quad SR = MCR \times PL$$

Metabolic clearance of hormones is accomplished by several mechanisms. Small amounts of hormones are excreted intact in urine or bile. The largest fraction is degraded and/or inactivated in target tissues and in the liver and kidneys. Peptide hormones are inactivated by proteases, largely in target tissues. Catabolism of steroid and thyroid hormone facilitates their excretion by rendering them soluble in urine or bile. Thyroid hormones are deiodinated, deaminated, and deconjugated largely by the liver. Steroid hormones are reduced, hydroxylated, and converted into water-soluble glucuronide and sulfate conjugates. Biliary conjugates may be hydrolyzed in the gastrointestinal tract and reabsorbed into the circulation. The degradative mechanisms for different hormones have one common feature, namely, that alternative pathways exist for the catabolism of all hormones described to date.

Because of the nature of feedback control of hormone secretion, changes in rates of hormone degradation alone, like changes in plasma protein binding, do not cause endocrine pathology, provided the feedback control mechanisms that regulate synthesis are intact. For example, in severe liver disease and in hypothyroidism, the degradation of glucocorticoids by the liver is impaired; as a consequence, the turnover of cortisol slows, but the plasma level does not rise above the normal range because secretion of ACTH is inhibited. Thus, a normal level of free hormone is maintained by a decrease in the rate of cortisol secretion. The opposite is the case when glucocorticoid degradation is enhanced (as in thyrotoxicosis); in this situation, cortisol secretion increases to keep the level of the hormone normal.

Although changes in hormone degradation rates alone do not cause hormone deficit or excess, they can alter endocrine pharmacology. For example, ordinary doses of glucocorticoids can cause Cushing's syndrome when glucocorticoid metabolism is impaired by hypothyroidism or liver disease, and consequently glucocorticoid dosage must be reduced appropriately in both states. Likewise, doses of glucocorticoids may have to be increased in patients with hyperthyroidism. In addition, the development of hyperthyroidism in a patient with inadequate adrenal reserve can precipitate an adrenal crisis by accelerating glucocorticoid metabolism. Thus, when the normal control mechanisms that regulate hormone synthesis are circumvented or inoperative, changes in rates of hormone degradation can cause or aggravate pathology.

REGULATION OF HORMONE PRODUCTION

As stated above, hormone levels are determined primarily by the rates of formation. A unifying feature of all endocrine systems is the fact that the production of most hormones is regulated directly or indirectly by the metabolic activity of the hormone itself. This regulation is accomplished through a series of negative (and positive) feedback loops (Fig. 327-1). For example, hormones produced under the control of pituitary trophic hormones (cortisol, thyroxine, gonadal steroids) feed back on the hypothalamic-pituitary system to regulate their own rates of secretion. Similarly, the secretion of parathyroid hormone and insulin is controlled by feedback signals from serum calcium and glucose levels, respectively. When the hormone itself acts as the direct regulator of feedback (testosterone on the hypothalamic-pituitary axis), the effect is mediated by the same receptor system by which the hormone acts in other target tissues. An example of positive feedback is the stimulation of LH release by estradiol prior to ovulation. Nonhormonal and environmental factors can alter both positive and negative feedback control mechanisms or the response to such control.

Most feedback control systems operate within minutes or hours in response to varying metabolic demands to maintain homeostatic control within a narrow range. The main exceptions relate to spermatogenesis (see Chap. 336). Spermatogenesis and sperm export require approximately 2.5 months from initiation of differentiation to ejaculation of mature sperm, so that changes in FSH levels may not alter the numbers of sperm in the ejaculate for long periods.

The fact that the secretion of hormones is under regulatory control has important clinical implications. First, the plasma levels of hormones may be interpretable only if the appropriate regulatory factors are taken into account (Fig. 327-2). The meaning of a borderline-low plasma thyroxine level may be clear only when TSH is measured simultaneously; likewise, plasma insulin and parathyroid hormone levels may be interpretable only in conjunction with simultaneous measurements of plasma glucose and calcium, respectively. Second, the finding of simultaneous elevation of a hormone pair (or of a hormone and its regulatory factor) in the absence of evidence of hormone excess suggests the presence of a hormone-resistance state. For example, simultaneous elevation of plasma glucose and insulin is characteristic of insulin resistance, and simultaneous elevation of LH and testosterone suggests androgen resistance. In contrast, simultaneous elevation of hormone pairs with signs of hormone excess suggests a hormone-secreting tumor. Third, the fact that hormone secretion is under regulatory control is the basis for the various dynamic tests of hormone reserve and hormone secretion for the evaluation of subtle derangements of endocrine pathology (see below).

MECHANISMS OF HORMONE ACTION

In some instances, the first step in hormone action is the metabolism of the circulating hormone into its active form, either in plasma (as in the formation of angiotensin II from angiotensin), in target tissues

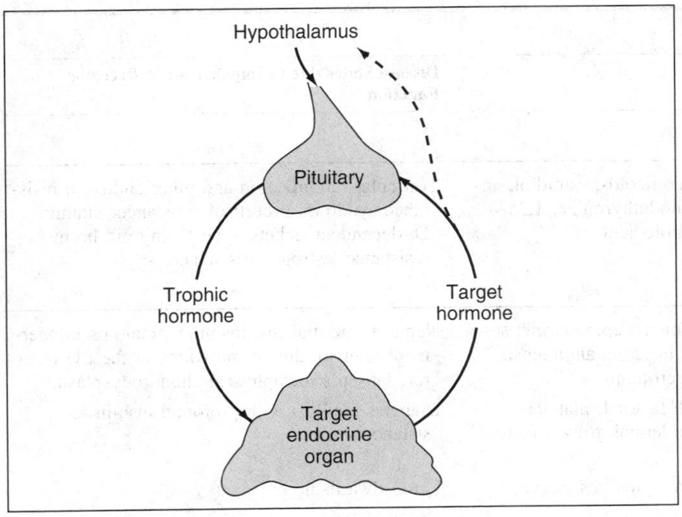

FIGURE 327-1 Feedback control of target endocrine organs such as the adrenal, thyroid, or gonads by the pituitary.

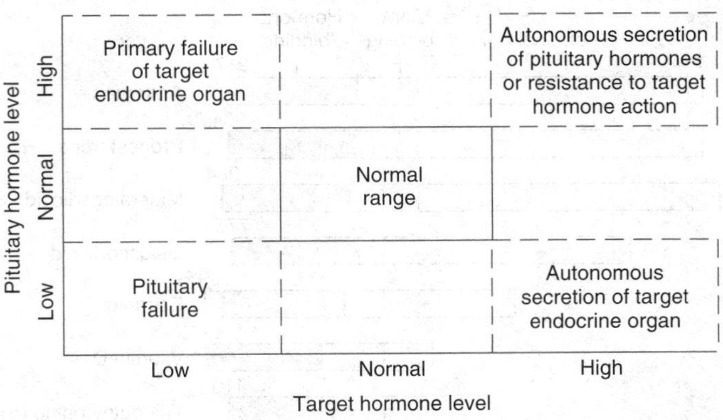

FIGURE 327-2 Relation between target hormone level and trophic hormone level in normal and disease states (e.g., TSH and thyroid hormones, ACTH and cortisol, LH and testosterone).

(as in the conversion of testosterone to dihydrotestosterone), or in secondary tissues for retransport back into plasma (as in the conversion of thyroxine to triiodothyronine and of testosterone to estradiol). All hormones then act by binding to receptors that are located either intracellularly or in the cell membrane.

INTRACELLULAR RECEPTORS Most intracellular hormones gain access to cell cytoplasm by what is believed to be a passive diffusion mechanism down an activity gradient and then bind to a specific receptor protein to form a hormone-receptor complex (Fig. 327-3). The hormone-receptor complex, which can either form in the cytoplasm and move into the nucleus or form within the nucleus itself, has the capacity to attach to specific regulatory sequences in DNA (so-called hormone regulatory elements) and acts to control the rate of RNA transcription from genes under the control of these regulatory elements. As the result, the synthesis of messenger RNA (mRNA) is either increased or decreased, and the synthesis of cytoplasmic proteins that mediate the effects of the hormone increases or decreases.

The receptors of this class bear a striking sequence homology to each other, suggesting that they evolved from a common ancestral transcription regulatory factor. Each contains a hormone-binding domain, a DNA-binding domain, and an *N*-terminal variable or immunodominant domain (Fig. 327-4). More than one receptor exists for certain hormones (thyroid hormones, retinoic acid). The hormone-receptor complexes are believed to act as dimers, and additional transcription regulatory factors are involved in their control of RNA transcription. Elucidation of the structures of these receptors made it possible to analyze the mutations that impair hormone action and cause hormone-resistance syndromes (see below).

MEMBRANE-BOUND RECEPTORS Membrane-bound hormone receptors can be divided into several classes, each of which

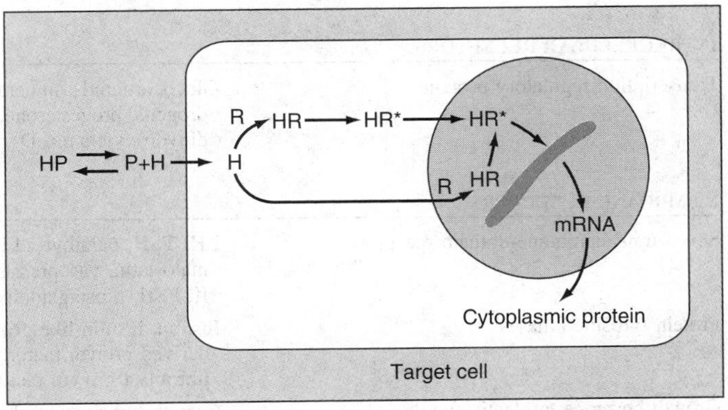

FIGURE 327-3 Mechanism of action of hormones with intracellular receptors. H, hormone; P, plasma transport protein; R, receptor; R*, activated receptor; mRNA, messenger RNA.

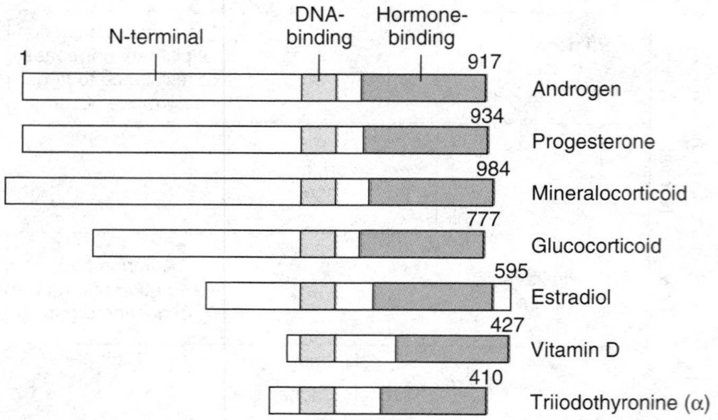

FIGURE 327-4 Intracellular receptors of the thyroid-steroid-retinoic acid class. The areas of greatest homology (DNA-binding domain) are shown by the light blue bars; the areas of intermediate homology (hormone-binding domain) are shown by the dark blue bars; and the areas with the least homology are shown by the open regions.

works by different mechanisms: seven-transmembrane-domain receptors, protein tyrosine kinase receptors, guanylyl cyclase receptors, and growth hormone/prolactin (cytokine family) receptors (Table 327-1 and Fig. 327-5).

Seven-Transmembrane-Domain Receptors This receptor family includes the α- and β-adrenergic receptors and receptors for parathyroid hormone, vasopressin, angiotensin II, glucagon, serotonin, dopamine, LH, FSH, TSH, and prostaglandins. Each of these receptors interacts within the plasma membrane with a member of another family of proteins, the guanine nucleotide–binding proteins (G proteins). The G protein family includes: G_s, which mediates adenyl cyclase stimulation; G_i, which mediates adenylyl cyclase inhibition; and G_q, which mediates phospholipase C activation. The G proteins are heterotrimers, composed of α, β, and γ subunits. The α subunits are unique to each G protein (some 15 different α subunits having been characterized), whereas the β and γ subunits of different G proteins are similar. The interaction of hormone-receptor complexes of this class with G proteins initiates reactions that cause the release of a variety of intracellular second messenger molecules that influence cellular metabolism. The classic second messenger is cyclic adenosine monophosphate (cyclic AMP), and many hormone actions are mediated by effects on adenylyl cyclase to increase or decrease cellular cyclic AMP, including actions of epinephrine and norepinephrine (the β-adrenergic receptor), vasopressin (V_2 receptors), glucagon, ACTH, LH, FSH, and TSH. Other hormone-receptor interactions activate phospholipase C to increase free cytosolic calcium and enhance protein kinase C, including epinephrine and norepinephrine (α-adrenergic receptors), vasopressin (V_1 receptors), and angiotensin II.

Protein Tyrosine Kinases Receptors of this class include the insulin receptor and receptors for epidermal growth factor (EGF), insulin-like growth factor I, fibroblast growth factor, and platelet-derived growth factor. The insulin receptor is a tetramer composed of two α and two β subunits, which are linked by sulfhydryl bonds (Fig. 327-5). The α subunits are extracellular and contain the insulin binding site, and the β subunits have one transmembrane domain and exhibit insulin-dependent tyrosine kinase activity; autophosphorylation of tyrosine residues on the receptor enhances the tyrosine kinase activity and enables the enzyme to phosphorylate other proteins that are components of downstream signaling pathways. The tyrosine kinase activity is essential for insulin action, as evidenced by the fact that point mutations in the coding sequence of the receptor gene that impair kinase activity cause profound resistance to insulin action (see below).

Receptors for Growth Hormone and Prolactin (the Cytokine Receptor Family) Receptors of this type do not have kinase domains, but ligand binding results in the rapid phosphorylation of tyrosine residues on the receptors themselves and on cellular proteins. This tyrosine phosphorylation is mediated by a family of cytoplasmic tyrosine kinases, the Janus kinases (JAK) (Fig. 327-5), which associate physically with intracellular domains of the receptors and are themselves activated to phosphorylate *s*ignal *t*ransducers and *a*ctivators of *t*ranscription (STATs), which mediate the actions of the hormones. The high-affinity growth hormone–binding protein in plasma corresponds to the extracellular hormone-binding domain of the growth hormone receptor and is believed to be cleaved from the receptor, but the role of the plasma protein in the regulation of growth is undefined. The growth hormone receptor has approximately 25 percent homology with the prolactin receptor, which suggests that the two receptors have evolved from a common ancestral gene. Mutations that impair the function of the growth hormone receptor are responsible for Laron dwarfism (see below).

Guanylyl Cyclase Receptors The receptor for atrial natriuretic peptide (ANP) is a guanylyl cyclase that spans the plasma membrane; the extracellular domain of the receptor binds the hormone, and the intracellular domain synthesizes guanosine-3′,5′-monophosphate (cyclic GMP) which serves as the second messenger for the hormone. The mechanism(s) by which cyclic GMP mediates the actions of ANP are not known, but in some cells cyclic GMP acts to maintain cation channels in an open configuration.

Table 327-1

Classification of Hormone Receptors

Type	Characteristic Hormones	Disease States due to Impairment of Receptor Function
INTRACELLULAR RECEPTORS		
Transcription regulatory proteins	Glucocorticoids, mineralocorticoids, estradiol, androgens, progesterone, triiodothyronine, 1,25-dihydroxyvitamin D, retinoic acid	Testicular feminization and other androgen resistance syndromes; cortisol resistance; vitamin D–dependent rickets, type II; thyroid hormone resistance; estrogen resistance
MEMBRANE RECEPTORS		
Seven-transmembrane-domain receptors	LH, TSH, parathyroid hormone, epinephrine, somatostatin, vasopressin, glucagon, angiotensin II, FSH, prostaglandins, serotonin	Nephrogenic diabetes insipidus, male pseudohermaphroditism due to mutations of the LH receptor, Jansen's metaphyseal chondrodysplasia
Protein tyrosine kinases	Insulin, insulin-like growth factor I, platelet-derived growth factor, epidermal growth factor, fibroblast growth factor	Diabetes mellitus with profound insulin resistance
Growth hormone–prolactin family	Growth hormone, prolactin, cytokines, nerve growth factor	Laron dwarfism
Guanylate cyclase	Atrial natriuretic peptide	—

Endocrinopathy can result from hormone deficiency, hormone excess, resistance to hormone action, or constititutive mutations that activate hormone response systems in the absence of ligand; abnormalities in more than one endocrine system may coexist in the same individual.

DEFICIENCY STATES With few exceptions (calcitonin), hormone deficiency results in pathologic manifestations. The investigation of clinical deficiency states played an important role in the evolution of the discipline of endocrinology. Recognition of the effects of hormone deficiency was followed by extraction of the responsible hormone from normal endocrine tissues, characterization of the chemical nature of the molecule (and, ultimately, organic synthesis of it), and administration of the hormone to replace the deficit. The treatment of hypothyroidism by the administration of thyroid hormone is probably as successful as any therapeutic measure in medicine. Because clinical deficiency states can be induced in experimental animals by destruction or removal of the endocrine organ, an enormous amount is known about the pathophysiology of deficiency states, such as diabetes mellitus, pituitary and adrenal insufficiency, hypothyroidism, and hypogonadism.

The destructive processes that cause failure of the endocrine organs are also understood in many instances and include infections (as in adrenal insufficiency due to tuberculosis), tissue death due to infarction (as in postpartum pituitary failure) or inflammation (as in diabetes mellitus secondary to pancreatitis), tumors (as in null cell tumors of the pituitary), autoimmune processes that either destroy endocrine organs (as in Hashimoto's thyroiditis) or block the binding of trophic hormones (as in idiopathic hypothyroidism), dietary inadequacy (as in hypothyroidism due to iodine deficiency), and hereditary defects in hormone synthesis (as in pituitary dwarfism). In type I diabetes mellitus, the cause may be a hereditary predisposition that renders the pancreas subject to destruction by several mechanisms (see Chap. 334). In some instances (congenital anorchia) the etiology of the defect is unknown.

HORMONE EXCESS With few exceptions (testosterone in men, progesterone in men and women) hormone excess causes pathologic effects. Four general types of hormone excess are recognized. In one, the hormone is overproduced by the gland that is the usual site of its production (hyperthyroidism, acromegaly, Cushing's disease). In this situation, excess hormone production is due to failure or circumvention of the feedback mechanisms that control normal production and can arise by several mechanisms, including autoantibodies that mimic the action of natural hormones (as in the case of thyroid-stimulating immunoglobulins in hyperthyroidism), mutations in receptor-effector mechanisms that impair feedback (as in mutation of G proteins in growth-hormone secreting pituitary adenomas), and development of tumors of uncertain provenance (such as Leydig cell tumors). A second type of hormone excess results when a hormone is produced by a tissue (usually malignant) that does not synthesize it ordinarily (for example, ACTH production by oat cell carcinoma of the lung, thyroid hormone secretion by struma ovarii). A third type of hormone excess involves the overproduction of hormones in peripheral tissues from circulating precursors, for example, overproduction of estrogen in liver disease because of diversion of the precursor androstenedione from its usual sites of catabolism in the liver to sites of extraglandular estrogen formation. Finally, hormone excess all too commonly results from iatrogenic causes (as in the complications resulting from glucocorticoid therapy; see Chap. 332) or from self-administration of hormones such as levothyroxine or insulin.

An excess of a given hormone may result from more than one cause. Thyrotoxicosis can result from overproduction of hormone by the thyroid as a result of overproduction of TSH (rare), from the action of thyroid-stimulating immunoglobulins on the thyroid, from autonomous thyroid hyperfunction, from leakage of preformed hormone due to an inflammatory injury of the thyroid, or from excess hormone arising from sources other than the thyroid itself, as in thyroid hormone overdosage, accidental ingestion of meats contaminated with thyroid tissue, or secretion by struma ovarii (see Chap. 331). The unraveling of the cause of specific hormone-excess states can be one of the most challenging problems of clinical endocrinology.

PRODUCTION OF ABNORMAL HORMONES In some instances abnormal hormones cause endocrine disease. One form of diabetes mellitus is the result of a single-gene mutation that results in the production of an abnormal insulin molecule that is ineffective because of defective binding to the insulin receptor. In other cases, hormone precursors, hormone subunits, or incompletely processed peptide hormones may be released into the circulation, as is common in so-called ectopic hormone production of neoplasia. Alternatively, immunoglobulins may bind to hormone receptors and thus exert hormonal actions, as is the case with the thyroid-stimulating immunoglobulins that exert TSH-like actions in hyperthyroidism (see Chap. 331) or the antibodies to the insulin receptor that have insulin-like actions (see Chap. 334).

HORMONE RESISTANCE The concept that an endocrinopathy can result because the tissues cannot respond to normal (or increased) levels of a hormone evolved from the deduction that pseudohypoparathyroidism is due to peripheral resistance to the action of parathyroid hormone (see Chap. 354). Diseases are now known to result from resistance to most hormones. Such hormone-resistance states frequently are due to mutations that impair hormone action, but they can be due to acquired defects in receptors and postreceptor effector mechanisms for hormones, to development of antibodies that block hormones or hormone receptors, or to the absence of target cells. Abnormalities of receptors also cause disease outside the endocrine domain, including familial hypercholesterolemia. Hormone resistance is not always the same in all tissues; selective resistance to thyroid hormone

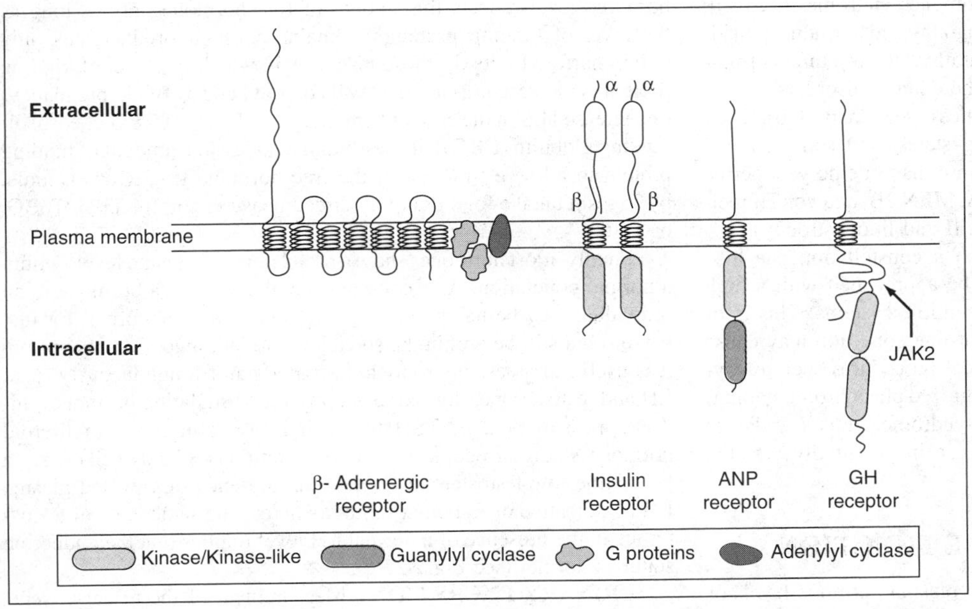

FIGURE 327-5 Schematic representation of different classes of hormone receptors on the cell surface. Seven-transmembrane-domain receptor (β-adrenergic receptor); protein tyrosine kinases (insulin receptor); guanylate cyclase receptor [atrial natriuretic peptide (ANP) receptor]; growth hormone-prolactin receptor family [growth hormone (GH) receptor].

can be restricted to the pituitary itself, and androgen resistance may be more severe in the testis than in other target tissues.

A common feature of hormone-resistance states is the presence of a normal or *elevated* level of the hormone in the circulation despite deficient hormone action. This feature is a consequence of the fact that hormones are normally under regulatory feedback control and that failure of hormone action leads to increased hormone production.

The elucidation of the structures of hormone receptors and the cloning of the cDNAs for these proteins has made it possible to define the molecular defects in many hormone-resistance states (Table 327-1). Several clinical implications of these studies are apparent. First, in the past it was only possible to identify receptor defects that caused profound hormone resistance, but now that subtle defects in receptor function can be identified, it is clear that hormone resistance is more common than previously recognized. Second, at the molecular level, disorders are genetically heterogeneous. Unrelated families with mutations of the insulin receptor, the growth hormone receptor, or the androgen receptor rarely have identical mutations. Furthermore, in regard to individual receptors such as the androgen receptor, mutations may be due to gross deletions or gene rearrangements that completely disrupt the coding sequence, but more commonly they are due to point mutations that cause single amino acid substitutions in the protein or create premature termination codons. It is thus necessary to analyze each family separately. Third, the analysis of these mutations has provided major insight into hormone action—for example, establishing the critical importance of the tyrosine kinase function of the insulin receptor and making it possible to define the various domains of the intracellular receptors.

GAIN-OF-FUNCTION MUTATIONS Mutations that cause constitutive activity of hormone receptors or cause hormone receptors to lose ligand-binding specificity can cause the manifestations of hormone excess even when the hormone itself is undetectable. For example, mutations that cause constitutive activation of the LH receptor cause testitoxicosis, the most common cause of premature puberty in boys, and mutations of the androgen receptor in advanced prostatic cancer may allow activation of the receptor by ligands that would normally be ineffective.

DISEASES AFFECTING MULTIPLE ENDOCRINE SYSTEMS The fact that disorders can affect more than one endocrine system has been known since the description of panhypopituitarism in the nineteenth century. Such disorders have diverse causes, including autoimmunity [as in polyglandular autoimmune syndromes (PGAs)], receptor abnormalities (as in resistance to parathyroid hormone, gonadotropins, and thyrotropin in pseudohypoparathyroidism), tumors [multiple endocrine neoplasia (MEN)], and hereditary disorders of unknown etiology (such as the lipodystrophies) (see Chap. 340). They include both hypo- and hyperfunctioning states, and some clinical syndromes may occur in the context of more than one polyendocrine state (e.g., pheochromocytoma in MEN 2A, MEN 2B, and von Hippel-Lindau disease; diabetes mellitus in PGA II and lipodystrophy).

Because each endocrinopathy in such a constellation can also occur alone, all endocrine patients must be approached with a high index of suspicion for abnormalities of multiple systems. This is of particular importance because treatment of one condition may cause worsening of another (for example, surgical procedures such as thyroidectomy can cause worsening of unrecognized pheochromocytoma) and because in certain of the familial syndromes it is mandatory to make systematic searches for the disease in potentially affected family members.

ASSESSMENT OF ENDOCRINE FUNCTION

Endocrine status is assessed by measuring plasma hormone levels or the urinary excretion of hormones or hormone metabolites, measuring hormone reserve and regulation by dynamic tests, measuring the levels of hormone receptors, assessing hormone actions in target tissues, or performing appropriate combinations of these tests.

MEASUREMENT OF PLASMA HORMONE LEVELS The plasma levels of steroid and thyroid hormones range between 1 nmol/L and 1 μmol/L, while those of peptide hormones are generally in the range of 1 pmol/L to 0.1 nmol/L. The application of chemical, chromatographic, bioassay, radioreceptor, radioimmunoassay, and immunometric techniques for the assessment of plasma levels has made clinical endocrinology one of the most quantitative of clinical disciplines. In the case of hormones whose plasma levels are relatively constant from moment to moment and day to day (such as thyroxine and triiodothyronine), single hormone level measurements provide a reliable assessment of the hormone status in most clinical situations.

In the case of hormones that undergo pulsatile secretion (such as LH or testosterone), a single value may not be representative of mean plasma levels. In such instances it is necessary either to measure levels in several samples drawn at random or to pool aliquots of three or more samples of plasma drawn at 20- to 30-min intervals for a single determination.

When plasma levels undergo a characteristic, predictable fluctuation, such as the diurnal variation of plasma cortisol, the timing of plasma sampling must be designed to provide a useful index of the hormone status. In women, appropriate interpretation of plasma levels of gonadotropins, progesterone, and estradiol during the reproductive years requires knowledge of the phase of the ovulatory and menstrual cycles in which the measurement was made, and it may be necessary to obtain sequential samples over many days to provide interpretable data. Seasonal variations also occur in the levels of certain hormones (such as thyroxine and testosterone), but these changes are generally so small that they do not affect the interpretation of individual values. In some situations, variation in hormone levels is not the result of any obvious rhythmicity but rather the consequence of waxing and waning of a disease process; repeated measurements of cortisol or of calcium and parathyroid hormone levels over many months may be necessary to establish the diagnosis of Cushing's syndrome or of hyperparathyroidism.

In the case of steroids, thyroid hormones, and some peptide hormones, such as growth hormone, that are transported in plasma largely bound to proteins, measurement of total hormone concentration provides an index of endocrine status *only* to the extent that it allows the level of the free or unbound hormone to be deduced. Methods for directly measuring the level of free hormone (usually 1 percent or less of the total level) are available for some of these hormones. Since the amount of free hormone is a function of the amount and binding affinity of the transport proteins and the amount of hormone, the total hormone level reflects the amount of free hormone only as long as the level of binding protein(s) remains constant or fluctuates only within narrow limits. In those instances in which the level of binding protein is increased (as are the levels of TBG and TeBG in pregnancy) or decreased [as in the case of hereditary low levels of TBG or cortisol-binding globulin (CBG)], it is essential to assess the amount of binding protein to allow estimation of the free hormone level (for example, by T_3 resin uptake for TBG or by direct measurement for TBG, TeBG, or CBG).

Finally, most hormones show a broad range of plasma levels within a normal population. As a consequence, the level of a hormone in an individual may be halved or doubled (and thus be abnormal for that person) but still be within the so-called normal range. For this reason, it is useful to assess appropriate hormone pairs simultaneously (e.g., LH and testosterone, thyroxine and thyroid-stimulating hormone); indeed, measurement of TSH by itself is a useful index of thyroid hormone status in people with normal pituitary glands. Likewise, a borderline low testosterone level in the presence of elevated plasma LH is indicative of testicular failure, whereas the same level of testosterone in the presence of a normal LH level implies that the endocrine status is normal (see Fig. 327-2).

URINARY EXCRETION Measurement of the urinary excretion rate of a hormone or a hormone metabolite that reflects plasma levels or secretory rates offers certain advantages over the measurement of isolated plasma levels; for example, urinary excretion reflects the average of the plasma levels over the time of collection. Thus, a 24-h urine free cortisol value may provide a better estimate of the function of the adrenal cortex than isolated measurements of plasma cortisol. Such measurements do have the following limitations, however.

1. Urinary creatinine should be measured routinely to document the adequacy of the urine collection. Women excrete on average about 1 g/d of creatinine, and men, about 1.8 g/d. The day-to-day variation in this quantity should not exceed 20 percent.
2. The amounts of individual metabolites in urine may not reflect changes in hormone secretion under all conditions. For example, the formation of the 18-oxo derivative of aldosterone may be influenced by drugs that do not alter secretion or plasma levels of the hormone.
3. Urine values are obviously meaningless for those hormones (thyroxine, triiodothyronine) that are excreted into bile. Peptide hormones such as gonadotropins may be metabolized differently in different individuals before being excreted in the urine, so that establishment of the range of normal is difficult.
4. Hormones from more than one source may be excreted as a given metabolite; urinary 17-ketosteroids are derived from both adrenal and gonadal androgens, and consequently their measurement is of little value in assessing testicular androgen production in men.
5. Changes in renal function may influence rates of hormone excretion into urine. Such changes can in part be corrected for by measurement of urine creatinine, but in the case of metabolites or conjugates formed in the kidney itself excretion patterns may be distorted out of proportion to the decrease in creatinine clearance.

DYNAMIC TESTS OF HORMONE RESERVE AND REGULATION When hypo- or hyperfunction is severe, measurement of the level of hormone in blood or urine may be satisfactory for making a diagnosis, particularly when the tests demonstrate appropriate feedback relationships; for example, low plasma testosterone coupled with high plasma LH indicates primary testicular failure. In less clear-cut instances, however, stimulation tests are useful in establishing the significance of borderline-low values. Likewise, suppression tests are used to demonstrate the presence of hyperfunction of endocrine systems. All such dynamic tests are designed to take advantage of the known feedback control mechanisms for various hormones (Fig. 327-1).

Two types of *stimulation tests* are in common use. In one, endogenous hormone production or action is blocked (e.g., cortisol production by metyrapone, estradiol action by clomiphene), and the capacity of the pituitary to respond by increasing endogenous production of the trophic hormone, and/or the capacity of the target tissue to respond, are then assessed; ideally, such tests measure the integrity of the hypothalamic-pituitary-target tissue loop. In the other type of stimulation test, the trophic hormone itself is administered under some standardized regimen, and the capacity of the target tissue to respond is determined (as in measurement of cortisol levels before and after ACTH administration). Stimulation tests are particularly useful in four situations: (1) in assessing hormone status when precise quantification of plasma levels is difficult or imperfect (as for ACTH), (2) in assessing endocrine status when static tests give borderline-low values, (3) in distinguishing primary from secondary (pituitary) causes of endocrine failure, and (4) in assessing gonadal reserve in prepubertal subjects in whom plasma levels of gonadotropins and gonadal steroids are difficult to interpret.

Suppression tests are useful for the diagnosis of endocrine hyperfunction, because, by definition, hyperfunctioning glands do not operate under normal control mechanisms. The suppression of endocrine function can be either quantitatively or qualitatively abnormal. For example, the feedback control of the pituitary may be reset to respond to high levels of the suppressing hormone (pituitary ACTH secretion in Cushing's disease), or secretion can be completely autonomous (ACTH secretion by carcinoma of the lung). In principle, the feedback regulator is administered, and the degree of inhibition of hormone secretion is assessed (e.g., by the change in radioactive iodine uptake after administration of thyroid hormones, the change in cortisol secretion after the administration of potent exogenous glucocorticoids, or the suppressibility of plasma growth hormone by glucose).

The clinical usefulness of all dynamic tests is limited by the fact that endocrine control systems are subject to influence by a multitude of secondary factors. Age, coexisting disease states, and concurrent drug regimens all interact to influence responsiveness and hence to limit the diagnostic specificity of such tests. For example, psychiatric disorders such as endogenous depression can impair responses to endocrine dynamic tests in the absence of specific endocrine pathology.

HORMONE RECEPTORS AND ANTIBODIES The measurement of hormone receptors in biopsy material from target tissues or in fibroblasts propagated from biopsy material is useful—for example, in the diagnosis of partial hormone-resistance states such as rickets due to vitamin D resistance, hyperglycemia and hyperinsulinemia associated with insulin resistance, and male pseudohermaphroditism due to androgen resistance. Certain laboratories can apply the techniques of molecular biology to provide specific information about the structure of mutant receptors. Likewise, measurement of antibodies to hormones (such as antibodies to thyroid hormones that can cause hypothyroidism) or antibodies to target tissues (adrenal gland, gonads, thyroid) may be essential for the assessment of endocrine status. With certain exceptions (e.g., assays for antibodies to thyroid tissue), these tests are not widely available.

TISSUE EFFECTS At the theoretical level, the ideal means of assessing endocrine function is to measure the result of hormone action in target tissues for the hormone. Such an assay would provide insight into hormone levels, hormone receptors, second messengers, and tissue responses. For example, demonstration of the capacity to concentrate urine maximally following water restriction indicates that the hypothalamic mechanisms that control the function of the posterior pituitary are intact, that the posterior pituitary has a normal capacity to secrete vasopressin, that the vasopressin receptor is intact, and that the postreceptor effector mechanisms for the hormone are operative. Ideally, such a test assesses the function of the entire pathway of hormone secretion and action. In practice, many such tests are imperfect. For example, even if vasopressin secretion is normal, intrinsic renal disease can cause a fixed low urine osmolality and thus distort the interpretation of the functional test of vasopressin action. In other instances, such tests are difficult to perform and subject both to artifacts and to influences from diverse parameters (for example, the metabolic rate is increased by fever even when thyroid function is normal). For these reasons, the identification of additional specific tissue markers for hormone action would be very useful.

IMAGING PROCEDURES Developments in imaging have made possible the noninvasive identification of abnormalities in almost every endocrine organ, including visualization of small lesions of the pituitary and hypothalamus, bone density assessments for metabolic bone disease, and localization of functioning parathyroid tissue in patients with persistent or recurrent hyperparathyroidism.

A major problem in imaging stems from the fact that small nodules of no functional significance are known from autopsy studies to occur in the pituitary, the adrenal, and, less commonly, the testes. The natural history of these nonfunctioning adenomas is not well understood; most appear to remain limited in size and nonfunctional for life, but in rare instances they evolve into autonomous and/or hyperfunctioning tumors. In addition, malignancies—both metastatic and primary—can occur in these tissues. As a consequence, adrenal and pituitary masses are common incidental findings in computed tomography (CT) and magnetic resonance imaging (MRI) scans performed for other reasons. Several types of criteria have been proposed for deciding whether a mass of the pituitary or adrenal is likely to be benign or should be removed. By one guideline, solid, endocrinologically silent lesions of the adrenal smaller than 3.5 cm may be followed safely with serial CT scans, whereas larger lesions deserve sonographically guided percutaneous needle biopsy or exploratory surgery. Additional experience will be required to establish the validity of these and other criteria for the assessment of such masses.

Another unresolved issue stems from the fact that it is not always clear which imaging procedure is best in a given clinical situation. In many instances, evidence has accumulated for the superiority of one or the other imaging procedure in a given situation. In other instances, definitive guidelines may be harder to develop, as in the choice between MRI and CT for delineation of the anatomy of the hypothalamic-pituitary system. In some patients, small lesions are best seen with MRI, whereas in others, lesions in the same areas—equally small and with similar histologic features—are better delineated with CT. In consequence, there is a tendency in the workup of suspected pituitary tumors to order both procedures routinely. Although this practice is justified in some cases, it inflates the cost of diagnostic workups.

An unexpected dividend of the developments in imaging is that it is now possible to chart the natural history of endocrine disease in a different way, as in the occasional documentation of hemorrhage into a pituitary tumor that eventuates in development of the empty sella syndrome or the uncovering of a functioning adrenal adenoma when biochemical or clinical evidence of Cushing's disease is minimal.

BIBLIOGRAPHY

BERRIDGE MJ: Inositol triphosphate and calcium signalling. Nature 361:315, 1993

BELLDEGRUN A et al: Incidentally discovered mass of the adrenal gland. Surg Gynecol Obstet 163:203, 1986

DOHLMAN HG et al: Model systems for the study of seven transmembrane segment receptors. Annu Rev Biochem 60:653, 1991

EXTON JH: Signalling through phosphatidyl choline breakdown. J Biol Chem 265:1, 1990

GODOWSKI PG et al: Characterization of the human growth hormone receptor gene and demonstration of a partial gene deletion in two patients with Laron-type dwarfism. Proc Natl Acad Sci USA 86:8083, 1989

GORDEN P, WEINTRAUB BD: Radioreceptor and other functional hormone assays, in *Williams Textbook of Endocrinology*, 8th ed, JD Wilson, DW Foster (eds). Philadelphia, Saunders, 1992, pp 1647–1661

GRIFFIN JE: Dynamic tests of endocrine function, in *Williams Textbook of Endocrinology*, 8th ed, JD Wilson, DW Foster (eds). Philadelphia, Saunders, 1992, pp 1663–1670

HAMPER UM et al: Primary adrenocortical carcinoma: Sonographic evaluation with clinical and pathologic correlation in 26 patients. Am J Roentgenol 148:915, 1987

KAHN CR, GOLDSTEIN BJ: Molecular defects in insulin action. Science 245:13, 1989

MENDELSON CR: Mechanisms of hormone action, in *Textbook of Endocrine Physiology*, 3d ed, JE Griffin, SR Ojeda (eds). New York, Oxford, 1996, pp 29–66

PARDRIDGE WM: Serum bioavailability of sex steroid hormones. Clin Endocrinol Metab 15:259, 1986

PEKARY AE, HERSHMAN JM: Hormone assays, in *Endocrinology and Metabolism*, 3d ed, P Felig et al (eds). New York, McGraw-Hill, 1995, p 201

QUIGLEY CA et al: Androgen receptor defects: Historical, clinical and molecular perspectives. Endocr Rev 16:271, 1991

REFETOFF S et al: The syndromes of resistance to thyroid hormone. Endocr Rev 14:348, 1993

TAYLOR SL et al: Mutations in the insulin receptor gene. Endocr Rev 13:566, 1992

TSAI MJ et al: Molecular mechanisms of action of steroid/thyroid receptor superfamily members. Annu Rev Biochem 63:451, 1994

328

Beverly M.K. Biller, Gilbert H. Daniels

NEUROENDOCRINE REGULATION AND DISEASES OF THE ANTERIOR PITUITARY AND HYPOTHALAMUS

The pituitary, appropriately titled the *master gland*, produces six major hormones and stores an additional two hormones (Fig. 328-1). Growth hormone (GH) regulates growth and has important influences on intermediary metabolism (see Chap. 329). Prolactin (PRL) is necessary for lactation (see Chap. 338). Luteinizing hormone (LH) and follicle-stimulating hormone (FSH) control the gonads in men and women. Thyroid-stimulating hormone (TSH, thyrotropin) regulates thyroid function. Adrenocorticotropin (ACTH) controls glucocorticoid function of the adrenal cortex. These hormones are all synthesized in the anterior pituitary. Vasopressin (AVP; also called antidiuretic hormone, ADH) and oxytocin are produced in neurons of the hypothalamus and stored in the posterior lobe of the pituitary (see Chap. 330). AVP controls water conservation by the kidneys; oxytocin is necessary for milk let-down during lactation and may aid in parturition.

A feedback relationship exists between the anterior pituitary and its three target endocrine glands—the gonads, the adrenal cortex, and the thyroid. When the gonads fail or are removed, the concentrations of LH and FSH rise, a condition known as *primary hypogonadism*. When the adrenal cortex is removed or destroyed, *primary adrenal insufficiency* (Addison's disease) results, and the serum ACTH concentration increases. Thyroid failure results in the characteristic rise in TSH of *primary hypothyroidism*.

When the pituitary gland is removed or destroyed, loss of the trophic hormones results in *secondary* hypogonadism, adrenal insufficiency, or hypothyroidism. Growth hormone and prolactin function are also lost. The functions of AVP and oxytocin are not affected by destruction of the pituitary, provided their site of origin in the hypothalamus is intact.

The pituitary is, in turn, under the control of the hypothalamus, which produces a number of chemical mediators. These hormones are synthesized in the hypothalamus and enter the portal vascular system, which carries them through the pituitary stalk to the anterior lobe (Fig. 328-1). Interruption of the pituitary stalk is followed by reduction in the release of GH, LH, FSH, TSH, and ACTH from the anterior pituitary. This fact implies that stimulatory influences from the hypothalamus are necessary for release of these hormones. In contrast, the level of prolactin rises after interruption of the stalk, implying that the normal hypothalamic influence on prolactin secretion is inhibitory. The rise in prolactin secretion also indicates that stalk section does not lead to pituitary destruction. If the stalk section is not at too high a level, AVP and oxytocin release continue, principally from axons that terminate in the median eminence of the hypothalamus. With

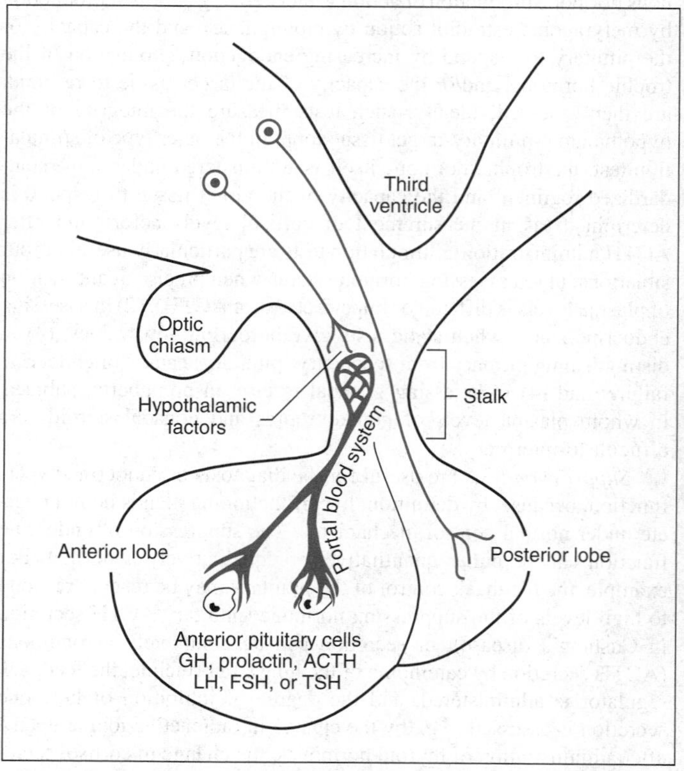

FIGURE 328-1 The relationship between the hypothalamus and the pituitary. See text for details.

Table 328-1

Anterior Pituitary and Hypophysiotropic Hormones

Pituitary Hormone	Hypophysiotropic Hormones: Name	Hypophysiotropic Hormones: Structure
Thyrotropin (TSH)	Thyrotropin-releasing hormone (TRH)	Tripeptide
Adrenocorticotropin (ACTH)	Corticotropin-releasing hormone (CRH)	41 amino acids
	Vasopressin (AVP)*	Peptide
Luteinizing hormone (LH)	Luteinizing hormone–releasing hormone (LHRH)	Decapeptide
Follicle-stimulating hormone (FSH)	LHRH	Decapeptide
Growth hormone (GH)	Growth hormone–releasing hormone (GHRH)	44 amino acids
	Growth hormone release–inhibiting hormone† (somatostatin, GIH)	14 amino acids
Prolactin	Prolactin release–inhibiting factor (PIF)	Dopamine
	Prolactin-releasing factor (PRF)‡	Peptide

* Other peptides are also important in ACTH release.
† Somatostatin also inhibits TRH-stimulated TSH release.
‡ TRH stimulates prolactin release.

hypothalamic ablation, the levels of GH, LH, FSH, TSH, ACTH, AVP, and oxytocin fall, whereas prolactin levels increase (Fig. 328-1).

Most hypothalamic factors that control secretion of the pituitary hormones are peptides (Table 328-1). Growth hormone–releasing hormone (GHRH) is the dominant influence on GH release, and somatostatin acts as an inhibitory hormone for GH release. Although LH and FSH levels vary independently in physiologic states, one releasing hormone [luteinizing hormone–releasing hormone (LHRH), also called gonadotropin-releasing hormone (GnRH)] plays a major role in controlling their release. Thyrotropin-releasing hormone (TRH) controls TSH release and also may influence prolactin release. Corticotropin-releasing hormone (CRH) and other factors control ACTH release. Dopamine acts as the major prolactin inhibitory factor (PIF).

Pituitary tumors may lead to hormonal over- or underproduction or may cause mechanical problems by impinging on neighboring structures. The most common syndromes produced by pituitary tumors are due to prolactin and GH excess. Prolactin excess leads to galactorrhea and/or hypogonadism; GH excess leads to gigantism and acromegaly. ACTH-secreting tumors produce Cushing's disease, and TSH-secreting tumors are a rare cause of hyperthyroidism. Paradoxically, gonadotropin-secreting tumors are most often associated with hypogonadism. Large pituitary tumors may cause partial or complete hypopituitarism by compression of the adjacent normal gland or pituitary stalk and are associated with visual field disturbances due to compression of the optic chiasm. Other neurologic disturbances occur if the tumor invades the cavernous sinuses or cranial fossae.

Hypothalamic disease may cause hypopituitarism, with the exception that secretion of prolactin may be increased. Diabetes insipidus due to AVP deficiency is virtually diagnostic of hypothalamic disease or of high interruption of the pituitary stalk. Disturbances of thirst, temperature regulation, appetite, and blood pressure may occur with hypothalamic disorders as well. Large hypothalamic masses may lead to visual field disturbances, obstruction of the third ventricle, and invasion of surrounding brain tissue.

ANATOMY AND EMBRYOLOGY

The pituitary gland (hypophysis) sits within the sella turcica ("Turkish saddle") of the sphenoid bone at the base of the skull and is composed principally of the anterior lobe (adenohypophysis) and posterior lobe (neurohypophysis). The intermediate lobe is rudimentary in humans. The normal adult pituitary gland weighs between 0.4 and 0.8 g.

The pituitary is separated from the brain by the diaphragma sella, an extension of the dura mater, and from the sphenoid sinus anteriorly and inferiorly by a thin layer of bone. The lateral walls of the sella abut on the cavernous sinuses, which contain the internal carotid arteries and cranial nerves III, IV, V, and VI. The optic chiasm is located slightly anterior to the pituitary stalk, just above the diaphragma sella. Thus, tumors of the pituitary may lead to visual field defects, to cranial nerve palsies, or to invasion of the sphenoid sinus (Fig. 328-2).

The hypothalamus extends anteriorly to the margin of the optic chiasm and posteriorly to include the mammillary bodies. Superiorly, the hypothalamic sulcus of the third ventricle separates the thalamus

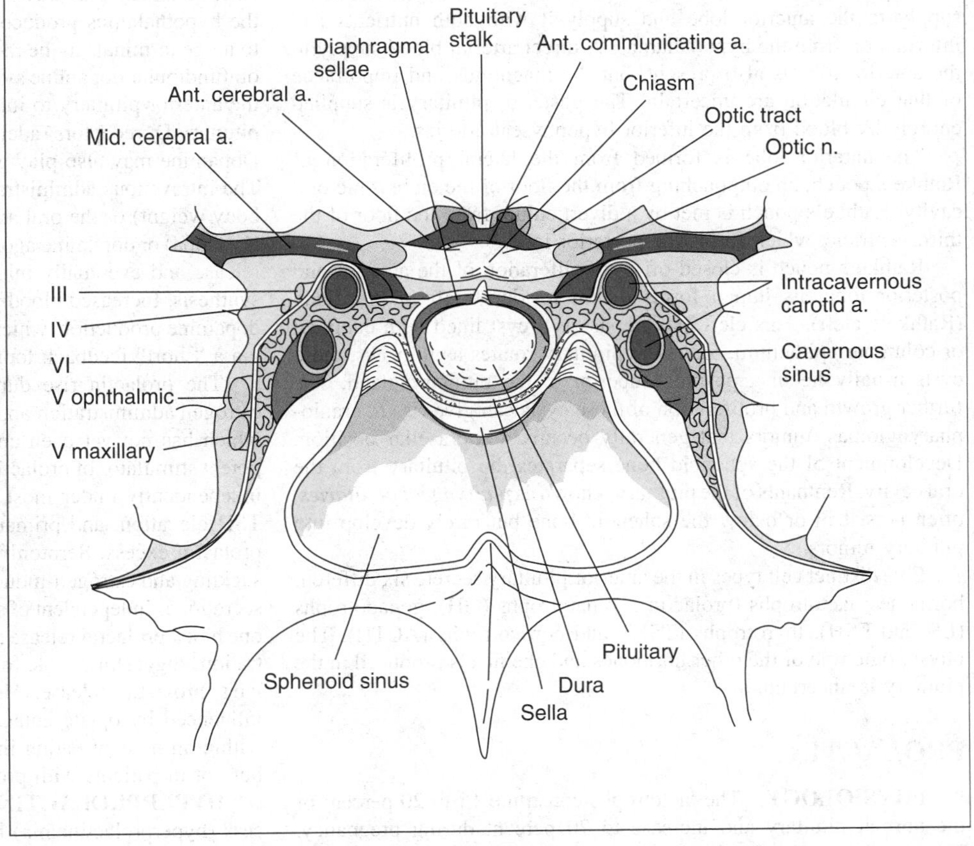

FIGURE 328-2 The relationship between the pituitary, the cranial nerves, and the cavernous sinus as viewed in a coronal section through the sella. *[From JA Taren, in Correlative Neurosurgery, 3d ed, RC Schneider et al (eds). Springfield, IL, Charles C Thomas, 1982.]*

from the hypothalamus. The rounded inferior base of the hypothalamus forms the tuber cinereum. The central portion of the base (termed the *infundibulum* or *median eminence*) is formed by the floor of the third ventricle and continues inferiorly to form the pituitary stalk. The releasing factors are synthesized in neurons situated along the margins of the third ventricle. They project fibers that terminate in the median eminence adjacent to the portal capillaries. The same releasing factors are produced by hypothalamic neurons that project to other parts of the brain.

The cell bodies of the supraoptic and paraventricular nuclei of the hypothalamus produce vasopressin and oxytocin, which travel down nerve axons in the supraopticohypophyseal and paraventriculohypophyseal tracts to reach the posterior lobe.

The communication between the hypothalamus and the anterior pituitary is chemical rather than physical. Releasing factors produced by hypothalamic neurons reach the anterior pituitary via the portal system to stimulate or inhibit hormone production. Some of the vasopressin-containing neurons also terminate in the median eminence, and vasopressin can stimulate release of ACTH and GH.

The anterior pituitary has the highest blood flow of any tissue in the body [0.8 (mL/g)/min]. The blood supply reaches the anterior pituitary by a circuitous route through the hypothalamus. Two derivatives of the internal carotid arteries, the superior hypophyseal arteries (SHA), branch in the subarachnoid space around the pituitary stalk and terminate in the capillary network of the median eminence. These capillaries have a fenestrated endothelium that allows easy access to the hypothalamic releasing hormones. Neurons containing vasoactive intestinal peptide (VIP) terminate on precapillary arterioles and may play a role in regulating blood flow. Transport of substances from the capillaries to the median eminence is also facilitated because the median eminence lies outside the blood-brain barrier. The capillaries then coalesce to form 6 to 10 straight veins known as the *hypothalamic-pituitary portal circulation*. These veins constitute the main blood supply to the anterior lobe and supply it with both nutrients and information from the hypothalamus. A direct arterial blood supply to the anterior lobe is also present, but the magnitude and importance of that circulation are uncertain. The posterior pituitary is supplied entirely by blood from the inferior hypophyseal arteries.

The anterior lobe is formed from the lateral proliferation of Rathke's pouch, an outpouching from the floor of the embryonic oral cavity. Rathke's pouch is met by a diverticulum from the floor of the third ventricle, which forms the posterior lobe.

Rathke's pouch is closed off by proliferation of the anterior and posterior lobe; its lumen forms a thin residual cleft in the gland (Rathke's cleft). This cleft may persist as a cyst lined with cuboidal or columnar epithelium. Since the pituitary rotates as it grows, these cysts usually lie in a position superior to the pituitary gland. The further growth and proliferation of these cysts can give rise to craniopharyngiomas, tumors that generally occupy a suprasellar position. Development of the sphenoid bone separates the pituitary from the oral cavity. Remnants of the pituitary, known as *pharyngeal pituitaries*, often persist in or below the sphenoid bone but rarely develop into pituitary tumors.

Five distinct cell types in the anterior pituitary secrete six different hormones: lactotrophs (prolactin), somatotrophs (GH), gonadotrophs (LH and FSH), thyrotrophs (TSH), and corticotrophs (ACTH). The physiologic role of the other hormones and chemicals produced in the pituitary is uncertain.

PROLACTIN

PHYSIOLOGY The lactotrophs constitute 15 to 20 percent of the normal pituitary and increase to 70 percent during pregnancy. These cells share many electrical characteristics with neurons. The prolactin gene on chromosome 6 codes for a precursor molecule that is larger than the circulating hormone. The predominant form of the processed hormone contains 198 amino acids (23,000 mol wt) in a single polypeptide chain containing three intrachain disulfide bonds. Higher-molecular-weight forms of prolactin represent dimers, polymers, aggregates, and protein-bound species. They may be present in small amounts in the circulation of normal persons and in larger amounts in patients with pituitary adenomas. These molecules have variable but generally decreased immunologic and biologic activity. The role of prolactin fragments and glycosylated forms is under investigation.

Prolactin is essential for lactation. Prolactin receptors are members of the cytokine receptor family and are found in breast, gonads, liver, kidney, and adrenal (see Chap. 327). Prolactin promotes breast cancer in rodents; a similar connection has not been established in human breast cancer (see Chap. 91). A possible role for prolactin in immune modulation has been suggested.

During pregnancy, increasing estrogen production stimulates the growth and replication of the pituitary lactotrophs and causes increased prolactin secretion. The pituitary doubles in size during pregnancy and returns to normal after delivery. Prolactin during pregnancy prepares the breast for postpartum lactation. High estrogen levels inhibit prolactin action at the breast, so that lactation does not commence until estrogen levels decline post partum. Prolactin levels rise in the fetus beginning at about 25 weeks, probably owing to maternal estrogen transfer and stimulation of the fetal pituitary. The level falls rapidly after delivery, reaching a nadir by 2 to 4 weeks post partum. High concentrations of prolactin are present in amniotic fluid, probably of both uterine and placental origin. The functional significance of this prolactin is unknown.

Under normal circumstances, prolactin secretion by the anterior pituitary is restrained by the hypothalamus. With hypothalamic destruction or pituitary stalk section, prolactin secretion increases, and serum concentrations rise. The release of prolactin from pituitary cells after stalk section in animals requires the autocrine release of VIP by pituitary cells. The major hypothalamic inhibitory factor for prolactin is dopamine, but peptide inhibitory factors such as endothelin and calcitonin may play a role. The arcuate and paraventricular nuclei of the hypothalamus produce dopamine; dopamine travels down axons to nerve terminals in the median eminence, where it is released (tuberoinfundibular dopamine system) into the portal circulation and reaches the anterior pituitary to inhibit prolactin release via interactions with pituitary D_2 receptors (adenylate cyclase–linked dopamine receptors). Dopamine may also play an important role in the posterior pituitary. The intravenous administration of dopamine (2 μg/min per kilogram body weight) or the oral administration of dopamine precursors (e.g., levodopa) or dopamine agonists (e.g., bromocriptine) inhibits prolactin release and eventually inhibits lactotrope proliferation and prolactin synthesis. Increased blood prolactin appears to increase hypothalamic dopamine production, which, in turn, partially inhibits prolactin release via a "short" feedback loop.

The prolactin rise during suckling, sleep, and stress and after estrogen administration appears to require a prolactin-releasing factor, which has not yet been conclusively identified. Although TRH is a potent stimulator of prolactin release, TSH and prolactin are controlled independently under most circumstances; lactation does not lead to TSH elevation, and primary hypothyroidism may or may not cause prolactin excess. Serotonin antagonists such as methysergide inhibit suckling and estrogen-induced prolactin increase, but resting prolactin secretion is independent of serotonin. Opiate antagonists such as naloxone block prolactin release after stress, suckling, and estrogen administration, suggesting a role for endogenous opiods, and morphine stimulates prolactin release. However, basal prolactin secretion is not influenced by opiate antagonists. An abrupt rise in prolactin occurs within an hour of eating in normal individuals and pregnant women but not in patients with prolactinomas. The mechanism is unknown.

HYPERPROLACTINEMIA Clinical Features Prolactin excess (hyperprolactinemia) has many causes, is often associated with hypogonadism and/or galactorrhea, and may indicate the presence of a pituitary adenoma or hypothalamic disease. Of women with amenorrhea, 10 to 40 percent have hyperprolactinemia, and about 30 percent of women with amenorrhea and galactorrhea have prolactin-secreting pituitary tumors.

The hypogonadism associated with hyperprolactinemia appears to be due to inhibition of hypothalamic release of LHRH, resulting in defective LH and FSH secretion. This functional hypogonadism can be regarded, in part, as a desirable physiologic mechanism whereby breast feeding causes decreased fertility and delayed resumption of menses. In general, the higher the plasma prolactin, the greater the likelihood of estrogen deficiency and amenorrhea. The wide variability in the clinical manifestations, despite similar degrees of hyperprolactinemia, is likely due to differing bioactivity of abnormal forms of prolactin produced by the tumors. Hyperprolactinemia in women can also cause either irregular menses or infertility despite regular menses, due at least in part to a shortened luteal phase. Prolactin excess in men can cause decreased libido, impotence, and infertility. In some series, 8 percent of men with impotence and 5 percent of men with infertility had hyperprolactinemia. With prolactin elevation, FSH and LH levels in men decline, and serum testosterone is often low.

Galactorrhea, defined as milk production in a patient who is not postpartum, is present in 30 to 90 percent of hyperprolactinemic women (see Chap. 338). The variation in incidence reflects, in part, variation in the intensity with which clinicians search for this finding. Galactorrhea may occur without hyperprolactinemia, particularly in parous women. However, galactorrhea is often a clue to prolactin excess; when galactorrhea is coupled with amenorrhea, hyperprolactinemia is present in 75 percent of patients. Hyperprolactinemia in men is a rare cause of gynecomastia or galactorrhea (see Chap. 338).

Differential Diagnosis Prolactin excess has many causes (Table 328-2) and several mechanisms: (1) autonomous production (pituitary adenomas), (2) decreased dopamine or dopamine inhibitory action (due, for example, to hypothalamic disease or to drugs that block the synthesis, release, or action of dopamine), (3) stimuli that overcome the normal dopaminergic inhibition (e.g., estrogens, possibly hypothyroidism), and (4) decreased clearance of prolactin (renal failure). No test can distinguish between physiologic and pharmacologic or pathologic causes of hyperprolactinemia.

Prolactin concentrations are slightly higher in women (<20 μg/L) than in men (<15 μg/L). During pregnancy, prolactin concentrations begin to increase during the second trimester and peak at term; maximal values are 100 to 300 μg/L, usually less than 200 μg/L. A pregnancy test is mandatory in all patients with hyperprolactinemic amenorrhea, as it is with amenorrhea alone. The mean prolactin level declines post partum but rises with each suckling episode. Over several months, basal and suckling-stimulated prolactin concentrations diminish; by 4 to 6 months post partum, basal prolactin levels are normal, and the suckling-induced rise is diminished or absent despite continued nursing. Prolactin levels rise within 1 h of eating and after seizures.

A careful drug history should be obtained in hyperprolactinemic patients. Dopamine-blocking drugs (e.g., phenothiazines, butyrophenones, metoclopramide, respiridone) and dopamine-depleting drugs (e.g., methyldopa and reserpine) are important causes of hyperprolactinemia. Chronic cocaine use causes modest hyperprolactinemia. In the absence of renal failure, prolactin levels are usually less than 100 μg/L with these agents (respiridone being a notable exception). However, concentrations as high as 275 μg/L have been reported. Although high-dose estrogens cause hyperprolactinemia, oral contraceptives containing low doses of estrogen do not.

End-stage renal failure is associated with elevated serum prolactin in 70 to 90 percent of women and 25 to 60 percent of men. This effect contributes to hypogonadism in some patients with renal failure. Both decreased prolactin clearance and increased prolactin secretion may contribute to this elevation. The increased serum prolactin level in cirrhosis of the liver has not been adequately explained.

Severe primary hypothyroidism may cause a mild elevation in serum prolactin level, due either to an elevation in the TRH level or to a decrease in dopaminergic tone. Since primary hypothyroidism also may cause enlargement of the sella turcica, mimicking a pituitary adenoma, thyroid function tests are essential in all patients with elevated serum prolactin. Rarely, primary adrenal insufficiency causes reversible serum prolactin elevation.

In 10,000 "normal" adults working at a single plant in Japan, the prevalence of hyperprolactinemia greater than 75 μg/L was 0.4 percent. Many different etiologies were found.

If a fasting hyperprolactinemic subject is not pregnant or in the postpartum period and is not cirrhotic, postictal, taking medications, hypothyroid, or in renal failure, disease of the pituitary or hypothalamus is likely. Ectopic production of prolactin by nonpituitary tumors occurs rarely if at all. Diseases of the hypothalamus or pituitary stalk cause moderate prolactin elevation (usually less than 150 μg/L). Hyperprolactinemia occurs in 20 to 50 percent of patients with hypothalamic tumors.

Prolactin-secreting pituitary adenomas (prolactinomas) are arbitrarily divided into microadenomas (<10 mm) and macroadenomas (≥10 mm). Large, nonfunctioning pituitary adenomas also may cause modest prolactin elevation, thought to be due to stalk compression and impairment of dopamine delivery to the gland. Some acromegalic persons (25 to 45 percent), some patients with Nelson's syndrome, and rare Cushing's patients have elevated serum prolactin levels due either to cosecretion of prolactin by the tumor or to stalk compression.

Laboratory Evaluation Serum prolactin levels should be measured in all people with unexplained hypogonadism, galactorrhea, or infertility. If a random prolactin concentration is elevated, further evaluation is warranted after it is established that the observed elevations are not simply normal minimal elevations (e.g., less than 30 μg/L) due to stress or food intake. Levels should be assessed after fasting or more than 1 h after eating. Although there is no simple test to distinguish the various causes of hyperprolactinemia, a serum prolactin level of over 300 μg/L is nearly always diagnostic of a

Table 328-2

Causes of Hyperprolactinemia

PHYSIOLOGIC STATES	
Pregnancy	Sleep
Nursing (early)	Nipple stimulation
"Stress"	Food ingestion
DRUGS	
Dopamine receptor antagonists	Dopamine-depleting agents
Phenothiazines	Methyldopa
Butyrophenones	Reserpine
Thioxanthenes	Hormones
Metoclopramide	Estrogens
Sulpiride	Antiandrogens
Respiradone	Opiates
	Verapamil
DISEASE STATES	
Pituitary tumors	
Prolactinomas	
Adenomas secreting GH and prolactin	
Adenomas secreting ACTH and prolactin (Nelson's syndrome and Cushing's disease)	
Nonfunctioning chromophobe adenomas with pituitary stalk compression	
Hypothalamic and pituitary stalk disease	
Granulomatous diseases, especially sarcoidosis	
Craniopharyngiomas and other tumors	
Cranial irradiation	
Stalk section	
Empty sella	
Vascular abnormalities, including aneurysm	
Lymphocytic hypophysitis	
Metastatic carcinoma	
Primary hypothyroidism	
Chronic renal failure	
Cirrhosis	
Chest wall trauma (including surgery, herpes zoster)	
Seizures	

prolactinoma; a serum prolactin of over 150 μg/L in a nonpregnant patient is usually caused by a pituitary adenoma. Administration of a dopamine agonist, such as bromocriptine, lowers the prolactin level regardless of the etiology and, therefore, is not useful as a differential test (Fig. 328-3). Most patients with prolactinomas show little or no rise in prolactin in response to TRH, as compared with the rise of 200 percent or more in normal individuals and the intermediate response (usually a doubling of serum prolactin) in patients with hypothalamic disease and in those taking dopamine-blocking agents. Unfortunately, the response to TRH is too variable to be of diagnostic value in individual patients. Antiprolactin antibodies may cause spuriously high (or low) prolactin levels in radioimmunoassays but not in immunoradiometric assays; the presence of normal menses in a woman with a serum prolactin level of >100 ng/dL suggests this phenomenon.

Patients with unexplained hyperprolactinemia require magnetic resonance imaging (MRI) of the hypothalamus and pituitary. Pituitary macroadenomas and most microadenomas are easily visualized on these scans, particularly with gadolinium enhancement. Any mass that impairs the flow of dopamine from the hypothalamus to the pituitary can cause hyperprolactinemia, a phenomenon termed "stalk hyperprolactinemia." MRI is essential to distinguish intrasellar lesions such as microprolactinomas and large "nonfunctioning" adenomas from suprasellar lesions such as craniopharyngiomas, germinomas, and meningiomas. When no radiologic abnormalities are found, the disorder is called *idiopathic hyperprolactinemia*, although a microadenoma may still be present.

Microprolactinomas do not cause hypopituitarism (except for hypogonadism). If a small pituitary lesion is seen in a patient with hypopituitarism and hyperprolactinemia, sarcoidosis or other lesions involving the pituitary stalk should be suspected, rather than a microprolactinoma. In patients with macroprolactinomas or hypothalamic lesions, evaluation of pituitary function and formal visual field examinations are essential.

Prolactinomas *Pathology* Prolactinomas are the most common functional pituitary adenomas. Small, unsuspected microadenomas are found in 6 to 24 percent of unselected autopsies; 40 percent of these small tumors contain prolactin by immunologic staining techniques, but the fraction that actually secrete prolactin is unknown. About 70 percent of macroadenomas previously thought to be nonfunctioning are, in fact, prolactinomas. Prolactin-secreting pituitary carcinomas are rare.

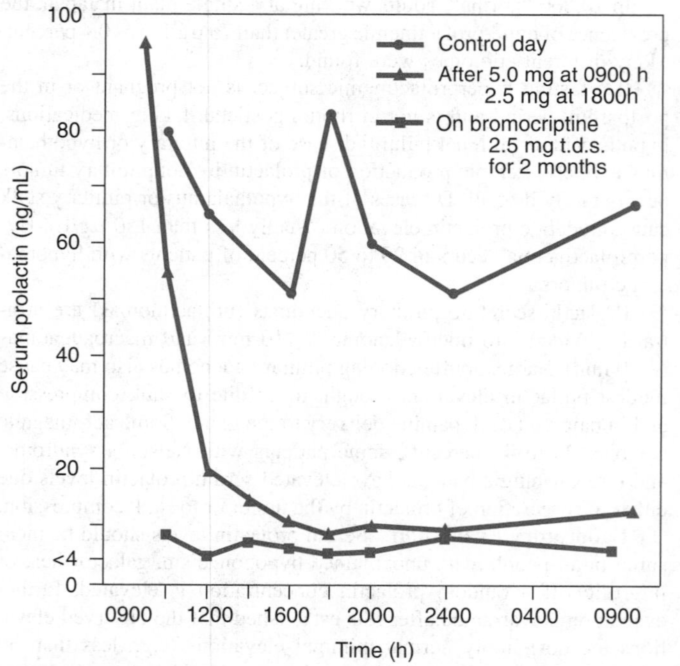

FIGURE 328-3 Changes in serum prolactin concentration in a woman with "idiopathic" hyperprolactinemia after an initial 5-mg dose of bromocriptine and when maintained on 7.5 mg daily. *(From GH Besser, MO Thorner, Postgrad Med J 52:66, 1976.)*

The size of a prolactinoma correlates with its hormone output; in general, the larger the tumor, the higher the prolactin levels. Large pituitary tumors accompanied by a modest prolactin elevation (50 to 100 μg/L) are not true prolactinomas and differ in their biologic behavior. Microprolactinomas cause only hyperprolactinemia and hypogonadotropism, whereas macroprolactinomas may influence other pituitary hormones and cause headaches, visual field disturbances, and other mass effects.

The pathophysiology of prolactinoma development is not understood. Known oncogenes do not play a role in most prolactinomas. However, a *ras* mutation may be important in rare, highly invasive prolactinomas and metastatic pituitary carcinomas.

Clinical presentation Microprolactinomas are more common than macroprolactinomas, and 90 percent of patients with microprolactinomas are women. In contrast, 60 percent of patients with macroprolactinomas are men. Irregular menses, amenorrhea, and galactorrhea are likely to result in early diagnosis, and this fact may partially explain the preponderance of microadenomas in women. Sexual dysfunction occurs in most men with prolactinomas, but this is the presenting complaint in 15 percent or less. Although a delay in seeking medical help probably explains the larger size of tumors in men, the possibility of more aggressive tumor behavior in men has not been excluded.

Estrogens promote the growth of lactotrophs, but an etiologic role has not been established for oral contraceptives in the pathogenesis of prolactinomas. Many women with prolactinomas first develop galactorrhea while on oral contraceptives or develop amenorrhea when the drug is discontinued. Some of these women may have been started on oral contraceptives for irregular menses that were the consequence of a prolactinoma. Although amenorrhea after discontinuance of oral contraceptives is rare (about 2 percent), about a third of patients with post-pill amenorrhea have a prolactinoma. Development of galactorrhea in a woman using oral contraceptives mandates a prolactin determination. About 5 to 7 percent of prolactinoma patients have never menstruated (primary amenorrhea), making prolactinoma an important treatable cause of primary amenorrhea. Prolactinomas may grow during pregnancy, and 15 percent of prolactinoma patients are first diagnosed in the postpartum period.

Women with prolactinomas who desire pregnancy need special consideration. Medical treatment of patients with microprolactinomas results in an uneventful pregnancy 95 to 98 percent of the time; the remaining patients may develop headaches or visual field disturbances due to tumor enlargement that rarely requires therapy. Asymptomatic enlargement of microprolactinomas, as ascertained by radiologic studies, occurs in about 5 percent of patients. With macroprolactinomas, the complications of tumor growth during pregnancy are more common. Symptomatic tumor enlargement occurs in about 15 percent of these patients, although prior therapy with bromocriptine may decrease this risk.

In prolactinoma patients, the effect of pregnancy on prolactin secretion is variable. A further rise in prolactin during pregnancy may not occur even in patients in whom tumor growth occurs. Rarely, macroprolactinomas in men grow during replacement testosterone therapy, presumably as a result of extraglandular conversion of testosterone to estrogen. The safety of oral contraceptives in women with microprolactinomas is uncertain, but some data suggest that such therapy is unlikely to cause a rise in prolactin levels or significant tumor growth.

℞ TREATMENT

The natural history of untreated hyperprolactinemia is incompletely understood. Although large pituitary adenomas must begin as small tumors, most microadenomas do not progress to macroadenomas. In general, 90 to 95 percent of untreated microprolactinomas remain stable or exhibit decreased serum prolactin concentrations over 7 years of follow-up. Serum prolactin returns to normal in a third of patients with idiopathic hyperprolactinemia (who may harbor microprolactinomas) who are followed for 5 years without therapy; this number increases to two-thirds if the basal prolactin is less than 40 μg/L. In 30 patients with varying degrees of hyperprolactinemia (30 to 260 μg/L) followed for a mean of 5.2 years, the prolactin level increased by more than 50 percent in one-fifth, and another fifth had signs of enlargement on computed tomography (CT) scans. The prolactin level decreased by more than 50 percent in one-third of the patients and returned to normal in one-fifth. The abnormal x-ray findings returned to normal in one-sixth of the patients.

Thus, not all patients with microprolactinomas need therapy. Women with microprolactinomas require therapy when they desire pregnancy or have amenorrhea (because of the risk of osteoporosis), acne or hirsutism, decreased libido, or troublesome galactorrhea. Men with microadenomas should be treated when they have hypogonadism (because of the risk of osteoporosis), decreased potency or libido, or infertility. Patients with macroprolactinomas require therapy to prevent or reverse the mass effects of the tumor.

The treatment of choice is medical therapy. Dopamine agonist drugs lower prolactin concentrations in virtually all hyperprolactinemic patients (Fig. 328-3). Bromocriptine, an ergot derivative with dopamine agonist actions, is the only effective prolactin-lowering agent licensed for this purpose in the United States. Bromocriptine should be given twice daily with food or a snack to prevent gastrointestinal irritation; in some patients, prolactin levels return to normal with once-daily dosing. Therapy should begin with a low dose of 0.625 to 1.25 mg with a snack at bedtime to minimize the side effects of nausea, vomiting, fatigue, nasal stuffiness, and postural hypotension. The dosage is gradually increased to an average of 2.5 mg twice daily. In some patients with microadenomas, control is achieved with 2.5 mg at bedtime, whereas up to 15 mg/d may be required with macroprolactinomas. Treatment success should be monitored by assessing clinical manifestations, prolactin levels in serum, and tumor size by MRI. Although the drug is expensive, it is effective in all forms of hyperprolactinemia and often abolishes nonhyperprolactinemic galactorrhea as well. Long-lasting parenteral and oral dopamine agonists and newer non-ergot-derived oral dopamine agonists are effective and in some cases better tolerated than bromocriptine; gastrointestinal intolerance to oral bromocriptine can be circumvented by vaginal administration. Neither the new agents nor vaginal administration is licensed in the United States.

Bromocriptine is the therapy of choice for patients with microprolactinomas who have one of the indications for treatment discussed above. Prolactin concentrations return to normal in almost all patients who tolerate the medication, usually within days of achieving the full therapeutic dosage (see Fig. 328-3). Menses usually resume within 2 months but may be delayed by up to a year. Since pregnancy may occur without resumption of menses, a barrier contraceptive is recommended until menses become regular. With this approach, bromocriptine can be stopped with the first missed period when pregnancy has occurred. Bromocriptine is not approved for use during pregnancy in the United States, but its use during pregnancy is not associated with an increased risk of congenital anomalies or fetal wastage. The effects of bromocriptine are usually not permanent, but one-sixth of microprolactinoma patients maintain normal prolactin concentrations after discontinuation of the drug.

In patients with macroprolactinomas, bromocriptine usually lowers the serum prolactin level and decreases tumor size (Fig. 328-4), but both effects may be incomplete. In men, testosterone concentrations usually begin to increase after 3 months of therapy, but they may remain subnormal. In some men sperm counts return to normal. Almost 90 percent of premenopausal women regain cyclic menses.

Tumor shrinkage is most rapid in the first 3 months of therapy. By 3 months 40 percent of tumors have shrunk by more than 50 percent. Of patients treated for a year 90 percent show tumor shrinkage of more than 50 percent. Most tumors shrink to some degree; more important, abnormal visual fields improve with medical therapy in 90 percent of patients. If the visual field defect does not resolve within a short period (1 to 3 months), surgery should be performed.

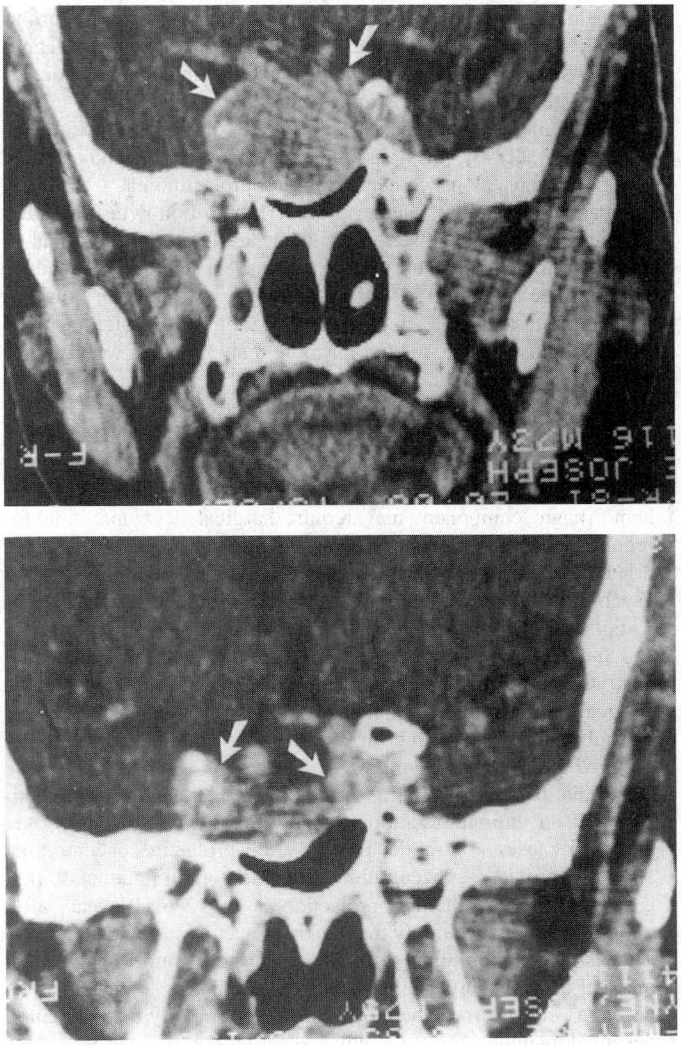

FIGURE 328-4 Frontal CT scan of a man with a large prolactin-secreting macroadenoma. *Top:* pretreatment scan. *Bottom:* scan after 1 year of treatment with bromocriptine. The upper border of the tumor is shown by arrows. *(From ME Molitch, 1987.)*

Prolactin levels fall to 20 percent of the baseline level in more than 90 percent of patients and return to normal in about a third. The dosage of bromocriptine can often be reduced after 2 years or more of therapy, but the drug rarely can be discontinued. In patients who have persistent symptomatic hyperprolactinemia despite a partial response to bromocriptine, surgical debulking or radiation therapy may be appropriate.

Although prolactin concentrations usually return rapidly to pretreatment levels when long-term bromocriptine treatment is stopped, tumor regrowth may be delayed for months or years. When pregnancy is considered by a patient with a macroprolactinoma, this slow regrowth should be kept in mind. Patients who conceive after prolonged bromocriptine therapy may be at less risk of tumor growth during pregnancy. In the United States, bromocriptine is generally stopped when pregnancy is confirmed; however, if tumor-related symptoms develop during pregnancy, bromocriptine should be reinstituted. Many physicians outside the United States use bromocriptine throughout pregnancy in patients with macroprolactinomas. There is no evidence that bromocriptine has an adverse effect on the fetus. Pregnant women with macroprolactinomas should have frequent testing of visual fields to monitor for tumor growth.

Patients who have large nonprolactinoma masses in the sella that cause stalk-compression hyperprolactinemia are sometimes treated mistakenly with bromocripitine. Although prolactin levels return to normal in such cases, the size of the mass is not affected. These patients should be treated surgically if debulking the mass or obtaining a tissue diagnosis is important.

While medical treatment is appropriate for most prolactinomas, surgery, usually by the transsphenoidal approach, is indicated in some situations, as in women with microprolactinomas who desire pregnancy and cannot tolerate bromocriptine. Following resection of microprolactinomas, serum prolactin levels return to normal in 80 to 90 percent of patients, usually within 24 h. However, recurrence rates may be as high as 40 percent within 6 years. Surgery may be more difficult and have a higher complication rate in microprolactinoma patients who are treated for more than 3 months with bromocriptine.

Surgery may also be necessary for macroprolactinoma patients in whom visual field defects persist despite bromocriptine treatment, who have tumor growth despite bromocriptine treatment, or who are intolerant of dopamine agonists. Tumors with a large cystic or hemorrhagic component may require surgical decompression for relief of visual symptoms or headaches. Surgery may also be appropriate for prolactinoma patients who need neuroleptic agents for psychiatric illness, because dopamine agonists counteract these medications and may precipitate psychotic episodes.

Surgery is rarely curative for macroprolactinomas. Prolactin concentrations return to normal in about 30 percent of patients treated surgically, but recurrence rates may be as high as 80 percent in this subgroup. Long-term bromocriptine therapy is therefore usually required after surgical therapy.

Radiation therapy plays a limited role in the treatment of prolactinomas. Conventional radiation therapy [4500 cGy (4500 rad) over 25 days] causes a slow decline in serum prolactin concentration. Although prolactin concentrations return to normal in about 30 percent of patients with microprolactinomas by 2 to 10 years after radiation therapy, we rarely treat microprolactinomas with radiation. The risks of hypopituitarism make this a poor fourth choice after medical therapy, surgery, or no therapy. Radiation therapy may be necessary for macroprolactinomas that grow rapidly or persistently despite dopamine agonist therapy and surgery or after surgery alone in patients intolerant of dopamine agonists. The respective roles of conventional radiation, focused gamma radiation ("gamma knife"), and heavy-particle (proton beam) radiation are not established.

PROLACTIN DEFICIENCY Prolactin deficiency is manifested as an inability to lactate. Failure of lactation is often the earliest clue to panhypopituitarism resulting from pituitary infarction during the peripartum period. The lateral wings of the pituitary, where most lactotrophs reside, have a precarious blood supply. During pregnancy, the hypertrophied and hyperplastic lactotrophs are at risk for necrosis. If systemic hypotension develops, as with postpartum hemorrhage, the pituitary may undergo infarction (Sheehan's syndrome). Patients with diabetes mellitus are susceptible to peripartum pituitary infarction even in the absence of significant hemorrhage. Autoimmune pituitary destruction (lymphocytic hypophysitis) also may occur during late pregnancy but often is associated with elevated prolactin levels.

Many prolactin radioimmunoassays cannot distinguish normal from low prolactin concentrations; hence, prolactin stimulation tests may be necessary to diagnose prolactin insufficiency. After administration of TRH or chlorpromazine, a rise in serum prolactin of less than 200 percent suggests prolactin deficiency. If prolactin deficiency is present, evaluation of other pituitary hormones is necessary to determine whether other manifestations of hypopituitarism are present.

GROWTH HORMONE

PHYSIOLOGY Growth hormone (GH, somatotropin) is secreted by somatotrophs, which make up about 50 percent of the anterior pituitary cells. The normal pituitary contains 3 to 5 mg of GH and secretes 500 to 875 μg of GH per day. GH shares an 85 percent structural identity with human placental lactogen (hPL, chorionic somatomammotropin). The GH and hPL genes are on chromosome 17 and appear to have originated by gene duplication. Human growth hormone consists of a single polypeptide chain of 191 amino acids (22,000 mol wt) with two intrachain disulfide bonds; it is cleaved from a larger precursor molecule (28,000 mol wt). Alternative splicing of this precursor yields a 20-kDa GH molecule with a lower biologic and immunologic activity. GH is stored in cytoplasmic granules in a high-molecular-weight polymeric form. A variant form of GH (GH-V) is found in the placenta, is the dominant form of GH circulating in the third trimester of pregnancy, and is a potent somatogen.

Multiple forms of GH exist in the circulation. The dominant form is monomeric GH (22 kDa), but larger, oligomeric forms (e.g., "big" GH, 44,000 mol wt) and smaller forms (e.g., the 20-kDa form) are present as well. All these variants contribute to the total circulating GH concentration. Several binding proteins for GH contribute to the heterogeneity of circulating GH. The high-affinity GH-binding protein, which is specific for the 22-kDa form of GH, appears to be a cleavage product of the extracellular domain of the GH receptor. A lower-affinity binding protein binds both the 22-kDa active and 20-kDa inactive forms of GH.

Pulsatile release of GH is characteristic. Circulating levels are immeasurably low for much of the day, and this base line level is punctuated by four to eight bursts, which occur after meals or exercise, during slow-wave sleep, or without an obvious cause. The half-life of the hormone in plasma is 20 to 30 min. GH secretion is low in infancy, slightly higher during early childhood, and dramatically increased during puberty. GH secretion is lower in adulthood than during puberty. After the third decade, a progressive (but individually variable) decline in GH secretion occurs.

GH is necessary for normal linear growth. GH deficiency causes short stature; GH excess (prior to epiphyseal closure) leads to gigantism. GH does not appear to be the principal direct stimulator of growth but rather acts indirectly by stimulating the formation of other hormones. These factors, known as *somatomedins* (SMs, somatotropin-mediating hormones) or *insulin-like growth factors* (IGFs), are GH-dependent and are responsible for growth stimulation (see also Chap. 329). IGF-I (formerly termed *somatomedin C*), the most important somatomedin for postnatal growth, is produced in the liver, chondrocytes, kidney, muscle, pituitary, and gastrointestinal tract. The liver is the main source of circulating IGF-I. IGF-I is a basic protein (7600 mol wt) that circulates bound to six distinct IGF binding proteins (IGF-BPs). IGF-BP3 is the major binding protein and is itself growth hormone–dependent. The net effect of the binding proteins is to increase the half-life of circulating IGF-I to 3 to 18 h, as compared with the half-life of 20 to 30 min for unbound hormone. The role of specific IGF-BPs in regulating IGF action is under investigation. Local tissue generation of IGF-I/SM-C, particularly in bone, may play an important role in growth mediation through its paracrine effects.

IGF-I is structurally similar to proinsulin and exerts some insulin-like actions. Furthermore, GH is a trophic factor for insulin release, facilitating release in response to various secretagogues, and GH-deficient individuals have impaired insulin release to glucose challenge. Technically, one might consider insulin a somatomedin.

During the prenatal and neonatal period, growth is independent of GH, as shown by the normal birth length of GH-deficient children born to GH-deficient mothers. Nevertheless, IGF-I levels are elevated during pregnancy; the concentration correlates with that of hPL, which may regulate IGF-I production. IGF-I levels at birth are lower than those of adults and rise gradually during childhood to reach the adult range by age 8 to 10 years. The levels also depend on nutritional status, declining in states of malnourishment. Serum IGF-I levels are elevated during the pubertal growth spurt, presumably accounting for pubertal growth acceleration.

Although IGF-I levels correlate with linear growth, the correlation is inexact, and, therefore, GH may have some direct influence on growth or cause somatomedin generation in target cells.

GH exerts additional metabolic effects, including stimulation of the incorporation of amino acids into protein. Although most of this action is IGF-mediated, GH can directly stimulate amino acid uptake in certain systems. Some amino acids, such as arginine, are potent stimuli for GH release.

GH may act as an insulin antagonist to inhibit glucose uptake by tissues. Patients with GH deficiency are prone to insulin-induced hypoglycemia; patients with GH excess develop insulin resistance. GH is one of the counterregulatory hormones that help restore a low blood sugar to normal (see Chap. 335). Hypoglycemia is a potent stimulus for GH release, and an acute rise in blood sugar inhibits GH release. Paradoxically, patients with type I diabetes mellitus have increased GH concentrations. GH increases the release of free fatty acids from adipocytes. The absence of this effect may be responsible for the pudgy appearance of children with GH deficiency and the high percentage of body fat in adults with GH deficiency. Increased serum free fatty acid concentrations tend to blunt GH release. GH opposes the action of insulin on sugar uptake and fatty acid release and complements the anabolic action of insulin on amino acid uptake.

GH is controlled by a dual hypothalamic regulation (Table 328-3). Secretion is stimulated by growth hormone–releasing hormone (GHRH, somatocrinin) and inhibited by somatostatin (growth hormone release–inhibiting hormone, somatotropin release–inhibiting factor, SRIF). GHRH appears to play the more important role, since pituitary stalk section leads to failure of GH release. Although GHRH and somatostatin are synthesized in separate neurons, these neurons have reciprocal interconnections.

Growth Hormone–Releasing Hormone GHRH has 44 amino acids, 29 of which are necessary for full potency. GHRH belongs to a family of molecules that includes secretin, glucagon, VIP, and gastric inhibitory peptide (GIP). The arcuate nucleus of the hypothalamus is the major site of GHRH production, although a few GHRH-producing neurons are found in the ventromedial nucleus. Axons containing the peptide project to the median eminence and terminate on the portal vessels. GHRH is also present in the mucosa of the small intestine.

The GHRH receptor is a G protein–coupled transmembrane receptor, and GHRH stimulates both the transcription of the GH gene and the synthesis and release of GH, an effect mediated by cyclic adenosine monophosphate (AMP). Intravenous injection of GHRH (0.1 to 3.3 μg/kg body weight) produces a peak GH response at 30 to 60 min with a return to baseline by 2 to 3 h after injection (Fig. 328-5).

Somatostatin Somatostatin, a cyclic tetradecapeptide, is the most widely distributed of the hypothalamic releasing hormones. The primary hypothalamic sources are the periventricular and medial preoptic areas of the anterior hypothalamus. Somatostatin is found in neurosecretory granules of axons that terminate in the median eminence. In addition to its function as a hormone, somatostatin is synthesized and distributed throughout the brain and serves as a neurotransmitter in many areas, including the spinal cord, brainstem, and cerebral cortex. Somatostatin is also present in the gastrointestinal tract and other organs. Somatostatin-secreting cells (D cells) of the pancreatic islets participate in the regulation of insulin and glucagon secretion, an example of paracrine regulation by this hormone (see Chap. 334). Somatostatin acts via a family of at least five G protein–coupled membrane receptors that utilize a number of different second messenger pathways.

Somatostatin is produced by processing of a larger precursor molecule and exists in both 28- and 14-amino-acid forms. The 28-amino-acid somatostatin has a longer half-life and is a more potent inhibitor of GH, TSH, and insulin secretion. Somatostatin 14 is the most abundant form but is less bioactive in inhibiting GH. It has a greater affinity for hypothalamic and cortical receptors and is more potent in inhibition of glucagon release, splanchnic blood flow, intestinal motility, and gastric exocrine secretion. Somatostatin analogues are effective in the therapy of acromegaly, TSH-secreting pituitary adenomas, secretory pancreatic tumors, carcinoid syndrome, and other conditions.

Somatostatin inhibits GH secretion and decreases the GH response to secretagogues without altering GH mRNA levels. Somatostatin also lowers serum TSH levels in normal and hypothyroid individuals and blunts TSH release in response to TRH. Somatostatin probably mediates the secondary hypothyroidism that may develop in GH-deficient children treated with GH. Somatostatin has no significant effect on the release of prolactin, gonadotropins, or ACTH in normal subjects but may lower ACTH concentrations in patients with Nelson's syndrome.

Table 328-3

Growth Hormone Regulation

Class of Agent	Stimulation	Inhibition
Hypothalamic factors	GHRH	Somatostatin
Amines	Alpha-2-adrenergic stimuli (norepinephrine, clonidine)	Beta-adrenergic stimuli
	Beta-adrenergic blockers (propranolol)	Alpha-2-adrenergic blockers (yohimbine)
	Dopaminergic stimuli (levodopa, bromocriptine, apomorphine)	Dopamine blockers (chlorpromazine)
	Serotonergic stimuli (L-tryptophan)	Serotonin blockers (methysergide, cyproheptadine)
Hormones	Decreased IGF-I/SM-C	Increased IGF-I/SM-C (obesity)
	Estrogen	Progestogens
	Vasopressin	Glucocorticoids*
	Glucagon†	
Fuels	Hypoglycemia‡	Increased blood sugar
	Decreased free fatty acids	Increased free fatty acids
	Amino acid (arginine)†	
Others	Exercise‡	Muscarinic cholinergic antagonists (atropine)
	Stress‡	
	Sleep†	
	Cholinergic (muscarinic stimuli) (pyridostigmine)	

* Acutely, glucocorticoids stimulate GH release.
† Probably mediated through cholinergic stimulation.
‡ Probably mediated through alpha-adrenergic stimulation.

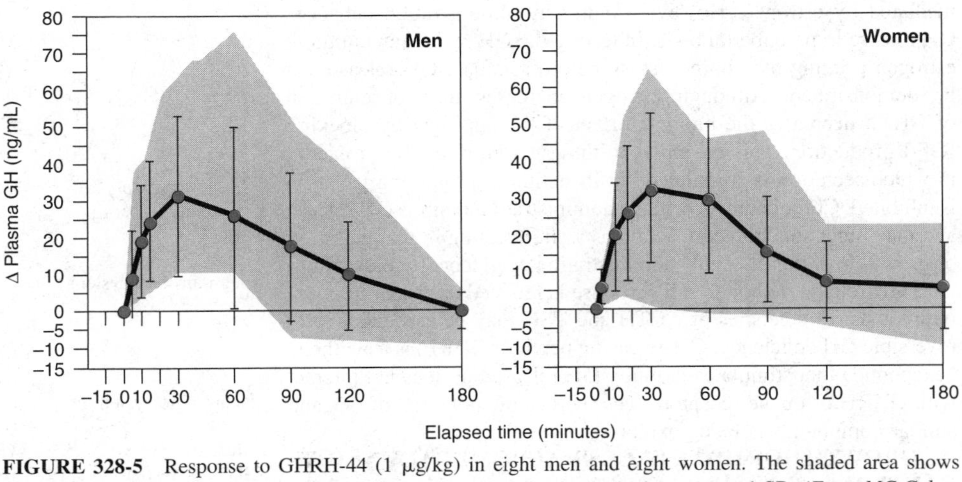

FIGURE 328-5 Response to GHRH-44 (1 μg/kg) in eight men and eight women. The shaded area shows the full range of responses at each time point, and the error bars indicate the mean ± 1 SD. *(From MC Gelato et al, J Clin Endocrinol Metab 59:200, 1984.)*

Somatostatinomas are rare pancreatic islet cell or duodenal tumors that secrete somatostatin (see Chap. 95).

Growth hormone release is under complex physiologic control (see Table 328-3). The various mediators appear to act through GHRH and somatostatin. IGF-I has an important feedback effect on GH secretion. An increased IGF-I concentration inhibits GH release both through increased somatostatin production and by a direct action on the pituitary. A decrease in IGF-I, as induced by starvation, leads to a compensatory increase in GH release.

A number of neurotransmitters influence GH release, as follows.

1. Alpha-adrenergic agonists such as clonidine stimulate GHRH and GH release, an effect probably mediated through decreased hypothalamic somatostatin secretion. Several stimuli for GH release, including insulin hypoglycemia, exercise, and galanin, act through alpha-adrenergic mechanisms. Beta-adrenergic blockers potentiate the GH stimulatory effect of clonidine and some other agents. $Alpha_2$-adrenergic blocking agents, such as yohimbine, decrease GH release.
2. Stimulation of muscarinic cholinergic receptors, for example with acetylcholinesterase inhibitors, facilitates GH release, and this effect also is thought to be due to inhibition of somatostatin release. The induction of GH release by arginine, glucagon, or sleep is inhibited by muscarinic receptor antagonists. Atropine is the most effective blocker of opioid peptide–mediated GH release.
3. Oral administration of dopamine precursors or agonists that cross the blood-brain barrier, such as levodopa, apomorphine, or bromocriptine, causes an increase in serum GH levels. Although these stimuli can be used to test the adequacy of GH secretion (the so-called GH reserve), the mechanism of dopamine stimulation remains controversial; it is probably mediated by GHRH. Dopamine agonists may inhibit GH release from growth hormone–secreting adenomas.
4. Although serotonin agonists stimulate GH release, the role of serotonin in the physiologic control of GH is uncertain.

Obesity blunts GH release in response to many stimuli, including GHRH itself. Weight reduction restores normal GH dynamics. In contrast, malnourished individuals, including women with anorexia nervosa, often have an increase in the secretion and plasma concentration of GH. This effect results partly from a decreased serum IGF-I level, which is possibly the result of resistance to GH at the cellular level. Oral glucose administration decreases serum GH and the GH response to GHRH. Arginine also stimulates GH release by inhibiting somatostatin release. Both basal and stimulated GH release are reduced in patients with major depression.

A number of hormones influence GH release. Most factors that stimulate GH release are more potent in women than in men, an effect mediated by estrogen. However, androgen administration enhances GH release in prepubertal boys. In testing the GH reserve in children, estrogen priming may be necessary before adequate GH release can be demonstrated. Although estrogen increases the concentration of GH, it decreases the biologic effect of the hormone by blocking IGF-I production. This is similar to the estrogen effect on prolactin, in which secretion is stimulated but its action in promoting lactation is inhibited. Chronic glucocorticoid administration inhibits GH release and may blunt somatomedin action as well, resulting in the inhibition of growth in children. Acute administration of glucocorticoids stimulates GH release, although this response is reduced or absent in obese individuals. Deficiencies of ACTH and TSH may be associated with reversible GH deficiency. GH-releasing peptide (GHRP) is a synthetic hexapeptide that stimulates pituitary GH release but does not interact with GHRH or opiate receptors. The therapeutic potential of this and similar compounds is being explored.

GROWTH HORMONE EXCESS: ACROMEGALY AND GIGANTISM **Clinical Features** GH excess results in acromegaly, an insidious, chronic, debilitating disease associated with bony and soft tissue overgrowth (Table 328-4). Acromegaly is equally prevalent in men and women and occurs most frequently in middle age. It is uncommon, with an estimated prevalence of 50 to 70 cases per million and an incidence of 3 to 4 cases per million per year. These figures may be an underestimation due to underdiagnosis of the disorder. When GH excess develops prior to epiphyseal closure in children, increased linear growth can cause gigantism. Tumors may be more aggressive and cause more rapid onset of acromegaly in younger patients.

Most patients have soft tissue and bone enlargement, which results in increased hand, foot, and hat size, prognathism, enlargement of the tongue, wide spacing of the teeth, and coarsening of facial features; these are rarely the presenting complaints. Acromegalics are said to look more like each other than like their own family members (Fig. 328-6). Laryngeal hypertrophy and sinus enlargement with hyperpneumatization of the skull lead to a hollow-sounding voice. A moist, doughy handshake, increased skin tags, acanthosis nigricans, and oily skin are common.

Acromegaly is more than a cosmetically disfiguring disease. Patients feel weak and tired. The basal metabolic rate increases, which, in turn, causes increased sweating. Obstructive sleep apnea may be an important cause of hypersomnolence. Most patients have neurologic and musculoskeletal symptoms, including headaches, nerve entrapments and paresthesias (often due to carpal tunnel syndrome), muscle weakness, and arthralgias (particularly involving the shoulders, back, and knees). The cartilage hypertrophy and osseous overgrowth often lead to degenerative arthritis, kyphoscoliosis, and on occasion spinal stenosis. Hypertension occurs in about one-third of patients and is characterized by suppressed renin and aldosterone secretion associated with expansion of plasma volume and an increase in total body sodium.

Table 328-4

Manifestations of Acromegaly

Location	Symptoms	Signs
General	Fatigue Increased sweating Heat intolerance Weight gain	
Skin and subcutaneous tissue	Enlarging hands, feet Coarsening facial features Oily skin Hypertrichosis	Moist, warm, fleshy, doughy handshake Skin tags Acanthosis nigricans Increased heel pad
Head	Headaches	Parotid enlargement, frontal bossing
Eyes	Decreased vision	Visual field defects
Ears		Otoscope speculum cannot be inserted
Nose, throat, paranasal sinuses	Sinus congestion	Enlarged, furrowed tongue
	Increased tongue size	Tooth marks on tongue
	Malocclusion Voice change	Widely spaced teeth Prognathism
Neck		Goiter Obstructive sleep apnea Enlarged sinuses
Cardiorespiratory system	Congestive heart failure	Hypertension Cardiomegaly Left ventricular hypertrophy
Genitourinary system	Decreased libido Impotence Oligomenorrhea Infertility Kidney stones	
Neurologic system	Paresthesias Hypersomnolence	Carpal tunnel syndrome
Muscles	Weakness	Proximal myopathy
Skeletal system	Joint pains (shoulders, back, knees)	Osteoarthritis

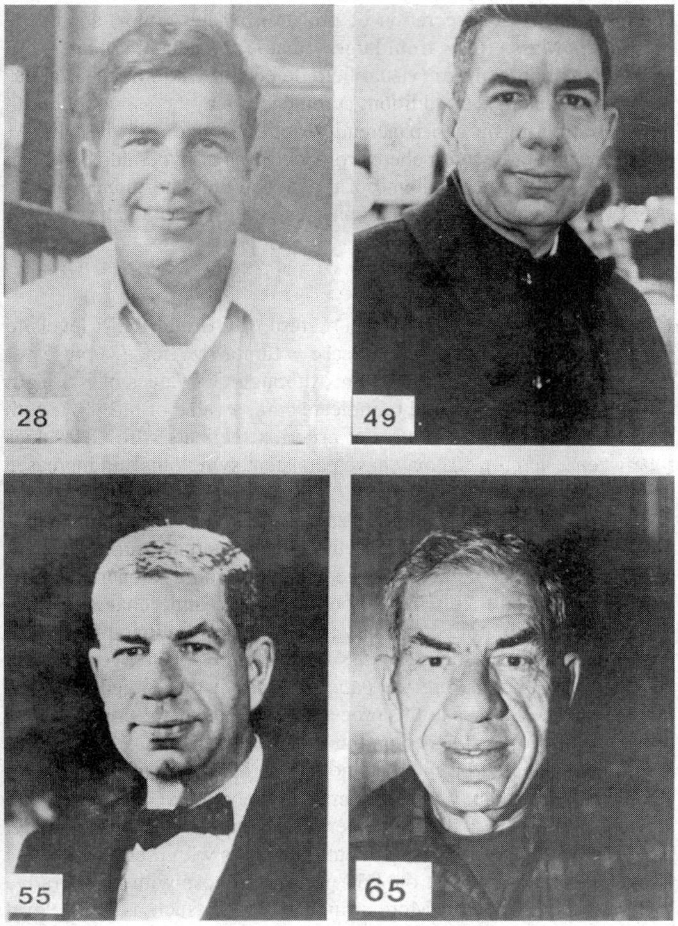

FIGURE 328-6 Serial photographs of a patient with acromegaly taken at ages 28, 49, 55, and 65 years, 6 months after removal of a GH-secreting adenoma. Note the gradual increase in the size of the nose, lips, and skin folds, particularly the nasolabial skin fold and forehead. *(From S Reichlin, Med Grand Rounds 1:9, 1982.)*

Almost all hypertensive acromegalics and about half of nonhypertensive acromegalics have increased left ventricular mass or left ventricular wall thickness. Although it is not established whether a specific cardiomyopathy occurs, acromegalics may develop congestive heart failure in the absence of another known underlying heart disease. Amenorrhea may occur with or without hyperprolactinemia, and hirsutism is often noted. Many organs, including the liver and kidneys, increase in size with no evidence of functional impairment. Goiter, which probably results from IGF-I stimulation of thyroid cell growth, occurs in about 40 percent of patients, and 3 to 7 percent of patients have hyperthyroidism. Some series report abdominal pain and inguinal hernias, each occurring in about one-third of patients, and nasal polyps in as many as 15 percent. Intracranial aneurysms coexist in 10 percent or fewer of patients.

Patients with untreated acromegaly have a shortened life expectancy with increased rates of death from cardiovascular, cerebrovascular, and respiratory disease and, in some studies, from malignancies. In studies in which modern therapy was available, deleterious effects on life expectancy were less striking. Patients with coexisting diabetes mellitus have increased mortality. Skin tags appear to correlate with increased prevalence of colonic polyps and possibly with an increased risk for carcinoma of the colon. Bowel surveillance by colonoscopy has been suggested.

Laboratory Investigations Insulin resistance occurs in 80 percent of patients, although abnormal glucose tolerance (20 to 40 percent) and clinical diabetes mellitus (13 to 20 percent) are less common. Hypercalciuria is frequent, apparently due to increased levels of circulating 1,25-dihydroxyvitamin D; renal stones occur in about one-fifth of patients. Hypercalcemia, when it occurs, is not due to acromegaly per se but suggests primary hyperparathyroidism as part of the multiple endocrine neoplasia 1 (MEN 1) syndrome (see Chap. 340). GH causes increased renal tubular reabsorption of phosphate by an undefined mechanism. Elevation of serum phosphate occurs in about one-half of patients. Hyperprolactinemia occurs in up to one-half of patients and is responsible for much of the associated galactorrhea, amenorrhea, and decreased libido.

Pathophysiology Well-defined pituitary adenomas are found in almost all patients with acromegaly and gigantism. The tumors tend to occur in the lateral wings of the sella, where somatotrophs normally are found in abundance. Occasionally, tumors are found in ectopic locations along the lines of migration of Rathke's pouch, such as the sphenoid sinus or parapharyngeal regions.

GH levels correlate, on average, with tumor size. Tumors tend to be larger and may be more aggressive in younger patients. At the time of diagnosis, 75 percent of somatotroph adenomas are macroadenomas; however, 70 percent are less than 20 mm in diameter at diagnosis. This feature is different than in prolactinomas, two-thirds of which are microadenomas at the time of diagnosis. Aggressive screening for acromegaly on the basis of subtle clinical clues might lead to early diagnosis while tumors are small and more easily curable.

Immunohistochemical staining and electron microscopy of somatotroph tumors help to predict their behavior. Densely granulated tumors have slower growth. GH-secreting carcinomas are rare and should be diagnosed only in the presence of distant metastases. Tumors that cause local invasion are called *invasive adenomas*.

Current evidence suggests a primary pituitary etiology for acromegaly. Most GH-secreting (and other pituitary) tumors are monoclonal in origin. A cellular mutation may lead to GH hypersecretion (and presumably tumor growth as well) in some patients. About 40 percent of somatotroph tumors have a mutation in the α subunit of a stimulatory G (G_s) protein. These G proteins normally couple surface signals to cyclic AMP production within the cells. Activation of G_s proteins is associated with binding of guanosine triphosphate (GTP) to the α subunit, which allows the α subunit to stimulate cyclic AMP production. The normal free subunit has intrinsic GTPase activity, which inactivates GTP, preventing continued cyclic AMP stimulation. The mutant α subunit in acromegalic patients does not possess GTPase activity; hence, continued cyclic AMP stimulation leads to autonomous GH production.

Another mechanism for tumor growth in somatotroph adenomas is deletion of the 11q13 region of chromosome 11, a loss believed to involve a normal suppressor gene. This loss occurs both as a part of the MEN 1 syndrome (see Chap. 340) and in sporadic tumors. Further evidence for a primary etiology of acromegaly is the fact that peripheral concentrations of GHRH are low, although this finding does not exclude the possibility that hypothalamic GHRH excess or somatostatin deficiency is the cause in some patients. Abnormal GH pulsations in some surgically "cured" acromegalics could be due to an underlying hypothalamic disorder, residual tumor, or previous GH excess.

GHRH-induced acromegaly is rare ($<$1 percent in one series) but is clinically indistinguishable from acromegaly caused by pituitary adenomas. This diagnosis should be considered when pituitary somatotroph hyperplasia, rather than an adenoma, is diagnosed histologically. Bronchial carcinoids and pancreatic islet cell tumors are the ones most likely to secrete GHRH ectopically, but small cell carcinoma of the lung, medullary thyroid carcinoma, and carcinoids of the small intestine and thymus contain GHRH as well. Many of the tumors associated with GHRH production also cause ectopic ACTH production. Hypothalamic gangliocytomas, hamartomas, and gliomas can produce GHRH (as well as somatostatin) and cause somatotroph hyperplasia and acromegaly. GHRH is not routinely measured in acromegalic patients unless somatotroph hyperplasia is present or an appropriate nonpituitary tumor is discovered.

Isolated ectopic production of GH has been described in a patient with a pancreatic islet cell tumor; the tumor size in this instance

(420 g) suggests inefficient GH production, since GH-secreting pituitary tumors are usually small.

Diagnosis Patients with acromegaly have symptoms for an average of 9 years and often see several physicians before the diagnosis is made. Suspecting the diagnosis is the most difficult step in the process. Newly consulted physicians are more likely to make the diagnosis than is one who has watched the insidious progress of the disease. When suggestive facial features are noted, a comparison with old pictures may be helpful (Fig. 328-6).

Once the diagnosis is suspected, confirmation is straightforward. Because basal or random GH determinations can yield elevated values in normal persons, particularly in women and people with uncontrolled diabetes mellitus, renal failure, or stress, they should not be used to screen for acromegaly. Two diagnostic tests are available: measurements of glucose-suppressed GH concentrations and measurement of IGF-I concentrations. GH concentrations are measured 60 to 120 min after the oral administration of 100 g glucose. Although a serum GH concentration of <5 μg/L was previously accepted as normal, a postsuppression value of <2 μg/L is a more rigorous criterion and should now be applied. Acromegalics usually have a GH concentration after glucose administration of >10 μg/L; in some the value is suppressed to below 5 μg/L but it is rarely below 2 μg/L. IGF-I concentrations also provide an excellent screening test for acromegaly. Pitfalls include unreliable commercial assays, failure to use age-adjusted normal values (especially during puberty), and possible false-negative results with starvation. Measurements of serum IGF-I concentration correlate with disease activity even in patients with basal GH concentrations below 10 μg/L. As GH values rise to >20 μg/L, IGF-I concentrations plateau, probably explaining why dramatic falls in GH after therapy do not necessarily cause clinical improvement. Although GH concentrations decline, IGF-I may remain nearly maximal until GH falls below 20 μg/L.

GH concentrations in acromegaly may vary during the day, although they are never undetectable, as they are in normal persons. GH levels increase in response to insulin-induced hypoglycemia and arginine infusion, and the response to GHRH is enhanced in most acromegalics. Somatostatin infusion lowers GH concentration but usually not to a normal value. In addition, GH-secreting pituitary tumors respond to stimuli that do not affect normal somatotrophs: TRH increases GH in 80 percent, and LHRH increases GH in about 10 to 15 percent of acromegalics. Dopamine agonists stimulate GH release in normal persons but inhibit it in most acromegalics.

The IGF binding proteins (IGF-BPs) are a family of proteins that bind IGF-I and modulate its action at the cellular level. IGF-BP-3 is an integrated marker of somatotroph function, and its measurement may prove to be a useful test of growth hormone levels.

All patients with large pituitary adenomas should have measurements of IGF-I levels or GH response to glucose ingestion. In rare cases, patients with large pituitaries and elevated serum levels of GH and IGF-I do not have clinical evidence of acromegaly. This syndrome, called *silent somatotroph adenoma*, is unexplained.

Radiologic investigation is necessary once the laboratory tests confirm the clinical suspicion of acromegaly. Although conventional skull x-rays or coned-down views of the sella turcica are abnormal in 90 percent of patients with acromegaly, MRI provides better definition of tumor size and is necessary for therapeutic planning. Additional clues to the diagnosis on conventional skull x-rays include thickening of the skull with increased bone density, enlargement of the paranasal sinuses and proliferation of the mastoid air cells, and prognathism. On bone x-rays, one may see enlarged vertebral bodies with anterior lipping, tufting of the distal phalanges of the hands and feet, increased thickness and lengthening of the ribs and clavicles, and bowing of the femur, tibia, and fibula. Soft tissue x-rays demonstrate increased thickness of the heel pad (>18 mm in women and >21 mm in men).

Testing for hypopituitarism (due to compression of the normal pituitary tissue) and for increased prolactin levels (due either to stalk compression or to cosecretion of prolactin by the tumor) should be performed. Mass effects from large somatotroph adenomas can cause neurologic abnormalities (visual field defects or oculomotor or abducens nerve lesions). In addition, acromegaly may be associated with hyperparathyroidism and pancreatic islet cell tumors in the MEN 1 syndrome and rarely with pheochromocytomas or hyperaldosteronism (see Chap. 340). The α subunit of the glycoprotein hormones may be oversecreted in acromegaly and may serve as an additional marker of tumor regrowth.

℞ TREATMENT

The objectives of therapy are (1) return of GH and IGF-I levels to normal, (2) stabilization or decrease in tumor size, and (3) preservation of normal pituitary function. Although GH values of <5 μg/L were formerly considered to indicate cure, a value of <2 μg/L with a normal IGF-I level is a better criterion; patients with GH values between 2 and 5 μg/L may have persistent symptoms and increased IGF-I concentrations.

Surgery Transsphenoidal surgery has the advantage of producing a rapid therapeutic response; it is potentially curative and is the treatment of choice. Anesthesiologists should be alerted to the potential of a difficult intubation due to anatomic changes in the jaw, tongue, epiglottis, and larynx. GH concentrations may fall to normal within hours, and soft tissue (but not bony) enlargement may melt away, even before the patient has been discharged from the hospital. The success of this procedure depends on the completeness of the resection and hence on the size of the tumor. Cure rates vary from 80 percent for microadenomas to less than 50 percent for tumors larger than 1 cm in diameter. Preoperative GH levels are also of predictive value. In expert hands, apparent cure rates (GH below 5 μg/L) average 75 percent in patients with preoperative GH levels of <40 μg/L but only 35 percent in those with preoperative GH levels >40 μg/L. More stringent criteria, such as a GH level of <2 μg/L and a normal IGF-I level, are rarely used in surgical series; the cure rate is probably closer to 20 to 40 percent when these criteria are applied. This may explain why tumor regrowth and recurrent acromegaly are more common than previously appreciated. Persistent GH response to TRH stimulation may have predictive value in assessing risk of relapse, even in those patients with "normal" postoperative GH concentrations. Postoperative hypopituitarism occurs in 10 to 20 percent of patients with large tumors, but up to 10 percent of patients with pituitary insufficiency prior to surgery regain normal function.

Radiation Heavy-particle pituitary irradiation is successful in lowering GH levels in acromegaly but is slow to accomplish this goal. Patients with suprasellar extension of the pituitary adenoma are generally excluded from this therapy. The Harvard cyclotron uses the Bragg peak with proton irradiation, achieving delivery of up to 12,000 cGy (12,000 rad) to the center of the pituitary adenoma. In patients with mean pretherapy GH concentration of 60 μg/L, GH concentrations are <5 μg/L in 29 percent of patients at 2 years, in 40 percent at 4 years, in 75 percent at 10 years, and in 92 percent by 20 years. The risk of hypopituitarism is at least 20 percent.

Conventional pituitary irradiation [4500 cGy (4500 rad) over 5 weeks] can cause a lowering of GH levels, but the effect may take years to develop. GH generally falls 50 percent after 2 ± 1 years. GH concentrations of <5 μg/L occur in 50 percent of patients at 5 years and in 70 percent at 10 years (after a mean pretherapy GH level of 60 μg/L). GH concentrations of <2.5 μg/L occur in 40 percent of patients, and values <1 μg/L are seen in 20 percent at 10 to 15 years. Hypopituitarism is a common sequela of radiation treatment, and up to 50 percent of patients require hormone replacement. The hypopituitarism is probably due to hypothalamic damage, which is possibly less common with focused heavy particles or gamma radiation. Higher doses of focused radiation [4000 to 7000 cGy (4000 to 7000 rad)] can be delivered with the cobalt 60 gamma unit ("gamma knife"), which delivers collimated radiation through multiple portals (over 200 in some units) that converge on the target. The radiation is delivered in a single session; radiation delivery to the tumor is the equivalent of two to three times the dosage of conventional radiation treatment. Reports to date do not suggest an advantage (apart from convenience) over conventional radiation treatment in terms of either efficacy or of the risk of hypopituitarism; however, the data are still preliminary. Rare complications of pituitary irradiation include development of malignancies in the radiation field, damage to the visual apparatus, brain necrosis, and cognitive impairment. Radiation treatment is advised for patients who have failed surgery and medical therapy, for tumors in an inoperable location, and when surgery is contraindicated or is refused by the patient. Because of the long delay between irradiation of the pituitary and response, medical therapy should be given in the interim.

Medical Treatment Bromocriptine is a useful adjunct to other modalities of therapy but rarely is successful alone. Clinical improvement is reported in up to 90 percent of patients with dosages of 20 to 60 mg/d. Objective decrease in hand and ring size as well as improvement in diabetes mellitus may occur in the absence of decreasing GH values. However, GH concentrations fall to <10 μg/L in only 35 percent of patients, and values of <5 μg/L are achieved in only 21 percent; IGF-I levels return to normal in only 8 percent. Tumor size decreases rarely.

The long-acting somatostatin analogue octreotide lowers GH to <5 μg/L and IGF-I to normal in half of acromegalics. Modest tumor regression occurs in 30 to 50 percent of patients. The drug must be administered subcutaneously several times a day. Dosages average 100 to 200 μg every 8 h but range from 50 to 250 μg every 6 to 12 h to a maximum of 1500 μg/d. Constant subcutaneous pump therapy also has been employed to prevent the rise in GH between injections. Temporary side effects are minimal and include local pain, steatorrhea, and abdominal cramps; the risk of cholelithiasis is substantial and may be due to decreased gallbladder contractility. Octreotide is 2000 times as potent as somatostatin in inhibiting GH secretion but only 1.5 to 2 times as potent an inhibitor of insulin secretion. Although impairment of glucose tolerance or worsening of diabetes mellitus may occur, the GH-lowering effects of the drug may improve glucose tolerance. Inhibition of TSH does not result in hypothyroidism. Headaches disappear quickly, possibly due to an effect on cerebral blood flow. The role of this agent as a primary treatment for acromegaly remains to be defined, but some patients have been treated successfully for over 5 years. It is likely that octreotide will be most useful as adjunctive therapy after unsuccessful surgery and/or radiation therapy. Studies suggesting that the success rate of surgery in acromegalic patients with invasive macroadenomas is higher after octreotide pretreatment have not been confirmed.

All acromegalic patients require long-term follow-up and evaluation for recurrent disease. Interlaboratory variation in GH determinations may be considerable; whenever possible, serial GH levels should be measured by the same laboratory. False elevations of GH concentrations in some acromegalics may be due to antibodies that displace GH in the radioimmunoassays used. Surveillance for colonic polyps and/or colon cancer, including colonoscopy, may be appropriate for all acromegalics; other workers advocate such surveillance only for those at higher risk: subjects over age 50, those with more than 10 years of acromegaly, and those with more than three skin tags.

GH DEFICIENCY AND PITUITARY DWARFISM GH is often the first hormone to be lost in pituitary and hypothalamic disorders. In adults, GH deficiency is usually cryptic and can only be diagnosed on the basis of stimulation tests for GH release. The consequences of GH deficiency and replacement in adults are being explored. GH deficiency may contribute to the increased cardiovascular mortality in hypopituitary adults; conversely, these patients have a decreased cancer mortality. Diabetics with GH deficiency show a reduction in insulin requirements and may develop hypoglycemia. In children GH deficiency leads to impaired growth and short stature and is often a consequence of hypothalamic GHRH deficiency (see Chap. 329). Short-term replacement therapy in GH-deficient adults results in improved exercise tolerance, decreased body fat, and increased lean body mass. Long-term studies of the benefits, risks, and optimal dosing of GH in adults are under way.

GONADOTROPINS

PHYSIOLOGY The gonadotropins, LH and FSH, are secreted by the gonadotrophs (see also Chaps. 336 and 337). These cells make up about 10 percent of the anterior pituitary and are dispersed throughout the lobe, often situated close to the lactotrophs. Most gonadotrophs produce both LH and FSH, although a few cells produce only one hormone.

LH and FSH are glycoproteins of similar size (about 30,000 mol wt) which share a common α subunit [also present in TSH and human chorionic gonadotropin (hCG)] but have unique β subunits. The α and β chains are encoded by separate genes, and α chains are often produced in excess. The carbohydrate components of the molecules influence the biologic behavior and duration of action and may vary during the menstrual cycle. Although both FSH and LH are secreted in pulsatile fashion, FSH has a longer half-life, so that FSH levels fluctuate less throughout the day. FSH and LH regulate ovarian and testicular function. hCG is also produced in the normal pituitary.

FSH stimulates the growth of the granulosa cells of the ovarian follicle and controls the aromatase responsible for estradiol formation in these cells. LH stimulates the ovarian theca cells to produce androgens, which diffuse to the granulosa cells, where they are converted to estrogens. The level of estradiol, the principal estrogen, peaks about 1 day prior to the LH surge, which, in turn, triggers ovulation. After ovulation LH contributes to corpus luteum formation. Once conception has occurred, pituitary gonadotropin function is no longer necessary to sustain pregnancy.

In the testis LH controls testosterone production by the Leydig cells. FSH, in conjunction with intratesticular testosterone, stimulates the seminiferous tubules to produce sperm. Thus, LH and FSH both are necessary for normal spermatogenesis, whereas testosterone production requires only LH.

Luteinizing hormone–releasing hormone [LHRH, also known as gonadotropin-releasing hormone (GnRH)], a decapeptide produced by the arcuate nuclei of the hypothalamus, is responsible for the release of both LH and FSH. Extrahypothalamic LHRH is present in other areas of the brain as well. Noradrenergic agonists appear to facilitate, whereas endogenous opioids inhibit, LHRH release.

LHRH acts on high-affinity pituitary receptors to stimulate LH and FSH production and release. The pituitary response to LHRH varies greatly throughout life. LHRH and the gonadotropins first appear in the fetus at about 10 weeks of gestation. During the first 3 months after birth, LHRH elicits a brisk gonadotropin rise. The sensitivity to LHRH then declines until the onset of puberty. Before puberty FSH levels increase to a greater extent after LHRH administration than does LH. With the onset of puberty, sensitivity to LHRH increases, and pulsatile LH secretion is first apparent during sleep. Later in puberty and during the reproductive years, pulsations are present throughout the day, with LH being more responsive to LHRH than is FSH. After menopause, FSH and LH levels rise, and postmenopausal FSH levels are higher than those of LH.

Pulsatile LHRH release results in pulsatile LH and FSH release. However, sustained infusion of LHRH and its analogues results in inhibition of LH and FSH release. This phenomenon has been used successfully in the treatment of gonadotropin-mediated precocious puberty by the sustained administration of LHRH or its analogues. Conversely, in people with LHRH deficiency, the pulsatile administration of LHRH can restore ovarian or testicular function.

The feedback relationship between the gonadal steroids and the hypothalamus and pituitary is detailed in Chaps. 336 and 337. Low doses of estrogens decrease the frequency of LHRH pulses and, more important, decrease the pituitary response to LHRH; this phenomenon is seen most clearly in postmenopausal women with elevated gonadotropin levels. However, sustained elevation of estrogens results in a positive-feedback signal that stimulates LHRH and LH release; this phenomenon is responsible, in part, for the LH surge that precedes ovulation. The sensitivity of LHRH to this positive feedback by estrogen increases during middle to late puberty. Although progesterone decreases LHRH pulse frequency, the progesterone rise in the late follicular phase augments the pituitary LH response to LHRH and contributes to the LH surge. In castrated men, testosterone administration usually suppresses LH to undetectable levels and less often lowers FSH to normal (but not undetectable) concentrations. Inhibin, a peptide hormone produced by the testicular Sertoli cell and ovarian granulosa cell, is a potent inhibitor of FSH (but not LH) release. Its physiologic role is under investigation. Testosterone decreases the frequency of LH pulsations, probably by a direct effect on LHRH release and is converted in many tissues, including the brain, to estradiol, which inhibits the pituitary response to LHRH.

Gonadotropin Measurements In evaluating gonadal failure associated with low testosterone concentrations in men or low estradiol levels in women, gonadotropin measurements help separate primary from central (secondary, hypogonadotropic) hypogonadism. High gonadotropin concentrations are indicative of primary gonadal failure; low or normal gonadotropin concentrations suggest hypothalamic or pituitary disease (see Chap. 330). Primary gonadal failure, as in women at menopause or after oophorectomy or in men with testicular failure, causes a marked increase in FSH and LH levels. Such elevated gonadotropin concentrations ensure the adequacy of pituitary gonadotroph function and establish that the disorder is at the gonadal level. On the other hand, gonadotropin measurements are rarely indicated in a woman with ovulatory menses and in men with normal sperm counts.

HYPOGONADOTROPIC (CENTRAL, SECONDARY) HYPOGONADISM Isolated gonadotropin deficiency may be a congenital or hereditary disorder. Kallmann's syndrome is a heterogeneous genetic disorder afflicting 1 in 10,000 to 60,000 individuals; X-linked as well as autosomal inheritance has been described. Kallmann's syndrome is characterized by gonadotropin deficiency due to LHRH deficiency in association with anosmia and midline anatomic defects. LHRH-secreting neurons migrate from the olfactory placode into the brain, along with the olfactory and other nerves. The mutation in X-linked Kallmann's syndrome results in a defect in neuronal migration. Most patients with Kallmann's syndrome secrete gonadotropins in response to LHRH administration after suitable priming. Mutations in the β subunit of LH are another cause of hypogonadism.

Acquired defects of LHRH production are common. Hyperprolactinemia causes amenorrhea due to inhibition of LHRH release, possibly mediated by increased hypothalamic dopamine. Amenorrhea that occurs with anorexia nervosa, starvation, intense exercise, and "stress" appears to be due to inhibition of LHRH release as well. Gonadotropin deficiency may be a relatively early defect in patients with large pituitary adenomas. Gonadotropin deficiency also occurs in patients with polyglandular endocrine deficiencies, presumably on an autoimmune basis (see Chap. 340), and in patients with hemochromatosis.

Patients with LHRH deficiency who desire fertility may respond to pulsatile therapy with LHRH or its agonists. When gonadotropin deficiency is due to pituitary disease, injections of FSH (menotropin) and chorionic gonadotropin (a hormone with LH-like activity) are necessary to achieve fertility.

ECTOPIC GONADOTROPIN SECRETION Ectopic gonadotropin production (usually of hCG) can be associated with germinomas of the nonseminoma type (see Chap. 98), lung carcinomas, hepatomas, and other tumors. Children may develop precocious puberty, and men may develop gynecomastia. No distinct clinical syndrome occurs in women.

GONADOTROPIN-SECRETING PITUITARY TUMORS Gonadotropin-secreting pituitary tumors, like other pituitary adenomas, are monoclonal in origin, implying that a somatic mutation in a single gonadotrope is responsible. The inhibin subunits that make up activin, a member of the transforming growth factor β family of peptides, are produced by these tumors and may play a role in their growth. Gonadotroph adenomas are generally large and are most commonly diagnosed in men with decreased libido, decreased serum testosterone levels, and normal or slightly elevated prolactin levels. Although 20 to 25 percent of pituitary macroadenomas are considered nonfunctioning (i.e., they do not cause a clinical syndrome of hormone overproduction), many of these tumors produce gonadotropin. Some produce high levels of intact gonadotropins (usually FSH or FSH in conjunction with LH, rarely LH alone), with or without a clinical syndrome. Testicular enlargement due to FSH excess and testosterone elevation due to elevated LH levels occur but are rare. The finding of an increased FSH concentration may be misinterpreted as primary hypogonadism if a pituitary adenoma is not suspected. Inhibin levels may be increased (as a consequence of FSH increase) in contrast to low inhibin levels in patients with primary hypogonadism. In some, the FSH has enhanced biologic activity, possibly because of altered glycosylation. In others, normal amounts of intact gonadotropins are associated with unbalanced production of gonadotropin subunits, particularly the α subunit of FSH or the LH β subunit. Although LH concentrations are often normal or elevated, testosterone levels are often low and respond normally to hCG administration. This suggests that the LH is biologically inactive (possibly because of abnormal glycosylation) or that the measured LH value represents immunologic cross-reactivity due to LH subunit overproduction. Some tumors secrete normal amounts of intact gonadotropins and gonadotropin subunits but demonstrate abnormal responses to TRH stimulation. FSH increase in response to TRH (e.g., 400 μg intravenously) occurs in 40 percent of patients with gonadotropin-secreting tumors but not in normal individuals, hypogonadal men, or postmenopausal women; an increased response of gonadotropin α and LH β subunits is common as well. Some tumors express gonadotropin gene mRNA and/or hormone production in vitro but do not cause in vivo abnormalities.

In postmenopausal women with macroadenomas, it may be difficult to ascertain whether a gonadotropin elevation is due to normal menopause or to a gonadotropin-secreting adenoma. TRH testing may provide a partial answer. Most such tumors produce increased LH β, FSH, or LH in response to TRH administration.

The therapy of nonfunctioning pituitary macroadenomas and gonadotropin-secreting adenomas is the same: surgery and/or radiation therapy. The response to bromocriptine, somatostatin analogues, or LHRH analogues is disappointing in terms of tumor shrinkage even when a hormonal response is achieved.

Men with primary hypogonadism (low testosterone level, elevated LH and FSH levels) are occasionally investigated for the presence of a gonadotropin-secreting tumor. There is no simple way of differentiating these two clinical situations. Primary hypogonadism is common; gonadotropin-secreting tumors are rare. The tumors are almost always large, but radiographic procedures may be necessary to exclude a tumor. A normal testicular response to hCG administration points toward a gonadotropin-secreting adenoma, but this test is cumbersome and poorly standardized.

THYROTROPIN

PHYSIOLOGY TSH is a glycoprotein hormone (28,000 mol wt) composed of an α subunit which it shares with LH, FSH, and hCG and a unique β subunit that confers specificity (also see Chap. 331). The individual subunits have no intrinsic biologic activity. TSH is produced by thyrotrophs, which constitute about 5 percent of the cells of the anterior pituitary. TSH regulates the biosynthesis, storage, and release of thyroid hormones and determines thyroid gland size. TSH first appears in the fetal pituitary at about 10 weeks of gestation. TSH levels in normal subjects average 0.5 to 5.0 mU/L, with a slight increase in the nocturnal hours. The nocturnal TSH rise is absent in patients with central hypothyroidism.

Thyrotropin-releasing hormone (TRH), the major hypothalamic mediator of TSH release, is a tripeptide found in highest concentrations in the medial division of the hypothalamic paraventricular nuclei and in the median eminence. Extrahypothalamic TRH is found in the posterior pituitary, in other parts of the brain and spinal cord, and in the gastrointestinal tract. TRH stimulates TSH secretion by increasing cytoplasmic free calcium; phosphatidylinositol and membrane phospholipids probably participate in TRH-stimulated TSH secretion. TRH stimulation increases the glycosylation and hence the biologic activity of secreted TSH. TRH stimulates the release of prolactin as well as that of TSH. The prolactin response is enhanced in hypothyroidism and diminished in hyperthyroidism. TRH-induced GH stimulation may occur in acromegaly, renal failure and depression; it also occurs in many normal children and in occasional normal adults.

The thyroid hormones thyroxine (T_4) and triiodothyronine (T_3) inhibit TSH production directly at the pituitary level. Both T_3 and T_4 bind to receptors on pituitary nuclei, but T_3 has a 40-fold greater affinity for these receptors than does T_4. Nevertheless, exogenous T_4 is more potent than T_3 in inhibiting TSH release because circulating T_4 is a more effective means of delivering T_3 to the pituitary than is T_3 itself. Half of intrapituitary T_3 is derived from T_4 conversion within the pituitary. The effects of T_4 and T_3 on hypothalamic TRH release in humans are unknown, but in animals they cause inhibition of TRH synthesis and release. In the usual causes of hyperthyroidism, TSH is suppressed, and the TSH response to TRH is absent; in primary hypothyroidism, the basal TSH concentration is elevated, and the response to TRH is exaggerated.

Somatostatin decreases basal TSH release, the TSH response to TRH, and the nocturnal TSH peak. Dopamine and glucocorticoids decrease the basal TSH concentration and the TSH response to TRH. Patients with untreated primary adrenal insufficiency may have slightly elevated TSH levels. TSH levels decline with severe illness.

TSH concentrations can be interpreted only when serum thyroid hormone concentrations are known (see Chap. 327). In the usual cases of hyperthyroidism, thyroid hormone levels are elevated, and TSH release is inhibited. TSH-induced hyperthyroidism is rare. Only sensitive TSH assays can differentiate between low and normal concentrations. A detectable serum TSH concentration by a sensitive assay excludes the common causes of hyperthyroidism. Low thyroid hormone and elevated serum TSH concentrations are characteristic of primary hypothyroidism. Low thyroid hormone concentrations with a "normal" or "low" TSH concentration are found in central (secondary) hypothyroidism. The TRH stimulation test (no TSH response in hyperthyroidism, exaggerated TSH response in primary hypothyroidism) has largely been supplanted by sensitive TSH measurements. The TRH stimulation test is also not useful in the diagnosis of secondary hypothyroidism or in differentiating pituitary from hypothalamic disease.

PRIMARY HYPOTHYROIDISM Thyroid gland failure (primary hypothyroidism) leads to compensatory hypertrophy of the thyrotrophs. With thyroid failure of long duration, the pituitary gland and the sella turcica may enlarge, occasionally causing visual field defects. Although TSH-secreting tumors may develop in animals after thyroid gland removal, the increased TSH and pituitary size in human hypothyroidism is not autonomous and decreases with thyroid hormone replacement. Since hyperprolactinemia also may occur in patients with primary hypothyroidism, pituitary enlargement (hyperplasia) may be incorrectly diagnosed as a prolactinoma; however, the return to normal of prolactin concentrations with thyroid hormone therapy excludes that diagnosis. Severe primary hypothyroidism occasionally causes impaired release of GH and ACTH after appropriate stimuli (so-called pituitary myxedema), and hypothyroid children may develop precocious puberty. These abnormalities are all corrected with thyroid hormone therapy.

SECONDARY HYPOTHYROIDISM Hypothyroidism due to pituitary or hypothalamic disease may be difficult to diagnose. With primary hypothyroidism, serum TSH commonly rises before thyroid hormone concentrations decline below the normal range. No similar early laboratory clue exists in secondary hypothyroidism. Patients with central hypothyroidism usually do not have goiter, and many have deficiencies of other pituitary trophic hormones.

Some patients with hypothalamic hypothyroidism have mild TSH elevations, rather than normal or low concentrations, as expected. Although the TSH elevations rarely exceed 10 mU/L, they are above the expected range for hypothyroidism due to TSH deficiency. Biologically inactive but immunologically active thyrotropin is present in such cases. After TRH injection, the TSH concentration rises, and the biologic potency of the TSH is increased. This suggests an additional role for TRH in controlling the biologic activity of the TSH molecule by controlling its rate of glycosylation. Although subclinical primary hypothyroidism is also characterized by mild TSH elevations, serum T_4 levels differ in the two states. Patients with central hypothyroidism and associated TSH elevations have very low T_4 concentrations; patients with subclinical hypothyroidism have normal or near-normal T_4 concentrations. TSH concentrations must not be used to guide replacement therapy in central hypothyroidism, because TSH concentrations fall before full replacement is achieved; rather, peripheral levels of T_4 and free T_4 should be monitored. Severe illness may cause laboratory changes indistinguishable from those of central hypothyroidism, part of the so-called euthyroid sick syndrome.

PITUITARY (TSH-INDUCED) HYPERTHYROIDISM Hyperthyroidism is not usually a disease of TSH overproduction. However, the following two types of TSH-mediated hyperthyroidism are recognized.

Pituitary Tumors These are usually macroadenomas with autonomous TSH secretion, unresponsive to thyroid hormone suppression or TRH stimulation. Patients with these tumors may appear to have Graves' disease with high free thyroxine levels and diffuse goiters with high radioiodine uptakes. However, they do not have the eye or skin changes of Graves' disease and do not have suppressed TSH levels. A hallmark of such tumors is overproduction of the glycoprotein hormone α subunit with a molar ratio of α to intact TSH of greater than 1:1 in serum. The free α subunit may be an important tumor marker and differs from the native α subunit in that one of its amino acids is carbohydrate-blocked and hence cannot combine with β subunits. These tumors may produce other pituitary hormones in addition to TSH, most commonly GH. In some patients TSH levels are within normal limits; increased TSH bioactivity is believed to explain the hyperthyroidism in such patients. Therapy is generally transsphenoidal surgery to remove the tumor, but control of hyperthyroidism may require radioactive iodine or antithyroid drugs. Octreotide may lower TSH levels when complete tumor removal is not possible.

Pituitary Resistance to Thyroid Hormone In this situation, thyroid hormone fails to inhibit TSH secretion appropriately in the absence of a pituitary adenoma. Since TSH secretion is not inhibited, TSH rises and stimulates thyroid hormone overproduction. The peripheral tissues are not resistant to thyroid hormone, and clinical hyperthyroidism results. The pituitary resistance to thyroid hormone is incomplete, since TSH can be suppressed with supraphysiologic levels of thyroid hormone and stimulated further with TRH; bromocriptine or octreotide may lower TSH as well. Pituitary resistance is usually diagnosed after thyroid gland ablation, when TSH cannot be lowered to normal values with the usual therapeutic doses of thyroid hormone. However, once the hyperthyroidism has been treated, pituitary resistance is of no clinical consequence, although the TSH measurements cannot be utilized to monitor adequacy of hormone replacement. In some patients the molecular defect in the thyroid hormone β receptor is the same as that in generalized resistance to thyroid hormone (see Chap. 331).

ADRENOCORTICOTROPIN

PHYSIOLOGY ACTH is produced by corticotrophs, which constitute about 15 percent of anterior pituitary cells and are located principally in the central portion of the gland. ACTH is synthesized as part of a large precursor molecule termed *pro-opiomelanocortin* (POMC, 265 amino acids). ACTH contains 39 amino acids, with nearly complete biologic activity residing in the *N*-terminal 26 amino acids. In the anterior pituitary, POMC is cleaved to yield ACTH, β-lipotropin, and an *N*-terminal precursor.

ACTH controls the release of cortisol from the adrenal cortex. Although aldosterone is primarily controlled by the renin-angiotensin system, ACTH also stimulates aldosterone release acutely. Other derivatives of the POMC molecule, such as γ melanocyte-stimulating hormone (γ-MSH), also influence aldosterone production and are found in increased levels in the plasma of patients with idiopathic hyperaldosteronism. Patients with ACTH deficiency have near-normal aldosterone production and do not require mineralocorticoid replacement.

Corticotropin-releasing hormone (CRH) is the major but not exclusive regulator of ACTH release. CRH contains 41 amino acids in a single polypeptide chain. It is synthesized primarily by neurons of the paraventricular nuclei of the hypothalamus but is also present in other areas of the brain, including the limbic system and cortex, and in the placenta, pancreas, gut, and adrenal medulla. Circulating CRH, which is largely of nonhypothalamic origin, is bound to a high-affinity binding protein. CRH stimulates cyclic AMP production, regulates intracellular calcium, and increases the concentration of POMC mRNA. Vasopressin potentiates the release of ACTH by CRH through a cyclic AMP–independent mechanism and may play a physiologic role in ACTH release. Naloxone, an opiate antagonist, causes release of CRH (and hence ACTH) in humans.

ACTH is released in pulses with an overriding circadian rhythm. With a normal sleeping pattern, ACTH concentration is highest in the early morning (around 4 A.M.) and lowest in late evening. The normal diurnal rhythm of plasma cortisol occurs in response to these ACTH changes. In primary adrenal insufficiency (Addison's disease), cortisol concentrations fall, and ACTH concentrations rise. This results in hyperpigmentation owing to the melanocyte-stimulating properties of ACTH. Cortisol administration inhibits ACTH release, a phenomenon dependent on both the rate of rise of cortisol and its absolute concentration. Increased plasma cortisol inhibits CRH-induced ACTH release and also may inhibit CRH release. When pharmacologic doses of glucocorticoids are given for prolonged periods, the hypothalamic-pituitary–adrenal cortex axis may remain suppressed for months after the drugs are stopped, probably as the result of prolonged hypothalamic CRH suppression (see Chap. 332).

Stress, including hypoglycemia, surgery, and psychic distress, stimulates ACTH release, in part via increased CRH release, but the magnitude of the ACTH release is greater than can be achieved with maximal doses of CRH. With severe illness, the requirements for cortisol may increase significantly; failure of cortisol secretion to be enhanced during such periods may cause clinical adrenal insufficiency when adrenal reserve is impaired.

The immune system is tightly linked to the hypothalamic-pituitary-adrenal (HPA) axis. Glucocorticoids inhibit immune function, and immune mediators such as interleukin 1 are potent stimulators of ACTH secretion. These mediators may explain at least part of the link between "stress" and activation of the HPA axis, the subsequent cortisol response serving to limit the immune response.

ACTH is present at low levels in normal serum [2 to 18 pmol/L (10 to 80 pg/mL)]. It is difficult to measure ACTH in plasma and often not possible to separate low from normal values using commercial assays. Random ACTH measurements have little clinical significance. Tests for adrenal insufficiency and excess rely primarily on measurements of cortisol and its metabolites rather than on measurement of ACTH.

ACTH EXCESS (CUSHING'S DISEASE AND NELSON'S SYNDROME) **Clinical Features** Cortisol excess is characterized by a central distribution of adipose tissue, muscle weakness, purplish striae, hypertension, amenorrhea, decreased libido, impotence, osteoporosis, fatigue, and psychiatric abnormalities. This syndrome may be caused by pituitary or ectopic ACTH overproduction, adrenal tumors, or exogenous glucocorticoid administration.

The presence of cortisol excess is suggested by the failure to suppress an 8 A.M. cortisol level to <140 nmol/L (<5 μg/dL) after an overnight dexamethasone suppression test (1 mg by mouth at midnight). Because there are many causes of false-positive failure of suppression, the diagnosis must be confirmed by the finding of increased excretion of urine free cortisol and/or 17-hydroxycorticosteroids that fails to decrease appropriately after 2-day low-dose dexamethasone administration (0.5 mg every 6 h for eight doses). Additional suppression (and occasionally stimulation) tests are required to determine whether the Cushing's syndrome is due to a pituitary lesion (Cushing's disease) or to some other cause. In patients with pituitary ACTH hypersecretion, high-dose overnight dexamethasone administration (8 mg at midnight) results in greater than 50 percent reduction in the 8 A.M. plasma cortisol level, and two-day dexamethasone administration (2 mg every 6 h for eight doses) should result in greater than 60 percent suppression of urine 17-hydroxycorticosteroids and more than 90 percent suppression of urine free cortisol. Urine 17-hydroxycorticosteroids increase after metyrapone administration in Cushing's disease. In contrast, most adrenal and ectopic tumors that produce cortisol and/or ACTH autonomously do not demonstrate suppression with dexamethasone or stimulation with metapyrone.

Plasma ACTH levels are normal or high-normal in Cushing's disease and show an exaggerated increase after CRH administration. ACTH levels are low in adrenal Cushing's disease and do not increase with CRH. In ectopic Cushing's disease ACTH levels can be extremely high but are often high normal, overlapping the levels in pituitary Cushing's disease. However, most patients with ectopic Cushing's disease do not exhibit a rise in ACTH with CRH administration. Pituitary Cushing's disease is caused by a corticotroph microadenoma in 90 percent of patients and by a macroadenoma in most of the rest. The microadenomas are often small (3 to 6 mm or less) and may be difficult to find even with the use of gadolinium-enhanced MRI. Corticotroph hyperplasia has been documented in a few cases. Previously, pituitary surgery was often recommended on the basis of dynamic testing alone. However, some ACTH-producing tumors, particularly bronchial carcinoids, give dynamic hormone test results similar to those in Cushing's disease, leading to misdiagnosis and inappropriate surgery. The technique of bilateral inferior petrosal sinus catheterization to localize the site of ACTH production is a major advance for confirming the pituitary source of ACTH production and for localizing adenomas when imaging studies are negative.

Nelson's syndrome (characterized by hyperpigmentation and high plasma ACTH levels despite adequate glucocorticoid replacement) is caused by growth of the residual pituitary tumor after bilateral adrenalectomy in patients with pituitary Cushing's disease. These tumors can cause mass effects such as bitemporal hemianopsia from optic chiasm compression or oculomotor nerve palsy from cavernous sinus invasion. The tumors are usually identified on MRI and may exhibit aggressive growth patterns.

℞ **TREATMENT**

Transsphenoidal microsurgery is successful in treating microadenomas in more than 80 percent of patients. When surgery is successful, plasma cortisol concentrations fall almost to zero and often remain low for many months owing to delayed recovery of CRH and ACTH secretion by the hypothalamus and normal remaining pituitary. Thus, glucocorticoid replacement is necessary until the hypothalamic-pituitary-adrenal axis recovers. Cushing's syndrome may recur, and long-term follow-up is important. Prior to the development of transsphenoidal surgery, bilateral adrenalectomy was the therapy of choice for pituitary Cushing's disease. Unfortunately, after this procedure Nelson's syndrome develops in 10 to 30 percent of patients, particularly in younger individuals.

Ectopic ACTH production is the cause of 10 to 15 percent of cases of Cushing's syndrome and may be difficult to diagnose (see Chaps. 102 and 332). When ACTH production is caused by a rapidly growing tumor such as small cell carcinoma of the lung, many of the symptoms of Cushing's syndrome may be absent. Rather, patients have hypokalemia, muscle weakness, weight loss, and hyperpigmentation. ACTH concentrations often exceed 66 pmol/L (300 pg/mL) and do not change with dexamethasone administration. ACTH concentrations may be lower in immunoradiometric assays that do not measure larger fragments of the POMC molecule. When slow-growing tumors such as thymic carcinoids, bronchial carcinoids, medullary carcinoma of the thyroid, and pancreatic islet cell tumors produce ACTH, the features of Cushing's syndrome are present. In the latter group, ACTH measurements and cortisol response to dexamethasone administration may mimic those found in patients with pituitary adenomas. When it is unclear whether ACTH production is pituitary or ectopic, bilateral inferior petrosal sinus catheterization for measurement of ACTH is necessary. Cushing's syndrome can rarely be caused by ectopic production of CRH itself.

ACTH DEFICIENCY (SECONDARY ADRENAL INSUFFICIENCY) ACTH deficiency may be isolated or occur in association with other anterior pituitary hormone deficiencies. Reversible isolated ACTH deficiency is common after long-term glucocorticoid administration. If glucocorticoids are withdrawn suddenly in this situation or continued at physiologic doses when severe illness is present, adrenal insufficiency may occur (see Chap. 332). Symptoms include nausea, vomiting, fatigue, joint discomfort, and dizziness, and there may be fever, hypotension, hyponatremia, and hypoglycemia. Reversible dementia may occur in the elderly. Although cortisol is necessary for free water excretion, it is not needed for potassium excretion. Hence, patients with ACTH deficiency are hyponatremic but not hyperkalemic, in contrast to patients with primary adrenal insufficiency. Hyperpigmentation does not occur. These factors make diagnosis of secondary adrenal insufficiency more difficult than that of primary adrenal insufficiency. Isolated ACTH deficiency may occur without prior glucocorticoid therapy and may be of hypothalamic or pituitary origin. The diagnosis is often missed.

In general, patients undergoing pituitary surgery need to be treated with "stress" doses of glucocorticoids until normal adrenal function can be demonstrated postoperatively. All patients with pituitary macroadenomas or hypothalamic disease require testing of the pituitary-adrenal axis, but when pituitary surgery is planned, testing can be limited in focus until after surgery is completed.

THE ENDOGENOUS OPIOID PEPTIDES

The endogenous opioid peptides bind to a family of opioid receptors. The endorphins, enkephalins, and dynorphins, although chemically related, arise by different biosynthetic pathways. In the pituitary, β-endorphin, the most abundant endorphin, is synthesized as part of a larger precursor molecule (proopiomelanocortin, POMC) that also contains the full sequences of ACTH, γ-MSH, β-MSH, and β-lipotropin (β-LPH) (Fig. 328-7). This biosynthetic pathway represents the

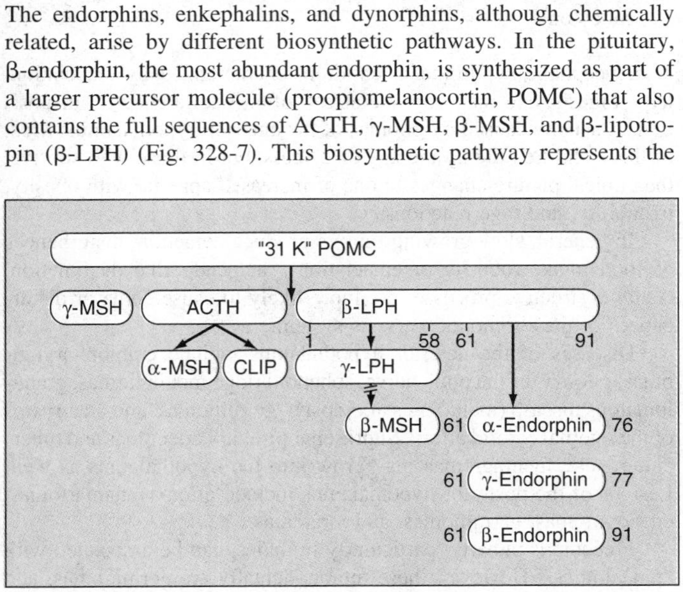

FIGURE 328-7 Biosynthetic pathway for β-endorphin in the pituitary gland. A single precursor protein, pro-opiomelanocortin (POMC) (molecular weight of approximately 31,000), is initially synthesized from translation of a gene that encodes the structure of adrenocorticotropin (ACTH), β-lipotropin (β-LPH), and β-endorphin. Prohormone-type cleavages can generate other hormones from the same precursor, although this occurs in tissues other than the pituitary. Abbreviations: MSH, melanocyte-stimulating hormone; LPH, lipotropin; CLIP, corticotropin-like intermediate peptide; ACTH, adrenocorticotropin.

only pathway for pituitary ACTH synthesis. In adrenal insufficiency and Nelson's syndrome and after CRH administration, plasma levels of ACTH and β-endorphin are elevated in parallel. Ectopic production of ACTH by tumors is also accompanied by β-endorphin and β-LPH excess. Unfortunately, differential processing of POMC by tumors does not usually allow separation of pituitary from ectopic ACTH production by analysis of metabolites. Production of "big" and "big-big" ACTH by tumors reflects the incomplete processing of the POMC precursor; the detection of higher ACTH levels by radioimmunoassay than by immunoradiometric assay also reflects this incomplete processing. The increased ratio of β-LPH to ACTH may be due to increased processing of ACTH to corticotropin-like intermediate lobe peptide (CLIP) by the tumor. Alternative processing of POMC occurs within other tissues. For example, hypothalamic neurons produce POMC, which serves as a precursor of β-endorphin in the brain; ACTH is not an end-product of POMC metabolism in these cells.

Two other opioid precursors give rise to potent endogenous opioids, including the enkephalins, dynorphins, and neoendorphins. These opioid precursors are produced in many parts of the brain, including various hypothalamic nuclei. Dynorphin often colocalizes with vasopressin in neurons.

The pituitary is the richest site of endorphin. ACTH- and endorphin-containing cells are found in the anteromedial region of the anterior lobe, at the posterior boundary of the anterior lobe, and in nerve fibers of the posterior lobe. The limbic system contains substantial quantities of immunoreactive endorphin, suggesting a role in memory, learning, and emotion.

Neurons containing the enkephalins are widely distributed in the central nervous system. Levels are particularly high in the dorsal horn of the spinal cord, a region that contains opiate receptors and is involved in the transmission of pain (see Chap. 12). Enkephalins may act at this location to inhibit pain transmission by sensory nerves. Euphoria produced by morphine may be related to enkephalin production in the locus coeruleus. Enkephalin concentrations are higher in the myenteric plexus of the longitudinal muscles of the gastrointestinal tract than in the brain. Enkephalin is released together with epinephrine and norepinephrine as part of the sympathetic response to stress and in patients with pheochromocytoma.

Two approaches have been employed to define the physiologic role of the endogenous opiates: assessment of the effects of administration of morphine or endogeneous opiate peptides and study of the effects of antagonists. Five opiate receptor types have been identified, making it difficult to draw general conclusions from the use of antagonists. Naloxone blocks the effects of endogenously secreted opiates on mu and epsilon receptors, revealing a tonic or physiologic role of opiate peptides. Endogenous opioids and exogenous opiates stimulate the release of GH and prolactin and inhibit the release of TSH and gonadotropin. Hence, amenorrhea is common in narcotic addicts. Opiates decrease the function of the pituitary-adrenal axis. Naloxone may prevent the stress-mediated rise in prolactin, stimulates LH and FSH release, and may reinitiate menses in some patients with hypothalamic amenorrhea. ACTH and cortisol are elevated only after high doses of naloxone. Naloxone may inhibit vasopressin release in some patients with the syndrome of inappropriate vasopressin secretion (SIADH).

Physiologic actions for these hormones may include (1) morphine-like analgesic properties, (2) euphoria and other behavioral effects, and (3) neurotransmitter and neuromodulator functions. The peptides may play a role in memory, learning, response to stress, reproduction, pain transmission, and regulation of appetite, temperature, and respiration. In addition, the placebo response, acupuncture-mediated analgesia, stress-induced amenorrhea, and the pathogenesis of shock may be mediated in part by enkephalins and the endorphins. Tranquilization, irritability, agitation, violent behavior, catalepsy, narcolepsy, catatonia, the smoking habit, alcoholism, and drug addiction may all be due to biochemical abnormalities of this system.

DISEASES OF THE HYPOTHALAMUS AND PITUITARY

Diseases that affect the hypothalamus and pituitary can have both endocrine and nonendocrine manifestations.

HYPOTHALAMUS The human hypothalamus weighs about 4 g; hypothalamic dysfunction occurs only when disease is bilateral. Tumors in this region are often slow-growing and may achieve large size before symptoms appear. Signs of hydrocephalus due to third ventricle obstruction may coexist with hypopituitarism and hypothalamic dysfunction. Neurologic symptoms and signs may be caused by compression of the optic nerve, chiasm, or tract. Large tumors may affect frontal or temporal lobe function.

Nonendocrine functions of the hypothalamus include the following:

1. *Food intake and feeding behavior*. The basal hypothalamus controls maintenance of a stable weight. Several regions of the hypothalamus are implicated in hunger and satiety. The ventromedial nucleus is thought to be involved in satiety, and there is a hunger center in the lateral hypothalamus. Stimulation of appetite and termination of food ingestion are affected by many neuropeptides and neurotransmitters. Appetite is stimulated by γ-aminobutyric acid (GABA), dopamine, β-endorphin, enkephalin, and neuropeptide Y; appetite is inhibited by serotonin, norepinephrine, cholecystokinin, neurotensin, TRH, bombesin, naloxone, somatostatin, and VIP. Hypothalamic obesity in humans is usually associated with lesions in the vicinity of the ventromedial nucleus; this obesity appears to involve a resetting of the weight set-point. With lesions in this area, aggressive behavior and marked hyperphagia (possibly related to rapid gastric emptying) occur until the new weight set-point is reached, at which time patients often demonstrate decreased activity and finicky eating. Animal models of obesity include the *ob/ob* mouse, in which deficiency of leptin prevents satiety, and the *db/db* mouse, in which the leptin receptor is deficient. Other factors, including thyroid and adrenal hormones, also influence feeding behavior. Acute hypothalamic damage often causes hyperglycemia, whereas chronic damage may rarely cause hypoglycemia.
2. *Temperature regulation*. The anterior hypothalamus contains warm- and cold-sensitive neurons that respond to local and environmental thermal gradients (see Chaps. 17 and 19). Serotonin released in this area stimulates hypothalamic heat production, an effect blocked by norepinephrine and epinephrine. The posterior hypothalamus, in response to input from the anterior hypothalamus, conserves heat by inducing shivering and vasoconstriction and controls heat dissipation by inducing vasodilation and sweating. Acetylcholine injection in this region results in hypothermia. The temperature increase associated with infections is generated by the hypothalamus. Phagocytic cells throughout the body produce a number of pyrogenic cytokines (including interleukin 1 and tumor necrosis factor) which stimulate the anterior hypothalamus to produce prostaglandin E_2. Prostaglandin E_2 raises the thermostat set point, leading to heat conservation and increased heat production until blood and core temperatures match the new hypothalamic set point.

   Abnormalities of temperature regulation may occur with hypothalamic disease. Poikilothermia (a change in body temperature of >1°C with change in enviromental temperature) is usually due to large posterior hypothalamic lesions. Hypothermia is a rare consequence of diffuse hypothalamic disease (see Chap. 19). Paroxysmal hypothermia due to sweating and vasodilation is accompanied by fatigue, decreased alertness, hypoventilation, and arrhythmias. This rare syndrome may be associated with agenesis of the corpus callosum; the therapeutic response to anticonvulsants, clonidine, and cyproheptadine is variable. Severe, acute hyperthermia may accompany acute pathologic processes such as hemorrhage into the third ventricle, hypothalamic surgery, or hypothalamic infarction. Such fever rarely lasts longer than 2 weeks. Paroxysmal hyperthermia with episodic shaking chills, spiking fevers, and autonomic phenomena is uncommon but may respond to anticonvulsants. It is important to remember that adrenal insufficiency can cause fever or hypothermia and that hypothyroidism can cause hypothermia.
3. *Sleep-wake cycle*. Lesions in the sleep center of the anterior hypothalamus result in insomnia and agitation, as in some patients with encephalitis. The posterior hypothalamus is important for arousal and maintenance of the waking state; posterior hypothalamic destruction due to ischemia, encephalitis, or trauma can result in a hypersomnolent state from which arousal is possible. Larger lesions extending to the reticular formation of the rostral midbrain cause coma (see Chap. 24).
4. *Memory and behavior*. Lesions of the ventromedial hypothalamus and premammillary region result in loss of short-term memory, often with Korsakoff's syndrome. However, dorsomedial thalamic lesions correlate best with memory loss (see Chap. 380). Longer-term memory is often intact. Large hypothalamic lesions also may cause symptoms and signs of dementia. The role of ACTH, ACTH fragments, vasopressin, and oxytocin in memory integration is under investigation. Rage reactions may result with ventromedial lesions, and lateral hypothalamic destruction may cause an apathetic state.
5. *Thirst*. The hypothalamus is the center for vasopressin production and for the control of thirst by serum osmolality. Impaired thirst may occur with hypothalamic lesions; rarely, primary polydipsia without diabetes insipidus is a consequence of hypothalamic lesions (see Chap. 330).
6. *Autonomic nervous system function*. Parasympathetic outputs are organized in the anterior hypothalamus; sympathetic pathways in the posterior hypothalamus. Subarachnoid hemorrhage may cause hypotension, bradycardia, electrocardiographic abnormalities and myocardial necrosis; the latter changes may be prevented by sympathetic blockade. Diencephalic epilepsy is a rare syndrome associated with paroxysms of autonomic hyperactivity. This syndrome is not clearly epileptic in nature and does not usually respond to anticonvulsants. The clinical picture may mimic that of pheochromocytoma.

A diencephalic syndrome in children, characterized by emaciation, hyperkinesis, and inappropriate affect, often with a cheerful disposition, is usually caused by gliomas of the anterior hypothalamus. Most of these children die by the age of 2 years, but in those who survive, the clinical picture changes to one of increased appetite with obesity, irritability, and rage reactions.

In general, slow-growing tumors produce dementia, disturbances of food intake (obesity or emaciation), and endocrine dysfunction. Acute destructive processes are more likely to cause coma or disturbances of the autonomic nervous system.

Diseases of the anterior hypothalamus include craniopharyngiomas, gliomas of the optic nerve, sphenoid ridge meningiomas, granulomatous disease (including sarcoidosis), germinomas, and aneurysms of the internal carotid artery. Suprasellar pituitary adenomas and tuberculum sella meningiomas may grow into the hypothalamus as well. Lesions of the posterior hypothalamus include gliomas, hamartomas, ependymomas, germinomas, and teratomas.

Precocious puberty, particularly in males, can be associated with "pinealomas." However, these tumors actually are germinomas, and the precocious puberty appears to result from the ectopic production of hCG by the tumors rather than from an effect on pituitary gonadotropins.

Craniopharyngiomas Craniopharyngiomas arise from remnants of Rathke's pouch and constitute 3 to 5 percent of all intracranial neoplasms. Most of these tumors are suprasellar, but about 15 percent are intrasellar. The tumors are usually cystic or partially cystic, often contain calcium, and are lined with stratified squamous epithelium. Although craniopharyngiomas are usually manifested in childhood,

45 percent of patients are over age 20, and 20 percent are over age 40 at the time of diagnosis.

Children usually present with signs of increased intracranial pressure due to hydrocephalus (80 percent), including headache, vomiting, and papilledema. Visual abnormalities such as loss of vision and field cuts occur in 60 percent. Short stature is found in 7 to 40 percent, and retarded bone age is even more common. Delayed sexual development occurs in about 20 percent, and diabetes insipidus may be present.

About 80 percent of adults present with visual complaints, and an additional 10 percent have visual abnormalities on careful testing. Papilledema is present in about 15 percent of adults. Headaches (40 percent), mental deterioration or personality change (26 percent), and hypogonadism (35 percent) are relatively common. Hyperprolactinemia is present in one-third to one-half of patients, but prolactin levels rarely exceed 100 to 150 μg/L. Diabetes insipidus (15 percent), weight gain (15 percent), and panhypopituitarism (7 percent) may occur as well. Rarely, the cyst contents spill into the cerebrospinal fluid, causing aseptic meningitis, and an inflammatory hypophysitis may occur when craniopharyngiomas extend into the sella. Craniopharyngiomas may enlarge and become symptomatic during pregnancy.

Suprasellar calcification (see Fig. 328-15) in a flocculent, granular, or curvilinear pattern is present on skull x-rays in most children and in some adults with craniopharyngioma. Calcification is evident on CT in most of these adults, however. Hypothalamic germinomas may calcify as well. Skull x-ray abnormalities include calcification, sellar enlargement, and signs of increased intracranial pressure in 90 percent of children and 60 percent of adults.

Therapy of craniopharyngiomas is often unsatisfactory. Total removal often results in major functional deficits. We generally favor biopsy and partial resection followed by conventional radiation therapy as a more conservative approach. Tumors less than 3 cm in diameter have a better prognosis.

Germ Cell Tumors Germinomas originate in the posterior third ventricle, in the anterior third ventricle (supra- or intrasellar), or in both locations (see also Chap. 98). Germinomas (also known as *atypical teratomas*) were previously confused with parenchymal tumors of the pineal (pinealomas); when located in the anterior third ventricle, they were known as "ectopic pinealomas." Germinomas often infiltrate the hypothalamus and occasionally metastasize to the cerebrospinal fluid or distant sites.

Most patients have diabetes insipidus and variable anterior pituitary insufficiency. Precocious puberty in boys is probably due to hCG production by these tumors. Diplopia, headache, vomiting, lethargy, weight loss, and hydrocephalus are common. The tumors begin in childhood but may be diagnosed in young adults. Because germinomas are radiosensitive, early recognition is important. Germinomas of the nonseminoma type may produce hCG and/or alpha fetoprotein, whereas pure seminomas rarely produce tumor markers (see Chap. 375). Elevated cerebrospinal fluid levels of hCG or alpha fetoprotein are virtually diagnostic; when elevated, a biopsy is generally unnecessary. When tumor markers are absent, a biopsy should be considered. When the tumor is located in the anterior third ventricle, biopsy by the transsphenoidal route is often possible. Tumors in the pineal region are more difficult to biopsy, leading some authors to recommend empirical radiation therapy or chemotherapy, whereas others prefer surgical biopsy or debulking followed by radiation and chemotherapy (see Chap. 375).

PITUITARY ADENOMAS Pituitary adenomas account for about 10 to 15 percent of intracranial neoplasms. They can cause either excess or deficiency of anterior pituitary hormones or structural problems related to invasion of surrounding structures. Small pituitary tumors are present in 6 to 24 percent of adults at autopsy. These incidental pituitary tumors (pituitary "incidentalomas") are recognized with increasing frequency now that cranial MRI and CT scans are commonly performed. Pituitary adenomas are monoclonal in origin. The mechanisms of tumorigenesis are unknown except for G protein mutations in some somatotroph adenomas and rare *ras* mutations in invasive pituitary adenomas.

Pathology Pituitary tumors were previously classified as basophilic, acidophilic, or chromophobic on the basis of hematoxylin and eosin staining. Corticotroph adenomas are generally basophilic; the more densely granulated prolactin-secreting tumors are acidophilic; the majority of prolactinomas, sparsely granulated GH-secreting tumors, TSH-secreting and gonadotropin-secreting tumors, and nonsecreting tumors are chromophobic. Because this classification provides little insight into hormone production, it has been abandoned. Many nonfunctioning pituitary tumors, however, are still referred to as "chromophobes." The current classification is based on immunohistochemical staining: corticotroph (ACTH and POMC), somatotroph (GH), thyrotroph (TSH), gonadotroph (LH, FSH, and their subunits), lactotroph (prolactin), and null cell.

Pituitary tumors have also been classified by Kovacs and Horvath according to size and invasive characteristics: Microadenomas are <10 mm, and macroadenomas are ≥ 10 mm in greatest diameter. Microadenomas may cause hormone overproduction but do not cause hypopituitarism, structural problems, or sellar enlargement. Intrapituitary adenomas are contained within the substance of the pituitary gland; intrasellar adenomas are confined to the sella. Diffuse adenomas may fill the sella and cause focal sellar wall erosions and be difficult to distinguish from intrasellar adenomas. Invasive adenomas erode through the sella into surrounding tissues, including but not limited to the sphenoid bone, cavernous sinuses, optic chiasm, third ventricle, and brain. Pituitary carcinomas are rare and are diagnosed when distant metastases are present.

Endocrine Manifestations Anterior pituitary hormone overproduction is suspected on clinical grounds and confirmed by appropriate laboratory evaluation (see Table 328-5). The most common secretory pituitary tumors are prolactinomas. They cause galactorrhea and hypogonadism, including amenorrhea, infertility, and impotence. GH-secreting tumors cause acromegaly or gigantism. Corticotroph adenomas cause cortisol excess (Cushing's disease). Although glycoprotein hormone–secreting pituitary adenomas are the second most common type, clinical syndromes of excess LH, FSH, or TSH are rare. Most patients with gonadotropin-secreting adenomas have clinically nonfunctioning tumors with hypogonadism, although testicular enlargement or testosterone excess may occur. TSH-secreting adenomas are a rare cause of hyperthyroidism.

About 15 percent of patients with tumors that come to surgery have adenomas that secrete more than one pituitary hormone. The most common combination is GH and prolactin, and other common patterns are GH-TSH, GH-prolactin-TSH, and ACTH-prolactin. Most of these tumors have one type of cell that secretes two hormones (unimorphous), but some tumors have two or more cell types, each producing a single hormone (polymorphous).

Prolactinomas in women and corticotroph adenomas in both sexes are usually microadenomas. In contrast, most patients with acromegaly and most men with prolactinomas have macroadenomas at diagnosis. Glycoprotein hormone–secreting tumors are also usually large at the time of diagnosis.

About 30 to 40 percent of pituitary adenomas that come to surgery are apparently nonsecretory, although most stain immunohistochemically for pituitary hormones. These statistics are influenced by the fact that most prolactinomas do not require surgery. In some cases, particularly with gonadotropin-secreting tumors, hormone secretion is overlooked. Some "nonfunctioning" pituitary tumors, as well as some functional ones, secrete part of the glycoprotein hormone molecule, most commonly the α subunit. An α subunit excess is a frequent finding in patients with TSH-secreting adenomas, and FSH α and β may be hypersecreted in patients with gonadotropin-secreting tumors.

Null cell tumors (no specific hormones identified by immunostaining) also are generally large when diagnosed, since no hormonal overproduction provides early clues to diagnosis. As with the glycoprotein-secreting tumors that are also clinically nonfunctioning, the presenting features usually relate to mass effects. Oncocytomas are nonsecretory pituitary adenomas with abundant mitochondria, commonly found in older men.

Pituitary adenomas are occasionally part of the MEN 1 syndrome (see Chap. 340). This dominantly inherited disease causes adenomas of the pituitary gland, secretory tumors of the endocrine pancreas, and hyperparathyroidism involving multiple parathyroid glands. Pituitary adenomas may be of any cell type. Insulinomas and gastrinomas are the most common pancreatic tumors in MEN-1. Pancreatic GHRH-secreting tumors can cause acromegaly and pituitary hyperplasia.

Mass Effects of Pituitary Tumors *Visual field defects* The optic chiasm lies anterior and superior to the pituitary, usually 8 to 13 mm above the diaphragma sella. In 80 percent of normal persons the chiasm overlies the pituitary fossa, in about 15 percent it is anterior to the tuberculum sella (prefixed), and in 5 percent it overlaps the dorsum sella posteriorly (postfixed). Since 90 percent of chiasmal axons originate in the macula, central vision is lost early. Foggy or dim vision is also described by many patients.

The most common visual field defect with pituitary adenomas is a bitemporal hemianopsia; about 8 percent of patients develop complete loss of vision in one eye and have a temporal defect in the other eye. Alternatively, patients may have bitemporal scotomas rather than hemianopsia, particularly with a rapidly growing lesion in a patient with a prefixed chiasm. For this reason, visual field examinations must assess more than the lateral fields of vision. Of those patients with visual field defects, about 9 percent have a single eye defect, most commonly a superior temporal defect. Occasionally, there is a monocular field loss, such as a central scotoma, that mimics a nonpituitary lesion. Pituitary adenomas causing visual field defects are macroadenomas with sellar enlargement and suprasellar extension.

Oculomotor palsies Pituitary adenomas may extend laterally, invade the cavernous sinuses, and cause oculomotor palsies. When this occurs, visual field defects are usually not present. Involvement of the third cranial nerve is most common and may mimic diabetic third nerve neuropathy in that pupillary reactivity is usually preserved. Additional findings with lateral extension of the adenoma may include involvement of the fourth and sixth cranial nerves, pain or numbness in the distribution of the fifth cranial nerve, and compression or obstruction of the carotid artery.

Headaches are common with larger tumors and are present in most patients with acromegaly. Headaches may be exacerbated by coughing. Headaches are thought to be due to stretching of the diaphragma sella but may be vascular in origin and can be referred to several locations, including the vertex of the skull and retroorbital, frontooccipital, frontotemporal, or occipital-cervical areas.

Very large pituitary tumors may invade the hypothalamus and cause hyperphagia, abnormal temperature regulation, loss of consciousness, and loss of hormonal input from the hypothalamus. Obstructive hydrocephalus that involves the third ventricle or causes diabetes insipidus is less common with pituitary adenomas than with craniopharyngiomas and other extrapituitary masses. Tumor invasion

Table 328-5

Pituitary Hormone Evaluation

Hormone	Excess	Deficiency
Growth hormone	A. Measurement of plasma growth hormone 1 h after glucose PO B. Measurement of IGF-I	A. Measurement of plasma growth hormone 30, 60, and 120 min after one of the following: 1. Regular insulin 0.1 to 0.15 unit/kg IV 2. Levodopa 10 mg/kg PO 3. L-Arginine 0.5 mg/kg intravenously over 30 min B. Measurement of IGF-I
Prolactin	A. Measurement of basal serum prolactin, preferably fasting	A. Measurement of serum prolactin 10 to 20 min after one of the following: 1. TRH 200 to 500 μg IV 2. Chlorpromazine 25 mg IM
TSH	A. Measurement of T_4, free T_4 index, T_3, TSH, TSH α	A. Measurement of T_4, free T_4, free T_4 index, TSH
Gonadotropins	A. Measurement of FSH, LH, LH β, testosterone, FSH β, FSH response to TRH	A. Measurement of basal LH, FSH in postmenopausal women; no measurements in menstruating, ovulating women B. Testosterone, FSH, and LH in men
ACTH	A. Measurement of urine free cortisol* B. Dexamethasone suppression by one of the following: 1. Measurement of 8 A.M. plasma cortisol after administration of 1 mg dexamethasone at midnight 2. Measurement of 8 A.M. plasma cortisol or 24-h urine 17-hydroxysteroids or free cortisol after 0.5 mg dexamethasone PO q 6 h for 8 doses C. High-dose dexamethasone suppression by one of the following: 1. Measurement of plasma cortisol after 8 mg dexamethasone PO at midnight 2. Measurement of 8 A.M. plasma cortisol or 24-h urine 17-hydroxysteroids or free cortisol after 2 mg dexamethasone q 6 h for 8 doses D. Metyrapone response (same protocol as for deficiency testing)† E. Response of plasma ACTH and cortisol to ovine corticotropin releasing hormone (1 μg/kg body wt)	A. Measurement of serum cortisol at 30 and 60 min after regular insulin 0.05 to 0.15 units per kilogram IV B. Metyrapone response by one of the following: 1. Measurement of plasma 11-deoxycortisol at 8 A.M. after 30 mg/kg body wt metyrapone at midnight (maximal dose 2 g)† 2. Measurement of 24-h urinary 17-hydroxycorticoids or plasma 11-deoxycortisol day of and day after 750 mg metyrapone q 4 h for 6 doses† 3. Measurement of 24-h urinary 17-hydroxycorticoids day of and day after 500 mg metyrapone q 2 h for 12 doses† C. ACTH stimulation test: Measurement of plasma cortisol and aldosterone at 0, 30, and 60 min after IM or IV administration of 0.25 mg cosyntropin D. ?Response of plasma ACTH and cortisol to ovine corticotropin-releasing hormone (1 μg/kg body weight)
Arginine vasopressin (AVP)	A. Measurement of serum sodium and osmolality, urine osmolality in presence of normal renal, adrenal, thyroid function B. Simultaneous measurement of serum osmolality and ADH levels	A. Comparison of urine osmolality and serum osmolality under conditions of increased AVP secretion‡ B. Simultaneous measurement of serum osmolality and AVP levels

* Tests 1 and 2 establish the diagnosis of Cushing's syndrome. Tests 3, 4, and 5 localize the Cushing's disease to the pituitary gland. Often bilateral inferior petrosal sinus catheterization will be necessary.

† Give food with metyrapone.

‡ May be achieved by water deprivation or saline administration.

of the temporal lobe may cause complex partial seizures; invasion of the posterior fossa may be associated with brainstem dysfunction; and invasion into the frontal lobes causes alterations in mental state and frontal release signs.

Pituitary apoplexy Acute hemorrhagic infarction of a pituitary adenoma may cause a dramatic syndrome including severe headache, nausea, vomiting, and depression of consciousness. Ophthalmoplegia, visual and pupillary disturbances, and meningismus may be present. Most of these symptoms are caused by direct pressure from the tumor, whereas meningismus results from blood in the cerebrospinal fluid. The syndrome may either evolve slowly over a period of 24 to 48 h or may lead to sudden death.

Pituitary apoplexy occurs most commonly in patients with somatotroph or corticotroph adenomas, but it may be the first clinical manifestation of a pituitary tumor; the diagnosis is often missed initially. Both anticoagulation and radiotherapy predispose to hemorrhagic infarction. Rarely, pituitary apoplexy produces "autohypophysectomy" with "cure" of acromegaly, Cushing's disease, or hyperprolactinemia. Hypopituitarism is a common sequela; although hormonal measurements may be normal acutely, cortisol deficiency can develop rapidly. Some of the morbidity and mortality with pituitary apoplexy is due to failure to recognize and treat acute adrenal insufficiency. Gonadal steroid levels decline over days, and thyroxine concentrations fall over weeks. Diabetes insipidus is rare.

It is important to differentiate between pituitary apoplexy and a leaking aneurysm; MRI may allow this distinction to be made, but angiography may be necessary. Acute pituitary apoplexy is usually a neurosurgical emergency and often requires acute decompression of the pituitary, generally via the transsphenoidal route. Many pituitary tumors contain small hemorrhagic foci that are clinically silent.

℞ TREATMENT

Ideal therapy for pituitary adenomas permanently corrects hormonal hypersecretion without causing hypopituitarism and shrinks or removes the tumor mass without morbidity or mortality. Therapy for microadenomas may achieve both these goals, whereas therapy for macroadenomas is usually less successful. In considering therapy, it is critical to weigh the disability caused by the tumor against the disability that could arise from the treatment. Regardless of tumor size, the therapy should not be worse than the disease. Potentially serious diseases such as Cushing's disease or acromegaly may require more aggressive treatment than do prolactinomas. (See also the sections on individual pituitary hormones in this chapter.)

Medical Treatment Bromocriptine, a dopamine agonist, is the therapy of choice in the United States for most patients with microprolactinomas who require therapy. Bromocriptine corrects hyperprolactinemia in most patients with microprolactinomas; however, when the drug is stopped, prolactin levels often return to pretreatment levels. More potent dopamine agonists are available outside the United States. Cabergoline, a dopamine agonist administered once or twice weekly, is under investigation in the United States.

The side effects of nausea, gastric irritation, and postural hypotension produced by bromocriptine can be minimized by initially giving a low dose (0.625 to 1.25 mg) at bedtime with a snack. Other side effects include headache, fatigue, abdominal cramps, nasal congestion, and constipation. The dosage is gradually increased to a twice-daily schedule (most commonly 2.5 mg bid) until prolactin levels and/or symptoms return to normal. In some patients, control can be achieved with a single bedtime dose. Vaginal administration of bromocriptine is better tolerated by some patients.

Bromocriptine is also effective for large prolactin-secreting macroadenomas. (Nonfunctioning macroadenomas causing minimal prolactin elevation must be excluded.) The prolactin level is lowered by at least 80 percent in 90 percent of patients, and normal values are achieved in about 40 percent of patients. Abnormal visual fields return to normal in most patients; the tumor shrinks by 50 percent in about 40 percent of patients within 3 months. Tumor shrinkage may be accompanied by reversal of hypopituitarism. With giant adenomas, bromocriptine-induced tumor shrinkage rarely causes a devastating intracranial hemorrhage or a cerebrospinal fluid leak. Prolactin levels quickly rise when bromocriptine is stopped; however, tumor regrowth may be delayed.

Surgery is required when visual field defects do not rapidly return to normal (e.g., after 1 to 3 months of bromocriptine). Symptomatic hyperprolactinemia with an inadequate response to bromocriptine requires further therapy with surgery and/or radiation. Additional indications for surgery include patients with cystic or hemorrhagic tumors and patients who require neuroleptic agents (bromocriptine may counteract the effectiveness of such drugs). In the United States, bromocriptine is usually stopped at the onset of pregnancy and reinstituted if tumor regrowth is symptomatic; alternatively, bromocriptine can be continued throughout pregnancy, although it is not licensed for this indication in the United States.

The somatostatin analogue octreotide is the most effective adjunctive therapy in acromegaly. IGF-I levels return to normal in more than half of treated patients. Bromocriptine is an effective adjunct in some patients with acromegaly, particularly those with coexisting hyperprolactinemia. GH and IGF-I levels rarely return to normal, but symptomatic improvement and tumor shrinkage may occur. While less effective bromocriptine is often tried in patients with persistent acromegaly after transsphenoidal surgery because it can be taken by mouth. Bromocriptine or octreotide can also be given to acromegalic subjects while waiting for radiation treatment to take effect. Octreotide also may be a useful adjunctive agent in patients with TSH-secreting adenomas. Nonfunctioning and gonadotropin-secreting adenomas usually shrink by 10 percent or less in response to high doses of octreotide or bromocriptine; the one instance in which medical therapy may be effective for these tumors may be tumors that secrete the α subunit.

Surgery Transsphenoidal surgery of pituitary microadenomas is safe and frequently corrects hormonal oversecretion. Hormonal overproduction is corrected within 24 h in over 75 percent of patients with Cushing's disease due to corticotroph microadenomas, acromegaly with GH levels of <40 μg/L, and microprolactinomas with serum prolactin levels of <200 μg/L. The surgical cure rate depends on the experience and skill of the neurosurgeon. Transsphenoidal surgery is the treatment of choice for Cushing's disease with high cure rates in many centers; when Cushing's disease is not cured by an initial operation, a second operation has a 75 percent cure rate. If the second operation is unsuccessful, additional options include bilateral adrenalectomy, radiation therapy, and/or medical therapy. Surgery is also the first line of therapy for acromegaly. The initial success rate for microprolactinomas varies among institutions from 50 to 95 percent. Unfortunately, after initially successful surgery, hyperprolactinemia recurs in about 17 percent of patients followed for 3 to 5 years, and possibly in 50 percent after 5 to 10 years. The recurrence rates after initially successful surgery in acromegaly and Cushing's disease are not well established.

We treat most patients with microadenomas with bromocriptine but recommend surgery for those patients who are intolerant of dopamine agonists. Surgery does not generally result in hypopituitarism. Surgery is also our treatment of choice in acromegaly and in Cushing's disease.

The mortality rate for transsphenoidal surgery of microadenomas is 0.27 percent, and the morbidity rate is about 1.7 percent. Major complications include cerebrospinal fluid rhinorrhea, oculomotor palsy, and visual loss.

Pituitary surgery is less successful at correcting hormonal hypersecretion with larger secretory tumors. In patients with serum prolactin levels of >200 μg/L, the levels return to normal in only 30 percent, and recurrence rates may be as high as 80 percent. These patients should be treated with a dopamine agonist. Surgery is successful in 40 to 60 percent of patients with Cushing's disease due to macroadenoma and 30 percent of acromegalics with GH levels of >40 μg/L. Whether pretreatment of patients with acromegaly due to invasive macroadenomas with octreotide improves the outcome is under study.

Patients with nonfunctioning macroadenomas require surgery if the tumor is symptomatic, is located near the optic chiasm, or is continuing to grow. In such cases the goal may be decompression of adjacent structures regardless of whether complete tumor resection is possible.

Although visual field abnormalities are usually reversible with surgery for macroadenomas, cure of the tumor is less likely than with microadenomas. The intrasellar portion of tumors invading the cavernous sinus may be debulked, but parasellar extension remains. Early series noted an 85 percent recurrence of symptoms (due to structural problems such as visual field defects) over 10 years in patients treated with surgery alone. When radiation therapy was used in combination with surgery, the 10-year recurrence rate was 15 percent. These series antedated modern radiologic techniques, hormone measurements, and medical therapy. Recurrence rates are now much lower, and in some patients with late recurrence a second operation may be successful.

Surgery for macroadenomas has a mortality rate of around 0.86 percent and a morbidity rate of about 6.3 percent. Hypopituitarism occurs in about 10 percent of patients, transient diabetes insipidus occurs in about 5 percent, and permanent diabetes insipidus occurs in 1 percent. Other complications of surgery for macroadenoma include cerebrospinal fluid rhinorrhea (3.3 percent), permanent visual loss (1.5 percent), permanent oculomotor palsy (0.6 percent), and meningitis (0.5 percent).

Radiation Conventional radiation therapy is effective in preventing tumor growth (70 to 90 percent) but is unsatisfactory in the acute management of pituitary hyperfunction. Therapy generally consists of 4500 cGy (4500 rad) at 1.8 Gy (180 rad) per day over 5 weeks using rotational techniques. GH values of <5 μg/L are achieved in half of acromegalics after 5 years and in 70 percent after 10 years; values of <2.5 μg/L are achieved in 40 percent, and values of <1 μg/L are achieved in only 20 percent by 10 to 15 years. Data on IGF-I are not readily available. Conventional radiation therapy alone is rarely successful in treating corticotroph adenomas in adults. The major complications of conventional radiation treatment are hypopituitarism in up to 50 percent of patients and post-therapy lassitude and fatigue lasting many months in the majority. Whether subtle cognitive defects occur is less certain. We generally use radiation treatment as an adjunct to surgery and medical therapy for patients with continued symptomatic hormonal oversecretion and for those with substantial residual tumor after surgery or when tumor regrowth is rapid. Slow tumor regrowth over 5 or 6 years is usually treated with repeat surgery.

The "gamma knife" delivers 4000 to 10,000 cGy (4000 to 10,000 rad) through several hundred portals in a single session, a dose thought to be equivalent to two to three times the total dose given by conventional radiation treatment. Preliminary results using 4000 to 7000 cGy for acromegaly are comparable to those achieved with conventional radiation treatment. Therapy for Cushing's disease with 7000 to 10,000 cGy is apparently successful in up to 75 percent of adults; this rate is comparable to that achieved with heavy-particle therapy (see below) and apparently represents a better result than achieved with conventional radiation therapy.

Heavy-particle therapy with proton beam or alpha particles is effective in treating secretory adenomas, but response is slow. Tumors with suprasellar extension or tissue invasion are generally excluded from such series. With proton beam therapy at the Harvard cyclotron, radiation doses of up to 14,000 cGy (14,000 rad) can be given safely without damage to surrounding structures. At 2 years, 28 percent of acromegalics achieve GH values of <5 μg/L; this response rate increases to 56 percent at 5 years and to 75 percent by 10 years. Values of IGF-I are not reported. With Cushing's disease proton beam irradiation corrects the hypercortisolism in 55 percent of patients at 2 years and in 80 percent by 5 years. Proton beam therapy effectively lowers ACTH and stops the growth of most corticotroph adenomas in patients with Nelson's syndrome, with the exception of adenomas that are invasive at the time of therapy. Long-term results for treatment of other tumors with proton beam therapy are not available.

Complications of heavy-particle therapy include hypopituitarism in at least 20 percent of patients, although the exact long-term prevalence of this complication is uncertain. Visual field defects and oculomotor dysfunction, usually temporary, have been reported in about 1.5 percent of patients. The major drawback of all forms of radiotherapy is the long delay before hormonal hypersecretion is corrected. Rare complications include malignancies in the radiation field, damage to the visual apparatus, cognitive impairment, and brain necrosis. Radiotherapy is an effective alternative to surgery in patients with acromegaly, Cushing's disease, or large intrasellar nonfunctioning tumors who have contraindications to or refuse surgery.

Pituitary adenomas may be discovered during MRI or CT scanning of the brain for other purposes (pituitary "incidentaloma"). With pituitary microadenomas, hormonal overproduction must be identified and treated; hypopituitarism and structural symptoms do not occur. If no hormone abnormalities are found in a patient with an incidentally discovered microadenoma, long-term monitoring for tumor growth is necessary. A follow-up scan at 6 months, then one yearly for 2 years, and subsequently one every 2 to 5 years seems reasonable.

Pituitary macroadenomas, however discovered, need to be evaluated for hormonal over- and underproduction and for mass effects, including visual field abnormalities. The approach to the hormonally active tumor has been described above. Should nonfunctioning tumors be treated with bromocriptine? Is prophylactic surgery or radiation therapy indicated? How often should the MRI and endocrine evaluations be repeated? The answers are unknown. We tend to recommend surgery for tumors directly abutting the optic chiasm. For other tumors, MRI scans should be repeated at 6 and 12 months and yearly thereafter. If growth occurs, surgery or radiation treatment with conventional radiation, the gamma knife, or protons may be indicated. Ten to fifteen percent of tumors shrink with bromocriptine therapy; how many stabilize without therapy is unknown.

HYPOPITUITARISM *Hypopituitarism* refers to deficiency of one or more pituitary hormones and has many causes (Table 328-6). Pituitary hormone deficiency may be congenital or acquired (see Chap. 329). Isolated GH or gonadotropin deficiency is common. Temporary ACTH deficiency as a consequence of long-term glucocorticoid therapy is also common, but permanent isolated deficiency of ACTH or TSH is rare. Deficiency of any of the anterior pituitary hormones may occur at the level of the pituitary gland or the hypothalamus. Mutations in Pit-1, a pituitary-specific transcription factor, cause a combined deficiency of GH, prolactin, and TSH. When diabetes insipidus is present, the primary defect is almost invariably in the hypothalamus or high in pituitary stalk; the diabetes insipidus often is accompanied by mild hyperprolactinemia and anterior pituitary hypofunction.

The manifestations of hypopituitarism depend on the specific pituitary hormones that are lacking. Growth failure due to GH deficiency is a common presenting complaint in children. GH deficiency in adults causes more subtle manifestations, such as fine wrinkling around the eyes and mouth and, in subjects with diabetes mellitus, increased sensitivity to insulin. Subcutaneous fat may be increased, and muscle mass is decreased. The mortality of GH-deficient individuals from cardiovascular disease is increased. Symptoms of gonadotropin deficiency include amenorrhea and infertility in women and testosterone deficiency and decreased libido, decreased beard and body hair, and preservation of a youthful scalp hairline in men. TSH deficiency causes hypothyroidism with fatigue, cold intolerance, and puffy skin in the absence of goiter. ACTH deficiency results in cortisol deficiency, manifested by fatigue; decreased appetite; weight loss; decreased skin and nipple pigmentation; an abnormal response to stress characterized

Table 328-6

Causes of Hypopituitarism

Isolated hormone deficiencies
- Congenital or acquired deficiencies including mutations in Pit-1

Tumors
- Large pituitary adenomas
- Pituitary apoplexy
- Hypothalamic tumors, e.g., craniopharyngiomas, germinomas, chordomas, meningiomas, gliomas, and others
- Metastatic carcinoma

Inflammatory diseases
- Granulomatous disease, e.g., sarcoidosis, tuberculosis, syphilis, granulomatous hypophysitis
- Eosinophilic granuloma
- Lymphocytic hypophysitis (autoimmune)

Vascular diseases
- Sheehan's postpartum necrosis
- ? Diabetic peripartum necrosis
- Carotid aneurysm

Destructive-traumatic events
- Surgery
- Stalk section
- Radiation (conventional—hypothalamus; heavy-particle—pituitary)
- Trauma

Developmental anomalies
- Pituitary aplasia
- Basal encephalocoele

Infiltration
- Hemochromatosis
- Amyloidosis

"Idiopathic" causes
- ? Autoimmune disease

by fever, hypotension, and hyponatremia; and a high mortality rate. Unlike primary adrenal insufficiency ACTH deficiency does not cause hyperpigmentation, hyperkalemia, or salt loss. With combined ACTH and gonadotropin deficiency, axillary and pubic hair may be lost. Children with combined GH and cortisol deficiency often develop hypoglycemia. Prolactin deficiency causes failure to lactate postpartum. AVP deficiency causes diabetes insipidus with polyuria and increased thirst. When pituitary adenomas impair anterior pituitary function, GH is often the first hormone to be compromised, followed by deficiencies of gonadotropins, TSH, and ACTH. Panhypopituitarism may be accompanied by inappropriate secretion of vasopressin (see Chap. 330).

Etiology Damage to the anterior pituitary can be due to a pituitary adenoma (with or without infarction), pituitary surgery or irradiation, closed head trauma, or infarction during the postpartum period (Sheehan's syndrome). Postpartum pituitary infarction occurs in the setting of hemorrhage with systemic hypotension; vasospasm is thought to mediate the pituitary destruction that ensues. The enlarged pituitary gland of pregnancy may be more vulnerable to ischemia. Inability to lactate is the most common initial clinical clue, and other symptoms of hypopituitarism may unfold over months or years. The condition is sometimes diagnosed years after the primary event. Although clinical diabetes insipidus is rare in this setting, a decreased vasopressin response to appropriate stimuli is common. Patients with diabetes mellitus are also prone to develop hypopituitarism late in pregnancy.

Lymphocytic hypophysitis that causes hypopituitarism is primarily a disease of women during pregnancy or in the postpartum period but occurs rarely in men and postmenopausal women. In this syndrome, a mass lesion is often seen on MRI or CT scanning which, when biopsied, consists of lymphocytic infiltration. Lymphocytic hypophysitis is due to autoimmune pituitary destruction and often occurs with other autoimmune diseases such as Hashimoto's (autoimmune) thyroiditis and gastric atrophy (see Chaps. 331 and 340). Circulating antibodies to lactotrophs have been identified in some patients. It is not clear whether autoimmune hypophysitis is a common cause of "idiopathic" hypopituitarism in adults.

Hypothalamic or pituitary stalk damage has many causes (Table 328-6). Certain lesions in this region, such as sarcoidosis, metastatic carcinoma, germinomas, histiocytosis, and craniopharyngiomas, commonly cause diabetes insipidus along with hypofunction of the anterior pituitary. Necrotizing infundibular hypophysitis is a rare entity associated with necrosis of the pituitary and stalk. Pituitary insufficiency, resulting from conventional radiation treatment to the brain or pituitary, is thought to be largely hypothalamic in origin, although diabetes insipidus generally does not occur.

"Functional" hypopituitarism is common. Anorexia nervosa, severe stress, and major illness are all associated with reversible LHRH deficiency. Emotional stress in children may cause GH deficiency and cessation of growth (*psychosocial dwarfism*). Severe illness may be associated with TSH and free T_4 deficiency (part of the "euthyroid sick" syndrome). ACTH deficiency occurs after long-term suppression of the hypothalamic-pituitary-adrenal axis.

Diagnosis (See Table 328-5) To diagnose GH deficiency, the most reliable GH stimulus is insulin-induced hypoglycemia in which the blood sugar declines to less than 2.2 pmol/L (40 mg/dL) (Fig. 328-8). Other pharmacologic agents that cause a rise in GH include arginine, which decreases the inhibitory effects of somatostatin, and levodopa and clonidine, which increase endogenous GHRH levels. A GH concentration of >10 μg/L after stimulation with hypoglycemia, levodopa, or arginine effectively excludes GH deficiency; it is unclear whether a cutoff point of 5 or 7 μg/dL should be used. Measurement of the basal GH or serum IGF-I level is a less reliable indicator,

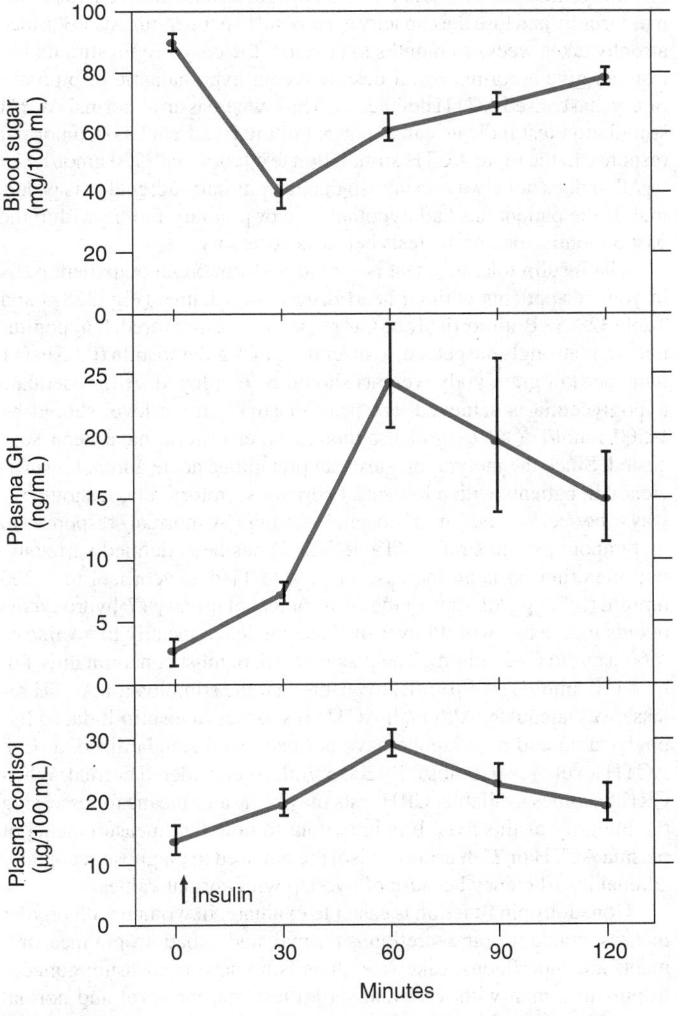

FIGURE 328-8 The insulin tolerance test. After an intravenous injection of regular insulin (0.1 unit per kilogram body weight) a fall in blood sugar and a rise in plasma GH and cortisol is expected. This test permits evaluation of both GH and ACTH in patients with pituitary disease. *(After KJ Catt, Lancet 1:933, 1970.)*

because GH levels are undetectable in normal persons for much of the day and because IGF-I levels in GH deficiency may overlap the normal range. Integrated 24-h GH secretion is low in some short children with a normal response to GH provocative stimuli. Few data are available about the best way to diagnose GH deficiency in adults; there is substantial overlap in the response to GH-provocative stimuli between normal and GH-deficient men.

ACTH deficiency results in cortisol deficiency and is potentially life-threatening. Basal cortisol function may be preserved in the face of extensive pituitary destruction; consequently, it is necessary to assess the ability of pituitary ACTH secretion to increase in response to "stress." A morning serum cortisol level of <3 μg/dL in this setting is always diagnostic of adrenal insufficiency; a level of >19 μg/dL establishes adequacy of the hypothalamic-pituitary-adrenal axis. Morning cortisol levels between these values mandate further testing. If chronic adrenal insufficiency is suspected, a rapid cosyntropin stimulation test is the best screening test. If hypothalamic or pituitary injury has occurred within a few months, an insulin tolerance test or metyrapone test is required.

The rapid ACTH stimulation test (Table 328-5) is the safest and most convenient screening test for determining the adequacy of the pituitary-adrenal axis if chronic deficiency is suspected. Although this test directly measures only the functional integrity of the adrenals, it indirectly assesses hypothalamic and pituitary function, because the adrenals depend on endogenous ACTH. When ACTH production is impaired, the adrenals atrophy and lose the capacity to respond to exogenous ACTH. Since atrophy takes weeks to months to develop, the cosyntropin stimulation test can give a normal result despite recent hypothalamic or pituitary injury that caused ACTH deficiency. Thus, whereas an abnormal ACTH stimulation test indicates an abnormal pituitary-adrenal axis, a normal response in the rapid ACTH stimulation test [cortisol >500 nmol/L (19 μg/dL)] does not always establish that the pituitary-adrenal axis is normal. If the patient has had hypothalamic or pituitary failure within the past 3 months, one of the tests below is necessary.

The insulin tolerance test is safe to perform on an outpatient basis in younger patients without heart disease or seizures (Fig. 328-8 and Table 328-5). Both cortisol and GH responses are measured. If hypopituitarism is strongly suspected, a lower dose of regular insulin (0.05 to 0.1 units per kilogram body weight) should be employed. After adequate hypoglycemia is achieved, the peak plasma cortisol level should be >500 nmol/L (>19 μg/dL), although other criteria have been suggested. Since the metyrapone test can precipitate acute adrenal insufficiency in patients with a low basal cortisol secretory rate, it should always be performed in a hospital setting. A normal response to metyrapone administration (Table 328-5) has been defined variously, but one criterion is an increase of plasma 11-deoxycortisol to >200 nmol/L (>7.5 μg/dL) and of the 24-h content of urinary 17-hydroxycorticoids to at least twofold over the baseline level, usually to a value of >60 μmol/d (>22 mg/d). The plasma cortisol must concomitantly fall to <110 nmol/L (<4 μg/dL) to ensure that the stimulus for ACTH release was adequate. Although ACTH responses to insulin-induced hypoglycemia and metyrapone have not been well standardized, a peak ACTH level of >40 pmol/L (>200 pg/mL) is considered normal. When CRH becomes available, CRH tests may be a safer means for assessing the integrity of this axis. It is important to note that measurements of plasma ACTH or 24-h urine cortisol are not used to diagnose secondary adrenal insufficiency because of overlap with normal values.

Gonadotropin function is easier to evaluate. In women with regular menses, gonadotropin secretion is normal, and gonadotropin measurements are superfluous. Likewise, there is no need to measure gonadotropins in a man with a normal serum testosterone level and normal spermatogenesis. In postmenopausal women, gonadotropin levels are elevated (the menopausal state effectively being an endogenous stimulation test); "normal" levels suggest gonadotropin deficiency. Estrogen deficiency in women and testosterone deficiency in men in the absence of elevated gonadotropins imply gonadotropin deficiency.

To diagnose central hypothyroidism (thyrotropin deficiency), the serum T_4 and free T_4 levels (or the free T_4 index) should first be measured. If these are in the mid-normal range, TSH function is likely to be normal. If the T_4 and free T_4 levels are low and the serum TSH level is not elevated, central hypothyroidism is present. Minimal TSH elevation (with bioinactive TSH) can occur in hypothalamic hypothyroidism, usually with low free T_4 concentrations. Mild central hypothyroidism, a consideration in patients with known pituitary disease who have low-normal serum T_4 and free T_4 concentrations, remains a clinical diagnosis. Before considering the diagnosis of isolated TSH deficiency in patients with the biochemical features of central hypothyroidism without evidence of other pituitary hormone deficiencies, it is important to exclude the syndrome of thyroxine-binding globulin (TBG) deficiency (low T_4, increased T_3 resin uptake, low to low-normal free T_4 index, normal TSH) and the "euthyroid sick" syndrome (low T_4, low free T_4 or free T_4 index, normal or low TSH) (see Chap. 331).

Several diagnostic tests utilize hypothalamic-releasing hormones to assess pituitary reserve. While these tests are generally *not helpful* in assessing the adequacy of anterior pituitary function, they can be useful in certain situations. In patients with isolated gonadotropin deficiency, the gonadotropin response to gonadorelin (synthetic LHRH) may be useful in predicting which patients will respond to therapy with gonadorelin. CRH testing may be useful in the differential diagnosis of Cushing's syndrome and has been suggested as a test for the pituitary-adrenal response to stress. TRH stimulation testing is useful in some patients in supporting a diagnosis of hyperthyroidism, recurrent acromegaly, or gonadotropin-secreting tumor and in those cases in which documentation of prolactin deficiency is necessary to support a diagnosis of more generalized anterior pituitary hormone deficiency (e.g., mild central hypothyroidism). TRH testing is not necessary in the evaluation of central hypothyroidism and cannot reliably separate pituitary from hypothalamic hypothyroidism. "Mega" tests with multiple releasing hormones have little clinical utility.

℞ TREATMENT

Multiple hormones must be replaced in patients with panhypopituitarism, but cortisol replacement is most important. We prefer using prednisone for reasons of convenience and cost, but many physicians use cortisone acetate or hydrocortisone (cortisol). Prednisone (5 to 7.5 mg) or cortisone acetate (20 to 37.5 mg) can be given to some patients as a single morning dosage, whereas others require divided doses (two-thirds at 8 A.M. and one-third at 3 P.M.). Hypopituitary patients may require lower daily glucocorticoid dosages than do patients with Addison's disease and do not require mineralocorticoid replacement. In stress situations or when these patients are being prepared for pituitary or other surgery, higher doses of glucocorticoids should be administered (e.g., for major surgery, hydrocortisone hemisuccinate 50 to 75 mg intramuscularly or intravenously every 6 h or methyl prednisolone sodium succinate 15 mg intramuscularly or intravenously every 6 h). Levothyroxine is the therapy of choice in central hypothyroidism (0.05 to 0.15 mg/d). The free T_4 level should be monitored, rather than the TSH level. Since thyroxine accelerates the degradation of cortisol and can precipitate adrenal crisis in patients with limited pituitary reserve, glucocorticoid replacement should always precede levothyroxine therapy in panhypopituitarism. Hypogonadism is treated in women with estrogen-progestogen combinations and in men with testosterone esters by injection or transdermal testosterone patch. To achieve fertility, gonadotropins must be administered by injection in patients with pituitary disease, whereas gonadorelin may be successful in those with hypothalamic disease. Therapy of GH deficiency in adults is under investigation; in children GH administration usually is required, but GHRH injections may be effective in those with hypothalamic disease (see Chap. 329). Diabetes insipidus is treated with nasal desmopressin (usually 0.05 to 0.1 mL twice a day) (see Chap. 330).

RADIOLOGY OF THE PITUITARY Conventional posteroanterior and lateral skull x-rays define the contours of the sella turcica (Fig. 328-9). Abnormalities that may be identified on these films

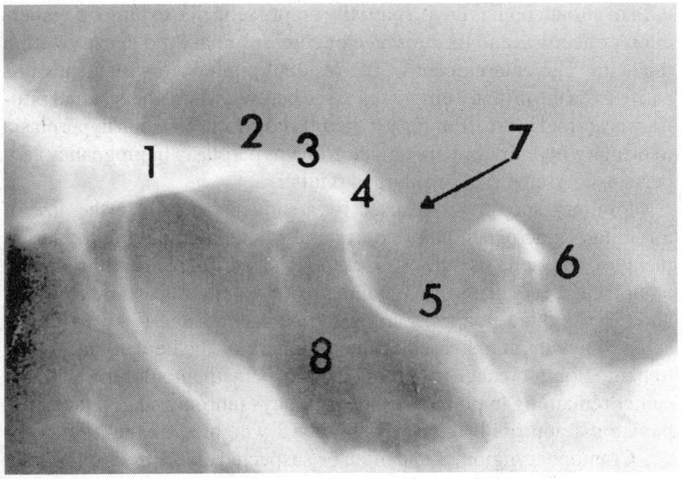

FIGURE 328-9 X-ray of the sella, lateral view. Note (1) planum sphenoidale, (2) limbus sphenoidale, (3) sulcus chiasmaticus, (4) tuberculum sellae, (5) sella floor with distinct lamina dura, (6) dorsum sellae, (7) anterior clinoid, and (8) sphenoid sinus. *[From SM Wolpert, in The Pituitary Adenoma, KD Post et al (eds). New York, Plenum, 1980.]*

include enlargement, erosions, hyperostosis, and calcification in the region of the sella. However, detailed study of pituitary and hypothalamic lesions requires MRI or CT scanning (Fig. 328-10). Anterior tomograms of the sella may be required to delineate the bony anatomy before transsphenoidal surgery; however, the high radiation doses and the limited information provided make routine tomography obsolete for diagnostic purposes. Angiography may be required when an aneurysm or vascular malformation is suspected as a cause of an enlarged sella; MRI often obviates the need for this study.

MRI (usually before and after intravenous injection of the contrast agent gadolinium; see Chap. 362) is the imaging study of choice for pituitary and hypothalamic abnormalities. Details of the optic chiasm, pituitary stalk, pituitary gland itself, intracavernous portion of the carotid artery, and relation to the cavernous sinus can be delineated on MRI (Figs. 328-10 and 328-11). Advantages over CT include lack of radiation, lack of iodinated contrast material, better tissue contrast, and direct multiplanar capability. MRI is clearly superior to CT in delineating microadenomas, visualizing the optic chiasm, and detecting cavernous sinus invasion. Patients with severe claustrophobia, those unable to remain still, and those with metallic implants (including ferrometallic aneurysm clips, pacemakers, and ossicular implants) require CT imaging. The use of sedatives and a prone position may allow patients with mild claustrophobia to tolerate MRI. MRI is less useful when details of bony erosion or calcification are desired. Specific problems with CT in this location include radiation to the lens of the eye, difficulty in obtaining direct coronal views, artifacts due to bone and dental amalgam, and limited soft tissue density resolution.

The normal pituitary has an appearance similar to brain white matter on most MR images; it has a height of 3 to 7 mm, although values up to 9 mm can be found, particularly in young women. The upper aspect is flat, concave, or, in younger patients, convex. The stalk is located in the midline and usually is less than 2 mm in diameter. The posterior pituitary usually has a bright signal on T1-weighted images; 10 percent of normal individuals lack this intense signal. Cerebrospinal fluid appears dark on T1-weighted images and bright on T2-weighted images and is easily visualized within the sella in patients with the empty sella syndrome (Fig. 328-12). The normal pituitary gland, stalk, and cavernous sinus all show an enhanced signal on T1-weighted images after intravenous gadolinium administration. Microadenomas do not enhance or have delayed enhancement, allowing improved resolution of these lesions (Fig. 328-11). Five minutes after gadolinium administration, this contrast may no longer be evident. Stalk deviation and upward bulging of the pituitary suggest a microadenoma but are not specific. Up to 20 percent of normal persons show pituitary abnormalities on contrast-enhanced CT scan or MRI. In random autopsies, up to one-fourth of individuals have small pituitary abnormalities (e.g., microadenomas, cysts, metastatic tumors, pituitary infarcts), but it is unclear whether such abnormalities correspond to the focal abnormalities on CT and MRI scanning.

Localization of corticotroph adenomas in patients with Cushing's disease may be helpful in directing the surgical approach. MRI in this situation may be negative in 30 percent or more of patients, and incidental nonfunctioning adenomas may be present in some patients with pituitary Cushing's disease. Bilateral inferior petrosal sinus catheterization for measuring ACTH (preferably with CRH administration) is useful when the MRI is negative and when the question of ectopic versus pituitary Cushing's disease is unresolved. Whether it is necessary in all cases of presumed pituitary Cushing's disease is uncertain. In patients with modest prolactin elevations, the purpose of pituitary and hypothalamic imaging is to exclude larger pathologic entities. Whether a microprolactinoma is actually visualized is less important, since this disorder is generally treated medically.

Pituitary macroadenomas causing sellar enlargement with or without bony erosion may be suspected on the basis of conventional radiography. However, these findings are not specific. Additional findings on skull x-rays in acromegaly may include prognathism, enlarged paranasal sinuses, hyperostosis of the external occipital protuberance, increased density of the central bone of the sella, and an enlarged, square sella with a tapered tuberculum. GH-secreting adenomas may calcify and regress to leave a calculus or stone.

Macroadenomas are well delineated on MRI. Coronal views are best (Fig. 328-13) for visualizing optic chiasm compromise, invasion of the cavernous sinus, vascular encasement, and invasion of the base of the skull. The medial wall of the cavernous sinus is thin and is not directly visualized. The lateral wall of the cavernous sinus is an important landmark; the presence of tissue between the lateral wall of the cavernous sinus and the internal carotid artery is a reliable sign of invasion. Macro-

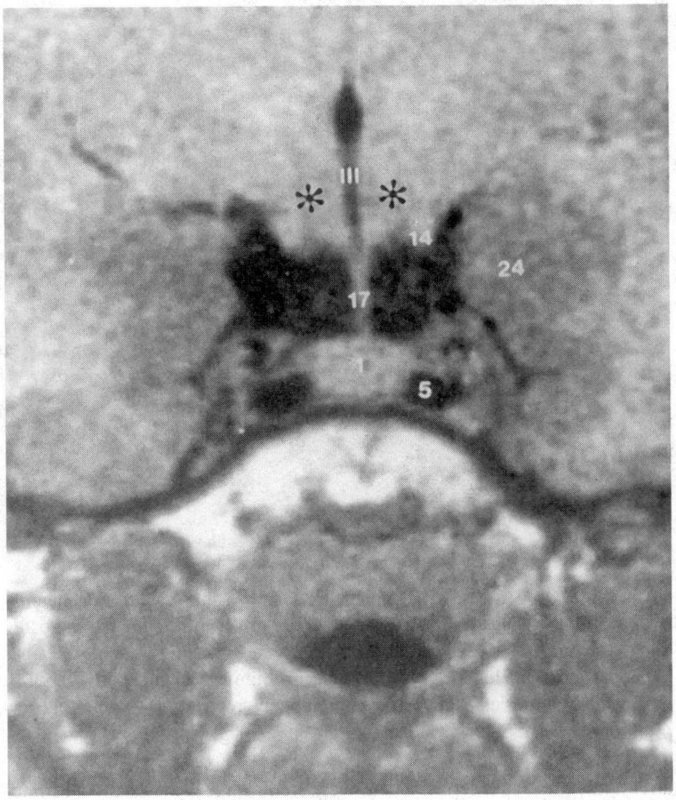

FIGURE 328-10 Coronal T1-weighted MRI scan through the posterior portion of the supraoptic hypothalamus (*). Note the anterior pituitary (1), cavernous sinus with internal carotid artery (5), proximal optic tracts (14), pituitary stalk (17), medial temporal lobes (24), and third ventricle (III). *(From DJ Quint, 1992.)*

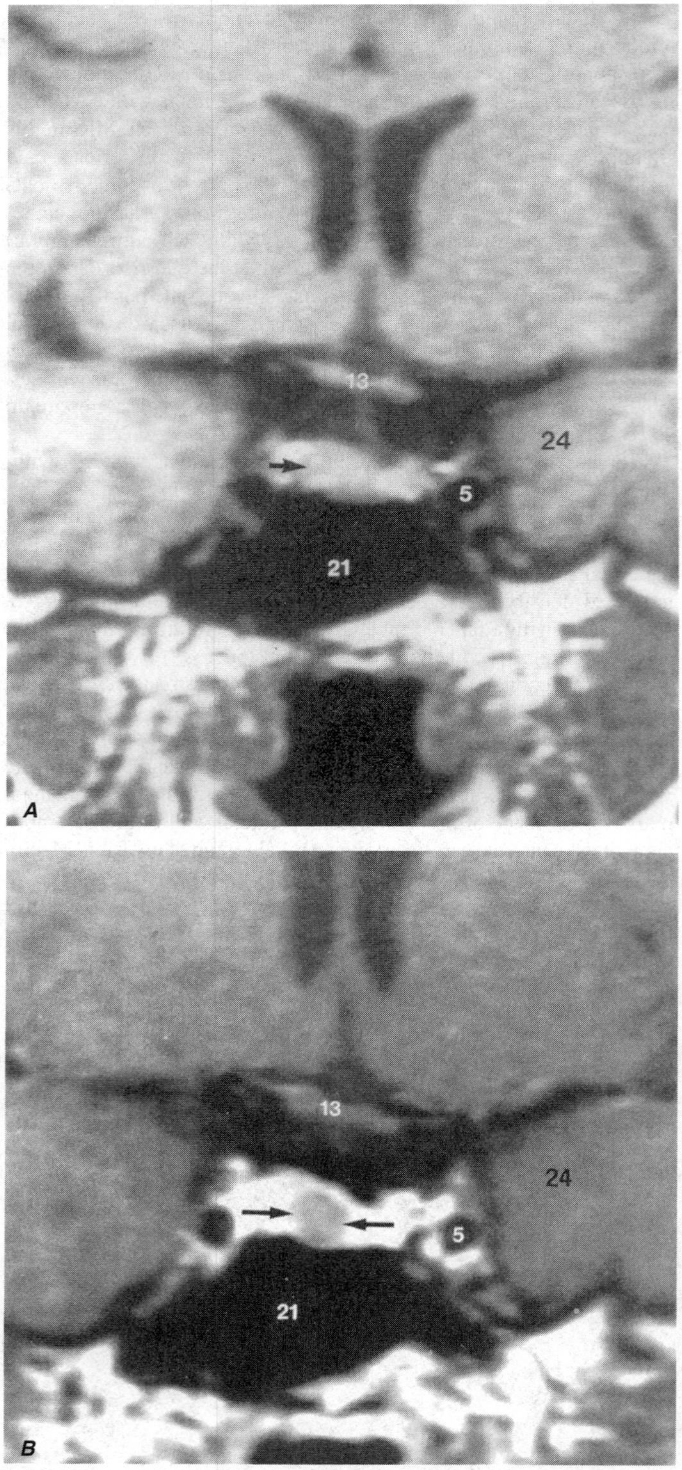

FIGURE 328-11 *A.* Coronal noncontrast T1-weighted MRI scan demonstrates pituitary gland asymmetry (*arrow*) compatible with a pituitary microadenoma. Cavernous internal carotid artery (5), optic chiasm (13), sphenoid sinus (21), and temporal lobe (24). *B.* Coronal gadolinium-enhanced T1-weighted MRI scan identifies a 4-mm right paramidline microadenoma (*arrows*). *(From DJ Quint, 1992.)*

adenomas are hyperdense on T2-weighted images in one-third to one-half of patients; in the remainder they are isointense. Old hemorrhage or cyst formation results in a focally hyperintense signal and may be seen in up to 22 percent of macroadenomas (see below). With hemorrhage, the signal is bright on T1 and T2; with fluid, the signal is of low intensity on T1 and bright on T2. Approximately one-fifth of patients with macroadenomas have a partially empty sella due to tumor degeneration or necrosis and the presence of cerebrospinal fluid density within the sella. The enlargement of the residual pituitary distinguishes this entity from the primary empty sella (see below), where the residual pituitary is normal in size. Pituitary hyperplasia (e.g., thyrotroph hyperplasia in primary hypothyroidism or lactotroph hyperplasia in pregnancy) appears as a symmetrically enlarged pituitary.

Pituitary apoplexy is caused by a sudden increase in the size of a pituitary macroadenoma due to hemorrhage or infarction; enlargement of the sella is almost always evident on plain films. Acute hemorrhage (<7 days) is hypointense or isointense to brain on T1- and T2-weighted images. During the subacute stage (7 to 14 days), signal intensity is increased in the periphery of the hematoma (owing to hemoglobin breakdown products such as methemoglobin), with the center remaining hypointense. After 14 days (chronic stage), the entire hematoma appears bright on T1- and T2-weighted images.

Craniopharyngiomas can often be suspected on the basis of nodular or curvilinear calcification in the suprasellar region on x-ray (Fig. 328-14). This calcification is visible in 80 to 90 percent of children and in about half of adults. On CT scanning, cystic components are present with ring or nodular calcification in most children and in 80 percent of adults. The findings on MRI are variable; some cysts resemble cerebrospinal fluid (CSF) in their behavior; some are less intense than CSF on T1 images but brighter than CSF on T2 images; and some mimic subacute hemorrhage, being hyperintense on T1 and T2 images. Calcification is usually not seen on MRI unless it is present in large amounts. Some craniopharyngiomas are primarily solid.

Most meningiomas of the sellar region cause abnormalities on routine skull films, including calcifications of the tumor and hyperostosis of the planum sphenoidale or of the chiasmatic sulcus. Meningiomas also may cause sella enlargement and thereby mimic pituitary adenomas. Meningiomas may be difficult to see on MRI without enhancement because they are isodense to gray matter. Almost all enhance with gadolinium, as they do on CT scans with iodine contrast. Delayed scanning (after 45 min) may be necessary with MRI to allow the normal enhancement of the pituitary gland and mucosal surfaces to

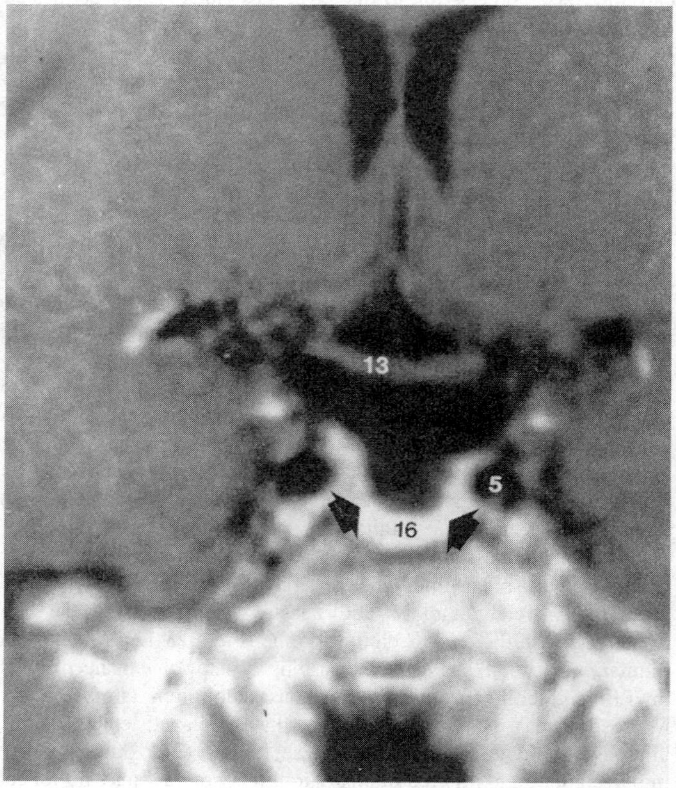

FIGURE 328-12 Empty sella. Coronal contrast-enhanced T1-weighted MRI scan through the pituitary region demonstrates an enlarged sella turcica (*arrows*) with normally enhancing pituitary tissue (16) displaced inferiorly. Note the optic chiasm (13) and intracavernous carotid artery (5). *(From DJ Quint, 1992.)*

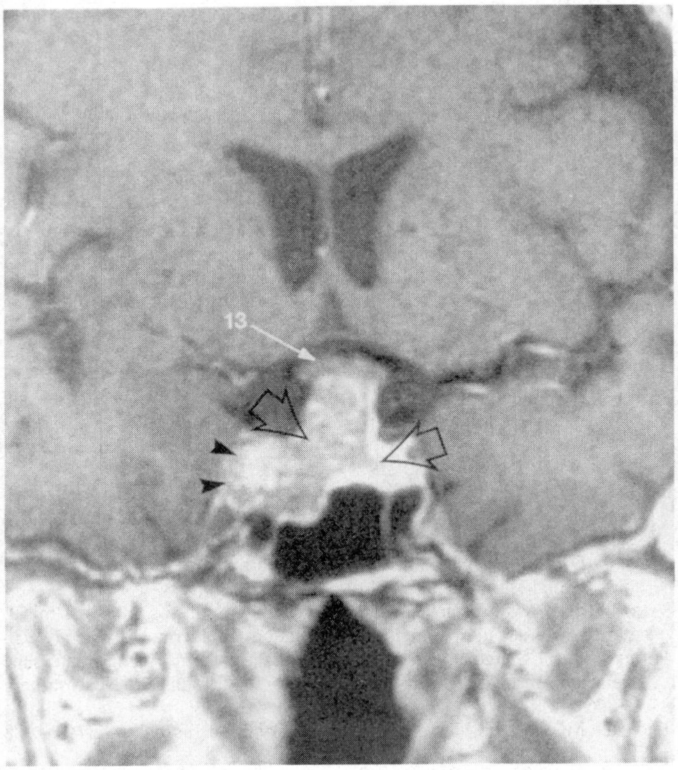

FIGURE 328-13 Macroadenoma. MRI scan through the pituitary region demonstrates a large sellar mass (*arrows*) elevating the optic chiasm (13) and invading the right cavernous sinus (*arrowheads*). The contrast-enhanced study differentiates the nonenhancing optic chiasm (13) from the enhancing tumor. *(From DJ Quint, 1992.)*

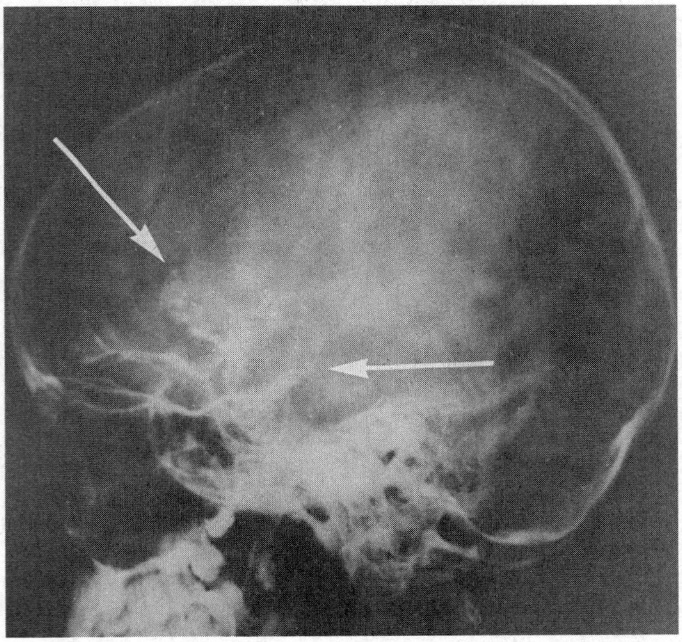

FIGURE 328-14 Lateral skull x-ray in a patient with a craniopharyngioma. Note dense calcification in suprasellar region (*arrow*).

dissipate. Vascular encasement of the carotid artery is common with meningiomas but rare with other sella-region tumors.

Aneurysms in the region of the sella contain concentric calcifications demonstrable on plain skull films in about 30 percent of patients. Aneurysms can cause sella enlargement, usually with lateral depression and erosion of the sella floor. On MRI, many aneurysms have the dark appearance of a flow void owing to blood flow through the lumen. Multilamellated thrombi appear as a high-intensity signal on T1 images; adjacent brain may show a low-intensity signal on T2 owing to hemosiderin deposition. In difficult cases, especially those with complete thrombosis, additional studies may be required, such as digital subtraction angiography, conventional angiography, and/or magnetic resonance angiography.

Other pathologic entities in the sellar region may be noted with MRI or CT. In hemochromatosis, the pituitary is dark, particularly on T2-weighted images, owing to iron deposition. Additional suprasellar masses include optic chiasm or hypothalamic gliomas, metastases to the hypothalamus or pituitary stalk, germinomas, sarcoid granulomas, histiocytosis, dermoid tumors, epidermoid tumors, and arachnoid cysts.

THE ENLARGED SELLA–EMPTY SELLA SYNDROME

Enlargement of the sella can be caused by pituitary adenomas, hypothalamic masses and cysts, aneurysms, primary hypothyroidism or hypogonadism, and increased intracranial pressure. It also can occur in patients with the primary empty sella syndrome (Fig. 328-15). In this situation, the sella tends to be symmetrically ballooned without bony erosion. The suprasellar subarachnoid space herniates through an incomplete diaphragma sella (Fig. 328-15) so that the sella is filled with CSF within an arachnoid-lined sac. An incomplete diaphragma sella is thought to be a prerequisite. It is not clear whether transiently or persistently increased CSF pressure is necessary to produce sella enlargement in these patients, but CSF pressure is generally normal when measured. The pituitary is flattened and pushed to one side but tends to function normally. The fact that CSF fills the sella can be demonstrated best with MRI scanning (see Fig. 328-12).

It is important to differentiate a primary empty sella from the enlarged, partially empty sella caused by a degenerated pituitary adenoma. In the former the pituitary volume is usually normal, whereas in the latter the pituitary volume is generally increased.

Most patients with the primary empty sella syndrome are obese, multiparous women with headaches; about 30 percent have hypertension. It is of interest that multiparity, obesity, and hypertension are associated with increases in CSF pressure. Selection bias cannot be excluded in case reports, since skull x-rays may be obtained in patients with headaches, which, in turn, uncovers the enlarged sella. Endocrine

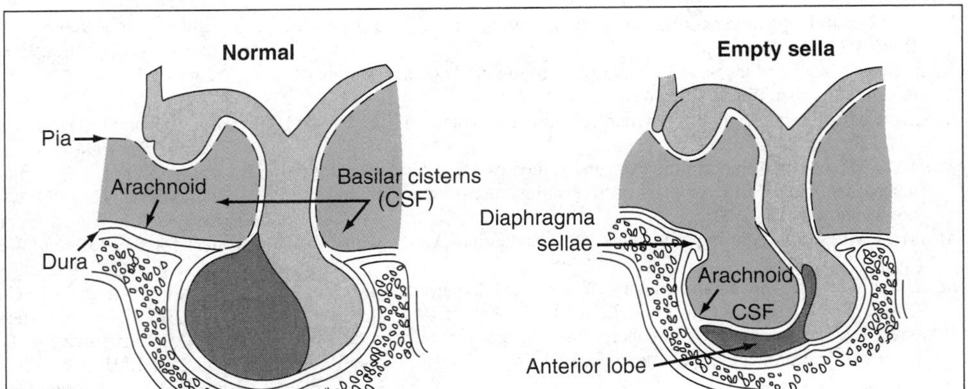

FIGURE 328-15 The findings in patients with the empty sella syndrome. *Left panel:* the normal anatomic relationships. With the empty sella syndrome *(right panel)*, ballooning of the sella results when an arachnoid diverticulum herniates through an incompetent diaphragma sellae. *(After RM Jordan et al, 1977.)*

abnormalities are uncommon. The report that antipituitary antibodies are present in 70 percent of these patients is therefore difficult to understand. Hyperprolactinemia occurs on occasion, possibly owing to stalk stretching or coincidental microprolactinomas. The GH secretory reserve is often abnormal in these patients, probably as a result of obesity. Spontaneous CSF rhinorrhea and pseudotumor cerebri have each been reported in about 10 percent of cases, but this association may represent an ascertainment bias. CSF rhinorrhea often necessitates surgical correction. Visual field defects have been reported and are thought to be caused by herniation of the optic chiasm into the sella turcica. Once the diagnosis of the empty sella syndrome is established by MRI or CT, further diagnostic studies should be performed to exclude hormone excess or deficiency; when hormone levels are normal, the therapy is reassurance.

Refer to Chap. 55, Adenohypophyseal hormones and their hypothalamic releasing factors, in Goodman & Gilman's The Pharmacological Basis of Therapeutics, *9th ed, New York, McGraw-Hill, 1996.*

BIBLIOGRAPHY

GENERAL

BLACK PMcL et al: *Secretory Tumors of the Pituitary Gland.* New York, Raven, 1984

CROWLEY WR, ARMSTRONG WE: Neurochemical regulation of oxytocin secretion in lactation. Endocrinol Rev 13:33, 1992

HOLLENHORST RW, YOUNGE BR: Ocular manifestations produced by adenoma of the pituitary gland. Analysis of 1000 cases, in *Diagnosis and Treatment of Pituitary Tumors,* PO Kohler, GT Ross (eds). Amsterdam, Excerpta Medica, 1973, p 53

JUNEAU P et al: Malignant tumors of the pituitary gland. Arch Neurol 49:555, 1992

KATZNELSON L et al: Clinically nonfunctioning pituitary adenomas. J Clin Endocrinol Metab 76:1089, 1993

KLIBANSKI A, ZERVAS NT: Diagnosis and management of hormone-secreting pituitary adenomas. N Engl J Med 324:822, 1991

KRENNING EP et al: Somatostatin receptor scintigraphy. Nucl Med Annu 1, 1995

KUPERSMITH MJ et al: Visual loss in pregnant women with pituitary adenomas. Ann Intern Med 121:473, 1994

LAMBERTS SWJ: The role of somatostatin and its analogues in the diagnosis and treatment of tumors. Endocrinol Rev 12:450, 1991

MINDERMANN T et al: Age-related and gender-related occurrence of pituitary adenomas. Clin Endocrinol 41:359, 1994

MOLITCH ME: Evaluation and treatment of the patient with a pituitary incidentaloma. J Clin Endocrinol Metab 80:3, 1995

SCHEITHAUER BW et al: The pituitary gland in pregnancy: A clinicopathologic and immunohistochemical study of 69 cases. Mayo Clin Proc 65:461, 1990

SNYDER PJ: Clinically nonfunctioning pituitary adenomas. Endocrinol Metab Clin North Am 22:163, 1993

PROLACTIN

BEVAN JS et al: Dopamine agonists and pituitary tumor shrinkage. Endocrinol Rev 13:220, 1992

KATZ E et al: Increased levels of bromocriptine following vaginal as compared to oral administration. Fertil Steril 55:882, 1991

MOLITCH ME: Pregnancy and the hyperprolactinemic woman. N Engl J Med 321:1364, 1985

MOLITCH ME et al: Bromocriptine as primary therapy for prolactin-secreting macroadenomas: Results of a prospective multicenter study. J Clin Endocrinol Metab 60:698, 1985

MOLITCH ME: Pathologic hyperprolactinemia. Endocrinol Metab Clin North Am 21:877, 1992

SCHLECTE J et al: The natural history of untreated hyperprolactinemia: A prospective analysis. J Clin Endocrinol Metab 68:412, 1989

WEBSTER J et al: A comparison of cabergoline and bromocriptine in the treatment of hyperprolactinemic amenorrhea. N Engl J Med 331:904, 1994

GROWTH HORMONE

ARIMURA A: Regulation of growth hormone secretion, in *The Pituitary Gland,* H Imura (ed). New York, Raven, 1994, p 217

ASA SL et al: A case for hypothalamic acromegaly: A clinicopathological study of six patients with hypothalamic gangliocytomas producing growth hormone-releasing factor. J Clin Endocrinol Metab 58:796, 1984

BATES AS et al: Assessment of GH status in adults with GH deficiency using serum growth hormone, serum insulin-like growth factor-1 and urinary growth hormone excretion. Clin Endocrinol 42:425, 1995

BAUMANN G: Growth hormone heterogeneity: Genes, isohormones, variants, and binding proteins. Endocrinol Rev 12:424, 1991

EZZAT S, MELMED S: Are patients with acromegaly at increased risk of neoplasia? J Clin Endocrinol Metab 72:245, 1991

EZZAT S et al: Octreotide treatment of acromegaly. A randomized, multicenter study. Ann Intern Med 117:711, 1992

MELMED S: Acromegaly. N Engl J Med 322:966, 1990

MELMED S et al: Consensus statement: Benefits versus risks of medical therapy for acromegaly. Am J Med 97:468, 1994

MELMED S et al: Clinical Review 75. Recent advances in pathogenesis, diagnosis, and management of acromegaly. J Clin Endocrinol Metab 80:3395, 1995

NEWMAN C et al: Safety and efficacy of long-term octreotide therapy of acromegaly and results of a multicenter trial in 103 patients. J Clin Endocrinol Metab 80:2768, 1995

PLOCKINGER U et al: Preoperative octreotide treatment of growth hormone-secreting and clinically nonfunctioning pituitary macroadenomas: Effect on tumor volume and lack of correlation with immunohistochemistry and somatostatin receptor scintigraphy. J Clin Endocrinol Metab 79:1416, 1994

RAJASOORYA C et al: Determinants of clinical outcome and survival in acromegaly. Clin Endocrinol 41:95, 1994

ROSS DA, WILSON CB: Results of transsphenoidal microsurgery for growth hormone-secreting pituitary adenomas in a series of 214 patients. J Neurosurg 68:854, 1988

RUDMAN D et al: Effects of human growth hormone in men over 60 years old. N Engl J Med 323:1, 1990

SANO T et al: Growth hormone–releasing hormone–producing tumors: Clinical, biochemical and morphological manifestations. Endocrinol Rev 9:357, 1988

THOREN M et al: Stereotactic radiosurgery with the cobalt-60 gamma unit in the treatment of growth hormone–producing pituitary tumors. Neurosurgery 29:663, 1991

THORNER MO, VANCE ML: Growth hormone 1988. J Clin Invest 82:745, 1988

TSH

BECK-PECCOZ P et al: Decreased receptor binding of biologically inactive thyrotropin in central hypothyroidism. Effect of treatment with thyrotropin-releasing hormone. N Engl J Med 312:1085, 1985

CHANSON P et al: Octreotide therapy for thyroid-stimulating hormone-secreting pituitary adenomas. Ann Intern Med 119:236, 1993

FAGLIA G et al: Inappropriate secretion of thyrotropin by the pituitary. Horm Res 26:79, 1987

JACKSON IMD: Regulation of thyrotropin secretion, in *The Pituitary Gland,* H Imura (ed). New York, Raven, 1994, p 179

GONADOTROPINS AND α SUBUNITS

DANESHDOOST L et al: Recognition of gonadotroph adenomas in women. N Engl J Med 324:589, 1991

HESELTINE DM et al: Testicular enlargement and elevated serum inhibin concentrations occur in patients with pituitary macroadenomas secreting follicle-stimulating hormone. Clin Endocrinol 31:411, 1989

KATZNELSON L et al: Imbalanced follicle-stimulating hormone β-subunit hormone biosynthesis in human pituitary adenomas. J Clin Endocrinol Metab 74:1343, 1992

MOGHISSI KS: Clinical applications of gonadotropin-releasing hormones in reproductive disorders. Endocrinol Metab Clin North Am 21:125, 1992

OPPENHEIM DS, KLIBANSKI A: Medical therapy of glycoprotein hormone–secreting pituitary tumors. Endocrinol Metab Clin North Am 18:339, 1989

OPPENHEIM DS et al: Prevalence of alpha-subunit hypersecretion in patients with pituitary tumors. J Clin Endocrinol Metab 64:1187, 1990

SNYDER PJ: Extensive personal experience: Gonadotroph adenomas. J Clin Endocrinol Metab 80:1059, 1995

TSATSOULIS A et al: Bioactive gonadotrophin secretion in man. Clin Endocrinol 35:193, 1991

ACTH

ARONS D, TYRELL B (eds): Cushing's syndrome. Endocrinol Metab Clin North Am 23(3): 1994

BATEMAN A et al: The immune-hypothalamic-pituitary-adrenal axis. Endocrinol Rev 10:92, 1989

FLACK MR et al: Urine free cortisol in the high-dose dexamethasone suppression test for the differential diagnosis of the Cushing syndrome. Ann Intern Med 116:211, 1992

LORIAUX DL, NIEMANN L: Corticotropin-releasing hormone testing in pituitary disease. Endocrinol Metab Clin North Am 20:363, 1991

ORME SM, BELCHETZ PE: Isolated ACTH deficiency. Clin Endocrinol (Oxf) 35:213, 1991

ORTH DN: Corticotropin-releasing hormone in humans. Endocrinol Rev 13:164, 1992

ORTH DN: Cushing's syndrome. N Engl J Med 332:79, 1995

SCHLAGHECKE R et al: The effect of long-term glucocorticoid therapy on pituitary response to exogenous corticotropin-releasing hormone. N Engl J Med 326:226, 1992

ENDORPHINS

BERTAGNA X: Proopiomelanocortin-derived peptides. Endocrinol Metab Clin North AM 23:467, 1994

HYPOTHALAMUS
BRAY GA, GALLAGHER TFJ: Manifestations of hypothalamic obesity in man: A comprehensive investigation of eight patients and a review of the literature. Medicine 54:301, 1974
DINARELLO CA: Interleukin-1 and the pathogenesis of the acute phase response. N Engl J Med 54:301, 1984
KLOOS RT: Spontaneous periodic hypothermia. Medicine 74:268, 1995
PLUM F, VAN UITERT R: Nonendocrine disease and disorders of the hypothalamus, in *The Hypothalamus*, S Reichlin et al (eds). New York, Raven, 1978, pp 415–473
CRANIOPHARYNGIOMAS
BANNA M: Craniopharyngioma: Based on 160 cases. Br J Radiol 49:206, 1976
PAJA M et al: Hypothalamic-pituitary dysfunction in patients with craniopharyngioma. Clin Endocrinol 42:467, 1995.
HYPOPITUITARISM
ARAFAH BM: Reversible hypopituitarism in patients with large nonfunctioning pituitary adenomas. J Clin Endocrinol Metab 62:1173, 1986
CONSTINE, LS et al: Hypothalamic-pituitary dysfunction after radiation for brain tumors. N Engl J Med 328:87, 1993
EDWARDS OM, CLARK JDA: Post-traumatic hypopituitarism. Medicine 62:281, 1986
GRINSPOON S, BILLER B: Laboratory assessment of adrenal insufficiency. J Clin Endocrinol Metab 79:923, 1994
JONES SL et al: An audit of the insulin tolerance test in adult subjects in an acute investigation unit over one year. Clin Endocrinol 41:123, 1994
MUIR A, MACLAREN NK: Autoimmune diseases of the adrenal glands, parathyroid glands, gonads and hypothalamic-pituitary axis. Endocrinol Metab Clin North Am 20:619, 1991
OELKERS W: Hyponatremia and inappropriate secretion of vasopressin (antidiuretic hormone) in patients with hypopituitarism. N Engl J Med 321:492, 1989
ROSEN T, BENGTSSON BA: Premature mortality due to cardiovascular disease in hypopituitarism. Lancet 336:285, 1990
VANCE ML: Hypopituitarism. N Engl J Med 330:1651, 1994
RADIOLOGY
CHAKERES DW et al: Magnetic resonance imaging of pituitary and parasellar abnormalities. Radiol Clin North Am 27:265, 1989
GLICK RP, TIESI JA: Subacute pituitary apoplexy: Clinical and magnetic resonance imaging characteristics. Neurosurgery 27:214, 1990
HALL WA et al: Pituitary magnetic resonance imaging in normal human volunteers: Occult adenomas in the general population. Ann Intern Med 120:817, 1994
JOHNSON MR et al: The evaluation of patients with a suspected pituitary microadenoma: Computed tomography compared to magnetic resonance imaging. Clin Endocrinol 36:335, 1992

329 DISORDERS OF GROWTH

Raymond L. Hintz

NORMAL GROWTH Children can grow rapidly over short periods of time, and the physician must be aware of normal standards for growth and development as a function of age. A record of these changes provides a sensitive indication of general health. Minimal aberrations in health may be reflected first in a deviation from the normal growth rate; conversely, an actively growing child seldom has a serious systemic disease. Thus, height and growth rate provide important information.

Both longitudinal and cross-sectional studies indicate that differences exist in growth among different ethnic groups. However, normal, well-nourished children have remarkably similar growth patterns. For example, the average length of children, which at birth is about 50 cm, increases by about 25 cm in the first year of life, 12.5 cm in the second year, and 6.0 cm per year thereafter until puberty. This formula can be used to estimate average height up to about age 10. Nomograms have been constructed to give a more accurate picture of average growth and the range of normal deviations from the mean (Figs. 329-1 and 329-2).

CONTROL OF GROWTH Growth involves an increase in both the number of cells and the size of individual cells. The relative importance of these processes varies from organ to organ and with age. The control and integration of growth also vary among tissues and with the stage of development.

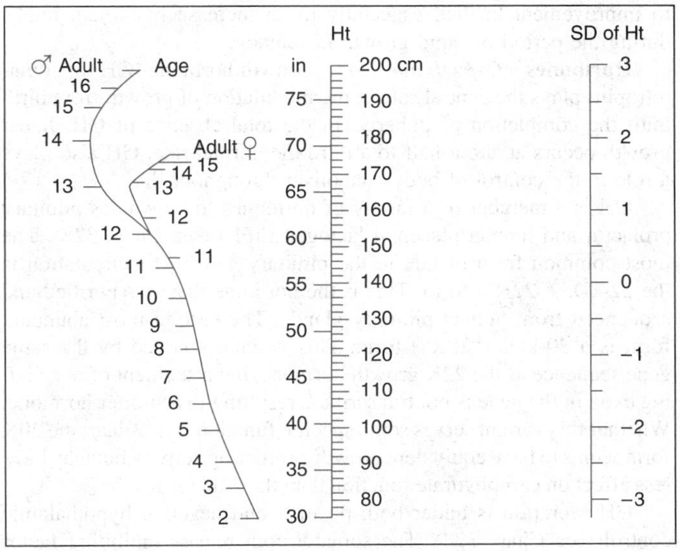

FIGURE 329-1 Nomogram for height of boys and girls.

Prenatal Growth Prenatal development exemplifies the complexities of the integration and control of growth. During this time, a single cell becomes a complex organism in which billions of cells work in harmonious concert. The growth rate is astounding; the most rapid growth rate occurs during the second trimester. Prenatal growth is controlled by different mechanisms than those that act in the postnatal period. Prenatal growth rates are dependent on uterine blood flow and other maternal influences and less on the factors that determine ultimate stature; growth hormone and thyroid hormone have relatively minor effects on prenatal growth. The correlation between body length at birth and adult height is weak ($r = 0.3$); by 2 years of age, the correlation between body length and adult height is stronger ($r = 0.7$), indicating that the factors influencing adult stature begin operating early in postnatal life.

Genetic Factors Stature is a polygenic trait (see Chap. 65), so there is no simple method of predicting the adult height of any given child. However, there is a correlation between the mean height of parents and the mean heights attained by their children.

Nutrition The next most important factor affecting growth is nutrition. Severe nutritional deprivation, as in marasmus or kwashiorkor (see Chap. 74), impairs growth, as may subclinical deficiencies of nutrients and selective deficiencies of vitamins and minerals. The trend toward increased adult stature over the last century may be due

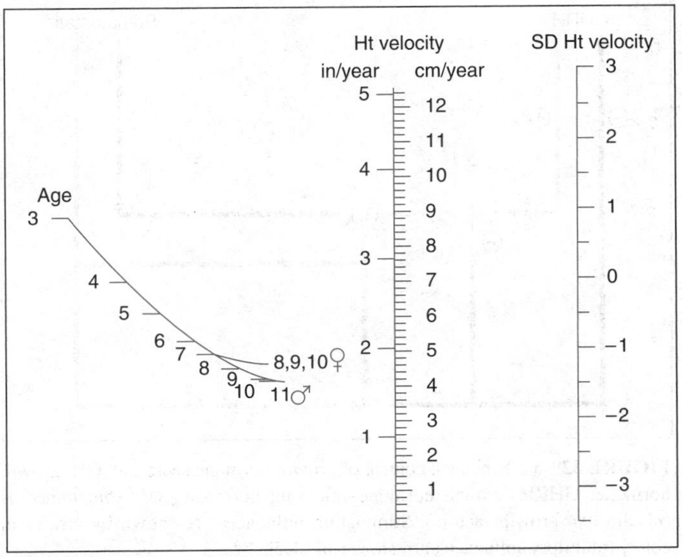

FIGURE 329-2 Nomogram for growth rate in boys and girls.

to improvement in diet, especially to an increase in protein intake during the period of rapid growth in infancy.

Hormones *Growth hormone* Growth hormone (GH, or somatotropin) plays the central role in the modulation of growth from birth until the completion of puberty. In the total absence of GH, linear growth occurs at about half to a third the normal rate. GH also plays a role in the control of body anabolism throughout life.

GH is a member of a family of hormones that includes pituitary prolactin and human placental lactogen (hPL) (see Chap. 328). The most common form of GH in the pituitary and in the circulation is the 22-kDa ("22K") form. This is the hormone that was purified and sequenced from human pituitary glands. The second most abundant form is a 20-kDa ("20K") form. This variant is coded by the same gene sequence as the 22K growth hormone, but a segment of one coding exon in the gene is not transcribed, resulting in a shorter hormone. Whether this variant serves some specific function is not clear; the 20K form seems to have equivalent growth-promoting activity but may have less effect on carbohydrate function than the 22K form.

GH secretion is under both positive and negative hypothalamic control (see Chap. 328). The somatotropin release-inhibiting factor (SRIF, somatostatin) is a 14-amino-acid peptide that is synthesized in the hypothalamus and is widely distributed in other tissues as well; it is a potent inhibitor of the secretion of many hormones, including insulin, glucagon, and gastrin.

The biologic action of GH-releasing hormone (GRH, somatocrinin) is contained in the first 29 amino acids of the 44-amino-acid peptide, and the amino-terminal amino acid is crucial for its biologic action. Patients with idiopathic GH deficiency may have a deficiency of GRH rather than an inability to make GH in the pituitary. Indeed, half or more of individuals with GH deficiency respond to prolonged pulsatile administration of GRH with an increase in plasma GH and an accelerated growth rate.

The secretion of somatostatin and GRH, and hence the release of GH, is under the influence of several factors (Fig. 329-3). Higher centers in the central nervous system have axons that terminate on hypothalamic cells that secrete somatostatin and GRH and exert both positive and negative effects. In addition, both GH and the GH-controlled insulin-like growth factors (IGFs) influence the secretion or action of GRH and somatostatin. The secretion of GH is episodic, and the hormone has a relatively short half-life (10 to 15 min) in plasma. A significant proportion of GH in serum is bound to a GH-binding protein (GHBP) that is structurally related to the GH receptor. Although small amounts of GH are secreted during waking periods, most GH secretion occurs during sleep, especially during third- and fourth-stage sleep.

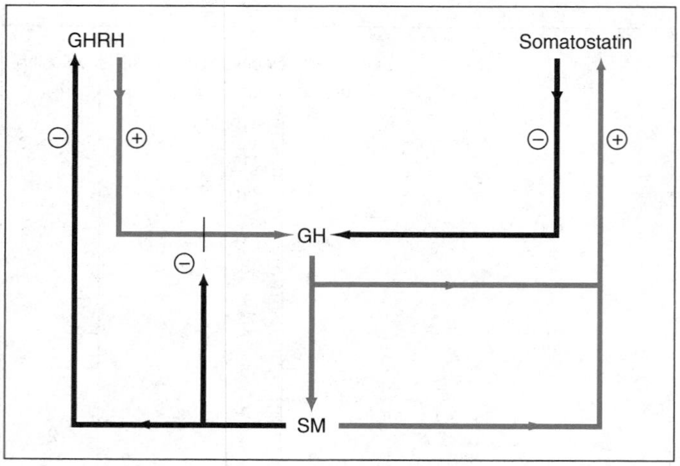

FIGURE 329-3 Feedback control of growth hormone secretion. GH, growth hormone; GHRH, growth hormone–releasing hormone; SM, somatomedins (insulin-like growth factors). Stimulating influences are shown by arrows in color. Inhibitory influences are shown in black.

Insulin-like growth factors Although GH may exert some direct effects on growth, most of its growth-promoting actions are mediated by the IGF or somatomedin peptides. Two human IGF peptides, IGF-I and IGF-II, have about 50 percent structural homology with human insulin and 70 percent homology with each other. Somatomedin C (SM-C) and IGF-I are structurally and functionally equivalent. The IGF peptides are bound tightly to six specific plasma IGF-binding proteins (IGFBPs) and have half-lives of hours rather than minutes. Levels of IGF-I and IGFBP-3 are dependent on GH secretion and consequently are high in acromegaly and low in hypopituitarism. Levels are also age-dependent, being low in early childhood, peaking during adolescence, and declining after age 50. The plasma levels of IGF-II also depend on the presence of a minimal amount of GH, but supraphysiologic levels of GH do not result in a further increase in IGF-II. Thus, the values of IGF-II are low in hypopituitarism but are not elevated in acromegaly. Plasma levels of IGF-II are constant from 1 year of age to beyond the eighth decade of life.

Thyroid hormone Unlike the pattern of growth with GH deficiency, the total absence of thyroid hormone causes an almost complete cessation of linear growth. Thus, adequate thyroid hormone appears to be an absolute prerequisite for normal growth. There are several potential mechanisms for this phenomenon. Thyroid hormones exert direct effects on cell metabolism, and thyroid hormone deficiency also results in diminished GH secretion in response to stimulation. In addition, the action of IGF-I on cartilage cells may be dependent on thyroid hormone.

Gonadal steroids Androgens and estrogens exert their major stimulation of growth at puberty. Much of the pubertal growth spurt is due to these hormones. Androgens directly stimulate the growth and maturation of bone, cartilage, and muscle. Estrogens appear to have a biphasic action, stimulating growth at low levels and inhibiting growth at high levels. In addition, estrogens are responsible for the closure of the epiphyses and the cessation of linear growth.

Insulin Insulin has anabolic actions that are separate from its effects on carbohydrate metabolism. These actions include stimulation of protein synthesis and cell division. The large size of infants of diabetic mothers may be the consequence of high levels of plasma insulin in the fetus. The close structural relationship of insulin to the IGF group of growth factors and the ability of insulin to bind to the IGF-I receptor may explain some of these effects of insulin at high levels. However, insulin also stimulates growth directly in some cell types.

Other factors Nerve growth factor, which is structurally related to the insulin-IGF family of peptides, has actions on the development of sympathetic neurons and possibly on the maintenance and repair of other neurons. Epidermal growth factor controls the maturation of the skin and also acts on other cell types. Platelet-derived growth factor is released from platelets upon clotting and is also a potent mitogen for many cells. The plasma levels, control mechanisms, interactions with other growth-stimulating peptides, and physiologic roles of these growth factors remain to be elucidated.

DIAGNOSIS OF GROWTH DISORDERS Most short people do not have a disease in the usual sense but exhibit some deviation from the normal growth pattern (Table 329-1). Thus, the first step in evaluating growth disorders is to identify those individuals with a normal variation in stature who presumably do not require treatment.

Table 329-1

Causes of Short Stature

Diagnosis	Usual Practice, %	Referral Center, %
Constitutional growth delay	98	80
GH deficiency	0.1	10
Hypothyroidism	0.2	4
Systemic disease	0.3	3
Chromosomal disorders	0.1	1
Bone-cartilage dysplasia	0.3	1
Psychosocial disorders	1	1

SOURCE: Modified from Horner et al.

Table 329-2

Physical Findings in Syndromes of Short Stature

Syndrome	Specific Physical Findings
GH deficiency	Frontal bossing, central obesity, high-pitched voice
Hypothyroidism	Dry skin, coarse hair, immature facies
Cushing's syndrome	Central obesity, striae, hypertension
Gonadal dysgenesis	Webbed neck, multiple pigmented nevi, shield chest, delayed sexual development
Pseudohypoparathyroidism	Moon facies and obesity, short metacarpals, mental retardation
Bone-cartilage dysplasia	Abnormal proportions, macrocephaly
Russell-Silver dwarfism	Small at birth, "pointed" facies, asymmetry

Height and Growth Rate An important factor in the differential diagnosis of short stature is the height percentile of the patient relative to others of the same age. This factor is determined using a nomogram such as the one shown in Fig. 329-1. A straightedge is placed on the points representing the patient's age and height. The value of the intercept with the right-hand scale is an estimate of the number of standard deviations (SDs) from the mean height for age. In general, the further the patient is from the mean height for age, the more likely it is that short stature is due to disease. A height above the −2-SD level indicates that the patient is likely normal. The growth rate also should be determined, if possible, either from existing growth data or by observation (see Fig. 329-2). A growth rate consistently below the mean is a cause for concern.

Because short stature is common, clinical judgment plays a large role in the approach to this problem. Individuals with severely short stature (−3 SD or greater for age) should undergo immediate evaluation, while those with a less severe abnormality may be observed serially so that the growth rate can be assessed. A consistently low growth rate should prompt further investigation. The diagnosis of constitutional delay is one of exclusion. In general, if hypothyroidism, GH deficiency, and the more common systemic diseases have been excluded, it is reasonable to observe the patient. However, the boundaries between "normal" and "disease" may be blurred, and the indications for treatment may change. Furthermore, continued failure to maintain a normal growth rate is an indication for reinvestigation.

History Important features in the history include the weight and gestational age at birth, growth and development in early infancy, and the presence of systemic disease. It is also crucial to assess the stature of the parents and first- and second-degree relatives and to review the growth and pubertal development patterns of parents, siblings, and other relatives. A family history of late pubertal development may be diagnostically helpful.

Physical Examination The body proportions must be evaluated. Limbs that are short relative to the trunk suggest either long-standing hypothyroidism or one of the chondrodystrophies, such as achondroplastic dwarfism; subtle forms of chondrodystrophy may be difficult to recognize (see also Chap. 348). It is also important to note the height-to-weight ratio. A short child who is underweight for height may have malnutrition or a systemic disease. On the other hand, a child who is short but overweight is more likely to have an endocrine disease. Patients with Cushing's syndrome, GH deficiency, or hypothyroidism may be overweight for their height. Specific physical findings may suggest specific syndromes (Table 329-2).

Table 329-3

Screening Laboratory Investigations in Short Stature

Test or X-Ray	Disorder
Serum thyroxine	Hypothyroidism
IGF-I and IGFBP-3	GH deficiency
GHBP	GH insensitivity syndromes
Bone age	Constitutional delay, hypothyroidism, GH deficiency
Magnetic resonance imaging	Craniopharyngioma or other central nervous system lesions
Serum calcium	Pseudohypoparathyroidism
Serum phosphate	Vitamin D–resistant rickets
Serum bicarbonate	Renal tubular acidosis
Blood urea nitrogen	Renal failure
Complete blood count	Anemia, nutritional disorder
Erythrocyte sedimentation rate	Inflammatory disease of bowel
Chromosomal karyotype	Gonadal dysgenesis or other abnormality

Laboratory Evaluation Assessment of bone age is useful to indicate possible pathology and to estimate final adult height. Because the manifestations of hypothyroidism may be minimal, thyroid function should be assessed routinely. Measurements of IGF-I and IGFGP-3 are also useful screening procedures, since most patients with GH deficiency have low values. Syndromes of GH resistance, such as Laron dwarfism, are characterized by low IGF-I levels, low GHBP levels, and high GH levels. Appropriate tests may be ordered to screen for other disease states (as summarized in Table 329-3). Any girl with unexplained short stature should have a chromosomal karyotype.

Testing of GH secretion Because GH secretion is episodic and therefore variable, random measurements of plasma GH are not an adequate test of GH deficiency. Some GH stimulation tests for screening for GH deficiency are summarized in Table 329-4 (also see Chap. 328). Because of the long half-life of IGF-I and IGFBP-3, a random measurement during the day is an accurate reflection of the mean

Table 329-4

Screening Tests for Assessing GH Secretion

IGF-I RADIOIMMUNOASSAY*

Age, years	Male Range, μg/L	Female Range, μg/L
1–2	31–160	11–206
3–4	45–230	75–320
5–6	51–288	70–320
7–8	157–385	125–396
9–10	136–308	123–330
11–12	180–440	191–462
13–14	220–616	286–660
15–16	200–836	242–660
17–18	286–627	240–506

IGFBP-3 RADIOIMMUNOASSAY*

Age	Range, mg/L	Mean, mg/L
1–12 months	0.5–1.2	1.3
1–5 years	1.4–3.0	2.1
5–7 years	1.5–3.4	2.4
7–9 years	2.1–4.2	3.0
9–11 years	2.0–4.8	3.3
11–13 years	2.1–6.2	3.8
13–15 years	2.2–5.9	4.2
15–18 years	2.5–4.8	3.8
Adults, 20–30 years	2.0–4.2	3.0

CLONIDINE TEST OF GH RELEASE

NPO after midnight
Administration of clonidine by mouth:

Body Weight, kg	Dose, mg
5–15	0.05
15–25	0.10
25–35	0.15
35–50	0.20
>50	0.25

Samples for measurement of GH at 0, 60, and 90 min
Side effects: Postural hypotension and somnolence
Keep patient supine until after postural hypotension is gone
Normal response: Greater than or equal to 10 μg/L (10 ng/mL) on any sample

* Values for age-related normal individuals (may vary with assay).

plasma concentration. If care is taken to use age-related standards, measurement of IGF-I and IGFBP-3 provide a reasonable screen for GH deficiency. Low levels of IGF-I or IGFBP-3 should prompt more extensive evaluation. The other tests listed are indirect and largely nonphysiologic ways of provoking the release of GH. In our clinic, a GH level of 10 μg/L (10 ng/mL) after a clonidine test is considered a normal response. If that level is not achieved, more definitive testing of the GH reserve should be carried out, as described in Chap. 328.

℞ TREATMENT

GH Deficiency The only established use of human GH is in the treatment of children who are GH-deficient. Between 1 in 4000 and 1 in 20,000 children have a GH deficiency; about half these cases are due to idiopathic GH deficiency, and the other half are secondary to tumor and/or radiation therapy. In approximately one-third of the latter cases, GH deficiency is isolated, and in the other two-thirds, there are multiple pituitary hormone deficiencies. Short stature due to chronic renal failure or gonadal dysgenesis is also an indication for GH treatment. If short stature is due to a systemic disease, treatment is directed toward the underlying disease state. Similarly, short stature due to hypothyroidism or cortisol excess is managed by treatment of the primary disorder. In general, the earlier the disorder is diagnosed and treated, the more successful is the growth response; if treatment of the underlying disease is delayed until after puberty, little or no improvement in stature can be expected.

Unlike the broad species specificity of peptide hormones such as insulin, GH exhibits a narrow species specificity. Human GH stimulates linear growth in children with GH deficiency, whereas the bovine hormone is ineffective in humans. The preparation of human GH from pituitary glands obtained from autopsy material did not supply enough hormone for the treatment of all children who had GH deficiency, let alone for the evaluation of the usefulness of GH treatment for other conditions. Furthermore, the distribution of human pituitary GH in the United States and several other countries was discontinued in 1985 because of the development of Creutzfeldt-Jakob disease in some patients who had been treated with human GH. The availability since 1985 of synthetic GH has relieved the supply problem. Hormone is readily available for patients with GH deficiency, and the potentially unlimited supply has allowed exploration of other therapeutic uses of GH, including the treatment of gonadal dysgenesis.

Most children with GH deficiency respond to GH treatment with an acceleration of growth to normal or above-normal rates. As with other hormones, there is a dose-response curve for GH administration. The doses that have been tested range from 0.01 to 0.1 mg per kilogram body weight as a subcutaneous injection daily. There is a wide variation in response, but the higher dosages usually result in higher average growth rates. Indeed, daily doses of 0.025 or 0.050 mg/kg cause a good growth response in most GH-deficient patients. If the patient fails to show an adequate growth rate, the dose can be increased until an adequate growth response is obtained or until the upper limit of 0.50 mg/kg per week is reached. GH doses above this level are associated with an increased risk of glucose intolerance and other complications.

An alternative method under study for the treatment of GH deficiency is the use of either GH-releasing hormone (GHRH) or GH-releasing peptide (GHRP). Since at least half of children with GH deficiency are able to secrete GH in response to GHRH, this approach may ultimately be useful for those patients.

Short Stature Of Other Causes *IDIOPATHIC SEVERE SHORT STATURE* Growth hormone has been given to some patients with growth failure not due to GH deficiency. Some children with severe short stature (more than 2.5 SDs below the mean for age) do not have GH deficiency but are responsive to GH treatment. Many of these patients have low IGF-I, IGFBP-3, and/or GHBP levels and may have a partial defect in the control of GH secretion. Many such children show a short-term increase in growth rate in response to GH therapy; whether their final height is greater than it would have been without GH treatment is not established. Furthermore, it is not known whether there are serious long-term side effects from GH treatment in this situation.

Gonadal Dysgenesis GH also may have a role in the treatment of gonadal dysgenesis (see Chap. 66). Most women with gonadal dysgenesis have an average adult height between 135 and 142 cm. Treatment with androgens can cause a short-term increase in the rate of growth of girls with this disorder but does not result in a greater final adult stature. The use of GH at modest doses is also associated with an increase in the rate of growth. Results of multicenter group studies in which synthetic GH was administered either alone or in combination with androgens are encouraging in terms of both initial growth response and increases in final height.

Skeletal Disorders Growth hormone also has been used to treat small numbers of subjects with a wide variety of other growth disorders, including bone-cartilage dysplasias and other genetic syndromes associated with short stature. It is not clear whether GH is of use in any of these disorders.

Please refer to Chap. 55 in Goodman & Gilman's The Pharmacological Basis of Therapeutics, *9th ed, McGraw-Hill, New York, 1996.*

BIBLIOGRAPHY

BAUMANN G: Growth hormone heterogeneity: Genes, isohormone, variants and binding proteins. Endocr Rev 12:424, 1991

BLUM WF et al: A specific radioimmunoassay for the growth hormone–dependent somatomedin binding protein: Its use for diagnosis of growth hormone deficiency. J Clin Endocrinol Metab 70:1291, 1990

BROWN P: Potential epidemic Creutzfeldt-Jakob disease from human growth hormone therapy. N Engl J Med 313:728, 1985

FRASIER SD: A review of growth hormone stimulation tests in children. Pediatrics 53:929, 1974

GRUMBACH M: Growth hormone therapy and the short end of the stick. N Engl J Med 319:238, 1988

HINDMARSH PC et al: Wider indications for treatment with biosynthetic human growth hormone in children. Clin Endocrinol 34:417, 1991

HINTZ RL: Growth factors. Curr Opin Pediatr 2:786, 1990

———: Untoward events in patients treated with GH in the USA. Horm Res 38(Suppl 1):44, 1992

——— et al: Efficacy of growth hormone therapy in patients without classically defined growth hormone deficiency. Growth Genet Horm 8(Suppl 1):10, 1992

———: The prismatic case of Creutzfeldt-Jakob disease associated with pituitary growth hormone treatment. J Clin Endocrinol Metab 80:2298, 1995.

HOPWOOD NJ et al: Growth response of non-growth hormone deficient children with marked short stature during three years of growth hormone therapy. J Pediatr 123:215, 1993

HORNER JM et al: Growth deceleration patterns in constitutional short stature: An aid to diagnosis. Pediatrics 62:529, 1978

LANTOS J et al: Ethical issues of growth hormone therapy. JAMA 261:1020, 1989

LEE PDK et al: Efficacy of insulin-like growth factor I levels in predicting the response to provocative growth hormone testing. Pediatr Res 27:45, 1990

ROSENFELD RG et al: Six-year results of a randomized, prospective trial of human growth hormone and oxandrolone in Turner's syndrome. J Pediatr 49:121, 1992

——— et al: The diagnosis of childhood growth hormone deficiency revisited. J Clin Endocrinol Metab 80:1532, 1995

TANNER JM, DAVIS PSW: Clinical longitudinal standards for height and height velocity for North American children. J Pediatr 107:317, 1985

———, ISREALSOHN WJ: Parent-child correlations for body measurements of children between the ages of one month and 7 years. Ann Hum Genet 26:245, 1963

——— et al: Effect of human growth hormone treatment for 1 to 7 years on growth of 100 children with growth hormone deficiency, inherited smallness, Turner's syndrome, and other complaints. Arch Dis Child 46:317, 1985

THORNER MO et al: Growth hormone–releasing hormone and growth hormone–releasing peptide as potential therapeutic modalities. Acta Paediatr Scand (Suppl) 376:29, 1990

VIPANI OV et al: Prevalence of severe growth hormone deficiency. Br Med J 2:427, 1977

330

Arnold M. Moses, David H. P. Streeten

DISORDERS OF THE NEUROHYPOPHYSIS

Axons from two largely independent hypothalamic-neurohypophyseal systems in the supraoptic and paraventricular nuclei extend through the pituitary stalk to the posterior pituitary. The hormones vasopressin and oxytocin are formed in separate ganglion cells and migrate down the axons as parts of precursor proteins. They are stored in secretory granules in the nerve terminals in the neurohypophysis and are released by exocytosis into the bloodstream in response to appropriate stimuli. Vasopressin (AVP; also called antidiuretic hormone, ADH) controls water conservation, and its release is coordinated with the activity of the thirst center that regulates fluid intake. Oxytocin stimulates uterine contractions and milk ejection.

VASOPRESSIN SYNTHESIS, RELEASE, AND ACTION

SYNTHESIS AVP is synthesized in the magnocellular neurons of the anterior hypothalamus as a preprohormone and is altered in the Golgi apparatus to form a prohormone that is packaged into neurosecretory vesicles. While it is being transported to axonal terminals, the prohormone is cleaved into AVP, a protein called *neurophysin* with a molecular weight of 10,000, and a 39-amino-acid glycopeptide. All three products are released into the peripheral circulation.

ACTIONS AVP initiates its action to conserve water and concentrate the urine by binding to the V_2 receptor on the basolateral surface of the principal cell of the renal conducting duct. AVP enhances the hydrosmotic flow of water from the lumen of the duct through the cell to the medullary interstitium and peritubular capillaries. AVP also increases the permeability of the collecting duct to urea and increases sodium absorption in the thick ascending limb of the loop of Henle. High concentrations of AVP acting on V_1 receptors can also cause vasoconstriction, as in response to severe hypotension or after infusion of vasopressin for treatment of bleeding esophageal varices.

AVP, perhaps from axons that terminate in the cerebrum, may play a role in learning and memory, and AVP from fibers in the median eminence participates in the stimulation of corticotropin secretion in response to stress.

NORMAL HORMONE LEVELS AVP concentrations in plasma and urine can be measured by radioimmunoassay. The results may be expressed either as units based on pressor activity in the rat or in terms of weight of purified vasopressin. Arginine vasopressin has a biologic activity of approximately 400 units/mg (1 mU = 2.5 ng = 2.3 pmol). The neurohypophysis under conditions of random fluid intake contains approximately 8 units of AVP. Under the same conditions, peripheral plasma AVP concentration ranges from 1.4 to 5.6 pmol/L (1.5 to 6 ng/L). At the latter plasma level and above, urine osmolality is maximal. The AVP concentration in plasma fluctuates, with a maximum late at night and in the early morning and a minimum in the early afternoon. Under conditions of normal hydration, healthy subjects release approximately 370 to 1400 pmol (400 to 1500 ng) from the pituitary and excrete 23 to 80 pmol (25 to 90 ng) AVP in urine in 24 h. During 24 to 28 h of dehydration, the amount released increases three to five times.

METABOLISM Inactivation of AVP occurs largely in liver and kidneys through cleavage of the terminal glycinamide to produce a biologically inactive substance. Approximately 7 to 10 percent of secreted AVP is excreted in the urine as active hormone.

CONTROL OF AVP RELEASE **Osmoregulation** Under normal conditions, AVP release is regulated primarily by osmoreceptors in the hypothalamus. Changes in the concentrations of plasma solutes to which the cellular membrane is impermeable cause alterations in the volume of the osmoreceptor cells, which in turn alter the electric activity of the neurons and control both the synthesis and release of AVP. As a consequence of this servomechanism between effective plasma osmolality and AVP release, plasma osmolality is normally maintained within a very narrow range. The mean plasma osmolality in a group of normal subjects following a water load of 20 mL/kg of body weight was 281.7 mmol/kg plasma water, and the osmolality that initiated AVP release following infusion of hypertonic saline solution into water-loaded subjects was 287.3 mmol/kg. Thus, the increase in plasma osmolality between full diuresis and the initiation of antidiuresis by hypertonic saline solution is only 5.6 mmol/kg or 2 percent.

The infusion of hypertonic saline solution into water-loaded subjects causes a linear rise in plasma osmolality with time. After an interval, there is an abrupt, progressive fall in free water clearance without a significant change in solute or creatinine excretion. We defined the osmotic threshold for AVP release as the plasma osmolality at the onset of antidiuresis under these conditions, which occurred at a mean plasma osmolality of 287 mmol/kg. The osmotic threshold for AVP release also may be determined, with very similar results, by constructing a linear regression line between simultaneously obtained plasma osmolality and either plasma or urine AVP concentration during hypertonic saline infusion and extrapolating the regression line to the *x*-axis intercept (plasma osmolality).

Volume Regulation Decreases in plasma volume, through effects on stretch receptors in the left atrium and perhaps in the pulmonary veins, stimulate the release of AVP by reducing the tonic inhibitory impulses from the left atrium to the hypothalamus. The neural impulses travel via the vagi to the reticular formation of the midbrain and diencephalon and then to the supraoptic and paraventricular nuclei, where they are integrated with the other stimuli that affect AVP release. Positive-pressure breathing, quiet standing, and vasodilation may activate this mechanism, which serves to restore plasma volume, even at times overriding osmotic inhibition of AVP release. Following volume contraction, plasma AVP levels may reach 10 times the levels induced by hypertonicity. Increased plasma volume inhibits AVP release by the reverse mechanisms, leading to a diuresis and correction of the hypervolemia. Negative-pressure breathing, recumbency, lack of gravitational force (as in space travel), submersion in water, and exposure to cold can activate this mechanism.

Baroreceptor Regulation Activation of carotid and aortic baroreceptors in response to hypotension causes release of AVP. Hypotension due to blood loss is the most potent stimulus and may at times raise plasma levels of AVP to 560 pmol/L (600 ng/L). These concentrations of AVP may cause vasoconstriction, which probably plays a role in the restoration of blood pressure.

Neural Regulation Several hypothalamic neurotransmitters and neuropeptides influence the release of AVP. Acetylcholine stimulates AVP release by its nicotinic action on supraoptic neurons. Angiotensin II, histamine, bradykinin, and neuropeptide Y probably stimulate AVP release. Norepinephrine, prostaglandins, and dopamine stimulate or inhibit AVP release, depending on the experimental conditions. Gamma-aminobutyric acid appears to act as an inhibitory neurotransmitter; serotonin and substance P are also present in the supraoptic nucleus, but their influence on AVP release is not clear. The regulatory action of opioid peptides on AVP release is also unclear, with reports indicating stimulation, inhibition, or no effect. Though the roles of these and other transmitters and peptides are incompletely defined, the antidiuretic actions of stress, emesis, and pain and the diuretic actions of hypnosis, psychological conditioning, and inhalation of carbon dioxide indicate that higher centers have an important influence on the release of AVP.

Aging Aging is associated with enhanced AVP release in response to a rising plasma osmolality and a progressive increase in plasma AVP concentration. These changes appear to place the older individual at greater risk of developing water retention and hyponatremia, despite a concomitant decline in maximal renal concentrating capacity in response to AVP, which is usually manifest after age 60.

Pharmacologic Influences Nicotine, morphine, vincristine, vinblastine, cyclophosphamide, clofibrate, chlorpropamide, and some tricyclic anticonvulsants and antidepressants stimulate AVP release. Ethanol exerts diuretic properties by inhibiting neurohypophyseal function under a variety of conditions. Some narcotic antagonists also inhibit AVP release. Experimentally, chlorpromazine, reserpine, and phenytoin all inhibit the secretion of AVP by the pituitary and the rise in urinary excretion of AVP after water deprivation. In humans, phenytoin and chlorpromazine may inhibit AVP release and produce diuresis.

AVP RESPONSE TO WATER DEPRIVATION AND TO WATER LOADING Water deprivation provides both an osmotic and a volume stimulus for vasopressin release by increasing plasma osmolality and decreasing plasma volume, but the maximum urinary osmolality after water deprivation depends on renal medullary osmolality and other intrarenal factors. In response to fluid deprivation for 18 to 24 h, plasma osmolality rarely rises above 292 mmol/kg in normal individuals. The resultant stimulation of AVP release increases plasma AVP concentration to 7.4 to 14 pmol/L (8 to 15 ng/L).

The administration of water lowers plasma osmolality and expands blood volume, inhibiting the release of AVP via both osmoreceptor and atrial volume receptor mechanisms. An oral water load of 20 mL/kg in normal adults causes a fall in plasma osmolality to a mean of 281.7 mmol/kg and a maximum diuresis in 1 to 1½ h with free water clearance rising to approximately 12 mL/min and urine osmolality falling to 40 to 60 mmol/kg. The delay in reaching maximal diuresis is accounted for by the time required for absorption of water from the gut, for metabolism of previously secreted vasopressin, and for renal recovery from the action of vasopressin.

INTERACTION OF OSMOTIC AND VOLUME INFLUENCES Under conditions of water deprivation and of water loading, volume and osmotic influences act in parallel to influence AVP release. In other circumstances, volume and osmotic influences may be competitive, and changes in plasma volume can modify the effects of hypertonic stimuli on AVP release. Osmotic factors ordinarily predominate to maintain plasma osmolality within a narrow range. Larger changes in blood volume, such as those induced by hemorrhage, may blunt and eventually overcome the osmotic influences, and hypotension can stimulate AVP secretion and override simultaneous inhibiting influences.

RELATION BETWEEN AVP RELEASE AND THIRST-INDUCED WATER INTAKE Under normal conditions, there is close coordination between AVP release and thirst, both of which are regulated by small changes in plasma osmolality. The perception of thirst generally becomes apparent when plasma osmolality exceeds 292 mmol/kg. Thus, thirst occurs only when the urine is maximally concentrated. Angiotensin II increases thirst and AVP release under conditions of extracellular volume depletion. Normally, therefore, water losses lead to slight hypernatremia, which increases thirst and fluid intake to restore and maintain normal plasma osmolality. In contrast, when thirst perception is impaired (adipsia), fluid losses are uncorrected, and hypernatremia occurs even though AVP release is adequate to concentrate the urine maximally.

EFFECTS OF GLUCOCORTICOIDS Glucocorticoids and the posterior pituitary have antagonistic effects on water excretion. Cortisol elevates the osmotic threshold for AVP release elicited by hypertonic saline infusion in water-loaded normal subjects and protects against water intoxication and overcomes the impaired response to water loading in adrenal insufficiency.

Although the impaired ability to dilute the urine in adrenal insufficiency may be due in part to excessive plasma AVP, glucocorticoids also can act directly on the renal tubules to decrease water permeability and increase free water excretion in the absence of AVP.

ANTIDIURETIC ACTION OF AVP The mechanism of action of AVP is demonstrated in Fig. 330-1: (1) AVP binds to a receptor (V_2) on the basolateral surface of the principal cell of the medullary collecting duct. This V_2 receptor has seven transmembrane domains.

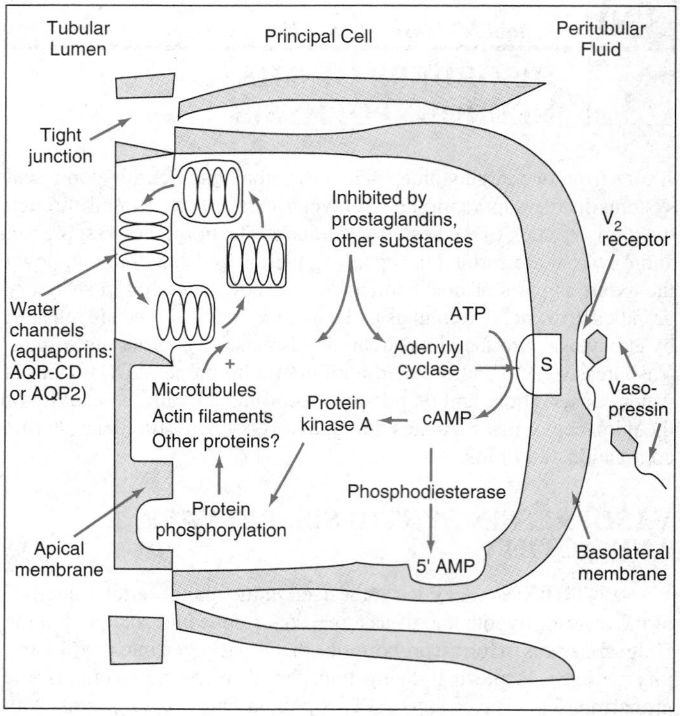

FIGURE 330-1 Schematic representation of the cellular mechanism for the antidiuretic action of vasopressin in the principal cell of the renal collecting duct. See text for the description of the mechanism. *(Modified from H Valtin, JA Schafer, Renal Function 3d ed, Boston, Little, Brown, 1955, with permission.)*

(2) The receptor-hormone complex activates a guanine nucleotide binding stimulatory protein (G_s). (3) This protein in turn activates adenylate cyclase in the membrane, which increases the concentration of cyclic AMP in the cytosol. AVP also stimulates prostaglandin E_2 production, which, in turn, acts as a feedback inhibitor of adenylate cyclase activity. (4) Cyclic AMP activates protein kinase A. (5) The activated protein kinase A causes the phosphorylation of unidentified proteins. (6) The phosphorylated protein stimulates exocytosis which causes the insertion of water channels, composed of proteins called aquaporins, into the apical membrane of the cell. This event coincides with the appearance of particle aggregates (Fig. 330-2). (7) As a consequence, the membrane becomes water permeable. (8) When AVP is removed, the water channels are reinternalized back into the cell, and the membrane particle aggregates disappear. Consequently, the membrane is again impermeable to water. (9) The basolateral membrane remains permeable to water, allowing water that has entered the cell under the influence of AVP to exit the cell along osmotic gradients into the medullary insterstitium and peritubular capillaries.

A variety of cations and drugs influence the action of AVP. Calcium and lithium inhibit the adenylate cyclase response to AVP. Lithium also interferes with a subsequent biochemical action, as does potassium deficiency. Demeclocycline inhibits adenylate cyclase stimulation by AVP and also inhibits the cyclic AMP–dependent protein kinase. In contrast, chlorpropamide increases AVP-induced activation of adenylate cyclase.

DEFICIENCY OF VASOPRESSIN: DIABETES INSIPIDUS

Diabetes insipidus refers to the passage through the body of a large quantity of dilute fluid. This state of excessive water intake and hypotonic polyuria may be due to failure of AVP release in response to normal physiologic stimuli (central or neurogenic diabetes insipidus) or failure of the kidney to respond to AVP (nephrogenic diabetes insipidus).

PATHOPHYSIOLOGY Deficiency of vasopressin release in response to the appropriate stimuli can result from lesions at several functional sites in the physiologic chain of events that regulates hor-

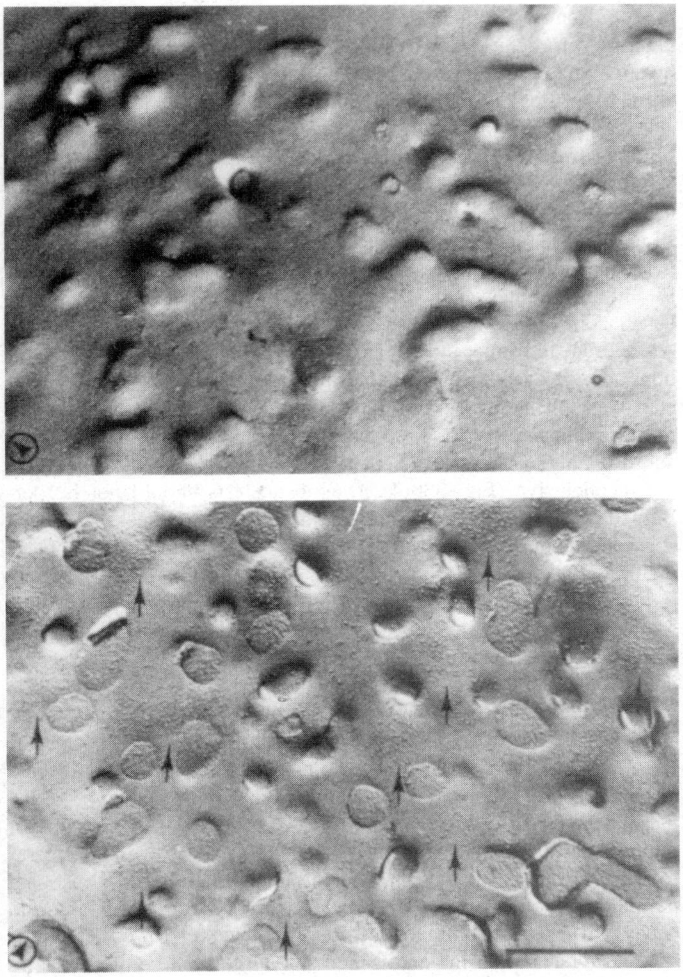

FIGURE 330-2 *Top*: Virtual absence of particle clusters in renal collecting duct luminal membrane obtained from untreated Brattleboro (congenital diabetes insipidus) rat. *Bottom*: Appearance of particle clusters (*arrows*) after treatment with AVP. The appearance of clusters coincides with the insertion of water channels into the cell membrane. *(From MC Harmanci et al, Am J Physiol 235:F440, 1978.)*

mone release. Four types of central diabetes insipidus can be defined. Patients with the first type show very little rise in urine osmolality, even with a marked increase in plasma osmolality (Fig. 330-3, line 1) and no evidence of AVP release during hypertonic saline infusion. They are essentially devoid of releasable AVP. In patients with the second type, there is an abrupt increase in urine osmolality during dehydration (Fig. 330-3, line 2), but there is no evidence of an osmotic threshold during saline infusion. These patients have a defective osmoreceptor mechanism but can release AVP in response to the hypovolemia of severe dehydration. Patients with the third type of disease have some rise in urine osmolality with increasing plasma osmolality (Fig. 330-3, line 3) and have an elevated osmotic threshold for AVP release. These patients have a sluggish release mechanism due to a high-set osmoreceptor. In patients with the fourth type of disease, urine and plasma osmolality coordinates are shifted to the right of normal (Fig. 330-3, line 4). AVP release in these patients is initiated at a normal plasma osmolality but is subnormal in amount.

Patients with the second to fourth types of disease may develop a good antidiuresis in response to nausea, nicotine, methacholine, chlorpropamide, or clofibrate, indicating that AVP formation is sufficient to allow for adequate urinary concentrating ability in the presence of an appropriate stimulus to release. In rare instances, patients with the second to fourth types of disease present with asymptomatic hypernatremia associated with mild or no polyuria.

ETIOLOGY The causes of central diabetes insipidus in 135 patients who satisfied the criteria described under "Diagnostic Tests" (below) and who had had the disorder for at least 6 months are shown

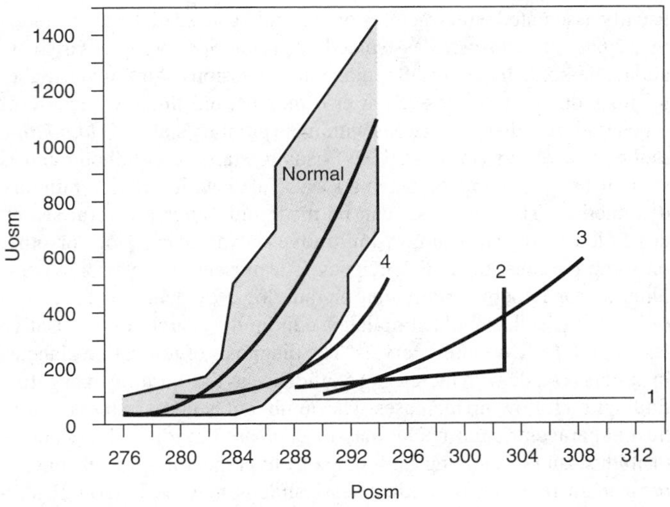

FIGURE 330-3 Relation of plasma and urinary osmolality during hydration and dehydration in normal adult subjects (*shaded area*) and in four types of patients with diabetes insipidus.

in Table 330-1. Diabetes insipidus frequently starts in childhood or early adult life (median age of onset, 24 years) and is more common in males than females. The major causes include the following: (1) *Neoplastic* or *infiltrative lesions* of the hypothalamus or pituitary, including pituitary adenomas, craniopharyngiomas, germinomas, pinealomas, metastatic tumors, leukemia, Langerhans cell granulomatosis (histiocytosis X), and sarcoidosis, caused diabetes insipidus in 37 patients. In approximately 60 percent of these patients partial or complete loss of anterior pituitary function was evident. (2) *Pituitary* or *hypothalamic surgery* caused diabetes insipidus in 32 patients and was usually associated with anterior hypopituitarism. Surgically induced diabetes insipidus usually develops 1 to 6 days after surgery and often disappears after a few days. It may recur and become chronic after an "interphase" of 1 to 5 days. Removal of the posterior lobe of the pituitary induces permanent diabetes insipidus only if the pituitary stalk is sectioned high enough to induce retrograde degeneration of most neurons of the supraoptic nucleus. (3) *Severe head injuries*,

Table 330-1

Characteristics of 135 Cases of Long-Standing* Central Diabetes Insipidus Diagnosed by the Authors at SUNY Health Science Center, Syracuse. Categories Are Arranged in Order of Increasing Median Age of Onset.

	Age of Onset, Years				
Cause	Median†	Range	Males	Females	Percent of Cases
Langerhans cell granulomatosis	2	1–30	3	2	4
Primary brain tumor					
Postoperative‡	15	6–50	9	11	15
Preoperative§	18	7–58	17	3	15
Idiopathic	20	<1–66	20	14	25
Head trauma	22	5–48	15	9	18
Nontraumatic encephalomalacia	43	15–73	3	4	5
Ruptured cerebral aneurysm	39		1	0	1
Post-hypophysectomy	42	24–68	4	8	9
Sarcoidosis	42		0	1	1
Metastatic cancer	56	32–72	6	5	8
			(58%)	(42%)	

* Longer than 6 months or until death.
† Median age of entire group = 24 years.
‡ 16 cases were of craniopharyngioma.
§ 5 cases were glioma, 7 germinoma, and 4 craniopharyngioma.

usually associated with fractures of the skull, caused diabetes insipidus in 24 patients and were associated with anterior hypopituitarism in about one-sixth of patients. Spontaneous remissions of traumatic diabetes insipidus may occur even after 6 months, presumably because of regeneration of disrupted axons within the pituitary stalk. (4) *Idiopathic diabetes insipidus* (in 34 patients) usually starts in childhood and is seldom (<20 percent of patients) associated with anterior pituitary dysfunction. This diagnosis can be made only after a careful search has failed to reveal a tumor, infiltrative or vascular lesion, or other presumptive cause of AVP deficiency. The presence of anterior hypopituitarism or hyperprolactinemia or radiologic evidence of lesions in or above the sella should stimulate a continuing search for a causative lesion at 3- to 12-month intervals. The diagnosis of idiopathic diabetes insipidus is made with increasing confidence as the duration of negative findings on follow-up increases. The number of neurons in the supraoptic and paraventricular nuclei may be decreased in idiopathic diabetes insipidus, and circulating antibodies to hypothalamic nuclei may be present. In rare instances, diabetes insipidus may be inherited as an isolated autosomal dominant defect or as part of an autosomal recessive syndrome (DIDMOAD) consisting of diabetes insipidus (DI), diabetes mellitus (DM), optic atrophy (OA), and deafness (D) (also called the *Wolfram syndrome*; see Chap. 340). (5) Seven patients had nontraumatic encephalomalacia from a variety of causes, including shock, cardiopulmonary arrest, hypertensive encephalopathy, poisoning, and meningitis; each was brain dead and maintained on total life support systems. Central diabetes insipidus has also been reported in patients with lymphocytic hypophysitis and AIDS. The diabetes insipidus in the latter group can be due to central nervous system (CNS) infection with herpes simplex virus, *Toxoplasma gondii*, or cytomegalovirus; lymphoma of the CNS has also been reported.

Diabetes insipidus may appear during pregnancy and cease a few days after delivery, or it may commence after parturition in women with Sheehan's syndrome, especially when cortisol deficiency is treated. Mild symptoms of diabetes insipidus may either worsen or improve during pregnancy. AVP-resistant diabetes insipidus also may develop during pregnancy, perhaps owing to increased circulating levels of placental vasopressinase. Fortunately, such patients respond to treatment with desmopressin.

CLINICAL MANIFESTATIONS *Polyuria, excessive thirst*, and *polydipsia* are invariably present in diabetes insipidus. Characteristically, these symptoms are sudden in onset, both when the disorder first becomes manifest and when the effects of administered vasopressin disappear during long-term therapy. In severe cases, the urine is pale in color, and the volume may be immense (up to 16 to 24 L/d), requiring micturition every 30 to 60 min throughout the day and night. More frequently, however, urine volume is only moderately increased (2.5 to 6 L/d) and causes no complaints in subjects who become accustomed to excessive water turnover. Urinary concentration of less than 290 mmol/kg (specific gravity less than 1.010) is usual, but the concentration may be higher than that of serum when subjects with mild disease are deprived of fluids.

The slight rise in serum osmolality resulting from hypotonic polyuria stimulates thirst. Large volumes of fluid are imbibed, and cold drinks are preferred, patients often going to great trouble to secure cold fluids. Although thirst is probably secondary to loss of water, the administration of vasopressin may relieve or reduce thirst, even in the absence of fluid intake.

Normal function of the thirst center ensures that polydipsia closely matches polyuria, so dehydration is seldom detectable except by a mild elevation of serum sodium. However, when replenishment of excreted water is inadequate, severe dehydration may cause weakness, fever, psychic disturbances, hypotension, tachycardia, prostration, and death. These features are associated with a rising serum osmolality and serum sodium concentration, the latter sometimes exceeding 175 mmol/L. Adipsia does not occur in idiopathic diabetes insipidus, but it may result from impairment of the hypothalamic thirst center because of extension of the same process that caused the diabetes insipidus. Alternatively, dehydration can occur during unconsciousness produced by surgical anesthesia, head trauma, or other causes.

Hydronephrosis and renal failure may complicate polyuria, especially in patients who fail to empty their bladders adequately because of bladder atony, urethral strictures, or other causes.

DIAGNOSTIC TESTS The cause of hypotonic polyuria can usually be recognized by a pragmatic clinical approach. Even though stimuli such as nausea, nicotine administration, hypoglycemia, and hypotension may release AVP, the results are clinically irrelevant. It is of little consequence to the patient with symptomatic diabetes insipidus that one or more nonosmotic stimuli retain their capacity to release AVP. Procedures that utilize plasma and urine osmolality determinations are readily available, reliable, and safe, and they allow the physician to establish the diagnosis and to initiate therapy rapidly. Measurements of plasma or urine AVP are expensive and time-consuming and are only occasionally needed, when osmolality measurements are inconclusive (Fig. 330-4). Diagnostic tests should not be performed in the presence of untreated thyroid or adrenocortical deficiency or when there is an osmotic diuresis (e.g., uncontrolled diabetes mellitus).

Assessment of the Relation of Plasma to Urine Osmolality The normal relationship between plasma osmolality (assuming no increase in blood urea or glucose) and urine osmolality is indicated in Fig. 330-3. If several simultaneously determined plasma and urine osmolalities in a patient with polyuria fall substantially to the right of the shaded area, the patient has central or nephrogenic diabetes insipidus. The latter diagnosis can be made if the response to injected vasopressin is subnormal (see "Dehydration Test," below) or if the plasma or urinary AVP concentration is increased. The practice of relating plasma to urine osmolality is useful, particularly in postoperative neurosurgical patients or after head trauma, where its use can permit quick differentiation of diabetes insipidus from parenteral fluid excess. If necessary, intravenous hydration can be slowed temporarily, and repeated plasma and urine osmolalities can be plotted as in Fig. 330-3, to determine whether the relationship is normal.

Dehydration Test Comparison of the urinary osmolality after dehydration with that after vasopressin administration is a simple and reliable way of diagnosing diabetes insipidus and of differentiating vasopressin deficiency from other causes of polyuria. This test should be combined with an assessment of the relationship between plasma and urine osmolality.

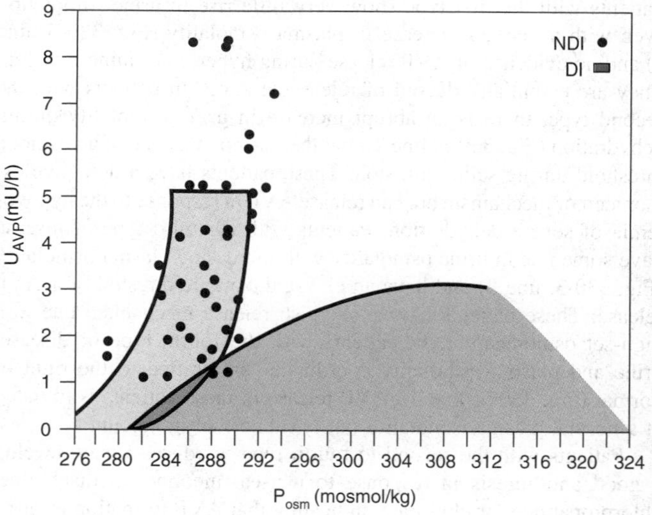

FIGURE 330-4 Relation between plasma osmolality (P_{osm}) and urinary AVP excretion (U_{AVP}) in normal subjects (*shaded area on left*), patients with central diabetes insipidus (*shaded area on right*), and patients with nephrogenic diabetes insipidus (*individual data points*). Correlates in patients with SIADH and with some other types of hyponatremia fall to the left of the normal range. *[From AM Moses, in Frontiers of Hormone Research, vol 13: Diabetes Insipidus in Man, P Czernichow, AG Robinson (eds). Basel, Karger, 1985.]*

The maximal urinary concentrating capacity varies among individuals, and no absolute lower limits of "normal" can be defined in patients with nonspecific illnesses in whom AVP is produced in adequate amounts. It is impossible to distinguish between deficiency and sufficiency of AVP release solely by the level of the urinary osmolality attained after specified periods of water deprivation. On the other hand, if after prolonged dehydration vasopressin administration induces a further rise in urinary osmolality, there is a strong implication that vasopressin deficiency exists.

Procedure

1. Fluids are withheld long enough to result in stable hourly urinary osmolalities (an hourly increase of <30 mmol/kg for at least three successive hours). This goal is usually associated with a loss in body weight of at least 1 kg. In patients whose daily urinary volume exceeds 10 liters, the fluid deprivation should begin between 4 A.M. and 6 A.M. so that the patient can be carefully watched and the test terminated if weight loss exceeds 2 kg or the clinical condition deteriorates. In patients whose urinary volumes are only mildly increased or who are hyponatremic, water deprivation may be started about midnight.
2. Urine specimens are collected hourly for osmolality measurements from 6 A.M. at least until noon and preferably until the osmolality remains stable for three consecutive hours.
3. After the third hour of stable urinary osmolality, the patient is given vasopressin as 5 units of aqueous arginine vasopressin or 1 μg of desmopressin by subcutaneous injection or 10 μg of desmopressin by nasal spray.
4. Plasma osmolality is determined immediately before the injection of vasopressin, and urinary osmolality is measured on the specimen collected between 30 and 60 min after the injection.

Vital signs should be monitored during the procedure, but when the test is performed as described adverse effects are rare.

Interpretation In subjects with normal pituitary function, urinary osmolality does not rise by more than 9 percent after the injection of vasopressin, whatever the maximal urinary osmolality achieved after dehydration alone. In central diabetes insipidus, the rise in urinary osmolality after vasopressin administration exceeds 9 percent. To ensure adequacy of dehydration, plasma osmolality before the vasopressin injection should be above 288 mmol/kg. Patients who have polyuria from renal diseases, potassium depletion, or nephrogenic diabetes insipidus (see below) usually show little rise in urinary osmolality with dehydration and no further rise after vasopressin injection. Patients with compulsive water drinking (primary polydipsia) often require prolonged water deprivation before plasma osmolality reaches 288 mmol/kg and before a plateau in urinary osmolality is reached; urinary osmolality rises by <9 percent after the administration of exogenous vasopressin.

Hypertonic Saline Infusion This test is sometimes necessary to differentiate between primary polydipsia and partial central diabetes insipidus. In the former condition the osmotic threshold is low, normal, or slightly increased, while in the latter it is substantially increased or absent. The saline infusion test is more precise and gives more quantitative data than dehydration. However, some patients cannot tolerate the saline, and the procedure is technically demanding. (See the bibliography for sources giving details.)

DIFFERENTIAL DIAGNOSIS Diabetes insipidus must be distinguished from other types of hypotonic polyuria (primary polydipsia and nephrogenic diabetes insipidus) and from states of osmotic diuresis (Table 330-2). Several types are recognizable by the history (e.g., types that occur following lithium or mannitol administration, surgery under methoxyflurane anesthesia, or renal transplantation). In other types, the physical examination or simple laboratory procedures will indicate the diagnosis (evidence of glycosuria, renal disease, sickle cell anemia, hypercalcemia, or potassium depletion, including primary aldosteronism).

Congenital nephrogenic diabetes insipidus is an X-linked recessive disorder resulting from mutations in the V_2 (antidiuretic) receptor gene located at the q28 region of the X chromosome. More than 50 V_2 receptor mutations have been characterized. Affected males are totally resistant to vasopressin, while heterozygote females are usually asymptomatic but may have varying degrees of polyuria, rarely severe. Females with severe symptoms are thought to have skewed X chromosome inactivation resulting in predominant expression of the mutant allele. Nephrogenic diabetes insipidus may also be inherited as an autosomal recessive defect due to mutations in the aquaporin gene that result in an absent or defective water channel resistant to the action of AVP. Some women with sporadic nephrogenic diabetes insipidus (defect unknown) respond to large doses of vasopressin. V_1 receptor–mediated functions are normal in patients with congenital nephrogenic diabetes insipidus.

Table 330-2

Major Polyuric Syndromes

Primary disorders of water intake or output
- A. Excessive water intake
  - 1. Psychogenic polydipsia
  - 2. Hypothalamic disease: histiocytosis X, sarcoidosis, trauma
  - 3. Drug-induced polydipsia
    - a. Thioridazine
    - b. Chlorpromazine
    - c. Anticholinergic drugs (dry mouth)
- B. Inadequate tubular reabsorption of filtered water
  - 1. Vasopressin deficiency
    - a. Central diabetes insipidus
    - b. Drug-induced inhibition of AVP release
      - (1) Narcotic antagonists
  - 2. Renal tubular unresponsiveness to AVP
    - a. Nephrogenic diabetes insipidus (congenital and familial)
    - b. Nephrogenic diabetes insipidus (acquired)
      - (1) Several chronic renal diseases, after obstructive uropathy, unilateral renal arterial stenosis, after renal transplantation, after acute tubular necrosis
      - (2) Potassium deficiencies, including primary aldosteronism
      - (3) Chronic hypercalcemias, including hyperparathyroidism
      - (4) Drug-induced: lithium, methoxyflurane anesthesia, demeclocycline
      - (5) Various systemic disorders: multiple myeloma, amyloidosis, sickle cell anemia, Sjögren's syndrome

Primary disorders of renal absorption of solutes (osmotic diuresis)
- A. Glucose: diabetes mellitus
- B. Salts, especially sodium chloride
  - 1. Various chronic renal diseases, especially chronic pyelonephritis
  - 2. After various diuretics, including mannitol

When patients with nephrogenic and central diabetes insipidus cannot be differentiated by simpler means, the documentation of a plasma or urinary AVP concentration that is elevated relative to plasma osmolality (Fig. 330-4) or of an AVP concentration that is high relative to urine osmolality will allow the diagnosis of nephrogenic diabetes insipidus.

Primary Polydipsia Primary or psychogenic polydipsia may be difficult to differentiate from diabetes insipidus when the polydipsia and polyuria are sustained throughout the day and night. At the other extreme, polydipsia may occur at intervals of weeks or months, a condition referred to as PIP (psychosis intermittent polydipsia). Between these extremes are individuals with various degrees of excessive water turnover. When polydipsia is extreme, dilution hyponatremia may occur even when urinary diluting capacity is normal. However, this phenomenon is rare because normal persons can excrete between 10 and 14 mL/min of solute-free water. Hyponatremia is more common when diluting capacity is impaired either by renal disease or by drugs such as nonsteroidal anti-inflammatory agents or thiazide diuretics.

We evaluated 22 women and 14 men (median age, 38) with symptomatic primary polydipsia. In 13 there was no definable cause, and 12 had a variety of psychiatric illnesses, often treated with medications having anticholinergic side effects such as dry mouth. Two had CNS

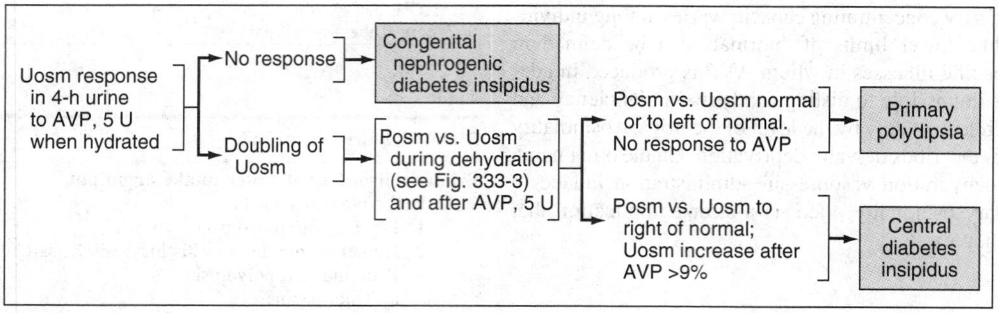

FIGURE 330-5 Approach to hypotonic polyurias.

sarcoidosis, two had antecedent head trauma, and two developed symptoms after becoming toxic from vitamin A or tretinoin. The disease in four was related to prolonged lactation, lithium therapy, chronic stomatitis, and hypertension. One was the sister of a subject with congenital nephrogenic diabetes insipidus.

The diagnosis of primary polydipsia is usually evident from the combination of low plasma and urinary osmolalities. The relationship between urine and plasma osmolality during water deprivation is typically normal or supranormal (to the left of normal in Fig. 330-3). There is little or no rise in urine osmolality after injection of vasopressin at the plateau of urine osmolality during dehydration. However, chronic overingestion of water may suppress release of AVP, and chronic polyuria may cause a wash-out of the medullary osmotic gradient, so that urine osmolality may be subnormal in relation to plasma osmolality (to the right of normal in Fig. 330-3). Therefore, it may be difficult, if not impossible, to differentiate primary polydipsia from partial central diabetes insipidus. Indeed, patients may have both problems. Treatment of these patients with vasopressin, even under close supervision, usually results in water intoxication.

A simple diagnostic approach to patients with hypotonic polyuria is shown in Fig. 330-5.

Determination of the Cause of Hypotonic Polyuria Once the type of the hypotonic polyuria is established, the cause must be determined (see "Etiology," above). Although treatment of the underlying disease rarely causes the polyuria to regress, the underlying disease may be treated with success (e.g., germinoma). In this sense, the development of the polyuria can be considered a tumor marker.

The history can reveal important clues, such as the age of onset and duration of disease, its presence in other members of the family, the constancy of symptoms, a preference for cold or lukewarm fluids, head trauma, evidence of anterior pituitary deficiency, or symptoms suggesting a space-occupying lesion. Examination may reveal evidence of endocrine deficiency or excess (particularly hyperprolactinemia) or of malignant, granulomatous, or infectious disease. Routine laboratory tests and chest radiographs may provide important information.

Most patients with newly diagnosed central diabetes insipidus and primary polydipsia should have a magnetic resonance imaging study of the pituitary-hypothalamic area. In addition to providing insight into the underlying pathologic abnormality, the presence or absence of the posterior pituitary hyperintense signal with appropriate T1-weighted imaging may confirm the diagnosis, since the signal is absent in central diabetes insipidus and present in primary polydipsia. Information obtained from lumbar puncture or even, at times, hypothalamic biopsy may diagnose lesions observed by magnetic resonance imaging. If magnetic resonance imaging is negative in patients with central diabetes insipidus, it should be repeated at increasing time intervals.

Rx TREATMENT

(See Table 330-3.) Aqueous arginine vasopressin may be administered subcutaneously in doses of 5 to 10 units and usually has a duration of action of 3 to 6 h. The main use of this preparation is in initial management of unconscious patients with acute onset of diabetes insipidus following head trauma or a neurosurgical procedure. The short duration of action of this agent allows recognition of the recovery of neurohypophyseal function and minimizes the development of water intoxication in patients receiving intravenous fluids.

Desmopressin has a prolonged antidiuretic activity and is almost completely devoid of pressor effects. When used intranasally in amounts between 10 and 20 μg (0.1 to 0.2 mL) or by subcutaneous or intravenous injection (1 to 4 μg), it exerts an antidiuretic action for 10 to 24 h in most patients. This analogue is the drug of choice in the treatment of most patients with diabetes insipidus. Lypressin is a nasal spray; a single application may result in an antidiuresis lasting approximately 4 to 6 h. Nasal absorption of both analogues may be decreased in the presence of an upper respiratory infection or allergic rhinitis. In such circumstances and in unconscious or uncooperative patients with diabetes insipidus, desmopressin should be given by subcutaneous or intravenous injection.

Patients with diabetes insipidus who have some residual releasable AVP (types 2 to 4 disease) may respond to oral treatment

Table 330-3

Agents Used in Treatment of Central Diabetes Insipidus

Route of Administration	Product Description	Chemical Composition	Concentration	Amount Administered and Mean Duration of Activity, h*
Intranasal	DDAVP or desmopressin acetate by rhinal tube or nasal spray	Desmopressin acetate	100 μg/mL	10 μg (0.1 mL) → 12 15 μg (0.15 mL) → 16 20 μg (0.2 mL) → 20
	Diapid nasal spray	Lypressin (lysine vasopressin)	50 USP units (185 μg)/mL	2–4 U → 4–6
Subcutaneous or intravenous	DDAVP injectable	Desmopressin acetate	4 μg/mL	0.5 μg → 10 1.0 μg → 14 2.0 μg → 18 4.0 μg → 22
Subcutaneous	Pitressin (aqueous)	Arginine vasopressin	50 μg (20 USP units)/mL	12.5 μg (5 U) → 4
Oral nonhormonal agents	Chlorpropamide		100- and 250-mg tablets	200–500 mg → 12–24
	Clofibrate		500-mg capsules	500 mg qid → 24 or more
	Carbamazepine		200-mg tablets	400–600 mg → 24

* All the listed durations of action are variable between patients but quite consistent in individual patients. Desmopressin acetate is also marketed in far higher concentrations (1.5 mg/mL) as Stimate for treatment of bleeding disorders.

with chlorpropamide, clofibrate, or carbamazepine. Chlorpropamide stimulates AVP release and potentiates the antidiuretic action of submaximal amounts of AVP. Doses of 200 to 500 mg, usually taken once daily, are sufficient for an antidiuretic response. The action of this agent starts within several hours of administration and usually lasts for 24 h. Chlorpropamide also may restore thirst perception and thus be useful in patients with thirst center defects. Oral agents are used rarely because of hypoglycemia and other undesirable side effects.

Primary polydipsia can be treated effectively only by eliminating the underlying problem. However, clozapine may improve the PIP syndrome in the subset of polydipsia patients with schizophrenia.

The only way to treat most patients with nephrogenic diabetes insipidus is by solute restriction and the administration of thiazides or other diuretics. The resulting sodium depletion causes a fall in glomerular filtration rate with enhanced reabsorption of fluid in the proximal portion of the nephron and decreased delivery of sodium to the ascending limb of the loop of Henle and consequently reduced capacity to dilute the urine. Some women with congenital nephrogenic diabetes insipidus and some patients with lithium-induced polyuria have been treated effectively by injecting large doses of desmopressin.

When antidiuretic therapy is initiated in patients with long-standing diabetes insipidus, care must be taken to avoid excessive drinking, which could result in water intoxication. Education about drinking water and other liquids according to thirst must be reinforced constantly in some patients. Excessive fluid intake may be more common and severe in subjects whose diabetes insipidus is due to sarcoidosis or lymphoma. Adipsic patients with diabetes insipidus are difficult to manage. Intake and output of fluids, body weight, vital signs, serum sodium, and renal function must be monitored closely. Fluid intake must approximate urine volume and fluid losses by other routes. Otherwise, such individuals can develop hypernatremia and circulatory collapse without becoming thirsty. Patients who are confused, obtunded, or unconscious must be monitored in the same way. Special care must be taken when patients with treated diabetes insipidus are subjected to procedures that require fluid restriction, as in preparation for an intravenous pyelogram, or hydration, as after administration of chemotherapy. In the former situation, fluid intake must be restricted to conform to urine output. In patients receiving antidiuretic therapy, fluids should not be administered beyond the amounts determined by thirst or urine output. If high urine flow rates are necessary, antidiuretic therapy can be discontinued, or furosemide may be administered while antidiuretic therapy is continued.

SYNDROMES ASSOCIATED WITH VASOPRESSIN EXCESS

Excessive blood levels or actions of vasopressin are associated with and probably cause water retention in several circumstances:

1. As a mechanism for *prevention of a rise in plasma osmolality*, which would otherwise result from sodium retention in edema associated with congestive heart failure, cirrhosis with ascites, nephrosis, orthostatic edema, myxedema, and treatment with sodium-retaining drugs (fludrocortisone, nonsteroidal anti-inflammatory agents, and others)
2. As a mechanism of *defense against hypovolemia and/or hypotension* in subjects with adrenal insufficiency, excessive fluid loss (from vomiting, diarrhea, drug-induced diuresis, or excessive sweating), fluid deprivation, and probably positive-pressure respiration
3. As a consequence of *drug- or disease-induced release of vasopressin from the neurohypophysis* caused by
   a. *Central nervous system disorders*: head trauma, subdural hematoma, subarachnoid hemorrhage, cerebral vascular thrombosis, brain tumor, cerebral atrophy, acute encephalitis, acute psychosis, tuberculous and other meningitides

Table 330-4

Causes of SIADH

Malignant neoplasms with autonomous AVP release	Cerebral atrophy
Small cell carcinoma of lung	Acute encephalitis
Carcinoma of pancreas	Tuberculous meningitis
Lymphoma, lymphocytic lymphoma, Hodgkin's disease	Purulent meningitis
Carcinoma of duodenum	Guillain-Barré syndrome
Thymoma	Lupus erythematosus
Nonmalignant pulmonary diseases	Acute intermittent porphyria
Tuberculosis	**Drugs**
Lung abscess	Chlorpropamide
Pneumonia	Vincristine
Viral pneumonitis	Vinblastine
Empyema	Cyclophosphamide
Chronic obstructive airways disease	Carbamazepine
Central nervous system disorders	Oxytocin
Skull fracture	General anesthesia
Subdural hematoma	Narcotics
Subarachnoid hemorrhage	Tricyclic antidepressants
Cerebral vascular thrombosis	**Miscellaneous causes**
	Hypothyroidism
	Positive pressure respiration

   b. *Drugs that release or potentiate the action of AVP*: chlorpropamide, vincristine, vinblastine, cyclophosphamide, carbamazepine, general anesthetics, tricyclic antidepressants
4. *In ectopic AVP production and release*:
   a. *From neoplastic tissue*: small cell carcinoma of lung, pancreatic carcinoma, lymphoma, Hodgkin's disease, lymphocytic lymphoma, thymoma, carcinoma of duodenum or bladder
   b. *From inflammatory lung diseases*: tuberculosis, lung abscess, pneumonias, empyema
5. *Other conditions*: Guillain-Barré syndrome, lupus erythematosus, acute intermittent porphyria, severe renovascular hypertension, and old age

SYNDROME OF INAPPROPRIATE AVP SECRETION

The syndrome of inappropriate AVP secretion [commonly termed the syndrome of inappropriate antidiuretic hormone (SIADH)] is applied to vasopressin excess of types 3 to 5 listed above, which are associated with hyponatremia without edema (Table 330-4). In these patients, the AVP excess is considered to be inappropriate because it occurs in the presence of plasma hyposmolality. SIADH is analogous to abnormalities produced by administration of vasopressin and water to normal subjects. Although it may be conceptually valid to consider the AVP excess to be inappropriate in adrenal insufficiency and in the edematous, hypovolemic, and hypotensive disorders listed in entries 1 and 2 above, the different pathogenic mechanisms and treatments make it advisable not to consider these disorders as variants of SIADH.

Pathogenesis of SIADH The ectopic origin of authentic AVP from neoplasms and pulmonary tissue of the types listed above has been documented by tissue analysis. Neoplastic cells obtained from the tumors of patients with SIADH can synthesize, store, and release AVP. Both AVP and its associated neurophysin are elevated in the plasma of over 60 percent of patients with small cell carcinoma of the lung. There is an excellent correlation between the increases in plasma AVP and neurophysin concentrations on the one hand and the clinical responses to treatment or the recurrences of disease on the other. Vasopressin also has been demonstrated in tuberculous lung tissue. Intracranial lesions (meningitis, encephalitis, trauma, vascular accidents) probably stimulate release of AVP from the neurohypophysis, possibly acting through cytokine-mediated mechanisms. Some drugs, such as vincristine, chlorpropamide, and carbamazepine, stimulate release of AVP from the neurohypophyseal system, and others (e.g., chlorpropamide and nonsteroidal anti-inflammatory agents) potentiate the antidiuretic action of secreted AVP.

Excessive release or an excessive renal tubular effect of vasopressin results in the excretion of a concentrated urine (with a urinary osmolality usually over 300 mmol/kg) despite a subnormal plasma osmolality and serum sodium concentration. Sodium excretion in the urine is maintained (usually above 20 mmol/L) by hypervolemia, suppression of the renin-angiotensin-aldosterone system, and an increased plasma concentration of atrial natriuretic peptide. However, the urinary sodium concentration may be below 20 mmol/L if sodium intake is low but is higher if sodium intake is unrestricted. Blood urea nitrogen and uric acid concentrations tend to fall because of plasma dilution and increased excretion of nitrogenous compounds. Because of the hypervolemia blood pressure shows no orthostatic fall, but in spite of hypervolemia there is no recumbent hypertension (except when plasma angiotensin II is simultaneously elevated) and no peripheral edema (for unknown reasons). The extracellular hypotonicity leads to intracellular swelling, and severe symptoms may result from cerebral edema.

Clinical Manifestations of SIADH In general, the rate of fall in serum sodium concentration is more important in producing the neurologic features of SIADH than the absolute magnitude of the fall. When SIADH is mild, with serum Na concentrations of 130 to 135 mmol/L, or develops gradually over several weeks, symptoms may be absent or limited to anorexia, nausea, and vomiting, as in other forms of hyponatremia. When hyponatremia is severe or acute in onset, body weight increases, and the symptoms of cerebral edema are predominant, including restlessness, irritability, confusion, coma, and convulsions associated with nonspecific electroencephalographic changes. Pitting edema is almost always absent.

Diagnosis SIADH should be suspected in patients who have hyponatremia and a concentrated urine (osmolality >300 mmol/kg) associated with lethargy and in the absence of edema, orthostatic hypotension, and features of dehydration. The diagnosis of SIADH is made when other causes of enhanced AVP release are excluded. The diagnosis is supported by the finding of blood urea nitrogen, serum uric acid, creatinine, and albumin concentrations in the low-normal or subnormal range. However, it is essential in making the diagnosis to differentiate SIADH from (1) the *dilutional hyponatremias* listed in entry 2 above, particularly adrenocortical insufficiency, in which orthostatic hypotension, tachycardia, and an elevated or high-normal blood urea nitrogen are characteristic; (2) the *edematous states* listed in entry 1 above, particularly hypothyroidism and congestive heart failure with hyponatremia; (3) *hypertensive states* associated with hyponatremia caused by renovascular stenosis or diuretic therapy; (4) *primary polydipsia*, which is always associated with a dilute urine (osmolality <150 mmol/kg); (5) *pseudohyponatremia* associated with excessive plasma glucose, triglyceride, or protein concentrations; and (6) the *"sick-cell" syndrome*, in which hyponatremia is due to a subnormal setting of the hypothalamic osmoreceptors, associated usually with a chronic, debilitating disease. Conditions (1) through (5) in this list are easily recognizable by the associated plasma abnormalities.

When the diagnosis of SIADH is not obvious after other causes of hyponatremia have been excluded, a positive diagnosis can usually be made with a *water-load test*. The water-load test is particularly useful in differentiating patients with a low-set osmoreceptor (who excrete the water normally) from all other hyponatremic states associated with a concentrated urine. This test should not be performed unless or until the serum sodium concentration has been elevated to a safe level (above 125 mmol/L) by restriction of water intake and/or, if necessary, by saline administration. The patient is asked to drink the water load (20 mL/kg of body weight up to 1500 mL) in 10 to 20 min, and urine is collected in hourly samples, with the patient recumbent between voidings, for 4 to 5 h in the morning. At least 65 percent of the water load should be excreted in 4 h or 80 percent in 5 h, and the lowest urinary osmolality, usually reached in the second hour, should be below 100 mmol/kg. It is essential to restrict further water intake for the rest of the day to prevent water intoxication in patients who fail to excrete the water load normally. Failure to excrete the water load may occur in adrenal insufficiency or renal insufficiency, as well as in SIADH. It is important to appreciate, too, that SIADH cannot be diagnosed in the presence of severe pain, nausea, "stress," hypovolemia, hypotension, or other conditions that can stimulate AVP release even in the presence of plasma hypotonicity.

Measurements of plasma or urinary AVP (P_{AVP}, U_{AVP}) are useful adjuncts in establishing the diagnosis of SIADH. Plasma AVP is often unmeasurable in hyponatremic states but is detectable, even after a water load, in SIADH. The correlates of plasma osmolality (P_{osm}) versus P_{AVP} or U_{AVP} concentration fall to the left of the normal values in SIADH (Fig. 330-4) and in the other hyponatremic states associated with a concentrated urine. Thus, in most patients with SIADH, P_{AVP} and U_{AVP} concentrations, which may fluctuate widely, are unrelated to concomitant changes in P_{osm} Occasionally, this lack of correlation between P_{osm} and P_{AVP} or U_{AVP} may be inconsistent. Rarely, for instance, the baseline, unstimulated AVP level may be inappropriately elevated and may fail to change as P_{osm} is raised until the P_{osm} reaches the normal range. Further increases in P_{osm} induced by hypertonic saline infusion or water deprivation may then result in normal or subnormal increases in P_{AVP} or U_{AVP}. This unusual phenomenon may reflect uncontrolled "leakage" of AVP into the circulation.

The diagnostic approach to SIADH is depicted in Fig. 330-6.

℞ TREATMENT

Restriction of fluid intake to 800 to 1000 mL daily is essential. Since this intake is almost always exceeded by urinary output plus insensible fluid loss, a negative water balance ensues that results in gradual, daily reduction in weight, a progressive rise in serum Na concentration and osmolality, and symptomatic improvement. It is useful to verify the effectiveness of fluid restriction by documenting the changes in weight and serum Na concentration daily, until serum Na exceeds 135 mmol/L.

Unless and until the underlying cause of the SIADH can be corrected, fluid intake should be restricted continuously, to maintain

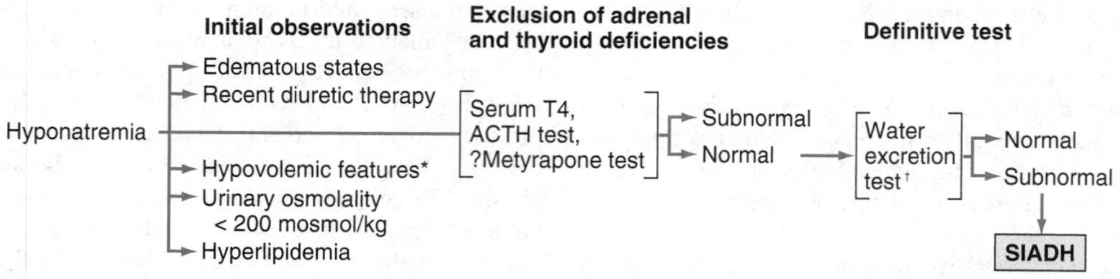

*Orthostatic hypotension and tachycardia, prerenal azotemia, etc.
†Water excretion test should only be performed when serum Na concentration has risen above 125 mEq/L, after water deprivation for as long as may be necessary.

FIGURE 330-6 Approach to diagnosis of SIADH in patients with hyponatremia.

normonatremia. In addition to restriction of fluid intake, 200 to 300 mL of 3% or 5% sodium chloride solution should be infused intravenously over 3 to 4 h in patients with severe confusion, convulsions, or coma. To avoid the possibility of inducing pontine myelinosis, the serum Na concentration should not be raised too rapidly. The possibility of causing congestive heart failure by infusing hypertonic saline is remote as long as fluid is restricted and may be further reduced by the simultaneous intravenous administration of furosemide.

Attempts should be made to identify and correct the cause of the SIADH as soon as possible. The administration of water-retaining drugs should be stopped. Treatment of hypothyroidism should be initiated. Pulmonary tuberculosis and other pulmonary infections should be treated appropriately, and meningitis or other CNS disorders should be treated, if present. When a malignant tumor is the source of autonomous AVP release and SIADH, surgery, radiation, and/or chemotherapy is often beneficial even if the underlying neoplasm cannot be cured.

Antagonism of the release or action of AVP is seldom successful. Although phenytoin inhibits AVP release, it is seldom effective in SIADH. Drugs that block the effect of AVP on the renal tubule are occasionally useful. Demeclocycline is the most potent inhibitor of AVP action available for chronic administration, in doses of 900 to 1200 mg/d. Patients receiving demeclocycline should be followed carefully to detect any evidence of renal failure, bacterial superinfection, or excessive drug-induced water loss. Lithium salts interfere with the action of AVP on tubular water reabsorption and can cause polyuria by this mechanism. Unfortunately, lithium can cause serious side effects in hyponatremic patients and, for this reason, is not recommended for treatment of SIADH.

Prognosis The prognosis of SIADH depends on the cause. Drug-induced SIADH is rapidly and completely corrected by withdrawal of the causative agent. Similarly, treatment of pulmonary or CNS infections can result in improvement and eventual cure of SIADH. Although SIADH resulting from small cell carcinoma of the lung or other malignancies can often be controlled with rigorous restriction of fluid intake, the underlying malignancy determines the prognosis.

PARAVENTRICULAR-NEUROHYPOPHYSEAL SYSTEM AND OXYTOCIN

CHEMISTRY AND PHYSIOLOGY Oxytocin, a nonapeptide that differs by two amino acids from vasopressin, is produced in the cell bodies of the paraventricular nuclei and to a lesser extent in those of the supraoptic nuclei. It is synthesized and transported in neurosecretory granules by way of neuronal axons to the neurohypophysis, where it is stored or released, in conjunction with an oxytocin-specific neurophysin. Oxytocin release is stimulated by nerve impulses from the hypothalamus that cause depolarization of the neurosecretory terminals of the posterior pituitary and subsequent release of oxytocin through a calcium-dependent process, similar to the mechanism for vasopressin release. Estrogen stimulates release of oxytocin and its neurophysin. The secretion of oxytocin, as well as of vasopressin, is inhibited by ethanol. Some stimuli such as pain apparently cause simultaneous release of oxytocin and vasopressin but most stimuli cause the two hormones to be released independently. Oxytocin is liberated during suckling, whereas vasopressin is released in much greater quantities than is oxytocin after an osmotic stimulus or hemorrhage. Manipulation or distention of the female genital tract, artificially or during parturition, is a more effective stimulus of oxytocin release than suckling.

Oxytocin acts on the membranes of myometrial and myoepithelial cells to cause an increased force of contraction. The sensitivity of the myometrium to oxytocin increases with the duration of pregnancy, and a role for oxytocin in the initiation and maintenance of labor is probable. Oxytocin may have survival value to the offspring, since it may hasten the final stages of birth and lessen the chances of anoxia. Oxytocin also exerts a contractile action on the myometrium post

partum and causes contraction of the myoepithelial cells of the mammary alveoli, causing them to expel milk from the secretory tissue to the nipple. In the human oxytocin is 100 times more potent than vasopressin in its milk-ejecting activity. In contrast, the antidiuretic potency of oxytocin is about 200 times less than that of vasopressin. Oxytocin probably does not exert any significant physiologic effects other than those on the uterus and breast.

One milligram of a purified oxytocin preparation contains 450 IU of hormone, and the amount of oxytocin in the posterior pituitary is similar to that of vasopressin. Even though oxytocin has no known role in the male, the male neural lobe stores oxytocin in amounts similar to those in the female. The plasma oxytocin concentration in both men and women exhibits episodic increases, with values ranging from about 1 to 4 pmol/L (1.25 to 5 ng/L) but with no diurnal variation. In normal women, there is a midcycle increase in plasma oxytocin concentration from a preovulatory value of about 2 pmol/L (2.5 ng/L) to a peak value of 4 to 8 pmol/L (5 to 10 ng/L) at the time of ovulation. During labor, plasma oxytocin concentrations increase and then fall rapidly after delivery to prepartum levels. During suckling, the plasma oxytocin levels of the mother are usually about 10 to 20 pmol/L (12 to 25 ng/L). The half-life of oxytocin in plasma is about 3 to 5 min. Oxytocin is removed from the circulation mainly by the kidneys and liver, although the uterus and mammary gland may remove some.

CLINICAL USE OF OXYTOCIN The clinical use of oxytocin is limited to the induction of labor, control of hemorrhage following incomplete abortion and curettage, and treatment of impaired milk ejection. For discussion of the obstetric uses of oxytocin, the reader is referred to textbooks on obstetrics. Care must be taken because oxytocin may cause uterine rupture and fetal death. The antidiuretic action of oxytocin can be elicited with single intravenous doses of as little as 100 mU. Maximal antidiuresis is reached with 40 to 50 mU/min. Since 10 to 40 units of oxytocin per liter of intravenous fluid may be used in obstetric practice, water intoxication may result. The vasodilatory action of oxytocin may cause hypotension, tachycardia, arrhythmias, and sudden death in obstetric patients with heart disease. Anesthetics may modify the cardiovascular responses to oxytocin. For instance, in patients under cyclopropane anesthesia, oxytocin causes more hypotension but less tachycardia than in unanesthetized subjects. The vasodilatory effect of oxytocin can be blocked by vasopressin.

Please refer to Chap. 30 in Goodman & Gilman's The Pharmacological Basis of Therapeutics, *9th ed, McGraw-Hill, New York, 1996.*

BIBLIOGRAPHY

Cross BA, Leng G: *Progress in Brain Research*, vol 60: *The Neurohypophysis: Structure, Function and Control*. Amsterdam, Elsevier, 1983

Czernichow P, Robinson AG: *Frontiers of Hormone Research*, vol 13: *Diabetes Insipidus in Man*. Basel, Karger, 1985

Durr JA: Diabetes insipidus in pregnancy. Am J Kidney Dis 9:276, 1987

Knoers NVAM et al: Inheritance of mutations in the V_2 receptor gene in thirteen families with nephrogenic diabetes insipidus. Kidney Int 46:170, 1994

Leadbetter RA, Shutty MS Jr: Differential effects of neuroleptics and clozapine on polydipsia and intermittent hyponatremia. J Clin Psychiatry 55:9(Suppl B), 1994

McLeod JF et al: Familial neurohypophyseal diabetes insipidus associated with a signal peptide mutation. J Clin Endocrinol Metab 77:599, 1993

Miller M et al: Recognition of partial defects in antidiuretic hormone secretion. Ann Intern Med 73:721, 1970

Moses AM: Osmotic thresholds for AVP release using plasma and urine AVP and free water clearance. Am J Physiol 256:R892, 1989

———, Clayton B: Impairment of osmotically stimulated AVP release in patients with primary polydipsia. Am J Physiol 265:R1247, 1993

———, Streeten DHP: Pathophysiologic and pharmacologic alterations in the release and action of ADH. Metabolism 25:697, 1976

——— et al: Marked hypotonic polyuria resulting from nephrogenic diabetes insipidus with partial sensitivity to vasopressin. J Clin Endocrinol Metab 59:1044, 1984

——— et al: Two distinct pathophysiological mechanisms in congenital nephrogenic diabetes insipidus. J Clin Endocrinol Metab 66:1259, 1988

——— et al: The use of T_1-weighted magnetic resonance imaging to differentiate between primary polydipsia and central diabetes insipidus. Am J Neuroradiol 13:1273, 1992

REICHLIN S: *The Neurohypophysis. Physiological and Clinical Aspects*. New York, Plenum, 1984

ROBERTSON GL: The regulation of vasopressin function in health and disease. Recent Prog Hormone Res 33:333, 1977

331 DISEASES OF THE THYROID*

Leonard Wartofsky

Normal function of the thyroid gland is directed to the secretion of L-thyroxine (T_4) and 3,5,3′-triiodo-L-thyronine (T_3), the active thyroid hormones that influence a diversity of metabolic processes (Fig. 331-1). Diseases of the thyroid are manifested by qualitative or quantitative alterations in hormone secretion, enlargement of the thyroid (goiter), or both. Insufficient hormone secretion results in *hypothyroidism* or *myxedema*, in which decreased caloric expenditure (hypometabolism) is a principal feature. Conversely, excessive secretion of hormone results in hypermetabolism and other features, together termed *hyperthyroidism* or *thyrotoxicosis*. Enlargement of the thyroid gland (which normally weighs 15 to 18 g in adults) may be generalized or focal. Generalized enlargements may not be symmetric, the right lobe tending to enlarge more than the left. Goiters may be associated with increased, normal, or decreased hormone secretion, depending on the underlying disturbance. Focal enlargement usually reflects neoplastic disease, either benign or malignant; the former sometimes is responsible for hypersecretion of hormone and hyperthyroidism, whereas the latter rarely causes hyperthyroidism. Any goiter may compress adjacent structures in the neck or mediastinum.

EMBRYOLOGY, ANATOMY, AND HISTOLOGY

The thyroid originates embryologically from an evagination of the pharyngeal epithelium with some contribution from the lateral pharyngeal pouches. Progressive descent of the midline thyroid anlage gives rise to the thyroglossal duct, which extends from the foramen cecum near the base of the tongue to the isthmus of the thyroid. Remnants of tissue may persist along the course of this tract as "lingual thyroid," thyroglossal cysts or nodules, or a structure contiguous with the thyroid isthmus called the *pyramidal lobe*. The latter is usually not discernible except when the remainder of the gland is enlarged. Rarely, lingual thyroid may be the sole functioning thyroid tissue. In such cases, its output may or may not be sufficient to maintain a normal metabolic (euthyroid) state. Thyroid aplasia and functional failure of ectopic thyroid tissue are causes of sporadic neonatal hypothyroidism (1 in every 4000 or 5000 newborns), which responds to early treatment.

The fetal thyroid acquires the capacity to concentrate and organify iodine at about 10 weeks of gestation. Both T_4 and thyroid-stimulating hormone (TSH, thyrotropin) are detectable in the blood soon thereafter and increase in concentration during the second trimester. The increase in serum T_4 is due both to increasing thyroid secretion and to the appearance in plasma of thyroxine-binding globulin (TBG), and the increase in TSH is a reflection of the maturation of the fetal hypothalamus with resulting secretion of thyrotropin-releasing hormone (TRH). Maternal TRH readily crosses the placenta and may play a role in the development of the fetal pituitary-thyroid axis. Maternal TSH, by contrast, does not cross the placenta. T_3 is detectable in the blood later during the second trimester, but its concentration in blood and amniotic fluid remains low until shortly after parturition. By contrast, the concentration of its analogue, 3,3′,5′-triiodo-L-thyronine (reverse T_3, rT_3), is increased in fetal blood and amniotic fluid relative to that in maternal blood (see Fig. 331-1). These differences are due to qualitative alterations in T_4 metabolism in the fetus. The low level of T_3 in fetal blood and amniotic fluid in the face of a high maternal concentration indicates that maternal-fetal transfer of T_3, while it occurs, is minimal, and the same is true for T_4. Hence T_4 from the fetal thyroid is the major thyroid hormone available to the fetus. Except for the possible effect of maternal TRH, therefore, the fetal pituitary-thyroid axis is a functional unit distinct from that of the mother.

The normal adult thyroid consists of two lobes joined by an isthmus and lies just anterior and caudal to the cartilages of the larynx. Fibrous septa divide the gland into pseudolobules which, in turn, are composed of vesicles, called *follicles* or *acini*, surrounded by a capillary network. Normally, the follicle walls are composed of cuboidal epithelium. The lumen is filled with a proteinaceous *colloid*, which contains a unique protein, *thyroglobulin*, within the peptide sequence of which T_4 and T_3 are synthesized and stored. The thyroid also contains a second, smaller population of cells, the C cells. They are the source of calcitonin and give rise to medullary thyroid carcinoma when they undergo malignant transformation.

* Revision and update of work by the late Sidney Ingbar.

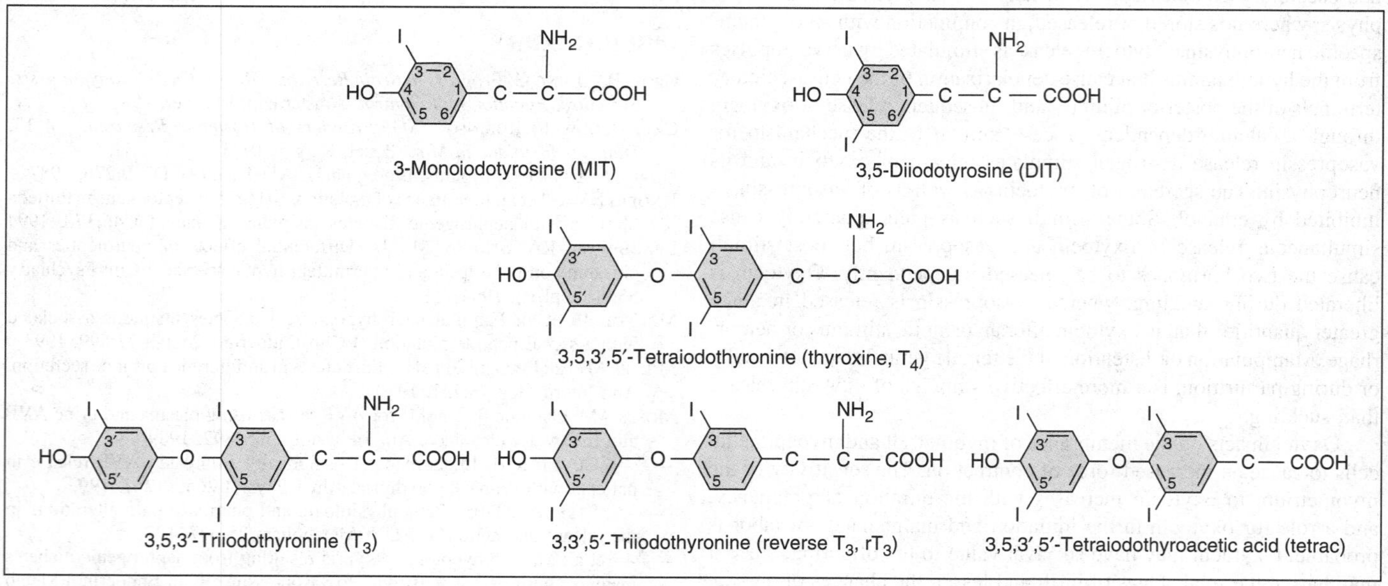

FIGURE 331-1 Structural formulas of thyroxine, its precursors, and certain of its metabolites.

THYROID HORMONE ECONOMY: NORMAL PHYSIOLOGY

The term *thyroid hormone economy* denotes the processes involved in the synthesis of hormones in the thyroid gland, their transport in the circulation, their action and metabolism in the peripheral tissues, and the regulatory mechanisms that maintain a normal supply of thyroid hormones.

TSH AND THE TSH RECEPTOR

The pituitary hormone thyrotropin (TSH) controls thyroid function and acts by binding to TSH receptors (TSH-R) on the basolateral membrane of thyroid follicular cells. Binding to TSH-R leads to activation of the adenylate cyclase and phospholipase C pathways of intracellular signaling that regulate thyroid function and growth. TSH-R is a member of the G protein–coupled receptor family and is organized into three domains: an extracellular domain of 398 amino acids, a membrane-spanning domain of 266 amino acids, and an 83-amino-acid intracellular carboxy-terminal domain. This protein is encoded by a single gene more than 60 kilobases long. Somatic mutations and clonal expansion of the TSH-R gene appear to account for chronic stimulation of the cyclic adenosine monophosphate (AMP) cascade leading to toxic follicular adenomas.

HORMONE SYNTHESIS AND SECRETION The synthesis of thyroid hormone depends on entry into the thyroid of adequate quantities of iodine, a constituent of T_4 and T_3; on normal iodine metabolism in the gland; and on the synthesis of thyroglobulin, a receptor protein for iodine. The structure of thyroglobulin favors iodination and particularly the formation of T_4 and T_3. Secretion of normal quantities of hormone requires both a normal rate of hormone synthesis and hydrolysis of thyroglobulin to liberate active hormones. Iodine enters the thyroid in the form of inorganic or ionic iodide, whose source is iodide derived either from the deiodination of thyroid hormones or from iodide ingested in food, water, or medication. Formerly, a dietary iodine intake of approximately 0.2 mg/d was considered normal in the United States, and this was sufficient to sustain a plasma iodide concentration of approximately 40 nmol/L (0.5 μg/dL). However, owing to iodine contamination of some foods and to the widespread use of iodine in drugs, vitamin preparations, and antiseptic agents, the average iodine intake has increased to about 0.5 to 1.0 mg/d, with corresponding increases in plasma iodide concentration. Iodide is removed from the plasma by the thyroid, kidneys, and salivary and gastrointestinal glands, but since iodide that enters gastrointestinal secretions is reabsorbed, net clearance is effected by the thyroid and kidneys. In effect, the thyroid and kidneys compete for plasma iodide. Renal clearance is largely a function of glomerular filtration rate and is not influenced by humoral factors or plasma iodide concentration. Hence, adjustments in the rate of iodide uptake by the thyroid relative to the rate of urinary excretion are mediated by changes in thyroid rather than renal avidity.

The synthesis and secretion of the active thyroid hormones can be divided into four sequential steps, each of which is under the control of TSH (Fig. 331-2). The first involves active transport of iodide into the thyroid cell, a process mediated by a protein in the plasma membrane of these cells termed the Na^+/I^- symporter. The rate of active iodide transport exceeds the rate of passive diffusion of iodide out of the gland, so that the thyroid maintains a concentration gradient for iodide (thyroid/plasma concentration ratio), which is usually around 25 but can be 500 or more under certain conditions. Energy for iodide transport depends on oxidative metabolism in the gland.

The second step involves oxidation of iodide to a higher-valence form that is capable of iodinating tyrosyl residues in thyroglobulin, a glycoprotein of approximately 660,000 mol wt that is synthesized in the follicular cell. Oxidation of iodide is effected by a peroxidase, which uses hydrogen peroxide generated during the course of oxidative metabolism in the gland. Organic iodinations occur at the cell-colloid interface, taking place largely in newly synthesized thyroglobulin undergoing exocytosis into the follicular lumen. The consequence is the formation of the peptide-bound precursors monoiodotyrosine (MIT) and diiodotyrosine (DIT).

In the third step, the iodotyrosines undergo oxidative condensation, again through the mediation of peroxidase. This coupling reaction occurs within the thyroglobulin molecule and yields a variety of iodothyronines, including T_4 and T_3. Although minute quantities of thyroglobulin are detectable in the blood, most thyroglobulin is retained for a time in the gland, serving as a storage vehicle for the thyroid hormones. Liberation of the active hormones into the blood involves pinocytosis of follicular colloid at the apical margin of the cells to form colloid droplets. The droplets fuse with thyroid lysosomes to form "phagolysosomes," in which thyroglobulin is hydrolyzed by proteases. The final step is release of the free iodothyronines T_4 and T_3 into the blood. The thyroid is the only source of endogenous T_4; in contrast, only about 20 percent of T_3 is produced in the thyroid, the remainder being generated in extraglandular tissues by the enzymatic removal of the 5′-iodine from the outer ring of T_4. Inactive iodotyrosines liberated by the hydrolysis of thyroglobulin are stripped of their iodine by an intrathyroid enzyme, iodotyrosine dehalogenase. Most iodide so liberated is reused in the synthesis of hormone, but a small proportion is lost into the blood (iodide leak); iodide leakage may become large under certain circumstances.

The thyroid also concentrates other monovalent anions such as pertechnetate, which is available as the radioactive isotope sodium [^{99m}Tc]pertechnetate. Unlike iodide, little pertechnetate is organically bound; hence, its duration of stay in the thyroid is short. This property, together with its short physical half-life, makes pertechnetate a valuable radionuclide for imaging the thyroid by scintillation scanning.

The foregoing reactions are subject to inhibition by a variety of agents, which are called *goitrogens* because their ability to inhibit hormone synthesis and indirectly stimulate TSH secretion enables them to induce goiter formation. Inorganic anions such as perchlorate and thiocyanate inhibit iodide transport and thereby reduce the supply of substrate for hormone formation. The goiter and hypothyroidism that follow, however, can be prevented or relieved by an amount of

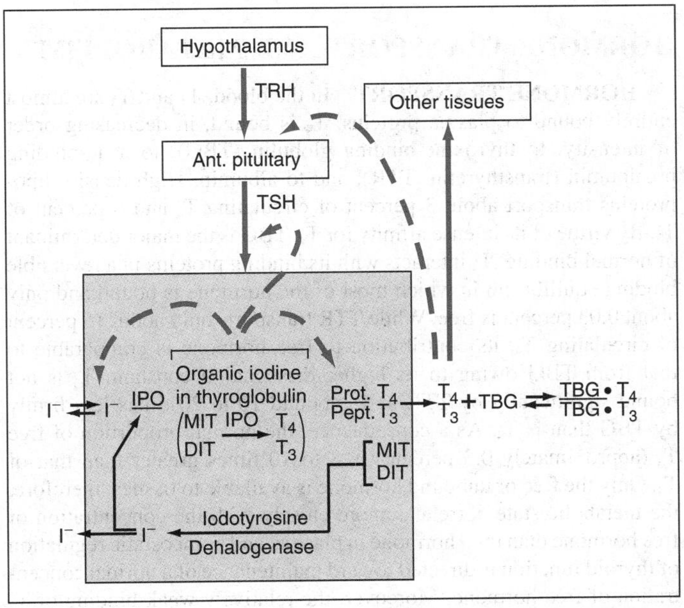

FIGURE 331-2 Schema depicting pathways in the synthesis and secretion of thyroid hormones and mechanisms for the suprathyroid and intrathyroid regulation of thyroid function. *Small, solid arrows* indicate pathways of iodine metabolism; *open arrows* indicate stimulation; *cross-hatched arrows* indicate inhibitory influences. TRH, thyrotropin-releasing hormone; TSH, thyroid-stimulating hormone; IPO, iodide peroxidase; prot., thyroid protease; peptid., thyroid peptidase; MIT, monoiodotyrosine; DIT, diiodotyrosine; T_4, thyroxine; T_3, 3,5,3′-triiodothyronine.

iodide large enough to enable adequate quantities to enter the gland by passive diffusion. The commonly employed antithyroid agents, such as the derivatives of thiourea and mercaptoimidazole, exert more complex actions on hormone biosynthesis. These agents inhibit the initial oxidation (organic binding) of iodide, decrease the proportion of DIT relative to MIT, and block coupling of iodotyrosines to form the hormonally active iodothyronines. The latter reaction is the most sensitive. Thus, the synthesis of hormonally active iodothyronines may be decreased, although the total incorporation of iodine by the thyroid is affected minimally. The goitrogenic action of thioureas is not overcome by large quantities of iodine. Indeed, certain weak goitrogens, such as sulfonamides and antipyrine, are more potent when given with iodide, an effect not understood. Iodine itself, when given acutely in large doses, blocks the organic binding and coupling reactions. This action (the Wolff-Chaikoff effect) is normally transient, but prolonged administration of iodide may be associated with continued inhibition of hormone synthesis and development of goiter, with or without hypothyroidism (iodide myxedema). Many patients with Graves' disease, especially after treatment with radioiodine or surgery, or with Hashimoto's disease are sensitive to the blocking effect of iodide and develop hypothyroidism when given iodides chronically. The fetal thyroid is similarly sensitive, and pregnant women should not ingest iodide in large amounts because of the danger of inducing goitrous hypothyroidism in the fetus. Iodide in large doses is capable of inhibiting proteolysis of thyroglobulin and hormone release, an effect responsible for the ameliorative action of iodides in hyperthyroidism. Excess iodide also may induce thyrotoxicosis in susceptible individuals, as discussed below. Lithium has several effects on intrathyroidal iodine metabolism, one of which is to inhibit hormone release. Glucocorticoids causes a decrease in serum thyroid hormone levels due to inhibition of TSH secretion and decreased binding of T_4 to TBG. Serum T_3 is also decreased, in part because of inhibition of the conversion of T_4 to T_3. A direct inhibitory action of glucocorticoids on the thyroid may occur in Graves' disease, possibly by inhibition of thyroid-stimulating immunoglobulins. Dexamethasone, in conjunction with iodide, can effect a rapid reduction in the degree of thyrotoxicosis.

HORMONE TRANSPORT AND METABOLISM

HORMONE TRANSPORT In the blood, T_4 and T_3 are almost entirely bound to plasma proteins. T_4 is bound, in decreasing order of intensity, to thyroxine-binding globulin (TBG), to a T_4-binding prealbumin (transthyretin, TTR), and to albumin. High-density lipoproteins transport about 3 percent of circulating T_4 and 6 percent of T_3. By virtue of its intense affinity for T_4, TBG is the major determinant of normal binding. T_4 interacts with its binding proteins in a reversible binding equilibrium in which most of the hormone is bound and only about 0.03 percent is free. While TTR transports only about 15 percent of circulating T_4, its contribution to free hormone is comparable to that from TBG owing to its higher dissociation constant. T_3 is not bound significantly by TTR and is bound 10 to 20 times less firmly by TBG than is T_4. As a consequence, the normal proportion of free T_3 (approximately 0.3 percent) is 8 to 10 times greater than that of T_4. Only the free or unbound hormone is available to tissues; therefore, the metabolic state correlates more closely with the concentration of free hormone than total hormone in plasma, and homeostatic regulation of thyroid function is directed toward maintenance of a normal concentration of free hormone. Moreover, the relatively weak binding of T_3 accounts for its more rapid onset and offset of action.

Disturbances of thyroid hormone–plasma protein interaction are of two general types (Table 331-1). In the first, the thyroid-pituitary axis is intrinsically normal, and the homeostatic control of thyroid hormone secretion is intact. In this situation, disordered binding interactions result from alterations in thyroid hormone binding. For example, an increase in the TBG concentration initially lowers the concentration of free hormone and thus diminishes the quantity of hormone available to tissues. The total hormone concentration in serum then increases until the concentration of free hormone is restored to normal. The increase in total hormone concentration counterbalances the decrease in the free proportion; as a result, the absolute concentration of free hormone is normal, and the metabolic state of the patient is normal. Opposite changes occur when the concentration of TBG declines. Table 331-2 summarizes the states associated with primary alterations in the concentration of TBG. Primary disturbances in thyroid hormone binding also occur when other binding proteins in blood are increased or when abnormal binding proteins appear. These are discussed below.

Table 331-1

Classification of the Varieties of Disordered Thyroid Hormone–Plasma Protein Interactions

Type of Abnormality	Serum T_4 and T_3 Levels	Percent FT_4 and FT_3 or RT_3U	FT_4 and FT_3 Levels or FT_4I and FT_3I
PRIMARY ABNORMALITY IN TBG			
Increased concentration	↑	↓	N
Decreased concentration	↓	↑	N
PRIMARY DISORDER OF THYROID FUNCTION			
Hypothyroidism	↓	↓	↓
Hyperthyroidism	↑	↑	↑

NOTE: FT_4, free T_4; FT_3, free T_3; FT_4I, free T_4 index; FT_3I, free T_3 index; N, normal; RT_3U, resin T_3 uptake; TBG, thyroid-binding globulin.

The second type of disturbance of thyroid hormone binding interactions results from a primary alteration in the concentration of thyroid hormones in the blood, as in hypothyroidism or thyrotoxicosis. Here, normal homeostatic control of thyroid hormone secretion is lost, either because of disease in the control mechanism or because an intact control mechanism is incapable of overcoming the effects of disease elsewhere. Under these circumstances, the concentration of TBG is changed little, if at all, and the concentration of free hormone varies directly with the total concentration of hormone. Since homeostatic mechanisms cannot restore the concentration of free hormone to normal, primary changes in thyroid function cause persistent changes in the concentration of total and free hormone and, consequently, alterations in the metabolic state.

HORMONE METABOLISM Following penetration into the cell, T_4 and T_3 undergo reactions that lead ultimately to their excretion or inactivation. Thyroid hormones undergo sequential removal of single iodine atoms (monodeiodinations), which ultimately yields the thyronine nucleus stripped of iodine. Deiodinative pathways account for approximately 70 percent of T_4 and T_3 disposal. In the case of T_4, the most important of these is the 5′-monodeiodination that leads to the generation of T_3. Since approximately 30 percent of T_4 is converted to T_3, and since T_3 has approximately three times the metabolic potency of T_4, virtually all the metabolic action of T_4 can be ascribed to the action of the T_3 that it gives rise to. Normally, extraglandular formation

Table 331-2

Circumstances Associated with Altered Concentrations of TBG

Increased TBG	Decreased TBG
Pregnancy	Androgen use
Newborn state	Use of large doses of glucocorticoid
Use of oral contraceptives and other sources of estrogen	Chronic liver disease
Use of tamoxifen	Severe systemic illness
Infectious and chronic active hepatitis	Active acromegaly
Biliary cirrhosis	Nephrosis
Acute intermittent porphyria	Genetic determination
Perphenazine	
Genetic determination	

accounts for about 80 percent of the T_3 in the blood and of overall T_3 production, the remainder coming from thyroid secretion. As a consequence, abnormal states and pharmacologic agents that impair T_3 formation lower the serum T_3 concentration (Table 331-3). When patients with thyroid hypofunction are treated with synthetic T_4 (levothyroxine) to sustain normal serum T_4 concentrations, normal or nearly normal serum T_3 concentrations are maintained. The generalization that the thyroid secretes relatively little T_3 does not apply when the thyroid is hyperfunctioning or is under increased stimulation by TSH. Under these conditions, the T_3/T_4 ratios of the secretory product and of the serum hormones are increased. In addition, when T_4 production is decreased, as in early thyroid failure or iodine deficiency, the T_3/T_4 concentration ratio in blood is increased still further by an autoregulatory mechanism that leads to an increase in the efficiency of T_3 formation.

Approximately 40 percent of T_4 disposal is accounted for by monodeiodination at the 5 position of its inner ring to yield reverse T_3 (rT_3); this process accounts for nearly all rT_3 produced. rT_3 has little, if any, metabolic potency; therefore, the relative rates of outer- and inner-ring monodeiodination of T_4 determine the availability of metabolically active hormone. Factors that impair T_3 formation almost invariably increase the serum rT_3 concentration. This increase is due not to an increase in the production of rT_3 from T_4, but rather to a decrease in the 5′-monodeiodination of rT_3 to yield 3,3′-diiodothyronine (3,3′T_2); i.e., both the decreased conversion of T_4 to T_3 and the decreased degradation of rT_3 result from a selective impairment of 5′-monodeiodination. There are two 5′-deiodinases. Most T_4 to T_3 conversion is effected by the type I isoenzyme in liver and kidney. The type II enzyme is localized in the pituitary, central nervous system, placenta, and brown fat and generates T_3 in these tissues. The type I enzyme is inactive during systemic illness and during normal fetal life, leading to low serum levels of T_3. An increase in type II activity in hypothyroidism allows continued T_3 formation in brain and pituitary as T_4 levels fall.

A second major pathway of metabolism of T_4, T_3, and their metabolites is conjugation in the liver, principally with glucuronate and sulfate. Conjugates either undergo deiodination locally or are secreted into the bile. The magnitude of the enterohepatic circulation of these compounds in humans is unknown. Reabsorption is incomplete at best, since the fecal excretion of T_4, T_3, and their iodine-containing metabolites accounts for approximately 20 percent of overall T_4 disposal. About 20 percent of T_4 and T_3 undergoes oxidative deamination and decarboxylation of the alanine side chain to yield tetraiodo- and triiodothyroacetic acid (*tetrac* and *triac*, respectively).

Both phenobarbital and phenytoin increase the metabolic clearance of thyroid hormones without increasing the proportion of free hormone in the blood. Indeed, in the case of phenytoin, both total and free T_4 concentrations are diminished. Nevertheless, in the presence of an intact thyroid gland a normal metabolic state is maintained, possibly because of an increase in T_3 formation.

HORMONE ACTION Thyroid hormones influence the growth and maturation of tissues, cell respiration and total energy expenditure, and the turnover of essentially all substrates, vitamins, and hormones, including the thyroid hormones themselves. Some actions of these hormones on cell metabolism may be mediated at the level of the mitochondrion to influence oxidative metabolism or at the level of the plasma membrane and endoplasmic reticulum to influence the activity of Ca^{2+}-ATPase and the transcellular flux of substrates and cations. However, the primary action of the hormone is exerted via binding to one or more intracellular receptor complexes, which, in turn, bind to specific regulatory sites in the chromosomes to influence genomic expression (see Chap. 327). Two classes of thyroid hormone receptor (TR), TRα and TRβ, are encoded by genes on chromosomes 17 and 3, respectively. By alternative splicing, these two genes generate additional isoforms (α_1, α_2, β_1, β_2, etc.). The TR proteins are part of a superfamily of genes encoded by mRNAs of cellular (c) homologues of the avian retroviral v-*erb* A proto-oncogene. The TR genes, c-*erb*-A-α (TRα) and c-*erb*-A-β (TRβ), encode receptor proteins with a T_3-binding domain and a DNA-binding domain. The DNA-binding domain attaches to regulatory sequences in those target genes with T_3-regulated transcription (e.g., the TSH, prolactin, and growth hormone genes). In an interaction stabilized by TR auxiliary proteins (TRAPs), the activation and modulation of rates of transcription are mediated by regulatory sequences called *thyroid response elements* (TREs). Thus, in the pituitary, the binding of T_3-TR complexes to TREs serves to inhibit the expression of genes for the synthesis of the α and β subunits of TSH. While the pituitary may contain the highest concentrations of TR, all tissues with high-affinity nuclear T_3 binding express TRα and TRβ receptors. High concentrations of c-*erb*-A-β_1 are found in brain, liver, heart, and kidney. The variable lack of T_3 responsiveness in different tissues ("resistance") is due to point mutations in the T_3-binding domain of the TRβ (see below).

THYROID HORMONE RESISTANCE Generalized thyroid hormone resistance (GTHR) is a syndrome characterized by reduced responsiveness to elevated levels of thyroid hormone. The resistance to thyroid hormone action is associated with elevated circulating levels of free T_4 and free T_3, inappropriately normal or elevated (i.e., nonsuppressed) serum TSH, and intact TSH responsiveness to TRH. Kindreds have been described whose members express variable patterns of resistance, and the responsiveness of target tissues may vary within the same individual. The varied phenotypes are due to a heterogeneous series of mutations of the TRβ. Clinical features include short stature, hyperactivity, attention deficits with mental deficiency or learning disability, and goiter. While GTHR patients are either euthyroid or hypothyroid, the differential diagnosis includes isolated pituitary resistance to thyroid hormone and a TSH-secreting pituitary tumor, disorders usually associated with hyperthyroidism. Indications for treatment of GTHR vary depending on the clinical features, but the presence of increased serum TSH reflects the need for supplemental thyroid hormone, the dosage requirement depending on parameters of tissue responses to thyroid hormone.

REGULATION OF THYROID FUNCTION Thyroid function is regulated by suprathyroid and intrathyroid mechanisms (Fig. 331-2). The mediator of suprathyroid regulation is TSH, a glycoprotein secreted by basophilic (thyrotropic) cells in the anterior pituitary. TSH stimulates thyroid hypertrophy and hyperplasia; accelerates most aspects of intermediary metabolism in the thyroid; enhances the synthesis of nucleic acids and proteins, including thyroglobulin; and stimulates the synthesis and secretion of thyroid hormones.

Regulation of TSH secretion, in turn, is controlled by two opposing influences at the level of the thyrotropic cell. Thyrotropin-releasing hormone (TRH), a tripeptide of hypothalamic origin, stimulates the secretion and synthesis of TSH, whereas thyroid hormones both inhibit the TSH secretory mechanism directly and antagonize the action of TRH. Thus, homeostatic control of TSH secretion is exerted in a negative-feedback manner by thyroid hormones, and the threshold for feedback inhibition is apparently set by TRH. TRH reaches the pituitary via the hypophyseal portal blood system and binds to specific high-affinity receptors on the plasma membrane of the thyrotropic cell. Either activation of the adenylate cyclase system or a concomitant translocation of extracellular calcium into the cell initiates release of

Table 331-3

States Associated with Decreased Peripheral Conversion of T_4 to T_3

Physiologic
Fetal and early neonatal life
? Old age
Pathologic
Fasting
Malnutrition
Systemic illness
Physical trauma
Postoperative state
Drugs (propylthiouracil, dexamethasone, propranolol, amiodarone)
Radiographic contrast agents (ipodate, iopanoate)

TSH. In addition to stimulating release of stored TSH, TRH enhances the synthesis of TSH via transcription and translation of the gene for the β subunit. TRH also plays a role in posttranslational processing of TSH, as indicated by the fact that TSH in patients with hypothalamic hypothyroidism has reduced biologic activity. The negative-feedback effect of the thyroid hormones appears to take place entirely at the level of the thyrotropic cell. Experimentally, thyroid hormones both inhibit production of TRH mRNA and TRH prohormone and reduce the number of TRH receptors on the thyrotropic cell, thus impairing the cell's responsiveness to TRH. The major negative-feedback action of the thyroid hormones is at the pituitary level, mediated by binding of the hormones to TR in the nucleus of the thyrotropic cell, resulting in reduced expression of the genes for the α and β subunits of TSH. The principal arbiter of thyroid hormone action in the pituitary is T_3, both that generated in the pituitary from T_4 and that derived from plasma. To what extent T_4 itself is effective in the pituitary is uncertain, but other factors also modify the secretion of TSH and its response to TRH. Both somatostatin and dopamine appear to be physiologic inhibitors of TSH secretion. Estrogens enhance responsiveness to TRH, whereas glucocorticoids inhibit this function. Catecholamines also play a role, with $alpha_1$-adrenergic pathways being inhibitory and $alpha_2$ pathways being stimulatory. Experimentally, tumor necrosis factor and interleukin 1 inhibit TSH secretion; these effects possibly play a role in the sick euthyroid syndrome.

Intrathyroid regulation of thyroid function is also important. In some manner, changes in glandular organic iodine content cause reciprocal changes in thyroid iodide transport activity and regulate growth, amino acid uptake, glucose metabolism, and nucleic acid synthesis. These influences are evident in the absence of TSH stimulation and hence may be termed *autoregulatory*, but their most important role is to modify the response to TSH (iodine-enrichment inhibiting and iodine-depletion enhancing), probably by influencing the generation of cyclic AMP consequent to TSH stimulation. Cytokines may exert stimulatory or inhibitory effects on thyroid hormone synthesis or secretion and on interactions with TSH, but the physiologic and pathophysiologic significance of these substances (e.g., atrial natriuretic peptide, tumor necrosis factor, transforming growth factor, epidermal growth factor, and endothelin) remains to be clarified.

LABORATORY TESTS

Laboratory tests of thyroid hormone economy can be divided into five general categories: direct tests of thyroid function, tests related to the concentration and binding of thyroid hormones in blood, metabolic indexes, tests of the homeostatic control of thyroid function, and miscellaneous tests.

DIRECT TESTS OF THYROID FUNCTION Those tests that involve in vivo administration of radioactive iodine test glandular function per se. Measurement of the *thyroid radioactive iodine uptake* (RAIU) is the most common of these. ^{131}I has been used for this purpose, but ^{123}I is preferable because it allows the use of a lower radiation dose. The administered radioiodine mixes uniformly with the endogenous iodide pool and, in the steady state, can be used to assess what percentage of the iodide entering and leaving the extracellular space per unit time is accumulated by the thyroid. The RAIU is measured 24 h after administration of the isotope, since it usually reaches a plateau value at this time, but in cases of severe thyroid hyperfunction it may peak early. The RAIU varies inversely with the plasma iodide concentration and directly with the functional state of the thyroid. At levels of iodine intake usual in the United States (up to 1 mg/d), the normal 24-h RAIU is approximately 10 to 30 percent of the administered dose. Consequently, this test discriminates poorly between normal and hypothyroid states. Values above the normal range, however, usually indicate thyroid hyperfunction and are useful in the diagnosis of hyperthyroidism. Measurement of the RAIU is also a part of the thyroid suppression test (see below).

One valuable application of the RAIU test occurs when thyrotoxicosis is associated with a low RAIU. Causes include iodine-induced hyperthyroidism, thyrotoxicosis factitia, inadvertent ingestion of ground meat containing thyroid glands ("hamburger toxicosis"), and the spontaneously resolving thyrotoxicosis associated with painless chronic thyroiditis, postpartum thyroiditis, or subacute thyroiditis.

TESTS RELATED TO HORMONE CONCENTRATION AND BINDING OF HORMONE IN BLOOD Prior to the evolution of highly sensitive assays for TSH, measurement of the concentration of T_4 and/or T_3 in serum, in conjunction with some assessment of hormone binding, was the traditional means of confirming a clinical diagnosis of hyperthyroidism or hypothyroidism. Highly specific and sensitive radioimmunoassays are used to measure *serum* T_4 and T_3 concentrations and rarely for the measurement of *serum* rT_3 concentration. The approximate normal ranges are 60 to 150 nmol/L (5 to 12 μg/dL) for T_4, 1 to 3 nmol/L (70 to 190 ng/dL) for T_3, and 0.2 to 0.6 nmol/L (10 to 40 ng/dL) for rT_3.

As mentioned above, alterations in hormone binding by plasma proteins, as well as alterations in the rate of hormone secretion, influence the concentration of hormone in the blood. However, only alterations in hormone secretion lead to steady-state alterations in free hormone levels. Because they most consistently reflect the rate of hormone production, free hormone concentrations usually correlate better with the metabolic state than do total levels. The free T_4 concentration (FT_4) can be measured directly by equilibrium dialysis of serum enriched with a tracer quantity of labeled T_4. The percent of T_4 that is dialyzable or free is thereby determined, and the product of this value and the total T_4 is the FT_4. However, since the dialysis technique is cumbersome, it has been replaced by indirect assays. The expression "free T_4 estimate" (FT_4E) may refer to a free T_4 fraction determined from equilibrium dialysis, to a derived free T_4 estimate, or to any other indirectly measured or calculated free T_4 concentration. One traditional indirect method, the in vitro uptake test, represents an assessment of hormone binding in which the serum is enriched with labeled T_4 or labeled T_3 and is then incubated with an insoluble particulate material, such as resin or charcoal, that binds free hormone (resin T_3 uptake, RT_3U). The percent of labeled hormone taken up by the particulate material varies inversely with both the concentration of unoccupied sites among the serum proteins and their affinity for the particular hormone being used. The RT_3U may be expressed as a thyroid hormone binding ratio (THBR), which serves to lessen confusion of the T_3 uptake with assays for T_3. Under most clinical conditions, values of the RT_3U, THBR, or FTE are proportionate to those of the percent of FT_4 and percent of free T_3 (FT_3). This proportionality reflects the fact that, in normal serum, T_4 and T_3 are mainly bound by a common binding site on TBG. Therefore, alterations in binding produced by an excess or deficiency of TBG or by an excessive or insufficient supply of T_4 do not seriously disturb the relationship between the intensity of T_4 binding and that of T_3. Under these conditions, therefore, one may calculate a *free* T_4 *index* (FT_4I) and a *free* T_3 *index* (FT_3I) as the product of the RT_3U and the total T_4 and T_3 concentrations, respectively; these quantities are proportional to the actual FT_4 and FT_3 concentrations.

Primary alterations in plasma TBG concentration (see Table 331-2) produce changes in the RT_3U that are inverse and approximately proportional to the changes in the serum T_4 and serum T_3 levels; as a result, the FT_4I and FT_3I remain normal. By contrast, alterations in T_4 secretion cause changes in the percent FT_4 and in the RT_3U that are in the same direction as those in serum T_4. As a result, the FT_4 and FT_4I deviate from normal values more markedly than do the percent FT_4 and RT_3U alone. Immunoradiometric assay (IRMA) and chemiluminescent assay methods for the direct measurement of FT_4 provide reliable results in a wide range of disorders and may replace measurement of total T_4, RT_3U, and FT_4I in the diagnosis of thyrotoxicosis and hypothyroidism. In spite of improvements in free T_4 assays, the highly sensitive TSH assay is the most sensitive test of thyroid function. The measurement of a TSH level and a FT_4E or FT_4I will provide effective diagnosis and management of most patients with thyroid disease.

As noted earlier, several disorders are characterized by increased plasma binding of T_4 in which, because the protein involved is not TBG, the intensity of T_4 binding relative to that of T_3 is abnormal. Most commonly, binding of T_4 is enhanced, while that of T_3 is increased little if at all. Included among these disorders is *familial dysalbuminemic hyperthyroxinemia* (FDH), inherited as an autosomal dominant trait, in which the plasma concentration of an albumin variant with an unusually high affinity for T_4 is increased. As a result, the serum T_4 is markedly elevated, but, in keeping with the euthyroid state, the FT_4 is normal. Because the RT_3U does not reflect the increase in the intensity of T_4 binding, calculated values of the FT_4I are increased, often leading to a mistaken diagnosis of thyrotoxicosis. Similar findings occur when there is *increased T_4 binding by transthyretin* or when *circulating antibodies* against T_4 are present.

In the foregoing disorders, serum T_4 is increased owing to an increase in T_4 binding, and the FT_4 and metabolic state are normal. These disorders therefore are classified among those that lead to a state of *euthyroid hyperthyroxinemia*, a term that implies the presence of hyperthyroxinemia not caused by intrinsic thyroid disease (Table 331-4). The mechanisms responsible are variable and in some cases uncertain. The increases in total T_4 do not appear to affect the metabolic state, but hyperthyroidism may be mistakenly diagnosed.

Some states are associated with an increased thyroid secretion of T_3, at least relative to the secretion of T_4. As a result, the serum T_3 concentration is disproportionately high relative to that of T_4. This situation apparently is caused by hyperfunction of the follicular cell, since it occurs in all varieties of hyperthyroidism and in early thyroid failure, when the gland is exposed to elevated TSH levels. Accordingly, the serum T_3 concentration and the derived value FT_3I are generally better for the diagnosis of hyperthyroidism than measurement of the T_4 concentration. In *early* hypothyroidism, by contrast, the serum T_3 concentration and the FT_3I are often normal despite subnormal values for the serum T_4 and FT_4I. Consequently, the serum T_3 concentration is not reliable for the diagnosis of hypothyroidism.

Measurement of the serum rT_3 concentration is valuable in differentiating the "low T_3 syndrome" (see below) from intrinsic hypothyroidism; in the former the serum rT_3 concentration is increased, whereas in the latter it is usually subnormal.

METABOLIC INDEXES Although measurements of the metabolic impact of thyroid hormones have value in the investigative setting, none is sufficiently sensitive, specific, and easily performed for routine use. Measurements of oxygen consumption in the basal state (basal metabolic rate, BMR) were once a mainstay in the diagnosis of thyroid disease but are now of historic interest. Several blood tests may yield abnormal results in patients with thyroid disease. For example, serum concentrations of creatine phosphokinase and, less frequently, lactate dehydrogenase and aspartate aminotransferase are increased in hypothyroidism and may be slightly decreased in hyperthyroidism. The changes are nonspecific, and the reason to be aware of them is to avoid making the inference that other diseases that produce similar changes are present. The concentrations in serum of testosterone-binding globulin (TeBG), the iron storage protein ferritin, and angiotensin-converting enzyme are thyroid hormone–dependent and are, therefore, increased in thyrotoxicosis, but they are of no value in the diagnosis of thyroid disease. Increases in the *serum cholesterol concentration* are common in hypothyroidism of thyroid origin, and decreases in serum cholesterol are common in thyrotoxicosis. *Systolic time indexes*, such as the preejection period and pulse-wave arrival time, are prolonged in hypothyroidism and shortened in hyperthyroidism. They may be of value in monitoring thyroid replacement therapy in elderly patients or in patients with coexisting heart disease.

TESTS OF HOMEOSTATIC CONTROL Measurement of the basal *serum TSH concentration* is useful in the diagnosis of both advanced and subclinical hypothyroidism. The latter state represents a stage in the evolution of hypothyroidism, in which a structural or functional abnormality that impairs hormone synthesis is compensated for by hypersecretion of TSH. In thyrotoxic states, the serum TSH concentration is almost always low or undetectable. While the original radioimmunoassays (RIAs) could not distinguish between normal and subnormal values, immunoradiometric or chemiluminescent techniques employing monoclonal antibodies now provide exquisite sensitivity. Thyrotoxic patients tend to have undetectable levels (<0.1 mU/L), while values in most normal subjects range between 0.3 and 3.0 mU/L in these assays (Fig. 331-3). Thus, these assays offer advantage over conventional RIAs and may be useful in the diagnosis of hyperthyroidism and hypothyroidism. Serum TSH concentrations are absolutely or inappropriately elevated relative to serum FT_4 and FT_3 values in patients with TSH-induced hyperthyroidism. This rare syndrome results either from a TSH-secreting pituitary adenoma or resistance of the TSH secretory mechanism to feedback inhibition by T_4 and T_3. Measurement of serum TSH is the best means of distinguishing between untreated hypothyroidism of thyroid origin, in which the values are invariably increased, and pituitary or hypothalamic hypothyroidism, in which the values are usually low or within the normal range. Occasional patients with hypothalamic or pituitary

Table 331-4

States Associated with Euthyroid Hyperthyroxinemia

Disorder	FT_4	FT_4I	T_3	TSH	Comments
Increased T_4 binding					
Increased TBG level	N	N	↑	N	See Tables 331-1 and 331-2
FDH	N	↑	N, Sl↑	N	Autosomal dominant inheritance
Increased TBPA binding	N	↑	N	N	Increased concentration (islet cell tumor) or affinity
Anti-T_4 antibody	N	↑	N	N	Anti-T_3 antibody may be present
Pituitary and peripheral thyroid hormone resistance	↑	↑	↑	↑	If only pituitary is resistant, patient will be thyrotoxic
Various disorders					
Sick euthyroid syndrome	↑, N	↑	↓	N,↓	Uncommon; poorly understood
Acute psychiatric illness	↑, N	↑	N,↑	N,↑	Remits without treatment in several weeks
Hyperemesis gravidarum	↑	↑	N	↓	Remits in several weeks
Drugs					
Inhibitors of T_3 formation	↑	↑	↓	↑	Particularly ipodate and iopanoate
Radiographic contrast agents					
Propranolol	↑	↑	↓	N,↑	Especially with large doses
Amiodarone	↑	↑	↓	↑	Increased TSH during first several months
Heparin	↑	↑	N	—	Requires only small intravenous doses
Levothyroxine	↑	↑	N	↓	Hyperthyroxinemia in about 50% of cases

NOTE: FDH, familial dysalbuminemic hyperthyroxinemia; FT_4, free T_4 concentration; FT_4I, free T_4 index calculated from an in vitro T_3 uptake test; TBPA, thyroxine-binding prealbumin; TSH, basal serum TSH concentration and response to TRH; N, normal; Sl, slightly.

hypothyroidism secrete a form of TSH that is immunoactive but not bioactive. Here, serum TSH concentrations may be elevated rather than depressed.

The *thyrotropin-releasing hormone stimulation test* assesses the TSH-secretory mechanism and has diagnostic value in diverse circumstances. Following the intravenous injection of TRH in normal subjects, the serum TSH level increases, reaches a maximum between 20 and 45 min, and then rapidly declines. The pituitary feedback mechanism is such that, when hypothalamic-pituitary function is normal, one would expect an increased response to TRH when the thyrotropic cell senses a deficiency of thyroid hormone, particularly T_3, and a decreased or absent response when thyroid hormone is in excess. Thus, except in the rare case of pituitary resistance to thyroid hormone, in which responses are usually normal, thyrotoxicosis is invariably accompanied by a blunted or absent TSH response to TRH. Owing to the extreme sensitivity of the TSH-secretory mechanism to feedback inhibition, diminished responses to TRH commonly occur in apparently euthyroid patients with serum T_4 or T_3 levels within the normal range but with marginally increased T_4 or T_3 output from autonomously functioning toxic adenomas or toxic multinodular goiters. Blunted TRH responses also may be seen in some patients with euthyroid Graves' disease. In addition, responses to TRH are often decreased in elderly individuals, especially men. Despite these exceptions, a subnormal or absent response to TRH is a useful confirmatory test for thyrotoxicosis. With the availability of highly sensitive TSH assays, the TRH test is rarely used for this purpose. TRH tests are of even less value in the diagnosis of hypothyroidism. Responses are increased in patients with primary hypothyroidism, but the magnitude of the increase is generally proportional to the extent of increase in basal serum TSH. Some patients with pituitary hypothyroidism have subnormal responses, and some with TRH deficiency due to hypothalamic disease have a near-normal response. Further, in about one-fourth of patients with hypothyroidism due to hypothalamic-pituitary disease, basal serum TSH levels are normal or slightly elevated, and the response to TRH is exaggerated, although some of this TSH may not be bioactive.

The *thyroid suppression test* is used to assess the homeostatic control of thyroid function. Normally, exogenous thyroid hormone suppresses pituitary TSH secretion, resulting in a decrease in the RAIU. Since liothyronine is usually employed for the test (100 μg/d for 7 to 10 days), the resulting decline in serum T_4, as well as in the RAIU, can serve as an index of suppression. A normal suppressive response is a decrease of the RAIU to less than half the control value and a decline of the serum T_4 to low-normal or subnormal values. A normal suppression test is incompatible with and excludes a diagnosis of hyperthyroidism, because liothyronine suppresses TSH rather than the thyroid directly and because TSH is unmeasurable in most hyperthyroid states. The suppression test always gives an abnormal result in hyperthyroidism, irrespective of the underlying cause; this finding usually indicates either autonomy of thyroid function or the presence of an abnormal (non-TSH) thyroid stimulator or, rarely, unremitting hypersecretion of TSH. An abnormal suppression test result is not pathognomonic of hyperthyroidism, however, since it may persist after treatment of hyperthyroidism in Graves' disease and is seen in about half the euthyroid patients with the ophthalmopathy of Graves' disease.

Because of the risk of adverse effects from exogenous thyroid hormone, especially liothyronine, in elderly patients and in those with cardiovascular disease, highly sensitive TSH measurements have almost entirely supplanted the thyroid suppression test in the diagnosis of hyperthyroidism.

MISCELLANEOUS TESTS Various tests that do not assess thyroid function are of value in defining the nature of the thyroid disorder or in planning therapy. For example, high titers of *antithyroid peroxidase* (anti-TPO or antimicrosomal) *antibodies* or *antithyroglobulin antibodies* are found in the serum of most patients with Hashimoto's disease and in many with primary thyroprivic hypothyroidism or Graves' disease. In the latter states, the serum also contains antibodies against the TSH receptor that are capable of inhibiting the receptor binding of TSH (TSH-binding inhibitory immunoglobulins, TBII) or of stimulating the production of cyclic AMP therein [thyroid-stimulating antibodies (TSAb) or thyroid-stimulating immunoglobulins (TSI)], respectively. The clinical utility of tests for TSI stems from the fact that the disappearance of these factors from the serum during a course of antithyroid therapy implies the likelihood of a long-term remission of hyperthyroidism when therapy is withdrawn. The analogous TBII antibodies have no intrinsic stimulatory effect but block the response to endogenous TSH and produce nongoitrous hypothyroidism. Both stimulatory and blocking anti-TSH receptor antibodies have the ability to cross the placenta and produce transient hyperthyroidism (neonatal Graves' disease) or hypothyroidism, respectively, in the newborn. Measurement of these antibodies during the last months of pregnancy makes it possible to assess the likelihood that these disorders will develop in the neonate.

Some patients, most commonly those with autoimmune thyroid disease, develop *circulating antibodies* against T_3, T_4, or both. In RIAs for these hormones, because the endogenous antibody competes with the exogenous antibody for binding of the added labeled ligand, spuriously high or low values for the concentration of the hormone are obtained, depending on the technique of RIA used. The true concentration of the hormone, as determined in extracts of the serum, is increased owing to the additional binding sites provided by the antibody, but antibody-bound hormone is unavailable for metabolic action. In the case of anti-T_3 antibodies, the usual values of the RT_3U are low because endogenous antibody competes with the resin for binding of the added labeled T_3. Such antibodies can be detected by adding labeled hormone to serum and demonstrating that immunoglobulins bind the labeled hormone.

Along with several other thyroid disorders, differentiated carcinomas of the thyroid release thyroglobulin into the bloodstream. As a consequence, measurements of the *serum thyroglobulin* by RIA have value not in the initial diagnosis of thyroid carcinoma but in assessing the adequacy of initial therapy and in monitoring for recurrence or dissemination of the disease; endogenous antithyroglobulin antibodies

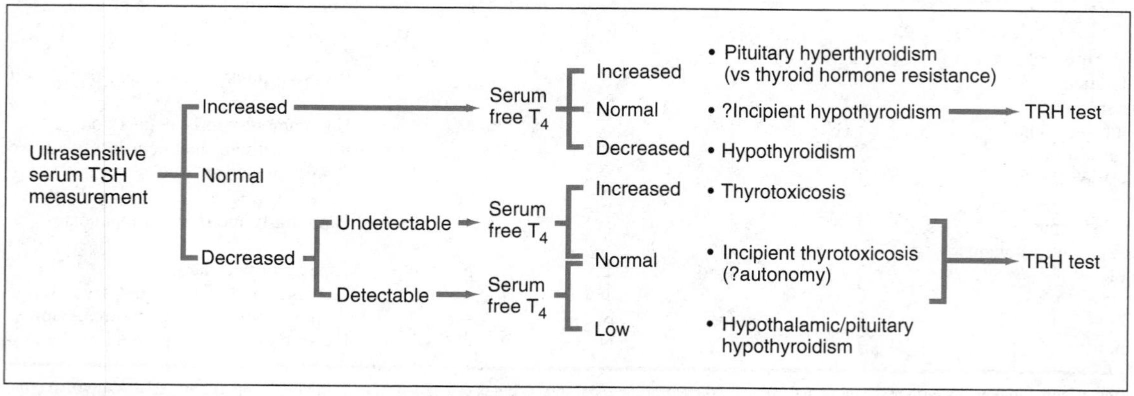

FIGURE 331-3 Utility of sensitive TSH assay in evaluation of suspected thyroid dysfunction in ambulatory patients.

can cause falsely low values. In patients with thyrotoxicosis, subnormal serum thyroglobulin concentrations together with decreased values of the RAIU suggest thyrotoxicosis factitia.

Imaging by *scintiscanning* permits localization of sites of accumulation of radioiodine or sodium [^{99m}Tc]pertechnetate. This technique is useful for defining areas of increased or decreased function within the thyroid and for detecting retrosternal goiter, ectopic thyroid tissue, hemiagenesis of the thyroid, and functioning metastases of thyroid carcinoma. Ultrasonic examination of the thyroid is also useful for differentiating cystic from solid nodules. Since ultrasonic scans provide an accurate indication of size, are noninvasive, and apparently have no injurious effects, sequential scans can be employed to assess changes in the size of the thyroid as a whole or of discrete nodules over time or in response to treatment.

SICK EUTHYROID SYNDROME

Severe illness, physical trauma, or physiologic stress can induce changes in one or more aspects of thyroid hormone economy, leading to findings referred to as the *sick euthyroid syndrome* (SES). Abnormalities in SES include alterations in the peripheral transport and metabolism of the thyroid hormones, in the regulation of TSH secretion, and, in some cases, in thyroid function itself. Acting alone or together, these alterations lead to changes in the concentrations of the circulating thyroid hormones, both total and free, which serve to define the several variants of SES. Because of the frequency and nonspecificity of the disorders that cause it, SES is probably a more common cause of abnormalities in the concentration of thyroid hormones in the blood than is intrinsic thyroid disease.

NORMAL-T_4 VARIANT OF SES Decreased production of T_3 owing to inhibition of the peripheral 5′-monodeiodination of T_4 is a consistent feature of SES. This effect is reflected in a decrease in the serum total T_3 concentration, which varies in severity with that of the illness. In moderately ill patients, serum total T_4 concentration is within the normal range. A decrease in the intensity of protein binding, greater for T_4 than for T_3, is also present. As a result, values of the RT_3U are moderately increased, and the percent FT_4 is increased to a proportionately greater extent. As a consequence, the values of the FT_4I and of the FT_4 concentration are often increased. Serum rT_3 concentrations are increased, owing to a decrease in the plasma clearance of rT_3 secondary to inhibition of the 5′-monodeiodination of T_3. The plasma clearance rate of T_4 is increased, probably as a result of decreased T_4 binding, and this alteration, in the face of normal T_4 concentrations, indicates that the overall rate of T_4 degradation and production is increased. Production rates for T_3 are decreased, and those for rT_3 are normal. The serum TSH concentration and the response of serum TSH to TRH are generally normal, although they may increase and then return to normal as recovery from the illness takes place. Despite the reduction in the serum T_3 level, this variant of SES can be separated from intrinsic thyroid disease because the serum T_4 and TSH levels are normal and because the serum T_3 level is not useful for diagnosing hypothyroidism.

LOW-T_4 VARIANT OF SES In more seriously ill patients, T_3 production rates and serum total and free T_3 concentrations decrease still further, and abnormalities in hormone binding increase in severity. As a consequence, serum T_4 concentrations decrease into the hypothyroid range. This effect is partly but not entirely due to decreased T_4 binding, since the FT_4 concentration is frequently subnormal. These changes are probably the result of decreased T_4 production in the most severely ill patients and are secondary to decreased secretion of TSH. Serum TSH concentrations appear normal by conventional assay but are low with sensitive TSH assays, and TRH responses are often blunted. Hence, in this variant of SES, there is an inappropriate hyposecretion of TSH, considering the low serum total and free T_4 and T_3 concentrations, and a diagnosis of pituitary hypothyroidism may be suggested. While the cause is unknown, the low TSH level may be due to the effects of somatostatin or cytokines such as interleukin 1 and tumor necrosis factor on the pituitary. With resolution of the underlying illness, TSH levels rise and may be transiently elevated

until T_4 and T_3 levels return to normal. Production rates for rT_3 are diminished owing to the decreased availability of the precursor T_4; nonetheless, serum rT_3 concentrations are increased due to slowing of rT_3 degradation, providing an important means of differentiating SES from pituitary hypothyroidism, in which serum rT_3 levels are low. In patients with primary hypothyroidism who have associated illness, serum TSH levels remain elevated, although generally they are lower than they otherwise would be.

HIGH-T_4 VARIANT OF SES An unusual variant of SES (approximately 1 percent of sick patients) is associated with increased serum total and free T_4 concentrations. This variant is most often seen in elderly women, many of whom have received medications that contain iodine. The principal source of diagnostic confusion is with the syndrome of "T_4 toxicosis," i.e., true thyrotoxicosis on which illness has been superimposed, so that serum T_4 levels are increased and serum T_3 concentrations are normal. In thyrotoxicosis, however, serum rT_3 concentrations are higher, the values of the serum total T_3 and of FT_3I are higher, TSH is usually undetectable, and TRH responses are blunted or absent.

ABNORMALITIES IN HORMONE BINDING IN SES Multiple factors are responsible for the decreased binding of T_4 and T_3 in SES. Illness is associated with decreased synthesis of TTR and a decrease in its serum concentration, but the extent to which this effect contributes to decreased T_4 binding is uncertain. In chronically ill patients, the serum TBG concentration is subnormal. Most often, however, the extent of decreased T_4 binding cannot be explained by decreases in serum TTR and TBG, and an inhibitor of hormone binding may be present. Its nature is uncertain, but one or more fatty acids may be responsible and may also cause diminished conversion of T_4 to T_3.

The importance of SES is that the changes in circulating thyroid hormone concentrations should not be confused with those due to intrinsic thyroid or pituitary disease. It is unclear whether the metabolic impact of thyroid hormone in peripheral tissues is decreased in SES and whether the syndrome is a beneficial or adverse response to illness. However, patients with low T_4 and T_3 levels due to SES do not appear to benefit from treatment with thyroid hormones.

AIDS AND THYROID FUNCTION Patients with AIDS may exhibit abnormal results on thyroid function tests that vary with the course of the illness. All but the most severely ill patients maintain normal levels of serum T_4 and T_3 (representing the normal-T_4 variant of SES). With falling CD4 counts and increasing frequency of systemic infections, serum T_3 falls in tandem with progressive cachexia (the low-T_4 variant of SES). Levels of rT_3 and serum TSH may remain normal. Rarely, AIDS patients develop hypothyroidism due to *Pneumocystis carinii* thyroiditis or involvement of the thyroid by Kaposi's sarcoma.

SIMPLE (NONTOXIC) GOITER

Endemic goiter has been defined as the presence of generalized or localized thyroid enlargement in more than 10 percent of the population. *Sporadic* goiter arises in nonendemic areas as a result of factors that do not affect the population generally. Since these terms fail to define the causes of goiter, and since thyroid enlargement of diverse etiologies may exist in both endemic and nonendemic regions, it is prudent to employ a general term such as *simple* or *nontoxic goiter*, which can be defined as any enlargement of the thyroid gland that does not result from an inflammatory or neoplastic process and that is not initially associated with thyrotoxicosis or myxedema.

ETIOLOGY AND PATHOGENESIS Simple goiter is sometimes due to a definable cause of impaired thyroid hormone synthesis, such as iodine deficiency, ingestion of a goitrogen, or a defect in a hormone biosynthetic pathway, but the cause is usually unknown. Whatever the cause, the clinical manifestations reflect the operation of a common pathophysiologic mechanism. Simple goiter occurs when one or more factors impair the capacity of the thyroid to secrete sufficient hormones to meet the needs of the peripheral tissues. Although this situation has been presumed to lead to increased secretion of TSH, concentrations of TSH in the serum of patients with established simple goiter are usually normal. Hence, other mechanisms of goitrogenesis may be operative. For example, depletion of organic iodine accompanying impaired hormone synthesis may increase the responsiveness to normal levels of TSH. The resulting increase in the functioning mass of the thyroid overcomes mild impairment of hormone synthesis, and the patient is metabolically normal, though goitrous. When the underlying disorder is severe, compensatory responses, now including hypersecretion of TSH, are inadequate to overcome the impairment, and the patient is both goitrous and hypothyroid. Thus, simple goiter cannot be clearly separated in the pathogenic sense from goitrous hypothyroidism. Specific causes of simple goiter may produce hypothyroidism in some cases (Table 331-5). Defective iodination of thyroglobulin may be a cause in many patients. Goiter may also be due to antibodies that stimulate the growth but not the function of the thyroid.

PATHOLOGY The histopathology of simple goiter varies with the etiology and the stage at which the examination is made. Initially, the gland exhibits a uniform hypertrophy, hyperplasia, and hypervascularity. As the disorder persists or undergoes exacerbations and remissions, the thyroidal architecture loses uniformity. Occasionally, most of the gland displays a uniform involution or hyperinvolution with colloid accumulation. More often, areas of involution are interspersed with areas of focal hyperplasia. Fibrosis may demarcate hyperplastic or involuted nodules, which may resemble true neoplasms (adenomas). Areas of hemorrhage and irregular calcification may be present. The evolution of the multinodular stage is usually accompanied by the development of functional autonomy. Indeed, heterogeneity of structure and function and a degree of functional autonomy are the hallmarks of the mature stage of this disorder.

CLINICAL MANIFESTATIONS In simple goiter, the manifestations arise solely from enlargement of the thyroid, since the metabolic state is normal. In goitrous hypothyroidism, symptoms caused by thyromegaly are accompanied by signs and symptoms of hormonal insufficiency. Mechanical sequelae include compression and displacement of the trachea or esophagus, occasionally with obstructive symptoms if the goiter becomes sufficiently large. Superior mediastinal obstruction may occur with large retrosternal goiters. Signs of compression can be induced with large retrosternal goiters when the patient's arms are raised above the head; they may include suffusion of the face, giddiness, and syncope (Pemberton's sign). Hoarseness due to compression of the recurrent laryngeal nerve is rare in simple goiter, and its presence suggests a neoplasm. Sudden hemorrhage into a nodule may lead to an acute, painful swelling in the neck and may produce or enhance compressive symptoms. Hyperthyroidism may supervene in long-standing multinodular goiter (toxic multinodular goiter). In both endemic and sporadic cases of multinodular goiter, the ingestion of excess iodide may result in the development of thyrotoxicosis (jodbasedow phenomenon).

In regions where iodine deficiency is severe, goitrous enlargement also may be associated with varying degrees of hypothyroidism. Cretinism, both goitrous and nongoitrous, occurs with increased frequency in the children of goitrous parents in many countries with endemic goiter. Although iodine deficiency is a factor in the etiology of endemic goiter, the frequency of goiter differs among persons with equally severe iodine deficiency. In such instances, dietary or waterborne goitrogens appear to be important conditioning factors. In some areas, goitrogens may cause goiter in the absence of iodine deficiency.

DIAGNOSIS The diagnosis of simple goiter requires demonstration of a euthyroid state and demonstration of normal serum T_4 and T_3 concentrations. The euthyroid state may be difficult to document because manifestations of thyrotoxicosis may be subtle or atypical, especially among the elderly (see the section "Toxic Multinodular Goiter"). Furthermore, serum T_4 and T_3 concentrations may be near the upper limit of the normal range, and the fact that serum T_3 concentrations may decrease in euthyroid elderly persons complicates the interpretation of this test. The RAIU is usually normal but may be increased in the presence of iodine deficiency or a biosynthetic defect. Thus, the presence of measurable concentration of TSH by a highly sensitive technique is the best index of euthyroidism. Indeed, subclinical thyrotoxicosis may be secondary to the functional autonomy of the goiter and consequently may cause a decrease in both the basal TSH level and the TSH response to TRH. Differentiation of nontoxic goiter from Hashimoto's disease is facilitated by the greater frequency of multinodularity in the former and by the presence of high titers of circulating antimicrosomal or antithyroglobulin antibodies in the latter. In some instances, emergence of a strongly dominant nodule may suggest the presence of a carcinoma, especially if bleeding has caused it to increase in size rapidly and to lose the ability to accumulate iodine or pertechnetate. Appropriate radiographic studies (computed tomography, magnetic resonance imaging) and respiratory flow measurements should be obtained when substernal extension has the potential to cause upper airway obstruction.

Rx TREATMENT

The object of treatment is to reduce the size of the goiter, either by relieving external encumbrances to hormone formation or by providing enough exogenous hormone to inhibit TSH secretion and thereby put the thyroid gland at rest. In disorders characterized by decreased thyroid iodide stores, such as iodine deficiency or impairment of the thyroid iodide-concentrating mechanism, small doses of iodide may prove effective. Occasionally, a known extrinsic goitrogen can be withdrawn. Most commonly, however, no specific etiologic factor can be detected, and thyroid hormone therapy is required. For this purpose, levothyroxine (L-thyroxine) is the agent of choice. In the younger patient with the early diffuse stage of simple goiter, treatment is instituted with 100 μg of levothyroxine daily, and the dose is increased over the next month or so to a maximum of 150 or 200 μg/d (the average dose being 1.7 μg/kg body weight per day). Complete suppression would imply reduction of serum TSH to levels of <0.1 mU/L as determined by an ultrasensitive assay. In patients at risk for loss of bone mineral (e.g., postmenopausal women not on estrogen replacement, patients with prior Graves' disease) thyroxine therapy should be titrated to slightly less than a fully suppressive dose. Adequacy of suppression also may be assessed by measuring the RAIU, which should decrease to less

Table 331-5

Classification of the Causes of Hypothyroidism

Thyroid
Thyroprivic
Congenital development defect
Primary idiopathic
Postablative (radioiodine, surgery)
Postradiation (e.g., for lymphoma)
Goitrous
Heritable biosynthetic defects
Maternally transmitted (iodides, antithyroid agents)
Iodine deficiency
Drug-elicited (aminosalicylic acid, iodides, phenylbutazone, iodoantipyrine, lithium)
Chronic thyroiditis (Hashimoto's disease)
Interleukin 2 and lymphokine-activated killer cells
Suprathyroid (Trophoprivic)
Pituitary
Panhypopituitarism
Isolated TSH deficiency
Hypothalamic
Congenital defects
Infection (encephalitis)
Neoplasm
Infiltrative (sarcoidosis)
Self-limited
Following withdrawal of suppressive thyroid therapy
Subacute thyroiditis and chronic thyroiditis with transient hypothyroidism (usually after a phase of thyrotoxicosis)

than 5 percent of the administered dose at 24 h. Lesser decreases indicate that suppression is only partial, which may reflect the presence of autonomous foci demonstrable by scanning techniques. In the elderly or in patients with long-standing multinodular goiter, TSH should be measured by an ultrasensitive assay before treatment with levothyroxine is initiated to determine whether significant functional autonomy is present. If such is indicated by the absence of a detectable basal TSH level, suppressive therapy with levothyroxine is contraindicated, as such patients are or will become thyrotoxic. Rather, consideration should be given to radioiodine ablation of the autonomous foci (see "Toxic Multinodular Goiter"). On the other hand, if the basal TSH level is normal (excluding autonomous hyperfunction) treatment with levothyroxine can be initiated. In elderly patients the initial dose should not exceed 50 μg/d, and the dosage should be increased gradually, the end point being partial rather than complete suppression of basal TSH and/or the RAIU. It is the usual practice to obtain a thyroid scan as part of the initial evaluation of all patients with multinodular goiter. In those patients in whom full suppressive doses of thyroxine are indicated, it is desirable to repeat the RAIU measurement and scan (suppression scan), when practical, to ascertain the efficacy of suppression and/or the presence of autonomous foci.

Results of therapy vary widely. Early diffuse, hyperplastic goiters respond well, with regression or disappearance in 3 to 6 months. In the author's experience, the later, nodular stage responds less well, and significant reduction in gland size is achieved only in about one-third of cases; however, in the remainder, suppressive treatment may forestall further glandular growth. Internodular tissue regresses more often than do nodules themselves. The latter may therefore appear to become more prominent during treatment. After maximum regression of the goiter has occurred, suppressive medication may be maintained for a prolonged period, reduced to a minimal level, or, in some cases, withdrawn. The goiter may stay regressed or may recur unpredictably. In the latter situation, if malignancy is ruled out by fine-needle biopsy, suppressive therapy should be reinstituted and continued indefinitely. In areas of endemic iodine deficiency, the size and prevalence of goiter and the frequency of cretinism can be reduced by the provision of iodized salt or water or the periodic injection of iodized oil.

Surgical therapy of simple goiter is physiologically unsound but may occasionally be necessary to relieve obstruction. Large substernal goiters with partial upper airway obstruction also have been treated by radioactive iodine with moderate success. Surgical exploration of nodular goiter also may be indicated in some individuals when evidence suggests carcinoma. However, the idea that subtotal resection of a multinodular nontoxic goiter affords effective prophylaxis against the development of thyroid carcinoma is unsound. If for some reason subtotal thyroidectomy has been performed, levothyroxine in a usual dose of about 1.7 μg/kg body weight per day is recommended to inhibit regenerative hyperplasia and further goitrogenesis.

HYPOTHYROIDISM

Hypothyroidism results from abnormalities that lead to insufficient synthesis of thyroid hormone. Hypothyroidism dating from birth and resulting in developmental abnormalities is termed *cretinism.* The term *myxedema* connotes severe hypothyroidism in which there is accumulation of hydrophilic mucopolysaccharides in the ground substance of the dermis and other tissues, leading to thickening of the facial features and doughy induration of the skin.

ETIOLOGY AND PATHOGENESIS A classification of hypothyroidism is presented in Table 331-5. The primary thyroid varieties account for the vast majority of cases, only 5 percent or fewer being suprathyroid in origin. In thyroprivic hypothyroidism, loss of thyroid tissue leads to inadequate synthesis of thyroid hormone, despite maximum stimulation of any thyroid remnant by TSH. The most common cause is surgical or radioiodine ablation of the thyroid gland for the treatment of Graves' disease. Thyroprivic hypothyroidism also may occur as a primary idiopathic disorder, which is usually due to autoimmunity and is associated with circulating cytotoxic antithyroid antibodies or, in some cases, antibodies that block the TSH receptor. This disorder may coexist with diabetes mellitus and other diseases in which circulating autoantibodies are found, such as pernicious anemia, systemic lupus erythematosus, rheumatoid arthritis, Sjögren's syndrome, and chronic hepatitis. In addition, hypothyroidism can be one manifestation of a polyglandular endocrine deficiency state in which autoantibodies cause variable insufficiency of thyroid, adrenal, parathyroid, and gonadal function (see Chap. 340). All these diseases, including isolated primary hypothyroidism, are associated with an increased frequency of specific HLA haplotypes. Finally, a developmental defect may result in failure of the gland to function adequately, leading to sporadic nongoitrous cretinism or juvenile hypothyroidism. A self-limited period of hypothyroidism is common in the course of subacute thyroiditis and in the syndrome of "painless thyroiditis," including the postpartum variant, and usually occurs after a temporary period of thyrotoxicosis. Owing to a persisting lack of TSH stimulation, intrinsically euthyroid subjects from whom chronic suppressive therapy is abruptly withdrawn experience a several-week period of thyroid hypofunction.

Inability to synthesize enough thyroid hormone leads to hypersecretion of TSH and hence goiter. If the compensatory response is inadequate, goitrous hypothyroidism ensues. The most common cause of goitrous hypothyroidism in North America is Hashimoto's disease, in which defective organic binding of iodide and abnormal secretion of iodoproteins are frequent. Iodide-induced goiter with or without hypothyroidism appears to arise from an intrinsic defect in the organic binding mechanism, which permits a persistent Wolff-Chaikoff effect. Euthyroid patients with Graves' disease, especially after surgery or radioiodine treatment, patients with Hashimoto's disease, and normal fetuses are particularly susceptible to iodide-induced goiter. In view of the susceptibility of the fetal thyroid to iodide, iodine in large doses should not be given during pregnancy. Less common causes of goitrous hypothyroidism are hereditary defects in hormone biosynthesis and ingestion of drugs that induce defects in hormone biosynthesis, such as aminosalicylic acid and lithium. Finally, in areas of environmental iodine deficiency, goitrous cretinism and hypothyroidism can be endemic. Diminished thyroid reserve occurs as a stage in the evolution of hypothyroidism.

Rarely, long-standing hypothyroidism leads to diffuse, nodular, or adenomatous thyrotroph hyperplasia. These patients may present with headache, visual field defects, abnormal pubertal development, galactorrhea, and pituitary enlargement, all of which disappear with levothyroxine therapy. Such patients have marked elevations in serum TSH levels, whereas in hypothyroidism of suprathyroid origin, the thyroid is intrinsically normal but is deprived of stimulation by TSH. Deprivation of TSH, most commonly the result of postpartum pituitary necrosis or a tumor of the pituitary, results in pituitary hypothyroidism. Hypothalamic hypothyroidism is less common and results from inadequate secretion of TRH.

CLINICAL PICTURE The manifestations of hypothyroidism in children depend on the age at which the deficiency began and the promptness with which replacement therapy is instituted. Cretinism may be manifest at birth but usually becomes evident within the first several months after birth, depending on the extent of thyroid failure. Hypothyroidism is present in approximately 1 in every 5000 neonates and manifests itself as persistence of physiologic jaundice, a hoarse cry, constipation, somnolence, and feeding problems; since clinical diagnosis is difficult and early treatment is crucial for normal intellectual development, all neonates should be screened for hypothyroidism with measurements of the serum T_4 or TSH. Later, delay in reaching the normal milestones of development becomes evident, and the physical characteristics of the cretin appear. These include short stature; coarse features with a protruding tongue, broad, flat nose, and widely set eyes; sparse hair; dry skin; a protuberant abdomen with an umbilical hernia; impaired mental development; retarded bone age; epiphyseal dysgenesis; and delayed dentition.

In the older child, the clinical manifestations of hypothyroidism include retardation of linear growth and delayed puberty. Poor performance at school may call attention to the diagnosis. Variable manifestations of adult hypothyroidism are present. X-ray examination reveals delayed union of the epiphyses.

In the adult, early symptoms of hypothyroidism are nonspecific and insidious in onset. In the elderly, symptoms may be erroneously attributed to aging itself, Parkinson's disease, depression, or Alzheimer's disease. They may include fatigue, lethargy, constipation, cold intolerance, stiffness and cramping of the muscles, carpal tunnel syndrome, and menorrhagia. Intellectual and motor activity slows, appetite declines, and weight increases. The hair becomes dry and tends to fall out, and the skin becomes dry. The voice becomes deeper and hoarse, and auditory acuity may deteriorate. Obstructive sleep apnea may occur. Ultimately, the clinical picture of florid myxedema appears, with a dull, expressionless facies, sparse hair, periorbital puffiness, large tongue, and pale, cool skin that feels rough and doughy. Thyroid tissue is usually not palpable, except in the goitrous variety. The heart is enlarged owing to both dilation and pericardial effusion; if the heart is small, pituitary hypothyroidism (with secondary adrenal insufficiency) or coincident primary adrenal insufficiency (Schmidt's syndrome) should be considered. Adynamic ileus may cause megacolon or intestinal obstruction. Rarely, psychiatric symptoms or cerebellar ataxia may dominate the clinical picture. The relaxation phase of the deep tendon reflexes is characteristically prolonged, the so-called hung-up reflex. If left untreated, the patient with long-standing hypothyroidism may pass into a hypothermic, stuporous state (*myxedema coma*) that may be fatal. Respiratory depression is an important component of this state, and hence arterial P_{CO_2} may be increased. Factors that predispose to myxedema coma include cold exposure, trauma, infection, and administration of central nervous system depressants. Hyponatremia may result from impaired water excretion and from disordered regulation of vasopressin secretion.

LABORATORY TESTS The single most useful measurement is the serum TSH, which is increased in the thyroprivic and goitrous varieties and is usually normal or undetectable in pituitary or hypothalamic hypothyroidism (see Fig. 331-3). In the latter instances, hyposecretion of TSH is usually accompanied by hyposecretion of other pituitary hormones (see Chap. 328). Decreases in serum T_4 and in the FT_4I are common to all varieties of hypothyroidism. In the primary varieties, the serum T_3 may be decreased less than the serum T_4, presumably because the compensatory hypersecretion of TSH leads to a relative preponderance of T_3 secretion. In thyroprivic hypothyroidism, the decreased RAIU is of limited diagnostic utility because of the low value for the lower limit of the normal range. In goitrous hypothyroidism, the RAIU may range from low to increased.

Manifestations of the hypothyroid state include an increased serum cholesterol level in hypothyroidism of thyroid (but not pituitary) origin and increased serum levels of creatine phosphokinase, aspartate transaminase, and lactate dehydrogenase. Systolic time intervals are altered in that the preejection period is prolonged and the ratio of the preejection period to the left ventricular ejection time is increased. Electrocardiographic changes include bradycardia, low-amplitude QRS complexes, and flattened or inverted T waves. In primary thyroprivic hypothyroidism, pernicious anemia occurs in about 12 percent of patients; histamine-fast achlorhydria and circulating antigastric parietal cell antibodies are more common.

Some patients who appear clinically euthyroid display laboratory evidence of early thyroid failure (subclinical hypothyroidism). In mild cases, serum TSH and its response to TRH administration are increased, while serum T_4 and T_3 levels are normal. When thyroid failure is more advanced, the serum T_4 concentration is decreased, but the serum T_3 concentration is normal or nearly so owing to TSH-induced hypersecretion of T_3 relative to T_4 and perhaps to more efficient conversion of T_4 to T_3. Subclinical hypothyroidism is most often seen in patients with Hashimoto's disease or those with Graves' disease who have been treated with ^{131}I or surgery; in the latter, subclinical hypothyroidism usually represents a stage in the evolution of frank hypothyroidism.

DIFFERENTIAL DIAGNOSIS It is not difficult to diagnose the classic picture of cretinism or juvenile and adult hypothyroidism. Occasionally, an infant with Down's syndrome may be confused with a cretin. Chronic nephritis and the nephrotic syndrome may simulate myxedema, particularly because of the facial puffiness and pallor. The nephrotic patient may have anemia, hypercholesterolemia, and anasarca, and the serum T_4 may be decreased if TBG is lost into the urine. However, the FT_4I is normal or increased, the serum T_3 concentration is often subnormal (as in any severe systemic illness, owing to impaired peripheral generation from T_4), and the serum TSH concentration is normal.

℞ TREATMENT

Hormones available for the treatment of hypothyroidism (Table 331-6) include the synthetic hormones levothyroxine (L-thyroxine), liothyronine (L-triiodothyronine), and liotrix (a combination of the two). A preparation of natural origin still occasionally used is thyroid extract, USP. Because of their uniform potency, the author prefers the synthetic preparations, specifically levothyroxine. Unlike liothyronine, liotrix, and even thyroid extract, ingestion of levothyroxine does not lead to an abrupt increase in serum T_3 level, which can cause adverse and sometimes dangerous effects in the older patient or the patient with coexisting heart disease. Rather, a stable T_3 concentration is attained through continuous generation from administered levothyroxine.

In most instances, a normal metabolic state should be restored gradually, especially in the elderly and in patients with heart disease, since a sudden increase in metabolic rate may tax cardiac or coronary reserve. In adults, an initial daily dose of 25 μg levothyroxine can be increased by 25- to 50-μg increments at 4-week intervals until a normal metabolic state is attained. Patients on levothyroxine who have autoimmume thyroid disease tend to require less levothyroxine than patients who have had total thyroidectomy, because some functioning tissue usually persists in the former group. Such patients require about 1.7 μg levothyroxine per kilogram body weight per day, whereas totally thyroidectomized patients require approximately 2.1 μg per kilogram body weight per day. Because of its long half-life, levothyroxine is administered as a single daily dose. While the serum T_3 may be superior to the serum T_4 as an indicator of the metabolic state in patients receiving levothyroxine, the optimal dose is best determined by clinical criteria and measurement of TSH by an ultrasensitive assay. An elevated TSH indicates that treatment is insufficient, and an elevated T_3 indicates that it is excessive. Serum T_3 is a particularly useful parameter in patients with pituitary or hypothalamic disease, in whom interpretation of serum TSH levels is more difficult.

In some circumstances a previously stable dosage of levothyroxine may need to be increased or decreased. Increases of 25 to 50 μg per day may be required during pregnancy, as evidenced by increases in serum TSH. Progressive increases in dose may be required as further atrophy of the gland occurs in patients with Hashi-

Table 331-6

Approximate Therapeutic Equivalence of Various Thyroid Hormone Preparations

Preparation	Average Daily Oral Maintenance Dose	Serum (T_4)	Undesirable Lability in Serum (T_3)
Levothyroxine	125 μg	Slightly increased	–
Liothyronine	50 μg	Decreased	+ +
Liotrix (T_4/T_3 = 4:1)	2 units	Normal	+
Thyroid extract, USP	120–180 mg	Normal	+

Table 331-7

Reasons for Changing Levothyroxine Requirements in Patients on a Previously Stable Dosage*

Requirement for increased dose
Pregnancy
Further decrease in thyroid function due to
Graves' disease after radioiodine administration
Hashimoto's thyroiditis
Impaired levothyroxine absorption due to
Cholestyramine, colestipol
Iron sulfate
Sucralfate
Aluminum hydroxide
Short bowel syndromes
Augmented levothyroxine metabolism due to
Phenytoin
Rifampin
Carbamazepine
Requirement for decreased dose
Spontaneous recovery from Hashimoto's thyroiditis due to disappearance of TSH receptor–blocking antibodies
Reactivation of Graves' disease
Emergence of autonomous nodules
Advanced age
Factitious ingestion of levothyroxine

* Exclusive of poor compliance

moto's disease or in patients with Graves' disease who have been treated with surgery or radioiodine. A number of drugs may interfere with gastrointestinal absorption or enhance the metabolic clearance of levothyroxine (Table 331-7). Similarly, decreases in dosage may be required with spontaneous disappearance of TSH receptor blocking antibodies in Hashimoto's disease, with increases in stimulatory antibodies to the TSH receptor causing reactivation of Graves' disease, or with the emergence of autonomy and hyperfunction in uninodular or multinodular goiter.

In neonatal, infantile, and juvenile hypothyroidism, full replacement therapy should be begun as soon as possible; otherwise, the chances of normal intellectual development and growth are poor. Infants and children require doses of levothyroxine that are disproportionately large in relation to body size. *In known or strongly suspected cases of pituitary and hypothalamic hypothyroidism, thyroid replacement should not be instituted until treatment with hydrocortisone has been initiated*, since acute adrenocortical insufficiency may be precipitated by an increase in metabolic rate and increased clearance of glucocorticoids.

In some adults, hypothyroidism should be treated rapidly. These include patients with myxedema coma and, because of the extreme sensitivity to central nervous system depressants, hypothyroid patients being prepared for emergency surgery. In these patients, intravenous administration of levothyroxine, in conjunction with the use of hydrocortisone, is indicated.

Patients with myxedema coma and associated systemic illness may have a reduced ability to convert T_4 to T_3, as in the sick euthyroid syndrome. Consequently, supplementary doses of liothyronine may be warranted, even though sole therapy with full doses of liothyronine is not recommended in view of the cardiovascular risk. For comatose patients, parenteral forms of both levothyroxine and liothyronine are available. A combined approach allows initial administration of 3 to 4 μg of levothyroxine per kilogram body weight intravenously followed by 100 μg/d thereafter, along with 10 μg of liothyronine every 8 h. Both parenteral preparations are discontinued when the patient becomes able to take oral medications.

THYROTOXICOSIS

The term *thyrotoxicosis* denotes the clinical, physiologic, and biochemical findings that result when the tissues are exposed to, and respond to, excess thyroid hormone. Rather than being a specific disease, thyrotoxicosis can originate in a variety of ways (Table 331-8). The most important of these disorders are those that lead to sustained overproduction of hormone by the thyroid gland itself. Rarely, this hyperfunction results from excessive secretion of TSH by a pituitary tumor or as a result of resistance to thyroid hormone in the pituitary but not in peripheral tissues. Other causes are the action of a homeostatically unregulated thyroid stimulator of extrapituitary origin, as in Graves' disease, Hashimoto's disease, and trophoblastic tumors, and the development of one or more areas of autonomous hyperfunction within the gland itself. Thyrotoxicosis not associated with thyroid hyperfunction includes that associated with subacute thyroiditis and the syndrome called chronic thyroiditis with transient thyrotoxicosis. In these disorders, an excess of preformed hormone leaks from the gland owing to the presence of inflammatory disease. New hormone formation is decreased because of the suppression of TSH secretion by the hormone excess and, in some cases, because of the inflammatory injury itself. Since the inflammatory disorders are transitory and since stores of preformed hormone are eventually depleted, the thyrotoxicosis in these disorders is self-limited and is often followed by a transient period of thyroid hormone insufficiency. Thyrotoxicosis can also occur when the source of excess hormone is outside of the thyroid gland, as in thyrotoxicosis factitia, the ingestion of meat contaminated with animal thyroids ("hamburger toxicosis"), the rare functioning metastatic thyroid carcinoma, and struma ovarii.

Table 331-8

Varieties of Thyrotoxicosis

Associated with thyroid hyperfunction*
Excess production of TSH (rare)
Abnormal thyroid stimulator
Graves' disease
Trophoblastic tumor
Intrinsic thyroid autonomy
Hyperfunctioning adenoma
Toxic multinodular goiter
Not associated with thyroid hyperfunction†
Disorders of hormone storage
Subacute thyroiditis
Chronic thyroiditis with transient thyrotoxicosis
Extrathyroid source of hormone
Thyrotoxicosis factitia
"Hamburger toxicosis"
Ectopic thyroid tissue
Struma ovarii
Functioning follicular carcinoma

* Associated with increased RAIU unless body iodine burden is excessive.
† Associated with decreased RAIU.

Not all of the foregoing disorders are associated with *hyperthyroidism*, a term that should be used to denote only those conditions in which sustained hyperfunction of the thyroid leads to thyrotoxicosis. This distinction has implications for diagnosis and for treatment. In hyperthyroidism, hyperfunction of the thyroid is reflected in an increased RAIU, whereas in the nonhyperthyroid thyrotoxic states, thyroid function (as reflected in the RAIU) is subnormal. Further, treatment of thyrotoxicosis by means intended to decrease hormone synthesis (antithyroid agents, surgery, or radioiodine) is appropriate in hyperthyroidism but is inappropriate and ineffective in other forms of thyrotoxicosis.

Although the diseases that cause thyrotoxicosis make their own imprint on the clinical picture, the manifestations of the thyrotoxic state are largely the same. For this reason, the common manifestations of thyrotoxicosis are described in relation to Graves' disease.

GRAVES' DISEASE

Graves' disease, also known as Parry's or Basedow's disease, is a disorder with three major manifestations: hyperthyroidism with diffuse goiter, ophthalmopathy, and dermopathy. These manifestations need not appear together. Indeed, one or two need never appear, and the three may run largely independent courses.

PREVALENCE Graves' disease is a relatively common disorder that can occur at any age but is especially common in the third and fourth decades. The disease is more frequent in women. In nongoitrous areas, the ratio of predominance in women may be as high as 7:1. In areas of endemic goiter, the ratio is lower. Genetic factors play an important role; there is an increased frequency of haplotypes HLA-B8 and -DRw3 in Caucasian, HLA-Bw36 in Japanese, and HLA-Bw46 in Chinese patients with the disease. Not surprisingly, there is a familial predisposition. In addition, among family members, a clinical and immunologic overlap exists with respect to Hashimoto's disease, primary thyroprivic hypothyroidism, and pernicious anemia and probably with respect to other autoimmune disorders as well. In occasional patients, the picture may change from Graves' disease to Hashimoto's disease or vice versa, and, rarely, patients with primary myxedema later become hyperthyroid. Thus, it is proper to consider Graves' disease, Hashimoto's disease, and primary myxedema as closely related autoimmune thyroid diseases.

ETIOLOGY AND PATHOGENESIS The cause of Graves' disease is unknown. In view of the variety of manifestations and courses, it is possible that no single factor is responsible for the entire syndrome. With respect to hyperthyroidism, the central disorder is a disruption of homeostatic mechanisms that normally control hormone secretion. This disruption results from the presence in plasma of thyroid-stimulating immunoglobulins (TSIs) of the IgG class that are elaborated by lymphocytes. When human thyroid tissue is used as the assay system, the end points are stimulation of colloid droplet or cyclic AMP generation (for thyroid-stimulating antibodies, TSAbs) and inhibition of the binding of TSH to its receptors in human thyroid tissue (TSH-binding inhibitory immunoglobulins, TBIIs). These factors represent antibodies against the thyroid TSH receptor (TRAbs). Activities of this type are also found in the serum of some patients with euthyroid ophthalmic Graves' disease, occasional patients with Hashimoto's disease, and some euthyroid relatives of patients with Graves' disease. Presumably, the absence of thyrotoxicosis in such instances reflects the predominance of blocking over stimulatory TRAbs or intrinsic thyroid disease that prevents a hyperthyroid response. Disappearance of stimulatory factors from the serum during antithyroid treatment augurs well for long-term remission after treatment is withdrawn. Thus, while the basic cause of Graves' disease is not understood, an immunoglobulin or family of immunoglobulins directed against the TSH receptor mediates the thyroid stimulation. An inherited abnormality in immune surveillance may permit particular lymphocytes to survive, proliferate, and secrete the stimulatory immunoglobulins in response to precipitating factors.

The pathogenesis of the ophthalmic component is more enigmatic. An antigen in orbital tissues that cross-reacts with the thyroid has been postulated, and fibroblasts from orbital tissues contain a material that reacts with antibodies to the TSH receptor. Both cellular and humoral immunity may play a role in the ophthalmopathy. Cytokines and/or growth factors released by T cells may lead to production of an inflammatory reaction with proliferation of more fibroblasts and glycosaminoglycan production, thereby initiating the edema and increase in muscle volume and retroorbital fat. Even less is known about the pathogenesis of the dermopathy.

PATHOLOGY The *thyroid gland* is diffusely enlarged, soft, and vascular. There is parenchymatous hypertrophy and hyperplasia, characterized by increased height of the epithelium and redundancy of the follicular wall, causing papillary infoldings, and cytologic evidence of increased activity. Such hyperplasia is usually accompanied by lymphocytic infiltration that reflects the immune nature of the disease and correlates with levels of antithyroid antibodies in the blood. Following iodine medication, there is colloid storage, which sometimes causes enlargement and increased firmness of the gland. Graves' disease is associated with generalized lymphoid hyperplasia and infiltration and occasionally with enlargement of the spleen or thymus. Thyrotoxicosis may lead to degeneration of skeletal muscle fibers, enlargement of the heart, fatty infiltration or diffuse fibrosis of the liver, decalcification of the skeleton, and loss of body tissue (including fat deposits, osteoid, and muscle).

The *ophthalmopathy* is characterized by an inflammatory infiltrate of the orbital contents, exclusive of the globe, with lymphocytes, mast cells, and plasma cells. The orbital musculature is often enlarged owing to infiltration with lymphocytes, mucopolysaccharides, and edema, which with fat largely account for the increased volume of the orbital contents that causes the globe to protrude. Muscle fibers show degeneration and loss of striations, with ultimate fibrosis.

The *dermopathy* of Graves' disease is characterized by thickening of the dermis, which is infiltrated with lymphocytes and with hydrophilic, metachromatically staining mucopolysaccharides.

CLINICAL MANIFESTATIONS The manifestations include those that reflect the associated thyrotoxicosis and those specifically related to Graves' disease.

Manifestations of Thyrotoxicosis Common manifestations include nervousness, emotional lability, inability to sleep, tremors, frequent bowel movements, excessive sweating, and heat intolerance. Weight loss is usual despite a well-maintained or increased appetite. Proximal muscle weakness with loss of strength is often manifested by difficulty in climbing stairs. In premenopausal women, oligomenorrhea and amenorrhea tend to occur. Dyspnea, palpitations, and, in older patients, enhancement of angina pectoris or cardiac failure may be present. In general, nervous symptoms dominate the clinical picture in younger individuals, whereas cardiovascular and myopathic symptoms predominate in older subjects.

Usually, the patient appears anxious, restless, and fidgety. The skin is warm and moist with a velvety texture, and palmar erythema is present. Separation of the fingernail from the nailbed (onycholysis; Plummer's nail) is common, especially on the ring finger. The hair is fine and silky. A fine tremor of the fingers and tongue, together with hyperreflexia, is characteristic. *Ocular signs* include a characteristic stare with widened palpebral fissures, infrequent blinking, lid lag, and failure to wrinkle the brow on upward gaze. These signs result from sympathetic overstimulation and usually subside when the thyrotoxicosis is corrected. They are to be distinguished from the *infiltrative ophthalmopathy* characteristic of Graves' disease, discussed below.

Cardiovascular features include a wide pulse pressure, sinus tachycardia, atrial arrhythmias (especially atrial fibrillation), systolic murmurs, increased intensity of the apical first sound, cardiac enlargement, and, at times, overt heart failure. A to-and-fro, high-pitched sound may be audible in the pulmonic area and may simulate a pericardial friction rub (Means-Lerman scratch).

Manifestations of Graves' Disease The distinctive manifestations—diffuse hyperfunctioning goiter, ophthalmopathy, and dermopathy—appear in varying combinations and in varying frequencies, goiter being the most common. Premature graying of the hair and patchy vitiligo are not specific for Graves' disease and are common in other autoimmune disorders.

The *diffuse toxic goiter* may be asymmetric and lobular. The presence of a bruit over the gland usually signifies that the patient is thyrotoxic, but this sign is present rarely in other forms of thyroid hyperplasia. Venous hums and carotid souffles should be distinguished from true thyroid bruits. An enlarged pyramidal lobe of the thyroid may be palpable.

The signs associated with the *ophthalmopathy* of Graves' disease may be divided into two components: the spastic and the mechanical. The former includes the stare, lid lag, and lid retraction that accompany thyrotoxicosis and account for the "frightened" facies and eye signs previously described. These findings need not be associated with proptosis, may be ameliorated by adrenergic antagonists, and usually return to normal after correction of thyrotoxicosis. The mechanical component includes proptosis of varying degrees with ophthalmoplegia and congestive oculopathy characterized by chemosis, conjunctivitis, periorbital swelling, and the potential complications of corneal ulceration, optic neuritis, and optic atrophy. When exophthalmos progresses rapidly and becomes the major concern in Graves' disease, it is termed *progressive* and, if severe, *malignant exophthalmos*. The term *exophthalmic ophthalmoplegia* refers to the ocular muscle weakness that results in impaired upward gaze and convergence and strabismus with varying degrees of diplopia. Exophthalmos may be unilateral early but usually becomes bilateral with time.

The *dermopathy* usually occurs over the dorsum of the legs or feet and is termed *localized* or *pretibial myxedema*. It is usually a late phenomenon but is not a manifestation of hyperthyroidism. About half of cases occur during the active stage of thyrotoxicosis, and virtually all have ophthalmopathy. The affected area is usually demarcated from normal skin by being raised and thickened and having a *peau d'orange* appearance; it may also be pruritic and hyperpigmented. The most common presentation is a nonpitting edema, but the lesions may be plaquelike, nodular, or polypoid in configuration. Clubbing of the fingers and toes with bony changes that differ from those of hypertrophic pulmonary osteoarthropathy may accompany the dermal changes (*thyroid acropachy*).

DIAGNOSIS When severe, Graves' disease presents little difficulty in diagnosis. Florid thyrotoxicosis is manifested by weakness, weight loss despite a good appetite, nervous instability, tremor, intolerance to heat, sweating, palpitations, and hyperdefecation. When associated with diffuse thyroid enlargement, often accompanied by a bruit, and particularly when associated with ophthalmopathy, the clinical picture is virtually unique. In such instances, laboratory tests documenting undetectable TSH and increased values of the RAIU, of serum T_4 and T_3 levels, of the RT_3U, and of the FT_4I serve as baselines for evaluation of therapy rather than necessary diagnostic aids. Occasionally, laboratory tests reveal a normal RAIU, a normal serum T_4 level and RT_3U, and an elevated serum T_3 level and FT_3I (T_3 toxicosis).

In less severe cases, particularly when ophthalmopathy is lacking, the diagnosis may be more difficult, since the symptoms of mild thyrotoxicosis are similar to those of other disorders (see "Differential Diagnosis," below). The presence of a goiter makes the diagnosis of hyperthyroidism likely, but careful palpation is necessary to determine whether toxic multinodular goiter, toxic adenoma, or subacute thyroiditis is present. Absence of thyroid enlargement makes the diagnosis of Graves' disease less likely but does not exclude it. In mild cases, confirmatory laboratory tests assume great importance. Unfortunately, mild thyrotoxicosis is often associated with marginal abnormalities in serum T_4 and T_3 values. In such instances, an ultrasensitive TSH assay or the TRH stimulation test assumes crucial importance.

In a few (usually older) patients, the clinical picture is one of apathy rather than hyperactivity, and evidence of hypermetabolism may be slight (*apathetic thyrotoxicosis*). In such patients, myopathic features may be pronounced. More often, cardiovascular manifestations predominate, since mild hyperthyroidism may produce severe disability in patients with underlying heart disease. Hence, *all patients with unexplained cardiac failure or atrial arrhythmias should be evaluated for thyrotoxicosis*.

DIFFERENTIAL DIAGNOSIS Signs and symptoms of several nonthyroid disorders may simulate certain aspects of the thyrotoxic syndrome. Anxiety is a prominent feature of thyrotoxicosis, and there is overlap in the symptomatology of thyrotoxicosis and of anxiety states. Tachycardia, tremulousness, irritability, weakness, and fatigue are common to both disorders. In anxiety, however, the peripheral manifestations of excessive thyroid hormones are absent; the skin is usually cold and clammy rather than warm and moist. Weight loss, when present in emotional anxiety, is characteristically accompanied by anorexia, whereas in thyrotoxicosis the appetite is increased. Thyrotoxicosis can occasionally be confused with such disorders as metastatic carcinoma, cirrhosis of the liver, hyperparathyroidism, sprue, myasthenia gravis, and muscular dystrophy. Hypokalemic periodic paralysis is more common in thyrotoxic patients, especially in Asian and Latin American men. Signs and symptoms of thyrotoxicosis may overlap with those of pheochromocytoma, which can cause heat intolerance, sweating, tachycardia with palpitations, and a hypermetabolic state. Laboratory tests usually make it possible to differentiate these various disorders from thyrotoxicosis.

When bilateral ophthalmopathy is accompanied by goiter and thyrotoxicosis, the diagnosis of Graves' ophthalmopathy is virtually certain. The presence of unilateral ophthalmopathy, even when associated with thyrotoxicosis, raises the possibility of some other intraorbital or intracranial disease. In the euthyroid patient with either unilateral or bilateral ophthalmopathy, other causes that must be excluded are cavernous sinus thrombosis, sphenoidal ridge meningioma, retrobulbar tumors, including leukemic deposits, and the rare granulomatous disorder pseudotumor oculi. Exophthalmos also may be seen in certain systemic disorders, such as uremia, accelerated hypertension, chronic alcoholism, chronic obstructive pulmonary disease, superior mediastinal obstruction, and Cushing's syndrome. Ophthalmoplegia in the absence of infiltrative manifestations can be confused with that in diabetes mellitus, myasthenia gravis, and myopathies. When doubt exists about the cause of ophthalmopathy, the demonstration of significant titers of TSI or TBII or of an abnormal result on a TRH stimulation or thyroid suppression test suggests that the cause is Graves' disease, though not all patients with "euthyroid Graves' disease" demonstrate abnormal responses. In such cases, ultrasonography, magnetic resonance imaging, or computed tomography of the orbits is valuable in demonstrating characteristic thickening of the extraocular muscles.

When a thyrotoxic state occurs in a patient lacking the ophthalmopathy of Graves' disease, other causes of thyrotoxicosis must be considered. Careful palpation of the thyroid and studies with radioactive iodine are important in this regard. A symmetric, diffuse goiter of moderate or large size suggests the diagnosis of Graves' disease, especially if a bruit is present. However, the uncommon patient whose hyperthyroidism is secondary to an excess of TSH (associated with a *pituitary tumor* or resistance to feedback suppression of TSH secretion) or an abnormal stimulator of trophoblastic origin (*hydatidiform mole* or *choriocarcinoma of the uterus* or *testis;* see Chap. 102) may present in this way. A single, prominent thyroid nodule or multiple nodules suggest *toxic adenoma* or *toxic multinodular goiter*, respectively. Tenderness of the thyroid associated with firm nodularity suggests *subacute thyroiditis*, while a small, firm, nontender goiter is consistent with chronic thyroiditis with spontaneously resolving thyrotoxicosis. The foregoing disorders are discussed in later sections. Absence of a palpable thyroid gland suggests an extrathyroid source of hormone, such as ectopic thyroid tissue (*struma ovarii*) or, more commonly, self-administration of hormone (*thyrotoxicosis factitia*). Studies with radioactive iodine are also helpful. Except when hormone overproduction is secondary to increased iodine intake, values of the RAIU are increased in all disorders producing hyperthyroidism. Conversely, thyrotoxicosis that is not the result of hyperthyroidism is characterized by subnormal values of the RAIU. Subacute thyroiditis and chronic thyroiditis with spontaneously resolving thyrotoxicosis are the most common. Ectopic thyroid tissue producing thyrotoxicosis is rare. Here, the RAIU, as measured over the thyroid, is low, since TSH secretion is suppressed, but urinary excretion of radioactive iodine is slowed, owing to accumulation by the ectopic tissue. Functioning ectopic tissue can be located by scintillation scanning.

Thyrotoxicosis factitia most frequently occurs in medical or paramedical personnel or in those who have easy access to thyroid hormone. The disorder resembles thyrotoxicosis caused by ectopic thyroid tissue in that the patient's thyroid is suppressed. Consequently, the RAIU is very low, and most of administered radioactive iodine is excreted promptly in the urine. When the disorder is caused by ingestion of preparations containing T_4, such as levothyroxine or thyroid extract, the serum T_4 is increased. On the other hand, when it is caused by liothyronine, the serum T_4 is subnormal. Irrespective of the preparation, the serum T_3 is increased, but more so when liothyronine is the offending agent. Measurement of serum thyroglobulin is useful to confirm thyrotoxicosis factitia. Levels are elevated in Graves' disease and thyroiditis but are subnormal with exogenous thyroid hormone suppression. The demonstration of elevated titers of thyroid-stimulating immunoglobulins in the blood also provides strong evidence that Graves' disease is the cause of thyrotoxicosis.

℞ TREATMENT

Hyperthyroidism Hyperthyroidism is often characterized by cyclic phases of exacerbation and remission, which are of unpredictable onset and duration. Moreover, long-standing disease may be associated with progressive thyroid failure, probably consequent to chronic thyroiditis, with the supervention of hypothyroidism or decreased thyroid reserve. These characteristics have important implications for the choice of and response to therapy.

The major treatments are directed to limiting the quantity of thyroid hormones the gland can produce. Antithyroid agents chemically block hormone synthesis—an effect that persists only as long as the drug is administered—and they may also enhance evolution to remission through their anti-immune effects. Their principal use is to control active thyrotoxicity while remission is awaited. The second major approach to limiting hormone production is ablation of thyroid tissue, either by surgery or by the use of radioactive iodine. Since these procedures permanently alter the thyroid anatomy, they can control the active phase of the disease and are more likely to prevent later exacerbation or recurrence. On the other hand, surgery or radiation is more likely to lead to hypothyroidism, either shortly after treatment or with the passage of years.

Each type of therapy has advantages and disadvantages, indications and contraindications, both relative and absolute. In general, a trial of long-term antithyroid therapy is desirable in children, adolescents, young adults, and pregnant women but also may be employed in older patients. Indications for ablative procedures include relapse or recurrence following drug therapy, a large goiter, drug toxicity, failure to follow a medical regimen, or failure to return for periodic examinations. Subtotal thyroidectomy may be elected for patients under the age of 30 in whom ablative therapy is required; however, opinions differ, and some authorities employ radioactive iodine in the treatment of patients in the second or third decade. Surgery is also preferable in patients with very large goiters or with a coincident nonfunctioning nodule, especially if there is a history of radiation to the head and neck. Radioactive iodine is the ablative procedure of choice in older patients, in patients with previous thyroid surgery, and in those in whom systemic disease contraindicates elective surgery.

In patients selected for *long-term antithyroid therapy*, satisfactory control can almost always be achieved if sufficient drug is administered. Most patients can be managed with propylthiouracil, 100 to 150 mg every 6 or 8 h. Larger doses may be required for initial control. Methimazole is at least as effective as propylthiouracil when administered at one-tenth the dosage. However, propylthiouracil has the advantage of inhibiting the peripheral conversion of T_4 to T_3, thereby bringing about more rapid symptomatic improvement. Once euthyroidism is achieved, the daily dosage may be reduced to the smallest amount that controls the thyrotoxicosis. In some clinics, the initial dose is continued and is supplemented with levothyroxine. This regimen avoids the risk of hypothyroidism from overdosage of antithyroid drugs and thus may forestall the undesirable consequences of hypothyroidism, such as enhancement of ophthalmopathy and enlargement of the goiter. The duration of antithyroid drug therapy is difficult to predict in the individual patient and may be a function of the natural course of the disease. The longer the course of therapy, the more likely it is that the patient will remain well when the drug is discontinued. In general, a 12- to 24-month course is employed, after which one-third to one-half of patients remain well for a prolonged period or indefinitely. The likelihood of a prolonged remission is increased by a decrease in goiter size, reversion of the results of the thyroid suppression test and TRH stimulation test to normal, or disappearance of TRAbs from the serum during treatment.

Leukopenia is the principal undesirable side effect of antithyroid drugs. A complete blood count should be obtained prior to initiating therapy to identify those patients with leukopenia related to Graves' disease. Mild transient leukopenia with antithyroid drugs may occur in an additional 10 percent of patients and is not necessarily an indication for discontinuing therapy. When the absolute number of polymorphonuclear leukocytes reaches $\leq 1500/\mu L$, antithyroid medication should be discontinued. Allergic rashes and drug sensitivity also occur on occasion. These may disappear with antihistamine therapy at the same or a reduced dosage of antithyroid agent, but when sensitivity reactions occur it is preferable to change to another drug. On rare occasions (in fewer than 0.2 percent of cases), agranulocytosis occurs. It may be sudden in onset. Hepatitis, drug fever, and arthralgias can also occur. In the author's view, severe sensitivity reactions, including agranulocytosis, mandate the abandonment of antithyroid therapy rather than recourse to an alternative drug.

Iodide inhibits the release of hormones from the hyperfunctioning thyroid gland, and its ameliorative effects occur more rapidly than those of agents that inhibit hormone synthesis. Hence, its main use is in patients with actual or impending thyrotoxic crisis and in patients with severe cardiac disease. The response to iodide alone is often incomplete and transient. Furthermore, by expanding the thyroid store of hormone, iodide may prolong the latency of response to antithyroid therapy. Therefore, iodide is safely used only in conjunction with the antithyroid agents. If the clinical course is sufficiently severe to require iodide administration, antithyroid drugs are usually the primary therapeutic agents and should be given in large doses prior to iodide. Iodide is also useful in controlling thyrotoxicosis following ^{131}I administration, during the period in which the therapeutic effect of radioiodine has not yet taken place. Large doses of *glucocorticoids* (2 mg dexamethasone every 6 h) reduce the serum T_4 concentration when relief of thyrotoxicosis is urgent. The iodinated x-ray contrast agent sodium ipodate has a similar effect. Iodine liberated from this agent inhibits thyroid secretion of T_4 and T_3, and serum T_3 is further reduced by the inhibition by ipodate of peripheral T_3 formation. Daily doses of 1 g orally are effective, but the same precautions that apply to the use of iodine therapy apply to ipodate.

Owing to the adrenergic component in thyrotoxicosis, various *adrenergic antagonists* have been employed in its management. Of these, propranolol is the agent of choice because of its relative freedom from side effects. In doses of 40 to 120 mg/d, propranolol alleviates such adrenergic manifestations as sweating, tremor, and tachycardia and may reduce to some extent the conversion of T_4 to T_3. However, propranolol should be used only as adjunctive therapy, since the underlying metabolic abnormalities are not affected. Moreover, although the diminution in heart rate and cardiac work may be beneficial, the blocking of adrenergic support of myocardial contractility necessitates caution in the use of this agent in patients with coexisting heart failure, unless the latter is rate- or rhythm-related. As an adjunctive agent, propranolol is useful while the response to conventional antithyroid agents or to radioiodine therapy is awaited and in the management of thyrotoxic crisis. It has been employed as the sole agent in preparation for thyroidectomy, but its use in this setting is not recommended, since it does not render the patient euthyroid, and thus probably does not minimize the risk of surgically induced crisis.

Radioactive iodine (^{131}I) affords a relatively simple, effective, and economical means of treating thyrotoxicosis. It can produce the ablative effects of surgery without the operative and postoperative complications. The principal disadvantage of ^{131}I therapy, in the dosage usually employed, is its tendency to produce hypothyroidism with a frequency that increases with time. As many as 40 to 70 percent of patients may develop this complication within 10 years after treatment. Although hypothyroidism is treatable once diagnosed, the insidious onset may obscure the diagnosis until serious complications develop. Hence, some workers recommend that all patients be treated with relatively large doses of ^{131}I to ensure relief of thyrotoxicosis and then placed on permanent physiologic replacement doses of thyroid hormone.

There is no evidence that radioiodine has carcinogenic or leukemogenic effects when given to adults in the doses commonly used in treating hyperthyroidism. However, the susceptibility to carcinogenesis may be increased in the thyroids of children. Mutagenic effects have not been reported and would be difficult to document. For these reasons, many physicians prefer to reserve radioiodine therapy for patients over 30 years of age or those unlikely to have children afterward. Moreover, the longer the life expectancy after ^{131}I therapy, the greater the likelihood that hypothyroidism will develop. Among younger patients, therefore, only those with recurrent thyrotoxicosis following surgery, those who refuse surgery, and those with a complicating illness that contraindicates surgery are candidates for radioiodine therapy. In elderly patients, treatment with large doses of radioiodine is the general method of choice, so that the undesirable effects of incomplete treatment or recurrence can be avoided. It is controversial whether radioiodine therapy worsens ophthalmopathy, but in patients with significant ophthalmopathy, it may be prudent to administer glucocorticoids for approximately 2 weeks before and 6 weeks after the ^{131}I dose to reduce the likelihood of exacerbation of eye disease. Other possible risk factors for worsening opthalmopathy include smoking and more severe thyrotoxicosis.

The usual therapeutic dose of ^{131}I [approximately 5.9 MBq (160 μCi) per gram of estimated gland weight] leads to a high frequency of hypothyroidism. As a result, some authorities who continue to use this dose regularly administer prophylactic replacement doses of thyroid hormone. Others have administered smaller doses [approximately 3.0 MBq/g (80 μCi/g)]. However, these smaller doses do not diminish the frequency of late hypothyroidism but merely delay its onset. Moreover, they are less likely to relieve thyrotoxicosis within a relatively short period. Antithyroid agents can be employed, however, to speed the attainment of a eumetabolic state, and propranolol can be given to relieve symptoms while the effect of the ^{131}I is taking hold. There is general agreement that patients with coexisting cardiac disease should receive ^{131}I in large doses in view of the hazard of persistent or recurrent thyrotoxicosis.

Radiation thyroiditis is an occasional early complication of ^{131}I therapy. It commonly appears within 7 to 10 days and is associated with accelerated release of hormone into the blood. Rarely, radiation thyroiditis causes thyrotoxic crisis (see below), most commonly in elderly thyrotoxic patients with other systemic illness. For these reasons, patients with severe hyperthyroidism or underlying heart disease should be rendered eumetabolic with antithyroid agents before ^{131}I is administered. Interruption of antithyroid therapy for 3 to 4 days before and after ^{131}I treatment suffices to permit adequate accumulation and retention of administered ^{131}I. Propranolol may be used as an adjunct both before and after ^{131}I administration but should not be relied on to provide adequate prophylaxis if given alone. The swelling that accompanies radiation thyroiditis may contraindicate the use of large doses of ^{131}I in patients with large retrosternal goiters.

Before radioactive iodine was introduced, *subtotal thyroidectomy* was the standard ablative therapy, and it is still employed in younger patients in whom antithyroid therapy is unsuccessful. Although precise preoperative programs differ, several general principles should be emphasized. Patients should first be rendered euthyroid by means of antithyroid agents. Only then should iodide (five drops of Lugol's solution a day for approximately 10 days) be administered concomitantly to effect an involutional response in the gland. Antithyroid drugs should not be discontinued merely because treatment with iodide is instituted. The response of the patient, and not the calendar, should dictate when surgery is performed.

Hazards of subtotal thyroidectomy include immediate complications, such as anesthetic accidents, hemorrhage sometimes leading to respiratory obstruction, and damage to the recurrent laryngeal nerve leading to vocal cord paralysis. Later complications include wound infection, hemorrhage, hypoparathyroidism, and hypothyroidism. Subtotal thyroidectomy should be performed by a surgeon experienced in this procedure; under this condition, surgery is effective and relatively safe. Postoperative recurrences are uncommon. However, carefully conducted follow-up studies reveal that hypothyroidism follows surgery more frequently than previously suspected, although not as often as with conventional doses of ^{131}I.

The *treatment of hyperthyroidism during pregnancy* is a subject of some disagreement. Most physicians believe that antithyroid therapy is preferable to surgery, which should not be performed in any event during the first and third trimesters. Antithyroid agents carry less risk to the patient and the pregnancy. Further, since they traverse the placental barrier, they have the theoretical advantage of preventing fetal and neonatal hyperthyroidism when maternal titers of TRAbs are high. As a clue to the risk of fetal hyperthyroidism, assays of such stimulators should be conducted in the third trimester in pregnant women with a history of Graves' disease, whether treated or not. On the other hand, the major disadvantage of antithyroid therapy is the possibility of inducing hypothyroidism in the fetus. T_4 and T_3 traverse the human placenta from mother to fetus only slowly, and simultaneous administration of thyroid hormone and antithyroid drugs to the mother will not protect the fetus from hypothyroidism. Hence, the cardinal rule in using the antithyroid agents in pregnancy is that the dosage should be the smallest necessary to control hyperthyroidism in the mother. From the laboratory standpoint, the physician should aim to keep the serum TSH and FT_4 concentrations within the normal limits, remembering that pregnancy is normally associated with some elevation of the serum total T_4 owing to an increase in serum TBG concentration. Since pregnancy appears to attenuate the severity of hyperthyroidism, control can often be achieved with maintenance doses of 200 mg of propylthiouracil daily or less. At this dose, fetal goiter and hypothyroidism have not been a problem. Patients who require doses of 300 mg/d or more during the first trimester should probably be treated by subtotal thyroidectomy during the middle trimester. The author believes that patients carried through pregnancy on antithyroid agents should not be given propranolol as adjunctive treatment, in view of reports that the agent may cause fetal growth retardation and neonatal respiratory depression. Propylthiouracil tends to be favored over methimazole, even though earlier reports of fetal anomalies with the latter agent have not been confirmed. Advantages of propylthiouracil include its effect on inhibiting conversion of T_4 to T_3 and its higher degree of protein binding, which retards its excretion into breast milk. Radioiodine should never be administered to a pregnant woman, and all women of childbearing age who are about to receive ^{131}I should have a pregnancy test performed first.

Ophthalmopathy, Dermopathy Severe and progressive ophthalmopathy is the most difficult component of Graves' disease to treat satisfactorily. Fortunately, in most patients the disorder runs a benign course that is largely independent of the hyperthyroidism, and even moderately severe disease usually improves with time, although some exophthalmos and ophthalmoplegia may persist. In mild disease, considerable benefit may be obtained from simple measures, such as elevating the head at night, administering diuretics to reduce edema, and providing tinted glasses for protection from sun, wind, and foreign bodies. A 1% solution of methylcellulose or plastic shields may prevent corneal drying in patients unable to close the lids during sleep. In more severe cases with progressive exophthalmos, chemosis, ophthalmoplegia, or loss of vision, large doses of prednisone (100 to 120 mg/d) are usually effective in reducing the edematous and infiltrative components. With improvement, the dosage is reduced to the lowest effective level to minimize glucocorticoid excess. Orbital radiation may be helpful in some patients with acute, severe infiltrative manifestations, particularly when administered concomitantly with glucocorticoids. In cases that progress despite these measures, orbital decompression—i.e., removal of part of the bony orbit—is required to relieve intraorbital pressure. The management must always be conducted in concert with an ophthalmologist.

Severe dermopathy can be alleviated by the topical application of glucocorticoids; only 10 percent of patients achieve complete remission, and 40 to 50 percent achieve partial remission.

TOXIC MULTINODULAR GOITER

Toxic multinodular goiter is an occasional consequence of long-standing simple goiter, although the frequency with which this complication arises is uncertain. In areas where goiter is not endemic, the cause of nontoxic multinodular goiter is usually indeterminate. Hence, it is unclear whether a specific factor underlies those cases of nontoxic multinodular goiter that progress to the thyrotoxic phase. A common feature of many nontoxic multinodular goiters, even in areas of iodine sufficiency, is a decreased iodine content of thyroglobulin, a finding that suggests either a conditioned deficiency of iodine or an impairment of the normal incorporation of iodine into the protein. There is no pathologic feature to distinguish nontoxic from toxic multinodular goiter. However, the transition from nontoxic to toxic nodular goiter involves the development of functional autonomy, i.e., independence from TSH stimulation in one or more areas of the gland. Scattered foci of functional autonomy are demonstrable early in the disease process, and they increase in size and number with time so that about a fourth of seemingly euthyroid patients with nontoxic nodular goiter display, as evidence of functional autonomy, subnormal or absent responses to TRH administration. As judged from scintillation scanning, functional patterns may be of two types. In the more common type, iodine accumulation occurs diffusely in patchy foci throughout the gland, whereas in the less common pattern, iodine accumulates in one or more discrete nodules within the gland, the remainder of the gland appearing to be essentially nonfunctional. Histologic and autoradiographic studies reveal marked heterogeneity of structure and function, the two being poorly correlated. In both endemic and sporadic nontoxic multinodular goiter, administration of iodides may lead to the development of thyrotoxicosis (jodbasedow), a complication consonant with the functional autonomy of this disorder.

Because it arises on a background of long-standing simple goiter, toxic multinodular goiter is a disease of the aging or elderly. For this reason, and because of the nature of the underlying disease, the clinical presentation differs from that of Graves' disease. Ophthalmopathy is rare and would signal the emergence of Graves' disease superimposed on simple goiter. Some patients have typical thyrotoxicosis. Often, however, the thyrotoxicosis is less severe than that in Graves' disease, although its physiologic impact on specific organ systems may be great. Notable among these is the cardiovascular system, in which arrhythmias or congestive failure may be precipitated or accentuated by thyrotoxicosis that may be manifested elsewhere by only subtle findings (apathetic hyperthyroidism). Weakness and wasting may predominate, frequently with loss of appetite rather than hyperphagia, suggesting the presence of malignancy.

In some patients, a definitive diagnosis of toxic nodular goiter is difficult to establish. On the one hand, enlargement or nodularity of the gland may escape detection because the patient has a short neck or is kyphotic or because the thyroid is substernal. When this is the case, and when the clinical findings suggest thyrotoxicosis, RAIU determination and scintiscan are particularly helpful. On the other hand, even when a nodular goiter is palpable, the presence of mild but clinically significant thyrotoxicosis may be difficult to confirm, since values of the serum total T_4 and T_3, the FT_4, and FT_4I are often only slightly above normal. For example, a serum T_3 value that would be normal for a young adult may represent an increase in the elderly patient, since serum T_3 usually declines with age. Despite their value in situations such as this, thyroid suppression tests should rarely be undertaken in elderly patients because of the hazard of adverse cardiovascular responses. Unfortunately, although a normal response to TRH would exclude a diagnosis of thyrotoxicosis in a patient with a nodular goiter, subnormal responses do not establish the diagnosis. Responses to TRH decline in the elderly, especially in men, and seemingly euthyroid patients with nodular goiter may respond subnormally to TRH as a reflection of at least partial functional autonomy of the gland. An undetectable basal TSH and absent response to TRH by an ultrasensitive assay imply thyrotoxicosis (see Fig. 331-3). When laboratory and clinical findings do not permit a clear diagnosis of thyrotoxicosis, a therapeutic trial of antithyroid drugs may be useful.

Radioactive iodine is the treatment of choice for toxic multinodular goiter. In contrast to Graves' disease, large doses [740 to 1110 MBq (20 to 30 mCi)] are usually required, owing to the generally lower RAIU and the variable degree of function throughout the gland. Moreover, the physiologic instability of the elderly patient makes definitive treatment urgent. For the same reason, it is usually wise to initiate therapy with antithyroid agents, withholding radioiodine until a euthyroid state is achieved, thereby forestalling an exacerbation of thyrotoxicosis should radiation thyroiditis occur. Unless contraindicated, propranolol is often useful in controlling manifestations of thyrotoxicosis both before and after radioiodine therapy, while its therapeutic effect is awaited. Hypothyroidism is an uncommon consequence of radioiodine treatment of toxic multinodular goiter owing to the variable activity of differing portions of the gland, which permits previously quiescent areas to function in place of those destroyed by ^{131}I.

UNUSUAL VARIETIES OF THYROTOXICOSIS

Thyrotoxicosis is also seen in other disorders, including follicular adenoma of the thyroid and various forms of thyroiditis, which are discussed in later sections. This section will consider still other unusual causes of thyrotoxicosis and unusual ways in which thyrotoxicosis may present.

UNUSUAL CAUSES OF THYROTOXICOSIS Rarely, hyperthyroidism and thyrotoxicosis are the result of sustained hypersecretion of TSH either from a *TSH-secreting pituitary adenoma* or owing to a selective *resistance of the TSH-secretory mechanism* to feedback inhibition by thyroid hormones. The various syndromes in which both the pituitary and peripheral tissues are relatively resistant to thyroid hormones are discussed above. TSH-secreting pituitary adenomas can be distinguished, in many cases, by radiologic evidence of a pituitary tumor, by the fact that the concentration of free α subunits of TSH in serum is elevated, and by the fact that the response of the serum TSH to TRH is negligible. In the variant caused by pituitary resistance, subunit concentrations are not grossly elevated, and the TSH response to TRH is usually normal.

Patients with *trophoblastic tumor*, either choriocarcinoma or hydatidiform mole, frequently display elevations, sometimes marked, of serum total and free T_4 and T_3 concentrations. In addition to signs of pregnancy, the usual manifestations of thyrotoxicosis may be present, but ophthalmopathy is absent. Thyroid hyperfunction is caused by a circulating thyroid stimulator of trophoblastic origin, which is human chorionic gonadotropin (hCG), and the diagnosis may be confirmed by the finding of extremely high blood or urine levels of βhCG. Abnormal thyroid function tests remit promptly after removal of the tumor.

Thyrotoxicosis factitia is a form of thyrotoxicosis without hyperthyroidism that results from purposeful or inadvertent ingestion of large amounts of thyroid hormone. The syndrome is usually a form of malingering and occurs most commonly in women with an underlying psychiatric disorder, usually paramedical personnel, or in patients who have taken thyroid hormones in the past or who have relatives who take thyroid hormones. In such patients, endogenous thyroid function is suppressed, as evidenced by subnormal values of the RAIU and serum thyroglobulin concentration. Serum TSH is suppressed, and both serum T_4 and T_3 concentrations are increased if the patient is taking a preparation that contains T_4, whereas the serum T_3 concentration is elevated and the serum T_4 depressed in patients taking T_3 alone. Factitious hyperthyroidism also has been described in people who ingest ground meats contaminated with thyroid tissue.

Very rarely, thyrotoxicosis with a low RAIU is the result of excess hormone secretion by *ectopic thyroid tissue*, either widespread functioning metastases of thyroid carcinoma or struma ovarii.

The *jodbasedow phenomenon* refers to the induction of thyrotoxicosis in a previously euthyroid patient as a result of exposure to iodine. It typically occurs in areas of endemic iodine deficiency when measures to increase iodine intake are implemented. The presumption is that the supplemental iodine permits functionally autonomous thyroid tissue to produce and secrete excessive hormone. A similar phenomenon can occur in patients with nontoxic multinodular goiter who receive large doses of iodide. Since such patients tend to be elderly, with the danger of serious cardiovascular manifestations should thyrotoxicosis ensue, large doses of iodine should not be given to those with multinodular goiter. Similarly, in such patients, pharmaceuticals containing iodine, such as x-ray contrast media, should be used only when indicated and with consideration of the possible hazard of the jodbasedow phenomenon. When a contrast study is indicated under these conditions, it may be judicious to administer large doses of propylthiouracil (450 to 600 mg/d) prior to and for a week after the procedure. Some patients develop hyperthyroidism following exposure to large quantities of iodine despite the fact that after the iodine is withdrawn, they recover, thyroid function appears to be entirely normal, and there is no evidence of functional autonomy.

The antiarrhythmic drug amiodarone has multiple effects on thyroid function, including inhibition of the deiodination of T_4 to T_3, induction of hypothyroidism, and induction of hyperthyroidism. The drug contains 37 percent iodine, and amiodarone-induced thyrotoxicosis in patients with underlying Graves' disease or autonomous adenomas is consistent with the jodbasedow phenomenon; this disorder is associated with goiter, measurable RAIU, and normal to slightly elevated interleukin-6 (IL-6) levels and is managed like other forms of jodbasedow. In contrast, a variant of amiodarone-induced thyrotoxicosis in nongoitrous individuals is a type of "chemical" thyroiditis marked by very low RAIU and high IL-6 levels. The latter disorder may require treatment with perchlorate and glucocorticoids in addition to symptomatic management.

UNUSUAL PRESENTATIONS OF THYROTOXICOSIS

T_3 Toxicosis Thyrotoxicosis in which serum T_4 is normal or low in the absence of a deficiency of TBG, while the serum T_3 is increased, is termed *T_3 toxicosis*. Although the production rate of T_3 is increased disproportionately relative to that of T_4 in all forms of hyperthyroidism, in some patients with Graves' disease, multinodular goiter, or hyperfunctioning adenoma this discrepancy is exaggerated. The diagnosis should be suspected in a patient with clinical manifestations of thyrotoxicosis in whom the serum T_4 and FT_4 are normal or low and the RAIU is normal or increased. These features, together with the goiter, serve to differentiate this disorder from liothyronine-induced thyrotoxicosis factitia. In contrast to nonthyroidal disorders that mimic thyrotoxicosis, patients with this disorder have nonsuppressible thyroid function in response to exogenous T_3, undetectable serum TSH, and absent responses to TRH. In many patients, thyrotoxicosis with increased serum T_3 and normal serum T_4 precedes emergence of typical increases in both, either during an initial episode of hyperthyroidism or, more commonly, during recurrence after previous treatment. In some patients in whom symptoms of thyrotoxicosis fail to regress during antithyroid therapy despite return of the serum T_4 level to normal, the serum T_3 concentration is persistently elevated. Such patients are likely to experience a recurrence of thyrotoxicosis when antithyroid therapy is withdrawn.

T_4 Toxicosis In most patients with hyperthyroidism, the serum T_3 is increased relatively more than is the serum T_4. This fact reflects the fact that in hyperthyroidism T_3 generated from T_4 peripherally is supplemented by release of substantial quantities of T_3 from the thyroid. However, thyrotoxicosis sometimes is associated with a clear elevation of serum T_4 and a seemingly normal serum T_3 concentration. This syndrome of *T_4 toxicosis* occurs most commonly in the setting of prior excess iodine exposure in patients who are elderly, ill, or both. Increased iodine intake favors T_4 biosynthesis. In the absence of a history of excess iodine, the combination of a high serum T_4 concentration and a normal serum T_3 concentration presumably reflects inhibition of peripheral generation of T_3 from T_4 combined with persistence of T_3 and T_4 secretion from the thyroid.

MAJOR COMPLICATIONS OF THYROTOXICOSIS

CARDIAC DISEASE Thyrotoxicosis causes increases in both systolic and diastolic cardiac function, probably secondary to effects on the expression of genes for the contractile protein myosin. Untreated, the increased work eventually progresses to decompensation. The increased cardiac output and the peripheral effects of thyroid hormone impose a variety of burdens on the heart. Hypermetabolism of the peripheral tissues increases both the metabolic and the nonmetabolic (heat-loss) circulatory load, while direct effects of thyroid hormone on the myocardium cause rapid filling and increase the force, velocity, and rate of ventricular contraction. As a result, cardiac work and cardiac output are increased. Moreover, atrial irritability is enhanced, leading to arrhythmias, most importantly atrial fibrillation. In patients with a normal heart, these burdens are usually tolerated. When there is underlying heart disease, however, cardiac insufficiency may be precipitated or aggravated. These complications are more common in elderly patients and in patients with toxic multinodular goiter and sometimes are the most prominent manifestation of the thyrotoxic state. In patients with cardiac insufficiency, clues to the presence of thyrotoxicosis include atrial fibrillation, relatively rapid circulation time, increased cardiac output (high-output failure), and resistance to the usual therapeutic doses of digitalis. In a 10-year follow-up of older individuals in the Framingham Heart Study, a low serum TSH level ("subclinical hyperthyroidism)" was associated with a threefold increase in the risk of developing atrial fibrillation.

Rx TREATMENT

Treatment is directed at rapid alleviation of thyrotoxicosis and restoration of cardiac compensation. The former objective is best met by administration of large doses of an antithyroid agent, followed by iodine if the clinical situation is urgent. In less severe cases, radioiodine treatment is preceded by antithyroid drug treatment alone. The cardiac decompensation is managed in the usual manner, employing larger than usual doses of digitalis but with care to avoid digitalis intoxication as thyrotoxicosis is alleviated. Adrenergic antagonists should be used with caution in the presence of cardiac failure, unless failure is the consequence primarily of a disturbance of cardiac rate or rhythm.

THYROTOXIC CRISIS Thyrotoxic crisis, or storm, involves a fulminating increase in the signs and symptoms of thyrotoxicosis. In the past, this disturbance usually occurred postoperatively in patients poorly prepared for surgery. However, with the preoperative use of antithyroid drugs and iodide and with appropriate therapy to control metabolic factors, weight, and nutritional status, postoperative thyrotoxic crisis should not occur. Now, so-called medical storm is more common and occurs in untreated or inadequately treated patients. It is precipitated by surgical emergency or complicating illness, usually sepsis. The syndrome is characterized by extreme irritability, delirium or coma, fever to 41°C or more, tachycardia, restlessness, hypotension, vomiting, and diarrhea. Rarely, the picture may be more subtle, with apathy, prostration, and coma, but with only slight elevation of temperature. Such postoperative complications as sepsis, septicemia, hemorrhage, and transfusion or drug reactions may mimic thyrotoxic crisis. The physiologic factor(s) that initiates thyrotoxic crisis is unknown. It does not appear to be an acute increase in the severity of thyroid hyperfunction. Rather, it may represent a shift from protein-bound to free hormone secondary to circulating inhibitors to binding in systemic illness.

Rx TREATMENT

Treatment consists of providing supportive therapy while undertaking measures to alleviate thyrotoxicosis as rapidly as possible. Supportive therapy includes treatment of dehydration and the intravenous administration of glucose and saline, vitamin B complex, and glucocorticoids. The latter are indicated because of the increased glucocorticoid requirements in thyrotoxicosis and because adrenal reserve may be reduced. Patients should be placed in a cooled, humidified oxygen tent, and if hyperpyrexia is present a cooling blanket should be used. Digitalization is required to control ventricular rate in those with atrial fibrillation. If shock exists, intravenous pressor agents should be employed. Therapy of the hyperthyroidism consists of blockade of hormone synthesis by the immediate and continued administration of large doses of an antithyroid agent (e.g., 100 mg propylthiouracil every 2 h). If the patient is unable to swallow the medication, the tablets should be triturated and given by nasogastric tube or per rectum, since parenteral preparations are unavailable. Following initiation of antithyroid therapy, hormone release is inhibited through the administration of large doses of iodine intravenously or by mouth. The iodinated x-ray contrast agent sodium ipodate can be administered instead of iodine and has the added action of inhibiting the peripheral conversion of T_4 to T_3. Doses of 1 g/d are effective. Adrenergic antagonists are an important, and perhaps critical, part of the therapeutic regimen in the absence of cardiac failure. Propranolol can be administered in doses of 40 to 80 mg every 6 h. If medications cannot be taken orally, 2 mg propranolol may be given intravenously, with careful electrocardiographic monitoring. Large doses of dexamethasone (e.g., 2 mg every 6 h) also should be administered, since they inhibit hormone release, impair the peripheral generation of T_3 from T_4, and provide adrenal support. Indeed, with the combined use of propylthiouracil, iodine, and dexamethasone, the serum T_3 concentration generally returns to normal within 24 to 48 h. Dexamethasone may be tapered thereafter, while antithyroid therapy and iodine must be continued until a normal metabolic state is approached, at which time iodine is progressively withdrawn and plans are made for definitive treatment.

NEOPLASMS

The prevalence of solitary nodules of the thyroid gland increases with age, averaging 6.4 percent of women and 1.5 percent of men. Many palpable thyroid nodules thought to be solitary are actually part of a multinodular thyroid gland. High-resolution ultrasound identifies nodules in a third of patients being evaluated for nonthyroid indications, and autopsy studies reveal thyroid nodules in as many as 50 percent of necropsies. In general, a nodule must reach a size of 1 cm in diameter to be detectable by palpation. In addition to thyroid neoplasms, the differential diagnosis of apparent thyroid nodules includes cysts, adenopathy, cystic hygroma, parathyroid tumors, and laryngocele. True intrathyroidal nodules usually represent colloid adenomas or simple follicular adenomas.

THYROID ADENOMAS True adenomas, as opposed to localized adenomatous areas, are encapsulated and compress contiguous tissue. Adenomas vary in size and are classified into three histologic types: papillary, follicular, and Hürthle cell. The follicular adenomas can be subdivided according to the size of the follicles into colloid or macrofollicular, fetal or microfollicular, and embryonal varieties. Adenomas vary in physiologic differentiation, as judged by their ability to concentrate radioiodine. The more highly differentiated adenomas (follicular) are the most common and are the most likely to mimic the function of normal thyroid tissue. Though the function may be responsive to TSH stimulation, it usually differs from that of normal thyroid tissue in being autonomous; i.e., the basal activity is independent of TSH stimulation. Adenomas of this type are usually unifocal, presenting as a single nodule. Often the patient reports that the nodule has grown slowly over many years. Initially, its function is insufficient to disturb hormonal equilibrium, although its capacity to accumulate radioiodine is evident in scintiscans as an area of increased density within the still-functioning extranodular tissue (a *"warm" nodule*). At this stage, demonstration of inherent autonomy requires scintiscanning while the patient is receiving suppressive doses of exogenous thyroid hormone (suppression scan). With time, the nodule grows larger, its function increasing until it is sufficient to suppress TSH secretion. Consequently, the remainder of the gland undergoes relative atrophy and loss of function, and the scintiscan reveals radioiodine accumulation only in the region of the nodule (a *"hot" nodule*). At this time, TSH is suppressed ("chemical" thyrotoxicosis), but the patient may or may not be overtly thyrotoxic. Frank thyrotoxicosis usually supervenes eventually (*toxic adenoma*) and may be precipitated by iodine exposure, such as from radiographic contrast dyes. Hyperfunctioning adenomas are a relatively frequent cause of T_3 toxicosis. They are amenable to ablation by surgery or by treatment with ^{131}I. Large doses of the latter are usually required to bring about a prompt cure. Although it has been thought that radiation damage would be confined solely to the hyperfunctioning nodule being treated with ^{131}I, the remaining tissue being spared, this may not always be the case, since some patients with hyperfunctioning adenoma become euthyroid after treatment with ^{131}I, only to become hypothyroid years later.

Although hyperfunctioning nodules are rarely the seat of carcinoma, one advantage of surgical excision (usually lobectomy) is the acquisition of definitive histologic diagnosis. Nevertheless, surgery is recommended infrequently for hyperfunctioning nodules because of its associated risks, the low incidence of cancer, and the efficacy of radiodine. One exception may be nodules >4 cm in diameter, for which the required dose of radiation is so large as to create a risk of radiation-induced neoplasia in the contralateral lobe.

Hyperfunctioning adenomas may undergo hemorrhagic necrosis. The resulting pain and nodularity may suggest subacute thyroiditis. With infarction of the hyperfunctioning nodule, the subsequent loss of function causes TSH levels to return to normal and the previously suppressed extranodular thyroid tissue to resume functioning. The previously hyperfunctioning nodule may then appear as a *"cold" nodule* on scintiscanning, which, together with the history of pain, could be misinterpreted to represent a carcinoma. Indeed, hypofunctioning, hemorrhagic adenomas and thyroid cysts account for most of the cold nodules initially suspected of being carcinoma.

MALIGNANT TUMORS OF THE THYROID Owing to its rich vascular supply, the thyroid is a common site of secondary or metastatic cancers from primary tumors elsewhere. Some common sources include malignant melanoma and carcinomas of the lung, breast, and esophagus. The thyroid also may be the site of lymphoproliferative disease, namely *thyroid lymphoma*, which constitutes about 5 percent of all thyroid malignancies. Of the latter, large cell histocytic (or immunoblastic) lymphoma is the most common and typically occurs in women between the ages of 55 and 75, who often have chronic lymphocytic thyroiditis with positive serum antithyroglobulin or anti-TPO antibodies. Indeed, the risk of this tumor is so much higher in elderly patients with Hashimoto's thyroiditis that an enlarging thyroid mass should be considered to be thyroid lymphoma until an appropriate evaluation rules out the diagnosis. The prognosis depends on the cell type and the extent of disease beyond the neck. Variable success rates have been reported with combinations of surgery, radiation, and chemotherapy.

Primary thyroid carcinomas may be classified into two varieties depending on whether the lesion arises in thyroid follicular epithelium or from the parafollicular or C cells. The latter disorder, *medullary thyroid carcinoma* (MTC), may occur in four presentations: a sporadic form, which accounts for 80 percent of cases, and three familial forms, which account for the remaining 20 percent. Two of these familial forms occur as part of types 2A and 2B, respectively, of the multiple endocrine neoplasia (MEN) syndrome, and the third occurs in a non-MEN setting. In familial forms, the disease may be diagnosed early in family members by means of screening measurements of serum calcitonin. This assay is not recommended for the routine evaluation of thyroid nodules, because MTC occurs in <0.5 percent of thyroid nodules. Calcitonin measurement may be useful when the diagnosis of carcinoma is suggested by fine-needle aspiration. The MEN syndromes are discussed in detail in Chap. 340. In brief, MEN 2A is characterized by MTC with pheochromocytoma and in some cases hyperparathyroidism. The MTC of MEN 2A is often preceded by C cell hyperplasia and contains multifocal tumors. MEN 2B includes MTC, pheochromocytoma, and mucosal neuromata. The *RET* proto-oncogene is responsible for MEN 2A and 2B, and heterogeneous mutations in *RET* have also been identified in sporadic MTC.

The incidence of the sporadic form peaks in the sixth and seventh decades of life, and patients usually have cervical lymph node metastases at presentation. The tendency of the tumor and involved lymph nodes to calcify may provide a clue to the diagnosis when calcification is noted on x-rays of the neck. Serum calcitonin serves as a tumor marker for residual disease after treatment, and the serum levels correlate with tumor burden. The status of the *RET* gene can be assessed in samples obtained by fine-needle aspiration of a thyroid nodule; differentiation between the mutations known for sporadic versus familial MTC makes it possible to decide whether preoperative screening for pheochromocytoma is necessary. The mainstay of therapy is surgical excision. Preoperative diagnosis of MTC will prepare the surgeon to search for metastases and perform extensive lymph node dissection. External radiation therapy and chemotherapy have a palliative role for recurrent or residual disease.

Carcinomas of Follicular Epithelium Of the three general histologic types, *papillary* and *follicular carcinomas*, which tend to be slow growing, account respectively for 70 and 15 percent of all thyroid cancers, while *anaplastic carcinoma* is the least common, constituting approximately 5 percent of thyroid cancers. *Anaplastic carcinoma* usually occurs in the sixth or seventh decade of life. The tumor is histologically undifferentiated, composed largely of spindle and giant cells, fast-growing, and highly malignant. Despite radical surgery, the prognosis is dismal, with survival in months rather than years, although survival is better in younger patients with early disease. The rapidly fatal character of the lesion is due to extensive local invasion that is refractory to both external radiation therapy and radioiodine therapy (because the tumor does not concentrate iodine). The fact that many patients have coexisting differentiated carcinoma suggests that anaplastic tumors arise from the former, and metastases of papillary or follicular carcinoma can undergo late malignant dedifferentiation. Anaplastic thyroid carcinoma may be confused with lymphoma or sarcoma, and positive immunocytochemical stains for keratin or the cytoskeletal protein vimentin help to confirm the diagnosis. While thyroglobulin staining may be positive owing to entrapped follicular cells or colloid, measurements of serum thyroglobulin are of no diagnostic value as a tumor marker for this tumor in contrast to the situation in well-differentiated thyroid cancer. The lack of calcitonin immunoreactivity differentiates anaplastic carcinoma from undifferentiated medullary thyroid carcinoma.

Follicular carcinoma tends to occur in older individuals, resembles normal thyroid epithelium histologically, is encapsulated, and differs from benign follicular adenoma only by the presence of capsular and/or vascular invasion. These tumors can be classified as minimally, moderately, or highly invasive, and prognosis varies accordingly. One subtype of follicular carcinoma, the Hürthle cell tumor, tends to be more invasive, to metastasize frequently to bone, and to have an unfavorable clinical course. Follicular carcinoma undergoes early hematogenous spread, and the patient may present with a distant metastasis, usually in lung, bone, or the central nervous system. Lesions in bone are osteolytic. As for papillary carcinoma, large primary lesions are associated with worse prognosis, but even small lesions may metastasize widely. Rarely, the functioning mass of metastatic follicular carcinoma is great enough to cause increased serum levels of T_4 and/or T_3 and clinical thyrotoxicosis. Follicular carcinoma or follicular elements in papillary carcinoma are responsible for the instances in which thyroid carcinoma, in situ or metastatic, accumulates significant quantities of ^{131}I. The third and most common type of tumor, *papillary carcinoma*, has a bimodal frequency—i.e., peaks occur in the second and third decades and again in later life. This lesion is slow-growing and usually unencapsulated, and it may spread through the thyroid capsule to structures in the surrounding neck, especially the regional lymph nodes, where it may remain indolent for many years. The prognosis depends on the size of the original lesion, with tumors less than 2 cm in diameter having a potentially excellent outcome. The presence of involved lymph nodes may be associated with a greater risk of recurrence but not, apparently, with increased mortality. Acceleration of the disease may take place at any time. Follicular elements are usually present in both the primary lesion and its metastases. Papillary carcinoma is the most common thyroid malignancy to develop after exposure of the head and neck to radiation in childhood. Tumors in this setting are usually multicentric, thereby meriting more extensive thyroidectomy, but they are associated with a good prognosis.

Diagnosis and treatment The diagnosis and treatment of thyroid carcinoma are interwoven with the management of the nodular goiter. In the past, there were a wide variety of views on this subject, stemming from seemingly contradictory data. On the one hand, surgically excised specimens of thyroid nodules, particularly solitary nodules, revealed a high frequency of carcinoma (as much as 20 percent in some series). On the other hand, despite the incidence of nodular goiter in the general population (approximately 4 percent), the frequency of thyroid carcinoma, either newly diagnosed or as a cause of death, is low. These two lines of data led to either vigorous or conservative approaches to the management of nodular goiter. The discordance can be explained by the ability of the physician to select for surgery those patients who are at high risk of harboring thyroid carcinoma, with consequent weighting of statistics from surgical series. With the advent of fine-needle aspiration biopsy, this capability has increased, bringing us closer to the as yet unrealized aim of operating only on those patients whose thyroids harbor carcinoma and avoiding surgery in patients whose thyroids do not.

Several features suggest the presence of carcinoma. Recent growth of a thyroid nodule or mass, especially if rapid and unaccompanied by tenderness and hoarseness, should prompt suspicion. Of particular importance is a history of radiation to the head or neck or upper mediastinum in infancy or childhood, because it is associated with a high incidence of thyroid disease, including carcinoma, later in life. Nodular disease develops in approximately 20 percent of patients so exposed and may not be apparent until 30 years or more after the exposure. Among patients in this group who have palpable nodules, approximately one-third have thyroid carcinoma at surgery, often multicentric and sometimes metastatic. The risk for neoplasia correlates directly with younger age at exposure, female sex, and radiation dose. Patients who do not undergo surgery should be followed indefinitely and may be candidates for levothyroxine therapy.

Skillful palpation of the thyroid provides important information. A nodule in an otherwise normal gland (a solitary nodule) should raise more suspicion of thyroid tumor than does one nodule among many, since the latter is likely to be part of a diffuse process, such as simple goiter. In addition, carcinomas are usually firm or hard in consistency and nontender. Fixation to surrounding structures and lymphadenopathy are late features, although patients may present with a midline mass above the thyroid isthmus (a Delphian node) or lateral cervical adenopathy. Since purely cystic lesions, especially cysts less than a few centimeters in diameter, are less likely to reflect malignancy than solid lesions, transillumination and/or ultrasonography is sometimes helpful. The age and sex of the patient also influence the clinical decision. Benign nodular lesions are more common in women than in men; malignant nodular lesions less so. Hence, nodular lesions create more suspicion of carcinoma in men than in women.

Laboratory tests are of little assistance in differentiating between malignant and nonmalignant thyroid nodules. Overall thyroid function is usually normal. Except in patients with medullary thyroid carcinoma, in whom serum calcitonin concentrations may be elevated, tumor markers are of little value. Serum thyroglobulin is elevated in many patients with differentiated thyroid carcinoma, but this feature is not useful in the initial diagnosis, as it may be present in patients with benign adenoma, simple goiter, or Graves' disease. Soft tissue x-rays of the neck may be of assistance, since finely stippled calcification in the thyroid suggests the presence of psammoma bodies within a papillary carcinoma, and more dense calcifications may signify medullary carcinoma.

Fine-needle aspiration for cytology is the initial procedure of choice in the evaluation of most patients (Fig. 331-4). The technique is simple to learn, free of complications, and applicable to most nodules. Success depends on obtaining a satisfactory specimen and on expert histopathologic interpretation. When the latter is available, aspiration biopsy provides a reliable means of differentiating between benign and malignant nodules in all except highly cellular lesions or follicular lesions, where evidence of vascular invasion may be required to differentiate benign from malignant forms. Needle aspirates of papillary carcinoma may reveal psammoma bodies, lymphocytes suggestive of Hashimoto's disease, and large pink follicular cells with large pale nuclei ("Orphan Annie cells") and numerous nucleoli. Despite the occasional occurrence of false-positive and false-negative results, the procedure can reduce the number of operations performed for nodules that prove to be benign. Further, a diagnosis of carcinoma permits the surgery to be planned preoperatively.

While fine-needle aspiration for cytology is the keystone of the approach to the management of the patient with nodular goiter, less specific measures such as ultrasonography or scintillation scanning also may be useful. Although only approximately 20 percent of nonfunctioning thyroid nodules prove to be malignant, the demonstration that a nodule is "cold" on scintiscan adds substantial weight to other factors suggesting carcinoma. Hyperfunctioning nodules are rarely malignant. Ultrasonograms of the thyroid have value in demonstrating whether nodules are cystic, solid, or a mixture of the two. Cystic nodules can be aspirated, a procedure that is often curative, and their contents should be subjected to cytopathologic examination. Solid or mixed lesions are consistent with tumor but may be either benign or malignant.

When the cytologic results are equivocal, the physician must decide whether to continue to observe the patient; to administer suppressive doses of thyroid hormone in the expectation that the suspect nodule will shrink or disappear—a hope that in the author's experience is usually unrealized; or to proceed to excisional biopsy and thyroidectomy. Patients in whom the author chooses the latter course include those with a history of radiation to the thyroid and one or more clearly palpable nodules, as well as young men and women with solitary cold nodules, particularly nodules that are hard, nontender, and changing rapidly in size. In the remainder, thyroid hormone therapy with repeat aspiration cytology in 3 to 6 months is recommended.

Regardless of the operative procedure planned, surgery for thyroid carcinoma should be performed by a surgeon experienced in the procedure. Should surgery be delayed, suppressive therapy with levothyroxine is often recommended preoperatively to facilitate the operative procedure and perhaps decrease the likelihood of tumor dissemination. In patients in whom a definitive preoperative diagnosis has not been made, the suspected lesion is removed en bloc with a wide margin of surrounding tissue and is examined by frozen section. Opinions vary as to the preferable procedure when carcinoma is found. For lesions 2 cm or less in size that are not multicentric and have not metastasized, some recommend ipsilateral lobectomy, isthmectomy, and possibly contralateral partial lobectomy. Despite its higher rate of morbidity, the author prefers a near-total thyroidectomy, especially for lesions >2 cm in size, in view of the frequency with which tumor is seeded throughout the gland by transglandular lymphatic spread and of evidence that both recurrence rates and subsequent mortality are lower after the more extensive operation. Regional lymph nodes should be explored and removed if there is evidence of involvement, but radical neck dissection is not justified. If permanent sections reveal carcinoma when frozen sections had failed to do so and the initial procedure was limited, secondary surgery should be undertaken to remove residual thyroid tissue, preferably within a few days. A more complete thyroidectomy is warranted for follicular carcinoma in view of its tendency to metastasize to distant sites. This is so because the metastases do not concentrate adequate ^{131}I in the presence of residual normal thyroid tissue, which both competes for the ^{131}I and prevents the increase in serum TSH required to stimulate uptake by tumor cells.

The need for postoperative ablation of the thyroid remnant with radioiodine and for subsequent periodic radioisotopic scanning for residual or recurrent disease varies with the histologic type of cancer, size of lesion, presence of metastases, and other indications of invasiveness or aggressiveness. Radioiodine treatment of known residual disease is associated with clinical improvement and reduced recurrence rates, but it is not clear whether mortality rates are improved by prophylactic postoperative ablation. Papillary cancers that are <1.5 cm in size and are unaccompanied by nodal metastases tend to have an excellent prognosis, and it is questionable whether ablation of the residual normal thyroid bed and subsequent scanning are necessary. The author favors a more conservative approach in such cases, only administering levothyroxine suppression with periodic follow-up determinations of serum thyroglobulin levels.

Total-body scintiscanning with ^{131}I is the method employed to evaluate for residual normal or malignant thyroid tissue in the neck and for distant metastases. Postoperatively, if replacement therapy is

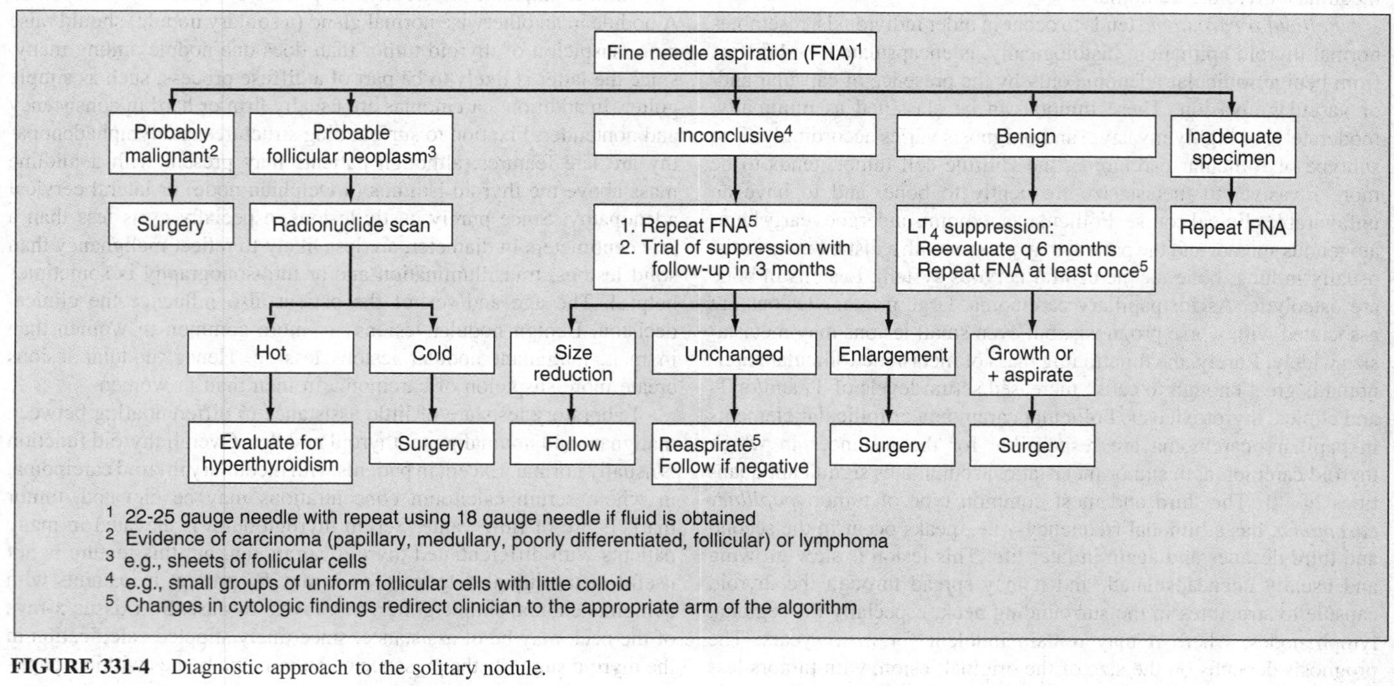

FIGURE 331-4 Diagnostic approach to the solitary nodule.

initiated with liothyronine (50 to 75 μg) rather than levothyroxine, a more rapid increase in TSH secretion is seen when the liothyronine is withdrawn some 3 weeks later. After an additional 2 or 3 weeks without any thyroid hormone replacement, when the serum TSH concentration has risen to the range of 50 mU/L, a large scanning dose of ^{131}I [185 to 370 MBq (5 to 10 mCi)] is administered and whole-body scans are obtained at 72 h. If residual thyroid tissue is found, as is usually the case, a thyroid-ablating dose of 1850 to 2220 MBq (50 to 60 mCi) of ^{131}I is administered; if functioning metastases are present, the dose is doubled. Suppressive therapy with levothyroxine is reinstituted 24 to 48 h later. Approximately 1 week after administration of the second (treatment) dose of ^{131}I, whole-body scans are repeated, since the larger dose of radioiodine may permit demonstration of functioning metastases not seen after the smaller initial dose. When metastases are found, some clinics withdraw suppressive therapy, administer an additional 3700 MBq (100 mCi) of ^{131}I, and then reinstitute suppressive therapy with levothyroxine. The future availability of recombinant human TSH for parenteral injection promises to make it unnecessary to discontinue thyroid hormone therapy for scanning. In some patients, only measurements of serum thyroglobulin before and after TSH injection might be performed, with follow-up scanning solely in those in whom a significant rise in thyroglobulin is seen. A practical consideration is whether the high doses of ^{131}I (a β-particle emitter) used for diagnostic scanning may have an adverse effect on the subsequent uptake of the therapeutic dose, a phenomenon that has been called "stunning." Pending an answer to this question, some centers employ ^{123}I (a pure γ-ray emitter) for initial scans and ^{131}I only when the ^{123}I scan is negative but residual disease is suspected on the basis of elevated serum thyroglobulin levels.

Patients are reexamined approximately 6 months after the initial operation and at least every 6 months for several years thereafter. At these examinations, the neck is palpated for evidence of recurrence of metastases, which often can be treated with selective surgical removal. Blood is drawn for a serum thyroglobulin measurement, since elevated values in patients receiving suppressive therapy signal the presence of metastatic disease. At the initial 6-month examination, patients in whom metastases had previously been found are prepared for a whole-body scan as described above. Those in whom no metastases have been demonstrated by earlier scans are not rescanned unless the serum thyroglobulin is elevated but are rescanned approximately 1 year after the initial surgery. Patients in whom whole-body scans are positive are reentered into the therapeutic algorithm, as described above. Those in whom scans are negative continue to be reexamined and have measurements of serum thyroglobulin concentrations at regular intervals. If both serum thyroglobulin concentrations and scans are unrevealing, patients are scanned for the last time after approximately 3 years, unless serum thyroglobulin concentrations rise. In some patients, serum thyroglobulin may be elevated despite the absence of demonstrable functioning metastases. Some patients treated with high-dose ^{131}I, irrespective of the fractional uptake, are said to exhibit a reduction in serum thyroglobulin, ostensibly reflecting therapeutic benefit. Alternatively, the patients can be imaged by CT or MRI to ascertain the site of the thyroglobulin-secreting metastases and to determine whether they may be amenable to external radiation.

A program of this nature, involving near-total thyroidectomy, long-term suppressive therapy, and treatment of functioning metastases with radioiodine, reduces the recurrence rate and prolongs survival in patients with papillary carcinoma of the thyroid. Follicular carcinoma should be treated with even greater vigor, since the results are generally less favorable. Because follicular carcinoma metastasizes to lung and bone, appropriate follow-up x-rays and measurements of serum thyroglobulin should be performed. Mixed differentiated tumors with both follicular and papillary elements tend to behave biologically as papillary tumors and should be so managed. Radioiodine treatment of medullary thyroid carcinoma is usually not successful; the cases that show some reduction in serum calcitonin possibly represent a rare variant of mixed medullary and follicular cancer. Treatment of anaplastic carcinoma is largely palliative; most patients die within 6 months of diagnosis.

THYROIDITIS

The term *thyroiditis* embraces disorders of differing etiology. *Pyogenic thyroiditis* and *chronic fibrosing (Riedel's) thyroiditis* are rare. Pyogenic thyroiditis is usually preceded by infection elsewhere and is characterized by tenderness and swelling of the thyroid, redness and warmth of the overlying skin, and constitutional signs of infection. Treatment consists of antibiotic therapy and incisional drainage of any fluctuant areas in the thyroid. Patients with AIDS may present with thyroiditis due to unusual organisms such as *Pneumocystis carinii*. Riedel's thyroiditis is a disorder in which intense fibrosis of the thyroid and surrounding structures causes induration of the neck and may be associated with mediastinal and retroperitoneal fibrosis. This disorder must be differentiated from thyroid neoplasia. The other forms of thyroiditis—subacute thyroiditis, chronic thyroiditis with transient thyrotoxicosis, and Hashimoto's thyroiditis—are more common. They are notable for their different clinical courses and for the fact that each can be associated, at one time or another, with a euthyroid, thyrotoxic, or hypothyroid state.

SUBACUTE THYROIDITIS This disorder, also termed *granulomatous, giant cell*, or *de Quervain's thyroiditis*, is viral in origin. Symptoms of thyroiditis usually follow those of an upper respiratory infection and include pronounced asthenia, malaise, and symptoms referable to stretching of the thyroid capsule, principally pain over the thyroid or pain referred to the lower jaw, ear, or occiput. Referred pain may predominate. These symptoms may smolder for weeks before the diagnosis is suspected. Less commonly, the onset is acute, with severe pain over the thyroid, fever, and occasionally symptoms of thyrotoxicosis. Physical findings include exquisite tenderness and nodularity of the thyroid, which may be unilateral but usually involves other areas of the gland. Although local or referred pain is usual, occasional patients have other features typical of the disease but no pain.

Two laboratory findings are characteristic: a high erythrocyte sedimentation rate (ESR) and a depressed RAIU. Values for the remaining tests depend on the stage of the disease at which they are obtained. Early, many patients are mildly thyrotoxic owing to leakage of hormone from the gland. The serum T_4 and T_3 are high, and TSH is undetectable. Later, as glandular hormone is depleted, the patient may pass through a hypothyroid phase, in which serum T_4 and T_3 are low and TSH is increased. Serum levels of the cytokine IL-6 increase during the thyrotoxic phase and return to normal with recovery. This phenomenon is presumed to relate to thyroid destruction; IL-6 levels are also elevated in amiodarone-induced thyroiditis, after radioiodine therapy, and after the therapeutic injection of ethanol into toxic adenomas. Diagnosis of the thyrotoxic phase is especially troublesome in the painless variant because the patient may be thought to have Graves' disease or toxic nodular goiter, and therapy inappropriate for subacute thyroiditis may be instituted. Demonstration of a low RAIU usually serves to differentiate subacute thyroiditis from these other causes of hyperthyroidism. Differentiation of painless subacute thyroiditis from chronic thyroiditis with transient thyrotoxicosis is discussed below.

The disorder may smolder for months but eventually subsides with a return of normal thyroid function. In mild cases, aspirin suffices to control the symptoms. In more severe cases, glucocorticoids (prednisone, 20 to 40 mg/d) are generally effective. Propranolol can be used to control associated thyrotoxicosis. When the RAIU and serum T_4 return to normal, therapy can be withdrawn without recurrence of symptoms.

CHRONIC THYROIDITIS WITH TRANSIENT THYROTOXICOSIS This term denotes a disorder in which a self-limited episode of thyrotoxicosis is associated with a histologic picture of chronic lymphocytic thyroiditis that differs from that of Hashimoto's disease. This syndrome has been variously designated as *painless thyroiditis, silent thyroiditis, hyperthyroiditis, chronic thyroiditis with spontaneously resolving hyperthyroidism*, or, as the author prefers, *chronic thyroiditis with transient thyrotoxicosis* (CT/TT). Designations that imply the existence of hyperthyroidism are inappropriate, since ongoing production of thyroid hormone is negligible and the RAIU is decreased.

The syndrome occurs in patients of any age and mainly in women. Manifestations of thyrotoxicosis are usually mild but may be severe. The thyroid is nontender, firm, symmetric, and slightly or moderately enlarged. Findings include elevations of the serum T_4 and T_3 levels consonant with the thyrotoxicosis and a depressed RAIU. The ESR is normal or slightly elevated, rarely exceeding 50 mm/h, and antithyroid antibodies, when present, are low in titer.

The etiology, pathogenesis, and pathophysiology of this disorder are unclear. Viral antibody titers show no characteristic patterns. It is presumed that thyrotoxicosis results from leakage of hormone from the gland, as in subacute thyroiditis. Low values for the RAIU, in turn, reflect hormonal suppression of TSH secretion and not increased plasma iodine, since urinary iodine excretion is not greatly elevated. Some degree of thyroid malfunction is indicated by failure of the RAIU to respond briskly to exogenous TSH stimulation.

Thyrotoxicosis in CT/TT usually abates within 2 to 5 months, and the thyrotoxic phase may be followed by a hypothyroid phase. The latter is usually self-limited and may be the only component of the disease recognized if the thyrotoxic phase is brief. Most patients recover completely; some have recurent episodes.

A variant of CT/TT after pregnancy is termed *postpartum thyroiditis*. This disorder develops within 2 to 6 months after delivery in 5 to 6 percent of otherwise normal women and in about one-fourth of women with insulin-dependent diabetes mellitus. Such patients usually have a small goiter and a family history of thyroid disease and may have postpartum depression. Within the first 2 to 3 months post partum, transient symptoms of thyrotoxicosis, such as fatigue, palpitations, emotional lability, and heat intolerance, are likely. Laboratory findings include elevated serum levels of T_4 and T_3, suppressed TSH, elevated titers of antithyroid antibodies, and a low RAIU. Patients may undergo a subsequent hypothyroid phase (from 4 to 8 months post partum) associated with a low serum T_4 level, elevated TSH, and high titers of autoantibodies. These patients require symptomatic management with levothyroxine until the thyroid recovers. Women who become pregnant again are at risk for recurrent postpartum thyroiditis.

In the thyrotoxic phase, this disorder can be differentiated from Graves' disease by demonstration of a depressed RAIU and the absence of increased urinary iodine excretion. The latter finding also excludes the jodbasedow syndrome. When these data are available, the disorder must be differentiated from other causes of thyrotoxicosis with a low RAIU, principally subacute thyroiditis. Lack of tenderness or nodularity of the thyroid and absence of marked elevation of the ESR tend to exclude the latter diagnosis. Patients with either functioning ectopic thyroid tissue or thyrotoxicosis factitia characteristically respond to exogenous TSH stimulation with a brisk increase in RAIU. Definitive diagnosis of CT/TT can be made by thyroid biopsy.

Since the thyroid is not hyperfunctioning in this disorder, measures used in the treatment of hyperthyroidism are useless. Propranolol may be administered until the thyrotoxicosis abates.

HASHIMOTO'S THYROIDITIS This disorder, also termed *lymphadenoid goiter*, is a common chronic inflammatory disease of the thyroid in which autoimmune factors play a prominent role. It occurs most frequently in women of middle age and is the most common cause of sporadic goiter in children. Evidence of the participation of autoimmune factors includes the lymphocytic infiltration of the gland and the presence in the serum of increased concentrations of immunoglobulins and antibodies against several components of thyroid tissue. Of these, the most important from the clinical standpoint are the antithyroglobulin antibody, detected by the tanned red cell agglutination test, and antithyroid peroxidase (anti-TPO or antimicrosomal) antibody, detected by immunofluorescence, complement fixation, or the more sensitive enzyme-linked immunosorbent assay (ELISA). These autoantibodies probably reflect but do not cause the thyroid destruction noted in autoimmune thyroid disease. The cloning and sequencing of the genes that encode the three major thyroid antigens—thyroglobulin, thyroid peroxidase, and the TSH receptor—have made possible detailed characterization of these autoantibodies. Hashimoto's thyroiditis also coexists with some frequency with other diseases of an autoimmune nature, including pernicious anemia, Sjögren's syndrome, chronic active hepatitis, systemic lupus erythematosus, rheumatoid arthritis, adrenal insufficiency, diabetes mellitus, and Graves' disease itself (see Chap. 340). These disorders, as well as Hashimoto's disease, also occur frequently in family members of patients with Hashimoto's disease. An association of HLA-DR3 and -DR5 with the atrophic and goitrous forms of Hashimoto's disease, respectively, has been noted. It is unclear whether Hashimoto's thyroiditis is a frequent precursor of the atrophic thyroid of primary hypothyroidism. The prevalence of Hashimoto's thyroiditis appears to be increasing, and the disorder is more common in the United States than in Europe. Increased iodine ingestion has been proposed as an explanation.

In the usual presentation of the disease, goiter is the outstanding feature. The enlargement involves the entire gland, but not necessarily symmetrically. Typically, the consistency is rubbery, the margins are scalloped, and the general outline of the gland is preserved. The pyramidal lobe may be prominent. Early in the disease the patient is metabolically normal; even then decreased thyroid reserve is often manifest in an increase in serum TSH. The RAIU may be elevated early, reflecting the secretion of physiologically inactive iodoproteins, but the serum T_4 and T_3 are normal, and the patient is euthyroid. As the disease progresses, thyroid failure, at first subclinical, may supervene owing to progressive replacement of thyroid parenchyma by lymphocytes or fibrous tissue. The thyroid failure is manifested first by a rise in serum TSH concentration. With time, the serum T_4 level declines, though the serum T_3 level remains normal. Eventually, the serum T_3 level falls, and frank hypothyroidism supervenes. Autoimmune thyroiditis, including Hashimoto's disease, may account for as many as 90 percent of cases of hypothyroidism. High titers of anti-TPO antibody are almost always present. High titers also may occur in other thyroid disorders, particularly primary thyroprivic hypothyroidism and Graves' disease, but with lesser frequency. Although the foregoing findings usually suffice to permit a diagnosis, histologic confirmation may be obtained by needle biopsy. An elevated serum TSH dictates that levothyroxine therapy be given. Treatment is probably also indicated in patients with marginally elevated TSH levels and positive antibody titers, in view of the frequency with which hypothyroidism eventually develops. In some patients, replacement therapy is associated with regression of goiter. Pregnant women with high antibody titers may be at a higher risk for miscarriage, independent of the thyroid status.

Occasional patients present with hyperthyroidism in association with a thyroid gland that is unusually firm and with high titers of circulating antithyroid antibodies, a combination that suggests, probably correctly, the concurrence of Graves' disease and Hashimoto's thyroiditis ("Hashitoxicosis"). In others, hyperthyroidism supervenes in a patient known to have Hashimoto's thyroiditis, presumably owing to the emergence of clones of lymphocytes that produce stimulatory anti-TSH receptor antibodies. Hyperthyroidism in association with Hashimoto's thyroiditis is treated in a conventional manner, but ablative therapy is less commonly employed, since the associated chronic thyroiditis tends to limit the duration of thyroid hyperfunction and also predisposes the patient to the development of hypothyroidism after surgical or radioiodine treatment.

Please refer to Chap. 57 in Goodman & Gilman's The Pharmacological Basis of Therapeutics, *9th ed, McGraw-Hill, New York, 1996.*

BIBLIOGRAPHY

AIN KB: Papillary thyroid carcinoma: Etiology, assessment, and therapy. Endocrin Metab Clin North Am 24:711, 1995

AYALA A, WARTOFSKY L: Minimally symptomatic (subclinical) hypothyroidism. The Endocrinologist 7:44, 1997

BRUCKER-DAVIS F et al: Genetic and clinical features of 42 kindreds with resistance to thyroid hormone. Ann Intern Med 123:572, 1995

BURCH HB: Evaluation and management of the solid thyroid nodule. Endocrin Metab Clin North Am 24:663, 1995

———, Wartofsky L: Graves' ophthalmopathy: Current concepts regarding pathogenesis and management. Endocr Rev 14:747, 1993
Burrow GN: Thyroid function and hyperfunction during gestation. Endocr Rev 14:194, 1993
DeGroot LJ et al: Therapeutic controversies: Radiation and Graves' ophthalmopathy. J Clin Endocrinol Metab 80:339, 1995
Fatourechi V et al: Dermopathy of Graves' disease (pretibial myxedema). Medicine 73:1, 1994
Franklin JA: The management of hyperthyroidism. N Engl J Med 330:1731, 1994
Grebe SKG, Hay ID: Follicular thyroid cancer. Endocrin Metab Clin North Am 24:761, 1995
Haden ST et al: Subclinical hyperthyroidism. The Endocrinologist 6:322, 1996
Levetan C, Wartofsky L: A clinical guide to the management of Graves' disease with radioactive iodine. Endocrine Practice 1:205, 1995
Mahoney KM, Wartofsky L: Significance of alterations in thyroid function tests in the critical care setting. J Intens Care Med 7:318, 1992
Marsh DJ et al: Medullary thyroid carcinoma: Recent advances and management update. Thyroid 5:407, 1995
Masters PA, Simons RJ: Clinical use of sensitive assays for thyroid-stimulating hormone. J Gen Intern Med 11:115, 1996
Mazzaferri EL, Jhiang SM: Long-term impact of initial surgical and medical therapy on papillary and follicular thyroid cancer. Am J Med 97:418, 1994
Oertel YC: Fine-needle aspiration and the diagnosis of thyroid cancer. Endocrin Metab Clin North Am 25:69, 1996
Oppenheimer JH et al: A therapeutic controversy. Thyroid hormone therapy: When and what? J Clin Endocrinol Metab 80:2873, 1995
Refetoff S et al: The syndromes of resistance to thyroid hormone. Endocr Rev 14:348, 1993; Update 1994, Endocr Rev Monographs 3:336, 1994
Sarne DH, Schneider AB: External radiation and thyroid neoplasia. Endocrin Metab Clin North Am 25:181, 1996
Singer PA: Thyroiditis: Acute, subacute, and chronic. Med Clin North Am 75:61, 1991
——— et al: Treatment guidelines for patients with hyperthyroidism and hypothyroidism. JAMA 273:808, 1995
Smallridge RC: Postpartum thyroid dysfunction: A frequently undiagnosed endocrine disorder. The Endocrinologist 6:44, 1996
Surks MI et al: American Thyroid Association guidelines for use of laboratory tests in thyroid disorders. JAMA 263:1529, 1990
———, Sievert R: Drugs and thyroid function. N Engl J Med 333:1688, 1995
Toft AD: Thyroxine therapy. N Engl J Med 331:174, 1994
Torrens JI, Burch HB: Serum thyroglobulin measurement: Utility in clinical practice. Endocrinologist 6:125, 1996
Van Sande J et al: Somatic and germline mutations of the TSH receptor gene in thyroid diseases. J Clin Endocrinol Metab 80:2577, 1995
Wartofsky L: Myxedema coma, in *The Thyroid*, 7th ed, LE Braverman, RD Utiger (eds). Philadelphia, Lippincott, 1996, p 871
———: Thyrotoxic storm, in *The Thyroid*, 7th ed, LE Braverman, RD Utiger (eds). Philadelphia, Lippincott, 1996, p 701
Weetman AP, McGregor AM: Autoimmune thyroid disease: Further developments in our understanding. Endocr Rev 15:788, 1994
Wohllk N et al: Application of genetic screening information to the management of medullary thyroid carcinoma and multiple endocrine neoplasia Type 2. Endocrin Metab Clin North Am 25:1, 1996

332

Gordon H. Williams, Robert G. Dluhy

DISEASES OF THE ADRENAL CORTEX

BIOCHEMISTRY AND PHYSIOLOGY

STEROID NOMENCLATURE Steroids contain as their basic structure a cyclopentenoperhydrophenanthrane nucleus consisting of three 6-carbon hexane rings and a single 5-carbon pentane ring (Fig. 332-1). The carbon atoms are numbered in a sequence beginning with ring A. Adrenal steroids contain either 19 or 21 carbon atoms. The C_{19} steroids have methyl groups at C-18 and C-19. C_{19} steroids with a ketone group at C-17 are termed *17-ketosteroids*. The C_{19} steroids have predominantly androgenic activity. The C_{21} steroids have a 2-carbon side chain (C-20 and C-21) attached at position 17 and methyl groups at C-18 and C-19. C_{21} steroids with a hydroxyl group at position 17 are termed *17-hydroxycorticosteroids*. The C_{21} steroids have either glucocorticoid or mineralocorticoid properties. A *glucocorticoid* is a C_{21} steroid that acts predominantly on intermediary metabolism; a *mineralocorticoid* is a C_{21} steroid that acts predominantly on the metabolism of sodium and potassium.

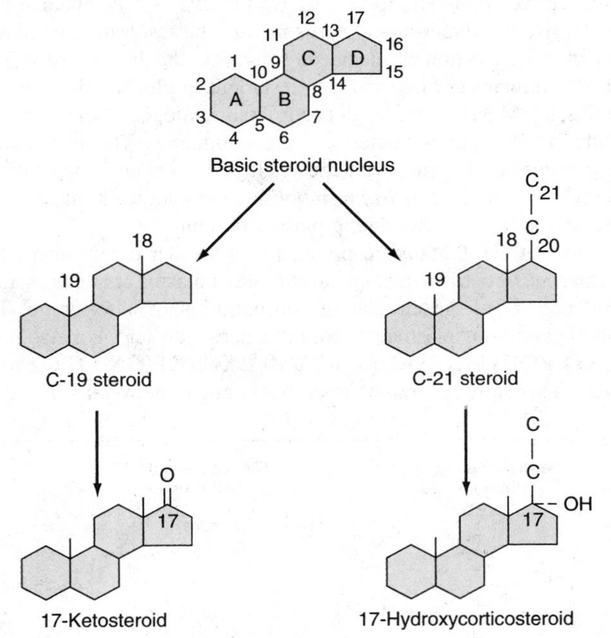

FIGURE 332-1 Basic steroid structure and nomenclature.

BIOSYNTHESIS OF ADRENAL STEROIDS Cholesterol, derived from the diet and from endogenous synthesis, is the substrate for steroidogenesis. Uptake of cholesterol by the adrenal cortex is mediated by the low-density lipoprotein (LDL) receptor. With long-term stimulation of the adrenal cortex by adrenocorticotropic hormone (ACTH), the number of LDL receptors increases. The three major adrenal biosynthetic pathways lead to the production of glucocorticoids (cortisol), mineralocorticoids (aldosterone), and adrenal androgens (dehydroepiandrosterone). Separate zones of the adrenal cortex synthesize specific hormones; this facts reflects the enzymatic capacity of each zone to carry out certain transformations and hydroxylations (Fig. 332-2). The outer (glomerulosa) zone contains the enzymes for aldosterone biosynthesis, and the inner (fasciculata-reticularis) zone is the site of cortisol and androgen biosynthesis.

STEROID TRANSPORT Some steroid hormones, e.g., testosterone and cortisol, circulate bound to a considerable extent to plasma proteins. Cortisol occurs in the plasma in three forms: free cortisol, protein-bound cortisol, and cortisol metabolites. *Free cortisol* is physiologically active hormone that is not protein-bound and, therefore, that can act directly on tissue sites. Normally, less than 5 percent of circulating cortisol is free. Only the unbound cortisol and its metabolites are filterable at the glomerulus. Increased quantities of free steroid are excreted in the urine in states characterized by hypersecretion of cortisol, because the unbound fraction of plasma cortisol rises. *Protein-bound cortisol* is bound reversibly to circulating plasma proteins. Plasma has two cortisol-binding systems. One is a high-affinity, low-capacity alpha$_2$ globulin termed *transcortin* or *cortisol-binding globulin* (CBG), and the other is a low-affinity, high-capacity protein, *albumin*. The binding affinity of CBG for cortisol is reduced in areas of inflammation, thus increasing the local concentration of free cortisol. CBG in normal human plasma can bind approximately 700 nmol of cortisol per liter (25 μg/dL). When the concentration of cortisol exceeds this level, part of the excess binds to albumin, and a greater proportion than usual circulates unbound. For example, when the total cortisol level is 1400 nmol/L (50 μg/dL), 25 percent is free. The CBG level is increased in high-estrogen states (e.g., pregnancy, oral contraceptive administration). The rise in CBG is accompanied by a parallel rise in protein-bound cortisol, with the result that the plasma cortisol concentration is elevated. However, the free cortisol level probably remains normal, and manifestations of glucocorticoid excess are absent. Most synthetic glucocorticoid analogues bind less efficiently to CBG (approximately 70 percent binding). This may explain the propensity of some synthetic analogues to produce cushingoid effects at low doses. *Cortisol metabolites* are biologically inactive and bind only weakly to circulating plasma proteins.

Aldosterone is bound to proteins to a smaller extent than either testosterone or cortisol, and an ultrafiltrate of plasma contains as much as 50 percent of the circulating concentration of aldosterone. This limited binding by plasma protein influences aldosterone metabolism.

STEROID METABOLISM AND EXCRETION **Glucocorticoids** The daily secretion of cortisol ranges between 40 and 80 μmol (15 and 30 mg), with a pronounced circadian cycle. Cortisol is distributed in a volume of body fluids approximating the total extracellular fluid space, with more than 90 percent in the protein-bound fraction. The plasma concentration of cortisol is determined by the rate of secretion, the rate of inactivation, and the rate of excretion of free cortisol. The liver is the major organ responsible for steroid inactivation. The major pathway is reduction of ring A and conjugation of the reduced products with glucuronic acid at position C-3 to form water-soluble compounds. The enzyme 11β-hydroxysteroid dehydrogenase converts cortisol to the inactive metabolite cortisone in the kidney. The activity of this enzyme is influenced by the level of circulating thyroid hormone, the oxidative reaction being increased in hyperthyroidism.

Mineralocorticoids In normal subjects with a normal salt intake, the average daily secretion of aldosterone ranges between 0.1 and 0.7 μmol (50 and 250 μg). Since aldosterone binds only weakly to proteins, its volume of distribution is larger than that of cortisol, being approximately 35 L. During a single passage through the liver, more than 75 percent of circulating aldosterone is normally inactivated by ring A reduction and conjugation with glucuronic acid. However, under certain conditions, such as congestive failure, this rate of inactivation is reduced.

From 7 to 15 percent of aldosterone is excreted in the urine as a glucuronide conjugate, from which free aldosterone is released on standing at pH 1. This *acid-labile conjugate* is formed in the liver and kidney. For persons with an average salt intake, the 24-h urine excretion of the acid-labile conjugate ranges from 15 to 50 nmol (5 to 19 μg), that of the reduced derivative ranges from 70 to 100 nmol (25 to 35 μg), and that of the nonconjugated, nonreduced free aldosterone ranges from 0.5 to 2 nmol (0.2 to 0.6 μg).

Adrenal Androgens The major androgen secreted by the adrenal is dehydroepiandrosterone (DHEA) and its C-3 sulfuric acid ester. From 15 to 30 mg of these compounds is secreted daily. Smaller amounts of androstenedione, 11β-hydroxyandrostenedione, and testosterone are secreted. DHEA is the major precursor of the urinary 17-ketosteroids. Two-thirds of the urine 17-ketosteroids in the male are derived from adrenal metabolites, and the remaining one-third comes from testicular androgens. In the female, almost all urine 17-ketosteroids are derived from the adrenal.

Steroids diffuse passively through the cell membrane and bind to intracellular receptors (see Chap. 327). These receptors are part of a superfamily of transcription regulatory factors that includes the thyroid hormone receptor. Glucocorticoid receptors are of two types: I and II. The type I receptor is the same as the mineralocorticoid receptor. Mineralocorticoids do not bind to the type II receptor, but most glucocorticoids bind to either receptor, although with different affinities. After the steroid binds to the receptor, the steroid-receptor complex is transported to the nucleus, where it binds

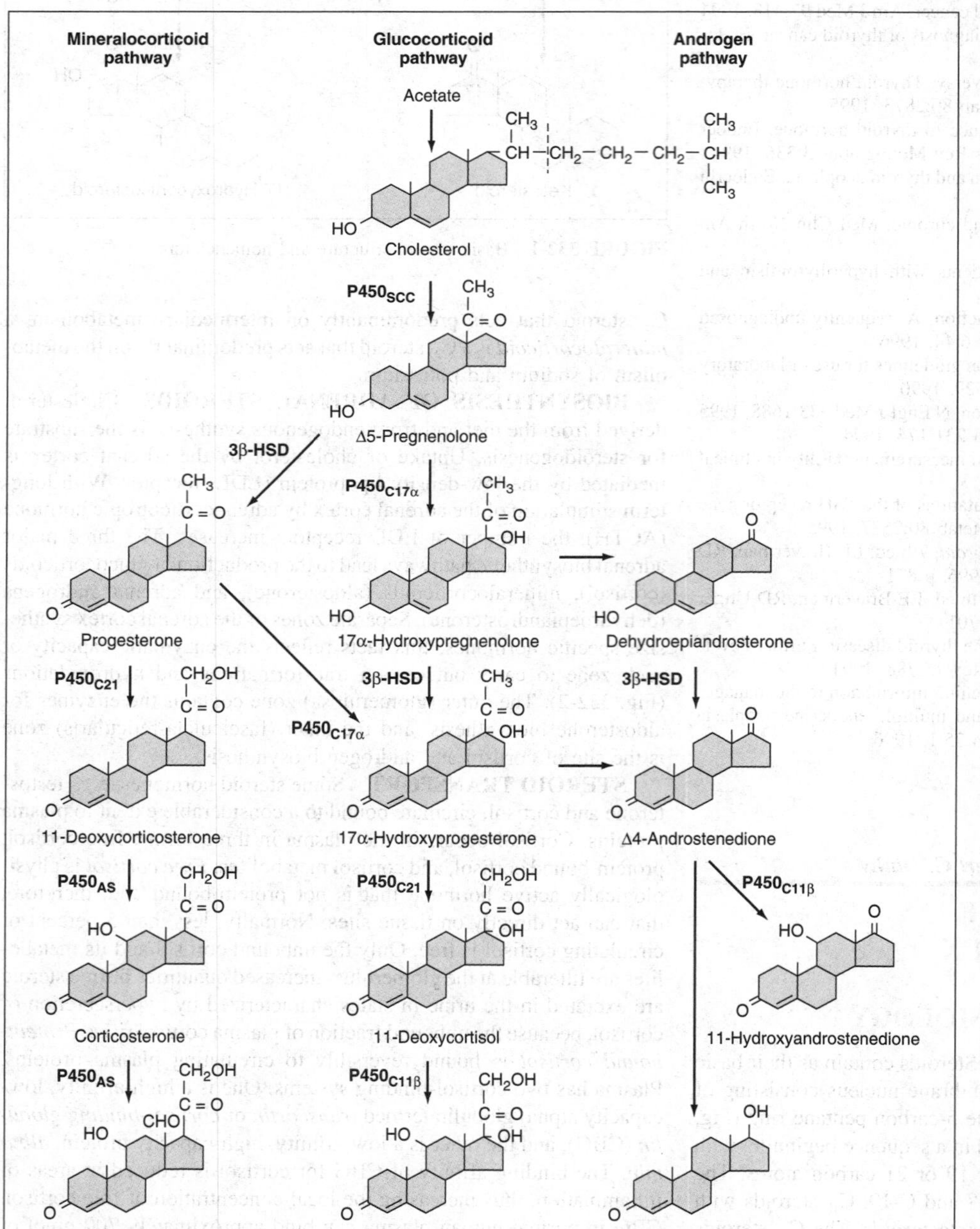

FIGURE 332-2 Biosynthetic pathways for adrenal steroid production; major pathways to mineralocorticoids, glucocorticoids, and androgens. Circled letters and numbers denote specific enzymes: $P450_{SCC}$, cholesterol side chain cleavage enzyme; 3β-HSD, 3β-hydroxysteroid dehydrogenase; $P450_{C11\beta}$, C-11 hydroxylase; $P450_{C17\alpha}$, C-17 hydroxylase; $P450_{C21}$, C-21 hydroxylase; $P450_{AS}$, aldosterone synthase.

to specific sites on steroid-regulated genes, modifying mRNA and protein synthesis. Because cortisol binds to the mineralocorticoid (type I glucocorticoid) receptor with the same affinity as aldosterone, mineralocorticoid specificity is achieved by local metabolism of cortisol to the inactive compound cortisone by 11β-hydroxysteroid dehydrogenase. Cortisone binds only minimally to the type I receptor. The glucocorticoid effects of other steroids, such as high-dose progesterone, correlate with their relative binding affinities for the type II glucocorticoid receptor. Inherited defects in the glucocorticoid receptor cause glucocorticoid resistance states. Individuals with type II receptor defects have high levels of cortisol but do not have manifestations of hypercortisolism.

ACTH PHYSIOLOGY ACTH (see Chap. 328) is an unbranched polypeptide containing 39 amino acids. ACTH and a number of other peptides (lipotropins, endorphins, and melanocyte-stimulating hormones) are processed from a larger precursor molecule of 31,000 mol wt—pro-opiomelanocortin (POMC) (see Chap. 328). POMC is made in a variety of tissues, including brain, anterior and posterior pituitary, and lymphocytes. The actual peptide secreted depends on the tissue. In the anterior pituitary, ACTH is synthesized and stored in basophilic cells. The basophilic staining of the corticotrophs is the result of the glycosylation of ACTH and related peptides. The *N*-terminal 18-amino-acid fragment of ACTH has full biologic potency, and shorter *N*-terminal fragments have partial biologic activity. Release of ACTH and related peptides from the anterior pituitary gland is governed by a "corticotropin-releasing center" in the median eminence of the hypothalamus, which, on stimulation, releases a 41-amino-acid peptide (corticotropin-releasing hormone, CRH) that travels via the portal vessels of the pituitary stalk to the anterior pituitary, where it stimulates the release of ACTH (Fig. 332-3). Some related peptides such as β-lipotropin (β-LPH) are released in equimolar concentrations with ACTH, suggesting that they are cleaved enzymatically from the parent POMC before or during the secretory process. However, β-endorphin levels may or may not correlate with circulating levels of ACTH, depending on the nature of the stimulus. The functions and regulation of secretion of the related peptides derived from POMC are poorly understood.

The major factors controlling ACTH release include CRH, the free cortisol concentration in plasma, stress, and the sleep-wake cycle (see Fig. 332-3). The plasma level of ACTH varies during the day as a result of its pulsatile secretion, and it follows a circadian pattern with a peak just prior to waking and a nadir before retiring. If a new sleep-wake cycle is adopted, the pattern changes over several days to conform to it. ACTH and cortisol levels also increase in response to eating. Stress (e.g., pyrogens, surgery, hypoglycemia, exercise, and severe emotional trauma) causes the release of CRH and arginine vasopressin (AVP) and activation of the sympathetic nervous system. These changes in turn enhance ACTH release, acting individually or in concert. For example, AVP release acts synergistically with CRH to amplify ACTH secretion; CRH also stimulates the locus coeruleus/sympathetic system. Stress-related secretion of ACTH abolishes the circadian periodicity of ACTH levels but is, in turn, suppressed by prior high-dose glucocorticoid administration. The normal pulsatile, circadian pattern of ACTH release is regulated by CRH; this mechanism is the so-called open feedback loop. CRH secretion, in turn, is influenced by hypothalamic neurotransmitters. For example, serotoninergic and cholinergic systems stimulate the secretion of CRH and ACTH; there is contradictory evidence regarding the inhibitory effects of alpha-adrenergic agonists and γ-aminobutyric acid (GABA) on CRH release. In addition, there may be direct pituitary effects of these neurotransmitters. There is also evidence for peptidergic regulation of ACTH release. For example, β-endorphin and enkephalin inhibit the secretion of ACTH, whereas vasopressin and angiotensin II augment it. The immune system also influences the hypothalamic-pituitary-adrenal axis (Fig. 332-4). For example, inflammatory cytokines [tumor necrosis factor (TNF)-α, interleukin (IL)-1α, IL-1β, and IL-6] produced by monocytes increase ACTH release by stimulating secretion of CRH and/or AVP. Finally, ACTH release is regulated by the level of free cortisol in plasma. Cortisol decreases the responsiveness of

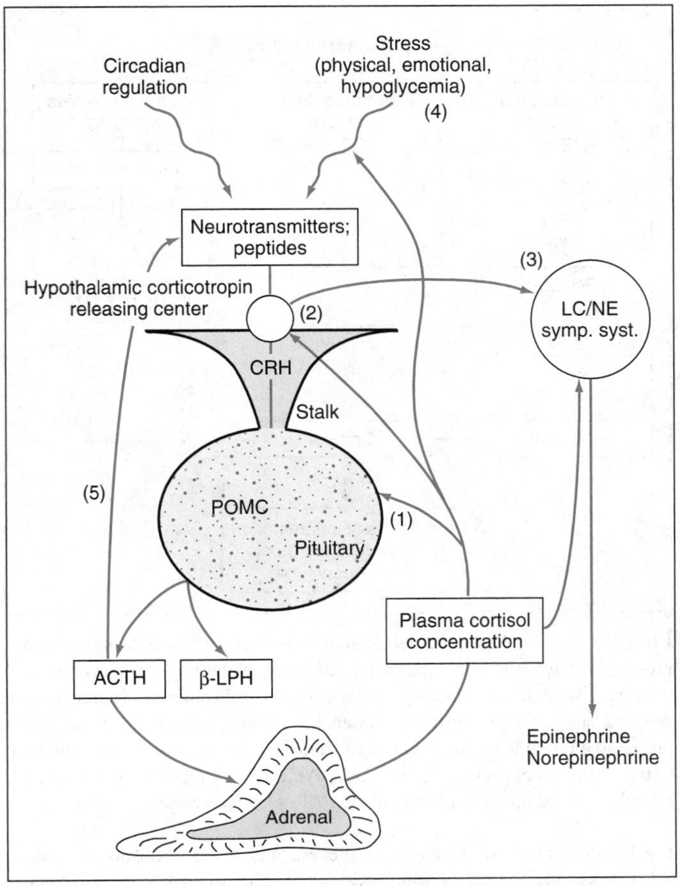

FIGURE 332-3 The hypothalamic-pituitary-adrenal axis. The main sites for feedback control by plasma cortisol are the pituitary gland (1) and the hypothalamic corticotropin-releasing center (2). Feedback control by plasma cortisol also occurs at the locus coeruleus/sympathetic system (3) and may involve higher nerve centers (4) as well. There also may be a short feedback loop involving inhibition of CRH by ACTH (5). Hypothalamic neurotransmitters influence CRH release; serotoninergic and cholinergic systems stimulate the secretion of CRH and ACTH; alpha-adrenergic agonists and γ-aminobutyric acid (GABA) probably inhibit CRH release. The opioid peptides β-endorphin and enkephalin inhibit, and vasopressin and angiotensin II augment, the secretion of CRH and ACTH. CRH, corticotropin-releasing hormone; β-LPH, β-lipotropin; POMC, pro-opiomelanocortin; LC, locus coeruleus; NE, norepinephrine.

pituitary corticotropic cells to CRH; that is, in the presence of cortisol, more CRH is required to produce a given increment of ACTH. The response of the POMC mRNA to CRH is also inhibited by glucocorticoids. In addition, glucocorticoids inhibit the locus coeruleus/sympathetic system and CRH release. The latter servomechanism establishes the primacy of cortisol in the control of ACTH secretion. The inhibition of ACTH occurs in two phases: (1) an early fast feedback, mediated via the type I glucocorticoid receptor, which lasts less than 10 min and depends on both the rate of increase of glucocorticoid levels and the specific glucocorticoid administered; and (2) a time-dependent, delayed feedback, likely mediated by the type II glucocorticoid receptor, which is probably due to inhibition of synthesis of the precursor protein. The suppression of ACTH secretion that results in adrenal atrophy following *prolonged* glucocorticoid therapy may be related primarily to suppression of hypothalamic CRH release, since exogenous CRH administration in this circumstance produces a rise in plasma ACTH. Cortisol also exerts feedback effects on higher brain centers (hippocampus, reticular system, and septum) and perhaps on the adrenal cortex (see Fig. 332-4).

The biologic half-life of ACTH in the circulation is less than 10 min. The action of ACTH is also rapid; within minutes of its release,

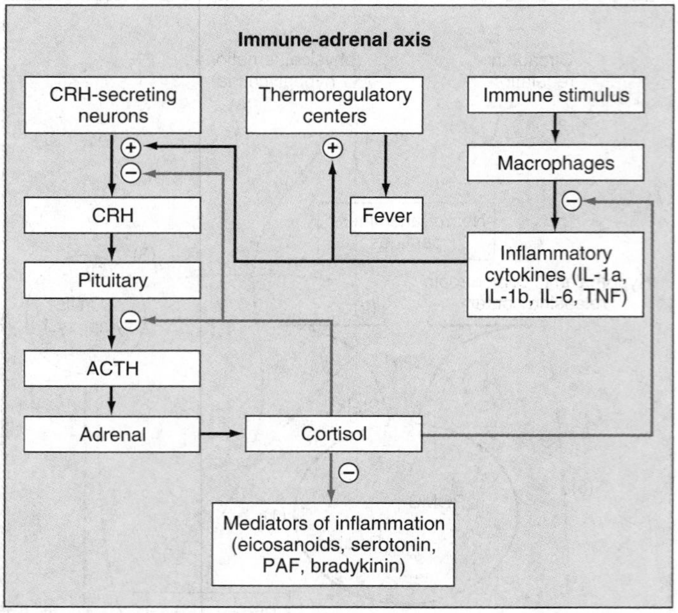

FIGURE 332-4 The immune-adrenal axis. Cortisol has anti-inflammatory properties that include effects on the microvasculature, cellular actions, and the suppression of inflammatory cytokines (the so-called immune-adrenal axis). A stress such as sepsis increases adrenal secretion, and cortisol in turn suppresses the immune response via this system. −, suppression; +, stimulation; CRH, corticotropin-releasing hormone; ACTH, adrenocorticotropin; IL, interleukin; TNF, tumor necrosis factor; PAF, platelet activating factor.

the concentration of steroids in the adrenal venous blood increases. ACTH stimulates steroidogenesis via activation of the membrane-bound adenyl cyclase. Adenosine-3′,5′-monophosphate (cyclic AMP), in turn, activates protein kinase enzymes, thereby resulting in the phosphorylation of proteins that activate steroid biosynthesis.

RENIN-ANGIOTENSIN PHYSIOLOGY (See also Chap. 246) Renin is a proteolytic enzyme that is produced and stored in the granules of the juxtaglomerular cells surrounding the afferent arterioles of glomeruli in the kidney. Renin exists in both active and inactive forms. Whether the inactive form is a precursor ("prorenin") or is a product formed after release is uncertain. The juxtaglomerular apparatus consists of both the juxtaglomerular cells and the cells of the macula densa. Renin acts on the basic substrate angiotensinogen (a circulating alpha$_2$ globulin made in the liver) to form the decapeptide angiotensin I (Fig. 332-5). Angiotensin I is then enzymatically transformed by angiotensin converting enzyme (converting enzyme), which is present in many tissues (particularly the pulmonary vascular endothelium), to the octapeptide angiotensin II by the removal of the two C-terminal amino acids. Angiotensin II is a potent pressor agent and exerts its action by a direct effect on arteriolar smooth muscle. In addition, angiotensin II stimulates production of aldosterone by the zona glomerulosa of the adrenal cortex; the heptapeptide angiotensin III also may stimulate aldosterone production. The two major classes of angiotensin receptors are termed AT1 and AT2; AT1 may exist as two subtypes α and β. Most of the effects of angiotensins II and III are mediated by the AT1 receptor. Angiotensinases rapidly destroy angiotensin II (half-life, approximately 1 min), while the half-life of renin is more prolonged (10 to 20 min). In addition to circulating renin-angiotensin, many tissues have a local renin-angiotensin system and the ability to produce angiotensin II. These tissues include the uterus, placenta, vascular tissue, heart, brain, and, particularly, the adrenal cortex and kidney. While the role of locally generated angiotensin II is not established, it may be involved in the growth and modulation of function of the adrenal cortex and vascular smooth muscle.

Renal renin release is controlled by four interdependent factors, and the amount of renin released reflects the combined effects of all four factors. The *juxtaglomerular cells*, which are specialized myoepithelial cells that cuff the afferent arterioles, act as miniature pressure transducers, sensing renal perfusion pressure and corresponding changes in afferent arteriolar perfusion pressures. For example, under conditions of a reduction in circulating blood volume, there is a corresponding reduction in renal perfusion pressure and, therefore, in afferent arteriolar pressure (see Fig. 332-5). This change is perceived by the juxtaglomerular cells as a decreased stretch exerted on the afferent arteriolar walls. The juxtaglomerular cells then release more renin into the kidney circulation. This results in the formation of angiotensin I, which is converted in the kidney and peripherally to angiotensin II by converting enzyme. Angiotensin II influences sodium homeostasis via two major mechanisms: it changes renal blood flow so as to maintain a constant glomerular filtration rate, thereby changing the filtration fraction of sodium, and it stimulates the adrenal cortex to release aldosterone. Increasing plasma levels of aldosterone lead to increasing renal sodium retention and thus result in expansion of the extracellular fluid volume, which, in turn, dampens the initiating signal for renin release. In this context, the renin-angiotensin-aldosterone system regulates volume by modifying renal hemodynamics and tubular sodium transport.

A second control mechanism for renin release is centered in the *macula densa* cells, a group of distal convoluted tubular epithelial cells directly apposed to the juxtaglomerular cells. They may function as chemoreceptors, monitoring the sodium (or chloride) load presented to the distal tubule, and such information may be conveyed to the juxtaglomerular cells, where appropriate modifications in renin release take place. Under conditions of increased delivery of filtered sodium to the macula densa, increasing release of renin is capable of decreasing the glomerular filtration rate, thereby reducing the filtered load of sodium.

The *sympathetic nervous system* regulates the release of renin in response to assumption of the upright posture. The mechanism is either a direct effect on the juxtaglomerular cell to increase adenyl cyclase activity or an indirect effect on either the juxtaglomerular or the macula densa cells via vasoconstriction of the afferent arteriole.

Finally, circulating factors influence renin release. Increased dietary intake of *potassium* decreases, and decreased potassium intake increases, renin release. The significance of these effects is unclear. *Angiotensin II* exerts negative feedback control on renin release that is independent of alterations in renal blood flow, blood pressure, or aldosterone secretion. *Atrial natriuretic peptides* also inhibit renin release. Thus, the control of renin release involves both *intrarenal* (pressor receptor and macula densa) and *extrarenal* (sympathetic nervous system,

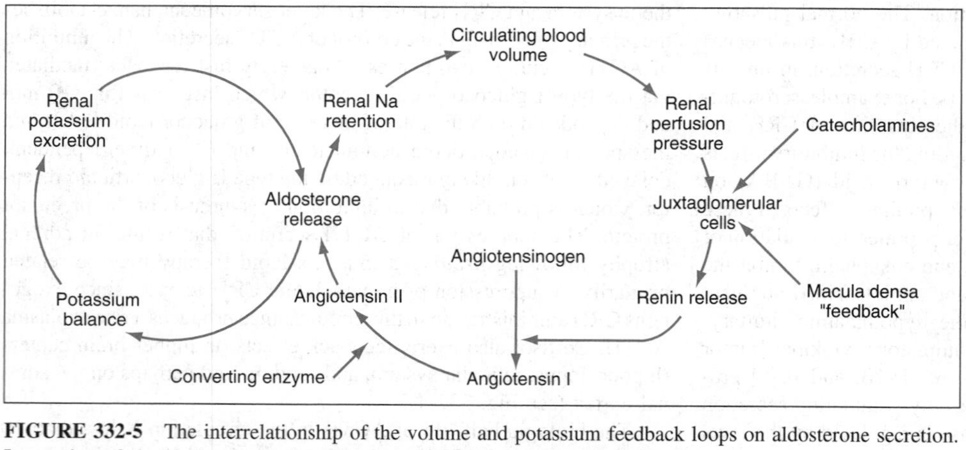

FIGURE 332-5 The interrelationship of the volume and potassium feedback loops on aldosterone secretion. Integration of signals from each loop determines the level of aldosterone secretion.

potassium, angiotensin, etc.) mechanisms. Steady-state renin levels reflect all these factors, with the intrarenal mechanism predominating.

GLUCOCORTICOID PHYSIOLOGY The division of adrenal steroids into glucocorticoids and mineralocorticoids is arbitrary in that most glucocorticoids have some mineralocorticoid-like properties. The descriptive term *glucocorticoid* is used for adrenal steroids whose predominant action is on intermediary metabolism. The principal glucocorticoid is cortisol (hydrocortisone). The effect of glucocorticoids on intermediary metabolism is mediated by the type II glucocorticoid receptor. Physiologic effects of glucocorticoids include the regulation of protein, carbohydrate, lipid, and nucleic acid metabolism. Glucocorticoids raise the blood glucose level by acting as an insulin antagonist and by suppressing the secretion of insulin, thereby inhibiting peripheral glucose uptake, which promotes hepatic glucose synthesis (gluconeogenesis) and increases hepatic glycogen content. The actions on protein metabolism are mainly catabolic in effect, resulting in an increase in protein breakdown and nitrogen excretion. In large part, these actions reflect a mobilization of glycogenic amino acid precursors from peripheral supporting structures, such as bone, skin, muscle, and connective tissue, due to protein breakdown and inhibition of protein synthesis and amino acid uptake. Hyperaminoacidemia also facilitates gluconeogenesis by stimulating glucagon secretion. Glucocorticoids act directly on the liver to stimulate the synthesis of certain enzymes, such as tyrosine aminotransferase and tryptophan pyrrolase. Glucocorticoids inhibit the synthesis of nucleic acids in most body tissues, but in the liver, RNA synthesis is stimulated. Glucocorticoids regulate fatty acid mobilization by enhancing the activation of cellular lipase by lipid-mobilizing hormones (e.g., catecholamines and pituitary peptides).

The actions of cortisol on protein and adipose tissue differ in different parts of the body. For example, pharmacologic doses of cortisol can deplete the protein matrix of the vertebral column (trabecular bone), but long bones (which are primarily compact bone) are affected only minimally; similarly, peripheral adipose tissue mass decreases, whereas abdominal and interscapular fat expand.

Glucocorticoids have anti-inflammatory properties, which are probably related to effects on the microvasculature and to suppression of inflammatory cytokines. In this sense, glucocorticoids modulate the immune response via the so-called immune-adrenal axis. This "loop" is one mechanism by which a stress, such as sepsis, increases adrenal hormone secretion, and the elevated cortisol level in turn suppresses the immune response. For example, cortisol maintains vascular responsiveness to circulating vasoconstrictors and opposes the increase in capillary permeability during acute inflammation. Glucocorticoids cause a leukocytosis due to release from the bone marrow of mature cells as well as to inhibition of their egress through the capillary wall. Glucocorticoids produce a depletion of circulating eosinophils and of lymphoid tissue, specifically T cells, by causing a redistribution from the circulation into other compartments. Thus, cortisol impairs cell-mediated immunity. Glucocorticoids also inhibit the production and action of the mediators of inflammation, such as the lymphokines and prostaglandins. These actions occur via the type II glucocorticoid receptor and are blocked by inhibitors of RNA and protein synthesis. Glucocorticoids inhibit the production and action of interferon by T lymphocytes and the production of IL-1 and IL-6 by macrophages. The antipyretic action of glucocorticoids may be explained by the effect on IL-1, which appears to be an endogenous pyrogen. Glucocorticoids also inhibit the production of T cell growth factor (IL-2) by T lymphocytes. Glucocorticoids reverse macrophage activation and antagonize the action of migration-inhibiting factor (MIF), leading to reduced adherence of macrophages to vascular endothelium. Glucocorticoids inhibit prostaglandin and leukotriene production by inhibiting the activity of phospholipase A_2, thus blocking release of arachidonic acid from phospholipids. Finally, glucocorticoids inhibit the production and inflammatory effects of bradykinin, platelet activating factor, and serotonin. It is probably only at pharmacologic dosages that antibody production is reduced and lysosomal membranes are stabilized, the latter effect suppressing the release of acid hydrolases.

Cortisol levels respond within minutes to stress, whether physical (trauma, surgery, exercise), psychological (anxiety, depression), or

physiologic (hypoglycemia, fever). The reasons why elevated glucocorticoid levels protect the organism under stress are not understood, but in conditions of glucocorticoid deficiency, such stresses may cause hypotension, shock, and death. Consequently, in individuals with adrenal insufficiency, glucocorticoid administration should be increased during stress.

Cortisol has major effects on body water. It helps regulate the extracellular fluid volume by retarding the migration of water into cells and by promoting renal water excretion, the latter effect mediated by suppression of vasopressin secretion, by an increase in the rate of glomerular filtration, and by a direct action on the renal tubule. The consequence is to prevent water intoxication by increasing solute-free water clearance. Glucocorticoids also have weak mineralocorticoid-like properties, and high doses promote renal tubular sodium reabsorption and increased urine potassium excretion. Glucocorticoids also can influence behavior; emotional disorders may occur with either an excess or a deficit of cortisol. Last, cortisol suppresses the secretion of pituitary POMC and its derivative peptides (ACTH, β-endorphin, and β-lipotropin) and the secretion of hypothalamic CRH and vasopressin.

MINERALOCORTICOID PHYSIOLOGY The major mineralocorticoid, aldosterone, has two important actions: It is a major regulator of extracellular fluid volume and a major determinant of potassium metabolism. These effects are mediated by the binding of aldosterone to the type I glucocorticoid (mineralocorticoid) receptor in target tissues (see Chap. 327). Volume is regulated through a direct effect on the collecting duct, where aldosterone causes a decrease in sodium excretion and an increase in potassium excretion. The reabsorption of sodium ions causes a fall in the transmembrane potential, thus enhancing the flow of positive ions, such as potassium, out of the cell into the lumen. The reabsorbed sodium ions are transported out of the tubular epithelium into the renal interstitial fluid and from there into the renal capillary circulation. Water passively follows the transported sodium.

Since the concentration of hydrogen ion is greater in the lumen than in the cell, hydrogen ion also is actively secreted. Mineralocorticoids also act on the epithelium of the salivary ducts, sweat glands, and gastrointestinal tract to cause reabsorption of sodium in exchange for potassium.

When normal individuals are given aldosterone, an initial period of sodium retention is followed by natriuresis, and sodium balance is reestablished after 3 to 5 days. As a result, edema does not develop. This process is referred to as the *escape phenomenon*, signifying an "escape" by the renal tubules from the sodium-retaining action of aldosterone. While renal hemodynamic factors may play a role in the escape, the level of atrial natriuretic peptide also increases. However, it is important to realize that there is no escape from the potassium-losing effects of mineralocorticoids. Aldosterone can also interact with a cell surface receptor, thereby possibly acting by a nongenomic mechanism.

Three primary mechanisms control aldosterone release—the renin-angiotensin system, potassium, and ACTH (Table 332-1). The renin-angiotensin system controls extracellular fluid volume via regulation of aldosterone secretion (see Fig. 332-1). In effect, the renin-angiotensin system maintains the circulating blood volume constant by causing aldosterone-induced sodium retention during volume deficiency and by decreasing aldosterone-dependent sodium retention when volume is ample.

Potassium ion directly regulates aldosterone secretion, independently of circulating renin-angiotensin (see Fig. 332-5). However, potassium stimulates the adrenal production of angiotensin II, and converting-enzyme inhibitors block the synthesis of angiotensin II and reduce the acute aldosterone response to potassium. Oral potassium loading increases aldosterone secretion, excretion, and plasma levels. In addition, an increase in serum potassium of as little as 0.1 mmol/L increases plasma aldosterone levels under certain circumstances.

Physiologic amounts of ACTH stimulate aldosterone secretion acutely, but this action is not sustained if ACTH is infused for longer

Table 332-1

Factors Regulating Aldosterone Biosynthesis

Factor	Effect
Renin-angiotensin system	Stimulation
Sodium ion	Inhibition (?physiologic)
Potassium ion	Stimulation
Neurotransmitters	
Dopamine	Inhibition
Serotonin	Stimulation
Pituitary hormones	
ACTH	Stimulation
Non-ACTH pituitary hormones (e.g., growth hormone)	Permissive (for optimal response to sodium restriction)
β-Endorphin	Stimulation
γ-MSH	Permissive
Atrial peptide	Inhibition
Ouabain-like factors	Inhibition

than 10 to 12 h. Most studies relegate ACTH to a minor role in the control of aldosterone. For example, subjects receiving high-dose glucocorticoid therapy and with presumed complete suppression of ACTH have normal aldosterone secretion in response to sodium restriction.

Prior dietary intake of both potassium and sodium can alter the magnitude of the aldosterone response to acute stimulation. This effect results from a change in aldosterone synthase. Increasing potassium intake or decreasing sodium intake sensitizes the response of the glomerulosa cells to acute stimulation by ACTH, angiotensin II, and/or potassium. Thus, regulation of aldosterone secretion occurs both early and late in the synthetic pathway.

Neurotransmitters (dopamine and serotonin) and some peptides, such as atrial natriuretic peptide, γ-melanocyte-stimulating hormone (γ-MSH), and β-endorphin, also participate in the regulation of aldosterone secretion (see Table 332-1). Thus, the control of aldosterone secretion involves both stimulatory and inhibitory factors.

ANDROGEN PHYSIOLOGY Androgens regulate male secondary sexual characteristics and can cause virilizing symptoms in women. Steroids with predominantly androgenic activity have 19 carbon atoms (see Fig. 332-1). The principal adrenal androgens are dehydroepiandrosterone (DHEA), androstenedione, and 11-hydroxyandrostenedione. DHEA and androstenedione are weak androgens and exert their effects via conversion to the potent androgen testosterone in extraglandular tissues. DHEA also has poorly understood effects on the immune and cardiovascular systems. Adrenal androgen formation is regulated by ACTH, not by gonadotropins. It follows that adrenal androgens are suppressed by exogenous glucocorticoid administration.

LABORATORY EVALUATION OF ADRENOCORTICAL FUNCTION

The basic assumption is that measurements of the plasma or urinary level of a given steroid reflects the rate of adrenal *secretion* of that steroid. However, urine *excretion* values may not truly reflect the secretion rate because of improper collection or altered metabolism. Measurement of the actual adrenal secretory rate of a given steroid is difficult, involving isotope dilution techniques following administration of a radioactive steroid. Plasma levels reflect the level of secretion only at the time of measurement. The plasma level (PL) depends on two factors: the secretion rate (SR) of the hormone and the rate at which it is metabolized, i.e., its metabolic clearance rate (MCR). These three factors can be related as follows:

$$PL = \frac{SR}{MCR} \quad \text{or} \quad SR = MCR \times PL$$

BLOOD LEVELS (See Table 332-2) **Peptides** The plasma levels of ACTH and angiotensin II can be measured by immunoassay techniques. ACTH levels fluctuate from moment to moment, and basal ACTH secretion shows a circadian rhythm, with lower levels in the early evening than in the morning. Angiotensin II levels also vary diurnally and are influenced by dietary sodium intake and posture. Both upright posture and sodium restriction elevate angiotensin II levels.

Most clinical determinations of the renin-angiotensin system, however, involve measurements of peripheral *plasma renin activity* (PRA) in which the renin activity is gauged by the generation of angiotensin I during a standardized incubation period. This method depends on the presence of sufficient angiotensinogen in the plasma as substrate. The generated angiotensin I is measured by radioimmunoassay. The plasma renin activity depends on the dietary sodium intake and on whether the patient is ambulatory. In normal humans, the PRA shows a diurnal rhythm characterized by peak values in the morning and decreases in activity in the afternoon.

Steroids Cortisol and aldosterone are both secreted episodically, and levels generally vary during the day, with peak values in the morning and low levels in the evening. In addition, the plasma level of aldosterone, but not of cortisol, is increased by dietary potassium loading, by sodium restriction, or by assumption of the upright posture. Measurement of the sulfate conjugate of DHEA may be a useful index of adrenal androgen secretion, since little DHEA sulfate is formed in the gonads and since the half-life of DHEA sulfate is 7 to 9 h. However, DHEA sulfate levels reflect both DHEA production and sulfatase activity.

URINE LEVELS For the assessment of glucocorticoid secretion, the urine *17-hydroxycorticosteroid* assay has been replaced largely by measurement of urinary free cortisol. Elevated levels of urinary free cortisol correlate with states of hypercortisolism, reflecting changes in the levels of unbound, physiologically active circulating cortisol. Normally, the rate of excretion is higher in the daytime (7 A.M. to 7 P.M.) than at night (7 P.M. to 7 A.M.).

Urinary *17-ketosteroids* contain a ketone group at C-17 (see Fig. 332-1). They originate in either the adrenal gland or the gonad. In normal women, 90 percent of urinary 17-ketosteroids is derived from the adrenal, and in men 60 to 70 percent is of adrenal origin. Urine 17-ketosteroid values are highest in young adults and decline with age.

Table 332-2

Range of Normal Values for Tests of Adrenal Function

Test	Normal Value, Range
Plasma cortisol, nmol/L (μg/dL):	
8 A.M.	140–690 (5–24)
4 P.M.	80–330 (3–12)
Cortisol secretory rate, μmol/d (mg/d)	14–69 (5–25)
Urinary free cortisol, nmol/d (μg/d)	55–275 (20–100)
17-Hydroxycorticosteroids, μmol/d (mg/d)	5.5–28 (2–10)
Plasma testosterone, nmol/L (ng/mL):	
Men	10–35 (3–10)
Women	<3.5 (<1)
Plasma dehydroepiandrosterone (DHEA), nmol/L (μg/L)	7–31 (2–9)
Plasma DHEA sulfate, μmol/L (μg/L)	1.3–6.7 (500–2500)
Plasma 11-deoxycortisol (S), nmol/L (μg/dL)	<30 (<1)
Plasma 17OH progesterone, nmol/L (μg/L):	
Women	
Follicular phase	0.6–3 (0.2–1)
Luteal phase	1.5–10.6 (0.5–3.5)
Men	0.2–9 (0.06–3)
Plasma aldosterone, pmol/L (ng/dL) (100 mmol Na^+, 60–100 mmol K^+, supine, 8 A.M.)	<240 (<8)
Aldosterone secretion, nmol/d (μg/d) (100 mmol Na^+, 60–100 mmol K^+)	140–690 (50–250)
Aldosterone excretion, nmol/d (μg/d) (100 mmol Na^+, 60–100 mmol K^+)	14–53 (5–19)
Plasma renin activity (μg/L)/h [(ng/mL)/h] (100 mmol Na^+, 60–100 mmol K^+, supine, 8 A.M.)	1–2.5 (1–2.5)
Plasma angiotensin II, ng/L (pg/mL) (100 mmol Na^+, 60–100 mmol K^+, supine, 8 A.M.)	10–30 (10–30)
Plasma ACTH, pmol/L (pg/mL) (8 A.M.)	2–14 (10–60)

A carefully timed urine collection is a prerequisite for all excretory determinations. Urinary creatinine should be measured simultaneously to determine the accuracy and adequacy of the collection procedure.

STIMULATION TESTS Stimulation tests are useful in the diagnosis of hormone deficiency states. A standardized and specific stimulus for the production and release of a given hormone is applied, and the amount of hormone released is then measured.

Tests of Glucocorticoid Reserve Within minutes after administration of ACTH, cortisol levels increase in adrenal venous blood. This responsiveness can be used as an index of the functional reserve of the adrenal gland for production of cortisol. Under maximal ACTH stimulation, cortisol secretion increases tenfold, to 800 µmol/d (300 mg/d), but maximal stimulation can be achieved only with prolonged ACTH infusions. For example, in normal subjects, cortisol levels exceed 1100 nmol/L (40 µg/dL) following a 24-h infusion of cosyntropin at a rate of 0.02 mg/h. In patients with secondary adrenal insufficiency, the maximal plasma cortisol value at 24 h ranges between 280 and 1100 nmol/L (10 and 40 µg/dL). Patients with primary adrenal insufficiency have smaller responses.

A screening test (the so-called rapid ACTH stimulation test) involves the administration of 25 units (0.25 mg) of cosyntropin intravenously or intramuscularly and measurement of plasma cortisol levels before and 30 and 60 min after administration; the test can be performed at any time of the day. The most clear-cut criterion for a normal response is a stimulated cortisol level of >500 nmol/L (>18 µg/dL), and the minimal stimulated normal increment of cortisol is >200 nmol/L (>7 µg/dL) above baseline. Severely ill patients with elevated basal cortisol levels may show no further increases following acute ACTH administration.

Tests of Mineralocorticoid Reserve and Stimulation of the Renin-Angiotensin System Stimulation tests use protocols designed to create a programmed volume depletion, such as sodium restriction, diuretic administration, or upright posture. A simple, potent test consists of severe sodium restriction and upright posture. After 3 to 5 days of a 10-mmol/d sodium intake, rates of aldosterone secretion or excretion should increase two- to threefold over the control values. Supine morning plasma aldosterone levels are usually increased three- to sixfold, and they increase a further two- to fourfold in response to 2 to 3 h of upright posture.

When the dietary sodium intake is normal, stimulation testing requires the administration of a potent diuretic, such as 40 to 80 mg furosemide, followed by 2 to 3 h of upright posture. The normal response is a two- to fourfold rise in plasma aldosterone levels.

SUPPRESSION TESTS Suppression tests to document hypersecretion of adrenal hormones involve measurement of the target hormone response after standardized suppression of its tropic hormone.

Tests of Pituitary-Adrenal Suppressibility The ACTH release mechanism is sensitive to the circulating glucocorticoid level. When blood levels of glucocorticoid are increased in normal individuals, less ACTH is released from the anterior pituitary, and less steroid is produced by the adrenal gland. The integrity of this feedback mechanism can be tested clinically by giving a glucocorticoid and judging the suppression of ACTH secretion by analysis of urine steroid levels and/or plasma cortisol and ACTH levels. A potent glucocorticoid such as dexamethasone is used, so that the agent can be given in an amount small enough not to contribute significantly to the pool of steroids to be analyzed.

The best *screening* procedure is the overnight dexamethasone suppression test. This involves the measurement of plasma cortisol levels at 8 A.M. following the oral administration of 1 mg dexamethasone the previous midnight. The 8 A.M. value for plasma cortisol in normal subjects should be less than 140 nmol/L (5 µg/dL).

The definitive test of adrenal suppressibility consists in administering 0.5 mg dexamethasone every 6 h for two successive days while collecting urine over a 24-h period for determination of creatinine and free cortisol and/or measuring plasma cortisol levels. In a patient with a normal hypothalamic-pituitary ACTH release mechanism, a fall in the urine free cortisol to less than 80 nmol/d (30 µg/d) or of plasma cortisol to less than 140 nmol/L (5 µg/dL) is seen on the second day of administration.

A normal response to either suppression test implies that the ACTH control of the adrenal glands is physiologically normal. However, an isolated abnormal result, particularly to the overnight suppression test, does not in itself imply pituitary and/or adrenal disease.

Tests of Mineralocorticoid Suppressibility These tests rely on an expansion of extracellular fluid volume, which should result in a decrease in renal renin release, a decrease in circulating plasma renin activity, and a decrease in the secretion and/or excretion of aldosterone. Various tests differ in the rate at which extracellular fluid volume is expanded. One convenient suppression test involves the intravenous infusion of 500 mL/h of normal saline solution for 4 h, which normally suppresses plasma aldosterone levels to <220 pmol/L (<8 ng/dL) on a sodium-restricted diet or to <140 pmol/L (<5 ng/dL) on a normal sodium intake. This test should not be performed in potassium-depleted subjects.

TESTS OF PITUITARY-ADRENAL RESPONSIVENESS Stimuli such as insulin hypoglycemia, arginine vasopressin, and pyrogens cause the release of ACTH from the pituitary by an action on higher neural centers or on the pituitary itself. Insulin-induced hypoglycemia is particularly useful, because it stimulates the release of both growth hormone and ACTH. In this test, 0.05 to 0.1 unit of regular insulin per kilogram body weight is given intravenously as a bolus to reduce the fasting glucose level to at least 50 percent below basal. The normal cortisol response is a rise to more than 500 nmol/L (18 µg/dL).

One of the best ways to test the integrity of the pituitary-adrenal axis is the metyrapone test. Metyrapone inhibits 11β-hydroxylase in the adrenal. As a result, the conversion of 11-deoxycortisol (compound S) to cortisol is impaired, causing 11-deoxycortisol to accumulate in the blood and the blood level of cortisol to decrease (see Fig. 332-2). The hypothalamic-pituitary axis responds to the declining cortisol blood levels by releasing more ACTH. *Note that assessment of the response depends on both an intact hypothalamic-pituitary axis and an intact adrenal gland.*

While modifications of the original metyrapone test have been described, we believe the best involves administering 750 mg of the drug by mouth every 4 h over a 24-h period and comparing the control and postmetyrapone plasma levels of 11-deoxycortisol, cortisol, and ACTH. In normal individuals, plasma 11-deoxycortisol levels should exceed 290 nmol/L (10 µg/dL) following metyrapone administration. The metyrapone test does not accurately reflect ACTH reserve if subjects are ingesting exogenous glucocorticoids or drugs that accelerate the metabolism of metyrapone (e.g., phenytoin).

A direct and selective test of the pituitary corticotrophs can be achieved with the investigational agent corticotropin-releasing hormone (CRH). The bolus injection of 1 µg of ovine CRH per kilogram of body weight stimulates secretion of ACTH and β-lipotropin in normal human subjects within 60 to 180 min. However, the magnitude of the ACTH response is less than that produced by the insulin tolerance test, which implies that additional factors (such as vasopressin) augment stress-induced increases in ACTH secretion.

Although the rapid ACTH stimulation test is useful for the diagnosis of primary adrenal insufficiency, normal cortisol responsiveness may be seen in some patients with a partial ACTH deficit and absence of adrenal atrophy. These patients have an inadequate pituitary ACTH reserve and fail to increase ACTH secretion in response to a stress such as surgery or hypoglycemia. Since the use of a bolus of exogenous ACTH does not invariably exclude a diagnosis of secondary adrenocortical insufficiency, direct tests of pituitary ACTH reserve (metyrapone test, insulin tolerance testing) may be required in the appropriate clinical setting. On the other hand, the rapid ACTH test can distinguish between primary and secondary adrenal insufficiency, because aldosterone secretion is preserved in secondary adrenal failure by the renin-angiotensin system and potassium. Cosyntropin (25 units) is given intravenously or intramuscularly, and plasma cortisol and aldosterone levels are measured before and 30 and 60 min after administration.

The cortisol response is abnormal in both groups, but patients with secondary insufficiency show an increase in aldosterone levels by at least 140 pmol/L (5 ng/dL). No aldosterone response is seen in patients in whom the adrenal cortex is destroyed.

HYPERFUNCTION OF THE ADRENAL CORTEX

Excess cortisol is associated with Cushing's syndrome; excess aldosterone causes aldosteronism; and excess adrenal androgens cause adrenal virilism. These syndromes do not always occur in the "pure" form but may have overlapping features.

CUSHING'S SYNDROME Etiology Cushing described a syndrome characterized by truncal obesity, hypertension, fatigability and weakness, amenorrhea, hirsutism, purplish abdominal striae, edema, glucosuria, osteoporosis, and a basophilic tumor of the pituitary. As awareness of this syndrome has increased, the diagnosis of Cushing's syndrome has been broadened into the classification shown in Table 332-3. Regardless of etiology, all cases of endogenous Cushing's syndrome are due to increased production of cortisol by the adrenal. In most cases the cause is *bilateral adrenal hyperplasia* due to hypersecretion of pituitary ACTH or production of ACTH by a nonendocrine tumor. The incidence of pituitary-dependent adrenal hyperplasia is three times greater in women than in men, and the most frequent age of onset is the third or fourth decade. The cause of the hypersecretion of pituitary ACTH is still debated. Some workers speculate that the primary defect is the de novo development of a pituitary adenoma, since in some reports tumors are found in over 90 percent of patients with pituitary-dependent adrenal hyperplasia. Alternatively, the defect may reside in the hypothalamus or in higher neural centers, leading to release of CRH inappropriate to the level of circulating cortisol. The consequence would be that a higher level of cortisol is required to reduce ACTH secretion to normal. This primary defect leads to hyperstimulation of the pituitary, resulting in hyperplasia or tumor formation. With time the pituitary tumor may become independent of the regulating influence of the central nervous system and/or circulating cortisol levels. In surgical series, most individuals with hypersecretion of pituitary ACTH are found to have a microadenoma ($<$10 mm in diameter; 50 percent are 5 mm or less in diameter), but a pituitary macroadenoma ($>$10 mm) or diffuse hyperplasia of the corticotropic cells may be found. The finding of a microadenoma in pituitary-dependent adrenal hyperplasia does not rule out dysregulation of hypothalamic CRH as the defect in Cushing's disease. Long-term follow-up to determine the rate of recurrence following successful surgical resection is necessary to answer this issue. In some studies, the recurrence rate is greater than 20 percent. Unfortunately, it may be difficult to distinguish between recurrence and inadequate primary therapy. Traditionally, only an individual who has an ACTH-producing pituitary tumor is defined as having *Cushing's disease*, but in some centers this designation is used for anyone who has hypersecretion of pituitary ACTH, regardless of whether a tumor is identified by radiography. In this chapter we will use the traditional definition, although these definitions may become less distinct as small tumors are more easily diagnosed by high-resolution scanning.

Nonendocrine tumors may secrete polypeptides that are biologically, chemically, and immunologically indistinguishable from either ACTH or CRH and that cause bilateral adrenal hyperplasia (see also Chap. 102). The ectopic production of CRH results in clinical, biochemical, and radiologic features indistinguishable from those caused by hypersecretion of pituitary ACTH. The typical signs and symptoms of Cushing's syndrome may be absent or minimal with ectopic ACTH production, and hypokalemic alkalosis is the prominent manifestation. Most of these cases are associated with the primitive small cell (oat cell) type of bronchogenic carcinoma or with tumors of the thymus, pancreas, or ovary; medullary carcinoma of the thyroid; or bronchial adenomas. The onset of Cushing's syndrome may be sudden, particularly in patients with carcinoma of the lung, and this feature accounts in part for the failure of these patients to exhibit the classic manifestations. On the other hand, patients with carcinoid tumors or pheochromocytomas have longer clinical courses and usually exhibit the typical cushingoid features. The secretion of ACTH by nonendocrine tumors is also accompanied by the accumulation of ACTH fragments in plasma and by elevated plasma levels of ACTH precursor molecules. Since such tumors may produce large amounts of ACTH, baseline steroid values are usually markedly elevated, and increased skin pigmentation may be present. Indeed, hyperpigmentation in patients with Cushing's syndrome almost always points to an extraadrenal tumor, either in an extracranial location or within the cranium.

Approximately 20 to 25 percent of patients with Cushing's syndrome have an adrenal neoplasm. These tumors are usually unilateral, and about half are malignant. Occasionally, patients have biochemical features both of hypersecretion of pituitary ACTH and of an adrenal adenoma. These individuals usually have micro- or macronodularity of both adrenal glands resulting in *nodular hyperplasia.* Two specific entities cause nodular hyperplasia: a familial autoimmune disorder in children or young adults (so-called pigmented multinodular cortical dysplasia) and hypersensitivity to gastric inhibitory polypeptide, probably secondary to enhanced expression of receptors for this peptide in the adrenal cortex.

The most common cause of Cushing's syndrome is *iatrogenic* administration of steroids for a variety of reasons. While the clinical features bear some resemblance to those seen with adrenal tumors, these patients are usually distinguishable on the basis of history and laboratory studies.

Clinical Signs, Symptoms, and Laboratory Findings Many of the signs and symptoms of Cushing's syndrome follow logically from the known action of glucocorticoids (Table 332-4). Mobilization of peripheral supportive tissue causes muscle weakness and fatigability, osteoporosis, cutaneous striae, and easy bruisability. The latter signs are secondary to weakening and rupture of collagen fibers in the dermis. Osteoporosis may cause collapse of vertebral bodies and pathologic fractures of other bones. Increased hepatic gluconeogenesis

Table 332-3

Causes of Cushing's Syndrome

Adrenal hyperplasia
- Secondary to pituitary ACTH overproduction
  - Pituitary-hypothalamic dysfunction
  - Pituitary ACTH-producing micro- or macroadenomas
- Secondary to ACTH or CRH-producing nonendocrine tumors (bronchogenic carcinoma, carcinoid of the thymus, pancreatic carcinoma, bronchial adenoma)

Adrenal nodular hyperplasia

Adrenal neoplasia
- Adenoma
- Carcinoma

Exogenous, iatrogenic causes
- Prolonged use of glucocorticoids
- Prolonged use of ACTH

Table 332-4

Frequency of Signs and Symptoms in Cushing's Syndrome

Sign or Symptom	Percent of Patients
Typical habitus	97
Increased body weight	94
Fatigability and weakness	87
Hypertension (blood pressure $>$150/90)	82
Hirsutism	80
Amenorrhea	77
Cutaneous striae	67
Personality changes	66
Ecchymoses	65
Edema	62
Polyuria, polydipsia	23
Hypertrophy of clitoris	19

and insulin resistance can cause impaired glucose tolerance. Overt diabetes mellitus occurs in fewer than 20 percent of patients, who probably are individuals with a predisposition to this disorder. Hypercortisolism promotes the deposition of adipose tissue in characteristic sites, notably the upper face (producing the typical "moon" facies), the interscapular area (producing the "buffalo hump"), and the mesenteric bed (producing "truncal" obesity) (Fig. 332-6). Rarely, episternal fatty tumors and mediastinal widening secondary to fat accumulation occur. The reason for this peculiar distribution of adipose tissue is not known, but it is associated with insulin resistance and/or elevated insulin levels. The face appears plethoric, even in the absence of any increase in red blood cell concentration. Hypertension is common, and emotional changes may be profound, ranging from irritability and emotional lability to severe depression, confusion, or even frank psychosis. In women, increased levels of adrenal androgens can cause acne, hirsutism, and oligomenorrhea or amenorrhea. Some signs and symptoms in patients with hypercortisolism—i.e., obesity, hypertension, osteoporosis, and diabetes—are nonspecific and therefore are less helpful in diagnosing the condition. On the other hand, easy bruising, typical striae, myopathy, and virilizing signs (although less frequent) are, if present, more suggestive of Cushing's syndrome.

Except in iatrogenic Cushing's syndrome, plasma and urine cortisol levels are variably elevated. Occasionally, hypokalemia, hypochloremia, and metabolic alkalosis are present, particularly with ectopic production of ACTH.

Diagnosis The diagnosis of Cushing's syndrome depends on the demonstration of increased cortisol production and failure to suppress cortisol secretion normally when dexamethasone is administered. Once the diagnosis is established, further testing is designed to determine the etiology (Fig. 332-7 and Table 332-5).

For initial screening, the overnight dexamethasone suppression test is recommended (see above). In difficult cases (e.g., in obese patients), measurement of a 24-h urine free cortisol also can be used as a screening test. A level greater than 275 nmol/d (100 μg/d) is suggestive of Cushing's syndrome. The definitive diagnosis is then established by failure of urinary cortisol to fall to less than 80 nmol/d (30 μg/d) or of plasma cortisol to fall to less than 140 nmol/L (5 μg/dL) after a standard low-dose dexamethasone suppression test (0.5 mg every 6 h for 48 h). Owing to circadian variability, plasma cortisol and, to a certain extent, ACTH determinations are not meaningful when performed in isolation, but demonstration that the normal fall in evening levels of plasma cortisol does not occur may be useful.

The task of determining the etiology of Cushing's syndrome is complicated by the fact that all the available tests lack specificity and by the fact that the tumors producing this syndrome are prone to spontaneous and often dramatic changes in hormone secretion (periodic hormonogenesis). No test has a specificity greater than 95 percent, and it may be necessary to use a combination of tests to arrive at the correct diagnosis. A useful step to distinguish patients with an ACTH-secreting pituitary microadenoma or hypothalamic-pituitary dysfunction from those with other forms of Cushing's syndrome is to determine the response of cortisol output to administration of high-dose dexamethasone (2 mg every 6 h for 2 days). Indeed, when the diagnosis of Cushing's syndrome is clear-cut on the basis of baseline urinary and plasma assays, the high-dose dexamethasone suppression test may

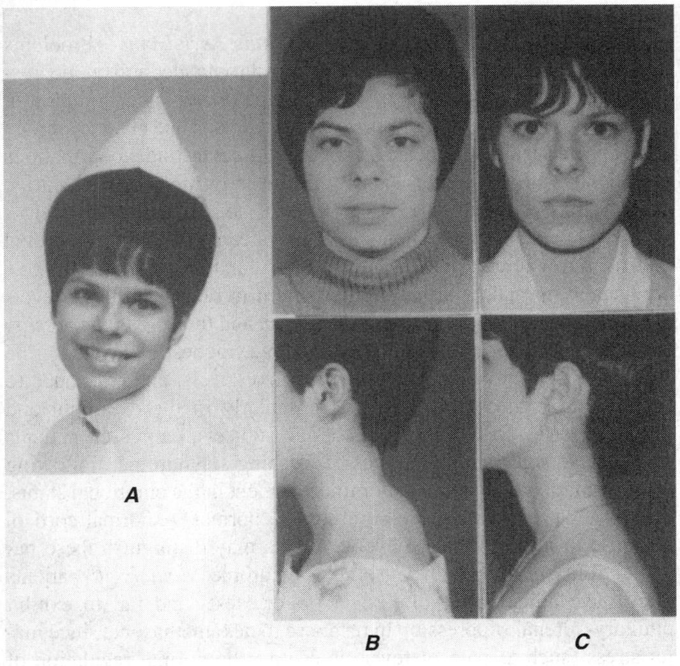

FIGURE 332-6 A woman with Cushing's syndrome due to a right adrenal cortical adenoma. *A.* Two years prior to surgery, age 18. *B.* One month prior to surgery, age 20. *C.* One year after surgery, age 21.

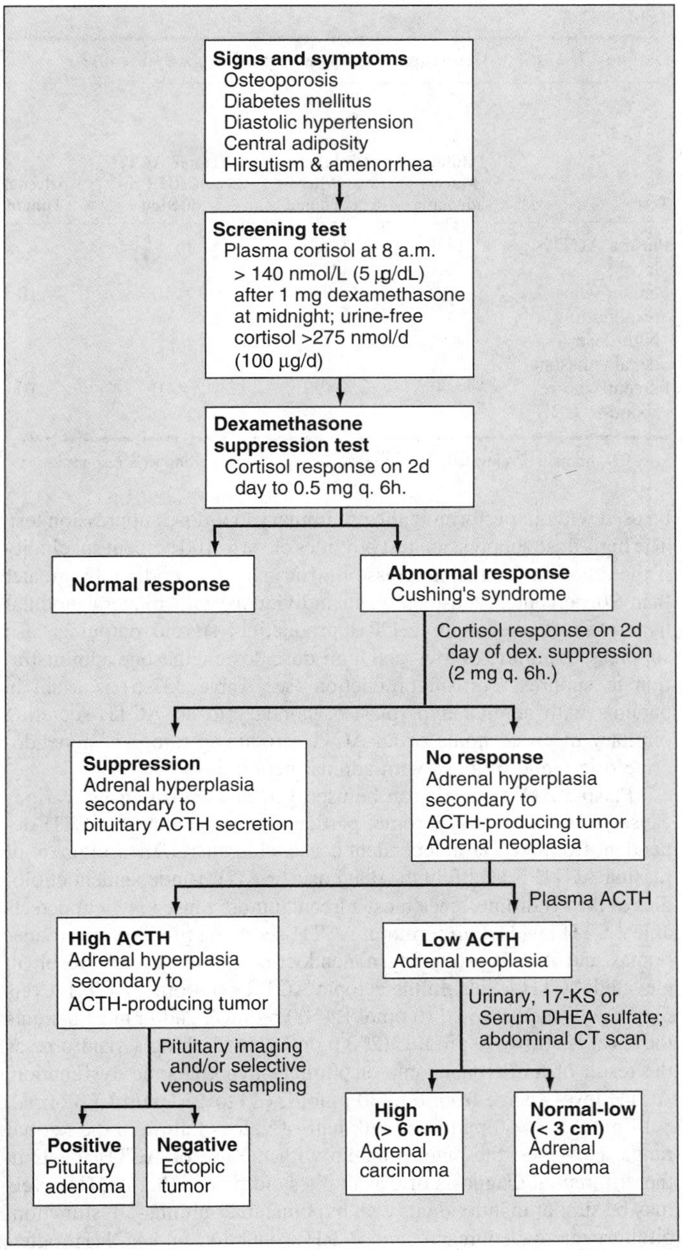

FIGURE 332-7 Diagnostic flowchart for evaluating patients suspected of having Cushing's syndrome. *This group probably includes some patients with pituitary-hypothalamic dysfunction and some with pituitary microadenomas. In some instances, a pituitary microadenoma may be visualized by MRI scanning of the sella turcica.

Table 332-5

Diagnostic Tests to Determine the Type of Cushing's Syndrome

Test	Pituitary Macro-adenoma	Pituitary-Hypothalamic Dysfunction or Micro-adenoma	Ectopic ACTH or CRH Production	Adrenal Tumor
Plasma ACTH level	↑ to ↑↑	N to ↑	↑ to ↑↑↑	↓
Percent who respond to high-dose dexamethasone	<10	95	<10	<10
Percent who respond to CRH	>90	>90	<10	<10

NOTE: N, normal; ↑, elevated; ↓, decreased. See text for definition of a response.

be used without performing the preliminary low-dose suppression test. The high-dose suppression test provides close to 100 percent specificity if the criterion used is suppression of urinary free cortisol by greater than 90 percent. Occasionally, in individuals with bilateral nodular hyperplasia and/or ectopic CRH production, steroid output is also suppressed. Failure of low- and high-dose dexamethasone administration to suppress cortisol production (see Table 332-5) is usual in patients with adrenal hyperplasia secondary to an ACTH-secreting pituitary macroadenoma or an ACTH-producing tumor of nonendocrine origin and in those with adrenal neoplasms.

Plasma ACTH levels can be useful in distinguishing the various causes of Cushing's syndrome, particularly in separating ACTH-dependent from ACTH-independent causes. In general, measurement of plasma ACTH is useful in the diagnosis of ACTH-independent etiologies of the syndrome, since most adrenal tumors cause low or undetectable ACTH levels. Furthermore, ACTH-secreting pituitary macroadenomas and ACTH-producing nonendocrine tumors usually result in elevated ACTH levels. In the ectopic ACTH syndrome, ACTH levels may be elevated above 110 pmol/L (500 pg/mL), and in most patients the level is above 40 pmol/L (200 pg/mL). In Cushing's syndrome as the result of a microadenoma or pituitary-hypothalamic dysfunction, ACTH levels range from 6 to 30 pmol/L (30 to 150 pg/mL) [normal, <14 pmol/L (<60 pg/mL)], with half of values falling in the normal range. However, the main problem with the use of ACTH levels in the differential diagnosis of Cushing's syndrome is that ACTH levels may be similar in individuals with hypothalamic-pituitary dysfunction, pituitary microadenomas, ectopic CRH production, and ACTH production from some nonendocrine tumors (especially carcinoid tumors) (see Table 332-5).

Because of these difficulties, several additional tests have been advocated, such as the metyrapone and CRH infusion tests. The rationale underlying these tests is that steroid hypersecretion by an adrenal tumor or the ectopic production of ACTH will suppress the hypothalamic-pituitary axis so that inhibition of pituitary ACTH release can be demonstrated by either test. Thus, most patients with pituitary-hypothalamic dysfunction and/or a microadenoma have an increase in steroid or ACTH secretion in response to metyrapone or CRH administration, while most patients with ectopic ACTH-producing tumors do not. Most pituitary macroadenomas also respond to CRH, while their response to metyrapone is variable. The usefulness of the CRH infusion test, however, is uncertain because only a limited number of studies have been performed and because CRH is not readily available. In addition, false-positive and false-negative CRH tests can occur in patients with nonendocrine and pituitary tumors.

The main diagnostic dilemma in Cushing's syndrome is to distinguish those instances due to microadenomas of the pituitary and/or pituitary-hypothalamic dysfunction from those due to tumors (e.g., carcinoids or pheochromocytoma) that produce CRH and/or ACTH ectopically. The clinical manifestations are similar unless the ectopic tumor produces other symptoms, such as diarrhea and flushing from a carcinoid tumor or episodic hypertension from a pheochromocytoma. Sometimes, one can distinguish between ectopic and pituitary ACTH production by using metyrapone or CRH tests, as noted above. In these situations, computed tomography (CT) of the pituitary gland is usually normal. Magnetic resonance imaging (MRI) with the enhancing agent gadolinium may be better than CT for this purpose but demonstrates pituitary microadenomas in only half of patients with Cushing's disease. In subjects with negative imaging studies, selective venous sampling for ACTH is employed in some centers. Demonstration of an ACTH gradient between the petrosal sinus and peripheral blood localizes the source of ACTH overproduction to the pituitary gland but does not distinguish pituitary-dependent adrenal hyperplasia from pituitary hyperplasia secondary to a tumor producing CRH. CRH levels should be measured in the peripheral blood prior to petrosal sinus sampling. No reliable test is available to make this distinction if the ectopic tumor is not seen or if it produces no other hormones.

The diagnosis of a *cortisol-producing adrenal adenoma* is suggested by disproportionate elevations in baseline urine free-cortisol levels with only modest changes in urinary 17-ketosteroids or plasma DHEA sulfate. Adrenal androgen secretion is usually reduced in these patients owing to the cortisol-induced suppression of ACTH and subsequent involution of the androgen-producing zona reticularis.

The diagnosis of *adrenal carcinoma* is suggested by a palpable abdominal mass and by *markedly* elevated baseline values of *both* urine 17-ketosteroids and plasma DHEA sulfate. Plasma and urine cortisol levels are variably elevated. Adrenal carcinoma is usually resistant to both ACTH stimulation and dexamethasone suppression. Elevated adrenal androgen secretion often leads to virilization in the female. Estrogen-producing adrenocortical carcinoma usually presents with gynecomastia in men and dysfunctional uterine bleeding in women. These adrenal tumors secrete increased amounts of androstenedione, which is converted peripherally to the estrogens estrone and estradiol (see Chap. 338). Adrenal carcinomas that produce Cushing's syndrome are most often associated with elevated levels of the intermediates of steroid biosynthesis (especially 11-deoxycortisol), suggesting inefficient conversion of the intermediates to the final product. Approximately 20 percent of adrenal carcinomas are not associated with endocrine syndromes and are presumed to be nonfunctioning or to produce biologically inactive steroid precursors. In addition, the excessive production of steroids is not always clinically evident (e.g., androgens in adult men).

Differential Diagnosis *Pseudo-Cushing's syndrome* Problems in diagnosis include patients with obesity, chronic alcoholism, depression, and acute illness of any type. Extreme *obesity* is uncommon in Cushing's syndrome; furthermore, with exogenous obesity, the adiposity is generalized, not truncal. On adrenocortical testing, abnormalities in patients with exogenous obesity are usually modest. Basal urine steroid excretion levels in obese patients are also either normal or slightly elevated. Some patients have elevated conversion of secreted cortisol into excreted metabolites. Urinary and blood cortisol levels are usually normal, and the diurnal pattern in blood and urine levels is normal. Patients with *chronic alcoholism* and those with *depression* share similar abnormalities in steroid output: modestly elevated urine cortisol, absent circadian rhythm of cortisol levels, and resistance to suppression with dexamethasone (particularly in the overnight and low-dose tests). In contrast to alcoholic subjects, depressed patients do not have signs and symptoms of Cushing's syndrome. Following discontinuation of alcohol and/or improvement in the emotional status, results of steroid testing usually return to normal. A normal cortisol response to insulin-induced hypoglycemia may distinguish these patients from subjects with Cushing's syndrome. *Acutely ill* patients often have abnormal results on laboratory tests and fail to exhibit pituitary-adrenal suppression in response to dexamethasone, since major stress (such as pain or fever) interrupts the normal regulation of ACTH secretion. A rare cause of hypercortisolism without cushingoid stigmata is *primary cortisol resistance* due to mutations in the type I glucocorticoid receptor; the resistance is incomplete because patients do not exhibit signs of adrenal insufficiency. *Iatrogenic Cushing's syndrome*, induced by the administration of glucocorticoids or other steroids such as megestrol that bind to the glucocorticoid receptor, is indistinguishable by physical findings from endogenous adrenocortical hyperfunction. The distinction can be made, however, by measuring blood or urine cortisol levels in a basal state; in the iatrogenic syndrome these levels are low secondary to suppression of the pituitary-adrenal axis. The severity of iatrogenic Cushing's syndrome is related to the total steroid dose, the biologic half-life of the steroid, and the duration of therapy. Also, individuals taking afternoon and evening doses of glucocorticoids develop Cushing's syndrome more readily and with a smaller total daily dose than do patients taking morning doses only. The enzymatic disposition and binding of administered steroids differ among patients.

Radiologic Evaluation for Cushing's Syndrome The preferred radiologic study for visualizing the adrenals is a CT scan of the abdomen (Fig. 332-8). CT is of value both for localizing adrenal tumors and for diagnosing bilateral hyperplasia. All patients believed to have hypersecretion of pituitary ACTH should have a pituitary MRI scan with the contrast agent gadolinium. Even with this technique, small microadenomas may be undetectable; alternatively, false-positive masses due to nonsecretory variations of the normal pituitary anatomy may be imaged. In patients with ectopic ACTH production, chest tomography is a useful first step.

Evaluation of Asymptomatic Adrenal Masses With abdominal CT scanning, many incidental adrenal masses (so-called incidentalomas) are discovered. This is not surprising, since 10 to 20 percent of subjects at autopsy have adrenocortical adenomas. The first step in evaluating such patients is to determine whether the tumor is functioning by means of appropriate screening tests, e.g., measurement of 24-h urine catecholamines and metabolites and serum potassium and assessment of adrenal cortical function by dexamethasone suppression testing. However, 90 percent of incidentalomas are nonfunctioning. If an extraadrenal malignancy is present, there is a 30 to 50 percent chance that the adrenal tumor is a metastasis. If the primary tumor is being treated and there are no other metastases, it is prudent to obtain a fine-needle aspirate of the adrenal mass to establish the diagnosis. In the absence of a known malignancy the next step is unclear. The probability of adrenal carcinoma is less than 0.01 percent, the vast majority of adrenal masses being benign adenomas. Features suggestive of malignancy include large size (a size greater than 4 to 6 cm

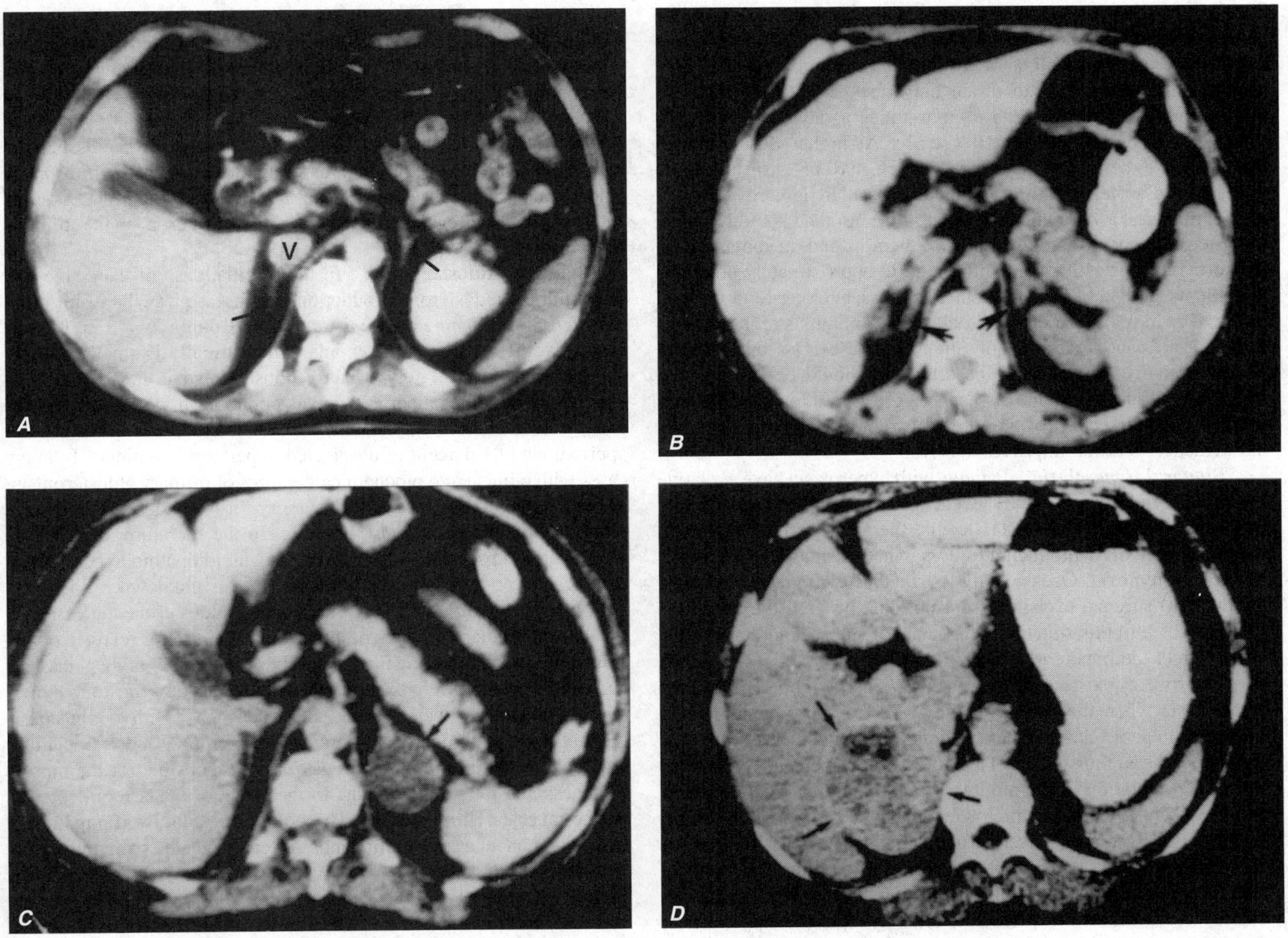

FIGURE 332-8 Computed tomography is the preferred method for visualizing the adrenal glands (*arrows*). *A*. The normal right adrenal gland is adjacent to the inferior vena cava (V) where it emerges from the liver. Approximately 90 percent of the right adrenal glands appear as linear structures extending posteriorly from the inferior vena cava into the space between the right lobe of the liver and the crus of the diaphragm. The normal left adrenal gland is lateral to the left crus of the diaphragm and below the stomach. Most left adrenal glands are shaped like an inverted V or Y. *B*. Adrenal CT scan of a patient with ectopic ACTH production. Both adrenal glands (*arrows*) are enlarged (compare with *A*). In contrast, only 50 percent of patients with bilateral adrenal hyperplasia secondary to pituitary ACTH hypersecretion show enlargement of the adrenals when imaged by CT scan. *C*. CT scan of a patient with Cushing's syndrome with biochemical evidence only of cortisol overproduction. The left adrenal has been replaced by a racquet-shaped 2-cm tumor (*arrow*). Attenuation of the tumor is low because of its high lipid content. *D*. CT scan in a patient with Cushing's syndrome and biochemical evidence of an adrenal carcinoma. In contrast to the tumor in *C*, the right-sided mass in this patient is large and has a heterogeneous appearance—usual characteristics of an adrenal carcinoma.

suggests carcinoma); irregular margins; and inhomogeneity, soft tissue calcifications visible on CT (see Fig. 332-8), and findings characteristic of malignancy on a chemical-shift MRI image. If surgery or fine-needle aspiration is not performed, a repeat CT scan should be obtained in 3 to 6 months.

Rx TREATMENT

Adrenal Neoplasm When an adenoma or carcinoma is diagnosed, adrenal exploration is performed with excision of the tumor. Because of the possibility of atrophy of the contralateral adrenal, the patient is treated pre- and postoperatively as if for total adrenalectomy, even when a unilateral lesion is suspected, the routine being similar to that for an Addisonian patient undergoing elective surgery (see Table 332-11).

Despite operative intervention, most patients with adrenal carcinoma die within 3 years of diagnosis. Metastases occur most often to liver and lung. The principal drug for the treatment of adrenocortical carcinoma is mitotane (*o,p'*-DDD), an isomer of the insecticide DDT. This drug suppresses cortisol production and decreases plasma and urine steroid levels. Although its cytotoxic action is relatively selective for the glucocorticoid-secreting zone of the adrenal cortex, the zona glomerulosa also may be inhibited. Because mitotane also alters the extraadrenal metabolism of cortisol, plasma and urinary cortisol levels must be assessed to titrate the effect. The drug is usually given in divided doses three to four times a day, with the dose increased gradually to 8 to 10 g daily. At higher doses, almost all patients experience side effects, which may be gastrointestinal (anorexia, diarrhea, vomiting) or neuromuscular (lethargy, somnolence, dizziness). All patients treated with mitotane should receive long-term glucocorticoid maintenance therapy, and, in some, mineralocorticoid replacement is appropriate. In approximately one-third of patients, both tumor and metastases regress, but long-term survival is limited. In many patients, mitotane only inhibits steroidogenesis and does not cause regression of tumor metastases. Osseous metastases are usually refractory to the drug and should be treated with radiation therapy. Mitotane also can be given as adjunctive therapy after surgical resection of an adrenal carcinoma, although there is no evidence that this improves survival.

Bilateral Hyperplasia Patients with hyperplasia have a relative or absolute increase in ACTH levels. Since therapy would logically be directed at reducing ACTH levels, the ideal primary treatment for ACTH- or CRH-producing tumors, whether pituitary or ectopic, is surgical removal. Occasionally (particularly with ectopic ACTH production) surgical excision is not possible because the disease is far advanced. In this situation, "medical" or surgical adrenalectomy may correct the hypercortisolism.

Controversy exists as to the proper treatment for bilateral adrenal hyperplasia when the source of the ACTH overproduction is not apparent. In some centers, these patients (especially those who suppress after the administration of a high-dose dexamethasone) undergo surgical exploration of the pituitary via a transsphenoidal approach in the expectation that a microadenoma will be found. However, in most circumstances selective petrosal sinus venous sampling is recommended, and the patient is referred to an appropriate center if the procedure is not available locally. If a microadenoma is not found at the time of exploration, total hypophysectomy may be needed. Complications of transsphenoidal surgery include cerebrospinal fluid rhinorrhea, diabetes insipidus, panhypopituitarism, and optic or cranial nerve injuries. Furthermore, these pituitary neoplasms may recur if the primary abnormality actually resides in the hypothalamus.

In other centers, total adrenalectomy is the treatment of choice. The cure rate with this procedure is close to 100 percent. The adverse effects include the certain need for lifelong mineralocorticoid and glucocorticoid replacement and a 10 to 20 percent probability of a pituitary tumor developing over the next 10 years (Nelson's syndrome; see Chap. 328). Many of these tumors require surgical therapy. It is uncertain whether they arise de novo in these patients or were present prior to adrenalectomy but were too small to be detected. Periodic radiologic evaluation of the pituitary gland by MRI as well as serial ACTH measurements should be performed in all individuals after bilateral adrenalectomy for Cushing's syndrome. Such pituitary tumors may become locally invasive and impinge on the optic chiasm or extend into the cavernous or sphenoid sinuses.

Except in children, pituitary irradiation is rarely used as primary treatment, being reserved rather for postoperative tumor recurrences. In some centers, high levels of gamma radiation can be focused on the desired site with less scattering to surrounding tissues by using stereotactic techniques. Side effects of radiation include ocular motor palsy and hypopituitarism. There is a long lag time between treatment and remission, and the remission rate is usually less than 50 percent.

Finally, in occasional patients in whom a surgical approach is not feasible, "medical" adrenalectomy may be indicated (Table 332-6). Inhibition of steroidogenesis also may be indicated in severely cushingoid subjects prior to surgical intervention. Chemical adrenalectomy may be accomplished by the administration of the inhibitor of steroidogenesis ketoconazole (600 to 1200 mg/d). In addition, mitotane (2 or 3 g/d) and/or the blockers of steroid synthesis aminoglutethimide (1 g/d) and metyrapone (2 or 3 g/d) may be effective either alone or in combination. Mitotane is slow to take effect (weeks). Mifepristone, a competitive inhibitor of the binding of glucocorticoid to its receptor, may be a treatment option. Adrenal insufficiency is a risk with all these agents, and replacement steroids may be required.

ALDOSTERONISM Aldosteronism is a syndrome associated with hypersecretion of the mineralocorticoid aldosterone. In *primary* aldosteronism the cause for the excessive aldosterone production resides within the adrenal gland; in *secondary* aldosteronism the stimulus is extraadrenal.

Primary Aldosteronism In the original case of excessive and inappropriate aldosterone production, the disease was the result of an *aldosterone-producing adrenal adenoma* (Conn's syndrome). Most cases involve a unilateral adenoma, which usually is small and may occur on either side. Rarely, primary aldosteronism is due to an adrenal carcinoma. Aldosteronism is twice as common in women as in men, usually occurs between the ages of 30 and 50, and is present in approximately 1 percent of unselected hypertensive patients. In many cases with clinical and biochemical features of primary aldosteronism, a solitary adenoma is not found at surgery. Instead, these patients have *bilateral cortical nodular hyperplasia.* In the literature, this disease is also termed pseudoprimary aldosteronism, idiopathic hyperaldosteronism, and nodular hyperplasia. The cause is unknown.

Signs and symptoms Hypersecretion of aldosterone increases the renal distal tubular exchange of intratubular sodium for secreted potassium and hydrogen ions, with progressive depletion of body potassium and development of hypokalemia. Most patients have diastolic hypertension, usually not very severe, and headaches. The hypertension is probably due to the increased sodium reabsorption and extracellular volume expansion. *Potassium depletion* is responsible for the muscle weakness and fatigue and is due to the effect of potassium depletion on the muscle cell membrane. The polyuria results from impairment of urinary concentrating ability and is often associated with polydipsia.

Table 332-6

Treatment Modalities for Patients with Adrenal Hyperplasia Secondary to Pituitary ACTH Hypersecretion

Treatments to reduce pituitary ACTH production
Transsphenoidal resection of microadenoma
Radiation therapy
Treatments to reduce or eliminate adrenocortical cortisol secretion
Bilateral adrenalectomy
Medical adrenalectomy (metyrapone, mitotane, aminoglutethimide, ketoconazole)*

* Not curative but effective as long as chronically administered in selected patients.

Electrocardiographic and roentgenographic signs of left ventricular enlargement are secondary to the hypertension. Electrocardiographic signs of potassium depletion include prominent U waves, cardiac arrhythmias, and premature contractions. In the absence of associated congestive heart failure, renal disease, or preexisting abnormalities (such as thrombophlebitis), edema is characteristically absent. In cases of long duration, nephropathy with azotemia may be associated with congestive heart failure and edema.

Laboratory findings Laboratory findings depend on both the duration and the severity of potassium depletion. An overnight concentration test often reveals impaired ability to concentrate the urine, probably secondary to the hypokalemia. Urine pH is neutral to alkaline because of excessive secretion of ammonium and bicarbonate ions to compensate for the metabolic alkalosis.

Hypokalemia may be severe (less than 3 mmol/L) and reflects body potassium depletion, usually in excess of 300 mmol. *Hypernatremia* is due to sodium retention, a concomitant water loss from polyuria, and a resetting of the osmostat. Metabolic alkalosis and elevation of serum bicarbonate are a result of hydrogen ion loss into the urine and migration into potassium-depleted cells. The alkalosis is perpetuated by potassium deficiency, which increases the capacity of the proximal convoluted tubule to reabsorb filtered bicarbonate. If hypokalemia is severe, serum magnesium levels are also reduced.

Total-body sodium content and total exchangeable sodium are usually increased, while total exchangeable body potassium is reduced. The expanded extracellular fluid volume may be responsible for the reversed circadian excretory pattern for salt and water, with salt and water excretion occurring predominantly during the night.

Diagnosis The diagnosis is suggested by persistent hypokalemia in a nonedematous patient with a normal sodium intake who is not receiving potassium-wasting diuretics (furosemide, ethacrynic acid, thiazides). If hypokalemia occurs in a hypertensive patient taking a potassium-wasting diuretic, the diuretic should be discontinued and the patient should be given potassium supplements. After 1 to 2 weeks, the potassium level should be remeasured, and if hypokalemia persists the patient should be evaluated for a mineralocorticoid excess syndrome (Fig. 332-9).

The criteria for the diagnosis of primary aldosteronism are (1) diastolic hypertension without edema, (2) hyposecretion of renin (as judged by low plasma renin activity levels) that fails to increase appropriately during volume depletion (upright posture, sodium depletion), and (3) hypersecretion of aldosterone that does not suppress appropriately in response to volume expansion (salt loading).

Patients with primary aldosteronism characteristically *do not have edema*, since they exhibit an "escape" phenomenon from the sodium-retaining aspects of mineralocorticoids. Rarely, pretibial edema is present in patients with associated nephropathy and azotemia.

The estimation of plasma renin activity is of limited value in separating patients with primary aldosteronism from those with hypertension of other causes. While failure of plasma renin activity to rise normally during volume-depletion maneuvers is a criterion for a diagnosis of primary aldosteronism, suppressed renin activity also occurs in about 25 percent of patients with essential hypertension.

Since the determination of plasma renin responsiveness is not sufficient, the demonstration of lack of suppression of aldosterone secretion is necessary to diagnose primary aldosteronism (see Fig. 332-9). The autonomy exhibited by aldosterone tumors in these patients refers only to the resistance to suppression of secretion during volume expansion; such tumors can and do respond in a normal or above-normal fashion to the stimulus of potassium loading or ACTH infusion.

Once hyposecretion of renin and failure of aldosterone secretion suppression are demonstrated, aldosterone-producing adenomas should be localized by abdominal CT scan, using a spiral, thin-slice technique since many aldosteronomas are less than 1 cm in size. If the CT scan is negative, percutaneous transfemoral bilateral adrenal vein catheterization with adrenal vein sampling may demonstrate a two- to threefold increase in plasma aldosterone concentration on the involved side. In cases of hyperaldosteronism secondary to cortical nodular hyperplasia, no localization is found. It is important for samples to be obtained simultaneously if possible and for cortisol levels to be measured to ensure that false localization does not reflect an ACTH- or stress-induced rise in aldosterone levels.

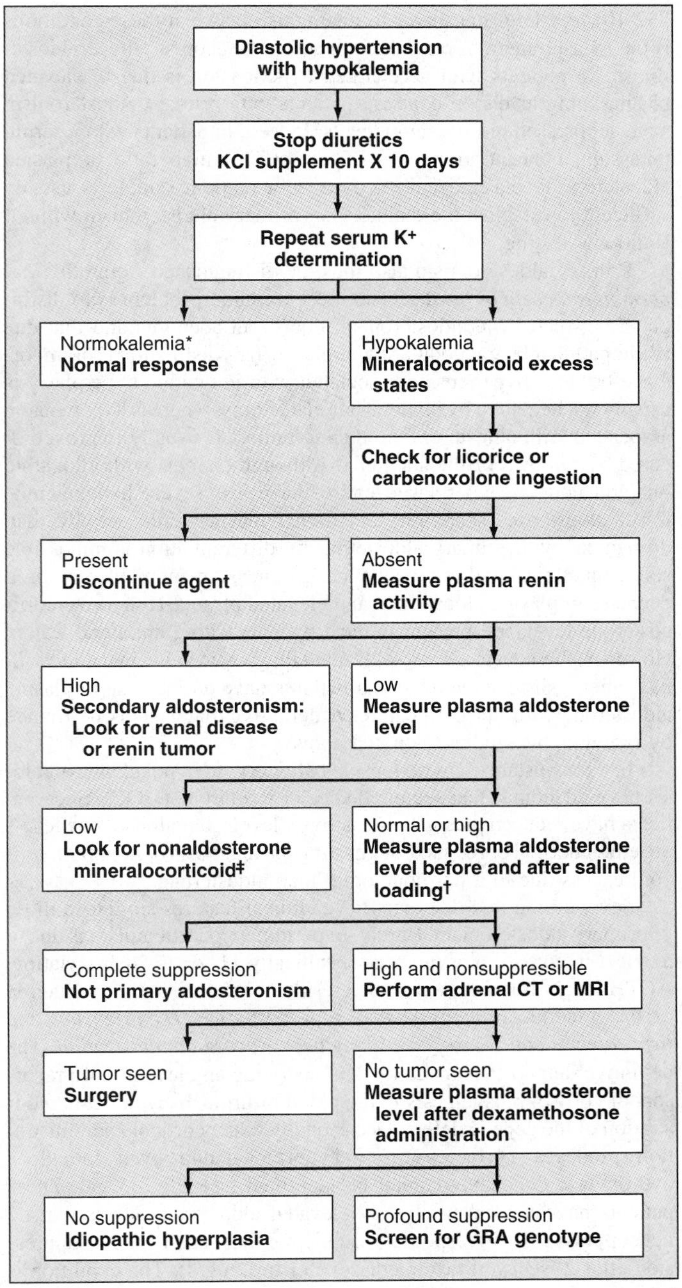

FIGURE 332-9 Diagnostic flowchart for evaluating patients with suspected primary aldosteronism. *Serum K^+ may be normal in some patients with hyperaldosteronism who are taking potassium-sparing diuretics (spironolactone, triamterene) or who have a low sodium intake and a high potassium intake. †This step should not be taken if hypertension is severe (diastolic pressure >115 mmHg) or if cardiac failure is present. Also, serum potassium levels should be corrected before the infusion of saline solution. Alternative methods that produce comparable suppression of aldosterone secretion include oral sodium loading (200 mmol/d for 3 days) or administration of 10 mg deoxycorticosterone acetate (DOCA) intramuscularly every 12 h for 3 days. (GRA, glucocorticoid-remediable aldosteronism.) ‡For example, Liddle's syndrome, apparent mineralocorticoid excess syndrome, or a deoxycorticosterone-secreting tumor.

Differential diagnosis Patients with hypertension and hypokalemia may have either primary or secondary hyperaldosteronism (Fig.

332-10). A useful maneuver to distinguish between these conditions is the measurement of plasma renin activity. Secondary hyperaldosteronism in patients with accelerated hypertension is due to elevated plasma renin levels; in contrast, patients with primary aldosteronism have suppressed plasma renin levels. Indeed, in patients with a serum potassium concentration of <2.5 mmol/L, a high ratio of plasma aldosterone to plasma renin activity in a random sample is usually sufficient to establish the diagnosis of primary aldosteronism without additional testing.

Primary aldosteronism also must be distinguished from other *hypermineralocorticoid states.* The most common problem is to distinguish between hyperaldosteronism due to an adenoma and that due to idiopathic bilateral nodular hyperplasia. This distinction is of importance because hypertension associated with idiopathic hyperplasia is usually not benefited by bilateral adrenalectomy, whereas hypertension associated with aldosterone-producing tumors is usually improved or cured by removal of the adenoma. Although patients with idiopathic bilateral nodular hyperplasia tend to have less severe hypokalemia, lower aldosterone secretion, and higher plasma renin activity than do patients with primary aldosteronism, differentiation is impossible solely on clinical and/or biochemical grounds. An anomalous postural decrease in plasma aldosterone and elevated plasma 18-hydroxycorticosterone levels are present in most patients with a unilateral lesion. However, these tests are also of limited diagnostic value in the individual patient, since some adenoma patients have an increase in plasma aldosterone with upright posture. A definitive diagnosis is best made by radiographic studies, as noted above.

In a few instances, hypertensive patients with hypokalemic alkalosis have adenomas that secrete deoxycorticosterone (DOC). Such patients have reduced plasma renin activity levels, but aldosterone levels are either normal or reduced, suggesting the diagnosis of mineralocorticoid excess due to a hormone other than aldosterone.

Several inherited disorders have clinical features similar to those of primary aldosteronism. Rarely, hypermineralocorticoidism is due to a defect in cortisol biosynthesis, specifically 11- or 17-hydroxylation. ACTH levels are increased, with a resultant increase in the production of the mineralocorticoid 11-deoxycorticosterone. *Hypertension and hypokalemia can be corrected by glucocorticoid administration.* The definitive diagnosis is made by demonstrating an elevation of precursors of cortisol biosynthesis in the blood or urine or by direct demonstration of the genetic defect. Occasionally, glucocorticoid administration produces normotension and normokalemia even though a hydroxylase deficiency cannot be identified (see Fig. 332-9). These patients have normal to slightly elevated aldosterone levels that do not suppress fully in response to saline but that usually show suppression after 2 weeks of dexamethasone (1 to 2 mg/d). The condition is inherited as an autosomal dominant trait and is termed *glucocorticoid-remediable aldosteronism* (GRA). This entity is secondary to a chimeric gene duplication whereby the 11β-hydroxylase gene promoter (which is under the control of ACTH) is fused to the aldosterone synthase coding sequence. Thus, aldosterone synthase activity is expressed in the zona fasciculata and is regulated only by ACTH, in a fashion similar to the regulation of cortisol secretion. Screening for this defect is best performed by assessing the presence or absence of the chimeric gene. Since the abnormal gene may be present in the absence of hypokalemia, its frequency as a cause of hypertension is unknown. Individuals with suppressed plasma renin levels and juvenile-onset hypertension or a history of early-onset hypertension in first-degree relatives should be screened for this disorder.

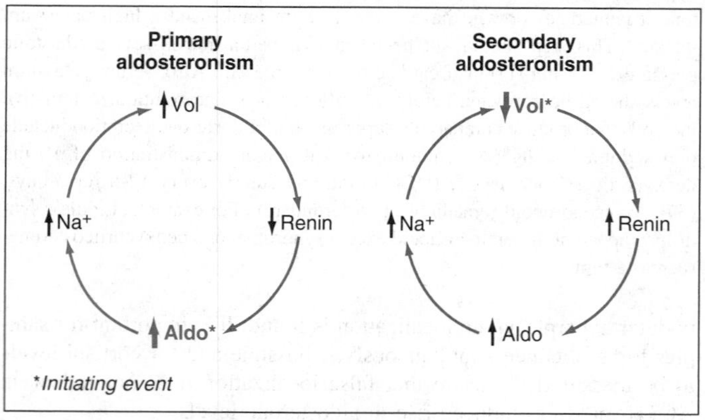

FIGURE 332-10 Responses of the renin-aldosterone volume control loop in primary versus secondary aldosteronism.

Liddle's syndrome is a rare autosomal dominant disorder that mimicks hyperaldosteronism. The defect is in the gene encoding the β subunit of the epithelial sodium channel. Both renin and aldosterone levels are low, owing to the continuously activated sodium channel and the resulting excess sodium reabsorption in the renal tubule.

A rare autosomal recessive cause of hypokalemia and hypertension is 11β-hydroxysteroid dehydrogenase deficiency, in which cortisol cannot be converted to cortisone and hence binds to the glucocorticoid type I (mineralocorticoid) receptor and acts as a mineralocorticoid. This condition, also termed *apparent mineralocorticoid excess syndrome,* is caused by a defect in the gene encoding the renal isoform of this enzyme. Patients can be identified either by documenting an increased ratio of cortisol to cortisone in the urine or by genetic analysis.

The ingestion of candies or chewing tobacco containing certain forms of licorice produces a syndrome that mimics primary aldosteronism. The component of such agents that causes sodium retention is glycyrrhizinic acid, which inhibits the 11β-hydroxysteroid dehydrogenase and hence allows cortisol to act as a mineralocorticoid and cause sodium retention, expansion of the extracellular fluid volume, hypertension, depressed plasma renin levels, and suppressed aldosterone levels. The diagnosis is established or excluded by a careful history.

Rx TREATMENT

Primary aldosteronism due to an adenoma is usually treated by surgical excision of the adenoma. Where possible a laparoscopic approach is favored. However, dietary sodium restriction and the administration of an aldosterone antagonist (spironolactone) are effective in many cases. Hypertension and hypokalemia are usually controlled by doses of 25 to 100 mg spironolactone every 8 h. In some patients medical management has been successful for years, but chronic therapy in men is usually limited by side effects of spironolactone such as gynecomastia, decreased libido, and impotence.

When idiopathic bilateral hyperplasia is suspected, surgery is indicated only when significant, symptomatic hypokalemia cannot be controlled with medical therapy, e.g., by spironolactone, triamterene, or amiloride. Hypertension associated with idiopathic hyperplasia is usually not benefited by bilateral adrenalectomy.

Glucocorticoid-remediable hyperaldosteronism documented by genetic analysis may be treated with glucocorticoid administration or antimineralocorticoids, e.g., spironolactone, triamterene, or amiloride. Glucocorticoids should be used only in small doses to avoid inducing iatrogenic Cushing's syndrome. A combination approach is often necessary. Patients with the 11β-hydroxysteroid dehydrogenase deficiency syndrome can be treated with small doses of dexamethasone. Although dexamethasone is a potent glucocorticoid that suppresses ACTH and endogenous cortisol production, it binds less well to the mineralocorticoid receptor than does cortisol.

Secondary Aldosteronism *Secondary aldosteronism* refers to an appropriately increased production of aldosterone in response to activation of the renin-angiotensin system (see Fig. 332-10). The production rate of aldosterone is often higher in patients with secondary aldosteronism than in those with primary aldosteronism. Secondary aldosteronism usually occurs in association with the accelerated phase of hypertension or on the basis of an underlying edema disorder. Secondary aldosteronism in pregnancy is a normal physiologic response to estrogen-induced increases in circulating levels of renin substrate and plasma renin activity and to the antialdosterone actions of progestogens.

Secondary aldosteronism in hypertensive states is due either to a primary overproduction of renin (primary reninism) or to an overproduction of renin secondary to a decrease in renal blood flow and/or perfusion pressure (see Fig. 332-10). Secondary hypersecretion of renin can be due to a narrowing of one or both of the major renal arteries by atherosclerosis or by fibromuscular hyperplasia. Overproduction of renin from both kidneys also occurs in severe arteriolar nephrosclerosis (malignant hypertension) or with profound renal vasoconstriction (the accelerated phase of hypertension). The secondary aldosteronism is characterized by hypokalemic alkalosis, moderate to severe increases in plasma renin activity, and moderate to marked increases in aldosterone levels (see Chap. 246).

Secondary aldosteronism with hypertension also can be caused by rare renin-producing tumors (primary reninism). These patients have the biochemical characteristics of renal vascular hypertension, but the primary defect is renin secretion by a juxtaglomerular cell tumor. The diagnosis can be made by demonstration of normal renal vasculature and/or demonstration of a space-occupying lesion in the kidney by radiographic techniques and documentation of a unilateral increase in renal vein renin activity. Rarely, these tumors arise in tissues such as the ovary.

Secondary aldosteronism is present in many forms of *edema*. The rate of aldosterone secretion is usually increased in patients with edema caused by either cirrhosis or the nephrotic syndrome. In congestive heart failure, elevated aldosterone secretion varies depending on the severity of cardiac failure. The stimulus for aldosterone release in these conditions appears to be *arterial hypovolemia* and/or hypotension. Thiazides and furosemide often exaggerate secondary aldosteronism via volume depletion; hypokalemia and, on occasion, alkalosis can then become prominent features.

On occasion secondary hyperaldosteronism occurs without edema or hypertension (Bartter's syndrome). This syndrome is characterized by severe hyperaldosteronism (hypokalemic alkalosis) with moderate to marked increases in renin activity but normal blood pressure and no edema. Renal biopsy shows juxtaglomerular hyperplasia. The pathogenesis may involve a defect in the renal conservation of sodium or chloride and/or an increased production of prostaglandins. The renal loss of sodium is thought to stimulate renin secretion and aldosterone production. Hyperaldosteronism produces potassium depletion, and hypokalemia further elevates prostaglandin production and plasma renin activity. In some cases, the hypokalemia may be potentiated by a defect in renal conservation of potassium. Increased production of prostaglandins is probably not a primary abnormality, since administration of inhibitors of prostaglandin synthesis reverses the features only temporarily (see Chap. 278).

SYNDROMES OF ADRENAL ANDROGEN EXCESS Adrenal androgen excess results from excess production of dehydroepiandrosterone and androstenedione, which are converted to testosterone in extraglandular tissues; elevated testosterone levels account for most of the virilization. Adrenal androgen excess may be associated with the secretion of greater or smaller amounts of other adrenal hormones and may, therefore, present as "pure" syndromes of virilization or as "mixed" syndromes associated with excessive glucocorticoids and Cushing's syndrome.

Clinical Signs and Symptoms The manifestations can be divided into four types: hirsutism, oligomenorrhea, acne, and virilization. Clinically, it is important to distinguish between hypertrichosis, simple hirsutism, and hirsutism associated with virilization. Hypertrichosis is an increased growth of hair in males or females anywhere on the body. In contrast, hirsutism is limited to females and is hair growth in a male pattern of distribution. Most cases of simple hirsutism have no known cause. However, if the patient is virilized as well as hirsute, increased levels of androgens are usually present (see Chap. 53). In general, the degree of virilization reflects both the duration and the degree of excess androgen secretion, although significant virilization can result from minimal changes in testosterone production, and a significant increase in testosterone production can cause minimal signs of virilization. The occurrence of oligomenorrhea in a hirsute patient increases the probability that androgen production is increased. Thus, the evaluation of the hirsute patient should include a careful history of the onset of menarche, past and present menstrual history, and reproductive capacity and examination for signs and symptoms of androgen excess.

Etiology As in other states of adrenocortical hyperfunction, the syndromes associated with androgen excess may result from hyperplasia, adenoma, or carcinoma (the latter two are discussed above). *Congenital adrenal hyperplasia* is the consequence of enzymatic defects. In these patients, increased adrenal androgen production is associated with either excessive or decreased secretion of mineralocorticoids or decreased production of glucocorticoids. Since cortisol is the principal adrenal steroid regulating ACTH elaboration and since ACTH stimulates production of both cortisol and adrenal androgen, a block in cortisol synthesis may result in the enhanced secretion of adrenal androgens. In severe congenital virilizing hyperplasia, the adrenal output of cortisol may be so compromised as to cause adrenal deficiency despite adrenal hyperplasia.

Congenital adrenal hyperplasia is the most common adrenal disorder of infancy and childhood and is the consequence of any of several autosomal recessive mutations (see Chap. 339). Partial enzyme deficiencies can be expressed after adolescence, predominantly in women with hirsutism and oligomenorrhea but minimal virilization. Late-onset adrenal hyperplasia may account for 5 to 25 percent of cases of hirsutism and oligomenorrhea in women, depending on the population.

Defects have been described in the $P450_{C21}$, $P450_{C18}$, $P450_{C17\alpha}$, and $P450_{C11\beta}$ hydroxylases and in 3β-hydroxysteroid dehydrogenase (3β-HSD) (see Fig. 332-2). While the cDNAs for these enzymes have been cloned, the diagnosis of specific enzyme deficiencies with genetic techniques is not practical for routine use. $P450_{C21}$ deficiency is closely linked to the histocompatibility leukocyte antigen (HLA)-B locus of chromosome 6 so that HLA typing and/or DNA polymorphism can be used to detect the heterozygous carriers and to diagnose affected individuals in some families (see Chap. 306). The clinical expression in the different disorders is variable, ranging from virilization of the female ($P450_{C21}$) to feminization of the male (3β-HSD) (see also Chap. 339).

Adrenal virilization in the female at birth is associated with ambiguous external genitalia (*female pseudohermaphroditism*). Virilization probably begins after the fifth month of intrauterine development. At birth there may be enlarged genitalia in the male infant and enlargement of the clitoris, partial or complete fusion of the labia, and sometimes a urogenital sinus in the female. If the labial fusion is nearly complete, the female infant has external genitalia resembling a penis with hypospadias. In the *postnatal* period, congenital adrenal hyperplasia is associated with virilization in the female and isosexual precocity in the male. The excessive androgen levels result in accelerated growth, so that bone age exceeds chronologic age. Since epiphyseal closure is hastened by excessive androgens, growth stops, but truncal development continues, the characteristic appearance being a short child with a well-developed trunk.

The most common form of congenital adrenal hyperplasia (95 percent of cases) is a result of impairment of $P450_{C21}$. In addition to cortisol deficiency, aldosterone secretion is decreased in approximately one-third of the patients. Thus, with $P450_{C21}$ deficiency, adrenal virilization occurs with or without a salt-losing tendency due to aldosterone deficiency (see Fig. 332-2).

$P450_{C11\beta}$ deficiency causes a "hypertensive" variant of congenital adrenal hyperplasia. Hypertension and hypokalemia occur because of the impaired conversion of 11-deoxycorticosterone to corticosterone, resulting in the accumulation of 11-deoxycorticosterone, a potent mineralocorticoid. The degree of hypertension is variable. Increased shunting again occurs into the androgen pathway.

$P450_{C17\alpha}$ deficiency is characterized by hypogonadism, hypokalemia, and hypertension. This rare disorder causes decreased production of cortisol and shunting of precursors into the mineralocorticoid pathway with hypokalemic alkalosis, hypertension, and suppressed plasma renin activity. Usually, 11-deoxycorticosterone production is elevated. Because $P450_{C17\alpha}$ hydroxylation is required for biosynthesis of both adrenal androgens and gonadal testosterone and estrogen, this defect is associated with sexual immaturity, high urinary gonadotropin levels, and low urinary 17-ketosteroid excretion. Female patients have primary amenorrhea and lack of development of secondary sexual characteristics. Because of deficient androgen production, male patients have either ambiguous external genitalia or a female phenotype *(male pseudohermaphroditism).* Exogenous glucocorticoids can correct the hypertensive syndrome, and treatment with appropriate gonadal steroids results in sexual maturation.

With 3β-HSD deficiency, conversion of pregnenolone to progesterone is impaired, so that the synthesis of both cortisol and aldosterone is blocked, with shunting into the adrenal androgen pathway via 17α-hydroxypregnenolone and DHEA. Because DHEA is a weak androgen, and because this enzyme deficiency is also present in the gonad, the genitalia of the male fetus may be incompletely virilized or feminized. Conversely, in the female, overproduction of DHEA may produce partial virilization.

Diagnosis The diagnosis of *congenital adrenal hyperplasia* should be considered in infants having episodes of acute adrenal insufficiency or salt wasting or with hypertension. The diagnosis is further suggested by the finding of hypertrophy of the clitoris, fused labia, or a urogenital sinus in the female or of isosexual precocity in the male. In infants and children with a *$P450_{C21}$ block*, increased urine 17-ketosteroid excretion and increased plasma DHEA sulfate levels are typically associated with an increase in the blood levels of 17-hydroxyprogesterone and the excretion of its urinary metabolite pregnanetriol. Demonstration of elevated levels of 17-hydroxyprogesterone in amniotic fluid at 14 to 16 weeks of gestation allows prenatal detection of affected female infants.

The diagnosis of a *salt-losing form of congenital adrenal hyperplasia* due to defects in $P450_{C21}$ is suggested by episodes of acute adrenal insufficiency with hyponatremia, hyperkalemia, dehydration, and vomiting. These infants and children often crave salt and have laboratory findings indicating deficits in both cortisol and aldosterone secretion.

With the *hypertensive form of congenital adrenal hyperplasia* due to $P450_{C11\beta}$ deficiency, 11-deoxycorticosterone and 11-deoxycortisol accumulate. The diagnosis is confirmed by demonstrating increased levels of 11-deoxycortisol in the blood or increased amounts of tetrahydro-11-deoxycortisol in the urine. Elevation of 17-hydroxyprogesterone levels does not imply a coexisting $P450_{C21}$ deficiency.

Very high levels of urine dehydroepiandrosterone with low levels of pregnanetriol and of cortisol metabolites in urine are characteristic of children with 3β-HSD deficiency. Marked salt wasting may also occur.

Adults with *late-onset adrenal hyperplasia* (partial deficiency of $P450_{C21}$, $P450_{C11\beta}$, or 3β-HSD) are characterized by normal or moderately elevated levels of urinary 17-ketosteroids and plasma DHEA sulfate. A high basal level of a precursor of cortisol biosynthesis (such as 17-hydroxyprogesterone, 17-hydroxypregnenolone, or 11-deoxycortisol), or elevation of such a precursor after ACTH stimulation, confirms the diagnosis of a partial deficiency. Measurement of steroid precursors 60 min after bolus administration of ACTH is usually sufficient. Adrenal androgen output is easily suppressed by the standard low-dose (2 mg) dexamethasone test.

Differential Diagnosis The causes of hirsutism can be divided into four broad categories: familial, idiopathic, androgen excess, and drugs. In general, hirsutism of the first two types is not associated with other signs of androgen excess (i.e., oligomenorrhea, significant acne, or virilization). Likewise, drug-induced hirsutism is usually not associated with other signs and symptoms of androgen excess, unless the drug is an androgen. The drugs that produce an increase in body hair include phenothiazines, minoxidil, and phenytoin. Each of these drugs, particularly minoxidil, produces a generalized increase in hair growth, not just an increase in male-pattern hair. The mechanism may be related to the ability of these drugs to convert vellus into terminal hair follicles.

If drugs are excluded, the only known cause of hirsutism amenable to treatment is excess production of androgens by either the adrenal or the ovary.

In the female, the differential diagnosis of hirsutism and virilization is between adrenal and ovarian etiologies (Table 332-7). *Sudden onset of progressive hirsutism and virilization* suggests an adrenal or ovarian neoplasm. *Adrenal adenomas and carcinomas* may cause a pure or mixed virilizing syndrome. Since adrenal androgens are weak androgens, adrenal virilization is characterized by a *markedly elevated urine 17-ketosteroid excretion.* Virilizing adrenal adenomas are rare. *Virilizing adrenal carcinomas*, the most common adrenal tumors causing virilization, are associated with high plasma levels of DHEA sulfate and high rates of urinary excretion of 17-ketosteroids; as a rule, the tumors exceed 6 cm in size. Cortisol levels in blood and urine are normal or moderately elevated. Failure of urinary 17-ketosteroid levels and plasma DHEA sulfate levels to fall to normal in response to dexamethasone suppression (0.5 mg given orally every 6 h for 2 days) supports a diagnosis of virilizing adrenal tumor and excludes congenital adrenal hyperplasia.

The most common virilizing *ovarian tumor* is the arrhenoblastoma, but other ovarian tumors, such as adrenal rest tumor, granulosa cell tumor, hilar cell tumor, and Brenner tumor, can be responsible. Virilization due to ovarian tumors is usually characterized by normal levels of urinary 17-ketosteroids and DHEA sulfate, since the neoplasm usually secretes the potent androgen testosterone. Increases in 17-ketosteroid excretion occur in some patients with ovarian neoplasms, but an excretion rate in excess of 100 μmol/d (30 mg/d) is rare, except in the case of adrenal rest tumors. As with adrenal neoplasms, steroid production by ovarian tumors is not suppressed by dexamethasone. With the exception of adrenal rest tumors, these tumors are largely independent of ACTH stimulation. Elevations of plasma testosterone do not localize the neoplasm to the ovary, since testosterone can be elevated owing to peripheral conversion of adrenal precursors, such as DHEA (see Chap. 337).

The most common ovarian cause of excess androgen production is ovarian hyperthecosis or polycystic ovaries (see Chap. 337). Virilization is less common with polycystic ovaries than with ovarian or adrenal tumors, whereas hirsutism is quite frequent. Many patients with this condition are obese and have hyperinsulinemia, glucose intolerance, and acanthosis nigricans. The rate of 17-ketosteroid excretion may be partially reduced by dexamethasone. Plasma levels and production rates of androstenedione and, to a lesser extent, testosterone are usually increased. Follicle-stimulating hormone (FSH) levels tend to be low, and luteinizing hormone (LH) levels may be tonically elevated, leading to an increased LH/FSH ratio. The laboratory findings in patients with hirsutism-virilizing syndromes are summarized in Table 332-8.

℞ TREATMENT

Treatment of adrenal virilism is dictated by the type of lesion. Patients with *congenital adrenal hyperplasia* have a fundamental defect of cortisol deficiency with resultant excessive ACTH secretion, producing hyperplasia of the adrenal glands and causing additional shunting into the adrenal androgen pathway. Therapy in these patients consists of daily administration of glucocorticoids to suppress pituitary ACTH secretion. Because of its cost and intermediate

Table 332-7

Causes of Hirsutism in Women

Familial
Idiopathic
Ovarian
  Polycystic ovaries; hilus cell hyperplasia
  Tumor: arrhenoblastoma, hilus cell, adrenal rest
Adrenal
  Congenital adrenal hyperplasia
  Noncongenital adrenal hyperplasia (Cushing's)
  Tumor: virilizing carcinoma or adenoma

half-life, prednisone is the drug of choice except in infants, in whom hydrocortisone is usually used. In adults with late-onset adrenal hyperplasia, the smallest single bedtime dose of a long- or intermediate-acting glucocorticoid that suppresses pituitary ACTH secretion should be administered. The amount of steroid required by children with congenital adrenal hyperplasia is approximately 1 to 1.5 times the normal cortisol production rate of 27 to 35 μmol (10 to 13 mg) of cortisol per square meter of body surface per day and is given in divided doses two or three times per day. The dosage schedule is governed by repetitive analysis of the urinary 17-ketosteroids, plasma DHEA sulfate, and/or precursors of cortisol biosynthesis. Skeletal growth and maturation also must be monitored closely, since overtreatment with glucocorticoid replacement therapy retards linear growth.

Table 332-8

Laboratory Evaluation of Hirsutism-Virilizing Syndromes

	Ovarian		Adrenal			
	PCO	Ovarian Tumor	CAH	Adrenal Neoplasm	Cushing's Syndrome	Idiopathic
Urinary 17-ketosteroids, plasma DHEA sulfate	N↑	N	N↑	↑↑↑	N↑	N
Plasma testosterone	N↑	↑↑	N↑	N↑	N↑	N
LH/FSH ratio	N↑	N	N	N	N	N
Precursors of cortisol biosynthesis:						
Basal	N	N	N↑	N↑	N	N
Following ACTH infusion	N	N	↑↑	N↑	N	N
Cortisol following overnight dexamethasone suppression test	N	N	N	↑	↑	N

NOTE: CAH, congenital adrenal hyperplasia; PCO, polycystic ovary syndrome; N, normal; ↑, elevated.

HYPOFUNCTION OF THE ADRENAL CORTEX

Cases of adrenal insufficiency can be divided into two general categories: (1) those associated with primary inability of the adrenal to elaborate sufficient quantities of hormone and (2) those associated with a secondary failure due to inadequate ACTH formation or release (Table 332-9).

PRIMARY ADRENOCORTICAL DEFICIENCY (ADDISON'S DISEASE) The original description of Addison's disease—"general languor and debility, feebleness of the heart's action, irritability of the stomach, and a peculiar change of the color of the skin"—summarizes the dominant clinical features. Advanced cases are usually easy to diagnose, but recognition of the early phases can be a real challenge.

Incidence Primary insufficiency is relatively rare, may occur at any age, and affects both sexes equally. Because of the common therapeutic use of steroids, secondary adrenal insufficiency is relatively common.

Etiology and Pathogenesis Addison's disease results from progressive destruction of the adrenals, which must involve more than 90 percent of the glands before adrenal insufficiency appears. The adrenal is a frequent site for chronic granulomatous diseases, predominantly tuberculosis but also histoplasmosis, coccidioidomycosis, and cryptococcosis. In early series, tuberculosis was responsible for 70 to 90 percent of cases, but the most frequent cause now is *idiopathic* atrophy, and an autoimmune mechanism is probably responsible. Rarely, other lesions are encountered, such as adrenoleukodystrophy, bilateral hemorrhage, tumor metastases, amyloidosis, adrenomyeloneuropathy, familial adrenal insufficiency, or sarcoidosis.

Half of patients have circulating adrenal antibodies. Specific adrenal antigens to which autoantibodies may be directed include $P450_{C21}$. While most antibodies cause adrenal destruction, some antibodies cause adrenal insufficiency by blocking the binding of ACTH to its receptors. Some patients also have antibodies to thyroid, parathyroid, and/or gonadal tissue (see also Chap. 340). There is also an increased incidence of chronic lymphocytic thyroiditis, premature ovarian failure, type I diabetes mellitus, and hypo- or hyperthyroidism. The presence of two or more of these autoimmune endocrine disorders in the same person defines the polyglandular autoimmune syndrome type II. Additional features include pernicious anemia, vitiligo, alopecia, nontropical sprue, and myasthenia gravis. Within families, multiple generations are affected by one or more of the above diseases. Type II polyglandular syndrome is the result of a mutant gene on chromosome 6 and is associated with the HLA alleles B8 and DR3.

The combination of parathyroid and adrenal insufficiency and chronic mucocutaneous moniliasis constitutes type I polyglandular autoimmune syndrome. Other autoimmune diseases in this disorder include pernicious anemia, chronic active hepatitis, alopecia, primary hypothyroidism, and premature gonadal failure. There is no HLA association; this syndrome is inherited as an autosomal recessive trait. The type I syndrome usually presents during childhood, whereas the type II syndrome is usually manifested in adulthood. The mechanisms by which genetic predisposition and/or autoimmunity interact in the pathogenesis of these disorders are unknown.

Clinical suspicion of adrenal insufficiency should be high in patients with AIDS (see Chap. 308). Cytomegalovirus regularly involves the adrenal glands [so-called cytomegalovirus (CMV) necrotizing adrenalitis], and involvement with *Mycobacterium avium-intracellulare*, *Cryptococcus*, and Kaposi's sarcoma has been reported. Adrenal insufficiency in AIDS patients may not be manifest, but tests of adrenal reserve frequently give abnormal results. When interpreting tests of adrenocortical function, it is important to remember that medications such as rifampin, phenytoin, ketoconazole, and opiates may cause or potentiate adrenal insufficiency.

Adrenoleukodystrophy causes severe demyelination and early death in children, and adrenomyeloneuropathy is associated with a mixed motor and sensory neuropathy with spastic paraplegia in adults; both disorders are associated with elevated circulating levels of very long chain fatty acids and cause adrenal insufficiency. Familial adrenal insufficiency is an autosomal recessive disorder that causes unresponsiveness to ACTH secondary to mutations in the ACTH receptor. Adrenal hemorrhage and infarction occur in patients on anticoagulants and in those with circulating anticoagulants and hypercoagulable states, such as the antiphospholipid syndrome.

Clinical Signs and Symptoms Adrenocortical insufficiency caused by gradual adrenal destruction is characterized by an insidious onset of fatigability, weakness, anorexia, nausea and vomiting, weight

Table 332-9

Classification of Adrenal Insufficiency

PRIMARY ADRENAL INSUFFICIENCY

- Anatomic destruction of gland (chronic or acute)
  - "Idiopathic" atrophy (autoimmune, adrenoleukodystrophy)
  - Surgical removal
  - Infection (tuberculous, fungal, viral—especially in AIDS patients)
  - Hemorrhage
  - Invasion: metastatic
- Metabolic failure in hormone production
  - Congenital adrenal hyperplasia
  - Enzyme inhibitors (metyrapone, ketoconazole, aminoglutethimide)
  - Cytotoxic agents (mitotane)
- ACTH-blocking antibodies
- Mutation in ACTH receptor gene

SECONDARY ADRENAL INSUFFICIENCY

- Hypopituitarism due to hypothalamic-pituitary disease
- Suppression of hypothalamic-pituitary axis
  - By exogenous steroid
  - By endogenous steroid from tumor

loss, cutaneous and mucosal pigmentation, hypotension, and occasionally hypoglycemia (Table 332-10). Depending on the duration and degree of adrenal hypofunction, the manifestations vary from mild chronic fatigue to fulminating shock associated with acute destruction of the glands, as described by Waterhouse and Friderichsen.

Asthenia is the cardinal symptom. Early it may be sporadic, usually most evident at times of stress; as adrenal function becomes more impaired, the patient is continuously fatigued, and bed rest is necessary.

Hyperpigmentation may be striking or absent. It commonly appears as a diffuse brown, tan, or bronze darkening of parts such as the elbows or creases of the hand and of areas that normally are pigmented such as the areolae about the nipples. Bluish-black patches may appear on the mucous membranes. Some patients develop dark freckles, and irregular areas of vitiligo may paradoxically be present. As an early sign, tanning following sun exposure may be persistent.

Arterial hypotension with postural accentuation is frequent, and blood pressure may be in the range of 80/50 or less.

Abnormalities of gastrointestinal function often are the presenting complaint. Symptoms vary from mild anorexia with weight loss to fulminating nausea, vomiting, diarrhea, and ill-defined abdominal pain, which may be so severe as to be confused with an acute abdomen. Patients may have personality changes, usually consisting of excessive irritability and restlessness. Enhancement of the sensory modalities of taste, olfaction, and hearing is reversible with therapy. Axillary and pubic hair may be decreased in women due to loss of adrenal androgens.

Laboratory Findings In the early phase of gradual adrenal destruction, there may be no demonstrable abnormalities in the routine laboratory parameters, but adrenal reserve is decreased—that is, while basal steroid output may be normal, a subnormal increase occurs after stress. Adrenal stimulation with ACTH uncovers abnormalities in this stage of the disease, eliciting a subnormal increase of cortisol levels or no increase at all. In more advanced stages of adrenal destruction, serum sodium, chloride, and bicarbonate levels are reduced, and the serum potassium level is elevated. The hyponatremia is due both to loss of sodium into the urine (due to aldosterone deficiency) and to movement into the intracellular compartment. This extravascular sodium loss depletes extracellular fluid volume and accentuates hypotension. Elevated plasma vasopressin and angiotensin II levels may contribute to the hyponatremia by impairing free water clearance. Hyperkalemia is due to a combination of aldosterone deficiency, impaired glomerular filtration, and acidosis. Basal levels of cortisol and aldosterone are subnormal and fail to increase following ACTH administration. Mild to moderate hypercalcemia occurs in 10 to 20 percent of patients for unclear reasons. The electrocardiogram may show nonspecific changes, and the electroencephalogram exhibits a generalized reduction and slowing. There may be a normocytic anemia, a relative lymphocytosis, and a moderate eosinophilia.

Diagnosis The diagnosis of adrenal insufficiency should be made only with ACTH stimulation testing to assess adrenal reserve capacity for steroid production (see above for ACTH test protocols). In *severe adrenal insufficiency*, the rate of cortisol secretion is markedly decreased, which may be ascertained indirectly by the finding of low to absent 24-h urine cortisol. With *mild adrenal insufficiency* (decreased adrenal reserve) urine and blood steroid values overlap the normal range; thus, the diagnosis of adrenal insufficiency should never be excluded solely on the basis of normal basal urine steroid determinations. Plasma cortisol values vary from zero to the lower range of normal and therefore have little diagnostic value. Aldosterone secretion is usually low, resulting in salt wasting and increases in plasma renin levels. In primary adrenal insufficiency, plasma ACTH and associated peptides (β-lipotropin) are elevated because of loss of the usual cortisol-hypothalamic-pituitary feedback relationship, whereas in secondary adrenal insufficiency, plasma ACTH values are low or "inappropriately" normal (Fig. 332-11).

Table 332-10

Frequency of Symptoms and Signs in Adrenal Insufficiency

Sign or Symptom	Percent of Patients
Weakness	99
Pigmentation of skin	98
Weight loss	97
Anorexia, nausea, and vomiting	90
Hypotension (<110/70)	87
Pigmentation of mucous membranes	82
Abdominal pain	34
Salt craving	22
Diarrhea	20
Constipation	19
Syncope	16
Vitiligo	9

Differential Diagnosis Since weakness and fatigue are common, diagnosis of early adrenocortical insufficiency may be difficult. However, the combination of mild gastrointestinal distress, weight loss, anorexia, and a suggestion of increased pigmentation makes it mandatory to perform ACTH stimulation testing to rule out adrenal insufficiency, particularly before steroid treatment is begun. Weight loss is useful in evaluating the significance of weakness and malaise. Racial pigmentation may be a problem, but a *recent* and progressive *increase* in pigmentation is usually reported by the patient with gradual adrenal destruction. Hyperpigmentation is usually absent when adrenal destruction is rapid, as in bilateral adrenal hemorrhage. The fact that hyperpigmentation occurs with other diseases also may present a problem, but the appearance and distribution of pigment in adrenal insufficiency are usually characteristic. When doubt exists, measurement of ACTH levels and testing of adrenal reserve with the infusion of ACTH provide clear-cut differentiation.

℞ TREATMENT

All patients with adrenal insufficiency should receive specific hormone replacement. Like diabetics, these patients require careful education about the disease. Replacement therapy should correct

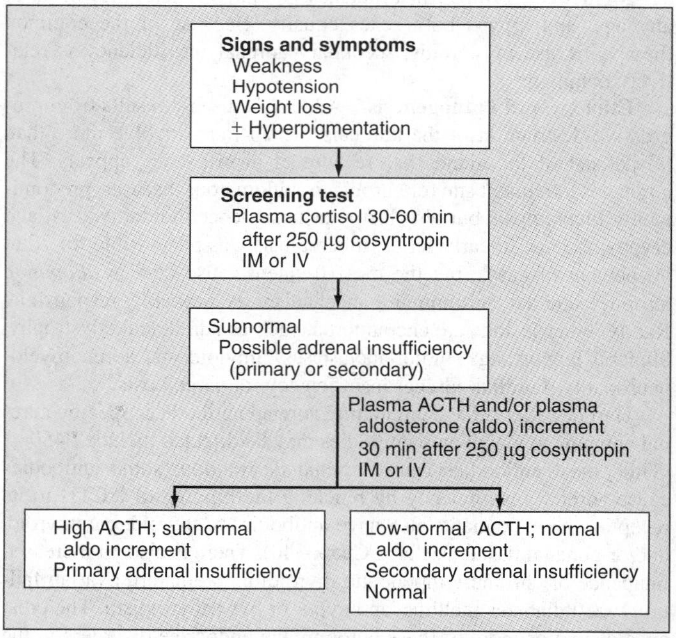

FIGURE 332-11 Diagnostic flowchart for evaluating patients with suspected adrenal insufficiency. Plasma ACTH levels are low in secondary adrenal insufficiency. In adrenal insufficiency secondary to pituitary tumors or idiopathic panhypopituitarism, other pituitary hormone deficiencies are present. On the other hand, ACTH deficiency may be isolated, as seen following prolonged use of exogenous glucocorticoids. Since the isolated blood levels obtained in these screening tests may not be definitive, the diagnosis may need to be confirmed by a continuous 24-h ACTH infusion. Normal subjects and patients with secondary adrenal insufficiency may be distinguished by insulin tolerance or metyrapone testing.

both glucocorticoid and mineralocorticoid deficiencies. Hydrocortisone (cortisol) is the mainstay of treatment. The dose for most adults (depending on size) is 20 to 30 mg/d. Patients are advised to take glucocorticoids with meals or, if that is impractical, with milk or an antacid, because the drugs may increase gastric acidity and exert direct toxic effects on the gastric mucosa. To simulate the normal diurnal adrenal rhythm, two-thirds of the dose is taken in the morning, and the remaining one-third is taken in the late afternoon. Some patients exhibit insomnia, irritability, and mental excitement after initiation of therapy; in these, the dosage should be reduced. Other situations that may necessitate smaller doses are hypertension and diabetes mellitus. Obese individuals and those on anticonvulsive medications may require increased dosages. Measurements of plasma ACTH or cortisol or of urine cortisol levels do not appear to be useful in determining optimal glucocorticoid dosages.

Since the replacement dosage of hydrocortisone does not replace the mineralocorticoid component of the adrenal hormones, mineralocorticoid supplementation is usually needed. This is usually accomplished by the administration of 0.05 to 0.1 mg fludrocortisone per day by mouth. Patients also should be instructed to maintain an ample intake of sodium (3 to 4 g/d).

The adequacy of mineralocorticoid therapy can be assessed by measurement of blood pressure and serum electrolytes. Blood pressure should be normal and without postural changes; serum sodium, potassium, creatinine, and urea nitrogen levels also should be normal. Measurement of plasma renin levels may also be useful in titrating the dose.

Complications of glucocorticoid therapy, with the exception of gastritis, are *rare* at the dosages recommended for treatment of adrenal insufficiency. Complications of mineralocorticoid therapy include hypokalemia, hypertension, cardiac enlargement, and even congestive heart failure due to sodium retention. Periodic measurements of body weight, serum potassium level, and blood pressure are useful. All patients with adrenal insufficiency should carry medical identification, should be instructed in the parenteral self-administration of steroids, and should be registered with a medical alerting system.

Special Therapeutic Problems During periods of intercurrent illness, especially in the setting of fever, the dose of hydrocortisone should be doubled. With severe illness it should be increased to 75 to 150 mg/d. When oral administration is not possible, parenteral routes should be employed. Likewise, before surgery or dental extractions, supplemental glucocorticoids should be administered. Patients also should be advised to increase the dose of fludrocortisone and to add salt to their otherwise normal diet during periods of strenuous exercise with sweating, during extremely hot weather, and with gastrointestinal upsets. A simple strategy is to supplement the diet one to three times daily with salty broth (1 cup of beef or chicken bouillon contains 35 mmol of sodium). For a representative program of steroid therapy for the patient with adrenal insufficiency who is undergoing major surgery, see Table 332-11. This schedule is designed so that on the day of surgery it will mimic the output of cortisol in normal individuals undergoing prolonged major stress (10 mg/h, 250 to 300 mg/d). Thereafter, if the patient is improving and is afebrile, the dose of hydrocortisone is tapered by 20 to 30 percent daily. Parenteral mineralocorticoid administration is unnecessary at hydrocortisone doses greater than 100 mg/d because of the mineralocorticoid effects of hydrocortisone at such dosages.

Table 332-11

Steroid Therapy Schedule for a Patient with Adrenal Insufficiency Undergoing Surgery*

	Hydrocortisone Infusion, Continuous, mg/h		Hydrocortisone (Orally)		Fludrocortisone (Orally),
			8 A.M.	4 P.M.	8 A.M.
Routine daily medication			20	10	0.1
Day before operation			20	10	0.1
Day of operation	10				
Postoperative					
Day 1	5–7.5				
Day 2	2.5–5				
Day 3	2.5–5	*or*	40	20	0.1
Day 4	2.5–5	*or*	40	20	0.1
Day 5			40	20	0.1
Day 6			20	20	0.1
Day 7			20	10	0.1

* All steroid doses are given in milligrams. An alternative approach is to give 100 mg hydrocortisone as an intravenous bolus injection every 6 h on the day of the operation (see text).

SECONDARY ADRENOCORTICAL INSUFFICIENCY ACTH deficiency causes *secondary* adrenocortical insufficiency; it may be a selective deficiency, as is seen following prolonged administration of excess glucocorticoids, or it may occur in association with deficiencies of multiple pituitary hormones (panhypopituitarism) (see Chap. 328). Patients with secondary adrenocortical hypofunction have many symptoms and signs in common with those having primary disease but are *characteristically not hyperpigmented*, since ACTH and related peptide levels are low. In fact, plasma ACTH levels distinguish between primary and secondary adrenal insufficiency, since they are elevated in the former and decreased to absent in the latter. Patients with total pituitary insufficiency have manifestations of multiple hormone deficiencies. An additional feature distinguishing primary adrenocortical insufficiency is the *near-normal level of aldosterone secretion* seen in pituitary and/or isolated ACTH deficiencies (see Fig. 332-11). Patients with pituitary insufficiency may have hyponatremia, which can be dilutional or secondary to a subnormal increase in aldosterone secretion in response to severe sodium restriction. However, severe *dehydration, hyponatremia*, and *hyperkalemia* are characteristic of severe mineralocorticoid insufficiency and favor a diagnosis of primary adrenocortical insufficiency.

Patients receiving long-term steroid therapy, despite physical findings of Cushing's syndrome, develop adrenal insufficiency because of prolonged pituitary-hypothalamic suppression and adrenal atrophy secondary to the loss of endogenous ACTH. These patients have two deficits, a loss of adrenal responsiveness to ACTH and a failure of pituitary ACTH release. They are characterized by low blood cortisol and ACTH levels, a low baseline rate of steroid excretion, and abnormal ACTH and metyrapone responses. Most patients with steroid-induced adrenal insufficiency eventually recover normal hypothalamic-pituitary-adrenal responsiveness, but recovery time varies from days to months. The rapid ACTH test provides a convenient assessment of recovery of hypothalamic-pituitary-adrenal function. Since the plasma cortisol concentrations after injection of cosyntropin and during insulin-induced hypoglycemia usually are similar, the rapid ACTH test assesses the integrated hypothalamic-pituitary-adrenal function (see "Tests of Pituitary-Adrenal Responsiveness," above). Additional tests to assess pituitary ACTH reserve include the standard metyrapone and insulin tolerance tests.

Glucocorticoid therapy in patients with secondary adrenocortical insufficiency does not differ from that for the primary disorder. Mineralocorticoid therapy is usually not necessary, since aldosterone secretion is preserved.

ACUTE ADRENOCORTICAL INSUFFICIENCY Acute adrenocortical insufficiency may result from several processes. On the one hand, *adrenal crisis* may be a rapid and overwhelming intensification of chronic adrenal insufficiency, usually precipitated by sepsis or surgical stress. Alternatively, acute hemorrhagic destruction of both adrenal glands can occur in previously well subjects. In children, this event is usually associated with septicemia with *Pseudomonas* or meningococcemia (Waterhouse-Friderichsen syndrome). In adults, anticoagulant therapy or a coagulation disorder may result in bilateral adrenal hemorrhage. Occasionally, bilateral adrenal hemorrhage in the newborn results from birth trauma. Hemorrhage has been observed during pregnancy, following idiopathic adrenal vein thrombosis, and as a complication of venography (e.g., infarction of an adenoma). The third and most frequent cause of acute insufficiency is the rapid withdrawal of steroids from patients with adrenal atrophy owing to chronic steroid administration. Acute adrenocortical insufficiency also may occur in patients with congenital adrenal hyperplasia or those with decreased adrenocortical reserve when they are given drugs capable of inhibiting steroid synthesis (mitotane, ketoconazole) or of increasing steroid metabolism (phenytoin, rifampin).

Adrenal Crisis The long-term survival of patients with adrenocortical insufficiency depends largely on the prevention and treatment of adrenal crisis. Consequently, the occurrence of infection, trauma (including surgery), gastrointestinal upsets, or other stresses necessitates an immediate increase in hormone. In untreated patients, preexisting symptoms are intensified. Nausea, vomiting, and abdominal pain may become intractable. Fever may be severe or absent. Lethargy deepens into somnolence, and hypovolemic vascular collapse ensues. In contrast, patients previously maintained on chronic glucocorticoid therapy may not exhibit dehydration or hypotension until they are in a preterminal state, since mineralocorticoid secretion is usually preserved. In all patients in crisis, a precipitating cause should be sought.

Rx TREATMENT

Treatment is directed primarily toward repletion of circulating glucocorticoids and replacement of the sodium and water deficits. Hence an intravenous infusion of 5% glucose in normal saline solution should be started with a bolus intravenous infusion of 100 mg hydrocortisone followed by a continuous infusion of hydrocortisone at a rate of 10 mg/h. An alternative approach is to administer a 100-mg bolus of hydrocortisone intravenously every 6 h. However, only continuous infusion maintains the plasma cortisol constantly at stress levels [>830 nmol/L (30 μg/dL)]. Effective treatment of hypotension requires glucocorticoid replacement and repletion of sodium and water deficits. If the crisis was preceded by prolonged nausea, vomiting, and dehydration, several liters of saline solution may be required in the first few hours. Vasoconstrictive agents (such as dopamine) may be indicated in extreme conditions as adjuncts to volume replacement. With large doses of steroid, e.g., 100 to 200 mg hydrocortisone, the patient receives a maximal mineralocorticoid effect, and supplementary mineralocorticoid is superfluous. Following improvement, the steroid dosage is tapered over the next few days to maintenance levels, and mineralocorticoid therapy is reinstituted if needed (see Table 332-11).

HYPOALDOSTERONISM

Isolated aldosterone deficiency accompanied by normal cortisol production occurs in association with hyporeninism, as an inherited biosynthetic defect, postoperatively following removal of aldosterone-secreting adenomas, during protracted heparin or heparinoid administration, in pretectal disease of the nervous system, and in severe postural hypotension.

The feature common to all forms hypoaldosteronism is the inability to increase aldosterone secretion appropriately in response to salt restriction. Most patients have unexplained hyperkalemia, which often is exacerbated by restriction of dietary sodium intake. In severe cases, urine sodium wastage occurs at a normal salt intake, whereas in milder forms, excessive loss of urine sodium occurs only with salt restriction.

Most cases of isolated hypoaldosteronism occur in patients with a deficiency in renin production (so-called hyporeninemic hypoaldosteronism), most commonly in adults with diabetes mellitus and mild renal failure and in whom hyperkalemia and metabolic acidosis are out of proportion to the degree of renal impairment. Plasma renin levels fail to rise normally following sodium restriction and postural changes. The pathogenesis is uncertain. Possibilities include renal disease (the most likely), autonomic neuropathy, extracellular fluid volume expansion, and defective conversion of renin precursors to active renin. Aldosterone levels also fail to rise normally after salt restriction and volume contraction; this effect is probably related to the hyporeninism, since biosynthetic defects in aldosterone secretion usually cannot be demonstrated. In these patients, aldosterone secretion increases promptly after ACTH stimulation, but it is uncertain whether the magnitude of the response is normal. On the other hand, the level of aldosterone appears to be subnormal in relationship to the hyperkalemia.

Hypoaldosteronism also can be associated with high renin levels. In many patients with this condition, the transformation of the C-18 methyl of corticosterone to the C-18 aldehyde of aldosterone is impaired, probably owing to a defect in corticosterone methyloxidase. These patients have low to absent aldosterone secretion, elevated plasma renin levels, and elevated levels of the intermediates of aldosterone biosynthesis (corticosterone and 18-hydroxycorticosterone). Severely ill patients also may have hyperreninemic hypoaldosteronism; such patients have a high mortality rate (80 percent). Hyperkalemia is not present. Possible explanations for the hypoaldosteronism include adrenal necrosis (uncommon) or a shift in steroidogenesis from mineralocorticoids to glucocorticoids, possibly related to prolonged ACTH stimulation.

Before the diagnosis of isolated hypoaldosteronism is considered for a patient with hyperkalemia, "pseudohyperkalemia" (e.g., hemolysis, thrombocytosis) should be excluded by measuring the plasma potassium level. The next step is to demonstrate a normal cortisol response to ACTH stimulation. Then, the response of renin and aldosterone levels to stimulation (upright posture, sodium restriction) should be measured. Low renin aldosterone levels establish the diagnosis of hyporeninemic hypoaldosteronism. A combination of high renin levels and low aldosterone levels is consistent with an aldosterone biosynthetic defect or a selective unresponsiveness to angiotensin II. Finally, elevated renin and aldosterone levels suggest primary renal unresponsiveness to aldosterone, so-called pseudohypoaldosteronism.

Rx TREATMENT

The treatment is to replace the mineralocorticoid deficiency. For practical purposes, the oral administration of 0.05 to 0.15 mg fludrocortisone daily should restore electrolyte balance if salt intake is adequate (e.g., 150 to 200 mmol/d). However, patients with hyporeninemic hypoaldosteronism may require higher doses of mineralocorticoid to correct hyperkalemia. This need poses a potential risk in patients with hypertension, mild renal insufficiency, or congestive heart failure. An alternative approach is to reduce salt intake and to administer furosemide, which can ameliorate acidosis and hyperkalemia. Occasionally, a combination of these two approaches is efficacious.

NONSPECIFIC CLINICAL USE OF ADRENAL STEROIDS

The widespread use of glucocorticoids emphasizes the need for a thorough understanding of the metabolic effects of these agents. Before adrenal hormone therapy is instituted, the expected gains should be weighed against undesirable effects.

HOW SERIOUS IS THE DISORDER? In a patient who has unexplained shock or in whom other measures have failed, the physician need not hesitate to employ high-dose steroid therapy. In contrast, one should exercise restraint in administering steroids to a patient with early rheumatoid arthritis for whom physiotherapy, analgesics, and general medical care have not been tried.

HOW LONG WILL GLUCOCORTICOID THERAPY BE REQUIRED? The use of intravenous steroids for 24 to 48 h for a life-threatening situation such as status asthmaticus or pseudotumor cerebri has few or no contraindications, in contrast to the initiation of chronic steroid therapy for asthma, arthritis, or psoriasis. In the latter instances, the almost certain development of some degree of Cushing's syndrome must be weighed against the potential benefit. These side effects should be minimized by a careful choice of steroid preparations, alternate-day or interrupted therapy, and the judicious use of supplementary adjuvants.

WHICH PREPARATION IS BEST? Several considerations should be taken into account in deciding which steroid preparation to use.

1. *The biologic half-life.* The rationale behind alternate-day therapy is to decrease the metabolic effects of the steroids for a significant part of each 48 h period while still producing a pharmacologic effect durable enough to be effective. Too long a half-life would defeat the first purpose, and too short a half-life would defeat the second. In general, the more potent the steroid, the longer its biologic half-life.
2. *The importance of the mineralocorticoid effects of the steroid.* Most synthetic steroids have less mineralocorticoid effect than hydrocortisone (Table 332-12).
3. *The biologically active form of the steroid.* Cortisone and prednisone have to be converted to biologically active metabolites before anti-inflammatory effects can occur. Because of this, in a condition for which steroids are known to be effective and when an adequate dose has been given without response, one should consider substituting hydrocortisone or prednisolone for cortisone or prednisone.
4. *The cost of the medication.* This is a serious consideration if chronic administration is planned. Prednisone is the least expensive of available steroid preparations.
5. *The type of formulation.* This factor may modify absorption, and patients whose steroid dosage has been standardized should use the same preparation consistently to avoid relapse or overdosage.

EVALUATION OF PATIENTS PRIOR TO INITIATING STEROID THERAPY (See Table 332-13) **Chronic Infection** Three issues demand attention: (1) Any active infection, particularly tuberculosis, should be identified. (2) If tuberculosis is present, steroid therapy should be employed only in conjunction with antituberculous chemotherapy. The chest film and tuberculin test provide baseline information for future comparison. Since high-dose steroids may impair the tuberculin reaction, serial chest roentgenograms may be necessary. (3) Infection due to opportunistic pathogens should be constantly considered in patients on steroid therapy, especially when combined with other immunosuppressive agents.

Diabetes Mellitus Prolonged glucocorticoid therapy may unmask or aggravate diabetes mellitus. The presence of diabetes mellitus or the demonstration of impaired glucose tolerance may affect the decision to institute adrenal hormone therapy.

Table 332-12

Glucocorticoid Preparations

	Estimated Potency†	
Commonly Used Name*	**Glucocorticoid**	**Mineralocorticoid**
SHORT-ACTING		
Hydrocortisone	1	1
Cortisone	0.8	0.8
INTERMEDIATE-ACTING		
Prednisone	4	0.25
Prednisolone	4	0.25
Methylprednisolone	5	<0.01
Triamcinolone	5	<0.01
LONG-ACTING		
Paramethasone	10	<0.01
Betamethasone	25	<0.01
Dexamethasone	30–40	<0.01

* The steroids are divided into three groups according to the duration of biologic activity. Short-acting preparations have a biologic half-life of less than 12 h; long-acting, greater than 48 h; and intermediate, between 12 and 36 h. Triamcinolone has the longest half-life of the intermediate-acting preparations.

† Relative milligram comparisons with hydrocortisone, setting the glucocorticoid and mineralocorticoid properties of hydrocortisone as 1. Sodium retention is insignificant for commonly employed doses of methylprednisolone, triamcinolone, paramethasone, betamethasone, and dexamethasone.

Table 332-13

A Checklist for Use Prior to the Administration of Glucocorticoids in Pharmacologic Doses

1. Presence of tuberculosis or other chronic infection (chest x-ray, tuberculin test)
2. Evidence of glucose intolerance or history of gestational diabetes mellitus
3. Evidence of preexisting osteoporosis (bone density assessment in postmenopausal patients)
4. History of peptic ulcer, gastritis, or esophagitis (stool guaiac test)
5. Evidence of hypertension or cardiovascular disease
6. History of psychological disorders

Osteoporosis Patients receiving long-term steroid therapy are at risk for osteoporosis. Indeed, osteoporosis with vertebral fractures or compression is a dreaded complication for patients at high risk (postmenopausal women, elderly men, and patients with restricted physical activity). Alternate-day or interrupted steroid therapy minimizes the risk of this complication (Table 332-14), and adjunctive therapies may be effective in treating the osteoporosis (see Chap. 355). Spine density should be assessed periodically with CT or digital radiography.

Peptic Ulcer, Gastric Hypersecretion, or Esophagitis In conventional doses (equivalent to 15 mg prednisone per day or less), glucocorticoids probably do not cause peptic ulceration; whether higher doses cause ulcer disease is not established and probably depends on duration and dose of treatment and predisposing factors such as hypoalbuminemia or cirrhosis. However, even at conventional doses, patients with a history of ulcer may experience aggravation of symptoms while receiving glucocorticoids. Consequently, all individuals with a positive history or with known risk factors should be managed with a vigorous antiulcer program (antacids, H_2 receptor antagonists, or ATPase inhibitors) along with glucocorticoids. *The development of anemia in a patient receiving glucocorticoids should suggest gastrointestinal bleeding as a cause.*

Hypertension or Cardiovascular Disease The capacity of many adrenal steroid preparations to promote sodium retention makes it necessary to exercise caution when using them in patients with preexisting hypertension or cardiovascular or renal disease. The use of preparations with minimal sodium-retaining activity, restriction of dietary sodium intake, and the use of diuretic agents and supplementary potassium salts minimize the mineralocorticoid effects of steroids. However, hypertension may be exacerbated by steroid-induced in-

Table 332-14

Supplementary Measures to Minimize Undesirable Metabolic Effects of Glucocorticoids

A. Monitor caloric intake to prevent weight gain.
B. Restrict sodium intake to prevent edema and minimize hypertension and potassium loss.
C. Provide supplementary potassium if necessary.
D. Provide antacid, H_2 receptor antagonist, and/or H^+,K^+-ATPase inhibitor therapy.
E. Institute alternate-day steroid schedule if possible. Patients receiving steroid therapy over a prolonged period should be protected by an appropriate increase in hormone level during periods of acute stress. A rule of thumb is to *double* the maintenance dose.
F. Minimize osteopenia by
    1. Administering gonadal hormone replacement therapy: 0.625–1.25 mg conjugated estrogens given cyclically with progesterone, unless the uterus is absent; testosterone replacement for hypogonadal men
    2. Ensuring high calcium intake (should be approximately 1200 mg/d)
    3. Administering supplemental vitamin D if blood levels of calciferol or $1,25(OH)_2$ vitamin D are reduced
    4. Administering calcitonin or diphosphonate if fractures occur even with the above treatments

creases in renin substrate and angiotensin II levels and by reduction in vasodilator prostaglandin production. Steroids also accelerate atherogenesis by induction of hypertension, glucose intolerance, and unfavorable lipid profiles. Glucocorticoid-associated lipid abnormalities include hypertriglyceridemia, hypercholesterolemia, and increased LDL cholesterol levels.

Psychological Difficulties Steroid therapy may cause psychological disturbances. In general, these disturbances correlate better with the patient's personality than with the dose of hormone, although larger doses cause more serious reactions. There is no reliable method of predicting the psychological reaction to steroid therapy; moreover, previous tolerance of steroids does not necessarily ensure immunity to subsequent courses. Likewise, untoward psychological reactions on one occasion do not invariably mean that the patient will respond unfavorably to a second course. However, patients with depressive symptoms during a first course of steroids may benefit from prophylactic lithium treatment prior to a second course.

Sleeplessness is common and can be minimized by using the shorter-acting steroids and by prescribing the total daily amount as a single early-morning dose.

ALTERNATE-DAY STEROID THERAPY The most effective way to minimize the cushingoid effects of glucocorticoids is to administer the total 48-h dose as a *single* dose of *intermediate-acting steroid* in the morning, *every other day*. If symptoms of the underlying disorder can be controlled by this technique, it offers distinct advantages. Three considerations deserve mention: (1) The alternate-day schedule may be approached through transition schedules that allow the patient to adjust gradually. (2) Supplementary nonsteroid medications may be needed on the "off" day to minimize symptoms of the underlying disorder. (3) Many symptoms that occur during the off day (e.g., fatigue, joint pain, muscle stiffness or tenderness, and fever) may represent relative adrenal insufficiency rather than exacerbation of the underlying disease.

The alternate-day approach capitalizes on the fact that cortisol secretion and plasma levels normally are highest in the early morning and lowest in the evening. The normal pattern is mimicked by administering an intermediate-acting steroid in the morning (7 to 8 A.M.) (see Table 332-12).

Initially, the steroid program often requires daily or more frequent doses of steroid to achieve the desired anti-inflammatory or immunity-suppressing action. *Only after this desired effect is achieved is an attempt made to switch to an alternate-day program.* A number of schedules can be used for transferring from a daily to an alternate-day program. The key points to be considered are flexibility in arranging a program and the use of supportive measures on the off day. One may attempt a gradual transition to the alternate-day schedule rather than an abrupt changeover. One approach is to keep the steroid dose constant on one day and gradually reduce it on the alternate day. Alternatively, the steroid dose can be increased on one day and reduced on the alternate day. In any case, it is important to anticipate that some increase in pain or discomfort may occur in the 36 to 48 h following the last dose.

The general principles advocated for the long-term use of steroids and for implementing an alternate-day schedule are as follows:

1. Utilize intermediate-acting steroids, such as prednisone or prednisolone.
2. Give the total daily amount of steroid as a single morning dose.
3. Begin a transition program as soon as the manifestations of the diseases are under reasonable control.
4. If possible, eliminate steroid medication on the alternate day.

WITHDRAWAL OF GLUCOCORTICOIDS FOLLOWING LONG-TERM USE It is possible to reduce gradually and eventually to discontinue a daily steroid dose, but under most circumstances withdrawal of steroids should be initiated by first implementing an alternate-day schedule. Patients who have been on an alternate-day program for a month or more experience less difficulty during termination regimens. The dosage is gradually reduced and finally discontinued after a replacement dosage has been reached (e.g., 5 to 7.5 mg prednisone). Complications rarely ensue unless undue stress is experienced, and patients should understand that for 1 year or longer after withdrawal from long-term high-dose steroid therapy, supplementary hormone should be given in the event of a serious infection, operation, or injury. A useful strategy in patients with symptoms of adrenal insufficiency on a tapering regimen is to measure plasma cortisol levels prior to the steroid dose. A level less than 140 nmol/L (5 μg/dL) indicates continuing suppression of the pituitary-adrenal axis and implies that a more cautious tapering of steroids is indicated.

In patients on high-dose daily steroid therapy, it is advised to reduce dosage to approximately 20 mg prednisone daily as a single morning dose before beginning the transition to alternate-day therapy. If a patient cannot tolerate an alternate-day program, consideration should be given to the possibility that the patient has developed primary adrenal insufficiency.

See Chap. 59, Adrenocorticotropic hormone; adrenocortical steroids and their synthetic analogs; inhibitors of the synthesis and actions of adrenocortical hormones, in Goodman & Gilman's The Pharmacological Basis of Therapeutics, *9th ed, New York, McGraw-Hill, 1996.*

BIBLIOGRAPHY

AZZIZ R et al: Nonclassic adrenal hyperplasia: Current concepts. Clinical review 56. J Clin Endocrinol Metab 78:810, 1994

BAMBERGER CM et al: The glucocorticoid receptor and RU 486 in man. Ann NY Acad Sci 761:296, 1995

BECKER M et al: Ectopic ACTH syndrome and CRH-mediated Cushing's syndrome. Endocrinol Metab Clin North Am 23:585, 1994

BERTAGNA X: Proopiomelanocortin-derived peptides. Endocrinol Metab Clin North Am 23:467, 1994

BONCHICCHIO D et al: Factors influencing the immediate and late outcome of Cushing's disease treated by transsphenoidal surgery: A retrospective study by the European Cushing's Disease Survey Group. J Clin Endocrinol Metab 80:3114, 1995

BRAVO EL: Primary aldosteronism. Issues in diagnosis and management. Endocrinol Metab Clin North Am 23:271, 1994

CONLIN PR et al: Disorders of the renin-angiotensin-aldosterone system, in *Renal and Electrolyte Disorders, 5th ed*, Schrier RW (ed). Boston, Little, Brown, 1997

DLUHY RG et al: Glucocorticoid-remediable aldosteronism. Endocrinol Metab Clin North Am 23:285, 1994

FERNANDEZ-REAL JM et al: Pre-clinical Cushing's syndrome: Report of three cases and literature review. Horm Res 41:230, 1994

GORDON RD et al: Primary aldosteronism—some genetic, morphological, and biochemical aspects of subtypes. Steroids 60:35, 1995

HATTNER RS: Practical considerations in the scintigraphic evaluation of endocrine hypertension. The adrenal cortex and medulla. Radiol Clin North Am 31:1029, 1993

HORTON R et al: Hypoaldosteronism. Curr Ther Endocrinol Metab 5:146, 1994

JORGE P et al: X-linked adrenoleukodystrophy in patients with idiopathic Addison disease. Eur J Pediatr 153:594, 1994

KATER GE et al: Disorders of steroid 17 alpha-hydroxylase deficiency. Endocrinol Metab Clin North Am 23:341, 1994

KONG MF et al: Eighty-six cases of Addison' disease. Clin Endocrinol 41:757, 1994

MCCANCE DR et al: Bilateral adrenalectomy: Low mortality and morbidity in Cushing's disease. Clin Endocrinol 39:315, 1993

MORTENSEN RM, WILLIAMS GH: Aldosterone action (physiology), in *Endocrinology*, 3d ed, DeGroot LJ et al (eds). Philadelphia, Saunders, 1994, p 1668

MUNE T et al: Human hypertension caused by mutations in the kidney isozyme of 11 beta-hydroxysteroid dehydrogenase. Nat Genet 10:394, 1995

NEW MI: Steroid 21-hydroxylase deficiency (congenital adrenal hyperplasia). Am J Med 98:2S, 1995

ORTH DN: Cushing's syndrome. N Engl J Med 332:791, 1995

OSELLA G et al: Endocrine evaluation of incidentally discovered adrenal masses (incidentalomas). J Clin Endocrinol Metab 79:1532, 1994

QUINN SJ, WILLIAMS GH: Regulation of aldosterone secretion, in *The Adrenal Gland*, 2d ed, VHT James (ed). New York, Raven, 1992, p 152

RAFF H: Interactions between neurohypophysial hormones and the ACTH adrenocortical axis. Ann NY Acad Sci 689:411, 1993

Sambrook P et al: Prevention of corticosteroid osteoporosis. A comparison of calcium, calcitriol, and calcitonin. N Engl J Med 328:1747, 1993
Savastano S et al: Hypothalamic-pituitary-adrenal axis and immune system. Acta Neurol 16:206, 1994
Shimket RA et al: Liddle's syndrome: Heritable human hypertension caused by mutations in the beta subunit of the epithelial sodium channel. Cell 79:407, 1994
Staren E et al: Selection of patients with adrenal incidentalomas for operation. Surg Clin North Am 75:499, 1995
Uibo R et al: Autoantibodies to cytochrome P450 enzymes P450scc, P450c17, and P450c21 in autoimmune polyglandular disease types I and II and in isolated Addison's disease. J Clin Endocrinol Metab 78:323, 1994
Ur E et al: Corticotropin-releasing hormone in health and disease: An update. Acta Endocrinol 127:193, 1992
White PC et al: Steroid 11 beta-hydroxylase deficiency and related disorders. Endocrinol Metab Clin North Am 23:325, 1994
Williams GH: Hirsutism, in: *Office Practice of Medicine*, 3d ed, Branch WT (ed). Philadelphia, Saunders, 1994, p 505

333

Lewis Landsberg, James B. Young

PHEOCHROMOCYTOMA

Pheochromocytomas produce, store, and secrete catecholamines. They are usually derived from the adrenal medulla but may develop from chromaffin cells in or about sympathetic ganglia (extraadrenal pheochromocytomas or paragangliomas). Related tumors that secrete catecholamines and produce similar clinical syndromes include chemodectomas derived from the carotid body and ganglioneuromas derived from the postganglionic sympathetic neurons.

The clinical features are due predominantly to the release of catecholamines and to a lesser extent to the secretion of other substances. Hypertension is the most common sign, and hypertensive paroxysms or crises, often spectacular and alarming, occur in over half the cases.

Pheochromocytoma occurs in approximately 0.1 percent of the hypertensive population but is, nevertheless, an important correctable cause of high blood pressure. Indeed, it is usually curable if properly diagnosed and treated, but it may be fatal if undiagnosed or mistreated. Postmortem series indicate that most pheochromocytomas are unsuspected clinically even when the tumor is related to the fatal outcome.

PATHOLOGY **Location and Morphology** In adults, approximately 80 percent of pheochromocytomas are unilateral and solitary, 10 percent are bilateral, and 10 percent are extraadrenal. In children, a fourth of tumors are bilateral, and an additional fourth are extraadrenal. Solitary lesions inexplicably favor the right side. Although pheochromocytomas may grow to large size (over 3 kg), most weigh less than 100 g and are less than 10 cm in diameter. The tumors are highly vascular.

The tumors are made up of large, polyhedral, pleomorphic chromaffin cells. Less than 10 percent of these tumors are malignant. As with other endocrine tumors, malignancy cannot be determined from the histologic appearance; tumors that contain large numbers of aneuploid or tetraploid cells, as determined by flow cytometry, are more likely to recur. Local invasion of surrounding tissues or distant metastases indicate malignancy.

Familial pheochromocytoma In approximately 5 percent of cases, pheochromocytoma is inherited as an autosomal dominant trait either alone or in combination with other abnormalities such as multiple endocrine neoplasia (MEN) type 2a (Sipple's syndrome) or type 2b (mucosal neuroma syndrome) (see Chap. 340), von Recklinghausen's neurofibromatosis, or von Hippel–Lindau's retinal cerebellar hemangioblastomatosis. Bilateral adrenal pheochromocytomas are common in the familial syndromes; within MEN kindreds, over half of pheochromocytomas are bilateral. A familial syndrome should be suspected in any patient with bilateral pheochromocytomas.

Extraadrenal pheochromocytomas Extraadrenal pheochromocytomas usually weigh 20 to 40 g and are less than 5 cm in diameter. Most are located within the abdomen in association with the celiac, superior mesenteric, and inferior mesenteric ganglia. Approximately 1 percent are in the thorax, 1 percent are within the urinary bladder, and less than 1 percent are in the neck, usually in association with the sympathetic ganglia or the extracranial branches of the ninth or tenth cranial nerves.

Catecholamine Synthesis, Storage, and Release Pheochromocytomas synthesize and store catecholamines by processes resembling those of the normal adrenal medulla (see Chap. 70). Little is known about the mechanisms of catecholamine release from pheochromocytomas, but changes in blood flow and necrosis within the tumor may be the cause in some instances. These tumors are not innervated, and catecholamine release does not result from neural stimulation. Pheochromocytomas also store and secrete a variety of peptides, including endogenous opioids, adrenomedullin, endothelin, erythropoietin, parathyroid hormone–related protein, neuropeptide Y, and chromagranin A (see Chap. 70). These peptides contribute to the clinical manifestations in selected cases, as noted below.

Epinephrine, norepinephrine, and dopamine Most pheochromocytomas contain and secrete both norepinephrine and epinephrine, and the percentage of norepinephrine is usually greater than in the normal adrenal. Most extraadrenal pheochromocytomas secrete norepinephrine exclusively. Rarely, pheochromocytomas produce epinephrine alone, particularly in association with MEN. Although epinephrine-producing tumors may cause a preponderance of metabolic and beta-receptor effects, in general the major catecholamine secreted cannot be predicted from the clinical presentation. Increased production of dopamine and homovanillic acid (HVA) is uncommon with benign lesions but may occur with malignant pheochromocytoma.

CLINICAL FEATURES Pheochromocytoma occurs at all ages but is most common in young to midadult life. Some series show a slight female preponderance. Most patients come to medical attention as a result of hypertensive crisis, paroxysmal symptoms suggestive of seizure disorder or anxiety attacks, or hypertension that responds poorly to conventional treatment. Less commonly, unexplained hypotension or shock in association with surgery or trauma will suggest the diagnosis. Most patients have hypertension in association with headaches, excessive sweating, and/or palpitations.

Hypertension Hypertension is the most common manifestation. In approximately 60 percent of cases the hypertension is sustained, although significant blood pressure lability is usually present, and half of patients with sustained hypertension have distinct crises or paroxysms. The other 40 percent have blood pressure elevations only during an attack. The hypertension is often severe, occasionally malignant, and may be resistant to treatment with standard antihypertensive drugs.

Paroxysms or Crises The paroxysm or crisis occurs in over half of patients. In an individual patient, the symptoms are often similar with each attack. The paroxysms may be frequent or sporadic, occurring at intervals as long as weeks or months. With time, the paroxysms usually increase in frequency, duration, and severity.

The attack usually has a sudden onset. It may last from a few minutes to several hours or longer. Headache, profuse sweating, palpitations, and apprehension, often with a sense of impending doom, are common. Pain in the chest or abdomen may be associated with nausea and vomiting. Either pallor or flushing may occur during the attack. The blood pressure is elevated, often to alarming levels, and the elevation is usually accompanied by tachycardia.

The paroxysm may be precipitated by any activity that displaces the abdominal contents. In some cases a particular stimulus may induce an attack in a characteristic fashion, but in others no clearly defined precipitating event can be found. Although anxiety may accompany the attacks, mental or psychological stress does not usually provoke a crisis.

Other Distinctive Clinical Features Symptoms and signs of an increased metabolic rate, such as profuse sweating and mild to moderate weight loss, are common. Orthostatic hypotension is a consequence of diminished plasma volume and blunted sympathetic reflexes. Both these factors predispose the patient with unsuspected pheochromocytoma to hypotension or shock during surgery or trauma. Secretion of the hypotensive peptide adrenomedullin may contribute to the hypotension in some patients.

Cardiac manifestations Sinus tachycardia, sinus bradycardia, supraventricular arrhythmias, and ventricular premature contractions all have been noted. Angina and acute myocardial infarction may occur even in the absence of coronary artery disease. A catecholamine-induced increase in myocardial oxygen consumption and, perhaps, coronary spasm may play a role in these ischemic events. Electrocardiographic changes, including nonspecific ST-T wave changes, prominent U waves, left ventricular strain patterns, and right and left bundle branch blocks may be present in the absence of demonstrable ischemia or infarction. Cardiomyopathy, either congestive with myocarditis and myocardial fibrosis or hypertrophic with concentric or asymmetric hypertrophy, may be associated with heart failure and cardiac arrhythmias. Multiorgan system failure with noncardiogenic pulmonary edema may be the presenting manifestation. Elevated levels of amylase, originating from damaged pulmonary endothelium, and abdominal pain may suggest acute pancreatitis, although serum lipase levels are normal.

Carbohydrate intolerance Over half of patients have impaired carbohydrate tolerance due to suppression of insulin and stimulation of hepatic glucose output. The impaired glucose tolerance rarely requires treatment with insulin and disappears after removal of the tumor.

Hematocrit The elevated hematocrit is secondary to diminished plasma volume. Rarely, production of erythropoietin by the tumor may cause a true erythrocytosis.

Other manifestations Hypercalcemia has been attributed to the ectopic secretion of parathyroid hormone–related protein. Fever and an elevated erythrocyte sedimentation rate have been reported in association with the production of interleukin 6. Elevated temperature more commonly reflects catecholamine-mediated increases in metabolic rate and diminished heat dissipation secondary to vasoconstriction. Polyuria is an occasional finding, and rhabdomyolysis with myoglobinuric renal failure may result from extreme vasoconstriction with muscle ischemia.

Pheochromocytoma of the urinary bladder Pheochromocytoma in the wall of the urinary bladder may result in typical paroxysms in relation to micturition. The location in the bladder wall is responsible for the occurrence of symptoms while the tumors are quite small, and, consequently, catecholamine excretion may be normal or minimally elevated. Hematuria is present in over half of patients, and the tumor can often be visualized at cystoscopy.

Adverse Drug Interactions Severe and occasionally fatal paroxysms have been induced by opiates, histamine, adrenocorticotropin, saralasin, and glucagon. These agents appear to release catecholamines directly from the tumor. Indirect-acting sympathomimetic amines, including methyldopa (when administered intravenously), may cause an increase in blood pressure by releasing catecholamines from the augmented stores within nerve endings. Drugs that block neuronal uptake of catecholamines, such as tricyclic antidepressants or guanethidine, may enhance the physiologic effects of circulating catecholamines. Indeed, all medications should be considered carefully and administered cautiously in patients with known or suspected pheochromocytoma.

Associated Diseases Pheochromocytoma is associated with medullary carcinoma of the thyroid in the MEN syndrome types 2a and 2b and with hyperparathyroidism in MEN 2a (see Chap. 340). Hypercalcemia, resolving after tumor resection, also has been described in the absence of parathyroid disease, as described above. Individuals at risk for MEN 2a and 2b should be screened periodically for pheochromocytoma by assay of a 24-h urine sample for catecholamines, including measurement of epinephrine. Pheochromocytoma should be excluded or removed before thyroid or parathyroid surgery.

The association of pheochromocytoma and neurofibromatosis is not common. Nevertheless, since incomplete forms of neurofibromatosis may be associated with pheochromocytoma, minor manifestations such as café au lait spots, vertebral abnormalities, or kyphoscoliosis should increase the suspicion of pheochromocytoma in a patient with hypertension. The incidence of pheochromocytoma in some kindreds with von Hippel–Lindau disease may be as high as 10 to 25 percent. Many of these are unsuspected clinically and diagnosed on a computed tomography (CT) scan or at postmortem.

The incidence of cholelithiasis is 15 to 20 percent. Cushing's syndrome is a rare association, usually a consequence of ectopic secretion of adrenocorticotropic hormone by the pheochromocytoma or, less commonly, by a coexistent medullary carcinoma of the thyroid.

Diagnosis The diagnosis is established by the demonstration of increased excretion of catecholamines or catecholamine metabolites. The diagnosis can usually be made by the analysis of a single 24-h urine sample, provided the patient is hypertensive or symptomatic at the time of collection.

Biochemical Tests The assays employed include those for vanillylmandelic acid (VMA), the metanephrines, and unconjugated or "free" catecholamines (see Chap. 70). The VMA assay is both less sensitive and less specific than assays of metanephrines or catecholamines. Accuracy of diagnosis is improved when two of the three determinations are employed. The following considerations apply to all the urinary tests: (1) Despite claims for the adequacy of determinations made on random urine samples, analysis of a full 24-h urine sample is preferable. Creatinine should be determined as well to assess the adequacy of collection. (2) Where possible, the collection should be made when the patient is at rest, on no medication, and without recent exposure to radiographic contrast media. When it is not practical to discontinue all medications, drugs known specifically to interfere with these assays (as noted below) should be avoided. (3) The urine should be acidified and refrigerated during and after collection. (4) With high-quality assays, dietary restrictions are minimal and should be specified by the laboratory performing the analyses. (5) Although most patients with pheochromocytoma excrete increased amounts of catecholamines and catecholamine metabolites, the yield is increased in patients with paroxysmal hypertension if a 24-h urine collection is initiated during a crisis.

Free catecholamines The upper limit of normal for total urinary catecholamines is between 590 and 885 nmol (100 and 150 μg) per 24 h. In most patients with pheochromocytoma, values in excess of 1480 nmol (250 μg) per day are obtained. Measurement of epinephrine is often of value, since increased epinephrine excretion [over 275 nmol (50 μg) per 24 h] is usually due to an adrenal lesion and may be the only abnormality in cases associated with MEN. False-positive increases in catecholamine excretion result from exogenous catecholamines and related drugs such as methyldopa, levodopa, labetalol, and sympathomimetic amines, which may elevate catecholamine excretion for up to 2 weeks. Endogenous catecholamines from stimulation of the sympathoadrenal system also may increase urinary catecholamine excretion. Relevant clinical situations that cause such increases include hypoglycemia, strenuous exertion, central nervous system disease with increased intracranial pressure, and clonidine withdrawal.

Metanephrines and VMA In most laboratories, the upper limit of normal is 7 μmol (1.3 mg) of total metanephrine and 35 μmol (7.0 mg) of VMA excretion per 24 h. In most patients with pheochromocytoma, the increase in these urinary metabolites is considerable, often to more than three times the normal range. Metanephrine excretion is increased by exogenous and endogenous catecholamines and by treatment with monoamine oxidase inhibitors; propranolol may cause a spurious increase in metanephrine excretion, since a propranolol metabolite interferes in the commonly used spectrophotometric assay. VMA is less affected by endogenous and exogenous catecholamines but is spuriously increased by a variety of drugs, including carbidopa. VMA excretion is decreased by monoamine oxidase inhibitors.

Plasma catecholamines Measurement of plasma catecholamines has a limited application. The care required in obtaining basal levels (see Chap. 70) and the satisfactory results with urinary determinations make measurement of plasma catecholamines unnecessary in most cases. Plasma catecholamine levels are affected by the same drugs and physiologic perturbations that increase urinary catecholamine excretion. In addition, alpha- and beta-adrenergic receptor blocking agents may elevate plasma catecholamines by impairing clearance.

When the clinical features suggest pheochromocytoma and the urinary assay results are borderline, measurement of plasma catecholamines may be worthwhile. Markedly elevated basal levels of total catecholamines support the diagnosis, although approximately one-third of patients with pheochromocytoma have normal or slightly elevated basal values. The usefulness of plasma catecholamine determinations may be increased by agents that suppress sympathetic nervous system activity. Clonidine and ganglionic blocking agents (see Chap. 70) reduce plasma catecholamine levels in normal subjects and in patients with essential hypertension. These drugs have little effect on catecholamine levels in patients with pheochromocytoma. In patients with elevated or borderline basal catecholamine values, failure to suppress plasma or urinary levels with clonidine supports the diagnosis of pheochromocytoma.

Pharmacologic Tests Reliable methods for the measurement of catecholamines and catecholamine metabolites in urine have rendered obsolete both the provocative and adrenolytic tests, which are nonspecific and entail considerable risk. A modified version of the adrenolytic test may be of some use, however, as a therapeutic trial in a patient in hypertensive crisis with features suggestive of pheochromocytoma. A positive response to phentolamine (5-mg bolus following a test dose of 0.5 mg) is a reduction in blood pressure of at least 35/25 mmHg that peaks after 2 min and persists for 10 to 15 min. The pharmacologic response is never diagnostic, and biochemical confirmation is essential. Provocative tests in normotensive patients are potentially dangerous and rarely indicated. However, a glucagon provocative test may be of use in patients with paroxysmal hypertension and nondiagnostic basal catecholamine levels. Glucagon has a negligible effect on blood pressure or plasma catecholamine levels in normal or hypertensive subjects. In patients with pheochromocytoma, on the other hand, glucagon may increase both blood pressure and circulating catecholamine levels. The elevation in plasma catecholamine concentration, moreover, may occur without a blood pressure response. It must be emphasized, however, that life-threatening pressor crises have occurred after administration of glucagon to patients with pheochromocytoma, so the test should never be performed casually. Careful continuous monitoring of the blood pressure is required, intravenous access must be adequate, and phentolamine must be at hand to terminate the test if a significant pressor reaction ensues.

Differential Diagnosis Since the manifestations of pheochromocytoma can be protean, the diagnosis must be considered and excluded in many patients with suggestive clinical features. In patients with essential hypertension and "hyperadrenergic" features such as tachycardia, sweating, and increased cardiac output, and in patients with anxiety attacks associated with blood pressure elevations, analysis of a 24-h urine collection is usually decisive in excluding the diagnosis. Repeated determinations on urine collected during attacks may be necessary, however, before the diagnosis can be excluded with certainty. The clonidine suppression and glucagon stimulation tests may be helpful in excluding the diagnosis in difficult cases. Pressor crises associated with clonidine withdrawal and the use of cocaine or monoamine oxidase inhibitors (Chap. 70) may mimic the paroxysms of pheochromocytoma. Factitious crises may be produced by self-administration of sympathomimetic amines in psychiatrically disturbed patients.

Intracranial lesions, particularly posterior fossa tumors or subarachnoid hemorrhage, may cause hypertension and increased excretion of catecholamines or catecholamine metabolites. While this is most common in patients with an obvious neurologic catastrophe, the possibility of subarachnoid or intracranial hemorrhage secondary to pheochromocytoma should be considered. Diencephalic or autonomic epilepsy may be associated with paroxysmal spells, hypertension, and increased plasma catecholamine levels. This rare entity may be difficult to distinguish from pheochromocytoma, but an aura, an abnormal electroencephalogram, and a beneficial response to anticonvulsant medications will often suggest the proper diagnosis.

Rx TREATMENT

Preoperative Management The induction of stable alpha-adrenergic blockade is the basis of preoperative management and provides the foundation for successful surgical treatment. Once the diagnosis is established, the patient should be placed on phenoxybenzamine to induce a long-lived, noncompetitive alpha-receptor blockade. The usual initial dose is 10 mg every 12 h with increments of 10 to 20 mg added every few days until the blood pressure is controlled and the paroxysms disappear. Because of the long duration of action, the therapeutic effects are cumulative, and the optimal dose must be achieved gradually with careful monitoring of supine and upright blood pressures. Most patients require between 40 and 80 mg phenoxybenzamine per day, although 200 mg or more may be necessary. Phenoxybenzamine should be administered for at least 10 to 14 days prior to surgery. Over this time, the combination of alpha-receptor blockade and a liberal salt intake will restore the contracted plasma volume to normal. Before adequate alpha-adrenergic blockade with phenoxybenzamine is achieved, paroxysms may be treated with intravenous phentolamine. Selective $alpha_1$ antagonists have been employed preoperatively, but their role in management has not been established. They may be useful as antihypertensive agents in patients with suspected pheochromocytoma while workup is in progress, since they are usually better tolerated than phenoxybenzamine and will prevent serious pressor crises if pheochromocytoma is present. Nitroprusside, calcium channel blocking agents, and possibly angiotensin converting enzyme inhibitors reduce blood pressure in patients with pheochromocytoma. Nitroprusside may be useful on occasion in the treatment of pressor crises.

Beta-adrenergic receptor blocking agents should be given only after alpha blockade has been induced, since administration of such agents by themselves may cause a paradoxic increase in blood pressure by antagonizing beta-mediated vasodilation in skeletal muscle. Beta blockade is usually initiated when tachycardia develops during the induction of alpha-adrenergic blockade. Low doses often suffice, and a reasonable starting dose is 10 mg propranolol three to four times per day, increased as needed to control the pulse rate. Beta blockade is effective for catecholamine-induced arrhythmias, particularly those potentiated by anesthetic agents.

Preoperative Localization of the Tumor Surgical removal of pheochromocytoma is facilitated if the location of the tumor or tumors can be established preoperatively. Once pheochromocytoma is diagnosed, localization should be undertaken while the patient is being prepared for surgery. CT or magnetic resonance imaging (MRI) of the adrenals is usually successful in identifying intraadrenal lesions. Extraadrenal tumors within the chest can frequently be identified by conventional chest films or CT. MRI is useful in identifying extraadrenal tumors in the abdomen. If these studies are negative, abdominal aortography (once alpha-adrenergic blockade is complete) may identify extraadrenal pheochromocytomas in the abdomen, since these lesions are often supplied by a large aberrant artery. If aortography and CT fail to localize the lesion, venous sampling at different levels of the inferior and superior vena cava may reveal catecholamine gradients in the region drained by the tumor; this area may then be restudied by selective angiography or scanning by CT or MRI. An additional localization technique involves a radionuclide scintiscan after administration of the radiopharmaceutical [^{131}I]metaiodobenzylguanidine (MIBG). This agent is concentrated by the amine uptake process and produces an external scintigraphic image at the site of the tumor. This type of scanning may be useful in characterizing lesions discovered by CT when biochemical confirmation is indeterminate, as well as in localizing extraadrenal pheochromocytomas. Percutaneous fine-needle aspiration of chromaffin tumors is contraindicated; indeed, pheochromocytoma should be considered before adrenal lesions are aspirated.

Surgery Surgical treatment of pheochromocytoma is best performed in centers with experience in the preoperative, anesthetic, and intraoperative management of pheochromocytoma. In experienced hands surgical mortality is 2 or 3 percent.

Monitoring during the surgical procedure should include continuous recording of arterial pressure and central venous pressure as well as electrocardiography; in the presence of cardiac disease or if congestive failure has been present, pulmonary capillary wedge pressure should be monitored. Adequate fluid replacement is crucial. Intraoperative hypotension responds better to volume replacement than to vasoconstrictors. Hypertension and cardiac arrhythmias are most likely during induction of anesthesia, intubation, and manipulation of the tumor. Intravenous phentolamine is usually sufficient to control the blood pressure, but nitroprusside may be required. Propranolol may be given in the treatment of tachycardia or ventricular ectopy.

PHEOCHROMOCYTOMA IN PREGNANCY Spontaneous labor and vaginal delivery in unprepared patients are usually disastrous for mother and fetus. In early pregnancy, the patient should be prepared with phenoxybenzamine, and the tumor should be removed as soon as the diagnosis is confirmed. The pregnancy need not be terminated, but the operative procedure itself may result in spontaneous abortion. In the third trimester treatment with adrenergic blocking agents should be undertaken; when the fetus is of sufficient size, cesarean section may be followed by extirpation of the tumor. Although the safety of adrenergic blocking drugs in pregnancy is not established, these agents have been administered in several cases without obvious adverse effect. Antepartum diagnosis and treatment lowers the maternal death rate, sometimes to zero, although fetal death still occurs on occasion.

UNRESECTABLE AND MALIGNANT TUMORS In cases of metastatic or locally invasive tumor or in patients with intercurrent illness that precludes surgery, long-term medical management is required. When the manifestations cannot be adequately controlled by adrenergic blocking agents, the concomitant administration of metyrosine may be required. This agent inhibits tyrosine hydroxylase, diminishes catecholamine production by the tumor, and often simplifies chronic management. Malignant pheochromocytoma frequently recurs in the retroperitoneum, and it metastasizes most commonly to bone and lung. Although these malignant tumors are resistant to radiotherapy, combination chemotherapy has had limited success in controlling them. Use of MIBG has had limited success in the treatment of malignant pheochromocytoma.

PROGNOSIS AND FOLLOW-UP The 5-year survival rate after surgery is usually over 95 percent, and the recurrence rate is less than 10 percent. After successful surgery, catecholamine excretion returns to normal in about 1 week and should be measured to ensure complete tumor removal. Catecholamine excretion should be assessed at the reappearance of suggestive symptoms or yearly for several years, if the patient remains asymptomatic. For malignant pheochromocytoma, the 5-year survival rate is less than 50 percent.

Complete removal cures the hypertension in approximately three-fourths of patients. In the remainder hypertension recurs but is usually well controlled by standard antihypertensive agents. In this group either underlying essential hypertension or irreversible vascular damage induced by catecholamines may cause the persistence of the hypertension.

See Chap. 10, Catecholamines, sympathomimetic drugs, and adrenergic receptor antagonists, in Goodman & Gilman's The Pharmacological Basis of Therapeutics, *9th ed, New York, McGraw-Hill, 1996.*

BIBLIOGRAPHY

AVERBUCH SD et al: Malignant pheochromocytoma: Effective treatment with a combination of cyclophosphamide, vincristine, and dacarbazine. Ann Intern Med 109:267, 1988

DALY PA, LANDSBERG L: Phaeochromocytoma: Diagnosis and management. Baillieres Clin Endocrinol Metab 6:143, 1992

FUDGE TL et al: Current surgical management of pheochromocytoma during pregnancy. Arch Surg 115:1224, 1980

FUKUMOTO S et al: Pheochromocytoma with pyrexia and marked inflammatory signs: A paraneoplastic syndrome with possible relation to interleukin-6 production. J Clin Endocrinol Metab 73:877, 1991

GAGNER M et al: Early experience with laparoscopic approach for adrenalectomy. Surgery 114:1120, 1993

GAN TJ et al: Phaeochromocytoma presenting as acute hyperamylasemia and multiple organ failure. Can J Anaesth 41:244, 1994

GRAHAM PE et al: Laboratory diagnosis of pheochromocytoma: Which analyses should we measure? Ann Clin Biochem 30:129, 1993

HORTON WA et al: von Hippel–Lindau disease: Clinical and pathological manifestations in nine families with 50 affected members. Arch Intern Med 136:769, 1976

KREMPF M et al: Use of m-(^{131}I) iodobenzylguanidine in the treatment of malignant pheochromocytoma. J Clin Endocrinol Metab 72:455, 1991

LANDSBERG L: Pheochromocytoma complicating pregnancy. Eur J Endocrinol 130:215, 1994

MACDOUGALL IC et al: Overnight clonidine suppression test in the diagnosis and exclusion of pheochromocytoma. Am J Med 84:993, 1988

MCCORKELL SJ, NILES NL: Fine-needle aspiration of catecholamine-producing adrenal masses: A possibly fatal mistake. Am J Roentgenol 145:113, 1985

MERIGIAN KS et al: Adrenergic crisis from crack cocaine ingestion: Report of five cases. J Emerg Med 12:485, 1994

NEUMANN HPH et al: Pheochromocytomas, multiple endocrine neoplasia type 2, and von Hippel-Lindau disease. N Engl J Med 329:1531, 1993

OISHI S et al: Elevated immunoreactive endothelin levels in patients with pheochromocytoma. Am J Hypertension 7:717, 1994

PANG L-C et al: Flow cytometric DNA analysis for the determination of malignant potential in adrenal and extra-adrenal pheochromocytomas or paragangliomas. Arch Pathol Lab Med 117:1142, 1993

PERRIER NA et al: Malignant pheochromocytoma masquerading as acute pancreatitis—a rare but potentially lethal occurrence. Mayo Clin Proc 69:366, 1994

REINIG JW, DOPPMAN JL: Magnetic resonance imaging of the adrenal. Radiologe 26:186, 1986

SANTIAGO JA et al: Synthetic human adrenomedullin and adrenomedullin 15-52 have potent short-lived vasodilator activity in the hindlimb vascular bed of the cat. Life Sci 55:Pl85, 1994

SHEMIN D et al: Pheochromocytoma presenting as rhabdomyolysis and acute myoglobinuric renal failure. Arch Intern Med 150:2384, 1990

STEWART AF et al: Hypercalcemia in pheochromocytoma. Ann Intern Med 102:776, 1985

334

Daniel W. Foster

DIABETES MELLITUS

Diabetes mellitus, the most common endocrine disease, is characterized by metabolic abnormalities and by long-term complications involving the eyes, kidneys, nerves, and blood vessels. The disorder is not homogeneous, and several distinct diabetic syndromes have been delineated.

DIAGNOSIS The diagnosis of symptomatic diabetes is not difficult. When a patient presents with signs and symptoms attributable to an osmotic diuresis and has hyperglycemia, the diagnosis is unequivocal. There is likewise no disagreement about an asymptomatic patient with persistently elevated fasting plasma glucose concentrations. The problem arises with the asymptomatic patient who for one reason or another is considered to be a potential diabetic but has a normal fasting glucose concentration in plasma. Such patients are often given an oral glucose tolerance test and, if abnormal values are found, are diagnosed as having impaired glucose tolerance or diabetes. There seems to be little question that normal glucose tolerance is strong evidence against the presence of diabetes; the predictive value of an abnormal test is less certain. Much evidence suggests that the standard oral glucose tolerance test overdiagnoses diabetes, probably because a variety of stresses can cause an abnormal response. The operative mechanism is thought to be epinephrine discharge. Epinephrine blocks insulin secretion, stimulates glucagon release, activates glycogen breakdown, and impairs insulin action in target tissues, so that hepatic glucose production is increased and the capacity to dispose of exogenous glucose is impaired. Even anxiety over venipunctures may generate enough epinephrine to produce an abnormal test. Coexisting illness, inadequate diet, and lack of physical exercise also contribute to false-positive tests.

In an attempt to deal with these problems, the National Diabetes Data Group of the National Institutes of Health in 1979 revised the criteria for the diagnosis of diabetes:

1. *Fasting (overnight):* Venous plasma glucose concentration ≥7.8 mmol/L (140 mg/dL) on at least two separate occasions.[1]
2. *Following ingestion of 75 g of glucose:* Venous plasma glucose concentration ≥11.1 mmol/L (200 mg/dL) at 2 h and on at least one other occasion during the 2-h test; i.e., *two* values ≥11.1 mmol/L (200 mg/dL) must be obtained for diagnosis.

If the 2-h value is between 7.8 and 11.1 mmol/L (140 and 200 mg/dL) and one other value during the 2-h test period is equal to or greater than 11.1 mmol/L (200 mg/dL), a diagnosis of "impaired glucose tolerance" is suggested. Persons in this category are at increased risk for the development of fasting hyperglycemia or symptomatic diabetes, but such progression is not predictable in an individual patient.

CLASSIFICATION A classification of diabetes is given in Table 334-1. The basic categories are those recommended by the National Diabetes Data Group, except for the division into primary and secondary types. *Primary* implies that no associated disease is present, while in the *secondary* category, some identifiable condition causes or allows a diabetic syndrome to develop. Insulin dependence in this classification is not equivalent to insulin therapy. Rather, the term means that the patient is at risk for diabetic ketoacidosis (DKA) in the absence of insulin. Many patients classified as non-insulin-dependent require insulin for control of hyperglycemia, although they do not become ketoacidotic if insulin is withdrawn.

The term *type 1 diabetes* is often used as a synonym for insulin-dependent diabetes mellitus (IDDM), and *type 2 diabetes* is considered equivalent to non-insulin-dependent diabetes mellitus (NIDDM). This linkage is not ideal, because a subset of patients with apparent non-insulin-dependent diabetes later become fully insulin-dependent and prone to ketoacidosis. These patients are nonobese and usually express HLA antigens associated with susceptibility to insulin-dependent diabetes and have evidence of an immune response to islet cell antigens (see "Pathogenesis," below). For this reason, it has been suggested that the classification shown in Table 334-1 be modified so that the terms *insulin-dependent* and *non-insulin-dependent* describe physiologic states (ketoacidosis-prone and ketoacidosis-resistant, respectively), while the terms *type 1* and *type 2* refer to pathogenetic mechanisms (immune-mediated and non-immune-mediated, respectively). Using such a classification, three major forms of primary diabetes would be recognized: (1) type 1 IDDM, (2) type 1 NIDDM, and (3) type 2 NIDDM. Category 2 is an intermediate stage of autoimmune destruction in which the capacity to produce insulin is sufficient to prevent ketoacidosis but not to maintain normal blood glucose; this variant likely occurs when the autoimmune process begins at an older age and progresses more slowly than usual. It is uncommon when IDDM appears in childhood or early adolescence. A subset of obese people with apparent non-insulin-dependent diabetes can become transiently insulin dependent and develop DKA. Such individuals do not have markers of autoimmunity suggestive of type 1 disease and may not require insulin permanently after recovery from DKA. Presumably, diminution of insulin reserve renders such subjects vulnerable to stress-induced metabolic decompensation and causes transient insulin dependence.

There are several secondary forms of diabetes. *Pancreatic disease*, particularly chronic pancreatitis in alcoholics, is a common cause. Destruction of the beta cell mass is the etiologic mechanism. *Hormonal* causes include pheochromocytoma, acromegaly, Cushing's syndrome, and administration of steroid hormones. "Stress hyperglycemia," associated with severe burns, acute myocardial infarctions, and other life-threatening illnesses, is due to endogenous release of glucagon and catecholamines. Hormonal hyperglycemia results from varying combinations of impairment of insulin release and induction of insulin resistance. A large number of *drugs* can lead to impaired glucose tolerance or hyperglycemia. Hyperglycemia and even ketoacidosis can be due to quantitative or qualitative defects in the *insulin receptor* or to antibodies directed against it. The mechanism is essentially pure insulin resistance. *Genetic syndromes* associated with impaired glucose tolerance or hyperglycemia include the lipodystrophies, myotonic dystrophy, and ataxia-telangiectasia. The final category, *other*, is poorly defined and is meant to include any condition that does not fit elsewhere in the etiologic scheme. The appearance of abnormal carbohydrate metabolism in association with any of these secondary causes does not necessarily indicate the presence of underlying diabetes, although, in some cases, mild, asymptomatic primary diabetes is made overt by the secondary illness.

PREVALENCE The prevalence of diabetes is difficult to determine because various standards, many no longer acceptable, have been used in diagnosis. If fasting hyperglycemia is the diagnostic standard, the prevalence in the United States is probably 1 to 2 percent. Using data from the National Health Interview Surveys, an estimate of 3.1 percent was made in 1993; the National Diabetes Data Group, using the response to a 75-g oral glucose tolerance test as the diagnostic criterion, estimated the prevalence of diabetes at 6.6 percent, with 11.2 percent of the population having impaired glucose tolerance. These figures are almost certainly too high. Most subjects who are diagnosed as having impaired glucose tolerance or diabetes on the basis of oral glucose tolerance testing never develop fasting hyperglycemia or symptomatic diabetes when followed longitudinally. For example, in a massive screening program (more than 300,000 subjects) carried out in Cleveland, Ohio, only 31 percent of persons who had 2-h glucose values of 10 mmol/L (180 mg/dL) or higher in the glucose tolerance test progressed to overt diabetes after 5 years. Other studies confirm the imprecision of oral glucose challenges in predicting or diagnosing diabetes—hence the estimates of 1 to 2 percent prevalence used here. Similar conclusions have been reached in Sweden, where the prevalence is around 1.5 percent. Estimates for IDDM are more reliable than for the NIDDM because most patients are diagnosed

Table 334-1

Classification of Diabetes Mellitus

PRIMARY
Autoimmune (type 1) diabetes mellitus
Non-insulin-dependent diabetes mellitus (type 1 NIDDM—*transient*)
Insulin-dependent diabetes mellitus (type 1 IDDM)
Non-autoimmune (type 2) diabetes mellitus
Insulin-dependent diabetes mellitus (type 2 IDDM—*transient*)
Non-insulin-dependent diabetes mellitus (type 2 NIDDM)
Maturity-onset diabetes of the young (MODY)
SECONDARY
Diabetes caused by pancreatic disease
Diabetes caused by hormonal abnormalities
Drug- or chemical-induced diabetes
Diabetes caused by insulin receptor abnormalities
Diabetes associated with genetic syndromes
Diabetes of other causes

[1] Venous whole blood concentrations of glucose are 15 percent lower than plasma values. Capillary whole blood, utilized in patient self-monitoring, is equivalent to venous plasma.

after the abrupt appearance of symptoms. In England, the prevalence of the type 1 disorder is estimated to be 0.22 percent by age 16, and a study in the United States suggested a prevalence of 0.26 percent by age 20. If the prevalence of diabetes is about 2 percent, it follows that NIDDM is seven to eight times more common than IDDM. The ratio of the frequency of IDDM to that of NIDDM varies with age, being higher if a young population is studied and lower in the older age range. The cited prevalences are for populations as a whole. Certain subsets have different rates. For example, more than 40 percent of Pima Indians in the United States have type 2 NIDDM.

The fact that persons with asymptomatic, undiagnosed diabetes occasionally develop complications despite the absence of fasting hyperglycemia has led to suggestions that large-scale screening with glucose tolerance tests be instituted. For the reasons given above, this course seems unwise.

PATHOGENESIS OF IDDM By the time IDDM appears, most of the beta cells in the pancreas have been destroyed. The destructive process is almost certainly autoimmune in nature, although details remain obscure. Pathogenesis begins with a genetic susceptibility to the disease, and some environmental event initiates the process in such susceptible individuals. Viral infection is one triggering mechanism, but noninfectious agents also may be involved. The best evidence that an environmental insult is required comes from studies in monozygotic twins, in whom the concordance rate for diabetes is less than 50 percent. If diabetes were a purely genetic illness, concordance rates should approximate 100 percent. Autoimmune attack then follows. Although the process is clinically silent, the islets become infiltrated by monocytes/macrophages and activated cytotoxic T cells. This infiltration is usually designated *insulitis* but is sometimes called *isletitis*. Multiple antibodies against beta cell antigens are present in blood. The patient's state while the immune attack is underway but unrecognized is termed *prediabetes*. The prediabetic state may be brief or prolonged and may be progressive and uninterrupted or intermittent. What is clear is that the insulin reserve steadily diminishes until it is insufficient to maintain blood glucose within normal bounds. At this point the diagnosis is diabetes.

Rarely, type 1 diabetes develops exclusively from an environmental insult, as from the ingestion of Vacor, a rat poison. It is also possible that autoimmune diabetes can develop in the absence of an environmental trigger, i.e., can be purely genetic. Usually, however, the pathogenetic sequence is genetic predisposition → environmental insult → autoimmune destruction of the beta cells → diabetes mellitus.

Genetics The mechanism of inheritance of IDDM is unclear. At various times, transmission has been postulated to be autosomal dominant, autosomal recessive, and mixed. While IDDM occurs with increased frequency in some families, familial aggregation is uncommon, so deduction of the mechanism of inheritance is difficult. The genetic predisposition is probably permissive and not causal.

Analysis of pedigrees shows a low prevalence of direct vertical transmission. In 493 families selected by the presence of a proband with IDDM, only 79 (16 percent) had a parent or sibling with diabetes. The risks for siblings is higher if the proband develops disease before age 10. Overall, the chance of a child developing type 1 diabetes when another first-degree relative has the disease is only 5 to 10 percent (Table 334-2). HLA identity in a sibling (see below) increases the risk; HLA nonidentity decreases it; and haploidentity (sharing of one HLA genotype) carries an intermediate risk. The presence of NIDDM in a parent increases the risk for IDDM in the offspring. It is not known whether the intermixing of IDDM and NIDDM in the same family represents the operation of a single genetic trait (i.e., the apparent NIDDM is really type 1 NIDDM) or whether two common genetic predispositions coexist in the family by chance, each perhaps influencing the expression of the other. While the low rates of transmission of IDDM make it difficult to discern mechanisms of inheritance through study of families, they are reassuring to diabetics who wish to have children.

Table 334-2

Relative Risk of Developing IDDM

Group	Percent Risk
US population	0.4
Relative of proband with IDDM	
Parent	3
Child	6
With affected father	8
With affected mother	3
Sibling	5
Identical twin	33
HLA-identical	15
HLA-haploidentical	5
HLA-nonidentical	1

SOURCE: Estimates from Atkinson and MacLaren.

Type 1 diabetes appears to be a disease in which *sexual imprinting* plays a role. The risk of diabetes is up to five times higher when the father has the disease than when the mother is diabetic. This paternity-related increased risk appears to be limited to fathers carrying an HLA DR4 susceptibility gene.

Genetic susceptibility to IDDM probably involves more than one gene. Candidate loci have been proposed on chromosomes 2, 6, 11, and 15. In NOD mice, which have an autoimmune form of diabetes resembling human IDDM, the number of susceptibility genes may be as high as 16. One (possibly the only) primary genetic site in humans is believed to be located in the major histocompatibility locus on the short arm of the 6th chromosome. There are strong associations between IDDM and certain human leukocyte antigens encoded by the major histocompatibility region. Four loci designated by the letters A, B, C, and D are recognized, with alleles at each site identified by numbers (e.g., HLA-DR3). A lowercase w indicates that identification is provisional. Gene products of the A, B, and C regions are called *class I molecules*, while D region products are called *class II molecules*. A map of the human major histocompatibility complex (MHC) is shown in Fig. 334-1. HLA gene products are glycoproteins located in the plasma membranes of cells and are believed to be recognition and/or programming signals for the initiation and amplification of immune responses in the body. These are two-chain molecules; the light chain in class I HLA is β_2-microglobulin, and the D region light chain encoded on chromosome 15 is a dimer composed of α and β chains. Class I molecules are present on all nucleated cells and function to defend against infections (especially viruses) and in immune surveillance against malignancy. Class II molecules are normally present on circulating and tissue macrophages, endothelial cells, B lymphocytes, and activated T lymphocytes. They function in the presentation of antigen to the regulatory T cell system. Activation of the immune system is "MHC-restricted," meaning that antigens are recognized only if they reach the cell surface in association with a "self" HLA allele that "fits" the receptor on the responding T cell. Thus, activation of cytotoxic T lymphocytes to fight a viral infection requires that a viral antigen be presented by a class I molecule recognized by the responding cytotoxic T cell. A similar restriction applies to antigen presentation by macrophages to helper T cells.

While definite associations exist between class I alleles and type 1 diabetes (B8, B15), the D locus is considered of primary importance. Class I loci are involved through nonrandom associations with D alleles (*linkage disequilibrium*). Because about 95 percent of white type 1 IDDM patients express either DR3 or DR4 or the heterozygous DR3/DR4 configuration, it was thought initially that a susceptibility gene might be located nearby. The focus has since shifted to the DQ locus. Typing of D regions is now carried out by analyzing DNA with allele-specific oligonucleotide probes. For example, $DQ\beta_1$*0301 and $DQ\beta_1$*0302 identify DR4 haplotypes, and $DQ\beta_1$*0201 segregates with DR3 haplotypes. $DQ\beta_1$*0502 and $DQ\beta_1$*0602 are associated with DR2 haplotypes. Some class II alleles predict susceptibility to IDDM, and others predict protection against it. Still others are apparently neutral. Susceptibility appears to be primarily vested in $DQ\beta_1$*0201 and DQβ$_1$*0302, with DQβ$_1$*0201/0302 heterozygosity portending a particularly high risk. DQβ$_1$*0602 is rarely present in persons with IDDM and is considered to be protective; i.e., it cancels the effects of a susceptibility gene when both are present. The DR2 allele, with which it is associated, is known to be protective. When IDDM occurs in a DR2/DR2 individual, it is due to a recombination event resulting in the presence of a susceptibility gene such as DQβ$_1$*0302. Terminology in the HLA field changes rapidly. DQβ$_1$*0301 was formerly known as DQw7 or DQw3.1; DQβ$_1$*0302 was previously known as DQw8 or DQw3.2; and DQβ$_1$*0602 was known as DQw1.2.

How might HLA alleles predispose to or protect from IDDM? Probably by exhibiting different affinities for diabetogenic peptides presented to the immune system. Thus HLA DQβ$_1$*0302 might bind a diabetogenic peptide with greater affinity for presentation on the cell surface than DQβ$_1$*0301. Conversely, a dominant protective allele (which presumably would not present antigen in such a way as to activate the immune system) might bind the diabetogenic peptide with such high affinity as to effectively "steal" it from a susceptibility gene even when both are present, thereby preventing the disease. Although the DQβ-chain alleles appear to predict risk for diabetes most precisely, they may well be influenced by interaction with α chains. Thus, T cell recognition of a DQβ$_1$*0302 chain is modified by the associated DQα chain. The situation is further complicated by the fact that α and β chains from different HLA molecules may interact to form new dimers, a process called *transcomplementation*. Susceptibility to autoimmune diabetes may be linked to decreased expression of class I HLA molecules on splenocytes and lymphocytes in NOD mice (which get autoimmune diabetes) and in humans. The meaning of this finding and its reproducibility are not clear.

Environmental Event As noted earlier, the fact that a significant proportion of monozygotic twins remains discordant for diabetes suggests that nongenetic factors are required for development of diabetes. Similarly, HLA identity or haploidentity does not ensure concordance.

The environmental factor in many cases is believed to be a viral infection of the beta cell. A viral etiology was originally suggested by seasonal variations in the onset of the disease and by what appeared to be more than a chance relationship between the appearance of diabetes and preceding episodes of mumps, hepatitis, infectious mononucleosis, congenital rubella, and coxsackievirus infections. Furthermore, certain strains of encephalomyocarditis virus cause diabetes in genetically susceptible mice. The isolation of a coxsackievirus B4 from the pancreas of a previously healthy boy who died after an episode of ketoacidosis, and the induction of diabetes in animals inoculated with the isolated virus, also suggested a viral etiology, and the fact that the titer of neutralizing antibody to coxsackievirus rose in this patient during the weeks prior to death indicated that the infection was recently acquired. Further support for the viral theory comes from the observation that about one-fifth of individuals with congenital rubella develop IDDM. The presence of an HLA susceptibility allele in the fetus may double the risk. Cytomegalovirus genes are present in the genome of one-fifth of patients with type 1 diabetes, and retroviral genes are present in the beta cells of NOD mice. Presumably, viral infections of the pancreas could induce diabetes by two mechanisms: direct inflammatory disruption of islets or induction of an immune response.

Despite its attractiveness, the viral theory should be treated with considerable caution. Serologic studies seeking evidence of recent viral infection in patients with new-onset IDDM are inconclusive at best.

It has been suggested that exposure to cow's milk or milk products early in life predisposes to autoimmune diabetes. The proposed environmental trigger is bovine albumin, operating through the mechanism of molecular mimicry. In the initial study, diabetic subjects were found to have antibodies to bovine albumin, and an antibody subset specific for a 17-amino-acid epitope showed the strongest association with the disease. The latter antibodies bind to a 69-kDa protein (p69) on the surface of the pancreatic beta cell. Exposure to cow's milk is presumed to induce an immune response to the 17-amino-acid fragment in some infants, and cross-reactivity of the antibody would destroy beta cells expressing the p69 antigen. Not universally present on beta cells, p69 can be induced through the action of interferon γ produced by intermittent viral infections. This hypothesis has not received wide support.

Insulitis/Isletitis In animals, macrophages and activated T lymphocytes infiltrate the pancreatic islets prior to or simultaneously with development of diabetes. Lymphocytes are also found in the islets of young persons dying from new-onset diabetes, and radioactively labeled lymphocytes localize in the pancreas in humans with IDDM. These findings are in accord with the fact that immune endocrinopathies are associated with lymphocytic infiltration of the affected tissue. It is not clear, however, that insulitis is central to the destructive sequence in autoimmune diabetes; the cellular infiltration may be an epiphenomenon.

Conversion of the Beta Cell from Self to Nonself and Activation of the Immune System There seems to be little doubt that the immune system mediates destruction of the beta cells in type 1 diabetes. The disease is frequently associated with other autoimmune endocrinopathies such as adrenal insufficiency and Hashimoto's thyroiditis; pancreatic tissue transplanted from a nondiabetic monozygotic twin into the diabetic twin is rapidly destroyed in the absence of immunosuppression, and temporary reversal of clinical symptoms occurs with early use of cyclosporine. Moreover, most patients have antibodies directed against insulin and other beta cell antigens. Since the immune

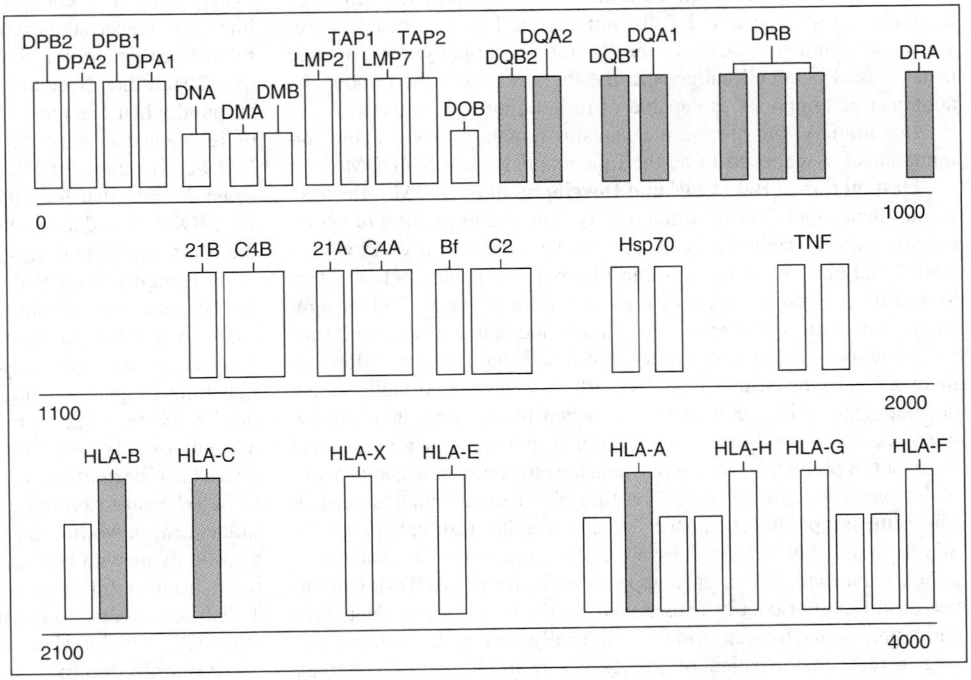

FIGURE 334-1 Schematized map of the human major histocompatibility complex. Primary sites of association with IDDM are shown as stippled bars. A1, A2, B1, and B2 in the DP and DQ regions refer to α and β chains. The top line (0 to 1000) represents the class II region; the middle line (1100 to 2000) represents the class III region (genes for some complement factors, heat shock protein 70S, and tumor necrosis factor), and the bottom line (2100 to 4000) represents the class I region. Unlabeled bars are pseudogenes. *(Map provided courtesy of Dr. Peter Stasny.)*

system normally does not attack self tissues, IDDM can be viewed as an autoimmune disease.

The mechanism behind this autoimmune destruction is not known. As noted earlier, an environmental trigger appears to be involved frequently. The putative environmental agent could be a virus, a toxin, or a food and might act in one of several ways. Direct destruction of beta cells by a virus or toxin might expose cryptic antigens to the immune system, evoking an immune response. Alternatively, destructive cytokines might be released by viruses to kill beta cells, or programmed cell death (*apoptosis*) might be induced. A relative deficiency of early complement components might impair the clearing of islet cell viruses (a mechanism analogous to the one responsible for persistent hepatitis B infection in some patients with chronic active hepatitis), thereby prolonging stimulation of the immune system by cryptic antigens. Another hypothesis is the aforementioned *molecular mimicry*, in which there is a chance homology between a foreign antigen and amino acid sequences in normal tissue. The best-known example occurs in acute rheumatic fever, where the immune response to group A streptococci results in cross-reacting attack on the heart. Once cytotoxic T cells and plasma cells are activated against a particular antigenic epitope (armed), they seek and destroy any cell bearing the epitope. The bovine milk albumin hypothesis presumes molecular mimicry, and homology exists between a coxsackievirus protein and glutamic acid decarboxylase (GAD). Antibodies against GAD are common in young people with type 1 diabetes.

A third possibility, currently less popular, is that viral infection, via cytokine release, induces expression of HLA D region molecules in the pancreas (where they are not normally present), converting one or more cell types into antigen-presenting cells.

Some patients may have a purely genetic form of the disease. In neonatal life, autoreactive T cells are normally destroyed in the thymus ("clonal deletion"). Any cells escaping the thymus are rendered anergic or suppressed in the periphery by regulatory T cells. Failure of either process could leave a repertoire of cells capable of responding to self antigens following cell injury. In support of the possibility that a contributing factor in autoimmune disease is suboptimal removal or regulation of autoreactive T cells, intrathymic injection of islets prevents autoimmune diabetes in the BB rat. Presumably, the presence of additional beta cell antigens in the thymus allows the removal of autoreactive lymphocytes capable of responding to islet tissue.

In summary, the precise mechanisms remain a mystery, but immune attack is believed to be the fundamental cause of IDDM.

Destruction of Beta Cells and Development of IDDM Because insulin-dependent diabetes often begins with an abrupt onset of symptomatic hyperglycemia, polyuria, and/or ketoacidosis, it was long assumed that beta cell damage occurred rapidly. It is now believed that loss of insulin reserve occurs over a few to many years. This insight came from studies of discordant monozygotic diabetic twins and triplets in whom one twin or triplet developed diabetes long after the index case. In the slow course, the earliest sign of abnormality is the development of islet cell antibodies when blood sugar and glucose tolerance are normal and when insulin responses to a glucose load are intact. A phase then ensues in which the only metabolic abnormality is decreased glucose tolerance. Fasting blood sugar remains normal. This is the last prediabetic phase. In the third stage, fasting hyperglycemia develops, but ketosis does not occur even when the diabetes is poorly controlled. The clinical appearance is that of NIDDM. Continued destruction of beta cells then leads to the insulin-dependent stage and a propensity for ketoacidosis, especially during stress. Once this stage is reached, the patient ordinarily requires lifelong insulin therapy unless a pancreatic transplant is performed. However, a few patients, after immunosuppression with cyclosporine, become insulin independent for months or years.

The immune-directed destruction of beta cells probably involves both humoral and cell-mediated mechanisms, the latter being more important. Islet cell antibodies include antibodies to insulin, proinsulin, two forms of glutamic acid decarboxylase (GAD 65 and GAD 67), carboxypeptidase H, two ganglioside antigens (GT3 and GM2-1), ICA 69 (the antigen that cross-reacts with antibody against bovine albumin), and ICA 512 (which may be a protein phosphatase). The presence of anti-GAD antibody may have modest predictive value for subsequent development of IDDM in persons who are at potential risk because of disease in a first-degree relative, but it does not definitively predict overt disease. A subset of anti-GAD antibodies appears to react with human and rat but not mouse islets. These "restricted" islet cell antibodies appear to be linked to the protective HLA allele DQβ_1*0602 and thus may protect against development of diabetes rather than predict its development.

Cells involved in the attack on the beta cell include natural killer cells, activated cytotoxic T lymphocytes (CD8+), and macrophages. Cell destruction may be at least partially due to release of cytokines such as interleukin 1 (IL-1) and tumor necrosis factor α (TNFα) from activated macrophages. Experimentally, mixtures of cytokines (IL-1, TNFα, interferon γ, and lymphotoxin) are more potent than single agents. Cytokines may work through induction of nitric oxide or of superoxide. Beta cells have a low capacity for free radical destruction and are especially vulnerable to oxygen toxicity.

By the time overt diabetes appears, most insulin-producing cells have disappeared. In one study, pancreatic weight at autopsy averaged 40 g in persons with type 1 diabetes versus 82 g in control individuals. Endocrine cell mass in subjects with IDDM decreased from 1395 mg to 413 mg, and the beta cell mass, which averaged 850 mg in normal individuals, was unmeasurable. Since alpha cells remained essentially intact, the ratio of glucagon- to insulin-producing cells approached infinity.

PATHOGENESIS OF NIDDM Although NIDDM is more common than IDDM and more frequently exhibits familial aggregation, its pathogenesis is less well understood. Nevertheless, both beta cell defects and insulin resistance are present in overt disease, and the major enviromental factor is obesity. The relation between the beta cell abnormality and insulin resistance is not resolved.

Genetics Although NIDDM occurs in families, modes of inheritance are not known except for the variant termed *maturity-onset diabetes of the young* (MODY). MODY is usually manifested by mild hyperglycemia in young persons who are resistant to ketosis. Three lines of evidence suggest transmission as an autosomal dominant trait. First, three-generation direct transmission has been demonstrated in over 20 families. Second, a 1:1 ratio of diabetic to nondiabetic children is found when one parent has the disease. Third, about 90 percent of obligate carriers have diabetes. Three different mutations can cause MODY. The gene for MODY 1 is located on the long arm of chromosome 20, and that for MODY 3 is on the long arm of chromosome 12. MODY 2 is due to mutations in the glucokinase gene located on the short arm of chromosome 7.

It is highly likely that ordinary NIDDM is polygenic. Much effort has been spent in evaluating candidate genes, with emphasis on molecules involved in glucose metabolism in the pancreatic beta cell, liver, muscle, and fat. A few cases of NIDDM appear to be associated with mutations in genes coding for insulin, mitochondrial components, the insulin receptor, glucokinase, and glycogen synthase. At best these account for only a fraction of NIDDM cases. More than 250 candidate genes have been examined by various groups, but none is established to be relevant to ordinary NIDDM. Whatever its nature, the genetic influence is powerful, since the concordance rate for diabetes in monozygotic twins with type 2 disease may be as high as 80 percent. Risk to offspring and siblings of patients with NIDDM is higher than in type 1 diabetes. Nearly four-tenths of siblings and one-third of offspring eventually develop abnormal glucose tolerance or frank diabetes.

Pathophysiology Patients with type 2 NIDDM have two physiologic defects: abnormal insulin secretion and resistance to insulin action in target tissues. Which of the abnormalities is primary is not known. Descriptively, three phases can be recognized in the usual clinical sequence. In the first phase, the plasma glucose remains normal despite demonstrable insulin resistance, because insulin levels are elevated. In the second phase, insulin resistance tends to worsen, so that postprandial hyperglycemia develops despite elevated insulin concentrations. In the third phase, insulin resistance does not change, but declining insulin secretion causes fasting hyperglycemia and overt diabetes. Most authorities believe that insulin resistance is primary and that hyperinsulinemia is secondary; i.e., insulin secretion increases to compensate for the resistance state. However, hypersecretion of insulin (and amylin?) may cause insulin resistance; i.e., a primary islet cell defect causes insulin hypersecretion, and insulin hypersecretion, in turn, leads to insulin resistance. Explanatory hypotheses involve increased fat synthesis in the liver and enhanced fat transport [via very low density lipoprotein (VLDL)] leading to secondary fat storage in muscle. Increased fat oxidation would impair glucose uptake and glycogen synthesis. Most patients with NIDDM are obese, and obesity per se causes insulin resistance. However, nonobese relatives of persons with NIDDM may have hyperinsulinemia and diminished insulin sensitivity, proving that obesity is not the sole cause of resistance. This statement is not to diminish the importance of excess fat, since a modest reduction in weight often results in major improvement in blood sugar control in obese subjects with NIDDM. The late decline in insulin release could be due to the underlying genetic defect or to metabolic toxicity in the beta cell. High levels of glucose or increased tissue levels of long-chain fatty acids ("lipotoxicity") could be the damaging molecules.

In summary, it is likely that an insulin secretory defect and insulin resistance are both required for diabetes to be expressed, since massively obese persons with marked insulin resistance may have normal glucose tolerance. Presumably, the beta cell lesion is not present in such persons. This fact might suggest that the primary defect resides in the insulin-producing cells. Beta cell mass is intact in type 2 NIDDM, in contrast to the situation with type 1 IDDM. The alpha cell population is increased, resulting in an elevated ratio of alpha to beta cells and in the excess of glucagon relative to insulin that characterizes all hyperglycemic states, including NIDDM.

Although insulin resistance in type 2 NIDDM is associated with decreased numbers of insulin receptors, most of the resistance is postreceptor in nature (see below). It has long been known that deposits of amyloid are found in the pancreas of patients with type 2 diabetes. This material is a 37-amino-acid peptide termed *amylin.* Amylin is normally copackaged with insulin in secretory granules and is released simultaneously with insulin in response to insulin secretagogues. In animals, amylin has been reported to induce insulin resistance, but in diabetic subjects an amylin derivative has hypoglycemic effects, apparently because it causes delayed absorption of nutrients from the gastrointestinal tract. Amylin deposition in the islets may be the consequence of overproduction secondary to the insulin resistance to which it contributes. Alternatively, accumulation of amylin in the islets might contribute to the late failure of insulin production with long-standing NIDDM. A definitive role for amylin is not established.

Regardless of the mechanism, the physiologic consequences of insulin resistance are clear. There is no major abnormality in either glucose uptake by the cell or its oxidative metabolism to CO_2, water, and lactate. Rather, the major metabolic block is in glycogen synthesis ("nonoxidative metabolism"). Impaired glycogen synthesis, like hyperinsulinemia and insulin resistance, may be seen in nonobese, normoglycemic relatives of subjects with NIDDM.

A rare form of type 2 NIDDM, clinically mild, is due to production of an abnormal insulin that does not bind well to insulin receptors. Persons with this variant of the disease respond normally to exogenous insulin.

CLINICAL FEATURES The manifestations of symptomatic diabetes mellitus vary from patient to patient. Most often, symptoms are due to hyperglycemia (polyuria, polydipsia, polyphagia), but the first event may be an acute metabolic decompensation resulting in diabetic coma. Occasionally, the initial expression is a degenerative complication, such as neuropathy, in the absence of symptomatic hyperglycemia. The metabolic derangements of diabetes are due to a relative or absolute deficiency of insulin and a relative or absolute excess of glucagon. Normally, a rise in the molar ratio of glucagon to insulin leads to metabolic decompensation. Changes in this ratio

can be caused by a fall in insulin or a rise in glucagon concentration, separately or together. Alteration in the biologic response to either hormone would have the same effect. Thus, insulin resistance could cause the metabolic effects expected of an elevated glucagon/insulin ratio, even if the ratio found by immunoassay of the two hormones in plasma were normal or even decreased (the glucagon being biologically active, the insulin relatively inactive). The relationship between metabolic abnormalities and degenerative complications will be discussed subsequently. Typically, the clinical features of IDDM and NIDDM are distinctive.

Insulin-Dependent Diabetes IDDM usually begins before age 40; in the United States, peak incidence is around age 14. Some patients develop type 1 diabetes late in life, with a first episode of ketoacidosis occurring at age 50 or even later in rare instances. The author has seen one patient with typical diabetic ketoacidosis as the initial event of IDDM at the age of 80. These patients, who on the basis of age should have type 2 NIDDM, are usually not obese. Onset of symptoms may be abrupt, with thirst, excessive urination, increased appetite, and weight loss developing over several days. In some cases, the disease is heralded by the appearance of ketoacidosis during an intercurrent illness or following surgery. As outlined in Table 334-3, type 1 patients may have normal weight or may be wasted, depending on the length of time between onset of symptoms and start of treatment. Characteristically, the plasma insulin level is low or unmeasurable. Glucagon levels are elevated but are suppressed by insulin administration. Once symptoms develop, insulin therapy is required. Occasionally, an initial episode of ketoacidosis is followed by a symptom-free interval (the "honeymoon" period), during which no treatment is required. The likely explanation for this phenomenon is shown in Fig. 334-2.

Non-Insulin-Dependent Diabetes NIDDM usually begins in middle life or later. The typical patient is overweight. Symptoms begin gradually, and the diagnosis is frequently made when an asymptomatic person is found to have an elevated plasma glucose level on routine laboratory examination. In contrast to IDDM, plasma insulin levels are normal to high in absolute terms, although they are lower than predicted for the level of the plasma glucose; i.e., relative insulin deficiency is present. Stated in another way, if plasma glucose concentrations in nondiabetic subjects were raised to levels equivalent to those found in NIDDM patients, insulin values would be higher in the normal group. This relative deficiency reflects the previously mentioned insulin secretory defect in NIDDM. Glucagon metabolism in NIDDM is complex. While the elevated fasting plasma concentrations can be lowered by large amounts of insulin, the exaggerated glucagon response to ingested nutrients cannot be suppressed; i.e., alpha cell function remains abnormal. For unknown reasons, patients with NIDDM do not develop ketoacidosis but are susceptible to development of hyperosmolar, nonketotic coma. One hypothesis to explain the absence of ketoacidosis during stress is that the liver is resistant

Table 334-3

General Characteristics of IDDM and NIDDM

Characteristic	IDDM	NIDDM
Genetic locus*	Chromosome 6	Unknown
Age of onset†	Usually <40	>40
Body habitus	Normal to wasted	Obese
Plasma insulin	Low to absent	Normal to high
Plasma glucagon	High, suppressible	High, resistant
Acute complication	Ketoacidosis	Hyperosmolar coma
Insulin therapy	Responsive	Responsive to resistant
Response to sulfonylurea therapy	Unresponsive	Responsive

* Both IDDM and NIDDM are polygenic (see text).
† Most cases of IDDM appear before age 20, but onset can be late in life.

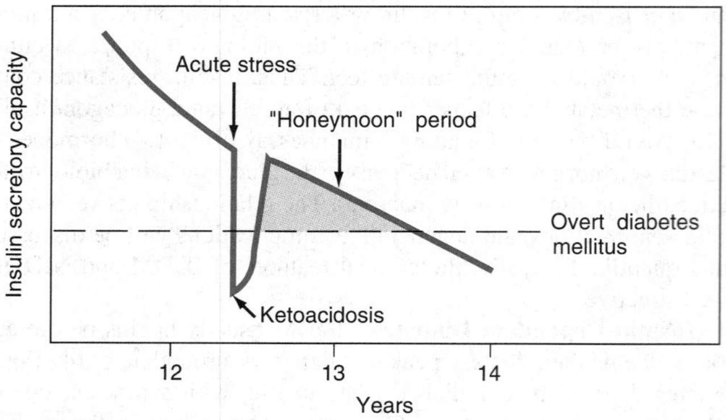

FIGURE 334-2 Schematic representation of the "honeymoon" period. The insulin secretory capacity is shown gradually decreasing in a patient destined to develop diabetes. At approximately 13½ years, insulin would become insufficient to maintain plasma glucose in the normal range. An initial episode of ketoacidosis—for example, in association with acute appendicitis—is shown occurring in the twelfth year. Presumably, stress-induced epinephrine release blocks insulin secretion and causes the syndrome. In normal subjects, insulin reserve is such that hormone release is adequate even in the face of stress. Following recovery from the stressful episode, insulin secretory capacity returns to the previous level and remains sufficient for an additional year, as indicated by the shaded area—the "honeymoon" period.

to glucagon, so that malonyl-CoA levels remain high, inhibiting the fatty acid oxidation–ketogenic pathway (see below). If weight loss can be induced, patients may be managed by diet alone. Most patients who fail dietary therapy respond to sulfonylureas or to combinations of sulfonylureas plus metformin, but, in many, the resulting improvement of hyperglycemia is not sufficient for control of diabetes. For this reason, a high percentage of patients with NIDDM are treated with insulin.

℞ TREATMENT

Diet For many years, dietary prescriptions for patients with diabetes were rigid and difficult to follow. "Exchange" lists of major foods were provided, listing calories and composition, and diets were constructed using the exchanges, such as the precalculated diets provided by the American Diabetes Association (ADA). This approach has now been abandoned by the ADA, whose policy for diet/nutrition is now as follows:

> Today there is no ONE 'diabetic' or 'ADA' diet. The recommended diet can only be defined as a dietary prescription based on nutrition assessment and treatment goals. Medical nutrition therapy for people with diabetes should be individualized, with consideration given to eating habits and other lifestyle factors. Nutrition recommendations are then developed to meet treatment goals and desired outcomes. Monitoring metabolic parameters, including blood glucose, glycated hemoglobin, lipids, blood pressure, and body weight, as well as quality of life, is crucial to ensure successful outcomes.

Flexibility in use of ordinary foods is important for patients and families. The first decision is the caloric content of the diet, based on the need to gain, lose, or maintain current weight. Caloric recommendations from the Food and Nutrition Board for adults carrying out "average" activity decrease with age and range from 175 kJ/kg of body weight (42 kcal/kg) in 18-year-old men to 140 kJ/kg (33 kcal/kg) for 75-year-old women. Intakes slightly less than the official recommendations are usually preferable; 150 kJ/kg (36 kcal/kg) for men and 140 kJ/kg (34 kcal/kg) for women are reasonable initial values in most patients.

The minimal protein requirement for good nutrition is about 0.9 g/kg of body weight per day, and the acceptable range is 1.0 to 1.5 g/kg per day. Since very low protein diets may slow the progression of nephropathy, protein content should probably be limited to 0.8 g/kg per day, or about 10 percent of daily calories, when this complication develops.

The distribution of calories between carbohydrate and fat must be determined individually. Restriction of fat is usually prudent if weight loss is desired because of the high energy content of fat relative to protein and carbohydrate. An average recommendation for nonobese patients and those without hyperlipidemias is that fat should make up 30 percent or less of total calories, with less than 10 percent as saturated fat. In hypercholesterolemic subjects, saturated fat should be lowered to less than 7 percent of calories, and cholesterol intake should be below 200 mg/day. An increase in polyunsaturated fats is usually recommended. Fat restriction is not recommended by all authors. For example, a 50 percent fat diet with 33 percent monounsaturated fatty acids and 35 percent carbohydrates was reported to lower glucose levels, insulin requirements, and VLDL levels while increasing the concentrations of high-density lipoprotein (HDL). Some authors recommend the addition of fish oils containing omega-3 fatty acids as beneficial, but this is not standard practice.

After the protein and fat content is chosen, the remaining calories are assigned to carbohydrate. Sucrose can be allowed in moderation as part of the carbohydrate component. Increasing the fiber content of the diet may be helpful. As in any dietary regimen, it is the long-term, overall dietary pattern that counts. Deviation for one or two meals does not matter much. Thus, a teenage diabetic may be allowed to eat a high-sugar, high-fat dessert, ordinarily forbidden, as a special treat with the understanding that resumption of the diet will be necessary the next day. Even in adults the "treat" technique often ensures better dietary cooperation than more rigid demands. Ideally, patients should be trained by dieticians in a formal teaching program. Such classes are available in most large hospitals. If a patient is from a smaller community, it will probably be helpful to refer him or her to a larger center for initial training.

In insulin-requiring patients, the distribution of calories is also important if hypoglycemia is to be avoided. A typical pattern might include 20 percent of the total for breakfast, 35 percent for lunch, 30 percent for dinner, and 15 percent as a late-evening feeding. Often, a midmorning and a midafternoon snack are necessary as well. Different distributions may be required for different life-styles; i.e., a person employed on a late-evening or night shift would not eat the major meal at noon. When regimes of meticulous control are attempted using multiple injections of insulin or insulin pumps, more frequent feedings are often prescribed. Thus one might recommend 20 percent of energy intake at both breakfast and lunch, 30 percent at dinner, and the remaining 30 percent as midmorning, midafternoon, and late-evening snacks, depending on the pattern of plasma glucose level during the day.

The importance of diet in the management of diabetes varies with the type of disease. In insulin-dependent patients, particularly those on intensive insulin regimens, the composition of the diet is not of critical importance, since adjustment of insulin can cover wide variations in food ingestion. In non-insulin-dependent patients not treated with exogenous insulin, more rigorous adherence to diet is required, since the endogenous insulin reserve is limited. Such patients cannot respond to the increased demand produced by excess calories or increased intake of rapidly absorbed carbohydrate.

Insulin Insulin is required for treatment of all patients with IDDM and many patients with NIDDM. If the physician does not use oral agents (see below), all diet-unresponsive NIDDM subjects must be given the hormone. It is fairly easy to control the symptoms of diabetes with insulin, but it is difficult to maintain a normal blood sugar throughout 24 h, even with the use of multiple injections of regular insulin or infusion pumps. In the Diabetes Control and Complications Trial (see below), where teams of health care workers attempted to return the blood glucose level to normal or near normal with much more frequent professional input than is usual in clinical situations, blood glucose levels and hemoglobin A_{1c} concentrations remained above normal in most subjects. It is even more difficult to maintain normal blood sugars by means of traditional insulin therapy given as one or two injections a day. Nondiabetic subjects maintain the plasma glucose concentration within a narrow range at all times despite episodic food intake. When a meal is eaten, a prompt rise in insulin release occurs, such that absorbed carbohydrate is rapidly taken up by the liver and other tissues. Even after meals, therefore, the plasma glucose level in normal subjects does not rise into the hyperglycemic or glycosuric range. As the plasma glucose level falls under the influence of insulin, release of the hormone is damped, and counterregulatory hormones enter the circulation to prevent hypoglycemia, ensuring smooth control of plasma glucose throughout the absorptive process. The patient treated with insulin by injection cannot reproduce these physiologic responses. If enough insulin is given to keep the postprandial glucose normal, too much insulin will inevitably be present during the postabsorptive phase, and hypoglycemia will result.

No single standard exists for patterns of administration of insulin, and treatment plans vary from physician to physician and, with a given physician, for different patients. Three treatment regimes will be described: conventional, multiple subcutaneous injections (MSI), and continuous subcutaneous insulin infusion (CSII). MSI or CSII is required in intensive treatment schedules designed to protect against complications. *Conventional insulin therapy* involves the administration of one or two injections a day of intermediate-acting insulin such as zinc insulin (lente insulin) or isophane insulin (NPH insulin) with or without the addition of small amounts of regular insulin. If the newly diagnosed subject is not in acute distress, therapy can be started on an outpatient basis, provided the patient has been instructed adequately on diet, insulin use, and monitoring and the physician or nurse-clinician can be reached by telephone for consultation. Adults of normal weight may be started on 15 to 20 units a day. (The estimated daily insulin production rate in nondiabetic subjects of normal size is about 25 units a day.) Obese patients, because of insulin resistance, may be started on 25 to 30 units a day. It is preferable to use the same quantity of insulin for several days before changing, the one exception being in a hypoglycemic patient, whose dose should be decreased immediately unless a nonrecurrent cause of hypoglycemia (such as excessive exercise) is present. Generally, changes should be no more than 5 or 10 units per step. It is probable that a single daily injection of insulin provides adequate control only in patients who have some residual capacity for insulin secretion. Patients with poorly controlled disease should be placed on split therapy, with about two-thirds of the total insulin given before breakfast and the remainder before supper. Two injections are almost always used when the total dose reaches 50 or 60 units a day but are helpful at smaller doses as well, since the peak action of intermediate insulins appears to be dose-related; i.e., a low dose may exhibit maximal activity earlier and disappear sooner than a large dose. Many physicians routinely add regular insulin to the intermediate dose even at initiation of therapy. Thus, in a single-dose schedule, one might begin with 20 units of intermediate and 5 units of regular insulin rather than 25 units of intermediate alone. This practice is based on the concept that the regular insulin lowers the plasma glucose level rapidly, after which the more slowly absorbed insulin maintains the lowered level. Most patients on twice-daily insulin injections are also treated with a mixture of intermediate and regular insulin; e.g., 25 units NPH plus 10 units of regular before breakfast and 10 units of NPH plus 5 units of regular before supper. Commercial premixed insulin (70/30 intermediate/regular) is acceptable and convenient for many patients. All patients should be taught to decrease insulin when significant extra activity or exercise is anticipated. The proper decrement must be determined by trial and error, although a reduction of 5 to 10 units is a reasonable first step. The blood glucose–lowering effect of exercise is due primarily to increased energy demands in previously noncontracting muscle. Extra regular insulin can be taken before a meal that contains extra calories or food ordinarily not allowed (e.g., when the diabetic must eat out at a banquet or the teenager goes out on a date). For patients willing to self-monitor plasma glucose level, an algorithm for adjusting insulin can be provided. A typical protocol is shown in Table 334-4. Patients with complicated control problems may require hospitalization, where frequent plasma glucose determinations can guide therapy.

The *multiple subcutaneous insulin injection technique* most commonly involves administration of intermediate- or long-acting insulin in the evening as a single dose together with regular insulin prior to each meal. Home glucose monitoring by the patient is necessary if the goal is the return of the plasma glucose level to normal. One approach to initiation of therapy involves administration of 25 percent of the previous daily insulin dose in the patient's conventional regimen at bedtime as intermediate insulin (NPH or lente insulin), with the other 75 percent given as regular insulin divided such that 40, 30, and 30 percent is given 30 min before breakfast, lunch, and supper, respectively. Alternatively, a three-injection schedule can be created by omitting the night intermediate insulin and giving a long-acting insulin, such as insulin zinc extended (ultralente insulin) or protamine zinc insulin (PZI insulin), before the evening meal. Adjustments of dosage depend on response of the plasma glucose. A number of different protocols have been used, all of which represent sliding scales of insulin based on the plasma glucose level. A typical schedule based on home monitoring of the plasma glucose level is shown in Table 334-5. Individual patients may require different dosages. For specific details, the reader should consult one of the published papers on the use of the technique (e.g., Schriffrin and Belmonte; Campbell and May). MSI can be effective in controlling the plasma glucose level, and in some studies it appears to match goals achieved with CSII.

Continuous subcutaneous insulin infusion involves the use of a small battery-driven pump that delivers insulin subcutaneously into the abdominal wall, usually through a 27-gauge butterfly needle. With CSII, insulin is delivered at a basal rate continuously throughout the day, with increases in rate programmed prior to meals. Adjustments in dosage are made in response to measured capillary glucose values in a fashion similar to that used in MSI. Ordinarily, about 40 percent of the total daily dose is given at the basal rate, the remainder being administered as preprandial boluses. There is little question that CSII can give better diabetic control than conventional therapy. Most patients report positive feelings of well-being as control improves. The danger of hypoglycemia is real, especially during the night in patients who maintain the plasma glucose consistently below 5.5 mmol/L (100 mg/dL). A fall in plasma glucose of 2.7 mmol/L (50 mg/dL) may not be important if the starting value is 8.3 mmol/L (150 mg/dL) but may be fatal if it occurs against a steady-state level of 3.3 mmol/L (60 mg/dL). Several deaths from hypoglycemia have occurred in pump users. There is also an increased frequency of diabetic ketoacidosis in persons using CSII.

Table 334-4

Adjusting Insulin Dosage in Conventional Insulin Therapy*

Blood Glucose		Regular Insulin, units	
		Breakfast	Supper
mmol/L	mg/dL	(To Be Mixed with Intermediate Dosage)	
2.8–5.5	51–100	8	4
5.6–8.3	101–150	10	5
8.4–11.1	151–200	12	6
11.2–13.9	201–250	14	7
14.0–16.6	251–300	16	8
>16.6	>300	20	10

* Once the patient's blood sugar level is in the reasonable range at most measurements, a prescription can be written for varying the regular insulin dosage as illustrated. The prescription in this case was for a patient in reasonable control on 25 units of NPH insulin plus 10 units of regular insulin before breakfast and 10 units of NPH insulin plus 5 units of regular insulin before supper. Change in metabolic status may require adjustments in both intermediate insulin and the sliding scale of regular insulin.

Table 334-5

Adjusting Insulin Dosage in a Multiple-Injection Schedule*

INITIATION OF THERAPY

1. 0.6 to 0.7 units insulin per kilogram body weight
2. 25% NPH insulin at 9 P.M.; 75% regular insulin in divided doses (40% before breakfast, 30% before lunch, 30% before supper)
3. Adjust NPH insulin every 48 h based on fasting blood glucose
   <3.3 mmol/L (<60 mg/dL): −2 units
   >5.0 mmol/L (>90 mg/dL): +2 units
4. Adjust regular insulin every 48 h based on 1-h postprandial glucose
   <3.3 mmol/L (<60 mg/dL): − 2 units
   >7.8 mmol/L (>140 mg/dL): + 2 units

DAILY THERAPY

Preprandial Glucose		
mmol/L	mg/dL	Regular Insulin, units
<3.3	<60	−2
3.4–5.0	61–90	No change
5.1–6.7	91–120	+1
6.8–8.3	121–150	+2
8.4–11.0	151–200	+3
11.1–13.9	201–250	+4
>13.9	>250	+6

* During the initiation of therapy, the insulin dosage is changed until the target range is reached (see Table 334-6). After initial stabilization, a variable insulin schedule is prescribed to maintain tight control. For example, if after initiation the patient is found generally to require 12 units of regular insulin before breakfast but has a prebreakfast blood sugar level of 8.9 mmol/L (160 mg/dL), 15 units of regular insulin instead of the usual 12 would be taken.

SOURCE: Adapted from Schiffrin and Belmonte.

Pumps should be prescribed only in disciplined and motivated patients who are under the care of a physician with extensive experience in their use.

In some centers, the catheters for insulin infusion pumps have been placed intravenously rather than subcutaneously. While few difficulties have been reported, this procedure appears unwise for routine use. Intraabdominal insulin pumps with reservoirs that are refillable from outside the body have been tried on experimental protocols. At present, no advantage is apparent except that a pump does not have to be worn externally.

For surgical procedures in diabetic patients, intermediate insulin is omitted, and treatment is carried out with regular insulin alone. An effective method is to add 10 to 20 units of insulin to a liter of 5% glucose in water with infusion at a rate of 100 to 150 mL/h. Measurement of plasma glucose in capillary blood allows the rate to be changed to avoid significant hypo- or hyperglycemia. It is also possible to administer 10 units of regular insulin subcutaneously and infuse 5% or 10% glucose at rates sufficient to avoid major changes in glucose concentration. Following surgery, a sliding scale can be constructed for use in postoperative management.

Types of Insulin A variety of insulins are available for use in the treatment of diabetes. Rapid-acting preparations are used in diabetic emergencies and in CSII and MSI programs. Intermediate-acting preparations are used in conventional and MSI regimens. Long-acting formulations are used almost exclusively in three-injection MSI schedules. Peak effects and duration vary from patient to patient and depend not only on route of administration but on dose. In patients treated for long periods, insulin action appears to be delayed, probably because of the presence of anti-insulin antibodies in plasma. In one study in diabetic subjects, the action of regular insulin given subcutaneously had its onset at about 1 h, reached a peak at 6 h, and remained measurable on average for 16 h, whereas in normal persons onset is within minutes, action peaks at around 2 h, and duration is only 6 to 8 h. With NPH insulin, diabetic patients exhibited an onset of action at 2.5 h, a peak at 11 h, and a total period of action of 25 h, more closely approximating values in normal subjects.

Commercial insulins are prepared in concentrations of 100 U/mL (U100), although higher concentrations can be obtained (e.g., U500). All animal insulins are purified so that proinsulin contamination is extremely low. Most patients are now treated with synthesized "human" insulin. The amino acid sequence is identical to that of the human hormone, and biologic activity appears to be equivalent. Complications of insulin therapy, such as insulin allergy, fat atrophy, and fat hypertrophy, are less common than with animal insulins but still occur.

Lente and NPH insulin are used in most conventional therapy and are roughly equivalent in biologic effects, although lente appears to be slightly more immunogenic and to mix less well with regular insulin than does NPH.

Self-Monitoring of Glucose Level For many years, the effectiveness of treatment for diabetes was followed by reviewing symptoms (such as frequency of nocturia) and measuring the glucose in urine by semiquantitative techniques. Since the renal threshold for glucose in normal persons is in the range of 10 to 11 mmol/L (180 to 200 mg/dL) plasma glucose and may increase with the appearance of renal disease, assessment of glycosuria is of little value. Most insulin-requiring patients now monitor control and alter therapy based on self-measurement of the capillary blood sugar. In addition to the fact that such measurements are necessary in all treatment schedules involving variable insulin dosage, the ability to assess the blood glucose as needed has other positive benefits. It gives the patient a sense of confidence and independence, has a reinforcing effect on therapeutic goals (e.g., the effect of dietary indiscretion can be immediately seen), serves to give early warning of incipient hypoglycemia, and allows verification of hypoglycemia when suggestive symptoms are present.

Although the blood glucose level can be estimated visually with the use of reagent strips, it is generally preferable to use an instrument for readings. This is so because it is difficult for many patients to extrapolate accurately between the color changes and because subjective wishes may influence the extrapolation. It is harder to ignore a number appearing in a machine. A variety of glucose analyzers are available. The cost of equipment is reasonable, and many insurance carriers reimburse for its purchase. The patient needs to have supervised training in the technique, and simultaneous checks of the blood sugar in a laboratory should be done periodically to test the accuracy of the self-analysis. Repeated studies show that patients can measure blood glucose accurately using these techniques.

Although urine testing for glucose is now rarely used to follow diabetes, the measurement of ketones in the urine remains important.

Goals of Therapy Intensive insulin therapy designed to keep the blood glucose level as near normal as possible has for many years been considered mandatory during pregnancy and after renal transplantation. Maintenance of a normal blood glucose level during pregnancy prevents fetal macrosomy, respiratory distress syndrome, and perinatal mortality. Prevention of congenital malformations probably requires that the blood glucose level be near normal at the time of conception, although one multicenter trial concluded that no relationship existed between control of diabetes and malformed fetuses. For maximal safety, however, intensive therapy should be started prior to conception, if at all possible. The issue of gestational diabetes, defined as carbohydrate intolerance first recognized in pregnancy, is controversial. Some authorities recommend screening of all women, while others test only those at high risk. Treatment is by diet, and insulin is rarely required.

The conclusion of the NIH-sponsored multicenter Diabetes Control and Complication Trial (DCCT) required broadening of the recommendation for intensive insulin therapy. This very large trial, involving more than 1400 patients with IDDM followed for 7 to 10 years, established that degenerative complications of diabetes are diminished by better control of the blood glucose level, although, as mentioned earlier, return of blood glucose level to normal was not achieved. Protection rates as high as 70 percent were seen in the case of retinopathy. It follows that many more patients and their physicians will desire intensive insulin therapy than has been the case in the past. To meet this demand will not necessarily be easy. It is clear from the DCCT that even with health care teams staffed with physicians, nutritionists, and experienced nurse-clinicians and with a dedicated group of participating volunteers, treatment goals were not met. Furthermore, there was a significant increase in the frequency and severity of hypoglycemia, so the therapy was not without risk. Patients with NIDDM were not studied. It thus remains to be seen whether the results of the DCCT can be applied widely under ordinary clinical circumstances.

If an experienced health care team familiar with both MSI and CSII is available and if the patient is physically, emotionally, intellectually, and financially able to undergo the rigors of intensive therapy, it should be tried. Intensive therapy should not be offered for patients under the age of 7 because of the danger of impairment of brain development by hypoglycemia. Older persons and those with comorbidity such as coronary artery disease or stroke should be excluded. Although subjects with NIDDM were not studied in the DCCT, it is likely that lowering the blood glucose level would be beneficial in the prevention of complications in these patients as well. Insulin resistance may prove a problem in NIDDM, especially if hyperinsulinemia proves to be a risk factor for atherosclerosis and hypertension, as some investigators believe. The treatment group in the DCCT also had significant weight gain, which likely will be a greater problem in NIDDM, since most patients are significantly overweight or obese. In short, persons with NIDDM should not be excluded, but considerable caution is required, especially in older persons with the disease.

Goals of therapy have not been defined. One set of standards for blood glucose is listed in Table 334-6. The "acceptable" category would apply in conventional therapy using a two-dose schedule of intermediate and regular insulin. The upper limit of 11.1 mmol/L (200 mg/dL) postprandially is arbitrary but is based on the finding in the Pima Indian population that complications of diabetes are rare if the 2-h value in the oral glucose tolerance test is less than 11.1 mmol/L. The "ideal" column represents values targeted in meticulous control regimens. Although some authors are more stringent and prefer the 1-h postprandial value to be no more than 7.8 mmol/L (140 mg/dL), the risk of hypoglycemia is greater under these circumstances. In general, avoidance of serious hypoglycemia is more important than avoidance of hyperglycemia, because the former has immediate consequences that may threaten the life of the patient or others (e.g., through an automobile accident), while the detrimental effects of hyperglycemia are long-term and less certain.

Hypoglycemia, the Somogyi Effect, and the Dawn Phenomenon (See also Chap. 335) The problem of hypoglycemia is common in insulin-dependent diabetics, particularly when aggressive efforts are made to keep both the fasting plasma glucose level and postprandial hyperglycemia within the normal range. Hypoglycemia may be caused by missing a meal or doing unexpected exercise but can occur in the absence of known precipitating events. Daytime episodes of hypoglycemia are usually recognized by autonomic symptoms, such as sweating, nervousness, tremor, and hunger. Hypoglycemia during sleep may produce no symptoms or cause night sweats, unpleasant dreams, and early-morning headache. In one study of insulin-dependent diabetic children monitored throughout 24 h, 18 percent had asymptomatic nocturnal hypoglycemia. If hypoglycemia is not aborted by counterregulatory hormone response or by ingestion of carbohydrate, central nervous system symptoms ensue: confusion, abnormal behavior, loss of consciousness, or convulsions.

Table 334-6

Goals for Blood Glucose Levels in the Control of Diabetes*

	Acceptable		Ideal	
Goal	mmol/L	mg/dL	mmol/L	mg/dL
Fasting	3.3–7.2	60–130	3.9–5.6	70–100
Preprandial	3.3–7.2	60–130	3.9–5.6	70–100
Postprandial (1 h)	<11.1	<200	<8.9	<160
3 A.M.	>3.6	>65	>3.6	>65

* Values for healthy patients below the age of 65. Goals may be shifted upward in older patients. *Acceptable* refers to goals for conventional therapy, while *ideal* indicates goals with intensive insulin therapy.

As blood glucose concentrations fall, protection against hypoglycemia is normally provided by two mechanisms: cessation of insulin release and mobilization of counterregulatory hormones. The latter increase hepatic glucose production and decrease glucose utilization in nonhepatic tissues. Glucagon is the primary counterregulatory hormone, while epinephrine and norepinephrine released from the adrenal medulla and the sympathetic nervous system serve as the major backup. Catecholamines are not required for maintenance of the blood glucose level, provided glucagon is available, but they become critical in the absence of glucagon. Cortisol and growth hormone do not function acutely but come into play with prolonged fasting or sustained hypoglycemia. Diabetic patients are vulnerable to hypoglycemia because of both insulin excess and counterregulatory failure. Since insulin is given by injection or infusion, the body does not have the capacity to decrease plasma concentrations of insulin as glucose levels fall. Very early on, patients with type 1 IDDM lose the capacity to increase glucagon release in response to hypoglycemia. Protection thus depends on epinephrine. Unfortunately, many patients subsequently also lose the capacity to release epinephrine and norepinephrine in response to hypoglycemia. Since the initial clinical signals of hypoglycemia are dependent on epinephrine (the other counterregulatory hormones are clinically silent), the loss of the catecholamine response results in the syndrome of *hypoglycemia unawareness*. This syndrome originally was thought to be due solely to autonomic neuropathy in patients with long-standing diabetes. It is now recognized that the syndrome may be *caused* by low blood glucose in the absence of neuropathy, with even a single episode of afternoon hypoglycemia having discernible effects the next day. Previous hypoglycemia does not prevent epinephrine release but lowers the level of glucose required to trigger the response. The end result is that potentially dangerous hypoglycemia is unrecognized, and the defense against hypoglycemia is impaired.

Both the hormonal defense against hypoglycemia and its warning symptoms are thought to originate in the hypothalamus. One explanation for the unawareness syndrome is an adaptive response to hypoglycemia that allows the brain to continue taking up a normal amount of glucose despite low glucose levels in the blood. Presumably, this effect is due to an increase in brain glucose transporter (GLUT 1) units. While there is evidence to support this concept in patients with IDDM, it would not explain the induction of next-day unawareness by a single episode of hypoglycemia. Hypoglycemia unawareness induced by hypoglycemia (as opposed to unawareness due to autonomic neuropathy) can be reversed by avoidance of hypoglycemia. Most patients with this syndrome are receiving intensive insulin therapy and have nearly normal hemoglobin A_{1c} levels. Relaxation of therapy sufficient to raise hemoglobin A_{1c} into the range of 7.0 to 7.5 percent is usually sufficient to restore warning signals in the absence of autonomic neuropathy.

An important question is whether hypoglycemic symptoms can occur in the absence of low plasma glucose levels. It was believed traditionally that counterregulatory hormone release and autonomic symptoms are not triggered until the plasma glucose level approaches 3 mmol/L (50 to 55 mg/dL). Careful studies in humans using auditory or visual evoked potentials as a measure of cortical function in the brain have shown that abnormalities can occur at a glucose level of 4 mmol/L (70 to 72 mg/dL). A drop in glucose level of only 0.5 mmol/L (10 mg/dL) resulted in a delay of the evoked potential and, with time, release of counterregulatory hormones. Thus, neuroglycopenic symptoms may occur in the presence of blood glucose levels not considered hypoglycemic.

From time to time, patients with diabetes report symptoms suggestive of catecholamine release in the presence of documented hyperglycemia. The cause is unknown, but possibilities include simple anxiety, insulin-induced vascular permeability with a hypotensive response, and activation of the sympathetic nervous system by insulin-enhanced carbohydrate utilization. Patients with poorly controlled disease release counterregulatory hormones at higher concentrations of blood glucose than do normal subjects or patients with tightly controlled diabetes. Thus, insulin treatment affects the counterregulatory response in two ways. With intensive therapy and tight control, especially with intermittent hypoglycemia, epinephrine release is impaired, and hypoglycemia unawareness may ensue. When control is less rigorous or is poor, symptoms of hypoglycemia may occur in the presence of normal blood glucose values, because of a shift upward in the counterregulatory glucose threshold.

Hypoglycemia can result from other mechanisms. Diabetic renal disease may be accompanied by diminished insulin requirements and may lead to frank hypoglycemia if adjustments in dosage are not made. The mechanism is not known. Although half-times for insulin in plasma are increased in such patients, other factors doubtless play a role. The impairment of gluconeogenesis by uremia may play a role.

Hypoglycemia may be due to the development of autoimmune adrenal insufficiency as part of polyglandular autoimmune deficiency (see Chap. 340), which is more frequent in persons with diabetes than in the population as a whole. Hypoglycemia can develop in association with high levels of circulating insulin antibodies. The exact mechanism is not known, but one possibility is dissociation of insulin from the antibody during the overnight fast. Occasionally, an insulinoma may develop in a diabetic patient. Very rarely, permanent remission of apparently typical diabetes occurs. The reason is not known, but the initial sign may be frequent hypoglycemia in a patient with previously well-controlled disease.

It must be emphasized that hypoglycemic attacks are dangerous and, if frequent, portend a serious or even fatal outcome. If the patient is conscious, sugar, candy, or a sugar-containing beverage can be given. If the patient is unarousable or unconscious, intravenous glucose is required. Patients should have a vial of glucagon available as well. If access to medical care is delayed, administration of 1 mg glucagon intramuscularly frequently aborts the attack.

The *Somogyi phenomenon* refers to rebound hyperglycemia following an episode of hypoglycemia due to counterregulatory hormone release. It should be suspected whenever wide swings in the plasma glucose occur over short time intervals, even if symptoms are not reported. Such rapid changes contrast with the changes after insulin withdrawal in previously well-controlled diabetic patients, in whom hyperglycemia and ketosis develop gradually and smoothly over a 12- to 24-h period. Excessive hunger and weight gain in the context of worsening hyperglycemia are clues that the insulin dosage may be too high, since poor control due to underinsulinization usually results in weight loss (because of osmotic diuresis and glucose wastage). If the Somogyi phenomenon is suspected, the insulin dose should be decreased as a trial, even when specific symptoms of overinsulinization are absent. The Somogyi phenomenon is probably rare in adults but may be more frequent in children.

The *dawn phenomenon* refers to an early morning rise in plasma glucose requiring increased amounts of insulin to maintain euglycemia. Although similar early morning hyperglycemia may result from hypoglycemia, as just described, the dawn phenomenon itself is thought to be independent of the Somogyi mechanism. The nocturnal surge of growth hormone release may be a factor. Increased clearance of insulin also occurs in the early morning hours, but the changes are probably not of major importance. Usually, the dawn phenomenon can be differentiated from posthypoglycemic hyperglycemia by measuring the blood glucose at 3 A.M. It is important to make this distinction, because the Somogyi phenomenon is avoided by decreasing insulin dosages for the critical time period, while the dawn phenomenon usually requires increased insulin to maintain glucose in the normal range.

Oral Agents NIDDM that cannot be controlled by dietary management often responds to sulfonylureas. The drugs are easy to use and appear to be safe. Nevertheless, use of oral agents has decreased in response to the emphasis on better control as a means of slowing the development of late complications. These drugs can bring plasma glucose back to normal in some patients with relatively mild disease, but in patients with significant hyperglycemia, plasma glucose tends to improve but not to approach the normal range in response to these agents. Thus, a high percentage of patients with NIDDM are now treated with insulin.

Sulfonylureas act primarily by stimulating release of insulin from the beta cell. The cDNA for the sulfonylurea receptor has been cloned and appears to be a subunit of the K_{ATP} channel that controls membrane potential in the beta cell. Binding of sulfonylureas to the receptor causes the channel to close and causes depolarization, calcium influx, and insulin secretion. Extrapancreatic actions of sulfonylureas include increasing the number of insulin receptors and enhancing the insulin-mediated glucose transport independent of increased insulin binding. The extrapancreatic effects are probably physiologically unimportant. Mean levels of plasma insulin do not increase following treatment with sulfonylureas, despite significantly improved mean plasma glucose concentrations. The paradox of improved glucose metabolism in the absence of higher steady state levels of insulin is explained by the fact that elevation of plasma glucose to pretreatment values results in a rise of plasma insulin to levels higher than those seen before treatment. Thus, the initial action of the drugs is to increase insulin release with lowering of the blood glucose level. As glucose levels fall, insulin levels also decrease, since blood glucose is the major stimulus to insulin release, thereby masking the initial stimulation of insulin secretion. The insulinogenic effect can then be unmasked by raising the blood glucose. The fact that sulfonylureas are ineffective in IDDM, where beta cell mass is diminished, supports the idea that the pancreatic effect is primary, although, as noted, extrapancreatic mechanisms may play a minor role.

Second-generation drugs, such as glipizide and glyburide, are effective in smaller doses but otherwise differ little from agents in long use, such as chlorpropamide and tolbutamide. First-generation agents are now infrequently prescribed, although in generic form they are less expensive. In patients with significant renal disease, it is preferable to use tolbutamide or tolazamide, since these agents are metabolized and inactivated exclusively by the liver. Chlorpropamide has the capacity to sensitize the renal tubule to antidiuretic hormone. It thus is helpful in some patients with partial diabetes insipidus but may cause water retention in patients with diabetes mellitus. Hypoglycemia occurs less often with oral agents than with insulin, but, when it occurs, it tends to be severe and prolonged. Some patients have required massive glucose infusions for days following the last dose of sulfonylurea. For this reason, hospitalization is mandatory in patients with sulfonylurea-induced hypoglycemia.

Metformin, a biguanide useful in NIDDM patients who are not responsive to diet and exercise, may be prescribed as monotherapy in obese diabetics but is usually added as an adjunctive agent in patients whose disease is not controlled by maximal doses of sulfonylureas (Table 334-7). The primary action of metformin is thought to be inhibition of hepatic gluconeogenesis, and it also may enhance glucose disposal in muscle and adipose tissue. In contrast to sulfonylureas, metformin does not cause hypoglycemia. Metformin can cause lactic acidosis, like the earlier biguanides, although it does so much less frequently. To avoid this complication, the drug should not be given to patients with renal disease. It should be stopped at once if nausea, vomiting, diarrhea, or intercurrent illness appears.

Thiazolidinedione derivatives such as troglitazone (Table 334-7) lower the blood levels of glucose, free fatty acids, and triglycerides and appears to reduce insulin resistance, possibly by increasing the activity of insulin receptor kinase. Troglitazone is approved for use

Table 334-7

Oral Hypoglycemic Agents

Agent	Daily Dose, mg	Doses per Day	Duration of Action, h
Sulfonylureas			
Acetohexamide	250–1500	1–2	12–18
Chlorpropamide	100–500	1–2	60
Tolazamide	100–1000	1–2	12–14
Tolbutamide	500–3000	2–3	6–12
Glimeripiride	4	1	Up to 24
Glyburide	1.25–20	1–2	Up to 24
Glipizide	2.5–40	1–2	Up to 24
Glibornuride	12.5–100	1–2	Up to 24
Biguanide			
Metformin	1500–2500	1–2	Up to 24
Thiazolidinedione			
Troglitazone	400–600	1	Up to 24

in obese patients with NIDDM who are poorly controlled on insulin and has been given by some physicians as an add-on agent in NIDDM patients who are on maximal doses of other oral agents.

Two peptides are under evaluation as adjunct treatments for NIDDM. Both insulin-like growth factor 1 (IGF-1, somatomedin C) and glucagon-like peptide 1 (GLP-1), a peptide derived from the proglucagon molecule, lower blood glucose levels in normal subjects and in patients with diabetes. GLP-1 (7-36) and (7-37) amides are the lead agents under trial. Their usefulness is not established.

Monitoring the Control of Diabetes As mentioned earlier, patients on intensive insulin therapy who keep accurate records of capillary blood glucose levels can easily monitor the adequacy of control of their disease and detect changing trends. It is also standard practice to measure hemoglobin A_{1c} levels quarterly in all patients. This step is particularly important in patients who do not measure glucose values frequently at home. Hemoglobin A_{1c} is an electrophoretically fast-moving hemoglobin component that is present in normal persons and increases in amount in the presence of hyperglycemia. It is formed by the nonenzymatic glycation of the amino acids valine and lysine on the beta chain of hemoglobin A. Some laboratories also report the level of total glycated hemoglobin. However, this quantity includes the level of the reversible Schiff base, which can change rapidly with alterations in blood glucose. Only hemoglobin A_{1c}, which is irreversibly glycated and thus stable, should be used for the assessment of glucose control. When properly assayed, the level of glycated hemoglobin gives an estimate of diabetic control for the preceding 3-month period. Normal values must be established for each laboratory; on average, nondiabetic subjects have hemoglobin A_{1c} values of less than 6 percent, while levels in patients with poorly controlled diabetes may be considerably above 10 percent. Measurement of glycated hemoglobin gives an objective assessment of metabolic control. Discrepancies between reported plasma glucose values and hemoglobin A_{1c} concentrations suggest that either the measurement or the reporting of the former is not accurate.

ACUTE METABOLIC COMPLICATIONS In addition to hypoglycemia, patients with diabetes are susceptible to two major acute metabolic complications: diabetic ketoacidosis and hyperosmolar, nonketotic coma. The former is a complication of IDDM, while the latter usually occurs in the setting of NIDDM. Ketoacidosis is rare in true NIDDM, although it can occur in that setting.

Diabetic Ketoacidosis Diabetic ketoacidosis appears to require insulin deficiency coupled with a relative or absolute increase in glucagon concentration. It is often caused by cessation of insulin intake, but it may result from physical (e.g., infection, surgery) or emotional stress despite continued insulin therapy. In the former case, the concentration of glucagon rises secondary to insulin withdrawal, while in stress, the stimulus for glucagon release is probably epinephrine. In addition to stimulating glucagon secretion, epinephrine presumably blocks the release of the small amount of residual insulin present in some subjects with IDDM and inhibits insulin-induced glucose transport in peripheral tissues. These hormonal changes have two critical effects: (1) They induce maximal gluconeogenesis and impair peripheral utilization of glucose, causing severe hyperglycemia. Glucagon facilitates gluconeogenesis by inducing a fall in fructose-2,6-bisphosphate, an intermediate that stimulates glycolysis and blocks gluconeogenesis. When fructose-2,6-bisphosphate levels fall, glycolysis is inhibited and gluconeogenesis is enhanced. The resulting hyperglycemia induces an osmotic diuresis that leads to the volume depletion and dehydration that characterize the ketoacidotic state. (2) They activate the ketogenic process and thus initiate the development of metabolic acidosis. For ketosis to occur, changes must be produced in both adipose tissue and the liver. Free fatty acids from adipose stores are the primary substrate for ketone body formation, and plasma levels of free fatty acids must rise if ketogenesis is to proceed at a high rate. However, fatty acids delivered to the liver are reesterified and stored as hepatic triglyceride or converted into VLDL and transported back into the circulation unless the hepatic oxidation of fatty acids is activated. While the release of free fatty acids is enhanced by insulin deficiency, accelerated fatty acid oxidation in the liver is induced primarily by glucagon, via its action on the carnitine palmitoyltransferase system of enzymes responsible for the transport of fatty acids into the mitochondria. When long-chain fatty acids reach the liver, they are first esterified to coenzyme A (CoA). The fatty acyl CoA cannot traverse the mitochondrial membranes until it is transesterified with carnitine. As shown in Fig. 334-3, carnitine palmitoyltransferase I transesterifies fatty acyl-CoA to fatty acylcarnitine, which then traverses the inner mitochondrial membrane via translocase. In the matrix the reverse reaction is then catalyzed by carnitine palmitoyltransferase II. In the fed state, carnitine palmitoyltransferase I is inactive, and, as a consequence, long-chain fatty acids cannot reach the β-oxidative

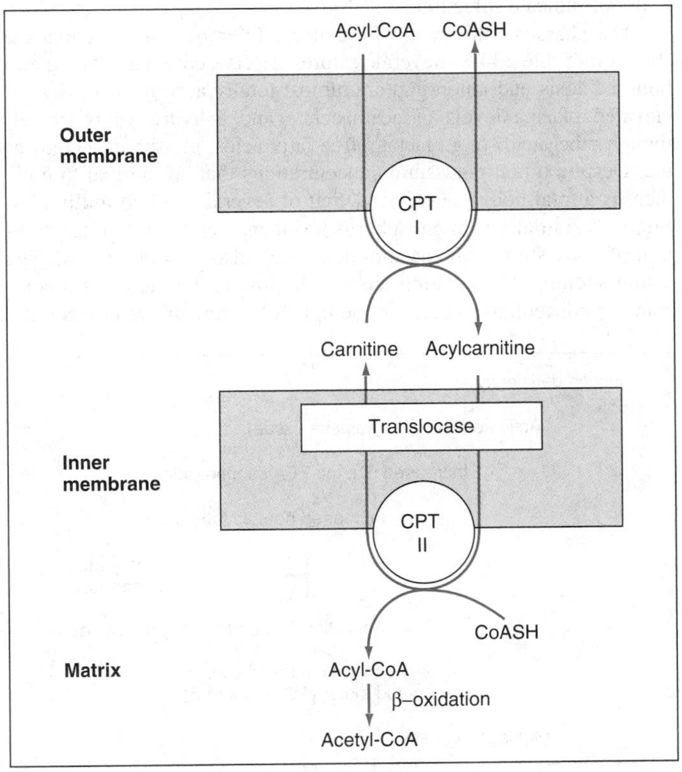

FIGURE 334-3 The carnitine palmitoyltransferase system. Long-chain fatty acyl-CoA molecules require transesterification to carnitine to traverse the inner mitochondrial membrane. Once across, the transesterification is reversed, and the fatty acyl-CoA is oxidized to either ketone bodies (liver) or CO_2 and water with the generation of ATP (nonhepatic tissues). CPT 1 is the rate-limiting step, controlled by malonyl-CoA levels in tissue. CPT 1, carnitine palmitoyltransferase 1; CPT II, carnitine palmitoyltransferase II.

enzymes for ketone body production. During starvation or uncontrolled diabetes, the system is activated; under these circumstances, the rate of ketogenesis is a first-order function of the concentration of fatty acids reaching carnitine palmitoyltransferase I.

Glucagon (or a change in the glucagon/insulin ratio) activates the transport system in two ways. First, it causes a rapid fall in hepatic malonyl-CoA content by interrupting the sequence glucose-6-phosphate → pyruvate → citrate → acetyl-CoA → malonyl-CoA by means of the previously mentioned decrease in fructose-2,6-bisphosphate. Glucagon also inhibits acetyl-CoA carboxylase, the enzyme that converts acetyl-CoA to malonyl-CoA. Malonyl-CoA, the first committed intermediate in the synthesis of fatty acids from glucose, is a competitive inhibitor of carnitine palmitoyltransferase I, and a fall in its concentration activates the enzyme. Second, glucagon causes a rise in hepatic carnitine concentration, which then drives the reaction toward fatty acylcarnitine formation by mass action. These events are summarized schematically in Fig. 334-4. At high plasma fatty acid concentrations, hepatic uptake of fatty acids is sufficient to saturate both oxidative and esterifying pathways, resulting in fatty liver, hypertriglyceridemia, and ketoacidosis. Overproduction of ketones by the liver is the primary event in ketotic states, but peripheral utilization is impaired at high levels of acetoacetate and β-hydroxybutyrate.

Clinically, ketoacidosis begins with anorexia, nausea, and vomiting, coupled with an increased rate of urine formation. Abdominal pain may be present. If the condition is not treated, altered consciousness or frank coma may occur. The initial examination usually shows Kussmaul respiration together with signs of volume depletion. Rarely, the latter is sufficient to cause vascular collapse and renal shutdown. Body temperature is normal or below normal in uncomplicated ketoacidosis; therefore, fever suggests the presence of infection. Leukocytosis, frequently very marked, is a feature of diabetic acidosis per se and may not indicate infection.

The characteristic metabolic abnormalities of diabetic coma are shown in Table 334-8. Several features deserve comment. The metabolic acidosis and anion gap are almost totally accounted for by the elevated plasma levels of acetoacetate and β-hydroxybutyrate, although other acids (e.g., lactate, free fatty acids, phosphates) contribute. Despite initial potassium concentrations that are normal to high, there is a total-body potassium deficit of several hundred millimoles. Similarly, initial serum phosphorus levels may be high despite depletion of body stores. Magnesium deficiency also may be present. The serum sodium concentration tends to be low in the face of a modest osmolar concentration because the hyperglycemia draws intracellular

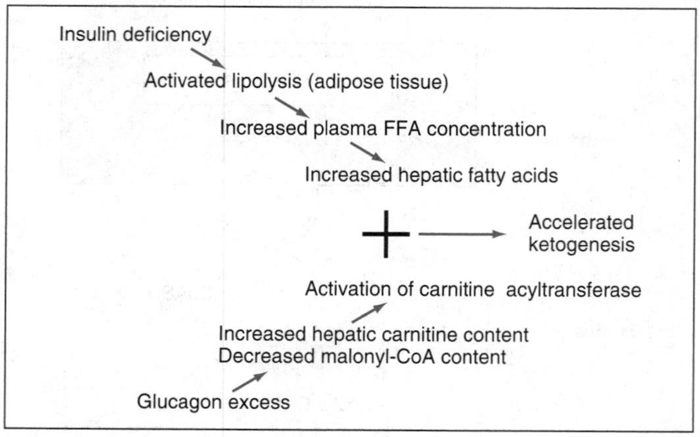

FIGURE 334-4 The regulation of ketogenesis. Significant production of acetoacetate and β-hydroxybutyrate by the liver requires provision of adequate free fatty acid substrate and activation of fatty acid oxidation. Lipolysis is increased primarily by insulin deficiency, while the fatty acid oxidative sequence is activated primarily by glucagon. The immediate signal for oxidation is a fall in malonyl-CoA content. *(After JD McGarry, DW Foster, Am J Med 61:9, 1976.)*

Table 334-8

Initial Laboratory Findings in Diabetic Ketoacidosis

Series:	Dallas*	Los Angeles†	Washington‡
Age, years:	38	36	43
Glucose, mmol/L (mg/dL)	26(475)	37(675)	41(733)
Sodium, mmol/L	132	131	132
Potassium, mmol/L	4.8	5.3	6.0
Bicarbonate, mmol/L	<10	6	10
BUN, mmol/L (mg/dL)	9(25)	11(32)	15(42)
Acetoacetate, mmol/L	4.8	—	—
β-Hydroxybutyrate, mmol/L	13.7	—	—
Free fatty acids, mmol/L	2.1	—	2.3
Lactate, mmol/L	4.6	—	—
Osmolality, mosmol/L	310	323	331

* Eighty-eight consecutive episodes of ketoacidosis at Parkland Memorial Hospital (DW Foster, unpublished observations).
† Mean data from 308 episodes of nonfatal ketoacidosis (PM Beigelman, Diabetes 20:490, 1971).
‡ Mean data from 10 episodes of ketoacidosis (JE Gerich et al, Diabetes 20:228, 1971).

water into the plasma space. A very low serum sodium level (e.g., 110 mmol/L) suggests vomiting with water drinking, or else pseudohyponatremia due to severe hypertriglyceridemia if the assays were done in autoanalyzers that do not remove fat prior to assay. Hypertriglyceridemia is common in ketoacidosis and is due both to impaired activity of lipoprotein lipase (a disposal defect) and to hepatic overproduction of VLDL. If a fatty meal has been ingested prior to the onset of ketoacidosis, chylomicrons may make up a major portion of the circulating fat. Hyperlipidemia is usually visible if the triglyceride concentration is above 4.5 mmol/L (400 mg/dL). Prerenal azotemia, reflecting volume depletion, is usually modest in degree and reverses with treatment. The serum amylase level may be elevated, and frank pancreatitis can occur.

The diagnosis of ketoacidosis in a patient known to have insulin-dependent diabetes is not difficult. Its appearance in a patient not known to be diabetic requires differentiation from the other common causes of metabolic acidosis with an anion gap: lactic acidosis, uremia, alcoholic ketoacidosis, and certain poisonings. The first step is to test the urine for glucose and ketones. If the urine is negative for ketones, another cause for the acidosis is likely. If it is positive, plasma examination is required to be certain that something more than starvation ketosis is present. Since quantitative assays of acetoacetate and β-hydroxybutyrate are not routinely available, semiquantitative tests must be done using ketone reagent strips. Serial dilutions of plasma can be made and tested. Undiluted plasma may give a strongly positive result when starvation alone is the problem; a strong reaction at a dilution exceeding 1:1 is presumptive evidence for ketoacidosis. Apart from diabetes, the only other common ketoacidotic state is alcoholic ketoacidosis. This syndrome, which by definition occurs in chronic alcoholics, usually follows a binge, but the patient may not have had alcohol for 24 h or longer. It never occurs in the absence of starvation and frequently is associated with severe vomiting and abdominal pain. Pancreatitis is present in up to 75 percent of patients. A plasma glucose level of less than 8.3 mmol/L (150 mg/dL) was found in three-fourths of cases in one series, and in 15 percent the level was less than 2.8 mmol/L (50 mg/dL) on arrival at the hospital. Hyperglycemia may occur but is usually mild and rarely, if ever, exceeds 17 mmol/L (300 mg/dL). Plasma free fatty acid concentrations are higher (mean, 2.9 mmol/L) than in normal starvation (range, 0.7 to 1.0 mmol/L), reaching levels seen in diabetic ketoacidosis. Presumably, the liver is activated for ketogenesis by starvation in these patients and is driven to maximal rates of ketone formation by the high fatty acid levels. Why some alcoholics mobilize fatty acids excessively is not known. In contrast to diabetic acidosis, the syndrome is rapidly reversed by the intravenous administration of glucose. As in all alcoholics given glucose, thiamine should be supplied to avoid precipitation of acute beriberi. (Other water-soluble vitamins, although not as critical, also should be infused.) Insulin is required only if hyperglycemia persists during therapy. True ketoacidosis can develop with fasting during the third trimester of pregnancy and in nursing mothers who do not eat, but the complication is rare.

Diabetic ketoacidosis cannot be reversed without insulin. For decades, 50 or more units of insulin was given per hour until ketosis was reversed, but now most patients are treated by "low-dose" insulin schedules in which 8 to 10 units of insulin are infused intravenously each hour. Most cases of diabetic acidosis can be reversed adequately with low-dose treatment, but some patients do not respond. Presumably, the insulin resistance that is characteristic of diabetic ketoacidosis is more pronounced in these patients than in responsive subjects. The problem is that resistant subjects cannot be identified prospectively. For this reason, it is probably preferable to give 25 to 50 units of insulin as an initial intravenous bolus, followed by an infusion of 15 to 25 units an hour until ketoacidosis is reversed. There are no known toxic effects of larger insulin doses, since the maximal physiologic response is obtained once the insulin receptors are saturated, regardless of how much insulin is given. The advantage of the higher dosage schedule is that it ensures saturation of the receptors in the face of competing antibodies or other resistance factors. High concentrations of insulin probably accelerate the reversal of ketoacidosis by acting via the IGF-1 receptor. Hormonal interaction with this receptor can lower the blood glucose level by a mechanism independent of the insulin receptor. Diabetic ketosis has been reversed by IGF-1 therapy in a patient with severe insulin resistance. If physicians choose to use the low-dose insulin schedule, they should be alert to the possibility of resistance. Should acidosis persist unabated after several hours of treatment, larger amounts of insulin are clearly indicated. Ketoacidosis also can be treated adequately with intramuscular (but not subcutaneous) insulin.

Therapy of ketoacidosis also requires intravenous fluids. The usual fluid deficit is 3 to 5 L, and both salt solutions and free water are needed. Between 1 and 2 L of isotonic saline or Ringer's lactate should be given rapidly intravenously on arrival, with additional amounts determined by urine output and clinical assessment of the fluid state. When the plasma glucose level falls to about 17 mmol/L (300 mg/dL), 5% glucose solutions should be added, both as a source of free water and as a prophylactic measure to prevent the late cerebral edema syndrome. The latter is a rare complication of ketoacidosis, occurring most often in children. It is suspected when the patient remains comatose or lapses into coma following reversal of acidosis.

Potassium replacement is always necessary, but the time of administration will vary. The initial potassium level is often high despite a total-body deficit because of the severe acidosis. In this case, the cation will ordinarily not be needed until 3 to 4 h after initiation of therapy, when reversal of acidosis and the action of insulin cause a shift of K^+ into intracellular water. On the other hand, if the admission value is normal or low, potassium should be given early, since plasma concentrations fall rapidly during therapy, predisposing the patient to cardiac arrhythmias or paralysis of the respiratory muscles. If the potassium is very low, insulin should be withheld for 60 to 90 min until 40 to 50 mmol of potassium can be given. In view of the phosphate depletion of ketoacidosis, potassium may be administered initially as the phosphate salt rather than as potassium chloride.

Bicarbonate therapy may be indicated in severely acidotic patients (pH 7.0 or below), especially if hypotension is present (acidosis itself can cause vascular collapse). It is not used routinely in less acutely ill subjects because rapid alkalinization may have detrimental effects on oxygen delivery to tissues. The hemoglobin-oxygen dissociation curve is normal in diabetic ketoacidosis because of the opposing effects of acidosis and deficiency of red blood cell 2,3-bisphosphoglycerate (2,3-BPG). If the acidosis is rapidly reversed, the deficiency of 2,3-BPG becomes manifest, increasing the avidity with which hemoglobin binds oxygen and impairing the release of oxygen in peripheral tissues. In a volume-depleted patient with poor tissue perfusion, such a change theoretically could predispose to the development of lactic acidosis. It is also thought that bicarbonate may impair left ventricular function through paradoxical acidification due to more rapid entry of CO_2 than bicarbonate into intracellular water. If bicarbonate is given, the infusion should be stopped when the pH reaches 7.2 to minimize possible detrimental side effects and to prevent metabolic alkalosis as circulating ketones are metabolized to bicarbonate with reversal of ketoacidosis.

Two points about following the response to treatment should be emphasized. (1) The plasma glucose level invariably falls more rapidly than the plasma ketone level. Insulin administration should not be stopped because glucose concentrations approach normal; rather, as mentioned, glucose should be infused and insulin continued until the ketosis has cleared. (2) Plasma ketone values are not very helpful in assessing clinical response. The testing materials measure acetoacetate and acetone but not β-hydroxybutyrate. Since β-hydroxybutyrate must be oxidized to acetoacetate prior to utilization, it is characteristic for the level of the plasma ketones measured by reagent strip to remain stable or even rise early in therapy at a time when total ketone concentration (acetoacetate plus β-hydroxybutyrate) is falling. Because β-hydroxybutyrate and acetoacetate represent a redox couple in equilibrium with mitochondrial NADH/NAD concentrations, vascular collapse or severe hypoxia may mask the presence of ketoacidosis because acetoacetate is reduced to β-hydroxybutyrate. Under these circumstances, the β-hydroxybutyrate/acetoacetate ratio, normally about 3:1, may reach 7:1 or 8:1. Paradoxically, in such a situation ketosis may seem to worsen as the patient gets better because of conversion of β-hydroxybutyrate to acetoacetate when the circulation is reestablished and tissue oxygenation is restored. The key parameters to follow are the pH and the calculated anion gap, since these give a more accurate assessment of response. The usual picture is for the pH to rise and the anion gap to narrow even though the plasma bicarbonate level remains low. The persistently low bicarbonate level is the consequence of hyperchloremia, which develops because of rapid infusion of sodium chloride, the loss of potential bicarbonate from the body in urine as ketones, and exchanges with intracellular buffers. Some patients demonstrate a persistent anion gap despite clinical improvement and a rising pH. Presumably, the unmeasured anion derives from tissue buffers. An anion gap that remains elevated and a pH that is persistently low indicate insulin resistance and mandate an aggressive increase in the amount of insulin administered. On the other hand, persistence of the anion gap does not indicate resistance when accompanied by clinical improvement, a rising pH, and clearing of urine ketones.

All patients should be followed with a flow sheet outlining amounts and timing of insulin and fluids together with a record of vital signs, urine volume, and blood chemistries. Without such a record, therapy tends to become chaotic.

Most patients with diabetic ketoacidosis recover when properly treated. While the mortality rate in large series is reported to be around 10 percent, most deaths result from late complications of ketoacidosis rather than from ketoacidosis itself. The major causes are myocardial infarction and infection, particularly pneumonia. Poor prognostic signs on admission include hypotension, azotemia, deep coma, and associated illness. In children, cerebral edema is a common cause of death (less frequent in adults). The cause of the brain swelling is not known. Theories include osmotic disequilibrium between brain and plasma as glucose is rapidly lowered, decreased plasma oncotic pressure due to infusion of large amounts of saline, and insulin-induced ion flux across the blood-brain barrier. Whatever the mechanism, mortality rates are high. Diagnosis is usually made by computed tomography. Treatment involves the bolus infusion of 1 g mannitol per kilogram of body weight in the form of a 20% solution. Although of questionable benefit, dexamethasone is also usually given: 12 mg initially, then 4 mg every 6 h. If there is no response, an anesthesiologist or pulmonary specialist should induce hyperventilation to an arterial P_{CO_2} of about 28 mmHg.

Other acute complications of ketoacidosis include vascular thrombosis and the adult respiratory distress syndrome. The former is induced by volume depletion, hyperosmolality, increased viscosity of blood, and changes in clotting factors favoring thrombosis. The cause of the pulmonary lesion is not known; it is probably not related to the metabolic acidosis, since respiratory distress syndrome occurs in hyperosmolar coma as well. Acute gastric dilation is another rare complication. An unusual infection associated with ketoacidosis is mucormycosis (see below). Table 334-9 summarizes the complications of diabetic ketoacidosis and their treatment.

Hyperosmolar Coma Hyperosmolar, nonketotic diabetic coma is usually a complication of NIDDM. It is a syndrome of profound dehydration resulting from a sustained hyperglycemic diuresis under circumstances in which the patient is unable to drink enough water to keep up with urinary fluid losses. Commonly, an elderly diabetic patient—often living alone or in a nursing home—develops a stroke or infection that worsens hyperglycemia and prevents adequate water intake. The full-blown syndrome probably does not occur until volume depletion is severe enough to decrease urine output. Hyperosmolar coma also can be precipitated by peritoneal dialysis or hemodialysis, tube feeding of high-protein formulas, high-carbohydrate infusion loads, and the use of osmotic agents such as mannitol and urea. Phenytoin, glucocorticoids, immunosuppressive agents, and diuretics also have been reported to initiate the disorder.

The absence of ketoacidosis is important in the pathophysiology of this condition. When ketoacidosis develops, nausea, vomiting, and air hunger bring the patient to the physician before extreme dehydration can occur. Such a protective mechanism is not operative in ketoacidosis-resistant, maturity-onset diabetes. Interestingly, hyperosmolar coma can occur in insulin-dependent diabetic patients who are given enough insulin to prevent ketosis but not enough to control hyperglycemia. Although it is unusual, the same person may present on one occasion with ketoacidosis and on the next with hyperosmolar coma.

The reason for the absence of ketoacidosis in maturity-onset diabetes is not known. The hepatic ketogenic machinery is not impaired, since the patients frequently have ketone concentrations in the starvation range (2 to 4 mmol/L). Free fatty acid levels are lower in hyperosmolar coma than in ketoacidosis, and substrate deficiency may limit ketone formation. However, some patients with hyperosmolar coma have high levels of free fatty acids in plasma. A more likely explanation is that insulin levels in the portal vein in NIDDM are higher than those of insulin-dependent subjects and prevent full activation of the hepatic carnitine palmitoyltransferase system. Other possibilities include glucagon resistance, previously mentioned, and maintenance of high malonyl-CoA levels via increased Cori cycle activity. The *Cori cycle* consists in the conversion of circulating glucose to lactate by peripheral tissues and the return of lactate to the liver for gluconeogenesis.

Clinically, patients present with extreme hyperglycemia, hyperosmolality, volume depletion, and central nervous system signs ranging from a clouded sensorium to coma. Seizure activity—sometimes Jacksonian in type—is not unusual, and transient hemiplegia may be seen. Infections, particularly pneumonia and gram-negative sepsis, are common and indicate a grave prognosis. Pneumonia is often due to gram-negative organisms. A high index of suspicion for infection should be maintained, and the blood and spinal fluid should be cultured. Because of the extreme dehydration, plasma viscosity is high, and widespread in situ thrombosis has been found at postmortem. Bleeding, probably caused by disseminated intravascular coagulation, and acute pancreatitis may occur.

The laboratory findings in two large series are shown in Table 334-10. Plasma glucose is generally around 55 mmol/L (1000 mg/dL), about twice the value seen in ketoacidosis. The serum osmolality is high, but because of the hyperglycemia, the absolute serum sodium concentration is often not elevated.[2] Prerenal azotemia causes marked elevation of blood urea nitrogen (BUN) and creatinine. Metabolic acidosis is mild, plasma bicarbonate on average being about 20 mmol/L. The acidosis is due to a combination of starvation ketosis, retention of inorganic acids secondary to renal hypoperfusion, and elevation of plasma lactate, the latter due to volume depletion. If the bicarbonate level is less than 10 mmol/L and plasma ketones are not elevated, lactic acidosis is assumed to be present.

The mortality rate in hyperosmolar coma is high (>50 percent). As a consequence, immediate treatment is urgent. The most important measure is rapid administration of large amounts of intravenous fluids to reestablish the circulation and urine flow. The average fluid deficit is 10 to 11 L. While free water is ultimately needed, initial therapy should be with isotonic salt solutions, and 2 to 3 L should be given over the first 1 to 2 h. Subsequently, half-strength saline can be used. As the glucose level approaches normal, 5% dextrose can be given as a vehicle for free water. While hyperosmolar coma may be reversed by fluids alone, insulin should be given to control the hyperglycemia more rapidly. Many authors recommend small doses of insulin, but larger amounts may be necessary, particularly in the obese patient. Potassium salts are usually required earlier in the treatment of hyperosmolar coma than in ketoacidosis because the intracellular shift of plasma K^+ during therapy is accelerated in the absence of acidosis. If lactic acidosis is present, sodium bicarbonate should be given until tissue perfusion can be reestablished. Antibiotics are required if infection is present.

LATE COMPLICATIONS OF DIABETES The diabetic patient is susceptible to a series of complications that cause morbidity and premature mortality. While some patients never develop these problems and in others they begin early, on average, symptoms develop 15 to 20 years after the appearance of overt hyperglycemia. Rare patients have complications at the time of diagnosis. A given patient may experience several complications simultaneously, or a single problem may dominate the picture.

Circulatory Abnormalities Atherosclerosis is more extensive and occurs earlier than in the general population. The cause of this accelerated course is not known, although, as discussed below, nonenzymatic glycation of lipoproteins may be important. The atherosclerotic lesion appears to be initiated by oxidized low-density lipoprotein (LDL) (not by native LDL) in a complicated cascade that operates through the acetyl-LDL or scavenger receptor. Both HDL and antioxi-

Table 334-9

Clues to Complications in Diabetic Ketoacidosis

Complication	Clues
Acute gastric dilatation or erosive gastritis	Vomiting of blood or "coffee-ground" material
Cerebral edema	Obtundation or coma with or without neurologic signs, especially if occurring after initial improvement
Hyperkalemia	Cardiac arrest
Hypoglycemia	Adrenergic or neurologic signs; rebound ketosis
Hypokalemia	Cardiac arrhythmias
Infection	Fever
Insulin resistance	Unremitting acidosis after 4–6 h of adequate therapy
Myocardial infarction	Chest pain, appearance of heart failure; appearance of hypotension despite adequate fluids
Mucormycosis	Facial pain, bloody nasal discharge, blackened nasal turbinates, blurred vision, proptosis
Respiratory distress syndrome	Hypoxemia in the absence of pneumonia, chronic pulmonary disease, or heart failure
Vascular thrombosis	Strokelike picture or signs of ischemia in nonnervous tissue

SOURCE: Adapted from DW Foster, in *Current Therapy in Endocrinology and Metabolism 1985–1986*, DT Krieger, CW Bardin (eds), Toronto/Philadelphia, Decker, 1985.

[2] Serum osmolality can be estimated from the following formula: Serum osmolality (mosmol/L) = $2([Na^+] + [K^+])$ + [glucose] (mmol/L) + BUN (mmol/L). Glucose and blood urea nitrogen (BUN) values in conventional units can be converted to mmol/L by dividing concentrations in milligrams per deciliter by 18 and 2.4, respectively. In practice, the contribution of the BUN is often ignored, since it contributes to total osmolality but does not reflect the free-water deficit. Situations in which an increased osmolality is not equivalent to dehydration include severe alcohol intoxication, the ethanol itself providing the unmeasured osmolyte.

Table 334-10

Initial Laboratory Findings in Hyperosmolar Coma

Series:	Brooklyn*	Washington†
Age, years:	60	57
Glucose, mmol/L (mg/dL)	65(1166)	54(976)
Sodium, mmol/L	144	142
Potassium, mmol/L	5	5
Chloride, mmol/L	99	98
Bicarbonate, mmol/L	17	22
BUN, mmol/L (mg/dL)	31(87)	23(65)
Creatinine, mmol/L (mg/dL)	490(5.5)	—
Free fatty acids, mmol/L	0.73	0.96
Osmolarity, mosmol/L	384	374

* Mean data from 33 episodes of hyperosmolar coma (AA Arieff, HJ Carroll, Medicine 51:73, 1972).
† Mean data from 20 episodes of hyperosmolar coma (JE Gerich et al, Diabetes 20:228, 1971).

dants have the capacity to impair LDL oxidation, thereby exerting an antiatherogenic action. In experimental animals, diabetes accelerates the oxidative process. Although lipoproteins are often in the normal range, HDL levels tend to be low, while LDL levels are high normal or high. A low HDL/LDL ratio favors atherosclerosis, presumably because reverse cholesterol transport out of arteries is impaired and because diminished antioxidant activity by the HDL-associated enzyme paraoxonase accelerates foam cell/plaque formation. Lipoprotein (a) levels are elevated in IDDM but not in NIDDM.

Other factors of potential importance are increased platelet adhesiveness, possibly due to enhanced thromboxane A_2 synthesis, and decreased prostacyclin synthesis. Hyperglycemia has been reported to increase secretion of endothelin-1 in vitro, and production of nitric oxide is diminished in aortas of diabetic rats and the coronary microvasculature of humans. Endothelin is a powerful vasoconstrictor and is mitogenic for vascular smooth muscle, while nitric oxide is a vasodilator, is antimitogenic in vascular smooth muscle, and inhibits platelet aggregation. Diabetes appears to be a procoagulant state with increased levels of tissue factor and deficiency of tissue factor pathway inhibitor type 1 playing major roles. Levels of factor VIII and von Willebrand factor are elevated. Fibrinolysis is impaired, probably due to elevated levels of tPA inhibitor, type 1.

Atherosclerosis produces symptoms in a variety of sites. Peripheral deposits may cause intermittent claudication, gangrene, and, in men, organic impotence on a vascular basis. Surgical repair of large-vessel lesions may be unsuccessful because of the simultaneous presence of widespread disease of the small vessels.

Coronary artery disease and stroke are common. Silent myocardial infarction occurs with increased frequency in diabetes and should be suspected whenever symptoms of left ventricular failure appear suddenly. Diabetes also may be associated with the clinical picture of cardiomyopathy, in which heart failure occurs in the face of apparently normal coronary arteries and in the absence of other identifiable causes of heart disease. As in nondiabetic subjects, smoking is a major risk for both coronary and peripheral vascular disease and should be avoided. Hypertension is a significant risk in many diabetic patients. An unusual ischemic lesion is focal infarction of muscle that causes painful lesions but not gangrene. This lesion may be confused with abscess.

Retinopathy Diabetic retinopathy is a leading cause of blindness in the United States. On the other hand, most diabetic patients never become blind. Retinopathic lesions are divided into two large categories, *simple* (background) and *proliferative* (Table 334-11). The earliest sign of retinal change is an increased capillary permeability that is evidenced by leakage of dye into the vitreous humor after fluorescein injection. Occlusion of retinal capillaries follows, with subsequent formation of saccular and fusiform aneurysms. Arteriovenous shunts also occur. The vascular lesions are accompanied by proliferation of lining endothelial cells and a loss of the pericytes that surround and support the vessels. Hemorrhages into the inner retinal areas are dot-shaped, while bleeding into the more superficial nerve fiber layer causes flame-shaped, blot-shaped, or linear lesions. Preretinal hemorrhages characteristically have a boat-shaped appearance. Exudates are of two types. Cotton-wool spots can be shown by angiography to be microinfarcts—nonperfused areas surrounded by a ring of dilated capillaries. A sudden increase in the number of cotton-wool spots is an ominous prognostic sign and may herald rapidly advancing retinopathy. Hard exudates are more common than cotton-wool spots and probably represent leakage of protein and lipids from damaged capillaries. Retinal edema due to the previously mentioned increase in vascular permeability is most often seen in the posterior pole of the eye, often in association with hard exudates. If the edema is in the macular region, visual acuity may be seriously and permanently impaired. Macular edema should be suspected when loss of visual acuity is not corrected by glasses, especially if posterior-pole exudates are seen. Edema is difficult to recognize without slit-lamp examination or stereoscopic fundal photographs. Consultation with a retinal surgeon should be sought early, since vision may be spared by laser therapy of the macular edema.

The fundamental characteristics of proliferative retinopathy are new vessel formation and scarring. The stimulus for neovascularization may be retinal hypoxia secondary to capillary or arteriolar occlusion. The primary angiogenic stimulus appears to be vascular endothelial growth factor (VEGF). Two serious complications of proliferative retinopathy are vitreal hemorrhage and retinal detachment. Either may cause a sudden loss of vision in one eye.

The frequency of diabetic retinopathy appears to vary with the age of onset as well as the duration of the disease. Approximately 85 percent of patients eventually develop the complication, but some never develop lesions even after 30 years of disease. Retinopathy appears to develop earlier in older patients, but proliferative retinopathy is less common. Some 10 to 18 percent of patients with simple retinopathy progress to proliferative disease in a 10-year period. About half of patients with proliferative disease progress to blindness within 5 years. Proliferative retinopathy appears to be more common in insulin-treated patients than in those not treated with insulin.

The treatment for diabetic retinopathy is photocoagulation. This treatment decreases the incidence of hemorrhage and scarring and is always indicated when new vessel formation occurs. Photocoagulation is also useful in treatment of microaneurysms, hemorrhages, and macular edema even if the proliferative stage has not begun. Panretinal photocoagulation is often used to diminish retinal demands for oxygen in the hope that the stimulus for neovascularization will be decreased. In this technique, several thousand lesions are produced over a 2-week period. Complications of photocoagulation are within the acceptable range. Some loss of peripheral vision is inevitable with extensive burns. Another surgical technique, pars plana vitrectomy, is used for treatment of nonresolving vitreal hemorrhage and retinal detachment. Postoperative complications are more frequent than with photocoagulation and include retinal tears, retinal detachment, cataracts, recurrent vitreal hemorrhage, glaucoma, infection, and loss of the eye. Hypophysectomy, once performed for diabetic retinopathy, is no longer recommended. There is hope that inhibition of angiogenesis by drugs such as the experimental heparin analogue beta-cyclodextrin tetradecasulfate

Table 334-11

Lesions of Diabetic Retinopathy

Background	Proliferative
Increased capillary permeability	New vessels
Capillary closure and dilatation	Scar (retinitis proliferans)
Microaneurysms	Vitreal hemorrhage
Arteriovenous shunts	Retinal detachment
Dilated veins	
Hemorrhages (dot and blot)	
Cotton-wool spots	
Hard exudates	

may prevent proliferative retinopathy. All patients with diabetic retinopathy should be followed by retinal specialists.

Diabetic Nephropathy Renal disease is a leading cause of death and disability in diabetes. About half of the cases of end-stage renal disease in the United States are now due to diabetic nephropathy. Approximately 35 percent of patients with IDDM develop this complication. The prevalence in NIDDM varies from 15 to 60 percent depending on ethnic background. Pima Indians have the highest rates, while Europeans have the lowest. Nephropathy, like other complications, is probably influenced by the genetic background of the patient. Some families with multiple diabetic members rarely have renal disease, while in others, more than 80 percent of persons at risk have nephropathy.

Diabetic nephropathy involves two distinct pathologic patterns, which may or may not coexist: diffuse and nodular. The former, which is more common, consists of widening of the glomerular basement membrane together with generalized mesangial thickening. In the nodular form, large accumulations of periodic acid–Schiff-positive material are deposited at the periphery of the glomerular tufts, the Kimmelstiel-Wilson lesion. In addition, there may be hyalinization of afferent and efferent arterioles, "drops" in Bowman's capsule, fibrin caps, and occlusion of glomeruli. Deposition of albumin and other proteins occurs in both glomeruli and tubules. The most specific lesions of diabetic glomerulosclerosis are hyalinization of afferent glomerular arterioles and the Kimmelstiel-Wilson nodules. Clinical renal dysfunction in diabetes does not correlate well with the histologic abnormalities.

Diabetic nephropathy may be functionally silent for long periods (10 to 15 years). At onset, the kidneys are usually enlarged and show "superfunction" (i.e., glomerular filtration rates may be 40 percent above normal). The next stage is the appearance of *microproteinuria* (microalbuminuria), the excretion of albumin in the range of 30 to 300 mg/d. Normal persons excrete less than 30 mg/d. Microalbuminuria is not detected by reagent sticks for urinary protein, which generally become positive only when proteinuria is greater than 550 mg/d, a degree of leakage termed *macroproteinuria*. Microalbuminuria appears to be due primarily to decreased concentration of anionic heparan sulfate–proteoglycan in the glomerular basement membrane. Since microalbuminuria is initially transient and can be induced by mechanisms other than diabetes, diagnosis requires an excretion rate of albumin greater than 30 mg/d in two of three samples collected in a 6-month period. Persistent leakage of protein greater than 50 mg/d is predictive of subsequent macroproteinuria. Interestingly, microalbuminuria also appears to predict cardiovascular mortality in diabetes. Once the macroproteinuric phase begins, there is a steady decline in renal function, with glomerular filtration rate falling, on average, by about 1 mL/min per month. A plot of the reciprocal of the serum creatinine level against time usually yields a straight line and allows prediction of the rate of deterioration. Ordinarily, azotemia begins about 12 years after diagnosis of diabetes. The nephrotic syndrome may occur prior to azotemia. Progression of renal disease is accelerated by hypertension.

There is no specific treatment for diabetic nephropathy. Meticulous control of diabetes can reverse microalbuminuria in some patients, and the progression of diabetic nephropathy may be slowed, as shown in the intensive treatment group of the DCCT. Hypertension must be treated aggressively whenever present. Angiotensin-converting enzyme inhibitors appear to slow progression of diabetic nephropathy. They should be used in hypertensive patients with diabetes and may have a role in normotensive subjects with microalbuminuria. Experimental studies in animals and humans indicate that low-protein diets may be useful. Once the azotemic phase is reached, treatment does not differ from that for other forms of renal failure. Chronic dialysis and renal transplantation are routine in patients with renal failure due to diabetes. Hyporeninemic hypoaldosteronism, which is associated with renal tubular acidosis, may require alkalinizing solutions (sodium bicarbonate or Shohl's solution) and avoidance of external potassium loads. Potassium tends to rise in parallel with hyperglycemia in the syndrome, since in the absence of aldosterone potassium loads must be disposed of intracellularly under the influence of insulin. Hyperglycemia, reflecting insulin deficiency, indicates impairment of the disposal pathway. Rarely, fludrocortisone may be required to control hyperkalemia.

Diabetic Neuropathy Diabetic neuropathy may affect every part of the nervous system, with the possible exception of the brain. While rarely a direct cause of death, neuropathy is a major cause of morbidity. Several distinct syndromes are recognized, and more than one type may be present in the same patient. The most common picture is that of *peripheral polyneuropathy*. Usually bilateral, the symptoms include numbness, paresthesias, severe hyperesthesias, and pain. The pain, which may be deep-seated and severe, is often worse at night. It is occasionally lancinating or lightning in type, resembling tabes dorsalis (pseudotabes). Fortunately, extreme pain syndromes are usually self-limited, lasting from a few months to a few years. Involvement of proprioceptive fibers leads to abnormalities of gait and development of typical Charcot joints, particularly in the feet. Loss of arch with multiple fractures of tarsal bones is a common finding by x-ray. On physical examination, absent stretch reflexes and loss of vibratory sense are early signs. Diabetic neuropathy also may cause delay in return of the ankle reflex identical to that seen in hypothyroidism. *Mononeuropathy*, though less common than polyneuropathy, also may occur. Characteristically, there is a sudden wrist drop, foot drop, or paralysis of the third, fourth, or sixth cranial nerves. Other single nerves, including the recurrent laryngeal, have been reported to be involved. Mononeuropathy is characterized by a high degree of spontaneous reversibility, usually over a several-week period. *Radiculopathy* is a sensory syndrome in which pain occurs over the distribution of one or more spinal nerves, usually in the chest wall or abdomen. The severe pain may mimic herpes zoster or an acute surgical abdomen. Like mononeuropathy, the lesion is usually self-limited. *Autonomic neuropathy* may present in a variety of ways. The gastrointestinal tract is a prime target, and there may be esophageal dysfunction with difficulty in swallowing, delayed gastric emptying, constipation, or diarrhea. The latter symptom is often nocturnal. Incompetence of the internal anal sphincter may mimic diabetic diarrhea. Orthostatic hypotension and frank syncope may occur. Cardiorespiratory arrest and sudden death, thought to be due solely to autonomic neuropathy, have been reported. Bladder dysfunction or paralysis is particularly distressing and often leads to the necessity of chronic catheter drainage. Impotence and retrograde ejaculation are additional manifestations in men. Erectile dysfunction is associated with a failure of nitric oxide generation in the penile vasculature. Deficiency of vasoactive intestinal polypeptide (VIP) may also be involved. Clues to autonomic neuropathy can be obtained by clinical tests such as measuring response of the heart rate to the Valsalva maneuver or standing. In both tests the subject has an electrocardiograph running for assessment of heart rate. In the former, the subject blows against an anaeroid or mercury manometer to 40 mmHg pressure for 15 s. The test is performed three times with a rest period of 1 min in between. Normally the heart rate speeds during Valsalva such that the ratio of the longest interval between beats after release to the shortest interval during the test is greater than 1.2. In autonomic neuropathy involving the parasympathetic system the ratio is less than 1.1. Similarly, the ratio at the thirtieth beat after standing relative to that at the fifteenth beat should be greater than 1.0. It is less than 1.0 in autonomic neuropathy. Diabetic *amyotrophy* is likely a form of neuropathy, although atrophy and weakness of the large muscles in the upper leg and pelvic girdle resemble primary muscle disease. Anorexia and depression may accompany amyotrophy. Because of the weight loss, such patients are often thought to have a paraneoplastic neuropathy.

Treatment of diabetic neuropathy is unsatisfactory in most respects. When pain is severe, it is easy for the patient to become habituated or addicted to narcotics or powerful nonnarcotic analgesics such as pentazocine. If the pain requires something stronger than aspirin, acetaminophen, or other nonsteroidal anti-inflammatory agents, codeine is the drug of choice. Phenytoin is used by some physicians, but others have not found it helpful. Combination therapy with amitriptyline and fluphenazine causes relief of pain in some patients and is worth trying. The recommended dosage is 75 mg amitriptyline at bedtime and 1 mg fluphenazine three times a day. Desipramine is as effective as amitriptyline; fluoxetine is no better than placebo. Mononeuropathies and radiculopathies usually require no specific therapy because they are self-limited. Diabetic diarrhea often responds to treatment with diphenoxylate and atropine or loperamide. Orthostatic hypotension is best treated by having the patient sleep with the head of the bed elevated, avoid sudden assumption of the upright position, and use full-length elastic stockings. Occasionally, volume expansion with fludrocortisone is required, as in other forms of orthostatic hypotension.

Experimental therapy with aldose reductase inhibitors and myoinositol has failed to provide significant clinical benefit, although enhanced regeneration of nerves has been reported in humans treated with an aldose reductase antagonist. Topical application of capsaicin is occasionally helpful with burning pain syndromes and hyperesthesia.

Diabetic Foot Ulcers A special problem in the diabetic patient is the development of ulcers of the feet and lower extremities. The ulcers appear to be due primarily to abnormal pressure distribution secondary to diabetic neuropathy. The problem is accentuated when there is bony distortion in the feet. Callus formation is usually the initial abnormality. Alternatively, the ulcer may be initiated by ill-fitting shoes that cause blister formation in patients whose sensory deficits preclude recognition of pain. Cuts and punctures from foreign bodies such as needles, tacks, and glass are common, and a foreign body of which the patient is unaware may be found in the soft tissue. For this reason, all patients with ulcers should have x-rays of the feet. Vascular disease with diminished blood supply contributes to development of ulcers, and infection is common, often with multiple organisms. While no specific therapy is available for diabetic ulcers, supportive treatment that minimizes weight bearing may make it possible to save the leg. One approach is simply to put the patient to bed, using hydrotherapy and debridement to remove nonviable tissue. Others recommend casting the leg with plaster to redistribute weight bearing and protect the lesion. Pending culture results, the initial antibiotic therapy for infected ulcers without systemic signs might be cefoxitin or ampicillin-sulbactam. If signs of sepsis are present, ampicillin-sulbactam plus gentamicin or aztreonam may be prescribed.

All patients should be instructed about proper foot care in an attempt to prevent ulcers. Feet should be kept clean and dry at all times. Patients with neuropathy should not walk barefoot, even in the home. Properly fitted shoes are essential. This is a particular problem with women, since an adequate shoe is not often stylish. The feet should be carefully inspected daily for callus, infection, abrasions, or blisters and the physician consulted about any potentially troublesome lesion. Transforming growth factor beta (TGFβ) improves the healing of decubitus ulcers and presumably would help for diabetic ulcers as well; it is not approved for clinical use.

What Causes the Complications of Diabetes? The cause of diabetic complications is not known and may be multifactorial. Major emphasis has been placed on the polyol pathway, wherein glucose is reduced to sorbitol by the enzyme aldol reductase. Sorbitol, which appears to function as a tissue toxin, has been implicated in the pathogenesis of retinopathy, neuropathy, cataracts, nephropathy, and aortic disease. The mechanism is perhaps best worked out in experimental diabetic neuropathy, where sorbitol accumulation is associated with a decrease in myoinositol content, abnormal phosphoinositide metabolism, and a decrease in Na^+,K^+-ATPase activity. In experimental models, the primacy of the polyol pathway in initiating neuropathy was proven by showing that inhibition of aldol reductase prevented the fall in tissue myoinositol content and the decrease in ATPase activity. Myoinositol deficiency was not found in sural nerve biopsy specimens from humans with diabetic neuropathy, in contrast to animals. Aldol reductase inhibition also has been shown to prevent experimental cataracts and retinopathy. It thus seems possible that neuropathy and retinopathy are due primarily to activation of the polyol pathway. This pathway also may play a role in diabetic nephropathy.

A second mechanism of potential pathogenetic importance is glycation of proteins. (Current terminology uses *glycation* for nonenzymatic addition of hexoses to proteins and *glycosylation* for enzymatic addition.) The effect of such glycation on hemoglobin has been mentioned, but multiple proteins in the body are altered in the same way, often with disturbance of their function. Examples include plasma albumin, lens protein, fibrin, collagen, lipoproteins, and the glycoprotein recognition system of hepatic endothelial cells. Particularly intriguing is the effect of glycation on lipoproteins. Glycated LDL is not recognized by the normal LDL receptor, and its plasma half-life is increased. Conversely, glycated HDL turns over more rapidly than native HDL. It also has been reported that glycated collagen traps LDL at rates two to three times that of normal collagen.

Glycated collagen is less soluble and more resistant to degradation by collagenase than native collagen, but it is not clear that these changes are related either to the basement membrane thickening or to the tight, waxy skin syndrome with limited joint mobility (scleroderma-like) seen in some patients with IDDM (see "Miscellaneous Abnormalities," below). However, evidence that nonenzymatic glycation of protein plays a role in some degenerative complications is less direct than with the polyol pathway. Linkage between the polyol pathway and the glycation sequence occurs as a result of the glycation of collagen and other proteins by fructose generated from sorbitol. The rate of glycation with fructose is seven or eight times that with glucose.

Glycated proteins also form cross-linked proteins termed *advanced glycation end products* (AGE) through a series of biochemical reactions that are poorly understood. An intermediate in the cross-linking is 3-deoxyglucose, which can be derived from either glucose or fructose. Receptors for AGE are present on macrophages and endothelial cells. Binding of AGE to its receptors may induce the synthesis or release of cytokines, vascular adhesion molecules, endothelin-1, and tissue factor. The latter plays a preeminent role in the initiation of coagulation, as mentioned earlier. The AGE also destroy endothelial-derived nitric oxide. Experimentally, AGE formation may be impaired or prevented by aminoguanidine, an agent currently in clinical trials. In animals, it has a beneficial effect in prevention of retinopathy, nephropathy, and neuropathy. In the past it has been common to attribute *microvascular complications* (retinopathy, nephropathy, neuropathy) to the polyol pathway and *macrovascular complications* (stroke, gangrene, myocardial infarction) to glycation and AGE. However, both pathways contribute to both sets of complications.

Increased blood flow may play an initiating role in diabetic complications, possibly by increasing the filtration of macromolecules that function as tissue toxins. There is supportive evidence for a role of hyperperfusion in diabetic nephropathy, but the hemodynamic hypothesis does not appear as attractive as the first two.

Can Diabetic Complications Be Prevented by Meticulous Control of Diabetes? As mentioned earlier, the strongest evidence that the answer is yes comes from the DCCT. Additional clinical evidence supports the view that metabolic environment per se influences or causes complications independent of genetic factors. For example, kidneys from donors who have neither diabetes nor a family history of diabetes develop characteristic lesions of diabetic nephropathy within 3 to 5 years after transplantation into a diabetic recipient. In contrast, diabetic nephropathy did not develop when a kidney was transplanted into a diabetic subject whose disease had been reversed by pancreatic transplantation prior to renal transplantation. It also has been reported that kidneys manifesting diabetic nephropathy demonstrated reversal of the lesion when transplanted into normal recipients. All these findings suggest that hyperglycemia or some other aspect of the abnormal metabolism of diabetes causes or influences the development of complications; additional factors, probably genetic, must also play a role. This follows from the fact that diabetic subjects with decades of poor control may escape the ravages of the late complications and from the fact that typical diabetic complications may be found in patients at the time of diagnosis of diabetes or even in the absence of fasting hyperglycemia.

Meticulous control with insulin infusion pumps has been reported to decrease microalbuminuria, improve motor nerve conduction velocity, lower plasma lipoproteins, and decrease capillary leakage of fluorescein in the retina. The width of the capillary basement membrane in skeletal muscle also has been decreased. The changes are small in general, however, and of questionable biologic significance. Thus, firm evidence does not exist to show that late complications can be *reversed* by long-term return of the plasma glucose to near-normal levels. Retinopathy can progress despite successful reversal of diabetes by pancreatic transplantation. The progression of diabetic complications after the return of the plasma glucose level to normal or near normal has been termed *hyperglycemic memory*. The mechanism may be formation of advanced glycation end products during hyperglycemia, which, being irreversible, continue their effects over the long term.

The question of intensive therapy for all patients with diabetes remains open, because it is uncertain that the results achieved in the DCCT can be matched in the general population. Persons with diabetes are often cared for by nonspecialists who do not have access to teams of support personnel like the ones used in the DCCT. There is no question, however, but that the thrust of treatment should be toward tighter control.

Miscellaneous Abnormalities of Diabetes Diabetes affects almost every system in the body. Space limitations preclude discussion of all associated features, but several deserve comment. *Infections* in persons with diabetes may not occur more frequently than in nondiabetics, but they tend to be more severe, possibly because of impaired leukocyte function, a frequent accompaniment of poor control. In addition to common infections of the skin, urinary tract, lungs, and bloodstream, four unusual infections appear to have a specific relationship with diabetes. *Malignant external otitis*, usually due to *Pseudomonas aeruginosa*, tends to occur in older patients and is characterized by severe pain in the ear, drainage, fever, and leukocytosis. Soft tissues around the ear are swollen and tender. A mound of granulation tissue is characteristically present internally at the junction of the osseous and cartilaginous portions of the ear. The facial nerve becomes paralyzed in half the cases, and other cranial nerves also may be involved. Facial nerve paralysis is a poor prognostic sign, and the mortality rate approximates 50 percent in this subset of patients. A 6-week course of ticarcillin or carbenicillin together with tobramycin is the treatment of choice. Ciprofloxacin, imipenem + cilastin, or third-generation parenteral antipseudomonal cephalosporin also may be used. Surgical debridement is often necessary. *Rhinocerebral mucormycosis* is a rare fungal infection that usually develops during or following an episode of diabetic ketoacidosis. Organisms are from the genera *Mucor*, *Rhizopus*, and *Absidia*. Onset is sudden, with periorbital and perinasal swelling, pain, bloody nasal discharge, and increased lacrimation. The nasal mucosa and underlying tissues become black and necrotic. Cranial nerve palsies and thrombosis of the internal jugular vein or sinuses of the brain may occur. Proptosis, chemosis, and retinal vein engorgement indicate cavernous sinus thrombosis. If the condition is untreated, death usually occurs in a week to 10 days. Amphotericin B and aggressive debridement are the indicated therapies. *Emphysematous cholecystitis* tends to affect diabetic men (in contrast to ordinary cholecystitis, a disease predominantly present in women). Gangrene of the gallbladder is 30 times more frequent than in the usual forms and accounts for high rates of perforation and higher mortality rates than in ordinary cholecystitis. Diagnosis is made when gas is seen in the gallbladder wall on plain films of the abdomen. Clostridial species are frequently cultured from bile, but other organisms may be present. Treatment is cholecystectomy and use of broad-spectrum antibiotics. Mezlocillin plus metronidazole provides adequate initial coverage. *Emphysematous pyelonephritis* is signaled by detection of gas in the kidney or perirenal space. Antibiotic therapy is usually ineffective, and nephrectomy may be required. Mortality rates of 80 percent have been reported.

Hypertriglyceridemia is common in diabetes and is due both to overproduction of VLDL in the liver and to a disposal defect in the periphery. The latter is a consequence of a deficiency of lipoprotein lipase, an insulin-dependent enzyme. Some patients exhibit hyperlipidemia even when diabetic control is adequate; these patients likely have a primary familial hyperlipoproteinemia that is independent of diabetes. Patients who do not respond to insulin and dietary therapy should be treated for hypertriglyceridemia and hypercholesterolemia with drugs, as in nondiabetic subjects (see Chap. 341).

A variety of skin lesions occur in diabetes. *Necrobiosis lipoidica diabeticorum* is a plaquelike lesion with a central yellowish area surrounded by a brownish border. It is usually found over the anterior surfaces of the legs. Ulceration may occur. *Diabetic dermopathy* ("shin spots") is also usually located over the anterior tibial surface. The lesions are small, rounded plaques with a raised border; they may crust at the edges and ulcerate centrally. Several plaques may be arranged in linear fashion. Pigmentation is not prominent early, but as the lesion heals, a depressed scar occurs with diffuse brown discoloration. A rarer abnormality is *bullosis diabeticorum*. The bullae may be superficial, with mildly hemorrhagic or clear serum. The cause is unknown. *Infestations of the skin* with *Candida* and dermatophytes are common, and bacterial infections of a variety of types occur. In women, *vaginal moniliasis* may be troublesome during hyperglycemic-glycosuric periods. While the symptoms respond to nystatin or gentian violet, recurrence is inevitable unless glycosuria is reversed. *Atrophy of adipose tissue* may occur at the site of insulin injections, even with recombinant human insulin. *Hypertrophy* of fat also may occur, producing a lipoma-like lesion visible on physical examination.

Hyperviscosity occurs in diabetes, and *platelet aggregation* is enhanced, possibly owing to increased thromboxane synthesis. *Wound healing* is impaired in experimental diabetes, but this effect probably is not a major factor clinically. An interesting accompaniment of IDDM is the presence of *joint contractures* (Dupuytren's contractures) coupled with *tight, waxy skin* over the dorsum of the hands. The hands resemble those in patients with scleroderma. The cause of the tendon contractures is unknown, although alterations of cross-linking in collagen has been proposed. Patients with the syndrome of joint contractures and waxy skin appear to have accelerated development of other diabetic complications. *Scleredema* is a common finding in diabetes. This benign lesion is a thickening of the skin over the shoulders and upper back that resembles scleroderma.

Patients with diabetes may have additional illnesses. For example, there is a significant prevalence of eating disorders in young women with IDDM.

NONROUTINE THERAPIES Transplantation with whole pancreas or pancreatic segments has cured diabetes but is usually performed only when kidney transplantation is required. There is no question that successful transplantation can return the blood glucose level to normal. If the kidney is transplanted simultaneously, immunosuppression is required, and the pancreatic transplantation is simply piggy-backed. The question of whether better diabetic control is worth the risks of immunosuppression when the pancreas alone is transplanted has not been addressed in clinical trials. Transplantation of islet cells (as opposed to whole pancreas) also has been attempted, but the results are poor. The use of nonpancreatic cells that have been genetically engineered to produce human insulin under glucose control is being studied.

Prevention of autoimmune diabetes by immunosuppressant agents is a desirable goal. Reversal of hyperglycemia without the need for insulin has been achieved in humans with new-onset diabetes using powerful drugs such as cyclosporine. The reversal is not permanent, however, and most physicians believe that prophylactic treatment with potent immunosuppressant agents is not warranted; i.e., the potential dangers are too great. Preventive trials are under way in which insulin is used as prophylaxis in subjects predicted to develop diabetes in the near future based on the presence of islet cell antibodies and diminished insulin response to an intravenous glucose load. Scattered positive results have been reported. Other trials are testing the effect of nicotinamide as a possible protective and repair agent.

INSULIN RESISTANCE Insulin resistance is defined arbitrarily as the requirement of 200 or more units of insulin per day to control hyperglycemia and prevent ketosis. Relative insulin resistance is present in most persons with diabetes when carefully sought using the glucose clamp technique. It is the consequence of near-complete insulin deficiency in IDDM, whereas in NIDDM the major cause is obesity.

The normal anabolic metabolism mediated by insulin requires the secretion of adequate amounts of insulin in response to meals. Insulin must then bind to a specific insulin receptor in target tissues (see Chap. 327). The insulin receptor is a tetrameric glycoprotein consisting of two α and two β subunits linked by disulfide bonds. The β subunit is a tyrosine kinase that is activated when insulin binds to the α subunit. The tyrosine kinase autophosphorylates the insulin receptor and initiates subsequent intracellular phosphorylations that mediate the multiple actions of insulin. The only such action that is reasonably understood is glucose transport. Glucose enters the cell by facilitated diffusion mediated by glucose transporter molecules. While some transporters are always present in the plasma membrane, the binding of insulin to the receptor initiates a rapid mobilization of intracellular stores of the transporter to the plasma membrane and activates units already in place. In poorly controlled diabetes, the number of stored transporters appears to be deficient.

Insulin resistance is characterized as *prereceptor* (abnormal insulin or anti-insulin antibodies), *receptor* (decreased receptor number or diminished binding of insulin), or *postreceptor* (abnormal signal transduction, especially failure to activate the receptor tyrosine kinase). Combinations may exist. The nature of the molecular defect is known in some forms of insulin resistance but has not been identified in many.

With full-blown insulin resistance (>200 units of insulin required per day), the problem is usually prereceptor resistance due to anti-insulin antibodies. Anti-insulin antibodies of the IgG class are present in most subjects within 60 days of the initiation of insulin therapy. The titer of these antibodies fluctuates for reasons that are not clear. Although the correlation between antibody titer and functional resistance is not close, binding of insulin by antibody is presumed to be the primary mechanism in most cases. Probably fewer than 0.1 percent of insulin-treated patients ever have significant resistance. The problem may appear within a few weeks of the start of therapy or many years later. The onset may be abrupt, resulting in ketoacidosis, but usually it is gradual, with uncontrollable hyperglycemia being the major problem. About 20 to 30 percent of patients have accompanying insulin allergy. Treatment requires glucocorticoids in large amounts—80 to 100 mg prednisone per day initially. Response often occurs in 48 to 72 h but may take longer. If no improvement has resulted after 3 to 4 weeks, it can be assumed that steroids will not be effective. Once insulin requirements begin to fall, the prednisone dosage can be decreased rapidly (by 10 to 20 mg every 3 to 7 days) until a maintenance level of 5 to 10 mg/d is reached. Maintenance therapy may be required for many months. Whether remission has occurred and therapy can be discontinued must be determined by trial. Sulfated insulin may be of benefit.

On rare occasions, insulin resistance appears to be due to enhanced destruction of the hormone at the subcutaneous injection site. Such patients tend to respond normally to insulin given intravenously or intraperitoneally. In some patients, addition of a protease inhibitor (aprotinin) to the insulin mixture is helpful. When resistance is extreme, U500 regular insulin should be used in order to control the volume of the injection.

Insulin resistance also occurs in the absence of overt diabetes. In such disorders, *acanthosis nigricans* is a physical sign of its presence. Acanthosis nigricans is a brown to black, velvety hyperpigmentation of the skin, usually present in the posterior and lateral folds of the neck, the axilla, groin, umbilicus, and other areas. Acanthosis nigricans occurred in about 7 percent of children in one study. The prevalence is higher in Hispanics and blacks than in whites. Although acanthosis nigricans may be a sign of occult malignancy, it is not associated with neoplasia in the insulin-resistance states. A list of the major syndromes of insulin resistance is given in Table 334-12.

Obesity is the most common cause of insulin resistance. It is associated with decreased receptor number, but the major problem is at the postreceptor level, where there is apparently a failure to activate the tyrosine kinase. *Werner's syndrome* is an autosomal recessive illness with a high incidence of hyperglycemia despite elevated concentrations of plasma insulin. There is little response to exogenous hormone. Other features include growth retardation, alopecia or premature graying of the hair, cataracts, hypogonadism, leg ulcers, atrophy of muscle, fat, and bone, soft tissue calcification, and a high frequency of sarcomas and meningiomas.

Of the rare conditions associated with acanthosis nigricans, the variants associated with *insulin receptor abnormalities* have attracted the greatest interest. Type A patients are tall young women with a tendency to hirsutism and abnormalities of the reproductive tract who have polycystic ovaries or other causes of ovarian androgen excess. Many mutations in the insulin receptor have been found in patients with the type A syndrome, most of them interfering with the activity of the receptor by blocking or diminishing its tyrosine kinase activity. Type B subjects are older women with immunologic disease. The clinical picture includes arthralgias, alopecia, enlarged salivary glands, proteinuria, leukopenia, and antinuclear and anti-DNA antibodies. Insulin resistance in these patients is due to blocking antibodies directed against the insulin receptor (not against insulin itself). Interestingly, antireceptor antibodies on occasion may cause hypoglycemia. Whether agonist (hypoglycemia) or antagonist (insulin resistance) activity occurs presumably depends on the site of binding to the insulin receptor. Both A and B patients have high plasma insulin concentrations.

Generalized and *partial lipodystrophies* are fat depletion syndromes that differ primarily in the extent of fat atrophy (see Chap. 352). In the generalized form, essentially all body fat is missing, while the more common partial type exhibits atrophy of fat in the face and trunk with normal or increased adiposity in the lower half of the body. The disease can be either congenital or acquired. Typically, the patients develop hyperglycemia at puberty, but ketoacidosis never occurs. Marked hypertriglyceridemia with eruptive xanthoma is common. Characteristic features are hepatomegaly, splenomegaly, cardiomegaly, hirsutism, lymphadenopathy, hypertrophy of the external genitalia, varicose veins, and (in the congenital forms) muscle hypertrophy. Mental retardation is common, and renal disease may develop. The term *lipoatrophic diabetes* is synonymous with total lipodystrophy. All patients have elevated plasma insulin levels. Resistance may be due to a decreased number of receptors, diminished affinity of the receptor for insulin, or a postreceptor defect.

The *pineal hypertrophy syndrome* is characterized by insulin resistance, early dentition with malformed teeth, dry skin, thick nails, hirsutism, and a peculiar sexual precocity with enlargement of the external genitalia. The latter may reach near adult size by age 3 or 4.

Table 334-12

Insulin-Resistant States
Prereceptor Resistance
Mutated insulins
Anti-insulin antibodies
Receptor and Postreceptor Resistance
Obesity
Type A syndrome (absent or dysfunctional receptor)
Type B syndrome (antibody to insulin receptor)
Lipodystrophic states (partial or generalized)
Leprechaunism
Ataxia-telangiectasia
Rabson-Mendenhall syndrome
Werner syndrome
Alström syndrome
Pineal hyperplasia syndrome

The insulin resistance is severe, and ketoacidosis may occur despite high endogenous insulin levels. The *Alström syndrome* is a rare autosomal recessive disease characterized by childhood blindness due to retinal degeneration, nerve deafness, vasopressin-resistant diabetes insipidus, and, in males, hypogonadism with high plasma gonadotropin levels. The patients thus appear to have end organ resistance to multiple hormones. Other features include baldness, hyperuricemia, hypertriglyceridemia, and aminoaciduria. Superficially, the patients may resemble subjects with the Laurence-Moon-Biedl syndrome but can be differentiated on initial examination by the absence of polydactyly and mental deficiency. Insulin resistance in the Alström syndrome is mild. *Ataxia-telangiectasia* is characterized by cerebellar ataxia, telangiectasia, a predisposition to breast cancer, and a variety of abnormalities in the immune system in addition to insulin resistance. The *Rabson-Mendenhall syndrome* consists of dental dysplasia, dystrophic nails, premature puberty, and acanthosis nigricans. The insulin resistance is probably due to an insulin receptor abnormality. *Leprechaunism* is characterized by an elfin appearance of the face, hirsutism, absence of subcutaneous fat, thickened skin, and insulin resistance. Defects are found in both the α and the β subunits of the insulin receptor, causing expression in plasma membranes to be markedly diminished. Not listed in Table 334-12 is insulin resistance due to hormone excess (acromegaly, Cushing's syndrome), myotonic dystrophy, and thalassemia major. The insulin resistance in these conditions usually is not clinically significant.

INSULIN ALLERGY Insulin allergy is due to IgE antibodies to insulin. Manifestations include immediate reactions with local stinging or itching, delayed local reactions with brawny swelling lasting up to 30 h, and generalized urticaria or frank anaphylaxis. Systemic reactions are usually seen in patients who have stopped insulin therapy for one reason or another and have then resumed treatment. The allergic reaction may occur as early as the second injection on resumption of therapy. Mild reactions can be treated with antihistamines. If the problem is severe, desensitization procedures are required. A 1-day insulin desensitization procedure is shown in Table 334-13. Once the patient is desensitized, insulin therapy should not be interrupted.

THE EMOTIONAL RESPONSE TO DIABETES It is difficult to accept that one has a chronic disease that requires a change in life-style. This is particularly true in the case of diabetes, since patients are usually aware that they are vulnerable to late complications and that their life expectancy is shortened. It is not surprising that the emotional response to diabetes often hampers treatment. The primary reaction can range from denial with an accompanying refusal to cooperate to excessive preoccupation with the illness. The physician should make every effort to bring the patient to a middle ground of acknowledging the disease and responding prudently without becoming obsessed. The goal is to live with diabetes, not for it. Patients with diabetes are no different from other patients, in that they may use their disease manipulatively with both family and physician. These problems are particularly acute with children and adolescents. While the psychiatric aspects of diabetes are not discussed here, most problems can be anticipated and handled if common sense is coupled with sympathy and firmness. It is also appropriate to offer cautious hope that the disease will be handled better in the future than is possible now.

Table 334-13

Insulin Desensitization*

Time, h	Dose, U	Route	Time, h	Dose, U	Route
0	0.001	Intradermal	3.5	0.2	Subcut.
0.5	0.002	Intradermal	4	0.5	Subcut.
1	0.004	Subcut.	4.5	1	Subcut.
1.5	0.01	Subcut.	5	2	Subcut.
2	0.02	Subcut.	5.5	4	Subcut.
2.5	0.04	Subcut.	6	8	Subcut.
3	0.1	Subcut.			

* Following desensitization, use 2 to 10 U of regular insulin every 4 to 6 h for 24 to 36 h after the 6-h injection before switching to intermediate-acting insulin.

SOURCE: *Schedule of JA Galloway*. For detailed information see JA Galloway, R Bressler, Med Clin North Am 62:663, 1978.

Please refer to Chap. 60, Insulin, oral hypoglycemic agents, and the pharmacology of the endocrine pancreas, in Goodman & Gilman's The Pharmacological Basis of Therapeutics, *9th ed., New York, McGraw-Hill*

BIBLIOGRAPHY

GENERAL REVIEW

UNGER RH, FOSTER DW: Diabetes mellitus, in *Williams' Textbook of Endocrinology*, 9th ed, JD Wilson, DW Foster (eds). Philadelphia, Saunders, 1997 (in press)

Report of the Expert Committee on the Diagnosis and Classification of Diabetes Mellitus. Diabetes Care 20:1183, 1997

GENETICS AND PATHOGENESIS

ATKINSON MA, MACLAREN NK: The pathogenesis of insulin-dependent diabetes mellitus. N Engl J Med 331:1428, 1994

BINGLY PJ et al: Can we really predict IDDM? Diabetes 42:213, 1993

COUSTAN DR et al: Gestational diabetes: Predictors of subsequent disordered glucose metabolism. Am J Obstet Gynecol 168:1139, 1993

GHOSH S, SCHORK NJ: Genetic analysis of NIDDM. The study of quantitative traits. Diabetes 45:1, 1996

HAGOPIAN WA et al: Glutamate decarboxylase-, insulin-, and islet cell-antibodies and HLA typing to detect diabetes in a general population-based study of Swedish children. J Clin Invest 95:1505, 1995

HARRISON LC et al: MHC molecules and β-cell destructive immune and nonimmune mechanisms. Diabetes 38:815, 1989

HYÖTY H et al: A prospective study of the role of coxsackie B and other enterovirus infections in the pathogenesis of IDDM. Diabetes 44:652, 1995

PALMER JP, MCCULLOCH DK: Prediction and prevention of IDDM—1991. Diabetes 40:943, 1991

PERMUTT MA et al: Glucokinase and NIDDM: A candidate gene that paid off. Diabetes 41:1367, 1992

POLONSKY KS et al: Non-insulin-dependent diabetes mellitus—a genetically programmed failure of the beta cell to compensate for insulin resistance. N Engl J Med 334:777, 1996

PUGLIESE A et al: HLA-DQB1*0602 is associated with dominant protection from diabetes even among islet cell antibody-positive first-degree relatives of patients with IDDM. Diabetes 44:608, 1995

THAI AC, EISENBARTH GS: Natural history of IDDM. Diabetes Rev 1:1, 1993

UMPIERREZ GE et al: Diabetic ketoacidosis in obese African-Americans. Diabetes 44:790, 1995

DIABETIC COMPLICATIONS

AIELLO LP et al: Vascular endothelial growth factor in ocular fluid of patients with diabetic retinopathy and other retinal disorders. N Engl J Med 331:1480, 1994

BEISSWENGER PJ et al: Formation of immunochemical advanced glycosylation end products precedes and correlates with early manifestations of renal and retinal disease in diabetes. Diabetes 44:824, 1994

BORG WP et al: Local ventromedial hypothalamus glucopenia triggers counterregulatory hormone release. Diabetes 44:180, 1995

BOYLE PJ et al: Brain glucose uptake and unawareness of hypoglycemia in patients with insulin-dependent diabetes mellitus. N Engl J Med 333:1726, 1995

BROWNLEE M: Glycation products and the pathogenesis of diabetic complications. Diabetes Care 15:1835, 1992

FOSTER DW, MCGARRY JD: The metabolic derangements and treatment of diabetic ketoacidosis. N Engl J Med 309:159, 1983

KROLEWSKI AS et al: Glycosylated hemoglobin and the risk of microalbuminuria in patients with insulin-dependent diabetes mellitus. N Engl J Med 332:1251, 1995

LEURS PB et al: Tissue factor pathway inhibitor activity in patients with IDDM. Diabetes 44:80, 1995

PARTANEN J et al: Natural history of peripheral neuropathy in patients with non-insulin-dependent diabetes mellitus. N Engl J Med 333:89, 1995

SEQUIST ER et al: Familial clustering of diabetic renal disease: Evidence for genetic susceptibility and diabetic nephropathy. N Engl J Med 320:1161, 1989

SIPERSTEIN MD: Diabetic ketoacidosis and hyperosmolar coma. Endocrinol Metab Clin North Am 21:915, 1992

TOWLER DA et al: Mechanism of awareness of hypoglycemia. Perception of neurogenic (predominantly cholinergic) rather than neuroglycopenic symptoms. Diabetes 42:1791, 1993

VIBERTI J et al: Diabetic nephropathy: Future avenue. Diabetes Care 15:1216, 1992

TREATMENT

AMERICAN DIABETES ASSOCIATION: Clinical Practice Recommendations 1996. Nutrition recommendations and principles for people with diabetes mellitus. Diabetes Care 19(Suppl 1):S16, 1996
BAILEY CJ et al: Metformin. N Engl J Med 334:574, 1996
CAMPBELL PJ, MAY ME: A practical guide to intensive insulin therapy. Am J Med Sci 310:24, 1995
RAVID M et al: Long-term stabilizing effect of angiotensin-converting enzyme inhibition on plasma creatinine and on proteinuria in normotensive type II diabetic patients. Ann Intern Med 118:577, 1993
ROBERTSON RP: Pancreatic and islet transplantation for diabetes—cures or curiosities? N Engl J Med 327:1861, 1992
SANTIAGO JV: Intensive management of insulin dependent diabetes: Risks, benefits, and unanswered questions. J Clin Endocrinol Metab 75:977, 1992
SKYLER JS: Insulin pharmacology. Med Clin North Am 72:1337, 1988
Troglitazone for non-insulin-dependent diabetes mellitus. Med Lett 39:49, 1997

INSULIN RESISTANCE

FLIER JS: Syndromes of insulin resistance: From patient to gene and back again. Diabetes 41:1207, 1992
TAYLOR SI: Molecular mechanisms of insulin resistance: Lessons from patients with mutations in the insulin receptor gene. Diabetes 41:1473, 1992

335

Daniel W. Foster, Arthur H. Rubenstein

HYPOGLYCEMIA

Maintenance of the plasma glucose concentration within narrow bounds is essential for health. Hypoglycemia is dangerous (in the short run more so than hyperglycemia) because glucose is the primary energy substrate of the brain. Its absence, like that of oxygen, produces deranged function, tissue damage, and death if the deficit is prolonged. The brain is vulnerable to hypoglycemia because it cannot utilize circulating free fatty acids as an energy source, in contrast to other tissues. The short-chain fatty acid metabolites acetoacetate and β-hydroxybutyrate (*ketone bodies, ketoacids*) are oxidized by the brain and can protect it from damage by hypoglycemia when present at moderate concentrations in plasma. However, development of ketosis requires a number of hours so that ketogenesis is ineffective in protecting against acute hypoglycemia. Preservation of central nervous system function in the early phases of fasting and during hypoglycemia thus requires a prompt increase in the production of glucose by the liver. At the same time, glucose utilization by other tissues is diminished by the availability of free fatty acids as an alternative substrate. These adaptive mechanisms are hormonally controlled and are effective under ordinary circumstances. When the system breaks down or is overwhelmed, hypoglycemia occurs.

DEFENSE AGAINST HYPOGLYCEMIA The hypoglycemic states can best be understood as derangements of normal fuel metabolism. Under ordinary circumstances, energy needs are met by exogenous substrate in the form of food. Oxidation of the constituent molecules of food to carbon dioxide and water generates adenosine triphosphate (ATP), the principal high-energy compound of the body. In one sense, life can be defined as the generation of ATP (and related high-energy nucleotides) for the preservation of cellular integrity. When caloric intake is greater than immediate oxidative needs, as after the usual meal, excess substrate is stored as fat, protein, and glycogen. In this *anabolic* phase of metabolism, the flux of substrate is from intestine to liver to utilization and storage sites. Insulin is the primary hormone mediating the anabolic phase, and counterregulatory hormone levels are suppressed.

The *catabolic* phase of metabolism begins about 5 to 6 h after a meal. Normally, the only significant catabolic period in the day is during the overnight fast, but under some circumstances, particularly serious illness, catabolic periods may be longer. During fasting/catabolism, the liver is activated to produce glucose and to maintain the plasma glucose level in a range safe for central nervous system function, and free fatty acids are mobilized to provide substrate for most other tissues of the body. Initially, glucose from the liver is derived almost exclusively from hepatic glycogen. However, since only about 70 g of glycogen are stored in the human liver, glycogenolysis ordinarily can sustain the plasma glucose only for 8 to 10 h. Exercise and the stress of severe illness may shorten this protective period. To compensate for glycogen depletion, gluconeogenesis increases early, with a flux of substrate from muscle and adipose tissue stores to liver and then to utilization sites.

The precursors for hepatic glucose synthesis (gluconeogenesis) are lactate/pyruvate and amino acids (primarily alanine and glutamine) derived from muscle and glycerol released from adipose tissue by lipolysis. Amino acids constitute the primary substrate for gluconeogenesis. Most of the lactate is recycled from preformed glucose (the *Cori cycle*), the only net contribution coming from the breakdown of muscle glycogen. Glycerol is initially a minor substrate but increases in importance with time. The liver is the primary source of glucose production after an overnight fast, but the kidney may contribute as much as half of glucose production in a prolonged fast, accounting for the frequent occurrence of hypoglycemia in renal failure. The rate of glucose production in the kidney is hormonally regulated, like that in the liver, and appears to be especially responsive to epinephrine. Proteolysis to provide amino acids for gluconeogenesis causes the negative nitrogen balance of starvation. The same mechanism is operative in the stress of trauma, surgery, and severe infection. In quantitative terms, the liver produces about 11 μmol/kg per minute (2 mg/kg per minute) of glucose in the initial phases of fasting. Higher rates of glucose production indicate increased utilization of glucose, an important consideration in the differential diagnosis of hypoglycemia.

The switch to fat metabolism is accomplished by activation in adipose tissue of the hormone-sensitive lipase, which hydrolyzes stored triglycerides to long-chain fatty acids and glycerol. The released fatty acids have two fates. Most (normally about 120 g/d) is used directly, and the remainder (about 40 g/d) is oxidized in the liver to acetoacetic and β-hydroxybutyric acids. Ketoacids can be used efficiently as an energy source by most tissues (liver uses them only minimally), but their primary importance is as backup substrate for the brain, as noted above. The shift of most tissues to lipid metabolism is important because the preferential oxidation of free fatty acids and ketones in place of glucose spares the latter for utilization by the central nervous system.

Catabolic metabolism is initiated by a fall in the concentration of insulin in plasma and secretion of the five counterregulatory hormones: glucagon, epinephrine, norepinephrine, cortisol, and growth hormone. Norepinephrine is released both from sympathetic neurons and from the adrenal medulla. Glucagon is the primary hormone of glucose maintenance, and epinephrine and norepinephrine play important backup roles. This backup function is particularly important in the defense against hypoglycemia in diabetes mellitus, where the glucagon response is lost early (see Chap. 334). Cortisol and growth hormone antagonize the action of insulin and promote the mobilization of substrate and activation of gluconeogenesis.

The anabolic and catabolic phases of metabolism are summarized in Table 335-1. Breakdown in any of the adaptive mechanisms can lead to hypoglycemia.

SYMPTOMATOLOGY Symptoms of hypoglycemia fall into two main categories: those induced by *excessive secretion of epinephrine/norepinephrine (autonomic response)* and those due to *dysfunction of the central nervous system (neuroglycopenia).* Rapid epinephrine release causes sweating, tremor, tachycardia, anxiety, and hunger. Central nervous system (CNS) symptoms worsen in severity with severe or prolonged hypoglycemia and include dizziness, headache, clouding of vision, blunted mental acuity, loss of fine motor skill, confusion, abnormal behavior, convulsions, and loss of consciousness. When the onset of hypoglycemia is gradual, the autonomic response may be masked so that CNS symptoms dominate the clinical picture. With a more rapid drop in plasma glucose (as in insulin reactions),

Table 335-1

The Feeding-Fasting Cycle

Phase	Primary Hormone	Plasma Substrates	Substrate Flux	Active Process
Anabolic*	Insulin	↑ Glucose ↑ Triglycerides ↑ Branched-chain amino acids ↓ Free fatty acids ↓ Ketones	Splanchnic bed → storage and utilization sites	Glycogen storage Protein synthesis Triglyceride formation
Catabolic†	Glucagon	↓ Glucose ↓ Triglycerides ↑ Alanine and glutamine‡ ↑ Free fatty acids ↑ Ketones	Storage sites → liver and utilization sites	Glycogenolysis Gluconeogenesis Proteolysis Lipolysis Ketogenesis

* Expected findings during the first several hours after ingestion of a mixed meal of fat, carbohydrate, and protein.
† The major daily catabolic phase occurs during the overnight fast, although partial catabolic cycles occur between meals.
‡ Arrows indicate plasma concentrations except for alanine and glutamine. While arterial concentrations of these amino acids are relatively constant, uptake by the liver and intestine is increased in the catabolic phase.

autonomic symptoms are prominent. In the diabetic subject, autonomic symptoms may not be manifest if severe neuropathy is present or if the syndrome of hypoglycemia unawareness is present.

The literature concerning the level of plasma glucose required to activate hormonal defenses and to produce symptoms is confusing because in many experimental studies, glucose is measured in "arterialized" venous blood samples (drawn from a hand vein in a heated box), while in clinical practice, glucose ordinarily is measured in plain venous blood, where its level may be as much as 1 mmol/L (18 mg/dL) lower than in an equivalent arterialized sample. Recognizable symptoms occur in persons without diabetes when the venous plasma glucose concentration falls below 2.5 mmol/L (45 mg/dL) if the plasma glucose is lowered acutely, as by insulin injection. With acute hypoglycemia, progressive defense responses occur as the glucose level falls. In one study (using arterialized venous samples), insulin secretion ceased at 4.6 mmol/L glucose (83 mg/dL), and glucagon and epinephrine were released at 3.8 mmol/L (68 mg/dL), growth hormone at 3.7 mmol/L (67 mg/dL), and cortisol at 3.2 mmol/L (58 mg/dL). Thus, protective mechanisms are activated before the symptomatic threshold is reached. Although overt symptoms are not present, CNS function may be impaired with minimal decrements of plasma glucose. In a study utilizing auditory evoked potentials as a sensitive indicator of CNS function, abnormalities were seen in normal persons with a drop of glucose in arterialized venous blood from 4.8 to 4.0 mmol/L (87 to 72 mg/dL). When blood glucose was sustained at 4.0 mmol/L (72 mg/dL), counterregulatory release eventually occurred (at 2 to 3 h) despite the fact that no symptoms were produced. Major CNS dysfunction may not develop until plasma glucose concentrations approximate 1 mmol/L (20 mg/dL) because cerebral blood flow increases enough to deliver some glucose to the brain even when glucose levels are low. Cerebral atherosclerosis, which reduces the elasticity of the nonelastic blood vessels, compromises this protective mechanism so that symptomatic distress occurs at higher glucose levels. Symptoms (autonomic or neuroglycopenic) due to hypoglycemia are unlikely to occur at a plasma glucose level above 2.8 mmol/L (50 mg/dL) in nondiabetic persons. As noted above, subtle CNS dysfunction occurs at higher glucose levels. Patients with poorly controlled diabetes mellitus appear to develop hypoglycemic symptoms at higher glucose concentrations than nondiabetic individuals, and patients with meticulously controlled diabetes have a lower symptomatic threshold and may exhibit the syndrome of *hypoglycemia unawareness* (see Chap. 334). In hypoglycemia unawareness the thresholds are reversed so that the autonomic response is not activated before the onset of neuroglycopenic symptoms. Some patients with insulinoma also have a lowering of the glucose threshold at which release of counterregulatory hormones is induced and thus experience hypoglycemia unawareness.

A rare syndrome that mimics the CNS manifestations of hypoglycemia has been described in which blood glucose is normal but the glucose level in cerebrospinal fluid (CSF) is low, presumably owing to a defect in the glucose transporter molecule GLUT 1. Seizures may result.

CLASSIFICATION It is traditional to classify hypoglycemia as either *postprandial* (reactive) or *fasting*. Pathologically low plasma glucose concentrations occur in the former type only in response to meals, while in the latter type they occur only after hours of fasting. Patients with fasting hypoglycemia (particularly those with insulinomas) may exhibit a reactive component, but reactive patients do not have symptoms when food is withdrawn. Fasting hypoglycemia usually means that a disease process is responsible, but symptoms suggestive of postprandial hypoglycemia may occur in the absence of recognizable disease.

CAUSES OF HYPOGLYCEMIA

Postprandial Hypoglycemia The most common cause of postprandial hypoglycemia is alimentary hyperinsulinism (Table 335-2). Patients who have undergone gastrectomy, gastrojejunostomy, pyloroplasty, or vagotomy are subject to hypoglycemia after meals, presumably because of rapid gastric emptying, brisk absorption of glucose, and excessive insulin release. Glucose levels fall more rapidly than insulin levels under these circumstances, and insulin-glucose imbalance leads to hypoglycemia. Ingestion of fructose or galactose causes hypoglycemia in children with fructose intolerance or galactosemia. Leucine intake rarely causes the syndrome in susceptible infants. The early phase of diabetes mellitus is usually listed as a cause of reactive hypoglycemia, but in our experience symptomatic hypoglycemia as a premonitory symptom of diabetes is uncommon. Prediabetics, who by definition are normoglycemic, may have a late fall in plasma glucose after oral glucose tolerance testing, but this pattern is similar to that frequently present in asymptomatic, healthy individuals (see below).

Idiopathic alimentary hypoglycemia consists of two syndromes: *true hypoglycemia* and *pseudohypoglycemia*. In the former, adrenergic symptoms appear postprandially and are accompanied by a low plasma glucose level. Symptoms appear spontaneously during everyday life and are relieved by ingestion of carbohydrate, which raises the plasma glucose. Such patients are rare. The mechanism of this disorder is unknown, although subtle dysfunction of the gastrointestinal tract might be operative. Some patients with true postprandial hypoglycemia turn out to have insulinomas (see below).

In pseudohypoglycemia, adrenergic symptoms suggestive of hypoglycemia appear 2 to 5 h after a meal, but plasma glucose concentrations are normal when symptoms are present. The condition is often self-diagnosed and "confirmed" when a 5-h glucose tolerance test reveals a lower than "normal" plasma glucose between 2 and 5 h.

Two questions have to be asked about pseudohypoglycemia. First, what causes the symptoms (which may be incapacitating)? Second, can a valid diagnosis of hypoglycemia be made by a glucose tolerance test? The symptoms of nervousness, weakness, tremor, tachycardia, dizziness, and sweating in this disorder are probably due to epinephrine release. Many normal people experience similar symptoms at some time in their lives and may even have gained relief by eating. Patients with pseudohypoglycemia, in contrast, develop the symptoms regularly and repetitively. In one study, 80 consecutive subjects with reproducible postprandial symptoms were studied by 5-h glucose tolerance testing. Hypoglycemia was considered to be present if (1) the plasma glucose fell below 3.3 mmol/L (60 mg/dL) during the test; (2) symptoms or signs compatible with hypoglycemia were present; and (3) at least a doubling of the plasma cortisol level occurred 30 to 90 min

Table 335-2

Causes of Postprandial (Reactive) Hypoglycemia

Alimentary hyperinsulinism	Leucine sensitivity
Hereditary fructose intolerance	Idiopathic
Galactosemia	

after the nadir of plasma glucose (indicating hypoglycemia severe enough to activate the hypothalamic-pituitary-adrenal axis). Only 18 of the 80 (23 percent) subjects whose history suggested postprandial hypoglycemia fulfilled these criteria. Twenty-five percent of asymptomatic matched normal controls also met all three criteria. When the patients and controls were tested after a mixed meal, no subject in either group had a plasma glucose below 3.3 mmol/L (60 mg/dL), yet 14 of the 18 patients (78 percent) had symptoms typical of those after glucose tolerance testing. The absence of hypoglycemia after mixed meals despite the presence of typical symptoms has been observed in other studies. *Pseudohypoglycemia* appears to be an accurate descriptive term for the syndrome and is preferable to "idiopathic postprandial syndrome," which also has been used. Many such patients are thought to have stress or anxiety as a predisposing factor. Presumably they have enhanced catecholamine release following a meal, or they may be abnormally sensitive to normal postprandial norepinephrine/epinephrine release. Insulin can stimulate epinephrine release in humans even if hypoglycemia is prevented. Whether enhanced insulin release plays a role in the pseudohypoglycemia syndrome is not known.

Fasting Hypoglycemia The causes of fasting hypoglycemia are many, but in all instances there is an imbalance between the production of glucose by the liver and its utilization in peripheral tissues. In some patients, hypoglycemia is due primarily to a defect in glucose production, while in others, the problem is excess glucose utilization. Both defects may be present. For example, with insulin excess enhanced glucose utilization is coupled with blunted hepatic glucose production. The latter is caused by blockade by insulin of the glycogenolytic/gluconeogenic effects of the counterregulatory hormones. Dual defects are probably operative in disorders of fat oxidation and non-insulin-producing tumors as well.

Supply-side hypoglycemia (*impaired production of glucose*) characteristically requires much less glucose during therapy than does demand-side hypoglycemia (*overutilization of glucose*) (Table 335-3). As noted above, in normal people glucose production during a fast approximates 11 μmol/kg per minute (2 mg/kg per minute), but with insulin-induced hypoglycemia, glucose utilization increases to about 67 μmol/kg per minute (12 mg/kg per minute). Thus, if more than 56 mmol (10 g) of glucose per hour is required to prevent or reverse hypoglycemia, it can be assumed that overutilization is present.

Underproduction of glucose As discussed earlier, the production of glucose by the liver initially involves breakdown of stored glycogen and subsequent gluconeogenesis, the synthesis of glucose from precursors delivered to the liver from peripheral tissues. Inadequate production of glucose during fasting can be due to five causes: (1) hormone deficiency, (2) defects in glycogenolytic or gluconeogenic enzymes, (3) inadequate substrate delivery, (4) liver disease, and (5) drugs. Hypopituitarism and adrenal insufficiency are the common hormonal causes of hypoglycemia. Defects in catecholamine or glucagon release are rare. Enzymatic abnormalities causing hypoglycemia are usually seen in children and not adults. Glucose-6-phosphatase deficiency is the classic example of a defect in glycogen breakdown, but hypoglycemia may occur in young children with deficiencies of hepatic glycogen phosphorylase and in other forms of glycogen storage disease (Chap. 347). The inability to make glycogen because of inadequate glycogen synthase activity also renders infants susceptible to fasting hypoglycemia. In addition to glucose-6-phosphatase, three other enzymes are necessary for gluconeogenesis: pyruvate carboxylase, phosphoenolpyruvate carboxykinase, and fructose-1,6-bisphosphatase (fructose-1,6-diphosphatase) (Fig. 335-1). Hypoglycemia can occur when any of these enzymes is deficient, often with associated lactic acidosis. The cause of lactic acidosis in this situation is not known, although impaired hepatic lactate uptake due to the gluconeogenic defect probably plays a role. Substrate deficiency appears to be one of the causes of ketotic hypoglycemia of infancy, since alanine turnover in such patients is low. Inadequate substrate supply also may contribute to hypoglycemia in malnutrition, muscle-wasting states, chronic renal failure, and late pregnancy. Acquired liver disease can cause serious hypoglycemia. Hepatic congestion due to right-sided heart failure is particularly troublesome, and severe viral hepatitis or cirrhosis also can cause hypoglycemia. Hypothermia, especially in association with alcohol ingestion, may cause very low levels of plasma glucose. Slowed enzymatic activity of the liver is the likely mechanism. The hypoglycemia of renal failure has multiple causes. Some patients have diminished release of alanine (and possibly of glutamine) from muscle, and uremic toxins may suppress hepatic gluconeogenesis. With end-stage renal disease, diminished kidney mass decreases the capacity for renal gluconeogenesis. Decreased insulin clearance, although present, is not thought to play a major role.

A number of drugs, in addition to insulin and sulfonylureas, cause hypoglycemia. Alcohol induces hypoglycemia only after a period of fasting sufficient to deplete liver glycogen stores. In this circumstance, hepatic glucose production is dependent on gluconeogenesis. The oxidation of ethanol in the liver generates high concentrations of NADH, the reduced form of nicotinamide adenine dinucleotide (NAD). The increased NADH/NAD ratio diverts oxaloacetate into malate formation, diminishing its availability to the gluconeogenic sequence via the action of phosphoenolpyruvate carboxykinase (see Fig. 335-1). Gluconeogenesis from pyruvate is thus blocked, leading to decreased hepatic glucose output and hypoglycemia. Large amounts of ethanol are not required to produce this syndrome, and plasma alcohol concentrations may be as low as 5.4 mmol/L (25 mg/dL) when symptoms occur. Ethanol-induced hypoglycemia usually occurs in adults but can occur in children who drink alcohol unknowingly. Many reports of the association between hypoglycemia and drugs are probably due to chance occurrence. Pentamidine, sulfonamides, salicylates (usually in children), propranolol, and quinine probably do cause hypoglycemia rarely. Pentamidine (no longer used commonly for prevention of *Pneumocystis* pneumonia in AIDS patients) induces β-cell cytolysis ("insulin leak"). The mechanism by which sulfonamides and salicylates induce hypoglycemia is unclear but may involve interaction of the agents with the sulfonylurea receptor (see below). Quinine has been reported to cause hyperinsulinemic hypoglycemia, but the issue

Table 335-3

Major Causes of Fasting Hypoglycemia

PRIMARILY DUE TO IMPAIRED PRODUCTION OF GLUCOSE	
Hormone deficiencies	**Liver disease**
Hypopituitarism	Hepatic congestion
Adrenal insufficiency	Severe hepatitis
Catecholamine deficiency	Cirrhosis
Glucagon deficiency	Uremia (probably multiple mechanisms)
Enzyme defects	Hypothermia
Glucose-6-phosphatase	**Drugs**
Liver phosphorylase	Alcohol
Pyruvate carboxylase	Propranolol
Phosphoenolpyruvate carboxykinase	Salicylates
Fructose-1,6-bisphosphatase	
Glycogen synthetase	
Substrate deficiency	
Ketotic hypoglycemia of infancy	
Severe malnutrition, muscle wasting	
Late pregnancy	
PRIMARILY DUE TO OVERUTILIZATION OF GLUCOSE	
Hyperinsulinism	
Insulinoma	
Exogenous insulin	
Sulfonylureas	
Immune disease with insulin or insulin receptor antibodies	
Drugs: quinine in falciparum malaria, disopyramide, pentamidine	
Sepsis	
Appropriate insulin levels	
Extrapancreatic tumors	
Systemic carnitine deficiency	
Deficiency in enzymes of fat oxidation	
3-Hydroxy-3-methylglutaryl-CoA lyase deficiency	
Cachexia with fat depletion	

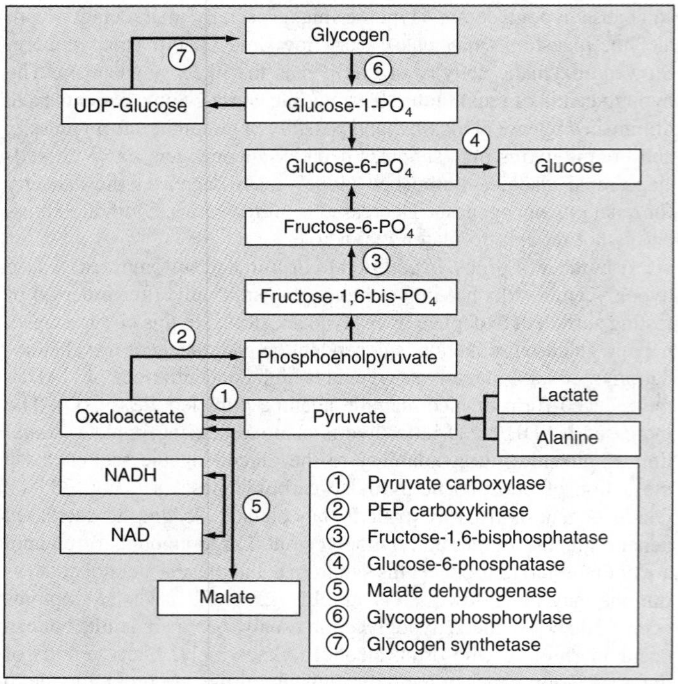

FIGURE 335-1 Scheme of hepatic carbohydrate metabolism. Only the sequences for gluconeogenesis, glycogen synthesis, and glycogenolysis are shown.

is clouded, because hypoglycemia also occurs in untreated malaria, possibly owing to malnutrition, liver involvement, or cytokine release.

Overutilization of glucose Overutilization of glucose occurs in two settings: when hyperinsulinism is present and when plasma insulin concentrations are low. There are four causes of hyperinsulinemic hypoglycemia: insulinoma, administration of exogenous insulin or of sulfonylureas, and a peculiar form of insulin autoimmunity. *Insulinoma* is used generically here to include single solid tumors, microadenomatosis, and islet cell hyperplasia (nesidioblastosis), a rare syndrome in adults. Familial hyperinsulinemic hypoglycemia of infancy is due to a gain-of-function mutation in the sulfonylurea receptor that causes constitutive, unregulated insulin secretion. Hypoglycemia in a diabetic taking prescribed insulin or oral agents is not a diagnostic problem. The difficulty occurs when a nondiabetic individual induces hypoglycemia deliberately and surreptitiously because of psychiatric disturbance, raising the possibility of an insulin-producing tumor. The diagnostic differentiation of insulinoma and factitious hypoglycemia is considered below. Rarely, hypoglycemia with hyperinsulinism is due to antibodies to endogenous insulin. The mechanisms underlying hypoglycemia in the latter condition are not well understood, although the most important is probably dissociation of free insulin from hormone-antibody complexes at inappropriate times. Idiotypic antibodies (antibodies against the anti-insulin antibodies) also might function as insulin agonists with the insulin receptor. By binding insulin, the antibodies also may induce excessive release of insulin from the pancreas. Some patients have alternating insulin resistance/hyperglycemia and hypoglycemia. Insulin autoantibodies have been seen most frequently in subjects with hyperthyroidism treated with methimazole but presumably can occur in any autoimmune syndrome. Antibodies directed against the insulin receptor, usually a cause of insulin resistance, also may induce hypoglycemia with high plasma insulin levels. Under these circumstances, the configuration of the antibody is thought to allow it to activate the insulin receptor, simultaneously blocking the clearance of insulin.

Sepsis with endotoxinemia causes hyperglycemia followed by hypoglycemia in experiment animals. Enhanced insulin release is thought to be caused by sepsis-associated cytokine release, probably acting directly on the β cells.

Hypoglycemia in the context of glucose overutilization and appropriately low plasma insulin concentrations occurs in two situations. The first is in association with solid extrapancreatic tumors, usually fibromas and sarcomas of large size but occasionally hepatomas, carcinomas of the gastrointestinal tract, renal cell carcinomas, or adrenal cancers. The mechanism of the hypoglycemia is not clear, although high levels of insulin-like growth factor (IGF)-2 are believed to play a role. The physiologic role of IGF-2 is not completely understood, although it is associated with organ hypertrophy (e.g., Beckwith-Wiedemann syndrome) and appears to function as an oncogene in Wilms' tumor of the kidney. IGF-2 could cause hypoglycemia through its own receptor or by interacting with the insulin receptor. One patient with tumor-associated hypoglycemia was reported to have an increased number of insulin receptors in liver, muscle, and circulating mononuclear cells, but the significance of the finding is not clear.

Hypoglycemia due to overutilization also may occur when fatty acids and ketones are not available for oxidation in muscle and other tissues. Patients with *systemic carnitine deficiency* can have severe hypoglycemia. In this condition, the level of carnitine, a metabolite that is necessary for the transportation of fatty acids into mitochondria for oxidation, is low in plasma, muscle, liver, and other tissues. As a consequence, peripheral tissues cannot utilize fatty acids for energy production, and the liver cannot make ketone bodies as alternative substrate. The result is that all tissues become glucose-dependent, and the liver's capacity to meet the demand is exceeded. Other features of systemic carnitine deficiency include nausea, vomiting, elevated blood ammonia levels, and hepatic encephalopathy. The illness thus constitutes one form of the Reye syndrome. (In *myopathic carnitine deficiency*, only muscle is involved, and a polymyositis-like syndrome without hypoglycemia is produced.) Nonketotic (or hypoketotic) hypoglycemia with secondary systemic carnitine deficiency and the Reye syndrome also accompany *deficiencies of medium- and long-chain acyl-CoA dehydrogenases and 3-hydroxy-3-methylglutaryl-CoA (HMG-CoA) lyase.* The first two enzymes operate in the fatty acid oxidative sequence, while HMG-CoA lyase catalyzes the conversion of HMG-CoA to acetoacetate and acetyl-CoA in the ketogenic cycle. Any time there is a block in fatty acid oxidation or ketone formation, a secondary carnitine deficiency may develop. Accumulated acyl-CoA is transesterified to form acyl carnitine, which is then lost in the urine. Systemic carnitine deficiency in the absence of an enzymic defect probably is due to a primary renal leak. It is not known whether the block in ketone production per se leads to hypoglycemia or whether secondary carnitine deficiency is required. If the former is the case, ketones must become a primary (necessary) substrate during an extended fast. Hypoglycemia is less common with deficiency of *carnitine palmitoyltransferases.* Presumably, the defect is not complete in most patients, so that some fatty acid oxidation occurs, and the tendency to hypoglycemia is minimized. The clinical picture is that of an exercise-induced myopathy with myoglobinuria. Hypoglycemia also occurs in patients with cachexia due to advanced cancer. At autopsy, no recognizable triglyceride stores are present in adipose tissue, suggesting that free fatty acid deficiency is the primary mechanism.

Hypoglycemia in Hospitalized Patients The frequency of this diagnosis varies in different series of hospitalized patients. Drugs are the most common cause, the three drugs most frequently implicated being insulin, sulfonylureas, and alcohol. It has been estimated that one of these three agents is involved in about 60 percent of the instances in which hypoglycemia is diagnosed in this population. Other causes include renal failure (about 15 percent), liver disease (about 15 percent), malnutrition (about 10 percent), and sepsis (about 5 percent). The finding of hypoglycemia in nondiabetic persons without uremia, liver disease, cachexia, or a history of alcohol intake should raise a high index of suspicion for insulinoma, solid tumors, enzymatic defects, or hormonal deficiencies.

DIAGNOSIS **Fasting Hypoglycemia** If a person with diabetes mellitus presents with symptoms of hypoglycemia, it is usually safe to conclude that no special diagnostic tests are needed because such hypoglycemia is almost always related to therapy. If a nondiabetic develops similar symptoms—particularly if confusion, loss of consciousness, or convulsions are present—a diagnostic workup is required. If the patient is seen in the office or emergency room with symptoms compatible with hypoglycemia, blood should be drawn for a glucose and hormone assay before intravenous glucose is administered. *The ideal time for a diagnosis is during an episode of spontaneous hypoglycemia.* The goal is to assess the plasma insulin level and the counterregulatory hormone response while the plasma glucose level is low. Assays should be carried out for glucose, insulin, insulin-connecting peptide (C peptide), cortisol, drugs, and toxins, especially sulfonylureas and alcohol. It is often wise to freeze a separate sample of plasma for subsequent tests (for example, for proinsulin, carnitine, insulin antibodies, or lactate) should the diagnosis not be clear from the initial evaluation. Demonstration that hypoglycemia is accompanied by inappropriate insulin levels sharply narrows the clinical possibilities.

If the patient is not seen during a hypoglycemic episode, the approach is somewhat different. The pattern of symptomatic episodes should be ascertained with an emphasis on the relation to food intake and the timing of symptom development (namely, during or after the overnight fast or after daytime meals). Obtaining a medication history is essential. Signs of heart failure and hepatic congestion should be sought, and the presence and thickness of the adipose tissue mass should be noted. Pigmentation of the skin may suggest adrenal insufficiency. The workup includes liver function studies and computed tomography (CT) or abdominal sonography (to look for solid tumors in the retroperitoneal space or abdominal cavity). Patients with enzyme defects and rare hormonal deficiencies (epinephrine, glucagon) usually require evaluation in referral centers, since assays for these hormones and enzymes are not routinely available. If hypoglycemia is severe or prolonged in a hospitalized patient, it is important to quantitate the amount of glucose required to prevent recurrent hypoglycemia during acute-phase therapy; if 8 to 10 g of glucose per hour is sufficient to prevent hypoglycemia, diminished glucose production is probably operative. A requirement for infusion rates higher than that suggests enhanced glucose utilization.

If the patient has a history compatible with recurrent unexplained hypoglycemia but does not have symptoms at the time of examination, hospitalization for fasting has traditionally been required. The fast should be carried out for at least 72 h unless symptoms develop. Plasma glucose, insulin, C peptide, and cortisol should be measured every 6 h. Occasionally, quantitation of plasma free fatty acids, glucagon, and total ketones is helpful. (For the glucagon assay, a protease inhibitor such as aprotinin must be added.) Two points are at issue. First, does the patient have fasting hypoglycemia? Second, is the hypoglycemia associated with hyperinsulinism? Neither question is easy to answer. There is no definitive lower limit of plasma glucose that unequivocally defines pathologic hypoglycemia during a 72-h fast. Values of the nadir in one study are shown in Table 335-4. Women usually develop lower levels than men. Another series reported mean minimal levels of 3.4 mmol/L (62 mg/dL) in men and 2.9 mmol/L (52 mg/dL) in women during a 72-h fast. However, values as low as 1.2 mmol/L (22 mg/dL) may occur in normal women without symptoms. On balance, a presumptive diagnosis of hypoglycemia is probably justified if the plasma glucose falls below 2.5 mmol/L (45 mg/dL) in venous blood at any time during the fast, provided typical symptoms are induced. The diagnosis of hypoglycemia is strengthened if symptoms are rapidly relieved by administration of glucose. If symptoms do not occur during a 72-h fast, the diagnosis of hypoglycemia should be made with caution.

Insulin measurements are not always helpful in diagnosing hyperinsulinism. In normal subjects when glucose concentrations rise, insulin levels also increase, and when plasma glucose concentrations fall, insulin release is inhibited. This relationship means that plasma insulin concentrations must be interpreted in the light of the simultaneously determined glucose value. Thus, a "normal" insulin level may be abnormal in the face of hypoglycemia, while high levels may be appropriate if the glucose level is elevated.

Plasma insulin levels generally reach background values for the assay when the plasma glucose falls below about 4.6 mmol/L (83 mg/dL), as noted earlier. While some studies have shown lower cutoff points, any measurable insulin level should probably be considered suspicious if the venous plasma glucose is below 2.5 mmol/L (45 mg/dL). If hyperinsulinism is not present, another cause of fasting hypoglycemia must be sought.

Some investigators screen for insulinoma in the outpatient setting. The C peptide suppression test is based on the fact that suppression of the release of endogenous insulin and C peptide during insulin infusion is impaired in persons with insulinomas. The results are influenced by age and obesity. Less well standardized tests involve intravenous tolbutamide infusion and rigorous exercise in the fasted state. However, the 72-h fast remains the gold standard when the patient cannot be studied during a spontaneous episode of hypoglycemia.

If hypoglycemia does not develop during fasting, an insulinoma or other hypoglycemia-producing organic disease is unlikely, although in rare cases (<2 percent) an insulinoma does not cause hypoglycemia during a prolonged fast. Insulinomas rarely cause only postprandial hypoglycemia. The diagnosis usually is suspected in such cases because insulin levels are inappropriately high during the postmeal episodes.

Postprandial Hypoglycemia In patients presumed to have postprandial hypoglycemia, the most widely used test in the past was the 5-h oral glucose tolerance test. Since normal persons may have chemical hypoglycemia without symptoms in the glucose tolerance test and since subjects with pseudohypoglycemia have symptoms in the absence of hypoglycemia following meals, the 5-h glucose tolerance test should be abandoned as a tool for diagnosis. The only unequivocal diagnostic test for true pseudohypoglycemia is the demonstration of a low plasma glucose concentration (less than 2.5 mmol/L, or 45 mg/dL) during the occurrence of spontaneous symptoms. Some physicians use a home glucose analyzer in diagnosis. If no hypoglycemia is demonstrated during 1 week of testing (on arising, 2 h after each meal, at bedtime, and during symptoms), the diagnosis of true postprandial hypoglycemia is rejected. Most authors consider home testing unreliable because of measurement inaccuracies in the hypoglycemic range. Patients with pseudohypoglycemia usually have slightly elevated glucose concentrations during spontaneous attacks because of the hyperglycemic action of epinephrine, the stress hormone that induces the symptoms.

Insulinoma versus Factitious Hypoglycemia The self-induction of hypoglycemia by the injection of insulin or the ingestion of sulfonylureas is probably as common as insulinoma. Therefore, the demonstration of hyperinsulinism during hypoglycemia is not definitive evidence for an islet cell tumor. Factitious disease should be suspected when hypoglycemic symptoms appear in medical personnel or relatives of diabetic patients. Several tests are helpful in distinguishing insulinoma from factitious hypoglycemia once hyperinsulinism is established. Patients with insulinoma tend to have high concentrations of proinsulin in plasma (>20 percent of total insulin). Plasma proinsulin is not elevated by the administration of insulin or sulfonylureas.

Table 335-4

Mean Plasma Glucose and Insulin during Fasting in Normal Individuals

Assay	Subjects	Hours of Fast: 0*	24	36	48	72
Glucose, mmol/L (mg/dL)	Men	4.7 (85)	4.6 (83)	4.3 (78)	4.3 (78)	3.9 (71)
	Women	4.6 (83)	3.5 (63)	2.8 (50)	2.6 (46)	2.7 (48)
Insulin, pmol/L (μU/mL)	Men	100 (14)	64 (9)	57 (8)	57 (8)	43 (6)
	Women	86 (12)	43 (6)	29 (4)	21 (3)	29 (4)

* Zero values were obtained after overnight fast. Results are mean values for 20 normal men and 60 normal women.

SOURCE: TJ Merimee, JE Tyson, Diabetes 26:161, 1977.

Table 335-5

Differential Diagnosis of Insulinoma and Factitious Hyperinsulinism

Test	Insulinoma	Exogenous Insulin	Sulfonylurea
Plasma insulin	High	Very high*	High
Insulin/glucose ratio	High	Very high	High
Proinsulin	Increased	Normal or low	Normal
C peptide	Increased	Normal or low†	Increased
Insulin antibodies	Absent	± Present‡	Absent
Plasma or urine sulfonylurea	Absent	Absent	Present

* Total plasma insulin in patients with insulinoma is rarely above 1435 pmol/L (200 μU/mL) in the basal state and often is much lower. Values greater than 7175 pmol/L (1000 μU/mL) are highly suggestive of exogenous insulin injection.

† C-peptide level may be normal in absolute terms but low in relation to the increased insulin value. See text for C-peptide suppression test.

‡ Insulin antibodies may not be present if only a few injections have been given, especially with purified insulin.

Measurement of the C-peptide level will indicate whether plasma insulin is of endogenous or exogenous origin. When insulin is cleaved from its precursor proinsulin molecule, C peptide is released into the portal vein in a 1:1 ratio with insulin. Thus, in patients with insulinoma, C-peptide levels should parallel plasma insulin values. The characteristic pattern in factitious hypoglycemia due to insulin injection is a high level of plasma insulin and a low plasma level of C peptide, because exogenous insulin, which does not contain C peptide, suppresses endogenous insulin release in normal persons, as described earlier. Antibodies to insulin are helpful if present because they usually indicate chronic insulin injection. Sulfonylureas elevate the concentrations of both C peptide and insulin in plasma. Therefore, factitious hypoglycemia due to oral agents can only be diagnosed by a high index of suspicion coupled with assay of the drug in plasma or urine. The features of insulinoma and the two types of factitious hypoglycemia are shown in Table 335-5.

℞ TREATMENT

The initial treatment of serious hypoglycemia (producing confusion or coma) is the intravenous administration of a bolus of 25 or 50 g glucose as a 50% solution followed by constant infusion of glucose until the patient is able to eat a meal. The importance of eating is due to the fact that repletion of hepatic glycogen is ineffective with small quantities of intravenous glucose. Patients in the overutilization-category may require large amounts of intravenous glucose to maintain consciousness. It is not enough to infuse 5% dextrose at a rate of 1 to 2 mL/min and assume the patient is protected (20% to 30% dextrose solutions may be required in some cases). Capillary glucose levels should be measured frequently during the acute treatment phase. Intravenous glucose usually can be stopped once the patient has eaten, but that can only be determined by trial. Adrenergic reactions without central nervous system abnormalities can be treated with oral carbohydrate and do not require parenteral therapy.

Hypoglycemia caused by sulfonylureas may last for prolonged periods (days) (Fig. 335-2), and patients may lapse back into coma if glucose infusions are stopped too soon. The reason for the prolonged effect is not always clear, though drug interactions, hepatic disease, and renal failure may play a role in some cases.

Surgery is the treatment of choice for insulinoma. The tumor is best localized by endoscopic ultrasonography. Intraoperative ultrasound may be useful if preoperative localization was unsuccessful. CT, magnetic resonance imaging, and arteriography are not as reliable. If the tumor cannot be found in the pancreas or in an extrapancreatic site at the time of surgery, stepwisepancreatectomy (from tail to head) should be carried out with examination of frozen sections of sequential slices. Capillary glucose should be measured at each stage of the resection if the tumor is not obvious. A rise in plasma glucose may indicate removal of a small, nonpalpable lesion. In general, resection is stopped with an 85 percent pancreatectomy, even if the tumor is not found, to avoid malabsorption. While most patients are cured by surgery, as many as 15 percent have persistent hypoglycemia. Postoperative complications include acute pancreatitis, peritonitis, fistulas, pseudocyst formation, and diabetes mellitus.

Medical treatment for insulinoma is indicated only in preparation for surgery or after failure to find the tumor at operation. Two drugs are available, diazoxide and octreotide, an analogue of somatostatin. Diazoxide can be given intravenously or orally in doses of 300 to 1200 mg/d. Because of its salt-retaining properties, it must be accompanied by a diuretic. Octreotide is given subcutaneously in divided doses of 100 to 600 μg/d. Chronic use may cause nausea and diarrhea and predispose to cholelithiasis. Treatment of insulin-producing carcinomas is unsatisfactory. It has been reported that streptozocin plus doxorubicin is superior to streptozocin plus fluorouracil (median survival 2.2 and 1.4 years, respectively). The use of chlorozotocin is currently under study; this agent appears to produce fewer toxic side effects than streptozocin. Despite the poor prognosis, occasional patients with islet cell carcinomas survive for long periods.

Therapy of other forms of recurrent hypoglycemia, apart from hormone replacement in cases of pituitary or adrenal insufficiency, is dietary. In most cases, avoidance of fasting is all that is required. This measure is critical in diseases of fat oxidation or ketone synthesis. If intercurrent illness prevents eating, hospitalization for intravenous glucose administration is absolutely required. A high-protein, low-carbohydrate diet may relieve symptoms in patients with pseudohypoglycemia. The most effective agents for pseudohypoglycemia are beta-adrenergic blockers, propranolol probably being the most effective. With true alimentary hypoglycemia, the size of the individual meals should be small. The practice of giving massive amounts of vitamin E, crude adrenocortical extract, and trace metals to patients with pseudohypoglycemia is useless even if harmless (which has not been established).

BIBLIOGRAPHY

Brackett JC et al: A novel mutation in medium chain acyl-CoA dehydrogenase causes sudden neonatal death. J Clin Invest 94:1477, 1994

Charles MA et al: Comparison of oral glucose tolerance tests and mixed meals in patients with apparent idiopathic postabsorptive hypoglycemia: Absence of hypoglycemia after meals. Diabetes 30:465, 1981

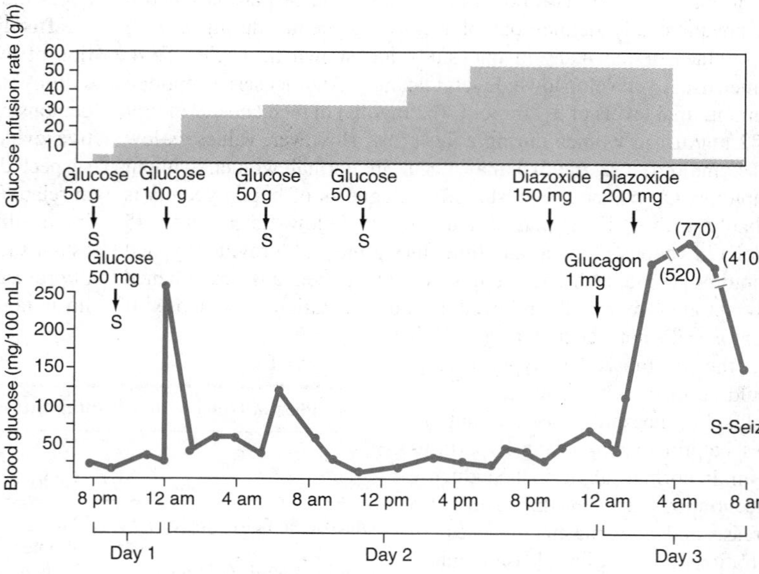

FIGURE 335-2 Prolonged and refractory hypoglycemia in factitious hypoglycemia due to chlorpropamide in an alcoholic. Note continued hypoglycemia despite the infusion of glucose at rates up to 50 g/h. *(From RM Jordan et al, Arch Intern Med 137:390, 1977. Copyright 1977, American Medical Association. Used by permission.)*

CRYER PE: Glucose counterregulation: Prevention and correction of hypoglycemia in humans. Am J Physiol 264:E149, 1993
——— et al: Hypoglycemia. Diabetes Care 17:734, 1994
DAUGHADAY WH: The pathophysiology of IGF-II hypersecretion in non-islet tumor hypoglycemia. Diabetes Rev 3:62, 1995
DE FEO P et al: Modest decrements in plasma glucose concentration cause early impairment in cognitive function and later activation of glucose counterregulation in the absence of hypoglycemic symptoms in normal man. J Clin Invest 82:436, 1988
GRUNBERGER G et al: Factitious hypoglycemia due to surreptitious administration of insulin: Diagnosis, treatment, and long-term follow-up. Ann Intern Med 108:252, 1988
KLONOFF DC et al: Hypoglycemia following inadvertent or factitious sulfonylurea overdosage. Diabetes Care 18:563, 1995
MERIMEE TJ: Insulin-like growth factors in patients with nonislet cell tumors and hypoglycemia. Metabolism 35:360, 1986
MOERTEL CG et al: Streptozocin-doxorubicin, streptozocin-fluorouracil, or chlorozotocin in the treatment of advanced islet-cell carcinoma. N Engl J Med 326:519, 1992
MORISON IM et al: Somatic overgrowth associated with overexpression of insulin-like growth factor II. Nature Med 2:321, 1996
PANDIT MK et al: Drug-induced disorders of glucose tolerance. Ann Intern Med 118:529, 1993
PHILIPSON LH, STEINER DF: Pas de deux or more: The sulfonylurea receptor and K^+ channels. Science 268:372, 1995
SERVICE FJ et al: C-peptide suppression test: Effects of gender, age, and body mass index; implications for the diagnosis of insulinoma. J Clin Endocrinol Metab 74:204, 1992
———: Hypoglycemic disorders. N Engl J Med 332:1144, 1995

336

James E. Griffin, Jean D. Wilson

DISORDERS OF THE TESTES

The testes produce sperm and the steroid hormones that regulate male sexual function. Both processes are under complex feedback control by the hypothalamic-pituitary system so that the testes have biosynthetic and regulatory features similar to those of the ovary and the adrenal. Testicular hormones are also responsible for the formation of the basic male phenotype during embryogenesis. The function of the embryonic testis and the disorders of sexual differentiation are described in Chap. 339.

PHYSIOLOGY AND REGULATION OF TESTICULAR FUNCTION The testis consists of two components—clusters of interstitial or Leydig cells, where androgenic steroids are synthesized, and a system of spermatogenic tubules for the production and transport of sperm.

THE LEYDIG CELL **Testosterone Synthesis** The biochemical pathway by which the 27-carbon sterol cholesterol is converted to androgens and estrogens is depicted in Fig. 336-1. Cholesterol can either be synthesized de novo in the Leydig cell or derived from plasma lipoproteins. Five enzymatic transformations are required for the conversion of cholesterol to testosterone. In this process, the side chain of cholesterol is cleaved in two steps to reduce the size of the molecule from 27 to 19 carbons, and the A ring of the steroid is converted to the Δ^4-3-keto configuration. The five enzyme reactions are cholesterol side chain cleavage ($P450_{SCC}$), 3β-hydroxysteroid dehydrogenase/isomerase (3β-HSD), 17α-hydroxylase ($P450_{17\alpha}$), 17,20-lyase ($P450_{17\alpha}$), and 17β-hydroxysteroid dehydrogenase (17β-HSD). Both the 17α-hydroxylase and the 17,20-lyase activities are present in a single cytochrome $P450_{17\alpha}$. The first four reactions take place in the adrenal as well as the testis.

The rate-limiting process in testosterone synthesis is the conversion of cholesterol to pregnenolone by $P450_{SCC}$; luteinizing hormone (LH) from the pituitary regulates the activity of this enzyme and of other enzymes in the pathway. Additional steroids including estradiol are synthesized in small amounts in the Leydig cell.

Testosterone Secretion and Transport Only about 70 nmol (20 μg) of testosterone is stored in the normal testes, so the total hormone content turns over about 200 times each day to provide the average of 17 to 20 μmol (5 to 6 mg) that is secreted into plasma in normal young men (Fig. 336-2). Testosterone is transported in plasma bound to protein, largely to albumin and to a specific transport protein, testosterone-binding globulin (TeBG, also called sex hormone–binding globulin, SHBG). The bound and unbound fractions in plasma are in dynamic equilibrium, only about 1 to 3 percent being unbound. The fraction of circulating testosterone available for entry into tissues approximates the sum of the free and albumin-bound fractions or about half the total plasma testosterone.

Peripheral Metabolism of Androgens Testosterone serves as a circulating precursor (or prohormone) for the formation of two other hormones that mediate many of the physiologic processes involved in androgen action (see Fig. 336-1). Testosterone can be 5α-reduced to dihydrotestosterone, which is responsible for many of the differentiative, growth-promoting, and functional aspects of male sexual differentiation and virilization. Circulating testosterone (and androstenedione) also can be converted to estrogens in extraglandular tissues. In males estrogens act in some instances in concert with androgens, but they also can have effects independent of or opposite to those of androgens. Thus the physiologic effects of testosterone are the result of the combined effects of testosterone itself plus those of the active androgen and estrogen metabolites of the parent molecule. (In normal men, small amounts of estradiol and dihydrotestosterone are also de-

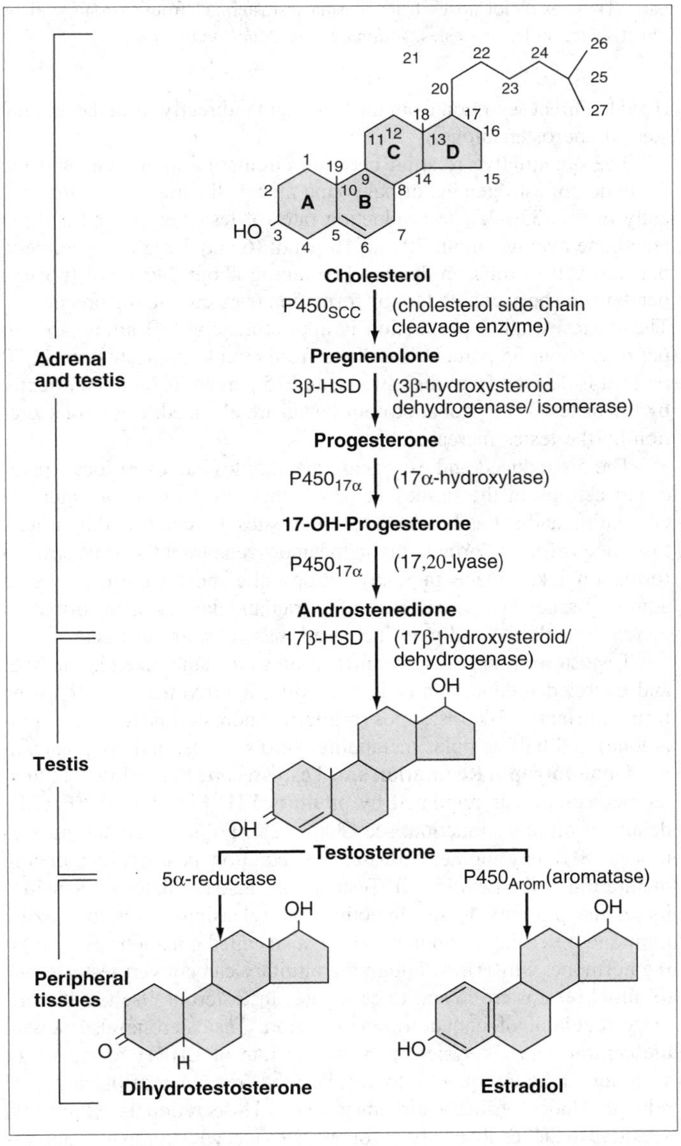

FIGURE 336-1 Pathways of androgen formation in the testis and the conversion of androgens to other active hormones in peripheral tissues.

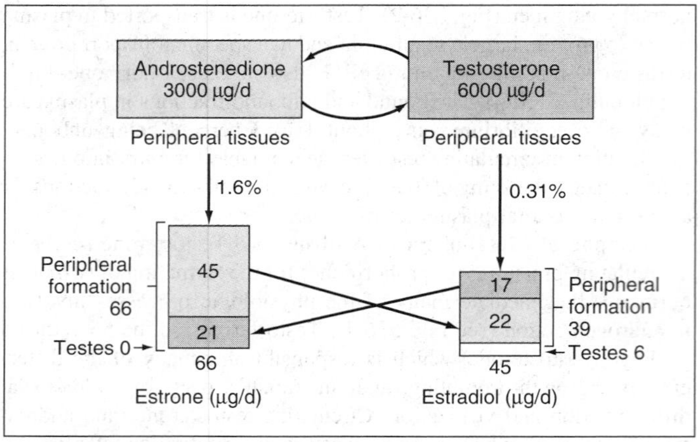

FIGURE 336-2 Androgen and estrogen production in normal young men. The average production of androstenedione and testosterone is shown in the top boxes, and the mean daily production of estrone and estradiol is shown in the lower boxes. Estrogen is formed by extraglandular aromatization (*braces*) or is secreted directly by the testes. *Vertical arrows* indicate the rates of extraglandular aromatization of androgens, and *horizontal arrows* indicate the interconversion of androgen and estrogens by 17β-hydroxysteroid dehydrogenase. Thus, estradiol arises from plasma testosterone, from estrone, and by direct secretion by the testes. *(Adapted from MacDonald et al.)*

rived by direct secretion from the testes and indirectly from the adrenal steroid androstenedione.)

The quantitative relation between circulating androgens and the formation of estrogen in normal young men is illustrated diagrammatically in Fig. 336-2. The production rates of testosterone and androstenedione average about 20 and 10 μmol (6 and 3 mg), respectively, per day. All estrone production [averaging about 240 nmol (66 μg) per day] can be accounted for by formation from circulating precursors. The mean estradiol production is approximately 170 nmol (45 μg) per day; about 35 percent is derived from circulating testosterone, 50 percent is derived from the estrone, and 15 percent is secreted directly by the testes. When gonadotropin levels are elevated, estradiol secretion by the testes increases.

The 5α-reduced and estrogenic metabolites can exert local (paracrine) actions in the tissues in which they are formed or enter the circulation and act as hormones at other sites. Circulating dihydrotestosterone is formed principally in the androgen target tissues; estrogen formation takes place in many tissues, the most significant being adipose tissue. The overall rate of extraglandular estrogen formation increases with age and with increased mass of adipose tissue.

Testosterone and its active metabolites are catabolized in the liver and excreted predominantly in the urine, approximately half in the form of urinary 17-ketosteroids (primarily androsterone and etiocholanolone) and half as polar metabolites (diols, triols, and conjugates).

Gonadotropin Regulation and Testosterone Secretion Testosterone secretion is regulated by pituitary LH (Fig. 336-3). (For the details of pituitary function, see Chap. 328.) Follicle-stimulating hormone (FSH) may augment testosterone secretion, possibly by inducing maturation of the Leydig cell. Testosterone also regulates the sensitivity of the pituitary to the hypothalamic-releasing factor luteinizing hormone–releasing hormone (LHRH, also called gonadotropin-releasing hormone, GnRH). Although the pituitary can convert testosterone to dihydrotestosterone and to estrogens, testosterone itself is the primary regulator of gonadotropin secretion. Testosterone also acts in the central nervous system to slow the rate of LHRH formation or secretion and consequently to decrease the frequency of pulsatile LH release. Under ordinary circumstances, LH secretion is exquisitely sensitive to the feedback effects of testosterone, with complete suppression after the administration of amounts of exogenous androgen that approximate the normal daily secretory rate of testosterone (about 20 μmol or 6 mg). However, prolonged elevation of plasma LH (as in testicular deficiency) renders the pituitary less sensitive to negative feedback control by androgen.

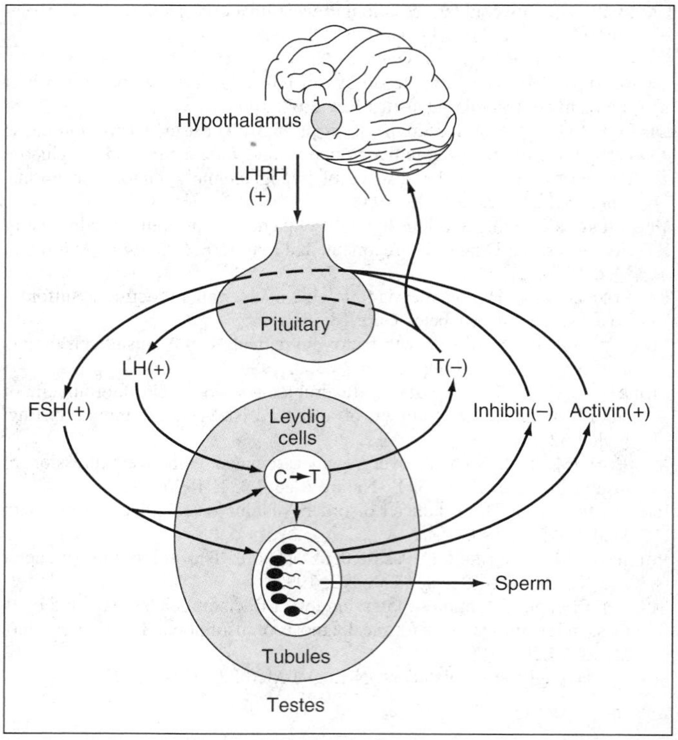

FIGURE 336-3 Regulation of testosterone and sperm production by LH and FSH. (C, cholesterol; T, testosterone.)

The plasma concentration of neither testosterone nor LH is constant, each fluctuating in a pulsatile manner that reflects changes in secretory rates (Fig. 336-4). Major sleep-related surges in the pulsatile secretion of both LH and testosterone signal the beginning of male puberty. In young adults the magnitude of episodic secretion of LH and testosterone varies diurnally, so that peak levels of testosterone are about 25 to 30 percent higher in the morning than in late afternoon.

Androgen Action The major functions of androgen are regulation of LH secretion, formation of the male phenotype during sexual differentiation, and induction of sexual maturation at puberty. The cellular process by which androgens perform these functions is schematized in Fig. 336-5. Testosterone enters the cell by passive diffusion and can be converted to dihydrotestosterone by either 5α-reductase 1 or 2; 5α-reductase 2 is responsible for dihydrotestosterone formation in most androgen target tissues. Testosterone or dihydrotestosterone is then bound to the androgen-receptor protein in the nucleus. The hormone-receptor complex attaches to specific chromosomal sites and regulates the transcription of messenger RNA and, ultimately, the

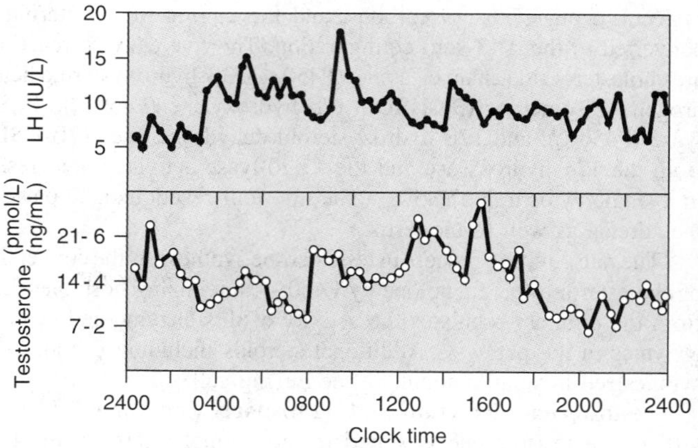

FIGURE 336-4 The 24-h pattern of plasma LH and testosterone in a normal man, as sampled every 20 min. *(From Griffin and Wilson.)*

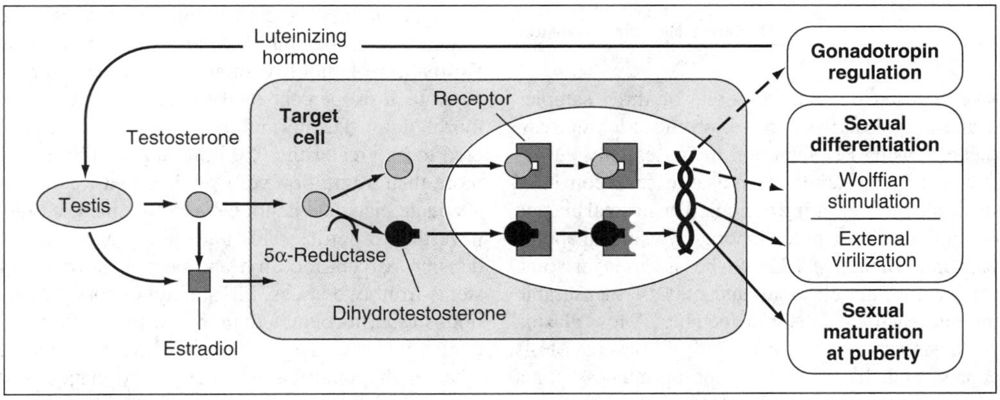

FIGURE 336-5 Current concepts of androgen action.

synthesis of cellular proteins. The androgen receptor is encoded by a gene on the long arm of the X chromosome; it contains 917 amino acids and has a molecular mass of about 110 kDa. It is similar in structure to other steroid hormone receptors and has distinct hormone-binding, DNA-binding, and functional domains (see Chap. 327). Estradiol acts by a mechanism similar to that of androgens but involving its own receptor (see Chap. 337).

Although testosterone and dihydrotestosterone bind to the same receptor, their physiologic roles differ. The testosterone-receptor complex regulates gonadotropin secretion, spermatogenesis, and the virilization of the wolffian ducts during sexual differentiation (see Chap. 339), whereas the dihydrotestosterone-receptor complex is responsible for external virilization during embryogenesis and for most androgen actions during sexual maturation and adult sexual life. The mechanism by which two hormones can interact with the same receptor but have different physiologic effects is also not well understood. Dihydrotestosterone binds to the receptor much more tightly than does testosterone, and hence its formation serves to amplify the hormonal signal.

THE SEMINIFEROUS TUBULE AND SPERMATOGENESIS Normal function of the seminiferous tubule is dependent on the pituitary and on the adjacent Leydig cells, both FSH and androgen being essential for spermatogenesis (see Fig. 336-3). The major site of FSH action is the Sertoli cell in the seminiferous tubules, and the seminiferous tubules also contain androgen receptors. Androgen appears to be essential for spermatogenesis, and FSH is required for spermatid maturation. Several cytokines and growth factors are also thought to be involved in the regulation of spermatogenesis by paracrine and autocrine mechanisms. The normal adult testes produce more than 100 million sperm per day.

The Sertoli cell cannot synthesize steroid hormones de novo and is dependent on testosterone that diffuses in from adjacent Leydig cells. Sertoli cells can convert testosterone to estradiol and to dihydrotestosterone. The seminiferous tubules also produce the peptide hormones inhibin, which exerts a negative feedback control, and activin, which feeds back positively on FSH secretion by the pituitary (see Fig. 336-3). Testosterone and estradiol also can inhibit FSH secretion.

The interlocking system in which two pituitary hormones regulate testicular function provides a precise dual-control mechanism in which hormonal signals from Leydig cells and the spermatogenic tubules feed back on the hypothalamic-pituitary system to regulate their own function (see Fig. 336-3).

ASSESSMENT OF TESTICULAR FUNCTION

LEYDIG CELL FUNCTION **History and Physical Examination** The assessment of Leydig cell function and androgen status should include inquiry about the presence of developmental abnormalities of the urogenital tract, the timing and extent of sexual maturation at puberty, the rate of beard growth, and the current libido, sexual function, strength, and energy. Inadequate Leydig cell function or androgen action during embryogenesis may cause hypospadias, cryptorchidism, or microphallus. If Leydig cell failure occurs prior to puberty, sexual maturation will not occur, and the individual will develop the features termed *eunuchoidism*, including an infantile amount and distribution of body hair, poor development of skeletal muscles, and failure of closure of the epiphyses, so that the arm span is more than 5 cm greater than the height and the lower body segment (heel to pubic bone) is more than 5 cm longer than the upper body segment (pubic bone to crown). Detection of postpubertal Leydig cell failure requires a high index of suspicion and appropriate laboratory assessment. One reason is that decreased sexual function in adult men may be caused by nonendocrine as well as endocrine factors. The second is that certain functions that require androgens for initiation continue unabated when Leydig cell failure occurs, and functions that eventually regress may do so very slowly. For example, the frequency of shaving may not decrease for months or years because of slow decline in the rate of beard growth once established.

Plasma Testosterone and Dihydrotestosterone Levels Plasma testosterone is measured by radioimmunoassay. Testosterone is secreted into plasma in a pulsatile fashion every 60 to 90 min (see Fig. 336-4); a single random sample provides a result within ±20 percent of the true mean value only two-thirds of the time, while three equally spaced samples 15 to 20 min apart provide a more accurate assessment. The samples do not need to be assayed separately, and aliquots of the three samples should be pooled for a single determination. The range of plasma testosterone in normal adult men is 10 to 35 nmol/L (3 to 10 ng/mL). In adult men, the plasma values vary somewhat throughout the day and at different times of the year. In young adult men the level of plasma testosterone is about 30 percent higher in the morning than in the evening. Estimation of TeBG concentration by radioimmunoassay is sometimes useful in the interpretation of total plasma testosterone levels. Bioavailable testosterone in plasma can be estimated by measuring the non-TeBG-bound fraction of testosterone.

The plasma testosterone value is slightly higher in prepubertal boys than in girls, the range in both being 0.2 to 0.7 nmol/L (0.05 to 0.2 ng/mL). The rise in plasma testosterone at the start of male puberty begins as a result of sleep-related nocturnal gonadotropin surges, so that plasma testosterone and LH are initially higher at night than during the day. Random daytime levels of plasma testosterone increase gradually as puberty progresses and reach adult levels at about age 17.

Dihydrotestosterone is also measured by radioimmunoassay. In young men the plasma dihydrotestosterone level is about one-tenth the value for testosterone and averages around 2 nmol/L (0.6 ng/mL). In older men with benign prostatic hyperplasia, plasma dihydrotestosterone levels average about 3 nmol/L (0.9 ng/mL).

Urinary 17-Ketosteroids The measurement of urinary 17-ketosteroids is not a valid way to assess testicular function because testosterone contributes only about 40 percent of urinary 17-ketosteroids in men, the bulk being derived from adrenal androgens.

Plasma LH Plasma LH is also measured by immunoassay. Dual-site immunometric assays have largely replaced competitive radioimmunoassays. LH is secreted in a pulsatile fashion and fluctuates widely so that in adult men a random plasma LH value is likely to be within ±20 percent of true mean value only a third of the time. Again, assay of a pool of plasma composed of equal portions of three samples drawn 15 to 20 min apart, as described above, provides a value approaching the true mean. Plasma LH secretion increases only during sleep in early puberty, but in the adult the pulsatile secretion is of similar magnitude during sleep and waking periods. The normal plasma LH values should be established for a given laboratory using an appropriate standard preparation. Bioactive LH can be assessed in some laboratories by the rat interstitial cell assay and may be measurable at times when the immunoreactive LH is undetectable. A low plasma testosterone level can be interpreted correctly only if plasma LH is measured simultaneously, and, likewise, the "appropriateness" of a given plasma LH value must be interpreted in relation to the plasma testosterone value. For example, a low plasma testosterone level coupled with a low LH level implies hypothalamic or pituitary disease, whereas the finding of a low plasma testosterone level and a high LH level suggests primary testicular insufficiency (see Chap. 327).

Response to Gonadotropin Stimulation Leydig cell function is difficult to assess prior to puberty when both LH and testosterone levels are low, and it is common to measure response of plasma testosterone to gonadotropin stimulation as an index of Leydig cell capacity. Normal prepubertal boys respond to 3 to 5 days of injection of 1000 to 2000 IU of human chorionic gonadotropin (hCG) with an increase in plasma testosterone to about 7 nmol/L (2 ng/mL); the response increases with the initiation of puberty and peaks in early puberty.

Response to Luteinizing Hormone–Releasing Hormone Prior to puberty, quantitative responses of plasma LH and FSH to the administration of LHRH are similar. With pubertal development, the LH response to acute administration of LHRH increases, while the FSH response remains the same. The amount of LH released following acute administration of LHRH probably reflects the amount of stored hormone in the pituitary. When 100 μg LHRH is given subcutaneously or intravenously to normal men, LH levels usually increase four- to fivefold, with the peak level at 30 min. However, the range of response is broad, some normal men having less than a doubling of LH levels. In primary testicular failure, measurement of basal LH is usually sufficient, and measurement of LHRH response is of little aid in diagnosis. Furthermore, since men with either pituitary or hypothalamic disease can have a normal or an abnormal LH response to acute administration of LHRH, a normal response is of no diagnostic value. A subnormal response is of value in establishing that an abnormality exists, even though the site is not determined. The LHRH test is most useful in men with secondary hypogonadism and subnormal LH response to acute administration of LHRH; if daily infusions of LHRH for a week lead to the development of a normal acute LH response, a hypothalamic etiology is likely. This test is rarely performed.

SEMINIFEROUS TUBULE FUNCTION Examination of the Testes Evaluation of the testes is an essential portion of the physical examination. The seminiferous tubules account for about 60 percent of testicular volume. The prepubertal testis measures about 2 cm in length and 2 mL in volume and grows during puberty to reach the adult proportions by age 16. When damage to the seminiferous tubules occurs prior to puberty, the testes are small and firm, whereas the testes are usually small and soft following postpubertal damage (the capsule, once enlarged, does not contract to its previous size). Testes in adults average 4.6 cm in length (range, 3.5 to 5.5 cm), corresponding to a volume of 12 to 25 mL. Advanced age does not influence testicular size, so the significance of small testes is the same at all ages in the adult. Testis size varies among ethnic groups. Asian men have smaller testes than western Europeans, independent of differences in body size. Because of its possible causal role in infertility, the presence of varicocele should be sought by palpation with the patient standing.

Semen Analysis Seminal fluid analysis is performed on samples obtained by masturbation into a glass container after 24 to 36 h of abstinence. Analysis should be performed within an hour. The normal ejaculate volume is 2 to 6 mL. Immediately after ejaculation, the seminal fluid coagulates, followed in 15 to 30 min by liquefaction. Estimation of motility should be made on undiluted seminal fluid; more than 60 percent of the sperm should be motile and of normal morphology. The normal range for sperm density is generally considered to be greater than 20 million per milliliter, with a total count of more than 60 million per ejaculate, but the definition of a minimally adequate ejaculate is not clear. Some men with low sperm counts are nevertheless fertile. This uncertainty as to the lower level of sperm density, percent motility, and percent normal forms in fertile semen stems from two issues. First, many factors produce temporary aberrations in sperm count, and in men who present with semen of equivocal quality it is necessary to examine three or more ejaculates to determine whether the abnormal findings are permanent or temporary. Second, the seminal fluid is routinely evaluated by tests that do not assess the functional capacity of sperm.

Plasma FSH Plasma FSH, as measured by immunoassay, usually correlates inversely with spermatogenesis. When damage to the germinal epithelium is severe, plasma levels of inhibin B fall, and plasma levels of FSH increase.

Testicular Biopsy Testicular biospy is useful in some patients with oligospermia and azoospermia both as an aid in diagnosis and as an indication of the feasibility of treatment. For example, normal findings on testicular biopsy and a normal FSH level in an azoospermic man suggest obstruction of the vas deferens, which may be correctable surgically.

ESTROGENIC FUNCTION Examination of the Breasts Breast enlargement (gynecomastia) is the most consistent feature of feminizing states in men (see Chap. 338). Gynecomastia is due to an increase in both glandular and adipose tissue. The presence of gynecomastia should be sought by examining the sitting patient, using the fingers to grasp glandular tissue. Palpation with the flat of the hand while the patient is supine may result in failure to detect early or minimal breast enlargement. In obese men it is important to try to define the rim of the glandular tissue where it meets the adipose tissue of the chest wall.

Plasma Estrogen As discussed above, most of the estradiol and all of the estrone produced in normal men is formed by extraglandular aromatization of circulating androgens. The plasma level of estradiol is usually less than 180 pmol/L (50 pg/mL) in normal men; the plasma estrone level is somewhat higher but usually is less than 300 pmol/L (80 pg/mL). Elevations in estrogen production and estrogen plasma levels can be due to elevations in plasma precursors (liver or adrenal disease), to increases in extraglandular aromatization (obesity), or to increased production by the testes (testicular tumors or androgen resistance).

PHASES OF NORMAL TESTICULAR FUNCTION

The phases of male sexual life can be defined in terms of the plasma testosterone value (Fig. 336-6). In the male embryo the production of testosterone by the testes commences at about 7 weeks of gestation. Shortly thereafter, plasma testosterone attains a high value that is maintained until late in gestation. The level then falls so that at the time of birth plasma testosterone is only slightly higher in males than in females. Shortly after birth, plasma testosterone in the male infant again begins to rise and remains elevated for approximately 3 months, falling to low levels by age 6 months to 1 year. The concentration then remains low (but slightly higher in boys than in girls) until the onset of puberty, when it begins to rise in boys, reaching adult levels by about age 17. The level of bioavailable testosterone remains constant until the 40s when it begins to decline at a rate of about 1.2 percent per year; the level of TeBG increases by about 1.2 percent per year so that there is little decline in total testosterone until the later decades of life. During the third, or adult, phase of male sexual life, sperm production becomes sufficient to allow reproduction to take place. The physiologic events during these various phases differ, as do the pathologic consequences of derangements in testicular func-

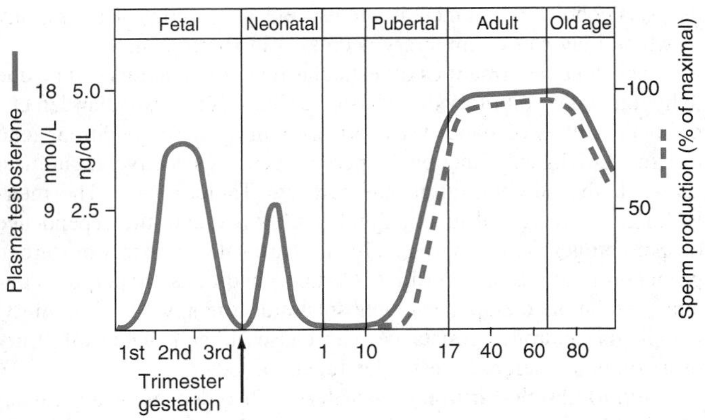

FIGURE 336-6 Phases of male sexual life. *(From Griffin and Wilson.)*

tion. Male sexual differentiation during embryogenesis is considered in Chap. 339. The role of the surge of testosterone formation during the first year of life is not certain. However, in primates, neonatal activation of the hypothalamic-pituitary-testicular axis is important for subsequent normal pubertal development. The focus of this chapter is on testicular pathophysiology during puberty, adulthood, and old age.

ABNORMALITIES OF TESTICULAR FUNCTION

PUBERTY The control of puberty is poorly understood and may reside in the hypothalamic-pituitary system, the testes, or the adrenals. Prior to the onset of puberty, gonadotropin secretion by the pituitary is low, but prepubertal castration results in a rise in plasma gonadotropin levels. This suggests that prior to puberty the negative feedback control of gonadotropin secretion is exquisitely sensitive to the small amount of circulating testosterone. The onset of puberty is heralded by sleep-associated surges in gonadotropin secretion. Later in puberty the rises in LH and FSH levels persist throughout the day. Thus, with maturation, the hypothalamic-pituitary system becomes less sensitive to negative feedback control, and the consequences are a higher mean plasma testosterone level, maturation of the testes, and the onset of spermatogenesis. The rise in gonadotropin secretion is the consequence of both an increase in LHRH secretion and an increase in the sensitivity of the pituitary to LHRH. Plasma levels of bioactive LH increase even more than those of immunoreactive hormone. The somatic changes at the time of puberty are secondary to the rise in plasma testosterone. Growth of the accessory organs of male reproduction (the penis, the prostate, the seminal vesicles, and the epididymides) accounts for about one-fourth of androgen-mediated nitrogen retention during puberty. Accelerated linear growth is accompanied by growth of muscle and connective tissue, accounting for the major portion of nitrogen retention at puberty. The principal androgen-sensitive muscles are those of the pectoral region and the shoulder. The characteristic hair growth of male puberty involves development of mustache and beard; regression of the scalp line; appearance of body, extremity, and perianal hair; and extension of the pubic hair upward into a diamond-shaped pattern. Growth of axillary and pubic hair is initiated under the control of adrenal androgens and is promoted by testicular androgens. The larynx enlarges, and the vocal cords thicken, resulting in a lowering of the pitch of the voice. Hemoglobin levels increase by about 10 g/L. These various androgen-mediated growth and maturation processes reach some limiting value so that once puberty is completed the administration of pharmacologic doses of androgen has no further effect. The entire process is heralded by testicular enlargement beginning at age 11 to 12 and is usually completed within 5 years, although some aspects of virilization, such as growth of the chest hair, may continue over a decade or more.

The events of normal male puberty are variable in onset, duration, and sequence. The central issue in dealing with disorders of puberty is separating true absence or precocity from the extremes of normal variation. The use of staging criteria that correlate developmental and anatomic landmarks with chronologic age is useful in making this distinction (see Marshall and Tanner).

Sexual Precocity Premature development of sexual characteristics that are phenotypically appropriate—i.e., virilization in boys—is termed *isosexual precocity. Heterosexual precocity* refers to feminizing syndromes in boys.

Isosexual precocity Sexual development prior to age 9 in boys is generally considered abnormal. *True precocious puberty* or *complete isosexual precocity* occurs when both virilization and spermatogenesis are premature, and *precocious pseudopuberty* or *incomplete isosexual precocity* refers to virilization unaccompanied by spermatogenesis. This distinction is blurred in practice, because pure virilizing syndromes may cause activation of gonadotropin secretion secondarily and thus be followed by development of spermatogenesis. Furthermore, local androgen production in the testis, as in Leydig cell tumors, can cause local areas of spermatogenesis and limited sperm production around the tumor. We therefore prefer a two-part classification: virilizing syndromes (in which hypothalamic-pituitary activity is appropriate for age) and premature activation of the hypothalamic-pituitary system.

Virilizing syndromes can result from Leydig cell tumors, hCG-secreting tumors, adrenal tumors, congenital adrenal hyperplasia (most commonly 21-hydroxylase deficiency), androgen administration, or Leydig cell hyperplasia. In these disorders plasma testosterone levels are inappropriately elevated for the age. Leydig cell tumors are rare in children but should be suspected when the testes are asymmetric in size (see Chap. 98). Virilizing adrenal tumors mainly secrete androstenedione and dehydroepiandrosterone, some of which is converted to testosterone; consequently, they cause elevated 17-ketosteroid excretion. Glucocorticoid administration does not suppress 17-ketosteroid excretion to normal in patients with testicular or adrenal tumors, in contrast to the prompt decrease that occurs after such treatment in congenital adrenal hyperplasia. Congenital adrenal hyperplasia leads to elevated 17-hydroxyprogesterone levels and, as a consequence, elevated androgen levels (see Chaps. 332 and 339). When this disorder is treated with glucocorticoids, true precocious puberty can then result if the increased androgen levels have caused sufficient hypothalamic maturation.

Gonadotropin-independent sexual precocity in boys may occur as a result of autonomous Leydig cell hyperplasia in the absence of a Leydig cell tumor. The disorder is inherited as a male-limited autosomal disorder either from affected fathers or from mothers who are unaffected carriers and is due to point mutations in the LH receptor that cause constitutive activation of the receptor in the absence of LH. Virilization begins usually by age 2. Testosterone levels are elevated, often to the adult male range; however, immunoreactive and bioactive LH levels and the LH response to LHRH are prepubertal. In the past many of these boys were mistakenly thought to have true precocious puberty because spermatogenesis may be present.

Premature activation of the hypothalamic-pituitary system may be "idiopathic" or due to central nervous system (CNS) tumors, infections, or injuries. Early hypothalamic-pituitary activation typically is associated with features of normal puberty, i.e., sleep-related gonadotropin secretion, elevated plasma bioactive LH, and enhanced gonadotropin response to LHRH. Since the diagnosis of idiopathic true precocious puberty is one of exclusion, patients may later prove to have been misclassified and to have a CNS abnormality. With improved means of diagnosis, such as magnetic resonance imaging, delays in diagnosis will probably be less frequent.

Management of sexual precocity due to steroid- or gonadotropin-producing tumors, congenital adrenal hyperplasia, or CNS abnormality is directed toward the primary disease. In boys with Leydig cell hyperplasia, attempts have been made to lower plasma testosterone with medroxyprogesterone acetate or ketoconazole, but the long-term effectiveness of these agents is unknown. Idiopathic true precocious puberty and true precocious puberty due to inoperable CNS lesions are treated with LHRH analogue therapy, which causes reversal of the pubertal maturation, including a decrease in the rate of skeletal development.

Heterosexual precocity Feminization in prepubertal boys can result from absolute or relative increases in estrogen due to a variety of causes (see Chap. 338).

Delayed or Incomplete Puberty The separation of failure of puberty from variants of normal development is one of the most difficult problems in endocrinology. Some boys fail to show the normal spurt of growth and sexual development at the usual time but eventually commence puberty by age 16 or older. Adolescence may then either progress rapidly, or a slow development and growth may continue until age 20 to 22. Many men with delayed onset of puberty attain heights within the normal adult range. At times the history reveals that a parent or sibling had a similar pattern of development. The major problem is to separate this group of boys with delayed puberty from those with organic disorders that impair puberty. Panhypopituitarism and hypothyroidism can cause pubertal failure (see Chaps. 328 and 331). Absent puberty also can result from primary testicular disease; this diagnosis is suspected on the basis of low plasma testosterone and elevated FSH and LH levels. Hereditary androgen resistance (in which plasma testosterone and LH levels are both high) usually causes male pseudohermaphroditism but in mild form may be manifested by absent or incomplete puberty (see Chap. 339).

Most boys with absent puberty have low plasma levels of both testosterone and gonadotropins; in these boys it is necessary to distinguish delayed puberty from isolated gonadotropin deficiency or idiopathic *hypogonadotropic hypogonadism* (*Kallman syndrome*). The manifestations of isolated gonadotropin deficiency vary from boys with eunuchoidal features and testes of prepubertal size to those with partial LH and/or FSH deficiency and some degree of testicular enlargement and pubertal development. Anosmia or hyposmia and cryptorchidism are common. The disorder is inherited as an X-linked recessive trait or as an autosomal dominant trait with variable expressivity. Serum FSH and LH levels are usually below the normal male range, and plasma testosterone levels are low for age. The secretion of other pituitary hormones is usually normal. The defect appears to be in the synthesis or release of LHRH. Defects have been identified in a neural cell adhesion molecule (KAL) involved in the migration of LHRH neurons into the olfactory bulb. The administration of synthetic LHRH corrects the endocrine abnormalities and initiates spermatogenesis. If untreated, these patients usually remain in the prepubertal state indefinitely. A prepubertal manifestation is microphallus, in which the size of the penis is below the fifth percentile for the age. Indeed, one-fourth or more of cases of isolated prepubertal microphallus are due to hypogonadotropic hypogonadism. Distinguishing between this disorder and delayed puberty is particularly difficult in patients of early or midpubertal age; the presence of microphallus, anosmia, or a family history of hypogonadotropic hypogonadism may suggest the diagnosis. In the absence of such evidence, it may take several years of observation before it becomes clear which of these states a patient has. Since delayed puberty is associated with a decreased bone mass, therapy should not be delayed too long. In some cases the response of plasma LH to LHRH stimulation may be helpful in suggesting that puberty is imminent.

ADULT ABNORMALITIES OF TESTICULAR FUNCTION At the completion of puberty, plasma testosterone levels reach the adult level of 10 to 35 nmol/L (3 to 10 ng/mL) throughout the day, plasma gonadotropins are in the normal adult range, and sperm production is sufficient to allow reproduction. The adult set of the complex regulatory system (see Fig. 336-3) is sustained in the normal man for more than 40 years. However, the system is subject to a variety of influences, at the level of both the testes and the hypothalamic-pituitary system. Spermatogenesis is exquisitely sensitive to alterations in temperature, and brief increases in either systemic or local temperature (as in a hot bath) can be followed by temporary decreases in sperm production. The system also is influenced by diet, drugs, alcohol, environmental agents, and psychological stress, any of which may cause temporary decreases in sperm count.

Persistent abnormalities of testicular function in adults can be due to hypothalamic-pituitary disorders (see Chap. 328), testicular defects, or abnormalities of sperm transport. Certain of these conditions tend to affect Leydig cell function or spermatogenesis selectively, but most impair both androgenization and fertility (Table 336-1). The interlocking of Leydig cell function and fertility is due to the dependence of spermatogenesis on androgen. Even a partial decrease in testosterone production can cause infertility. Certain conditions (hyperprolactinemia, radiation therapy, cyclophosphamide therapy, autoimmunity, paraplegia, androgen resistance) can cause either isolated infertility or a combined defect in testicular function.

Hypothalamic-Pituitary Disorders Disorders of the hypothalamus and pituitary can impair the secretion of gonadotropins either as one manifestation of a generalized disease of the anterior pituitary (see Chap. 328) or as an isolated defect. In the latter case the cause is usually hypogonadotropic hypogonadism, in which secretion of both LH and FSH are impaired. This disorder usually is congenital but rarely is an acquired defect. Alternatively, gonadotropin secretion can be altered by factors other than hypothalamic-pituitary pathology. For example, elevation of plasma cortisol in the *Cushing syndrome* can depress LH secretion independent of a space-occupying lesion of the pituitary. Some patients with *congenital adrenal hyperplasia* have suppressed gonadotropin secretion and consequent infertility. *Hyperprolactinemia* (as the consequence either of pituitary adenomas or of

Table 336-1

Abnormalities of Adult Testicular Function

Infertility with Underandrogenization	Infertility with Normal Virilization
HYPOTHALAMIC-PITUITARY	
Panhypopituitarism	
Isolated gonadotropin deficiency	Isolated FSH deficiency
Cushing's syndrome	Congenital adrenal hyperplasia
Hyperprolactinemia	Hyperprolactinemia
Hemochromatosis	Androgen use
TESTICULAR	
Developmental and structural defects	
Klinefelter's syndrome*	Germinal cell aplasia
XX male	Cryptorchidism
	Varicocele
	Immotile cilia syndrome
Acquired defects	
Viral orchitis*	*Mycoplasma* infection
Trauma	
Radiation	Radiation
Drugs (spironolactone, alcohol, ketoconazole, cyclophosphamide)	Drugs (cyclophosphamide)
Environmental toxins	Environmental toxins
Autoimmunity	Autoimmunity
Granulomatous disease	
Associated with systemic diseases	
Liver disease	Febrile illness
Renal failure	Celiac disease
Sickle cell disease	
Immune disease (AIDS, rheumatoid arthritis)	
Neurologic disease (myotonic dystrophy, spinobulbar muscular atrophy, and paraplegia)	Neurologic disease (paraplegia)
Androgen resistance	Androgen resistance
SPERM TRANSPORT	
	Obstruction of the epididymis or vas deferens (cystic fibrosis, diethylstilbesterol exposure, congenital absence)

* The common testicular causes of underandrogenization and infertility in adults—Klinefelter's syndrome and viral orchitis—are associated with small testes.

drugs such as phenothiazines) can cause combined Leydig cell and seminiferous tubule dysfunction, presumably due to inhibition of LH and FSH secretion by prolactin. Occasionally, impaired fertility in hyperprolactinemia is associated with normal gonadotropin and androgen levels and is presumed to result from direct inhibition of spermatogenesis by prolactin. *Hemochromatosis* usually impairs testicular function as the result of effects on the pituitary; less often it affects the testis directly (see Chap. 342). The use of *androgens* for purposes other than replacement therapy is often associated with impaired sperm production (see below). In some conditions, testosterone levels may be decreased in association with normal LH levels, and the mechanism is less clear. Men with massive obesity have decreased levels of TeBG and of total and bioavailable testosterone, which return toward normal with weight loss. Obesity may be part of the mechanism for decreased testosterone levels in the subset of such men with Pickwickian syndrome (see Chap. 263). Some men with temporal lobe seizures also have hypogonadotropic hypogonadism.

Testicular Defects Abnormalities of testicular function in the adult can be grouped into several categories: developmental and structural defects of the testes, acquired testicular defects, and disorders secondary to systemic disease.

Developmental abnormalities The *Klinefelter syndrome* (both the classic and the mosaic forms) and the *XX male syndrome* are usually not recognized until after the time of expected puberty (see Chap. 339). Some developmental defects cause infertility in the presence of normal androgen production. These include varicocele, germinal cell aplasia, and cryptorchidism. *Varicocele* may be of etiologic importance in as much as one-third of all cases of male infertility. It is caused by retrograde flow of blood into the internal spermatic vein that eventuates in progressive, often palpable dilation of the peritesticular pampiniform plexus of veins. Varicocele occurs in about 10 to 15 percent of men in the general population and in 20 to 40 percent of men with infertility and is thought to result from incompetence of the valve between the internal spermatic vein and the renal vein. It is more common on the left side (85 percent). Unilateral varicocele increases the blood flow and the temperature of both testes as a result of the extensive anastomoses of the venous systems. The increased scrotal (and testicular) temperature is believed to be the cause of the poor-quality semen and infertility (the testes no longer are 2°C cooler than the abdominal cavity, as they normally are). The findings on semen analysis are usually nonspecific, with all parameters showing some abnormality. Surgical resection results in fertility in about half of men, with the best results (70 percent pregnancy rate) in those whose preoperative sperm counts are over 10 million per milliliter.

Some patients with *germinal cell aplasia* (the Sertoli cell–only syndrome) have a positive family history and may constitute a specific group in whom the germinal epithelium is missing with resulting azoospermia; plasma testosterone and LH values are normal, and plasma FSH levels are elevated. Other patients with identical histologic and clinical findings have androgen resistance or a history of viral orchitis or cryptorchidism; as many as 18 percent of men with idiopathic azoospermia or severe oligospermia have microdeletions in the Yq interval 6 region, and more than one gene has been proposed as an azoospermia factor (AZF) gene.

Unilateral *cryptorchidism*, even when corrected prior to puberty, is associated with abnormal semen in many individuals. This observation suggests that even in unilateral cryptorchidism the testicular abnormality is usually bilateral.

The *immotile cilia syndrome* is an autosomal recessive defect characterized by immotility or poor motility of the cilia of the airways and of the sperm. Kartagener's syndrome is a subgroup of the immotile cilia syndrome associated with situs inversus, chronic sinusitis, and bronchiectasis (see Chap. 256). The immotile sperm cannot fertilize. The structural abnormality leading to impaired motility of cilia can usually be defined by the electron-microscopic appearance. The specific defects that are known to cause the syndrome include defects in the dynein arms, spokes, or microtubule doublets. Cilia from epithelia and sperm tails from the same individual exhibit the same defects, but the pulmonary manifestations may be minor. *Other less well understood structural defects of sperm* can cause immotility without involvement of cilia in the lung.

Acquired testicular defects Acquired testicular failure in the adult can be due to *viral orchitis*. The responsible viruses include mumps virus, echovirus, lymphocytic choriomeningitis virus, and group B arboviruses. The orchitis is due to actual infection of the tissue by virus rather than to indirect effects of infection. Orchitis occurs in as many as one-fourth of adult men with mumps; in about two-thirds the orchitis is unilateral, and in the remainder it is bilateral. Orchitis usually develops a few days after the onset of parotitis but may precede it. The testis may return to normal size and function or undergo atrophy. Atrophy is believed to be due both to direct effects of the virus on the seminiferous tubules and to ischemia secondary to pressure and edema within the taut tunica albuginea. Semen analysis returns to normal in three-fourths of men with unilateral involvement and in only one-third of men with bilateral orchitis. Atrophy is usually perceptible within 1 to 6 months after the acute illness, and the degree of atrophy is not necessarily proportional to the severity of the acute orchitis. Unilateral atrophy occurs in about one-third of patients, and bilateral atrophy occurs in about one-tenth.

Trauma can also cause secondary atrophy of the testes. The exposed position of the testes in the scrotum renders them susceptible to both thermal and physical trauma—particularly in individuals with hazardous occupations.

The testes are sensitive to *radiation damage;* decreased secretion of testosterone appears to be a consequence of diminished testicular blood flow. Doses higher than 200 mGy (20 rad) cause increases in plasma FSH and LH levels and damage to the spermatogonia. After about 800 mGy (80 rad), oligospermia or azoospermia develops, and higher doses may obliterate the germinal epithelium, except for occasional stem and Sertoli cells. Fractionated radiation may have a more profound effect than single-dose radiation. Recovery of sperm density occurs in a dose-related fashion, and complete recovery of sperm density may require as long as 5 years. Permanent infertility can occur after radiation therapy for malignant lymphoma despite shielding of the testes. Permanent androgen deficiency in adult men is uncommon after therapeutic radiation; however, most boys given direct testicular radiation therapy for acute lymphoblastic leukemia have permanently low plasma testosterone levels.

In general, *drugs* interfere with testicular function in one of four ways—inhibition of testosterone synthesis, blockade of androgen action, enhancement of estrogen levels, or direct inhibition of spermatogenesis. Some drugs have multiple effects, and agents such as guanethidine that block the sympathetic nervous system can impair sexual function in men whose pituitary-testicular axis is normal.

Spironolactone and ketoconazole block the synthesis of androgen by interfering with the late steps in androgen biosynthesis. Spironolactone and cimetidine compete with androgen for binding to the androgen receptor and thus block androgen action in target cells. Testosterone levels may be low, and estradiol levels may be elevated in persons using marijuana, heroin, or methadone, although the exact reasons are unclear. Alcohol, when consumed in excess for prolonged periods, causes decreased plasma testosterone, independent of liver disease or malnutrition. Elevated plasma estradiol and decreased plasma testosterone levels have been reported in men taking digitalis.

Antineoplastic and chemotherapeutic agents commonly interfere with spermatogenesis. Cyclophosphamide causes azoospermia or extreme oligospermia within a few weeks after the initiation of therapy. Cessation of therapy is followed by a return of spermatogenesis within 3 years in about half of patients. Combination chemotherapy for acute leukemia, Hodgkin's disease, and other malignancies also may impair Leydig cell function. In pubertal boys this is manifested by decreased serum testosterone and elevated LH levels; in adult men, testosterone levels do not decline, and the impaired Leydig cell function may only be detected as an enhanced LH response to LHRH. The alkylating agents in the chemotherapeutic regimens seem to be responsible for Leydig cell toxicity.

Because of the potentially toxic effects of many physical and chemical agents on spermatogenesis, the occupational and recreational history should be carefully evaluated in all men with infertility. Known environmental hazards include microwaves and ultrasound and chemicals such as the nematocide dibromochloropropane, cadmium, and lead. In some populations, sperm density is said to have declined by as much as 40 percent in the past 50 years, and it has been postulated that environmental estrogens or antiandrogens may be responsible.

Testicular failure also occurs as a part of *polyglandular autoimmune insufficiency* (see Chap. 340). Sperm antibodies are also a cause of isolated male infertility. In some instances, such antibodies may be secondary phenomena resulting from duct obstruction or vasectomy. *Granulomatous diseases* such as leprosy can destroy the testes, and testicular atrophy occurs in 10 to 20 percent of men with lepromatous leprosy owing to direct invasion of the tissue by the mycobacteria. The tubules are involved initially, followed by endarteritis and destruction of Leydig cells.

Testicular abnormalities associated with systemic disease The common systemic diseases that cause underandrogenization and infertility are liver disease and renal failure. In *cirrhosis of the liver*, a combined testicular and pituitary abnormality leads to decreased testosterone production independent of the direct toxic effects of ethanol. Although plasma LH is elevated, the level may be below the expected range given the degree of androgen deficiency. This situation most likely results from the inhibition of LH secretion by estrogen in patients with chronic liver disease. Increased estrogen production results from impaired hepatic extraction of adrenal androstenedione and subsequent increased extraglandular conversion to estrone and estradiol. In effect, estrogen precursors are shunted to sites of extraglandular aromatization. Testicular atrophy and gynecomastia are present in about half of men with cirrhosis, and many such men are impotent. Successful liver transplantation reverses the effects of cirrhosis on the pituitary-testicular axis.

In chronic *renal failure*, androgen synthesis and sperm production decrease in the setting of elevated plasma gonadotropins. The elevated LH level is due to increased production and reduced clearance but is incapable of effecting normal testosterone production. In addition, about one-fourth of men with renal failure have hyperprolactinemia; the role of hyperprolactinemia in decreasing testosterone production is unclear. Low testosterone coupled with normal or increased plasma estrogen levels cause gynecomastia in about half of men on chronic hemodialysis, and about half of men on dialysis have decreased libido and/or impotence. The etiology of the testicular abnormalities in renal failure is not well understood. Improvement in testosterone production with hemodialysis is incomplete, but successful transplantation may return testicular function to normal.

Men with *sickle cell anemia* usually have impaired secondary sexual development, and testicular atrophy is present in one-third of them. The defect may be at either the testicular or the hypothalamic-pituitary level. Abnormalities in Leydig cell function, frequently accompanied by decreased sperm density, have been noted in a variety of chronic systemic diseases, including protein-energy *malnutrition*, advanced *Hodgkin's disease* and *cancer* prior to chemotherapy, and *amyloidosis*. Most of these disorders cause a lowered plasma testosterone level coupled with a normal to increased plasma LH level, suggesting combined hypothalamic-pituitary and testicular defects. Similar hormone changes occur following *surgery, myocardial infarction*, and severe *burns* and thus may be a nonspecific effect of illness. Men with AIDS may have decreased testosterone levels without an appropriate elevation of gonadotropins; although human immunodeficiency virus (HIV) may infect the testes, the hormonal changes are likely nonspecific and related to severe illness. Whether testosterone deficiency contributes to muscle wasting in this disorder is unclear.

The temporary decrease in sperm density after *acute febrile illness* usually occurs in the absence of any changes in testosterone production. Infertility in men with *celiac disease* is associated with a hormonal pattern typical of androgen resistance, namely elevated testosterone and LH levels. *Neurologic diseases* associated with altered testicular function include myotonic dystrophy, spinobulbar muscular atrophy, and paraplegia. In myotonic dystrophy, small testes may be associated with abnormalities of both spermatogenesis and Leydig cell function. Men with spinobulbar muscular atrophy often have as a late manifestation underandrogenization and infertility and the hormonal features of androgen resistance (see Chap. 339). Expansion of the glutamine repeat sequences in the amino-terminal region of the androgen receptor impairs its function, but it is unclear whether altered androgen receptor function is related to the neurologic disorder. Spinal cord lesions that cause paraplegia lead to a temporary decrease in testosterone levels and persistent defects in spermatogenesis; some patients retain the capacity to obtain erection and to ejaculate.

Androgen resistance Defects of the androgen receptor cause resistance to the action of androgen, usually associated with defective male phenotypic development, infertility, and underandrogenization (see Chap. 339). A less severe form of androgen resistance, associated with infertility due to oligo- or azoospermia in otherwise phenotypically normal men, may be the cause of a significant fraction of cases of infertility previously classified as idiopathic azoospermia. Point mutations in the hormone-binding domain of the androgen receptor have been reported in idiopathic infertility.

Impairment of Sperm Transport Disorders of sperm transport may cause infertility in as many as 6 percent of infertile men with normal virilization. The obstruction may be unilateral or bilateral, congenital or acquired. In men with unilateral obstruction of sperm transport, the infertility may result from antisperm antibodies. Obstructive azoospermia at the level of the epididymis also occurs in association with chronic infections of the paranasal sinuses and lungs. Tuberculosis, leprosy, and gonorrhea are rare causes of acquired obstruction of ejaculatory structures. Congenital defects of the vas deferens can occur as an isolated abnormality associated with absence of the seminal vesicles (and consequently absence of fructose in the ejaculate), in men whose mothers received *diethylstilbestrol* during pregnancy, and in patients with *cystic fibrosis*. Furthermore, congenital bilateral absence of the vas deferens can be due to mutations in the cystic fibrosis conductance regulator different than the mutations that cause full-blown cystic fibrosis. Thus, isolated congenital absence of the vas and cystic fibrosis represent a spectrum of defects that have a similar molecular basis.

Empirical Therapy of Male Infertility The management of male infertility is usually unsatisfactory. Disorders for which there are logical or effective treatments (genital tract obstruction, sperm autoimmunity, gonadotropin deficiency) account for only 10 percent of infertile men, and pregnancies are infrequent with genital tract obstruction or sperm autoimmunity. Severe oligospermia/azoospermia of other causes accounts for about a fourth of cases of male infertility and has largely been considered untreatable. The other two-thirds of infertile men have a partial reduction in semen parameters and subfertility of a variable degree, and in this group spontaneous fertility may occur in untreated men (as high as 25 percent in one year). In the past a variety of empirical therapies (e.g., testosterone rebound, gonadotropins, antiestrogens) have been unsuccessful. The only successful empirical therapy for men with mild to moderate defects in semen quality is in vitro fertilization. However, standard in vitro fertilization does not provide a good outcome with severely abnormal semen parameters, such as a sperm density of <5 million/mL, poor motility, and many abnormal forms. For such men the technique of intracytoplasmic sperm injection makes in vitro fertilization more successful; indeed fertilization and pregnancy rates with this technique are similar to those for standard in vitro techniques in couples with fallopian tube pathology, i.e., a 50 to 70 percent fertilization rate and a 30 percent pregnancy rate per cycle.

Fertility Control in Men A variety of approaches to fertility control in men have been tried, including use of the condom as an effective barrier that also prevents sexually transmitted diseases. Another widely used technique is ligation of the vas deferens, a procedure that has been successful in large numbers of men and can be performed on an outpatient basis. The time required for azoospermia to occur following the operation depends on the number of sperm in the terminal vas deferens and ejaculatory ducts at the time of surgery but is usually less than 40 days. Azoospermia should be documented in each case to prove effectiveness. No deleterious effects on either testosterone production or the hypothalamic-pituitary axis have been documented. Despite reports of immune-complex–associated accelerated atherosclerosis in vasectomized nonhuman primates, there does not appear to be any association between vasectomy and atherosclerosis in men. Vasectomy should only be recommended for men requesting permanent sterilization. Only about 30 to 40 percent of men subjected to vasovasostomy for reanastomosis of the vas subsequently achieve fertility.

OLD AGE Beginning at about age 40, mean plasma bioavailable testosterone concentrations decline gradually, and about 40 percent of elderly men have low bioavailable testosterone levels. Nevertheless, although statistically lower than the levels in young men, the concentrations of total testosterone even in elderly men usually remain within the normal range. The cause of the decreased testosterone level is likely a decreased number of Leydig cells in the testes. There is also a decline in seminiferous tubule function and decreased sperm production in older men. Plasma LH and FSH levels are usually increased in elderly men, and an increase in the rate of conversion of androgen to estrogen in peripheral tissues results in a decrease in the effective ratio of androgen to estrogen. These latter endocrine changes may play a role in the development of prostatic hyperplasia and possibly in the development of gynecomastia in aging men (see Chaps. 97 and 338). Male sexual function gradually declines after early adulthood, but there is no convincing evidence that hormonal changes have any direct bearing on changes in sexual function with age in healthy men.

Prostatic Hyperplasia See Chap. 97

Cancer of the Prostate See Chap. 97

DISORDERS OF ALL AGES **Testicular Tumors** (See Chap. 98) Chorionic gonadotropin is present in normal testes, and it is not surprising that plasma gonadotropins may be elevated in persons with testicular tumors. Indeed, an elevated plasma level of the β subunit of human chorionic gonadotropin (hCG-β) is a sensitive and specific marker of tumor activity in some men with germ cell tumors. Plasma levels of hCG-β are elevated in all men with choriocarcinoma, in one-third of those with embryonal carcinomas and teratocarcinomas, and rarely in those with seminomas. Changes in hCG-β levels correlate with response to therapy.

Testicular tumors can give rise to elevated estradiol and testosterone levels by at least two mechanisms. Trophoblastic tumors and Leydig and Sertoli cell tumors produce both hormones autonomously; plasma gonadotropin levels and hormone production by the uninvolved portions of the testes are depressed, and azoospermia is common. However, secretion of gonadotropins by the tumor increases estradiol and testosterone production in the unaffected areas of the testes, and azoospermia is uncommon with such tumors. When estrogens and androgens are formed (directly or indirectly) by the tumors, feminization, virilization, or no obvious change may result, depending on the hormones produced and the age of the patient. Other cellular markers of testicular tumor activity include alpha fetoprotein.

Gynecomastia See Chap. 338

℞ TREATMENT

Androgens PHARMACOLOGIC PREPARATIONS When testosterone itself is ingested, it is absorbed into the portal blood and degraded promptly by the liver, so that only insignificant amounts reach the systemic circulation; when administered parenterally, testosterone is rapidly absorbed from the injection vehicle and rapidly degraded. As a consequence, effective androgen therapy requires either the administration of a slowly absorbed form of testosterone (dermal patches or micronized oral preparation) or the administration of modified analogues. Such chemical modifications either retard absorption or catabolism, so as to sustain effective blood levels, or enhance the androgenic potency of each molecule, so that full effects can be achieved at a lower blood level of drug. Three types of modification have had widespread clinical application (Fig. 336-7): esterification of the 17β-hydroxyl group, alkylation at the 17α position, and alteration of the ring structure, particularly by substitutions at the 2, 9, and 11 positions. Most agents actually have combinations of ring structure alterations and either 17α-alkylation or esterification of the 17β-hydroxyl group. Esterification serves to decrease the polarity of the molecule so that the steroid is more soluble in the fat vehicles used for injection and is released into the circulation more slowly. Most esters must be injected parenterally. The larger the acid esterified, the more prolonged is the action. Esters such as testosterone cypionate and testosterone enanthate can be injected every 1 to 3 weeks. Because the esters are hydrolyzed before the hormones act, the effectiveness of therapy can be monitored by assaying plasma testosterone level with time after administration.

The oral effectiveness of 17α-alkylated androgens (such as methyltestosterone and methandrostenolone) is due to slower hepatic catabolism, which allows the alkylated derivatives to escape degradation by the liver and reach the systemic circulation. For this reason, 17α-methyl or -ethyl substitution is a feature of most orally active androgens. Unfortunately, all 17α-alkylated steroids can cause abnormal liver function, and for this reason they have a limited role in medicine.

Other alterations of the ring structure have been adopted empirically; some slow the rate of inactivation, others enhance the potency of a given molecule, and some alter the conversion to other active metabolites. For example, the potency of fluoxymesterone may be due to the fact that, unlike most androgens, it is a poor precursor for conversion to estrogens in peripheral tissues. Two transdermal preparations in which a testosterone-loaded patch is applied each day are available. One is a single scrotal patch applied each morning;

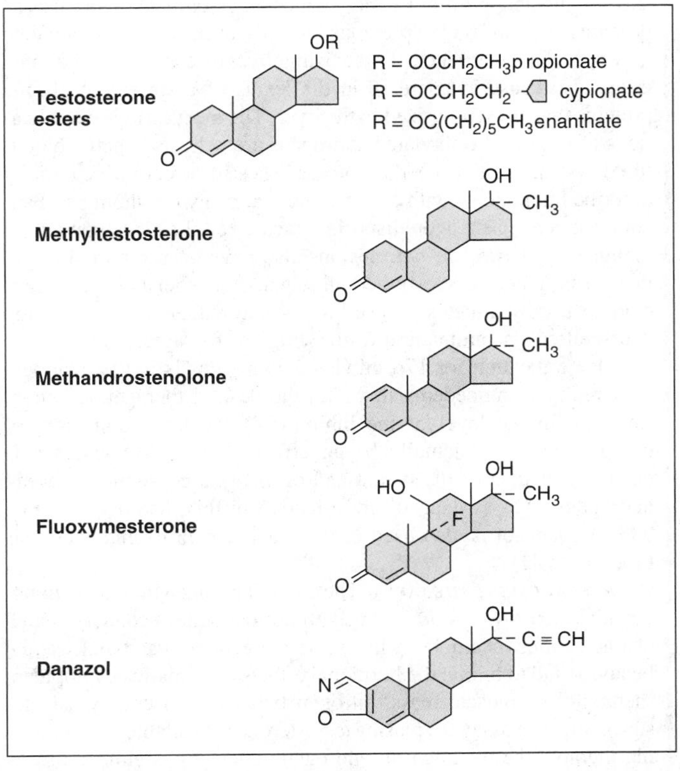

FIGURE 336-7 Some of the androgen preparations available for pharmacologic use.

the other system involves two nonscrotal patches applied at bedtime. Both preparations produce physiologic testosterone levels and avoid the wide swings in serum testosterone values that occur between injections of testosterone esters.

SIDE EFFECTS OF ANDROGENS All androgens carry the risk of inducing virilization in women. Early manifestations include acne, coarsening of the voice, hirsutism, and menstrual irregularities. If treatment is discontinued as soon as these effects develop, the manifestations may slowly subside. Long-term side effects such as male-pattern baldness, worsening of the hirsutism and voice changes, and hypertrophy of the clitoris are largely irreversible. At physiologic replacement doses, testosterone esters have no known toxic effects in mature men. At supraphysiologic doses, however, gonadotropin secretion is inhibited, the testes shrink, and the sperm count falls (indeed, low sperm counts may persist for as long as 9 months after cessation of androgen abuse).

The so-called toxic side effects differ among the different agents and with the clinical setting in which they are used. Retention of a limited amount of sodium is an inevitable consequence of androgen therapy, but in patients with underlying heart disease or renal failure or when androgens are administered in enormous amounts, sodium retention may lead to edema. Although androgens do not cause malignancy, they may promote the growth of and intensify pain from carcinomas of the prostate and breast in men.

The feminizing side effects of androgen therapy in men are poorly understood. Testosterone (but not 5α-reduced androgens) can be converted (aromatized) in extraglandular tissues to estradiol. The most common manifestation of feminization is the development of gynecomastia. Such breast enlargement is common in children given androgens, possibly because of a greater capacity to convert androgens to estrogens in childhood. The administration of testosterone esters to men results in an increase in plasma estrogen levels, but in men with normal liver function gynecomastia usually develops only after use of high doses.

All 17α-alkylated androgens can produce liver function abnormalities such as elevation of plasma levels of alkaline phosphatase and conjugated bilirubin. The incidence of clinical liver disease probably depends on the previous integrity of the liver, but jaundice may occur in the absence of preexisting liver disease. 17α-Alkylated drugs also cause an increase in the levels of a variety of plasma proteins that are synthesized in the liver. The most serious complications of use of 17α-alkylated androgens are peliosis hepatis (blood-filled cysts in the liver) and hepatoma. These disorders were initially described in patients with aplastic anemia, many of whom had Fanconi anemia, itself a predisposing factor for the development of malignancy. However, both lesions also have been reported in patients who received substituted androgens for other indications, including use by athletes. These tumors may either follow a benign course after discontinuation of the drugs or be rapidly fatal.

One indication for 17α-alkylated androgens is in the treatment of hereditary angioedema in which the desired therapeutic benefit (increase in the level of the inhibitor of the first component of complement) may actually be an effect of the 17-alkylated side chain rather than of the parent androgen. As a consequence, weak androgens such as danazol are effective in this disorder (see Fig. 336-7). Danazol is also used in the management of endometriosis (see Chap. 52).

REPLACEMENT THERAPY The aim of androgen therapy in hypogonadal men is to restore or bring to normal male secondary sexual characteristics (beard, body hair, external genitalia) and male sexual behavior and to mimic the hormonal effects on somatic development (hemoglobin, muscle mass, nitrogen balance, and epiphyseal closure). Since an assay for plasma testosterone is available for monitoring therapy, the treatment of androgen deficiency is almost universally successful. The parenteral administration of a long-acting testosterone ester such as 100 to 200 mg testosterone enanthate at 1- to 2-week intervals results in a sustained increase in plasma testosterone to the normal male range. Such esters act only through the release of testosterone itself into the circulation. Alternatively, testosterone may be administered transdermally. If the hypogonadism is primary and of long duration (as in the Klinefelter syndrome), suppression of plasma LH to the normal range may not occur for many weeks, if at all. There is considerable variability in the relation between plasma testosterone and male sexual behavior, but in cases of postpubertal testicular failure (even of many years duration), normal sexual activity usually is resumed after adequate replacement. Androgen administration does not restore spermatogenesis in hypogonadal states, but the volume of the ejaculate (derived largely from the prostate and seminal vesicles) and other male secondary sex characteristics return to normal. The effects of endogenous androgen on hemoglobin, nitrogen retention, and skeletal development are also reproduced.

In men of all ages in whom hypogonadism developed prior to expected puberty (such as men with isolated gonadotropin deficiency), it is appropriate to bring plasma testosterone slowly into the adult range. When therapy is commenced at the time of expected puberty in such men, the normal events of puberty proceed in the usual fashion. If therapy is delayed until after the time of usual puberty, the degree to which normal virilization will occur is variable, but many patients undergo a relatively complete anatomic and functional maturation. Intermittent low-dose androgen therapy is indicated in prepubertal hypogonadal boys with microphallus to bring the external genitalia into the normal range. If such patients are monitored closely and given androgens only for short periods, such therapy usually has no adverse effects on somatic growth.

In boys of pubertal age with either isolated gonadotropin deficiency or primary testicular disease, the usual practice is to institute androgen therapy between the ages of 12 and 14 years, depending on the subjective need for sexual development. The initial administration of small doses of testosterone esters followed by a gradual increase to 100 to 150 mg/m^2 of body surface area every 1 to 3 weeks should result in a normal pubertal growth spurt. The time from the start of treatment to the appearance of secondary sex characteristics is variable. Penile development, deepening of the voice, and the appearance of other secondary sexual characteristics usually commence during the first year of treatment. In normal boys, puberty extends over several years, and treatment designed to replicate normal development does not shorten the process greatly.

Testosterone exerts its full action only in the presence of a balanced hormonal environment and, particularly, in the presence of adequate levels of growth hormone. Consequently, prepubertal boys with coexisting growth hormone and androgen deficiency respond poorly to androgens unless growth hormone is given simultaneously.

PHARMACOLOGIC USES Androgens have been used for a variety of disorders unassociated with hypogonadism, in the hope that potential benefits from the nonvirilizing actions of the agents (such as increase in nitrogen retention and muscle mass, increased hemoglobin, etc.) would outweigh any deleterious actions of the drugs. The most common nonreplacement uses of androgen have been attempts to improve nitrogen balance in catabolic states, self-administration by athletes in the belief that muscle mass and/or athletic performance will be improved, attempts to enhance erythropoiesis in refractory anemias (including the anemia of renal failure), treatment of hereditary angioedema and endometriosis, and management of growth retardation of various etiologies. Most of the expected benefits in these disorders did not materialize, for two reasons. First, modest pharmacologic doses of androgens do little, if anything, in men beyond the normal testicular androgen, and in women the virilizing side effects of androgens are formidable. Second, no androgen has been devised that exhibits only the nonvirilizing effects of the hormone. This is not surprising in view of the fact that the physiologic actions of androgens are mediated by a single, high-affinity receptor protein in the cytoplasm (see Fig. 336-5).

The most pervasive form of androgen abuse is by male athletes in the expectation that muscle development and athletic performance will be improved. In controlled studies using modest pharmacologic doses (two to four times the usual replacement doses), these agents do not improve performance consistently. However, at the doses frequently taken by athletes (which sometimes exceed 10 times the replacement dose), these agents do enhance nitrogen balance and muscle mass; since the drugs have multiple side effects at high doses, these putative benefits do not outweigh the risks associated with androgen abuse, a practice that cannot be condemned too harshly. The only established indications for androgen therapy outside of male hypogonadism are in selected patients with anemia due to bone marrow failure or hereditary angioedema and as an adjunct to growth hormone therapy.

Gonadotropins Gonadotropin therapy is used to establish or restore fertility in patients with gonadotropin deficiency of any cause. Two gonadotropin preparations are available: human menopausal gonadotropins (hMG) (purified from the urine of postmenopausal women) and human chorionic gonadotropin (hCG) (purified from the urine of pregnant women). hMG contains 75 IU FSH and 75 IU LH per vial. hCG has little FSH activity and resembles LH in its ability to stimulate testosterone production by Leydig cells. Because of the expense of hMG, treatment is usually begun with hCG alone, and hMG is added later to promote the FSH-dependent stages of spermatid development. A high ratio of LH to FSH activity and a long duration of treatment (3 to 6 months) are necessary to bring about maturation of the prepubertal testes. Once spermatogenesis is restored in hypophysectomized patients or initiated in hypogonadotropic hypogonadal men by combined therapy, it can usually be maintained with hCG alone.

The dosage of hCG required to maintain a normal testosterone level varies from 1000 to 5000 IU weekly. A number of regimens have been used to induce maturation of spermatogenesis. Most involve starting with 2000 IU hCG three or more times a week until most of the clinical parameters, including plasma testosterone levels, are normal. hMG (usually one ampul) is then added three times a week to complete the development of spermatogenesis. After spermatogenesis has regressed, the length of therapy required to restore spermatogenesis may be as long as 12 months.

Luteinizing Hormone–Releasing Hormone And LHRH Analogues LHRH (gonadorelin) is available for endocrine testing. LHRH therapy is used by some physicians for chronic therapy of the infertility of hypogonadotropic hypogonadism. It is necessary to administer LHRH in frequent boluses (25 to 200 ng/kg of body weight every 2 h), which necessitates the use of portable infusion pumps. In general, LHRH does not appear to be more efficacious than gonadotropin in returning sperm counts to normal. LHRH analogues (leuprolide and nafarelin) are available for the suppression of gonadotropin secretion and the induction of hypogonadism. In prostatic cancer, testicular androgen production can be blocked by monthly injection of 7.5 mg leuprolide in depot form.

See Chap. 58, Androgens, in Goodman & Gilman's The Pharmacological Basis of Therapeutics, *9th ed, New York, McGraw-Hill, 1996.*

BIBLIOGRAPHY

Baker HWG: Male infertility, in *Endocrinology*, 3d ed, LLJ deGroot (ed). Philadelphia, Saunders, 1995, pp 2404–2433

Carr BR, Griffin JE: Fertility control and its complications, in *Williams Textbook of Endocrinology*, 8th ed, JD Wilson, DW Foster (eds). Philadelphia, Saunders, 1992, pp 1007–1031

———, Robertson DM: The isolation and physiology of inhibin and related proteins. Biol Reprod 40:33, 1989

Chillon M et al: Mutations in the cystic fibrosis gene in patients with congenital absence of the vas deferens. N Engl J Med 332:1475, 1995

de Kretser DM: Declining sperm counts. BMJ 312:457, 1996

Goldzieher JW et al: Improving the diagnostic reliability of rapidly fluctuating plasma hormone levels by optimized multiple-sampling techniques. J Clin Endocrinol Metab 43:824, 1976

Gray A et al: Age, disease and changing sex hormone levels in middle-aged men: Results of the Massachusetts male aging study. J Clin Endocrinol Metab 73:1016, 1991

Griffin JE, Wilson JD: Disorders of the testes and male reproductive tract, in *Williams Textbook of Endocrinology*, 8th ed, JD Wilson, DW Foster (eds). Philadelphia, Saunders, 1992, pp 799–852

Grumbach MM, Styne DM: Puberty: Ontogeny, neuroendocrinology, physiology, and disorders, in *Williams Textbook of Endocrinology*, 8th ed, JD Wilson, DW Foster (eds). Philadelphia, Saunders, 1992, pp 1139–1221

Handlesman DJ: Testicular dysfunction in systemic disease. Endocrinol Metab Clin North Am 23:839, 1994

Illingworth PJ et al: Inhibin-B: A likely candidate for the physiologically important form of inhibin in men. J Clin Endocrinol Metab 81:1321, 1996

Laue L et al: Treatment of familial male precocious puberty with spironolactone and testolactone. N Engl J Med 320:496, 1989

MacDonald PC et al: Origin of estrogen in normal men and in women with testicular feminization. J Clin Endocrinol Metab 49:905, 1979

Marshall WA, Tanner JM: Variation in the pattern of pubertal changes in boys. Arch Dis Child 45:13, 1970

Meikle AW et al: Enhanced transdermal delivery of testosterone across nonscrotal skin produces physiological concentrations of testosterone and its metabolites in hypogonadal men. J Clin Endocrinol Metab 74:623, 1992

Najmabadi H et al: Substantial prevalence of microdeletions of the Y-chromosome in infertile men with idiopathic azoospermia and oligospermia detected using a sequence-tagged site-based mapping strategy. J Clin Endocrinol Metab 81:1347, 1996

Palermo GD et al: Intracytoplasmic sperm injection: A novel treatment for all forms of male factor infertility. Fertil Steril 63:1231, 1995

Pescovitz OH et al: Paracrine control of spermatogenesis. Trends Endocrinol Metab 3:126, 1994

Poretsky L et al: Testicular dysfunction in human immunodeficiency virus-infected men. Metabolism 44:946, 1995

Rugarli EI, Ballabio A: Kallmann syndrome. JAMA 270:2173, 1993

Snyder PJ: Hypogonadotropic hypogonadism: Gonadotropin therapy, in *Current Therapy in Endocrinology and Metabolism*, 5th ed, CW Bardin (ed). St Louis, Mosby, 1994, pp 300–303

Snyder PF, Lawrence DA: Treatment of male hypogonadism with testosterone enanthate. J Clin Endocrinol Metab 51:1335, 1980

Whitcomb RW, Crowley WF Jr: Hypogonadotropic hypogonadism: Gonadotropin-releasing hormone therapy, in *Current Therapy in Endocrinology and Metabolism*, 5th ed, CW Bardin (ed). St Louis, Mosby, 1994, pp 303–305

337

Bruce R. Carr, Karen D. Bradshaw

DISORDERS OF THE OVARY AND FEMALE REPRODUCTIVE TRACT

The ovary is the source of ova for reproduction and of the hormones that regulate female sexual life. The anatomic structure, response to hormonal stimuli, and secretory capacity of the ovary differ at different periods of life. This chapter will review normal ovarian physiology as a background for understanding ovarian abnormalities and will consider other disorders of the female reproductive tract.

DEVELOPMENT, STRUCTURE, AND FUNCTION OF THE OVARY

EMBRYOLOGY During the third week of gestation, the primordial germ cells differentiate from the endoderm lining the yolk sac at the caudal end of the embryo. The germ cells migrate to the genital ridge adjacent to the mesonephric kidney by the fifth week of gestation and undergo mitotic division. The gonads exist in an undifferentiated state until the seventh week of fetal life, at which time the primitive ovary can be distinguished from the testis (see Chap. 339). Estrogen formation in the ovary commences between weeks 8 and 10, and by 10 to 11 weeks of gestation, oogonia in the ovarian cortex begin developing into primary oocytes. The ovary contains a finite number of germ cells, the number peaking at about 7 million oogonia by the fifth to sixth month of gestation. Subsequently, the germ cells decrease in number through a process of atresia so that only 1 million remain at birth, 400,000 are present at menarche, and only a few remain at menopause. Two X chromosomes are required for normal development of the ovary; in individuals with a 45,X karyotype, ovarian development occurs, but the rate of atresia is accelerated so that only a fibrous streak remains at birth (see Chap. 339).

After the oogonia cease to proliferate, meiosis commences, continues until the diplotene stage of the first meiotic division is completed and then is arrested until the onset of ovulation at puberty. From the fifth month of fetal life, the primordial follicle consists of the primary oocyte arrested in meiosis, a single surrounding layer of granulosa cells, and a basement membrane that separates the primordial follicle from surrounding stromal (interstitial) tissues.

PUBERTAL MATURATION The final maturation of ovarian follicles commences during puberty. The two major hormones that regulate follicular development are the pituitary gonadotropins—follicle-stimulating hormone (FSH) and luteinizing hormone (LH) (Fig. 337-1). During the second trimester of fetal development, the plasma gonadotropins rise to levels similar to those at menopause. This peak in gonadotropin levels may be responsible for the simultaneous peak in oocyte replication. After the second trimester, the hypothalamic-pituitary axis (the so-called gonadostat) becomes functional and is sensitive to negative feedback by steroid hormones, particularly estrogen and progesterone produced in the placenta. The levels of circulating gonadotropins consequently decrease, and gonadotropins are almost undetectable at the time of birth. In the neonate, concomitant with the decrease in estrogen and progesterone levels caused by separation from the placenta, there is a rebound increase in gonadotropin secretion for the first few months of life. With continued maturation of the hypothalamic-pituitary system, the gonadostat becomes sensitive to negative feedback by low levels of circulating steroid hormones, and plasma gonadotropins again decrease.

As the time of puberty nears, a decrease in the sensitivity of the gonadostat allows for increased secretion of FSH and LH, possibly secondary to increased episodic or pulsatile secretion of luteinizing hormone–releasing hormone (LHRH) by the hypothalamus (see Chap. 328). A sleep-induced, pulsatile pattern of LH secretion then ensues, the first step in the development of a cyclic pattern of gonadotropin secretion (see Fig. 337-1). The increase in estrogen secretion exerts a positive feedback, which leads to an exaggeration of the pulsatile release of LH and eventually to ovulation and the menarche, after which plasma gonadotropin concentrations reach adult values in which day and night levels are similar. After the menopause, plasma gonadotropin levels rise, then plateau 5 to 10 years after menopause and remain fairly constant until the eighth to ninth decade of life when the levels may fall. Although ovarian function is regulated primarily by LH and FSH, the ovary is a source of peptide and protein hormones and growth factors that may play a role in ovarian function.

With puberty the sensitivity of the hypothalamic-pituitary centers to circulating steroid hormones is decreased, LHRH release by the hypothalamus increases, gonadotropin secretion by the pituitary is enhanced, ovarian estrogen secretion increases, and the anatomic changes of puberty ensue. At age 10 to 11, the first secondary sexual characteristics begin to appear in girls, namely, development of the breast buds (thelarche), followed by the development of pubic hair (pubarche), and later by the development of axillary hair (adrenarche). Pubic and axillary hair are believed to be controlled by adrenal androgens, the levels of which begin to rise at approximately 6 to 8 years of age. A growth spurt ensues, and peak growth rate is attained by age 12.

The culmination of puberty is the onset of predictable, cyclic menses. The average time between the beginning of breast development and the onset of menses (menarche) is 2 years. During the first few years after menarche, menstrual cycles are often irregular and unpredictable due to anovulation. The age of menarche is variable and is influenced by socioeconomic and genetic factors and by general health. In the United States, the mean age of menarche is believed to have decreased at a rate of 3 to 4 months per decade over the past 100 years and is now around 13 years, a change believed to be due to improved nutrition. A body weight of around 48 kg or some critical combination of weight, body water, and body fat is associated with development of hypothalamic insensitivity to feedback by steroids that leads to increased secretion of gonadotropins and finally to menarche. Obese girls have earlier menarche than girls with normal weights. In contrast, participation in sports or ballet, malnutrition, and chronic debilitating disease can delay menarche.

MATURE OVARY **Morphology** The anatomic components and function of the adult ovary are illustrated schematically in Fig. 337-2. Under the influence of gonadotropins, a group of primary follicles are recruited, and by day 6 to 8 of the menstrual cycle, one

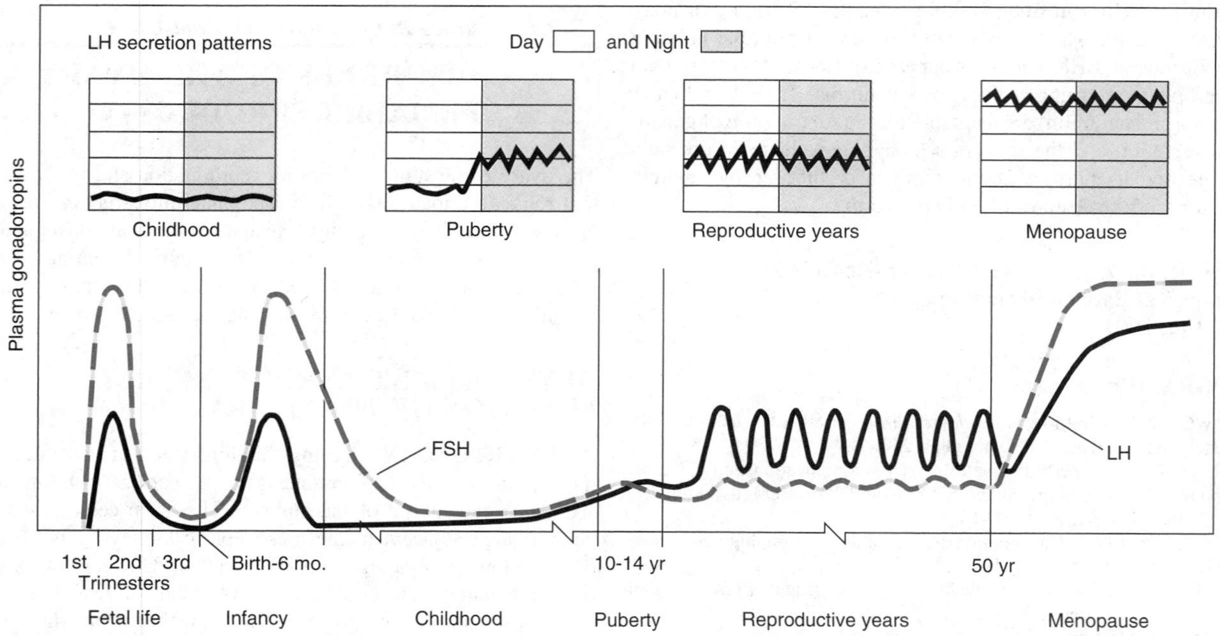

FIGURE 337-1 Pattern of gonadotropin secretion during different stages of life in women. FSH, follicle-stimulating hormone; LH, luteinizing hormone. The secretory patterns of LH during the waking hours (clear area) and night (stippled area) for each stage are indicated in the upper insets. *(After Faiman et al.)*

follicle becomes mature or "dominant," a process characterized by accelerated growth of granulosa cells and enlargement of the fluid-filled antrum. The recruited follicles not destined to ovulate undergo degeneration, similar to the atresia that occurs in other follicles during embryogenesis. Just prior to ovulation, meiosis resumes in the ovum of the dominant follicle, and the first meiotic division results in formation of the first polar body. The antrum rapidly enlarges (up to 10 to 25 mm in size), follicular fluid increases in amount, and the follicular surface thins and forms a conical stigma. Ovulation from the dominant follicle occurs some 16 to 23 h after the LH peak and some 24 to 38 h after the onset of the LH surge as the result of rupture of the follicular wall at the area of the stigma. The ovum is then expelled together with a mass of surrounding granulosa cells called *cumulus cells*. The rupture is believed to result from the action of hydrolytic enzymes on the surface of the follicle, possibly under the control of prostaglandins. The second meiotic division occurs after the egg is fertilized by a sperm, and the second polar body is then extruded. The formation of the corpus luteum begins in the retained remnant of the ovulated follicle; the remaining granulosa and theca cells increase in size and accumulate lipids and a yellow pigment, lutein, to become "luteinized." The basement membrane that separated the granulosa cells from the stroma and blood vessels breaks, and capillaries, fibroblasts, and lymphatics from the theca invade the granulosa cells and reach the central cavity, thereby filling it with blood. After a period of 14 $\pm$ 2 days (the functional life of the corpus luteum), vessels regress, and the corpus luteum begins to atrophy, to be replaced in time by a fibrous scar, the corpus albicans. The factors that limit the life span of the human corpus luteum are not known, but if pregnancy occurs, the corpus luteum persists under the influence of placental or chorionic gonadotropins, and progesterone is produced by the corpus luteum for the support of pregnancy.

Hormone Formation *Steroid hormones* Like other steroid hormones, ovarian steroids are derived from cholesterol (Fig. 337-3). The ovary can synthesize cholesterol de novo and also can utilize cholesterol obtained from circulating lipoproteins as substrate for steroid hormone formation (Fig. 337-4). Virtually all ovarian cells are believed to possess the complete complement of enzymes required for the synthesis of estradiol from cholesterol (see Fig. 337-3); however, different cell types in the ovary contain different amounts of these enzymes so that the main steroids produced differ in different compartments. For example, the corpus luteum forms mainly progesterone and 17-hydroxyprogesterone, whereas theca and stromal cells convert cholesterol to androstenedione and testosterone. Granulosa cells are particularly rich in the aromatase responsible for estrogen synthesis and utilize as substrates for this process androgens synthesized in the granulosa cells and the adjacent theca cells.

The principal sites of action of LH and FSH are also illustrated in Figs. 337-3 and 337-4. LH acts primarily to regulate the first step in steroid hormone biosynthesis, namely, the conversion of cholesterol to pregnenolone, and also induces subsequent enzymes in the pathway. FSH acts to regulate the final process by which androgens are aromatized to estrogens. As a consequence, LH enhances substrate flow and the formation of androgens and/or progesterone in the absence of FSH, whereas FSH action is impeded in the absence of LH because of diminished substrate for aromatization.

ESTROGENS Naturally occurring estrogens are 18-carbon steroids characterized by an aromatic A ring, a phenolic hydroxyl group at C-3, and either a hydroxyl group (estradiol) or a ketone (estrone) at C-17 (see Fig. 337-3). (For the numbering of the steroid ring, see Fig. 336-1.) The principal estrogen secreted by the ovary and the most potent estrogen is estradiol. Estrone is also secreted by the ovary, but most estrone is formed by extraglandular conversion of androstenedione in peripheral tissues. Estriol (16-hydroxyestradiol), the main estrogen in urine, arises from the 16-hydroxylation of estrone and estradiol. Catechol estrogens are formed by hydroxylation of estrogens at the C-2 or C-4 position and may act as the intracellular mediators of some estrogen action. Estrogens promote development of the secondary sexual characteristics in women and cause uterine growth, thickening of the vaginal mucosa, thinning of the cervical mucus, and development of the ductule system of the breasts. The mechanism of estrogen action in target tissues is similar to that for other steroid hormones and involves binding to a nuclear steroid receptor and enhancement of the transcription of messenger RNA, which in turn causes increased protein synthesis in the cell cytoplasm (see Chap. 327).

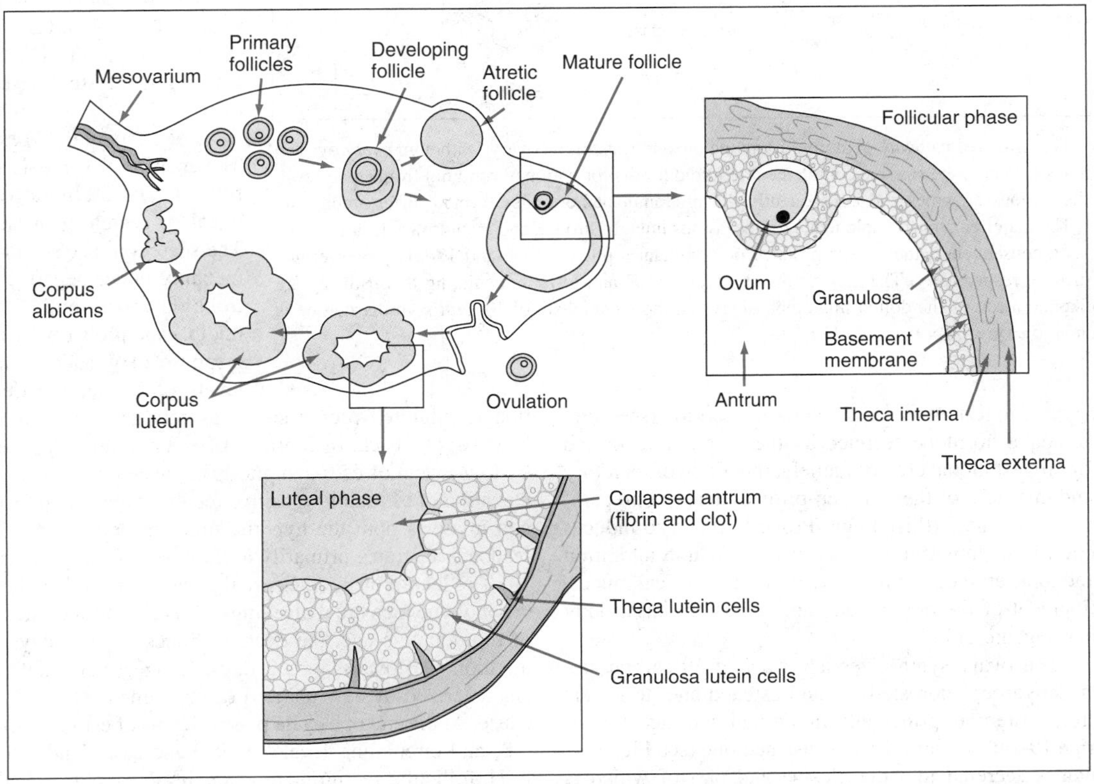

FIGURE 337-2 Developmental changes in the adult ovary during a complete 28-day cycle.

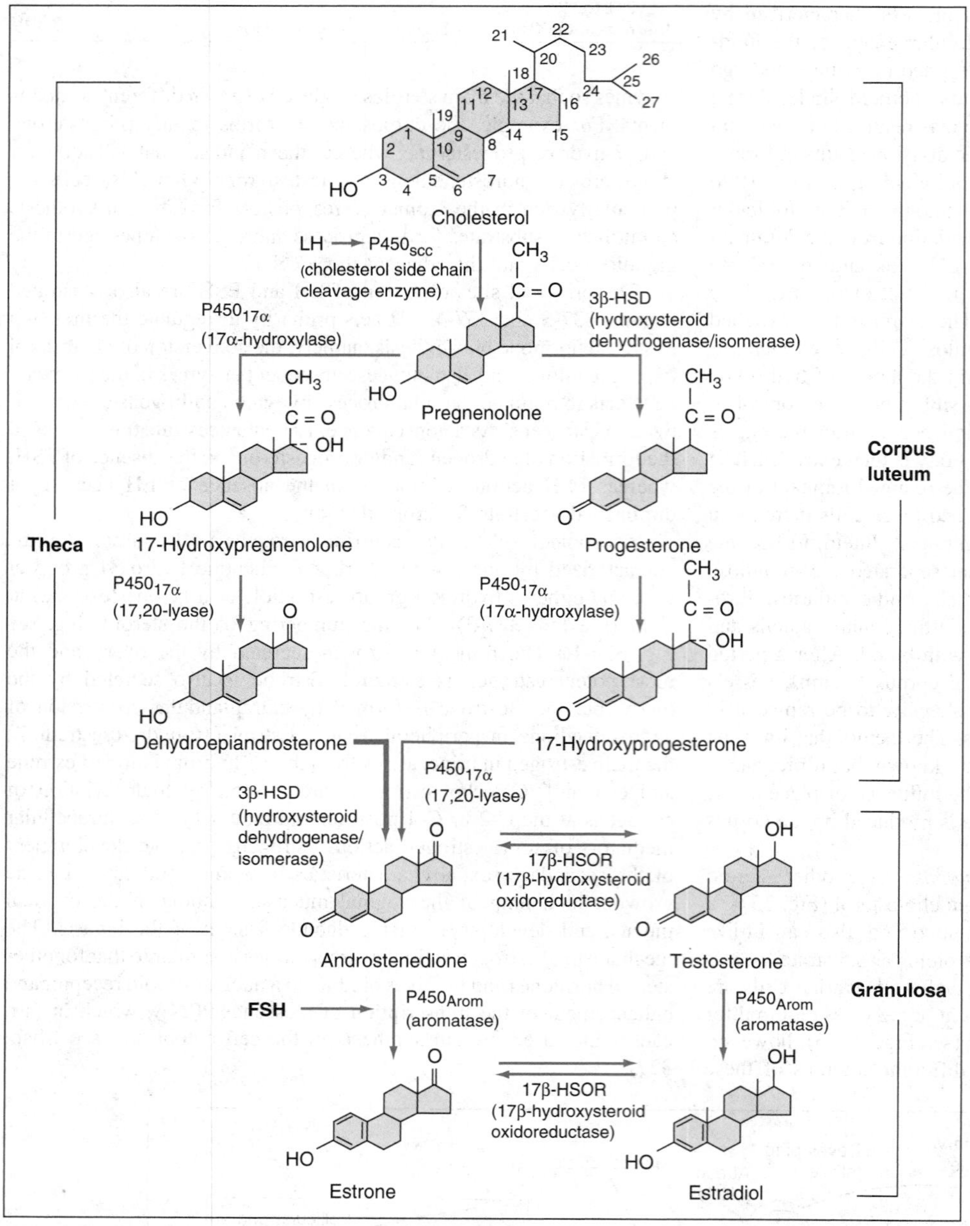

FIGURE 337-3 The principal pathway of steroid hormone biosynthesis in the ovary. Although every ovarian cell probably contains the complete enzyme complement required for the formation of estradiol from cholesterol, the amounts of the various enzymes and consequently the predominant hormones formed differ among the various cell types. The major enzyme complements for the corpus luteum, stroma, and granulosa cells are shown by the brackets; as a consequence, these cells produce predominantly progesterone and 17-OH progesterone, androgen, and estrogen, respectively. The major sites of action of LH and FSH in mediating this pathway are shown in the horizontal arrows. The dotted line emphasizes that the metabolism of 17-hydroxyprogesterone is limited in the human ovary. *(From Carr, 1992.)*

PROGESTERONE Progesterone, a 21-carbon steroid (see Fig. 337-3), is the principal hormone secreted by the corpus luteum and is responsible for progestational effects, namely, induction of secretory activity in the endometrium of the estrogen-primed uterus in preparation for implantation of the fertilized egg. Progesterone also induces a decidual reaction in endometrium. Other effects include inhibition of uterine contractions, an increase in the viscosity of cervical mucus, glandular development of the breasts, and an increase in basal body temperature (thermogenic effect).

ANDROGENS The ovary synthesizes a variety of 19-carbon steroids, including dehydroepiandrosterone, androstenedione, testosterone, and dihydrotestosterone, principally in stromal and thecal cells. The major ovarian 19-carbon steroid is androstenedione (see Fig. 337-3), part of which is secreted into the plasma and part of which is converted to estrogen in granulosa cells or to testosterone in the interstitium. Androstenedione also can be converted to testosterone and estrogens in peripheral tissues. Only testosterone and dihydrotestosterone are true androgens that interact with the androgen receptor and induce virilizing signs in women (see Chaps. 53 and 336).

Other hormones Some ovarian hormones play an uncertain role in human physiology. *Relaxin*, a polypeptide hormone produced by the human corpus luteum and by the decidua, causes softening of the cervix and loosening of the symphysis pubis in preparation for parturition in animals. *Oxytocin, vasopressin*, and other hypothalamic and pituitary hormones are also present in granulosa and/or luteal cells, but their function in these cells is unknown. *Follicular inhibin*, or *folliculostatin* (the equivalent of testicular inhibin), is secreted by the follicle and is believed to inhibit the release of FSH by the hypothalamic-pituitary unit. *Activin* is also secreted by the follicle and may enhance FSH secretion. *Follicle regulatory protein* (FRP), found in human follicular fluid, inhibits granulosa secretion and growth. *Gonadocrinins*, peptides purified from rat follicular fluid, stimulate the release of both FSH and LH from the pituitary in vitro and in vivo. Granulosa cells secrete *oocyte maturation inhibitor* (OMI), a factor that prevents premature ovulation. In addition, in the gonads of both sexes a *meiosis-inducing substance* (MIS) triggers the onset of meiosis, an event that occurs earlier in ovarian than in testicular development. Local growth factors [including insulin-like growth factors (IGFs) 1 and 2 and transforming growth factors (TGFs) α and β] may also influence steroid secretion by the ovary.

The Normal Menstrual Cycle The menstrual cycle is divided into a follicular or proliferative phase and a luteal or secretory phase (Fig. 337-5). The secretion of FSH and LH is fundamentally under negative feedback control by ovarian steroids (particularly estradiol) and probably by inhibin, but the response of gonadotropins to different levels of estradiol varies. FSH secretion is inhibited progressively as estrogen levels increase—typical negative feedback. In contrast, LH secretion is suppressed maximally by low levels of estrogen and is enhanced by a rising and sustained elevation of estradiol—positive feedback. Negative feedback of estrogen involves both the hypothalamus and pituitary, whereas positive feedback operates primarily at the level of the pituitary.

The length of the menstrual cycle is defined as the time from the onset of one menstrual bleeding episode to onset of the next. In women of reproductive age, the cycle averages 28 ± 3 days, and the mean duration of flow is 4 ± 2 days. Longer menstrual cycles (usually characterized by anovulation) occur at menarche and prior to menopause. At the end of a cycle plasma levels of estrogen and progesterone fall, and circulating levels of FSH increase. Under the influence of FSH, follicular recruitment results in development of the follicle that will be dominant during the next cycle.

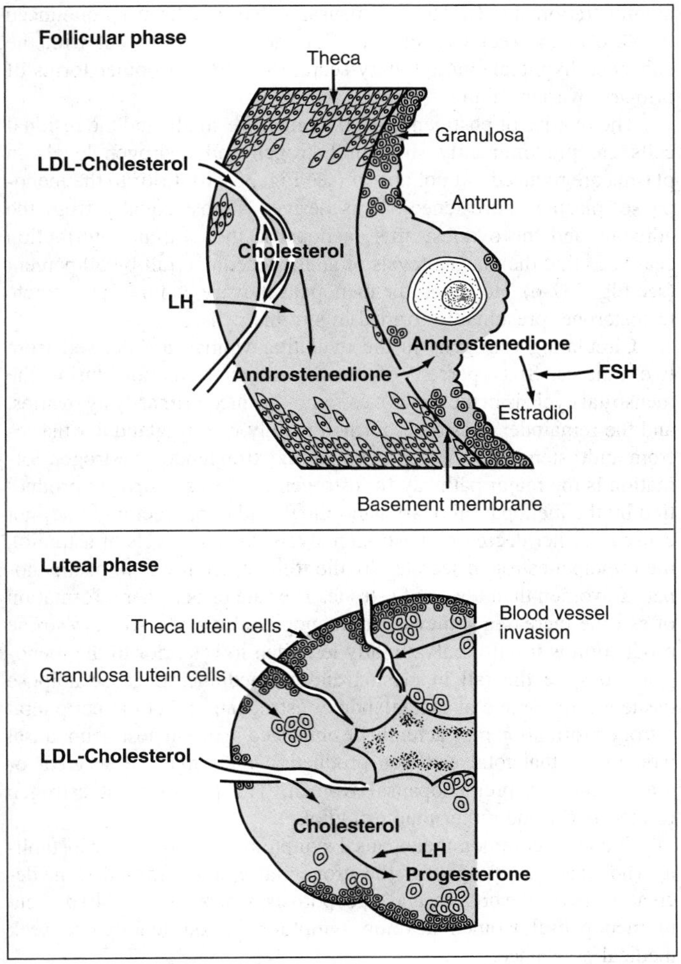

FIGURE 337-4 Cellular interactions in the ovary during the follicular phase (*top*) and luteal phase (*bottom*). LDL, low-density lipoprotein; FSH, follicle-stimulating hormone; LH, luteinizing hormone. *(From Carr et al, 1982.)*

After the onset of menses, follicular development continues, but FSH levels decrease. Approximately 8 to 10 days prior to the midcycle LH surge, plasma estradiol levels begin to rise as the result of estradiol formation by the granulosa cells of the dominant follicle. During the second half of the follicular phase, LH levels also begin to rise (owing to positive feedback). Just before ovulation, estradiol secretion reaches a peak and then falls. Immediately thereafter, a further rise in the plasma level of LH mediates the final maturation of the follicle, followed by follicular rupture and ovulation 16 to 23 h after the LH peak. The rise in LH is accompanied by a smaller increase in the level of plasma FSH, the physiologic significance of which is unclear. The plasma progesterone level also begins to rise just prior to midcycle and facilitates the positive feedback action of estradiol on LH secretion.

At the onset of the luteal phase, plasma gonadotropins decrease, and plasma progesterone increases. A secondary rise in estrogens causes further gonadotropin suppression. Near the end of the luteal phase, progesterone and estrogen levels fall, and FSH levels begin to rise to initiate the development of the next follicle (usually in the contralateral ovary) and the next menstrual cycle.

The endometrium lining the uterine cavity undergoes marked alterations in response to the changing plasma levels of ovarian hormones (see Fig. 337-5). Concurrent with the decrease in plasma estrogen and progesterone and the decline of corpus luteum function in the late luteal phase, intense vasospasm occurs in the spiral arterioles supplying blood to the endometrium, causing ischemic necrosis, endometrial desquamation, and bleeding. This vasospasm is caused by locally synthesized prostaglandins. The onset of bleeding marks the first day of the menstrual cycle. By the fourth to fifth day of the cycle, the endometrium is thin. During the proliferative phase, glandular growth of the endometrium is mediated by estrogen. After ovulation, increased progesterone levels lead to further thickening of the endometrium, but the rapid growth slows. The endometrium then enters the secretory phase, characterized by tortuosity of the glands, curling of the spiral arterioles, and glandular secretion. As corpus luteum function begins to wane in the absence of conception, the sequence of events leading to menstruation is again set into action.

Biphasic changes in basal body temperature are characteristic of the ovulatory cycle and are mediated by alterations in progesterone levels (see Fig. 337-5). An increase in basal body temperature by 0.3 to 0.5°C begins after ovulation, persists during the luteal phase, and returns to the normal baseline (36.2 to 36.4°C) after the onset of the subsequent menses.

Cellular Interactions in the Ovary during the Normal Cycle LH stimulates thecal cells surrounding the follicle to form androgens, and androstenedione diffuses across the basement membrane of the follicle into granulosa cells, where it is aromatized to estrogen (see Figs. 337-3 and 337-4).

The increase of FSH late in the preceding menstrual cycle stimulates growth and recruitment of the primary follicles by enhancing granulosa cell proliferation, resulting ultimately in the formation of the dominant follicle. In the granulosa cells, FSH also stimulates estrogen synthesis. Enhanced secretion of estradiol causes an increase in the number of estradiol receptors and further proliferation of granulosa cells. In the late follicular phase, FSH, in concert with estradiol, causes induction of LH receptors on the granulosa cells. LH acts via these receptors to increase progesterone secretion at midcycle. The amount of progesterone formed by the follicle is believed to be limited by the availability of cholesterol to serve as substrate for steroidogene-

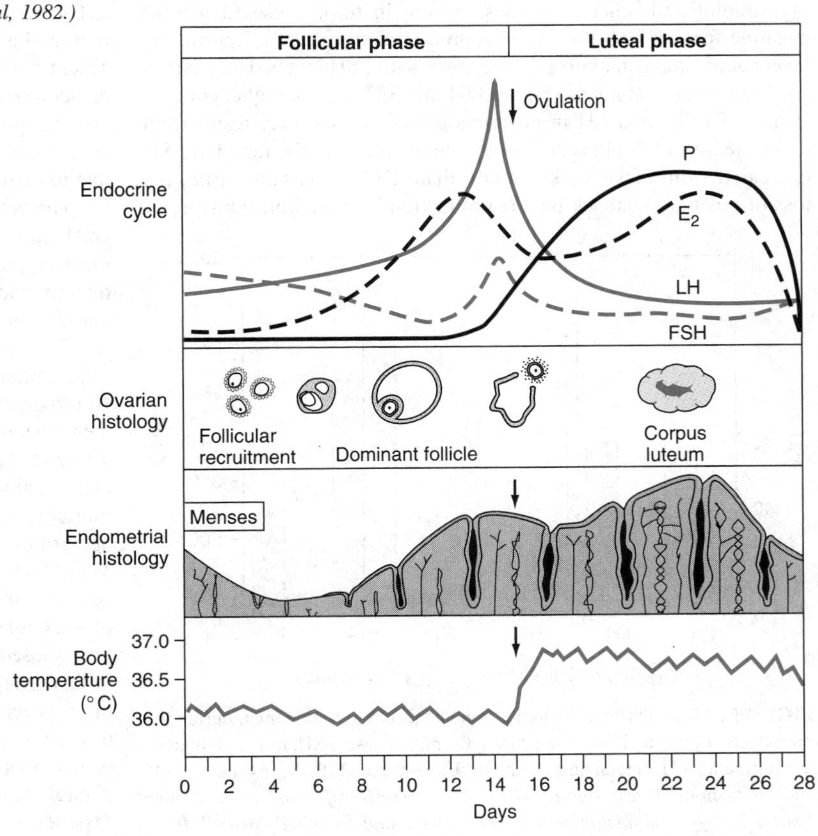

FIGURE 337-5 The hormonal, ovarian, endometrial, and basal body temperature changes and relationships throughout the normal menstrual cycle.

sis and by the fact that most of the progesterone is converted to androstenedione by thecal cells. Prior to ovulation, the granulosa cells of the follicle are bathed in follicular fluid but have limited access to circulating blood and consequently to plasma low-density lipoprotein (LDL). As depicted in Fig. 337-4, the granulosa cells become vascularized after ovulation, and plasma cholesterol is made available to serve as the major substrate for progesterone synthesis by the corpus luteum. Thus, increased progesterone synthesis by the corpus luteum is the consequence of increased substrate availability. The peak in progesterone secretion by the corpus luteum occurs 8 days after ovulation at the time of maximal vascularization of the granulosa cells.

MENOPAUSE The *menopause* is defined as the final episode of menstrual bleeding in women. However, the term is used commonly to refer to the period that encompasses the transitional period between the reproductive years up to and after the last episode of menstrual bleeding. During this period, there is a progressive loss of ovarian function and a variety of endocrine, somatic, and psychological changes.

The median age of women at the time of cessation of menstrual bleeding is 50 to 51 years. Since the life expectancy of women is close to 80 years, approximately one-third of life occurs after cessation of reproductive function. Preceding the menopause, the pattern of menstrual cycles is variable, but the interval between menses usually becomes longer. In addition, there is an increase in the mean levels of plasma FSH and LH, despite the continuation of ovulatory cycles. Thus, the ovary appears to become less responsive to gonadotropins prior to the menopause.

The menopause is the consequence of the exhaustion of ovarian follicles. The decrease in the number of ova begins in intrauterine life; by the time of the menopause, few ova remain, and these appear to be nonfunctional. Only a small number of ova are lost as the result of ovulation during reproductive life; the majority are lost by atresia. The cessation of follicular development results in decreased production of estradiol and other hormones, which, in turn, causes a loss of negative feedback on the hypothalamic-pituitary centers. In turn, the levels of plasma gonadotropins increase, with FSH levels rising earlier and higher than LH levels (Figs. 337-1 and 337-6). The higher concentration of FSH than LH in postmenopausal women may result from the decrease in inhibin secretion by the ovary, from the fact that FSH is cleared from plasma less rapidly than LH, and possibly from the loss of positive feedback on LH production by estradiol. Intravenous administration of LHRH to menopausal women results in a pronounced increase in the secretion of both FSH and LH, consistent with the enhanced hypothalamic-pituitary secretory activity in other forms of primary ovarian failure.

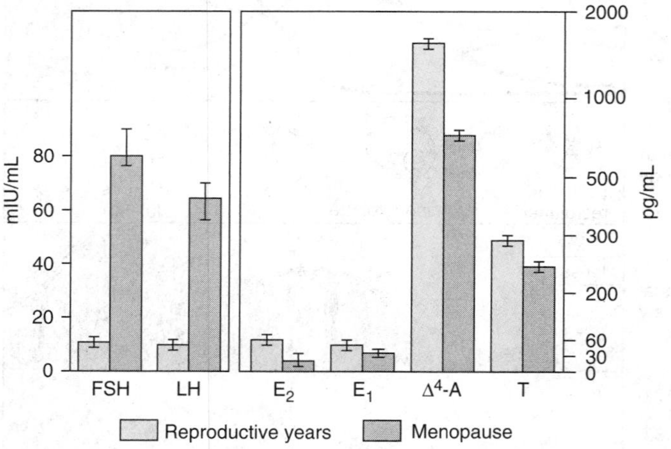

FIGURE 337-6 Differences in hormone concentration in women during the reproductive years and in women during the menopause. FSH, follicle-stimulating hormone; LH, luteinizing hormone; E_2, estradiol-17β; E_1, estrone; Δ^4-A, androstenedione; T, testosterone. *[From SSC Yen, RB Jaffe (eds), Reproductive Endocrinology. Philadelphia, Saunders, 1986; and from DR Mishell Jr, V Dajavan (eds), Reproductive Endocrinology, Infertility, and Contraception, 2d ed, Philadelphia, Davis, 1986.]*

The ovaries of postmenopausal women are small, and the residual cells are predominantly stromal. Estrogen and androgen levels in plasma are reduced but not absent (see Fig. 337-6). Prior to the menopause, plasma androstenedione is derived almost equally from the adrenals and the ovaries; after menopause the ovarian contribution ceases so that the plasma levels of androstenedione fall by 50 percent (see Fig. 337-6). However, the menopausal ovary continues to secrete testosterone, presumably formed in stromal cells.

Circulating estrogens in the ovulating woman are derived from two sources. Sixty percent of mean estrogen formation during the menstrual cycle is in the form of estradiol, formed primarily by ovaries, and the remainder is estrone, formed mainly in extraglandular tissues from androstenedione. After menopause, extraglandular estrogen formation is the major pathway for estrogen synthesis. Estrogen production by the menopausal ovary is minimal, and oophorectomy does not cause a further decrease in estrogen levels. Plasma levels of estradiol, the principal estrogen secreted by the follicle, are lower in postmenopausal women than levels of estrone. The rate of peripheral formation of estrone increases somewhat in menopausal women so that estrone production is usually only slightly less than it was prior to the menopause despite the fall in plasma androstenedione. Because adipose tissue is a major site of extraglandular estrogen production, peripheral estrogen formation may actually be enhanced in obese postmenopausal women, so that total estrogen production rates may be as great or greater than in premenopausal women. The predominant estrogen formed is estrone rather than estradiol.

The most common menopausal symptoms are vasomotor instability (hot flashes), atrophy of the urogenital epithelium and skin, decreased size of the breasts, and osteoporosis. Approximately 40 percent of menopausal women develop symptoms serious enough to seek medical assistance.

The pathogenesis of the hot flash is uncertain. There is a close temporal relationship between the onset of the hot flash and pulses of LH secretion; however, hot flashes occur in women with hypopituitarism and after treatment with LHRH analogues, when LH levels are absent or low. Alterations in catecholamine, prostaglandin, endorphin, or neurotensin metabolism may play a role in conjunction with low estrogen production. Symptoms associated with the hot flash, including nervousness, anxiety, irritability, and depression, may or may not be due to estrogen deficiency.

The decrease in size of the tissues of the female reproductive tract and breasts in the menopause is due to estrogen deficiency. The vaginal mucosa and the endometrium usually become thin and atrophic (although endometrial hyperplasia occurs in one-fifth of postmenopausal women).

Osteoporosis is one of the dread afflictions of aging, and there is a close relationship between estrogen deprivation and its development. Approximately one-fourth of aging women and one-tenth of elderly men sustain a vertebral or hip fracture between the ages of 60 and 90, and the incidence is highest in elderly white women. Such fractures are a major cause of death and morbidity, and the fracture-related mortality increases from less than 10 percent in the 60- to 64-year age group to 30 percent or more in patients over 80 (see Chap. 355). Many factors affect the development of osteoporosis, including diet, activity, smoking, and general health, and estrogen deprivation is of particular importance. White postmenopausal women are more predisposed to osteoporosis and its consequences because bone density in this group is lower prior to menopause, so loss in bone density has more severe consequences. Further evidence that osteoporosis is a disease of estrogen deprivation is suggested by the early development of osteoporosis in women with premature menopause due to either natural causes or surgical castration. After the menopause women experience an increase in the incidence of cardiovascular disease, possibly as the result of a decrease in the level of high-density lipoprotein (HDL) cholesterol.

LABORATORY AND CLINICAL ASSESSMENT OF HORMONAL STATUS

The hormonal status of women can usually be assessed by history and physical examination. In general, the presence of secondary sexual characteristics such as normal female breast development indicates adequate estrogen secretion in the past, and the presence of regular, predictable, cyclic menses implies that ovulation and the production of gonadotropins, estrogen, progesterone, and androgens are adequate and that the outflow tract is intact. Such a history may be more valuable than laboratory tests in evaluating ovarian hormone status. However, laboratory tests provide valuable ancillary information in the workup of women with endocrine dysfunction or infertility.

PITUITARY GONADOTROPINS Plasma gonadotropins are assessed by radioimmunoassay (RIA), fluoroimmunoassay (FIA), or enzyme-linked immunosorbent assay (ELISA). Because both FSH and LH are secreted in a pulsatile manner, the results obtained from a single serum sample may be difficult to interpret. Consequently, multiple samples taken at 20-min intervals over 2 h may be pooled to obtain a mean value. Serum gonadotropin measurements are of the most use in evaluating women with suspected ovarian failure and in supporting the diagnosis of polycystic ovarian disease and hypogonadotropic hypogonadism. The normal ranges for serum LH and FSH in ovulating women are 0.8 to 57 and 1.4 to 21 IU/L, respectively. FSH levels that are persistently above 34 IU/L are diagnostic of ovarian failure, and an LH value of less than 0.8 IU/L suggests hypogonadotropic hypogonadism. In practice, however, gonadotropin values may be equivocal and must be interpreted in light of the remainder of the findings.

OVARIAN HORMONES The mean plasma levels and production rates of the principal ovarian hormones are presented in Table 337-1. The production rate of a hormone is the sum of the amount of hormone formed by direct glandular secretion and by extraglandular conversion of prohormones.

Estrogen The presence of normal secondary sexual characteristics implies that estrogen production was adequate in the past. The current estrogen status can be estimated by pelvic examination. The presence of a moist, rugated vagina with copious, clear, thin cervical mucus that can be stretched and that exhibits arborization or ferning when spread on a slide is strong evidence of adequate estrogen production. Cytologic demonstration of mature vaginal epithelial cells and abundant cornified squamous epithelial cells with pyknotic nuclei confirms the presence of adequate estrogen levels.

The progesterone-withdrawal test provides a functional assessment of estrogen status. If menses appear within a week to 10 days after the end of a trial of medroxyprogesterone acetate (10 mg by mouth once or twice a day for 5 days) or after a single intramuscular injection of progesterone (100 mg), then prior estrogen priming was adequate to allow withdrawal bleeding.

Owing to its variable level in plasma during the normal cycle and the difficulty of estimating the day of the cycle in women with abnormal cycles, the measurement of estrogen levels in plasma or urine is of little use in the routine assessment of estrogen status. Measurement of plasma estradiol is useful during attempts to induce ovulation with human menopausal gonadotropins to prevent the development of the ovarian hyperstimulation syndrome and is used along with ultrasound assessment to monitor follicular growth in women who are to undergo in vitro fertilization.

Progesterone Cyclic, predictable menses also imply that adequate progesterone is secreted during the luteal phase of the menstrual cycle. Assessment of progesterone is useful to detect ovulation, to evaluate the adequacy of the luteal phase in infertile women, and to distinguish women with müllerian agenesis from those with testicular feminization. Several functional assays of progesterone can be used. The least expensive and most useful is the daily measurement of basal body temperature throughout a cycle. Owing to the thermogenic properties of progesterone, a normal biphasic monthly curve showing a temperature elevation lasting for approximately 2 weeks after ovulation is a valid indication of progesterone secretion during the luteal phase (see Fig. 337-5). The presence of viscous cervical mucus that does not stretch or fern and of predominantly intermediate cells on vaginal cytology or demonstration of a secretory epithelium in an endometrial biopsy during the luteal phase on days 20 to 22 of the cycle provides additional assessment of progesterone secretion. In addition, serum progesterone can be measured by RIA, FIA, or ELISA to assess the function of the corpus luteum.

Androgen Under normal conditions, the ovary secretes androstenedione, testosterone, and dehydroepiandrosterone. In conditions of androgen excess, hirsutism and/or virilization are common. The evaluation of androgen excess is discussed in Chap. 53.

DIAGNOSIS OF PREGNANCY Pregnancy is usually recognized on the basis of the history and physical examination. That is, a woman with previously cyclic, predictable menses develops amenorrhea accompanied by breast tenderness, malaise, lassitude, and nausea, and on physical examination the uterus is soft and enlarged.

Assays of placental products facilitate the diagnosis of pregnancy. Human chorionic gonadotropin (hCG) is secreted by the trophoblastic cells of the placenta into the maternal plasma and excreted in the urine. Assays of the hCG content of serum or urine use either antibody against hCG or the LH/hCG receptor and make it possible to detect pregnancies 8 to 10 days after ovulation, before the first missed menstrual period and long before pregnancy can be diagnosed by clinical assessments. Assay of the β subunit of hCG in serum or urine makes it possible to differentiate between excess LH and hCG, an important distinction in evaluating women with trophoblastic disease such as hydatidiform mole or choriocarcinoma.

DISORDERS OF OVARIAN FUNCTION

PREPUBERTAL YEARS Puberty is said to be *precocious* if breast budding begins before age 8 or if menarche occurs before age 9. Those disorders in which the developing sexual characteristics are appropriate for the genetic and gonadal sex—i.e., feminization in girls or virilization in boys—are termed *isosexual precocity*, whereas *heterosexual precocity* occurs when sexual characteristics are not in accord with the genetic sex, namely, virilization in girls or feminization in boys. Pubertal disorders of boys are described in Chap. 336.

Isosexual Precocious Puberty Isosexual precocious puberty in girls can be divided into three major categories (Table 337-2).

True precocious puberty True precocious puberty is characterized by an early but otherwise normal sequence of pubertal development, including increased secretion of gonadotropins and ovulatory

Table 337-1

Concentrations, Metabolic Clearance Rates, and Production Rates of the Major Ovarian Steroid Hormones in Blood of Ovulatory Women

Steroid	Binding*	Phase of Menstrual Cycle	Plasma Concentration, nmol/L, ng/ml	Production Rate, μmol/d, mg/d
Estradiol	TeBG and albumin	Follicular	0.07–2.6 (0.02–0.7)	0.3–3.6 (0.08–1.0)
		Luteal	0.7 (0.2)	0.9 (0.25)
Estrone	Albumin	Follicular	0.2–1.1 (0.05–0.3)	0.4–2.6 (0.1–0.7)
		Luteal	0.4 (0.1)	0.9 (0.24)
Progesterone	CBG and albumin	Follicular	3 (1)	6.4 (2)
		Luteal	16–80 (5–25)	80 (25)
Androstenedione	Albumin	—	5.6 (1.6)	10 (3)
Testosterone	TeBG and albumin	—	1.4 (0.4)	0.9 (0.25)

* TeBG, testosterone-binding globulin; CBG, cortisol-binding globulin.

SOURCE: Modified from MB Lipsett, in *Reproductive Endocrinology*, SSC Yen, RB Jaffe (eds). Philadelphia, Saunders, 1986.

Table 337-2

Differential Diagnosis of Sexual Precocity

Isosexual precocity
- A. True precocious puberty
  1. Constitutional
  2. Organic brain disease
  3. Congenital adrenal hyperplasia
- B. Precocious pseudopuberty
  1. Ovarian tumors
  2. Adrenal tumors
  3. McCune-Albright syndrome
  4. Hypothyroidism
  5. Russell-Silver syndrome
  6. Estrogen-containing medications
- C. Incomplete sexual precocity
  1. Premature thelarche
  2. Premature adrenarche
  3. Premature pubarche

Heterosexual precocity
- A. Ovarian tumors
- B. Adrenal tumors
- C. Congenital adrenal hyperplasia

menstrual cycles. Constitutional or idiopathic precocious puberty accounts for 90 percent of cases. In these individuals, no cause for the premature maturation of the central nervous system–hypothalamic-pituitary axis can be identified, and the diagnosis is one of exclusion. As many as half these individuals have abnormal findings on electroencephalograms. Premature appearance of secondary sexual characteristics and of ovulatory cycles with the accompanying risk of fertility may cause significant emotional disturbance. Therefore, prompt initiation of therapy is imperative. LHRH analogues inhibit estrogen synthesis and thus reverse precocious puberty; they may also prevent premature closure of the epiphyses and the resulting short stature.

About 10 percent of cases are due to organic brain diseases, including brain tumors (hypothalamic gliomas, astrocytomas, ependymomas, germinomas, and hamartomas), encephalitis, meningitis, hydrocephalus, head injury, tuberous sclerosis, and neurofibromatosis. It is essential to distinguish this group of patients from those with the idiopathic disorder, and patients whose disorder is designated as idiopathic occasionally prove to have such tumors. Fortunately, most patients with organic lesions serious enough to cause precocious puberty have obvious neurologic signs and symptoms. Evaluation of all patients with precocious puberty should include, at a minimum, skull films and computed tomography (CT) or magnetic resonance imaging (MRI) of the brain. The success of treatment depends on the nature of the lesion, but surgical and radiation treatment of well-localized tumors is occasionally successful.

A rare cause of isosexual precocity is congenital adrenal hyperplasia due to 21-hydroxylase deficiency in girls in whom treatment is delayed until 4 to 8 years of age. After initiation of glucocorticoid replacement, such individuals may undergo isosexual precocious puberty (see Chap. 332).

Precocious pseudopuberty Precocious pseudopuberty occurs when girls undergo feminization as a consequence of enhanced estrogen formation but do not ovulate or develop cyclic menses. Ovarian cysts or tumors that secrete estrogen (granulosa-theca cell tumors) are the most frequent cause of precocious pseudopuberty. Granulosa-theca cell tumors associated with intestinal polyps and pigmentation of the mucous membranes occur in the Peutz-Jeghers syndrome. Other ovarian tumors that secrete estrogens (or androgens that can be converted to estrogens at extraglandular sites) include dysgerminomas, teratomas, cystadenomas, and ovarian carcinomas (also see Chap. 99). Ovarian tumors usually can be detected by rectoabdominal examination or by sonography, CT, MRI, and/or laparoscopy. Ovarian teratomas and choriocarcinomas and other carcinomas that secrete hCG do not cause precocious puberty in girls unless they also secrete estrogen (hCG or LH in the absence of FSH does not induce ovarian estrogen production). Rarely, feminizing tumors of the adrenal cause isosexual precocious puberty by direct formation of estrogens or by secretion of weak androgens, which are converted to estrogens in extraglandular tissues.

Other causes of precocious pseudopuberty include the following:

1. The McCune-Albright syndrome (polyostotic fibrous dysplasia) is due to a G-protein defect that causes gonadotropin receptor activation in the absence of ligand, leading to autonomous ovarian follicle development and estrogen formation. It is characterized by café au lait spots, cystic fibrous dysplasia of bones, and sexual precocity. Occasionally, this disorder leads to true precocious puberty (see Chap. 340).
2. Primary hypothyroidism is associated with enhanced secretion of thyrotropin-releasing hormone (TRH) and, occasionally, of other hypothalamic hormones as well, leading to increased FSH levels and ovarian estrogen secretion, frequently with galactorrhea.
3. The Russell-Silver syndrome, or congenital asymmetry, is associated with short stature and precocious feminization.
4. Estrogen-containing medications, including use of estrogen-containing creams for diaper rash or the ingestion of meat from estrogen-treated animals or poultry or of any estrogen by mouth, can cause this disorder.

Incomplete isosexual precocity This term is used to describe the premature development of a single pubertal event and encompasses several entities. Breast budding prior to age 8 (*premature thelarche*) without other evidence of estrogen secretion and without premature bone maturation is believed to be due to a transient increase in estrogen secretion or to a temporary increase in sensitivity to the small amounts of circulating estrogens formed prior to puberty. Usually, the disorder is self-limited and resolves spontaneously. Occasionally, axillary hair and/or pubic hair (*premature adrenarche* and *pubarche*) appear without any other secondary sexual development. The phenomenon is associated with adrenal androgen secretion in the range of normal puberty and can be distinguished from syndromes of virilization by the absence of clitoromegaly. It requires no treatment, and patients enter puberty at about the average time.

Heterosexual Precocity Virilization in a prepubertal female is usually due to congenital adrenal hyperplasia or to androgen secretion by an ovarian or adrenal tumor. The manifestations of virilization are described in Chaps. 53 and 332. Virilization in girls with congenital adrenal hyperplasia usually takes place in a background of variable sexual ambiguity (see Chap. 339).

Evaluation of Sexual Precocity The evaluation of sexual precocity involves a careful history and physical examination, including rectoabdominal examination, abdominal sonography, determination of bone age, and measurement of thyroid hormones, thyroid-stimulating hormone (TSH), and gonadotropins (and androgen or estrogen levels when appropriate). MRI and/or CT scans should be obtained if a neurologic disorder is suspected and no evidence of ovarian or adrenal tumor is found.

REPRODUCTIVE YEARS Disorders of the Menstrual Cycle *Abnormal uterine bleeding* Between menarche and the menopause, almost every woman experiences one or more episodes of abnormal uterine bleeding, here defined as any bleeding pattern that differs in frequency, duration, or amount from the pattern observed during a normal menstrual cycle. A variety of descriptive terms (such as *menorrhagia*, *metrorrhagia*, and *menometrorrhagia*) have been used to characterize patterns of abnormal uterine bleeding. A more logical approach is to divide abnormal uterine bleeding into those patterns associated with ovulatory cycles and those associated with anovulatory cycles.

Ovulatory cycles Normal menstrual bleeding with ovulatory cycles is spontaneous, regular, cyclic, and predictable and frequently is associated with discomfort (dysmenorrhea). Deviations from this pattern associated with cycles that are still regular and predictable are most often due to organic disease of the outflow tract. For example, regular but prolonged and excessive bleeding episodes unassociated with bleeding dyscrasias (hypermenorrhea or menorrhagia) can result from abnormalities of the uterus such as submucous leiomyomas, adenomyosis, or endometrial polyps. Regular, cyclic, predictable menstruation characterized by spotting or light bleeding is termed *hypomenorrhea* and is due to obstruction of the outflow tract as from intrauterine synechiae or scarring of the cervix. Intermenstrual bleeding between episodes of regular, ovulatory menstruation is also often due to cervical or endometrial lesions. An exception to the association between organic disease and abnormal uterine bleeding is the occurrence of regular menstruation more frequently than 21 days apart (polymenorrhea). Such cycles may be a normal variant.

Anovulatory cycles Uterine bleeding that is unpredictable with respect to amount, onset, and duration and is usually painless is described as *dysfunctional uterine bleeding*. This disorder is not due to abnormalities of the uterus but rather to chronic anovulation and occurs when there is interruption of the normal sequence of follicular and luteal phases under the influence of a dominant follicle and its resulting corpus luteum. As discussed above, uterine bleeding in ovulatory cycles is due to progesterone withdrawal and requires that the endometrium first be primed with estrogen. (When castrates or postmenopausal women are given progesterone, withdrawal bleeding usually does not occur.)

Dysfunctional uterine bleeding can occur in women who have a transient disruption of the synchronous hypothalamic-pituitary-ovarian patterns necessary for ovulatory cycles, most often at the extremes of the reproductive life—in the early menarche and in the perimenopausal period—but also after temporary stress or intercurrent illness.

Primary *dysfunctional uterine bleeding* can result from three disorders.

1. *Estrogen withdrawal bleeding* occurs when estrogen is given to a castrated or postmenopausal woman and then withdrawn. As in other types of dysfunctional uterine bleeding, this form of menstrual bleeding is usually painless.
2. *Estrogen breakthrough bleeding* occurs when there is continuous estrogen stimulation of the endometrium not interrupted by cyclic progesterone secretion and withdrawal. This is the most common type of dysfunctional uterine bleeding and is usually due to anovulation associated with chronic acyclic estrogen production, as in women with polycystic ovarian disease. Such women may have histories of irregular, unpredictable menses, oligomenorrhea, or amenorrhea (see below). Alternatively, estrogen breakthrough bleeding can occur in hypogonadal women given estrogens chronically rather than intermittently and in women with estrogen-secreting tumors of the ovary. Estrogen breakthrough bleeding may be profuse and is unpredictable with respect to duration, amount of flow, and time of occurrence. The endometrium is typically thin because its repair between episodes of bleeding is incomplete.
3. *Progesterone breakthrough bleeding* occurs in the presence of abnormally high ratios of progesterone to estrogen, e.g., in women using continuous low-dose oral contraceptives.

The approach to a patient with dysfunctional uterine bleeding begins with a careful history of menstrual patterns and prior hormonal therapy. Since not all urogenital tract bleeding is from the uterus, rectal, bladder, and vaginal or cervical sources must be excluded by physical examination. If the bleeding is from the uterus, a pregnancy-related disorder such as abortion or ectopic pregnancy must be ruled out. Once the diagnosis of dysfunctional uterine bleeding is established, a rational approach to management is as follows: During a first episode of dysfunctional bleeding the patient can simply be observed, provided the bleeding is not copious and no evidence of bleeding dyscrasia is present. If bleeding is moderately severe, control can be achieved with relatively high dose estrogen oral contraceptives for 3 weeks. Alternatively, a regimen of three or four low-dose oral contraceptive pills per day for 1 week followed by tapering to the usual dosage for up to 3 weeks is also effective. If uterine bleeding is more severe, hospitalization, bed rest, and intramuscular injections of estradiol valerate (10 mg) and hydroxyprogesterone caproate (500 mg) or intravenous or intramuscular conjugated estrogens (25 mg) usually control the bleeding. After initial treatment, iron replacement should be instituted, and recurrence can be prevented by cyclic oral contraceptives for 2 to 3 months (or more if pregnancy is not desired). Alternatively, menses can be induced every 2 to 3 months with medroxyprogesterone acetate, 10 mg by mouth once or twice a day for 10 days. If hormone therapy fails to control uterine bleeding, an endometrial biopsy, hysteroscopy, or dilatation and curettage may be required for diagnosis and therapy. Indeed, uterine sampling should be performed prior to hormone therapy in women at risk for endometrial cancer (i.e., in women who are approaching the age of menopause or are massively obese); endometrial cancer is rare in ovulatory women of reproductive age.

Amenorrhea An acceptable definition of amenorrhea is failure of menarche by age 16, irrespective of the presence or absence of secondary sexual characteristics, or the absence of menstruation for 6 months in a woman with previous periodic menses. However, women who do not fulfill these criteria should be evaluated if (1) the subject and/or her family are greatly concerned, (2) no breast development has occurred by age 14, or (3) any sexual ambiguity or virilization is present (Chap. 339). Amenorrhea is commonly categorized as either primary (the woman has never menstruated) or secondary (when menstruation has been present for a variable period of time in the past and has ceased). However, some disorders can cause either primary or secondary amenorrhea. For example, most women with gonadal dysgenesis have primary amenorrhea, but some have some follicles and ovulate for short periods so that pregnancy occurs rarely. Furthermore, patients with chronic anovulation (polycystic ovarian disease) usually have secondary amenorrhea but on occasion have primary amenorrhea. For these reasons, categorization of amenorrhea into primary and secondary types is less helpful than a classification based on the underlying physiologic derangements: (1) anatomic defects, (2) ovarian failure, and (3) chronic anovulation with or without estrogen present.

ANATOMIC DEFECTS Anatomic or structural defects of the genital tract can preclude menstrual bleeding. Starting from the caudal end of the female genital tract, labial agglutination or fusion is often associated with disorders of sexual development, particularly female pseudohermaphroditism (congenital adrenal hyperplasia or exposure to maternal androgens in utero) (see Chap. 339). Congenital defects of the vagina, imperforate hymen, and transverse vaginal septae also can cause amenorrhea. These women frequently have accumulation of menstrual blood behind the obstruction and may have cyclic, predictable episodes of abdominal pain.

More severe müllerian anomalies include müllerian agenesis (the Mayer-Rokitansky-Küster-Hauser syndrome; see Chap. 339), second in frequency only to gonadal dysgenesis as a cause of primary amenorrhea. Women with this syndrome have a 46,XX karyotype, female secondary sex characteristics, and normal ovarian function, including cyclic ovulation, but have absence or hypoplasia of the vagina. The uterus usually consists of only rudimentary bicornuate cords, but if the uterus contains endometrium, cyclic abdominal pain and accumulation of blood may occur, as in other forms of outlet obstruction. One-third of women with this syndrome have abnormalities of the urogenital tract, and one-tenth have skeletal anomalies, usually involving the spine. The major diagnostic problem is distinguishing müllerian agenesis from complete testicular feminization, in which 46,XY genetic males with testes differentiate as phenotypic women but with a blind vaginal pouch and no uterus. Women with testicular feminization have feminized breasts but a paucity of pubic and axillary hair. The disorder is due to a defect in the androgen receptor that causes profound resistance to the action of testosterone (see Chap. 339). Testicular feminization can be diagnosed by demonstrating a male level of serum testosterone or a 46,XY karyotype, whereas demonstration of a 46,XX karyotype, the biphasic basal body temperature curve characteristic of ovulation, and elevated levels of progesterone during the luteal phase establish the diagnosis of müllerian agenesis.

A rare cause of absence of the uterus in 46,XY phenotypic women who are sexually infantile is the so-called testicular regression syndrome or testicular agenesis (see Chap. 339).

Other abnormalities of the uterus that cause amenorrhea include obstruction due to scarring or stenosis of the cervix, often resulting from surgery, electrocautery, laser therapy, or cryosurgery. Such destruction of the endometrium (Asherman's syndrome) usually follows vigorous curettage for postpartum hemorrhage or after therapeutic abortion complicated by infection. This diagnosis is confirmed by hysterosalpingography or by direct visual examination of the endometrial scarring or synechiae using a hysteroscope.

Treatment of disorders of the outflow tract is surgical.

OVARIAN FAILURE Primary ovarian failure is associated with elevated plasma gonadotropin levels and can result from several causes. The most frequent cause is *gonadal dysgenesis*, in which the germ cells are absent and the ovary is replaced by a fibrous streak (also see Chaps. 65 and 339). Women with gonadal dysgenesis can be divided into two broad groups on the basis of chromosomal karyotype. The most common type is due to deletion of genetic material in the X chromosomes and accounts for about two-thirds of cases of gonadal dysgenesis. A 45,X karyotype is found in about half of women with this disorder, and most have somatic defects, including short stature, webbed neck, shield chest, and cardiovascular defects, collectively termed the *Turner phenotype*. The remainder of women with X chromosome abnormalities have chromosomal mosaicism with or without associated structural abnormalities of the X. The most common form of mosaicism is 45,X/46,XX. Gonadal tumors are rare in 45,X patients, but gonadal malignancies may occur in women with chromosomal mosaicism involving the Y chromosome. Therefore, chromosomal analysis should be performed in all cases of amenorrhea associated with ovarian failure, and the streak gonad should be removed if a Y chromosome is present. One means of identifying the presence of a Y chromosome is to amplify the sex-determining regions of the Y chromosome (SRY) by means of the polymerase chain reaction (see Chap. 339). Approximately 90 percent of women with gonadal dysgenesis due to partial or complete deletion of the X never have menstrual bleeding, and the remaining 10 percent have sufficient follicles to experience menses and, rarely, fertility; the menstrual and reproductive lives of such individuals are invariably brief.

One-tenth of individuals identified as having bilateral streak gonads have a normal 46,XX or 46,XY karyotype and are said to have *pure gonadal dysgenesis*. These individuals have either normal or above-average stature, owing to failure of estrogen-mediated epiphyseal closure in the presence of a normal chromosomal constitution. Pure gonadal dysgenesis does not constitute a phenotypic or chromosomally homogeneous disorder (see Chap. 339). Occasional women with a 46,XY karyotype develop signs of virilization, including clitoromegaly, and have an increased incidence of tumors in the gonadal streaks; as a consequence, gonadal streaks should be removed prophylactically, as discussed above, when a Y chromosome is present. Approximately two-thirds of women with 46,XX gonadal dysgenesis experience no menses, while the remainder have one or more menstrual episodes and are occasionally fertile.

Other causes of ovarian failure and amenorrhea include deficiency of the $P450_{17\alpha}$ gene that encodes 17α-hydroxylase and 17,20-lyase activities, premature ovarian failure, the resistant-ovary syndrome, and ovarian failure secondary to chemotherapy or radiation therapy for malignancy. *17α-Hydroxylase deficiency* is characterized by primary amenorrhea, sexual infantilism, and hypertension, the latter due to increased production of desoxycorticosterone (DOC); whereas women with *17,20-lyase deficiency* have primary amenorrhea and sexual infantilism with normal blood pressure (see Chaps. 332 and 339). The diagnosis of *premature ovarian failure* or *premature menopause* is applied to women who cease menstruating prior to age 40. The ovaries in such women are similar to the ovaries of postmenopausal women, containing few or no follicles as the result of accelerated follicular atresia. Premature ovarian failure due to ovarian antibodies may be one component of polyglandular failure, together with adrenal insufficiency, hypothyroidism, and other autoimmune disorders (see Chap. 340). A rare form of ovarian failure is the *resistant-ovary syndrome*, in which the ovaries contain many follicles that are arrested in development prior to the antral stage, possibly because of resistance to the action of FSH in the ovary. To differentiate this disorder from the 46,XX variety of pure gonadal dysgenesis, which also is associated with sexual immaturity, it is necessary to perform ovarian biopsy. However, it is not clinically useful to make this distinction, since the conventional treatment of infertility in both conditions is usually unsuccessful. Women with ovarian failure who desire pregnancy have been treated with hormone replacement and transfer of donor embryos to the uterine cavity or fallopian tubes.

Chronic anovulation At least 80 percent or more of gynecologic endocrine disorders result form chronic anovulation. Women with chronic anovulation fail to ovulate spontaneously but may ovulate with appropriate therapy. The ovaries of such women do not secrete estrogen in a normal cyclic pattern; it is clinically useful to differentiate those women who produce enough estrogen to have withdrawal bleeding after progestogen therapy from those who do not; the latter often have hypothalamic-pituitary dysfunction.

CHRONIC ANOVULATION WITH ESTROGEN PRESENT Women with chronic anovulation who experience withdrawal bleeding after progestogen administration are said to be in a state of "estrus" due to the acyclic production of estrogen, largely estrone, by extraglandular aromatization of circulating androstenedione. This disorder is commonly termed *polycystic ovarian disease* (PCOD) and is characterized by infertility, hirsutism, obesity, and amenorrhea or oligomenorrhea. When spontaneous uterine bleeding occurs in women with PCOD, it is unpredictable as to time of onset, duration, and amount; on occasion the bleeding can be severe. The dysfunctional uterine bleeding is usually due to estrogen breakthrough (see above).

The disorder, as originally described by Stein and Leventhal, was characterized by enlarged, polycystic ovaries, but it is now known to be associated with a variety of pathologic findings in the ovaries, only some of which result in enlargement and none of which are pathognomonic. The most common finding is a white, smooth, sclerotic ovary with a thickened capsule, multiple follicular cysts in various stages of atresia, a hyperplastic theca and stroma, and rare or absent corpora albicans. Other ovaries have hyperthecosis in which the ovarian stroma is hyperplastic and may contain lipid-laden luteal cells. Thus, the diagnosis of PCOD is a clinical one, based on the coexistence of chronic anovulation and varying degrees of androgen excess.

In most women with PCOD, menarche occurs at the expected time, but uterine bleeding is unpredictable in onset, duration, and amount. Amenorrhea ensues after a variable period, although primary amenorrhea occurs in some women. Signs of androgen excess (hirsutism) usually become evident around the time of menarche. One scenario suggests that this disorder originates as an exaggerated adrenarche in obese girls (Fig. 337-7). The combination of elevated levels of adrenal androgens and obesity leads to increased formation of extraglandular estrogen. This estrogen exerts a positive feedback on LH secretion and negative feedback on FSH secretion, resulting in a ratio of LH to FSH levels in plasma that is characteristically greater than 2. The increased LH levels can then lead to hyperplasia of the ovarian stroma and theca cells and increased androgen production, which in turn provides more substrate for peripheral aromatization and perpetuates the chronic anovulation. In the advanced stage of the disorder, the ovary is the major site of androgen production, but the adrenal may continue to secrete excess androgen as well. The greater the obesity, the more strongly this sequence would be perpetuated because more androgen is converted to estrogen by adipose tissue stromal cells, which in turn exaggerates inappropriate LH release by positive feedback.

Thus, the fundamental defect in PCOD is viewed as inappropriate signals to the hypothalamus and pituitary. In turn, the hypothalamic-pituitary axis responds appropriately to high levels of estrogen, and ovulation can be induced with antiestrogen agents such as clomiphene

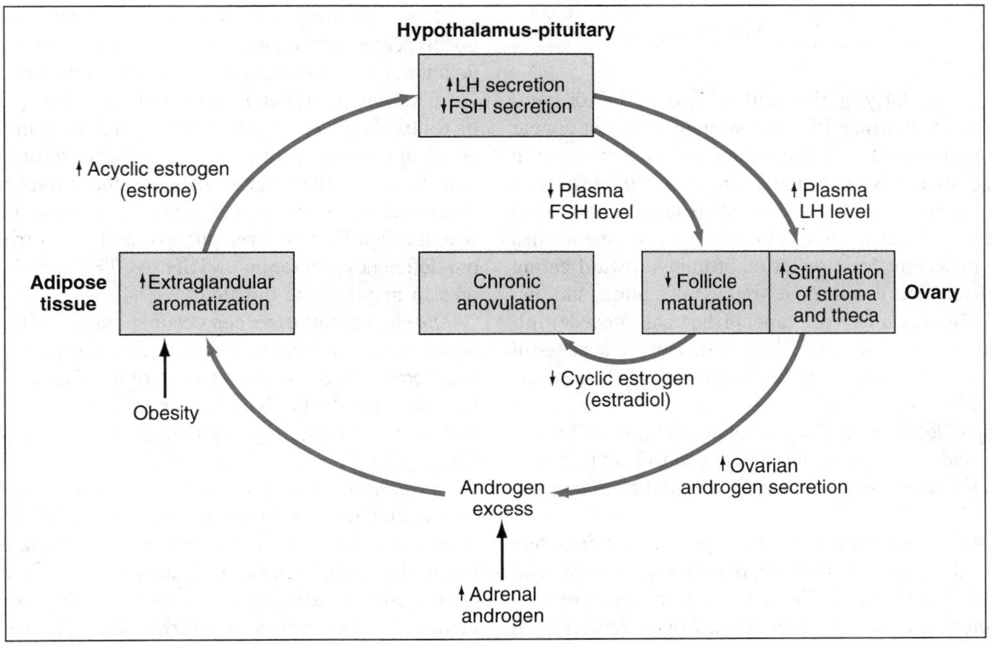

FIGURE 337-7 Proposed mechanism for the initiation and perpetuation of chronic anovulation in polycystic ovarian disease (PCOD). This cycle may be entered or initiated via adrenal androgen excess or obesity, both of which result in enhanced extraglandular formation of estrogens. The therapy of PCOD involves interruption of the cycle at any of several steps. *[From SSC Yen, RB Jaffe (eds), Reproductive Endocrinology. Philadelphia, Saunders, 1986; and from U Goebelmann, in Reproductive Endocrinology, Infertility, and Contraception, 2d ed, DR Mishell Jr, V Davajan (eds), Philadelphia, Davis, 1986.]*

citrate. Increased levels of plasma endorphins and inhibin may contribute to the perpetuation of the defect. The concept that the fundamental defect is one of inappropriate signals is supported by the findings in the ovary itself. Ovarian follicles from women with PCOD have low aromatase activity, but normal aromatase can be induced by treatment with FSH. In short, the anovulation is not due to an intrinsic abnormality in the ovary but rather results from a deficiency of FSH and an excess of LH. An association exists between PCOD/hyperthecosis, virilization, acanthosis nigricans, and insulin resistance; in the ovary, insulin may interact via the insulin-like growth factor receptors to enhance androgen synthesis in insulin-resistant states.

Rx TREATMENT

Treatment of PCOD is directed toward interrupting the self-perpetuating cycle and can be accomplished in several ways, such as by decreasing ovarian androgen secretion (by wedge resection or the use of oral contraceptive agents), decreasing peripheral estrogen formation (by weight reduction), or enhancing FSH secretion [by administration of clomiphene, human menopausal gonadotropin (hMG), LHRH (gonadorelin) by portable infusion pump, or purified FSH (urofollitropin)]. The choice of therapy depends on the clinical findings and the needs of the patient. An attempt at weight reduction is appropriate in all who are obese. If the woman is not hirsute and does not desire pregnancy, periodic withdrawal menses can be induced with medroxyprogesterone acetate 10 days per month; such treatment prevents the development of endometrial hyperplasia. If the woman is hirsute and does not desire pregnancy, the ovarian (and possibly the adrenal) component of androgen production can be suppressed with combined estrogen-progestogen oral contraceptive agents. Combined oral contraceptives are also indicated if prolonged or excessive menstrual bleeding is present. Once androgen excess is controlled, treatment of previously existing hair growth by shaving, depilatories, or electrolysis may be indicated (see Chap. 53). If pregnancy is desired ovulation must be induced. The drug of choice for this purpose is clomiphene, which promotes ovulation in three-fourths of cases, or hMG, urofollitropin, or gonadorelin. Pretreatment with LHRH analogues prior to use of hMG, urofollitropin, or gonadorelin may improve the rates of ovulation and pregnancy. An alternative therapy is ovarian drilling by laser or cautery performed at laparoscopy in women in whom hormonal therapy is not effective; however, the procedure is associated with a high incidence of ovarian adhesions.

Chronic anovulation with estrogen present also may occur with tumors of the ovary. These include granulosa-theca cell tumors, Brenner tumors, cystic teratomas, mucous cystadenomas, and Krukenberg tumors (also see Chap. 99). Such tumors can either secrete excess estrogen themselves or produce androgens that are aromatized in extraglandular sites. Chronic anovulation and the clinical features of PCOD result. Occasionally, areas of the ovary not involved with tumors show the characteristic histologic changes of PCOD. Other causes of chronic anovulation with estrogen present include adrenal production of excess androgen (usually adult-onset adrenal hyperplasia due to partial $P450_{C21}$ deficiency) and various thyroid disorders.

CHRONIC ANOVULATION WITH ESTROGEN ABSENT Women with chronic anovulation who have low or absent estrogen production and do not experience withdrawal bleeding after progestogen treatment usually have hypogonadotropic hypogonadism due to disease of either the pituitary or the central nervous system.

Isolated hypogonadotropic hypogonadism associated with defects of smell (olfactory bulb defects) is known as the *Kallmann syndrome* (see Chaps. 328 and 336). Affected women are sexually infantile and have a defect in the synthesis and/or release of LHRH. Hypothalamic lesions that impair LHRH production and cause hypogonadotropic hypogonadism include craniopharyngioma, germinoma (pinealoma), glioma, Hand-Schüller-Christian disease, teratomas, endodermal-sinus tumors, tuberculosis, sarcoidosis, and metastatic tumors that cause suppression or destruction of the hypothalamus. Central nervous system trauma and irradiation also can cause hypothalamic amenorrhea and deficiencies in secretion of growth hormone, adrenocorticotropic hormone (ACTH), vasopressin, and thyroid hormone.

More commonly, gonadotropin deficiency leading to chronic anovulation is believed to arise from functional disorders of the hypothalamus or higher centers. A history of a stressful event in a young woman is frequent. For example, chronic anovulation can begin suddenly in a woman who leaves home for the first time or experiences the death of a loved one. Gonadotropin and estrogen levels are in the low to low-normal range as compared with normal women in the early follicular phase of the cycle. In addition, rigorous exercise such as jogging or ballet and diets that result in excessive weight loss may lead to chronic anovulation, particularly in girls with a history of prior menstrual irregularity. The amenorrhea in these women does not appear to be due to weight loss alone but to a combination of a decrease in body fat and chronic stress. An extreme form of weight loss with chronic anovulation occurs in anorexia nervosa. Anorexia nervosa is characterized by the development in a young woman of amenorrhea with associated severe weight loss, distorted attitudes toward eating and weight gain, self-induced vomiting, extreme emaciation, and distorted body image. In anorexia nervosa amenorrhea can precede, follow, or coincide with weight loss (see Chap. 76). During successful therapy, gonadotropin changes recapitulate those observed during normal puberty (see Fig. 337-1).

In addition, chronic debilitating diseases such as end-stage kidney disease, malignancy, and malabsorption are believed to lead to development of hypogonadotropic hypogonadism via a hypothalamic mechanism.

Treatment of chronic anovulation due to hypothalamic disorders includes ameliorating the stressful situation, decreasing exercise, and correcting weight loss if appropriate. These women appear to be susceptible to the development of osteoporosis; estrogen replacement therapy is recommended to induce and maintain normal secondary sexual characteristics and prevent bone loss in those who do not desire pregnancy, and gonadotropin or gonadorelin therapy is indicated when pregnancy is desired (see "Treatment," below). When appropriate, therapy is directed at the primary disease of the hypothalamus.

Disorders of the pituitary can lead to the estrogen-deficient form of chronic anovulation by at least two mechanisms—direct interference with gonadotropin secretion by lesions that either obliterate or interfere with the gonadotropic cells (chromophobe adenomas, Sheehan's syndrome) or inhibition of gonadotropin secretion in association with excess prolactin (prolactinoma). *Pituitary tumors* make up approximately 10 percent of all intracranial tumors and may secrete no hormone, one hormone, or more than one hormone (see Chap. 328). Prolactin levels are elevated in 50 to 70 percent of patients with pituitary tumors, either because of prolactin secretion by the tumor itself (in the case of prolactinomas) or because the tumor mass interferes with the normal hypothalamic inhibition of prolactin secretion.

Prolactinomas can be divided into microadenomas (less than 10 mm in diameter) and macroadenomas (greater than 10 mm). Prolactin excess associated with low levels of LH and FSH constitutes a specific subtype of hypogonadotropic hypogonadism. One-tenth or more of amenorrheic women have increased levels of serum prolactin, and more than half of women with both galactorrhea and amenorrhea have elevated prolactin levels. The amenorrhea is most often associated with decreased or absent estrogen production, but prolactin-secreting tumors on occasion are associated with normal ovulatory menses or chronic anovulation with estrogen present. Most prolactin-secreting adenomas grow slowly, and some cease to grow after attaining a certain size. The increased frequency of diagnosis of prolactin-secreting adenomas is probably due to several factors, including increased awareness, improved radiographic detection methods, and availability of radioimmunoassays for prolactin. Since in older autopsy series a 9 to 23 percent prevalence of pituitary adenomas was observed in asymptomatic women, the clinical and prognostic significance of small microadenomas in asymptomatic individuals is unclear. However, when tumors of any size are associated with symptoms of amenorrhea or galactorrhea, particularly when visual field defects or severe headaches are present, bromocriptine therapy or neurosurgical evaluation is indicated. The evaluation, differential diagnosis, and management of hyperprolactinemia are described in Chap. 328. In the latter half of pregnancy, prolactin-secreting pituitary tumors may expand, leading to headaches, compression of the optic chiasm, and blindness. Therefore, before inducing ovulation for the purposes of achieving pregnancy, it is mandatory to exclude the presence of a pituitary tumor.

Large pituitary tumors such as null cell adenomas—whether or not hyperprolactinemia is present—are likely to be associated with deficiency of hormones in addition to gonadotropins (Chap. 328).

Craniopharyngiomas, which are thought to arise from remnants of Rathke's pouch, account for 3 percent of intracranial neoplasms, occur most frequently in the second decade of life, and may extend into the suprasellar region. Many of these tumors calcify and can be diagnosed by conventional skull films. Patients often present with sexual infantilism, delayed puberty, and amenorrhea due to gonadotropin deficiency; secretion of TSH, ACTH, growth hormone, and vasopressin may also be impaired.

Panhypopituitarism can occur spontaneously, result from surgical or radiation treatment of pituitary adenomas, or develop after postpartum hemorrhage (Sheehan's syndrome). Patients with the latter disorder characteristically have failure to lactate or ovulate, loss of genital and axillary hair, hypothyroidism, and adrenal insufficiency (see Chap. 328).

Evaluation of amenorrhea A general scheme for the evaluation of women with amenorrhea is given in Fig. 337-8. On physical examination, attention should be given to three features: (1) the degree of maturation of the breasts, pubic and axillary hair, and external genitalia; (2) the current estrogen status; and (3) the presence or absence of a uterus. All women with amenorrhea should be assumed to be pregnant until proven otherwise; it is prudent to exclude pregnancy by a suitable screening test even when the history and physical examination are not suggestive. Once that is done, the cause of amenorrhea can frequently be diagnosed clinically. For example, Asherman's syndrome is suggested by a history of curettage in a woman who previously menstruated; in women with primary amenorrhea and sexual infantilism, the essential differential diagnosis is between gonadal dysgenesis and hypopituitarism, and the diagnosis of gonadal dysgenesis (Turner's syndrome) or of anatomic defects of the outflow tract (müllerian agenesis, testicular feminization, and cervical stenosis) is frequently suggested on the basis of physical findings. When a specific cause is suspected, it is appropriate to proceed directly to confirm the diagnosis (as by obtaining a chromosomal karyotype or measurement of plasma gonadotropins). It is also useful to measure serum prolactin and FSH levels during the initial evaluation.

Estrogen status is evaluated by determining if the vaginal mucosa is moist and rugated and if the cervical mucus can be stretched and shown to fern upon drying. If these criteria are indeterminate, a progestational challenge is indicated, most often the administration of 10 mg medroxyprogesterone acetate by mouth once or twice daily for 5 days or 100 mg progesterone in oil intramuscularly. (It should be emphasized that progestogen should never be administered until pregnancy is excluded.) If estrogen levels are adequate (and the outflow tract is intact), menstrual bleeding should occur within 1 week of ending the progestogen treatment. If withdrawal bleeding occurs, the diagnosis is chronic anovulation with estrogen present, usually caused by polycystic ovarian disease.

If no withdrawal bleeding or only minimal vaginal spotting occurs, the nature of the subsequent workup depends on the results of the initial prolactin assay. If plasma prolactin is elevated, or if galactorrhea is present, radiography of the pituitary should be undertaken. When the plasma prolactin level is normal in an anovulatory woman with estrogen absent and with elevated FSH levels, the diagnosis is ovarian failure. If the gonadotropins are in the low or normal range, the diagnosis is either hypothalamic-pituitary disorder or an anatomic defect of the outflow tract. As indicated previously, the diagnosis of outflow tract disorder is usually suspected or established on the basis of the history and physical findings. When the physical findings are not clear-cut, it is useful to administer cyclic estrogen plus progestogen (1.25 mg oral conjugated estrogens per day for 3 weeks, with 10 mg medroxyprogesterone acetate added for the last 7 to 10 days of estrogen treatment), followed by 10 days of observation. If no bleeding occurs, the diagnosis of Asherman's syndrome or another anatomic defect of the outflow tract is confirmed by hysterosalpingography or hysteroscopy. If withdrawal bleeding occurs following the estrogen-progestogen combination, the diagnosis of chronic anovulation with estrogen absent (functional hypothalamic amenorrhea) is suggested. Radiologic evaluations of the pituitary-hypothalamic areas may be indicated in the latter cases—irrespective of the prolactin level—because of the danger of overlooking a pituitary-hypothalamic tumor and because the diagnosis of functional hypothalamic amenorrhea is one of exclusion (see Chap. 328).

Infertility Infertility, the failure to become pregnant after 1 year of unprotected intercourse, affects approximately 10 to 15 percent of couples and is a common reason for seeking gynecologic assistance. Male factors account for 40 percent of infertility problems (see Chap. 336). In women, failure of ovulation accounts for 30 percent of cases; pelvic factors, such as tubal disease or endometriosis, account for half; and a cervical factor is implicated in about one-tenth. In 10 to 20 percent of infertile women no etiology is found. An immunologic cause may underlie some of these cases. Finally, infertility in women may be due to *luteal-phase dysfunction*, in which ovulation is assumed to occur but progesterone formation is insufficient to allow preparation of the endometrium for implantation; the disorder is believed to be due to inadequate secretion or action of FSH and consequent inadequate formation of estrogen by the dominant follicle during the follicular phase.

The first diagnostic step in evaluation of the infertile couple is to determine whether the man or woman is the infertile partner, ordinarily by first performing a semen analysis in the man (see Chap. 336) and looking for signs of presumed ovulation in the woman. Documentation of ovulatory cycles is obtained by daily measurement of basal body temperatures throughout the month. Occasionally, accurate basal body temperature records are not obtained, and demonstration of elevated serum progesterone levels during the luteal phase may be used as evidence of ovulation. Dating of endometrium by histologic examination of a biopsy sample is also useful for establishing ovulation or luteal phase dysfunction.

If the infertility is associated with amenorrhea, then the workup is that described in Fig. 337-8. If polycystic ovarian disease is the basis for infertility, ovulation can be induced with clomiphene, gonadotropins, gonadorelin, or, on occasion, ovarian drilling. Bromocriptine is used to induce ovulation in cases of hyperprolactinemia. The appropriate therapy for prolactinomas in women who do not desire pregnancy is discussed in Chap. 328.

To evaluate the fallopian tubes and uterine cavity, hysterosalpingograms may be obtained, followed when appropriate by diagnostic laparoscopy and the demonstration of dye spillage from the fimbria after transcervical injection of dye during laparoscopy. Microsurgical repair of damaged or previously ligated fallopian tubes is followed by an apparent increase in pregnancy rates. Removal of peritubular and fimbrial adhesions by means of laparoscopic surgery plus laser beam therapy is an alternative treatment. Endometriosis can be diagnosed by laparoscopy, and treatment includes surgical resection of the endometrial implants or temporary gonadotropin suppression using danazol (400 to 800 mg orally in divided doses for 4 to 6 months), LHRH analogues given by nasal spray or subcutaneous or depot injection, or continuous low-dose oral contraceptive agents to promote regression of the implants.

The cervical factor in infertility is evaluated by study of cervical mucus at an appropriate time after coitus, preferably just prior to ovulation (day 12 to 13) when cervical mucus is thin and stretchy; such an examination provides information as to the penetration and survival of the sperm in the female genital tract. The preferred treatment of infertility due to such abnormality is intrauterine insemination with washed sperm.

When other treatment modalities are unsuccessful, in vitro fertilization and embryo transfer (IVF-ET) may be tried. Indications for the use of IVF-ET in infertile couples include tubal obstructive disease, cervical factors, endometriosis, oligospermia, and unexplained infertility. Multiple follicles are induced with clomiphene and/or gonadotropins, and follicles are usually obtained by transvaginal aspiration with ultrasound monitoring. After fertilization and cleavage, embryos are transferred to the uterine cavity. Although pregnancy rates vary, successful pregnancy has been reported in as many as 30 percent of cases after IVF-ET. Other techniques include a modification of IVF-ET known as *gamete-intrafallopian transfer* (GIFT), in which a mixture of sperm and ova are introduced into the end of the fallopian tube at laparoscopy, and intrauterine insemination after gonadotropin stimulation.

Medical Aspects of Pregnancy The possibility of pregnancy should be considered in all women of reproductive age who are evaluated for medical illness or considered for surgery. Procedures such as x-ray exposure, drugs, and anesthetics may be harmful to the developing fetus, and a variety of medical problems may worsen during pregnancy, including hypertension; diseases of the heart, lungs, kidney, and liver; and metabolic and endocrine disorders. Indeed, all women who present with abnormal vaginal bleeding or amenorrhea during the reproductive years should be assumed to have a complication of pregnancy, such as incomplete abortion, ectopic pregnancy, or trophoblastic disease (hydatidiform mole or choriocarcinoma). Women who present with these complications of pregnancy often have histories of abdominal pain and vaginal bleeding and may have evidence of intraabdominal hemorrhage.

Choriocarcinoma is a particular problem because of its protean manifestations. Half these malignancies follow pregnancies complicated by hydatidiform mole, and the remainder occur after spontaneous abortion, ectopic pregnancy, or normal deliveries. Patients may present with intraabdominal bleeding due to rupture of the uterus, liver, or

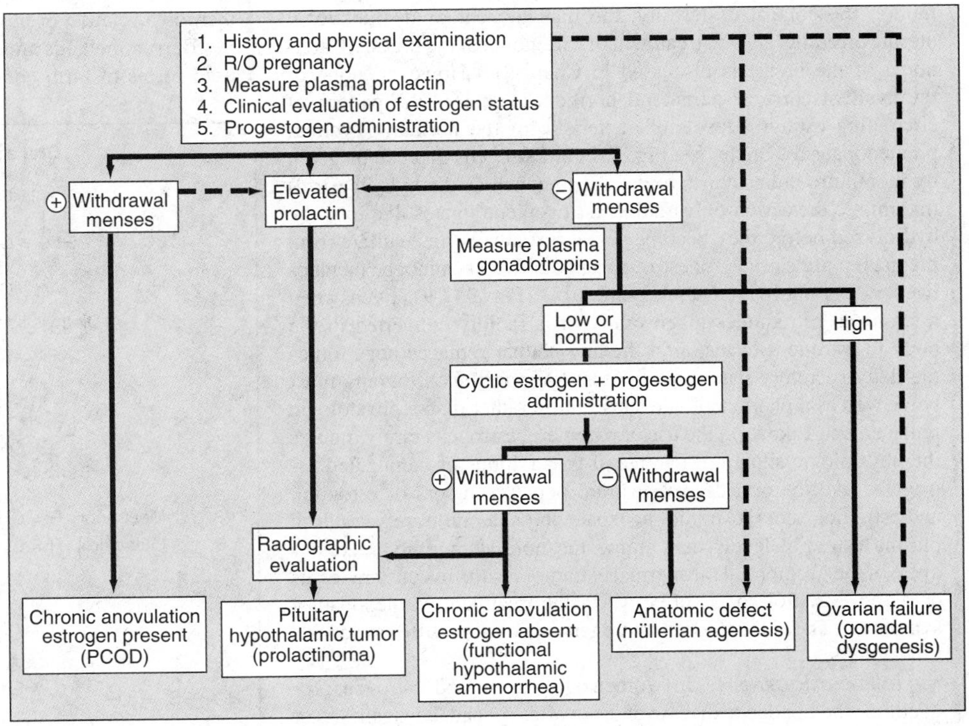

FIGURE 337-8 Flow diagram for the evaluation of women with amenorrhea. The most common diagnosis for each category is shown in parentheses. The dotted lines indicate that in some instances a correct diagnosis can be reached on the basis of history and physical examination alone.

ovary, with pulmonary manifestations (cough, hemoptysis, pleuritic pain, dyspnea, and respiratory failure) or gastrointestinal symptoms, usually chronic blood loss or melena. In addition, patients can present with cerebral metastases or renal involvement. The diagnosis can be established by demonstrating an elevated level of the β subunit of hCG in plasma. Treatment and cure are possible with chemotherapeutic agents (dactinomycin and/or methotrexate). →*For manifestations of choriocarcinoma in men, see Chap. 98.*

Ovarian Tumors See Chap. 99

TREATMENT

Progestogens The major use of progestogens is in conjunction with estrogen to ensure the full maturation of the endometrium, both in combination birth control pills and in the therapy of hypogonadal states. In certain circumstances, however, progestogen therapy is appropriate by itself—to induce a progestational effect on the estrogen-primed endometrium (in diagnostic tests for the evaluation of amenorrhea), to inhibit pituitary gonadotropins for contraception (the progestogen-only birth control pill or progestogen-containing implants), for prophylaxis to prevent hyperplasia in PCOD, for palliation in cases of endometrial and breast carcinoma, and for treatment of endometriosis. Even when a direct progestational effect is desired, the available oral drugs substitute a synthetic derivative for the naturally occurring hormone. Oral progestogens include medroxyprogesterone acetate, megestrol acetate, norethindrone, norgestrel, and micronized progesterone. Parenteral agents include progesterone in oil, medroxyprogesterone acetate suspension, and 17-hydroxyprogesterone caproate. Vaginal progesterone suppositories are used for treatment of luteal-phase defects, and progestogen implants are available for long-term contraception.

The most common undesirable side effect is breakthrough bleeding, which occurs when progestogens are used continuously. Other complications include nausea, vomiting, and hirsutism. Abnormal liver function is a side effect of those derivatives with alkyl substitution in the 17α position. Synthetic progestogens are contraindicated if pregnancy is known or suspected, because of the risk of birth defects.

Estrogens Estrogens are used for the treatment of gonadal failure, the control of fertility, the management of dysfunctional uterine bleeding, and the treatment of carcinoma of the breast. (Carcinoma of the breast is discussed in Chap. 91.) However, none of the available oral or parenteral hormones replaces the pattern of circulating estradiol levels characteristic of the normally cycling, premenopausal woman (see Fig. 337-5). Estrogens that can be given by mouth are either nonsteroidal agents (such as diethylstilbestrol) that mimic the action of estradiol, estrogen conjugates that must be hydrolyzed before they become active (usually estrone sulfate from pregnant mare's urine), or estrogen analogues that cannot be metabolized to estradiol (mestranol, quinestrol) (Fig. 337-9). Even when micronized estradiol is given orally, it is rapidly converted in the body to estrone. Because oral therapy neither replaces nor mimics the daily secretory pattern of the lost hormone, such therapy must be viewed as a pharmacologic substitution rather than a physiologic replacement. Likewise, the use of parenteral estrogens rarely mimics the physiologic situation. Parenteral preparations of conjugated estrogens, like the oral derivatives, are poor precursors of estradiol, and estradiol esters (estradiol benzoate and valerate) rarely result in plasma estradiol levels that mimic the normal monthly secretory cycle of the hormone. Transdermal estradiol results in constant levels of blood estradiol and is effective in the treatment of menopausal symptoms. The side effects of estrogen substitution differ at various times of life.

HYPOESTROGENISM In women with decreased estrogen production, whether due to disease of the ovaries (gonadal dysgenesis) or to hypogonadotropic hypogonadism, treatment with cyclic estrogens should be instituted at the time of expected puberty to induce the development and maintenance of female secondary sexual characteristics and to prevent osteoporosis. The most commonly used medications are conjugated estrogens (0.625 to 1.25 mg/d by mouth) together with medroxyprogesterone acetate (2.5 mg/d or 5 to 10 mg during the last several days of monthly estrogen treatment to prevent development of endometrial hyperplasia). Alternatively, oral contraceptives may be given. Abnormal bleeding in women receiving estrogen replacement mandates histologic evaluation of the endometrium. Such substitution therapy or the use of oral contraceptives (see below) also may be used for the purpose of suppressing pituitary gonadotropins, as in women with PCOD, in whom the major therapeutic aim is suppression of ovarian androgen production prior to the time when fertility is desired.

Temporary administration of estrogens in larger quantities (up to two times the usual adult maintenance dose) may be necessary to induce the full development of secondary sexual characteristics in girls and for the control of menopausal symptoms. Even larger doses of parenteral estrogens (10 mg estradiol valerate or 25 mg conjugated estrogen) in conjunction with progestogen may be required in some instances of dysfunctional uterine bleeding. In addition to the potential long-term side effects of all estrogens (see below), high doses may cause nausea, vomiting, and edema.

Fertility Control An understanding of the use, mechanisms of actions, and consequences of contraceptive agents is important to all physicians. Furthermore, since pregnancy may aggravate a variety of chronic illnesses, fertility control is an essential feature of the management of many disorders.

To be effective, fertility control requires patient compliance. Widely used methods include (1) rhythm and withdrawal techniques; (2) barrier methods, including the condom, jellies, foam, suppositories, and diaphragms; (3) intrauterine devices (IUDs); (4) hormonal contraceptives; (5) sterilization; and (6) abortion.

The rhythm and withdrawal techniques and the barrier methods are effective if used correctly and consistently, but in practice they have high failure rates because of imperfect compliance. Nevertheless, these methods carry the lowest incidence of side effects, and the side effects, when produced, are minor except for local allergic reactions. When the rhythm method is combined with self-evaluation of the preovulatory part of the menstrual cycle (i.e., evaluation of cervical mucus) plus home LH testing, it is an effective method of contraception. Use of these methods should be recommended when there is a relative or absolute contraindication to other methods.

Barrier methods are among the oldest, simplest, and most widely used forms of birth control. The term *barrier* originally implied a

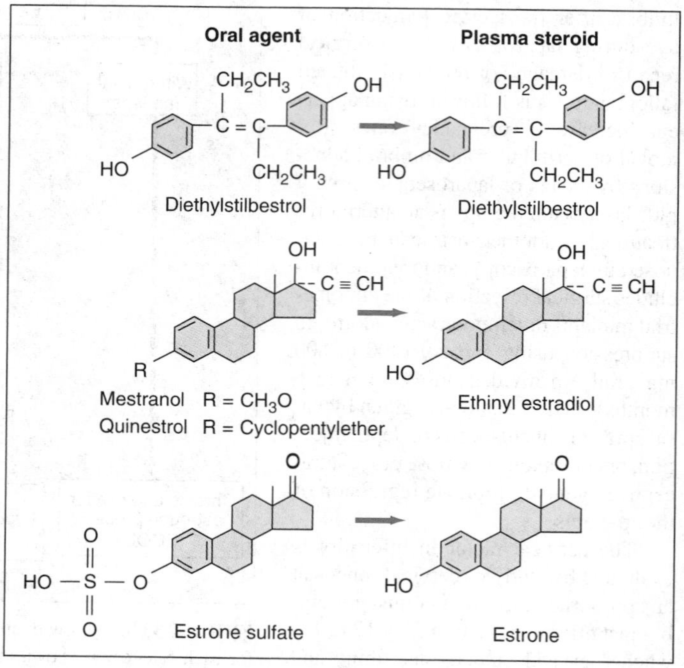

FIGURE 337-9 The circulating forms of administered estrogenic drugs.

physical barrier that prevents the sperm from reaching the egg, but the definition has been broaded to include biologic, chemical, and physical means of preventing fertilization. Barrier contraceptives are often underutilized, but if used correctly and continuously they provide adequete contraception and some protection against sexually transmitted diseases. All barrier methods require prior planning and motivation.

The most widely used nonsurgical methods of contraception, the IUD and oral contraceptive agents, are effective but may be associated with significant side effects.

IUD The success rates of most IUDs are 95 to 98 percent. Only two devices are marketed in the United States. Both are T-shaped, cause minimal pain at insertion, and are associated with low expulsion rates. One contains copper, which enhances effectiveness, and is replaced at 8-year intervals. The other contains slow-release progesterone, which makes annual replacement necessary. The IUD is believed to prevent pregnancy by inducing a chronic inflammatory reaction in the endometrium, resulting in an unfavorable environment for the implantation of the blastocyst, although some evidence suggests that IUDs prevent fertilization.

Once the IUD is inserted, it is necessary to check periodically to be certain that the device is in place. Both minor and serious side effects can occur. Intermenstrual spotting and increased bleeding and pain or cramps at the time of menses are frequent causes of discontinuation of IUD use. In addition, the device may be expelled spontaneously during a menstrual period without the user noticing. The most serious side effect is pelvic infection, occasionally leading to the development of tuboovarian abscess and subsequent infertility. Pelvic infection is more frequent than in users of oral or barrier contraceptives but no more common than in women using no contraception. Women with multiple sex partners are at the greatest risk for pelvic infection. For this reason, use of IUDs by nulligravid women is not advocated by many gynecologists. In addition, pregnancy with an IUD in place is more likely to be ectopic, because intrauterine but not extrauterine pregnancies are inhibited. Because of the increased incidence of spontaneous and septic abortions when IUDs are in place, the device should be removed if pregnancy is detected. When persistent, severe bleeding, lower abdominal pain, fever, or discharge develops, the IUD should be removed.

ORAL CONTRACEPTIVES Oral contraceptive agents have been used by over 200 million women worldwide and by 1 of 4 women in the United States under age 45. The agents are popular because of ease of administration, low pregnancy rates (less than 1 percent), and relatively infrequent side effects.

The most widely used oral contraceptives are either combination tablets or triphasic formulations. A list of oral contraceptives marketed in the United States is given in Table 337-3. Combination oral contraceptive tablets contain one of two synthetic estrogens (mestranol or ethinyl estradiol) and one of seven synthetic progestogens (norethindrone, norethindrone acetate, norethynodrel, norgestrel, ethynodiol diacetate, desogestrel, and norgestimate). The available agents contain no more than 50 μg of ethinyl estradiol or its equivalent. The combination or triphasic tablets are taken for 21 consecutive days followed by 7 days of rest. Progestogen-only tablets are taken continuously on a daily basis. Presumably, the best contraceptive—i.e., one that is effective while producing the fewest side effects—is the one that contains the lowest amount of steroid that is sufficient to prevent pregnancy or breakthrough bleeding. The triphasic tablets,

Table 337-3

Composition of Currently Marketed Oral Contraceptives

Name	Estrogen	μg	Progestogen	mg
COMBINATION-TYPE				
Fixed type				
Estrogen content = 50 μg:				
Ortho-Novum 1/50	Mestranol	50	Norethindrone	1.0
Norinyl 1/50	Mestranol	50	Norethindrone	1.0
Ovcon 50	Ethinyl estradiol	50	Norethindrone	1.0
Ovral	Ethinyl estradiol	50	Norgestrel	0.5
Demulen	Ethinyl estradiol	50	Ethynodiol diacetate	1.0
Norlestrin 2.5/50	Ethinyl estradiol	50	Norethindrone acetate	2.5
Norlestrin 1/50	Ethinyl estradiol	50	Norethindrone acetate	1.0
Estrogen content <50 μg:				
Ortho-Novum 1/35	Ethinyl estradiol	35	Norethindrone	1.0
Norinyl 1+35	Ethinyl estradiol	35	Norethindrone	1.0
Modicon	Ethinyl estradiol	35	Norethindrone	0.5
Brevicon	Ethinyl estradiol	35	Norethindrone	0.5
Ovcon 35	Ethinyl estradiol	35	Norethindrone	0.4
Demulen 1/35	Ethinyl estradiol	35	Ethynodiol diacetate	1.0
Loestrin 1.5/30	Ethinyl estradiol	30	Norethindrone acetate	1.5
Loestrin 1/20	Ethinyl estradiol	20	Norethindrone acetate	1.0
Nordette	Ethinyl estradiol	30	Levonorgestrel	0.15
Lo-Ovral	Ethinyl estradiol	30	Norgestrel	0.3
Desogen	Ethinyl estradiol	30	Desogestrel	0.15
Ortho-cept	Ethinyl estradiol	30	Desogestrel	0.15
Ortho-cyclen	Ethinyl estradiol	35	Norgestamate	0.25
Biphasic type				
Ortho-Novum 10/11				
First 10 days	Ethinyl estradiol	35	Norethindrone	0.5
Next 11 days	Ethinyl estradiol	35	Norethindrone	1.0
Triphasic type				
Ortho-Novum 7/7/7				
First 7 days	Ethinyl estradiol	35	Norethindrone	0.5
Second 7 days	Ethinyl estradiol	35	Norethindrone	0.75
Third 7 days	Ethinyl estradiol	35	Norethindrone	1.0
Tri-Norinyl				
First 7 days	Ethinyl estradiol	35	Norethindrone	0.5
Next 9 days	Ethinyl estradiol	35	Norethindrone	1.0
Next 5 days	Ethinyl estradiol	35	Norethindrone	0.5
Triphasil				
First 6 days	Ethinyl estradiol	30	Levonorgestrel	0.05
Second 5 days	Ethinyl estradiol	40	Levonorgestrel	0.075
Third 10 days	Ethinyl estradiol	30	Levonorgestrel	0.125
Tri-Levein				
First 6 days	Ethinyl estradiol	30	Levonorgestrel	0.05
Second 5 days	Ethinyl estradiol	40	Levonorgestrel	0.075
Third 10 days	Ethinyl estradiol	30	Levonorgestrel	0.125
Ortho Tri-Cyclen				
First 7 days	Ethinyl estradiol	35	Norgestimate	0.18
Second 7 days	Ethinyl estradiol	35	Norgestimate	0.215
Third 7 days	Ethinyl estradiol	35	Norgestimate	0.25
PROGESTOGEN ONLY				
Micronor	None		Norethindrone	0.35
Nor Q.D.	None		Norethindrone	0.35
Ovrette	None		Norgestrel	0.075

containing 35 μg or less of estrogen and less than 1 mg progestogen, come closest to this goal.

Oral contraceptives inhibit ovulation by suppressing FSH and LH secretion. In consequence, the secretion of all ovarian steroids, including estrogen, progesterone, and androgen, is also suppressed (Fig. 337-10). These agents also exert minor direct inhibitory effects on the reproductive tract, altering the cervical mucus and thereby decreasing sperm penetration, and decreasing the motility and secretions of the fallopian tubes and uterus.

The death rates associated with oral contraceptives and other forms of birth control are summarized in Table 337-4. Up to age 40, the mortality rates in women using oral contraceptives and IUDs are lower than in women using no contraception (this difference results from the increased risk of death with pregnancy). The decrease in death rate below age 40 is even more striking in nonsmokers than in smokers using contraceptives. In fact, the death rates in nonsmoking women aged 15 to 24 who use oral agents are lower than those with other forms of fertility control. The increased death rates in women using rhythm or barrier techniques probably results from the higher failure rate and the consequent risk of pregnancy in such women. Oral contraceptive agents are not recommended for smoking women after age 35 and for women of any ages who are at increased risk for myocardial infarction.

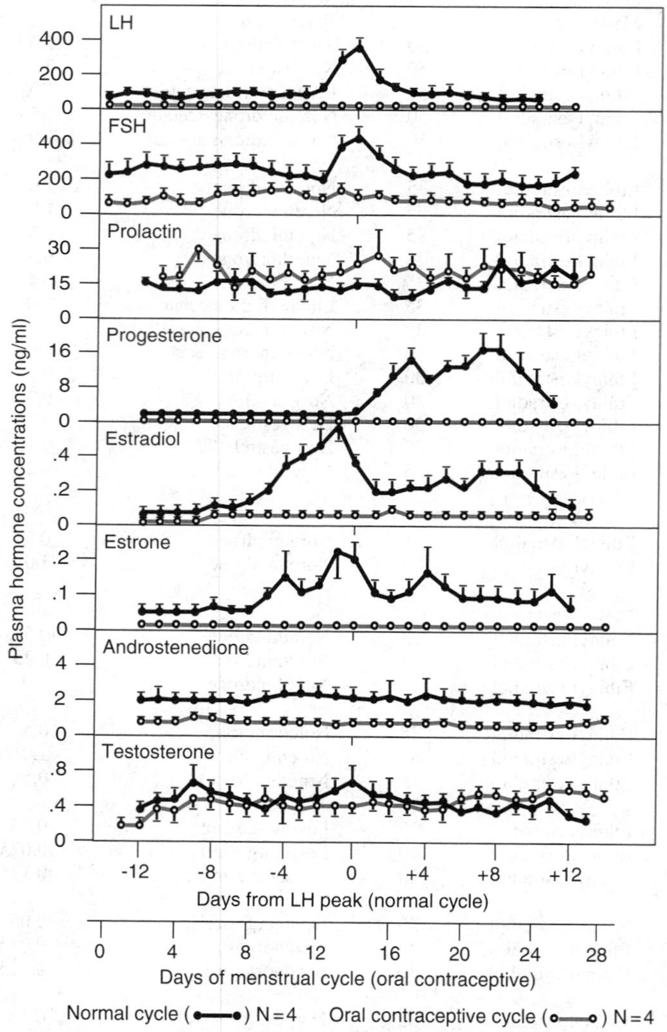

FIGURE 337-10 The mechanism of action of oral contraceptives. Mean daily plasma hormone concentrations during the ovarian cycle are shown for four ovulating women and four women treated with combination-type oral contraceptives. Data for the normal ovarian cycle are presented in relationship to the day of the LH peak; day 1 of the contraceptive cycle corresponds to the first day of uterine bleeding. The values are the mean ± SE obtained from four women. *(From Carr et al, 1979.)*

Despite the overall safety of these agents, users are at risk for serious side effects. In most retrospective and prospective studies, there is an increased incidence of *deep vein thrombosis* and *pulmonary embolism.* The increased risk varies from two- to twelvefold and is greater for women taking tablets containing more than 50 μg estrogen. The use of oral contraceptives is also associated with an increased risk of thromboembolism after surgery, and for this reason, the agents should be discontinued at least 1 month prior to elective surgery. In retrospective studies there is a three- to ninefold increase in the risk for *thromboembolic stroke* and a twofold increase in the risk for *hemorrhagic stroke* in oral contraceptive users. However, three large prospective studies of contraceptive use demonstrated only a slight increase in the rate of hemorrhagic stroke. Nevertheless, the drugs should be discontinued in women who experience visual complaints or severe headaches. Smoking and age increase the risk for stroke and the frequency of death from deep venous thrombosis, pulmonary emboli, and myocardial infarction.

A small rise in blood pressure is common, and 5 percent of women develop significant *hypertension* (blood pressure greater than 140/90) after 5 years of oral contraceptive use. Estrogens induce the synthesis of a variety of proteins by the liver, including the renin substrate angiotensinogen. The resulting increased formation of angiotensin is believed to be involved in the development of hypertension. Alternatively, the progestogen component of oral contraceptives may be associated with increased risk of hypertension. In most cases, blood pressure returns to normal when the agents are discontinued.

Serum lipids and lipoproteins are altered in women on oral contraceptives, the nature of the change depending on the specific contraceptive. In general, estrogens increase serum levels of HDL and of very low density lipoprotein (VLDL), and progestogens decrease the concentration of HDL. However, with oral contraceptives containing less than 35 μg estrogen, lipoprotein levels change little if at all.

A few women taking oral contraceptives develop *impairment of glucose tolerance* as manifested by abnormal glucose levels and elevated plasma insulin levels after an oral glucose load; both indices usually return to normal after discontinuing the agents. Because juvenile-onset and adult-onset diabetes may be associated with increased incidence of cardiovascular disease, it is preferable to use other forms of contraception in these individuals.

Oral contraceptives should not be used by women with abnormal results on liver function tests or with acute or chronic liver disease. A rare complication is the development of peliosis hepatis, which can cause death due to sudden rupture and hemorrhage of the liver. Cholestatic jaundice may occur in those women predisposed to the development of the recurrent jaundice of pregnancy.

Oral contraceptives cause an increased concentration of cholesterol in the bile, which is probably the cause for the twofold increase in *cholelithiasis* and cholecystitis in women on oral contraceptives.

Estrogens induce elevated levels of a variety of proteins secreted by the liver, including cortisol-binding globulin (CBG), testosterone-binding globulin (TeBG), and thyroxine-binding globulin (TBG). Consequently, results of various laboratory tests of adrenal and thyroid function may be altered, and these tests must be interpreted with caution (see Chap. 331). Oral contraceptives also slightly lower plasma ACTH levels possibly owing to an inhibitory effect on ACTH secretion or cortisol catabolism. Finally, serum prolactin levels are slightly elevated in women using oral contraceptives, but such treatment is not believed to play a role in the development of pituitary prolactinomas.

Other effects of oral contraceptive pills include minor dyspepsia, breast discomfort, weight gain, development of pigmentation of the face (chloasma), which is augmented by exposure to the sun, and a variety of psychological effects, such as depression and changes in libido. There is no convincing evidence that oral contraceptive use is associated with a significant increase in the incidence of cancer of the uterus, cervix, or breast. In fact, oral contraceptives have many beneficial effects including control of dysmenorrhea and anovulatory bleeding, prevention of sexually transmitted diseases, and a decreased incidence of endometrial and ovarian cancer.

The absolute contraindications to the use of oral contraceptives include previous thromboembolic disorders, cerebral vascular or coronary artery disease, known or suspected carcinoma of the breast or estrogen-dependent neoplasia, undiagnosed abnormal genital bleeding, or known or suspected pregnancy. Relative contraindications must be weighed against the potential benefits and include hypertension, migraine headaches, diabetes mellitus, uterine leiomyomas, sickle cell anemia, hyperlipidemia, and elective surgery.

OTHER STEROID CONTRACEPTIVES Types of steroid contraception other than the conventional oral contraceptives include injectable steroids, such as progestogen-containing implants and depot medroxyprogesterone acetate (150 mg by injection every 3 months). Alternatively, postcoital contraception can be effective, such as ingestion of high-dose estrogen for 5 days during the fertile part of the cycle (the morning-after pill) but is associated with significant side effects, particularly nausea.

Estrogen Treatment of the Menopause The rationale for use of estrogens in postmenopausal women is the belief that such therapy may relieve some of the complications of the postmenopausal state, including osteoporosis, and some manifestations of aging itself. In some parts of the United States, by the mid-1970s as many as half of women in the menopausal age group used one or more forms of estrogen replacement for a median period of 5 years, accounting for more than 30 million prescriptions per year.

The menopause is not a state of simple estrogen deprivation, since some estrogens continue to be produced but is instead a state of altered estrogen metabolism; the predominant estrogen becomes estrone, which is formed by extraglandular conversion of prehormone, rather than estradiol secreted by the ovary. As is true for all estrogen therapy, the estrogen treatment of the menopause is actually a pharmacologic substitution of one or another estrogen analogue for estradiol rather than a physiologic replacement of the missing steroid. The estrogens available for replacement therapy include conjugated estrogens, estrogen substitutes (diethylstilbestrol), synthetic estrogen (ethinyl estradiol or derivatives), micronized estradiol, estrogen-containing vaginal creams, and estrogen-containing dermal patches. Regimens associated with a low risk of complications include (1) cyclic estrogen therapy in the lowest effective dose for 25 days per month or continuous estrogens given each day of the month and (2) estrogens plus the addition of progestogen during the last 10 to 14 days of estrogen therapy, or low-dose continuous progestogen plus estrogen given daily.

The most clear-cut early benefit of estrogen therapy in the menopause is the relief of vasomotor instability (hot flashes) and of atrophy of the urogenital epithelium and skin. Estrogen therapy ameliorates these symptoms in most cases. When estrogen therapy is intended to treat hot flashes alone, it should be continued for only a few years, since hot flashes tend to diminish after 3 to 4 years in untreated women.

Several lines of evidence indicate that routine estrogen therapy is beneficial in preventing the complications of menopausal osteoporosis, especially in high-risk women (i.e., thin white women). First, in women undergoing premature menopause, the incidence and complication rates of osteoporosis are increased, and long-term estrogen replacement appears to be beneficial. Second, estrogen therapy has short-term positive effects on calcium balance and long-term beneficial effects on bone density. Third, in women given estrogen therapy, the incidence of fractures is decreased.

Of the potential side effects, the possibility of an increased risk of endometrial carcinoma is perhaps most worrisome. The relative risk of developing endometrial adenocarcinoma in estrogen users is between six and eight times the risk in nonusers. This risk increases with increasing duration and dosage of estrogen but is smaller in women given combination estrogen-progestogen therapy.

Despite the large body of evidence linking endometrial carcinoma and estrogen use, doubts have been raised about the clinical significance of the association. First, some epidemiologists have argued that the increased risk associated with estrogens has been exaggerated because of problems inherent in inadequate controls in retrospective analyses. Second, despite the increased incidence of endometrial carcinoma in the United States, there was no concomitant increased mortality from this disease. In fact, the increased incidence apparently involves low-grade malignancies that may be difficult to distinguish histologically from hyperplasia. These forms of malignancy have little effect on life expectancy.

Apprehension concerning worsening of hypertension and thromboembolic disease appears to be due to reports of the effects of estrogen-progestogen oral contraceptives during the reproductive years and not to estrogen use in postmenopausal women. There is no conclusive evidence that low-dose estrogen therapy after menopause increases the incidence or the severity of thromboembolic disease, breast cancer, or hypertension. Low-dose estrogen treatment after menopause does not appear to influence the development of atherosclerosis, myocardial infarction, or stroke. Strong evidence suggests that, in fact, estrogens may decrease the incidence of death from myocardial infarction. There is a slightly increased risk for the development of gallbladder disease with postmenopausal estrogen use.

A reasonable approach to the postmenopausal use of estrogens is as follows: (1) For long-term use, estrogens should be given in the minimal effective doses (0.625 mg conjugated estrogen orally or 1.0 mg micronized estradiol or transdermal estradiol 0.05 to 1.0 mg in a formulation that is changed every 3.5 days or every week). For women with an intact uterus, it is the practice in some clinics to give estrogens alone for 15 days and estrogen plus a daily progestogen dose for the remainder of the month. The most common regimens involve continuous estrogen plus low-dose continuous progestogen. (2) Such replacement therapy is indicated routinely in women undergoing premature menopause (surgically induced or spontaneous). (3) Estrogen therapy is also indicated routinely in women of all ages who have severe hot flashes or symptomatic atrophy of the urogenital epithelium. Hot flashes rarely persist for longer than 7 years, so, if therapy is given for this purpose, its duration can be limited. (4) In women who have had a hysterectomy, the potential benefits of treatment appear to outweigh the dangers, and in such women cyclic or continuous estrogen without progestogen is recommended. Whether estrogens should be given routinely to all women with intact uteri is an unsettled question, but the authors prescribe it routinely in the absence of contraindications in hopes of ameliorating

Table 337-4

Annual Death Rates Associated with Fertility Control per 100,000 Women

	Age Group					
Contraceptive Techniques	**15–19**	**20–24**	**25–29**	**30–34**	**35–39**	**40–44**
None (birth-related)	7.0	7.4	9.1	14.8	25.7	28.2
Oral contraceptives						
Smokers	2.4	3.6	6.8	13.7	51.4	117.6
Nonsmokers	0.5	0.7	1.1	2.1	14.1	32.0
IUD	1.3	1.1	1.3	1.3	1.9	2.1
Abortion	0.5	1.1	1.3	1.9	1.8	1.1
Barrier methods (birth-related)	1.5	1.4	1.0	0.8	1.3	7.6

SOURCE: Adapted from HW Ory, Fam Plann Perspect 15:57, 1983.

osteoporosis. (5) Each woman receiving estrogens must be monitored indefinitely at yearly intervals.

Induction of Ovulation The most common treatment for ovulation induction in women with PCOD is *clomiphene*. This agent is believed to act as an antiestrogen in the hypothalamus and thus to allow FSH levels to rise, stimulating follicular development and resulting in ovulation. Clomiphene therapy is usually begun with a dose of 50 mg by mouth daily for 5 days commencing on the fifth day of progestogen-induced uterine bleeding. If ovulation does not occur, the dose may be increased to 100 or 150 mg/d. Such treatment results in ovulatory cycles in 60 percent of women with PCOD. Additional regimens include clomiphene in combination with human menopausal gonadotropins (hMG), glucocorticoids, or human chorionic gonadotropin (hCG).

The most commonly used gonadotropins for induction of ovulation are hMG, urofollitropin, and hCG. These agents are indicated in women who fail to ovulate on clomiphene. (For women with hypogonadotropic hypogonadism, urofollitropin is not recommended.) The usual treatment regimen requires 1 to 3 ampuls of hMG or urofollitropin per day over an 8- to 12-day period to achieve adequate follicular stimulation and growth, followed by a single injection of 10,000 units of hCG 12 to 24 h after the last injection of hMG. For women with PCOD, pretreatment with LHRH analogues prior to hMG or urofollitropin appears to improve ovulation and pregnancy rates. Ovulation is successful in 90 percent of women, and pregnancy rates exceed 50 to 60 percent. Measurement of daily estrogen levels and frequent evaluation of ovarian size by ultrasound are indicated to prevent ovarian hyperstimulation. Ovarian hyperstimulation syndrome results from excessive stimulation of ovarian follicles with resulting enlargement of the ovaries; it may progress to the development of ascites, hypotension, and shock. Therapy using hMG, urofollitropin, and hCG also carries a 20 percent risk of multiple pregnancies.

Bromocriptine is a dopamine agonist that is effective in inducing ovulation in women with elevated prolactin levels. Treatment is instituted at a usual dosage of 2.5 mg by mouth two or three times a day. Treatment should be discontinued as soon as pregnancy is diagnosed. → ***The management of prolactin-secreting pituitary tumors is discussed in Chap. 328.***

LUTEINIZING HORMONE–RELEASING HORMONE (GONADORELIN) AND ANALOGUES Gonadorelin has been used successfully to induce ovulation in infertile women. The agent is infused subcutaneously or intravenously by a portable infusion pump which administers pulses at 90- to 120-min intervals for 10 to 20 days. After ovulation has occurred, hCG is given to maintain corpus luteum function.

LHRH analogues that block ovulation have been used to treat a variety of gynecologic disorders; ovulation and ovarian steroidogenesis are inhibited owing to the down-regulation of LHRH receptors with a resulting decreased release of gonadotropins. Conditions for which these agents are under trial include fertility control, true precocious puberty, endometriosis, uterine leiomyomas, hirsutism, and, in combination with gonadotropins, ovulation induction and in vitro fertilization.

OTHER DISORDERS OF THE FEMALE REPRODUCTIVE TRACT

VULVA Most disorders of the vulva are due to venereal disease, most commonly syphilis (painless chancre), condylomata acuminata (venereal warts), and herpes vulvitis (painful ulcers) (see Chap. 129). All other lesions of the vulva, particularly in older women, must be biopsied. Early biopsy of cancer of the vulva is mandatory, because when it becomes symptomatic (pruritus and bleeding), it has often progressed to an advanced stage.

VAGINA Infections of the vagina usually present as vaginal discharge and pruritus. The most frequent organisms are *Trichomonas*, *Candida albicans*, and *Gardnerella vaginalis* (see also Chap. 129). The diagnosis is made by microscopic examination of the discharge, and appropriate therapy can be instituted using vaginal or oral antibiotics.

Abnormalities of the vagina and cervix in female offspring of women given diethylstilbestrol during pregnancy include adenosis of the vagina and structural abnormalities of the vagina, cervix, and uterus; the risk of developing a rare vaginal cancer (adenocarcinoma, clear cell type) is increased (2 per 10,000 exposed women). Periodic examination of women at risk should begin at age 12 to 14, and reexamination should be done after any episode of abnormal bleeding.

CERVIX Preinvasive lesions of the cervix (also known as *cervical intraepithelial neoplasia*) and invasive carcinoma of the cervix can be detected reliably by obtaining a Papanicolaou smear (Pap smear).

Evaluation of the Pap Smear The incidence of invasive cervical cancer has declined as a result of Pap smear screening. In the United States, approximately 2 to 3 million abnormal Pap smears are found each year. Most represent low-grade lesions but require appropriate follow-up. The follow-up of abnormal Pap smears requires an understanding of the Bethesda System for evaluating such smears and of the limitations of cytologic screening systems. Further evaluation may require repeat cytologic examination, colposcopy, or both.

Current Screening Recommendations Risk factors for cervical neoplasia include a history of multiple sexual partners, coitus beginning at an early age, a history of infection with human papillomavirus, infection with human immunodeficiency virus (HIV) or another immunosuppressed state, and a history of cancer of the lower genital tract. Cervical cancer screening is recommended annually beginning at 18 years of age or when the woman becomes sexually active, if earlier than age 18. "Less frequent" screening is performed when three consecutive, negative, satisfactory annual Pap smears have been obtained or if the woman is in a low-risk category. There is no upper age limit for screening, because the prevalence of invasive cancer shows a linear increase with age, most of these cancers being diagnosed after age 50. Even after hysterectomy, annual screening should be performed if there is a history of abnormal Pap smears or other lower genital tract neoplasia.

The Bethesda System of Cytologic Examination Pap smears are evaluated in regard to the adequacy of the specimen (satisfactory for evaluation, satisfactory but limited, or unsatisfactory for evaluation because of a stated reason), the general diagnosis (normal or abnormal), and a descriptive diagnosis if the smear is abnormal. The descriptive diagnoses include benign cellular changes, reactive cellular changes, and epithelial cell abnormalities, the latter including (1) atypical squamous cells of undetermined significance (ASCUS); (2) low-grade squamous intraepithelial lesion (LSIL), which is further categorized to include human papillomavirus (HPV) infection, cervical intraepithelial neoplasia (CIN 1), and high-grade squamous intraepithelial lesion (HSIL, which is itself subdivided into CIN 2 and CIN 3); and (3) squamous cell carcinoma.

Guidelines for the Management of Women with Abnormal Pap Smears For ASCUS smears that are unqualified or suggest a reactive process, a repeat smear should be obtained every 4 to 6 months for 2 years until three consecutive negative smears have been obtained. For ASCUS smears that are unqualified but have severe inflammation, any specific cause should be treated, and the smear should be repeated in 2 to 3 months; because invasive carcinoma can be obscured by severe inflammation, clinical evaluation is mandatory. For postmenopausal women not using hormone replacement, a course of topical estrogen should be given before the test is repeated. For LSIL smears, the Pap test is repeated every 4 to 6 months for 2 years until three consecutive negative smears have been obtained; treatment of HPV is of no established benefit, and there is a high rate of regression of LSIL, so that in compliant, low-risk individuals, the outcome is usually favorable. If LSIL is persistent, colposcopy with directed biopsy is performed, and endocervical curettage is undertaken if a specific diagnosis is made by biopsy. Cervical cone biopsy or loop electrosurgical excision procedures are performed for higher-grade lesions such as HSIL. If cervical cancer is diagnosed by biopsy, clinical staging is performed, and the patient is treated with radiation therapy or surgery.

UTERUS Only 40 percent of cases of endometrial adenocarcinoma are detected by Pap smear. In women at high risk for endometrial carcinoma (because of obesity, a history of chronic anovulatory cycles, diabetes mellitus, hypertension, or estrogen treatment), yearly endometrial sampling should be performed. Low-dose oral estrogen therapy rarely causes breakthrough or withdrawal bleeding in postmenopausal women. Therefore, irrespective of whether the patient is using estrogen therapy, the occurrence of postmenopausal bleeding makes it mandatory to obtain a tissue diagnosis by either endometrial sampling or curettage to exclude endometrial cancer.

One of the most common disorders of the uterus and the most frequent tumor of women (one of four women affected) is the uterine leiomyoma, or fibroid tumor. Three-fourths of women with leiomyoma are asymptomatic, and the diagnosis is made on routine pelvic examination. When the tumor is associated with excessive menstrual blood loss, is large or fast-gowing, or causes significant pelvic pain (see Chap. 52), the preferred treatment is hysterectomy if there is no desire for further childbearing. In young women, myomectomy is sometimes indicated when infertility or repeated fetal wastage is a manifestation or where future childbearing is desired.

FALLOPIAN TUBES AND OVARIES Infectious pelvic inflammatory disease is a common disorder of the fallopian tubes and usually becomes symptomatic after a menstrual period; the symptoms include fever, chills, abdominal pain, and vaginal discharge, and pelvic tenderness on physical examination is common. The initiating organism most often is *Chlamydia trachomatis* or *Neisseria gonorrhoeae*, but tuboovarian abscess and sterility are probably caused by mixed aerobic and anaerobic superinfections and require wide-spectrum antibiotic treatment (see Chap. 130).

Endometriosis is a benign disorder characterized by the presence and proliferation of endometrial tissue (stroma and glands) outside the endometrial cavity. The clinical manifestations are variable. Endometriosis occurs most commonly between the ages of 30 and 40 and is found incidentally at the time of surgery in approximately one-fifth of all gynecologic operations. The fertility rate is reduced in affected women. The disorder usually involves the posterior cul-de-sac or the ovaries and can give rise to ovarian enlargement (endometriomas), although it may involve distant sites (lung, umbilicus). The major symptom is pelvic pain, characteristically dysmenorrhea (see Chap. 52). However, the frequency and severity of symptoms correlate poorly with the extent of disease. Other manifestations include dyspareunia, pain with defecation, and infertility. The characteristic physical findings are multiple tender nodules palpable along the uterosacral ligament at the time of rectal-vaginal examination, a posteriorly fixed uterus, or enlarged, cystic ovaries. The diagnosis can only be confirmed by direct visualization, usually at diagnostic laparoscopy. Treatment depends on the degree of involvement and the desires of the patient and includes observation for mild disease with no associated infertility or pain, hormonal suppressive therapy (see "Infertility," above), conservative surgery if fertility is desired, or removal of the uterus, tubes, and ovaries in severe disease. Endometriosis is rare after the menopause.

Any adnexal mass that persists for more than 6 weeks or is larger than 6 cm must be evaluated. Although ovarian cysts and neoplasms are the most common pelvic adnexal masses (see above), tumors of the fallopian tubes, uterus, gastrointestinal tract, or urinary tract also should be considered. Sonography or radiographic evaluation is often helpful in identifying the nature of the adnexal mass prior to surgical exploration.

See Chap. 57, Estrogens and progestins, in Goodman & Gilman's The Pharmacological Basis of Therapeutics, *9th ed, New York, McGraw-Hill, 1996.*

BIBLIOGRAPHY

ADASHI EV, LEUNG PCK: *The Ovary*. New York, Raven Press, 1993

CARR BR: Disorders of the ovary and reproductive tract, in *Williams Textbook of Endocrinology*, 8th ed, JD Wilson, DW Foster (eds). Philadelphia, Saunders, 1992, pp 733–798

———, BLACKWELL RE (eds): *Textbook of Reproductive Medicine*. Norwalk, CT, Appleton & Lange, 1993

———, GRIFFIN JE: Fertility control and its complications, in *Williams Textbook of Endocrinology*, 8th ed, JD Wilson, DW Foster (eds). Philadelphia, Saunders, 1992, pp 1007–1031

CUNNINGHAM FG et al: *Williams' Obstetrics*, 19th ed. Norwalk, CT, Appleton & Lange, 1993

FUTTERWEIT W: *Polycystic Ovarian Disease*. New York, Springer-Verlag, 1984

GRAVE GD, CUTLER GB: *Sexual Precocity*. New York, Raven Press, 1993

GRUMBACH MM, CONTE FA: Disorders of sex differentiation, in *Williams Textbook of Endocrinology*, 8th ed, JD Wilson, DW Foster (eds). Philadelphia, Saunders, 1992, pp 853–952

———, STYNE DM: Puberty: Ontogeny, neuroendocrinology, physiology and disorders, in *Williams Textbook of Endocrinology*, 8th ed, JD Wilson, DW Foster (eds). Philadelphia, Saunders, 1992, pp 1139–1222

HATCHER RA et al: *Contraceptive Technology 1994–1996*. New York, Irvington, 1996

HERBST AL et al: *Comprehensive Gynecology*, 2d ed. St. Louis, Mosby, 1992

KAPLAN SA (ed): *Clinical Pediatric Endocrinology*. Philadelphia, Saunders, 1990

KNOBIL E, NEILL JD (eds): *The Physiology of Reproduction*, 2d ed. New York, Raven Press, 1994

LOBO RA: *Treatment of the Menopausal Woman*. New York, Raven Press, 1993

ROCK JA et al: *Female Reproductive Surgery*. Baltimore, Williams & Wilkins, 1992

SEIBEL MM: A new era in reproductive technology. N Engl J Med 318:828, 1988

SODERSTROM RM: *Operative Laparoscopy*. New York, Raven Press, 1993

SPEROFF L et al: *Clinical Gynecologic Endocrinology and Infertility*, 5th ed. Baltimore, Williams & Wilkins, 1994

STUDD JWW, WHITEHEAD MI (eds): *The Menopause*. Oxford, Blackwell, 1988

STYNE DM, GRUMBACH MM: Disorders of puberty in the male and female, in *Reproductive Endocrinology*, SSC Yen, RB Jaffe (eds). Philadelphia, Saunders, 1991, pp 11–54

THOMPSON JD, ROCK JA: *Te Lindes Operative Gynecology*. Philadelphia, Lippincott, 1992

YEN SSC, JAFFE RB (eds): *Reproductive Endocrinology*, 3d ed. Philadelphia, Saunders, 1991

338

Jean D. Wilson

ENDOCRINE DISORDERS OF THE BREAST

Examination of the breasts is an important part of the physical examination. The breasts are the site of fatal and preventable disease in women and provide clues to underlying systemic illness in both men and women. It is the duty of every physician to distinguish the abnormal from the normal at the earliest possible stage and to call for assistance if there is any doubt. → ***For further discussion of cancer of the breast, see Chap. 91***

ENDOCRINE CONTROL OF THE BREAST There is no histologic or functional difference in the breasts of boys and girls prior to the onset of puberty, but a profound sexual dimorphism in breast development ensues at the time of puberty. The endocrine control of female breast development is illustrated in Fig. 338-1. The pubertal growth of the female breast is dependent primarily on the action of estradiol, which induces the growth, division, and elongation of the tubular duct system and maturation of the nipples. In men the administration of estrogen is equally effective in this regard. To produce true alveolar development at the ends of the ducts, however, the synergistic action of progesterone is required, a ratio of estrogen to progesterone of 1:20 to 1:100 being optimal. Within the gland a variety of mediators influence cell division and differentiation, including stimulatory factors such as the insulin-like growth factors and epidermal growth factor and inhibitory factors such as transforming growth factor beta. Once the anatomic development of the ducts and alveoli is complete, the continued action of estrogen and progesterone is not required for lactation itself.

The endocrine control of milk formation is complex, requiring, in addition to appropriate priming by estrogen and progesterone, specific lactogenic hormone and the permissive action of glucocorticoid, insulin, thyroxine, and, in some species, growth hormone. There are two lactogenic hormones. Human placental lactogen (hPL, or chorionic somatomammotropin) is secreted in large amounts by the placenta during the latter part of gestation and prepares the breast for milk production. hPL disappears from the maternal (and fetal) circulation shortly after termination of pregnancy. The secretion of pituitary prolactin (see Chap. 328) rises during pregnancy and plays the critical role in the initiation and maintenance of lactation in the puerperium; during late pregnancy and lactation, 60 to 80 percent of the anterior pituitary may consist of prolactin-secreting cells.

Unlike most pituitary hormones, the predominant regulation of prolactin secretion is negative, i.e., under ordinary basal conditions inhibitory hypothalamic hormones, the most important being dopamine, are delivered from the central nervous system to the pituitary via the hypothalamic portal system and inhibit the release of prolactin into the blood (see Chap. 328). Most factors that influence prolactin secretion do so by affecting the synthesis or release of the inhibitory factor(s). Basal prolactin levels fall following delivery, but prolactin secretion is enhanced by stimulation of the breasts, such as the act of nursing (the so-called sucking reflex), a phenomenon that is probably mediated by the reflex release of oxytocin. Prolactin binds to a specific receptor on the cell surface of the breast acinar cells to enhance the synthesis of milk constituents via a tyrosine kinase–mediated process. In the postgestational state, the normal lactating woman forms about a liter of milk per day containing 38 g fat, 70 g lactose, and 12 g protein. Lactation can be suppressed by the administration of estrogens or diethylstilbestrol, which inhibit milk production by direct effects on the breast, or dopaminergic agents such as bromocriptine, which inhibit prolactin secretion by the pituitary. Alternatively, if a woman does not nurse or empty her breasts postpartum, lactation usually ceases in 1 to 2 weeks.

GALACTORRHEA Exactly what constitutes nonpuerperal or inappropriate lactation is not always clearly defined in the literature. According to the studies of Friedman and Goldfein, no breast secretions whatsoever are detectable in normal, regularly menstruating nulligravid women, but breast secretions can be demonstrated in a fourth of normal women who have been pregnant in the past; thus breast secretions in small amounts may be of no clinical significance in these instances. Spontaneous leakage of milk from the breasts is usually of more importance than milk that must be expressed. A second problem is related to the composition of the breast secretions. When the secretion is milky or white, it is safe to assume that it contains fat, casein, and lactose and is in fact milk; however, when the secretion is brown or greenish, it rarely contains normal milk constituents and consequently may not result from an underlying endocrinopathy. Milk also must be distinguished from blood or bloody discharges that may be due to neoplasms of the breast. It also should be remembered that the composition of milk constituents may increase upon repeated sampling, from low, colostrum-like values to those typical of milk. With these problems in mind, galactorrhea can be defined as inappropriate production of milk that is persistent or worrisome to the patient, recognizing that in some instances no underlying pathology may be demonstrated.

Since the action of a lactogenic hormone is necessary for the initiation of milk production, it is logical to consider galactorrhea as a consequence of deranged prolactin physiology. However, as indicated above, a complex endocrinologic milieu is necessary for lactation, and in many instances in which prolactin is elevated, both in women who have not been appropriately primed and in men, no production of milk takes place. As a consequence, hyperprolactinemia is more common than galactorrhea. Furthermore, while enhanced prolactin secretion is necessary for the initiation of lactation, continued production can be maintained in the presence of minimally or intermittently elevated prolactin levels so that basal plasma prolactin levels are not always elevated in patients with galactorrhea. In some such women prolactin levels may be elevated only during sleep; in others, hyperprolactinemia is believed to have been present transiently. Perhaps the strongest evidence for a critical role for prolactin in galactorrhea is the fact that administration of dopaminergic agents that suppress plasma prolactin levels causes a disappearance of galactorrhea even when the basal plasma prolactin levels are normal.

Differential Diagnosis Galactorrhea is due either to a failure of the normal hypothalamic inhibition of prolactin release, to increased prolactin-releasing factor(s), or to autonomous prolactin secretion by tumors (Table 338-1). Pituitary stalk section results in a striking increase in prolactin secretion, as the result of the interruption of the delivery of prolactin inhibitory factors to the pituitary. Likewise, many drugs that influence the central nervous system (including virtually all psychotropic agents, methyldopa, reserpine, and antiemetics) cause enhanced prolactin release, presumably by inhibiting synthesis or release of prolactin inhibitory factors such as dopamine. Estrogens on the one hand increase prolactin secretion, and on the other estrogen withdrawal (as in the discontinuation of oral contraceptives) may trigger the onset of galactorrhea. Central nervous system diseases outside the pituitary presumably cause galactorrhea by interfering with delivery of the inhibitory factors to the pituitary (central nervous system sarcoidosis, craniopharyngioma, pinealoma, encephalitis, meningitis, hydrocephalus, hypothalamic tumors).

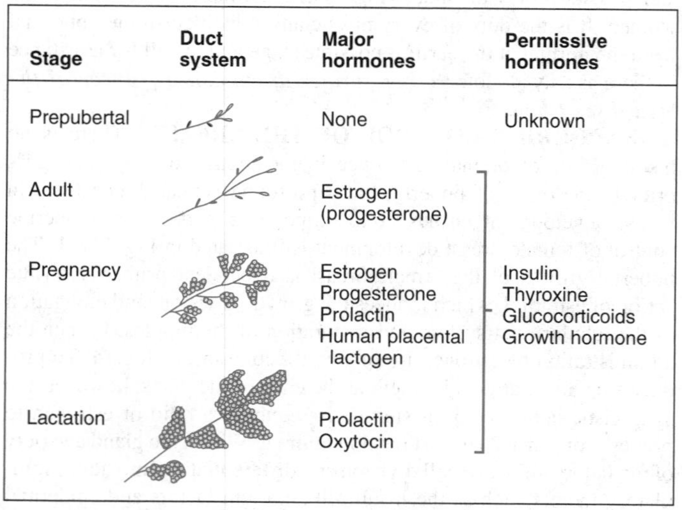

Stage
Duct system
Major hormones
Permissive hormones
Prepubertal
None
Unknown
Adult
Estrogen (progesterone)
Pregnancy
Estrogen
Progesterone
Prolactin
Human placental lactogen
Insulin
Thyroxine
Glucocorticoids
Growth hormone
Lactation
Prolactin
Oxytocin

FIGURE 338-1 Endocrine control of female breast development and function at various stages of life.

Table 338-1

Classification of Galactorrhea

A. Failure of normal hypothalamic inhibition of prolactin release
   1. Pituitary stalk section
   2. Drugs (phenothiazines, butyrophenones, methyldopa, tricyclic antidepressants, opiates, reserpine, verapamil)
   3. Central nervous system disease, including extrapituitary tumors and null cell adenomas of the pituitary
B. Enhanced prolactin-release
   1. Hypothyroidism
   2. Sucking reflex and breast trauma
C. Autonomous prolactin release
   1. Pituitary tumors
      a. Prolactin-secreting tumors
      b. Mixed growth hormone and prolactin-secreting tumors
      c. Null cell adenomas
   2. Ectopic production of human placental lactogen and/or prolactin
      a. Hydatidiform moles and choriocarcinomas
      b. Bronchogenic carcinoma and hypernephroma
D. Idiopathic

In primary hypothyroidism, galactorrhea results from enhanced prolactin-releasing activity. Thyrotropin-releasing hormone (TRH) stimulates prolactin release, and thyroid hormone replacement cures the galactorrhea. A similar mechanism, as the result of enhanced secretion of oxytocin, may cause the galactorrhea that follows breast surgery or breast trauma.

Enhanced prolactin release also can occur from pituitary or nonpituitary tumors. Three types of pituitary tumors (see Chap. 328) may be associated with galactorrhea: pure prolactin-secreting tumors (micro- or macroadenomas), mixed tumors that secrete both growth hormone and prolactin and cause acromegaly with galactorrhea, and some null cell adenomas. The latter may interfere with the delivery of inhibitory factors to the pituitary. Excess growth hormone secretion in the absence of hyperprolactinemia may on occasion cause galactorrhea. Prolactin also can be secreted by other malignancies such as bronchogenic carcinoma, and hydatidiform moles and choriocarcinomas may secrete placental lactogen.

In series involving several hundred patients, a pituitary tumor was identified in about one-fourth, other known causes could be identified in another fourth or fifth, and the remaining half fell into the idiopathic category. Many of the latter group ultimately developed prolactin-secreting pituitary tumors, some probably had subtle disorders of hypothalamic function, and in others a drug-related cause may have been missed; but the fact remains that no satisfactory diagnosis is reached in many patients. When normal menses and galactorrhea coexist, the likelihood of establishing a diagnosis is poor.

Galactorrhea is unusual in men, even in the presence of profound elevations of plasma prolactin; when it does occur, it is usually upon the background of a feminizing state (see below).

Diagnostic Evaluation If hyperprolactinemia is present, the workup is fundamentally that of a pituitary tumor once drug causes and hypothyroidism are excluded (see Chap. 328). Even when a specific cause cannot be identified and the diagnosis of idiopathic galactorrhea is made by exclusion, it is necessary to remember that pituitary tumors may subsequently become manifest. The higher the prolactin values and the more persistent the galactorrhea, the greater is the likelihood of such a development.

℞ TREATMENT

Breast binders can be effective in patients with mild galactorrhea of unknown etiology, presumably by preventing stimulation of the nipple and the consequent perpetuation of lactation. The aim of treatment in other instances is to correct the elevated prolactin, and treatment of a pituitary tumor, cessation of causative drugs, or correction of hypothyroidism is often followed by the disappearance of galactorrhea. Dopaminergic agents that suppress plasma prolactin have been used to treat idiopathic hyperprolactinemia, prolactin-secreting tumors of the pituitary (see Chap. 328), and even normoprolactinemic galactorrhea. These drugs not only suppress lactation but also may cause resumption of menstrual cycles (and even fertility) in patients with amenorrhea and galactorrhea.

GYNECOMASTIA A central issue in the evaluation of breast tissue in adult men is the separation of the normal from the abnormal. The incidence of active gynecomastia in autopsy series is between 5 and 9 percent, but Nuttall and colleagues have reported that approximately 40 percent of normal men and up to 70 percent of hospitalized men have palpable breast tissue. The reason for this discrepancy is not clear. On the one hand, it may be difficult to distinguish true breast tissue from masses of adipose tissue without true breast enlargement (lipomastia); in such cases, true gynecomastia can be separated from lipomastia by mammography or ultrasonography. Alternatively, the incidence of gynecomastia may have increased (possibly due to exposure to environmental or plant estrogens), or the autopsy data may underestimate the frequency of palpable breast tissue. Regardless, we are left with major uncertainties; the finding of gynecomastia (distinct from lipomastia) may indicate underlying pathology or a normal variant. In this discussion, we shall assume that any palpable breast tissue in men (except for the three physiologic states; see below) can be due to an underlying endocrinopathy and deserves, at a minimum, a limited evaluation.

Early gynecomastia is characterized by proliferation in the breast of both the fibroblastic stroma and the duct system, which elongates, buds, and duplicates. As gynecomastia persists, progressive fibrosis and hyalinization are associated with regression of epithelial proliferation and, eventually, a decrease in the number of ducts. When the cause of the gynecomastia is corrected early in the course, resolution occurs by reduction in size and epithelial content with gradual disappearance of the ducts, leaving hyaline bands that eventually disappear.

Growth of the breast in men, as in women, is mediated by estrogen and results from disturbances of the normal ratio of active androgen to estrogen. As described in Chap. 336, estradiol formation in normal men occurs principally by the conversion of circulating androgen to estrogen in extraglandular tissues; the normal ratio of production of testosterone to estradiol in adult men is approximately 100:1 (6 mg versus 45 μg/day), and the normal ratio of the two hormones in plasma is about 300:1. Growth of the breast ensues in men when the normal ratio decreases as the result of diminished testosterone production or action, enhanced estrogen formation, or both processes occurring simultaneously.

Enlargement of the male breast can be a normal physiologic phenomenon at certain times of life or the result of several pathologic states (Table 338-2).

Table 338-2

Differential Diagnosis of Gynecomastia

PHYSIOLOGIC GYNECOMASTIA

Newborn
Adolescence
Aging

PATHOLOGIC GYNECOMASTIA

A. Deficient production or action of testosterone
  1. Congenital anorchia
  2. Androgen resistance (testicular feminization and Reifenstein syndrome)
  3. Defects of testosterone synthesis
  4. Klinefelter syndrome
  5. Viral orchitis
  6. Trauma
  7. Castration
  8. Neurologic and granulomatous diseases
  9. Renal failure
B. Increased estrogen production
  1. Increased estrogen secretion
    a. Testicular tumors
    b. True hermaphroditism
    c. Carcinoma of the lung and other tumors producing hCG
  2. Increased substrate for extraglandular aromatase
    a. Adrenal disease
    b. Liver disease
    c. Malnutrition
    d. Hyperthyroidism
  3. Increase in extraglandular aromatase
C. Drugs
  1. Estrogens (diethylstilbestrol, birth control pills, digitalis, estrogen-containing cosmetics, estrogen-contaminated foods, phytoestrogens)
  2. Drugs that enhance endogenous estrogen secretion (gonadotropins, clomiphene)
  3. Inhibitors of testosterone synthesis and/or action (ketoconazole, metronidazole, alkylating agents, cisplatin, spironolactone, cimetidine, flutamide, etomidate)
  4. Unknown mechanisms (busulfan, isoniazid, methyldopa, tricyclic antidepressants, penicillamine, diazepam, omeprazole, calcium channel blockers, angiotensin-converting enzyme inhibitors, marijuana, heroin, finasteride)
D. Idiopathic

Physiologic Gynecomastia In the *newborn*, transient enlargement of the breast is due to the action of maternal and/or placental estrogens. The enlargement usually disappears in a few weeks but may persist longer. *Adolescent* gynecomastia is common at some time during puberty. The median age of onset is 14; it is often asymmetric, occasionally unilateral for a portion of its course, and frequently tender, and it regresses so that by age 20 only a small number of men have palpable vestiges of gynecomastia in one or both breasts. Although the origin of the excess estrogen has not been identified, the onset of gynecomastia correlates with transient elevations of plasma estradiol prior to the completion of puberty so that the androgen/estrogen ratio is low. *Gynecomastia of aging* also occurs in otherwise healthy men. Forty percent or more of aged men have gynecomastia. A likely explanation is the increase with age in the conversion of androgens to estrogens in extraglandular tissues. Abnormal liver function or drug therapy may be contributing causes in such men.

Pathologic Gynecomastia Pathologic gynecomastia can result from one of three basic mechanisms: deficiency in testosterone production or action (with or without a secondary increase in estrogen production), increase in estrogen production, or drugs (Table 338-2). Most of the individual disorders that cause primary and secondary testicular failure are discussed in Chap. 336. The fact that a deficiency in testosterone production by itself can cause gynecomastia is illustrated by the syndrome of congenital anorchia in which normal (or slightly low) estradiol production in the presence of profoundly decreased testosterone production results in florid gynecomastia. Decreased testosterone production is also responsible in some patients with Klinefelter syndrome and in men with testicular failure from other causes. In the disorders of androgen resistance, such as testicular feminization, deficient androgen action and increased testicular estrogen production are both present.

A primary increase in estrogen production can result from a variety of causes. Increased secretion of testicular estrogen may result from elevations in plasma gonadotropins, for example, in cases of aberrant production of chorionic gonadotropin by testicular tumors or by bronchogenic carcinoma, from the ovarian elements in the gonads of men with true hermaphroditism, or as the result of formation by testicular tumors (particularly Leydig cell and Sertoli cell tumors). Increased conversion of androgen to estrogens in extraglandular tissues can be due either to increased availability of substrate for extraglandular estrogen formation, for example, from increased production of androstenedione (congenital adrenal hyperplasia, hyperthyroidism, and most feminizing adrenal tumors), or to diminished catabolism of androstenedione (liver disease). Increased amounts of extraglandular aromatase can be caused by a rare hereditary abnormality or by tumors of the liver or adrenal gland.

Drugs can cause gynecomastia by several mechanisms. Many drugs either act directly as estrogens or cause an increase in plasma estrogen activity, for example, in men receiving diethylstilbestrol for prostatic carcinoma and in transsexuals in preparation for sex-change operations. Boys and young men are particularly sensitive to estrogen and can develop gynecomastia after the use of dermal ointments containing estrogen or after the ingestion of milk or meat from estrogen-treated animals. The gynecomastia of digitalis ingestion is usually attributed to an estrogen-like side effect of the drug, but in the experience of the author it usually occurs in men with abnormal liver function. A second mechanism of drug-induced gynecomastia is illustrated by clomiphene and human chorionic gonadotropin (hCG), which cause enhanced testicular secretion of estrogen. Other drugs cause gynecomastia by interfering with testosterone synthesis (ketoconazole and alkylating agents) and/or testosterone action, for instance, by blocking the binding of androgen to its receptor protein in target tissues (spironolactone and cimetidine). Finally, drugs that cause gynecomastia by mechanisms that have not been defined include busulfan, ethionamide, isoniazid, methyldopa, tricyclic antidepressants, penicillamine, omeprazole, calcium channel blocking agents, angiotensin-converting enzyme inhibitors, diazepam, marijuana, and heroin. In some instances, the feminization is due to effects of drugs on liver function.

Diagnostic Evaluation The evaluation of patients with gynecomastia should include: (1) a careful drug history; (2) measurement and examination of the testes (if both are small, a chromosomal karyotype should be obtained; if they are asymmetric, a workup for testicular tumor should be instituted); (3) evaluation of liver function; and (4) endocrine evaluation to include measurement of serum androstenedione or 24-h urinary 17-ketosteroids (usually elevated in feminizing adrenal states), measurement of plasma estradiol and hCG (helpful if elevated but usually normal), and measurement of plasma luteinizing hormone (LH) and testosterone. If LH is high and testosterone is low, the diagnosis is usually testicular failure; if LH and testosterone are both low, the diagnosis is most likely increased primary estrogen production (e.g., a Sertoli cell tumor of the testis); and if both LH and testosterone are elevated, the diagnosis is either an androgen-resistance state or a gonadotropin-secreting tumor.

A satisfactory diagnosis can be made in only half or fewer of patients referred for gynecomastia. This implies either that the diagnostic techniques are not sufficiently refined to recognize mild disturbances, that many causes of gynecomastia are as yet undefined, that the causes may be transient and difficult to diagnose, or, as suggested by Nuttall, that gynecomastia may in some instances be normal rather than due to a pathologic state. Because of the problem of separating the normal from the abnormal, gynecomastia should probably be routinely worked up only if the drug history is negative, the breast is tender (indicating rapid growth), or the breast mass is larger than 4 cm in diameter. In other instances, a decision to perform an endocrine evaluation depends on the clinical context. For example, gynecomastia associated with signs of underandrogenization should always be evaluated.

Rx TREATMENT

When the primary cause can be identified and corrected, the breast enlargement usually subsides promptly and eventually disappears. For example, androgen replacement therapy may produce dramatic improvement in men with testicular insufficiency. However, if the gynecomastia is of long duration (and fibrosis has replaced the original ductal hyperplasia), correction of the primary defect may not be followed by resolution. In such instances and when the primary cause cannot be corrected, surgery is the only effective therapy. Indications for surgery include several psychologic and/or cosmetic problems, continued growth, or a suspected malignancy. Although the relative risk of carcinoma of the breast is increased in men with gynecomastia, it is rare nevertheless. Prophylactic radiation of the breasts prior to the institution of diethylstilbestrol therapy is effective in preventing gynecomastia and has a low complication rate in elderly men. In rare patients who have painful gynecomastia and who are not candidates for other therapy, treatment with antiestrogens such as tamoxifen may be indicated.

BIBLIOGRAPHY

GALACTORRHEA

ABDEL GADIN A et al: The etiology of galactorrhea in women with regular menstruation and normal prolactin levels. Human Reprod 7:912, 1992

BENJAMIN F: Normal lactation and galactorrhea. Clin Obstet Gynecol 37:887, 1994

CAVANAUGH J et al: Gynecomastia and cirrhosis of the liver. Arch Intern Med 150:563, 1990

CHOTINER HC et al: Lactose and casein content of nonpuerperal breast secretion. J Reprod Med 22:267, 1979

FRANTZ AG, WILSON JD: Endocrine disorders of the breast, in *Williams Textbook of Endocrinology*, 8th ed, JD Wilson, DW Foster (eds). Philadelphia, Saunders, 1992, p 593

FRIEDMAN S, GOLDFEIN A: Breast secretions in normal women. Am J Obstet Gynecol 104:846, 1969

JOHNSON DG et al: Prolactin secretion and biological activity in females with galactorrhoea and normal circulating prolactin concentrations at rest. Clin Endocrinol 22:661, 1985

KLEINBERG DL: Galactorrhea. Curr Ther Endocrinol Metab 5:360, 1994

KOPPELMAN MCS et al: Hyperprolactinemia, amenorrhea, and galactorrhea. A retrospective assessment of twenty-five cases. Ann Intern Med 100:115, 1984
KULSKI JK et al: Changes in the milk composition of nonpuerperal women. Am J Obstet Gynecol 139:597, 1981
LAMBERTS SW, QUIK RF: A comparison of the efficacy and safety of pergolide and bromocriptine in the treatment of hyperprolactinemia. J Clin Endocrinol Metab 72:635, 1991
LAURENCE DJ, MONAGHAN P, GUSTERSON BA: The development of the normal human breast. Oxf Rev Reprod Biol 13:149, 1991
RUIZ-VELASCO V: Hyperprolactinemia and mammary prostheses. A report of eight cases. J Reprod Med 31:267, 1986
SAUER HJ: Physiology of lactation and factors affecting lactation. Obstet Gynecol Clin North Am 14:615, 1987
TURKSOY RN et al: Diagnostic and therapeutic modalities in women with galactorrhea. Obstet Gynecol 56:323, 1980
YAMAGUCHI M et al: Effects of nocturnal hyperprolactinemia on ovarian luteal function and galactorrhea. Eur J Obstet Gynecol 39:187, 1991

GYNECOMASTIA

ANDERSON JA, GROOM JB: Male breast at autopsy. Acta Pathol Microbiol Immunol Scand 90:191, 1982
CIMORA GA et al: Percutaneous oestrogen-induced gynecomastia: A case report. Br J Plast Surg 35:209, 1982
DE GASPARO M et al: Antialdosterones: Incidence and prevention of sexual side effects. J Steroid Biochem 32:223, 1989
FASS D et al: Radiotherapeutic prophylaxis of estrogen-induced gynecomastia: A study of late sequela. Int J Radiat Oncol Biol Phys 12:407, 1986
FELDMAN D: Ketoconazole and other imidazole derivatives as inhibitors of steroidogenesis. Endocr Rev 7:409, 1986
FRANTZ AG, WILSON JD: Endocrine disorders of the breast, in *Williams Textbook of Endocrinology*, 8th ed, JD Wilson, DW Foster (eds). Philadelphia, Saunders, 1992, p 953
GEORGIADIS E et al: Incidence of gynaecomastia in 954 young males and its relationship to somatometric parameters. Ann Hum Biol 21:579, 1994
KORENMAN SG: The endocrinology of the abnormal male breast. Ann NY Acad Sci 464:400, 1986
MABUCHI K et al: Risk factors for male breast cancer. J Natl Cancer Inst 74:371, 1985
MAHONEY CP: Adolescent gynecomastia: Differential diagnosis and management. Pediatr Clin North Am 37:1389, 1990
MCDERMOTT MT et al: Tamoxifen therapy for painful idiopathic gynecomastia. South Med J 83:1283, 1990
NIEWOEHNER CV, NUTTALL FQ: Gynecomastia in a hospitalized male population. Am J Med 77:633, 1984
NUTTALL FQ: Gynecomastia as a physical finding in normal men. J Clin Endocrinol Metab 48:338, 1979
ROSE DP: Endocrine epidemiology of male breast cancer (review). Anticancer Res 8:845, 1988
THOMPSON DF, CARTER R: Drug-induced gynecomastia. Pharmacotherapy 13:37, 1993

339

Jean D. Wilson, James E. Griffin

DISORDERS OF SEXUAL DIFFERENTIATION

Sexual differentiation is a sequential and ordered process. *Chromosomal sex*, established at the moment of fertilization, determines *gonadal sex*, and gonadal sex, in turn, causes the development of *phenotypic sex*, in which the male or female urogenital tract is formed (Table 339-1). A disturbance of any step in this process during embryogenesis may impair sexual differentiation. Known causes of such disorders include environmental insults as in the ingestion of a virilizing drug during pregnancy, nonfamilial aberrations of the sex chromosomes as in 45,X gonadal dysgenesis, birth defects of multifactorial etiology as in most cases of hypospadias, and disorders due to single gene mutations as in the testicular feminization syndrome.

Limitations of knowledge make it necessary to make empirical assignments as to the nature of the derangement in certain disorders, but specific diagnoses usually can be made as the result of genetic, endocrine, phenotypic, and chromosomal assessment. As a conse-

quence, appropriate gender assignment can be made, even in extreme instances of ambiguous genitalia, and tailoring of the phenotype can be undertaken when appropriate.

NORMAL SEXUAL DIFFERENTIATION

The first event in sexual differentiation is the establishment of chromosomal sex, the heterogametic sex (XY) being male and the homogametic sex (XX) female. The embryos of both sexes then develop in an identical fashion until approximately 40 days of gestation. The second phase of sexual differentiation is the conversion of the indifferent gonad into a testis or an ovary. No matter how many X chromosomes are present (as in 47,XXY, 48,XXXY, etc.), a testis will develop as long as a normal Y chromosome is present. Differentiation of the indifferent gonad into a testis is mediated by a single gene on the short arm of the Y chromosome (SRY); insertion of a transgene containing this gene into female mice causes them to develop as males. The gene encodes a DNA-binding protein, but the mechanism by which it promotes testicular development is unknown. The final process, the translation of gonadal sex into phenotypic sex, is the consequence of the type of gonad formed and the endocrine secretions of the fetal gonads and results in the formation of the male and female urogenital tracts.

The internal urogenital tract is derived from the wolffian and müllerian ducts that exist side by side in early embryos of both sexes (Fig. 339-1*A*). In the male the wolffian ducts give rise to the epididymides, vasa deferentia, and seminal vesicles, and the müllerian ducts disappear. In the female the fallopian tubes, uterus, and upper vagina are derived from the müllerian ducts, and the wolffian ducts regress. The external genitalia and urethra in the two sexes develop from common anlage—the urogenital sinus and the genital tubercle, folds, and swellings (Fig. 339-1*B*). The urogenital sinus gives rise to the prostate and prostatic urethra in the male and to the urethra and lower portion of the vagina in the female. The genital tubercle gives rise to the glans penis in the male and the clitoris in the female. The urogenital swellings become the scrotum or the labia majora, and the urethral folds develop into the labia minora or fuse to form the shaft of the penis and the male urethra.

In the absence of the testis, as in the normal female or in the male embryo castrated prior to the onset of gonadal differentiation, phenotypic sex develops along female lines. Thus, masculinization of the fetus is induced by hormones from the fetal testes, whereas female development does not require the presence of the ovary. Phenotypic sex normally conforms to chromosomal sex. That is, chromosomal sex determines gonadal sex, and gonadal sex, in turn, controls phenotypic sex.

Table 339-1

Classification of Disorders of Sexual Development

Disorders of Chromosomal Sex
Klinefelter syndrome
XX male
Gonadal dysgenesis
Mixed gonadal dysgenesis
True hermaphroditism
Disorders of Gonadal Sex
Pure gonadal dysgenesis
Absent testis syndrome
Disorders of Phenotypic Sex
Female pseudohermaphroditism
Congenital adrenal hyperplasia
Nonadrenal female pseudohermaphroditism
Developmental disorders of müllerian ducts
Male pseudohermaphroditism
Abnormalities in androgen synthesis
Abnormalities in androgen action
Persistent müllerian duct syndrome
Development defects of male genitalia

The formation of the male phenotype is vested in the action of three hormones. Two—müllerian duct inhibitor and testosterone—are secreted by the fetal testis. Müllerian duct inhibitor [(MDI), also termed müllerian-inhibiting substance or antimüllerian hormone] is a protein that suppresses the müllerian ducts and prevents development of the uterus and fallopian tubes in the male. Testosterone acts directly to virilize the wolffian duct and is the precursor for the third embryonic male hormone, dihydrotestosterone (see Chap. 336), which promotes development of the male urethra and prostate and formation of the penis and scrotum. Testosterone and dihydrotestosterone induce formation of the male urogenital tract during fetal life by the same intracellular machinery by which they act in postembryonic life (Chap. 336).

The secretion of testosterone by the fetal testes approaches a maximum by the tenth week of gestation, and formation of the sexual phenotypes is largely completed by the end of the first trimester. During the latter phases of gestation, the ovarian follicles develop and the vagina matures in the female, and descent of the testes and growth of the external genitalia take place in the male.

DISORDERS OF CHROMOSOMAL SEX

Disorders of chromosomal sex (Table 339-2) occur when the number or structure of the X or Y chromosomes is abnormal (see Chap. 66).

KLINEFELTER SYNDROME Clinical Features Klinefelter syndrome is characterized by small, firm testes, azoospermia, gynecomastia, and elevated levels of plasma gonadotropins in men with two or more X chromosomes. The common karyotype is either a 47,XXY chromosomal pattern (the classic form) or 46,XY/47,XXY mosaicism. It is the most frequent major abnormality of sexual differentiation, the incidence being around 1 in 500 men.

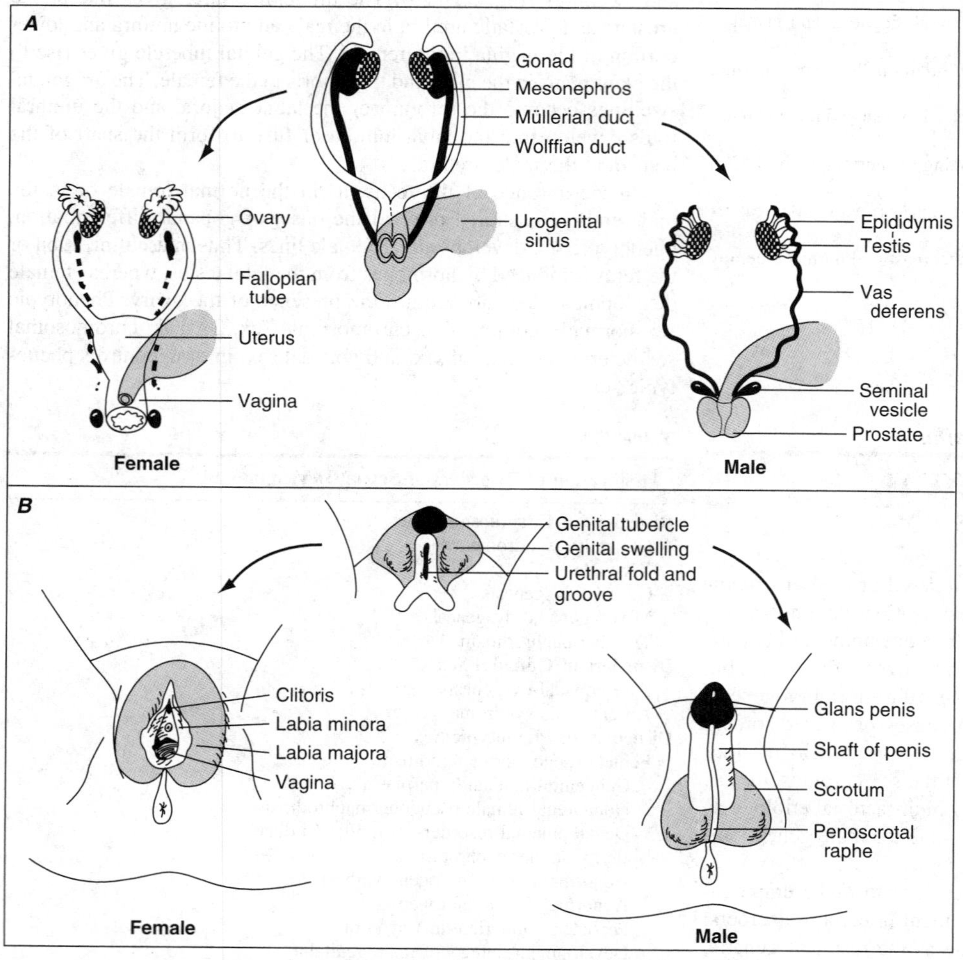

FIGURE 339-1 Normal sexual differentiation. *A.* Internal urogenital tract. *B.* External genitalia.

Prepubertally, the testes are small but otherwise appear normal. After puberty, the disorder is manifest as infertility, gynecomastia, or occasionally underandrogenization (Table 339-3). Hyalinization of the seminiferous tubules and azoospermia are consistent features of the 47,XXY variety. The small, firm testes are usually <2 cm and always <3.5 cm in length (corresponding to 2- and 12-mL volume, respectively). The increased mean body height results from longer legs. Gynecomastia ordinarily develops during adolescence, is generally bilateral and painless, and may become disfiguring (see Chap. 338). Obesity and varicose veins occur in one-third to one-half, and mild mental deficiency, social maladjustment, abnormalities of thyroid function, diabetes mellitus, and pulmonary disease may be present. The risk of breast cancer is 20 times that of normal men (but only about a fifth that in women). Most have male psychosexual orientation and function sexually as normal men.

The mosaic variant comprises about 10 percent of the patients, as estimated by chromosomal karyotypes on peripheral blood leukocytes. The frequency of this variant may be underestimated, since chromosomal mosaicism may be present in the testes when the peripheral leukocyte karyotype is normal. The mosaic form is usually not as severe as the 47,XXY variety, and the testes may be normal in size (see Table 339-3). The endocrine abnormalities are less severe, and gynecomastia and azoospermia are less common. Indeed, occasional mosaic individuals are fertile. In some the diagnosis may not even be suspected because of the minor manifestations.

Approximately 30 additional variants of Klinefelter syndrome have been described, including those with uniform cell lines (such as 48,XXYY, 48,XXXY, and 49,XXXXY) and a variety of mosaicisms of the X chromosome with or without associated structural abnormalities of the X. In general, the greater the chromosomal abnormality the more severe are the manifestations.

Pathophysiology The classic form is due to meiotic nondisjunction of the chromosomes during gametogenesis (Fig. 339-2). About 40 percent of the responsible meiotic nondisjunctions occur during spermatogenesis, and 60 percent occur during oogenesis. Advanced maternal age is a predisposing factor. The mosaic form is thought to result from chromosomal mitotic nondisjunction after fertilization of the zygote and can take place in either a 46,XY zygote (see Fig. 339-2) or a 47,XXY zygote. The latter situation, double nondisjunction (meiotic and mitotic), may be the usual cause and thus explain why the mosaic form is less frequent than the classic disorder.

Plasma follicle stimulating hormone (FSH) and luteinizing hormone (LH) levels are usually high; FSH shows the best discrimination, little overlap occurring with normal individuals, because of the consistent damage to the seminiferous tubules. The plasma testosterone level averages half normal but may overlap the normal range. Mean plasma estradiol levels are elevated; early, estradiol secretion by the testes may be increased in response to the elevated plasma LH level, but the testicular secretion of estradiol and testosterone eventually declines. Elevated plasma estradiol late in the course is probably due both to decreased metabolic clearance rate and to increased conversion of testosterone to estradiol in extragonadal tissues. The net result both early and late is a variable degree of feminization and virilization. The feminization, including gynecomastia, depends

Table 339-2

Clinical Features of the Disorders of Chromosomal Sex

Disorder	Common Chromosomal Complement	Gonadal Development	External Genitalia	Internal Genitalia	Breast Development	Comment
Klinefelter syndrome	47,XXY *or* 46,XY/47,XXY	Hyalinized testes	Normal male	Normal male	Gynecomastia	Most common disorder of sexual differentiation; tall stature.
XX male	46,XX	Hyalinized testes	Normal male	Normal male	Gynecomastia	Shorter than normal men; increased incidence of hypospadias. Similar to Klinefelter syndrome. May be familial.
Gonadal dysgenesis (Turner syndrome)	45,X *or* 46,XX/45,X	Streak gonads	Immature female	Hypoplastic female	Immature female	Short stature and multiple somatic abnormalities. May be 46,XX with structurally abnormal X chromosome.
Mixed gonadal dysgenesis	46,XY/45,X *or* 46,XY	Testis and streak gonad	Variable but almost always ambiguous; 60% reared as female	Uterus, vagina, and one fallopian tube	Usually male	Second most common cause of ambiguous genitalia in the newborn; tumors common.
True hermaphroditism	46,XX *or* 46,XY *or* mosaics	Testis and ovary or ovotestis	Variable but usually ambiguous; 60% reared as males	Usually a uterus and urogenital sinus; ducts correspond to gonad	Gynecomastia in 75%	May be familial.

on the ratio of circulating estrogen to androgen (relative or absolute), and individuals with lower plasma testosterone and higher plasma estradiol levels are more likely to develop gynecomastia (see Chap. 338). The normal feedback inhibition of testosterone on pituitary LH secretion is diminished. Men with untreated Klinefelter syndrome may have enlarged or abnormal sella turcicas, presumably due to hyperplasia of the gonadotrophs because of inadequate testosterone feedback.

℞ **TREATMENT**

In men with some sperm production fertility might be achieved with in vitro fertilization (see Chap. 336). Gynecomastia should be treated surgically. Some underandrogenized patients benefit from supplemental androgen, but such treatment may worsen the gynecomastia, presumably by providing increased substrate estrogen formation in peripheral tissues. Testosterone should be injected in the form of testosterone cypionate or testosterone enanthate or administered via the transdermal route (see Chap. 336). Following the administration of testosterone, the plasma LH level returns to normal only after several months, if at all.

XX MALE SYNDROME A 46,XX karyotype is found in approximately 1 in 20,000 phenotypic males. The findings resemble those in Klinefelter syndrome: the testes are small and firm (generally less than 2 cm), gynecomastia is frequent, the penis is normal to small in size, azoospermia and hyalinization of the seminiferous tubules are usual, no female urogenital structures are present, psychosexual identification is male, mean plasma testosterone level is low, plasma estradiol level is elevated, and plasma gonadotropin levels are high. Affected individuals differ from typical Klinefelter patients only in that average height is less than in normal men, the incidence of cognitive problems is not increased, and the incidence of hypospadias is increased.

Table 339-3

Characteristics of Patients with Classic versus Mosaic Klinefelter Syndrome*

	47,XXY, %	46,XY/47,XXY, %
Abnormal testicular histology	100	94†
Decreased length of testis	99	73†
Azoospermia	93	50†
Decreased testosterone	79	33
Decreased facial hair	77	64
Increased gonadotropins	75	33†
Decreased sexual function	68	56
Gynecomastia	55	33†
Decreased axillary hair	49	46
Decreased length of penis	41	21

* Table based on 519 XXY patients and 51 XY/XXY patients.
† Significantly different at $p < .05$ or better.
SOURCE: After Gordon et al.

The majority of XX males whose DNA is probed with Y-chromosome DNA fragments containing the SRY gene are positive for Y-related DNA; thus an X-Y or Y-autosome translocation appears to be the common cause. Some 46,XX males are negative for all Y-specific DNA, suggesting that the disorder is due to mutation in a downstream, autosomal or X-linked gene involved in development of the testes. The management is similar to that of Klinefelter syndrome.

GONADAL DYSGENESIS (TURNER SYNDROME) Clinical Features Gonadal dysgenesis is characterized by primary amenorrhea, sexual infantilism, short stature, multiple congenital anomalies, and bilateral streak gonads in phenotypic women with any of several defects of the X chromosome. This condition should be distinguished from (1) mixed gonadal dysgenesis in which a unilateral testis and a contralateral streak gonad may be present; (2) pure gonadal dysgenesis in which bilateral streak gonads are associated with a normal 46,XX or 46,XY karyotype, normal stature, and primary amenorrhea; and (3) the Noonan syndrome, an autosomal dominant disorder in both sexes characterized by webbed neck, short stature, congenital heart disease, cubitus valgus, and other congenital defects despite normal karyotypes and normal gonads.

The incidence is estimated at 1 in 3000 newborn females; the prenatal incidence may be as high as 2 percent of all human conceptuses, only a small fraction of whom survive to term. The diagnosis is made either at birth because of the associated anomalies or at puberty when amenorrhea and failure of sexual development are noted in conjunction with the associated anomalies. Gonadal dysgenesis is the most common cause of primary amenorrhea, accounting for a third of such patients. The external genitalia are unambiguously female but remain immature, and there is no breast development unless exogenous estrogen is given. The fallopian tubes and uterus are immature, and bilateral streak gonads are present in the broad ligaments. Primordial germ cells are present transiently during embryogenesis but disappear because of an accelerated rate of atresia (see Chap. 337). After the age of expected puberty, these streaks lack identifiable follicles and ova and consist of fibrous tissue that is indistinguishable from normal ovarian stroma.

The associated somatic anomalies primarily involve the skeleton and connective tissue. Lymphedema of the hands and feet, webbing of the neck, low hairline, redundant skin folds on the back of the neck, a shieldlike chest with widely spaced nipples, and growth retardation are features that suggest the diagnosis in infancy. Micrognathia, epicanthal folds, prominent low-set or deformed ears, a fishlike mouth, and ptosis may be present. Short fourth metacarpals are present in half, and 10 to 20 percent have coarctation of the aorta. In adults, the average height rarely exceeds 150 cm. Associated conditions include renal malformations, pigmented nevi, hypoplastic nails, tendency to keloid formation, perceptive hearing loss, unexplained hypertension, glucose intolerance, and autoimmune thyroid disease.

Pathophysiology About half have a 45,X karyotype, approximately one-fourth have mosaicism with no structural abnormality (46,XX/45,X), and the remainder have a structurally abnormal X chromosome with or without mosaicism (see Chap. 66). The mechanism of chromosome loss is unknown but may occur during gametogenesis in either parent or as a mitotic error during one of the early cleavage divisions of the fertilized zygote (see Fig. 339-2). Short stature and other somatic features result from loss of genetic material on the short arm of the X chromosome. Streak gonads result when genetic material is missing from either the long or short arm of the X. In individuals with mosaicism or structural abnormalities of the X, phenotypes on average are intermediate in severity between that seen in the 45,X variety and the normal. In some patients with hypertrophy of the clitoris, there is an unidentified fragment of a chromosome present in addition to the X chromosome, assumed to be an abnormal Y; gonadoblastoma may develop in the streak gonads in this subset of patients. The Y-linked genes that predispose to gonadoblastoma are believed to be distinct from SRY because XY women with SRY deletions or mutations are at risk. Rarely, familial transmission of gonadal dysgenesis can be the result of a balanced X-autosome translocation (see Chap. 66). Analysis of chromosomal karyotype is necessary to establish the diagnosis and to identify the group with Y chromosomal elements and a high chance of developing malignancy in the streak gonads.

After the time of expected puberty pubic and axillary hair remain sparse, the breasts are infantile, and no menses occur. Serum FSH is elevated in infancy, falls during midchildhood to the normal range, and increases to castrate levels at the age of 9 or 10. At this time, the serum LH level is also elevated, and plasma estradiol levels are low [<40 pmol/L (<10 pg/mL)]. Approximately 2 percent of 45,X and 12 percent of mosaic women have sufficient residual follicles to allow some menstruation. Indeed, occasionally minimally affected women become pregnant; the reproductive life in such individuals is brief.

℞ TREATMENT

At the anticipated time of puberty, replacement therapy with estrogen should be instituted to induce maturation of the breasts, labia, vagina, uterus, and fallopian tubes (see Chap. 337). Linear growth and bone maturation rates are approximately doubled during the first year of treatment with estradiol, but the eventual height rarely approaches the predicted level. Combination therapy with oxandrolone and/or growth hormone accelerates growth and increases final height (see Chap. 329).

Gonadal tumors are rare in 45,X patients but do occur in women carrying Y chromosome fragments or with mosaicism of the Y chromosome; consequently, streak gonads should be removed in all women with evidence of virilization or with Y-chromosome sequences.

MIXED GONADAL DYSGENESIS **Clinical Features** Mosaicism for a Y-bearing cell line, usually the 45,X/46,XY karyotype, is responsible for most instances of mixed gonadal dysgenesis. Affected individuals usually have a testis on one side and a streak gonad on the other, but bilateral dysgenetic testes or bilateral streak gonads may be present. The incidence is unknown, but in most hospitals the disorder is the second most common cause of ambiguous genitalia in the neonate after congenital adrenal hyperplasia.

The phenotype varies depending on the proportion of XY cells and their distribution. About two-thirds of such children are reared as females. Many have ambiguous genitalia, including phallic enlargement, a urogenital sinus, and some labioscrotal fusion. In most the testis is located intraabdominally; individuals with a testis in the inguinal or scrotal position are usually reared as males. A uterus, vagina, and at least one fallopian tube are almost invariably present.

The prepubertal testis appears relatively normal. The postpubertal testis contains abundant Leydig cells, but the seminiferous tubules lack germinal elements and contain only Sertoli cells. The streak gonad, a thin, pale, elongated structure located either in the broad ligament or along the pelvic wall, is composed of ovarian stroma. At puberty the testis secretes androgen, causing virilization and phallic enlargement. Feminization is rare; when it occurs, estrogen secretion from a gonadal tumor should be suspected.

Approximately a third of such individuals exhibit somatic features of 45,X gonadal dysgenesis, i.e., low posterior hairline, shield chest, multiple pigmented nevi, cubitus valgus, webbing of the neck, and short stature (height less than 150 cm).

Approximately two-thirds have the 45,X/46,XY karyotype, and the remainder have a 46,XY karyotype or a variant mosaicism. The origin of 45,X/46,XY mosaicism is best explained by the loss of a Y chromosome during an early mitotic division of an XY zygote similar to the postulated loss of the X chromosome in the 46,XY/47,XXY mosaicism shown in Fig. 339-2.

Pathophysiology It is assumed (but has been difficult to prove) that the 46,XY cell line stimulates testicular differentiation, whereas the 45,X stem leads to the development of the contralateral streak gonad.

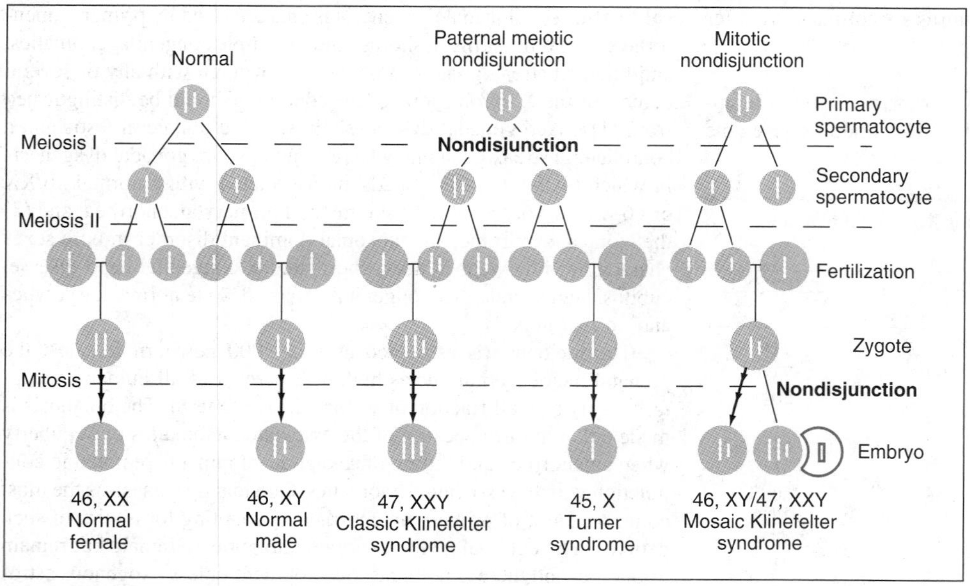

FIGURE 339-2 Schema for normal spermatogenesis and fertilization showing effects of meiotic and mitotic nondisjunction leading to classic Klinefelter syndrome, Turner syndrome, and mosaic Klinefelter. The schema would be similar if the abnormal events took place during oogenesis.

Both masculinization and müllerian duct regression in utero are incomplete. Since Leydig cell function is normal at puberty, inadequate virilization in utero may be due to delayed development of a testis that is ultimately capable of normal Leydig cell function.

℞ TREATMENT

For the older child or adult in whom gender is fixed prior to diagnosis, the central issue in management is the possibility of tumor development in the gonads, which may occur prior to puberty. The overall incidence of seminomas and gonadoblastomas may be as high as 25 percent. Such tumors occur most frequently in subjects with a female phenotype who lack the somatic features of 45,X gonadal dysgenesis and are more common in testes than in the streak gonad. When the diagnosis is established in phenotypic females, prophylactic gonadectomy should be performed because gonadal tumors may occur in childhood and because the testes secrete androgen at puberty and thus cause virilization. Such women, like those with gonadal dysgenesis, are then given estrogen to induce and maintain feminization.

When the diagnosis is established in phenotypic males during late childhood or in adults, the management is more complicated. Men with mixed gonadal dysgenesis are infertile (no germinal elements are present in the testes) and have a high risk of developing gonadal tumors. In deciding which testes can be safely conserved the following observations apply: (1) tumors develop in scrotal streak gonads but not in scrotal testes, (2) tumors that develop in intraabdominal testes are always associated with ipsilateral müllerian duct structures, and (3) tumors in streak gonads are always associated with tumors in the contralateral abdominal testis. Based on these observations, it is recommended that (1) all streak gonads should be removed, (2) scrotal testes should be preserved, and (3) intraabdominal testes should be excised unless they can be relocated in the scrotum and are not associated with ipsilateral müllerian duct structures. Reconstructive surgery of the phallus should be performed when appropriate.

When the diagnosis is established in early infancy and the genitalia are ambiguous, gender assignment is usually female, and resection of the phallus and gonadectomy can be performed in infancy, sometimes in one procedure. If the decision is for male gender assignment, the same criteria apply as to which testes should be removed as in older males.

TRUE HERMAPHRODITISM **Clinical Features** True hermaphroditism is a condition in which both an ovary and a testis or one or more gonads with features of both (ovotestis) are present. To justify the diagnosis, both types of gonadal epithelium must be documented histologically, the presence of ovarian stroma without oocytes not being sufficient. The incidence is unknown, but more than 400 cases have been reported. Three categories are recognized: (1) one-fifth are bilateral—testicular and ovarian tissue (ovotestes) on each side, (2) two-fifths are unilateral—an ovotestis on one side and an ovary or a testis on the other, and (3) the remainder are lateral—a testis on one side and an ovary on the other.

The external genitalia exhibit all gradations of the male-to-female spectrum. Two-thirds are sufficiently masculinized to be reared as males, but less than one-tenth have normal male external genitalia; most have hypospadias and incomplete labioscrotal fusion. Two-thirds of phenotypic females have an enlarged clitoris, and most have a urogenital sinus. Differentiation of the internal ducts usually corresponds to the adjacent gonad. Although an epididymis usually develops adjacent to a testis, the vas deferens is complete in only one-third. Of the patients with an ovotestis, three-fourths have an epididymis, two-thirds have a fallopian tube, one-tenth have a vas deferens, and one-tenth have both a vas deferens and a fallopian tube. The uterus may be hypoplastic or unicornuate. The ovary is usually in the normal position, but the testis or ovotestis may be found at any level along the route of embryonic testicular descent, frequently associated with an inguinal hernia. Testicular tissue is present in the scrotum or the labioscrotal fold in one-third, in the inguinal canal in one-third, and in the abdomen in one-third.

Variable feminization and virilization ensue at puberty, three-fourths develop gynecomastia, and about half menstruate. In phenotypic men, menstruation may cause cyclic hematuria. Ovulation occurs in approximately one-fourth and is more common than spermatogenesis. In men, ovulation may cause testicular pain. Fertility has been reported in women and more rarely in men. Congenital malformations of other systems are rare.

Pathophysiology About two-thirds of individuals have a 46,XX karyotype, a tenth have a 46,XY karyotype, and the remainder are chimeras or mosaics in whom a Y cell line is present. The mechanism responsible for the gonadal development is unknown. Only 10 percent of 46,XX true hermaphrodites are SRY positive and are believed to have either mosaicism or translocation involving a portion of the Y chromosome; the remainder are believed to result from gain of function mutations in downstream genes involved in SRY action. In rare instances, multiple sibs with a 46,XX karyotype are affected, possibly the result of an autosomal or X-linked mutation.

Because corpora lutea are frequently present in the ovaries, it is presumed that the female neuroendocrine axis functions normally in such individuals. Feminization (gynecomastia and menstruation) is the result of secretion of estradiol by ovarian tissue. In masculinized patients, secretion of androgen predominates, and some produce sperm.

℞ TREATMENT

When the diagnosis is made in early infancy, gender assignment depends on the anatomic features. In older children and adults, gonads and internal duct structures that are contradictory to the predominant phenotype (and the gender of rearing) should be removed, and the external genitalia should be modified when appropriate. Gonadal tumors are rare but have been reported in true hermaphrodites who carry Y chromosome sequences. Consequently, the possibility of future tumor development must be taken into account when the decision regarding conservation of gonadal tissue is made.

DISORDERS OF GONADAL SEX

Disorders of gonadal sex result when chromosomal sex is normal, but for one of several reasons differentiation of the gonads is abnormal. Thus, gonadal sex does not correspond to chromosomal sex.

PURE GONADAL DYSGENESIS **Clinical Features** Pure gonadal dysgenesis is a disorder in which phenotypic females with gonads and genitalia characteristic of gonadal dysgenesis (bilateral streaks, infantile uterus and fallopian tubes, and sexual infantilism) have normal height, few if any somatic anomalies, and either a normal 46,XX or 46,XY karyotype. This disorder is about one-tenth as common as gonadal dysgenesis. It is genetically distinct but cannot be distinguished clinically from those instances of gonadal dysgenesis with minimal somatic abnormalities. The height is normal or greater than normal, some individuals being over 170 cm. Estrogen levels vary from profound deficiency typical of 45,X gonadal dysgenesis to some breast development and menses that terminate in an early menopause. About 40 percent have some feminization. Axillary and pubic hair are scanty, and the internal genitalia consist of müllerian derivatives only.

Tumors may develop in the streak gonads, particularly dysgerminoma or gonadoblastoma in the 46,XY disorder. Such tumors may be heralded by the development of virilizing signs or a pelvic mass.

Pathophysiology Although chromosomal mosaicisms have been described under this nosology, the designation here is restricted to women with uniform 46,XX or 46,XY karyotypes. (Those with mosaicism are variants of gonadal dysgenesis or mixed gonadal dysgenesis, as described above.) The rationale for this restricted definition is based on the fact that both the XX and XY varieties can result from single gene mutations that are presumed to involve gene(s) essential for gonadal development. Several sibships have been reported in which more than one individual is affected with the 46,XX disorder, frequently the result of consanguineous matings, suggesting an autosomal recessive inheritance. Familial occurrence of the 46,XY variety also has been described; in some the disorder appears to be inherited as an X-linked trait, and in others the pattern suggests a male-limited autosomal recessive inheritance. About 15 percent of the 46,XY women have either a deletion or a mutation in the SRY coding sequence. Other instances could be due to mutations in SRY outside the coding sequence, in the downstream genes that are controlled by SRY, or in other genes that influence SRY expression. One of these downstream genes is the SOX 9 gene; mutations of this gene are associated with 46,XY gonadal dysgenesis and skeletal abnormalities (campomelic dysplasia). In both the 46,XX and the 46,XY forms the disorder prevents differentiation of ovary or testis, respectively; the development of the female phenotype and the elevation of gonadotropin secretion are due to failure of gonadal development.

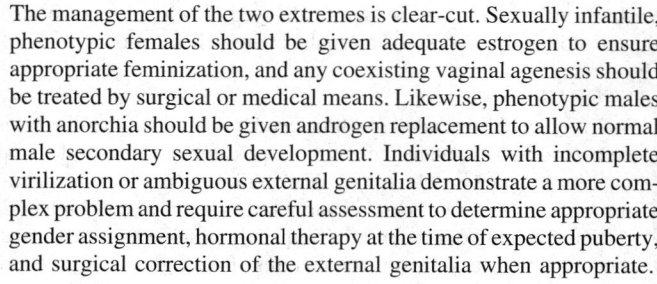

℞ TREATMENT

The management of the estrogen deficiency is identical to that in gonadal dysgenesis; namely, appropriate estrogen replacement therapy is initiated at the time of expected puberty and maintained in adult life (see Chap. 337). Because of the high frequency of gonadal tumors in the 46,XY variety, the streak gonads should be removed once the diagnosis is made; development of virilizing signs is indication for immediate surgery. The natural history of the gonadal tumors is uncertain, but the prognosis after surgical removal is usually good.

THE ABSENT TESTES SYNDROME (ANORCHIA, TESTICULAR REGRESSION, GONADAL AGENESIS, AGONADISM) Clinical Features A spectrum of phenotypes occurs in 46,XY males with absent or rudimentary testes but in whom unequivocal evidence exists that endocrine function of the testis (e.g., consistent müllerian duct regression and variable testosterone synthesis) was present at some time during embryonic life. In pure gonadal dysgenesis, in contrast, no evidence can be inferred for gonadal function during embryonic development. The manifestations vary from complete failure of virilization to incomplete virilization of the external genitalia to otherwise normal men with bilateral anorchia.

The purest form is represented by 46,XY females with absent testes, sexual infantilism, and absence of both müllerian duct derivatives and accessory organs of male reproduction. Such individuals differ from those with 46,XY pure gonadal dysgenesis in that no gonadal remnant can be identified, including no streak gonad and no müllerian derivatives. Testicular failure must have occurred between the onset of MDI synthesis and the onset of testosterone secretion, i.e., after development of Sertoli cells but before the onset of Leydig cell function.

In others, testicular failure occurred later in gestation, and these individuals may constitute problems in gender assignment. In some, failure of müllerian regression is more pronounced than failure of testosterone secretion, but none exhibit normal müllerian development. In those with more extensive virilization, the external genitalia are phenotypically male, but rudimentary oviducts and vasa deferentia may coexist internally.

At the final extreme is the syndrome of bilateral anorchia in which phenotypic men have absence of müllerian structures and gonads but male wolffian duct derivatives and external genitalia. Microphallus implies that failure of testosterone secretion occurred late in embryogenesis after anatomic development of the male urethra was complete. Gynecomastia may or may not be present.

Pathophysiology The pathogenesis is not understood. Testicular regression could be the result of mutant genes, teratogen, or trauma, and the disorder may well be heterogeneous in origin. Sibships with multiple affected individuals have been described, and several instances of agonadism have occurred in the same family, some unilateral and others bilateral. Some subjects in whom no testes can be identified at laparotomy have blood testosterone values above the castrate range, presumably derived from remnant testes.

℞ TREATMENT

The management of the two extremes is clear-cut. Sexually infantile, phenotypic females should be given adequate estrogen to ensure appropriate feminization, and any coexisting vaginal agenesis should be treated by surgical or medical means. Likewise, phenotypic males with anorchia should be given androgen replacement to allow normal male secondary sexual development. Individuals with incomplete virilization or ambiguous external genitalia demonstrate a more complex problem and require careful assessment to determine appropriate gender assignment, hormonal therapy at the time of expected puberty, and surgical correction of the external genitalia when appropriate.

DISORDERS OF PHENOTYPIC SEX

FEMALE PSEUDOHERMAPHRODITISM Congenital Adrenal Hyperplasia *Clinical features* The pathways by which glucocorticoids are synthesized in the adrenal gland and androgens are formed in the testis and adrenal are summarized in Fig. 339-3. Three reactions are common to both pathways (cholesterol side chain-cleavage, 3β-hydroxysteroid dehydrogenase/isomerase, and 17α-hydroxylase); impairment of any of these reactions results in deficiency of glucocorticoid and androgen synthesis and consequently in both congenital adrenal hyperplasia (due to enhanced ACTH levels) and defective virilization of the male embryo (male pseudohermaphroditism). Two reactions are involved exclusively in androgen synthesis (17,20-lyase and 17β-hydroxysteroid dehydrogenase); deficiency in either results in pure male pseudohermaphroditism with normal glucocorticoid synthesis. Deficiency of either of the terminal two enzymes of glucocorticoid synthesis (21-hydroxylase and 11β-hydroxylase) impairs formation of hydrocortisone; the compensatory increase in ACTH secretion causes adrenal hyperplasia and a secondary increase in androgen formation that causes virilization in the female and precocious masculinization in the male.

The major features of congenital adrenal hyperplasia are listed in Table 339-4. The *adrenal insufficiency* can be equally severe and life-threatening in both sexes and is described in Chap. 332. From the standpoint of *abnormal sexual development*, some defects in steroidogenesis result in female pseudohermaphroditism, and some cause male pseudohermaphroditism. (3β-Hydroxysteroid dehydrogenase/isomerase deficiency can cause either male or female pseudohermaphroditism, but since incomplete virilization of the male is more common, the disorder will be discussed under male pseudohermaphroditism.)

Congenital adrenal hyperplasia due to classic 21-hydroxylase deficiency is the most common cause of ambiguous genitalia in the newborn, with an incidence of between 1 in 5000 and 1 in 15,000 live births in Europe and the United States; it may or may not be associated with mineralocorticoid deficiency (salt loss) (see Table 339-4). Virilization is usually apparent at birth in the female and within the first 2 to 3 years of life in the male. Manifestations in females include hypertrophy of the clitoris with ventral binding (chordee), partial fusion of the labioscrotal folds, and variable virilization of the urethra. The uterus, fallopian tubes, and ovaries are normal, and the wolffian ducts do not virilize, probably because adrenal function begins relatively late in embryogenesis. The external appearance of an affected female newborn is similar to that of a male with bilateral cryptorchidism and hypospadias. The labioscrotal folds are bulbous and rugated and resemble a scrotum. Rarely, the virilization is so severe that development of a complete penile urethra and prostate results in errors in sex assignment at birth. Radiography following the injection of radiopaque dye into the external genital orifice is helpful in demonstrating the presence of vagina, uterus, and (sometimes) fallopian tubes. Occasionally, virilization of the female is slight or absent at birth and becomes evident in later infancy, adolescence, or adulthood (the so-called nonclassic or late-onset form of the disorder). In both sexes, rapid somatic maturation results in premature epiphyseal closure and a short adult height. The untreated female with the classic disorder grows rapidly during the first year of life and has progressive virilization. At the time of expected puberty there is a failure of normal female sexual development and absence of menstruation.

Since male phenotypic differentiation is normal, the condition is usually not recognized at birth in boys in the absence of adrenal insufficiency. However, early maturation of the external genitalia, development of secondary sex characteristics, coarsening of the voice, frequent erections, and excessive muscular development are noticeable during the first few years of life. Virilization in the male can follow two patterns. Excessive adrenal androgens can inhibit gonadotropin production so that the testes remain infantile in size despite the acceleration of masculinization. Such untreated adult men are capable of erection and ejaculation but have no spermatogenesis. Alternatively, adrenal androgen secretion can induce premature maturation of the hypothalamic-pituitary axis and initiate a true precocious puberty including early maturation of spermatogenesis (see Chap. 336). The untreated male is also subject to the development of ACTH-dependent "tumors" of the adrenal rest cells of the testes.

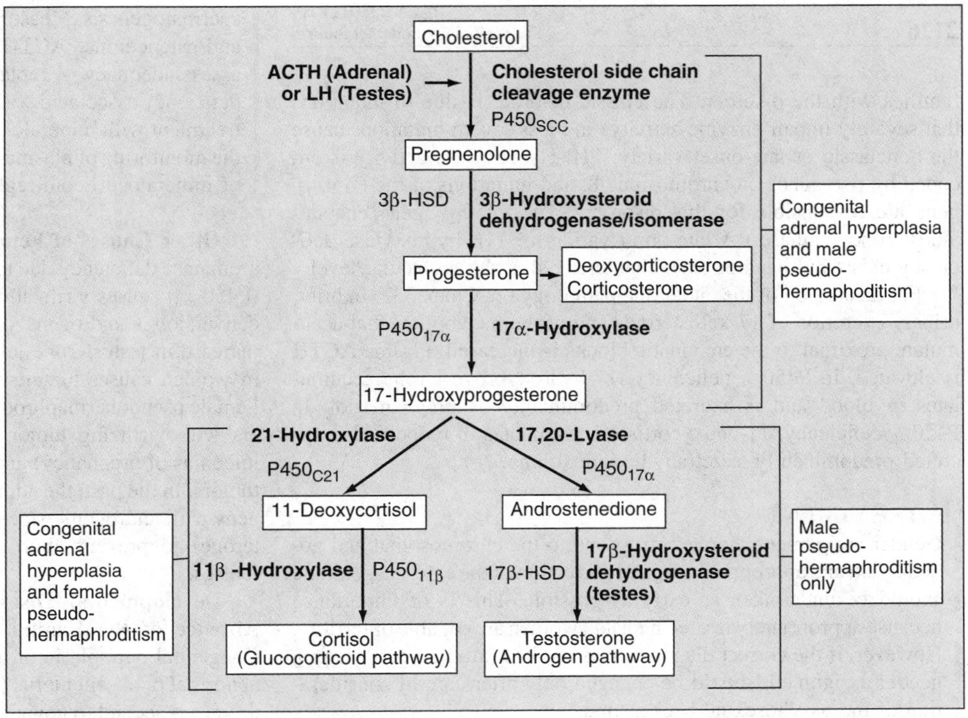

FIGURE 339-3 Pathways of glucocorticoid and androgen synthesis. Note abnormal conditions corresponding to impaired enzyme reactions.

In classic 21-hydroxylase deficiency, which accounts for about 95 percent of congenital adrenal hyperplasia, decreased production of hydrocortisone leads to increased release of ACTH, enlargement of the adrenal glands, and partial or complete compensation of the defect in the secretion of hydrocortisone. In about half, the enzyme defect appears to be partial, and cortisol secretion is normal. This form is termed *simple virilizing*. When deficiency of the enzyme is more complete, the so-called salt-losing form of 21-hydroxylase deficiency, production of cortisol and aldosterone is inadequate, and severe salt wastage with anorexia, vomiting, volume depletion, and collapse occurs within the first few weeks of life. In untreated patients, overproduction of the cortisol precursors prior to the 21-hydroxylase step leads to increase in plasma progesterone and 17-hydroxyprogesterone. These steroids are weak aldosterone antagonists at the receptor level, and in the compensated state aldosterone production increases to attempt to maintain normal sodium balance. Increased substrate availability is also responsible for the increase in androgen synthesis and hence for the virilization.

Female pseudohermaphroditism also occurs in 11β-hydroxylase deficiency. In this disorder, a block in hydroxylation at the 11 carbon results in the accumulation of 11-deoxycortisol and deoxycorticosterone (DOC), a potent salt-retaining hormone that causes hypertension rather than salt loss. The clinical features that stem from glucocorticoid deficiency and androgen excess are similar to those in 21-hydroxylase deficiency.

Pathophysiology Both disorders are due to autosomal recessive mutations. The carrier frequency for $P450_{C21}$ deficiency is about 1 in 50. Because the gene is located on the sixth chromosome close to the HLA-B locus, carriers of the disorder (as well as homozygotes) within a given family can be identified on the basis of the HLA haplotype. At the molecular level the mutations that give rise to 21-hydroxylase deficiency are even more polymorphic; indeed, deletions of portions of the gene (10 to 30 percent), conversion of the gene from a functional state to a form that is not transcribed normally (10 percent), and point mutations (60 to 75 percent) have been characterized in different

Table 339-4

Forms of Congenital Adrenal Hyperplasia

Deficiency	Cortisol	Aldosterone	Degree of Virilization of Females	Failure of Virilization in Males	Dominant Steroid Secreted	Comment
Classic 21-hydroxylase:						
Partial (simple virilizing or compensated)	Normal	↑	+ + + +	0	17-Hydroxy-progesterone	Most common type (95% of total); from one- to two-thirds salt losers
Severe (salt-losing)	↓	↓	+ + + +	0	17-Hydroxy-progesterone	
11β-Hydroxylase (hypertension)	↓	↓	+ + + +	0	11-Deoxycortisol and 11-deoxy-corticosterone	Hypertension
3β-Hydroxysteroid dehydrogenase/isomerase	0	0	+	+ + + +	Δ^5-3β-OH compounds (dehy-droepiandrost-erone)	Probably second most common, usually salt loss
17α-Hydroxylase	↓	↓	0	+ + + +	Corticosterone and 11-deoxy-corticosterone	No feminization of female, hypertension
Cholesterol side chain cleavage	0	0	0	+ + + +	Cholesterol(?)	Rare, usually salt loss

families with the disorder. The classic disorder is due to mutations that severely impair enzyme activity, and less severe mutations cause the nonclassic or late-onset variety. 11β-Hydroxylase activity is encoded by two genes on chromosome 8, and mutations of the $P450_{11\beta 1}$ gene are responsible for this disorder. (The $P450_{11\beta 2}$ gene encodes aldosterone synthase.) A late-onset variant of 11β-hydroxylase deficiency exists but has not been characterized at the molecular level.

For discussion of the endocrine pathology see Chap. 332. In brief, urinary excretion of 17-ketosteroids and of the metabolites that accumulate proximal to the enzymatic blocks is increased. Plasma ACTH is elevated. In $P450_{C21}$ deficiency, 17-hydroxyprogesterone accumulates in blood and is excreted predominantly as pregnanetriol. In $P450_{11\beta}$ deficiency, 11-deoxycortisol accumulates in blood and is excreted predominantly as tetrahydrocortexolone.

℞ TREATMENT

Gender assignment should correspond to the chromosomal and gonadal sex, and appropriate surgical correction of the external genitalia should be undertaken as early as possible. This is of importance because appropriately treated men and women are capable of fertility. However, if the correct diagnosis is made late (after 3 years of age), gender assignment should be changed only after careful consideration of the psychosexual background.

Treatment with appropriate glucocorticoids prevents the consequences of hydrocortisone deficiency, arrests the rapid virilization, and prevents premature somatic and epiphyseal maturation. The suppression of the abnormal steroid secretion corrects the hypertension in $P450_{11\beta}$ deficiency and in both disorders allows normal onset of menses and development of female secondary sex characteristics. In males, glucocorticoid therapy suppresses adrenal androgens and results in normal gonadotropin secretion, testicular development, and spermatogenesis. Measurements of plasma 17-hydroxyprogesterone, androstenedione, ACTH, and renin levels have all been used to assess adequacy of replacement therapy. In severe 21-hydroxylase deficiency associated with salt loss or elevated plasma renin activity, treatment with mineralocorticoids is also indicated. In such patients, the monitoring of plasma renin is useful for determining the adequacy of mineralocorticoid replacement.

Other Causes of Female Pseudohermaphroditism Placental aromatase deficiency due to mutations in the gene encoding aromatase ($P450_{arom}$) causes virilization of female embryos because of defective conversion of androgens to estrogens in the placenta and the secondary increase in testosterone levels; in postnatal life aromatase deficiency in women causes hirsutism and development of polycystic ovaries. Female pseudohermaphroditism can also occur in babies born to mothers with virilizing tumors of the ovary (e.g., arrhenoblastomas or luteomas of pregnancy) and, rarely, to mothers with virilizing adrenal tumors. In the past, the administration to pregnant women of progestogens with androgenic side effects (such as 17α-ethinyl-19-nor-testosterone) to prevent abortion resulted in masculinization of female fetuses.

Developmental Disorders of Müllerian Ducts (Congenital Absence of the Vagina, Müllerian Agenesis) *Clinical features* Congenital hypoplasia or absence of the vagina in combination with abnormal or absent uterus (the Mayer-Rokitansky-Kuster-Hauser syndrome) is second to gonadal dysgenesis as a cause of primary amenorrhea. Most patients are ascertained after the time of expected puberty because of failure to menstruate. The height is normal, and the breasts, axillary and pubic hair, and habitus are feminine in character. The uterus can vary from almost normal, lacking only a conduit to the introitus, to the characteristic rudimentary bicornuate cords with or without a lumen. In some patients cyclic abdominal pain indicates that sufficient functional endometrium is present to result in retrograde menstruation and/or hematometra.

Table 339-5

Anatomic, Genetic, and Endocrine Profile of Hereditary Male Pseudohermaphroditism

		Phenotype					
Disorder	**Inheritance**	**Müllerian Ducts**	**Wolffian Ducts**	**Spermatogenesis**	**Urogenital Sinus**	**External Genitalia**	**Breast**
DEFECTS IN TESTOSTERONE SYNTHESIS							
Five enzyme deficiencies	Autosomal or X-linked recessive	Absent	Variable development	Normal or decreased	Variable from male to female	Generally female	Usually male
DEFECTS IN ANDROGEN ACTION							
Steroid 5α-reductase 2 deficiency	Autosomal recessive	Absent	Male	Normal or decreased	Female	Clitoromegaly	Male
Receptor disorders:							
Complete testicular feminization	X-linked recessive	Absent	Absent	Absent	Female	Female	Female
Incomplete testicular feminization	X-linked recessive	Absent	Male	Absent	Female	Clitoromegaly and posterior fusion	Female
Reifenstein syndrome	X-linked recessive	Absent	Variable development	Absent	Variable from male to female	Incomplete male development	Female
Infertile male syndrome	X-linked recessive	Absent	Male	Absent or decreased	Male	Male	Usually male
Undervirilized fertile male	X-linked recessive	Absent	Male	Normal or decreased	Male	Male	Usually male
DEFECTS IN MÜLLERIAN REGRESSION							
Persistent müllerian duct syndrome	Autosomal or X-linked recessive	Rudimentary uterus and fallopian tubes	Male	Normal	Male	Male	Male

About one-third have abnormal kidneys, most commonly agenesis, ectopy, fused kidneys of the horseshoe type, or solitary ectopic kidneys in the pelvis. Skeletal abnormalities are present in one-tenth; most involve the spine, and limb and rib defects account for the rest. Specific abnormalities include wedge vertebrae, fused rudimentary or asymmetric vertebral bodies, supernumerary vertebrae, and the Klippel-Feil syndrome (congenital fusion of the cervical spine, short neck, low posterior hairline, and painless limitation of cervical movement).

Pathophysiology The karyotype is 46,XX. Familial occurrence has been described, and the pattern of inheritance in most is consistent with a sex-limited autosomal dominant mutation. Sporadic cases may represent new mutations of the type responsible for the familial disorder or be multifactorial in etiology. In the familial cases, expressivity is variable; some have skeletal or renal abnormalities only, and some have other abnormalities of müllerian derivatives such as a double uterus. Bilateral renal aplasia in stillborn infants is commonly associated with absence of the uterus and vagina. Thus, the family history should be probed for isolated skeletal and renal abnormalities and for stillbirths that might result from congenital absence of both kidneys. Ovarian function is normal, and successful pregnancies have occurred after corrective vaginal surgery in patients with a normal uterus.

℞ TREATMENT

Vaginal agenesis can be treated by surgical or nonsurgical means. Surgical repair generally utilizes a split-thickness skin graft around a solid rubber mold to create an artificial vagina. Medical therapy involves the repeated application of pressure against the vaginal dimple with a simple dilator to force development of adequate vaginal depth. In view of complication rates of 5 to 10 percent in surgical series, surgery should be reserved for patients in whom a well-formed uterus is present and the possibility of fertility exists. Frequent coitus or instrumental dilatation is essential for maintaining patency of neovaginas formed by either technique.

Endocrine Profile Relative to Normal Male		
Testosterone Production	**Estrogen Production**	**LH**
Normal to decreased	Variable	High
Normal	Normal	Normal or increased
High	High	High
High	High	High
High	High	High
Normal or high	Normal or high	Normal or high
Normal or high	Normal or high	Normal or high
Normal	Normal	Normal

MALE PSEUDOHERMAPHRODITISM Defective virilization of the male embryo (male pseudohermaphroditism) can result from defects in androgen synthesis, defects in androgen action, defects in müllerian duct regression, and uncertain causes.

Abnormalities in Androgen Synthesis *Clinical features* Enzymatic defects that result in defective testosterone synthesis (see Fig. 339-3) account for only about a fifth of cases of male pseudohermaphroditism (Tables 339-4 and 339-5). Each of the defects blocks a step in the conversion of cholesterol to testosterone. Three are common to the synthesis of other adrenal hormones as well: cholesterol side chain cleavage, 3β-hydroxysteroid dehydrogenase/isomerase, and 17α-hydroxylase or $P450_{17\alpha}$. Consequently, their deficiency results in congenital adrenal hyperplasia (see Table 339-4) as well as male pseudohermaphroditism. Two others (17,20-lyase and 17β-hydroxysteroid dehydrogenase) are unique to the pathway of androgen synthesis, and their deficiency results only in male pseudohermaphroditism. Since androgens are obligatory precursors of estrogens, synthesis of estrogen is also low in all but the terminal defect (17β-hydroxysteroid dehydrogenase deficiency).

The adrenal dysfunction is described in Chap. 332, and the present discussion concerns the abnormal sexual development. In genetic males with defective testosterone synthesis, absence of the uterus and fallopian tubes indicates that müllerian duct inhibition was normal during embryogenesis. Masculinization of the urogenital tract and external genitalia and virilization at puberty vary from almost normal to absent, and, therefore, the manifestations vary from men with mild hypospadias to phenotypic women who prior to puberty resemble patients with complete testicular feminization. This variability is the consequence of varying severity of the enzymatic defects, varying effects of the steroids that accumulate proximal to the various metabolic blocks, and the presence of alternative enzymatic pathways in some disorders. In patients with partial defects in whom the plasma testosterone level is normal, the diagnosis can only be made by measuring the steroids that accumulate proximal to the metabolic block.

Cholesterol side chain cleavage deficiency (lipoid adrenal hyperplasia) is an autosomal recessive disorder in which virtually no urinary steroids (either 17-ketosteroids or 17-hydroxycorticoids) can be detected. The defect is an inability to convert cholesterol to pregnenolone, a step catalyzed by a single cholesterol side chain cleavage enzyme ($P450_{SCC}$). Manifestations of this disorder include salt wasting and profound adrenal insufficiency, and most affected individuals die during infancy. At autopsy, the adrenals and testes are enlarged and infiltrated with lipid. Affected males are incompletely masculinized, whereas affected female infants have normal genital development. The coding sequence of the $P450_{SCC}$ gene is normal in several affected individuals, and the nature of the molecular defect is unknown.

3β-Hydroxysteroid dehydrogenase/isomerase deficiency causes varying failure of masculinization and development of a vagina in male infants. Female infants may be modestly virilized at birth due to the weak androgenic potency of dehydroepiandrosterone, the major steroid secreted. If the enzyme is absent in both the adrenal and testis, no urinary steroids contain a Δ^4-3-keto configuration, whereas in patients in whom the defect is partial or affects only the testis, the urine may contain normal or elevated levels of Δ^4-3-ketosteroids. Most patients have marked salt wasting and profound adrenal insufficiency, and long-term survival in untreated cases occurs only in states of partial deficiency. Minimally affected males may experience an otherwise normal male puberty except for profound gynecomastia. In these boys, a low-normal blood testosterone level is accompanied by elevated Δ^5 precursors. 3β-Hydroxysteroid dehydrogenase is catalyzed by more than one isoenzyme. The type 1 gene is expressed in many tissues, and type 2 is expressed in adrenals and gonads. The human deficiency is due to any of several mutations in the type 2 enzyme, but the coding sequence of this gene is said to be normal in several individuals with the late-onset variant of the disease.

17α-Hydroxylase-17,20-lyase ($P450_{17\alpha}$) *deficiency* impairs the introduction of the 17-hydroxyl and the scission of the C-17,20 carbon bond that convert pregnenolone and progesterone to dehydroepiandrosterone and androstenedione, respectively, which are mediated by a single enzyme, $P450_{17\alpha}$, encoded on chromosome 10; it is unclear why both reactions occur in the ovary and testis, whereas in the adrenal 17-hydroxyprogesterone is largely converted to glucocorticoids and mineralocorticoids rather than the 19-carbon steroids. Likewise, it is unclear why some patients appear to have selective impairment of either 17α-hydroxylase or 17,20-lyase activity; the distinction between these activities must be functional and may involve the relative concentration of steroid substrates and competing enzymes. Whatever the explanation, the consequences of 17α-hydroxylase and 17,20-lyase deficiencies are different.

17α-Hydroxylase deficiency is characterized by hypogonadism, absence of secondary sex characteristics, hypokalemic alkalosis, hypertension, and virtually undetectable hydrocortisone secretion in phenotypic women. Formation of both corticosterone and DOC by the adrenal is elevated, and urinary 17-ketosteroids are low. Aldosterone secretion is low due to high plasma DOC and depressed angiotensin levels and returns to normal after suppressive doses of glucocorticoids. In 46,XX individuals, amenorrhea, absent sexual hair, and hypertension are common, but the phenotype is that of a normal prepubertal woman. In males, the deficiency results in defective virilization that varies from complete male pseudohermaphroditism to ambiguous genitalia with perineoscrotal hypospadias and, in some, gynecomastia. Adrenal insufficiency does not develop, since the secretion of both corticosterone (a weak glucocorticoid) and DOC (a mineralocorticoid) is elevated. Hypertension and hypokalemia are prominent (even in the neonatal period) and remit after suppression of the DOC secretion by glucocorticoid replacement. A variety of point mutations, deletions, and insertions in the $P450_{17\alpha}$ gene on chromosome 10 have been characterized in affected individuals.

17,20-Lyase deficiency in males is associated with normal function of the adrenal cortex and a variable pattern of male pseudohermaphroditism. In the majority there is genital ambiguity at birth, with some virilization at the time of expected puberty. Rare 46,XY patients have had a female phenotype and no virilization at the time of expected puberty. The disorder has been recognized in one 46,XX woman with sexual infantilism. The molecular defect in this disorder has not been described but is presumed to involve less severe mutations of the $P450_{17\alpha}$ gene.

17β-Hydroxysteroid dehydrogenase (17β-HSD-3) *deficiency* involves the final step in testosterone biosynthesis, reduction of the 17-keto group of androstenedione. This is the most common enzymatic defect in testosterone synthesis. Affected 46,XY males usually have a female phenotype with a blind-ending vagina and absence of müllerian derivatives, but inguinal or abdominal testes and virilized wolffian duct structures are present. At the time of expected puberty, both virilization (with phallic enlargement and development of facial and body hair) and a variable degree of feminization take place. In some untreated patients, reversal of gender behavior from female to male occurs at puberty. Plasma testosterone level may be in the low-normal range, making it essential to document elevation in plasma androstenedione to make the diagnosis. Isoenzymes encoded by several different genes possess 17β-hydroxysteroid dehydrogenase activity, but the isoenzyme 3 is expressed in the testes. A variety of mutations have been characterized in the 17β-HSD-3 gene in affected individuals.

Pathophysiology These various disorders are inherited as autosomal recessive traits. The pattern of steroid secretion and excretion depends on the site of the various metabolic blocks (see Fig. 339-3). In general, gonadotropin secretion is high, and many individuals with incomplete defects are able to compensate so that the steady state levels of testosterone may be normal or almost normal.

In rare cases of male pseudohermaphroditism, testosterone formation is deficient for reasons other than a single enzyme defect in androgen synthesis. These include disorders in which Leydig cell agenesis is due to autosomal recessive loss-of-function mutations of the LH receptor or to the secretion of a biologically inactive LH molecule. In addition, as described above, several disorders, including familial 46,XY pure gonadal dysgenesis, sporadic dysgenetic testes, and the absent testis syndrome, are characterized by deficient testosterone production due to abnormal gonadal development.

℞ TREATMENT

Therapy with glucocorticoids and in some instances mineralocorticoids is indicated in those disorders causing adrenal hyperplasia. The management of the genital abnormalities depends on the individual case. Fertility has not been reported, and its consideration does not enter into sex assignment. In genetic females there is no problem (except in diagnosis), in that affected individuals are raised appropriately as females and estrogen therapy is begun at the time of expected puberty to promote development of female secondary sex characteristics. Whether newborn males with ambiguous genitalia should be raised as males or females depends on the anatomic defect; in general, the more severely affected should be raised as females, and corrective surgery of the genitalia and removal of the testes should be undertaken as early as possible. In such women estrogen therapy is begun at the appropriate age to allow development of normal female secondary sex characteristics. In individuals raised as males, corrective surgery is indicated for any coexisting hypospadias, and plasma androgens should be monitored at the time of expected puberty to determine whether testosterone therapy is appropriate.

Abnormalities in Androgen Action Several disorders of male phenotypic development result from abnormalities of androgen action. The spectrum of phenotypes is described in Tables 329-4 and 329-5. In these disorders, testosterone formation and müllerian regression are normal, but male development is impaired because of resistance to androgen action in target tissues.

Steroid 5α-reductase 2 deficiency This autosomal recessive disorder is characterized by (1) severe perineoscrotal hypospadias; (2) a blind vaginal pouch of variable size opening either into the urogenital sinus or into the urethra; (3) testes with normal epididymides, vasa deferentia, and seminal vesicles, and termination of the ejaculatory ducts in the blind-ending vagina; (4) a female habitus with normal axillary and pubic hair but without female breast development; (5) the absence of uterus and fallopian tubes; (6) normal male plasma testosterone; and (7) masculinization to a variable degree at the time of puberty.

The realization that virilization during embryogenesis is defective only in the urogenital sinus and the external genitalia provided insight into the fundamental abnormality. Testosterone, the androgen secreted by the fetal testis, is responsible for conversion of the wolffian duct into the epididymis, vas deferens, and seminal vesicle, whereas dihydrotestosterone mediates virilization of the urogenital sinus and the external genitalia. Consequently, impairment of dihydrotestosterone formation in a male embryo would be expected to cause the phenotype in this disorder—normal male wolffian duct derivatives with defective masculinization of the external genitalia and urogenital sinus. Since testosterone itself regulates LH secretion (see Chap. 336), plasma LH level is normal or minimally elevated. As a result, testosterone and estrogen production rates are those of normal men, and gynecomastia does not develop.

The fact that 5α-reductase 2 enzyme is deficient in this disorder was established by assay of biopsied tissues and cultured fibroblasts from affected individuals. Deletions or point mutations in the gene encoding steroid 5α-reductase 2 have been identified in most families studied. Approximately 40 percent are compound heterozygotes.

Receptor disorders The androgen receptor is a typical member of the steroid/thyroid family of receptors with steroid-binding, DNA-binding, and functional domains and is encoded by a gene on the long arm of the X chromosome. Mutations of this gene impair receptor function and hence impair male phenotypic differentiation and/or virilization.

CLINICAL FEATURES *Complete testicular feminization* is a common form of male pseudohermaphroditism; estimates of frequency vary from 1 in 20,000 to 1 in 64,000 male births. It is the third most common cause of primary amenorrhea after gonadal dysgenesis and congenital absence of the vagina. The features are characteristic. Namely, a woman is ascertained either because of inguinal hernia (prepubertal) or primary amenorrhea (postpubertal). The development of the breasts, the habitus, and the distribution of body fat are female in character so that most have a truly feminine appearance. Axillary and pubic hair is absent or scanty, but some vulval hair is usually present. Scalp hair is that of a normal woman, and facial hair is absent. The external genitalia are unambiguously female, and the clitoris is normal. The vagina is short and blind-ending and may be absent or rudimentary. All internal genitalia are absent except for testes that contain normal Leydig cells and seminiferous tubules without spermatogenesis. The testes may be located in the abdomen, along the course of the inguinal canal, or in the labia majora. Occasionally, remnants of müllerian or wolffian duct origin are present in the paratesticular fascia or in fibrous bands extending from the testis. Patients tend to be rather tall, and bone age is normal. Psychosexual development is unmistakably female with regard to behavior, outlook, and maternal instincts.

The major complication of undescended testes in this disorder, as in all forms of cryptorchidism, is the development of tumors (Chap. 98). Since affected individuals undergo normal pubertal growth and feminize at the time of expected puberty and since testicular tumors rarely develop until after puberty, it is usual to delay castration until after the time of expected puberty. Prepubertal castration is indicated if the testes are present in the inguinal region or labia majora and result in discomfort or hernia formation. (If hernia repair is indicated prepubertally, most physicians prefer to remove the testes at the same time to limit the number of operative procedures.) If the testes are removed prepubertally, estrogen therapy is required at the appropriate age to ensure normal growth and breast development. When castration is performed postpubertally, menopausal symptoms and other evidence of estrogen withdrawal supervene, and suitable estrogen replacement is indicated (see Chap. 337).

Incomplete testicular feminization is about one-tenth as frequent as the complete form. In this disorder there is minor virilization of the external genitalia (partial fusion of the labioscrotal folds and/or some degree of clitoromegaly), normal pubic hair, and mixed virilization and feminization at the time of expected puberty. The vagina is short and blind-ending, but in contrast to the complete form, the wolffian duct derivatives are often partially developed. Since women with the incomplete disorder virilize at the time of expected puberty, gonadectomy should be performed before the expected time of puberty in all prepubertal patients with clitoromegaly or posterior labial fusion.

Reifenstein syndrome is the term applied to forms of incomplete male pseudohermaphroditism initially described by a number of eponyms (Reifenstein syndrome, Gilbert-Dreyfus syndrome, Lubs syndrome). These syndromes are mutations that partially impair the function of the androgen receptor. The most common phenotype is a man with perineoscrotal hypospadias and gynecomastia, but the spectrum of defective virilization in affected families ranges from men with azoospermia to phenotypic women with pseudovaginas. Axillary and pubic hair is normal, but chest and facial hair is scanty. Cryptorchidism is common, the testes are small, and azoospermia is present. Some have defects in wolffian duct derivatives such as absence or hypoplasia of the vas deferens. Since the psychological development in most is unequivocally male, the hypospadias and cryptorchidism should be corrected surgically. The treatment of the gynecomastia is surgical removal.

The *infertile male syndrome* may be the most common disorder of the androgen receptor and is not actually a form of male pseudohermaphroditism. Some such individuals are minimally affected subjects in families with Reifenstein syndrome in whom azoospermia is the only manifestation of the receptor defect. More commonly, subjects with negative family histories present with male infertility. The *undervirilized fertile male* is another manifestation of an androgen receptor defect. In these families, affected men have gynecomastia and undervirilization, and some are fertile.

PATHOPHYSIOLOGY The karyotype is 46,XY, and the mutation is X-linked. The frequency of a positive family history varies from about two-thirds of patients with testicular feminization and Reifenstein syndrome to only occasional patients with the infertile male syndrome. The patients with a negative family history are believed to be the result of new mutations.

Hormone dynamics are similar in all disorders of the androgen receptor. Plasma testosterone levels and rates of testosterone production by the testes are normal or high. Elevated testosterone production is caused by the high mean plasma level of LH, which, in turn, is due to defective feedback regulation caused by resistance to the action of androgen at the hypothalamic-pituitary level. Elevated LH concentration is responsible also for the increased estrogen production by the testes (see Chap. 338). (In normal men, most estrogen is derived from peripheral formation from circulating androgens, but when the plasma LH level is elevated, the testes secrete increased amounts of estrogen into the circulation.) Thus resistance to the feedback regulation of LH secretion by circulating androgen results in elevated plasma LH levels, and this, in turn, results in the enhanced secretion of both testosterone and estradiol by the testes. Gonadotropin levels rise even higher (and menopausal symptoms may develop) when the testes are removed, indicating that gonadotropin secretion is under partial feedback control. Presumably, in the steady state and in the absence of an androgen effect, estrogen alone regulates LH secretion, a control purchased at the expense of an elevated plasma estrogen concentration for a male. The hormonal changes in the infertile male syndrome are similar to those in the other receptor disorders but less marked. Some men with this syndrome do not have an elevation of plasma LH or plasma testosterone level.

Feminization in these disorders is the result of two interlocking phenomena. First, androgens and estrogens have antagonistic effects, and in the absence of androgen action, the cellular effect of estrogen is unopposed. Second, the testicular production of estradiol is greater than that of the normal male (although less than that of the normal female). Variable degrees of androgen resistance and enhanced estradiol production result in different degrees of defective virilization and enhanced feminization in the four clinical syndromes.

Each of these syndromes is the result of defects in the androgen receptor. In most families, the fundamental defect is due to point mutations in the coding sequence leading to premature termination codons or to amino acid substitutions in the hormone-binding domain. Such mutations impair receptor function to variable degrees. Some families with clinical syndromes typical of an androgen receptor disorder have normal androgen binding in fibroblasts; in most, point mutations in the DNA-binding domain of the androgen receptor are responsible for the androgen resistance.

℞ TREATMENT

Individuals with 5α-reductase deficiency who are raised as females but elect at the time of expected puberty to change social sex to male or who are raised from the first as males should be monitored carefully and given supplemental androgens, preferably androgens such as nandrolone decanoate that do not require 5α-reduction for activation, when virilization is incomplete. Fertility has been reported in such an individual. Subjects with 5α-reductase deficiency who continue to function as females should be gonadectomized, given feminizing doses of estrogens indefinitely, and receive surgical correction of the introitus when appropriate. The management of subjects with androgen receptor defects depends on the phenotypic manifestations. Women with testicular feminization should be castrated (preferably after the completion of the pubertal growth spurt and the feminization of the breasts) to prevent tumor development in the testes, receive estrogen replacement to maintain feminization, prevent hot flashes, and protect the bones; shallow vaginal depth can usually be treated medically with the Frank technique. Men with the Reifenstein phenotype should have surgical correction of the hypospadias and may require surgery for gynecomastia; supplemental androgen therapy in these men rarely improves the incomplete virilization.

Persistent Müllerian Duct Syndrome Men with this uncommon disorder have testes and male phenotypic development and in addition have fallopian tubes and a uterus. In some, one or both testes are descended and the uterus and ipsilateral fallopian tube are in the inguinal canal or scrotum; both testes and fallopian tubes may be present in the hernia sac or can be drawn into it. In others, the testes are located high in the abdomen and hernias are not present. In both types, the vasa deferentia are embedded in the wall of the uterus, a feature that complicates surgical procedures designed to preserve potential fertility. Most patients have uninformative family histories, but in some the condition is inherited as an autosomal recessive trait. Because the external genitalia are well developed and the patients masculinize normally at puberty, it is assumed that during the critical stage of embryonic differentiation the fetal testes produce a normal amount of androgen. However, müllerian regression does not occur. Two types of mutations have been described in this disorder. In one the gene that encodes MDI is defective, and blood levels of MDI are usually low or undetectable; in the other the MDI receptor is defective, and blood levels of MDI are elevated. To minimize the chance of tumor development and to maintain virilization, orchiopexy should be performed. Malignancy in the uterus or vagina has not been described, and because the vasa deferentia are closely associated with the broad ligaments, the uterus and vagina should be left in place to avoid disruption of the vasa deferentia during removal and consequently to preserve possible fertility.

Developmental Defects of the Male Genitalia *Hypospadias* Hypospadias is a congenital anomaly in which the urethra terminates in an abnormal position along the ventral midline of the penis at some site between the normal urethral meatus and the perineum. This malformation occurs in 0.5 to 0.8 percent of male births in the United States and is often associated with ventral contraction and bowing of the penis (chordee). It is common to categorize hypospadias as glandular (involving the glans penis), penile, or perineoscrotal. Since androgens control penile development, hypospadias is generally assumed to result from some unidentified defect in androgen formation or action during embryogenesis. Indeed, hypospadias occurs in most disorders of male sexual differentiation, and a rare cause of hypospadias is maternal ingestion of progestational agents early in pregnancy. However, the known causes (single-gene defects, chromosomal abnormalities, and maternal drug ingestion) account for only about one-fourth of cases, and the etiology of most is unknown. The management is surgical.

Cryptorchidism The control of testicular descent is poorly understood, both in regard to the nature of the forces that cause the movement and to the hormonal factors that regulate the process. In anatomic terms, testicular descent can be divided into three phases: (1) transabdominal movement of the testis from its site of origin above the kidney to the inguinal ring, (2) formation of the opening in the inguinal canal (processus vaginalis) through which the testis exits the abdominal cavity, and (3) actual movement of the testis through the inguinal canal to its permanent site in the scrotum. This process occurs over a 6- to 7-month period during gestation, beginning at about the sixth week and not completed in some until after birth. Impairment at any stage in this process can impair descent of one or both testes. About 3 percent of full-term and 30 percent of premature male infants have at least one cryptorchid testis at birth, but descent is usually completed within the first few weeks of life, so that the incidence of failure of descent by 6 to 9 months of age is only 0.6 to 0.7 percent. It is this latter category of maldescent that requires intervention.

Permanent cryptorchidism can be classified as intraabdominal (10 percent), canalicular (in the inguinal canal) (20 percent), high scrotal (40 percent), or obstructed (30 percent), in which maldescent is due to a physical barrier between the inguinal pouch and the inlet of the scrotum. These disorders must be distinguished from the temporarily retracted normal testis.

The cryptorchid testis functions poorly after puberty, but the extent to which maldescent is the result of an abnormality of the testis or the cause of abnormal function is unknown. Two general theories have been advanced as to the etiology—inadequate intraabdominal pressure and deficient endocrine function of the testis either because of deficient testosterone synthesis or inadequate formation of MDI. Indeed, defects that result in inadequate development of intraabdominal pressure or inadequate development of the testes can cause cryptorchidism. As in hypospadias, however, the known causes of cryptorchidism constitute only a small fraction of the cases, and the etiology in most remains to be identified. Two complications of cryptorchidism are important; spermatogenesis cannot occur at the temperature of the abdominal cavity, and it is necessary to correct the process as early as possible to allow possible fertility. The fact that infertility is common in men who have been treated for unilateral as well as bilateral cryptorchidism suggests that maldescent is usually the consequence rather than the cause of the testicular malfunction. There is also a greater frequency of malignancy in undescended testes, and all should be surgically corrected for this reason (see Chap. 98).

BIBLIOGRAPHY

Affara NA et al: Analysis of the SRY gene in 22 sex-reversed XY females identifies four new point mutations in the conserved DNA binding domain. Am J Hum Genet 2:785, 1993

Andersson S et al: 17β-Hydroxysteroid dehydrogenase 3 deficiency. Trends Endocrinol Metab 7:121, 1996

Behringer RR et al: Müllerian-inhibiting substance function during mammalian sexual development. Cell 79:415, 1994

Berta P et al: Genetic evidence equating SRY and the testis-determining factor. Nature 348:448, 1990

Boucekkine C et al: Clinical and anatomical spectrum in XX sex reversed patients. Relationship to the presence of Y-specific DNA sequences. Clin Endocrinol 40:733, 1994

Conte FA et al: A syndrome of female pseudohermaphroditism, hypergonadotropic hypogonadism, and multicystic ovaries associated with missense mutations in the gene encoding aromatase ($P450_{arom}$). J Clin Endocrinol Metab 78:1287, 1994

De La Chapelle A: The etiology of maleness in XX men. Hum Genet 58:105, 1981

Donahoe PK et al: Mixed gonadal dysgenesis, pathogenesis and management. J Pediatr Surg 14:287, 1979

——— et al: Congenital adrenal hyperplasia, in *The Metabolic and Molecular Bases of Inherited Disease*, 7th ed, CR Sriver et al (eds). New York, McGraw-Hill, 1995, p 2929

Edman CD et al: Embryonic testicular regression: A clinical spectrum of XY agonadal individuals. Obstet Gynecol 49:208, 1977

Foster JW et al: Campomelic dysplasia and autosomal sex reversal caused by mutations in an SRY-related gene. Nature 372:525, 1994

George FW, Wilson JD: Sex determination and differentiation, in *The Physiology of Reproduction*, 2d ed, E Knobil, JD Neill (eds). New York, Raven Press, 1994, vol 1, pp 3–28

Gordon DL et al: Pathologic testicular findings in Klinefelter's syndrome. 47,XXY vs 46,XY/47,XXY. Arch Intern Med 130:726, 1972

Griffin JE, Wilson JD: Disorder of sexual differentiation, in *Campbell's Textbook of Urology,* 6th ed, PC Walsh et al (eds). Philadelphia, Saunders, 1992, pp 1509–1542

——— et al: Congenital absence of the vagina. The Mayer-Rokitansky-Kuster-Hauser syndrome. Ann Intern Med 85:224, 1976

——— et al: The androgen resistance syndromes: 5α-Reductase deficiency, and related disorders, in *The Metabolic and Molecular Bases of Inherited Disease,* 7th ed, CR Scriver et al (eds). New York, McGraw-Hill, p. 2967, 1995

Grumbach MM, Conte FA: Disorders of sexual differentiation, in *Williams Textbook of Endocrinology,* 8th ed, JD Wilson, DW Foster (eds). Philadelphia, Saunders, 1992, pp 853–951

Imbeaud S et al: Insensitivity to anti-Müllerian hormone due to a mutation in the human anti-Müllerian hormone receptor. Nat Genet 11:679, 1995

Josso N et al: Anti-müllerian hormone and intersex states. Trends Endocrinol Metabol 2:227, 1991

Latronico AC et al: Testicular and ovarian resistance to luteinizing hormone caused by inactivating mutations of the luteinizing hormone-receptor gene. N Engl J Med 334:507, 1996

Leonard JM et al: The classification of Klinefelter's syndrome, in *Genetic Mechanism of Sexual Development,* HL Vallet, IH Porter (eds). New York, Academic Press, 1979, p 407

Miller WL: Molecular biology of steroid hormone synthesis. Endocrinol Rev 9:295, 1988

Ramsay M et al: XX True hermaphroditism in Southern African blacks: An enigma of primary sexual differentiation. Am J Hum Genet 43:4, 1988

Rheaume E et al: Molecular basis of congenital adrenal hyperplasia in two siblings with classical nonsalt-losing 3β-hydroxysteroid dehydrogenase deficiency. J Clin Endocrinol Metab 79:1012, 1994

SAKAI Y et al: No mutation in cytochrome P450 side chain cleavage in a patient with congenital lipoid adrenal hyperplasia. J Clin Endocrinol Metab 79:1198, 1994

SIMPSON JL: Gonadal dysgenesis and sex chromosome abnormalities: Phenotypic-karyotypic correlations, in *Genetic Mechanisms of Sexual Development,* HL Vallet, IH Porter (eds). New York, Academic Press, 1979, p 365

WILSON JD et al: Steroid 5α-reductase 2 deficiency. Endocrinol Rev 14:577, 1993

YANASE T et al: 17α-Hydroxylase/17,20-lyase deficiency: From clinical investigation to molecular definition. Endocrinol Rev 12:91, 1991

340

Steven I. Sherman, Robert F. Gagel

DISORDERS AFFECTING MULTIPLE ENDOCRINE SYSTEMS

NEOPLASTIC DISORDERS AFFECTING MULTIPLE ENDOCRINE ORGANS

In several familial disorders, neoplasia of multiple endocrine organs causes syndromes of hormone excess. Management of these disorders requires an understanding of endocrine neoplasia and of the unique features associated with the manifestations of multiple hormone excess in a single patient. Genetic loci for the two major syndromes and several others have been identified, and DNA-based genetic screening is now available for these disorders.

MULTIPLE ENDOCRINE NEOPLASIA (MEN) TYPE 1

Clinical Manifestations MEN 1, or Wermer's syndrome, is characterized by neoplasia of parathyroid, pituitary, and pancreatic islet cells (Table 340-1). The syndrome is inherited as an autosomal dominant trait so that each child of an affected parent has a 50 percent chance of inheriting the predisposing gene.

Several features of this syndrome have an impact on management. First, the disease process within a single organ is multicentric. Each of the tumors is derived from a single cell, and any endocrine cell within the affected organs can become transformed. Second, hyperplasia is the initiating lesion, followed later by adenomatous or carcinomatous changes. Third, neoplasia in one organ may affect the progression of disease in another organ. For example, hormone production by a pancreatic tumor may stimulate growth of a pituitary tumor. Fourth, this syndrome generally evolves over a 30- to 40-year period, and the manifestations depend in part on when the disorder is identified.

Hyperparathyroidism is the most common manifestation. Hypercalcemia may be present during the teenage years, and most individuals are affected by age 40. Screening for hyperparathyroidism involves measurement of either an albumin-adjusted or ionized serum calcium level. The diagnosis is established by demonstrating elevated levels of serum calcium and intact parathyroid hormone. Manifestations of hyperparathyroidism in MEN 1 do not differ substantially from those in sporadic hyperparathyroidism and include calcium-containing kidney stones, bone abnormalities, and gastrointestinal and musculoskeletal complaints (see Chap. 354).

Other familial disorders associated with hypercalcemia include familial parathyroid hyperplasia, familial adenomatous hyperparathyroidism, and familial hypocalciuric hypercalcemia (FHH). Calcium excretion is usually elevated in the patient with MEN 1 or other forms of primary hyperparathyroidism and low in FHH. Another distinguishing feature is that the serum calcium level is rarely elevated at birth in patients with MEN 1 and frequently elevated at birth in patients with FHH. Differentiation of hyperparathyroidism of MEN 1 from other forms of familial primary hyperparathyroidism is usually based on family history, histologic features of resected parathyroid tissue, and, sometimes, long-term observation to determine whether other manifestations of MEN 1 develop. FHH is due to inactivating mutations of the calcium sensor, a transmembrane G-protein normally present in parathyroid tissue and kidney (see Chap. 354).

Parathyroid hyperplasia is the common cause of hyperparathyroidism in MEN 1, although single and multiple adenomas have been described. Hyperplasia of one or more parathyroid glands is common in younger patients; adenomas are usually found in older patients or those with long-standing disease.

Neoplasia of the pancreatic islets is the second most common manifestation of MEN 1 and tends to occur in parallel with hyperparathyroidism. The syndromes of pancreatic islet cell hormone excess cause increases in levels of pancreatic polypeptide (75 to 85 percent), gastrin (60 percent, Zollinger-Ellison syndrome), insulin (25 to 35 percent), vasoactive intestinal peptide (VIP) (3 to 5 percent, Verner-Morrison or watery diarrhea syndrome), glucagon (5 to 10 percent), and somatostatin (1 to 5 percent). The tumors rarely produce adrenocorticotropin (ACTH), corticotropin-releasing hormone (CRH), growth hormone–releasing hormone (GHRH), calcitonin gene products, neurotensin, gastric inhibitory peptide, and others. Many of the tumors produce more than one peptide. The pancreatic neoplasms differ from the other components of MEN 1 in that approximately one-third of the tumors display malignant features, including hepatic metastases.

Pancreatic islet cell tumors are diagnosed by identification of a characteristic clinical syndrome, hormonal assays with or without provocative stimuli, or radiographic techniques. One approach involves annual screening of people at risk with measurement of basal and meal-stimulated levels of pancreatic polypeptide to identify the tumors as early as possible; the rationale of this screening strategy is the concept that surgical removal of islet cell tumors at an early stage will be curative. Other approaches to screening include measurement of serum gastrin and pancreatic polypeptide levels every 2 to 3 years, with the rationale that pancreatic neoplasms will be detected at a later stage but can be managed medically, if possible, or by surgery. High resolution computed tomography (CT) scanning provides the best noninvasive technique for identification of these tumors, but intraoperative ultrasonography is the most sensitive method for detection of small tumors.

Table 340-1

Disease Associations in the Multiple Endocrine Neoplasia (MEN) Syndromes

	MEN 2		
MEN 1	**MEN 2A**	**MEN 2B**	**Mixed Syndromes**
Parathyroid hyperplasia or adenoma	MTC	MTC	Familial pheochromocytoma and islet cell tumor
Islet cell hyperplasia, adenoma, or carcinoma	Pheochromocytoma	Pheochromocytoma	von Hippel–Lindau syndrome, pheochromocytoma, and islet cell tumor
Pituitary hyperplasia or adenoma	Parathyroid hyperplasia or adenoma	Mucosal and gastrointestinal neuromas	Neurofibromatosis with features of MEN 1 or 2
Other less common manifestations: foregut carcinoid, pheochromocytoma, subcutaneous or visceral lipomas	With cutaneous lichen amyloidosis	Marfanoid features	Myxomas, spotty pigmentation, and generalized endocrine overactivity in a single family
	With Hirschsprung disease		
	FMTC		

NOTE: MTC, medullary thyroid carcinoma; FMTC, familial MTC.

Zollinger-Ellison syndrome (ZES) is caused by excessive gastrin production and occurs in more than half of MEN 1 patients with pancreatic islet cell tumors (see Chap. 95). Clinical features include increased gastric acid production, recurrent peptic ulcers, diarrhea, and esophagitis. The ulcer diathesis is refractory to conservative therapy such as antacids. The diagnosis is made by finding increased gastric acid secretion, elevated basal gastrin levels in serum [generally >115 pmol/L (200 pg/mL)], and an exaggerated response of serum gastrin to either secretin or calcium. Other causes of elevated serum gastrin levels, such as achlorhydria, treatment with H_2 receptor antagonists or omeprazole, retained gastric antrum, small-bowel resection, gastric outlet obstruction, and hypercalcemia, should be excluded. Gastrin-producing carcinoid-like tumors may be present in the duodenal wall.

Insulinoma causes hypoglycemia in about one-third of MEN 1 patients with pancreatic islet cell tumors (see Chap. 335). The tumors may be benign or malignant (25 percent). On occasion, the diagnosis can be established by documenting hypoglycemia during a short fast with simultaneous inappropriate elevation of serum insulin and C-peptide levels. More commonly, it is necessary to subject the patient to a supervised 72-h fast to provoke hypoglycemia (see Chap. 335). Large insulin-secreting tumors may be localized by CT scanning, and small tumors not detected by radiographic techniques may be localized by selective arteriographic injection of calcium into each of the arteries that supply the pancreas and sampling the hepatic vein to determine the anatomic region containing the tumor. Intraoperative ultrasonography can also be used to localize these tumors, but preoperative calcium injection data are helpful in guiding the subtotal pancreatectomy if multiple or no abnormalities are detected by intraoperative ultrasonography.

Glucagonoma in occasional MEN 1 patients causes a syndrome of hyperglycemia, skin rash (necrolytic migratory erythema), anorexia, glossitis, anemia, depression, diarrhea, and venous thrombosis. In about half of these patients the plasma glucagon level is high, leading to its designation as the *glucagonoma syndrome*, although elevation of plasma glucagon level in MEN 1 patients is not necessarily associated with these symptoms. The glucagonoma syndrome may represent a complex interaction between glucagon overproduction and the nutritional status of the patient, although continuous infusion of glucagon sometimes reproduces the syndrome.

The *Verner-Morrison* or *watery diarrhea syndrome* consists of watery diarrhea, hypokalemia, hypochlorhydria, and metabolic acidosis. The diarrhea can be voluminous and is almost always found in association with an islet cell tumor, prompting use of the term *pancreatic cholera*, although the syndrome is not restricted to pancreatic islet tumors and has been observed with carcinoids or other tumors. This syndrome is believed to be due to overproduction of VIP, although plasma VIP levels may not be elevated. Hypercalcemia is believed to be caused by the effects of VIP on bone.

Pituitary tumors occur in more than half of MEN 1 patients and tend to be multicentric, making them difficult to resect (see Chap. 328). The most common tumors are prolactinomas, which are diagnosed by finding serum prolactin levels >200 μg/L with or without a pituitary mass evident by magnetic resonance imaging (MRI). Values less than 200 μg/L may be due to a prolactin-secreting neoplasm or to compression of the pituitary stalk. Acromegaly due to excessive growth hormone production is the second most common syndrome caused by pituitary tumors in MEN 1 (see Chap. 328) but can rarely be due to production of GHRH by an islet cell tumor. Cushing's disease can be caused by ACTH-producing pituitary tumors or by ectopic production of ACTH or CRH by other tumors in the MEN 1 syndrome. Diagnosis of pituitary Cushing's disease is generally best accomplished by a high-dose dexamethasone suppression test or by petrosal venous sinus sampling for ACTH after intravenous injection of CRH (see Chap. 328). Differentiation of a primary pituitary tumor from an ectopic CRH-producing tumor may be difficult because the pituitary is the source of ACTH in both disorders; documentation of CRH production by a pancreatic islet or carcinoid tumor may be the only method of proving ectopic CRH production.

Unusual manifestations of MEN 1 The rare carcinoid tumors in MEN 1 are of the foregut type and are derived from thymus, lung, stomach, or duodenum; they may metastasize or be locally invasive. These tumors usually produce serotonin, calcitonin, or CRH; the typical carcinoid syndrome with flushing, diarrhea, and bronchospasm is rare (see Chap. 95). Subcutaneous or visceral lipomas and cutaneous leiomyomas also may be present but rarely undergo malignant transformation.

Genetics and Pathophysiology The mutation responsible for MEN 1 is believed to involve a *tumor suppressor gene* that plays an important role in the regulation of cell growth. The disorder is inherited as an autosomal dominant trait, and the responsible gene on chromosome 11q13 encodes a protein termed menin. A second possible mechanism for development of MEN 1 tumors is that elevated levels of fibroblast growth factor may stimulate epithelial growth in the parathyroid glands.

℞ TREATMENT

Almost everyone who inherits a mutant MEN 1 gene develops at least one of the manifestations. Most develop hyperparathyroidism, 80 percent develop pancreatic islet cell tumors, and more than half develop pituitary tumors. In most cases, surgery is not curative; most patients require surgery on two or more endocrine glands during a lifetime, and many require multiple surgical procedures. For this reason, it is essential to establish clear goals for management of these patients rather than to recommend surgery casually each time a tumor is discovered. Ranges for acceptable management are discussed below.

Hyperparathyroidism Hyperparathyroid individuals with serum calcium levels >3.0 mmol/L (12 mg/dL), evidence of calcium nephrolithiasis or renal dysfunction, neuropathic or muscular symptoms, or bone involvement (including osteopenia) should undergo parathyroid exploration. In MEN 1 an additional criterion for parathyroid surgery is hypercalcemia associated with elevated gastrin levels, because elevated serum calcium may stimulate gastrin production and ZES, a condition that may be reversed by return of calcium levels to normal. There is less agreement regarding the necessity for parathyroid exploration in individuals who do not meet these criteria, and observation may be appropriate in the MEN 1 patient with asymptomatic hyperparathyroidism.

When parathyroid surgery is indicated in MEN 1, all parathyroid tissue should be identified and removed at the time of primary operation, and parathyroid tissue should be implanted in the nondominant forearm. If reoperation is necessary, transplanted tissue can be resected under local anesthesia with titration of tissue removal to return the serum calcium level to normal. A less desirable approach is to remove 3 to 3½ parathyroid glands from the neck, carefully marking the location of residual tissue so that the remaining tissue can be located easily during subsequent surgery.

Pancreatic Islet Tumors (See Chap. 95 for discussion of pancreatic islet tumors not associated with MEN 1.) Two features of pancreatic islet cell tumors in MEN 1 complicate the management. First, the pancreatic islet cell tumors are multicentric, malignant about a third of the time, and cause death in 10 to 20 percent of patients. Second, removal of all pancreatic islets to prevent malignancy causes diabetes mellitus, a disease with severe long-term complications. These features make it difficult to formulate clear-cut guidelines, but some general concepts appear to be valid. First, islet cell tumors producing insulin, glucagon, VIP, GHRH, or CRH should be resected because medical therapy is ineffective. Second, gastrin-producing islet cell tumors that cause ZES are frequently multicentric, and the surgical cure rate is low. If a single tumor can be identified, a surgical approach seems reasonable, and duodenal wall carcinoid tumors that cause ZES can also be successfully resected in most cases. Treatment with H_2 receptor antagonists (cimetidine or ranitidine) and the H^+,K^+-ATPase inhibitor omeprazole provides an effective alternative to surgery for control of the ulcers in patients with multicentric tumors or with hepatic metastases. Third, in families in which there is a high incidence of malignant islet cell tumors that cause death, total pancreatectomy at an early age may be justified to prevent malignancy.

Management of metastatic islet cell carcinoma is unsatisfactory. Hormonal abnormalities can sometimes be controlled. For example, ZES can be treated with H_2 receptor antagonists or omeprazole, and the somatostatin analogue octreotide is useful in the management of carcinoid and the watery diarrhea syndrome. Bilateral adrenalectomy may be required for ectopic ACTH syndrome if medical therapy is ineffective (see Chap. 332). Islet cell carcinomas frequently metastasize to the liver but may grow slowly. Hepatic artery embolization or chemotherapy (5-fluorouracil, streptozocin, chlorozotocin, doxorubicin, or dacarbazine) may reduce tumor mass, control symptoms of hormone excess, and prolong life but are never curative.

Pituitary Tumors Treatment of prolactinomas with bromocriptine usually returns the serum prolactin level to normal and prevents further tumor growth (see Chap. 328). Surgical resection of a prolactinoma is rarely curative but may relieve mass effects. Transsphenoidal resection is appropriate for neoplasms that secrete ACTH, growth hormone (GH), or the α-subunit of the pituitary glycoprotein hormones. Octreotide reduces tumor mass in one-third of tumors and reduces GH and insulin-like growth factor I levels in more than 75 percent of patients with postoperative elevations in GH levels. Radiation therapy may be useful for large or recurrent tumors.

MULTIPLE ENDOCRINE NEOPLASIA TYPE 2 Clinical Manifestations Thyroid carcinoma and pheochromocytoma are associated in two major syndromes (see Table 340-1). MEN type 2A is the combination of medullary thyroid carcinoma, hyperparathyroidism, and pheochromocytoma. Three subvariants of MEN 2A are familial medullary thyroid carcinoma (FMTC), MEN 2A with cutaneous lichen amyloidosis, and MEN 2A with Hirschsprung disease. MEN type 2B is the combination of medullary thyroid carcinoma, pheochromocytoma, mucosal neuromas, intestinal ganglioneuromatosis, and marfanoid-like features.

Multiple endocrine neoplasia type 2A Medullary thyroid carcinoma is the most common manifestation. The fully developed neoplasm is typically located at the junction of the upper one-third and lower two-thirds of each lobe of the thyroid and appears grossly as chalky white to yellow lesions; tumors greater than 1 cm in size are frequently associated with local or distant metastases. This tumor usually develops in childhood, beginning as hyperplasia of the calcitonin-producing cells (C cells) of the thyroid. Measurement of the serum calcitonin level after injection of a stimulator of release such as calcium or pentagastrin makes it possible to diagnose this disorder when the likelihood of metastasis is low.

Pheochromocytoma occurs in approximately 50 percent of MEN 2A patients and causes palpitations, nervousness, headaches, and sometimes sweating. About half the tumors are bilateral, and more than 50 percent of patients who have had unilateral adrenalectomy develop a pheochromocytoma in the contralateral gland within a decade. A second feature of these tumors is a disproportionate increase in the secretion of epinephrine relative to norepinephrine. Patients with minimal abnormalities of epinephrine secretion may be asymptomatic. Capsular invasion is common, but malignant behavior is uncommon.

Hyperparathyroidism occurs in 15 to 20 percent of patients, with the peak incidence in the third or fourth decade. Hyperparathyroidism may occur early. The manifestations of hyperparathyroidism do not differ from those in other forms of primary hyperparathyroidism (see Chap. 354), with nephrolithiasis being common. Diagnosis is established by finding hypercalcemia, hypophosphatemia, hypercalciuria, and an inappropriately high serum level of intact parathyroid hormone. Multiglandular parathyroid hyperplasia is the most common histologic finding, although withlong-standing disease adenomatous changes may be superimposed on hyperplasia.

Multiple endocrine neoplasia type 2B The association of medullary thyroid carcinoma, pheochromocytoma, mucosal neuromas, and a marfanoid habitus in the absence of hyperparathyroidism is designated MEN 2B. Medullary thyroid carcinoma in MEN 2B develops earlier and is more aggressive than in MEN 2A. Metastatic disease has been described prior to 1 year of age, and death commonly occurs in the second or third decade of life. However, the prognosis is not invariably bad even in patients with metastatic disease, as evidenced by a number of multigenerational families with this disease.

Pheochromocytoma occurs in more than half of MEN 2B patients and does not differ from that in MEN 2A. Hypercalcemia is rare in MEN 2B, and there are no well-documented examples of hyperparathyroidism.

The mucosal neuromas and marfanoid body habitus are the most distinctive features and are recognizable in childhood. Neuromas are present on the tip of the tongue, under the eyelids, and throughout the gastrointestinal tract and are true neuromas, distinct from neurofibromas. Children may present with gastrointestinal symptoms, including increased gas, intermittent obstruction, and diarrhea caused by neuromas.

Genetics and Pathophysiology Mutations of the *c-ret* protooncogene have been identified in 93 to 95 percent of patients with MEN 2. Two regions of the Ret tyrosine kinase receptor are mutated (Fig. 340-1). The first is a cysteine-rich extracellular domain; point mutations in the coding sequence for one of five cysteines (codons 609,

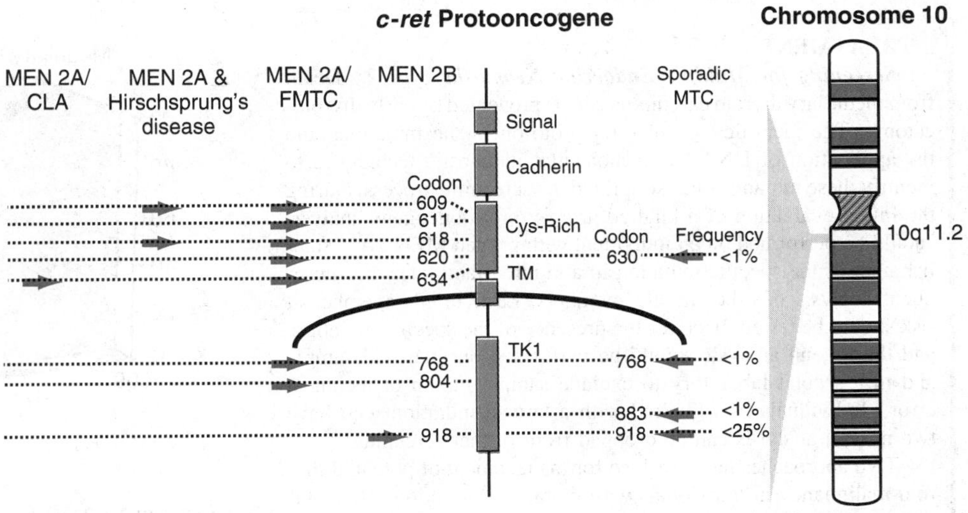

FIGURE 340-1 Schematic diagram of the *c-ret* proto-oncogene showing mutations found in multiple endocrine neoplasia type 2 and sporadic medullary thyroid carcinoma. The *c-ret* proto-oncogene is located on the proximal arm of chromosome 10q (10q11.2). Activating mutations of two functional domains of Ret tyrosine kinase receptor have been identified. The first affects a cysteine-rich (Cys-Rich) region in the extracellular portion of the receptor. Each germline mutation changes a cysteine at codons 609, 611, 618, 620, or 634 to another amino acid. The second region is the intracellular tyrosine kinase (TK) domain. Germline mutations of codons 768, 804, and 918 have been identified. Codon 634 mutations account for approximately 80 percent of all germline mutations. Mutations of codons 630, 768, 883, and 918 have been identified as somatic (nongermline) mutations that occur in a single parafollicular or C cell within the thyroid gland in sporadic medullary thyroid carcinoma. A codon 918 mutation is the most common somatic mutation. Abbreviations: MEN 2, multiple endocrine neoplasia type 2; CLA, cutaneous lichen amyloidosis; FMTC, familial medullary thyroid carcinoma; Signal, the signal peptide; Cadherin, a cadherin-like region in the extracellular domain; TM, transmembrane domain; TK, tyrosine kinase domain; MTC, medullary thyroid carcinoma.

611, 618, 620, or 634) cause amino acid substitutions that activate the receptor and initiate transformation. Codon 634 mutations occur in 80 to 90 percent of MEN 2A kindreds and are most commonly associated with classic MEN 2A features (Figs. 340-1 and 340-2); an arginine substitution at this codon accounts for half of all MEN 2A mutations. All reported families with MEN 2A and cutaneous lichen amyloidosis have a codon 634 mutation (Fig. 340-1). Mutations of codons 609, 611, 618, or 620 occur in 10 to 15 percent of MEN 2A kindreds and are more commonly associated with FMTC (Fig. 340-2). Mutations in codons 609, 618, and 620 have also been identified in the MEN 2A and Hirschsprung variant (Fig. 340-1). Although a codon 634 mutation is most commonly associated with classic MEN 2A and mutations in codons 609, 611, 618, or 620 with FMTC, overlap exists (Fig. 340-2).

The second region of the Ret tyrosine kinase that is mutated in MEN 2 is in the substrate recognition pocket at codon 918 (Fig. 340-1). This activating mutation is present in approximately 95 percent of MEN 2B patients and accounts for 10 to 15 percent of all *c-ret* proto-oncogene mutations in MEN 2.

Approximately 5 percent of kindreds with FMTC have no identifiable mutation of either of these regions. In a few such kindreds a point mutation of codon 768 or 804 has been identified. The glial-cell-line–derived neurotropic factor is a ligand for the Ret tyrosine kinase receptor, and it seems likely that mutations of this peptide might also cause either MEN 2 or Hirschsprung disease.

Somatic mutations (mutations found only in the tumor and not transmitted in the germline) of the *c-ret* proto-oncogene have been identified in sporadic medullary thyroid carcinoma; 25 to 50 percent of sporadic tumors have codon 918 mutations, and a few somatic codon 630, 768, and 804 mutations have been identified (Fig. 340-1). Germline mutations of the *c-ret* proto-oncogene are present in about 6 percent of patients with apparent sporadic medullary thyroid carcinoma, indicating that other family members may be at risk for development of this disease. This finding suggests that all patients with sporadic medullary thyroid carcinoma should have a peripheral blood *c-ret* proto-oncogene analysis.

℞ TREATMENT

Screening for Multiple Endocrine Neoplasia Type 2 Death from medullary thyroid carcinoma can be prevented by early thyroidectomy. The identification of *c-ret* proto-oncogene mutations and the application of DNA-based molecular diagnostic techniques to identify these mutations has simplified the screening process. During the initial evaluation of a kindred, a *c-ret* proto-oncogene analysis should be performed on an individual with proven MEN 2A. Establishment of the specific mutation in a kindred facilitates the subsequent analysis of other family members. Each family member at risk should be tested twice for the presence of the specific mutation, and the second analysis should be performed on a second sample and in a second laboratory to exclude sample mixup or technical error.[1] Individuals in a kindred with a known mutation who have two normal analyses can be dropped from further screening.

Two approaches have evolved for management of potential thyroid malignancy in individuals with mutations of codons 609, 611, 620, or 634. The first is to perform a total thyroidectomy in early childhood, usually before the age of 6 years. More than 90 percent of affected individuals will develop medullary thyroid carcinoma (Fig. 340-2), and metastases have occurred in MEN 2A by age 6. This approach eliminates the need for annual pentagastrin screening. Risks of thyroidectomy include hypoparathyroidism and recurrent laryngeal nerve damage, although the frequency of these complications is no greater in children.

A second approach, based on many years of experience in MEN 2A screening, is to measure each year the release of calcitonin into the bloodstream after the administration of pentagastrin or combined pentagastrin-calcium to carriers of the mutations to identify medullary thyroid carcinoma or its precursor lesion, C-cell hyperplasia, before development of metastatic disease. Screening of individuals at risk should begin in early childhood, preferably before age 5. The

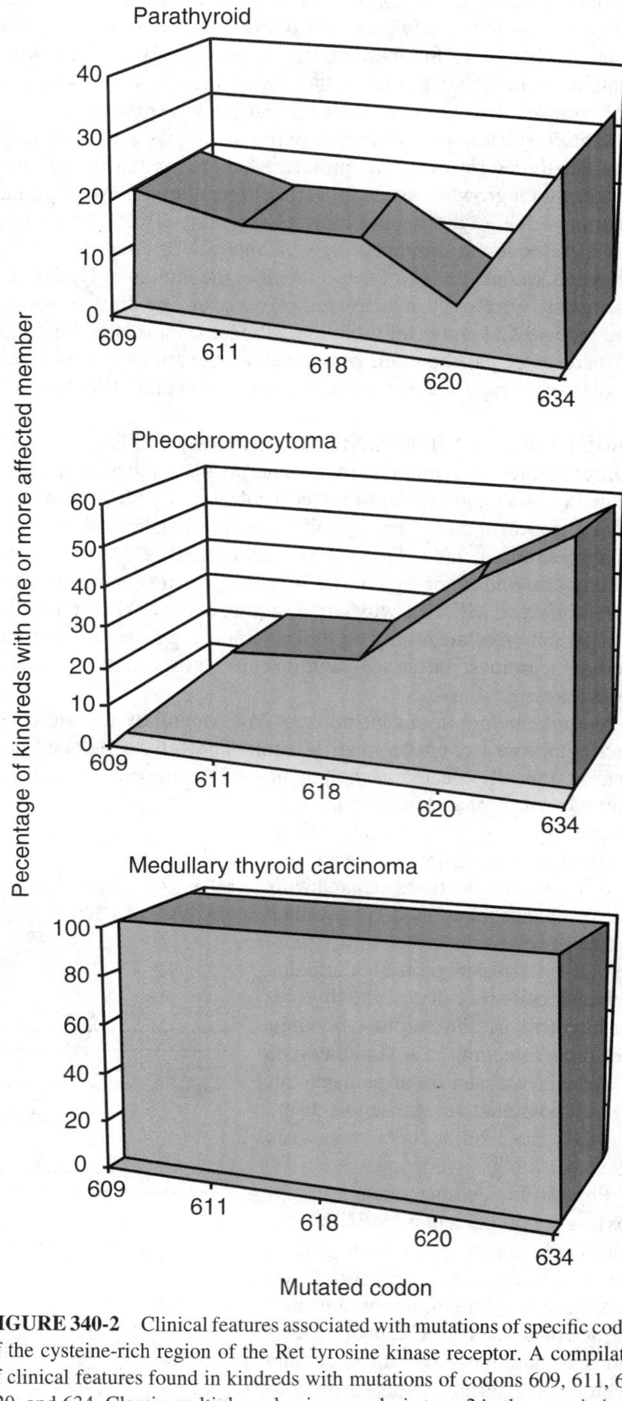

FIGURE 340-2 Clinical features associated with mutations of specific codons of the cysteine-rich region of the Ret tyrosine kinase receptor. A compilation of clinical features found in kindreds with mutations of codons 609, 611, 618, 620, and 634. Classic multiple endocrine neoplasia type 2A, the association of medullary thyroid carcinoma, pheochromocytoma, and parathyroid neoplasia, is most commonly found in association with a codon 634 mutation. However, this compilation clearly makes the point that parathyroid neoplasia has been identified in 10 to 20 percent of kindreds with mutations of codons 609, 611, 618, and 620, and pheochromocytoma has been identified in 20 to 40 percent of kindreds with codon 611, 618, and 620 mutations. Pheochromocytoma has not been identified in a kindred with a codon 609 mutation, although the infrequency of this mutation (fewer than 10 reported kindreds) suggests additional experience is needed. The data in this figure have been accumulated from published information from over 300 kindreds.

[1] A list of laboratories that perform *c-ret* proto-oncogene testing can be found on the University of Texas M.D. Anderson Cancer Center Web site at: http://endrcr06.mda.uth.tmc.edu. A pamphlet for patients with MEN 2A and FMTC that provides a description of clinical features and diagnostic testing is also available at the same Web site.

pentagastrin test involves measurement of serum calcitonin basally and 2, 5, 10, and 15 min after bolus injection of 5 μg pentagastrin/kg body weight. Patients should be warned before injection of epigastric tightness, nausea, warmth, and tingling of extremities and reassured that the symptoms will last approximately 2 min. Thyroidectomy should be performed when an abnormal pentagastrin test is identified. A follow-up of children identified with this approach indicates that 90 percent have no recurrence of disease 15 to 20 years later. The advantage of this approach is a delay of thyroidectomy, on average, until 10 years of age. The disadvantages include the cost and discomfort of annual testing and the small possibility that metastases could occur before thyroidectomy is performed.

There is no consensus on which of these approaches is better, although the excellent results with early thyroidectomy; the potential for improvement of cure rate; and the avoidance of the cost, discomfort, and parental anxiety associated with annual pentagastrin testing suggest that early total thyroidectomy will become accepted with time.

The *c-ret* proto-oncogene analysis should be performed in patients with suspected MEN 2B to detect codon 918 mutations, especially in newborn children where the diagnosis is suspected but the clinical phenotype not fully developed. Other family members at risk may also be tested if the diagnosis is not clear because the mucosal neuromas can be subtle and not always identified. In the occasional families with proven germline transmission of medullary thyroid carcinoma but no identifiable *c-ret* proto-oncogene mutation, annual pentagastrin or calcium-pentagastrin testing should be performed on members at risk.

Annual screening for pheochromocytoma in subjects with germline *c-ret* mutations should be performed by measuring basal plasma or 12-h urine catecholamines. The goal is to identify a pheochromocytoma before it causes significant symptoms or is likely to cause sudden death, an event most commonly associated with large tumors. Radiographic studies, such as MRI or CT scans, are generally reserved for individuals with abnormal screening tests or with symptoms suggestive of pheochromocytoma (see Chap. 333). Women should be tested during pregnancy because undetected pheochromocytoma can cause maternal death during childbirth.

Measurement of serum calcium and parathyroid hormone levels every 2 to 3 years provides an adequate screen for hyperparathyroidism, except in those families in which hyperparathyroidism is a prominent component, where measurements should be made annually.

Treatment of Medullary Thyroid Carcinoma FMTC is a multicentric disorder. Total thyroidectomy with a central lymph node dissection should be performed in children who carry the mutant genes. Long-term follow-up studies indicate an excellent outcome with approximately 90 percent of children free of disease 15 to 20 years after surgery. In contrast, 15 to 25 percent of patients in whom the diagnosis is made on the basis of a palpable thyroid nodule die from the disease within 15 years.

In adults with medullary thyroid cancer greater than 1 cm in size, metastases to regional lymph nodes are common. Total thyroidectomy with central lymph node dissection and selective dissection of other regional chains provides the best chance for cure. In patients with extensive local metastatic disease in the neck, external radiation may prevent local recurrence or reduce tumor mass but is not curative. Chemotherapy with combinations of adriamycin, vincristine, cyclophosphamide, and dacarbazine may provide palliation.

Treatment of Pheochromocytoma The long-term goal for management of pheochromocytoma is to prevent death and cardiovascular complications. Improvements in radiographic imaging of the adrenals make direct examination of the apparently normal contralateral gland during surgery less important, making a posterior approach practical for unilateral adrenalectomy. The major question is whether to remove both adrenal glands or to remove only the affected adrenal at the time of primary surgery. Issues to be considered in making this decision include the possibility of malignancy (fewer than 15 reported cases), the likelihood of development of pheochromocytoma in the apparently unaffected gland over an 8- to 10-year period, and the risks of adrenal insufficiency caused by removal of both glands (two deaths related to adrenal insufficiency in MEN 2 patients). Most but not all clinicians recommend removal only of the affected gland and leave the contralateral gland. If both adrenals are removed, glucocorticoid and mineralocorticoid replacement is mandatory. An alternative approach is to remove the pheochromocytoma and adrenal medulla, leaving the adrenal cortex behind. If successful, this approach eliminates the necessity for steroid hormone replacement, although the pheochromocytoma recurs in some.

Treatment of Hyperparathyroidism Hyperparathyroidism has been managed by one of two approaches. Removal of 3½ glands with maintenance of the remaining half gland in the neck is the usual procedure. In families in whom hyperparathyroidism is a prominent manifestation and recurrence is common, total parathyroidectomy with transplantation of parathyroid tissue into the nondominant forearm is preferred. This approach is discussed above in the context of hyperparathyroidism associated with MEN 1.

OTHER GENETIC TUMOR SYNDROMES A number of mixed syndromes exist in which the neoplastic associations differ from those in MEN 1 or 2 (see Table 340-1).

von Hippel–Lindau (VHL) syndrome, the association of central nervous system tumors, renal cell carcinoma, pheochromocytoma, and islet cell neoplasms, is caused by mutations in a tumor-suppressor gene. Germline-inactivating mutations of the VHL gene cause tumor formation when there is additional loss or somatic mutation of the normal VHL allele in brain, kidney, pancreatic islet, or adrenal medullary cells. A specific subset of mutations is more common in families with pheochromocytomas.

The molecular defect in type 1 neurofibromatosis inactivates neurofibromin, a cell membrane–associated protein that normally activates a GTPase. Inactivation of this protein impairs GTPase and causes continuous activation of p21 Ras and its downstream tyrosine kinase pathway.

IMMUNOLOGIC SYNDROMES AFFECTING MULTIPLE ENDOCRINE ORGANS

When immune dysfunction affects two or more endocrine glands and other nonendocrine immune disorders are present, the polyglandular autoimmune (PGA) syndromes should be considered. These syndromes are designated PGA types I, II, and III (Table 340-2). The type I syndrome starts in childhood and is characterized by mucocutaneous candidiasis, hypoparathyroidism, and adrenal insufficiency. Patients with the type II (or Schmidt) syndrome are more likely to present as adults and typically have adrenal insufficiency, thyroiditis, and type 1 diabetes mellitus. The type III syndrome is heterogeneous and consists of autoimmune thyroid disease along with any autoimmune glandular dysfunction other than adrenal insufficiency.

POLYGLANDULAR AUTOIMMUNE SYNDROME TYPE I PGA type I usually is recognized in the first decade of life and requires two of three components for diagnosis: mucocutaneous candi-

Table 340-2

Disease Associations in Polyglandular Autoimmune (PGA) Syndromes

PGA I	PGA II	PGA III
Mucocutaneous candidiasis	Adrenal insufficiency	Type 1 diabetes and autoimmune thyroid disease or adrenal insufficiency and autoimmune thyroid disease
Hypoparathyroidism	Hypothyroidism	
Adrenal insufficiency	Graves' disease	
Hypogonadism	Type 1 diabetes	
Alopecia	Hypogonadism	
Hypothyroidism	Myasthenia gravis	
Malabsorption	Vitiligo	
Chronic active hepatitis	Alopecia	
Vitiligo	Pernicious anemia	
Pernicious anemia	Celiac disease	

diasis, hypoparathyroidism, and adrenal insufficiency. Mineralocorticoids and glucocorticoids may be lost simultaneously or sequentially. This disorder is also called *autoimmune polyendocrinopathy-candidiasis-ectodermal dystrophy* (APECED). Other endocrine defects can include gonadal failure, hypothyroidism, and, less commonly, destruction of the β cells of the pancreatic islets and development of insulin-dependent (type 1) diabetes mellitus. Additional features include hypoplasia of the dental enamel, ungual dystrophy, tympanic membrane sclerosis, vitiligo, keratopathy, and gastric parietal cell dysfunction resulting in pernicious anemia. Some patients develop autoimmune hepatitis, malabsorption (variably attributed to intestinal lymphangiectasia, IgA deficiency, bacterial overgrowth, or hypoparathyroidism), asplenism, achalasia, and cholelithiasis. At the outset, only one organ may be involved, but the number increases with time so that patients eventually manifest two to five components of the syndrome. In one variant among Iranian Jews, hypoparathyroidism frequently occurs by itself.

In a Finnish series, 78 percent of patients had a nonendocrine presentation, most commonly oral candidiasis. Although candidiasis occurs in most patients, is poorly responsive to treatment, and relapses frequently, the symptoms are often mild and can easily be missed. Involvement of the parathyroid glands usually occurs before adrenal insufficiency develops. More than 60 percent of postpubertal women develop premature hypogonadism. The endocrine components, including adrenal insufficiency and hypoparathyroidism, may not develop until the fourth decade, making continued surveillance necessary.

POLYGLANDULAR AUTOIMMUNE SYNDROME TYPE II Lymphocytic infiltration of the adrenal and thyroid glands along with type 1 diabetes mellitus and hypogonadism are characteristic of PGA type II, or Schmidt, syndrome. Type 1 diabetes mellitus occurs in approximately half of affected families. The autoimmune thyroid disease causes either Hashimoto's thyroiditis or hyperthyroidism; however, many patients with antimicrosomal and antithyroglobulin antibodies never develop abnormalities of thyroid function. Thus these antibodies alone are poor predictors of future disease. Dermatologic manifestations include vitiligo, caused by antibodies against the melanocyte, and alopecia and are less common than in the type I syndrome. Mucocutaneous candidiasis does not occur. A few patients develop a late-onset, usually transient hypoparathyroidism caused by antibodies that compete with parathyroid hormone for binding to the parathyroid hormone receptor. Up to 25 percent of patients with myasthenia gravis and an even higher percentage who have myasthenia and a thymoma have PGA type II (see Chap. 382).

POLYGLANDULAR AUTOIMMUNE SYNDROME TYPE III In rare families, hereditary abnormalities of the thyroid and adrenal or the thyroid and pancreatic islets occur in the absence of other autoimmune disorders. These families either have diabetes mellitus and autoimmune thyroid disease or adrenal insufficiency and Hashimoto's thyroiditis.

GENETICS AND PATHOGENESIS The underlying defects in these disorders are unknown but probably include inherited and acquired components. Type I PGA syndrome shows no HLA associations and is inherited as an autosomal recessive trait. The Finnish variant of PGA type I is linked to chromosome 21q22.3 and has been mapped to a 500 kb segment. The type II and III syndromes are usually associated with the DR3 or DR4 HLA haplotypes, or both, and are inherited as autosomal dominant traits with variable expressivity. Epidemiologic studies of twins with either type 1 diabetes mellitus or Graves' disease showed development of disease in both twins only about half of the time. Thus, additional factors must contribute to the immune dysregulation. Putative precipitants for either type 1 diabetes mellitus or thyroiditis include viral infections (rubella, Coxsackie B, mumps, and cytomegalovirus) and dietary antigens such as milk proteins.

Patients with the PGA syndromes may have a variety of autoantibodies directed against organ-specific antigens. Some of the antibodies are specific markers of autoimmunity and recognize cytoplasmic components of various endocrine cells, e.g., antibodies against thyroid peroxidase, adrenal side chain cleavage enzyme, or pancreatic glutamic acid decarboxylase. Other antibodies may interact directly with cell-surface receptors such as those for thyroid-stimulating hormone (TSH), adrenocorticotropin, or insulin and impair normal function. Still others bind to complement and lead to cytotoxicity. The role of cytokines such as interferon and of impairment of cell-mediated immunity in the pathogenesis of the PGA syndromes is unclear.

DIAGNOSIS The clinical manifestations of adrenal insufficiency often develop slowly, may be difficult to detect, and can be fatal if not diagnosed and treated appropriately. Thus, prospective screening should be performed routinely in all patients and family members at risk for PGA I and II. The most effective screening test for adrenal disease is a cosyntropin stimulation test (see Chap. 332). A fasting blood glucose level can be obtained to screen for hyperglycemia. Additional screening tests should include measurements of TSH, luteinizing hormone, follicle-stimulating hormone, and, in men, testosterone levels. In families with suspected type I PGA syndrome, calcium and phosphorus levels are also measured. These screening studies should be performed every 1 to 2 years up to about age 50 in families with PGA type II and III syndrome and until about age 40 in patients with type I syndrome. Screening measurements of autoantibodies against potentially affected endocrine organs are of uncertain prognostic value. The differential diagnosis of PGA should include the DiGeorge syndrome (hypoparathyroidism due to glandular agenesis and mucocutaneous candidiasis), Kearns-Sayre syndrome (hypoparathyroidism, primary hypogonadism, type 1 diabetes mellitus, and panhypopituitarism), Wolfram's syndrome (congenital diabetes insipidus and diabetes mellitus), and congenital rubella (type 1 diabetes mellitus and hypothyroidism).

℞ TREATMENT

With the exception of Graves' disease, the management of each of the endocrine components of the disease involves hormone replacement and is covered in detail in the chapters on adrenal, thyroid, gonadal, and parathyroid disease (Chaps. 332, 331, 336, 337, and 354). One aspect of therapy deserves special emphasis. Namely, primary hypothyroidism can mask adrenal insufficiency by prolonging the half-life of cortisol, and consequently administration of thyroid hormone to a patient with unsuspected adrenal insufficiency can precipitate adrenal crisis. Thus, all patients with hypothyroidism in the context of PGA should be screened for adrenal disease and, if present, be treated with glucocorticoids prior to or concurrently with thyroid hormone therapy.

OTHER AUTOIMMUNE ENDOCRINE SYNDROMES Insulin Receptor Antibodies Insulin resistance, defined as a decrease in the biologic response to a given amount of insulin, occurs commonly in patients with obesity, severe infections, trauma, or surgery, as well as in individuals with acromegaly or Cushing's syndrome, in whom growth hormone or cortisol excess can antagonize the action of insulin. Rare insulin-resistance syndromes occur in patients who develop spontaneous antibodies directed against insulin receptor, thereby preventing interaction of insulin with the insulin receptor. Conversely, other classes of anti-insulin receptor antibodies can activate the receptor and can cause hypoglycemia and must be considered in the differential diagnosis of fasting hypoglycemia (see Chap. 335).

Patients with insulin receptor antibodies and acanthosis nigricans are often middle-aged women who acquire insulin resistance in association with other autoimmune disorders such as systemic lupus erythematosus or Sjögren's syndrome. Vitiligo, alopecia, Raynaud's phenomenon, and arthritis also may be seen. Other autoimmune endocrine disorders, including thyrotoxicosis, hypothyroidism, and hypogonadism, occur rarely. Acanthosis nigricans, a velvety, hyperpigmented, thickened skin lesion, is prominent on the dorsum of the neck and other skin fold areas in the axillae or groin and often heralds the diagnosis in these patients. However, acanthosis nigricans also occurs in patients with obesity or polycystic ovarian syndrome, in which insulin resistance appears to be due to a postreceptor defect, and thus acanthosis nigricans itself is not diagnostic of the immunologic form of insulin resistance. This syndrome is called the *type B insulin resistance syndrome* and must be differentiated from type A insulin resistance syndromes, which are secondary to mutations in the gene that encodes the insulin receptor and impair insulin receptor signaling.

Anti-insulin receptor antibodies block the interaction of the hormone with its receptor and impair its action to varying degrees. Activation of the receptor by the antibodies also may result in receptor downregulation and desensitization. The degree of insulin resistance can be quite variable. Some patients with acanthosis nigricans show normal to mild glucose intolerance, with a compensatory increase in insulin secretion that is only detected when insulin levels are measured. Others have severe diabetes mellitus requiring massive doses of insulin (several thousand units per day) to lower the blood glucose levels. The nature of the antibodies determines the manifestations. Although insulin resistance is more common, fasting hypoglycemia can be the presenting symptom or develop during the course of the disease. The hypoglycemia results from the interaction of insulinomimetic antibodies with insulin receptor.

Ataxia telangiectasia is an autosomal recessive disorder with insulin-resistant diabetes mellitus, ataxia, telangiectasia, immune abnormalities, and an increased incidence of malignancies. This disorder is also associated with anti-insulin antibodies.

Autoimmune Insulin Syndrome with Hypoglycemia In this disorder polyclonal insulin-binding autoantibodies, typically found in patients with other autoimmune disorders, bind to endogenously synthesized insulin. If the insulin dissociates from the antibodies several hours or more after a meal, hypoglycemia can result. Most cases of the syndrome have been described from Japan, and there may be a genetic component. The anti-insulin antibodies may interfere in the insulin assay and falsely elevate measured insulin levels. A finding of normal C-peptide levels in this situation suggests a false-positive insulin measurement. In plasma cell dyscrasias such as multiple myeloma, the plasma cells may produce monoclonal antibodies against insulin and cause hypoglycemia by a similar mechanism.

Antithyroxine Antibodies and Hypothyroidism Circulating autoantibodies against thyroid hormones in patients with both immune thyroid disease and plasma cell dyscrasias such as Waldenström's macroglobulinemia can bind thyroid hormones, decrease their biologic activity, and result in primary hypothyroidism. In other patients the antibodies simply interfere with thyroid hormone immunoassays and cause false elevations or decreases in measured hormone levels.

Crow-Fukase Syndrome The features of this syndrome are highlighted by an acronym that emphasizes its important features: *p*olyneuropathy, *o*rganomegaly, *e*ndocrinopathy, *M*-proteins, and *s*kin changes (POEMS). The most important feature is a severe, progressive sensorimotor polyneuropathy associated with a plasma cell dyscrasia. Localized collections of plasma cells (plasmacytomas) can cause sclerotic bone lesions and produce monoclonal IgG or IgA proteins. Endocrine manifestations include amenorrhea in women and impotence and gynecomastia in men, hypogonadism, hyperprolactinemia, type 2 diabetes mellitus, primary hypothyroidism, and adrenal insufficiency. Skin changes include hyperpigmentation, thickening of the dermis, hirsutism, and hyperhidrosis. Hepatomegaly and lymphadenopathy occur in about two-thirds of patients, and splenomegaly is seen in about one-third. Other manifestations include increased cerebrospinal fluid pressure with papilledema, peripheral edema, ascites, pleural effusions, glomerulonephritis, and fever.

Table 340-3

Other Disorders with Common Polyglandular Manifestations

		Type of Endocrine Involvement						
Condition	**Clinical Features**	**Hypothalamic-Pituitary**	**Thyroid**	**Parathyroid**	**Pancreas**	**Adrenal**	**Gonads**	**Inheritance/ Molecular Defect**
Ataxia-telangiectasia	Early ataxia Oculocutaneous telangiectasia Immunologic deficiency	Occasional diminished pituitary reserve			Diabetes mellitus	Cortical hypoplasia	Dysgenetic gonads: gonado-blastomas later in females	Autosomal recessive
Pseudo-hypoparathyroidism	Short stature Short metacarpals and metatarsals Round facies Ectopic calcification	Variable deficiency of all pituitary hormones including prolactin	Hypo- or hyper-thyroidism	Elevated parathyroid hormone levels with normo- or hypocalcemia	Diabetes mellitus		Ovarian failure	Mutation of the $G_{\alpha s}$
Myotonic dystrophy	Muscular dystrophy Premature baldness Mental retardation	Gonadotropin and growth hormone abnormalities, ? related to central integrative defect	Hypo-thyroidism		Diabetes mellitus		Primary gonadal failure	Insertion of unstable CTG repeat in myotonic dystrophy gene on chromosome 19
Noonan syndrome	Short stature Ptosis Webbed neck Pulmonary stenosis	Gonadotropin deficiency	Thyroiditis				Primary gonadal failure	Autosomal dominant
Fanconi syndrome	Short stature Bone marrow hypoplasia Abnormal skin pigmentation Radius malformations	Panhypo-pituitarism			Diabetes mellitus	Adrenal atrophy	Gonadal atrophy	Autosomal recessive
Werner syndrome	Premature aging Atropic skin Cataracts Early osteopenia		Papillary thyroid carcinoma		Diabetes mellitus		Gonadal atrophy	Autosomal recessive

The systemic nature of the disorder may cause confusion with other connective tissue diseases. The endocrine manifestations suggest an autoimmune basis of the disorder, but circulating antibodies against endocrine cells have not been demonstrated. Increased serum and tissue levels of interleukin 6 are present, but the pathophysiologic basis for the POEMS syndrome is uncertain. Therapy directed against the plasma cell dyscrasia such as local radiation of bony lesions or chemotherapy may result in endocrine improvement.

MISCELLANEOUS DISORDERS WITH ENDOCRINE MANIFESTATIONS

A variety of other clinical and genetic disorders are associated with multiple endocrine manifestations (Table 340-3). The molecular and genetic defects for several of these disorders are now known. One example is the McCune-Albright syndrome, in which a constitutively activating mutation of the α subunit of the stimulatory G-protein causes overactivity of adenyl cyclase in a variety of glands. The clinical syndrome can include precocious puberty, acromegaly, thyrotoxicosis, and Cushing's syndrome, all reflecting autonomous hyperfunction of glands usually regulated by a G protein–dependent receptor.

BIBLIOGRAPHY

AALTONEN J et al: An autosomal locus causing autoimmune disease: Autoimmune polyglandular disease type I assigned to chromosome 21. Nat Genet 8:83, 1994

AHONEN P et al: Clinical variation of autoimmune polyendocrinopathy-candidiasis-ectodermal dystrophy (APECED) in a series of 68 patients. N Engl J Med 322:1829, 1990

BARDWICK PA et al: Plasma cell dyscrasia with polyneuropathy, organomegaly, endocrinopathy, M protein, and skin changes: The POEMS syndrome. Medicine 59:311, 1980

CHANDRASEKHARAPPA SC et al: Positional cloning of the gene for multiple endocrine neoplasia-type 1. Science 276:404, 1997

DURBEC P et al: GDNF signalling through the Ret receptor tyrosine kinase. Nature 381:789, 1996

GAGEL RF: Multiple endocrine neoplasia, in *Williams Textbook of Endocrinology*, 9th ed, JD Wilson, DW Foster (eds). Philadelphia, Saunders, in press

——— et al: The clinical outcome of prospective screening for multiple endocrine neoplasia type 2a. An 18-year experience. N Engl J Med 318:478, 1988

KAHN CR et al: The syndromes of insulin resistance and acanthosis nigricans: Insulin-receptor disorders in man. N Engl J Med 294:739, 1976

LATIF F et al: Identification of the von Hippel-Lindau disease tumor suppressor gene. Science 260:1317, 1993

LIPS CJM et al: Clinical screening as compared with DNA analysis in families with multiple endocrine neoplasia type 2A. N Engl J Med 331:828, 1994

MULLIGAN LM et al: Germline mutations of the RET proto-oncogene in multiple endocrine neoplasia type 2A (MEN 2A). Nature 363:458, 1993

NEUFELD M et al: Two types of autoimmune Addison's disease associated with different polyglandular autoimmune (PGA) syndromes. Medicine 60:355, 1981

RIZZOLI R et al: Primary hyperparathyroidism in familial multiple endocrine neoplasia type I. Long-term follow-up of serum calcium levels after parathyroidectomy. Am J Med 78:467, 1985

SHERMAN SI, LADENSON PW: Octreotide therapy of growth hormone excess in the McCune-Albright syndrome. J Endocrinol Invest 15:185, 1992

SKOGSEID B et al: Multiple endocrine neoplasia type 1: A 10-year prospective screening study in four kindreds. J Clin Endocrinol Metab 73:281, 1991

THAKKER RV: Multiple endocrine neoplasia type 1, in *Endocrinology*, 3d ed, LJ DeGroot (ed). Philadelphia, Saunders, 1995, pp 2815–2831

WELLS SA JR et al: Predictive DNA testing and prophylactic thyroidectomy in patients at risk for multiple endocrine neoplasia type 2A. Ann Surg 220:237, 1994

WOHLLK N et al: Application of genetic screening information to the management of medullary thyroid carcinoma and multiple endocrine neoplasia type 2. Endocrinol Metab Clin North Am 25:1, 1996

SECTION 2

DISORDERS OF INTERMEDIARY METABOLISM

341 DISORDERS OF LIPOPROTEIN METABOLISM

Henry N. Ginsberg, Ira J. Goldberg

Lipoproteins are macromolecular complexes that carry hydrophobic plasma lipids, particularly cholesterol and triglyceride, in the plasma. More than half of the coronary heart disease (CHD) in the United States is attributable to abnormalities in the levels and metabolism of plasma lipids and lipoproteins. Some premature CHD is due to mutations in major genes involved in lipoprotein metabolism, but elevated lipoprotein levels in most patients with CHD reflect the adverse impact of a sedentary lifestyle, excess body weight, and diets high in total and saturated fat on a less-than-perfect genetic background. Primary care providers and subspecialists need to understand the pathophysiology of and available therapies for these disorders. This chapter is focused on the major lipid disorders, both the dyslipoproteinemias caused by single-gene defects and the disorders that are likely to be polygenic in origin. We will then provide a practical approach to assist in the identification, evaluation, and treatment of patients with increased risk of CHD.

LIPID AND LIPOPROTEIN TRANSPORT

LIPOPROTEIN STRUCTURE Lipoproteins are spherical particles made up of hundreds of lipid and protein molecules. They are smaller than red blood cells and visible only by electron microscopy. However, when the larger, triglyceride-rich lipoproteins are present in high concentration, plasma can appear turbid or milky to the naked eye. The major lipids of the lipoproteins are cholesterol, triglycerides, and phospholipids. Triglycerides and the esterified form of cholesterol (cholesteryl esters) are nonpolar lipids that are insoluble in aqueous environments (hydrophobic) and comprise the core of the lipoproteins. Phospholipids and a small quantity of free (unesterified) cholesterol, which are soluble in both lipid and aqueous environments (amphipathic), cover the surface of the particles, where they act as the interface between the plasma and core components. A family of proteins, the apolipoproteins, also occupies the surface of the lipoproteins to serve as an additional interface between lipid and aqueous environments. These proteins play crucial roles in the regulation of lipid transport and lipoprotein metabolism.

Lipoproteins have been classified on the basis of their densities into five major classes: chylomicrons, very low density lipoproteins (VLDL), intermediate-density lipoproteins (IDL), low-density lipoproteins (LDL), and high-density lipoproteins (HDL). The physical-chemical characteristics of the major lipoprotein classes are presented in Table 341-1.

APOLIPOPROTEINS The apolipoproteins (apos) provide structural stability to the lipoproteins and determine the metabolic fate of the particles upon which they reside. They were named in an arbitrary alphabetical order and, for the purposes of this discussion, will be described in relation to their association with lipoprotein classes (Table 341-2.)

Table 341-1

Physical-Chemical Characteristics of the Major Lipoprotein Classes

Lipoprotein	Density, g/dL	Molecular Mass, kDa	Diameter, nm	Lipid, % TG	Lipid, % Chol	Lipid, % PL
Chylomicrons	0.95	400×10^3	75–1200	80–95	2–7	3–9
VLDL	0.95–1.006	$10–80 \times 10^3$	30–80	55–80	5–15	10–20
IDL	1.006–1.019	$5–10 \times 10^3$	25–35	20–50	20–40	15–25
LDL	1.019–1.063	2.3×10^3	18–25	5–15	40–50	20–25
HDL	1.063–1.210	$1.7–3.6 \times 10^2$	5–12	5–10	15–25	20–30

NOTE: TG, triglyceride; Chol, the sum of free and esterified cholesterol; PL, phospholipid. The remaining percent composition is made up of the apoproteins.

There are two forms of apo B—apo B100 and apo B48. Apo B100 is the major apolipoprotein of VLDL, IDL, and LDL, comprising approximately 30, 60, and 95 percent of the proteins in these lipoproteins respectively. Apo B100 has a molecular mass of about 545 kDa and is synthesized in the liver. It is essential for the assembly and secretion of VLDL from the liver and is the ligand for the removal of LDL by the LDL receptor. The LDL receptor is a cell-surface protein that binds and internalizes lipoproteins that contain apo B100 or apo E. The LDL receptor binding domain of apo B100 is the sequence between amino acids 3200 and 3600, a region that is absent in apo B48.

Apo B48 is essential for the assembly and secretion of chylomicrons. Apo B48 is encoded by the same gene and the same messenger ribonucleic acid (mRNA) as Apo B100, but in the intestine the mRNA is edited in an unusual way: A cytidine deaminase in the intestine changes a cytidine to a uridine in base 6666 of the apo B100 mRNA to produce a nonsense codon so that apo B48 contains only the N-terminal 48 percent of the full-length apo B100. In contrast, the apo B100 mRNA in human liver is not edited. The role of apo B48 in the metabolism of chylomicrons in plasma is unclear. Individuals with mutations that interfere with the normal synthesis of apo B have absent or very low levels of chylomicrons, VLDL, IDL and LDL.

The apolipoproteins of the C series are synthesized in the liver and are present in all plasma lipoproteins (trace amounts in LDL). Individual apo C's have different metabolic roles, but all inhibit the removal of plasma chylomicrons and VLDL remnants by the liver. Overexpression of apo CI in transgenic mice inhibits the uptake of chylomicron and VLDL remnants by the liver. Apo CI under- or overexpression has not been described in humans. Apo CII is an essential activator of the enzyme lipoprotein lipase (LPL), which hydrolyzes triglycerides in chylomicrons and VLDL, and individuals lacking apo CII have severe hypertriglyceridemia. Apo CIII inhibits LPL, and apo CIII overexpression in transgenic mice causes severe hypertriglyceridemia. Two humans who lacked apo CIII had accelerated rates of lipolysis of VLDL triglyceride.

Apo E is synthesized mainly in hepatocytes but is also made in other cells, including macrophages, neurons, and glial cells. It is found in chylomicrons, IDL, VLDL, and HDL and mediates the uptake of these lipoproteins in liver both by the LDL receptor and by the LDL receptor–related protein (LRP). Apo E can also bind to heparin-like proteoglycan molecules on the surface of all cells. Three major alleles of the apo E gene encode E2, E3, and E4, isoforms that differ in sequence at two positions and have frequencies of about 0.12, 0.75, and 0.13 in the general population. Apo E2 binds to the LDL receptor with lower affinity than apo E3 or E4. Individuals who are homozygous for apo E2 may develop severe hyperlipidemia (type III dyslipoproteinemia), and complete absence of apo E causes elevations of plasma levels of chylomicron and VLDL remnants and early atherosclerosis.

Apo AI, apo AII, and apo AIV are found primarily on HDL. Apo AI and apo AII are synthesized in the small intestine and the liver; apo AIV is made only in the intestine. Apo AI comprises about 70 to 80 percent of the protein of HDL and plays a critical role in maintaining the integrity of HDL particles. Individuals with a profound deficiency of apo AI also lack HDL. Apo AI also activates the enzyme lecithin:cholesterol acyltransferase (LCAT), which esterifies free cholesterol in plasma. Plasma levels of HDL cholesterol and apo AI are inversely related to risk for CHD, and some patients with apo AI deficiency develop early, severe atherosclerosis. Transgenic mice overexpressing human apo AI are resistant to atherosclerosis. Apo AII is the second most abundant apoprotein in HDL, and its function has not been determined; transgenic mice that overexpress apo AII have high plasma levels of both HDL cholesterol and triglycerides and may be susceptible to atherosclerosis. Apo AII knockout mice have low levels of HDL, indicating that apo AII is also necessary for the integrity of HDL particles. Apo AIV, a minor component of HDL and chylomicrons, may play a role in the activation of LCAT.

Apoprotein(a), a large glycoprotein that shares a high degree of sequence homology with the plasma zymogen plasminogen, is made by hepatocytes and is secreted into plasma where it forms a covalent linkage with the apo B100 of LDL to form lipoprotein(a). The physiologic role of lipoprotein(a) is not known, but elevated levels are associated with an increased risk for atherosclerosis.

LIPOPROTEIN METABOLISM LPL is synthesized in fat and muscle, secreted into the interstitial space, transported across endothelial cells, and binds to proteoglycans on the luminal surfaces in the adjacent capillary beds. LPL mediates the hydrolysis of the triglycerides of chylomicrons and VLDL to generate free fatty acids

Table 341-2

Characteristics of the Major Apolipoproteins

Apolipoprotein	Molecular Mass, Da	Lipoproteins	Metabolic Functions
Apo AI	28,016	HDL, chylomicrons	Structural component of HDL; LCAT activator
Apo AII	17,414	HDL, chylomicrons	Unknown
Apo AIV	46,465	HDL, chylomicrons	Unknown: possibly facilitates transfer of other apos between HDL and chylomicrons
Apo B48	264,000	Chylomicrons	Necessary for assembly and secretion of chylomicrons from the small intestine
Apo B100	540,000	VLDL, IDL, LDL	Necessary for assembly and secretion of VLDL from the liver; structural protein of VLDL, IDL, LDL; ligand for LDL receptor
Apo CI	6630	Chylomicrons, VLDL, IDL, HDL	May inhibit hepatic uptake of chylomicron and VLDL remnants
Apo CII	8900	Chylomicrons, VLDL, IDL, HDL	Activator of lipoprotein lipase
Apo CIII	8800	Chylomicrons, VLDL, IDL, HDL	Inhibitor of lipoprotein lipase; may inhibit hepatic uptake of chylomicron and VLDL remnants
Apo E	34,145	Chylomicrons, VLDL, IDL, HDL	Ligand for binding of several lipoproteins to the LDL receptor, to LRP, and possibly to a separate hepatic apo E receptor

and glycerol. The free fatty acids diffuse into adjacent tissues to be burned for energy or stored as fat. Most circulating LPL is associated with LDL. Insulin stimulates the synthesis and secretion of LPL, and reduced LPL activity in diabetes mellitus can lead to impaired triglyceride clearance. Homozygotes for mutations that impair LPL have severe hypertriglyceridemia that is usually manifested in childhood (type I hyperlipidemia), and heterozygotes for LPL defects have mild to moderate fasting hypertriglyceridemia but may have marked hypertriglyceridemia after consuming a high-fat meal. LPL is also expressed in macrophages, including cholesteryl ester–laden macrophages (foam cells) in atherosclerotic lesions. In this setting, secreted LPL may associate with LDL, causing retention of the lipoprotein in the subendothelial space.

Hepatic triglyceride lipase (HTGL), a member of a family of enzymes that includes LPL and pancreatic lipase, is synthesized in the liver and interacts with lipoproteins in hepatic sinusoids. HTGL can remove triglycerides from VLDL remnants (IDL), thus promoting the conversion of VLDL to LDL, and may also play a role in the clearance of chylomicron remnants and in the conversion of HDL_2 to HDL_3 in the liver by hydrolyzing the triglyceride and phospholipid in HDL (see below). Severe hypertriglyceridemia in individuals with genetic deficiency of HTGL is due to accumulation of chylomicron and VLDL remnants in plasma. In contrast to most patients with hypertriglyceridemia, however, subjects with HTGL deficiency have normal levels of HDL.

LCAT is synthesized in the liver and secreted into plasma where it is bound predominantly to HDL. LCAT mediates the transfer of linoleate from lecithin to free cholesterol on the surface of HDL to form cholesteryl esters that are then transferred to VLDL and eventually LDL. Apo AI is a cofactor for esterification of free cholesterol by LCAT.

Cholesteryl ester transfer protein (CETP) is synthesized primarily in the liver and circulates in plasma in association with HDL. CETP mediates the exchange of cholesteryl esters from HDL with triglyceride from chylomicrons or VLDL. LDL cholesteryl ester can also be exchanged with triglyceride from chylomicrons and VLDL, leading to small, dense LDL. Individuals who are homozygotes for mutations in the CETP gene have marked elevations of HDL cholesterol and apo AI, and heterozygotes for these mutations have slight elevations of HDL, indicating that CETP plays an important role in the removal of cholesteryl esters from HDL.

TRANSPORT OF EXOGENOUS (DIETARY) LIPIDS Exogenous lipid transport in chylomicrons and chylomicron remnants is depicted in Fig. 341-1*A*. In western societies, where individuals ordinarily consume 50 to 100 g of fat and 0.5 g of cholesterol during three or four meals, transport of dietary fats is essentially continual. Normolipidemic individuals dispose of most dietary fat in the bloodstream within 8 h of the last meal, but some individuals with dyslipidemia, particularly those with elevated fasting levels of VLDL triglyceride, have measurable levels of intestinally derived lipoproteins in the circulation as long as 24 h after the last meal.

In the intestinal mucosa dietary triglyceride and cholesterol are incorporated into the core of nascent chylomicrons. The surface coat of the chylomicron is composed of phospholipid, free cholesterol, apo B48, apo AI, apo AII, and apo AIV. The chylomicron, essentially a fat droplet containing 80 to 95 percent triglycerides, is secreted into lacteals and transported to the circulation via the thoracic duct. In the plasma, apo C proteins are transferred to the chylomicron from HDL. Apo CII is required for hydrolysis of triglycerides by LPL on capillary endothelial cells in fat and muscle, and apo CIII may modulate core triglyceride hydrolysis by regulating LPL activity. The addition of apo E allows the chylomicron remnant to bind to hepatic LDL receptors and/or LRP after the triglyceride core has been hydrolyzed and after apo CII and apo CIII have recirculated back to HDL. As a consequence, dietary triglyceride is delivered to adipocytes and muscle cells as fatty acids, and dietary cholesterol is taken up by the liver where it can be used for bile acid formation, incorporated into membranes, resecreted as lipoprotein cholesterol back into the circulation, or excreted as cholesterol into bile. Dietary cholesterol also regulates endogenous hepatic cholesterol synthesis.

Abnormal transport and metabolism of chylomicrons may predispose to atherosclerosis, and postprandial hyperlipidemia may be a risk

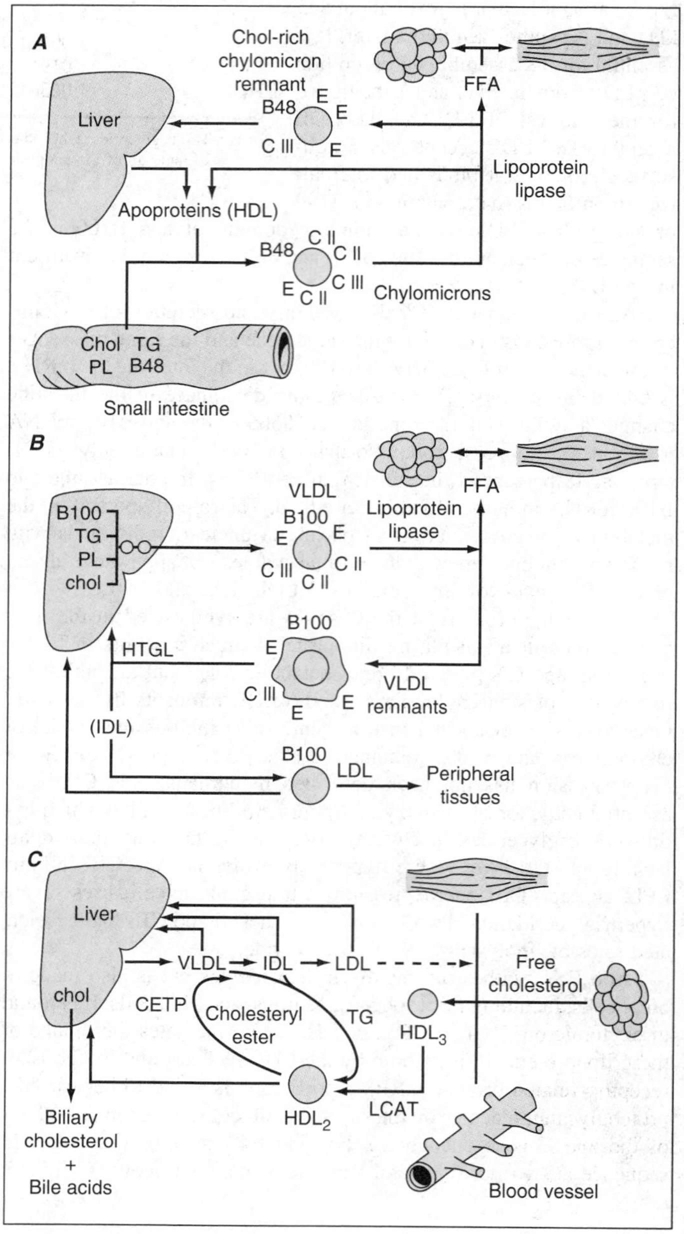

FIGURE 341-1 *A.* Transport of endogenous hepatic lipids via VLDL, IDL, and LDL. Note the relative and absolute changes in apoproteins, other than apo B100, as VLDL is converted to IDL and LDL. The sites of action of the two lipases, LPL and HTGL, are denoted as well, although the role of HTGL has not been completely defined. *B.* A schematic depiction of the transport of exogenously derived lipids from the intestine to peripheral tissues and liver via the chylomicron system. The cyclic movement of several apoproteins between HDL and chylomicrons is represented also. *C.* Simplified representation of HDL metabolism and the role of HDL in reverse cholesterol transport. Free cholesterol is accepted from peripheral tissues by HDL_3 and, after esterification, may be transferred to apo B100 lipoproteins. Cholesteryl ester also may be delivered to the liver by HDL itself. The significance of each of the three possible transport systems for cholesterol in overall reverse cholesterol transport is unknown. CETP, cholesteryl ester transfer protein; FFA, free fatty acids; HDL, high-density lipoprotein; HTGL, hepatic triglyceride lipase; IDL, intermediate-density lipoprotein; LDL, low-density lipoprotein; LPL, lipoprotein lipase; PL, phospholipase; TG, triglyceride; VLDL, very low density lipoprotein. *[From HN Ginsberg, Endocrinol Metab Clin North Am 19(2): 211, 1990.]*

factor for CHD. Chylomicrons and their remnants can be taken up by cells of the vessel wall, including monocyte-derived macrophages that migrate into the vessel wall from plasma. Cholesteryl ester accumulation by these macrophages transforms them into foam cells, the earliest cellular lesion of the atherosclerotic plaque. If the postprandial levels of chylomicrons or their remnants are elevated or if their removal from plasma is prolonged, cholesterol delivery to the artery wall may be increased.

TRANSPORT OF ENDOGENOUS LIPIDS The endogenous lipid transport system, which conveys lipids from the liver to peripheral tissues and from peripheral tissues back to the liver, can be separated into two subsystems: the apo B-100 lipoprotein system (VLDL, IDL, and LDL) and the apo AI lipoprotein system (HDL).

The apo B100 Lipoprotein System (See Fig. 341-1*B*) In the liver, triglycerides are made from fatty acids that are either taken up from plasma or synthesized de novo within the liver. Cholesterol can also be synthesized by the liver or delivered to the liver via chylomicron remnants. These core lipids are packaged together with apo B100 and phospholipids into VLDL and secreted into plasma where apos CI, CII, CIII, and E are added to the VLDL particles. Triglycerides make up the bulk of the VLDL (55 to 80 percent by weight), and the size of the VLDL is determined by the amount of triglyceride available. Hence, very large triglyceride-rich VLDL is secreted in situations where excess triglycerides are synthesized, such as in states of caloric excess, in diabetes mellitus, and with alcohol consumption. Small VLDL is secreted when fewer triglycerides are available. Although VLDL is normally the principal hepatic lipoprotein secreted by most individuals, VLDL and cholesteryl ester–enriched IDL and/or LDL-like particles may be secreted by the liver in individuals with combined hyperlipidemia (see below).

In the plasma, VLDL interacts with LPL, and as the triglycerides are hydrolyzed, VLDL particles become smaller and more dense and are converted to VLDL remnants (IDL). In contrast to chylomicron remnants, VLDL remnants can either enter the liver or give rise to LDL. Larger VLDL particles carry more triglycerides and are likely to be removed directly from plasma without being converted to LDL; apo E in the VLDL remnants is the ligand that binds the remnants to the LDL receptor for removal from the plasma. Smaller, more dense VLDL particles are efficiently converted to LDL, and apo E and HTGL play important roles in this process. Individuals with deficiency of either apo E2 or HTGL accumulate IDL in plasma. Apo B100 is the only protein remaining on the surface of the LDL particle.

The half-life of LDL in plasma is determined principally by the availability (or "activity") of LDL receptors. Most plasma LDL is taken up by the liver, and the remainder is delivered to peripheral tissues, including the adrenals and gonads, which utilize cholesterol as a precursor for steroid hormone synthesis. The adrenals have the highest concentration of LDL receptors per cell in the body. Overall, about 70 to 80 percent of LDL catabolism occurs via LDL receptors, and the remainder is removed by fluid endocytosis and possibly by other receptors.

The LDL receptor, a glycoprotein with a molecular mass of approximately 160 kDa, is present on the surfaces of nearly all cells in the body. Goldstein and Brown characterized the molecular genetics and cell biology of the LDL receptor and defined its role in cholesterol metabolism by showing that cholesterol delivered to the cytoplasm by LDL regulates both the rate of cholesterol synthesis in the liver and the number of LDL receptors on the surface of hepatocytes. These feedback mechanisms allow cells to maintain cholesterol homeostasis. While the LDL receptor is a major factor in determining plasma LDL cholesterol levels, the rates of entry of VLDL into plasma and the efficiency with which VLDL is converted to LDL also influence steady-state LDL concentrations in plasma.

Increased levels of plasma LDL cholesterol and apo B100 are risk factors for atherosclerosis. Normal LDL does not cause foam cell formation when incubated with cultured macrophages or smooth-muscle cells, but when LDL undergoes lipid peroxidation it becomes a ligand for an alternative, scavenger receptor pathway. Scavenger receptors are present on endothelial cells and macrophages, and uptake of modified (oxidized) lipoproteins by these receptors in macrophages results in formation of cholesterol-laden foam cells. In addition to inducing foam cell formation, oxidized LDL acts in the vessel wall to stimulate the secretion of cytokines and growth factors by endothelial cells, smooth-muscle cells, and monocyte-derived macrophages. The consequence is recruitment of more monocytes to the lesion and proliferation of smooth-muscle cells, which synthesize and secrete increased amounts of extracellular matrix, such as collagen. The critical role of LDL in atherosclerosis has been confirmed in genetically altered mice. Although mice are normally resistant to atherosclerosis, increased plasma levels of remnant lipoproteins or LDL lead to atherosclerosis in this species.

The role of VLDL in atherogenesis is uncertain. The major reason for this uncertainty derives from the inverse relationship between elevated levels of triglyceride-rich lipoproteins and reduced levels of the antiatherogenic HDL cholesterol, and it is possible that hypertriglyceridemia may not be directly atherogenic but the surrogate of other lipoprotein abnormalities. Hence, if postprandial hyperlipidemia is a risk factor for CHD, individuals who have normal fasting plasma triglyceride levels but develop postprandial hypertriglyceridemia after consumption of a fat load would be misclassified as normal in studies in which only fasting blood samples are analyzed. It is clear that cholesteryl ester–enriched VLDL, isolated from cholesterol-fed animals, can be taken up by receptors on macrophages and smooth-muscle cells and cause foam cell formation. These cholesteryl ester–rich VLDL are enriched in apo E and are probably representative of VLDL remnants. Thus, the risk of atherosclerosis from hypertriglyceridemia and elevated VLDL levels may be determined by the level of cholesteryl ester–enriched VLDL remnants within the plasma VLDL. The atherogenic potential of IDL is probably similar to that of VLDL remnants.

Apo AI–Containing Lipoproteins (See Fig. 341-1*C*) In contrast to atherogenic apo B lipoproteins, the apo AI–containing HDL appear to be antiatherogenic. In fact, in some studies, HDL cholesterol levels are as strong an indicator of protection from CHD as LDL cholesterol levels are an indicator of risk. Although a great deal is known about the HDL transport system, the mechanism by which these lipoproteins protect against atherosclerosis is poorly defined.

HDL particles are formed in plasma from the coalescence of individual phospholipid-apolipoprotein complexes. Apo AI appears to be the crucial, structural apoprotein for HDL, and apo AI/phospholipid complexes probably fuse with other phospholipid vesicles containing apo AII and apo AIV to form the various types of HDL. The C apoproteins can be added to HDL after their secretion as phospholipid complexes or by transfer from triglyceride-rich lipoproteins. These small, cholesterol-poor nascent HDL particles are heterogeneous in size and content and are referred to as HDL_3. Free cholesterol is transferred from cell membranes to HDL_3 and converted by LCAT to cholesteryl ester, which moves into the core of the particle. Formation of cholesteryl ester increases the capacity of the HDL_3 to accept more free cholesterol and enlarge to form the more buoyant class of HDL particles termed *HDL_2*. HDL_2 can be metabolized by two pathways: (1) cholesteryl esters can be transferred from HDL_2 to apo B lipoproteins or cells, or (2) the entire HDL_2 particle can be removed from plasma. The transfer of cholesteryl ester from HDL to triglyceride-rich, apo B lipoproteins (chylomicrons and VLDL in the fed and fasted states, respectively) is mediated by CETP. Triglyceride is transferred to HDL in this process and is a substrate for lipolysis by LPL and/or HTGL. As a result, HDL_2 is converted back into HDL_3. HDL-mediated reverse cholesterol transport (from peripheral tissues to the liver) is thought to be the primary mechanism by which HDL protects against atherosclerosis. When the apo B lipoproteins are removed by the liver, reverse cholesterol transfer is complete. HDL cholesteryl ester may also be transferred selectively to cells via interaction of HDL with cell membranes. Alternatively, the subset of HDL particles that contains apo E can be taken up in toto via LDL receptors or LRP.

In rare cases low plasma HDL is due to a genetic deficiency of one of the structural components of HDL (such as apo AI), but low HDL cholesterol levels are usually the secondary consequence of increased plasma levels of VLDL and IDL (or chylomicrons and their remnants). Low levels of HDL cholesterol and apo AI may increase atherosclerosis risk by any of several mechanisms. HDL could remove cholesterol from foam cells in atherosclerotic lesions or protect LDL from oxidative-modification. Alternatively, the atherosclerotic risk of low HDL may be due to the commonly associated elevations of apo B–containing lipoproteins, which both accept HDL cholesteryl ester and deliver cholesteryl esters to the vessel wall.

THE HYPERLIPOPROTEINEMIAS (See Table 341-3)

HYPERCHOLESTEROLEMIA Elevated levels of fasting plasma total cholesterol in the presence of normal levels of triglycerides are almost always associated with increased concentrations of plasma LDL cholesterol (type IIa), since LDL carries about 65 to 75 percent of total plasma cholesterol. The rare patient with markedly elevated HDL cholesterol may also have increased plasma total cholesterol levels. Elevations of LDL cholesterol can result from single-gene defects, polygenic disorders, and secondary effects of other disease states.

Familial Hypercholesterolemia FH is a codominant genetic disorder that occurs in the heterozygous form in approximately 1 in 500 individuals. FH is due to mutations in the gene for the LDL receptor and is genetically heterogeneous, more than 200 different mutations in the gene having been described. Plasma levels of total and LDL cholesterol are elevated at birth and remain so throughout life. In untreated adults, total cholesterol levels range from 7 to 13 mmol/L (275 to 500 mg/dL). Plasma triglyceride levels are typically normal, and HDL cholesterol levels are normal or reduced. As would be expected with a decreased number of LDL receptors, the fractional clearance of LDL apo B is decreased. LDL production is increased because more VLDL and more IDL are secreted by the liver and more IDL particles are converted to LDL rather than taken up by the hepatic LDL receptors. *Tendon xanthomas*, which are due to both intracellular and extracellular deposits of cholesterol, most commonly involve the Achilles tendons and the extensor tendons of the knuckles and are found in about 75 percent of adults with FH. *Tuberous xanthomas*, which are softer, painless nodules on the elbows and buttocks, and *xanthelasmas*, which are barely elevated deposits of cholesterol on the eyelids, are common in heterozygous FH. In men CHD develops by the fourth decade of life (or earlier).

The homozygous form of FH occurs in one out of 1 million individuals and is associated with plasma cholesterol levels >13 mmol/L (>500 mg/dL), large xanthelesmas, and prominent tendon and planar xanthomas. These individuals have an aggressive, premature CHD that can be manifested in childhood.

Familial Defective Apo B100 This autosomal dominant disorder is a phenocopy of FH and is due to a missense mutation at amino acid 3500 that reduces the affinity of LDL for the LDL receptor and thus impairs LDL catabolism. The prevalence and manifestations of both the heterozygous and homozygous forms are similar to those produced by mutations of the LDL receptor.

Polygenic Hypercholesterolemia Most moderate hypercholesterolemia [plasma cholesterol levels between 6.5 and 9 mmol/L (240 and 350 mg/dL)] is polygenic in origin. Multiple genes interact with environmental factors to contribute to the hypercholesterolemia, and both overproduction and reduced catabolism of LDL are thought to play roles in the pathophysiology. The severity is probably affected by the consumption of saturated fat and cholesterol, by age, and by the level of physical activity. Plasma triglyceride and HDL cholesterol levels are usually normal. Tendon xanthomas are not present. Genes involved in cholesterol and bile acid metabolism may be involved in the pathogenesis.

HYPERTRIGLYCERIDEMIA The diagnosis of hypertriglyceridemia is made by determining levels of plasma lipids after an overnight fast. Because of the less certain association of triglycerides with CHD (compared to LDL cholesterol), plasma concentrations

Table 341-3

Characteristics of Common Hyperlipidemias

Lipid Phenotype	Plasma Lipid Levels, mmol/L (mg/dL)	Lipoproteins Elevated	Phenotype	Clinical Signs
ISOLATED HYPERCHOLESTEROLEMIA				
Familial hypercholesterolemia	Heterozygotes: total chol = 7–13 (275–500)	LDL	IIa	Usually develop xanthomas in adulthood and vascular disease at 30–50 years
	Homozygotes: total chol > 13 (>500)	LDL	IIa	Usually develop xanthomas and vascular disease in childhood
Familial defective apo B100	Heterozygotes: total chol = 7–13 (275–500)	LDL	IIa	
Polygenic hypercholesterolemia	Total chol = 6.5–9.0 (250–350)	LDL	IIa	Usually asymptomatic until vascular disease develops; no xanthomas
ISOLATED HYPERTRIGLYCERIDEMIA				
Familial hypertriglyceridemia	TG = 2.8–8.5 (250–750) (plasma may be cloudy)	VLDL	IV	Asymptomatic; may be associated with increased risk of vascular disease
Familial lipoprotein lipase deficiency	TG > 8.5 (>750) (plasma may be milky)	Chylomicrons	I, V	May be asymptomatic; may be associated with pancreatitis, abdominal pain, hepatosplenomegaly
Familial apo CII deficiency	TG > 8.5 (>750) (plasma may be milky)	Chylomicrons	I, V	As above
HYPERTRIGLYCERIDEMIA AND HYPERCHOLESTEROLEMIA				
Combined hyperlipidemia	TG = 2.8–8.5 (250–750) Total chol = 6.5–13.0 (250–500)	VLDL, LDL	IIb	Usually asymptomatic until vascular disease develops; familial form may also present as isolated high TG or an isolated high LDL cholesterol
Dysbetalipoproteinemia	TG = 2.8–5.6 (250–500) Total chol = 6.5–13.0 (250–500)	VLDL, IDL; LDL normal	III	Usually asymptomatic until vascular disease develops; may have palmar or tuboeruptive xanthomas

NOTE: total chol, the sum of free and esterified cholesterol; LDL, low-density lipoprotein; TG, triglycerides; VLDL, very low density lipoproteins; IDL, intermediate-density lipoprotein.

greater than the 90th or 95th percentile for age and sex have been used to define hypertriglyceridemia. Isolated elevations of plasma triglycerides can be due to increased levels of VLDL (type IV) or combinations of VLDL and chylomicrons (type V). Rarely, only chylomicron levels are elevated (type I). Plasma is usually clear when triglyceride levels are <4.5 mmol/L (<400 mg/dL) and becomes cloudy when levels are higher and VLDL (and/or chylomicron) particles become large enough to diffuse light. When chylomicrons are present, a creamy layer floats to the top of plasma after storage in the cold for several hours. Tendon xanthomas and xanthelasma do not occur with isolated hypertriglyceridemia, but eruptive xanthomas, small orange-red papules, can appear on the trunk and extremities when triglyceride levels are >11 mmol/L (>1000 mg/dL) (i.e., when chylomicronemia is present). At these high levels of triglycerides, the retinal vessels can appear to be orange-yellow in color (lipemia retinalis). Pancreatitis is the major risk associated with plasma triglyceride concentrations >11 mmol/L (>1000 mg/dL).

Elevations in plasma triglycerides are usually associated with increased synthesis and secretion of VLDL triglycerides by the liver. Hepatic triglyceride synthesis is regulated by substrate flow (the availability of free fatty acids), energy balance (the level of glycogen stores in the liver), and hormonal status (the balance between insulin and glucagon). Obesity, excessive consumption of simple sugars and saturated fats, inactivity, alcohol consumption, and insulin resistance are commonly associated with hypertriglyceridemia. In most of these situations, increased free fatty acid flux from adipose tissue to the liver stimulates the assembly and secretion of VLDL. When VLDL triglyceride levels are markedly elevated [>11 mmol/L (>1000 mg/dL)], LPL may be saturated so that even if there is no underlying genetic disorder an acquired LPL deficiency develops during the postprandial period. The addition of chylomicrons to the circulation may cause dramatic increases in plasma triglycerides.

Familial Hypertriglyceridemia Familial hypertriglyceridemia appears to be transmitted as an autosomal dominant disorder, but the underlying mutation(s) have not been identified. The pathophysiology is complex; both reduced catabolism of triglyceride-rich lipoproteins and overproduction of VLDL have been reported. Elevated levels of fasting plasma triglycerides in the range of 2.3 to 8.5 mmol/L (200 to 750 mg/dL) are usually associated with increased levels of VLDL triglycerides only. When VLDL triglyceride levels are markedly elevated (regardless of etiology), chylomicron triglycerides can also be present, even after a 14-h fast. This disorder does not appear to increase risk for CHD, either because large triglyceride-rich lipoproteins are not atherogenic or because only normal amounts of LDL can be generated.

Familial Lipoprotein Lipase Deficiency This autosomal recessive disorder is due to the impairment or absence of LPL, as a consequence of which chylomicrons accumulate to massive levels in plasma. Manifestations begin in infancy and include pancreatitis, eruptive xanthomas, hepatomegaly, splenomegaly, foam cell infiltration of the bone marrow, and, when the level of triglycerides is greater than 11 mmol/L (1000 mg/dL), lipemia retinalis. Atherosclerosis is not accelerated. The diagnosis is suspected by finding a layer of cream (chylomicrons) at the top of plasma that has incubated overnight at 4°C and confirmed by demonstrating that LPL levels in plasma do not increase after the administration of heparin (which normally releases LPL from endothelial surfaces). Manifestations recede dramatically when patients are placed on fat-free diets.

LPL levels are within the normal range in most patients with moderate hypertriglyceridemia [2.8 to 5.6 mmol/L (250 to 500 mg/dL)], but heterozygous mutations in the LPL gene are present in 5 to 10 percent of hypertriglyceridemic individuals; LPL activity may be reduced by 20 to 50 percent in these heterozygotes.

Familial Apoprotein CII Deficiency This rare autosomal recessive disorder causes a functional deficiency of LPL and clinical manifestations that are similar to those of familial LPL deficiency. Deficiency of apoprotein CII impairs hydrolysis of chylomicrons and VLDL so that either or both lipoproteins accumulate in blood. The diagnosis is suspected in children or adults with recurrent attacks of pancreatitis and confirmed by demonstrating absence of apo CII on gel electrophoresis and demonstrating that the transfusion of plasma (which contains abundant apo CII) causes a dramatic fall in plasma triglycerides. Heterozygotes have half normal levels of apo CII, may have mild elevations of triglycerides, and are asymptomatic. Dietary fat restriction should be life-long.

Hepatic Lipase Deficiency Total deficiency of HTGL is a rare autosomal recessive disorder that impairs the final catabolism and/or remodeling of small VLDL and IDL. Subjects with HTGL deficiency often have elevated levels of VLDL remnants, and HDL_2 levels may be elevated since HTGL participates in the conversion of HDL_2 to HDL_3. HTGL activity is frequently elevated in hypertriglyceridemic subjects, but the meaning of this association is unclear.

HYPERCHOLESTEROLEMIA WITH HYPERTRIGLYCERIDEMIA Concomitant hypercholesterolemia and hypertriglyceridemia occurs in two disorders.

Familial Combined Hyperlipidemia (FCHL) FCHL is inherited as an autosomal dominant disorder, and probands (the initial case discovered within a family) may have combined hyperlipidemia, isolated hypertriglyceridemia, or isolated elevated levels of LDL cholesterol. The diagnosis requires documentation at some time of combined hyperlipidemia in the proband or, if the proband has isolated hypercholesterolemia or hypertriglyceridemia, the various lipid phenotypes in first-degree relatives at risk. In affected individuals the lipoprotein phenotype may change with time. The underlying defect in this disorder is not known, although mutations or polymorphisms in the gene for LPL and in the gene cluster for apo AI, apo CIII, and apo AIV may contribute to the disorder in some families. Insulin resistance is present in many individuals with FCHL; the link may be via increased free fatty acid flux driving assembly and secretion of apo B100 lipoproteins.

FCHL is associated with increased secretion of VLDL particles, as determined by the flux of VLDL apo B. The lipoprotein patterns associated with the disorder are most likely determined by genetic polymorphisms in genes that regulate the metabolism of VLDL. For example, if the affected individual also has a defect in LPL, hypertriglyceridemia will be present. Since the hydrolysis of VLDL triglycerides also regulates the generation of LDL in plasma, individuals with FCHL who have inefficient catabolism of VLDL may have reduced levels of LDL cholesterol and high VLDL cholesterol. Finally, individuals with FCHL who synthesize normal quantities of triglycerides and secrete VLDL that carries normal amounts of triglyceride generate increased numbers of LDL particles and present with isolated elevations of plasma LDL cholesterol. These variations in VLDL catabolism, together with additional genetic heterogeneity and environmental variability, are the basis for the variable phenotype in this disorder. FCHL may occur in as many as 0.5 to 1.0 percent of Americans and is the most common familial lipid disorder in survivors of myocardial infarction. The increased risk for atherosclerosis is due to the presence of increased numbers of small, atherogenic VLDL and the conversion of VLDL to the more atherogenic IDL and LDL. Subjects with FCHL usually have clear plasma and do not have xanthomas or xanthelasma.

Dysbetalipoproteinemia This rare disorder affects 1 in 10,000 persons and is due to homozygosity for apo E2, the binding-defective form of apo E. Because apo E plays a crucial role in the catabolism of chylomicron and VLDL remnants, affected individuals have elevations in both VLDL triglyceride and VLDL cholesterol, and chylomicron remnants are present in fasting plasma. The ratio of total cholesterol to triglyceride approximates 1.0 and the ratio of VLDL cholesterol to triglyceride is greater than 0.25. LDL and HDL cholesterol levels are usually low. Although 1 percent of the population is homozygous for apo E2, most have normal plasma triglyceride and cholesterol levels. Thus, a second defect in lipid metabolism must be present in the 0.01 percent of individuals with dysbetalipoproteinemia. These individuals can have tuberous xanthomas and deposits of cholesterol in the palmar creases (striae palmaris); the latter, appearing as yellow-orange lines, are specific for dysbetalipoproteinemia. Risk for atherosclerosis and its complications is increased, with onset in the fourth and fifth decades. The incidence of peripheral vascular disease is higher than in familial hypercholesterolemia.

REDUCED HDL CHOLESTEROL Low levels of HDL cholesterol can be defined as <0.9 mmol/L (<35 mg/dL) in men and <1 to 1.2 mmol/L (<40 to 45 mg/dL) in women. Low concentrations of HDL cholesterol are usually associated with coexistent hypertriglyceridemia, although "primary hypoalphalipoproteinemia" has been identified in both individuals and families. The relationship between hypertriglyceridemia and low HDL levels probably derives from (1) CETP-mediated transfer of cholesteryl ester from the core of HDL to VLDL; (2) shift of surface components, particularly phospholipids, apo C-II, and apo C-III, from HDL to VLDL; and (3) increased fractional catabolism of the cholesteryl ester–poor HDL that results from the first two processes. The complexity of the relationship between HDL and triglyceride levels is highlighted by the fact that HDL levels do not return to normal when fasting plasma triglycerides are reduced in most persons with hypertriglyceridemia and low HDL cholesterol levels. Low HDL is clinically silent, and the plasma is usually clear (it can be cloudy or creamy if there is concomitant hypertriglyceridemia).

Primary hypoalphalipoproteinemia refers to the state where HDL cholesterol concentrations are markedly reduced but plasma triglyceride concentrations are normal. Although this disorder certainly exists, many individuals with this phenotype have had hypertriglyceridemia in the past or have an older (or more obese) first-degree relative who has both low HDL and increased triglyceride levels. Hence, both family studies and long-term follow-up may be required to identify individuals with primary reductions in HDL cholesterol. Rare mutations have been described in the apo AI gene that lead to reductions in apo AI synthesis or increases in catabolism. One mutation that is common in Italy, apo AI-Milano, is associated with a high fractional clearance rate of apo AI but is not associated with increased risk for atherosclerosis.

Some rare genetic disorders of lipid metabolism are summarized in Table 341-4.

SECONDARY CAUSES OF HYPERLIPOPROTEINEMIA (See Table 341-5) **Diabetes Mellitus** Diabetes can affect lipid and lipoprotein metabolism through several mechanisms. In insulin-dependent diabetes mellitus (IDDM), plasma lipids are usually normal when control of diabetes with insulin is adequate. In diabetic ketoacidosis, hypertriglyceridemia can be severe due to increases in both VLDL and chylomicrons; these abnormalities are associated with overproduction of VLDL and LPL deficiency secondary to insulinopenia and usually improve with tight control of the diabetes. In non-insulin-dependent diabetes mellitus (NIDDM), insulin resistance and obesity combine to cause mild to moderate hypertriglyceridemia and low HDL cholesterol levels. In general, this pattern of dyslipidemia is due to overproduction of VLDL. LDL cholesterol is usually normal in NIDDM, although the LDL are small, dense, and perhaps more atherogenic. Treatment of NIDDM and weight reduction improve but usually do not cure the dyslipidemia, particularly the low HDL cholesterol

Table 341-4

Rare Genetic Disorders of Lipid Metabolism

Disorder	Typical Age of Onset	Plasma Lipid Abnormality	Major Clinical Manifestations	Pathogenesis	Treatment
Hypobetalipoproteinemia, Abetalipoproteinemia	Early childhood	Very low cholesterol and triglyceride levels	Malabsorption of fat, ataxia, neuropathy, retinitis pigmentosa, acanthocytosis	Defective synthesis or secretion of apoprotein B leads to low or absent chylomicrons, VLDL, and LDL in plasma	Vitamin E
Tangier disease	Childhood	Low cholesterol; triglycerides, normal to slightly elevated	Large orange tonsils, corneal opacities, relapsing polyneuropathy No premature atherosclerosis	Abnormal cholesterol uptake into and/or efflux from macrophages; increased Apo AI clearance	None
Lecithin:cholesterol acyltransferase (LCAT) deficiency (fish-eye disease)	Young adult	Total plasma cholesterol level variable with marked decrease in esterified cholesterol and increase in unesterified cholesterol; elevated VLDL level; structure of all lipoproteins is abnormal	Corneal opacities, hemolytic anemia, renal insufficiency, premature atherosclerosis	Decreased LCAT activity in plasma leads to accumulation of excess unesterified cholesterol in plasma and body tissues	Fat-restricted diet, kidney transplantation
Cerebrotendinous xanthomatosis	Young adult	None	Progressive cerebellar ataxia, dementia and spinal cord paresis, subnormal intelligence, tendon xanthomas, cataracts	Defective synthesis of primary bile acids in liver leads to increased hepatic synthesis of cholesterol and cholestanol, which accumulate in brain, tendons, and other tissues	None
Sitosterolemia	Childhood	Elevated levels of plant sterols in plasma, elevated or normal levels of cholesterol, normal triglyceride levels	Tendon xanthomas	Increased intestinal absorption of dietary cholesterol, sitosterol, and other plant sterols with accumulation in plasma and tendons	Diet low in plant sterols and cholesterol

NOTE: VLDL, very low density lipoprotein; LDL, low-density lipoprotein; HDL, high-density lipoprotein; LCAT, lecithin:cholesterol acyltransferase.

SOURCE: Modified from MS Brown and JL Goldstein in *Harrison's Principles of Internal Medicine,* 13th ed, KJ Isselbacher et al (eds), New York, McGraw-Hill, 1994.

levels. Therapy of hyperlipidemia should not be delayed in patients with NIDDM, who are at increased risk for CHD.

Hypothyroidism Hypothyroidism accounts for about 2 percent of all cases of hyperlipidemia and is second only to diabetes mellitus as a cause of secondary hyperlipidemia. Levels of LDL cholesterol can be elevated, even in patients with subclinical disease in whom thyroid-stimulating hormone (TSH) levels are elevated but other thyroid function tests are normal. Hypertriglyceridemia can occur if obesity is also present. Hypothyroidism is also associated with increased levels of HDL cholesterol, probably because of reduced HTGL activity. Correction of hypothyroidism reverses the lipid abnormalities.

Renal Disease Renal disease causes a wide range of lipid abnormalities. The nephrotic syndrome can be accompanied by elevations in LDL, VLDL, or both, the severity of the hyperlipidemia correlating with the degree of hypoproteinemia. Renal failure is associated with hypertriglyceridemia and low HDL cholesterol concentrations.

Ethanol The metabolism of ethanol enhances the level of NADH in the liver, which in turn stimulates the synthesis of fatty acids and their incorporation into triglycerides. Moderate ethanol consumption raises plasma VLDL levels, with the degree of elevation dependent on the baseline level. Severe hypertriglyceridemia and pancreatitis usually develop on the background of a genetic hyperlipidemia and heavy alcohol intake. Because ethanol also stimulates the synthesis of apo AI and inhibits CETP, ethanol-associated hypertriglyceridemia is usually accompanied by normal or elevated levels of HDL cholesterol.

Liver Disease Primary biliary cirrhosis and extrahepatic biliary obstruction can cause hypercholesterolemia and elevated levels of plasma phospholipids associated with elevated levels of an abnormal lipoprotein (lipoprotein X) (see Chap. 293). Severe liver injury often leads to a decrease in levels of both cholesterol and triglyceride. Acute hepatitis can cause elevated levels of VLDL and impairment of LCAT formation.

DIAGNOSIS Although the initial indication of an abnormality in lipoprotein metabolism is via blood measurements of triglyceride and cholesterol, the disorders are due to abnormalities of specific lipoproteins. Thus, lipoprotein analysis should assess VLDL, LDL, and HDL levels. Direct measurements of plasma LDL require laborious centrifugation techniques, but LDL cholesterol concentrations can be estimated indirectly in individuals with triglyceride levels <4.5 mmol/L (<400 mg/dL) by subtracting the HDL and VLDL cholesterol from the total plasma cholesterol. HDL cholesterol is determined after chemical precipitation of VLDL and LDL. VLDL cholesterol is estimated to be the plasma triglyceride level divided by five. Therefore

$$\text{LDL cholesterol} = \text{total cholesterol} - (\text{HDL} + \text{triglycerides}/5)$$

where all values are measured in milligrams per deciliter.

In subjects with triglyceride levels >4.5 mmol/L (>400 mg/dL), the ratio of triglyceride to cholesterol in VLDL is >5 so this equation cannot be used to calculate the plasma LDL cholesterol level. The other disorder that is not detected with this method is dysbetalipoproteinemia, because the ratio of triglyceride to cholesterol in the VLDL is <<5. In these two situations, direct measurement of LDL cholesterol must be performed in ultracentrifuged plasma.

Since plasma triglyceride levels rise and since both HDL and LDL cholesterol levels fall modestly (due to the action of CETP) after a fat-containing meal, it is preferable to measure plasma lipids after a 12-h fast. Since measuring only cholesterol levels will not detect individuals with isolated low HDL, screening for CHD should include measurement of HDL. Since serum lipid levels vary from day to day, at least two to three measurements should be made days or weeks apart before initiating therapy. Some experts advocate the use of total cholesterol/HDL ratios as a better assessment of individual risk, a reasonable approach provided both the patient and physician are aware that the treatment goal is to reduce LDL. In addition, physicians must be aware of the absolute values of each because rare patients with very high or very low levels of both LDL and HDL have ratios that are not interpretable on the basis of population studies. Although research and clinical laboratories often offer measurements of individual apoproteins, e.g., apo B-100 and apo AI, this information is generally not helpful in decision-making. Lipoprotein electrophoresis is also not useful except for the diagnosis of dysbetalipoproteinemia, which otherwise requires ultracentrifugation methods. Genotyping of apo E is available in some laboratories and is helpful in the diagnosis of dysbetalipoproteinemia (although rarely the disorder can be due to other defects in the apo E gene).

Both LDL and HDL cholesterol levels are temporarily decreased for several weeks after myocardial infarction or acute inflammatory states but can be accurately measured if blood is obtained within 8 h of the event.

Table 341-5

Secondary Causes of Lipoprotein Abnormalities

HYPERCHOLESTEROLEMIA	
Hypothyroidism	Acute intermittent porphyria
Obstructive liver disease	Drugs: progestogens, cyclosporine, thiazides
Nephrotic syndrome	
Anorexia nervosa	
HYPERTRIGLYCERIDEMIA	
Obesity	Pregnancy
Diabetes mellitus	Drugs: estrogen, isotretinoin, beta blockers, glucocorticoids, bile acid–binding resins, thiazides
Chronic renal failure	
Lipodystrophy	
Glycogen storage disease	Acute hepatitis
Alcohol	Systemic lupus erythematosus
Ileal bypass surgery	Monoclonal gammopathy: multiple myeloma, lymphomas
Stress	
Sepsis	
HYPOCHOLESTEROLEMIA	
Malnutrition	Monoclonal gammopathy
Malabsorption	Chronic liver disease
Myeloproliferative diseases	
Chronic infectious diseases: AIDS, tuberculosis	
LOW HDL	
Malnutrition	Beta blockers
Obesity	Anabolic steroids
Cigarette smoking	

NOTE: HDL, high-density lipoprotein.

TREATMENT

Elevated LDL Cholesterol Treatment can have either of two aims—primary prevention of the complications of atherosclerosis or secondary treatment after complications have occurred. The rationale for primary prevention is based on the large body of data linking elevated levels of LDL cholesterol with increased CHD risk and an impressive body of clinical and experimental data demonstrating that reducing LDL cholesterol slows progression and may actually induce regression of CHD. Both primary and secondary intervention trials indicate that total mortality can be reduced when the LDL cholesterol is lowered.

For primary prevention the National Cholesterol Education Program (NCEP) Adult Treatment Panel recommends aggressive therapy for patients with multiple risk factors. Risk factors include family history of premature CHD (below the age of 55 years in a male parent or sibling or below 65 in female relatives), hypertension (even if it is controlled with medications), cigarette smoking (>10 cigarettes per day), diabetes mellitus, and low HDL [<0.9 mmol/L (<35 mg/dL)]. In addition, since CHD is more prevalent in older individuals, age (men >45 years, women >55 years, or younger women with premature menopause without estrogen replacement) are also at risk. HDL cholesterol >1.6 mmol/L (>60 mg/dL) is a negative risk factor, i.e., one other risk factor can be negated by a high HDL cholesterol level.

Table 341-6

LDL Cholesterol Treatment Guidelines

	Levels of LDL for Beginning Therapy, mmol/L (mg/dL)		
	Diet	Drugs	Goal
No CHD and less than two risk factors	≥4.1(≥160)	≥4.9(≥190)	<4.1(<160)
No CHD but two or more risk factors	≥3.4(≥130)	≥4.1(≥160)	<3.4(<130)
Presence of CHD	>2.6(>100)	>3.4(>130)	<2.6(<100)

The NCEP guidelines are stringent for the secondary treatment of patients with CHD. Patients with CHD should be screened for lipid abnormalities during and after their initial diagnoses. A goal of lowering plasma LDL concentrations to <2.6 mmol/L (<100 mg/dL) is advocated for such individuals (Table 341-6).

ALTERATIONS IN LIFE-STYLE The typical American diet derives about 35 percent of its calories from fat (14 to 15 percent from saturated fat) and contains 400 to 500 mg/d of cholesterol. Individuals with hyperlipidemia should be encouraged to eat a diet lower in cholesterol and saturated fat. The NCEP Step 1 diet, which is recommended for all Americans above age 2, provides 30 percent of calories from fat, fewer than 10 percent calories from saturated fat, and less than 300 mg/d of cholesterol. Carbohydrate is the typical nutrient used to replace fat in patients with isolated hypercholesterolemia. In general, whole-milk dairy products, egg yolks, meats, palm oil, and coconut oil should be replaced with fresh fruits and vegetables, complex carbohydrates (especially whole-grain products), and low-fat dairy products. Shellfish are low in fat content and, except for shrimp, also have low cholesterol levels; shrimp, in moderation, is acceptable. Portion size needs to be stressed; the protein and fat-rich portion of meat in a given meal should be less than 115 g (4 oz), the size of a deck of cards. Substitutions with any food low in saturated fat such as bran, nuts, and olive oil will have positive effects on LDL. Hydrogenation of vegetable oils increases the saturation of the fatty acids and is not advantageous. In particular, trans-fatty acids, mainly found in commercially hydrogenated vegetable oils, raise LDL and can lower HDL cholesterol levels. When further diet therapy is indicated, the NCEP Step 2 diet provide 30 percent calories as fat but fewer than 5 percent calories from saturated fat, and less than 200 mg/d of cholesterol. The NCEP recommendations for the Step 1 and Step 2 diets are presented in Table 341-7. (See also Chap. 77.) The response in LDL cholesterol upon changing from the average American diet to the Step 1 diet is a drop of 8 to 10 percent; an additional reduction of 5 to 7 percent can be achieved by moving to the Step 2 diet. There is, however, great individual variability in diet responsiveness, and several values should be obtained before judging efficacy of any diet treatment.

Table 341-7

The Two-Step Approach to Treating Hypercholesterolemia*

Nutrient	Step 1 Diet	Step 2 Diet
Total fat	<30% calories	<30% calories
Fatty acids		
Saturated	<10% calories	<7% calories
Polyunsaturated	≤10% calories	≤10% calories
Monounsaturated	10–15% calories	10–15% calories
Carbohydrates	50–60% calories	50–60% calories
Protein	10–20% calories	10–20% calories
Cholesterol	<300 mg/d	<200 mg/d

* Total calories: to achieve and maintain desirable body weight.

The decision as to how long diet therapy be attempted as the sole form of therapy should be based on the severity of the hyperlipidemia and the goals of treatment as determined by the risk factors for CHD. If a patient with CHD has only a modestly elevated LDL cholesterol level [i.e., <3.4 mmol/L (<130 mg/dL)] and the goal is an LDL cholesterol level <2.6 mmol/L (<100 mg/dL), a 4- to 6-week period of Step 1 diet therapy can precede the addition of drugs. If the patient is elderly, has no CHD, and has only one other risk factor besides a high LDL level, long-term diet therapy alone may be sufficient. In such a patient, moving to the Step 2 diet, which provides the same total fat but fewer than 5 percent of calories from saturated fat, can be useful. If, however, the LDL cholesterol is very high, if multiple risk factors are present, or if CHD is documented, drug therapy should be instituted along with diet therapy.

DRUG THERAPY (See Table 341-8) Three classes of lipid-lowering agents are recommended as first-line therapy against hypercholesterolemia: the bile acid sequestrants or –binding resins; niacin; and the 3-hydroxy-3-methylglutaryl-coenzyme A (HMG-CoA) reductase inhibitors. Fibric acid derivatives such as gemfibrozil are second-line agents for hypercholesterolemia and are most effective for lowering of triglycerides.

1. *Bile acid–binding resins.* The bile acid–binding resins cholestyramine and colestipol have been in use as lipid-lowering agents for almost three decades. These drugs interfere with reabsorption of bile acids in the intestine, resulting in a compensatory increase in bile acid synthesis and upregulation of LDL receptors in hepatocytes. The bile acid sequestrants are primary agents in the treatment

Table 341-8

Hypolipidemic Agents

Class	Mode of Action	Lipoprotein Class Affected	Dose
Bile acid–binding resins	Interrupts enterohepatic circulation of bile acids; ↑ Synthesis of new bile acids and LDL receptors	↓ LDL cholesterol 20–30% ↑ HDL cholesterol and triglycerides	Cholestyramine 8–12 g bid or tid Cholestipol 10–15 g bid or tid
Nicotinic acid	↓ Synthesis of VLDL and LDL	↓ Triglycerides 25–85% ↓ VLDL cholesterol 25–35% ↓ LDL cholesterol 15–25% HDL may ↑	Niacin 50–100 mg tid initially then increase to 1.0–2.5 g tid
HMG-CoA reductase inhibitors	↓ Cholesterol synthesis ↑ LDL receptors	↓ LDL cholesterol 25–40% ↓ VLDL	Lovastatin 10–80 mg/d Pravastatin 10–40 mg/d Simvastatin 5–40 mg/d Fluvastatin 20–40 mg/d Atorvastatin 10–80 mg/d
Fibric acid derivatives	↑ LPL and ↑ triglyceride hydrolysis ↓ VLDL synthesis ↑ LDL catabolism	↓ Triglycerides 25–40% ↑ or ↓ LDL cholesterol ↑ HDL	Gemfibrozil 600 mg bid

NOTE: LDL, low-density lipoprotein; HMG-CoA, 3-hydroxy-3-methylglutaryl-coenzyme A; HDL, high-density lipoprotein; VLDL, very low density lipoprotein; LPL, lipoprotein lipase.

of patients with elevated levels of LDL cholesterol and normal triglycerides. Sequestrants produce dose-dependent decreases on the order of 15 to 25 percent in total cholesterol and of 20 to 35 percent in LDL cholesterol. The agents cause modest increases in HDL cholesterol. A limitation of the sequestrants is their tendency to raise triglyceride levels through compensatory increases in hepatic synthesis of VLDL, and they should not be given to hypertriglyceridemic individuals. Bile acid–binding resins are efficacious and safe and are recommended for young adult men and premenopausal women with moderate cholesterol elevations. Patient compliance is low, in part because of the need to dissolve these powdered agents in fluid; the availability of colestipol as a tablet may alleviate this problem. Gastrointestinal side effects include constipation, bloating, and gas.

2. *Niacin.* The mechanism of action of niacin is not fully understood, but it appears to inhibit the secretion of lipoproteins containing apo B100 from the liver. Niacin decreases both total and LDL cholesterol approximately 15 to 25 percent, reduces VLDL levels by 25 to 35 percent, and raises HDL cholesterol levels by as much as 15 to 25 percent. Thus, on the basis of its effects on three major lipoproteins, VLDL, LDL, and HDL, niacin would appear to be an optimal agent. Efficacy of monotherapy was confirmed in a long-term secondary prevention trial in which niacin significantly reduced the incidence of myocardial infarction. An even longer-term follow-up of that study (15 years total) showed an 11 percent decrease in all-cause mortality among patients randomized to niacin. Like the bile acid–binding resins, niacin is safe, having been in use for almost 30 years. Niacin, however, has unpleasant side effects that limit patient acceptability, including uncomfortable and potentially dose-limiting cutaneous flushing with or without pruritus. However, the cutaneous symptoms tend to subside after several weeks and may be minimized by initiating therapy at low doses. Less common adverse effects include elevations of liver enzymes, gastrointestinal distress, impaired glucose tolerance, and elevated serum uric acid levels with or without gouty arthritis. Liver enzymes may be elevated in 3 to 5 percent of patients on full doses of niacin (>2 g/d).

3. *HMG-CoA reductase inhibitors.* HMG-CoA reductase inhibitors, which include lovastatin, simvastatin, pravastatin, fluvastatin, and atorvastatin inhibit the rate-limiting step in hepatic cholesterol biosynthesis (the conversion of HMG-CoA to mevalonate), which causes a rise in LDL receptor levels in hepatocytes and enhanced receptor-mediated clearance of LDL cholesterol from the circulation. At usual doses, the HMG-CoA reductase inhibitors decrease total cholesterol by 20 to 30 percent and LDL cholesterol by 25 to 40 percent. Larger reductions may be achieved with higher doses. Treatment with reductase inhibitors often produces reductions in triglycerides of 10 to 20 percent, possibly due to reduced secretion of VLDL by the liver. HDL cholesterol levels rise about 5 to 10 percent. In comparison with other lipid-lowering agents, HMG-CoA reductase inhibitors are relatively free of side effects, which have been reported by fewer than 5 percent of patients. Mild, transient elevations in liver enzymes occur with all of the agents at the highest doses, but elevations in serum aminotransferases to more than three times the upper limits of normal occur in fewer than 2 percent of patients. Therapy should be discontinued when elevations of this magnitude occur. A rare but potentially serious adverse effect of HMG-CoA reductase inhibitors is myopathy, with elevations of serum creatine phosphokinase (CPK) more than 10 times the upper limit of normal; this occurs in fewer than 1 percent of patients treated with reductase inhibitors alone but is more common (about 5 percent) when used in combination with gemfibrozil, niacin, or cyclosporine.

4. *Combination therapy.* Combinations of bile acid–binding resins and reductase inhibitors are effective for the treatment of severe, isolated elevations of LDL cholesterol. Combinations of either resins and niacin or reductase inhibitors and niacin are useful for the treatment of high LDL and low HDL cholesterol levels, although the latter combination carries an increased risk of myositis (2 to 3 percent). If triglyceride and LDL levels are both elevated (HDL is usually reduced as well), resins and niacin are an excellent combination, with resins and gemfibrozil as an alternative. The combination of a reductase inhibitor and gemfibrozil can be useful when LDL cholesterol is very high in the face of concomitant hypertriglyceridemia, but the risk of myositis (about 5 percent) must be considered. Combinations of reductase inhibitors with either niacin or gemfibrozil might best be reserved for patients with CHD and combined hyperlipidemia.

5. *LDL apheresis.* In patients with homozygous FH and in ordinary FH patients who respond poorly to diet and drug therapy or who cannot tolerate drugs, apheresis at 7- to 14-day intervals can cause profound lowering of LDL cholesterol levels. Diet and drug regimens are continued during treatment. The long-term efficacy/safety of such therapy is not established, but the therapy should be considered for patients with few therapeutic options.

High Triglycerides and Low HDL The evidence that treatment to reduce plasma triglyceride levels or increase levels of HDL cholesterol leads to long-term health benefits is less compelling than that for treatment of high LDL levels. There have been no intervention trials in which only increases in HDL cholesterol concentrations have been achieved. However, treatment of hypercholesterolemic patients with gemfibrozil led to a decrease in CHD events that was greater than that expected with the observed decreases in LDL. Beneficial effects of niacin have been attributed, in part, to its HDL-raising action as well as the lowering of triglycerides and LDL. Even with drugs that primarily

Side Effects	Contraindications	Drug Interactions	Combined Use with
Constipation, gastric discomfort, nausea, hemorrhoidal bleeding	Biliary track obstruction, gastric outlet obstruction, hypertriglyceridemia	↓ Absorption of phenylbutazone, phenobarbital, thyroid hormones, digitalis, warfarin, thiazide diuretics, some antibiotics	Nicotinic acid, HMG-CoA reductase inhibitors, gemfibrozil
Flushing, tachycardia, atrial arrhythmias, pruritus, dry skin, nausea, diarrhea, hyperuricemia, peptic ulcer disease, glucose intolerance, hepatic dysfunction	Peptic ulcer disease, cardiac arrhythmias, liver disease, gout, diabetes mellitus	Synergistic with ganglionic blocking agents	Bile acid–binding resins, HMG-CoA reductase inhibitors, gemfibrozil
Abnormal liver function, myositis	↑ Myositis in patients with renal failure and in patients on gemfibrozil, nicotinic acid, or cyclosporine	Gemfibrozil, ketoconazole, cyclosporine, warfarin, niacin	Bile acid–binding resins
↑ Lithogenicity of bile, nausea, abnormal liver functions, myositis	Hepatic or biliary disease; ↓ dose in renal insufficiency	↑ Anticoagulant activity of warfarin	Bile acid–binding resins

affect LDL cholesterol levels, such as bile acid–binding resins and HMG-CoA reductase inhibitors, some of the benefits achieved may be related to increases in HDL cholesterol levels.

Efforts should be made to reduce triglycerides when they are at levels that may precipitate pancreatitis. Thus, triglyceride levels >5.6 mmol/L (>500 mg/dL) are generally treated whereas lower levels [2.2 to 5.6 mmol/L (200 to 500 mg/dL)] are not treated unless other CHD risk factors are present.

ALTERATIONS IN LIFESTYLE (See above under "Hypercholesterolemia"). In patients with isolated elevations of triglyceride levels or with hypertriglyceridemia and high LDL cholesterol, weight reduction should be strongly encouraged if obesity is present. Also, fat intake should be decreased, but the concomitant increase in the intake of carbohydrate may raise triglyceride and lower HDL cholesterol levels. If this occurs, replacing some of the saturated fat with monounsaturated fat, which will not raise LDL cholesterol, may be valuable. Severe hypertriglyceridemia and hyperchylomicronemia require very low fat diets, avoidance of free sugars, and decreased alcohol intake. Patients with genetic LPL deficiency are instructed to prepare their food using medium-chain triglycerides, which are not incorporated into chylomicrons. Fish oils decrease triglyceride synthesis and in high doses may be used for severe hypertriglyceridemia.

DRUG THERAPY The recommendations for evaluating and treating hypertriglyceridemia focus on the associated LDL and HDL concentrations as guidelines for therapy. Thus, the overall risk profile can be used to set goals for LDL cholesterol, using a low HDL level (commonly associated with hypertriglyceridemia) as a concomitant major risk factor for atherosclerosis. However, when triglyceride levels are >5.6 mmol/L (>500 mg/dL), the risk of developing pancreatitis increases, and a direct focus on lowering triglycerides is recommended.

1. *Niacin.* Niacin is a first-line drug for hypertriglyceridemia. The positive and negative characteristics of niacin were outlined above, but it is relevant to note that since LDL cholesterol is the target of intervention in many patients with elevated plasma triglyceride levels, the potency of niacin against both triglycerides and LDL cholesterol makes it a top choice. The ability of niacin to raise HDL cholesterol further enhances its usefulness. Because of its propensity to worsen the control of blood sugar, niacin should be used with caution in patients with diabetes mellitus.

2. *Gemfibrozil.* The only fibric acid derivative widely used in the United States is gemfibrozil. The mechanism of action of the fibrates is only partially understood, but they appear to stimulate the enzyme LPL, probably the basis for much of the triglyceride-lowering effect. However, fibrates may also reduce VLDL triglyceride entry into plasma and reduce synthesis of apo CIII by impairing gene transcription, which might improve LPL-induced lipolysis or reduce VLDL secretion. Stimulation of peroxisomal fatty acid oxidation by fibrates may also contribute to the triglyceride-lowering actions. In any event, gemfibrozil treatment is associated with 25 to 40 percent reductions in plasma triglyceride levels. Postprandial triglyceride levels, which are linked to fasting concentrations, are also reduced. Gemfibrozil and a low-fat diet are particularly useful in the treatment of dysbetalipoproteinemia and are the first line of therapy for this disorder except in postmenopausal women, who should initially be given estrogen replacement.

Significant increases in LDL cholesterol can accompany otherwise potentially beneficial falls in triglycerides and increases in HDL cholesterol during fibrate therapy. Such rises may require a change to another drug or addition of a second agent.

In the short term, these drugs are well tolerated, with mild gastrointestinal distress in the form of epigastric pain as the major side effect. Mild elevations of liver enzymes occur in 2 to 3 percent of patients but do not usually require cessation of treatment. Rarely, hepatitis can occur. Fibrates appear to make the bile more lithogenic, and long-term use is probably associated with a twofold increase in gallstone formation. Myopathy with myositis is a rare occurrence with the fibrates, alone or in combination. The long-term safety issues have been the source of controversy; in a meta-analysis of several studies in which fibrates were used, overall mortality was slightly increased despite reductions in CHD events and CHD deaths.

3. *Combination therapy.* (See above)

HYPOCHOLESTEROLEMIA

A low total cholesterol concentration [<2.6 mmol/L (<100 mg/dL)] in an adult can be due to rare hereditary traits or secondary to a number of diseases. As described earlier, mutations in the gene for apo B100 that disrupt synthesis or produce truncated forms of apo B100 are associated with hypobetalipoproteinemia. These mutations are inherited as codominant traits, and heterozygotes have plasma cholesterol levels in the range of 1.3 to 2.6 mmol/L (50 to 100 mg/dL), with reduced LDL cholesterol levels but normal plasma HDL cholesterol levels. Heterozygotes are asymptomatic, whereas hypolipoproteinemia homozygotes (or compound heterozygotes) have even lower total and LDL cholesterol concentrations and may have malabsorption of fats and fat-soluble vitamins similar to that in abetalipoproteinemia.

Abetalipoproteinemia (Table 341-4) is a rare, autosomal recessive disorder in which the microsomal triglyceride transfer protein (MTP) is absent because of mutations in the MTP gene. Individuals who are homozygous for this disorder have total cholesterol levels <1.3 mmol/L (<50 mg/dL) and essentially no VLDL, IDL, LDL, or chylomicrons. Because dietary fat as well as vitamins A and E are transported from the intestine in chylomicrons, these patients may have malabsorption of fat and fat-soluble vitamins. Vitamin E deficiency in infancy and early childhood can result in neurologic problems (see also Chap. 79). If vitamin replacement is adequate, individuals with abetalipoproteinemia can live normal, healthy lives.

Moderately low levels of total cholesterol may also be associated with extreme reductions in HDL cholesterol; as noted above, these are almost always secondary to mutations in the gene for apo AI and a lack of apo AI in plasma.

A number of systemic diseases can cause low cholesterol concentrations. Malnutrition, often associated with alcoholism or gastrointestinal disease, can cause low levels of total and LDL cholesterol. Patients with AIDS may have total cholesterol levels <2.1 mmol/L (<80 mg/dL), usually associated with severe wasting, diarrhea, and a poor prognosis. Several neoplasms, particularly those involving the hematopoietic system, are associated with hypocholesterolemia. Patients with acute and chronic myelogenous leukemia and myeloid metaplasia with splenomegaly can have severe reductions in both LDL and HDL levels. Other diseases with concomitant splenomegaly, including lipid storage diseases such as Gaucher's disease and Niemann-Pick disease, can cause very low LDL and HDL cholesterol concentrations due to increased lipoprotein catabolism.

See Chap. 36, Drugs used in the treatment of hyperlipoproteinemia, in Goodman & Gilman's The Pharmacological Basis of Therapeutics, *9th ed, New York, McGraw-Hill, 1996.*

BIBLIOGRAPHY

FRUCHART JC, SHEPHERD J: *Human Plasma Lipoproteins: Clinical Biochemistry, Principles, Methods, Applications.* Berlin, Walter De Gruyter, 1989

GINSBERG HN: Treatment of hypertriglyceridemia, in *Lipoproteins and Coronary Artery Disease*, RA Kreisberg, JA Segrest (eds). Cambridge, MA, Blackwell Scientific, 1992, pp 331–356

GOLDBERG IJ: American College of Physicians Medical Knowledge Self-Assessment Program 10. Endocrinology and Metabolism Syllabus. Philadelphia, American College of Physicians, 1994, pp 1075–1079

GOLDSTEIN JL et al: Familial hypercholesterolemia, in *The Metabolic and Molecular Bases of Inherited Disease*, 7th ed, CR Scriver et al (eds). New York, McGraw-Hill, 1995, p 1981

GORDON BR et al: Treatment of refractory familial hypercholesterolemia by low-density lipoprotein apheresis using an automated dextran sulfate cellulose absorption system. Am J Cardiol 70:1010, 1992

HUNNINGHAKE D (ed): Lipid disorders. Med Clin North Am vol 78, no. 1, January 1994

Report of the National Cholesterol Education Program Expert Panel on Detection, Evaluation and Treatment of High Blood Cholesterol in Adults. Arch Intern Med 148:36, 1988

Summary of the Second Report of the National Cholesterol Education Program Expert Panel on Detection, Evaluation, and Treatment of High Blood Cholesterol in Adults. JAMA 269:3015, 1993

342

Lawrie W. Powell, Kurt J. Isselbacher

HEMOCHROMATOSIS

DEFINITION Hemochromatosis is a common disorder of iron storage in which inappropriate increase in intestinal iron absorption results in deposition of excessive amounts of iron in parenchymal cells with eventual tissue damage and impaired function of organs, especially the liver, pancreas, heart, and pituitary. The disease was termed *hemochromatosis* and the iron-storage pigment was called *hemosiderin* because it was believed that the pigment was derived from the blood. The terms *hemosiderosis* and *siderosis* are often used to describe the presence of stainable iron in tissues, but tissue iron must be quantified to assess body iron status (see below and Chap. 106). *Hemochromatosis* implies present or potentially severe progressive iron overload leading to fibrosis and organ failure. Cirrhosis of the liver, diabetes mellitus, arthritis, cardiomyopathy, and hypogonadotrophic hypogonadism are common manifestations. Although there is debate about definitions, it seems logical to use the following terminology: (1) *hereditary* or *genetic hemochromatosis*—the disorder due to the inheritance of a mutant gene that is tightly linked to the HLA-A6 locus of the major histocompatibility complex on chromosome 6p, and (2) *secondary iron overload*—with tissue injury usually secondary to an iron-loading anemia such as thalassemia or sideroblastic anemia, in which increased erythropoiesis is ineffective. In the acquired iron-loading disorders, massive iron deposits in parenchymal tissues can lead to the same clinical and pathologic features as in hemochromatosis.

The metabolic defect leading to increased iron absorption in hemochromatosis is unknown. The genetic disease can be recognized during its early stages when the iron overload and organ damage are minimal. At this stage the disease is best referred to as *early* or *precirrhotic hemochromatosis* (see Fig. 342-1).

PREVALENCE Hemochromatosis is one of the most common autosomal recessive disorders. The mutation is believed to be of Celtic origin. In European populations, approximately 1 in 10 persons is a heterozygous carrier, and 0.3 percent of persons are homozygotes. However, expression of the disease is modified by several factors, especially dietary iron intake, blood loss associated with menstruation and pregnancy, and blood donation. The clinical expression is 5 to 10 times more frequent in men than in women. Nearly 70 percent of patients develop the first symptoms between ages 40 and 60. The disease is rarely evident below age 20, although with family screening (see below) and periodic health examinations asymptomatic subjects with iron overload can be identified, including young menstruating women.

GENETICS AND MODE OF INHERITANCE The gene for hemochromatosis is closely linked to the HLA-A locus on chromosome 6. Discovery of this linkage made it possible to clarify the mode of inheritance and prevalence of the disorder. For example, the fact that siblings with hemochromatosis usually share the same HLA haplotypes implied that they are homozygotes for the same autosomal recessive mutation. A candidate gene in this region of chromosome 6 termed HLA-H encodes a 343 amino acid MHC class 1 protein, and 83 percent of affected subjects have a homozygous Cys282Tyr substitution in the protein. The role in the remainder of the patients of a second variant in the HLA-H protein His63Asp is unclear. The function of the normal HLA-H protein in iron metabolism is also not known.

PATHOGENESIS Normally, the body iron content of 3 to 4 g is maintained such that intestinal mucosal absorption of iron is equal to iron loss. This amount is approximately 1 mg/d in men and 1.5 mg/d in menstruating women. In hemochromatosis, mucosal absorption is inappropriate to body needs and amounts to 4 mg/d or more. The resulting progressive accumulation of iron causes an early elevation in plasma iron, an increased saturation of transferrin, and progressive elevation of plasma ferritin level. The basic defect causing increased iron absorption is unknown. In hemochromatosis the coordinate regulation of the synthesis of ferritin and the transferrin receptor is intact and responds normally to the usual influences, e.g., blood loss. An abnormally fast transport of iron out of intestinal and reticuloendothelial cells has been postulated, but the mechanism is not known. Either the demonstration of normal function or location of the encoding genes on chromosomes other than chromosome 6 makes it possible to exclude a primary role in the pathogenesis for ferritin, the transferrin receptor, and the iron regulatory protein involved in the coordinate regulation of ferritin and the transferrin receptor.

In advanced disease the body may contain 20 g or more of iron deposited mainly in parenchymal cells of the liver, pancreas, and heart. Iron in the liver and pancreas may increase 50 to 100 times and in the heart 5 to 25 times. Iron deposition in the pituitary causes hypogonadotrophic hypogonadism in both men and women. Tissue injury may result from disruption of iron-laden lysosomes, from lipid peroxidation of subcellular organelles by excess iron, or from stimulation of collagen synthesis by activated stellate cells.

Parenchymal iron overload leading to *secondary iron overload* occurs in chronic disorders of erythropoiesis, particularly in those due to defects in hemoglobin synthesis or ineffective erythropoiesis such as sideroblastic anemia and thalassemia. In these disorders, the absorption of iron is increased, and such patients are also frequently treated with iron and blood transfusions. Porphyria cutanea tarda (PCT), a disorder characterized by a defect in porphyrin biosynthesis (Chap. 343), is also sometimes associated with excessive parenchymal iron deposits; however, the magnitude of the iron load is usually insufficient to produce tissue damage. The exact relationship between these two disorders is unclear, although iron may accentuate the inherited enzyme deficiency in PCT. Another cause of hepatic parenchymal iron overload is hereditary aceruloplasminemia. In this disorder impairment of iron

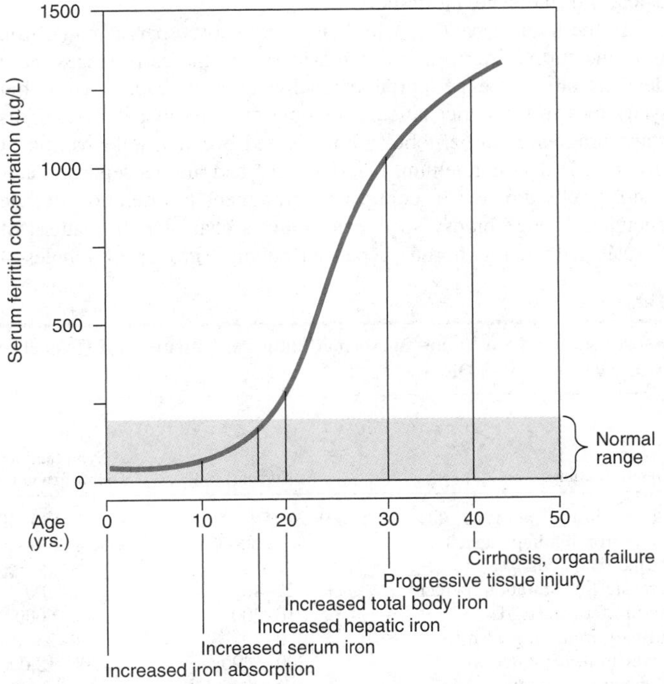

FIGURE 342-1 Sequence of events in genetic hemochromatosis and their correlation with the serum ferritin concentration. Increased iron absorption is present throughout life. Overt, symptomatic disease usually develops between ages 40 and 60, but latent precirrhotic disease can be detected long before this.

mobilization due to deficiency of ceruloplasmin (a ferroxidase) causes iron overload in hepatocytes.

Alcoholic subjects with chronic liver disease and increased tissue iron stores can be divided into two groups. The first comprises patients with a moderate increase in stainable hepatic iron but relatively normal body iron. These patients have alcoholic liver disease (usually cirrhosis) but not hemochromatosis. The increased iron may be due in part to cell death and uptake of released iron. The second (less common) group of alcoholics with increased hepatic iron have gross iron deposition and increased body iron stores and usually prove to have hemochromatosis with or without superimposed alcoholic liver disease. Hemochromatosis in a heavy drinker may be distinguished from alcoholic liver disease in two ways: (1) measurement of hepatic iron concentration and hepatic iron index (see below and Table 342-1) and (2) studying relatives for evidence of the disease, including HLA typing.

Excessive iron ingestion over many years rarely, if ever, results in hemochromatosis. The one important exception is South African blacks, in whom the intake of excessive iron in an alcoholic beverage has been due to the practice of brewing fermented beverages in vessels made of iron. In other populations hemochromatosis has on occasion been described in apparently normal subjects who have taken medicinal iron over many years, but such individuals probably have the genetic disorder. Family studies may be helpful.

The common denominator in all patients with hemochromatosis is *excessive amounts of iron in parenchymal tissues*. Parenteral administration of iron in the form of blood transfusions or iron preparations results predominantly in *reticuloendothelial cell* iron overload. This appears to lead to less tissue damage than iron loading of parenchymal cells.

PATHOLOGY At autopsy, the enlarged, nodular liver and pancreas are rusty in color. Histologically, iron is increased in amount in many organs, particularly in the liver, heart, and pancreas and to a lesser extent in the endocrine glands. The epidermis of the skin is thin, and *melanin* is increased in the cells of the basal layer. Deposits of iron are present around the synovial lining cells of the joints, and calcium pyrophosphate crystals may be present within deposits of calcium in the synovial tissue.

In the liver of patients with hemochromatosis, parenchymal iron is in the form of ferritin and hemosiderin. In the early stages these deposits are in the periportal parenchymal cells, especially within lysosomes in the pericanalicular cytoplasm of the hepatocytes. This stage progresses to perilobular fibrosis and eventually deposition of iron in bile duct epithelium, Kupffer cells, and fibrous septa. Inflammatory cells are few in contrast to prominent proliferation of bile ductules. Wedge biopsy specimens show a characteristic pattern of fibrosis with dense fibrous septa surrounding groups of lobules—somewhat analogous to the findings in the liver in chronic biliary tract disease. In the advanced stage, a macronodular or mixed macro- and micronodular cirrhosis develops.

CLINICAL MANIFESTATIONS The symptoms and signs include skin pigmentation, diabetes mellitus, liver and cardiac impairment, arthropathy, and hypogonadism. Initial symptoms include weakness, lassitude, weight loss, change in skin color, abdominal pain, loss of libido, and symptoms of diabetes mellitus. Hepatomegaly, pigmentation, spider angiomas, splenomegaly, arthropathy, ascites, cardiac arrhythmias, congestive heart failure, loss of body hair, testicular atrophy, and jaundice are prominent in advanced disease.

The *liver* is usually the first organ to be affected, and hepatomegaly is present in more than 95 percent of symptomatic patients. Hepatic enlargement may exist in the absence of symptoms or of abnormal liver function tests. Indeed, over half the patients with symptomatic hemochromatosis have little laboratory evidence of functional impairment of the liver, in spite of hepatomegaly and fibrosis. Loss of body hair, palmar erythema, testicular atrophy, and gynecomastia are common. Manifestations of portal hypertension and esophageal varices occur less commonly than in cirrhosis from other causes. *Hepatocellular carcinoma* develops in about 30 percent of patients with cirrhosis. Its incidence increases with age, and it is the most common cause of death in treated patients. However, it occurs almost exclusively in cirrhotic patients; hence the importance of early diagnosis and therapy. Splenomegaly occurs in approximately half of symptomatic cases.

Excessive *skin pigmentation* is present in over 90 percent of symptomatic patients at the time of diagnosis due to melanin deposition in the skin; this usually gives rise to bronzing. The characteristic metallic or slate gray hue is believed to result from increased melanin or of both melanin and iron in the dermis. Pigmentation usually is diffuse and generalized, but it may be more pronounced on the face, neck, extensor aspects of the lower forearms, dorsa of the hands, lower legs, genital regions, and in scars. In rare cases pigmentation is demonstrable in the oral mucosa.

Diabetes mellitus occurs in about 65 percent of patients and is more likely to develop in those with a family history of diabetes. The genetic predisposition and direct damage to the pancreas by iron deposition both contribute to the development of diabetes. The management is similar to that of other forms of diabetes except for a higher incidence of insulin resistance. Late degenerative sequelae are the same as in ordinary diabetes mellitus.

Arthropathy develops in 25 to 50 percent of patients. It usually occurs after age 50 but may occur as a first manifestation or long after therapy. The joints of the hands, especially the second and third metacarpophalangeal joints, are usually the first joints involved, a feature that helps to distinguish this chondrocalcinosis from the idiopathic form. A progressive polyarthritis involving wrists, hips, ankles, and knees also may ensue. Acute brief attacks of synovitis may be associated with deposition of calcium pyrophosphate (chondrocalcinosis or pseudogout), chiefly in the knees. Radiologic manifestations

Table 342-1

Representative Iron Values in Normal Subjects, Patients with Hemochromatosis, and Patients with Alcoholic Liver Disease

Determination	Normal	Symptomatic Hemochromatosis	Homozygotes with Early, Asymptomatic Hemochromatosis	Heterozygotes	Alcoholic Liver Disease
Plasma iron, μmol/L (μg/dL)	9–27 (50–150)	32–54 (180–300)	Usually elevated	Elevated or normal	Often elevated
Total iron-binding capacity, μmol/L (μg/dL)	45–66 (250–370)	36–54 (200–300)	36–54 (200–300)	Elevated or normal	45–66 (250–370)
Transferrin saturation, percent	22–46	50–100	50–100	Normal or elevated	27–60
Serum ferritin, μg/L	10–200	900–6000	200–500	Usually <500	10–500
Urinary iron,* mg/24 h	0–2	9–23	2–5	2–5	Usually <5
Liver iron, μg/g dry wt	300–1400	6000–18,000	2000–4000	300–3000	300–2000
Hepatic iron index $\frac{(\mu g/g \text{ dry wt})}{56 \times \text{age}}$	<1.0	>2	Usually >2	<2	<2

* After intramuscular administration of 0.5 g deferoxamine.

include cystic changes of sclerosis of the subchondral bones, loss of articular cartilage with narrowing of the joint space, diffuse demineralization, hypertrophic bone proliferation, and calcification of the synovium. The arthropathy tends to progress despite removal of iron by phlebotomy. Although the relation of these abnormalities to iron metabolism is not known, the fact that similar changes occur in other forms of iron overload suggests that iron is a critical factor.

Cardiac involvement is the presenting manifestation in about 15 percent of patients, the most common manifestation being congestive heart failure in about 10 percent of young adults with the disease. Symptoms of congestive failure may develop suddenly, with rapid progression to death if untreated. The heart is diffusely enlarged and may be misdiagnosed as idiopathic cardiomyopathy if other overt manifestations are absent. Cardiac arrhythmias include premature supraventricular beats, paroxysmal tachyarrhythmias, atrial flutter, atrial fibrillation, and varying degrees of atrioventricular block.

Hypogonadism occurs in both sexes and may antedate other clinical features. Manifestations include loss of libido, impotence, amenorrhea, testicular atrophy, and sparse body hair. Gynecomastia is less common than in other forms of cirrhosis. These changes are due to the decreased production of gonadotropins due to impairment of hypothalamic-pituitary function by iron deposition. Adrenal insufficiency, hypothyroidism, and hypoparathyroidism occur on occasion.

DIAGNOSIS The association of (1) hepatomegaly, (2) skin pigmentation, (3) diabetes mellitus, (4) heart disease, (5) arthritis, and (6) hypogonadism should suggest the diagnosis. However, a parenchymal iron overload of comparatively short duration or modest degree may exist with none or only some of these manifestations [e.g., in young subjects (see Fig. 342-1)]. Therefore, a high index of suspicion is needed to make the diagnosis early, and hemochromatosis should be considered in any patient with unexplained hepatomegaly, cardiomyopathy, abnormal skin pigmentation, loss of libido, diabetes mellitus, or arthritis. This is particularly important because treatment before there is permanent organ damage can reverse the iron toxicity and restore life expectancy to normal (see below).

The history should be particularly detailed in regard to disease in other family members, alcohol ingestion, iron intake, and ingestion of large doses of ascorbic acid, which promotes iron absorption. Appropriate tests should be performed to exclude the iron deposition of hematologic disease. The presence of liver, pancreatic, cardiac, and joint disease should be confirmed by physical examination, roentgenography, and standard function tests of these organs. Then it must be demonstrated that there is an increase in total-body iron stores and, in particular, an increase in parenchymal iron concentration with or without tissue damage.

The methods available for assessing parenchymal iron stores include (1) measurement of serum iron and the percent saturation of transferrin, (2) measurement of serum ferritin concentration, (3) liver biopsy with measurement of the iron concentration and calculation of the hepatic iron index (Table 342-1), (4) estimation of chelatable iron stores following the administration of deferoxamine, and (5) computed tomography and/or magnetic resonance imaging of the liver. Each has its advantages and limitations. The serum iron level and percent saturation of transferrin are elevated early in the course, but their specificity is reduced by significant false-positive and false-negative rates. For example, serum iron concentration may be increased in patients with alcoholic liver disease without iron overload; in this situation, however, the hepatic iron index is usually not increased as in hemochromatosis (Table 342-1). In otherwise healthy persons, a fasting serum transferrin saturation greater than 62 percent suggests homozygosity for hemochromatosis.

The serum ferritin concentration is usually a good index of body iron stores, whether decreased or increased. In fact, an increase of 1 μg/L in serum ferritin level reflects an increase of some 65 mg in body stores. In most untreated patients with hemochromatosis, the serum ferritin level is greatly increased (Fig. 342-1 and Table 342-1).

These tests have generally replaced the more cumbersome screening tests involving measurement of urinary iron excretion after the administration of the iron chelator deferoxamine. However, in patients with inflammation and hepatocellular necrosis, serum ferritin levels may be elevated out of proportion to body iron stores due to increased release from tissues. A repeat determination of serum ferritin should therefore be carried out when any concurrent acute hepatocellular damage has subsided, e.g., in alcoholic liver disease. Ordinarily, the *combined measurements* of the percent transferrin saturation and serum ferritin level provide a simple and reliable screening test for hemochromatosis, including the precirrhotic phase of the disease. If either of these tests is abnormal, liver biopsy should be performed, since it is the *definitive* diagnostic test. It permits histochemical estimation of tissue iron, measurement of hepatic iron concentration, and the presence or absence of cirrhosis. In addition, calculation of the hepatic iron index (hepatic iron concentration ÷ age in years) helps to distinguish early homozygous subjects from heterozygotes and from patients with alcoholic liver disease (see Table 342-1). Increased density of the liver due to iron deposition can be demonstrated by computed tomography. Magnetic resonance imaging also may detect increased tissue iron, but its sensitivity requires further evaluation. A retrospective assessment of body iron storage is also provided by performing *weekly phlebotomy* and calculating the amount of iron removed before iron stores are exhausted (1 mL blood = approximately 0.5 mg iron).

When the diagnosis of hemochromatosis is established, it is of importance to examine family members. Asymptomatic as well as symptomatic family members with the disease usually have an increased saturation of transferrin and an increased serum ferritin concentration. These changes occur even before the iron stores are greatly increased (see Fig. 342-1). A liver biopsy should then be performed, since it is imperative to confirm the diagnosis, confirm or exclude the presence of cirrhosis, and begin therapy as early as possible. As stated above, HLA typing is helpful in evaluating families with the disease. Affected siblings (homozygotes) usually have both HLA haplotypes identical with those of the proband. When children of a proband are affected, a homozygote-heterozygote mating has probably occurred. Siblings sharing only one HLA haplotype with a patient (heterozygotes) will probably not develop progressive iron overload. Thus HLA typing helps in predicting the probability of a sibling later developing the disease and therefore in determining the desirable frequency of screening.

The distinction between hemochromatosis and alcoholic cirrhosis with increased tissue iron is usually not difficult if liver iron concentration and hepatic iron index are measured (Table 342-1). Where biopsy is not possible, the deferoxamine excretion test can provide diagnostic information. It should be reemphasized that subjects with a history of excessive alcohol consumption and who have increased hepatic iron concentration are usually homozygous for hemochromatosis.

℞ TREATMENT

The therapy of hemochromatosis involves removal of the excess body iron and supportive treatment of damaged organs. Iron removal is best begun by weekly or twice-weekly phlebotomy of 500 mL. Although there is an initial modest decline in the volume of packed red blood cells to about 35 mL/dL, the level stabilizes after several weeks. The plasma transferrin saturation remains increased until the available iron stores are depleted. In contrast, the plasma ferritin concentration falls progressively, reflecting the gradual decrease in body iron stores. Since one 500-mL unit of blood contains from 200 to 250 mg iron and about 25 g iron should be removed, weekly phlebotomy may be required for 1 or 2 years. When the transferrin saturation and ferritin level become normal, phlebotomies are performed at intervals as required to maintain levels within the normal range. The measurements promptly become abnormal with iron reaccumulation. Usually one phlebotomy every 3 months will suffice.

Chelating agents such as deferoxamine, when given parenterally, remove 10 to 20 mg iron per day, a fraction of that mobilized by once weekly phlebotomy. Phlebotomy is also less expensive, more convenient, and safer for most patients. However, chelating agents are indicated when anemia or hypoproteinemia is severe enough to preclude phlebotomy. Subcutaneous infusion of deferoxamine using a portable pump is the most effective means of administration.

The management of the hepatic failure, cardiac failure, and diabetes mellitus is similar to conventional therapy for these conditions. Loss of libido and change in secondary sex characteristics are partially relieved by parenteral testosterone or gonadotropin therapy (see Chap. 336).

PROGNOSIS The principal causes of death in *untreated* patients are cardiac failure (30 percent), hepatocellular failure or portal hypertension (25 percent), and hepatocellular carcinoma (30 percent).

Life expectancy is improved by removal of the excessive stores of iron and maintenance of these stores at near-normal levels. The 5-year survival rate with therapy increases from 33 to 89 percent. With repeated phlebotomy, the liver and spleen decrease in size, liver function improves, pigmentation of skin decreases, and cardiac failure may be reversed. Diabetes improves in about 40 percent, but removal of excess iron has little effect on hypogonadism or arthropathy. Hepatic fibrosis may decrease, but cirrhosis is irreversible. End-stage liver disease can be treated with orthotopic liver transplantation, but the results are suboptimal unless excess iron stores are first corrected. Hepatocellular carcinoma occurs as a late sequela in about one-third of patients who are cirrhotic at presentation despite adequate iron removal. The apparent increase in its incidence in treated patients is probably related in part to the increased life span. Hepatocellular carcinoma does not appear to develop if the disease is treated in the precirrhotic stage. Indeed, the life expectancy of homozygotes treated before the development of cirrhosis is normal.

The importance of family screening and early therapy cannot be emphasized too strongly. Asymptomatic subjects detected by family studies should have phlebotomy therapy if iron stores are moderately to severely increased. Assessment of iron stores at appropriate intervals is also important. With this management approach, most manifestations of the disease can be prevented.

BIBLIOGRAPHY

BROCK J et al: *Iron Metabolism in Health and Disease.* London, Saunders, 1994

EDWARDS CQ et al: Prevalence of hemochromatosis among 11,065 presumably healthy blood donors. N Engl J Med 318:1355, 1988

FEDER JN et al: A novel MHC class I-like gene is mutated in patients with hereditary hemochromatosis. Nat Gen 13:399, 1996

GUALDI R et al: Excess iron into hepatocytes is required for activation of collagen Type 1 gene during experimental siderosis. Gastroenterology 107:1118, 1994

HARRIS ZL et al: Aceruloplasminemia: Molecular characterization of this disorder of iron metabolism. Proc Natl Acad Sci USA 92:2539, 1995

JAZWINSKA EC et al: Localization of the hemochromatosis gene close to D6S105. Am J Hum Genet 53:347, 1993

KLAUSNER RD, HARFORD JB: Cis-trans models for post-transcriptional gene regulation. Science 246:870, 1989

NEIDERAU C et al: Long-term survival in patients with hereditary hemochromatosis. Gastroenterology, 110:1107, 1996

RAMM GA et al: Chronic iron overload causes activation of rat lipocytes in vivo. Am J Physiol 268:G451, 1995

343

Robert J. Desnick

THE PORPHYRIAS

The porphyrias are inherited or acquired disorders of specific enzymes in the heme biosynthetic pathway (Fig. 343-1). These disorders are classified as either *hepatic* or *erythropoietic* depending on the primary site of overproduction and accumulation of the porphyrin precursor or porphyrin (Tables 343-1 and 343-2), but some have overlapping features. The major manifestations of the hepatic porphyrias are neurologic, including abdominal pain, neuropathy, and mental disturbances, whereas the erythropoietic porphyrias characteristically cause cutaneous photosensitivity. The reason for neurologic involvement in the hepatic porphyrias is poorly understood. Cutaneous sensitivity to sunlight is due to the fact that excitation of excess porphyrins in the skin by long-wave ultraviolet light leads to cell damage, scarring, and deformation. Steroid hormones, drugs, and nutrition influence the production of porphyrin precursors and porphyrins, thereby precipitating or increasing the severity of some porphyrias. Thus, the porphyrias are actually *ecogenic* disorders, in which environmental, physiologic, and genetic factors interact to cause disease.

Many symptoms of the porphyrias are nonspecific, and diagnosis is often delayed. Laboratory testing can confirm or exclude the diagnosis of a porphyria. Table 343-2 summarizes the major metabolites that accumulate in each porphyria. Urinary δ-aminolevulinic acid (ALA) and porphobilinogen (PBG) are easily quantitated by chemical methods, and the urinary porphyrin isomers can be separated and quantitated by high-performance liquid chromatography. The diagnostic profile of accumulated precursors and/or porphyrins in each disorder can also be defined by extraction and thin-layer chromatography of fecal porphyrins. However, a definite diagnosis requires demonstration of the specific enzyme deficiency. The isolation and characterization of the cDNAs encoding the heme biosynthetic enzymes have permitted the definition of the molecular lesions that cause each porphyria. Molecular analyses that take advantage of this information make it possible to provide prenatal diagnoses in families with known mutations or with informative polymorphisms.

HEME BIOSYNTHESIS The first and last three enzymes in the heme biosynthetic pathway are located in the mitochondrion, whereas the other four are in the cytosol (see Fig. 343-1). The first enzyme, δ-aminolevulinate synthase (ALA synthase), catalyzes the condensation of glycine, activated by pyridoxal phosphate and succinyl coenzyme A, to form ALA. In the liver, this rate-limiting enzyme can be induced by a variety of drugs, steroids, and other chemicals. Distinct erythroid-specific and nonerythroid (i.e., housekeeping) forms of ALA synthase are encoded by separate genes. The two ALA synthase genes provide the basis for tissue-specific regulation of this pathway.

The second enzyme, δ-aminolevulinate dehydratase (ALA dehydratase), catalyzes the condensation of two molecules of ALA to form PBG. Four molecules of PBG condense to form the tetrapyrrole uroporphyrinogen III by a two-step process catalyzed by hydroxymethylbilane (HMB) synthase (also known as PBG deaminase or uroporphyrinogen I synthase) and uroporphyrinogen III (URO) synthase. HMB synthase catalyzes the head-to-tail condensation of four PBG molecules by a series of deaminations to form the linear tetrapyrrole hydroxymethylbilane. URO synthase catalyzes the rearrangement and rapid cyclization of HMB to form the asymmetric, physiologic, octacarboxylate porphyrinogen uroporphyrinogen III.

The fifth enzyme in the pathway, uroporphyrinogen decarboxylase (URO decarboxylase), catalyzes the sequential removal of the four carboxyl groups from the acetic acid side chains of uroporphyrinogen III to form coproporphyrinogen III, a tetracarboxylate porphyrinogen. This compound then enters the mitochondrion, where coproporphyrinogen (COPRO) oxidase, the sixth enzyme, catalyzes the decarboxylation of two of the four propionic acid groups to form the two vinyl groups of protoporphyrinogen IX, a dicarboxylate porphyrinogen. Next, protoporphyrinogen (PROTO) oxidase oxidizes protoporphyrinogen IX to protoporphyrin IX by the removal of six hydrogen atoms. The product of the reaction is a porphyrin (oxidized form), in contrast to the preceding tetrapyrrole intermediates, which are porphyrinogens (reduced forms). Finally, ferrous iron is inserted into protoporphyrin IX to form heme, a reaction catalyzed by the eighth enzyme in the pathway, ferrochelatase (also known as heme synthetase or protoheme ferrolyase).

Each of the heme biosynthetic enzymes is encoded by a separate gene. Full-length human cDNAs for each of the enzymes, including those for both forms of ALA synthase, have been isolated and sequenced, and the chromosomal locations of the genes have been identified (Table 343-3).

REGULATION OF HEME BIOSYNTHESIS About 85 percent of the heme produced in the body is synthesized in erythroid cells to provide heme for hemoglobin, and most of the remainder is produced in the liver, where the biosynthetic pathway is under negative feedback control. "Free" heme in the liver regulates the synthesis and mitochondrial translocation of the housekeeping form of ALA synthase. Heme represses the synthesis of the ALA synthase mRNA and interferes with the transport of the enzyme from the cysotol into mitochondria. ALA synthase is inducible by many of the same chemicals that induce the cytochrome P450 enzymes in the endoplasmic reticulum of the liver. Because most of the heme in the liver is used for the synthesis of cytochrome P450 enzymes, hepatic ALA synthase and the cytochrome P450s are regulated in a coordinated fashion.

Different regulatory mechanisms control production of heme for hemoglobin. The erythroid-specific ALA synthase encoded on the X chromosome is expressed at higher levels than the hepatic enzyme, and an erythroid-specific control mechanism regulates iron transport into erythroid cells. During erythroid differentiation, the activities of the heme biosynthetic enzymes increase in a coordinated fashion.

THE HEPATIC PORPHYRIAS

The acute hepatic porphyrias are characterized by the rapid onset of neurologic manifestations. During the acute attack, individuals have

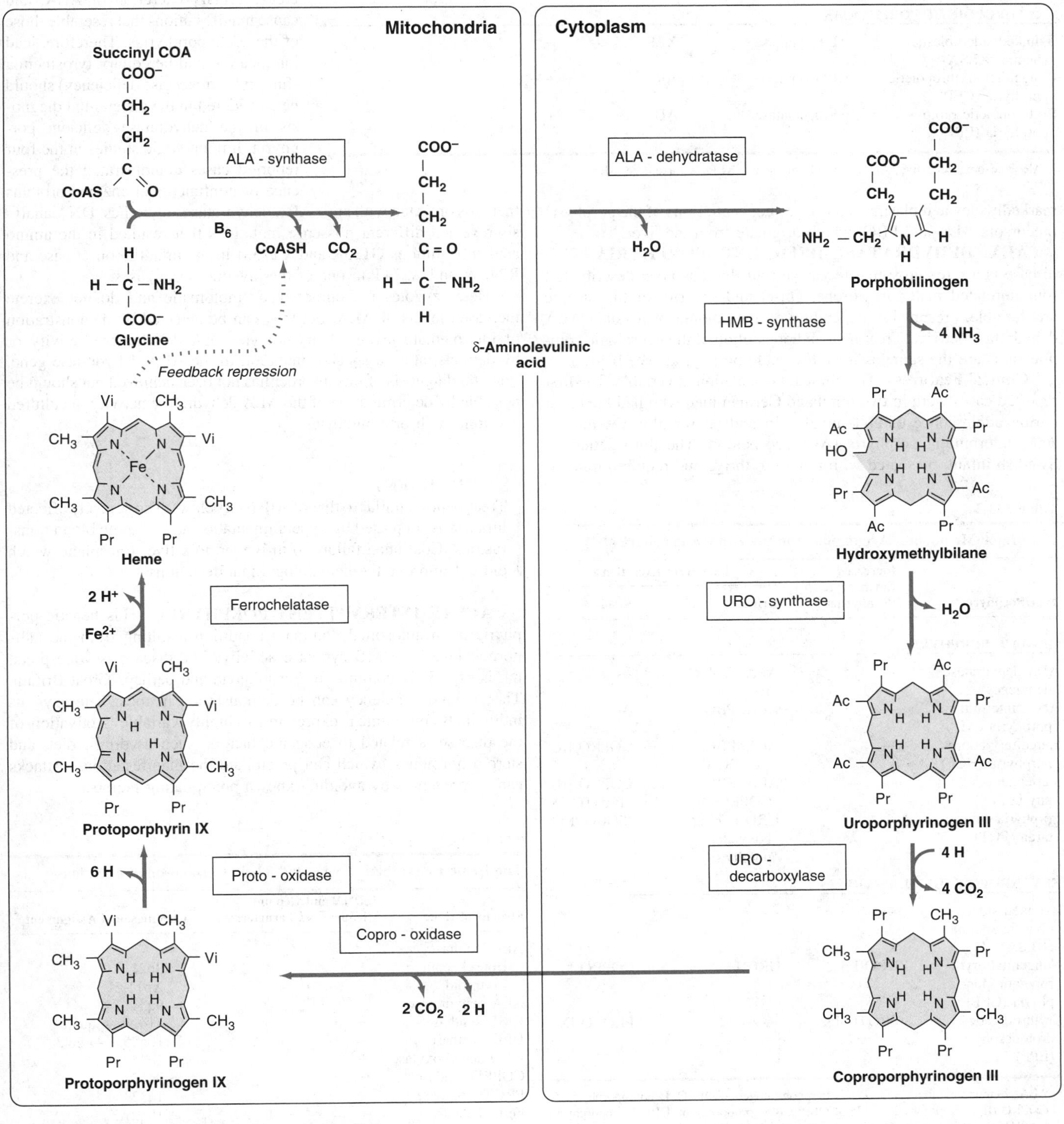

FIGURE 343-1 The human heme biosynthetic pathway.

Table 343-1

Classification of the Human Porphyrias

Type/Porphyria	Deficient Enzyme	Inheritance*	Photosensitivity	Neurovisceral Symptoms
HEPATIC PORPHYRIAS				
ALA dehydratase deficiency	ALA dehydratase	AR	−	+
Acute intermittent porphyria (AIP)	HMB synthase	AD	−	+
Hereditary coproporphyria (HCP)	COPRO oxidase	AD	+	+
Variegate porphyria (VP)	PROTO oxidase	AD	+	+
Porphyria cutanea tarda (PCT)	URO decarboxylase	AD	+	−
ERYTHROPOIETIC PORPHYRIAS				
X-linked sideroblastic anemia (XLSA)	ALA synthase	XLR	−	−
Congenital erythropoietic porphyria (CEP)	URO synthase	AR	+ + +	−
Erythropoietic protoporphyria (EPP)	Ferrochelatase	AD	+	−

* AR, autosomal recessive; AD, autosomal dominant; XLR, X-linked recessive.

markedly elevated plasma and urinary concentrations of the porphyrin precursors ALA and PBG, which originate from the liver.

ALA DEHYDRATASE–DEFICIENT PORPHYRIA This disease is a rare autosomal recessive trait that has been described in four unrelated males in Europe. Onset and severity of the disease are variable, presumably depending on the amount of residual ALA dehydratase activity. Treatment and prevention of the neurologic complications are the same as for other acute porphyrias (see below).

Clinical Features The clinical presentation is variable. The first reported cases were in two unrelated German men who had the onset during adolescence of abdominal pain and neuropathy, resembling acute intermittent porphyria (AIP; see below). The third patient, a Swedish infant, presented with failure to thrive and required transfusions and parenteral nutrition. Presumably, the earlier age of onset and more severe manifestations reflect a more complete enzyme deficiency. The fourth patient, a Belgian man, developed an acute motor polyneuropathy and polycythemia at age 63.

Diagnosis All four patients had increased urinary levels of ALA and coproporphyrin. ALA dehydratase activity in erythrocytes was <5 percent of normal. Both succinylacetone (which accumulates in hereditary tyrosinemia and is structurally similar to ALA) and lead can inhibit ALA dehydratase, increase urinary excretion of ALA, and cause manifestations that resemble those of the acute porphyrias. Therefore, lead intoxication and hereditary tyrosinemia (fumarylacetoacetase deficiency) should be considered in the differential diagnosis of the dehydratase-deficient porphyria. Immunologic studies in the four reported cases demonstrated the presence of nonfunctional enzyme proteins that cross-reacted with anti–ALA dehydratase antibodies. DNA analysis revealed different missense mutations that resulted in the amino acid substitutions G133R and V275M in the infantile-onset case and R240W and A274T in one of the juvenile-onset cases.

Heterozygotes are clinically asymptomatic and do not excrete increased levels of ALA, but they can be detected by demonstration of intermediate levels of erythrocyte ALA dehydratase activity or by demonstrating a specific mutation in the ALA dehydratase gene. Prenatal diagnosis of this disorder has not been achieved but should be possible by determination of the ALA dehydratase activity in cultured chorionic villi or amniocytes.

Table 343-2

The Major Metabolites Accumulated in the Human Porphyrias

Type/Porphyria	Increased Erythrocyte Porphyrins	Porphyrin Excretion*: Urine	Porphyrin Excretion*: Stool
HEPATIC PORPHYRIAS			
ALA dehydratase deficiency	—	ALA, COPRO III	—
Acute intermittent porphyria (AIP)	—	ALA, PBG	—
Hereditary coproporphyria (HCP)	—	ALA, PBG, COPRO III	COPRO III
Variegate porphyria (VP)	—	ALA, PBG COPRO III	COPRO III, PROTO IX
Porphyria cutanea tarda (PCT)	—	URO I, 7-carboxylate, porphyrin	ISOCOPRO
ERYTHROPOIETIC PORPHYRIAS			
X-linked sideroblastic anemia (XLSA)	—	—	—
Congenital erythropoietic porphyria (CEP)	URO I	URO I	COPRO I
Erythropoietic protoporphyria (EPP)	PROTO IX	—	PROTO IX

* ALA, δ-aminolevulinic acid; PBG, porphobilinogen; COPRO I, coproporphyrin I; COPRO III, coproporphyrin III; ISOCOPRO, isocoproporphyrin; URO I, uroporphyrin I; URO III, uroporphyrin III; PROTO, protoporphyrin IX

℞ TREATMENT

Treatment is similar to that of AIP (see below). The severely affected infant was supported by hyperalimentation and periodic blood transfusions. Continued failure to thrive led to a liver transplant, which did not improve the hematologic manifestations.

ACUTE INTERMITTENT PORPHYRIA This hepatic porphyria is an autosomal dominant condition resulting from the half-normal level of HMB synthase activity. The disease is widespread but is especially common in Scandinavia and perhaps Great Britain. The enzyme deficiency can be demonstrated in most heterozygous individuals, but clinical expression is highly variable. Activation of the disease is related to ecogenic factors, such as drugs, diet, and steroid hormones, which can precipitate the manifestations. Attacks can be prevented by avoiding known precipitating factors.

Table 343-3

The Heme Biosynthetic Genes and Their Chromosomal Locations

Structural Gene	cDNA and Genomic Sequences Characterized	Chromosomal Assignment
ALA synthase		
Housekeeping	+	3p21
Erythroid	+	Xp11.21
ALA dehydratase	+	9q34
HMB synthase	+	11q23 → qter
URO synthase	+	10q25.3 → 26.3
URO decarboxylase	+	1p34
COPRO oxidase	−	3q12
PROTO oxidase	−	1q32
Ferrochelatase	+	18q21.3

Table 343-4

Categories of Unsafe and Safe Drugs in AIP, HCP, and VP

Unsafe	Safe
Barbiturates	Narcotic analgesics
Sulfonamide antibiotics	Aspirin
Meprobamate	Acetaminophen
Glutethimide	Phenothiazines
Methyprylon	Penicillin and derivatives
Ethchlorvynol	Streptomycin
Mephenytoin	Glucocorticoids
Succinimides	Bromides
Carbamazepine	Insulin
Valproic acid	Atropine
Pyrazolones	
Griseofulvin	
Ergots	
Synthetic estrogens and progestogens	
Danazol	
Alcohol	

Clinical Features Most heterozygotes remain clinically asymptomatic (latent) unless exposed to factors that increase the production of porphyrins. Endogenous and exogenous gonadal steroids, porphyrinogenic drugs, alcohol ingestion, and low-calorie diets, usually instituted to produce weight loss, are common precipitating factors. Table 343-4 lists the major drugs that are harmful in AIP [and also in hereditary coproporphyria (HCP) and variegate porphyria (VP)] and some drugs and anesthetic agents known to be safe. More extensive lists of drugs considered harmful or safe are available (see the bibliography), but information is incomplete for many of them. Attacks also can be provoked by infections and by surgery.

Because the neurovisceral symptoms rarely occur before puberty and are often nonspecific, a high index of suspicion is required to make the diagnosis. The disease can be disabling but is rarely fatal. Abdominal pain, the most common symptom, is usually steady and poorly localized but may be cramping. Ileus, abdominal distention, and decreased bowel sounds are common. However, increased bowel sounds and diarrhea may occur. Abdominal tenderness, fever, and leukocytosis are usually absent or mild because the symptoms are neurologic rather than inflammatory. Nausea, vomiting, constipation, tachycardia, hypertension, mental symptoms, pain in the limbs, head, neck, or chest, muscle weakness, sensory loss, dysuria, and urinary retention are characteristic. Tachycardia, hypertension, restlessness, tremors, and excess sweating are due to sympathetic overactivity.

The peripheral neuropathy is due to axonal degeneration (rather than demyelinization) and affects primarily motor neurons. Significant neuropathy does not occur with all acute attacks; abdominal symptoms are usually more prominent. Motor neuropathy affects the proximal muscles initially, more often in the shoulders and arms. The course and degree of involvement are variable. Deep tendon reflexes may be normal or hyperactive but are usually decreased or absent with advanced neuropathy. Motor weakness can be asymmetric and focal and may involve cranial nerves. Sensory changes such as paresthesias and loss of sensation are less prominent. Progressive muscle weakness can lead to respiratory and bulbar paralysis and death when diagnosis and treatment are delayed. Sudden death may result from sympathetic overactivity and cardiac arrhythmia.

Mental symptoms such as anxiety, insomnia, depression, disorientation, hallucinations, and paranoia can occur in acute attacks. Seizures can be due to neurologic effects or to hyponatremia. Treatment of seizures is difficult because virtually all antiseizure drugs (except bromides) may exacerbate AIP (clonazepam may be safer than phenytoin or barbiturates). Hyponatremia results from hypothalamic involvement and inappropriate vasopressin secretion or from electrolyte depletion due to vomiting, diarrhea, poor intake, or excess renal sodium loss. Persistent hypertension and impaired renal function may occur. When an attack resolves, abdominal pain may disappear within hours, and paresis begins to improve within days and may continue to improve over several years.

Diagnosis ALA and PBG levels are increased in plasma and urine during acute attacks. Urinary PBG excretion is usually 220 to 880 μmol/d (50 to 200 mg/d) [normal, 0 to 18 μmol/d (0 to 4 mg/d)], and urinary ALA excretion is 150 to 760 μmol/d (20 to 100 mg/d) (normal, 8 to 53 μmol/d [1 to 7 mg/d]). The excretion of these compounds generally decreases with clinical improvement, particularly after hematin infusions (see below). A normal urinary PBG level effectively excludes AIP as a cause for current symptoms. Fecal porphyrins are usually normal or minimally increased in AIP, in contrast to HCP and VP. Most asymptomatic ("latent") heterozygotes with HMB synthase deficiency have normal urinary excretion of ALA and PBG. Therefore, measurement of HMB synthase in erythrocytes is useful to confirm the diagnosis and to screen asymptomatic family members.

The enzyme deficiency is detectable in erythrocytes from most AIP heterozygotes (*classic AIP*). However, the activity is higher in young erythrocytes and may increase into the normal range in AIP when erythropoiesis is increased due to a concurrent condition. However, patients with the rare erythroid form of AIP (*erythroid AIP*) have normal enzyme levels in erythrocytes and deficient activity in nonerythroid tissues (see below). The erythroid and housekeeping forms of HMB synthase are encoded by a single gene, which has two promoters. One promotes transcription of messenger RNA for the housekeeping form found in all tissues, and the other promotes formation of the erythroid-specific transcript. Several deletions and over 45 different point mutations in the coding region of the gene have been found in unrelated AIP families (Fig. 343-2). These mutations alter the kinetic properties and/or stability of the mutant enzymes or create premature termination codons. Mutations that cause erythroid AIP variants with half-normal enzyme in nonerythroid tissues but normal activity in erythrocytes include point mutations in the initiation methionine codon (that prevent translation) or in the 5′ splice site

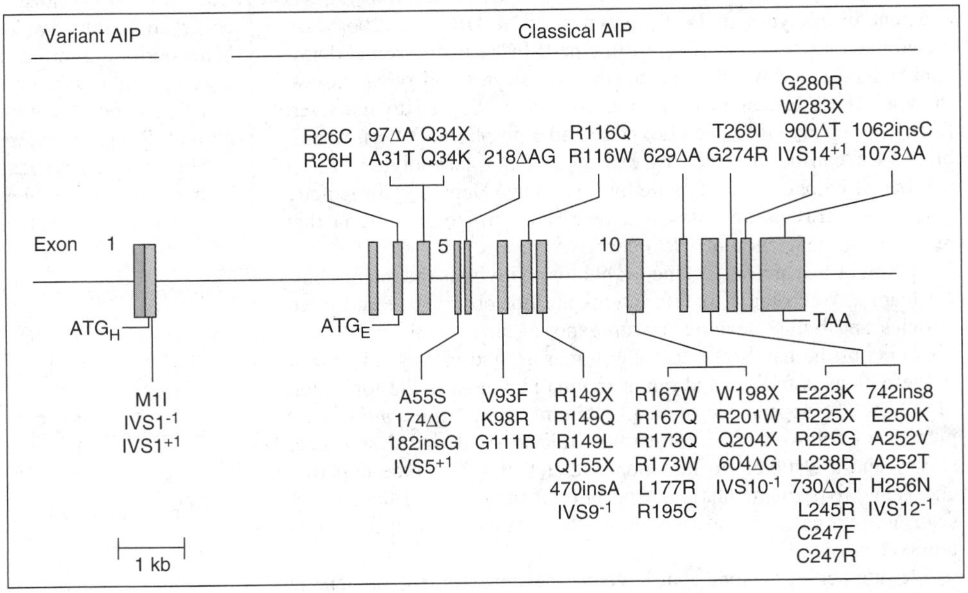

FIGURE 343-2 Mutations in the HMB synthase gene causing AIP. Mutation nomenclature: letters, one-letter code for amino acids; numbers, codon positions.

of intron 1 (that cause abnormal splicing of the HMB synthase transcript).

Heterozygotes can be identified by restriction fragment length polymorphism (RFLP) studies in informative families using various polymorphic sites in the HMB synthase gene. Efforts are now under way to identify the specific mutations in the HMB synthase gene in all AIP families; this information will make it possible to identify all heterozygotes in affected families and to advise them to avoid the factors known to cause acute attacks. The prenatal diagnosis of a fetus at risk can be made with cultured amniotic cells or chorionic villi.

℞ TREATMENT

During acute attacks, narcotic analgesics may be required for abdominal pain, and phenothiazines are useful for nausea, vomiting, anxiety, and restlessness. Chloral hydrate can be given for insomnia, and benzodiazepines in low doses are probably safe if a minor tranquilizer is required. Although intravenous glucose (at least 300 g/d) has been given for acute attacks of porphyria, a more complete parenteral nutritional regimen may be beneficial if oral feeding is not possible for a prolonged period. However, intravenous heme is more effective than glucose in reducing porphyrin precursor excretion and probably leads to more rapid recovery. The response to heme therapy is reduced if therapy is delayed. Therefore, 3 to 4 mg of heme, in the form of hematin (Abbott Laboratories), heme albumin, or heme arginate (Leiras Oy, Turku, Finland), may be infused daily for 4 days beginning as soon as possible after onset of an attack. Heme arginate and heme albumin are chemically stable and are less likely than hematin to produce phlebitis or an anticoagulant effect. The rate of recovery from an acute attack depends on the degree of neuronal damage and may be rapid (1 to 2 days) with prompt therapy. Recovery from severe motor neuropathy may continue for months or years. Identification and avoidance of inciting factors can hasten recovery from an attack and prevent future attacks. Multiple inciting factors may contribute to a symptomatic episode. Frequent clear-cut cyclical attacks occur in some women and can be prevented with a luteinizing hormone–releasing hormone analogue (this indication is not approved by the U.S. Food and Drug Administration).

PORPHYRIA CUTANEA TARDA Porphyria cutanea tarda (PCT), the most common of the porphyrias, can be sporadic (type I) or familial (types II and III) and also can develop after exposure to halogenated aromatic hydrocarbons. Hepatic URO decarboxylase is deficient in all types of PCT. In type I PCT, URO decarboxylase activity is normal in erythrocytes. In type II PCT, an autosomal dominant trait, the enzyme is deficient in erythrocytes and other tissues. In type III PCT, deficiency of the enzyme is limited to the liver. Deficient hepatic URO decarboxylase and a porphyrin pattern resembling PCT can be produced by exposure of normal individuals to a number of halogenated aromatic hydrocarbons. Hepatoerythropoietic porphyria (HEP) is an autosomal recessive form of porphyria that results from deficiency of URO decarboxylase.

Clinical Features Cutaneous photosensitivity is the major clinical feature. Neurologic manifestations are not observed. Fluid-filled vesicles and bullae develop on sun-exposed areas such as the face, the dorsa of the hands and feet, the forearms, and the legs. The skin in these areas is friable, and minor trauma may lead to the formation of bullae. The appearance of small white plaques, termed *milia*, may precede or follow vesicle formation. Bullae and denuded skin heal slowly and are subject to infection. Other features include hypertrichosis and hyperpigmentation, especially of the face, and thickening, scarring, and calcification resembling the cutaneous changes of systemic sclerosis.

A number of factors contribute to the development of hepatic URO decarboxylase deficiency, including excess alcohol, iron, and estrogens. PCT also can be induced by various chemicals; an epidemic of PCT occurred in eastern Turkey in the 1950s as a result of consumption of wheat contaminated with the fungicide hexachlorobenzene. Hexachlorobenzene produces a disorder similar to PCT and induces hepatic URO decarboxylase deficiency in animals. PCT in humans has occurred after exposure to other chemicals, including di- and trichlorophenols and 2,3,7,8-tetrachlorodibenzo-(p)-dioxin (TCDD, dioxin). Patients with PCT characteristically have liver damage and are at risk for hepatocellular carcinoma. These carcinomas do not produce porphyrins.

Hepatoerythropoietic porphyria (HEP) resembles congenital erythropoietic porphyria (CEP) but also has erythropoietic features and usually presents with blistering skin lesions, hypertrichosis, scarring, and red urine in infancy or childhood.

Diagnosis Porphyrins are increased in the liver, plasma, urine, and stool. The urinary ALA level may be slightly increased, but the PBG level is normal. Urinary porphyrins consist mostly of uroporphyrin and 7-carboxylate porphyrin, with lesser amounts of coproporphyrin and 5- and 6-carboxylate porphyrins. Plasma porphyrins also are increased in a pattern that resembles that in urine. Isocoproporphyrins are increased in feces and sometimes also in plasma and urine. The finding of increased isocoproporphyrins is diagnostic for a deficiency of hepatic URO decarboxylase.

Type II PCT and HEP can be distinguished by finding low activity of URO decarboxylase in erythrocytes. URO decarboxylase activity in liver, erythrocytes, and cultured skin fibroblasts in type II PCT is approximately 50 percent of normal in affected individuals and in family members with latent disease. In HEP, the URO decarboxylase activity is 3 to 28 percent of normal. Several point mutations have been identified in the coding region of the URO decarboxylase gene from unrelated type II PCT and HEP patients (Fig. 343-3). Hepatic iron contributes to development of sporadic and familial forms of PCT. In the familial forms (types II and III), iron inhibits the residual normal enzyme, so that enzymatic activity in liver is less than 50 percent of normal. In type I PCT the decreased hepatic URO decarboxylase activity is not accompanied by a decrease in the amount of enzyme protein, suggesting that the enzyme is present in an inactive form, and hepatic URO decarboxylase activity gradually increases after a remission is induced by phlebotomy.

℞ TREATMENT

Alcohol, estrogens, iron supplements, and, if possible, any drugs that may exacerbate the disease should be discontinued, but this step does not always lead to improvement. A complete response can almost always be achieved by repeated phlebotomy to reduce hepatic iron. A unit (450 mL) of blood can be removed every 1 to 2 weeks. Because iron overload is not marked in most cases, remission may occur after only five or six phlebotomies. Hemoglobin levels or hematocrits and serum ferritin should be followed closely to prevent development of iron deficiency and anemia. After remission, continued phlebotomy may not be needed even if ferritin levels return to normal. Relapses are treated by additional phlebotomy.

PCT also can be treated with chloroquine or hydroxychloroquine, both of which complex with the excess porphyrins and promote their excretion. Small doses (e.g., 125 mg chloroquine phosphate

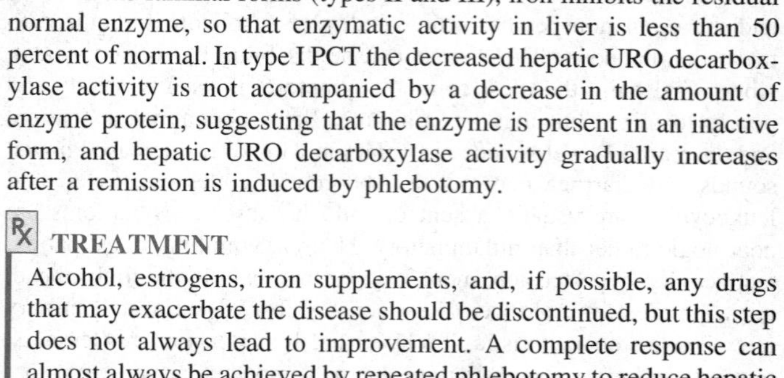

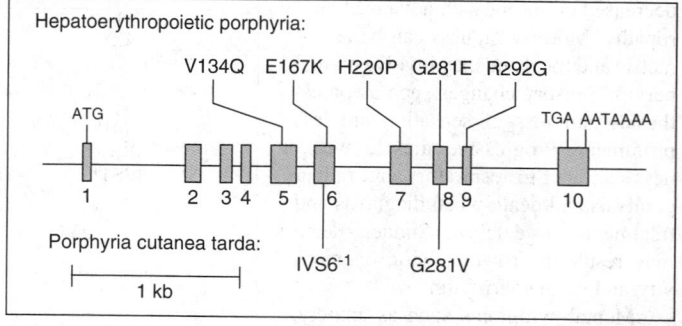

FIGURE 343-3 Mutations in the URO synthase gene causing familial PCP and HEP. Mutation nomenclature as in Fig. 343-2.

twice weekly) should be given, because standard doses can induce transient, sometimes marked increases in photosensitivity and hepatocellular damage. Hepatic imaging may be advisable to exclude complicating hepatocellular carcinoma. Treatment of PCT in patients with end-stage renal disease is facilitated by administration of erythropoietin.

HEREDITARY COPROPORPHYRIA Hereditary coproporphyria (HCP) is an autosomal dominant form of hepatic porphyria that results from deficiency of COPRO oxidase. Photosensitivity may occur. A few cases of homozygous HCP have been reported.

Clinical Features HCP is influenced by the same factors that cause attacks in AIP. The disease is latent before puberty, and symptoms are more common in women. Neurovisceral symptoms and other manifestations are virtually identical to those of AIP. Photosensitivity may resemble that in PCT and VP. Cutaneous lesions may begin in childhood in homozygous cases.

Diagnosis Coproporphyrin is markedly increased in the urine and feces in symptomatic disease and sometimes when there are no symptoms. Urinary ALA and PBG levels are increased during acute attacks but may return to normal when symptoms resolve. Although the diagnosis can be confirmed by measuring COPRO oxidase activity, these assays are not widely available and require cells other than erythrocytes.

℞ TREATMENT

Neurologic symptoms are treated as in AIP (see above). Phlebotomy and chloroquine are ineffective when cutaneous lesions are present.

VARIEGATE PORPHYRIA VP is a hepatic porphyria that results from the deficient activity of PROTO oxidase, is inherited as an autosomal dominant trait, and can present with neurologic symptoms, photosensitivity, or both.

Clinical Features Neurovisceral signs and symptoms develop after puberty and are similar to those of AIP or HCP (see above). Attacks are provoked by the same drugs, steroids, and nutritional factors that are detrimental in AIP. Skin manifestations are more common than in HCP but usually occur apart from the neurovisceral symptoms. Since the skin lesions in VP, HCP, and PCT are not distinguishable by clinical examination or biopsy, these conditions must be diagnosed by assay of porphyrins and porphyrin precursors in blood, urine, and feces.

VP is particularly common in South Africa, where 3 of every 1000 whites have the disorder. Most are descendants of a couple who emigrated from Holland to South Africa in 1688. Homozygous VP is associated with photosensitivity, neurologic symptoms, and developmental disturbances, including growth retardation, in infancy or childhood; all cases had increased erythrocyte levels of zinc protoporphyrin, a characteristic finding in all homozygous porphyrias so far described.

Dual porphyria, the simultaneous occurrence of VP and familial PCT, has been documented in several kindreds. *Chester porphyria* was described in a large British family in which individuals had acute porphyric attacks and deficiency of both PROTO oxidase and HMB synthase. Photosensitivity was not observed. It is unclear whether Chester porphyria is a variant of VP or AIP.

Diagnosis When VP is symptomatic, levels of fecal protoporphyrin and coproporphyrin and of urinary coproporphyrin are increased. Urinary ALA and PBG levels are increased during acute attacks. Plasma levels of porphyrins are increased, particularly when there are cutaneous lesions. VP can be distinguished rapidly from all other porphyrias by examining the fluorescence emission spectrum of porphyrins in plasma at neutral pH. This test is particularly useful for differentiating VP from PCT.

Assays of PROTO oxidase activity in cultured fibroblasts or lymphocytes are not widely available. Some latent cases of VP can be diagnosed by measurement of fecal porphyrins in relatives of VP patients.

℞ TREATMENT

Acute attacks are treated with hematin as in AIP. Other than avoiding sun exposure, there are few effective measures for treating the skin lesions. β-Carotene, phlebotomy, and chloroquine are not helpful.

THE ERYTHROPOIETIC PORPHYRIAS

In the erythropoietic porphyrias, porphyrins from bone marrow erythrocytes and plasma are deposited in the skin and lead to cutaneous photosensitivity.

X-LINKED SIDEROBLASTIC ANEMIA X-linked sideroblastic anemia (XLSA) results from the deficient activity of the erythroid form of ALA synthase and is associated with ineffective erythropoiesis, weakness, and pallor.

Clinical Features Males with XLSA develop refractory hemolytic anemia, pallor, and weakness during infancy. They have secondary hypersplenism, become iron overloaded, and can develop hemosiderosis. The severity depends on the level of residual erythroid ALA synthase activity and on the responsiveness of the specific mutation to pyridoxal 5′-phosphate supplementation (see below). Peripheral blood smears reveal a hypochromic, microcytic anemia with striking anisocytosis, poikilocytosis, and polychromasia; the leukocytes and platelets appear normal. Hemoglobin content is reduced, and the mean corpuscular volume and mean corpuscular hemoglobin concentration are decreased.

Diagnosis Bone marrow examination reveals a hypercellular marrow with a left shift and megaloblastic erythropoiesis with an abnormal maturation. A variety of Prussian blue–staining sideroblasts are observed. Levels of urinary porphyrin precursors and of both urinary and fecal porphyrins are normal. The level of erythroid ALA synthase is decreased in bone marrow, but this enzyme is difficult to measure in the presence of the normal housekeeping enzyme. Definitive diagnosis requires the demonstration of mutations in the erythroid ALA synthase gene.

℞ TREATMENT

The severe anemia may respond to pyridoxine supplementation. This cofactor is essential for ALA synthase activity, and mutations in the pyridoxine binding site of the enzyme have been found in several responsive patients. Cofactor supplementation may make it possible to eliminate or reduce the frequency of transfusion. Unresponsive patients may be transfusion-dependent and require chelation therapy.

CONGENITAL ERYTHROPOIETIC PORPHYRIA Congenital erythropoietic porphyria (CEP) is an autosomal recessive disorder, also known as *Gunther's disease*, that is due to deficiency of URO synthase activity and is associated with hemolytic anemia and cutaneous lesions. CEP is characterized by accumulation of the type I isomers of uroporphyrin and coproporphyrin.

Clinical Features Severe cutaneous photosensitivity begins in early infancy. The skin over sun-exposed areas is friable, and bullae and vesicles are prone to rupture and infection. Skin thickening, focal hypo- and hyperpigmentation, and hypertrichosis of the face and extremities are characteristic. Secondary infection can lead to disfiguring of the face and hands. Porphyrins are deposited in teeth and in bones. As a result, the teeth are reddish brown and fluoresce on exposure to long-wave ultraviolet light. Hemolysis is probably due to the marked increase in erythrocyte porphyrins and leads to splenomegaly. A milder form of the disease begins in adulthood.

Diagnosis Uroporphyrin and coproporphyrin (mostly isomer I) accumulate in the bone marrow, erythrocytes, plasma, urine, and feces. The diagnosis should be confirmed by demonstration of markedly deficient URO synthase activity. The disease can be detected in utero by measuring porphyrins in amniotic fluid and URO synthase activity in cultured amniotic cells or chorionic villi. Molecular analyses of the mutant alleles from over 20 unrelated patients have revealed the presence of gene rearrangements, an mRNA processing defect, and several point mutations that cause amino acid substitutions.

℞ **TREATMENT**

The transfusion of sufficient blood to suppress erythropoiesis is effective but results in iron overload. Splenectomy may reduce hemolysis and decrease transfusion requirements. Protection from sunlight and from minor skin trauma is important. β-Carotene may be of some value. Complicating bacterial infections should be treated promptly. Bone marrow transplantation was tried in one patient, who died from transplant complications.

ERYTHROPOIETIC PROTOPORPHYRIA Erythropoietic protoporphyria (EPP) is due to the partial deficiency of ferrochelatase and is inherited as an autosomal dominant trait. Protoporphyrin accumulates in erythroid cells and plasma and is excreted in bile and feces. EPP is the most common erythropoietic porphyria and, after PCT, the second most common porphyria.

Clinical Features Skin photosensitivity usually begins in childhood. The skin manifestations differ from those of other porphyrias. Vesicular lesions are uncommon. Redness, swelling, burning, and itching can develop within minutes of sun exposure and resemble angioedema. Symptoms may seem out of proportion to the visible skin lesions. Sparse vesicles and bullae occur in 10 percent of cases. Chronic skin changes may include lichenification, leathery pseudovesicles, labial grooving, and nail changes. Severe scarring is rare, as are pigment changes, friability, and hirsutism.

The primary source of excess protoporphyrin is the bone marrow reticulocyte. Erythrocyte protoporphyrin is free (not complexed with zinc) and is mostly bound to hemoglobin. In plasma protoporphyrin is bound to albumin. Hemolysis and anemia are usually absent or mild.

Liver function is usually normal, but in some patients accumulation of protoporphyrin causes chronic liver disease that can progress to liver failure and death. The hepatic complications are often preceded by increasing levels of erythrocyte and plasma protoporphyrin and probably result, in part, from protoporphyrin accumulation in the liver. Protoporphyrin is insoluble, forms crystalline structures in liver cells, and can decrease hepatic bile flow. Gallstones composed at least in part of protoporphyrin occur in some patients.

Some obligate heterozygotes are asymptomatic and have little or no increase in erythrocyte protoporphyrin. Thus there is phenotypic variation in this disease.

Diagnosis Protoporphyrin levels are increased in bone marrow, circulating erythrocytes, plasma, bile, and feces. Urinary levels of porphyrin and porphyrin precursors are normal. Ferrochelatase activity in cultured lymphocytes or fibroblasts is decreased.

℞ **TREATMENT**

Oral β-carotene (Hoffmann-LaRoche) (120 to 180 mg/d) improves tolerance to sunlight in many patients. The dosage may need to be adjusted to maintain serum carotene levels in the recommended range of 10 to 15 μmol/L (600 to 800 μg/dL). Mild skin discoloration due to carotenemia is the only significant side effect. The beneficial effects of β-carotene may involve quenching of singlet oxygen or free radicals. Unfortunately, this drug is less effective in other forms of porphyria associated with photosensitivity.

Treatment of hepatic complications is difficult. However, cholestyramine and other porphyrin absorbents such as activated charcoal may interrupt the enterohepatic circulation of protoporphyrin and promote its fecal excretion, leading to some improvement. Splenectomy may be helpful when the disease is accompanied by hemolysis and significant splenomegaly. Caloric restriction and drugs or hormones that may induce the heme pathway or impair hepatic excretory function should be avoided. Iron deficiency should be prevented or treated. Transfusions or intravenous heme therapy may suppress erythroid and hepatic protoporphyrin production and are sometimes beneficial. Liver transplantation has been carried out in some patients with severe liver complications.

BIBLIOGRAPHY

Anderson KE et al: A GnRH analogue prevents cyclical attacks of porphyria. Arch Intern Med 150:1469, 1990

Astrin KH, Desnick RJ: Molecular basis of acute intermittent porphyria. Hum Mutation 4:243, 1994

Cotter PD et al: Enzymatic defect in "X-linked" sideroblastic anemia: Molecular evidence for erythroid δ-aminolevulinate synthase deficiency. Proc Natl Acad Sci USA 89:4028, 1992

Desnick RJ, Anderson KE: Heme biosynthesis and its disorders: Porphyrias and sideroblastic anemias, in *Hematology: Basic Principles and Practices,* 2d ed, R Hoffman et al (eds). New York, Churchill Livingstone, 1995, pp 523–545

Kappas A et al: The porphyrias, in *The Metabolic and Molecular Bases of Inherited Disease,* 7th ed, CR Scriver et al (eds). New York, McGraw-Hill, 1995, pp 2103–2159

Moore MR et al: *Disorders of Porphyrin Metabolism.* New York, Plenum, 1987

Mustajoki P, Nordmann Y: Early administration of heme arginate for acute porphyric attacks. Ann Intern Med 153:2004, 1993

Plewinska M et al: δ-Aminolevulinate dehydratase deficient porphyria: Identification of the molecular lesions in a severely affected homozygote. Am J Hum Genet 49:167, 1991

Xu W et al: Congenital erythropoietic porphyria: Identification and expression of 10 mutations in the uroporphyrinogen III synthase gene. J Clin Invest 95:905, 1995

344

Robert L. Wortmann

GOUT AND OTHER DISORDERS OF PURINE METABOLISM

Gout encompasses a group of disorders that occur alone or in combination and include (1) hyperuricemia, (2) attacks of acute, typically monarticular, inflammatory arthritis, (3) tophaceous deposition of urate crystals in and around joints, (4) interstitial deposition of urate crystals in renal parenchyma, and (5) urolithiasis. *Hyperuricemia,* the cardinal feature and prerequisite for gout, is defined as a plasma urate level greater than 420 μmol/L (7.0 mg/dL) and indicates that total-body urate is increased. Hyperuricemia can result from increased production or decreased excretion of uric acid or from a combination of the two processes. When hyperuricemia exists, plasma and extracellular fluids are supersaturated with respect to urate, and conditions favor crystal formation and tissue deposition. These conditions cause the clinical manifestations included in the term *gout.*

URIC ACID METABOLISM Uric acid is the final breakdown product of purine degradation in humans. It is a weak acid with pK_as of 5.75 and 10.3. Urates, the ionized forms of uric acid, predominate in plasma, extracellular fluid, and synovial fluid, with approximately 98 percent existing as monosodium urate at pH 7.4. Monosodium urate is easily ultrafiltered and dialyzed from plasma. Binding of urate to plasma proteins has little physiologic significance.

Plasma is saturated with monosodium urate at a concentration of 415 μmol/L (6.8 mg/dL) at 37°C. At higher concentrations, plasma is therefore supersaturated, and potential exists for urate crystal precipitation. However, precipitation does not occur even at plasma urate concentrations as high as 4800 μmol/L (80 mg/dL), perhaps because of the presence of solubilizing substances in plasma.

Uric acid is more soluble in urine than in water, possibly because of the presence of urea, proteins, and mucopolysaccharides. The pH of urine greatly influences its solubility. At pH 5.0, urine is saturated with uric acid at concentrations ranging from 360 to 900 μmol/L (6 to 15 mg/dL). At pH 7.0, saturation is reached at concentrations between 9480 and 12,000 μmol/L (158 and 200 mg/dL). Ionized forms of uric acid in urine include mono- and disodium, potassium, ammonium, and calcium urates.

Although purine nucleotides are synthesized and degraded in all tissues, urate is produced only in tissues that contain xanthine oxidase, primarily liver and small intestine. The amount of urate in the body is the net result of the amount produced and the amount excreted (Fig. 344-1). Urate production varies with the purine content of the diet and the rates of purine biosynthesis, degradation, and salvage. Normally, two-thirds to three-fourths of urate is excreted by the kidneys, and most of the remainder is eliminated through the intestines. A three-component model that includes glomerular filtration and both tubular secretion and reabsorption is proposed for the renal handling of uric acid in humans (Fig. 344-2). Approximately 8 to 12 percent of urate filtered by the glomeruli is excreted in the urine as uric acid. After filtration, 98 to 100 percent of the urate is reabsorbed, about half the reabsorbed urate is secreted back into the proximal tubule, and about 40 percent of that is again reabsorbed.

Serum urate levels vary with age and sex. Most children have serum urate concentrations of 180 to 240 μmol/L (3.0 to 4.0 mg/dL). Levels begin to rise during puberty in males but remain low in females until menopause. Although the cause of this gender variation is not completely understood, it is in part due to higher excretion of urate in females and is attributable to hormonal influences. Mean serum urate values for adult men and premenopausal women are 415 and 360 μmol/L (6.8 and 6.0 mg/dL), respectively. After menopause, values for women increase to approximate those of men. Adult concentrations rise steadily over time and vary with height, body weight, blood pressure, renal function, and alcohol intake.

HYPERURICEMIA

Hyperuricemia may be defined as a plasma (or serum) urate concentration greater than 420 μmol/L (7.0 mg/dL). This definition is based on physicochemical, epidemiologic, and disease-related criteria. Physicochemically, hyperuricemia is the concentration of urate in the blood that exceeds the solubility limits of monosodium urate in plasma, 415 μmol/L (6.8 mg/dL). In epidemiologic studies, hyperuricemia is defined as the mean plus 2 standard deviations of values determined from a randomly selected healthy population. When measured in unselected individuals, 95 percent have serum urate concentrations below 420 μmol/L (7.0 mg/dL). Finally, hyperuricemia can be defined in relation to the risk of disease. The risk of developing gout or urolithiasis increases with urate levels greater than 420 μmol/L (7.0 mg/dL) and escalates in proportion to the degree of elevation. Hyperuricemia is present in between 2.0 and 13.2 percent of ambulatory adults and somewhat more frequently in hospitalized individuals.

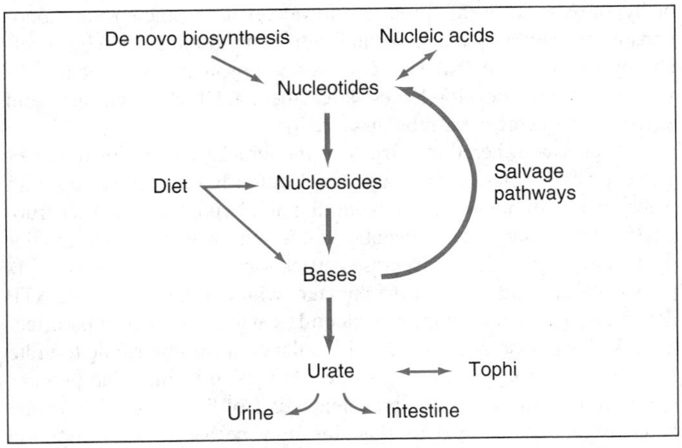

FIGURE 344-1 The total-body urate pool is the net result between urate production and excretion. Urate production is influenced by dietary intake of purines and the rates of de novo biosynthesis of purines from nonpurine precursors, nucleic acid turnover, and salvage by phosphoribosyltransferase activities. The formed urate is normally excreted by urinary and intestinal routes. Hyperuricemia can result from increased production, decreased excretion, or a combination of both mechanisms. When hyperuricemia exists, urate can precipitate and deposit in tissues as tophi.

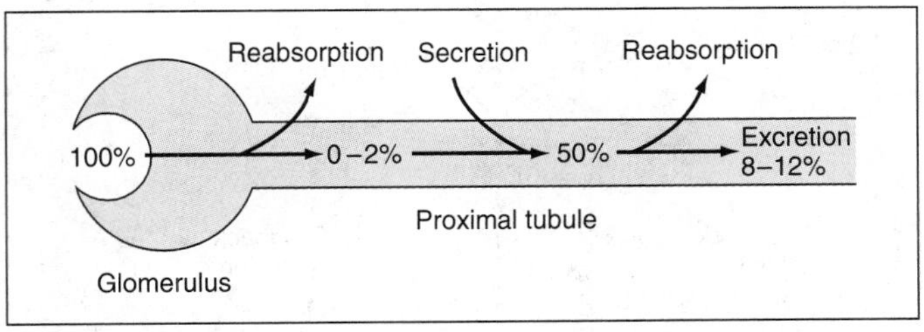

FIGURE 344-2 Schematic for handling of uric acid by the kidney. Components are illustrated with the percentage of filtered urate.

CAUSES OF HYPERURICEMIA It is useful to classify hyperuricemia in relation to the underlying physiology, i.e., whether the hyperuricemia results from increased production, decreased excretion, or a combination of the two (Fig. 344-1, Table 344-1).

Increased Urate Production Diet provides an exogenous source of purines and, accordingly, contributes to the serum urate in proportion to its purine content. Strict restriction of purine intake reduces the mean serum urate level by as little as 60 μmol/L (1.0 mg/dL) and urinary uric acid excretion by approximately 1.2 mmol/d (200 mg/d). Because about 50 percent of ingested RNA purine and 25 percent of ingested DNA purine appear in the urine as uric acid, foods high in nucleic acid content have a significant effect on the serum urate level. Such foods include liver, "sweetbreads" (i.e., thymus and pancreas), kidney, and anchovy.

Endogenous sources of purine production also influence the serum urate level (Fig. 344-3). De novo purine biosynthesis, the formation of a purine ring from nonring structures, is an 11-step process that results in formation of inosine monophosphate (IMP). The first step combines phosphoribosylpyrophosphate (PRPP) and glutamine and is catalyzed by amidophosphoribosyltransferase (amidoPRT). The rates of purine biosynthesis and urate production are determined, for the most part, by this enzyme. AmidoPRT is regulated by the substrate PRPP, which drives the reaction forward, and by the end products of biosynthesis (IMP and other ribonucleotides), which provide feedback inhibition. A second regulatory pathway is the salvage of purine bases by hypoxanthine phosphoribosyltransferase (HPRT). HPRT catalyzes the combination of the purine bases hypoxanthine and guanine with PRPP to form the respective ribonucleotides IMP and guanosine mono-

Table 344-1

Classification of Hyperuricemia

URATE OVERPRODUCTION		
Primary idiopathic HPRT deficiency PRPP synthetase overactivity Hemolytic processes Lymphoproliferative diseases	Myeloproliferative diseases Polycythemia vera Psoriasis Paget's disease Glycogenosis III, V, and VII	Rhabdomyolysis Exercise Alcohol Obesity Purine-rich diet
DECREASED URIC ACID EXCRETION		

Primary idiopathic
Renal insufficiency
Polycystic kidney disease
Diabetes insipidus
Hypertension
Acidosis
  Lactic acidosis
  Diabetic ketoacidosis
	Starvation ketosis
	Berylliosis
	Sarcoidosis
	Lead intoxication
	Hyperparathyroidism
	Hypothyroidism
	Toxemia of pregnancy
	Bartter's syndrome
	Down syndrome
		Drug ingestion
		  Salicylates (>2 g/d)
		  Diuretics
		  Alcohol
		  Levodopa
		  Ethambutol
		  Pyrazinamide
		  Nicotinic acid
		  Cyclosporine

COMBINED MECHANISM		
Glucose-6-phosphatase deficiency	Fructose-1-phosphate aldolase deficiency	Alcohol Shock

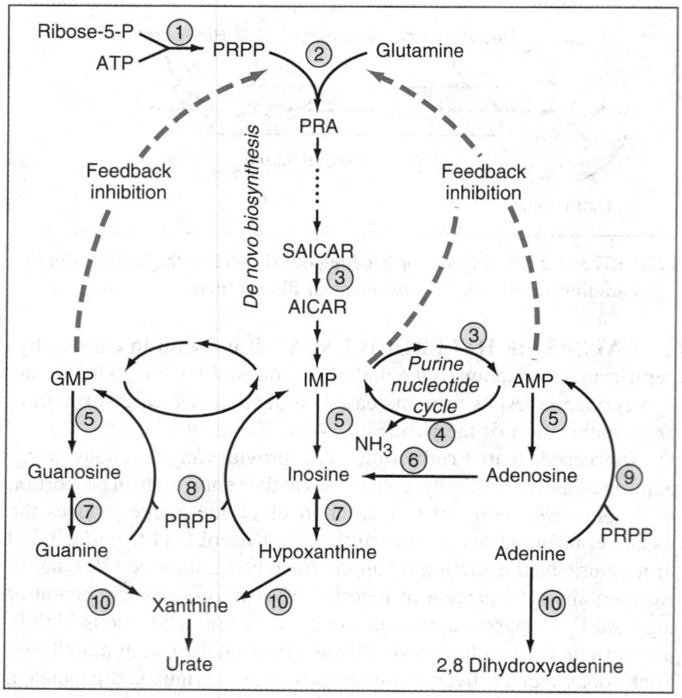

FIGURE 344-3 Abbreviated scheme of purine metabolism. (1) Phosphoribosylpyrophosphate (PRPP) synthetase, (2) amidophosphoribosyltransferase (amidoPRT), (3) adenylosuccinate lyase, (4) adenylate (AMP) deaminase, (5) 5′-nucleotidase, (6) adenosine deaminase, (7) purine nucleoside phosphorylase, (8) hypoxanthine phosphoribosyltransferase (HPRT), (9) adenine phosphoribosyltransferase (APRT), and (10) xanthine oxidase. PRPP, phosphoribosylpyrophosphate; PRA, phosphoribosylamine; SAICAR, succinylaminoimidazole carboxamide ribotide; AICAR, aminoimidazole carboxamide ribotide; GMP, guanylate; IMP, inosinate; AMP, adenylate.

phosphate (GMP). Increased salvage activity thus retards de novo synthesis by reducing PRPP levels and increasing concentrations of inhibitory ribonucleotides.

Serum urate levels are closely coupled to the rates of de novo purine biosynthesis. An X-linked disorder that causes an increase in activity of the enzyme PRPP synthetase causes increased PRPP production and accelerated de novo biosynthesis. PRPP is a substrate and allosteric activator of amidoPRT, the first enzyme in the de novo pathway. Individuals with this inborn error of metabolism have overproduction of purines, hyperuricemia, and hyperuricaciduria and develop uric acid calculi and gout before age 20.

Similarly, individuals deficient in HPRT have hyperuricemia, hyperuricaciduria, uric acid calculi, and gout because of urate overproduction. HPRT deficiency is also X-linked. A complete deficiency of HPRT, the Lesch-Nyhan syndrome, is also associated with self-mutilation, choreoathetosis, and other neurologic problems. Individuals with partial HPRT deficiency, the Kelley-Seegmiller syndrome, develop gout and renal calculi only. HPRT deficiency enhances urate biosynthesis in two ways. PRPP is accumulated as a result of decreased utilization in the salvage pathway and, in turn, provides increased substrate for amidoPRT and de novo biosynthesis. In addition, decreased formation of the nucleoside monophosphates IMP and GMP via the salvage pathway impairs feedback inhibition on amidoPRT, further enhancing de novo biosynthesis.

Accelerated purine nucleotide degradation also can cause hyperuricemia, e.g., with conditions of rapid cell turnover, proliferation, or cell death, as in leukemic blast crises, cytotoxic therapy for malignancy, hemolysis, or rhabdomyolysis. Nucleic acids released from cells are hydrolyzed by the sequential activities of nucleases and phosphodiesterases, forming nucleoside monophosphates, and then are degraded to nucleosides, bases, and urate. Hyperuricemia can result from excessive degradation of skeletal muscle ATP after strenuous physical exercise or status epilepticus and in glycogen storage diseases types III, V, and VII (see Chap. 347). The hyperuricemia of myocardial infarction, smoke inhalation, and acute respiratory failure also may be related to accelerated breakdown of ATP.

Decreased Uric Acid Excretion As many as 98 percent of individuals with primary hyperuricemia and gout have a defect in the renal handling of uric acid. This is evidenced as a lower than normal ratio of urate clearance to glomerular filtration rate (or urate to inulin clearance rate) over a wide range of filtered loads. As a result, gouty individuals excrete approximately 40 percent less uric acid than nongouty individuals for any given plasma urate concentration. Uric acid excretion increases in gouty and nongouty individuals when plasma urate levels are raised by purine ingestion or infusion, but in those with gout, plasma urate concentrations must be 60 to 120 μmol/L (1 to 2 mg/dL) higher than normal to achieve equivalent uric acid excretion rates.

Altered uric acid excretion could theoretically result from decreased glomerular filtration, decreased tubular secretion, or enhanced tubular reabsorption. Decreased urate filtration does not appear to cause primary hyperuricemia but does contribute to the hyperuricemia of renal insufficiency. Although hyperuricemia is invariably present in chronic renal disease, the correlation between serum creatinine, urea nitrogen, and urate concentration is poor because although uric acid excretion per unit of glomerular filtration rate increases progressively with chronic renal insufficiency, tubular secretory capacity tends to be preserved, tubular reabsorptive capacity is reduced, and extrarenal clearance of uric acid increases as renal damage becomes more severe.

Decreased proximal tubular secretion of urate may cause the hyperuricemia in individuals with gout and no evidence of urate overproduction. Decreased tubular secretion of urate also causes the secondary hyperuricemia of acidosis. Diabetic ketoacidosis, starvation, ethanol intoxication, lactic acidosis, and salicylate intoxication are accompanied by accumulations of organic acids (β-hydroxybutyrate, acetoacetate, lactate, or salicylates) that compete with urate for tubular secretion. In some individuals with gout, hyperuricemia may be due to enhanced reabsorption of uric acid distal to the site of secretion, a mechanism known to be responsible for the hyperuricemia of extracellular volume depletion such as with diabetes insipidus or diuretic therapy.

Combined Mechanisms Both increased urate production and decreased uric acid excretion may contribute to hyperuricemia. Individuals with a deficiency of glucose-6-phosphatase, the enzyme that hydrolyzes glucose-6-phosphate to glucose, are hyperuricemic from infancy and develop gout early in life (see Chap. 347). Increased urate production results from accelerated ATP degradation during fasting or hypoglycemia. In addition, the lower levels of nucleoside monophosphates decrease feedback inhibition of amidoPRT, thereby accelerating de novo biosynthesis. Glucose-6-phosphatase–deficient individuals also may develop hyperlacticacidemia, which blocks uric acid excretion by decreasing tubular secretion.

Patients with hereditary fructose intolerance caused by fructose-1-phosphate aldolase deficiency also develop hyperuricemia by both mechanisms. In homozygotes, vomiting and hypoglycemia after fructose ingestion can lead to hepatic failure and proximal renal tubular dysfunction. Ingestion of fructose causes accumulation of fructose-1-phosphate, the substrate for the enzyme, which in turn results in ATP depletion, accelerated purine nucleotide catabolism, and hyperuricemia. Both lactic acidosis and renal tubular acidosis contribute to urate retention. Heterozygous carriers develop hyperuricemia, and perhaps one-third develop gout. The prevalence of 1 of 80 to 1 of 250 for the heterozygous state suggests that this may be a relatively common cause of familial gout.

Alcohol also promotes hyperuricemia by both mechanisms. Excessive alcohol consumption causes accelerated hepatic breakdown of ATP and increased urate production and may cause hyperlacticacidemia, which blocks uric acid secretion. The higher purine content in some alcoholic beverages such as beer may be a factor.

EVALUATION OF HYPERURICEMIA Hyperuricemia does not necessarily represent a disease, nor is it a specific indication for therapy. Rather, the finding of hyperuricemia is an indication to determine its cause. The decision to treat depends on the cause and the potential consequences of the hyperuricemia in each individual.

Quantification of the uric acid excretion can be used to determine whether hyperuricemia is caused by overproduction or decreased excretion. On a purine-free diet, men with normal renal function excrete less than 3.6 mmol/d (600 mg/d). Thus, the hyperuricemia of individuals who excrete more uric acid while on a purine-free diet is due to purine overproduction, and that in those excreting less is due to decreased excretion. If the assessment is performed while the patient is on a regular diet, the level of 4.2 mmol/d (800 mg/d) can be used as the discriminating value. With renal insufficiency, less urate is filtered in the glomeruli and less uric acid appears in the urine. Consequently, a lower 24-h urinary uric acid value in the presence of renal insufficiency does not necessarily rule out urate overproduction, but an elevated value provides strong evidence of urate overproduction. Spuriously high values can occur if a uricosuric agent is being taken at the time of urine collection. Glucocorticoids, ascorbic acid, salicylates in doses greater than 2 g/d, and other agents that promote urate excretion interfere with the interpretation of results.

Assessment of the ratio of uric acid to creatinine (or the ratio of uric acid clearance to creatinine clearance) in spot or random urine samples is not a reliable method to screen for urate overproduction. However, this is a useful tool for evaluating individuals with acute renal failure suspected of having acute uric acid nephropathy (see below).

COMPLICATIONS OF HYPERURICEMIA Although the manifestations of gout can occur in almost any combination, the typical sequence involves progression through asymptomatic hyperuricemia, acute gouty arthritis, interval or intercritical gout, and chronic or tophaceous gout. Nephrolithiasis can occur before or after the first attack of gouty arthritis.

The prevalence of hyperuricemia ranges between 2.0 and 13.2 percent, and the prevalence of gout is between 1.3 and 3.7 percent of the general population. The higher the serum urate level, the more likely an individual is to develop gout. In one study, the incidence of gout was 4.9 percent for individuals with serum urate concentrations of 540 μmol/L (9.0 mg/dL) or more compared with 0.5 percent for those with values between 415 and 535 μmol/L (7.0 and 8.9 mg/dL). The complications of gout correlate with both the duration and severity of hyperuricemia. Most first attacks of gouty arthritis follow 20 to 40 years of sustained hyperuricemia; the peak age of onset is between 40 and 60 years for men and after menopause for women.

Gouty Arthritis The benchmark feature of gout is acute monarticular arthritis. The first attack begins explosively and is very painful. Occasionally, individuals report a prodrome or previous episodes of milder pain lasting hours. The agonizing pain of acute gout is accompanied by signs of intense inflammation: swelling, erythema, warmth, exquisite tenderness, and on occasion low-grade fever. If untreated, the attack usually peaks 24 to 48 h after the first symptoms and subsides within 7 to 10 days. The skin over the involved part may desquamate as the episode resolves.

The initial attack usually affects a single joint, although polyarticular onsets occur and may be more common in women. Gouty arthritis primarily affects peripheral joints, particularly those of the lower extremities, but periarticular sites such as plantar fascia, Achilles tendon insertions, Heberden's nodes, or other tenosynovia can be affected. The first metatarsophalangeal joint is involved in over 50 percent of first attacks and in 90 percent of individuals at some time. Sacroiliac, sternomanubrial, and spinal involvement is rare.

Any factor that causes either an abrupt increase or decrease in the serum urate level may provoke an acute attack, the best correlations being with factors that cause a rapid fall. In theory, sudden increases in urate concentration may cause new crystals to form, whereas a drop in serum and extracellular urate concentrations may lead to partial dissolution and shedding of previously formed crystals. Other provocative factors include stress, trauma, infection, hospitalization, surgery, starvation, weight reduction, hyperalimentation, excessive food intake, alcohol, and medications (Table 344-2). Of these, hospitalization and medications are probably the most significant. Acute gouty attacks occur in 20 to 86 percent of individuals with a history of gout when they are hospitalized for medical or surgical reasons. The stress of a severe illness, changes in medication, shifts in fluid status or electrolytes, and general anesthesia probably contribute to the exacerbations. Attacks can follow the use of thiazide diuretics that cause hyperuricemia or after initiation of allopurinol or other therapies to lower serum urate.

Table 344-2

Medications with Uricosuric Activity

Acetohexamide	Glyceryl guaiacolate
ACTH	Glycopyrrolate
Ascorbic acid	Halofenate
Azauridine	Meclofenamate
Benzbromarone	Phenolsulfonphthalein
Calcitonin	Phenylbutazone
Chlorprothixene	Probenecid
Citrate	Radiographic contrast agents
Dicumarol	Salicylates (>2 g/2d)
Diflunisal	Sulfinpyrazone
Estrogens	Tetracycline that is outdated
Glucocorticoids	Zoxazolamine

Occasional attacks of acute gouty arthritis occur in the absence of hyperuricemia. Presumably most such attacks can be explained by factors that lower serum concentrations, temporarily altering the usual hyperuricemic state (and that perhaps triggered the attack). Occasionally, hyperuricemia cannot be documented despite repeated attempts. Gout could theoretically develop anytime synovial fluid is supersaturated with urate. Free water is cleared from the joint space more rapidly than urate, and if the amount of synovial fluid containing a normal level of urate increases because of trauma or edema, then the urate level within the joint would temporarily increase as the problem resolved and the water was more rapidly cleared. Supersaturated concentrations of urate could cause the formation of crystals and precipitate an attack.

Some individuals have only a single gouty attack in their lifetime; others experience recurrence. Although the interval between first and second attacks may be over 40 years, three-fourths have a second attack within 2 years. The terms *interval gout* or *intercritical gout* describe the periods between attacks of acute arthritis when the individual has no joint complaints. In severe cases, unless therapeutic intervention occurs, chronic gouty arthritis develops with time. The pain-free intercritical periods shorten, and acute attacks occur with increased frequency, last longer, and involve more joints. The intensity of attacks may lessen somewhat, and involvement becomes polyarticular. Chronic gout is characterized by persistent polyarticular low-grade pain with acute or subacute inflammation. During this stage, tophi become apparent on physical examination (Fig. 344-4). The rates of urate deposition in joint tissues and of articular destruction correlate with the duration and severity of hyperuricemia. Approximately 10 years usually elapse between the first attack of arthritis and appearance of tophi. During the interim, however, destruction of cartilage and bone occurs, as evidenced by the radiographic changes (Fig. 344-5).

Pathogenesis Acute gout results from the interaction between urate crystals and polymorphonuclear leukocytes (Fig. 344-6) and involves activation of humoral and cellular inflammatory mechanisms. Urate crystals activate complement through both the classic and alternate pathways. Factor XII (Hageman factor) and the contact system of coagulation are also activated and result in generation of bradykinin, kallikrein, and plasmin. Urate crystals interact with neutrophils to cause the release of lysosomal enzymes, oxygen-derived free radicals, leukotriene and prostaglandin metabolites, collagenase, and protease. Phagocytosis of crystals by neutrophils causes release of crystal-induced chemotactic factor. Chemotactic factor, leukotriene B_4, and the activated complement component C5a are all chemotactic and contribute to the marked polymorphonuclear leukocyte response in the initial phase of acute arthritis. With time, phagocytic mononuclear cells replace the

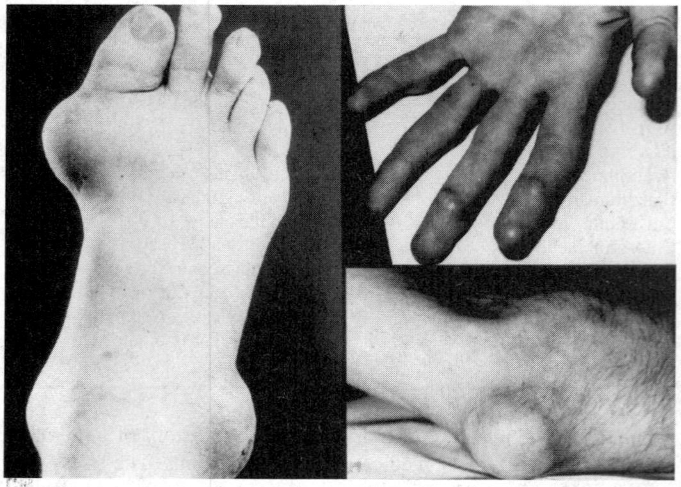

FIGURE 344-4 Chronic tophaceous gout. The left panel shows deformities of the foot in a 65-year-old man with a long history of gouty arthritis. On the right are tophi in an olecranon bursa and in the fingers of a 25-year-old man with Kelley-Seegmiller syndrome (partial HPRT deficiency).

polymorphonuclear cells. Urate crystals cause these cells to release prostaglandins (PGE_2), lysosomal enzymes, tumor necrosis factor α, and interleukin (IL) 1 and IL-6. Synovial lining cells participate in the inflammation by releasing inflammatory mediators such as IL-8.

The inflammatory potential of urate crystals is affected by the presence of absorbed proteins. Absorbed purified IgG causes enhanced crystal-induced platelet secretion, increased superoxide generation, and increased lysosomal enzyme release from polymorphonuclear leukocytes. On the other hand, apoprotein B, a component of very low density, low-density, and intermediate-density lipoproteins, inhibits urate crystal–induced stimulation of neutrophils. Apoprotein B is not normally present in synovial fluid and probably does not have access to that compartment under normal conditions because of its size. When synovitis develops, larger molecules, including lipoproteins, enter the joint space, bind to urate crystals, and, perhaps, play a role in terminating the attack.

Tophi are aggregates of monosodium urate monohydrate crystals and are generally surrounded by a giant cell, foreign body–type mononuclear cell inflammatory reaction. They can form in extraarticular and articular structures and cause deformity and destruction of hard and soft tissues. In joints, they lead to destruction of cartilage and bone, triggering secondary degeneration.

Renal Disease Despite the invariable hyperuricemia in renal failure, gouty arthritis occurs in fewer than 1 percent of patients with chronic renal failure. Since most gouty arthritis follows many years of sustained hyperuricemia, most patients with renal failure are probably not hyperuricemic long enough to accumulate the necessary urate load. In addition, individuals with chronic renal insufficiency have diminished inflammatory responses to urate crystals injected subcutaneously. Polycystic disease of the kidneys is an exception, with a prevalence of gout between 24 and 36 percent. The mechanism for this association is unknown.

Chronic renal failure patients on long-term hemodialysis can experience recurrent acute arthritis or periarthritis. Some of these attacks are gout due to urate crystal deposition, and others are caused by crystals of calcium phosphate (apatite) or calcium oxalate.

Gout is an important cause of morbidity in recipients of renal allografts. From 7 to 12 percent of individuals who receive cyclosporine and glucocorticoids for immunosuppression develop acute gouty arthritis, an occurrence that is even more common when diuretics are given concomitantly; there is a mean duration of about 17 months between transplantation and first attack. In contrast, gouty attacks are rare in transplant recipients maintained with azathioprine and glucocorticoids. In cyclosporine-treated transplant recipients, urate synthesis is normal, and urate clearance is decreased compared with azathioprine-treated controls.

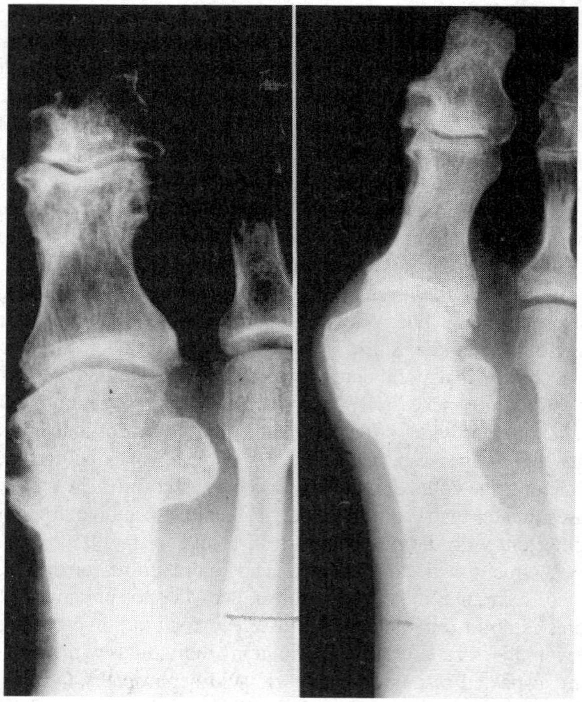

FIGURE 344-5 Radiographic changes in gout are the result of urate deposition. At first deposits are microscopic and are undetectable by x-ray. With persistent hyperuricemia, tophi enlarges to involve juxtaarticular bone and are apparent radiographically but not on physical examination. If unaltered by therapy, tophi continue to enlarge and become obvious in physical examination. The classic radiographic change of gout is a bony erosion. The location can be intraarticular, paraarticular, or at a distance from the joint. The erosions tend to be round and surrounded by a sclerotic border, giving a "punched out" appearance. There may be an "overhanging margin or lip." Nodular soft tissue prominence develops as the tophi enlarge. Joint spaces are typically preserved until late in the disease when secondary degenerative changes may occur. The left panel shows classic advanced changes of tophaceous gout including soft tissue distortion and erosion with sclerotic margins and overhanging edges. The right panel shows an erosive lesion in the interphalangeal joint in a patient with no tophi found on physical examination.

Hyperuricemia causes several renal problems: (1) nephrolithiasis; (2) urate nephropathy, a rare cause of renal insufficiency attributed to monosodium urate crystal deposition in the renal interstitium; and (3) uric acid nephropathy, a reversible cause of acute renal failure resulting from deposition of large amounts of uric acid crystals in the renal collecting ducts, pelvis, and ureters.

Nephrolithiasis Nephrolithiasis may precede the onset of gouty arthritis in 40 percent of individuals with both conditions. In gout, the prevalence of nephrolithiasis correlates with the serum and urinary uric acid levels, reaching approximately 50 percent with serum urate levels of 770 μmol/L (13 mg/dL) or urinary uric acid excretion over 6.5 mmol/d (1100 mg/d).

Not all kidney stones in individuals with gout are composed of uric acid. Stones of calcium oxalate, calcium phosphate, or those salts combined with uric acid occur in approximately 15 percent of cases. Uric acid may act as a nidus on which calcium oxalate can precipitate or lower the formation product for calcium oxalate crystallization. Furthermore, uric acid stones can develop in individuals with no other manifestations of gout, only 20 percent of whom are hyperuricemic. Some nongouty individuals with calcium oxalate stones have hyperuricemia or hyperuricaciduria.

Urate nephropathy Urate nephropathy, sometimes referred to as *urate nephrosis*, is a late manifestation of severe gout and is characterized histologically by deposits of monosodium urate crystals surrounded by a giant cell inflammatory reaction in the medullary intersti-

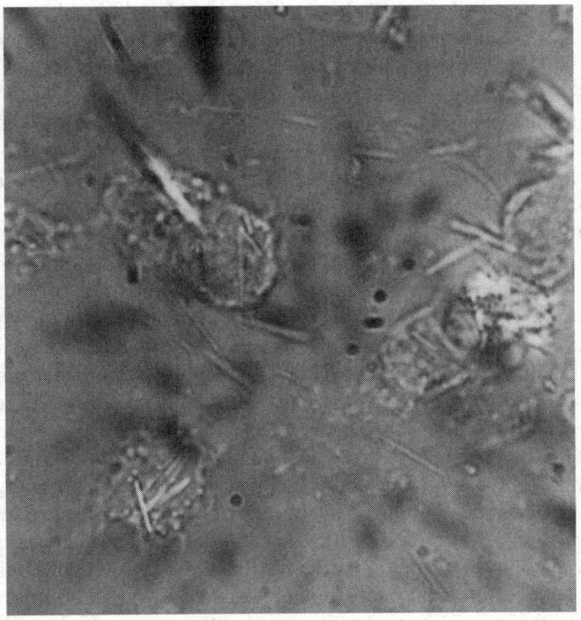

FIGURE 344-6 Crystals of monosodium urate in polymorphonuclear leukocytes and synovial fluid.

tium and pyramids and can cause chronic renal insufficiency. The disorder is now rare and cannot be diagnosed in the absence of gouty arthritis. The lesions may be clinically silent or cause proteinuria, hypertension, and renal insufficiency.

Prior to the advent of antihyperuricemic agents and aggressive treatment for asymptomatic hypertension, renal failure was the cause of death in up to 25 percent of individuals with gout. Postmortem evaluations of kidneys from patients with gout frequently revealed urate crystals, pyelonephritis, and vascular changes. At present, aging or coexisting diseases that cause nephropathy, such as cardiovascular disease, hypertension, or independently occurring renal disease, are usually responsible for decreased renal function in gout.

Uric acid nephropathy This reversible cause of acute renal failure is due to precipitation of uric acid in renal tubules and collecting ducts that causes obstruction to urine flow. Uric acid nephropathy develops following sudden urate overproduction and marked hyperuricaciduria. Factors that favor uric acid crystal formation include dehydration and acidosis. This form of acute renal failure occurs most often during an aggressive "blastic" phase of leukemia or lymphoma prior to or coincident with cytolytic therapy but also has been observed in individuals with other neoplasms, following epileptic seizures, and after vigorous exercise with heat stress. Autopsy studies have demonstrated intraluminal precipitates of uric acid, dilated proximal tubules, and normal glomeruli. The initial pathogenic events are believed to include obstruction of collecting ducts with uric acid and obstruction of distal renal vasculature.

If recognized, uric acid nephropathy is potentially reversible. Appropriate therapy has reduced the mortality from about 50 percent to practically nil. Serum levels cannot be relied on for diagnosis because this condition has developed in the presence of urate concentrations varying from 720 to 4800 μmol/L (12 to 80 mg/dL). The distinctive feature is the urinary uric acid concentration. In most forms of acute renal failure with decreased urine output, urinary uric acid content is either normal or reduced, and the ratio of uric acid to creatinine is less than 1. In acute uric acid nephropathy the ratio of uric acid to creatinine in a random urine sample or 24-h specimen is greater than 1, and a value that high is essentially diagnostic.

℞ TREATMENT

Asymptomatic Hyperuricemia For many years, fear of adverse outcomes caused physicians to prescribe urate-lowering agents for asymptomatic hyperuricemia. Today, treatment of asymptomatic hyperuricemia is not generally cost-effective or beneficial. The exception is in individuals with neoplastic disease who are about to receive cytolytic therapy and are at risk for acute uric acid nephropathy.

Although hyperuricemic individuals are at risk for gouty arthritis, especially those with higher serum urate levels, treatment of asymptomatic hyperuricemia to prevent the first attack of gouty arthritis is not appropriate because most hyperuricemic people never develop gout. Furthermore, neither structural kidney damage nor tophi are identifiable before the first attack. Reduced renal function cannot be attributed to asymptomatic hyperuricemia, and treatment of asymptomatic hyperuricemia does not alter the progression of renal dysfunction in patients with renal disease. Although nephrolithiasis is common in gouty patients and although a number of individuals with nephrolithiasis are hyperuricemic, the risk of stone formation in people with asymptomatic hyperuricemia is not established. Nor is hyperuricemia an independent risk factor for atherosclerotic cardiovascular disease.

Thus, because treatment with antihyperuricemic agents entails inconvenience, cost, and potential toxicity, routine treatment of asymptomatic hyperuricemia cannot be justified other than for prevention of acute uric acid nephropathy. In addition, routine screening for asymptomatic hyperuricemia is not recommended. If hyperuricemia is diagnosed, however, the cause should be determined. Causal factors should be corrected if the condition is secondary, and associated problems such as hypertension, hypercholesterolemia, diabetes mellitus, and obesity should be treated.

Symptomatic Hyperuricemia Initially, therapy should be directed toward relieving symptoms. Both gouty arthritis and nephrolithiasis are excruciatingly painful. Once the presenting symptoms are controlled, a decision must be made whether to initiate antihyperuricemic therapy.

Acute Gouty Arthritis As with any disease, appropriate and effective treatment requires accurate diagnosis. Few conditions can be diagnosed with more certainty or treated more successfully than gout. A definitive diagnosis requires aspiration of the involved joint or tissue and demonstration of intracellular monosodium urate crystals in synovial fluid polymorphonuclear leukocytes or in tophaceous aggregates. Using polarized light microscopy with a first-order red compensator, the strong negative birefringence of the needle-shaped crystals can be demonstrated easily. The triad of acute monarticular arthritis, hyperuricemia, and a dramatic response to colchicine provides presumptive evidence for gouty arthritis. These criteria, however, are a poor substitute for crystal identification, because some patients with gout are not hyperuricemic at the time of the attack. In addition, colchicine may be effective for other disorders, especially pseudogout (calcium pyrophosphate dehydrate crystal deposition disease) and calcific (basic calcium phosphate or apatite) tendinitis. These diseases that mimic acute gout may occur in individuals who happen to be hyperuricemic. Finally, acute gouty arthritis can coexist with septic arthritis, psoriatic arthritis, systemic lupus erythematosus, rheumatoid arthritis, osteoarthritis, and pseudogout.

Once the diagnosis of gouty arthritis is secure, the choice of therapeutic agents includes colchicine, nonsteroidal anti-inflammatory drugs (NSAIDs), or intraarticular glucocorticoids. Regardless of the choice, the effectiveness of the agent is dependent on when it is used. Each will work if started early; none works quickly if initiated late in the attack.

Colchicine, the traditional agent used, inhibits neutrophil activation by inhibiting crystal-induced protein tyrosine phosphorylation. Oral doses of 0.6 mg are given every hour until improvement occurs, gastrointestinal side effects develop, or 10 doses have been taken without relief (in which case the diagnosis may be questioned). Although highly effective, oral colchicine cannot be tolerated by up to 80 percent of people because of abdominal pain, diarrhea, and nausea. Colchicine also can be given intravenously, but administration by this route is potentially dangerous and should be used with extreme caution despite the fact that this route of administration can eliminate the gastrointestinal side effects (provided the drug is not also being taken orally). A single dose of 1 or 2 mg diluted in 20 mL normal saline is usually adequate. A second dose of 1 mg can be repeated 6 to 12 h later. Absolute contraindications for intravenous colchicine include depressed bone marrow function, renal disease (creatinine clearance less than 10 mL/min, oliguria, or anuria), liver disease (liver function tests over twice the upper limit of normal), and sepsis.

Because of its relative specificity for acute gouty arthritis, oral colchicine is the agent of choice for the ambulatory patient in whom the diagnosis is not certain. If the diagnosis is certain, NSAIDs may be more appropriate because of better tolerance. Indomethacin is the usual agent, but ibuprofen, naproxen, tolmetin, sulindac, piroxicam, ketoprofen, flurbiprofen, and other NSAIDs have been effective. These agents are less specific for gout than colchicine, but they are effective, especially if used early in the attack. Treatment is begun with the highest approved dose of the selected agent and is continued until 3 to 4 days after all signs of inflammation have resolved. These agents are contraindicated in patients with active peptic ulcer disease; should be used with caution in patients with heart failure, other edematous states, or hypertension because of potential problems from sodium retention; and may precipitate hyperkalemia and renal insufficiency.

Intraarticular injection of glucocorticoids also may be used for acute gout. This is most useful when the patient cannot take oral medications, when colchicine and NSAIDs are contraindicated, or in refractory cases. A single intramuscular injection of ACTH (40 or 50 units) has also been employed for acute gouty arthritis.

INTERCRITICAL AND CHRONIC GOUT The term *intercritical* (or *interval*) *gout* applies to the period after the acute gouty attack when the patient is asymptomatic. At that time the decision must be made whether to initiate antihyperuricemic therapy. All authors agree that hyperuricemia should be treated in patients with recurrent attacks, those with chronic gout or evidence of tophi, and those with gouty arthritis and nephrolithiasis. Some maintain that the first attack of acute gouty arthritis alone is sufficient indication. Others argue that first attacks are easily, inexpensively, and effectively treated and postpone urate-lowering therapy until one or more additional attacks occur.

Sustained hyperuricemia provides a definite risk to bone and cartilage for those with gouty arthritis. If hyperuricemia is not controlled, urate deposits enlarge and become radiographically evident before subcutaneous tophi develop. In a study of patients with intercritical gout, 42 percent had radiographic changes characteristic of bony tophi despite no evidence of tophi on physical examination (see Fig. 344-5). One cannot predict from the frequency of acute attacks, the history of therapy, or the serum urate levels at the time of evaluation which patients will show bony changes.

Before starting treatment with urate-lowering agents, the patient should be free of all signs of inflammation and have begun colchicine for prophylaxis. The sudden drop in serum urate with the initiation of allopurinol or uricosuric therapy may prolong or precipitate an acute attack. Colchicine, at a dose of 0.6 mg orally one to three times a day, is about 90 percent effective in preventing subsequent gout attacks. Rarely, a reversible colchicine-induced toxicity may be manifested by subacute myopathy and axonal neuropathy with elevated serum creatinine kinase levels. This toxicity is most common in individuals with renal insufficiency and is reversible when colchicine is discontinued.

Once antihyperuricemic therapy is initiated, the dosage used should maintain the serum urate at or below 300 μmol/L (5.0 mg/dL). Extracellular fluid is saturated with urate at a concentration of approximately 415 μmol/L (6.8 mg/dL). If the serum urate remains above this level, tissue deposition of urate crystals will continue. A reduction of the serum urate concentration from 600 to 480 μmol/L (10 to 8 mg/dL), for example, will not reduce the total-body urate pool but will slow the rate at which the pool increases. If, on the other hand, the urate concentration is reduced below 415 μmol/L (6.8 mg/dL), urate crystals can dissolve, and the urate pool will decrease. Successful therapy will prevent future attacks of gout and cause resolution of tophi.

Treatment of hyperuricemia includes diet and specific urate-lowering agents. Diet now plays a minor role in the treatment of hyperuricemia because modern therapeutic agents are so effective, but dietary counseling is important and should address obesity, hyperlipidemia, diabetes mellitus, hypertension, and the use of alcohol.

Allopurinol, a substrate and competitive inhibitor of xanthine oxidase, is the most widely used antihyperuricemic agent. Oxypurinol, the major metabolite of allopurinol, is also an effective inhibitor of xanthine oxidase. Allopurinol is efficiently absorbed from the gastrointestinal tract and has a half-life of 3 h. Oxypurinol excretion is enhanced by uricosuric agents and is reduced in renal insufficiency. Allopurinol is effective in the treatment of all types of hyperuricemia but is specifically indicated for the following: (1) Patients with gout and (a) evidence of urate overproduction [24-h urinary uric acid greater than 4.8 mmol (800 mg) on a general diet or greater than 3.6 mmol (600 mg) on a purine-restricted diet], (b) nephrolithiasis, (c) renal insufficiency (creatinine clearance less than 80 mL/min), (d) tophaceous deposits, (e) age over 60 years, or (f) inability to take uricosuric agents because of ineffectiveness or intolerance; (2) patients with nephrolithiasis of any type plus urinary uric acid excretion greater than 3.6 mmol/d (600 mg/d); (3) patients with renal calculi composed of 2,8-dihydroxyadenine; and (4) patients with, or at risk for, acute uric acid nephropathy

Allopurinol administration decreases the serum urate concentration and the urinary excretion of uric acid in the first 24 h, with a maximum reduction occurring within 2 weeks. The average effective dose of allopurinol is 300 mg/d. However, the dosage required to control the serum urate concentration depends on the severity of the tophaceous disease and on renal function. Failure of a 400-mg dose to produce an adequate antihyperuricemic effect is rare and suggests noncompliance. Allopurinol can be given once a day because of the long half-life (18 h) of its active metabolite oxypurinol. The drug is effective in patients with renal insufficiency, but the dose should be reduced.

Side effects, serious complications, and toxicity of allopurinol are unusual. The most frequent side effects are skin rash, gastrointestinal distress, diarrhea, and headache. The rash is usually maculopapular and erythematous, but exfoliative dermatitis and toxic epidermal necrolysis may occur. Desensitization with low doses of allopurinol may be useful in individuals with demonstrated hypersensitivity.

Serious adverse effects include alopecia, fever, lymphadenopathy, bone marrow suppression, hepatic toxicity, interstitial nephritis, renal failure, hypersensitivity vasculitis, and death. Such toxicity is fortunately rare but does occur in patients with renal insufficiency or in those taking thiazide diuretics.

Potential drug interactions must be considered when allopurinol is prescribed. Because 6-mercaptopurine and azathioprine are inactivated by xanthine oxidase, allopurinol prolongs the half-life of these agents and thus potentiates their therapeutic and toxic effects. Cyclophosphamide toxicity also may be enhanced by concomitant use. A threefold increase in ampicillin- and amoxicillin-related skin rashes has been reported in patients taking allopurinol.

Uricosuric agents also can effectively lower serum urate concentrations by the partial inhibition of proximal tubular reabsorption of filtered and secreted urate from the luminal side of the tubule at a site distal to the point of uric acid secretion. Candidates for these agents are gouty patients who meet all the following criteria: (1) hyperuricemia attributable to decreased uric acid excretion [less than 4.8 mmol (800 mg) urinary uric acid per day while taking a regular diet or less than 3.6 mmol (600 mg) with a purine-restricted diet], (2) age under 60 years, (3) satisfactory renal function (a creatinine clearance greater than 80 mL/min), and (4) no history of nephrolithiasis.

Uricosuric agents are effective in 70 to 80 percent of patients. Failure to control the serum urate concentration may be attributed to drug intolerance, poor compliance, concomitant salicylate ingestion, or impaired renal function. Salicylates block the uricosuric effects of these agents, probably by inhibiting urate secretion. Uricosuric agents lose effectiveness as the creatinine clearance falls and are ineffective when glomerular filtration falls below 30 mL/min. The most commonly used uricosuric agents are probenecid and sulfinpyrazone. Probenecid therapy is begun at 250 mg twice a day and is increased as necessary up to 3.0 g/d. Because the half-life is 6 to 12 h, probenecid should be taken in two to three evenly spaced doses. Sulfinpyrazone therapy is initiated at a dose of 50 mg twice a day. The usual maintenance level is 300 to 400 mg/d in three or four divided doses.

By promoting uric acid excretion, uricosuric agents may precipitate nephrolithiasis. This rare complication can occur early in the course of treatment and may be prevented by initiating therapy at low doses, forcing hydration, and, possibly, alkalinizing the urine. Hypersensitivity, skin rash, and gastrointestinal complaints are the major side effects. Serious toxicity is rare, but hepatic necrosis and the nephrotic syndrome have been reported.

Nephrolithiasis Antihyperuricemic therapy is recommended for the individual who has both gouty arthritis and either uric acid– or calcium-containing stones, both of which may occur in association with hyperuricaciduria. Regardless of the nature of the calculi, fluid ingestion should be sufficient to produce a daily urine volume greater than 2 L. Alkalinization of the urine with sodium bicarbonate or acetazolamide may be justified to increase the solubility of uric acid. Specific treatment of uric acid calculi requires reducing the urine uric acid concentration with allopurinol. Allopurinol is also useful in reducing the recurrence of calcium oxalate stones in gouty subjects and in nongouty individuals with hyperuricemia or hyperuricaciduria. Potassium citrate (30 to 80 mmol/d orally in divided doses) is an alternative therapy for patients with uric acid stones alone or mixed calcium/uric acid stones. Allopurinol is also indicated for the treatment of 2,8-dihydroxyadenine kidney stones.

Uric Acid Nephropathy Uric acid nephropathy is often preventable, and immediate, appropriate therapy has reduced the mortality rate to practically nil. Vigorous intravenous hydration and diuresis with furosemide dilute the uric acid in the tubules and promote urine flow to 100 mL/h or more. The administration of acetazolamide, 240 to 500 mg every 6 to 8 h, and sodium bicarbonate, 89 mmol/L, intravenously enhances urine alkalinity and thereby solubilizes more uric acid. It is important to ensure that the urine pH remains above 7.0 and to watch for circulatory overload. In addition, antihyperuricemic therapy in the form of allopurinol in a single dose of 8 mg/kg is administered to reduce the amount of urate that reaches the kidney. If renal insufficiency persists, subsequent daily doses should be reduced to 100 to 200 mg because oxypurinol, the active metabolite of allopurinol, accumulates in renal failure. Despite these measures, hemodialysis may be required.

HYPOURICEMIA

Hypouricemia, defined as a serum urate concentration less than 120 μmol/L (2.0 mg/dL), can result from decreased production of urate, increased excretion of uric acid, or a combination of both mechanisms. It occurs in fewer than 0.2 percent of the general population and fewer than 0.8 percent of hospitalized individuals. Hypouricemia causes no symptoms or pathology and therefore requires no therapy. It is, however, a sign of potential pathology, and its cause should be determined.

Most hypouricemia results from increased renal uric acid excretion. The finding of normal amounts of uric acid in a 24-h urine collection in an individual with hypouricemia is evidence for a renal cause. Medications with uricosuric properties (see Table 344-2) include aspirin (at doses over 2.0 g/d), x-ray contrast materials, and glycerylguaiacholate. Total parenteral hyperalimentation also can cause hypouricemia, possibly a result of the high glycine content of the infusion formula. Other causes of an increased urate clearance include neoplastic disease, hepatic cirrhosis, diabetes mellitus, inappropriate secretion of vasopressin, and defects in renal tubular transport such as primary Fanconi syndrome and Fanconi syndromes caused by Wilson's disease, cystinosis, multiple myeloma, and heavy metal toxicity, and as isolated congenital defects in the bidirectional transport of uric acid.

Hypouricemia from decreased production of urate is accompanied by very low urinary uric acid levels. Accumulation of other purine nucleosides and bases may occur depending on the specific defect. Individuals treated with allopurinol and some subjects with neoplastic disease or severe hepatic dysfunction are hypouricemic and excrete increased quantities of hypoxanthine and xanthine in the urine. Xanthine oxidase deficiency can be inherited or acquired. Inherited forms include isolated xanthine oxidase deficiency and combined xanthine oxidase and sulfite oxidase deficiencies. Both cause hypouricemia and xanthinuria. Affected individuals excrete essentially no uric acid and may develop xanthine nephrolithiasis. Individuals with purine nucleoside phosphorylase deficiency, an inborn error of metabolism causing T cell–deficient immune dysfunction, are hypouricemic and excrete increased quantities of guanosine, deoxyguanosine, inosine, and deoxyinosine in the urine.

INBORN ERRORS OF PURINE METABOLISM

(See also Table 344-3, Fig. 344-3)

HPRT DEFICIENCY A complete deficiency of HPRT, the Lesch-Nyhan syndrome, is characterized by hyperuricemia, self-mutilative behavior, choreoathetosis, spasticity, and mental retardation. A partial deficiency of HPRT, the Kelley-Seegmiller syndrome, is associated with hyperuricemia but no central nervous system manifestations. In both disorders, the hyperuricemia results from urate overpro-

Table 344-3

Inborn Errors of Purine Metabolism

Enzyme	Activity	Inheritance	Clinical Features
Hypoxanthine phosphoribosyltransferase	Complete deficiency	X-linked	Self-mutilation, choreoathetosis, hyperuricemia, gout, and uric acid lithiasis
	Partial deficiency	X-linked	Hyperuricemia, gout, and uric acid lithiasis
Phosphoribosylpyrophosphate synthetase	Overactivity	X-linked	Hyperuricemia, gout, uric acid lithiasis, and deafness
Adenine phosphoribosyltransferase	Deficiency	Autosomal recessive	2,8-Dihydroxyadenine lithiasis
Xanthine oxidase	Deficiency	Autosomal recessive	Xanthinuria and xanthine lithiasis
Adenylosuccinate lyase	Deficiency	Autosomal recessive	Autism and psychomotor retardation
Myoadenylate deaminase	Deficiency	Autosomal recessive	Myopathy with exercise intolerance or asymptomatic
Adenosine deaminase	Deficiency	Autosomal recessive	Severe combined immunodeficiency disease and chrondro-osseous dysplasia
Purine nucleoside phosphorylase	Deficiency	Autosomal recessive	T cell–mediated immunodeficiency

duction and can cause uric acid crystalluria, nephrolithiasis, obstructive uropathy, and gouty arthritis. Early diagnosis and appropriate therapy with allopurinol can prevent or eliminate all the problems attributable to hyperuricemia but have no effect on the behavioral or neurologic abnormalities.

HPRT catalyzes the reaction that combines PRPP and the purine bases hypoxanthine and guanine to form the respective nucleoside monophosphate IMP or GMP and pyrophosphate. The enzyme is encoded by a single gene located on the X chromosome. Consequently, affected males are hemizygous for the trait and inherit the mutant allele from their asymptomatic mother, who is a carrier, or are the result of spontaneous gene mutations. The deficiency state is generally the result of point mutations, deletions, insertions, or endoduplication of exons rather than major gene alterations.

INCREASED PRPP SYNTHETASE ACTIVITY Cells from individuals with increased PRPP synthetase activity contain elevated levels of PRPP. The high substrate content drives de novo purine synthesis causing overproduction of uric acid. Similar to the HPRT deficiency states, PRPP synthetase overactivity is X-linked and results in gouty arthritis and uric acid nephrolithiasis. Nerve deafness occurs in some families.

ADENINE PHOSPHORIBOSYLTRANSFERASE (APRT) DEFICIENCY Individuals with a deficiency of APRT develop kidney stones composed of 2,8-dihydroxyadenine. APRT catalyzes the conversion of adenine to adenosine monophosphate (AMP). In the absence of APRT, adenine is converted by xanthine oxidase to 2,8-dihydroxyadenine, which is insoluble in urine. Reports of 2,8-dihydroxyadenine stones are rare, most likely because of its chemical similarity to uric acid. Analysis by x-ray powder diffraction is necessary for correct identification. Because this technique is rarely employed, many 2,8-dihydroxyadenine stones are incorrectly called uric acid. The consequence of this misidentification is not too severe, because allopurinol therapy is the correct treatment for each type of stone.

APRT deficiency is inherited as an autosomal recessive trait. Caucasians with the deficiency have a complete deficiency (type I), whereas Japanese subjects have some measurable enzyme activity (type II). Expression of the defect is similar in the two populations, as is the frequency of the heterozygous state (0.4 to 1.1 per 100).

HEREDITARY XANTHINURIA A deficiency of xanthine oxidase causes all purine in the urine to occur in the form of hypoxanthine and xanthine. About two-thirds of deficient individuals are asymptomatic. The remainder develop kidney stones composed of xanthine. A very small number of symptomatic individuals also have myopathy or recurrent polyarteritis. Xanthinuria appears to be inherited in an autosomal recessive pattern.

In a second form of inherited xanthinuria, the deficiency of xanthine oxidase is associated with a deficiency of sulfite oxidase. Neurologic symptoms attributable to the sulfite oxidase deficiency predominate over those of xanthinuria in individuals with the combined deficiency.

MYOADENYLATE DEAMINASE DEFICIENCY Adenylate deaminase (AMP deaminase) catalyzes the conversion of AMP to IMP with the release of ammonia and is an integral component of the purine nucleotide cycle, which plays an important role in skeletal muscle energy metabolism. A deficiency of myoadenylate deaminase, the isoform of AMP deaminase in skeletal muscle, is associated with myopathic syndromes.

Both primary (inherited) and secondary (acquired) forms of myoadenylate deaminase deficiency have been described. Myoadenylate deaminase is the only activity affected in the inherited form, whereas other muscle enzymes (creatine kinase and myokinase) are also decreased in the acquired deficiencies. Inherited deficiency is probably the result of point mutations, small deletions, or rearrangements. A single nonsense mutation has been identified in 11 unrelated families. In contrast, mRNA abundance is low in muscle from patients with acquired deficiencies, suggesting a different molecular basis for this form. The primary form is inherited as an autosomal recessive trait. Clinically, this form tends to be a relatively benign disorder characterized by easy fatigability and postexercise cramps and myalgias. Most individuals with this defect may be asymptomatic, and some believe that other explanations for the myopathy should be sought in symptomatic patients.

The acquired deficiency occurs in association with a wide variety of neuromuscular diseases, including muscular dystrophies, neuropathies, inflammatory myopathies, and collagen vascular diseases. Measurement of plasma lactate and ammonia levels after ischemic exercise of the forearm can be used to screen for this disorder. Under these conditions, subjects deficient in myoadenylate can generate lactate but not ammonia. The diagnosis can be made only by documenting the enzyme deficiency in a muscle biopsy specimen.

ADENYLOSUCCINATE LYASE DEFICIENCY Adenylosuccinate lyase participates in the synthesis of purine nucleotides in two ways. It catalyzes the conversion of succinylaminoimidazole carboxamide ribotide (SAICAR) to aminoimidazole carboxamide ribotide (AICAR) in the de novo pathway and in the conversion of AMP succinate to AMP in the purine nucleotide cycle. Deficiency of this enzyme is due to an autosomal recessive trait and causes profound psychomotor retardation, seizures, and other movement disorders. All individuals with this deficiency are mentally retarded, and most are autistic.

ADENOSINE DEAMINASE DEFICIENCY AND PURINE NUCLEOSIDE PHOSPHORYLASE DEFICIENCY See Chap. 307.

See Chap. 27, Drugs used in the treatment of gout, in Goodman & Gilman's The Pharmacological Basis of Therapeutics, *9th ed. New York, McGraw-Hill, 1996.*

BIBLIOGRAPHY

Becker MA et al: Purines and pyrimidines, in *The Molecular and Metabolic Bases of Inherited Disease,* 7th ed, CR Scriver et al (eds). New York, McGraw-Hill, 1995, pp 1655–1841

Kelley WN, Wortmann RL: Gout and hyperuricemia, in *Textbook of Rheumatology,* 5th ed, WN Kelley et al (eds). Philadelphia, Saunders, 1996, p 1313

McCarthy GM et al: Influence of antihyperuricemic therapy on the clinical and radiographic progression of gout. Arthritis Rheum 34:1489, 1991

Rosenthal AK, Ryan LM: Treatment of refractory crystal-associated arthritis. Rheum Clin North Am 21:151, 1995

Wortmann RL: Management of hyperuricemia, in *Arthritis and Allied Conditions,* 13th ed, DJ McCarty, WJ Koopman (eds). Philadelphia, Lea & Febiger, 1996, p 1807

Wyngaarden JB, Kelley WN: *Gout and Hyperuricemia.* New York, Grune & Stratton, 1976

345 WILSON'S DISEASE

I. Herbert Scheinberg

Wilson's disease is an inherited disorder of copper metabolism in individuals with two mutant ATP7B genes. Impairment of the normal excretion of hepatic copper results in toxic accumulations of the metal in liver, brain, and other organs. The disease occurs in every ethnic and geographic population, with a worldwide prevalence of about 1 in 30,000, and the frequency of heterozygous carriers of the mutation is about 1 in 90.

NATURAL HISTORY The average low concentration of ceruloplasmin and high concentration of hepatic copper in normal neonates are indistinguishable from the concentrations exhibited by neonates with Wilson's disease. In normal infants, the ceruloplasmin concentration increases and the hepatic copper concentration falls to adult levels during the first year of life. However, in infants with Wilson's disease, the neonatal deficiency of ceruloplasmin and excess of hepatic copper persist indefinitely. Clinical manifestations are rare before age 6, occur most frequently in mid-adolescence, and eventually develop in all untreated patients.

In about half of patients any of four types of hepatic disturbances may herald the clinical onset. *Acute hepatitis* is usually self-limited and often mistaken for viral hepatitis or infectious mononucleosis. It may be overlooked later in life when a diagnosis of Wilson's disease is entertained unless the patient is carefully questioned. *Parenchymal liver disease* may persist after acute hepatitis or develop insidiously without prior acute disease into a histologic and clinical picture indistinguishable from chronic active hepatitis and cirrhosis. In other patients *cirrhosis* may develop insidiously after a lapse of decades with no sign or symptom of liver disease. *Fulminant hepatitis*, generally fatal, is characterized by progressive jaundice, ascites, encephalopathy, hypoalbuminemia, hypoprothrombinemia, moderately elevated plasma levels of liver enzymes, and Coombs-negative hemolytic anemia.

In most other patients neurologic or psychiatric disturbances are the first clinical signs and are always accompanied by Kayser-Fleischer rings **(see Plate III-16)**. These golden deposits of copper in Descemet's membrane of the cornea do not interfere with vision but indicate that copper has been released from the liver and has probably caused brain damage. If a patient with frank neurologic or psychiatric disease does not have Kayser-Fleischer rings when examined by a trained observer using a slit lamp, the diagnosis of Wilson's disease can be excluded. Rarely, Kayser-Fleischer rings may be accompanied by sunflower cataracts.

The neurologic manifestations include resting and intention tremors, spasticity, rigidity, chorea, drooling, dysphagia, and dysarthria. Babinski responses may be present, and abdominal reflexes are often absent. Inexplicably—in view of the ubiquity of copper excess in the brain—sensory changes, save for headache, never occur.

Psychiatric disturbances are present in most patients with neurologic symptoms. Schizophrenia, manic-depressive psychoses, and classic neuroses may occur, but the commonest disturbances are bizarre behavioral patterns that defy classification. Improvement in the psychiatric state can occur with pharmacologic reduction of the copper excess, but psychotherapy and additional pharmacotherapy may be required.

In about 5 percent of patients the clinical onset reflects neither a hepatic nor a central nervous system disturbance. The first manifestation may be primary or secondary amenorrhea or repeated and unexplained spontaneous abortions, perhaps due to excess free copper in intrauterine secretions. Kayser-Fleischer rings may occasionally first be discovered during routine ophthalmologic examination.

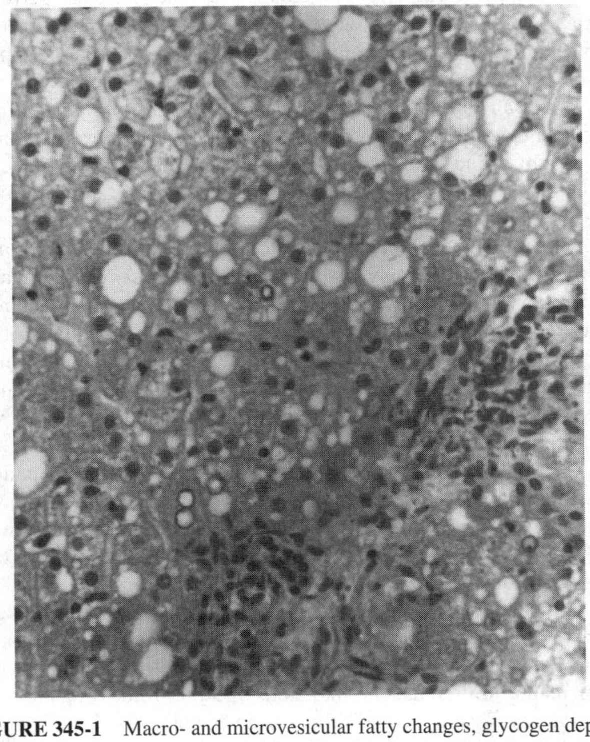

FIGURE 345-1 Macro- and microvesicular fatty changes, glycogen deposits in nuclei, and cellular infiltrates in a hematoxylin- and eosin-stained section of liver from an asymptomatic boy with Wilson's disease.

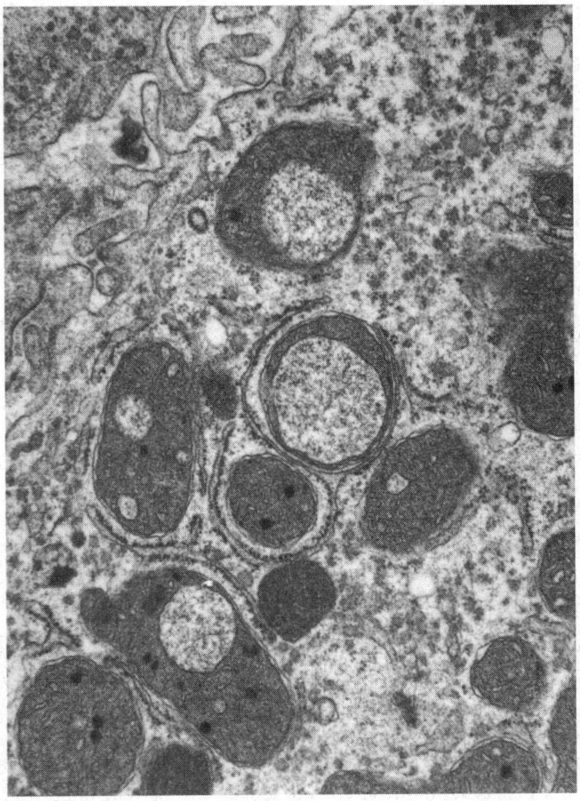

FIGURE 345-2 Electron micrograph of a liver biopsy sample from a 6-year-old asymptomatic boy. There are prominent vacuoles, containing granular material, in mitochondria (M). P, peroxisome; PM, plasma membrane.

PATHOGENESIS The metabolic defect in Wilson's disease is an inability to maintain a near-zero balance of copper. Dietary copper is generally in excess of the small amount that is essential to life. Normally any excess copper that is absorbed is excreted by the liver, but in patients with Wilson's disease copper accumulates in the liver.

Fatty infiltration of the hepatic parenchyma and nuclear glycogen deposits are the earliest findings by light microscopy (Fig. 345-1). With electron microscopy, characteristic mitochondrial abnormalities appear to be specific for Wilson's disease (Fig. 345-2). Later, necrosis, inflammation, fibrosis, bile duct proliferation, and cirrhosis ensue. Abnormalities in liver chemistries, particularly elevations in aminotransferases, may be seen at any stage. The capacity of hepatocytes to store copper is eventually exceeded, and copper is released into blood and taken up into extrahepatic tissues with disastrous effects in the brain (Table 345-1).

With magnetic resonance imaging, the effects of copper toxicity in the brain are seen most frequently in the lenticular nuclei and less commonly in the pons, medulla, thalamus, cerebellum, and cerebral cortex. Opalski and Alzheimer type II cells are present early in the course, although neither is specific for Wilson's disease, and neuronal necrosis and cavitation develop later.

Increased copper in the kidney produces little, if any, structural change and usually does not alter renal function. Microscopic hematuria and/or minimal proteinuria occur occasionally, and nephrocalcinosis, renal calculi, and renal tubular acidosis are rare. Pathologic effects in other organs and tissues are minor.

GENETICS The ATP7B gene on chromosome 13 that is mutated in this disease has been cloned and sequenced, and the protein product has been identified as a P type, copper-transporting ATPase.

Table 345-1

Summary of Analytic Data in Patients with Wilson's Disease, Heterozygous Carriers, and Control Subjects

	Serum Ceruloplasmin		Hepatic Copper Concentration	
Group	No. of Patients	Mean ± SD, mg/L	No. of Patients	Mean ± SD, μg/g Dry Weight
Wilson's disease:				
Asymptomatic	31	36 ± 53	36	983.5 ± 368
Symptomatic	84	59 ± 71	33	588.3 ± 304
Heterozygous carriers	95*	284 ± 85	14	117.0 ± 51
Normal subjects	180	307 ± 35	16	31.5 ± 6.8

* 71 parents of patients with Wilson's disease and 24 children, each of whom had one parent with Wilson's disease.

SOURCE: Sternlieb and Scheinberg, 1968.

More than 40 mutant forms of the normal gene have been identified, and the disease can develop either in homozygotes or individuals who are compound heterozygotes for these mutant genes. As a consequence, molecular diagnosis is only practical in family members of patients in whom the genetic defect has already been identified. The mechanism by which the normal ATP7B protein promotes the excretion of hepatic copper is not yet established, nor is it clear whether the secondary decrease in ceruloplasmin in this disorder plays a role in the pathogenesis of the disease.

DIAGNOSIS *The diagnosis is easy provided it is suspected.* Wilson's disease should be considered in any patient under the age of 40 with an unexplained disorder of the central nervous system, signs or symptoms of hepatitis, chronic active hepatitis, unexplained persistent elevations of serum aminotransferase, hemolytic anemia in the presence of hepatitis, or unexplained cirrhosis and in any patient who has a near blood relative with Wilson's disease.

The diagnosis is confirmed by the demonstration of either: (1) a serum ceruloplasmin level less than 200 mg/L *and* Kayser-Fleischer rings or (2) a serum ceruloplasmin level less than 200 mg/L *and* a concentration of copper in liver biopsy greater than 250 μg/g dry weight. Most symptomatic patients excrete more than 100 μg copper per day in urine and have histologic abnormalities on liver biopsy.

About 5 percent of patients have a serum ceruloplasmin level greater than 200 mg/L, and some patients with other hepatic disorders, usually primary biliary cirrhosis, have elevated hepatic copper levels and, rarely, Kayser-Fleischer rings. In either circumstance, measurement of the ability to incorporate isotopic copper into ceruloplasmin is useful as a discriminating test. Even in the presence of a normal concentration of ceruloplasmin, patients with Wilson's disease incorporate little or no isotope into the protein, while patients with other liver disorders incorporate the isotope normally.

℞ TREATMENT

Treatment consists of removing and detoxifying the deposits of copper as rapidly as possible and must be instituted once the diagnosis is secure whether the patient is ill or asymptomatic. Penicillamine is administered orally in an initial dose of 1 g daily in a single or divided doses at least 30 min before and 2 h after eating. Because penicillamine has an antipyridoxine effect, 25 mg/d of pyridoxine is also given. In about 10 percent of patients sensitivity to penicillamine develops early, making it necessary to monitor the body temperature and skin daily and to assess white blood cell and platelet counts and perform urinalysis several times during the first month of treatment. Penicillamine should be discontinued if rash, fever, leukopenia, thrombocytopenia, lymphadenopathy, or proteinuria develops. After subsidence of the reaction, the drug can usually be resumed in small and gradually increasing dosage. Reactions are less likely to recur if 20 mg/d of prednisone is given during the first 2 weeks after penicillamine therapy is reinstituted, but prednisone should not be used for isolated leukopenia. Allergic reactions requiring a desensitizing regimen may recur several times before penicillamine can be administered without a glucocorticoid.

After therapy with penicillamine has been successfully instituted, the patient should be seen at 1- to 3-month intervals to assess the effectiveness of therapy and monitor for late drug toxicity. The history and the physical examination should focus on hepatic, neurologic, and psychiatric signs and symptoms; slit-lamp examination of the cornea should be performed by an ophthalmologist at least yearly. White blood cell and platelet counts, transaminase levels, albumin, bilirubin, and free serum copper (total serum copper minus ceruloplasmin-bound copper) should be measured, the aim being a concentration of free copper less than about 2 μmol/L (10 μg/dL). A persistent concentration greater than 4 μmol/L (20 μg/dL) indicates that the dose of penicillamine is too low or that the patient is noncompliant. In patients who are asymptomatic or who have improved maximally after several years on 1 g/d of penicillamine, the usual effective maintenance dose is 0.75 g/d taken 45 min before breakfast.

At any time, even after years of uneventful penicillamine administration, granulocytopenia, thrombocytopenia, the nephrotic syndrome, Goodpasture's syndrome, systemic lupus erythematosus, severe arthralgias, myasthenia, mammary gigantism, or elastosis perforans serpiginosa may supervene. The toxicity is sometimes dose-related, and it may be possible to reduce the dose to a level that is effective but nontoxic. Glucocorticoids may control penicillamine-associated lupus or arthralgias.

In two situations penicillamine should be replaced by trientine. First, although irreversible intolerance to penicillamine is rare, some types of toxicity such as significant, persistent proteinuria may make discontinuation necessary. Second, in occasional patients the commencement of penicillamine treatment may cause the appearance or worsening of neurologic manifestations. Substitution of trientine for penicillamine is indicated if neurologic symptoms persist or worsen over a 4- to 6-week period.

The dose of trientine is 1g/d in divided doses given on an empty stomach. Pyridoxine need not be given. Although the only reported toxic reaction to trientine is sideroblastic anemia, the same parameters should be followed during its administration as with penicillamine therapy. Except for systemic lupus and elastosis perforans serpiginosa, the other late penicillamine-induced toxic reactions disappear or improve with trientine therapy. Moreover, trientine appears to be as effective as penicillamine.

Zinc salts are effective at doses of 150 mg/d of elemental zinc in patients whose copper stores have been reduced by penicillamine or trientine. Zinc must *not*, however, be given together with penicillamine or trientine since zinc can chelate either drug and form complexes that are ineffective.

Treatment must be continual and lifelong. Inadequate treatment or interruption of therapy can be fatal or cause irreversible relapse. Indeed, of 11 patients who voluntarily discontinued penicillamine after years of successful treatment, 8 died after an average of 2.6 years of noncompliance. In contrast, of 13 patients in whom trientine was substituted because of an adverse reaction to penicillamine, 1 died accidentally, 5 were lost to follow-up, and 7 are alive and well 11 to 23 years later.

Prophylactic treatment of more than 100 asymptomatic patients with a documented diagnosis of Wilson's disease has shown that continual therapy with penicillamine or trientine can maintain the asymptomatic state indefinitely; several such patients having been followed for over 30 years.

Patients with severe neurologic disease who do not improve on penicillamine or trientine therapy that has reduced serum free copper to less than 2 μmol/L (10 μg/dL) may benefit from treatment with dimercaprol. Intramuscular injections of 3 mL of the drug are given on five successive days. Therapy is interrupted for 2 to 3 weeks, and if neurologic improvement occurs during this intermission, the courses should be repeated until no further improvement is noted.

The simultaneous occurrence of fulminant hepatitis and Coombs-negative hemolytic anemia may be the initial clinical manifestation of Wilson's disease or may occur in a noncompliant patient. The syndrome is almost always fatal, usually within a week or two, unless liver transplantation is performed. Of 55 patients who received liver transplants, 43 had survived for from 3 months to 20 years at last follow-up.

BIBLIOGRAPHY

Brewer GJ et al: Treatment of Wilson's disease with zinc: XI. Interaction with other anticopper agents. J Am Coll Nutr 12:26, 1993

Hoogenraad TU et al: Management of Wilson's disease with zinc sulfate: Experience in a series of 27 patients. J Neurol Sci 77:137, 1987

Petrukhin K et al: Mapping, cloning and genetic characterization of the region containing the Wilson disease gene. Nature (Genetics) 5:338, 1993

Scheinberg IH, Sternlieb I: Wilson's disease, in *Major Problems in Internal Medicine.* Philadelphia, Saunders, 1984

———, ———1994.: Treatment of the neurological manifestations of Wilson's disease. Arch Neurol 52:339, 1995

——— et al: The use of trientine in preventing the effects of interrupting penicillamine therapy in Wilson's disease. N Engl J Med 317:209, 1987

——— et al: Penicillamine may detoxify copper in Wilson's disease. Lancet 2:95, 1987

Schilsky ML et al: Liver transplantation for Wilson's disease: Indications and outcome. Hepatology 19:583, 1994

Sternlieb I: Evolution of the hepatic lesion in Wilson's disease (hepatolenticular degeneration), in *Progress in Liver Diseases*, H Popper et al (eds). New York, Grune & Stratton, 1972, vol IV, pp 511–526

———, Scheinberg IH: Prevention of Wilson's disease in asymptomatic patients. N Engl J Med 278:352, 1968

———, ———: Chronic hepatitis as a first manifestation of Wilson's disease. Ann Intern Med 76:59, 1972

Walshe JM: Wilson's disease, in *Handbook of Clinical Neurology*, PJ Vinken et al (eds). New York, American Elsevier, 1986, vol 5 (49)

346

Margaret M. McGovern

LYSOSOMAL STORAGE DISEASES

GENERAL FEATURES

DEFINITION The lysosomal storage diseases are a family of over 30 disorders that result from different defects in lysosomal function. Lysosomes are cytoplasmic organelles containing acid hydrolases that degrade macromolecules to their basic building blocks: peptides, amino acids, monosaccharides, nucleic acids, and fatty acids (Fig. 346-1). Lysosomal enzymes are synthesized in the endoplasmic reticulum, usually as precursor forms that undergo posttranslational processing (proteolytic cleavage, the addition of N-linked oligosaccharide chains, and the synthesis of recognition markers such as mannose-6-phosphate) prior to packaging in primary lysosomes. The primary lysosomes may fuse with other vesicles, including phagosomes or autophagosomes that contain macromolecules, cell debris, and cellular organelles to form secondary lysosomes where degradation of macromolecules occurs. Through absorptive endocytosis, lysosomes also function in the uptake of vitamin B_{12}, lipoproteins, peptide hormones, and growth factors.

Disorders of lysosomal function are traditionally classified according to the nature of the primary stored material and include mucopolysaccharidoses, lipid storage diseases, mucolipidoses, glycoprotein storage diseases, and others (Table 346-1). The first delineation of the pathophysiology of a lysosomal disorder came from the observation that accumulation of glycogen in lysosomes in Pompe's disease [glycogen storage disease (GSD) type II] is due to deficiency of a specific enzyme, α-glucosidase. Based on this finding and observations in other disorders, Hers defined the lysosomal storage diseases as disorders characterized by deficiency of a single lysosomal enzyme and the consequent accumulation of its substrates in lysosomes. Subsequently, the definition was expanded to include disorders such as the mucolipidoses and multiple sulfatase deficiency, in which single-gene defects impair the function of more than one lysosomal enzyme, and the deficiency of other proteins required for normal lysosomal function such as cofactors or protective proteins.

The clinical features of the lysosomal storage diseases can be predicted by knowing the normal site of degradation of the deficient enzyme's substrate and are dependent on the rate and magnitude of accumulation of undegraded material. Thus, defects of myelin degradation cause white matter disease; defective glycolipid degradation causes organomegaly; and defects in the degradation of mucopolysaccharides, which are ubiquitous, cause abnormalities in numerous tissues. The disorders are progressive, and most affected individuals appear normal at birth and develop manifestations after months or years. Many of the disorders are fatal in childhood or adolescence, although there is extensive phenotypic variability.

DIAGNOSIS The lysosomal storage diseases should be included in the differential diagnosis for any patient with progressive neurologic dysfunction, hepatosplenomegaly, and/or skeletal dysostosis. In particular, progression of disease and neurologic degeneration suggest a storage disease. The evaluation of a patient suspected of having one of these disorders should include a three-generation pedigree to detect consanguinity and/or the presence of an X-linked pattern of inheritance and determination of the ethnic background, because there is an increased frequency of Tay-Sachs disease, Niemann-Pick disease (NPD), and Gaucher's disease in Ashkenazi Jews; mannosidosis and aspartylglucosaminuria in Scandinavians; and the juvenile form of sialidosis in Japanese. The history should include the developmental milestones, which may be characterized by a period of normal development followed by slowing of development and then regression. Particular attention should be given to neurologic symptoms including seizures, visual loss and auditory impairment, the presence of umbilical hernias, a delayed or aberrant growth pattern, and joint limitations or pain.

Physical findings include coarse features, enlarged tongue, corneal clouding, exaggerated startle response (hyperacusis), hepatosplenomegaly, limited joint mobility and contractures, and umbilical hernias. Gigantism is a feature early in the course for the mucopolysaccharide and glycoprotein storage diseases, whereas short stature is characteristic for many of the other disorders. Neurologic examination should focus on determining the extent of involvement of gray matter, white matter, and peripheral nerves. Cutaneous features, when present, are distinctive and include angiokeratomas in Fabry's disease and fucosidosis, ichthyosis in multiple sulfatase deficiency, and papular, pebbly lesions of the shoulders and trunk in Hunter's syndrome. Funduscopic and slit-lamp examinations may reveal corneal clouding or the presence of a cherry red macule. Laboratory evaluation should include examination of the peripheral smear for vacuolated lymphocytes, analysis of the urine for mucopolysaccharides, and radiography of the spine and tubular bones to determine skeletal involvement. In some patients light- and electron-microscopic examination of biopsies of skin, conjunctivae, rectum, bone marrow, liver, or peripheral nerves may demonstrate engorgement of lysosomes. However, on the basis of clinical findings, skeletal survey, and the analysis of mucopolysaccharides in urine, it is usually possible to select a small number of enzyme assays in serum, leukocytes, or cultured skin fibroblasts to provide a definitive diagnosis.

GENETICS AND HETEROGENEITY The lysosomal storage diseases are inherited as autosomal recessive traits, with the exceptions of Hunter's syndrome [mucopolysaccharidosis (MPS) type II, or MPS II] and Fabry's disease, which are X-linked. Most of the conditions are characterized by clinical, biochemical, and genetic heterogeneity. In some cases, different mutations in the lysosomal structural genes account for the observed heterogeneity. For example, one mutation in a gene that encodes a lysosomal enzyme may cause total loss of the enzyme activity, whereas another mutation in the same gene may result in only partial impairment of enzyme activity and a less severe clinical course. Other mutations alter posttransitional modification or the affinity for various substrates. Heterogeneity in these disorders is further increased by the fact that patients with autosomal recessive traits are frequently compound heterozygotes and inherit two different mutant alleles, one from each carrier parent. The different mutant alleles may cause different properties, further increasing biochemical diversity among affected individuals. A typical example of heterogeneity among the lysosomal storage diseases is MPS I, which is discussed in detail below. A different type of genetic heterogeneity is demonstrated by the Sanfilippo syndromes (MPS III A, B, C, and D), in which similar phenotypes are caused by mutations in different genes.

The molecular pathology and specific mutations have been elucidated for many of the lysosomal diseases, and in some instances informative correlations can be made between genotype and the resulting phenotype. For example, in Gaucher's disease one mutation in the β-glucosidase gene, N370S, is protective against the development of neurologic disease. Similarly, in NPD the 608 mutation does not occur in patients with neurologic disease but is associated with variable somatic manifestations including organomegaly. Such genotype-phenotype correlations, when informative, are useful in prognosis and permit genetic counseling that allows families to make decisions about future pregnancies.

MANAGEMENT AND PREVENTION Most lysosomal storage diseases are characterized by a progressive course with severe morbidity and early mortality. Treatment is largely symptomatic, a notable exception being Gaucher's disease which is amenable to therapy with recombinantly produced acid β-glucosidase. However, such therapy has not been evaluated in patients with Gaucher's disease who have central nervous system (CNS) involvement. There is also a limited experience with bone marrow transplantation in the mucopolysaccharidoses, NPD, and Gaucher's disease. The results have been variable but with no appreciable effect on CNS involvement.

Because of the lack of effective therapy, prevention is of central importance. Couples who have had one affected child should be offered prenatal diagnosis in future pregnancies, since all the lysosomal storage diseases in which the enzymatic deficiency is known can be diagnosed in utero. Heterozygote identification for at-risk family members is also available for many of these disorders, both by enzymatic assays and by the identification of specific alleles in families that have been genotyped. Another approach to prevention is by the prospective identification of carrier couples at risk through heterozygote screening programs, such as the one for Tay-Sachs disease. However, these programs require the availability of a rapid and inexpensive carrier detection method and are usually targeted at populations known to be at increased risk, such as Ashkenazi Jews in whom Tay-Sachs disease, Gaucher's disease, and NPD occur with increased frequency. In other groups carrier screening would be less cost effective because of the low frequency of the mutant alleles in the general population.

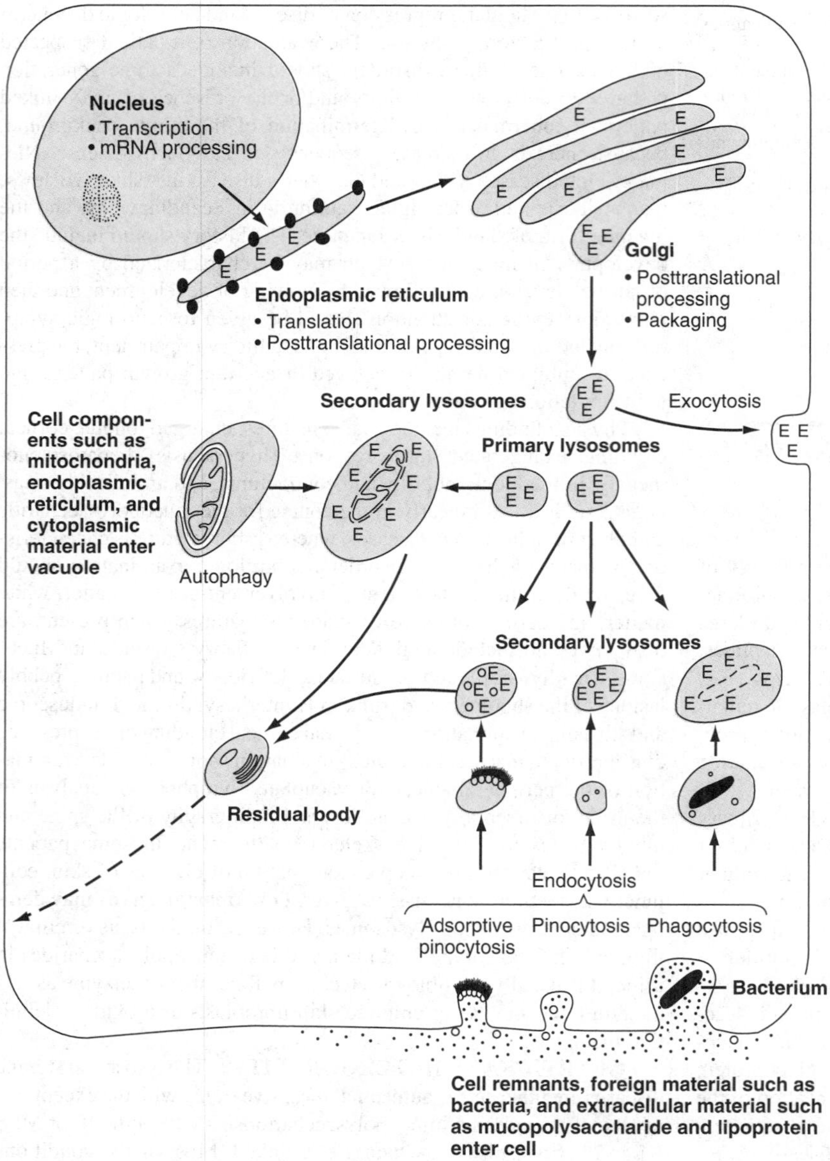

FIGURE 346-1 Biology of lysosomes. Lysosomal enzymes are synthesized in the endoplasmic reticulum and undergo posttranslational processing in the Golgi prior to packaging in the primary lysosome. Primary lysosomes can then participate in the process of autophagy or form secondary lysosomes as depicted. E, precursor and mature forms of lysosomal enzymes. [*From A Beaudet: Liposomal storage diseases, in KJ Isselbacher et al (ed), Harrison's Principles of Internal Medicine, 13th ed. New York, McGraw-Hill, p 2091, 1994.*]

SPECIFIC DISORDERS

The Mucopolysaccharidoses MPS results from the deficiency of one of the lysosomal enzymes required for glycosaminoglycan (GAG) catabolism. GAGs, which are major constituents of connective tissue, are long-chain, complex carbohydrates that are usually linked to proteins to form proteoglycans and include chondroitin-4-sulfate, chondroitin-6-sulfate, heparan sulfate, dermatan sulfate, keratan sulfate, and hyaluronic acid. The clinical features of the mucopolysaccharidoses result from the lysosomal accumulation of partially degraded or undegraded GAGs and typically include coarse facies, corneal clouding, organomegaly, joint stiffness, bony abnormalities, hernias, short stature, and, in some disorders, mental retardation. The phenotype of each disorder is determined by the specific enzymatic deficiency and the resultant pattern of accumulation of GAG degradation products; dermatan, keratan, and chondroitin sulfate degradation products are associated with visceral manifestations, and accumulation of heparan sulfate degradation products causes mental deficiency.

Laboratory findings include the presence of vacuolated lymphocytes in the peripheral smear and the presence of GAGs in urine. Since some features of the mucopolysaccharidoses also occur with the mucolipidoses, glycoprotein storage diseases, and other lysosomal storage diseases, definitive diagnosis is made by specific enzyme assays in leukocytes and/or cultured skin fibroblasts. Prenatal diagnosis by enzyme assays in fetal cells and/or by isotopic studies of GAG formation in cultured amniotic cells is available for each MPS, and carrier identification is possible in individuals with a positive family history by appropriate enzyme assay in leukocytes or serum. In addition, molecular identification of carriers is possible after the mutant alleles have been characterized in the family.

MPS IH (Hurler's disease) is one of the more severe forms and results from the deficiency of α-L-iduronidase. It is characterized by progressive organ involvement and mental retardation and causes death, usually in the first decade. Patients appear normal at birth and have accelerated growth in the first year, followed by slowing of growth and eventual short stature. The diagnosis is usually made by 2 years of age when organomegaly, corneal clouding, coarse features, large tongue, and joint stiffness are apparent. Developmental delay appears between 12 and 28 months, and subsequently there is regression in mental function. Other features include hearing loss, chronic respiratory infections, valvular heart disease, and increased intracranial pressure. MPS IS (Scheie's disease) and MPS I H/S (Hurler-Scheie disease) result from allelic mutations in the α-L-iduronidase gene and are characterized by a less severe clinical course, presumably due to the presence of residual α-L-iduronidase activity.

MPS II (Hunter's syndrome) is inherited as an X-linked recessive trait and is notable for the absence of corneal clouding and the presence of severe and mild forms with and without mental impairment. MPS IIIA, IIIB, IIIC, and IIID (the Sanfilippo syndromes) result from one of four enzymatic deficiencies and are characterized by behavioral problems and seizures, moderately severe somatic manifestations, and survival into the third decade. Individuals with MPS IV (Morquio's syndrome) have normal intelligence and severe skeletal findings sometimes confused with the spondyloepiphyseal dysplasias. The most serious complication is upper cervical spinal cord compression due to atlantoaxial instability. Patients with MPS VI (Maroteaux-Lamy disease) have a phenotype similar to Hurler's disease but with normal intelligence.

Treatment of the mucopolysaccharidoses is symptomatic and may include corneal transplantation, correction of nerve entrapments in the hands, and heart valve replacement. In MPS III, control of the behavioral problems may require psychotropic medications. For patients with MPS IV, cervical myelopathy should be prevented by surgery of the cervical spine. Attempts at enzyme replacement in various forms of MPS have not been successful, and bone marrow transplantation has produced variable results.

The GM_2 Gangliosidoses The GM_2 gangliosidoses include Tay-Sachs disease and Sandhoff's disease, each of which results from deficiency of hexosaminidase and the accumulation in lysosomes of GM_2 gangliosides, particularly in the CNS. Both disorders have infantile, juvenile, and adult-onset forms, depending on the age of onset and clinical features. Hexosaminidase A is composed of one α and one β subunit, and hexosaminidase B has two β subunits. Hexosaminidase A deficiency (Tay-Sachs disease) results from mutations in the α subunit, and mutations in the β subunit gene result in the deficiency of both hexosaminidase A and B and cause Sandhoff's disease. Both disorders are inherited as autosomal recessive traits; the carrier frequency of Tay-Sachs disease in Ashkenazi Jews is known 1 in 25.

The cDNAs for both the α and β subunits of hexosaminidase have been cloned. To date, over 50 mutations have been identified, most associated with the infantile forms of disease. Three mutations account for over 95 percent of mutant alleles among Ashkenazi Jews, including one allele associated with the adult-onset form. Mutations that cause the subacute or chronic forms have resulted in higher residual enzymatic activity levels that correlate with the severity of the disease.

The infantile form of Tay-Sachs disease causes loss of motor skills, increased startle reaction, and macular pallor (cherry red spot) on slit-lamp examination; it causes death by age 4. The juvenile-onset form is associated with ataxia and dementia and progresses to death by age 10 to 15. The adult-onset disorder is characterized by clumsiness in childhood and motor weakness in adolescence. Although spinocerebellar and lower motor neuron symptoms predominate in the adult form, some patients are psychotic. Intelligence and vision are typically normal. The infantile form of Sandhoff's disease is nearly identical in course to infantile Tay-Sachs, but two distinguishing features are the presence of organomegaly and occasional bony changes. Treatment is supportive.

The diagnosis of infantile Tay-Sachs and Sandhoff's disease is usually suspected during infancy on the basis of neurologic features and the finding of a cherry red spot and is confirmed by measurement of hexosaminidase levels in blood leukocytes. Future at-risk pregnancies can be monitored by prenatal diagnosis by amniocentesis or chorionic villus sampling, and identification of carriers within the family can be by hexosaminidase assays. Indeed, carrier screening of all couples in whom at least one member is an Ashkenazi Jew is recommended prior to the beginning of pregnancy to identify couples at risk. Since the introduction of such carrier screening programs for Ashkenazi Jews, the incidence of Tay-Sachs disease in this population has decreased.

The Lipid Storage Disorders The lipid storage diseases include Fabry's disease, Gaucher's disease, and NPD. For each of these disorders affected individuals may survive into adulthood.

Fabry's disease Fabry's disease is an inborn error of glycosphingolipid metabolism characterized by angiokeratomas (telangiectatic skin lesions), hypohidrosis, corneal and lenticular opacities, acroparesthesia, and vascular disease of the kidney, heart, and/or brain. The disease is an X-linked recessive trait that is manifested in affected hemizygous males and has an estimated prevalence of 1 in 40,000. Atypical hemizygous males with residual α-galactosidase A activity may be asymptomatic or have late-onset, mild manifestations, usually limited to the heart. Heterozygous females are usually asymptomatic or exhibit mild manifestations.

The disease results from the deficient activity of α-galactosidase A, which is encoded by a gene on the long arm of the X chromosome (Xq22). The defect leads to the accumulation of neutral glycosphingolipids, primarily globotriaosylceramide, in the plasma and lysosomes of vascular endothelial and smooth-muscle cells. The progressive deposition of glycosphingolipid in vessel walls results in ischemia and infarction, the major disease manifestations. Affected males who have blood group B or AB have a more severe course due to accumulation of blood group B substance, which is normally degraded by α-galactosidase A. The cDNA and genomic sequences encoding α-galactosidase A have been characterized, and known mutations responsible for this disease include amino acid substitutions, gene rearrangements, and mRNA splicing defects.

The angiokeratomas in Fabry's disease usually appear in childhood and may lead to early diagnosis. The lesions are punctate, dark red to blue-black, and flat or slightly raised. They do not blanch with pressure, and the larger ones may show slight hyperkeratosis. They increase in size and number with age and range from barely visible to several millimeters in diameter. Characteristically, the lesions are most dense between the umbilicus and knees, in the "bathing trunk area," but may occur anywhere, including the oral mucosa. The hips, thighs, buttocks, umbilicus, lower abdomen, scrotum, and penis are common sites, and there is a tendency toward bilateral symmetry. Skin lesions are not invariably present. Sweating is usually decreased or absent. Corneal opacities and characteristic lenticular lesions, observed in slit-lamp examination, are present in affected men and in about 70 percent of asymptomatic heterozygotes. Tortuosity of the conjunctival and retinal vessels is common.

Pain is the most debilitating symptom in childhood and adolescence. Fabry crises, lasting from minutes to days, consist of agonizing, burning pain in the hands, feet, and proximal extremities and are usually precipitated by exercise, fatigue, or fever. These painful acroparesthesias usually become less frequent in the third and fourth decades of life but on occasion become more frequent and more severe. Abdominal or flank pain may simulate appendicitis or renal colic.

With age the major morbidity is caused by progressive involvement of the vascular system. Early in the course casts, red cells, and lipid inclusions with characteristic birefringent "Maltese crosses" appear in the urinary sediment. Proteinuria, isosthenuria, and deterioration of

Table 346-1

Summary of Lysosomal Storage Diseases

Disorder	Enzyme Deficiency	Stored Material	Clinical Subtypes (Onset)	Inheritance	Neurologic
MUCOPOLYSACCHARIDOSES (MPS)					
MPS I H, Hurler (78) MPS I H/S, Hurler/Scheie MPS I S, Scheie	α-L-Iduronidase	Dermatan sulfate Heparan sulfate	Infantile Intermediate Adult	AR	Mental retardation, except in Scheie
MPS II, Hunter (78)	Iduronate sulfatase	Dermatan sulfate Heparan sulfate	Severe infantile Mild juvenile	X-linked	Mental retardation, less in mild form
MPS III A, Sanfilippo A (78)	Heparan-*N*-sulfatase	Heparan sulfate	Late infantile	AR	Severe mental retardation
MPS III B, Sanfilippo B	*N*-Acetyl-α-glucosaminidase	Heparan sulfate	Late infantile	AR	Severe mental retardation
MPS III C, Sanfilippo C	Acetyl-CoA: α-glucosaminide *N*-acetyltransferase	Heparan sulfate	Late infantile	AR	Severe mental retardation
MPS III D, Sanfilippo D	*N*-Acetylglucosamine-6-sulfate sulfatase	Heparan sulfate	Late infantile	AR	Severe mental retardation
MPS IV, Morquio (78)	*N*-Acetylgalactosamine-6-sulfate sulfatase	Keratan sulfate Chondroitin-6 sulfate	Childhood	AR	0
MPS VI, Maroteaux-Lamy (78)	Arylsulfatase B	Dermatan sulfate	Late infantile	AR	0
MPS VII (78)	β-Glucuoronidase	Dermatan sulfate Heparan sulfate	Neonatal Infantile Adult	AR	Mental retardation, absent in some adults
GM_2 GANGLIOSIDOSES					
Tay-Sachs' disease (92)	Hexosaminidase A	GM_2 gangliosides	Infantile Juvenile	AR	Mental retardation, seizures, later juvenile form
Sandhoff's disease (92)	Hexosaminidases A and B	GM_2 gangliosides	Infantile	AR	Mental retardation, seizures
LIPID STORAGE DISORDERS					
Fabry's disease (89)	α-Galactosidase A	Trihexosylceramide	Childhood	X-linked	Painful neuropathy
Gaucher's disease (86)	Acid β-Glucosidase	Glucosylceramide	Adult, type 1 Infantile, type 2 Juvenile, type 3	AR	Mental retardation in infantile, ataxia in juvenile, no symptoms in adult
Niemann-Pick's disease (84)	Sphingomyelinase	Sphingomyelin	Infantile neuronopathic, type A Nonneuronopathic, type B	AR	Mental retardation and seizures in type A
GLYCOPROTEINOSES					
Fucosidosis (81)	α-Fucosidase	Glycopeptides, oligosaccharides	Infantile Juvenile	AR	Mental retardation
α-Mannosidosis (81)	α-Mannosidase	Oligosaccharides	Infantile Milder variant	AR	Mental retardation
β-Mannosidosis (81)	β-Mannosidase	Oligosaccharides		AR	Seizures, mental retardation
Aspartylglucosaminuria (81)	Aspartylglucosaminidase	Aspartylglucosamine, glycopeptides	Young adult onset	AR	Mental retardation
Sialidosis (81)	Neuraminidase	Sialyloligosaccharides	Type I, congenital Type II, infantile and juvenile forms	AR	Myoclonus, mental retardation
MUCOLIPIDOSES (ML)					
ML-II, I-cell disease (78)	UDP-*N*-Acetylglucosamine-1-phosphotransferase	Glycoprotein, glycolipids	Infantile	AR	Mental retardation
ML-III, pseudo-Hurler polydystrophy (79)	UDP-*N*-Acetylglucosamine-1-phosphotransferase	Glycoprotein, glycolipids	Late infantile	AR	Mild mental retardation
LEUKODYSTROPHIES					
Krabbe's disease (87)	Galactosylceramidase	Galactocerebroside	Infantile	AR	Mental retardation
Metachromatic leukodystrophy (88)	Arylsulfatase A	Cerebroside sulfate	Infantile Juvenile Adult	AR	Mental retardation, dementia, and psychosis in adult
Multiple sulfatase deficiency (88)	Arylsulfatases A, B, and C	Sulfatides, mucopolysaccharides	Late infantile	AR	Mental retardation
Wolman's disease (82)	Acid lipase	Cholesterol ester, triglycerides	Infantile	AR	Mild mental retardation
Cholesterol ester storage disease (82)	Acid lipase	Cholesterol ester, triglycerides	Adult	AR	0
Farber's disease (83)	Acid ceramidase	Ceramide	Infantile Juvenile	AR	Occasional mental retardation

NOTE: Numbers in parentheses refer to the chapters in Scriver et al, 7th edition, in which the disorders are discussed.

Clinical Features				
Liver and/or Spleen Enlargement	**Skeletal Dysplasia**	**Ophthalmologic**	**Hematologic**	**Unique Features**
+ + +	+ + + +	Corneal clouding	Vacuolated lymphocytes	Coarse facies, cardiovascular involvement, joint stiffness
+ + +	+ + + +	Retinal degeneration, no corneal clouding	Granuolated lymphocytes	Coarse facies, cardiovascular, joint stiffness, distinctive pebbly skin lesions
+	+	0	Granuolated lymphocytes	Mild coarse facies
+	+	0	Granuolated lymphocytes	Mild coarse facies
+	+	0	Granuolated lymphocytes	Mild coarse facies
+	+	0	Granuolated lymphocytes	Mild coarse facies
+	+ + + +	Corneal clouding	Granuolated neutrophils	Distinctive skeletal deformity, odontoid hypoplasia, aortic valve disease
+ +	+ + + +	Corneal clouding	Granuolated neutrophils and lymphocytes	Coarse facies, valvular heart disease
+ + +	+ + +	Corneal clouding	Granuolated neutrophils	Coarse facies, vascular involvement, hydrops fetalis in neonatal form
0	0	Cherry red spot in infantile form	0	Macrocephaly, hyperacusis in infantile
0	0	Cherry red spot	0	Macrocephaly, hyperacusis
0	0	Corneal dystrophy, vascular lesions	0	Cutaneous angiokeratoses, hypohydrosis
+ + + +	+ +	0	Foam cells	Adult form includes pathologic fractures
+ + + +	0	Macular degeneration and cherry red spot in type A	Foam cells	Pulmonary infiltrates
+ +	+ +	0	Vacuolated lymphocytes, foam cells	Coarse facies, angiokeratomas in juvenile form
+ + +	+ +	Cataracts, corneal clouding	Vacuolated lymphocytes, granuolated neutrophils	Coarse facies, enlarged tongue
	+ +	0	Vacuolated lymphocytes, foam cells	Angiokeratomas
0	+ +	0	Vacuolated lymphocytes, foam cells	Coarse facies
+ +, less in type I	+ + less in type I	Cherry red spot	Vacuolated lymphocytes	MPS phenotype in type II
0/+	+ + + +	Corneal clouding	Vacuolated and granuolated neutrophils	Coarse facies, absence of mucopolysacchariduria, gingival hypoplasia
0	+ + +	Corneal clouding, mild retinopathy, hyperopic astigmatism		Coarse facies, stiffness of hands and shoulders
0	0	0	0	White matter globoid cells
0	0	Optic atrophy	0	Gait abnormalities in late infantile
+	+ +	Retinal degeneration	Vacuolated and granuolated cells	Ichthyosis
+ + +	0	0		Adrenal calcification
0	0	0		Premature atherosclerosis
+/−	0	Macular degeneration	0	Arthropathy, subcutaneous nodules

renal function are apparent by the second to fourth decades of life. Cardiovascular manifestations may include hypertension, left ventricular hypertrophy, anginal chest pain, myocardial ischemia or infarction, and congestive heart failure, frequently due to mitral insufficiency. Electrocardiographic and echocardiographic abnormalities are common. Cerebrovascular manifestations are due to multifocal small vessel involvement. Other features include chronic bronchitis and dyspnea, lymphedema of the legs without hypoproteinemia, episodic diarrhea, osteoporosis, growth retardation, and delayed puberty. Death is due to renal failure or vascular disease of the heart or brain. Prior to hemodialysis or renal transplantation, the mean age of death was 41 years. Atypical patients with residual α-galactosidase A activity may be asymptomatic or mildly affected, and patients with no early manifestations can develop late-onset cardiac or cardiopulmonary disease. In these "cardiac variants," cardiomegaly usually involves the left ventricular wall and interventricular septum, and electrocardiographic abnormalities are consistent with cardiomyopathy. Hypertrophic cardiomyopathy and/or myocardial infarction have been described.

The diagnosis is typically made from the history of painful acroparesthesias and the presence of hypohidrosis, characteristic skin lesions, and typical corneal opacities and lenticular lesions. The disorder is often misdiagnosed as rheumatic fever, erythromyalgia, or neurosis. The skin lesions must be differentiated from the benign angiokeratomas of the scrotum (Fordyce's disease) and from angiokeratoma circumscriptum. Angiokeratomas identical to those of Fabry's disease have been reported in fucosidosis, aspartylglycosaminuria, late-onset GM_1 gangliosidosis, galactosialidosis, α-*N*-acetylgalactosaminidase deficiency, and sialidosis. The diagnosis of the mild cardiac variants should be considered in individuals with left ventricular hypertrophy and/or cardiomyopathy of unknown etiology. The diagnosis is confirmed by demonstration of decreased α-galactosidase A activity in plasma, leukocytes, or cultured lymphoblasts or skin fibroblasts.

Heterozygous females may have corneal opacities, isolated skin lesions, and intermediate levels of α-galactosidase A in plasma or cells. Rare heterozygous women have manifestations as severe as those in men. Even asymptomatic at-risk women in families with Fabry's disease should be diagnosed by the direct analysis of the specific family mutation. Affected males can be diagnosed prenatally by demonstration of deficient α-galactosidase A activity or of the specific family mutation in chorionic villi in the first trimester or in cultured amniocytes in the second trimester of pregnancy.

Phenytoin and carbamazepine decrease the frequency and severity of the chronic acroparesthesias and of the periodic crises of excruciating pain. Otherwise, treatment is supportive and nonspecific. Renal transplantation and chronic hemodialysis can be lifesaving. Replacement therapy using partially purified human enzyme has been biochemically effective in short-term pilot trials, but sufficient enzyme is not available to evaluate the clinical effectiveness of long-term therapy. The availability of the cDNA encoding human α-galactosidase A may make possible the production of recombinant enzyme for long-term trials.

Gaucher's disease Gaucher's disease is a multisystemic lipidosis characterized by hematologic problems, organomegaly, and skeletal involvement, usually manifested as bone pain and pathologic fractures. It is the most common lysosomal storage disease and the most common genetic defect in Ashkenazi Jews. The three clinical subtypes are delineated by the absence or presence and progression of neurologic manifestations: type 1, the adult, nonneuronopathic form; type 2, the infantile or acute neuronopathic form; and type 3, the juvenile or Norrbotten form. All three are inherited as autosomal recessive traits. Type 1, which accounts for 99 percent of cases, has an incidence of about 1 in 1000 and a carrier frequency of 1 in 18 in Ashkenazi Jews.

Gaucher's disease results from deficiency of the lysosomal hydrolase, acid β-glucosidase, which is encoded by a gene on chromosome 1 (q21 to q31). The defect causes progressive accumulation of undegraded glycolipid substrates, particularly glucosylceramide, in reticuloendothelial cells and results in infiltration of the bone marrow, hepatosplenomegaly, and skeletal complications. The cDNA for acid β-glucosidase has been cloned, and the more than 35 identified mutant alleles include missense, insertion, and deletion mutations. Four of these mutations, N370S, L444P, 84insG, and IVS2, account for 90 to 95 percent of mutations among Ashkenazi Jews, making screening practical in this population. The molecular basis of the clinical heterogeneity in Gaucher's disease type 1 is partially understood. For example, homozygotes for the N370S mutation tend to have later onset of manifestations and a more indolent course than patients with one copy of N370S and another common allele.

Manifestations of Gaucher's disease type 1 have a variable age of onset, from early childhood to late adulthood, but most patients are symptomatic by adolescence; manifestations include easy bruisability due to thrombocytopenia, chronic fatigue secondary to anemia, hepatomegaly with or without elevated liver function tests, splenomegaly, bone pain, and occasional pulmonary involvement. Patients presenting in the first decade are frequently non-Jewish, have growth retardation, and have a more malignant course. Other patients are discovered fortuitously and have a benign course. In symptomatic patients, splenomegaly is progressive and can become massive. Bone involvement, which occurs in over 20 percent of patients, can cause pain or pathologic fractures or be manifested only by radiologic findings, including Erlenmeyer flask deformities of the distal femur. With symptomatic bone disease, lytic lesions in the femur, ribs, and pelvis and osteosclerosis may be evident at an early age, and bone crises with pain and swelling can be severe. Bleeding secondary to thrombocytopenia may manifest as epistaxis and bruising and is frequently overlooked until other symptoms become apparent. With the exception of the child with severe growth retardation and developmental delay secondary to the effects of chronic disease, development and intelligence are normal. The pathologic hallmark of the disease is the Gaucher cell in the reticuloendothelial system, particularly in the bone marrow. These cells are 20 to 100 μm in diameter and have a characteristic "wrinkled paper" appearance resulting from intracytoplasmic inclusions of substrate. The cytoplasm of the Gaucher cell reacts strongly positive with the periodic acid Schiff stain, and the presence of this cell in bone marrow and tissue biopsy specimens is suggestive of Gaucher's disease, although similar cells may be found in patients with granulocytic leukemia and myeloma.

Gaucher's disease type 2 is less common, does not have a striking ethnic predilection, and is characterized by a rapid neurodegenerative course with extensive visceral involvement and death within the first 2 years. It presents in infancy with increased tone, strabismus, organomegaly, failure to thrive, and stridor due to laryngospasm. After a period of psychomotor retrogression, death is usually due to respiratory complications. Gaucher's disease type 3 has clinical manifestations that are intermediate to those in types 1 and 2; they begin in childhood and cause death by age 10 to 15. Type 3 disease has a predilection for the Swedish Norbotten population where the incidence is 1 in 50,000. Neurologic involvement begins later and is less severe than in type 2 disease. Type 3 is further classified as type 3a and 3b, based on whether there is progressive myotonia and dementia (type 3a) or isolated supranuclear gaze palsy (type 3b).

The diagnosis should be considered in any patient with unexplained organomegaly, easy bruisability, and/or bone pain. Bone marrow examination usually reveals the presence of Gaucher cells, but the diagnosis should be confirmed by measurement of acid β-glucosidase activity in isolated leukocytes or cultured fibroblasts. Heterozygous carriers can be identified by enzyme and/or by molecular testing in many families. Testing should be offered to all family members, recognizing that heterogeneity even among members of the same kindred can be so great that asymptomatic affected individuals may be diagnosed during such testing. Prenatal diagnosis is available by determination of enzyme activity in chorionic villi or cultured amniotic fluid cells.

In the past, symptomatic management included blood transfusions for anemia, partial or total splenectomy for mechanical cardiopulmonary compromise or hypersplenism, analgesics for bone pain, and orthopedic procedures or joint replacement for severe bony involvement. A small number of patients have been cured by bone marrow transplantation, but the morbidity and mortality of the procedure limit its usefulness. It is now established that enzyme replacement with purified placental acid β-glucosidase is safe and efficaceous. Most extraskeletal manifestations are reversed by administration of 30 to 60 IU/kg of enzyme intravenously every other week. The effectiveness of this therapy in reversing and preventing bony manifestations is under study, but some data suggest that it is efficacious in this regard as well. An enzyme made by recombinant DNA technology is being studied in clinical trials. Once the efficacy of the recombinant enzyme is documented, enzyme therapy for Gaucher's disease will be implemented more widely.

Niemann-Pick disease The original report of NPD described what is now known as type A NPD, a fatal disorder of infancy characterized by failure to thrive, hepatosplenomegaly, a rapidly progressive neurodegenerative course, and death by 2 to 3 years of age. Six subtypes of NPD are now recognized, including type B, which is a nonneuronopathic form in adults, and other, rarer forms that result from defects in cholesterol metabolism. All six subtypes are inherited as autosomal recessive traits and display variable clinical features.

Types A and B NPD result from the deficient activity of sphingomyelinase, a lysosomal enzyme encoded by a gene on chromosome 11 (11p15.1 to p15.4). The defect results in accumulation of sphingomyelin, a ceramide phospholipid, and other lipids in the monocyte-macrophage system. The progressive deposition of sphingomyelin in the CNS causes the neurodegenerative manifestations in type A and in the systemic manifestations of type B, including progressive lung disease in some. The sphingomyelinase gene has been sequenced, and 12 mutations that cause types A and B NPD have been identified, including 9 single-base substitutions and 3 small deletions.

The manifestations and course of type A NPD are relatively uniform and are characterized by normal appearance at birth (although the newborn period is sometimes complicated by prolonged jaundice); hepatosplenomegaly, moderate lymphadenopathy, and psychomotor retardation are evident by 6 months of age, followed thereafter by regression. The loss of motor function and the deterioration of intellectual capabilities become progressively debilitating and eventuate in spasticity, rigidity, and loss of contact with the environment. In contrast, the manifestations and course of type B disease are more variable. Most patients are diagnosed in infancy or childhood when enlargement of the liver and/or spleen is detected during a routine physical examination, and evidence of mild pulmonary involvement is usually evident as a diffuse reticular or finely nodular infiltrate on the chest roentgenogram. Although hepatosplenomegaly is prominent in childhood, the abdominal protuberance decreases and becomes less conspicuous with time. In mildly affected patients, the splenomegaly may not be noted until adulthood, and disease manifestations may be minimal.

In most type B patients, pulmonary diffusion is decreased due to alveolar infiltration during childhood and worsens with age. Pulmonary compromise may be severe by 15 to 20 years of age. Such patients have low P_{O_2} levels and dyspnea on exertion. Bronchopneumonia and cor pulmonale may occur. Liver involvement can lead to cirrhosis of the liver, portal hypertension, and ascites. Pancytopenia due to secondary hypersplenism may respond to partial or complete splenectomy. Type B patients usually do not have neurologic involvement and are intellectually intact.

Type C NPD patients may have prolonged neonatal jaundice, appear normal for 1 to 2 years, and then undergo a slowly progressive and variable neurodegeneration. The hepatosplenomegaly is less severe than with types A or B NPD, and these patients may survive into adulthood. The underlying biochemical defect in type C NPD is an abnormality in cholesterol transport, leading to the accumulation of sphingomyelin and cholesterol in lysosomes and a secondary reduction in sphingomyelinase activity. Type D NPD patients develop neurologic symptoms later in childhood and have a slower course of neurodegeneration than type C patients. Most individuals with type D disease share a common ancestry traceable to Acadians from Yarmouth County, Nova Scotia. These patients also have an abnormality in cholesterol metabolism, and the defect may be allelic to the defect in type C NPD.

In type B NPD patients, splenomegaly is usually noted in early childhood, but in mild cases detection of splenic enlargement may be delayed into adolescence or adulthood. The presence of the characteristic NPD cells in the bone marrow aspirates supports the diagnosis of type B NPD. However, patients with types C and D NPD also have NPD cells in the bone marrow, and the suspected diagnosis should be confirmed by measuring sphingomyelinase in peripheral leukocytes, cultured fibroblasts, and/or lymphoblasts. Patients with types A and B NPD have markedly decreased levels (1 to 10 percent), whereas patients with types C and D NPD have intermediate levels and patients with Gaucher's disease and other storage disorders that cause hepatosplenomegaly and/or neurologic involvement have normal or near-normal levels of sphingomyelinase. The enzymatic identification of NPD carriers is problematic, but in families in whom the specific molecular defect has been identified, heterozygotes can be identified by DNA analysis. Prenatal diagnosis of NPD can be made by measurement of sphingomyelinase in cultured amniocytes or chorionic villi, and molecular studies of fetal DNA can provide the diagnosis or serve as a confirmatory test.

There is no specific treatment for NPD. Orthotopic liver transplantation in an infant with type A disease and amniotic cell transplantation in several type B NPD patients have had little or no success. Bone marrow transplantation in one type B NPD patient reduced the spleen and liver volumes, the sphingomyelin content in the liver, the number of NPD cells in the marrow, and the radiologic infiltration of the lungs, but the patient died 3 months after transplantation. To date, lung transplantation has not been performed.

The Glycoproteinoses The glycoproteinoses, or oligosaccharidoses, are disorders of impaired glycoprotein degradation and include fucosidosis, mannosidosis, sialidosis, and aspartylglucosaminuria. These disorders, each of which is inherited as an autosomal recessive trait, share features with both the mucopolysaccharidoses and the sphingolipidoses and are characterized by neurologic manifestations and varying somatic features. *Fucosidosis* is a rare disorder that results from the deficient activity of α-fucosidase. Although the disorder is panethnic, most described patients have been from Italy or the United States. Within the first year it causes developmental delay, somatic features similar to those in MPS, sweat electrolyte abnormalities, and development of angiokeratomas. Most severely affected patients have a relentless neurodegenerative course with death in childhood, although a mild variant is compatible with longer survival. *Mannosidosis*, resulting from α-mannosidase deficiency, includes a severe infantile form characterized by progressive mental retardation, facial coarsening, dysostosis multiplex, and organomegaly with death in childhood. A juvenile–adult-onset phenotype with survival into adulthood is characterized by normal early development and the later appearance of neurologic symptoms and mental retardation in childhood or adolescence. *Aspartylglucosaminuria*, which has its highest incidence in Finland, presents later in childhood with progressive mental deterioration, coarsening of the facies, and behavioral problems. The deficiency of aspartylglucosaminidase results in the excretion of aspartylglucosamine in urine in diagnostic quantities. *Sialidosis* results from sialidase deficiency and includes a neonatal form that presents with hydrops and an infantile form characterized by glomerular nephropathy. A childhood form shares somatic features with Hurler's syndrome, including coarse facies; the juvenile form (the cherry red spot myoclonus syndrome) is characterized by the development of ocular cherry red spots and generalized myoclonus in the second decade. Combined deficiencies of sialidase and β-galactosidase are due to defects in a glycoprotein required for the protection of both enzymes from degradation.

No treatment is available for the glycoproteinoses, although one patient with α-mannosidosis had some improvement in somatic manifestations after bone marrow transplantation. Prenatal diagnosis is available for each disorder using either chorionic villi or cultured amniocytes, and molecular identification of the specific mutation in some of these disorders makes prenatal diagnosis and carrier detection possible.

The Leukodystrophies The leukodystrophies are disorders of the white matter of the brain and include Krabbe's disease (or globoid cell leukodystrophy) and metachromatic leukodystrophy (MLD). Krabbe's disease, a rapidly progressive, fatal disorder of infancy that results from galactosylceramidase deficiency, is characterized by the presence of multinucleated globoid cells, almost complete loss of myelin, and astrocytic gliosis in the white matter. Manifestations are confined to the nervous system, and patients rarely survive beyond the second year. Diagnosis is by the demonstration of the enzymatic defect, and treatment is supportive. In contrast, MLD may present at any age and has been divided into late infantile, juvenile, and adult forms. The disease results from the deficient activity of arylsulfatase A and the accumulation of galactosyl sulfatide in the white matter of the CNS and peripheral nervous system. The infantile form typically presents in the second year and is fatal, whereas the juvenile and adult forms are more variable and include gait disturbances, mental regression, peripheral neuropathy, seizures, and, in adults, behavioral disturbances and dementia. Treatment of late-onset disease by bone marrow transplantation has yielded variable results. Each of these disorders can be detected by prenatal diagnosis.

Glycogen Storage Disease Type II (See also Chap. 347) GSDII or Pompe's disease is due to deficiency of acid α-glucosidase and the accumulation of glycogen in lysosomes, particularly in cardiac and skeletal muscle. The infantile form is a rapidly fatal disorder associated with cardiomegaly, macroglossia, and hypotonia. The juvenile form is characterized by progressive proximal muscle weakness, including impairment of respiratory function. Electromyography can be helpful in making the diagnosis, but in adult patients the abnormalities vary among different muscles. Treatment is supportive. Prenatal diagnosis is available.

The Mucolipidoses The mucolipidoses include I-cell disease or mucolipidosis (ML) II and pseudohurler polydystrophy or ML-III. I-cell disease shares many phenotypic features with Hurler's syndrome, whereas ML-III is a milder disorder that presents later. Both disorders result from abnormal transport of the lysosomal enzymes, which results in decreased levels of several enzymes in the cell and excretion of the enzymes into the extracellular compartment. The specific defect is in the lysosomal enzyme *N*-acetylglucosamine-1-phosphotransferase, an essential enzyme for the synthesis of a mannose-6-phosphate recognition marker that targets lysosomal enzymes to the lysosome. The diagnosis is by demonstrating elevated serum levels of the lysosomal enzymes or by demonstration of the phosphotransferase deficiency. Treatment is supportive, and carrier identification and prenatal diagnosis are possible.

BIBLIOGRAPHY

BEIGHTON P (ed): *Heritable Disorders of Connective Tissue*, 5th ed. St. Louis, Mosby, 1993

HERS HG, VAN HOOF F (eds): *Lysosomes and Storage Diseases*. New York, Academic Press, 1973

SCRIVER CR et al (eds): *The Metabolic and Molecular Bases of Inherited Diseases*, 7th ed. New York, McGraw-Hill, 1995

WATTS RWE, GIBBS DA (eds): *Lysosomal Storage Diseases: Biochemical and Clinical Aspects*. Philadelphia, Taylor and Francis, 1986

347 GLYCOGEN STORAGE DISEASES

Yuan-Tsong Chen

Glycogen, the storage form of glucose in animal cells, is composed of glucose residues joined in straight chains by α1-4 linkages and branched at intervals of 4 to 10 residues with α1-6 linkages. The treelike molecule can have a molecular weight of many millions and may aggregate to form structures recognizable by electron microscopy. In muscle, glycogen forms β particles, which are spherical and contain up to 60,000 glucose residues. Each β particle contains a covalently linked protein called *glycogenin*. Liver contains β particles and rosettes of glycogen called α *particles*, which appear to be aggregated β particles.

The primary function of glycogen varies in different tissues. In skeletal muscle, stored glycogen is a source of fuel that is used for short-term, high-energy consumption during muscle activity; in the brain, the small amount of stored glycogen is used during brief periods of hypoglycemia or hypoxia as an emergency supply of energy. In contrast, the liver takes up glucose from the bloodstream after a meal and stores it as glycogen. When blood glucose levels start to fall, the liver converts glycogen back into glucose and releases it into the blood for use by tissues such as brain and erythrocytes that cannot store significant amounts of glycogen.

Glycogen storage diseases are inherited disorders that affect glycogen metabolism. Disorders in virtually every enzyme involved in the synthesis or degradation of glycogen and its regulation cause some type of glycogen storage disease (Fig. 347-1) in which glycogen is abnormal in quantity, quality, or both. Excluded from this chapter are those conditions in which tissue glycogen accumulation is secondary, such as overtreatment of diabetes mellitus with insulin or administration of pharmacologic amounts of glucocorticoids.

Historically, the glycogen storage diseases were categorized numerically in the order in which the enzymatic defects were identified, up to number VII. They can also be classified by the organs involved and clinical manifestations, the system followed in this chapter (Table 347-1).

Because liver and muscle have abundant glycogen, they are the most commonly and seriously affected tissues. The hepatic glycogen storage diseases can be divided into two groups, with some overlap. The first is characterized by hepatomegaly and hypoglycemia. Because carbohydrate metabolism in the liver controls plasma glucose levels, the disorders of hepatic glycogen degradation and glucose release cause fasting hypoglycemia. Diseases in this group include glucose-6-phosphatase deficiency (type I), debranching enzyme deficiency (type III), liver phosphorylase deficiency (type VI), and phosphorylase kinase deficiency (formerly type VIa or IX). The second group, characterized by cirrhosis of the liver and hepatomegaly, is associated with accumulation of abnormal forms of glycogen, which may be the cause of the hepatocellular injury. This group includes branching enzyme deficiency (type IV) and debranching enzyme deficiency (type III).

The role of glycogen in muscle is to provide substrates for the generation of sufficient ATP for muscle contraction. The muscle glycogen storage diseases can also be divided into two groups. The first is a muscle-energy disorder characterized by muscle pain, exercise intolerance, myoglobinuria, and susceptibility to fatigue. This group includes type V (McArdle disease), a muscle phosphorylase deficiency, and deficiencies of phosphofructokinase (type VII), phosphoglycerate kinase, phosphoglycerate mutase, or lactate dehydrogenase. Some of these latter enzyme deficiencies are associated with a compensated hemolysis, suggesting a more generalized defect in glucose metabolism. The second group of muscle disorders is characterized by progressive skeletal muscle weakness and atrophy and/or cardiomyopathy and includes a lysosomal enzyme deficiency (acid α-glucosidase, type II), muscle debranching enzyme deficiency (type IIIa), a form of branching enzyme deficiency (type IV), and deficiency of cardiac-specific phosphorylase kinase.

The overall frequency of all forms of glycogen storage disease is approximately 1 in 20,000 to 25,000 live births. The most common childhood disorders are glucose-6-phosphatase deficiency (type I), lysosomal acid α-glucosidase deficiency (type II), debrancher deficiency (type III), and liver phosphorylase kinase deficiency (formerly type VIa or IX). The most common adult disorder is myophosphorylase deficiency (type V, or McArdle disease). In the past, the prognosis for many glycogen storage diseases was guarded. Early diagnosis and better management have improved the survival rates, and many affected children are now adults.

The majority of the glycogen storage diseases are inherited as autosomal recessive traits, but phosphoglycerate kinase deficiency and

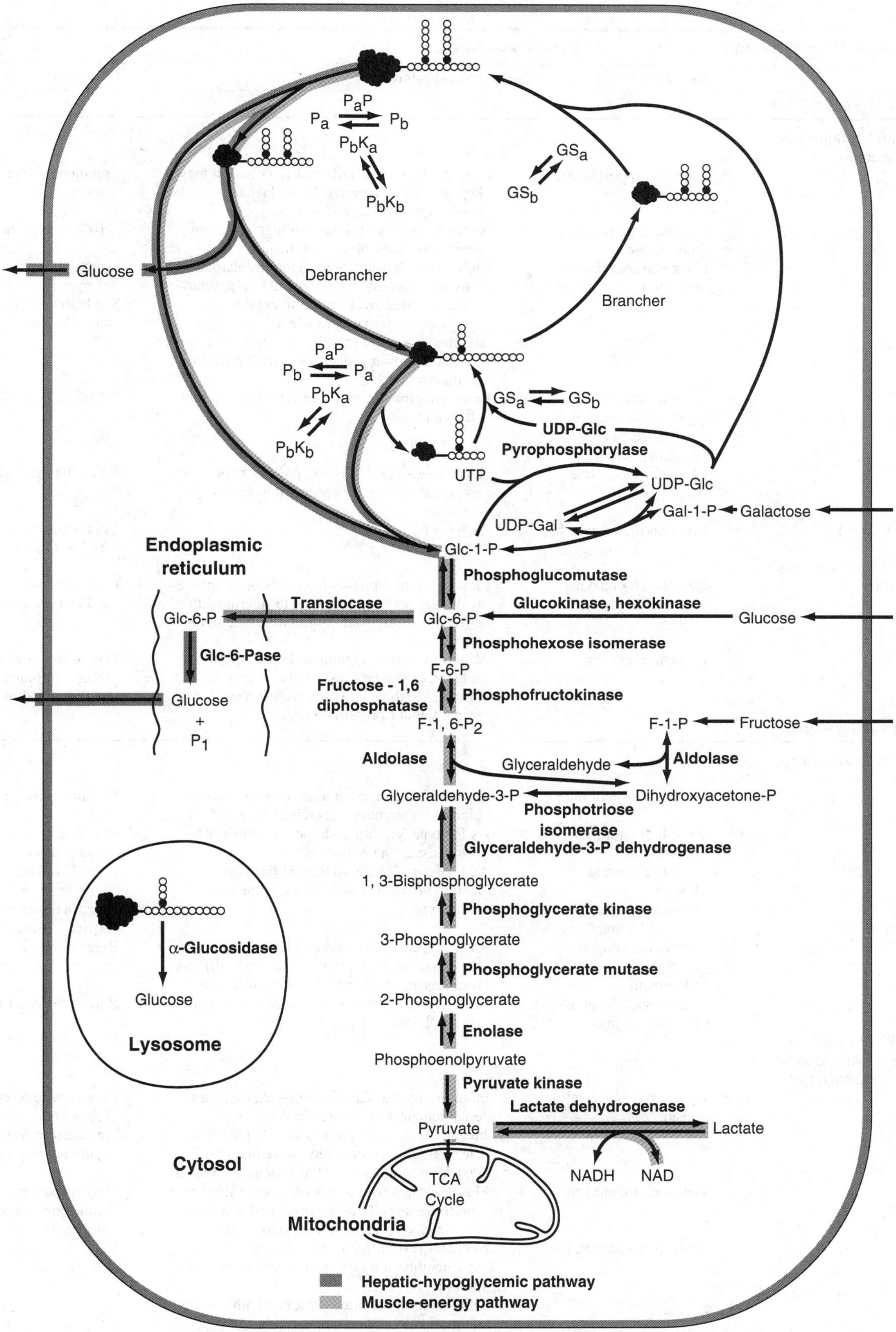

FIGURE 347-1 Metabolic pathways related to glycogen storage disease. A hypothetical composite cell is shown depicting both hepatic and muscle pathways. The shaded areas depict pathways that are blocked in the hepatic-hypoglycemic diseases or in the muscle-energy diseases. Nonstandard abbreviations are as follows: GS_a, active glycogen synthase; GS_b, inactive glycogen synthase; P_a, active phosphorylase; P_b, inactive phosphorylase; P_aP, phosphorylase *a* phosphatase; P_bK_a, active phosphorylase *b* kinase; P_bK_b, inactive phosphorylase *b* kinase. [*From AR Beaudet: Glycogen storage diseases, in KJ Isselbacher et al. (ed): Harrison's Principles of Internal Medicine, 13th ed., New York, McGraw-Hill, 1994, p 1855.*]

Table 347-1

Glycogen Storage Diseases by Organ Involvement and Clinical Features

Type	Basic Defect	Clinical Features	Comments
LIVER GLYCOGENOSES			
Disorders with hepatomegaly and hypoglycemia			
Ia	Glucose-6-phosphatase	Growth retardation, enlarged liver and kidney, hypoglycemia, elevated blood lactate, cholesterol, triglycerides, and uric acid	Common, severe hypoglycemia
Ib	Glucose-6-phosphate translocase	As for Ia, with additional findings of neutropenia and neutrophils dysfunction	~10% of type Ia
IIIa	Liver and muscle debranching enzyme	Childhood: Hepatomegaly, growth retardation, muscle weakness, hypoglycemia, hyperlipidemia, elevated liver transaminases; liver symptoms improve with age Adulthood: muscle atrophy and weakness; onset: third to fourth decades; variable cardiomyopathy	Common, intermediate severity of hypoglycemia See below for liver cirrhosis and myopathy
IIIb	Liver debranching enzyme deficiency, normal muscle debrancher activity	Liver symptoms same as in type IIIa; no muscle symptoms	~15% of type III
VI	Liver phosphorylase	Hepatomegaly, mild hypoglycemia, hyperlipidemia and ketosis; symptoms improve with age	Rare, "benign" glycogenosis.
Formerly VIa or IX	Liver phosphorylase kinase α subunit	As for VI	Common, "benign glycogenosis," X-linked
Disorders with liver cirrhosis			
IIIa and IIIb	Debranching enzyme	Elevated transaminases in childhood, improve with age; periportal fibrosis to micronodular cirrhosis, mostly nonprogressive, rare overt cirrhosis	Overt cirrhosis frequently seen in Japanese patients
IV	Branching enzyme	Failure to thrive, hypotonia, hepatomegaly, splenomegaly, progressive liver cirrhosis and failure (death usually before fifth year); some without progression	One of the rarer glycogenoses; other neuromuscular variants exist, see below
MUSCLE GLYCOGENOSES			
Disorders with muscle-energy impairment			
V	Muscle phosphorylase	Exercise intolerance, muscle cramps, myoglobinuria on strenuous exercise, increased CK	Common, male predominance
VII	Phosphofructokinase—M subunit	As for type V, with additional findings of a compensated hemolysis	Prevalent in Japanese and Ashkenazi Jews
	Phosphoglycerate kinase	As for type V, with additional findings of a hemolytic anemia and CNS dysfunction	Rare, X-linked
	Phosphoglycerate mutase—M subunit	As for type V	Rare; majority of patients are African-American
	Lactate dehydrogenase—M subunit	As for type V, with additional findings of erythematous skin eruption and uterine stiffness resulting in childbirth difficulty in female	Rare
	Muscle-specific phosphorylase kinase	As for type V, some patients may have muscle weakness and atrophy	Rare, autosomal recessive
Disorders with progressive skeletal muscle weakness, atrophy, and/or cardiomyopathy			
II	Lysosomal acid α-glucosidase	Infantile: hypotonia, muscle weakness, cardiac enlargement and failure, fatal early Juvenile and adult: progressive skeletal muscle weakness and atrophy, proximal muscle and respiratory muscle are seriously affected	Common, undetectable, or very low level of enzyme activity in infantile form; residual enzyme activity in late-onset
IIIa	Debranching enzyme	Muscle weakness and atrophy; onset third to fourth decades; both proximal and distal muscles involved; variable cardiomyopathy	Only in patients with debranching enzyme deficiency in muscle
IV	Branching enzyme	Neonatal severe hypotonia, muscle atrophy, and neuronal involvement; death in neonatal period Childhood presentation with myopathy or cardiomyopathy Adult with central and peripheral nervous system dysfunction	Very rare
	Cardiac-specific phosphorylase kinase	Severe cardiomyopathy and failure; fatal early	Very rare

NOTE: CK, creatine kinase; M, muscle; CNS, central nervous system.

one form of phosphorylase kinase deficiency are X-linked disorders. For most glycogen storage diseases, the genes that encode the defective enzymes have been characterized at the molecular level, including genes for glucose-6-phosphatase, lysosomal α-1,4-glucosidase, debrancher enzyme, branching enzyme, phosphorylase, phosphorylase kinase, phosphofructokinase, phosphoglycerate mutase, phosphoglycerate kinase, and lactate dehydrogenase—muscle subunit. Genetic heterogeneity is present at the protein, mRNA, and DNA levels. Advances in understanding the molecular basis of the disease are being used to improve the diagnosis and management of the disorders, and some are candidates for early trials of gene therapy.

LIVER GLYCOGENOSES

DISORDERS WITH HEPATOMEGALY AND HYPOGLYCEMIA Type I Glycogen Storage Disease (Glucose-6-Phosphatase or Translocase Deficiency, von Gierke Disease) Type I glycogen storage disease is due to a defect in glucose-6-phosphatase in liver, kidney, and intestinal mucosa. It can be divided into two subtypes: type Ia, in which the glucose-6-phosphatase enzyme is defective, and type Ib, which is due to a defect in the translocase that transports glucose-6-phosphate across the microsomal membrane. The defects in both type Ia and Ib lead to inadequate conversion in liver of glucose-6-phosphate to glucoses and thus make affected individuals susceptible to fasting hypoglycemia.

Clinical and laboratory findings Patients with type I disease may develop hypoglycemia and lactic acidosis during the neonatal period but more commonly present at 3 to 4 months of age with hepatomegaly and/or hypoglycemia. These children may have doll-like faces with fat cheeks, relatively thin extremities, short stature, and a protuberant abdomen that is due to massive hepatomegaly; the kidneys are enlarged, and the spleen and heart are of normal size.

The hallmarks of the disease are hypoglycemia, lactic acid acidosis, hyperuricemia, and hyperlipidemia. Hypoglycemia and lactic acid acidosis can develop after a short fast. Hyperuricemia is present in young children, but gout rarely develops before puberty. Despite hepatomegaly, liver enzymes are usually normal or near normal. Intermittent diarrhea may occur (the mechanism is not known). Easy bruising and epistaxis are associated with a prolonged bleeding time as a result of impaired platelet aggregation/adhesion.

Hypertriglyceridemia may cause the plasma to appear "milky," and cholesterol and phospholipids are also elevated. The lipid abnormality resembles type IV hyperlipidemia and is characterized by increased levels of very low density lipoprotein (VLDL); low-density lipoprotein (LDL); increased levels of apoliproteins B, C, and E; and normal or reduced levels of apoliproteins A and D. The hepatocytes are distended by glycogen and fat with large and prominent lipid vacuoles. There is no associated fibrosis.

All these findings apply to both type Ia and Ib glycogen storage diseases, but type Ib has the additional feature of recurrent bacterial infections due to neutropenia and impaired neutrophil function. Oral and intestinal mucosa ulcerations are common, and inflammatory bowel disease may occur.

Long-term complications Although type I glycogen storage disease mainly affects the liver, multiple organ systems are also involved. Gout usually becomes symptomatic around puberty as a result of the long-term hyperuricemia. Puberty is often delayed, but fertility appears to be normal. Hypertriglyceridemia causes an increased risk of pancreatitis, but premature atherosclerosis has not been documented. Impaired platelet aggregation may reduce the risk of atherosclerosis.

By the second or third decade of life, most patients with type I glycogen storage disease develop hepatic adenomas that can hemorrhage and, in rare cases, may become malignant. Other complications include pulmonary hypertension and osteoporosis.

Renal disease is a late complication, and almost all patients above age 20 have proteinuria. Many have hypertension, kidney stones, nephrocalcinosis, and altered creatinine clearance. Glomerular hyperfiltration, increased renal plasma flow, and microalbuminuria can occur before the onset of gross proteinuria. In young patients, hyperfiltration and hyperperfusion may be the only signs of renal abnormalities. With advanced renal disease, focal segmental glomerulosclerosis and interstitial fibrosis are evident on biopsy. In some patients, renal function deteriorates and progresses to failure, requiring dialysis or transplantation. Other abnormalities in renal function include amyloidosis, Fanconi-like syndrome, and distal renal tubular acidification defect. The increases in renal perfusion and maternal blood volume that normally occur in pregnancy can exacerbate renal problems. In addition, hypoglycemia may also become more difficult to control.

Diagnosis The diagnosis of type I disease can be suspected on the basis of clinical presentation and abnormal plasma lactate and lipid values. In addition, administration of glucagon or epinephrine causes little or no rise in blood glucose but increases lactate levels significantly. A definitive diagnosis, however, requires a liver biopsy to demonstrate a deficiency of either glucose-6-phosphatase or translocase. Molecular diagnoses can now be made for the majority of type Ia glycogen storage disease patients.

℞ TREATMENT

Treatment is designed to maintain normal blood glucose levels and is achieved by continuous nasogastric infusion of glucose or oral administration of uncooked cornstarch. Nasogastric drip feeding in early infancy may consist of an elemental enteral formula or may contain only glucose to maintain normoglycemia during the night; frequent feedings with a high-carbohydrate content are given during the day.

Uncooked cornstarch acts as a slow-release form of glucose and can be given at a dose of 1.6 g/kg every 4 h for infants under the age of 2 years. As the child grows older, the cornstarch regimen can be changed to every 6 h, and it can be given by mouth as a liquid (1:2, weight:volume) at a dose of 1.75 to 2.5 g/kg of body weight. Because fructose and galactose cannot be converted to free glucose, their dietary intake should be restricted, and dietary supplements of multivitamins and calcium are required. Allopurinol is given to lower the levels of uric acid. In patients with type Ib glycogen storage disease, granulocyte and granulocyte-macrophage colony stimulating factors have been used successfully to correct the neutropenia, decrease the severity of bacterial infection, and improve the chronic inflammatory bowel disease.

Prior to surgery, the bleeding status should be evaluated, and good metabolic control should be established. Prolonged bleeding time can be corrected by the administration of a constant intravenous glucose infusion for 24 to 48 h prior to surgery. Vasopressin can be given during surgery to reduce bleeding complications, and normal glucose levels should be maintained throughout surgery.

Prognosis In the past, many patients with type I glycogen storage disease died, and the prognosis was guarded for those who survived. The long-term complications discussed above occur mostly in adults whose disease was not adequately treated during childhood. Early diagnosis and initiation of effective treatment have improved the outcome, but it is not known if all long-term complications can be avoided through good metabolic control.

Genetics Type I glycogen storage disease is an autosomal recessive disorder. Both type Ia and Ib diseases have been reported in many ethnic groups, but type Ia is rarely seen in blacks. The structural gene for glucose-6-phosphatase is located on chromosome 17; three common mutations (R83C, 130X, Q347X) are responsible for 70 percent of the known disease alleles. Carrier detection and prenatal diagnosis are possible with the use of molecular techniques.

Type III Glycogen Storage Disease (Debrancher Deficiency, Limit Dextrinosis) Type III glycogen storage disease is caused by a deficiency of glycogen debranching enzyme. Debranching enzyme and phosphorylase are responsible for complete degradation of glycogen; when debranching enzyme is defective, glycogen breakdown is incomplete, and an abnormal glycogen that has short outer chains and that resembles limit dextrin accumulates.

Clinical and laboratory findings Deficiency of glycogen debranching enzyme causes hepatomegaly, hypoglycemia, short stature, variable skeletal myopathy, and cardiomyopathy. The disorder usually involves both liver and muscle and is termed *type IIIa glycogen storage disease*. However, in about 15 percent of patients, the disease appears to involve only the liver and is classified as *type IIIb*.

During infancy and childhood, the disease may be almost indistinguishable from type I disease because hepatomegaly, hypoglycemia, hyperlipidemia, and growth retardation are common features of both. Splenomegaly may be present, but kidneys are not enlarged in type III. Remarkably, hepatomegaly and hepatic symptoms in most of type III patients improve with age and usually disappear after puberty. Overt liver cirrhosis is rare except in Japanese patients.

In patients with muscle involvement (type IIIa), muscle weakness is usually minimal during childhood but can become severe during the third or fourth decade of life, as evidenced by slowly progressive weakness and muscle wasting. Electromyographic (EMG) changes are consistent with a widespread myopathy, and nerve conduction may be abnormal. Ventricular hypertrophy is frequent, but overt cardiac dysfunction is rare. Hepatic symptoms may be so mild that the diagnosis is not made until adulthood, when neuromuscular disease becomes manifest.

Hypoglycemia, hyperlipidemia, and elevated liver transaminases occur in childhood. In contrast to type I disease, fasting ketosis is prominent, and blood lactate and uric acid concentrations are usually normal. The administration of glucagon 2 h after a carbohydrate meal causes a normal rise of blood glucose, but after an overnight fast glucagon may provoke no change in blood glucose. Serum creatine kinase levels can sometimes be used to identify patients with muscle involvement, but normal levels do not rule out muscle enzyme deficiency.

The histology of the liver is characterized by a universal distention of hepatocytes by glycogen and by the presence of fibrous septa. The fibrosis and the paucity of fat distinguish type III from type I glycogenosis. The fibrosis can range from minimal periportal fibrosis to micronodular cirrhosis and appears, in most cases, to be nonprogressive.

Diagnosis In glycogen storage disease type IIIa, deficient debranching enzyme activity can be demonstrated in liver, skeletal muscle, and heart. In contrast, type IIIb patients have debranching enzyme deficiency only in the liver and not in muscle. Definitive diagnosis and assignment of subtype in this disorder require enzyme assays in both liver and muscle.

℞ TREATMENT

Dietary management of type III disease is less demanding than in type I. If hypoglycemia is present, frequent high-carbohydrate meals with cornstarch supplements or nocturnal gastric drip feedings are usually effective. A high-protein diet during the daytime plus overnight protein enteral infusion may be tried in patients with myopathy, but it is not established whether such a regimen is effective. Patients do not need to restrict dietary intake of fructose and galactose, as do those with type I disease.

Prognosis Liver symptoms improve with age and usually disappear after puberty. Cirrhosis of the liver is rare. In type IIIa disease muscle weakness and atrophy worsen during adulthood.

Genetics The type III glycogenoses are inherited as autosomal recessive traits. The disease has been reported in many different ethnic groups, and the frequency is relatively high in non-Ashkenazi Jews of North African descent. The gene for debranching enzyme is located on chromosome 1p21. Carrier detection and prenatal diagnosis are possible using DNA-based linkage or mutation analysis.

Type VI Glycogen Storage Disease [Liver Phosphorylase Deficiency (Hers Disease) and Phosphorylase Kinase Deficiency] Defects of the phosphorylase system cause a heterogeneous group of glycogenoses. The heterogeneity is due to the complexity of the reactions involved in glycogenolysis. A cascade of enzymatic reactions, involving adenylate cyclase, cyclic adenosine monophosphate–dependent protein kinase (protein kinase A), and phosphorylase kinase, activate phosphorylase, the rate-limiting enzyme of glycogenolysis. Theoretically, glycogen storage disease can result from any enzyme deficiency along this pathway, but phosphorylase kinase deficiency is the most common. Phosphorylase kinase has four subunits (α, β, γ, and δ), each encoded by different genes and differentially expressed in various tissues.

The numerical classification of this group of glycogenoses is confusing, ranging from type VI, VIa, to IX. It is advisable to refrain from such a designation and to classify the various disorders according to organ involvement and mode of inheritance.

Clinical and laboratory findings LIVER PHOSPHORYLASE DEFICIENCY Liver phosphorylase deficiency has been documented in only a small number of patients. It appears to be a benign disorder. The patients present with hepatomegaly and growth retardation early in childhood. Hypoglycemia, hyperlipidemia, and hyperketosis are usually mild, if present. Lactate and uric acid levels are normal. The heart and skeletal muscles are not involved. The hepatomegaly improves with age and usually disappears around puberty. The liver phosphorylase gene has been cloned and mapped to chromosome 14.

X-linked liver phosphorylase kinase deficiency X-linked liver phosphorylase kinase deficiency is one of the most common liver glycogenoses. Phosphorylase kinase activity may also be deficient in erythrocytes and leukocytes but is normal in muscle. Typically, a child between the ages of 1 and 5 years presents with growth retardation and hepatomegaly. Levels of cholesterol, triglycerides, and liver enzymes are mildly elevated. Ketosis may occur after fasting. Lactate and uric acid levels are normal. Hypoglycemia is mild, if present. The rise in blood glucose following the administration of glucagon is normal. Hepatomegaly and abnormal blood chemistries gradually return to normal with age. Most adults achieve a normal final height and are practically asymptomatic, despite a persistent phosphorylase kinase deficiency.

Liver histology shows glycogen-distended hepatocytes. The accumulated glycogen (α particles, rosette form) has a frayed or burst appearance and is less compact than in type I or III disease. Fibrous septae and low-grade inflammatory changes may be present.

The structural gene for the liver isoform of the phosphorylase kinase α-subunit is located on chromosome Xp22, and mutations of this gene have been found in the disorder.

AUTOSOMAL LIVER AND MUSCLE PHOSPHORYLASE KINASE DEFICIENCY An autosomal recessive form of liver and muscle phosphorylase kinase deficiency has been reported in several patients. As in the X-linked form of the disorder, hepatomegaly and growth retardation are the predominant symptoms in early childhood. Some patients also exhibit muscle hypotonia and have reduced activity of phosphorylase kinase in muscle. Because of the autosomal recessive mode of inheritance, mutations are likely to be found in the genes that encode the β and/or γ subunits of the phosphorylase kinase.

MUSCLE-SPECIFIC PHOSPHORYLASE KINASE DEFICIENCY Muscle-specific phosphorylase kinase deficiency causes cramps and myoglobinuria on exercise or progressive muscle weakness and atrophy. The activity of the enzyme is decreased in muscle but (when determined) normal in liver and blood cells. There is no hepatomegaly or cardiomegaly. The disorder is presumed to be an autosomal recessive trait.

CARDIAC-SPECIFIC PHOSPHORYLASE KINASE DEFICIENCY Phosphorylase kinase deficiency limited to the heart has been reported in only two cases. Both patients died during infancy from cardiac failure due to massive glycogen deposition in the myocardium.

Diagnosis Definitive diagnosis of phosphorylase kinase deficiency requires demonstration of the enzymatic defect in affected tissues. Although phosphorylase kinase can be measured in leukocytes and erythrocytes, the enzyme has many tissue-specific isozymes, and the diagnosis can be missed without studies of the liver, muscle, or heart.

℞ TREATMENT

The treatment for liver phosphorylase or phosphorylase kinase deficiency is based on symptoms. A high-carbohydrate diet and frequent feedings are effective in preventing hypoglycemia, but most patients require no specific treatment. Prognosis is usually good; adult patients have normal stature and minimal hepatomegaly. There is no treatment for the fatal form of isolated cardiac phosphorylase kinase deficiency.

Genetics Carrier detection is possible using DNA-based linkage or mutation analysis for the common form of X-linked phosphorylase kinase deficiency.

DISORDERS WITH LIVER CIRRHOSIS **Type IV Glycogen Storage Disease (Branching Enzyme Deficiency, Amylopectinosis, or Andersen Disease)** Deficiency of branching enzyme activity results in accumulation of an abnormal glycogen with poor solubility. The disease is referred to as *type IV glycogen storage disease* or *amylopectinosis*, because the abnormal glycogen has fewer branch points, more α1-4 linked glucose units, and longer outer chains, resulting in a structure resembling amylopectin.

Clinical and laboratory findings This disorder is clinically variable. The most common form is characterized by progressive cirrhosis of the liver and is manifest in the first 18 months of life as hepatosplenomegaly and failure to thrive. The cirrhosis progresses to cause portal hypertension, ascites, esophageal varices, and liver failure that leads to death by age 5. Rare patients survive without progression of liver disease.

Tissue deposition of amylopectin-like materials can be demonstrated in liver, heart, muscle, skin, intestine, brain, spinal cord, and peripheral nerve. The histologic findings in the liver are characterized by both micronodular cirrhosis and faintly stained basophilic inclusions in the hepatocytes. The inclusions consist of coarsely clumped, stored material that is periodic acid Schiff–positive and partially resistant to diastase digestion. Electron microscopy shows, in addition to the conventional α and β glycogen particles, an accumulation of fibrillar aggregations typical of amylopectin. Definitive diagnosis requires demonstration that branching enzyme activity is deficient in liver, muscle, cultured skin fibroblasts, or leukocytes.

A neuromuscular form of type IV glycogen storage disease has also been reported. These patients may (1) present at birth with severe hypotonia, muscle atrophy, and neuronal involvement and die during the neonatal period; (2) present in late childhood with myopathy or cardiopathy; or (3) present as adults with diffuse central and peripheral nervous system dysfunction accompanied by accumulation of polyglucosan bodies in the nervous system (so-called adult polyglucosan body disease). Definitive diagnosis of the adult disease requires assay of branching enzyme in leukocytes or nerve biopsy, as the deficiency is limited to those tissues.

℞ TREATMENT

There is no specific treatment for type IV glycogen storage disease. For progressive hepatic failure, liver transplantation has been performed, but because it is a multisystem disorder the long-term success of liver transplantation is not known.

Genetics Type IV glycogen storage disease is a rare autosomal recessive disease. Prenatal diagnosis is available by using cultured aminocytes or chorionic villi to measure the level of enzymatic activity. The glycogen branching enzyme gene is located on chromosome 3p14. Mutations responsible for type IV glycogen storage disease have been identified, and their characterization in individual patients may be useful in predicting the clinical course.

MUSCLE GLYCOGENOSES

DISORDERS WITH MUSCLE-ENERGY IMPAIRMENT **Type V Glycogen Storage Disease (Muscle Phosphorylase Deficiency, McArdle Disease)** Deficiency of muscle phosphorylase is the prototype muscle-energy disorder. Deficiency of this enzyme in muscle limits ATP generation by glycogenolysis and results in glycogen accumulation.

Clinical and laboratory findings Symptoms usually develop first in adulthood and are characterized by exercise intolerance with muscle cramps. Two types of activity tend to cause symptoms: (1) brief exercise of great intensity, such as sprinting or carrying heavy loads; and (2) less intense but sustained activity, such as climbing stairs or walking uphill. Moderate exercise, such as walking on level ground, can be performed by most patients for long periods. Many patients experience a characteristic "second wind" phenomenon; if they rest briefly at the first appearance of muscle pain, they can resume exercise with more ease. About half report burgundy-colored urine after exercise, the consequence of myoglobinuria secondary to the rhabdomyolysis. Intense myoglobinuria after vigorous exercise may cause renal failure. Although most patients are diagnosed in the second or third decade, many report weakness and lack of endurance since childhood. In rare cases, EMG findings may suggest an inflammatory myopathy, and the diagnosis can be confused with polymyositis.

The level of serum creatine kinase is usually elevated at rest and increases more after exercise. Exercise also increases the levels of blood ammonia, inosine, hypoxanthine, and uric acid. The latter abnormalities are attributed to accelerated recycling of muscle purine nucleotides in the face of insufficient ATP production.

Clinical heterogeneity is not common, but late-onset disease with no symptoms as late as the eighth decade and an early-onset, fatal form with hypotonia, generalized muscle weakness, and progressive respiratory insufficiency have been reported.

Diagnosis Lack of an increase in blood lactate and exaggerated blood ammonia elevations after an ischemic exercise test are indicative of muscle glycogenosis and suggest a defect in the conversion of glycogen or glucose to lactate. The abnormal exercise response, however, is not limited to type V disease and can occur with other defects in glycogenolysis or glycolysis, such as deficiencies of muscle phosphofructokinase or debranching enzyme (when the test is done after fasting). Definitive diagnosis is made by enzymatic assay of muscle.

℞ TREATMENT

Exercise tolerance can be augmented by oral administration of glucose or fructose or by injection of glucagon. A high-protein diet may increase exercise endurance in some patients. In general, avoidance of strenuous exercise prevents the symptoms, and there is no need for a specific therapy. Longevity does not appear to be affected.

Genetics Type V glycogen storage disease is an autosomal recessive disorder that does not appear to have ethnic predilection. The gene for muscle phosphorylase is located on chromosome 11q13-qter. The most common mutation in U.S. patients is a nonsense mutation that changes an arginine to a stop at codon 49 (R49X), and the most common mutation in the Japanese is deletion of a single codon (ΔF708). This allows DNA-based diagnosis and carrier detection for the two populations.

Type VII Glycogen Storage Disease (Muscle Phosphofructokinase Deficiency, Tarui Disease) Type VII disease is caused by a deficiency of muscle phosphofructokinase, which catalyzes the conversion of fructose-6-phosphate to fructose-1,6-diphosphate and is a key regulatory enzyme of glycolysis.

Phosphofructokinase is composed of three isozyme subunits (M, muscle; L, liver; and P, platelet), which are encoded by different genes and are differentially expressed in tissues. Skeletal muscle contains only M subunit, and red blood cells contain a hybrid of L and M forms. Type VII disease is due to defective M isoenzyme, which causes complete enzyme deficiency in muscle and partial deficiency in red blood cells.

Clinical and laboratory findings The features are similar to those in type V disease, namely, early onset of fatigue and pain with exercise.

Vigorous exercise causes severe muscle cramps and myoglobinuria. However, several features of type VII disease are distinctive. (1) Exercise intolerance is usually evident in childhood, is more severe than in type V disease, and may be associated with nausea and vomiting. (2) A compensated hemolysis occurs as evidenced by an increased level of serum bilirubin and reticulocyte count. (3) Hyperuricemia is common and becomes more marked after exercise. (4) An abnormal glycogen resembling amylopectin is present in muscle fibers; it is periodic acid Schiff–positive and resistant to diastase digestion. (5) Exercise intolerance is particularly acute following meals rich in carbohydrate because glucose cannot be utilized in muscle and because the ingested glucose inhibits lipolysis and thus deprives muscle of fatty acid and ketone substrates. In contrast, patients with type V disease can metabolize glucose derived from either liver glycogenolysis or exogenous glucose. Indeed, glucose infusion improves exercise tolerance in type V patients.

Two rare type VII variants have been reported. One presents in infancy with hypotonia and limb weakness, and a rapidly progressive myopathy leads to death by age 4. The other presents in adults and is characterized by a slowly progressive, fixed muscle weakness rather than by cramps and myoglobinuria.

Diagnosis The M isoenzyme defect must be demonstrated in muscle, red blood cells, or cultured skin fibroblasts by biochemical or histochemical techniques.

℞ TREATMENT

There is no specific treatment. Avoidance of strenuous exercise prevents acute attacks of muscle cramps and myoglobinuria.

Genetics Type VII glycogen storage disease is inherited as an autosomal recessive trait. The disease appears to be rare, and most reported patients are either Japanese or Ashkenazi Jews. The gene for the M isoenzyme is located on chromosome 1 cen-1q32. In Ashkenazi Jews 95 percent of mutant alleles are either a splicing defect or a nucleotide deletion.

Other Muscle Glycogenoses with Muscle-Energy Impairment Three additional enzyme defects produce muscle glycogenoses, namely, deficiencies in phosphoglycerate kinase, phosphoglycerate mutase, and lactate dehydrogenase. All three enzymes affect terminal glycolysis, and deficiency causes muscle-energy impairment similar to that in type V and VII disease. The failure of blood lactate to increase in response to exercise can be used to separate muscle glycogenoses from disorders of lipid metabolism, such as carnitine palmitoyl transferase II deficiency and very long chain acyl–coenzyme A dehydrogenase deficiency, which also cause muscle cramps and myoglobinuria. Muscle glycogen levels may be normal in the disorders affecting terminal glycolysis, and definitive diagnosis is made by assaying the enzymatic activity in muscle.

DISORDERS WITH PROGRESSIVE SKELETAL MUSCLE WEAKNESS, ATROPHY, AND/OR CARDIOMYOPATHY

Glycogen Storage Disease Type II (α1,4-Glucosidase Deficiency, Pompe Disease) (See also Chap. 346) GSD II is caused by a deficiency of lysosomal acid α1,4 glucosidase (acid maltase), an enzyme responsible for the degradation of glycogen in lysosomal vacuoles. This disease is characterized by accumulation of glycogen in lysosomes as opposed to its accumulation in cytoplasm in the other glycogenoses.

Clinical and laboratory findings The disorder encompasses a range of phenotypes, each including myopathy but differing in age of onset, organ involvement, and clinical severity. The most severe is the infantile-onset disease with cardiomegaly, hypotonia, and death prior to 2 years of age. Infants appear normal at birth but soon develop generalized muscle weakness with feeding difficulties, macroglossia, hepatomegaly, and congestive heart failure due to a hypertrophic cardiomyopathy. Electrocardiographic findings include a high-voltage QRS complex and a shortened PR interval. Death usually occurs from cardiorespiratory failure or aspiration pneumonia.

The juvenile or late-childhood form is characterized by skeletal muscle manifestations, usually without cardiac involvement, and a slowly progressive course. The juvenile form typically presents as delayed motor milestones (if age of onset is early enough) and difficulty in walking and is followed by swallowing difficulties, proximal muscle weakness, and respiratory muscle involvement; it can cause death before the end of the second decade.

An adult form of type II disease presents as a slowly progressive myopathy without cardiac involvement and has its onset between the second and seventh decades. The clinical picture is dominated by slowly progressive proximal muscle weakness with truncal involvement and greater involvement of the lower than the upper limbs. Pelvic girdle, paraspinal muscle, and diaphragm are most seriously affected. The initial symptoms may be respiratory insufficiency manifested by somnolence, morning headache, orthopnea, and exertional dyspnea.

Laboratory findings include elevated levels of serum creatine kinase, aspartate transaminase, and lactate dehydrogenase, particularly in infants. Muscle biopsy shows the presence of vacuoles that stain positively for glycogen, and muscle acid phosphatase is increased, presumably from a compensatory increase of lysosomal enzymes. Electron microscopy reveals the glycogen accumulation. EMG reveals myopathic features with irritability of muscle fibers and pseudomyotonic discharges. Serum creatine kinase is not always elevated in adults, and, depending on the muscle biopsied or tested, muscle histology or EMG may not be abnormal. It is prudent to examine affected muscle.

Diagnosis Diagnosis can be established by demonstration of absence or reduced levels of acid α-glucosidase activity in muscle or cultured skin fibroblasts. Deficiency is usually more severe in the infantile form than in the juvenile and adult disorders.

℞ TREATMENT

No effective treatment for the infantile form is available. A high-protein diet may be useful for the juvenile and adult forms. Nocturnal ventilatory support in adults may improve the quality of life and have dramatic effects during respiratory decompensation.

Genetics Pompe disease is an autosomal recessive disorder and does not appear to have an ethnic predilection. The gene for acid α-glucosidase is on chromosome 17q23. A splice site mutation (IVS1-13T→G) is commonly seen in patients with adult-onset disease. Prenatal diagnosis using amniocytes or chorionic villi is available in the fatal infantile form.

BIBLIOGRAPHY

CHEN Y-T, BURCHELL A: Glycogen storage diseases, in *The Metabolic and Molecular Bases of Inherited Disease*, 7th ed, CR Scriver et al (eds). New York, McGraw-Hill, 1995, pp 935–965

——— et al: Renal disease in Type I glycogen storage disease. N Engl J Med 318:7, 1988

FERNANDEZ J et al: Glycogen storage disease. Recommendations for treatment. Eur J Pediatr 147:226, 1988

HIRSCHHORN R: Glycogen storage disease type II: Acid α-glucosidase (acid maltase) deficiency, in *The Metabolic and Molecular Bases of Inherited Disease*, 7th ed, CR Scriver et al (eds). New York, McGraw-Hill, 1995, pp 2243–2464

LEI K-J et al: Mutations in the glucose-6-phosphatase gene that cause glycogen storage disease type Ia. Science 262:580, 1993

TALENTE GM et al: Glycogen storage disease in adults: A retrospective study of clinical and laboratory findings in types Ia, Ib, and III. Ann Intern Med 120:218, 1994

TSUJINO S et al: Molecular genetic heterogeneity of myophosphorylase deficiency (McArdle's disease). N Engl J Med 329:241, 1993

348 *Darwin J. Prockop, Helena Kuivaniemi, Gerard Tromp*

INHERITED DISORDERS OF CONNECTIVE TISSUE

Heritable disorders that involve the major connective tissues of the body such as bone, skin, cartilage, blood vessels, and basement membranes are among the most common genetic diseases in human beings. Such diseases include many clinical entities that were not previously recognized either as involving specific components of connective tissue or being inherited. Here we will focus primarily on those disorders that can have severe manifestations, are relatively common, and are sufficiently understood at the molecular level to provide useful paradigms: osteogenesis imperfecta (OI), the Ehlers-Danlos syndrome (EDS), chondrodysplasias (CDs), the Marfan syndrome (MS), epidermolysis bullosa (EB), and the Alport syndrome (AS).

THE CHALLENGE OF CLASSIFYING THE DISEASES The first comprehensive effort to classify diseases of connective tissue was made by McKusick in a series of reports and then in the monograph *Heritable Disorders of Connective Tissue*, in which he drew attention to patients and families with connective tissue disorders in whom the changes appeared to be inherited as single-gene traits. He subsequently expanded the classification to include more than 12 major diseases of connective tissue that were likely to be caused by single-gene defects on the basis of the pattern of inheritance, the cluster of signs and symptoms, the histologic changes in tissues, and limited information about the molecular defects involved. This classification was extended by other investigators so that about a dozen types and subtypes were defined for OI, about the same number for the EDS, and over 150 for the CDs.

For some of the original disease categories, most patients with the classic features of the disease have a mutation in a gene or genes coding for a single protein. For example, the majority of patients with OI have a mutation in one of the two genes coding for type I procollagen. Similarly, most patients with MS have mutations in a gene for fibrillin. For other disease categories, the situation is more complex. In EDS, for example, the type IV variant is usually due to mutations in the gene for type III procollagen, the type VI variant to defects in the gene for lysyl hydroxylase, and the type VII variant to defects that impair the processing of type I procollagen to type I collagen.

Several limitations in the original classifications are now apparent. One is that the same mutation does not always produce the same disease phenotype in terms of severity of the condition or its clinical course. Such phenotypic variation occurs in many genetic diseases, including the connective tissue disorders, in which some members of a family are severely affected, whereas others with the same mutation have a mild disorder.

Classifications of these disorders also tend to overemphasize the etiologic differences between severe genetic diseases that are apparent in infants and the more common diseases that appear much later in life. Single-gene defects can cause subsets of late-onset diseases such as osteoporosis, aneurysms, and osteoarthritis. For example, a small subset of patients with postmenopausal osteoporosis have mutations in the genes for procollagen I similar to the mutations in the same genes that produce lethal variants of OI. Likewise, a subset of patients with familial aortic aneurysms have mutations in the gene for procollagen III similar to the mutations in the same gene that cause lethal variants of type IV EDS, and occasional patients with osteoarthritis have mutations in the gene for procollagen II similar to the mutations in the same gene that cause lethal CDs. There is disagreement as to the best diagnosis for such patients in that some investigators feel that after a mutation similar to those seen in the early-onset diseases is identified, the patients should be reclassified as having mild forms of OI, EDS, or CD, even though they do not have definitive evidence of the early-onset diseases or seek medical attention until adulthood. The debate is fueled by the fact that many of the classification systems are based on clusters of signs and symptoms for which there are few objective criteria. However, some patients with late-onset diseases of connective tissue such as osteoporosis, osteoarthritis, and aneurysms inherit the disorders in a manner suggesting single-gene defects. Therefore, the category of diseases referred to as *inherited disorders of connective tissue* may have to be expanded.

DEFINITION AND COMPOSITION OF CONNECTIVE TISSUES Connective tissues are composed of specific macromolecules, many of which are also constituents of the lung, the kidney, the walls of blood vessels, the vitreous gel of the eye, and the synovial fluid. Indeed, most organs and tissues contain small amounts of the same macromolecules assembled into membranes and septa. Therefore, virtually all structures contain connective tissue.

The distinguishing feature of connective tissues is that the component macromolecules are assembled into an insoluble extracellular matrix (Table 348-1). The macromolecules include at least 19 different

Table 348-1

Constituents of Various Connective Tissues

Connective Tissue	Known Constituents	Approximate Amounts, % dry wt	Characteristics or Functions
Skin, ligaments, tendons	Type I collagen	80	Bundles of fibrils
	Type III collagen	5–15	Thin fibrils
	Type IV collagen, laminin, nidogen	<5	In basal laminae under epithelium and in blood vessels
	Types V, VI, and VII collagens	<5	Functions unclear
	Elastin, fibrillin	<5	Provide elasticity
	Fibronectin	<5	Associated with collagen fibers and cell surfaces
	Proteoglycans* and hyaluronate	0.5	Provide resiliency
Bone (demineralized)	Type I collagen	90	Complex fibril network
	Type VI collagen	1–2	Function unclear
	Proteoglycans	1	Function unclear
	Osteonectin, osteocalcin, osteopontin, α2-glycoprotein, sialoproteins	1–5	Probably initial or regulate mineralization
Aorta	Type I collagen	20–40	Fibril network
	Type III collagen	20–40	Thin fibrils
	Elastin, fibrillin	20–40	Provide elasticity
	Type IV collagen, laminin, nidogen	<5	Form basal lamina
	Types V and VI collagens	<2	Functions unclear
	Proteoglycans	<3	Provide resiliency
Cartilage	Type II collagen	40–50	Arcades of thin fibrils
	Type IX collagen	5–10	Links type II fibrils
	Type X collagen	5–10	Surrounds hypertrophic cells
	Type XI collagen	<10	Function unclear
	Proteoglycans and hyaluronate	15–50	Provide resiliency

* As discussed in text, at least five proteoglycans have now been identified. They differ in the structures of their core proteins and their contents of mucopolysaccharide side chains of chondroitin-4-sulfate, chondroitin-6-sulfate, dermatan sulfate, and keratan sulfate. Basil lamina contain a proteoglycan with a side chain of heparan sulfate that resembles heparin.

types of collagens, the related fibrous proteins known as *elastin* and *fibrillin*, a series of proteoglycans, and components whose structure and function are only partially defined.

Differences in the connective tissues of bone, skin, and cartilage are in part explained by differences in the content of specific components (see Table 348-1). For example, tendons and ligaments consist primarily of type I collagen fibrils and small amounts of other components that help organize the type I fibrils into fibers and fiber bundles. Cartilage consists primarily of fibrils of type II collagen in the form of arcades that are distended by highly charged proteoglycans. The extracellular matrix of the aorta contains collagens that provide tensile strength and elastin that provides elasticity. Differences among the connective tissues also depend on the three-dimensional organization of the molecular components. The type I collagen fibrils in tendon are packed into thick, parallel bundles of fibers, whereas type I collagen fibrils in skin are randomly oriented. In cortical bone, helical arrays of type I collagen fibrils are deposited around haversian canals.

BIOSYNTHESIS OF CONNECTIVE TISSUE Connective tissues largely form by self-assembly, in which a molecule of the correct size, shape, and surface properties binds to other molecules with the same or similar structure in a spontaneous but ordered manner. The molecular mechanisms and driving forces are similar to those involved in crystal formation.

The self-assembly of connective tissue is illustrated by the assembly of collagen into fibrils. The fibril that forms collagen is a long, thin rod consisting of three polypeptide α chains wrapped into a rigid, ropelike triple helix (Fig. 348-1). The fibril has a triple-helical conformation, because each of the three α chains has a simple, repetitive amino acid sequence of about 1000 amino acids in which glycine (Gly) appears as every third amino acid. Therefore, the sequence of each α chain can be designated as $(\text{-Gly-X-Y-})_{333}$, where X and Y represent amino acids other than glycine. To fold into a triple helix, every third amino acid in an α chain must be glycine, the smallest amino acid, since this residue must fit in a sterically restricted space where the three chains of the triple helix come together. Many of the X- and Y-position amino acids are proline and hydroxyproline, which provide rigidity to the triple helix. The remaining amino acids form clusters of hydrophobic and charged regions on the surface of the molecule that direct how one molecule spontaneously binds to other collagen molecules and thereby self-assembles into the large collagen fibrils in tissues (see Fig. 348-1).

More than 19 different collagens have been identified. Most are minor constituents that probably have highly specialized functions. The fibrillar collagens are found in tissues as long, highly ordered fibrils with a characteristic banding pattern by electron microscopy. Type I collagen, the most abundant, is found as cross-striated fibrils in a large number of tissues (see Table 348-1). It is composed of two identical α chains called α1(I) and one α2(I) chain. Type II collagen, a fibrillar collagen of cartilage, is composed of three identical α chains called α1(II). Type III collagen is found in small amounts in many tissues that contain type I collagen and in large amounts in large blood vessels; it is composed of three identical chains called α1(III). The nonfibrillar collagens are similar to the fibrillar collagens in that they contain -Gly-X-Y- sequences of amino acids that form triple-helical domains, but they also contain large globular domains. Self-assembly of most of the nonfibrillar collagens usually involves binding between the globular domains to form networks. For example, the type IV collagen in basement membranes self-assembles into a complex three-dimensional network that provides a diffusion barrier in the renal glomerulus and pulmonary alveolus and provides support for epithelial and endothelial cells in these tissues and in skin, the gastrointestinal tract, and blood vessels. Some nonfibrillar collagens bind to the surface of fibrils formed by the more abundant collagens and alter the lateral growth of the fibrillar collagens or prevent the fibrils from coalescing into fiber bundles.

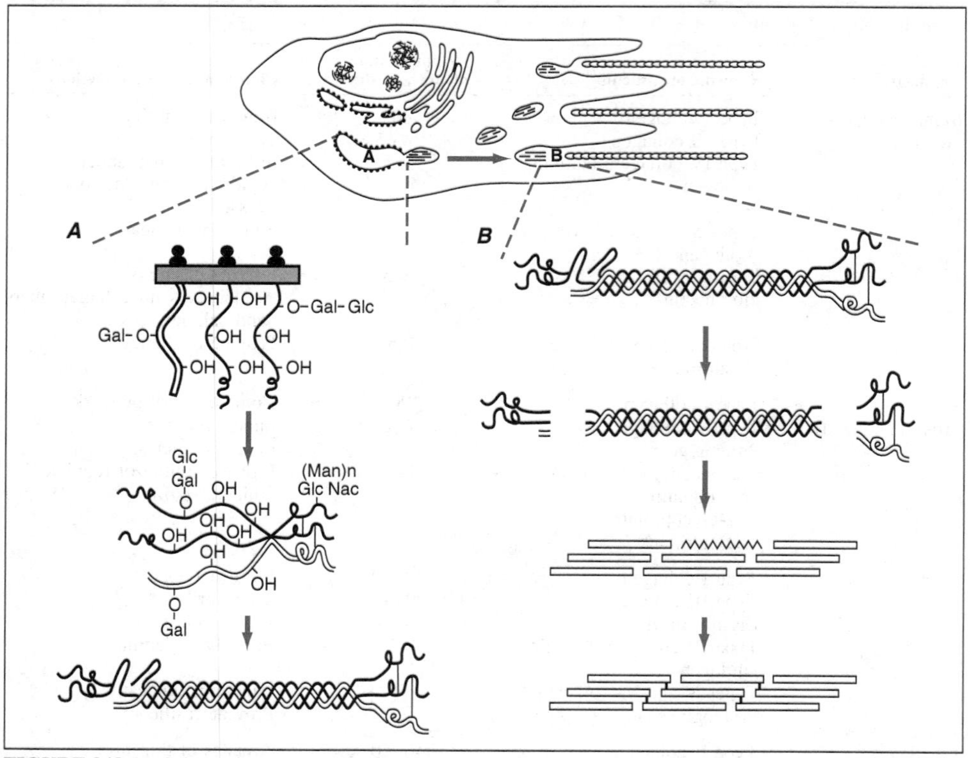

FIGURE 348-1 Schematic representation of synthesis of a type I collagen fibril by a fibroblast. *A.* Intracellular steps in the assembly of the procollagen molecule. Hydroxylations and glycosylations of the proα chains begin soon after the amino termini pass into the cisternae of the rough endoplasmic reticulum and continue after the three chains associate through their carboxy-terminal propeptides and become disulfide linked. *B.* Cleavage of procollagen to collagen, self-assembly of the collagen molecule into quarter-staggered fibrils, and cross-linking of the molecules in the fibrils. Cleavage of the propeptides may occur within crypts of the fibroblast, as shown here, or some distance from the cell. *(From DJ Prockop and KI Kivirikko, N Engl J Med 311:376, 1984, with permission.)*

Because fibrillar collagens spontaneously self-assemble into fibrils, they are first synthesized as larger and more soluble precursors called *procollagens*. The procollagen forms of type I, II, and III collagens are 1.5 times the mass of the mature collagens because of the presence of amino acid sequences (*propeptides*) located at both the N and C termini of the proα chains of the procollagens.

The biosynthesis of procollagens involves complex intracellular processing (see Fig. 348-1) and an unusual self-assembly whereby the three chains fold into a triple helix. As the proα chains of procollagen are synthesized on ribosomes, the free ends move into the cisternae of the rough endoplasmic reticulum. Hydrophobic signal peptides at the N terminus are cleaved, and additional posttranslational reactions begin. Proline residues in the Y position of the repeating -Gly-X-Y- sequences are converted to hydroxyproline by prolyl hydroxylase in a reaction requiring ascorbic acid. Lysine residues in the Y position are similarly hydroxylated to hydroxylysine by lysyl hydroxylase. Many of the hydroxylysine residues are glycosylated with galactose or with galactose and glucose. A large mannose-rich oligosaccharide is assembled on the C-terminal propeptide of each chain. As the last amino acids are incorporated into the proα chains, they are released into the cisternae of the rough endoplasmic reticulum. At this stage two proα1(I) and one proα2(I) chains are associated through their C-propeptides. The association of the proα chains is directed by the structure and the surface properties of the globular C-propeptides. After the C-propeptides assemble correctly, the structure is locked in place by the formation of interchain disulfide bonds. Posttranslational modifications of the proα chains continue until each chain acquires about 100 hydroxyproline residues. Then a few of the hydroxyproline-rich -Gly-X-Y- sequences at the C terminus of the protein fold into a triple helix. The short region of triple helix becomes a nucleus for self-assembly of the triple helix of the whole protein, much like a nucleus for crystallization, in that the triple-helical conformation in one -Gly-X-Y- sequence induces the next -Gly-X-Y- sequence to fold into the same conformation. As a result, the conformation is propagated in a zipper-like fashion from the C terminus to the N terminus of the molecule, and the entire α-chain domain becomes a continuous triple helix. The protein then passes from the rough endoplasmic reticulum to other compartments and is secreted. The requirement for ascorbic acid in the hydroxylation of prolyl residues explains why wounds fail to heal in scurvy (see Chap. 79). If sufficient proline residues are not converted to hydroxyproline, collagen cannot fold into a triple helix that is stable at body temperature. The abnormal protein accumulates in the cisternae of the rough endoplasmic reticulum and is slowly degraded.

After secretion, procollagen is processed to collagen by cleavage of the N-propeptides by procollagen N-proteinase and of the C-propeptides by procollagen C-proteinase. The processing of type I procollagen by the two proteinases converts the soluble precursor to type I collagen, whose solubility is less than 1 μg/mL under the same conditions. The 1000-fold decrease in solubility as procollagen is converted to collagen provides the entropic energy that drives the spontaneous self-assembly of the collagen into fibrils, a process that is again similar to crystal formation. Collagen monomers first assemble into a nucleus that grows by addition of monomers as determined by the structure of the nucleus. The initial nucleus for fibril assembly probably involves few molecules and has been difficult to define. However, structures intermediate between the initial nucleus and the final fibrils have pointed and highly symmetrical tips and grow by addition of monomers to the pointed tips. The nucleus, the intermediate structures, and the final fibril can all be assembled spontaneously from a single kind of collagen such as type I or type II, but other fibrils are assembled as copolymers in which two or more collagens are incorporated into the same fibril simultaneously. Alternatively, a second collagen or a proteoglycan can bind to the surface of a growing fibril or to a fully formed fibril and thereby influence the final structure and the functional properties of the fibrils. The final structure of the fibrils in tissues is also influenced by the pressure and tensions on the fibrils, particularly after their tips are inserted into muscle and bone. The tension on tendons, for example, probably makes the initial thin fibrils coalesce into large fiber bundles. The initial self-assembly of collagen into fibrils, however, involves a large number of specific interactions along the surface of each rodlike molecule and therefore can only be altered by molecules that bind either to the surface of the large, rodlike monomer or to the surfaces of the growing fibrils.

Self-assembled collagen fibers have considerable tensile strength, which is increased by cross-linking reactions that form covalent bonds between α chains in one molecule and α chains in adjacent molecules. The first step in cross-linking is oxidation by lysyl oxidase of amino groups on a few lysine or hydroxylysine residues to form aldehydes. The aldehydes then interact to form stable covalent bonds that may or may not involve enzymic reactions.

Collagen fibers in most tissues of normal adults undergo very little metabolic turnover. One exception to this is the collagen fibrils that are degraded and resynthesized as part of the continual remodeling of bone. During growth and development the collagen fibrils in all tissues undergo repeated synthesis, degradation, and resynthesis. The degradation of collagen fibers in tissues is initiated by specific collagenases in leukocytes, fibroblasts, synovial cells, or related cell types. The collagenases cleave the collagen molecule at a point about three-quarters of the distance from its N terminus. The cleavage apparently triggers unfolding of the molecules on the surface of a fibril and further degradation by other proteinases.

Although the collagen in many adult tissues is metabolically stable, the rate of turnover changes under some circumstances. In starvation, a large fraction of the collagen in skin and other connective tissues is degraded, thus providing amino acids for gluconeogenesis. Large losses of collagen also occur in most connective tissues during immobilization or prolonged periods of low-gravitational stress. In rheumatoid arthritis, pannus invasion causes a rapid degradation of collagen in the articular cartilage, and glucocorticoid excess decreases the collagen content of most connective tissues, including bone, by decreasing the rate of collagen synthesis. Decrease in collagen weakens the tissues. In many pathologic states, however, collagen is deposited in excess. With injury to tissue, inflammation is usually followed by increased deposition primarily of type I collagen fibrils in the form of fibrotic tissue and scars. The deposition of collagen fibrils during the repair process is largely irreversible and is a major feature of the pathologic changes in hepatic cirrhosis, pulmonary fibrosis, atherosclerosis, and nephrosclerosis and in the scarring in skin and ligaments after surgery or trauma.

The biosynthesis of all collagens involves essentially the same steps of assembly and processing. Assembly of nonfibrillar collagens such as the type IV of basement membranes does not, however, involve cleavage of the globular domains at the ends of the protein, since the globular domains are required for the self-assembly of the proteins. Elastin assembly appears to be closely related to that of collagen, since a few of the prolines in the protein are hydroxylated to hydroxyproline by prolyl hydroxylase. The elastin monomer, however, is a single polypeptide that does not fold into a defined three-dimensional structure and is not synthesized as a larger precursor molecule. Instead, it is slowly secreted from cells into extracellular compartments, where it forms amorphous deposits around previously deposited microfibrils. The elastin deposits then become covalently cross-linked through oxidation of lysine residues to aldehydes by the lysyl oxidase that initiates the cross-linking of collagen. The microfibrils in elastin deposits are largely composed of fibrillin, a large protein that forms beadlike strands. The amorphous deposits of elastin and fibrillin also may contain additional components that have not been identified.

The synthesis of proteoglycans begins in the cisternae of the rough endoplasmic reticulum with assembly of a core protein that then undergoes modification by sugar and sulfate transferases that generate large side chains of glycosaminoglycans. At least five proteoglycans have been identified by differences in the structures of their core proteins. The major proteoglycan of cartilage, called *aggrecan*, has a core protein of about 2000 amino acids to which are bound multiple side chains of chondroitin sulfate and keratin sulfate, mucopolysaccharides consisting of highly charged and repetitive disaccharide sequences. After secretion from cells, the aggrecan monomer binds to a smaller protein called a *link protein*. The complex of core protein and link protein then spontaneously binds to a long chain of hyaluronic acid to form a huge copolymer called a *proteoglycan aggregate*. The highly charged proteoglycan aggregate binds water and small ions and thereby provides a large swelling pressure and resiliency to cartilage. Smaller proteoglycans such as decorin, biglycan, and fibromodulin have smaller core proteins with different mucopolysaccharide side chains. They do not form large aggregates with hyaluronate but bind to fibrils of collagen or fibronectin and may thereby help regulate the assembly or spatial orientation of fibrils. One group of small proteoglycans known as *syndecans* binds to the plasma membranes of cells and may have a role in cell migration along fibrils or in signal transduction.

The assembly of bone follows much the same principles as the assembly of other connective tissues (see also Chap. 353). The first step is deposition of osteoid tissue that consists largely of type I collagen fibrils (see Fig. 348-1). Mineralization of osteoid occurs by steps that are still incompletely defined; proteins such as osteopontin and osteocalcin probably bind to the collagen fibrils and chelate calcium to initiate mineralization. Small proteoglycans such as decorin or fibromodulin also may play a role.

MUTATIONS THAT PRODUCE DISEASES OF CONNECTIVE TISSUES Because of the large number of tissue-specific macromolecules present in connective tissues, a large number of gene-protein systems are candidates for mutations that might cause disease. The situation is somewhat simplified by the fact that most of the disease-causing mutations identified to date are in genes that encode collagen or collagen-associated proteins. Therefore, the molecular mechanisms by which the mutations cause their deleterious effects can be related to a single paradigm. However, achondroplasia is caused by mutations in a fibroblast growth factor receptor, and mutations in genes involved in embryonic patterning such as homeo box genes may cause abnormalities of the skeletal system. Therefore, the number of mutant genes that can cause connective tissue diseases is likely to increase.

The most complete data on mutations causing heritable disorders of connective tissue are available on OI. Most patients with severe OI (types II and III) have mutations in either the gene for the proα1(I) chain or the gene for the proα2(I) chain of type I procollagen (the COL1A1 and COL1A2 genes). In patients with mild disease, some of the mutations decrease expression of protein from one allele of the genes. Most of the mutations in patients with severe OI cause synthesis of a structurally abnormal but partially functional proα chain (Figs. 348-2 and 348-3). Mutations that cause synthesis of structurally abnormal proα chains include partial gene deletions, partial gene duplications, and RNA splicing mutations. The most common mutations, however, cause the substitution of single amino acids with bulky side chains for the glycine residues that appear as every third amino acid in the triple helix of a proα chain (Fig. 348-4). The structurally abnormal proα chains exert their effects primarily through one of three mechanisms (see Fig. 348-2). First, the presence of an abnormal proα chain in a procollagen molecule containing two normal proα chains can prevent folding of the protein into a triple-helical conformation and lead to degradation of the whole molecule in a process called *procollagen suicide*. Similar dominant negative mutations are seen with other multisubunit proteins. The net result of procollagen suicide is a reduction in the amount of collagen available for fibril assembly. Second, the presence of one abnormal proα chain in a procollagen molecule can interfere with cleavage of the N-propeptide from the protein. The persistence of the N-propeptide on a fraction of the molecules interferes with the self-assembly of normal collagen so that thin and irregular collagen fibrils are formed. Third, the substitution of a bulkier amino acid for glycine can produce a change in the conformation of the molecule and result in the assembly of collagen fibrils that are abnormally branched (see Fig. 348-3) or abnormally thick and short. Also, copolymerization of the mutated collagen with normal collagen can slow fibril assembly and decrease the total amount of collagen incorporated into fibrils.

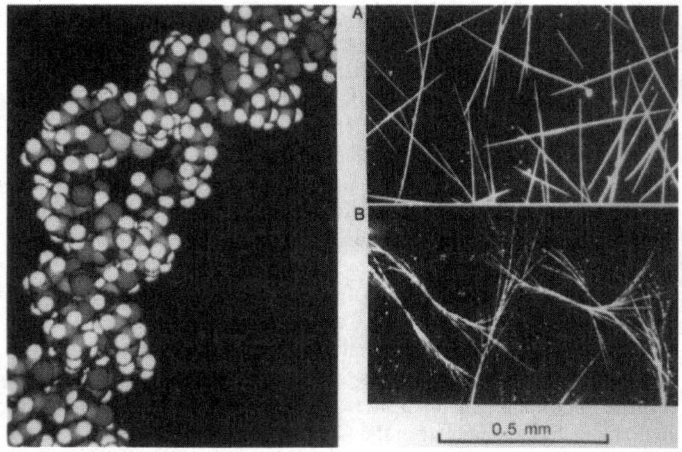

FIGURE 348-3 Space-filling model showing a cysteine substitution of glycine α1-748 of type I procollagen (*on the left*) and dark-field light micrographs (*on the right*) of fibrils formed from control type I collagen at 32°C (*A*) and from the mixture of normal and mutated type I collagen containing the same cysteine substitution (*B*). *(From A Vogel et al, J Biol Chem 263:19249, 1988; and KE Kadler et al, Biochemistry 30:5081, 1991, with permission.)*

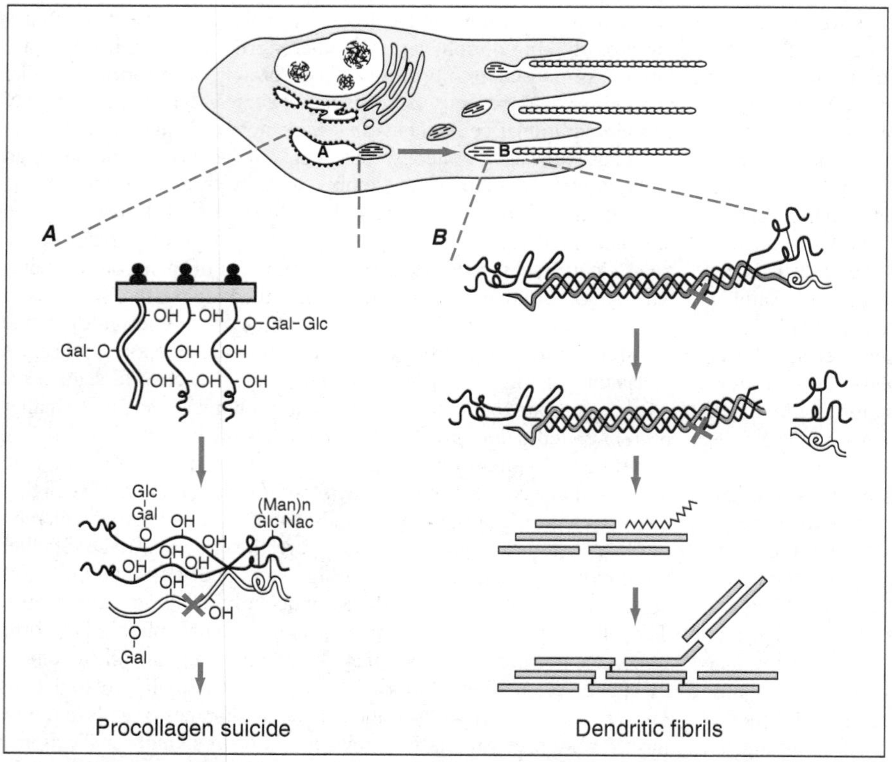

FIGURE 348-2 Schematic summary of three mechanisms (see text) whereby mutations that cause biosynthesis of structurally abnormal proα1(I) or proα2(I) chains of type I procollagen interfere with either the assembly of the protein (*A*) or its processing to normal collagen fibrils (*B*). *(From DJ Prockop et al, Am J Med Genet 34:60, 1989, with permission.)*

There are several reasons why most of the mutations that cause OI are in the type I procollagen genes. One, because collagen fibrils are a principal source of the strength of bone, the structure is weakened by any mutation that reduces the amount or distorts the normal geometry of collagen. The self-assembly of collagen fibrils is easily disrupted when a defective subunit can participate in the assembly process but has the wrong structure. For example, the substitution of a bulky amino acid for a single glycine in one proα chain can interfere with the zipper-like formation of the triple helix and trigger degradation of both the normal and abnormal proα chains. In a similar manner, the presence of a few incompletely processed or flawed collagen monomers can interfere with the self-assembly of normal collagen into fibrils. Hence a mutation at any one of a large number of different sites can either decrease the amount of collagen available for fibril assembly or interfere with the process of fibril assembly so as to markedly decrease the strength of bone and other connective tissues.

Over 150 mutations in the two genes for type I procollagen have been found in patients with OI (see Fig. 348-4). Initially, there was concern that many of the mutations might be neutral variations in the structure of the genes and not the cause of the disease phenotypes. However, the causal relationship between most of the mutations and the disease has been established by several kinds of evidence: (1) DNA linkage studies in families with mild variants of OI showed that specific mutated alleles were coinherited with the disease phenotypes. (2) Probands with lethal variants of OI were shown to have new mutations not found in the normal parents or in only a few cells from a mosaic parent (see below). (3) Studies with cultured skin fibroblasts from patients demonstrated that the mutations either produced specific disruptions in the biosynthesis of type I procollagen or caused synthesis of a type I procollagen that formed abnormal collagen fibrils (see Fig. 348-2). (4) The mutations in probands with OI were not found in normal alleles for the genes. (5) Expression of several of the mutated genes for type I procollagen in transgenic mice generates disease phenotypes similar to those seen in patients who inherited the mutated genes (Fig. 348-5).

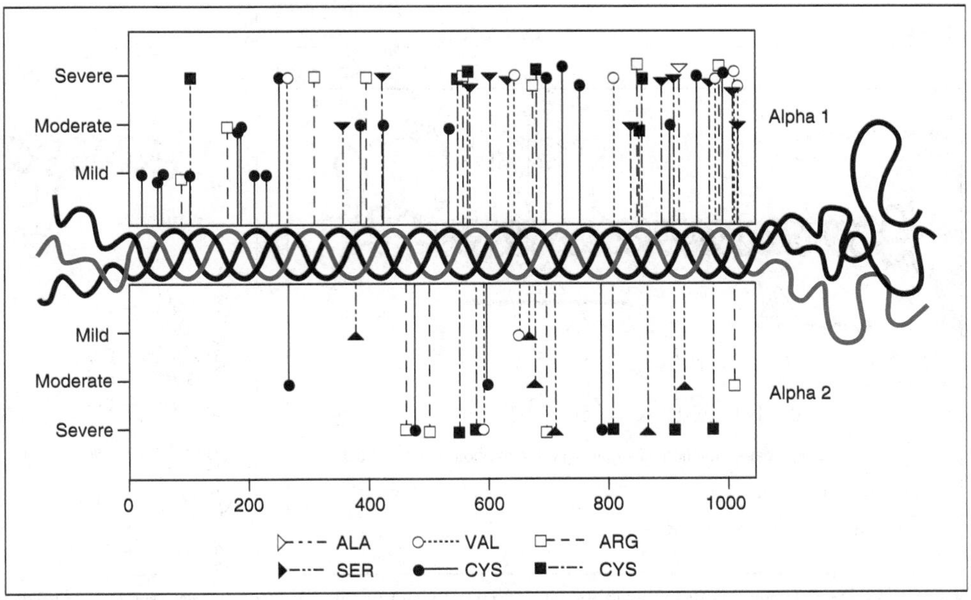

FIGURE 348-4 Single-base mutations found in type I procollagen in patients with OI and osteoporosis. Mild refers to type I OI, severe to type II OI, and moderate to type III or type IV OI.

The data on mutations in type I procollagen that cause OI have been used as a paradigm for defining other mutations in collagen and procollagen genes that cause other disorders of connective tissue. For example, similar mutations in the gene for type III procollagen occur in patients with the type IV variant of EDS, which causes early death because of rupture of the aorta or other hollow organs (Fig. 348-6). Also, similar mutations in the gene for type II procollagen (COL2A1) are found in about half of patients with the CDs (Fig. 348-7). In addition, transgenic mice expressing mutated genes for type II procollagen develop phenotypes resembling the CDs. Similar mutations in the gene for type VII collagen (COL7A1) are found in patients with the dystrophic form of EB, and mutations in the genes for type IV collagen are found in many patients with AS. As discussed below, the paradigm for defining the consequences of mutations in procollagen genes also helps explain findings on mutations in a fibrillin gene that cause MS and mutations in keratin genes that cause the simplex variant of EB.

Several generalizations can be made about mutations in collagen genes. One is that unrelated patients rarely have the same mutation in the same gene. Another is that mutations that cause the most severe disease are usually new mutations in one allele that occur either during the generation of the germline in one of the parents or during meiosis in the fertilized egg. Still another is that most mild variants are caused by mutations that are specific or "private" to a given family. Indeed, the number of recurrent mutations in structural genes are so infrequent that there are, in effect, no common mutations responsible for the disorders in unrelated patients and no "hot spots" that contain most of the mutations.

Another general trend is that similar mutations in the same gene can produce different disease syndromes in terms of both severity and the major tissues involved. One reason for heterogeneity in pathologic manifestations is that different regions of a large molecule may be more important for its function in some connective tissues than in others. For example, some regions of the type I collagen molecule may be essential for the binding of mineralizing proteins in bone so that mutations in these regions cause fragile bones but do not impair function in skin and other nonmineralizing tissues. It is more difficult, however, to explain how the same mutation can produce a severe phenotype in some and a mild phenotype in other members of the same family. Such phenotypic variation appears to be characteristic of OI, where some subjects are short and have multiple fractures from minor trauma, whereas others in the same family can be of normal stature and free of fractures. In the past, such phenotypic variation was explained by undefined variations in the genetic background of different family members. Studies in transgenic mice, however, demonstrated similar phenotypic variation with expression of a mutated collagen gene in an inbred strain of mice in whom the genetic background is uniform. Therefore, the phenotypic variation is probably caused by undefined stochastic or chance events during embryonic and fetal development. Although dramatic phenotypic variation is relatively rare in OI and related disorders, it is important to consider in counseling families about the consequences of inherited mutations.

OSTEOGENESIS IMPERFECTA OI is an inherited disorder that causes a generalized decrease in bone mass (osteopenia) and makes the bones brittle. The disorder is frequently associated with blue sclerae, dental abnormalities (dentinogenesis imperfecta), progressive hearing loss, and a positive family history. The most severe forms cause death in utero, at birth, or shortly thereafter. The course of mild and moderate forms is more variable. Some patients appear normal at birth and become progressively worse. Some have multiple fractures in infancy and childhood, improve after puberty, and fracture more frequently later in life. Women are particularly prone to fracture during pregnancy and after menopause. A few women from families with mild variants of OI do not develop fractures until after menopause, and their disease may be difficult to distinguish from postmenopausal osteoporosis.

Classification The most common classification for OI was developed by Sillence (Table 348-2). Type I, the mildest form, is inherited as an autosomal dominant trait. Most patients have distinctly blue

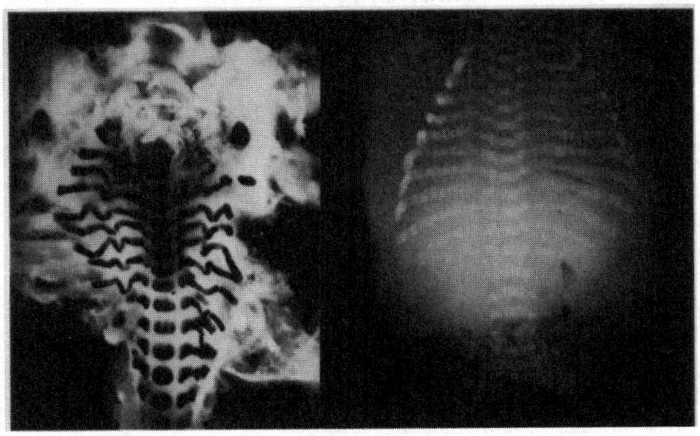

FIGURE 348-5 Similarities of the phenotypes in transgenic mice with mutated type I procollagen and in an OI child. Note in both pictures the waviness of the ribs due to fractures in utero.

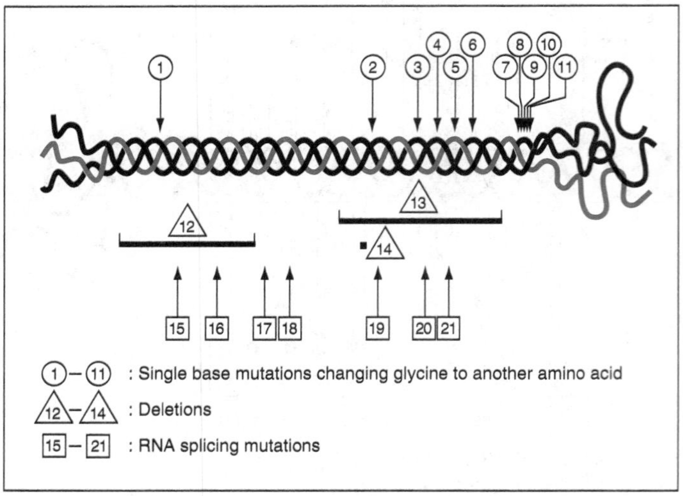

FIGURE 348-6 Mutations in the gene for the proα1(III) chain of type III procollagen that cause EDS IV and familial aneurysms.

sclerae. Type I is subdivided into types IA and IB depending on whether or not dentinogenesis imperfecta is present. Type II is lethal in utero or shortly after birth. Radiographic criteria can be used to subdivide type II into five groups, with subgroup 1 showing the most severe changes and subgroup 5 the least. Types III and IV OI are intermediate in severity between types I and II. They differ from type I because of lesser severity and because the sclerae are only slightly bluish in infancy and white in adulthood. Type III differs from type IV in that it tends to become more severe with age. Also, type III can be inherited either as an autosomal recessive or autosomal dominant trait, whereas type IV is always dominant. The clinical courses are variable, and the mode of inheritance in types III and IV may be difficult to ascertain because many patients have sporadic mutations and because many couples with one severely affected OI child do not have additional children. For these and related reasons, the distinction between type IV OI and other severe variants of OI may not be helpful. Therefore, it may be sufficient to classify patients simply as mild (type I), lethal (type II), and moderately severe (type III).

Incidence Type I OI has a frequency of about 1 in 30,000. Type II OI has a reported incidence at birth of about 1 in 60,000, but the incidence of the three severe forms recognizable at birth (types II, III, and IV) may be as high as 1 in 20,000.

Skeletal Changes In type I OI, the fragility of bones may be severe enough to limit physical activity or so mild that individuals are unaware of any disability. Radiographs of the skull of patients with mild disease may show a mottled appearance, because of small islands of irregular ossification. In type II OI bones and other connective tissues are so fragile that massive injuries can occur in utero or during delivery (see Fig. 348-5). Ossification of many bones is frequently incomplete. Continuously beaded or broken ribs and crumpled long bones (accordina femora) may be present. For unclear reasons, the long bones may be either thick or thin. In types III and IV, multiple fractures from minor physical stress can produce severe deformities. Kyphoscoliosis can impair respiration, cause cor pulmonale, and predispose to pulmonary infections. The appearance on radiographs of "popcorn-like" deposits of mineral on the ends of long bones is an ominous sign. Progressive neurologic symptoms may result from basilar compression and communicating hydrocephalus.

In all forms of OI, bone mineral density in unfractured bone is decreased.

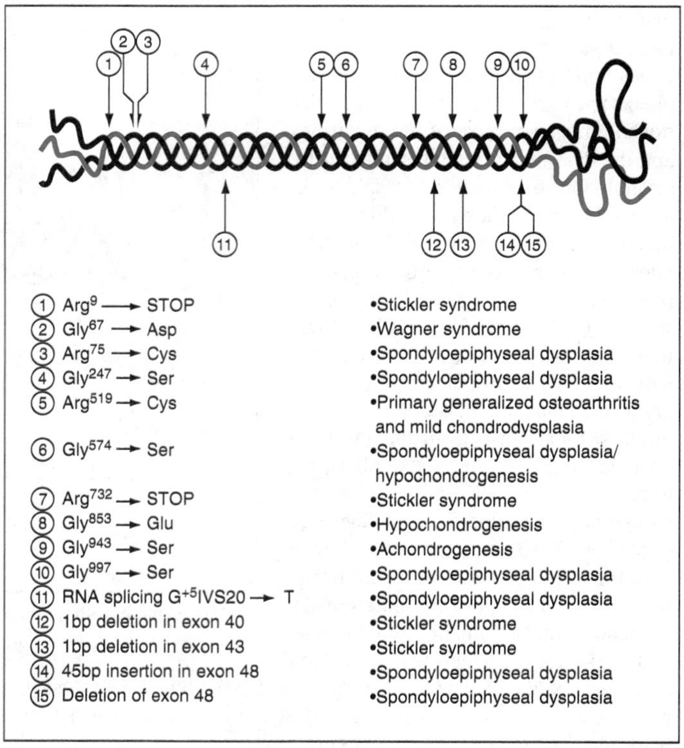

FIGURE 348-7 Mutations in the gene for the proα1(II) chain of type II procollagen that cause CD and related disorders.

However, the degree of osteopenia may be difficult to evaluate because recurrent fractures limit exercise and thereby worsen the decrease in bone mass. Surprisingly, fractures appear to heal normally.

Ocular Changes The sclerae can be normal, slightly bluish, or bright blue. The color is probably caused by a thinness of the collagen layers of the sclerae that allows the choroid layers to be seen. Blue sclerae, however, are an inherited trait in some families who do not have increased bone fragility.

Dentinogenesis Imperfecta The teeth may be normal, moderately discolored, or grossly abnormal. The enamel generally appears normal, but the teeth may have a characteristic amber, yellowish brown, or translucent bluish gray color because of improper deposition or deficiency of dentin. The deciduous teeth are usually smaller than normal, whereas permanent teeth are frequently bell-shaped and restricted at the base. In some patients, the teeth readily fracture and need to be extracted. The defect in dentin is directly attributable to the fact that normal dentin is rich in type I collagen. Similar tooth defects, however, can occur without any evidence of OI.

Hearing Loss Hearing loss usually begins during the second decade of life and occurs in 90 percent of subjects over age 30. The loss can be conductive, sensorineural, or mixed and varies in severity. The middle ear usually exhibits maldevelopment, deficient ossification, persistence of cartilage in areas that are normally ossified, and abnormal calcium deposits.

Associated Features Other connective tissue involvement can include thin skin that scars extensively, joint laxity with permanent

Table 348-2

Classification of Osteogenesis Imperfecta (OI)

Type	Bone Fragility	Blue Sclerae	Abnormal Dentition	Hearing Loss	Inheritance*
I	Mild	Present	Absent in IA, present in IB	Present in most	AD
II	Extreme	Present	Present in some	Unknown	S, rarely AR
III	Severe	Bluish at birth	Present in some	High incidence	AR or AD
IV	Variable	Absent	Absent in IVA, present in IVB	High incidence	AD

* AD, autosomal dominant; AR, autosomal recessive; S, sporadic.

dislocations indistinguishable from those of EDS, and, occasionally, cardiovascular manifestations such as aortic regurgitation, floppy mitral valves, mitral incompetence, and fragility of large blood vessels. For unknown reasons, some patients develop a hypermetabolic state with elevated serum thyroxine levels, hyperthermia, and excessive sweating.

Molecular Defects Most patients with OI have mutations in one of the two genes that encode type I procollagen. A third or more of the patients with type I OI have as yet undefined mutations in the proα1(I) gene that decrease the steady-state levels of the mRNA for proα1(I) chains and decrease the rates of synthesis of proα1(I) chains relative to those for proα2(I) chains. In more severe forms (types II, III, and IV), the effects of mutations that cause synthesis of abnormal proα chains are amplified by the three mechanisms discussed above (see Fig. 348-2). Mutations that change the structure of the protein near the N-proteinase cleavage site cause accumulation of a partially processed procollagen and produce lax joints similar to those in type VII EDS. Mutations that change the structure in the middle or near the C terminus of the molecule tend to cause severe or lethal variants of OI. It is difficult, however, to correlate the site or nature of the mutation and the clinical phenotype (see Fig. 348-4). Rare patients are homozygotes with two mutated alleles for proα1(I) or proα2(I) chains.

Mosaicism in Germ Line Cells and in Somatic Cells Most lethal OI is the result of new autosomal dominant mutations. The frequency of a second child with lethal OI in the same family, however, is about 7 percent because of germ line mosaicism in one of the parents. The presence of germ line mosaicism has been demonstrated in several fathers of patients with type II OI by demonstrating the mutated gene in a fraction of their sperm. Apparently normal parents of children with severe OI also may have somatic cell mosaicism in which the mutated allele is present in a fraction of somatic cells such as fibroblasts, leukocytes, and hair root cells. Because of the possibility of germ line mosaicism, asymptomatic parents of a child with severe OI should be counseled that recurrence can occur.

Diagnosis The diagnosis is usually made on the basis of clinical criteria. The presence of fractures together with blue sclerae, dentinogenesis imperfecta, or family history of the disease is usually sufficient to make the diagnosis. Other causes of pathologic fractures must be excluded, including the battered child syndrome, nutritional deficiencies, malignancies, and other inherited disorders such as CDs and hypophosphatasia (Table 348-3). X-rays usually reveal a decrease in bone density that can be verified by photon or x-ray absorptiometry. There is no consensus, however, as to whether the diagnosis can be made by microscopy of bone. With research procedures, a molecular defect in type I procollagen can be demonstrated in half or more of patients by incubating skin fibroblasts with radioactive amino acids and then analyzing the proα chains by polyacrylamide gel electrophoresis. The analysis detects decreases in the rate of synthesis of proα1(I) chains relative to proα2(I) chains, abnormally long proα chains, abnormally short proα chains, and proα chains with abnormal posttranslational modification because of an amino acid substitution that impairs folding of the triple helix. The mutations themselves can be defined in most patients by sequencing of cDNA or genomic DNA. Because each proband and family usually has a "private" mutation, extensive analysis of 5000 or more bases in each of the two genes is required to identify the exact mutation. After a mutation in a type I procollagen gene is identified, a test based on the polymerase chain reaction can be used to screen family members at risk and for prenatal diagnosis.

Table 348-3

Differential Diagnosis of OI

Age	Diagnosis	Distinguishing Features
At birth	Hypophosphatasia	Unmineralized skull
	Achondrogenesis	Unmineralized vertebrae
	Thanatophoric dwarfism	H-shaped vertebrae
	Asphyxiating thoracic dystrophy	Cylindrical thorax
	Achondroplasia	Large head, short, tubular bones
Infancy	Battered child syndrome	Skull and rib fractures more common
	Immobilization osteogenesis	
	Scurvy	
	Congenital syphilis	
Childhood	Homocystinuria	Marfanoid appearance and mental deficiency
	Celiac disease	Steatorrhea, anemia
	Adrenal cortical tumor	
	Glucocorticoid therapy	

SOURCE: After R Smith et al, *The Brittle Bone Syndrome: Osteogenesis Imperfecta*, London, Butterworth, 1983, p 128.

Rx TREATMENT

Treatment is ineffective, but many subjects have successful careers despite severe deformities. Those with mild disorder may need little treatment when fractures decrease after puberty, but women require special attention during pregnancy and after menopause, when fractures again increase. More severely affected children require a comprehensive program of physical therapy, surgical management of fractures and skeletal deformities, and vocational education.

Many of the fractures are only slightly displaced and have little soft tissue swelling. Therefore, they can be treated with minimal support or traction for a week or two followed by a light cast. If fractures are relatively painless, physical therapy can be initiated early. A judicious amount of exercise prevents loss of bone mass secondary to physical inactivity. Some physicians advocate insertion of steel rods into long bones to correct limb deformities; the risk/benefits and cost/benefits of such procedures are difficult to evaluate. Aggressive conventional intervention is usually warranted for pneumonia and cor pulmonale. For severe hearing loss, stapedectomy or replacement of the stapes with a prosthesis may be successful. Moderately to severely affected patients should be evaluated periodically to anticipate possible neurologic problems. About half of children have a substantial increase in growth when given growth hormone. Treatment with bisphosphorates to decrease bone loss has been discussed, but no controlled studies have been reported.

A program for careful orthotic management developed by Bleck and a program for compressive management developed by Marini are useful. Counseling and emotional support is important for patients and parents, and lay organizations in some countries provide help in these areas. Prenatal ultrasonography will detect severely affected fetuses at about 16 weeks of pregnancy. Diagnosis by demonstrating synthesis of abnormal proα chains or by DNA sequencing can be carried out in chorionic villa biopsies at 8 to 12 weeks of pregnancy.

EHLERS-DANLOS SYNDROME EDS is characterized by hyperelasticity of the skin and hypermobile joints (Fig. 348-8).

Classification Beighton initially identified five types of EDS based primarily on the extent to which the skin, joints, and other tissues are involved, but the classification has now been extended (Table 348-4). Type I is the classic, severe form of the disease, with both severe joint hypermobility and skin that is velvety in texture, hyperextensible, and easily scarred. Type II is similar to type I but milder. In type III joint hypermobility is more prominent than skin changes, and the skin changes in type IV are more prominent than joint changes. However, type IV patients are predisposed to sudden death from rupture of large blood vessels or the large bowel. Type V is similar to type II but is inherited as an X-linked trait. Type VI is characterized by scoliosis, ocular fragility, and a cone-shaped deformity of the cornea (keratoconus). Type VII is characterized by marked joint hypermobility that is difficult to distinguish from type III except by the specific molecular defects in the processing of type I procollagen to collagen. Type VIII is distinguished by periodontal changes. Types IX, X, and XI were defined on the basis of preliminary biochemical

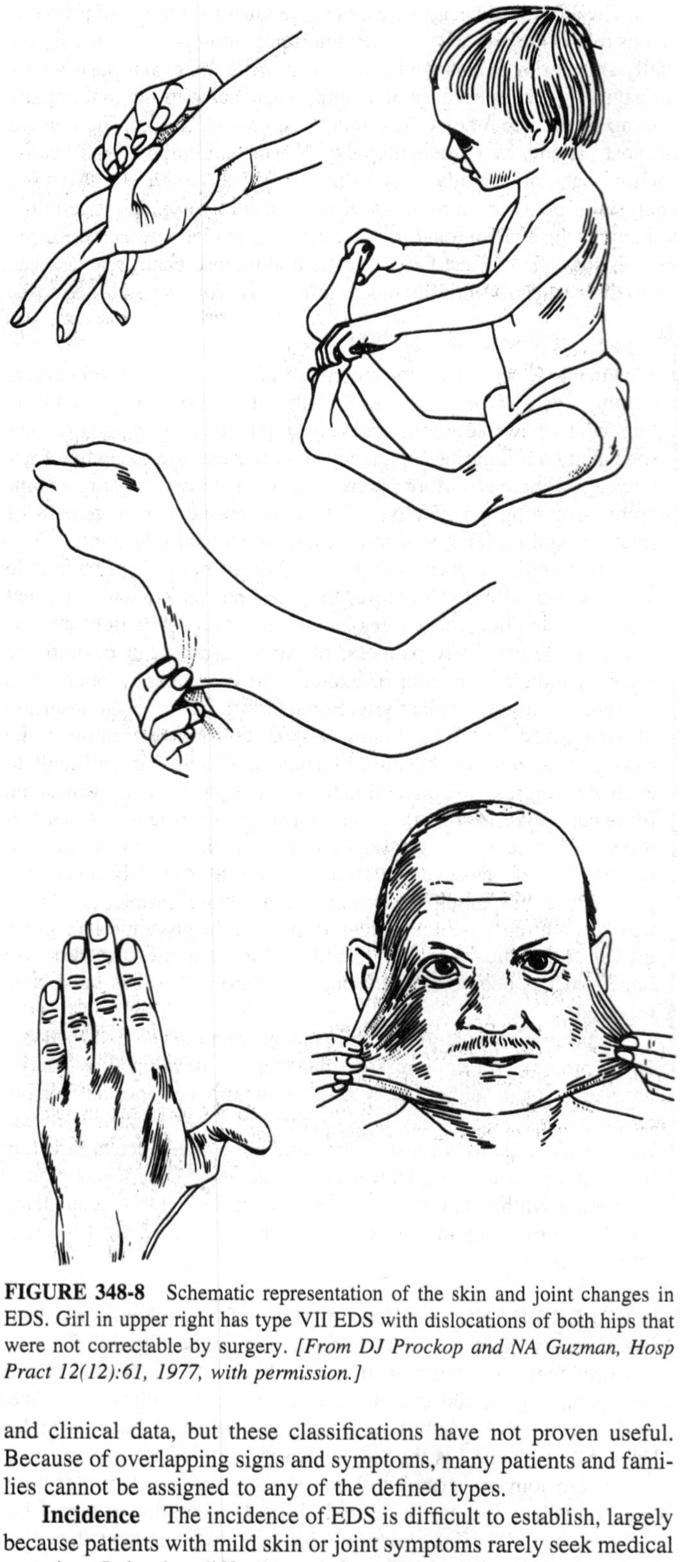

FIGURE 348-8 Schematic representation of the skin and joint changes in EDS. Girl in upper right has type VII EDS with dislocations of both hips that were not correctable by surgery. *[From DJ Prockop and NA Guzman, Hosp Pract 12(12):61, 1977, with permission.]*

and clinical data, but these classifications have not proven useful. Because of overlapping signs and symptoms, many patients and families cannot be assigned to any of the defined types.

Incidence The incidence of EDS is difficult to establish, largely because patients with mild skin or joint symptoms rarely seek medical attention. It is also difficult to define the normal range of variation for joint mobility or skin elasticity. The incidence may be about 1 in 5000 births, although a higher value has been reported for blacks. Types I, II, and III account for most diagnoses.

Skin The changes vary from thin and velvety skin to skin that is either dramatically hyperextensible ("rubber man" syndrome) or easily torn or scarred. Type I patients develop characteristic "cigarette-paper" scars. In type IV extensive scars and hyperpigmentation develop over bony prominences, and the skin may be so thin that subcutaneous blood vessels are visible. In type VIII the skin is more fragile than hyperextensible, and it heals with atrophic, pigmented scars. Easy bruisability occurs in several types of EDS.

Ligament and Joint Changes Laxity and hypermobility of joints vary from mild to unreducible dislocations of hips and other large joints. In mild forms patients learn to reduce dislocations themselves and to avoid them by limiting physical activity. In more severe forms, surgical repair may be required. Some patients have progressive difficulty with age, but severe joint laxity is compatible with a normal life span.

Associated Changes Mitral valve prolapse and hernias occur, particularly in type I. Pes planus and mild to moderate scoliosis are common. Extreme joint laxity and repeated dislocations may lead to degenerative arthritis. In type VI the eye may rupture with minimal trauma, and kyphoscoliosis can cause respiratory impairment. Sclerae may be blue in type VI.

Molecular Defects The molecular defects in most patients with the type I, II, and III forms of EDS are unknown, but the responsible gene has been identified in three families. In one there is a mutation in the COL5A1 gene for the $\alpha 1(V)$ chain of type V collagen, a collagen found in small amounts in association with type I collagen. Linkage to the same gene was present in a second family with type II EDS, but mutation in this gene has been excluded in other families with types I or II EDS. One type III EDS family had a mutation in the COL3A1 gene that caused replacement of an obligate glycine in type III procollagen. Electron microscopy of skin from some patients with types I, II, or III EDS are consistent with mutations in a low-abundance collagen such as types III or V that either copolymerize with or bind to the surface of type I fibrils. However, irregular fibrils are not seen in all patients, and similar irregular fibrils can be seen in normal skin.

Most patients with type IV EDS have a defect either in the synthesis or structure of type III procollagen, a finding consistent with the fact that these patients are prone to spontaneous rupture of the aorta and intestines, tissues rich in type III collagen. The thinness and scarring of skin are more difficult to explain, since type III constitutes a small fraction of the collagen in skin (see Table 348-1). The more than 50 mutations identified in the type III procollagen gene include partial gene deletions, RNA splicing mutations, and single-base mutations that cause substitution of amino acids with bulkier side chains for glycine (see Fig. 348-6). In brief, most of the mutations lead to synthesis of abnormal but partially functional pro$\alpha 1(III)$ chains that produce procollagen suicide or alter fibril formation by the same mechanisms that amplify the effects of mutations in the genes for type I procollagen. Similar mutations in type III procollagen can cause aortic aneurysms in some individuals without other evidence of EDS type IV, MS, or other inherited disorders of connective tissue.

Type VI EDS is caused by a deficiency of lysyl hydroxylase. Mutations in the gene for this enzyme have been defined in several patients. One was a compound heterozygote, and two probands were homozygotes for the same large deletion and rearrangement of the gene; the mutations in the four alleles from these two patients were identical even though the parents were not thought to be related. Both types of mutation caused profound deficiency of lysyl hydroxylase, a decrease in the hydroxylysine content of collagen, and a decrease in the cross-links in collagen fibers.

Type VII EDS is due to a defect in the conversion of procollagen to collagen caused either by mutations that make type I procollagen resistant to cleavage by procollagen N-proteinase or by mutations that decrease the activity of the enzyme. The type VIIA mutations alter the cleavage site in the pro$\alpha 1(I)$ chain, and the type VIIB mutations alter the cleavage site in the pro$\alpha 2(I)$ chain. Both types are dominantly inherited. Type VIIC is caused by mutations that decrease the activity of procollagen N-proteinase and is inherited as an autosomal recessive trait. In all three forms of type VII EDS, the persistence of the N-propeptide causes the formation of collagen fibrils that are thin and irregular. Since most patients do not have clinical osteopenia, the thin and irregular fibrils apparently suffice for the mineralization of bone but do not provide the necessary tensile strength for ligaments and joint capsules.

The cause of type VIII EDS is unknown. Type IX is a disorder of copper transport. The syndrome, also referred to as *Menkes' syn-*

drome, is due to an X-linked defect and is associated with cutis laxa, hypopigmentation, unusual hair ("kinky"), vascular aneurysms, neurologic degeneration, and mental retardation. Mutations in a gene coding for a copper-transporting ATPase cause the disease. Type X EDS may be caused by defects in fibronectin, but no specific mutations have been defined. (See also Chaps. 80 and 350.)

Diagnosis The diagnosis is based on clinical criteria. Biochemical assays and gene analyses for known molecular defects in EDS are difficult and time-consuming, but specific diagnostic tests should be available in the future for families in which the mutations have been defined.

℞ TREATMENT

There is no specific therapy. Surgical repair and tightening of joint ligaments require careful evaluation of individual patients, since the ligaments frequently do not hold sutures. Patients with easy bruisability should be evaluated for other bleeding disorders. Patients with type IV EDS and members of their families probably should be evaluated at regular intervals by sonography and related techniques for early detection of aneurysms. Surgical repair of aneurysms may be difficult because of increased friability of tissues, and there is limited experience with elective surgery in such patients. Also, women with type IV EDS should be counseled about the increased risk of uterine rupture, bleeding, and other complications of pregnancy.

CHONDRODYSPLASIAS The chondrodysplasias are inherited skeletal disorders that cause dwarfism and abnormal body proportions. The category also includes some individuals with normal stature and body proportions who have features such as typical ocular changes or cleft palate that are common in more severe CDs. Many patients develop degenerative joint changes, and mild CD in adults may be difficult to differentiate from primary generalized osteoarthritis. Some authors refer to the disorders as "skeletal dysplasias," but CD is a more widely used term.

Classification Over 150 distinct types and 8 major subtypes have been defined (Table 348-5) based on criteria such as "bringing death" (thanatophoric), causing "twisted" bones (diastrophic), affecting metaphyses (metaphyseal), affecting epiphyses (epiphyseal), and producing histologic changes such as an apparent increase in the fibrous material in the epiphyses (fibrochondrogenesis). Also, a number of eponyms are based on the first or most comprehensive case reports. Severe forms of the diseases produce gross distortions of most cartilaginous structures and of the eye (see Table 348-1). Mild forms are more difficult to classify. Among the features are cataracts, degeneration of the vitreous and retinal detachment, high forehead, hypoplastic facies, cleft palate, short and thin extremities, and gross distortions of the epiphyses, metaphyses, and joint surfaces.

Incidence Data on the frequency of most CDs are not available, but the incidence of the Stickler syndrome may be as high as 1 in 10,000. Therefore, the diseases are probably among the more common heritable disorders of connective tissue.

Molecular Defects The first mutations shown to cause CDs were in the COL2A1 gene for type II collagen, the most abundant protein in cartilage. Over 40 mutations in this gene have now been reported in variants of CD ranging from mild to lethal (Fig. 348-7). About 20 percent of patients with severe or moderate CD and about 2 percent of families with early-onset generalized osteoarthritis have mutations in the same gene. However, similar phenotypes can also be caused by mutations in other genes, including genes for three other collagens, additional components of the cartilage matrix, growth factors, growth factor receptors, and transcription factors (Table 348-6). The number of mutated genes reported does not necessarily reflect the incidence of such mutations in the diseases themselves but rather the complexity of the genes and the technical difficulties in searching the complete gene for mutations. Also, it reflects the availability of large families for DNA linkage analysis and the vigor with which investigators have pursued their interest in a given gene. It is likely that mutations in additional genes will be found.

Most of the 40 or so mutations identified in the COL2A1 gene are in patients with severe CD and cause gross deformities of bones and cartilage such as hypochondrogenesis/achondrogenesis II and the Kniest syndrome. However, mutations in the COL2A1 gene have been found in a few families in which few if any symptoms are present in childhood but in which joint stiffness, joint pain, and degenerative changes of osteoarthritis develop in midlife. The mutations in the COL2A1 gene are similar to the mutations in the genes for types I and III procollagens (Fig. 348-7), and the correlations between genotype and phenotype are equally difficult. However, the first four mutations identified to cause premature termination signals for a collagen gene were in the COL2A1 gene and were in patients with the Stickler syndrome. In addition, mutations that change a codon for a Y-position amino acid in the -Gly-X-Y- repeat sequence from an arginine to

Table 348-4

Clinical Features, Mode of Inheritance, and Biochemical Defects in EDS

Type	Clinical Features	Inheritance*	Biochemical Defect
I, gravis	Soft, velvety, hyperextensible skin; easy bruising; "cigarette paper" scars; hypermobile joints; varicose veins; prematurity	AD	Some in type V collagen
II, mitis	Similar to EDS type I but less severe	AD	Some in type I collagen
III, familial hypermobility	Soft skin, no scarring, marked hypermobility	AD	Some in type II procollagen
IV, acrogeric, ecchymotic, vascular	Thin, translucent skin with visible veins; increased bruisability, skin and joints have normal extensibility; arterial, bowel, and uterine rupture	AD	Mutations in type III procollagen (see Fig. 348-6)
V, X-linked	Similar to EDS type II	XLR	Not known
VI, ocular-scoliotic	Soft, velvety, hyperextensible skin; hypermobile joints; scoliosis; ocular fragility and keratoconus	AR	Lysyl hydroxylase deficiency
VII, arthrochalasis multiplex congenita	Marked joint hypermobility, soft skin with normal scarring	AD	A. Structural defect in the proα1(I) chain
		AD	B. Structural defect in the proα2(I) chain
		AR	C. Procollagen *N*-proteinase deficiency
VIII, periodontal	Generalized periodontitis, skin similar to EDS type II	AD	Not known
IX, cutis laxa occipital horn syndrome	Vacant, now recategorized as a disorder of copper transport		
X	Similar to EDS type II	AR	Possible defect in fibronectin
XI, familial joint instability	Vacant, now recategorized with familial articular hypermobility syndromes		

* AD, autosomal dominant; AR, autosomal recessive; XLR, X-linked recessive.

SOURCE: After PH Byers, in *Clinical Medicine*, Philadelphia, Harper & Row, 1983, p. 1; and P Beighton et al, Am J Med Genet 29:581, 1988.

Table 348-5

Classifications of Chondrodysplasias

Achondrodysplasia family
Achondroplasia
Hypochondroplasia
Thanatophoric dysplasia
Spondyloepiphyseal dysplasia (SED) family
Achondrogenesis type IA
Achondrogenesis type IB
Achondrogenesis type II
Hypochondrogenesis
SED congenita
Strudwick syndrome
Stickler syndrome
Kniest dysplasia
Chondrodysplasia punctata family
Rhizomelic chondrodysplasia punctata
Conradi-Hünermann disease
X-linked dominant chondrodysplasia punctata
Chondrodysplasia punctata associated with Xp
Short rib (-polydactyly) family
Ellis–van Creveld syndrome
Asphyxiating thoracic dysplasia
Short rib–polydactyly syndrome type I
Short rib–polydactyly syndrome type II
Metatropic dysplasia family
Metatropic dysplasia
Metatropic-like dysplasia
Metaphyseal chondrodysplasia family
Metaphyseal chondrodysplasia, Jansen type
Metaphyseal chondrodysplasia, Schmid type
Metaphyseal chondrodysplasia, McKusick type
Brachyolmia family
Brachyolmia, Hobaek type
Brachyolmia, Maroteaux type
Brachyolmia, autosomal dominant type
Acromelic dysplasia family
Peripheral dysostosis
Achodysplasia
Trichorhinophalangeal syndrome type I
Trichorhinophalangeal syndrome type II

SOURCE: After J Spranger, Eur J Pediatr 151:407, 1992; WA Horton and JT Hecht.

cystine were found in families with early-onset osteoarthritis and minimal evidence of CDs.

Many individuals with the Schmid metaphyseal CD, characterized by short stature, *coxa vara*, flaring metaphyses, and waddling gait, have mutations in the gene for the type X collagen, a short, network-forming collagen found primarily in the hypertrophic zone of endochondral cartilage. A few patients with the nonocular variants of the Stickler syndrome have mutations in the gene for the α2(XI) chain of type XI collagen, a low-abundance collagen in cartilage and other tissues.

Mutations in the receptor for fibroblast growth factor (FGFR) 3 are present in most patients with achondroplasia, the most common cause of short-limbed dwarfism accompanied by macrocephaly and dysplasias of the metaphyses of long bones. The same single-base mutation in the gene that converts glycine to arginine at position 380 is present in more than 90 percent of patients. Most patients represent sporadic new mutations, and this nucleotide change must be one of the most common recurring mutations in the human genome. The mutation causes unregulated signal transduction through the receptor and inappropriate development of cartilage. Mutations that alter other domains of FGFR-3 have been found in patients with the more severe disorders hypochondroplasia and thanatophoric dysplasia and in a few families with a variant of craniosynostosis. However, most patients with craniosynostosis appear to have mutations in the related gene FGFR-2.

Mutations in the gene for the cartilage oligomeric matrix protein (COMP) have been found in patients with multiple epiphyseal dysplasia or pseudoachondroplasia, related syndromes characterized by short limbs and degenerative arthritis. However, one family with multiple epiphyseal dysplasia had a mutation in the gene for the α2(IX) chain of type IX collagen (COL9A1).

Diagnosis The diagnosis of severe forms of CD is made on the basis of analysis of the physical appearance, x-ray findings, histologic changes, and clinical course (Table 348-5).

℞ TREATMENT

No definitive therapy is available. Symptomatic treatment is directed to secondary features such as degenerative arthritis. Many patients require joint replacement surgery and corrective surgery for cleft palates. The eyes should be monitored carefully for the development of cataracts and for the need for laser therapy to prevent retinal detachment. Patients probably should be advised to avoid obesity and contact sports. Counseling for the psychological problems of short stature is critical, and support groups have formed in many countries. Ultrasonography is sometimes successful for prenatal diagnosis but less frequently than with OI. Specific tests should be available in the future for the CDs caused by mutations in the COL2A1 gene.

MARFAN SYNDROME Severe MS is characterized by a triad of features: (1) long, thin extremities frequently associated with other skeletal changes; (2) reduced vision as the result of dislocations of the lenses (ectopia lentis); and (3) aortic aneurysms that typically begin at the base of the aorta. Mild forms of the disorder, particularly those with only the skeletal changes, are difficult to classify.

Classification The severe form is usually caused by a mutation in a single allele of the fibrillin gene (FBN1). At the same time, MS must be distinguished from related syndromes: (1) homocystinuria, which can cause ectopia lentis and the same skeletal changes as MS; (2) congenital contractural arachnodactyly that causes similar skeletal changes but none of the other features of MS and is caused by mutations in a related fibrillin gene (FBN2); (3) familial ectopia lentis not associated with other features of MS; and (4) familial aortic aneurysms that result from a more common autosomal dominant disorder not associated with other features of MS, type IV EDS, or other known disorders of connective tissue.

Incidence and Inheritance MS has an incidence of about 1 in 10,000 in most racial and ethnic groups. The disorder is inherited as an autosomal dominant trait; at least one-fourth of patients do not have an affected parent, and their cases are probably due to new mutations.

Skeletal Changes Patients are usually tall compared with other members of the same family and have long limbs. The ratio of the upper segment (top of the head to top of the pubic ramus) to the lower segment (top of the pubic ramus to the floor) is usually 2 standard deviations below mean for age, race, and sex. The fingers and hands are long and slender and have a spider-like appearance (arachnodactyly). Many patients have severe chest deformities, including depression (pectus excavatum), protrusion (pectus carinatum), or asymmetry. Scoliosis is usually accompanied by kyphosis. High-arched palate and high pedal arches or pes planus are common. A few patients have joint hypermobility similar to that in mild EDS, but joint mobility is usually normal.

Cardiovascular Changes Cardiovascular abnormalities are the major source of morbidity and mortality. Mitral valve prolapse develops early in life and in about one-quarter progresses to mitral valve regurgitation of increasing severity because of redundancy of the leaflets, stretching of the chordae tendineae, and dilatation of the valvulae annulus. Dilatation of the root of the aorta and the sinuses of Valsalva may be detected by echocardiography in utero. The rate of dilatation is unpredictable, but the dilatation can cause aortic regurgitation, dissection of the aorta, and rupture. Dilatation is probably accelerated by physical and emotional stress, as well as by pregnancy.

Ocular Changes The dislocation of the lens may be readily apparent, but diagnosis usually requires pupillary dilatation and slit-lamp examination. The displacement is usually not progressive but may contribute to the formation of cataracts. The ocular globe is frequently elongated, most patients are myopic, and some develop retinal detachment. A few patients have lattice degeneration and retinal tears; most have adequate vision.

Associated Changes Striae may occur over the shoulders and buttocks. Otherwise the skin is normal. A number of patients develop spontaneous pneumothorax. Inguinal and incisional hernias are common. Marked dilatation of the dural sac is seen frequently in computed tomography scans, but the condition is usually asymptomatic. Patients are typically thin with little subcutaneous fat, but adults may develop centripetal obesity.

Molecular Defects Most patients with the classic features of MS are heterozygotes for mutations in a gene on chromosome 15 that encodes fibrillin, a glycoprotein of 350 kDa that is a major component of elastin-associated microfibrils. These microfibrils are abundant in large blood vessels and the suspensory ligaments of the lens. About one-third of the mutations cause premature termination of translation, and most of the remainder cause single amino acid substitutions in the epidermal growth factor–like domains of the molecule that may be involved in calcium binding. The function of fibrillin has not been defined, but the data suggest that fibrillin self-assembles into a fibrillar structure and that the conformation and surface properties of the entire molecule are critical for normal assembly. Therefore, the functional consequences of mutations that change the amino acid sequence of fibrillin may be similar to the effects of mutations that change the conformation of a fibrillar collagen (see Figs. 348-2, 348-4, 348-6, and 348-7). DNA linkage studies indicate that the gene that causes familial ectopia lentis without any other signs of MS is also located on chromosome 15, but it is unclear whether the gene is identical with FBN1. Several families with a Marfan-related syndrome characterized by congenital contractural arachnodactyly demonstrate linkage to a second fibrillin gene located on chromosome 5 (FBN2). A third fibrillin gene (FBN3) is present on chromosome 17, but no defect has yet been linked to the gene. Also, two patients with atypical forms of MS have defects in the proα2(I) chain of type I procollagen.

Diagnosis The diagnosis is easily established if the patient and other members of the family have dislocated lenses, aortic dilatation, and long and thin extremities together with kyphoscoliosis or other chest deformities. The diagnosis is frequently made if ectopia lentis and an aneurysm of the ascending aorta occur in the absence of a Marfan habitus or a positive family history. All patients in whom the diagnosis is suspected should have a slit-lamp examination and an echocardiogram. Also, homocystinuria (see Table 348-3) should be ruled out by a negative cyanide-nitroprusside test for disulfides in the urine. A few patients with types I, II, and III EDS have ectopia lentis but lack the Marfan habitus and instead have characteristic skin changes not present in MS. Patients with familial aortic aneurysms tend to develop aneurysms at the base of the abdominal aorta. The location of the aneurysms, however, is variable, and the high incidence of aortic aneurysms (1 in 100) makes the differential diagnosis difficult unless other features of MS are clearly present. A few families with familial aortic aneurysms have mutations in the gene for type III procollagen (see Fig. 348-6).

Rx TREATMENT

There is no established treatment, but several investigators have recommended use of propranolol or other beta-adrenergic blocking agents to delay or prevent aortic dilatation. Surgical replacement of the aorta, aortic valve, and mitral valve has been successful in some patients, and all patients should be followed carefully with echocardiography and other techniques for evaluation of cardiovascular changes. Patients probably should be advised of the risks of severe physical and emotional stress and of pregnancy.

The scoliosis tends to be progressive and should be treated by mechanical bracing and physical therapy if greater than 20 degrees or by surgery if it progresses to greater than 45 degrees. Estrogen has been tried in girls with scoliosis, but the results are inconclusive. Dislocated lenses rarely require surgical removal, but patients should be followed closely for retinal detachment. Pyeritz has summarized current protocols for the management of patients.

Diagnostic tests based on detection of fibrillin defects in cultured skin fibroblasts or DNA analysis of the gene may be available in the near future.

EPIDERMOLYSIS BULLOSA Epidermolysis bullosa (EB) is the name given to a group of disorders in which the skin and related epithelial tissues break and blister as the result of minor trauma. As with most heritable disorders of connective tissues, the clinical manifestations range from lethal to mild disorders.

Classification Three categories are defined on the basis of the level at which blistering occurs: EB simplex for blistering in the epidermis, EB junctional for blistering in the dermal-epidermal junction, and EB dystrophica for blistering in the dermis. More than 20 subtypes have been separated on the basis of the clinical findings together with ultrastructural and immunohistologic changes in skin.

Incidence The incidence of EB in the United States is estimated to be 1 in 50,000.

Molecular Defects The molecular basis of several specific variants of EB has been defined. Some of the first information came from experiments with transgenic mice in which mice expressing a gene for a truncated keratin (keratin 14) developed intraepidermal blistering similar to that seen in patients with EB simplex. Subsequently, a series of patients with EB simplex were found to have mutations in either keratin 14 or keratin 5, two of the major keratins in basal epithelial cells. Patients with the related syndrome, epidermolytic icthyosis, have mutations in keratin 1 and keratin 10. Some patients with the more severe dystrophic EB have mutations in type VII collagen (COL7A1),

Table 348-6

Reported Gene Mutations in Chondrodysplasias*

	Mutated Gene (Number Reported)					
Disease	COL2A1	COL9A2	COL10A1	COL11A2	FGFR-3	COMP
Achondrodysplasia family						
Achondrodysplasia					>250	
Hypochondroplasia					3	
Thanatophoric dysplasia					9	
SED family						
Achondrogenesis II/ hypochondrogenesis	13					
SED congenita	11					
Stickler syndrome						
Classic	6					
Nonocular				2		
Kniest dysplasia	5					
Metaphyseal CD family						
Schmid type			17			
Multiple epiphyseal dysplasia or pseudo-chondroplasia		1				23
Osteoarthritis with mild CD	3					

* Additional mutations reported: A series of patients with craniosynostoses (Crouzon, Apert, Jackson-Weiss, and Pfeiffer syndromes) had mutations in the FGFR-2 gene, but three families with the Crouzon syndrome and acanthosis nigricans had mutations in the FGFR-3 gene.

NOTE: FGFR, fibroblast growth factor; COMP, cartilage oligomeric matrix protein; SED, spondyloepiphyseal dysplasia.

the collagen that forms strandlike fibrils that anchor the basal lamina to the type I collagen and other collagens of the dermis. Patients with junctional EB have mutations in the gene for laminin 5, one of a family of large, cross-shaped proteins in basal membranes.

Diagnosis The diagnosis is based on skin that readily breaks and forms blisters. EB simplex, which affects only the epidermis, is generally milder than EB junctional or EB dystrophica. EB dystrophica variants usually cause large and prominent scars. Classification within subtypes usually requires electron microscopy.

℞ TREATMENT

The treatment is symptomatic. Bruckner-Tuderman has reviewed the diagnostic criteria and management.

ALPORT SYNDROME (See also Chap. 275) AS is an inherited disorder characterized by hematuria. Four forms of the disease are now recognized: (1) classic AS, which is inherited as an X-linked disorder with hematuria, sensorineural deafness, and conical deformation of the anterior surface of the lens (lenticonus); (2) a second X-linked form associated with diffuse leiomyomatosis; (3) an autosomal recessive form; and (4) an autosomal dominant form. The two autosomal forms can cause renal disease without deafness or lenticonus.

Incidence The incidence of AS is about 1 in 10,000 in the general population and as high as 1 in 5000 in some ethnic groups.

Molecular Defects Electron microscopy of kidneys from patients with classic AS demonstrated that the glomerular basement membrane was up to five times thicker than normal and that the lamina densa was distorted and split. The X-linked and autosomal recessive forms are caused primarily by mutations in genes for the α2(IV), α4(IV), α5(IV), or α6(IV) chains of type IV collagen, a major component of basement membranes. The type IV collagen in most membranes consists primarily of α1(IV) and α2(IV) chains folded into a large, rodlike molecule with globular ends and a long triple-helical domain that is interrupted by short sequences that do not form triple helices. The molecules self-assemble through both the globular ends and the long triple-helical domain to form a complex three-dimensional network. The four additional α chains of type IV collagen are similar in structure and are probably incorporated into the same or similar molecules. The six genes for the proteins are arranged in tandem pairs on different chromosomes in a head-to-head orientation and with overlapping promoters, i.e., the α1(IV) and α2(IV) genes are head-to-head on chromosome 13q34, the α3(IV) and α4(IV) genes are on chromosome 2q35-37, and the α5(IV) and α6(IV) genes are on chromosome Xq22. An X-linked variant is caused by mutations in the COL4A6 gene, and the X-linked variant associated with leiomyomatosis is caused by deletions that involve both the COL4A5 gene and the nearby COL4A6 gene. The autosomal recessive variants are caused by mutations in either the COL4A3 or COL4A4 genes, and the mutations responsible for the autosomal dominant variants are still unknown.

Diagnosis The diagnosis of classic AS is based on X-linked inheritance of hematuria, sensorineural deafness, and lenticonus. Because of the X-linked transmission, women are usually less severely affected than men and are generally underdiagnosed. The hematuria progresses to nephritis and may cause renal failure in late adolescence in affected males and at older ages in some women. The sensorineural deafness is primarily in the high-tone range. It frequently can be detected only by an audiogram and usually is not progressive. The lenticonus rarely occurs without nephritis and is considered to be pathognomonic of classic AS.

℞ TREATMENT

There is no known treatment.

BIBLIOGRAPHY

BRUCKNER-TUDERMAN L: Epidermolysis bullosa, in *Connective Tissue and Its Heritable Disorders*, PM Royce, B Steinmann (eds). New York, Wiley-Liss, 1993, p 507

BYERS PH: Osteogenesis imperfecta, in *Connective Tissue and Its Heritable Disorders*, PM Royce, B Steinmann (eds). New York, Wiley-Liss, 1993, p 317

CHRISTIANO AM, UITTO J: Molecular complexity of the cutaneous basement membrane zone. Revelations from the paradigms of epidermolysis bullosa. Exp Dermatol 5:1, 1996

DIETZ HC, PYERITZ RE: Mutations in the human gene for fibrillin-1 (FBN1) in the Marfan syndrome and related disorders. Hum Mol Genet 4:1799, 1995

FLINTER FA et al: Genetics of classic Alport's syndrome. Lancet 2:1005, 1988

HORTON WA, HECHT JT: The chondrodysplasias, in *Connective Tissue and Its Heritable Disorders*, PM Royce, B Steinmann (eds). New York, Wiley-Liss, 1993, p 641

KASHTAN CE: Clinical and molecular diagnosis of Alport syndrome. Proc Assoc Am Physicians 107:306, 1995

KUIVANIEMI H et al: Mutations in the fibrillar collagens (types I, II, III, IX and XI), and fibril-associated collagen, and the network-forming collagen (type X) cause a spectrum of diseases of bone, cartilage and blood vessels. Hum Mutat, 1997

MARINI JC: Osteogenesis imperfecta. Comprehensive management. Adv Pediatr 35:391, 1988

——— et al: Evaluation of growth hormone axis and responsiveness to growth stimulation of short children with osteogenesis imperfecta. Am J Med Genet 45:261, 1993

MCKUSICK VA: *Heritable Disorders of Connective Tissue*, 4th ed. St Louis, Mosby, 1972

MEYERS GA: FGFR2 exon IIIa and IIIc mutations in Crouzon, Jackson-Weiss, and Pfeiffer syndromes: Evidence for missense changes, insertions, and a deletion due to alternative RNA splicing. Am J Med Genet 58:491, 1996

PROCKOP DJ: Mutations in collagen genes as a cause of connective-tissue diseases. N Engl J Med 326:540, 1992

———, KIVIRIKKO KI: Collagen: Molecular biology, diseases and potentials for therapy. Annu Rev Biochem 64:403, 1996

PYERITZ RE: The Marfan syndrome, in *Connective Tissue and Its Heritable Disorders*, PM Royce, B Steinmann (eds). New York, Wiley-Liss, 1993, p 437

SILLENCE DO: Osteogenesis imperfecta: An expanding panorama of variance. Clin Orthop 191:11, 1981

STEINMANN et al: The Ehlers-Danlos syndrome, in *Connective Tissue and Its Heritable Disorders*, PM Royce, B Steinmann (eds). New York, Wiley-Liss, 1993, p 351

349

Louis J. Elsas, Nicola Longo, Leon E. Rosenberg

INHERITED DISORDERS OF AMINO ACID METABOLISM AND STORAGE

All polypeptides and proteins are polymers of amino acids. Eight amino acids, referred to as *essential*, cannot be synthesized by humans and must be obtained from dietary sources. The others are formed endogenously. Although most of the body's amino acids are "tied up" in proteins, small intracellular pools of *free* amino acids are in equilibrium with extracellular reservoirs in plasma, cerebrospinal fluid, and the lumina of the gut and kidney. Physiologically, amino acids are more than mere "building blocks." Some (glycine, glutamate, gamma-aminobutyric acid) are neurotransmitters. Others (phenylalanine, tyrosine, tryptophan, glycine) are precursors of hormones, coenzymes, pigments, purines, or pyrimidines. Each has a unique degradative pathway by which its nitrogen and carbon components are used for the synthesis of other amino acids, carbohydrates, and lipids.

More than 70 disorders of amino acid metabolism are now known, the catabolic and storage defects (approximately 60) discussed in this chapter far outnumbering the transport abnormalities (approximately 10) considered in Chap. 350. Each of these disorders is rare—the incidences range from 1 in 10,000 for cystinuria or phenylketonuria to 1 in 200,000 for homocystinuria or alkaptonuria. Collectively, however, they occur in perhaps 1 in 500 to 1 in 1000 live births.

The features of inherited disorders of amino acid catabolism are summarized in Table 349-1. In general, these disorders are named for the compound that accumulates to highest concentration in blood (*-emias*) or urine (*-urias*). For many conditions (often called *amino-*

Table 349-1

Inherited Disorders of Amino Acid Catabolism

Amino Acid(s) Affected	Disorder or Condition	Enzyme Defect	Clinical Manifestations*: Mental Retardation	Neuropsychiatric Dysfunction	Protein Intolerance	Metabolic Ketoacidosis	Ammonia Intoxication	Other	Inheritance Pattern†
AROMATIC—HETEROCYCLIC									
Phenylalanine	Phenylketonuria type I (severe to mild)	Phenylalanine hydroxylase	+	+	−	−	−	Hypopigmented skin and hair, eczema	AR
	Phenylketonuria type II	Dihydropteridine reductase	+	+	−	−	−		AR
	Phenylketonuria type III	Dihydrobiopterin synthesis	+	+	−	−	−		AR
	Malignant hyperphenylalaninemia	GTP cyclohydrolase	+	+	−	−	−		AR
Tyrosine	Tyrosinemia type I (hepatorenal)	Fumarylacetoacetate hydrolase	−	−	±	−	−	Cirrhosis, hepatic failure, renal tubular defects, rickets	AR
	Tyrosinemia type II (oculocutaneous)	Tyrosine transaminase	±	−	−	−	−	Palmoplantar keratosis, painful corneal erosions with photophobia	AR
	Tyrosinemia type III	4-Hydroxyphenylpyruvate dioxygenase	−	−	−	−	−		AR
	Hawkinsinuria	4-Hydroxyphenylpyruvate dioxygenase	−	−	−	−	−	Failure to thrive, metabolic acidosis in infancy, fine hairs	AD
	Alkaptonuria	Homogentisic acid oxidase	−	−	−	−	−	Ochronosis, arthritis	AR
	Albinism (oculocutaneous)	Tyrosinase	−	−	−	−	−	Hypopigmentation of hair, skin, and optic fundus	AR
	Albinism (ocular)	Unknown	−	−	−	−	−	Hypopigmentation of optic fundus	XL, AR
Tryptophan	Tryptophanuria	Unknown	+	+	−	−	−	Photosensitive skin rash	AR
	Xanthurenic aciduria	Kynureninase	?	−	−	−	−		?
Histidine	Histidinemia	Histidine-ammonia lyase	±	±	−	−	−	Hearing and speech deficit	AR
	Urocanic aciduria	Urocanase	+	+	−	−	−		?
	Formiminoglutamic aciduria	Formiminotransferase	?	+	−	−	−		(AR)
GLYCINE-IMINO ACIDS									
Glycine	Hyperglycinemia	Glycine cleavage	+	+	−	−	−		AR
	Sarcosinemia	Sarcosine dehydrogenase	−	−	−	−	−		AR
	Hyperoxaluria (type I)	Alanine: glyoxylate amino-transferase	−	−	−	−	−	Calcium oxalate nephrolithiasis, renal failure	AR
	Hyperoxaluria (type II)	D-Glyceric acid dehydrogenase/glyoxylate reductase	−	−	−	−	−	Calcium oxalate nephrolithiasis, renal failure	AR
Imino acids	Hyperprolinemia (type I)	Proline oxidase	−	−	−	−	−		AR
	Hyperprolinemia (type II)	Δ'-Pyrroline dehydrogenase	−	−	−	−	−		AR
	Hyperhydroxyprolinemia	Hydroxyproline reductase	−	−	−	−	−		AR
	Iminopeptiduria	Prolidase	+	−	−	−	−	Crusting erythematous, ecchymotic dermatitis, recurrent infections	AR

(continued)

Inherited Disorders of Amino Acid Catabolism

			Clinical Manifestations*						
Amino Acid(s) Affected	**Disorder or Condition**	**Enzyme Defect**	**Mental Retardation**	**Neuropsychiatric Dysfunction**	**Protein Intolerance**	**Metabolic Ketoacidosis**	**Ammonia Intoxication**	**Other**	**Inheritance Pattern†**
SULFUR-CONTAINING									
Methionine	Hypermethioninemia	Methionine adenosyltransferase	−	−	−	−	−		?
Homocystine	Homocystinuria	Cystathionine β-synthase	±	±	−	−	−	Dislocated lenses, osteoporosis, thrombotic vascular disease	AR
	Homocystinuria	5,10-Methylenetetrahydrofolate reductase	+	+	−	−	−		AR
	Homocystinuria and methylmalonic acidemia (cblC, -D)‡	Cobalamin (vitamin B_{12}) reductase (cytosol)	+	+	−	−	−	Megaloblastic anemia	AR
	Homocystinuria and methylmalonic acidemia (cblF)	Lysosomal efflux	+	+	−	−	−		(?)
	Homocystinuria (cblE, -G)	Methyltransferase-associated cobalamin reductase (?)	+	+	−	−	−	Megaloblastic anemia	AR
Cystathionine	Cystathioninuria	Cystathionase	−	−	−	−	−		AR
Cystine	Cystinosis	Lysosomal efflux	−	−	−	−	−	Fanconi syndrome, renal failure, photophobia	AR
S-Sulfo-L-cysteine	*S*-Sulfo-L-cysteine, sulfite, and thiosulfaturia	Sulfite oxidase	+	+	−	−	−	Dislocated lenses	AR
CATIONIC									
Lysine	Hyperlysinemia	α-Aminoadipic semialdehyde synthase			−	−	−		AR
	Saccharopinuria	δ-Aminoadipic semialdehyde synthase	−	−	−	−	−		?
	α-Ketoadipic aciduria	α-Ketoadipic acid dehydrogenase			−	−	−		?
	Glutaric aciduria (type I)	Glutaryl CoA dehydrogenase	−	+	−	−	−	Progressive dystonia and athetosis	AR
	Glutaric aciduria (type II)	Electron transfer flavoprotein; or ETF-ubiquinone oxidoreductase	−	+	−	+	−	Hypoglycemia, acidosis, "sweaty feet" odor, hypotonia, fatty degeneration of liver and kidney	AR
Ornithine	Hyperornithinemia, hyperammonemia, homocitrullinuria	Mitochondrial ornithine translocator (?)	+	+	+	−	+		AR
	Hyperornithinemia	Ornithine-D-aminotransferase	−	−	−	−	−	Gyrate atrophy of choroid and retina	AR
UREA CYCLE									
Carbamylphosphate	Hyperammonemia (type I)	Carbamylphosphate synthetase I	+	+	+	−	+		AR
N-acetylglutamate	Hyperammonemia (type IA)	*N*-acetylglutamate synthetase	?	+	+	−	+		AR
Ornithine	Hyperammonemia (type II)	Ornithine transcarbamylase	±	+	+	−	+		XL
Citrulline	Citrullinemia	Argininosuccinate synthetase	+	+	+	−	+		AR
Argininosuccinic acid	Argininosuccinic aciduria	Argininosuccinase	+	+	+	−	+		AR
Arginine	Argininemia	Arginase	+	+	+	−	+		AR

(continued)

Table 349-1—*(Continued)*

Inherited Disorders of Amino Acid Catabolism

Amino Acid(s) Affected	Disorder or Condition	Enzyme Defect	Clinical Manifestations* Mental Retardation	Neuropsychiatric Dysfunction	Protein Intolerance	Metabolic Ketoacidosis	Ammonia Intoxication	Other	Inheritance Pattern†
BRANCHED-CHAIN									
Valine	Hypervalinemia	Valine aminotransferase	+	+	+	−	−		AR
Leucine, isoleucine	Hyperleucine-isoleucinemia	Leucine-isoleucine aminotransferase	+	+	+	−	−		?
Valine, leucine, isoleucine	Classic branched-chain ketoaciduria	Branched-chain ketoacid dehydrogenase	+	+	+		−	"Maple syrup" odor	AR
	Intermittent branched-chain ketoaciduria	Branched-chain ketoacid dehydrogenase	±	−	+	+	−		AR
Leucine	Isovaleric acidemia	Isovaleryl CoA dehydrogenase	±	±	+	+	±	"Sweaty feet" odor	AR
	β-Methylcrotonyl glycinuria	β-Methylcrotonyl CoA carboxylase	+	+	−	+	−	"Cat's urine" odor	AR
	β-Hydroxy-β-methylglutaric aciduria	β-Hydroxy-β-methylglutaryl CoA lyase	−	+	+	+	−		?
Isoleucine, valine	α-Methylacetoacetic aciduria	β-Ketothiolase	±	±	+	+	+		AR
	Propionic acidemia (pcc A, B, C)‡	Propionyl CoA carboxylase	±	±	+	+	+		AR
	Propionic acidemia (bio)‡	Holocarboxylase synthetase; biotinidase	+	±	+	+	−		AR
	Methylmalonic acidemia (mut)‡	Methylmalonyl CoA mutase	±	±	+	+	+		AR
	Methylmalonic acidemia (cbl A)‡	Cobalamin (vitamin B_{12}) reductase (mitochondrial) (?)	±	±	+	+	+		AR
	Methylmalonic acidemia (cbl B)‡	Cobalamin (vitamin B_{12}): ATP adenosyltransferase	±	±	+	+	+		AR

* +, Regularly present; ±, sometimes present; −, absent; ?, uncertain; all designations refer to manifestations in untreated disorder.
† AR, autosomal recessive; XL, X-linked; (AR), probably autosomal recessive.
‡ Designations in parentheses refer to complementation groups assigned by genetic analysis with cultured cells.

acidopathies), the parent amino acid is found in excess; for others, generally referred to as *organic acidemias*, products in the catabolic pathway accumulate. Which compound(s) accumulates depends, of course, on the site of the enzymatic block, the reversibility of the reactions proximal to the lesion, and the availability of alternative pathways of metabolic "runoff." For some amino acids, such as the sulfur-containing or branched-chain molecules, defects have been described at nearly each step in the catabolic pathway. For others, only small numbers of defective reactions have been described. Biochemical and genetic heterogeneity is common. Four distinct forms of hyperphenylalaninemia, seven forms of homocystinuria, and seven types of methylmalonic acidemia are recognized. Such heterogeneity reflects the presence of an even larger array of molecular defects.

The manifestations of these conditions differ widely (see Table 349-1). Some, such as sarcosinemia or hyperprolinemia, produce no clinical consequences. At the other extreme, complete deficiency of ornithine transcarbamylase or of branched-chain keto acid dehydrogenase is lethal in the untreated neonate. Central nervous system (CNS) dysfunction, in the form of developmental retardation, seizures, alterations in sensorium, or behavioral disturbances, is present in more than half the disorders. Protein-induced vomiting, neurologic dysfunction, and hyperammonemia occur in many disorders of urea cycle intermediates. Metabolic ketoacidosis, often accompanied by hyperammonemia, is a frequent presenting finding in the disorders of branched-chain amino acid metabolism. Occasional disorders produce focal tissue or organ involvement such as liver disease, renal failure, cutaneous abnormalities, or ocular lesions.

The clinical manifestations in many of these conditions can be prevented or mitigated if diagnosis is achieved early and appropriate treatment (i.e., dietary protein or amino acid restriction or vitamin supplementation) is instituted promptly. For this reason, several aminoacidopathies and organic acidemias are screened for in mass newborn surveys that analyze blood or urine with an array of chemical and microbiologic techniques. Once a presumptive diagnosis is made, confirmation can be provided by direct enzyme assay on extracts of leukocytes, erythrocytes, or cultured fibroblasts. DNA-based diagnostic capability is possible for several disorders. For example, substitutions, deletions, and insertions can be utilized to diagnose and characterize phenylketonuria, ornithine transcarbamylase deficiency, citrullinemia, gyrate atrophy of the retina, propionic acidemia, and methylmalonic acidemia (see also Chap. 65). As additional mutations are defined, DNA-based analysis will be used to predict outcome and the therapeutic plan.

Several of these disorders (including branched-chain ketoaciduria, isovaleric acidemia, propionic acidemia, methylmalonic acidemia, homocystinuria, cystinosis, phenylketonuria, ornithine transcarbamylase deficiency, citrullinemia, argininosuccinic aciduria) can be diagnosed prenatally by chemical analysis of amniotic fluid or by chemical, enzymatic, or DNA-based studies of fresh or cultured amniotic fluid cells. In addition to predicting genotype and alleviating parental anxiety, prenatal diagnosis has led to improved treatment of affected newborns.

The focus in this chapter is on selected disorders that illustrate the principles, properties, and problems presented by the disorders of amino acid metabolism.

THE HYPERPHENYLALANINEMIAS

DEFINITION The hyperphenylalaninemias (see Table 349-1) result from impaired conversion of phenylalanine to tyrosine. The most common and clinically important is phenylketonuria, which is characterized by an increased concentration of phenylalanine in blood, increased concentrations of phenylalanine and its by-products (notably phenylpyruvate, phenylacetate, phenyllactate, and phenylacetylglutamine) in urine, and severe mental retardation if untreated in infancy.

ETIOLOGY AND PATHOGENESIS Each of the hyperphenylalaninemias results from reduced activity of *phenylalanine hydroxylase*. In humans, the complete enzyme system is expressed only in liver. Phenylalanine and molecular oxygen are substrates, and a reduced pteridine, tetrahydrobiopterin, is cofactor (Fig. 349-1). Tyrosine and dihydrobiopterin are the products of this catalytic system, the latter being reconverted to tetrahydrobiopterin by a second enzyme, dihydropteridine reductase. In the most severe forms of phenylketonuria type I, activity of the hydroxylase apoenzyme, encoded by a gene on chromosome 12q22-q24.1, is almost totally deficient. More than 200 mutations in this gene have been identified in patients with phenylketonuria. The prevalence of these mutations varies widely among different ethnic groups. Mutations causing a complete impairment of enzyme activity, such as the R408W, are associated with more severe outcome, requiring stringent dietary restriction of phenylalanine. Mutations causing a less complete deficiency of the enzyme, such as the I65T, are associated with milder forms of type I phenylketonuria. Transient hyperphenylalaninemia (sometimes called *transient phenylketonuria*)

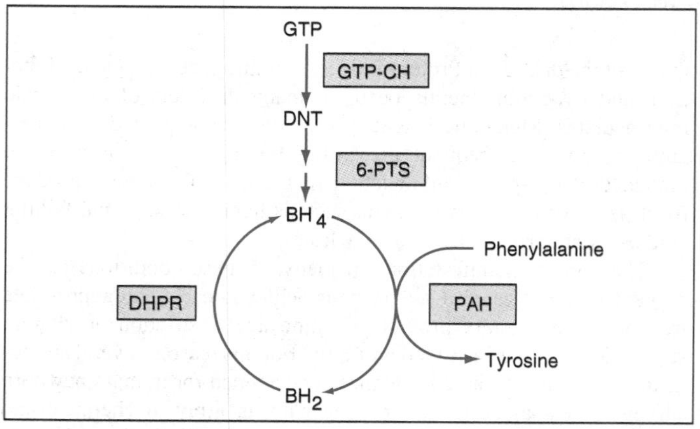

FIGURE 349-1 Pathways, enzymes, and coenzymes involved in the hyperphenylalaninemias. Blocked-in symbols highlight points of etiologic or therapeutic significance to the various genetic defects underlying these disorders. Abbreviations: GTP, guanosine triphosphate; GTP-CH, guanosine triphosphate cyclohydrolase; DNT, dihydroneopterin triphosphate; 6-PTS, 6-pyruvoyltetrahydropterin synthase; BH_4, tetrahydrobiopterin; BH_2, dihydrobiopterin; DHPR, dihydropteridine reductase; PAH, phenylalanine hydroxylase.

is caused by a delayed maturation of the hydroxylase apoenzyme. In "malignant" hyperphenylalaninemia, however, persistent impairment of hydroxylating activity results not from abnormality in the apohydroxylase but from tetrahydrobiopterin deficiency due to blocks in the pathway by which tetrahydrobiopterin is synthesized from GTP (phenylketonuria type III and malignant hyperphenylalaninemia) or deficiency of dihydropteridine reductase (phenylketonuria type II), the enzyme that regenerates tetrahydrobiopterin from dihydrobiopterin (see Fig. 349-1). Tyrosine hydroxylase and tryptophan hydroxylase also require tetrahydrobiopterin, and their products (L-dopa and 5-hydroxytryptophan) are essential for the synthesis of neurotransmitters.

Abnormalities in phenylalanine metabolism are autosomal recessive traits that occur in about 1 in 10,000 births. Phenylketonuria type I, which accounts for nearly two-thirds of these, is widely distributed among whites and Asians. It is rare in blacks. Phenylalanine hydroxylase activity in obligate heterozygotes is low but higher than in affected homozygotes. Adult heterozygous carriers are clinically well but can be identified by an increased ratio of phenylalanine/tyrosine in plasma in the semifasting state. They may have transient cognitive impairment after phenylalanine loads.

Phenylalanine accumulation in blood and urine and reduced tyrosine formation are direct consequences of the impaired hydroxylation. In untreated phenylketonuria and in its tetrahydrobiopterin-deficient variants, plasma concentrations of phenylalanine become sufficiently high [>1 mmol/L (16 mg/dL)] to activate alternative pathways of metabolism and lead to formation of phenylpyruvate, phenylacetate, phenyllactate, and other derivatives that are rapidly cleared by the kidney and excreted in urine. Plasma concentrations of several other amino acids are moderately reduced, probably secondary to inhibition of gastrointestinal absorption or impairment of renal tubular reabsorption by excess phenylalanine. The severe brain damage is due to several consequences of phenylalanine accumulation: competitive inhibition of transport of other amino acids required for protein synthesis, impaired polyribosome formation or stabilization, reduced synthesis and increased degradation of myelin, and inadequate formation of norepinephrine and serotonin. Phenylalanine is a competitive inhibitor of tyrosinase, a key enzyme in the pathway of melanin synthesis. This block, plus reduced availability of the melanin precursor tyrosine, accounts for the hypopigmentation of hair and skin.

CLINICAL MANIFESTATIONS No abnormalities are apparent at birth, but untreated children with classic phenylketonuria fail to attain early developmental milestones, develop microcephaly, and demonstrate progressive impairment of cerebral function. Hyperactivity, seizures, and severe mental retardation are major clinical problems later in life. Electroencephalographic abnormalities, "mousy" odor of skin, hair, and urine (due to phenylacetate accumulation), and a tendency to hypopigmentation and eczema complete the devastating clinical picture. In contrast, affected children who are detected at birth and treated promptly show none of these abnormalities. Children with tetrahydrobiopterin deficiency, however, are the most unfortunate. Seizures appear early, followed by progressive cerebral and basal ganglia dysfunction (rigidity, chorea, spasms, hypotonia). Most succumb to secondary infection within a few years despite early diagnosis and vigorous treatment.

A number of women with phenylketonuria who have been treated since infancy have reached adulthood and become pregnant. If phenylalanine levels are not strictly controlled before and during pregnancy, the offspring is at risk from *maternal phenylketonemia*. At birth, such children have microcephaly and an increased risk of congenital defects. After birth, these children have severe neurodevelopmental delay and growth retardation. Since these children are heterozygous, not homozygous, carriers of a mutation in the phenylalanine hydroxylase gene, the clinical manifestations must be attributed to damage produced by the elevated maternal concentrations of phenylalanine to which they have been exposed in utero.

DIAGNOSIS Plasma phenylalanine concentrations are usually normal at birth in the hyperphenylalaninemias but rise rapidly after institution of protein feedings. To prevent mental retardation, diagnosis and initiation of dietary treatment of classic phenylketonuria must occur before the child is 3 weeks of age. For this reason, most newborns in North America and Europe are screened by determinations of blood phenylalanine concentration using the Guthrie bacterial inhibition assay. Abnormal values are confirmed with more quantitative fluorometric or chromatographic assays. In newborns with type I phenylketonuria, plasma levels depend on the amount of phenylalanine to which the infant has been exposed and the degree of impaired phenylalanine hydroxylase. Dietary phenylalanine restriction is usually instituted if blood phenylalanine levels are above 250 μmol/L (4 mg/dL). Careful monitoring of these infants reveals the degree of phenylalanine hydroxylase impairment and dictates the degree of dietary phenylalanine restriction. Deficiency of tetrahydrobiopterin, which occurs in 1 to 5 percent of newborns with increased blood phenylalanine, is excluded by screening the urinary pteridine profile and by assay of dihydropteridine reductase activity on dried blood specimens. Tetrahydrobiopterin deficiency manifests with hyperphenylalaninemia and progressive neurologic impairment despite prompt restriction of dietary phenylalanine. Prenatal diagnosis of type I phenylketonuria is now feasible using DNA-based tests capable of detecting specific mutations or restriction fragment length polymorphisms of the phenylalanine hydroxylase gene. Dihydropteridine reductase deficiency and the blocks in tetrahydrobiopterin synthesis also can be detected in utero using assays on cultured amniocytes.

℞ TREATMENT

Phenylketonuria is the first inherited metabolic disease in which prevention of the accumulation of the offending metabolite prevented the dire clinical consequences. This was accomplished by a special diet low in phenylalanine and supplemented with tyrosine. Tyrosine becomes an essential amino acid in phenylalanine hydroxylase deficiency. Sufficient phenylalanine is provided for new protein synthesis and normal growth. This amount varies with age and requires frequent adjustments, especially early in life. Ordinarily, plasma phenylalanine concentrations are maintained between 120 and 360 μmol/L (2 and 6 mg/dL).

Such diet therapy must be instituted during the first 3 weeks of life. Even then, modest CNS dysfunction may occur with more deleterious mutations or after excess protein intake. Because uncontrolled hyperphenylalaninemia results in brain damage throughout childhood (and perhaps in adults), dietary restriction should usually be continued and monitored indefinitely, recognizing that transient phenylketonuria may not require lifelong therapy. Children with tetrahydrobiopterin deficiency deteriorate despite dietary phenylalanine restriction; efficacy of pteridine cofactor replacement is under study. Such patients may be helped, however, by a regimen in which dietary phenylalanine restriction is combined with supplements of levodopa and 5-hydroxytryptophan. Finally, the deleterious consequences of maternal phenylketonuria can be minimized by continuing lifelong phenylalanine-restricted diets in females with phenylketonuria and assuring even stricter phenylalanine restriction prior to conception and throughout gestation.

THE HOMOCYSTINURIAS (HYPERHOMOCYSTEINEMIAS)

The homocystinurias are seven biochemically and clinically distinct disorders (see Table 349-1), each characterized by increased concentration of the sulfur-containing amino acid homocystine in blood and urine. The most common form results from reduced activity of cystathionine β-synthase, an enzyme in the transsulfuration pathway that converts methionine to cysteine (Fig. 349-2). The other forms are the result of impaired conversion of homocysteine to methionine, a reaction catalyzed by homocysteine:-methyltetrahydrofolate methyltransferase and two essential cofactors, methyltetrahydrofolate and methylcobalamin (methyl-vitamin B_{12}). Depending on the underlying disorder, some patients show chemical and, in some instances, clinical improvement following administration of specific vitamin supplements (pyridoxine, folate, or cobalamin). In classic homocystinuria, the levels of free homocystine in plasma increase and result in homocystinuria. Hyperhomocysteinemia refers to increased total plasma concentration of homocysteine and homocystine, free and protein-bound. Hyperhomocysteinemia in the absence of significant homocystinuria is found in heterozygotes and homozygotes for variant forms involving impaired folate or vitamin B_{12} metabolism and cystathionine synthase deficiency. Elevation of total plasma homocysteine is an independent risk factor for premature vascular disease.

CYSTATHIONINE β-SYNTHASE DEFICIENCY Definition Deficiency of this enzyme leads to increased concentrations of methionine and homocystine in body fluids and to decreased concentrations of cysteine and cystine. Clinical hallmarks include dislocation of optic lenses (usually downward and medially), mental retardation, marfanoid habitus, osteoporosis, and thrombotic vascular disease.

Etiology and Pathogenesis The sulfur atom of the essential amino acid methionine is transferred ultimately to cysteine by the transsulfuration pathway (Fig. 349-2). In one of these steps, homocysteine condenses with serine to form cystathionine. This reaction is catalyzed by the pyridoxal phosphate–dependent enzyme cystathionine β-synthase. The gene for this homodimeric enzyme has been mapped to chromosome 21q22.3. Heterogeneous mutations in this gene are present in different families. The G307S mutation is associated with lack of response to pyridoxine, while the I278T mutation correlates with pyridoxine-responsiveness and a milder clinical phenotype. Homocystinuria is relatively common in Ireland (1 in 60,000 births) but rare elsewhere (less than 1 in 200,000 births).

Homocysteine and methionine accumulate in cells and body fluids; cysteine synthesis is impaired, resulting in reduced concentrations of this amino acid and its disulfide form cystine. In approximately half of patients, synthase activity in liver, brain, leukocytes, and cultured fibroblasts is undetectable. In the remaining patients, tissues retain 1 to 5 percent of normal activity, and this residual activity often can be stimulated by pyridoxine supplementation. Heterozygosity for cystathionine β-synthase deficiency is a cause of hyperhomocyst(e)inemia, which increases the risk for thrombotic vascular disease.

Homocysteine interferes with the normal cross-linking of collagen, an effect that likely plays an important role in the ocular, skeletal, and vascular complications. Altered collagen in the suspensory ligament of

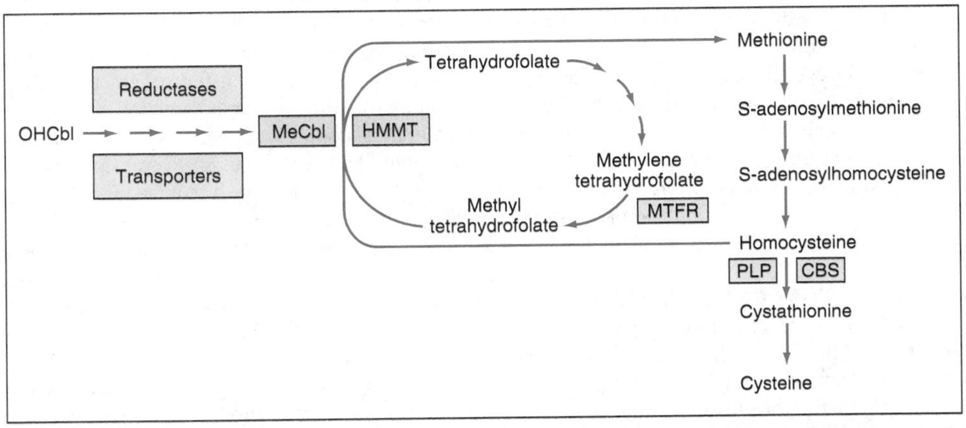

FIGURE 349-2 Pathways, enzymes, and coenzymes involved in the homocystinurias. Blocked-in symbols highlight specific moieties of particular etiologic or therapeutic significance to the various genetic defects underlying these disorders. Abbreviations: OHCbl, hydroxocobalamin (hydroxo B_{12}); MeCbl, methylcobalamin; MTFR, methylene tetrahydrofolate reductase; PLP, pyridoxal phosphate; CBS, cystathionine β-synthase.

the optic lens and in bone matrix may account for the dislocated lenses and osteoporosis. Similarly, interference with normal ground substance metabolism in vascular walls may predispose to the arterial and venous thrombotic diathesis. Increased platelet adhesiveness may result from homocysteine accumulation, thereby contributing to the thrombotic occlusive disease so often observed. Recurrent cerebrovascular accidents secondary to thrombotic disease may account for the mental retardation, but direct chemical effects on cerebral cell metabolism have not been excluded.

Clinical Manifestations More than 80 percent of homozygotes for complete cystathionine synthase deficiency develop dislocated optic lenses. This abnormality usually appears by 3 to 4 years of age and often results in glaucoma and impaired visual acuity. Mental retardation occurs in about half of such patients, often accompanied by ill-defined behavioral disturbances. Osteoporosis is a common radiologic finding (seen in two-thirds of patients by age 15) but rarely causes clinical disease. Life-threatening vascular complications, probably initiated by damage to vascular endothelium, are the major cause of morbidity and mortality. Occlusion of coronary, renal, and cerebral arteries with attendant tissue infarction can occur during the first decade of life. Nearly a fourth of patients die of vascular disease before age 30. These vascular complications seem to be exacerbated by angiographic procedures. Importantly, pyridoxine-responsive patients have milder clinical manifestations and may escape newborn screening and present with ectopia lentis or premature vascular occlusion. Heterozygous carriers for synthase deficiency (about 1 in 70 in the population) and others with high concentrations of plasma homocystine are at increased risk for premature coronary, peripheral, and cerebral vascular disease.

Diagnosis The cyanide-nitroprusside test is a simple way of demonstrating increased excretion of sulfhydryl-containing compounds in urine. The diagnosis is confirmed by measurement of free plasma methionine and homocystine. Plasma methionine tends to be increased in synthase-deficient patients and normal or low in those with other causes of homocystinuria and impaired methionine formation (see below). Diagnostic confirmation depends on measurements of cystathionine β-synthase activity in tissue extracts or cells cultured from patients. Heterozygotes can be identified by measurement of peak serum homocystine after an oral methionine load and by measurement of tissue synthase activity.

℞ TREATMENT

As with classic phenylketonuria, effective treatment depends on early diagnosis. A number of infants diagnosed in the newborn period have been treated successfully with methionine-restricted, cystine-supplemented diets. Their clinical course is benign compared with that of untreated affected siblings. In approximately half of patients, oral pyridoxine (25 to 500 mg/d) produces a fall in plasma and urinary methionine and homocystine and an increase in cystine concentration in body fluids. This effect probably reflects a modest increase in cystathionine β-synthase activity in cells of patients in whom the defect is characterized either by reduced affinity for cofactor or by accelerated degradation of mutant enzyme. Vitamin supplementation at these doses is apparently harmless and should be tried in all patients. There are no reports of the effect of the initiation of pyridoxine supplementation soon after birth. Similarly, there are no data regarding pyridoxine supplements in heterozygous carriers.

5,10-METHYLENETETRAHYDROFOLATE REDUCTASE DEFICIENCY **Definition** Hyperhomocysteinemia with normal or decreased methionine levels is caused by deficiency of 5,10-methylenetetrahydrofolate reductase, the enzyme involved in the synthesis of 5-methyltetrahydrofolate, a cofactor in the enzymatic formation of methionine from homocysteine (Fig. 349-2). CNS dysfunction and premature vascular occlusion may occur.

Etiology and Pathogenesis 5-Methyltetrahydrofolate:homocysteine methyltransferase catalyzes the conversion of homocysteine to methionine. The methyl group transferred in this reaction comes from 5-methyltetrahydrofolate, which is converted to tetrahydrofolate in the process. 5-Methyltetrahydrofolate, in turn, is synthesized enzymatically from 5,10-methylenetetrahydrofolate by 5,10-methylenetetrahydrofolate reductase. Thus reductase activity controls both methionine synthesis and tetrahydrofolate generation. This series of reactions is critical to normal DNA and RNA synthesis. A primary defect in the reductase activity results, secondarily, in deficient methyltransferase activity and impaired conversion of homocysteine to methionine. Methionine deficiency and impaired nucleic acid synthesis may contribute to the CNS dysfunction, while homocystine accumulation may predispose to thrombosis. The disorder appears to be inherited as an autosomal recessive trait. The gene for methylenetetrahydrofolate reductase maps to chromosome 1p36.3, and mutations have been identified in patients with hyperhomocysteinemia due to deficiency of this gene. A thermolabile variant form of this enzyme has reduced activity and may be a common cause of hyperhomocysteinemia associated with increased risk of vascular disease in young adults.

Clinical Manifestations More than 25 children with homocystinuria due to methylenetetrahydrofolate reductase deficiency have been reported. The most severely affected have developmental retardation and cerebral atrophy early in life. Others have behavioral disturbances (catatonia) during the second decade or mild retardation. The severity of the clinical manifestations reflects the severity of the reductase deficiency.

Diagnosis Increased concentrations of free homocystine in body fluids with normal or decreased concentrations of methionine should suggest severe methylenetetrahydrofolate reductase deficiency. Total plasma homocysteine levels slightly above the normal range suggest milder dysfunction of this enzyme. Serum folate concentrations are low in some patients. Confirmation requires direct assay of methylenetetrahydrofolate reductase in tissue extracts (brain, liver, cultured fibroblasts).

℞ TREATMENT

Therapeutic experience is limited. Folate, methionine, or betaine supplementation decreases urinary homocystine excretion and improves the clinical manifestations in some patients.

DEFICIENCY OF COBALAMIN (VITAMIN B_{12}) COENZYME SYNTHESIS **Definition** Five other forms of homocystinuria also reflect impaired conversion of homocysteine to methionine. The primary defects in these entities, however, are in the synthesis of methylcobalamin, a cobalamin (vitamin B_{12}) coenzyme required by methyltetrahydrofolate:homocysteine methyltransferase (see Fig. 349-2). In some, methylmalonic acid accumulates in body fluids because of impaired synthesis of a second coenzyme, adenosylcobalamin, required for isomerization of methylmalonyl coenzyme A (CoA) to succinyl CoA. These disorders are designated cblC, -D, -E, -F, and -G.

Etiology and Pathogenesis As with 5,10-methylenetetrahydrofolate reductase deficiency, each disorder impairs remethylation of homocysteine. Since methylcobalamin is required for methyl-group transfer from methyltetrahydrofolate to homocysteine, impaired cobalamin metabolism leads to deficient methyltransferase activity. The defects responsible for impaired synthesis of methylcobalamin involve one of several steps in lysosomal or cytosolic activation of the vitamin precursor (see Fig. 349-2). In the cblF disorder, the transport of cobalamins out of lysosomes is impaired. In cblC and -D, a reductase needed for formation of both methylcobalamin and adenosylcobalamin is deficient. In cblE and -G, some component required to maintain a reduced form of cobalamin on the methyltransferase apoenzyme is impaired. Somatic cell genetic studies indicate that each of these abnormalities is distinct and imply that all are inherited as autosomal recessive traits.

Clinical Manifestations More than 45 patients—mostly children—have been described. Although clinical manifestations vary, abnormalities include developmental delay, dementia, spasticity, megaloblastic anemia, and pancytopenia. It is not possible to define a specific clinical syndrome for each of the defects in cobalamin metabolism.

Diagnosis Homocystinuria, homocystinemia, and hypomethioninemia are the chemical hallmarks. Methylmalonic acidemia, too, has been noted in those defects resulting from defective synthesis of both cobalamin coenzymes. These findings also may be present in juvenile- or adult-onset pernicious anemia in which intestinal cobalamin absorption is impaired. Measurement of serum cobalamin concentrations, low in pernicious anemia and normal in patients with defective conversion of cobalamin vitamin to coenzymes, helps in the differential diagnosis. Definitive diagnosis depends on demonstrating impaired coenzyme synthesis in cultured cells.

℞ TREATMENT

Treatment of affected children with cobalamin supplements (1 to 2 mg/d) causes homocystine and methylmalonate excretion to fall to near normal values; the hematologic and neurologic deficits also improve to a variable degree in some patients. Intervention early in life seems to offer the best long-term prognosis.

ALKAPTONURIA

DEFINITION Alkaptonuria is a rare disorder of tyrosine catabolism in which deficiency of homogentisic acid oxidase leads to excretion of large amounts of homogentisic acid in urine and accumulation of oxidized homogentisic acid pigment in connective tissues (*ochronosis*). After many years, ochronosis produces a distinctive form of degenerative arthritis.

ETIOLOGY AND PATHOGENESIS Homogentisic acid is an intermediate in the catabolism of tyrosine. Activity of homogentisic acid oxidase, the enzyme that catalyzes the opening of the phenolic ring yielding maleylacetoacetic acid, is deficient in the liver and kidneys of patients with alkaptonuria, and homogentisic acid accumulates in cells and body fluids. The gene for this enzyme has been mapped to chromosome 3q2. Patients have minimally increased concentrations of homogentisic acid in blood because it is rapidly cleared by the kidney. The excretion of as much as 3 to 7 g of homogentisic acid in the urine per day is of little pathophysiologic significance. However, homogentisic acid and its oxidized polymers bind to collagen, leading to the progressive deposition of a gray to bluish-black pigment. The mechanism(s) by which this deposition causes degenerative changes in cartilage, intervertebral disks, and other connective tissues is unknown but may involve direct chemical irritation, impaired collagen cross-linking, disturbed articular chondrocyte metabolism, or some combination of factors.

Alkaptonuria was the first human disease shown to be inherited as an autosomal recessive trait. Affected homozygotes occur with a frequency around 1 in 200,000. Heterozygous carriers are clinically well and excrete no homogentisic acid in urine, even after loading doses of tyrosine.

CLINICAL MANIFESTATIONS Alkaptonuria may go unrecognized until middle life when degenerative joint disease develops. Prior to this time, the tendency of the patient's urine to darken on standing may go unnoticed, as may slight discoloration of the sclerae and ears. The latter manifestations are generally the earliest external evidence of the disorder and develop after age 20 to 30. Foci of gray-brown scleral pigment and generalized darkening of the concha, anthelix, and finally, helix of the ear are typical. Ear cartilages may be irregular and thickened. *Ochronotic arthritis* is heralded by pain, stiffness, and some limitation of motion of the hips, knees, and shoulders. Acute arthritis may resemble rheumatoid arthritis, but small joints are usually spared. Limitation of motion and ankylosis of the lumbosacral spine are common late manifestations. Pigmentation of heart valves, larynx, tympanic membranes, and skin occurs, and occasional patients develop pigmented renal or prostatic calculi. Degenerative cardiovascular disease may be increased in older patients.

DIAGNOSIS A patient whose urine darkens to blackness on standing must be suspected of having alkaptonuria but, because of modern plumbing conditions, this change is not often observed. The diagnosis is usually made from the triad of degenerative arthritis, ochronotic pigmentation, and urine that turns black upon alkalinization. Homogentisic acid in urine may be identified presumptively by other tests: upon addition of ferric chloride, a purple-black color is observed; treatment with Benedict's reagent yields a brown color; addition of a saturated silver nitrate solution produces an intermediate black color. These screening tests can be confirmed by chromatographic, enzymatic, or spectrophotometric determinations of homogentisic acid. X-rays of the lumbar spine are virtually pathognomonic. They show degeneration and dense calcification of the intervertebral disks and narrowing of the intervertebral spaces.

℞ TREATMENT

There is no specific treatment for ochronotic arthritis. Joint manifestations might be mitigated if homogentisic acid accumulation and deposition could be curbed by dietary restriction of phenylalanine and tyrosine, but the long-term course of the disease discourages such therapeutic attempts. Ascorbic acid impedes oxidation and polymerization of homogentisic acid in vitro, but the efficacy of this form of treatment has not been established. Symptomatic treatment is similar to that for osteoarthritis (Chap. 322).

CYSTINOSIS

DEFINITION Cystinosis is a rare disorder characterized by the intralysosomal accumulation of free cystine in body tissues. This results in the appearance of cystine crystals in the cornea, conjunctiva, bone marrow, lymph nodes, leukocytes, and internal organs. Three variants have been identified: an infantile (nephropathic) form leading to the Fanconi syndrome and renal insufficiency in the first decade, a juvenile (intermediate) form in which renal disease is manifest during the second decade, and an adult (benign) form characterized by deposition of cystine in the cornea but not in the kidney.

ETIOLOGY AND PATHOGENESIS The basic defect involves impaired efflux of cystine from lysosomes rather than an abnormality in cystine catabolism. Lysosomal cystine efflux is an active, ATP-dependent process. The cystine content of tissues may be more than 100 times normal in the infantile form and more than 30 times normal in the adult form. Intracellular cystine in lysosomes does not exchange with other intracellular or extracellular pools of this amino acid. Neither plasma nor urinary concentrations of cystine are particularly elevated.

The extent of crystal deposition varies from patient to patient, depending on the form of the disease and on the methods used to prepare pathologic specimens. Cystine accumulation in the kidney causes renal insufficiency in the infantile and juvenile forms. The kidneys are pale and shrunken, the capsule is adherent, and the corticomedullary junction is obscured. Microscopically, nephron organization is interrupted, glomeruli are hyalinized, connective tissue is increased, and the normal epithelium of the tubules is replaced by cuboidal cells. Narrowing and shortening of the proximal tubule produce the swan-neck deformity that is characteristic of but not specific for cystinosis. Patchy depigmentation and degeneration of the peripheral retina occur in the infantile and juvenile forms. Cystine crystals also may be deposited in the cornea, ocular conjunctiva, or uvea.

All types of the disorder are inherited as autosomal recessive traits. In 24 families with infantile and juvenile forms of cystinosis, the mutant gene was mapped to chromosome 17p. Obligate heterozygotes have intracellular cystine concentrations intermediate between those of normal persons and affected patients but are free of clinical abnormalities.

CLINICAL MANIFESTATIONS In the infantile form, abnormalities are usually apparent by 4 to 6 months of age. Growth retardation, vomiting, fever, vitamin D–resistant rickets, polyuria, dehydration, and metabolic acidosis are prominent. Generalized proximal tubular dysfunction (the Fanconi syndrome) leads to hyperphosphaturia and hypophosphatemia, renal glycosuria, generalized amino aciduria, hypouricemia, and often hypokalemia. Pyelonephritis may contribute, along with interstitial fibrosis, to progressive glomerular insufficiency. Death due to uremia or intercurrent infection usually occurs before age 10. Ocular manifestations are prominent. Photophobia is usually demonstrable within the first years of life due to cystine deposits in the cornea, and retinal degeneration may appear even earlier.

In contrast, patients with the adult form have only ocular abnormalities. Photophobia, headache, and burning or itching of the eyes are major complaints. Glomerular and tubular function and the integrity of the retina are preserved. The findings in the juvenile variant fall between these extremes. Ocular and renal manifestations do not become significant until the second decade. The renal lesion, albeit milder than that in the infantile form, eventually leads to renal insufficiency.

DIAGNOSIS Cystinosis must be considered in any child with vitamin D–resistant rickets, the Fanconi syndrome, or glomerular insufficiency. Hexagonal or rectangular cystine crystals can be detected in the cornea (by slit-lamp examination), in leukocytes from peripheral blood or bone marrow, or in biopsies of rectal mucosa. Diagnosis can be confirmed by quantification of cystine in peripheral blood leukocytes or cultured fibroblasts. The infantile form has been diagnosed prenatally by the demonstration of increased cystine content in cultured amniotic fluid cells.

℞ TREATMENT

The adult form is benign and requires no treatment. Treatment of renal disease in the infantile or juvenile form does not differ from that of other forms of chronic renal failure: maintenance of adequate fluid intake to prevent dehydration; correction of the metabolic acidosis; and administration of supplementary calcium, phosphate, and vitamin D to heal the rickets. Such measures are effective in maintaining growth, development, and well-being in affected children for a time. One specific therapy has been useful. Administration of the free thiol cysteamine slows the progression of renal dysfunction, improves growth, and dissolves corneal cystine crystals. This compound acts in lysosomes by forming a mixed disulfide with cysteine that can be transported out of the organelle by a different transporter than the one deficient in the disease. Although cysteamine causes a definite improvement during the first few years, gradual loss of kidney function continues.

Children with nephropathic cystinosis and end-stage renal disease benefit from kidney transplantation. Those patients who tolerated the procedure and do not develop immunologic problems have return of kidney function toward normal. The transplanted kidneys have not developed the functional abnormalities typical of cystinosis (i.e., the Fanconi syndrome or glomerular insufficiency). However, patients may continue to accumulate cystine in the cornea and other ocular tissues. Because the usual life span of a transplanted kidney is generally 15 to 20 years, some patients with the infantile form of cystinosis have received two or more transplanted kidneys.

PRIMARY HYPEROXALURIA

DEFINITION Primary hyperoxaluria is the designation for two rare disorders characterized by chronic excessive urinary excretion of oxalic acid and by calcium oxalate nephrolithiasis and nephrocalcinosis. Typically, patients with both forms develop renal insufficiency early in life and die of uremia. At postmortem examination, calcium oxalate deposits are widespread in renal and extrarenal tissues, a condition referred to as *oxalosis*.

ETIOLOGY AND PATHOGENESIS The metabolic basis for the primary hyperoxalurias involves pathways of glyoxylate metabolism. In type I hyperoxaluria, urinary excretion of oxalate and of the oxidized and reduced forms of glyoxylate is increased. The excessive synthesis of these substances results from a block in glyoxylate metabolism. The primary defect in most patients is deficiency of the hepatic peroxisomal enzyme alanine:glyoxylate amino transferase. The gene for this enzyme maps to chromosome 2q36→37, and several distinct mutations have been defined in patients with type I hyperoxaluria. Some of these mutations misdirect the enzyme to mitochondria and render it nonfunctional. Expansion of the glyoxylate pool leads to enhanced oxidation of glyoxylate to oxalate and to enhanced reduction of glyoxylate to glycolate. Each of these 2-carbon acids is then excreted in excess in the urine. In type II hyperoxaluria, L-glyceric acid is excreted in excess along with oxalate. In this condition, activity of D-glyceric acid dehydrogenase, which catalyzes the reduction of hydroxypyruvate to D-glyceric acid in the catabolic pathway of serine metabolism, is absent in leukocytes (and presumably other tissues). The accumulated hydroxypyruvate is instead reduced by lactic dehydrogenase to the L-isomer of glycerate, which is excreted in the urine. The same enzyme possesses glyoxylate reductase activity, and its deficiency promotes the oxidation of glyoxylate to oxalate, thus causing the formation of increased oxalate. Both disorders are inherited as autosomal recessive traits. Heterozygotes are asymptomatic.

Stone formation, nephrocalcinosis, and oxalosis are due to insolubility of calcium oxalate. Extrarenal deposits of oxalate are prominent in the heart, walls of arteries and veins, male urogenital tract, and bone, particularly in type I hyperoxaluria.

CLINICAL MANIFESTATIONS Nephrolithiasis and oxalosis may be manifest during the first year of life. Most patients experience renal colic or hematuria between ages 2 and 10 and succumb to uremia before age 20. With the onset of uremia, patients may develop severe peripheral arterial spasm and necrosis with resulting vascular insufficiency. Oxalate excretion falls as renal failure worsens. In patients with delayed onset of symptoms, survival to age 50 or 60 has been reported, despite recurrent nephrolithiasis. Type II hyperoxaluria is a milder disease with less involvement of extrarenal organs and delayed impairment of kidney function.

DIAGNOSIS Oxalate excretion in normal children or adults is less than 0.5 mmol (60 mg) per 1.73 m^2 surface area per day. Patients with type I or type II hyperoxaluria excrete two to four times this amount. Distinction between the two types depends on the identification of the other organic acids that identify them: glycolic acid in type I and L-glyceric acid in type II. Since patients with pyridoxine deficiency or chronic ileal disease may excrete excessive amounts of oxalate, these conditions must be excluded.

℞ TREATMENT

There is no satisfactory treatment. Urinary oxalate concentration can be transiently reduced by increasing the urinary flow rate. Large doses of pyridoxine (100 mg/d) may reduce urinary oxalate in some patients, but long-term effects are not dramatic. A diet high in phosphate content seems to reduce the frequency of renal colic, but oxalate excretion is unaffected. Combined liver-kidney transplantation can correct the enzyme deficiency and replace the damaged organs and warrants further study.

BIBLIOGRAPHY

Boushley CJ et al: A quantitative assessment of plasma homocysteine as a risk factor for vascular disease. Probable benefit of increasing folic acid intakes. JAMA 274:1049, 1995

Danpure CJ, Purdue PE: Primary hyperoxaluria, in *The Molecular and Metabolic Bases of Inherited Disease*, 7th ed, CR Scriver et al (eds). New York, McGraw-Hill, 1995, p 2385

Elsas LJ, Acosta PB: Nutritional support of inherited metabolic diseases, in *Modern Nutrition in Health and Disease*, 8th ed, ME Shils et al (eds). Philadelphia, Lea & Febiger, 1994, p 1147

Fenton WA, Rosenberg LE: Inherited disorders of cobalamin transport and metabolism, in *The Molecular and Metabolic Bases of Inherited Disease*, 7th ed, CR Scriver et al (eds). New York, McGraw-Hill, 1995, p 3129

Frosst P et al: A candidate genetic risk factor for vascular disease: A common mutation in methylenetetrahydrofolate reductase. Nature (Genetics) 10:111, 1995

Gahl WA et al: Lysosomal transport disorders: Cystinosis and sialic acid storage disorders, in *The Molecular and Metabolic Bases of Inherited Disease*, 7th ed, CR Scriver et al (eds). New York, McGraw-Hill, 1995, p 3763

La Du BN: Alkaptonuria, in *The Molecular and Metabolic Bases of Inherited Disease*, 7th ed, CR Scriver et al (eds). New York, McGraw-Hill, 1995, p 1371
Mudd SH et al: Disorders of transsulfuration, in *The Molecular and Metabolic Bases of Inherited Disease*, 7th ed, CR Scriver et al (eds). New York, McGraw-Hill, 1995, p 1279
Rosenberg LE, Scriver CR: Disorders of amino acid metabolism, in *Metabolic Control and Disease*, 8th ed, PK Bondy, LE Rosenberg (eds). Philadelphia, Saunders, 1980, p 583
Rosenblatt DS: Inherited disorders of folate transport and metabolism, in *The Molecular and Metabolic Bases of Inherited Disease*, 7th ed, CR Scriver et al (eds). New York, McGraw-Hill, 1995, p 3111
Scriver CR et al: The hyperphenylalaninemias, in *The Molecular and Metabolic Bases of Inherited Disease*, 7th ed, CR Scriver et al (eds). New York, McGraw-Hill, 1995, p 1015

350

Louis J. Elsas, Nicola Longo, Leon E. Rosenberg

INHERITED DEFECTS OF MEMBRANE TRANSPORT

The passage of many molecules across plasma cell membranes depends on transport systems that owe their specificity to membrane receptor and "carrier" proteins. These membrane constituents recognize individual molecules or structurally related substances and catalyze their transmembrane movement. The disorders considered in this chapter have three features in common: each is characterized by a specific defect in the transport of one or more compounds; each is inherited as a dominant or recessive trait, implying that variation in a single genetic locus is involved; and each is presumed to reflect a primary alteration in a specific membrane protein. Some of these defects have been well characterized physiologically and genetically, and the genes and/or cDNAs encoding several of these transporters have been identified.

More than 20 inherited disorders of membrane transport have been described (Table 350-1). Most affect the gut and/or kidney only. Classes of substrates represented include amino acids, sugars, cations, anions, vitamins, and water. Some are discussed elsewhere in this text. Those impairing the transport of amino acids, hexoses, urate, and chloride are discussed here as examples of the abnormalities encountered.

DISORDERS OF AMINO ACID TRANSPORT

As noted in Table 350-1, ten disorders of amino acid transport have been described. Five (cystinuria, dibasicaminoaciduria, Hartnup disease, iminoglycinuria, and dicarboxylicaminoaciduria) show transport abnormalities for structurally related amino acids, thereby implying the existence of group-specific membrane receptors or carriers. With the exception of iminoglycinuria and dicarboxylicaminoaciduria, the defects have important clinical consequences. The remaining five disorders affect the transport of only one amino acid, implying the existence of substrate-specific transport systems. Each of these conditions affects transport in the kidney, gut, or both; none has been shown to alter transport in other tissues.

CYSTINURIA Definition Cystinuria, the most common inborn error of amino acid transport, is characterized by impaired tubular reabsorption and excessive urinary excretion of the dibasic amino acids lysine, arginine, ornithine, and cystine. A similar transport defect exists in the intestinal mucosa. Because cystine is the least soluble of the naturally occurring amino acids, its overexcretion predisposes to the formation of renal, ureteral, and bladder stones. Such stones are responsible for the signs and symptoms of the disorder.

Etiology and Pathogenesis Massive excretion of cystine and the other dibasic amino acids occurs in homozygotes for classic cystinuria. The disorder, inherited as an autosomal recessive trait, results from impaired function of membrane carrier proteins essential for transport of this group of amino acids in the apical brush border of proximal renal tubule and small intestinal cells. Although the renal clearance of all four amino acids is increased in homozygotes, the presence of some residual transport capacity for these compounds plus the existence of three other disorders marked by selective excretion of members of this group (dibasicaminoaciduria, hypercystinuria, lysinuria) argues for the existence of at least three discrete renal transport systems for these amino acids: one for each amino acid alone; one shared by lysine, arginine, and ornithine; and one for all four amino acids.

Whereas urinary excretion patterns and renal clearance abnormalities in all homozygotes are similar, evidence for three variants has come from studies of intestinal transport in homozygotes and of urinary excretion in heterozygotes. Type I homozygotes lack mediated intestinal transport of cystine, lysine, arginine, and ornithine; heterozygotes have normal urinary amino acid excretion patterns. Type II homozygotes lack mediated lysine transport in the gut but retain some capacity for cystine transport; heterozygotes have moderately increased urinary excretion of each of the four amino acids. Type III homozygotes retain some capacity for mediated intestinal transport of the four involved substrates; heterozygotes have modestly increased urinary lysine and cystine. The gene for type I cystinuria, solute carrier family 3 (SLC3A1), has been mapped to 2p16.3. Heterogeneous mutations in this gene cause the type I disorder. Some of the mutations virtually abolish cystine transport when the mutant cDNAs are expressed in reporter cells.

Clinical Manifestations Cystinuria is among the most common inborn errors, with a frequency of 1 in 10,000 to 1 in 15,000 in many ethnic groups. Two-thirds of adults with cystinuria are type I homozygotes. Cystine stones account for 1 to 2 percent of all urinary tract calculi but are the most common cause of stones in children. The maximum solubility of cystine in the physiologic urinary pH range of 4.5 to 7.0 is about 1200 μmol/L (300 mg/L). Since affected homozygotes regularly excrete 2400 to 7200 μmol (600 to 1800 mg) daily, crystalluria and stone formation are a constant threat. Stone formation usually becomes manifest in the second or third decade but may occur in the first year of life or as bladder calculi in the newborn. Symptoms and signs are those typical of urolithiasis: hematuria, flank pain, renal colic, obstructive uropathy, and infection (see Chap. 279). Recurrent urolithiasis may lead to progressive renal insufficiency.

Diagnosis The presence of cystine in a urinary tract stone is pathognomonic of cystinuria. However, since half the stones in cystinuric subjects are of mixed composition and since as many as 10 percent may have a cystine core that is not detected, a urinary nitroprusside test should be done on all patients with urolithiasis to exclude this diagnosis. The nitroprusside test is also positive (appearance of a cherry red color) in some heterozygotes for cystinuria and in patients with hypercystinuria, homocystinuria, and mercaptolactate-cystine disulfiduria. When cystine content exceeds 1000 μmol/L (250 mg/L), cystine crystals may be seen in the sediment of acidified, concentrated, chilled urine. These hexagonal crystals are pathognomonic of cystine overexcretion in patients not taking sulfonamides.

Diagnostic confirmation of cystinuria depends on demonstration of the characteristic amino acid excretion pattern in the urine. Selective overexcretion of cystine, lysine, arginine, and ornithine can be demonstrated by qualitative and quantitative chromatography. Quantitation is important for differentiating some heterozygotes from homozygotes and for following free cystine excretion during therapy.

Rx TREATMENT

Management is aimed at preventing cystine crystal formation by reducing the concentration of cystine in urine. This aim is accomplished by increasing urinary volume and by maintaining an alkaline urine pH. Fluid ingestion in excess of 4 L/d is essential, and 5 to 7 L/d is optimal. Urinary cystine concentration should be less than 1000 to 1200 μmol/L (250 to 300 mg/L). The daily fluid ingestion necessary to maintain this dilution of excreted cystine should be

Table 350-1

Genetic Disorders of Membrane Transport

Class of Substance and Disorder	Individual Substrates	Tissues Manifesting Transport Defect	Proposed Molecular Basis of Defect	Major Clinical Manifestations	Mode of Inheritance	Location of Discussion
AMINO ACIDS						
Classic cystinuria	Cystine, lysine, arginine, ornithine	Proximal renal tubule, jejunal mucosa	Mutation of shared dibasic-cystine transport protein	Cystine nephrolithiasis	Autosomal recessive	Chap. 350
Dibasicamino-aciduria	Lysine, arginine, ornithine	Proximal renal tubule, jejunal mucosa	Mutation of dibasic transport protein	Type I: Benign Type II: Protein intolerance, hyperammonemia, retardation	Autosomal recessive	Chap. 350
Hypercystinuria	Cystine	Proximal renal tubule	Mutation of cystine transport protein	Some risk of cystine nephrolithiasis	Autosomal recessive	Chap. 350
Lysinuria	Lysine	Proximal renal tubule, jejunal mucosa	Mutation of lysine transport protein	Seizures, physical and mental retardation	Possible autosomal recessive	Chap. 350
Hartnup disease	Neutral amino acids	Proximal renal tubule, jejunal mucosa	Mutation of shared neutral amino acid transport protein	Constant neutral aminoaciduria, intermittent symptoms of pellagra	Autosomal recessive	Chap. 350
Tryptophan malabsorption	Tryptophan	Jejunal mucosa	Mutation of tryptophan transport protein	Indoluria, ?hypercalcemia, ?nephrocalcinosis	Probable autosomal recessive	Chap. 350
Methionine malabsorption	Methionine	Jejunal mucosa	Mutation of methionine transport protein	α-Hydroxybutyricaciduria, white hair, mental retardation, convulsions, hyperpneic attacks, edema	Probable autosomal recessive	Chap. 350
Histidinuria	Histidine	Proximal renal tubule, jejunal mucosa	Mutation of histidine transport protein	Mental retardation	Autosomal recessive	Chap. 350
Iminoglycinuria	Glycine, proline, hydroxyproline	Proximal renal tubule, jejunal mucosa	Mutation of shared glycine–imino acid transport protein	None	Autosomal recessive	Chap. 350
Dicarboxylic-aminoaciduria	Glutamic acid, aspartic acid	Proximal renal tubule, jejunal mucosa	Mutation of shared dicarboxylic amino acid transport protein	None	Probable autosomal recessive	Chap. 350
Cystinosis	Cystine	Lysosomal membranes	Mutation of cystine transport protein	Renal failure, hypothyroidism, blindness	Autosomal recessive	Chap. 349
HEXOSES						
Renal glycosuria	D-Glucose	Proximal renal tubule	Mutation of D-glucose transport protein	Glycosuria with normal blood glucose	Autosomal recessive	Chap. 350
Glucose-galactose malabsorption	D-Glucose D-Galactose	Jejunal mucosa, proximal renal tubule	Mutation of shared Na^+-dependent glucose-galactose transport protein	Watery diarrhea on feeding glucose, lactose, sucrose, or galactose	Autosomal recessive	Chaps. 285, 350
LIPIDS						
Familial hypercholesterolemia	Cholesterol	Fibroblasts, lymphoid lines, leukocytes	Mutation of membrane LDL–cholesterol receptor protein	Hypercholesterolemia, tendon xanthomas, arcus corneae, coronary artery atherosclerosis	Autosomal dominant	Chap. 341
URATE						
Hypouricemia	Uric acid	Proximal renal tubule	Mutation of urate transport protein	Hypouricemia, hyperuricosuria, ?hypercalcinuria	Autosomal recessive	Chap. 350

(continued)

Table 350-1—*(Continued)*

Genetic Disorders of Membrane Transport

Class of Substance and Disorder	Individual Substrates	Tissues Manifesting Transport Defect	Proposed Molecular Basis of Defect	Major Clinical Manifestations	Mode of Inheritance	Location of Discussion
ANIONS						
Familial hypophosphatemic rickets	Inorganic phosphate	Proximal renal tubule, jejunal mucosa	Mutation of inorganic phosphate transport protein	Hypophosphatemia, phosphaturia, phosphatopenic rickets/osteomalacia	X-linked dominant	Chap. 355
Congenital chloridorrhea	Chloride	Ileal and colonic mucosa	Mutation of Cl^-/H^+ uptake pump of Cl^-/HCO_3 exchange pump carrier protein	Hydramnios, watery diarrhea, elevated fecal chloride, achloriduria, metabolic alkalosis with volume depletion, hyperaldosteronism	Autosomal recessive	Chaps. 285, 350
Cystic fibrosis	Chloride	Lung, pancreas, sweat gland	Mutation of ion channel protein	Pulmonary, pancreatic destruction	Autosomal recessive	Chap. 257
Familial goiter	Inorganic iodide	Thyroid gland, salivary gland, gastric mucosa	Mutation of iodide transport protein	Congenital hypothyroidism (cretinism), goiter	Probable autosomal recessive	Chap. 331
CATIONS						
Distal renal tubular acidosis (type I—gradient)	Hydrogen ion	Distal renal tubule	Mutation of distal tubule H^+ pump carrier protein	Hyperchloremic acidosis, hypokalemia, acquired nephrocalcinosis, and hypercalcinuria	Autosomal dominant	Chap. 278
Proximal renal tubular acidosis (type II—HCO_3^- wasting)	Hydrogen ion	Proximal renal tubule	Mutation of proximal tubule H^+ pump carrier protein	Hyperchloremic acidosis, bicarbonate wasting	Probable autosomal recessive	Chap. 278
Menkes' disease	Copper	Most tissues except liver	Mutation of copper-transporting ATPase (ATP7B)	Severe mental retardation, pili torti (kinky hair), typical facies, arterial tortuosity, excess Wormian bones, thermal instability	X-linked recessive	Chap. 80
Wilson's disease	Copper	Liver and kidney	Mutation in copper-transporting ATPase (ATP7B)	Motor and psychiatric disturbances, hepatolenticular degeneration	Autosomal recessive	Chap. 345
Lethal diarrhea	Sodium ion	Jejunal intestinal cells	Mutation of Na^+/H^+ proton exchange pump	Watery diarrhea, severe sodium depletion, and acidosis	Recessive?	Chap. 285
WATER						
Nephrogenic diabetes insipidus (AVP-resistant)	Water	Distal renal tubule	Lack of activation of AVP-responsive luminal membrane adenylate cyclase, possible defect in receptor or enzyme protein	Polyuria, polydipsia, hyposthenuria	X-linked recessive	Chap. 278
VITAMINS						
Juvenile pernicious anemia	Cobalamin (vitamin B_{12})	Ileal mucosa	Mutation of receptor for intrinsic factor–cobalamin complex	Megaloblastic anemia	Autosomal recessive	Chap. 108
Folate malabsorption	Folic acid	Small bowel	Mutation of folate transport protein	Megaloblastic anemia	Autosomal recessive	Chap. 108
OTHER						
Sialic acid storage	Sialic acid (monosaccharide)	Lysosomes	Mutation of sialic acid transport protein	Retardation	Autosomal recessive	Chap. 346
Carnitine transport	Carnitine	Muscle, kidney leukocytes, fibroblasts	Mutation of high-affinity carnitine transporter	Hypoketotic hypoglycemia, cardiomyopathy, hypotonia	Autosomal recessive	Chap. 335

spaced over 24 h, with one-third of the total volume ingested between bedtime and 2 to 3 A.M. Stones can be prevented and even dissolved by such hydration. It must be made clear to cystinuric subjects that for them water is a necessary drug. Solubility of cystine rises sharply in urine above pH 7.5, and urinary alkalinization can be therapeutic in some situations. Vigorous administration of sodium bicarbonate, acetazolamide, and polycitrates is required to maintain a persistently alkaline pH, but this measure introduces the danger of inducing formation of calcium oxalate, calcium phosphate, and magnesium ammonium phosphate stones and of producing nephrocalcinosis.

Another treatment involves administration of penicillamine, which undergoes sulfhydryl-disulfide exchange with cystine to form the mixed disulfide of penicillamine and cysteine. Since this disulfide is more than 50 times as soluble as cystine, penicillamine (in doses of 1 to 3 g/d) reduces free cystine excretion markedly, thereby preventing new stone formation and promoting dissolution of existing calculi. Unfortunately, side effects include acute serum sickness, agranulocytosis, pancytopenia, immune glomerulitis, and the Goodpasture syndrome. Thus its use should be reserved for patients who fail to respond to hydration alone or who are in a high-risk category (one remaining kidney, renal insufficiency). Those patients unable to tolerate penicillamine may benefit from α-mercaptopropionylglycine, an experimental drug whose mechanism of action is similar to that of penicillamine but whose structure, and hence toxicity, is different. As many as two-thirds of patients unable to tolerate penicillamine may take α-mercaptopropionylglycine without ill effects. Captopril, a sulfhydryl-containing antihypertensive agent, is ineffective in reducing cystine excretion. When medical management fails, urologic surgery is required but should be considered a last resort since cystine stones reform more easily in scarred epithelium. Lithotripsy is not useful and may produce smaller fragments that cause severe colic. Occasional patients may require renal transplantation.

DIBASICAMINOACIDURIA This disorder is characterized by a defect in renal tubular reabsorption of lysine, arginine, and ornithine but *not* of cystine. The disorder almost surely reflects mutations in the gene(s) coding for a widely distributed transport protein used solely by the three dibasic amino acids. Two variants are each apparently inherited as an autosomal recessive trait. Manifestations are related to the losses of ornithine, arginine, and perhaps lysine.

In the common form of dibasicaminoaciduria (type II), also known as *lysinuric protein intolerance* and more common in Finland (1 in 60,000) than elsewhere, homozygotes show defective intestinal transport of dibasic amino acids as well as exaggerated renal losses. The transport defect affects basolateral rather than luminal membrane transport and is associated with impairment of the urea cycle. Affected individuals present in childhood with hepatosplenomegaly, protein intolerance, and episodic ammonia intoxication. Older subjects may present with severe osteoporosis, impairment of kidney function, or interstitial changes in the lungs. Plasma concentrations of lysine, arginine, and ornithine are reduced, and urinary excretion of lysine is increased. Hyperammonemia may develop after the ingestion of protein loads or with infections and is believed to be due to insufficient amounts of arginine and ornithine to maintain proper function of the urea cycle. The clinical features have been attributed to the hyperammonemia and to insufficient amounts of lysine to support synthesis of protein and carnitine during growth. Obligate heterozygotes are healthy and show no excess urinary loss of dibasic amino acids.

Type I dibasicaminoaciduria has been described in a large French-Canadian kindred. These patients have profound mental retardation without hyperammonemia or protein intolerance. The condition also differs from type II by the presence of modest excesses of dibasic amino acids in urine of asymptomatic heterozygotes. Type I disease may involve the same transport system as that impaired in the more common type II disorder.

℞ TREATMENT

Treatment includes dietary protein restriction and supplementation with citrulline, a neutral amino acid whose intestinal and hepatic transport are unimpaired, and which, when metabolized to arginine and ornithine, fuels the urea cycle. With 2.0 to 8.0 g of oral citrulline daily, dietary protein intake can be increased and growth improved in children. Carnitine supplements may improve growth by sparing lysine and by enhancing fatty acid oxidation.

HARTNUP DISEASE Pellagra-like skin lesions, variable neurologic manifestations, and neutral or aromatic aminoaciduria characterize this disease. Alanine, serine, threonine, valine, leucine, isoleucine, phenylalanine, tyrosine, tryptophan, glutamine, asparagine, and histidine are excreted in urine in quantities 5 to 10 times normal, and intestinal transport for these same amino acids is defective. The clinical manifestations result from nutritional deficiency of the essential amino acid tryptophan, caused by intestinal and renal malabsorption. Manifestations are episodic, related, at least in part, to metabolic demands for tryptophan. Only a small fraction of patients with the chemical findings of this disorder develop a pellagra-like syndrome, implying that manifestations depend on factors over and above the transport defect.

The major pathway of tryptophan metabolism leads to the synthesis of niacin and nicotinamide-adenine dinucleotide. This pathway supplies about half the daily niacin needs. In patients with Hartnup disease, the renal and intestinal transport defect for tryptophan leads to niacin deficiency. The transport defect likely reflects abnormalities of a group-specific system for neutral amino acids. Some residual reabsorptive capacity persists for each involved amino acid. This suggests that they are transported by other carrier systems as well, a conclusion supported by the identification of patients with substrate-specific transport errors for tryptophan, methionine, and histidine.

Hartnup disease is inherited as an autosomal recessive trait. Homozygotes occur with a frequency of about 1 in 24,000 births. Heterozygotes exhibit no clinical or chemical abnormalities.

Pellagra is the clinical syndrome produced by dietary niacin deficiency, and its features are those of Hartnup disease (see Chap. 79). The diagnosis of Hartnup disease should be suspected in any patient with pellagra without a history of dietary niacin deficiency. The neurologic and psychiatric manifestations range from attacks of cerebellar ataxia to mild emotional lability to frank delirium and usually accompany exacerbations of the erythematous, eczematoid skin rash. Fever, sunlight, stress, and sulfonamide therapy provoke clinical relapses. Diagnosis is made by detection of the neutral aminoaciduria that does not occur in dietary niacin deficiency. Treatment is directed at niacin repletion and includes a high-protein diet and daily nicotinamide supplementation (50 to 250 mg). Tryptophan ethyl esters also can bypass the absorption defect.

IMINOGLYCINURIA This benign autosomal recessive trait is characterized by excessive urinary excretion of glycine and the imino acids proline and hydroxyproline. Homozygotes occur with a frequency of about 1 in 16,000. The enhanced excretion of glycine, proline, and hydroxyproline reflects a defect in the tubular transport system shared by these three compounds. An intestinal transport defect also may be present. This suggests that more than one mutation may lead to iminoglycinuria, a thesis corroborated by the demonstration that obligate heterozygotes from some but not all families have glycinuria. No consistent clinical abnormalities have been reported in homozygotes, who are usually detected by urinary amino acid screening programs.

DICARBOXYLICAMINOACIDURIA Selective urinary loss and exaggerated endogenous renal clearance of glutamic and aspartic acids have been described in two unrelated children. Intestinal absorption of these dicarboxylic amino acids was impaired in one. This child had recurrent hypoglycemia; the other was asymptomatic.

SUBSTRATE-SPECIFIC DEFECTS IN AMINO ACID TRANSPORT Rare pedigrees exist in which individuals have defective renal tubular reabsorption and/or impaired intestinal absorption of a single free amino acid. These disorders, each apparently inherited as an autosomal recessive trait, suggest that transport of amino acids is catalyzed by substrate-specific as well as group-specific transport mechanisms.

Hypercystinuria Two siblings exhibited modest cystinuria without excessive urinary excretion of lysine, arginine, or ornithine. Fractional tubular reabsorption of cystine was reduced to about 80 percent of the filtered load, and up to 250 mg/d was excreted in the urine. Intestinal absorption of cystine was normal. Both were clinically well, although the cystine excretion places them at risk for cystine urolithiasis. Cystine excretion by the parents was normal.

Lysinuria A child with selective impairment of renal tubular reabsorption of lysine has been described. Endogenous lysine clearance was increased; intestinal transport was impaired; plasma lysine was reduced. Mental and growth retardation and seizures were present. A lysine-supplemented diet stimulated growth. Carnitine requires lysine for biosynthesis and may be deficient in this condition.

Histidinuria Two siblings, each with mental retardation, exhibited a selective renal transport defect for histidine. Urinary loss of histidine approached 40 to 50 percent of the filtered load, and intestinal transport of histidine also was defective. The clinically normal parents had normal urinary excretion but a modest defect in intestinal absorption of histidine. In two additional cases of isolated histidinuria myoclonic seizures occurred.

Methionine Malabsorption Children from two pedigrees have shown an intestinal transport defect for methionine. One may have had a renal transport defect as well. This disorder was detected because of urinary excretion of α-hydroxybutyric acid, a by-product of the intestinal bacterial breakdown of the unabsorbed methionine. This compound, which gives an odor resembling malt or dried celery to the urine, appears to be responsible for the white hair, attacks of hyperpnea, convulsions, edema, and mental retardation. Treatment of one of these children with a methionine-restricted diet caused improvement in all clinical manifestations. Transient methioninuria in early childhood has been associated with colic that improved with dietary methionine restriction.

Tryptophan Malabsorption An isolated defect in intestinal absorption of tryptophan has been described in two siblings. The renal tubular reabsorption of tryptophan was normal. A number of indoles were excreted in stool and urine. These compounds result from chemical degradation of unabsorbed tryptophan by intestinal bacteria and may be present in patients with Hartnup disease as well. Because of concomitant renal disease, hydrolytic enzymes were released into the urine, acted on the indoles found there, and led to the formation of a blue pigment, indigotin. This sequence of events earned this condition the sobriquet "blue-diaper syndrome." No pellagra-like symptoms were described. The mother also excreted indole compounds, suggesting that she is a carrier of this trait.

DISORDERS OF HEXOSE TRANSPORT

Nondiabetic melituria occurs in a number of conditions. Pentoses, hexoses, heptoses, and disaccharides have been identified in the urine; all except sucrose yield a positive test for reducing substances. Some meliturias result from diffuse renal injury, others from ingestion of nonmetabolizable sugars. In still others the sugars accumulate in blood owing to deficient activity of catabolizing enzyme systems and "spill" into the urine. Only among the hexoses have specific inherited disorders of sugar transport been identified. The existence of renal glycosuria and intestinal glucose-galactose malabsorption as heritable, autosomal recessive disorders points to the existence of at least two specific carrier proteins for hexoses in human jejunal and renal brush border membranes: one for glucose and one shared by glucose and galactose.

RENAL GLYCOSURIA Renal glycosuria is characterized by the urinary excretion of glucose at normal concentrations of blood glucose. The renal tubular malabsorption is specific for glucose. Unlike generalized tubular dysfunction, other compounds such as phosphate and amino acids are transported normally. The condition is benign, but occasionally glycosuria may be great enough to cause polyuria and polydipsia. Even more rarely, dehydration or ketosis may develop under conditions of stress such as pregnancy or starvation.

In normal persons, glucose is present in the glomerular filtrate at a concentration equal to that in plasma water and is reabsorbed throughout the proximal renal tubule by a sodium-dependent, phlorizin-inhibitable transport process. Reabsorptive capacity exceeds normal plasma glucose concentration. Thus glucose does not appear in the urine until the threshold for reabsorption is reached. The plasma concentration at which filtered glucose begins to escape proximal tubular reabsorption is usually around 10 mmol/L (200 mg/dL). Maximal renal reabsorptive capacity is exceeded at a filtered load of around 2 mmol (325 mg)/min per 1.73 m^2 body surface area, and this value is defined as the tubular maximum for glucose (TmG).

Two patterns of glycosuria are recognized: type A, characterized by a reduced tubular maximum reabsorptive capacity, and type B, showing a reduced threshold for glycosuria, an increased "splay" in the titration curve, and a normal TmG. Renal glycosuria occurs in homozygotes for either of these recessively inherited mutations and in compound heterozygotes for these presumably allelic mutations. Modest reduction in renal threshold or TmG is present in heterozygotes in some families; modest glycosuria occurs in such family members when plasma glucose is elevated. In the few patients studied, renal glycosuria was not associated with impaired intestinal transport.

GLUCOSE-GALACTOSE MALABSORPTION In this condition, infants develop a profuse, watery diarrhea when fed milk or foods containing lactose, sucrose, glucose, or galactose. Fructose or carbohydrate-free formulas are well tolerated. A specific defect in intestinal absorption of glucose and galactose can be demonstrated by oral tolerance tests that produce little or no increase in plasma glucose or galactose. The primary defect involves the sodium/hexose cotransporter in the intestinal and renal brush border. Active D-glucose and D-galactose transport is absent in affected children, and intermediate transport capacity is present in their parents. These findings confirm the specificity and the autosomal recessive inheritance of the disorder. Treatment with a glucose- and galactose-free diet leads to resolution of symptoms in childhood. Although the basic transport defect is present throughout life, most patients show an improved tolerance for glucose and galactose with age.

A number of these patients have renal glycosuria at normal plasma glucose concentrations. Renal titration studies generally demonstrate a reduced threshold for glucose reabsorption (type B renal glycosuria) and a normal TmG. Urinary glucose loss is not as severe as in isolated renal glycosuria. This finding suggests the presence of multiple glucose transport proteins in the kidney. One, whose gene remains to be identified, is responsible for the bulk of glucose reabsorption, is located in the proximal convoluted tubule, and is believed to be abnormal in renal glycosuria. Another (SGLT1) is shared by glucose and galactose and is responsible for the reabsorption of the last traces of glucose in the late proximal straight tubule. SGLT1 is abnormal in glucose-galactose malabsorption, and heterogeneous mutations have been demonstrated in the encoding gene on chromosome 22q. In glucose-galactose malabsorption, as in renal glycosuria, transport of sugars in other tissues is normal, reflecting the multiplicity and tissue specificity of hexose transporters.

DEFECTIVE URATE TRANSPORT: HYPOURICEMIA

Individuals with a selective defect in renal tubular reabsorption of sodium urate have marked hypouricemia with serum urate levels ranging from 12 to 110 μmol/L (0.2 to 1.8 mg/dL). Moderate uricosuria is present, and 25 percent of patients have renal calculi, which is the only known adverse manifestation of this condition.

Renal urate clearance normally averages 15 percent of glomerular filtration rate, and the excreted urate is composed both of filtered urate that has escaped reabsorption and of secreted urate. Subjects with isolated hypouricemia have urate clearances averaging from 33 to 85 percent of the filtration rate; in some, urate clearance exceeds the glomerular filtration rate. Studies with probenecid, which blocks tubular reabsorption of urate, and pyrazinamide, which blocks tubular secretion, reveal that 11 of the 16 families described have a presecretory urate reabsorptive defect, and 5 have defective transport affecting the entire tubule. In four families hypercalciuria due to enhanced intestinal calcium absorption is also present, but in others only uricosuria has been demonstrated. The defect is inherited as an autosomal recessive trait. Urate transport appears to be normal in nonrenal tissue. Obligate heterozygotes have moderately increased urate clearance. The defect is presumed to reflect mutation of one or both of the proximal renal tubular membrane proteins that transport sodium urate. The findings in these families support the hypothesis that renal urate reabsorption is controlled by more than one transport protein.

DEFECTIVE ANION TRANSPORT: CHLORIDORRHEA

This rare, autosomal recessive disease results from impairment of active transport of chloride in the ileum and colon. Absence of chloride-bicarbonate ion exchange causes profound symptoms even before birth (polyhydramnios and absence of meconium). Massive watery diarrhea is apparent from the first days of life. This fluid loss, with its attendant impairment of electrolyte homeostasis, is life-threatening. A hypokalemic, hypochloremic, hyponatremic metabolic alkalosis develops with dehydration and secondary hyperaldosteronism. Fecal fluid contains an excess of chloride ion over the sum of the accompanying cations sodium and potassium. Fecal chloride concentration always exceeds 90 mmol/L when volume and serum electrolyte disturbances are corrected, and this chloridorrhea is diagnostic. Renal chloride transport is normal. Decreased urine chloride results from the kidney's attempts to conserve salt and water. The gene for this condition maps to chromosome 7q and is distinct from the gene that is mutated in cystic fibrosis.

℞ TREATMENT

Treatment requires adequate, lifelong repletion of electrolyte and fluid losses. Exact replacement of water, sodium chloride, and potassium chloride can prevent the growth and psychomotor retardation and the development of progressive renal damage. The renal lesion, with hyalinized glomeruli, juxtaglomerular hyperplasia, calcifications, and arteriolar changes, is probably a result of chronic volume depletion. Treatment of hyperreninemia and hypokalemia with prostaglandin inhibitors may reduce renal damage but does not alter intestinal symptoms or the need for chronic sodium chloride repletion.

BIBLIOGRAPHY

Desjeux JF: Congenital selective Na^+ D-glucose cotransport defects leading to renal glycosuria and congenital selective intestinal malabsorption of glucose and galactose, in *The Molecular and Metabolic Bases of Inherited Disease*, 7th ed, CR Scriver et al (eds). New York, McGraw-Hill, 1995, p 3563

Elsas LJ, Rosenberg LE: Renal glycosuria, in *Strauss and Welt's Diseases of the Kidney*, 3d ed, LE Earley, CW Gottschalk (eds). Boston, Little, Brown, 1979, pp 1021–1028

———, Longo N: Glucose transporters: Human disorders and insulin receptor regulation. Int Pediatr 10:57,1995

Gasparini P et al: Molecular genetics of cystinuria: Identification of four new mutations and seven polymorphisms and evidence for genetic heterogeneity. Am J Hum Genet 57:781, 1995

Levy HL: Hartnup disorder, in *The Molecular and Metabolic Bases of Inherited Disease*, 7th ed, CR Scriver et al (eds). New York, McGraw-Hill, 1995, p 3629

Segal S, Thier SO: Cystinuria, in *The Molecular and Metabolic Bases of Inherited Disease*, 7th ed, CR Scriver et al (eds). New York, McGraw-Hill, 1995, p 3581

Short EM, Rosenberg LE: Renal aminoaciduria, in *Strauss and Welt's Diseases of the Kidney*, 3d ed, LE Earley, CW Gottschalk (eds). Boston, Little, Brown, 1979, pp 975–1020

Simell O: Lysinuric protein intolerance and other cationic aminoacidurias, in *The Molecular and Metabolic Bases of Inherited Disease*, 7th ed, CR Scriver et al (eds). New York, McGraw-Hill, 1995, p 3603

Sperling O: Hereditary renal hypouricemia, in *The Molecular and Metabolic Bases of Inherited Disease*, 7th ed, CR Scriver et al (eds). New York, McGraw-Hill, 1995, p 3747

351

Kurt J. Isselbacher

GALACTOSEMIA, GALACTOKINASE DEFICIENCY, AND OTHER RARE DISORDERS OF CARBOHYDRATE METABOLISM

DEFINITION *Galactosemia* refers to any of three inborn errors of galactose metabolism. *Classic galactosemia* is due to the deficiency of galactose-1-phosphate uridyl transferase (GALT) and is typically associated with cataract formation, mental retardation, and cirrhosis. The second disorder, *galactokinase deficiency*, leads primarily to cataract formation. The third, *UDP-galactose-4-epimerase deficiency*, is the rarest of the group; few cases have been described, and the eventual outcome is uncertain.

PATHOGENESIS Lactose, the main carbohydrate in milk, is a disaccharide containing galactose and glucose; when ingested, it is hydrolyzed by intestinal lactase. Normally, the absorbed galactose is converted to glucose in the liver. The first reaction in this pathway is the phosphorylation of galactose to galactose-1-phosphate by galactokinase (specified by a gene on chromosome 17):

$$\text{Galactose} + \text{ATP} \xrightarrow{\text{galactokinase}} \text{galactose-1-phosphate}$$

The next step involves the conversion of galactose-1-phosphate to glucose-1-phosphate by GALT (the gene for which is on chromosome 9):

$$\text{Galactose-1-phosphate} + \text{UDP-glucose}$$

$$\xrightarrow{\text{GALT}} \text{UDP-galactose} + \text{glucose-1-phosphate}$$

The uridine diphosphate (UDP) sugars can be reversibly interconverted by an epimerase reaction (UDP-galactose-4-epimerase):

$$\text{UDP-galactose} \rightleftharpoons \text{UDP-glucose}$$

Galactose also can be metabolized by alternative pathways. It can be converted (reduced) in the presence of NADPH (or NADH) to galactitol (dulcitol) by aldose reductase. It also can be oxidized to a limited extent by galactose dehydrogenase, leading to the formation of galactonic acid, xyulose, and CO_2. These pathways account for limited galactose metabolism in patients with galactosemia.

In galactokinase deficiency, galactose accumulates in the blood and tissues. In the lens, galactose is converted by aldose reductase to galactitol, a sugar to which the lens is impermeable. As a consequence, excessive hydration occurs which, together with a decrease in glutathione in the lens, leads to cataract formation.

In classic galactosemia, GALT deficiency results in tissue accumulation of galactose-1-phosphate and galactose. As in galactokinase deficiency, cataracts develop secondary to galactitol accumulation in the lens. It is assumed that the cirrhosis and mental retardation of classic galactosemia are related to increased amounts of galactose-1-phosphate in these tissues. Elevated blood galactose levels may lead to a decreased hepatic output of glucose and hence to hypoglycemia. In the kidney and intestine, accumulation of galactose and galactose-1-phosphate appears to lead to an inhibition of amino acid transport. In female homozygotes there is an increased incidence of hypergonadotrophic hypogonadism in which ovarian failure develops at an early age, and this complication may persist despite dietary therapy.

Both galactokinase and GALT deficiencies are transmitted as autosomal recessive traits. Heterozygotes for these disorders have half-normal enzyme levels but are asymptomatic. Maternal deficiency of galactokinase, together with lactose intake during pregnancy, may contribute to cataract formation during fetal development. However, not all persons with decreased GALT enzyme activity in their cells are carriers of classic galactosemia. GALT is a polymorphic enzyme, and the most common variant, called the *Duarte variant* (D), has reduced activity. In addition, the D allele has numerous isoforms.

The most common mutation of the GALT gene that causes classic galactosemia is the Q188R substitution (G); the homozygous form of this disorder (GG) has a frequency of about 1 per 40,000 births in the white population. The Duarte phenotypes (D/N, D/D, and D/G) have approximately 75, 50, and 25 percent of normal GALT activity, respectively, and occur with an overall prevalence of about 6 percent in whites. Such individuals are clinically asymptomatic.

CLINICAL FEATURES Symptoms of classic galactosemia usually begin within days to weeks after birth. The infant usually is reluctant to ingest breast milk or milk formulas, develops vomiting, shows poor nutrition, and fails to thrive. Jaundice, hepatomegaly, and evidence of liver disease may develop. Cataracts are usually not present at birth but develop gradually over weeks to months. Mental retardation becomes evident after 6 to 12 months and is usually not reversible. Infants with classic galactosemia are subject to bacterial sepsis (especially with *Escherichia coli*), and this may be the leading cause of death in the neonatal period. The only consistent feature of galactokinase deficiency is cataract formation.

DIAGNOSIS Galactokinase deficiency should be suspected in infants or children with cataract formation who have non-glucose-reducing substances in the urine. The diagnosis is made by demonstrating the deficiency of galactokinase in red blood cells.

Classic galactosemia must be considered when one or more of the clinical features described above are found. If the patient is ingesting milk, reducing sugar is present in the urine but gives a negative glucose oxidase reaction (i.e., is not glucose) and is identified as galactose by other techniques, such as chromatography. If the child is vomiting, has a poor food intake, or is on intravenous glucose feedings, galactose may not be present in the urine. The definitive diagnosis is made by demonstrating a lack or deficiency of red cell GALT by one of several techniques. The disease also can be diagnosed prenatally by enzyme studies on cultured amniocentesis cells or by demonstrating increased galactitol in amniotic fluid. A nonenzymatic glycosylation of hemoglobin, analogous to that in diabetes mellitus, can be detected in patients with galactosemia as manifested by increased concentrations in the blood of Hb A_{lab} rather than Hb A_{lc}.

In the neonatal period galactosemia needs to be differentiated from primary liver disease. With liver damage, galactose removal from the blood is impaired, and elevated blood galactose levels and galactosuria may be present. However, GALT levels are normal in patients with liver damage.

℞ TREATMENT

The treatment of galactosemia consists of the removal of galactose-containing foods from the diet, especially milk. Milk substitutes such as Nutramigen are often used. Although soybean preparations contain polysaccharide-bound galactose, they appear to be well tolerated because the bound galactose is not readily liberated. In general, the red cell levels of galactose-1-phosphate are not increased in affected infants fed soybean formulas.

The institution of a galactose-free diet usually leads to a dramatic improvement in all clinical features except for mental retardation. Patients should be kept on galactose-free diets indefinitely or at least until they have attained adequate physical and neurologic development.

OTHER DISORDERS OF CARBOHYDRATE METABOLISM Features of hereditary fructose intolerance and fructose-1,6-diphosphatase deficiency, two autosomal recessive disorders of fructose metabolism that lead to hypoglycemia, are summarized in Table 351-1 (also see Chaps. 335 and 347).

Table 351-1

Some Other Disorders of Carbohydrate Metabolism

Metabolic Defect	Manifestations
HEREDITARY FRUCTOSE INTOLERANCE	
Deficiency of fructose-1-phosphate aldolase leads to accumulation of fructose-1-PO_4 in tissues.	Liver disease, renal tubular damage, and hypoglycemia.
FRUCTOSE-1,6-DIPHOSPHATASE DEFICIENCY	
Deficiency of the enzyme prevents gluconeogenesis from its normal precursors, lactate, glycerol, and alanine. Thus maintenance of blood sugar is dependent on exogenous glucose.	Lactic acidosis leads to hyperventilation, somnolence, and coma, usually with hypoglycemia and ketosis.

BIBLIOGRAPHY

BEUTLER E: Galactosemia: Screening and diagnosis. Clin Biochem 24:293, 1991

ELIAS LJ et al: A common mutation associated with the Duarte galactosemia allele. Am J Hum Genet 54:1030, 1994

GITZELMANN R et al: Disorders of fructose metabolism, in *The Metabolic and Molecular Bases of Inherited Disease*, 7th ed, CR Scriver et al (eds). New York, McGraw-Hill, 1995, p 905

KAUFMAN FR et al: Correlation of ovarian function with galactose-1-phosphate uridyl transferase levels in galactosemia. J Pediatr 112:754, 1988

NG WG et al: Biochemical and molecular studies of 132 patients with galactosemia. Hum Genet 94:359, 1994

REICHARDT JKV, WOO SLC: Molecular basis of galactosemia: Mutations and polymorphisms in the gene encoding human galactose-1-phosphate uridyltransferase. Proc Natl Acad Sci USA 88:2633, 1991

SEGAL S, BERRY GT: Disorders of galactose metabolism, in *The Metabolic and Molecular Bases of Inherited Disease*, 7th ed, CR Scriver et al (eds). New York, McGraw-Hill, 1995, p 967

WAGGONER D et al: Long-term prognosis in galactosemia: Results of a survey of 350 cases. J Inherited Metab Dis 13:802, 1990

352

Daniel W. Foster

THE LIPODYSTROPHIES AND OTHER RARE DISORDERS OF ADIPOSE TISSUE

This chapter is concerned with rare abnormalities in adipose tissue. In most instances, the pathophysiology is not clear.

THE LIPODYSTROPHIES

The lipodystrophies are characterized by generalized or partial loss of body fat and metabolic abnormalities, including insulin resistance, hyperglycemia, and hypertriglyceridemia. A classification is shown in Table 352-1. In *generalized lipodystrophy* essentially all body fat is lost, while in *partial lipodystrophy* fat atrophy is limited. The common acquired form of partial lipodystrophy ordinarily involves the upper half of the body, whereas dominantly transmitted partial lipodystrophy tends to spare the face. One variant is associated with eye and tooth malformations, the Rieger anomaly. *Localized lipodystrophy* may be either inflammatory or noninflammatory. The best-studied localized disorder is *centrifugal lipodystrophy*, in which fat atrophy begins in

Table 352-1

The Lipodystrophies

I. Generalized lipodystrophy	III. Localized lipodystrophy
A. Congenital (familial or sporadic)	A. Inflammatory
B. Acquired (sporadic)	B. Noninflammatory
II. Partial lipodystrophy	
A. Common (sporadic)	
B. Dominant (familial)	
1. Limb and trunk	
2. With Rieger anomaly	

the groins or axillae of children under the age of 3 and spreads centrally to involve the entire abdomen. Occasionally, the disorder begins outside the abdomen. The edge of the lesion is red and scaly, with an inflammatory infiltrate demonstrable on histologic examination. Fat atrophy usually disappears spontaneously by about 13 years of age.

GENERALIZED LIPODYSTROPHY Generalized lipodystrophy (also called *lipoatrophic diabetes*) may be either congenital or acquired. The congenital form is an autosomal recessive disorder that affects both sexes equally. Parental consanguinity is common. Loss of fat is usually obvious at birth, but other manifestations may not appear until later (up to 30 years). The acquired form often develops after some other illness such as measles, chicken pox, whooping cough, and infectious mononucleosis; hypothyroidism, hyperthyroidism, and pregnancy have also been implicated. Some cases begin with painful nodular swellings of adipose tissue that resemble acute panniculitis (see below). The manifestations of the congenital and acquired forms are similar (Table 352-2).

Fat Atrophy Loss of body fat is the central feature. In congenital cases the skin of the face is tightly drawn, and the entire body appears to be devoid of adipose tissue on physical examination. However, with whole-body magnetic resonance imaging (MRI) some fat can be demonstrated in the orbits, palms, soles, and juxtaarticular and epidural regions where the cushioning functions of adipose tissue are critical. Thus, mechanical (supportive or cushioning) fat is spared while metabolic fat disappears. In the acquired form the face may be spared. In atrophic areas adipocytes devoid of triglyceride stores can be identified microscopically. Paradoxically, the liver is engorged with fat, and the reticuloendothelial system contains lipid-laden macrophages (foam cells). The cause of the fat atrophy is not known. Fat-mobilizing polypeptides have been described in the urine of patients with generalized lipodystrophy, but their role in the disease is uncertain.

A candidate molecule for the induction of lipodystrophy would be a compound similar to tumor necrosis factor α (TNFα), a potent inhibitor of lipoprotein lipase that causes fat depletion and hypertriglyceridemia when injected into animals. Lipoprotein lipase activity is low in generalized lipodystrophy, as would be predicted if TNFα or a similar cytokine were the cause. However, plasma levels of TNF were normal in two of the author's patients. Hepatic lipase is not impaired. Since triglyceride content of the adipocyte is the result of a balance between fat synthesis and fat breakdown, an alternative mechanism might involve activation of the hormone-sensitive lipase that catalyzes hydrolysis of triglycerides in the fat cell. For example, a defect in a natural inhibitor of the lipase, such as adenosine, could enhance the response to normal levels of lipolytic hormones. Enhanced lipolysis also could be due to sympathetic nervous system activity. Release of free fatty acids into plasma following norepinephrine infusion is impaired, but this may simply reflect the depleted triglyceride stores.

A mutation or deletion of an adipocyte developmental gene might also be involved. For example, the transcription factor PPARγ2 (peroxisome proliferator activated receptor-γ2) can transform fibroblasts to fat cells in tissue culture and, if mutated, might thwart adipocyte development. In the acquired form, one would have to postulate another mechanism that could cause dedifferentiation of the adipocyte, perhaps the indirect consequence of a viral infection or other insult.

Growth and Maturation Linear growth is accelerated in the first few years of life in the congenital disorder and in acquired disease that begins early in childhood. Epiphyses close early, however, so that the final height is usually normal. Muscular hypertrophy is present, and patients may have an acromegalic appearance with coarse facial features and large hands and feet. The ears tend to be prominent in the congenital form. Many viscera are enlarged, and generalized lymphadenopathy may be present. The cause of the growth disorder is not known. Levels of growth hormone and insulin-like growth factor (IGF) I are normal or low. IGF-II has not been systematically assessed. Abnormal growth and pseudoacromegaly might be due to high concentrations of insulin in plasma secondary to insulin resistance (see below). Insulin binds to the IGF-I receptor and at high concentrations could cause acromegalic features by activating the IGF-I receptor.

Liver Fatty engorgement of the liver causes protuberance of the abdomen and may progress to cirrhosis, especially in the acquired disorder. Portal hypertension can cause splenomegaly and bleeding esophageal varices.

Kidneys The kidneys are usually enlarged. Subjects with the acquired disorder may have proteinuria and the nephrotic syndrome, although not as frequently as in partial lipodystrophy. Moderate hypertension is common.

Genitalia The external genitalia (penis and testes in males, clitoris and labia majora in females) are usually enlarged in children with the congenital disease. In women, polycystic ovaries can cause the clinical picture of Stein-Leventhal syndrome. The cause of the genital abnormalities is not known.

Skin Acanthosis nigricans is present in most. Hypertrichosis of face, neck, trunk, and limbs is frequent. Scalp hair is usually thick and curly, particularly early in life.

Central Nervous System Mental retardation is present in about half the congenital cases. It appears to be less common in the acquired form. Early studies suggesting that structural abnormalities are present in brain have not been confirmed by computed tomography (CT) and MRI studies.

Table 352-2

Characteristics of the Lipodystrophies

Feature	Congenital General	Acquired General	Acquired Partial	Dominant Partial
Inheritance	Autosomal recessive	Sporadic	Usually sporadic	Autosomal dominant
Age of onset	Infancy	Childhood to adult	Childhood to adult	Puberty
Sex incidence	Males and females equal	Female preponderance	Female preponderance	Female preponderance
Lipoatrophy	Face, trunk, limbs	Face, trunk, limbs	Face, upper trunk, upper limbs	Trunk and limbs
Liver involvement	+	+ +	Rare	0
Renal disease	+	+	+ +	0
Insulin resistance	+	+	+	+
Hyperglycemia	+	+	+	+
Hypertriglyceridemia	+	+	+	+
Acanthosis nigricans	+	+	Rare	+
Genital hypertrophy	+	+	Rare	+
Bone age	Accelerated	Normal to accelerated	Normal	Normal

Other Abnormalities Osteolytic lesions may cause bone cysts, and the skeleton occasionally appears sclerotic. Cystic bone lesions also occur in membranous lipodystrophy (Nasu disease), which is associated with presenile dementia; despite its name, membranous lipodystrophy is associated with fat necrosis and is actually a form of panniculitis (see below). Cardiomegaly is common but rarely leads to heart failure. Goiter is frequent. The associated abnormalities in generalized lipodystrophy are summarized in Table 352-3.

Metabolic and Endocrine Abnormalities Three major metabolic disturbances are characteristic.

1. *Insulin-resistant diabetes mellitus (lipoatrophic diabetes).* Insulin resistance may be mild or severe, and, when severe, the diabetes may be difficult to control. Insulin and C-peptide concentrations are relatively or absolutely elevated, and response to exogenous insulin is impaired. The cause of the insulin resistance is not known, but mutations in the insulin receptor gene have been excluded as a major factor. It is possible that elevated levels of free fatty acids may induce insulin resistance in muscle and fat and stimulate insulin secretion; increased free fatty acid turnover is believed to cause insulin resistance by impairing glucose transport into cells. Insulin in the plasma of affected individuals is biologically active. Although glucagon levels are high (indicating insulin resistance in the alpha cell of the islets of Langerhans) and free fatty acid concentrations are elevated, ketoacidosis is unusual.

True ketoacidosis may be infrequent because insulin resistance is less severe in liver and skeletal muscle than in adipose tissue. Glycogen levels in the liver are high (insulin stimulates glycogen synthesis), and levels of branched-chain amino acids fall normally in response to injected insulin. Elevated insulin levels in portal vein plasma would counteract the actions of glucagon in the insulin-responsive hepatocyte (see Chap. 335), prevent activation of ketone body synthesis in liver, and ensure utilization of fatty acids for triglyceride/very low density lipoproteins (VLDL) synthesis. The long-chain fatty acids in the plasma are of dietary origin and fall toward normal with restriction of dietary fat. Diabetes mellitus of lipodystrophy appears to be typical apart from insulin resistance, including a propensity to develop late degenerative complications. High levels of insulin in plasma and resistance to ketoacidosis distinguish this condition from type I (autoimmune) insulin-dependent diabetes mellitus, although both conditions begin in childhood or early adult life.

2. *Hypertriglyceridemia with accumulation of both chylomicrons and VLDL in the blood.* Eruptive xanthomas, lipemia retinalis, and recurrent pancreatitis may be seen. Although lipoprotein lipase is low and the disposal of triglycerides in the atrophied fat tissue is defective, the major cause for the hypertriglyceridemia is overproduction of VLDL in the liver, probably driven by the elevated free fatty acids in blood, since dietary fat restriction returns VLDL production rates toward normal. Hyperinsulinemia may contribute by enhancing hepatic fat synthesis.

3. *High metabolic rate despite normal thyroid function.* Basal metabolic rates are usually elevated, although thyroid function is normal. Patients do not gain weight with excessive caloric intake, indicating a facile capacity to waste calories as heat. Daily food intakes as high as 21,000 kJ (5000 kcal) are not unusual. One 16-month-old child ate 10,000 kJ (2400 kcal) daily. Following thyroidectomy in one patient, the basal metabolic rate decreased but did not return to normal; symptomatic hypothyroidism developed and required treatment with thyroid hormone despite continued high metabolic rates. It thus seems clear that hypermetabolism is not due to hyperthyroidism. There is also no evidence of mitochondrial defects. The most likely explanation for the increased metabolic rate is enhanced "futile" cycles with wastage of ATP, possibly due to increased sympathetic nervous system activity. Function of the adrenal medulla is normal.

Table 352-3

Accompanying Abnormalities of Lipodystrophy

Bone	Sclerosis, cystic angiomatosis
Brain	Mental retardation, third ventricle dilatation
Genitalia	Clitoromegaly, polycystic ovaries, penile hypertrophy
Heart	Cardiomegaly
Kidneys	Hypertrophy without renal failure
Liver	Hepatomegaly, fatty liver, cirrhosis, hepatic failure
Lymph nodes	Generalized lymphadenopathy
Skin	Acanthosis nigricans, hypertrichosis
Thyroid	Goiter, euthyroid state

Course Patients with generalized lipodystrophy may die at an early age from hepatic failure, hemorrhage from esophageal varices, renal failure, or recurrent pancreatitis. Despite longstanding hypertriglyceridemia, symptomatic coronary artery disease is rare.

℞ TREATMENT

There is no specific treatment for lipodystrophy, although dietary fat restriction is generally recommended. Medium-chain triglyceride supplementation has been reported to be of benefit. Because of insulin resistance, large amounts of insulin are often required to control the plasma glucose. Gemfibrozil is usually prescribed to lower triglycerides but is often ineffective. In patients with recurrent pancreatitis, nicotinic acid may lower triglycerides.

ACQUIRED PARTIAL LIPODYSTROPHY This is the most common of the lipodystrophies and usually affects women. The cause is unknown. Transplantation of tissue from atrophic areas to unaffected areas is said to restore the retention of triglycerides, whereas transplantation of normal tissue to atrophic areas causes atrophy of adipocytes, suggesting a local lesion as the cause of fat atrophy. Fat atrophy occurs in the upper half of the body, including the face, and spares the lower extremities. Rarely, the lower half of the body is affected, and the upper torso is intact. Occasionally, the lesion is unilateral. The anatomic features of generalized lipodystrophy are usually absent, and liver disease is unusual. Proteinuria, with or without the nephrotic syndrome, occurs more frequently than in other forms. The complement system is abnormal, and C3 levels tend to be low. C3 nephritic factor, a polyclonal IgG immunoglobulin that interacts with alternative pathway convertase (C3bBb) to augment C3 activation, is present in serum, and lupus erythematosus can develop after many years. In unaffected first-degree relatives C3 levels may be low, but C3 nephritic factor is not present. Complement abnormalities disappeared after renal transplantation in one subject. Dermatomyositis and Sjögren's syndrome may occur. Rarely, partial lipodystrophy progresses to the generalized form of the disease.

An unusual form of partial lipodystrophy is mandibuloacral dysplasia, a syndrome with typical features of lipodystrophy, including insulin resistance, hypermetabolism, and increased glucose production. Other features include hypoplasia of the mandibles and clavicles with lytic bone lesions, wrinkled skin, and joint contractures. Some patients have hypogonadism, short stature, and alopecia.

LIPODYSTROPHY WITH DOMINANT TRANSMISSION This variant is characterized by fat atrophy of the limbs and trunk and with sparing of the face, which may actually be rounded, and neck. The disease usually begins at puberty but may not appear until middle age. Males are rarely affected. In families with the Rieger anomaly, onset tends to be in infancy. Insulin resistance and hyperglycemia are usual, and severe hypertriglyceridemia may cause eruptive xanthomas. The labia majora are hypertrophied, and polycystic ovaries may be seen. Acanthosis nigricans is usually present, but liver and renal disease do not occur.

LOCALIZED LIPODYSTROPHY Localized lipodystrophy takes several patterns. Centrifugal lipodystrophy (*lipodystrophia centrifugalis abdominalis infantilis*) has been mentioned. *Annular lipoatrophy* is a bandlike ring of fat atrophy encircling a limb or the ankles. Occasionally, only half the limb is involved, in which case the term often used is *lipoatrophia semicircularis*. On biopsy, inflammatory infiltrates in the areas of fat atrophy suggest that this condition is actually a form of panniculitis. Localized lipodystrophy also may occur secondary to injection of insulin, iron dextrans, triamcinolone, and diphtheria/pertussis/tetanus vaccine.

DIAGNOSIS The diagnosis of the lipodystrophies is clinical. Taut stretching of the skin of the face may suggest scleroderma. The hypertrophied muscles appear "cleaved" as in body builders, because of absence of the usual fat between muscles. The finding of fat atrophy together with acanthosis nigricans, eruptive xanthomas, and typical laboratory findings usually render diagnosis straightforward.

MULTIPLE SYMMETRIC LIPOMATOSIS

Multiple symmetric lipomatosis usually occurs in men and is characterized by formation of nonencapsulated lipomas in two patterns of distribution: In the *type I* variant, lipomas are primarily in the nape of the neck and in the supraclavicular and deltoid regions, resulting in an extraordinary bull-necked appearance (*Madelung collar*). Extension of the lipomas into the mediastinum may obstruct the trachea or vena cava. Fat over the remainder of the body appears normal. In the *type II* pattern, lipomas extend over the body, giving the appearance of simple obesity. Diagnosis requires recognition that the fat masses are symmetric and that the distal arms and legs are spared. Deep lipomatosis is absent in type II disease, and vena caval and tracheal compression do not occur.

Multiple symmetric lipomatosis may occur sporadically or in families. Autosomal dominant transmission has been postulated in the latter. Alcoholism is common and may cause coexisting folate deficiency, macrocytic anemia, and abnormal liver function. Neuropathy may be sensory, motor, or autonomic, and neuropathic foot ulcers can develop. Histologic evidence from sural nerve biopsies suggests that neuropathy is integral to the disease, namely, a chronic distal atrophy without the axonal degeneration and demyelination of alcohol injury. Central nervous system abnormalities include defects in evoked potentials.

Metabolic abnormalities include hyperuricemia, hypertriglyceridemia (VLDL, chylomicrons), and paradoxically, elevated high-density lipoproteins (HDL). Diabetes mellitus has not been reported, although hyperinsulinism may be present. Renal tubular acidosis has occurred.

The cause is not known. The lipomas do not contain brown fat, and the fat cells are slightly smaller than normal, suggesting hyperplasia. Isolated adipocytes have increased lipoprotein lipase activity and a defect in adrenergic lipolysis. Lipolytic response to cyclic AMP is intact, suggesting an abnormality at the hormone receptor/adenylate cyclase unit. The biochemical abnormalities are not present in all cases.

There is no treatment except for surgical removal of lipomas that cause compression or for cosmetic reasons.

OTHER LIPOMATOSES

MEDIASTINOABDOMINAL This disorder may be a variant of multiple symmetric lipomatosis. The syndrome comprises (1) exertional dyspnea due to compression of airways by lipomas of the mediastinum, (2) massive enlargement of the abdomen (pseudoascites) due to intraperitoneal and retroperitoneal fat, and (3) abnormal glucose tolerance or diabetes mellitus. The metabolic abnormalities and enzymic changes in adipocytes are identical with those in multiple symmetric lipomatosis except that HDL levels are not elevated.

PELVIC Pelvic lipomatosis is characterized by overgrowth of dense, unencapsulated fat in pelvic spaces enveloping the pelvic viscera. The male-to-female ratio is 18:1. Symptoms include bladder dysfunction (frequency, dysuria, hematuria), constipation, and vague abdominal pain. Bilateral ureteral obstruction may cause hydronephrosis and renal failure. Hypertension is common. Radiographic studies show a deformed bladder, deviation of the ureters, displacement of rectosigmoid junction, and hydronephrosis in advanced cases. MRI or CT defines the compressing fat. There is no treatment except surgery to remove the fat and relieve upper urinary tract obstruction.

EPIDURAL Epidural lipomatosis is a syndrome of spinal cord compression due to adipose tissue. It causes back pain, radicular pain, or compression of the cord. The disorder is most often seen with chronic glucocorticoid therapy and may occur in Cushing's syndrome. Cord compression requires laminectomy, but otherwise a trial of decreased steroid dosage should be undertaken.

ACUTE PANNICULITIS (NODULAR FAT NECROSIS)

The appearance of single or multiple crops of tender nodules in subcutaneous fat with a histologic picture of fat cell necrosis, infiltration of inflammatory cells, and development of fat-filled macrophages (foam cells) is the hallmark of acute panniculitis. The nodules range in size from 0.5 to 10 cm and may be firm or fluctuant. They are usually tender. On occasion they drain an oily solution, and suppuration may occur. Individual lesions last from 1 to 8 weeks before disappearing, sometimes leaving a pigmented depressed area at the involved site. While some patients have only panniculitis, which may or may not be relapsing, others develop fever, abnormal liver function, a leukemoid white blood cell response, bleeding tendencies, nodular lung lesions, and pancreatic dysfunction with elevated amylase and lipase levels. In the past this constellation of findings was called *Weber-Christian disease*. However, painful or nonpainful panniculitis may result from a variety of conditions, and the term should probably be abandoned.

It is not possible to develop a firm classification of acute panniculitis since the lesions may appear in sporadic fashion with many conditions. One classification system is given in Table 352-4.

Panniculitis without systemic disease is usually due to trauma (sometimes factitiously induced) or cold. For example, in equestrian cold panniculitis the lesions appear in the outer thighs of persons riding horseback for several hours in cold weather. Subcutaneous fat necrosis of the newborn may be due to a combination of obstetric trauma and hypothermia.

Panniculitis with systemic disease can be divided into several large categories. Collagen vascular diseases such as lupus and scleroderma are a frequent cause. Indeed, nodular fat necrosis occurs in about 2 to 3 percent of patients with lupus and is more common in discoid than in systemic lupus. Lymphomas and histiocytosis represent a second category. Histiocytic cytophagic panniculitis (HCP) is characterized by fever, pleural effusions, hepatosplenomegaly, panniculitis, anemia, leukopenia, thrombocytopenia, and coagulation defects. The characteristic lesion is the "beanbag" histiocyte containing ingested lymphocytes, red cells, and platelets. While some patients have a benign course, most die from hemorrhagic complications. Malignant T cell lymphoma may involve subcutaneous tissue directly and can mimic HCP. Infiltrating T lymphocytes in HCP are of clonal origin, suggesting that subcutaneous T cell lymphomas are a malignant, late transformation phase of HCP. Panniculitis with systemic symptoms also occurs in lymphoplasmatic lymphoma with crystal-laden histiocytes. Deficiencies of α_1-antitrypsin have been found in a number of patients with acute panniculitis. It is postulated that the α_1-antitrypsin deficiency

Table 352-4

Causes of Panniculitis

Panniculitis without systemic disease
Trauma
Cold
Subcutaneous fat necrosis of the newborn
Panniculitis with systemic disease
Connective tissue disorders (lupus erythematosus, scleroderma)
Lymphoproliferative disease (lymphoma, histiocytosis)
α_1-Antitrypsin deficiency
Pancreatic disease (cancer, pancreatitis)
Generalized lipodystrophy
Paraproteinemia with C1 inhibitor deficiency
Fasciitis-panniculitis syndrome
Miscellaneous (see text)

predisposes to panniculitis after trauma and induces a hyperactive immune response. Panniculitis with systemic symptoms, including fever and hepatitis, also occurs with light chain paraproteinemia and acquired deficiency of C_1 inhibitor in the classic complement-generating sequence. Severe pancreatic disease also can cause acute panniculitis. One variant, *disseminated fat necrosis,* is described below. Panniculitis rarely may be associated with generalized lipodystrophy, especially the acquired type. Other rare causes of panniculitis include gout, familial Mediterranean fever, Nasu disease (see above), drugs (glucocorticoids, aspartame), renal failure, atheromatous emboli, and infection. Eosinophilic panniculitis may occur with vasculitis, parasitic infestation, lymphomas, and atopic dermatitis. Eosinophilic panniculitis can also be a variant of the fasciitis-panniculitis syndrome characterized by chronic inflammation, induration of the skin, and eosinophilic fasciitis, resulting in fibrosis of subcutaneous and muscle septae, and may follow Sweet's syndrome.

Acute panniculitis can only be diagnosed histologically, and then a search for the cause must be made. If systemic symptoms are present and the course is rapidly downhill, the primary differential diagnosis is between collagen vascular disease, lymphoproliferative disorder, and pancreatitis or pancreatic cancer. Milder cases raise the possibility of α_1-antitrypsin deficiency.

℞ TREATMENT

Treatment is often unsatisfactory. Some patients with histiocytic cytophagic panniculitis respond to combined chemotherapy with cyclophosphamide, bleomycin, and prednisone. Patients with α_1-antitrypsin deficiency may respond to dapsone and may be given α_1-antiprotease concentrate (60 mg/kg body weight weekly) if this fails.

DISSEMINATED FAT NECROSIS

Disseminated fat necrosis (also called *metastatic fat necrosis*) is a disorder in which patients with pancreatitis (two-thirds) or carcinoma of the pancreas (one-third) develop lesions that are characteristic of nodular panniculitis and that have a predilection for periarticular sites. Fever is usual. Arthritis occurs in about 60 percent of cases and may cause joint destruction. Sinus tracts may extend from the site of subcutaneous fat necrosis to the joint space, leading to deposition of necrotic material. Lytic bone lesions may underlie the site of fat necrosis. Polyserositis and vasculitis may be present. Since complement levels are low and immunofluorescent staining shows deposition of complement and IgG, the syndrome resembles, in some respects, lupus-associated panniculitis. Serologic studies for lupus have not been reported systematically, but antinuclear antibody (ANA) and rheumatoid factor have been undetectable in some patients.

Release of pancreatic enzymes into blood may cause disseminated fat necrosis at distal sites in some patients. Presumably, free fatty acids released by pancreatic lipase and phospholipase A_2, both of which may be elevated in serum, induce tissue necrosis, with trypsin playing an ancillary role. Experimentally, necrosis can be induced in pericardial, subpleural, and subcutaneous fat by ligation of pancreatic ducts. Amylase and lipase levels may be elevated in pleural, pericardial, and ascitic fluid. These enzymes also have been found in fluid aspirated from subcutaneous nodules. The possibility that release of pancreatic enzymes is causal is supported by the occurrence of disseminated fat necrosis in patients with pancreatic–portal vein fistulas. The relation of pancreatic enzyme leakage to autoimmune mechanisms, if any, and the meaning of the eosinophilia that frequently accompanies disseminated fat necrosis are not known.

Mortality rates are high (even in the absence of pancreatic carcinoma), and death may occur in weeks to months. No treatment is known. Infusion of the protease inhibitor aprotinin appeared to have beneficial effects in one patient.

ADIPOSIS DOLOROSA

Adiposis dolorosa (Dercum's disease) occurs in women (30:1) and is characterized by painful circumscribed adipose tissue deposits in

subcutaneous tissues of the extremities and of other parts of the body. Juxtaarticular areas, particularly the knees, are the most common sites. Lesions vary from 0.5 to 5.0 cm. Pain and paresthesia may occur spontaneously or result from pressure. Affected individuals are usually obese. The disorder is associated with weakness, fatigue, emotional instability, and occasional dementia and rarely begins before menopause. Most cases are sporadic, but familial occurrence has been noted with a presumed dominant inheritance. Most reported associations are probably chance phenomena. Autopsy reports from early in the century suggested abnormalities of the pituitary and other endocrine glands, but modern endocrinologic evaluations have not been undertaken.

Biopsy of affected sites may show no abnormalities, but granulomas with giant cell formations are usually seen. Fat necrosis is rare, thus separating the condition from acute panniculitis.

Treatment is unsatisfactory, although intravenous lidocaine, glucocorticoids, surgical excision, and liposuction have been tried.

BIBLIOGRAPHY

LIPODYSTROPHY

Chandalia M et al: Postmortem findings in congenital generalized lipodystrophy. J Clin Endocrinol Metab 80:3077, 1995

Chun SI et al: Membranous lipodystrophy: Primary idiopathic type. J Am Acad Dermatol 24:844, 1991

Cutler DL et al: Insulin-resistant diabetes mellitus and hypermetabolism in mandibulo-acral dysplasia: A newly recognized form of partial lipodystrophy. J Clin Endocrinol Metab 73:1056, 1991

Desbois-Mouthou C et al: Lipoatrophic diabetes: Genetic exclusion of the insulin receptor gene. J Clin Endocrinol Metab 80:314, 1995

Garg A et al: Peculiar distribution of adipose tissue in patients with congenital generalized lipodystrophy. J Clin Endocrinol Metab 75:358, 1991

Klein S et al: Generalized lipodystrophy: In vivo evidence for hypermetabolism and insulin-resistant lipid, glucose, and amino acid kinetics. Metabolism 41:893, 1992

Morison IM et al: Somatic overgrowth associated with overexpression of insulin-like growth factor II. Nature Med 2:321, 1996

Seip M: Generalized lipodystrophy, in *Ergebnisse der Inneren Medizin und Kinderheilkunde*, P Frick et al (eds). Berlin, Springer-Verlag, 1971, pp 59–95

MULTIPLE SYMMETRIC LIPOMATOSIS

Enzi G: Multiple symmetric lipomatosis: An updated clinical report. Medicine 63:56, 1984

Kazumi T et al: Failure to detect brown adipose tissue uncoupling protein mRNA in benign symmetric lipomatosis (Madelung's disease). Endocr J 41:315, 1994

Naumann M et al: Neurological multisystem manifestation in multiple symmetric lipomatosis: A clinical and electrophysiological study. Muscle Nerve 18:693, 1995

MEDIASTINOABDOMINAL LIPOMATOSIS, PELVIC LIPOMATOSIS, AND EPIDURAL LIPOMATOSIS

Fessler RG et al: Epidural lipomatosis in steroid-treated patients. Spine 17:183, 1992

Heyns CF: Pelvic lipomatosis: A review of its diagnosis and management. J Urol 146:267, 1991

ACUTE PANNICULITIS

Alegre VA, Winkelmann RK: Histiocytic cytophagic panniculitis. J Am Acad Dermatol 20:177, 1989

Attias D et al: Acute neutrophilic myositis in Sweet's syndrome: Late transformation into fibrosing myositis and panniculitis. Hum Pathol 26:687, 1995

Harada M et al: Crystal-storing histiocytosis associated with lymphoplasmacytic lymphoma mimicking Weber-Christian disease: Immunohistochemical, ultrastructural and gene-rearrangement studies. Hum Pathol 27:84, 1996

Hytiroglou P et al: Histiocytic cytophagic panniculitis: Molecular evidence for a clonal T-cell disorder. J Am Acad Dermatol 27:333, 1992

Naschitz JE et al: The fasciitis-panniculitis syndromes. Clinical and pathologic features. Medicine 75:6, 1996

Peters MS, Su WPD: Panniculitis. Dermatol Clin 10:37, 1992

SMITH KC et al: Panniculitis associated with severe α_1-antitrypsin deficiency: Treatment and review of the literature. Arch Dermatol 123:1655, 1987

DISSEMINATED FAT NECROSIS

POTTS JR: Pancreatic–portal vein fistula with disseminated fat necrosis treated by pancreaticoduodenectomy. South Med J 84:632, 1991

WILSON HA et al: Pancreatitis with arthropathy and subcutaneous fat necrosis. Evidence for the pathogenicity of lipolytic enzymes. Arthritis Rheum 26:121, 1983

ADIPOSIS DOLOROSA

BRODOVSKY J et al: Adiposis dolorosa (Dercum's disease): 10 year follow-up. Ann Plast Surg 33:664, 1994

SECTION 3

DISORDERS OF BONE AND MINERAL METABOLISM

353

Michael F. Holick, Stephen M. Krane, John T. Potts, Jr.

CALCIUM, PHOSPHORUS, AND BONE METABOLISM: CALCIUM-REGULATING HORMONES

BONE STRUCTURE AND METABOLISM (See also Chap. 355) Bone is a dynamic tissue that is remodeled constantly throughout life. The arrangement of compact and cancellous bone provides a strength and density suitable for mobility. In addition, bone provides a reservoir for calcium, magnesium, phosphorus, sodium, and other ions necessary for homeostatic functions. The skeleton is highly vascular and receives about 10 percent of the cardiac output.

The properties of bone are a function of its extracellular components. The structure consists of a solid mineral phase in close association with an organic matrix, of which 90 to 95 percent is type I collagen (see Chap. 348). The noncollagenous portion of the organic matrix contains proteins derived from serum (albumin and α_2-HS glycoproteins), proteins containing α-carboxyglutamic acid (GLA) [*bone GLA protein* (BGP), *osteocalcin*, and a matrix GLA protein], the glycoprotein *osteonectin*, the phosphoprotein *osteopontin*, sialoproteins, *thrombospondin*, and other less well characterized proteins. Some of these proteins may function in initiating mineralization and in binding of the mineral phase to the matrix. The mineral phase is made up of calcium and phosphate and is best characterized as a poorly crystalline hydroxyapatite, although the calcium/phosphate molar ratio is less than the 1.67 molar ratio of hydroxyapatite [empirical formula $Ca_{10}(PO_4)_6(OH)_2$]. Additional ions are present, particularly in the surface layers. The mineral phase of bone is deposited initially in intimate relation to the collagen fibrils and is found in specific locations in the "holes" between the collagen fibrils. This architectural arrangement of mineral and matrix results in a two-phase material well suited to withstand mechanical stresses. The formation and localization of the inorganic phase are determined in part by the organic matrix.

Cells of mesenchymal origin—*osteoblasts*—synthesize and secrete the organic matrix. Mineralization of the matrix, largely in *osteons* (haversian systems), begins soon after the matrix is secreted (primary mineralization) but is not completed until after several weeks (secondary mineralization). Osteoblasts are characterized by their location and morphology, the presence of a specific skeletal form of alkaline phosphatase, the presence of receptors for parathyroid hormone (PTH) and 1,25-dihydroxyvitamin D [$1,25(OH)_2D$], and the ability to synthesize specific matrix proteins, such as type I collagen, osteocalcin, and osteopontin. As an osteoblast secretes matrix, which is then mineralized, the cell becomes surrounded by matrix and becomes an *osteocyte*, still connected with its blood supply through a series of canaliculi. Resorption of bone is carried out mainly by *osteoclasts*, multinucleated cells that are formed by fusion of hematopoietic stem cells related to the mononuclear phagocyte series. Resorption of bone takes place in scalloped spaces (Howship's lacunae) where the osteoclasts are attached through a specific $\alpha v\beta 3$ integrin to components of the bone matrix such as osteopontin. This zone (clear zone) contains contractile proteins. The resorbing end of the cell forms a specialized ruffled border. Mineral and matrix are removed in this space where the ruffled border is folded and is in contact with the bone. Proteins, including a specialized proton-pump ATPase, are found in the ruffled border membrane, which contributes to the production in the enclosed extracellular compartment of an acid environment, which solubilizes the mineral phase. This area is also rich in protein encoded by the oncogene c-*src* and in the Src phosphorylation substrate p80/85. In addition to the proton pump, carbonic anhydrase (type II isoenzyme) is required to maintain the acid pH. Other features of osteoclasts include the presence of tartrate-resistant acid phosphatase, cell-surface receptors for calcitonin, sodium pumps of the kidney type, a bicarbonate/chloride exchanger of the band 3 family, and an ability to resorb mineralized bone. The bone matrix is resorbed in the acid environment adjacent to the ruffled border by acid hydrolyases following solubilization of the mineral phase. Several soluble ligands modulate the differentiation of osteoblasts or osteoclasts from precursor cells and modulate the function of the differentiated cells; prominent among these substances are the colony stimulating factors and interleukins (ILs) 6 and 11. Bone is a storehouse for growth-regulatory factors. Some that affect osteoblast function include transforming growth factor (TGF) β types I and II, acidic fibroblast growth factor (aFGF) and basic fibroblast growth factor (bFGF), platelet-derived growth factor (PDGF), and insulin-like growth factors (IGFs) I and II. In addition, several proteins that induce ectopic bone formation may have a role in bone remodeling, e.g., osteoinductive factor, osteogenin, and bone morphogenic proteins. Other cytokines modulate resorption through effects on osteoclasts, e.g., IL-1, tumor necrosis factor (TNF), interferon γ, and colony stimulating factors (CSFs). Some of these effects on osteoclasts are mediated by osteoblasts and adjacent stromal fibroblasts in the marrow. For example, PTH receptors are not found on mature osteoclasts, and PTH increases osteoclastic bone resorption by first acting on osteoblasts or stromal fibroblasts. $1,25(OH)_2D$ receptors are found in precursor cells that can differentiate into monocytes or osteoclasts, and $1,25(OH)_2D$ promotes differentiation along the osteoclast pathway. Some cytokines, such as IL-1 and TGFα, may induce local production of prostaglandins and other cytokines, such as IL-6 and CSFs. What was initially termed *osteoclast-activating factor* is currently thought to reflect the presence of cytokines such as IL-1, TNFα, TNFβ (lymphotoxin), and probably others as well.

In the embryo and in the growing child, bone develops by remodeling and replacing previously calcified cartilage (endochondral bone formation) or is formed without a cartilage matrix (intramembranous bone formation). New bone, whether formed in infants or in adults during repair, has a relatively high ratio of cells to matrix and is characterized by coarse fiber bundles of collagen that are interlaced and randomly dispersed (woven bone). In adults, the more mature bone is organized with fiber bundles regularly arranged in parallel or concentric sheets (lamellar bone). In long bones, deposition of lamellar bone in a concentric arrangement around blood vessels forms the haversian systems. Growth in length of bones is dependent on proliferation of cartilage cells and on the endochondral sequence at the growth plate. Growth in width and thickness is accomplished by formation of bone at the periosteal surface and by resorption at the endosteal surface, with the rate of formation exceeding that of resorption. In adults, after the epiphyses close, growth in length and endochondral bone formation cease, except for some activity in the cartilage cells beneath the articular surface. Even in adults, however, remodeling of bone (remodeling of haversian systems as well as trabecular bone) continues through life. Newly forming surfaces are characterized by smooth character, by uptake of tetracycline, and by relatively low mineral density and are covered by active osteoblasts. The osteoid seam that results from the lag in mineralization of the newly formed organic matrix is about 12 μm in width. An index of the rate of bone formation can be obtained by examination of undemineralized sections of bone biopsy specimens from individuals who have received tetracycline for two periods separated by a drug-free interval. The distance between the fluorescent bands on the sections reflects the amount of new bone formed. Resorption areas are characterized by irregular configurations and the presence of osteoclasts (Fig. 353-1). Resorption precedes formation and is more intense, but it does not persist as long as formation. In adults, approximately 4 percent of the surface of trabecular bone (such as iliac crest) is involved in active resorption, whereas 10 to 15 percent of trabecular surfaces is covered with osteoid. Radioisotope studies indicate that as much as 18 percent of the total skeletal calcium is deposited and removed each year. Thus, bone is an active metabolizing tissue that requires an intact blood supply. The remodeling of bone is somehow related to the mechanical stresses to which it is subjected. Bone also serves as an important reservoir of mineral ions such as calcium, which are critical for a variety of processes.

The response of bone to fractures, infection, and interruption of blood supply and to expanding lesions is relatively limited. Dead bone must be resorbed, and new bone must be formed, a process carried out in association with growth of new blood vessels into the involved area. In injuries that disrupt the organization of the tissue, such as a fracture in which apposition of fragments is poor and motion exists at the fracture site, the progenitor stromal cells differentiate into cells with functional capacities different from those of osteoblasts, and varying amounts of fibrous tissue and cartilage are formed. When there is good apposition with fixation and little motion at the fracture site, repair occurs predominantly by formation of new bone without other scar tissue. Remodeling of this bone occurs along lines of force determined by mechanical stresses that are somehow translated into biologic response.

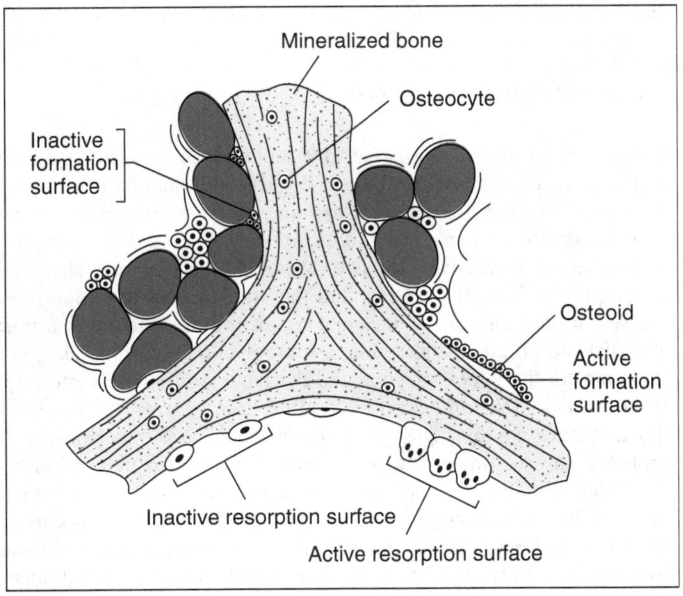

FIGURE 353-1 Schematic representation of bone remodeling surfaces in trabecular bone. Most bone surfaces in adults are involved in neither formation nor resorption. Such surfaces are usually smooth, have no osteoid seam, and are covered either by no visible cells or by flattened cells. Active formation surfaces are smooth and covered by osteoblasts which have an osteoid seam (*solid blue*), normally no thicker than 12 μm. The calcification front is located at the junction of the osteoid seam and mineralized bone (*stippled*). Inactive formation surfaces are not covered by osteoblasts but by only a few flattened cells. Active resorption surfaces are irregular or scalloped and contain multinucleated osteoclasts. The latter are not seen on inactive resorption surfaces.

Expanding lesions in bone, such as tumors, induce resorption at the surface in contact with the tumor. A bowing deformity causes increased new bone formation at the concave surface and resorption at the convex surface, all seemingly designed to produce the strongest mechanical structure. Even in a disorder as architecturally disruptive as Paget's disease, remodeling is dictated by mechanical forces. Thus, the plasticity of bone is due to the interaction of cells with each other and with the environment.

Mechanisms of Bone Formation and Resorption Bone formation is an orderly process in which deposition of inorganic mineral is controlled by an organic matrix. The mineral phase is composed of calcium and phosphorus, and the concentration of these ions in the plasma and extracellular fluid (ECF) influences the rate at which mineral is formed. In vitro, mineralization can proceed, and crystals of hydroxyapatite can grow, at concentrations of calcium and phosphorus similar to those in an ultrafiltrate of plasma. However, the concentration of these ions at the sites of mineralization is unknown, and the cells involved (osteoblasts, osteocytes) may influence the local ion concentrations. Collagens from a variety of sources can catalyze the nucleation of a mineral phase of calcium and phosphorus from solutions of these ions, and the initial mineral phase is deposited in specific locations in the "holes" produced by the packing arrangement of the collagen molecules. The organization of collagen probably influences the amount and type of mineral phase formed in bone. The primary structures of type I collagen in skin and bone tissues are similar. There are differences, however, in posttranslational modifications of type I collagen, such as hydroxylations, glycosylations, and the type, number, and distribution of intermolecular cross-links. In addition, the holes in the packing structure of the collagen are larger in mineralized collagen of bone and dentin than in unmineralized collagens such as tendon. The fact that single-amino-acid substitutions in the helical portion of either the α1 or α2 chain of type I collagen due to mutations in the *COL*1A1 or *COL*1A2 genes in osteogenesis imperfecta disrupt the organization of bone indicates the importance of the fibrillar matrix in the structure of bone (see also Chap. 348). The noncollagenous organic components such as osteocalcin, osteonectin, and osteopontin also may play a role in the mineralization of bone. Alkaline phosphatase is a marker for osteoblasts, and cellular levels of this enzyme correlate with mineralization potential of osteoblasts. Although mineralization defects occur in individuals with mutations that cause decreased alkaline phosphatase activity (hypophosphatasia), the function of alkaline phosphatase in mineralization is not completely understood. Inorganic pyrophosphate is a potent inhibitor of mineralization at levels below those necessary to bind calcium ions. Since alkaline phosphatase in osteoblasts and other cells can catalyze the hydrolysis of inorganic pyrophosphate at neutral pH, this enzyme could regulate mineralization by controlling the concentrations of pyrophosphate. In addition, macromolecular inhibitors such as proteoglycan aggregates also may influence mineralization. In cartilage undergoing calcification, mineralization may be initiated in membrane-bound vesicles outside the cells.

In bone, the calcium phosphate solid phase at the inception of mineralization is brushite ($CaHPO_4 \cdot 2H_2O$). As mineralization progresses, the solid phase is a poorly crystalline hydroxyapatite with a relatively low (~1.2) calcium/phosphate molar ratio. With age and maturation, the perfection of the crystals and the calcium/phosphate ratio increase. Fluoride ions, when incorporated into the mineral phase, decrease the proportion of amorphous calcium phosphate and enhance the crystal structure.

There is a limit for the concentration of calcium and phosphorus ions in the ECF below which mineralization does not occur. A "solubility product" for bone mineral is difficult to calculate because the mineral phase itself is of variable composition and because the various components in ECF that regulate this solubility product are not known. Nevertheless, when the concentrations of calcium and phosphorus in ECF are excessive, a mineral phase may form in areas that are not normally mineralized.

When bone is resorbed, calcium and phosphorus ions are released into the ECF, and the organic matrix is resorbed. The fact that bone resorption takes place in the region of the osteoclast adjacent to the bone surface, where the extracellular pH is low, suggests that an acid environment is required for solubilization of bone mineral. The alkaline phosphatase of bone cells is an ectoenzyme that is released into the ECF. Increased circulating levels of the bone-derived enzyme are correlated with rates of bone formation. Other circulating markers of bone formation include osteocalcin and type I procollagen carboxy-terminal peptides. Urinary markers for bone resorption are hydroxyproline, hydroxylysine and its glycosides, and the bone-specific hydroxypyridinium collagen cross-links.

CALCIUM METABOLISM A total of 1 to 2 kg of calcium is present in the average adult, over 98 percent of it in the skeleton. The calcium of the mineral phase at the surface of the crystals is in equilibrium with that in the ECF, but only a minor fraction of the total pool (about 0.5 percent) is exchangeable. The calcium in ECF is critical for a variety of functions and is remarkably constant. In normal adults plasma levels range from 2.2 to 2.6 mmol/L (8.8 to 10.4 mg/dL). The calcium in plasma is present as three forms: free ions, ions bound to plasma proteins, and, to a small extent, diffusible complexes. The concentration of free calcium ions, averaging 1.2 mmol/L (4.8 mg/dL), influences many cellular functions and is subjected to tight hormonal control, especially through PTH, as described below. The concentration of serum proteins is an important determinant of calcium ion concentration; most calcium ion is bound to albumin. Ionized calcium can be measured directly with the use of calcium-specific electrodes. If ionized calcium cannot be measured, certain approximations can be used to distinguish the protein-bound and ionized fractions. One formula that approximates the amount of calcium bound to protein is

$$\% \text{ protein-bound Ca} = 0.8 \times \text{albumin (g/L)} + 0.2 \times \text{globulin (g/L)} + 3$$

A simplified correction is sometimes used to indicate whether a stated total serum calcium concentration is abnormal when serum proteins are low. The correction is to add 1 mg/dL to the serum calcium level for every 1 g/dL by which the serum albumin level is below 4.0 g/dL. If the serum calcium level, for example, is 7.8 mg/dL (a subnormal value) and the serum albumin level is only 3.0 mg/dL, then the stated serum calcium level is corrected by adding 1 mg/dL; the corrected value of 8.8 mg/dL is within the normal range. These rough approximations generally agree with measurements of ionized calcium in patients with subnormal serum proteins.

Calcium ions inside the cell mediate a variety of cellular functions. Most intracellular calcium is in the form of insoluble complexes. The level of free calcium in the cell, which is critical for functional regulation, is low, approximately 0.1 μmol/L; thus, the gradient between plasma and intracellular free calcium is about 10,000 to 1. This gradient is tightly regulated. The concentration of calcium ions in the ECF is kept constant by processes that constantly add and remove calcium. Calcium enters the plasma via absorption from the intestinal tract and resorption of ions from the bone mineral. Calcium leaves the ECF via secretion into the gastrointestinal tract (~100 to 200 mg/d), urinary excretion (~50 to 300 mg/d), deposition in bone mineral, and losses in sweat (up to 100 mg/d). Bone resorption and formation are tightly coupled, approximately 12 mmol (500 mg) calcium entering and leaving the skeleton daily (Fig. 353-2).

The average dietary calcium intake for most adults in the United States is approximately 15 to 20 mmol/d (0.6 to 0.8 g/d). However, with heightened awareness of the role of adequate calcium intake for

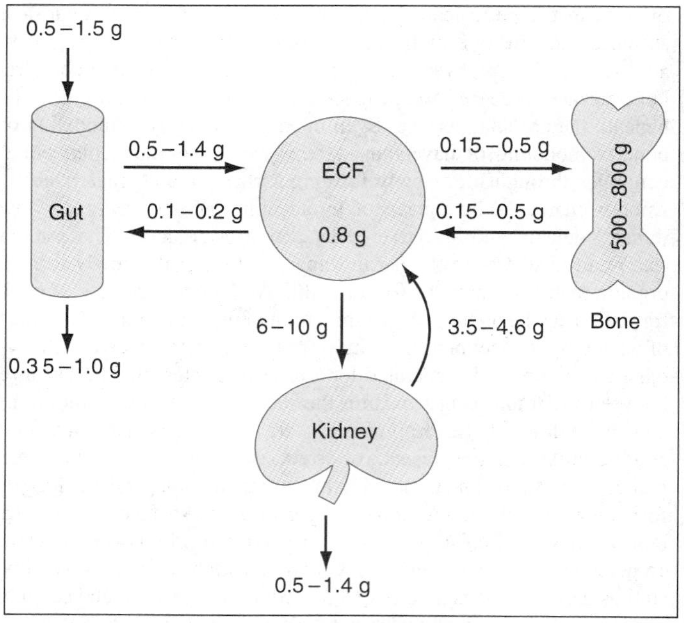

FIGURE 353-2 Calcium homeostasis. Schematic illustration of calcium content of extracellular fluid (ECF) and bone as well as of diet and feces; magnitude of calcium flux per day as calculated by various methods is shown at sites of transport in intestine, kidney, and bone. Ranges of values shown are approximate and chosen to illustrate certain points discussed in text. In intestine, absorption efficiency varies inversely with dietary calcium (chronic adaptation). This is reflected in typical quantities absorbed and excreted in feces; with 0.5-g intake, 50 percent absorption is depicted to occur (0.25 g), but at 1.5 g, only 30 percent (0.5 g). Endogenous fecal calcium, the 0.1 to 0.2 g secreted into the intestinal lumen daily, is constant and does not vary with calcium intake or absorption. Quantities of calcium depicted as filtered, reabsorbed, and excreted at the kidney are chosen arbitrarily to indicate that at lower rates of filtration of calcium (expected at lower glomerular filtration rates), most is reabsorbed (e.g., 5.85 of 6 g), leading to urinary excretion of 150 mg; at higher rates of filtration (at high dietary calcium intake), slightly less is reabsorbed (e.g., 9.7 of 10 g), leading to a higher urinary excretion, 300 mg. In all situations, renal calcium reabsorption exceeds 95 percent of filtered load. Urinary calcium excretion is seen, therefore, to increase by only 150 mg despite a 1-g increase in dietary intake. In conditions of calcium balance, rates of calcium release from and uptake into bone are equal.

the prevention of osteoporosis, many adults on supplements have an intake of 20 to 37 mmol/d (0.8 to 1.5 g/d). Less than half of dietary calcium is absorbed in adults. Calcium absorption increases during periods of rapid growth in children, in pregnancy, and in lactation and decreases with advancing age. Most of the calcium is absorbed in the proximal small intestine, and the efficiency of absorption decreases in the more distal intestinal segments. Both active transport and diffusion-limited absorption are involved; the former is more important in the upper intestine and the latter in the lower intestine. Both processes are influenced by vitamin D. All forms of calcium in the diet may not be equally absorbed; calcium as the chloride is probably absorbed more efficiently than that in other preparations.

Calcium is also secreted into the lumen of the gastrointestinal tract. When radioactive calcium is administered intravenously, it appears in the feces, making possible calculations of *endogenous fecal calcium* (see Fig. 353-2). Higher estimates of calcium losses in intestinal juices have been made by other techniques. Secretion of calcium into the intestinal lumen is constant and independent of absorption. If calcium availability in the diet is low [<12 mmol/d (500 mg/d)], a positive calcium balance requires an efficiency of absorption greater than 30 to 40 percent.

The urinary calcium excretion of normal adults having an average calcium intake ranges between 2.5 and 10 mmol/d (100 and 400 mg/d). When the dietary calcium level is below 5 mmol/d (200 mg/d), urinary calcium excretion is usually less than 5 mmol/d (200 mg/d). However, in most normal individuals, wide variations in dietary intake have little effect on urinary calcium. Hence, when the diet is low in calcium, the relative inefficiency of renal calcium conservation leads to a negative calcium balance unless calcium absorption is maximal (see Fig. 353-2).

The amount of calcium in the urine is small compared with that filtered by the glomerulus [about 150 to 250 mmol/d (6 to 10 g/d)] because the rates of reabsorption of the filtered calcium are high. Reabsorption takes place predominantly in the proximal tubule (~60 percent) and in Henle's loop (~25 percent) and to a small extent in the distal tubule. It is not clear whether non-protein-bound, nonionic calcium such as calcium citrate is cleared at different rates. The excretion of other electrolytes affects the urinary excretion of calcium. For example, urinary calcium is usually proportional to urinary sodium; sulfate also increases calcium excretion.

Maintenance of the calcium balance depends on the efficiency of intestinal absorption (see Fig. 353-2). A deficiency of PTH or vitamin D, intestinal disease, or severe dietary calcium deprivation may provide challenges to calcium homeostasis that cannot be compensated adequately by renal calcium conservation, resulting in a negative calcium balance. Increased bone resorption may protect against ECF calcium depletion even in states of chronic negative calcium balance but only at the expense of progressive bone loss.

Pathophysiology A decrease in the concentration of free calcium ions in plasma results in increased neuromuscular irritability and tetany. This syndrome is characterized by peripheral and perioral paresthesias, carpal spasm, pedal spasm, anxiety, seizures, bronchospasm, laryngospasm, Chvostek's, Trousseau's, and Erb's signs, and lengthening of the QT interval of the electrocardiogram. In infants tetany may be manifested only by irritability and lethargy. The level of calcium ions that determines which features of tetany will be manifested varies among individuals. Tetany is also influenced by other components of the ECF. For example, hypomagnesemia and alkalosis lower whereas hypokalemia and acidosis raise the threshold for tetany.

Increases in total serum calcium are usually accompanied by increases in free calcium levels and may be associated with anorexia, nausea, vomiting, constipation, hypotonia, depression, and occasionally lethargy and coma. Persistent hypercalcemia, especially when accompanied by normal or elevated levels of serum phosphate, may cause ectopic deposition of a solid phase of calcium and phosphate in walls of blood vessels, connective tissue about the joints, gastric mucosa, cornea, and renal parenchyma. Hypercalcemia per se alters renal function in addition to the pathologic effects of calcium phosphate deposition.

PHOSPHORUS METABOLISM Phosphorus is a major component of bone and of all other tissues and in some form is involved in almost all metabolic processes. About 32 mol (1 kg) of phosphorus is present in the normal adult, of which about 85 percent is in the skeleton.

In fasting plasma, most of the phosphorus is present as inorganic orthophosphate in concentrations of approximately 0.9 to 1.3 mmol/L (2.8 to 4 mg/dL). In contrast to calcium, of which about 50 percent is bound, only about 12 percent of the phosphorus in plasma is bound to proteins. Free HPO_4^{2-} and $NaHPO_4^-$ normally accounts for about 75 percent of the total phosphorus, and free $H_2PO_4^-$ accounts for 10 percent. Since so many species are present, depending on pH and other factors, concentrations are usually expressed in terms of elemental phosphorus, in units of mmol/L or mg/dL. Total phosphorus levels are higher in children and in women after menopause. There is a circadian variation in phosphorus levels even during a 24-h fast, mediated in part by the adrenal cortex. The nadir occurs between 9 A.M. and 12 noon, followed by an increase to a plateau in the afternoon and another small peak after midnight. The magnitudes of the peaks and troughs vary with phosphorus intake but occur regardless of whether the intake is high or low. Dietary restriction of phosphorus that only modestly decreases the morning fasting levels may abolish the afternoon rise. Even with twofold changes in serum phosphorus levels, levels of serum ionized calcium do not change significantly.

During phosphate depletion, phosphaturia decreases before serum phosphorus declines. This adaptive response of increasing tubular transport when luminal concentrations are decreasing is an intrinsic property of tubular cells. There is also heterogeneity of phosphorus transport among different segments of proximal renal tubules. Tubular fluxes of phosphorus, rather than hypophosphatemia per se, may be critical in modulating effects of hypophosphatemia such as the stimulation of 25(OH)D-1α-hydroxylase. Conversely, increased phosphorus loads and increased renal tubular phosphorus fluxes result in decreased renal tubular reabsorption and increased clearance of phosphorus and suppress the activity of 25(OH)D-1α-hydroxylase (see below). Ingestion of carbohydrate depresses serum phosphorus acutely by 0.3 to 0.5 mmol/L (1 to 1.5 mg/dL), presumably owing to cellular uptake and formation of phosphate esters. Ingestion of phosphorus per se increases serum levels. Therefore, for the interpretation of serum levels and urinary clearances, samples should be obtained in the fasting state. Decreases in plasma phosphorus also occur during induction of alkalosis.

Whereas dietary calcium is absorbed inefficiently from the intestine, phosphorus absorption is remarkably efficient. At levels of intake less than 2 mg/kg of body weight per day, 80 to 90 percent of ingested phosphorus is absorbed. Even with levels of intake greater than 10 mg/kg of body weight per day in the form of dairy products, cereals, eggs, and meat, absorption is about 70 percent. Hypophosphatemia due to deficient intestinal absorption is unusual except when nonabsorbable antacids are administered; the antacids bind phosphorus and prevent absorption from the intestinal lumen.

The major control of phosphorus economy is exerted at the level of the kidney. Phosphorus filtered through the glomerulus is reabsorbed largely in the proximal tubule (there is homeostatically important distal reabsorption as well) so that only about 10 to 15 percent of the filtered load is normally excreted. When filtered loads of phosphorus decrease, proximal tubular reabsorption increases. Conversely, when phosphorus loads are increased, tubular reabsorption decreases, and clearance rises. Thus, the urinary excretion of phosphorus normally reflects dietary intake, and conservation or elimination of excessive amounts depends on adequate renal handling (Fig. 353-3). There is no good evidence for renal tubular phosphate secretion. Proximal reabsorption of phosphorus is dependent on parallel sodium reabsorption, but whereas the sodium rejected by the proximal tubule may be reabsorbed distally, the rejected phosphorus is not. Therefore, volume expansion and decreased sodium reabsorption increase phosphorus clearance; similarly, diuretics that act proximally, such as acetazolamide, are phosphaturic to a degree that parallels the degree to which they are natriuretic.

Pathophysiology No direct symptoms result from hyperphosphatemia. When high levels are maintained for long periods, however, mineralization is enhanced, and calcium phosphate may be deposited in abnormal sites. Ectopic calcification occurs in untreated chronic renal failure, with severe hypercalcemia, and in vitamin D intoxication. *Tumoral calcinosis* is a rare heritable disorder in which ectopic calcification is associated with hyperphosphatemia and a normal glomerular filtration rate (GFR). The disorder is characterized by a high ratio of phosphorus tubule maximum (TmP) to GFR and increased serum levels of $1,25(OH)_2D$. The latter is a paradoxical finding and presumably is related to the abnormal renal tubular phosphate fluxes. In contrast, severe acute hypophosphatemia may cause anorexia, dizziness, bone pain, proximal muscular weakness, and waddling gait. Significant hypophosphatemia is encountered in severe alcoholics and may be aggravated after repletion of nutrients, in the course of therapy of diabetic ketoacidosis, and for various reasons in severely ill, hospitalized elderly patients (see also Chap. 356). Myopathy in hypophosphatemia may be accompanied by elevations in serum creatinine kinase levels and by rhabdomyolysis. Severe congestive cardiomyopathy can occur with chronic hypophosphatemia, and restoration of phosphorus deficits leads to prompt reversal. Respiratory muscle weakness in severe hypophosphatemia also may improve with phosphate repletion. The bone pain and waddling gait are attributed to the osteomalacia that occurs with phosphate depletion. The muscular weakness may be due either to direct effects of hypophosphatemia on nerves and muscle

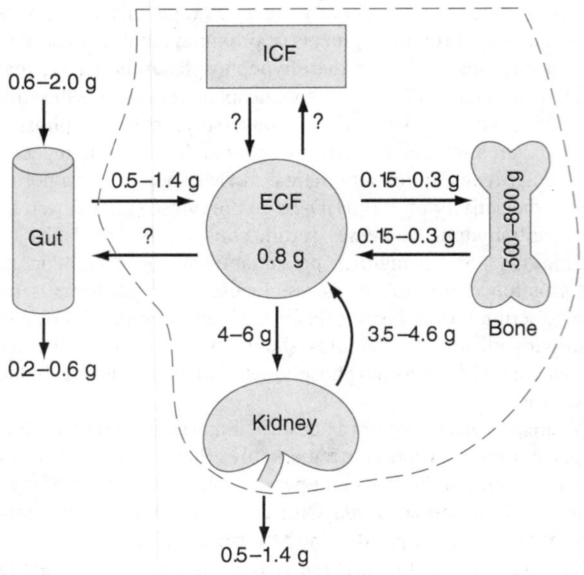

FIGURE 353-3 Phosphate homeostasis. Schematic illustration of inorganic phosphorus content (termed here *phosphate*) in extracellular fluid (ECF) and bone as well as diet and feces; magnitude of phosphorus flux per day as estimated by various methods is shown at transport sites in intestine, kidney, and bone. Range of values shown illustrates special features of phosphorus metabolism discussed in text. Intestinal phosphorus absorption is highly efficient, 85 percent at a lower intake (0.5 g of a 0.6-g intake) and 70 percent at a higher intake (1.4 g of a 2.0-g intake). Estimates of magnitude of endogenous fecal phosphate are less well established than for calcium. Contribution of at least 0.15 g is estimated to be added to the nonabsorbed phosphorus to provide a total of 0.2 g fecal phosphorus at the low intake level. At high phosphorus dietary intakes, no correction for endogenous fecal phosphate is calculated. Higher quantities of phosphorus are excreted in urine at all levels of dietary intake than for corresponding intakes of calcium; quantities excreted match closely the quantities absorbed, thereby maintaining phosphorus balance (no correction in this illustration is made for endogenous fecal phosphorus). Note that renal phosphorus reabsorption, in contrast to high and relatively invariant renal calcium reabsorption, varies from a low of 75 percent of filtered load to greater than 85 percent. The compartment labeled ICF refers to intracellular phosphorus, both organic and inorganic; rapid shifts of phosphorus into cells (and corresponding, possibly slower, efflux of phosphorus from cells) contribute to changes in ECF phosphorus. These shifts between ECF and ICF and phosphorus release from and uptake by bone are equal in conditions of phosphorus balance.

or, occasionally, to the effects of hyperparathyroidism (either primary or secondary), which may have a role in the etiology of the hypophosphatemia. Phosphorus depletion in children may impair growth. Hypophosphatemia causes decreased levels of 2,3-diphosphoglyceric acid and ATP in erythrocytes, which in turn alter the dissociation of oxyhemoglobin so that less oxygen is delivered to tissues. Hemolytic anemia may result from impairment of the ability of erythrocytes to deform in small vessels.

VITAMIN D

Vitamin D is a hormone rather than a vitamin. With adequate exposure to sunlight, no dietary supplements are needed. The active principle of vitamin D is synthesized under metabolic control via successive hydroxylations in the liver and kidney and is transported through the blood to its target tissues (the small intestine and bone), where it regulates calcium homeostasis. Calcium and phosphate ions, parathyroid hormone, and possibly other peptide and steroid hormones regulate the renal metabolism of vitamin D. Analysis of hereditary and acquired defects in these processes has provided new insights into the pathophysiology of several disorders involving calcium, phosphorus, and bone metabolism. These discoveries culminated in the chemical synthesis of active vitamin D metabolites and analogues, the clinical use of 1,25-dihydroxyvitamin D, [1,25$(OH)_2$D] (calcitriol) in many vitamin D–resistant states, and the development of assays for measuring vitamin D metabolites in blood to define abnormalities in vitamin D metabolism.

PHOTOBIOGENESIS OF VITAMIN D Vitamin D_3 is a derivative of 7-dehydrocholesterol (provitamin D_3), the immediate precursor of cholesterol. When skin is exposed to sunlight or certain artificial light sources, the ultraviolet radiation enters the epidermis and causes transformation of 7-dehydrocholesterol to vitamin D_3. Wavelengths between 290 and 315 nm are absorbed by the conjugated double bonds at C_5 and C_7 of 7-dehydrocholesterol and fragment the B ring between C_9 and C_{10} to yield a 9,10-secosterol (*seco* means "split"), previtamin D_3 (Fig. 353-4). Previtamin D_3 is biologically inert but undergoes a spontaneous temperature-dependent molecular rearrangement of its conjugated triene system (three double bonds) to form the thermally stable 9,10-secosterol, vitamin D_3 (see Fig. 353-4). At body temperature it takes approximately 24 h for previtamin D_3 to convert completely into vitamin D_3. Wide changes in skin surface temperature do not affect the rate of this conversion because the process occurs in the actively growing layers of the epidermis, where the temperature is relatively constant; changes in the core body temperature also have little effect on this reaction. Once vitamin D_3 is synthesized, it is translocated from the epidermis into the circulation by the vitamin D–binding protein. Thus, vitamin D is made in the skin from the previtamin for many hours after a single sun exposure (see Fig. 353-4). Although melanin in the skin competes with 7-dehydrocholesterol for ultraviolet photons and thus can limit the synthesis of previtamin D_3, the photochemical isomerization of previtamin D_3 and vitamin D_3 to biologically inert products appears to be more important in preventing excessive production of previtamin D_3 and vitamin D_3 during prolonged exposure to the sun.

Aging decreases the capacity of the skin to produce vitamin D_3; this capacity is reduced more than fourfold after age 70. Topical sunscreens can reduce or prevent cutaneous production of vitamin D_3 by absorbing the solar radiation responsible for previtamin D_3 synthesis in the skin. Other factors that affect the cutaneous synthesis of vitamin D_3 include altitude, geographic location, time of day, and area exposed. Latitude has profound effects on the cutaneous synthesis of vitamin D_3. As the zenith angle of the sun increases with approaching winter, more of the high-energy ultraviolet photons responsible for formation of the previtamin are absorbed by the ozone layer. In Boston (42°N) and in Edmonton (52°N), the absorption of these photons is so complete that essentially no vitamin D_3 is made in the skin between the months of November through February and October through March, respectively. When the entire body is exposed to sufficient sunlight to cause mild erythema, the increase in the blood vitamin D is about equivalent to consuming an oral dose of 10,000 to 25,000 international units (1 IU = 0.025 μg) of vitamin D. Only when skin irradiation is insufficient to produce the required quantities of vitamin D_3 is dietary supplementation needed to prevent skeletal mineralization defects. Fish liver oils, a natural source of vitamin D, were used widely for the treatment of rickets early in this century. The fortification of milk and some cereals with either crystalline vitamin D_2 (see Fig. 353-4) or vitamin D_3 prevents rickets and osteomalacia. However, a survey of the vitamin D content in milk from the United States and western Canada revealed that 71 percent did not contain 80 to 120 percent of the amount of vitamin D on the label and that approximately 15 percent of skim milk did not contain detectable vitamin D. Although the National Research Council of the United States recommends an intake of 200 IU/d for adults, this amount may be inadequate if there is little cutaneous production of vitamin D_3. In the absence of sunlight, between 400 and 600 IU of vitamin D is required to satisfy the daily requirement.

METABOLISM OF VITAMIN D Once vitamin D enters the circulation, either by absorption from the diet or through synthesis in the skin, it is transported to the liver bound to a specific alpha$_1$ globulin (vitamin D–binding protein). In the liver, vitamin D is metabolized to 25-hydroxyvitamin D [25(OH)D] by hepatic mitochondrial and/or microsomal enzyme(s) (see Fig. 353-4). 25(OH)D is one of the major circulating metabolites, and its half-life is about 21 days. The concentrations of 25(OH)D and some of its metabolites in the serum are measured using competitive binding assays. The normal serum 25(OH)D concentration varies among different laboratories from 20 to 200 nmol/L (8 to 80 ng/mL). Individuals exposed to excessive sunlight may have concentrations of 25(OH)D up to 250 nmol/L (100 ng/mL) without adverse effects on calcium metabolism. The normal range is lower in Great Britain, where additions of vitamin D to foods are not routine and where exposure to sunlight is less than in most regions of the United States. The serum 25(OH)D levels usually reflect both 25-hydroxyvitamin D_2 [25(OH)D_2] and 25-hydroxyvitamin D_3 [25(OH)D_3]. The ratio of these two 25-hydroxylated derivatives depends on the relative amounts of vitamins D_2 or D_3 present in the diet and the amount of previtamin D_3 produced by exposure to sunlight.

The hepatic 25-hydroxylation of vitamin D is regulated by a product feedback mechanism. This regulation, however, is not tight; an increase in dietary intake or endogenous production of vitamin D_3 causes increases in 25(OH)D levels in the serum. The levels can rise to greater than 1200 nmol/L (500 ng/mL) when the intake of vitamin D is excessive. Serum 25(OH)D levels are reduced in severe chronic liver disease (Table 353-1).

25(OH)D is not biologically active at physiologic levels in vivo but is active in vitro at high concentrations. After formation in the liver, 25(OH)D is bound by the vitamin D–binding protein and transported to the kidney for an additional stereospecific hydroxylation on either C_1 or C_{24} (see Fig. 353-4). The kidney plays a pivotal role in the metabolism of 25(OH)D to the biologically active metabolite. The renal mitochondrial 25(OH)D-1-hydroxylase activity is enhanced by hypocalcemia, so that hypocalcemia causes the rate of conversion of 25(OH)D to 1,25(OH)$_2$D to increase. Hypocalcemia may not control this hydroxylation directly, however. Any decrease in the serum concentration of calcium below normal is a stimulus for increased secretion of PTH, which increases the synthesis of 1,25(OH)$_2$D in the renal proximal convoluted tubule. The renal production of 1,25(OH)$_2$D enhances the effects of PTH in lowering circulating concentrations (and presumably renal intracellular concentrations) of phosphate (Fig. 353-5). 1,25(OH)$_2$D also influences the renal metabolism of 25(OH)D by diminishing 25(OH)D-1α-hydroxylase activity and enhancing the metabolism of 25(OH)D to 24*R*,25-dihydroxyvitamin D [24,25(OH)$_2$D].

24,25(OH)$_2$D is normally present in serum at a concentration of 1 to 10 nmol/L (0.5 to 5.0 ng/mL). 24,25(OH)$_2$D is also a substrate for renal 25(OH)D-1α-hydroxylase and is converted to 1α,24*R*,25-trihydroxyvitamin D [1,24,25(OH)$_3$D], which, in turn, is metabolized to the biologically inactive substance calcitroic acid (see Fig. 353-4). Cultured cells that possess nuclear receptors for 1,25(OH)$_2$D, such as chondrocytes, skin keratinocytes and fibroblasts, and intestinal and melanoma cells, also metabolize 25(OH)D to 24,25(OH)$_2$D. Although 24,25(OH)$_2$D may play a role in the expression of vitamin D action, it is more likely that the C_{24} hydroxylation is the first step in the degradation of both 25(OH)D and 1,25(OH)$_2$D to water-soluble inactive metabolites, including calcitroic acid; 25(OH)D and 1,25(OH)$_2$D are converted to more than 35 metabolites, most of which appear to be degradation products.

PHYSIOLOGY OF VITAMIN D 1,25(OH)$_2$D, produced by the kidney and the placenta, is the only known important metabolite of vitamin D; the potential roles of other metabolites have not been clarified. 1,25(OH)$_2$D bound to a vitamin D–binding protein is deliv-

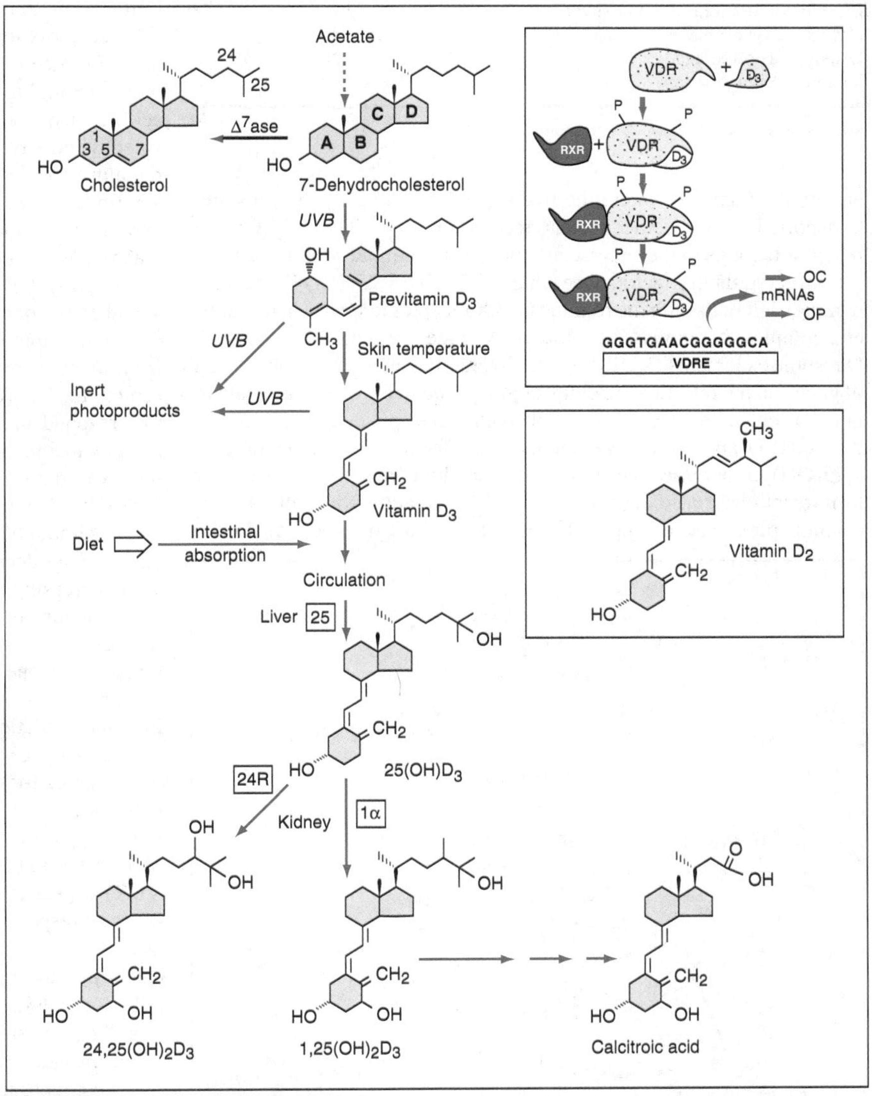

FIGURE 353-4 The photobiogenesis and metabolism of vitamin D. 7-Dehydrocholesterol either can be reduced by 7-dehydrocholesterol reductase (Δ^7ase) to cholesterol or photolyzed in the skin by solar ultraviolet B radiation (UVB) to previtamin D_3. Once formed, previtamin D_3 thermally isomerizes to vitamin D_3. Exposure of previtamin D_3 and vitamin D_3 to UVB radiation results in the generation of a variety of biologically inert photoproducts. Vitamin D_3 enters the circulation and is hydroxylated by the hepatic vitamin D-25-hydroxylase (step 25) to 25-hydroxyvitamin D_3, shown as 25(OH)D_3. 25-Hydroxyvitamin D_3 can be metabolized by a 25(OH)D-24-hydroxylase (step 24R) to 24,25-dihydroxyvitamin D_3, i.e., 24,25-(OH)$_2D_3$. 25-Hydroxyvitamin D_3 is converted in the kidney by the 25-OH-D-1α-hydroxylase (step 1α) to its biologically active form, 1,25-dihydroxyvitamin D_3, i.e., 1,25(OH)$_2D_3$. This form enters the circulation and is ultimately recognized by target tissues that possess a specific nuclear receptor (VDR) for it.

As shown in the top two inserts, the VDR, a member of the steroid superfamily of receptors, interacts with 1,25(OH)$_2D_3$ (identified as D_3), resulting in the phosphorylation of the 1,25(OH)$_2D_3$–VDR complex. This complex interacts with the retinoic acid X receptor (RXR) to form a heterodimer which, in turn, interacts with the vitamin D–responsive element (VDRE) in the targeted nuclei. In the bone, this interaction increases the expression of mRNAs for osteocalcin (OC) and osteopontin (OP).

1,25-Dihydroxyvitamin D_3 can undergo multiple hydroxylations in its side chain that may ultimately result in the formation of the water-soluble biologically inactive calcitroic acid.

The lower insert is the structure for vitamin D_2. It is structurally different from vitamin D_3 in having a double bond between C_{22} and C_{23} and a methyl group on C_{24}.

Table 353-1

Serum Concentrations of 25(OH)D in Disorders of Calcium, Phosphorus, and Bone Metabolism

Disease States	Serum 25(OH)D
Vitamin D deficiency	↓
Intestinal malabsorption syndromes	↓
Liver disorders (chronic and severe)	↓
Nephrotic syndrome	↓
Osteopenia in the aged	N or ↓
Vitamin D intoxication	↑

NOTE: ↓, decreased; N, normal; ↑, increased.

ered to the intestine, where the free form is taken up by the cells and transported to a specific nuclear receptor protein. The $1,25(OH)_2D$ receptor belongs to the superfamily of steroid-retinoid-vitamin D transcription regulatory factors (see Chap. 327). The $1,25(OH)_2D$-receptor complex interacts with the retinoic acid X receptor to form a heterodimeric complex that binds to specific DNA sequences, termed the vitamin D response elements (VDREs). This interaction alters the transcription of genes; in the intestine, calcium-binding protein is synthesized, and in bone, osteocalcin, osteopontin, and alkaline phosphatase are produced. $1,25(OH)_2D$ also may have nonnuclear effects on its target tissues; $1,25(OH)_2D$ increases the transport of calcium from the extracellular to intracellular space, and it can mobilize calcium from intracellular calcium pools and enhance phosphatidylinositol metabolism. In the

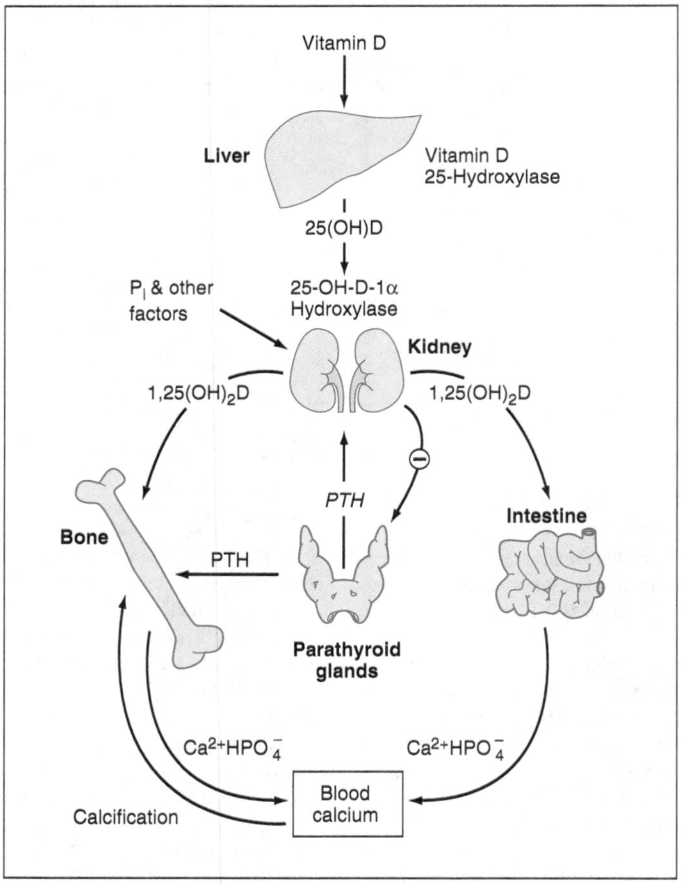

FIGURE 353-5 Schematic representation of the hormonal control loop for vitamin D metabolism and function. A reduction in the serum calcium below approximately 2.2 mmol/L (8.8 mg/dL) prompts a proportional increase in the secretion of PTH and so mobilizes additional calcium from the bone. PTH promotes the synthesis of $1,25(OH)_2D$ in the kidney, which, in turn, stimulates the mobilization of calcium from bone and intestine and regulates the synthesis of PTH by negative feedback.

intestine, the net effect of $1,25(OH)_2D$ is to stimulate calcium and phosphate transport from the lumen of the small intestine into the circulation (see Fig. 353-5). The effect of $1,25(OH)_2D$ on the enhancement of bone resorption is believed to be synergistic with that of PTH. Mature osteoclasts do not possess receptors either for PTH or for $1,25(OH)_2D$, and the two hormones may increase bone resorption activity by stimulating immature osteoclastic precursors that possess receptors for both to become mature osteoclasts and/or by interacting with osteoblasts and bone marrow stromal cells to produce cytokines that enhance the activity of mature osteoclasts. The role of $1,25(OH)_2D$ in the renal handling of calcium and phosphorus remains uncertain.

Receptors for $1,25(OH)_2D$ are present in intestine, bone, and kidney and in cells not classically considered target organs for this hormone, including skin, breast, pituitary, parathyroids, pancreatic beta cells, gonads, brain, skeletal muscle, circulating monocytes, and activated B and T lymphocytes. Although its physiologic role in these cells remains to be determined, in vitro, $1,25(OH)_2D$ inhibits proliferation of keratinocytes and fibroblasts, stimulates terminal differentiation of keratinocytes, induces monocytes to produce IL-1 and to mature into macrophages and osteoclast-like cells, inhibits the production of PTH, and inhibits the production of IL-2 and immunoglobulin by activated T and B lymphocytes, respectively.

In addition, a variety of tumor cell lines, including lines derived from breast carcinomas, melanomas, and promyeloblasts, possess receptors for $1,25(OH)_2D$. Tumor cell lines that have $1,25(OH)_2D$ receptors respond to the hormone by decreasing the rate of proliferation and enhancing differentiation. For example, when malignant receptor-positive human promyelocytic cells (HL-60) are exposed to $1,25(OH)_2D$, the cells mature into functioning macrophages within 1 week. Although the mechanism of induction of maturation is unknown, $1,25(OH)_2D$ decreases the expression of c-*myc* oncogene coincident with decreasing replication. This effect, however, is not a lasting one; when the metabolite is removed from maturing HL-60 promyelocytes, the cells revert to their original malignant state, and expression of c-*myc* oncogene is no longer suppressed.

The role of $1,25(OH)_2D$ in the regulation of differentiation and immunoregulation is also unknown. However, it may regulate PTH synthesis by negative feedback (see Fig. 353-5). This possibility is the rationale for giving $1,25(OH)_2D_3$ intravenously to suppress PTH in patients with chronic renal failure. Patients with vitamin D–dependent rickets type II who are unable to respond to physiologic concentrations of $1,25(OH)_2D$ (because of mutations that impair the function of the VDR) appear to have no demonstrable in vivo defects in the cellular immune response and in the growth of skin (with the exception of the associated alopecia) and other tissues. Administration of intravenous calcium infusions to these patients reverses the metabolic bone disease. Although calcitriol [$1,25(OH)_2D$] is not useful for the treatment of leukemia, the antiproliferative effects of calcitriol and its analogue calcipotriene provide the rationale for their use in the treatment of psoriasis.

Most measurements of circulating $1,25(OH)_2D$ in various physiologic or pathologic states utilize a receptor/competitive binding assay (Table 353-2). Serum levels of vitamin D and 25(OH)D vary with the season and with vitamin D intake, whereas levels of $1,25(OH)_2D$ appear to be unaltered by seasonal variation, by increases in dietary vitamin D, or by exposure to sunlight (Table 353-2); as long as vitamin D supplies and circulating concentrations of 25(OH)D are sufficient, metabolic influences control the renal 25(OH)D-1α-hydroxylase to ensure a closely regulated circulating concentration of $1,25(OH)_2D$. The serum concentration of $1,25(OH)_2D$ ranges from 40 to 160 pmol/L (16 to 65 pg/mL), and its serum half-life is from 3 to 6 h.

The principal physiologic mechanism regulating the production of $1,25(OH)_2D$ appears to involve changes in serum extracellular calcium concentrations that result in reciprocal changes in secretion of PTH, the latter controlling, possibly through actions on serum or tissue phosphorus levels, the rate of $1,25(OH)_2D$ production. Other factors that enhance $1,25(OH)_2D$ production include estrogen, prolactin, and growth hormone. Humans adapt to increased calcium requirements during growth, pregnancy, and lactation by increasing the efficiency of intestinal calcium absorption, possibly by enhancing 25(OH)D-1-

Table 353-2

Serum Concentrations of $1,25(OH)_2D$ in Disorders of Calcium, Phosphorus, and Bone Metabolism

Disease States	Serum $1,25(OH)_2D$
Vitamin D deficiency	↓*
Renal failure:	
GFR > 30 (mL/min)/1.7 m^2	↓ or N
GFR < 30 (mL/min)/1.7 m^2	↓
Hypoparathyroidism	↓ or N
Pseudohypoparathyroidism	↓ or N
Vitamin D–dependent rickets:	
Type I	↓
Type II	↑
X-linked vitamin D–resistant rickets	↓ or N
Tumor-induced osteomalacia	↓
Oncogenic hypercalcemia	↓
Some lymphomas	↑
Hyperparathyroidism	↑
Sarcoidosis, tuberculosis, silicosis	↑
Idiopathic hypercalciuria	N or ↑
Williams' syndrome	↑
Vitamin D intoxication	N or ↑

* Serum $1,25(OH)_2D$ concentrations are normal or elevated in occasional patients with biopsy-proven osteomalacia and undetectable or low circulating concentrations of 25(OH)D. These patients also have secondary hyperparathyroidism, and they may represent a partially treated state; if a small amount of vitamin D is obtained from the diet or generated in the skin in these patients, the vitamin is efficiently converted to $1,25(OH)_2D$. The net effect is low or undetectable circulating concentrations of 25(OH)D along with normal or elevated concentrations of $1,25(OH)_2D$. However, in extreme vitamin D deficiency, circulating concentrations of $1,25(OH)_2D$ are low or undetectable.

NOTE: ↓, decreased; N, normal; ↑, increased; GFR, glomerular filtration rate.

hydroxylase activity. During the first two trimesters of pregnancy, the levels of $1,25(OH)_2D$ increase in proportion to the concentration of the vitamin D–binding protein; levels of free $1,25(OH)_2D$ do not change. During the last trimester, the need for calcium for mineralization of the fetal skeleton is met by an increase in the concentrations of free $1,25(OH)_2D$ and enhanced maternal intestinal calcium absorption.

PATHOPHYSIOLOGY OF DISORDERS OF VITAMIN D NUTRITION AND METABOLISM *Hypovitaminosis D* results from inadequate endogenous production of vitamin D_3 in the skin, from insufficient dietary supplementation, and/or from an inability of the small intestine to absorb adequate amounts of the vitamin from the diet. Resistance to the effects of vitamin D can result from (1) use of drugs that antagonize vitamin D action, (2) alterations in the metabolism of vitamin D, or (3) deficient or defective receptors for $1,25(OH)_2D$. The consequences of hypovitaminosis D include (1) disturbances of mineral ion metabolism and secretion of PTH and (2) mineralization defects in the skeleton (e.g., rickets in children, osteomalacia in adults). The changes in the skeleton are described in Chap. 355. With regard to calcium metabolism, lack of vitamin D action leads to insufficient intestinal calcium absorption and hypocalcemia. The latter stimulates the secretion of PTH (secondary hyperparathyroidism), which enhances calcium release from bone and decreases calcium clearance by the kidney and tends to blunt the hypocalcemia; as a consequence most patients have a normal or low-normal serum calcium level. (Late in the course of untreated hypovitaminosis D, severe hypocalcemia develops.) Hypophosphatemia is more marked than hypocalcemia, especially in early stages of the deficiency. The efficiency of intestinal phosphate absorption is also decreased. The increased secretion of PTH, although partially effective in minimizing hypocalcemia, leads to urinary phosphate wasting through decreases in renal tubular reabsorption. This latter effect is the most significant factor in causing hypophosphatemia. With an adequate GFR, the main changes are hypophosphatemia, normal or near-normal serum calcium levels, increased levels of PTH, and low levels of 25(OH)D (see Table 353-1). As discussed in Chap. 355, defects in skeletal mineralization may accompany these disturbances in mineral ion metabolism.

Although the conversion of vitamin D to 25(OH)D is impaired in severe chronic liver disease, there is no strong correlation between low serum 25(OH)D levels and osteopenia. Patients with nephrotic syndrome with more than 4 g/d of proteinuria may have low 25(OH)D levels owing to loss in the urine of the vitamin D–binding protein with its associated tightly bound 25(OH)D. Circulating levels of 25(OH)D also may be decreased when the metabolism of 25(OH)D to $1,25(OH)_2D$ is increased, as in sarcoidosis and hyperparathyroidism. Chronic anticonvulsant therapy also can cause the development of osteomalacia or rickets; mineralization defects are worse in patients receiving multiple drug therapy and when vitamin D intake or exposure to sunlight is inadequate. Anticonvulsant drugs have multiple effects on calcium metabolism. Phenobarbital induces hepatic microsomal enzymes, alters the kinetics of the vitamin D-25-hydroxylase, and stimulates bile secretion, resulting in decreased serum concentrations of vitamin D and 25(OH)D. Phenytoin and phenobarbital inhibit intestinal calcium transport and bone mineral mobilization, independent of effects of vitamin D metabolism.

Glucocorticoids in high doses cause osteoporosis but do not induce osteomalacia and rickets. Glucocorticoids directly inhibit vitamin D–mediated intestinal calcium absorption and bone mineral mobilization and enhance the sensitivity of bone cells to $1,25(OH)_2D$ by stabilizing the $1,25(OH)_2D$ receptor or by increasing the affinity or number of receptors. Patients receiving glucocorticoids chronically may have depressed circulating levels of $1,25(OH)_2D$; the mechanism(s) is unknown.

A genetic defect in the hepatic 25-hydroxylation of vitamin D has not been described, but in one inherited disorder of calcium and bone metabolism renal production of $1,25(OH)_2D$ is defective. In the syndrome of pseudovitamin D–deficient rickets (also known as vitamin D–dependent rickets type I; see Chap. 355), renal production of $1,25(OH)_2D$ is impaired, circulating levels of $1,25(OH)_2D$ are low, but the therapeutic response to physiologic doses of calcitriol (0.25 to 1.0 μg/d) is normal. These findings are accounted for by a deficiency in renal 25(OH)D-1α-hydroxylase activity. In patients with a similar phenotype, pseudovitamin D–resistant rickets (vitamin D–dependent rickets type II), mutations impair the function of the $1,25(OH)_2D$ receptor by altering the binding of the hormone to the receptor or the binding of the hormone-heterodimer complex to DNA. Individuals with this disorder have high circulating levels of $1,25(OH)_2D$; administration of high doses of vitamin D produces further increases in the levels of $1,25(OH)_2D$.

In patients with X-linked hypophosphatemic rickets, serum concentrations of $1,25(OH)_2D$ are normal or low. Since hypophosphatemia is a potent stimulator of the renal 25(OH)D-1α-hydroxylase, levels of $1,25(OH)_2D$ should be high. In this syndrome there is a functional defect in the 25(OH)D-1-hydrolase. Therefore, the combination of calcitriol and phosphate supplements is more effective than therapy with phosphate supplements alone (Chap. 355). In patients with mild to moderate chronic renal failure [GFR > 0.5 mL/s (> 30 mL/min)] and decreased phosphate clearance, hyperphosphatemia and acidosis play important roles in suppressing the renal production of $1,25(OH)_2D$ despite high circulating concentrations of PTH. With progressive destruction of the renal cortex, the reserves of the 25(OH)D-1α-hydroxylase are depleted to a point at which the kidney is unable to produce sufficient $1,25(OH)_2D$ to maintain calcium homeostasis, even when serum phosphorus concentrations are normal. Under these circumstances, replacement therapy with calcitriol is most beneficial (Chap. 355). Aging decreases the responsiveness of the renal 25(OH)D-1-hydroxylase to PTH, results in small decreases in circulating levels of $1,25(OH)_2D$, and may contribute to decreased calcium absorption in the elderly.

Patients with hypocalcemia due to hypoparathyroidism or pseudohypoparathyroidism have lower-than-normal mean serum concentrations of $1,25(OH)_2D$, although individual values may be in the normal range. In these patients, small replacement doses of calcitriol (0.25 to 1.0 μg/d; see Chap. 354) are effective even when the serum 25(OH)D concentrations are elevated. These observations suggest that absent or ineffective action of PTH decreases the activity of renal 25(OH)D-1-

hydroxylase. It is not known whether serum 1,25$(OH)_2$D levels would be restored if the hyperphosphatemia were controlled.

Patients with tumor-induced (oncogenic) osteomalacia have low levels of serum phosphorus and 1,25$(OH)_2$D. These tumors presumably secrete a substance(s) that causes renal phosphorus wasting and inhibits the synthesis of 1,25$(OH)_2$D; after removal of the tumor, the serum phosphorus and 1,25$(OH)_2$D levels return to normal.

In disorders such as sarcoidosis (and other chronic granulomatous disorders), lymphomas, idiopathic hypercalciuria, and Williams' syndrome there is enhanced synthesis of 1,25$(OH)_2$D from 25(OH)D (see Table 353-2). Hypercalcemia and hypercalciuria in sarcoidosis are associated with elevated circulating concentrations of 1,25$(OH)_2$D; granulomas and pulmonary alveolar macrophages from patients with sarcoidosis synthesize 1,25$(OH)_2$D. Normal pulmonary macrophages also can be induced to metabolize 25(OH)D to 1,25$(OH)_2$D in vitro when exposed to lipopolysaccharides from the cell wall of gram-negative bacteria or to interferon γ. Most patients with tumor-induced hypercalcemia have low circulating levels of 1,25$(OH)_2$D (see Table 353-2). The exceptions are patients with several types of lymphoma (including T cell, mixed histiocytic-lymphocytic, and B cell immunoblastic lymphomas) where hypercalcemia is associated with elevated concentrations of 1,25$(OH)_2$D. In one report, surgical excision of a solitary splenic lymphoma resulted in rapid return of elevated serum 1,25$(OH)_2$D and calcium levels to normal, suggesting that the lymphoma metabolized 25(OH)D to 1,25$(OH)_2$D in an unregulated manner. Patients with hypercalcemia and elevated blood levels of 1,25$(OH)_2$D due to unregulated extrarenal production of the hormone respond to glucocorticoids with a decrease in the circulating concentrations of 1,25$(OH)_2$D and calcium. Patients with primary hyperparathyroidisim, hypercalciuria, and renal stones usually have elevated circulating levels of 1,25$(OH)_2$D. Similarly, in some instances of idiopathic hypercalciuria, intestinal calcium absorption is increased inappropriately. Approximately one-third of these patients have high-normal or elevated circulating 1,25$(OH)_2$D. These findings are consistent with the hypothesis that excessive 1,25$(OH)_2$D production is responsible for the hyperabsorption of calcium by the small intestine. Infants with hypercalcemia associated with supravalvular aortic stenosis, mental retardation, and elfin facies (*Williams' syndrome*) also have elevated serum concentrations of 1,25$(OH)_2$D. It is not clear whether the increased levels result from abnormal synthesis or degradation of 1,25$(OH)_2$D.

It has been suggested that alteration of vitamin D receptor levels in target tissues (such as intestine) could affect calcium and bone metabolism, and bone mineral density appears to be associated with specific polymorphism of the VDR gene. These polymorphisms affect the noncoding intervening DNA sequences (introns) or the coding sequence in a way that does not alter the amino acid sequence of the VDR; specifically, polymorphisms involving the endonucleases Bsm-I and Taq-I (bb, TT) have been associated with higher bone mineral density.

PHARMACOLOGY AND SOURCES OF VITAMIN D AND ITS METABOLITES Casual exposure to sunlight provides most humans with their vitamin D requirement. For the elderly who wish to take advantage of this natural source of vitamin D, exposure of hands, face, and arms to a suberythemal dose of sunlight two to three times a week is usually adequate. If the patient plans to remain outdoors in sunlight after the initial exposure, a sunscreen with a protection factor of at least 15 (SPF-15) should be applied to help prevent the damaging effects caused by excessive chronic overexposure to sunlight. A variety of over-the-counter vitamin preparations contain 400 IU of either vitamin D_2 or vitamin D_3. More potent preparations of vitamin D (calciferol) are available in capsule and tablet form (50,000 IU), as oil (500,000 IU/mL), and in oral solution (8000 IU/mL). A single oral dose of 50,000 IU of vitamin D_2 increases the circulating concentrations of vitamin D from less than 25 nmol/L (10 ng/mL) to 130 to 260 nmol/L (50 to 100 ng/mL) within 12 to 24 h; the plasma half-life is about 2 d. Serum concentrations of 25(OH)D and 1,25$(OH)_2$D are not changed by these doses of vitamin D. For treatment of vitamin D deficiency, 50,000 IU of vitamin D once a week for 8 weeks raises the circulating concentration of 25(OH)D into the normal range; in the presence of secondary hyperparathyroidism, the circulating concentrations of 1,25$(OH)_2$D can increase to supranormal levels [up to 600 pmol/L (250 pg/mL)]. 25(OH)D_2 (calcifediol) is available in capsules containing either 20 or 50 μg. This drug may be useful in treating vitamin D deficiency [low 25(OH)D concentrations] in patients with severe liver dysfunction. Pharmacologic doses are used to treat disorders of 25(OH)D metabolism; in pharmacologic doses, 25(OH)D_3 is believed to act via interaction with the VDR. Calcitriol is available in capsules containing 0.25 or 0.5 μg and as a solution for intravenous use (1.0 and 2.0 μg/mL). Calcitriol is efficacious in a variety of disorders (see Chap. 354). 1α-Hydroxyvitamin D_3 [1(OH)D_3] is a potent 1,25$(OH)_2D_3$ agonist that is used in Europe and Japan. The structure of this analogue is identical to that of the natural renal hormone with the exception that it lacks a C_{25} OH (Fig. 353-6). In humans, this analogue is rapidly metabolized by the liver to 1,25$(OH)_2D_3$. Topical preparations of calcitriol (3 μg/g) in Europe and calcipotriene (50 μg/g) in Europe and the United States are used for the treatment of psoriasis. When used over a large surface area, both potentially could cause hypercalcemia and hypercalciuria. Oral calcitriol is also effective for psoriasis and psoriatic arthritis.

When vitamin D is chemically manipulated to rotate the A ring through 180 degrees, the C_3 β-OH assumes a geometric position that mimics the C_1 α-OH (see Fig. 353-6). These compounds, called *pseudo-1α-hydroxyvitamin D analogues*, include the clinically useful dihydrotachysterol (DHT). This analogue is less effective in stimulating intestinal calcium transport on a weight basis than either vitamin

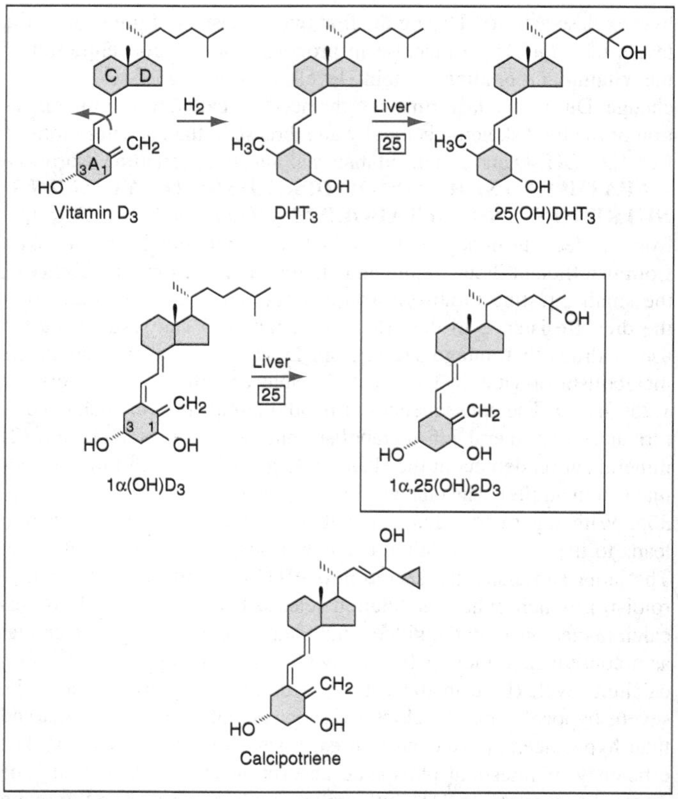

FIGURE 353-6 Structure of 1,25-dihydroxyvitamin D_3, i.e., 1α,25$(OH)_2D_3$, and some of its clinically important analogues. When vitamin D_3 is hydrogenated, its A ring is rotated 180°, placing the 3β-OH in a pseudo 1α spatial orientation. This analogue, dihydrotachysterol (DHT_3) is metabolized by a liver 25-hydroxylase (step 25) to 25-hydroxydihydrotachysterol, i.e., 25(OH)DHT_3. It is believed that 25(OH)DHT_3 is the biologically active form that mimics 1,25$(OH)_2D_3$ in its activity. Two clinically important analogues of 1α,25$(OH)_2D_3$ include its 25-deoxy derivative 1α-hydroxyvitamin D_3, i.e., 1α(OH)D_3, and calcipotriene. 1α(OH)D_3 is metabolized in the liver by 25-hydroxylase to 1α,25(OH)D_3. Calcipotriene is an analogue that is currently being used in Europe for the topical treatment of psoriasis.

D or 1,25$(OH)_2$D, but because it does not require 1-hydroxylation to be active on intestinal calcium transport, it is 3 to 10 times more potent than vitamin D in disease states that impair renal 25(OH)D-1-hydroxylase, such as hypoparathyroidism and chronic renal failure. Dihydrotachysterol is efficiently metabolized in the liver to 25-hydroxy-DHT, which is the biologically active form.

PARATHYROID HORMONE **Physiology** The function of PTH is to maintain the ECF calcium concentration. The hormone acts directly on bone and kidney and indirectly on intestine through its effects on synthesis of 1,25$(OH)_2$D to increase serum calcium concentrations; in turn, PTH production is closely regulated by the concentration of serum ionized calcium. This feedback system is the critical homeostatic mechanism for maintenance of ECF calcium. Any tendency toward hypocalcemia, as might be induced by calcium-deficient diets, is counteracted by an increased secretion of PTH. This in turn (1) acts to increase the rate of dissolution of bone mineral, thereby increasing the flow of calcium from bone into blood; (2) reduces the renal clearance of calcium, returning more of the calcium filtered at the glomerulus into ECF; and (3) increases the efficiency of calcium absorption in the intestine. The relative physiologic importance in minute-to-minute calcium homeostasis of stimulation of calcium transport in bone, kidney, and intestine is not established, but immediate control of blood calcium is probably due to effects of the hormone on bone and, to a lesser extent, on renal calcium clearance. Maintenance of steady-state calcium balance, on the other hand, probably results from the effects of the hormone on 1,25$(OH)_2$D levels and hence on the efficiency of intestinal calcium absorption. As much as 12 mmol (500 mg) calcium is transferred between the ECF and bone each day (a large amount in relation to the total ECF calcium pool), and PTH has a major effect on this transfer. The homeostatic role of the hormone serves to preserve calcium concentration in blood acutely at the cost of bone destruction. The action of PTH on kidney to increase the reabsorption of filtered calcium also may contribute to rapid regulation of blood calcium concentration.

PTH has multiple actions on bone, some direct and some indirect. There is an increased rate of release of calcium from bone into blood after administration of PTH, the time needed to observe the change varying with the dose of hormone and the overall metabolic status (influenced by age, diet, etc.). Usually 30 min to 1 h is required to detect a significant increase in blood calcium, but with the use of radioisotopes, changes in bone calcium release can be seen within minutes. When the phenomenon is studied carefully, there is even a rapid efflux of calcium out of blood into bone, presumably into bone cells, that precedes the release of calcium from bone. The chronic effects of PTH cause an increase in the number of bone cells, especially osteoclasts, and an increase in the remodeling of bone; these effects are apparent within hours after the hormone is given and persist for hours after PTH is withdrawn. Continuous exposure to elevated levels of PTH for days (as in hyperparathyroidism or the long-term infusions in animals) leads to osteoclast-mediated bone resorption. However, the administration of PTH intermittently over days in animals leads to a net stimulation of bone formation rather than bone breakdown. Studies in humans confirm that chronic *intermittent* hormone administration can lead to anabolic actions in skeleton rather than merely increased turnover. This skeletal anabolic action of PTH is being evaluated in clinical trials (see Chap. 355). Osteoblasts are thought to be crucial to this bone-forming effect of PTH, and osteoclasts are thought to mediate bone breakdown. Osteoblasts, which have PTH receptors, stimulate osteoclasts indirectly. Osteoclasts are believed to lack PTH receptors.

The action of PTH on osteoclasts is believed to be indirect, through cytokines released from osteoblasts to activate osteoclasts; in experimental studies of bone resorption in vitro osteoblasts must be present along with osteoclasts for PTH to activate osteoclasts to resorb bone. The nature of the cytokines that stimulate osteoclasts is a subject of major interest. IGF-1, interleukin-6, granulocyte-macrophage colony stimulating factor (GM-CSF), and possibly other agents are candidates, but the definitive messenger(s) has not been determined.

Chemistry The complete amino acid sequences of PTH from cow, pig, rat, and human have been defined. The peptides consist of a single-chain structure composed of 84 amino acids. The molecules lack cysteine or cystine; the sequences of the four forms of the hormone are similar. The sequence of chicken PTH has been deduced from the nucleotide sequence of the cloned cDNA. This molecule differs from the mammalian hormones. One large sequence deletion in the middle of the molecule and a larger addition near the carboxyl terminus result in a molecule of 88 rather than 84 amino acids. There is, however, marked conservation in the amino-terminal portion needed for biologic actions of the molecule.

Some structural requirements for the binding of the hormone to receptors and hence for its biologic activity have been defined. Synthetic fragments containing the amino-terminal sequence residues 1–34 (or even shorter sequences, 2–26 being minimally active) exert the known biologic actions of the hormone on mineral ion transport in kidney and bone and, by stimulating the renal 25-hydroxyvitamin D-1α-hydroxylase, stimulate intestinal calcium absorption. The biologic role of the carboxyl-terminal region of PTH is under investigation; a separate receptor may exist for this region of the molecule.

Fragments shortened at the amino terminus bind to the PTH receptor but have lost the capacity to stimulate biologic response. The peptide composed of sequences 7–34 is a competitive inhibitor of the binding of active hormone to receptors in vitro but is a weak inhibitor in vivo.

Biosynthesis, Secretion, and Metabolism and Mode of Action Several larger molecular forms have been identified in the biosynthetic sequence leading from gene transcription and translation to final packaging of the 84-amino-acid peptide in secretory granules prior to secretion. The earliest detected precursor, *preproparathyroid hormone*, consists of 115 amino acids; this molecular form is converted to an intermediate form of 90 amino acids termed *proparathyroid hormone* and then to the secreted product of 84 amino acids, PTH. PTH shares with other polypeptides and proteins destined for secretion from cells this complex pattern of initial synthesis as a larger molecule, which is then reduced in size by several cleavages prior to secretion; there is close analogy with the regulatory steps in biosynthesis, transport, and packaging of other proteins destined for secretion. The hydrophobic regions of the preproparathyroid hormone are similar to preprotein-specific regions of other cell-secreted proteins and serve a role in guiding transport of the polypeptide from sites of synthesis on polyribosomes through the endoplasmic reticulum to secretory granules. The degree and nature of the regulation of these sequential steps in PTH biosynthesis is poorly understood. In one kindred with hypoparathyroidism, a mutation in the preprotein region of the gene disrupts the critical hydrophobic sequence and interferes with hormone secretion.

The genes for bovine, rat, and human PTH have been cloned, and the gene structures from these three species are highly homologous. Studies with cloned and expressed PTH genes in vitro have demonstrated regions for control of gene expression at the transcriptional level, including sites for interaction and regulation by 1,25$(OH)_2$D and its receptor and "upstream" silencer elements as well as sites in which ambient calcium concentration regulates transcription. These in vitro observations are not well understood in terms of physiologic regulation of PTH biosynthesis and secretion; the rate of processing of hormone precursors and the proteolytic destruction and turnover of the hormone itself (posttranslational regulation of hormone production) may be more central to hormone availability than changes in rates of transcription. It does not appear that changes in transcriptional activity of the PTH gene in the normal physiologic range of levels of blood calcium and 1,25$(OH)_2$D nor in short-term environmental stresses (e.g., fasting for 24 h) are important in control of blood levels of the hormone. Control over hormone stores is exerted by variation in the rates of proteolytic destruction of preformed hormone under the control of ECF calcium; high calcium increases and low calcium inhibits the proteolytic destruction of hormone stores.

Blood calcium concentration over wide ranges controls the secretion of PTH; the ionized fraction of blood calcium is the important determinant of hormone secretion. Hormone secretion increases steeply to a maximum value of five times the basal rate of secretion as calcium concentration falls from normal to the range of 1.9 to 2.0 mmol/L (7.5 to 8.0 mg/dL) (measured as total calcium). Beta-adrenergic agonists such as epinephrine and H_2 agonists also may increase hormone secretion, but the physiologic significance of these secretagogues is not established. Furthermore, drugs such as propranolol or cimetidine do not reproducibly decrease circulating PTH levels.

Magnesium may influence hormone secretion in the same direction as calcium but is a less potent secretagogue. It is unlikely that physiologic variations in magnesium concentration affect PTH secretion, but severe intracellular magnesium deficiency impairs PTH secretion.

ECF calcium level controls PTH secretion by interaction with a calcium sensor, a G protein–linked receptor for which Ca^{2+} ions act as the ligand. Stimulation of the receptor by high calcium levels leads to a suppression of the rate of PTH secretion via intracellular signals generated by the active receptor. The intracellular signals appear to be inositol triphosphate and diacylglycerol formed by activation of phospholipase by the calcium sensor. This receptor is a member of a subfamily of the G protein receptor superfamily that is characterized by a large extracellular domain suitable for "clamping" the small-molecule ligand. The receptor is present in parathyroid glands, the calcitonin-secreting cells (C cells) of the thyroid, brain, and kidney. The biologic role of the receptor in tissues other than the parathyroid gland is not known. As discussed in Chap. 354, the physiologic role of the calcium sensor as the mediator of the response of the gland was substantiated by demonstrating that point mutations that impair function of the receptor lead to distinctive phenotypes, hyperparathyroidism or hypoparathyroidism.

The hormone secreted in vivo by normal bovine and human parathyroid glands and from parathyroid adenomas is indistinguishable by immunologic criteria and by molecular size from the 84-amino-acid peptide (molecular weight 9500) extracted from glands. However, much of the immunoreactive material found in the circulation of humans and animals (cow, dog) is smaller than the extracted or secreted hormone. The principal circulating fragments of immunoreactive hormone (approximate molecular weight 7000) lack a portion of the critical amino-terminal sequence required for biologic activity and, hence, may be biologically inactive fragments (so-called middle- and carboxyl-terminal fragments). Study of these fragments suggests that an endopeptidase cleaves the molecule into at least two types of pieces. Much of the proteolysis of hormone occurs in the liver and kidney.

The proteolytic process should result in formation of a second fragment (molecular weight 2000 to 3000) representing the amino-terminal, biologically active portion of the hormone. Hormone fragments as well as intact hormone are also released from the gland. However, fragments corresponding only to the middle- and carboxyl-terminal portions have been detected so far in effluent blood. If biologically active fragments do actually survive hormone proteolysis within the gland or in peripheral sites, such amino-terminal fragments could be alternative active hormonal species. After much study, certain conclusions can be drawn. There is no convincing evidence for circulating amino-terminal fragments. Circulating biologically active fragments are also not detected after analysis of products produced by peripheral metabolism. Peripheral metabolism of PTH does not appear to be regulated by physiologic states (high versus low calcium, etc.); hence peripheral metabolism of hormone, although responsible for rapid clearance of secreted hormone, appears to be a high-capacity, metabolically invariant catabolic process.

The rate of clearance of the secreted 84-amino-acid peptide from blood is more rapid than the rate of clearance of the biologically inactive fragment(s) corresponding to the middle- and carboxyl-terminal regions of the molecules that result from peripheral metabolism or glandular secretion. Hence measurements of PTH in blood by most earlier immunoassays provided only an overall index of parathyroid gland activity rather than a direct measure of biologically active hormone. Changes in the rate of production or clearance of fragments can change the concentration of immunoreactive hormone without influencing the rate of hormone secretion. Such discordance between concentrations of immunoreactive hormone and biologically active peptide occurs, for example, in renal failure, since the kidney seems to be the principal route of excretion of inactive hormone fragments. The problems inherent in accurate measurements of PTH in blood due to the heterogeneity of circulating forms of the molecule are circumvented by use of double-antibody assays that detect only the intact molecule. → *This is discussed in Chap. 354).*

Parathyroid Hormone–Related Protein The hormone termed parathyroid hormone–related protein (PTHrP) is responsible for hypercalcemia in cancer patients, a syndrome that resembles hyperparathyroidism. This hormone, now appreciated to be principally a paracrine or autocrine factor, plays a role both in fetal development and in adult physiology. Many different cell types produce PTHrP, including brain, pancreas, heart, lung, mammary tissue, placenta, endothelial cells, and smooth muscle.

PTH and PTHrP, although distinctive proteins and products of different genes, share considerable functional and structural homology (Fig. 353-7) and may have evolved from an ancestral gene. The structure of the gene for human PTHrP, however, is more complex than that of PTH, containing multiple exons and multiple sites for alternate splicing patterns during formation of the messenger RNA. Protein products of 141, 139, and 173 amino acids are produced. The varying molecular forms have multiple potential internal cleavage sites, and the biologic roles of these various molecular species and the nature of the circulating forms of PTHrP are unclear. The assays currently available are based on a variety of immunologic methods. Furthermore, multiple PTHrP products are synthesized, and other molecular forms

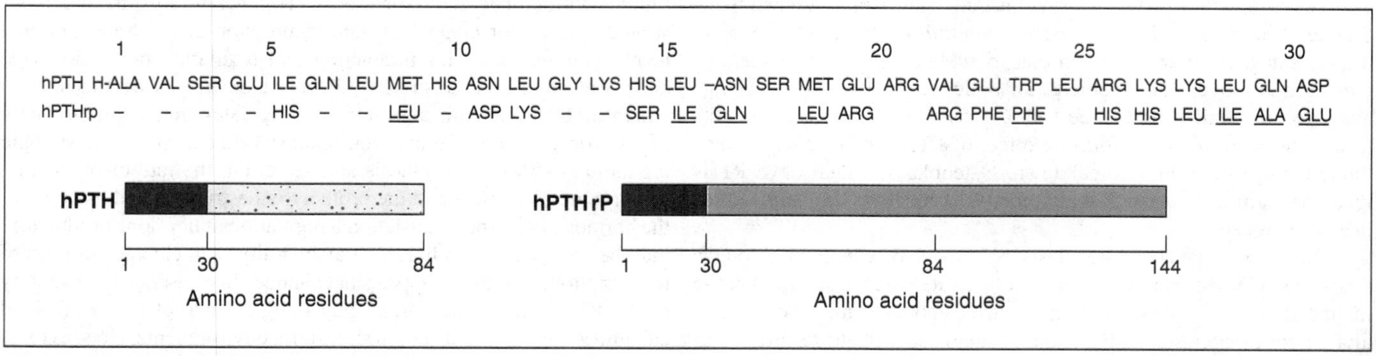

FIGURE 353-7 Schematic diagram to illustrate similarities and differences in structure of human PTH and human PTHrP. Close structural (and functional) homology exists between the first 30 amino acids of hPTH and hPTHrP. The PTHrP sequence may be 144 amino acid residues in length or longer. PTH is only 84 residues long; after residue 30, there is little structural homology between the two. Dashed lines in the PTHrP sequence indicate homology; underlined residues, although different from those of PTH, still represent conservative changes (charge or polarity preserved). Eleven amino acids are identical, and a total of 21 of 30 are homologues.

may result from tissue-specific degradation at accessible internal cleavage sites. In fact, it is uncertain whether PTHrP circulates at all in normal human adults; as a paracrine factor, PTHrP may be produced, act within, and be destroyed locally within tissues.

In adults PTHrP may have little to do with calcium homeostasis, except in disease states (Chap. 354), when large tumors, especially of the squamous cell type, lead to massive overproduction of PTHrP, which then circulates. PTHrP (see Fig. 353-7) shares a significant homology with PTH in the critical amino terminus that allows it to bind to the PTH receptor; synthetic molecules corresponding to the first 34 amino acids of PTHrP bind to and activate the PTH receptor indistinguishably from effects seen with PTH.

PTHrP exerts important developmental influences in calcium and bone biology. Homozygous knockout of the PTHrP gene in mice causes a lethal deformity in which animals are born with severe skeletal deformities resembling chondrodysplasia. In fetal animals, PTHrP directs transplacental calcium transfer, and high concentrations of PTHrP are produced in mammary tissue and secreted into milk. Human and bovine milk, for example, contain very high concentrations of the hormone. The biologic significance of the latter is unknown. PTHrP also may play a role in uterine contraction.

Hormone Action The action of PTH at the biochemical level involves receptor-mediated effects on second messengers in target cells. Stimulation of enzyme activity (adenyl cyclase, phospholipase C) during hormone–target cell membrane interaction leads to an increase in second messengers, including intracellular cyclic AMP, products of polyphosphoinositol metabolism, and transmembrane and intracellular fluxes of calcium. PTH interacts with a specific receptor/adenylate cyclase complex on plasma membranes of target cells consisting of hormone receptor, enzyme catalytic unit (adenylate cyclase), and a guanyl nucleotide (GTP or GDP)–binding regulatory protein (G protein). The latter protein consists of α subunits that bind GTP and dissociate from the remainder of the G protein complex. The α subunit with bound GTP complexes with adenylate cyclase, thereby activating the enzyme to increase the rate of cyclic AMP production from ATP. Hydrolysis of the GTP to GDP on the α subunit leads to reassociation of the G units and reduction in adenylate cyclase activity. The receptor, when activated by hormone binding, drives the G protein cycle by binding the α subunit portion and catalyzing the GDP/GTP exchange. Other G proteins link hormone action to phospholipase C; rapid changes in intracellular calcium concentrations within cells may be independent of phospholipase C stimulation.

The multiplicity of PTH actions on target cells in kidney and bone and the variety of second messengers—cyclic AMP, inositol 1,4,5-triphosphate (IP_3), diacylglycerol (DAG), and Ca^{2+}—raise obvious questions as to the mechanism whereby specific responses are mediated. With many other hormonal systems, different receptor subtypes modulate different hormone responses.

However, only one species of PTH receptor (PTH2 receptor) has been detected so far in PTH target cells in kidney and bone in human, rat, and other animal species; studies involving the cloned PTH receptor indicate that a single PTH receptor (Fig. 353-8*B*) can be coupled to more than one G protein second-messenger kinase pathway. The receptors for PTH and calcitonin (the two receptors share close homology) are polypeptides of 500 to 600 amino acids. These receptors belong to a family of structurally related receptors that includes those for glucagon, secretin, and vasoactive intestinal peptide. Receptors of this type share limited amino acid sequence homology (Fig. 353-9) but no sequence homology with other membrane receptors. The primary amino acid sequence predicts the structures illustrated in Fig. 356-9: an extracellular domain, seven hydrophobic membrane-spanning domains connected by three extracellular and three intracellular loops, and a carboxyl-terminal intracellular domain. The extracellular regions are involved in hormone binding, and the intracellular domains, after hormone activation, bind G protein subunits to transduce hormone signaling into cellular responses through stimulation of second messengers by activated G protein subunits.

A second PTH receptor (PTH2 receptor) is expressed in brain. Its amino acid sequence and the pattern of its binding and stimulatory

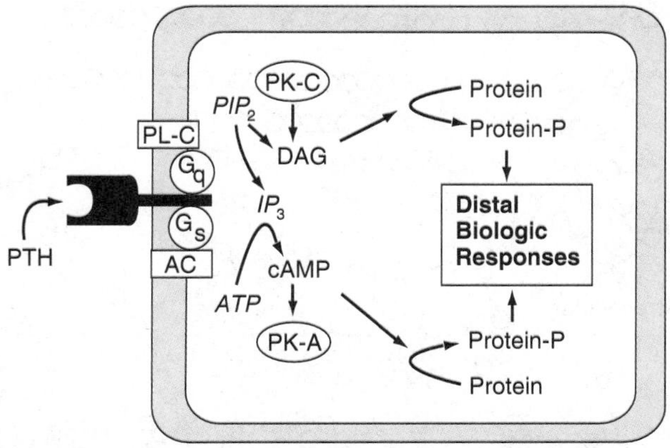

FIGURE 353-8 Schematic model of PTH action. Only one PTH receptor has been identified in bone and kidney. Different G proteins—G_s, G_q, etc.—activate a cellular second messenger pathway involving either an effect on adenyl cyclase (AC) to enhance cyclic AMP (cAMP) or phospholipase C (PL-C) activation of diacylglycerol (DAG) and inositol triphosphate (IP_3). These second messengers then activate protein kinase A (PK-A) or protein kinase C (PK-C). Phosphorylation of specific proteins mostly still unidentified leads to distal biologic responses. Cellular specificity or other factors, such as hormone levels, receptor expression levels, must determine which pathway is activated predominantly in a given cell type. Although only one form of receptor appears to be present in kidney and bone, another receptor (PTH2 receptor) has been described in brain, and others may exist.

response to PTH and PTHrP indicate that it is structurally distinct from the PTH1 receptor. The tissue distribution of PTH2 receptor is also different. The endogenous ligand and the physiologic significance of this receptor are not defined.

The details of the biochemical steps by which an increased intracellular concentration of cyclic AMP, IP_3, or DAG lead to changes in calcium and phosphate ion translocation are unknown. Stimulation of protein kinases (protein kinase A, cyclic AMP; protein kinase C, DAG) and calcium transport channels is associated with a variety of hormone-specific tissue responses, some of which are cyclic AMP–dependent and others cyclic AMP–independent. These responses include inhibition of phosphate and bicarbonate transport and stimulation of calcium transport and renal 1α-hydroxylase in the kidney. The responses in bone include effects on collagen synthesis; alkaline phosphatase activity; ornithine decarboxylase, citrate decarboxylase, and glucose-6-phosphate dehydrogenase activity; DNA, protein, and phospholipid synthesis; and calcium and phosphate transport. Ultimately, these cellular biochemical events lead to an integrated hormonal response in bone turnover and calcium homeostasis.

Pathophysiology In hyperparathyroidism, PTH is overproduced by tumors of the parathyroid or by hyperplasia involving all glands. The excess hormone results in hypercalcemia secondary to increased intestinal calcium absorption [increased synthesis of $1,25(OH)_2D$], reduced renal calcium clearance, and increased bone calcium release. Bone turnover increases in all patients, and resorption exceeds formation in many. Individual patients respond to the excess hormone variably at intestinal, renal, and bone target sites; the factors influencing the response from patient to patient are not known.

Hypophosphatemia results from the actions of the excessive PTH on renal tubular phosphate reabsorption. Hypophosphatemia in turn aggravates the hypercalcemia by increasing the synthesis of $1,25(OH)_2D$ and by increasing the sensitivity of the bone to PTH. Hypophosphatemia also may interfere with the normal mineralization of bone, leading to a mixed picture of increased resorption and deficient mineralization in adjacent skeletal sites.

Hypoparathyroidism causes hypocalcemia and hyperphosphatemia, a reversal of the response seen with hormone excess. See Chap. 354 for details of the clinical syndromes.

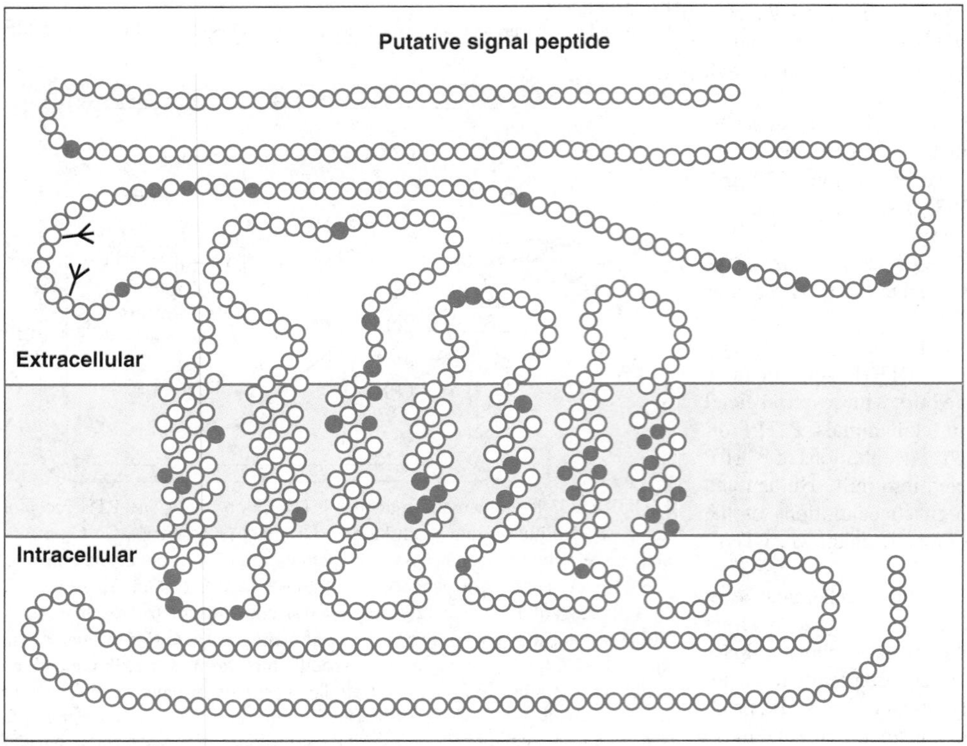

FIGURE 353-9 Schematic illustration of predicted structure of the PTH and calcitonin receptors contains one large extracellular domain, seven membrane-spanning domains, three extracellular loops connecting the membrane-spanning domains on the cell surface, one large intracellular domain, and three intracellular loops. Backbone structure is of the PTH receptor; solid residues are common between PTH and the CT receptor.

CALCITONIN (See also Chap. 340) Calcitonin is a hypocalcemic peptide hormone that, in many ways, acts as the physiologic antagonist to parathyroid hormone. The hypocalcemic activity is accounted for primarily by inhibition of osteoclast-mediated bone resorption and secondarily by stimulation of renal calcium clearance. These effects are mediated by receptors on osteoclasts and renal tubular cells. Calcitonin exerts additional effects presumably through binding to receptors present in brain, gastrointestinal tract, and the immune system (Fig. 353-9). The hormone, for example, exerts analgesic effects directly on cells in the hypothalamus and related structures, possibly by interacting with receptors for related peptide hormones, such as calcitonin gene–related peptide (CGRP) or amylin. The latter ligands have specific high-affinity receptors and also can bind to and trigger calcitonin receptors. The calcitonin receptors, as deduced from the nucleotide sequences of the cDNA, contain seven transmembrane α-helical domains, like G protein–coupled receptors. The calcitonin, PTH, and PTHrP receptors are sufficiently different from other G protein–coupled receptors to constitute a distinct subfamily. Other members of this subfamily include receptors for secretin, vasoactive intestinal peptide, growth hormone–releasing hormone, and gastric inhibitory peptide. Interaction of calcitonin with its receptors activates signal transduction pathways that, like those for PTH, involve distinct G proteins. Thus calcitonin can stimulate adenylyl cyclase and protein kinase A as well as protein kinase C and can induce calcium transients a well. These specific G protein interactions probably involve distinct amino acid sequences in a single receptor protein.

The thyroid is the major source of the hormone, and the cells involved in calcitonin synthesis arise from neural crest tissue. During embryogenesis, these cells migrate into the ultimobranchial body, derived from the last branchial pouch. In submammalian vertebrates, the ultimobranchial body constitutes a discrete organ, anatomically separate from the thyroid gland, but in mammals the ultimobranchial gland fuses with and is incorporated into the thyroid gland.

The naturally occurring calcitonins consist of a peptide chain of 32 amino acids. There is considerable sequence variability among species. The entire chain of 32 amino acids appears to be required for biologic activity in the intact animal, although fragments function in in vitro systems. Calcitonin from salmon is 10 to 100 times more potent than mammalian forms in lowering serum calcium in animals; eel calcitonin is also potent. Slow turnover may in part explain the greater potency of salmon calcitonin, but the hormone binds more tightly to receptor sites as well. Calcitonin is synthesized as a precursor molecule that is four times larger than calcitonin itself. Analysis of the sequence of the coding portions of the gene for rat calcitonin indicates that at least two peptides flank calcitonin, from which they are separated by basic residues. It is likely (by analogy with the common precursor for adrenocorticotropic hormone and endorphin) that these peptides are released along with calcitonin. They have no known biologic function.

There are two calcitonin genes, α and β, located on chromosome 11 in the general region of the β globulin and parathyroid hormone genes. The two genes are sometimes called calcitonin/CGRP-1 and /CGRP-2. The transcription of these genes is complex. Two different messenger RNA molecules are transcribed from the α gene; one is translated into the precursor for calcitonin, and the other message is transcribed into an alternative product, CGRP. CGRP is synthesized wherever the calcitonin message is expressed, e.g., in medullary carcinoma of the thyroid. The β, or CGRP-2, gene is transcribed into the messenger RNA for CGRP in the central nervous system (CNS) in animals; this gene is silent for calcitonin production. CGRP has cardiovascular actions and may serve a neurotransmitter or developmental role in CNS.

The secretion of calcitonin is under the direct control of blood calcium: An increase in the blood calcium level causes an increase in the calcitonin level, and a decrease in the blood calcium level causes a decrease in the calcitonin level. Once secreted, calcitonin disappears from the circulation with a half-life of 2 to 15 min.

The circulating level of calcitonin in humans is lower than that in many other species. Basal and stimulated immunoreactive calcitonin levels are lower in women than in men and tend to decrease with age to a greater extent in women.

In animals calcitonin acts to lower both blood calcium and blood phosphate levels by inhibiting bone resorption and by increasing urinary calcium and phosphate clearance. The actions of calcitonin on kidney and bone are in turn modulated by the regulation of calcitonin production by serum calcium. The view that calcitonin serves to protect against hypercalcemia is thus explained by the hypocalcemic effects of calcitonin triggered in response to hypercalcemia.

In humans changes in calcium and phosphate metabolism are not seen despite extreme variations in calcitonin production; no definite effects are attributable to calcitonin deficiency (totally thyroidectomized patients receiving only replacement thyroxine) or excess (patients with medullary carcinoma of the thyroid, a calcitonin-secreting tumor) (see Chap. 340). Although there are no obvious abnormalities in calcium metabolism in patients with elevated calcitonin levels, bone remodeling is chronically suppressed. Calcitonin is a useful pharmacologic agent to suppress bone resorption in Paget's disease (Chap. 358) and osteoporosis (Chap. 355).

BIBLIOGRAPHY

CALCIUM, PHOSPHOROUS, AND BONE METABOLISM

ANDERSON JB: Nutritional biochemistry of calcium and phosphorus. J Nutr Biochem 2:300, 1991

AVIOLI LV, KRANE SM (eds): *Metabolic Bone Disease and Clinically Related Disorders*. Philadelphia, Saunders, 1990
BRINGHURST FR: Calcium and phosphate distribution, turnover, and metabolic actions, in *Endocrinology*, 3d ed, LJ DeGroot et al (eds). Philadelphia, Saunders, 1995, p 1015
CANALIS E et al: Growth factors and cytokines in bone cell metabolism. Annu Rev Med 42:17, 1991
COHN DV et al (eds): *Calcium Regulating Hormones and Bone Metabolism: Bone and Clinical Aspects*. Amsterdam, Excerpta Medica, 1992
DELMAS PD: Clinical use of biochemical markers of bone remodeling in osteoporosis. Bone 13:S17, 1992
HEANEY RP: Thinking straight about calcium. N Engl J Med 328:503, 1993
HOROWITZ MC: Cytokines and estrogen in bone: Anti-osteoporotic effects. Science 260:626, 1993
MATKOVIC V: Calcium intake and peak bone mass. N Engl J Med 327:119, 1992
PORTALE AA et al: Physiologic regulation of the serum concentration of 1,25-dihydroxyvitamin D by phosphorus in normal men. J Clin Invest 83:1494, 1989
ROODMAN GD: Interleukin-6: An osteotropic factor? J Bone Miner Res 7:474, 1992
SAGE EH, BORNSTEIN P: Extracellular proteins that modulate cell-matrix interactions. SPARC, tenascin, and thrombospondin. J Biol Chem 266:14831, 1991
SLAVKIN H, PRICE P (eds): *Chemistry and Biology of Mineralized Tissues*. Amsterdam, Excerpta Medica, 1992
SORIANO P et al: Targeted disruption of the *c-src* proto-oncogene leads to osteopetrosis in mice. Cell 64:693, 1991
SUDA T et al: Modulation of osteoclast differentiation. Endocr Rev 13:66, 1992
UEBELHART D et al: Urinary excretion of pyridinium crosslinks: A new marker of bone resorption in metabolic bone disease. Bone Miner 8:87, 1990

VITAMIN D

DARWIN H, DELUCA H: Vitamin D-regulated gene expression. Crit Rev Eukaryotic Gene Expr 3:89, 1993
DEMAY M: Hereditary defects in vitamin D metabolism and vitamin D receptor defects, in *Endocrinology*, 3d ed, LJ DeGroot et al (eds). Philadelphia, Saunders, 1995, p 1173
HOLICK MF: McCollum Award Lecture 1994: Vitamin D—new horizons for the 21st century. Am J Clin Nutr 60:617, 1994
———: Vitamin D: Biosynthesis, metabolism, and mode of action, in *Endocrinology*, 3d ed, LJ DeGroot et al (eds). Philadelphia, Saunders, 1995 p 990
PIKE JW: Vitamin D_3 receptors: Structure and function in transcription. Annu Rev Nutr 11:189, 1991
TILYARD MW et al: Treatment of postmenopausal osteoporosis with calcitriol or calcium. N Engl J Med 326:356, 1992

PARATHYROID HORMONE AND CALCITONIN

ABOU-SAMRA AB et al: Expression cloning of a common receptor for parathyroid hormone and parathyroid hormone–related peptide from rat osteoblast-like cells: A single receptor stimulates intracellular accumulation of both cAMP and inositol triphosphates and increases intracellular free calcium. Proc Natl Acad Sci USA 89:2732, 1992
ARNOLD A et al: Mutation of the signal peptide-encoding region of the preproparathyroid hormone gene in familial isolated hypoparathyroidism. J Clin Invest 86:1094, 1990
DEMAY MB et al: Sequences in the human parathyroid hormone gene that bind the 1,25-dihydroxyvitamin D_2 receptor and mediate transcriptional repression in response to 1,25-dihydroxyvitamin D_3. Proc Natl Acad Sci USA 89:8097, 1992
FITZPATRICK LA, ARNOLD A: Hypoparathyroidism, in *Endocrinology*, 3d ed, LJ DeGroot et al (eds). Philadelphia, Saunders, 1995, p 1123
GORN AH et al: The cloning characterization and expression of a human calcitonin receptor from an ovarian carcinoma cell line. J Clin Invest 90:1726, 1992
KARAPLIS AC et al: Disruption of parathyroid hormone–related peptide gene leads to a multitude of skeletal abnormalities and perinatal mortality. J Bone Miner Res 7(Suppl 1):abst 1, 1992
LEVINE MA, SPIEGEL AM: Pseudohypoparathyroidism, in *Endocrinology*, 3d ed, LJ DeGroot et al (eds). Philadelphia, Saunders, 1995, p 1136
MACINTYRE I: Calcitonin: Physiology, biosynthesis, secretion, metabolism, and mode of action, in *Endocrinology*, 3d ed, LJ DeGroot et al (eds). Philadelphia, Saunders, 1995, p 1123
MARTIN TJ, MOSELEY JM: Parathyroid hormone-related protein, in *Endocrinology*, 3d ed, LJ DeGroot et al (eds). Philadelphia, Saunders, 1995, p 967
MIRIC A et al: Heterogenous mutations in the gene encoding the alpha subunit of the stimulating G protein of adenylyl cyclase in Albright hereditary osteodystrophy. J Clin Endocrinol Metab 76:1560, 1993
POTTS JT JR et al: Parathyroid hormone: Physiology, chemistry, biosynthesis, secretion, metabolism, and mode of action, in *Endocrinology*, 3d ed, LJ DeGroot et al (eds). Philadelphia, Saunders, 1995, p 920

SCHIPANI E et al: Identical complementary deoxyribonucleic acids encode a human renal and bone parathyroid hormone (PTH)/PTH–related peptide receptor. Endocrinology 132:2157, 1993
USDIN TB et al: Identification and functional expression of a receptor selectively recognizing parathyroid hormone, the PTH2 receptor. J Biol Chem 270:15455, 1995

354

John T. Potts, Jr

DISEASES OF THE PARATHYROID GLAND AND OTHER HYPER- AND HYPOCALCEMIC DISORDERS

HYPERCALCEMIA

Hypercalcemia can be a manifestation of a serious illness such as malignancy or can be detected coincidentally by laboratory testing in a patient with no obvious illness. The number of patients recognized with asymptomatic hypercalcemia has increased severalfold in the past 25 years, and management is a particular problem in the asymptomatic patient.

Whenever hypercalcemia is confirmed, a definitive diagnosis must be established. Although hyperparathyroidism, a frequent cause of asymptomatic hypercalcemia, is a chronic disorder in which manifestations, if any, may be expressed only over months or years, hypercalcemia also can be the earliest manifestation of malignancy, the second most common cause of hypercalcemia in the adult. The causes of hypercalcemia are numerous (Table 354-1), but hyperparathyroidism and cancer account for 90 percent of cases. Diagnosis can usually be established, but the appropriate management of hypercalcemia is sometimes unclear. Whether all asymptomatic hyperparathyroidism should be corrected surgically is unsettled, but there is now a consensus that simple medical surveillance is appropriate for patients over age 50 when bone and renal status are satisfactory.

Before undertaking a workup, it is essential to be sure that true hypercalcemia, not a false-positive laboratory test, is present. Hypercalcemia is a chronic problem, and it is cost-effective to obtain several

Table 354-1

Classification of Causes of Hypercalcemia

I. Parathyroid-related
   A. Primary hyperparathyroidism
      1. Solitary adenomas
      2. Multiple endocrine neoplasia
   B. Lithium therapy
   C. Familial hypocalciuric hypercalcemia
II. Malignancy-related
   A. Solid tumor with metastases (breast)
   B. Solid tumor with humoral mediation of hypercalcemia (lung, kidney)
   C. Hematologic malignancies (multiple myeloma, lymphoma, leukemia)
III. Vitamin D–related
   A. Vitamin D intoxication
   B. ↑ $1,25(OH)_2D$; sarcoidosis and other granulomatous diseases
   C. Idiopathic hypercalcemia of infancy
IV. Associated with high bone turnover
   A. Hyperthyroidism
   B. Immobilization
   C. Thiazides
   D. Vitamin A intoxication
V. Associated with renal failure:
   A. Severe secondary hyperparathyroidism
   B. Aluminum intoxication
   C. Milk-alkali syndrome

serum calcium measurements; these tests need not be in the fasting state. False-positive hypercalcemia is usually the result of inadvertent hemoconcentration during blood collection or elevation in serum proteins such as albumin. There is no advantage, except in research applications, to measurement of ionized rather than total calcium.

Clinical features are helpful in differential diagnosis. Hypercalcemia in an adult who is asymptomatic is usually due to primary hyperparathyroidism. In malignancy-associated hypercalcemia the disease is usually not occult; rather, symptoms of malignancy bring the patient to the physician, and hypercalcemia is discovered during the workup. In such patients the interval between detection of hypercalcemia and death is often less than 6 months. Accordingly, if an asymptomatic individual has had hypercalcemia or some manifestation of hypercalcemia, such as kidney stones, for more than 1 or 2 years, it is unlikely that malignancy is the cause. Nevertheless, differentiating primary hyperparathyroidism from *occult* malignancy can occasionally be difficult, and careful evaluation is required, particularly when the duration of the hypercalcemia is unknown.

Hypercalcemia not due to hyperparathyroidism or malignancy can result from excessive vitamin D action, high bone turnover from any of several causes, or from renal failure (Table 354-1). The sensitivity and specificity of various diagnostic tests for the differential diagnosis previously were not optimal, but parathyroid hormone (PTH) immunoassays based on double-antibody methods are reliable. Dietary history and a history of ingestion of vitamins and drugs are often helpful in diagnosing some of the less frequent causes. Except in malignancy-associated hypercalcemia, acute management of the hypercalcemia is usually successful prior to definitive therapy. The type of treatment is based on the severity of the hypercalcemia and the nature of associated symptoms.

Hypercalcemia from any cause can result in fatigue, depression, mental confusion, anorexia, nausea, vomiting, constipation, reversible renal tubular defects, increased urination, a short QT interval in the electrocardiogram, and, in some patients, cardiac arrhythmias. There is a variable relation from one patient to the next between the severity of hypercalcemia and the symptoms. Generally, symptoms are more common at calcium levels above 2.9 to 3 mmol/L (11.5 to 12.0 mg/dL), but some patients, even at this level, are asymptomatic. When calcium exceeds 3.2 mmol/L (13 mg/dL), calcification in kidneys, skin, vessels, lungs, heart, and stomach and renal insufficiency may develop, particularly if blood phosphate levels are normal or elevated due to impaired renal function. Severe hypercalcemia, usually defined as 3.7 mmol/L (15 mg/dL) or above, is a medical emergency. When serum calcium is 3.7 to 4.5 mmol/L (15 to 18 mg/dL) or higher, coma and cardiac arrest can occur.

PARATHYROID-RELATED HYPERCALCEMIA Primary Hyperparathyroidism *Natural history and incidence* Primary hyperparathyroidism is a generalized disorder of calcium, phosphate, and bone metabolism due to an increased secretion of parathyroid hormone. The elevation of circulating hormone usually leads to hypercalcemia and hypophosphatemia. There is great variation in the manifestations. Patients may present with multiple signs and symptoms, including recurrent nephrolithiasis, peptic ulcers, mental changes, and, less frequently, extensive bone resorption. However, with greater awareness of the disease and wider use of multiphasic screening tests, including blood calcium assays, the diagnosis is frequently made in patients who have no symptoms and minimal, if any, signs of the disease other than hypercalcemia and elevated levels of parathyroid hormone. The annual incidence of the disease is estimated to be as high as 0.2 percent in patients over age 60, with an estimated prevalence including undiscovered asymptomatic patients of 1 percent or higher. The manifestations may be subtle, and the disease may have a benign course for many years or a lifetime. Rarely, the disease develops or worsens abruptly and causes severe complications, such as marked dehydration and coma, so-called hypercalcemic parathyroid crisis. The disease has a peak incidence between the third and fifth decades but occurs in young children and in the elderly.

Etiology and pathology SOLITARY ADENOMAS The cause of hyperparathyroidism is one or more hyperfunctioning glands. The traditional view has been that a single abnormal gland is the cause in approximately 80 percent of patients; the abnormality in the gland is usually a benign neoplasm or adenoma and rarely a parathyroid carcinoma. In approximately 15 percent all glands are hyperfunctioning; this is termed *chief cell parathyroid hyperplasia* and is usually hereditary and frequently associated with other endocrine abnormalities. Some surgeons and pathologists report that the enlargement of multiple glands is common.

MULTIPLE ENDOCRINE NEOPLASIA Hereditary hyperparathyroidism can occur without other endocrine abnormalities but is usually part of a multiple endocrine neoplasia (MEN) (see Chap. 340). MEN 1 (Wermer's syndrome) consists of hyperparathyroidism and tumors of the pituitary and pancreas, often associated with gastric hypersecretion and peptic ulcer disease (Zollinger-Ellison syndrome). MEN 2A consists of hyperparathyroidism, pheochromocytoma, and medullary carcinoma of the thyroid. Both disorders are inherited as autosomal dominant defects. Since the various endocrine tumors can develop at widely separated intervals, management of these patients is a formidable challenge, and in MEN 2A a screening technique makes it possible to identify (or exclude) first-degree relatives at risk.

MOLECULAR DEFECTS IN HYPERPARATHYROIDISM Analyses of kindreds with MEN 1 and MEN 2A and cytogenetic studies of tumor tissue from patients with solitary adenomas have documented that at least two molecular defects are involved in the hyperparathyroid state, namely, overactivity of a proto-oncogene, or growth-promoting gene, and loss of function of a growth-regarding gene, or antioncogene.

A gene locus on chromosome 11 appears to be responsible for MEN 1, and the normal allele of this gene may be an antioncogene. The loss of one allele is inherited as an autosomal trait, and loss of the other allele via somatic cell mutation leads to monoclonal expansion and tumor development in tissues such as the parathyroids. In approximately 25 percent of sporadic parathyroid adenomas, the same locus on chromosome 11 appears to be lost, implying that the same defect responsible for MEN 1 can also cause the common disease. In MEN 1 there is a defect in one allele at birth, and in patients with sporadic adenomas one copy is lost as a silent somatic mutation; in both disorders, the second allele becomes mutated or deleted in some cell, resulting in a monoclonal outgrowth (Fig. 354-1*A*).

In other parathyroid adenomas, a second mechanism of abnormal growth is operative, namely, activation of a proto-oncogene (Fig. 354-1*B*). The synthesis of parathyoid hormone is under the control of a promoter that, in the presence of a reciprocal translocation involving chromosome 11, can also drive the expression of a gene product termed PRAD-1, a D-cyclin protein that plays a role in cell division. If overexpressed (or mutated), cyclins contribute to abnormal cell replication. This translocation is found in 5 percent or more of parathyroid adenomas, usually in larger glands. These findings also explain why hyperparathyroidism develops earlier in the MEN syndromes (germ line defect) than with parathyroid adenomas (two somatic mutations required). Proliferation of parathyroid cells may favor such somatic mutations because more than 60 percent of patients operated on for secondary hyperparathyroidism due to renal failure appear to have monoclonal proliferation associated with loss of a portion of the X chromosome.

Additional genetic abnormalities are probably involved in the etiology of hyperparathyroidism, because allelic loss of a portion of chromosome 1 is found in 40 percent of parathyroid adenomas. Still different mechanisms appear to be operative in parathyroid carcinoma, namely, loss of both copies of the retinoblastoma gene. Hence, unlike the situation with some cancers in which there appears to be progression from benign to malignant neoplasms as cellular genetic defects accumulate, parathyroid adenomas do not seem to be precursors of parathyroid carcinoma.

In MEN 2A the frequency of hyperparathyroidism is less common than in MEN 1 and varies within families and between families. The mutation in MEN 2A is one of several activating mutations in a tyrosine kinase–type proto-oncogene RET (see Chap. 340). The mutation is carried in all cells as a germ line defect and can be detected by diagnostic genetic techniques. The principal practical utility of this assay is that it makes it possible to make the diagnosis and operate early to prevent development of medullary thyroid cancer.

Adenomas are most often located in the inferior parathyroid gland, but in 6 to 10 percent of patients, parathyroid adenomas may be located in the thymus, the thyroid, the pericardium, or behind the esophagus. Adenomas are usually 0.5 to 5 g in size but may be as large as 10 to 20 g (normal glands weigh 25 mg on average). Chief cells are predominant in both hyperplasia and adenoma. The adenoma is sometimes encapsulated by a rim of normal tissue. With chief cell hyperplasia, the enlargement may be so asymmetric that some involved glands appear grossly normal. If hyperplasia is present, histologic examination reveals a uniform pattern of chief cells and disappearance of fat even in the absence of an increase in gland weight. Thus, microscopic examination of biopsy specimens of several glands is essential to interpret findings at surgery. When an adenoma is present, the other glands are usually normal and contain a normal distribution of all cell types (rather than only chief cells) and normal amounts of fat.

Parathyroid carcinoma is usually not aggressive in character. Long-term survival without recurrence is common if at initial surgery the entire gland is removed without rupture of the capsule. Even recurrent parathyroid carcinoma is usually slow-growing with local spread in the neck, and surgical correction of recurrent disease may be feasible. Occasionally, however, parathyroid carcinoma is more aggressive, with distant metastases (lung, liver, and bone) found at the time of initial operation. It may be difficult to appreciate initially that a primary tumor is carcinoma; increased numbers of mitotic figures and increased fibrosis of the gland stroma may precede invasion. The diagnosis of carcinoma is often made in retrospect. Hyperparathyroidism from a parathyroid carcinoma may be indistinguishable from other forms of primary hyperparathyroidism; a potential clue to the diagnosis, however, is provided by the degree of calcium elevation. Calcium values of 3.5 to 3.7 mmol/L (14 to 15 mg/dL) are frequent with carcinoma and may alert the surgeon to remove the abnormal gland with care to avoid capsular rupture.

Signs and symptoms Half or more of patients with hyperparathyroidism are asymptomatic. In series in which patients are followed without operation, as many as 80 percent are classified as without symptoms; the number may be smaller if mild manifestations, such as silent bone deterioration or reduced renal function, are included. Manifestations of hyperparathyroidism involve primarily the kidneys and the skeletal system. Kidney involvement, due either to deposition of calcium in the renal parenchyma or to recurrent nephrolithiasis, was present in 60 to 70 percent of patients prior to 1970. With earlier detection, renal complications are less common.

Renal stones are usually composed of either calcium oxalate or calcium phosphate. In occasional patients repeated episodes of nephrolithiasis or the formation of large calculi may lead to urinary tract obstruction, infection, and loss of renal function. Nephrocalcinosis also may cause decreased renal function and phosphate retention.

The unique bone manifestation of hyperparathyroidism is osteitis fibrosa cystica, which in the past occurred in 10 to 25 percent of patients. Histologically, the pathognomonic features are a reduction in the number of trabeculae, an increase in the giant multinucleated osteoclasts in scalloped areas on the surface of the bone (Howship's lacunae), and a replacement of the normal cellular and marrow elements by fibrous tissues. Other bone changes include resorption of the phalangeal tufts and replacement of the usually sharp cortical outline of the bone in the digits by an irregular outline (subperiosteal resorption). Loss of the lamina dura of the teeth is less specific. Tiny "punched-out" lesions may cause the so-called salt-and-pepper appearance in the skull.

Osteitis fibrosa cystica is now uncommon, even though hyperparathyroidism may be of long standing. The reduced frequency is unexplained. Other bone disorders, however, are frequent. The rate of bone mineral turnover is enhanced in most patients, even in those who do not have a decrease in bone mass; in such patients, rates of bone formation and bone restoration must be increased but balanced. In some patients, however, rates of formation and resorption are not

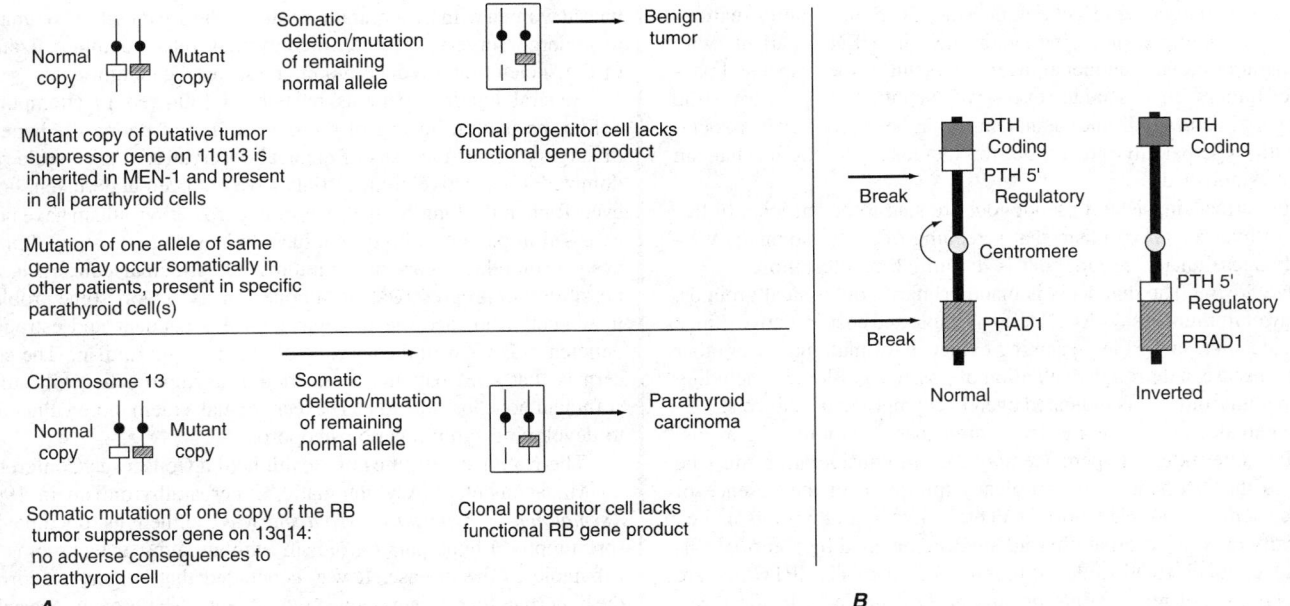

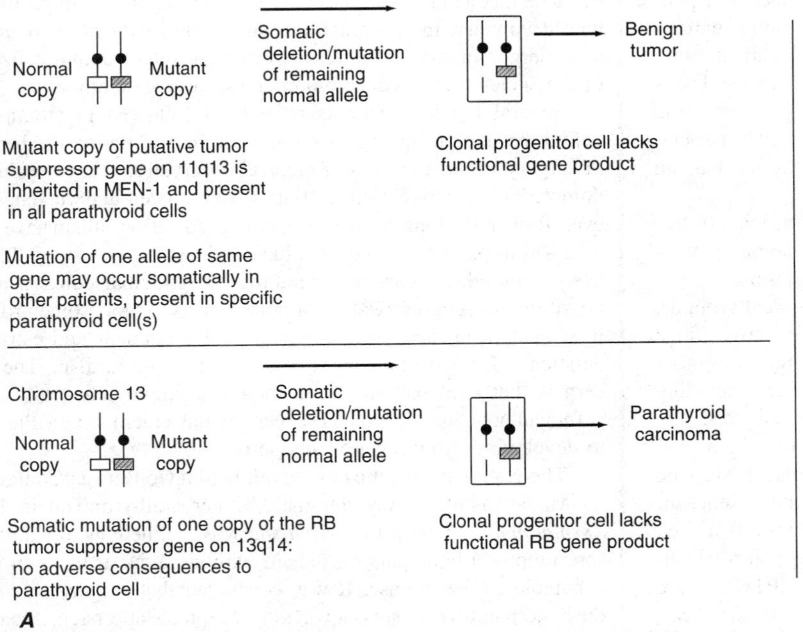

FIGURE 354-1 *A.* Schematic diagram indicating concept of autosomal recessive rather than autosomal dominant inheritance of tumor susceptibility. The patient with the hereditary abnormality (multiple endocrine neoplasia, or MEN) is envisioned as having one defective gene (mutant receptor) inherited from the affected parent on chromosome 11, but one copy of the normal gene is present from the other parent. In the monoclonal tumor (benign tumor), a somatic event, here partial chromosomal deletion, removes the normal gene from a cell. The cell, deprived of growth-regulating influence from this gene, has unregulated growth and becomes a tumor. A different genetic locus also involving loss of an anti-oncogene, or growth-regulating gene, on chromosome 13 is involved in the pathogenesis of parathyroid carcinoma. *B.* Schematic illustration of the mechanism and consequences of gene rearrangement and overexpression of the PRAD 1 proto-oncogene (pericentromeric inversion of chromosome 11) in parathryoid adenomas. The excessive expression by the highly active PTH gene promoter in the parathyroid cell of PRAD 1, which is a cell cycle control protein, contributes to excess cellular proliferation, thereby activating the receptor, increasing activity of PLC through Gq. *(From Habener et al, with permission.)*

balanced so that a progressive loss of bone mineral mass causes osteopenia. There are no pathognomonic criteria to separate unequivocally parathyroid-dependent osteopenia from "high-turnover" osteoporosis, as can occur in patients who are not hyperparathyroid.

Improved techniques are now available for monitoring bone mineral density. Computed tomography (CT) and quantitative digital radiography (DEXA) of the spine provide reproducible quantitative estimates (within a few percent) of spinal bone density. Similarly, cortical bone density in the extremities can be quantified by single-photon densitometry. Serial measurements with these techniques can provide early evidence as to whether osteopenia is progressive. Most studies indicate that in hyperparathyroidism cortical rather than trabecular bone tends to be lost selectively.

In symptomatic patients, dysfunctions of the central nervous system, peripheral nerve and muscle, the gastrointestinal tract, and the joints also occur. An awareness of the signs and symptoms of hyperparathyroidism may give the initial clue to the diagnosis. It has been reported that severe neuropsychiatric manifestations may be reversed by parathyroidectomy; it is not clear that this improvement is a defined cause-and-effect relationship in the absence of controlled studies, however. Generally, the fact that hyperparathyroidism is common in elderly patients, in whom there are often other problems, suggests the possibility that such coexisting problems as hypertension, renal deterioration, and depression may not be parathyroid-related and suggests caution in recommending parathyroid surgery as a cure for these conditions. It is not apparent why some patients with hyperparathyroidism have no symptoms, while others with similar biochemical abnormalities develop symptomatic disease.

Neuromuscular manifestations may include proximal muscle weakness, easy fatigability, and atrophy of muscles and may be so striking as to suggest a primary neuromuscular disorder. The distinguishing feature is the complete regression of neuromuscular disease after surgical correction of the hyperparathyroidism.

Gastrointestinal manifestations are sometimes subtle and include vague abdominal complaints and disorders of the stomach and pancreas. Again, cause and effect are unclear, except in certain situations such as the multiple endocrine syndromes. In MEN 1 patients with hyperparathyroidism, duodenal ulcer is a result of the associated pancreatic tumors that secrete excessive quantities of gastrin (the Zollinger-Ellison syndrome). Pancreatitis has been reported in association with hyperparathyroidism, but the incidence and the mechanism are not established.

Chondrocalcinosis and pseudogout are said to be sufficiently frequent in hyperparathyroidism that screening of such patients is warranted. Occasionally, pseudogout is the initial manifestation.

Diagnosis The diagnosis is made primarily on clinical grounds. The newer immunoassays for PTH are reliable and cost-effective. Since hypercalcemia can be the presenting evidence for malignancy or other serious disease, a thorough evaluation of possible etiologies, including hyperparathyroidism, is indicated even in asymptomatic subjects.

Hypercalcemia is the most common manifestation—either sustained or intermittent hypercalcemia. Careful consideration must be given to the justification for surgical exploration in the absence of hypercalcemia. So-called normocalcemic hyperparathyroidism, i.e., surgically proven hyperparathyroidism accompanied by a normal calcium level but elevated values of immunoreactive PTH (iPTH), is rare in the absence of renal failure or vitamin D deficiency. If normocalcemic patients have coexisting conditions that interfere with the calcium-elevating actions of PTH, such as chronic renal failure, severe malabsorption, or vitamin D deficiency, then the lack of calcium elevation need not mitigate against the presence of hyperparathyroidism. Confusing situations can arise, however, in patients with recurrent kidney stones who are suspected of having hyperparathyroidism because of elevated iPTH levels but who have normal serum calcium. These patients may have true normocalcemic hyperparathyroidism. In such situations in which the symptoms call for early definitive diagnosis and treatment, it may be useful to search for postabsorptive hypercalcemia (detectable in certain patients when fasting hypercalcemia is absent) or to use a provocative test with benzothiadiazides (see below).

Hypercalciuria is common in hyperparathyroidism. However, PTH actually reduces calcium clearance, and the daily excretion of calcium in urine is lower than in patients with equivalent degrees of hypercalcemia from nonparathyroid causes.

Serum phosphate is usually low but may be normal, especially if renal failure has developed. Hypophosphatemia is a less specific diagnostic finding than hypercalcemia for two reasons. First, phosphate levels are influenced by dietary intake, diurnal variations, and other factors; to be useful, samples must be obtained in the morning under fasting conditions. Second, patients with severe hypercalcemia of any cause may have a low serum phosphate.

Many tests based on renal responses to excess parathyroid hormone (renal calcium and phosphate clearance; blood phosphate, chloride, magnesium; urinary or nephrogenous cyclic AMP) have been used in the past. These tests have low specificity for hyperparathyroidism, are not cost-effective, and have been replaced by PTH immunoassays.

℞ TREATMENT

Medical Treatment Management of hyperparathyroidism involves two separate issues. The critical question is whether the disease should be treated surgically (see below). If surgery is indicated, the serum calcium may need to be lowered prior to surgery. However, since surgery is the quickest method of lowering serum calcium in hyperparathyroidism, operation should be performed promptly when hypercalcemia is severe. Hypercalcemia is not symptomatic in most patients with hyperparathyroidism, and it is usually not difficult to control the hypercalcemia. Simple hydration often suffices to lower the calcium concentration to values below 2.9 mmol/L (11.5 mg/dL). There have been discussions in the past as to whether the hypercalcemia of hyperparathyroidism should be treated chronically with oral phosphate. Lowering the calcium level by phosphate is accompanied by an increase in iPTH levels in blood; it is unclear whether the increased PTH levels would cause more or less organ deterioration. There have been no controlled trials to evaluate medical therapy for hyperparathyroidism, but in postmenopausal women with hyperparathyroidism who are unwilling or unable to undergo surgery, estrogen therapy may retard demineralization of the skeleton and reduce blood and urinary calcium levels.

Several hundred patients have been followed in attempts to define the natural history of the disease and to define the benefits of surgery versus the risks of medical observation. Large-scale randomized, prospective clinical trials have not been undertaken, however. Rather, the long-term effects of hyperparathyroidism have been assessed in patients who do not have kidney stones, osteitis fibrosa cystica, or other clear-cut symptoms. Of principal concern is the possibility of progressive loss of bone density, a worrisome problem in women who face the problem of age-dependent and estrogen-deficient bone loss in the absence of hyperparathyroidism. The concern is that such patients, even though asymptomatic, will suffer sufficient bone loss due to PTH excess to make them more vulnerable to developing symptomatic osteoporosis.

The National Institutes of Health held a Consensus Conference on Management of Asymptomatic Hyperparathyroidism in 1991. *Asymptomatic hyperparathyroidism* was defined as documented (presumptive) hyperparathyroidism without signs or symptoms attributable to the disease. It was concluded that surgery to correct the hyperparathyroidism is always an acceptable approach, if feasible medically, but surveillance may be justified in patients over the age of 50 with minimal calcium elevation when renal function and bone mass are close to normal and remain so during careful monitoring.

The recommendation was that the diagnosis of primary hyperparathyroidism can best be established by demonstrating persistent hypercalcemia (artifactual elevation in serum calcium concentration must be excluded) and an elevated serum iPTH level. The panel agreed that the PTH assay is now sensitive, specific, and reliable and that other tests are usually unnecessary.

As to which asymptomatic patients should be followed medically, the consensus was that a subgroup of patients over age 50 is appropriate for medical monitoring if certain criteria are met and the patients wish to avoid surgery.

Patients under age 50 should be routinely operated on, given the long surveillance that would be required. Other guidelines for recommending surgery in patients with asymptomatic hyperparathyroidism include the following:

1. Elevation of serum calcium, more than 0.25 to 0.40 mmol/L (1 to 1.6 mg/dL) above the upper limit of normal for the laboratory.
2. History of an episode of life-threatening hypercalcemia, such as an episode induced by dehydration and recurring illness.
3. Reduction of creatinine clearance by greater than 30 percent compared with age-matched controls (the author finds it difficult to use this criterion as an absolute, given the multiplicity of factors that affect creatinine clearance with age).
4. Presence of kidney stones detected by abdominal radiograph even if they are asymptomatic.
5. Elevation of 24-h urinary calcium excretion above 400 mg.
6. Reduction of bone mass more than 2 standard deviations below normal by one of several noninvasive methods of measuring bone mass.

Other considerations that favor surgery include concern that consistent follow-up would be unlikely or that coexistent illness would complicate management. Asymptomatic patients should be monitored regularly. Surgical correction of hyperparathyroidism can always be undertaken when indicated, since the success rate is high (>90 percent), mortality is low, morbidity is minimal, and cure is common. The goals of monitoring are early detection of worsening hypercalcemia, deteriorating bone or renal status, or other complications of hyperparathyroidism. Cortical bone mass is principally at risk in untreated primary hyperparathyroidism. Indeed, reports that vertebral bone fractures are increased in patients with untreated hyperparathyroidism have been challenged, and cancellous bone loss may be a problem only when vitamin D and calcium intakes are low.

Although patients have reduced bone mass at the time of initial detection, there may be little further loss over years of subsequent follow-up. The use of single-photon absorptiometry to follow cortical bone mass is relatively easy and inexpensive; increased loss of cancellous bone and increased risk of vertebral fractures are unusual, and the monitoring of spinal bone mass by dual-energy x-ray absorptiometry need not be undertaken. The consensus panel did not make a recommendation as to estrogen use in patients for whom surgery was not elected because there was insufficient cumulative experience with such therapy. It has been reported that untreated hyperparathyroidism is a risk factor for increased cardiovascular mortality, leading some to recommend surgery for all patients. The majority view is that medical surveillance is justified since the reports of increased cardiovascular risk are retrospective in nature.

Surgical Treatment Parathyroid exploration is best undertaken by an experienced surgeon with the help of an experienced pathologist. Certain features help in predicting the pathology; for example, in familial cases multiple abnormal glands are likely. However, some critical decisions regarding management can be made only during the operation. The examination by frozen section of tissue removed at surgery helps direct the subsequent course of the operation.

As discussed under "Etiology and Pathogenesis," there are many unresolved issues to consider in surgery for this disease. At the extreme of conservatism, the surgical approach is based on the view that typically only one gland (the adenoma) is abnormal. If an enlarged gland is found, a normal gland should be sought. If a biopsy of a normal-sized second gland confirms its histologic (and presumed functional) normality, no further exploration, biopsy, or excision is needed. At the other extreme is the minority viewpoint that all four glands be sought and that most of the total parathyroid tissue mass should be removed.

The concern with the former approach is that the rate of recurrence of hyperparathyroidism may be high if a second abnormal gland is missed; the latter approach could involve unnecessary surgery and an unacceptable rate of hypoparathyroidism.

The majority viewpoint, judged by surgical reviews, is in favor of conservative surgery, i.e., removal of what is usually only one enlarged gland but only after four-gland exploration to eliminate the possibility that more than one gland is abnormal. When normal glands are found in association with one enlarged gland, excision of the single adenoma usually leads to cure or symptom-free disease, although long-term follow-up studies are limited.

Multiple gland hyperplasia, as predicted in familial cases, poses more difficult questions of surgical management. Once a diagnosis of hyperplasia is established, all the glands must be identified, and two schemes have been proposed for surgical management. One is that three glands be totally removed and the fourth gland be partially excised; care is taken to leave a good blood supply for the remaining gland. Other surgeons advocate total parathyroidectomy with immediate transplantation of a portion of a removed, minced parathyroid gland into the muscles of the forearm with the view that even if recurrence of residual gland enlargement and hyperfunction is seen, surgical excision is easier from the ectopic site in the arm. When parathyroid carcinoma is encountered, the tissue should be widely excised; care must be taken to avoid rupture of the capsule to prevent local seeding of tumor cells.

If no abnormal parathyroid glands are found in the neck, the issue of further exploration must be decided. There are documented cases of five or six parathyroid glands and, therefore, of unusual locations for adenomas. A variety of techniques have been developed to aid in the preoperative localization of the abnormal parathyroid tissue. Noninvasive or minimally invasive techniques include ultrasound, CT of the neck and mediastinum, and differential scanning after technetium-sestamibi administration. Usually these techniques are recommended only in patients with initial unsuccessful neck explorations, since the combined success of the localization techniques is not better than that of an experienced parathyroid surgeon in finding the abnormal tissue at the first operation.

When a second parathyroid exploration is indicated, the minimally invasive techniques such as ultrasound, CT, and isotope scanning should probably be combined with selective digital arteriography in one of the centers specializing in these techniques. At one center, long-term cures have been achieved with selective embolization or injection of large amounts of contrast material into the end-arterial circulation feeding the parathyroid tumor.

A decline in serum calcium occurs within 24 h after successful surgery; usually blood calcium falls to low-normal values for 3 to 5 days until the remaining parathyroid tissue resumes hormone secretion. Intraoperative monitoring of PTH levels by rapid PTH immunoassays may be useful in guiding the surgery, especially in patients who are reexplored after an initial unsuccessful operation. Severe postoperative hypocalcemia is likely only if osteitis cystica is present or if injury to all the normal parathyroid glands occurs during surgery.

In general, patients who do not have symptomatic bone disease or a large deficit in bone mineral and who have good renal and gastrointestinal function have few problems with postoperative hypocalcemia. The extent of postoperative hypocalcemia varies with the surgical approach. If all glands are biopsied, hypocalcemia may be transiently symptomatic and more prolonged. Hypocalcemia is more likely to be symptomatic after second parathyroid explorations, particularly when normal parathyroid tissue was removed at the initial operation and when the manipulation and/or biopsy of the remaining normal glands is more extensive in the search for the missing adenoma. Patients with hyperparathyroidism have efficient intestinal calcium absorption due to the increased levels of 1,25-dihydroxyvitamin D [$1,25(OH)_2D$] stimulated by parathyroid excess. Once hypocalcemia signifies successful surgery, patients can be put on a high-calcium intake or be given oral calcium supplements. Despite mild hypocalcemia, most patients do not require parenteral therapy. If the serum calcium falls below 2 mmol/L (8 mg/dL), *in particular if the phosphate level simultaneously rises*, the possibility that surgery has caused hypoparathyroidism must be considered. Coexistent hypomagnesemia should be checked for, since it interferes with PTH secretion and causes a relative hypoparathyroidism. Parenteral calcium replacement at a low level should be instituted when hypocalcemia is symptomatic. Such indications include a general sense of anxiety and positive Chvostek and Trousseau signs coupled with serum calcium consistently below 2 mmol/L (8 mg/dL). For parenteral therapy, calcium (gluconate or chloride) solutions are prepared at a concentration of 1 mg/mL in 5% dextrose in water. The rate and duration of intravenous therapy are determined by the severity of the symptoms and the response of the serum calcium. A rate of infusion of 0.5 to 2 (mg/kg)/h or 30 to 100 mL/h of a 1-mg/mL solution usually suffices to relieve symptoms. Usually, parenteral therapy is required for only a few days. If symptoms worsen or if parenteral calcium is needed for more than 2 to 3 days, therapy with a vitamin D analogue and/or oral calcium (2 to 4 g/d) should be started (see below). It is cost-effective to use calcitriol (doses of 0.5 to 1.0 μg/d) because of the rapidity of onset and rapidity of cessation of action, in contrast to vitamin D per se (see below). A sudden rise in blood calcium after several months of vitamin D replacement may indicate restoration of parathyroid function to normal. It is also appropriate to monitor serum PTH serially to estimate gland function in such patients.

Magnesium deficiency also may complicate the postoperative course. Magnesium deficiency impairs the secretion of PTH, and therefore, hypomagnesemia should be corrected whenever detected. Magnesium chloride is effective by mouth, but this compound is not widely available. Accordingly, repletion is usually parenteral. Since the depressant effect of magnesium on central and peripheral nerve functions does not occur below 2 mmol/L (normal range 0.8 to 1.2 mmol/L), parenteral replacement can be given rapidly. A cumulative dose as great as 0.5 to 1 mmol/kg of body weight can be administered if severe hypomagnesemia is present; often, however, total doses of 20 to 40 mmol are sufficient. The magnesium is given either as an intravenous infusion over 8 to 12 h or in divided doses intramuscularly (magnesium sulfate, USP).

Lithium Therapy Lithium, used in the management of bipolar depression and other psychiatric disorders, causes hypercalcemia in approximately 10 percent of patients. The parathyroids are involved in mediation of the hypercalcemia, and PTH levels may be elevated. The hypercalcemia is dependent on continued lithium treatment, remitting and recurring when lithium is stopped and restarted. In a few patients, parathyroid adenomas were present. Histologic findings in the remaining parathyroid glands in these patients have not been described, but the implication is that there is a single abnormal gland.

The presence of hypercalcemia does not correlate with plasma lithium level, but the frequency with which hypercalcemia occurs is sufficiently high to support a causal relationship between lithium and the hypercalcemia, particularly the dependence of the hypercalcemia on the continuation of the lithium. It is presumed that in most cases an adenoma is not present, merely hyperfunctioning glands. Lithium, at the levels achieved in blood in treated patients, can be shown in vitro to shift the curve describing PTH secretion by parathyroid glands as a function of calcium level to the right; i.e., higher calcium levels are required to lower PTH secretion. It is logical to assume that this effect can cause elevated PTH levels and consequent hypercalcemia in otherwise normal individuals. If careful studies were done, elevated PTH levels might be found in even more patients treated with lithium than the 10 percent in whom hypercalcemia is symptomatic. The adenomas reported in some hypercalcemic patients with lithium therapy may reflect the presence of an independently occurring parathyroid tumor; a permanent effect of lithium on parathyroid gland growth need not be implicated since most patients have complete reversal of hypercalcemia when lithium is stopped. However, long-standing stimulation of parathyroid cell replication may predispose to development of adenomas such as those seen in primary hyperparathyroidism, and it is possible that chronic lithium stimulation of the parathyroids may be a risk factor for adenoma formation. Some hypercalcemic patients are continued on lithium because of psychiatric indications. These patients are presumably best managed according to the principles used in asymptomatic hypercalcemia independent of lithium administration. If troubling symptoms or signs such as rising blood calcium levels, progressive bone demineralization, or kidney stones develop, it may be necessary to try alternative psychotropic medication. Parathyroid surgery should not be recommended unless hypercalcemia and elevated PTH levels persist after lithium is discontinued.

Familial Hypocalciuric Hypercalcemia (FHH) FHH (also called familial benign hypercalcemia) is inherited as an autosomal dominant trait. Affected individuals are discovered because of asymptomatic hypercalcemia. This disorder and Jansen's disease (discussed below) are variants of hyperparathyroidism. FHH involves excessive secretion of parathyroid hormone, and Jansen's disease excessive biological activity of the parathyroid hormone receptor in target tissues. Neither disorder, however, involves a primary growth disorder of the parathyroid glands and hence cannot be cured by parathyroidectomy.

The pathophysiology of FHH is now understood. The primary defect is abnormal sensing of the blood calcium by the parathyroid gland and renal tubule, causing inappropriate secretion of parathyroid hormone and excessive renal reabsorption of calcium (Fig. 354-2*A*). As discussed in Chap. 353, the calcium sensor consists of a member of the G protein family of receptor proteins tightly coupled to a transmembrane calcium channel. More than a dozen different point mutations in the calcium-sensing receptor have been identified in patients with FHH (Fig. 354-2*B*). These mutations lower the capacity of the sensor to bind calcium, and the mutant receptors function as though blood calcium were low; excessive secretion of parathyroid hormone occurs from an otherwise normal gland. The mutations act in a dominant negative fashion so that one abnormal copy of the receptor impairs the function of the normal allele. Other affected individuals and kindreds do not appear to have mutations in the coding sequence of this gene but may have mutations outside the coding sequence or mutations in other components of the calcium sensor.

Prior to the elucidation of the pathophysiology, abundant clinical evidence served to separate FHH from primary hyperparathyroidism. Most patients with primary hyperparathyroidism have less than 99 percent renal calcium reabsorption, and most patients with FHH exceed 99 percent reabsorption. The hypercalcemia in FHH is often detectable in affected members of the kindreds in the first decade of life, whereas hypercalcemia rarely occurs in patients with primary hyperparathyroidism and the MEN syndromes under the age of 10 years. The iPTH values may be elevated in FHH, but the values are usually normal or lower for the same degree of calcium elevation than in patients with primary hyperparathyroidism. Parathyroid surgery in a few patients led to permanent hypoparathyroidism, but hypocalciuria persisted nevertheless; the hypocalciuria, therefore, is not PTH-dependent but due to the abnormal calcium sensor in the kidney. Serum magnesium levels are, on average, higher in FHH than in primary hyperparathyroidism.

Few clinical signs or symptoms are present in patients with FHH. Unlike the MEN syndromes, other endocrine abnormalities are not present in FHH kindreds. Most patients are detected as a result of family screening after the diagnosis of hyperparathyroidism is made in one member of the kindred. All too commonly, the initial patient is operated on, and extensive parathyroid resection does not result in reversal of the hypercalcemia. At operation, the parathyroids appear normal or moderately hyperplasic. No patient has had reversal of hypercalcemia by surgery unless all the parathyroid tissue has been inadvertently removed, rendering the patient hypoparathyroid, a most undesirable outcome. The natural history of this disorder is not clear, but since the parathyroid glands are permissive rather than responsible

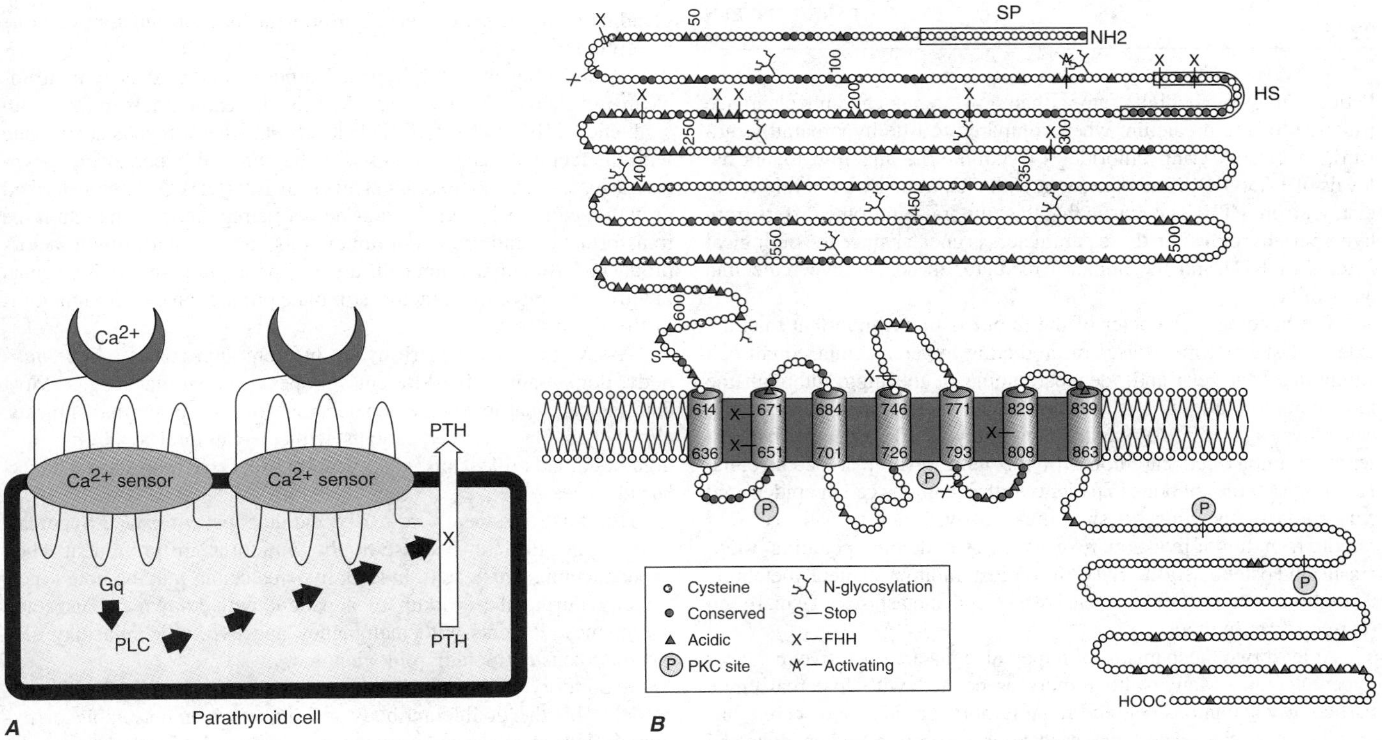

FIGURE 354-2 *A.* The calcium sensor's role in PTH secretion and calcium homeostasis. The extracellular domain is shown closing upon binding to calcium. PLC, phospholipase C; the G protein is shown as Gq (the subclass of G protein thought to activate PLC). When calcium in the blood is low, the sensor is less active and suppression of PTH secretion is lowered (i.e., more PTH is secreted). *(From Conklin and Bourne, with permission.) B.* Schematic two-dimensional diagram illustrating multiple points in the amino acid sequence of the calcium sensor (receptor) due to point mutations in the gene. The identified sequence alterations (X) cause loss of function and lead to inadequate suppression of PTH release and, therefore, mild hypercalcemia (FHH); ✯, a gain-of-function mutation that causes hypocalcemia; S, a stop codon that is a loss of function mutation; ●, conserved residues; ▲, acidic residues. *(From Brown et al, with permission.)*

for the syndrome, parathyroid surgery is not appropriate, nor, in view of the lack of symptoms, does medical treatment seem needed to lower the calcium. Organic compounds that bind to and activate the calcium sensor (calcimimetic agents) are under trial.

The characteristic mild elevation in blood calcium reflects a moderate excess in PTH levels; the hormone acts on target cells in bone and elsewhere to increase blood calcium levels until a new steady state is achieved between blood calcium and PTH secretion. A homozygous offspring of a consanguineous marriage has been identified in one FHH kindred, resulting in a profound neonatal hyperparathyroidism.

Jansen's Disease Children with this rare disorder often do not survive to adulthood. There are multiple developmental defects of the skeleton, including short stature, bowed legs, and multiple cystic resorptive areas in bones, associated with hypercalcemia and hypophosphatemia. PTH levels are undetectable, and the disorder is due to mutations that cause constitutive activation of the PTH receptor; two principle mutations have been identified in patients (Fig. 354-3). When these mutant receptors are expressed in vitro, they exhibit high levels of PTH-independent activity, indicating that the disease is due to excessive biological effects mimicking those of the hormone itself.

MALIGNANCY-RELATED HYPERCALCEMIA Clinical Syndromes and Mechanisms of Hypercalcemia Hypercalcemia due to malignancy is common (occurring with 10 to 15 percent of certain types of tumor, such as lung carcinoma), often severe and difficult to manage, confusing as to etiology, and sometimes difficult to distinguish from primary hyperparathyroidism. Traditionally, hypercalcemia in malignancy was thought to be due to a local invasion and destruction of bone by tumor cells; many cases are now known to result from the elaboration by the malignant cells of humoral mediators of hypercalcemia.

Although malignancy is often clinically obvious, hypercalcemia can occasionally be due to an occult tumor. With occult malignancy, diagnosis and definitive treatment must be accomplished quickly if the patient is to be protected from the complications of the underlying malignancy.

Humoral hypercalcemia of malignancy occurs with certain types of cancer of the lung and kidney, in which bone metastases are absent, minimal, or not detectable clinically. The clinical picture resembles primary hyperparathyroidism (hypophosphatemia accompanies hypercalcemia), and elimination or regression of the primary tumor leads to disappearance of the hypercalcemia. The disorder is due to secretion by the tumors of parathyroid hormone–like factors chemically distinct from PTH.

Many patients with the humoral hypercalcemia of malignancy have elevated urinary nephrogenous cyclic AMP excretion, hypophosphatemia, and increased urinary phosphate clearance, findings compatible with the actions of a humoral agent that emulates PTH action. However, with second-generation immunoassays, patients with the hypercalcemia of malignancy have either undetectable or suppressed immunoreactive PTH levels, making the differential diagnosis easier. Other features of the disorder differ from true hyperparathyroidism.

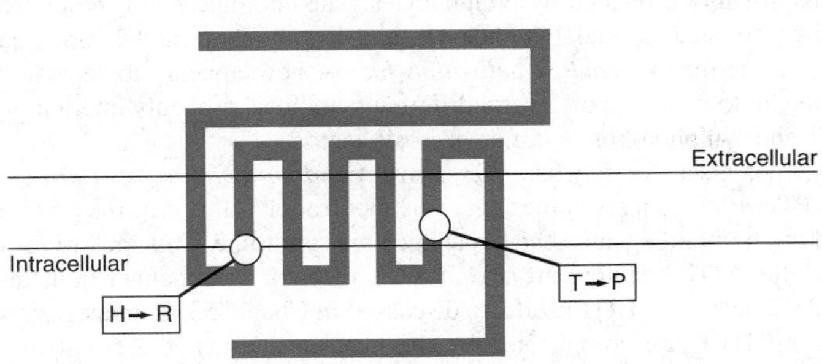

FIGURE 354-3 Pathogenesis of hypercalcemia in Jansen's disease is due to mutations at two sites in the PHT receptor, illustrated schematically with seven transmembrane-spanning domains. Histidine (H) found invariably in all members of the receptor family to which the PTH receptor belongs is mutated to arginine (R) in one locus; in the other, threonine (T) is mutated to proline (P). The resulting mutated receptors are constantly (constitutively) active without requiring PTH for simulation, thereby causing hypercalcemia and a condition simulating hyperparathyroidism. *(From Schipani et al, with permission.)*

Patients may have high, rather than low, renal calcium clearance (relative to serum calcium when compared to true hyperparathyroidism), levels of serum chloride <103 mmol/L, and low to normal levels of 1,25$(OH)_2$D, all consistent with mediation by humoral factors distinct from PTH. The reason that the humoral syndrome differs from hyperparathyroidism in these parameters is unclear since the biological actions of PTH and the humoral mediator in cancer hypercalcemia are similar.

The histologic character of the tumor is more important than the extent of skeletal metastases in predicting hypercalcemia. Small cell carcinoma (oat cell) and adenocarcinoma of the lung, although the most common lung tumors associated with skeletal metastases, rarely cause hypercalcemia. By contrast, as many as 10 percent of patients with squamous cell carcinoma of the lung develop hypercalcemia. Histologic studies of bone in patients with squamous cell or epidermoid carcinoma of the lung, in sites invaded by tumor as well as areas remote from tumor invasion, reveal bone remodeling, including osteoclastic and osteoblastic activity. In contrast, minimal skeletal metabolic activation occurs despite extensive skeletal metastases of small cell (oat cell) carcinoma.

At least two mechanisms of hypercalcemia are operative in cancer hypercalcemia. Many solid tumors associated with hypercalcemia, particularly squamous cell and renal tumors, produce and secrete humoral factors that cause increased bone resorption and mediate the hypercalcemia through systemic actions on the skeleton. Alternatively, direct bone marrow invasion occurs with hematologic malignancies such as leukemia, lymphoma, and multiple myeloma and with solid tumors such as breast carcinoma. Lymphokines and cytokines produced by cells involved in the marrow response to the tumors promote resorption of bone through local destruction.

Disorders of the latter class include myeloma and other hematologic malignancies involving the bone marrow that cause bone destruction and hypercalcemia through local mechanisms of malignant cells in the marrow spaces. Breast carcinoma is typical of solid tumors that cause hypercalcemia through *localized osteolytic destruction*, probably mediated by locally secreted tumor products that may differ from those involved in multiple myeloma or lymphoma.

In some patients with the humoral hypercalcemia of malignancy, osteoclastic resorption is unaccompanied by an osteoblastic or bone-forming response to bone resorption, implying some inhibition of the normal coupling of formation and resorption. Thus the interaction of more than one substance may determine whether hypercalcemia develops in a particular patient.

Several hormones, hormone analogues, cytokines, and growth factors have been implicated as the result of clinical assays, in vitro tests, or chemical isolation. In some lymphomas, typically B cell lymphomas, there is an increased blood level of 1,25$(OH)_2$D, which is probably produced by lymphocytes. The etiologic factor produced by activated normal lymphocytes and by myeloma and lymphoma cells, termed *osteoclast activation factor*, now appears to represent the biologic action of several different cytokines, probably interleukin 1 and lymphotoxin or tumor necrosis factor.

As discussed in Chap. 353, *parathyroid hormone–related protein* (PTHrP), which resembles but is distinct from PTH, fulfills the criteria for a humoral agent in the hypercalcemia syndrome. This factor binds to the PTH receptor and activates the receptor in a manner indistinguishable from PTH itself. As discussed in Chap. 353, immunoassays for PTHrP are complicated by the heterogeneity of the circulating forms of the peptide, but nonetheless, elevated levels of PTHrP are present in patients with the typical syndrome of humoral hypercalcemia of malignancy. The complexity of the etiologic mechanisms in cancer hypercalcemia are illustrated by the fact that some breast carcinoma cells and a distinctive type of T cell lymphoma/leukemia due to human T cell lymphotropic virus I infection produce PTHrP so that these tumors may produce hypercalcemia both by humoral and local mechanisms. Breast carcinoma cells also produce and secrete prostaglandins of the E series, which are potent local stimulators of bone resorption.

Several aspects of the hypercalcemia of malignancy remain unclear. Levels of urinary cyclic AMP rise in test animals treated with synthetic PTHrP, but 1,25$(OH)_2$D levels also rise, which is at variance with the fact that many patients with the humoral hypercalcemic syndrome have normal or depressed levels of 1,25$(OH)_2$D. Tumor-derived growth factors, believed to act as autocrine regulators to maintain the transformation and growth of tumor cells, and cellular growth factors produced by nonmalignant cells are also potent bone-resorbing agents in vitro. Several of these factors stimulate production of prostaglandins of the E_2 type.

Assays to detect PTHrP using different approaches (single-antibody, double-antibody, different epitopes) give similar results. Most data indicate that levels are undetectable (or low) in normal subjects, elevated in many cancer patients with the humoral syndrome, and high in human milk. Thus, identification of PTHrP represents a singular advance.

Diagnostic Issues Ordinarily, the diagnosis of cancer hypercalcemia is not difficult because tumor symptoms are prominent when hypercalcemia is detected. Indeed, hypercalcemia may be noted incidentally during the workup of a patient with known or suspected malignancy. Patients with malignancy and hypercalcemia may also have a coexistent parathyroid adenoma.

Laboratory testing is critical to exclude occult carcinoma. Levels of iPTH by the double-antibody technique are undetectable or extremely low in tumor hypercalcemia, as would be expected with the mediation of the hypercalcemia by a factor other than PTH (the hypercalcemia suppressing the normal parathyroid glands). Improvement in the usefulness of the PTH assay is a significant advance in laboratory diagnosis. (Earlier assays gave equivocal results.) Assays for PTHrP should be helpful; low or undetectable PTH and elevated PTHrP would focus attention on occult malignancy.

Clinical suspicion that malignancy is the cause of the hypercalcemia is heightened when symptoms associated with neoplasia, such as weight loss, fatigue, muscle weakness, and unexplained skin rash, or symptoms specific for a particular tumor are present. Squamous cell tumors are most frequently associated with hypercalcemia, particularly tumors of the lung, kidney, and urogenital tract. Radiologic examinations can focus on these areas when clinical evidence is unclear. Bone scans with technetium-labeled bisphosphonate are useful for detection of osteolytic metastases; the sensitivity is high, but specificity is low; results must be confirmed by conventional x-rays to be certain that areas of increased uptake are due to osteolytic metastases per se. Bone marrow biopsies are helpful in patients with anemia or abnormal peripheral blood smears.

Rx TREATMENT

Treatment of the hypercalcemia of malignancy is directed to control of the tumor, and reduction of tumor mass usually corrects hypercalcemia. If a patient has severe hypercalcemia yet has an excellent chance for effective tumor therapy, treatment of the hypercalcemia should be vigorous while awaiting the results of definitive therapy. If hypercalcemia, on the other hand, occurs in the late stages of a tumor that is resistant to therapy, the treatment of the hypercalcemia should be judicious, since hypercalcemia can have a mild sedating effect. Standard therapies for hypercalcemia (discussed below) are applicable to patients with malignancy.

VITAMIN D–RELATED HYPERCALCEMIA Hypercalcemia related to abnormal vitamin D action can be due to *excessive ingestion* of vitamin D or *abnormal metabolism* of the vitamin. Abnormal metabolism of the vitamin is usually acquired in association with some widespread granulomatous disorder, but one rare hereditary form of vitamin D sensitivity in infants is associated with other developmental anomalies. As discussed in Chap. 353, vitamin D metabolism is carefully regulated, particularly the activity of the renal 1α-hydroxylase responsible for the production of 1,25$(OH)_2$D. The regulation of 1α-hydroxylase and the normal feedback suppression by 1,25$(OH)_2$D on the kidney enzyme seem to work less well in infants than in adults and to operate poorly, if at all, in sites other than the renal tubule; these phenomena explain the occurrence of hypercalcemia secondary to excessive $1,25(OH)_2D_3$ production in infants with Williams' syndrome and adults with sarcoidosis or lymphoma.

Vitamin D Intoxication The chronic ingestion of 50 to 100 times the normal physiologic requirement of vitamin D (amounts in excess of 50,000 to 100,000 U/d) is required to produce hypercalcemia in normal individuals. In animals, vitamin D intoxication causes increased bone resorption and increased intestinal calcium absorption. In humans, vitamin D excess increases intestinal calcium absorption, but it is not known whether bone resorption is increased.

The mechanism for the hypercalcemia is an excessive production of $1,25(OH)_2D$ as a consequence of an increase in the substrate for the renal 1α-hydroxylase, namely, 25(OH)D. The production of 25(OH)D is less tightly regulated than is the production of $1,25(OH)_2D$. Hence concentrations of 25(OH)D are elevated 5- to 10-fold on average in patients on high-dose vitamin D. 25(OH)D has a definite, if low, biologic activity in intestine and bone, and part of vitamin D intoxication may be due to high levels of both 25(OH)D and $1,25(OH)_2D$.

The diagnosis is substantiated by documenting elevated levels of 25(OH)D. Hypercalcemia is usually controlled by restriction of dietary calcium intake and appropriate attention to hydration. These measures, plus discontinuation of vitamin D, usually lead to resolution of hypercalcemia. However, vitamin D stores in fat may be substantial, and vitamin D intoxication may persist for weeks after vitamin D ingestion is terminated. Such patients are responsive to glucocorticoids, which in doses of 100 mg of hydrocortisone per day, or its equivalent, usually return serum calcium levels to normal over several days; severe intoxication may require intensive therapy.

Sarcoidosis and Other Granulomatous Diseases In patients with sarcoidosis, $1,25(OH)_2D$ is believed to be synthesized in macrophages or other cells in the granulomas. Indeed, hypercalcemia has been reported in an anephric sarcoidosis patient in association with increased $1,25(OH)_2D$ levels. Macrophages obtained from granulomatous tissue convert 25(OH)D to $1,25(OH)_2D$ at an increased rate. There is a positive correlation in patients with sarcoidosis between 25(OH)D levels (reflecting vitamin D intake) and the circulating concentrations of $1,25(OH)_2D$, whereas normally there is no increase in $1,25(OH)_2D$ with increasing 25(OH)D levels due to multiple feedback controls on the renal 1α-hydroxylase (see Chap. 353). The usual regulation of active metabolite production by calcium or PTH does not operate in these patients; hypercalcemia does not lead to a reduction in the blood levels of $1,25(OH)_2D$ in patients with sarcoidosis. The PTH independence of $1,25(OH)_2D$ production in this disorder is indicated by reports of normal $1,25(OH)_2D$ production in a patient with sarcoidosis and hypoparathyroidism. Clearance of $1,25(OH)_2D$ from blood may be decreased in sarcoidosis as well.

Even normocalcemic patients with sarcoidosis have unregulated production of $1,25(OH)_2D$ in response to vitamin D loading. Exposure to sunlight or administration of as little as 9000 units of vitamin D daily is followed by increased levels of the active metabolite. Administration of moderate doses of glucocorticoids leads to a reversal of the hypercalcemia, as in other cases of excessive vitamin D action such as vitamin D intoxication, and reversal of the abnormal responsiveness of $1,25(OH)_2D$ levels to vitamin D challenge. Presumably, glucocorticoids have multiple effects in the disease and block both excessive production of the metabolite and the response to it in target organs.

Variation in reported frequency of hypercalcemia in sarcoidosis (10 percent or less in recent reports, 60 percent or more in older reports) is probably explained in part by the common use of glucocorticoids to control pulmonary complications and other manifestations of the granulomatous disease. Lytic lesions also occur in bone so that increased bone resorption may play a role in some cases. In most, however, hypercalcemia is directly related to an increased intestinal calcium absorption. Hypercalcemia is usually a manifestation of disseminated disease. Hence pulmonary involvement is usually evident; chest x-ray may reveal a diffuse fibronodular infiltrate and/or prominent hilar adenopathy. Levels of angiotensin-converting enzyme are elevated; blood gamma globulin also may be elevated. The most useful diagnostic procedure is demonstration of noncaseating granulomas in liver or lymph node biopsy. Hypercalcemia due to sarcoidosis can be elusive when the typical features of the disease are lacking (see "Differential Diagnosis: Special Tests").

Management of the hypercalcemia can be accomplished by avoiding excessive sunlight exposure and by limiting vitamin D and calcium intake; glucocorticoids in the equivalent of 100 mg hydrocortisone per day or less usually are sufficient to control hypercalcemia. Presumably, however, the abnormal sensitivity to vitamin D and abnormal regulation of $1,25(OH)_2D$ synthesis will persist as long as the disease is active. PTH levels are usually low and $1,25(OH)_2D$ levels are elevated, but primary hyperparathyroidism and sarcoidosis may coexist in some patients.

Idiopathic Hypercalcemia of Infancy This rare disorder, also referred to as *Williams' syndrome*, consists of multiple congenital development defects, including supravalvular aortic stenosis, mental retardation, and an elfin facies, in association with hypercalcemia due to abnormal sensitivity to vitamin D. The syndrome was first recognized in England after the fortification of milk with vitamin D. Hypercalcemia develops with vitamin D intakes as small as 2000 to 4000 U/d. Levels of $1,25(OH)_2D$ are elevated, ranging from 46 to 120 nmol/L (150 to 500 pg/mL). The mechanism of the abnormal sensitivity to vitamin D and of the increased circulating levels of $1,25(OH)_2D$ is unclear. Hypercalcemia is due to excessive intestinal calcium absorption. The abnormality in vitamin D metabolism and the increased sensitivity to vitamin D intake disappear after the first year of life. Treatment is restriction of calcium intake. When the hypercalcemia is severe, glucocorticoids in the doses used for vitamin D intoxication or sarcoidosis, adjusted for body weight, are effective.

HYPERCALCEMIA ASSOCIATED WITH HIGH BONE TURNOVER Hyperthyroidism As many as 20 percent of hyperthyroid patients have high-normal or mildly elevated serum calcium concentrations; hypercalciuria is even more common. The hypercalcemia is due to increased bone turnover, with bone resorption exceeding bone formation. Severe calcium elevations are not typical, and the presence of such suggests a concomitant disease such as hyperparathyroidism. Indeed, patients with thyrotoxicosis are more sensitive to the hypercalcemic effects of PTH. Usually, the diagnosis is obvious, but signs of hyperthyroidism may occasionally be occult, particularly in the elderly. Hypercalcemia is managed by treatment of the hyperthyroidism.

Immobilization Immobilization is a rare cause of hypercalcemia in adults in the absence of an associated disease but may cause hypercalcemia in children and adolescents, particularly after spinal cord injury and paraplegia or quadriplegia. With resumption of some ambulation, the hypercalcemia in children usually returns to normal.

The mechanism appears to involve a disproportion between bone formation and bone resorption. Hypercalciuria and increased mobilization of skeletal calcium can develop in normal volunteers subjected to extensive bed rest, although hypercalcemia is unusual. Immobilization of an adult with a disease associated with high bone turnover, such as Paget's disease, may cause hypercalcemia.

Thiazides Administration of benzothiadiazines (thiazides) can cause hypercalcemia in patients with high rates of bone turnover, such as patients with hypoparathyroidism treated with high doses of vitamin D. Traditionally, thiazides are associated with aggravation of hypercalcemia in primary hyperparathyroidism, but this effect can be seen in other high-bone-turnover states as well. The mechanism of action of thiazides is complex, but the result seems to be to impose a challenge to calcium homeostasis by actions on renal calcium excretion, bone-calcium turnover, and parathyroid action. Thiazide administration to normal individuals causes a transient increase in blood calcium (usually within the high-normal range) that reverts to preexisting levels after a week or more of continued administration. If hormonal function and calcium and bone metabolism are normal, homeostatic controls are reset to counteract the calcium-elevating effect of the thiazides. In the presence of hyperparathyroidism or increased bone turnover from another cause, homeostatic mechanisms are ineffective. The abnormal effects of the thiazide on calcium metabolism disappear within days of cessation of the drug.

Many aspects of thiazide action on calcium metabolism are unclear. The drugs augment PTH responsiveness of bone and renal tubule. Chronic thiazide administration leads to reduction in urinary calcium; the hypocalciuric effect appears to reflect the enhancement of proximal tubular resorption of sodium and calcium in response to sodium depletion. Some of this renal action is due to augmentation of PTH action and is more pronounced in individuals with intact parathyroid secretion. However, thiazides cause hypocalciuria in hypoparathyroid patients on high-dose vitamin D and oral calcium replacement if sodium intake is restricted. This finding is the rationale for the use of thiazides as an adjunct to therapy in hypoparathyroid patients as discussed below.

Vitamin A Intoxication Vitamin A intoxication is a rare cause of hypercalcemia. Most vitamin A intoxication is a side effect of dietary faddism (see Chap. 79). Calcium levels can be elevated into the 3 to 3.5 mmol/L (12 to 14 mg/dL) range after the ingestion of 50,000 to 100,000 units of vitamin A daily (10 to 20 times the minimum daily requirement). Typical features of severe hypercalcemia include fatigue, anorexia, and in some severe muscle and bone pain. Vitamin A intake excess is presumed to increase bone resorption.

Diagnosis can be established by history and by measurement of vitamin A levels in serum, which may be severalfold above normal. Occasionally, skeletal x-rays reveal periosteal calcifications, particularly in the hands. Withdrawal of the vitamin is usually associated with the prompt disappearance of the hypercalcemia and reversal of the skeletal changes. As in vitamin D intoxication, administration of 100 mg/d hydrocortisone or its equivalent leads to a rapid return of the serum calcium to normal.

HYPERCALCEMIA ASSOCIATED WITH RENAL FAILURE Severe Secondary Hyperparathyroidism Secondary hyperparathyroidism occurs when partial resistance to the metabolic actions of the hormone leads to excessive PTH production. Parathyroid gland hyperplasia occurs because resistance to the normal level of the hormone leads to hypocalcemia, which, in turn, is a stimulus to enlargement of the parathyroid glands with resultant increased secretion of PTH. This concept is based on studies in experimental animals with renal failure and phosphate retention and studies of the treatment of patients with bisphosphonates that block skeletal resorptive response. When the parathyroid secretory reserve is tested by deliberately lowering blood calcium, the extent of rise in PTH for each decrement of plasma calcium is greater with hyperplastic than with normal parathyroids. There is, therefore, a higher concentration of iPTH at any given level of calcium concentration. Since a portion of PTH secretion by each parathyroid cell is not suppressible by any degree of elevation of blood calcium, larger glands (more cells) have a higher hormone output at the hypercalcemic end of the dose-response curve.

Secondary hyperparathyroidism occurs in patients with renal failure, osteomalacia (vitamin D deficiency), and pseudohypoparathyroidism (deficient response to PTH at the level of the receptor). The clinical manifestations of secondary hyperparathyroidism vary in these states. Hypocalcemia seems to be the common denominator in secondary hyperparathyroidism. Primary and secondary hyperparathyroidism can be distinguished conceptually by the autonomous growth of the parathyroid glands in primary hyperparathyroidism (presumably irreversible) and the adaptive growth of the parathyroids in secondary hyperparathyroidism (presumably reversible). In fact, reversal over weeks from an abnormal pattern of secretion, presumably accompanied by involution of parathyroid gland mass to normal, occurs in patients who have been treated medically to reverse the resistance to PTH.

In progressive renal failure, the initial tendency to hypocalcemia is attributable to phosphate retention due to the reduced excretion of phosphate and reduced production of $1,25(OH)_2D$ by the failing kidney. The net consequence is reduced skeletal responsiveness to PTH. $1,25(OH)_2D$ deficiency also interferes with calcium absorption from the intestine, already impaired in uremia. The consequence in any given patient with chronic renal failure represents the outcome of competing physiologic adaptations, stimuli that cause parathyroid gland hyperplasia (tendency toward hypercalcemia and excessive bone resorption) versus those that modify the responsiveness of the end organs—bone, gut, and residual renal tubules (tendency toward hypocalcemia, hyperphosphatemia, and reduced bone resorption). Typically patients with renal failure exhibit hyperphosphatemia (renal retention and increased bone breakdown) and a low-normal or moderately low blood calcium level (calcium-lowering action of the phosphate level and reduced availability of calcium from bone and gut). In patients with severe secondary hyperparathyroidism, hypercalcemia and hyperphosphatemia both develop due to an increase in bone resorption; parathyroid hypersecretion "overshoots" the degree of resistance to hormone action; monoclonal expansion of parathyroid gland mass may contribute to the "overshoot" and hypercalcemia.

In addition to hypercalcemia and hyperphosphatemia, patients with secondary hyperparathyroidism may develop bone pain, ectopic calcification, and pruritus. The bone disease in patients with secondary hyperparathyroidism and renal failure is usually termed *renal osteodystrophy*. Concomitant osteomalacia (vitamin D and calcium deficiency) and osteitis fibrosa cystica (excessive PTH action on bone) may occur. In fact, osteitis fibrosa cystica is now more common in untreated renal failure than in primary hyperparathyroidism.

Two other skeletal disorders are associated with long-term dialysis in patients with renal failure. Aluminum deposition (see below) is associated with an osteomalacia-like picture. The other entity is a low bone turnover state termed "aplastic" or "adynamic" bone disease; PTH levels are lower than in typical secondary hyperparathyroidism. The adynamic state responds to measures that stimulate PTH secretion, implying that the cause is excessive involution of the hyperparathyroidism by calcium carbonate.

℞ TREATMENT

Medical therapy to reverse secondary hyperparathyroidism includes reduction of excessive blood phosphate by restriction of dietary phosphate, the use of nonabsorbable antacids, and careful, selective addition of calcitriol (0.25 to 2.0 μg/d); calcium carbonate is preferred over aluminum-containing antacids to prevent aluminum toxicity. Intravenous administration of calcitriol, sometimes administered as several pulses each week, has been reported to cause long-term involution of secondary hyperparathyroidism. Involution of the parathyroids often occurs; reduction of the increased parathyroid mass causes the exaggerated secretory response to return to normal. The level of PTH at any given level of blood calcium is now more appropriate, and excessive parathyroid action is reversed. Somewhat paradoxically, during successful medical reversal of secondary hyperparathyroidism, elevated serum calcium (and phosphate) levels may return to normal despite the administration of increased amounts of calcium and vitamin D metabolites that might have been expected to aggravate the hypercalcemia.

Occasional patients develop severe manifestations of secondary hyperparathyroidism, including hypercalcemia, pruritus, extraskeletal calcifications, and painful bones, despite aggressive medical efforts to suppress the hyperparathyroidism. Parathyroid surgery may be necessary to control the condition. Since one or more of the enlarged glands may be monoclonal in nature, this phenomenon must be due to conversion of the parathyroids from a state of reversible hyperplasia to an irreversible growth defect and state of PTH hypersecretion no longer responsive to medical therapy. This state of severe hyperparathyroidism in patients with renal failure that requires surgery has been referred to as *tertiary hyperparathyroidism*.

Aluminum Intoxication Aluminum intoxication may occur in patients on chronic dialysis; manifestations include acute dementia and unresponsive and severe osteomalacia. Bone pain, multiple nonhealing fractures, particularly of the ribs and pelvis, and a proximal myopathy may occur. Hypercalcemia develops when these patients are treated with vitamin D or calcitriol, as in the typical patient with severe secondary hyperparathyroidism and renal osteodystrophy, as discussed above. Acute hypercalcemia occurs after administration of vitamin D because of impaired skeletal responsiveness. Aluminum is present at the site of osteoid mineralization, osteoblastic activity is minimal, and calcium incorporation into the skeleton is impaired. Prevention is accomplished by avoidance of aluminum excess in the dialysis regimen; treatment involves mobilizing aluminum through the use of the chelating agent deferoxamine. Aluminum is mobilized from bone and, being tightly bound to the chelating agent, can be removed via dialysis. After aluminum toxicity is reversed, patients may show typical features of renal osteodystrophy and secondary hyperparathyroidism and are managed like other patients with secondary hyperparathyroidism due to renal disease. Failure to recognize the syndrome is associated with persistence of the disabling bone disease and with hypercalcemia inadvertently induced by treatment with vitamin D. The iPTH levels may not increase to the normal hyperparathyroid range as a result of the aluminum toxicity.

Milk-Alkali Syndrome The milk-alkali syndrome can cause several clinical presentations—acute, subacute, and chronic—all of which feature hypercalcemia, alkalosis, and renal failure. The disorder is due to an excessive ingestion of calcium and absorbable antacids such as milk or calcium carbonate and is less frequent since nonabsorbable antacids and other treatments became available for peptic ulcer disease.

Individual susceptibility must be important in the pathogenesis, since many patients are treated with calcium carbonate without developing the syndrome. One variable is the fractional calcium absorption as a function of calcium intake. Some individuals absorb a high fraction of calcium, even with intakes as high as 2 g and more of elemental calcium per day, instead of reducing calcium absorption with high intake, as occurs in most normal individuals. Resultant mild hypercalcemia after meals in such patients is postulated to contribute to the generation of alkalosis. Development of hypercalcemia causes increased sodium excretion and some depletion of total-body water. These phenomena and perhaps some suppression of endogenous PTH secretion due to mild hypercalcemia lead to increased bicarbonate resorption and to alkalosis in the face of continued calcium carbonate ingestion. Alkalosis per se selectively enhances calcium resorption in the distal nephron, thus aggravating the hypercalcemia. The cycle of mild hypercalcemia → bicarbonate retention → alkalosis → renal calcium retention → severe hypercalcemia perpetuates and aggravates hypercalcemia and alkalosis as long as calcium and absorbable alkali are ingested.

Acute hypercalcemia and alkalosis occurring within days of beginning calcium and alkali ingestion, *acute milk-alkali syndrome*, is manifested by weakness, myalgia, irritability, and apathy. The impairment of renal function, including reduced renal concentrating ability and tubular dysfunction, hypercalcemia, and alkalosis reverse rapidly upon stopping the intake of calcium and alkali.

The far-advanced milk-alkali syndrome, sometimes referred to as *Burnett's syndrome*, is due to long-standing calcium and alkali ingestion. Severe hypercalcemia, irreversible renal failure, and phosphate retention may be accompanied by ectopic calcification. Some improvement may result when the ingestion of calcium and alkali is reduced, but prior to the availability of renal dialysis renal failure led to death. There is an intermediate or subacute form in which the renal failure is reversible over a period of weeks after withdrawal of excessive calcium and alkali intake.

DIFFERENTIAL DIAGNOSIS: SPECIAL TESTS Differential diagnosis of hypercalcemia is best achieved by using clinical criteria, but the radioimmunoassay for PTH is useful in distinguishing among major causes. The clinical features that deserve major emphasis are the presence or absence of symptoms or signs of disease and evidence of chronicity. If one discounts fatigue or depression, more than 90 percent of patients with *asymptomatic hypercalcemia* have primary hyperparathyroidism; symptoms of malignancy are usually present in cancer hypercalcemia. Disorders other than hyperparathyroidism and malignancy cause no more than 10 percent of cases of hypercalcemia, and some of the nonparathyroid causes are associated with clear-cut manifestations such as renal failure.

Table 354-2

Differential Diagnosis of Hypercalcemia

Criterion	Conclusion
Clinical issues alone	
>90% caused by hyperparathyroidism or cancer	
If asymptomatic or chronic:	Hyperparathyroidism most likely
Level of PTH measured by PTH assay	
Increased or normal (despite hypercalcemia):	Hyperparathyroidism confirmed
Decreased or undetectable:	Acute presentation with or without symptoms—screen carefully for malignancy Chronic—malignancy unlikely, sarcoidosis or other rarer cause

Chronicity is the second most important clinical criterion. If hypercalcemia has been manifest for more than 1 year, malignancy can usually be excluded as the cause. A striking feature of malignancy-associated hypercalcemia is the rapidity of the course, whereby signs and symptoms of the underlying malignancy are evident within months of the detection of hypercalcemia. Hyperparathyroidism is the likely diagnosis in patients with *chronic hypercalcemia*. Diseases such as sarcoidosis are rare causes of chronic hypercalcemia. A careful *history* of dietary supplements and drug use may suggest intoxication with vitamins D or A or the use of thiazides.

Although clinical considerations are helpful in arriving at the correct diagnosis of the cause of hypercalcemia, appropriate laboratory testing is essential for definitive diagnosis (Table 354-2). Theoretically, the radioimmunoassay for PTH should separate hyperparathyroidism from all other causes of hypercalcemia, those with hyperparathyroidism having elevated levels of iPTH despite hypercalcemia and patients with malignancy and the other causes of hypercalcemia (except for disorders mediated by PTH such as lithium-induced hypercalcemia) having levels of hormone below normal or undetectable. Assays based on the double-antibody method separate those with primary hyperparathyroidism from the hypercalcemia of malignancy (Fig. 354-4 and Table 354-2). $1,25(OH)_2D$ levels are elevated in many (but not all) patients with primary hyperparathyroidism and are increased in states of vitamin D intoxication, particularly sarcoidosis. In other disorders associated with hypercalcemia, concentrations of $1,25(OH)_2D$ are low or, at the most, normal. Since not all patients with hyperparathyroidism have elevated $1,25(OH)_2D$ levels, and since not all nonparathyroid hypercalcemic patients have suppressed $1,25(OH)_2D$, the test is of low specificity and not cost-effective in differential diagnosis; measurement of $1,25(OH)_2D$ is of critical value in establishing the cause of hypercalcemia in sarcoidosis and certain B cell lymphomas.

PTH levels are elevated in chronic renal failure; the elevation seen in early assays reflects, in part, accumulation of fragments secondary to renal failure rather than true parathyroid oversecretion. Results with the double-antibody assay correlate well with independent evidence for parathyroid gland overactivity. Patients with sarcoidosis have low or undetectable levels of iPTH. No systematic surveys have been reported of the results of double-antibody PTH radioimmunoassays in many of the other non-parathyroid-related causes of hypercalcemia largely because of the infrequency of the disorders, but it is predicted that they will be low or undetectable.

In summary, iPTH values are elevated in more than 90 percent of parathyroid-related causes of hypercalcemia, undetectable or low in malignancy-related hypercalcemia, and undetectable or normal in vitamin D–related and high-bone-turnover causes of hypercalcemia (although there is little data for these latter categories).

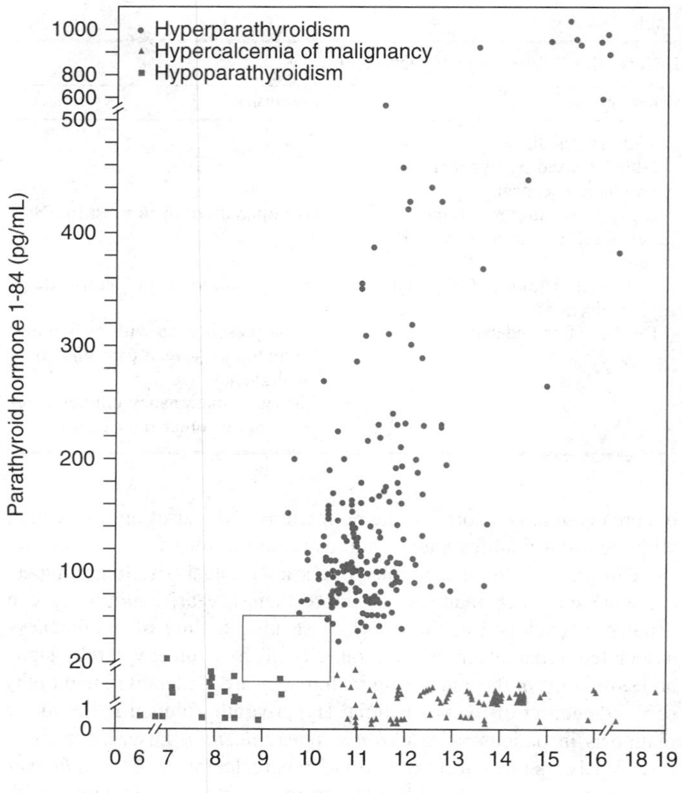

FIGURE 354-4 Levels of iPTH detected in patients with primary hyperparathyroidism, hypercalcemia of malignancy, and hypoparathyroidism. Boxed area represents the upper and normal limits of blood calcium and/or iPTH. *(From Nussbaum and Potts, with permission.)*

Measurements of nephrogenous cyclic AMP are of limited value in distinguishing primary hyperparathyroidism and malignancy because nephrogenous cyclic AMP is elevated in some patients with malignancy as well as in most patients with primary hyperparathyroidism. Specific laboratory tests are of utility in diagnosing particular disorders (such as thyrotoxicosis), and the newer immunoassays for PTH-rP are helpful in diagnosing certain types of malignancy-associated hypercalcemia.

Some general conclusions are warranted as to the differential diagnosis of hypercalcemia. Two independent causes of hypercalcemia in the same person, although reported, are rare. If a specific disease traditionally associated with hypercalcemia is clinically evident, it is reasonable to assume that the disease is responsible for the hypercalcemia. In view of the specificity of the PTH immunoassay and the high frequency of hyperparathyroidism in hypercalcemic patients, it is cost-effective to measure the iPTH level in all hypercalcemic patients unless malignancy or a specific nonparathyroid disease is obvious. If hypercalcemia disappears in response to control of hyperthyroidism or after reduction of excessive intake of fat-soluble vitamins or alkali and calcium, in the cases of vitamin D intoxication and milk-alkali syndrome, respectively, there is no need to search for a second cause of hypercalcemia. If specific treatment does not lead to a reversal of the hypercalcemia, a search for an additional cause must be undertaken. It also follows that the management of the hypercalcemia of malignancy focuses on treatment of the malignancy.

When the diagnosis is unclear, either because the patient is asymptomatic or because chronic illness obscures manifestations that might indicate the presence of malignancy, the following general approach can be used: If the patient is *asymptomatic* and there is evidence by history of *chronicity* to the hypercalcemia, hyperparathyroidism is almost certainly the cause. If iPTH levels (usually measured at least twice) are elevated, little additional evaluation is necessary. Hyperparathyroidism is never confirmed until abnormal parathyroid tissue is removed surgically and hypercalcemia is corrected, but the presumptive diagnosis can be made in patients with asymptomatic hypercalcemia on the basis of elevated concentration of iPTH. If there is a family history suggestive of other endocrine abnormalities, screening for MEN should be undertaken in the patient and family.

If the patient does not have clear-cut symptoms and there is only a short history or no clue as to the duration of the hypercalcemia, *occult malignancy* must be considered. If the iPTH levels with the double-antibody technique are increased, the diagnosis of asymptomatic hyperparathyroidism is established.

If patients with recent-onset hypercalcemia have clear-cut systemic symptoms and/or the iPTH levels are not elevated, then a thorough workup must be undertaken for malignancy, including chest x-ray, CT of chest and abdomen, and bone scan. Attention also should be paid to clues for underlying hematologic disorders such as anemia, increased plasma globulin, and abnormal serum immunoelectrophoresis; bone scans can be negative in patients with multiple myeloma.

Finally, if a patient with *chronic hypercalcemia* is *asymptomatic* but iPTH values are not elevated, and if malignancy seems unlikely on clinical grounds (chronicity), it is useful to search for other chronic causes of hypercalcemia, such as occult sarcoidosis. Table 354-2 summarizes the approach.

℞ TREATMENT

Hypercalcemic States The acute treatment of hypercalcemia is usually successful. The serum calcium concentration can be decreased by 0.7 to 2.2 mmol/L (3 to 9 mg/dL) within 24 to 48 h in most patients, enough to relieve acute symptoms, prevent death from hypercalcemic crisis, and permit diagnostic evaluation. However, the chronic medical management of hypercalcemia is less satisfactory unless the underlying cause can be corrected because available therapies are inconvenient and may be toxic.

Hypercalcemia develops because of excessive skeletal calcium release, increased intestinal calcium absorption, or inadequate renal calcium excretion. Understanding the particular pathogenesis helps guide therapy. For example, hypercalcemia in patients with osteolytic metastases or acute immobilization is primarily due to excessive skeletal calcium release and is, therefore, minimally improved by restriction of dietary calcium. On the other hand, patients with vitamin D hypersensitivity or vitamin D intoxication have excessive intestinal calcium absorption, and restriction of dietary calcium is beneficial. Decreased renal function or extracellular fluid depletion decreases urinary calcium excretion. If additional abnormalities, such as increased bone breakdown, are present, hypercalcemia will develop. This may happen, for example, when patients with resorptive bone disease become dehydrated. In such situations, rehydration may rapidly reduce or reverse the hypercalcemia, even though bone resorption and urinary calcium excretion are increased.

HYDRATION, INCREASED SALT INTAKE, MILD AND FORCED DIURESIS The first principle of treatment is to restore *normal hydration.* Many hypercalcemic patients are dehydrated because of vomiting, inanition, and/or hypercalcemia-induced defects in urinary concentrating ability. The resultant drop in glomerular filtration rate is accompanied by an additional decrease in renal tubular sodium and calcium clearance. Restoring a normal extracellular fluid volume corrects these abnormalities and increases urine calcium excretion by 2.5 to 7.5 mmol/d (100 to 300 mg/d). Increasing urinary sodium excretion to 400 to 500 mmol/d increases urinary calcium excretion even further than simple rehydration. After rehydration has been achieved, saline can be administered or furosemide or ethacrynic acid can be given twice daily to depress the tubular reabsorptive mechanism for calcium (care must be taken to prevent dehydration). The combined use of these therapies can increase urinary calcium excretion to 12.5 mmol/d (500 mg/d) or higher in most hypercalcemic patients. Since this is a substantial percentage of the exchangeable calcium pool, the serum calcium concentration usually falls 0.25 to 0.75 mmol/L (1 to 3 mg/dL) within 24 h. Precautions should be taken to prevent potassium and magnesium depletion; calcium-containing renal calculi are a potential complication.

Under life-threatening circumstances, the preceding approach can be pursued more aggressively, giving as much as 6 L isotonic saline (900 mmol sodium) daily plus furosemide or equivalent in doses up to 100 mg every 1 to 2 h or ethacrynic acid in doses to 40 mg every 1 to 2 h. Urinary calcium excretion may exceed 25 mmol/d (1000 mg/d), and the serum calcium may decrease by 1 mmol/L (4 mg/dL) or more within 24 h. Depletion of potassium and magnesium is inevitable unless replacements are given; pulmonary edema can be precipitated. The potential complications can be reduced by careful monitoring of central venous pressure and plasma or urine electrolytes; catheterization of the bladder may be necessary. This treatment approach should be supplemented with agents to block bone resorption that become effective within a few days, since forced diuresis is difficult to sustain even in patients with good cardiopulmonary and renal function.

BISPHOSPHONATES The bisphosphonates are analogues of pyrophosphate, with high affinity for bone, especially in areas of increased bone turnover. These bone-seeking compounds are stable in vivo because phosphatase enzymes cannot hydrolyze the central carbon-phosphorus-carbon bond. The bisphosphonates are concentrated in areas of high bone turnover and are taken up by and inhibit osteoclast action; the mechanism of action is not well understood. Bisphosphonates may alter proton pump function or impair the release of acid hydrolases into the extracellular lysosomes contiguous with mineralized bone. They also may inhibit the differentiation of monocyte-macrophage precursors into osteoclasts and possibly have effects on osteoblasts as well.

Etidronate, a first-generation bisphosphonate, is poorly absorbed and, like most bisphosphonates, generally must be given intravenously to be effective. At times, the continuation of oral etidronate after intravenous therapy may be useful to control hypercalcemia.

A newer class of bisphosphonates has more favorable efficacy and longer duration of action (Table 354-3). Pamidronate is a potent inhibitor of osteoclast-mediated skeletal resorption yet does not cause mineralization defects at ordinary doses. Several additional bisphosphonates (alendronate, tiludronate, and risedronate) are highly potent and have a favorable ratio of blocking resorption over inhibiting bone formation. The potency of the compounds for inhibition of bone resorption varies a thousandfold in the order of etidronate, tiludronate, pamidronate, alendronate, and risedronate. Oral alendronate is approved for the therapy of osteoporosis in the United States, and in Europe oral preparations of these bisphosphonates are used in the chronic treatment of hypercalcemia. Only the intravenous use of pamidronate is approved for this purpose in the United States; between 60 and 90 mg pamidronate, given as a single intravenous dose, returns serum calcium to normal for weeks in 80 to 100 percent of patients.

While the bisphosphonates have similar structures, efficacy, toxicity, and side effects vary. Etidronate causes hyperphosphatemia, through a direct renal mechanism, whereas hypophosphatemia is seen following therapy with other bisphosphonates. Pamidronate causes low-grade fever in as many as 20 percent of patients, likely related to release of cytokines from osteoclasts, monocytes, and macrophages (Table 354-3). Overall, second-generation bisphosphonates are now the agents of choice in severe hypercalcemia, particularly that associated with malignancy.

CALCITONIN Calcitonin acts within minutes of its administration, through receptors on osteoclasts, to decrease the release of skeletal calcium, phosphorus, and hydroxyproline. In addition, inhibition of renal tubular calcium reabsorption may, in part, contribute to its rapid onset of action. In various reports, however, the adminis-

Table 354-3

Therapies for Severe Hypercalcemia

Treatment	Onset of Action	Duration of Action	Advantages	Disadvantages
MOST USEFUL THERAPIES				
Hydration with saline	Hours	During infusion	Rehydration invariably needed	
Forced diuresis; saline + loop diuretic	Hours	During treatment	Rapid action	Cardiac decompensation, intensive monitoring electrolyte disturbance, hypokalemia, hypomagnesemia
Bisphosphonates				
1st generation: etidronate	1–2 days	5–7 days in doses used	First available bisphosphonate; intermediate onset of action	Hyperphosphatemia; 3-day infusion
2d generation: pamidronate	1–2 days	10–14 days after high dose	High potency; intermediate onset; prolonged duration of action	Fever in 20%; hypophosphatemia, hypocalcemia, hypomagnesemia
Calcitonin	Hours	2–3 days	Rapid onset of action; useful as adjunct in severe hypercalcemia	Often limited calcium lowering, rapid tachyphylaxis
OTHER THERAPIES				
Gallium nitrate	Day after 5-day administration	7–10 days	High potency	Length of IV administration; cannot be used with renal failure
Plicamycin	3–4 days	Days	Potent antiresorptive	Liver, kidney, and marrow toxicity; bleeding
Phosphate				
Oral	24 h	During use	Low toxicity if $P < 4$ mg/dL	Limited use except as adjuvant or chronic therapy
Intravenous	Hours	During use and 24–48 h afterward	Rapid action, highly potent	Ectopic calcification; severe hypocalcemia
Glucocorticoids	Days	Days, weeks	Oral therapy, antitumor agent	Active only in certain malignancies; glucocorticoid side effects
Dialysis	Hours	During use and 24–48 h afterward	Useful in renal failure; onset of effect in hours; can immediately reverse life-threatening hypercalcemia	Complex procedure, reserved for extreme or special circumstances

tration of 2 to 8 U/kg of body weight intravenously, subcutaneously, or intramuscularly every 6 to 12 h caused variable and minimal lowering of calcium in some patients. Tachyphylaxis, a known phenomenon with this drug, may explain the variable results. This escape from the hypocalcemic effects of calcitonin can be prevented by glucocorticoids in vitro. In vivo in humans, administration of glucocorticoids in combination with calcitonin may augment or prolong the action of calcitonin; in some patients, particularly those with lymphoproliferative malignancies, lowering of calcium may persist for as long as 10 days. In other studies, however, glucocorticoids did not prevent tachyphylaxis. Calcitonin therapy with the salmon, porcine, and human sequences, as currently used, rarely returns serum calcium to normal and can best be viewed as a nontoxic therapy with a very rapid onset of action and limited efficacy. However, in life-threatening hypercalcemia, calcitonin can be used while waiting for more sustained effects from plicamycin, gallium, or bisphosphonate. Calcitonin therapy may be associated with transient nausea, cramping, abdominal pain, and flushing.

PLICAMYCIN For the acute management of hypercalcemia, plicamycin (mithramycin), which inhibits bone resorption, has been a useful therapeutic agent. Plicamycin must be given intravenously, either as a bolus injection or by slow infusion. The usual dose is 25 μg/kg of body weight. In some patients, 10 μg/kg of body weight can be given twice a week for chronic therapy. Treatment should not be repeated until hypercalcemia recurs, because toxicity is dependent on the frequency of treatment and the total dosage. Careful monitoring is needed if repeated doses are used. The major side effects are thrombocytopenia, hepatocellular necrosis with increased lactic acid dehydrogenase (LDH) and aspartate aminotransferase (AST) levels, and decreased levels of clotting factors with resultant epistaxis, bruising, hemorrhage, and bleeding gums. Azotemia, proteinuria, hypocalcemia, hypophosphatemia, hypokalemia, nausea, vomiting, stomatitis, and facial swelling may occur. Toxicity is rare when only one or two doses are used and can be minimized by repeating single doses only when hypercalcemia recurs. Toxic effects other than hemorrhage can usually be reversed by stopping the drug. Use of plicamycin has been largely replaced by the less toxic second-generation bisphosphonates.

GALLIUM NITRATE Gallium nitrate exerts a hypocalcemic action by inhibiting bone resorption and altering the structure of bone crystals. Major disadvantages include the 5-day duration of infusion and the potential for nephrotoxicity. Alternative, shorter-dosage regimens have not been reported. (Its use is approved by the FDA for the treatment of hypercalcemia; further experience should define its ultimate role.)

OTHER THERAPIES Glucocorticoids increase urinary calcium excretion and decrease intestinal calcium absorption when given in pharmacologic doses (e.g., 40 to 200 mg prednisone daily in divided doses), but they also cause negative skeletal calcium balance. In normal subjects and in patients with primary hyperparathyroidism, glucocorticoids neither increase nor decrease the serum calcium concentration. In patients with hypercalcemia due to certain osteolytic malignancies, however, glucocorticoids may be effective as a result of antitumor effects. The malignancies in which hypercalcemia responds to glucocorticoids include multiple myeloma, leukemia, Hodgkin's disease, other lymphomas, and carcinoma of the breast, at least early in the course. Glucocorticoids are also effective in treating hypercalcemia due to vitamin D intoxication and sarcoidosis. In all the preceding situations, the hypocalcemic effect develops over several days, and the usual glucocorticoid dosage is 40 to 100 mg prednisone (or its equivalent) daily in four divided doses. The side effects of chronic glucocorticoid therapy may be acceptable in some circumstances.

Hypercalcemia complicated by renal failure is difficult to manage; dialysis is often the treatment of choice. Peritoneal dialysis with calcium-free dialysis fluid can remove 5 to 12.5 mmol (200 to 500 mg) of calcium in 24 to 48 h and lower the serum calcium concentration by 0.7 to 3 mmol/L (3 to 12 mg/dL). Large quantities of phosphate are lost during dialysis, and serum inorganic phosphate concentrations usually fall, thus aggravating hypercalcemia. Therefore, the serum inorganic phosphate concentration should be measured after dialysis, and phosphate supplements should be added to the diet or to dialysis fluids if necessary.

Phosphate therapy, oral or intravenous, has a role in certain circumstances. Patients with primary hyperparathyroidism are frequently hypophosphatemic, and hypercalcemia of other causes also may be complicated by hypophosphatemia. Hypophosphatemia decreases the rate of calcium uptake into bone, increases intestinal calcium absorption, and directly and indirectly stimulates bone breakdown. These effects aggravate hypercalcemia, and correcting hypophosphatemia lowers the serum calcium concentration. The usual treatment is 1 to 1.5 g phosphorus per day for several days, given in four divided doses to minimize the chances of developing hyperphosphatemia. Such therapy has been administered for prolonged periods in selected patients. It is generally believed but not established that toxicity does not occur if therapy is limited to restoring serum inorganic phosphate concentrations to normal.

Raising the serum inorganic phosphate concentration above normal does decrease serum calcium levels, sometimes strikingly. Intravenous phosphate is one of the most dramatically effective treatments available for severe hypercalcemia but is toxic and even dangerous so that it is used rarely and only in severely hypercalcemic patients with cardiac or renal failure. A dose of 1500 mg phosphate phosphorus or more intravenously over 6 to 8 h leads to a prompt decrease in serum calcium of as much as 1.2 to 2.5 mmol/L (5 to 10 mg/dL) in patients with initially normal serum inorganic phosphate concentrations. This therapy should be employed only in extreme emergencies for two reasons. First, fatal hypocalcemia can be produced by excessive dosage; serum calcium should be measured frequently if intravenous phosphate is administered. Second, unlike sodium chloride, sodium phosphate does not remove calcium from the body. In fact, urine calcium generally declines, and fecal calcium declines or remains the same. The decline in serum calcium reflects a redistribution of calcium within the body. There is a rapid efflux of calcium with no change in calcium influx to the circulation, findings indicative of precipitation of calcium phosphate salt. The calcium precipitates in bone, and metastatic calcification also may occur in patients receiving oral or intravenous phosphate therapy for hypercalcemia. Indeed, hyperphosphatemia can cause metastatic calcification in normocalcemic animals. Thus administration of intravenous phosphate in patients with compromised renal function who cannot have diuretic therapy is justifiable only as an emergency treatment.

Inorganic phosphate is commercially available for oral use in liquid, powder, and capsule form and as a liquid for intravenous use. It is important to calculate doses in terms of phosphate phosphorus.

SUMMARY The various therapies for hypercalcemia are listed in Table 354-3. The choice depends on the underlying disease, the severity of the hypercalcemia, the serum inorganic phosphate level, and the renal, hepatic, and bone marrow function. Mild hypercalcemia [3 mmol/L (12 mg/dL) or less] can usually be managed by the sequence of hydration followed by intravenous sodium chloride and, if needed, small doses of furosemide or ethacrynic acid. Severe hypercalcemia [3.7 mmol/L (15 mg/dL)] requires rapid correction. Calcitonin should be given for its rapid, albeit short-lived, blockade of bone resorption, and intravenous pamidronate should be administered, although its onset of action is delayed for 1 to 2 days. Hence aggressive sodium-calcium diuresis with intravenous saline and large doses of furosemide and ethacrynic acid works but should be initiated only if appropriate monitoring is available and cardiac function is adequate.

There is a role for oral phosphate therapy in chronic management of hypercalcemia, but its utility may be superseded by the bisphosphonates. Phosphate should only be given if hyperphosphatemia is not present.

Dietary calcium should be restricted and glucocorticoids should be administered if intestinal absorption is enhanced (in sarcoidosis, vitamin D intoxication). Dialysis is appropriate for hypercalcemia complicating acute or chronic renal failure.

Chronic therapy of hypercalcemia poses greater problems of toxicity. One satisfactory regimen for chronic use is a combination of dietary calcium restriction, administration of sodium chloride with or without furosemide or ethacrynic acid to maintain high urinary calcium, and moderate-dose oral phosphate (the patient is kept normophosphatemic). Some of the effective remedies (plicamycin, glucocorticoids, high-dose oral phosphate) may have significant toxicity when used chronically. Oral bisphosphonates, if proven nontoxic, may become the chronic treatment of choice in hypercalcemia where increased bone resorption is present.

HYPOCALCEMIA

PATHOPHYSIOLOGY OF HYPOCALCEMIA: CLASSIFICATION BASED ON MECHANISM *Chronic hypocalcemia* is less common than hypercalcemia; causes include chronic renal failure, hereditary and acquired hypoparathyroidism, vitamin D deficiency, pseudohypoparathyroidism (PHP), and hypomagnesemia.

Critically ill patients may have transient hypocalcemia with severe sepsis, burns, acute renal failure, and extensive transfusions with citrated blood. Acute hypocalcemia with certain medications is also usually transient and may have no symptoms. Although as many as half of patients in an intensive care setting are reported to have calcium concentrations below 2.1 mmol/L (8.5 mg/dL), fewer than 10 percent have a reduction in ionized calcium. Patients with severe sepsis may have a decrease in ionized calcium (true hypocalcemia), but in other severely ill subjects, hypoalbuminemia is the cause of the reduced total calcium concentration. Alkalosis increases calcium binding to proteins, and in this setting direct measurements of ionized calcium should be made.

Medications such as protamine, heparin, and glucagon may cause transient hypocalcemia. These forms of hypocalcemia are usually not associated with tetany and resolve with improvement in the overall medical condition. The hypocalcemia after repeated transfusions of citrated blood also usually resolves quickly.

Patients with acute *pancreatitis* have hypocalcemia that persists during the acute inflammation and varies in degree with the severity of the pancreatitis. The cause of hypocalcemia remains unclear. PTH values are reported to be low, normal, or elevated, and both resistance to PTH and impaired PTH secretion have been postulated. Occasionally, a chronic low total-blood calcium and low ionized calcium concentration are detected in an elderly patient without obvious cause and with a paucity of symptoms; the pathogenesis is unclear.

Chronic hypocalcemia, however, is usually symptomatic and requires treatment. Neuromuscular and neurologic manifestations of chronic hypocalcemia include muscle spasms, carpopedal spasm, facial grimacing, and, in extreme cases, laryngeal spasm and convulsions. Respiratory arrest may occur. Increased intracranial pressure occurs in some patients with long-standing hypocalcemia, often in association with papilledema. Mental changes include irritability, depression, and psychosis. The QT interval on the electrocardiogram is prolonged, in contrast to its shortening with hypercalcemia. Arrhythmias occur, and digitalis effectiveness may be reduced. Intestinal cramps and chronic malabsorption may occur. Chvostek's or Trousseau's sign can be used to confirm latent tetany.

The classification of hypocalcemia shown in Table 354-4 is based on the premise that PTH is responsible for minute-to-minute regulation of plasma calcium concentration within narrow limits and, therefore, that the occurrence of hypocalcemia must mean a failure of the homeostatic action of PTH. Failure of the PTH response can occur due to hereditary or acquired parathyroid gland failure, if PTH is ineffective in target organs, or if the action of the hormone is overwhelmed by the loss of calcium from the extracellular fluid at a rate faster than it can be replaced.

PTH ABSENT Hypoparathyroidism, whether hereditary or acquired, has a number of common components. Acute and chronic symptoms of untreated hypocalcemia are shared by both types of

Table 354-4

Functional Classification of Hypocalcemia (Excluding Neonatal Conditions)

PTH ABSENT	
Hereditary hypoparathyroidism	Hypomagnesemia
Acquired hypoparathyroidism	
PTH INEFFECTIVE	
Chronic renal failure	Active vitamin D ineffective
Active vitamin D lacking	Intestinal malabsorption
↓ Dietary intake or sunlight	Vitamin D–dependent rickets type II
Defective metabolism:	Pseudohypoparathyroidism
Anticonvulsant therapy	
Vitamin D–dependent rickets type I	
PTH OVERWHELMED	
Severe, acute hyperphosphatemia	Osteitis fibrosa after parathyroidectomy
Tumor lysis	
Acute renal failure	
Rhabdomyolysis	

hypoparathyroidism, although typically the onset of hereditary hypoparathyroidism is more gradual and hereditary hypoparathyroidism is associated with developmental defects. In earlier decades, acquired hypoparathyroidism secondary to surgery in the neck was more common than hereditary hypoparathyroidism, but the frequency of surgically induced parathyroid failure has diminished as a result of improved surgical techniques that spare the parathyroid glands and increased use of nonsurgical therapy for hyperthyroidism. Basal ganglia calcification and extrapyramidal syndromes are more common and earlier in onset in hereditary hypoparathyroidism. PHP, an example of ineffective PTH action rather than a failure of parathyroid gland production, shares several features with hypoparathyroidism, including extraosseous calcification and extrapyramidal manifestations such as choreoathetotic movements and dystonia. Papilledema and raised intracranial pressure occur in both states, as do chronic changes in fingernails and hair and lenticular cataracts, the latter usually reversible with treatment of hypocalcemia. Certain skin manifestations, including alopecia and candidiasis, occur exclusively in hereditary hypoparathyroidism.

Hypocalcemia associated with hypomagnesemia is associated with both deficient PTH release and impaired responsiveness to the hormone (see also Chap. 357). Patients with hypocalcemia secondary to hypomagnesemia have absent or low levels of circulating PTH, indicative of diminished hormone release despite maximum physiologic stimulus by hypocalcemia. Plasma PTH levels return to normal with correction of the hypomagnesemia. Thus hypoparathyroidism with low levels of PTH in blood can be due to hereditary gland failure, acquired gland failure, or acute but reversible gland dysfunction (hypomagnesemia). Patients with acquired or hereditary hypoparathyroidism also have hyperphosphatemia and absent or low levels of $1,25(OH)_2D$.

Hereditary Hypoparathyroidism Hereditary hypoparathyroidism can occur as an isolated entity without other endocrine or dermatologic manifestations (idiopathic hypoparathyroidism) or, more typically, in association with other abnormalities such as defective development of the thymus or failure of function of other endocrine organs such as the adrenal thyroid or ovary (see also Chap. 340). Idiopathic and hereditary hypoparathyroidisms are often manifest within the first decade but may appear later.

A rare form of hypoparathyroidism associated with defective development of both the thymus and the parathyroid glands is termed the *DiGeorge syndrome*, or the *third and fourth branchial pouch syndrome*. Congenital cardiovascular and other developmental defects are present, and most patients die in early childhood with severe infections, hypocalcemia and seizures, or cardiovascular complications. Some survive into adulthood, and milder, incomplete forms occur. Most cases are sporadic, and cytogenetic abnormalities involving chromosome 22 are reported.

Hypoparathyroidism can occur in association with other diverse developmental defects or as part of a complex hereditary autoimmune syndrome involving failure of the adrenals, the ovaries, and the parathyroids in association with recurrent mucocutaneous candidiasis, alopecia, vitiligo, and pernicious anemia (see Chap. 340). In many cases, antibodies to endocrine organs are present; there is, in addition, a failure of cell-mediated immunity. The autoimmune disorder is inherited as an autosomal recessive trait, and some unaffected family members show antibodies to endocrine tissue without evidence of endocrine failure. The disorder is usually referred to as *autoimmune polyglandular deficiency*.

Hereditary hypoparathyroidism occurs also as an isolated entity without any other defects. The pattern of inheritance varies from one kindred to another, including autosomal dominant, autosomal recessive, and X-linked inheritance patterns. In one family in which the disorder was transmitted as an autosomal dominant trait, a structural abnormality in the PTH gene has been identified. The defect in the signal sequence needed for processing of the hormone before secretion impairs PTH secretion. In another kindred with autosomal recessive inheritance, the mutant allele in the first intron of the PTH gene causes a splicing defect in mRNA production. Gain-of-function mutations in the calcium sensor are the cause of autosomal dominant hypoparathyroidism in at least three families; the exaggerated responsiveness of the calcium sensor to calcium causes inappropriate suppression of PTH secretion. In most kindreds, however, the genetic basis of the hypoparathyroidism is not known.

Acquired Hypoparathyroidism *Acquired chronic hypoparathyroidism* is usually the result of inadvertent surgical removal of all the parathyroid glands; in some instances, not all the tissue is removed, but the remainder undergoes compromise of vascular supply secondary to fibrotic changes in the neck after surgery. In the past, the most frequent cause of acquired hypoparathyroidism was surgery for hyperthyroidism. Hypoparathyroidism now usually occurs after surgery for hyperparathyroidism when the surgeon, facing the dilemma of removing too little tissue and thus not curing the hyperparathyroidism, removes too much.

Parathyroid function may not be totally absent in all patients with postoperative hypoparathyroidism, but suitable therapy varies greatly from patient to patient irrespective of the type of hypoparathyroidism or the question of residual parathyroid activity.

Even rarer causes of acquired chronic hypoparathyroidism include radiation-induced damage subsequent to radioiodine therapy of hyperthyroidism and glandular damage in patients with hemochromatosis or hemosiderosis after repeated blood transfusions. Infection may involve one or more of the parathyroids but usually does not cause hypoparathyroidism because all four glands are rarely involved.

Transient hypoparathyroidism is frequent following surgery for hyperparathyroidism. After a variable period of hypoparathyroidism, normal parathyroid function may return due to hyperplasia or recovery of remaining tissue. Occasionally, recovery occurs months after surgery. The management of transient postoperative hypoparathyroidism is discussed under the surgical treatment of hyperparathyroidism. The treatment of chronic acquired hypoparathyroidism is similar to that of idiopathic hypoparathyroidism: replacement with calcitriol and oral calcium.

℞ TREATMENT

Treatment of acquired and hereditary hypoparathyroidism is similar to that for PHP, although specific features of each disease require specific treatments. Replacement therapy with vitamin D or calcitriol combined with a high oral calcium intake usually suffices to regulate blood calcium and phosphate levels satisfactorily. Oral calcium and vitamin D restore the overall calcium-phosphate balance but do not reverse the lowered urinary calcium reabsorption typical of hypoparathyroidism. Therefore, care must be taken to avoid excessive urinary calcium excretion after vitamin D and calcium replacement therapy; otherwise, kidney stones can develop. Thiazide diuretics lower urine calcium by as much as 100 mg/d in hypoparathyroid patients on vitamin D, provided they are maintained on a low-sodium diet. Use of thiazides seems to be of benefit in mitigating hypercalciuria.

Hypomagnesemia Severe hypomagnesemia is associated with severe hypocalcemia (see also Chap. 357). Restoration of the total-body magnesium deficit leads to rapid reversal of hypocalcemia. There are at least two causes of the hypocalcemia—impaired PTH secretion and reduced responsiveness to PTH.

Hypomagnesemia is generally classified as primary or secondary; primary hypomagnesemia is due to hereditary defects in intestinal absorption or renal reabsorption of magnesium. Secondary hypomagnesemia, a more common condition, occurs on a nutritional basis or as a result of acquired intestinal or renal disorders. The most common causes of the secondary disorder are chronic alcoholism with poor nutritional intake, intestinal malabsorption syndromes, and parenteral nutrition when magnesium replacement is omitted.

The effects of magnesium on PTH secretion are similar to those of calcium; hypermagnesemia suppresses and hypomagnesemia stimulates PTH secretion. The effects of magnesium on PTH secretion are normally of little significance, however, because the calcium effects dominate. Greater change in magnesium than in calcium is needed to influence hormone secretion. Nonetheless, hypomagnesemia might be expected to increase hormone secretion. It is therefore surprising to find that severe hypomagnesemia is associated with blunted secretion of PTH. The explanation for the paradox is that severe, chronic hypomagnesemia reflects intracellular magnesium deficiency, which interferes with secretion and peripheral responses to PTH. The mechanism of the cellular defects of hypomagnesemia is unknown, although a defective adenylate cyclase (for which magnesium may serve as a cofactor) has been proposed.

In most cases in which hypomagnesemia is associated with hypocalcemia, serum magnesium is below 0.4 mmol/L (1.0 mg/dL). PTH levels are usually undetectable or inappropriately low despite the stimulus of severe hypocalcemia, and acute repletion of magnesium leads to a rapid increase in PTH level. Since PTH secretion is blunted in virtually all patients with severe hypomagnesemia, absolute or relative hypoparathyroidism is present in most patients with hypocalcemia secondary to hypomagnesemia.

In addition, diminished peripheral responsiveness to administered PTH occurs in some patients, as manifested by subnormal response in urinary phosphorus and urinary cyclic AMP excretion after administration of exogenous PTH to patients who are hypocalcemic and hypomagnesemic. Both blunted PTH secretion and lack of renal response to administered PTH can occur in the same patient. When acute magnesium repletion is undertaken, the restoration of PTH levels to normal or supranormal may precede by several days restoration of normal serum calcium.

Blunted PTH secretory response in hypomagnesemia seems the main cause of hypocalcemia. The fact that impaired peripheral responsiveness, particularly renal response, is more variable from patient to patient suggests that an even greater degree of magnesium deficiency is required to induce end-organ resistance than to impair hormone secretion.

Several other features have been noted. The brisk increase in PTH secretion following magnesium repletion, sometimes demonstrable within minutes of giving parenteral magnesium, indicates that hormone biosynthesis is not impaired, only secretion. Serum phosphate levels are often not elevated, in contrast to the situation with acquired or idiopathic hypoparathyroidism, probably because phosphate deficiency is a frequent accompaniment of hypomagnesemia. Magnesium wasting may occur in chronic renal disease; magnesium may be elevated in acute renal failure but is usually normal in chronic renal failure.

℞ TREATMENT

Repletion of magnesium cures the condition, and attention must be given to restoring the intracellular deficiency, which may be considerable. After intravenous magnesium administration, serum magnesium may return transiently to the normal range, but unless replacement therapy is adequate serum magnesium will again fall. If renal function is normal, a useful indicator of restoration of magnesium deficiency is the urinary magnesium excretion; magnesium is retained by the kidney until magnesium deficiency is repleted. Intracellular deficits can be as great as 50 mmol or more. Parenteral administration of 10 to 14 mmol magnesium usually reverses the signs of magnesium deficiency. If the cause of the hypomagnesemia is renal magnesium wasting, magnesium may have to be given chronically to prevent recurrence.

PTH INEFFECTIVE PTH is considered ineffective when the hormone receptor–guanyl nucleotide–binding protein complex is defective, when PTH action to promote calcium absorption from the diet is impaired because of vitamin D deficiency or because vitamin D is ineffective (receptor or synthesis defects), or in chronic renal failure in which the calcium-elevating action of PTH is impaired.

Despite diverse pathophysiologic mechanisms, these latter conditions involving ineffectiveness of PTH (excluding the rare condition of defective PTH-receptor response) often involve the unavailability of vitamin D as a cofactor for PTH. Hypocalcemia is usually mild and is accompanied by hypophosphatemia. Typically, hypophosphatemia is more severe than hypocalcemia because of the increased secretion of PTH, which is only partly effective in elevating blood calcium but is capable of promoting renal phosphate excretion in vitamin D deficiency, so that phosphaturia leads to hypophosphatemia. Varying degrees of bone disease with impaired mineralization and/or frank osteomalacia are the consequence of chronic renal failure and/or impairment of vitamin D action by the hypophosphatemia.

PHP, on the other hand, has a pathophysiology different from the other disorders of ineffective PTH action. PHP resembles conditions in which PTH synthesis is deficient and is manifested by hypocalcemia and hyperphosphatemia. The cause of the disorder is defective hormone binding to the receptor or deficient activation of guanyl nucleotide–binding proteins, resulting in failure of PTH to increase intracellular cyclic AMP (see below).

Chronic Renal Failure Severe abnormalities in mineral and bone metabolism occur in chronic renal failure, and improved medical management of chronic renal failure and/or a more indolent course of the renal disease allow many patients to survive long enough for renal osteodystrophy, the bone disease associated with renal failure, to become manifest. Phosphate retention and impaired production of $1,25(OH)_2D$ are the principal factors that cause calcium deficiency, secondary hyperparathyroidism, and bone disease. The uremic state also causes impairment of intestinal absorption by mechanisms other than defects in vitamin D metabolism. Nonetheless, treatment with supraphysiologic amounts of vitamin D or calcitriol corrects the calcium absorption.

Hyperphosphatemia in renal failure lowers blood calcium levels by several mechanisms, including extraosseous deposition of calcium and phosphate, impairment of the bone-resorbing action of PTH, reduction in $1,25(OH)_2D$ production by surviving renal tissue, and reduction in calcium absorption due to trapping of calcium in insoluble form as calcium phosphate complexes. In animals, prevention of hyperphosphatemia by dietary means can block the development of secondary hyperparathyroidism, emphasizing the importance of phosphate retention in the pathogenesis of secondary hyperparathyroidism and the associated disorders of mineral and bone metabolism in renal failure. Low levels of $1,25(OH)_2D$ are due to hyperphosphatemia and to destruction of renal tissue and are critical in the hypocalcemia.

℞ TREATMENT

Therapy of chronic renal failure (see Chaps. 271 and 272) involves appropriate management of patients prior to dialysis and adjustment of regimens once dialysis becomes necessary. Attention should be paid to restriction of phosphate in the diet; use of phosphate-binding antacids such as those based on aluminum hydroxide or calcium-containing salts, which avoid the problem of aluminum intoxication; provision of an adequate calcium intake by mouth, usually 1 to 2 g/d; and supplementation with 0.25 to 1.0 μg/d calcitriol. Each patient must be monitored closely. The aim of therapy is to restore normal calcium balance to prevent osteomalacia and secondary hyperparathyroidism. Reduction of hyperphosphatemia and restoration of normal intestinal calcium absorption by calcitriol can improve blood calcium levels and reduce the manifestations of secondary hyperparathyroidism. Since adynamic bone disease can occur in association with low PTH levels, it is important to avoid excessive suppression of the parathyroid glands while recognizing the beneficial effects of controlling the secondary hyperparathyroidism.

Vitamin D Deficiency Due to Inadequate Diet and/or Sunlight Vitamin D deficiency is more common in the United States than previously recognized. Biopsies of bone in elderly patients with hip fracture (documenting osteomalacia) and abnormal levels of vitamin D metabolites, PTH, calcium, and phosphate indicate that vitamin D deficiency may occur in as many as 25 percent of elderly patients, particularly in areas where there is little ambient sunlight. Concentrations of 25(OH)D are low or low normal in these patients. Quantitative histomorphometry of bone biopsy specimens reveals widened osteoid seams consistent with osteomalacia. PTH hypersecretion compensates for the tendency for the blood calcium to fall but also induces renal phosphate wasting and results in osteomalacia.

The genesis of vitamin D deficiency is inadequate intake of dairy products enriched with vitamin D, lack of vitamin supplementation, and reduced sunlight exposure in the elderly, particularly during winter in northern latitudes.

Treatment involves the administration of vitamin D and provision of 1 to 1.5 g calcium in the diet. Vitamin D supplementation should aim to provide several times the recommended daily requirement in younger people; a dosage of 1000 to 2000 units of vitamin D per day is satisfactory. Vitamin D is usually not available in small-dose forms. Hence the administration of a capsule containing 50,000 units of vitamin D once monthly is safe in elderly patients who have osteomalacia. The increased awareness of the importance of calcium supplementation, particularly in women, even without supplementation of vitamin D, may lessen the frequency of this problem. Severe hypocalcemia rarely occurs in moderately severe vitamin D deficiency of the elderly, but vitamin D deficiency must be considered in the differential diagnosis of mild hypocalcemia.

Defective Vitamin D Metabolism *Anticonvulsant therapy* Anticonvulsant therapy with any of several agents induces acquired vitamin D deficiency by increasing the conversion of vitamin D to inactive compounds. The more marginal the vitamin D intake in the diet, the more likely that anticonvulsant therapy will lead to abnormal mineral and bone metabolism. Manifestations may include severe rickets with bone fractures, hypocalcemia, hypophosphatemia, and, on occasion, proximal myopathy. More often, hypocalcemia is minimal, and mild osteomalacia is the only sign. In other patients on long-term anticonvulsant therapy, no symptoms or signs are present, but bone density is low and responds to vitamin D supplementation.

Anticonvulsants stimulate the hepatic microsomal mixed-oxidase enzymes and hence increase the rate of clearance of vitamin D and its metabolites. Phenytoin also impairs intestinal calcium absorption independent of effects on vitamin D and has deleterious effects on bone cell function in vitro, including inhibition of collagen synthesis.

Although $1,25(OH)_2D$ levels are lower in patients treated with chronic anticonvulsants than in the normal population, there is a great deal of variation. The greater prevalence of the disorder in some European populations and in the mentally retarded probably reflects the lower vitamin D intake of those groups. Restoration of bone mineral mass and reversal of hypocalcemia can be accomplished with vitamin D replacement plus oral calcium. Adjustments in dose are indicated depending on the age and size of the patient, but approximately 50,000 units of vitamin D weekly plus 1 g elemental calcium per day for several months is usually sufficient. Alternatively, administration of administration of 50,000 units of vitamin D monthly may be preventive if anticonvulsant therapy is given chronically.

Vitamin D–dependent rickets type I Rickets can be due to *resistance to the action* of vitamin D as well as to vitamin D deficiency. Vitamin D–dependent rickets type I, previously termed *pseudo-vitamin D–dependent rickets*, differs from vitamin D–resistant rickets in that it is less severe and the biochemical and radiographic abnormalities can be reversed with large doses of the vitamin.

Clinical features include hypocalcemia, often with tetany or convulsions, hypophosphatemia, secondary hyperparathyroidism, and osteomalacia, often associated with skeletal deformities and increased alkaline phosphatase. Doses of vitamin D or calcifediol, 100 to 1000 times above the usual amounts, are required to heal the bone disease, whereas physiologic amounts of calcitriol cure the disease. This finding fits with the pathophysiology. The disorder is due to an autosomal recessive defect in conversion of 25(OH)D to $1,25(OH)_2D$. Plasma levels of $1,25(OH)_2D$ are low or undetectable even after administration of large doses of vitamin D or calcifediol. Response to high doses of vitamin D or calcifediol is probably due to direct effects of 25(OH)D at high levels. Treatment requires careful adjustment of calcitriol dose, particularly during growth periods.

Vitamin D Ineffective *Intestinal malabsorption* Mild hypocalcemia, secondary hyperparathyroidism, severe hypophosphatemia, and a variety of nutritional deficiencies occur with gastrointestinal diseases. Hepatocellular dysfunction can lead to reduction in 25(OH)D levels, as in portal or biliary cirrhosis of the liver, and malabsorption of vitamin D and its metabolites, including $1,25(OH)_2D$, may occur in a variety of bowel diseases, hereditary or acquired. Hypocalcemia itself can lead to steatorrhea, due to deficient production of pancreatic enzymes and bile salts. Depending on the disorder, vitamin D or its metabolites can be given parenterally, guaranteeing adequate blood levels of active metabolites.

Vitamin D–dependent rickets type II Pseudo-vitamin D–dependent rickets can be due to defective response to $1,25(OH)_2D$. This disorder, vitamin D–dependent rickets type II, results from any of several types of end-organ resistance to the active metabolite, including absence or qualitative defects of the intracellular vitamin D receptor and postreceptor blocks in hormone action (see Chap. 327). The clinical features resemble those of the type I disorder and include hypocalcemia, hypophosphatemia, secondary hyperparathryoidism, and rickets. Plasma levels of $1,25(OH)_2D$ are at least three times normal, in keeping with the refractoriness of the end organs. Alopecia totalis may be severe early in life. Patients require much higher doses of vitamin D or vitamin D metabolites than with the type I disorder.

Pseudohypoparathyroidism PHP is a hereditary disorder characterized by symptoms and signs of hypoparathyroidism, typically in association with distinctive skeletal and developmental defects. The hypoparathyroidism is due to a deficient end-organ response to PTH. Hyperplasia of the parathyroids, a response to the resistance to hormone action, causes elevation of PTH levels. Studies, both clinical and basic, have clarified some aspects of this syndrome, including the variable spectrum of the clinical features, the pathophysiology, the genetic defects, and the inheritance.

Most patients show a characteristic phenotype termed *Albright's hereditary osteodystrophy* (AHO), consisting of short stature, round face, skeletal anomalies (brachydactyly), and heterotopic calcification. Patients have low calcium and high phosphate levels, as with true hypoparathyroidism. PTH levels, however, are elevated, and resistance to hormone action can be demonstrated by defective urinary cyclic AMP response to PTH administration. The disorder is usually familial; some kindreds do not show the AHO phenotype but only abnormal mineral metabolism. A few patients are resistant to PTH but have normal urinary cyclic AMP response (responses in calcium and phosphate seemingly blocked after the adenyl cyclase step).

At least part of the defect in most patients (those with the AHO phenotype) is due to inheritance of one defective allele that encodes the α subunit of the guanyl nucleotide–binding protein ($G_{s\alpha}$). This defect causes a diminished response to PTH (approximately 50 percent of normal, consistent with one defective allele). However, in some kindreds individuals with a distinctive AHO phenotype who, while unaffected with symptoms or signs of defective mineral metabolism, still have a demonstrable 50 percent reduction in assays of $G_{s\alpha}$ subunits (so-called pseudopseudohypoparathyroidism). Hence the defective guanyl nucleotide subunit is not itself sufficient to explain the pathophysiology. Perhaps another independently inherited allelic defect so far undetected is needed to provide full expression of the disordered mineral metabolism.

Since the defective $G_{s\alpha}$ subunit function was recognized, attention has focused on the molecular mechanism of the defective guanyl nucleotide–binding protein function. The gene encoding this subunit has been cloned (chromosome 20); multiple defects have now been identified, including abnormalities in splice junctions associated with deficient mRNA production and point mutations that result in a protein unit with defective function. The view that the disease is an X-linked disorder has given way, with a combination of careful family and molecular genetic studies, to recognition that the subset with hereditary osteodystrophy is due to an autosomal dominant mode of inheritance (chromosome 20). The inheritance of the variant disorder in which individuals do not have hereditary osteodystrophy is not understood.

A working classification of the various forms of PHP is given in Table 354-5. The classification scheme is based on the signs of ineffective PTH action (low calcium and high phosphate), urinary cyclic AMP response to exogenous PTH, the presence or absence of AHO, and assays of the concentration of the $G_{s\alpha}$ subunit of the adenylate cyclase enzyme. Using these criteria, there are four types: PHP type I, subdivided into a and b categories; PHP-II; and pseudopseudohypoparathyroidism (PPHP). Individuals with PHP-I, the most common of the disorders, show a deficient response in urinary cyclic AMP to administration of exogenous PTH. PHP-II refers to patients with hypocalcemia and hyperphosphatemia who have a normal urinary cyclic AMP response to PTH. These patients are assumed to have a defect in the response to PTH at a lcous beyond that of cyclic AMP production, although at least some patients may instead have occult vitamin D deficiency. It is disputed whether PHP-II is a discrete phenotypic and genotypic entity because vitamin D deficiency and an associated hypocalcemia can cause an enhanced cyclic AMP response yet a blunted phosphatemic response to administered PTH (the hallmark of PHP-II). Patients with PHP-I are divided into type a, who have reduced amounts of $G_{s\alpha}$ in in vitro assays, and type b, with normal amounts of $G_{s\alpha}$ in erythrocytes. Subjects with PHP-Ia have shortened metacarpals and metatarsals and the other features of AHO and commonly show resistance to hormones in addition to PTH. Patients with PHP-Ib have a normal phenotype without the AHO syndrome. Fibroblasts cultured from the skin of some patients with PHP-Ib show a much reduced response of cyclic AMP accumulation to PTH, consistent with the presence of a defective receptor. A subset of these patients,

Table 354-5

Classification of Pseudohypoparathyroidism (PHP) and Pseudopseudohypoparathyroidism (PPHP)

Type	Hypocalcemia, Hyperphosphatemia	Response of Urinary cAMP to PTH	Serum PTH	$G_{s\alpha}$ Subunit Deficiency	AHO	Resistance to Hormones in Addition to PTH
PHP-Ia	Yes	↓	↑	Yes	Yes	Yes
PHP-Ib	Yes	↓	↑	No	No	No
PHP-II	Yes	Normal	↑	No	No	No
PPHP	No	Normal	Normal	Yes	Yes	±

NOTE: ↓, decreased; ↑, increased; AHO, Albright's hereditary osteodystrophy.

however, has a normal response to cyclic AMP production fibroblasts in vitro, and no structural defects in the PTH receptor have been identified in these patients to date.

Patients with PPHP have typical features of the hereditary osteodystrophy syndrome despite normal serum calcium levels and normal response of urinary cyclic AMP to exogenous PTH. These individuals are usually first-degree relatives of patients with PHP-Ia, and patients initially classified as having PPHP occasionally develop mild hypocalcemia. Patients with PPHP on average have levels of $G_{s\alpha}$ subunits that are half normal, suggesting that PPHP is a mild variant of PHP-Ia.

The mineral deposits in ectopic sites may include true bone, whereas bone formation never occurs in ectopic sites in idiopathic hypoparathyroidism. Amorphous deposits of calcium and phosphate are found in the basal ganglia in about half of patients. The defects in metacarpal and metatarsal bones are sometimes accompanied by short phalanges as well, possibly reflecting premature closing of the epiphyses. The typical findings are short fourth and fifth metacarpals and metatarsals. The defects are usually bilateral. Exostoses and radius curvus are frequent. Impairments in olfaction and taste and unusual dermatoglyphic abnormalities have been reported. There is little improvement in mental status even after adequate therapy with calcium and vitamin D.

The diagnosis can usually be made without difficulty. Positive family history for developmental defects and/or the presence of developmental defects characteristic of PHP-Ia, including brachydactyly, in association with the signs of hypoparathyroidism, low calcium, and high phosphate, make the diagnosis likely on clinical grounds. However, patients with PHP-Ib or PHP-II do not have phenotypic abnormalities but have hypocalcemia with high PTH levels. In PHP-Ib, the response of urinary cyclic AMP to the administration of exogenous PTH is blunted; such tests are useful to confirm the diagnosis even in PHP-Ia. Low levels of $G_{s\alpha}$ subunits in erythrocyte membranes can also distinguish patients with PHP-Ia from those with PHP-Ib. In both categories serum PTH levels are elevated, particularly in hypocalcemic patients. The diagnosis of PHP-II is more complex, in that cyclic AMP responses in urine are, by definition, normal. Since vitamin D deficiency itself can result in dissociation between phosphaturic and urinary cyclic AMP responses to exogenous PTH, vitamin D deficiency must be excluded before diagnosis of PHP-II can be made.

℞ TREATMENT

Treatment of PHP is similar to that of hypoparathyroidism, except that the doses of vitamin D and calcium are usually lower than those required in true hypoparathyroidism, presumably because the defect in PHP is only partial (a 50 percent reduction in $G_{s\alpha}$). Variability in response makes it necessary to establish the optimal regimen for each patient, based on maintining the appropriate blood calcium level and urinary calcium excretion.

PTH Overwhelmed Occasionally, loss of calcium from the extracellular fluid is so severe that PTH cannot compensate. Such situations include acute pancreatitis and severe, acute hyperphosphatemia, often in association with renal failure, conditions in which there is rapid efflux of calcium from extracellular fluid. Severe hypocalcemia can occur quickly; PTH rises in response to hypocalcemia but does not return blood calcium to normal. The chance of hypocalcemia is enhanced when renal failure is present.

Severe, Acute Hyperphosphatemia Severe hyperphosphatemia is associated with extensive tissue damage or cell destruction (see Chap. 356). The combination of increased release of phosphate from muscle and impaired ability to excrete phosphorus because of renal failure causes moderate to severe hyperphosphatemia, the latter causing calcium loss from the blood and mild to moderate hypocalcemia. Hypocalcemia is usually reversed with tissue repair and restoration of renal function as phosphorus and creatinine values return to normal. There may even be a mild hypercalcemic period in the oliguric phase of recovery of renal function. This sequence, severe hypocalcemia followed by mild hypercalcemia, reflects widespread deposition of

calcium in muscle and subsequent redistribution of some of the calcium to the extracellular fluid after return of phosphate levels to normal.

Other causes of hyperphosphatemia include hypothermia, massive hepatic failure, and hematologic malignancies, either because of high cell turnover of malignancy or because of cell destruction with chemotherapy.

℞ TREATMENT

Treatment is directed toward lowering of blood phosphate by the administration of phosphate-binding antacids or dialysis, often needed for the management of renal failure. Although calcium replacement may be necessary if hypocalcemia is severe and symptomatic, calcium administration during the hyperphosphatemic period tends to increase extraosseous calcium deposition and aggravate tissue damage. Although the levels of $1,25(OH)_2D$ may be low during the hyperphosphatemic phase and return to normal during the oliguric phase of recovery, mineral ion imbalance per se seems to be the principal pathophysiologic mechanism.

Osteitis Fibrosis after Parathyroidectomy Severe hypocalcemia after parathyroid surgery is less common now that osteitis fibrosa cystica is an infrequent manifestation of hyperparathyroidism. When osteitis fibrosa cystica is severe, however, bone mineral deficits can be large, and after parathyroidectomy hypocalcemia can persist for days if calcium replacement is inadequate. The mechanism of the hypocalcemia is complex. Increased cellularity of bone in osteitis fibrosa cystica involves both osteoblasts and osteoclasts, but high levels of PTH enhance resorption more than formation; an abrupt decrease in PTH levels with surgery leaves bone formation favored over resorption. Calcium loss from blood is increased, and temporary hyporesponsiveness of bone to the bone-resorbing actions of PTH (lowered hormone levels after parathyroid surgery in the presence of receptor down-regulation) may add to the imbalance between bone resorption and bone formation. Treatment may require parenteral administration of calcium; addition of calcitriol and oral calcium supplementation make it possible to discontinue parenteral calcium and/or reduce the amount.

DIFFERENTIAL DIAGNOSIS Care must be taken to ensure that true hypocalcemia is present; in addition, acute transient hypocalcemia can be a manifestation of a variety of severe, acute illnesses, as discussed above. *Chronic hypocalcemia*, however, can usually be ascribed to a few disorders associated with absent or ineffective PTH. Important clinical criteria include the duration of the illness, signs or symptoms of associated disorders, and the presence of features that suggest a hereditary abnormality. A nutritional history can be helpful in recognizing a low intake of vitamin D and calcium in the elderly, and a history of excessive alcohol intake can be the clue to magnesium deficiency.

Hypoparathyroidism and PHP are typically lifelong illnesses; hence a recent onset of hypocalcemia in an adult is usually due to nutritional deficiencies, renal failure, or intestinal disorders that result in deficient or ineffective vitamin D. A history of seizure disorder raises the issue of anticonvulsive medication. Neck surgery, even long past, can be associated with a delayed onset of postoperative hypoparathyroidism. Developmental defects, particularly in childhood and adolescence, may point to the diagnosis of PHP. Rickets and a variety of neuromuscular syndromes and deformities may indicate ineffective vitamin D action, either due to defects in vitamin D metabolism or to vitamin D deficiency.

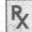

A pattern of *low calcium with high phosphorus* in the absence of renal failure or massive tissue destruction almost invariably means hypoparathyroidism or PHP. A *low calcium and low phosphorus* points to absent or ineffective vitamin D, thereby impairing the action of PTH on calcium metabolism. The relative ineffectiveness of PTH in vitamin D deficiency, anticonvulsant therapy, gastrointestinal disorders, and hereditary defects in vitamin D metabolism leads to secondary hyperparathyroidism as a compensation. The relatively unopposed action of the excess PTH on renal tubule phosphate transport, which is less dependent on vitamin D than calcium transport, accounts for renal phosphate wasting and hypophosphatemia.

Exceptions to these patterns may occur. Most forms of hypomagnesemia are due to long-standing nutritional deficiency, and despite the fact that the hypocalcemia is due principally to an acute absence of PTH, phosphate levels are usually low rather than elevated as in hypoparathyroidism. Chronic renal failure is often associated with hypocalcemia and hyperphosphatemia, despite secondary hyperparathyroidism.

Diagnosis is usually established by application of the PTH radioimmunoassay, tests for vitamin D metabolites, and measurements of the urinary cyclic AMP response to exogenous PTH. In hereditary and acquired hypoparathyroidism and in severe hypomagnesemia, PTH is either undetectable or in the normal range, and this finding in a hypocalcemic patient is supportive of hypoparathyroidism, as distinct from ineffective PTH action, in which even mild hypocalcemia is associated with elevated PTH levels. Hence a failure to detect elevated PTH levels establishes the diagnosis of hypoparathyroidism; elevated levels suggest the presence of secondary hyperparathyroidism, as found in many of the situations in which the hormone is ineffective due to associated abnormalities in vitamin D action. Assays for 25(OH)D and $1,25(OH)_2D$ can be helpful. Low or low normal 25(OH)D indicates vitamin D deficiency due to lack of sunlight, inadequate vitamin D intake, or intestinal malabsorption. A low level of $1,25(OH)_2D$ in the presence of elevated concentrations of PTH suggests ineffective PTH action; include the causes chronic renal failure, severe vitamin D deficiency, vitamin D–dependent rickets type I, and PHP. Recognition that mild hypocalcemia, rickets, and hypophosphatemia are due to anticonvulsant therapy is made by history.

℞ TREATMENT

Hypocalcemic States The management of hypoparathyroidism, PHP, chronic renal failure, and hereditary defects in vitamin D metabolism involves the use of vitamin D or vitamin D metabolites and calcium supplementation. Vitamin D itself is the least expensive form of vitamin D replacement and is frequently used in the management of uncomplicated hypoparathyroidism and disorders associated with ineffective vitamin D action. When vitamin D is used prophylactically, as in the elderly or in those with chronic anticonvulsant therapy, there is a wider margin of safety than with the more potent metabolites. However, most of the conditions in which vitamin D is administered chronically for hypocalcemia require amounts 50 to 100 times the daily replacement dose because the formation of $1,25(OH)_2D$ is deficient. In such situations, vitamin D is no safer than the active metabolite because intoxication can occur with high-dose therapy. Calcitriol is more rapid in onset of action and also has a short biologic half-life; in high doses, vitamin D is stored in body tissues and is cleared slowly.

From 1 to 5 μg/d of vitamin D or calcifediol and lower doses of calcitriol (0.25 to 1.0 μg/d) are required to prevent rickets in normal subjects. In contrast, 500 to 3000 μg of vitamin D_2 or D_3 is typically required in hypoparathyroidism; doses of calcifediol are also high (several hundred micrograms per day). The dose of calcitriol is unchanged in hypoparathyroidism, since the defect is in hydroxylation by the 1α-hydroxylase.

The greater therapeutic efficacy of calcifediol than vitamin D_3 when the metabolism of the vitamin is impaired may be due to superior metabolic availability for the renal 1α-hydroxylase or to direct action directly by 25(OH)D at receptors in target tissues. Vitamin D is metabolized to a variety of compounds other than the principal product, 25(OH)D. Calcifediol bypasses these alternative pathways and is directly available for metabolism to $1,25(OH)_2D$. In hypoparathyroidism and in hereditary defects in renal 1α-hydroxylase, the formation of $1,25(OH)_2D$ from 25(OH)D is impaired, but some formation occurs at high substrate levels. Calcifediol has about 1 percent of the potency of calcitriol in vivo and in vitro.

Unless a loading dose is given, 2 to 4 weeks or even longer are required to achieve the maximum calcium replacement action of vitamin D or calcifediol; the onset of action of calcifediol is more rapid. Calcitriol can be given for hypoparathyroidism at the same dose required for the prevention of rickets in euparathyroid individuals, 0.2 to 1.0 μg/d. Its onset of action is days rather than weeks. When vitamin D or calcifediol is withdrawn, weeks are required for the disappearance of the biologic effects, compared with a few days for calcitriol.

Patients with hypoparathyroidism should be given 2 to 3 g elemental calcium by mouth each day. The two agents, vitamin D (or vitamin D metabolites) and oral calcium, can be varied independently. Higher doses of vitamin D or its metabolites increase the efficiency of intestinal calcium absorption; higher intakes of oral calcium permit adequate calcium assimilation despite a lower efficiency of intestinal calcium absorption. When hypercalcemia occurs during the treatment of chronic hypocalcemia, discontinuation of the calcium lowers calcium within 24 h, even more rapidly than withdrawal of calcitriol. Most patients with hypoparathyroidism can be managed with high-dose vitamin D therapy and 2 to 3 g oral calcium per day. If hypocalcemia alternates with episodes of hypercalcemia, administration of calcitriol often makes management easier.

The administration of thiazide diuretics in the usual antihypertensive doses and sodium restriction in patients with hypoparathyroidism lowers urinary calcium excretion and makes it possible to reduce the doses of calcium and vitamin D. Patients have a lower urinary calcium excretion at any given level of blood calcium on thiazides. Thiazides also may protect against the development of kidney stones, a potential complication of the management of hypoparathyroidism. If on dialysis, patients with chronic renal failure and hypocalcemia can have adjustments in dialysate calcium concentrations as an alternative to vitamin D and calcium supplementation. The doses of vitamin D and calcium required for the management of PHP are usually lower than those required for hypoparathyroidism, reflecting incomplete resistance to the action of PTH in PHP. The acute treatment of hypomagnesemia is discussed above.

BIBLIOGRAPHY

AHN TG et al: Familial isolated hypoparathyroidism: A molecular genetic analysis of 8 families with 23 affected persons. Medicine 65:73, 1986

ARNOLD A et al: Monoclonality of parathyroid tumors in chronic renal failure and in primary parathyroid hyperplasia. J Clin Invest 95:2047, 1995

BENSON L et al: Hyperparathyroidism presenting as the first lesion in multiple endocrine neoplasia type 1. Am J Med 82:731, 1987

BROWN EM et al: The cloning of extracellular Ca^{2+}-sensing receptors from parathyroid and kidney: Molecular mechanisms of extracellular Ca^{2+}-sensing. J Nutr 125:1965S, 1995

CHOU Y-H W et al: Mutations in the human Ca^{2+}-sensing-receptor gene that cause hypocalciuric hypercalcemia. Am J Hum Genet 56:1075, 1995

CONKLIN BR, BOURNE HR: Marriage of the flytrap and the serpent. Nature 367:22, 1994

CRYNS VL et al: Frequent loss of chromosome arm Ip DNA in parathyroid adenomas. Genes Chromosom Cancer 13:9, 1995

DIRKS JH: The kidney and magnesium regulation. Kidney Int 23:771, 1983

FIBISON WJ et al: Molecular studies of DiGeorge syndrome. Am J Hum Genet 46:888, 1990

FITCH N: The identification and inheritance of Albright's hereditary osteodystrophy. Am J Med Genet 11:11, 1982

FITZPATRICK LA, ARNOLD A: Hypoparathyroidism in *Endocrinology*, L DeGroot et al (eds). Philadelphia, Saunders, 1995, p 1123

FLEISCH H: Bisphosphonates: Pharmacology and use in the treatment of tumor-induced hypercalcemia and metastatic bone disease. Drugs 42:919, 1991

FRIEDMAN E et al: Clonality of parathyroid tumors in familial multiple endocrine neoplasia type 1. N Engl J Med 321:213, 1989

FUKAGAWA M et al: Suppression of parathyroid gland hyperplasia by $1,25(OH)_2D_3$ pulse therapy. N Engl J Med 315:421, 1990

GRILL V et al: PTH-related protein: Elevated levels in both humoral hypercalcemia of malignancy and hypercalcemia complicating metastatic breast cancer. J Clin Endocrinol 73:1309, 1991

GUISE TA, MUNDY GR: Breast cancer and bone. Curr Opin Endocrinol Diab 2:548, 1995

HABENER J et al: Hyperparathyroidism, in *Endocrinology*, L DeGroot et al (eds). Philadelphia, Saunders, 1995, p 1044

HINDIE E et al: Primary hyperparathyroidism: Is technetium-99m–sestamibi/iodine-123 subtraction scanning the best procedure to locate enlarged glands before surgery? J Clin Endocrinol Metab 80:302, 1994

HOWE JR et al: Prevalence of pheochromoctyoma and hyperparathyroidism in multiple endocrine neoplasia type 2A: Results of long-term follow-up. Surgery 114:1070, 1993

JAMESON JL, ARNOLD A: Recombinant DNA strategies for determining the molecular basis of endocrine disorders. J Endocrinol Metab 70:301, 1990

KRUSE K, SCHÜTZ C: Calcium metabolism in the Jansen type of metaphyseal dysplasia. Eur J Pediatr 152:912, 1993

LEDGER GA et al: Genetic testing in the diagnosis and management of multiple endocrine neoplasia type II. Ann Intern Med 122:118, 1995

LEVINE MA, SPIEGEL AM: Pseudohypoparathyroidism, in *Endocrinology*, L DeGroot et al (eds). Philadelphia, Saunders, 1995, p 1136

LIPS CJM et al: Clinical screening as compared with DNA analysis in families with multiple endocrine neoplasia type 2A. N Engl J Med 331:828, 1994

MALLETTE LE, EICHORN E: Effects of lithium carbonate on human calcium metabolism. Arch Intern Med 146:770, 1986

MARCUS R: Editorial: Bones of contention: The problem of mild hyperparathyroidism. J Clin Endocrinol Metab 80:720, 1995

MARX SJ: Familial hypocalciuric hypercalcemia, in *Primer on the Metabolic Bone Diseases and Disorders of Mineral Metabolism*, MJ Favus (ed). Richmond, VA, William Byrd Press, 1990, p 113

MAYNARD FM: Immobilization hypercalcemia following spinal cord injury. Arch Phys Med Rehabil 67:41, 1986

MITCHELL BK et al: Primary hyperparathyroidism: Preoperative localization using technetium-sestamibi scanning. J Clin Endocrinol Metab 80:7, 1995

MOTOKURA T et al: Cloning and characterization of human cyclin D3, a cDNA closely related in sequence to the PRAD1/cyclin D1 proto-oncogene. J Biol Chem 267:20412, 1992.

MUDDE AH et al: Ectopic product of 1,25-dihydroxyvitamin D by B-cell lymphoma as a cause of hypercalcemia. Cancer 59:1543, 1987

NEMETH EF, HEATH H III: The calcium receptor and familial benign hypocalciuric hypercalcemia. Curr Opin Endocrinol Diab 2:556, 1995

NEUFELD M et al: Autoimmune polyglandular syndromes. Pediatr Ann 9:43, 1980

NUSSBAUM SR, POTTS JT JR: Immunoassays for parathyroid hormone 1-84 in the diagnosis of hyperparathyroidism. J Bone Miner Res 6 (Suppl 2):S43, 1991

——— et al: Medical management of hyperparathyroidism and hypercalcemia, in *Endocrinology*, DeGroot L et al (eds). Philadelphia, Saunders, 1995, p 1094

O'RIORDAN DS et al: Surgical management of primary hyperparathyroidism in multiple endocrine neoplasia types 1 and 2. Surgery 114:1031, 1993

ORWOLL ES: The milk-alkali syndrome: Current concepts. Ann Intern Med 97:242, 1982

PARFITT AM et al: Asymptomatic primary hyperparathyroidism discovered by multichannel biochemical screening: Clinical course and considerations bearing on the need for surgical intervention. J Bone Miner Res 6 (Suppl 2):S97, 1991

PARKINSON DB, THAKKER RV: A donor splice site mutation in the parathyroid hormone gene is associated with autosomal recessive hypoparathyroidism. Nature Genet 1:149, 1992

PATTEN JL et al: Mutation in the gene encoding the stimulatory G protein of adenylyl cyclase in Albright's hereditary osteodystrophy. N Engl J Med 322:1412, 1990

POLLAK MR et al: Mutations in the human Ca^{2+}-sensing receptor gene cause familial hypocalciuric hypercalcemia and neonatal severe hyperparathyroidism. Cell 75:1297, 1993

POTTS JT JR et al (eds): Proceedings of the NIH Consensus Development Conference on Diagnosis and Management of Asymptomatic Primary Hyperparathyroidism. J Bone Miner Res 6 (Suppl 2):S1, 1991

RALSTON SH et al: Cancer-associated hypercalcemia: Morbidity and mortality. Ann Intern Med 12:499, 1990

RATCLIFFE WA et al: Immunoreactivity of plasma parathyrin-related peptide. Clin Chem 37:1781, 1991

ROSENBERG CL et al: Coding sequence of the overexpressed transcript of the putative oncogene PRAD1/cyclin D1 in two primary human tumors. Oncogene 8:519, 1993

SALUSKY IB et al: The renal osteodystrophies, in *Endocrinology*, L DeGroot et al (eds). Philadelphia, Saunders, 1995, p 1151

SCHIPANI E et al: Constitutively activated receptors for parathyroid hormone and parathyroid hormone-related peptide in Jansen's metaphyseal chondrodysplasia. N Engl J Med 335:708, 1996

SEGRE GV, POTTS JT JR: Differential diagnosis of hypercalcemia, in *Endocrinology*, DeGroot L et al (eds). Philadelphia, Saunders, 1995, p 1075

SILVERBERG SJ et al: Longitudinal measurements of bone density and biochemical indices in untreated primary hyperparathyroidism. J Clin Endocrinol Metab 80:723, 1995

——— et al: Increased bone mineral density after parathyroidectomy in primary hyperparathyroidism. J Clin Endocrinol Metab 80:729, 1995

STEFENELLI T et al: Primary hyperparathyroidism: Incidence of cardiac abnormalities and partial reversibiity after successful parathyroidectomy. Am J Med 95:197, 1993

STEWART AF et al: Malignancy-associated hypercalcemia, in *Endocrinology*, DeGroot L et al (eds). Philadelphia, Saunders, 1995, p 1061

STUCKEY BGA et al: Fasting calcium excretion and parathyroid hormone together distinguish familial hypocalciuric hypercalcaemia from primary hyperparathyroidism. Clin Endocrinol 27:525, 1987

THAKKER RV et al: Association of parathyroid tumors in multiple endocrine neoplasia type 1 with loss of alleles on chromosome 11. N Engl J Med 321:218, 1989

——— et al: Mapping the gene causing X-linked recessive idiopathic hypoparathyroidism to Xq26–Xq27 by linkage studies. J Clin Invest 86:40, 1990

WARRELL RP et al: A randomized double-blind study of gallium nitrate compared with etidronate for acute control of cancer related hypercalcemia. J Clin Oncol 9:1467, 1991

WILSON DI et al: A prospective cytogenetic study of 36 cases of DiGeorge syndrome. Am J Hum Genet 51:957, 1992

355 METABOLIC BONE DISEASE

Stephen M. Krane, Michael F. Holick

OSTEOPOROSIS

GENERAL CONSIDERATIONS *Osteoporosis* is the term used for diseases that cause a reduction in the mass of bone per unit volume. It is used to define any degree of skeletal fragility sufficient to increase the risk of fracture. The reduction in mass results from an imbalance in the processes that influence the acquisition and maintenance of skeletal mass and is not accompanied by a change in the ratio of the mineral phase to the organic phase or by any abnormality in bone mineral or organic matrix. Histologically, the disorder is characterized by a decrease in cortical thickness and in the number and size of the trabeculae of cancellous bone. Individual trabecular plates are abnormally perforated and may be fractured, and trabecular connectivity is reduced. The osteoid seams, however, are of normal width. Osteoporosis, the most common of the metabolic bone diseases (disorders in which all the skeleton is involved), is an important cause of morbidity in the elderly.

The remodeling of bone (its formation and resorption) is a continuous process. Since the bone mass is decreased in osteoporosis, the affected individual either failed to attain optimal skeletal mass during the first 3 decades of life, and/or the rate of bone resorption exceeded that of bone formation after peak skeletal mass was attained. Bone formation is higher in cortical than in cancellous bone. This difference is exaggerated by the normal menopause and exaggerated further in patients with osteoporosis, because rates of formation of cancellous bone tend to be lower in patients with osteoporosis, particularly in women after the menopause. The fact that about a third of postmenopausal women have high skeletal turnover, as assessed by histomorphometry, retention of bone-seeking markers such as ^{99m}Tc-methylene diphosphonate, and biochemical markers, could reflect the greater relative contribution of cortical remodeling in these women. After closure of epiphyses and cessation of longitudinal growth, there is a period of consolidation with a decrease in cortical porosity. When peak adult bone mass is reached at about age 30 to 35 for cortical bone and probably earlier for trabecular bone, rates of bone formation and resorption are relatively low (compared with the period of growth spurt) and approximately equal. The normal balance between bone formation and bone resorption maintains skeletal mass. The rates of remodeling differ, however, not only between cortical and trabecular bone but also in individual bones or portions of bones. Most of the in formation or resorption. Active surfaces may be distributed randomly, but formation and resorption are locally coupled as units. Resorption areas are covered by osteoclasts if active; bone formation surfaces are characterized by the presence of osteoid seams and are covered by active osteoblasts. Resorption precedes formation and is probably more intense, but it does not last as long as formation. As a consequence, there are more sites of active formation than of resorption. Bone turnover is high when many units are active and low when few are active. Unless formation compensates for resorption, bone mass decreases. After age 40 to 50, cortical bone is lost at a rate of about 0.3 to 0.5 percent per year in both sexes. Around the menopause in women, an accelerated loss of cortical bone is superimposed on the age-related loss. Loss of trabecular bone begins at an earlier age in both sexes but is probably greater in women. The cumulative losses of bone mass range from 20 to 30 percent in men and 40 to 50 percent in some women. Bone loss involves predominantly trabecular bone in the spine and distal radius in women and the spine and hip in both women and men. The fact that loss is not uniform has been documented with techniques such as single- and dual-photon absorptiometry, quantitative computed tomography, dual-energy x-ray densitometry (DEXA), and neutron activation analysis of total-body calcium. For example, the rate of loss is greater in the metacarpals, the femoral neck, and the vertebral bodies than in the midshaft of the femur, the tibia, and the skull.

Remodeling activity is increased in most women with postmenopausal osteoporosis as compared with age-matched controls. These differences are even more marked when the comparison is with healthy premenopausal women in whom rates of remodeling are lower than in healthy postmenopausal women. Even in those individuals with increased bone resorption, however, bone formation does not compensate. At some critical point if the difference between rates of formation and resorption is maintained, loss of bone substance may become so marked that the bone can no longer resist the normal mechanical forces to which it is subjected, and fracture results. The template for formation of new bone is lost, and loss of bone accelerates as bone resorption continues and is even more uncoupled from formation. Osteoporosis may only be recognized as a clinical problem when fractures occur. Although the level of reduction in bone mass required to cause fractures after minimal trauma varies, the bone mineral density as measured by DEXA is an excellent predictor of fracture risk. The strength of bones such as vertebrae depends on "quality" (e.g., trabecular connectivity and arrangement) and on mineral density. For example, the horizontal trabeculae of the cancellous bone of vertebrae are preferentially lost in osteoporosis. Additional factors that influence the susceptibility to fracture include the adequacy of ligamentous support and age-related changes in the intervertebral disks. Microfractures are frequent. Age- or drug-related impairments of vision, hearing, and other neurologic and intellectual functions are additional contributors to the occurrence of fractures.

In the remodeling of lamellar bone in adults, most of the net resorption occurs at the corticoendosteal surface. The abnormal remodeling in osteoporosis follows the same pattern; the loss of cancellous bone, cortical bone at the endosteal surface, and intracortical bone results in enlargement of the medullary cavity and thinning of the cortex. Since bone formation at the periosteum continues at a slow rate, the diameter of the bone does not decrease, and the periosteal surface remains smooth. The cancellous bone also undergoes progressive resorption, some trabeculae being resorbed faster than others, particularly horizontal vertebral trabeculae.

The age-related loss of bone begins earlier and proceeds more rapidly in women and tends to accelerate before the menopause. All the factors responsible for bone loss with age are not known, although some risk factors have been identified. In general, white women have a greater risk than black women, and white men have a greater risk than black men. One explanation for these ethnic differences is that the bone mass at skeletal maturity is one determinant of the bone mass at subsequent ages. The lower incidence of osteoporosis and hip fracture in black men and women has been attributed to a higher bone mineral content in blacks than in whites, despite the fact that bone formation is lower in blacks. Since formation and resorption are usually coupled and since bone mass is increased, bone resorption (and turnover) also must be reduced. Osteoporotic subjects are frequently less muscular and have lower average body weight, and exercise may have a beneficial effect in maintaining bone mass. Patients who are kept at complete bed rest and astronauts in microgravity can lose approximately 1 percent of the bone mass each month. The facts that accelerated bone loss accompanies the menopause in some women and that premature osteoporosis occurs after premature surgical menopause suggest that estrogens play a major role in preventing bone loss. Osteoporotic women also have a higher incidence of cigarette smoking, which might affect bone remodeling directly or have secondary effects on ovarian function. Excessive alcohol consumption can decrease bone formation and is a risk factor for osteoporosis. Dietary calcium intake during the first 3 decades of life influences the ultimate peak bone mass, and calcium intake during adult life also has a small effect on bone mass and risk of fracture. Inability to synthesize adequate amounts of 1α,25-dihydroxyvitamin D [1,25(OH)$_2$D] may play a role in the decreased calcium absorption, possibly because of decreased sensitivity of the 25(OH)D-1α-hydroxylase to parathyroid hormone or impaired activity of the renal 25(OH)D-1α-hydroxylase.

Genetic factors influence bone mass. Indeed, in identical twins, as much as 80 percent of age-specific variation in bone mass can be accounted for on a genetic basis. Several reports suggest that the presence of a specific polymorphism (termed *b* and *B*) in the vitamin D receptor correlates with bone mineral density in some populations; specifically, the homozygous *bb* genotype is associated with higher lumbar and femoral bone mineral density than the *Bb* or *BB* genotypes. Other gene loci also probably influence bone density and strength.

Local production of cytokines appears to mediate the enhanced osteoclast-mediated bone resorption of estrogen deficiency. Peripheral blood monocytes from patients with osteoporosis secrete more interleukin (IL) 1, and the increased production of IL-1 in women with postmenopausal osteoporosis is suppressed by estrogen treatment. IL-1 and other cytokines such as tumor necrosis factor α (TNFα) stimulate production of IL-6 by osteoblasts and other mesenchymal cells. IL-6 is probably the most important cytokine in the recruitment of osteoclasts in the abnormal bone remodeling in postmenopausal osteoporosis. Although osteoporosis occurs with Cushing's syndrome, there is no established role for adrenal steroids in the osteoporosis associated with the menopause or advanced age.

Excessive acid intake, particularly in the form of high-protein diets, may contribute to "dissolution" of bone as the body attempts to buffer the extra acid. Acidosis also may increase osteoclast function directly. Prolonged use of heparin as an anticoagulant is also associated with osteoporosis, and heparin potentiates bone resorption in vitro. The bone marrows of subjects with osteoporosis have increased numbers of mast cells, which presumably are capable of producing heparin and other substances that modulate bone cell function. Circumscribed and diffuse areas of osteoporosis occur in patients with systemic mastocytosis.

As mentioned earlier, the remodeling of bone is responsive to mechanical forces. Immobilization initially causes an increase in bone resorption, while bone formation remains normal or is decreased; later, there is a compensatory increase in bone formation. In osteoporosis, immobilization tends to aggravate the defect by increasing the gap between formation and resorption. A sedentary life-style may reduce mechanical forces exerted on the skeleton and increase the tendency to bone loss.

CLASSIFICATION (See Table 355-1) In some instances, osteoporosis is a manifestation of another disease, such as Cushing's syndrome or osteogenesis imperfecta (see Chap. 348). In most cases of osteoporosis, however, no other disease is apparent. One form occurs in children or young adults of both sexes and with normal gonadal function and is frequently termed *idiopathic osteoporosis*, although most of the other forms are also of unknown pathogenesis. *Type I osteoporosis* occurs in a subset of postmenopausal women who are between 51 and 75 years of age and is characterized by an acceler-

Table 355-1

Classification of Osteoporosis

Common forms, unassociated with other disease	
	Idiopathic osteoporosis (juvenile and adult)
	Type I osteoporosis
	Type II osteoporosis
Disorders in which osteoporosis is a common feature	
	Hypogonadism
	Hyperadrenocorticism
	Chronic glucocorticoid administration
	Hyperparathyroidism
	Thyrotoxicosis
	Malabsorption
	Scurvy
	Calcium deficiency
	Immobilization
	Chronic heparin administration
	Systemic mastocytosis
	Adult hypophosphatasia
	Other metabolic bone diseases
Heritable disorders of connective tissue in which osteoporosis is a feature	
	Osteogenesis imperfecta
	Homocystinuria due to cystathionine synthase deficiency
	Ehlers-Danlos syndrome
	Marfan's syndrome
Disorders in which the pathogenesis of associated osteoporosis is not understood	
	Rheumatoid arthritis
	Malnutrition
	Alcoholism
	Epilepsy
	Primary biliary cirrhosis
	Chronic obstructive pulmonary disease
	Menkes' syndrome

ated and disproportionate loss of trabecular bone. Fractures of vertebral bodies and the distal forearm are common complications. Decreased parathyroid gland function may be compensatory to increased bone resorption. *Type II osteoporosis* occurs in women and men over the age of 70 and is associated with fractures of the femoral neck, proximal humerus, proximal tibia, and pelvis, sites that contain both cortical and trabecular bone. Circulating levels of parathyroid hormone (PTH) tend to be high. Both groups have decreased mean circulating levels of 1,25$(OH)_2$D.

GENERAL CLINICAL FEATURES Although osteoporosis is a generalized disorder of the skeleton, the major sequelae result from fractures of the vertebrae, wrist, hip, humerus, and tibia. The most frequent symptoms from vertebral body fractures are pain in the back and deformity of the spine. Pain usually results from collapse of the vertebrae, especially in the dorsal and lumbar regions, is typically acute in onset, and often radiates around the flank into the abdomen. Such episodes may occur after sudden bending, lifting, or jumping movements that may have seemed trivial; on some occasions they cannot be related to trauma. The pain may be increased with even slight movements such as turning in bed or the Valsalva maneuver. Bed rest may relieve the pain temporarily, only for it to recur in spasms of variable duration. Radiation of pain down one leg is uncommon, and symptoms or signs of spinal cord compression are rare. The acute episodes of pain also may be accompanied by abdominal distention and ileus, thought to be due to retroperitoneal hemorrhage, but the use of narcotics also contributes to the ileus. Loss of appetite and muscular weakness also may be present. Episodes of pain usually subside after several days to a week, and by 4 to 6 weeks patients may be fully ambulatory and able to resume normal activities. Although acute pain may be minimal, nagging, deep, dull, uncomfortable sensations may be localized to the area of fracture and brought about by straining or sudden changes in position. Patients may be unable to sit up in bed and may have to arise by rolling over on the side and then propping themselves up, but the pain usually disappears or decreases between episodes of vertebral body collapse. Other patients do not have acute episodes but complain of backache that is made worse by standing or sudden movement. Tenderness is common over involved areas of the spinous processes or rib cage. Some patients have an associated disease such as osteoarthritis of facet joints to account for chronic back pain. Vertebral bodies usually collapse anteriorly, producing a wedge-shaped deformity and contributing to loss in height. This is particularly common in the middorsal region, where collapse may not be associated with pain but may result in a dorsal kyphosis and exaggerated cervical lordosis described as a "dowager's" or "widow's" hump. Postural slumping with increase in existing curves contributes to the loss of height. Scoliosis is also common. Generalized skeletal pain is uncommon, and between fractures most patients are free of pain. Although recurrent episodes of vertebral collapse, increasing spine deformity, and loss of height are common, the course in any one person is not predictable, and there may be intervals of several years between fractures.

Hip fractures are the most severe complication. They may be the consequence of trauma, most resulting from a fall from standing height. The likelihood of fracture in a particular location is related in part to the site where the bond density is most reduced, such as the femoral neck or intertrochanteric region. The incidence of hip fractures in both men and women increases with age.

RADIOLOGIC FEATURES Prior to fracture and collapse, the osteoporotic vertebral body shows a decrease in mineral density, an increase in the prominence of vertical striations due to a relatively greater loss of the horizontally oriented trabeculae, and prominence of the end plates. The bodies may become increasingly biconcave because of weakening of the subchondral plates, microfractures, and expansion of the intervertebral disks, resulting in so-called codfish vertebrae. When collapse occurs, it usually produces a decrease in the anterior height of the vertebral body and irregularity in the anterior cortex (Fig. 355-1). Older compression fractures may show reactive changes and osteophytes about the anterior margins. Most osteoporotic fractures occur in the middle and lower thoracic and upper lumbar

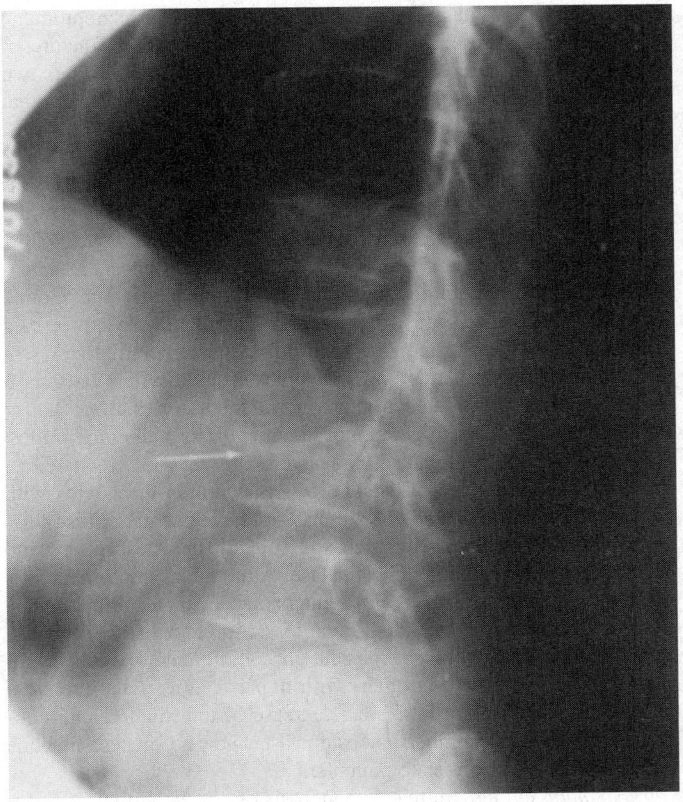

FIGURE 355-1 Lateral views of the lumbar spine of a 54-year-old man with idiopathic osteoporosis. A typical anterior compression fracture is indicated by the arrow.

vertebral bodies. Fractures of isolated vertebral bodies at T4 or higher suggest malignancy. Although the cortices of long bones may be thin because of excessive endosteal resorption, the outer margins are sharp, in contrast to the typical effects of the subperiosteal resorption of hyperparathyroidism. Pseudofractures or Looser's zones do not occur in the absence of osteomalacia, but it may be impossible to distinguish osteoporosis from osteomalacia on radiologic grounds alone. In the absence of fractures, standard roentgenograms are insensitive indicators of bone loss, since a decrease by as much as 30 percent in bone mass may not be appreciated. Other procedures are required to establish whether a given individual has a sufficient decrease in bone mass to be at risk for fracture. DEXA is an excellent technique because of its sensitivity, ability to scan the entire skeleton, low radiation exposure, and short scanning time. Single- and dual-photon absorptiometry and quantitative computed tomography (CT) also can detect small (1 to 2 percent) changes in the bone mineral density of the hip and lumbar spine.

LABORATORY FINDINGS The concentrations of calcium and inorganic phosphorus in the blood are usually normal. Slight hyperphosphatemia occurs in women who are past the menopause. The alkaline phosphatase level in uncomplicated instances is normal, but it may increase after fractures. About 20 percent of postmenopausal women with osteoporosis have hypercalciuria. Biochemical indices of bone resorption are, on the average, increased. Immunoassays for urinary excretion of type I collagen–derived pyridinoline cross-links such as free and total pyridinolines and *N*-telopeptide cross-links are better than assays of hydroxyproline. Such assays and serum assays of bone-specific alkaline phosphatase, osteocalcin, and C-terminal procollagen peptides are particularly useful in monitoring the effects of therapy.

DIFFERENTIAL DIAGNOSIS Since decrease in skeletal mass is a universal feature of aging, it is difficult to evaluate asymptomatic decreased bone density, determined radiographically, in older women, especially when not accompanied by marked increase in biconcavity of vertebral bodies or fractures. Quantitative measurement of bone mass is, however, a predictor of future fractures, and measurements of vertebral height may reveal the presence of asymptomatic fractures. In the presence of bone pain with or without fracture or deformity, it is important to establish the presence or absence of known causes of osteoporosis as listed in Table 355-1 and to be certain that osteoporosis is the correct diagnosis. Malignancies of various types, particularly *multiple myeloma, lymphoma, leukemia*, and *metastatic carcinoma*, may result in diffuse loss of bone, especially the trabecular bone of the vertebral column, even in the absence of hypercalcemia. The absence of anemia, elevated erythrocyte sedimentation rate, abnormal electrophoretic patterns of serum proteins, and Bence Jones proteinuria is helpful in eliminating the possibility of multiple myeloma. However, needle bone biopsy or marrow aspiration may be appropriate in instances of severe osteoporosis with fractures. Quantitative histomorphometry on standard biopsy samples from the iliac crest is a research tool but is available in some referral laboratories. Bone biopsy samples must be properly fixed, not demineralized, and embedded in plastic to rule out osteomalacia, however.

Radiologic evidence of osteoporosis is common in patients with primary *hyperparathyroidism*, who may not have osteitis fibrosa (discrete lytic lesions of varying size and subperiosteal resorption) and elevation of serum alkaline phosphatase. Although asymptomatic primary hyperparathyroidism is not a major risk factor in osteoporosis, it does contribute to accelerated bone loss. An element of secondary hyperparathyroidism may be present in some elderly patients with type II osteoporosis and in others with impairment of renal function, inadequate oral calcium intake, or decrease of intestinal calcium absorption. Increased numbers of osteoclasts may be present in bone biopsy specimens from such patients.

Osteomalacia may mimic osteoporosis or coexist with it, yet specific radiologic signs of osteomalacia are not always present. Although the presence of abnormalities such as low or undetectable circulating levels of 25-hydroxyvitamin D[25(OH)D] and PTH with or without hypophosphatemia suggests the possibility of osteomalacia, bone biopsy may be essential for diagnosis, as discussed below. Since osteomalacia is more responsive to therapy (e.g., vitamin D in hypovitaminosis D or phosphate supplements in phosphate depletion) than is the usual case of osteoporosis, such diagnostic procedures are often warranted. Subclinical vitamin D deficiency with associated secondary hyperparathyroidism may be more common in elderly women than previously recognized, and treatment of postmenopausal women with small doses of vitamin D (20 μg or 800 IU daily) may reduce the risk of hip fractures and other nonvertebral fractures.

In an occasional patient with *Paget's disease*, pure lytic radiologic features may be confused with osteoporosis. High alkaline phosphatase levels and increased urinary excretion of pyridinoline cross-links are clues to the presence of Paget's disease. Scanning procedures with bone-seeking isotopes are not helpful in differential diagnosis if fractures are present because fractures cause preferential uptake of isotope. In the absence of fractures "hot spots" are more suggestive of tumor or early Paget's disease, particularly if present in the appendicular skeleton.

IDIOPATHIC OSTEOPOROSIS *Idiopathic osteoporosis* occurs in younger men and in premenopausal women in whom no other etiologic factor is detected. These patients probably have a number of different disorders with superficial resemblances. Occasionally, osteoporosis appears in young women during or shortly after pregnancy. Such women have decreases in trabecular bone, and bone mass may remain low for many years. The etiology is unknown. Some patients have low levels of serum alkaline phosphatase, though not low enough to fulfill diagnostic criteria for *hypophosphatasia*. Estrogens are ineffective in this form of osteoporosis. Losses of calcium and phosphorus are probably excessive, and it is unwise to permit women with osteoporosis to breast-feed, because calcium losses via lactation are appreciable. Some patients have a disorder similar to mild forms of osteogenesis imperfecta and may thus have defects in type I collagen genes, although such features as family history, blue sclerae, and deafness are lacking. The course is variable; although recurrent episodes of fractures are characteristic, progressive deterioration does not occur in all patients, and in some the clinical problem is benign. Juvenile osteoporosis is a rare disorder, with onset usually between the ages of 8 and 14 years; it is characterized by the abrupt appearance of bone pain and fractures after minimal trauma. In many cases the disorder is self-limited, and recovery takes place spontaneously within 4 or 5 years.

GLUCOCORTICOID EXCESS Glucocorticoid excess does not appear to be involved in idiopathic osteoporosis or in the type I or II disorder. Osteoporosis, however, commonly accompanies Cushing's syndrome, both endogenous and exogenous, and in some instances is rapidly progressive, especially in children and in women over age 50. Bone loss is usually most rapid in the first 6 to 12 months of therapy with glucocorticoids but continues indefinitely with prolonged therapy. The skeletal pathophysiology is probably accounted for by a combination of low rates of bone formation (depressed osteoblastic function) and high rates of bone resorption reflected in the hypercalciuria that accompanies increased activation frequency of bone remodeling units. A part of the latter may be the result of glucocorticoid-induced secondary hyperparathyroidism, although increases in circulating PTH are not found consistently. Glucocorticoids, however, potentiate the effects of PTH and $1,25(OH)_2D$ on bone cells in vitro. Glucocorticoids depress collagen synthesis in many tissues, as evidenced by delayed wound healing, thinning of the dermis, striae, and tendency to blue sclerae. In some disorders in which glucocorticoids are administered in pharmacologic doses, such as rheumatoid arthritis, a tendency to osteoporosis is present beforehand, and the skeletal effects of the glucocorticoids may be particularly severe. Even low doses of glucocorticoids can accelerate bone loss in postmenopausal women and men with rheumatoid arthritis. Blood levels of 25(OH)D are normal or slightly decreased, and blood levels of $1,25(OH_2)D$ are usually normal. Glucocorticoids inhibit intestinal calcium absorption by a direct, vitamin D–independent action on the intestine, but osteomalacia does not occur. Once osteoporosis develops in adults with Cushing's syndrome, the abnormality may persist indefinitely following alleviation of the glucocorticoid excess. In children, however, cure of the Cushing's syndrome can result in striking improvement in the appearance of the spine due to new endochondral bone formation around the less dense, older osteoporotic bone. Likewise, increase in bone mass, increase in serum osteocalcin levels (indicative of increased osteoblastic function), and decrease in urinary excretion of markers of bone resorption may occur in young adults following treatment of Cushing's syndrome. Withdrawal of glucocorticoids or a decrease of the dose by use of an alternate-day schedule is important to halt progression of the osteoporosis. Anabolic steroids are not effective in this regard. The defect in intestinal calcium absorption may be overcome by administering calcitriol [$1,25(OH)_2D$] in oral doses of 0.5 to 1.0 μg/d plus 1 g supplemental oral calcium daily. Such regimens with or without calcitonin (e.g., 400 IU/d intranasally) are effective in preventing glucocorticoid-induced bone loss. Vitamin D metabolites such as calcifediol [25(OH)D] also may be effective. It is important to monitor serum and urinary calcium levels at intervals of 2 to 4 months. In Cushing's syndrome, spontaneous, symptomless fractures may occur in ribs and pubic and ischial rami even in the absence of marked osteoporosis of the spine. These fractures often heal partially with an exuberant calcified callus surrounding a radiolucent zone of nonunion, superficially resembling the pseudofractures of osteomalacia. If they appear in the thorax superimposed on the lungs, they may be confused with nodules suggesting primary or metastatic tumor.

GONADAL DEFICIENCY Osteoblasts have receptors for estrogens, and estrogens may function in these cells by stimulating production of substances that are anabolic for bone such as insulin-like growth factor I or by reducing the production of catabolic cytokines by osteoblasts and mononuclear phagocytes. Estrogen is deficient in the postmenopausal woman, and the administration of estrogen to such an individual reduces the negative calcium balance and decreases urinary excretion of markers of bone resorption. Estrogens are particularly useful in retarding the bone loss in women who have oophorectomy at an early age and in preventing the development of osteoporosis following the menopause. Bone mass is also decreased in women athletes who are amenorrheic, such as marathon runners. Such women are particularly prone to tibial stress fractures. In patients of either sex castrated at an early age, the adult skeleton is smaller to begin with, and, therefore, age-related losses are more significant. Bone density is also decreased in women with hyperprolactinemia and in men with hypogonadism of all types. Estrogens also play a critical role in skeletal growth and the attainment and maintenance of peak bone mass, as evidenced by the presence of severe osteopenia in a man with tall stature, marked osteoporosis, and increased urinary excretion of the markers of bone resorption associated with a loss-of-function mutation in the estrogen receptor.

THYROTOXICOSIS In many patients with hyperthyroidism, including some with mild or subclinical hyperthyroidism, excessive bone resorption, occasionally marked in degree and far exceeding that in the usual patient with osteoporosis, can be associated with increased excretion of calcium and phosphorus in urine and feces. The excessive bone resorption is usually accompanied by a compensatory increase in bone formation. PTH secretion is decreased, intestinal calcium absorption is low, and levels of $1,25(OH)_2D$ are normal or low. If the hyperthyroidism is of short duration, skeletal losses are inconsequential. In patients with chronic hyperthyroidism, however, especially in women after the menopause, this accelerated bone loss becomes significant, and it is important to eliminate hyperthyroidism as a contributing cause of osteoporosis. Mild or subclinical hyperthyroidism due to the use of excessive replacement doses of levothyroxine causes decrease in cortical bone, particularly in estrogen-deficient women. The treatment of hypothyroid patients with replacement doses of levothyroxine decreases bone mass to values found in normal individuals, and excessive doses of levothyroxine in these patients can result in accelerated bone loss. Although typical osteitis fibrosa (resorption lacunae containing osteoclasts and a fibrous stroma) may be seen on biopsy, the skeletal lesions have the radiologic appearance of osteoporosis.

ACROMEGALY Hypercalciuria and overall net negative calcium balance occur in acromegaly, and, occasionally, osteoporosis is an associated finding. The secondary panhypopituitarism and the associated gonadal insufficiency may be factors in production of the osteoporosis. In adult animals, growth hormone decreases endosteal resorption and stimulates bone formation, and it is therefore unlikely that excessive secretion of growth hormone in itself produces osteoporosis.

DIABETES MELLITUS Individuals with juvenile or adult-onset diabetes mellitus have a decreased bone mass. In some series, the incidence of hip fractures is increased, but studies of large groups of diabetic subjects have not revealed abnormal calcium metabolism or significant bone disease specifically attributable to the diabetes.

CALCIUM DEFICIENCY AND MALABSORPTION Adequate calcium intake is an important influence in the attainment of peak bone mass. Calcium deficiency is not a major factor in the pathogenesis of postmenopausal osteoporosis or the osteoporosis of aging in both sexes. However, osteoporosis is present in many patients with steatorrhea, prolonged obstructive jaundice, and lactose intolerance and in patients following gastrectomy. Other patients may have a specific defect in calcium absorption or a failure to adapt adequately to a low-calcium diet either by increasing the percentage of dietary calcium absorbed or by decreasing urinary calcium excretion. Presumably, vitamin D is adequate in these instances to prevent osteomalacia.

HERITABLE DISORDERS OF CONNECTIVE TISSUE In the strict sense, the bone disease of osteogenesis imperfecta is osteoporosis (see Chap. 348). *Osteogenesis imperfecta* is clinically, genetically, and biochemically heterogeneous. Type I osteogenesis imperfecta is the autosomal dominant form, characterized by mild to moderate bone fragility, blue sclerae, and premature deafness. The frequency of fractures tends to decrease around puberty, and another period of increased incidence occurs in women after the menopause. Type II is the lethal perinatal disorder. Type III is characterized by severe bone fragility, progressive bone deformity, and white sclerae. In type IV, sclerae are white, but other features are similar to those of type I disease. Many instances of osteogenesis imperfecta of all types have been linked to mutations in the *COL*1A1 and *COL*1A2 genes that encode type I collagen. It is unlikely, however, that mutations in the coding region of the type I collagen genes are important in controlling bone mass in individuals with postmenopausal osteoporosis. Osteoporosis also occurs in patients with *homocystinuria* due to cystathionine synthase deficiency, an autosomal recessive trait associated with ectopia lentis, various deformities of the extremities, mental retardation, decreased pigmentation of hair and skin, and thromboembolism. The diagnosis is established by the finding of homocystine in urine. Homocystine has effects on the cross-linking of collagen, but it is not known how homocystinuria causes osteoporosis.

Rx TREATMENT

Potent agents are now available for preventing bone loss and for treating established osteoporosis. The ability to measure bone density and predict fracture in osteoporosis has changed the approach to treatment. Clinical benefit can be documented not only in the form of improved bone mass but as a decreased incidence of fractures. Although most available drugs are inhibitors of bone resorption, some agents, such as sodium fluoride, increase bone formation.

General Measures After Fractures Have Occurred Patients with acute pain secondary to fracture of vertebral bodies frequently require rest in bed in a position of maximum comfort, local heat, adequate analgesics, and avoidance of constipation. Use of traction or plaster jacket splints is not indicated. As soon as pain permits, the patient should attempt to move out of bed, slowly at first, perhaps with the support of a walker or crutches. Braces are commonly employed, but their efficacy in preventing progression of spinal deformity is not established. A well-made corset may provide support and comfort. Exercises to correct postural deformity and increase muscle tone are useful. Patients should be taught to avoid sudden painful movements such as jumping, and how to lift and carry objects with minimal back strain. After the fractures have healed, a supervised exercise program that includes daily walking may be helpful in preventing further skeletal losses.

Acute mortality after hip fracture is relatively low (around 3 to 4 percent), but mortality within a year is relatively high (20 to 25 percent). Morbidity is also high; only about one-half of patients return to prefracture activity levels within a year.

Estrogens and Androgens The administration of estrogens to postmenopausal women causes a decrease in urinary excretion of calcium and markers of bone resorption, especially during the first few months of treatment (see Chap. 337). Estrogens may have direct effects on osteoblasts and mononuclear phagocytes and can decrease the rate of bone resorption, but bone formation usually does not increase and eventually decreases. Nevertheless, estrogens produce significant calcium retention, decrease the difference between the rates of bone formation and resorption, and retard bone loss. Although any restoration of skeletal mass is minimal, the use of estrogens effectively prevents bone loss following castration and after the menopause and decreases the incidence of osteoporotic fracture in postmenopausal women. The major role of estrogens is in preventing osteoporosis in menopausal women rather than treating clinical disease already developed, although they also may be effective in mild or moderate disease during the first 10 years following cessation of ovarian function. The common dosage is 0.625 mg/d as conjugated estrogens, usually given in a cyclic fashion for the first 25 days of each month. (Lower doses are usually ineffective.) Estradiol also can be administered in a percutaneous patch or gel for transdermal absorption (see Chap. 337). In women after hysterectomy, progestogens are not necessary, but in women with a uterus, a progestogen (e.g., medroxyprogesterone, 5 mg/d) may be added for the last 12 days of estrogen administration (see Chap. 337). Estrogen (e.g., conjugated estrogens, 0.625 mg/d) and a progestogen (e.g., medroxyprogesterone, 2.5 mg/d) also may be administered continuously and will prevent the menstrual cycle. Patient compliance is a major problem in the use of estrogens in postmenopausal women. Many women are reluctant to use estrogens to prevent bone loss and/or treat established osteoporosis because of issues such as return of menstrual bleeding and fear of breast cancer. The estrogen antagonist tamoxifen retains agonist activity in the skeleton and prevents bone loss in the spine and femoral neck. Unfortunately, tamoxifen can also induce uterine bleeding. Testosterone preparations are useful in the treatment of osteoporotic men with gonadal deficiency, but there is no evidence of efficacy in men with normal gonadal function. There is also no proven advantage to combinations of estrogens and androgens in either sex.

Calcium Supplements, Vitamin D Metabolites, and Thiazide Diuretics Women who are estrogen-deprived require an average oral intake of 1500 mg/d of elemental calcium to remain in calcium equilibrium. The recommendation of the National Institutes of Health of 1000 mg elemental calcium per day for women on estrogen replacement and for men is reasonable. In postmenopausal women unable to take estrogens, the use of 1500 mg/d of oral calcium may have a minor benefit in preserving cortical bone but has no effects on trabecular bone mass. Adequate calcium intake before age 30 to 35 may enhance peak bone mass, however. The content of elemental calcium of available preparations varies depending on the accompanying anion and the composition (Table 355-2). Vitamin D preparations have been used in osteoporosis because calcium absorption is impaired and serum levels of $1,25(OH)_2D$ are marginally low.

Subclinical vitamin D deficiency and associated secondary hyperparathyroidism are common in elderly women, particularly those confined to nursing homes. In these women, low doses of vitamin D (20 μg or 800 IU daily) combined with calcium supplements (1 to 1.5 g elemental calcium daily) are effective in maintaining bone mass and decreasing the incidence of hip fractures. Oral administration of calcitriol also may improve intestinal calcium absorption, suppress bone resorption, and prevent bone loss in postmenopausal osteoporosis. Bone formation is not increased, however, and at the doses suggested (an average of 0.8 μg/d) hypercalcemia and hypercalciuria may occur. Thiazide diuretics are useful in patients with high-turnover osteoporosis associated with hypercalciuria and secondary hyperparathyroidism. In the absence of secondary hyperparathyroidism, the thiazide diuretics lower urinary calcium excretion, suppress parathyroid gland function, inhibit the synthesis of $1,25(OH)_2D$, and reduce intestinal calcium absorption.

Table 355-2

Elemental Calcium Content of Various Oral Calcium Preparations

Calcium Preparation	Elemental Calcium Content
Calcium citrate	40 mg/300 mg
Calcium lactate	80 mg/600 mg
Calcium gluconate	40 mg/500 mg
Calcium carbonate	400 mg/g
Calcium carbonate + 5 μg vitamin D_2 (OsCal 250)	250 mg/tablet
Calcium carbonate (Tums 500)	500 mg/tablet

Calcitonin Calcitonin decreases bone resorption, and the use of salmon calcitonin in established osteoporosis has been recommended in doses of 50 U subcutaneously every other day. Patients with high-turnover osteoporosis (elevated levels of serum osteocalcin, increased urinary excretion of markers of bone absorption, and increased total-body retention of ^{99m}Tc-methylene diphosphonate) appear to respond best with improvement in bone mass. Calcitonin can also be administered by nasal spray (200 U/d) to avoid parenteral administration. Calcitonin may have beneficial effects on bone pain owing to a central analgesic effect.

Bisphosphonates The first bisphosphonate approved as an antiresorptive agent was etidronate, which was administered cyclically in alternation with calcium and vitamin D supplements, to prevent mineralization defects. This regimen caused increases in the density of spinal bone and possibly decreases in the incidence of fractures.

Newer bisphosphonates such as alendronate, pamidronate, and tiludronate are more potent inhibitors of bone resorption and therefore do not cause osteomalacia at effective antiresorptive doses. In two large multicenter studies alendronate at a dose of 10 mg/d was effective over a 3-year period at increasing the mineral density of spinal bone by about 10 percent, increasing the density of femoral neck bone by about 5 percent, and decreasing the incidence of spine and hip fracture by about one-half. The agent is approved for use in the United States for established osteoporosis. Although there was no increased incidence of gastrointestinal side effects during the trials, it was recommended that to reduce the potential for esophageal irritation the agent be taken first thing on arising with a full glass of water [180 to 240 mL (6 to 8 oz)] at least 30 min before the first meal or beverage and that the patient should avoid lying down for at least 30 min after ingesting the medication. Esophagitis has been reported in postmarketing surveillance, and strict adherence to the dosing recommendations is essential to reduce the risk of this complication.

Fluoride Fluoride ions are deposited in the skeleton, where they are incorporated into the crystal lattice of hydroxyapatite, substituting for hydroxyl ions. This process results in a mineral phase of greater crystallinity. Sodium fluoride or intermittent low doses of PTH (currently in therapeutic trials) are the only agents that can stimulate osteoblastic proliferation and function and increase bone formation. Indeed, chronic ingestion of high amounts of fluoride, usually in areas where the fluoride content of drinking water is high, produces a form of hyperostosis, with dense bones, exostoses, neurologic complications due to bony overgrowth, and ligament ossification. An increased amount of bone with excessive osteoid is evidence of stimulation of bone formation. When sodium fluoride is used to treat osteoporosis, there is a continuous increase in the bone mass of the spine. In some series this increase in bone mass is accompanied by a decreased incidence of spinal fractures, but the therapy may result in an increased risk of fractures of the hip as well as other nonvertebral fractures. Even in series in which a satisfactory effect of sodium fluoride is observed, some patients do not respond at all. Some patients develop side effects, including knee, foot, and ankle pain attributed to microfractures; other patients cannot tolerate the drug because of nausea.

Parathyroid Hormone PTH stimulates bone resorption, but under some circumstances PTH is anabolic. Whereas high-dose, continuous administration results in lower bone mass, low-dose, intermittent administration can increase bone mass. In several studies, PTH prevented bone loss in young women treated with a luteinizing hormone–releasing hormone analogue for endometriosis and increased trabecular bone mass in postmenopausal women. Although not approved for use, this regimen may provide an additional approach for therapy.

RICKETS AND OSTEOMALACIA

Rickets and *osteomalacia* are disorders in which mineralization of the organic matrix of the skeleton is defective (Table 355-3). In *rickets* the growing skeleton is involved; defective mineralization occurs both in bone and in the cartilaginous matrix of the growth plate. The term *osteomalacia* is usually reserved for the disorder in the adult, in whom the epiphyseal growth plates are closed. A number of conditions result in rickets and/or osteomalacia, such as inadequate dietary intake of vitamin D, inadequate exposure to solar ultraviolet radiation with resulting inadequate formation of endogenous vitamin D, intestinal malabsorption of vitamin D, acquired and inherited disorders of vitamin D metabolism, inherited defects in the receptor for $1,25(OH)_2D$ in target tissues, chronic acidosis, renal tubular defects that produce hypophosphatemia or acidosis, aluminum intoxication, and chronic administration of anticonvulsants. In the renal tubular disorders, rickets and osteomalacia develop in the presence of normal intestinal function and are not cured by treatment with doses of vitamin D adequate to cure deficiency rickets. Thus, the term *vitamin D–resistant* (or *refractory*) *rickets* has been applied in these instances. Renal insufficiency, especially in children, and chronic hemodialysis per se are also associated with rickets or osteomalacia.

PATHOGENESIS AND HISTOPATHOLOGY For skeletal mineralization, sufficient calcium and phosphate must be present at the mineralization sites. Other conditions required for normal mineralization include intact metabolic and transport functions of osteoblasts and chondrocytes, adequate collagen matrix, possibly phosphorylation or other modifications of matrix components, and low concentrations of inhibitory substances such as proteoglycan aggregates or inorganic pyrophosphate. A specific function in the mineralization process for the noncollagenous matrix proteins synthesized by bone cells (e.g., osteocalcin, osteonectin, and phosphosialoproteins) has not been demonstrated, although they bind calcium ions. In cartilage the initial mineral phase is enclosed in membrane-bound extracellular vesicles. If the osteoblast continues to produce matrix components that cannot be mineralized adequately, rickets and osteomalacia result. If calcification continues to be inadequate, the production of organic matrix (osteoid) also gradually decreases. In bone there will be an increase in the fraction of the forming surface covered by incompletely mineralized osteoid, an increase in osteoid volume and thickness (the latter being normally less than 12 to 14 μm), and a decrease in the calcification or mineralization front. The latter is detected in undemineralized sections by the fluorescence of previously ingested tetracycline or by special stains. There is a marked decrease in the rate of apposition of mineralized bone. A number of methods are available to measure the thickness of the osteoid seams and the calcification front. In histologic sections stained with hematoxylin and eosin, the more heavily mineralized areas tend to appear violet or blue, whereas the osteoid seams appear pink. Subtle degrees of osteomalacia may not be appreciated with routine preparations, and undecalcified, thin sections (3 to 5 μm) stained, for example, with Goldner's trichrome method are necessary to establish its presence (Fig. 355-2). Rickets is also characterized by inadequate mineralization of the matrix of cartilage in the growing

Table 355-3

Classification of Rickets and Osteomalacia

- **Vitamin D deficiency**
  - Dietary deficiency
  - Deficient endogenous synthesis
- **Gastrointestinal disorders**
  - Small-intestinal diseases with malabsorption
  - Partial or total gastrectomy
  - Hepatobiliary disease
  - Chronic pancreatic insufficiency
- **Disorders of vitamin D metabolism**
  - Hereditary: pseudovitamin D deficiency or vitamin D dependency types I and II
  - Acquired
    - Anticonvulsants
    - Chronic renal failure
    - Tumor-associated (oncogenic) rickets and osteomalacia
- **Acidosis**
  - Distal renal tubular acidosis (classic or type I)
  - Secondary forms of renal acidosis
  - Ureterosigmoidostomy
  - Drug-induced disease
    - Chronic acetazolamide ingestion
    - Chronic ammonium chloride ingestion
- **Chronic renal failure**
- **Phosphate depletion**
  - Dietary: low phosphate intake plus ingestion of nonabsorbable antacids
  - Impaired renal tubular phosphate reabsorption
    - Hereditary
      - X-linked hypophosphatemic rickets (vitamin D–resistant rickets)
      - Adult-onset vitamin D–resistant hypophosphatemic osteomalacia
    - Acquired
      - Sporadic hypophosphatemic osteomalacia (phosphate diabetes)
      - Tumor-associated (oncogenic) rickets and osteomalacia
      - Neurofibromatosis
      - Fibrous dysplasia
- **Generalized renal tubular disorders (Fanconi's syndrome)**
  - Primary renal
  - Associated with systemic metabolic abnormality
    - Cystinosis
    - Glycogenosis
    - Lowe's syndrome
  - Systemic disorder with associated renal disease
    - Hereditary
      - Inborn errors
        - Wilson's disease
        - Tyrosinemia
      - Neurofibromatosis
    - Acquired
      - Multiple myeloma
      - Nephrotic syndrome
      - Transplanted kidney
    - Intoxications
      - Cadmium
      - Lead
      - Outdated tetracycline
- **Primary mineralization defects**
  - Hereditary: hypophosphatasia
  - Acquired
    - Disodium etidronate treatment (Note: Of the bisphosphonates, only etidronate has this effect)
    - Fluoride treatment
- **States of rapid bone formation with or without a relative defect in bone resorption**
  - Postoperative hyperparathyroidism with osteitis fibrosa cystica
  - Osteopetrosis
- **Defective matrix synthesis: fibrogenesis imperfecta ossium**
- **Miscellaneous**
  - Magnesium-dependent conditions
  - Axial osteomalacia
  - Parenteral alimentation
  - Aluminum intoxication

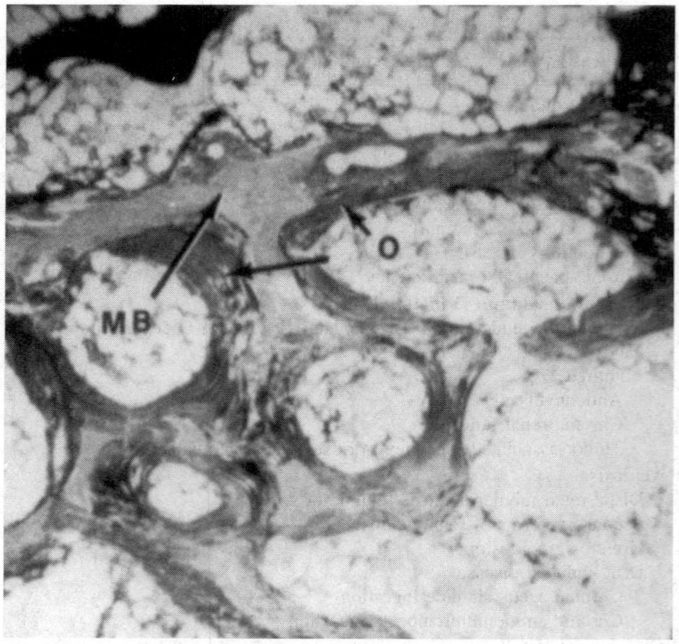

FIGURE 355-2 Photomicrograph of an undemineralized section stained with Goldner method of an iliac crest bone biopsy from a 45-year-old man with chronic renal failure maintained on hemodialysis. Almost the entire surface is covered by osteoid (O), which is readily distinguished from mineralized bone (MB). The thickness of the osteoid seams exceeds 100 μm in several areas.

epiphyseal plate. Calcification in the interstitial regions of the hypertrophic zone is defective, the growth plate increases in thickness, the columns of cartilage cells (which normally are highly ordered) are disorganized, and there is a variable cupping of the epiphyses. The rachitic bones are often incapable of withstanding usual mechanical stresses and tend to undergo bowing deformities. If rickets is untreated, growth at the epiphyseal plates is slowed, and the eventual length of the long bones is diminished.

It is not known whether vitamin D, through one of its metabolites, has a major direct effect on mineralization as long as the supply of mineral ions is adequate. Its primary roles after metabolic conversion to 25(OH)D and 1,25$(OH)_2$D are to regulate and enhance absorption of calcium ions from the intestinal lumen and, possibly, to enhance differentiation of stem cells to form osteoclasts. Insufficiency of the active metabolites of vitamin D leads to decreased intestinal absorption of calcium and decreased mobilization of calcium from bone, resulting in hypocalcemia. This stimulates increased synthesis and secretion of PTH and hyperplasia of the parathyroid glands. The increased circulating concentration of PTH tends to increase plasma levels of calcium to normal and to enhance renal phosphate clearance, which, in turn, produces hypophosphatemia. When the concentration of phosphorus in the extracellular fluid falls below a critical level, mineralization cannot proceed normally. In severe vitamin D deficiency, normal levels of serum calcium cannot be maintained, and the driving force for mineralization is further decreased. The absence of a metabolite of vitamin D such as 24,25$(OH)_2$D that acts directly on the skeleton also may play a role in the defective mineralization of rickets and osteomalacia.

Phosphate depletion alone can produce osteomalacia, as in patients consuming large amounts of nonabsorbable antacids and in persons with excessive renal loss of phosphate due to decreased tubular reabsorption. Secondary hyperparathyroidism is usually not present in these patients. Hypophosphatemia per se produces mineralization defects despite its effect of increasing the activity of the renal 25(OH)D-1α-hydroxylase, but it cannot account for the osteomalacia in all the disorders listed in Table 355-3. In chronic renal failure, for example, plasma phosphate levels are not decreased and usually are increased. Similarly, plasma phosphorus levels are not depressed in infants and children with osteomalacia secondary to hypophosphatasia, a hereditary deficiency in alkaline phosphatase. Osteomalacia in some patients with chronic renal failure is associated with accumulation of aluminum in bone, and the aluminum probably plays a role in production of the mineralization defect.

CLINICAL FINDINGS The clinical manifestations of rickets are the result of skeletal deformities, susceptibility to fractures, weakness and hypotonia, and disturbances in growth. In extreme instances of vitamin D–deficiency rickets, hypocalcemia causes tetany, which, when severe, may be accompanied by laryngeal spasm and seizures. In infants and young children, features include listlessness, irritability, and often profound hypotonia and muscular weakness. As the disorder progresses, children become unable to walk without support. Abnormal parietal flattening and frontal bossing develop in the skull. The calvariae are softened (craniotabes), and sutures may be widened. Prominence of the costochondral junctions is called the "rachitic rosary," and the indentation of the lower ribs at the site of attachment of the diaphragm is known as *Harrison's groove*. If untreated, deformities of the pelvis and extremities progress, with bowing being particularly common in the tibia, femur, radius, and ulna. Fractures are frequent, dental eruption is often delayed, and enamel defects are common.

The presentation of osteomalacia in adults is usually more insidious. The skeletal deformities may be overlooked, and the features of the underlying disorder may dominate, as, for example, in the vitamin D deficiency of adult celiac disease. Symptoms, when they occur, include diffuse skeletal pain and bony tenderness. Pain about the hips may result in an antalgic gait. Muscular weakness may be difficult to distinguish from hesitancy to move because of skeletal pain. Proximal weakness may mimic that of primary muscle disorders and contribute to the waddling gait. Pain and weakness may cause patients to be confined to bed and chair. Many factors, including secondary hyperparathyroidism, contribute to the myopathy. Clinical improvement in the myopathy usually results from specific therapy such as vitamin D repletion in nutritional osteomalacia, phosphate replacement in renal hypophosphatemia, or correction of acidosis. Fractures of the involved bones may occur with minimal trauma. When the ribs are involved, severe deformities may develop in the thoracic cage, and the collapse of vertebral bodies may produce loss of height.

RADIOLOGIC FEATURES In rickets, radiologic alterations are most evident at the epiphyseal growth plate, which is increased in thickness, cupped, and hazy at the metaphyseal border owing to decreased calcification of the hypertrophic zone and inadequate mineralization of the primary spongiosa. The trabecular pattern of the metaphyses is abnormal, the cortices of the diaphyses may be thinned, and the shafts may be bowed.

In osteomalacia, a decrease in bone density is usually associated with loss of trabeculae and thinning of the cortices. The radiologic changes may be indistinguishable from those in osteoporosis. Trabecular patterns may be blurred, producing a homogeneous ground glass appearance. The specific finding that suggests osteomalacia is the presence of radiolucent bands ranging from a few millimeters to several centimeters in length, usually oriented perpendicular to the surface of the bones. They are particularly common at the inner aspects of the femur, especially near the femoral neck, in the pelvis, in the outer edge of the scapula, in the upper fibula, and in the metatarsals (Figs. 355-3 and 355-4). These radiolucent bands, called *pseudofractures* or *Looser's zones*, occur most often at sites where major arteries cross the bones and are thought to be due to the mechanical stress of the pulsation of these vessels. On radionuclide bone scans, the pseudofractures appear as hot spots. Subperiosteal erosions along the diaphyseal cortices are sometimes seen in secondary hyperparathyroidism.

Increased rather than decreased density of bones may be observed in patients who have renal tubular disorders rather than vitamin D deficiency and may produce a striking thickening of the cortices and trabeculae of spongy bone. Despite the increase in bone mass per unit volume, the trabeculae are covered with thickened osteoid seams typical of osteomalacia. Similar findings may occur in patients with chronic renal failure. The reason for the hyperostosis is unknown; the bone is architecturally abnormal and is subject to fracture with minimal trauma.

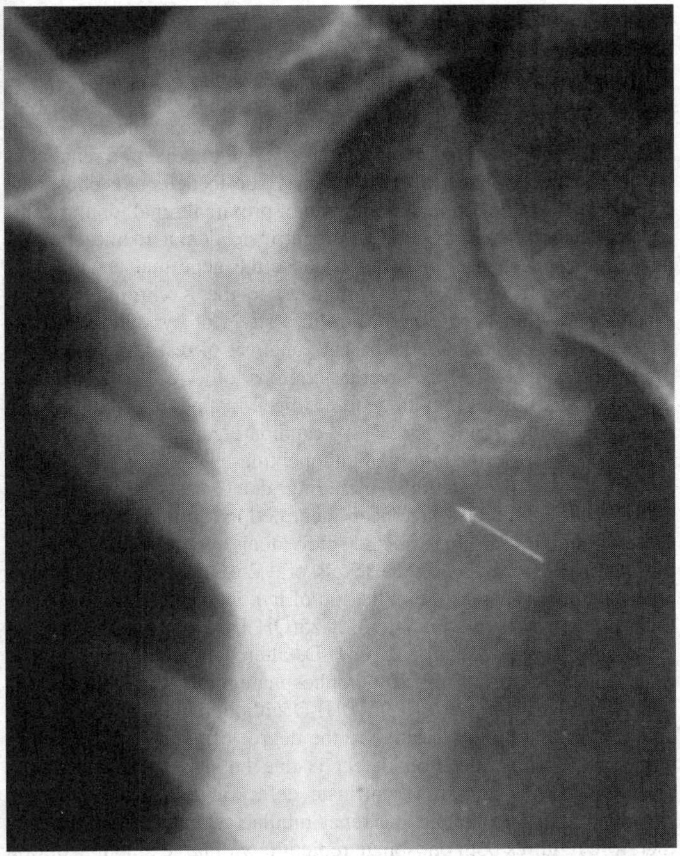

FIGURE 355-3 Radiographs of the scapula of a 58-year-old woman with phosphate diabetes. The presence of a pseudofracture or Looser's zone is indicated by the arrow.

LABORATORY FINDINGS Changes in serum concentrations of calcium, inorganic phosphorus, 25(OH)D, and 1,25$(OH)_2$D vary with the different disorders (see Chap. 353). In vitamin D deficiency, whether due to dietary lack, inadequate sunlight exposure, or intestinal malabsorption, serum calcium levels are normal or low, whereas phosphorus and 25(OH)D levels are consistently low, the latter usually <20 nmol/L (<8 ng/mL) depending on the assay used. In contrast, levels of 1,25$(OH)_2$D may be normal or elevated owing to secondary hyperparathyroidism. Eventually, when levels of 25(OH)D become so low that there is inadequate substrate for the renal 25(OH)D-1α-hydroxylase, then the serum level of 1,25$(OH)_2$D also declines. In adults, the lower limit of serum phosphorus concentration is around 0.9 mmol/L (2.8 mg/dL); in children, the lower limit of normal is closer to 1.3 to 1.5 mmol/L (4.0 to 4.5 mg/dL). In *severe* vitamin D depletion, hypocalcemia may be sufficient to produce tetany. Mild acidosis and generalized aminoaciduria result from secondary hyperparathyroidism. As a rule, patients with renal tubular disorders have normal serum calcium levels and hypophosphatemia. Other laboratory findings, such as glucosuria, aminoaciduria, acidosis, and hypouricemia, reflect variable degrees of disturbance of proximal tubular function or are features of the underlying disease (e.g., low plasma ceruloplasmin in Wilson's disease or abnormalities of immunoglobulins in multiple myeloma). In chronic renal failure, hyperphosphatemia and hypocalcemia are usually accompanied by normal 25(OH)D and low 1,25$(OH)_2$D levels. In nephrotic syndrome, serum 25(OH)D levels can be low owing primarily to urinary losses of protein-bound 25(OH)D. Serum phosphorus levels are also normal or elevated in hypophosphatasia. Increased urinary excretion of markers of bone resorption occurs when secondary hyperparathyroidism and excessive bone resorption are associated with the defect in mineralization. Alkaline phosphatase levels in plasma are usually elevated in rickets or osteomalacia, but typical and even severe osteomalacia, especially that due to renal tubular disorders, may be accompanied by normal levels or borderline elevations. Levels may increase during the early phases of therapy.

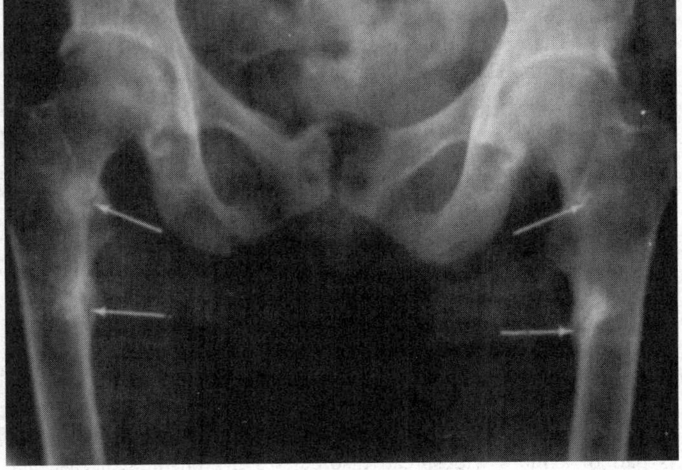

FIGURE 355-4 Radiograph of the femurs of a 47-year-old woman with Fanconi's syndrome of adult onset. The presence of multiple pseudofractures is indicated by the arrows.

DIETARY VITAMIN D DEFICIENCY AND INADEQUATE ENDOGENOUS SYNTHESIS Most foods unfortified with vitamin D contain too little of the vitamin to prevent rickets in growing children or osteomalacia in adults living in temperate-zone cities. As discussed in Chap. 353, in the absence of supplements, vitamin D must be formed endogenously through the ultraviolet irradiation of precursor 7-dehydrocholesterol in the skin. Many factors decrease the formation of vitamin D_3 from its precursor: increased melanin pigmentation, hyperkeratosis, sunscreens, limited exposure of the body, increase in the angle of sunlight, especially during the winter, and factors in the atmosphere, such as smog, which prevent adequate penetration of solar ultraviolet radiation. Since fortification of milk and routine use of vitamin D supplements for infants have been in effect, deficiency is unusual in the United States. Poor, dark-skinned infants living in crowded northern cities are most susceptible. Furthermore, elderly individuals with insufficient sun exposure, particularly those who are housebound or in nursing homes, drink no milk, and receive no vitamin D supplements, may have low serum levels of 25(OH)D, secondary hyperparathyroidism, and increased frequency of hip fractures. Intestinal absorption of vitamin D is normal in the elderly.

VITAMIN D LOSS AND INTESTINAL MALABSORPTION Osteomalacia may occur with intestinal malabsorption, as in adult celiac disease and regional enteritis. Prior to the discovery of gluten sensitivity in some of these cases, celiac disease was among the more common disorders underlying osteomalacia. Vitamin D absorption, which normally occurs via chylomicrons, is impaired in diseases that cause steatorrhea, such as chronic biliary obstruction. Patients with cholestatic liver disease or extrahepatic biliary obstruction may have low serum levels of 25(OH)D and osteomalacia owing not only to poor vitamin D absorption but also to decreased hepatic production of 25(OH)D. Osteomalacia is less frequent in chronic pancreatic insufficiency. Patients who have had gastric surgery for peptic ulcer disease or gastric bypass for obesity also may develop osteomalacia, possibly owing to malfunction of the proximal small bowel. Additional factors may contribute to the osteomalacia in patients with small-bowel disease, such as inadequate absorbing surface and failure of intestinal cells to respond to the active metabolites of vitamin D. Secondary hyperparathyroidism is usually present in patients with intestinal malabsorption and in those with a dietary lack of vitamin D and may be particularly severe in patients who develop osteomalacia following intestinal bypass surgery. Some patients who lack vitamin D, usually owing to intestinal malabsorption, have normal circulating levels of 1,25$(OH)_2$D despite low or undetectable levels of 25(OH)D.

In these individuals the normal levels of 1,25$(OH)_2$D may be accounted for by ingestion of sufficient vitamin D in hospital diets to produce substrate 25(OH)D for 1α-hydroxylation by the renal enzyme, the activity of which is increased owing to secondary hyperparathyroidism. In other patients circulating 1,25$(OH)_2$D levels may not reflect levels at critical target cells.

ABNORMAL METABOLISM OF VITAMIN D Serum 25(OH)D levels are reduced in some instances of parenchymal and obstructive liver disease, but these findings have not been correlated with quantitative histologic studies of bone. Patients consuming anticonvulsant drugs such as phenobarbital, phenytoin, or carbamazepine may develop rickets or osteomalacia. The problem is most severe in patients taking multiple anticonvulsant drugs and in those who are institutionalized, not ambulatory, or confined indoors. The major laboratory abnormality is a low or undetectable serum level of 25(OH)D. Treatment with vitamin D (1000 IU/d) will return the serum level of 25(OH)D to normal. As discussed in Chap. 353, the anticonvulsant drugs have multiple actions on calcium homeostasis.

Two autosomal recessive syndromes associated with rickets have been termed *vitamin D–dependent rickets* (see also Chap. 353). Features of *type I vitamin D–dependent rickets* include hypocalcemia, hypophosphatemia, short stature, skeletal deformities of rickets, dental enamel hypoplasia, frequently marked elevations of serum alkaline phosphatase activity, generalized aminoaciduria, and secondary hyperparathyroidism. Circulating levels of 1,25$(OH)_2$D are low or undetectable. Treatment with massive doses of vitamin D or small doses of calcitriol reverses the abnormal biochemical findings, induces healing of the rickets, and restores the rate of skeletal growth. The abnormalities are due to mutations that impair the renal 25(OH)D-lα-hydroxylase. By linkage analysis, the disorder has been mapped to chromosome 12q14. Lifelong replacement therapy with calcitriol is required. *Type II vitamin D–dependent rickets*, also termed *hereditary resistance to 1,25(OH)$_2$D*, has many clinical features of the type I syndrome. Rickets is usually of early onset but varies in severity in different kindreds. Distinguishing features include alopecia, which may develop during the first few months of life, and multiple milia and epidermal cysts. The type II disorder is due to mutations that impair the structure and function of the 1,25$(OH)_2$D receptor. Different molecular abnormalities in different kindreds include mutations that impair binding of the receptor to DNA, mutations that cause the formation of incomplete receptor molecules, and mutations that cause single amino acid substitutions in the protein. This disorder also maps by linkage analysis to chromosome 12 in a locus close to but distinct from that for type I vitamin D–dependent rickets.

Both osteomalacia and acquired abnormalities in vitamin D metabolism may develop in patients receiving long-term total parenteral nutrition. Some of these individuals have secondary hypoparathyroidism, but hypoparathyroidism cannot account for the osteomalacia. Serum levels of 25(OH)D are normal, although levels of 1,25$(OH)_2$D may be low. Aluminum has been detected in increased amounts in plasma, urine, and bone and may play a role in the genesis of the osteomalacia similar to its postulated role in patients with renal failure on chronic hemodialysis.

RENAL TUBULAR DISORDERS Rickets and osteomalacia occur in association with a variety of disorders of proximal renal tubular function. These disorders have in common increased renal clearance of inorganic phosphorus and hypophosphatemia with a normal or near-normal glomerular filtration rate. Increased phosphate clearance with resultant hypophosphatemia is usually an isolated defect accompanied by no other abnormalities except for increased urinary glycine excretion (hyperglycinuria). X-linked hypophosphatemia (also called *phosphate diabetes* or *vitamin D–resistant rickets*) is an X-linked dominant disorder characterized by rickets in an otherwise well-nourished, healthy-appearing child. When the child begins to walk and bear weight, lower limb deformities appear and become progressively worse. The rate of linear growth is at first normal and then slowed. Many of these individuals develop a unique disorder of tendons, ligaments, and joint capsules characterized by calcification or, more probably, ossification of insertions of tendons and ligaments and joint capsules (enthesopathy). In some patients, spontaneous remissions may be followed by recurrences in adult life, for example, with pregnancy and lactation. Hypophosphatemia is due to defective renal conservation of phosphate, which in turn is due to defective phosphate transport across the luminal membrane of proximal renal tubular cells, but the defect cannot be due to an intrinsic defect in the sodium-dependent phosphate transporter because the gene that encodes this protein maps to chromosome 5 and not to the X chromosome. (A model of the human disease occurs in a strain of hypophosphatemic mice designated Hyp). On the basis of analysis of restriction fragment polymorphism studies in several kindreds of X-linked hypophosphatemia, the mutant human gene has been mapped to the short arm of the X chromosome (Xp22.1). A candidate gene, called *PEX*, that exhibits homology to a family of endopeptidase genes has been identified, and several mutations, including deletions, frameshifts, and splice-junction defects, have been identified in kindreds with vitamin D–resistant rickets. In affected individuals, the serum levels of 25(OH)D are normal, and the levels of 1,25$(OH)_2$D are in the low-normal range. Whereas the induction of hypophosphatemia in normal individuals results in stimulation of 25(OH)D-lα-hydroxylase and an increase in the levels of 1,25$(OH)_2$D, altered renal tubular cellular phosphate fluxes in X-linked hypophosphatemia fail to stimulate the hydroxylase. Thus levels of 1,25$(OH)_2$D, although in the normal range, are inappropriately low relative to the degree of phosphate depletion. The skeletal mineralization defect is due both to the low ambient phosphate levels and to an intrinsic defect in osteoblast function, possibly related to that in the renal tubular cells. Effective therapy therefore requires both phosphate repletion with large amounts of oral phosphate and treatment with calcitriol (see below). Such combined therapy reverses the osteomalacia of trabecular bone surfaces, corrects the microscopic periosteocytic mineralization defects, and results in improvement in longitudinal growth. The patients who are shortest at the inception of therapy tend to have the poorest growth response to therapy. After the rickets is healed, defects in phosphate clearance and hypophosphatemia persist, and medical therapy is still required. The effects of excessive calcitriol administration, such as nephrocalcinosis and nephrolithiasis, must be avoided. Adults with X-linked hypophosphatemia frequently have pseudofractures; osteoarthritis in the sacroiliac joints, wrists, knees, hips, and feet; and marked enthesopathy. Another variant of hereditary rickets has been termed *hereditary hypophosphatemic rickets with hypercalciuria*. Muscular weakness, not a feature of X-linked hypophosphatemia, may be present. These individuals, whose disorder is probably inherited as an autosomal recessive trait, have normocalcemia, hypophosphatemia, and striking absorptive hypercalciuria; the latter disappears after fasting and returns after oral calcium loading. Levels of 1,25$(OH)_2$D in serum are elevated, in contrast to the low-normal levels found in X-linked hypophosphatemia. These elevations of serum 1,25$(OH)_2$D are an appropriate response of the 25(OH)D-lα-hydroxylase to phosphate depletion. Phosphate replacement induces healing of the rachitic lesions.

Sporadic cases of hypophosphatemia also have been described in adults in whom family histories are negative and proximal muscle weakness is a prominent feature (see also Chap. 356). These patients also are best treated with a combination of calcitriol and inorganic phosphorus. As mentioned above, secondary hyperparathyroidism is not present in most untreated patients with renal tubular disorders associated with rickets and osteomalacia.

In other patients the disorder in tubular function may be more widespread, involving (besides phosphorus) glucose, potassium, amino acids, and uric acid; the various combinations are termed the *de Toni-Debré-Fanconi syndrome*. The more complete renal tubular defects may occur sporadically or in families. In some instances, the lesion is part of a more widespread disorder, as in Wilson's disease and cystinosis. Fanconi's syndrome also may be a feature of plasma cell myeloma, where it is attributed to toxic effects of deposited Bence Jones protein. Similarly, osteomalacia and renal tubular acidosis have been observed in Sjögren's syndrome with increased urinary excretion of beta$_2$-microglobulin and retinol-binding protein. The acidosis of proximal tubular defects also plays a role in the development of osteomalacia, possibly by altering the metabolism of vitamin D or the renal handling of calcium and phosphorus. In this regard, osteomalacia has accompanied the hyperchloremic acidosis or ureterocolic anastomosis.

TUMOR-ASSOCIATED (ONCOGENOUS) OSTEOMALACIA Osteomalacia and hypophosphatemia with high renal phosphate clearance occur with a variety of mesenchymal tumors, including giant cell tumors (benign or malignant), reparative granulomas, hemangiomas, fibromas, and other mesenchymal neoplasms. A similar syndrome occurs in patients with prostatic carcinoma. In some instances, removal of the tumor resulted in return of renal phosphorus clearance to normal, a rise in serum phosphorus levels, and healing of the osteomalacia (or rickets in children). Serum 1,25(OH)$_2$D levels are low or undetectable, although chronic administration of sufficient calcitriol to raise circulating levels of this metabolite to normal does not alter renal phosphorus clearance or serum phosphorus concentrations. Humoral factors released by these tumors may impair proximal tubular functions such as 1α-hydroxylation of 25(OH)D *and* act as inhibitors of phosphate transport.

CHRONIC RENAL FAILURE Osteomalacia is common in patients with chronic renal failure; it tends to be the predominant type of renal osteodystrophy in younger patients and is more frequent in those with the lower plasma levels of calcium and phosphorus. A component of secondary hyperparathyroidism and osteitis fibrosa is almost always present. The defect itself probably involves a decreased conversion of 25(OH)D to 1,25(OH)$_2$D either because of insufficient viable renal cortical tissue or the inhibitory effect of hyperphosphatemia on renal 25(OH)D-1α-hydroxylase activity. In addition, there may be a primary defect in intestinal calcium absorption. Part of the secondary hyperparathyroidism also may be due to decreased phosphate clearance and subsequent hyperphosphatemia. Under circumstances of hyperphosphatemia and a near-normal plasma concentration of calcium, the presence of inhibitors probably causes the defective mineralization. In some patients, the osteomalacia responds to large doses of vitamin D or dihydrotachysterol or to small doses of calcitriol or calcifediol. In some patients, however, renal osteodystrophy does not respond to pharmacologic doses of vitamin D or to calcitriol. In others, accumulation of aluminum in the bone accounts for the vitamin D–refractory osteomalacia. Aluminum deposits can be identified at the mineralization fronts, and bone apposition rates are low. These individuals have high levels of aluminum and uncoupling of matrix deposition and mineralization. Individuals with lower amounts of aluminum develop a form of "aplastic" bone disease in which matrix deposition and mineralization are more closely coupled. Deferoxamine can mobilize aluminum from bone and other tissues and is effective therapy. In some patients with renal osteodystrophy, the total bone mass may be increased (osteosclerosis), resulting in increased density of bone. This is particularly evident in the spine, where a characteristic appearance is that of dense bone at the superior and inferior margins of the vertebral bodies with more radiolucent central portions ("rugger jersey sign"). Histologically, although there is more bone per unit area, each trabecula is covered by a wide osteoid seam.

HYPOPHOSPHATASIA Rickets is a feature of a deficiency of alkaline phosphatase in infants and children termed *hypophosphatasia*. There are four forms of hypophosphatasia: lethal perinatal, infantile, childhood, and adult. Rickets occurs in the infantile and childhood forms. In adults, the disorder may not be recognized until middle age, but there is frequently a history of early loss of deciduous or permanent teeth. Osteomalacia and calcium pyrophosphate deposition disease occur in the adult form. The severe perinatal and infantile forms are inherited as autosomal recessive traits; the pattern of inheritance in the other forms is uncertain. The low levels of circulating alkaline phosphatase activity are explained by a deficiency of the tissue-nonspecific enzyme (bone-liver-kidney). Missense mutations have been demonstrated in the alkaline phosphatase gene.

Although alkaline phosphatase is abundant in osteoclasts, its function in mineralization is not established. In hypophosphatasia, there is increased urinary excretion of phosphoethanolamine and increased circulating levels of pyridoxal-5′-phosphate. The metabolic origin of the phosphoethanolamine is not established. Concentrations of pyridoxal-5′-phosphate are not elevated intracellularly, and the extracellular increases are consistent with the function of alkaline phosphatase as an ectoenzyme; whether alterations of pyridoxal-5′-phosphate metabolism contribute to the clinical abnormalities is not known. Inorganic pyrophosphate (PPi) is a substrate for alkaline phosphatase, which accounts for increased levels of PPi in urine and plasma and for the increased incidence of calcium pyrophosphate deposition disease in hypophosphatasia. Since PPi also can function to inhibit growth of the calcium-phosphate mineral phase, excessive concentrations of PPi may cause the rickets and osteomalacia. There is no effective therapy.

OTHER DISORDERS ASSOCIATED WITH DEFECTIVE MINERALIZATION Disturbances in mineralization may be seen in patients consuming high doses of fluoride ion and in patients with Paget's disease treated with etidronate. Some decrease in mineralization of newly forming matrix, increase in surface covered by osteoid, and increase in the width of the osteoid seams may occur in conditions that are not usually considered as osteomalacia except by these criteria. Examples include patients with the osteitis fibrosa of hyperparathyroidism following surgical cure. In these circumstances, there is a temporary imbalance between the rate at which mineral is supplied to bone and the rate at which bone matrix is formed. Biopsies in some of these conditions show a normal calcification front. Wide osteoid seams and hypophosphatemia are also seen in children with osteopetrosis, in whom there is inadequate resorption of bone and calcified cartilage but active bone formation.

A condition that resembles osteomalacia and is associated with a coarsened, mottled bony trabecular pattern, pseudofractures, and bone pain but normal plasma levels of calcium and phosphorus is *fibrogenesis imperfecta ossium*. The bone has a distinctive histologic appearance, with wide osteoid seams, distortion of the birefringent pattern of normal bone, and abnormal collagen fibers by electron microscopy. The nature of the abnormality is not known.

℞ TREATMENT

In rickets and osteomalacia due to dietary absence of vitamin D or inadequate exposure to sunlight, vitamin D$_2$ (ergocalciferol) or vitamin D$_3$ (cholecalciferol) is given orally in doses of 800 to 4000 IU (0.02 to 0.1 mg) daily for 6 to 12 weeks, followed by daily supplements of 200 to 400 IU, which are adequate to prevent the development of the disorder in otherwise normal persons. In elderly persons with vitamin D deficiency, the administration of vitamin D, 50,000 IU by mouth once each week for 8 weeks, raises the serum levels of 25(OH)D into the mid-normal range. In infants and children, such treatment causes improvement in muscle tone and strength, an increase in serum calcium and phosphorus levels, and a decrease in alkaline phosphatase levels after several weeks. Radiologic evidence of healing appears within weeks, and healing may be complete by a few months. Calcium supplements and larger initial doses of vitamin D may be necessary in infants and children with tetany. In adults with nutritional osteomalacia, healing of pseudofractures may be evident within 3 to 4 weeks after therapy with as little as 2000 IU (0.5 mg) vitamin D daily. Healing is complete usually by 6 months.

Patients with osteomalacia due to intestinal malabsorption do not respond to small doses of vitamin D. In the presence of active steatorrhea, daily oral doses of vitamin D of 50,000 to 100,000 IU (1.25 to 2.5 mg) and large doses of calcium (e.g., 15 g calcium lactate or 4 g calcium carbonate orally per day) may be required. In some instances, oral vitamin D is ineffective, and the parenteral route is required (e.g., 10,000 IU/d intramuscularly). Another approach is the use of artificial ultraviolet B radiation or exposure to sunlight in addition to supplemental calcium. Small doses of calcitriol (0.5 to 1.0 μg daily) are also usually effective in this form of osteomalacia. Inorganic phosphate therapy is not indicated either in deficiency or in intestinal malabsorption of the vitamin, since hypocalcemia will develop and intestinal calcium absorption will remain inadequate. In all patients in whom large doses of vitamin D are used, serum calcium and 25(OH)D levels should be monitored periodically. Semiquantitative urinary calcium measurements are inadequate.

In patients treated with multiple anticonvulsant agents, it is usually necessary to continue the drugs while adding 1000 IU/d of vitamin D and to monitor levels of serum calcium and serum 25(OH)D until a therapeutic response (evidence of radiologic healing, improvement in symptoms) is obtained.

Treatment of rickets and osteomalacia in the presence of renal tubular disorders is more difficult. In the past, the X-linked form of hypophosphatemic osteomalacia was treated with large doses of vitamin D (from 50,000 to several hundred thousand IU per day), but skeletal responses were rarely complete. Currently, oral supplements of inorganic phosphate in divided doses of phosphorus, 1.0 to 3.6 g/d (50 mg/kg body weight per day for children), and calcitriol, 0.5 to 2.0 μg/d (30 ng/kg body weight per day for children), constitute the best regimen to restore skeletal growth and heal the bone disease. In some adults, therapy with inorganic phosphate alone abolishes muscle weakness and bone pain and produces radiologic and histologic healing. The addition of calcitriol improves calcium balance and helps decrease secondary hyperparathyroidism and maintain a sufficient level of serum phosphorus to permit complete healing. In some patients there may be a temporary increase in bone pain and rise in serum alkaline phosphatase during the early phases of treatment. In the osteomalacia associated with the chronic acidosis of renal tubular disorders, the use of alkali may be of value in supplementing therapy with phosphate and calcitriol. In patients with ureterosigmoidostomy, oral sodium bicarbonate can reverse acidosis, improve the serum phosphate level, and heal the bone disease; with maintenance doses of alkali, recurrence of symptoms can be prevented.

Patients with nephrotic syndrome and low serum 25(OH)D levels benefit from modest vitamin D supplementation (800 to 1000 IU/d). Small doses of calcitriol are equally effective in treating hypocalcemia and osteodystrophy resulting from chronic renal failure. The recommended initial dose of calcitriol is 0.25 μg/d. If after 2 to 4 weeks on this dose the biochemical parameters are unaltered, the dose is increased by 0.25 μg/d every 2 to 4 weeks until a satisfactory clinical biochemical response (including elevation of serum calcium levels and decrease in PTH levels) is obtained. The usual dose is 0.5 to 1.0 μg/d. Calcitriol also may be administered intravenously (1.0 to 2.5 μg three times weekly) in patients on dialysis, particularly to treat refractory osteitis fibrosa. Because there are no regulatory mechanisms to control the biologic responses to calcitriol, there is a high incidence of transient hypercalciuria and hypercalcemia, especially initially. Thus, serum calcium levels should be monitored frequently during the first 1 to 2 months of therapy and less frequently once a stable dose has been established. Some patients treated with calcitriol have an apparent increase in serum creatinine levels and a decrease in creatinine clearance; these changes are due to altered metabolism of creatinine rather than a decrease in renal function. Since calcitriol has a short duration of action and is not stored in fat depots, hypercalcemia usually resolves in 2 to 7 days after the dose is discontinued or decreased. Phosphate supplements are, of course, contraindicated in the usual patient with chronic renal failure. Occasionally, however, hypophosphatemia may result from the excessive use of nonabsorbable antacids or from excessive removal of phosphate through hemodialysis.

In patients who have had rickets in childhood, the abnormal mechanical stress of severe deformities may contribute to the development of degenerative joint disease, particularly in the hips and knees. Osteotomies at the proper time after healing may prevent this complication and the requirement for more extensive arthroplasties later in life.

See Chap. 61, Agents affecting calcification and bone turnover, in Goodman & Gilman's The Pharmacological Basis of Therapeutics, *9th ed, New York, McGraw-Hill, 1996.*

BIBLIOGRAPHY

OSTEOPOROSIS

ALOIA JF et al: Calcium supplementation with and without hormone replacement therapy to prevent postmenopausal bone loss. Ann Intern Med 120:97, 1994

AVIOLI LV, KRANE SM(*eds*)*: Metabolic Bone Disease and Clinically Related Disorders*. Philadelphia, Saunders, 1990

BACHRACH LK et al: Osteopenia in adults with cystic fibrosis. Am J Med 96:27, 1994

CALVO MS et al: Molecular basis and clinical application of biological markers of bone turnover. Endocr Rev 17:333, 1996

CANALIS E: Insulin-like growth factors and their role in osteoporosis. Calcif Tissue Int 58:133, 1996

CHAPUY MC et al: Vitamin D_3 and calcium to prevent hip fractures in elderly women. N Engl J Med 327:1637, 1992

COLLINS JA: Hormone replacement therapy and breast cancer: What is happening? J Surg Obstet Gynecol Can 17:837, 1995

COSMAN F et al: Estrogen protection against bone resorbing effects of parathyroid hormone infusion. Ann Intern Med 118:337, 1993

CUMMINGS SR et al: Risk factors for hip fracture in white women. N Engl J Med 332:767, 1995

DE GROEN PC et al: Esophagitis associated with the use of alendronate. N Engl J Med 335:1016, 1996

DEMPSTER DW, LINDSAY R: Pathogenesis of osteoporosis. Lancet 341:797, 1993

EISMAN JA: Vitamin D receptor gene alleles and osteoporosis: An affirmative view. Editorial. J Bond Miner Res 10:1289, 1995

EPSTEIN FH: Mechanisms of disease. N Engl J Med 332:305, 1995

FINKELSTEIN JS et al: Parathyroid hormone for the prevention of bone loss induced by estrogen deficiency. N Engl J Med 331:1618, 1994

GREENSPAN SL et al: Fall severity and bone mineral density as risk factors for hip fracture in ambulatory elderly. JAMA 271:128, 1994

GREY AB et al: The effect of the antiestrogen tamoxifen on bone mineral density in normal late postmenopausal women. Am J Med 99:636, 1995

HEANEY RP: Fluoride and osteoporosis. Ann Intern Med 120:689, 1994

HOPPER JL et al: The bone density of female twins discordant for tobacco use. N Engl J Med 330:387, 1994

KRALL EA et al: Walking is related to bone density and rates of bone loss. Am J Med 96:20, 1994

LANDMAN JO et al: Skeletal metabolism in patients with osteoporosis after discontinuation of long term treatment with oral pamidronate. J Clin Endocrinol Metab 80:3465, 1995

LEE AH et al: Osteoporosis and bone morbidity in cardiac transplant recipients. Am J Med 96:35, 1994

LIBERMAN UA et al: Effect of oral alendronate on bone mineral density and the incidence of fractures in postmenopausal osteoporosis. N Engl J Med 333:1437, 1995

LINDSAY R: Prevention and treatment of osteoporosis. Lancet 341:801, 1993

MARCUS R et al: (eds): *Osteoporosis*. San Diego, Academic Press, 1996

NABULSI AA et al: Association of hormone-replacement therapy with various cardiovascular risk factors in postmenopausal women. N Engl J Med 328:1069, 1993

PAK CYC et al: Treatment of postmenopausal osteoporosis with slow-release sodium fluoride. Final report of a randomized controlled trial. Ann Intern Med 123:401, 1995

PEACOCK M: Vitamin D receptor gene alleles and osteoporosis: A contrasting view. Editorial. J Bone Miner Res 10:1294, 1995

REID IR et al: Effect of calcium supplementation of bone loss in postmenopausal women. N Engl J Med 328:460, 1993

RIGOTTI NA et al: The clinical course of osteoporosis in anorexia nervosa. A longitudinal study of cortical bone mass. JAMA 265:1133, 1991

RIGGS BL, MELTON LJ III: The prevention and treatment of osteoporosis. N Engl J Med 327:620, 1992

ROSEN HN et al: Specificity of urinary excretion of cross-linked N-telopeptides of type I collagen as a marker of bone turnover. Calcif Tissue Int 54:26, 1994

RYAN PJ et al: Osteoporosis and chronic back pain: A study with single-photon emission computed tomography bone scintigraphy. J Bone Miner Res 7:1455, 1992

SAMBROOK P et al: Prevention of corticosteroid osteoporosis: A comparison of calcium, calcitriol, and calcitonin. N Engl J Med 328:1747, 1993

SMITH EP et al: Estrogen resistance caused by a mutation in the estrogen-receptor gene in a man. N Engl J Med 331:1056, 1994

STEPAN JJ et al: Castrated men exhibit bone loss: Effect of calcitonin treatment on biochemical indices of bone remodeling. J Clin Endocrinol Metab 69:523, 1989

STEWART AF: PTHrP(1-36) as a skeletal anabolic agent for the treatment of osteoporosis. Bone 19:303, 1996

TILYARD MW et al: Treatment of postmenopausal osteoporosis with calcitriol or calcium. N Engl J Med 326:357, 1992

YAMAMOTO N et al: Bone mineral density and bone histomorphometric assessments of postpregnancy osteoporosis: A report of five patients. Calcif Tissue Int 54:20, 1994

OSTEOMALACIA

BONKOVSKY HL et al: Prevalence and prediction of osteopenia in chronic liver disease. Hepatology 12:273, 1990

CHINES A, PACIFICI R: Antacid and sucralfate-induced hypophosphatemic osteomalacia: A case report and review of the literature. Calcif Tissue Int 47:291, 1990

COLLINS N et al: A prospective study to evaluate the dose of vitamin D required to correct low 25-hydroxyvitamin D levels, calcium, and alkaline phosphatase in patients at risk of developing antiepileptic drug-induced osteomalacia. Q J Med 78:113, 1991

DAWSON-HUGHES B et al: Effect of vitamin D supplementation on wintertime and overall bone loss in healthy postmenopausal women. Ann Intern Med 115:505, 1991

FEDDE KN et al: Aberrant properties of alkaline phosphatase in patient fibroblasts correlate with clinical expressivity in severe forms of hypophosphatasia. J Clin Endocrinol Metab 81:2587, 1996

FRIEDMAN NE et al: Effects of calcitriol and phosphorus therapy on the growth of patients with X-linked hypophosphatemia. J Clin Endocrinol Metab 76:839, 1993

GALLAGHER JC: Vitamin D metabolism and therapy in elderly subjects. South Med J 85:2S43, 1992

GLORIEUX FH: Rickets, the continuing challenge. N Engl J Med 325:1875, 1991

HENDERSON JB et al: Blunted seasonal variation in serum 25-hydroxy vitamin D and increased risk of osteomalacia in vegetarian London Asians. Eur J Clin Nutr 46:509, 1992

HENTHORN PS et al: Different missense mutations at the tissue-nonspecific alkaline phosphatase gene locus in autosomal recessively inherited forms of mild and severe hypophosphatasia. Proc Natl Acad Sci USA 89:9924, 1992

HRUSKA KA et al: X-linked hypophosphatemic rickets and the murine Hyp homologue. Editorial. Am J Physiol 268:F357, 1995

HUTCHISON FN, BELL NH: Osteomalacia and rickets. Semin Nephrol 12:127, 1992

KLEIN GL, COLVURN JW: Bone disease in burn patients. J Bone Miner Res 8:337, 1993

KONISHI K et al: Hypophosphatemic osteomalacia in von Recklinghausen neurofibromatosis. Am J Med Sci 301:322, 1991

KUMAR R et al: Inhibitors of renal epithelial phosphate transport in tumor-induced osteomalacia and uremia. Proc Assoc Am Physicians 107:296, 1995

LABUDA M et al: Two hereditary defects related to vitamin D metabolism map to the same region of human chromosome 12q13–14. J Bone Miner Res 7:1447, 1992

LEICHT E et al: Tumor-induced osteomalacia: Pre- and postoperative biochemical findings. Horm Metab Res 22:640, 1990

MONTE NESTO JT et al: Osteomalacia secondary to renal tubular acidosis in a patient with primary Sjögren's syndrome. Clin Exp Rheumatol 9:625, 1991

NIJHAWAN R et al: Antiepileptic drugs, hepatic enzyme induction and raised serum alkaline phosphatase isoenzymes. Int J Clin Pharmacol Res 10:319, 1990

PETERSON DJ et al: X-linked hypophosphatemic rickets: A study (with literature review) of linear growth response to calcitrol and phosphate therapy. J Bone Miner Res 7:583, 1992

SCRIVER CR et al: X-linked hypophosphatemia: An appreciation of a classic paper and a survey of progress since 1958. Medicine 70:218, 1991

STONE MD et al: A neuroendocrine cause of oncogenic osteomalacia. J Pathol 167:181, 1992

SULLIVAN W et al: A prospective trial of phosphate and 1,25-dihydroxyvitamin D_3 therapy in symptomatic adults with x-linked hypophosphatemic rickets. J Clin Endocrinol Metab 75:879, 1992

THE HYP CONSORTIUM: A gene (*PEX*) with homologies to endopeptidases is mutated in patients with X-linked hypophosphatemic rickets. Nature Genet 11:130, 1995

VILLAREAL DT et al: Subclinical vitamin D deficiency in postmenopausal women with low vertebral bone mass. J Clin Endocrinol Metab 72:6281, 1991

WEIDNER N: Review and update: Oncogenic osteomalacia-rickets. Ultrastruct Pathol 15:317, 1991

WHYTE MP: Hypophosphatasia, in *The Molecular and Metabolic Bases of Inherited Disease*, 7th ed, CR Scriver et al (eds). New York, McGraw-Hill, 1995, p 4113

356

James P. Knochel

DISORDERS OF PHOSPHORUS METABOLISM

Phosphorus is the most abundant intracellular anion and is critical for membrane structure, transport, and energy storage. The role of phosphate ions in tissues explains the systemic nature of cellular injury consequent to phosphorus deficiency.

At a plasma pH of 7.4, inorganic phosphate in plasma is a 4:1 mixture of HPO_4^{2-} and $H_2PO_4^{2-}$. The sum of the products of the valences of these ions $(4 \times 2^- + 1 \times 1^-)$ divided by the sum of the ions $(4 + 1)$ is equal to 9/5, or an average valence of 1.8. Of the average 700 g of phosphorus in the body, 85 percent is in the skeleton, about 15 percent is in soft tissues, and 0.1 percent is in extracellular fluid. The phosphorus in extracellular fluid is in a freely diffusible form that (1) permits excretion of hydrogen ions as phosphate buffer into the urine and (2) is in diffusion equilibrium with cytosolic inorganic phosphate in cells.

A normal adult consumes approximately 1 g phosphorus each day. Soluble phosphates in dairy products and meat are almost completely absorbed, predominantly in the midjejunum. Insoluble phosphates, in vegetables and seeds, are absorbable provided the phosphate can be digested from its ligand. For example, phosphorus in corn and oats is partly in the form of phytic acid; these foods contain little phytase, which splits phytic acid (inositol hexaphosphate) into phosphate and inositol, and hence phosphorus from this source may be poorly absorbed. Thus corn and oats may be rachitogenic in children if they are the major components of the diet. Addition of rye bran, which contains phytase, to the diet increases the bioavailability of phosphorus from these sources.

Phosphorus absorption is under the influence of vitamin D, and phosphorus excretion is under the control of parathyroid hormone (PTH). PTH decreases tubular phosphate reabsorption and increases excretion into the urine. The effect of vitamin D on phosphate reabsorption by the kidney is relatively minor. The quantity of soluble phosphorus available for absorption from the diet varies, and excretion of phosphorus in the urine on a given day depends directly on absorption. Accordingly, the range for phosphorus excretion in health is very broad.

HYPOPHOSPHATEMIA

CAUSES Hypophosphatemia has many causes (Table 356-1). The finding of hypophosphatemia is not always a reliable indicator of deficiency, since a total-body deficit of phosphorus may exist in the face of hyperphosphatemia, such as, for example, in diabetic ketoacidosis.

Hypophosphatemia can be moderate or severe. Decreased dietary intake is an unusual cause of hypophosphatemia because of the ubiquitous and abundant distribution of the mineral in foods. Decreased absorption of phosphorus from the small intestine occurs in a variety of malabsorptive states, but simple diarrhea is usually not a cause. One of the most common causes of hypophosphatemia is respiratory alkalosis. Indeed, discovery of hypophosphatemia should lead to a search for potentially serious causes of hyperventilation such as sepsis or otherwise unsuspected alcohol withdrawal. Reduction of intracellular PCO_2 and elevation of pH increase the activity of phosphofructokinase, the rate-limiting enzyme of glycolysis. Phosphorylation of glucose intermediates causes cellular uptake of phosphorus and hypophosphatemia. Administration of insulin and consumption of nutrients that stimulate insulin release are also common causes of hypophosphatemia. Insulin stimulates phosphorus uptake by cells. Cellular phosphorus uptake also occurs in patients recovering from hypothermia as a result of reactivation of metabolism. Certain rapidly growing

Table 356-1

Causes of Hypophosphatemia

I. Decreased dietary intake
II. Decreased intestinal absorption
  A. Vitamin D deficiency
  B. Malabsorption
  C. Steatorrhea
  D. Secretory diarrhea
  E. Vomiting
  F. PO_4-binding antacids
III. Shifts from extracellular fluid into cells
  A. Respiratory alkalosis
    1. Sepsis
    2. Alcohol withdrawal
    3. Heat stroke
    4. Neuroleptic malignant syndrome
    5. Hepatic coma
    6. Salicylate poisoning
    7. Gout
    8. Panic attacks
    9. Psychiatric depression
  B. Hormone effects
    1. Insulin
    2. Glucagon
    3. Epinephrine
    4. Androgens
    5. Glucocorticoids
    6. Oral contraceptives
  C. Nutritional effects
    1. Glucose
    2. Fructose
    3. Glycerol
    4. Lactate
    5. Amino acids
    6. Xylitol
  D. Cellular uptake syndromes
    1. Recovery from hypothermia
    2. Burkitt's lymphoma
    3. Histiocytic lymphoma
    4. Acute myelomonocytic leukemia
    5. Acute myelogenous leukemia
    6. Treatment of pernicious anemia
    7. "Hungry bone" syndrome
      a. Following parathyroidectomy
      b. Acute leukemia
IV. Increased excretion into the urine
  A. Hyperparathyroidism
  B. Renal tubular defects
    1. Renal rickets
      a. Fanconi syndrome
      b. Familial hypophosphatemia
    2. Polyostotic fibrous dysplasia
    3. Metaphyseal chondrodysplasia
    4. After kidney transplantation
    5. Oncogenic osteomalacia
    6. Recovery from hemolytic uremic syndrome
  C. Aldosteronism
  D. Licorice ingestion
  E. Volume expansion
  F. Inappropriate secretion of vasopressin
  G. Mineralocorticoid administration
  H. Glucocorticoid administration
  I. Diuretic therapy

malignancies may take up enough phosphate to cause hypophosphatemia. Deposition of bone mineral following parathyroidectomy also may be a cause (the "hungry bone syndrome"). Certain tumors secrete a substance that not only reduces renal tubular reabsorption of phosphorus but also reduces production of 1,25-dihydroxy vitamin D [$1{,}25(OH)_2D$] by the kidney, resulting in a condition called *oncogenic osteomalacia*. Reduction of vitamin D synthesis is paradoxical since hypophosphatemia usually increases D production. Benign, often small, mesenchymal tumors have usually been responsible. Fibrosarcomas, prostatic cancers, and possibly small cell cancers of the lung have been reported as additional causes. Removal of the tumor may be curative. Hypocalcemia consequent to saline infusion causes release of PTH. Thus volume expansion and PTH both reduce tubular reabsorption of phosphorus. A number of other conditions associated with chronic volume expansion may cause hypophosphatemia.

Severe hypophosphatemia is defined as phosphorus levels in serum below 0.3 mmol/L (1.0 mg/dL). Many of the conditions that result in such low levels are associated with prolonged hyperventilation with respiratory alkalosis or reflect rapid cellular uptake (Table 356-2). Respiratory alkalosis does not cause phosphorus deficiency but may reduce serum phosphorus values to 0.1 mmol/L (0.3 mg/dL) and urinary phosphorus excretion to virtually undetectable levels. Severe hypophosphatemia and severe total-body deficiency of phosphorus occur in patients with poor dietary intake who consume phosphate-binding antacids. Similarly, treatment of diabetic ketoacidosis results in hypophosphatemia. Reduction of serum phosphorus below 0.3 mmol/L (1.0 mg/dL) suggests, but does not prove, the existence of serious phosphorus depletion. In chronic alcoholics, reduction of phosphorus content of skeletal muscle may occur because of the toxic effects of alcohol per se or because of a renal phosphate leak. In the case of ethanol, it is possible that negatively charged acetate ions, produced in the metabolism of ethanol, may enter the muscle cell and displace negatively charged phosphate ions from the cell. This, in conjunction with reduced capacity to reabsorb phosphate in the renal tubule, could well result in net phosphorus loss into the urine. The resulting phosphorus deficiency may cause a reduction of muscle magnesium and potassium and accumulations of calcium, sodium, chloride, and water. These findings are not necessarily associated with elevations of creatine phosphokinase activity that would reflect acute muscle damage. However, during withdrawal from alcohol, phosphorus is often taken up rapidly into skeletal muscle or liver, resulting in severe hypophosphatemia, and in this instance hypophosphatemia may precipitate acute rhabdomyolysis.

Table 356-2

Causes of Severe Hypophosphatemia

Chronic alcoholism and alcohol withdrawal
Dietary deficiency
Ingestion of phosphate-binding antacids
Severe burns
Recovery from diabetic ketoacidosis
Hyperalimentation
Nutritional recovery syndrome
Respiratory alkalosis
Therapeutic hyperthermia
Neuroleptic malignant syndrome
Recovery from exhaustive exercise
Renal transplantation
Acute renal failure

Most patients with diabetic ketoacidosis are not severely depleted of phosphorus. Although, on the one hand, metabolic acidosis and insulin deficiency mobilize intracellular phosphate stores and lead to their excretion into the urine, most patients have not been sick long enough for severe phosphorus deficiency to occur. On the other hand, patients with hypophosphatemia and hypokalemia, in the presence of severe diabetic ketoacidosis, are likely severely depleted of phosphorus and potassium and require treatment. The history usually shows that this type of patient with diabetic ketoacidosis has been sick for many days, has not had significant vomiting, has maintained a good intake of fluids, and has excreted phosphorus briskly for a period of many days, thus establishing severe deficiency. Such patients probably represent no more than 5 percent of cases of diabetic ketoacidosis.

MANIFESTATIONS The manifestations of phosphorus deficiency are listed in Table 356-3; many of these can occur simultaneously.

Phosphate trapping is an acute disorder resulting from reduction of intracellular inorganic phosphate concentration. The most common cause is administration of intravenous fructose. Fructose is metabolized by only three tissues in the body—the liver, the small bowel epithelium, and the proximal tubule of the kidney. When glucose is taken up into liver cells and phosphorylated by hexokinase, the resulting glucose-6-phosphate inhibits hexokinase, producing a smoothly regulated uptake of glucose that does not deplete or trap stores of inorganic phosphate. When fructose is administered intravenously, it is taken up into liver cells, where it is converted to fructose-1-phosphate by the enzyme fructokinase. Fructose-1-phosphate does not inhibit fructokinase, thus permitting rapid uptake of fructose into liver cells and consumption or trapping of available stores of inorganic phosphate.

Table 356-3

Hypophosphatemic Syndromes

Phosphate trapping	Leukocyte dysfunction
Rhabdomyolysis	Skeletal demineralization
Cardiomyopathy	Metabolic acidosis
Respiratory insufficiency	Nervous system dysfunction
Erythrocyte dysfunction	

Reduced intracellular phosphate concentration activates AMP deaminase and nucleotidase. The consequent reduction of adenylate compounds is reflected by increased uric acid production and hyperuricemia. Acute reduction of ATP, which is bound to magnesium, is heralded by a modest rise of magnesium in serum. Acute liver cell damage may occur. Disturbances of renal function also may occur after intravenous fructose. Hepatic and renal metabolic disturbances that follow fructose administration are preventable by infusing inorganic phosphate. Whether oral fructose affects intestinal epithelium in a similar manner is not known.

Rhabdomyolysis predictably occurs in chronic alcoholics who become acutely hypophosphatemic during the course of alcohol withdrawal. Hypophosphatemic rhabdomyolysis also occurs rarely during treatment for diabetic ketoacidosis, during the course of hyperalimentation, or while refeeding patients with malnutrition. In normal individuals, in contrast, acute hypophosphatemia does not appear to damage skeletal muscle, and rhabdomyolysis only occurs if there is preexisting muscle damage. Virtually all severe, chronic alcoholics have a subclinical myopathy characterized by biochemical abnormalities and ultrastructural damage. In these patients, the incidence and severity of rhabdomyolyis appear to be reduced if hypophosphatemia is prevented during realimentation.

Cardiomyopathy occurs in severe phosphorus depletion. The manifestations include reduction in cardiac output, hypotension, impaired pressor responsiveness to catecholamines, and a reduced threshold to ventricular arrhythmias. Patients in septic shock treated with catecholamines showed a 22 percent elevation of left ventricular stroke work index and a 12 percent elevation of systolic blood pressure without change of filling pressure when their hypophosphatemia [serum phosphorus below 0.6 mmol/L (2.0 mg/dL)] was treated by infusing 20 mmol (0.62 g) of elemental phosphorus over 60 min.

Respiratory insufficiency occurs in malnourished patients receiving intravenous nutrients with inadequate phosphorus who become progressively hypophosphatemic over 8 or 10 days. Profound weakness causes failure of diaphragm function, hypoxia, and respiratory acidosis. Despite severe hypophosphatemia, these patients rarely develop rhabdomyolysis, presumably because they had no preexistent muscle damage. The initial clue may be an inability to extubate a patient from a ventilator at the anticipated time. This syndrome is seldom seen in chronic alcoholics because rhabdomyolysis in such patients may correct hypophosphatemia spontaneously. Rapid correction of chronic respiratory acidosis also may cause hypophosphatemia and diaphragm weakness. In these patients, administration of phosphorus rapidly corrects muscle weakness and respiratory insufficiency. Fifty percent of patients with chronic obstructive pulmonary disease show abnormally low phosphorus content in both intercostal and peripheral skeletal muscle. This can be explained by chronic respiratory acidosis and/or the combined effects of treatment with glucocorticoids, xanthine derivatives, and diuretics.

Erythrocyte dysfunction is due to a decrease in 2,3-bisphosphoglycerate (2,3-BPG) content. The red cell is the only tissue in the body that produces this substance. Both 2,3-BPG and ATP facilitate dissociation of oxyhemoglobin and promote oxygen delivery to tissue. Reduced 2,3-BPG and ATP both enhance affinity of oxygen for hemoglobin and reduce tissue oxygenation. This mechanism may explain central nervous system dysfunction in hypophosphatemia. Hemolysis due to phosphorus deficiency probably does not occur.

Leukocyte dysfunction due to phosphorus deficiency results in impaired phagocytosis and opsonization. As a result, chronic hypophosphatemia increases susceptibility to bacterial and fungal infections.

Skeletal demineralization is an important effect of phosphorus deficiency, especially in patients with poor dietary intake who simultaneously ingest phosphate-binding antacids. Under conditions of increased bone turnover, in normal children or in adults with Paget's disease, hyperparathyroidism, or bony metastases, demineralization may occur at such a rate as to cause hypercalcemia. Osteopenia, bone pain, and a syndrome resembling osteomalacia occur in chronic phosphorus deficiency.

Phosphorus deficiency normally causes increased production of $1,25(OH)_2D$ by the kidney, which serves to increase intestinal absorption of phosphorus. In phosphorus-deficient normal volunteers, the normal rise of plasma $1,25(OH)_2D$ levels is reduced by superimposed metabolic acidosis by about 50 percent. One-half of the reduction is explained by increased metabolism of $1,25(OH)_2D$ and the remaining one-half by decreased vitamin D synthesis.

Metabolic acidosis may occur in children or adults with phosphorus deficiency due to vitamin D deficiency. Reduced phosphorus intake results in mobilization of hydroxyapatite from bone that serves to maintain normal levels of serum phosphorus. Hypercalciuria occurs normally as a result of phosphorus deprivation, which is also explained by hydroxyapatite mobilization. Severe hypophosphatemia has three important metabolic effects on the kidney. First, as hypophosphatemia becomes severe, inorganic phosphate excretion into the urine falls so that hydrogen excretion as NaH_2PO_4 into the urine is eliminated. Second, based upon experimental evidence, there is a marked reduction of the Na^+/H^+ antiporter activity in the proximal tubule, which by reducing H^+ secretion into the tubular lumen, prevents reabsorption of filtered HCO_3^- ions. Third, phosphorus deficiency also decreases ammonia production. The reduction in ammonia production eliminates hydrogen excretion as ammonium ions (NH_4^+). Since excretion of hydrogen as phosphate buffer or ammonium accounts for nearly all the kidney's capacity to secrete acid, it is surprising that phosphorus deficiency is only rarely associated with metabolic acidosis. The explanation lies in the fact that mobilization of hydroxyapatite from bone provides carbonate ions, which, in turn, buffer the retained hydrogen ions that otherwise would be excreted in the urine. Under conditions in which hydroxyapatite cannot be mobilized during phosphorus deprivation (e.g., vitamin D deficiency, severe magnesium deficiency, perhaps aluminum poisoning, and experimentally by administration of colchicine), buffer cannot be mobilized adequately, and metabolic acidosis ensues.

Nervous system dysfunction is a distinctive and predictable feature of severe hypophosphatemia and phosphorus deficiency. This syndrome usually occurs in the setting of refeeding or hyperalimentation-induced hypophosphatemia that develops over the course of 8 to 10 days. Such patients become irritable and apprehensive and hyperventilate sufficiently to cause paresthesia and numbness. Profound muscular weakness is followed by dysarthria, confusion, obtundation, convulsive seizures, coma, and death. Alternatively, ascending motor paralysis with or without sensory disturbances may resemble the Guillain-Barré syndrome. In such cases, the cerebrospinal fluid is normal. Ophthalmoplegia, diplopia, and dysphagia suggest botulism, and poorly defined defects in color perception (metachromatopsia) suggests cerebral cortical dysfunction. In these patients, as in those with respiratory failure, spontaneous rhabdomyolysis does not occur despite severe hypophosphatemia.

Compared to normal persons of advanced age, patients with multi-infarct dementia or Alzheimer's type dementia show reduced concentrations of phosphorus and ionized calcium in cerebrospinal fluid. There is no known explanation for this observation.

℞ TREATMENT

Before initiating treatment for hypophosphatemia, the cause should be ascertained. Measurement of arterial pH and and blood gases of phosphorus concentration in the urine is helpful.

Milk is an excellent source of phosphorus, containing 33 mmol/L (100 mg/dL). Phosphate salts are also available for oral use. They are less likely to cause diarrhea in phosphorus-deficient patients than in a normal person. Phosphorus salts cannot be given by intramuscular or subcutaneous injection, but sodium phosphate and potassium phosphate are available for intravenous use. Intravenous sodium or potassium phosphate, 15 mmol (0.465 g of elemental phosphorus), given in 100 ml of 0.9% saline over 60 min elevated serum phosphorus from an average value of 0.6 to 1.2 mmol/L (1.75 to 3.8 mg/dL). The potassium salt should be given when hypokalemia and hypophosphatemia coexist. A safe dosage regimen for treatment of alcoholics who are hypophosphatemic, hypokalemic, and hypomagnesemic is the infusion each 8 to 12 h of 1 L of 0.5 normal NaCl in 5% glucose containing 9 mmol of potassium phosphate and 4.2 mmol $MgSO_4$ (2.0 mL of 50% $MgSO_4$ solution). Serum concentrations of potassium, magnesium, and phosphate should be monitored closely. Such infusions should be stopped when oral intake becomes possible.

PTH reduces renal tubular reabsorption of phosphorus by stimulating degradation of cyclic AMP to adenosine. Adenosine, in turn, inhibits Na^+/P_i transport. Dipyridamole inhibits adenosine uptake by the cell and reduces phosphaturia. Preliminary studies suggest that dipyridamole may be of use in treatment of PTH-mediated phosphaturia and familial hyperphosphaturic hypophosphatemia.

During treatment of hypophosphatemia, hyperphosphatemia should be avoided because it can cause severe hypocalcemia and crystal deposition in important structures, including blood vessels of the eye, lung, heart, and kidney. Fatal alveolar diffusion block has occurred, especially if the patient is alkalotic.

HYPERPHOSPHATEMIA

CAUSES Defined in adults as an elevation of serum phosphorus above 1.67 mmol/L (5 mg/dL), hyperphosphatemia is a common finding with many causes (Table 356-4). Spurious hyperphosphatemia may occur in patients with thrombocytosis when blood is allowed to clot to obtain serum. Undelayed collection of plasma from heparinized samples will show lower values. Certain autoanalyzers cause spurious hyperphosphatemia because of chemical interference. Abnormal positively charged serum proteins, as in plasma cell dyscrasias, may cause marked elevations of phosphorus. In one instance, the serum concentration was 4.5 mmol/L (13.5 mg/dL), and each millimole of myeloma protein bound 15 molecules of phosphate.

Decreased renal excretion of phosphorus is the most common cause of hyperphosphatemia. Since PTH is phosphaturic, hyperphosphatemia is a cardinal feature of hypoparathyroidism, either as a primary disorder or in patients whose renal cyclic AMP response to PTH is abnormal (pseudohypoparathyroidism type I) or those whose phosphaturic response to PTH is suppressed (pseudohypoparathyroidism type II).

Of interest, severe hypomagnesemia causes marked suppression of PTH in plasma despite hypocalcemia but does not cause hyperphosphatemia. Hyperphosphatemia occurs in tumoral calcinosis, pseudoxanthoma elasticum, infantile hypophosphatasia, and hyperostosis because of decreased renal excretion. Untreated severe hyperthyroidism apparently increases cellular catabolism sufficiently to elevate serum phosphorus despite increased phosphorus loss in the urine. Acromegaly or administration of growth hormone causes modest hyperphosphatemia. Presumably, the higher phosphorus levels in children partly reflect growth hormone activity. Hyperphosphatemia occurs in untreated adrenal insufficiency because of volume contraction, metabolic acidosis, and possibly reduced glomerular permeability. Mild hyperphosphatemia may occur with bisphosphonate therapy because of increased tubular reabsorption of phosphorus.

Hyperphosphatemia, sometimes with levels up to 15 mmol/L (46 mg/dL), has occurred secondary to increased absorption from the gut following administration of excess phosphate salts by mouth or from the colon as a result of enemas that contain phosphorus. Overmedication with vitamin D and production of vitamin D by granulomatous tissue in diseases such as sarcoidosis and tuberculosis can cause hyperphosphatemia. Both acute metabolic and acute respiratory acidosis may decompose cellular organic phosphates, reduce phosphorylation, and result in diffusion of phosphorus from the cell and hyperphosphatemia. Lactic acidosis is especially important as a cause of hyperphosphatemia. Reduced insulin levels or clonidine administration also can cause hyperphosphatemia. Cellular release of phosphorus may cause hyperphosphatemia, particularly in rhabdomyolysis, infarction of other tissues, or hemolysis. The tumor lysis syndrome, usually seen in patients whose tumor responds briskly to chemotherapy, consists of hyperphosphatemia, hypocalcemia, hyperkalemia, metabolic acidosis, hyperuricemia, and, in many cases, acute renal failure. Severe hyperphosphatemia after intravenous infusion of phosphate salts is a particular danger in patients who are acidotic or oliguric. Finally, infusion of compounds containing phospholipids for parenteral nutrition has caused hyperphosphatemia.

Table 356-4

Causes of Hyperphosphatemia

Binding to serum proteins	**Internal redistribution**
Plasma cell dyscrasias	Acute metabolic acidosis
Decreased renal excretion	Lactic acidosis
Renal insufficiency	Acute respiratory acidosis
Hypoparathyroidism	Lactic acid infusion
Pseudohypoparathyroidism, types I and II	Reduced insulin level
Tumoral calcinosis	Clonidine administration
Pseudoxanthoma elasticum	**Cellular release**
Infantile hypophosphatasia	Rhabdomyolysis
Hyperostosis	Organ infarction
Hyperthyroidism	Tumor lysis
Growth hormone activity	Burkitt's lymphoma
Adrenal insufficiency	Lymphoblastic lymphoma
Bisphosphonate therapy	Metastatic small cell carcinoma
Increased intestinal absorption	Thyrotoxicosis
Phosphorus-containing cathartics	Acute hemolysis
Vitamin D ingestion	**Parenteral administration**
Granulomatous diseases producing vitamin D	Intravenous phosphate salts
Sarcoidosis	Lipid (phospholipid) infusion
Tuberculosis	**Spurious hyperphosphatemia**
	Thrombocytosis
	Hyperlipidemia

℞ TREATMENT

Hyperphosphatemia is potentially dangerous because of metastatic calcification. Before initiating treatment the cause should be identified and corrected whenever possible. Although only an approximate guide, a calcium-phosphorus product [serum Ca (mg/dL) X serum P (mg/dL)] greater than 70 indicates a potential threat of calcification. Calcification is more likely to occur in the presence of an elevated blood pH or an elevated level of serum PTH.

In the absence of renal insufficiency, hydration or volume expansion by the infusion of hypotonic saline increases the fractional clearance of phosphorus by the kidney. Aluminum-based antacids bind phosphorus in the lumen of the gastrointestinal tract and prevent its absorption. Although long-term use of these compounds may cause aluminum toxicity, short-term use may be very helpful in acute hyperphosphatemia. Hyperphosphatemia in the presence of renal insufficiency usually requires either peritoneal dialysis or hemodialysis.

BIBLIOGRAPHY

AGARWAL R, KNOCHEL JP: Fluid and electrolyte disorders associated with alcoholism and liver disease, in *Fluid and Electrolytes*, 3d ed, JP Kokko, R Tannen (eds). Philadelphia, Saunders, 1996, p 449

BOLLAERT PE et al: Hemodynamic and metabolic effects of rapid correction of hypophosphatemia in patients with septic shock. Chest 107:1698, 1995

CAI Q et al: Brief report: Inhibition of renal phosphate transport by a tumor product in a patient with oncogenic osteomalacia. N Engl J Med 330:1645, 1994

DEMARCHI S et al: Renal tubular dysfunction in chronic alcohol abuse—effects of abstinence. N Engl J Med 329:1927, 1993

EMMETT M et al: The pathophysiology of acid-base changes in chronically phosphate-depleted rats. J Clin Invest 59:291, 1977

FERGUSON ER et al: Derangements of muscle composition, ion transport, and oxygen consumption in chronically alcoholic dogs. Am J Physiol 246:F700, 1984

FIACCADORI E et al: Hypophosphatemia and phosphorus depletion in respiratory and peripheral muscles of patients with respiratory failure due to COPD. Chest 105:1392, 1994

FULLER TJ et al: Reversible depression in myocardial performance in dogs with experimental phosphorus deficiency. J Clin Invest 62:1194, 1978
GREEN J et al: Acute phosphate depletion inhibits the Na^+/H^+ antiporter in a cultured renal cell line. Am J Physiol 265:F440, 1993
JOHNSON MA et al: Adenosine triphosphate turnover in humans. J Clin Invest 84:990, 1989
KNOCHEL JP: Central nervous system manifestations of hypophosphatemia and phosphorus depletion, in *Metabolic Brain Dysfunction in System Disorders*, AC Arieff, RC Griggs (eds). Boston, Little, Brown, 1992, chap 10, p 183
———: Hypophosphatemia and rhabdomyolysis. Am J Med 92:455, 1992
——— et al: Hypophosphatemia and phosphorus deficiency, in *The Kidney*, 5th ed, B Brenner, F Rector (eds). Philadelphia, Saunders, 1996, chap 25, p 1086
KOTANKO P: Hyperphosphatemia in multiple myeloma. N Engl J Med 326:1781, 1992
LEVI M et al: Disorders of phosphate and magnesium metabolism, in *Disorders of Bone and Mineral Metabolism*, FC Coe, MJ Favus (eds). New York, Raven Press, 1992, chap 28, p 587
LUTOMSKI DM et al: The effect of thrombocytosis on serum potassium and phosphorus concentrations. Am J Med Sci 307:255, 1994
MICHAUT P et al: Dipyridamole for renal phosphate leak? N Engl J Med 331:58, 1994
OSTER JR et al: Pathogenesis of hyperphosphatemia in lactic acidosis: Disparate effects of racemic (DL-) and levo (L-) lactic acid on plasma phosphorus concentration. Can J Physiol Pharmacol 63:1599, 1985
PORTALE AA et al: Metabolic acidosis reverses the increase in serum 1,25(OH)2D in phosphorus-restricted normal men. Am J Physiol 263:E1164, 1992
ROSEN GH et al: Intravenous phosphate repletion regimen for critically ill patients with moderate hypophosphatemia. Crit Care Med 23:1204, 1995
SUBHASH MN et al: Calcium and phosphorus levels in serum and CSF in dementia. Neurobiol Aging 12:267, 1991
THATTE L et al: Review of the literature: Severe hyperphosphatemia. Am J Med Sci 310:167, 1995
VEECH RL et al: Cystolic phosphorylation potential. J Biol Chem 254:6538, 1979
——— et al: Metabolic hyperpolarization of liver by ethanol: The importance of Mg^{2+} and H^+ in determining impermeant intracellular anionic charge and energy of metabolic reactions. Alcohol Clin Exper Res 18:1040, 1994

357 DISORDERS OF MAGNESIUM METABOLISM

James P. Knochel

Magnesium is the most abundant intracellular divalent cation. The total magnesium content of a normal man is 12.4 mmol (0.3 g) per kilogram of body weight. Of this, 1 percent is extracellular, 31 percent is in cells, and 67 percent is in bone. Serum magnesium ranges between 0.7 and 1.0 mmol/L (1.8 and 2.5 mg/dL). Of this, the unbound diffusible fraction is about 0.6 mmol/L (1.4 mg/dL). It exists in two forms in cells, one in solution in equilibrium with the diffusible form in plasma and a larger quantity bound to organic components. Since most magnesium inside cells is bound to ATP, MgATP is in equilibrium with free magnesium ions. Thus, shifts in free magnesium concentration may help regulate stores of ATP. From the opposite viewpoint, when the ATP concentration in cells is acutely reduced, e.g., by infusion of intravenous fructose, magnesium ions diffuse from the cell, and serum magnesium rises. Since ATP is critical to nearly all metabolic transformations, normal stores of magnesium are essential to sustain life.

The optimal intake of magnesium for an adult is 15 to 20 mmol/d (36 to 48 mg/d). Foods rich in magnesium include green vegetables, seed grains, nuts, peas, beans, and coca derivatives. Fresh meat, fish, and most fresh fruits contain relatively small amounts of magnesium. Magnesium is absorbed primarily in the jejunum and ileum, and healthy persons absorb about 30 to 40 percent of dietary magnesium. Absorption may increase to 70 percent when intake is low or magnesium deficiency exists. Vitamin D plays a minor role in magnesium absorption. When magnesium intake is restricted, fecal excretion becomes negligible, and urinary excretion decreases. Thus, magnesium retention by the kidney is very efficient. Magnesium excretion depends on glomerular filtration of the unbound fraction, of which 25 percent is reabsorbed in the proximal tubule and 50 to 60 percent is reabsorbed in the loop of Henle. Loop diuretics, such as ethacrynic acid, bumetanide, or furosemide, cause greater excretion of magnesium than do diuretics, such as thiazides, that act on the distal tubule. Magnesium excretion is increased when extracellular fluid volume is expanded by ingestion of water and salt, and aldosterone decreases reabsorption of magnesium by the renal tubule. Magnesium excretion increases sharply when the concentration in serum exceeds 0.8 mmol/L (2 mg/dL).

Slight hypomagnesemia occurs in athletically trained individuals, in hypermetabolic states such as pregnancy and cold acclimatization, and after administration of thyroid hormone.

MAGNESIUM DEFICIENCY

When any of the three major intracellular elements—magnesium, potassium, or phosphorus—is deprived or lost, deficiencies of the others usually follow. For this reason, deficiency of a single intracellular component almost never occurs. A diet devoid of magnesium causes depletion of phosphorus and potassium in skeletal muscle. Selective potassium deficiency may cause reductions in magnesium and phosphorus. Phosphorus deficiency may cause reductions in potassium and magnesium contents of tissue. The usual somatic responses to selective deprivation of one major intracellular element are anorexia, cellular atrophy, a negative nitrogen balance, and net loss of the other two major intracellular elements. Shrinkage of cell mass and expulsion of the elements not deprived help to maintain a normal intracellular composition.

During hyperalimentation a different situation prevails. Provision of a diet that is otherwise replete but deficient in one major intracellular element promotes an anabolic state, and newly synthesized protoplasm will be deficient in the deprived ion. Serious derangements of cellular composition ensue, including accumulations of sodium, chloride, calcium, and water. Indeed, elevation of cellular calcium may be an important cause of cellular injury in this situation by activating proteases and phospholipases.

As in deficiencies of other major intracellular elements, deficiency of body magnesium can be present when serum values are normal. In addition, certain tissues become deficient before others. The definition of a true deficit of an intracellular element is reduction of its ratio to nitrogen in the tissue. In muscle, this ratio is about 0.3 mmol (7 mg) magnesium per gram of nitrogen. Red cell magnesium content decreases consistently in magnesium deficiency, whereas muscle magnesium content may remain normal.

THE CLINICAL PHYSIOLOGY OF MAGNESIUM DEFICIENCY Within 3 to 7 days after reducing dietary magnesium intake to less than 0.5 mmol/d (12 mg/d), renal excretion of magnesium decreases to <0.5 mmol/d (12 mg/d). Anorexia, nausea, vomiting, lethargy, and weakness develop within weeks. Symptoms of severe magnesium deficiency, including paresthesia, muscular cramps, irritability, decreased attention span, and mental confusion, may require months to appear.

The physical findings are largely due to the associated hypocalcemia and include positive Trousseau and Chvostek signs, peculiar movements of the fingers best described as athetoid tetany, and, on occasion, convulsions. Fasciculations may be precipitated by a tap to muscle with a neurologic hammer. About half of patients with selective magnesium depletion become hypokalemic, the etiology of which is poorly understood. Aldosterone production may be enhanced, thus increasing potassium excretion into the urine. It is difficult to correct the potassium deficiency with supplemental potassium salts. However, correction of hypomagnesemia promptly reduces potassium excretion and corrects the hypokalemia. For this reason, it should be kept in mind that hypokalemia refractory to potassium supplements may be due to magnesium deficiency. Cardiac arrhythmias, disturbances of conduction, ventricular fibrillation, and cardiac arrest can occur in patients with coexisting hypokalemia and hypomagnesemia. Magnesium plays a critical role in maintenance of intracellular potassium concentration by regulating potassium movement through myocardial cell membranes. This property is known as *inward rectification.* In the sinus and atrioventricular nodule tissue, magnesium ions also affect transsarcolemmal calcium inflow and modulate intracellular handling of calcium in the sarcoplasmic reticulum. Indeed, the actions of magnesium resemble those of calcium channel blocking agents. Levels of magnesium below 0.7 mmol/L cause electrocardiographic changes similar to those of hypokalemia, including depression of ST segments, flattening of T waves, QT/QT_c prolongation, and enhanced atrial and ventricular excitability; these changes in magnesium deficiency may be secondary to intracellular potassium deficiency. Either magnesium or potassium deficiency can cause a substantial reduction in myocardial Na,K-Mg-dependent ATPase. Since this enzyme is the site of digitalis binding, reduction in ATPase may explain the propensity for digitalis poisoning in both magnesium and potassium deficiency. In addition, magnesium deficiency itself increases the liklihood of cardiac arrhythmias. Because of QT prolongation, potentially dangerous arrhythmias, in particular torsade de pointes, are more likely to occur. The causes of magnesium deficiency are summarized in Table 357-1.

Hypocalcemia usually does not develop until serum magnesium falls below 0.5 mmol/L (1.2 mg/dL). Although mild magnesium deficiency may enhance release of parathyroid hormone (PTH), severe hypomagnesemia [levels below 0.4 mmol/L (1 mg/dL)] blocks release of PTH. In addition, magnesium deficiency impairs the normal calcemic response to PTH at the level of the skeleton. Hypocalcemia can become sufficiently severe to cause tetany. Although tetany has been reported in hypomagnesemia independently of hypocalcemia, both conditions usually coexist with this finding. In most cases the tetany with hypomagnesemia does not respond to infusions of calcium alone and requires correction of magnesium levels. In addition, the hypocalcemia may respond only to magnesium replacement, usually requiring 2 to 7 days for correction. When hypomagnesemia is caused by steatorrhea, administration of magnesium salts intravenously can cause prompt and sometimes marked release of PTH. In rare instances, acute hypercalcemia can occur.

GASTROINTESTINAL CAUSES OF MAGNESIUM DEFICIENCY Familial hypomagnesemia is manifested during childhood and is due to diminished absorption of dietary magnesium. The most common cause of magnesium deficiency in adults is intestinal malabsorption and steatorrhea, as in nontropical sprue, the short bowel syndrome, chronic pancreatic insufficiency, or biliary diversion. Because of unabsorbed fat, nonabsorbable magnesium–fatty acid soaps form in the intestinal lumen. When long-standing, hypomagnesemia is often associated with hypocalcemia, hypokalemia, and hypophosphatemia. Because of steatorrhea, malabsorption of fat-soluble vitamins, especially vitamins K, A, and D, may coexist. Vitamin D deficiency and osteomalacia can cause weakness due to proximal myopathy in association with pain in the lower back and hips. Secondary hyperparathyroidism, sometimes severe, almost always coexists.

Magnesium deficiency can also occur after ingestion of cellulose phosphate to reduce calcium absorption or after prolonged nasogastric suction in patients who have not received adequate magnesium supplementation. Acute hypomagnesemia, along with acute hypocalcemia, can occur in acute hemorrhagic pancreatitis when magnesium– and calcium–fatty acid soaps form in sites of tissue necrosis.

ENDOCRINE CAUSES OF HYPOMAGNESEMIA Hypomagnesemia occurs in poorly controlled diabetes mellitus and may be more severe after diabetic ketoacidosis. Moderate hypomagnesemia may occur in hyperparathyroidism, hypoparathyroidism, hyperthyroidism, and primary hyperaldosteronism. In primary hyperaldosteronism, aldosterone acts both directly and via volume expansion to enhance magnesium excretion. These effects can be reversed by spironolactone, triamterene, or amiloride. Hypomagnesemia may occur in patients with the syndrome of inappropriate vasopressin secretion (commonly termed the syndrome of inappropriate antidiuretic hormone, SIADH) (see Chap. 330), presumably the result of increased aldosterone production and overexpansion of extracellular volume. Epinephrine and other potent beta agonists may cause transient hypomagnesemia as the result of uptake of magnesium into adipose tissue as fatty acids are released. Furthermore, release of fatty acids into the blood can cause the formation of insoluble fatty acid–magnesium and –calcium complexes in serum. If serum is centrifuged, the precipitates settle to the bottom of the tube, and spurious hypomagnesemia and hypocalcemia can be diagnosed. Hypomagnesemia has also been observed after multiple blood transfusions, possibly secondary to complex formation with sodium citrate. Transient hypomagnesemia occurs commonly after cardiopulmonary bypass surgery.

Table 357-1

Causes of Hypomagnesemia

I. Primary nutritional disturbances
  A. Inadequate intake
  B. Total parenteral nutrition
  C. Refeeding syndrome
II. Gastrointestinal disorders
  A. Specific absorptive defects
  B. Malabsorption syndromes
    1. Enteric fistulas
    2. Nontropical sprue
    3. Whipple's disease
    4. Intestinal lymphoma
    5. Chronic pancreatic insufficiency
    6. Biliary diversion
    7. Giardiasis
    8. Short bowel syndrome
  C. Prolonged diarrhea
  D. Prolonged nasogastric suction
  E. Pancreatitis
  G. Cellulose phosphate ingestion
III. Endocrine disorders
  A. Hyperparathyroidism
  B. Hypoparathyroidism
  C. Hyperthyroidism
  D. Primary hyperaldosteronism
  E. Bartter's syndrome
  G. Gitelman's syndrome
  H. Diabetic ketoacidosis
  I. Alcoholic ketoacidosis
IV. Cellular uptake or redistribution
  A. Administration of epinephrine
  B. Acute pancreatitis
  C. Following correction of respiratory acidosis
  D. "Hungry bone" syndrome after parathyroidectomy
  E. Massive blood transfusions
V. Chronic alcoholism, alcoholic withdrawal
VI. Increased renal excretion
  A. Ethanol ingestion
  B. Idiopathic
  C. Following renal transplantation
  D. Cyclosporine therapy
  E. Cisplatin therapy
  F. Aminoglycoside therapy
  G. Amphotericin B therapy
  H. Capreomycin therapy
  I. Viomycin therapy
  J. Syndrome of inappropriate vasopressin secretion (SIADH)
  K. Diuretic administration
    1. Furosemide
    2. Ethacrynic acid
    3. Bumetanide
    4. Acetazolamide
    5. Thiazides
    6. Chlorthalidone
    7. Osmotic agents
  J. Recovery phase of acute tubular necrosis
  K. Pentamidine therapy
  L. Theophylline toxicity
  M. Colony stimulating factor therapy

HYPOMAGNESEMIA ASSOCIATED WITH ALCOHOLISM Ethanol causes a transient loss of magnesium into the urine. Alcoholics with a reasonably normal nutrient intake and normal intestinal function usually have normal or only slightly depressed magnesium levels in blood. The total-body deficit of magnesium in chronic alcoholics is modest, amounting to 100 to 150 mmol (2.4 to 3.6 g). However, during alcohol withdrawal, hypomagnesemia may occur in association with acute hypophosphatemia and acute hypokalemia. Simultaneously, urinary excretion of magnesium, phosphate, and potassium decreases. Thus, hypomagnesemia occurs both because of net deficit and because of a shift into cells during withdrawal. In animals, sustained ethanol administration in intoxicating doses causes severe depletion of phosphorus, moderate depletion of magnesium and potassium, and increases in intracellular sodium, chloride, water, and calcium. Selective depletion of phosphorus also causes magnesium wasting and muscle magnesium deficiency. The same findings occur in muscle of severely alcoholic humans. In acute alcohol withdrawal, respiratory alkalosis and insulin release stimulated by administration of nutrients act in concert to move phosphate into cells. Increased ATP synthesis as a result of phosphate movement into cells may cause increased magnesium binding and worsen hypomagnesemia.

In alcoholic patients with intestinal malabsorption and steatorrhea, severe hypomagnesemia can be associated with hypocalcemia, hypophosphatemia, and hypokalemia. Although a relationship between hypomagnesemia and alcohol withdrawal seizures has been suggested, alcoholics in a withdrawal state also have prominent respiratory alkalosis, which lowers the threshold for seizure activity. Thus, the relationship of hypomagnesemia to seizures in this setting is not clear. Furthermore, correction of hypomagnesemia appears to have no favorable effect on the course of the alcohol withdrawal syndrome.

However, magnesium deficiency may play a role in the temporary hypertension that occurs during alcohol withdrawal. Independently of alcohol, magnesium deficiency causes accumulation of calcium in smooth muscle and increases vascular tone. Magnesium salts reduce arteriolar tone by reducing cytosolic calcium. Accumulation of calcium potentiates the pressor response to circulating catecholamines. Withdrawing alcoholics usually have elevations of circulating catecholamines and enhanced sympathetic nerve activity. Thus, the combined effects of magnesium depletion, calcium accumulation in cells, and elevated levels of catecholamines may cause the hypertension and explain the favorable effect of calcium channel blocking drugs under such circumstances.

MAGNESIUM DEFICIENCY DUE TO INCREASED RENAL EXCRETION Hypomagnesemia also can result from impaired renal tubular reabsorption, usually in association with renal potassium wasting and hypokalemia. Some patients, especially those with Bartter's syndrome, may be hypercalciuric. Gitelman's syndrome, resembling Bartter's syndrome, is also associated with hypokalemic metabolic alkalosis, hypermagnesuria, and hypomagnesemia, but calcium excretion is low. However, in these patients, calcium excretion is abnormally low. Transient hypomagnesemia due to reduced renal tubular reabsorption may follow renal transplantation.

Aminoglycosides, cisplatin, diuretics, foscarnet, and cyclosporine can cause magnesium wasting in the urine. Hypomagnesemia and hypokalemia as a result of impaired tubular reabsorption occur after prolonged aminoglycoside treatment, usually in patients who have received more than 8.0 g of the drug. Total recovery is the rule after the drug is stopped. Hypomagnesemia in patients treated with cisplatin can be severe; hypokalemia is less common. Renal tubular mitochondrial injury may be responsible. Even after cisplatin is withdrawn, the renal defect may persist indefinitely. Of interest, calcitriol may enhance magnesium wasting in patients with cisplatin nephrotoxicity who are also hypomagnesemic and hypocalcemic. About a fourth of patients treated with cyclosporine and prednisone after renal transplantation develop serum magnesium levels below 0.5 mmol/L (1.2 mg/dL). Although loop diuretics are potent magnesuric agents, hypomagnesemia is infrequent except in patients who receive large doses or who receive two or more diuretics that act at different sites in the nephron. Treatment with pentamidine, theophylline, and granulocyte-macrophage colony stimulating factor can on occasion cause hypermagnesuria and hypomagnesemia.

℞ TREATMENT

Treatment of hypomagnesemia should focus on correcting the cause. Hypomagnesemia due to inadequate dietary intake or to disorders that reduce intestinal absorption or cause excessive losses into the urine can often be corrected by oral administration of magnesium salts. Patients with potentially serious cardiac arrhythmias or with nausea and vomiting should be given intravenous magnesium sulfate. One mL of 50% magnesium sulfate heptahydrate ($MgSo_4 \cdot 7\ H_2O$) contains 2.1 mmol (50 mg) of magnesium. The usual adult dose of magnesium sulfate is 2 mL of a 50% solution by mouth every 6 h on the first day and half this quantity for the following 3 to 4 days. Magnesium sulfate may be given intramuscularly, but this is painful and may cause elevation of creatine phosphokinase levels, reflecting muscle damage and thus blunting the value of measurements of the enzyme to detect rhabdomyolysis. When parenteral administration is indicated it is preferable to infuse magnesium in a dose of 4.2 mmol magnesium sulfate (1 g) every 6 h. Patients who require intravenous magnesium are often hypokalemic and hypophosphatemic. Potassium phosphate and potassium chloride may be included with magnesium sulfate in 0.5 *N* saline containing 5% glucose. The total potassium content in each infusion bottle should represent one-fourth of the daily requirement. In patients with adequate urine flow, such solutions can be given in a quantity of 750 mL every 6 h until nausea and vomiting cease and oral intake becomes possible. In patients with tetany due to magnesium deficiency, although hypocalcemia coexists, calcium is generally ineffective, and infusions of magnesium salts usually require 2 h or more to relieve the tetany. Up to a full day may be required for all signs of latent tetany, such as Chvostek and Trousseau signs, to disappear completely. Several oral preparations of magnesium salts are available. Thus, 5 mL of magnesium hydroxide–containing antacids (Maalox, Gelusil, Mylanta) contains 14 mmol (340 mg) of magnesium. However, there are two theoretical objections to the use of these preparations: they contain aluminum salts that may be hazardous if renal impairment is present, and they bind phosphate in the gut, which by itself promotes loss of magnesium. Other preparations include magnesium chloride tablets, magnesium gluconate tablets, and commercially available magnesium oxide powder. Since both spironolactone and triamterene cause retention of magnesium and potassium, these drugs may be useful adjuncts to maintain normal serum magnesium balance in patients taking diuretics.

The recommended dose of magnesium salts for treatment of torsade de pointes or ventricular arrhythmias is unsettled. In general, 4.0 mL of 50% $MgSO_4 \cdot 7H_2O$ (8 mmol) may be safely infused over 1 to 2 min, which results in a serum magnesium concentration of 1.0 to 1.7 mmol/L (2.4 to 4.1 mg/dL). This is followed by infusions of 8 to 12 mmol/h (200 to 300 mg/h) for 4 to 8 h and smaller doses thereafter. Although this regimen may cause transient facial flushing and warmth, the resulting concentration in serum does not exceed 1.8 mmol/L (4.4 mg/dL). Magnesium salts should be administered with great caution in patients with renal insufficiency.

Several studies suggest that administration of magnesium salts to patients with acute myocardial infarction who are neither hypomagnesemic nor hypokalemic causes a reduction in mortality. However, in a more recent prospective study (ISIS-4) involving 58,050 patients who were given a loading dose of 8 mmol (200 mg) of magnesium followed by an additional 72 mmol (1800 mg) over the following 24 h, no benefit was observed. Thus, in the patient with uncomplicated myocardial infarction, there is no clear indication to administer magnesium.

Magnesium salts have also been proposed as an adjunct in the treatment of asthma to relax bronchial smooth muscle. There is not sufficient evidence at this time to establish efficacy of this treatment.

HYPERMAGNESEMIA

Patients with end-stage renal disease frequently have modest hypermagnesemia that is aggravated by ingesting magnesium-containing compounds such as antacids or cathartics. Surreptitious ingestion of magnesium salts as a cathartic can be diagnosed by demonstration of hypermagnesemia in serum and of fecal magnesium concentrations above 25 mmol/L (60 mg/dL). Rhabdomyolysis causes hypermagnesemia because of release from injured muscle. Adrenal insufficiency may cause hypermagnesemia. Half of patients with familial benign hypocalciuric hypercalcemia have hypermagnesemia. Pronounced hypermagnesemia [>6.5 mmol/L (16 mg/dL)] has been described in patients with near-drowning in the Dead Sea in Jordan or Basque Lake in British Columbia. Magnesium levels in water from these sources average 164 and 178 mmol/L (400 and 435 mg/dL), respectively. Survival in many near-drowning victims in the Dead Sea has been attributed to pronounced hypercalcemia because of the high calcium levels in this water.

Symptomatic hypermagnesemia is uncommon and is usually precipitated by inadvertent overdosage with magnesium salts or is deliberately induced to treat patients with eclampsia. Infants born of eclamptic mothers treated with magnesium may be hypermagnesemic. Magnesium can reduce neuromuscular transmission and act as a central nervous system depressant. Symptoms of hypermagnesemia correspond poorly to serum levels. However, the toxicity of any given level will be exaggerated in the presence of hypocalcemia, hyperkalemia, and uremia. Nausea and facial paresthesia usually appear between 2 and 4 mmol/L (5 and 10 mg/dL). Sedation, hypoventilation with respiratory acidosis, decreased deep tendon reflexes, and muscle weakness may appear at levels above 5 mmol/L (12 mg/dL). Hypotension, bradycardia, and diffuse vasodilatation appear at levels of 7.5 mmol/L. Areflexia, coma, and respiratory paralysis occur at higher levels. Patients treated for eclampsia must be observed very carefully for signs of magnesium intoxication. If this occurs, symptoms and findings can generally be reversed promptly by infusion of calcium salts, since these ions electrically oppose one another at their sites of action. Administration of saline and furosemide may help promote excretion of magnesium. Hemodialysis is also effective.

BIBLIOGRAPHY

ALFREY AC et al: Evaluation of body magnesium stores. J Lab Clin Med 84:153, 1974

AL-GHAMDI S et al: Magnesium deficiency: Pathophysiologic and clinical overview. Am J Kid Dis 24:737, 1994

ANDERSON R et al: Skeletal muscle phosphorus and magnesium deficiency in alcoholic myopathy. Miner Electrolyte Metab 4:106, 1980

BRITTON J: Dietary magnesium, lung function, wheezing, and airway hyperreactivity in a random adult population sample. Lancet 344:357, 1994

CLAUSEN T: Correlation between magnesium and potassium contents in muscle: Role of Na^+-K^+ pump. Am J Physiol 264:C457, 1993

CRONIN RE et al: Skeletal muscle injury after magnesium depletion in the dog. Am J Physiol 243:F113, 1982

D'ANGELO EKG et al: Magnesium relaxes arterial smooth muscle by decreasing intracellular Ca^{2+} without changing intracellular Mg^{2+}. J Clin Invest 89:1988, 1992

FAZEKAS T et al: Magnesium and the heart: Antiarrhythmic therapy with magnesium. Clin Cardiol 16:768, 1993

FERGUSON ER et al: Derangements of muscle composition, ion transport, and oxygen consumption in chronically alcoholic dogs. Am J Physiol 246:F700, 1984

FINE KD et al: Diagnosis of magnesium-induced diarrhea. N Engl J Med 324:1012, 1991

HAMPTON E et al: Intravenous magnesium therapy in acute myocardial infarction. Ann Pharmacother 28:212, 1994

ISIS-4 (FOURTH INTERNATIONAL STUDY OF INFARCT SURVIVAL) COLLABORATIVE GROUP: A randomised factorial trial assessing early oral captopril, oral mononitrate, and intravenous magnesium sulphate in 58,050 patients with suspected acute myocardial infarction: ISIS-4. Lancet 345:669, 1995

KNOCHEL JP: Hypophosphatemia in the alcoholic. Arch Intern Med 140:613, 1980

———: Hypophosphatemia and rhabdomyolysis. Am J Med 92:455, 1992

KROENKE K et al: The value of serum magnesium determination in hypertensive patients receiving diuretics. Arch Intern Med 147:1553, 1987

MCLEAN RM: Magnesium and its therapeutic uses: A review. Am J Med 96:63, 1994

PORATH A et al: Dead Sea water poisoning. Ann Emerg Med 18:121, 1989

RALSTON MA et al: Serum and tissue magnesium concentrations in patients with heart failure and serious ventricular arrhythmias. Ann Intern Med 113:841, 1990

SHILS ME: Experimental human magnesium depletion. Medicine 48:61, 1969

VICTOR M: The role of hypomagnesemia and respiratory alkalosis in the genesis of alcohol withdrawal symptoms. Ann NY Acad Sci 215:235, 1973

WEISS M et al: Should magnesium therapy be considered for the treatment of coronary heart disease? I. A critical appraisal of current facts and hypotheses. Magnesium Res 7:135, 1994

WHANG R: Magnesium homeostasis and clinical disorders of magnesium deficiency. Ann Pharmacother 28:220, 1994

358

Stephen M. Krane

PAGET'S DISEASE OF BONE

Paget's disease of bone (osteitis deformans) is usually focal but may be widespread. The initial event is excessive resorption of bone by osteoclasts, followed by the replacement of normal marrow by vascular, fibrous connective tissue. At some stage and to a variable degree, the resorbed bone is replaced by coarse-fibered, dense trabecular bone organized in haphazard fashion. The irregular and often rapid deposition of this new bone, to a great extent still lamellar, results in an increase in the number of prominent, irregular cement lines that give the bone its characteristic "mosaic" pattern. Most lesions show both excessive resorption and chaotic new bone formation.

INCIDENCE The prevalence is difficult to determine because the disease is often asymptomatic and is frequently detected when roentgenograms are obtained for other reasons or because of a high level of alkaline phosphatase on routine blood screening. On the basis of autopsy examination, the incidence is estimated to be about 3 percent in individuals over age 40; the likelihood of occurrence increases with age. The incidence varies in different parts of the world. Radiologic surveys indicate that the frequency in adults is less than 1 percent in the United States, Great Britain, and Australia. In India, Japan, the Middle East, and Scandinavia, the disease is rare.

ETIOLOGY The cause is unknown. No convincing evidence of endocrine abnormality has been produced. Likewise, although pagetic bone can be exceedingly vascular, the vascular abnormality may not be primary. Some of the manifestations can be suppressed with glucocorticoids, salicylates, and cytotoxic drugs, but there is no convincing evidence that the fundamental lesion is inflammatory. Intranuclear inclusions have been found by electron microscopy in osteoclasts in pagetic bone but not in osteoclasts or other bone cells in normal persons or patients with other bone diseases with the exception of pyknodysostosis. Some of the inclusions resemble nucleocapsids of viruses belonging to the measles group. Indirect immunofluorescence and immunoperoxidase studies using antibodies to measles virus suggest that the inclusions are indeed measles virus nucleocapsids. Measles virus nucleocapsid mRNA has been detected in some but not all in situ hybridization studies of bone cells from patients with Paget's disease, and measles virus nucleocapsid mRNA has been identified in bone marrow mononuclear cells using the polymerase chain reaction. The presence of mutations in specific regions of the viral genome is consistent with persistent infection. In some individuals with Paget's disease, osteoclasts and bone marrow mononuclear cells contain nucleocapsids of respiratory syncytial virus alone or in addition to nucleocapsids of measles virus, and in some areas of Britain canine distemper virus sequences have been identified in pagetic bone cells. Thus, different paramyxoviruses may have roles in the initiation or propagation of Paget's disease.

PATHOPHYSIOLOGY The characteristic feature is increased resorption of bone accompanied by an increase in bone formation, which is usually adequate to compensate. In the early phase bone resorption predominates (e.g., in the variant *osteoporosis circumscripta*), and the bones are very vascular. This has been termed the *osteoporotic*, *osteolytic*, or *destructive phase* of disease in which body calcium balance may be negative. Commonly, the excessive resorption is followed closely by formation of new pagetic bone. In this so-called mixed phase of the disease, the rate of bone formation is so geared to that of bone resorption that the magnitude of the increase in bone turnover is not reflected in the overall calcium balance.

As the activity decreases, the resorptive rate may decline progressively relative to formation, eventually leading to development of hard, dense, less vascular bone (the so-called *osteoplastic* or *sclerotic phase*) and a positive calcium balance. The rates of bone turnover may be increased enormously in the early phases of the disease, occasionally more than 20 times normal. Quantitative histomorphometry of bone biopsies confirms the extent of remodeling with marked increase in resorption surfaces and deep scalloped lacunae containing osteoclasts and increased numbers of osteoblasts lining the edges. Increased generation and overactivity of osteoclasts are considered the major abnormality. The osteoclasts are larger than normal and contain multiple pleomorphic nuclei. Increased numbers of osteoclast-like multinucleated cells are generated from hematopoietic precursors in long-term marrow cultures from individuals with Paget's disease compared with normal individuals. Production of the cytokine interleukin (IL) 6 by the pagetic bone and marrow cells is increased, and levels of the IL-6 receptor are high. Thus, IL-6 could act locally to contribute to the increased osteoclast formation. The calcification rate is also increased. The normal hematopoietic marrow is replaced by a loose stroma which may be highly vascular. The increase in bone turnover varies with the extent and activity of the disease. Bone turnover correlates with the increased plasma levels of bone alkaline phosphatase, which are higher in Paget's disease than in any other condition except for hereditary hyperphosphatasia. Although increased bone resorption enhances release of calcium and phosphate ions from bone, utilization of these ions for new bone formation and, presumably, feedback control of parathyroid hormone secretion usually maintain the concentration of calcium ions in the plasma at normal levels. The concentration of phosphate in the plasma is normal or slightly elevated. When the imbalance between bone formation and resorption favors resorption, as after prolonged immobilization or fractures, urinary calcium excretion may be increased, and on occasion hypercalcemia may occur. If, on the other hand, bone formation exceeds resorption (relatively uncommon), circulating levels of parathyroid hormone may be increased. Significant increases in trabecular bone resorption and osteoid surfaces in normal bone from patients with Paget's disease may be due to compensatory, secondary hyperparathyroidism. Resorption involves both the organic and mineral phases of bone. While the inorganic ions of the mineral phase are reutilized for bone formation, amino acids such as hydroxyproline and hydroxylysine and the hydroxypyridinium cross-link compounds are released during resorption of the collagen matrix of bone and are not reutilized for collagen biosynthesis. The increased urinary excretion of small peptides containing hydroxyproline reflects increased bone resorption. The pyridinium cross-link compounds pyridinoline (Pyr) and deoxypyridinoline (D-Pyr) are released from bone collagen during osteoclastic bone resorption and can be measured in urine by high-performance liquid chromatography and immunoassays. In some of the immunoassays the reacting antigen includes peptide sequences, whereas in others free Pyr or D-Pyr are measured. In Paget's disease measurement of the excretion of the bound forms correlates better with the extent and activity of the disease, and changes in excretion of the bound form are better indicators of responses to therapy than free Pyr or D-Pyr.

RADIOLOGIC CHANGES The radiologic findings reflect the underlying pathology and the phase of the disease that predominates at the time of the examination. The pelvic bones are most commonly involved, followed by the femur, skull, tibia, lumbosacral spine, dorsal spine, clavicles, and ribs; small bones are not as frequently diseased. The lytic phase of the disease may be overlooked except when it occurs in the skull as osteoporosis circumscripta, with areas of sharply demarcated radiolucency in the frontal, parietal, and occipital bones. In the long bones, the lytic areas are usually first seen at one end and progress toward the other end with a V-shaped advancing edge. The lesion may cause expansion of the cortex and exhibit features suggesting malignancy. Usually lysis is followed by a zone of increased density, representing the new bone formation of the mixed phase of the disease. In general, the bone enlarges with an irregularly widened cortex in a coarse, striated pattern and with increased density, occasionally focal in distribution. Perpendicular lines of radiolucency (cortical infractions) are frequent and occur on the convex side of bowed long bones, particularly the femur and tibia. Transverse fractures may occur, some at the sites of these cortical infractions. The remodeling of the pagetic bone usually follows the lines of stress produced by muscle pull or gravity, accounting for the characteristic lateral bowing of the femur or anterior bowing of the tibia and the tendency for most of the dense bone to be deposited on the concave side of the bowed bone. In the mixed stage, there is enlargement and thickening of the skull, especially of the outer table, with irregular areas of increased density, often spotty (Fig. 358-1). Basilar invagination is common with involvement of the base of the skull. The changes in the pelvis reflect the varying degrees of bone resorption and new bone formation and are frequently accompanied by a characteristic thickening of the pelvic brim. In the sclerotic phase of the disease, the bone may show uniform increase in density, often in the absence of striations. This is common in the facial bones but occasionally occurs in the vertebrae, where a homogeneous, dense pattern gives an "ivory" appearance similar to that typical of Hodgkin's disease, although the involved vertebrae in Hodgkin's disease are not enlarged. Computed tomography and magnetic resonance imaging are useful in defining atypical lesions, particularly where neoplastic involvement is suspected. Technetium 99m diphosphonate bone scans are useful in documenting the extent of disease when therapy is contemplated or to confirm the diagnosis when radiologic findings are inconclusive.

CLINICAL PICTURE The clinical presentation is a function of the extent of the disease, the particular bones involved, and the presence of complications. Many patients are asymptomatic. In these

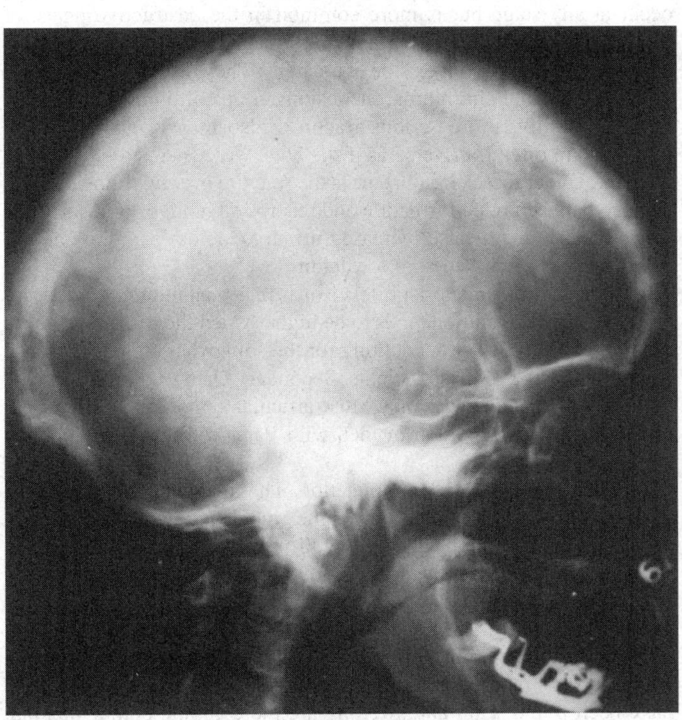

FIGURE 358-1 Lateral roentgenogram of the skull from a 58-year-old woman with Paget's disease of bone.

individuals the disorder is discovered during radiologic examination of the pelvis or spine for an unrelated disease or complaint or because of the finding of an elevated level of plasma alkaline phosphatase. Other individuals may gradually become aware of a swelling or deformity of a long bone or develop a disturbance in gait due to unequal length of the lower extremities. Enlargement of the skull is often not noticed by the patients, except by awareness of increasing hat size. Facial pain and headache are initial complaints in some; backache and leg pain are common. The pain is usually dull but may be shooting or knifelike. Back pain is most common in the lumbar region and may radiate into the buttocks or lower extremities. This pain can be due to the pagetic process itself, to distortion of articular facets, or to secondary osteoarthritis. Pain in the lower extremities may be associated with the transverse cortical infractions along the convex lateral surface of the femur or the anterior surface of the tibia. New lytic lesions detected on bone scan may be the most painful. Pain also may be due to involvement of the hip joint resembling degenerative joint disease and characterized by narrowing of the joint space, bony lipping at the margin of the acetabulum, and deepening of the acetabulum. Angioid streaks may be present in the retina. Hearing loss is due to direct involvement of the ossicles of the inner ear or of bone in the region of the cochlea or to impingement by bone on the eighth cranial nerve in the auditory foramen. More serious neurologic complications can result from overgrowth of bone at the base of the skull (platybasia) and compression of the brainstem. Compression of the spinal cord can cause paraplegia, particularly with involvement of the middorsal spine. Pathologic fractures of vertebrae also may produce spinal cord lesions.

COMPLICATIONS Blood flow may be markedly increased in extremities involved with Paget's disease. There is proliferation of blood vessels in pagetic bone, but anatomic and functional studies have not confirmed the presence of arteriovenous fistulas. Although blood flow is increased in bone, cutaneous vasodilatation in the pagetic extremities accounts for the increased warmth noted clinically. When the disease is widespread, involving one-third or more of the skeleton, the increased blood flow may be associated with *high cardiac output* and rarely with high-output heart failure. However, heart disease in individuals with Paget's disease is usually due to the same conditions that occur in other patients of similar age. *Pathologic fracture* may occur at any stage but is more common in the destructive phase of the disease. In the weight-bearing bones fractures are often incomplete, multiple, and on the convex side of the bone. They may occur spontaneously or follow slight trauma; the lesions are painful but heal with no major disability. More serious fractures also may occur. Complete fractures are often transverse as if the bone were snapped like a piece of chalk. Under these circumstances the fracture may upset the delicate balance between bone formation and resorption in favor of resorption; the imbalance may cause increased urinary calcium excretion and in rare instances increased serum calcium level.

There is no characteristic level of urinary calcium excretion, although calcium excretion tends to be higher when the resorptive phase predominates, possibly accounting for the somewhat higher incidence of *urinary stones* in these patients. Secondary changes in the cartilage of the hip joints and knees may cause articular symptoms. Hyperuricemia and gout are common in men with Paget's disease, and calcific periarthritis may occur.

Sarcoma is the dread complication. The incidence is probably no greater than 1 percent, although higher incidence has been noted in series that include many patients with polyostotic involvement. The sarcomas most frequently arise in the femur, humerus, skull, facial bones, and pelvis and rarely in the vertebrae. Pagetic osteosarcomas are lytic in appearance on radiographs in contrast to the sclerotic appearance of radiation-induced osteosarcomas. In about 20 percent the tumors are multicentric. Fibrosarcomas and chondrosarcomas also have been found. Pain and swelling are the common complaints that lead to recognition of the sarcomas. The extent and character of the neoplastic involvement are established by computed tomography and/or magnetic resonance imaging. The level of alkaline phosphatase in the serum of patients with sarcomas usually reflects the activity and extent of the Paget's disease. In occasional patients, an "explosive rise" of the phosphatase level may accompany the growth of the sarcoma, whereas in patients with limited Paget's disease, phosphatase levels may be only slightly elevated and give no clue to the development of the malignant lesion. The prognosis is poor following the development of sarcomas, and ablative surgery is rarely successful. In contrast to the successful treatment of some osteosarcomas in children, chemotherapy has little effect on survival of patients with pagetic osteosarcomas. Reparative granulomas resembling giant cell tumors may cause local destruction, but they do not metastasize.

℞ TREATMENT

Most patients require no treatment, since the disease is localized and does not cause symptoms. Indications for therapy include persistent pain in involved bones, neural compression, rapidly progressive deformity resulting in disabling disturbance of posture and/or gait, high-output congestive heart failure, hypercalcemia, severe hypercalciuria with or without formation of renal stones, repeated fractures or nonunion, and preparation for major orthopedic surgery. Nonsteroidal anti-inflammatory drugs such as *indomethacin*, 25 mg three or four times daily, may relieve pain, especially in the presence of hip involvement. Patients with severe hip or knee pain, unrelieved by analgesics and not responsive to therapy with agents that inhibit bone resorption, are candidates for total joint replacement. Results of the latter procedures are often excellent, although patients with Paget's disease have an increased risk of ectopic bone formation around the operative site. Osteotomies are also useful in patients with bowing deformities of the tibia. In patients who have undergone surgical procedures, early ambulation and adequate fluid intake are important to prevent the development of hypercalciuria and hypercalcemia.

Potent bisphosphonates can inhibit bone resorption and are safe and usually well tolerated. Cytotoxic drugs such as plicamycin and dactinomycin no longer have a place in therapy. Of the bisphosphonates etidronate, in dosages up to 20 mg/kg body weight per day, is moderately effective in reducing bone resorption and producing clinical improvement, but in many patients responses are incomplete. Furthermore, osteomalacia may occur as a complication of therapy. Etidronate is no longer the bisphosphonate of choice. The newer bisphosphonates such as alendronate, pamidronate, risendronate, and tiludronate are more potent than etidronate and do not produce mineralization defects. Two of these compounds, pamidronate for intravenous use and alendronate for oral administration, are approved for use in the United States. Alendronate is approximately 700-fold more potent than etidronate. All bisphosphonates act to inhibit bone resorption, possibly by adsorbing to the surface of the calcium/phosphate mineral phase of bone and inhibiting osteoclast function. Alternatively, the bisphosphonates may inhibit osteoclasts indirectly through actions on osteoblasts.

The bisphosphonates as a class are poorly absorbed from the gastrointestinal tract, and alendronate should be given orally with water after an overnight fast 30 to 60 min before breakfast; the dose is 40 mg/d for 6 months. Gastric irritability and rarely esophageal ulcerations may occur. Pamidronate is given intravenously at a dose of 30 mg/d as an infusion in 5% glucose in water or normal saline over 4 h on three successive days. Responses are usually rapid with decreases in urinary excretion of hydroxyproline and pyridinium cross-link compounds within days to weeks, followed by a fall in levels of serum alkaline phosphatase. Flulike symptoms accompanied by fever may occur but usually subside rapidly.

Patients given bisphosphonates should also be given daily calcium supplements of 1 to 1.5 g and approximately 400 IU of vitamin D. Clinical and biochemical improvement often lasts for more than a year after bisphosphonate therapy. Clinical evaluation and assessment of alkaline phosphatase levels at 3-month intervals are useful for assessing the need for retreatment. Radiographs at 6-month intervals may be indicated for evaluation of lytic lesions, which usually heal with these agents.

It is almost certain that calcitonin has been or will be replaced by bisphosphonates such as alendronate or pamidronate for primary treatment of severe disease, but calcitonin may still be useful in patients who cannot tolerate alendronate because of gastrointestinal side effects or who prefer to avoid intravenous therapy with pamidronate. The administration of porcine, salmon, and human *calcitonins* for prolonged periods to pagetic patients causes a decrease in plasma alkaline phosphatase and in urinary hydroxyproline excretion. Treatment with calcitonin causes variable decrease in bone pain due to suppression of the pagetic lesion, replacement of pagetic bone with normal lamellar bone, and an independent, centrally mediated analgesic effect. Calcitonin also induces improvement in neurologic symptoms and a decrease in elevated cardiac output. Some patients have not continued to respond to porcine and salmon calcitonins, possibly because of the development of neutralizing antibodies. These individuals usually continue to exhibit a satisfactory response to human calcitonin. In others, the development of secondary hyperparathyroidism has been postulated as the cause for a diminished response, although this cannot account for resistance in all cases. The calcitonins are probably most useful in patients with pain in areas of pagetic involvement not due to associated joint disease. The dose of salmon calcitonin is 50 to 100 MRC units daily given subcutaneously. In most cases, it is possible to reduce the dose to three times weekly. In severe cases, alkaline phosphatase levels decrease, but not to the normal range. The disorder relapses after weeks or months when the calcitonin is discontinued. Some patients develop a sensation of warmth and/or nausea 30 min to several hours after injection. This may occur after initiating treatment or after months or years of therapy. The etiology is unknown, but the symptoms may be severe enough to discontinue the medication. Nasal spray formulations of calcitonin can be administered at doses of 200 IU/d.

Although the bisphosphonates and calcitonins act primarily to decrease bone resorption, the rate of new bone formation subsequently falls. As a result, the state of high bone turnover is shifted to a state of lower turnover, where rates of formation and resorption are still apparently geared to each other. In this lower turnover state, collagen fibers of the bone matrix are deposited in a more orderly fashion similar to normal bone.

See Chap 61, Agents affecting calcification and bone turnover, in Goodman & Gilman's The Pharmacological Basis of Therapeutics, *9th ed, New York, McGraw-Hill, 1996.*

BIBLIOGRAPHY

BONE HG, KLEEREKOPER M: Clinical review 39: Paget's disease of bone. J Clin Endocrinol Metab 75:1179, 1992
GARNERO P et al: Different effects of bisphosphonate and estrogen therapy on free and peptide-bound bone cross-links excretion. J Bone Mineral Res 10:641, 1995
HARINCK HIJ et al: Relation between signs and symptoms in Paget's disease of bone. Q J Med 226:133, 1986
HEALEY JH, BUSS D: Radiation and pagetic osteogenic sarcoma. Clin Orthop Rel Res 270:128, 1991
HUVOS AG et al: Osteogenic sarcoma associated with Paget's disease of bone: A clinicopathologic study of 65 patients. Cancer 52:1489, 1983
KHAN SA et al: Paget's disease of bone and unvaccinated dogs. Bone 19:47, 1996
LIN JH: Bisphosphonates: A review of their pharmacokinetic properties. Bone 18:75, 1996
MCDONALD DJ, SIM FH: Total hip arthroplasty in Paget's disease. J Bone Joint Surg 69A:766, 1987
MEE AP et al: Generation of multinucleated osteoclast-like cells from canine bone marrow: Effects of canine distemper virus. Bone 17:47, 1995
NAGANT DE DEUXCHAISNES C, KRANE SM: Paget's disease of bone: Clinical and metabolic observations. Medicine 43:233, 1964
REBEL A*(ed): Symposium on Paget's disease. Clin Orthop 217:1, 1987*
ROODMAN GR et al: Interleukin 6: A potential autocrine/paracrine factor in Paget's disease of bone. J Clin Invest 89:46, 1992
SINGER FR, KRANE SM: Paget's disease of bone, in *Metabolic Bone Disease,* LV Avioli, SM Krane (eds). Philadelphia, Saunders, 1990, pp 546–615
SIRIS E et al: Comparative study of alendronate versus etidronate for the treatment of Paget's disease of bone. J Clin Endocrinol Metab 81:961, 1996
WALLACH S (ed): *Paget's Disease of Bone.* New York, Elsevier 1991, pp 1–313

359

Stephen M. Krane, Alan L. Schiller

HYPEROSTOSIS, FIBROUS DYSPLASIA, AND OTHER DYSPLASIAS OF BONE AND CARTILAGE

HYPEROSTOSIS

A number of disease states have in common an increase in the mass of bone per unit volume (hyperostosis) (Table 359-1). Such increase in bone mass is detected radiologically as increased density of the bone, often associated with disturbance in the architecture of the tissue. In the absence of quantitative histomorphometric data, it is usually not possible to distinguish an increase in bone mass due to excessive formation of new bone from that due to decreased resorption of bone already formed. When bone deposition is rapid, the new bone may be of the woven type, but if the process is more chronic, true lamellar bone is formed. The additional bone may be located at the periosteum, within the compact bone of the cortex, or in the trabeculae of the cancellous regions. In the medullary area, the new bone is deposited on and between the trabeculae and encroaches on the medullary spaces. Such responses are seen in areas adjacent to tumors or in association with infection. In some diseases, the increase in bone mass may be spotty, as in osteopoikilosis, whereas in others, most of the skeleton may be involved, as in the malignant form of osteopetrosis in children. The increase in mass usually is not due to an excessive amount of

Table 359-1

Causes of Hyperostosis
Endocrine disorders
Primary hyperparathyroidism
Hypothyroidism
Acromegaly
Radiation osteitis
Chemical poisoning
Fluoride
Elemental phosphorus
Beryllium
Arsenic
Vitamin A intoxication
Lead
Bismuth
Osteomalacia
Renal tubular osteomalacia (vitamin D resistance or phosphate diabetes)
Chronic renal glomerular failure
Osteosclerosis (localized) associated with chronic infection
Osteosclerotic phase of Paget's disease
Osteosclerosis associated with carcinomatous metastases, malignant lymphoma, and hematologic disorders (myeloproliferative disorders, sickle cell disease, leukemia, multiple myeloma, systemic mastocytosis)
Osteosclerosis of erythroblastosis fetalis
Osteopetrosis
Infantile (malignant, autosomal recessive form)
Adult (benign, dominant form)
Intermediate form with carbonic anhydrase II deficiency and renal tubular acidosis
Unclassified disorders
Pyknodysostosis
Osteomyelosclerosis
Hyperostosis corticalis generalisata
Hyperostosis generalisata with pachydermia
Hereditary hyperphosphatasia
Progressive diaphyseal dysplasia (osteopathia hyperostotica multiplex infantilis; Camurati-Engelmann disease)
Melorheostosis
Osteopoikilosis
Hyperostosis frontalis interna

mineral relative to matrix, except in disorders where islands of calcified cartilage may persist such as osteopetrosis. (The mineral density of calcified cartilage is greater than that of bone.) In some diseases, such as the osteosclerosis of untreated renal insufficiency, the bone mass and radiodensity may be increased, even though the new bone formed is poorly mineralized and contains widened osteoid seams. Although hyperostosis usually is due to decreased osteoclast function, dysfunction of osteoblasts can also occur. For example, an engineered null mutation of the osteocalcin gene in mice results in a higher bone mass due to increased bone formation without change in bone resorption. It is also of interest that infection of newborn mice produces an osteopetrosis-like phenotype in which osteoblast progenitors appear to induce increased bone formation. In human osteopetrosis of the relatively benign and sporadic type, viral nucleocapsid particles have been found in osteoclasts, and it is possible that viral infection accounts for the excessive bone mass.

Several of these conditions are discussed in more detail in other chapters, although some generalizations are pertinent. Bone that is denser than normal may be seen in the osteitis fibrosa associated with hyperparathyroidism. When the hyperparathyroidism is successfully treated, an abrupt decrease in the rate of bone resorption may lead to the development of areas of bone density greater than in the surrounding skeleton, especially in the healing of brown tumors. In addition, intermittent low levels of parathyroid hormone act directly on osteoblasts to increase bone formation. In hypothyroidism, the rates of both bone formation and resorption may be decreased, but when the balance is in favor of formation bones are of increased density but normal architecture. Increased bone density also occurs in some instances of osteomalacia associated with disturbances in renal tubular function. The increased mass of bone is accompanied by widened osteoid seams, as in untreated chronic renal glomerular insufficiency. In the vertebral bodies the bone appears denser in transverse bands at the upper and lower margins, with a relatively radiolucent center. This "sandwich" appearance is similar to that in osteopetrosis and has been termed by the British the *rugger jersey sign*. Skeletal hyperostosis, including cortical hyperostoses, periostitis, and tendon and ligament ossification, is also a complication of long-term therapy with synthetic retinoids such as isotretinoin.

OSTEOPETROSIS Osteopetrosis (Albers-Schönberg or marble bone disease) is clinically, biochemically, and genetically heterogeneous. Although osteopetrosis has many causes, a defect in bone resorption is always the underlying mechanism. Several inherited forms of osteopetrosis occur in rodents, some of which can be cured by bone marrow transplantation from a normal littermate and are probably due to stem cell defects. The osteopetrosis in *op/op* mice and in *tl/tl* toothless rats is not cured by bone marrow transplantation, however. These animals have few osteoclasts, and those that are present appear to be defective. The *op/op* mice have a defect in the coding region of the gene for colony stimulating factor 1 (CSF-1, also known as M-CSF, the M standing for macrophage), and the skeletal defects in these animals and in *tl/tl* rats can be reversed by treatment with CSF-1. Another form of osteopetrosis has been produced in mice by targeted disruption of the c-*src* gene, which is normally expressed at high levels in osteoclasts; these *src* −/− mice have osteoclasts on bone surfaces but fail to form a ruffled border at the bone-resorbing surface of the cells. Disruption of the c-*fos* gene results in osteopetrosis in which osteoclasts are absent. Human homologues of these rodent diseases have not been described, but the most severe osteopetrosis in human infants is also due to defects in the formation and/or function of osteoclasts. Infantile osteopetrosis is an autosomal recessive trait that is manifested in utero and progresses after birth with anemia, hepatosplenomegaly, hydrocephalus, cranial nerve involvement, and death, often due to infections. Transplantation of bone marrow from normal donors to provide normal osteoclast precursor cells has been successful in several patients, in whom osteopetrotic bone was repopulated with donor osteoclasts that produced radiologic and/or bone-biopsy evidence of bone resorption. One infant received a bone marrow transplant from a brother and had a successful response lasting more than 4 years, although vision was not restored. In other individuals with osteopetrosis, peripheral blood monocyte function is defective. Attempts to stimulate osteoclast formation and/or activity with calcitriol or recombinant interferon γ have resulted in some clinical improvement.

Less fulminant forms of osteopetrosis occur in older children and adults. In some the disorder appears to be sporadic, and in others the osteopetrosis is inherited as an autosomal dominant trait and progresses with age; anemia is not as severe, neurologic abnormalities are not as frequent, and recurrent pathologic fractures are the main feature. Although most common in infants and children, the diagnosis may be made in adults when roentgenograms are obtained because of fractures or unrelated diseases. There is no sex predilection. The inherited adult disorder is heterogeneous. Type I is characterized by increased thickness of the cranial vault, whereas the rugger jersey sign and "endo bones" in the pelvis are features of type II. A defect in modeling of endosteal bone is present in both types, and the remodeling of trabecular bone is also defective in type II osteopetrosis.

An "intermediate" form of autosomal recessive osteopetrosis has been described in kindreds in which the skeletal abnormality is associated with renal tubular acidosis and cerebral calcification. This form is compatible with long survival and is associated with profound impairment of one of the isoenzymes of carbonic anhydrase (carbonic anhydrase II). Carbonic anhydrase II is a major component of the system that generates the acid environment adjacent to the ruffled border of the osteoclast, and deficiency of the enzyme impairs bone resorption. In some instances islands of unresorbed calcified cartilage are encased in bone. The defect in remodeling results in disorganization of bone structure, with thickened cortices and lack of funnelization of metaphyses. Despite increased density, the bone may be abnormal mechanically and can fracture readily. Osteomalacia or rickets is sometimes a component of osteopetrosis in children (Fig. 359-1).

The histologic changes are reflected in roentgenograms (Fig. 359-2), which reveal uniformly dense, sclerotic bone, often with no distinction between the cortical and cancellous regions. In the severe infantile form, there is persistence of the primary spongiosa with central calcified cartilage cores surrounded by woven bone. Osteoclasts may be increased in number but apparently do not function properly. Osteoclasts may be morphologically normal or have loss of the ruffled borders, suggesting that a spectrum of changes may occur. The variability may reflect heterogeneity in this syndrome, as in the osteopetrosis in rodents. The long bones are usually involved, with increased density along the entire shaft. Foci of increased density in the epiphyses may correspond to regions of unresorbed calcified cartilage. The metaphyses have a characteristic clubbed or splayed appearance. Alternating horizontal bands of increased and decreased density in the long bones and vertebrae suggest that the defect is intermittent during periods of growth. The skull, pelvis, ribs, and other bones may be involved. The phalanges and the distal humerus are usually spared.

Encroachment of bone on the marrow cavity, particularly in the severe infantile disorder, is associated with anemia of the myelo-

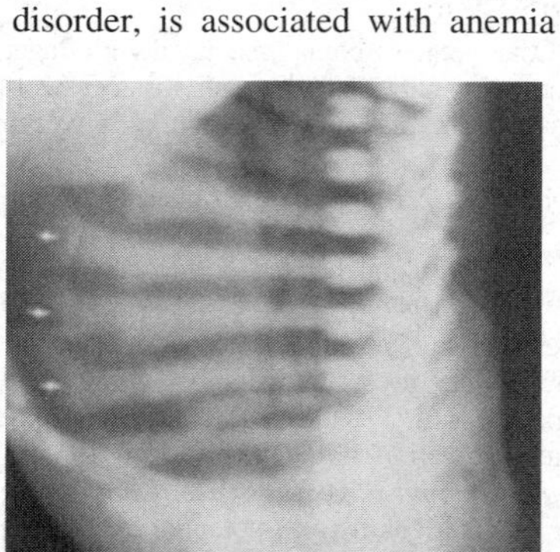

FIGURE 359-1 Lateral roentgenogram of the thorax of a 9-month-old boy with the "malignant" form of osteopetrosis. Note the uniform increase in mineral density of the vertebral bodies and the marked flaring of the ends of the ribs (*arrows*), indicative of rickets.

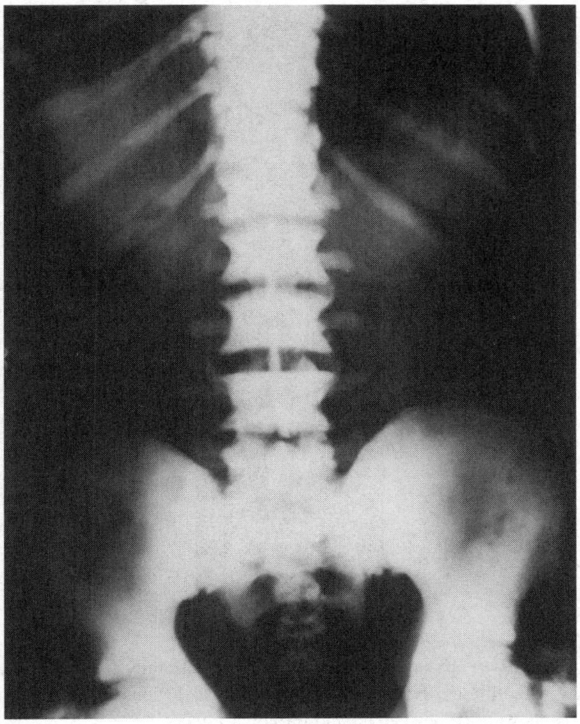

FIGURE 359-2 Roentgenogram of the spine and pelvis of a 55-year-old man with the more benign, dominant form of osteopetrosis.

phthisic type with extramedullary hematopoiesis in liver, spleen, and lymph nodes and enlargement of these organs. Neurologic abnormalities caused by encroachment on cranial nerves include optic atrophy, nystagmus, papilledema, exophthalmos, and impairment of extraocular muscles. Facial paralysis and deafness are frequent; trigeminal lesions and anosmia are less common. In infants, macrocephaly, hydrocephalus, and convulsions may occur, and infections such as osteomyelitis are frequent. Renal tubular acidosis is a feature of the osteopetrosis associated with a deficiency in carbonic anhydrase II.

In the less severe forms, about half of patients have no symptoms, and the disorder is discovered incidentally on roentgenograms. Others present with fractures, bone pain, osteomyelitis, and cranial nerve palsies.

Fractures may occur with trivial trauma. Healing of such fractures is usually slow but satisfactory. When the disease is manifested first in adult life, fractures may be the only clinical problem. Levels of calcium and alkaline phosphatase in the plasma are usually normal in adults, but hypophosphatemia and moderate hypocalcemia may occur in children. Serum acid phosphatase levels are usually increased.

The skeletal defect is not the same in all forms of osteopetrosis, and genetic and biochemical heterogeneity are common. As mentioned, in children with severe osteopetrosis, bone marrow transplantation from HLA-identical siblings has resulted in histologic and radiologic increases in bone resorption and variable improvement in anemia, vision, hearing, and growth and development.

Unfortunately, it is not always possible to find appropriate donors, or patients may not be good candidates for bone marrow transplantation. In patients with the lethal forms of the disorder, calcitriol therapy is associated with the appearance of osteoclasts with normal ruffled borders and other evidence for increased bone resorption.

PYKNODYSOSTOSIS *Pyknodysostosis* is an autosomal recessive form of osteosclerosis that superficially resembles osteopetrosis. It is one of the types of short-limbed dwarfism associated with bone fragility and a tendency to fracture with minimal trauma. Nevertheless, life span is usually normal. In addition to a generalized increase in bone density, features include short stature, separated cranial sutures, hypoplasia of the mandible, kyphoscoliosis and deformities of the trunk, persistence of deciduous teeth, progressive acroosteolysis of the terminal phalanges, high, arched palate, proptosis, blue sclerae,

and a pointed, beaked nose. Patients usually present because of frequent fractures. The responsible gene is located on chromosome 1q21 and encodes cathepsin K, a cysteine proteinase that is expressed in normal osteoclasts and that is mutated in patients with pynknodystostosis.

OSTEOMYELOSCLEROSIS *Osteomyelosclerosis* is a disorder in which the marrow cells are replaced by diffuse fibroplasia, occasionally accompanied by osseous metaplasia and increased skeletal density on roentgenograms. In early stages woven bone may be found in intratrabecular locations, whereas in more advanced stages, woven bone is observed in the medulla. The disorder is probably a phase in the course of the myeloproliferative disorders and is characteristically accompanied by extramedullary hematopoiesis.

Hyperostosis corticalis generalisata (van Buchem's disease) is characterized by osteosclerosis of the skull (base and calvaria), lower jaw, clavicles, and ribs and thickening of the diaphyseal cortices of the long and short bones. Alkaline phosphatase levels in the serum are elevated, and the disorder may be due to increased formation of bone of normal structure. The major manifestations are due to neural compression and consist of optic atrophy, facial paralysis, and perception deafness. In *hyperostosis generalisata with pachydermia* (Uehlinger), the sclerosis is due to increased formation of subperiosteal spongy bone and involves the epiphyses, metaphyses, and diaphyses. Pain, swelling of joints, and thickening of the skin of the lower arms are common.

HEREDITARY HYPERPHOSPHATASIA This disorder is characterized by structural deformities of the skeleton with increased thickness of the calvaria, increased density at the base of the skull, and widening and loss of normal architecture of the shafts and the epiphyses of the long and short bones. The failure to deposit normal bone and the haphazard orientation of lamellae suggest active remodeling that resembles that of Paget's disease. Osteoclasts with multiple nuclei characteristic of Paget's disease and the typical "mosaic" pattern of faceted units of lamellar bone are not found, however. Levels of plasma alkaline phosphatase and urinary excretion of hydroxyproline peptides and other collagen degradation products are increased. The disorder is apparently inherited as an autosomal recessive trait. Calcitonin therapy may be of value.

PROGRESSIVE DIAPHYSEAL DYSPLASIA A disorder in which a symmetric thickening and increased diameter of the diaphyses of long bones occurs, particularly in femurs, tibias, fibulas, radii, and ulnas, has been termed *progressive diaphyseal dysplasia* (Camurati-Engelmann disease). Pain over affected areas, fatigue, abnormal gait, and muscle wasting are the major manifestations. Serum alkaline phosphatase levels may be elevated, and, on occasion, hypocalcemia and hyperphosphatemia may be found. Other abnormalities include anemia, leukopenia, and an elevated erythrocyte sedimentation rate. Clinical and biochemical improvement may result from the use of glucocorticoids.

MELORHEOSTOSIS This rare condition usually begins in childhood and is characterized by a slowly progressive linear hyperostosis in one or more bones of one limb, usually in a lower extremity. All segments of the bone may be involved, with sclerotic areas that have a "flowing" distribution. The involved limb is often extremely painful. Soft tissue masses, not connected to bone, are often mineralized and are composed of osseous or cartilaginous tissue. Other types of soft tissue masses are associated with joint contractures or consist of fibrofatty, lymphatic, or vascular tissue.

OSTEOPOIKILOSIS This benign autosomal dominant trait is usually discovered by chance. It is characterized by dense spots of trabecular bone less than a centimeter in diameter, usually of uniform density, located in the epiphyses and adjacent parts of the metaphyses. All bones may be involved except the skull, ribs, and vertebrae.

HYPEROSTOSIS FRONTALIS INTERNA *Hyperostosis frontalis interna* is an abnormality of the inner table of the frontal bones of the skull consisting of smooth, rounded enostoses covered by dura and projecting into the cranial cavity. These enostoses are usually less than 1 cm at their greatest diameter and usually do not extend posteriorly beyond the coronal suture. The abnormality is found almost exclusively in women, who are frequently obese, hirsute, and have a variety of neuropsychiatric complaints (Morgagni-Stewart-Morel syndrome). The disorder also occurs in women with no obvious illness or particular associated disease. The finding in the skull may be a manifestation of a generalized metabolic disorder.

FIBROUS DYSPLASIA (McCUNE-ALBRIGHT SYNDROME)

The bony lesions of fibrous dysplasia are characterized by proliferation of fibroblast-like cells that in some areas have features of osteoblasts, with production of an extracellular matrix that may be calcified and have the appearance of woven bone. In other areas the cells have features of chondrocytes and produce a cartilage-like extracellular matrix. The lesions of fibrous dysplasia are usually focal and have a radiolucent appearance; they may be monostotic or polyostotic. The disorder occurs with equal frequency in both sexes. Some individuals have distinctive areas of skin pigmentation and precocious puberty (McCune-Albright syndrome). These diverse manifestations are the consequence of postzygotic mutations in the gene encoding the regulatory $G_{\alpha s}$ proteins.

Incidence The monostotic form is the most common type of fibrous dysplasia. The lesions can be asymptomatic, can be associated with local pain, or can predispose to pathologic fracture. Most of the lesions are in the ribs or in the craniofacial bones, especially the maxillas. Other bones that may be affected include metaphyseal or diaphyseal portions of the proximal femurs or tibias. Monostotic fibrous dysplasia is most often diagnosed between 20 and 30 years of age. There are usually no associated skin lesions. Approximately one-quarter of the individuals with the polyostotic form have more than half the skeleton involved by disease. One side of the body may be affected, and the lesions may be distributed segmentally in a limb, particularly in the lower extremities. Craniofacial lesions are present in approximately half of patients with the polyostotic form. Whereas the monostotic form is usually detected in young adults, fractures and skeletal deformities occur in childhood in the polyostotic form; early-onset disease is generally more severe. Lesions, especially monostotic lesions, can become quiescent at puberty and worsen during pregnancy. McCune-Albright syndrome (polyostotic fibrous dysplasia, multiple café au lait spots, and sexual precocity) is more common (10:1) in females. Short stature is due to premature closure of the epiphyses.

Pathology The skeletal lesions of the various forms of fibrous dysplasia are similar, although cartilaginous elements are more common in the polyostotic form. The marrow cavity is filled by gritty, gray-pink, rubbery tissue that replaces the normal cancellous bone. Often, the endosteal cortical surface is scalloped. Histologically, the lesions contain benign-appearing fibroblastic tissue arranged in a loose whorled pattern (Fig. 359-3). The grittiness is due to the presence in the fibrous tissue of irregularly arranged woven bone spicules, most of which lack osteoblastic palisading or rimming but which may contain prominent cement lines. In approximately 10 percent of cases islands

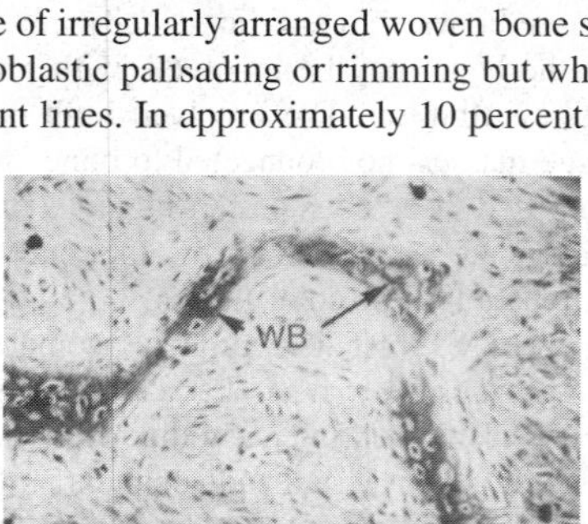

FIGURE 359-3 Photomicrograph of the lesion of fibrous dysplasia. Note spicules of dark-staining woven bone (WB) surrounded by loose fibroblastic tissue.

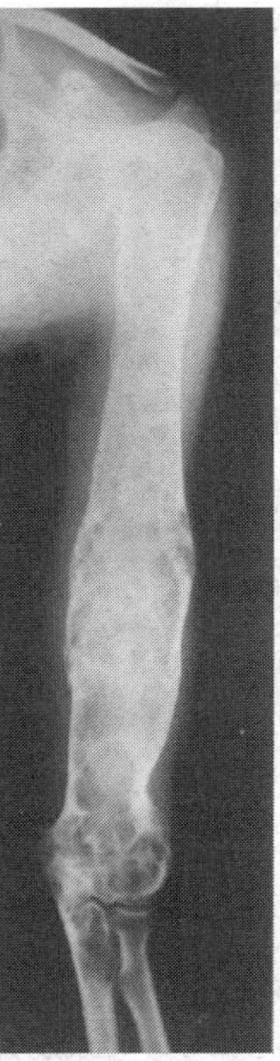

FIGURE 359-4 Roentgenogram of the upper extremity from a 33-year-old woman with fibrous dysplasia of bone. Typical lesions involve the entire humerus as well as the scapula and proximal ulna.

of hyaline cartilage are present, and myxoid tissue may predominate in young patients. Examination by polarized light and with the use of special stains indicates a contiguity of collagen fibers of the osseous and marrow tissue. In the polyostotic form, cystic degeneration may be characterized by the presence of hemorrhage, with hemosiderin-containing macrophages and osteoclast-type giant cells in the periphery of the cyst. Malignant transformation of either monostotic or polyostotic fibrous dysplasia occurs with a frequency of less than 1 percent. The malignant change is usually detected in the third or fourth decade in individuals who have had lesions first identified in childhood. In about one-third of the cases the neoplasms arise in previously irradiated lesions. Ossifying fibroma of long bones is a peculiar fibroosseous cortical lesion that may be a variant of fibrous dysplasia. It is most common in the tibial shaft in teenagers. Although benign, the lesion has a tendency to recur if not adequately excised.

Radiologic Changes The roentgenographic appearance of the lesions is that of a radiolucent area with a well-delineated, smooth or scalloped border, typically associated with focal thinning of the cortex of the bone (Fig. 359-4). Fibrous dysplasia and Paget's disease of bone can cause bones to become larger than normal. The lesions of fibrous dysplasia are not usually cysts in the strict sense, since they are not fluid-filled cavities. They occasionally appear multiloculated. The ground-glass appearance is due to the thin spicules of calcified woven bone. Deformities can include coxa vara, shepherd's-crook deformity of the femur, bowing of the tibia, Harrison's grooves, and protrusio acetabuli. Involvement of facial bones, usually with lesions of increased radiodensity, may create a leonine appearance (leontiasis ossea). Fibrous dysplasia of the temporal bones can cause progressive loss of hearing and obliteration of the external ear canal. Advanced skeletal age in girls is correlated with sexual precocity but can occur in boys without sexual precocity. The lesions tend to spare the epiphyseal regions before puberty, but in older individuals fibrous dysplasia may develop in the epiphyses. Occasionally, a focus of fibrous dysplasia may undergo cystic degeneration with an enormous distortion of the shape of the bone and mimic the so-called aneurysmal bone cyst.

Clinical Picture The clinical course is variable. Skeletal lesions are usually detected because of localized pain, deformities, or fractures. Other symptoms ascribable to bone involvement are headache, seizures, cranial nerve abnormalities, hearing loss, narrowing of the external ear canal, or even spontaneous scalp hemorrhages if there is craniofacial bone disease. On rare occasions the onset of sexual precocity is the first clinical manifestation of the McCune-Albright syndrome. Serum calcium and phosphorus values are usually normal. In approximately one-third of patients with the polyostotic form, bone turnover is increased, as reflected in high levels of serum alkaline phosphatase and increased urinary excretion of collagen breakdown products. In some subjects high cardiac output resembles that in extensive Paget's disease. Widespread disease is usually evident when the disorder is detected, whereas widespread disease usually does not develop when the disease is mild at the outset.

The cutaneous pigmentation in most patients with McCune-Albright syndrome consists of isolated dark-brown to light-brown macules that tend to be located on one side of the midline (Fig. 359-5). The border is usually, although not always, irregular or jagged ("coast of Maine"), in contrast to the smooth borders of the pigmented macules of neurofibromatosis ("coast of California"). As a rule, there are fewer than six of the lesions, which range in size from 1 cm to very large lesions, covering areas such as the back, buttocks, or sacral regions. When the lesions are in the scalp, the overlying hair may be more deeply pigmented than the other hair. Localized alopecia is associated with osteomas of the skin, and such lesions tend to overly skeletal lesions. The pigmentation also tends to be on the same side as the skeletal lesions and actually to overlie them. Occasionally, neurofibromatosis and fibrous dysplasia coexist.

Sexual precocity occurs more commonly in girls than in boys (see also Chaps. 336 and 337). Premature vaginal bleeding and development of axillary and pubic hair and of breasts are the usual features. In the few ovaries that have been examined, no corpora lutea have been seen. When measurements have been reported, the girls have high estrogen levels and low or undetectable gonadotropins. Estrogen receptors have been detected in the bone lesions, and it is therefore not surprising that precocious puberty is not limited to patients with cranial involvement. The characteristic pigmented macules are usual but not invariable. Hyperthyroidism occurs with increased frequency, and rare associations include Cushing's syndrome, acromegaly, hypogonadotropic hypogonadism, and soft tissue myxomas. Hypophosphatemic osteomalacia also may accompany fibrous dysplasia and resembles the disorder associated with other skeletal and nonskeletal tumors. Sexual precocity and adrenal and thyroid hyperfunction in association with fibrous dysplasia are due to autonomous end-organ activity, not to pituitary or hypothalamic dysfunction. Thus, luteinizing hormone (LH) and follicle-stimulating hormone (FSH) levels are low, do not show the expected early pubertal nocturnal rise, and are not responsive to luteinizing hormone–releasing hormone (LHRH). Furthermore, continuous treatment with LHRH agonists does not suppress gonadal steroid secretion or reverse sexual precocity.

As mentioned earlier, this disorder is due to postzygotic mutations in the genes encoding $G_{\alpha s}$ proteins. These mutations cause constitutive activation of the cyclic AMP–protein kinase A signal transduction pathway. Such postzygotic mutations are mosaic and are not present in all cells. In the monostotic disorder, the $G_{\alpha s}$ mutations are present only in the skeletal lesions, whereas with more extensive disease, the mosaicism is more generalized. It has been proposed that the constitutively activated $G_{\alpha s}$ proteins trigger increased expression of the c-*fos* proto-oncogene in bone cells. Animals that overexpress a c-*fos* transgene develop skeletal lesions that resemble those of fibrous dysplasia. It is of interest that the error in Albright's hereditary osteodystrophy (pseudohypoparathyroidism) is the opposite of that found in the McCune-Albright syndrome (fibrous dysplasia). In the former, inactivating mutations in $G_{\alpha s}$ proteins result in *deficient* activity and decreased responsiveness to hormones that function through cyclic AMP–mediated signal transduction pathways.

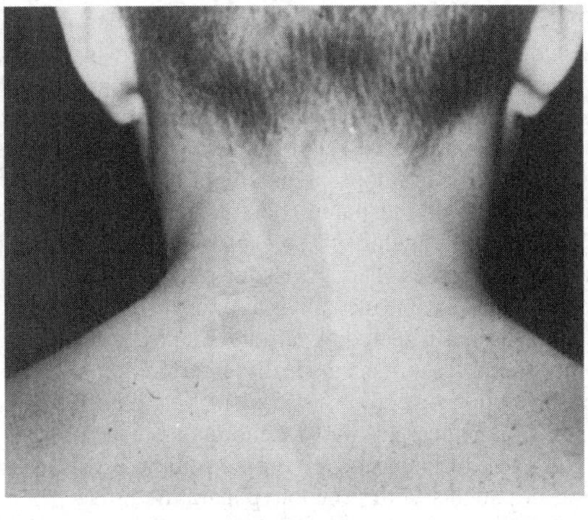

FIGURE 359-5 Typical pigmented café au lait lesion of the skin in an 11-year-old boy with polyostotic fibrous dysplasia. The border has the jagged "coast of Maine" appearance that is characteristic of McCune-Albright's syndrome. Note that the lesion is limited to one side (left) of the body.

Although the lytic lesions of fibrous dysplasia resemble the brown tumors of hyperparathyroidism, the age of the patient, normal calcium levels, increased density of bone in the skull, and areas of cutaneous pigmentation identify the former condition. Fibrous dysplasia and hyperparathyroidism may coexist, however. Neurofibromas may involve bone and produce cutaneous pigmentation as well as nodules in the skin. The pigmented macules of neurofibromatosis are more numerous and more widely distributed than in fibrous dysplasia, usually have smooth borders, and tend to involve areas such as the axillary folds. Other lesions that have roentgenographic features similar to those of isolated fibrous dysplasia are unicameral bone cysts, aneurysmal bone cysts, and nonossifying fibromas. Leontiasis ossea is most often due to fibrous dysplasia, although other disorders also may produce this appearance, such as craniometaphyseal dysplasia, hyperphosphatasia, and, in adults, Paget's disease.

℞ TREATMENT

Fibrous dysplasia is not curable. The skeletal lesions, however, can be improved by orthopedic procedures such as casting, osteotomy with internal fixation, curettage, and bone grafting, depending on the lesion and the age of the patient. Indications for such procedures include progressive deformity, nonunion of fractures, and pain unresponsive to conservative treatment. Calcitonin may be effective in treatment of widespread disease associated with bone pain and high serum alkaline phosphatase levels (see Chap. 358).

OTHER DYSPLASIAS OF BONE AND CARTILAGE

A variety of diseases of bone and cartilage have been called *dystrophies* or *dysplasias*. The *osteochondrodysplasias* are heritable disorders of connective tissue that are characterized by primary abnormalities of cartilage that lead to disturbances in cartilage and bone growth and development. They comprise several hundred distinct entities, which can be distinguished on the basis of clinical, genetic, and radiologic features. The molecular defects in a number of these disorders have been identified utilizing positional cloning and screening of candidate genes. Several of the disorders are due to mutations in collagen genes (see also Chap. 348). For example, mutations in *COL2A1*, the gene that encodes type II collagen, have been identified in Stickler syndrome, Kniest dysplasia, chondrodysplasias associated with osteoarthritis, and spondyloepiphyseal dysplasia. A deletion in *COL10A1*, the gene that encodes type X collagen, has been identified in the Schmid form of metaphyseal chondrodysplasia. A mutation in *COL9A2*, the gene that encodes one chain of the type IX collagen heterotrimer, has been identified in another variant of the Stickler syndrome. Mutations in genes that encode other extracellular matrix proteins can also cause chondrodysplasia. For example, the gene that encodes cartilage oligomeric matrix protein (COMP), a relative of thrombospondin, is the site of mutations in pseudochondrodysplasia. In the Jansen type of chondrodysplasia, a mutation in the PTH receptor gene causes constitutive activity of the receptor, manifested by disordered growth plates and hypercalcemia. Eventually, it should be possible to classify these disorders on the basis of the genetic and biochemical defects. At present, however, a useful clinical classification has been formulated by Rubin based on the consideration of errors in modeling of bone and cartilage (Table 359-2). Other clinical and genetic features form the basis of a classification by Rimoin. Pathologic processes in the skeletal dysplasias may be expressed as a deficiency (hypoplasia) or excess (hyperplasia) in relation to normal development.

SPONDYLOEPIPHYSEAL DYSPLASIA The *spondyloepiphyseal dysplasias* are disorders in which abnormalities of growth occur in various bones, including the vertebrae, pelvis, carpal and tarsal bones, and the epiphyses of tabular bones. On the basis of roentgenographic findings, this group can be divided into (1) those with generalized platyspondyly, (2) those with multiple epiphyseal dysplasias, and (3) those with epiphysometaphyseal dysplasias. *Morquio's syndrome*, in which there is a defect in degradation of glycosaminoglycans (therefore, a "mucopolysaccharidosis"), is inherited as an autosomal recessive trait and is associated with corneal opacities, dental defects, variable disturbances in intellect, and increased urinary excretion of keratosulfate; it belongs in the first group (see also Chap. 347). Other forms of spondyloepiphyseal dysplasia, some of which are accounted for by defects in type II collagen, may not be recognized until late in childhood or young adult life. Flat vertebral bodies are associated with other abnormalities in shape and alignment. The disordered development of the capital femoral epiphyses leads to irregularities in shape and flattening of the femoral heads and early onset of osteoarthritis of the hips.

ACHONDROPLASIA *Achondroplasia* is a physeal dysplasia in which dwarfism results from a decrease in the proliferation of cartilage in the growth plate. This disorder is among the more common types of dwarfism and is inherited as an autosomal dominant trait, although most cases are sporadic and due to new mutations. Histologic sections through the growth plate show a thin zone of cartilage cells with absence or abbreviation of the normal columnar arrangement and zone of provisional calcification, although endochondral ossification may not be completely disorganized. Formation of the primary spongiosa is reduced, since there is often a transverse bar of bone sealing off the plate from further endochondral ossification. Formation and maturation of the secondary ossification centers and articular cartilage are not disturbed. Appositional growth at the metaphysis continues, with resulting flare in this region of the bone; intramembranous bone formation at the periosteum is normal. The abnormal proliferation at the growth plate, leaving other areas relatively unaffected in the tubular bones, causes production of short bones that are proportionately thick. The length of the spine is almost always normal. The appearance of short limbs, particularly the proximal portions, with a normal trunk is characteristically accompanied by a large head, a saddle nose, and an exaggerated lumbar lordosis. The disease is usually recognized at birth. Those who survive infancy usually have normal mental and sexual development, and life span may be normal. Spinal deformity nevertheless may lead to a cord compression and nerve root encroachment, especially in those with kyphoscoliosis. Homozygous achondroplasia is a more serious disorder and a cause of neonatal death.

The gene for achondroplasia has been mapped to chromosome 4p, and the responsible gene encodes the fibroblast growth factor (FGF) receptor 3 (FGFR3). The responsible mutation causes the substitution of an arginine for a glycine in the transmembrane domain of FGFR3 and is believed to cause a gain of function, implying that FGF normally acts via the FGFR3 to inhibit chondrocyte proliferation in the growth plate. Indeed, construction of a null mutation in the *FGFR3* gene in mice causes increased growth in the physis. Mutations in other domains of the *FGFR3* gene have been described in lethal thanaphoric dwarfism. In several types of the so-called craniosynostosis syndromes (Pfeiffer, Crouzon, Jackson-Weiss, and Apert syndromes), mutations have been identified in the *FGFR1* or *FGFR2* genes.

ENCHONDROMATOSIS (DYSCHONDROPLASIA, OLLIER'S DISEASE) This is also a disorder of the growth plate in which the hypertrophic cartilage is not resorbed and ossified normally. It results in masses of cartilage with disorderly arrangement of the chondrocytes showing variable proliferative and hypertrophic changes. These masses are located in the metaphyses in close association with the growth plate in children but may be diaphyseal in teenagers and young adults. The disorder is usually recognized in childhood by the appearance of deformities or retardation in growth. The most common sites of involvement are the ends of long bones, usually in the region where rate of growth is most marked. The pelvis is often involved, but ribs, sternum, and skull are seldom affected. There is also a tendency toward unilateral involvement. Chondrosarcoma develops occasionally in the enchondromata. Granulosa cell tumors of the ovary may occur. The association of enchondromatosis and cavernous hemangiomata in the soft tissues including the skin is known as *Maffucci's syndrome*.

MULTIPLE EXOSTOSES (DIAPHYSEAL ACLASIS OR OSTEOCHONDROMATOSIS) This is a disorder of the metaphysis, inherited as an autosomal dominant character, in which areas of the growth plate become displaced, presumably by growing through a defect in the perichondrium or so-called ring of Ranvier. The spongiosa forms within the mass as vessels invade the cartilage. Therefore, the diagnostic radiographic finding is the direct continuity of the mass to the marrow cavity of the parent bone with absence of underlying cortex. Usually the growth of these exostoses ceases when growth of the adjacent plate ceases. The lesions may be solitary or multiple and are usually located in the metaphyseal areas of long bones, with the apex of the exostosis directed toward the diaphysis. Often the lesions produce no symptoms, but occasionally, interference with the function of a joint or tendon or compression of nerves may result. Dwarfism may occur. The metacarpals may be shortened, resembling those seen in Albright's hereditary osteodystrophy. Multiple exostoses are sometimes seen in patients with pseudohypoparathyroidism.

An exostosis may suddenly begin to enlarge long after growth should have ceased, and rarely, chondrosarcomas may develop from the cartilage cap of an exostosis. Although pregnancy may stimulate growth of an exostosis that clinically may mimic malignancy, the lesion

Table 359-2

Working Classification of Bone Dysplasias

Epiphyseal dysplasias
Epiphyseal hypoplasias
Failure of articular cartilage: spondyloepiphyseal dysplasia congenita and tarda
Failure of ossification of center: multiple epiphyseal dysplasia congenita and tarda
Epiphyseal hyperplasia
Excess of articular cartilage: dysplasia epiphysialis hemimelica
Physeal (growth plate) dysplasias
Cartilage hypoplasias
Failure of proliferating cartilage: achondroplasia congenita and tarda
Failure of hypertrophic cartilage: metaphyseal dysostosis congenita and tarda
Cartilage hyperplasias
Excess of proliferating cartilage: hyperchondroplasia
Excess of hypertrophic cartilage: enchondromatosis
Metaphyseal dysplasias
Metaphyseal hypoplasias
Failure to form primary spongiosa: hypophosphatasia congenita and tarda
Failure to absorb primary spongiosa: osteopetrosis congenita and tarda
Failure to absorb secondary spongiosa: craniometaphyseal dysplasia congenita and tarda
Metaphyseal hyperplasia
Excessive spongiosa: familial exostosis
Diaphyseal dysplasias
Diaphyseal hypoplasias
Failure of periosteal bone formation: osteogenesis imperfecta congenita and tarda
Failure of endosteal bone formation: idiopathic osteoporosis
Diaphyseal hyperplasias
Excessive periosteal bone formation: Engelmann's disease
Excessive periosteal bone formation: hyperphosphatasia

merely undergoes exuberant endochondral ossification and cartilage hyperplasia without malignant changes.

A gene that covers a chromosomal breakpoint has been identified in two families with multiple exostoses. The *EXT* gene probably functions normally as a tumor suppressor, and mutations in *EXT* could contribute both to the development of the exostoses and to malignant transformation to chondrosarcoma that sometimes occurs.

RELAPSING POLYCHONDRITIS See Chap. 326.

TIETZE'S SYNDROME (COSTOCHONDRAL SYNDROME) See Chap. 326.

BIBLIOGRAPHY

HYPEROSTOSIS

Benli IT et al: Epidemiological, clinical and radiological aspects of osteopoikilosis. J Bone Joint Surg 74B:504, 1992

Bollersley J et al: Structural and histomorphometric studies of iliac crest trabecular and cortical bone in autosomal dominant osteopetrosis: A study of two radiological types. Bone 10:19, 1989

Byers PH et al: Research perspectives in heritable disorders of connective tissue. Matrix 12:333, 1992

Caudle RJ et al: Melorheostosis of the hand: A case report with long-term follow-up. J Bone Joint Surg 69A:1229, 1987

Chan Y-L et al: Dialysis osteodystrophy: A study involving 94 patients. Medicine 64:296, 1985

Coindre JM et al: Histomorphometric analysis of sclerotic bone from idiopathic myeloid metaplasia (nine cases). J Pathol 144:163, 1984

Crisp AJ, Brenton DP: Engelmann's disease of bone—a systemic disorder? Ann Rheum Dis 41:183, 1982

DiGiovanna JJ et al: Extraspinal tendon and ligament calcification associated with long-term therapy with etretinate. N Engl J Med 315:1177, 1986

Edelson JG et al: Pycnodysostosis: Orthopedic aspects with a description of 14 new cases. Clin Orthop 280:263, 1992

Einhorn TA et al: Hyperphosphatasemia in an adult: Clinical, roentgenographic, and histomorphometric findings and comparison to classical Paget's disease. Clin Orthop 204:253, 1986

Genant HK et al: Osteosclerosis in primary hyperparathyroidism. Am J Med 59:104, 1975

Goldman AB et al: Case report 778. Skeletal Radiol 22:206, 1993

Jaccobson HG: Dense bone—too much bone: Radiological considerations and differential diagnosis, part II. Skeletal Radiol 13:97, 1985

Johnson CC et al: Osteopetrosis: A clinical, genetic, metabolic and morphologic study of the dominantly inherited benign form. Medicine 47:149, 1968

Kaplan FS et al: Successful treatment of infantile malignant osteopetrosis by bone-marrow transplantation. J Bone Joint Surg 70A:617, 1988

Kraemer KH et al: Prevention of skin cancer in xeroderma pigmentosum with the use of oral isotretinoin. N Engl J Med 318:1633, 1988

Kuivaniemi H et al: Mutations in collagen genes; causes of rare and some common diseases in humans. FASEB J 5:2052, 1991

Shapiro F et al: Variable osteoclast appearance in human infantile osteopetrosis. Calcif Tissue Int 43:67, 1988

Sheldon J et al: Engelmann's disease (progressive diaphyseal dysplasia): A review and presentation of two cases with abnormal phosphate retention. Metab Bone Dis Rel Res 2:307, 1981

Silve C: Hereditary hypophosphatasia and hyperphosphatasia. Curr Opin Rheumatol 6:336, 1994

Singer FR: Osteopetrosis. Semin Nephrol 12:191, 1992

Sly WS et al: Carbonic anhydrase II deficiency in 12 families with the autosomal recessive syndrome of osteopetrosis with renal tubular acidosis and cerebral calcification. N Engl J Med 313:139, 1985

Thompson RC Jr et al: Hereditary hyperphosphatasia. Am J Med 47:209, 1969

Van Buchem FSP et al: Hyperostosis corticalis generalisata. Am J Med 33:387, 1962

Whyte MP, Murphy WA: Osteopetrosis and other sclerosing bone disorders, in *Metabolic Bone Disease*, LV Avioloi, SM Krane (eds). Philadelphia, Saunders, 1990, pp 616–658

Wulfsberg EA et al: Chondrodysplasia punctata: A boy with X-linked recessive chondrodysplasia punctata due to an inherited X-Y translocation with a current classification of these disorders. Am J Med Genet 43:823, 1992

FIBROUS DYSPLASIA

Albright FA et al: Syndrome characterized by osteitis fibrosa disseminata, areas of pigmentation and endocrine dysfunction, with precocious puberty in females. Report of five cases. N Engl J Med 216:727, 1937

Benedict PH et al: Melanotic macules in Albright's syndrome and in neurofibromatosis. JAMA 205:618, 1968

Candeliere GA et al: Increased expression of the c-fos proto-oncogene in bone from patients with fibrous dysplasia. N Engl J Med 332:1546, 1995

Grabias SL, Campbell CJ: Fibrous dysplasia. Orthop Clin North Am 8:771, 1977

Harris WH et al: The natural history of fibrous dysplasia: An orthopaedic, pathological and roentgenographic study. J Bone Joint Surg 44A:207, 1962

Ringel MD et al: Clinical implications of genetic defects in G proteins. The molecular basis of McCune-Albright syndrome and Albright hereditary osteodystrophy. Medicine 75:171, 1996

Stephenson RB et al: Fibrous dysplasia. An analysis of options for treatment. J Bone Joint Surg 69A:409, 1987

Weinstein LS et al: Activating mutations of the stimulatory G protein in the McCune-Albright syndrome. N Engl J Med 325:1688, 1991

Yabul SM et al: Malignant transformation of fibrous dysplasia. A case report and review of the literature. Clin Orthop 281, 1988

OTHER DYSPLASIAS OF BONE AND CARTILAGE

Ahn J et al: Cloning of the putative tumour suppressor gene for hereditary multiple exostoses (EXT1). Nature Genet 2:137, 1995

Akeson WH et al: *Symposium on Heritable Disorders of Connective Tissue.* St. Louis, Mosby, 1982

Erlebacher A et al: Toward a molecular understanding of skeletal development. Cell 80:371, 1995

Gelb BD et al: Pycnodysostosis, a lysosomal disease caused by cathepsin K deficiency. Science 273:1236, 1996

Lee B et al: Identification of the molecular defect in a family with spondyloepiphyseal dysplasia. Science 244: 978, 1989

Mulvihill JJ: Craniofacial syndromes: No such thing as a single gene disease. Nature Genetics 9:101, 1995

Rimoin DL: The chondrodystrophies. Adv Hum Genet 5:1, 1975

Rubin P: *Dynamic Classification of Bone Dysplasias.* Chicago, Year Book, 1964

Sambrook PN et al: Synovial complications of spondylepiphyseal dysplasia of late onset. Arthritis Rheum 31:282, 1988

Shiang R et al: Mutations in the transmembrane domain of FGFR 3 cause the most common genetic form of dwarfism, achondroplasia. Cell 78:335, 1994

Sillence DO et al: Neonatal dwarfism. Pediatr Clin North Am 25:431, 1978

Wicklund CL et al: Natural history study of hereditary multiple exostoses. Am J Med Genet 55:43, 1995

COLOR ATLASES

I. Atlas of Dermatology

Stephen F. Templeton / Thomas J. Lawley

A. Common Skin Diseases and Lesions

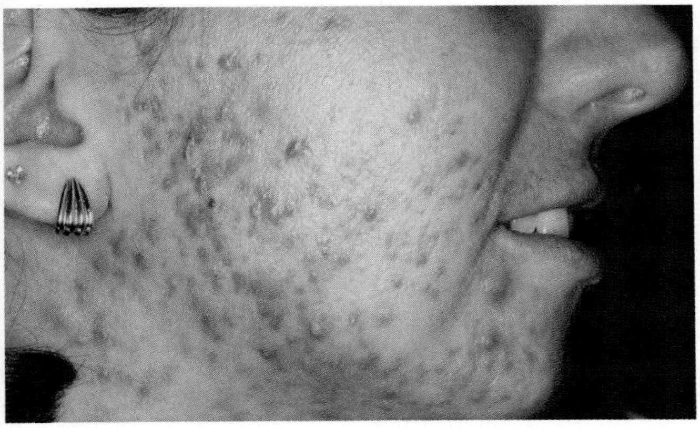

IA-1 **Acne vulgaris** with inflammatory papules, pustules, and comedones

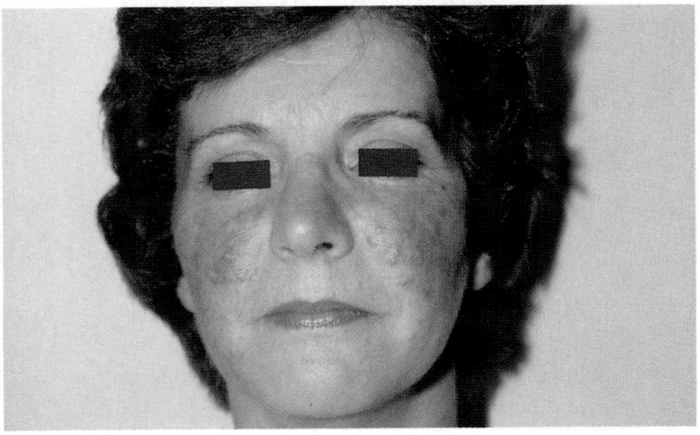

IA-2 **Acne rosacea** with prominent facial erythema, telangiectasias, scattered papules, and small pustules

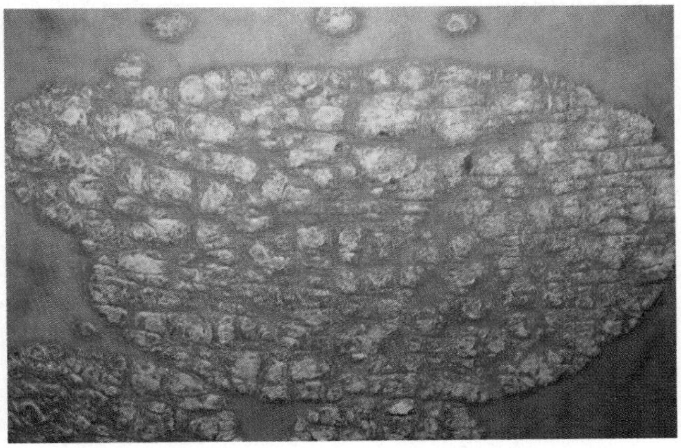

IA-3 **Psoriasis** is characterized by small and large erythematous plaques with adherent silvery scale.

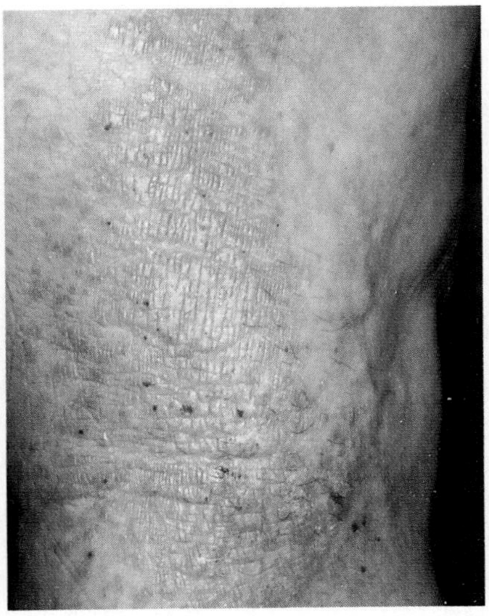

IA-4 **Atopic dermatitis** with excoriated, lichenified plaques in the popliteal fossa

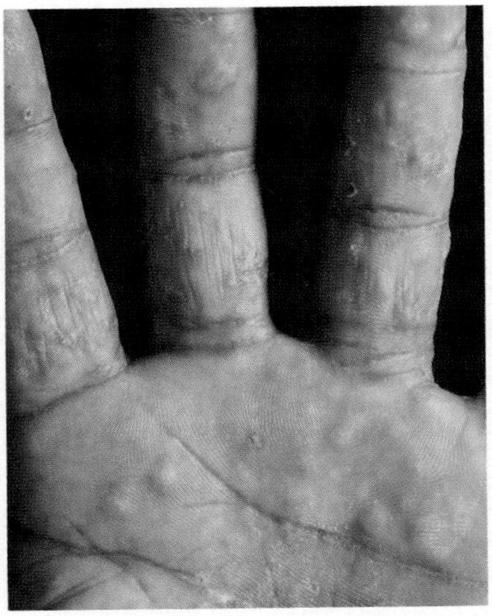

IA-5 **Dyshidrotic eczema,** characterized by deep-seated vesicles and scaling on palms and lateral fingers, is often associated with an atopic diathesis.

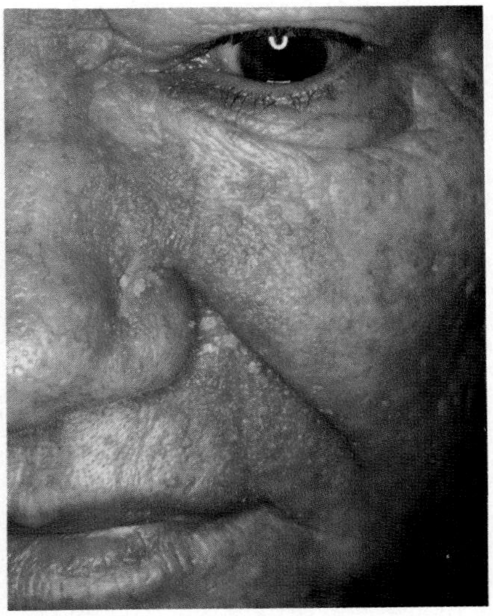

IA-6 **Seborrheic dermatitis** showing central facial erythema with overlying greasy, yellowish scale

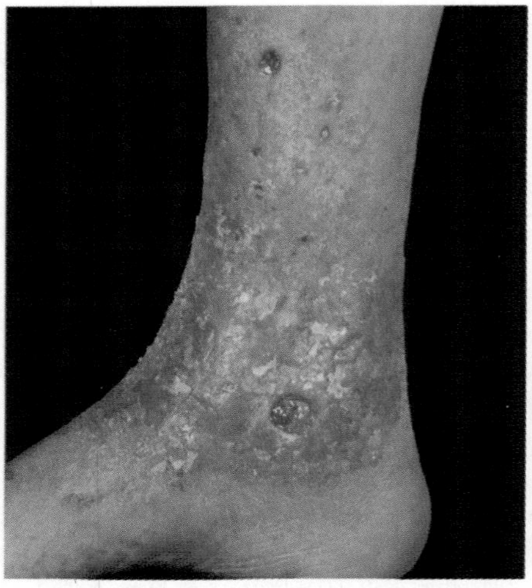

IA-7 **Stasis dermatitis** showing erythematous, scaly, and oozing patches over the lower leg. Several stasis ulcers are also seen in this patient.

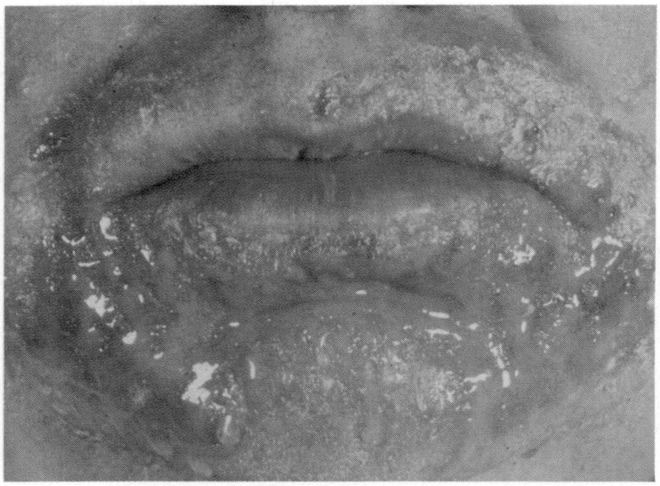

IA-8 **Allergic contact dermatitis,** acute phase, with sharply demarcated, weeping, eczematous plaques in a perioral distribution

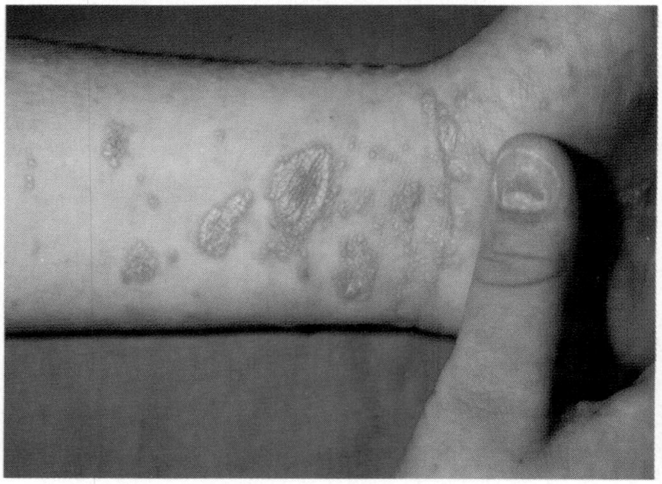

IA-9 **Lichen planus** showing multiple flat-topped, violaceous papules and plaques. Nail dystrophy as seen in this patient's thumbnail may also be a feature.

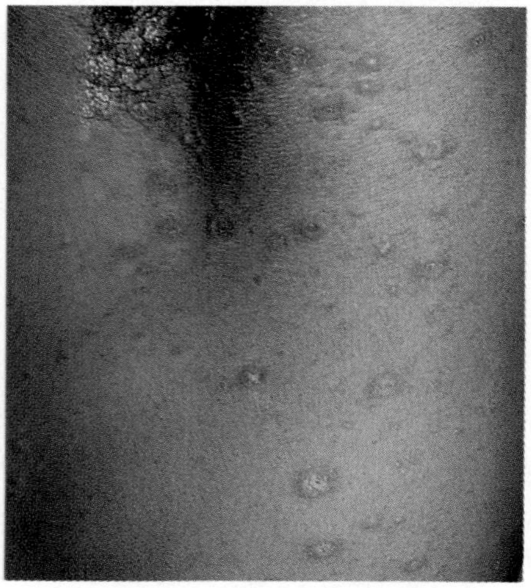

IA-10 **Pityriasis rosea** Multiple round to oval erythematous patches with fine central scale are distributed along the skin tension lines on the trunk.

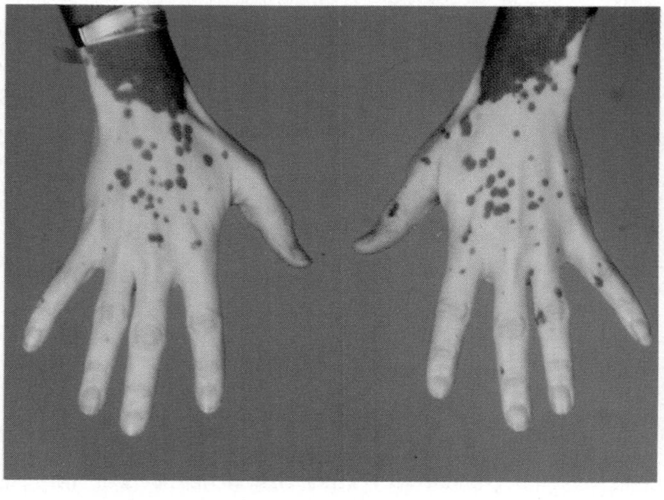

IA-11 **Vitiligo** in a typical acral distribution demonstrating striking cutaneous depigmentation, as a result of loss of melanocytes

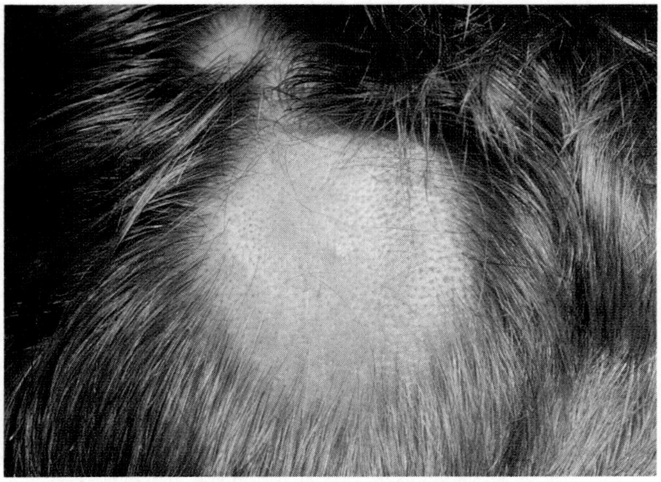

IA-12 **Alopecia areata** characterized by a sharply demarcated circular patch of scalp completely devoid of hairs. Follicular orifices are preserved, indicating a nonscarring alopecia.

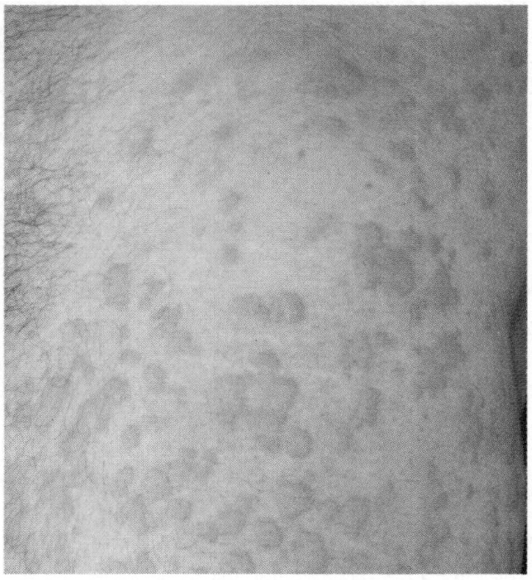

IA-13 **Urticaria** showing characteristic discrete and confluent, edematous, erythematous papules and plaques

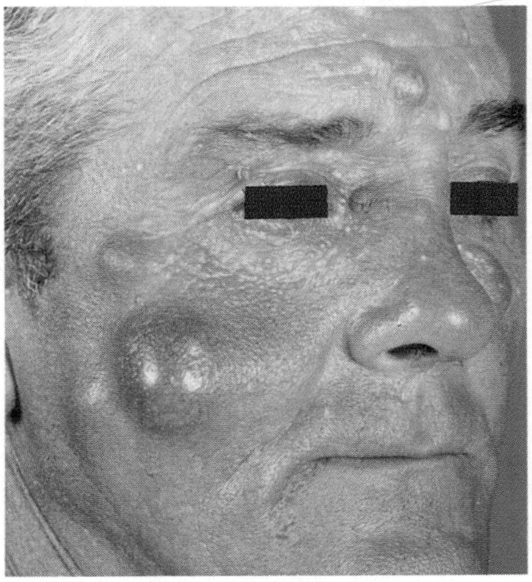

IA-14 **Epidermoid cysts** Several inflamed and noninflamed firm, cystic nodules are seen in this patient. Often a patulous follicular punctum is observed on the overlying epidermal surface.

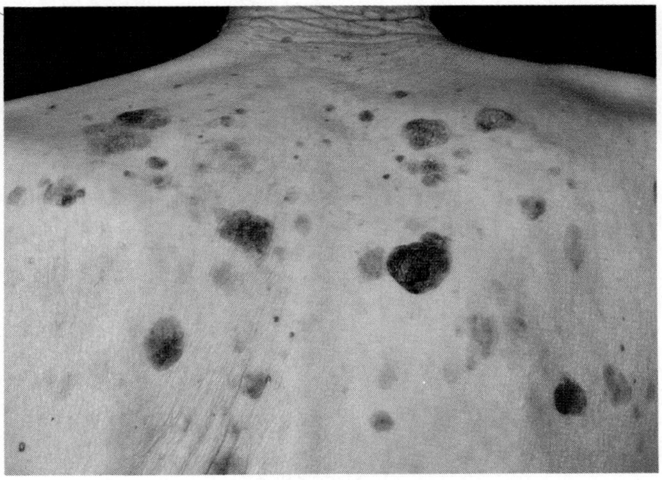

IA-15 **Seborrheic keratoses** are seen as "stuck on," waxy, verrucous papules and plaques with a variety of colors ranging from light tan to black.

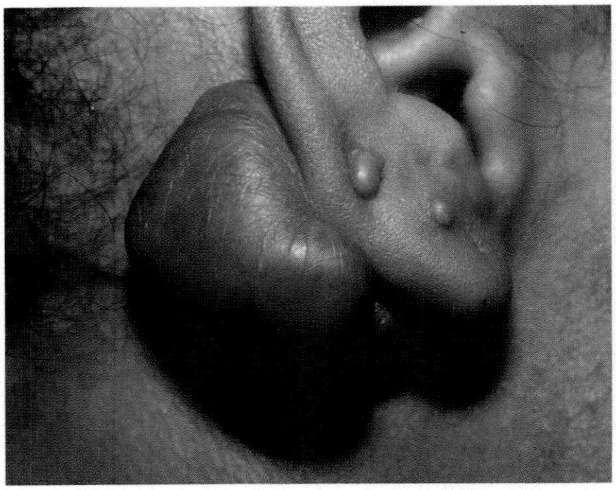

IA-16 **Keloids** resulting from ear piercing, with firm exophytic flesh-colored to erythematous nodules of scar tissue.

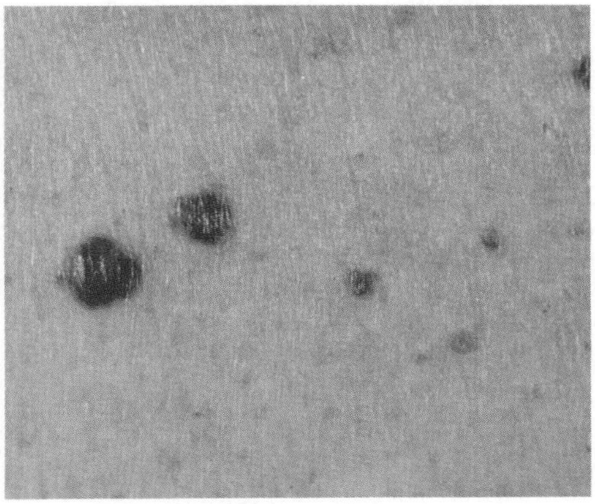

IA-17 **Cherry hemangiomas** are very common and arise in middle-aged to older adults. They are characterized by multiple erythematous to dark-purple papules usually located on the trunk.

B. Cutaneous Neoplasms

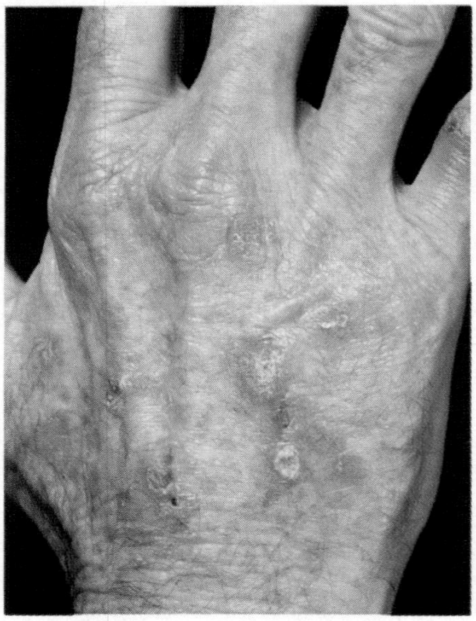

IB-18 **Actinic keratoses** consist of hyperkeratotic erythematous papules and patches on sun-exposed skin. They arise in middle-aged to older adults and have some potential for malignant transformation.

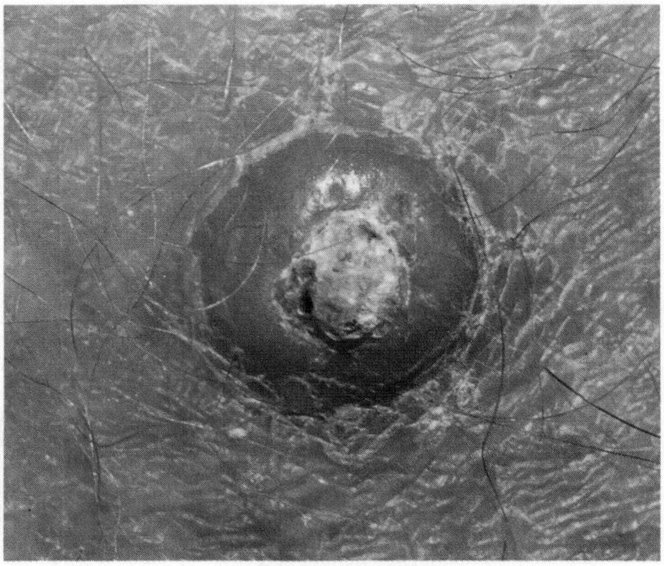

IB-19 **Keratoacanthoma** is a low-grade squamous cell carcinoma that presents as an exophytic nodule with central keratinous debris.

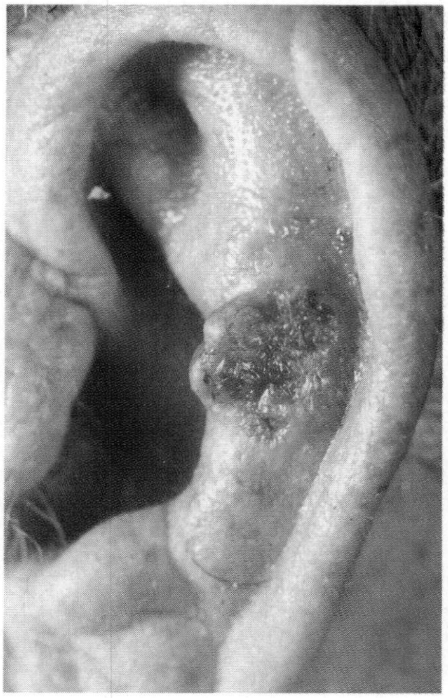

IB-20 **Basal cell carcinoma** showing central ulceration and a pearly, rolled, telangiectatic tumor border

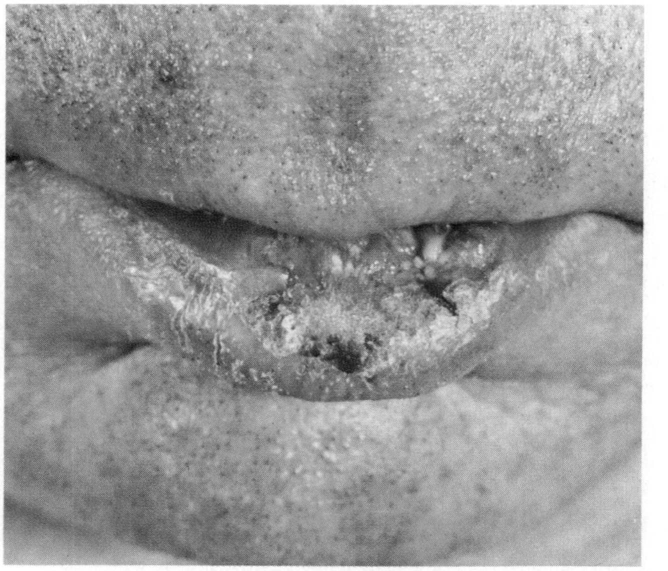

IB-21 **Squamous cell carcinoma** seen here as a hyperkeratotic crusted and somewhat eroded plaque on the lower lip. Sun-exposed skin such as the head, neck, hands, and arms are other typical sites of involvement.

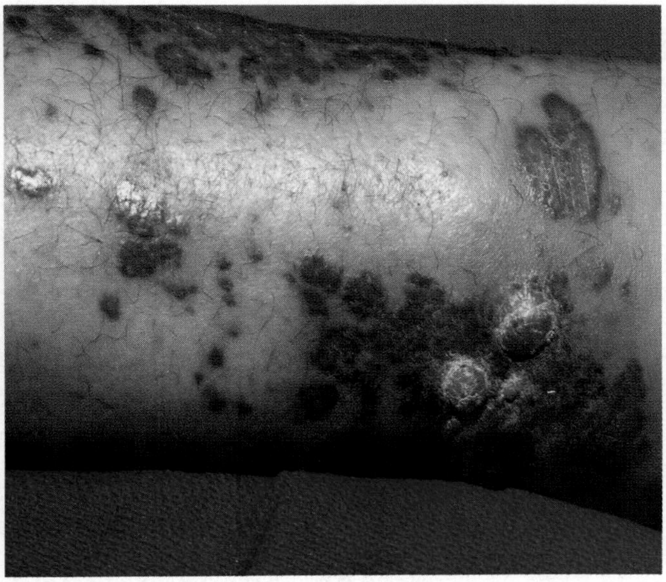

IB-22 **Kaposi's sarcoma** in a patient with AIDS demonstrating patch, plaque, and tumor stages

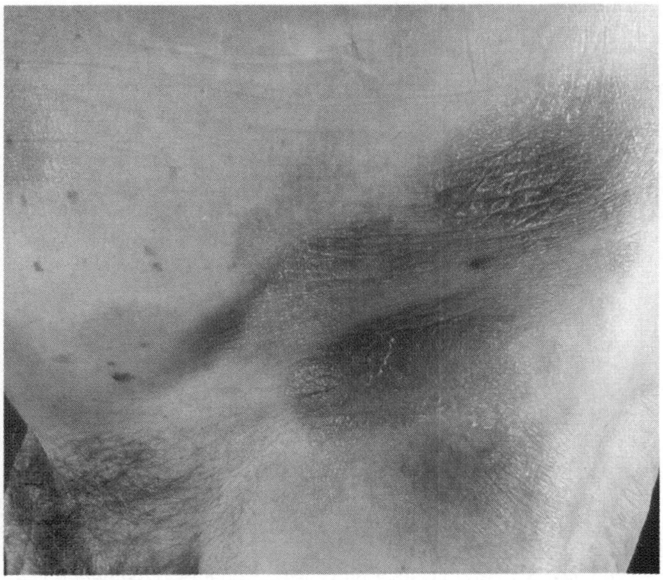

IB-23 **Mycosis fungoides** is a cutaneous T cell lymphoma, and plaque stage lesions are seen in this patient.

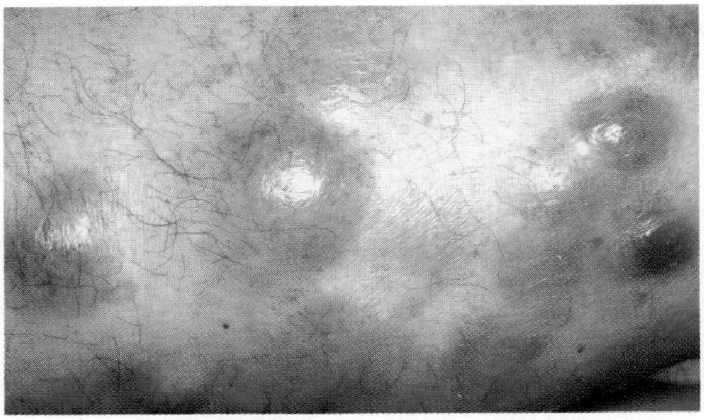

IB-24 **Non-Hodgkin's lymphoma** involving the skin with typical violaceous, "plum-colored" nodules

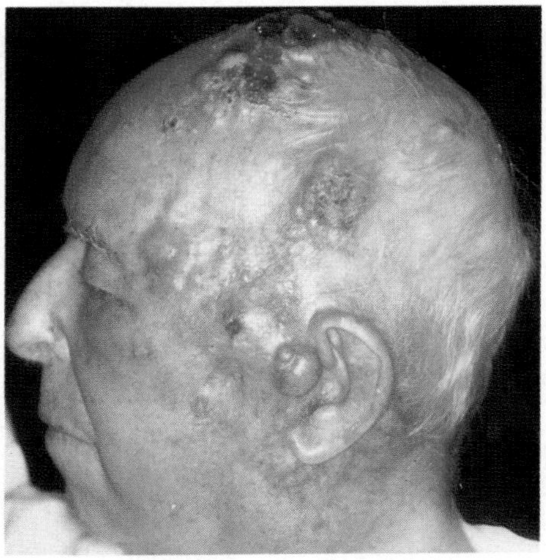

IB-25 **Metastatic carcinoma** to the skin is characterized by inflammatory, often ulcerated dermal nodules.

C. Pigmented Lesions—Benign and Malignant

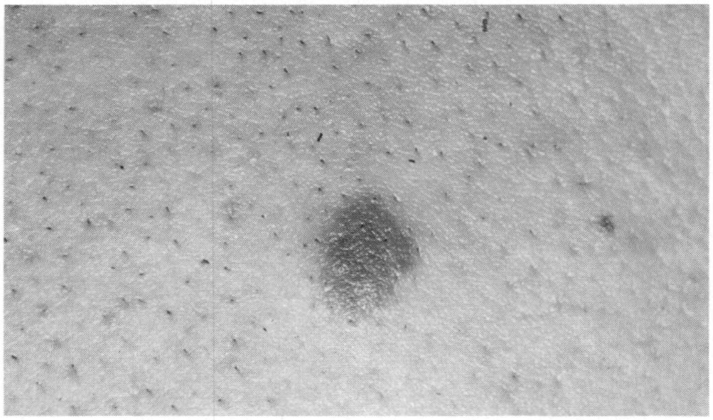

IC-26 **Nevus** Nevi are benign proliferations of nevomelanocytes characterized by regularly shaped hyperpigmented macules or papules of a uniform color.

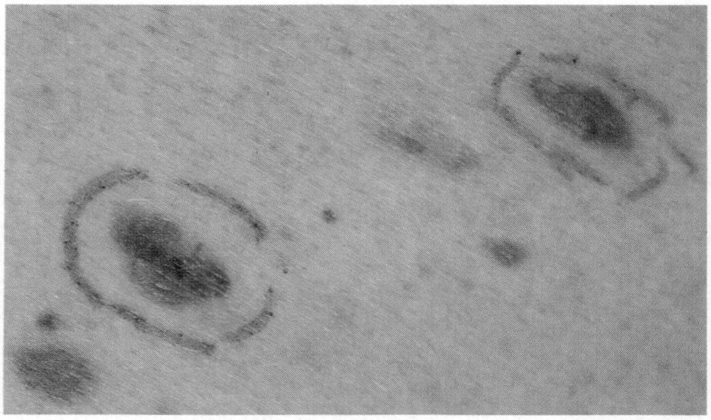

IC-27 **Dysplastic nevi** are irregularly pigmented and shaped nevomelanocytic lesions that may be associated with familial melanoma.

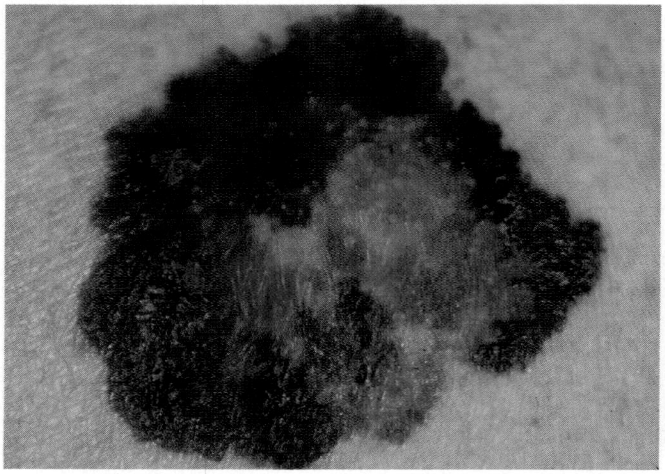

IC-28 **Superficial spreading melanoma** is the most common type of malignant melanoma and demonstrates color variegation (black, blue, brown, pink, and white) and irregular borders.

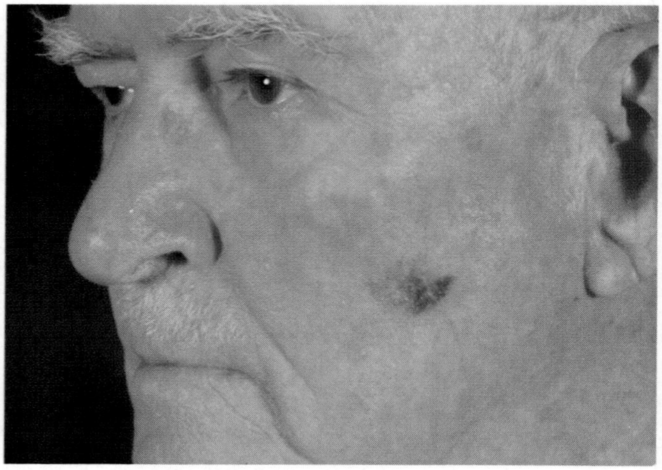

IC-29 **Lentigo maligna melanoma** occurs on sun-exposed skin as a large, hyperpigmented macule or plaque with irregular borders and variable pigmentation.

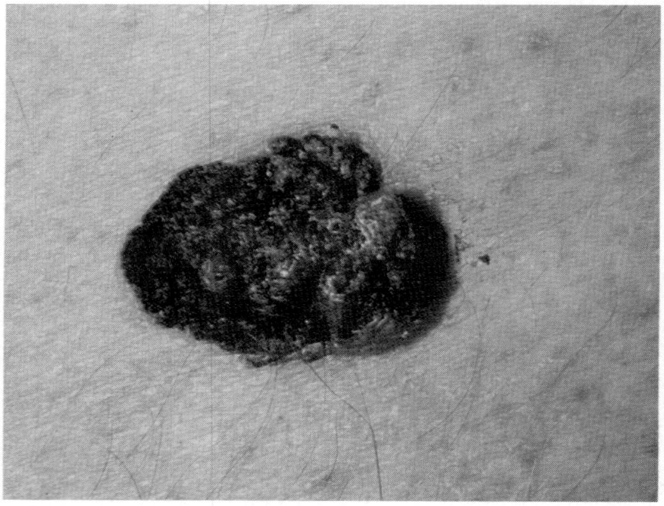

IC-30 **Nodular melanoma** most commonly manifests itself as a rapidly growing, often ulcerated or crusted black nodule.

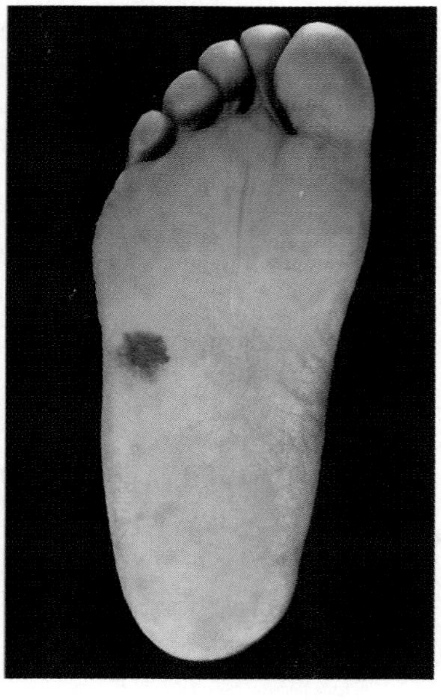

IC-31 **Acral lentiginous melanoma** is more common in blacks, Asians, and Hispanics and occurs as an enlarging hyperpigmented macule or plaque on the palms and soles. Lateral pigment diffusion is present.

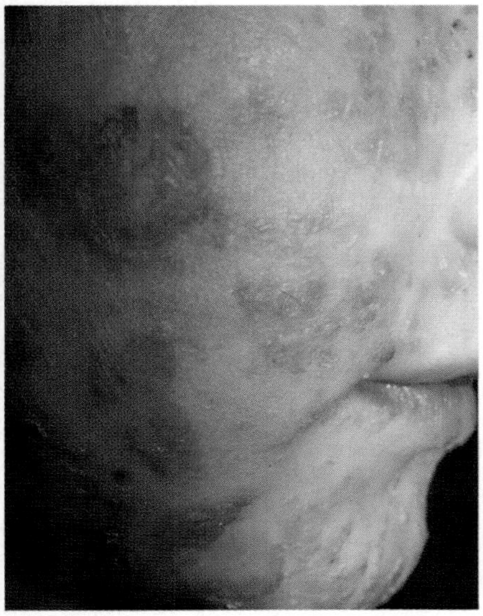

ID-32 **Impetigo contagiosa** is a superficial streptococcal or *S. aureus* infection consisting of honey-colored crusts and erythematous weeping erosions. Occasionally bullous lesions may be seen.

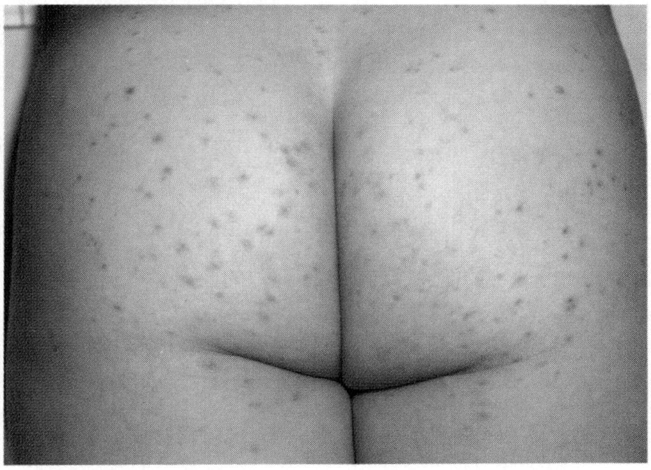

ID-33 **Folliculitis** is a bacterial infection of hair follicles and is seen as erythematous follicular papules and pustules.

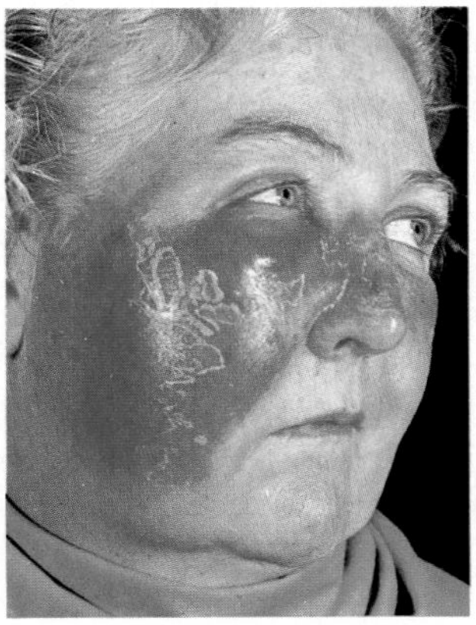

ID-34 **Erysipelas** is a streptococcal infection of the superficial dermis and consists of well-demarcated, erythematous, edematous, warm plaques.

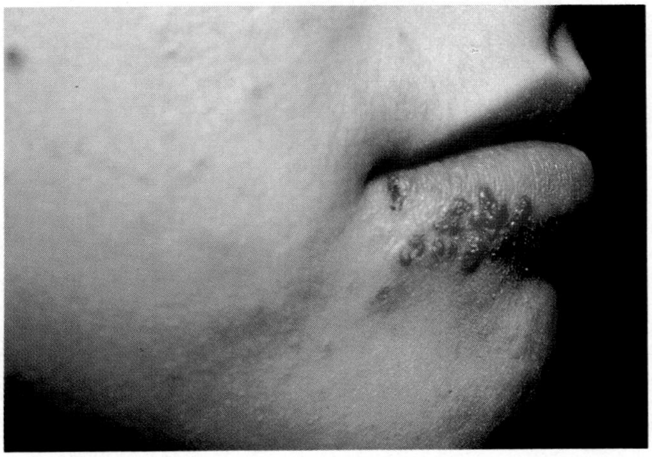

ID-35 **Herpes simplex** Grouped vesiculopustules on an erythematous base characterize primary HSV infections.

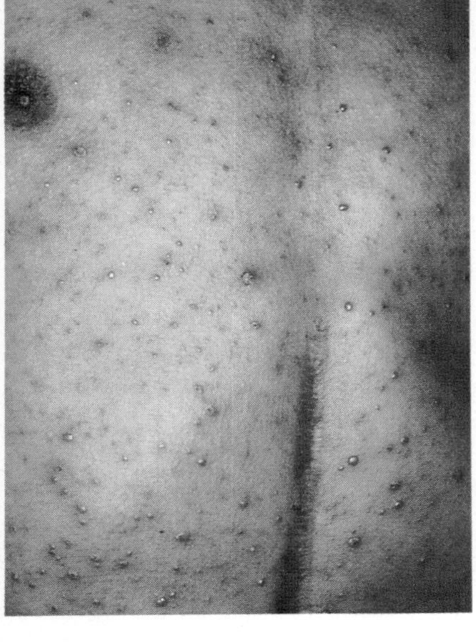

ID-36 **Varicella** showing numerous lesions in various stages of evolution: vesicles on an erythematous base, umbilicated vesicles, and crusts

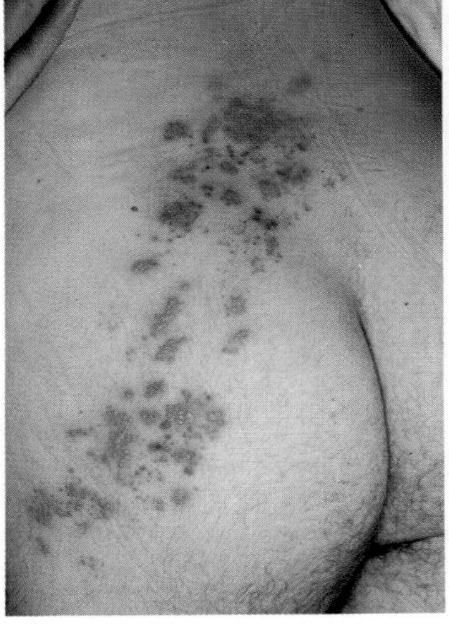

ID-37 **Herpes zoster** is seen in this HIV-infected patient as hemorrhagic vesicles and pustules on an erythematous base grouped in a dermatomal distribution.

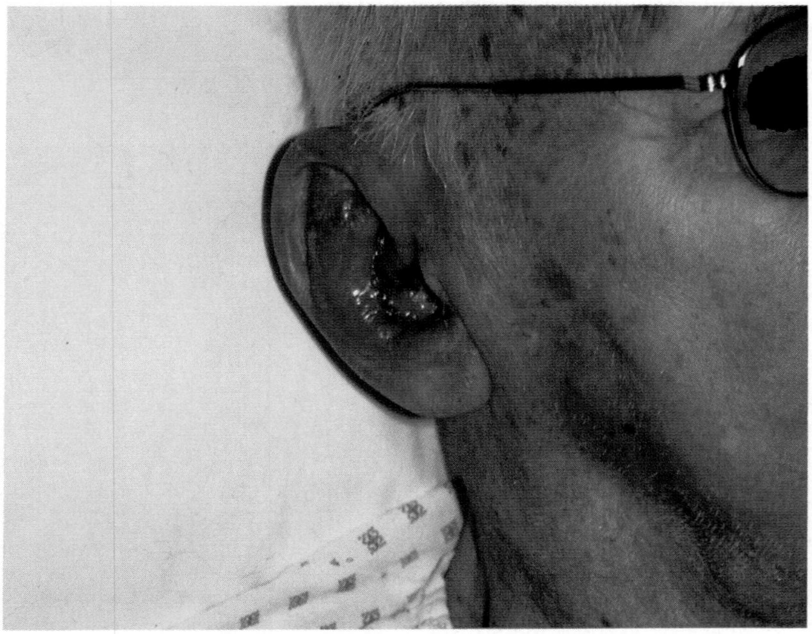

ID-38 **Spread of herpes zoster with chemotherapy**

A. The patient reported external ear pain. A vesicular rash on the concha and antihelix suggested Ramsay Hunt syndrome.

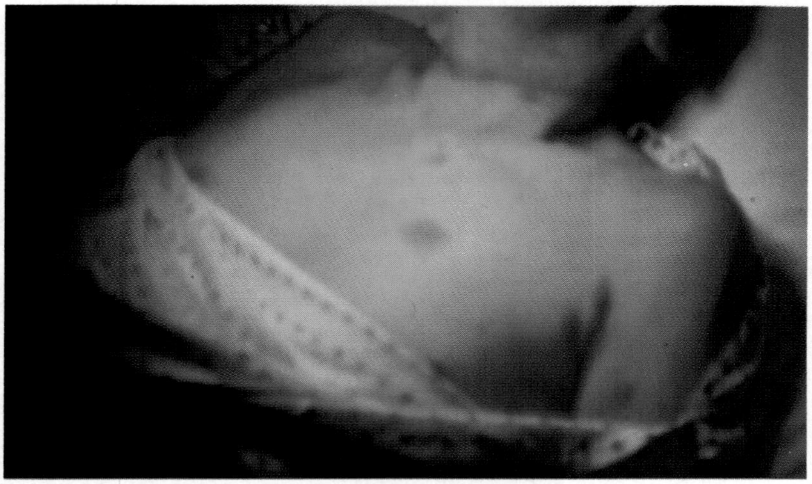

B. After chemotherapy for prostate cancer, the patient developed disseminated zoster, which was eventually controlled with acyclovir.

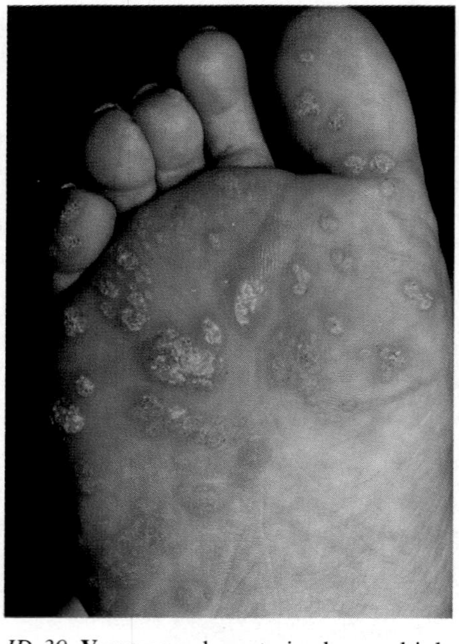

ID-39 **Verrucae** characterized as multiple hyperkeratotic verrucous papules

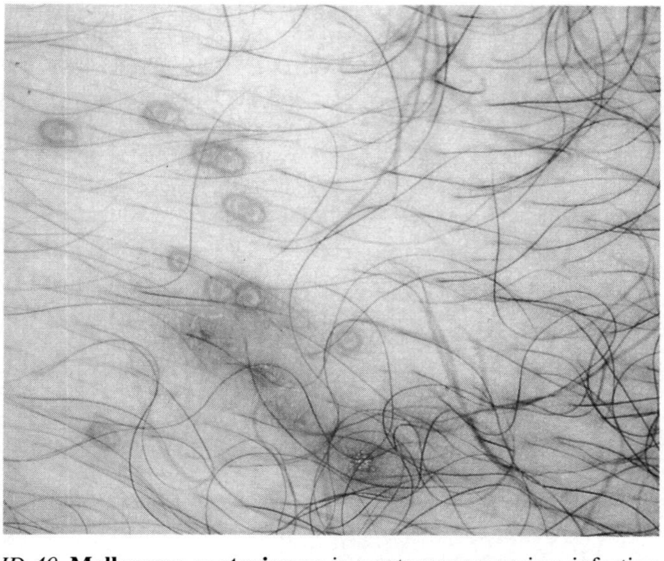

ID-40 **Molluscum contagiosum** is a cutaneous poxvirus infection characterized by multiple umbilicated flesh-colored or hypopigmented papules.

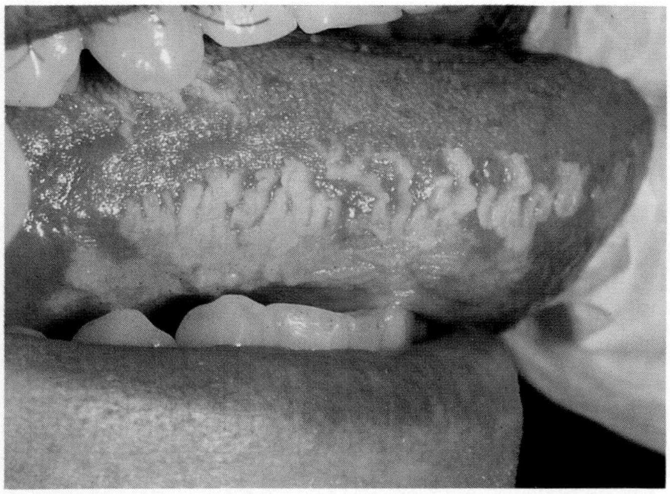

ID-41 **Oral hairy leukoplakia** often presents as white plaques on the lateral tongue and is associated with Epstein-Barr virus infection.

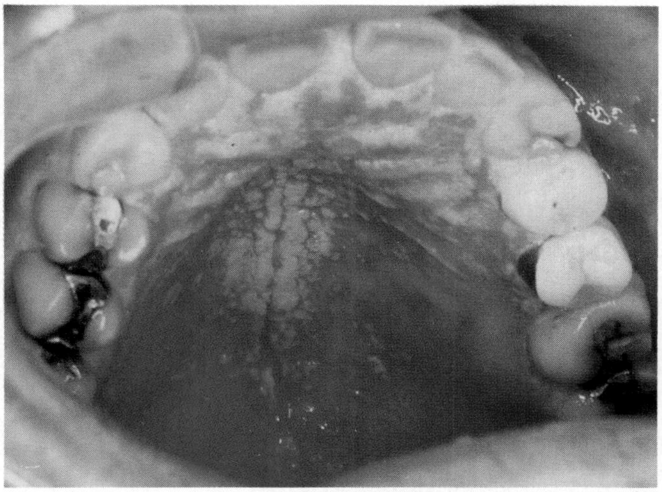

ID-42 **Pseudomembranous oral candidiasis** Adherent white, mucoid plaques with an erythematous halo seen here on the palate often indicate an immunocompromised state.

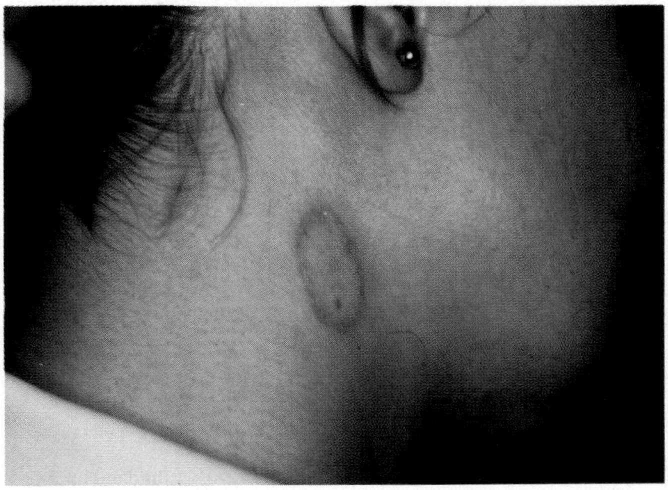

ID-43 **Tinea corporis** is a superficial fungal infection seen here as an erythematous annular scaly plaque with central clearing.

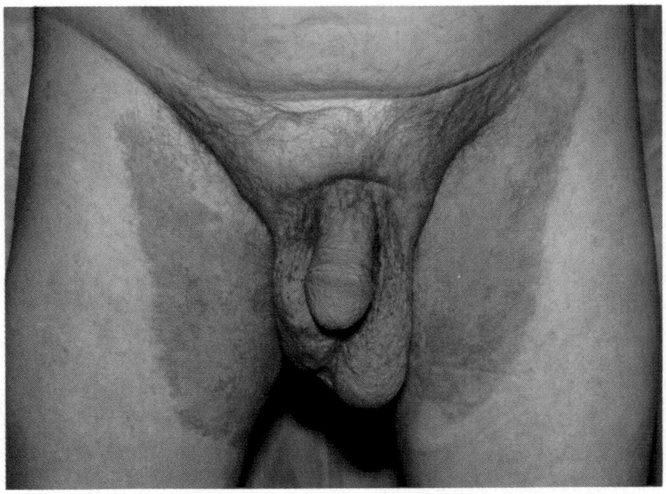

ID-44 **Tinea cruris** is a superficial dermatophyte infection with bilateral scaly, erythematous, annular plaques extending from the inguinal crease to the upper thighs.

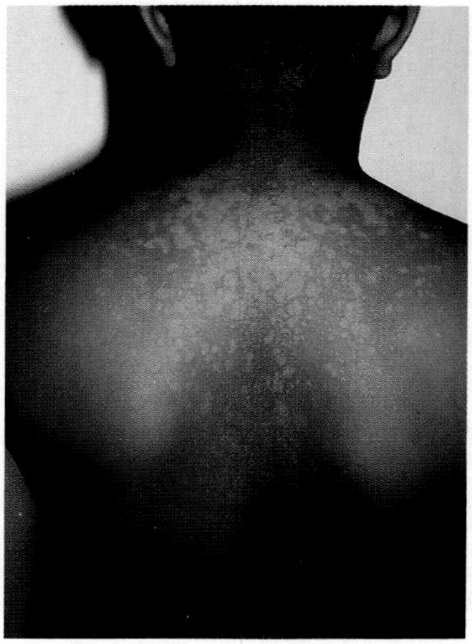

ID-45 **Tinea versicolor** is a superficial cutaneous fungal infection showing a wide variety of lesions. Finely scaling patches may be small or large, hyperpigmented or hypopigmented.

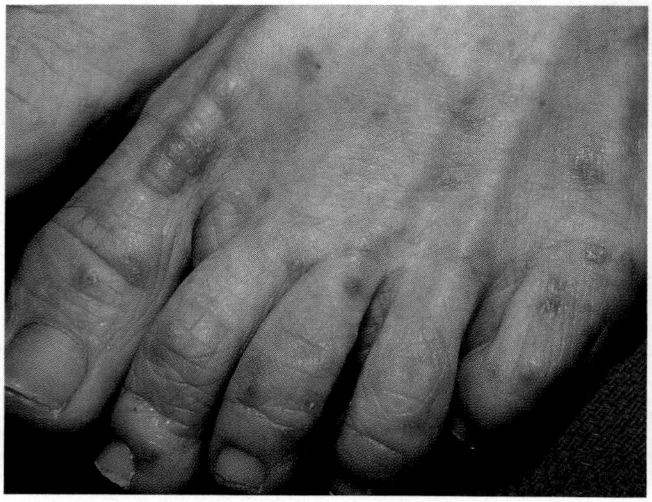

ID-46 **Scabies** showing typical scaling erythematous papules and few linear burrows

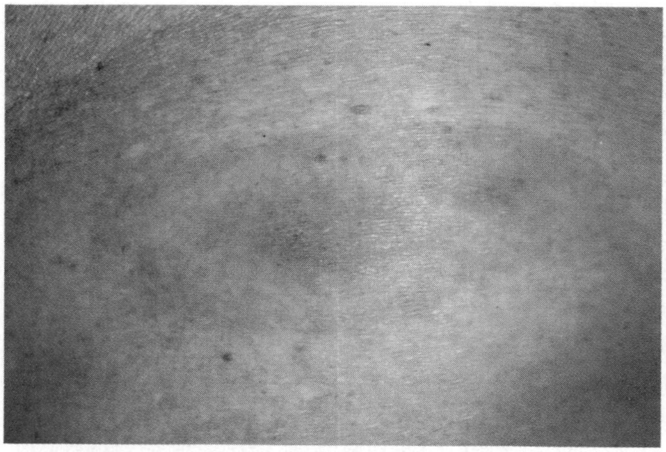

ID-47 **Erythema chronicum migrans** is the early cutaneous manifestation of Lyme disease and is characterized by erythematous annular patches, often with a central erythematous papule at the tick bite site.

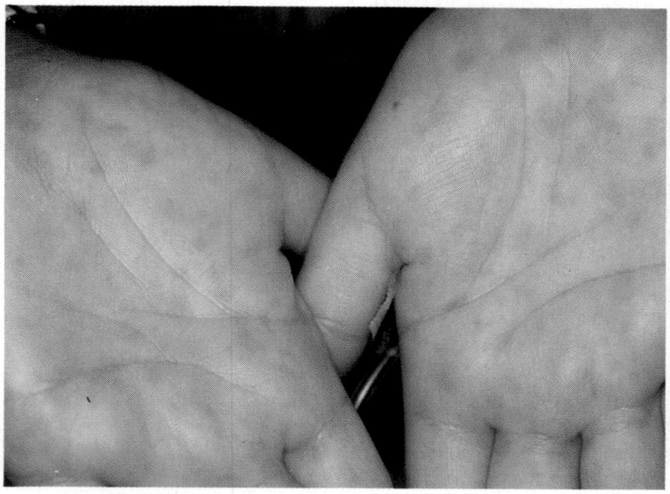

ID-48 **Rocky Mountain spotted fever** demonstrating faint erythematous palmar macules in the early phase of the disease. Lesions may become hemorrhagic (purpuric) as the disease progresses.

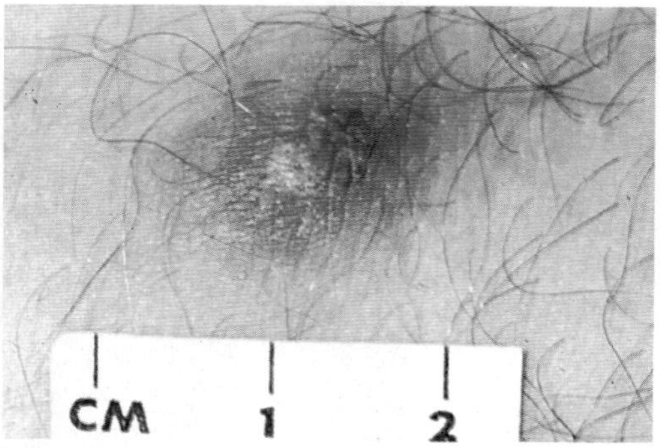

ID-49 **Disseminated gonococcemia** in the skin is seen as hemorrhagic papules and pustules with purpuric centers in an acral distribution.

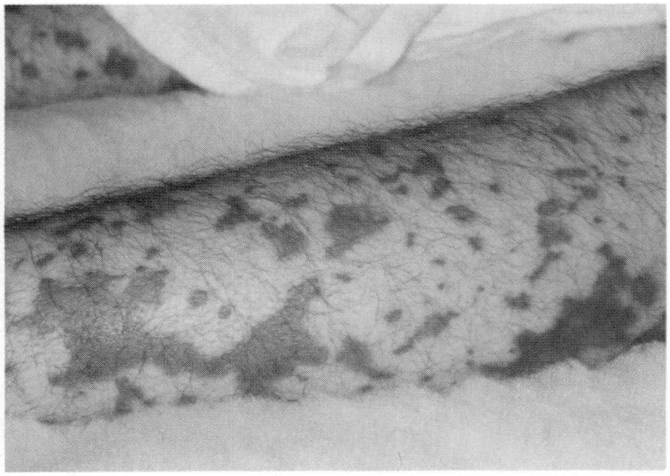

ID-50 **Fulminant meningococcemia** with extensive angular purpuric patches

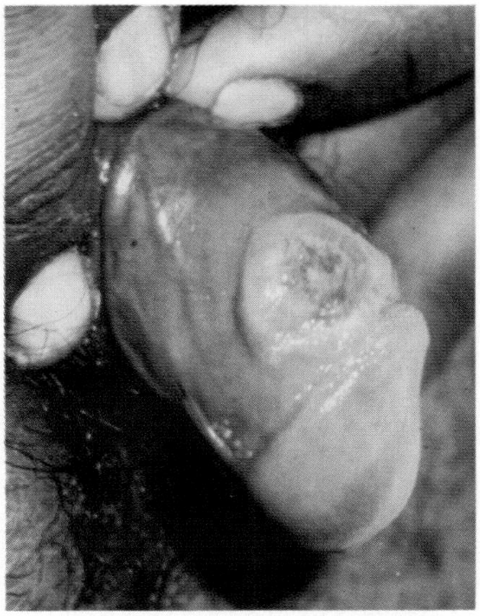

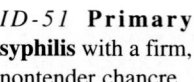

ID-51 **Primary syphilis** with a firm, nontender chancre

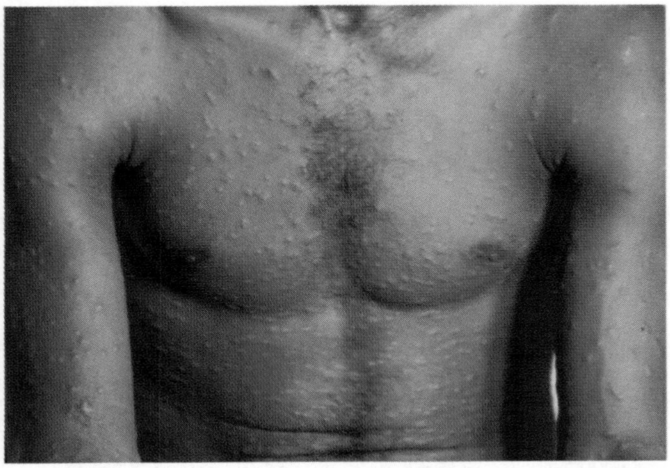

ID-52 **Secondary syphilis** demonstrating the papulosquamous truncal eruption

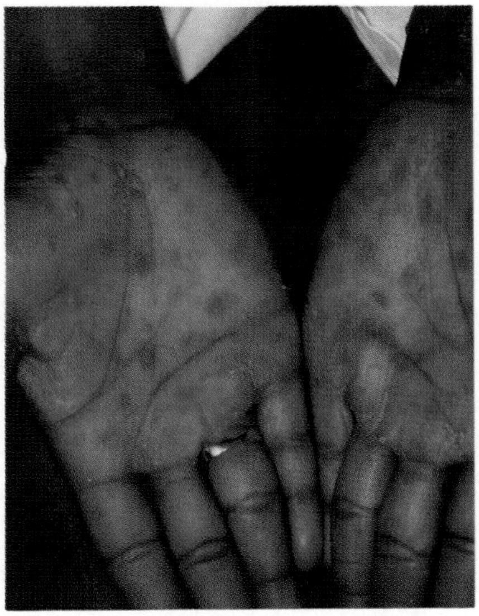

ID-53 **Secondary syphilis** commonly affects the palms and soles with scaling, firm, red-brown papules.

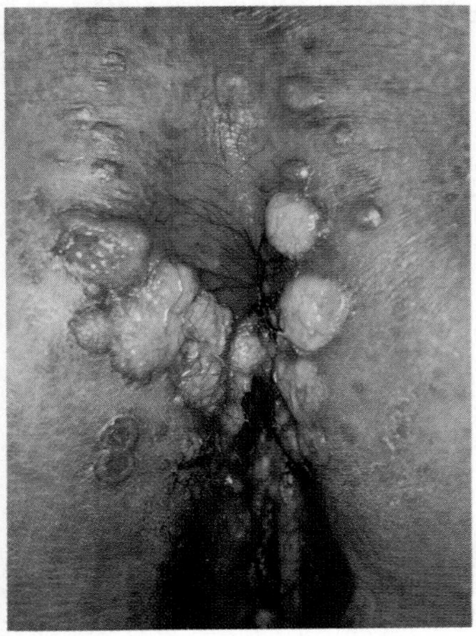

ID-54 **Condylomata lata** are moist, somewhat verrucous intertriginous plaques seen in secondary syphilis.

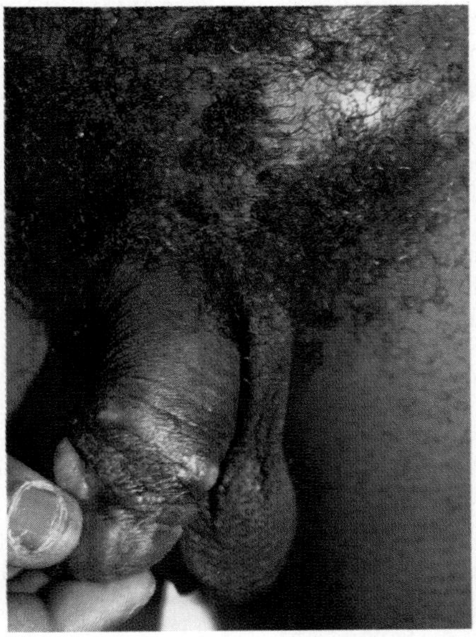

ID-55 **Chancroid** with characteristic penile ulcers and associated left inguinal adenitis (bubo)

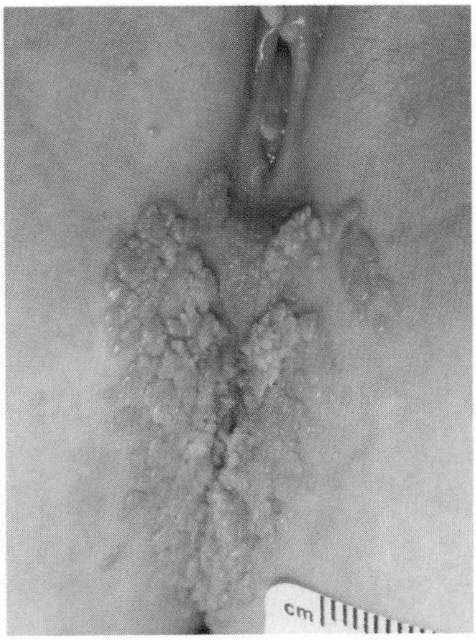

ID-56 **Condylomata acuminata** are lesions induced by human papillomavirus (HPV) and in this patient are seen as multiple verrucous papules coalescing into plaques.

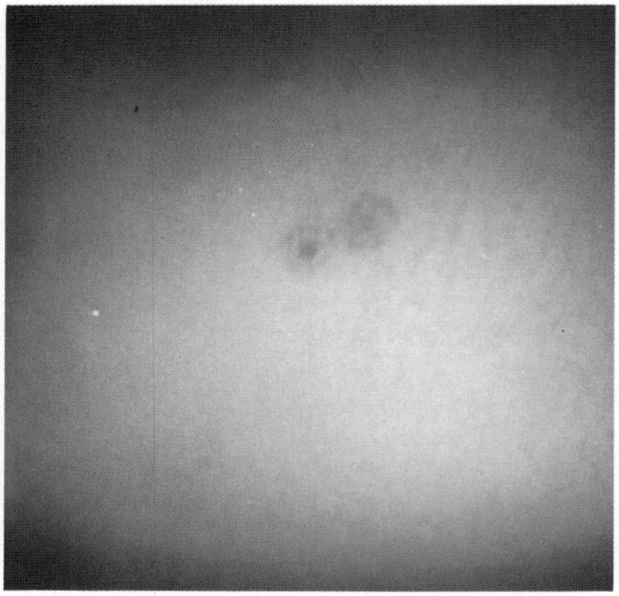

A

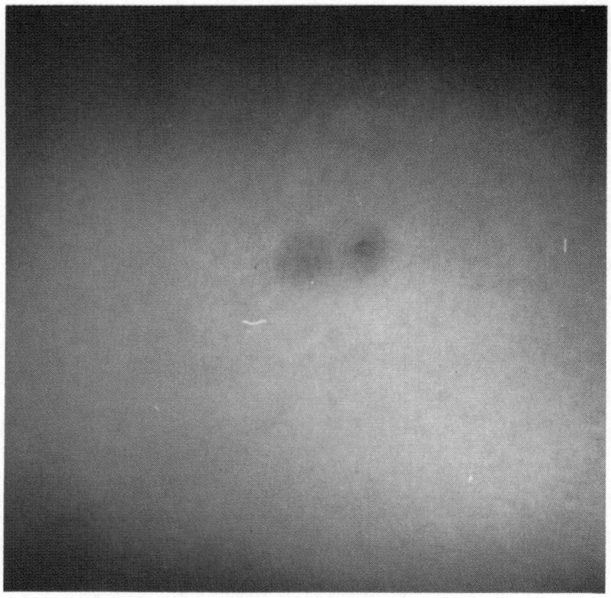

B

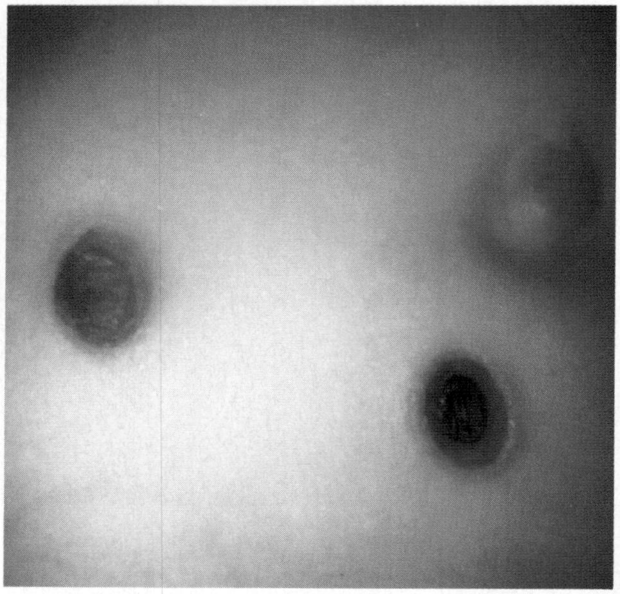

C

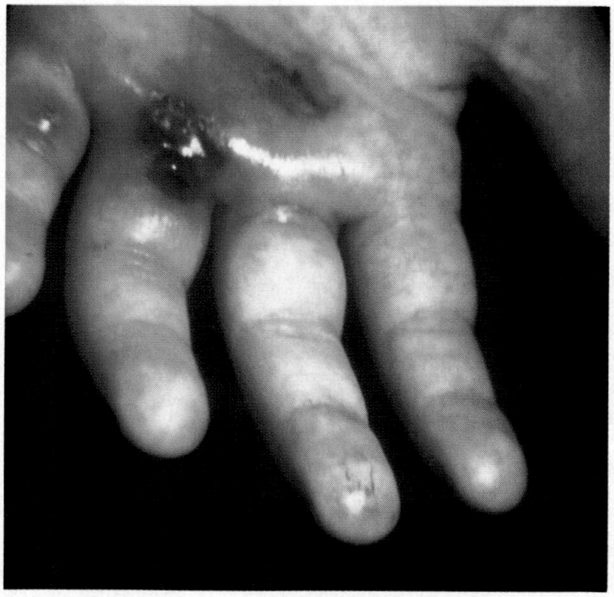

D

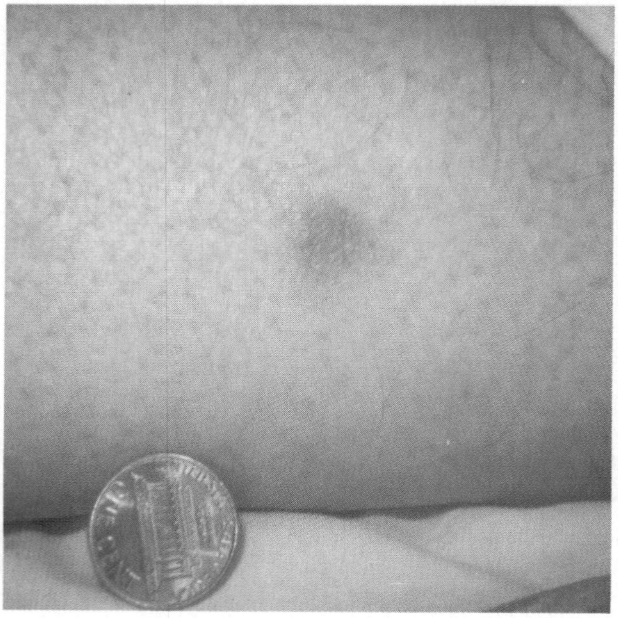

E

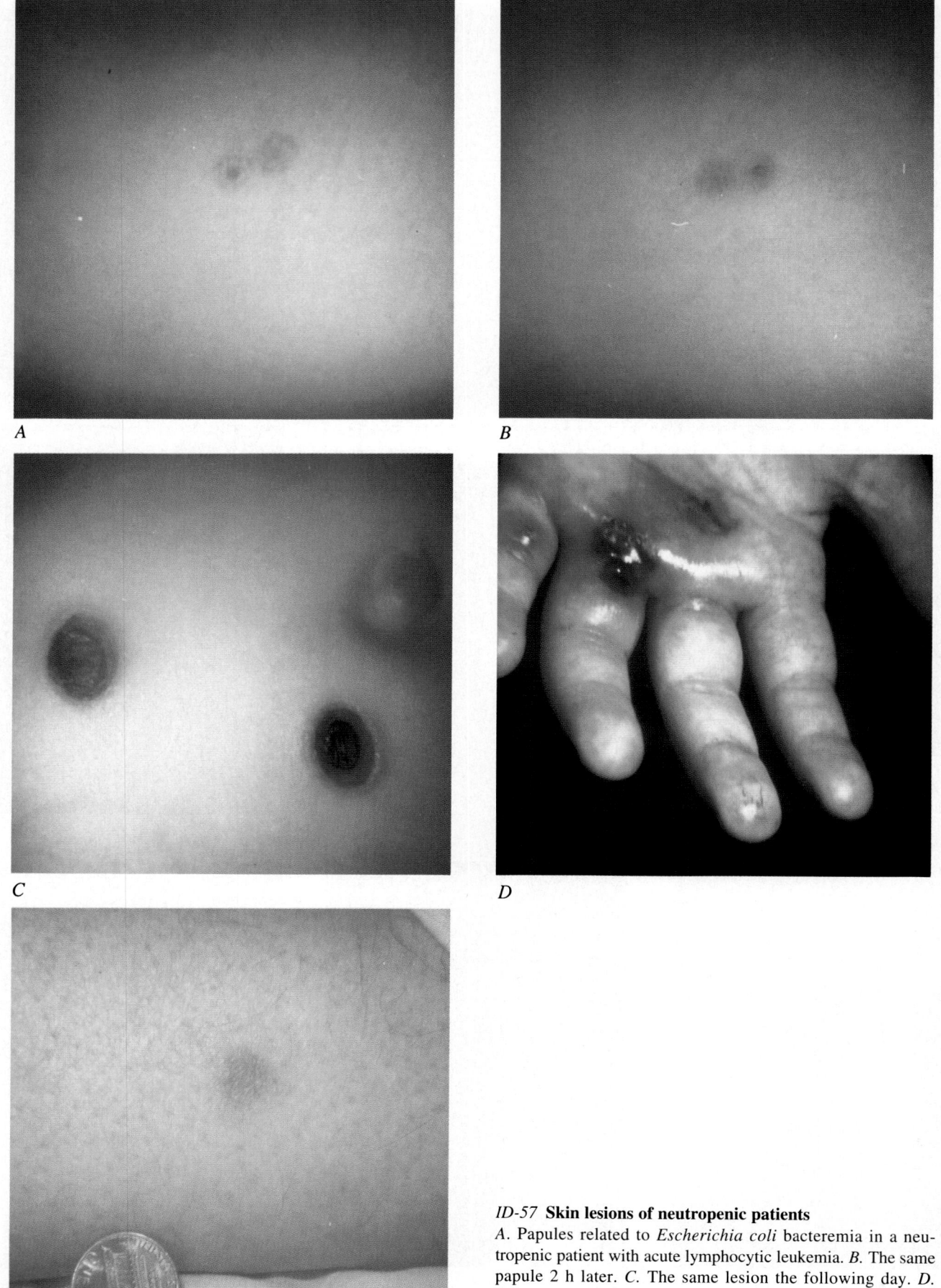

ID-57 **Skin lesions of neutropenic patients**

A. Papules related to *Escherichia coli* bacteremia in a neutropenic patient with acute lymphocytic leukemia. *B*. The same papule 2 h later. *C*. The same lesion the following day. *D*. Ecthyma gangrenosum in a neutropenic patient with *Pseudomonas aeruginosa* bacteremia. *E*. Papule in a neutropenic patient with *Candida tropicalis* fungemia.

E. Immunologically Mediated Skin Disease

IE-58 **Systemic lupus erythematosus** showing prominent, scaly, malar erythema. Involvement of other sun-exposed sites is also common.

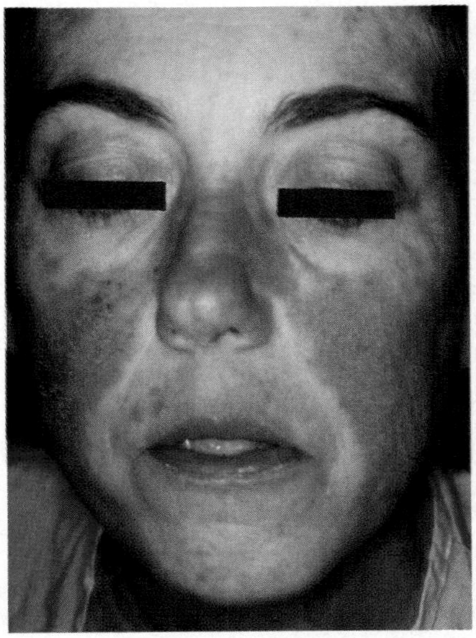

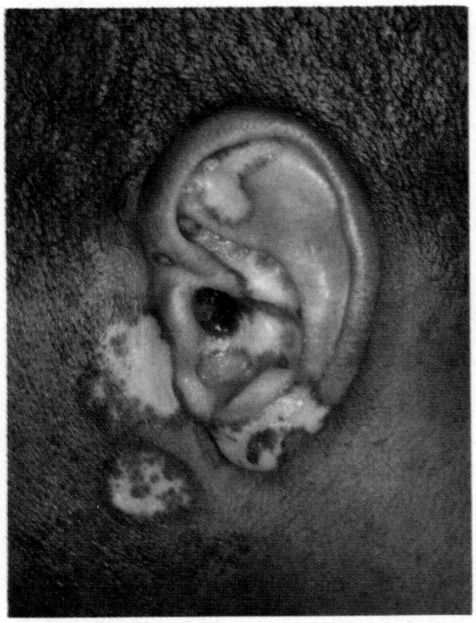

IE-59 **Discoid lupus erythematosus** Violaceous, hyperpigmented, atrophic plaques, often with evidence of follicular plugging, which may result in scarring, are characteristic of this cutaneous form of lupus.

IE-60 **Dermatomyositis** Periorbital violaceous erythema characterizes the classic heliotrope rash.

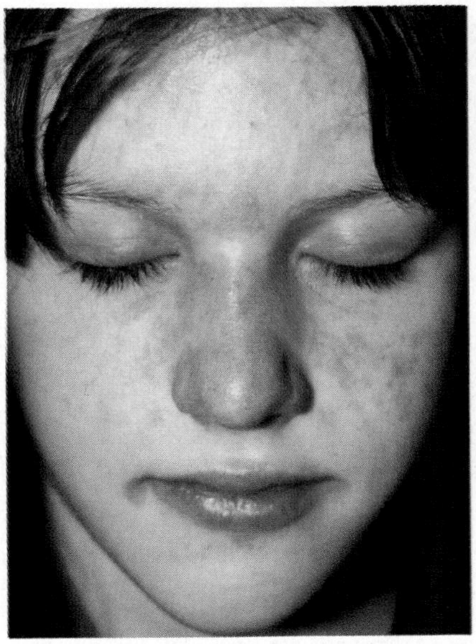

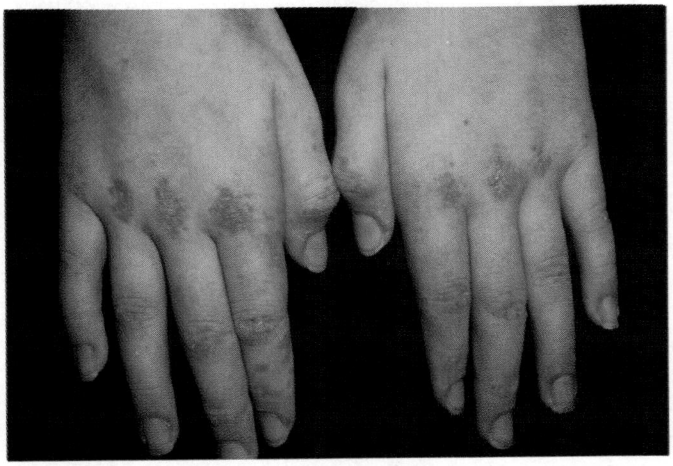

IE-61 **Dermatomyositis** often involves the hands as erythematous flat-topped papules over the knuckles (Gottron's sign) and periungal telangiectasias.

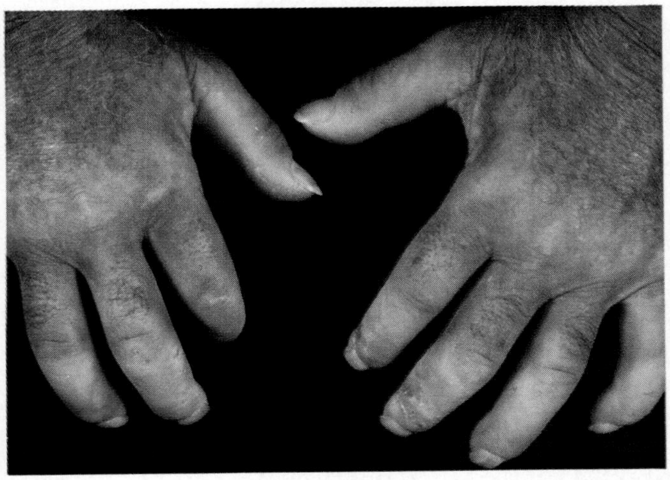

IE-62 **Scleroderma** showing acral sclerosis and focal digital ulcers

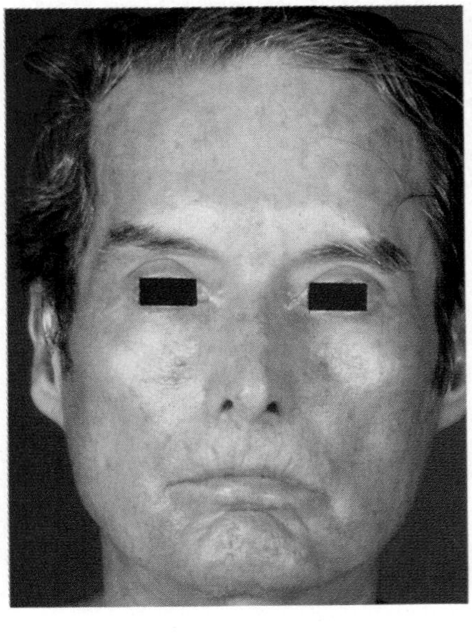

IE-63 **Scleroderma** is characterized by typical expressionless, mask-like facies.

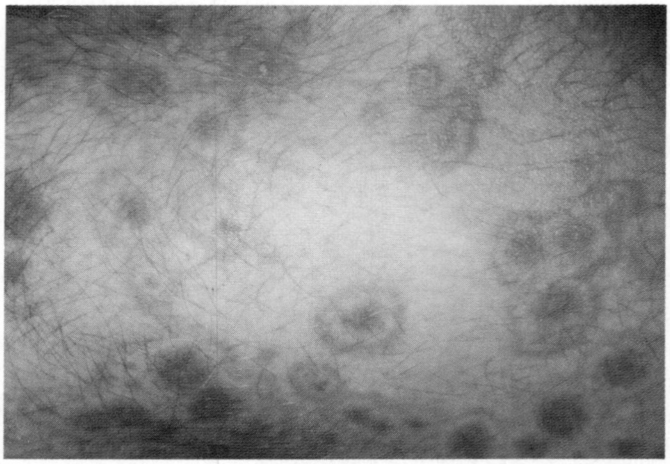

IE-64 **Erythema multiforme** is characterized by multiple erythematous plaques with a target or iris morphology and usually represents a hypersensitivity reaction to drugs or infections (especially herpes simplex virus).

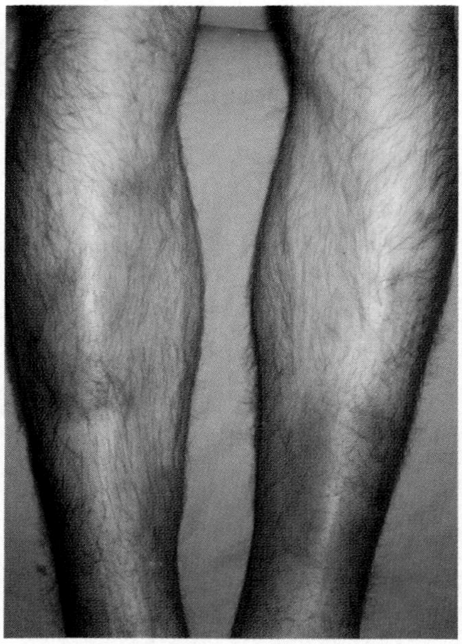

IE-65 **Erythema nodosum** is a panniculitis characterized by tender deep-seated nodules and plaques usually located on the lower extremities.

IE-66 **Vasculitis** Palpable purpuric papules on the lower legs are seen in this patient with cutaneous small vessel vasculitis.

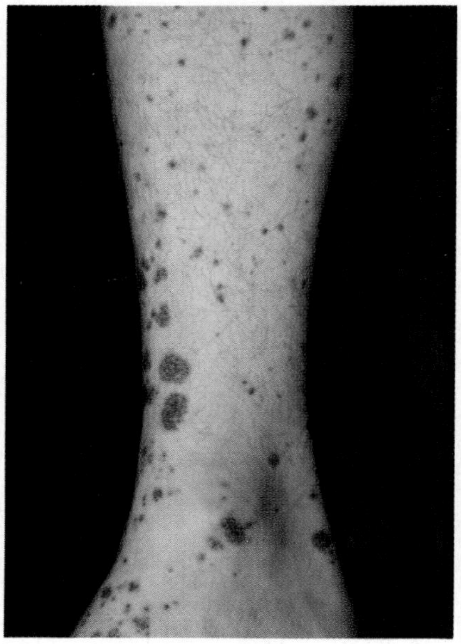

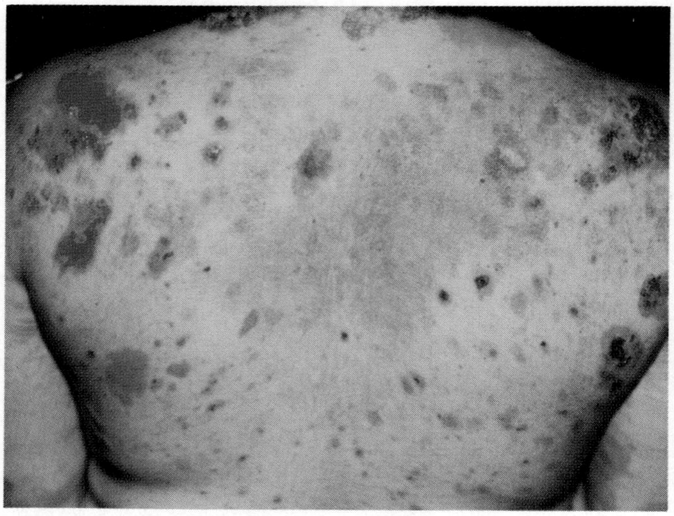

IE-67 **Pemphigus vulgaris** demonstrating flaccid bullae that are easily ruptured, resulting in multiple erosions and crusted plaques

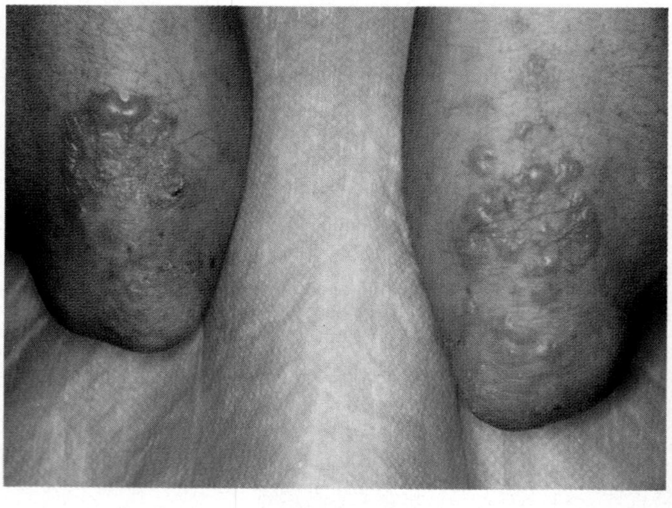

IE-68 **Dermatitis herpetiformis** manifested by pruritic, grouped vesicles in a typical location. The vesicles are often excoriated and may occur on knees, buttocks, and posterior scalp.

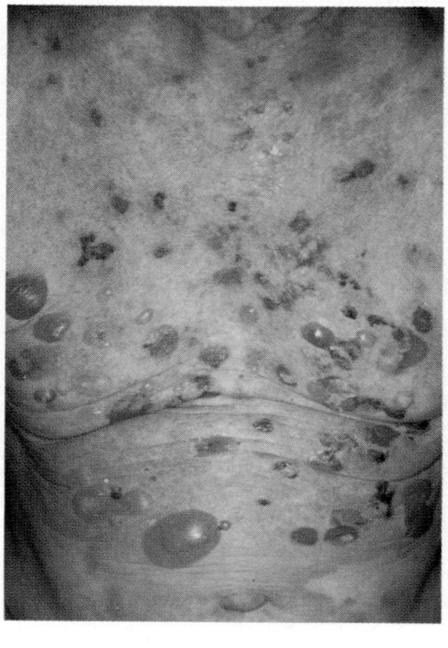

IE-69 **Bullous pemphigoid** with tense vesicles and bullae on an erythematous, urticarial base

F. Skin Manifestations of Internal Disease

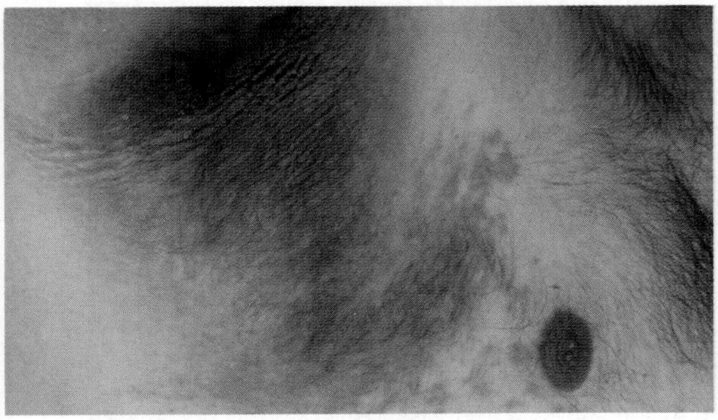

IF-70 **Acanthosis nigricans** demonstrating typical hyperpigmented axillary plaques with a velvet-like, verrucous surface

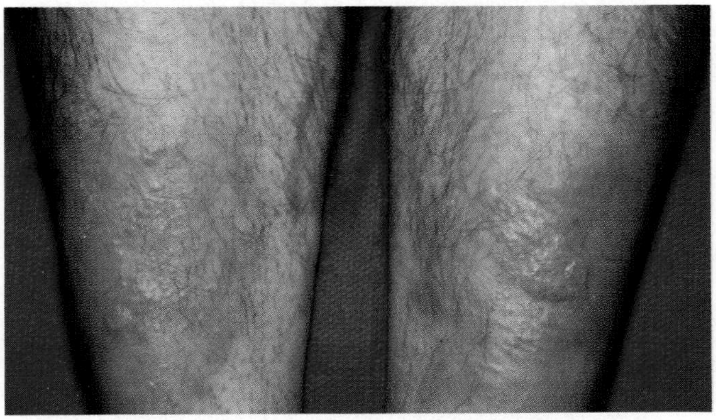

IF-71 **Pretibial myxedema** manifesting as waxy, infiltrated plaques in a patient with Graves' disease

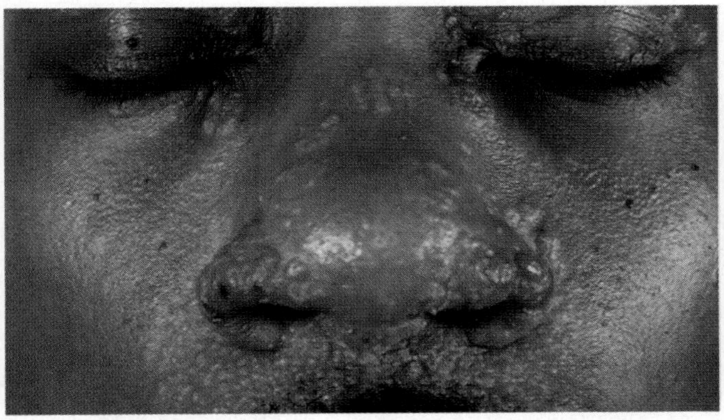

IF-72 **Sarcoid** Infiltrated papules and plaques of variable color are seen in a typical paranasal and periorbital location.

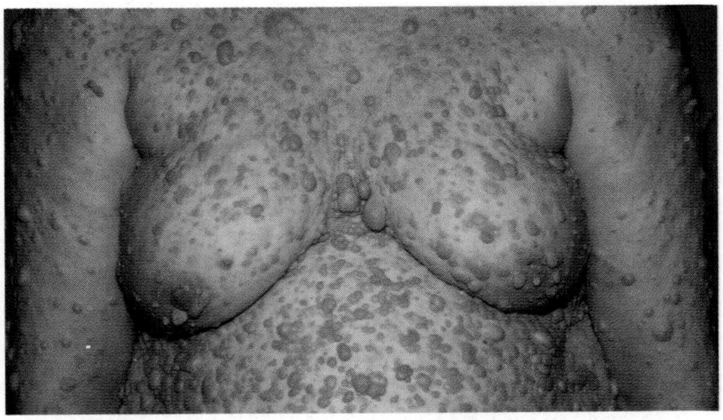

IF-73 **Neurofibromatosis** demonstrating numerous flesh-colored cutaneous neurofibromas

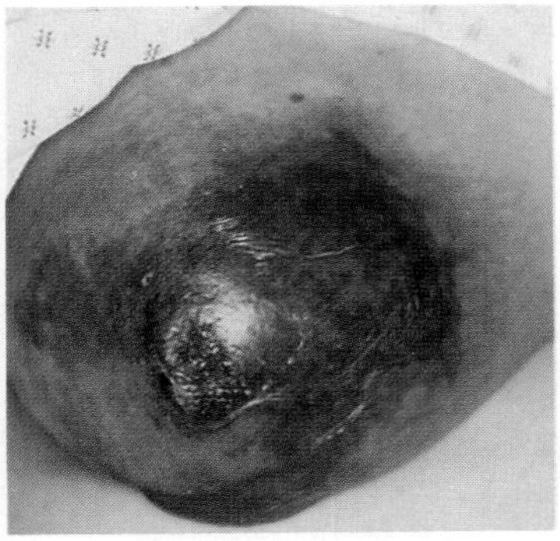

IF-74 **Coumarin necrosis** showing cutaneous and subcutaneous necrosis of a breast. Other fatty areas such as buttocks and thighs are also common sites of involvement.

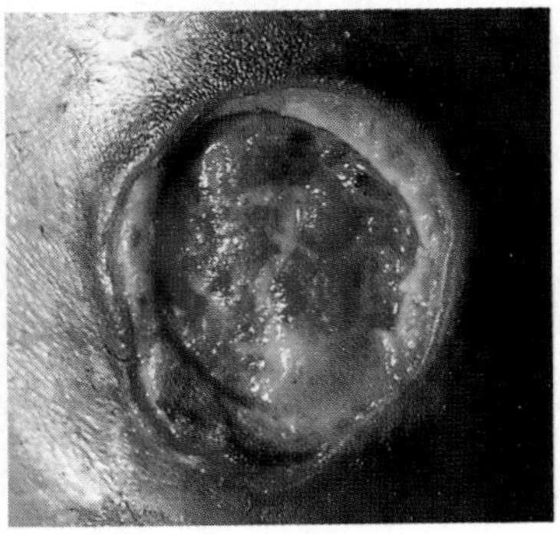

IF-75 **Pyoderma gangrenosum** showing a somewhat purulent ulcer with violaceous and undermined wound edges

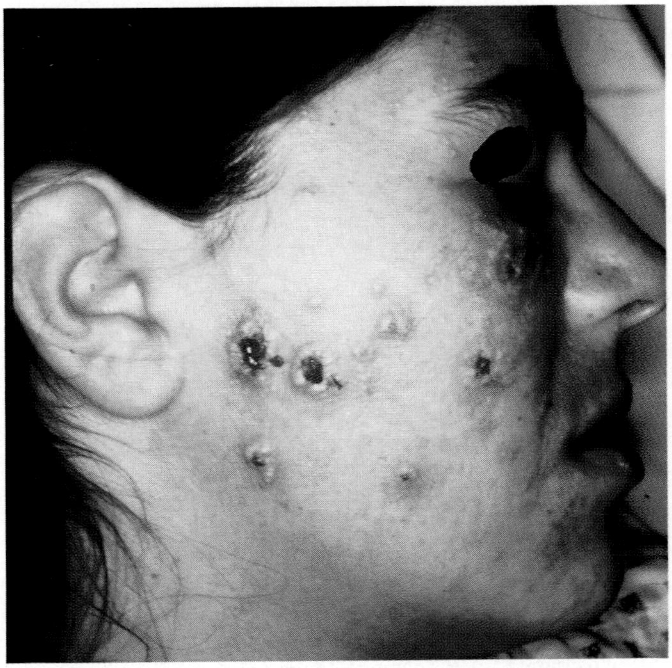

IF-76 **Plaques of Sweet's syndrome** in a patient with acute myelocytic leukemia.

II. Atlas of Endoscopic Findings

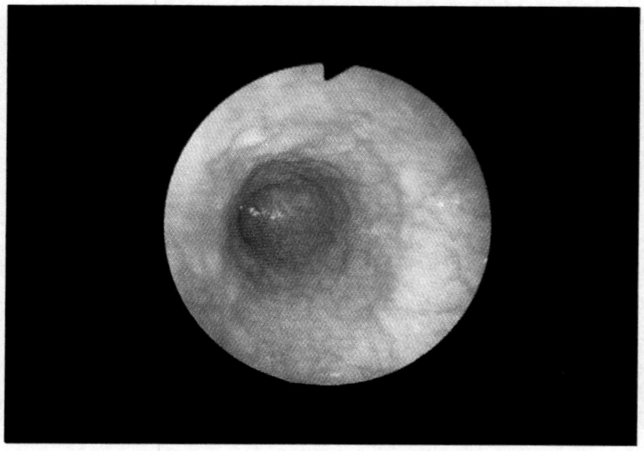

II-1 **Normal esophagus** Fine vasculature can be seen

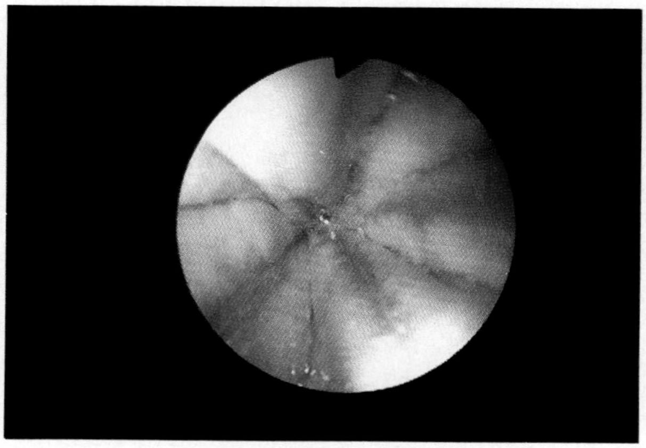

II-2 **Peptic regurgitant esophagitis** Linear red streaks with a central white streak extend up the esophagus

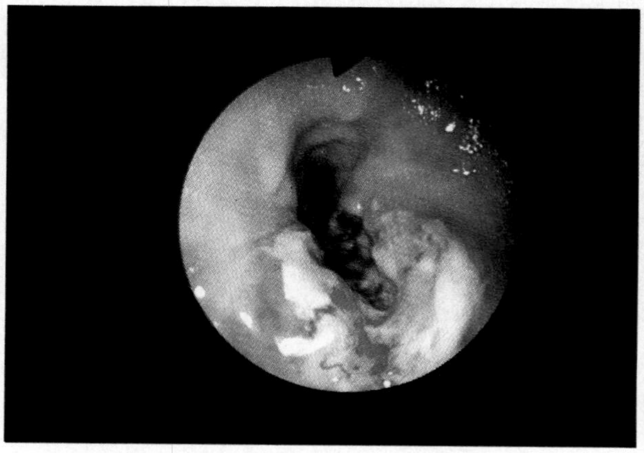

II-3 **Ulcerated squamous cell carcinoma,** with a depressed center, involving one wall of the esophagus

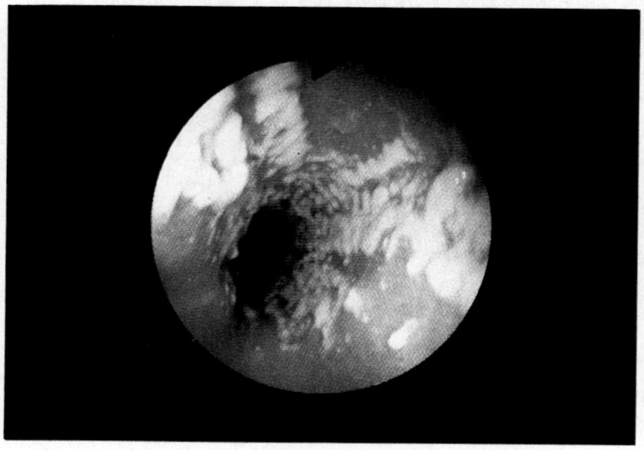

II-4 **Moniliasis of the esophagus** A white exudate is seen with underlying erythematous mucosa

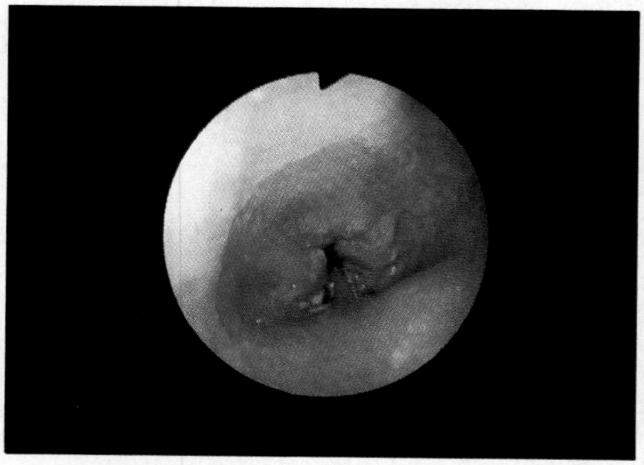

II-5 **Barrett's metaplasia of the esophagus with an adenocarcinoma** The squamocolumnar junction is noted in the proximal esophagus. A mucosal irregularity in the center of the photograph was an adenocarcinoma.

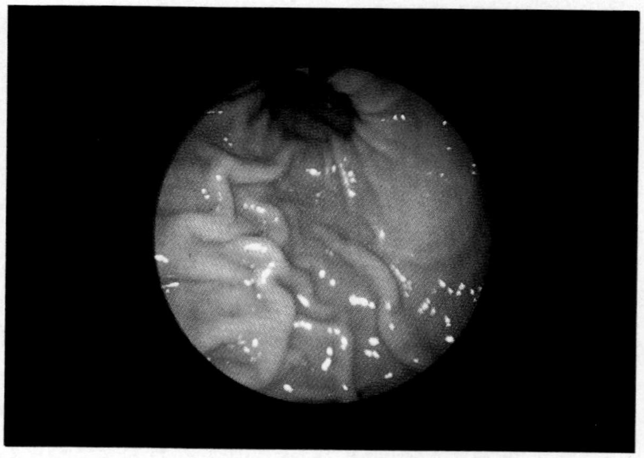

II-6 **Normal body of the stomach with rugal folds**

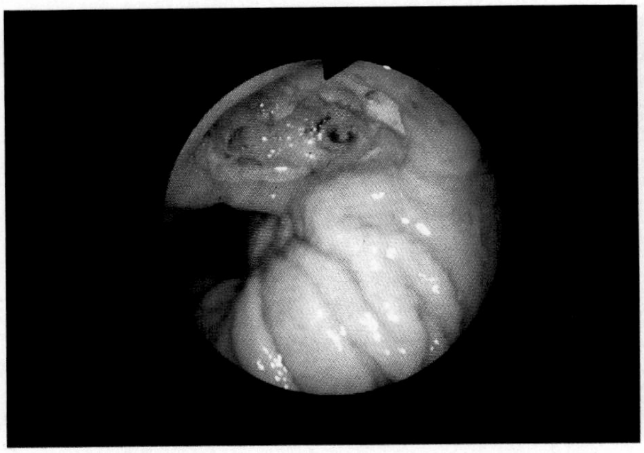

II-7 **Large, benign, lesser curve gastric ulcer** The folds end at the ulcer margin.

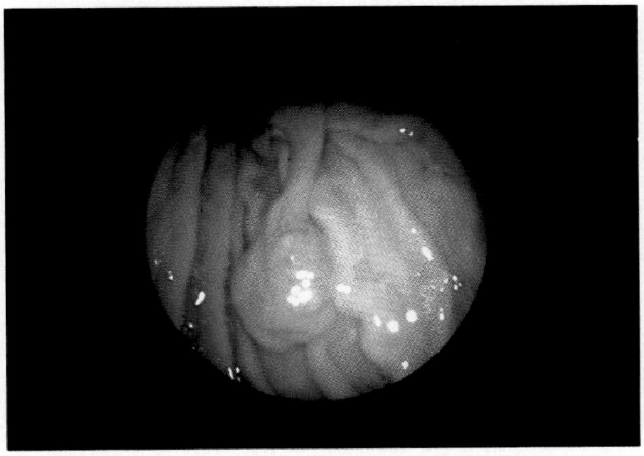

II-8 **Gastric polyp** The histologic type must be determined by excision and pathologic examination.

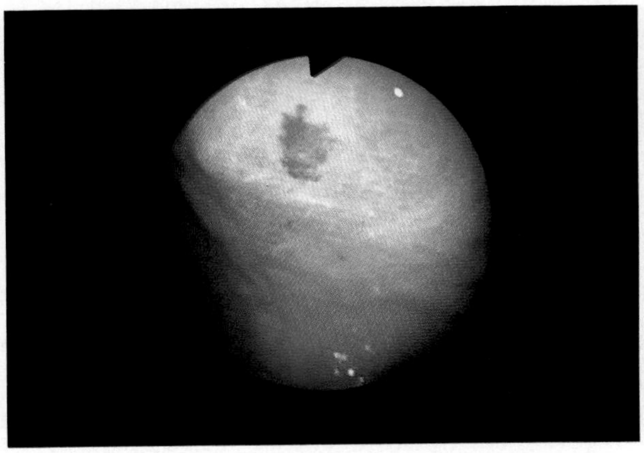

II-9 **Arteriovenous malformation of the gastric mucosa**

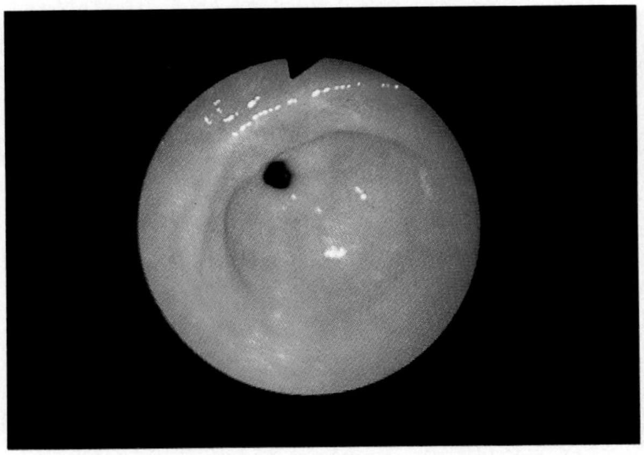

II-10 **Normal pylorus** Note the absence of gastric rugal folds in the antrum proximal to the pylorus.

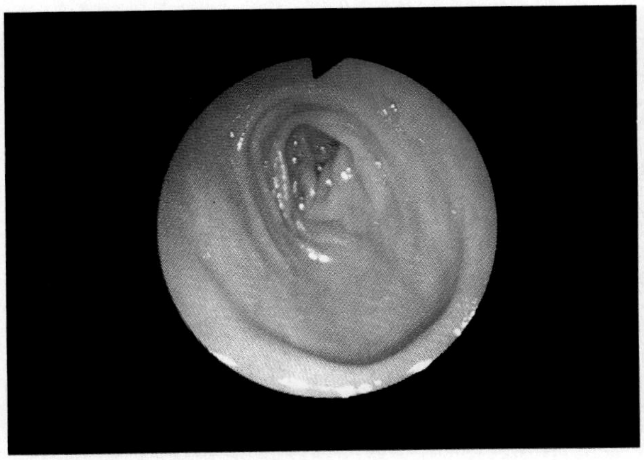

II-11 **Normal duodenal bulb**

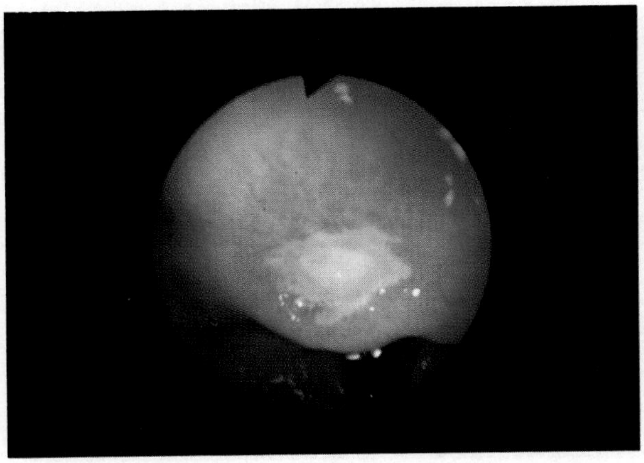

II-12 **Duodenal ulcer** A typical ulcer with a clean base is seen on the anterior surface of the duodenal bulb.

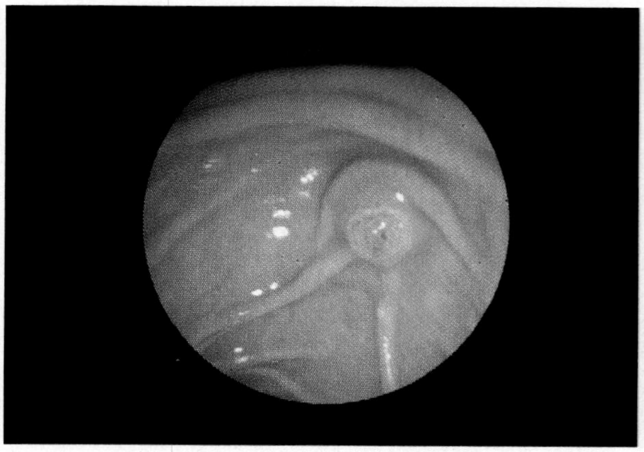

II-13 **Normal papilla of Vater** The fold pattern surrounding the papilla is normal; bile is seen adjacent to the papilla.

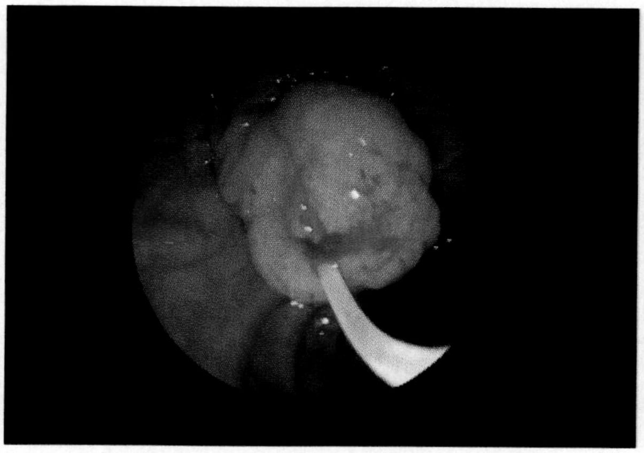

II-14 **Periampullary carcinoma** The mass at the papilla of Vater has been catheterized during ERCP.

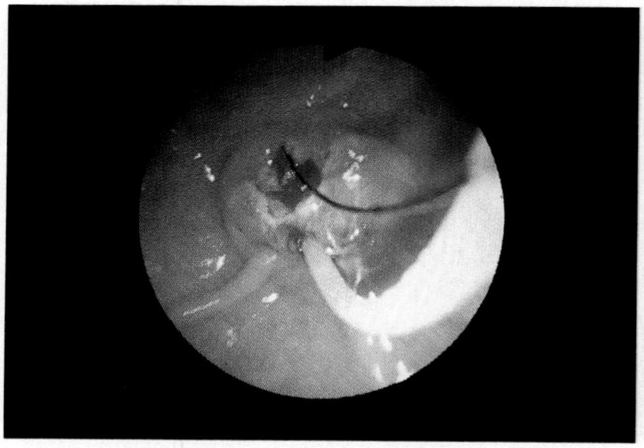

II-15 **Endoscopic papillotomy** A papillotome has been passed into the papilla, the wire bowed, and an incision made, with electrosurgical current, in the superior aspect of the papilla.

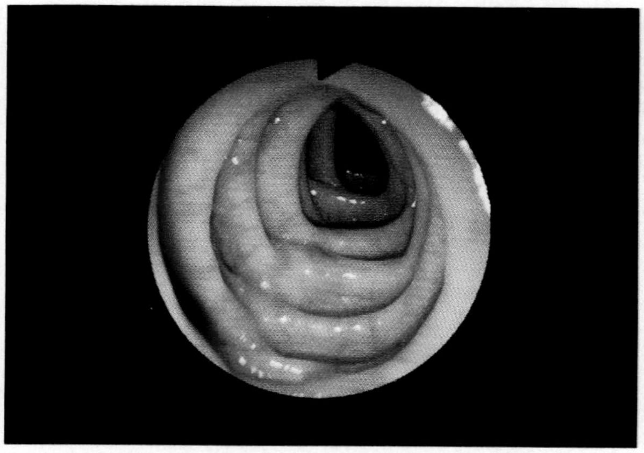

II-16 **Normal colon** Typical folds and vascular pattern can be seen.

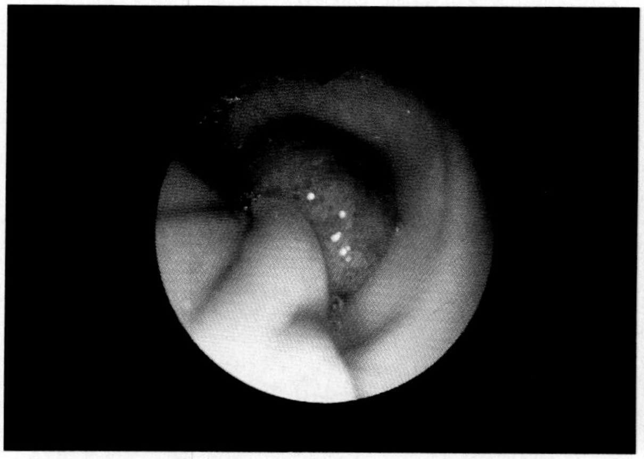

II-17 **Colonic adenomatous polyp** The polyp is erythematous; a stalk is seen covered with normal mucosa.

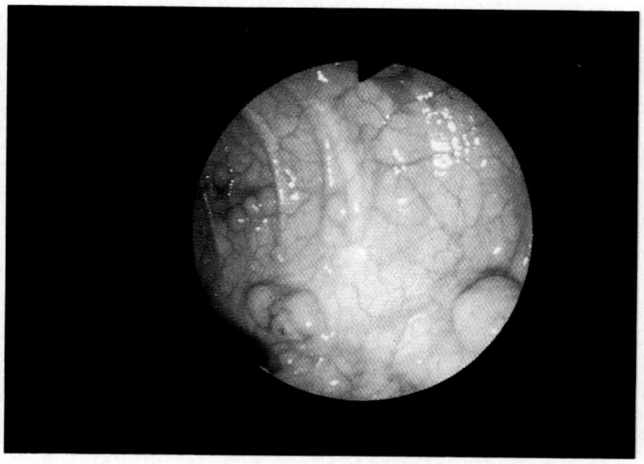

II-18 **Multiple, small, colonic adenomatous polyps** in a case of familial polyposis coli. This colon must be removed to prevent the development of cancer.

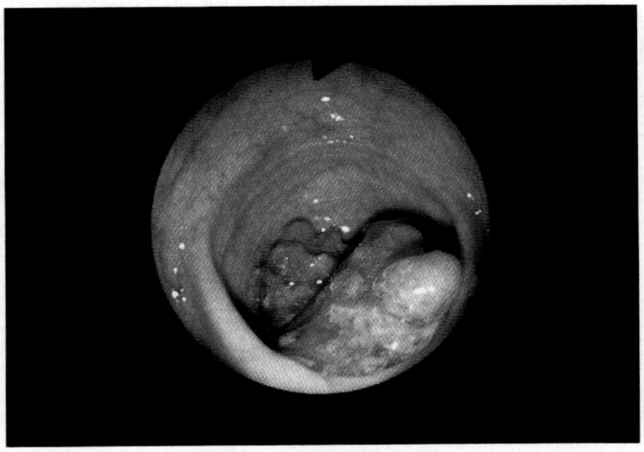

II-19 **Colon adenocarcinoma** The cancer is multilobed and growing into the lumen.

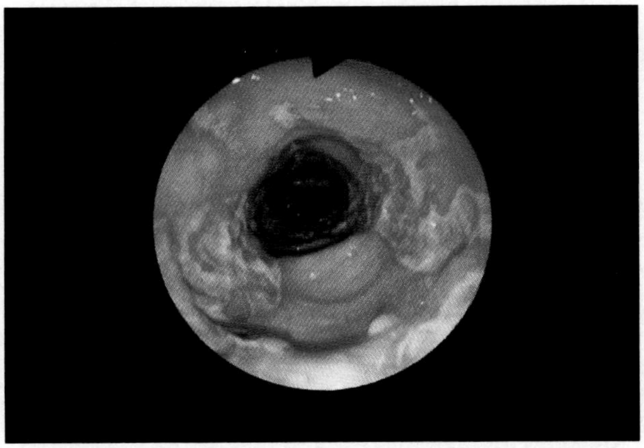

II-20 **Crohn's colitis** with linear, serpiginous, white-based ulcers surrounded by colonic mucosa that is relatively normal

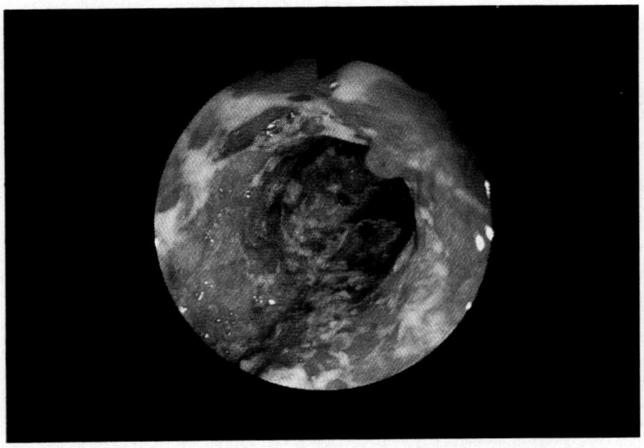

II-21 **Severe ulcerative colitis** with diffuse ulceration, bleeding, and exudation

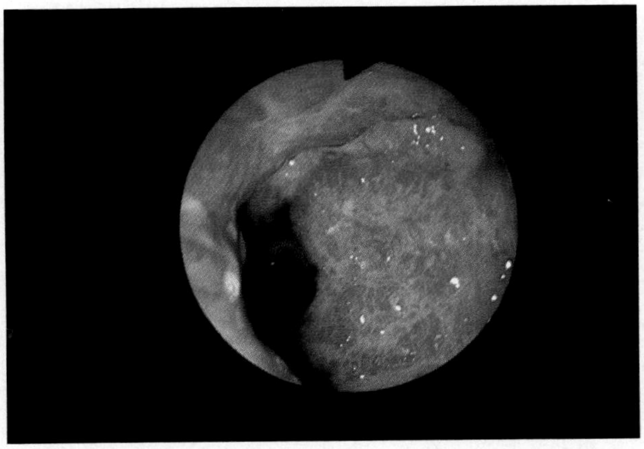

II-22 **Kaposi's sarcoma involving the colon** in a patient with AIDS. The erythematous lesions involve most of the colonic mucosa in the photograph.

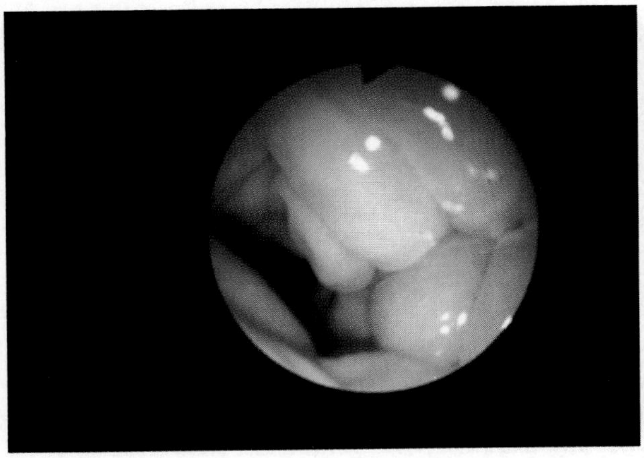

II-23 **Colonic varices** Multiple, serpiginous, subepithelial structures impinge on the colonic lumen.

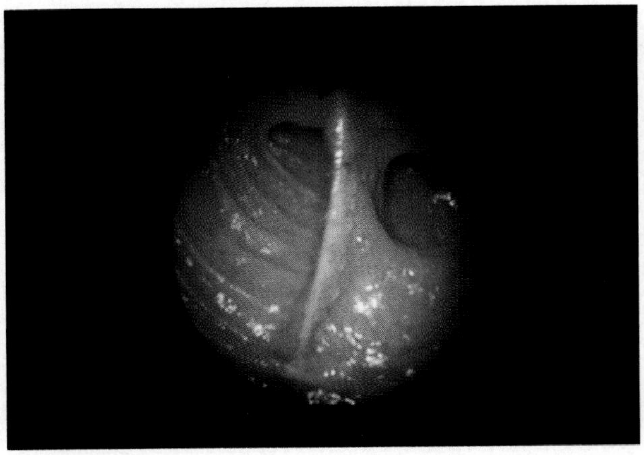

II-24 **Ileal pouch** The mucosa appears normal in this pouch reconstructed from ileum to provide a reservoir after total proctocolectomy and ileoanal anastomosis.

III. Atlas of Funduscopic Examination

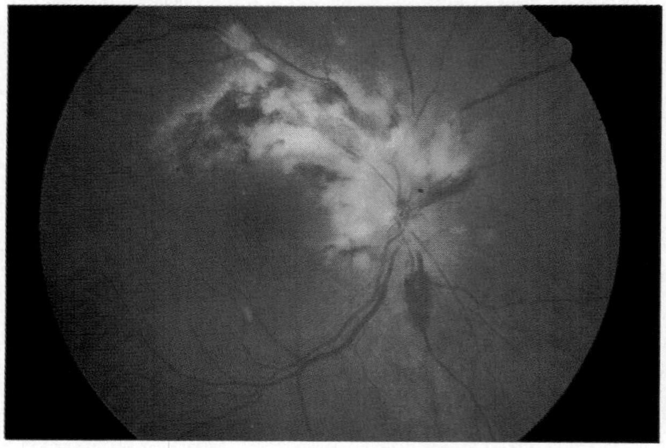

III-1 **Cytomegalovirus** in a patient with AIDS appears as an arcuate zone of retinitis with hemorrhages and optic disc swelling. Often CMV is confined to the retinal periphery, beyond view of the direct ophthalmoscope.

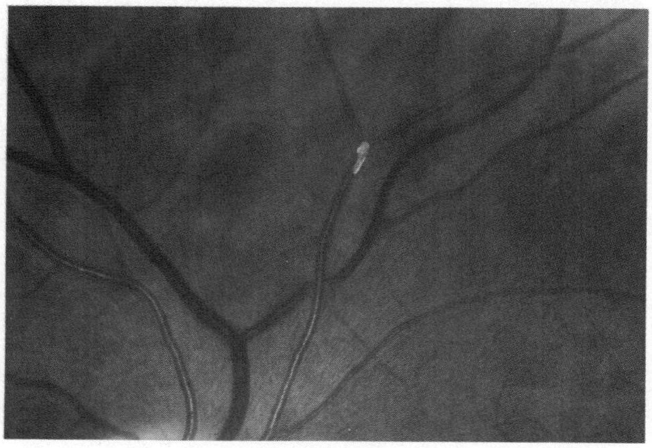

III-2 **Hollenhorst plaque** lodged at the bifurcation of a retinal arteriole proves that a patient is shedding emboli from either the carotid artery, great vessels, or heart.

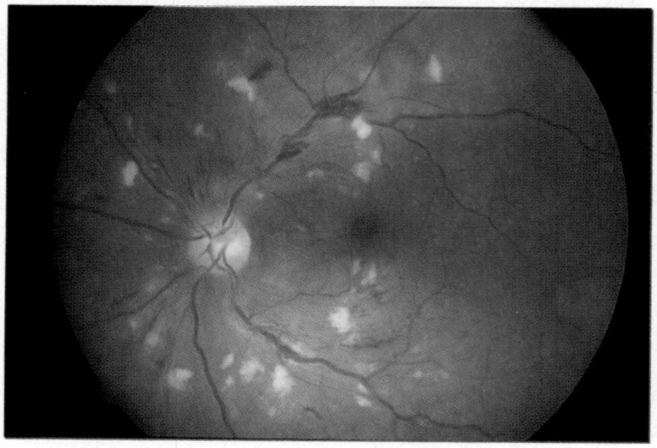

III-3 **Hypertensive retinopathy** with scattered flame (splinter) hemorrhages and cotton wool spots (nerve fiber layer infarcts) in a patient with headache and a blood pressure of 234/120

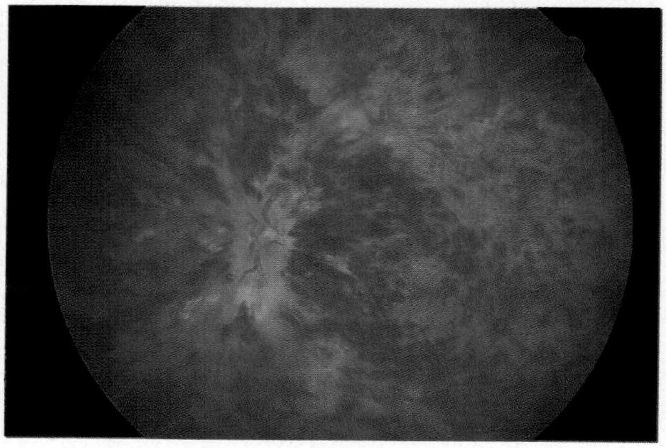

III-4 **Central retinal vein occlusion** can produce massive retinal hemorrhage ("blood and thunder"), ischemia, and vision loss.

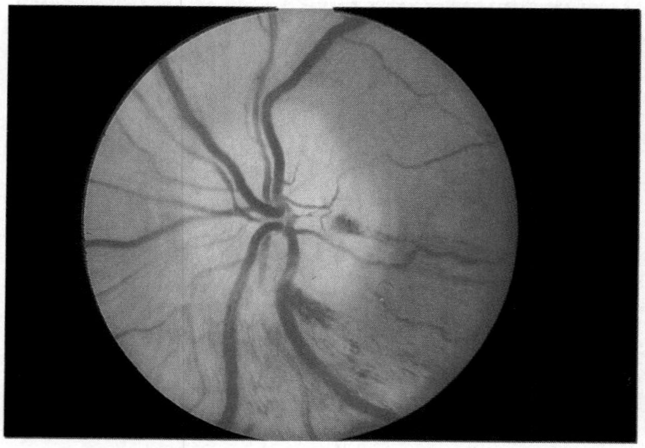

III-5 **Anterior ischemic optic neuropathy** from temporal arteritis in a 78-year old woman with pallid disc swelling, hemorrhage, visual loss, myalgia, and an erythrocyte sedimentation rate of 86 mm/h

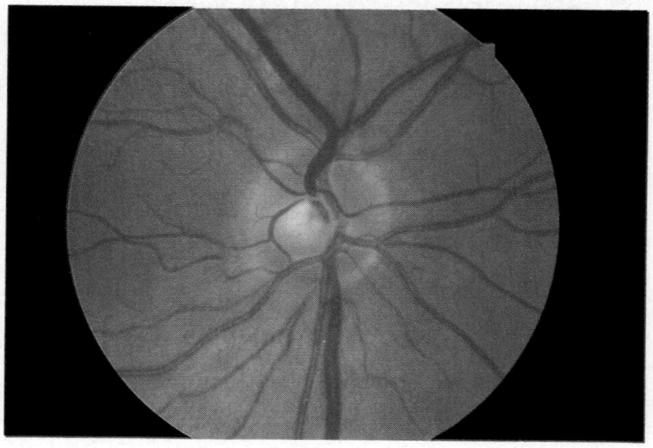

III-6 **Retrobulbar optic neuritis** is characterized by a normal fundus examination initially, hence the rubric, "the doctor sees nothing, and the patient sees nothing." Optic atrophy develops after severe or repeated attacks.

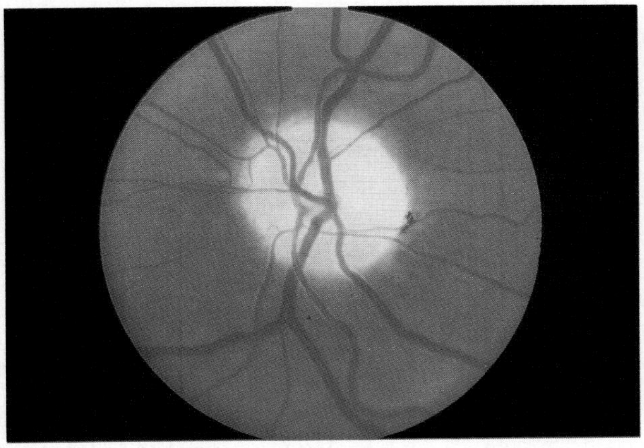

III-7 **Optic atrophy** is not a specific diagnosis but refers to the combination of optic disc pallor, arteriolar narrowing, and nerve fiber layer destruction produced by a host of eye diseases, especially optic neuropathies.

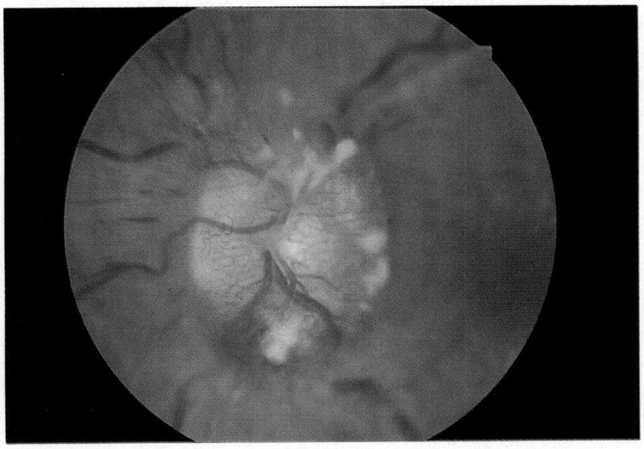

III-8 **Papilledema** means optic disc edema from raised intracranial pressure. This obese young woman with pseudotumor cerebri was misdiagnosed as a migraineur until fundus examination was performed, showing optic disc elevation, hemorrhages, and cotton wool spots.

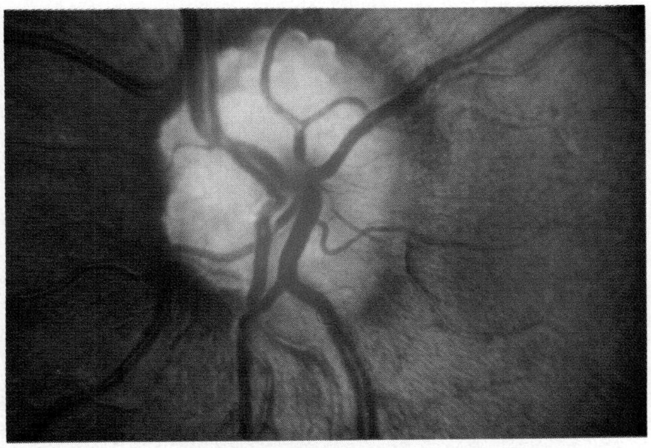

III-9 **Optic disc drusen** are calcified deposits of unknown etiology within the optic disc. They are sometimes confused with papilledema.

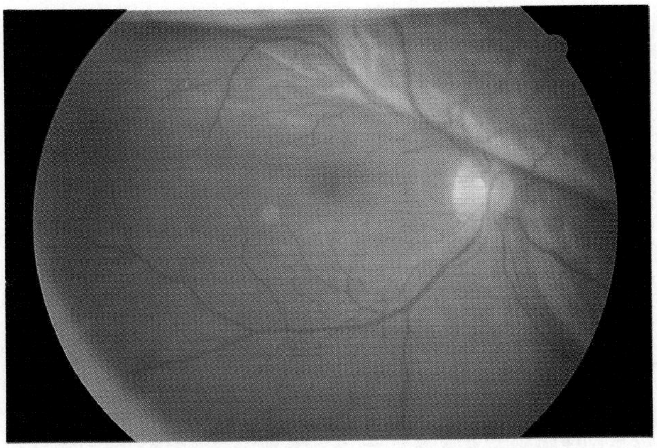

III-10 **Retinal detachment** appears as an elevated sheet of retinal tissue with folds. In this patient the fovea was spared, so acuity was normal, but a superior detachment produced an inferior scotoma.

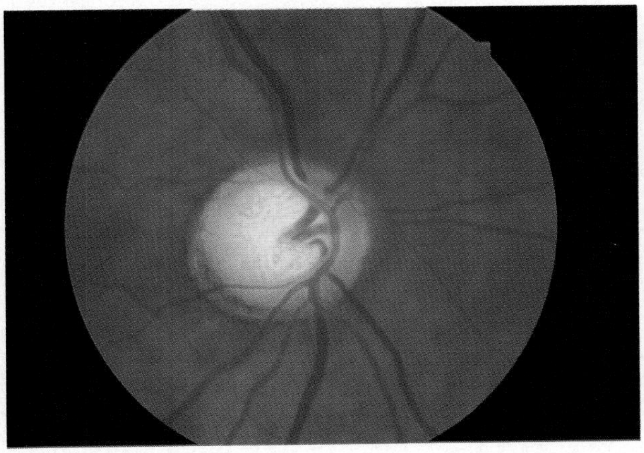

III-11 **Glaucoma** results in "cupping" as the neural rim is destroyed and the central cup becomes enlarged and excavated. The cup-to-disc ratio is about 0.7/1.0 in this patient.

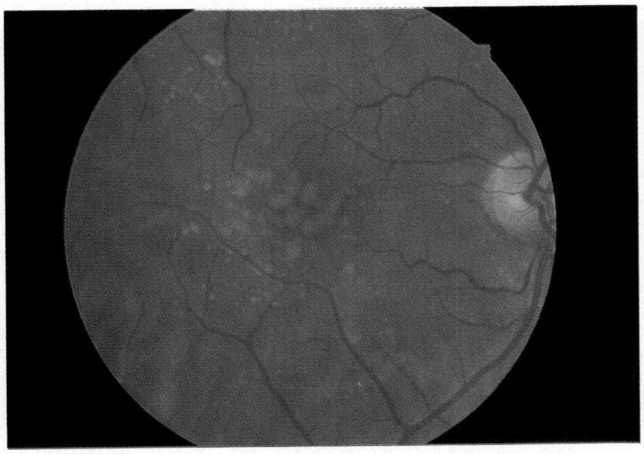

III-12 **Age-related macular degeneration** begins with the accumulation of drusen within the macula. They appear as scattered yellow subretinal deposits.

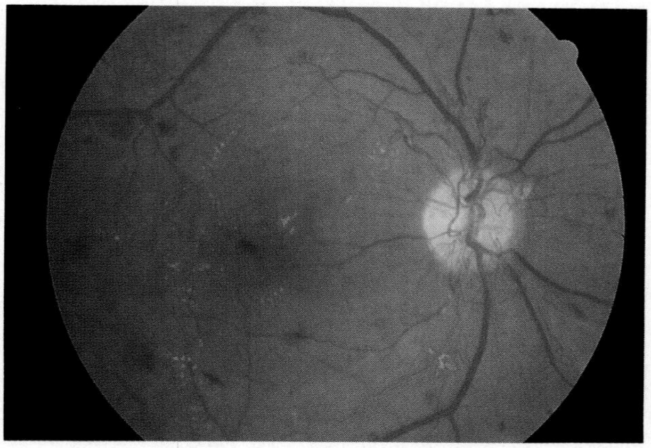

III-13 **Diabetic retinopathy** results in scattered hemorrhages and yellow exudates. This patient has neovascular vessels proliferating from the optic disc, requiring urgent pan retinal laser photocoagulation.

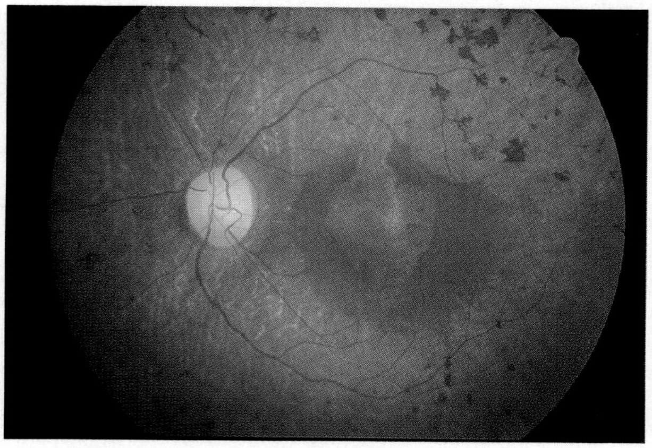

III-14 **Retinitis pigmentosa** with black clumps of pigment in the retinal periphery known as "bone spicules." There is also atrophy of the retinal pigment epithelium, making the vasculature of the choroid easily visible.

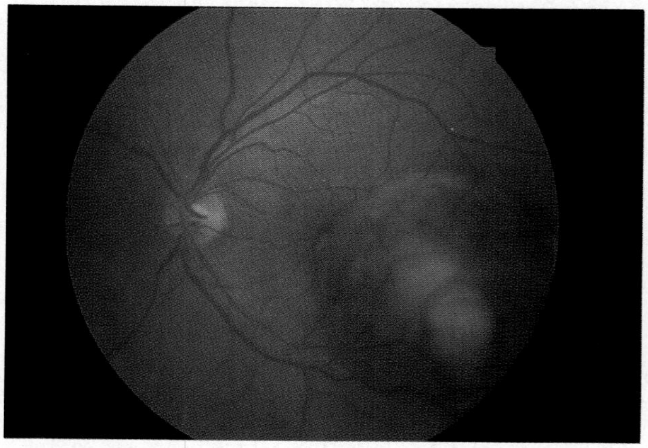

III-15 **Melanoma** of the choroid, appearing as an elevated dark mass in the inferior temporal fundus, just encroaching upon the fovea.

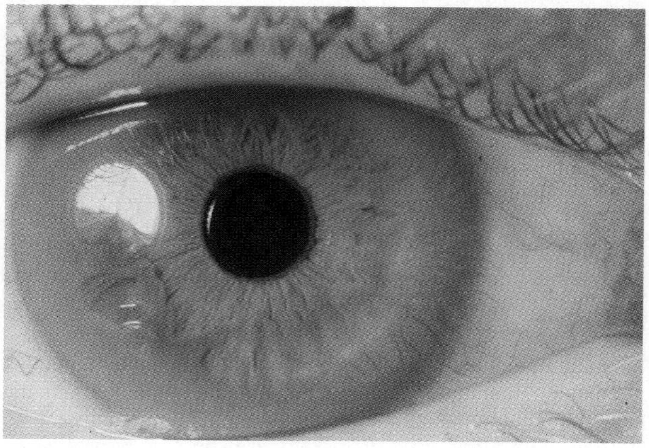

III-16 **Kayser-Fleischer ring** develops in Wilson's disease from copper deposition in Descemet's membrane, producing brownish discoloration of the peripheral cornea. It should not be confused with the yellow-white lipid ring of arcus senilis, which is common in the elderly and occasionally signifies hyperlipidemia, especially when it appears at a young age.

IV. Atlas of Hematology

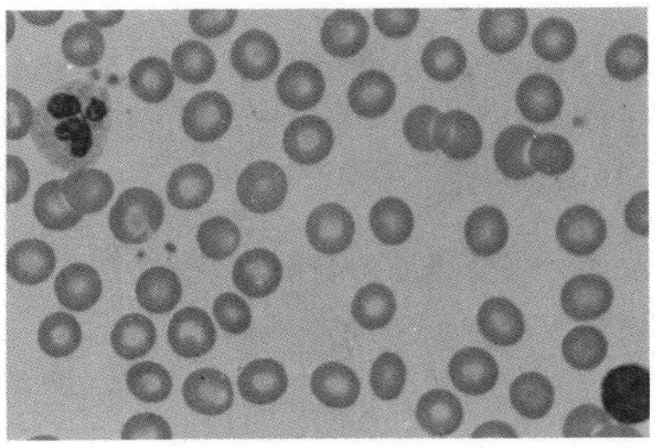

IV-1 **Normal blood smear** Normal red blood cells are round, possess an area of central pallor, appear slightly smaller than the nucleus of a mature lymphocyte, and vary little in size (anisocytosis) or in shape (poikilocytosis).

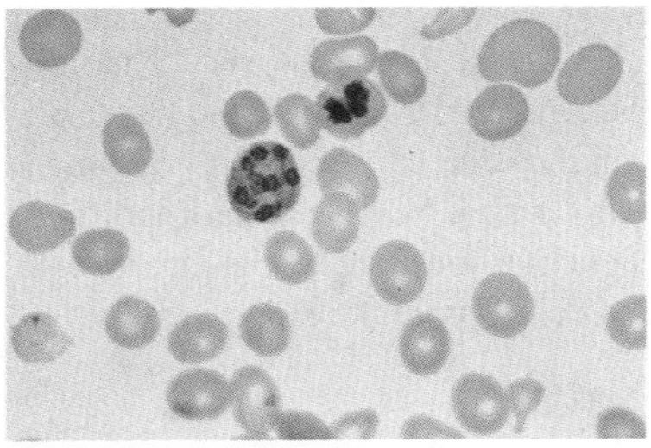

IV-2 **Megaloblastic anemia** Oval macrocytes, well filled with hemoglobin, are admixed with lesser numbers of small teardrop-shaped red blood cells. Note also hypersegmented granulocyte.

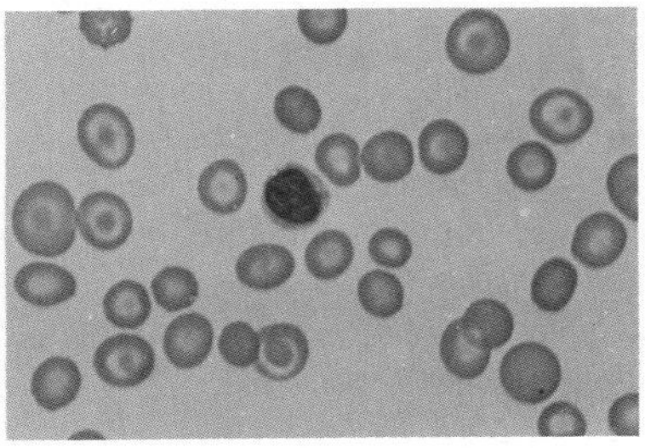

IV-3 **Liver disease** Round macrocytes of rather uniform size are seen. Many of the macrocytes are also target cells.

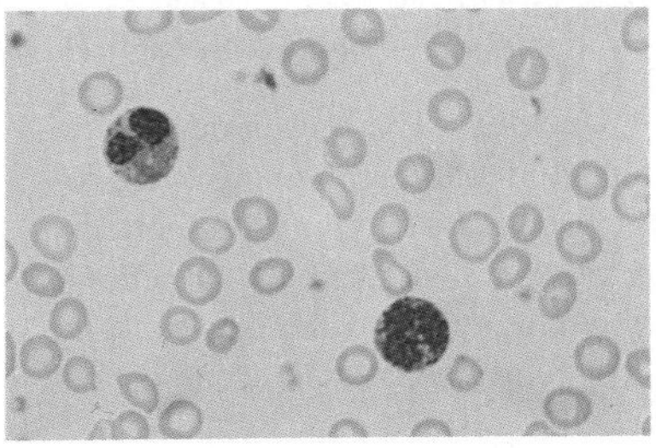

IV-4 **Iron-deficiency anemia** In severe iron deficiency, the red blood cells are smaller than normal (microcytosis), and their central area of pallor is expanded (hypochromia) so that the cells appear to have only a thin rim of hemoglobin.

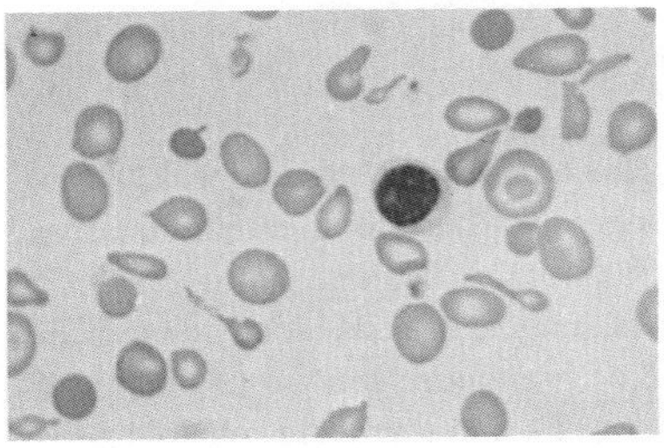

IV-5 **ß Thalassemia intermedia** Microcytic and hypochromic red blood cells are seen that resemble the red blood cells of severe iron deficiency anemia shown in Fig. IV-4. Many elliptical and teardrop-shaped red blood cells are noted.

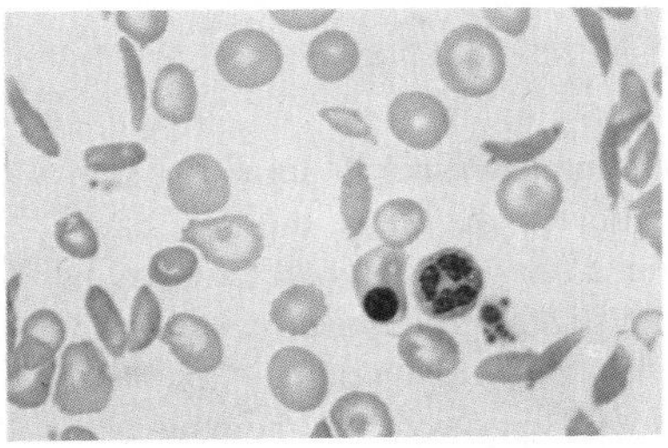

IV-6 **Sickle cell anemia** The elongated and crescent-shaped red blood cells seen on this smear represent circulating irreversibly sickled cells. Target cells and a nucleated red blood cell are also seen.

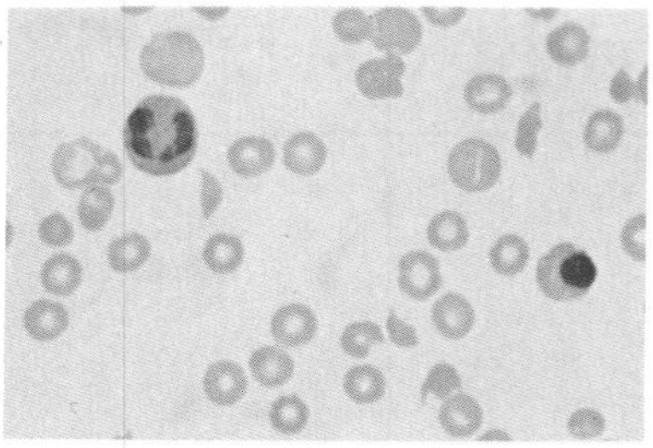

IV-7 **Traumatic hemolysis** The helmet-shaped red blood cell and the small triangular-shaped red blood cells seen on this smear represent morphologic evidence of mechanical damage to red blood cells within the blood vessels.

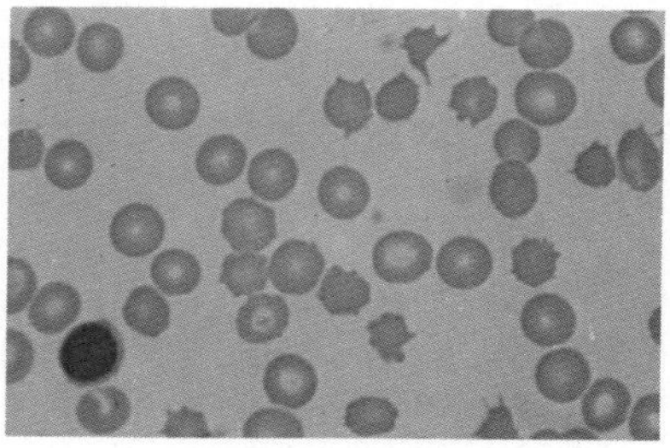

IV-8 **Spur cell anemia** Spur cells are recognized as distorted red blood cells containing several irregularly distributed thornlike projections. Cells with this morphologic abnormality are also called acanthocytes.

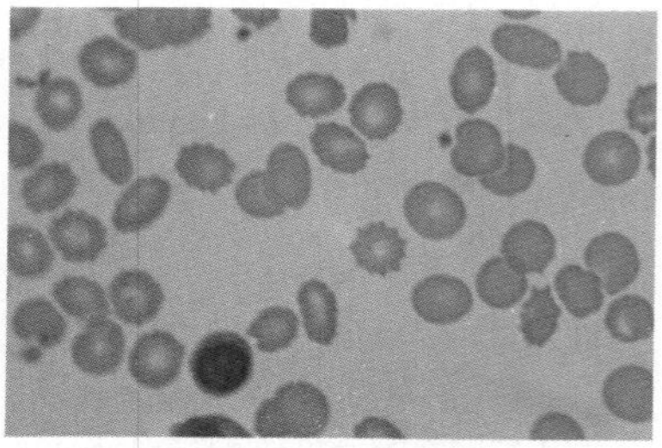

IV-9 **Uremia** The red blood cells in uremia may acquire numerous, regularly spaced, small spiny projections. Such cells, called burr cells or echinocytes, are readily distinguishable from the irregularly spiculated acanthocytes shown in Fig. IV-8.

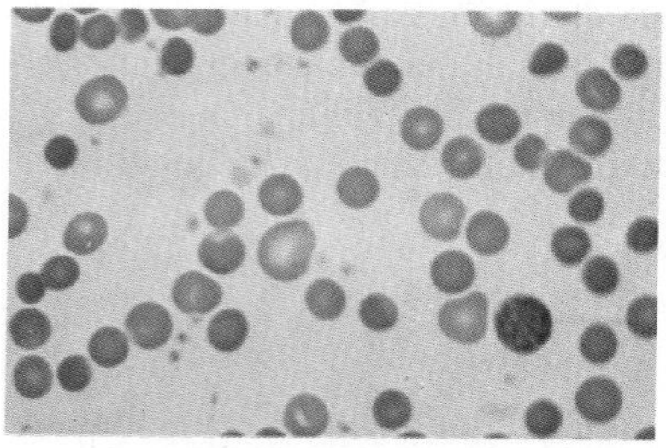

IV-10 **Hereditary spherocytosis** Small, densely staining red blood cells are seen that have lost their central area of pallor (microspherocytes). Microspherocytes may also be found in other hemolytic disorders (Fig. IV-11).

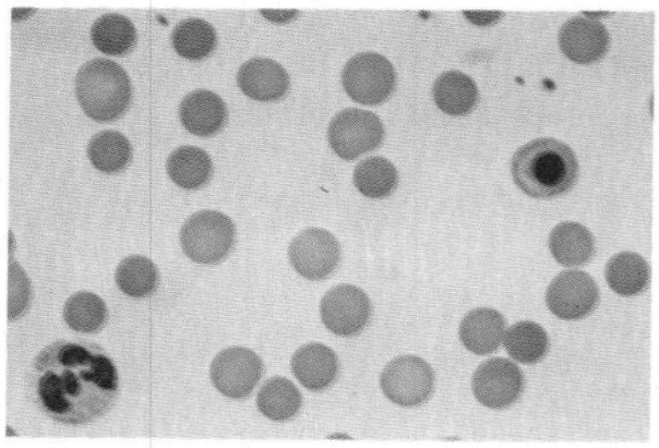

IV-11 **Immunohemolytic anemia** Microspherocytes are seen on this blood smear along with several macrocytes with a slight purple tinge (polychromasia). The latter represent new red blood cells released early from the bone marrow. The microspherocytes seen in immunohemolytic anemia may be indistinguishable from the microspherocytes seen in hereditary spherocytosis (Fig. IV-10).

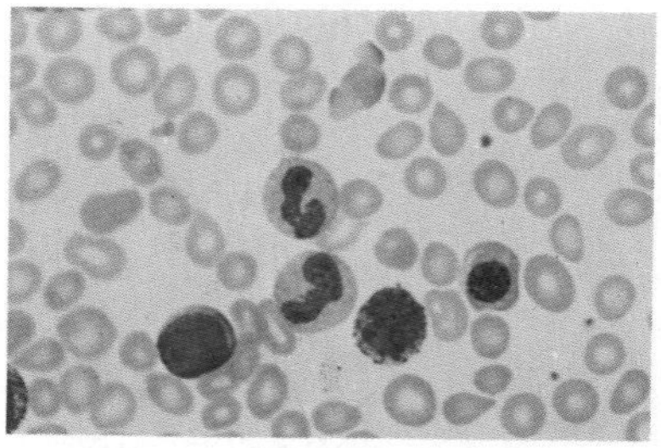

IV-12 **Leukoerythroblastic smear** Teardrop-shaped red blood cells indicative of membrane damage from collagen fibers, a nucleated red blood cell indicative of premature release of erythroid precursors, and immature myeloid cells indicative of extramedullary hematopoiesis are noted. This peripheral blood smear is related to marrow fibrosis, either primary myelofibrosis or secondary myelophthisis.

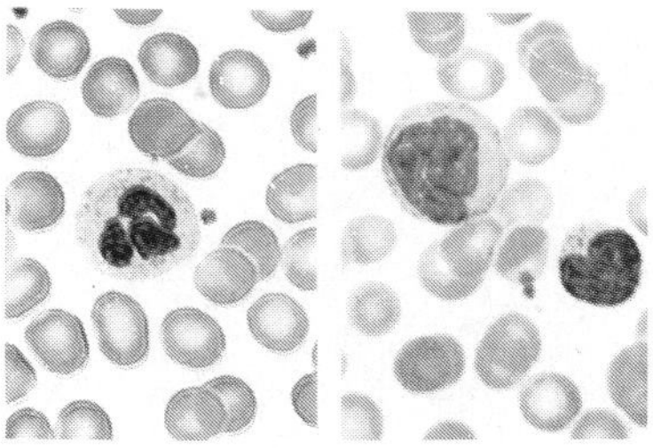

A *B*

IV-13 A. **Normal granulocyte** The normal granulocyte has a segmented nucleus with heavy, clumped chromatin; fine neutrophilic granules are dispersed throughout its cytoplasm.

B. **Normal monocyte and lymphocyte** The normal monocyte is a large cell with an indented or folded nucleus containing loose, strand-like chromatin; the cytoplasm is a blue-gray color and usually contains fine azurophilic granules. The normal lymphocyte is a smaller cell. Its nucleus is usually round but may be indented, as in the cell shown in this plate. The nuclear chromatin has a smudgy appearance; the cytoplasm is blue.

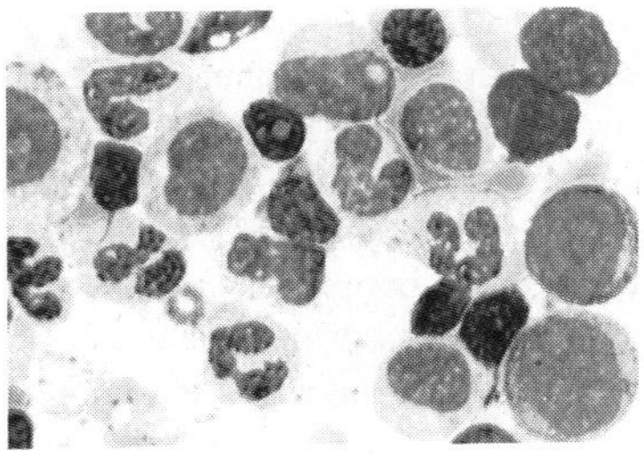

IV-15 **Normal granulocyte precursors in marrow** The earliest granulocytic precursor (myeloblast) possesses a round nucleus with fine, punctate chromatin and one or more nucleoli; the cytoplasm is blue. As nuclear differentiation proceeds, the nucleoli disappear, the chromatin coarsens, and the nucleus becomes increasingly indented and finally segmented. As cytoplasmic differentiation proceeds, azurophilic granules appear and the cytoplasm changes color from blue to the yellow-pink-gray hue of the mature granulocyte, and as this occurs the azurophilic granules become obscured by fine neutrophilic granules.

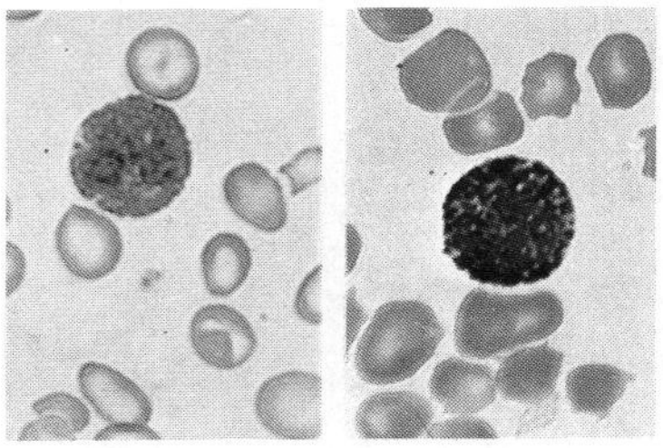

A *B*

IV-14 A. **Normal eosinophil** The eosinophil contains large, bright-orange granules; the nucleus is bilobed.

B. **Basophil** The basophil contains large purple-black granules that fill the cell and obscure the nucleus.

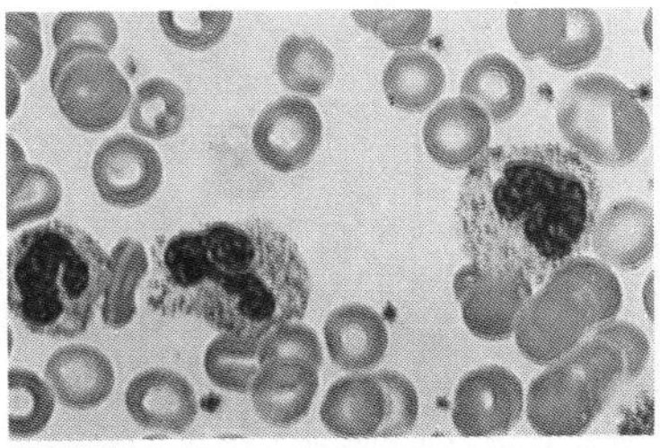

IV-16 **Neutrophils with toxic granulation** In infection and other toxic states, azurophilic granules may become visible in mature granulocytes as coarse, dark-staining cytoplasmic granules.

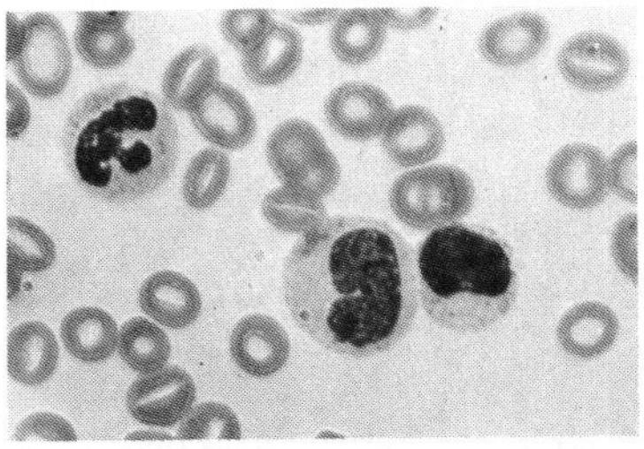

IV-17 **Band with Döhle body** *(center)* Döhle bodies are discrete, blue-staining non-granular areas found in the periphery of the cytoplasm of the neutrophil in infections and other toxic states. They represent aggregates of rough endoplasmic reticulum.

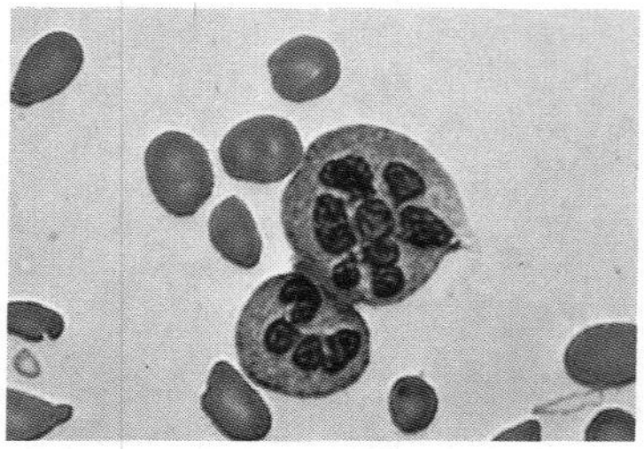

IV-18 **Hypersegmentation** Frequent five-lobed granulocytes on a blood smear or granulocytes with more than five lobes are evidence of hypersegmentation, an important clue to the diagnosis of megaloblastic anemia.

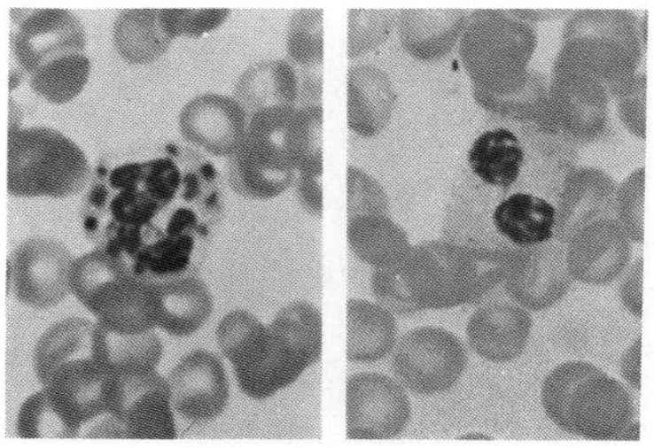

A *B*

IV-19 A. **Chédiak-Higashi anomaly** In this ultimately fatal disorder, the granulocytes contain huge cytoplasmic granules, formed from aggregation and fusion of azurophilic and specific granules. Large, abnormal granules are found in other granule-containing cells throughout the body. *B.* **Pelger-Hüet anomaly** In this benign disorder, the majority of granulocytes are bilobed. The nucleus frequently has a spectacle-like or "pince-nez" configuration.

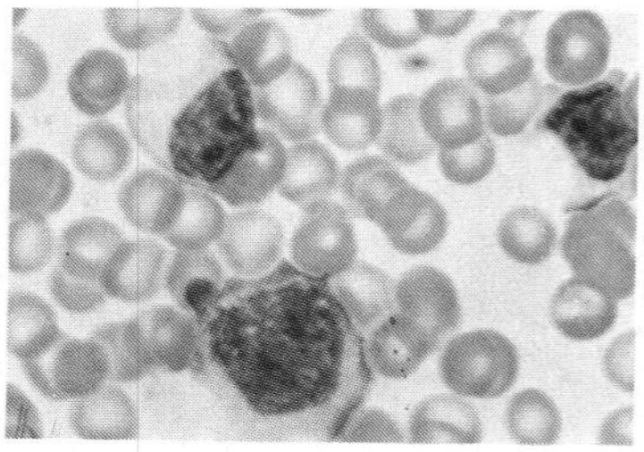

IV-20 **Reactive lymphocytes** (infectious mononucleosis) Reactive lymphocytes are usually large, and contain abundant cytoplasm. The nucleus may be eccentrically placed and may have irregular borders and indentations (not seen on this plate). The cytoplasm contains areas that stain a darker blue due to their increased content of RNA. The cytoplasm may be indented where it abuts against a red blood cell.

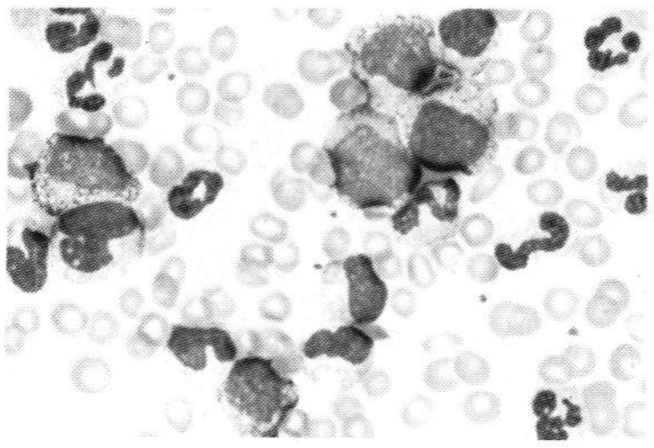

IV-21 **Chronic granulocytic leukemia** The peripheral WBC count is high due to increased numbers of granulocytes and their precursors. The majority of the WBCs are segmented granulocytes or band forms, but myelocytes (as seen on this plate) and promyeloblasts (not seen on this plate) may also be found on review of the blood smear.

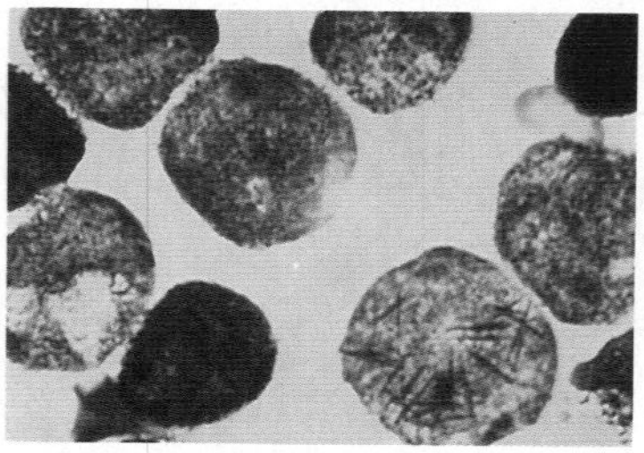

IV-22 **Leukemic cell in acute promyelocytic leukemia** Note multiple Auer rods.

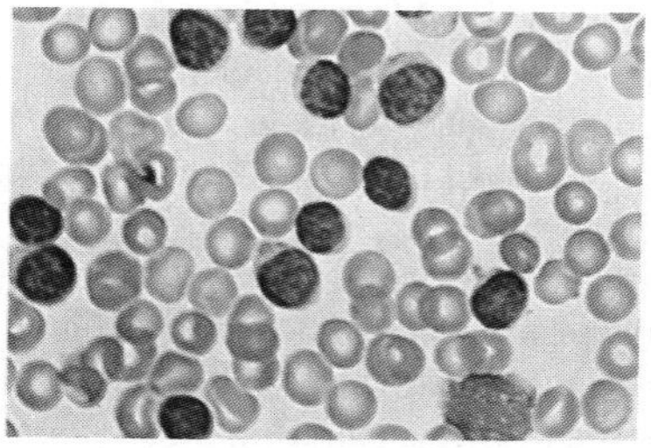

IV-23 **Chronic lymphocytic leukemia** The peripheral WBC count is high due to increased numbers of small, well-differentiated lymphocytes. However, the leukemic lymphocytes are fragile, and substantial numbers of broken, smudged cells are usually also present on the blood smear.

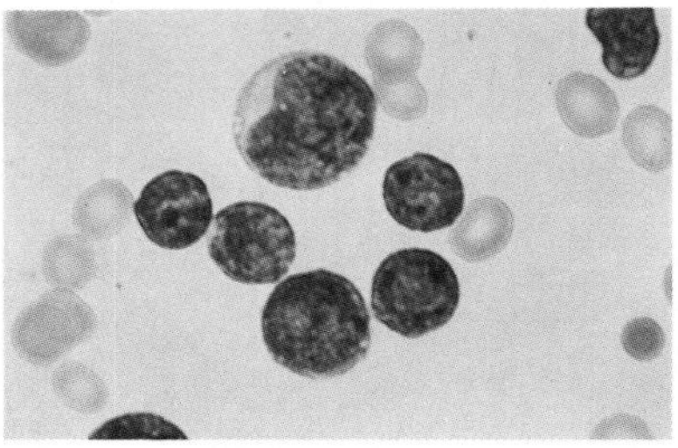

IV-24 **Leukemic cells in acute lymphoblastic leukemia** characterized by round or convoluted nuclei, high nuclear/cytoplasmic ratio and absence of cytoplasmic granules

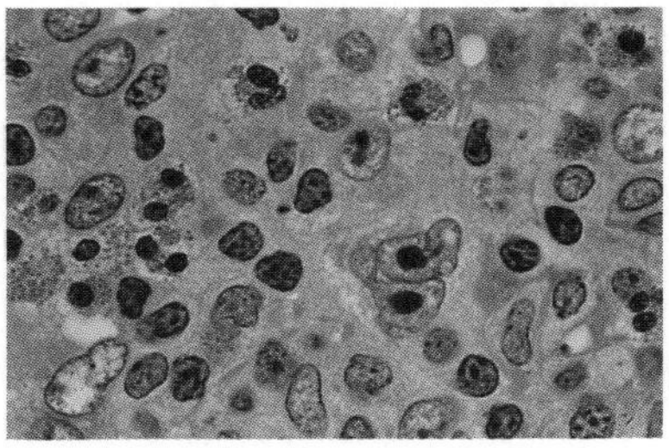

IV-25 **Hodgkin's disease, mixed cellularity** A Reed-Sternberg cell is present near the center of the field; a large cell with a bilobed nucleus and prominent nucleoli. The majority of the cells are normal lymphocytes, neutrophils, and eosinophils that form a pleiomorphic cellular infiltrate.

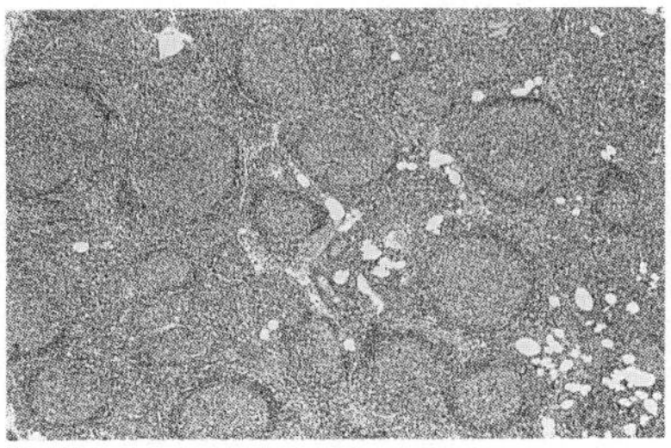

IV-26 **Follicular lymphoma** The normal nodal architecture is effaced by nodular expansions of tumor cells. Nodules vary in size and mimic normal lymphoid follicles.

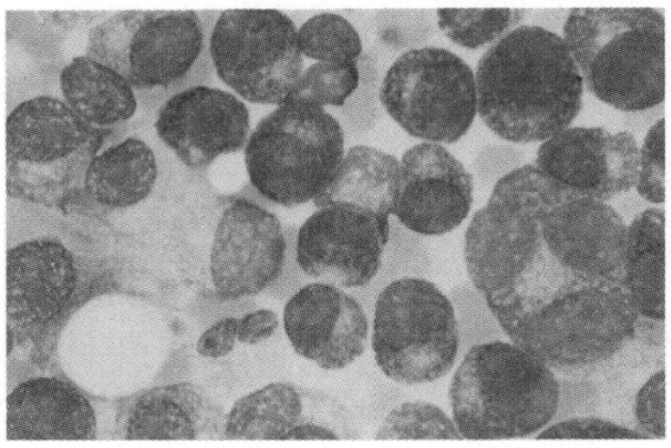

IV-27 **Multiple myeloma** (marrow) The cells bear the characteristic morphologic features of plasma cells, round or oval cells with an eccentric nucleus composed of coarsely clumped chromatin, a densely basophilic cytoplasm, and a perinuclear clear zone (hof) containing the Golgi apparatus. Binucleate and multinucleate malignant plasma cells also can be seen.

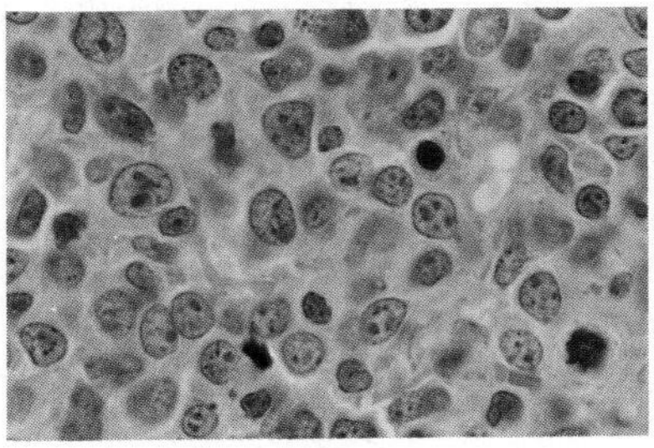

IV-28 **Diffuse large B cell lymphoma** The neoplastic cells are large with vesicular nuclear chromatin and prominent nucleoli.

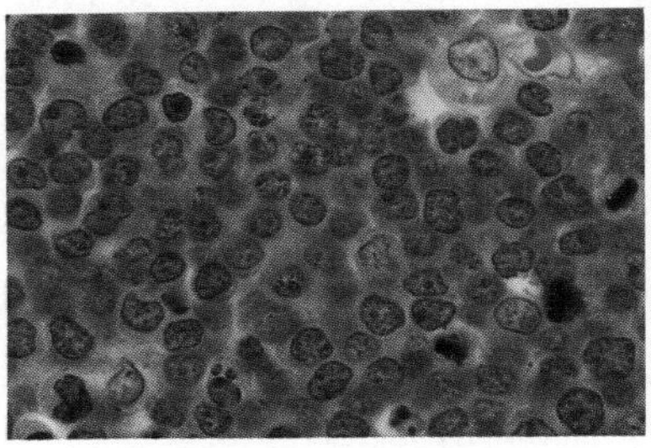

IV-29 **Burkitt's lymphoma** The neoplastic cells are homogeneous, medium-sized B cells with frequent mitotic figures, a morphologic correlate of high growth fraction. Reactive macrophages are scattered through the tumor and their pale cytoplasm in a background of blue-staining tumor cells gives the tumor a so-called "starry sky" appearance.

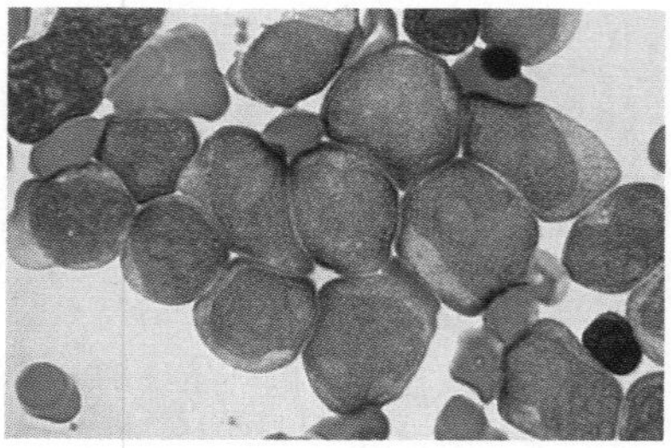

IV-30 **Acute myelocytic leukemia** This marrow section shows sheets of primitive myeloblasts with numerous large nucleoli.

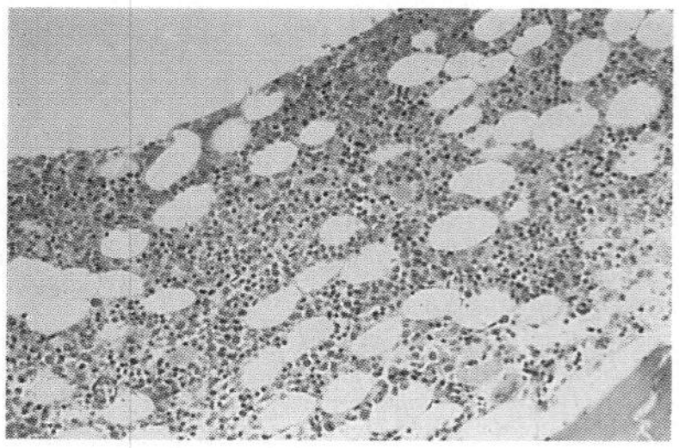

IV-32 **Normal bone marrow biopsy** This is a low power view of an H&E-stained section of normal marrow. Note that the nucleated cellular elements account for about 40 to 50 percent and the fat *(clear areas)* accounts for about 50 to 60 percent of the area.

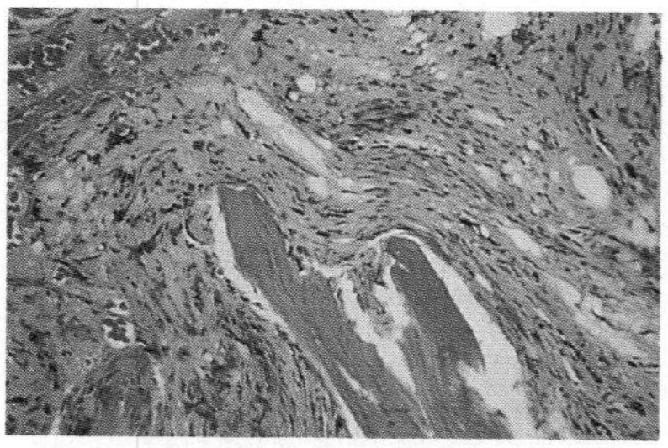

IV-34 **Marrow fibrosis** This marrow section shows the marrow cavity replaced by fibrous tissue composed of reticulin fibers and collagen. When this fibrosis is due to a primary hematologic process, it is called *myelofibrosis.* When the fibrosis is secondary to a tumor or a granulomatous process, it is called *myelophthisis.*

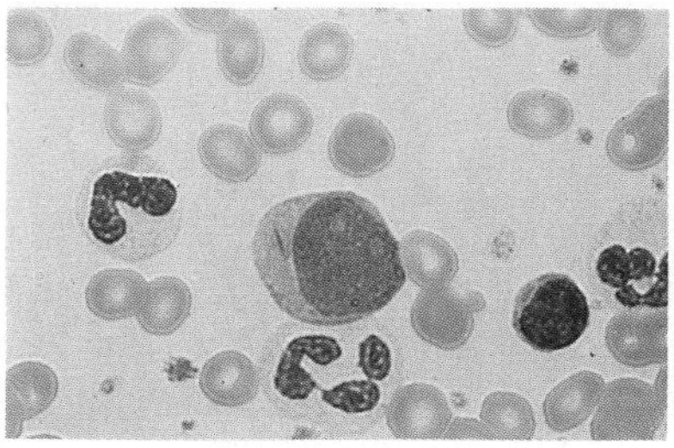

IV-31 **Auer rod** This peripheral blood smear shows a myeloblast with a single Auer rod in the cytoplasm. Auer rods, when present, are usually seen in acute myelocytic leukemia.

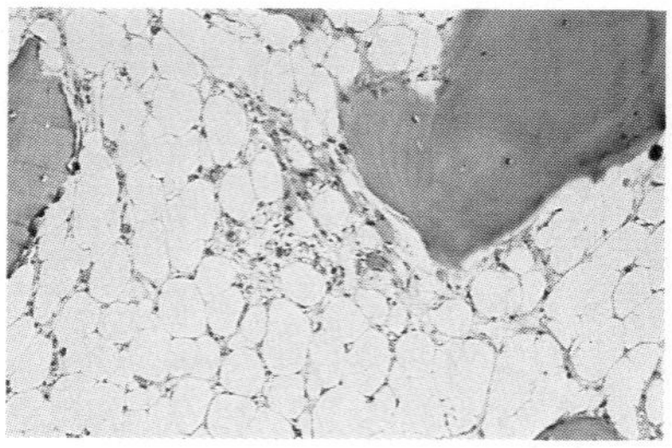

IV-33 **Aplastic anemia** This marrow section shows only fat with nearly complete absence of hematopoietic tissue.

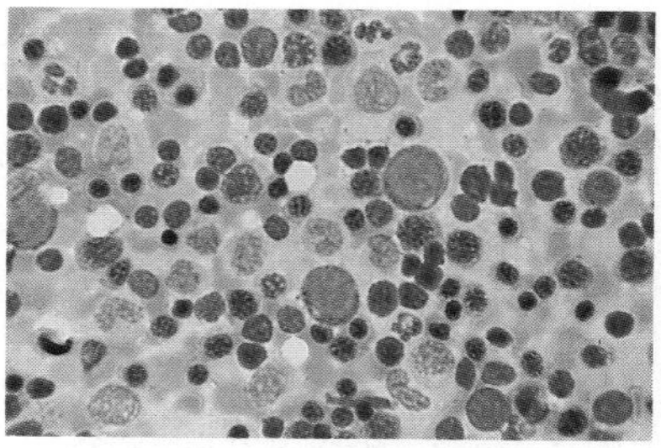

IV-35 **Erythroid hyperplasia** This marrow section shows an increase in the fraction of cells in the erythroid lineage as might be seen in a healthy marrow compensating for acute blood loss or hemolysis. The E/G ratio is greater than 1/1.

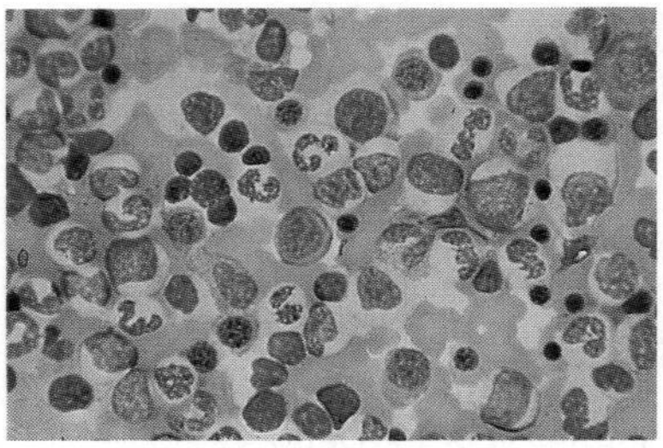

IV-36 **Granulocytic hyperplasia** This marrow section shows an increase in the fraction of cells in the myeloid or granulocytic lineage as might be seen in a healthy marrow responding to infection. The E/G ratio is less than 1/3.

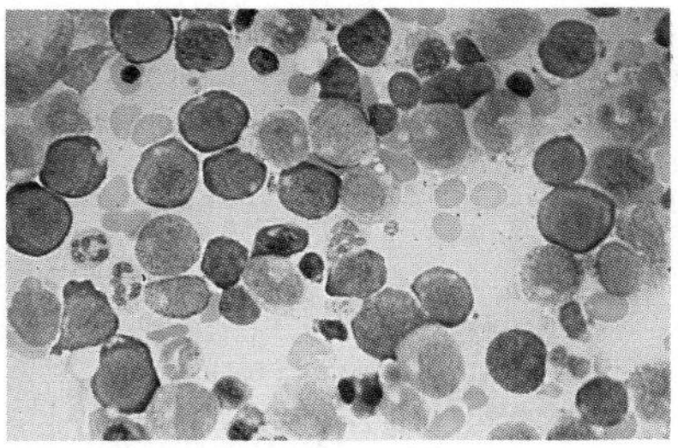

IV-37 **Megaloblastic erythropoiesis** This marrow section demonstrates so-called nuclear-cytoplasmic dissociation; the cytoplasm of erythroblasts is filled with hemoglobin demonstrating nearly complete maturation while the nuclei have loose chromatin characteristic of more immature erythroid cells. The slow nuclear maturation is related to a decrease in DNA synthesis related to an insufficient supply of reduced folate to synthesize thymidylate. DNA synthesis inhibitors can produce this picture, as can folate and B_{12} deficiency.

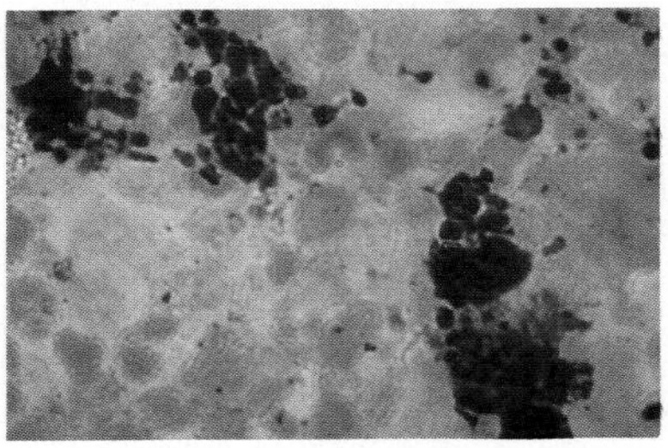

IV-38 **Marrow iron stores** This marrow section is stained with Prussian blue. Iron takes up the stain and is concentrated in reticuloendothelial cells. This picture shows normal iron stores. In iron deficiency states, no stainable iron is detectable. In the anemia of chronic disease, iron is present but cytokines prevent its mobilization and utilization in heme synthesis.

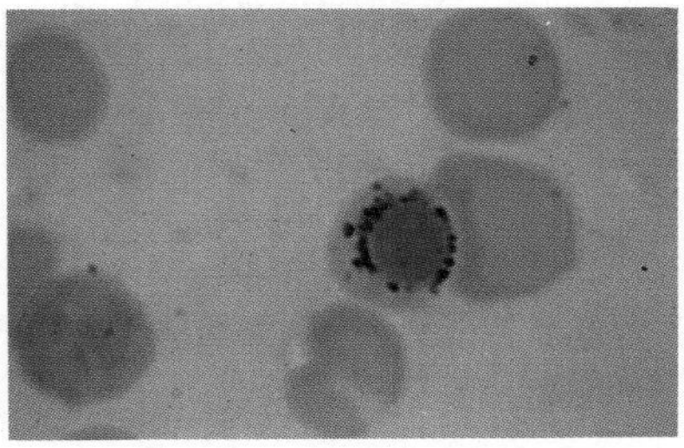

IV-39 **Ringed sideroblast** Refractory anemia with ringed sideroblasts (RARS) is in the spectrum of myelodysplastic syndromes. This marrow Prussian blue stain shows an orthochromatic normoblast with a collar of blue granules surrounding the nucleus. The blue granules represent iron-laden mitochondria.

SOURCES OF PHOTOGRAPHS

I. DERMATOLOGY

Robert Swerlick, M.D. IA-1 Acne rosacea; IA-9 Lichen planus; IA-12 Alopecia areata; ID-33 Folliculitis; IE-65 Erythema nodosum; IE-66 Vasculitis

S. Wright Caughman, M.D. IC-30 Nodular melanoma; ID-35 Herpes simplex; ID-50 Fulminant meningococcemia; ID-58 Condylomata acuminatum

Alvin Solomon, M.D. IC-29 Lentigo maligna melanoma; ID-53 Secondary syphilis of the palms

Mary Spraker, M.D. ID-32 Impetigo contagiosa

Kim Yancey, M.D. IF-74 Coumarin necrosis

John Greenspan, Ph.D. ID-41 Oral hairy leukoplakia; ID-42 Pseudomembranous oral candidiasis

Gregory Cox, M.D. ID-51 Primary syphilis

Marilynne McKay, M.D. IE-59 Discoid lupus erythematosus

James Krell, M.D. IE-60 Dermatomyositis

Yale Resident's Slide Collection ID-40 Molluscum contagiosum; ID-48 Rocky Mountain spotted fever; ID-69 Bullous pemphigoid; ID-47 Erythema chronicum migrans; ID-54 Condylomata lata; ID-64 Erythema multiforme

Kalman Watsky, M.D. IA-1 Acne vulgaris

Jean Bolognia, M.D. IA-6 Seborrheic dermatitis; IB-24 Non-Hodgkin's lymphoma

Robert Hartman, M.D. ID-36 Varicella

Irwin Braverman, M.D. IA-4 Atopic dermatitis

II. ENDOSCOPIC FINDINGS

FE Silverstein and **GN Tytgat** *Atlas of Gastrointestinal Endoscopy,* New York, Gower Medical Publishing, 1987 All photographs except II-12, II-23, II-24

GN Tytgat II-12, II-23, II-24

III. FUNDUSCOPIC FINDINGS

Jonathan C. Horton, M.D., Ph.D. All photographs, III-1 to III-16

IV. HEMATOLOGY

Elaine Jaffe, M.D. IV-25 to IV-29

Robert S. Hillman, M.D., and **Kenneth A. Ault, M.D.** *Hematology in General Practice,* New York, McGraw-Hill, 1995. Courtesy of the American Society of Hematology Slide Bank. IV-30 to IV-39

PART FOURTEEN

NEUROLOGIC DISORDERS

SECTION 1
DIAGNOSIS OF NEUROLOGIC DISORDERS

360

Joseph B. Martin, Stephen L. Hauser

APPROACH TO THE PATIENT WITH NEUROLOGIC DISEASE

Neurologic disorders are frequent in clinical medicine, yet many physicians are uncomfortable with the diagnosis of nervous system disease and unprepared to manage neurologic conditions efficiently. Neurologic disorders may produce a bewildering array of symptoms and signs or disturb a patient's ability to communicate normally with the examiner. The examination may be time-consuming, and correct diagnosis requires a working knowledge of relevant neuroanatomic principles. Finally, many physicians are disadvantaged by limited formal training in neurology, due to the growth of the field as an independent specialty with separate clinical services that sequester neurologic problems from general medical services.

Most patients with neurologic symptoms seek care from internists and other generalists rather than neurologists. This situation is likely to continue in the future as primary care–based health care systems become increasingly prevalent and the number of specialists, including neurologists, is reduced. For all practitioners, the importance of a level of competence in neurology cannot be overstated, as the explosive increase in the number of useful therapies for many neurologic disorders makes correct diagnosis an ethical imperative. In subsequent chapters, various algorithms are presented as aids to diagnosis and therapy of various neurologic disorders. Appropriate use of these algorithms requires that the physician first correctly assess and interpret the presenting symptoms and signs of these conditions.

The goal of the neurologic method is to define the patient's illness, first in anatomic and then in pathophysiologic terms. Arrival at a diagnosis permits the physician to institute therapy and to inform and counsel patients and their families as to the expected disease course.

THE NEUROLOGIC METHOD OF CLINICAL EVALUATION

The strategy used in evaluating a patient with neurologic illness is to begin with the question, "What portion of the neural axis is likely to be involved in causing the neurologic symptoms?" The first clues to defining the anatomic area of involvement appear in the history, and the examination is then directed to confirm or rule out these impressions and to clarify uncertainties suggested by the history. A more detailed examination of a particular region of the central nervous system (CNS) or peripheral nervous system is often indicated. For example, optokinetic nystagmus may be an important part of the examination in a patient with a left hemiparesis and dressing apraxia but irrelevant to the examination of a patient complaining of burning feet. In a patient who presents with a history of ascending paresthesia and weakness, the examination should be *directed* toward deciding, among other things, if the location of the lesion is the spinal cord or peripheral nerves. Notations regarding muscle stamina or endurance might be crucial to the examination of a patient with myasthenia gravis, as opposed to the usual tests of peak muscle power. What one does in the neurologic examination depends on what the questions are; the questions are formulated by a properly taken history.

Deciding "where the lesion is" accomplishes the task of delimiting the number of possible etiologies to a manageable, finite size. In addition, this strategy safeguards against making really tragic errors. Symptoms of recurrent vertigo, diplopia, and nystagmus should not trigger "multiple sclerosis" as an answer (etiology) but "brainstem" or "pons" (location); then a diagnosis of brainstem arteriovenous malformation will not be missed because it is not considered. Similarly, the combination of optic neuritis and spastic ataxic paraparesis should not suggest only multiple sclerosis; CNS syphilis and vitamin B_{12} deficiency (both treatable) also can cause these findings. When the question, "Where is the lesion?" is answered, then the question, "What is the lesion?" can be addressed.

THE NEUROLOGIC HISTORY Careful attention to the description of the symptoms as experienced by the patient and substantiated by family members or friends permits, in many instances, an accurate localization and determination of the probable cause of the complaints even before the neurologic examination is undertaken. Two principles should be followed. First, each complaint should be pursued as far as possible in an effort to delineate where the lesion might be or, more important, *to formulate a set of questions to be answered by the examination.* A patient complains of weakness of the right arm. What are the associated features? Is this weakness for brushing the hair or opening a twist-top bottle? Second, in neurology—where many of the diseases are due to *anatomically restricted* lesions—*negative* associations may be crucial. A patient with a right hemiparesis without a language deficit likely has a different lesion (and likely etiology) than a patient with a right hemiparesis and aphasia. Additional important factors that aid in defining the nature of the neurologic disorder include the following:

1. *Temporal course of the illness.* It is important to ascertain the precise time of appearance and rate of progression of the symptoms experienced by the patient. The rapid onset of a neurologic complaint, occurring within seconds or minutes, usually indicates a vascular event or a seizure. Attention to the temporal march of symptoms may help define a focal seizure, a cerebral transient ischemic attack (TIA), or the onset of a migraine. For example, the onset of sensory symptoms located in one extremity that spread over a few seconds to adjacent portions of that extremity and then to the other limb or to the face suggests a seizure. A more gradual onset involving less discrete regions of the extremities points to the possibility of a TIA. A similar but slower progression of sensory change occurring in a young person together with other symptoms of headache, nausea, or visual disturbance suggests migraine. In general, the march of a migraine is slower than that of seizure, and a TIA tends to be more generalized in location on the side of the body or extremities. The presence of "positive" sensory symptoms (e.g., buzzing) or motor movements suggests a seizure; in contrast, transient loss of a function (negative symptom) suggests a TIA. A stuttering onset where symptoms appear, stabilize, and then progress over hours or days also suggests the presence of cerebrovascular disease. In acute vascular disease, a history of transient remission or regression indicates that the process is likely ischemic and not hemorrhagic. In some cases, a demyelinating process may also produce new symptoms that evolve rapidly over the course of a few hours. Progressing symptoms associated with the systemic manifestations of fever, stiff neck, and altered level of consciousness or awareness suggest the possibility of an infectious process. The course of the illness over years in terms of remissions and exacerbations offers additional clues to the nature of the process. Recurrent neurologic symptoms involving different levels of the neuraxis with partial or complete recovery suggest the possibility of multiple sclerosis. Slowly progressive symptoms without remissions tend to be characteristic of a neurodegenerative disorder.

Achilles tendon. Occasional normal individuals will have two or three beats of physiologic ankle clonus, but sustained ankle clonus is an abnormal finding that signifies hyperactivity of the motor unit resulting from an upper motor neuron lesion.

In addition to the stretch reflexes, assessment of the superficial cutaneous reflexes provides confirmatory and localizing data. The plantar reflex is elicited by stroking, with a blunt object (i.e., a key or tongue blade), the lateral surface of the foot beginning near the heel and moving toward the toes. The normal reflex consists of plantar flexion of the toes. With upper motor neuron lesions above the S1 level of the spinal cord, a paradoxical extension of the great toe is noted, associated with fanning and extension of the other toes (extensor plantar response or Babinski sign); a prominent extensor plantar response may be accompanied by triple flexion at the ankle, knee, and hip. In some patients with corticospinal tract lesions, the great toe on the involved side may assume an extensor posture at rest or following movement of the foot. Some patients may voluntarily withdraw from the plantar stroke, simulating an extensor response. In these situations, the direction of the plantar response may be determined by pressure applied to the anterior tibia, stroking towards the ankle (Oppenheim sign), pressure applied to the calf (Gordon sign) or ankle (Schaefer sign), or pricking of the dorsum of the great toe (Bing sign).

Superficial abdominal reflexes are often neglected but can be of diagnostic value, particularly in localization of spinal cord disease. These are elicited by lightly stroking the abdominal wall with a sharp object (e.g., a pin) and observing movement of the umbilicus. The upper abdominal reflex (spinal cord level T9) is elicited by stroking the lateral upper corner of the abdomen towards the umbilicus, whereas the lower abdominal reflex (T12) is stimulated by a stimulus beginning at the lower lateral abdomen. The normal response consists of diagonal deviation of the umbilicus toward the origin of the stimulus. With upper motor neuron lesions, these reflexes are absent. They are most helpful when there is preservation of upper but not lower abdominal reflexes, indicating a spinal lesion between T9 and T12, or when the response is asymmetric. Obese individuals or multiparous women may not have visible superficial abdominal reflexes. Many other useful cutaneous reflexes have been described, including the sacral cremasteric (ipsilateral elevation of the testicle following stroking of the medial thigh), anal (contraction of the anal sphincter following pinprick stimulation of the perianal region), and bulbocavernosus (contraction of urethra and anal sphincter following a stimulus to the glans penis) reflexes.

Finally, in patients with suspected frontal lobe disease, hydrocephalus, or dementia, several primitive reflexes, not normally present in the adult, may appear. These include the suck, root, grasp, and palmomental reflexes. The suck response is elicited by lightly touching the center of the lips, and the root reponse the corner of the lips, with a tongue blade; the patient will move the lips to suck or root in the direction of the stimulus. The grasp reflex is elicited by touching the palm, and in particular the area between the thumb and index finger, with the examiner's fingers; a positive (abnormal) response consists of a forced grasp of the stimulated hand. The palmomental response consists of contraction of the chin ipsilateral to a scratch stimulus diagonally applied to the palm.

Sensory Examination (See also Chap. 23) Five primary sensory modalities—vibration, joint position, light touch, pinprick, and temperature—are routinely tested in each limb. Unlike reflex testing, the evaluation of sensation requires cooperation and concentration by the patient. The examiner should provide a brief introduction to the purpose and methods of each sensory test prior to performing the examination. Assessment of vibration and position sense is usually performed first. Vibration testing generally utilizes a 128-Hz weighted tuning fork, but some physicians prefer the smaller 256-Hz fork. The vibrating tuning fork is applied to the terminal phalynx of the great toe or middle finger just below the nail bed. The examiner compares the patient's threshold of vibration perception with his or her own or compares distal and proximal thresholds in the patient. For joint position testing, the examiner grasps the limb laterally and distal to the joint to be assessed. Light touch is best assessed with a wisp of cotton, pinprick with a clean pin (compare sharp versus blunt end), and temperature initially with a tuning fork immersed in cold and hot water. Patients with lesions above the level of the thalamus may have disorders of "discriminative sensation," resulting in an inability to perceive double simultaneous stimuli, to localize stimuli accurately, to identify closely approximated stimuli as separate (two-point discrimination), to identify objects by touch alone (stereognosis), or to judge weights, evaluate texture, or identify letters or numbers written on the skin surface (graphesthesia). Although difficult to master, facility with sensory examination skills is of great value in many clinical situations. In peripheral neuropathy, a gradient of distal more than proximal sensory loss may be present. In early stages of spinal cord disease, a sensory level may be detected to pinprick and temperature as the examiner moves up and down each side of the back. A tumor of the conus medullaris may present with focal sensory loss in a sacral distribution. In systemic vasculitis, identification of a mononeuropathy may signal involvement of the vasa nervorum (mononeuritis multiplex).

Coordination (See also Chap. 21) The patient is asked to touch his or her index finger repetitively to the nose and then to the examiner's outstretched finger; the examiner's finger can be moved with each repetition. Another useful test is to ask the patient to alternate tapping the palm then the back of one hand on the thigh. To test coordination in the legs, in the supine position the patient is asked to slide the heel (not the arch!) of each foot from the knee down the shin of the other leg, and to raise the leg and touch with the great toe the examiner's index finger. For all these movements, the accuracy, speed, and rhythm are noted.

Gait (See also Chap. 21) Gait is easily tested and highly informative, and observation of gait is an essential component of the neurologic examination. Unexpected abnormalities may be detected that prompt the examiner to return, in more detail, to other aspects of the examination. Normal gait requires that multiple systems—including power, sensation, coordination, and praxis—function in a coordinated fashion. The ability to rise from the sitting or lying position, to stand with eyes closed and feet together (Romberg test), and to walk, turn, and heel-toe walk along a straight line should be noted. The examination may reveal decreased arm swing on one side (corticospinal tract disease), a stooped posture and short-stepped gait (Parkinson's syndrome), a broad-based unstable gait (ataxia), scissoring (spasticity), or a high-stepped, slapping gait (posterior column or peripheral nerve disease) or the patient may appear to be stuck in place (apraxia).

This detailed neurologic examination is undertaken only if there are symptoms of disturbed nervous system functioning. If none are present, it suffices to do an abbreviated examination that includes evaluation only of pupils, ocular movements, optic fundi, facial movements, speech, strength of arm and leg muscles, tendon and plantar reflexes, pain and vibratory sensation in hands and feet, and gait. All this can be completed in 3 to 5 min. The findings, even in the short examination, should be recorded in the patient's record for future reference.

Two additional points about the examination are worth noting. First, in recording observations, it is important for the physician to describe what is found rather than to apply a poorly defined medical term (i.e., "patient groans to sternal rub" rather than "obtunded"). Second, if the patient's complaint is brought out by some activity, reproduce the activity in the office. If the complaint is of dizziness when raising the right arm and turning the head to the left, have the patient do it. If pain occurs after walking two blocks, have the patient demonstrate it, and repeat the examination.

Experience teaches that the neurologic examination may be normal even in patients with a serious neurologic disease, such as one that causes seizures or syncope. Or the patient may arrive in a coma with no available history, and the examination proceeds along the lines described in Chap. 24. An inadequate history may be compensated to some extent by a succession of examinations from which the course of the illness may be plotted.

FORMULATION OF THE PROBLEM AND ESTABLISHMENT OF AN ETIOLOGIC DIAGNOSIS The clinical data obtained from the history and the examination are assembled into one of the known syndromes and are interpreted and translated in terms of neuroanatomy and neurophysiology. From the syndrome the physician should be able to determine the anatomic localization(s) that best explains the clinical findings. The anatomic localization, mode of onset and course of illness, other medical data, and laboratory findings are then integrated. Finally, the etiologic diagnosis is reached, and therapy appropriate for the disorder is proposed.

LABORATORY TESTS The proper selection of tests is important to arrive at an anatomic, but more particularly an etiologic, diagnosis. The laboratory assessment of a patient with positive neurologic findings may include (1) serum electrolytes, complete blood count, and renal, liver, and endocrine studies; (2) cerebrospinal fluid (CSF) examination; (3) imaging studies of the CNS (see Chap. 362); or (4) electrophysiologic studies (see Chap. 361).

LUMBAR PUNCTURE The clinical indications for lumbar puncture are listed in Table 360-2. In experienced hands, lumbar puncture is a safe procedure. It should always be performed under sterile conditions. The patient is asked to lie on his or her side facing away from the examiner. The back is positioned at the edge of the bed or table near the examiner. The patient is asked to "roll up into a ball"—the neck is gently flexed and the knees drawn up to the abdomen. Proper positioning is essential for success; the examiner should ensure that the shoulders and pelvis are aligned in a perfect vertical position without forward or backward tilt. A pillow is placed under the neck for comfort and a blanket offered for warmth. Because the spinal cord terminates at approximately the L1 vertebral level, the puncture is performed below this level; i.e., at or below the L2–L3 interspace. A useful anatomic guidepost is the posterior iliac crest that corresponds to the L3–L4 interspace. The interspace is chosen following gentle palpation to identify the spinous processes at each lumbar level. The area is draped and cleansed by multiple washings with antiseptic ointment and alcohol. Local anesthetic, typically 1% lidocaine, is injected into the subcutaneous tissue; a topical anesthetic cream (lidocaine 2.5%/prilocaine 2.5%) applied 90 min prior to the procedure can eliminate pain associated with injection. About 5 min after the lidocaine injection, the lumbar puncture needle (typically 22 gauge) is inserted in the midline between two spinous processes and slowly advanced at a slightly caudal angle aiming at the umbilicus. It is important that the bevel of the needle be maintained in a horizontal position, parallel to the direction of the dural fibers; this minimizes injury to the fibers as the dura is penetrated. In most adults, the needle is advanced 4 to 5 cm (1 1/2 to 2 in.) before the subarachnoid space is reached, and the examiner usually recognizes entry as a sudden release of resistance. Some examiners prefer to remove the stylet periodically as the needle is advanced to look for CSF flow. If the needle cannot be advanced because bone is hit, if the patient experiences sharp radiating pain down one leg, or if the tap is "dry," the needle is removed completely and repositioned.

Table 360-2

Indications for Lumbar Puncture

ABSOLUTE INDICATIONS	
Meningitis	
Encephalitis	
Meningeal cancer	
Acute inflammatory polyneuritis (Guillain-Barré syndrome)	
Acute demyelinating disorders	
	Acute disseminated encephalomyelitis
	Transverse myelitis
	Brainstem encephalomyelitis
Benign intracranial hypertension (pseudotumor cerebri)	
Unexplained neurologic disorders	
	Seizure
	Stroke
	Polyneuropathy
	Dementia
	Altered level of consciousness
Therapeutic administration of antibiotics or antineoplastic agents	
Diagnostic injections of dyes (myelography) or radioisotopes (CSF leak)	
POSSIBLE INDICATIONS (Depending on the Clinical Situation)	
Multiple sclerosis	
Subarachnoid hemorrhage	

Once the subarachnoid space is reached, a manometer is attached to the needle and pressure measured. The examiner should look for normal oscillations in CSF pressure associated with pulse and respirations. Depending on the clinical indication, fluid is then obtained for studies including: (1) cell count, differential, and presence of microorganisms—it is often useful to repeat the cell count in the first and last tube; (2) protein, sugar, and other chemical measurements; (3) cytology; (4) VDRL, cryptococcal antigen, and serologic and genetic tests for other microorganisms as appropriate; (5) immunoelectrophoresis for determination of gamma globulin level (paired serum sample essential), oligoclonal banding, and other special biochemical tests (for NH_3, pH, CO_2, enzymes, etc.); and (6) bacteriologic cultures and virus isolation. Normal values of CSF constituents are shown in Appendix A. Under most conditions, the physician should not be concerned about removing too large a quantity of CSF. A sufficient volume to obtain all the data required is essential. In particular, adequate volumes for cytology, when indicated, should be removed.

Failure to enter the lumbar subarachnoid space after two or three trials can usually be corrected by repositioning patients in the sitting position and then assisting them to lie on their side for pressure measurements and fluid removal. The "dry tap" is more often due to an improperly placed needle than to a pathologic obliteration of subarachnoid space by a compressive lesion of the spinal cord or by chronic adhesive arachnoiditis. A bloody tap due to penetration of a meningeal vessel may result in confusion with subarachnoid hemorrhage. In these situations it is essential that a specimen of CSF be centrifuged immediately after it is obtained; clear supernatant CSF following centrifugation supports the diagnosis of a bloody tap, whereas xanthochromic supernatant suggests subarachnoid hemorrhage. In general, bloody CSF due to a meningeal vessel puncture clears gradually in successive tubes, whereas blood due to a subarachnoid hemorrhage does not. Xanthochromic CSF not due to blood products may also be present in patients with liver disease or when the level of CSF protein is elevated [>1.5 to 2.0 g/L (150 to 200 mg/dL)].

There are several absolute or relative contraindications to lumbar puncture. Lumbar puncture should be undertaken with particular care in patients with thrombocytopenia or disorders of blood coagulation because serious hemorrhage into the extradural or intradural space may occur. In these situations, it is prudent whenever possible to transfuse platelets, administer fresh frozen plasma, or reverse therapeutic anticoagulation prior to the procedure. The presence of local skin or soft tissue infections along the needle tract may result in spread of infection to the meninges; thus lumbar puncture at these sites should be avoided.

Lumbar puncture also carries a risk if the CSF pressure is high (evidenced by headache and papilledema), for it increases the possibility of fatal cerebellar or tentorial herniation. If this possibility exists and if CSF examination is required, it is wise first to obtain a computed tomography (CT) or magnetic resonance imaging (MRI) scan to exclude a mass lesion before proceeding to lumbar puncture. An exception to this rule is suspected meningitis, where CSF examination is always indicated. In this situation, the lumbar puncture may be performed with a fine-bore (24-gauge) needle. If the pressure is over 400 mmHg, the minimum required sample of fluid should be obtained, the needle removed, and, according to the suspected clinical disease and the patient's condition, mannitol administered in a dose of 0.75 to 1.0 mg/kg. Unless contraindicated, dexamethasone may be started in a dose of 4 to 6 mg every 6 h.

Cisternal puncture and lateral cervical puncture (C1–C2) are safe procedures in the hands of the expert but should not be performed by those without experience. Cisternal puncture is sometimes necessary in instances of spinal block to perform myelography above a lesion.

Following lumbar puncture, the patient should be positioned in a comfortable, recumbant position for 1 h before rising. The principal complication of lumbar puncture is a headache, occurring in 5 to 10 percent of patients, caused by a drop in CSF pressure related to persistent leakage of CSF. Such headaches typically begin 12 to 48 h after the procedure and may last from several days to 2 weeks. These headaches are strikingly positional in character; they are worsened by an upright posture and are relieved by lying flat. → *Therapy is discussed in Chap. 15.*

BIBLIOGRAPHY

ADAMS RD, VICTOR M: *Principles of Neurology*, 6th ed. New York, McGraw-Hill, 1997

FISHMAN RA: *Cerebrospinal Fluid in Diseases of the Nervous System*, 2d ed. Philadelphia, Saunders, 1992

HAERER AF: *DeJong's The Neurologic Examination*. Philadelphia, Lippincott, 1992

SWANSON PD: *Symptoms and Signs in Neurology*. Philadelphia, Lippincott, 1984

361

Michael J. Aminoff

ELECTROPHYSIOLOGIC STUDIES OF THE CENTRAL AND PERIPHERAL NERVOUS SYSTEMS

ELECTROENCEPHALOGRAPHY

The electrical activity of the brain [the electroencephalogram (EEG)] is easily recorded from electrodes placed on the scalp. The potential difference between pairs of electrodes on the scalp (bipolar derivation) or between individual scalp electrodes and a relatively inactive common reference point (referential derivation) is amplified and displayed on paper or the screen of an oscilloscope. The findings depend on the patient's age and level of arousal. The rhythmic activity normally recorded represents the postsynaptic potentials of vertically oriented pyramidal cells of the cerebral cortex and is characterized by its frequency. In normal awake adults lying quietly with the eyes closed, an 8- to 13-Hz alpha rhythm is seen posteriorly in the EEG, intermixed with a variable amount of generalized faster (beta) activity, and it is attenuated when the eyes are opened (Fig. 361-1). During drowsiness, the alpha rhythm is also attenuated; with light sleep, slower activity in the theta (4 to 7 Hz) and delta (<4 Hz) ranges becomes more conspicuous.

The EEG is best recorded from several different electrode arrangements (montages) in turn, and activating procedures are generally undertaken in an attempt to provoke abnormalities. Such procedures commonly include hyperventilation (for 3 or 4 min), photic stimulation, sleep, and the deprivation of sleep on the night prior to the recording.

Electroencephalography is relatively inexpensive and may aid clinical management in several different contexts.

THE EEG AND EPILEPSY The EEG is most useful in evaluating patients with suspected epilepsy. The presence of *electrographic seizure activity*, i.e., of abnormal, repetitive, rhythmic activity having an abrupt onset and termination, clearly establishes the diagnosis. The absence of such electrocerebral accompaniment does not exclude a seizure disorder, however, because there may be no change in the scalp-recorded EEG during simple or complex partial seizures. It is often not possible to obtain an EEG during clinical events that may represent seizures, especially when such events occur unpredictably or infrequently. The development of portable equipment to record the EEG continuously on cassettes for 24 h or longer in ambulatory patients has made it easier to capture the electrocerebral accompaniments of such clinical episodes, and monitoring by this means is sometimes helpful in confirming that seizures are occurring, characterizing the nature of clinically equivocal episodes, and determining the frequency of epileptic events.

The EEG findings may also be helpful in the interictal period by showing certain abnormalities that are strongly supportive of a diagnosis of epilepsy. Such *epileptiform activity* consists of bursts of abnormal discharges containing spikes or sharp waves. The presence of epileptiform activity is not specific for epilepsy, but it has a much greater prevalence in epileptic patients than in normal individuals. When epileptiform activity is found in the EEG of a patient with episodic behavioral disturbances that clinically might be epileptic in nature, the likelihood that epilepsy is the correct diagnosis is markedly increased.

The EEG findings also have been used in classifying seizure disorders and selecting appropriate anticonvulsant medication for individual patients (Fig. 361-2). The episodic generalized spike-wave activity that occurs both during and between seizures in patients with typical absences (petit mal epilepsy) contrasts with the normal findings, focal interictal epileptiform discharges, or ictal patterns found in patients with complex partial seizures. These latter seizures may have no correlates in the scalp-recorded EEG or may be associated with abnormal rhythmic activity of variable frequency, a localized or generalized distribution, and a stereotyped pattern that varies with the patient. Focal or lateralized epileptogenic lesions are important to recognize, especially if surgical treatment is contemplated. Intensive long-term monitoring of clinical behavior and the EEG is required for operative candidates, however, and this generally also involves recording from intracranially placed electrodes (which may be subdural, extradural, or intracerebral in location).

The findings in the routine scalp-recorded EEG may indicate the prognosis of seizure disorders: in general, a normal EEG implies a better prognosis than otherwise, whereas an abnormal background or profuse epileptiform activity suggests a poor outlook. The EEG findings are not helpful in determining which patients with head injuries, stroke, or brain tumors will go on to develop seizures, because in such circumstances epileptiform activity is commonly encountered regardless of whether seizures occur. The EEG findings are sometimes used to determine whether anticonvulsant medication can be discontinued in epileptic patients who have been seizure-free for several years, but the findings provide only a general guide to prognosis: further seizures may occur after withdrawal of anticonvulsant medication despite a normal EEG or, conversely, may not occur despite a continuing EEG abnormality. The decision to discontinue anticonvulsant medication is made on clinical grounds, and the EEG does not have a useful role in this context except for providing guidance when there is clinical ambiguity or the patient requires reassurance about a particular course of action.

The EEG has no role in the management of tonic-clonic status epilepticus except when there is clinical uncertainty whether seizures are continuing in a comatose patient. In patients treated by pentobarbital-induced coma for refractory status epilepticus, the EEG findings are useful in indicating the level of anesthesia and whether seizures are occurring. During status epilepticus, the EEG shows repeated electrographic seizures or continuous spike-wave discharges. In nonconvulsive status epilepticus, a disorder that may not be recognized unless an EEG is performed, the EEG may also show continuous spike-wave activity ("spike-wave stupor") or, less commonly, repetitive electrographic seizures (complex partial status epilepticus).

THE EEG AND COMA The EEG tends to become slower as consciousness is depressed, regardless of the underlying cause (Fig. 361-1). Other findings may also be present and may suggest diagnostic possibilities, as when electrographic seizures are found or there is a focal abnormality indicating a structural lesion. The response of the EEG to external stimulation is helpful prognostically because electrocerebral responsiveness implies a lighter level of coma than a nonreactive EEG. Serial records provide a better guide to prognosis than a single record and supplement the clinical examination in following the course of events. As the depth of coma increases, the EEG becomes nonreactive and may show a burst-suppression pattern, with bursts of mixed-frequency activity separated by intervals of relative cerebral inactivity. In other instances there is a reduction in amplitude of the EEG until eventually electrocerebral activity cannot be detected. Such electrocerebral silence does not necessarily reflect irreversible brain damage, because it may occur in hypothermic patients or with drug overdose. The prognosis of electrocerebral silence, when recorded using an adequate technique, depends upon the clinical context in which it is found. In patients with severe cerebral anoxia, for example, electrocerebral silence in a technically satisfactory record implies that useful cognitive recovery will not occur.

The EEG is usually normal in patients with locked-in syndrome and helps in distinguishing this disorder from the comatose state with which it is sometimes confused clinically.

THE EEG IN OTHER NEUROLOGIC DISORDERS In the developed countries, computed tomography (CT) scanning and magnetic resonance imaging (MRI) have taken the place of EEG as a noninvasive means of screening for focal structural abnormalities of the brain, such as tumors, infarcts, or hematomas (Fig. 361-1). Nonetheless, the EEG is still used for this purpose in many parts of the world, although infratentorial or slowly expanding lesions may fail to cause any abnormalities. Focal slow-wave disturbances, a localized loss of electrocerebral activity, or more generalized electrocerebral disturbances are common findings but provide no reliable indication about the nature of the underlying pathology.

The EEG is also helpful for diagnostic purposes when it reveals the characteristic but nonspecific abnormalities found in certain neurologic disorders. The presence of complexes occurring with a regular repetition rate (so-called periodic complexes) in dementing disorders, for example, supports a diagnosis of Creutzfeldt-Jakob disease (Fig. 361-1) or subacute sclerosing panencephalitis, depending upon the appearance and frequency of the complexes and the clinical context. Focal or lateralized periodic slow-wave complexes, sometimes with a sharpened outline, in patients with an acute encephalopathy suggest a diagnosis of herpes simplex encephalitis, and periodic lateralized epileptiform discharges are commonly found with acute hemispheric pathology such as a hematoma, abscess, or rapidly expanding tumor.

The EEG generally slows in metabolic encephalopathies, and triphasic waves may be present. The findings do not permit differentiation of the underlying metabolic disturbance but help to exclude other encephalopathic processes by indicating the diffuse extent of cerebral dysfunction.

The EEG findings in dementia are nonspecific and usually do not distinguish between the different causes of cognitive decline except in rare instances when Creutzfeldt-Jakob disease or subacute sclerosing panencephalitis is responsible. The EEG may be normal or diffusely slowed, and the EEG findings alone cannot indicate whether a patient is demented or distinguish between dementia and pseudodementia.

EVOKED POTENTIALS

SENSORY EVOKED POTENTIALS The noninvasive recording of spinal or cerebral potentials elicited by stimulation of specific afferent pathways is an important means of monitoring the functional integrity of these pathways but does not indicate the pathologic basis of lesions involving them. Such evoked potentials (EPs) are so small compared to the background EEG activity that the responses to a number of stimuli have to be recorded and averaged with a computer in order to permit their recognition and definition. The background EEG activity, which has no fixed temporal relationship to the stimulus, is averaged out by this procedure.

Visual evoked potentials (VEPs) are elicited by monocular stimulation with a reversing checkerboard pattern and are recorded from the occipital region in the midline and on either side of the scalp. The component of major clinical importance is the so-called P100 response, a positive peak having a latency of approximately 100 ms. Its presence, latency, and symmetry over the two sides of the scalp are noted. Amplitude may also be measured, but changes in size are much less helpful for the recognition of pathology. VEPs are most useful in detecting dysfunction of the visual pathways anterior to the optic chiasm. In patients with acute severe optic neuritis, the P100 is frequently lost or grossly attenuated; as clinical recovery occurs and visual acuity improves, the P100 is restored but with an increased latency that generally remains abnormally prolonged indefinitely. The VEP findings are therefore helpful in indicating previous or subclinical optic neuritis. They may also be abnormal with ocular abnormalities and with other causes of optic nerve disease, such as ischemia or compression by a tumor. Normal VEPs may be elicited by flash stimuli in patients with cortical blindness.

Brainstem auditory evoked potentials (BAEPs) are elicited by monaural stimulation with repetitive clicks and are recorded between the vertex of the scalp and the mastoid process or earlobe. A series of potentials, designated by roman numerals, occur in the first 10 ms after the stimulus and represent in part the sequential activation of different structures in the pathway between the auditory nerve (wave I) and the inferior colliculus (wave V) in the midbrain. The presence, latency, and interpeak latency of the first five positive potentials recorded at the vertex are

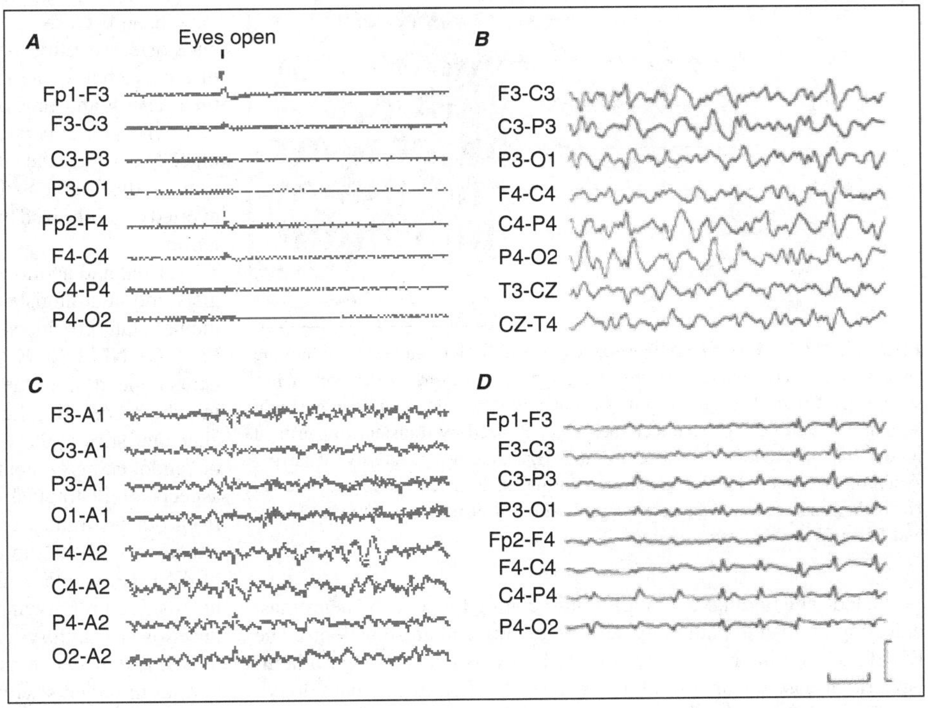

FIGURE 361-1 *A.* Normal EEG showing a posteriorly situated 9-Hz alpha rhythm that attenuates with eye opening. *B.* Abnormal EEG showing irregular diffuse slow activity in an obtunded patient with encephalitis. *C.* Irregular slow activity in the right central region, on a diffusely slowed background, in a patient with a right parietal glioma. *D.* Periodic complexes occurring once every second in a patient with Creutzfeldt-Jakob disease. Horizontal calibration: 1 s; vertical calibration: 200 μV in A, 300 μV in other panels. *(From Aminoff, 1992.)* In this and the following figure, electrode placements are indicated at the left of each panel and accord with the international 10:20 system. A, earlobe; C, central; F, frontal; Fp, frontal polar; P, parietal; T, temporal; O, occipital. Right-sided placements are indicated by even numbers, left-sided placements by odd numbers, and midline placements by Z.

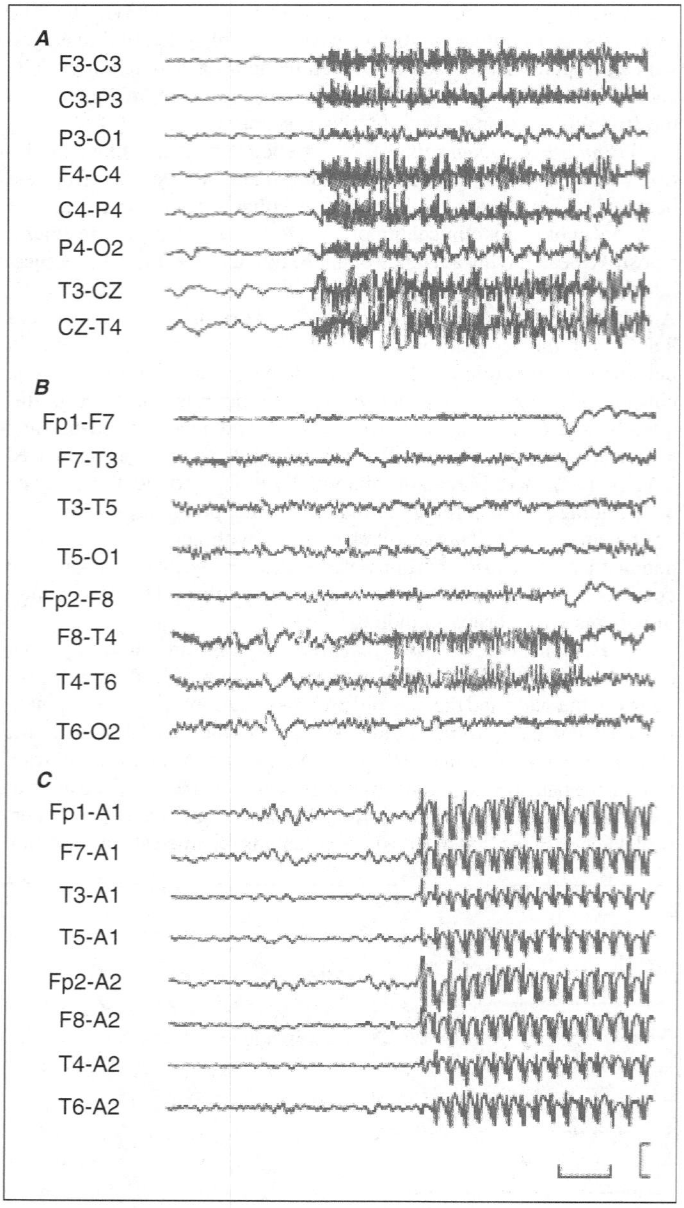

FIGURE 361-2 Electrographic seizures. *A.* Onset of a tonic seizure showing generalized repetitive sharp activity with synchronous onset over both hemispheres. *B.* Burst of repetitive spikes occurring with sudden onset in the right temporal region during a clinical spell characterized by transient impairment of external awareness. *C.* Generalized 3-Hz spike-wave activity occurring synchronously over both hemispheres during an absence (petit mal) attack. Horizontal calibration: 1 s; vertical calibration: 400 μV in A, 200 μV in B, and 750 μV in C. *(From Aminoff, 1992.)*

evaluated. The findings are helpful in screening for acoustic neuromas, detecting brainstem pathology, and evaluating comatose patients. The BAEPs are normal in coma due to metabolic/toxic disorders or bihemispheric disease but abnormal in the presence of brainstem pathology.

Somatosensory evoked potentials (SEPs) are recorded over the scalp and spine in response to electrical stimulation of a peripheral (mixed or cutaneous) nerve. The configuration, polarity, and latency of the responses depend on the nerve that is stimulated and on the recording arrangements. SEPs are used to evaluate proximal (otherwise inaccessible) portions of the peripheral nervous system and the integrity of the central somatosensory pathways.

Clinical Utility of Sensory Evoked Potentials EP studies may detect and localize lesions in afferent pathways in the central nervous system (CNS). They have been used particularly to investigate patients with suspected multiple sclerosis (MS), the diagnosis of which requires the recognition of lesions involving several different regions of the central white matter. In patients with clinical evidence of only one lesion, the electrophysiologic recognition of abnormalities in other sites helps to suggest or support the diagnosis but does not establish it unequivocally. In patients with suspected MS (or other neurologic disorders) who have vague, ill-defined complaints, the organic basis of symptoms may be supported by the presence of EP abnormalities in the appropriate afferent pathway. MRI is also helpful in detecting lesions in patients with possible MS, but electrophysiologic studies are cheaper and monitor the functional rather than anatomic status of the afferent pathways under study. Moreover, the electrophysiologic studies occasionally reveal abnormalities missed by MRI or vice versa. The two techniques therefore complement each other. Normal electrophysiologic (or imaging) findings do not exclude MS when this is a clinical possibility. In established MS, the use of EP studies to follow the disorder or its response to treatment is of uncertain value and unjustified at the present time.

EP abnormalities occur in disorders other than MS that involve the afferent pathways under test. Even multimodality EP abnormalities are not specific for MS; they may occur in AIDS, Lyme disease, systemic lupus erythematosus, neurosyphilis, spinocerebellar degenerations, familial spastic paraplegia, and deficiency of vitamin E or B_{12}. The diagnostic utility of the electrophysiologic findings therefore depends upon the circumstances in which they are found. Abnormalities may aid in the localization of lesions to broad areas of the CNS, but attempts at precise localization on electrophysiologic grounds are misleading because the generators of many components of the EP are unknown.

The EP findings are sometimes of prognostic relevance. Bilateral loss of those SEP components that are generated in the cerebral cortex implies that cognition may not be regained in posttraumatic or postanoxic coma, and EP studies may also be useful in evaluating patients with suspected brain death. In patients with spinal cord injuries, SEPs have been used to indicate the completeness of the lesion—the presence or early return of a cortically generated response to stimulation of a nerve below the injured segment of the cord indicates an incomplete lesion and thus a better prognosis for functional recovery than otherwise. Intraoperative monitoring of function in neural structures placed at risk by the surgical procedure may permit the early recognition of dysfunction. This may enable any permanent deficit to be averted or minimized by alteration of the responsible operative manipulation.

Visual and auditory acuity have been determined by ophthalmologists and audiologists using EP techniques in patients whose age or mental state precludes their cooperation for behavioral testing.

COGNITIVE EVOKED POTENTIALS Certain EP components depend upon the mental attention of the subject and the setting in which the stimulus occurs, rather than simply on the physical characteristics of the stimulus. Such "event-related" potentials (ERPs) or "endogenous" potentials are related in some manner to the cognitive aspects of distinguishing an infrequently occurring target stimulus from other stimuli occurring more frequently. For clinical purposes, attention has been directed particularly at the so-called P3 component of the ERP, which is also designated the P300 component because of its positive polarity and latency of approximately 300 to 400 ms after onset of an auditory target stimulus. The P3 component is prolonged in latency in many patients with dementia, whereas it is generally normal in patients with depression or other psychiatric disorders that might be mistaken for dementia. ERPs are therefore sometimes helpful in making this distinction when there is clinical uncertainty, although a response of normal latency does not exclude a dementing disorder.

MOTOR EVOKED POTENTIALS The electrical potentials recorded from muscle or the spinal cord following stimulation of the motor cortex or central motor pathways are referred to as motor evoked potentials. For clinical purposes such responses are recorded most often as the compound muscle action potentials elicited by transcutaneous magnetic stimulation of the motor cortex. A strong but brief magnetic field is produced by passing a current through a coil, and this induces stimulating currents in the subjacent neural tissue. The procedure is painless and apparently safe. Abnormalities have been described in several neurologic disorders with clinical or subclinical involvement of central motor pathways, including MS and motor neuron disease. The clinical utility of the technique is still being examined. In addition to a possible role in the diagnosis of neurologic disorders or in evaluating the extent of pathologic involvement, the technique may provide information of prognostic relevance (for example, in suggesting the likelihood of recovery of motor function after stroke) and may be useful as a means of monitoring intraoperatively the functional integrity of central motor tracts.

ELECTROPHYSIOLOGIC STUDIES OF MUSCLE AND NERVE

The motor unit is the basic element subserving motor function. It is defined as an anterior horn cell, its axon and neuromuscular junctions, and all the muscle fibers innervated by the axon. The number of motor units in a muscle ranges from approximately 10 in the extraocular muscles to several thousand in the large muscles of the legs. There is considerable variation in the average number of muscle fibers within the motor units of an individual muscle, i.e., in the innervation ratio of different muscles. Thus the innervation ratio is less than 25 in the human external rectus or platysma muscle and between 1600 and 1700 in the medial head of the gastrocnemius muscle. The muscle fibers of individual motor units are divided into two general types by distinctive contractile properties, histochemical stains, and characteristic responses to fatigue. Within each motor unit, all of the muscle fibers are of the same type.

ELECTROMYOGRAPHY The pattern of electrical activity in muscle [i.e., the *electromyogram* (EMG)], both at rest and during activity, may be recorded from a needle electrode inserted into the muscle. The nature and pattern of abnormalities relate to disorders at different levels of the motor unit.

Relaxed muscle normally is electrically silent except in the endplate region, but abnormal spontaneous activity (Fig. 361-3) occurs in various neuromuscular disorders, especially those associated with denervation or inflammatory changes in affected muscle. Fibrillation potentials and positive sharp waves (which reflect muscle fiber irritability) and complex repetitive discharges are most often—but not always—found in denervated muscle and may also occur after muscle injury and in certain myopathic disorders, especially inflammatory disorders such as polymyositis. After an acute neuropathic lesion they are found earlier in proximal rather than distal muscles and sometimes do not develop distally in the extremities for 4 to 6 weeks; once present, they may persist indefinitely unless reinnervation occurs or the muscle degenerates so completely that no viable tissue remains. Fasciculation potentials (which reflect the spontaneous activity of individual motor units) are characteristic of slowly progressive neuropathic disorders, especially those with degeneration of anterior horn cells (such as amyotrophic lateral sclerosis). Myotonic discharges—high-frequency discharges of potentials derived from single muscle fibers that wax and wane in amplitude and frequency—are the signature of myotonic disorders such as myotonic dystrophy or myotonia congenita but occur occasionally in polymyositis or other, rarer, disorders.

Slight voluntary contraction of a muscle leads to activation of a small number of motor units. The potentials generated by any muscle fibers of these units that are within the pick-up range of the needle electrode will be recorded (Fig. 361-3). The parameters of normal motor unit action potentials depend on the muscle under study and age of the patient, but their duration is normally between 5 and 15 ms, amplitude is between 200 μV and 2 mV, and most are bi- or triphasic. The number of units activated depends on the degree of voluntary activity. An increase in muscle contraction is associated with an increase in the number of motor units that are activated (recruited) and in the frequency with which they discharge. With a full contraction, so many motor units are normally activated that individual motor unit action potentials can no longer be distinguished, and a complete interference pattern is said to have been produced.

The incidence of small, short-duration, polyphasic motor unit action potentials (i.e., having more than four phases) is usually increased in myopathic muscle, and an excessive number of units is activated for a specified degree of voluntary activity. By contrast the loss of motor units that occurs in neuropathic disorders leads to a reduction in number of units activated during a maximal contraction and an increase in their firing rate, i.e., there is an incomplete or reduced interference pattern; the configuration and dimensions of the potentials may also be abnormal depending on the duration of the neuropathic process and on whether reinnervation has occurred. The surviving motor units are initially normal in configuration but, as reinnervation occurs, they increase in amplitude and duration and become polyphasic (Fig. 361-3).

Action potentials from the same motor unit sometimes fire with a consistent temporal relationship to each other, so that double, triple, or multiple discharges are recorded, especially in tetany, hemifacial spasm, or myokymia.

Electrical silence characterizes the involuntary, sustained muscle contraction that occurs in phosphorylase deficiency, which is designated a *contracture*.

EMG enables disorders of the motor units to be detected and characterized as either neurogenic or myopathic. In neurogenic disorders, the pattern of affected muscles may localize the lesion to the anterior horn cells or to a specific site as the axons traverse a nerve root, limb plexus, and peripheral nerve to their terminal arborizations.

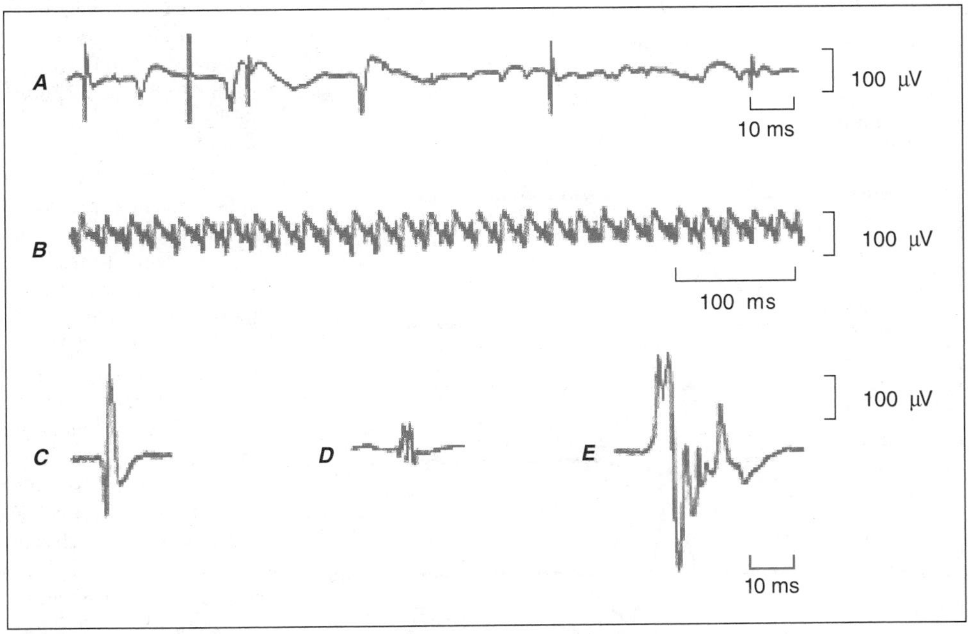

FIGURE 361-3 Activity recorded during EMG. *A.* Spontaneous fibrillation potentials and positive sharp waves. *B.* Complex repetitive discharges recorded in partially denervated muscle at rest. *C.* Normal triphasic motor unit action potential. *D.* Small, short-duration, polyphasic motor unit action potential such as is commonly encountered in myopathic disorders. *E.* Long-duration polyphasic motor unit action potential such as may be seen in neuropathic disorders.

The findings do not enable a specific etiologic diagnosis to be made, however, except in conjunction with the clinical findings and results of other laboratory studies.

The findings may provide a guide to the severity of an acute disorder of a peripheral or cranial nerve (by indicating whether denervation has occurred and the completeness of the lesion), and whether the pathologic process is active or progressive in chronic or degenerative disorders such as amyotrophic lateral sclerosis. Such information is important for prognostic purposes.

Various quantitative EMG approaches have been developed. The most common is to determine the mean duration and amplitude of 20 motor unit action potentials using a standardized technique. The technique of macro-EMG provides information about the number and size of muscle fibers in a larger volume of the motor unit territory and has also been used to estimate the number of motor units in a muscle. Scanning EMG is a computer-based technique that has been used to study the topography of motor unit action potentials and, in particular, the spatial and temporal distribution of activity in individual units. Both of these latter approaches are of limited interest except to specialists and merit no further discussion. The technique of single-fiber EMG is of immediate clinical relevance, however, and is discussed separately below.

NERVE CONDUCTION STUDIES Recording of the electrical response of a muscle to stimulation of its motor nerve at two or more points along its course (Fig. 361-4) permits conduction velocity to be determined in the fastest-conducting motor fibers between the points of stimulation. The latency and amplitude of the electrical response of muscle (i.e., of the compound muscle action potential) to stimulation of its motor nerve at a distal site are also compared with values defined in normal subjects. Sensory nerve conduction studies are performed by determining the conduction velocity and amplitude of action potentials in sensory fibers when these fibers are stimulated at one point and the responses are recorded at another point along the course of the nerve. In adults, conduction velocity in the arms is normally between 50 and 70 m/s, and in the legs is between 40 and 60 m/s.

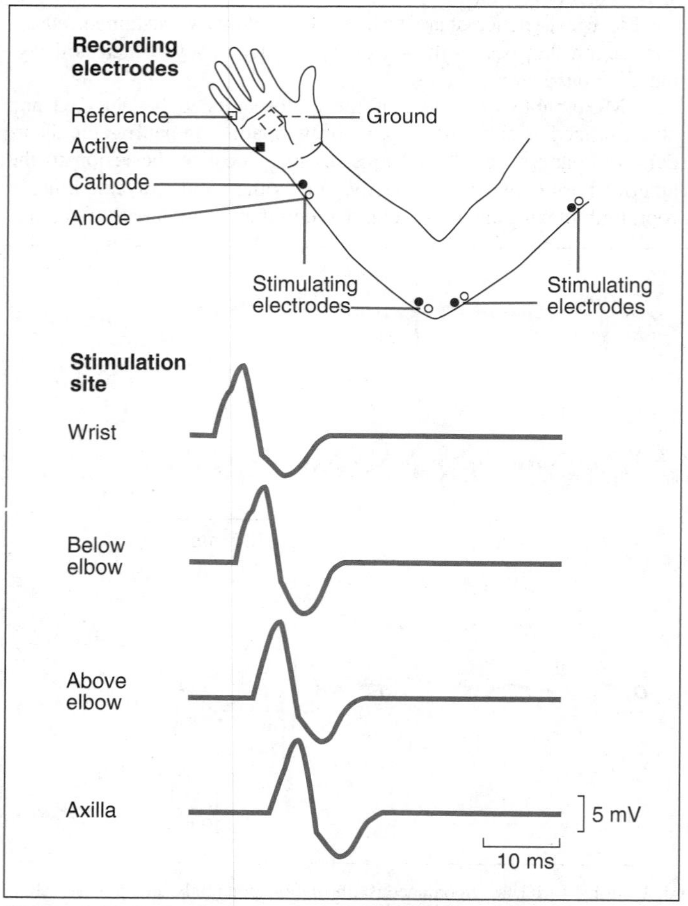

FIGURE 361-4 Arrangement for motor conduction studies of the ulnar nerve. Responses are recorded with a surface electrode from the abductor digiti minimi muscle to supramaximal stimulation of the nerve at different sites, and are shown in the lower panel. *(From Aminoff, 1987.)*

Nerve conduction studies complement the EMG examination, enabling the presence and extent of peripheral nerve pathology to be determined. They are particularly helpful in determining whether sensory symptoms are arising from pathology proximal or distal to the dorsal root ganglia (in the former instance, peripheral sensory conduction studies will be normal) and whether neuromuscular dysfunction relates to peripheral nerve disease. In patients with a mononeuropathy, they are invaluable as a means of localizing a focal lesion, determining the extent and severity of the underlying pathology, providing a guide to prognosis, and detecting subclinical involvement of other peripheral nerves. They enable a polyneuropathy to be distinguished from a mononeuropathy multiplex when this is not possible clinically, an important distinction because of the etiologic implications. Nerve conduction studies provide a means of following the progression and therapeutic response of peripheral nerve disorders and may suggest the underlying pathologic basis in individual cases. Conduction velocity is often markedly slowed, terminal motor latencies are prolonged, and compound motor and sensory nerve action potentials may be dispersed in the demyelinative neuropathies (such as in chronic inflammatory polyneuropathy, metachromatic leukodystrophy, or certain hereditary neuropathies); conduction block is frequent in acquired varieties of these neuropathies (see Chap. 381). By contrast, conduction velocity is normal or slowed only mildly, sensory nerve action potentials are small or absent, and there is EMG evidence of denervation in axonal neuropathies such as occur in association with metabolic or toxic disorders.

The utility and complementary role of EMG and nerve conduction studies are best illustrated by reference to a common clinical problem. Numbness and paresthesia of the little finger and associated wasting of the intrinsic muscles of the hand may result from a spinal cord lesion, C8/T1 radiculopathy, brachial plexopathy (lower trunk or medial cord), or a lesion of the ulnar nerve. If sensory nerve action potentials can be recorded normally at the wrist following stimulation of the digital fibers in the affected finger, the pathology is probably proximal to the dorsal root ganglia, i.e., there is a radiculopathy or more central lesion; absence of the sensory potentials, by contrast, suggests distal pathology. EMG examination will indicate whether the pattern of affected muscles conforms to radicular or ulnar nerve territory, or is more extensive (thereby favoring a plexopathy); ulnar motor conduction studies will generally also distinguish between a radiculopathy (normal findings) and ulnar neuropathy (abnormal findings) and will often identify the site of an ulnar nerve lesion—the nerve is stimulated at several points along its course to determine whether the compound action potential recorded from a distal muscle that it supplies shows a marked alteration in size or area, or a disproportionate change in latency, with stimulation at a particular site. The electrophysiologic findings thus permit a definitive diagnosis to be made and specific treatment instituted in circumstances where there is clinical ambiguity.

F WAVE STUDIES Stimulation of a motor nerve causes impulses to travel antidromically toward the spinal cord (as well as orthodromically to the nerve terminals). Such antidromic impulses cause a few of the anterior horn cells to discharge, producing a small motor response that occurs considerably later than the direct response elicited by nerve stimulation. The F wave so elicited is sometimes abnormal (absent or delayed) with proximal pathology of the peripheral nervous system, such as a radiculopathy, and may therefore be helpful in detecting abnormalities when conventional nerve conduction studies are normal. In general, however, the clinical utility of F wave studies has been disappointing, except perhaps in Guillain-Barré syndrome, where they are often absent or delayed.

H REFLEX STUDIES The H reflex is easily recorded only from the soleus muscle in normal adults. It is elicited by low-intensity stimulation of the tibial nerve, and represents a monosynaptic reflex in which spindle (Ia) afferent fibers constitute the afferent arc and alpha motor axons the efferent pathway. The H reflexes are often absent bilaterally in elderly patients or with polyneuropathies and may be lost unilaterally in S1 radiculopathies.

MUSCLE RESPONSE TO REPETITIVE NERVE STIMULATION The size of the electrical response of a muscle to supramaximal electrical stimulation of its motor nerve relates to the number of muscle fibers that are activated. Neuromuscular transmission can be tested by several different protocols, but the most helpful is to record with surface electrodes the electrical response of a muscle to supramaximal stimulation of its motor nerve by repetitive (2 to 3 Hz) shocks delivered before and at selected intervals after a maximal voluntary contraction.

There is normally little or no change in size of the compound muscle action potential following repetitive stimulation of a motor nerve at 2 to 3 Hz with stimuli delivered at intervals after voluntary contraction of the muscle for about 20 to 30 s, even though preceding activity in the junctional region influences the release of acetylcholine and thus the size of the endplate potentials elicited by a test stimulus. This is because more acetylcholine is normally released than is required to bring the motor endplate potentials to the threshold for generating muscle fiber action potentials. In disorders of neuromuscular transmission this safety factor is reduced. Thus, in myasthenia gravis repetitive stimulation, particularly at a rate of between 2 and 5 Hz, may lead to a depression of neuromuscular transmission, with a decrement in size of the response recorded from affected muscles. Similarly, immediately after a period of maximal voluntary activity, single or repetitive stimuli of the motor nerve may elicit larger muscle responses than before, indicating that more muscle fibers are responding. This postactivation facilitation of neuromuscular transmission is followed by a longer-lasting period of depression, maximal between 2 and 4 min after the conditioning period and lasting for as long as 10 min or so, during which responses are reduced in size.

Decrementing responses to repetitive stimulation at 2 to 5 Hz are common in myasthenia gravis but may also occur in the congenital myasthenic syndromes. In Lambert-Eaton myasthenic syndrome, in which there is defective release of acetylcholine at the neuromuscular junction, the compound muscle action potential elicited by a single stimulus is generally very small. With repetitive stimulation at rates of up to 10 Hz, the first few responses may decline in size, but subsequent responses increase. If faster rates of stimulation are used (20 to 50 Hz), the increment may be dramatic so that the amplitude of compound muscle action potentials eventually reaches a size that is several times larger than the initial response. In patients with botulism, the response to repetitive stimulation is similar to that in Lambert-Eaton syndrome, although the findings are somewhat more variable and not all muscles are affected.

SINGLE-FIBER ELECTROMYOGRAPHY The technique of single-fiber EMG is particularly helpful in detecting disorders of neuromuscular transmission. A special needle electrode is placed within a muscle and positioned to record action potentials from two muscle fibers belonging to the same motor unit. The time interval between the two potentials will vary in consecutive discharges, and this is called the *neuromuscular jitter*. The jitter can be quantified as the mean difference between consecutive interpotential intervals and is normally between 10 and 50 μs. This value is increased when neuromuscular transmission is disturbed for any reason, and in some instances impulses in individual muscle fibers may fail to occur because of impulse blocking at the neuromuscular junction. Single-fiber EMG is more sensitive than repetitive nerve stimulation or determination of acetylcholine receptor antibody levels in diagnosing myasthenia gravis.

Single-fiber EMG can also be used to determine mean fiber density of motor units (i.e., mean number of muscle fibers per motor unit within the recording area) and to estimate the number of motor units in a muscle, but this is of less immediate clinical relevance.

BLINK REFLEXES Electrical or mechanical stimulation of the supraorbital nerve on one side leads to two separate reflex responses of the orbicularis oculi—an ipsilateral R1 response having a latency of approximately 10 ms and a bilateral R2 response with a latency in the order of 30 ms. The trigeminal and facial nerves constitute the afferent and efferent arcs of the reflex, respectively. Abnormalities of either nerve or intrinsic lesions of the medulla or pons may lead to uni- or bilateral loss of the response, and the findings may therefore be helpful in identifying or localizing such pathology.

TESTS OF AUTONOMIC FUNCTION

Noninvasive tests of autonomic function are becoming increasingly important for the recognition of small-fiber peripheral neuropathies and in defining central dysautonomias, such as the Shy-Drager syndrome. Invasive tests, such as microneurography, provide information of considerable academic importance, but because of their specialized nature and limited clinical utility they are not discussed further. → *For further discussion, see Chap. 371*.

Heart-rate responses and the Valsalva maneuver are described in Chap. 371. Heart-rate increases with changes from a supine to erect posture are considered normal if the heart rate increases in the first 15 s or so and then slows. Assessment of sudomotor function is also discussed in Chap. 371.

BIBLIOGRAPHY

AMINOFF MJ: *Electromyography in Clinical Practice: Electrodiagnostic Aspects of Neuromuscular Disease*, 2d ed. New York, Churchill Livingstone, 1987

——— (ed): *Electrodiagnosis in Clinical Neurology*, 3d ed. New York, Churchill Livingstone, 1992

DALY DD, PEDLEY TA (eds): *Current Practice of Clinical Electroencephalography*, 2d ed. New York, Raven Press, 1990

DUMITRU D: *Electrodiagnostic Medicine*. Philadelphia, Hanley and Belfus, 1995

EBERSOLE JS (ed): *Ambulatory EEG Monitoring*. New York, Raven Press, 1988

KIMURA J: *Electrodiagnosis in Diseases of Nerve and Muscle*, 2d ed. Philadelphia, Davis, 1989

NIEDERMEYER E, LOPES DA SILVA F (eds): *Electroencephalography*, 3d ed. Baltimore, Urban & Schwarzenberg, 1993

362

William P. Dillon

NEUROIMAGING IN NEUROLOGIC DISORDERS

A dramatic increase in the role of imaging in diagnosis of neurologic diseases occurred with the development of computed tomography (CT) in the early 1970s and of magnetic resonance imaging (MRI) in the 1980s. MRI has gradually replaced CT for many indications and has also replaced many of the invasive neuroimaging techniques, such as myelography and angiography. Guidelines for the use of new imaging technologies are difficult to develop during a period of rapid advance. In general, MRI is more sensitive than CT for the evaluation of most lesions affecting the brain and spinal cord parenchyma. CT is more sensitive than MRI for visualizing osseous detail and brain hemorrhage (parenchymal or subarachnoid). Conventional angiography is reserved for cases in which small-vessel detail is essential for diagnosis (Table 362-1). Recent developments, such as helical CT, CT angiography (CTA), MR angiography (MRA), positron emission tomography, Doppler ultrasound, and interventional angiography have continued to advance diagnosis and therapy.

COMPUTED TOMOGRAPHY **Technique** The CT image is a computer-generated cross-sectional representation of anatomy created by an analysis of the attenuation of x-ray beams passed through various points around a section of the body. As the x-ray source, collimated to the desired slice thickness, rotates around the patient, sensitive x-ray detectors aligned 180° from the source detect x-rays attenuated by the patient's anatomy. A computer calculates a "back projection" image from the 360° x-ray attenuation profile. Greater x-ray attenuation, as caused by bone, results in areas of high "density," while soft tissue structures, which attenuate x-rays less, are lower in density. The resolution of an image depends on the radiation dose, the collimation (slice thickness), the field of view, and the matrix size of the display. A typical modern CT scanner is capable of obtaining sections 1 to 2, 5, and 10 mm thick at a speed of 1 to 3 s per section; complete studies of the brain can be completed in 2 to 3 min.

Intravenous contrast is often administered prior to or during a CT study to identify vascular structures and to detect defects in the blood-brain barrier (BBB) associated with pathologies such as tumors, infarcts, and infections. An intact BBB prevents contrast molecules, which are large, from exiting the intravascular compartment. In the normal central nervous system (CNS), only vessels and those structures not having a BBB (e.g., the pituitary gland, choroid plexus, and dura) enhance. The use of contrast agents carries a risk of allergic reaction, increases the dose of radiation when both noncontrast and contrast CT scans are to be obtained, adds expense, and may mask hemorrhage; thus before contrast is administered, the indication for its use should always be considered carefully.

Helical CT is a new technique in which continuous three-dimensional CT information is obtained. In the helical scan mode, the table moves continuously through the rotating x-ray beam, generating a "helix" of information which can be reformatted into various slice thicknesses. Advantages include shorter scan times, reduced patient and organ motion, and the ability to acquire images during the infusion of intravenous contrast. The contrast images can be used to construct CT angiograms of vascular structures. CTA images require a workstation to threshold and segment CT images for display (Fig. 362-1). CTA has proven useful in assessing the carotid bifurcation and intracranial arterial anatomy in selected instances in which a contraindication to MR angiography exists.

Indications The indications for CT have diminished since the development of MRI. While MRI gives greater soft tissue contrast and is more sensitive than CT in detecting early brain damage, CT is useful in imaging osseous structures of the spine, skull base, and temporal bones. CT is also more sensitive and specific than MRI for acute parenchymal and subarachnoid hemorrhage. In the spine, CT is often useful in evaluating patients with osseous spinal stenosis and spondylosis, but MRI is often preferred in those with neurologic deficits.

Complications CT is safe and reliable. Radiation levels are between 3 and 5 cGy per examination. The most frequent complications are associated with use of intravenous contrast agents. Two broad categories of contrast media, ionic and nonionic, are in use. Ionic agents are relatively safe and inexpensive but cause a higher incidence of toxicity reactions than nonionic agents.

Nephrotoxicity resulting from contrast administration (*contrast nephropathy*) may result from hemodynamic changes, tubular obstruction and cell damage, or immunologic reactions to contrast agents. A rise in serum creatinine of at least 1 mg/dL within 48 h of contrast administration is often used as a definition of contrast nephropathy, although other causes of acute renal failure must be excluded. The prognosis is usually favorable, with serum creatinine levels returning to baseline within 1 to 2 weeks. Risk factors for contrast nephropathy include advanced age, chronic renal insufficiency, diabetes, dehydration, and high contrast dose. Preexisting renal disease, diabetes, and cardiac disease indicate a worse prognosis. Diabetics and those with mild renal failure should be well hydrated prior to the administration of nonionic agents. Nonionic, low-osmolar media produce fewer abnormalities in renal blood flow and less endothelial cell damage than ionic agents (Table 362-2).

A sensation of heat, pain, nausea, and vomiting are well-known side effects following intravenous administration of ionic contrast media, and they become more important as studies require longer imaging times and repeated contrast injections. Pain and the sensation of heat are probably due to the osmolality of the agent and vasodilation. These side effects are less intense or nonexistent with nonionic contrast media.

Anaphylactoid reactions to intravenous contrast media range from mild hives to bronchospasm to acute anaphylaxis and death. The pathogenesis of these allergic reactions is not fully understood, but it is thought to include the release of mediators such as histamine, antibody-antigen reactions, and complement activation. Severe allergic

Table 362-1

Guidelines for the Use of CT, Ultrasound, and MRI

Condition	Recommended Technique
Hemorrhage	
Acute parenchymal	CT > MRI
Subacute/chronic	MRI
Subarachnoid hemorrhage	CT, lumbar puncture → angiography
Aneurysm	Angiography > ?MRA
Ischemic infarction	
Hemorrhagic infarction	CT or MRI
Bland infarction	MRI > CT
Carotid or vertebral dissection	MRI/MRA
Vertebral basilar insufficiency	MRI/MRA
Carotid stenosis	Doppler ultrasound, MRA
Suspected mass lesions	
Neoplasm, primary or metastatic	MRI + contrast
Infection/abscess	MRI + contrast
Immunosuppression with focal findings	MRI + contrast
Vascular malformations	MRI ± angiography
White matter disorders	MRI
Demyelinating disease	MRI ± contrast
Dementia	MRI or CT
Trauma	
Acute trauma	CT (noncontrast)
Shear injury/chronic hemorrhage	MRI
Headache/migraine	CT (noncontrast) or MRI
Seizure	
First time, no focal neurologic deficits	MRI > CT as screen
Partial complex/refractory	MRI + coronal T2W imaging
Cranial neuropathy	MRI + contrast
Meningeal disease	MRI + contrast
SPINE	
Low back pain	
No neurologic deficits	Conservative therapy, consider MRI or CT after 4 weeks
With focal deficits	MRI > CT
Spinal stenosis	MRI or CT
Cervical spondylosis	MRI or CT myelography
Infection	MRI + contrast, CT
Myelopathy	MRI + contrast, consider myelography if MRI negative
Arteriovenous malformations	MRI, myelography/angiography

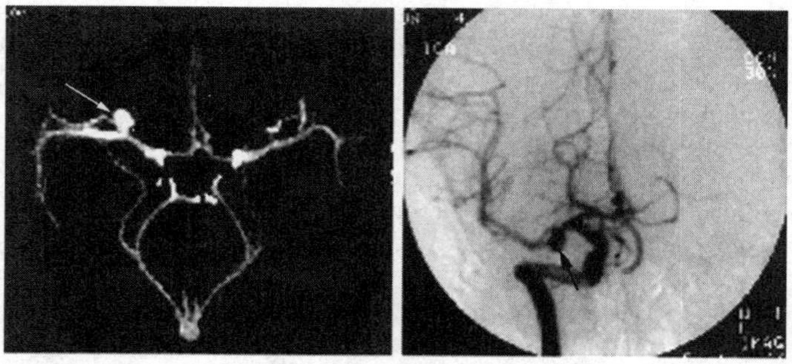

FIGURE 362-1 CT angiography of middle cerebral aneurysm. A right middle cerebral aneurysm (*arrow*) is shown on CTA (*left image*) and confirmed by conventional internal carotid angiography (*right image*). CTA image is produced by helical scans or 1-mm CT scans performed during a rapid bolus infusion of intravenous contrast medium. Subtraction of background nonenhancing brain results in the CTA image. *(From RA Alberico et al, Am J Neuroradiol 16:1571, 1995.)*

Table 362-2

Guidelines for Use of Intravenous Contrast in Patients with Impaired Renal Function

Serum Creatinine Level, μmol/L (mg/dL)*	Guideline
<133 (<1.5)	Use either ionic or nonionic contrast at 2 mL/kg to 150 mL total
133–177 (1.5–2.0)	Use nonionic contrast; hydrate diabetics
>177 (>2.0)	Consider noncontrast CT or MRI; use nonionic contrast if required
177–221 (2.0–2.5)	Use nonionic contrast only if required (as above); contraindicated in diabetics
>265 (>3.0)	Nonionic contrast given only to patients undergoing dialysis within 24 h

* Note risk is greatest in patients with rising creatinine levels.

Table 362-4

Guidelines for the Premedication of Patients with Prior Allergic Reaction to Contrast Agents

12 h before examination
Prednisone, 40 mg PO *or* methylprednisolone (Medrol), 32 mg PO

2 h before examination
Prednisone, 40 mg PO *or* methylprednisolone (Medrol), 32 mg PO
and
Cimetidine, 300 mg PO *or* ranitidine, 150 mg PO

Immediately before examination
Benadryl, 50 mg IV (alternatively, can be given PO 2 h before exam)

reactions occur in approximately 0.04 percent of patients receiving nonionic media, sixfold fewer than with ionic media. Risk factors include a history of prior contrast reaction, allergy (asthma and hay fever), and cardiac disease. In these patients, an alternative noncontrast CT or MRI procedure should be considered, or nonionic agents should be used in conjunction with pretreatment with glucocorticoids and antihistamines (Tables 362-3 and 362-4). Patients with allergic reactions to iodinated contrast material do not usually react against gadolinium-based MR contrast material, although it would be wise to pretreat in a similar fashion prior to MR contrast administration.

MAGNETIC RESONANCE IMAGING Technique The phenomenon of magnetic resonance is a complex interaction between protons in biologic tissues, a static and alternating magnetic field (the magnet), and energy in the form of radiofrequency waves of a specific frequency (Rf), introduced by coils placed next to the body part of interest. The energy state of the hydrogen protons is transiently excited. The subsequent return to equilibrium (relaxation) of the protons results in a release of Rf energy (the echo) which can be measured by the same surface coils that delivered the Rf pulses. The complex Rf signal or echo is transformed by Fourier analysis into the information used to form an MR image.

T1 and T2 relaxation times The rate of return to equilibrium of perturbed protons is called the *relaxation rate*. The relaxation rate is different for different normal and pathologic tissues. The relaxation rate of a hydrogen proton in a tissue is influenced by surrounding molecular environment and atomic neighbors. Two relaxation rates, the T1 and T2 relaxation times, are measurable. The T1 relaxation rate is the time for 63 percent of the protons to return to their normal equilibrium state, while the T2 relaxation rate is the time for 63 percent of the protons to become dephased owing to interactions among adjacent protons. The intensity of the signal and thus the image contrast can be modulated by altering certain parameters, such as the interval between Rf pulses (TR) and the time between the Rf pulse and the signal reception (TE). So-called T1-weighted (T1W) images are produced by keeping the TR and TE relatively short. Under these conditions, contrast between structures is based primarily on their T1 relaxation differences. T2-weighted (T2W) images are produced by using longer TR and TE times (Fig. 362-2). Fat and subacute hemorrhage have short T1 relaxation rates and have a high signal intensity on T1W images. Watery media, such as cerebrospinal fluid (CSF) and edematous tissue, have long T1 and T2 relaxation rates and have a low signal intensity on T1W images and a high signal intensity on T2W images (Table 362-5). Gray matter contains 10 to 15 percent more water than white matter, and white matter contains more lipid (due to myelin) than gray matter. These two chemical differences account for much of the contrast difference between gray and white matter on MRI (Fig. 362-2). T2W images are more sensitive than T1W images to edema or myelin destruction (see Fig. 376-2).

Table 362-3

Indications for the Use of Nonionic Contrast Media

- Prior adverse reaction to contrast media, with the exception of heat, flushing, or an episode of nausea or vomiting
- Asthma or other serious lung disease
- History of atopic allergies (pretreatment with glucocorticoids and antihistamines recommended)
- Age under 2 years old
- Renal failure or a creatinine level >177 μmol/L (>2.0 mg/dL)
- Cardiac dysfunction, including cardiac failure, severe arrhythmias, unstable angina pectoris, recent myocardial infarction, or pulmonary hypertension
- Diabetes
- Severe debilitation

MR images can be generated in sagittal, coronal, axial, and oblique planes without changing the patient's position. Each plane obtained requires a separate sequence lasting 5 to 10 minutes. Unlike CT, movement of the patient during a sequence will distort *all* the images; therefore, patient cooperation is important. Approximately 5 percent of the population experience claustrophobia in the MR environment. This can be reduced by mild sedation. Three-dimensional volumetric imaging is also possible with MR, resulting in a volume of data that can be reformatted in any plane and manipulated in a real-time fashion to highlight certain disease processes.

Contrast material The heavy-metal element *gadolinium* forms the basis of all current intravenous MR contrast agents. Gadolinium is a paramagnetic substance, which means that it reduces the T1 and T2 relaxation times of nearby water protons, resulting in a high signal on T1W images. The metal is chelated to an agent such as DTPA, which allows renal excretion without toxicity. Approximately 0.2 mL/kg body weight is administered intravenously (10 to 15 mL for the average-sized adult); the cost is approximately $100. Gadolinium contrast does not cross a normal BBB, and thus it causes enhancement of brain tissue only at sites of abnormalities in the BBB (see Fig. 376-2*C*) and in areas of the brain that normally have no BBB, such as the pituitary gland. Allergic reactions are extremely rare; renal failure does not occur. These agents can be administered safely to children as well as adults.

MAGNETIC RESONANCE ANGIOGRAPHY Flowing blood exhibits complex MR signals that range from bright to dark relative to background stationary tissue (Fig. 362-2). Fast-flowing blood, such as arterial blood, shows no signal on routine MR images. Slower flow, as in veins or distal to arterial stenoses, may appear high in signal. It is possible, by varying the MR image parameters, to assess blood flow either qualitatively or quantitatively. This is the basis of

Table 362-5

Some Common Intensities on T1- and T2-Weighted MRI Sequences

			Signal Intensity			
Image	TR	TE	CSF	Fat	Brain	Edema Fluid
T1W	Short	Short	Low	High	Low	Low
T2W	Long	Long	High	Low	High	High

ABBREVIATIONS: T1W, T1-weighted; T2W, T2-weighted.

MR angiography which capitalizes on the differences in signal between moving blood and stationary tissue on gradient echo images (Fig. 362-3). *Gradient echo images* differ from standard spin echo images in being more sensitive to blood products, calcification, and other susceptibility artifacts. The suppression of background signal achieved in short-flip-angle gradient echo images provides the contrast needed for flowing blood to appear bright in signal on MRA images.

It is important to understand that MRA provides a *vascular flow map* rather than the anatomic map given by conventional angiography. Two MRA techniques, time-of-flight (TOF) and phase-contrast, are currently used. TOF, currently the technique used most frequently, relies on the suppression of nonmoving tissue to provide a background for the high signal intensity of flowing blood. A typical TOF angiography sequence results in a series of contiguous thin MR sections (0.9 mm thick), which can be viewed as a stack to create an angiographic image data set that can be reformatted or viewed in various planes and angles to reveal the vascular relationships (Fig. 362-3). Either arterial or venous structures may be highlighted.

Phase-contrast MRA has a longer acquisition time than TOF MRA but reveals the velocity and direction of blood flow in addition to providing anatomic information similar to that of TOF imaging. Through the selection of different imaging parameters, differing blood velocities can be highlighted; selective venous and arterial MRA images thus can be obtained. One advantage of phase-contrast MRA is the excellent suppression of background signal.

MRA has lower resolution than conventional angiography and therefore cannot detect small-vessel detail, such as is needed in the workup of vasculitis. It is also less sensitive to slow flow and thus may not differentiate occlusive disease from near-occlusive disease. Motion, either by the patient or by anatomic structures, may distort the images, creating artifacts that may be misinterpreted as stenoses or occlusions. These limitations notwithstanding, MRA has proved useful in evaluation of the cervical carotid artery and larger-caliber intracranial arterial and venous structures. It has also proved useful in the noninvasive detection of intracranial aneurysms (Fig. 366-13) and vascular malformations.

ECHO-PLANAR MR IMAGING Recent improvements in gradients, software, and high-speed computer processors now permit MR imaging of the brain on the order of milliseconds. With echo-planar MRI (EPI), fast gradients are switched on and off at high speeds to create the information used to form an image. In routine spin echo imaging, images of the brain can be obtained in 5 to 10 min. With EPI, all of the information required for processing an image is accumulated in 50 to 150 ms, and the information for the entire brain is obtained in 5 to 10 s (Fig. 362-4*A*). EPI allows motion-free imaging, as well as perfusion imaging, diffusion imaging (Fig. 362-4*B*), functional MRI (Fig. 362-5), and kinematic motion studies.

EPI techniques are just now making their way into clinical practice. The hope for these techniques is that they can provide useful functional data in addition to exquisite anatomic images. Early indications suggest a possible role for EPI perfusion and diffusion imaging in early detection of ischemic injury of the brain and in the characterization of white matter tracts (Fig. 362-4*B*). *Functional MRI* of the brain is a technique that localizes regions of activity in the brain following task activation. EPI or gradient echo techniques can be used for somatosensory localization with tasks that alter the balance of oxyhemoglobin and deoxyhemoglobin. Repetitive actions such as finger tapping elicit an increase in the amount of blood flow delivered to a specific region of the brain, resulting in a slight increase in oxyhemoglobin and a 2 to 3 percent change in signal intensity (Fig. 362-5). Further work will determine whether these techniques are cost effective or clinically useful.

Complications of MRI and Patient Safety MRI is considered safe for patients at magnetic field levels up to 3 T. However, serious injuries have been caused by the high magnetic fields used. Ferromagnetic (metal) objects can be attracted to the magnet and act as missiles if brought into the magnet room. Likewise, ferromagnetic aneurysm clips may torque within the magnet, causing hemorrhage and even death. Metallic foreign bodies in the eye have moved and caused hemorrhage, so screening for ocular metallic fragments is indicated in those with a history of metalwork. Implanted cardiac pacemakers are a contraindication to MRI owing to the risk of induced arrhythmias. All personnel and patients must be screened thoroughly to prevent such disasters. Table 362-6 lists several of the more common contraindications for MRI.

POSITRON EMISSION TOMOGRAPHY Positron emission tomography (PET) relies on the detection of positrons emitted during the decay of a radionuclide that has been injected into a patient. The most frequently used moiety is 2-[^{18}F]fluoro-2-deoxy-D-glucose (FDG), which is an analogue of glucose and is taken up by cells competitively with 2-deoxyglucose. Multiple images of glucose uptake activity are formed after 45 to 60 min. Images reveal differences in regional glucose activity among normal and pathologic brain structures. FDG PET scanning has been used to assist in differentiating radiation necrosis from active neoplasm following therapy, in localizing temporal lobe

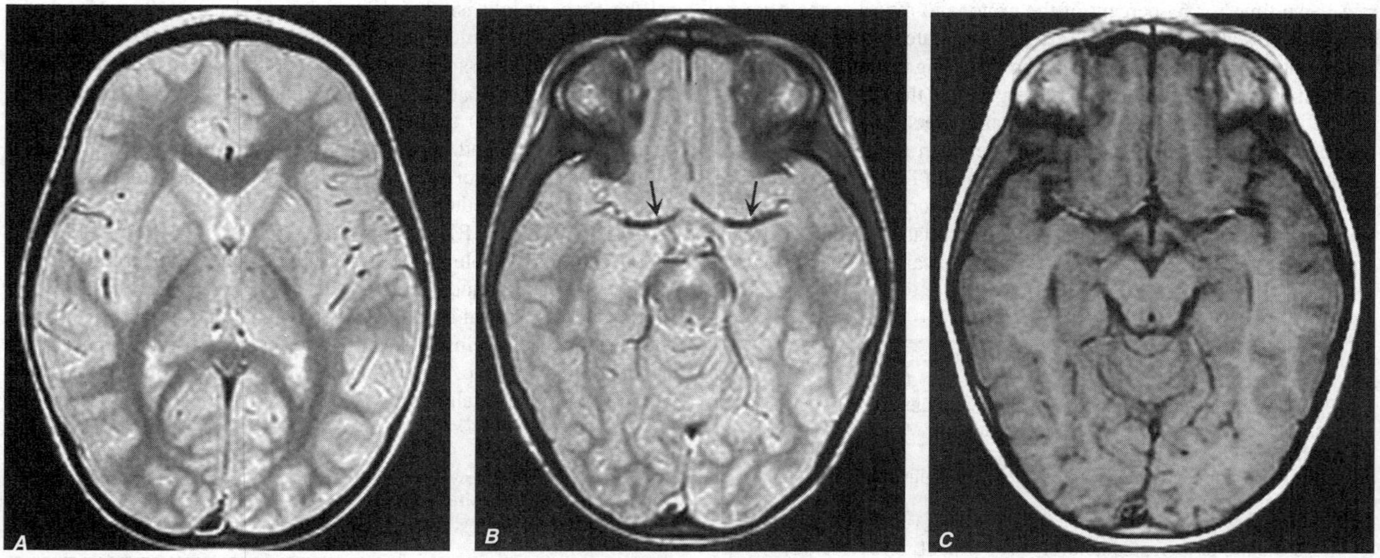

FIGURE 362-2 Normal MRI scans of the brain. *A, B.* Axial T2-weighted images through (*A*) the lateral ventricles and (*B*) the circle of Willis. Note that gray matter is slightly higher in signal intensity than white matter. CSF has a bright signal intensity owing to its free mobile water content. Moving protons in arterial structures demonstrate a signal void (*arrows*). *C.* T1-weighted image. Less contrast is visible between gray and white matter structures; however white matter appears slightly higher in signal intensity than gray matter owing to a shorter T1 relaxation time. Signal flow voids are seen in arterial structures and CSF spaces.

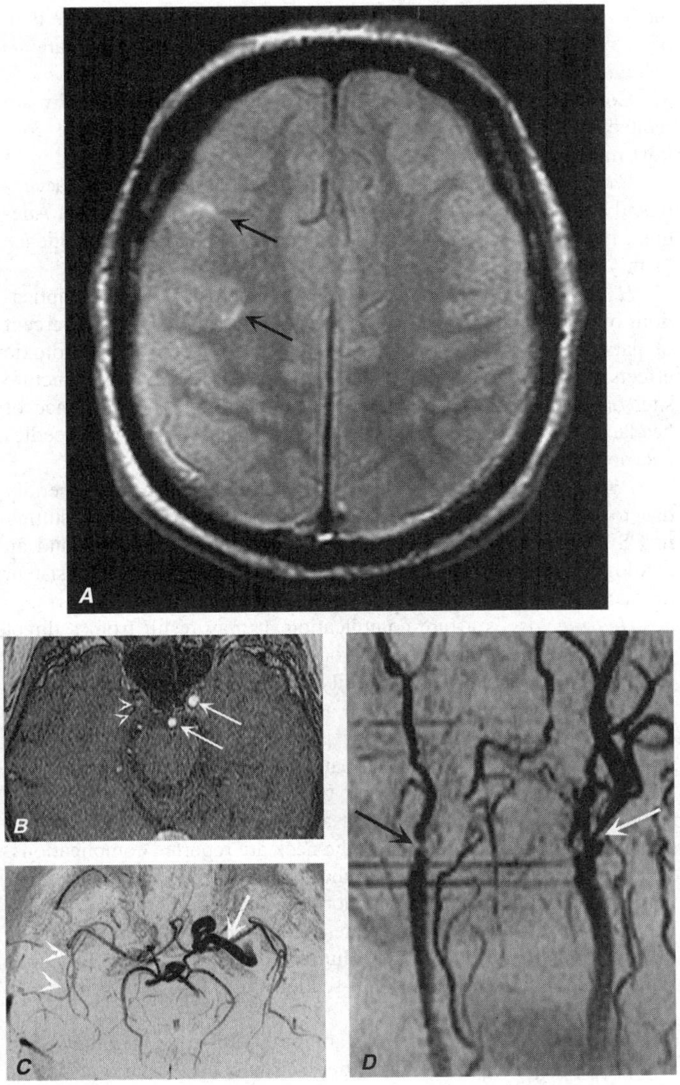

FIGURE 362-3 Use of MR angiography in cerebral ischemia. *A.* Axial proton density–weighted image demonstrates two focal areas of increased signal intensity in the right frontal lobe consistent with subcortical infarction (*arrows*). *B.* One of 90 sections from a 3-D time-of-flight gradient echo MR angiogram sequence in which flowing blood produces high signal intensity. The left internal carotid and basilar arteries show normal flow-related enhancement (*arrows*). The absence of signal in the right internal carotid artery (*arrowheads*) indicates either occlusion or high-grade stenosis with extremely slow flow in the internal carotid artery system. *C.* Maximum intensity projection, collapsed (submento-vertex) view, MRA. This image is obtained from the summation of the 90 partitions, one of which is shown in *B.* The left internal carotid artery is patent (*arrow*). Flow is absent in the right internal carotid artery. The right middle cerebral artery (*arrowheads*) is perfused by collateral flow across the anterior communicating artery as well as through the posterior communicating arteries. *D.* A 15° projection from a 2-D time-of-flight MR angiogram sequence through the cervical carotid arteries. The right internal carotid artery is occluded at the carotid bifurcation (*black arrow*). A high-grade (70 to 80 percent) stenosis is also present at the origin of the left internal carotid artery (*white arrow*).

epileptic foci, and in detecting metastatic disease and determining cardiac viability. A lower activity of FDG in the parietal lobes has been associated with Alzheimer's disease (see Fig. 367-1).

MYELOGRAPHY **Technique** Myelography involves the intrathecal instillation of 8 to 15 mL of water-soluble iodinated contrast medium (180 to 300 mg%) into the lumbar or cervical subarachnoid space via a percutaneously placed spinal needle (22 gauge or smaller). Contrast is maneuvered into the area of interest by fluoroscopic guidance and patient rotation. *Conventional myelography* involves a relatively high concentration and volume of contrast material and visualization by x-ray "spot films" and formal "overhead" plain films. The radiation exposure during conventional myelography is 4 to 8 cGy, making it one of the more radiation-intense procedures. The gonads should be shielded if possible, although doing so is sometimes difficult. CT scanning is often performed after myelography (*CT myelography*), in which case it demonstrates the spinal cord and roots as filling defects in the opacified subarachnoid space. CT myelography alone, in which CT is performed after the subarachnoid injection of a relatively small amount of relatively dilute contrast material, has replaced conventional myelography for many indications, thereby reducing exposure to radiation and contrast media. CT slices 3 to 5 mm thick are routinely obtained through the area of interest.

Indications For diagnosis of diseases of the spinal canal and cord, myelography has been largely replaced by CT, CT myelography, and MRI (Table 362-1). The remaining indications for conventional plain film myelography include the evaluation of suspected meningeal

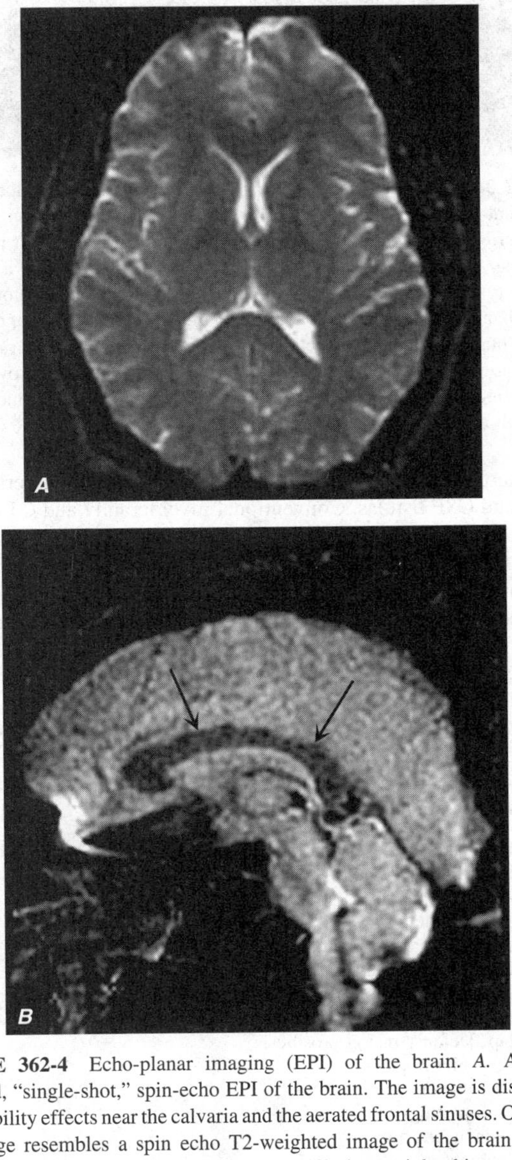

FIGURE 362-4 Echo-planar imaging (EPI) of the brain. *A.* Axial T2-weighted, "single-shot," spin-echo EPI of the brain. The image is distorted by susceptibility effects near the calvaria and the aerated frontal sinuses. Otherwise, this image resembles a spin echo T2-weighted image of the brain, but was obtained in 100 ms. *B.* Sagittal echo planar diffusion-weighted image. Restriction of microscopic water motion, such as occurs within axons coursing in one plane, results in increased signal intensity. So-called diffusion anisotropy is demonstrated in the corpus callosum (*arrows*). Diffusion of water protons is restricted in the corpus callosum to the left-to-right direction along the axonal fibers. This technique is also very sensitive to early infarction.

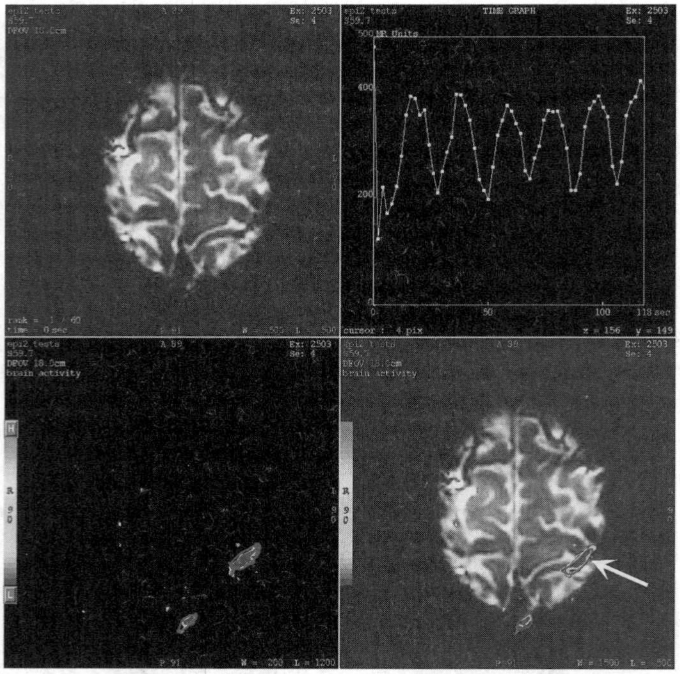

FIGURE 362-5 Functional EPI imaging with somatosensory localization. The patient was asked to repetitively touch his right index finger to thumb with a periodicity of 2 Hz for 10 s intervals alternating with rest periods of 10 s (*upper right image*). Echo planar images were obtained with a TE of 26 and 60 ms (*upper left image*). Subtraction of task-on and task-off images reveals changes in signal intensity related to increases in the level of oxyhemoglobin brought to the site of activation (*lower left image*). Superimposition shows that the increase in oxyhemoglobin during task activation overlies the anatomic region of the central sulcus corresponding to the right index finger and thumb regions (*arrow, lower right image*).

or arachnoid cysts and the localization of spinal dural arteriovenous fistulas and CSF fistulas. Conventional myelography and CT myelography provide the most precise information in patients with prior spinal fusion and spinal fixation hardware.

Contraindications Myelography is relative safe. However, it should be performed with caution in any patient with suspected herniation, elevated intracranial pressure, or a history of allergic reaction to intrathecal contrast media. In patients with a suspected spinal block, only a small amount of contrast medium should be instilled below the level of the block to prevent deterioration. Lumbar puncture is to be avoided in patients with bleeding disorders, including patients receiving anticoagulant therapy.

Table 362-6

Common Contraindications for MRI*
Cardiac pacemaker or permanent pacemaker leads
Internal defibrillatory devices
Cochlear prostheses
Bone growth stimulators
Implanted spinal cord stimulators
Electronic infusion devices
Intracranial aneurysm clips (some but not all)
Ocular implants (some) or ocular metallic foreign body
McGee stapedectomy piston prosthesis
Omniphase penile implant
Swan-Ganz catheter
Magnetic stoma plugs
Magnetic dental implants
Magnetic sphincters
Ferromagnetic IVC filters, coils, stents—considered safe at 6 weeks after implantation
Tattooed eyeliner (contains ferromagnetic material and may result in eye irritation)

* For a complete list, see Shellock and Kanal.

Complications Complications resulting from myelography are related to the needle puncture and to reactions to intrathecal contrast material.

Vasovagal syncope may occur during lumbar puncture; it is accentuated by the upright position used during lumbar myelography. Adequate hydration before and after myelography will reduce the incidence of this complication.

Headache, nausea, and vomiting are the most frequent complications of dural puncture and myelography, occurring in up to 38 percent of patients. These symptoms are thought to result from neurotoxic effects of the contrast agent, persistent leakage of CSF at the puncture site, or psychological reactions to the procedure. The incidence of headache has been reduced with the use of smaller-gauge spinal needles and nonionic, water-soluble contrast agents.

Postural headache (post–lumbar puncture headache) is generally due to prolonged leakage of CSF from the puncture site, resulting in CSF hypotension. Intravenous hydration may be helpful, and an autologous epidural blood patch is indicated in patients with persistent headache 48 h after myelography (see also Chap. 15).

Hearing loss is a rare complication. It may result from a direct toxic effect of the contrast medium or from an alteration of the pressure equilibrium between CSF and perilymph in the inner ear.

Puncture of the spinal cord is a rare but serious complication of cervical (C1-2) and high lumbar puncture. The cervical approach requires proper alignment of the patient and is best performed in the prone position using fluoroscopy guidance. Direct puncture of the spinal cord, laceration of epidural and vertebral venous and arterial structures, and hyperextension of the neck are reported complications. Injection of contrast material into the spinal cord can precipitate acute neurologic decline or subacute hemorrhagic necrosis of the gray matter. The risk of cord puncture is greatest in patients with spinal stenosis or conditions that reduce CSF volume. In these settings, a low-dose lumbar injection followed by thin-section CT is a safer alternative to cervical puncture.

Intrathecal contrast reactions are rare, but aseptic meningitis and encephalopathy may occur. The latter is usually dose-related and associated with contrast entering the intracranial subarachnoid space. *Seizures* occur following myelography in 0.1 to 0.3 percent of patients. Risk factors include a preexisting seizure disorder and the use of a total iodine dose of >4500 mg. Other reported symptoms include headache, hyperthermia, hallucinations, depression, and anxiety states. These neurotoxic side effects have been reduced by the development of nonionic, water-soluble contrast agents, as well as by head elevation and generous hydration following myelography.

Arachnoiditis, or inflammation of the leptomeninges, has also been ascribed to the use of contrast agents for myelography. Pantopaque, an oil-soluble contrast agent no longer used, was first noted to cause arachnoiditis, especially in cases where myelography results in subarachnoid bleeding (i.e., traumatic tap). The incidence of arachnoiditis with new water-soluble, nonionic contrast agents is much lower than with Pantopaque and with ionic, water-soluble agents (metrizamide). Other variables that increase the likelihood of arachnoiditis include trauma, infection, and subarachnoid hemorrhage.

ANGIOGRAPHY Technique Angiography is essential in the diagnostic evaluation of many patients with vascular pathology. However, it carries the greatest risk of morbidity of all diagnostic imaging procedures, owing to the necessity of inserting a catheter into a blood vessel, directing the catheter to the required location, injecting contrast material to visualize the vessel, and removing the catheter while maintaining hemostasis. Therapeutic transcatheter procedures (see below) have become important options for the treatment of some cerebrovascular diseases. The decision to undertake a diagnostic or therapeutic angiographic procedure requires careful assessment of the goals of the investigation and its attendant risks.

Patients undergoing angiography should be well hydrated before and after the procedure to better tolerate the contrast agents. Since the femoral route is used most commonly, the femoral artery must be compressed after the procedure to prevent a hematoma from developing. The puncture site and distal pulses should be evaluated carefully after the procedure in search of complications such as thigh hematoma or distal emboli.

Indications Table 362-1 lists some of the indications for conventional angiography. Over the past 20 years, angiography has been replaced for many indications by CT or MRI. However, it is still used today for evaluating intracranial small-vessel pathology, such as vasculitis, for assessing vascular malformations and aneurysms, and in intravascular therapeutic procedures.

Complications The vast majority of aortic arch, carotid, and vertebral arteriograms are carried out via transfemoral arterial access. A common femoral arterial puncture provides retrograde access via the aorta to the aortic arch and great vessels. The most feared complication of cerebral angiography is stroke. Thrombus can form on or inside the tip of the catheter, and atherosclerotic thrombus or plaque can be dislodged by the catheter or guidewire or by the force of injection and can embolize distally in the cerebral circulation. The duration and extent of the resulting ischemic neurologic deficit depends on the size and length of the embolus, its composition (fresh thrombus is thought to fragment more readily), its location, and the available collateral circulation. Risk factors for ischemic complications include limited experience on the part of the angiographer, atherosclerosis, vasospasm, low cardiac output, decreased oxygen-carrying capacity, advanced age, and possibly migraine. The risk of a neurologic complication varies but is approximately 4 percent for transient ischemic attack and stroke, 1 percent for permanent deficit, and very low ($<$0.1 percent) for death.

Ionic contrast material injected into the cerebral vasculature can be neurotoxic if the BBB is breached, either by an underlying disease or by the injection of hyperosmolar contrast agent. Ionic contrast media are less well tolerated than nonionic media, probably because they can induce changes in cell membrane electrical potentials. Patients with dolichoectasia of the basilar artery can suffer reversible brainstem dysfunction and acute short-term memory loss during angiography owing to the slow percolation of the contrast material and the consequent prolonged exposure of the brain. Rarely, an intracranial aneurysm ruptures during an angiographic contrast injection, causing subarachnoid hemorrhage, perhaps as a result of injection under high pressure.

Spinal Angiography Spinal angiography may be indicated to evaluate vascular malformations and tumors and to identify the artery of Adamkiewicz prior to aortic aneurysm repair. The procedure is lengthy and requires the use of relatively large volumes of contrast; the incidence of serious complications, including paraparesis, subjective visual blurring, and altered speech, is approximately 2 percent.

Interventional Neuroradiology This rapidly developing field is providing new therapeutic options for patients with difficult neurovascular problems. Available procedures include detachable coil therapy for aneurysms, particulate or liquid adhesive embolization of arteriovenous malformations, balloon angioplasty of stenosis or vasospasm, transarterial or transvenous embolization of dural arteriovenous fistulas, balloon occlusion of carotid-cavernous and vertebral fistulas, endovascular treatment of vein of Galen malformations, preoperative embolization of tumors, and thrombolysis of acute arterial or venous thrombosis. Many of these diseases place the patient at high risk of cerebral hemorrhage, stroke, or death. The therapeutic risks are comparable to those of neurosurgery rather than radiology.

The highest complication rates are found with the therapies geared to treating the highest-risk diseases. In a large series of surgically difficult intracranial aneurysms treated with detachable balloons, Higashida and colleagues reported a 7.4 percent incidence of stroke and a 9.8 percent death rate. These figures must be considered in light of the high morbidity and mortality associated with untreated and surgically unapproachable aneurysms (Chap. 366). The advent of the electrolytically detachable coil may reduce these rates, but endovascular therapy is still reserved largely for treatment of aneurysms not amenable to standard craniotomy and surgical clipping.

BIBLIOGRAPHY

Berg KJ, Jacobsen JA: Nephrotoxicity related to contrast media, in *Patient Safety and Adverse Events in Contrast Medium Examinations. International Congress Series 816,* I Enge, J Edgren (eds). Amsterdam, Excerpta Medica, 1989

Donaghy M et al: Encephalopathy after iohexol myelography. Letter. Lancet 2:887, 1985

Earnest F, 4th et al: Complications of cerebral angiography: Prospective assessment of risk. Am J Roentgenol 142:247, 1984

Gaa J et al: Noninvasive perfusion imaging of human brain tumors with EPISTAR. Eur Radiol 6(4):518, 1996

Guglielmi G: Embolization of intracranial aneurysms with detachable coils and electrothrombosis, in *Interventional Neuroradiology: Endovascular Therapy of the Central Nervous System,* F Viñuela et al (eds). New York, Raven Press, 1992, p 63

——— et al: Electrothrombosis of saccular aneurysms via endovascular approach. Part 2: Preliminary clinical experience. J Neurosurg 75:8, 1991

Higashida RT et al: Intracranial aneurysms: Interventional neurovascular treatment with detachable balloons—results in 215 cases. Radiology 178:663, 1991

Katayama H: Report of the Japanese Committee on Safety of Contrast Media. Presented at the Radiological Society of North America Meeting, Chicago, IL, November 1988

Mani RL, Eisenberg RL: Complications of catheter cerebral arteriography: Analysis of 5,000 procedures. II. Relation of complication rates to clinical and arteriographic diagnoses. Am J Roentgenol 131:867, 1978

Mattay VS et al: Whole-brain functional mapping with isotropic MR imaging. Radiology 201(2):399, 1996

Pan XM et al: Assessment of carotid artery stenosis by ultrasonography, conventional angiography, and magnetic resonance angiography: Correlation with ex vivo measurement of plaque stenosis. J Vasc Surg 21(1):82, 88, 1995

Riederer SJ et al: New technical developments in magnetic resonance imaging of epilepsy. Magn Reson Imaging 13(8):1095, 1995

Shellock FG, Kanal E: Policies, guidelines, and recommendations for MR imaging safety and patient management. SMRI Safety Committee. J Magn Reson Imaging 1:97, 1991

Sorensen AG et al: Hyperacute stroke: Evaluation with combined multisection diffusion-weighted and hemodynamically weighted echo-planar MR imaging. Radiology 199(2):391, 1996

Wilton NC et al: Epidural blood patch for postdural puncture headache: It's never too late. Anesth Analg 65:895, 1986

363

Joseph B. Martin, Frank M. Longo

MOLECULAR DIAGNOSIS OF NEUROLOGIC DISORDERS

The accelerating progress in the Human Genome Project will continue to increase the rate at which genes responsible for neurologic disorders are discovered. The widespread availability of DNA testing has already changed traditional diagnostic approaches and raised novel ethical issues. For example, the discovery of "susceptibility" genes that do not directly cause disease but modify the age of disease onset or rate of disease progression creates complexity in the application of molecular diagnosis, particularly in guiding the use of preventative therapies. In this chapter we will review molecular diagnostic approaches relevant to neurologic disease and illustrate how they contribute to patient care.

DNA-BASED DIAGNOSIS OF NEUROLOGIC DISORDERS As in other laboratory applications, appropriate use of DNA testing in the clinical setting requires that the clinician have a general understanding of the available molecular diagnostic approaches. The majority of disorders listed in Table 363-1 have been mapped to specific chromosomal regions, although for many the specific gene affected by mutations has not been identified. Presymptomatic testing or DNA diagnosis in some disorders is possible by family linkage

Table 363-1

Classification of Neurologic Disorders

Disorder	Chromosomal Localization	Principal Clinical Findings—Phenotype	Mode of Inheritance	Genotype/Gene Products/ Functions/Disease Mechanisms	Genetic Testing Available	Reference or Chapter
NEURODEGENERATIVE DISEASE						
Dementia						
Alzheimer's disease, early onset	AD4: 1q31-42	Dementia, memory loss, typical Alzheimer's disease	AD	Mutations in presenilin-2 gene (*SM2*); product is a putative membrane protein which may be involved in intracellular protein transport		367
Alzheimer's disease, early onset	AD3: 14q24.3	Dementia, memory loss, typical Alzheimer's disease; accounts for majority of familial Alzheimer's disease cases	AD	Mutations in presenilin-1 gene (*S182*); product is a putative membrane protein which may be involved in intracellular protein transport		367
Alzheimer's disease, late onset familial, and sporadic	AD2: 19q13.2	Memory loss, dementia	Codominant	Apolipoprotein E4 associated with increased risk and earlier age of onset; ApoE is secreted by astrocytes and internalized by neurons, where it supports cellular functions requiring lipoprotein mobilization	Yes	367
Familial Alzheimer's disease with amyloid precursor protein (APP) mutation	AD1: 21q21.3-22.05	Rare cause of early-onset Alzheimer's disease	AD	Point mutations in APP gene alter APP metabolism	Possible	367
Huntington's disease*	4p16.3	Chorea, depression, dementia; rigidity and epilepsy in juvenile patients	AD	CAG triplet repeats in gene that encodes a novel protein huntingtin → expanded polyglutamate tract in protein, which may cause gain of toxic functions	Yes	367
Familial Creutzfeldt-Jakob disease	20pter-p12	Spongiform encephalopathy with dementia, myoclonus	AD	Prion protein gene mutation		379
Fatal familial insomnia	20pter-p12	Adult-onset insomnia	AD	Prion protein gene mutation		27
Gerstmann-Straüssler-Scheinker disease	20pter-p12	Spongiform encephalopathy with dementia, myoclonus	AD	Prion protein gene mutation		379
Movement disorders						
Ataxia telangiectasia	11q22.3	Cerebellar degeneration, choreoathetosis, ocular apraxia, oculocutaneous telangiectasia, immunodeficiency, endocrinopathy	AR	Mutations in *ATM* gene, which codes for protein with domains similar to phosphatidylinositol 3′ kinase, an intracellular growth and differentiation factor signal transduction mediator, and rad3, a DNA repair monitor/cell cycle checkpoint regulator protein		369
Autosomal dominant cerebellar ataxia with pigmentary macular dystrophy (ADCAII)	3p12-21.1	Cerebellar ataxia, decreased vision, ophthalmoplegia, decreased vibration sense, increased deep tendon reflexes	AD	Unknown; mapped to within 8 cM		Holmberg et al.
Dentatorubral-pallidoluysian atrophy (DRPLA)	12p12.3-13.1	Ataxia, choreoathetosis, dementia, progressive myoclonus epilepsy (PME), psychiatric disorder	AD	CAG repeat expansions in DRPLA gene—unknown function; PME more common with larger expansions	Yes	369
Episodic ataxia type 1 (EA-1)	12p13	Ataxic episodes lasting seconds to minutes, myokymia, paroxysmal kinesogenic choreoathetosis, acetazolamide and phenytoin responsive	AD	Potassium channel (KCNA1) gene mutations		369

(*continued*)

Classification of Neurologic Disorders

Disorder	Chromosomal Localization	Principal Clinical Findings—Phenotype	Mode of Inheritance	Genotype/Gene Products/ Functions/Disease Mechanisms	Genetic Testing Available	Reference or Chapter
Episodic ataxia type 2 (EA-2)	19p13	Ataxic episodes lasting hours to days, downgaze nystagmus, headache, progressive cerebellar signs and atrophy, acetazolamide responsive	AD	Unknown		369
Friedreich's ataxia	9q13-21.1	Onset during puberty; ataxia, dysarthria, absent reflexes, decreased vibration, joint position sense, cardiomyopathy, diabetes mellitus	AR	GAA repeat expansion of *X25* (*frataxin*) gene	Possible	369; Campuzano et al.
Ataxia with vitamin E deficiency, Friedreich-like (AVED)	8q13	Same as Friedreich's ataxia but with severe vitamin E deficiency	AR	Mutations in α-tocopherol transfer protein gene (α*TTP*) → impaired binding of vitamin E to VLDL		369
Hereditary progressive dystonia with marked diurnal fluctuation (HPD)	14q22.1-22.2	Distal lower extremity dystonia in first decade, spreads to other limbs over years; symptoms greatest in evening, decreased in morning; responds markedly to levodopa	AD? female predominance	Mutations in GTP cyclohydrolase I gene → biopterin deficiency → decreased tyrosine hydroxylase activity → decreased dopamine		Ichinose et al.
Machado-Joseph disease (MJD)	14q24.3-31	Ataxia, ophthalmoparesis, corticospinal signs, dystonia-rigidity, amyotrophy	AD	CAG repeat expansions in *MJD1* gene	Yes	369
Spinocerebellar ataxia-1 (SCA1)	6p22-23	Ataxia, progressive dementia, spasticity, onset 3d or 4th decade; anticipation in successive generations	AD	Expansion of trinucleotide repeat (CAG) in ataxin-1; *SCA1* gene encoding ataxin-1	Yes	369
Spinocerebellar ataxia-2 (SCA2)	12q23-24.1	Features extensively overlap with SCA1, but more common hypotonia and ophthalmoplegia	AD	Unknown; anticipation observed, suggesting possibility of trinucleotide repeat expansion		369
Spinocerebellar ataxia-3(SCA3)	14qter-24.3	Similar to MJD	AD	CAG repeat expansions in *MJD1* gene	Yes	369
Spinocerebellar ataxia-4(SCA4)	16qter-24	Ataxia, axonal neuropathy, corticospinal signs, normal eye movements	AD	Unknown		369
Spinocerebellar ataxia-5(SCA5)	11 centromeric	Ataxia, dysarthria	AD	Unknown		369
Torsion dystonia	9q34	Early onset, generalized dystonia, occurs in both Ashkenazi Jewish (AJ) and non-Jewish pedigrees	AD	DYT1 locus; unknown gene	Yes	367
Wilson's disease	13q14.3	Disorder of copper transport into liver: extrapyramidal signs, psychiatric disorders	AR	Mutations in gene *ATP7B*, encoding a putative copper-transporting P-type membrane ATPase, 57% similar to that associated with Menkes' syndrome (MNK)		345
Retinitis pigmentosa						
Retinitis pigmentosa-1	3q21-24	Night blindness, peripheral field loss, blindness, abnormal ERG	AD	Mutations in gene that encodes rhodopsin → interference in maturational processing of wild-type protein		28

(*continued*)

Classification of Neurologic Disorders

Disorder	Chromosomal Localization	Principal Clinical Findings—Phenotype	Mode of Inheritance	Genotype/Gene Products/ Functions/Disease Mechanisms	Genetic Testing Available	Reference or Chapter
Retinitis pigmentosa, peripherin-related	6p21.1-cen	Night blindness, peripheral visual loss leading to blindness	AD	Mutations in RDS/peripherin gene, a rod photoreceptor membrane protein		28
Spastic paraplegia						
Autosomal dominant familial spastic paraplegia (SPG3, SPG4, SPG6)	SPG3: 14q SPG4: 2p21-24 SPG6: 15q11.1	Pure spastic paraplegia	AD	Unknown		370
Autosomal recessive familial spastic paraplegia	8q	Pure spastic paraplegia	AR	Unknown		370
X-linked familial spastic paraplegia-2 (SPG2)	Xq21-22	Initial pure spastic paraplegia; involvement of entire CNS over years	X-LR	Myelin proteolipid protein gene mutation; allelic with Pelizaeus-Merzbacher		367
Vascular diseases						
Cerebral autosomal dominant arteriopathy with subcortical infarcts (CADASIL)	19q12	Multiple subcortical infarcts, dementia	AD	Unknown		Tournier-Lasserve et al.
Familial cerebral amyloid angiopathy (Dutch type)	21q21.3-22.05	Cerebral hemorrhage	AD	Point mutations in APP gene	Possible	Levy et al.
Familial hemiplegic migraine	19p13	Onset 5–30 years, aura with unilateral paresis and other focal symptoms lasting 30–60 min; followed by headache, may have persistent cerebellar signs	AD	Unknown, may be related to episodic ataxia - type 2		364
Hereditary cystatin C amyloid angiopathy (HCCAA) (Icelandic)	20p11.2	Cerebral hemorrhage	AD	Mutations in cystatin C gene, product is a cysteine protease inhibitor; forms amyloid, which deposits in the walls of cerebral vessels		Levy et al.
Miscellaneous						
Abetalipoproteinemia (Bassen-Kornzwieg)	4q24	Vitamin E deficiency; neuropathy, ataxia, retinitis pigmentosa, acanthocytosis	AR	Mutations in gene coding large subunit of microsomal triglyceride transfer protein (MTP) → impairment of synthesis of VLDL		Narcisi et al.
Adrenoleukodystrophy	Xq28	Leukodystrophy, hypoadrenalism, mild neuropathy, baldness, hypogonadism	X-LR	Mutations in ALD protein gene, a peroxisomal membrane transporter; associated with impaired β-oxidation of unbranched saturated very long chain fatty acids in peroxisomes		380
Menkes' syndrome (kinky hair disease, steely hair disease)	Xq13.3	Abnormal whitish kinky hair, growth and mental retardation, spastic quadriparesis, seizures	X-LR	Mutations in *ATP7A*, encoding MNK, a protein very similar to P-type cation-transporting membrane ATPases; may be involved in copper transport across membranes; mutations may lead to copper deficiency.		Das et al.
EPILEPSY SYNDROMES						
Awakening grand mal (AGM)	6p	Adolescent onset, pure grand mal occurring on awakening	?	Also linked to EJM1—may be allelic with juvenile myoclonic epilepsy		365

(continued)

Table 363-1—*(Continued)*

Classification of Neurologic Disorders

Disorder	Chromosomal Localization	Principal Clinical Findings—Phenotype	Mode of Inheritance	Genotype/Gene Products/ Functions/Disease Mechanisms	Genetic Testing Available	Reference or Chapter
Benign neonatal epilepsy-1 (EBN1)	20q13.2-13.3	Generalized seizures, neonatal onset, benign course, usually resolving at 6–12 months, 10–15% have seizures later in life	AD	Mutations in the α-4 subunit of the neuronal nicotinic acetylcholine receptor gene		365
Benign neonatal epilepsy-2 (EBN2)	8q	Clinically indistinguishable from EBN1	AD	Unknown		365
Familial partial epilepsy	10q	Simple partial seizures, normal intelligence	AD, reduced penetrance	Unknown; mapped to within 10 cM		365
Juvenile myoclonic epilepsy (JME)	6p11-21.2	Onset in adolescence, myoclonic jerks, generalized tonic-clonic seizures	Uncertain	Gene locus named EJM1		365
Nocturnal frontal lobe epilepsy (ADNFLE)	20q13.2-13.3	Nocturnal seizures	AD	May be allelic with EBN1, also with a normal low voltage electroencephalogram variant		365
Progressive epilepsy with mental retardation (EPMR)	8pter-p22	Normal at birth, generalized seizures onset age 5–10 years, severe mental retardation 2–5 years after seizure onset	AR	Unknown; mapped to within 7 cM		365
Progressive myoclonus epilepsy, Unverricht-Lundborg type (EPM1)	21q22.3	Generalized seizures, stimulus-reactive myoclonus, onset age 6–15, progressive	AD	Unknown; EPM1 mapped to within about 300 kb		365
NEUROMUSCULAR DISORDERS						
Motor neuron diseases						
Familial amyotrophic lateral sclerosis, adult, dominant (ALS1)	21q22.1	Weakness, muscle atrophy, spasticity, increased deep tendon reflexes; about 10% of cases are familial, indistinguishable clinically from sporadic form	AD	Point mutations in Cu, Zn-superoxide dismutase (SOD1) in some families (20%); heterogeneity exists → motor neuron injury possibly due to defective detoxification of reactive oxygen species	Yes	370
Familial amyotrophic lateral sclerosis, juvenile recessive (ALS2)	2q33-35	Earlier onset and slower progression than ALS1	AR	Unknown		370
Familial amyotrophic lateral sclerosis, adult, dominant (ALS3)	11	Similar to ALS1	AD	Mutations in neurofilament protein heavy chain gene → disruption of neurofilament crosslinking		370
Spinal muscular atrophy (SMA) I–III	5q11.2-13.3	SMA I: infantile (Werdnig-Hoffman) disease—present by 3 months, hypotonia, proximal limb weakness, areflexia SMA II: childhood onset, limb/girdle weakness, areflexia, 70% never ambulate independently SMA III: juvenile (Kugelberg-Welander) disease—onset after age 2, slowly progressive symmetric proximal muscle weakness sparing bulbar muscles	AR	Mapped to about 1 Mb region; region is unstable and highly polymorphic making reconciliation of mapping data difficult; two candidate genes have been identified: "neuronal apoptosis inhibitory protein" (NAIP) gene, with amino acid homology to baculovirus apoptosis inhibitory proteins and survival motor neuron (SMN) gene coding a novel 294 aa protein	Yes	370

(*continued*)

Table 363-1—*(Continued)*

Classification of Neurologic Disorders

Disorder	Chromosomal Localization	Principal Clinical Findings—Phenotype	Mode of Inheritance	Genotype/Gene Products/ Functions/Disease Mechanisms	Genetic Testing Available	Reference or Chapter
Spinobulbar muscular atrophy (Kennedy syndrome)	Xq12	Muscular weakness and atrophy	X-LR	Trinucleotide repeats in androgen receptor gene → expanded polyglutamate tract in protein may cause partial loss of some physiologic functions and gain of other functions	Yes	370
Muscle diseases						
Becker myotonia (recessive myotonia congenita)	7q35	Similar to myotonia congenita	AR	Known *ClC-1* mutations present in about 16% unrelated cases		383
Central core disease (CCD)	19q13.1	Nonprogressive primarily proximal myopathy, onset in infancy	AD	Mutation in ryanodine receptor gene (*RYR1*); allelic with MHS1		383
Congenital muscular dystrophy (merosin deficient) (CMD)	6q2	Weakness and hypotonia at birth, limb contractures at birth or later	AR	Probable mutations in merosin gene		383
Congenital myasthenic syndromes/ "slow-channel" syndrome (SCS)	2q,17p	Weakness, fatigability, hypotonia, muscle atrophy	AD (?)	Mutations in genes encoding subunits of the acetylcholine receptor → altered channel kinetics		Sine et al.
Duchenne/Becker muscular dystrophy (DMD/BMD)	Xp21.2	DMD: onset of muscular weakness early in life, progressive; BMD form is later onset, less severe	X-LR	Mutations in dystrophin gene resulting in complete absence or major deletions of dystrophin (DMD), or less severe derangements of dystrophin structure (BMD) → disruption of linkage between microfilaments and the trans-sarcolemmal glycoprotein complex mediating adhesion to the extracellular matrix protein merosin → may lead to membrane damage with contraction	Yes	383
Emery-Dreifuss muscular dystrophy	Xq28	Childhood onset, benign course with early contractures, progressive muscle wasting with humeral/peroneal predominance, cardiac conduction defects—arrhythmias, heart block	X-LR	Mutations in emerin gene; codes a 254 aa serine-rich protein which may be membrane-anchored and has unknown function		383
Facioscapulohumeral dystrophy	4q35	Weakness, atrophy; face and shoulder muscles	AD	Unknown; exhibits anticipation, which may be associated with successive deletions in a region of tandem repeats		383
Fukuyama-type congenital muscular dystrophy (FCMD)	9q31-33	Weakness and hypotonia at birth, cerebral and cerebellar polymicrogyria and cerebellar cysts, ocular anomalies; overlaps with Walker-Warburg syndrome	AR	Unknown; proposed allelic with Walker-Warburg syndrome		383
Hereditary myoglobinuria	1p32	Episodic myalgia, rhabdomyolysis, myoglobinuria presenting 2nd and 3rd decades	AR	Mutations in gene coding carnitine palmitoyltransferase II → diminished import of long-chain fatty acids into mitochondria → mitochondrial dysfunction		Taroni et al.

(*continued*)

Classification of Neurologic Disorders

Disorder	Chromosomal Localization	Principal Clinical Findings—Phenotype	Mode of Inheritance	Genotype/Gene Products/ Functions/Disease Mechanisms	Genetic Testing Available	Reference or Chapter
Hyperkalemic periodic paralysis (HYPP)	17q23.1-25.3	Myotonia, periodic areflexic paralysis	AD	Point mutation in α subunit, sodium channel (SCN4A) → impairment of sodium current inactivation; normokalemic variants occur (normoPP)		383
Hypokalemic periodic paralysis (HOKPP)	1q32	Similar to HYPP, but attacks accompanied by hypokalemia, triggered by insulin and epinephrine, last longer and patients have no myotonia	AD	Loss of function mutations in α-1 subunit of the dihydropyridine (DHP) receptor gene, a slow voltage-gated L-type calcium channel → ? dominant negative disruption of channel function (decreased Ca^{2+} current); predominant expression in males may be hormone effect		383
Limb-girdle muscular dystrophy, autosomal dominant 1A (LGMD1A)	5q22.3-31.3	Late (third decade) onset muscular dystrophy, sparing the face; slow progression	AD	Unknown; mapped to within 7 cM		383
Limb-girdle muscular dystrophy, autosomal recessive 2A (LGMD2A)	15q15.1-21.1	Progressive symmetric atrophy of proximal limb muscles, beginning in first two decades	AR	Mutations in calcium-activated neutral protease 3 (CANP3) gene, large subunit gene important, but probably requires another as-yet-unidentified mutation for disease expression (digenic model)		383
Limb-girdle muscular dystrophy, autosomal recessive 2B (LGMD2B)	2p13-16	Pelvic girdle affected earliest; onset in late 2d decade	AR	Unknown		383
Malignant hyperthermia (MHS1) and central core disease (CCD)	19q13.1	Sensitivity to volatile anesthetics, muscle contraction	AD	Mutation in ryanodine receptor gene (*RYR1*) at 19q13.1 → ? disturbance of Ca^{2+} release; when mild → excessive contraction; when severe (as in CCD) → Ca^{2+} mediated mitochondrial toxicity		MacLennan
Malignant hyperthermia (MHS2,3,4)	MHS2: 17q11.2-24 MHS3: 7q21-22 MHS4: 3q13.1	Sensitivity to volatile anesthetics, muscle contraction	AD	Unknown		MacLennan
Myotonia congenita (dominant MC, Thomsen's disease)	7q35	Onset first decade, muscle stiffness/myotonia, muscle hypertrophy without weakness	AD	Known mutations in the chloride channel gene (*ClC-1*) account for about 15% of MC cases. Mutations cause loss of function and functional channel is likely homooligomer → dominant-negative mechanism		383
Myotonic dystrophy	19q13.3	Multisystem disorder: cataracts, myotonia, weakness, frontal baldness, mental retardation	AD, anticipation	CTG repeats at 3′ end of myotonin protein kinase gene—product is membrane associated and localized primarily to neuromuscular and myotendinous junctions; expression of adjacent genes may also be affected	Yes	383

(continued)

Classification of Neurologic Disorders

Disorder	Chromosomal Localization	Principal Clinical Findings—Phenotype	Mode of Inheritance	Genotype/Gene Products/ Functions/Disease Mechanisms	Genetic Testing Available	Reference or Chapter
Nemaline myopathy	1p13-q25	Most commonly congenital non- or slowly progressive myopathy; forms range from severe congenital to mild adult	AD (other forms AR)	Dominant form associated with α-tropomyosin gene (*TPM3*) mutation. Met9Arg mutation may increase tropomyosin-actin affinity → rod body formation		383
Oculopharyngeal muscular dystrophy (OPMD)	14q11.2-13	Onset usually after age 50, ptosis, dysphagia	AD	Gene unknown; maps near cardiac β-myosin		383
Paramyotonia congenita (PC)	17q23.1-25.3	Cold-induced muscle stiffness (myotonia) and weakness, occasional periodic paralysis	AD	SCN4A mutations; allelic with HYPP		383
Potassium-aggravated myotonia (PAM)	17q23.1-25.3	Potassium-sensitive muscle stiffness (myotonia) and weakness, occasional periodic paralysis	AD	SCN4A mutations; allelic with HYPP [other variants occur ("sodium-channel myotonias")]		Hoffman et al.
Severe childhood autosomal recessive muscular dystrophy (SCARMD, LGMD2C, LGMD2D)	13q12, 17q21	Similar to DMD or BMD	AR	17q21-linked form: mutations of adhalin gene; adhalin is a component of the membrane glycoprotein complex noted above; 13q12-linked form: gene unknown		383
Startle disease (hyperekplexia)	5q21-31	Exaggerated startle, neonatal hypertonia, nocturnal myoclonus	AD, AR	Mutations in the α-1 subunit of the inhibitory glycine receptor → mechanisms unknown, though Arg271 mutations seen in some human cases causes decreased agonist sensitivity in a mouse model		22; Rees et al.
X-linked myotubular myopathy	Xq28	Severe neonatal hypotonia, apnea, common perinatal death	X-LR	Unknown		Wallgren-Pettersson et al.
Peripheral neuropathies						
Charcot-Marie-Tooth disease, type 1A (CMT1A)	17p11.2	HMSNI: Variable onset, motor > sensory neuropathy, distal muscle atrophy, absent reflexes, high arches in feet, decreased nerve conduction velocities, +/- nerve enlargement	AD	Mutations or 1.5 Mb duplication in peripheral myelin protein (PMP-22) gene, product is a component of compact myelin	Yes	381
Charcot-Marie-Tooth disease, type 1B (CMT1B)	1q22	HMSNI	AD	Mutations in P_o gene, product is a component of compact myelin		381
Charcot-Marie-Tooth disease, type 1, X-linked (CMTX1,2,3)	CMTX1: Xq13.1 CMTX2: Xp22.2 CMTX3: Xq26	HMSNI	X-linked dominant	CMTX1: mutations in connexin32 gene coding a gap junction protein localized to uncompacted peripheral myelin at the nodes of Ranvier and Schmidt-Lanterman clefts; CMTX2,3: genes unknown	Yes	381
Charcot-Marie-Tooth disease, type 2A (CMT2A)	1p35-36	HMSNII: Later onset, sensorimotor axonal neuropathy, near normal nerve conduction velocities	AD	Unknown		381

(*continued*)

Table 363-1—*(Continued)*

Classification of Neurologic Disorders

Disorder	Chromosomal Localization	Principal Clinical Findings—Phenotype	Mode of Inheritance	Genotype/Gene Products/ Functions/Disease Mechanisms	Genetic Testing Available	Reference or Chapter
Charcot-Marie-Tooth disease, type 4A (CMT4A)	8q13-21.1	HMSNI	AR	Unknown		381
Dejerine-Sottas disease, type A (DSDA)	17p11.2-12	HMSNIII: Onset birth/infancy, slowly progressive sensorimotor deficits, high arches, scoliosis, ataxia, enlarged nerves, markedly decreased conduction velocities	AD	*PMP-22* mutations (see above)		362
Dejerine-Sottas disease, type B (DSDB)	1q22-23	HMSNIII	?	P_O mutations (see above)		362
Familial amyloidotic polyneuropathy (FAP)	18q11.2-12.1	Sensory/autonomic peripheral neuropathy, cardiomyopathy	AD	Mutations in transthyretin gene → formation of amyloid	Yes	381
Hereditary neuropathy with pressure palsies, type A (HNPPA)	17p11.2	Recurrent entrapment/pressure neuropathies, segmental demyelination	?AD	*PMP-22* deletions; CMT1A and HNPPA may result from reciprocal products of unequal crossover	Yes	381
CENTRAL NERVOUS SYSTEM TUMORS						
Neurofibromatosis, type 1 (Von Recklinghausen) (NF1)	17q11.2	Multiple neurofibromas, 1:3500 individuals, café au lait spots, malignant gliomas, Lisch nodules in iris	AD	Disruption of *NF1* gene; encodes neurofibromin, a member of the Ras-GTPase activating protein (GAP) family		375
Neurofibromatosis, type 2 (NF2)	22q12.2	Acoustic neuromas, bilateral meningiomas	AD	Deletions in the *NF2* gene that encodes for merlin/schwannomin, a tumor suppressor protein with sequence similarity to tyrosine phosphatase and cytoskeleton linkage protein	Yes	375
Retinoblastoma	13q14.1-14.2	40% hereditary, 60% nonhereditary, multiple tumors in inherited form	AR	*Rb* gene mutations or deletions cause disease; Rb protein is 105-kDa tumor suppressor, DNA-binding protein	Possible	28, 65
Von Hippel-Lindau type 1, 2 (VHL1, VHL2)	3p25-26	Type 1: retinal angiomas, CNS hemangioblastomas, pancreatic cysts in some Type 2: identical to type 1 plus pheochromocytoma	AD	Type 1: 56% microdeletions, deletions, insertions, nonsense mutations in *VHL* gene, a tumor suppressor of otherwise unknown function Type 2: 96% missense mutations in *VHL* gene	Yes	375
DEFECTS OF NEURONAL MIGRATION AND DIFFERENTIATION						
Familial cavernous malformations of the brain	7q11.2-21	Seizures, headache, intracerebral hemorrhage, neurologic deficits	AD	Unknown		Dubovsky et al.
Fragile X syndrome-A (FRAXA)	Xq27.3	Mental retardation, decreased head size, large forehead, macroorchidism	X-LR	CGG trinucleotide repeat expansions in 5′ region of *FMR-1* gene → transcriptional inhibition of gene due to overmethylation, as well as translational inhibition. *FMR-1* product contains KH domains and RGG box, motifs found in RNA binding proteins	Yes	Feng et al.

(continued)

Classification of Neurologic Disorders

Disorder	Chromosomal Localization	Principal Clinical Findings—Phenotype	Mode of Inheritance	Genotype/Gene Products/ Functions/Disease Mechanisms	Genetic Testing Available	Reference or Chapter
Fragile X syndrome-E (FRAXE)	Xq28	Mild mental retardation	X-LR	CGG/CCG repeat expansions, 600 kb distal to FRAXA site; developmentally regulated transcript recently found in region	Yes	Knight et al.
Hydrocephalus due to stenosis of the aqueduct of Sylvius (HSAS)	Xq28	Hydrocephalus with moderate to severe mental retardation, adducted hypoplastic thumbs (25% of cases), spastic paraparesis, aplasia or hypoplasia of the corticospinal tract and corpus callosum	X-LR	Mutations in L1 gene—product is a multifunctional/ multidomain cell adhesion molecule		Wong et al.
MASA syndrome (Gareis-Mason syndrome)	Xq28	Mental retardation, aphasia, shuffling gait (due to spastic paraparesis) and adducted thumbs (due to absent or hypoplastic extensor pollicis brevis and/or longus); may also have hydrocephalus	X-LR	L1 gene mutations		Wong et al.
Spastic paraplegia, X-linked, type 1 (SPXL or SPG1)	Xq28	Spastic paraplegia, ataxia, absent extensor pollicis longus	X-LR	L1 gene mutations		367; Wong et al.
Kallmann syndrome	Xp22.3	Anosmia with hypogonadism (GnRH deficiency); syndrome due to failure of olfactory neuronal migration	X-LR	Mutations in gene (*KALIG-1*) that encodes protein with homology to neural-cell adhesion (N-CAM) molecules		337
Miller-Dieker lissencephaly syndrome	17p13.3	Microcephaly, micrognathia, epilepsy, agyria due to failure of cortical neuronal migration	AD	Mutation in *LIS-1* gene coding the 45-kDa (regulatory) subunit of platelet-activating factor (PAF) acetylhydrolase; part of heterotrimeric enzyme which inactivates PAF; PAF proposed to modulate neuronal differentiation or migration; effect of mutation on PAF unknown	Yes	Hattori et al.
Norrie disease (ND)	Xp11.4	Retinal malformation, hearing loss, mental retardation	X-LR	Mutations in *ND*; sequence comparisons and modeling suggest similarity to transforming growth factor β family/ cysteine-knot motif growth factors		Chen et al; Berger
Tuberous sclerosis, type 1	9q34	1:10,000 births, mental retardation, seizures, adenoma sebaceum	AD	Unknown; may be a growth suppressor		White
Tuberous sclerosis, type 2	16p13.3	Hamartomas, epilepsy, mental retardation	AD	Gene encodes tuberin, which has homology to GTPase activating protein GAP3; effects of mutations on protein function unknown		Rouleau et al.

(continued)

Table 363-1—*(Continued)*

Classification of Neurologic Disorders

Disorder	Chromosomal Localization	Principal Clinical Findings—Phenotype	Mode of Inheritance	Genotype/Gene Products/ Functions/Disease Mechanisms	Genetic Testing Available	Reference or Chapter
Waardenburg syndrome-1 (WS1)	2q35	Deafness, white forelock, dystopia canthorum, pigmentary abnormalities	AD	Mutation in paired box-containing *(PAX-3)* gene; product is a transcription factor involved in embryonic patterning/neural crest migration; heterozygotes have WS1, homozygotes have WS3, which is more severe and includes upper limb abnormalities		Tassabehji
Waardenburg syndrome-2 (WS2)	3p12.3-14.1	Deafness, white forelock, dystopia canthorum, heterochromia irides, early graying	AD	Mutations in microphthalmia *(MITF)* gene encoding a putative basic helix-loop-helix-leucine-zipper transcription factor		Tassabehji
Walker-Warburg syndrome (WWS)	9q31-33	Lissencephaly, ocular anomalies, hydrocephalus, callosal hypoplasia, septal agenesis, congenital muscular dystrophy	AR	Unknown; proposed allelic with FCMD		Arahata et al.

* HD causes both dementia and movement disorder.

NOTE: AD, autosomal dominant; AR, autosomal recessive; CNS, central nervous system; ERG, electroretinogram; GnRH, gonadotropin-releasing hormone; HMSN, hereditary motor and sensory neuropathy; Rb, retinoblastoma; VLDL, very low density lipoprotein; X-LR, X-linked recessive.

analysis. Linkage analysis requires that family relationships (such as paternity) are correctly established, that the clinical status of family members is accurate, that informative markers are available, and that an adequate number of family members are genotyped. For many patients, these requirements often eliminate application of DNA diagnosis.

Direct DNA diagnosis can be used in a large number of disorders. Most disease-causing mutations consist of single base substitutions leading to amino acid substitutions (missense mutations), premature translation stop signals (nonsense mutations), or abnormal RNA transcript splicing. Other mutations result from DNA deletions or instability of trinucleotide repeats. For genetic diseases in which the pathologic phenotype is caused by only one or a small number of well-defined mutations within a given gene, detection of the mutation can be used for diagnosis. The ability to detect a mutation eliminates the need for diagnosis by physical examination and the need for linkage studies.

Approaches for Detection of DNA Mutations *Direct sequencing of patient DNA* These methods generally require amplification of DNA by the polymerase chain reaction (PCR). With most current methods, only 300 to 400 DNA bases are sequenced; therefore, sequencing-based strategies are best applied when a limited region contains the majority of potential mutation sites. Direct DNA sequencing allows novel mutations to be detected and decreases the chances of a "false-negative" result. In some cases, the significance of previously uncharacterized missense mutations will be difficult to interpret. They might code for harmless amino acid polymorphisms or in other cases constitute the cause of the disease. The segregation of the same mutation with the disease phenotype within a family or the substitution of nonconserved amino acids, especially in critical protein regions, would suggest the latter.

Allele-specific oligonucleotide hybridization This technique, in which sequence-specific oligonucleotides differentially recognize DNA segments with normal sequence or mutated sequence, is best suited for detecting known mutations and can be applied to a large number of samples.

Differential restriction endonuclease patterns of PCR-amplified DNA DNA is digested with restriction enzymes that recognize either normal or mutated DNA sequence; the size pattern of resulting DNA fragments indicates whether the DNA sample contains normal or variant sequence (see Chap. 65). This method is also directed toward detecting known mutations.

Analysis of single-stranded conformation polymorphisms Segments of the gene of interest of several hundred bases in length are PCR amplified and electrophoresed under denaturing conditions. Mutation-induced alterations of DNA structure lead to altered electrophoretic patterns. This approach can detect novel mutations directly. Large numbers of samples either covering many exons of a large gene or from many patients can be analyzed.

Detection of DNA deletions by fluorescence in situ hybridization DNA deletions are detected by hybridizing chromosomes with a fluorescent probe corresponding to the gene of interest. Fluorescence in situ hybridization (FISH) can detect deletions smaller than the 2000- to 3000-kb minimum detected by banding techniques.

Cytogenetic testing Chromosomes isolated from peripheral blood lymphocytes or tissue are stained allowing identification of insertions, deletions, other chromosome imbalances, and assessment of chromosomal number (see Chap. 66).

Some disorders such as muscular dystrophy (DM), neurofibromatosis (type 1 and 2), and familial amyotrophic lateral sclerosis (ALS) can be caused by dozens of different mutations within one gene. Genetic heterogeneity over a wide region of a given gene is common for many genes involved in metabolic diseases. Many methods of DNA analysis focus on recurring point mutations or relatively short segments of DNA. Using such focused DNA analysis, mutations are found in only about two-thirds of Duchenne muscular dystrophy (DMD), Becker muscular dystrophy (BMD), and neurofibromatosis type 2 patients and in less than half of those with neurofibromatosis type 1. Advances in multiplex PCR and single-strand chain polymorphism analysis have increased this yield, but the clinician should be aware of the "sensitivity" of each DNA analysis.

Detection of Protein Abnormalities For some applications, diagnostic methods based on protein properties or function are more effective and efficient than DNA-based tests. Traditional enzyme activity–based assays continue to be useful for diagnosis of many metabolic diseases, and additional protein functions can be used to detect other disorders. For example, immunologic assays may reveal decreased protein levels or aberrant distribution of dystrophin in a muscle biopsy of a patient in whom no DNA mutations are detected.

COMPLICATIONS AND LIMITATIONS OF GENETIC TESTING The limitations of DNA testing must also be considered. If the presumed diagnosis is in error or if the phenotype overlaps with other disorders, the detection of normal alleles of the gene tested is of limited value. Different mutations in the same gene can result in different phenotypes (*allelic heterogeneity*), and mutations in different genes can result in the same phenotype (*nonallelic genetic heterogeneity*). Other phenomena such as phenocopies, incomplete penetrance, age-dependent onset of phenotype, polygenic inheritance, imprinting mitochondrial inheritance, and dynamic mutations (trinucleotide repeats) may also make interpretation of genetic testing difficult.

Nonallelic Genetic Heterogeneity Nonallelic genetic heterogeneity (also known as genetic heterogeneity) describes the occurrence of individuals or families with similar pathologic and/or clinical syndromes who have mutations in different genes, as in the multiple demyelinating forms of Charcot-Marie-Tooth disease (CMT; see Table 363-1). For CMT type 1A the locus is 17p11.2, and the affected gene encodes the peripheral myelin protein (PMP-22) gene. CMT type 1B, which is clinically similar to CMT 1A but less common, is caused by a mutation on chromosome 1q that results from a mutation in the gene for P_0, a component of compact myelin. Familial Alzheimer's disease (AD) is caused by mutations in genes located on chromosome 14 (*presenilin 1*, causing 70 to 80 percent of early-onset AD), chromosome 1 (*presenilin 2*), and chromosome 21 (*amyloid precursor protein*). Several forms of type I autosomal dominant spinocerebellar ataxias (SCA) including SCA1 and SCA3/Machado-Joseph disease (MJD) are caused by expansions of CAG repeats in genes located at 6p23 (*SCA1*) and 14q32 (*SCA3/MJD1*), respectively. Familial ALS can be caused by mutations in the gene encoding cytosolic copper/zinc superoxide dismutase 1 (SOD1) or, less commonly, the gene for the heavy neurofilament subunit, and retinitis pigmentosa can be caused by mutations in more than 10 different genes.

Allelic Heterogeneity Different mutations in the same gene (allelic mutations) cause DMD and BMD (dystrophin gene, Xp21.2) and infantile and juvenile onset spinal muscular atrophies (5q11.2-13.3). Familial Creutzfeldt-Jakob disease, fatal familial insomnia, and Gerstmann-Sträussler-Scheinker disease are all caused by allelic mutations in the prion protein gene (20pter-p12), each of which results in distinct aberrant protein isoforms or alterations in expression.

Phenocopies Patients may have a clinical presentation that resembles a disease phenotype but that has a nongenetic cause. Examples include vascular dementia appearing as familial AD, toxin- or drug-induced chorea mimicking Huntington's disease (HD), and vitamin E deficiency resembling Friedreich's ataxia.

Variable Expressivity Variable expressivity occurs when the severity of a trait resulting from a mutant allele varies from mild to severe. Expression of the disease phenotype can be modified by other factors such as predisposing alleles of other genes, environmental agents, sex, and age. Variation in expression can also occur following somatic variations in trinucleotide repeats, as occurs in DM.

Incomplete Penetrance Penetrance refers to the all-or-none expression of a mutant genotype. If a disease is expressed in fewer than 100 percent of individuals carrying the abnormal allele, it is said to have incomplete penetrance.

Polygenic Inheritance Some diseases are caused by concomitant mutations in multiple genes. In one form of retinitis pigmentosa mutations are present in both the RDS/peripherin and *ROM1* genes. Similarly, some forms of Hirschsprung disease may result from simultaneous mutations in loci at 13q22 and 21q22.

INFLUENCE OF GENETIC BACKGROUND MJD and SCA3 are autosomal dominant ataxias originally described in different ethnic backgrounds and described as having distinct features. MJD occurs in families, often of Portuguese-Azorean origin, and is manifest as hereditary ataxia with dystonia, rigidity, faciolingual fasciculation, and bulging eyes. In French families with progressive ataxia and dysarthria, the SCA3 gene was mapped to a site on chromosome 14q near the MJD locus. It is now clear that MJD and SCA3 are both caused by expansion of the same tract of CAG repeats in the same gene (*MJD1*) at 14q32.1. Although expansions in *MJD1* are the most common mutations in German SCA patients, the diagnosis of MJD has not previously been considered in this population. The extent to which different genetic backgrounds causes phenotypical heterogeneity will require further studies.

SUSCEPTIBILITY GENES Allelic variations or mutations can cause increased susceptibility to specific diseases. Detection of such DNA polymorphisms can influence differential diagnosis, as in the genotyping of *APOE* alleles in the diagnosis of AD. Apolipoprotein E (apoE) is a 299-amino-acid protein involved in mobilization and reutilization of lipoprotein cholesterol. ApoE secreted by astrocytes appears to be internalized by neurons via low-density, lipoprotein-related receptors where it contributes to neuronal function. The three isoforms of apoE (apoE2, apoE3, and apoE4) are derived from three corresponding alleles of the *APOE* gene located at 19q13.2; the apoE4 allele is overrepresented in sporadic and familial AD, and its presence is a significant risk factor for the disease. In contrast, the apoE2 allele is underrepresented and thus may have a "protective" effect (see Chap. 367).

The increased incidence of the *APOE4/4* genotype in AD patients has raised the possibility that ascertainment of *APOE* genotype might be useful in the diagnostic assessment of patients with dementia. For example, since AD accounts for some two-thirds of late-onset dementia, the prior probability of an elderly patient with dementia having AD is approximately 0.66. Based on preliminary studies, it appears that the probability of a demented patient with the *APOE4/4* genotype having AD increases to 0.94 and in a patient with *APOE3/4* to 0.81.

As a research tool, *APOE* genotyping is likely to contribute substantially to the neurobiologic understanding of AD and to be an important stratification variable for future clinical trials. On the other hand, current data do not, for several reasons, support its routine application in the clinical assessment of dementia. First, available *APOE* genotype data are not derived from age-specific epidemiologic studies. If a 25-year-old presents with dementia and has the *APOE4/4* genotype, it nevertheless is very unlikely that this patient has AD. Second, since individuals with all *APOE* genotypes can have AD, genotypes cannot absolutely rule in or rule out this diagnosis. Even if genotyping increases the odds that a given patient has AD, it does not rule out the possibility that a treatable cause of dementia is present. Since current diagnostic studies for demented patients are focused on detecting reversible causes of dementia, it can be argued that *APOE* genotype results would not change the diagnostic evaluation and therefore should not be ordered on a routine basis. Nevertheless, *APOE* genotyping might eventually be combined with other diagnostic tests such as cerebrospinal fluid β-amyloid or τ protein levels to form a "panel" of data with acceptable sensitivity and specificity for diagnosis (see Chap. 367).

The issue of predictive *APOE* genotyping for asymptomatic individuals must also be considered. Until genotyping can contribute to identifying individuals who might benefit from preventive therapy, many clinicians would consider predictive testing to be unethical. Moreover, useful predictions of age of onset based solely on *APOE* genotyping are not possible. For the 2 percent of the population with the high-risk *E4/E4* genotype, the period of risk extends from the fifties to beyond the nineties.

APPROACH TO GENETIC TESTING One indication for DNA analysis is confirmatory diagnosis for a specific disease already suggested by clinical assessment. DNA testing can also be useful in narrowing a differential diagnosis in situations where multiple diagnostic possibilities are present. DNA testing for HD often allows patients to avoid neuroimaging and other diagnostic studies. Another application of genetic analysis is presymptomatic testing in members of families known or suspected to have a specific disorder. In these cases the most common reasons for individuals desiring testing are life management issues, reproductive planning decisions, and eliminating the stress of not knowing one's own carrier status. Development of new therapies that delay onset or progression of neurodegenerative diseases will provide additional indication for presymptomatic testing.

Genetic testing should be conducted only in the context of comprehensive genetic counseling, in which the implications of potential test results are fully understood and adequate support services are available. Clinicians ordering genetic studies should be familiar with issues regarding informed consent, suicide risk, ongoing patient support, insurance, employment discrimination, testing of minors, and testing of fetal tissue.

A computerized directory of laboratories offering DNA diagnostic services, known as Helix, is accessible to health care professionals, and information on access and/or listing of new laboratories can be obtained at the Helix office [(206) 527-5742]. Many university centers offer testing for multiple neurogenetic disorders.

CLINICAL AND GENETIC CLASSIFICATION OF GENE DISORDERS Neurogenetic disorders have traditionally been classified and subtyped on the basis of clinical and pathophysiologic concepts. The complexity, variability in phenotype, and overlapping features limit the resolution of phenotype-based classification and confound disease nosology. Identification of tightly linked disease markers and discovery of disease-causing mutations have provided a basis for refining such classifications. For example, the distinction between neurofibromatosis type 1 and type 2 has been upheld by the discovery that they are caused by mutations in different genes belonging to distinct gene families: GTPase-activating protein and the merlin (schwannomin) cytoskeletal protein, respectively. In contrast, the finding that DMD and BMD are caused by mutations in the same gene points to shared pathophysiologic mechanisms and blurs the distinctions between these disorders. Mutations in different genes can lead to overlapping clinical syndromes in the case of the inherited ataxias. In other instances, phenotypically dissimilar disorders are caused by mutations in the same gene; both X-linked spastic paraparesis and X-linked hereditary hydrocephalus are caused by mutations in the gene encoding the L1 cell adhesion molecule.

Neurogenetic disorders with known chromosomal gene localization are organized primarily by clinical-pathologic phenotype in Table 363-1. Neurogenetic diseases resulting from mutations in mitochondrial DNA are reviewed in Chap. 383. Chromosomal disorders involving gross structural aberrations or alterations in number (aneuploidy) cause a large number of syndromes, many of which include mental retardation (see Chap. 383).

In the classification used in Table 363-1, the first group is the neurodegenerative disorders, which implies that deterioration and death of neurons occurs after normal development. These diseases may affect any portion of the nervous system. The second group is the epilepsy syndromes. The third group is the neuromuscular diseases, which affect the peripheral nervous system, the neuromuscular junction, or muscle. The fourth group is tumors of the central nervous system. The fifth group is abnormalities of development characterized by defects in neuronal development and migration. The availability of testing by DNA diagnostic laboratories is indicated.

Different modes of inheritance occur in each of these categories. Neurologic genetic disorders inherited in Mendelian autosomal dominant mutations include HD, familial AD, ALS, DM, CMT, familial hyperkalemic periodic paralysis, SCA, and tuberous sclerosis. Autosomal recessive disorders include Friedreich's ataxia (FA), Wilson's disease, ataxia telangiectasia, Tay-Sach's disease, and other lysosomal disorders, whereas DMD, spinobulbar muscular atrophy (Kennedy syndrome), Kallmann's syndrome, and fragile X syndrome are X-linked recessive traits. Non-Mendelian patterns of transmission such as maternal inheritance can result from mitochondrial mutations (see Chap. 383) and unstable trinucleotide repeats (see below).

The types of mutations causing neurologic genetic disorders include gene deletions (the most common finding in DMD), insertions (e.g., Von Hippel-Lindau, type 1), duplications (e.g., CMT1A), translocations that interrupt the gene (neurofibromatosis type 1), and point mutations (e.g., in the superoxide dismutase gene in ALS). Point mutations can substitute an alternative base and thereby alter the amino acid sequence (missense mutations) or introduce stop codons leading to premature truncation of protein translation (nonsense mutations). These DNA alterations are considered "static" mutations because they generally remain stable during meiosis and provide the basis for classic Mendelian inheritance. Unstable trinucleotide repeats cause "dynamic" mutations and account for the clinical phenomenon of anticipation.

GENETICALLY INDUCED MECHANISMS OF CELL DEATH Three general mechanisms for cell death in genetic disorders have been proposed: (1) loss of function, (2) dominant-negative effects, and (3) gain of function.

In *loss-of-function disorders*, the mutation causes a deficiency in an enzyme or protein resulting in cellular dysfunction. The best defined examples are the lysosomal storage disorders in which enzymatic deficiencies in complex lipid metabolism lead to accumulation of normal or abnormal cellular constituents. The mode of inheritance in these disorders is most often autosomal recessive, but it can also be X-linked or the result of a combined inherited germ cell mutation and an acquired somatic mutation ("second hit") that knocks out both alleles (such as the loss of a growth suppressor gene as occurs in tumors like retinoblastoma). It is less common for loss-of-function disorders to result from autosomal dominant mutations. One example is the mutation of one allele of the low-density lipoprotein receptor gene ("haplo-insufficiency") with insufficient compensation by the normal allele causing familial hypercholesterolemia.

In the case of a *dominant-negative effect*, the abnormal mutation competes with or abolishes the normal allelic function at either the DNA, RNA, or protein level. This mechanism has been postulated to be an important example of cellular dysfunction in osteogenesis imperfecta in which abnormal collagen protein causes destruction of collagen fibrils. A dominant-negative mechanism in DM has been suggested by observations that RNA transcripts with expanded CTG repeats precipitate normal RNA transcripts. True dominant disorders such as HD and SCA1, in which the heterozygote genotype elicits the full spectrum of the disease phenotype, could be the result of either dominant-negative or true toxic gain-of-function effects. In the former, proteins with expanded polyglutamine tracts would form oligomers with normal protein isoforms and thereby interfere with their function. In the case of *gain-of-function effects*, the abnormal cellular function exerted by the mutation at one allele would in some way render the cell susceptible to toxic effects, whether or not the normal allele is expressed.

DISORDERS ASSOCIATED WITH TRINUCLEOTIDE REPEATS At least 10 neurologic disorders are caused by abnormal expansions of trinucleotide repeats (Table 363-2). A useful way of organizing repeat diseases and understanding their mechanisms can be based on the location of the repeat expansions within the gene. Expansions can occur in the 5′ untranslated region (UTR), within the open reading frame (translated portion of the gene), within the 3′ UTR, or within introns.

Four fragile X sites located on the long arm of the X chromosome (FRAXA, FRAXE, FRAXF, and FRA16A) are associated with expansions of CGG or CCG trinucleotide repeats (see also Chap. 66). The FRAXA site is associated with the fragile X syndrome, the most common cause of inherited mental retardation. FRAXA is located in the 5′ UTR of the *FMR1* gene, which encodes a protein identified as FMRP. Loss of FMRP is responsible for the fragile X phenotype. One proposed mechanism to account for the defect in fragile X syndrome is that expanded CGG repeats become methylated and become targets of methyl CpG binding proteins that act to inhibit transcription. A loss-of-function model is suggested by studies showing decreased *FMR1* RNA and FMRP protein in fragile X patients and by the identification of two patients with classic features of fragile X with intragenic loss-of-function deletions. In expansions of more than 200 repeats, inhibition of transcript translation also affects FMRP levels. Expansions at the FRAXE locus are associated with a mild form of mental retardation.

The second category of trinucleotide expansion diseases consists of six neurodegenerative disorders in which expansion of a CAG repeat in the open reading frame encodes an aberrant protein with an expanded polyglutamine tract. The stretches of CAG repeats, which vary between 5 and 37 in the normal alleles of each condition, are increased by two- to fourfold in the mutation. Earlier age of onset and increased severity of the neurologic disorder demonstrate a striking correlation with larger numbers of repeats. Normal alleles identified to date never contain more than 38 CAG repeats. One possible disease mechanism is that the expanded polyglutamine tract causes a loss of protein function. HD patients homozygous for the disease allele have phenotypes similar to heterozygous patients.

These observations suggest a model in which a gain of function is toxic to neurons. One possibility is that expanded polyglutamine tracts provide a substrate for transglutaminases causing abnormal cross-linking of proteins. Expanded polyglutamine tracts might also acquire the function of "polar zippers" via hydrogen bond formation between main-chain and side-chain amides of interacting proteins. In both models, loss of the function of a critical protein(s), inhibited or depleted by aberrant interaction with expanded polyglutamine tracts, would lead to neuronal degeneration. Several lines of evidence support such a protein-based hypothesis. Open reading frame CAG repeats are indeed translated into protein. Transgenic mice expressing a human *SCA1* gene with an expanded CAG repeat develop the characteristic phenotype only when the transgene is expressed. One study has suggested that polyglutamine tracts of the proteins that cause HD and dentatorubral-pallidoluysian atrophy (DRPLA) interact with glyceraldehyde-3-phosphate dehydrogenase and thereby might have a deleterious effect on neuronal energy metabolism.

Gain-of-function models of polyglutamine tract diseases must also reconcile the observations that each neurodegenerative disease affects only regionally specific populations of neurons, yet proteins associated with these disorders are widely expressed. One possibility is that each of these polyglutamine tract proteins interacts with yet-to-be discovered proteins that are indeed cell-type specific. The huntingtin-associated protein (HAP1) is one such candidate. HAP1 is selectively expressed in brain tissue and demonstrates enhanced association with forms of huntingtin protein with increased lengths of glutamine repeats. Another potential mechanism of cell-type specificity is that somatic instability of CAG repeats leads to greater expansions in specific cell populations. The relatively small variations of three to five in the number of triplet repeats in the HD gene in different regions of the brain makes this explanation less likely.

In the third category of trinucleotide repeat disorders, repeat expansion occurs in the 3′ UTR. So far, only one disease demonstrates expansion in this region. In DM, a GTC (CAG in the antisense) repeat in the 3′ UTR of the DM kinase gene expands manyfold from 5 to 40 repeats in normal alleles to several kilobases in severe cases. The repeat expansion is variable in different tissues, indicating that errors in DNA replication can occur during meiosis and during somatic cell mitosis. Since DNA sequence motifs in the 3′ UTR of RNA transcripts regulate transcript stability and processing, expansions in this region might affect transcript levels and alter DM kinase protein levels. Quantitative analysis of messenger RNA in muscle biopsies demonstrated marked disease-specific decreases in DM kinase mRNA in adult-onset DM patients. Levels of normal DM transcripts as well as mutant transcripts were decreased, suggesting a novel mechanism of a dominant-negative mutation occurring at the RNA level.

A second potential mechanism in DM is that expansion of the GTC repeat could inhibit expression of nearby genes. The *DMR-N9* gene is located immediately upstream (telomeric) from the DM kinase gene and the highest expression of *DMR-N9* is in neural tissue and testis; therefore alterations in its expression might cause pathology at these sites. A novel homeodomain-encoding gene (DM-locus-associated homeodomain protein) is located immediately downstream (centromeric) of the GTC repeat. The disruption of adjacent chromatin structure by repeat expansion is one mechanism by which expression of adjacent genes could be inhibited. Alternatively, repeat expansions at one locus might affect expression of more than one gene by a *cis*-acting effect, and expansion-containing transcripts may alter levels of transcripts derived from a separate allele by a *trans*-acting effect.

A fourth category of trinucleotide repeat disease occurs with repeat expansion in an intron. FA is caused by the expansion of a GAA triplet in intron 1 of the *X25* gene. Decreased mRNA levels due to either inhibition of transcription or disrupted RNA splicing occurs. Consistent with an autosomal recessive pattern of inheritance and a loss-of-function disease mechanism, the majority of

Table 363-2

Neurologic Diseases Caused by Expansion of Trinucleotide Repeats

Disorders	Site of Repeat	Effect on Gene Expression
Fragile X-A	CGG repeat 5′ to translation initiation site; point mutation identified in some patients	Failure of expression of FMR-1
Fragile X-E	CGG/CCG repeats; relationship to genes unknown	Unknown
Dentatorubral-pallidoluysian atrophy (DRPLA)	CAG repeat within ORF	Normal gene expression
Huntington's disease	CAG repeat within ORF	IT15 transcript shows normal expression without cellular selectivity; expanded polyglutamine tract may alter huntingtin protein intersection with huntingtin-associated protein-1 (HAP-1) or GAPDH
Kennedy syndrome	CAG repeat within ORF of androgen receptor gene	Normal gene expression; polyglutamine tract in androgen receptor
Spinocerebellar ataxia type 1 (SCA1)	CAG repeat within ORF	Normal gene expression
Spinocerebellar ataxia type 2 (SCA2)	CAG repeat within ORF	Normal gene expression
Spinocerebellar ataxia type 3 (SCA3): also called Machado-Joseph disease	CAG repeat within ORF	Normal gene expression
Myotonic dystrophy	CTG repeat in 3′ untranslated region of *DM*-1 gene, 5′ end of DM-associated homeodomain protein gene; cases without repeats also described	Gene expression decreased; possible dominant-negative effect at RNA level
Friedreich's ataxia	GAA repeat in intron 1 of *X25* gene	Decreased mRNA levels due to inhibition of transcription or disrupted RNA splicing

NOTE: ORF, open reading frame.

FA patients tested to date demonstrate homozygosity for expanded alleles, while some are heterozygous with a combination of one expanded allele and point mutations in the other allele. FA is not associated with anticipation (see below) and manifests more often during adolescence rather than middle age, characteristics that are different from other trinucleotide repeat diseases identified.

The discovery of triplet repeats has given molecular precision to old concepts such as *anticipation* (earlier onset of the disease in successive generations, which is associated with further expansion of the abnormal repeats in those individuals who are more severely affected) and has helped to account for variations in gene expression. Variations in trinucleotide repeats in HD (and particularly in DM) have given a molecular explanation for concepts of *variable expression* (where variations in repeats occurring among individual members of the family can lead to earlier onset or more severe symptoms and signs, as occurs in juvenile HD). Studies suggesting that other neurologic and psychiatric disorders involve anticipation raise the possibility that additional trinucleotide repeat diseases will be discovered.

ONLINE MENDELIAN INHERITANCE IN MAN (OMIM) The OMIM catalogue contains a frequently updated listing of all genetic traits. For each disease one can obtain information on clinical manifestations, mapping studies and identity (if available) of the relevant gene, and status of genetic testing. OMIM is located at the National Center for Biotechnologic Information and can be accessed via the Internet. The OMIM Home Page is http://www3.ncbi.nlm.nih.gov/omim/.

BIBLIOGRAPHY

BIRD TD: Apolipoprotein E genotyping in the diagnosis of Alzheimer's disease: A cautionary view. Ann Neurol 38:2, 1995

———, BENNETT RL: Why do DNA testing? Practical and ethical implications of new neurogenetic tests. Ann Neurol 38:141, 1995

BURKE JR et al: Huntingtin and DRPLA proteins selectively interact with the enzyme GAPDH. Nat Med 2:347, 1996

CAMPUZANO V et al: Friedreich's ataxia: Autosomal recessive disease caused by an intronic GAA triplet repeat expansion. Science 271:1423, 1996

DAS S et al: Diverse mutations in patients with Menkes disease often lead to exon skipping. Am J Hum Genet 55:883, 1994

DOERFLINGER N et al: Ataxia with vitamin E deficiency: Refinement of genetic localization and analysis of linkage disequilibrium by using new markers in 14 families. Am J Hum Genet 56:1116, 1995

DUBOVSKY J et al: A gene responsible for cavernous malformations of the brain maps to chromosome 7q. Hum Mol Genet 4:453, 1995

FENG Y et al: Translational suppression by trinucleotide repeat expansion at *FMR1*. Science 268:731, 1995

FINK JK et al: Autosomal dominant, familial spastic paraplegia, type I: Clinical and genetic analysis of a large North American family. Neurology 45:325, 1995

FU Y-H et al: An unstable triplet repeat in a gene related to myotonic dystrophy. Science 255:1256, 1992

HARDING AE: Clinical features and classification of inherited ataxias. Adv Neurol 61:1, 1993

HOFFMAN EP et al: Overexcited or inactive: Ion channels in muscle disease. Cell 80:681, 1995

HOLMBERG M et al: Localization of autosomal dominant cerebellar ataxia associated with retinal degeneration and anticipation to chromosome 3p12-p21.1. Hum Mol Genet 4:1441, 1995

HUNTINGTON'S DISEASE COLLABORATIVE RESEARCH GROUP: A novel gene containing a trinucleotide repeat that is expanded and unstable on Huntington's disease chromosomes. Cell 72:971, 1993

ICHINOSE H et al: Hereditary progressive dystonia with marked diurnal fluctuation caused by mutations in the GTP cyclohydrolase I gene. Nat Genet 8:236, 1994

INTERNATIONAL HUNTINGTON ASSOCIATION (IHA) AND THE WORLD FEDERATION OF NEUROLOGY (WFN) RESEARCH GROUP ON HUNTINGTON'S CHOREA: Guidelines for the molecular genetics predictive test in Huntington's disease. Neurology 44:1533, 1994

KNIGHT SJL et al: Trinucleotide repeat amplification and hypermethylation of a CpG island in *FRAXE* mental retardation. Cell 74:127, 1993

LANDER ES, SCHORK NJ: Genetic dissection of complex traits. Science 265:2037, 1994

LA SPADA AR et al: Meiotic stability and genotype-phenotype correlation of the trinucleotide repeat in X-linked spinal and bulbar muscular atrophy. Nat Genet 2:301, 1992

LEVY E et al: Mutation of the Alzheimer's disease amyloid gene in hereditary cerebral hemorrhage, Dutch type. Science 248:1124, 1990

LONGO FM: Transgenic mice: What are we learning about gene function and neurological disease? Neuroscientist 1:309, 1995

MACLENNAN DH: Discordance between phenotype and genotype in malignant hyperthermia. Curr Opin Neurol 8:397, 1995

NARCISI TM et al: Mutations of the microsomal triglyceride-transfer-protein gene in abetalipoproteinemia. Am J Hum Genet 57:1298, 1995

REES MI et al: Evidence for recessive as well as dominant forms of startle disease (hyperekplexia) caused by mutations in the $\alpha 1$ subunit of the inhibitory glycine receptor. Hum Mol Genet 3:2175, 1994

ROSES AD: Apolipoprotein E genotyping in the differential diagnosis, not prediction, of Alzheimer's disease. Ann Neurol 38:6, 1995

SERVADIO A et al: Expression analysis of the ataxin-1 protein in tissues from normal and spinocerebellar ataxia type 1 individuals. Nat Genet 10:94, 1995

SINE SM et al: Mutation of the acetylcholine receptor alpha subunit causes a slow-channel myasthenic syndrome by enhancing agonist binding affinity. Neuron 15:229, 1995

TARONI F et al: Identification of a common mutation in the carnitine palmitoyltransferase II gene in familial recurrent myoglobinuria patients. Nat Genet 4:314, 1993

TOURNIER-LASSERVE E et al: Cerebral autosomal dominant arteriopathy with subcortical infarcts and leukoencephalopathy maps to chromosome 19q12. Nat Genet 3:256, 1993

WALLGREN-PETTERSSON C et al: The myotubular myopathies: Differential diagnosis of the X-linked recessive, autosomal dominant, and autosomal recessive forms and present state of DNA studies. J Med Genet 32: 673, 1995

WONG EV et al: Mutations in the cell adhesion molecule L1 cause mental retardation. Trends Neurosci 18:168, 1995

SECTION 2

DISEASES OF THE CENTRAL NERVOUS SYSTEM

364

Neil H. Raskin

MIGRAINE AND THE CLUSTER HEADACHE SYNDROME

MIGRAINE

The term *migraine* stems from Galen's usage of *hemicrania* to describe a periodic disorder consisting of paroxysmal blinding hemicranial pain, vomiting, photophobia, recurrence at regular intervals, and relief by dark surroundings and sleep. *Hemicrania* was later corrupted into low Latin as *hemigranea* and *migranea*; eventually the French cognate, *migraine*, gained acceptance in the eighteenth century and has prevailed ever since. Time has proved this to be a misleading designation for the condition, however, as it is manifested by lateralized head pain in less than 60 percent of those affected. Furthermore, undue emphasis on the dramatic features of migraine has often led to the illogical conclusion that periodic headache lacking such features is not migrainous in mechanism. It has become clear that severe headache attacks, regardless of cause, are more likely to be described as throbbing and associated with vomiting and scalp tenderness. Milder headaches tend to be nondescript—tight, band-like discomfort often involving the entire head—the profile of "tension headache." These differing clinical profiles of headaches that are not caused by an intracranial structural anomaly or systemic disease probably represent different points on a continuum rather than disparate clinical entities. Whether a single common mechanism underlies these various headache profiles is currently not known. A working definition of migraine offered here is benign recurring headache and/or neurologic dysfunction usually attended by pain-free interludes and often provoked by stereotyped stimuli. Migraine may be identified by its activators (red wine, menses, hunger, lack of sleep, glare, perfumes, periods of letdown) and its deactivators (sleep, pregnancy, exhilaration, sumatriptan). It is by far more common in women; there is a hereditary predisposition toward attacks; and the cranial circulatory phenomena that attend attacks appear to be secondary to a primary central nervous system (CNS) disorder.

CLINICAL SUBTYPES The designation *classic migraine* (migraine with aura) denotes the syndrome of headache associated with characteristic premonitory sensory, motor, or visual symptoms; *common migraine* (migraine without aura) denotes one in which no focal neurologic disturbance precedes the headache. Common migraine is by far the more frequent clinical problem, and focal neurologic disturbances are more common during headache attacks than as prodromal symptoms. Focal neurologic disturbances without headache or vomiting have come to be known as *migraine equivalents* or *accompaniments* and appear to occur more commonly in patients between the ages of 40 and 70 years. The term *complicated migraine* has generally been used to describe migraine with dramatic focal neurologic features, thus overlapping with *classic migraine*; it has also been used to describe a migraine attack that leaves a persisting residual neurologic deficit.

Common Migraine Benign periodic headache of several hours' duration, often attributed to "tension" by its sufferers, is the most liberal definition of common migraine. Traditional definitions of migraine often identify only patients with severe attacks, not those with more modest head pain; thus, in various combinations, unilateral pain, attendant nausea or vomiting, a positive family history, responsiveness to ergotamine, and scalp tenderness have been considered necessary to establish a diagnosis of migraine. However, the validity of using such clinical features to diagnose migraine has never been formally established (Table 364-1). Common migraine is the most frequent headache type reported by patients.

Classic Migraine The most common premonitory symptoms reported by migraineurs are visual, arising from dysfunction of occipital lobe neurons. Scotomas and/or hallucinations occur in about one-third of migraineurs and usually appear in the central portions of the visual fields. A highly characteristic syndrome occurs in about 10 percent of patients; it usually begins as a small paracentral scotoma, which slowly expands into a "C" shape. Luminous angles appear at the enlarging outer edge, becoming colored as the scintillating scotoma expands and moves toward the periphery of the involved half of the visual field. It eventually disappears over the horizon of peripheral vision, the entire process taking 20 to 25 min. This phenomenon never occurs *during* the headache phase of an attack and is pathognomonic for migraine, never having been described in association with a cerebral structural anomaly. It is commonly referred to as a *fortification spectrum* because the serrated edges of the hallucinated "C" seemed to Dr. Hubert Airy to resemble a "fortified town with bastions all round it"; "spectrum" is used in the sense of an apparition or specter.

Table 364-1

Symptoms Accompanying Severe Migraine Attacks in a Group of 500 Patients

Symptom	Percent of Patients Affected
Nausea	87
Vomiting	56
Diarrhea	16
Photophobia	82
Visual disturbances	36
Fortification spectra	10
Photopsia	26
Paresthesia	33
Scalp tenderness	65
Lightheadedness	72
Vertigo	33
Alteration of consciousness	18
Seizure	4
Syncope	10
Confusional state	4

SOURCE: NH Raskin: *Headache*, 2d ed, New York, Churchill Livingstone, 1988.

Basilar Migraine Symptoms referable to a disturbance in brainstem function, such as vertigo, dysarthria, or diplopia, occur as the only neurologic symptoms of the attack in about 25 percent of patients. Bickerstaff called attention to a stereotyped sequence of dramatic neurologic events, often comprising total blindness and sensorial clouding, that is common among but not restricted to adolescent women. These episodes begin with total blindness accompanied or followed by admixtures of vertigo, ataxia, dysarthria, tinnitus, and distal and perioral paresthesia. In about one-quarter of patients, a confusional state supervenes. The neurologic symptoms usually persist for 20 to 30 min and are generally followed by a throbbing occipital headache. This basilar migraine syndrome is now known also to occur in children and in adults over age 50. An altered sensorium may persist for as long as 5 days and may take the form of confusional states superficially resembling psychotic reactions. Full recovery after the episode is the rule.

Carotidynia The carotidynia syndrome, sometimes called *lower-half headache* or *facial migraine*, is most common among older patients, with the incidence peaking in the fourth through sixth decades. Pain is usually located at the jaw or neck, although sometimes periorbital or maxillary pain occurs; it may be continuous, deep, dull, and aching, and it becomes pounding or throbbing episodically. There are often superimposed sharp, ice pick–like jabs. Attacks occur one to several times per week, each lasting several minutes to hours. Tenderness and prominent pulsations of the cervical carotid artery, and soft tissue swelling overlying the carotid, usually are present ipsilateral to the pain; many patients also report throbbing ipsilateral headache concurrent with carotidynia attacks as well as between attacks. Dental trauma is a common precipitant of this syndrome. Carotid artery involvement appears also to be common in the more traditional forms of migraine; over 50 percent of patients with frequent migraine attacks are found to have carotid tenderness at several points on the side most often involved during their hemicranial migraine attacks.

PATHOGENESIS Modern orientations toward migraine began with the publication by Liveing in 1873 of the first major treatise devoted to the subject of migraine, *A Contribution to the Pathology of Nerve Storms*. Liveing believed that the analogy of migraine to epilepsy was obvious and that the clinically apparent circulatory phenomena that occurred during migrainous attacks were secondary to cerebral discharges, or "nerve storms." Attention was focused on the vascular features of migraine by Graham and Wolff in the 1930s, who showed that the administration of ergotamine reduced the amplitude of the pulsations of the temporal artery in patients with headache, and that this effect was often, although *not consistently*, associated with a decrease in head pain. Because of these observations and other less substantial lines of evidence, it was widely held for many years that the headache phase of migrainous attacks was caused by extracranial vasodilation and that the neurologic symptoms were produced by intracranial vasoconstriction, the "vascular" hypothesis of migraine.

K.S. Lashley, physiologic psychologist at Harvard, in 1941 was among the first to chart his own migrainous fortification spectrum in detail and at brief intervals. He was able to estimate that the evolution of his own scotoma proceeded across the occipital cortex at a rate of 3 mm/min. He speculated that a wavefront of intense excitation followed by a wave of complete inhibition of activity were propagated across the visual cortex. In 1944, the phenomenon that has come to be known as *spreading depression* was described by the Brazilian physiologist, Leão, in the cerebral cortex of laboratory animals. It is a slowly moving (2 to 3 mm/min), potassium-liberating depression of cortical activity, preceded by a wavefront of increased metabolic activity that can be produced by a variety of experimental stimuli, including hypoxia, mechanical trauma, and the topical application of potassium. These observations could not easily be integrated into a simple vascular model of migraine.

Current concepts of the pathogenesis of migraine focus on three mechanisms and anatomic regions. First, there is a vasomotor component mediated by constriction or dilation of arteries within and outside the brain. Second, there is a midbrain trigger, perhaps in serotonergic neurons of the dorsal raphe. Third, there is activation of a trigeminal-vascular system, consisting of medullary neurons in the trigeminal nucleus caudalis that terminate on the walls of arteries and release vasoactive neuropeptides. The role of each of these systems in the production of specific symptoms of migraine is unknown; it is possible that activation of any of the three may be *sufficient* for headache production, and that one mechanism may dominate in a particular migrainous syndrome. For example, the evolution of the fortification spectrum may be entirely neurogenic, requiring only activation of the dorsal raphe system.

Vasomotor Component Regional cerebral blood flow studies have shown that in patients with classic migraine there is, during attacks, a modest cortical hypoperfusion that begins in the visual cortex and spreads forward at a rate of 2 to 3 mm/min. The decrease in blood flow averages 25 to 30 percent (insufficient to explain symptoms on the basis of ischemia) and progresses anteriorly in a wave-like fashion independent of the topography of cerebral arteries. The wave of hypoperfusion persists for 4 to 6 h, appears to follow the convolutions of the cortex, and does not cross the central or lateral sulcus, progressing to the frontal lobe via the insula. Perfusion of subcortical structures is normal. Contralateral neurologic symptoms appear during temporoparietal hypoperfusion; at times, hypoperfusion persists in these regions after symptoms cease. More often, frontal spread continues as the headache phase begins. A few patients with classic migraine show no flow abnormalities; an occasional patient has developed focal ischemia sufficient to cause symptoms. However, focal ischemia does not appear to be *necessary* for focal symptoms to occur. During common migraine, no flow abnormalities are usually seen.

Serotonergic Projections and the Dorsal Raphe Taken together, the pharmacologic data on migraine point to involvement of serotonin receptors. About 35 years ago, methysergide was found to antagonize certain peripheral actions of serotonin [5-hydroxytryptamine (5-HT)] and was introduced as the first drug capable of preventing migraine attacks. Subsequently, it was found that platelet levels of serotonin fall consistently at the onset of headache and that migrainous episodes may be triggered by drugs that cause serotonin to be released. Such changes in circulating levels proved to be pharmacologically trivial, however, and interest in the humoral role of serotonin in migraine declined. Currently, there is renewed interest, due almost entirely to the introduction of the drug sumatriptan, which is remarkably effective for migraine attacks. Of still greater interest is the fact that sumatriptan is a designer drug, synthesized to activate selectively a particular subpopulation of serotonin receptors.

There are four main families of 5-HT receptors—types 1, 2, 3, and 4; receptor subtypes have been found for each type. Many of the drugs effective in migraine prophylaxis are type 2 antagonists, whereas the abortive agents are type 1 agonists. Sumatriptan is most potent as an agonist of 5-HT_{1D} receptors, and is less potent at 5-HT_{1A} and 5-HT_{1B} receptors. By contrast, dihydroergotamine, another drug that is highly effective in aborting migraine attacks, is most potent as an agonist of 5-HT_{1A} receptors and is an order of magnitude less potent at 5-HT_{1D} receptors. After systemic administration, dihydroergotamine in the brain is found in the highest concentrations in the midbrain dorsal raphe. The dorsal raphe is a good candidate as a generator of migraine and as a site of antimigraine drug action; the highest concentration of serotonin receptors in brain tissue is found there. They are mainly of the 5-HT_{1A} variety, but 5-HT_{1D} receptors also are present.

Electrical stimulation near dorsal raphe neurons can result in migraine-like headaches (see also Chap. 15). Blood flow in the pons and midbrain increases focally during migraine headache episodes; this alteration probably results from increased activity of cells in the dorsal raphe and locus ceruleus. There are projections from the dorsal raphe that terminate on cerebral arteries and alter cerebral blood flow. There are also major projections from the dorsal raphe to important visual centers, including the lateral geniculate body, superior colliculus, retina, and visual cortex. These various serotonergic projections may represent the neural substrate for the circulatory and visual characteristics of migraine. The dorsal raphe cells stop firing during deep sleep, and sleep is known to ameliorate migraine; the antimigraine prophylactic drugs also inhibit activity of the dorsal raphe cells through a direct or indirect agonist effect (Fig. 364-1).

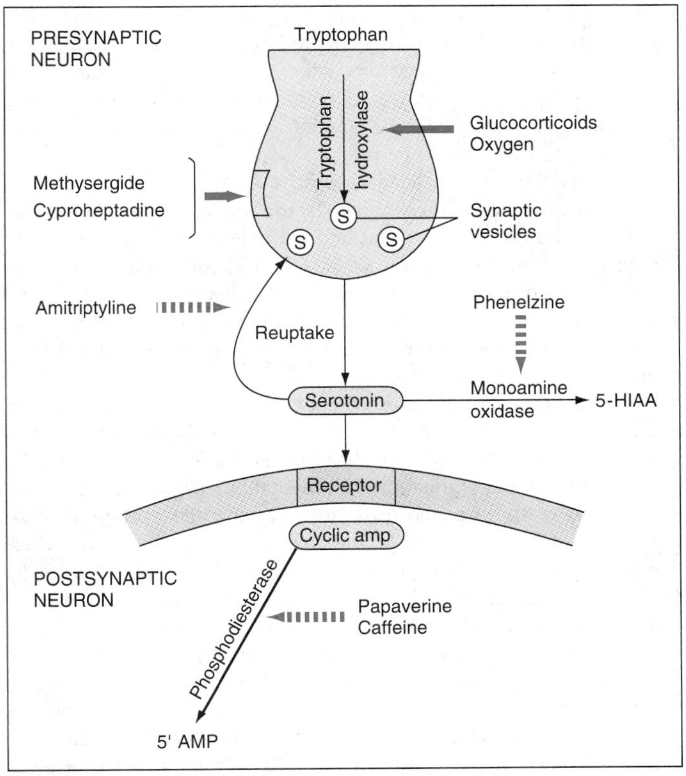

FIGURE 364-1 The actions of the antimigraine drugs at brainstem and forebrain synapses. The solid arrows indicate stimulative or agonist properties, and the segmented arrows indicate inhibitory properties. 5-HIAA, 5-hydroxyindoleacetic acid. *(From NH Raskin: Headache, 2d ed, New York, Churchill Livingstone, 1988.)*

Trigeminal-Vascular System Activation of cells in the trigeminal nucleus caudalis in the medulla (a pain processing center for the head and face region) results in the release of vasoactive neuropeptides, including substance P and calcitonin gene–related peptide, at vascular terminations of the trigeminal nerve. Moskowitz and colleagues have proposed that these peptide neurotransmitters induce a sterile inflammation that activates trigeminal nociceptive afferents originating on the vessel wall, further contributing to the production of pain. This mechanism also provides a potential mechanism for the soft tissue swelling and tenderness of blood vessels that attend migraine attacks.

The genetic basis of migraine is largely unknown. Family studies indicate that genetic heterogeneity—i.e., independent migraine genes—is likely to be present. Genetic linkage analysis has been successful in one rare migraine syndrome, autosomal dominant familial hemiplegic migraine (see Chap. 363). In this disorder, hemiplegia and hemisensory loss develop and persist for hours to days, after which headache supervenes. In approximately one-half of families, a mutation in a P/Q-type calcium channel α1-subunit gene located on chromosome 19 has been found.

℞ TREATMENT

The mainstay of therapy is the judicious use of one or more of the many drugs that are relatively specific for migraine.

Acute Treatment In general, an adequate dose of whichever agent is chosen should be used at the onset of an attack. If additional medication is required in 30 to 60 min because symptoms return or have not abated, the initial dose should be increased for subsequent attacks. Drug absorption is impaired during migrainous attacks because of reduced gastrointestinal motility. Delayed absorption occurs in the absence of nausea and is related to the severity of the attack and not its duration. Therefore, when oral agents fail, alternative therapies, including rectal ergotamine, subcutaneous sumatriptan, parenteral dihydroergotamine, and intravenous chlorpromazine and prochlorperazine, should be tried.

For patients whose headaches have a prolonged buildup, oral agents may indeed suffice. When aspirin and acetaminophen alone fail, the addition of butalbital and caffeine to these analgesics is highly effective; ibuprofen (600 to 800 mg) and naproxen (375 to 750 mg) are often useful. Isometheptene compound, 1 to 2 capsules, is effective for mild to moderate "common migraine." When these measures fail, more aggressive therapy should be considered (Table 364-2).

A subnauseating dose of ergotamine should be sought; a dose that provokes nausea—probably a centrally mediated side effect—is too high and may intensify head pain. The average oral dose is 3 mg (three 1-mg ergotamine-caffeine tablets taken together). The drug also exists in suppository form (2 mg); the average dose is one-half of a suppository (1 mg), and many patients achieve an excellent result with one-quarter of a suppository (0.5 mg). Sumatriptan may be given as a 50-mg oral dose or a 6-mg subcutaneous dose; there is a high recurrence rate because of the short half-life of this drug (2 h), so that a second dose may be necessary.

Dihydroergotamine is available as a parenteral preparation and as a nasal spray. Peak plasma levels of dihydroergotamine are achieved 45 min after subcutaneous dosing, 30 min after intramuscular dosing, and 3 min after intravenous dosing. If an attack has not already peaked, subcutaneous or intramuscular administration of 1 mg suffices for about 90 percent of patients. The nasal spray results in substantial blood levels in 45 to 60 min. A common intravenous protocol is the administration over 2 min of a mixture of 5 mg of prochlorperazine and 0.5 mg of dihydroergotamine (they are miscible).

If a patient's headache profile transforms into a chronic daily headache syndrome, opiate-type analgesics should be restricted to 2 days out of 7. The mainstay of therapy for these patients is daily amitriptyline (30 to 100 mg) or nortriptyline (40 to 120 mg). If the syndrome is recalcitrant, valproic acid (500 to 2000 mg) or phenelzine (45 to 90 mg) may be necessary

Prophylaxis A substantial number of drugs are now available that have the capacity to stabilize migraine (Table 364-3). They must be taken daily. The decision of whether to use this approach depends on the frequency of attacks and on how well acute treatment is working. The occurrence of at least two or three attacks per month could be an indication for this approach. There is usually a lag of 2 weeks before an effect is seen. The major drugs and recommended daily doses are as follows: propranolol (60 to 320 mg), amitriptyline (10 to 175 mg), valproate (500 to 1500 mg), verapamil (160 to 480 mg), phenelzine (30 to 75 mg), and methysergide (2 to 8 mg). Phenelzine and methysergide are usually reserved for recalcitrant cases because of their serious potential side effects. Phenelzine is a monoamine oxidase inhibitor; therefore, tyramine-containing foods, decongestants, and meperidine are contraindicated. Methysergide may cause retroperitoneal or cardiac valvular fibrosis when it is used for more than 8 months, so monitoring is required for patients using this drug; the risk of the fibrotic complication is about 1:1500 and is likely to reverse after the drug is stopped.

The probability of success with any one of the antimigraine drugs is 60 to 75 percent; if one drug is assessed each month, there is a good chance that effective stabilization will be achieved within a few months. The large majority of patients are successfully managed with propranolol or amitriptyline; for more urgent resolution, valproate, methysergide, or phenelzine can be used. Once effective stabilization is achieved, the drug is continued for 5 to 6 months and then slowly tapered to assess the continued need for it. Many patients are able to discontinue medication and experience fewer and milder attacks for long periods, suggesting that these drugs may alter the natural history of migraine.

Nonpharmacologic Approaches Patients with migraine do not encounter more stress than headache-free individuals; over-responsiveness to stress appears to be the issue. Since the stresses of everyday living cannot be eliminated, lessening one's response to stress by various techniques is helpful for many patients, as long as these methods are practiced continually. They include yoga, transcendental meditation, hypnosis, and conditioning techniques such as biofeedback. For most patients, this approach is, at best, an adjunct to pharmacotherapy.

CLUSTER HEADACHE

In the past, a variety of names have been used for this condition, including *Raeder's syndrome*, *histamine cephalalgia*, and *sphenopalatine neuralgia*. *Cluster headache* is now firmly established as a distinctive syndrome, whose recognition is important since it is likely to be responsive to treatment. The episodic type is most common, and is characterized by one to three short-lived attacks of periorbital pain per day over a 4- to 8-week period, followed by a pain-free interval that averages 1 year. The chronic form, which may begin de novo or several years after an episodic pattern has become established, is characterized by the absence of sustained periods of remission. Each type may transform into the other. Men are affected seven to eight times more often than women; hereditary factors are usually absent. Although the onset is generally between ages 20 and 50, it may occur as early as the first decade of life. Propranolol and amitriptyline are largely ineffective. Lithium is beneficial for cluster headache and ineffective in migraine. The cluster syndrome is thus clinically, genetically, and therapeutically different from migraine. Nevertheless, mixed features of the two disorders are occasionally present, suggesting some common elements to their pathogenesis.

CLINICAL FEATURES Periorbital, or, less commonly, temporal, pain begins without warning and reaches a crescendo within 5 min. It is often excruciating in intensity and is deep, nonfluctuating, and explosive in quality; only rarely is it pulsatile. Pain is strictly unilateral and usually affects the same side in subsequent months. Attacks last from 30 min to 2 h; there are often associated symptoms of homolateral lacrimation, reddening of the eye, nasal stuffiness, lid ptosis, and nausea. Alcohol provokes attacks in about 70 percent of patients but ceases to be provocative when the bout remits; this on-off vulnerability to alcohol is pathognomonic of cluster headache. Only rarely do foods or emotional factors precipitate pain, in contrast to migraine.

There is a striking periodicity of attacks in at least 85 percent of patients. At least one of the daily attacks of pain recurs at about the same hour each day for the duration of a cluster bout. Onset is nocturnal in about 50 percent of the cases, and in that case the pain usually awakens the patient within 2 h of falling asleep.

PATHOGENESIS No consistent cerebral blood flow changes accompany attacks of pain. Perhaps the strongest evidence for a central mechanism is the periodicity of attacks; the existence of a central mechanism also is suggested by the observation that autonomic symptoms that accompany the pain are bilateral and are more severe on the painful side. The hypothalamus may be the site of activation in this disorder. The posterior hypothalamus contains cells that regulate autonomic functions, and the anterior hypothalamus contains cells (in the suprachiasmatic nuclei) that constitute the principal circadian pacemaker in mammals. Activation of both is necessary to explain the symptoms of cluster headache. The pacemaker is modulated via serotonergic dorsal raphe projections. It can be concluded tentatively that both migraine and cluster headache result from abnormal serotonergic neurotransmission, albeit at different loci.

℞ TREATMENT

The most satisfactory treatment is the administration of drugs to prevent cluster attacks until the bout is over. Effective prophylactic drugs are prednisone, lithium, methysergide, ergotamine, and vera-

Table 364-2

Treatments Used to Abort Migraine Headaches

Time to Peak Head Pain,* h	Treatment Option 1	Treatment Option 2	Treatment Option 3
>3	Ergotamine tablets (Wigraine), 2–3 tablets	Isometheptene compound (Midrin), 1–2 capsules	Butalbital compound with aspirin or acetaminophen (Fiorinal, Floricet, Esgic), 1–2 tablets
1–3	Dihydroergotamine nasal spray (Migranal), one dose (2 mg)	1/2 ergotamine suppository (= 1 mg) (Cafergot, Wigraine)	Sumatriptan (Imitrex), 1 tablet, 25 *or* 50 mg
<1	Sumatriptan (Imitrex), 6 mg SC	Dihydroergotamine (DHE-45), 1 mg IM or SC	Nasal butorphanol (Stadol), 1–2 mg

* The time required for head pain to reach its peak intensity after first being perceived by the patient.

Table 364-3

Drugs Effective for the Prophylaxis of Migraine

Drug	Daily Dosage Range (mg)	Most Common Side Effects
Amitriptyline	10–175	Sedation, dry mouth, weight gain
Propranolol	60–320	
Nadolol	40–160	
Atenolol	50–200	Lethargy, insomnia, lightheadedness, impotence
Timolol	20–60	
Metoprolol	50–200	
Papaverine	300–900	Nausea
Cyproheptadine	8–32	Sedation, weight gain
Verapamil	160–480	Constipation, nausea, fluid retention, lightheadedness, hypotension
Phenelzine	30–75	Insomnia, lightheadedness, slowed bladder emptying, weight gain
Valproic acid	500–1500	Nausea, weight gain, tremor, hair loss
Methysergide	2–8	Nausea, muscle cramps, insomnia, weight gain, peripheral vasoconstriction; retroperitoneal fibrosis with prolonged use (>6 months)

pamil. Lithium (600 to 900 mg daily) appears to be particularly useful for the chronic form of the disorder. A 10-day course of prednisone, beginning at 60 mg daily for 7 days followed by a rapid taper, may interrupt the pain bout for many patients. When ergotamine is used, it is most effective when given 1 to 2 h before an expected attack; for patients who have a single nocturnal episode, 1 mg of ergotamine in suppository form taken at bedtime may be all that is necessary. Patients must be educated regarding the early symptoms of ergotism when ergotamine is used daily; a weekly limit of 14 mg should be adhered to.

For the attacks themselves, oxygen inhalation (9 L/min via a loose mask) is the most effective modality; 15 min of inhalation of 100% oxygen is often necessary. The self-administration of intranasal lidocaine, either 4% topical or 2% viscous, to the most caudal aspect of the inferior nasal turbinate can produce a sphenopalatine ganglionic block that is usually remarkably effective in terminating an attack. Sumatriptan, 6 mg subcutaneously, will usually shorten an attack to 10 to 15 min.

BIBLIOGRAPHY

Bates D et al: Subcutaneous sumatriptan during the migraine aura. Neurology 44:1587, 1994

Davidoff RA: *Migraine*. Philadelphia, Davis, 1995

Ferrari MD, Saxena PR: On serotonin and migraine; a clinical and pharmacological review. Cephalalgia 13:151, 1993

Goadsby PJ, Edvinsson L: Human in vivo evidence for trigeminovascular activation in cluster headache. Brain 117:427, 1994

Joutel A et al: Genetic heterogeneity of familial hemiplegic migraine. Am J Hum Genet 55:1166, 1994

Kelly K: Cardiac arrest following use of sumatriptan. Neurology 45:1211, 1995

Lauritzen M: Pathophysiology of the migraine aura: The spreading depression theory. Brain 117:199, 1994

McLachlan RS, Girvin JP: Spreading depression of Leão in rodent and human cortex. Brain Research 666:133, 1994

Moskowitz MA: The visceral organ brain: Implications for the pathophysiology of vascular head pain. Neurology 41:182, 1991

Olesen J: Cerebral and extracranial circulatory disturbances in migraine: Pathophysiological implications. Cerebrovasc Brain Metab Rev 3:1, 1991

——— et al (eds): *The Headaches*. New York, Raven, 1993

Ophoff RA et al: Familial hemiplegic migraine and episodic ataxia type-2 are caused by mutations in the Ca^{2+} channel gene CACNL1A4. Cell 87:543, 1996

Plosker GL, McTavish D: Sumatriptan: A reappraisal of its pharmacology and therapeutic efficacy in the acute treatment of migraine and cluster headache. Drugs 47:622, 1994

Report of the Quality Standards Subcommittee of the American Academy of Neurology: Practice parameter: Appropriate use of ergotamine tartrate and dihydroergotamine in the treatment of migraine and status migrainosus. (Summary statement.) Neurology 45:585, 1995

Weiller C et al: Brain stem activation in spontaneous human migraine attacks. Nature Med 1:658, 1995

Welch KMA: Drug therapy of migraine. N Engl J Med 329:1476, 1993

Winner P et al: A double-blind study of subcutaneous dihydroergotamine vs subcutaneous sumatriptan in the treatment of acute migraine. Arch Neurol 53:180, 1996

Woods RP et al: Bilateral spreading cerebral hypoperfusion during spontaneous migraine headache. N Engl J Med 331:1689, 1994

365 SEIZURES AND EPILEPSY

Daniel H. Lowenstein

A *seizure* (from the Latin *sacire*, "to take possession of") is a paroxysmal event due to abnormal, excessive, hypersynchronous discharges from an aggregate of central nervous system (CNS) neurons. Depending on the distribution of discharges, this abnormal CNS activity can have various manifestations, ranging from dramatic convulsive activity to experiential phenomena not readily discernible by an observer. Although a variety of factors influence the incidence and prevalence of seizures, approximately 5 to 10 percent of the population will have at least one seizure during their lifetime, with the highest incidence occurring in early childhood and late adulthood. Because seizures are common, this clinical problem is encountered frequently during medical practice in a variety of settings.

The meaning of the term seizure needs to be carefully distinguished from that of epilepsy. *Epilepsy* describes a condition in which a person has *recurrent* seizures due to a chronic, underlying process. This definition implies that a person with a single seizure, or recurrent seizures due to correctable or avoidable circumstances, does not necessarily have epilepsy. Epilepsy refers to a clinical phenomenon rather than a single disease entity, since there are many forms and causes of epilepsy. However, among the many causes of epilepsy there are various *epilepsy syndromes* in which the clinical and pathologic characteristics are distinctive and suggest a specific underlying etiology.

Using the definition of epilepsy as two or more unprovoked seizures, the incidence of epilepsy is approximately 0.3 to 0.5 percent in different populations throughout the world, and the prevalence of epilepsy has been estimated at 5 to 10 people per 1000.

CLASSIFICATION OF SEIZURES

An essential step in the evaluation and management of a patient with a seizure is to determine the type of seizure that has occurred. The importance of this cannot be over emphasized—classifying the seizure is essential for focusing the diagnostic approach on particular etiologies, selecting the appropriate therapy, and providing potentially vital information regarding prognosis. In 1981, the International League Against Epilepsy (ILAE) published a modified version of the International Classification of Epileptic Seizures that has continued to be a useful classification system (Table 365-1). This system is based on the clinical features of seizures and associated electroencephalographic (EEG) findings. Other potentially distinctive features such as etiology or cellular substrate are not factored into the classification system, although this will probably change in the future as more is learned about the pathophysiologic mechanisms that underlie specific seizure types.

The main characteristic that distinguishes the different categories of seizures is whether the seizure activity is *partial* (synonymous with *focal*) or *generalized*. Partial seizures are those in which the seizure activity is restricted to discrete areas of the cerebral cortex. Generalized seizures involve diffuse regions of the brain simultaneously in a bilaterally symmetric fashion. As a rule, partial seizures are typically associated with structural abnormalities of the brain. In contrast, generalized seizures may result from cellular, biochemical, or structural abnormalities that have a more widespread distribution. Other aspects of seizure classification and semiology (phenomenology) continue to be debated among epileptologists, including the definition of altered consciousness, use of the terms "partial" versus "focal," and the concept of aura.

PARTIAL SEIZURES Partial seizures occur within discrete regions of the brain. If consciousness is fully preserved during the seizure, the clinical manifestations are considered relatively simple and the seizure is termed a *simple-partial seizure*. If consciousness is impaired, the symptomatology is more complex and the seizure is termed a *complex-partial seizure*. An important additional subgroup comprises those seizures that begin as partial seizures and then spread diffusely throughout the cortex, i.e., *partial seizures with secondary generalization*.

Simple-Partial Seizures Simple-partial seizures cause motor, sensory, autonomic, or psychic symptoms without an obvious alteration in consciousness. For example, a patient having a partial motor seizure arising from the right primary motor cortex in the vicinity controlling hand movement will note the onset of involuntary movements of the contralateral, left hand. These movements are typically clonic (i.e., repetitive, flexion/extension movements) at a frequency of approximately 2 to 3 Hz; pure tonic posturing may be seen as well. Since the cortical region controlling hand movement is immediately adjacent to the region for facial expression, the seizure may also cause abnormal movements of the face synchronous with the movements of the hand. The EEG recorded with scalp electrodes during the seizure (i.e., an ictal EEG) may show abnormal discharges in a very limited region over the appropriate area of cerebral cortex if the seizure focus involves the cerebral convexity. Seizure activity occurring within deeper brain structures is often not recorded by the standard EEG, however, and may require intracranial electrodes for its detection.

Table 365-1

Classification of Seizures

1. Partial seizures
   A. Simple-partial seizures (with motor, sensory, autonomic, or psychic signs)
   B. Complex-partial seizures
   C. Partial seizures with secondary generalization
2. Primarily generalized seizures
   A. Absence (petit mal)
   B. Tonic-clonic (grand mal)
   C. Tonic
   D. Atonic
   E. Myoclonic
3. Unclassified seizures
   A. Neonatal seizures
   B. Infantile spasms

Three additional features of partial motor seizures are worth noting. First, in some patients the abnormal motor movements may begin in a very restricted region such as the fingers and gradually progress (over seconds to minutes) to include a larger portion of the extremity. This phenomenon was originally described by Hughlings Jackson and is known as a "Jacksonian march," representing the spread of seizure activity over a progressively larger region of motor cortex. Second, patients may experience a localized paresis (Todd's paralysis) for minutes to many hours in the involved region following the seizure. Third, in rare instances the seizure may continue for hours or days. This condition, termed *epilepsia partialis continua*, is often quite refractory to medical therapy.

Other forms of simple-partial seizures include those that cause changes in somatic sensation (e.g., paresthesia), vision (flashing lights or formed hallucinations), equilibrium (sensation of falling or vertigo), or autonomic function (flushing, sweating, piloerection). Simple-partial seizures arising from the temporal or frontal cortex may also cause alterations in hearing, olfaction, or higher cortical function (psychic symptoms). This includes the sensation of unusual, intense odors (e.g., burning rubber or kerosene) or sounds (crude or highly complex sounds), or an epigastric sensation that rises from the stomach or chest to the head. Some patients describe odd, internal feelings such as fear, a sense of impending change, detachment, depersonalization, déja vu, or illusions that objects are growing smaller (micropsia) or larger (macropsia). When such symptoms precede a complex-partial or secondarily generalized seizure, these simple-partial seizures serve as a warning, or *aura*.

Complex-Partial Seizures Complex-partial seizures are characterized by focal seizure activity accompanied by a transient impairment of the patient's ability to maintain normal contact with the environment. Operationally this means that the patient is unable to respond to visual or verbal commands during the seizure and has impaired recollection or awareness of the ictal phase. The seizures frequently begin with an aura (i.e., a simple-partial seizure) that is stereotypic for the patient. The start of the ictal phase is often a sudden behavioral arrest or motionless stare, and this marks the onset of the event for which the patient will be amnestic. The behavioral arrest is usually accompanied by automatisms, which are involuntary, automatic behaviors that have a wide range of manifestations. Automatisms may consist of very basic behaviors such as chewing, lip smacking, swallowing, or "picking" movements of the hands, or more elaborate behaviors such as a display of emotion or running. The patient is typically confused following the seizure, and the transition to full recovery of consciousness may range from seconds up to an hour. Careful examination of the patient immediately following the seizure may show an anterograde amnesia or, in cases involving the dominant hemisphere, a postictal aphasia.

The routine, interictal (i.e., between seizures) EEG in patients with complex-partial seizures is often normal, or may show brief discharges termed *epileptiform spikes*, or *sharp waves*. Since complex-partial seizures often arise from the medial temporal lobe or inferior frontal lobe, i.e., regions distant from the scalp, the EEG recorded during the seizure may be non–localizing. However, the seizure focus is often detected using special electrodes such as sphenoidal or surgically-placed intracranial electrodes.

The range of potential clinical behaviors linked to complex-partial seizures is so broad that extreme caution is advised before concluding that stereotypic episodes of bizarre or atypical behavior are not due to seizure activity. In such cases it is imperative to consider more detailed EEG studies in order to determine whether the behaviors are caused by a seizure disorder.

Partial Seizures with Secondary Generalization Partial seizures can spread to involve both cerebral hemispheres and produce a generalized seizure, usually of the tonic-clonic variety (discussed below). Secondary generalization is observed frequently following simple-partial seizures, especially those with a focus in the frontal lobe, but may also be associated with partial seizures occurring elsewhere in the brain. A partial seizure with secondary generalization is often difficult to distinguish from a primarily generalized tonic-clonic seizure, since bystanders tend to emphasize the more dramatic, generalized convulsive phase of the seizure and overlook the more subtle, focal symptoms present at onset. In some cases, the focal onset of the seizure becomes apparent only when a careful history identifies a preceding aura (i.e., simple-partial seizure). Often, however, the focal onset is not clinically evident and may be established only through careful EEG analysis. Nonetheless, distinguishing between these two entities is extremely important, as there may be substantial differences in the evaluation and treatment of partial versus generalized seizure disorders.

GENERALIZED SEIZURES By definition, generalized seizures arise from both cerebral hemispheres simultaneously. However, it is currently impossible to exclude entirely the existence of a focal region of abnormal activity that initiates the seizure prior to rapid secondary generalization. For this reason, generalized seizures may be practically defined as bilateral clinical and electrographic events without any detectable focal onset. Fortunately, a number of the subtypes of generalized seizures have distinctive features that facilitate clinical diagnosis.

Absence Seizures (Petit Mal) Absence seizures are characterized by sudden, brief lapses of consciousness without loss of postural control. The seizure typically lasts for only seconds, consciousness returns as suddenly as it was lost, and there is no postictal confusion. Although the brief loss of consciousness may be clinically inapparent or the sole manifestation of the seizure discharge, absence seizures are usually accompanied by subtle, bilateral motor signs such as rapid blinking of the eyelids, chewing movements, or small-amplitude, clonic movements of the hands.

Absence seizures almost always begin in childhood (ages 4 to 8) or early adolescence and are the main seizure type in 15 to 20 percent of children with epilepsy. The seizures can occur hundreds of times per day, but the child may be unaware of or unable to convey their existence. This can lead to a situation in which the patient is constantly struggling to piece together experiences that have been interrupted by the seizures. Since the clinical signs of the seizures are subtle, especially to new parents, it is not surprising that the first clue to absence epilepsy is often unexplained "daydreaming" and a decline in school performance recognized by a teacher.

The electrophysiologic hallmark of typical absence seizures is a generalized, symmetric, 3 Hz spike-and-wave discharge that begins and ends suddenly on a normal EEG background. Periods of spike-and-wave discharges lasting more than a few seconds usually correlate with the clinical signs, but the EEG often shows many more periods of abnormal cortical activity than were suspected clinically. Hyperventilation tends to provoke these electrographic discharges and even the seizures themselves and is routinely used when recording the EEG.

Typical absence seizures are not associated with other neurologic problems and respond well to treatment with specific anticonvulsants. Although estimates vary, approximately 60 to 70 percent of such patients will have a spontaneous remission during adolescence. Unfortunately, a significant number of the nonremitting patients have associated generalized, tonic-clonic seizures and suffer from the problems of chronic epilepsy.

Atypical Absence Seizures Atypical absence seizures have features that deviate from both the clinical and EEG features of typical absence seizures. For example, the lapse of consciousness is usually of longer duration and less abrupt in onset and cessation, and the seizure is accompanied by more obvious motor signs that may include focal or lateralizing features. The EEG shows a generalized, slow

spike-and-wave pattern with a frequency of 2.5 per second or less, as well as other abnormal activity. Atypical absence seizures are usually associated with diffuse or multifocal structural abnormalities of the brain and therefore may accompany other signs of neurologic dysfunction such as mental retardation. Furthermore, the seizures are less responsive to anticonvulsants compared to typical absence seizures.

Generalized, Tonic-Clonic Seizures (Grand Mal) Primarily generalized, tonic-clonic seizures are the main seizure type in approximately 10 percent of all persons with epilepsy. They are also the most common seizure type resulting from metabolic derangements and are therefore frequently encountered in many different clinical settings. The seizure usually begins abruptly without warning, although some patients describe vague premonitory symptoms in the hours leading up to the seizure. This prodrome should be distinguished from the stereotypic auras associated with focal seizures that secondarily generalize. The initial phase of the seizure is usually tonic contraction of muscles throughout the body, accounting for a number of the classic features of the event. Tonic contraction of the muscles of expiration and the larynx at the onset will produce a loud moan or cry. Respirations are impaired, secretions pool in the oropharynx, and the patient becomes cyanotic. Contraction of the jaw muscles may cause biting of the tongue. A marked enhancement of sympathetic tone leads to increases in heart rate, blood pressure, and pupillary size. After 10 to 20 s, the tonic phase of the seizure typically evolves into the clonic phase, produced by the superimposition of periods of muscle relaxation on the tonic muscle contraction. The periods of relaxation progressively increase until the end of the ictal phase, which usually lasts no more than 1 min. The postictal phase is characterized by unresponsiveness, muscular flaccidity, and excessive salivation that can cause stridorous breathing and partial airway obstruction. Bladder or bowel incontinence may occur at this point as well. Patients gradually regain consciousness over minutes to hours, and during this transition there is typically a period of postictal confusion. Patients will subsequently complain of headache, fatigue, and muscle ache that can last for many hours. The duration of impaired consciousness in the postictal phase can be extremely long, i.e., many hours, in patients with prolonged seizures or underlying CNS diseases such as alcoholic cerebral atrophy.

The EEG during the tonic phase of the seizure shows a progressive increase in generalized low-voltage fast activity, followed by generalized high-amplitude, polyspike discharges. In the clonic phase, the high-amplitude activity is typically interrupted by slow waves to create a spike-and-wave pattern. The postictal EEG shows diffuse slowing that gradually recovers as the patient awakens.

There are many variants of the generalized tonic-clonic seizure, including pure tonic and pure clonic seizures. Brief tonic seizures lasting only a few seconds are especially noteworthy since they are usually associated with known epileptic syndromes having mixed seizure phenotypes, such as the Lennox-Gastaut syndrome (discussed below).

Atonic Seizures Atonic seizures are characterized by sudden loss of postural muscle tone lasting 1 to 2 s. Consciousness is briefly impaired, but there is usually no postictal confusion. A very brief seizure may cause only a quick head drop or nodding movement, while a longer seizure will cause the patient to collapse. This can be quite dramatic and extremely dangerous, since there is a substantial risk of direct head injury with the fall. The EEG shows brief, generalized spike-and-wave discharges followed immediately by diffuse slow waves that correlate with the loss of muscle tone. Similar to pure tonic seizures, atonic seizures are usually seen in association with known epileptic syndromes.

Myoclonic Seizures Myoclonus is a sudden and brief muscle contraction that may involve one part of the body or the entire body. A normal, common physiologic form of myoclonus is the sudden jerking movement observed while falling asleep. Pathologic myoclonus is most commonly seen in association with metabolic disorders, degenerative CNS diseases, or anoxic brain injury (see Chap. 21).

Although the distinction from other forms of myoclonus is imprecise, myoclonic seizures are considered to be true epileptic events since they are caused by cortical (versus subcortical or spinal) dysfunction. The EEG shows bilaterally synchronous spike-and-wave discharges. Myoclonic seizures usually coexist with other forms of generalized seizure disorders but are the predominant feature of juvenile myoclonic epilepsy (discussed below).

UNCLASSIFIED SEIZURES Not all seizure types can be classified as partial or generalized. This appears to be especially true of seizures that occur in neonates (i.e., less than 1 month of age) and infants (younger than 1 year). The distinctive phenotypes of seizures at these early ages likely result, in part, from differences in neuronal function and connectivity in the immature versus mature CNS.

Neonatal Seizures Neonatal seizures are characteristically very subtle (especially to the nonneonatologist) and may consist of brief episodes of apnea, eye deviation, eye blinking, or repetitive movements of the arms and legs. An EEG is critical for diagnosis in such cases. Generalized tonic-clonic seizures, multifocal clonic seizures, and myoclonus can also be observed in some patients, but these are the exception rather than the rule.

Infantile Spasms Infantile spasms are usually seen in infants under 12 months of age and are characterized by abrupt movements of the head, trunk, or limbs that often occur in clusters of 10 to 20 movements per episode. The classic spasm is a sudden flexion of the neck and abdomen with extension of the limbs ("jackknife" seizure), although other combinations of flexion and extension are described. Infantile spasms are often quite subtle and can appear strikingly similar to the signs of discomfort in a baby with colic. The EEG usually shows *hypsarrythmia*, which consists of high-voltage slowing, multifocal spikes, and a variety of other pleiomorphic abnormalities. Infantile spasms are often seen in association with other signs of CNS dysfunction, including developmental delay and mental retardation.

EPILEPSY SYNDROMES

In addition to recognizing the patterns of different types of seizures, it is also useful to be familiar with some of the more common epilepsy syndromes, since this often helps in the determination of therapy and prognosis. Epilepsy syndromes are disorders in which epilepsy is a predominant feature, and there is sufficient evidence (e.g., through clinical, EEG, radiologic, or genetic observations) to suggest a common underlying mechanism. Some examples are listed below.

IDIOPATHIC (PRIMARY) EPILEPSY SYNDROMES Benign Neonatal Convulsions Benign neonatal convulsions is an idiopathic, generalized seizure disorder observed in otherwise normal newborn infants typically between the second to sixth day of life. The seizures are usually tonic or manifest as short apneic spells and spontaneously remit within days to weeks; the infants have no further problems. A subgroup of patients have an inherited form of this syndrome known as *benign familial neonatal convulsions*. A mutation in chromosome 20 has been shown to be associated with the disease in at least one family.

Juvenile Myoclonic Epilepsy Juvenile myoclonic epilepsy (JME) is a generalized seizure disorder of unknown cause that appears in early adolescence and is usually characterized by bilateral myoclonic jerks that may be single or repetitive. The myoclonic seizures are most frequent in the morning after awakening and can be provoked by sleep deprivation. Consciousness is preserved unless the myoclonus is especially severe. Many patients also experience generalized tonic-clonic seizures, and up to one-third have absence seizures. The condition is otherwise benign, and although complete remission is uncommon, the seizures respond well to appropriate anticonvulsant medication. There is often a family history of epilepsy, and genetic linkage studies suggest a polygenic cause (see Chap. 363).

Benign Childhood Epilepsy with Centrotemporal Spikes This is an idiopathic, focal epilepsy that appears in otherwise normal children between ages 3 and 13 and may account for 25 percent of all epilepsies in childhood. Patients have brief, simple-partial seizures characterized by hemifacial sensory or motor symptoms that can spread to the limbs or become generalized. Most seizures, especially those that generalize, occur during sleep. The interictal EEG shows a distinctive pattern of high-voltage spikes or sharp waves in the centrotemporal region that may shift from one side to the other. The seizures are easily treated with anticonvulsant medications and almost always remit by age 15. The disorder has an autosomal dominant inheritance pattern with variable penetrance, and many clinically unaffected family members are found to have the EEG abnormality.

SYMPTOMATIC (SECONDARY) EPILEPSY SYNDROMES Lennox-Gastaut Syndrome Lennox-Gastaut syndrome occurs in children (ages 1 to 8) and is defined by the following triad: (1) multiple seizure types (usually including generalized tonic-clonic, atonic, and atypical absence seizures); (2) an EEG showing slow (<3 Hz) spike-and-wave discharges and a variety of other abnormalities; and (3) impaired cognitive function in most but not all cases. Lennox-Gastaut syndrome is associated with CNS disease or dysfunction from a variety of causes, including developmental abnormalities, perinatal hypoxia/ischemia, trauma, infection, and other acquired lesions. The multifactorial nature of this syndrome suggests that it is a nonspecific response of the brain to diffuse neural injury. Unfortunately, many patients have a poor prognosis due to the underlying CNS disease and the physical and psychosocial consequences of severe, poorly controlled epilepsy. A similar syndrome in infancy that often evolves into Lennox-Gastaut syndrome is *West syndrome*, characterized by infantile spasms, other findings of cerebral dysfunction, and a characteristic EEG pattern.

Mesial Temporal Lobe Epilepsy Syndrome Mesial temporal lobe epilepsy (MTLE) is the most common syndrome associated with complex-partial seizures and is an example of a symptomatic, partial epilepsy. Distinctive clinical, electroencephalographic, and pathologic features define this syndrome (Table 365-2). High-resolution magnetic resonance imaging (MRI) can detect the characteristic hippocampal sclerosis that appears to be an essential element in the pathophysiology of MTLE for many patients (Fig. 365-1). Recognition of this syndrome is especially important because it tends to be refractory to treatment with anticonvulsants but responds extremely well to surgical interven-

Table 365-2

Characteristics of the Mesial Temporal Lobe Epilepsy (MTLE) Syndrome

HISTORY	
History of febrile seizures	Seizures may remit and reappear
Positive family history of epilepsy	Seizures often intractable
Early onset	
Rare secondarily generalized seizures	
CLINICAL OBSERVATIONS	
Aura common	Postictal disorientation, memory loss, dysphasia (with focus in dominant hemisphere)
Behavioral arrest/stare	
Complex automatisms	
Unilateral posturing	
LABORATORY STUDIES	
Unilateral or bilateral anterior temporal spikes on EEG	
Hypometabolism on interictal PET	
Hypoperfusion on interictal SPECT	
Material-specific memory deficits on intracranial amobarbital (Wada's) test	
MRI findings:	
Small hippocampus with increased signal on T2-weighted sequences	
Small temporal lobe	
Enlarged temporal horn	
Pathologic findings:	
Highly selective loss of specific cell populations within hippocampus in most cases	

ABBREVIATIONS: PET, positron emission tomography; SPECT, single photon emission computed tomography

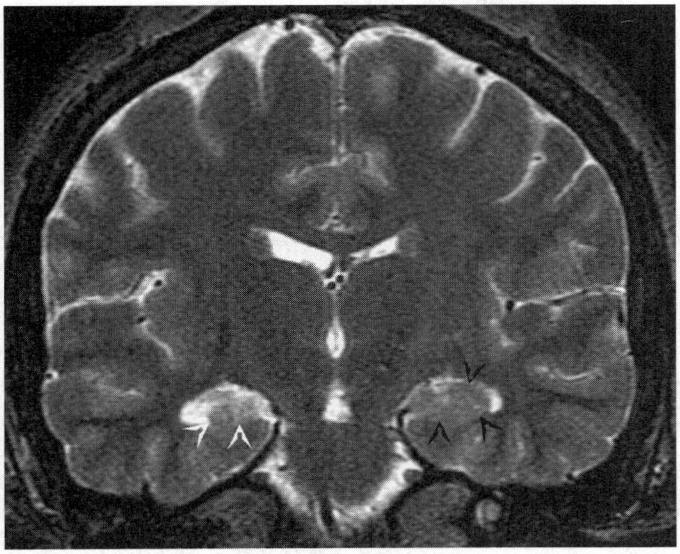

FIGURE 365-1 Mesial temporal lobe epilepsy. The EEG suggested a right temporal lobe focus. Coronal high-resolution T2-weighted fast spin echo magnetic resonance image obtained through the body of the hippocampus demonstrates abnormal high signal intensity in the right hippocampus (white arrows; compare with the normal hippocampus on the left, black arrows) consistent with mesial temporal sclerosis.

tion. Major advances in the understanding of basic mechanisms of epilepsy have come through studies of experimental models of MTLE, discussed below.

THE CAUSES OF SEIZURES AND EPILEPSY

Seizures are a result of a shift in the normal balance of excitation and inhibition within the CNS. Given the numerous properties that control neuronal excitability, it is not surprising that there are many different ways to perturb this normal balance, and therefore many different causes of both seizures and epilepsy. Our understanding of the basic mechanisms involved remains very limited, and consequently there is not a rigorous, mechanistic-based framework for organizing all the etiologies. Conceptually, however, three important clinical observations emphasize how a variety of factors determine why certain conditions may cause seizures or epilepsy in a given patient.

1. *The normal brain is capable of having a seizure under the appropriate circumstances, and there are differences between individuals in the susceptibility or threshold for seizures.* For example, seizures may be induced by high fevers in children who are otherwise normal and who never develop other neurologic problems, including epilepsy. However, febrile seizures occur only in approximately 3 to 5 percent of children. This implies there are various underlying, *endogenous factors* that influence the threshold for having a seizure. Some of these factors are clearly genetic, as it has been shown that a family history of epilepsy will influence the likelihood of seizures occurring in otherwise normal individuals. Normal development also plays an important role, since the brain appears to have different seizure thresholds at different maturational stages.

2. *There are a variety of conditions that have an extremely high likelihood of resulting in a chronic seizure disorder.* One of the best examples of this is severe, penetrating head trauma, which is associated with up to a 50 percent risk of leading to epilepsy. The high propensity for severe traumatic brain injury to lead to epilepsy suggests that the injury results in a long-lasting, pathologic change in the CNS that transforms a presumably normal neural network into one that is abnormally hyperexcitable. This process is known as *epileptogenesis*, and the specific changes that result in a lowered seizure threshold can be considered *epileptogenic factors*. Other processes associated with epileptogenesis include stroke, infections, and abnormalities of CNS development. Likewise, the genetic abnormalities associated with epilepsy, such as the gene mutations linked to benign familial neonatal convulsions or JME, likely involve processes that trigger the appearance of specific sets of epileptogenic factors.

3. *Seizures are episodic.* Patients with epilepsy have seizures intermittently and, depending on the underlying cause, many patients are completely normal for months or even years between seizures. This implies there are important provocative or *precipitating factors* that induce seizures in patients with epilepsy. Similarly, precipitating factors are responsible for causing the single seizure in someone without epilepsy. Precipitants include those due to intrinsic physiologic processes, such as psychological or physical stress, sleep deprivation, or hormonal changes associated with the menstrual cycle. They also include exogenous factors such as exposure to toxic substances and certain medications.

These observations emphasize the concept that the many causes of seizures and epilepsy result from a dynamic interplay between endogenous factors, epileptogenic factors, and precipitating factors. The potential role of each needs to be carefully considered when determining the appropriate management of a patient with seizures. For example, the identification of predisposing factors (e.g., family history of epilepsy) in a patient with febrile seizures may increase the necessity for closer follow-up and a more aggressive diagnostic evaluation. Finding an epileptogenic lesion may help in the estimation of seizure recurrence and duration of therapy. Finally, removal or modification of a precipitating factor may be an effective and safer method for preventing further seizures than the prophylactic use of anticonvulsant drugs.

CAUSES ACCORDING TO AGE In practice, it is useful to consider the etiologies of seizures based on the age of the patient, as age is one of the most important factors determining both the incidence and likely causes of seizures or epilepsy (Table 365-3). During the *neonatal period and early infancy*, potential causes include hypoxic-ischemic encephalopathy, trauma, CNS infection, congenital CNS abnormalities, and metabolic disorders. Babies born to mothers using neurotoxic drugs such as cocaine, heroin, or ethanol are susceptible to drug-withdrawal seizures in the first few days after delivery. Hypoglycemia and hypocalcemia, which can occur as secondary complications of perinatal injury, are also causes of seizures early after delivery. Seizures due to inborn errors of metabolism usually present once regular feeding begins, typically 2 to 3 days after birth. Pyridoxine (vitamin B_6) deficiency, an important cause of neonatal seizures, can be effectively treated with pyridoxine replacement. The idiopathic or inherited forms of benign neonatal convulsions are also seen during this time period.

The most common seizures arising in *late infancy and early childhood* are febrile seizures, which are seizures associated with fevers but without evidence of CNS infection or other defined causes. The overall prevalence is 3 to 5 percent and even higher in some parts of the world, such as Asia. Patients often have a family history of febrile seizures or epilepsy. Febrile seizures usually occur between 3 months and 5 years of age and have a peak incidence between 18 and 24 months. The typical scenario is a child who has a generalized, tonic-clonic seizure during a febrile illness in the setting of a common childhood infection such as otitis media, respiratory infection, or gastroenteritis. The seizure is likely to occur during the rising phase of the temperature curve (i.e., during the first day) rather than well into the course of the illness. A *simple* febrile seizure is a single, isolated event, brief, and symmetric in appearance. *Complex* febrile seizures have repeated seizure activity, last more than 15 minutes, or have focal features. Approximately one-third of patients with febrile seizures will have a recurrence, but fewer than 10 percent have three or more episodes. Recurrences are much more likely when the febrile seizure occurs in the first year of life. Simple febrile seizures are not associated with an increase in the risk of developing epilepsy, while complex febrile seizures have a risk of 2 to 5 percent; other risk factors include the presence of preexisting neurologic deficits and a family history of nonfebrile seizures.

Table 365-3

The Causes of Seizures

Neonates (<1 month)	Perinatal hypoxia and ischemia Intracranial hemorrhage and trauma Acute CNS infection (bacterial and viral meningitis) Metabolic disturbances (hypoglycemia, hypocalcemia, hypomagnesemia, pyridoxine deficiency) Drug withdrawal Developmental disorders (acquired and genetic) Genetic disorders
Infants and children (>1 mo and <12 years)	Febrile seizures Genetic disorders (metabolic, degenerative, primary epilepsy syndromes) CNS infection Developmental disorders (acquired and genetic) Trauma Idiopathic
Adolescents (12–18 years)	Trauma Genetic disorders Infection Brain tumor Illicit drug use Idiopathic
Young adults (18–35 years)	Trauma Alcohol withdrawal Illicit drug use Brain tumor Idiopathic
Older adults (>35 years)	Cerebrovascular disease Brain tumor Alcohol withdrawal Metabolic disorders (uremia, hepatic failure, electrolyte abnormalities, hypoglycemia) Alzheimer's disease and other degenerative CNS diseases Idiopathic

Childhood marks the age at which many of the well-defined epilepsy syndromes present, including typical childhood absence epilepsy and benign childhood epilepsy with centrotemporal spikes. Some children who are otherwise normal develop idiopathic, generalized tonic-clonic seizures without other features that fit into specific syndromes. Temporal lobe epilepsy usually presents in childhood and may be related to mesial temporal lobe sclerosis (as part of the MTLE syndrome) or other focal abnormalities such as cortical dysgenesis. Other types of partial seizures, including those with secondary generalization, may be the relatively late manifestation of a developmental disorder, an acquired lesion such as head trauma, CNS infection (especially viral encephalitis), or very rarely a CNS tumor. This is also the period that Lennox-Gastaut syndrome is identified, almost always in the child who has other neurologic problems such as static encephalopathy.

The period of adolescence and early adulthood is one of transition during which the idiopathic or genetically based epilepsy syndromes, including JME and juvenile absence epilepsy, become less common, while epilepsies secondary to acquired CNS lesions begin to predominate. Seizures in patients in this age range can be associated with head trauma, CNS infections (including parasitic infections such as cysticercosis), brain tumors, congenital CNS abnormalities, illicit drug use, or alcohol withdrawal.

Head trauma is a common cause of epilepsy in adolescents and adults. The head injury can be caused by a variety of mechanisms, and the likelihood of developing epilepsy is strongly correlated with the severity of the injury. A patient with a penetrating head wound, depressed skull fracture, intracranial hemorrhage, or prolonged post-traumatic coma or amnesia has a 40 to 50 percent risk of developing

Table 365-4

Drugs and Other Substances that Can Cause Seizures

Antimicrobials β-lactam and related compounds Quinolones Isoniazid Ganciclovir Anesthetic and antiarrhythmics Beta-adrenergic antagonists Local anesthetics Class 1B agents Immunosuppressants Cyclosporine OKT3 (monoclonal antibodies to T cells) Psychotropics Antidepressants Antipsychotics Lithium	Radiographic contrast agents Theophylline Sedative-hypnotic drug withdrawal Alcohol Barbiturates Benzodiazepines Drugs of abuse Amphetamine Cocaine Phencyclidine Methylphenidate

epilepsy, while a patient with a closed head injury and cerebral contusion has a 5 to 25 percent risk. Recurrent seizures usually develop within 1 year after head trauma, although intervals of 10 years or longer are well known. In controlled studies, mild head injury, defined as a concussion with amnesia or loss of consciousness of less than ½ h, was not found to be associated with an increased likelihood of epilepsy. Nonetheless, most epileptologists know of patients who have partial seizures within hours or days of a mild head injury and subsequently develop chronic seizures of the same type; such cases may represent rare examples of chronic epilepsy resulting from mild head injury.

The causes of seizures in *older adults* include cerebrovascular disease, trauma (including subdural hematoma), CNS tumors, and degenerative diseases. Cerebrovascular disease may account for approximately 50 percent of new cases of epilepsy in patients older than 65. Acute seizures (i.e., occurring at the time of the stroke) are seen more often with embolic rather than hemorrhagic or thrombotic stroke. Chronic seizures typically appear months to years after the initial event and are associated with all forms of stroke.

Metabolic disturbances such as electrolyte imbalance, hypo- or hyperglycemia, renal failure, and hepatic failure may cause seizures at any age. Similarly, endocrine disorders, hematologic disorders, vasculitides, and many other systemic diseases may cause seizures over a broad age range. A wide variety of medications and abused substances are known to precipitate seizures as well (Table 365-4).

BASIC MECHANISMS

MECHANISMS OF SEIZURE INITIATION AND PROPAGATION Partial seizure activity can begin in a very discrete region of cortex and then spread to neighboring regions, i.e., there is a *seizure initiation* phase and a *seizure propagation* phase. Studies of experimental models of these phases suggest that the initiation phase is characterized by two concurrent events in an aggregate of neurons: (1) high-frequency bursts of action potentials, and (2) hypersynchronization. The bursting activity is caused by a relatively long-lasting depolarization of the neuronal membrane due to influx of extracellular calcium (Ca^{2+}), which leads to the opening of voltage-dependent sodium (Na^+) channels; influx of Na^+; and generation of repetitive action potentials. This is followed by a hyperpolarizing afterpotential mediated by γ-aminobutyric acid (GABA) receptors or potassium (K^+) channels, depending on the cell type. The synchronized bursts from a sufficient number of neurons result in a so-called spike discharge on the EEG.

Normally, the spread of the bursting activity is prevented by intact hyperpolarization and a region of surrounding inhibition created by inhibitory neurons. With sufficient activation there is a recruitment of surrounding neurons via a number of mechanisms. Repetitive discharges lead to the following: (1) an increase in extracellular K^+, which blunts the extent of hyperpolarization and depolarizes neighboring neurons; (2) accumulation of Ca^{2+} in presynaptic terminals, leading to enhanced neurotransmitter release; and (3) depolarization-induced activation of the *N*-methyl-D-aspartate (NMDA) subtype of the excitatory amino acid receptor, which causes more Ca^{2+} influx and neuronal activation. The recruitment of a sufficient number of neurons leads to a loss of the surrounding inhibition and propagation of seizure activity into contiguous areas via local cortical connections, and to more distant areas via long commissural pathways such as the corpus callosum.

Many factors control neuronal excitability, and thus there are many potential mechanisms for altering a neuron's propensity to have bursting activity. Examples of mechanisms *intrinsic* to the neuron include changes in the conductance of ion channels, response characteristics of membrane receptors, cytoplasmic buffering, second-messenger systems, and protein expression as determined by gene transcription, translation, and posttranslational modification. Mechanisms *extrinsic* to the neuron include changes in the amount or type of neurotransmitters present at the synapse, modulation of receptors by extracellular ions and other molecules, and temporal and spatial properties of both synaptic and nonsynaptic input. Nonneural cells, such as astrocytes and oligodendrocytes, have an important role in many of these mechanisms as well.

Certain known causes of seizures are explained by these mechanisms. For example, accidental ingestion of domoic acid, which is an analogue of glutamate (the principal excitatory neurotransmitter in the brain), causes profound seizures via direct activation of excitatory amino acid receptors throughout the CNS. Penicillin, which can lower the seizure threshold in humans and is a potent convulsant in experimental models, reduces inhibition by antagonizing the effects of GABA and its receptor. The basic mechanisms of other precipitating factors of seizures, such as sleep deprivation, fever, alcohol withdrawal, hypoxia, and infection, are not as well understood but presumably involve analogous perturbations in neuronal excitability. Similarly, the endogenous factors that determine an individual's seizure threshold may relate to these properties as well.

Knowledge of the mechanisms responsible for the initiation and propagation of most generalized seizures (including tonic-clonic, myoclonic, and atonic types) remains rudimentary and reflects the limited understanding of the connectivity of the brain at a systems level. Much more is understood about the origin of generalized spike-and-wave discharges in absence seizures. These appear to be related to oscillatory rhythms that are normally generated during sleep by circuits connecting the thalamus and cortex. This oscillatory behavior involves an interaction between $GABA_B$ receptors, T-type Ca^{2+} channels, and K^+ channels located within the thalamus. Pharmacologic studies indicate that modulation of these receptors and channels can induce absence seizures, and there is speculation that the genetic forms of absence epilepsy may be associated with mutations of components of this system.

MECHANISMS OF EPILEPTOGENESIS Epileptogenesis refers to the transformation of a normal neuronal network into one that is chronically hyperexcitable. For example, there is often a delay of months to years between an initial CNS injury such as trauma, stroke, or infection and the first seizure. The injury appears to initiate a process that gradually lowers the seizure threshold in the affected region until a spontaneous seizure occurs. In many genetic and idiopathic forms of epilepsy, epileptogenesis is presumably determined by developmentally regulated events.

Pathologic studies of the hippocampus from patients with temporal lobe epilepsy have led to the suggestion that some forms of epileptogenesis are related to *structural changes in neuronal networks*. For example, many patients with MTLE syndrome have a highly selective loss of neurons that has been proposed to contribute to inhibition of the main excitatory neurons within the dentate gyrus. There is also evidence that, in response to the loss of neurons, there is reorganization or "sprouting" of surviving neurons in a way that affects the excitability of the network. Some of these changes can be seen in experimental models of prolonged electrical seizures or traumatic brain injury. Thus, an initial injury such as head injury may lead to a very focal, confined region of structural change that causes local hyperexcitability. The local hyperexcitability leads to further structural changes that evolve over time until the focal lesion produces clinically evident seizures. Similar models have also provided strong evidence for long-term alterations in *intrinsic, biochemical properties of cells* within the network, such as chronic changes in glutamate receptor function. Recent studies of a rare childhood epilepsy syndrome (Rasmussen's syndrome) have also raised the possibility that some forms of epileptogenesis may be caused by an immune response in which autoantibodies against glutamate receptors lead to receptor activation, depolarization, seizures, and excitotoxic cell injury.

GENETIC CAUSES OF EPILEPSY The genetic causes of a few epilepsy syndromes have recently been discovered. Myoclonic epilepsy with ragged red fibers (MERRF) syndrome is associated with a mutation of mitochondrial tRNA-lysine. Mutations in the cystatin B gene may cause another form of progressive myoclonus epilepsy (Unverricht-Lundborg type), and a mutation within the gene encoding the β_4 subunit of the acetylcholine receptor appears responsible for a frontal lobe epilepsy syndrome consisting of nocturnal partial seizures (see Chap. 363). A number of other epilepsy syndromes have been mapped to chromosomal locations. Epilepsy has been produced in transgenic mice having a wide range of genetically engineered mutations, suggesting that many potential genetic abnormalities can result in a change in the seizure threshold.

MECHANISMS OF ACTION OF ANTIEPILEPTIC DRUGS Currently available antiepileptic drugs appear to act primarily by blocking the initiation or spread of seizures. Phenytoin, carbamazepine, valproic acid, and lamotrigine inhibit Na^+-dependent action potentials in a frequency-dependent manner, resulting in a preferential blockade of the sustained high-frequency activity that is characteristic of burst-firing neurons in a seizure focus. Phenytoin also appears to suppress seizure spread through inhibition of specific voltage-gated Ca^{2+} channels. Benzodiazepines and barbiturates augment inhibition by distinct interactions with GABA receptors. Valproic acid elevates the concentration of GABA in the brain, perhaps through interaction with enzymes involved in the synthesis (glutamic acid decarboxylase) and catabolism (GABA transaminase) of GABA. Gabapentin, which is a structural analogue of GABA, appears to increase GABA levels by enhancing GABA synthesis and release and may also cause a decrease in glutamate synthesis. The two most effective drugs for absence seizures, ethosuximide and valproic acid, probably act by inhibiting T-type Ca^{2+} channels in thalamic neurons.

In contrast to the relatively large number of antiepileptic drugs that can attenuate seizure activity, there are currently no drugs known to prevent the formation of a seizure focus following CNS injury in humans. The eventual development of such "antiepileptogenic" drugs will provide an important means of preventing the emergence of epilepsy following injuries such as head trauma, stroke, and CNS infection.

EVALUATION OF THE PATIENT WITH A SEIZURE

When a patient presents shortly after a seizure, the first priorities are attention to vital signs, respiratory and cardiovascular support, and treatment of seizures if they resume (see "Treatment"). Life-threatening conditions such as CNS infection, metabolic derangement or drug toxicity must be recognized and managed appropriately.

When the patient is not acutely ill, the evaluation will initially focus on whether or not there is a history of earlier seizures (Fig. 365-2). If this is the patient's first seizure, then the emphasis will be to (1) establish whether the reported episode was a seizure rather than another paroxysmal event, (2) determine the cause of the seizure by identifying risk factors and precipitating events, and (3) decide whether anticonvulsant therapy is required in addition to treatment for any underlying illness.

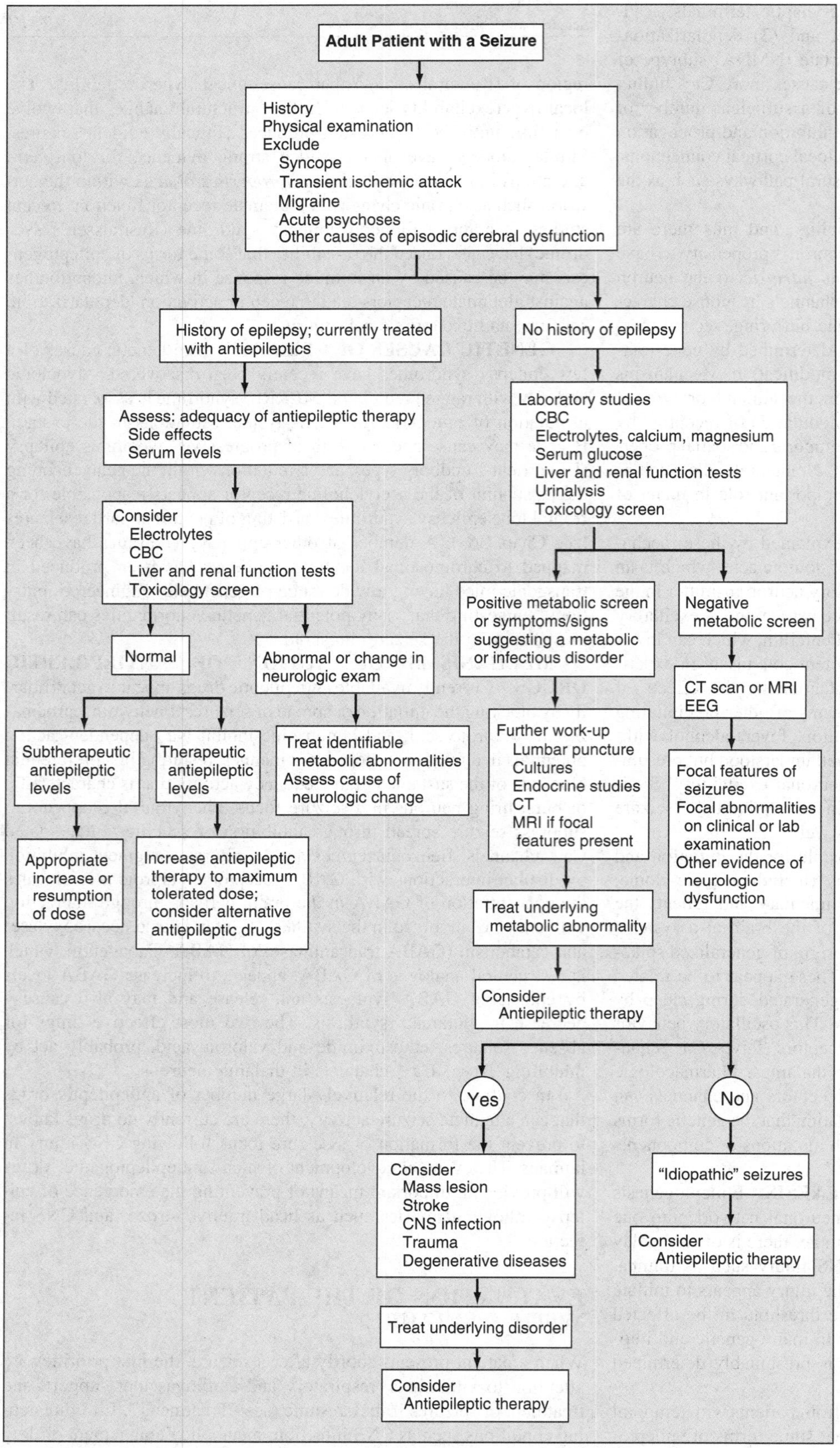

FIGURE 365-2 Evaluation of the adult patient with a seizure. CBC, complete blood count; CT, computed tomography; MRI, magnetic resonance imaging; EEG, electroencephalogram; CNS, central nervous system.

In the patient with prior seizures or a known history of epilepsy, the evaluation is directed toward (1) identification of the underlying cause and precipitating factors, and (2) determination of the adequacy of the patient's current therapy.

HISTORY AND EXAMINATION The history should first determine whether the event was truly a seizure. It is essential to take the time to gather an in-depth history, for *in many cases the diagnosis of a seizure is based solely on clinical grounds—the examination and laboratory studies are often normal*. Keeping in mind the characteristics of different seizure types, questions need to focus precisely on the symptoms before, during, and after the episode in order to discriminate a seizure from other paroxysmal events (see "Differential Diagnosis of Seizures"). Seizures frequently occur out-of-hospital, and the patient may be unaware of the ictal and immediate postictal phases; thus witnesses to the event should be interviewed carefully.

The history should also focus on risk factors and predisposing events. Clues for a predisposition to seizures include a history of febrile seizures, earlier auras or brief seizures not recognized as such, and a family history of seizures. Epileptogenic factors such as prior head trauma, stroke, tumor, or vascular malformation should be identified. In children, a careful assessment of developmental milestones may provide evidence for underlying CNS disease., Precipitating factors such as sleep deprivation, systemic diseases, electrolyte or metabolic derangements, acute infection, drugs that lower the seizurem threshold (see Table 365-4), or alcohol or illicit drug use should also be identified.

The general physical examination includes a search for signs of infection or systemic illness. Careful examination of the skin may reveal signs of tuberous sclerosis (adenoma sebaceum, "ash-leaf" spots), neurofibromatosis (café au lait spots, peripheral neurofibromas), Sturge-Weber syndrome (facial angioma), or chronic liver or renal disease. A finding of organomegaly may indicate a metabolic storage disease, and limb asymmetry may provide a clue for brain injury early in development. Signs of head trauma and use of alcohol or illicit drugs should be sought. Auscultation of the heart and carotid arteries may identify an abnormality that predisposes to cerebrovascular disease.

All patients require a complete neurologic examination, with particular emphasis on eliciting signs of cerebral hemispheric disease (see Chap. 360). Careful assessment of mental status (including memory, language function, and abstract thinking) may suggest lesions in the anterior frontal, parietal, or temporal lobes. Testing of visual fields will help screen for lesions in the optic pathways and occipital lobes. Screening tests of motor function such as pronator drift, deep tendon reflexes, gait, and coordination may suggest lesions in motor (frontal) cortex, and cortical sensory testing (e.g., double simultaneous stimulation) may detect lesions in the parietal cortex.

LABORATORY STUDIES Routine blood studies are indicated to identify the more common metabolic causes of seizures, such as abnormalities in electrolytes, glucose, calcium, or magnesium, and hepatic or renal disease. A screen for toxins in blood and urine should also be obtained from all patients in the appropriate risk groups, especially when no clear precipitating factor has been identified. A lumbar puncture is indicated if there is any suspicion of meningitis or encephalitis and is mandatory in all patients infected with the human immunodeficiency virus, even in the absence of symptoms or signs suggesting infection.

All patients who have a possible seizure disorder should be evaluated with an EEG (see Chap. 361) as soon as possible. The EEG may help to establish the diagnosis of epilepsy, classify the seizure type, and provide evidence for the existence of a particular epilepsy syndrome. If the patient is having frequent seizures, such as a child with absence epilepsy, the EEG may confirm the presence of seizures and help to identify the seizure type. In patients with infrequent seizures, the EEG may reveal potentially abnormal interictal activity that, when combined with clinical or radiologic data, aids in establishing the diagnosis. However, the existence of epileptiform patterns such as spikes or sharp waves are not diagnostic in themselves, since similar patterns can be seen in 1 to 2 percent of normal individuals. Ideally, the EEG should be performed after sleep deprivation to increase the potential diagnostic yield of the study.

Almost all patients with new-onset seizures should have a brain imaging study to determine whether there is an underlying structural abnormality that is responsible. The main exception to this rule is children who have an unambiguous history and examination suggestive of a benign, generalized seizure disorder such as absence epilepsy. MRI has been shown to be superior to computed tomography (CT) in scanning for the detection of cerebral lesions associated with epilepsy. In some cases MRI will identify lesions such as tumors, vascular malformations, or other pathologies that need immediate therapy. The use of newer MRI methods has increased the sensitivity for detection of abnormalities of cortical architecture, including hippocampal atrophy associated with mesial temporal sclerosis, and abnormalities of cortical neuronal migration. In such cases the findings may not lead to immediate therapy, but they do provide an explanation for the patient's seizures and point to the need for chronic anticonvulsant therapy or possible resective surgery.

In the patient with suspected CNS infection or mass lesions, CT scanning should be performed emergently when MRI is not immediately available. Otherwise, it is usually appropriate to obtain an MRI study within a few days of the initial evaluation. Functional imaging procedures such as positron emission tomography (PET) and single photon emission computed tomography (SPECT) are also used to evaluate certain patients with medically refractory seizures (discussed below).

DIFFERENTIAL DIAGNOSIS OF SEIZURES

The various disorders that may mimic seizures are listed in Table 365-5. In most cases seizures can be distinguished from these other conditions by meticulous attention to the history and relevant laboratory studies. On occasion, additional studies, such as video-EEG monitoring, sleep studies, tilt table analysis, or cardiac electrophysiology may be required to reach a correct diagnosis. Two of the more common syndromes in the differential diagnosis are detailed below.

Syncope The diagnostic dilemma encountered most frequently is the distinction between a generalized seizure and syncope. Observations by the patient and bystanders that can help discriminate between the two are listed in Table 365-6. Characteristics of a seizure include the presence of an aura, cyanosis, unconsciousness, motor manifestations lasting more than 30 s, postictal disorientation, muscle soreness, and sleepiness. In contrast, a syncopal episode is more likely if the event was provoked by acute pain or anxiety or occurred immediately after arising from the lying or sitting position. Patients with syncope often describe a stereotyped transition from consciousness to unconsciousness that includes tiredness, sweating, nausea, and tunneling of vision, and they experience a relatively brief loss of consciousness. Headache or incontinence may be observed following either a seizure or syncope and are thus not useful distinguishing features. A brief period (i.e., 1 to 10 s) of convulsive motor activity is frequently seen immediately at the onset of a syncopal episode, especially if the patient remains in an upright posture after fainting (e.g., in a dentist's chair) and therefore has a sustained decrease in cerebral perfusion. Rarely, a syncopal episode can induce a full tonic-clonic seizure. In such cases the evaluation must focus on both the cause of the syncopal event as well as the possibility that the patient has a propensity for recurrent seizures.

Psychogenic Seizures Psychogenic seizures are nonepileptic behaviors that resemble seizures. The behavior is often part of a conversion reaction precipitated by underlying psychological distress. Certain behaviors, such as side-to-side turning of the head, asymmetric and large amplitude shaking movements of the limbs, twitching of all four extremities without loss of consciousness, pelvic thrusting, and screaming or talking during the event, are more commonly associated

Table 365-5

The Differential Diagnosis of Seizures

1. Syncope	5. Transient ischemic attack (TIA)
Vasovagal syncope	Basilar artery TIA
Cardiac arrhythmia	6. Sleep disorders
Valvular heart disease	Narcolepsy/cataplexy
Cardiac failure	Benign sleep myoclonus
Orthostatic hypotension	7. Movement disorders
2. Psychological disorders	Tics
Psychogenic seizure	Nonepileptic myoclonus
Hyperventilation	Paroxysmal choreoathetosis
Panic attack	8. Special considerations in children
3. Metabolic disturbances	Breath-holding spells
Alcoholic blackouts	Migraine with recurrent abdominal pain and cyclic vomiting
Delirium tremens	Benign paroxysmal vertigo
Hypoglycemia	Apnea
Hypoxia	Night terrors
Psychoactive drugs (e.g., hallucinogens)	Sleepwalking
4. Migraine	
Confusional migraine	
Basilar migraine	

Table 365-6

Clinical Features of a Generalized Tonic-Clonic Seizure Versus Syncope

Features	Seizure	Syncope
Immediate precipitating factors	Usually none	Emotional stress, Valsalva, other specific causes
Premonitory symptoms	None or aura (e.g., odd odor)	Tiredness, nausea, diaphoresis, tunneling of vision
Posture at onset	Variable	Usually erect
Transition to unconsciousness	Often immediate	Gradual over seconds*
Duration of unconsciousness	Minutes	Seconds
Duration of tonic or clonic movements	30–60 s	Never more than 15 s
Facial appearance during event	Cyanosis, frothing at mouth	Pallor
Disorientation and sleepiness after event	Many minutes to hours	<5 min
Aching of muscles after event	Often	Sometimes
Biting of tongue	Sometimes	Rarely
Incontinence	Sometimes	Sometimes

* May be sudden with certain cardiac arrhythmias.

with psychogenic rather than epileptic seizures. However, the distinction is sometimes difficult on clinical grounds alone, and there are many examples of diagnostic errors made by experienced epileptologists. This is especially true for psychogenic seizures that resemble complex-partial seizures, since the behavioral manifestations of complex-partial seizures (especially of frontal lobe origin) can be extremely unusual, and in both cases the routine surface EEG may be normal. Video-EEG monitoring is often useful when the clinical observations are nondiagnostic. Generalized tonic-clonic seizures always produce marked EEG abnormalities during and after the seizure. For suspected complex-partial seizures of temporal lobe origin, the use of additional electrodes beyond the standard scalp locations (e.g., sphenoidal electrodes) may be required to detect a seizure focus. Measurement of serum prolactin levels may also help to discriminate between organic and psychogenic seizures, since most generalized seizures and many complex-partial seizures are accompanied by rises in serum prolactin (during the immediate 30-min postictal period), whereas psychogenic seizures are not. It is important to note that the diagnosis of psychogenic seizures does not exclude a concurrent diagnosis of epilepsy, since the two often coexist.

℞ TREATMENT

Therapy for a patient with a seizure disorder is almost always multimodal and includes treatment of underlying conditions that cause or contribute to the seizures, avoidance of precipitating factors, suppression of recurrent seizures by prophylactic therapy with antiepileptic medications or surgery, and addressing a variety of psychological and social issues. Treatment plans must be individualized, given the many different types and causes of seizures as well as the differences in efficacy and toxicity of antiepileptic medications for each patient. In almost all cases a neurologist with experience in the treatment of epilepsy should design and oversee implementation of the treatment strategy. Furthermore, patients with refractory epilepsy or those who require polypharmacy with antiepileptic drugs should remain under the regular care of a neurologist.

Treatment of Underlying Conditions If the sole cause of a seizure is a metabolic disturbance such as an abnormality of serum electrolytes or glucose, then treatment is aimed at reversing the metabolic problem and preventing its recurrence. Therapy with antiepileptic drugs is usually unnecessary unless the metabolic disorder cannot be corrected promptly and the patient is at risk of having further seizures. If the apparent cause of a seizure was a medication (e.g., theophylline) or illicit drug use (e.g., cocaine), then appropriate therapy is avoidance of the drug and there is usually no need for antiepileptic medications unless subsequent seizures occur.

Seizures caused by a structural CNS lesion such as a brain tumor, vascular malformation, or brain abscess may not recur after appropriate treatment of the underlying lesion. However, despite removal of the structural lesion, there is a risk that the seizure focus will remain in the surrounding tissue or develop *de novo* as a result of gliosis and other processes induced by surgery, radiation, or other therapies. Most patients are therefore maintained on an antiepileptic medication for at least 1 year, and an attempt is made to withdraw medications only if the patient has been completely seizure-free. If the seizures are refractory to medication, the patient may benefit from surgical removal of the epileptic brain region (see "Surgical Treatment of Refractory Epilepsy").

Avoidance of Precipitating Factors Unfortunately, little is known about the specific factors that determine precisely when a seizure will occur in a patient with epilepsy. Some patients can identify particular situations that appear to lower their seizure threshold; these situations should be avoided. For example, a patient who has seizures in the setting of sleep deprivation should be advised to maintain a normal sleep schedule. Many patients note an association between alcohol intake and seizures, and they should be encouraged to modify their drinking habits accordingly. There are also relatively rare cases of patients with seizures that are induced by highly specific stimuli such as a video game monitor, music, or an individual's voice ("reflex epilepsy"). If there is an association between stress and seizures, stress reduction techniques such as physical exercise, meditation, or counseling may be helpful.

Antiepileptic Drug Therapy Antiepileptic drug therapy is the mainstay of treatment for most patients with epilepsy. The overall goal is to completely prevent seizures without causing any untoward side effects, preferably with a single medication and a dosing schedule that is easy for the patient to follow. Seizure classification is an important element in designing the treatment plan, since some antiepileptic drugs have different activities against various seizure types. However, there is considerable overlap between many antiepileptic drugs, such that the choice of therapy is often determined more by specific needs of the patient, especially the patient's subjective assessment of side effects.

WHEN TO INITIATE ANTIEPILEPTIC DRUG THERAPY Antiepileptic drug therapy should be started in any patient with recurrent seizures of unknown etiology or a known cause that cannot be reversed. Whether to initiate therapy in a patient with a single seizure is controversial. Patients with a single seizure due to an identified lesion such as a CNS tumor, infection, or trauma, in which there is strong evidence that the lesion is epileptogenic, should be treated. The risk of seizure recurrence in a patient with an apparently unprovoked or idiopathic seizure is uncertain, with estimates ranging from 31 to 71 percent in the first 12 months after the initial seizure. This uncertainty arises from differences in the underlying seizure types and etiologies in various published epidemiologic studies. Generally accepted risk factors associated with recurrent seizures include the following: (1) an abnormal neurologic examination, (2) seizures presenting as status epilepticus, (3) postictal Todd's paralysis, (4) a strong family history of seizures, or (5) an abnormal EEG. Most patients with one or more of these risk factors should be treated. Issues such as employment or driving may influence the decision whether or not to start medications as well. For example, a patient with a single, idiopathic seizure and whose job depends on driving may prefer taking antiepileptic drugs rather than risking a seizure recurrence and the potential loss of driving privileges.

SELECTION OF ANTIEPILEPTIC DRUGS The choices of antiepileptic drugs in the United States for different seizure types are shown in Table 365-7, and the main pharmacologic characteristics of commonly used drugs are listed in Table 365-8. Older medications such as phenytoin, valproic acid, carbamazepine, and ethosuximide are

Table 365-7

Antiepileptic Drugs of Choice

	Generalized Seizures			
Focal-Onset Seizures*	Generalized Tonic-Clonic	Absence	Myoclonic	Atonic
FIRST-LINE				
Carbamazepine Phenytoin Valproic acid	Valproic acid Carbamazepine Phenytoin	Ethosuximide Valproic acid	Valproic acid	Valproic acid
ALTERNATIVES				
Lamotrigine Gabapentin Phenobarbital Primidone	Phenobarbital Primidone	Acetazolamide Clonazepam Phenobarbital	Clonazepam Acetazolamide	Clonazepam

* Simple-partial, complex-partial, and secondarily generalized tonic-clonic seizures.

Table 365-8

Commonly Used Antiepileptic Drugs

Generic Name	Trade Name	Principal Uses	Typical Dosage and Dosing Intervals	Half-Life	Therapeutic Range	Adverse Effects		Drug Interactions
						Neurologic	Systemic	
Phenytoin (diphenylhydantoin	Dilantin	Tonic-clonic (grand mal) Focal-onset	300–400 mg/d (3–6 mg/kg, adult; 4–8 mg/kg, child) qd-bid	24 h (wide variation, dose-dependent)	10–20 μg/mL	Ataxia Incoordination Confusion Cerebellar	Gum hyperplasia Lymphadenopathy Hirsutism Osteomalacia Facial coarsening Skin rash	Level increased by isoniazid, sulfonamides Level decreased by carbamazepine, phenobarbital Altered folate metabolism
Carbamazepine	Tegretol	Tonic-clonic Focal-onset	600–1800 mg/d (15–35 mg/kg, child) bid-qid	13–17 h	4–12 μg/mL	Ataxia Dizziness Diplopia Vertigo	Aplastic anemia Leukopenia Gastrointestinal irritation Hepatotoxicity	Level decreased by phenobarbital, phenytoin Level increased by erythromycin, propoxyphene, isoniazid, cimetidine
Valproic acid	Depakane Depakote	Tonic-clonic Absence Atypical absence Myoclonic Focal-onset	750–2000 mg/d (20–60 mg/kg) bid-qid	15 h	50–150 μg/mL	Ataxia Sedation Tremor	Hepatotoxicity Thrombocytopenia Gastrointestinal irritation Weight gain Transient alopecia Hyperammonemia	Level decreased by carbamazepine, phenobarbital, phenytoin
Phenobarbital	Luminol	Tonic-clonic Focal-onset	60–180 mg/d (1–4 mg/kg, adult); (3–6 mg/kg, child) qd	90 h (70 h in children)	10–40 μg/mL	Sedation Ataxia Confusion Dizziness Decreased libido Depression	Skin rash	Level increased by valproic acid, phenytoin Enhances metabolism of other drugs via liver enzyme induction
Primidone	Mysoline	Tonic-clonic Focal-onset	750–1000 mg/d (10–25 mg/kg) bid-tid	Primidone, 8–15 h Phenobarbital, 90 h	Primidone, 4–12 μg/mL Phenobarbital, 10–40 μg/mL	Same as phenobarbital		
Ethosuximide	Zarontin	Absence (petit mal)	750–1250 mg/d (20-40 mg/kg) qd-bid	60 h, adult 30 h, child	40–100 μg/mL	Ataxia Lethargy Headache	Gastrointestinal irritation Skin rash Bone marrow suppression	
Gabapentin	Neurontin	Focal-onset	900–2400 mg/d tid-qid	5–9 h	Not established	Sedation Dizziness Ataxia Fatigue	Gastrointestinal irritation	No known significant interactions
Lamotrigine	Lamictal	Focal-onset Lennox-Gastaut syndrome	150–500 mg/d bid	25 h 14 h (with enzyme-inducers) 59 h (with valproic acid)	Not established	Dizziness Diplopia Sedation Ataxia Headache	Skin rash Stevens-Johnson syndrome	Level decreased by carbamazepine, phenobarbital, phenytoin Level increased by valproic acid
Clonazepam	Klonopin	Absence Atypical absence Myoclonic	1–12 mg/d (0.1–0.2 mg/kg) qd-tid	24–48 h	10–70 ng/mL	Ataxia Sedation Lethargy	Anorexia	Level decreased by carbamazepine, phenobarbital
Felbamate	Felbatol	Focal-onset Lennox-Gastaut syndrome	2400–3600 mg/d, (45 mg/kg, child) tid-qid	16–22 h	Not established	Insomnia Dizziness Sedation Headache	Aplastic anemia Hepatic failure Weight loss Gastrointestinal irritation	Increases phenytoin, valproic acid, active carbamazepine metabolite

generally used as first-line therapy for most seizure disorders since, overall, they are as effective as recently marketed drugs and significantly less expensive. Experience with newer drugs such as gabapentin and lamotrigine is comparatively limited in the United States, and their use is predominantly as add-on or alternative therapy. Felbamate, introduced in 1993, was found to be associated with a relatively high incidence of irreversible aplastic anemia and hepatic failure and is currently recommended only for medically refractory patients.

In addition to efficacy, other factors influencing the specific choice of an initial medication for a patient include the relative convenience of dosing schedule (e.g., once daily versus three or four times daily) and potential side effects. Almost all of the commonly used antiepileptic drugs can cause similar, dose-related side effects such as sedation, ataxia, and diplopia. Close follow-up is required to insure these are promptly recognized and reversed. Most of the drugs may also cause idiosyncratic toxicity such as rash, bone marrow suppression, or hepatotoxicity. Although rare, these side effects need to be carefully considered during drug selection, and patients require laboratory tests (e.g., complete blood count and liver function tests) prior to the institution of a drug (to establish baseline values) and during initial dosing and titration of the agent.

1. *Antiepileptic drug selection for partial seizures.* Carbamazepine or phenytoin is currently the initial drug of choice for the treatment of partial seizures, including those that secondarily generalize. Overall they have very similar efficacy, but differences in pharmacokinetics and toxicity are the main determinants for use in a given patient. Phenytoin has a relatively long half-life and offers the advantage of once or twice daily dosing compared to two or three times daily dosing for carbamazepine. An advantage of carbamazepine is that its metabolism follows first-order pharmacokinetics, and the relationship between drug dose, serum levels, and toxicity is linear. By contrast, phenytoin shows properties of saturation kinetics, such that small increases in phenytoin doses above a standard maintenance dose can precipitate marked side effects. This is one of the main causes of acute phenytoin toxicity. Long-term use of phenytoin is associated with untoward cosmetic effects (e.g., hirsutism, coarsening of facial features, and gingival hypertrophy), so it is often avoided in young patients who are likely to require the drug for many years. Carbamazepine can cause leukopenia, aplastic anemia, or hepatotoxicity and would therefore be contraindicated in patients with predispositions to these problems.

Valproic acid is an effective alternative for some patients with partial seizures, especially when the seizures secondarily generalize. Gastrointestinal side effects are fewer when using the valproate semisodium formulation (Depakote). Valproic acid also rarely causes reversible bone marrow suppression and hepatotoxicity, and laboratory testing is required to monitor toxicity. This drug should generally be avoided in patients with preexisting bone marrow or liver disease. Irreversible, fatal hepatic failure appearing as an idiosyncratic rather than dose-related side-effect is a relatively rare complication; its risk is highest in children younger than 2 years old, especially those taking other antiepileptic drugs or with inborn errors of metabolism. Valproic acid therapy should therefore only be used in infants and young children when the benefits clearly exceed this risk.

Lamotrigine, gabapentin, and phenobarbital are additional drugs currently used for the treatment of partial seizures with or without secondary generalization. Lamotrigine appears to have an overall efficacy profile similar to the more standard drugs but may cause severe rash or Stevens-Johnson syndrome, particularly in children. Lamotrigine must be started very slowly when used as add-on therapy with valproic acid, since its inhibition of lamotrigine metabolism causes a substantial prolongation of its half-life. Gabapentin is unique among the standard antiepileptic drugs in not having any significant drug interactions. This makes it potentially useful as add-on therapy, especially in patients who are particularly susceptible to side effects of other medications. Gabapentin is also useful in patients with severe liver disease since its clearance is exclusively renal. Until recently, phenobarbital and other barbiturate compounds were commonly used as first-line therapy for many forms of epilepsy. However, the barbiturates frequently cause sedation in adults, hyperactivity in children, and other more subtle cognitive changes; thus, their use should be limited to situations in which no other suitable treatment alternatives exist.

2. *Antiepileptic drug selection for generalized seizures.* Valproic acid is currently considered the best initial choice for the treatment of primarily generalized, tonic-clonic seizures, and carbamazepine and phenytoin are suitable alternatives. Valproic acid is also particularly effective in absence, myoclonic, and atonic seizures and is therefore the drug of choice in patients with epilepsy syndromes having mixed seizure types. Ethosuximide remains the preferred drug for the treatment of uncomplicated absence seizures, but it is not effective against tonic-clonic or partial seizures. Ethosuximide rarely causes bone marrow suppression, so that periodic monitoring of blood cell counts is required. Clonazepam is an alternative for the treatment of myoclonic, atonic, and absence seizures, but it is not indicated for the treatment of most other seizure types. This is especially important since the drug is sometimes abused due to its sedative-hypnotic qualities rather than its antiepileptic effect. Although approved for use in partial seizure disorders, lamotrigine is proving to be effective in epilepsy syndromes with mixed, generalized seizure types such as JME and Lennox-Gastaut syndrome.

INITIATION AND MONITORING OF THERAPY Because the response to any antiepileptic drug is unpredictable, patients should be carefully educated about the approach to therapy. Patients need to understand that the goal is to prevent seizures and minimize the side effects of therapy; determination of the optimal dose is often a matter of trial and error. This process may take months or longer if the baseline seizure frequency is low. Most anticonvulsant drugs need to be introduced relatively slowly to minimize side effects, and patients should expect that minor side effects such as mild sedation, slight changes in cognition, or imbalance will typically resolve within a few days. Starting doses are usually the lowest value listed under the dosage column in Table 365-8. Subsequent increases should only be made after achieving a steady state with the previous dose (i.e., after an interval of five or more half-lives).

Monitoring of serum antiepileptic drug levels can be very useful for establishing the initial dosing schedule. However, the published therapeutic ranges of serum drug concentrations are only an approximate guide for determining the proper dose for a given patient. The key determinants are the clinical measures of seizure frequency and presence of side effects, not the laboratory values. Conventional assays of serum drug levels measure the total drug (i.e., both free and protein-bound), yet it is the concentration of free drug that reflects extracellular levels in the brain and correlates best with efficacy. Thus, patients with decreased levels of serum proteins (e.g., decreased serum albumin due to impaired liver or renal function) may have an increased ratio of free to bound drug, yet the concentration of free drug may be adequate for seizure control. These patients may have a "subtherapeutic" drug level, but the dose should be altered only if seizures remain uncontrolled, not just to achieve a "therapeutic" level. In practice, other than during the initiation or modification of therapy, monitoring of antiepileptic drug levels is most useful for documenting compliance.

If seizures continue despite gradual increases to the maximum tolerated dose and documented compliance, then it becomes necessary to switch to another antiepileptic drug. This is usually done by maintaining the patient on the first drug while a second drug is added. The dose of the second drug should be adjusted to decrease seizure frequency without causing toxicity. Once this is achieved, the first drug can be gradually withdrawn (usually over weeks unless there is significant toxicity). The dose of the second drug is then further optimized based on seizure response and side effects.

WHEN TO DISCONTINUE THERAPY Overall, about 70 percent of children and 60 percent of adults who have their seizures completely controlled with antiepileptic drugs can eventually discontinue therapy. Clinical studies suggest that the following patient profile yields the greatest chance of remaining seizure-free after drug withdrawal: (1) complete medical control of seizures for 1 to 5 years; (2) single seizure type, either partial or generalized; (3) normal neurologic examination, including intelligence; and (4) a normal EEG. The appropriate seizure-free interval is unknown and undoubtedly varies for different forms of epilepsy. However, it seems reasonable to attempt withdrawal of therapy after 2 years in a patient who meets all of the above criteria, is motivated to discontinue the medication, and clearly understands the potential risks and benefits. In most cases it is preferable to reduce the dose of the drug gradually over 2 to 3 months. Most recurrences occur in the first 3 months after discontinuing therapy, and patients should be advised to avoid potentially dangerous situations such as driving or unsupervised swimming during this period.

TREATMENT OF REFRACTORY EPILEPSY Approximately one-third of patients with epilepsy do not respond to treatment with a single antiepileptic drug, and it becomes necessary to try a combination of drugs to control seizures. Patients who have focal epilepsy related to an underlying structural lesion, or those with multiple seizure types and developmental delay are particularly likely to require multiple drugs. There are currently no clear guidelines for rational polypharmacy, but in most cases the initial combination therapy is with two of the three first-line drugs, i.e., carbamazepine, phenytoin, and valproic acid. If these drugs are unsuccessful, then the addition of a newer drug such as lamotrigine or gabapentin is indicated. Patients with myoclonic seizures resistant to valproic acid may benefit from the addition of clonazepam, and those with absence seizures may respond to a combination of valproic acid and ethosuximide. The same principles concerning the monitoring of therapeutic response, toxicity, and serum levels for monotherapy apply to polypharmacy, and potential drug interactions need to be recognized. If there is no improvement, a third drug can be added while the first two are maintained. If there is a response, the least effective of the first two drugs should be gradually withdrawn.

Surgical Treatment of Refractory Epilepsy Twenty percent of patients with epilepsy are resistant to medical therapy despite efforts to find an effective combination of antiepileptic drugs. For some, surgery can be extremely effective in substantially reducing seizure frequency and even providing complete seizure control. Understanding the potential value of surgery is especially important when, at the time of diagnosis, a patient has an epilepsy syndrome that is considered likely to be drug-resistant. Rather than submitting the patient to years of unsuccessful medical therapy and the associated psychosocial trauma of ongoing seizures, the patient should have an efficient but relatively brief attempt at medical therapy and then be referred for surgical evaluation.

The most common surgical procedure for patients with temporal lobe epilepsy involves resection of the anteromedial temporal lobe (temporal lobectomy) or a more limited removal of the underlying hippocampus and amygdala. Focal seizures arising from extratemporal regions may be suppressed by a focal neocortical resection or precise removal of an identified lesion (lesionectomy). When the cortical region cannot be removed, multiple subpial transection, which disrupts intracortical connections, is sometimes used to prevent seizure spread. Hemispherectomy or multilobar resection is useful for some patients with severe seizures due to hemispheric abnormalities such as hemimegaloencephaly or other dysplastic abnormalities, and corpus callosotomy has been shown to be effective for disabling tonic or atonic seizures, usually when they are part of a mixed-seizure syndrome (e.g., Lennox-Gastaut syndrome).

Presurgical evaluation is designed to identify the functional and structural basis of the patient's seizure disorder. Inpatient video-EEG monitoring is used to define the anatomic location of the seizure focus and to correlate the abnormal electrophysiologic activity with behavioral manifestations of the seizure. Routine scalp or scalp-sphenoidal recordings are usually sufficient for localization, and advances in neuroimaging have made the use of invasive electrophysiologic monitoring such as implanted depth electrodes or subdural electrodes much less common. A high-resolution MRI scan is routinely used to identify structural lesions. Functional imaging studies such as SPECT and PET are adjunctive tests that may help verify the localization of an apparent epileptogenic region with an anatomic abnormality. Once the presumed location of the seizure onset is identified, additional studies, including neuropsychological testing and the intracarotid amobarbital test (Wada's test) may be used to assess language and memory localization and to determine the possible functional consequences of surgical removal of the epileptogenic region. In some cases, the exact extent of the resection to be undertaken is determined by performing cortical mapping at the time of the surgical procedure. This involves electrophysiologic recordings and cortical stimulation in the awake patient to identify the extent of epileptiform disturbances and the function of cortical regions in question.

Advances in presurgical evaluation and microsurgical techniques have led to a steady increase in the success of epilepsy surgery. Clinically significant complications of surgery are less than 5 percent, and the use of functional mapping procedures has markedly reduced the neurologic sequelae due to removal or sectioning of brain tissue. For example, about 70 percent of patients treated with temporal lobectomy will become seizure-free, and another 15 to 25 percent will have at least a 90 percent reduction in seizure frequency. Marked improvement is also usually seen in patients treated with hemispherectomy for catastrophic seizure disorders due to large hemispheric abnormalities. Postoperatively, patients generally need to remain on antiepileptic drug therapy, but the marked reduction of seizures following surgery can have a dramatic, beneficial effect on their quality of life.

STATUS EPILEPTICUS Status epilepticus refers to continuous seizures or repetitive, discrete seizures with impaired consciousness in the interictal period. The duration of seizure activity sufficient to meet the definition of status epilepticus has traditionally been specified as 15 to 30 min. However, a more practical definition is to consider status epilepticus as a situation in which the duration of seizures prompts the acute use of anticonvulsant therapy, typically when seizures last beyond 5 min.

Status epilepticus is an emergency, since cardiorespiratory dysfunction, hyperthermia, and metabolic derangements can develop as a consequence of prolonged seizures, and these can lead to irreversible neuronal injury after approximately 2 h. Furthermore, CNS injury can occur even when the patient is paralyzed with neuromuscular blockade but continues to have electrographic seizures. The most common causes of status epilepticus are anticonvulsant withdrawal or noncompliance, metabolic disturbances, drug toxicity, CNS infection, CNS tumors, refractory epilepsy, and head trauma.

Generalized status epilepticus is obvious when the patient is having overt convulsions. However, after 30 to 45 min of uninterrupted seizures, the signs may become increasingly subtle. Patients may have mild clonic movements of only the fingers, or fine, rapid movements of the eyes. There may be paroxysmal episodes of tachycardia, hypertension, and pupillary dilation. In such cases, the EEG may be the only method of establishing the diagnosis. Thus, if the patient stops having overt seizures, yet remains comatose, an EEG should be performed to rule out ongoing status epilepticus.

The first step in the management of a patient in status epilepticus is to attend to any acute cardiorespiratory problems or hyperthermia, perform a brief medical and neurologic examination, establish venous access, and send samples for laboratory studies aimed at identifying metabolic abnormalities. Anticonvulsant therapy should then begin without delay; a suggested treatment approach is shown in Fig. 365-3.

BEYOND SEIZURES: OTHER MANAGEMENT ISSUES

Interictal Behavior The adverse effects of epilepsy often go beyond the occurrence of clinical seizures, and the extent of these effects depends largely upon the etiology of the seizure disorder, the degree to which the seizures are controlled, and the presence of side effects from antiepileptic therapy. Many patients with epilepsy are completely normal between seizures and able to live highly successful and productive lives. In contrast, patients with seizures secondary to developmental abnormalities or acquired brain injury may have impaired cognitive function and other neurologic deficits. Frequent interictal EEG abnormalities have been shown to be associated with subtle dysfunction of memory and attention. Patients with many seizures, especially those emanating from the temporal lobe, often note an impairment of short-term memory that may progress over time.

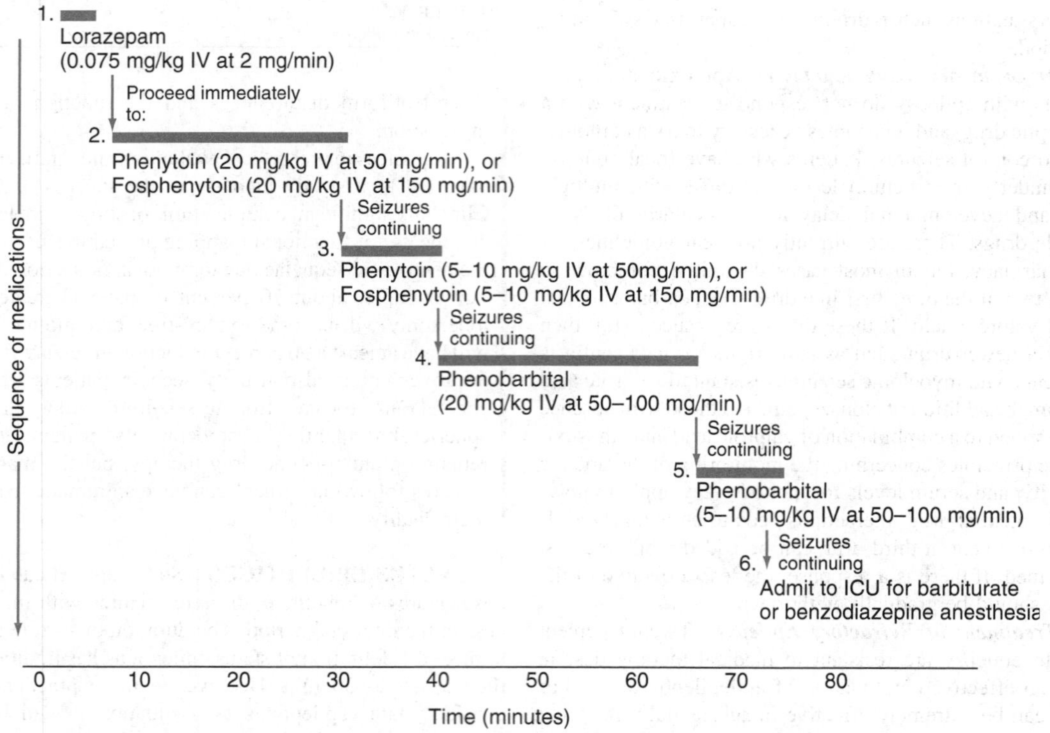

FIGURE 365-3 Pharmacologic treatment of generalized tonic-clonic status epilepticus in adults.

Patients with epilepsy are at risk of developing a variety of psychiatric problems including depression, anxiety, and psychosis. This risk varies considerably depending on many factors, including the etiology, frequency, and severity of seizures and the patient's age and previous history. Depression occurs in approximately 20 percent of patients, and the incidence of suicide is higher in epileptic patients than in the general population. Depression should be treated through counseling or antidepressant medication. The selective serotonin reuptake inhibitors typically have no effect on seizures, while the tricyclic antidepressants may lower the seizure threshold. Anxiety can appear as a manifestation of a seizure, and anxious or psychotic behavior can sometimes be observed as part of a postictal delirium. Interictal psychosis is a rare phenomenon that typically occurs after a period of increased seizure frequency. There is usually a brief lucid interval lasting up to a week, followed by days to weeks of agitated, psychotic behavior. The psychosis will usually resolve spontaneously but may require treatment with antipsychotic or anxiolytic medications.

There is ongoing controversy as to whether some patients with epilepsy (especially partial-complex epilepsy) have a stereotypical "interictal personality." The predominant view is that the unusual or abnormal personality traits observed in such patients are, in most cases, not due to epilepsy but result from an underlying structural brain lesion, the effects of antiepileptic drugs, or psychosocial factors.

Psychosocial Issues There continues to be a cultural stigma about epilepsy, although it is slowly declining in societies with effective health education programs. Because of this stigma, many patients with epilepsy harbor fears, such as the fear of becoming mentally retarded or dying during a seizure. These issues need to be carefully addressed by educating the patient about epilepsy and by ensuring that family members, teachers, fellow employees, and other associates are equally well informed. The Epilepsy Foundation of America (1-800-EFA-1000) is a patient advocacy organization and a useful source of educational material.

Employment and Driving Many patients with epilepsy face difficulty in obtaining or maintaining employment, even when their seizures are well controlled. Federal and state legislation is designed to prevent employers from discriminating against patients with epilepsy, and patients should be encouraged to understand and claim their legal rights. Patients in these circumstances also benefit greatly from the assistance of health providers who act as strong patient advocates.

Loss of driving privileges is one of the most disruptive social consequences of epilepsy. Physicians should be very clear about local regulations concerning driving and epilepsy, since the laws vary considerably among states and countries. In all cases, it is the physician's responsibility to warn patients of the danger imposed on themselves and others while driving if their seizures are uncontrolled (unless the seizures are not associated with impairment of consciousness or motor control). In general, most states allow patients to drive after a seizure-free interval (on or off medications) between 6 months and 2 years.

SPECIAL ISSUES RELATED TO WOMEN AND EPILEPSY

Catamenial Epilepsy Some women experience a marked increase in seizure frequency around the time of menses. This is thought to reflect either the effects of estrogen and progesterone on neuronal excitability or changes in antiepileptic drug levels due to altered protein binding. Acetazolamide (250 to 500 mg/d) has been found effective as adjunctive therapy when started 7 to 10 days prior to the onset of menses and continued until bleeding stops. Some patients may benefit from increases in antiepileptic drug dosages during this time or from control of the menstrual cycle through the use of oral contraceptives.

Pregnancy Most women with epilepsy who become pregnant will have an uncomplicated gestation and deliver a normal baby. However, epilepsy poses some important risks to a pregnancy. Seizure frequency during pregnancy will remain unchanged in approximately 50 percent of women, increase in 30 percent, and decrease in 20 percent. Changes in seizure frequency are attributed to endocrine effects on the CNS, variations in antiepileptic drug pharmacokinetics (such as acceleration of hepatic drug metabolism or effects on plasma protein binding), and changes in medication compliance. It is therefore useful to see patients at more frequent intervals during pregnancy and monitor serum antiepileptic drug levels. Measurement of the unbound drug concentrations may be useful if there is an increase in seizure frequency or worsening of side effects of antiepileptic drugs.

The overall incidence of fetal abnormalities in children born to mothers with epilepsy is 5 to 6 percent, compared to 2 to 3 percent in healthy women. Part of the higher incidence is due to teratogenic effects of antiepileptic drugs, and the risk increases with the number of medications used (e.g., 10 percent risk of malformations with three drugs). A syndrome comprising facial dysmorphism, cleft lip, cleft palate, cardiac defects, digital hypoplasia, and nail dysplasia was originally ascribed to phenytoin therapy, but it is now known to occur with other first-line antiepileptic drugs (i.e., carbamazepine and valproic acid) as well. Also, valproic acid and carbamazepine are associated with a 1 to 2 percent incidence of neural tube defects compared with a baseline of 0.5 to 1 percent. Little is currently known about the safety of newer drugs.

Since the potential harm of uncontrolled seizures on the mother and fetus is considered greater than the teratogenic effects of antiepileptic drugs, it is currently recommended that pregnant women be maintained on effective drug therapy. When possible, it seems prudent to have the patient on monotherapy at the lowest effective dose, especially during the first trimester. Patients should also take folate (1–4 mg), since the antifolate effects of anticonvulsants are thought to play a role in the development of neural tube defects, although the benefits of this treatment remain unproved in this setting.

Enzyme-inducing drugs such as phenytoin, phenobarbital, and primidone cause a transient and reversible deficiency of vitamin K–dependent clotting factors in approximately 50 percent of newborn infants. Although neonatal hemorrhage is uncommon, the mother should be treated with oral vitamin K (20 mg daily) in the last 2 weeks of pregnancy, and the infant should receive an intramuscular injection of vitamin K (1 mg) at birth.

Breast Feeding Antiepileptic medications are excreted into breast milk to a variable degree. The ratio of drug concentration in breast milk relative to serum is approximately 80 percent for ethosuximide, 40 to 60 percent for phenobarbital, 40 percent for carbamazepine, 15 percent for phenytoin, and 5 percent for valproic acid. Given the overall benefits of breast feeding and the lack of evidence for long-term harm to the infant by being exposed to antiepileptic drugs, mothers with epilepsy should not be discouraged from breast feeding. This should be reconsidered, however, if there is any evidence of drug effects on the infant, such as lethargy or poor feeding.

BIBLIOGRAPHY

Brodie MJ, Dichter MA: Antiepileptic drugs. N Engl J Med 334:168, 1996

Engel J Jr: *Seizures and Epilepsy.* Philadelphia, FA Davis, 1989

Engel J Jr: Surgery for seizures. N Engl J Med 334:647, 1996

Hopkins A, Shorvon S, Cascino G (eds): *Epilepsy,* 2d ed. London, Chapman and Hall Medical, 1995

McNamara JO: Cellular and molecular basis of epilepsy. J Neuroscience 14:3413, 1994

Noebels JL: Targeting epilepsy genes. Neuron 16:241, 1996

Sackellares JC, Berent S (eds): *Psychological Disturbances in Epilepsy.* Boston, Butterworth-Heinemann, 1996

Steinlein OK et al: A missense mutation in the neuronal nicotinic acetylcholine receptor alpha 4 subunit is associated with autosomal dominant nocturnal frontal lobe epilepsy. Nat Genet 11:201, 1995

Wyllie E (ed): *The Treatment of Epilepsy,* 2d ed. Baltimore, Williams & Wilkins, 1997

366 CEREBROVASCULAR DISEASES

J. Donald Easton, Stephen L. Hauser, Joseph B. Martin

Cerebrovascular diseases predominate in the middle and late years of life. They cause approximately 200,000 deaths in the United States each year as well as considerable neurologic disability. The incidence of stroke increases with age and affects many people in their "golden years," a rapidly growing segment of the population. These diseases cause either ischemia-infarction or intracranial hemorrhage (Table 366-1). Ischemia and infarction constitute 85 to 90 percent of the total group in western countries, while 10 to 15 percent are intracranial hemorrhages; hemorrhage constitutes a larger percentage in Asia. The morbidity and mortality from cerebrovascular diseases has been diminishing in recent years, due largely to better recognition and treatment of the underlying arterial and cardiac diseases, including hypertension.

Table 366-1

Classification of Cerebrovascular Diseases

Cerebral Ischemia-Infarction	Intracranial Hemorrhage
Thrombotic occlusion	Intracerebral
Embolic occlusion	Subarachnoid
Artery-to-artery	Subdural (usually traumatic)
Cardiogenic	Epidural (traumatic)

Most cerebrovascular diseases present as the abrupt onset of a focal neurologic deficit. The deficit may remain fixed, or it may rapidly improve or progressively worsen. It is this abrupt onset of a nonconvulsive and focal neurologic deficit that is referred to as a stroke, a cerebrovascular accident (CVA), or apoplexy. In the United States, the term *stroke* is generally used specifically to mean cerebral infarction. It is always preferable to use the more precise terms: cerebral ischemia, cerebral infarction, intracerebral hemorrhage, etc.

Cerebral ischemia is caused by a reduction in blood flow that lasts for several seconds or a few minutes. If the cessation of flow lasts for more than a few minutes, *infarction* of brain tissue results. A *generalized* reduction in cerebral blood flow due to systemic hypotension (e.g., cardiac arrhythmia, myocardial infarction, or hemorrhagic shock) usually produces syncope (see Chap. 20), infarction in the border zones between the major cerebral artery distributions, or widespread brain necrosis, depending on the duration of hypotension. *Focal* ischemia or infarction, on the other hand, is usually caused by disease in the cerebral vessels themselves or by emboli from a proximal arterial source or the heart.

Intracranial hemorrhage may occur into the brain parenchyma, the subarachnoid space, or the subdural or epidural space. Subdural and epidural hematomas are usually the result of trauma, not cerebrovascular disease, and are discussed elsewhere (see Chap. 374). The majority of intracerebral hemorrhages are associated with hypertension; spontaneous hemorrhage, arteriovenous malformation (AVM), and bleeding into a neoplasm are less common causes. Subarachnoid hemorrhage (SAH) is usually due to a ruptured saccular aneurysm or, less commonly, an AVM. Sometimes, no source for the hemorrhage can be found.

GENERAL PATHOPHYSIOLOGY OF CEREBRAL ISCHEMIA AND INFARCTION Within 10 s after cerebral blood flow ceases, metabolic failure of brain tissue occurs. The electroencephalogram shows slowing of electrical activity, and the brain dysfunction becomes clinically manifest. If the circulation is immediately restored, there is abrupt and complete recovery of function. If the perfusion abnormality persists for a few minutes, neuronal injury results. With restoration of flow, the recovery of function takes several minutes or hours and may be incomplete. In addition, during the circulatory failure, the blood elements may sludge, the capillary endothelium may swell, and the blood flow may not reestablish itself, even when the primary cause of the flow failure is corrected (the "no-reflow" phenomenon). More prolonged periods of ischemia result in frank tissue necrosis. Cerebral edema follows and progresses over the subsequent 2 to 4 days. If the region of infarction is large, the edema may produce considerable mass effect with all of its attendant consequences (see Chap. 374).

The commonest causes of cerebral ischemia and infarction are *atherosclerosis with thromboembolism* and *cardiogenic embolism* (see Table 366-2).

ATHEROSCLEROTIC ISCHEMIA AND INFARCTION

Ischemic cerebrovascular disease is divided into two broad categories: thrombotic and embolic. The precise cause of ischemia often cannot be determined. When it occurs in elderly patients, especially those with

Table 366-2

Causes of Ischemic Stroke

Thrombosis
- Atherosclerosis
- Vasculitis
  - Collagen vascular diseases: temporal (giant cell) arteritis, polyarteritis nodosa, Wegener's granulomatosis, Takayasu's arteritis, syphilis
  - Meningitis: tuberculosis, fungi, syphilis, bacteria, herpes zoster
- Arterial dissection: carotid, vertebral, intracranial arteries at the base of the brain (spontaneous or traumatic)
- Hematologic disorders: polycythemia, thrombocytosis, thrombotic thrombocytopenic purpura, disseminated intravascular coagulation, dysproteinemias, hemoglobinopathies (sickle cell disease)
- Miscellaneous: cocaine, amphetamines, moyamoya disease, fibromuscular dysplasia, Binswanger's disease

Embolism
- Cardiac source: see Table 366-4
- Atherothrombotic arterial source: bifurcation of common carotid artery, carotid siphon, distal vertebral artery, aortic arch
- Unknown source: may be associated with a hypercoagulable state secondary to systemic disease, carcinoma (especially pancreatic), eclampsia, oral contraceptives, lupus, factor C or S deficiency, factor V mutation, etc.

Vasoconstriction
- Vasospasm: cerebral vasospasm following subarachnoid hemorrhage
- Reversible cerebral vasoconstriction: idiopathic, migraine, eclampsia, trauma

Venous
- Dehydration, pericranial infection, postpartum and postoperative states, systemic cancer

other manifestations of atherosclerosis, the term *atherothrombotic*, or *atherothromboembolic*, is used when it seems likely that atherosclerosis-induced thrombosis occurred and the thrombus then lysed or embolized distally and fragmented. Thrombotic strokes occur without warning symptoms in 80 to 90 percent of patients. Between 10 and 20 percent are heralded by one or more transient ischemic attacks (TIAs). Thrombotic strokes often present with stuttering, fluctuating symptoms that worsen over several minutes or hours. Embolic strokes usually present with a neurologic deficit that is maximum at onset.

PATHOPHYSIOLOGY Atherosclerosis is usually maximal at arterial bifurcations, and it commonly affects the origin of the internal carotid artery in the neck and the origin of major and minor arterial branches inside the head. Although individuals with the most atherosclerosis are the ones most likely to have a stroke, the correlation is only approximate. Some patients with large infarcts have minimal disease, and others have no ischemic symptoms but one or more major cerebral artery occlusions. The integrity of the extracranial and intracranial collateral circulation, the state of systemic cardiovascular function, and, possibly, hematologic factors play a role in determining whether a given atherosclerotic lesion will cause ischemia or infarction.

Atherosclerotic plaques can cause an arterial stenosis that produces a *hemodynamic obstruction to flow*. If this regional decrease in cerebral blood flow falls below a critical level, it will cause a transient or permanent ischemic event. In addition, *artery-to-artery emboli* appear to be an important cause of retinal and hemispheric ischemia and infarction. When an atherosclerotic plaque on the arterial wall ulcerates, the necrotic material (cholesterol crystals, calcified connective tissue debris, etc.) may dislodge and serve as emboli or may provide a surface on which aggregation of platelets and coagulation of fibrin occurs. The resulting fibrin clot also may dislodge into the arterial circulation, or it may enlarge and produce thrombotic occlusion of the artery. The contribution of vasospasm in cerebral ischemia or infarction is not known. *Lacunar infarcts* are small infarcts in the deep white matter of the hemisphere or brainstem. They are usually due to hypertension-induced lipohyalinosis or arteriosclerosis of small penetrating arteries, rather than to large artery atherosclerosis or cardioembolism.

Although the exact cause of ischemia or infarction in a given patient with atherosclerosis is not always known, the primary abnormality is clearly atherosclerosis with its complicating lesion, the fibrous plaque. The plaque contains various degrees of degeneration that may result in *stenosis* or *ulceration*, with subsequent *thrombosis* or *embolization*.

Frequently, however, cerebral infarction occurs in elderly people without an obvious source. The term *cerebral atherothromboembolism of unknown source* is used. Some authors presume the event is embolic when a sudden stroke occurs and cardiac monitoring, echocardiography, and carotid, vertebral, and transcranial Doppler studies fail to disclose an obvious source. About 40 percent of ischemic strokes fall into this category, one of the most perplexing problems in cerebrovascular disease. Sophisticated analyses of activity of the hemostatic system, blood coagulation factors, and autoantibodies show that patients with hypercoagulable states are prone to cerebral embolism. Hypercoagulability may be induced by antiphospholipid antibodies, factor V mutations, protein C deficiency, protein S deficiency, antithrombin III deficiency, systemic neoplasm, and traumatic and surgical tissue injury. These pathophysiologic conditions undoubtedly contribute to cerebral atherothromboembolism, but their importance is uncertain.

CEREBRAL EDEMA At the cellular level, several types of brain edema have been described: cytotoxic, vasogenic, interstitial and ischemic. The various types differ in cause, time of development, region of the brain affected, and response to various methods of prevention or treatment.

Cytotoxic edema is caused by swelling of glia, neurons, and endothelial cells and begins within minutes after an insult such as hypoxia. Because of failure of the energy-dependent sodium pump in the cellular membrane, sodium accumulates intracellularly, and water moves from the extracellular to the intracellular space to maintain osmotic equilibrium. Cytotoxic edema affects predominantly the gray matter.

Vasogenic edema, the most common type of brain edema, results from increased permeability of the capillary endothelial cells; the white matter is primarily affected. Breakdown in the blood-brain barrier allows movement of proteins from the intravascular space through the capillary wall into the extracellular space. This same mechanism permits the leakage of contrast agents which cause computed tomography (CT) and magnetic resonance (MR) brain scans to "contrast enhance." This is in contrast to cytotoxic edema, in which the permeability of the brain vasculature is unaltered.

Interstitial edema is seen in hydrocephalus when outflow of cerebrospinal fluid (CSF) is obstructed and intraventricular pressure increases. The result is movement of sodium and water across the ventricular wall into the paraventricular space.

Cerebral ischemia results initially in cytotoxic, and subsequently vasogenic, edema. The pathophysiology is sufficiently characteristic that many authors propose that it be designated "ischemic edema." Within several minutes of the onset of ischemia, cells begin to swell, particularly those surrounding capillaries. Swelling is more prominent in astrocytes than in neurons. If circulation is restored quickly, these changes may be reversible. If it is not, a series of additional changes is superimposed on the initial cytotoxic edema. As swelling occurs in the glia surrounding the capillaries and in the endothelial cells, the capillary lumen is progressively compressed. Thus, even if circulation is reestablished, the compressed capillaries may not perfuse. This no-reflow phenomenon may contribute to further development of ischemia and necrosis.

In the vasogenic phase, permeability of capillary membranes increases. Some studies indicate that this increased permeability is due both to enhanced pinocytotic transport across the endothelium and to disruption of the tight junctions between endothelial cells. Permeability of the blood-brain barrier tends to increase after return of flow to the ischemic area, and the rapidity with which edema occurs depends on the duration and severity of the ischemia. As in other forms of vasogenic edema, white matter is predominantly affected.

Necrosis develops simultaneously with cytotoxic and vasogenic edema. Glia and neurons are particularly susceptible to necrosis, whereas the capillary endothelium is relatively resistant. With degradation of these cellular elements, osmolarity increases, and this promotes the further accumulation of water.

Ischemic edema reaches its maximum 2 to 4 days after infarction and subsides by the end of the second week. If the infarction and edema are not sufficient to cause death, inflammatory changes and phagocytosis occur in the area of necrosis during the days and weeks that follow, resulting in removal of necrotic debris and resolution of the edema. It is possible that edema itself contributes to ischemia and, thus, to a progressively enlarging infarct.

CELLULAR MECHANISMS OF ISCHEMIC NEURONAL INJURY Experimental studies of focal ischemic stroke support the concept that there is a core of severe ischemia, the "ischemic core," that is surrounded by an area of reduced perfusion, the "ischemic penumbra," where cells may remain viable for several hours. Within the ischemic core, failure of glucose and oxygen delivery leads to rapid depletion of energy stores and cell death. The etiology of progressive cell injury and death in the ischemic penumbra has been clarified to some extent. *Acidosis* results from the anaerobic metabolism of glucose into lactic acid; blood normally carries far more glucose than oxygen, hence in hypoxic tissue glucose delivery may still be adequate to support anaerobic metabolism. *Excitotoxicity* results from excessive release and impaired (astrocyte) uptake of the excitatory neurotransmitter glutamate (Chap. 380). Glutamate activates the *N*-methyl-D-aspartate (NMDA) receptor, increasing levels of intracellular calcium leading to activation of proteases, lipases, and other mediators of cell injury; it also results in membrane depolarization and spreading depression (Chap. 365), further increasing energy demands and levels of extracellular glutamate. *Free radicals* (partially reduced oxygen species) are generated that damage DNA, proteins, and fatty acids. Induction of *programmed cell death* (*apoptosis*) may also occur as a mechanism of cell death. Neuroprotective drugs that interfere with these processes of cell injury represent important potential new therapies for cerebrovascular disease.

CLINICAL MANIFESTATIONS OF ISCHEMIC STROKE The typical ischemic stroke presents with the abrupt onset of a focal neurologic deficit and is characterized clinically by its mode of onset and subsequent course. A *TIA* is manifested by a neurologic deficit lasting less than 24 h (usually 5 to 20 min). It is often referred to as a mini-, warning, or transient stroke, because it quickly resolves but often portends an impending stroke. The deficit is focal and confined to an area of the brain perfused by a specific artery. This definition of TIA excludes presyncope and syncope, which are due to diffuse, not focal, cerebral ischemia.

The presumed pathophysiologic mechanisms responsible for TIAs are: (1) low flow in an artery due to tight stenosis or occlusion, or (2) embolism from the heart or proximal arterial or atherosclerotic plaque debris or thrombus. Any obstructive vascular process in the extra- or intracranial arteries can cause a low-flow TIA if collateral flow to the potentially ischemic brain is also impaired (see Figs. 366-1 and 366-2), and can lead to arterial thrombosis. If symptoms or signs persist beyond 24 h, infarction has occurred. Even symptoms that last only an hour or so may be associated with infarction.

Because presyncope and syncope often are confused with focal cerebral ischemia, it is necessary to distinguish these conditions and their pathophysiology from focal cerebral ischemia (see Chap. 20).

Reversible ischemic neurologic deficit is an infrequently used term that defines an ischemic event in which the deficit usually recovers over a 24- to 72-h period, but which may take as long as 1 week to resolve.

A *completed stroke*, or cerebral infarction, of the thrombotic type is generally nonhemorrhagic. It typically evolves to its maximal deficit within a few hours. Often, the patient awakens with a completed deficit. A completed stroke is sometimes heralded by one or more TIAs in the preceding days, weeks, or months. This is most likely when a tight arterial stenosis is causative. Ischemic strokes are produced by the same pathophysiologic mechanism responsible for TIAs. Thrombosis complicating atherosclerosis accounts for most thrombotic strokes, and embolism from proximal atherosclerosis or the heart accounts for most embolic strokes.

In *progressing stroke*, or stroke-in-evolution, the focal ischemia worsens from minute to minute or hour to hour. There are usually stepwise incremental increases in neurologic deficit occurring over a several-hour period. In the posterior circulation, however, the stroke may evolve over 2, 3, or even several days. Many clinicians include *crescendo TIA*, i.e., the sudden onset of a series of ischemic attacks over a few hours or days, in this category. While there may be several pathogenic mechanisms producing a progressing stroke, one such appears to be a thrombus-in-evolution, with a thrombus extending from its site of origin in a primary artery and progressively obliterating collateral branches, thereby interfering with anastomotic vessels.

The symptoms and signs of an ischemic stroke vary depending on the location of the occlusion and the extent of the spared collateral flow. The hallmark presentation is the abrupt onset of a hemiparesis in an individual in the atherosclerotic age group. Virtually any symptom of brain dysfunction may occur, however. Symptoms and signs of carotid system disease most commonly affect the distribution of the middle cerebral artery, and the patient may exhibit a contralateral hemiparesis, hemisensory deficit, and hemianopia. If the dominant

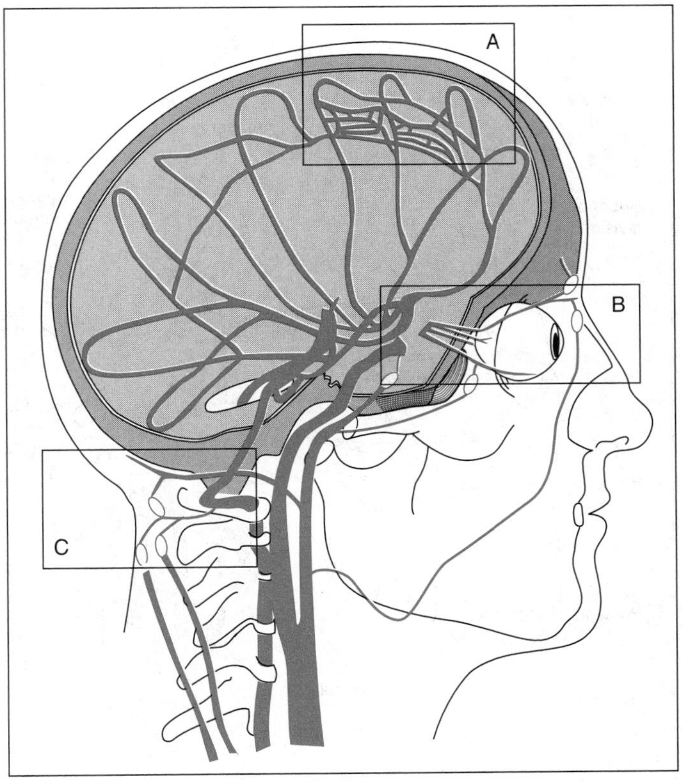

FIGURE 366-1 Arrangement of the major arteries of the right side carrying blood from the heart to the brain. Also shown are vessels of collateral circulation that may modify the effects of cerebral ischemia (*A, B, C*). Not shown is the circle of Willis, which also provides a source for collateral circulation. *A.* The anastomotic channels between the distal branches of the anterior and middle cerebral artery, termed border-zone or watershed anastomotic channels. Note that they also occur between the posterior and middle cerebral arteries and the anterior and posterior cerebral arteries. *B.* Anastomotic channels occurring through the orbit between branches of the external carotid artery and ophthalmic branch of the internal carotid artery. *C.* Wholly extracranial anastomotic channels between the muscular branches of the ascending cervical arteries and muscular branches of the occipital artery that anastomose with the distal vertebral artery. Note that the occipital artery arises from the external carotid artery, thereby allowing reconstitution of flow in the vertebral from the carotid circulation. *(Courtesy of CM Fisher, M.D.)*

hemisphere is involved, there is usually some degree of aphasia. Lacunar infarction is common in the distribution of the lenticulostriate branches of the middle cerebral artery.

Either the anterior (carotid) or posterior (vertebrobasilar) circulation may be involved. The following descriptions apply to ischemia and infarction in specific arteries due to atherothrombosis, although similar syndromes may occur with other types of arterial pathology, after embolic stroke, and occasionally after intracerebral hemorrhage.

Atherothrombotic Disease of the Internal Carotid Artery and Its Branches *Pathophysiology* The origin of the internal carotid artery is the most common site of atherosclerosis and superimposed atherothrombosis that leads to TIA or stroke. Less often, disease at the siphon (S-shaped portion of the internal carotid artery in the cavernous sinus) or in the proximal segment of the middle or anterior cerebral arteries may be responsible. These intracranial sites predominate in African Americans and Asians. Rarely, the origin of the common carotid artery may be the site.

INTERNAL CAROTID ARTERY Atherosclerosis in the proximal internal carotid artery is usually most severe in the first 2 cm and arises from the posterior wall, often extending downward into the common carotid artery. Atherosclerosis at this site is often heralded by a TIA or minor stroke, presumably caused by embolism or, less frequently, low flow.

Emboli arising from a stenotic or ulcerated atherosclerotic plaque at the origin of the internal carotid artery may cause occlusion of the ophthalmic artery, the proximal middle cerebral artery or one of its branches, or, less often, the anterior cerebral artery. Small platelet emboli that occlude the ophthalmic artery branches cause transient monocular blindness (TMB; amaurosis fugax). Larger emboli composed of platelet-fibrin thrombus may occlude the primary and secondary branches of the middle cerebral territory (e.g., lenticular nucleus, deep white matter, and cortical surface). In some instances, only deep infarction occurs because collateral flow through leptomeningeal artery collaterals over the cortical surface are sufficient (see Fig. 366-1*A*). Large emboli may partially occlude a major artery or may migrate or lyse and disperse, causing a neurologic deficit that fluctuates (stroke-in-evolution) or resolves.

In some patients, an ulcerated plaque may be the only lesion in the carotid bifurcation, but more often there is an accompanying stenosis of 50 percent or more. A nonstenotic or slightly stenotic carotid lesion in conjunction with a stroke or a single prolonged TIA suggests the heart as the source of the embolus. Atheromatous lesions at the origin of the great vessels in the aortic arch also can produce cerebral emboli that cause ischemia or infarction, but the incidence of this mechanism is thought to be low.

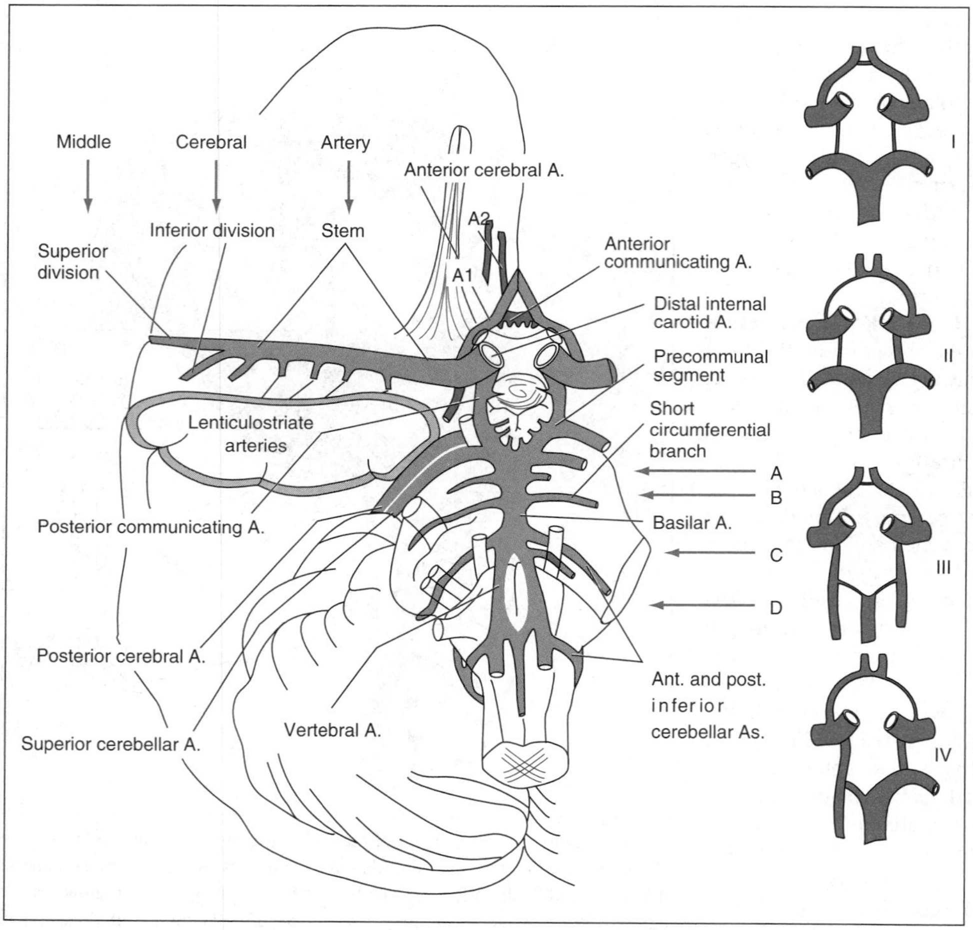

FIGURE 366-2 Diagram of the brainstem, cerebellum, inferior right frontal lobe, and transected temporal lobe. Principal branches of the vertebral basilar arterial system are pictured. The stem of the middle cerebral artery with its small, deep penetrating lenticulostriate arteries and the circle of Willis with its small, deep penetrating branches are shown. Roman numerals I, II, III, and IV represent some of the possible variations of the circle of Willis due to atresia of one or more of its arterial components. *A*, *B*, *C*, and *D* arrows point to the four cross sections of the brainstem diagrammed below (*D*, Fig. 366-7; *A*, Fig. 366-8; *B*, Fig. 366-9; *C*, Fig. 366-10). Although typical vascular syndromes of the pons and medulla have been designated by the shaded areas in Figs. 366-7 to 366-10, the shading is approximate only. Great variability in infarct size and location occurs when the basilar or vertebral arteries or one of their penetrating branches becomes occluded. This variability is because of variation in arterial anatomic location and available collateral circulation. Thus the stroke syndromes produced are often atypical, incomplete, or merge with one another. *(Courtesy of CM Fisher, M.D.)*

When *low flow* is the mechanism, there is presumably inadequate collateral flow through the circle of Willis.

INTRACRANIAL INTERNAL CAROTID ARTERY Although less common, lesions in the siphon can cause strokes and TIAs whose pathophysiologic and clinical features duplicate those discussed above.

MIDDLE CEREBRAL ARTERY In contrast to the internal carotid artery, occlusion of the proximal middle cerebral artery or one of its major branches is usually due to embolus (artery-to-artery, cardiac, or of unknown source) rather than intracranial atherothrombosis, though intracranial atherothrombosis is common in African Americans and Asians. Symptomatic atheroma are rarely located distal to the first bifurcation of the middle cerebral artery. Because the circle of Willis is proximal to the origin of the middle cerebral artery, collateral blood flow to the distal middle cerebral artery territory must arise from small cortical surface border zones and anastomotic (leptomeningeal) arteries of the anterior and posterior cerebral arteries.

ANTERIOR CEREBRAL ARTERY Atheromatous deposits in the proximal segment of the anterior cerebral artery rarely cause symptoms because the effects of occlusion are usually mitigated by collateral circulation through the anterior communicating artery. If the anterior communicating artery is congenitally atretic, or the atheromatous lesion occurs distal in the anterior cerebral artery, TIAs and stroke may occur.

Clinical manifestations *MIDDLE CEREBRAL ARTERY* The cortical branches of the middle cerebral artery supply the lateral surface of the hemisphere except for (1) the frontal pole and a strip along the superomedial border of the frontal lobe supplied by the anterior cerebral artery, and (2) the lower temporal and occipital pole convolutions, which are in the territory of the posterior cerebral artery (Fig. 366-3).

The proximal middle cerebral artery gives rise to penetrating branches that supply the putamen, outer globus pallidus, posterior limb of the internal capsule above the plane of the upper border of the globus pallidus, the adjacent corona radiata, and the body and upper and lateral head of the caudate nucleus. In the sylvian fissure, the middle cerebral artery in most patients divides into *superior* and *inferior* divisions. Branches of the inferior division supply the inferior parietal and temporal cortex, and those from the superior division supply the frontal and superior parietal cortex (Fig. 366-4). There is considerable variability in the parietal lobe supply between the two divisions, with about two-thirds of individuals having an inferior division that supplies regions above the angular gyrus.

If the entire middle cerebral artery is occluded at its origin, blocking both its penetrating and cortical branches, and the distal collaterals are limited, the clinical findings are contralateral hemiplegia, hemianesthesia, and homonymous hemianopia. When the dominant hemisphere is involved, global aphasia is present also, and when the nondominant hemisphere is affected, apractagnosia and anosognosia are found (see Fig. 366-4). Dysarthria also may occur.

Complete middle cerebral territory syndromes occur most often when a thromboembolus occludes the stem of the artery. Cortical collateral blood flow and differing arterial configurations are probably responsible for the development of partial middle cerebral artery syndromes. Partial middle cerebral territory syndromes also may be due to an embolus that enters the proximal middle cerebral artery without complete occlusion or that lyses and moves distally. Symptoms and signs may fluctuate in such patients (stroke-in-evolution).

Partial syndromes resulting from embolic occlusion of a single branch include hand, or arm and hand, weakness alone (brachial syndrome) or facial weakness with motor aphasia, with or without arm weakness (frontal opercular syndrome). A combination of sensory disturbance, motor weakness, and motor aphasia suggests that an embolus has occluded the proximal superior division and infarcted large portions of the frontal and parietal cortices (see Fig. 366-4). If Wernicke's aphasia occurs without weakness, the inferior division of the middle cerebral artery supplying the posterior part (temporal cortex) of the dominant hemisphere is probably involved (see Fig. 366-4). Jargon speech and an inability to comprehend written and spoken language are prominent features, often accompanied by a contralateral, homonymous inferior quadrantanopia or hemianopia (see Chap. 25). Hemineglect or spatial agnosia without weakness indicates that the inferior division of the middle cerebral artery in the nondominant hemisphere is involved.

ANTERIOR CEREBRAL ARTERY The anterior cerebral artery is divided into two segments: the precommunal (A1) circle of Willis, or stem, which connects the internal carotid artery to the anterior communicating artery, and the postcommunal (A2) segment distal to the anterior communicating artery (see Fig. 366-2). The A1 segment of the anterior cerebral artery gives rise to several deep penetrating branches that supply the anterior limb of the internal capsule, the anterior perforate substance, amygdala, anterior hypothalamus, and the inferior part of the head of the caudate nucleus (see Fig. 366-3).

Occlusion of the proximal anterior cerebral artery is usually well tolerated because of collateral flow. Occlusion of a single A2 segment results in the contralateral symptoms noted in the legend of Fig. 366-5. If both A2 segments arise from a single anterior cerebral stem (contralateral A1 segment atresia), the occlusion affects both hemispheres. Profound abulia (a delay in verbal and motor response) and bilateral pyramidal signs with paraparesis and urinary incontinence result.

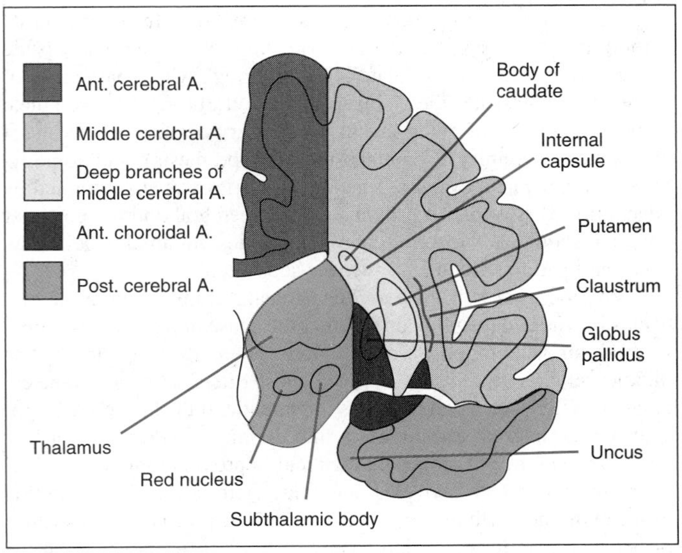

FIGURE 366-3 Diagram of a cerebral hemisphere in coronal section showing the territories of the major cerebral vessels. *(Courtesy of C M Fisher, M.D.)*

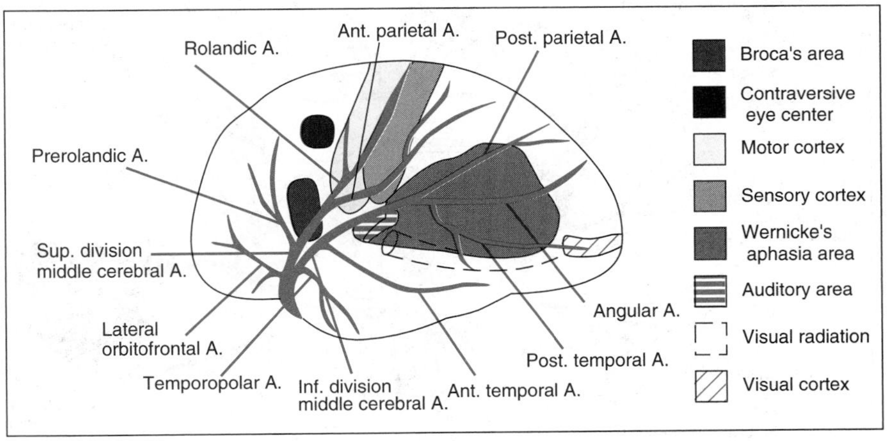

FIGURE 366-4 Diagram of a cerebral hemisphere, lateral aspect, showing the branches and distribution of the middle cerebral artery and the principal regions of cerebral localization. Note the bifurcation of the middle cerebral artery into a superior and inferior division. *(Courtesy of CM Fisher, M.D.)*

Signs and symptoms: *Structures involved*

Paralysis of the contralateral face, arm, and leg; sensory impairment over the same area (pinprick, cotton touch, vibration, position, two-point discrimination, stereognosis, tactile localization, barognosis, cutaneographia): *Somatic motor area for face and arm and the fibers descending from the leg area to enter the corona radiata and corresponding somatic sensory system*

Motor aphasia: *Motor speech area of the dominant hemisphere*

Central aphasia, word deafness, anomia, jargon speech, sensory agraphia, acalculia, alexia, finger agnosia, right-left confusion (the last four comprise the Gerstmann syndrome): *Central, suprasylvian speech area and parietooccipital cortex of the dominant hemisphere*

Conduction aphasia: *Central speech area (parietal operculum)*

Apractognosia of the minor hemisphere (amorphosynthesis), anosognosia, hemiasomatognosia, unilateral neglect, agnosia for the left half of external space, dressing "apraxia," constructional "apraxia," distortion of visual coordinates, inaccurate localization in the half field, impaired ability to judge distance, upside-down reading, visual illusions (e.g., it may appear that another person walks through a table): *Nondominant parietal lobe (area corresponding to speech area in dominant hemisphere); loss of topographic memory is usually due to a nondominant lesion, occasionally to a dominant one*

Homonymous hemianopia (often homonymous inferior quadrantonopia): *Optic radiation deep to second temporal convolution*

Paralysis of conjugate gaze to the opposite side: *Frontal contraversive field or projecting fibers*

ANTERIOR CHOROIDAL ARTERY This artery arises from the internal carotid artery and supplies the posterior limb of the internal capsule and the white matter posterolateral to it, through which pass some of the geniculocalcarine fibers (Figs. 366-3 and 366-6). The complete clinical syndrome of anterior choroidal artery occlusion consists of contralateral hemiplegia, hemianesthesia (hypesthesia), and homonymous hemianopia. However, because this territory is also supplied by penetrating vessels of the proximal middle cerebral and the posterior communicating and posterior choroidal arteries, minimal deficits may occur and patients frequently recover substantially.

INTERNAL CAROTID ARTERY The clinical picture of internal carotid occlusion varies depending on whether the cause of ischemia is propagated thrombus, embolism, or low flow. The cortex supplied by the middle cerebral territory is affected most often. With a competent circle of Willis, occlusion can be asymptomatic. If the thrombus propagates up the internal carotid artery into the middle cerebral artery, or embolizes into it, symptoms are identical to proximal middle cerebral artery occlusion (see above). Sometimes there is massive infarction of the entire deep white matter and cortical surface. When the origins of both the anterior and middle cerebral arteries are occluded at the top of the carotid artery, abulia or stupor occurs with hemiplegia, hemianesthesia, and aphasia or anosognosia. When the posterior cerebral artery arises from the internal carotid artery (an unusual configuration called a *fetal posterior cerebral artery*), it also may become occluded and give rise to symptoms referable to its peripheral territory (see Figs. 366-5 and 366-6).

In addition to supplying the ipsilateral brain, the internal carotid artery perfuses the optic nerve and retina via the ophthalmic artery. In about 25 percent of symptomatic internal carotid disease, recurrent TMB warns of the lesion. Patients typically describe a shade that sweeps down or up across the field of vision. They also may complain that their vision was blurred in that eye or that the upper or lower half of vision disappeared. In most cases, these symptoms last only a few minutes. Rarely, ophthalmic or central retinal artery ischemia or infarction occurs at the time of cerebral TIA or infarction.

The natural history of asymptomatic atherosclerotic lesions of the carotid bifurcation that produce a bruit is uncertain. There is evidence that the tighter the stenotic lesion, the more likely symptoms are to occur over time. Patients with tightly stenotic lesions that are hemodynamically significant (approximately 75 percent diameter stenosis) are at higher risk of embolic stroke. Although such patients have reduced flow in the distal internal carotid artery, they remain asymptomatic because of adequate collateral flow in the circle of Willis. However, thrombus may form in the low-flow carotid and cause occlusion or artery-to-artery embolism.

A high-pitched prolonged carotid bruit fading into diastole is often associated with such tightly stenotic lesions. As the stenosis grows tighter and flow distal to the stenosis becomes reduced, the bruit becomes fainter and may disappear when occlusion is imminent.

COMMON CAROTID ARTERY All the neurologic symptoms and signs of internal carotid occlusion also may be present with occlusion of the common carotid artery. Bilateral common carotid artery occlusion at their origin may occur in Takayasu's arteritis or the aortic arch syndrome (see Chap. 319). An incomplete aortic arch syndrome has been reported consisting of various combinations of carotid, subclavian, or innominate stenosis or occlusion (see below).

Atherothrombotic Disease of the Vertebrobasilar–Posterior Cerebral Artery System The two vertebral arteries join to form the basilar artery at the pontomedullary junction. The basilar artery divides into two posterior cerebral arteries in the interpeduncular fossa (see Fig. 366-2). Each of these major arteries gives rise to long and short circumferential branches and to smaller deep penetrating branches that supply the cerebellum, medulla, pons, midbrain, subthalamus, thalamus, hippocampus, and medial temporal and occipital lobes. Atherosclerosis has a predilection for the origin and the distal segments of the vertebral arteries, the proximal basilar artery, and the origin of the major and minor branches of the vertebral, basilar, and posterior cerebral arteries. Predictably, atheromatous disease at each site produces its own clinical syndromes.

Pathophysiology *POSTERIOR CEREBRAL ARTERY* In 75 percent of patients, both posterior cerebral arteries arise from the bifurcation of the basilar artery; in 20 percent, one or the other comes from the ipsilateral internal carotid artery; in 5 percent, both come from the ipsilateral internal carotid artery via the

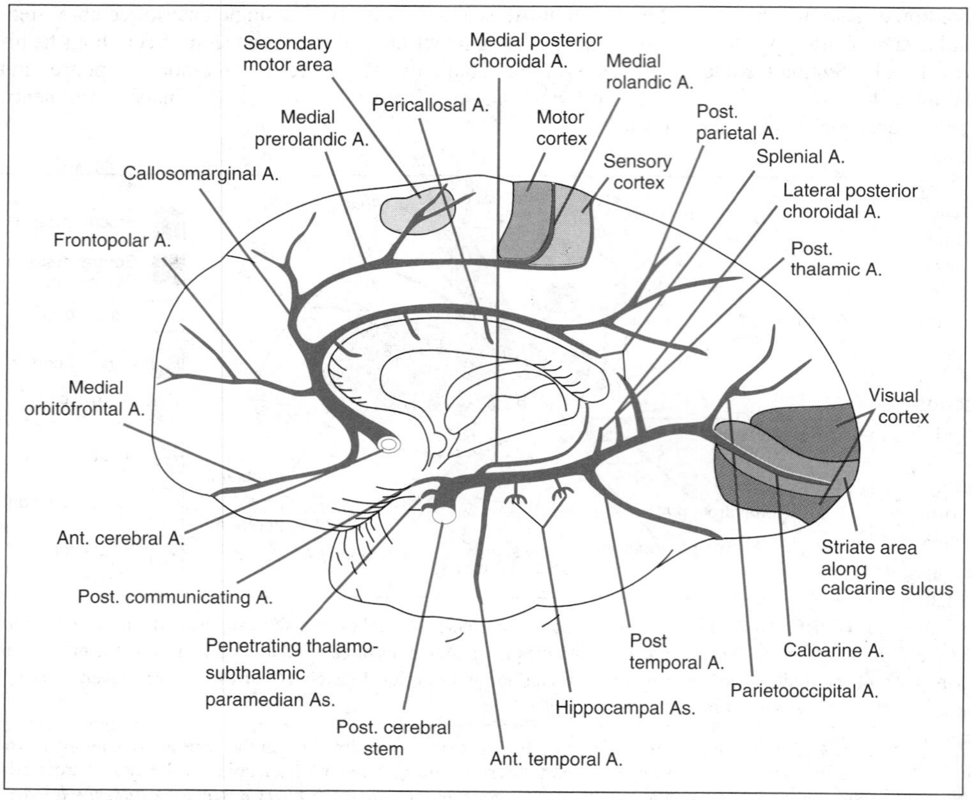

FIGURE 366-5 Diagram of a cerebral hemisphere, medial aspect, showing the branches and distribution of the anterior cerebral artery and the principal regions of cerebral localization. *(Courtesy of CM Fisher, M.D.)*

Signs and symptoms: *Structures involved*

Paralysis of opposite foot and leg: *Motor leg area*
A lesser degree of paresis of opposite arm: *Arm area of cortex or fibers descending to corona radiata*
Cortical sensory loss over toes, foot, and leg: *Sensory area for foot and leg*
Urinary incontinence: *Sensorimotor area in paracentral lobule*
Contralateral grasp reflex, sucking reflex, gegenhalten (paratonic rigidity): *Medial surface of the posterior frontal lobe (?) supplemental motor area*
Abulia (akinetic mutism), slowness, delay, intermittent interruption, lack of spontaneity, whispering, reflex distraction to sights and sounds: *Uncertain localization—probably cingulate gyrus and medial inferior portion of frontal, parietal, and temporal lobes*
Impairment of gait and stance (gait apraxia): *Frontal cortex near leg motor area*
Dyspraxia of left limbs, tactile aphasia in left limbs: *Corpus callosum*

posterior communicating arteries. The precommunal segment (mesencephalic portion) of the true posterior cerebral artery is atretic in such cases.

Atheroma formation at the top of the basilar artery or along the precommunal segment of the posterior cerebral artery may cause symptoms by narrowing one or more of the small brainstem-penetrating branches (see Figs. 366-2 and 366-6) that supply the middle cerebral peduncles, the substantia nigra, red nucleus, oculomotor nuclei, midbrain reticular formation, subthalamic nucleus, decussation of the superior cerebellar peduncles, the medial longitudinal fasciculus, and the medial lemniscus. The artery of Percheron (the posterior thalamosubthalamoparamedian artery) is a single artery that arises from either the right or the left precommunal segment of the posterior cerebral artery. It divides in the subthalamus to supply the inferomedial and anterior portions of the thalamus and subthalamus bilaterally. The thalamogeniculate branches, which also originate from the precommunal portion of the posterior cerebral artery, supply the dorsal, dorsomedial, anterior and inferior thalamus, and the medial geniculate body. The medial posterior choroidal artery supplies the superior dorsomedial and dorsoanterior thalamus and the medial geniculate body in addition to the tela choroidea of the third ventricle. The lateral posterior choroidal artery supplies the choroid plexus of the lateral ventricle.

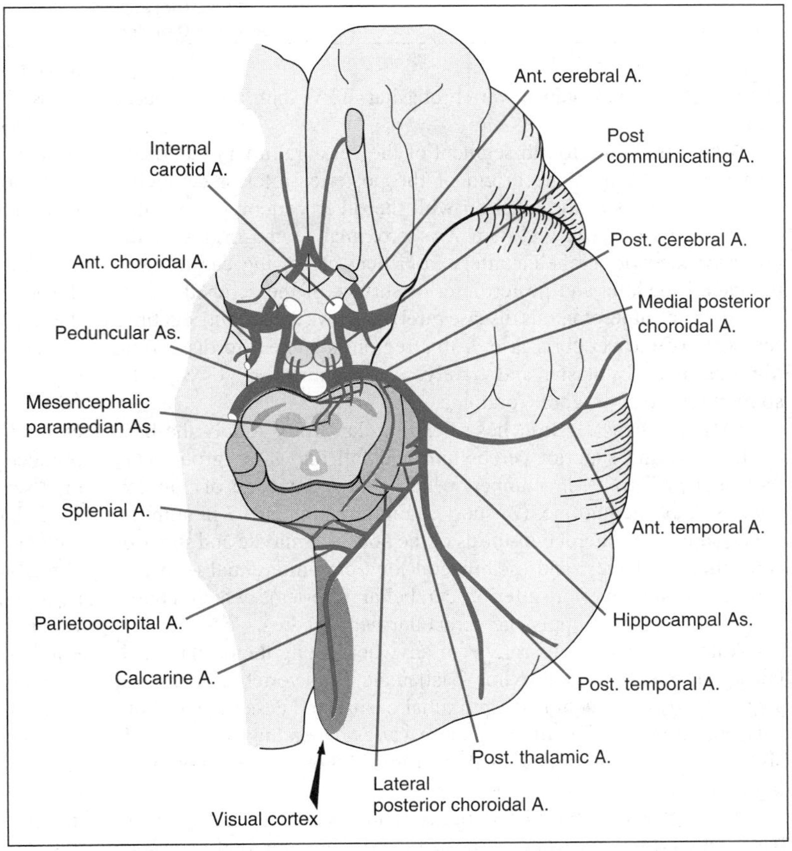

FIGURE 366-6 Inferior aspect of the brain with the branches and distribution of the posterior cerebral artery and the principal anatomic structures shown. *(Courtesy of CM Fisher, M.D.)*

Signs and symptoms: *Structures involved*

1. Peripheral territory (see also Fig. 366-5)
   - Homonymous hemianopia (often upper quadrantic): *Calcarine cortex or optic radiation nearby*
   - Bilateral homonymous hemianopia, cortical blindness, awareness or denial of blindness; tactile naming, achromatopsia (color blindness), failure to see to-and-fro movements, inability to perceive objects not centrally located, apraxia of ocular movements, inability to count or enumerate objects, tendency to run into things that the patient sees and tries to avoid: *Bilateral occipital lobe with possibly the parietal lobe involved*
   - Verbal dyslexia without agraphia, color anomia: *Dominant calcarine lesion and posterior part of corpus callosum*
   - Memory defect: *Hippocampal lesion bilaterally or on the dominant side only*
   - Topographic disorientation and prosopagnosia: *Usually with lesions of nondominant, calcarine, and lingual gyrus*
   - Simultagnosia, hemivisual neglect: *Dominant visual cortex, contralateral hemisphere*
   - Unformed visual hallucinations, peduncular hallucinosis, metamorphopsia, teleopsia, illusory visual spread, paliopsia, distortion of outlines, central photophobia: *Calcarine cortex*
   - Complex hallucinations: *Usually nondominant hemisphere*
2. Central territory
   - Thalamic syndrome: sensory loss (all modalities), spontaneous pain and dysesthesias, choreoathetosis, intention tremor, spasms of hand, mild hemiparesis: *Posteroventral nucleus of thalamus; involvement of the adjacent subthalamus body or its afferent tracts*
   - Thalamoperforate syndrome: crossed cerebellar ataxia with ipsilateral third nerve palsy (Claude's syndrome): *Dentatothalamic tract and issuing third nerve*
   - Weber's syndrome: third nerve palsy and contralateral hemiplegia: *Third nerve and cerebral peduncle*
   - Contralateral hemiplegia: *Cerebral peduncle*
   - Paralysis or paresis of vertical eye movement, skew deviation, sluggish pupillary responses to light, slight miosis and ptosis (retraction nystagmus and "tucking" of the eyelids may be associated): *Supranuclear fibers to third nerve, interstitial nucleus of Cajal, nucleus of Darkschewitsch, and posterior commissure*
   - Contralateral rhythmic, ataxic action tremor; rhythmic postural or "holding" tremor (rubral tremor): *Dentatothalamic tract (?)*

Atheroma in the posterior cerebral artery distal to the junction with the posterior communicating artery (see Fig. 366-6) may occlude small circumferential branches that course around the midbrain to supply the lateral part of the cerebral peduncles, medial lemniscus, tegmentum of the midbrain, superior colliculi, lateral geniculate body and posterolateral nucleus of the thalamus, choroid plexus, and hippocampus. On the rare occasions when atheroma occur more distally in the posterior cerebral artery, occlusion may produce ischemia in the inferomedial temporal lobe, parahippocampal and hippocampal gyri, and occipital lobe—including the calcarine cortex and the visual association areas 18 and 19.

VERTEBRAL AND POSTERIOR INFERIOR CEREBELLAR ARTERIES Each *vertebral artery* arises from the respective subclavian artery and divides into four anatomic segments. The first extends from its origin to its entrance into the sixth or fifth transverse vertebral foramen. The second transverses the vertebral foramina from C6 to C2. The third passes through the transverse foramen and circles around the arch of the atlas to pierce the dura at the foramen magnum. The fourth segment courses upward to join the other vertebral artery to form the basilar artery; only the fourth segment gives rise to branches that supply the brainstem and cerebellum. The *posterior inferior cerebellar artery* in its proximal segment supplies the lateral medulla and, in its distal branches, the inferior surface of the cerebellum. Anastomotic channels exist among the ascending cervical arteries, the thyrocervical arteries, the occipital artery (branch of the external carotid artery), and the second segment of the vertebral artery.

Atherothrombotic lesions have a predilection for the first and fourth segments of the vertebral artery. Although the atheromatous narrowing in the first segment may be significant, it seldom produces strokes. Collateral flow from the contralateral vertebral artery or the ascending cervical and ascending thyrocervical or occipital arteries is usually sufficient to prevent ischemia. When one vertebral artery is atretic and an atherothrombotic lesion threatens the origin of the other, the collateral circulation is through the ascending cervical artery, the thyrocervical artery, and the occipital artery or by retrograde flow down the basilar artery via the posterior communicating artery (see Figs. 366-2 and 366-6). In this setting, low flow in the vertebrobasilar system and TIAs may occur. In addition, thrombosis in the proximal basilar or distal vertebral system may occur. If the subclavian is blocked proximal to the origin of the vertebral artery, exercise of the left arm may draw blood in a retrograde fashion down the vertebral artery to the distal subclavian artery. This "subclavian steal" may cause vertebrobasilar TIAs but rarely causes stroke.

Atheroma in the fourth segment of the vertebral artery can occur proximal or distal to the origin of the posterior inferior cerebellar artery, as well as at the junction with the other vertebral artery that forms the basilar artery. When it is proximal to the origin of the posterior inferior cerebellar artery, a critical narrowing can threaten the lateral medulla and posteroinferior surface of the cerebellum.

Although atheromatous disease rarely narrows the second and third segments of the vertebral artery, this region is subject to dissection, fibromuscular dysplasia, and, rarely, encroachment by osteophytic spurs within the vertebral foramina.

BASILAR ARTERY Branches of the basilar artery supply the base of the pons and superior cerebellum and fall into three groups: (1) paramedian, 7 to 10 in number, which supply a wedge of pons on either side of the midline; (2) short circumferential, 5 to 7 in number, which supply the lateral two-thirds of the pons and middle and superior cerebellar peduncles; and (3) bilateral long circumferential (superior cerebellar and anterior inferior cerebellar arteries), which course around the pons to supply the cerebellar hemispheres.

Atheromatous lesions can occur anywhere along the basilar trunk but are most often in the proximal basilar and distal vertebral segments. Typically, lesions occlude the proximal basilar and either one or both vertebral arteries. The clinical picture varies depending on the availability of retrograde collateral flow from the posterior communicating arteries.

Although atherothrombosis occasionally occludes the top of the basilar artery, emboli from the heart or proximal vertebral or basilar segments are more common.

Clinical manifestations POSTERIOR CEREBRAL ARTERY The site of atheromas and the degree of narrowing determine the clinical syndrome. Although factors of collateral circulation or serum viscosity may play a role in some cases, embolic occlusion is the usual cause of stroke in this vascular territory. Two syndromes are commonly observed: (1) midbrain, subthalamic, and thalamic signs, which are due to disease of the precommunal segment or of its penetrating branches; and (2) cortical temporal and occipital lobe syndromes, due to occlusion of the postcommunal segment.

1. *Proximal precommunal syndromes (central territory).* If the proximal posterior cerebral artery is occluded, infarction usually occurs in the ipsilateral subthalamus, medial thalamus and midbrain (Fig. 366-6). Hemiplegia secondary to infarction of the cerebral peduncle may occur. Involvement of the red nucleus and/or dentatorubrothalamic tract can produce contralateral ataxia. A third nerve palsy may be combined with contralateral ataxia (Claude's syndrome) or with contralateral hemiplegia (Weber's syndrome). If the subthalamic nucleus is involved, contralateral hemiballismus may occur. Occlusion of the artery of Percheron produces paresis of upward gaze and drowsiness and is often associated with abulia. Extensive infarction in the midbrain and subthalamus occurring with bilateral proximal posterior cerebral artery occlusion is usually secondary to embolism. Coma, bilateral pyramidal signs, and decerebrate rigidity occur in this setting.

Atheromatous occlusion of the penetrating branches of thalamic and thalamogeniculate arteries produces less extensive thalamic and thalamocapsular lacunar syndromes. The *thalamic syndrome of Déjérine and Roussy* is the best known. Its main feature is contralateral hemisensory loss of both superficial sensation (pain and temperature) and deep sensation (touch and proprioception). Occasionally, it may affect only pain and temperature or vibration and joint position sense. After a few weeks or months, an agonizing, searing or burning pain may develop in the affected areas. It is persistent and responds poorly to analgesics. Anticonvulsants or tricyclic drugs may be beneficial. If the posterior limb of the internal capsule is involved, hemiparesis may accompany the hemisensory syndrome. Other associated motor signs include hemiballismus, choreoathetosis, intention tremor, incoordination, and posturing of the hand and arm, particularly while walking.

2. *Postcommunal syndromes (peripheral or cortical territory)* (see also Fig. 366-6). Occlusion of the posterior cerebral artery causes infarction of the cortical surface of the medial temporal and occipital lobes. Contralateral homonymous hemianopia is the usual manifestation. Occasionally, only the upper quadrant of visual field is involved. If the visual association areas are spared and only the calcarine cortex is involved, the patient is aware of visual defects. Medial temporal lobe and hippocampal involvement may cause an acute disturbance in memory, particularly if it occurs in the dominant hemisphere. The defect usually clears because memory has bilateral representation. If the dominant hemisphere is affected and the infarct extends to involve the splenium of the corpus callosum, the patient may demonstrate alexia without agraphia (see Chap. 25). Visual agnosia for faces, objects, mathematical symbols, and colors and anomia with paraphasic errors (amnestic aphasia) also may occur in this setting, even without callosal involvement. Occlusion of the posterior cerebral artery can produce *peduncular hallucinosis* (visual hallucinations of brightly colored scenes and objects).

Bilateral infarction in the distal posterior cerebral arteries produces cortical blindness. The patient is often unaware of the blindness. The clinical clue to the site is a finding of normal pupillary reaction to light. Tiny islands of vision may persist, and the patient reports that vision fluctuates as images are captured in the preserved portions. Rarely, only peripheral vision is lost and central vision is spared, resulting in "gun-barrel" vision. A constellation of symptoms termed *Balint's syndrome* can occur with unilateral or bilateral visual association area lesions (see Chap. 25). It includes optic ataxia, (inability to visually guide limb movements), ocular ataxia (inability to direct eyes to a precise point in the visual field), inability to enumerate objects in a picture or extract meaning from a picture, and inability to avoid objects seen in one's path. Balint's syndrome is seen most often with bilateral infarctions secondary to low flow in the "watershed" between the distal posterior and middle cerebral artery territories, as occurs after cardiac arrest. Embolic occlusion of the top of the basilar artery can produce a clinical picture that includes any or all of the central or peripheral territory symptoms; its hallmark is suddenness of onset and bilaterality of symptoms, including ptosis and somnolence (see above in the discussion of the artery of Percheron).

VERTEBRAL AND POSTERIOR INFERIOR CEREBELLAR ARTERIES TIAs resulting from vertebral artery insufficiency cause dizziness or vertigo, numbness of the ipsilateral face and contralateral limbs, diplopia, hoarseness, dysarthria, and dysphagia. Hemiparesis is rare.

When *infarction* ensues, it most often affects the lateral medulla with or without the posteroinferior cerebellum (Wallenberg's syndrome). Its features are listed in Fig. 366-7. In the majority of cases, the syndrome occurs after ipsilateral vertebral artery occlusion; in the remainder, it results from posterior inferior cerebellar artery occlusion. Atherothrombotic occlusion of the medullary penetrating branches of the vertebral or posterior inferior cerebellar artery results in partial syndromes of the ipsilateral medulla.

Rarely, a medial medullary syndrome occurs in which the pyramid becomes infarcted, causing a contralateral hemiparesis of the arm and leg and sparing the face. If the medial lemniscus and emerging hypoglossal nerve fibers are involved, contralateral loss of joint position sense and ipsilateral tongue weakness occur.

Cerebellar infarction with edema formation can lead to *sudden respiratory arrest* due to raised intracranial pressure in the posterior fossa. Drowsiness, Babinski signs, dysarthria, and bifacial weakness may be absent, or present only briefly, before respiratory arrest ensues. Gait unsteadiness, dizziness, nausea, and vomiting may be the only early symptoms and signs of this impending complication.

BASILAR ARTERY Because the brainstem contains many structures in close proximity, a diversity of clinical syndromes may emerge with ischemia. Involvement of the corticospinal tracts, corticobulbar tracts, and cranial nerve nuclei causes the common symptoms and signs (Figs. 366-8 to 366-10).

Unfortunately, the symptoms of transient ischemia or infarction in the territory of the basilar artery often do not indicate whether the basilar artery itself or one of its branches is diseased, yet the distinction has important implications for therapy. The picture of complete basilar insufficiency, however, is easy to recognize. A combination of bilateral long tract signs (sensory and motor) with signs of cranial nerve and cerebellar dysfunction suggests this diagnosis. A "locked-in" state of awake quadriplegia, bifacial and oropharyngeal palsy, and paralysis of horizontal gaze occurs with bilateral basis pontis infarction. Stupor indicates dysfunction of the reticular activating system, and when combined with third cranial nerve palsies it suggests devastating upper midbrain infarction (see Chap. 24). The therapeutic goal, however, is to recognize *impending* basilar occlusion before devastating infarction occurs. A series of TIAs or a slowly progressive, fluctuating stroke are extremely significant as they often herald an atherothrombotic occlusion of the distal vertebral or proximal basilar artery.

TIAs in the proximal basilar distribution may produce dizziness (often described by patients as "swimming," "swaying," "moving," "unsteadiness" or "light-headedness"). Other symptoms that warn of basilar thrombosis include diplopia, dysarthria, facial or circumoral numbness, and hemisensory symptoms. In general, symptoms of basilar branch TIAs affect one side of the brainstem, whereas symptoms of basilar artery TIAs usually affect both sides, though a "herald" hemiparesis has been emphasized as an initial symptom of basilar occlusion. Most often TIAs, whether due to impending occlusion of the basilar artery or a basilar branch, are short-lived (5 to 30 min) and repetitive, occurring several times a day. The pattern suggests intermittent reduction of flow.

Atherothrombotic occlusion of the basilar artery with *brainstem infarction* usually causes *bilateral* brainstem signs. For example, gaze paresis or internuclear ophthalmoplegia may be associated with ipsilateral hemiparesis. By contrast, occlusion of a branch of the basilar artery usually causes *unilateral* symptoms and signs involving motor, sensory, and cranial nerves.

SUPERIOR CEREBELLAR ARTERY Occlusion of this artery results in severe ipsilateral cerebellar ataxia, nausea and vomiting, dysarthria, and contralateral loss of pain and temperature sensation over the extremities, body, and face. Partial deafness, ataxic tremor of the ipsilateral upper extremity, Horner's syndrome, and palatal myoclonus may also occur. Partial syndromes are common (Fig. 366-8).

ANTERIOR INFERIOR CEREBELLAR ARTERY Occlusion produces variable degrees of infarction because the size of this artery and the territory it supplies vary inversely with those of the posterior inferior cerebellar artery. The principal symptoms include ipsilateral deafness, facial weakness, true vertigo (whirling dizziness), nausea and vomiting, nystagmus, tinnitus, cerebellar ataxia, Horner's syndrome, and paresis of conjugate lateral gaze. The opposite side of the body loses pain and temperature sensation. An occlusion close to the origin of the artery may cause corticospinal tract signs (see Fig. 366-10).

Occlusion of one of the five to seven short circumferential branches of the basilar artery affects the lateral two-thirds of the pons and middle or superior cerebellar peduncle, whereas occlusion of one of the 7 to 10 paramedian branches affects a wedge-shaped area on either side of the medial pons (Figs. 366-8 to 366-10).

Lacunar Disease The term *lacunar infarction* refers to infarction following atherothrombotic or lipohyalinotic occlusion of one of the penetrating branches of the circle of Willis, middle cerebral artery stem, or vertebral and basilar arteries.

Pathophysiology The middle cerebral artery stem, the arteries comprising the circle of Willis (A1 segment of the anterior cerebral artery, anterior and posterior communicating arteries, precommunal segment of the posterior cerebral arteries), and the basilar and vertebral

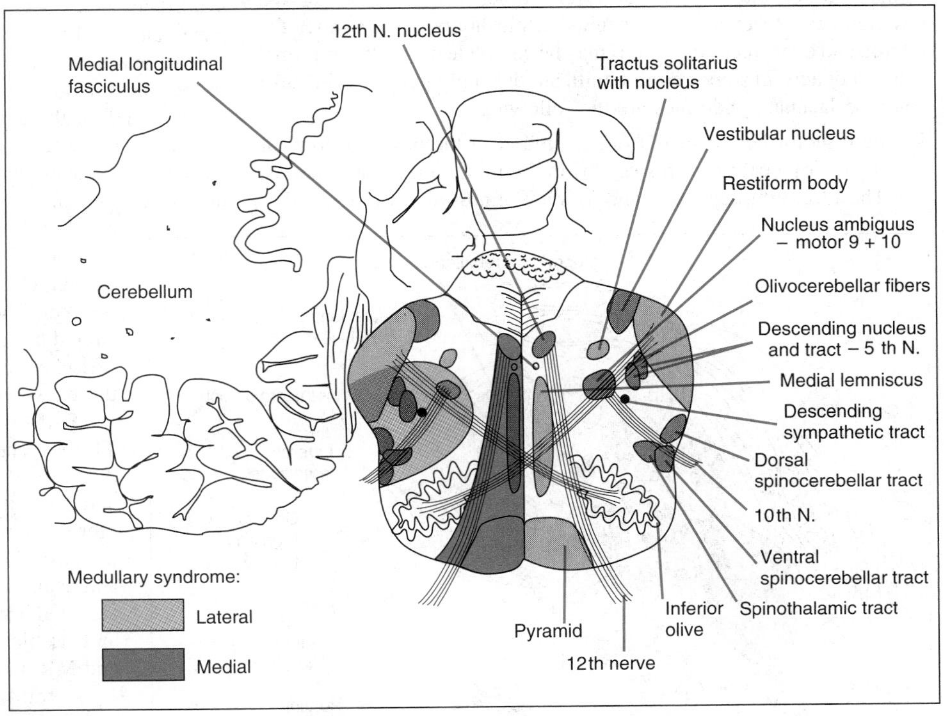

FIGURE 366-7 *(Courtesy of CM Fisher, M.D.)*

Signs and symptoms: *Structures involved*

1. Medial medullary syndrome (occlusion of vertebral artery or of branch of vertebral or lower basilar artery)
   On side of lesion
   Paralysis with atrophy of half the tongue: *Ipsilateral twelfth nerve*
   On side opposite lesion
   Paralysis of arm and leg sparing face; impaired tactile and proprioceptive sense over half the body: *Contralateral pyramidal tract and medial lemniscus*
2. Lateral medullary syndrome (occlusion of any of five vessels may be responsible—vertebral, posterior inferior cerebellar, superior, middle, or inferior lateral medullary arteries)
   On side of lesion
   Pain, numbness, impaired sensation over half the face: *Descending tract and nucleus fifth nerve*
   Ataxia of limbs, falling to side of lesion: *Uncertain—restiform body, cerebellar hemisphere, cerebellar fibers, spinocerebellar tract (?)*
   Nystagmus, diplopia, oscillopsia, vertigo, nausea, vomiting: *Vestibular nucleus*
   Horner's syndrome (miosis, ptosis, decreased sweating): *Descending sympathetic tract*
   Dysphagia, hoarseness, paralysis of palate, paralysis of vocal cord, diminished gag reflex: *Issuing fibers ninth and tenth nerves*
   Loss of taste: *Nucleus and tractus solitarius*
   Numbness of ipsilateral arm, trunk, or leg: *Cuneate and gracile nuclei*
   On side opposite lesion
   Impaired pain and thermal sense over half the body, sometimes face: *Spinothalamic tract*
3. Total unilateral medullary syndrome (occlusion of vertebral artery): Combination of medial and lateral syndromes
4. Lateral pontomedullary syndrome (occlusion of vertebral artery): Combination of lateral medullary and lateral inferior pontine syndromes
5. Basilar artery syndrome (the syndrome of the lone vertebral artery is equivalent): A combination of the various brainstem syndromes plus those arising in the posterior cerebral artery distribution
   Bilateral long tract signs (sensory and motor; cerebellar and peripheral cranial nerve abnormalities): *Bilateral long tract; cerebellar and peripheral cranial nerves*
   Paralysis or weakness of all extremities, plus all bulbar musculature: *Corticobulbar and corticospinal tracts bilaterally*

arteries all give rise to 100- to 300-μm diameter branches that penetrate the deep gray and white matter of the cerebrum or brainstem (see Fig. 366-2). Each of these small branches can thrombose either by atherothrombotic disease at its origin or by the development of lipohyalinotic thickening. Thrombosis of these vessels causes small infarcts that are referred to as *lacunes*. They range in size from as small as 3 or 4 mm to 1 or 2 cm. Hypertension is the principal risk factor for such small-vessel disease. Lacunar infarcts cause approximately 20 percent of all strokes.

Clinical manifestations Lacunar infarcts cause recognizable stroke syndromes. Transient symptoms (lacunar TIAs) may herald a lacunar infarct; they may occur several times a day and last only a few minutes. Recovery often begins within hours or days after the infarct, and over weeks or months may be complete or result in minimal residual deficit. In some cases, significant disability persists. The most common lacunar syndromes are the following:

1. Pure motor hemiparesis from an infarct in the posterior limb of the internal capsule, crus cerebri in the midbrain, or basis pontis. The face, arm, leg, foot, and toes are almost always involved.
2. Pure sensory stroke from an infarct in the ventrolateral thalamus.
3. Ataxic hemiparesis from an infarct in the base of the pons.
4. Dysarthria and a clumsy hand or arm due to infarction in the base of the pons or in the genu of the internal capsule.
5. Pure motor hemiparesis with "motor aphasia" due to thrombotic occlusion of a lenticulostriate branch supplying the genu and anterior limb of the internal capsule and adjacent white matter of the corona radiata.

Syndromes resulting from occlusion of the penetrating arteries of the proximal posterior cerebral artery were discussed above. Syndromes resulting from occlusion of the penetrating arteries of the basilar artery (see Figs. 366-8 to 366-10) include ipsilateral ataxia and crural (leg) paresis, pure motor hemiparesis with horizontal gaze palsy, and hemiparesis with a contralateral sixth nerve palsy. Lower basilar branch syndromes include sudden internuclear ophthalmoplegia, horizontal gaze palsy, and appendicular cerebellar ataxia.

An anarthric pseudobulbar syndrome due to bilateral infarctions in the internal capsule can occur from disease in the lenticulostriate arteries. Before the advent of antihypertensive therapy, multiple lacunes often caused pseudobulbar palsy with emotional instability, a slowed abulic state, and bilateral pyramidal signs; this syndrome is now less common.

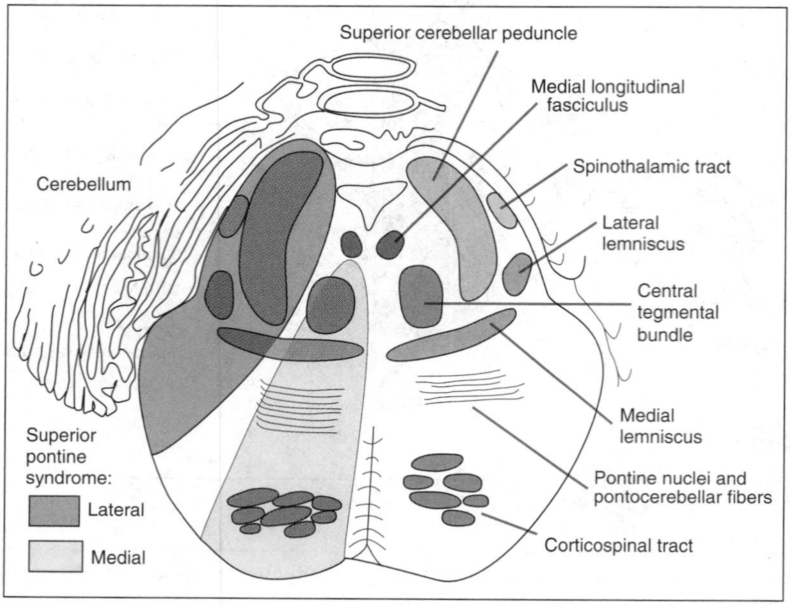

FIGURE 366-8 *(Courtesy of CM Fisher, M.D.)*
Signs and symptoms: *Structures involved*

1. Medial superior pontine syndrome (paramedian branches of upper basilar artery)
   - On side of lesion
     - Cerebellar ataxia (probably): *Superior and/or middle cerebellar peduncle*
     - Internuclear ophthalmoplegia: *Medial longitudinal fasciculus*
     - Myoclonic syndrome, palate, pharynx, vocal cords, respiratory apparatus, face, oculomotor apparatus, etc.: *Localization uncertain—central tegmental bundle (?), dentate projection (?), inferior olivary nucleus (?)*
   - On side opposite lesion
     - Paralysis of face, arm, and leg: *Corticobulbar and corticospinal tract*
     - Rarely touch, vibration, and position are affected: *Medial lemniscus*
2. Lateral superior pontine syndrome (syndrome of superior cerebellar artery)
   - On side of lesion
     - Ataxia of limbs and gait, falling to side of lesion: *Middle and superior cerebellar peduncles, superior surface of cerebellum, dentate nucleus*
     - Dizziness, nausea, vomiting; horizontal nystagmus: *Vestibular nucleus*
     - Paresis of conjugate gaze (ipsilateral): *Pontine contralateral gaze*
     - Skew deviation: *Uncertain*
     - Miosis, ptosis, decreased sweating over face (Horner's syndrome): *Descending sympathetic fibers*
     - Static tremor reported in one case: *Dentate nucleus (?), superior cerebellar peduncle (?)*
   - On side opposite lesion
     - Impaired pain and thermal sense on face, limbs, and trunk: *Spinothalamic tract*
     - Impaired touch, vibration, and position sense, more in leg than arm (there is a tendency to incongruity of pain and touch deficits): *Medial lemniscus (lateral portion)*

Aortic Atheromatous Disease Atherosclerotic disease of the ascending aorta is a potential source of cerebral emboli. One study found a strong, independent association between atherosclerotic disease of the aortic arch, demonstrated by transesophageal echocardiography, and the risk of ischemic stroke. The incidence and natural history of these lesions are uncertain.

LABORATORY AND IMAGING EVALUATION Therapy in ischemic stroke is aided by a precise diagnosis that determines the primary vascular pathology and the extent and location of the stroke. The clinical presentation and temporal profile of a stroke often suggest its cause. Accurate diagnosis is based largely on the history and examination, supplemented by judicious use of blood tests and imaging of the brain [CT and MR imaging (MRI)] and its blood vessels (arterial Doppler ultrasonography, and MR and x-ray angiography).

Careful auscultation for bruits of the carotid arteries and their extracranial branches may add supporting evidence for a diagnosis. Ancillary diagnostic studies generally should be used to confirm or exclude other conditions, rather than to search for evidence of every possible diagnosis. Chest x-rays, urinalysis, complete blood count, erythrocyte sedimentation rate, serum electrolytes, blood urea nitrogen, blood sugar, serologic tests for syphilis, serum lipid profile, serum uric acid, blood clotting studies, and thyroid function studies all may be helpful in detecting precipitating causes of vascular thrombosis or intracranial hemorrhage. An electrocardiogram (ECG) may demonstrate conduction abnormalities and arrhythmias or reveal evidence of recent myocardial infarction. A CT scan will often demonstrate an area of infarction and will confirm or exclude the presence of an intracerebral, subdural, or epidural hemorrhage or other mass lesion. Moreover, it may demonstrate large aneurysms and AVMs and subarachnoid or intraventricular blood. A lumbar puncture (LP) will confirm or exclude subarachnoid hemorrhage or meningitis due to syphilis or other chronic infections. An LP should not be performed on patients with intracranial mass lesions (Chap. 360).

Atherothrombotic Disease of the Internal Carotid Artery and its Branches Several diagnostic techniques are available for evaluating patients with carotid bruits, TIA, and stroke. Positive findings must be interpreted in the appropriate clinical context. For example, a carotid artery bruit in the neck or an ulcerated plaque at the origin of the internal carotid artery detected by ultrasonography or contrast angiography in a patient with dizzy spells or syncopal episodes is almost certainly an incidental finding. Inappropriate reliance on an isolated clinical finding (e.g., a bruit) or on a vascular abnormality detected in an ancillary study may result in incorrect diagnosis and inappropriate therapy.

Brain imaging (Figs. 366-11 and 362-3) Brain imaging is important in assessing the patient who has just experienced a TIA or stroke.

CT scans identify or exclude hemorrhage as the cause of stroke, and they identify extraparenchymal hemorrhages, neoplasms, abscesses, and other conditions masquerading as a stroke. Scans obtained in the first several hours after an infarction generally show no abnormality, and the infarct may not be seen reliably for 24 to 48 h (see Chap. 362). Even later, they may fail to show small ischemic strokes in the posterior fossa because of bone artifact. Also, they may miss small infarcts on the cortical surface. Contrast-enhanced CT scans add specificity by showing contrast enhancement of subacute infarcts.

MRI reliably documents the extent and location of infarction within 1 h of onset in all areas of the brain, including the posterior fossa and cortical surface. It also identifies intracranial hemorrhage and other abnormalities. The higher the field strength, the more reliable and precise the image.

Xenon-blood-flow and *positron emission tomography* (PET) can assess cerebral blood flow, and PET scanning can measure metabolism. These two methods are generally used for research (see Chap. 362).

Artery imaging *X-RAY ANGIOGRAPHY* Cerebral angiography, performed by injection of x-ray contrast dye into selected extracranial arteries after transfemoral catheterization, remains the most accurate method of assessing the cerebrovascular system. It can detect atherosclerotic plaque stenoses and ulcers, intralumenal thrombi, arterial dissections, arteritis and vasospasm, collateral circulation around the circle of Willis and on the cortical surface, and occlusion of large and small arteries.

The advantages of selective cerebral angiography must be balanced in each patient against complications that occur in 0.5 to 3 percent. The principal risks are stroke, allergic reactions to the dye, and renal failure. Because of the risks of invasive angiography, ultrasonography and MR angiography are supplanting it in many situations.

ULTRASONOGRAPHY Stenoses at the origin of the internal carotid artery can be reliably identified and quantified by ultrasonography, utilizing a B-mode ultrasound image combined with a Doppler ultrasound assessment of flow. Transcranial Doppler can also assess flow in middle, anterior, and posterior cerebral arteries and in the vertebrobasilar systems. It can detect stenotic lesions in the middle cerebral stem, the distal vertebral arteries, and the basilar artery because such lesions increase systolic flow velocity. When there is an occlusion or a hemodynamically significant stenosis at the origin of the internal carotid artery or in the carotid siphon, transcranial Doppler assesses collateral flow across the anterior or posterior circle of Willis. Ultrasound cannot distinguish reliably between complete and near-complete carotid occlusion, a very important distinction in some clinical situations. The distinction can be made reliably only by x-ray angiography.

Noninvasive techniques are increasingly used to evaluate asymptomatic patients found to have a carotid bruit in the neck on routine physical examination. The role of these techniques in the management of cerebral vascular disease is uncertain because the treatment for asymptomatic carotid artery stenosis is controversial (see below). Noninvasive carotid testing is a useful and risk-free method to document progression of stenosis.

MR ANGIOGRAPHY This rapidly developing and noninvasive technique provides images of arterial flow. It is particularly valuable for identifying lesions of the extracranial carotid circulation. These images tend to overestimate the degree of stenosis and also cannot distinguish reliably between complete and near-complete carotid occlusion. Using high field strengths (1.5 tesla) and different pulse sequencing, blood flow also may be imaged in the large intracranial arteries. MR angiography does not reliably detect carotid siphon and middle cerebral stem lesions.

In many cases, MR angiography combined with carotid and transcranial ultrasound studies eliminates the need for x-ray angiography in evaluating carotid artery lesions. The combination of the two studies is less expensive than x-ray angiography.

Atherothrombotic Disease of the Vertebrobasilar System CT scanning may detect a large cerebellar infarction in the territory of the posterior inferior cerebellar artery. MRI is more sensitive than CT; it detects cerebellar infarction earlier and can also detect lateral medullary infarction. MR angiography can detect patency of the vertebral artery and occasionally the posterior inferior cerebellar artery. Cerebral angiography is rarely necessary to evaluate stroke in this territory if MR angiography is available. Transcranial Doppler analysis of flow in the vertebral artery determines its patency, but its sensitivity in detecting distal vertebral artery stenotic lesions is limited.

Infarction in the peripheral territory of the posterior cerebral artery can be documented easily by CT or MRI. Infarction in the central territory of the posterior cerebral artery, particularly in territories supplied by the penetrating branches of the posterior cerebral artery, is not reliably detected by CT, but generally is with MRI. MR angiography and intracranial Doppler may identify atherosclerosis stenotic lesions in the proximal posterior cerebral artery.

MRI scanning can detect brainstem infarction due to either basilar artery or basilar branch occlusion. MR angiography combined with transcranial Doppler analysis may eventually replace conventional

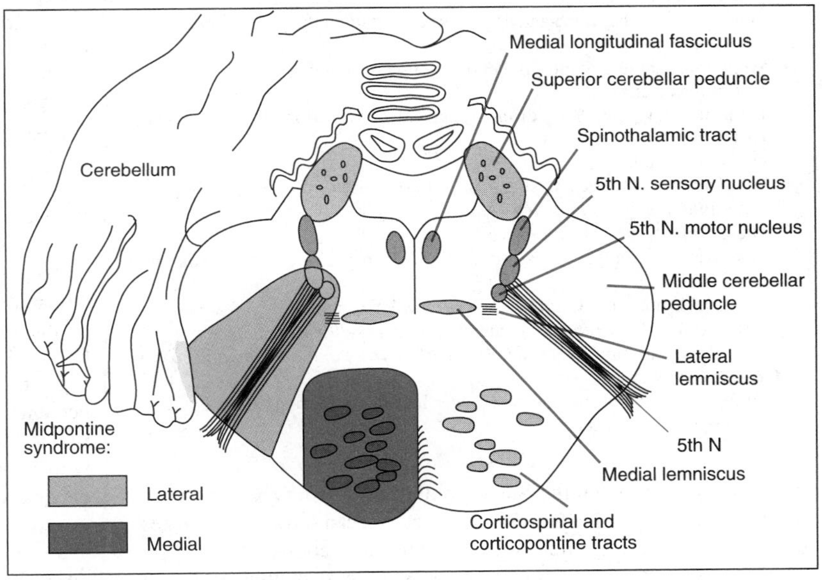

FIGURE 366-9 *(Courtesy of CM Fisher, M.D.)*

Signs and symptoms: *Structures involved*

1. Medial midpontine syndrome (paramedian branch of midbasilar artery)
   - On side of lesion
     - Ataxia of limbs and gait (more prominent in bilateral involvement): *Pontine nuclei*
   - On side opposite lesion
     - Paralysis of face, arm, and leg: *Corticobulbar and corticospinal tract*
     - Variable impaired touch and proprioception when lesion extends posteriorly: *Medial lemniscus*
2. Lateral midpontine syndrome (short circumferential artery)
   - On side of lesion
     - Ataxia of limbs: *Middle cerebellar peduncle*
     - Paralysis of muscles of mastication: *Motor fibers or nucleus of fifth nerve*
     - Impaired sensation over side of face: *Sensory fibers or nucleus of fifth nerve*
   - On side opposite lesion
     - Impaired pain and thermal sense on limbs and trunk: *Spinothalamic tract*

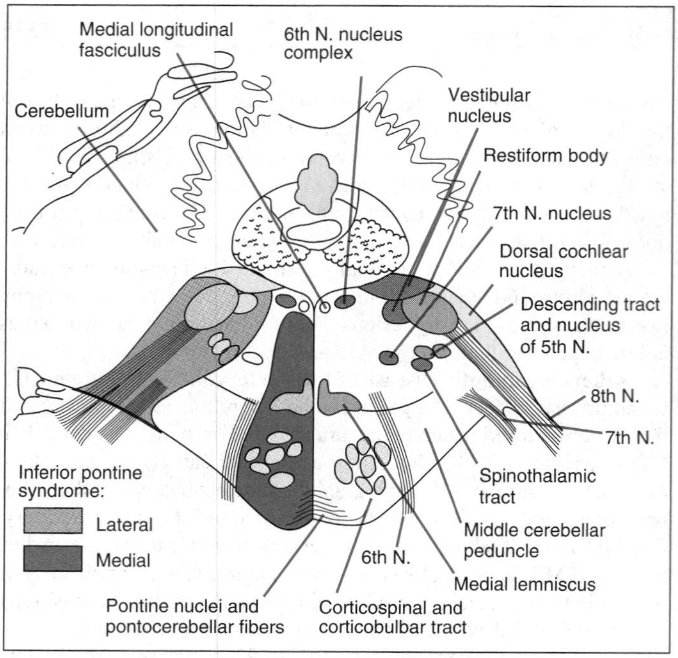

FIGURE 366-10 *(Courtesy of CM Fisher, M.D.)*

Signs and symptoms: *Structures involved*

1. Medial inferior pontine syndrome (occlusion of paramedian branch of basilar artery)
   - On side of lesion
     - Paralysis of conjugate gaze to side of lesion (preservation of convergence): *"Center" for conjugate lateral gaze*
     - Nystagmus: *Vestibular nucleus*
     - Ataxia of limbs and gait: *Middle cerebellar peduncle (?)*
     - Diplopia on lateral gaze: *Abducens nerve*
   - On side opposite lesion
     - Paralysis of face, arm, and leg: *Corticobulbar and corticospinal tract in lower pons*
     - Impaired tactile and proprioceptive sense over half of the body: *Medial lemniscus*
2. Lateral inferior pontine syndrome (occlusion of anterior inferior cerebellar artery)
   - On side of lesion
     - Horizontal and vertical nystagmus, vertigo, nausea, vomiting, oscillopsia: *Vestibular nerve or nucleus*
     - Facial paralysis: *Seventh nerve*
     - Paralysis of conjugate gaze to side of lesion: *"Center" for conjugate lateral gaze*
     - Deafness, tinnitus: *Auditory nerve or cochlear nucleus*
     - Ataxia: *Middle cerebellar peduncle and cerebellar hemisphere*
     - Impaired sensation over face: *Descending tract and nucleus fifth nerve*
   - On side opposite lesion
     - Impaired pain and thermal sense over half the body (may include face): *Spinothalamic tract*

angiography in documenting patency of the basilar artery. CT scanning is not reliable in detecting brainstem infarcts but can show hemorrhages and assess mass effect after large cerebellar infarctions.

Selective x-ray arteriography remains the best method to define atherothrombotic disease of the basilar artery. Arteriography entails potential morbidity and may precipitate the very stroke one is seeking to prevent. It is recommended only when MR angiography fails to detect the clinically suspected basilar arterial lesion that, if known, would influence patient management. Occasionally, injection of angiographic dye in the posterior circulation precipitates a delirious state sometimes associated with cortical blindness. This reversible state can last for 1 or 2 or, rarely, several days.

Lacunes The CT scan detects most supratentorial lacunar infarcts, and MRI detects both supratentorial and infratentorial infarctions when the lacunes are 5 mm or greater. Lacunar infarction can be diagnosed when the infarct size is less than 2 cm and its location is attributable to occlusion of a small penetrating arterial branch of a major parent vessel at the base of the brain.

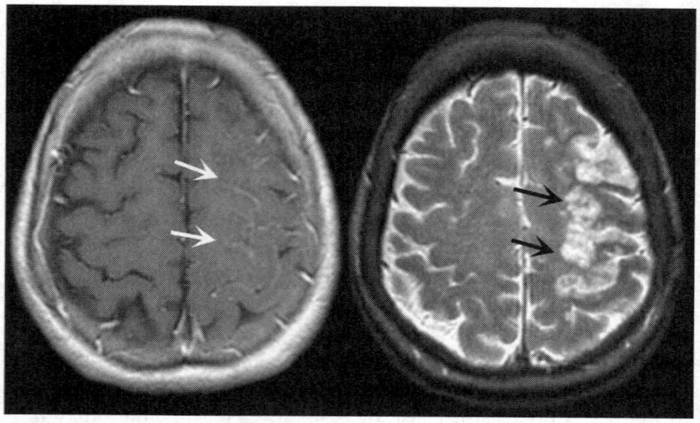

FIGURE 366-11 MRI findings in acute cerebral infarction. Acute onset of right hemiparesis. The axial postcontrast T1-weighted image (*left*) demonstrates contrast enhancement within the vascular bed (*white arrows*) distal to a high-grade stenosis or occlusion. Gadolinium percolates slowly into these vessels through collaterals resulting in enhancement of vessels distal to the occlusion. 24 h later, abnormal prolongation of T2-weighted signal is seen in the cortex supplied by the middle cerebral occlusion (*right image, black arrows*).

℞ TREATMENT

Treatments for atherothrombotic stroke can be divided into those for prevention and those for acute management.

Prevention GENERAL PRINCIPLES Many means are now available for preventing stroke. Some can be applied widely across large populations of people because they are effective, cost little, and carry minimal risk. Other measures are expensive and carry substantial risk; these cannot be applied broadly across the population but may be valuable in selected high-risk patients for whom the benefits substantially outweigh the cost and risk. Some may be indicated only for secondary prevention in patients with preexisting cerebrovascular or cardiovascular disease.

The concept of a *clinical risk profile* is well known but often not articulated. One study analyzed data from pooled published studies to determine whether one can reliably predict, based on clinical manifestations of cerebrovascular atherosclerosis (e.g., cervical bruit, TIA, stroke), the annual risk of stroke (Table 366-3). It revealed that the annual stroke rates are low for patients with asymptomatic carotid stenosis and high for patients who have had a major stroke. The analysis suggested that a hierarchical profile of worsening clinical characteristics mirrors a hierarchical progression of increasing risk for stroke. The North American Symptomatic Carotid Endarterectomy Trial (NASCET; see below) found that even in patients with the same degree of carotid artery stenosis (70 to 99 percent), nine prospectively selected risk factors predicted stroke risk in the medically treated patients. In the high-risk group (those with more than six risk factors), 39 percent of medically treated patients experienced an ipsilateral stroke within 2 years. The rate

Table 366-3

Annual Vascular Event Rates for Individuals with Various Features of Atherothrombotic Cerebral Vascular Disease

	Annual Probability, %, of		
Cerebrovascular Features	**Stroke**	**Vascular Death**	**All Death**
Asymptomatic carotid disease	1.3	3.4	6.0
Transient monocular blindness	2.2	3.5	4.3
Transient ischemic attack	3.7	2.3	4.0
Minor stroke	6.1	3.2	4.9
Major stroke	9.0	3.5	7.6
>70% Symptomatic carotid stenosis	15.0	2.0	

NOTE: The annual probability of stroke in the general elderly male population is 0.6%.
SOURCE: Modified with permission from Wilterdink and Easton, 1992.

for the low-risk group (fewer than six risk factors) was less than half but was still 17 percent. Patients with six risk factors had an intermediate risk of 23 percent. These data support the view that there is a clinical risk profile, in addition to the conventional atherosclerosis risk factor profile, that estimates the likelihood of stroke.

ATHEROSCLEROSIS RISK FACTORS Chapter 242 describes the relationship of various factors to the risk of atherosclerosis. Older age, family history of thrombotic stroke, diabetes mellitus, hypertension, tobacco smoking, elevated blood cholesterol, and other factors are either proven or probable risk factors for ischemic stroke, largely by their link to atherosclerosis. Whether or not tight control of blood sugars in patients with diabetes and other general care measures lower stroke risk is uncertain. Tobacco smoking should be discouraged in everyone.

Of the atherosclerosis factors, hypertension is of the greatest importance. In general, all hypertension should be treated. The first lines of treatment are dietary and life-style modification. All stages of hypertension are associated with increased risk of nonfatal and fatal cardiovascular disease events and renal disease. The higher the blood pressure, the greater the risk. High blood pressure stage 1, previously termed "mild," is the most common form of high blood pressure in the adult population and is therefore responsible for a large proportion of the excess morbidity, disability, and mortality attributable to hypertension. The presence of cerebrovascular disease is not a contraindication to treatment aimed at achieving normotension. Also, the value of treating systolic hypertension in older patients has been clearly established. Care must be taken to avoid overtreatment of hypertension, as these patients may have focal vascular stenoses and impaired vasomotor reactivity. The treatment goal should be gradually to achieve normotension.

Recommendations regarding the treatment of hyperlipidemia are complicated. There are strong data regarding the value of treating hypercholesterolemia to prevent coronary artery disease and consequent myocardial infarction and vascular death. While the treatment benefits regarding stroke are less clear, coronary artery disease is the commonest cause of death in patients with cerebrovascular disease. As with treatment of hypertension, the first line of treatment is dietary and life-style modification. Drug treatment generally should be reserved for those at highest risk for coronary heart disease.

ANTIPLATELET AGENTS *Platelet antiaggregation agents* prevent atherothrombotic events, including TIA and stroke. They inhibit the formation of intraarterial platelet aggregates that can form on diseased arteries, induce thrombus formation, and occlude the artery or embolize into the distal circulation. Aspirin and ticlopidine are the antiplatelet agents used most for this purpose.

Aspirin is the most widely studied antiplatelet agent. Its antiplatelet effect is accomplished by acetylating the cyclooxygenase enzyme in platelets. This irreversibly inhibits the formation in platelets of thromboxane A_2, a platelet aggregating and vasoconstricting prostaglandin. This effect is permanent and lasts for the usual 8-d life of the platelet. Paradoxically, aspirin also inhibits the formation in endothelial cells of prostacyclin, an antiaggregating and vasodilating prostaglandin. This effect is transient. As soon as the aspirin is cleared from the blood, the nucleated endothelial cells again produce prostacyclin. Aspirin in low doses given once daily inhibits the production of thromboxane A_2 in platelets without substantially inhibiting prostacyclin formation. Therefore, many physicians recommend aspirin in doses of 300 mg or less per day.

Ticlopidine blocks the ADP receptor on platelets and thus prevents the cascade resulting in activation of the glycoprotein IIb/IIIa receptor that leads to fibrinogen binding to the platelet and consequent platelet aggregation (see Chap. 60). Ticlopidine is more effective than aspirin. However, it has the disadvantage of causing a small incidence of neutropenia, diarrhea, and skin rash. It commonly is recommended for use as an antiplatelet agent only if aspirin is contraindicated or fails. Dipyridamole is an antiplatelet agent that acts by inhibiting platelet phosphodiesterase, which is responsible for the breakdown of cyclic AMP. The resulting elevation in cyclic AMP inhibits aggregation of platelets. Dipyridamole has not been proven more effective than aspirin, and there is no proof of an additional antiplatelet benefit when added to aspirin.

Many large clinical trials have demonstrated clearly that antiplatelet agents reduce vascular atherothrombotic events (ischemic stroke, myocardial infarction, and death due to all vascular causes) in at-risk patients. The overall *relative* reduction in risk of nonfatal stroke is 25 to 30 percent and of overall vascular events is 25 percent. The *absolute* reduction varies considerably depending on the particular patient's risk. Individuals at very low risk for stroke seem to experience the same relative reduction, but their risk may be so low that the "benefit" is meaningless. On the other hand, someone with a 10 to 15 percent risk per year can reduce the risk to between 7.5 and 11 percent.

Aspirin is inexpensive, can be given in low doses as infrequently as every other day, and could be recommended for all adults to prevent both stroke and myocardial infarction. However, it causes adverse effects including epigastric discomfort, gastric ulceration, and gastrointestinal hemorrhage. The gastric bleeding may be asymptomatic and detectable only by regular stool examinations. A life-threatening hemorrhage may occur without warning. Consequently, not every 20- or 30-year-old should be advised to take aspirin regularly because the risk of atherothrombotic stroke is extremely low and is outweighed by the risk of adverse side effects. Conversely, every patient who has experienced an atherothrombotic stroke and has no contraindication should be taking an antiplatelet agent regularly because the average annual risk of another stroke is 8 to 10 percent, and another few percent will experience a myocardial infarction or vascular death. In this setting, the likelihood of benefit far outweighs the risks of treatment.

The choice of antiplatelet agent, and dose, similarly must balance the risk of stroke against the benefit, risk, and cost of the treatments. These data are less definitive, and opinions therefore vary. Many authorities believe low-dose (30 to 75 mg daily) and high-dose (650 to 1300 mg daily) aspirin are equally effective. Most physicians in North America recommend 325 to 1300 mg daily, while most Europeans recommend 30 to 325 mg. Similarly, the choice of aspirin or ticlopidine must balance the fact that ticlopidine is more effective than aspirin but the cost and risk of adverse effects are higher.

ANTICOAGULATION THERAPY The role of anticoagulation in atherothrombotic cerebral disease is uncertain. Four randomized prospective studies comparing anticoagulant-treated patients with TIA to controls showed no significant difference in the incidence of stroke or death in the two groups. All of these early randomized trials involved inadequate numbers of patients to provide definitive results.

Heparin is widely used for "unstable TIA" (i.e., crescendo or recent-onset TIA). There are almost no data from controlled studies regarding the systematic use of heparin for these patients. It has been largely for theoretical reasons, and by extrapolation from the results of studies of anticoagulation for progressing stroke and myocardial infarction, that anticoagulation is used.

In progressing stroke, the focal ischemia worsens over several hours or a day or two. Progressing stroke is common; approximately 20 percent of carotid territory strokes, and a higher percentage of posterior circulation strokes, progress. For example, a few hours after the onset of a stroke a patient may appear to have a stable deficit such as a mild aphasia and right hemiparesis, but the following morning a severe aphasia and right hemiplegia are noted. It is difficult to predict or monitor for progression; thus many physicians heparinize all patients with recent mild ischemic stroke in order to prevent some of the worsening that will occur in 20 percent. Results of a recent small randomized, controlled trial of heparin for the prevention of progression in acute partial thrombotic stroke did not support the use of heparin. Nevertheless, heparin continues to be used for many of these patients. The bleeding complication rate for 7 days of heparin is about 10 percent, with a serious bleed rate of about 2 percent. Clearly the value of this approach must be clarified.

A recent study found a substantial reduction in death and disability from acute ischemic stroke with a new low-molecular-weight heparin, nadroparin, administered subcutaneously for 10 days. Confirmation will be required before the results are accepted and widely applied. The International Stroke Trial (IST) and Trial of Organon 10172 in Acute Stroke Treatment (TOAST) are two large trials currently addressing the role of heparin and a low-molecular-weight heparinoid in acute ischemic stroke.

When used, heparinization generally is accomplished by giving 3000 to 5000 units of heparin intravenously, followed with 600 to 1000 units per hour by intravenous drip infusion, monitored to maintain the activated partial thromboplastin time at approximately twice normal. This regimen is maintained for 2 to 5 days. During this time the patient is monitored for hemorrhagic complications and a decision is made regarding the need for carotid endarterectomy and long-term warfarin or antiplatelet therapy. If long-term anticoagulation is chosen, warfarin is administered. When the international normalized ratio (INR) (see Chap. 119) is about 3.0, the heparin is discontinued.

There also are few data to support the use of long-term warfarin for preventing atherothrombotic stroke. Two large trials in progress, The Stroke Prevention in Reversible Ischemia Trial (SPIRIT) and The Warfarin Aspirin Recurrent Stroke Study (WARSS), should clarify the role of anticoagulation in the prevention and progression of ischemic stroke. It may be some time before data become available to decide the optimal preventive treatment for specific groups of patients at risk.

SURGICAL THERAPY Surgery for atherosclerotic occlusive disease is largely limited to *carotid endarterectomy* for plaques located at the origin of the internal carotid artery in the neck. About 100,000 carotid endarterectomies are done annually in the United States. Surgery in the proximal common carotid, the subclavian, and the vertebral arteries is uncommon. Anastomosing extracranial scalp arteries to major intracranial arteries to bypass inoperable obstructions in the internal carotid artery is of no value.

Carotid endarterectomy is valuable for some individuals with carotid stenosis, but not all. The benefits vary greatly, depending on the clinical profiles of the patients and the operative complication rates of the surgeons. In many communities the perioperative stroke and death rates are as high as 6 to 8 percent and 1 to 3 percent respectively, in which case the operation is not beneficial.

1. *Symptomatic patients*. Both the NASCET and the European Carotid Surgery Trial (ECST) showed a substantial benefit for surgery in patients with a symptomatic carotid artery stenosis of greater than 70 percent. In NASCET, the average cumulative ipsilateral stroke rate at 2 years was 26 percent for patients treated medically and 9 percent for those receiving the same medical treatment plus a carotid endarterectomy, corresponding to a 65 percent *relative* risk reduction favoring surgery. For every 100 patients treated surgically, 17 were spared an ipsilateral stroke over the next 2 years. The perioperative stroke plus death rate was 5.8 percent in the surgical group and 3.3 percent in the medical group in the same 1-month period, in spite of optimal medical therapy. Thus the excess morbidity and mortality attributable to the surgery was 2.5 percent. If minor ischemic events are excluded from the analyses, the excess major stroke and death rate for the surgical patients was 1.2 percent (2.1 less 0.9 percent) and the excess fatality rate was 0.3 percent (0.6 less 0.3 percent). The NASCET and ECST investigators concluded that their patients with a 70 to 99 percent stenosis clearly benefited from carotid endarterectomy. Results in community hospitals should be similar if patients are properly selected and the perioperative morbidity and mortality are comparably low.

Analysis of several subgroups yielded important information. The cumulative risk of ipsilateral stroke correlated with the degree of stenosis. While the absolute risk reduction favoring the entire surgical group was 17 percent in NASCET, the risk reduction favoring those with a 90 to 99 percent stenosis was 26 percent, and this decreased to 12 percent for those with a 70 to 79 percent stenosis. The overall 26 percent cumulative risk of an ipsilateral stroke at 2 years for this group of patients with "high-grade" stenosis calculates to an annual risk of 13 percent. The operative morbidity and mortality were similar for patients with different degrees of stenosis.

The presence of retinal versus hemispheric symptoms, degree of arterial stenosis, extent of associated medical conditions, surgical morbidity and mortality in the patients' institution, and other factors are all important in estimating an individual patient's risk of stroke and therefore magnitude of benefit from surgery. A patient with multiple atherosclerosis risk factors, symptomatic hemispheric ischemia, very high grade stenosis in the appropriate internal carotid artery, and an institutional perioperative morbidity and mortality rate of less than 6 percent generally should undergo carotid endarterectomy. The spontaneous risk of stroke is much higher than the operative risk, and surgery confers a long-term benefit. On the other hand, a patient with few atherosclerosis risk factors, an asymptomatic moderate-grade stenosis in one internal carotid artery, and an institutional perioperative morbidity and mortality rate of 6 percent should not undergo carotid endarterectomy (see below).

In summary, it is now clear that about one in four recently symptomatic patients with a high-grade carotid stenosis will have an ipsilateral stroke in the next 2 years, even while receiving good risk factor management and aspirin. These patients clearly will benefit from carotid endarterectomy, provided it is done by a surgeon with proven good results. However, there are patients within this ≥70 percent stenosis group whose risk of stroke, and risk of surgical complications, is substantially higher or lower than the group's average.

The ECST additionally showed that patients with a 0 to 29 percent stenosis have a low risk of ipsilateral stroke and are not helped by surgery. The value of carotid endarterectomy for patients with a 30 to 69 percent carotid stenosis remains uncertain, and the NASCET and ECST are continuing to study this group.

2. *Asymptomatic patients*. The Asymptomatic Carotid Atherosclerosis Study (ACAS) demonstrated that asymptomatic people with internal carotid artery stenoses greater than 60 percent are at low risk for stroke. More than 1600 patients were randomized to treatment with the best medical therapies available versus the same medical treatment plus carotid endarterectomy. Patients in the nonsurgical group had a risk over 5 years for ipsilateral stroke (and any perioperative stroke or death) of 5.1 percent, whereas the risk for the nonsurgical group was 11 percent. While this demonstrates a 53 percent *relative* risk reduction, the *absolute* risk reduction is only 5.9 percent over 5 years, or 1.2 percent annually. If only major strokes and death are counted, the comparable numbers are 43 percent relative risk reduction, and an absolute risk reduction of only 2.6 percent over 5 years, or 0.5 percent annually. This latter result was not statistically significant. There was no clear difference in benefit for those with moderate (60 to 80 percent) compared with severe (80 to 99 percent) stenosis.

Many of the strokes in the surgery group were caused by preoperative angiograms. If carotid artery ultrasonography and MR angiography replace catheter angiography, this morbidity and mortality will be obviated.

While there are benefits for carotid endarterectomy in patients with asymptomatic carotid stenosis, the benefits are very small. Medical therapy for reduction of atherosclerosis risk factors in addition to aspirin (325 mg/d) generally are recommended for patients with asymptomatic carotid stenosis.

3. *Conclusions*. From a public health point of view, it is important to consider the magnitude of any benefits demonstrated in clinical trials, particularly if the intervention is costly. In the NASCET, there was a 17 percent absolute reduction in ipsilateral stroke, meaning that six endarterectomies need to be performed in order to prevent one ipsilateral stroke. There was a 10.1 percent

absolute reduction in the most significant outcomes of major stroke and death, meaning that 10 operations need to be performed in order to prevent 1 of these disasters. Most people probably find these trade-offs acceptable. However, at some point the cost may become too high. In the ACAS, surgery reduced the absolute risk of stroke by only 1.2 percent annually; thus 85 endarterectomies need to be performed to prevent 1 stroke annually in a group of patients with these characteristics. The same calculation for preventing 1 major or fatal stroke annually would require that 192 endarterectomies be performed.

As the average carotid endarterectomy in the United States likely costs more than $15,000, and about 100,000 are done annually, the total cost to the nation is about $1.5 billion. At some level, these costs must be considered in decisions regarding treatment of this common disease. Obviously, the higher the expected event rate and the lower the surgical morbidity, the fewer the number of patients who need to be treated to prevent one event. Additionally, the more serious the event and the cheaper the treatment, the greater the overall benefits.

Finally, the results of the carotid endarterectomy trials emphasize the fact that carotid artery disease is a marker for cardiovascular disease. One-half to two-thirds of all deaths in these patients are due to heart disease, and a much smaller proportion are due to stroke (about 5 percent in asymptomatic patients and nearly 20 percent in symptomatic patients). This is despite appropriate treatment for atherosclerotic risk factors and with aspirin. The optimal cardiac evaluation and management of these patients has not been determined.

ANGIOPLASTY Angioplasty is an experimental procedure in the prevention of stroke.

Acute Management *GENERAL PRINCIPLES* When cerebral infarction occurs, the immediate goal is to optimize cerebral perfusion of the ischemic area. Also, attention is directed toward preventing the common complications of bedridden patients, namely, infections (pneumonia, urinary tract, and skin) and deep venous thrombosis with pulmonary embolism.

Elevated blood pressure should not be lowered unless there is malignant hypertension (see Chap. 246). If the blood pressure is low, raising it is advisable. Fever is detrimental and should be avoided.

Between 5 and 10 percent of patients develop symptomatic cerebral edema, resulting in obtundation with its attendant consequences or brain herniation. Edema peaks on the second or third day but causes mass effect for 10 days. The larger the infarct, the more likely edema will be a problem. Even small amounts of edema from a cerebellar stroke can raise intracranial pressure in the posterior fossa. The resulting brainstem compression may result in coma and respiratory arrest requiring emergency surgical decompression. Restriction of free water and intravenous mannitol may be used to raise the serum osmolarity. Intravascular volume should be maintained.

Other treatments for cerebral ischemia-infarction have not been proved beneficial. These include use of mannitol and low-molecular-weight dextran to lower blood viscosity, vasodilating agents to increase cerebral blood flow, hypothermia and barbiturates to decrease the metabolic demands of ischemic tissue, and hyperoxygenation to reduce hypoxic damage.

THROMBOLYSIS The role of thrombolysis in acute cerebral infarction is not entirely clear. Several studies have shown that occlusions in arteries appropriate to the symptoms are very frequently found if angiography is carried out within a few hours of acute infarction. It is this association of atherothromboembolic arterial occlusion with acute neurologic symptoms that prompted the use of thrombolytic agents in stroke patients. In 1992, a meta-analysis reviewed the 60 published reports of thrombolytic therapy for stroke. It was not possible to conclude anything about benefit or safety because there were no controls. Nevertheless, the overall recanalization rate at 24 h reported in these limited studies was about 60 percent, as compared to the spontaneous rate of 20 percent. These results were encouraging, if tentative.

Three recent trials of streptokinase were stopped because of safety concerns in the streptokinase-treated patients. The death rate was higher in the thrombolysis groups, mainly due to symptomatic intracranial bleeds. In one trial, there was a significant increase in death and disability at 3 months, whereas in another moderate disability was reduced in a selected subgroup of patients.

The European Cooperative Acute Stroke Study (ECASS) reported results of a randomized trial using intravenous recombinant tissue plasminogen activator (rt-PA), alteplase, (1.1 mg/kg to a 100-mg maximum; 10 percent as a bolus, then the remainder over 60 min) versus placebo in patients with ischemic stroke within 6 h of onset. The median time to treatment was 4 h. Overall, thrombolysis was not beneficial because of an excess of cerebral hemorrhage. However, in those patients who had no signs of major infarction on the initial CT scan the functional outcome was improved. The investigators emphasized that identification of this subgroup is difficult and depends on recognition of early CT findings of major infarction.

The National Institute of Neurological Disorders and Stroke (NINDS) rt-PA Stroke Study showed a clear benefit for rt-PA in selected patients with acute stroke. The NINDS rt-PA trial used intravenous rt-PA alteplase (0.9 mg/kg to a 90-mg maximum; 10 percent as a bolus, then the remainder over 60 min) versus placebo in patients with ischemic stroke within 3 h of onset. Symptomatic intracerebral hemorrhage occurred in 6.4 percent of patients on rt-PA and 0.6 percent on placebo. There was a 4 percent reduction in mortality on rt-PA (21 percent on placebo and 17 percent on rt-PA), and a 12 percent increase in the number of patients with only minimal disability (32 percent on placebo and 44 percent on rt-PA). Thus, despite an increased incidence of symptomatic intracerebral hemorrhage, treatment with intravenous rt-PA within 3 h of the onset of ischemic stroke improved clinical outcome. A lower dose of rt-PA was used than in ECASS, and half of the patients were treated within 90 min of stroke onset and the other half between 90 and 180 min. These two features may account for much of the increase in benefit and decrease in bleeding hazard compared to the results seen in ECASS.

It seems clear that thrombolysis works. However, the therapeutic window is narrow, and the selection of patients and timing and dose of drug are key determinants of the therapeutic response. Thrombolysis should only be administered using the strict protocol of the NINDS rt-PA study, with adequate protection of patients by full disclosure of the possible risks. Additional trials in progress will further clarify the overall role for thrombolysis in acute ischemic stroke.

REHABILITATION Rehabilitation of the stroke patient is important, and it includes early physical, occupational, and speech therapy. It is directed toward educating the patient and family about the patient's neurologic deficit, preventing the complications of immobility (e.g., pneumonia, pressure sores of the skin, muscle contractures), and providing encouragement and instruction in overcoming the deficit.

CEREBRAL EMBOLISM

PATHOPHYSIOLOGY OF CARDIOGENIC CEREBRAL EMBOLISM Cardioembolism causes about 15 percent of all strokes. Stroke caused by heart disease is primarily due to embolism of thrombotic material forming on the atrial or ventricular wall or the left heart valves. These thrombi then detach and embolize into the arterial circulation where they may fragment or lyse, and the circulation may be restored quickly. Alternatively, the arterial occlusion may be permanent, and thrombosis distal to the obstruction may occur with consequent disruption of the distal collateral circulation.

Emboli from the heart most often lodge in the middle cerebral artery or one of its branches. They infrequently cause infarcts in the anterior cerebral artery territory. Emboli large enough to occlude the stem of the middle cerebral artery (3 to 4 mm) lead to a large stroke that involves both deep gray and white matter and some portions of the cortical surface and its underlying white matter. A smaller embolus may occlude a small cortical or penetrating arterial branch. The location and size of an infarct also depend on the extent of the spared collateral circulation.

Cardiogenic cerebral embolism is presumed to have occurred when cardiac arrhythmias or structural abnormalities are found or known to be present. The commonest causes of cardioembolic stroke are nonrheumatic (often called nonvalvular) atrial fibrillation (AF), myocardial infarction, prosthetic valves, rheumatic heart disease (RHD), and ischemic cardiomyopathy (see Table 366-4). Many clinical trials in recent years have evaluated treatments for stroke prevention in nonrheumatic AF. A smaller number of good studies in the treatment of prosthetic heart valves and myocardial infarction have been done. Most of the other conditions causing cardioembolic stroke have been less well studied.

Nonrheumatic AF is the commonest cause of cerebral embolism. Patients with AF have an average annual risk of stroke of about 5 percent. However, the risk varies according to the presence of certain risk factors, including old age, hypertension, poor left ventricular function, prior cardioembolism, and diabetes mellitus. Patients less than 60 years of age with none of these risk factors have an annual risk for stroke of about 0.5 percent. Those with most of these risks have a rate of about 15 percent. The presumed stroke mechanism is thrombus formation in the fibrillating atrium or atrial appendage, with subsequent embolization.

Recent *myocardial infarction*, especially when transmural and involving the anteroapical ventricular wall, is an important risk for embolus, particularly in the first few weeks.

Cardiomyopathies with poor left ventricular function are frequently associated with left ventricular thrombus formation.

Prosthetic heart valves, especially mechanical ones, are a common cause of cerebral embolism.

RHD usually causes ischemic stroke when there is prominent mitral stenosis or AF; left atrial enlargement and congestive heart failure are further risk factors for formation of atrial thrombi.

Mitral valve prolapse can be a source of emboli. This common disorder probably causes cerebral embolism only when severe.

Congenital septal defects are associated with cerebral embolism. Usually they are major defects, but a small foramen ovale or septal aneurysm may occasionally be causative. It is presumed that the deep peripheral venous system is usually the source of *paradoxical emboli*. Transesophageal and bubble echocardiographic techniques can demonstrate a patent foramen ovale. Other causes, such as fat and tumor in the blood, marantic endocarditis, and air and amniotic fluid emboli associated with parturition, may occasionally be responsible.

Infectious endocarditis (see Chap. 126) causes vegetations that give rise to multiple septic emboli. The appearance of multifocal or diffuse symptoms and signs in a patient with stroke should raise the possibility of underlying bacterial endocarditis. Infarcts may be microscopic in size or large, and septic emboli may produce brain abscess, mycotic aneurysms, and subarachnoid hemorrhage (SAH) or intracerebral hemorrhage.

Nonbacterial thrombotic (marantic) endocarditis, mitral annulus calcification, chronic sinoatrial disorder, systemic lupus erythematosus (Libman-Sacks vegetations), atrial myxoma, and thrombus in a pulmonary vein also increase the risk of cerebral embolism.

Table 366-4

Causes of Cardiogenic Cerebral Embolism

Dysrhythmia
Atrial fibrillation, sick sinus syndrome
Coronary heart disease
Myocardial infarction
Ischemic cardiomyopathy
Rheumatic heart disease
Mitral stenosis with or without atrial fibrillation
Other
Nonischemic cardiomyopathies
Prosthetic valve
Congenital heart disease: patent foramen ovale, mitral valve prolapse, etc.
Septic endocarditis
Mitral annulus calcification
Atrial myxoma
Fat emboli
Nonbacterial thrombotic endocarditis
Hypercoagulable states: cancer, systemic diseases, oral contraceptives

PATHOLOGY Cerebral infarcts may be pale (nonhemorrhagic) or red (hemorrhagic). Vascular congestion of varying degree is common in all infarcts, but extravasation of blood is usually associated with embolic infarcts. Because emboli migrate and lyse, recirculation into the infarcted brain may cause petechial hemorrhages. Sometimes there is enough seepage of blood into the infarct to cause visible *hemorrhagic infarction* on a CT scan. *Hemorrhagic transformation* of a pale infarct typically occurs from 12 to 36 h after embolization and is often asymptomatic. Frank hemorrhage into the infarct almost always causes clinical worsening. This is more likely to occur when the stem of the middle cerebral artery is occluded and a large infarct develops in the territory of the lenticulostriate arteries before recirculation occurs.

Infarcts in the distribution of small, penetrating arteries ultimately leave small cavities or lacunes (lacunar infarcts), whereas major arterial occlusions may produce a wide area of necrosis that ultimately leaves a large, fluid-filled cavity in the brain.

Edema invariably accompanies the tissue necrosis. In small infarcts it may be relatively insignificant. In large infarcts, however, massive edema compresses adjacent tissue and adds to the ischemic process; it also increases intracranial pressure and may cause herniation of the brain from one intracranial compartment to another.

CLINICAL MANIFESTATIONS An embolus to the brain usually causes the sudden onset of a focal neurologic deficit that is maximum at the onset. Deficits correspond to the areas of cerebral cortex supplied by the affected artery and resemble those caused by occlusive atheromatous lesions (see sections on atherothrombosis and lacunar stroke). Certain neurologic syndromes suggest embolism as their cause. In the middle cerebral artery territory these include the following: (1) the frontal opercular syndrome, in which there is facial weakness and severe aphasia or dysarthria; (2) the brachial or hand plegia syndrome, in which the arm or hand is paralyzed, with or without cortical sensory abnormalities; (3) Broca's or Wernicke's aphasia alone; or (4) left visual neglect, when the nondominant parietal lobe is involved. Sudden hemianopia suggests a posterior cerebral artery embolus, and sudden foot and shoulder weakness suggests an anterior cerebral artery embolus. Sudden sleepiness and inability to look up associated with bilateral ptosis suggest an embolus to the top of the basilar artery, specifically to the artery of Percheron (the small artery supplying both sides of the medial subthalamus and thalamus arising from the top of the basilar artery).

Seizures at the time of stroke occur in 3 to 5 percent of infarctions. They occur more often after embolism than thrombosis. They usually are associated with supratentorial cortical surface infarctions. Another 3 to 5 percent of patients develop epilepsy from 6 to 18 months after their stroke. Many cases of idiopathic epilepsy in the elderly are probably the result of silent cortical infarction.

LABORATORY AND IMAGING EVALUATION Although early CT scanning is usually negative in the first several hours after an embolic stroke, it excludes hemorrhage. Later it visualizes the location and extent of infarction, and it can support the diagnosis of embolism by demonstrating hemorrhagic infarction or multiple infarcts. However, embolic injury may appear as a single low-density area compatible with pale infarction. Petechial hemorrhages within the area may not visualize as increased tissue density because when superimposed on the low-density infarct, the average tissue density is near that of normal brain. MRI scanning is the most sensitive method to detect embolic infarction.

A thorough cardiac evaluation should be undertaken when embolism is suspected, including young patients and those with a history of heart disease, multifocal or hemorrhagic infarcts, or seizures at onset. Continuous ECG monitoring may demonstrate an intermittent arrhythmia. An echocardiogram may disclose mitral valve disease, an intracardiac thrombus or tumor, and akinetic myocardium. Transesophageal and bubble echocardiography can demonstrate a patent foramen ovale.

In patients with myocardial infarction, the clinical and ECG findings, together with echocardiography, may identify those patients with large anteroapical infarcts, ventricular aneurysms, mural thrombi, and other factors that predispose to peripheral embolism.

Cerebral angiography is rarely indicated. When performed in the first day or two it often shows occlusion of one or more vessels. Complete lysis of emboli often occurs, and angiography performed after several days may be normal.

CSF obtained immediately after a cerebral embolism is usually normal. The presence of more than a few white or red blood cells makes bacterial endocarditis more likely.

℞ TREATMENT

Treatment of patients with embolic infarction consists of managing the stroke itself, in both the acute and chronic phases, and of preventing further emboli.

Prevention Virtually every type of cardiac disease is associated with increased risk for stroke, and the best treatment for cerebral embolism is prevention. Consequently, prophylactic treatment of patients with thrombus-prone heart disease is indicated.

ANTICOAGULATION THERAPY Several recent clinical trials demonstrated that anticoagulation (INR of 2.0 to 3.0) in patients with chronic nonvalvular (nonrheumatic) AF prevents cerebral embolism and is safe. Anticoagulation with warfarin reduces the risk by about 65 percent and is generally recommended for these patients.

Anticoagulation also reduces the risk of embolism in acute myocardial infarction. Most clinicians recommend anticoagulation when there is substantial left ventricular dysfunction or a major, focal wall-motion abnormality.

Patients with prominent RHD are at risk of systemic embolism and should be anticoagulated indefinitely. This category includes mitral stenosis, a large left atrium, congestive heart failure, AF, and echocardiographically demonstrated atrial thrombi. Whether the benefit of long-term anticoagulation outweighs the risk in patients with lesser degrees of RHD is unclear.

Thromboembolism has been recognized as one of the most serious complications of prosthetic heart valve implantation since the procedure became feasible in 1960. Anticoagulation with warfarin has been proven effective for preventing strokes in this situation, while antiplatelet therapy alone has not; concomitant therapy with aspirin adds substantially to the beneficial effect of warfarin prophylaxis. Higher intensities of anticoagulation (INR of 3.5) are recommended for prosthetic heart valve patients compared to those with AF.

ANTIPLATELET AGENTS Warfarin is more effective than aspirin in preventing ischemic stroke associated with AF. However, some patients with AF have a low rate of ischemic stroke and do not need warfarin. Others have a high risk of hemorrhage and thus lose the benefit of anticoagulation. Still others are at such high risk for ischemic stroke that the benefits of warfarin override even the high hemorrhage rate. The use of any preventive treatment is based upon the relative risks and benefits for a particular patient.

Three clinical trials conducted in recent years systematically compared aspirin to placebo for prevention of cerebral infarction in patients with nonrheumatic AF. In aggregate, they showed about a 25 percent relative reduction in stroke with aspirin, compared to the reduction by warfarin of 65 percent. Still, not every patient with AF requires treatment with warfarin to prevent stroke. The Stroke Prevention in Atrial Fibrillation II trial showed that in low-risk patients (those without hypertension, recent heart failure, or prior thromboembolism) younger than 75 years old given aspirin, the thromboembolism rate was only 0.5 percent per year. Consequently, one could reasonably recommend that patients younger than 75 years old with no risk factors be treated with aspirin only.

Acute Management The acute management is basically the same as for thrombotic infarction. If the indications are appropriate, the patient should receive thrombolytic therapy. Since the embolic source generally persists at least temporarily, these patients are at substantial risk for early reembolization. For most of the causes, the risk is about 0.5 to 1 percent daily for the first week or two. Consequently, prompt anticoagulation is desirable. However, heparin is generally avoided for about a week when the infarct is large, as the risk of serious hemorrhage increases with increasing infarct size. It is also avoided if bacterial endocarditis is likely. The duration of anticoagulation is determined by the causative heart lesion and its associated continuing risk of future embolization. If the embolic source is self-limited or treatable, anticoagulation should be discontinued when the high-risk period has passed. For myocardial infarction, this is after 2 or 3 months; for a reversible cardiomyopathy it may be several weeks after cardiac function has recovered. After conversion of nonvalvular AF, the high-risk period may comprise the few weeks after the appearance of a stable sinus rhythm.

Generally, if the embolic source cannot be eliminated, anticoagulation should be continued indefinitely. This includes any patient with RHD, even if the mitral valve is replaced or the AF is successfully converted to normal sinus rhythm. It also includes the patient who has had one or more systemic emboli and who has nonvalvular AF, persistent cardiomyopathy with chronic ventricular failure, and, possibly, severe mitral valve prolapse.

OTHER CAUSES OF CEREBRAL INFARCTION

Dissection of the Cervicocerebral Arteries Dissection of the large extracranial arteries may cause cerebral infarction and is a frequent cause of stroke in children and young adults. A small tear in the intima allows blood to dissect into the media of the artery or separate the intima from the media. TIAs and infarction occur when the artery is critically narrowed or occluded or when thromboembolism results. Trauma, either severe or trivial, accounts for most cases.

The internal carotid artery high in the neck is the most common site. There are usually pain in the ipsilateral neck, face, or head and an oculosympathetic palsy (partial Horner's syndrome). A self-audible bruit may appear, and tenderness over the upper neck may be present. Dissection of a vertebral artery may produce posterior lateralized neck pain, accompanied by signs of lateral medullary ischemia or other brainstem syndromes.

TIAs, or TMB in carotid dissections, often precede infarction, leaving time for therapeutic intervention. When the patient has only oculosympathetic palsy, TIAs, or a minor stroke, anticoagulation with heparin is recommended. After the patient's symptoms have stabilized, anticoagulation with warfarin is recommended for 4 months. MR angiography with MRI of the dissection site often makes the diagnosis. X-ray angiography is sometimes required. Repeat imaging in 6 to 10 weeks often demonstrates a reestablished lumen in the formerly occluded vessel.

Fibromuscular Dysplasia Fibromuscular dysplasia rarely causes stroke. It affects the cervical arteries and occurs mainly in women. The carotid or vertebral arteries show multiple rings of segmental narrowing alternating with dilatation. Occlusion is usually incomplete. The process is often asymptomatic but occasionally is associated with an audible bruit, TIAs, or stroke. The cause and natural history of fibromuscular dysplasia is unknown (see Chap. 248). TIA or stroke generally occurs only when the artery is severely narrowed. Anticoagulation or antiplatelet therapy may be helpful.

Temporal Arteritis (Giant Cell Arteritis) This is a relatively common affliction of mainly elderly persons in which the external carotid system, particularly the temporal arteries, is the site of a subacute granulomatous inflammation with giant cells (Chap. 319). Occlusion of posterior choroidal branches of the ophthalmic artery results in blindness in one or both eyes in many patients. It rarely causes stroke.

Other Arteritides Arteritis due to bacterial or syphilitic infection is no longer a common cause of cerebral thrombosis in developed countries. Other arteritides are rare but can cause cerebral thrombosis (see below and Chaps. 312 and 319). Necrotizing or granulomatous arteritis, occurring alone or in association with generalized polyarteritis nodosa or Wegener's granulomatosis, involves the distal small branches (<2 mm diameter) of the main intracranial arteries and produces small ischemic infarcts in the brain, optic nerve, and spinal cord. The CSF often has inflammatory changes. Idiopathic giant cell arteritis involving the great vessels arising from the aortic arch (Takayasu's syndrome) may, on rare occasions, cause carotid or vertebral thrombosis. It is an infrequent cause of the aortic arch syndrome in the western hemisphere (see Chap. 319).

Moyamoya Disease Moyamoya disease is a poorly understood occlusive disease involving large intracranial arteries, especially the distal internal carotid artery and the stem of the middle and anterior cerebral arteries. The lenticulostriate arteries develop a rich collateral circulation around the middle cerebral occlusive lesion that on angiography gives the impression of a puff of smoke (*moyamoya*). Other collaterals include transdural anastomoses between the cortical surface branches of the middle cerebral artery and the scalp arteries. The disease mainly occurs in Asian children or young adults. Its etiology is unknown. Because of the occurrence of SAH from rupture of the transdural anastomotic channels, anticoagulation is risky.

Hypercoagulable States Certain diseases have been associated with ischemic infarction through a mechanism of a hypercoagulable state (see Chaps. 117 and 118). They include polycythemia vera, thrombotic thrombocytopenic purpura, idiopathic thrombocytosis, hyperproteinemia, sickle cell anemia, and inherited clotting abnormalities, e.g., protein C deficiency. Circulating antiphospholipid antibodies (including "lupus anticoagulants") have been associated with stroke in young adults.

Reversible Segmental Vasoconstriction Reversible, widespread cerebral segmental vasoconstriction occurs in patients with headache and fluctuating neurologic symptoms and signs. Sometimes cerebral infarction ensues. The cause is unknown. Head injury, migraine, sympathomimetic intoxication, eclampsia, and the postpartum period have all been associated with this entity. Angiography is the only means of establishing the diagnosis. The CSF is usually normal, but an elevated protein and slight lymphocytic pleocytosis occur. No effective therapy is known. Maintenance of normal systemic arterial pressure with adequate hydration seems prudent. Glucocorticoids and vasodilators may be considered.

Binswanger's Disease Binswanger's disease (diffuse white matter disease) is a rare condition in which infarction of the subcortical white matter occurs subacutely (see Chap. 367). CT or MRI scan detects periventricular areas of white matter disruption and gliosis. There is lipohyalinosis in the small arteries of the deep white matter, as in hypertension. There are usually associated lacunar infarcts. Binswanger's disease may represent a type of border-zone ischemic infarction in the deep white matter between the penetrating arteries of the circle of Willis and cortical vessels. The pathophysiologic basis of the disease is unclear, but it typically occurs in older patients with severe long-standing hypertension.

Oral Contraceptive Agents Oral contraceptives are associated with an increased incidence of stroke in young women, but the incidence is minimal unless there is associated hypertension, cigarette smoking, or migraine. Hypercoagulability may be the mechanism predisposing to thrombosis.

Venous Thrombosis Lateral or sagittal sinus thrombosis, or thrombosis of small cortical veins, occurs as a complication of pregnancy and the postpartum period, sepsis, intracranial infections (meningitis), and hypercoagulable states such as polycythemia and sickle cell anemia. Venous thrombosis may cause an increase in intracranial pressure, headaches, focal seizures, and infarction primarily affecting the parasagittal cortex. Paraparesis is common. Massive venous infarction with secondary edema may be fatal. The CT and MR scans show hemorrhagic infarction underlying the occluded veins and may show thrombus in the involved veins and sinuses. MR angiography makes the diagnosis. Because the primary abnormality is thrombosis, anticoagulation is recommended unless hemorrhage is prominent.

℞ TREATMENT

Anticoagulation is often recommended as preventive treatment in patients with extracranial cervicocerebral artery dissection, severe mitral valve prolapse, antiphospholipid antibody syndrome, cortical vein–dural sinus thrombosis, and other situations associated with stroke. It will be difficult to obtain definitive information about the proper preventive treatment of many of these conditions. Arterial dissections provide an example of the difficulty. Even if the stroke rate were as high as 5 percent after initiating treatment of a cervical dissection, a sample size of approximately 1600 patients would be required to compare two treatments with an 80 percent chance of detecting a 50 percent reduction in events ($\alpha = 0.05$; 2-tailed). It seems unlikely that such a definitive randomized trial will be carried out to evaluate the value of anticoagulation or any other treatment.

Antiplatelet therapy also is often recommended for patients with extracranial cervicocerebral artery dissection, mitral valve prolapse, vasculitis, and other conditions associated with arterial thromboembolism; definitive trials have not been conducted for any of these indications.

INTRACEREBRAL HEMORRHAGE

Intracerebral hemorrhage is the most common type of nontraumatic intracranial hemorrhage (Table 366-5). It is an important cause of stroke, especially in Asians and blacks. Hypertension and cerebral amyloid angiopathy cause the majority of these hemorrhages. Advanced age and heavy alcohol consumption increase the risk. Cocaine-induced hemorrhage is one of the most important causes in the young.

HYPERTENSIVE INTRACEREBRAL HEMORRHAGE

Pathophysiology and Pathology Intracerebral hemorrhage usually results from spontaneous rupture of a small penetrating artery deep in the brain. The most common sites are (1) the basal ganglia (putamen, thalamus, and adjacent deep white matter), (2) the deep cerebellum, and (3) the pons. When hemorrhages occur in other brain areas or in nonhypertensive patients, greater consideration should be given to hemorrhagic disorders, neoplasms, and other causes. The small arteries in these areas seem most prone to hypertension-induced vascular injury. The leak may be small, or a large clot may form and compress adjacent tissue, causing herniation and death. Rupture or seepage into the ventricular system often occurs. Primary intraventricular hemorrhage is rare. If the patient survives, the clot liquefies, is absorbed, and leaves only a small residual cleft.

Most hypertensive intracerebral hemorrhages develop over 30 to 90 min, whereas those associated with anticoagulant therapy may evolve for as long as 24 to 48 h. Once bleeding stops, it generally

Table 366-5

Causes of Intracranial Hemorrhage

Spontaneous intracerebral hemorrhage	Ruptured arteriovenous malformation
Hypertensive	Cocaine, amphetamines
Amyloid angiopathy	Trauma (see Chap. 374)
Ruptured aneurysm	Bleeding with brain tumors
Saccular	Systemic bleeding disorders, including anticoagulation therapy
Mycotic	Hemorrhagic infarction

Table 366-6

Common Symptoms and Signs of Intracerebral Hemorrhage

Location	Neurologic Signs
Basal ganglia	Contralateral hemiparesis, hemisensory loss, and homonymous hemianopia
	Aphasia with dominant hemisphere
	Conjugate deviation of eyes downward or toward the side of the hematoma
	Obtundation, stupor, or coma
Cerebellum	Vomiting and ataxia
	Skew deviation of eyes and small pupils
	Deviation of eyes toward the opposite side
	Obtundation, late-developing stupor, or coma
Pons	Abrupt onset of coma
	Pinpoint, reactive pupils
	Skew deviation of eyes and gaze paresis
	Decerebration or flaccidity
	Ataxic respiration

does not start again. Within 48 h macrophages begin to phagocytize the hemorrhage at its outer surface. After 1 to 6 months, the hemorrhage is generally resolved to a slitlike orange cavity lined with glial scar and hemosiderin-laden macrophages.

Clinical Manifestations Although not particularly associated with exertion, intracerebral hemorrhages almost always occur while the patient is awake and sometimes when stressed. The clinical presentation is generally that of an abrupt onset of a focal neurologic deficit that typically worsens steadily over 30 to 90 min. The common clinical presentations are shown in Table 366-6.

The putamen is the most common site for hypertensive hemorrhage, and the adjacent internal capsule is invariably damaged. Contralateral hemiparesis is therefore the sentinel sign. When mild, the face sags on one side, speech becomes slurred, the arm and leg gradually weaken, and the eyes deviate away from the side of the hemiparesis. The paralysis may worsen until the affected limbs become flaccid or extend rigidly with a Babinski sign on the same side. When hemorrhages are large, drowsiness gives way to stupor as signs of upper brainstem compression appear. Coma ensues, accompanied by deep, irregular, or intermittent respiration; a dilated and fixed ipsilateral pupil; bilateral Babinski signs; and decerebrate rigidity. In milder cases, edema in adjacent brain tissue may cause progressive deterioration over 12 to 72 h.

Thalamic hemorrhages also produce a hemiplegia or hemiparesis from pressure on, or dissection into, the adjacent internal capsule. A prominent sensory deficit involving all modalities is usually present. Aphasia, often with preserved verbal repetition, may occur after hemorrhage into the dominant (left) thalamus, and apractognosia or mutism occurs in some cases of nondominant hemorrhage. There also may be a transient homonymous visual field defect. Thalamic hemorrhages cause several typical ocular disturbances by virtue of extension medially into the upper midbrain. These include deviation of the eyes downward and inward so that they appear to be looking at the nose, unequal pupils with absence of light reaction, skew deviation with the eye opposite the hemorrhage displaced downward and medially, ipsilateral Horner's syndrome, absence of convergence, paralysis of vertical gaze, and retraction nystagmus.

In pontine hemorrhages, deep coma with quadriplegia usually occurs over a few minutes. There is often prominent decerebrate rigidity and "pin-point" (1 mm) pupils that react to light. There is impairment of reflex horizontal eye movements evoked by head turning (doll's-head or oculocephalic maneuver) or by irrigation of the ears with ice water (see Chap. 24). Hyperpnea, severe hypertension, and hyperhidrosis are common. Death usually occurs within a few hours, but there are exceptional survivors.

Cerebellar hemorrhages usually develop over several hours and are characterized by occipital headache, repeated vomiting, and ataxia of gait. In mild cases there may be no other neurologic signs; therefore it is imperative to test gait. Dizziness or vertigo may be prominent. There is often paresis of conjugate lateral gaze toward the side of the hemorrhage, forced deviation of the eyes to the opposite side, or an ipsilateral sixth nerve palsy. Less frequent ocular signs include blepharospasm, involuntary closure of one eye, ocular bobbing, and skew deviation. There may be little or no evidence of the usual signs of cerebellar disease, and only a minority of patients show nystagmus or limb ataxia. A mild ipsilateral facial weakness and a diminished corneal reflex are common. Dysarthria and dysphagia may occur. There are no Babinski signs until late in the evolution of the hemorrhage as it compresses or dissects into the ventral brainstem. As the hours pass, the patient often becomes stuporous and then comatose from brainstem compression.

In summary, ocular signs have been highlighted as a method of rapidly localizing hemorrhages. In putamenal hemorrhage, the eyes are deviated to the side opposite the paralysis; in thalamic hemorrhage, the eyes are deviated downward and the pupils may be 2 to 3 mm and minimally reactive; in pontine hemorrhage, the reflex lateral eye movements are impaired and the pupils are <1 mm yet reactive; and in cerebellar hemorrhage, the eyes may be deviated laterally (to the side opposite the lesion) in the absence of paralysis.

Laboratory and Imaging Evaluation The CT scan reliably detects acute focal hemorrhages of 1 cm or more in diameter (Fig. 366-12). Small pontine hemorrhages may not be identified because of motion and bone artifact that obscure structures in the posterior fossa. After the first 2 weeks, x-ray attenuation values of clotted blood diminish until they become isodense with surrounding brain. Mass effect and edema may remain. In some cases, a surrounding rim of contrast enhancement appears after 2 to 4 weeks and may persist for months. MRI, though more sensitive for delineating posterior fossa lesions, is not necessary in most instances. Images of flowing blood on MRI scan may identify AVMs as the cause of the hemorrhage. Angiography is used when the cause of intracranial hemorrhage is uncertain, particularly if the patient is not hypertensive and the hematoma is not in one of the four usual sites for hypertensive hemorrhage.

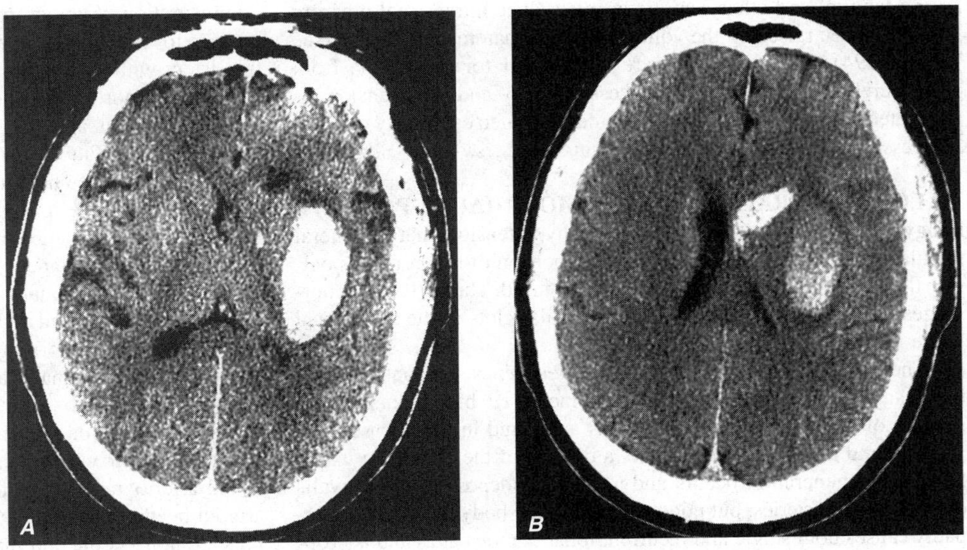

FIGURE 366-12 Acute onset of right hemiparesis. Transaxial noncontrast CT scans through the region of the basal ganglia reveals a hematoma involving the left putamen with extension into the left frontal horn of the lateral ventricle (B). This is a typical hypertensive hemorrhage.

For example, hemorrhage into the temporal lobe suggests rupture of a middle cerebral artery saccular aneurysm.

Since these patients typically have focal neurologic signs and obtundation, and often show signs of increased intracranial pressure, an LP should be avoided as it may induce cerebral herniation. Although the CSF usually will be bloody several hours after the hemorrhage, especially in large hemorrhages, it is sometimes normal initially. In either case, it does not provide definitive diagnostic information.

℞ TREATMENT

Prevention Hypertension is the leading cause of primary cerebral hemorrhage. Prevention is primarily aimed at reducing hypertension, excessive alcohol use, and use of illicit drugs such as cocaine and amphetamines.

Acute Management Approximately 75 percent of patients with a hypertensive intracerebral hemorrhage die. The size and location of the hematoma determine the prognosis. Supratentorial hematomas >5 cm in largest diameter have a poor prognosis, and infratentorial pontine hematomas >3 cm are usually fatal. Except possibly in patients with a bleeding disorder, nothing can be done about the hemorrhage itself. Treating severe hypertension seems reasonable, but harmful hypotension is a risk. Generally, the bleeding has stopped by the time the patient comes under medical care. General measures for treating intracranial hypertension secondary to mass effect are warranted.

Evacuation of the hematoma usually is not helpful, except in cerebellar hemorrhages. For cerebellar hemorrhages, a neurosurgeon should be consulted immediately to assist with the evaluation, with a view to possible surgery. Most hematomas >3 cm in diameter will require surgical evacuation. If the patient is alert without focal brainstem signs and if the hematoma is <1 cm in diameter, surgical removal usually will not be necessary. Patients with hematomas between 1 and 3 cm require careful observation for signs of impaired consciousness, which usually mean surgery is required.

If a patient survives the initial hemorrhage without signs of severe brain injury and subsequently fails to improve or insidiously worsens, surgical evacuation of the hematoma also should be considered.

Tissue surrounding hematomas is displaced and compressed but not necessarily infarcted. Hence, in survivors, major improvement commonly results as the hematoma is reabsorbed and the adjacent tissue regains its function. Careful management of the patient during the acute phase of the hemorrhage can lead to considerable recovery.

Mannitol and other osmotic agents reduce intracranial pressure that has been raised by the volume of the hematoma and edema (see Chap. 374). Glucocorticoids are not helpful for the edema from intracerebral hematoma. Both excessive hypo- and hypertension associated with acute hemorrhage should be treated cautiously to avoid excessive or precipitous blood pressure changes.

LOBAR INTRACEREBRAL HEMORRHAGE Pathophysiology and Pathology As control of hypertension in the general population has improved, the relative proportion of hemorrhages outside the basal ganglia and thalamus has increased. These "lobar hemorrhages" appear on CT scan as oval or circular clots in the subcortical white matter.

The role of chronic hypertension in their genesis is controversial, but many occur without a history of increased blood pressure. A number of other underlying conditions are found in many cases.

Cerebral *amyloid angiopathy* is a disease of the elderly in which arteriolar degeneration occurs and amyloid is deposited in the walls of the cerebral arteries, but not elsewhere in the body. Amyloid angiopathy causes both single and recurrent lobar hemorrhages and is probably the commonest cause of lobar hemorrhage in the elderly. This disorder can be diagnosed only by postmortem demonstration of Congo red staining of amyloid in cerebral vessels. Patients may have multiple hemorrhages over several months or years. Rarely, genetic causes are found as in mutation of the amyloid precursor peptide (see Chap. 363).

Other causes are bleeding diatheses (often associated with warfarin administration), AVM, aneurysm, and tumor (often a melanoma or glioma). Often the cause remains undetermined even after extensive study, though amyloid angiopathy can not be excluded in the absence of brain histology. Some lobar hemorrhages may result from AVMs or venous angiomas that are obliterated by the hemorrhage or are angiographically occult.

Clinical Manifestations The neurologic symptoms and signs of lobar hemorrhage appear over several minutes. Most hemorrhages are small and cause a restricted clinical syndrome that simulates an embolus to an artery supplying one lobe. For example, the major neurologic deficit of occipital hemorrhage is hemianopia; of left temporal hemorrhage, aphasia and delirium; of parietal hemorrhage, thalamic-like hemisensory loss; and of frontal hemorrhage, arm weakness. Large hemorrhages may be associated with stupor or coma if they secondarily compress the thalamus or midbrain. Most patients with lobar hemorrhages have focal headaches. More than half the patients vomit or are drowsy, while stiff neck and seizures are uncommon.

Laboratory and Imaging Evaluation CT scanning reliably detects all but the smallest lobar hemorrhages. MRI is more sensitive for delineating associated abnormalities, such as aneurysm, vascular malformation, and neoplasm. Angiography is used when the cause of intracranial hemorrhage is uncertain, especially in the young and the middle-aged in whom amyloid angiopathy is not a consideration.

℞ TREATMENT

The recommendations for management of hypertensive intracerebral hemorrhage generally apply in this condition. If a causative lesion is found, it is treated appropriately.

COCAINE-RELATED INTRACEREBRAL HEMORRHAGE Pathophysiology and Pathology Cocaine elevates the heart rate, blood pressure, body temperature, and metabolic rate and is associated with ischemia of the myocardium, kidney, intestines, and brain.

Cocaine-induced stroke is one of the most important causes of stroke in the young. Most cocaine-related strokes occur in individuals under 40 years of age. Intracerebral hemorrhage, ischemic stroke, and SAH are all associated with cocaine use; they occur with all routes of administration and in both first-time and chronic users. Hemorrhagic stroke occurs twice as often as ischemic stroke, especially with cocaine hydrochloride. With the use of crack cocaine, hemorrhagic and ischemic complications occur with nearly equal frequency.

The strokes typically occur within minutes to hours of cocaine administration. Angiographic findings vary from completely normal arteries to large vessel occlusion or stenosis, vasospasm, or changes consistent with vasculitis.

Slightly more than half of cocaine-related intracranial hemorrhages are intracerebral and the rest are subarachnoid. Cocaine enhances sympathetic activity causing acute, sometimes severe, hypertension, and this may lead to hemorrhage. In patients with intracranial hemorrhage, underlying lesions are found in approximately half. In cases of SAH, a saccular aneurysm is usually identified; presumably, acute hypertension causes aneurysmal rupture. In the patients in whom no underlying lesion is found, approximately half have lobar hemorrhages or hematomas localized to the subcortical white matter. This is atypical for hypertensive hemorrhages, yet hypertension may still be responsible. These patients may have undetected underlying lesions such as cryptic AVMs, and some may have ischemic infarcts secondary to vasospasm followed by reperfusion and bleeding.

It is unclear whether cocaine can induce vasculitis. While occasional arteriograms of patients with cocaine-associated stroke show arterial beading or irregularities consistent with vasculitis, these findings are nonspecific and may be seen with vasospasm, fibromuscular dysplasia, and other disorders

Amphetamines cause stroke on the basis of acute hypertension and drug-induced vasculitis. Other stimulant drugs, including phenylephrine and ephedrine, are also reported to rarely induce intracerebral hemorrhage.

SUBARACHNOID HEMORRHAGE

The commonest cause of spontaneous SAH is a ruptured saccular aneurysm. Other causes are bleeding from an AVM or extension into the subarachnoid space from a primary intracerebral hemorrhage. Some cases are idiopathic, and these are often localized to the perimesencephalic cisterns and have an excellent prognosis. They probably have a venous or capillary, rather than arterial, source.

SACCULAR ANEURYSM Autopsy studies have found that 3 to 4 percent of the population harbor aneurysms, for a prevalence of 8 to 10 million in the United States. The incidence of bleeding is only 25,000 to 30,000 cases per year. The mortality rate for patients who arrive alive at hospital is about 50 percent during the first month. Of those who survive, more than half are left with major neurologic deficits as a result of the initial hemorrhage, cerebral vasospasm with infarction, or hydrocephalus. If the patient survives but the aneurysm is not obliterated, the annual rebleed rate is about 3 percent. Given these alarming figures, the major therapeutic emphasis is on preventing the predictable early complications of the rupture. Also, studies are in progress to assess the value of identifying and treating incidentally discovered aneurysms before they rupture.

Pathophysiology and Pathology Saccular aneurysms occur at the bifurcations of the large arteries at the base of the brain and rupture into the subarachnoid space in the basal cisterns. Approximately 85 percent of aneurysms occur on the anterior circulation, mostly on the circle of Willis. The common sites include the junction of the anterior communicating artery with the anterior cerebral artery, the junction of the posterior communicating artery with the internal carotid artery, and the bifurcation of the middle cerebral artery. The top of the basilar artery, the junction of the basilar artery and the superior cerebellar artery or the anterior inferior cerebellar artery, and the junction of the vertebral artery and the posterior inferior cerebellar artery comprise most of the remainder. About 20 percent of patients have multiple aneurysms, many at mirror sites bilaterally. As an aneurysm develops, it often forms a neck with a dome. The arterial internal elastic lamina disappears at the base of the neck. The media thins, and connective tissue replaces smooth-muscle cells. At the site of rupture (most often the dome), the wall thins, and the tear that allows bleeding is often no more than 0.5 mm long.

It is not possible to predict which aneurysms are likely to rupture, but limited data suggest that most ruptured aneurysms are large, e.g., average 7 mm in diameter.

Clinical Manifestations Most aneurysms present without warning as sudden SAH.

Occasionally, prodromal symptoms suggest the location of a progressively enlarging unruptured aneurysm. A third cranial nerve palsy, particularly when associated with pupillary dilatation, loss of light reflex, and focal pain above or behind the eye, may occur with an expanding aneurysm at the junction of the posterior communicating artery and the internal carotid artery. A sixth nerve palsy may indicate an aneurysm in the cavernous sinus, and visual field defects can occur with an expanding supraclinoid carotid aneurysm. Occipital and posterior cervical pain may signal a posterior inferior cerebellar artery (PICA) or anterior inferior cerebellar artery (AICA) aneurysm. Pain in or behind the eye and in the low temple can occur with an expanding middle cerebral aneurysm. Head pains in the absence of neurologic symptoms and signs are rarely caused by growing aneurysms.

Aneurysms can undergo small ruptures and leaks of blood into the subarachnoid space, so-called warning leaks. Sudden unexplained headache at any location should raise suspicion of SAH and be investigated because a major hemorrhage may be imminent.

At the moment of aneurysmal rupture with major SAH, the intracranial pressure suddenly rises. Abrupt, severe, and generalized vasospasm may occur transiently. These events may account for the sudden transient loss of consciousness that occurs in nearly half of patients. Sudden loss of consciousness may be preceded by a brief moment of excruciating headache, but most patients first complain of headache upon regaining consciousness. In 10 percent of patients, aneurysmal bleeding is severe enough to cause loss of consciousness for several days. In about 45 percent of cases, severe headache associated with exertion is the presenting complaint. The headache is often called by the patient "the worst headache of my life," even in those who do not lose consciousness. The headache is usually generalized. Vomiting is common and when coupled with sudden headache should always raise the suspicion of SAH.

Although sudden headache in the absence of focal neurologic symptoms is the hallmark of aneurysmal rupture, focal neurologic deficits may occur (in addition to direct cranial nerve compression by the enlarging aneurysm as noted above). Anterior communicating artery or middle cerebral bifurcation aneurysms may rupture into the adjacent brain and form a hematoma large enough to produce mass effect. The common deficits that result include hemiparesis, aphasia, and abulia.

Delayed neurologic deficits There are three major causes of delayed neurologic deficits: rerupture, hydrocephalus, and vasospasm.

Rerupture The incidence of rerupture in the first month following subarachnoid hemorrhage is about 30 percent, with the peak at 7 days. It is associated with a 60 percent mortality and poor outcome. Early surgery eliminates this risk.

Hydrocephalus Acute hydrocephalus can cause stupor and coma. More often, subacute hydrocephalus develops over a few days or weeks and causes progressive drowsiness or abulia with incontinence. Differentiating hydrocephalus from symptomatic cerebral vasospasm in the anterior communicating arteries is often difficult. Hydrocephalus may clear spontaneously or require temporary ventricular drainage. Chronic hydrocephalus may appear a few weeks to months after SAH. It presents with gait difficulty, incontinence, or slowed mentation (abulia). The clue to the diagnosis may be a lack of initiative in conversation or a failure to recover independence.

Vasospasm Narrowing of the arteries at the base of the brain following SAH regularly occurs. This vasospasm causes symptomatic ischemia and infarction in approximately 30 percent of patients and is the major cause of delayed morbidity or death. Signs of ischemia appear 4 to 14 days after the hemorrhage, most frequently at about 7 days. The severity and distribution of vasospasm determine whether infarction will occur.

Although the precise mechanism of delayed vasospasm is uncertain, it seems related to direct effects of clotted blood and its breakdown products on the artery. In general, the more blood there is surrounding the arteries, the more likely there will be symptomatic vasospasm.

Symptomatic severe vasospasm presents with symptoms referable to the specific arterial territories involved. However, even severe vasospasm may not produce ischemic symptoms if sufficient collateral blood flow develops through border zone anastomotic channels (see Fig. 366-1*A*). Spasm of the middle cerebral artery typically causes contralateral hemiparesis and dysphasia (dominant hemisphere). Proximal anterior cerebral artery vasospasm causes abulia and incontinence, while severe vasospasm of the posterior cerebral artery causes hemianopia. Severe spasm of the basilar or vertebral arteries occasionally produces focal brainstem ischemia. All these focal neurologic symptoms may develop over a few days, fluctuate, or present abruptly.

Severe cerebral edema in patients with infarction from vasospasm may increase the intracranial pressure enough to reduce cerebral perfusion pressure.

Laboratory and Imaging Evaluation (Figs. 366-13 and 362-1) The hallmark of aneurysmal rupture is blood in the CSF. About 80 percent have enough blood to be visualized on a noncontrast CT scan obtained within 72 h. A small hemorrhage may not be seen by CT scan. If the scan neither establishes the diagnosis of SAH nor demonstrates a mass lesion or obstructive hydrocephalus, an LP should be performed to establish the presence of subarachnoid blood.

The extent and location of subarachnoid blood on CT scan help locate the underlying aneurysm and identify the cause of any neurologic deficit. The clot also will help predict delayed vasospasm. A noncontrast CT scan should be done first, because on an enhanced scan normal arteries in the basal cisterns may be mistaken for clotted blood. A high incidence of symptomatic vasospasm in the middle and anterior cerebral arteries has been found when early CT scans show subarachnoid clots larger than 5 × 3 mm in the basal cisterns, or layers of blood more than 1 mm thick in the cerebral fissures. CT scans less reliably predict vasospasm in the vertebral, basilar, or posterior cerebral arteries.

LP prior to scanning is indicated only if a CT scan is not available at the time of the suspected SAH. Once the diagnosis of hemorrhage from ruptured saccular aneurysm has been established, four-vessel angiography (both carotids and vertebrals) is generally performed to localize and define the anatomic details of the aneurysm and to determine if other unruptured aneurysms exist.

The ECG frequently shows ST-segment and T-wave changes similar to those associated with cardiac ischemia. Prolonged QRS complex, increased QT interval, and prominent "peaked" or deeply inverted symmetric T waves, although suggesting primary cardiac disease, are usually secondary to the intracranial hemorrhage. The cause of these changes is debated, but there is evidence that structural myocardial lesions may occur after SAH.

Serum electrolyte levels should be measured because hyponatremia may develop.

Transcranial Doppler ultrasound assessment of proximal middle, anterior, and posterior cerebral and basilar artery flow is helpful in detecting the onset of vasospasm, even prior to symptoms, and following its course and response to therapy.

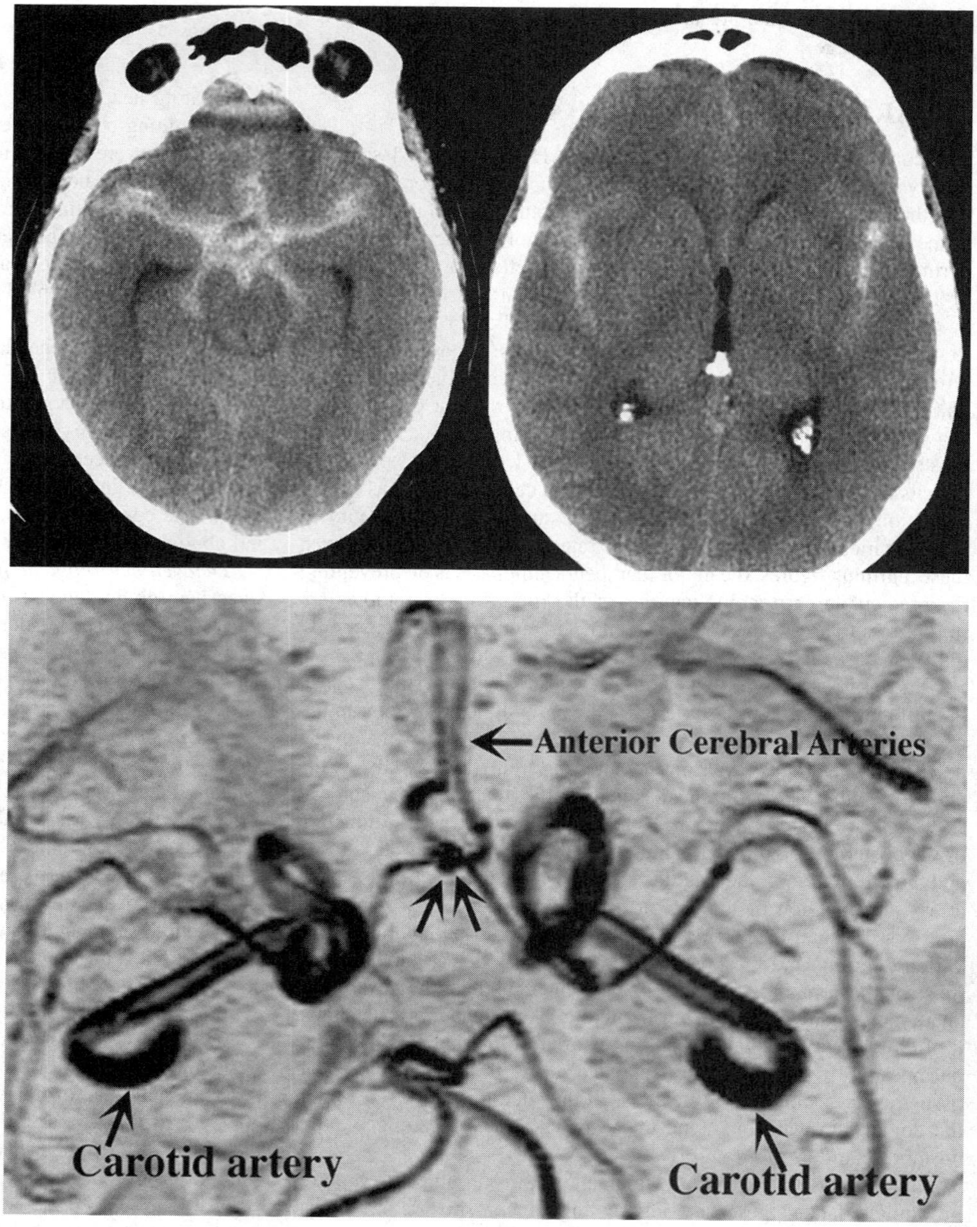

FIGURE 366-13 Cerebral aneurysm. *Top.* Sudden onset of headache and reduced mental status. Noncontrast CT scan at the level of the suprasellar cistern (*left*) and the third ventricle (*right*) revealed subarachnoid hemorrhage within the suprasellar cistern and middle cerebral cisterns also extending along the sylvian fissures bilaterally. Communicating hydrocephalus is present, indicated by dilation of the temporal horns of the lateral ventricle (*left image*). Angiography demonstrated an aneurysm of the anterior communicating artery, which had ruptured. *Bottom.* MR angiogram of an unruptured aneurysm demonstrates the anterior communicating artery aneurysm (*paired arrows*) as well as the internal carotid arteries and the anterior cerebral arteries.

℞ TREATMENT

Aneurysm rerupture is common in the early days after SAH and is associated with a 60 percent incidence of death or poor outcome. Consequently, patients who are alert or only mildly drowsy, have no major neurologic deficit, and have a surgically accessible aneurysm should undergo prompt microsurgical clipping of their aneurysm. Early aneurysm repair prevents future hemorrhage and allows the safe application of techniques to improve blood flow (e.g., induced hypertension and hypervolemia) should symptomatic vasospasm develop. Patients who are not candidates for early surgery should be managed medically to minimize the complications of obtundation, rebleeding, vasospasm, and hydrocephalus. Promising new techniques, such as endovascular placement of intraaneurysmal coils, are currently being evaluated in these patients.

Following aneurysmal rupture, intracranial hypertension can occur secondary to the presence of subarachnoid blood or parenchymal hematoma, acute hydrocephalus, or loss of vascular autoregulation. Emergency ventriculostomy is indicated for patients who are lethargic, have neurologic deficits, or have radiographic evidence of mass effect. Medical therapies to reduce intracranial pressure (e.g., mild hyperventilation, mannitol, and sedation) also can be used as needed.

Care is required to maintain adequate cerebral perfusion pressure while avoiding excessive elevation of arterial pressure. Occasionally an intracranial hematoma causing neurologic deterioration requires removal.

Because rebleeding is common, all patients who are not candidates for early surgical treatment are put on bed rest in a quiet, preferably darkened, room and are given adequate stool softeners to prevent constipation. If headache or neck pain is severe, mild sedation and analgesia are prescribed. Aspirin, an antiplatelet agent, is inappropriate, but acetaminophen may be used. Extreme sedation is generally avoided because it can obscure the assessment for neurologic deficits. Adequate hydration is necessary since patients with a decreased blood volume are especially prone to brain ischemia.

Seizures are uncommon at the onset of aneurysmal rupture. The quivering, jerking, and extensor posturing that often accompany loss of consciousness are probably related to the sharp rise in intracranial pressure and perhaps acute generalized vasospasm. However, phenytoin or phenobarbital are usually given as prophylactic therapy, since a seizure may promote rebleeding.

Glucocorticoids may help reduce the head and neck ache caused by the irritative effect of the subarachnoid blood. There is no good evidence that they reduce the cerebral edema that sometimes develops or are neuroprotective or reduce vascular injury, and their routine use therefore is controversial.

Antifibrinolytic agents may be used in patients in whom treatment is delayed. They are associated with a reduced incidence of aneurysmal rerupture but also are associated with an increased incidence of delayed cerebral infarction. This is especially true in patients who develop vasospasm and is presumably due to thrombosis induced by the antifibrinolytic agent. Because of the increased risk of ischemic complications, antifibrinolytics are not routinely given to patients who are at risk for developing vasospasm.

Although vasospasm remains the leading cause of morbidity and mortality following aneurysmal SAH, therapies to prevent or treat symptomatic arterial narrowing have been disappointing. Treatment with the calcium channel antagonist nimodipine has been reported to have beneficial effects, but the effect seems to be modest.

The most commonly accepted therapy for symptomatic cerebral vasospasm is to increase the cerebral perfusion pressure by raising mean arterial pressure through plasma volume expansion and the judicious use of pressor agents, ordinarily phenylephrine or dopamine. Raised perfusion pressure has been associated with symptomatic improvement in many patients, but high arterial pressure may promote rebleeding in unprotected aneurysms. Therefore, this treatment is reserved for patients whose aneurysm has been obliterated. Treatment with induced hypertension and hypervolemia generally requires monitoring the arterial and central venous pressure and, in severe cases, the intracranial and pulmonary artery wedge pressure. If symptomatic vasospasm persists despite optimal medical therapy, intraarterial papaverine and percutaneous intraarterial angioplasty are considered. They can relieve focal symptomatic vasospasm in the arteries at the base of the brain but also can precipitate further ischemia or arterial rupture.

Acute hydrocephalus can cause stupor or coma; it may clear spontaneously or require temporary ventricular drainage. When chronic hydrocephalus develops, ventricular shunting is the treatment of choice.

Giant aneurysms, those larger than 2.5 cm in diameter, occur at the same sites as small aneurysms and account for 5 percent of cases. The three most common locations are the terminal internal carotid, middle cerebral bifurcation, and top of the basilar arteries. Although they can bleed, they usually cause symptoms by compressing the adjacent brain or cranial nerves.

Incidentally discovered aneurysms that have not previously hemorrhaged have a 2 to 3 percent annual risk of bleeding. The risk of surgery, typically 5 percent morbidity and mortality, is modified by the patients' age and medical condition. The overall role of prophylactic surgical excision of incidentally discovered asymptomatic aneurysms and other lesions with potential for bleeding is being studied.

Mycotic aneurysms are located distal to the first bifurcation of major arteries of the circle of Willis. Most result from infected emboli due to bacterial endocarditis causing septic degeneration of arteries and subsequent dilatation and rupture. Whether these lesions should be sought and treated prior to rupture, or left to heal spontaneously, is controversial.

ARTERIOVENOUS MALFORMATION

Vascular malformations, or angiomas, may be tiny and cryptic or massive anomalies that cause headaches, brain damage, seizures, and hemorrhages. AVMs are the most important vascular malformations of the nervous system and consist of a tangle of abnormal vessels forming an abnormal communication between the arterial and venous systems. Most are developmental arteriovenous fistulas in which the involved vessels enlarge with the passage of time. AVMs vary in size from a small blemish a few millimeters in diameter to a huge mass of tortuous channels composing an arteriovenous shunt of sufficient magnitude to raise the cardiac output. Hypertrophic and dilated arterial feeders approach the main lesion, disappear below the cortex, and break up into a network of thin-walled blood vessels that connect directly with draining veins. These often form huge, dilated, pulsating channels carrying away arterial blood. The blood vessels forming the tangle interposed between arteries and veins are usually abnormally thin and do not have a normal structure. AVMs occur in all parts of the brain, brainstem, and spinal cord, but the largest ones are most frequently in the posterior half of the hemispheres, commonly forming a wedge-shaped lesion extending from the cortex to the ventricle.

AVMs are more frequent in men and may occur in more than one member of a family in the same or successive generations. Although the lesion is present from birth, bleeding or other problems are most common between the ages of 10 and 30, occasionally as late as the fifties.

The chief clinical symptoms and signs are headache, seizures, and those associated with rupture. When headache occurs (without bleeding), it may be hemicranial and throbbing, like migraine, or diffuse. Focal seizures, with or without generalization, occur in about 30 percent of cases. In half of patients, AVMs become evident as intracerebral hemorrhages, and in most of these patients, the hemorrhage is mainly intraparenchymal with a small amount of spillage into the subarachnoid space. Blood is usually not deposited in the basal cisterns, and symptomatic cerebral vasospasm is therefore rare. The threat of rerupture in the early weeks is low, so antifibrinolytic agents are not used. Hemorrhages may be massive, leading to death, or may be as small as 1 cm in diameter, leading to minor focal symptoms or no deficit. In either case, the hematoma may compress the AVM so completely that angiography cannot detect it. Hence, when an AVM is suspected, angiography is best postponed until the hematoma has resolved, i.e., after 6 to 8 weeks. Rarely the AVM is large enough to steal blood away from adjacent normal brain tissue, rendering the surrounding brain ischemic. This is seen most often when large AVMs in the middle cerebral territory extend from the cortical surface to the ventricular system. Hydrocephalus may result if the vein of Galen enlarges as a channel for drainage from the AVM.

Large AVMs of the carotid–middle cerebral system may be associated with systolic and diastolic bruits (sometimes self-audible) over the eye, forehead, or neck where a bounding carotid pulse may be perceived. Headache at the onset of AVM rupture is not generally as explosive as with aneurysmal rupture. Contrast CT scanning often detects the channels of an AVM prior to rupture, and new MRI techniques are even more sensitive.

AVMs less than 0.5 cm in diameter are usually low-pressure venous angiomas that bleed infrequently and minimally. If they bleed, surgical or gamma-knife resection or obliteration should be considered.

Most data suggest that patients with asymptomatic AVMs have a low risk for hemorrhage, which increases after a first hemorrhage to about 2 to 3 percent annually. Smaller lesions seem to have a higher hemorrhage rate, and the mortality rate with each bleed is about 15 percent.

The management of patients with arterial AVMs is best accomplished by a team approach. Surgical excision, interventional radiologic obliteration techniques, and radiotherapy all have a role. Intraarterial occlusion of feeding arteries is often used to shrink the lesion and make surgical excision less formidable.

OTHER CAUSES OF INTRACRANIAL HEMORRHAGE

Trauma Head injury often causes intracranial bleeding. The common sites are intracerebral (especially temporal and inferior frontal lobes), subarachnoid, subdural, and epidural. Trauma must be considered in any patient with an unexplained acute neurologic deficit (hemiparesis, stupor, or confusion), particularly if the deficit occurred in the context of a fall. These entities are discussed more fully in Chap. 374.

Hematologic Intracerebral hemorrhage associated with hematologic disorders (leukemia, aplastic anemia, thrombocytopenic purpura) can occur at any site and may present as multiple intracerebral hemorrhages. Skin and mucous membrane bleeding is usually evident and offers a diagnostic clue. Intracranial hemorrhage associated with anticoagulant therapy can occur at any location but is often lobar or subdural. Anticoagulant-related intracerebral hemorrhages may evolve slowly, over 24 to 48 h. Fresh frozen plasma and vitamin K may be required. When intracerebral hemorrhage is associated with platelet deficiencies, platelet transfusion may be required.

Brain Tumors Hemorrhage into a brain tumor may be the first manifestation of neoplasm (Chap. 375). Choriocarcinoma, malignant melanoma, renal cell carcinoma, and bronchogenic carcinoma are among the most common metastatic tumors associated with intracerebral hemorrhage. Glioblastoma multiforme in adults and medulloblastoma in children also may have areas of intracerebral hemorrhage.

Hypertensive Encephalopathy (See Chap. 246) Hypertensive encephalopathy is a complication of malignant hypertension. In this acute syndrome, severe hypertension is associated with headache, nausea, vomiting, convulsions, confusion, stupor, and coma. Focal or lateralizing neurologic signs, either transitory or lasting, may occur but are infrequent and therefore suggest some other vascular disease (hemorrhage, embolism, or atherosclerotic thrombosis). Retinal hemorrhages, exudates, papilledema (hypertensive retinopathy grade IV), and evidence of renal and cardiac disease may be present. In most cases the CSF pressure and protein levels are elevated. Lowering the blood pressure reverses the process, but permanent damage may have occurred. Neuropathologic examination reveals multifocal or diffuse cerebral edema with hemorrhages that vary in size from petechial to massive. Microscopically, necrosis of arterioles, minute cerebral infarcts, and hemorrhages are noted.

The term *hypertensive encephalopathy* should be reserved for this syndrome and not for chronic recurrent headaches, dizziness, epileptic seizures, recurrent TIAs, or small strokes that often occur in association with high blood pressure.

Other Causes Primary intraventricular hemorrhage is rare. It usually begins intraparenchymally and dissects into the ventricular system without leaving signs of intraparenchymal hemorrhage. Inflammatory disease of the arteries and veins, especially polyarteritis nodosa and lupus erythematosus, can produce hemorrhage into the central nervous system, most often in association with hypertension. Sepsis can cause small petechial hemorrhages throughout the cerebral white matter. There is no blood in the spinal fluid. Moyamoya disease most commonly causes ischemic symptoms but may on occasion produce multiple small aneurysms that rupture. Hemorrhages into the spinal cord are usually the result of an AVM or metastatic tumor (see Chap. 373).

BIBLIOGRAPHY

Antiplatelet Trialists' Collaboration: Collaborative overview of randomised trials of antiplatelet therapy—I: Prevention of death, myocardial infarction, and stroke by prolonged antiplatelet therapy in various categories of patients. BMJ 308:81, 1994

Atrial Fibrillation Investigators: Risk factors for stroke and efficacy of antithrombotic therapy in atrial fibrillation. Analysis of pooled data from five randomized controlled trials. Arch Intern Med 154:1449, 1994 [Erratum: ibid, p 2254]

Easton JD, Wilterdink JL: Carotid endarterectomy: Trials and tribulations. Ann Neurol 35:5, 1994

European Carotid Surgery Trialists' Collaborative Group: MRC European Carotid Surgery Trial: Interim results for symptomatic patients with severe (70–99%) or with mild (0–29%) carotid stenosis. Lancet 337:1235, 1991

Executive Committee for the Asymptomatic Carotid Atherosclerosis Study: Endarterectomy for asymptomatic carotid artery stenosis. JAMA 273:1421, 1995

Moore WS et al: Guidelines for carotid endarterectomy: A multidisciplinary consensus statement from the Ad Hoc Committee, American Heart Association. Stroke 26:188, 1995

North American Symptomatic Carotid Endarterectomy Trial Collaborators: Beneficial effect of carotid endarterectomy in symptomatic patients with high-grade carotid stenosis. N Engl J Med 325:445, 1991

Stroke Prevention in Atrial Fibrillation Investigators: Warfarin versus aspirin for prevention of thromboembolism in atrial fibrillation: Stroke Prevention in Atrial Fibrillation II Study. Lancet 343:687, 1994

The European Atrial Fibrillation Trial Study Group: Optimal oral anticoagulant therapy in patients with nonrheumatic atrial fibrillation and recent cerebral ischemia. The European Atrial Fibrillation Trial Study Group. N Engl J Med 333:5, 1995

The National Institute of Neurological Disorders and Stroke rt-PA Stroke Study Group: Tissue plasminogen activator for acute ischemic stroke. N Engl J Med 333:1581, 1995

van Gijn J et al: Major ongoing stroke trials: Anticoagulants versus aspirin in patients with transient ischemic attacks or nondisabling ischemic stroke: SPIRIT (Stroke Prevention In Reversible Ischemia Trial) (in progress). Stroke 26:1140, 1995

Wilterdink JL, Easton JD: Vascular event rates in patients with atherosclerotic cerebrovascular disease. Arch Neurol 49:857, 1992

367 ALZHEIMER'S DISEASE AND OTHER PRIMARY DEMENTIAS

Thomas D. Bird

ALZHEIMER'S DISEASE Alzheimer's disease (AD) is the most common cause of dementia in western countries. Approximately 10 percent of all persons over the age of 70 have significant memory loss, and more than half is the result of AD. This translates into approximately 3 to 4 million persons with AD in the United States, with a total health care cost of more than 50 billion dollars per year. It is estimated that the annual total cost of caring for a single AD patient in an advanced stage of the disease is $47,000. The disease also exacts a heavy emotional toll on family members and caregivers. AD was first described in 1907 in a 55-year-old woman by Professor Alois Alzheimer in Germany. The condition was initially thought to represent a relatively uncommon form of presenile dementia. However, it has become clear that AD can occur in any decade of adulthood and is the most common cause of dementia in the elderly. The disease is defined as a clinical-pathologic entity. Clinically, AD most often presents with subtle onset of memory loss followed by a slowly progressive dementia that has a course of several years. Pathologically there is gross, diffuse atrophy of the cerebral cortex with secondary enlargement of the ventricular system. Microscopically there are neuritic plaques containing Aβ amyloid, silver-staining neurofibrillary tangles in neuronal cytoplasm, and accumulation of Aβ amyloid in arterial walls of cerebral blood vessels (see "Pathogenesis," below). The recent identification of four different susceptibility genes for AD has provided a foundation for rapid progress in understanding the biologic basis of the disease.

Clinical Manifestations In the early stages of the disease, the memory loss may go unrecognized or may be ascribed to benign forgetfulness. Slowly the cognitive problems begin to interfere with daily activities, such as keeping track of finances, following instructions on the job, driving, shopping, and housekeeping. Some patients are unaware of these difficulties (agnosognosia) and others have considerable insight, resulting in frustration and anxiety. These major differences in insight have no clear explanation. Change of environment may be bewildering, and the patient may become lost on walks or while driving an automobile. In the middle stages of the disease, the patient is unable to work, is easily lost and confused, and requires daily supervision. Social graces, routine behavior, and superficial conversation may be surprisingly retained. Language may be impaired, especially comprehension and naming of objects. In some patients, aphasia is an early and prominent feature. Word-finding difficulties and circumlocution may be a problem even when formal testing demonstrates intact naming and fluency. Although confrontation naming is frequently deficient, there are often other language deficits as well, including impairments in fluency, comprehension, and repetition. Various apraxias are also common, that is, deficits in performing sequential motor tasks such as dressing, eating, solving simple puzzles, and copying geometric figures. Patients may be unable to do simple calculations or tell time. Rarely, AD patients may have a form of cortical blindness in which they deny their inability to see. This correlates at autopsy with severe neuropathologic changes in the visual cortex. In the late stages of the disease, some persons remain ambulatory but wander aimlessly and may have complete loss of judgment, reason, and cognitive abilities. Hallucinations and delusions are common; they are usually concrete and not too complex or bizarre. For example, patients may falsely accuse a spouse of infidelity, not recognize an old friend, think a visitor is a burglar, or become frightened of their own image in a mirror. Loss of inhibitions and belligerence may occur and may even alternate with passivity and social withdrawal. Sleep-wake patterns may be disturbed, and nighttime wandering may be very disruptive to the household. Some patients develop a shuffling gait with generalized muscle rigidity associated with slowness and awkwardness of movement. The patients often look parkinsonian but rarely have a rapid, rhythmic, resting tremor. In end-stage AD, patients frequently, but not always, become rigid, mute, incontinent, and bedridden. Help may be needed with the simplest tasks, such as eating, dressing, and toilet function. They may show hyperactive tendon reflexes and primitive sucking and snouting reflexes. Myoclonic jerks (sudden brief contractions of various muscles or the whole body) may occur spontaneously or in response to physical or auditory stimulation. This phenomenon raises the possibility of Creutzfeldt-Jakob disease (CJD) (Chap. 379), but the course of AD is much more prolonged. Generalized seizures may also occur. Death usually results from malnutrition, secondary infections, or heart disease. The typical duration of AD is 8 to 10 years, but the course can range from 1 to 25 years. For unknown reasons, some AD patients show a steady downhill decline in function, while others have prolonged plateaus without major deterioration.

Differential Diagnosis Early in the disease course, other etiologies of dementia should be excluded. These include treatable entities such as thyroid disease, vitamin deficiencies, brain tumor, drug and medication intoxication, chronic infection, and severe depression (pseudodementia) (see Chap. 26). Neuroimaging studies [computed tomography (CT) and magnetic resonance imaging (MRI)] are not specific for AD and may be normal early in the course of the disease. However, neuroimaging helps to exclude other disorders, such as primary and secondary neoplasms, multi-infarct dementia, diffuse white matter disease, and normal-pressure hydrocephalus. As AD progresses, diffuse cortical atrophy becomes apparent, and detailed MRI scans show atrophy of the hippocampus (Fig. 367-1*A*). The electroencephalogram (EEG) in AD may be normal or show nonspecific slowing. Routine spinal fluid examination gives normal results. Research studies have indicated a general decrease in cerebrospinal fluid (CSF) acetylcholine and Aβ amyloid levels with an increase in tau protein. There is considerable overlap of these levels with those of the normal aged population, and the usefulness of these measurements in diagnosis remains unclear. The use of blood apolipoprotein (Apo) E genotyping is discussed under "Pathogenesis," below. A report has appeared that the pupillary reaction in patients with AD is hypersensitive to tropicamide and that this response could form the basis of a diagnostic test. There has been no confirmation of the clinical utility of this phenomenon, and its use is not presently recommended. Slowly progressive decline, normal results on laboratory tests, and an MRI or CT scan showing only diffuse cortical atrophy including the hippocampus is highly suggestive of AD. A clinical diagnosis of AD reached after careful evaluation is confirmed at autopsy about 85 to 90 percent of the time. The misdiagnosed cases usually represent one of the other dementing disorders described later in this chapter. Relatively simple clinical clues are useful in the differential diagnosis. Early prominent gait disturbance with only mild memory loss suggests normal-pressure hydrocephalus (see below). Resting tremor with stooped posture, bradykinesia, and mask facies suggests Parkinson's disease (Chap. 368). Chronic alcoholism suggests vitamin deficiency. Loss of sensibility to position and vibration stimuli accompanied by Babinski responses suggests vitamin B_{12} deficiency (Chaps. 373 and 380). Early onset of a seizure suggests a metastatic or primary brain neoplasm (Chap. 375). A past history of long-term depression suggests pseudodementia (see below). A history of treatment for insomnia, anxiety, psychiatric disturbance, or epilepsy suggests chronic drug intoxication. Rapid progression over a few weeks or months associated with rigidity and myoclonus suggests CJD (Chap. 379). A positive family history of dementia suggests either one of the familial forms of AD or one of the other genetic disorders associated with dementia, such as Huntington's disease (see below), Pick's disease (see below), familial forms of prion diseases (Chap. 379), or rare forms of hereditary ataxias (Chap. 369).

Pathogenesis The most important risk factors for AD are old age and a positive family history. The frequency of AD increases with each decade of adult life to reach 20 to 40 percent of the population over the age of 85. A positive family history of dementia suggests a genetic cause of AD, as discussed below. Female gender may also be a risk factor independent of the greater longevity of women. Unconfirmed studies have suggested that postmenopausal estrogen use is associated with a decreased frequency of AD. Some AD patients have a past history of head trauma with concussion, but this appears to be a relatively minor risk factor. There is some suggestion that AD is more common in groups with lower educational attainment, but education influences test-taking ability, and it is clear that AD can affect persons of all intellectual levels. A recent unconfirmed study found that the capacity to express complex written language in early adulthood correlated with a decreased risk for AD. Numerous environmental factors, including aluminum, mercury, viruses, and prions, have been proposed as causes of AD, but none has been proved to play a role. Preliminary studies have suggested that the use of nonsteroidal anti-inflammatory agents is associated with a decreased risk of AD. Such reports require careful confirmation. Vascular disease does not seem to be a direct cause of AD, even though there is an associated amyloid angiopathy.

Positron emission tomography (PET) has indicated that the earliest metabolic changes in AD occur in parietal cortex (Fig. 367-1*B*). At autopsy, the most severe pathology is usually seen in the hippocampus, temporal cortex, and nucleus basalis. The most important microscopic findings are neuritic "senile" plaques and neurofibrillary tangles (NFTs). These two lesions accumulate in small numbers during normal aging of the brain but occur in quantitative excess in the dementia of AD. The neuritic plaques contain a central core that includes Aβ amyloid, proteoglycans, Apo E, α_1 antichymotrypsin, and other proteins. Aβ amyloid is a 4.2 kDa protein of 39 to 42 amino acids that is derived proteolytically from a larger transmembrane protein (amyloid precursor protein, APP). The normal function of Aβ amyloid is unknown. APP has been shown to have neurotrophic and neuroprotective activities. The plaque core is surrounded by the debris of

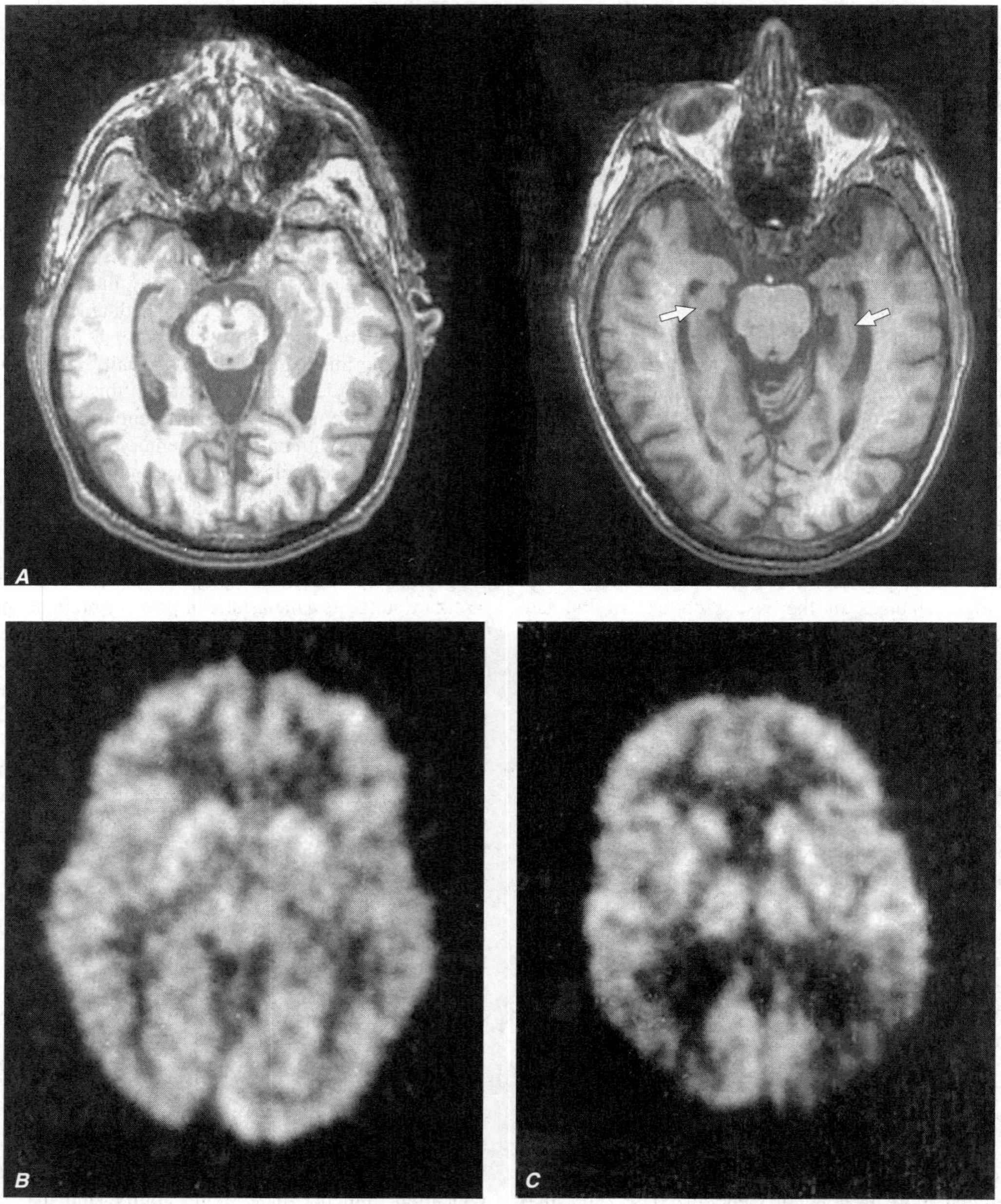

FIGURE 367-1 Alzheimer's disease. *A.* Axial T1-weighted MR images through the midbrain of a normal 86-year-old athlete (*left*) and a 77-year-old male (*right*) with Alzheimer's disease. Note that both individuals have prominent sulci and slight dilatation of the lateral ventricles. However, there is a reduction in the volume of the hippocampus of the patient with Alzheimer's disease (*arrows*) compared with that of the normal-aged athlete. *B*, C. Fluorodeoxyglucose PET scans of a normal-aged control (*left*) and a patient with Alzheimer's disease (*right*). Note that the patient with Alzheimer's disease has decreased activity in the parietal lobes bilaterally (*arrows*), a typical finding in this condition. (Images courtesy of TF Budinger, University of California.)

degenerating neurons and macrophages. The accumulation of Aβ amyloid in cerebral arterioles is termed *amyloid angiopathy*. The NFTs were first noted by Alzheimer. They are silver-staining, twisted neurofilaments in neuronal cytoplasm that represent abnormally phosphorylated tau (τ) protein and appear as paired helical filaments by electron microscopy. Tau is a microtubule-associated protein that may function to assemble and stabilize the microtubules that convey cell organelles, glycoproteins, and other important materials through the neuron. The ability of tau protein to bind to microtubule segments is determined partly by the number of phosphate groups attached to it. Increased phosphorylation of tau protein may disturb this normal process. Biochemically, AD is associated with a decrease in the cerebral cortical levels of several proteins and neurotransmitters, especially acetylcholine, its synthetic enzyme choline acetyltransferase (CAT), and nicotinic cholinergic receptors. Reduction of acetylcholine may be related in part to degeneration in the nucleus basalis of Meynert of cholinergic neurons that project to many areas of cortex. There is also reduction in norepinephrine levels in brainstem nuclei such as the locus coeruleus.

Several genetic factors are known to play important roles in the pathogenesis of at least some cases of AD. One is the amyloid precursor protein gene on chromosome 21. Adults with trisomy 21 (Down's syndrome) consistently develop the typical neuropathologic hallmarks of AD if they survive beyond age 40. Many also develop a progressive dementia superimposed on their baseline mental retardation. APP is a membrane-spanning protein that is subsequently processed into smaller units, including the Aβ amyloid that is deposited in the neuritic plaques of AD. Presumably the extra dose of the APP gene on chromosome 21 is the initiating cause of AD in adult Down's syndrome and eventually results in an excess of cerebral Aβ amyloid. Furthermore, a few families with early-onset familial AD (FAD) have been discovered to have point mutations in the APP gene. Although very rare, these families were the first indication of a single-gene autosomal dominant genetic transmission of AD. The most frequent of these APP mutations is substitution of valine for isoleucine at position 717.

Investigation of large families with multigenerational FAD led subsequently to the discovery of two additional AD genes, termed the *presenilins*. Presenilin-1 (*PS-1*) is on chromosome 14 and encodes a protein called S182. Mutations in this gene cause an early-onset AD (onset before age 60 and often before age 50) that is transmitted in an autosomal dominant, highly penetrant fashion. More than 20 different mutations have been found in the *PS-1* gene in families from a wide range of ethnic backgrounds. Presenilin-2 (*PS-2*) is on chromosome 1 and encodes a protein called STM2. A mutation in the *PS-2* gene was first found in a group of American families with Volga German ethnic background. The two genes (*PS-1* and *PS-2*) are highly homologous and encode similar proteins that at first appeared to have seven transmembrane domains (hence the designation *STM*, but subsequent studies have suggested eight such domains with a ninth submembrane region). The normal function of these proteins and the means by which mutations affecting them result in AD is unknown. Both S182 and STM2 are cytoplasmic neuronal proteins that are widely expressed throughout the nervous system. They are homologous to a cell-trafficking protein, sel 12, that is found in the nematode *Coenorhabditis elegans*. Patients with mutations in these genes have elevated plasma levels of Aβ41-42 amyloid, suggesting a possible link between the presenilins and APP. Mutations in the chromosome-14 gene have thus far proved to be the most common cause of early-onset FAD, representing perhaps 70 percent of this relatively rare syndrome. Mutations in *PS-1* tend to produce AD with an earlier age of onset (mean, 45 years) and a shorter, more rapidly progressive course (mean duration, 6 to 7 years) than the disease caused by mutations in *PS-2* (onset, 53 years; duration, 11 years). Some carriers of uncommon *PS-2* mutations have had onset of dementia after the age of 70. It is not yet clear whether presenilins are involved in the more common sporadic cases of late-onset AD occurring in the general population. Molecular DNA blood testing for these uncommon mutations is now possible on a research basis. Any testing of asymptomatic persons at risk must be done in the context of formal, thoughtful genetic counseling (see Chap. 363).

A discovery of great importance has implicated the Apo E gene on chromosome 19 in the pathogenesis of late-onset familial and sporadic forms of AD. Apo E is involved in cholesterol transport (Chap. 341) and has three alleles: ε2, ε3, and ε4. The ε4 allele of Apo E shows a strong association with AD in the general population, including sporadic and late-onset familial cases. Approximately 24 to 30 percent of the normal white population has at least one ε4 allele (12 to 15 percent allele frequency), and about 2 percent are ε4/4 homozygotes. In a group of AD patients, approximately 40 to 65 percent have at least one ε4 allele, a highly significant difference compared with controls. On the other hand, many AD patients have no ε4 allele, and individuals with ε4 may never develop AD. Therefore, ε4 is neither necessary nor sufficient as a cause of AD. Nevertheless, it is clear that the Apo E ε4 allele, especially in the homozygous 4/4 state, is an important risk factor for AD. It appears to act as a dose-dependent modifier of age of onset, with the earliest onset associated with the ε4/4 homozygous state. It is unknown how Apo E functions as a risk factor modifying age of onset. Apo E is present in the neuritic amyloid plaques of AD, and it may also be involved in neurofibrillary tangle formation, because it binds to tau protein. Apo E4 decreases neurite outgrowth in cultures of dorsal root ganglion neurons. There is some evidence that the ε2 allele may be "protective," but that remains to be clarified. Interesting but unconfirmed reports suggest that AD patients with an ε4 allele may be less responsive to tacrine. There is also preliminary evidence that the A allele of α_1 antichymotrypsin increases the risk of AD in carriers of the Apo E ε4 genotype. The use of Apo E testing in the diagnosis of AD is controversial. It is not indicated as a predictive test in normal persons, because its precise predictive value is unclear, and many individuals with the ε4 allele never develop dementia. However, some cognitively normal ε4/4 homozygotes have been found by PET to have decreased cerebral cortical metabolic rates, suggesting possible presymptomatic abnormalities compatible with the earliest stage of AD. It has also been proposed that in elderly demented persons, the finding of the Apo E ε4/4 homozygous state strongly confirms the diagnosis of AD, at about the 96 to 98 percent certainty level. Unfortunately, only a minority of persons are ε4/4 homozygotes, and even they may have other causes of dementia, such that a search for treatable causes is still necessary. Nevertheless, Apo E remains the single most important biologic marker associated with risk for AD, and studies of its functional role and diagnostic usefulness are progressing rapidly. Its association (or lack thereof) with other dementing illnesses needs to be fully evaluated. The ε4 allele is not associated with the dementia of Parkinson's disease or CJD.

℞ TREATMENT

The management of Alzheimer's disease is difficult and frustrating, because there is no specific treatment and the primary focus is on long-term amelioration of associated behavioral and neurologic problems. Building rapport with the patient, family members, and other caregivers is essential to successful management.

Tacrine (tetrahydroaminoacridine), 80 to 160 mg/d, is the only drug presently approved by the Food and Drug Administration (FDA) for treatment of AD. Its pharmacologic action is presumed to be inhibition of cholinesterase, with a resulting increase in cerebral levels of acetylcholine. Double-blind, placebo-controlled, crossover studies with tacrine have shown its use to be associated with improved caregiver ratings of patients' functioning and with an apparent decreased rate of decline in cognitive test scores over periods of up to 2 years. Such studies are difficult to perform because of the subjective nature of many of the observations and the lack of a uniform rate of decline among patients. Nevertheless, a small but important minority of AD patients (approximately 10 to 20 percent) appear to show a modest response to tacrine and tolerate its side effects (which include dose-related nausea, vomiting, and diarrhea). Tacrine gives no benefit in the late stages of AD. The medication is expensive and hepatotoxic, necessitating frequent testing of liver function and adjustment of the dose. Numerous other drugs, such as estrogen, anti-inflammatory agents, and anti-cholinesterases, are currently undergoing therapeutic trials.

Mild to moderate depression is common in the early stages of AD and may respond to antidepressant medication. Selective serotonin reuptake inhibitors (SSRIs) are commonly used, as are tricyclic antidepressants with low anticholinergic side effects (desipramine and nortriptyline). Generalized seizures should be treated with an appropriate anticonvulsant, such as phenytoin or carbamazepine. Agitation, insomnia, hallucinations, and belligerence are especially troublesome characteristics of some AD patients and often are responsible for nursing home placement. Mild sedation with benadryl may help insomnia, and agitation has been variously treated with phenothiazines (such as thioridazine), haloperidol, and benzodiazepines (such as lorazepam). These medications frequently have untoward side effects, including sedation, confusion, increased muscle tone, and adventitious movements. Low-dose haloperidol (0.5 to 2 mg), trazodone, buspirone, and propranolol may be the most helpful and have the least side effects. The few controlled studies comparing drugs with behavioral intervention in the treatment of agitation suggest that both approaches are equally effective. However, careful, daily, non-drug behavior management is often not available, rendering medication necessary. In the early stages of AD, memory aids such as notebooks and posted daily reminders are helpful. Common sense and clinical studies have shown that family members should emphasize activities that are pleasant and deemphasize those that are unpleasant. Kitchens, bathrooms, and bedrooms need to be made safe, and patients eventually must stop driving. Loss of independence and change of environment may worsen confusion, agitation, and anger. Communication and repeated calm reassurance are necessary. Caregiver "burnout" is common, often resulting in nursing home placement of the patient, and respite breaks for the caregiver help to maintain successful long-term management of the patient. Use of adult daycare centers can be most helpful. Local and national support groups, such as the Alzheimer's Disease and Related Disorders Association, are valuable resources.

VASCULAR DEMENTIA Dementia associated with cerebral vascular disease can be divided into two general categories: multi-infarct dementia and diffuse white matter dementia (also called subcortical arteriosclerotic encephalopathy or Binswanger's disease). Cerebral vascular disease appears to be a more common cause of dementia in Asia than in Europe and North America. Individuals who have had several strokes may develop chronic cognitive deficits, commonly called *multi-infarct dementia*. The strokes may be large or small (sometimes lacunar) and usually involve several different brain regions. The occurrence of dementia seems to depend partly on the total volume of damaged cortex, but it is also more common in individuals with left-hemisphere lesions, independent of any language disturbance. The patients give a history of episodes of sudden neurologic deterioration. Multi-infarct dementia patients usually also have a history of hypertension, diabetes, coronary artery disease, or other manifestations of diffuse atherosclerosis. Physical examination usually shows focal neurologic deficits such as hemiparesis, unilateral Babinski reflex, a visual field defect, or pseudobulbar palsy. The recurrent strokes result in a stepwise progression of disease. Neuroimaging studies clearly show the multiple areas of infarction. Thus, the history and neuroimaging findings differentiate this condition from AD. However, AD and multiple infarctions are both common and sometimes occur together. With normal aging, there is also an accumulation of amyloid in cerebral blood vessels, leading to a condition called *cerebral amyloid angiopathy of aging* (not associated with dementia), which predisposes older persons to hemorrhagic lobar stroke. AD patients with amyloid angiopathy and hypertension also appear to be at increased risk of cerebral infarction. Apo E ϵ4 has been reported to be a risk factor for amyloid angiopathy independent of AD.

Some persons with dementia are discovered on MRI studies to have bilateral abnormalities of subcortical white matter, termed diffuse white matter disease (or leukoaraiosis) (Fig. 367-2). The dementia may be of subtle onset and slow progression, features that distinguish it from multi-infarct dementia. (A few such patients have been described with apparently sudden onset of cognitive impairment.) Early symptoms are mild confusion, apathy, change in personality, and memory deficit. Marked difficulties in judgment and orientation and dependence on others for daily activities develop later. Euphoria, elation, or aggressive behavior are common. A mixed picture of pyramidal and cerebellar signs may be present in the same patient. Lateralizing motor signs are uncommon. A gait disorder appears in at least half the patients. In advanced cases, urinary incontinence and dysarthria with or without pseudobulbar features are frequent. Seizures and myoclonic jerks appear in a minority of patients. This disorder appears to be the result of chronic ischemia due to occlusive disease of small penetrating cerebral arteries and arterioles (microangiopathy). The patients usually, but not always, have a history of hypertension, but any disease causing stenosis of small cerebral vessels may be the critical underlying factor. Binswanger described several patients with this condition, but the term *Binswanger's disease* should be used with caution, because it does not really identify a single entity. Other rare causes of white matter disease may also present with dementia, such as adult metachromatic leukodystrophy and progressive multifocal leukoencephalopathy (papovavirus infection).

Treatment of vascular dementia must be focused on the underlying causes, such as hypertension, atherosclerosis, and diabetes. Recovery of lost cognitive function is not likely to occur.

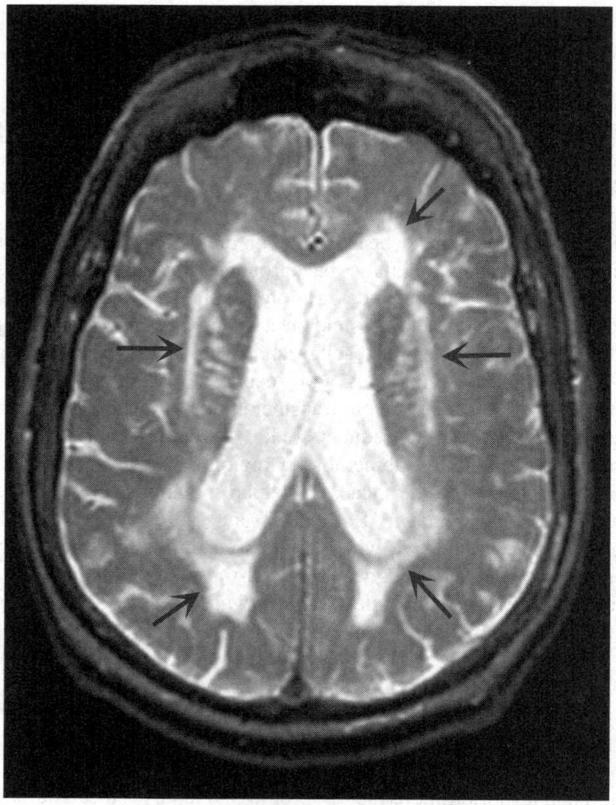

FIGURE 367-2 Diffuse white matter disease (Binswanger's disease). Axial T2-weighted MR image through the lateral ventricles reveals multiple areas of abnormal high signal intensity involving the periventricular white matter as well as the corona radiata and lentiform nuclei (*arrows*). While seen in some individuals with normal cognition, this appearance is more pronounced in patients with dementia of a vascular etiology.

PICK'S DISEASE Pick's disease is a commonly discussed disorder that is difficult to differentiate clinically from AD and is less well defined as a distinct entity. The major distinguishing hallmarks are marked symmetric lobar atrophy of temporal and/or frontal lobes, which can be visualized by neuroimaging studies and is readily apparent at autopsy. For this reason, the diagnosis of frontotemporal dementia overlaps with Pick's disease. The atrophy is sometimes asymmetric and may involve the basal ganglia. Microscopic findings include gliosis, neuronal loss, and swollen or ballooned neurons, which frequently contain silver-staining cytoplasmic inclusions referred to as *Pick bodies*. Pick bodies consist of straight and constricted fibrils that share antigenic determinants with the NFTs of AD, including the microtubule-associated protein tau, suggesting that Pick bodies derive from altered components of the neuronal cytoskeleton. Onset is usually in the fifth through seventh decades. Clinically, there is a slowly progressive dementia often associated with hyper-oral behavior, bulimia, language disturbance, emotional disinhibition, irritability, and persistent aimless wandering. The language disturbance may be aphasia or forced repetitive speech patterns, sometimes progressing to echolalia, language impoverishment, and mutism. Unfortunately, each of these clinical characteristics, as well as relative lobar atrophy, may occur in AD, so that the clinical diagnosis of Pick's disease is simply an educated guess that must be confirmed at autopsy. Furthermore, brains containing Pick bodies may also have varying quantities of amyloid plaques and neurofibrillary tangles, again blurring the distinction from AD. Examples of familial Pick's disease that display an autosomal dominant-like pattern of inheritance have been reported. There is no specific treatment.

DIFFUSE LEWY BODY DISEASE Lewy bodies are intraneuronal cytoplasmic inclusions that stain with periodic acid–Schiff (PAS)

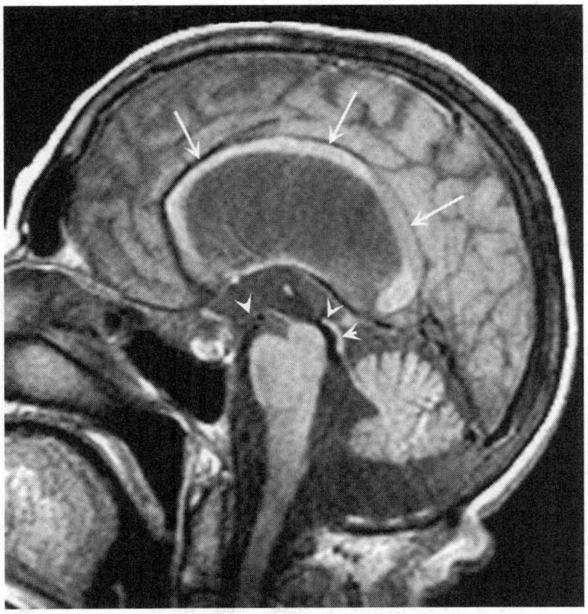

A

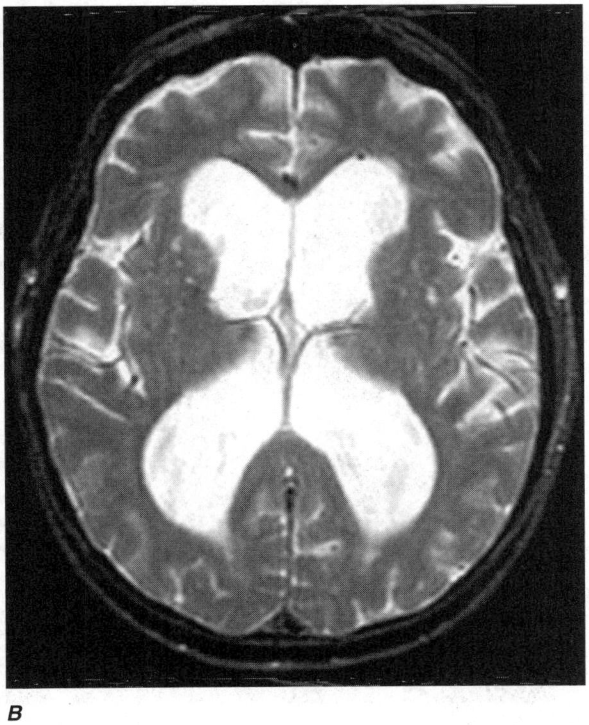

B

FIGURE 367-3 Normal pressure hydrocephalus. *A*. Sagittal T1-weighted MR image demonstrates dilatation of the lateral ventricle and stretching of the corpus callosum (*arrows*), depression of the floor of the third ventricle (*single arrowhead*), and enlargement of the aqueduct (*double arrowheads*). Note the diffuse dilatation of the lateral, third, and fourth ventricles with a patent aqueduct, typical of communicating hydrocephalus. *B*. Axial T2-weighted MR images demonstrate dilatation of the lateral ventricles. This patient underwent successful ventriculoperitoneal shunting.

and ubiquitin. They are composed of straight neurofilaments 7 to 20 nm long with surrounding amorphous material. They contain epitopes recognized by antibodies against phosphorylated and nonphosphorylated neurofilament proteins as well as ubiquitin. Lewy bodies are traditionally found in the substantia nigra of patients with idiopathic Parkinson's disease. Large numbers of such inclusions have also been discovered in cortical neurons in patients with dementia. In patients

without other pathologic features, the condition is referred to as *diffuse Lewy body disease*. In patients whose brains also contain amyloid plaques and neurofibrillary tangles, the condition is called the *diffuse Lewy body type of Alzheimer's disease*. The quantity of Lewy bodies required to establish the diagnosis is not agreed on. Nevertheless, the diagnosis is primarily a neuropathologic entity. However, there is some evidence that there is a characteristic clinical syndrome. In addition to chronic progressive dementia, these patients often also have Parkinsonian features, especially rigidity sometimes combined with an intention tremor. There may be frequent fluctuations of behavior, cognitive ability, and level of alertness. These fluctuations can be marked, with the occurrence of episodic confusion and lucid intervals suggesting delirium. However, despite the fluctuating pattern, the clinical features persist over a long period, unlike a typical transient delirium. Delusions and visual hallucinations are common, and auditory hallucinations may also occur. Repeated unexplained falls are often noted. Frequently there is an unusual sensitivity to neuroleptic medications and benzodiazepines, with exaggerated adverse responses to standard doses. In most patients, this condition is difficult to distinguish from AD or Parkinson's disease with dementia. The population prevalence of diffuse Lewy body disease is unclear, but it is more commonly diagnosed nowadays with the use of ubiquitin staining during neuropathologic studies. At autopsy, 10 to 30 percent of demented patients may show cortical Lewy bodies. It is not yet clear what role Apo E may play in Lewy body disease without AD changes. There is no specific treatment.

NORMAL-PRESSURE HYDROCEPHALUS Normal-pressure hydrocephalus (NPH) is a syndrome with several clinical, physiologic, and neuroimaging characteristics. The clinical triad includes an abnormal gait (ataxic or apractic), dementia (usually mild to moderate), and urinary incontinence. Neuroimaging studies of the brain reveal enlarged lateral ventricles (hydrocephalus) with little or no cortical atrophy. This is a communicating hydrocephalus with a patent aqueduct of Sylvius (Fig. 367-3). Lumbar puncture opening pressure is in the high normal range, and the CSF protein and sugar concentrations and cell count are normal. NPH is presumed to be caused by obstruction to normal flow of CSF over the cerebral convexity and delayed absorption into the venous system. The indolent nature of the process results in enlarged lateral ventricles but relatively little increase in CSF pressure. There is presumably stretching and distortion of white matter tracts in the corona radiata, but the exact physiologic cause of the clinical syndrome is unclear. Some patients with NPH have a history of conditions producing scarring of the basilar meninges (blocking upward flow of CSF) such as previous meningitis, subarachnoid hemorrhage, or head trauma. Most patients seem to have no pertinent past history. In contrast to patients with AD, the patient with NPH has an early and prominent gait disturbance and no evidence of cortical atrophy on CT or MRI. A number of attempts have been made to use various special studies to improve the diagnosis of NPH and predict the success of ventricular shunting. These include radionuclide cisternography (showing a delay in CSF absorption over the convexity) and various attempts to monitor and alter CSF flow dynamics, including a constant-pressure infusion test. None of these studies has proven to be specific or consistently useful. There is sometimes a transient improvement in gait or cognition following lumbar puncture (or serial punctures) with removal of 30 to 50 mL of CSF, but this finding also has not proved to be consistently predictive of post-shunt improvement. One study determined that no more than 1 to 2 percent of a large group of demented patients had NPH. AD often masquerades as NPH, because the gait may be abnormal in AD and cortical atrophy sometimes is difficult to determine by CT or MRI early in the disease. Hippocampal atrophy on MRI may be a clue favoring AD. Approximately 30 to 50 percent of patients identified by careful diagnosis as having NPH will show improvement with a ventricular shunting procedure.

Gait may improve more than memory. Transient, short-lasting improvement is common. Patients should be carefully selected for this operation, because subdural hematoma and infection are known complications.

HUNTINGTON'S DISEASE Huntington's disease (HD) is a genetic, autosomal dominant, degenerative brain disorder. It has a population frequency of about 10/100,000. The two clinical hallmarks of the disease are chorea and behavioral disturbance. The illness may begin with either or both of these symptoms predominating. Onset is usually in the fourth or fifth decade, but there is a wide range in age of onset, from childhood to greater than 70 years. The chorea begins as subtle fidgeting that may be unrecognized by the patient and family. However, the movement disorder is usually slowly progressive and eventually may become disabling. There are frequent, irregular, sudden jerks and movements of any of the limbs or trunk. Grimacing, grunting, and poor articulation of speech may be prominent. The gait is disjointed and poorly coordinated and has a so-called dancing (choreic) quality. Memory is frequently not impaired until late in the disease, but attention, judgment, and executive functions may be seriously deficient at an early stage. Depression, apathy, social withdrawal, irritability, and intermittent disinhibition are common. Delusions and obsessive-compulsive behavior may occur. Schizophrenia is occasionally the initial diagnosis. The disease duration is typically about 15 years but also shows a wide range. Early onset before the age of 20 (juvenile HD) is associated with rigidity, ataxia, cognitive decline, and more rapid progression, with a typical duration of about 8 years. Seizures are rare with adult-onset HD but more common with juvenile-onset disease. There is no specific treatment, but the adventitious movements and behavioral changes may partially respond to phenothiazines, haloperidol, or benzodiazepines.

Neuropathologically, the disease predominantly strikes the striatum. Atrophy of the caudate nuclei, which form the lateral margins of the lateral ventricles, can be visualized on neuroimaging studies in the middle and late stages of the disease (Fig. 367-4). Microscopically there are no dramatic pathologic characteristics, such as the plaques and tangles seen with AD. However, there is gliosis and neuronal loss, especially of medium-sized spiny neurons in the caudate and putamen. There is relative sparing of large cholinergic aspiny neurons. (Treatment with 3-nitroproprionic acid, a succinate dehydrogenase inhibitor, has produced HD-like pathologic changes in experimental animals). Neurochemically there is a marked decrease of gamma-aminobutyric acid (GABA) and its synthetic enzyme glutamic acid decarboxylase throughout the basal ganglia. The levels of other neurotransmitters, including substance P and enkephalins, are also reduced. Nuclear magnetic resonance (NMR) spectroscopy in living subjects with HD has shown elevated levels of lactate in the basal ganglia.

The HD gene, called *IT15*, is located on chromosome 4p, contains a CAG trinucleotide repeat expansion, and codes for a protein called huntingtin. The protein is found in neurons throughout the brain; its normal function is unknown. Inactivation of the homologous gene in mice causes embryonic death in homozygotes, but heterozygotes are phenotypically normal. Transgenic mice with an expanded CAG repeat in the HD gene develop a progressive movement disorder. The CAG repeat codes for a long polyglutamine domain in the expressed protein. The disease process may result from a toxic gain of function (Chap. 363). One hypothesis is that these polyglutamine tracts cause abnormal protein binding reactions which then interfere with other cell processes, such as mitochondrial activity. Abnormal binding of IT15 to glyceraldehyde 3-phosphate dehydrogenase has been reported. There is also evidence for inappropriate neuronal apoptosis in HD.

The DNA repeat expansion forms the basis of a diagnostic blood test for the disease gene. Persons having 38 or more CAG repeats in the HD gene have inherited the disease mutation and will eventually develop symptoms if they live to an advanced age. Each of their children has a 50 percent risk of also inheriting the abnormal gene. There is a rough correlation between a larger number of repeats and an earlier age of onset, but most patients fall into a range of intermediate repeat numbers (40 to 49 repeats) in which this correlation is not clinically useful. For unclear reasons, juvenile onset with a large repeat expansion most often occurs when the father is the affected parent (a form of genetic anticipation). Asymptomatic adult children at risk for HD should receive careful genetic counseling prior to DNA testing, because a positive result may have serious emotional and social consequences. Detailed testing and counseling protocols have been published. In addition

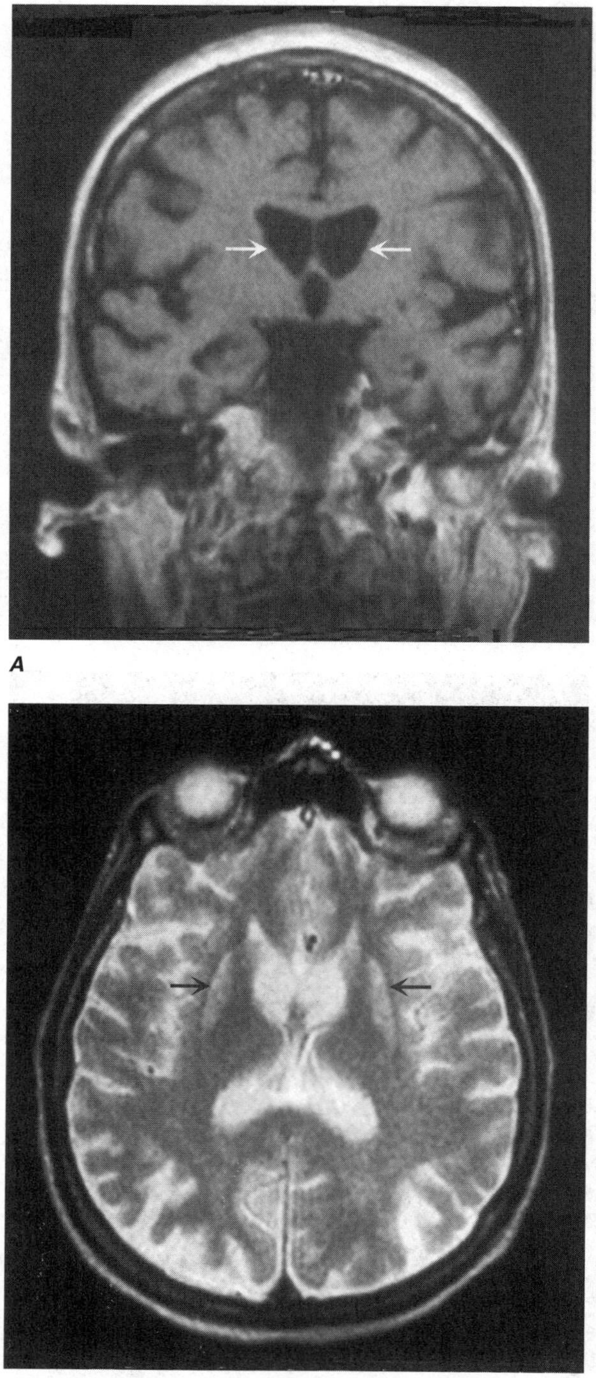

A

B

FIGURE 367-4 Huntington's disease *A*. Sagittal T1-weighted MRI shows enlargement of the lateral ventricles reflecting typical caudate atrophy (*arrows*). *B*. Axial T2-weighted image demonstrates abnormal high signal intensity in the putamen (*arrows*).

to use in genetic counseling of persons at risk for HD, the DNA test can also be used in differential diagnosis. For example, some persons with late-onset, apparently sporadic "senile" chorea have been found to carry the HD mutation. Also, disorders that may mimic HD, such as schizophrenia, benign familial chorea, inherited ataxias, neural acanthocytosis and familial AD, will not show the CAG expansion in the HD gene.

OTHER DEGENERATIVE DEMENTIAS Several other primary neurologic disorders have been associated with dementia and are the result of various poorly understood degenerative neuronal processes. These conditions include so-called frontal lobe dementia, cortical basal degeneration, progressive supranuclear palsy, and primary progressive aphasia. These are progressive dementing illnesses of unknown cause whose names are descriptive of the typical clinical signs or the anatomic brain areas that are involved with nonspecific atrophy and neuronal degeneration.

One such condition is *progressive supranuclear palsy* (see also Chap. 368). This is a degenerative disease that involves both the brainstem and neocortex with diffuse NFTs. Clinically, this disorder begins with vertical supranuclear gaze paresis and progresses slowly to include rigidity and dementia. Stiff posture with hyperextension of the neck and slow gait with frequent falls are common. Early in the disease, the patients have difficulty with down-gaze and lose vertical opticokinetic nystagmus on downward movement of the target. Although the patients have very limited voluntary eye movements, their eyes still retain oculocephalic reflexes (doll's head maneuver). The dementia is considered to be of the subcortical type, with slowed thought processes, impaired verbal fluency, and difficulty with sequential actions and with shifting from one task to another. Seizures and sleep apnea may occur. There is only a limited response to L-dopa, and there is no other effective treatment. Death occurs within 5 to 10 years. At autopsy, the NFTs are found in multiple subcortical structures (including the subthalamus, globus pallidus, substantia nigra, locus coeruleus, periaqueductal gray, superior colliculi, and oculomotor nuclei) as well as in the neocortex. The NFTs have similar staining characteristics to those of AD, but on electron microscopy they generally are seen to consist of straight tubules rather than the paired helical filaments found in AD.

Progressive supranuclear palsy is often confused with idiopathic *Parkinson's disease*. Although elderly Parkinson's patients may have some difficulty with upgaze, they do not develop significant downgaze paresis or progressive supernuclear palsy. However, dementia does occur in approximately 20 percent of Parkinson's patients. The occurrence of dementia in Parkinson's disease is more likely with increasing age, increasing severity of extrapyramidal signs, and the presence of depression. These patients may also show cortical atrophy on brain imaging. Neuropathologically, there may be Alzheimer changes in the cortex (amyloid plaques and NFTs), neuronal Lewy body inclusions in both the substantia nigra and the cortex, or no specific microscopic changes other than gliosis and neuronal loss.

Some authors refer to a condition called *frontal lobe* or *frontotemporal dementia* (see Chap. 25). In addition to progressive memory loss and confusion, the patients are often irritable and have loss of inhibitions. These patients may do better than those with AD on construction and calculation tasks. Imaging studies reveal atrophy confined to the frontal or frontal and temporal lobes. The condition is not a specific entity, and the designation usually includes Pick's disease. Frontal lobe dementia represents as much as 10 percent of dementia cases in some autopsy series.

Cortical basal degeneration is a slowly progressive dementing illness associated with severe gliosis and neuronal loss in both the neocortex and basal ganglia (substantia nigra and striatum). There is often a unilateral onset with rigidity, dystonia, and apraxia of one arm and hand. Eventually the condition becomes bilateral and includes dysarthria, slow gait, action tremor, and dementia. The microscopic features include enlarged, achromatic neurons in the cortex, and there may also be NFTs and amyloid plaques. The condition is rarely familial; the cause is unknown; and there is no specific treatment.

Another entity is *primary progressive aphasia* (see Chap. 25). Patients with this disorder have aphasia associated with asymmetric atrophy of the left hemisphere and occasionally go on to develop dementia. Neuroimaging studies show the left hemisphere atrophy. Some patients are nonfluent, with hesitant, telegraphic speech associated with impaired comprehension and naming. Neuropathologic studies have shown a heterogeneous group of abnormalities, including Pick's disease, AD, CJD, and nonspecific gliosis.

A rare degenerative disease has also occurred in the Chamorro natives on the island of Guam and is referred to as the *ALS/parkinsonian/dementia complex of Guam* (see Chap. 370). Individual patients may have any combination of parkinsonian features, dementia, and motor neuron disease. The most characteristic pathologic features are the presence of NFTs in degenerating neurons of the cortex and substantia nigra and loss of motor neurons in the spinal cord. Epidemiologic evidence supports a probable environmental cause, such as exposure to a neurotoxin with a long latency period. One interesting but unproven candidate neurotoxin occurs in the seed of the false palm tree, which Guamanians traditionally used to make flour. The ALS syndrome is decreasing in frequency on Guam, but a dementing illness continues to be seen.

Finally, a rare autosomal dominant genetic form of dementia with nonspecific neuropathologic findings has been linked to DNA markers on chromosome 17. The specific gene has not been identified. Some of these families have dementia associated with motor neuron disease, others with parkinsonian features. This condition is now referred to as frontotemporal dementia with parkinsonism linked to chromosome 17 (FTDP-17).

BIBLIOGRAPHY

American College of Medical Genetics/American Society of Human Genetics Working Group on APOE and Alzheimer Disease: Consensus statement on use of apolipoprotein E testing for Alzheimer disease. JAMA 274:1627, 1995

Bird TD, Bennett RL: Why do DNA testing? Practical and ethical implications of new neurogenetic tests. Ann Neurol 38:141, 1995

Caplan LR: Binswanger's disease—revisited. Neurology 45:626, 1995

Daniel SE et al: The clinical and pathological spectrum of Steele-Richardson-Olszewski syndrome (progressive supranuclear palsy): A reappraisal. Brain 118:759, 1995

Davis KL, Powchik P: Tacrine. Lancet 345:625, 1995

del Ser T et al: Vascular dementia: A clinicopathological study. J Neurol Sci 96:1, 1990

Kertesz A et al: The pathology and nosology of primary progressive aphasia. Neurology 44:2065, 1994

Levy-Lahad E et al: Candidate gene for the chromosome 1 familial Alzheimer's disease locus. Science 269:973, 1995

———, Bird TD: Genetic factors in Alzheimer's disease: A review of recent advances. Ann Neurol 40:829, 1996

Lynch T et al: Clinical characteristics of a family with chromosome 17-linked disinhibition-dementia-parkinsonism-amyotrophy complex. Neurology 44:1878, 1994

Malm J et al: The predictive value of cerebrospinal fluid dynamic tests in patients with the idiopathic adult hydrocephalus syndrome. Arch Neurol 52:783, 1995

McKeith IG et al: An evaluation of the predictive validity and inter-rater reliability of clinical diagnostic criteria for senile dementia of Lewy body type. Neurology 44:872, 1994

Mendez MF et al: Pick's disease versus Alzheimer's disease: A comparison of clinical characteristics. Neurology 43:289, 1993

Raftopoulos C et al: Cognitive recovery in idiopathic normal pressure hydrocephalus: A prospective study. Neurosurgery 35:397, 1994

Reiman EM et al: Preclinical evidence of Alzheimer's disease in persons homozygous for the $\epsilon 4$ allele for apolipoprotein E. N Engl J Med 334:752, 1996

Sherrington R et al: Cloning of a gene bearing missense mutations in early-onset familial Alzheimer's disease. Nature 375:754, 1995

Tatemichi TK et al: Dementia after stroke: Baseline frequency, risks, and clinical features in a hospitalized cohort. Neurology 42:1185, 1992

Terry RD et al: *Alzheimer Disease.* New York, Raven Press, 1994

Tison F et al: Dementia in Parkinson's disease: A population-based study in ambulatory and institutionalized individuals. Neurology 45:705, 1995

Van Broeckhoven CJ: Molecular genetics of Alzheimer disease: Identification of genes and gene mutations. Eur Neurol 35:8, 1995

Vanneste JAL: Three decades of normal pressure hydrocephalus: Are we wiser now? J Neurol Neurosurg Psychiatr 57:1021, 1994

Wiggins S et al: The psychological consequences of predictive testing for Huntington's disease. N Engl J Med 237:1401, 1992

368

Michael J. Aminoff

PARKINSON'S DISEASE AND OTHER EXTRAPYRAMIDAL DISORDERS

PARKINSON'S DISEASE Parkinsonism is a syndrome consisting of a variable combination of tremor, rigidity, bradykinesia, and a characteristic disturbance of gait and posture. Parkinson's disease is a chronic, progressive disorder in which idiopathic parkinsonism occurs without evidence of more widespread neurologic involvement.

Parkinson's disease generally commences in middle or late life and leads to progressive disability with time. The disease occurs in all ethnic groups, has an equal sex distribution, and is common, with a prevalence of 1 to 2 per 1000 of the general population and 1 per 100 among people older than 65 years. Signs of parkinsonism are extremely common in the elderly; a recent survey indicated that 15 percent of individuals between 65 and 74 years of age, and more than half of all individuals after age 85, have abnormalities on examination consistent with the presence of an extrapyramidal disorder.

Neuroanatomy Symptoms of Parkinson's disease are caused by loss of nerve cells in the pigmented substantia nigra pars compacta and the locus coeruleus in the midbrain. Cell loss also occurs in the globus pallidus and putamen. Eosinophilic intraneural inclusion granules (Lewy bodies) are present in the basal ganglia, brainstem, spinal cord, and sympathetic ganglia; they do not occur in other disorders in which parkinsonism is a feature.

The neural pathways that modulate motor activity are considered in detail in Chap. 21. Pars compacta neurons of the substantia nigra provide dopaminergic input to the striatum, which is part of the basal ganglia (Fig. 21-4*A*). These dopaminergic neurons, and also cholinergic striatal interneurons, modulate a monosynaptic gamma-aminobutyric acid (GABA-ergic) inhibitory output to the globus pallidus interna and pars reticulata of the substantia nigra, which project in turn by a GABA-ergic inhibitory pathway to the ventroanterior and ventrolateral nuclei of the thalamus. Stimulation of this "direct" pathway in the striatum disinhibits these thalamic nuclei so that their excitatory output to the motor region of the cerebral cortex is increased. An alternative, polysynaptic ("indirect") pathway from the striatum reduces the excitatory output from these thalamic nuclei to the motor cortex, as shown in Fig. 21-4*A*. This latter pathway involves striatal GABA-ergic inhibitory neurons that project to the globus pallidus externa, which has an inhibitory effect on the subthalamic nucleus. This nucleus has excitatory glutamatergic connections with the globus pallidus interna and pars reticulata of the substantia nigra.

In Parkinson's disease, loss of dopaminergic cells in the substantia nigra leads to striatal dopamine depletion. Because dopamine activates excitatory D1 receptors in the direct pathway and represses inhibitory D2 receptors in the indirect pathway, this depletion results in decreased activity of the direct pathway and increased activity of the indirect pathway and so in reduced thalamic excitation of the motor cortex (Fig. 21-4*B*). Other neurotransmitters, such as norepinephrine, are also depleted, with clinical consequences that are uncertain but perhaps contribute to depression.

Pathogenesis Parkinsonism can be induced in primates by exposure to 1-methyl-4-phenyl-1,2,3,6-tetrahydropyridine (MPTP), which is converted by monoamine oxidase B to *N*-methyl-4-phenylpyridinium (MPP^+), an active toxin. MPP^+ is taken up by dopaminergic nigral neurons through an active transport system that is normally involved in dopamine reuptake, and then inhibits oxidative phosphorylation, possibly at the level of complex I in the respiratory chain. This results in the death of nigrostriatal neurons, dopamine depletion in the basal ganglia, and parkinsonism. In addition to energy failure, MPP^+ may also generate free radicals and oxidative stress.

The cause of Parkinson's disease is unknown. One suggested cause is exposure to an unrecognized environmental toxin, perhaps structurally similar to MPTP. Such exposure may have occurred years before the onset of any clinical disturbance, because symptoms will not develop until the cumulative cell loss from toxin exposure and natural aging approximates 80 percent of the original cell population. Alternatively or additionally, endogenous toxins may be responsible. In particular, the normal neurotransmitter dopamine readily oxidizes to produce free radicals, which can cause cell death by oxidizing various cellular constituents. Although the precise role of dopamine itself remains unclear, the evidence relating Parkinson's disease to damage by free radicals remains compelling.

It is not clear whether there is a significant genetic component in the etiology of Parkinson's disease. Studies in monozygotic and dizygotic twins initially suggested that the disease rarely had a genetic basis. More recent work involving positron emission tomography (PET) studies have shown, however, that asymptomatic twins of parkinsonian patients commonly have abnormalities of striatal dopamine uptake; this suggests that genetic factors are important, although this finding was present equally in monozygotic and dizygotic twins. Attempts to identify the responsible gene or genes contributing to the development of Parkinson's disease are currently in progress; linkage to chromosome 4q21-23 was recently reported in a large Italian family with autosomal dominant parkinsonism.

Clinical Manifestations The 4- to 6-Hz tremor is typically most conspicuous at rest and worsens with emotional stress. It often begins with rhythmic flexion-extension of the fingers, hand, or foot, or with rhythmic pronation-supination of the forearm, and may be confined initially to one limb or to the two limbs on one side before becoming more generalized. It may also involve the mouth and chin. In 10 to 15 percent of patients, however, the tremor is faster (7 to 8 Hz) and postural, resembling essential tremor (see below) both clinically and in its response to pharmacotherapy.

Rigidity, defined as an increase in resistance to passive movement (Chap. 21), is a common clinical feature that accounts for the flexed posture of many patients. The most disabling feature, however, is bradykinesia (or, in its most severe form, akinesia), a slowness of voluntary movement and an associated reduction in automatic movements, such as swinging of the arms when walking. There is a fixity of facial expression, with widened palpebral fissures and infrequent blinking. There may be blepharoclonus (fluttering of the closed eyelids), blepharospasm (involuntary closure of the eyelids), and drooling of saliva from the mouth. The voice is hypophonic and poorly modulated. Power is preserved, but fine or rapidly alternating movements are impaired. The combination of tremor, rigidity, and bradykinesia results in small, tremulous, and often illegible handwriting. Patients have difficulty in rising from bed or an easy chair and tend to assume a flexed posture when erect. Walking is often difficult to initiate, and patients may have to lean forward increasingly until they can advance. They walk with small, shuffling steps, have no arm-swing, are unsteady (especially on turning), and may have difficulty in stopping. Some patients walk with a festinating gait, i.e., at an increasing speed to prevent themselves from falling because of their abnormal center of gravity.

The tendon reflexes are unaltered, and the plantar responses are flexor. Repetitive tapping (at about 2 Hz) over the glabella produces a sustained blink response (Myerson's sign), in contrast to the response of normal subjects. A depressed mood is common, and an impairment of cognitive function—sometimes amounting to a frank dementia—is frequently evident in advanced cases.

Differential Diagnosis Parkinsonism is simulated by certain disorders. *Depression* is associated with changes in the voice and facial appearance and a poverty of spontaneous activity, such as occur in Parkinson's disease. A trial of treatment with antidepressant drugs helps to clarify the diagnosis if uncertainty persists and other signs of parkinsonism are absent. *Essential (benign, familial) tremor* may be mistaken for parkinsonian tremor, but a family history of tremor is common; alcohol in small quantities may ameliorate the tremor, and other neurologic signs are lacking. Moreover, essential tremor commonly involves the head (with a nodding or no-no tremor), whereas parkinsonism spares the head but affects the face and lips. *Normal-pressure hydrocephalus* (see Chap. 367) causes an apraxic gait disturbance (sometimes resembling the gait of parkinsonism), urinary incontinence, and dementia. Imaging studies reveal dilation of the ventricular system without cortical atrophy, and surgical shunting procedures to bypass any obstruction to the flow of cerebrospinal fluid (CSF) may be helpful.

Parkinsonism may occur as part of various neurologic diseases that are important to distinguish from Parkinson's disease for prognostic and therapeutic purposes. In *Wilson's disease* (see Chap. 345), other abnormal movements are also usually present. The family history, early age of onset, associated Kayser-Fleischer rings, and low serum copper and ceruloplasmin levels distinguish it from Parkinson's disease. *Huntington's disease* (see Chap. 367) sometimes presents with rigidity and akinesia, but the family history and any accompanying dementia point to the correct diagnosis, which can be confirmed by genetic studies. The *Shy-Drager syndrome* (see also Chap. 371) is a degenerative disorder characterized by parkinsonism, impaired autonomic function (resulting in postural hypotension, abnormal thermoregulatory sweating, disturbances of bladder and bowel control, impotence, and gastroparesis) and by signs of more widespread neurologic involvement (pyramidal, cerebellar, or lower motor neuron signs). There is generally no treatment except for the postural hypotension, which may respond to the measures discussed in Chap. 371. The response to antiparkinsonian agents is usually disappointing. *Striatonigral degeneration* (see below) leads to bradykinesia and rigidity, but tremor is usually inconspicuous. Cerebellar deficits sometimes occur (multisystem atrophy), and there may be autonomic insufficiency (Shy-Drager syndrome). Antiparkinsonian drugs are generally ineffective. *Progressive supranuclear palsy* (discussed separately, below) causes bradykinesia and rigidity, but conspicuous abnormalities of voluntary eye movements (especially vertical gaze), dementia, pseudobulbar palsy, and axial dystonia distinguish it from Parkinson's disease. There is little or no response to antiparkinsonian drugs. *Cortical-basal ganglionic degeneration* may be mistaken for Parkinson's disease, but intellectual decline, aphasia, apraxia, sensory neglect, and other evidence of cortical dysfunction should suggest the correct diagnosis. In *diffuse Lewy body disease*, parkinsonism is joined with a conspicuous dementia and with evidence of more widespread neurologic involvement. In *Creutzfeldt-Jakob disease*, any parkinsonian features are overshadowed by the rapidly progressive dementia; myoclonus is common, ataxia or pyramidal signs may occur, visual disturbances are sometimes conspicuous, and the electroencephalographic findings are often characteristic. Similarly, in *Alzheimer's disease* there may be minor extrapyramidal deficits, but these are generally inconsequential compared with the marked cognitive impairment that characterizes the disorder. → ***Alzheimer's disease and diffuse Lewy body disease are considered in Chap. 367, and Creutzfeldt-Jakob disease is discussed in Chap. 379.***

Parkinsonism sometimes occurs as a consequence of a systemic disorder. Drug-induced *secondary parkinsonism* is especially common (discussed below). MPTP-induced parkinsonism has occurred in several humans who inadvertently took this meperidine analogue for recreational purposes. The mechanisms involved are discussed above, and the history of exposure, unusually early age of onset, and rapid progression should suggest the correct diagnosis. Exposure to various toxins, such as manganese dust or carbon disulfide, also causes parkinsonism, and the diagnosis is suggested by an accurate occupational history. Parkinsonism sometimes occurs as a result of severe carbon monoxide poisoning or develops after an encephalitic illness. Postencephalitic parkinsonism was especially common after the outbreak of encephalitis lethargica that occurred in an early part of the twentieth century.

℞ TREATMENT

Approaches to treatment are summarized in Fig. 368-1.

Symptomatic Pharmacologic Treatment Nonselective muscarinic antagonists (*anticholinergic drugs*) are sometimes helpful, especially in relieving tremor. Various preparations are available, including trihexyphenidyl, benztropine, procyclidine, and orphenadrine. The usual starting and maintenance doses are shown in Table

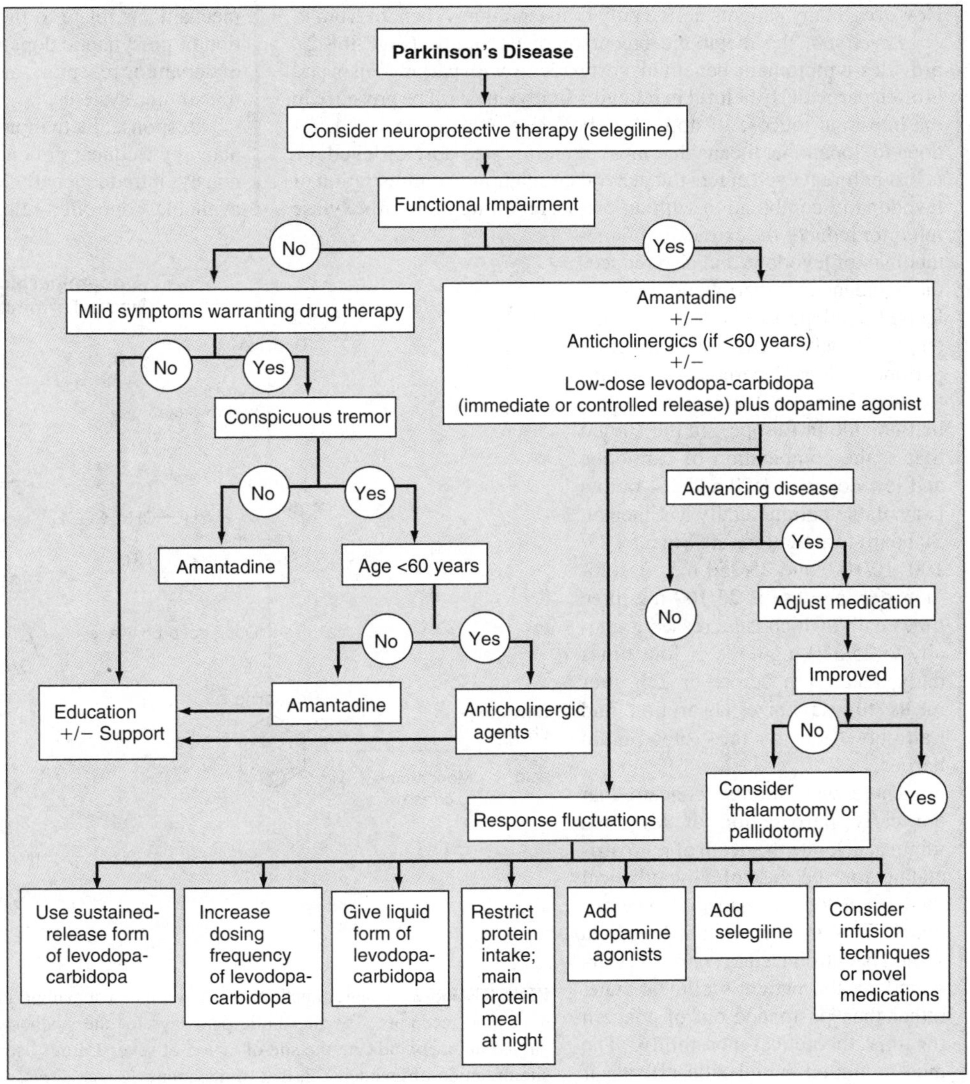

FIGURE 368-1 Algorithm for the management of patients with Parkinson's disease.

Table 368-1

Commonly Used Muscarinic Antagonists (Anticholinergic Drugs) for the Treatment of Parkinson's Disease

Generic Name	Proprietary Name	Tablet Strength	Usual Dose, mg
Benztropine	Cogentin	0.5, 1, 2	0.5–2 tid
Biperiden	Akineton	2	1–3 qid
Orphenadrine	Disipal	100	100 tid
Procyclidine	Kemadrin	5	2.5–10 tid
Trihexyphenidyl	Artane	2, 5	2–5 tid

368-1. Common side effects include dryness of the mouth, constipation, urinary retention, and blurred vision. Narrow-angle glaucoma may be aggravated. Confusion and hallucinations are especially troublesome in the elderly. Treatment is started with the preparation of choice in a small initial dose that is gradually increased depending on response and tolerance. If the drug is unhelpful, another anticholinergic preparation is substituted.

Amantadine, either alone or combined with an anticholinergic agent, is sometimes helpful for mild parkinsonism; it acts by potentiating the release of endogenous dopamine. It may improve all major clinical features of the disorder, has relatively uncommon side effects (restlessness, confusion, skin rashes, edema, disturbances of cardiac rhythm), and is given in a standard dose (100 mg twice daily). However, many patients derive only transient, if any, benefit from it.

Levodopa, the metabolic precursor of dopamine (Fig. 368-2), provides symptomatic benefit in most patients with parkinsonism and is often particularly helpful in relieving bradykinesia. The presence in the intestinal mucosa of dopa decarboxylase, which converts levodopa to dopamine, means that most of an ingested dose of levodopa is lost before it even enters the general circulation. Administration of levodopa in combination with an extracerebral dopa-decarboxylase inhibitor reduces the extracerebral metabolism of levodopa and also reduces the incidence of peripheral side effects. Levodopa is therefore administered routinely in combination with a peripheral dopa-decarboxylase inhibitor (carbidopa in the United States; benserazide in Europe). In the United States, the combination of carbidopa and levodopa (in 1:10 and 1:4 ratios) is available commercially as Sinemet. Standard formulations are Sinemet 25/100, 10/100, and 25/250 mg. A common starting dose is 25/100 mg three times daily, which is increased gradually to 25/250 mg three or four times daily, taken 1 h before or 2 h after meals to maximize absorption and transport across the blood-brain barrier.

There was initially concern that the early introduction of levodopa might accelerate the death of nigrostriatal neurons because of a hypothetical increase in dopamine-mediated neurotoxity. It is now clear that levodopa should be introduced as soon as is warranted by the patient's clinical state, rather than postponed out of concern for this theoretical possibility. The most common initial side effects of levodopa are nausea, vomiting, postural hypotension, and, occasionally, cardiac arrhythmias. Abnormal movements (dyskinesias), restlessness (akathisia), and confusion tend to occur somewhat later and are dose-related. Dyskinesias probably result from denervation supersensitivity of postsynaptic dopamine receptors. They may be present during most of the day, occur only when plasma levodopa levels peak, or develop when the plasma levodopa concentration reaches a certain submaximal level. Management depends on distinguishing these possibilities by the temporal profile of the dyskinesia. When dyskinesias occur only at a certain submaximal blood level of levodopa, adjustment of the daily dose to produce higher or lower blood levels may alleviate them; dyskinesias related to peak blood levels of levodopa are helped by a reduction in dose.

Important late complications of levodopa therapy are the wearing-off effect (transient deterioration shortly before the next dose is due) and the "on-off" phenomenon—abrupt but transient fluctuations in clinical state that occur frequently during the day, without warning or an obvious relationship to dosing schedule, resulting in alternating periods of marked akinesia or greater mobility accompanied by iatrogenic dyskinesias. The on-off phenomenon can be controlled in part by reducing dosing intervals, administering levodopa 1 h before meals and restricting dietary protein intake (to reduce any competition by various amino acids with levodopa for the active carrier system that transports it into the blood and from the blood into the brain), or treatment with dopamine agonists. The addition of selegiline (5 mg at breakfast and lunch), a monoamine oxidase B inhibitor, reduces the metabolic breakdown of dopamine and may also be helpful (see "Neuroprotective Treatment" below). The pathogenesis of the on-off phenomenon is obscure, but proposed mechanisms relate to the pharmacokinetics of levodopa, degeneration of presynaptic dopaminergic nerve terminals, altered sensitivity of dopamine receptors, and abnormalities of nondopaminergic neurotransmitter systems.

Response fluctuations to oral levodopa may be reduced or eliminated by frequent or continuous administration of levodopa intravenously, intraduodenally, or by intragastric infusion. A commercially available controlled-release formulation of Sinemet (Sinemet CR

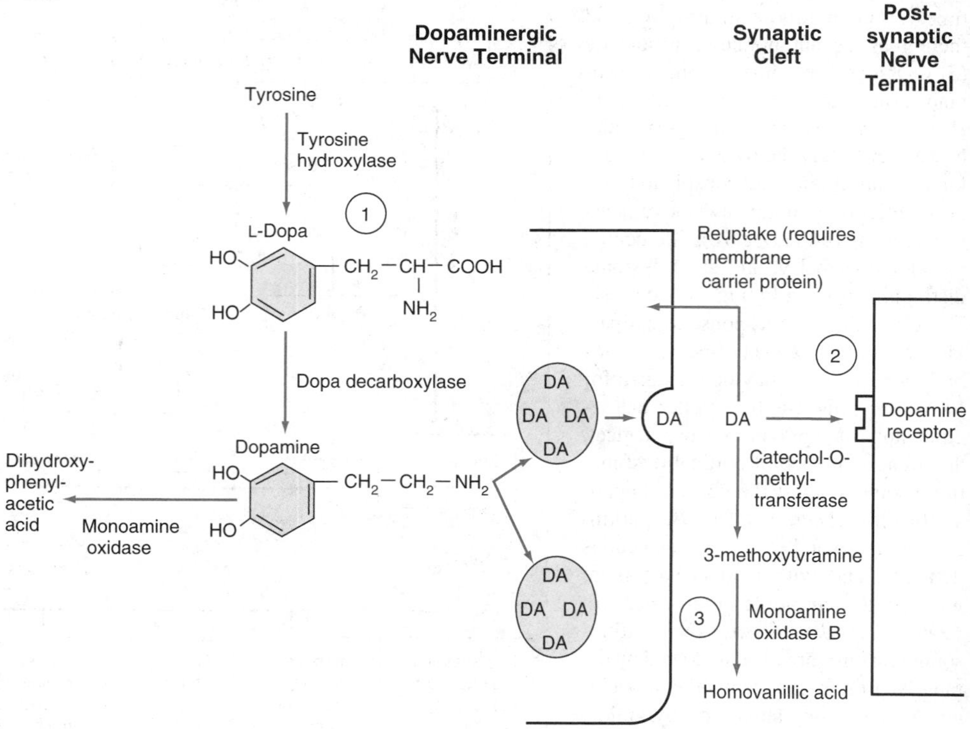

FIGURE 368-2 Diagrammatic representation of a dopaminergic nerve terminal and the associated postsynaptic dopamine receptors. The metabolic pathways for the synthesis and breakdown of dopamine are shown. The circled numbers indicate the site of action of several drugs used in the treatment of Parkinson's disease: *1*, the site of action of levodopa; *2*, that of dopamine agonist drugs, such as bromocriptine and pergolide; and *3*, that of selegiline. DA, dopamine.

25/100 or 50/200 mg) sometimes helps in reducing the dosing frequency and maintaining steady blood levels of levodopa, but it is of only limited benefit in reducing response fluctuations.

Dopamine agonist drugs, such as the ergot derivatives bromocriptine and pergolide, may produce symptomatic benefit by direct stimulation of dopamine receptors (Fig. 368-2), although the benefit may not be sustained unless levodopa is also taken. Their absorption and cerebral distribution are less erratic than those of levodopa, and they do not require enzymatic conversion to an active metabolite. Their early introduction in conjunction with low-dose Sinemet therapy (25/100 mg three times daily) yields sustained benefit and a lower incidence of late complications (such as response fluctuations and dyskinesias) than when levodopa is used alone and in a higher dose.

Bromocriptine, which stimulates dopamine D2 receptors, is introduced in a dose of 1.25 mg/d for one week and 2.5 mg/d for the next week, after which the daily dose is increased by 2.5-mg increments every 2 weeks, depending on response and tolerance. Maintenance doses range between 2.5 and 10 mg three times daily when the drug is taken with Sinemet. Pergolide activates both D1 and D2 dopamine receptors. It is introduced in a dose of 0.05 mg daily for 2 days; the dose is then increased by 0.1 to 0.15 mg/d every 3 days for 12 days and by 0.25 mg/d every 3 days thereafter. The usual maintenance dose is 1 mg three times daily. The side effects of these agonists are similar to those of levodopa, but psychiatric effects such as delusions or hallucinations are more common, and dyskinesias are less common, than with levodopa. Dopamine agonists are contraindicated in patients with psychotic disorders and are best avoided in those with recent myocardial infarction, severe peripheral vascular disease, or active peptic ulceration.

Various new dopamine agonists are being evaluated, and new means of administering them (e.g., by subcutaneous infusion pump or transdermally) may lead to a steadier clinical response.

Novel symptomatic therapies currently being evaluated or developed include selective catechol-*O*-methyltransferase (COMT) inhibitors, which may enhance the benefits of levodopa therapy by reducing the conversion of levodopa to 3-*O*-methyldopa (which competes with levodopa for an active carrier mechanism) and by increasing the availability in the brain of levodopa. Experimental studies suggest that glutamate antagonists may benefit patients with Parkinson's disease, and clinical studies of such agents are planned. G_{M1} ganglioside and various neurotrophic factors influence dopaminergic nigrostriatal cells, and work is in progress to develop delivery systems that will permit their use in the treatment of Parkinson's disease.

Surgical Treatment Destructive neurosurgical procedures were used for some years to treat parkinsonism, but their use declined with the advent of levodopa. Unilateral posteroventral pallidotomy or thalamotomy has recently been resurrected as a therapeutic approach for relieving rigidity, bradykinesia, and tremor in patients with advanced disease in whom antiparkinsonian medication is ineffective or poorly tolerated. A positive (but incomplete) response to surgery is reported in preliminary studies to occur in more than 90 percent of patients; the beneficial effect predominates on the side contralateral to the procedure.

There has been recent interest in transplantation of fetal midbrain dopaminergic (nigral) cells into the putamen of patients with Parkinson's disease. Survival of engrafted cells has been documented by enhancement of fluorodopa uptake as visualized by PET, and in one autopsy study there was extensive striatal reinnervation by the transplanted cells. Fetal nigral transplantation remains an experimental procedure, and the nature of any long-term benefit is uncertain. Transplantation of autologous adrenal medullary tissue has also been attempted for Parkinson's disease, with mixed results; benefit seems most likely to occur in individuals younger than 50 years of age.

Neuroprotective Treatment Selective inhibitors of monoamine oxidase B such as selegiline (Eldepryl; Deprenyl) may reduce oxidative damage and thus slow disease progression, but the evidence for this effect is incomplete. In a large multicenter study, treatment with selegiline delayed the need for symptomatic therapy in patients with untreated parkinsonism, suggesting that progression of the disease had been retarded, but it was subsequently found that selegiline itself has a mild effect on symptoms. Thus, the basis of the observed effect is uncertain. The use of selegiline for protective purposes should probably be discussed with all patients unless they have end-stage disease or are very elderly, but the uncertainty of any benefit should be indicated. Selegiline in a standard dose (5 mg with breakfast and 5 mg with lunch) is not associated with the hypertensive ("cheese") effect of nonselective monoamine oxidase inhibitors. Acute toxic interactions may, however, occur with meperidine, tricyclic drugs, or serotonin reuptake inhibitors, and selegiline should not be prescribed to patients receiving those medications. Selegiline is metabolized to amphetamine and methamphetamine, so some patients may experience anxiety or insomnia. Moreover, an increased mortality rate has recently been found among patients receiving selegiline, raising concerns about its long-term safety. Patients must understand that selegiline is not intended to relieve symptoms and that there is no means of determining whether it is affecting disease progression in individual cases. Other inhibitors of monamine oxidase B, such as lazabemide, are currently being evaluated for their effect on the natural history of Parkinson's disease and may clarify the issue.

Tocopherol (vitamin E) is an important scavenger of free radicals, but in a large study it failed to provide any protective benefit when taken in a dose of 2000 units daily. The extent to which it penetrates the brain, however, is not clear.

General Measures Physical therapy and speech therapy may help patients with moderately severe parkinsonism. In advanced cases, the quality of life can be improved by certain aids to daily living, such as extra rails or banisters placed in the home, table cutlery with large handles, nonslip table mats, voice amplifiers, and chairs that can gently eject the occupant.

FAMILIAL OR BENIGN ESSENTIAL TREMOR A postural tremor (Chap. 21) may develop in otherwise normal subjects, sometimes on a familial basis with autosomal dominant inheritance. The pathophysiologic basis of the disorder is unknown.

Symptoms can develop at any age but often do not appear until middle or later life. Typically one or both hands, the head, and the voice are affected in any combination; the legs are generally spared. Apart from the tremor, no other abnormalities are present on neurologic examination. The tremor may worsen with time and ultimately become an embarrassment, but it generally causes no disability except when it disturbs handwriting or performance of fine tasks with the hands. A small quantity of alcohol sometimes relieves the tremor for a short period.

Rx TREATMENT

Treatment is often unnecessary and is best delayed for as long as possible because, once initiated, it generally needs to be continued indefinitely. Propranolol, 40 to 120 mg orally twice daily, may reduce the amplitude of the tremor. A single oral dose (40 to 120 mg) may be taken in anticipation of known precipitating circumstances. Primidone is also effective but has to be introduced gradually.

PROGRESSIVE SUPRANUCLEAR PALSY Progressive supranuclear palsy (also referred to as Steele-Richardson-Olszewski syndrome) is a sporadic degenerative disorder characterized pathologically by neuronal loss, gliosis, and neurofibrillary tangles in the midbrain, pons, basal ganglia, and dentate nuclei of the cerebellum. The neurofibrillary tangles of this disorder are distinct from those of Alzheimer's disease in that they are composed of straight filaments rather than paired helical filaments. There are decreased concentrations of dopamine and homovanillic acid in the caudate nucleus and putamen.

Clinical Manifestations This uncommon disorder generally begins between the ages of 45 and 75 years; it affects men twice as frequently as women. Supranuclear ophthalmoplegia is characteristic. There is conspicuous failure of voluntary saccadic gaze (and of the fast phase of optokinetic nystagmus) in a vertical plane, especially downward, with later involvement of horizontal gaze. Eventually, smooth pursuit movements are also affected. Oculocephalic (e.g., doll's-head) and oculovestibular (caloric) reflexes are intact. Axial dystonia in extension, especially of the neck, is common and is frequently accompanied by limb rigidity and bradykinesia that may mimic Parkinson's disease. Tremor, however, is unusual. The combination of supranuclear ophthalmoplegia and axial rigidity accounts for the common presenting complaint of frequent falls. There may be facial weakness, dysarthria, dysphagia, and exaggerated jaw jerk and gag reflexes (pseudobulbar palsy) as well as exaggerated and inappropriate emotional responses (pseudobulbar affect). Brisk tendon reflexes, extensor plantar responses, and cerebellar signs are sometimes encountered. A global impairment of intellectual function is frequent, but focal cortical dysfunction is rare.

Progressive supranuclear palsy should be considered whenever a middle-aged or elderly person with repeated falls has an extrapyramidal syndrome accompanied by nuchal dystonia and paralysis of voluntary downgaze. The marked impairment of voluntary downward and horizontal gaze distinguishes this disorder from Parkinson's disease, as does the extended rather than flexed dystonic posturing of the axial musculature, the absence of tremor, and the poor response to antiparkinsonian medications.

℞ TREATMENT

The course is generally progressive, with aspiration or inanition leading to a fatal outcome within 10 years. The response to pharmacotherapy is usually disappointing. Dopaminergic preparations sometimes reduce rigidity and bradykinesia, and anticholinergic (trihexyphenidyl, 6 to 15 mg/d) or tricyclic drugs (amitriptyline, 50 to 75 mg at bedtime) may benefit speech, gait, and pseudobulbar affect.

CORTICAL-BASAL GANGLIONIC DEGENERATION This rare sporadic disorder typically begins in middle or later life with functional impairment of one or more limbs. Examination reveals signs of parkinsonism, but the extrapyramidal abnormalities are generally insufficient to account for the clinical deficit, which results from apraxia. As the disorder progresses, other evidence of cortical dysfunction also appears, such as aphasia, agnosias, sensory inattention, and mild dementia. Pathologically there is cell loss and gliosis in the cerebral cortex as well as the substantia nigra. The response to antiparkinsonian medication is disappointing, and the course is generally progressive, with increasing disability and dependence leading ultimately to death.

STRIATONIGRAL DEGENERATION In a few patients with seemingly classic Parkinson's disease, there is little or no response to dopaminergic medication, and pathologic study at autopsy reveals neuronal loss and gliosis in the putamen, globus pallidus, caudate and subthalamic nuclei, and substantia nigra. This disorder has therefore been called striatonigral degeneration. It has an age and gender distribution similar to those of Parkinson's disease. Clinical examination reveals the findings of parkinsonism, but tremor is usually relatively inconspicuous. Cognitive function is preserved.

There may be an accompanying impairment of autonomic function (Shy-Drager syndrome; Chap. 371), and examination in such cases often reveals that a combination of pyramidal and cerebellar signs is also present. Indeed, in some cases the cerebellar findings are so conspicuous that the disorder is more properly called spinocerebellar ataxia type 1 (olivopontocerebellar atrophy; Chap. 369).

The management of patients with striatonigral degeneration is difficult. Antiparkinsonian medications generally are prescribed but usually are ineffective.

MACHADO-JOSEPH DISEASE / SPINOCEREBELLAR ATAXIA TYPE 3 Machado-Joseph disease is an autosomal dominant form of striatonigral degeneration that generally begins in the third or fourth decade. Most affected individuals are of Portuguese ancestry. There may be only mild parkinsonian signs, whereas spasticity, hyperreflexia, extensor plantar responses, cerebellar findings, external ophthalmoplegia and, sometimes, peripheral neuropathy are conspicuous. Cognitive function is preserved. Pathologically the findings are similar to those of striatonigral degeneration, but the dentate nucleus of the cerebellum is also involved. There is no specific treatment. → ***The different clinical subtypes of the disease, their genetic basis, and related autosomal dominant ataxias with some extrapyramidal features are discussed in Chap. 369.***

IDIOPATHIC TORSION DYSTONIA The occurrence of dystonic movements and postures without other neurologic signs in patients with a normal birth and developmental history is designated *idiopathic torsion dystonia.* The pathophysiologic and biochemical basis of this entity is unknown. Pathologic examination reveals no specific abnormalities, but the disorder is attributed to basal ganglia dysfunction partly because of observations made in cases of secondary dystonia. Other possible causes of dystonia (Chap. 21) should be excluded before this diagnosis is made. The disorder may occur on a sporadic or hereditary basis. Inheritance can be either autosomal dominant (with the gene localized to 9q32-34 in some families), autosomal recessive, or X-linked recessive (Xq21.3). Onset in childhood is associated with a positive family history, symptoms that begin in the legs, and greater disability than with later onset. About one-third of patients eventually become chair- or bedbound.

Examination reveals the abnormal movements and sustained postures that characterize the disorder. There may be involvement of the neck, trunk, limbs, and face (blepharospasm or oromandibular dystonia). A description of these various motor abnormalities is provided in Chap. 21. Initially they may be brought out by voluntary activity, but eventually they are present constantly, leading to deformity and disability.

Occasional patients have *dopa-responsive dystonia*, which is inherited in an autosomal dominant manner with incomplete penetrance. The responsible gene maps to chromosome 14q. Onset is usually in childhood, and examination typically reveals associated bradykinesia and rigidity. The response to low-dose levodopa therapy is dramatic.

℞ TREATMENT

Treatment is purely symptomatic and is often unsatisfactory. Anticholinergic drugs in high doses (e.g., trihexyphenidyl, 40 to 50 mg/d) are probably the most effective means of providing some relief of the abnormal movements and postures. They are introduced in a low dose and built up gradually, depending on response and tolerance. Phenothiazines or haloperidol are sometimes helpful but usually cause mild parkinsonism. Diazepam, baclofen, and carbamazepine are helpful occasionally. Stereotactic thalamotomy may be beneficial when dystonia is predominantly unilateral and involves the limbs.

FOCAL TORSION DYSTONIA Dystonia may occur as an isolated phenomenon affecting a discrete part of the body, rather than having the more generalized distribution described above. Such focal or segmental dystonias probably represent variants of idiopathic torsion dystonia. Both *blepharospasm* (spontaneous, involuntary forced closure of the eyelids) and *oromandibular dystonia* can occur as isolated focal dystonias. Oromandibular dystonia consists of involuntary contractions of the masticatory, lingual, and perioral muscles, leading to opening or closure of the mouth; pouting, pursing, or retraction of the lips; and roving or protruding movements of the tongue. The combination of blepharospasm and oromandibular dystonia is called *Meige syndrome*.

Spasmodic torticollis is characterized by a tendency for the head to turn to one side. The designation *anterocollis* indicates that the head is flexed forward, and *retrocollis* that it is pulled backward. These cervical dystonias are often intermittent initially, but eventually the head is held continuously in the abnormal position. Spontaneous remission occurs occasionally, especially in the first few months after onset, but thereafter the disorder is likely to be permanent and may worsen with time.

TREATMENT

Pharmacotherapy is usually unrewarding, but the drugs used in treating idiopathic torsion dystonia are helpful in some patients. Local injection of botulinum toxin into the overactive muscles often produces a benefit lasting several weeks or months by producing a temporary presynaptic block of neuromuscular transmission, and injections can be repeated as needed. This is the most effective treatment available for most focal dystonias. Selective section of the spinal accessory nerve (cranial nerve XI) and the upper cervical nerve roots is sometimes helpful for patients with cervical dystonia unresponsive to other measures.

TASK-SPECIFIC FOCAL DYSTONIA Writer's cramp is a task-specific dystonia in which abnormal posturing of the hand and forearm occurs when the hand is used for writing. As the disorder worsens, abnormal posturing may also occur with other tasks, such as applying cosmetics, shaving, or using table cutlery. Drug treatment is usually unrewarding, and it is often necessary for patients to learn to use the other hand for these tasks. Injections of botulinum toxin into the involved muscles are sometimes helpful, but function usually remains impaired. Other task-specific dystonias include violinist's cramp, barber's cramp, and telegrapher's cramp, in each of which dystonic posturing occurs when the hand is used for a skilled, occupationally related function. The pathophysiologic basis of these disorders is uncertain, but recent work relates it to abnormal processing of sensory input from the affected extremity during the activity.

DRUG-INDUCED MOVEMENT DISORDERS **Parkinsonism** Parkinsonism is a frequent complication of treatment with dopamine-depleting agents such as reserpine or antipsychotic dopamine antagonists such as the phenothiazines or butyrophenones. The antipsychotic drugs most likely to cause parkinsonism are those that are potent D2 receptor antagonists having little anticholinergic effect, such as piperazine phenothiazines, haloperidol, and thiothixene. Women and the elderly have an increased risk of this complication. In comparison with Parkinson's disease, tremor is less common and bradykinesia is typically symmetric, but the two disorders are sometimes impossible to distinguish except by the history of drug ingestion. Signs usually develop within 3 months of starting the causal agent and may persist for several months (or longer) after its withdrawal. Drug-induced parkinsonism is best managed by discontinuing the antipsychotic drug when possible, substituting an antipsychotic with greater anticholinergic potency, or adding an anticholinergic drug such as trihexyphenidyl. Levodopa should not be prescribed—it is of no help if the offending neuroleptic agent is continued, and it may worsen the underlying psychotic disorder.

Acute Dystonia or Dyskinesia Acute dystonia (such as blepharospasm or torticollis) or dyskinesia (such as chorea or facial grimacing) may complicate treatment with a dopamine receptor antagonist. It typically commences within 1 week of the introduction of such medication, usually in the first 48 h, and is more common in young patients. Its pathophysiologic basis is uncertain. Treatment with an anticholinergic drug (e.g., benztropine, 2 mg, or diphenhydramine, 50 mg intravenously) is usually helpful.

Tardive Akathisia *Akathisia* denotes a motor restlessness. Patients are unable to sit still but feel obliged to move about. It is commonly induced by chronic antipsychotic drug treatment, especially in women, and is treated like drug-induced parkinsonism.

Tardive Dyskinesia or Dystonia Tardive dyskinesia or dystonia is a common complication of long-term antipsychotic drug treatment (with dopamine receptor antagonists). The risk of its development increases with advancing age, but its pathogenesis is unclear. One suggestion is that it is related to drug-induced supersensitivity of striatal dopamine receptors. However, although supersensitivity is an inevitable accompaniment of chronic antipsychotic drug treatment, tardive dyskinesia does not always occur. Moreover, the time courses of the two phenomena are different. Supersensitivity occurs relatively early during treatment and reverses when medication is withdrawn, whereas tardive dyskinesia usually requires exposure for at least 6 months before it develops and may persist indefinitely. Another suggestion is that it involves an abnormality of GABA-ergic neurons. This is supported by observations that GABA and glutamic acid decarboxylase (its synthesizing enzyme) are depleted in the basal ganglia by long-term administration of antipsychotic drugs to animals and that CSF levels of GABA are reduced in patients with tardive dyskinesia.

The clinical features of tardive dyskinesia include abnormal choreoathetoid movements, especially involving the face and mouth in adults and the limbs in children. Tardive dystonia may be focal, producing, for example, blepharospasm, torticollis, or oromandibular dystonia, or it may affect contiguous body parts (e.g., the face and neck or arm and trunk). Generalized dystonia is uncommon, especially in older patients. It may be impossible to distinguish these disturbances from those of Huntington's disease (Chap. 367), Sydenham's chorea (Chap. 236), or idiopathic torsion dystonia except by the history of drug exposure. The iatrogenic disorder often resolves spontaneously in children or young adults but frequently persists in middle-aged or older individuals.

TREATMENT

Treatment of the established disorder is often unsatisfactory. It is therefore important that antipsychotic drugs be prescribed only when necessary and that their long-term use be accompanied by periodic drug holidays to determine whether treatment is still required. Drug holidays may actually unmask incipient dyskinesias, which often worsen on withdrawal of the causal agent. In such circumstances, permanent withdrawal of the antipsychotic medication, if this is possible, may lead to remission of the dyskinesia. Treatment with antidopaminergic agents such as haloperidol or phenothiazines (which cause the disorder) often suppresses the dyskinesias at least for a period, but these agents are best avoided, because they may exacerbate the underlying problem. Treatment with dopamine-depleting agents, such as reserpine, 0.25 mg gradually increased to 2 to 4 mg/d, or tetrabenazine (in countries where it is available), 12.5 mg gradually increased to as much as 200 mg/d, is sometimes worthwhile in reducing the severity of the dyskinesia. Other pharmacologic approaches are unrewarding in most instances. Tardive dystonia may respond to tetrabenazine (if available) or to anticholinergic drugs used as for idiopathic torsion dystonia.

Tardive tic resembles Gilles de la Tourette's syndrome (see below) and is best treated with clonidine or clonazepam.

Neuroleptic Malignant Syndrome Rigidity, hyperthermia, altered mental status resembling catatonia, labile blood pressure, and autonomic dysfunction characterize this serious complication of treatment with antipsychotic (neuroleptic) agents, especially haloperidol. Associated clinical features include tachycardia, tachypnea, metabolic acidosis, and myoglobinuria that may be fatal. The cause is unknown, but antagonism of dopamine is a likely contributor. The prevalence of this syndrome among patients receiving neuroleptics is less than 2 percent, with the disorder occurring must commonly in young adults. Symptoms evolve over 1 to 2 days. The syndrome can develop at any time during exposure to the medication, but usually it occurs within the first 30 days of use.

The differential diagnosis includes infection, malignant hyperthermia, and alcohol- or drug-withdrawal states. Drug-induced parkinsonism may be similar but is not associated with fever or the autonomic features described above.

TREATMENT

Treatment includes immediate withdrawal of antipsychotic drugs and also of lithium and anticholinergic agents, which may increase the risk of developing the disorder. Symptomatic treatment is also necessary and includes antipyretics and artificial cooling, rehydration, and measures to maintain the blood pressure. Serum potassium should be monitored. Dantrolene, bromocriptine or another dopamine agonist, levodopa, amantadine, or benzodiazepines are sometimes helpful, but the mortality rate is on the order of 5 to 20 percent. Subcutaneous heparin administration reduces the risk of venous thrombosis. Most survivors recover completely, but potential complications include renal failure, pulmonary embolism, and a chronic cerebellar syndrome (related to the hyperthermia). Recovery generally occurs over 2 to 3 weeks.

Other Drug-Induced Movement Disorders Dyskinesia or dystonia may complicate therapy with levodopa or dopamine agonists as a dose-related phenomenon that is reversed by withdrawal of the medication or reduction of the dose. Reversible chorea may also complicate treatment with anticholinergic drugs, phenytoin, carbamazepine, amphetamines, lithium, and oral contraceptives; dystonia from lithium, carbamazepine, and metoclopramide; and postural tremor from theophylline, caffeine, lithium, thyroid hormone, tricyclic antidepressants, valproic acid, and isoproterenol.

GILLES DE LA TOURETTE'S SYNDROME Gilles de la Tourette's syndrome, which has a prevalence in the United States of approximately 0.05 percent, consists of chronic multiple motor and phonic tics that have no known cause. The disorder is not related to social or ethnic background or to perinatal abnormalities. Symptoms typically begin between 5 and 15 years of age and follow a relapsing and remitting course. A family history is sometimes obtained, and partial expression of the trait may occur in siblings or offspring of patients. In most families with chronic tic disorders, there is an autosomal dominant mode of inheritance with variable penetrance that is gender related. Boys are affected much more commonly than girls.

The pathophysiology is obscure, and no structural pathology has been recognized. A dopaminergic excess has been suggested by the clinical observation that the tics may respond to treatment with dopamine-blocking drugs.

Clinical Manifestations The first signs consist of single or multiple motor tics in 80 percent of cases and of phonic tics in 20 percent. Motor tics commonly affect the face and may consist of repetitive sniffing, winking, blinking, elevation of the eyelids, eye closure, pursing of the lips, or facial twitching. Patients eventually develop several different motor and phonic tics, the latter frequently taking the form of grunts, barks, hisses, sighs, throat-clearing, coughing, and verbal utterances that may involve coprolalia (involuntary and inappropriate swearing or obscene speech), echolalia (involuntary repetition of the phrases of others), and palilalia (repetition of words or phrases). The tics may change in location, severity, complexity, and character with time, are worsened by emotional stress, and can be suppressed voluntarily for short periods. In some cases, tics are complex (such as jumping up in the air) or involve repetitive self-mutilating activities (such as nail-biting, hair-pulling, or lip-biting). Tics that involve repetitive sensory phenomena, such as pressure, tickle, or thermal sensations, also occur. Many patients have associated behavioral abnormalities, especially obsessive-compulsive disorder and attention deficit hyperactivity disorder.

Apart from the presence of tics, physical examination typically reveals no other abnormalities, but the incidence of left-handedness or ambidexterity is greater than among normal persons, and many patients have nonspecific electroencephalographic abnormalities of no diagnostic significance.

The diagnosis is often delayed for years, the symptoms sometimes being attributed to psychiatric illness. Patients may be subjected to unnecessary and expensive treatment before the correct diagnosis is made. Depression, sometimes leading to suicide, may result from social embarrassment caused by the tics.

Differential Diagnosis Many children develop transient or chronic simple tics, and these have a benign prognosis and require no treatment. In some instances, simple or multiple tics persist for several years but resolve in late adolescence. Wilson's disease, a treatable cause of dyskinesias and tics, is generally associated with hepatic and renal involvement, Kayser-Fleischer corneal rings, low serum copper and ceruloplasmin levels, and increased 24-h urinary copper excretion (Chap. 345). The associated dementia, the character of the abnormal movements, and genetic studies distinguish Huntington's disease (Chap. 367). Sydenham's chorea (Chap. 236) may be confused with Gilles de la Tourette's syndrome when a history of rheumatic fever or polyarthritis is lacking and there is no cardiac involvement, but it usually resolves over 3 to 6 months. Tics may also occur in postencephalitic syndromes and as a side effect of stimulant or neuroleptic medication.

℞ TREATMENT

Treatment is symptomatic and may need to be continued indefinitely.

Clonidine alleviates motor and phonic tics in approximately 50 percent of children, possibly by reducing activity in noradrenergic neurons of the locus coeruleus. The initial dose is 2 to 3 μg/kg per day, increased after 2 weeks to 4 μg/kg per day and then, if required, to 5 μg/kg per day. There may be a transient fall in blood pressure when this agent is introduced. Other side effects are sedation, reduced or excessive salivation, and diarrhea.

Haloperidol has been used widely for many years. It is introduced in a low daily dose (0.25 mg), which is gradually increased by 0.25 mg every 5 days, depending on response and tolerance. The optimal dose is usually 2 to 8 mg/d. Side effects include extrapyramidal movement disorders, sedation, xerostomia, blurred vision, and gastrointestinal disturbances. Pimozide, another dopaminergic-receptor antagonist, may be of benefit when haloperidol is unhelpful or poorly tolerated. It may produce widening of the QT interval and sudden death at high doses, so the electrocardiogram should be monitored routinely. Its long-term safety is unknown. It is introduced in a dose of 1 mg/d, and the dose is then increased by 2 mg every 10 days; most patients require 7 to 16 mg/d. The total dose should not exceed 0.3 mg/kg per day. Phenothiazines such as fluphenazine sometimes help, but patients unresponsive to haloperidol do not usually benefit from these drugs. Clonazepam or carbamazepine can also be tried. Family counseling and psychotherapy are sometimes helpful.

RESTLESS LEGS SYNDROME The restless legs syndrome is a common, chronic disorder that often has a familial basis, with evidence of autosomal dominant inheritance. It is characterized by a need to move because of unpleasant creeping sensations that arise deep within the legs and occasionally also in the arms, especially when patients are relaxed. For this reason, there is often difficulty in settling down to sleep at night. Periodic leg movements may also occur during sleep and can be documented by polysomnography. The cause is unknown, although the disorder is common during pregnancy and is sometimes associated with uremic or diabetic neuropathy, primary amyloidosis, or malignancy. Clinical examination may reveal evidence of underlying systemic disease or mild peripheral neuropathy but is more often normal. Symptoms may respond to correction of coexisting iron-deficiency anemia or to treatment with dopaminergic medication (such as levodopa or bromocriptine), benzodiazepines (diazepam or clonazepam), or opiates (codeine, propoxyphene, or oxycodone).

BIBLIOGRAPHY

AMINOFF MJ: Treatment of Parkinson's disease. West J Med 161:303, 1994

BENNETT DA et al: Prevalence of parkinsonian signs and associated mortality in a community population of older people. N Engl J Med 334:771, 1996

CLEETER MWJ et al: Irreversible inhibition of mitochondrial complex I by 1-methyl-4-phenylpyridinium: Evidence for free radical involvement. J Neurochem 58:786, 1992

DOGALI M et al: Stereotactic ventral pallidotomy for Parkinson's disease. Neurology 45:753, 1995

EDWARDS RH: Neural degeneration and the transport of neurotransmitters. Ann Neurol 34:638, 1993

GRATZ SS, SIMPSON GM: Neuroleptic malignant syndrome. Diagnosis, epidemiology and treatment. CNS Drugs 2:429, 1994

HYDE TM, WEINBERGER DR: Tourette's syndrome: A model neuropsychiatric disorder. JAMA 273:498, 1995
IANNACCONE S et al: Evidence of peripheral axonal neuropathy in primary restless legs syndrome. Mov Disord 10:2, 1995
KORDOWER JH et al: Neuropathological evidence of graft survival and striatal reinnervation after the transplantation of fetal mesencephalic tissue in a patient with Parkinson's disease. N Engl J Med 332:1118, 1995
LOZANO AM et al: Effect of GPi pallidotomy on motor function in Parkinson's disease. Lancet 346:1383, 1995
MOURADIAN MM et al: Modification of central dopaminergic mechanisms by continuous levodopa therapy for advanced Parkinson's disease. Ann Neurol 27:18, 1990
NYGAARD TG et al: Linkage mapping of dopa-responsive dystonia (DRD) to chromosome 14q. Nature Genet 5:386, 1993
PARKINSON STUDY GROUP: Effects of tocopherol and deprenyl on the progression of disability in early Parkinson's disease. N Engl J Med 328:176, 1993
———: Impact of deprenyl and tocopherol treatment on Parkinson's disease in DATATOP subjects not requiring levodopa. Ann Neurol 39:29, 1996
POLYMEROPOULOS MH et al: Mapping of a gene for Parkinson's disease to chromosome 4q21-q23. Science 274:1197, 1996
REMY P et al: Clinical correlates of [^{18}F]fluorodopa uptake in five grafted parkinsonian patients. Ann Neurol 38:580, 1995
QUINN N: Drug treatment of Parkinson's disease. BMJ 310:575, 1995
SCHULZER M et al: The antiparkinson efficacy of deprenyl derives from transient improvement that is likely to be symptomatic. Ann Neurol 32:795, 1992
WICHMANN T et al: Parkinson's disease and the basal ganglia: Lessons from the laboratory and from neurosurgery. Neuroscientist 1:236, 1995

369 ATAXIC DISORDERS

Roger N. Rosenberg

The inherited and acquired ataxic disorders comprise a series of clinical phenotypes that include ataxia, dysarthria, dysmetria, and intention tremor resulting from the involvement of the cerebellum and its afferent and efferent pathways.

Approach to the Patient

With Ataxic Disorders Ataxia is a common and important neurologic sign. Patients manifest symptoms and signs of ataxia with gait impairment, unclear speech, blurred vision, altered hand coordination, and tremor with movement. The rate and pattern of these cerebellar symptoms are important in determining the differential diagnostic possibilities (Table 369-1). A slow, regular, and progressive increase in symptoms with bilateral and symmetric involvement suggests a biochemical, metabolic, immunologic, or toxicity-induced cause of symptoms. Conversely, a focal, unilateral symptomatology with headache and impaired level of consciousness, possibly accompanied by ipsilateral cranial nerve palsies and contralateral weakness, implies a space-occupying cerebellar lesion, such as a primary or metastatic cerebellar tumor, abscess, large infarction, hemorrhage, or subdural hematoma in the posterior fossa.

Progressive, symmetrical ataxia can be further classified as acute in onset (onset over hours or days), subacute in onset (weeks or months), or chronic, developing over months to years. The acute and reversible types of ataxia include those caused by intoxication with alcohol, diphenylhydantoin, barbiturates, and other agents. Intoxication caused by toluene exposure, gasoline sniffing, glue sniffing, spray painting, or exposure to mercury are examples. Children with a postinfectious syndrome can develop gait ataxia and mild dysarthria, which are both reversible. Subacute development of ataxia over weeks to months may be the combined direct effect of alcoholism and nutrition impairment, particularly for vitamins B_1 and B_{12}. A paraneoplastic syndrome, which may be associated with myoclonus and opsoclonus, is associated with incapacitating gait ataxia. Specific autoantibodies (Yo, Ri, and PCD) have been identified that are responsible for cerebellar degeneration involving principally the midline or vermis (see Chap. 103). Female patients may present with cerebellar ataxia prior to the identification of a breast or ovarian carcinoma. Removal of the tumor may prevent further progression of symptoms and in some patients results in gait improvement. Chronic gait ataxia of months' to years' duration suggests a metabolic or inherited ataxia. Hypothyroidism must be considered as a readily treatable and reversible form of gait ataxia.

In patients with focal, increasing signs of ataxia of an acute nature, it is important to consider vascular lesions, including acute cerebellar infarction with edema, cerebellar hemorrhage, and a posterior fossa subdural hematoma. Computed tomography (CT) will reveal clinically significant processes of this type, which may require surgical decompression. Similarly, a primary cerebellar glioma or a metastatic tumor to the cerebellar hemisphere may present with increasing focal deficits associated with an impaired level of consciousness. Herniation rostrally onto the brainstem or a sudden caudal herniation of cerebellar tonsils must be considered and an urgent evaluation implemented (see Chap. 366). A primary cerebellar abscess may present in a similar manner. Lymphoma or progressive multifocal leukoencephalopathy (PML) in a patient with AIDS may present with acute focal cerebellar signs. Patients with acute multiple sclerosis may present with significant focal and ipsilateral cerebellar deficits due to a large demyelinating plaque. A history of previous neurologic deficits and an examination of cerebrospinal fluid (CSF) may be highly diagnostic for multiple sclerosis.

Table 369-1

Etiology of Cerebellar Ataxia

Symmetrical and Progressive Signs			Focal and Ipsilateral Cerebellar Signs		
Acute (Hours to Days)	**Subacute (Days to Weeks)**	**Chronic (Months to Years)**	**Acute (Hours to Days)**	**Subacute (Days to Weeks)**	**Chronic (Months to Years)**
Alcohol, lithium, diphenylhydantoin, barbiturates (positive history and toxicology screen) Acute viral cerebellitis (cerebrospinal fluid supportive of acute viral infection) Postinfection syndrome	Intoxication: mercury, solvents, gasoline, glue; cytotoxic chemotherapeutic drugs Alcoholic-nutritional (vitamin B_1 and B_{12} deficiency) Lyme disease	Paraneoplastic syndrome Hypothyroidism Inherited diseases Tabes dorsalis (tertiary syphilis)	Vascular: Cerebellar infarction, hemorrhage, or subdural hematoma Infectious: cerebellar abscess (positive mass lesion on MRI/CT, positive history in support of lesion)	Neoplastic: cerebellar glioma or metastatic tumor (positive for neoplasm on MRI/CT) Demyelinating: Multiple sclerosis (history, CSF and MRI are consistent) AIDS-related progressive multifocal leukoencephalopathy (positive HIV test and CD4+ cell count for AIDS)	Stable gliosis secondary to vascular lesion or demyelinating plaque (stable lesion on MRI/CT older than several months) Congenital lesion: Dandy-Walker or Arnold-Chiari malformations (malformation noted on MRI/CT)

ABBREVIATIONS: CSF, cerebrospinal fluid; CT, computed tomography; HIV, human immunodeficiency virus; MRI, magnetic resonance imaging.

True cerebellar ataxia needs to be separated from vertiginous ataxia, as the latter is a disorder of gait associated with a significant degree of dizziness, light-headedness, or the perception of movement (see Chap. 20). True cerebellar ataxia is devoid of these vertiginous complaints and is clearly an unsteady gait due to imbalance. Weakness of proximal leg muscles and a variant of acute idiopathic polyneuritis (Miller-Fisher syndrome) can simulate the imbalance of cerebellar disease.

ACQUIRED ATAXIAS

The cerebellar circuit comprising the cerebellum, spinocerebellar pathways, and the frontopontocerebellar pathway originating in the rostral frontal lobe (Brodmann's area 10) are also involved in a variety of acquired diseases. Cerebrovascular disease producing acute and subacute infarctions, hemorrhagic infarctions, and hemorrhages may result in an acute ataxic syndrome. Lesions of these types will result in cerebellar symptoms ipsilateral to the injured cerebellum and may be associated with impaired levels of consciousness due to increased intracranial pressure and ipsilateral pontine signs, including sixth and seventh nerve palsies due to direct pontine compression. Similarly, cerebellar tumors, demyelinating plaques of multiple sclerosis, and abscess formation produce progressive deficits ipsilateral to the cerebellar lesion. Two other important entities are paraneoplastic disease due to neoplasms outside the brain and causing acute bilateral cerebellar deficits by an antibody-mediated process (see Chap. 103) and subacute cerebellar degeneration of the vermis with gait ataxia, due to chronic alcoholism.

Patients with AIDS may develop an acute ataxic syndrome due to progressive multifocal leukoencephalopathy, which causes a rapid demyelinating process, as a result of the JC virus (see Chap. 379). Progressive ataxia of gait and extremities may also be caused by toxic or metabolic disorders, including hypothyroidism, hyponatremia, vitamin B_1 deficiency, vitamin B_{12} deficiency, toxic levels of phenytoin, lithium, bismuth, germanium, methyl mercury, and organic solvents, and treatment with cytotoxic chemotherapeutic drugs (see Chap. 380). Rarely, congenital lesions, such as the Chiari type I malformation with cerebellar tonsillar compression of the brainstem, and congenital dilation of the fourth ventricle into a large cyst owing to impaired drainage of CSF (Dandy-Walker syndrome), present in adults as a progressive diffuse ataxic syndrome. Specific infectious diseases that can present with ataxia are meningovascular syphilis in patients recently infected and tabes dorsalis due to degeneration of the spinocerebellar pathway in chronically infected patients. Lyme disease may cause ataxic symptoms.

Other rare infectious causes of acquired ataxia include poliovirus, coxsackievirus, echovirus, Epstein-Barr virus, toxoplasmosis, *Legionella*, and the prion protein mediating Creutzfeldt-Jakob disease (see Chaps. 153 and 379).

THE INHERITED ATAXIAS

Of the syndromes that constitute the inherited ataxias, some show autosomal dominant or autosomal recessive inheritance, and some are caused by mitochondrial mutations and thus show maternal inheritance. Significant progress has been made in recent years in identifying the molecular basis of these syndromes (Table 369-2), so that a genomic classification is superseding previous ones based on clinical expression alone.

Although the clinical manifestations and neuropathologic findings of cerebellar disease dominate the clinical picture, there may also be characteristic changes in the basal ganglia, brainstem, spinal cord, optic nerves, retina, and peripheral nerves. In large families with dominantly inherited disease, there are many gradations from purely cerebellar manifestations to mixed cerebellar and brainstem disorders, cerebellar and basal ganglia syndromes, and spinal cord or peripheral nerve disease. Rarely, dementia is present as well. The clinical picture may be consistent within a family with dominantly inherited ataxia, but sometimes most affected family members show one characteristic syndrome, while one or several members have an entirely different phenotype.

The problem posed by dominantly inherited diseases of the nervous system, such as the inherited cerebellar degenerations, is the lack of a known primary metabolic clue, or primary storage product, to indicate a potential molecular basis for disease. In these cerebellar disorders, there is a patterned neuronal degeneration with variable secondary gliosis. Even the findings of specific protein abnormalities on two-dimensional gels or specific changes in messenger RNA on northern blots obtained from brain samples of patients having a dominantly inherited cerebellar disease do not warrant the conclusion that these products are due to primary gene mutations rather than being a result of the disease. Therefore, new research strategies must be employed to determine the molecular basis of autosomal dominant disorders and the molecular explanation for phenotypic variation within and between families. Linkage analysis has proved to be a powerful tool with which to map the chromosomal location of a series of dominantly inherited ataxic neurologic diseases for which no biochemical basis was known, and these new findings have aided the classification of the various clinical phenotypes (see Table 369-2).

AUTOSOMAL DOMINANT ATAXIAS As presented in Table 369-2, the new genomic classification of the dominantly inherited ataxias includes spinocerebellar ataxia (SCA) type 1, SCA2, SCA3/Machado-Joseph disease, SCA4, SCA5, dentatorubropallidoluysian atrophy (DRPLA), spinocerebellar degeneration with retinal degeneration (SCA7), and episodic ataxia (EA) types I and II (EA-1 and EA-2). The use of SCA6 has been for those autosomal dominant families with ataxia that have not been assigned a chromosomal locus.

SCA1 SCA1 was previously referred to as *olivopontocerebellar atrophy*, but the new genomic data has shown that that entity represents several different genotypes with overlapping clinical features.

Symptoms and signs The clinical syndrome of SCA1 is characterized by the development in adult or late middle life of progressive cerebellar ataxia of the trunk and limbs, impairment of equilibrium and gait, slowness of voluntary movements, scanning speech, nystagmoid jerks, and oscillatory tremor of the head and trunk. Dysarthria, dysphagia, and oculomotor and facial palsies may also occur. Extrapyramidal symptoms include rigidity, immobile facies, and parkinsonian tremor. The reflexes are usually normal, but knee and ankle jerks may be lost, and extensor plantar responses may occur. Dementia may occur but is usually mild. Impairment of sphincter function is common, with urinary and sometimes fecal incontinence.

Marked shrinkage of the ventral half of the pons, disappearance of the olivary eminence on the ventral surface of the medulla, and atrophy of the cerebellum are evident on gross postmortem inspection of the brain. Variable loss of Purkinje cells, reduction in the number of cells in the molecular and granular layer, demyelination of the middle cerebellar peduncle and the cerebellar hemispheres, and severe loss of cells in the pontine nuclei and olives are found on histologic examination. Degenerative changes in the striatum, especially the putamen, and loss of the pigmented cells of the substantia nigra may be found in cases with extrapyramidal features. More widespread degeneration in the central nervous system (CNS), including involvement of the posterior columns and the spinocerebellar fibers, is often present, especially in the cases with autosomal dominant inheritance.

Genetics SCA1 was mapped positionally to chromosome 6 (6p22-p23), and the causal gene was found to contain CAG expanded DNA repeats (see Chap. 363). The mutant allele has more than 43 CAG repeats, whereas alleles from control subjects have 36 or fewer repeats. There is a direct correlation between a larger number of repeats and a younger age of onset for SCA1. Juvenile cases have higher repeat numbers, and anticipation is present in subsequent generations. The SCA1 gene is 450 kilobases (kb) long and has nine exons, with the first seven exons located in a 5′ untranslated region and the last two exons containing the coding region. The SCA1 transcript contains

10,660 bases and is transcribed from both the wild-type allele and SCA1 alleles. The CAG repeat, which codes for a polyglutamine tract, lies within the coding region. The SCA1 gene product, called ataxin-1, is a novel protein of unknown function. It will be of great interest to discover how variable CAG repeat expansions, coding for polyglutamine tract lengths, can lead to selective neuronal degeneration accompanied by clinical anticipation (see Chap. 363).

SCA2 *Symptoms and signs* Another clinical phenotype, SCA2, has been described in Cubans. These patients probably are descendants of a common ancestor, and the population may be the largest homogeneous group of ataxic patients yet described. The age of onset ranges from 2 to 65 years, and there is considerable clinical variability within various families. Assuming these patients have a common ancestry, the frequency of the disease in the population represents a founder effect. Although neuropathologic and clinical findings are compatible with a diagnosis of SCA1 (including parkinsonian rigidity, optic disk pallor, spasticity, and retinal degeneration), it appears that SCA2 is a unique form of cerebellar degenerative disease.

Genetics The gene in SCA2 families has been mapped to 12q23-q24.1. Thus, the similar clinical phenotypes of SCA1 and SCA2, mapped respectively to 6p and 12q, represent different genotypes. The gene has just been identified, and it also contains CAG repeat expansions. Dominant spinocerebellar atrophy with retinal disease is a separate genotype and maps to 3p12-p21.1.

Machado-Joseph Disease/SCA3 Machado-Joseph disease (MJD) is an autosomal dominant spinocerebellar degenerative disease first described among the Portuguese and their descendants in New England and California. Subsequently, MJD has been found in families from Portugal, Australia, Brazil, Canada, China, England, France, India, Israel, Italy, Japan, Spain, Taiwan, and the United States.

Symptoms and signs MJD has been classified into three clinical types. In type I MJD (amyotrophic lateral sclerosis–parkinsonism–dystonia type), neurologic deficits appear in the first two decades and involve weakness and spasticity of extremities, especially the legs, often with dystonia of the face, neck, trunk, and extremities. Patellar and ankle clonus are common, as are extensor plantar responses. The gait is slow and stiff, with a slightly broadened base and lurching

Table 369-2

Genotype Classification of the Spinocerebellar Ataxias

Name	Locus	Phenotype
SCA1 (autosomal dominant type 1)	6p22-p23 with CAG repeats	Ataxia with ophthalmoparesis, pyramidal and extrapyramidal findings
SCA2 (autosomal dominant type 2)	12q-23-24.1 with CAG repeats	Ataxia with slow saccades and minimal pyramidal and extrapyramidal findings
Machado-Joseph disease/SCA3 (autosomal dominant type 3)	14q24.3-q32 with CAG repeats in open reading frame	Ataxia with ophthalmoparesis and variable pyramidal, extrapyramidal, and amyotrophic signs
SCA4 (autosomal dominant type 4)	16q24-ter	Ataxia with normal eye movements, sensory axonal neuropathy, and pyramidal signs
SCA5 (autosomal dominant type 5)	Centromeric region of chromosome 11	Ataxia and dysarthria
SCA6 (autosomal dominant type 6)	Polymorphic CAG repeats in α_{1A}-voltage-dependent calcium channel	Ataxia, dysarthria, nystagmus, mild proprioceptive sensory loss
Dentatorubropallidoluysian atrophy (autosomal dominant)	12p12-ter with CAG repeats	Ataxia, choreoathetosis, dystonia, seizures, myoclonus, dementia
Spinocerebellar degeneration with retinal degeneration (autosomal dominant)	3p12-p21.1	Ataxia with retinal degeneration
Friedreich's ataxia (autosomal recessive)	9q with intronic GAA repeats	Ataxia, areflexia, extensor plantar responses, position sense deficits, cardiomyopathy, diabetes mellitus, scoliosis, foot deformities
Friedreich's ataxia (autosomal recessive)	8q13, α-TTP deficiency	Same as phenotype that maps to 9q but associated with vitamin E deficiency
Kearns-Sayre syndrome (sporadic)	mtDNA deletion and duplication mutations	Ptosis, ophthalmoplegia, pigmentary retinal degeneration, cardiomyopathy, diabetes mellitus, deafness, heart block, increased CSF protein, ataxia
Myoclonus epilepsy and ragged red fiber syndrome (MERRF) (maternal inheritance)	Mutation in mtDNA of $tRNA^{lys}$ at 8344; also a mutation at 8356	Myoclonic epilepsy, ragged red fiber myopathy, ataxia
Mitochondrial encephalopathy, lactic acidosis, and stroke syndrome (MELAS) (maternal inheritance)	$tRNA^{leu}$ mutation at 3243; also at 3271 and 3252	Headache, stroke, lactic acidosis, ataxia
Leigh's disease; subacute necrotizing encephalopathy (maternal inheritance or autosomal recessive)	mtDNA complex V defect (ATPase gene at 8993) or mitochondrial protein synthesis defect (both maternally inherited); or complex IV defect (autosomal recessive)	Obtundation, hypotonia, cranial nerve defects, respiratory failure, hyperintense signals on T2-weighted magnetic resonance images in basal ganglia, cerebellum, or brainstem; ataxia
Episodic ataxia, type I (EA-1) (autosomal dominant)	12p; potassium channel gene, KcNA1	Episodic ataxia for minutes; provoked by startle or exercise; with facial and hand myokymia; cerebellar signs are not progressive; responds to phenytoin
Episodic ataxia, type II (EA-2) (autosomal dominant)	19p; gene not known	Episodic ataxia for days; provoked by stress, fatigue; with down-gaze nystagmus; cerebellar atrophy results; progressive cerebellar signs; responds to acetazolamide
Ataxia telangiectasia (autosomal recessive)	11q22-23; *ATM* gene for regulation of cell cycle, mitogenic signal transduction, and meiotic recombination	Telangiectasia, ataxia, dysarthria, pulmonary infections, neoplasms of lymphatic system; IgA and IgG deficiencies; diabetes mellitus, breast cancer
Infantile-onset spinocerebellar ataxia of Nikali et al. (autosomal recessive)	10q23.3-q24.1	Infantile ataxia, sensory neuropathy; athetosis, hearing deficit, ophthalmoplegia, optic atrophy; primary hypogonadism in females

SOURCE: Modified from Rosenberg (1995).

from side to side; this gait results from spasticity, not true ataxia. There is no truncal titubation. Pharyngeal weakness and spasticity cause difficulty with speech and swallowing. Of note is the prominence of horizontal and vertical nystagmus, loss of fast saccadic eye movements, hypermetric and hypometric saccades, and impairment of upward vertical gaze. Facial fasciculations, facial myokymia, lingual fasciculations without atrophy, ophthalmoparesis, and ocular prominence are common and early manifestations.

In type II MJD (ataxic type), true cerebellar deficits appear, including dysarthria, gait, and extremity ataxia, beginning in the second to fourth decades, along with corticospinal and extrapyramidal deficits of spasticity, rigidity, and dystonia. Type II is the most common form of the disease. Ophthalmoparesis, upward vertical gaze deficits, and facial and lingual fasciculations are also present. Type II MJD must be distinguished from SCA1 and SCA2 degeneration, which share features with it.

Type III MJD (ataxic-amyotrophic type) presents in the fifth to the seventh decades with a pancerebellar disorder that includes dysarthria, gait, and extremity ataxia. Distal sensory loss involving pain, touch, vibration, and position senses and distal atrophy are prominent, indicating the presence of peripheral neuropathy. The deep tendon reflexes are depressed to absent, and no corticospinal or extrapyramidal findings occur.

The mean age of onset of symptoms in MJD is 25 years. Neurologic deficits invariably progress and lead to death from debilitation within 15 years of onset, especially in patients with types I and II disease. Patients retain full intellectual function.

The major pathologic findings are variable loss of neurons and glial replacement in the corpus striatum and severe loss in the zona compacta portion of the substantia nigra. A moderate loss of neurons occurs in the dentate nucleus of the cerebellum and in the red nucleus. Purkinje cell loss and granule cell loss is found in the cerebellar cortex. Cell loss also occurs in the dentate nucleus and in the cranial nerve motor nuclei. Sparing of the inferior olives distinguishes MJD from other dominantly inherited ataxias.

Genetics The gene locus for MJD has been assigned to 14q24.3-q32 by genetic linkage. The genes from families with MJD in Japan and North and South America all map to the same chromosome locus. Unstable CAG repeat expansions are present in the MJD gene, and earlier age of onset is associated with longer repeats. Normal control subjects have between 12 and 37 CAG repeats, and MJD alleles have 62 to 84 CAG repeats.

SCA4 One family with progressive ataxia, pyramidal tract deficits, normal eye movements, and prominent sensory axonal neuropathy is described in which the trait has autosomal dominant transmission and is mapped to chromosome 16q24-ter.

SCA5 Finally, another family is reported (which has two major branches, both descended from the paternal grandparents of President Abraham Lincoln) in which dominantly inherited spinocerebellar ataxia (SCA5) is mapped to chromosome 11.

SCA6 Genomic screening for CAG repeats in other families with autosomal dominant ataxia have yielded another locus (see Table 369-2).

Dentatorubropallidoluysian Atrophy (DRPLA) DRPLA is a disorder of variable clinical presentation that is characterized by progressive ataxia, choreoathetosis, dystonia, seizures, myoclonus, and dementia. The syndrome of DRPLA is due to unstable CAG triplet repeats in the open reading frame of a gene located on chromosome 12p12-ter. Larger expansions are found in patients with earlier onset. The number of repeats is $\geq$49 in patients with DRPLA; it is $\leq$26 in control individuals. Anticipation occurs; successive generations in individual families show progressively earlier onset of disease in association with an increasing CAG repeat number. Larger expansions occur in children who inherit the disease from their father.

SCA with Retinal Degeneration (SCA7) Dominantly inherited spinocerebellar degeneration with associated pyramidal abnormalities has also been described with retinal degeneration, including loss of color discrimination and macular degeneration. Anticipation is present in several families with this syndrome, suggesting that it may be due to a trinucleotide repeat expansion. This syndrome has been mapped to chromosome 3p12-p21.1, but the gene has not been cloned and identified.

EPISODIC ATAXIA TYPES 1 AND 2 These are two rare dominantly inherited disorders that have been mapped to chromosomes 12p (a potassium channel gene) for type 1 and to 19p for type 2. See Table 369-2 for more details.

AUTOSOMAL RECESSIVE ATAXIAS Friedreich's Ataxia This is the most common form of inherited ataxia, comprising one-half of all hereditary ataxias. It can occur in a classic form or in association with a genetically determined vitamin E deficiency syndrome.

Symptoms and signs Friedreich's ataxia presents before 25 years of age with progressive staggering gait, frequent falling, and titubation. The lower extremities are more severely involved than the upper ones. Dysarthria occasionally is the presenting symptom, and rarely progressive scoliosis, foot deformity, nystagmus, or cardiopathy are initial signs.

The neurologic examination reveals nystagmus, loss of fast saccadic eye movements, truncal titubation, dysarthria, dysmetria, and ataxia of extremity and truncal movements. Extensor plantar responses (with normal tone in trunk and extremities), absent deep tendon reflexes, and weakness (greater distally than proximally) are usually found. Loss of vibratory and proprioceptive sensation occurs. The median age of death is 35 years. Women have a significantly better prognosis, with 20-year survival being 100 percent in women versus 63 percent in men.

Cardiac involvement occurs in 90 percent of patients with Friedreich's ataxia. Cardiomegaly, symmetrical hypertrophy, murmurs, and conduction defects are reported. Moderate mental retardation or psychiatric syndromes are present in a small percentage of patients. An unusually high incidence of diabetes (20 percent) is found and is associated with insulin resistance, pancreatic beta-cell dysfunction, and type 1 diabetes. However, no linkage is reported between the Friedreich's ataxia gene and loci predisposing to diabetes mellitus. Musculoskeletal deformities are common and include pes cavus, pes equinovarus, and scoliosis.

The primary site of pathology is the spinal cord and the peripheral nerves. Slight atrophy of the cerebellum and cerebral gyri may occur. Sclerosis and degeneration are seen predominantly in the spinocerebellar tracts, lateral corticospinal tracts, and posterior columns. Degeneration of the glossopharyngeal, vagus, hypoglossal, and deep cerebellar nuclei is described. The cerebral cortex is histologically normal except for loss of Betz cells in the precentral gyri.

Peripheral nerves are extensively involved, with a loss of large myelinated fibers. The density of small myelinated fibers is normal, but axonal size and myelin thickness are diminished.

Cardiac pathology consists of myocytic hypertrophy and fibrosis, focal vascular fibromuscular dysplasia with subintimal or medial deposition of periodic acid–Schiff (PAS)-positive material, myocytopathy with unusual pleomorphic nuclei, and focal degeneration of myelinated and unmyelinated nerves and cardiac ganglia.

Genetics The classic form of Friedreich's ataxia has been mapped to 9q13-q21, and the mutant gene contains expanded GAA triplet repeats in the first intron of the "frataxin gene." There is homozygosity for expanded GAA repeats in most patients. Normal persons have 7 to 22 GAA repeats and patients have 200 to 900 GAA repeats. Patients with Friedreich's ataxia have undetectable or extremely low levels of mRNA, as compared with carriers and unrelated controls, and thus, disease is caused by a loss of function of the frataxin protein. Classic Friedreich's ataxia must be compared and contrasted with Friedreich's ataxia associated with vitamin E deficiency. The clinical features of classic Friedreich's ataxia are indistinguishable from those of the form associated with vitamin E deficiency.

Two forms of hereditary ataxia associated with abnormalities in the interactions of vitamin E (α-tocopherol) with very-low-density lipoprotein (VLDL) have been delineated. Ataxia of the Friedreich's phenotype with vitamin E deficiency (AVED) and abetalipoproteinemia (Bassen-Kornzweig syndrome) have both been clarified at the molecular genetic level. Abetalipoproteinemia is caused by mutations in the gene coding for the larger subunit of the microsomal triglyceride transfer protein (MTP). Defects in MTP result in impairment of formation and secretion of VLDL in liver. This defect results in a deficiency of delivery of vitamin E to tissues, including the central and peripheral nervous system, as VLDL is the transport molecule for vitamin E and other fat-soluble substitutes. AVED is due to mutations in the gene for α-tocopherol transfer protein (α-TTP) on chromosome 8 (8q13). These patients have an impaired ability to bind vitamin E into the VLDL produced and secreted by the liver, resulting in a deficiency of vitamin E in peripheral tissues. Hence, either absence of VLDL (abetalipoproteinemia) or impaired binding of vitamin E to VLDL (AVED) causes an ataxic syndrome. The classic form of Friedreich's ataxia may also be related to impairment of VLDL or vitamin E metabolism. Once again, a genotype classification has proved to be essential in sorting out the various clinical forms of the Friedreich's disease syndrome.

Ataxia Telangiectasia *Symptoms and signs* Patients present in the first decade of life with progressive telangiectatic lesions associated with deficits in cerebellar function and nystagmus. The neurologic manifestations correspond to those seen in Friedreich's disease, and this entity should be included in that differential diagnosis. Truncal ataxia, extremity ataxia, dysarthria, extensor plantar responses, myoclonic jerks, areflexia, and distal sensory deficits may develop. There is a high incidence of recurrent pulmonary infections and neoplasms of the lymphatic and reticuloendothelial system in patients with ataxia-telangiectasia (AT). There is an increased incidence of cancer. Thymic hypoplasia with cellular and humoral (IgA and IgG2) immunodeficiencies, premature aging, and endocrine disorders such as insulin-dependent diabetes mellitus are described. There is an increased incidence of lymphomas, Hodgkin's disease, and acute leukemias. The acute leukemias are of T cell type. There is an increased incidence of breast cancer in women who are also heterozygous for AT.

The immunologic defects and increased susceptibility to cancer have been causally linked to cellular disorders in AT. Exposure of cultured cells to ionizing radiation slows the rate of DNA replication and increases the frequency of chromosomal aberrations.

The most striking neuropathologic changes include loss of Purkinje, granule, and basket cells in the cerebellar cortex as well as of neurons in the deep cerebellar nuclei. The inferior olives of the medulla also may have neuronal loss. There is a loss of anterior horn neurons in the spinal cord and of dorsal root ganglion cells associated with posterior column spinal cord demyelination. A poorly developed or absent thymus gland is the most consistent defect of the lymphoid system.

Genetics The gene for AT (the *ATM* gene) has been positionally mapped to chromosome 11q22-q23. *ATM*, which has a 12-kb transcript, was mutated in AT patients from all complementation groups described previously. A partial *ATM* cDNA clone of 5.9 kb encodes a protein that is similar to several yeast and mammalian phosphatidylinositol-3′-kinases involved in mitogenic signal transduction, meiotic recombination, and cell cycle control. The discovery of *ATM* will make possible the identification of heterozygotes who are at risk for cancer (e.g., breast cancer) and permit early diagnosis.

Mitochondrial Ataxias Spinocerebellar syndromes have been identified with mutations in mitochondrial DNA (mtDNA). Thirty pathogenic mtDNA point mutations and over 60 different types of mtDNA deletions are known, and several of these mutations cause or are associated with ataxia (see Chaps. 380 and 383).

Xeroderma Pigmentosum Xeroderma pigmentosum is a rare autosomal recessive neurocutaneous disorder caused by inability to repair damage to DNA, such as that produced by ultraviolet radiation. In addition to skin lesions, patients may show progressive mental deterioration, microcephaly, ataxia, spasticity, choreoathetosis, and hypogonadism. Nerve deafness, peripheral neuropathy (predominantly axonal), electroencephalographic abnormalities, and seizures are reported. Neuronal death is noted in pyramidal cells, cerebellar Purkinje cells, the deep nuclei of the cerebellum, the brainstem, the spinal cord, and peripheral nerves.

Cockayne Syndrome This is a rare autosomal recessive disorder first described by Cockayne in 1936. Clinical features are mental retardation, optic atrophy, dwarfism, neural deafness, hypersensitivity of skin to sunlight, cataracts, and retinal pigmentary degeneration. Cerebellar, pyramidal, and extrapyramidal deficits and peripheral neuropathy may occur, with bird-headed facies and normal-pressure hydrocephalus. Skin fibroblasts show defective DNA repair when exposed to an ultraviolet light.

Marinesco-Sjögren Syndrome This rare syndrome, in which progressive cerebellar deficits begin early in childhood, is another rare example in which a Friedreich's syndrome is associated with additional specific features. In this case, cataracts, mental retardation, multiple skeletal abnormalities, hypogonadotropic hypogonadism, and severe cerebellar atrophy are associated. The syndrome is likely a lysosomal storage disorder caused by an enzymatic defect, but the pathophysiology is unknown.

Rx TREATMENT

There is no proven therapy for the dominant ataxias (SCA1-5). The physician's task is to identify treatable disease entities resembling these disorders. Malignancies may present with chronic progressive ataxia either directly with a mass effect in the posterior fossa or indirectly by paraneoplastic degeneration (see Chap. 103). Malabsorption syndromes leading to vitamin E deficiency may lead to ataxia. The vitamin E deficiency form of Friedreich's ataxia must be considered, and serum vitamin E levels measured. Vitamin E therapy is indicated for these rare patients. Vitamin B_1 and B_{12} levels in serum must be measured, and the vitamin administered to patients having deficient levels. The deleterious effects of diphenylhydantoin and alcohol on the cerebellum are well known. Hypothyroidism may also produce ataxia. Aminoacidopathies, leukodystrophies, urea-cycle abnormalities, and mitochondrial encephalomyopathies may produce ataxia, and some dietary or metabolic therapies are available (see Chap. 380). The cerebrospinal fluid should be tested for a syphilitic infection in patients with progressive ataxia and other features of tabes dorsalis. Similarly, antibody titers for Lyme disease and *Legionella* should be measured, and appropriate antibiotic therapy should be instituted in antibody-positive patients. The identification of gene defects will, it is hoped, lead to specific pharmacologic therapy. At present, identification of an at-risk person's genotype, together with appropriate family and genetic counseling, can reduce the incidence of these cerebellar syndromes (see Chap. 363).

BIBLIOGRAPHY

Conner KE, Rosenberg RN: The hereditary ataxias, in *The Molecular and Genetic Basis of Neurological Disease*, RN Rosenberg et al (eds). Boston, Butterworth-Heinemann, 1993, pp 697–736

Dürr A et al: Clinical and genetic abnormalities in patients with Friedreich's ataxia. N Engl J Med 335:1169, 1996

Harding AE: Clinical features and classification of inherited ataxias. Adv Neurol 61:1, 1993

Kawaguchi Y et al: CAG expansions in a novel gene for Machado-Joseph disease at chromosome 14q32.1. Nat Genet 8:221, 1994

Matilla T et al: Molecular and clinical correlations in spinocerebellar ataxia type 3 and Machado-Joseph disease. Ann Neurol 38:68, 1995

Orr HT et al: Expansion of an unstable trinucleotide CAG repeat in spinocerebellar ataxia type 1. Nat Genet 4:221, 1993

Ouahchi K et al: Ataxia with isolated vitamin E deficiency is caused by mutations in the alpha-tocopherol transfer protein. Nat Genet 9:141, 1995

Servadio A et al: Expression analysis of the ataxin-1 protein in tissues from normal and spinocerebellar ataxia type 1 individuals. Nat Genet 10:94, 1995

Rosenberg RN: Autosomal dominant cerebellar phenotypes: The genotype has settled the issue. Neurology 45:1, 1995

———: DNA triplet repeats and neurologic disease. N Engl J Med 335:1222, 1996

———: The genetic basis of ataxia. Clin Neurosci 3:1, 1995
———: Spinocerebellar ataxias and ataxins. N Engl J Med 333:1351, 1995
———, IANNACCONE ST: The prevention of neurogenetic disease. Arch Neurol 52:356, 1995
TERRY JB, ROSENBERG RN: Frontal lobe ataxia. Surg Neurol 44:583, 1995
ZHUCHENKO O et al: Autosomal dominant cerebellar ataxia (SCA6) associated with small polyglutamine expansions in the α_{1A}-voltage-dependent calcium channel. Nat Genet 15:62, 1997
ZOGHBI H: Spinocerebellar ataxia and other disorders of trinucleotide repeats, in *Textbook of Molecular Medicine*, JL Jameson (ed). Cambridge, MA, Blackwell Science, 1997 (in press)

370

Robert H. Brown, Jr.

THE MOTOR NEURON DISEASES

AMYOTROPHIC LATERAL SCLEROSIS Amyotrophic lateral sclerosis (ALS) is the most common form of progressive motor neuron disease. It is a prime example of a neuronal system disease and is arguably the most devastating of the neurodegenerative disorders.

Pathology The pathology of motor neuron degenerative disorders involves lower motor neurons (consisting of anterior horn cells in spinal cord and their brainstem homologues innervating bulbar muscles) and upper or corticospinal motor neurons (emanating from layer five of motor cortex to descend via the pyramidal tract to synapse with lower motor neurons, either directly or indirectly via interneurons) (see Chap. 21). Although at its onset ALS may involve selective loss of function of only upper or lower motor neurons, it ultimately causes progressive loss of both categories of motor neurons (Tables 370-1 and 370-2). Indeed, in the absence of clear involvement of both motor neuron types, the diagnosis of ALS is questionable.

Other motor neuron diseases involve only particular subsets of motor neurons (Tables 370-1 and 370-2). Thus, in *bulbar palsy* and *spinal muscular atrophy* (also called progressive muscular atrophy), the lower motor neurons of brainstem and spinal cord, respectively, are most severely involved. By contrast, *pseudobulbar palsy*, *primary lateral sclerosis*, and *familial spastic paraplegia* affect only upper motor neurons innervating the brainstem and spinal cord.

In each of these diseases, the affected motor neurons undergo shrinkage, often with accumulation of the pigmented lipid (lipofuscin) that normally develops in these cells with advancing age. In ALS, the motor neuron cytoskeleton is typically affected early in the illness. Focal enlargements are frequent in proximal motor axons; ultrastructurally, these "spheroids" are composed of accumulations of neurofilaments. Beyond some astroglial proliferation, which is the inevitable accompaniment of all degenerative processes in the central nervous system (CNS), the interstitial and supportive tissues and the macrophage system remain largely inactive, and there is no inflammation.

The death of the peripheral motor neurons in the brainstem and spinal cord leads to denervation and consequent atrophy of the corresponding muscle fibers. Histochemical and electrophysiologic evidence indicates that in the early phases of the illness denervated muscle can be reinnervated by sprouting of nearby distal motor nerve terminals, although reinnervation in this disease is considerably less extensive than in most other disorders affecting motor neurons (e.g., poliomyelitis, peripheral neuropathy). As denervation progresses, muscle atrophy is readily recognized in muscle biopsies and on clinical examination. This is the basis for the term *amyotrophy* in the name for the disease. The loss of cortical motor neurons results in thinning of the corticospinal tracts that travel via the internal capsule and brainstem to the lateral (and anterior) white matter columns of the spinal cord. The loss of fibers in the lateral columns and resulting fibrillary gliosis impart a particular firmness (*lateral sclerosis*) to the affected tissues (Fig. 370-1). A remarkable feature of the disease is the selectivity of neuronal cell death. By light microscopy, the entire sensory apparatus, the regulatory mechanisms for the control and coordination of movement, and the components of the brain that are needed for cognitive processes, remain intact. However, immunostaining indicates that neurons bearing ubiquitin, a marker for degeneration, are also detected in nonmotor systems. Moreover, studies of glucose metabolism early in the illness also indicate that there is neuronal dysfunction outside of the motor system. Within the motor system, there is some selectivity of involvement. Thus, motor neurons required for ocular motility remain unaffected, as do the parasympathetic neurons in the sacral spinal cord (the nucleus of Onufrowicz or Onuf) that innervate the sphincters of the bowel and bladder.

Clinical Manifestations The manifestations of ALS are somewhat variable depending on whether corticospinal or lower motor neurons in the brainstem and spinal cord are more prominently involved. With lower motor neuron dysfunction and early denervation, the first evidence of the disease typically is insidiously developing asymmetric weakness, usually first evident distally in one of the limbs. A detailed history often discloses recent development of cramping with volitional movements, typically in the early hours of the morning (e.g., while stretching in bed). Weakness caused by denervation is associated with progressive wasting and atrophy of muscles and, particularly early in the illness, spontaneous twitching of motor units, or fasciculations. In the hands, a preponderance of extensor over flexor weakness is common. When the initial denervation involves bulbar rather than limb muscles, the problem at onset is difficulty with chewing, swallowing, and movements of the face and tongue. Early involvement of the muscles of respiration may lead to death before the disease is far advanced elsewhere.

With prominent corticospinal involvement, there is hyperactivity of the muscle-stretch reflexes (tendon jerks) and, often, spastic resistance to passive movements of the affected limbs.

Patients with significant reflex hyperactivity complain of muscle stiffness often out of proportion to weakness. Degeneration of the corticobulbar projections innervating the brainstem results in dysarthria and exaggeration of the motor expressions of emotion. The latter leads to involuntary excess in weeping or laughing (so-called *pseudobulbar affect*).

Virtually any muscle group may be the first to show signs of the disease, but, as time passes, more and more muscles become involved until ultimately the disorder takes on a symmetric distribution in all regions. It is characteristic of ALS that, regardless of whether the initial disease involves upper or lower motor neurons, both will eventually be implicated. Even in the late stages of the illness, sensory, bowel and

Table 370-1

Sporadic Motor Neuron Diseases

CHRONIC
Upper and lower motor neurons
Amyotrophic lateral sclerosis
Predominantly upper motor neurons
Primary lateral sclerosis
Predominantly lower motor neurons
Multifocal motor neuropathy with conduction block
Motor neuropathy with paraproteinemia or cancer
Motor-predominant peripheral neuropathies
Other
Associated with other degenerative disorders
Secondary motor neuron disorders (See Table 370-3)
ACUTE
Poliomyelitis
Herpes zoster
Coxsackie virus

Table 370-2

Genetic Motor Neuron Diseases

Disease	Loci	Gene
I. Upper and lower motor neurons (familial ALS)		
A. Autosomal dominant	21q	Superoxide dismutase
	22q	Neurofilament heavy subunit
B. Autosomal recessive (juvenile)	2q	
II. Lower motor neurons		
A. Spinal muscular atrophies I, II, III	5q	Survival motor neuron
1. Infantile: Werdnig-Hoffmann disease, I		Neuronal apoptosis inhibitory protein
2. Childhood, II		
3. Adolescent: Kugelberg-Welander disease, III		
B. X-linked spinobulbar muscular atrophy	Xq	Androgen receptor
C. GM2 gangliosidosis		
1. Adult Tay-Sach's disease	15q	Hexosaminidase A
2. Sandhoff disease	5q	Hexosaminidase B
3. AB variant	5q	GM_2 activator protein
III. Upper motor neurons Familial spastic paraplegia (FSP)		
A. Autosomal dominant	2p, 14q	
B. Autosomal recessive	8p	
C. X-linked	Xq21	Proteolipid protein
	Xq28	*L1 CAM*

bladder, and cognitive functions are preserved. Dementia is not a component of sporadic ALS, although in some families with the inherited form dementia may be present. Similarly, even when there is severe brainstem disease, ocular motility is spared until the very late stages of the illness.

Epidemiology The illness is relentlessly progressive, leading to death from respiratory paralysis; the median survival is from 3 to 5 years. There are very rare reports of stabilization or even regression of ALS. In most societies there is an incidence of 1 to 3 per 100,000 and a prevalence of 3 to 5 per 100,000. Several endemic foci of higher prevalence exist in the western Pacific (e.g., in specific regions of Guam or Papua New Guinea). In the United States and Europe, males are somewhat more frequently affected than females. While ALS is overwhelmingly a sporadic disorder, some 5 to 10 percent of cases are inherited as an autosomal dominant trait.

Familial ALS Several forms of selective motor neuron disease are heritable (Table 370-2). Two involve both corticospinal and lower motor neurons. The most common is familial ALS (FALS). Apart from its inheritance as an autosomal dominant trait, it is clinically indistinguishable from sporadic ALS. Genetic studies have identified mutations in the gene encoding the cytosolic enzyme superoxide dismutase (SOD) 1 as the cause of one form of FALS. However, this accounts for only 20 percent of inherited cases of ALS; there clearly are other ALS genes to be identified. There is also a recessive form of hereditary ALS that, unlike sporadic or dominantly inherited ALS, begins in childhood and is associated with prolonged survival. A locus for this disease has been mapped to the long arm of chromosome 2. Another familial, adult-onset disorder that may mimic aspects of ALS is Kennedy's syndrome, described below.

Differential Diagnosis Because ALS is currently untreatable, it is imperative that potentially remediable causes of motor neuron dysfunction be excluded (see Table 370-3). This is particularly true in cases that are atypical by virtue of (1) restriction to either upper or lower motor neurons, (2) involvement of neurons other than motor neurons, and (3) evidence of motor neuronal conduction block on electrophysiologic testing. Compression of the cervical spinal cord or cervicomedullary junction from tumors in the cervical regions or at the foramen magnum or from cervical spondylosis with osteophytes projecting into the vertebral canal can produce weakness, wasting, and fasciculations in the upper limbs and spasticity in the legs, closely resembling ALS. The absence of cranial nerve involvement may be helpful in differentiation, although some foramen magnum lesions may compress the twelfth cranial (hypoglossal) nerve, with resulting paralysis of the tongue. Absence of pain or of sensory changes, normal bowel and bladder function, normal roentgenographic studies of the spine, and normal cerebrospinal fluid (CSF) all favor ALS. Where doubt exists, magnetic resonance imaging (MRI) scans and contrast myelography should be performed to visualize the cervical spinal cord.

Another important entity in the differential diagnosis of ALS is *multifocal motor neuropathy with conduction block* (MMCB), discussed below. A diffuse, lower motor axonal neuropathy mimicking ALS sometimes evolves in association with hematopoietic disorders such as lymphoma. The underlying marrow pathology is often signaled by the presence of an M-component in serum which, in this clinical setting, should prompt consideration of a bone marrow biopsy. Lyme infection may also cause an axonal, lower motor neuropathy.

Other treatable disorders that occasionally mimic ALS are chronic lead poisoning and thyrotoxicosis. These disorders may be suggested by the patient's social or occupational history or by unusual clinical features. When the family history is positive, enzyme disorders involv-

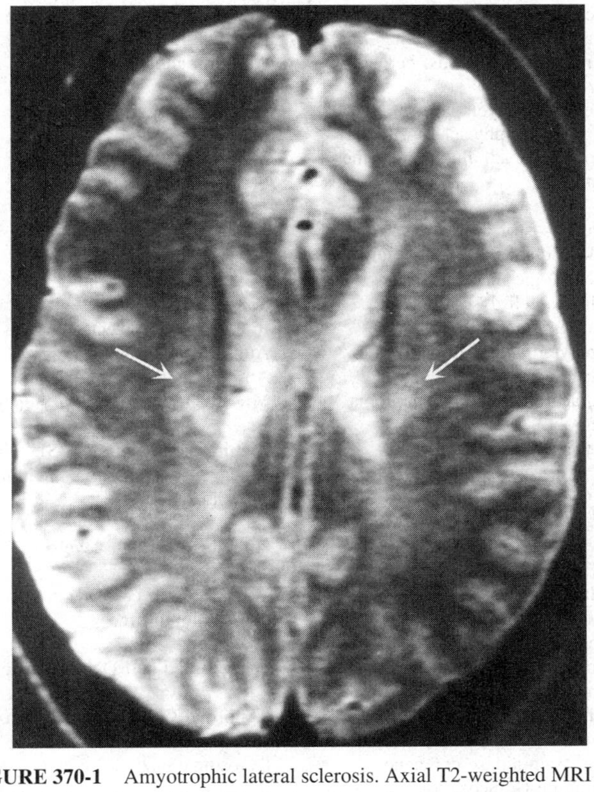

FIGURE 370-1 Amyotrophic lateral sclerosis. Axial T2-weighted MRI scan through the lateral ventricles of the brain reveals abnormal high signal intensity within the corticospinal tracts (*arrows*). This MRI feature represents an increase in water content in myelin tracts undergoing Wallerian degeneration secondary to cortical neuronal loss. This finding is commonly present in ALS, but can also be seen in AIDS-related encephalopathy, infarction, or other disease processes that produce neuronal loss in a symmetric fashion.

ing SOD1, hexosaminidase A, or α-glucosidase deficiency must be excluded (see Chap. 346). These are readily identified by appropriate laboratory tests. Benign fasciculations are occasionally a source of concern because on inspection they resemble the fascicular twitchings that accompany motor neuron degeneration. The absence of weakness, atrophy, or denervation phenomena on electrophysiologic examination usually excludes ALS or other serious neurologic disease. Patients who have recovered from poliomyelitis may experience a delayed deterioration of motor neurons that presents clinically with progressive weakness, atrophy, and fasciculations. Its cause is unknown but is thought to reflect sublethal prior injury to motor neurons by poliovirus (see Chap. 379).

Rarely, ALS develops concurrently with features indicative of more widespread neurodegeneration. Thus, one infrequently encounters otherwise typical ALS patients with a Parkinsonian movement disorder or dementia. It remains unclear whether this reflects the unlikely simultaneous occurrence of two disorders or a primary defect triggering two forms of neurodegeneration. The latter is suggested by the observation that multisystem neurodegenerative diseases may be inherited; rare families are reported with ALS and parkinsonism, or ALS and dementia with features of Pick's disease (see Chap. 368).

Pathogenesis The cause of sporadic ALS is not well defined. Some data suggest that excitotoxic neurotransmitters such as glutamate may participate in the death of motor neurons in ALS. It is striking that one cellular defense against such excitotoxicity is the enzyme SOD1, which detoxifies the free radical superoxide anion. Because SOD1 is mutated in some familial cases of ALS, it may be that glutamate excitotoxicity and ALS result from free radical accumulations in motor neurons. Precisely why the SOD1 mutations are toxic to motor nerves is not established, although it is clear that the effect is not simply loss of normal scavenging of the superoxide anion.

Table 370-3

Etiology and Investigation of Motor Neuron Disorders

Diagnostic Categories	Investigations
Structural lesions	MRI scan of head (including foramen magnum), cervical spine
Parasagittal or foramen magnum tumors	
Cervical spondylosis	
Chiari malformation or syrinx	
Spinal cord arteriovenous malformation	
Infections	CSF exam, culture
Bacterial—tetanus, Lyme	Lyme antibody titer
Viral—poliomyelitis, herpes zoster	Antiviral antibody titers
Retroviral myelopathy	HTLV-I titer
Intoxications, physical agents	
Toxins—lead, aluminum, other metals	24-h urine for heavy metals Serum and urine for lead, aluminum
Drugs—strychnine, phenytoin	
Electric shock, x-irradiation	
Immunologic mechanisms	Complete blood count
Plasma cell dyscrasias	Sedimentation rate
Autoimmune	Immunoprotein electrophoresis
polyradiculoneuropathy	Anti-GM_1 antibodies
Paraneoplastic	Anti-Hu antibody
Paracarcinomatous/lymphoma	MRI scan, bone marrow biopsy
Metabolic	
Hypoglycemia	Fasting blood sugar (FBS), routine chemistries including calcium
Hyperparathyroidism	Thyroid functions
Hyperthyroidism	
Deficiency of folate, vitamins B_{12}, E, and folate	Vitamin B_{12}, folate levels
Malabsorption	24-h stool fat, carotene, prothrombin time
Hereditary biochemical disorders	
Superoxide dismutase 1 mutation	White blood cell DNA analysis
Androgen receptor defect (Kennedy's disease)	Abnormal CAG insert in androgen receptor gene
Hexosaminidase deficiency	Lysosomal enzyme screen
Infantile (-glucosidase deficiency (Pompe's disease)	
Hyperlipidemia	Lipid electrophoresis
Hyperglycinuria	Urine and serum amino acids
Methylcrotonylglycinuria	CSF amino acids

NOTE: CSF, cerebrospinal fluid; MRI, magnetic resonance imaging.

℞ TREATMENT

There is no treatment capable of arresting the underlying pathologic process in ALS. Recently, the drug riluzole was approved for use in ALS because it produces a modest lengthening of survival. In one trial, the survival rate at 18 months with riluzole was similar to placebo at 15 months. The mechanism of this effect is not known with certainty; it may reduce excitotoxicity by diminishing glutamate release. There are encouraging preliminary results with other excitotoxin inhibitors or growth factors in ALS, and phase III clinical trials of several agents are in progress.

By contrast with ALS, several of the disorders (see Table 370-2) that bear some clinical resemblance to ALS are treatable; for this reason, a careful search for such forms of secondary motor neuron disease is warranted. In the absence of a primary therapy for ALS, a variety of rehabilitative aids may substantially assist ALS patients. Foot-drop splints facilitate ambulation by avoiding tripping on a floppy foot and obviating excessive hip flexion. Finger-extension splints can potentiate grip. Respiratory support may be life-sustaining. For patients electing against long-term ventilation by tracheostomy, positive-pressure ventilation by mouth or nose may provide transient (several weeks) relief from hypercarbia and hypoxia.

SELECTED LOWER MOTOR NEURON DISORDERS In the varieties of motor neuron disease grouped under this heading, the peripheral motor neurons are affected without evidence of involvement of the corticospinal motor system (Table 370-1).

X-linked Spinobulbar Muscular Atrophy (Kennedy's Disease) This is an X-linked lower motor neuron disorder in which progressive weakness and wasting of limb and bulbar muscles begins in males in midadult life and is conjoined with androgen insensitivity manifested by gynecomastia and reduced fertility (see Chap. 336). In addition to gynecomastia, which may be subtle, two findings distinguishing this disorder from ALS are the absence of signs of pyramidal tract disease (spasticity) and the presence of a subtle sensory neuropathy in some patients. The underlying molecular defect is an expanded trinucleotide repeat (-CAG-) in the first exon of the androgen receptor gene on the X chromosome; this may be readily screened from DNA from blood. An inverse correlation appears to exist between the number of -CAG- repeats and the age of onset of the disease (see Chap. 363).

Adult Tay-Sach's Disease Several reports have described adult-onset, predominantly lower motor neuropathies arising from deficiency of the enzyme β-hexosaminidase (hex A). These tend to be distinguishable from ALS because they are very slowly progressive; dysarthria and radiographically evident cerebellar atrophy may be prominent. In rare cases, spasticity may also be present, although it is generally absent (see Chap. 346).

Spinal Muscular Atrophy The spinal muscular atrophies (SMAs) are a family of selective lower motor neuron diseases of early onset. Despite some phenotypic variability (largely in age of onset), the defect in the majority of families with SMA is genetically linked to a locus on the proximal long arm of chromosome 5. Two candidate genes have been identified at this locus: a putative motor neuron survival protein (SMN for *s*urvival *m*otor *n*euron) and a protein that may be an inhibitor of apoptotic cell death (NAIP for *n*euronal *a*poptosis *i*nhibitory *p*rotein). All types of SMA are transmitted as autosomal recessive traits. Neuropathologically these disorders are characterized by extensive loss of large motor neurons; muscle biopsy reveals evidence of denervation atrophy. Several clinical forms are described.

Infantile SMA (SMA I, Werdnig-Hoffmann Disease) has the earliest onset and most rapidly fatal course. In some instances it is apparent even before birth, as indicated by decreased fetal movements late in the third trimester. Though alert, afflicted infants are weak and floppy (hypotonic) and lack muscle stretch reflexes. Death generally ensues within the first year of life. When the family history is unclear, it is difficult in the early weeks and months to distinguish SMA I from benign congenital hypotonia. An electromyogram is often particularly helpful as SMA I usually demonstrates fulminant denervation, while in congenital hypotonia the electromyogram is often myopathic or normal.

Chronic childhood SMA (SMA II) begins later in childhood and evolves with a more slowly progressive course. *Juvenile SMA (SMA III, Wohlfart-Kugelberg-Welander disease)* manifests during late childhood and runs a slow, indolent course. Unlike most denervating diseases, in this chronic disorder weakness is greatest in the proximal muscles; indeed, the pattern of clinical weakness can suggest a primary myopathy such as limb-girdle dystrophy. Electrophysiologic and muscle biopsy evidence of denervation distinguish SMA III from the myopathic syndromes.

Multifocal Motor Neuropathy with Conduction Block In this disorder, lower motor neuron function is regionally and chronically disrupted by remarkably focal blocks in conduction. Many cases have elevated serum titers of mono- and polyclonal antibodies to ganglioside GM_1; it is hypothesized that the antibodies produce selective, focal, paranodal demyelination of motor neurons. MMCB is not typically associated with corticospinal signs. In contrast with ALS, MMCB may respond dramatically to therapy such as intravenous gamma globulin or chemotherapy; it is thus imperative that MMCB be excluded when considering a diagnosis of ALS.

Other Forms of Lower Motor Neuron Disease In individual families, other syndromes characterized by selective lower motor neuron dysfunction in an SMA-like pattern have been described. There are rare X-linked and autosomal dominant forms of apparent SMA. There is an ALS variant of juvenile onset, the Fazio-Londe syndrome, which involves mainly the musculature innervated by the brainstem. A component of lower motor neuron dysfunction is also found in some multisystem degenerative disorders such as Machado-Joseph disease and the related olivopontocerebellar degenerations (see Chap. 369).

SELECTED DISORDERS OF THE UPPER MOTOR NEURON **Primary Lateral Sclerosis (PLS)** This exceedingly rare disorder arises sporadically in adults in mid- to late life. Clinically it is characterized by progressive spastic weakness of the limbs, preceded or followed by spastic dysarthria and dysphagia, indicating combined involvement of the corticospinal and corticobulbar tracts. Fasciculations, amyotrophy, and sensory changes are absent; neither electromyography nor muscle biopsy shows denervation. On neuropathologic examination, there is selective loss of the large pyramidal cells in the precentral gyrus and degeneration of the corticospinal and corticobulbar projections. The peripheral motor neurons and other neuronal systems are spared. The course of PLS is variable; while long-term survival is documented, the course may be as aggressive as in ALS, with approximately 3-year survival from onset to death. Early in its course, PLS raises the question of multiple sclerosis or other demyelinating diseases such as adrenoleukodystrophy as diagnostic considerations. A myelopathy suggestive of PLS is infrequently seen with infection with the retrovirus HTLV-I (see Chap. 373). The clinical course and laboratory testing will distinguish these possibilities.

Familial Spastic Paraplegia (FSP) In its pure form, this disorder, usually transmitted in families as an autosomal dominant trait, is characterized by progressive spastic weakness beginning in the distal lower extremities. It arises in the third or fourth decade and typically has long survival, presumably because respiratory function is spared. Late in the illness there may be urinary urgency and incontinence, and sometimes fecal incontinence; sexual function tends to be preserved. In pure forms of FSP, ataxia, posterior column sensory loss, and amyotrophy are absent or minimal; however, in some patients, minor sensory changes (impaired vibration and position sense) may be observed in late stages. Some family members may show spasticity without clinical symptoms. Neuropathologically, in FSP there is degeneration of the corticospinal tracts, which appear nearly normal in the brainstem but show increasing atrophy at more caudal levels in the spinal cord. It is now apparent that defects at several different loci underlie both dominantly and recessively inherited forms of FSPs (Table 370-2). With one exception, the primary gene defects causing FSP have not been described. The exception is an infantile-onset form of X-linked, recessive FSP arising from mutations in the gene for proteolipid protein. This is an example of rather striking allelic variation, as most other mutations in the same gene cause not FSP but Pelizaeus-Merzbacher disease, a disorder of CNS myelin.

Rarely, FSP may arise concomitantly with significant involvement of other regions of the nervous system. Thus, it has been described concurrently with amyotrophy, mental retardation, mental retardation with skin thickening, optic atrophy, and sensory neuropathy. In some cases there is loss of fibers in the ascending posterior columns and the spinocerebellar tracts, features reminiscent of Friedreich's ataxia. These complicated forms of FSP emphasize the challenge inherent in classifying the neurodegenerative disorders; there may be considerable overlap of the clinical phenotypes in diseases otherwise classified as distinct. Fortunately, it is likely that increasingly available genetic testing will clarify these nosologic difficulties.

BIBLIOGRAPHY

Bensimon G et al: A controlled trial of riluzole in amyotrophic lateral sclerosis. N Engl J Med 330:585, 1994

Brooks BP, Fischbeck KH: Spinal and bulbar muscular atrophy: A trinucleotide-repeat expansion neurodegenerative disease. Trends Neurosci 18:459, 1995

Crawford TO: From enigmatic to problematic: The new molecular genetics of childhood spinal muscular atrophy. Neurology 46:335, 1996

Dalakas MC: The post-polio syndrome as an evolved clinical entity. Definition and clinical description. Ann N Y Acad Sci 753:68, 1995

Ikeda M et al: Variable clinical symptoms in familial amyotrophic lateral sclerosis with a novel point mutation in the Cu/Zn superoxide dismutase gene. Neurology 45:2038, 1995

Kunst CB et al: Mutations in SOD1 associated with amyotrophic lateral sclerosis cause novel protein interactions. Nat Genet 15:91, 1997

Lacomblez L et al: Dose-ranging study of riluzole in amyotrophic lateral sclerosis. Lancet 347:1425, 1996

La Spada AR et al: Androgen receptor gene mutations in X-linked spinal muscular atrophy. Nature 352:77, 1991

Martin JB: CNS genetic disorders: Loss of function, gain of function, or something else? Curr Opin Neurobiol 5:669, 1995

Navon R et al: A new mutation in the HEXA gene associated with a spinal muscular atrophy phenotype. Neurology 45:539, 1995

Parano E et al: Molecular basis of phenotypic heterogeneity in siblings with spinal muscular atrophy. Ann Neurol 40:247, 1996

Rosen DR et al: Mutations in Cu/Zn superoxide dismutase gene are associated with familial amyotrophic lateral sclerosis. Nature 362:59, 1993

Smith RA (ed): *Handbook of Amyotrophic Lateral Sclerosis*. New York, Marcel Dekker, 1992

Vechio JD: Sequence variants in human neurofilament proteins: Absence of linkage to familial amyotrophic lateral sclerosis. Ann Neurol 40:603, 1996

371 John Engstrom, Joseph B. Martin

DISORDERS OF THE AUTONOMIC NERVOUS SYSTEM

The regulation of homeostatic functions is accomplished by the autonomic nervous system (ANS). An extensive peripheral innervation network combined with central vigilance provides rapid adjustments in vital physiologic mechanisms that are critical to survival. The importance of this regulation is emphasized by the extent and severity of disability resulting from compromised ANS function. This chapter describes the clinical manifestations, diagnosis, and treatment of ANS disorders. → ***The functional anatomy and relevant pharmacology of the sympathetic and parasympathetic components of the ANS are discussed in Chap. 70. Hypothalamic disorders that cause disturbances in homeostasis are discussed in Chaps. 17 and 328.***

CLINICAL MANIFESTATIONS **Classification** Disorders of the ANS may result from central nervous system (CNS) or peripheral nervous system (PNS) causes; they may be generalized, segmental, or focal. In many instances, the clinical signs and symptoms are due to interruption of the reflex arc controlling autonomic responses. The interruption can occur in the afferent limb, CNS processing centers, or efferent limb of the reflex arc. For example, posterior fossa tumors and syringobulbia can produce lesions of the medulla that impair blood pressure (BP) responses to postural changes and result in orthostatic hypotension. Hypotension can also follow lesions of vasomotor nerve fibers to blood vessels (as in diabetes mellitus or spinal cord disease) or afferent connections (as in tabes dorsalis or Guillain-Barré syndrome). Segmental disorders or focal deficits occur in spinal cord disease, reflex sympathetic dystrophy (causalgia), and Horner's syndrome (Table 371-1). Diagnosis of the site of reflex interruption is dependent on associated clinical findings, autonomic nervous system tests, and neuroimaging.

Another approach to the classification of ANS disorders is based on the presence or absence of CNS signs. The primary value of this approach is that pathophysiology and prognosis differ between these two groups. Subcategories of disease are differentiated on the basis of characteristics such as the presence of a positive family history, pathologic findings, and the association with sensory or motor neuropathy. Unfortunately, some syndromes do not fit easily into any classification scheme and little is known about their causes, pathology, or treatment (see Table 371-1).

Symptoms of Autonomic Dysfunction The clinical manifestations of autonomic lesions are influenced by the organ involved, the normal balance of sympathetic-parasympathetic innervation, the nature of the underlying illness, and the severity and stage of progression (Table 371-2). *Impotence* often heralds autonomic failure in men and may precede other symptoms by more than a decade, making its relevance apparent only in retrospect (see Chap. 51). A decrease in the frequency of spontaneous early morning erections may occur months before loss of nocturnal penile tumescence and development of total impotence. *Bladder dysfunction* also appears early in men and women, particularly in those with CNS involvement. Brain and spinal cord disease above the level of the lumbar spine (upper motor neuron or spastic bladder) results first in urinary frequency and small bladder volumes and eventually in incontinence. Disease of autonomic nerve fibers to the bladder (lower motor neuron bladder) or sensory denervation results in large bladder volumes, urinary frequency, and overflow incontinence. Measurements of bladder volume (postvoid residual volume) can be useful in distinguishing between upper and lower motor neuron bladder dysfunction. *Gastrointestinal dysfunction* is typically manifested as severe constipation. Diarrhea occurs occasionally (as in diabetes mellitus) due to rapid transit of contents or uncoordinated small bowel motor activity, or on an osmotic basis from bacterial overgrowth associated with small bowel stasis. Impairment of glandular secretory function may cause difficulty with food intake (due to decreased salivation) and eye irritation (due to decreased lacrimation). Occasionally, temperature elevation and vasodilation can result from *anhidrosis*, since sweating is an important form of heat dissipation (see Chap. 17).

Orthostatic hypotension is the most disabling feature of autonomic dysfunction. Generally accepted criteria for diagnosis are a postural decrease from the supine to standing position of at least 20 mmHg in systolic or 10 mmHg in diastolic BP sustained for at least 3 min; the latter criterion differentiates autonomic failure from sluggish baroreflex responses that are common in the elderly. Postural hypotension can cause a variety of symptoms, including dimming or loss of vision, lightheadedness, diaphoresis, diminished hearing, pallor, and weakness. Syncope results when the drop in BP impairs cerebral perfusion and metabolism (see Chap. 20). Other manifestations of impaired cardiovascular control from baroreflex dysfunction include supine hypertension, a heart rate that is fixed regardless of posture, and postprandial hypotension.

Approach to the Patient

The most common, clinically significant autonomic disorders present with symptoms of orthostatic hypotension. Suggestive symptoms that may appear on standing include lightheadedness, dimming of vision, nausea, diminished hearing, sweating, pallor, and weakness. The results of the history and examination are essential to distinguish the types of syncope or near-syncope from each other—neurocardiogenic, cardiogenic, autonomic failure, and autonomic failure associated with neurologic disease (see Fig. 20-1). → ***Neurocardiogenic and cardiac syncope are considered in Chap. 20.***

As a practical matter, the first step in the evaluation of symptomatic orthostasis is the exclusion of treatable causes for postural hypotension.

Table 371-1

Classification of ANS Disorders

Generalized ANS disorders
With CNS signs
Multiple system atrophy
Shy-Drager syndrome
Olivopontocerebellar degeneration
Striatonigral degeneration
Parkinson's disease
Huntington's disease
Hypothalamic disorders
Without CNS signs
Pure autonomic failure (as described by Bradbury and Eggleston)
Guillain-Barré syndrome (occasionally accompanied by CNS signs)
Chronic idiopathic anhidrosis
Postural orthostatic tachycardia syndrome
Raynaud's syndrome
Familial dysautonomia—Riley-Day syndrome
Segmental or peripheral ANS disorders
Diabetes mellitus
Spinal cord and root disorders
Peripheral neuropathy (amyloidosis, porphyria, alcoholism)
Guillain-Barré syndrome
Tabes dorsalis
Lambert-Eaton syndrome
Postprandial hypotension
Focal ANS disorders
Complex regional pain syndrome type I (RSD)
Shoulder–hand syndrome
Complex regional pain syndrome type II (causalgia)
Horner's syndrome
Reinnervation anomalies
"Crocodile" tears

The history should include an adequate review of patient medications (i.e., diuretics, antihypertensives, antidepressants, phenothiazines, ethanol, narcotics, insulin, barbiturates, and beta-adrenergic and calcium channel blockers), which may cause postural hypotension. Although medications may be responsible for symptoms, it is important to remember that exaggerated responses to medications may be the first sign of an underlying autonomic disorder. A complete list of patient medical problems may reveal a potential underlying cause for symptoms (i.e., diabetes, Parkinson's disease). The relationship of symptoms to meals (due to splanchnic shunting of blood) and awakening in the morning (due to relative intravascular volume depletion) should be sought.

The examination includes measurement of supine and standing pulse and blood pressure, with a gap of at least 2 min between positions. Sustained drops in systolic (>20 mmHg) or diastolic (>10 mmHg) blood pressure after standing for at least 2 min (unassociated with an appropriate increase in pulse rate) are suggestive of an autonomic deficit. Neurologic evaluation should include a mental status examination (to exclude neurodegenerative disorders), cranial nerve examination (to detect the impaired downgaze found with progressive supranuclear palsy), motor examination (for Parkinson's disease and parkinsonian syndromes), and sensory examination (for polyneuropathies). In patients without a clear initial diagnosis, follow-up neurologic evaluations performed at long intervals will often reveal an evolution of neurologic findings that makes it possible to reach a specific diagnosis. Autonomic function tests can be useful in selected circumstances to detect subclinical involvement, to evaluate the extent of abnormalities revealed by autonomic test results, and to monitor the effect of therapy on autonomic function.

Pharmacologic therapy is discussed below. It is helpful to remember that postural hypotension is a severely disabling disorder. Patients often lose their source of livelihood as a result, and families assume a tremendous burden for outpatient care. Adequate home health support for patients and psychological support for caregiving families is essential to maximize patient function.

Disorders of autonomic function need to be considered in the differential diagnosis of patients with symptoms of altered sweating (hyperhidrosis or hypohidrosis), constipation, impotence, or bladder dysfunction (urinary frequency, hesitancy, or incontinence). A review of concurrent medical illnesses, medications, and symptoms suggestive of autonomic or neurologic dysfunction will allow the examiner to decide which patients require further autonomic or neurologic evaluation.

Autonomic Testing (See also Chap. 361) The functional characteristics of the ANS can be assessed by physiologic and pharmacologic tests. Commonly used physiologic tests primarily assess autonomic aspects of cardiovascular function. These tests are noninvasive, easy to use, and provide quantitative or regional information about autonomic function. Interpretation of results requires collection of data under controlled circumstances. Pharmacologic tests can elucidate pathophysiologic abnormalities and guide the development of rational therapy.

HEART RATE VARIATION WITH DEEP BREATHING This is a test of parasympathetic influence on cardiovascular function. The test results are influenced by the subject's posture, rate and depth of respiration [5 to 6 breaths/min and a forced vital capacity (FVC) of >1.5 L are optimal], age, and medications and hypocapnea. Interpretation of results requires comparison of test data with results from normal control individuals collected under the same test conditions. For example, the lower limit of normal heart rate variation with deep breathing in persons younger than 20 years is more than 15 to 20 beats/min, but in persons over age 60 it is 5 to 8 beats/min. Heart rate variation with deep breathing (respiratory sinus arrhythmia) is abolished by the administration of atropine.

VALSALVA RESPONSE This response assesses integrity of the afferent limb, central processing, and efferent limb of the baroreceptor reflex. The response is obtained with the subject sitting or supine. A constant expiratory pressure of 40 mmHg is maintained for 15 s while changes in heart rate and beat-to-beat BP are measured. There are four phases of BP and heart rate response to the Valsalva maneuver (Table 371-3). Phases I and III are mechanical, related to changes in intrathoracic and intraabdominal pressure, and will not be discussed further. In the first portion of phase II, reduced stroke volume and venous return results in a fall in BP, tachycardia, and increased total peripheral resistance. Increased total peripheral resistance arrests the BP drop approximately 5 to 8 s after the onset of the maneuver. The BP nadir normally is followed by a progressive rise in BP toward baseline by the end of the maneuver. Venous return and cardiac output return to normal in phase IV. Persistent peripheral arteriolar resistance results in the temporary BP overshoot and phase IV bradycardia (mediated by the baroreceptor reflex).

Autonomic function during the Valsalva maneuver can be measured in several ways. The *Valsalva ratio* is calculated from heart rate changes during the maneuver and is defined as the maximum phase II tachycardia divided by the minimum phase IV bradycardia. The ratio reflects the integrity of the entire baroreceptor reflex arc and of sympathetic efferents to blood vessels; sympathetic efferent function is assessed in the phase II BP response and the BP overshoot. Test results depend on the age and posture of the

Table 371-2

Major Clinical Manifestations in Some Generalized Autonomic Failure Syndromes*

Disorder	Postural Hypotension	Genitourinary Dysfunction	Gastrointestinal Involvement	Sweating Deficit	Other Manifestations
Aging	+ +	+	+	+/−	Postprandial hypotension
Alcoholism	+	+			Tachycardia
Amyloidosis	+ + +	+	+ +	+ +	Dissociated sensory loss
Diabetes mellitus	+ + +	+ +	+ + + +	+	Distal neuropathy
Familial dysautonomia	+ +	+	+ + +	+	Abdominal crises, fevers, reduced sensitivity to pain
Holmes-Adie syndrome	+ +		+ +	+	Tonic pupils, areflexia, supine hypertension
Multiple system atrophy	+ + + +	+ + +	+ + +	+ + +	Parkinsonian and/or cerebellar dysfunction
Parkinson's disease	+ +	+	+ +	+/−	Sweating may be increased
Progressive supranuclear palsy	+	+ +	+ + +	+	Rigidity, gaze palsies
Pure autonomic failure	+ + + +	+	+ + +	+ + +	

* Dr. Ronald Polinsky contributed to this table in the 13th edition.

ABBREVIATIONS: ±, inconsistent or minimal; +, mild; + +, moderate; + + +, severe; + + + +, disabling lack of adrenergic output. Also, insulin can cause profound hypotensive effects.

subject, the expiratory pressure, the duration of expiration, the FVC, and medications. Noninvasive recording of beat-to-beat BP changes provides a direct measure of sympathetic efferent input to blood vessels that does not depend on the presence of a normal baroreceptor reflex arc.

SUDOMOTOR FUNCTION The capacity to produce sweat can be assessed quantitatively or qualitatively. Sweating is induced by release of acetylcholine from sympathetic postganglionic fibers. The *quantitative sudomotor axon reflex test* (QSART) allows for quantification of acetylcholine-induced sweating. A reduced or absent response indicates a lesion of the postganglionic sudomotor axon. The test provides a *quantitative* measure of regional autonomic function. For example, sweating may be reduced in the legs as a result of peripheral neuropathy (e.g., in diabetes) before other signs of autonomic dysfunction emerge. The *thermoregulatory sweat test* (TST) is a *qualitative* measure of regional sweat production in response to an elevation of body temperature. An indicator powder placed on the anterior body surface changes color with sweat production during temperature elevation. The pattern of color changes is a measure of regional sweat secretion. The pattern of sweat abnormality may suggest a peripheral or central cause for the deficit. For example, a unilateral decrease over half the body suggests a central lesion. Measurement of galvanic skin responses in the limbs following an induced electrical potential is another qualitative test used for detecting the presence or absence of sweating. The response is simple to measure but habituates easily.

ORTHOSTATIC BLOOD PRESSURE RECORDINGS Beat-to-beat BP measurements determined in supine, 80° tilt, and tilt-back positions are useful to quantitate orthostatic failure in BP control. It is important to allow a 20-min period of supine rest before assessing changes in BP during tilting. The test can be useful for the evaluation of patients with unexplained syncope and to detect vagally mediated syncope.

COLD PRESSOR TEST The cold pressor test assesses sympathetic function by having the subject immerse one hand in ice water (1 to 4°C) and then measuring BP at 30 s and 1 min. The systolic and diastolic pressures normally rise by 10 to 20 mmHg. The afferent pathway is spinothalamic and thus is distinct from the afferent limb of the baroreceptor reflex arc. When spinothalamic pathways are intact, an abnormal response indicates an abnormality of autonomic central processing or sympathetic efferent function. When the response to cold pressor test is normal and the Valsalva response is abnormal, then the lesion is located in the afferent limb of the baroreceptor reflex arc.

PHARMACOLOGIC TESTS Pharmacologic assessments can help localize an autonomic defect to the central or peripheral nervous system. For example, very low supine plasma norepinephrine (NE) levels reflect postganglionic (PNS) involvement, as seen in diabetes mellitus and pure autonomic failure. Specific abnormalities in noradrenergic neuronal function can be defined by using drugs with pressor activity. Tyramine, an indirect sympathomimetic, increases BP if neuronal NE stores are adequate and uptake mechanisms are intact. Up-regulation of postsynaptic noradrenergic receptors, a manifestation of denervating lesions, can be demonstrated by measuring the BP response to NE. Denervation supersensitivity is reflected as a specific exaggerated pressor response to NE infusion (but not to tyramine), while a CNS lesion (decentralization) results in a nonspecific increase in BP responsiveness to sympathomimetic agents (i.e., to NE *and* tyramine).

SPECIFIC SYNDROMES OF ANS DYSFUNCTION Two neurodegenerative disorders, pure autonomic failure (PAF) and multiple system atrophy (MSA), have been studied intensively in an effort to clarify the distinction between central and peripheral ANS lesions (see Table 371-1).

Pure Autonomic Failure This syndrome of postural hypotension, impotence, bladder dysfunction, and defective sweating was described by Bradbury and Eggleston in 1925; it is also called *chronic postganglionic autonomic insufficiency*. The etiology is unknown. The disease is not inherited and occurs in the absence of peripheral neuropathy. The disorder generally begins insidiously in the middle decades and affects women more than men. The symptoms, particularly postural hypotension, can be disabling. The disease does not appear to shorten the life span. The clinical and neuropharmacologic characteristics suggest primary involvement of postganglionic sympathetic neurons. There is a severe reduction in the density of neurons within sympathetic ganglia. Low supine plasma NE levels, a reduced NE response to tyramine, decreased neuronal uptake of NE, and noradrenergic supersensitivity reflect the peripheral sympathetic noradrenergic dysfunction. The clinical diagnosis is tentative in the early stages because patients may present with just postural hypotension and only later develop signs of multiple system atrophy.

Multiple System Atrophy MSA comprises several overlapping clinical syndromes, including striatonigral degeneration, Shy-Drager syndrome, and olivopontocerebellar atrophy (see Chap. 370). The full clinical syndrome includes the postural hypotension, impotence, bladder and bowel dysfunction, and defective sweating seen in PAF; rigidity, tremor, loss of associative movements, or abnormal eye movements are additional clinical findings seen in MSA. The pathologic and neurochemical features of MSA differ also.

Shy-Drager syndrome is a well-characterized severe form of MSA that is accompanied by autonomic failure. Most patients present with autonomic dysfunction alone, and other neurologic manifestations usually develop within 5 years. Patients with the striatonigral variant exhibit a form of parkinsonism in which bradykinesia and rigidity are more prominent than tremor. Patients with either a pure cerebellar syndrome or striatonigral degeneration may also develop pyramidal tract involvement. Some patients have features of both subtypes (see Chap. 370).

These disorders progress relentlessly to death 7 to 10 years after onset. Normal or elevated plasma NE and low monoamine metabolite levels in cerebrospinal fluid (CSF) (norepinephrine/methoxyhydroxyphenylglycol, serotonin/5-hydroxyindoleacetic acid, and

Table 371-3

Normal Blood Pressure and Heart Rate Changes during the Valsalva Maneuver

Phase	Maneuver	Blood Pressure	Heart Rate	Comments
I	Onset of expiration against a partially closed glottis	Rises due to aortic compression	Decreases	
II*e**	Continued expiration	Falls due to decreased venous return	Increases	
II*l**	Continued expiration	Total peripheral vascular resistance increases (increased sympathetic discharge and plasma epinephrine)	Increases at slower rate	Requires efferent sympathetic response
III	End of expiration	Falls due to increased capacitance of pulmonary bed	Increases further	
IV	Recovery	Increases ("overshoot") due to vasoconstriction and increased cardiac output	Compensatory bradycardia	Requires efferent sympathetic response

* *e*, early; *l*, late.

dopamine/homovanillic acid) are consistent with CNS involvement in this syndrome. Neuropathologic changes include primary neuronal degeneration with loss of neurons and gliosis in many CNS regions, including the brainstem, the cerebellum, the striatum, and the intermediolateral cell column of the thoracolumbar spinal cord. Both PAF and MSA are relatively uncommon. Autonomic nervous system disorders occurring in Parkinson's disease, Huntington's disease, and progressive supranuclear palsy are more common (see Chap. 368).

Peripheral Nerve Disorders Peripheral neuropathies are the most common cause of chronic autonomic insufficiency (see Chap. 381). Neuropathies that affect small myelinated and unmyelinated fibers of the sympathetic and parasympathetic nerves occur in diabetes mellitus, amyloidosis, chronic alcoholism, porphyria, and Guillain-Barré syndrome.

Diabetes mellitus Autonomic involvement in diabetes may begin at any stage in the disease and often presents with asymptomatic abnormal vagal function (see Chap. 334) that can be detected as reduced heart rate variation with deep breathing. Loss of small myelinated and unmyelinated nerve fibers in the splanchnic distribution, carotid sinus, and vagus nerves characterize the disorder. Widespread enteric neuropathy can cause profound disturbances in gut motility (gastroparesis), nausea and vomiting, malnutrition, achlorhydria, and bowel incontinence. Other symptoms include impotence, urinary incontinence, pupillary abnormalities, and postural hypotension. Typical symptoms and signs of hypoglycemia may fail to appear because damage to the sympathetic innervation of the adrenal gland results in a lack of epinephrine release. Insulin excess may also cause profound hypotension. Autonomic dysfunction may lengthen the QT interval and enhance the risk of sudden death. The cause of the neuropathy in diabetes is unknown. Hyperglycemia appears to be one risk factor for autonomic involvement. Biochemical and pharmacologic studies in diabetic neuropathy are compatible with autonomic failure localized to the PNS and reveal low supine plasma NE levels, a decreased BP response to tyramine, and enhanced pressor responsiveness to phenylephrine.

Amyloid polyneuropathy Autonomic neuropathy occurs in both sporadic and familial forms of amyloidosis (see Chap. 381). Although patients usually present with a distal painful neuropathy accompanied by sensory loss, autonomic insufficiency can precede the development of the sensorimotor neuropathy. Cardiac and renal impairment are the usual causes of death. Postmortem studies reveal amyloid deposition in many organs, including two sites that contribute to autonomic failure: intraneural blood vessels and neurons in autonomic ganglia. Pathologic examination reveals a loss of unmyelinated and myelinated nerve fibers.

Alcoholic neuropathy Abnormal parasympathetic vagal and efferent sympathetic function occur in chronic alcoholics. Pathologic changes can be demonstrated in the vagus nerves, sympathetic fibers, and ganglia. Impotence is a major problem, but concurrent abnormalities in gonadal hormones may obscure the parasympathetic contribution to this symptom. Clinical symptoms of autonomic failure generally appear only when peripheral neuropathy is severe; however, orthostatic hypotension may be prominent in Wernicke's encephalopathy. Alcoholics with liver disease are more likely to develop autonomic neuropathy. Autonomic involvement may contribute to the high mortality rates associated with alcoholism.

Porphyria Although each of the porphyrias can cause autonomic dysfunction, the condition is most extensively documented in the acute intermittent type (see Chap. 343). Autonomic symptoms include tachycardia, sweating, urinary retention, hypertension, and, less commonly, hypotension. Other prominent symptoms include anxiety, abdominal pain, nausea, and vomiting. Abnormal autonomic function can occur both during acute attacks and during remissions. Elevated catecholamine levels during acute attacks correlate with the degree of tachycardia and hypertension. Interestingly, several heme precursors inhibit NE uptake in platelets from patients with acute porphyria.

Guillain-Barré syndrome Blood pressure fluctuation and arrhythmias can be severe in acute inflammatory demyelinating polyradiculoneuropathy. It is estimated that 2 to 10 percent of seriously ill patients with Guillain-Barré syndrome suffer fatal cardiovascular collapse. Abnormal sweating, sphincter disturbance, and pupillary dysfunction also occur. Demyelination has been described in the vagus and glossopharyngeal nerves, the sympathetic chain, and the white rami communicantes. The presence of autonomic involvement is not clearly related to the severity of motor or sensory involvement.

Spinal cord lesions Descending pathways from the brain normally coordinate organized patterns of sympathetic activity and modulate segmental autonomic reflexes necessary for homeostasis. Spinal cord transection may be attended by autonomic hyperreflexia affecting bowel, bladder, sexual, temperature-regulation, and cardiovascular functions. Dangerous increases or decreases in body temperature are the result of inability to experience the sensory accompaniments of heat or cold exposure below the level of the injury. Quadriparetic patients exhibit both orthostatic hypotension and supine hypertension after upward tilting. Markedly increased autonomic discharge (autonomic dysreflexia) can be elicited by bladder pressure or stimulation of the skin or muscles. This phenomenon affects 85 percent of patients with a spinal cord lesion above the C6 level. Suprapubic palpation of the bladder, catheter insertion, catheter obstruction, or urinary infection are common and correctable underlying causes. Blood pressure can often be lowered by tilting the head upward. Vasodilator drugs may be used to treat acute elevations in BP, and clonidine is used prophylactically to reduce the hypertension resulting from bladder stimulation. Sudden, dramatic increases in BP can lead to intracranial hemorrhage and death.

Multiple sclerosis The abnormalities in autonomic function that occur in patients with multiple sclerosis are the result of multifocal CNS disease. Abnormal sweating occurs in approximately 40 percent of cases. Impairment of cardiovascular control is less common (measured most consistently as reduced heart rate variation with deep breathing) and usually minor. There does not appear to be any relationship between the severity of the disease and the degree of autonomic involvement. However, the sympathetic nervous system can modulate immune mechanisms that could contribute to disease progression.

Reflex Sympathetic Dystrophy and Causalgia The role of the autonomic nervous system in the pathogenesis of these disorders is highly controversial. The lack of an accepted cause or mechanism to explain their cause has resulted in a change in nomenclature for reflex sympathetic dystrophy (RSD) and causalgia by the International Association for the Study of Pain. The terms *complex regional pain syndrome* (CRPS) *types I* and *II* are now substituted for *RSD* and *causalgia*, respectively.

CRPS type I (reflex sympathetic dystrophy) is a regional pain syndrome that usually develops after tissue trauma. Types of associated trauma include myocardial infarction, minor shoulder or limb injury, stroke, or medications. Spontaneous pain, *allodynia* (the perception of a nonpainful stimulus as painful), and *hyperpathia* (an exaggerated pain response to a mildly painful stimulus) are out of proportion to the initial trauma and are not confined to the distribution of a single peripheral nerve. CRPS type II (causalgia) is a regional pain syndrome that develops after injury to a peripheral nerve, as first described by the Civil War surgeon Weir Mitchell. Spontaneous pain develops in the territory of the affected nerve; it may spread beyond that region, but the initially affected area remains involved. Vasomotor abnormalities, sudomotor abnormalities, and focal edema may occur alone or in combination in both CRPS types I and II. Other conditions that can account for the observed degree of limb pain or dysfunction must be excluded before making the diagnosis of CRPS.

Pain is the primary clinical feature of CRPS. Vasomotor, sudomotor, or edematous changes must also be present to satisfy criteria for diagnosis. Limb pain syndromes that do not meet these criteria are best classified as "limb pain—not otherwise specified (NOS)" to avoid diagnostic and therapeutic confusion.

CRPS type I (RSD) is divided into three clinical phases. Phase I consists of pain and swelling in the distal extremity occurring within weeks to 3 months after the precipitating event. The pain is diffuse, spontaneous, and either burning, throbbing, or aching in quality. The involved extremity is warm and edematous, and the joints are tender. Increased sweating and hair growth are present. In phase II (3 to 6 months after injury), thin, shiny, cool skin appears. After 3 to 6 additional months (phase III), atrophy of the skin and subcutaneous tissue plus flexion contractures complete the clinical picture. A recent, large prospective study provides evidence for a more variable presentation and course.

Abnormalities of autonomic function are present in both CRPS types I and II. Autonomic dysfunction results in localized sweating (increased resting sweat output) and changes in blood flow that may result in temperature asymmetries between affected and unaffected limbs. The changes in blood flow and sweating may result from localized noradrenergic and cholinergic supersensitivity.

Therapy for both disorders is not entirely satisfactory. Limitations of treatment study designs include use of variable diagnostic criteria, lack of placebo-treated groups, failure to control for symptom duration, and small patient numbers. Despite these flaws, the desire to provide relief for these severely disabling pain syndromes has yielded a variety of surgical and medical treatments with conflicting reports of efficacy. Clinical trials suggest that early mobilization with physical therapy or a brief course of steroids may be helpful for CRPS type I (RSD). The long-term results of this treatment are unclear. Other medical treatments have included the use of adrenergic blockers, nonsteroidal anti-inflammatory drugs (NSAIDs), calcium channel blockers, phenytoin, opioids, and calcitonin. Stellate ganglion and regional intravenous blockade are commonly used invasive therapeutic techniques. A recent study found no difference in pain relief between patients with early RSD treated with placebo and those treated with intravenous regional blockade with guanethidine. Although stellate ganglion blocks often provide temporary pain relief, the efficacy of repetitive use of these blocks is controversial.

Postprandial Hypotension The importance of postprandial hypotension among healthy elderly persons, hypertensive patients, and elderly patients in nursing homes has probably been underestimated, as compared to the well-accepted association with diabetes, Parkinson's disease, renal failure treated with hemodialysis, cardiovascular disease, paraplegia, and autonomic failure. The wisdom of administering cardiovascular medications that have hypotensive effects at mealtimes to healthy and hypertensive elderly patients needs reassessment. Abnormally reduced peripheral vasoconstriction in response to shunting of blood to the splanchnic circulation after a meal often contributes to postprandial hypotension.

Inherited Disorders Riley-Day syndrome (familial dysautonomia) is an autosomal recessive disorder of infants and children which occurs among Ashkenazi Jews. The defective gene has not been identified. Decreased tearing, hyperhidrosis, reduced sensitivity to pain, areflexia, absent fungiform papillae on the tongue, and labile BP may be present. Episodic abdominal crises and fever are common. Increased sensitivity to intraocular methacholine and absent axon flare response to intradermal histamine injection are useful diagnostic markers. Normal resting plasma NE levels that do not increase upon standing are consistent with an afferent lesion. Pathologic examination of nerves reveals a loss of small myelinated and unmyelinated nerve fibers (see Chap. 363).

Miscellaneous Other conditions associated with autonomic failure include autoimmune disease, infections, exposure to toxins (botulinum), poisoning (organophosphates), malignancy, and aging. Disorders of the hypothalamus can affect autonomic function and produce abnormalities in temperature control, satiety, sexual function, and circadian rhythms (see Chap. 328).

Rx TREATMENT

In most conditions, management of autonomic failure is limited to alleviating the disability caused by the symptoms. If possible, the primary disorder should be treated, but that will not generally improve autonomic function. Treatment of orthostatic hypotension is important, because the hypotension can drastically impair function. The history is key to the identification of easily reversible conditions contributing to symptomatic hypotension. A review of patient medications, the relationship of symptoms to meals, medical illnesses, and other symptoms of possible autonomic origin is mandatory.

Orthostatic hypotension only requires treatment if it causes symptoms. In the early stages, patients can maintain normal function by using good judgment and a few precautions. For example, small meals are better tolerated by patients with postprandial hypotension. Alcohol intake and excessive environmental temperatures should be avoided, because vasodilation can precipitously lower BP in patients with deficient baroreflex activity. Drugs that affect BP should be used with caution; many nonprescription medicines contain sympathomimetic agents that may result in severe hypertension in the setting of autonomic failure accompanied by denervation supersensitivity.

Salt intake should be increased to the maximum tolerated. Sleeping in a reverse Trendelenburg position (head-up tilt) reduces nocturnal diuresis, morning postural hypotension, hypovolemia, and helps to minimize supine hypertension. Compressive garments are of questionable value but may be tried; they present a number of practical problems, particularly for individuals with neurogenic bladder and/or neurologic impairment.

Eventually, most patients require drug therapy for management of hypotension. Fludrocortisone, which enhances renal sodium conservation and increases the sensitivity of arterioles to norepinephrine, is the initial drug of choice; potassium supplements are often necessary with chronic administration. Inhibitors of prostaglandin synthesis (e.g., ibuprofen) have potent pressor effects in patients with autonomic dysfunction. Other pharmacologic agents have been used with variable success to elevate BP. These include beta-blockers (propranolol, pindolol, xamoterol), sympathomimetics (ephedrine, midodrine), dopamine antagonists (metoclopramide), and venoconstrictors (dihydroergotamine). The supine hypertension seen in many patients with autonomic failure often limits pharmacotherapy.

Other approaches include the vasopressin analogue desmopressin (DDAVP) and the somatostatin analogue octreotide. Long-term or short-term therapy with desmopressin minimizes fluid loss, which may play an important role in exacerbating the hypotension in patients with autonomic failure. Single intranasal doses at bedtime help prevent nocturia and morning postural hypotension. Octreotide is administered parenterally and inhibits release of gut peptides, some of which have profound vasodilator and hypotensive effects. Since these substances are typically released after a meal, octreotide is most effective in alleviating postprandial hypotension.

Novel approaches have been studied to treat orthostatic hypotension. A pilot study found that erythropoietin administration increased standing systolic pressure by 20 mmHg and improved orthostatic symptoms. Erythropoietin is administered subcutaneously or intravenously at doses of 25 to 75 U/kg three times a week. The hematocrit increases after 2 to 6 weeks. Moclobemide, a selective monoamine oxidase (MAO)-A inhibitor, has been combined with tyramine to provide a dose-dependent, graded activation of MAO-B receptors to treat orthostatic hypotension. Midodrine, an α_1 receptor agonist, has also been shown to be effective.

Many patients with ANS failure exhibit exaggerated sensitivity to various drugs. Compounds with hypotensive actions should generally be avoided. For example, anticholinergic agents are a better initial choice than dopaminergic compounds for parkinsonism. Anesthetic management poses unique problems since these patients may have abnormal baroreceptor reflexes, sympathetic innervation of peripheral arterioles, pharmacologic responses, abnormal fluid balance, and adrenal medullary insufficiency. More important than the choice of anesthetic is awareness by the physician of the implications autonomic failure may have for peri- and postoperative monitoring and management.

BIBLIOGRAPHY

Bannister R (ed): *Autonomic Failure*, 3d ed. London, Oxford University Press, 1992

Braus DF et al: The shoulder-hand syndrome after stroke: A prospective clinical trial. Ann Neurol 36:728, 1994

Bradbury S, Eggleston C: Postural hypotension: A report of three cases. Am Heart J 1:73, 1925

Dyck P et al (eds): *Peripheral Neuropathy*, 3d ed. Philadelphia, Saunders, 1993

Jansen RW, Lipsitz LA: Postprandial hypotension: Epidemiology, pathophysiology, and clinical management. Ann Intern Med 122:286, 1995

Kozin F et al: The reflex sympathetic dystrophy syndrome. I. Clinical and histological studies: Evidence for bilaterality, response to corticosteroids and articular involvement. Am J Med 60:321, 1976

Low PA, Pfeifer MA: Standardization of autonomic function, in *Clinical Autonomic Disorders: Evaluation and Management*, PA Low (ed). Boston, Little, Brown, 1992

——— et al: Efficacy of midodrine vs. placebo in neurogenia orthostatic hypotension. JAMA 277:1046, 1997

Mathias CJ: Orthostatic hypotension: Causes, mechanisms, and influencing factors. Neurology 45(Suppl 5):S6, 1995

McLeod JG: Autonomic dysfunction in peripheral nerve disease. Invited review. Muscle Nerve 15:3, 1992

Polinsky RJ: Clinical autonomic neuropharmacology. Neurol Clin 8:77, 1990

Robertson D, Davis TL: Recent advances in the treatment of orthostatic hypotension. Neurology 45(Suppl 5):S26, 1995

Shy GM, Drager GA: A neurological syndrome associated with orthostatic hypotension. Arch Neurol 2:511, 1960

Stanton-Hicks M et al: Reflex sympathetic dystrophy: Changing concepts and taxonomy. Pain 63:127, 1995

Veldman PHJM et al: Signs and symptoms of reflex sympathetic dystrophy: Prospective study of 829 patients. Lancet 342:1012, 1993

372

*Joseph B. Martin, M. Flint Beal**

DISORDERS OF THE CRANIAL NERVES

The cranial nerves are susceptible to disorders that rarely affect the spinal peripheral nerves and, for this reason, deserve to be considered separately. This chapter describes the principal syndromes of disordered cranial nerve function and the diseases that cause them. → ***Disorders of taste and smell, vision and ocular movement, and hearing and balance are discussed in Chaps. 20, 28, and 29.***

OLFACTORY NERVE See Chap. 29

OPTIC NERVE See Chap. 28

OCULOMOTOR, TROCHLEAR, AND ABDUCENS NERVES See Chap. 28

TRIGEMINAL NERVE

The trigeminal nerve supplies sensation to the skin of the face and anterior half of the head. Its motor part innervates the masseter and pterygoid masticatory muscles.

PAROXYSMAL FACIAL PAIN (TRIGEMINAL NEURALGIA, TIC DOULOUREUX) The most striking disorder of trigeminal nerve function is tic douloureux, a condition characterized by excruciating paroxysms of pain in the lips, gums, cheek, or chin and, very rarely, in the distribution of the ophthalmic division of the fifth nerve. The disorder occurs almost exclusively in middle-aged and elderly persons. The pain seldom lasts more than a few seconds or a minute or two but may be so intense that the patient winces, hence

* The authors acknowledge the contributions of Maurice Victor to this chapter in previous editions.

the term *tic*. The paroxysms recur frequently, both day and night, for several weeks at a time. Another characteristic feature is the initiation of pain by stimuli applied to certain areas on the face, lips, or tongue ("trigger zones") or by movement of these parts. Sensory loss cannot be demonstrated. The adequate stimulus to a trigger zone for precipitating an attack is a tactile one and possibly tickle, rather than a noxious or thermal stimulus. Usually a spatial and temporal summation of impulses is necessary to trigger an attack, which is followed by a refractory period of up to 2 or 3 min.

The *diagnosis* of this disorder rests on these strict clinical criteria, and the condition must be distinguished from other forms of facial and cephalic neuralgia and pain arising from diseases of the jaw, teeth, or sinuses (see Chap. 15). Tic douloureux is usually without assignable cause; occasionally, when it appears in younger adults, it may be due to a demyelinative plaque at the root entry zone of the fifth nerve. Very rarely it occurs with herpes zoster or a tumor. To a degree that remains uncertain, pain of tic douloureux may be caused by a redundant or tortuous blood vessel in the posterior fossa, causing an irritative lesion of the nerve or its root. Usually, however, lesions such as aneurysms, neurofibromas, or meningiomas affecting the nerve produce a loss of sensation (trigeminal neuropathy, see below).

Rx TREATMENT

The initial treatment of tic douloureux is pharmacologic. Carbamazepine is the drug of choice and is effective initially in 75 percent of patients. Carbamazepine should be started gradually, as a single daily dose of 100 mg taken with food, and increased to 200 mg qid. Doses greater than 1200 mg daily provide no additional benefit. Unfortunately, not all patients can tolerate the drug in the doses required to alleviate pain, in which case phenytoin, 300 to 400 mg daily, can be substituted. Baclofen may also be administered, either alone or in combination with carbamazepine or phenytoin. The initial dose is 5 to 10 mg tid gradually increasing as needed to 20 mg qid.

If drug treatment fails, surgical therapy should be offered. The most widely applied procedure is percutaneous retrogasserian rhizotomy accomplished by radiofrequency lesions. Injection of glycerol in Meckel's cave is a method preferred by some surgeons. Either procedure produces relief in more than 95 percent of patients. The pain recurs in 7 to 31 percent of patients. Complications and morbidity are infrequent in experienced hands. These procedures result in partial numbness of the face and carry a risk of corneal denervation with secondary keratitis when used for the rare instances of first-division trigeminal neuralgia.

A third treatment, microvascular decompression, requires a suboccipital craniectomy, a major procedure requiring several days of hospitalization. It has an 80 percent efficacy rate, but the pain may recur, and, in a small number of cases, there is damage to the eighth or seventh nerve.

TRIGEMINAL NEUROPATHY A variety of diseases in addition to those mentioned above may affect the trigeminal nerve. Most present with sensory loss on the face or with weakness of the jaw muscles. Deviation of the jaw on opening indicates weakness of the pterygoids on the side to which the jaw deviates. Tumors of the middle cranial fossa (meningiomas), of the trigeminal nerve (schwannomas), or of the base of the skull (metastatic tumors) may cause a combination of motor and sensory signs. Lesions in the cavernous sinus can affect the first and second divisions of the trigeminal nerve, and lesions of the superior orbital fissure can affect the first (ophthalmic) division. The accompanying corneal anesthesia increases the risk of ulceration (neurokeratitis).

Loss of sensation over the chin can be the only manifestation of systemic malignancy. Rarely, an idiopathic form of trigeminal neuropathy is observed. It is characterized by feelings of numbness and paresthesias, sometimes bilaterally, with loss of sensation in the territory of the trigeminal nerve but without weakness of the jaw. Recovery is the rule, but the symptoms may be troublesome for many months, or even years. Leprosy may involve the trigeminal nerves.

Tonic spasm of the masticatory muscles, known as *trismus*, is symptomatic of tetanus (see Chap. 146). It also may occur as an idiosyncratic reaction in patients treated with phenothiazine drugs; lesser degrees may be associated with disease of the pharynx, temporomandibular joint, teeth, and gums.

FACIAL NERVE

FACIAL PALSY AND FACIAL SPASM The seventh cranial nerve supplies all the muscles concerned with facial expression. The sensory component is small (the nervus intermedius of Wrisberg); it conveys taste sensation from the anterior two-thirds of the tongue and probably cutaneous impulses from the anterior wall of the external auditory canal. The motor nucleus of the seventh nerve lies anterior and lateral to the abducens nucleus. After leaving the pons, the seventh nerve enters the internal auditory meatus with the acoustic nerve. The nerve continues its course in its own bony channel, the facial canal, and exits from the skull via the stylomastoid foramen. It then passes through the parotid gland and subdivides to supply the facial muscles.

A complete interruption of the facial nerve at the stylomastoid foramen paralyzes all muscles of facial expression. The corner of the mouth droops, the creases and skin folds are effaced, the forehead is unfurrowed, and the eyelids will not close. Upon attempted closure of the lids, the eye on the paralyzed side is seen to roll upward (Bell's phenomenon). The lower lid sags also, and the punctum falls away from the conjunctiva, permitting tears to spill over the cheek. Food collects between the teeth and lips, and saliva may dribble from the corner of the mouth. The patient complains of a heaviness or numbness in the face, but sensory loss is rarely demonstrable and taste is intact.

If the lesion is in the middle ear portion, taste is lost over the anterior two-thirds of the tongue on the same side. If the nerve to the stapedius is interrupted, there is hyperacusis (painful sensitivity to loud sounds). Lesions in the internal auditory meatus also may affect the adjacent auditory and vestibular nerves, causing deafness, tinnitus, or dizziness. Intrapontine lesions that paralyze the face usually affect the abducens nucleus as well, and often the corticospinal and sensory tracts.

If the peripheral facial paralysis has existed for some time and recovery of motor function has begun but is incomplete, a kind of contracture (actually a continuous diffuse contraction) of facial muscles may appear. The palpebral fissure becomes narrowed, and the nasolabial fold deepens. With the passage of time, the face and even the tip of the nose become pulled to the unaffected side. Attempts to move one group of facial muscles may result in contraction of all of them (associated movements, or *synkinesis*). Facial spasms may develop and persist indefinitely, being initiated by every facial movement (*hemifacial spasm*). This condition may represent a transient or permanent sequela to a Bell's palsy but also may be due to an irritative lesion of the facial nerve (e.g., an acoustic neuroma, an aberrant artery that compresses the nerve and is relieved by surgery, or a basilar artery aneurysm). However, in the most common form of hemifacial spasm, the cause and pathology are unknown. Anomalous regeneration of the seventh nerve fibers may result in other troublesome phenomena. If fibers originally connected with the orbicularis oculi come to innervate the orbicularis oris, closure of the lids may cause a retraction of the mouth, or if fibers originally connected with muscles of the face later innervate the lacrimal gland, anomalous tearing ("crocodile tears") may occur with any activity of the facial muscles, such as eating. Yet another unusual facial synkinesia is one in which jaw opening causes a closure of the eyelids on the side of the facial palsy (jaw-winking).

BELL'S PALSY The most common form of facial paralysis is idiopathic, i.e., *Bell's palsy*. The incidence rate of this disorder is about 23 per 100,000 annually, or about 1 in 60 or 70 persons in a lifetime. The pathogenesis of the paralysis is unknown. The few autopsied cases of this disease have shown only nondescript changes in the facial nerve and not inflammatory changes, as is commonly presumed.

Clinical Manifestations The onset of Bell's palsy is fairly abrupt, maximal weakness being attained by 48 h as a general rule. Pain behind the ear may precede the paralysis for a day or two. Taste sensation may be lost unilaterally, and hyperacusis may be present. In some cases there is mild cerebrospinal fluid (CSF) lymphocytosis. Fully 80 percent of patients recover within a few weeks or months. Electromyography may be of value in distinguishing a temporary conduction defect from a pathologic interruption in the continuity of nerve fibers. Evidence of denervation after 10 days indicates that there has been axonal degeneration and that there will be a long delay (3 months, as a rule) before regeneration occurs and that it may be incomplete. The presence of incomplete paralysis in the first week is the most favorable prognostic sign.

℞ TREATMENT

Protection of the eye during sleep, massage of the weakened muscles, and a splint to prevent drooping of the lower part of the face are the measures generally employed in the management of such cases. A course of prednisone beginning with 60 to 80 mg daily during the first 5 days and then tapered over the next 5 days may be beneficial and appears to shorten the recovery period.

Differential Diagnosis There are many other causes of facial palsy. Tumors that invade the temporal bone (carotid body, cholesteatoma, dermoid) may produce a facial palsy, but the onset is insidious and the course progressive. The *Ramsay Hunt syndrome*, presumably due to herpes zoster of the geniculate ganglion, consists of a severe facial palsy associated with a vesicular eruption in the pharynx, external auditory canal, and other parts of the cranial integument; often the eighth cranial nerve is affected as well. *Acoustic neuromas* frequently involve the facial nerve by local compression. Infarcts and tumors are the common pontine lesions that interrupt the facial nerve fibers. Bilateral facial paralysis (facial diplegia) occurs in acute inflammatory polyradiculoneuritis (*Guillain-Barré syndrome*) and in a variety of sarcoidosis known as *uveoparotid fever* (*Heerfordt syndrome*). The patient should be screened for Lyme disease, which is a frequent cause of facial palsies in endemic areas. The *Melkersson-Rosenthal syndrome* consists of a rarely encountered triad of recurrent facial paralysis, recurrent—and eventually permanent—facial (particularly labial) edema, and less constantly, plication of the tongue; many causes of this rare syndrome have been suggested, but none has been established. Leprosy frequently involves the facial nerve.

A puzzling disorder is the *facial hemiatrophy of Romberg*. It occurs mainly in females and is characterized by a disappearance of fat in the dermal and subcutaneous tissues on one side of the face. It usually begins in adolescence or early adult years and is slowly progressive. In its advanced form, the affected side of the face is gaunt, and the skin is thin, wrinkled, and rather brown. The facial hair may turn white and fall out, and the sebaceous glands become atrophic. The muscles and bones are not involved as a rule. Sometimes the atrophy becomes bilateral. The condition is a form of lipodystrophy. There is no treatment other than transplantation of skin and subcutaneous fat by a plastic surgeon.

Facial myokymia refers to a fine rippling activity of the facial muscles; it may be caused by a plaque of multiple sclerosis. *Blepharospasm* is an involuntary recurrent spasm of both eyelids that occurs in elderly persons as an isolated phenomenon or with varying degrees of spasm of other facial muscles. Severe, persistent cases of blepharospasm or hemifacial spasm are now successfully treated by local injection of botulinus toxin into the orbicularis oculi; the spasms are relieved for 3 to 4 months, and the injections can be repeated without morbidity.

All these forms of nuclear or peripheral facial palsy must be distinguished from the supranuclear type. In the latter, the frontalis and orbicularis oculi muscles are involved less than those of the lower part of the face, since the upper facial muscles are innervated by corticobulbar pathways from both motor cortices, whereas the lower facial muscles are innervated only by the opposite hemisphere. In supranuclear lesions there may be a dissociation of emotional and voluntary facial movements, and often some degree of paralysis of the arm and leg or an aphasia (in dominant hemisphere lesions) is conjoined.

VESTIBULAR NERVE

The eighth cranial nerve has two components, vestibular and auditory. Symptoms and signs of involvement of the vestibular portion are discussed in Chap. 20 and in this section. The auditory nerve and its disorders are discussed in Chap. 29.

MÉNIÈRE'S SYNDROME Ménière's disease, or Ménière's syndrome, is the name applied to recurrent vertigo associated with tinnitus and progressive deafness. Tinnitus and/or deafness may be absent during the initial attack(s) of vertigo, but they invariably appear as the disease progresses and are increased in severity during an acute attack. With milder forms of the syndrome, the patient may complain more of head discomfort, slight instability, and difficulty in concentration than of vertigo and may be considered to be anxious or depressed. Provided that deafness is not complete, the recruitment phenomenon can be demonstrated (see Chap. 29).

Ménière's disease has its onset most frequently in the fifth decade of life, although younger adults and the elderly are not spared. The pathologic changes are said to consist of a dilation of the endolymphatic system that leads to a degeneration of the delicate vestibular and cochlear hair cells. The relation of these pathologic changes to the paroxysmal disorder of labyrinthine function is unknown.

℞ TREATMENT

During an acute attack, rest in bed is the most effective treatment, since the patient can usually find a position in which vertigo is minimal. Dimenhydrinate, cyclizine, or meclizine in doses of 25 to 50 mg tid is useful in treating more protracted attacks. A low-salt diet is still used in treatment, but its value is difficult to judge. Mild sedative drugs may help the anxious patient between attacks. Usually the deafness is unilateral and progressive, and when it is complete, the vertiginous attacks cease. However, the course is variable, and if the attacks persist in a severe manner, permanent relief can be obtained by surgical destruction of the labyrinth or section of the vestibular portion of the eighth nerve intracranially.

BENIGN POSITIONAL VERTIGO Another disorder of labyrinthine function is characterized by the occurrence of paroxysmal vertigo and nystagmus when the head assumes certain critical positions. This is the positional vertigo of Bárány, of the so-called benign paroxysmal type (see Chap. 20). In refractory cases, in which attacks continue, vestibular exercises may be beneficial.

DIFFERENTIAL DIAGNOSIS OF VERTIGO There are many other causes of acute vertigo, such as purulent labyrinthitis complicating meningitis, serous labyrinthitis due to infection of the middle ear, "toxic labyrinthitis" due to drug intoxication (e.g., with alcohol, quinine, streptomycin, gentamicin, and other antibiotics), motion sickness, trauma, and hemorrhage into the internal ear. In these instances, the attacks of vertigo tend to last longer than in the recurrent form, but in other respects the symptoms are similar. Aminoglycoside antibiotics may damage the fine hair cells of the vestibular end organs and cause a permanent disorder of equilibrium (as well as hearing), especially in older patients (see also Chap. 20).

There has been described a dramatic clinical syndrome, characterized by the abrupt onset of severe vertigo, nausea, and vomiting without tinnitus or hearing loss. The vertigo persists for several days or weeks, and labyrinthine function is permanently ablated on one side. Occlusion of the labyrinthine division of the internal auditory artery would logically explain this syndrome, but pathologic or angiographic confirmation of this hypothesis has so far not been obtained.

Vertigo of vestibular nerve origin may occur with diseases that involve the nerve in the petrous bone or the cerebellopontine angle. Except that it is less severe and is less frequently paroxysmal, it has many of the characteristics of labyrinthine vertigo. The adjacent auditory division of the eighth cranial nerve also may be affected, which explains the frequent association of vertigo with tinnitus and deafness. The function of the eighth cranial nerve may be disturbed by tumors of the lateral recess (especially acoustic neuroma), less frequently by meningeal inflammation in this region and, rarely, by an abnormal vessel that compresses the nerve.

Vestibular neuronitis and *benign recurrent vertigo* are the names applied to a clinical syndrome that occurs mainly in middle-aged and young adults (sometimes in children) and is characterized by the abrupt onset of vertigo, nausea, and vomiting without impairment of hearing. The attacks are brief and leave the patient for some days with a mild positional vertigo. They may occur only once or recur in varying degrees of severity. The cause is unknown. The medical treatment is the same as for Ménière's disease.

GLOSSOPHARYNGEAL NERVE

GLOSSOPHARYNGEAL NEURALGIA This form of neuralgia resembles trigeminal neuralgia in many respects but is much less common. The pain is intense and paroxysmal; it originates in the throat, approximately in the tonsillar fossa. In some cases the pain is localized in the ear or may radiate from the throat to the ear because of involvement of the tympanic branch of the glossopharyngeal nerve. Spasms of pain may be initiated by swallowing. There is no demonstrable sensory or motor deficit. Cardiac symptoms—bradycardia, hypotension, and fainting—have been reported. A trial of carbamazepine or phenytoin is the recommended therapy, but if that is unsuccessful, division of the glossopharyngeal nerve near the medulla is the definitive treatment. Percutaneous rhizotomy of glossopharyngeal and vagal fibers in the jugular foramen alleviates pain in some patients.

Very rarely, herpes zoster involves the glossopharyngeal nerve. Glossopharyngeal neuropathy in conjunction with vagus and accessory nerve palsies may occur with a tumor or aneurysm in the posterior fossa or in the jugular foramen. Hoarseness due to vocal cord paralysis, some difficulty in swallowing, deviation of the soft palate to the intact side, anesthesia of the posterior wall of the pharynx, and weakness of the upper part of the trapezius and sternocleidomastoid muscles make up the syndrome (see Table 372-1, jugular foramen syndrome).

VAGUS NERVE

DYSPHAGIA AND DYSPHONIA Complete interruption of the intracranial portion of one vagus nerve results in a characteristic paralysis. The soft palate droops ipsilaterally and does not rise in phonation. There is loss of the gag reflex on the affected side, as well as of the "curtain movement" of the lateral wall of the pharynx, whereby the faucial pillars move medially as the palate rises in saying "ah." The voice is hoarse and slightly nasal, and the vocal cord lies immobile in the cadaveric position, i.e., midway between abduction and adduction. There also may be a loss of sensibility at the external auditory meatus and back of the pinna. Usually no change in visceral function can be demonstrated.

The pharyngeal branches of both vagi may be affected in diphtheria; the voice has a nasal quality, and regurgitation of liquids through the nose occurs during the act of swallowing.

The vagus nerve may be involved at the meningeal level by neoplastic and infectious processes and within the medulla by tumors, vascular lesions (e.g., the lateral medullary syndrome of Wallenberg), and motor neuron disease. This nerve may be involved by the inflammatory lesion of herpes zoster. Polymyositis and dermatomyositis, which cause hoarseness and dysphagia by direct involvement of laryngeal and pharyngeal muscles, may be confused with diseases of the vagus nerves. Also, dysphagia is a symptom in some patients with myotonic dystrophy. → *See Chap. 40 for discussion of nonneurologic forms of dysphagia.*

The recurrent laryngeal nerves, especially the left, are most often damaged as a result of intrathoracic disease. Aneurysm of the aortic arch, an enlarged left atrium, and tumors of the mediastinum and bronchi are much more frequent causes of an isolated vocal cord palsy than are intracranial disorders.

When confronted with a case of laryngeal palsy, the physician must attempt to determine the site of the lesion. If it is intramedullary, there are usually other signs, such as ipsilateral cerebellar dysfunction, loss of pain and temperature sensation over the ipsilateral face and contralateral arm and leg, and an ipsilateral Horner syndrome. If the lesion is extramedullary, the glossopharyngeal and spinal accessory nerves are frequently involved (see jugular foramen syndrome, Table 372-1). If it is extracranial in the posterior laterocondylar or retroparotid space, there may be a combination of ninth, tenth, eleventh, and twelfth cranial nerve palsies and a Horner syndrome. Combinations of these lower cranial nerve palsies have a variety of eponymic designations, listed in Table 372-1. If there is no sensory loss over the palate and pharynx and no palatal weakness or dysphagia, the lesion is below the origin of the pharyngeal branches, which leave the vagus nerve high in the cervical region; the usual site of disease is then the mediastinum.

Table 372-1

Cranial Nerve Syndromes

Site	Cranial Nerves Involved	Eponymic Syndrome	Usual Cause
Sphenoid fissure (superior orbital)	III, IV, first division V, VI	Foix	Invasive tumors of sphenoid bone; aneurysms
Lateral wall of cavernous sinus	III, IV, first division V, VI, often with proptosis	Foix Tolosa-Hunt	Aneurysms or thrombosis of cavernous sinus; invasive tumors from sinuses and sella turcica; benign granuloma responsive to steroids
Retrosphenoid space	II, III, IV, V, VI	Jacod	Large tumors of middle cranial fossa
Apex of petrous bone	V, VI	Gradenigo	Petrositis; tumors of petrous bone
Internal auditory meatus	VII, VIII		Tumors of petrous bone (dermoids, etc.); infectious processes; acoustic neuroma
Pontocerebellar angle	V, VII, VIII, and sometimes IX		Acoustic neuroma; meningioma
Jugular foramen	IX, X, XI	Vernet	Tumors and aneurysms
Posterior laterocondylar space	IX, X, XI, XII	Collet-Sicard	Tumors of parotid gland and carotid body and metastatic tumors
Posterior retroparotid space	IX, X, XI, XII and Horner syndrome	Villaret Mackenzie Tapia	Tumors of parotid gland, carotid body, lymph nodes; metastatic tumor; tuberculous adenitis

ACCESSORY NERVE

Isolated involvement of the accessory, or eleventh cranial, nerve can occur anywhere along its route, resulting in partial or complete paralysis of the sternocleidomastoid and trapezius muscles. More commonly, involvement occurs in combination with deficits of the ninth and tenth cranial nerves in the jugular foramen or after exit from the skull (see Table 372-1). An idiopathic form of accessory neuropathy, akin to Bell's palsy, has been described, and it may be recurrent in some cases. Most but not all patients recover.

HYPOGLOSSAL NERVE

The twelfth cranial nerve supplies the ipsilateral muscles of the tongue. The nucleus of the nerve or its fibers of exit may be involved by intramedullary lesions such as tumor, poliomyelitis, or most often motor neuron disease. Lesions of the basal meninges and the occipital bones (platybasia, invagination of occipital condyles, Paget's disease) may compress the nerve in its extramedullary course or in the hypoglossal canal. Isolated lesions of unknown cause can occur. Atrophy and fasciculation of the tongue develop weeks to months after interruption of the nerve.

MULTIPLE CRANIAL NERVE PALSIES

Several cranial nerves may be affected by the same disease process. In this situation, the main clinical problem is to determine whether the lesion lies within the brainstem or outside it. Lesions that lie on the surface of the brainstem are characterized by involvement of adjacent cranial nerves (often occurring in succession) and late and rather slight involvement of the long sensory and motor pathways and segmental structures lying within the brainstem. The opposite is true of intramedullary, intrapontine, and intramesencephalic lesions. The extramedullary lesion is more likely to cause bone erosion or enlargement of the foramens of exit of cranial nerves. The intramedullary lesion involving cranial nerves often produces a crossed sensory or motor paralysis (cranial nerve signs on one side of the body and tract signs on the opposite side).

Involvement of multiple cranial nerves outside the brainstem is frequently the result of diabetes or trauma (sudden onset), localized infections such as herpes zoster (acute onset), granulomatous disease such as Wegener's granulomatosis (subacute onset), Behçet's disease, or tumors and enlarging saccular aneurysms (chronic development). Of the tumors, lymphomas, neurofibromas, meningiomas, chordomas, cholesteatomas, carcinomas, and sarcomas have all been observed to involve a succession of lower cranial nerves. Owing to their anatomic relationships, the multiple cranial nerve palsies form a number of distinctive syndromes, listed in Table 372-1. Sarcoidosis has been found to be the cause of some cases of multiple cranial neuropathy, and chronic glandular tuberculosis (scrofula) the cause of a few others. Malignant granuloma of the nasopharynx also may affect multiple cranial nerves, as do nasopharyngeal tumors, platybasia, basilar invagination of the skull, and the Chiari malformation that becomes evident in adult life. A purely motor disorder without atrophy always raises the question of myasthenia gravis (see Chap. 382). Guillain-Barré syndrome commonly affects the facial nerves bilaterally (facial diplegia). In the Fisher variant of the Guillain-Barré syndrome, oculomotor paresis occurs with ataxia and areflexia in the limbs. Wernicke encephalopathy can cause a severe ophthalmoplegia combined with other brainstem signs.

An idiopathic form of multiple cranial nerve involvement on one or both sides of the face is occasionally seen (see Juncos and Beal). The syndrome consists of a subacute onset of boring facial pain, followed by paralysis of motor cranial nerves. The clinical features overlap those of the Tolosa-Hunt orbitocavernous sinus syndrome. The syndrome is frequently responsive to steroids.

BIBLIOGRAPHY

ADAMS RD, VICTOR M: *Principles of Neurology*, 6th ed. New York, McGraw-Hill, 1997, chap 47, pp 1370–1385

Adour KK: Medical management of idiopathic (Bell's) palsy. Otolaryngol Clin North Am 24:663, 1991
Beck RW et al: The effect of corticosteroids for acute optic neuritis on the subsequent development of multiple sclerosis. N Engl J Med 329:1764, 1993
Brodal A: The cranial nerves, in *Neurological Anatomy in Relation to Clinical Medicine*, 3d ed. New York, Oxford, 1980, chap 7, pp 448–577
Chalk C, Isaacs H: Recurrent spontaneous accessory neuropathy. J Neurol Neurosurg Psychiatry 53:621, 1990
Dallessio DJ: Medical treatment of the major neuralgias. Semin Neurol 8:286, 1988
Durelli L et al: The Melkersson-Rosenthal syndrome: A case with increased CNS IgG synthesis. Ann Neurol 18:623, 1985
Fromm GH et al: Baclofen in the treatment of refractory trigeminal neuralgia. Neurology 29:550, 1979
Jankovic J, Brin MF: Therapeutic uses of botulinum toxin. N Engl J Med 324:1186, 1991
Juncos JL, Beal MF: Idiopathic cranial polyneuropathy. Brain 110:197, 1987
Karnes WE: Diseases of the seventh cranial nerve, in *Peripheral Neuropathy*, 3d ed, PJ Dyck et al (eds). Philadelphia, Saunders, 1993, chap 43, pp 818–836
Keane JR: Bilateral seventh nerve palsy: Analysis of 43 cases and review of the literature. Neurology 44:1198, 1994
———: Fourth nerve palsy: Historical review and study of 215 inpatients. Neurology 43:2439, 1993
Kroenke K et al: Causes of persistent dizzyness: A prospective study of 100 patients in ambulatory care. Ann Intern Med 117:898, 1992
Lachance DH et al: Primary leptomeningeal lymphoma: Report of 9 cases, diagnosis with immunocytochemical analysis, and review of the literature. Neurology 41:95, 1991
Lecky BRF et al: Trigeminal sensory neuropathy. Brain 110:1463, 1987
Lossos A, Siegal T: Numb chin syndrome in cancer patients: Etiology, response to treatment, and prognostic significance. Neurology 42:1181, 1992
Mayo Clinic and Mayo Foundation: *Clinical Examinations in Neurology*, 6th ed. St. Louis, Mosby Year Book, 1991
Sawle GV et al: The natural history of non-arteritic anterior ischemic optic neuropathy. J Neurol Neurosurg Psychiatry 53:830, 1990
Selby G: Diseases of the fifth cranial nerve, in *Peripheral Neuropathy*, 3d ed, PJ Dyck et al (eds). Philadelphia, Saunders, 1993, chap 42, pp 801–817
Sweet WH: The treatment of trigeminal neuralgia (tic douloureux). N Engl J Med 315:174, 1986
———: Percutaneous methods for the treatment of trigeminal neuralgia and other faciocephalic pain; comparison with microvascular decompression. Semin Neurol 8:272, 1988
Troost BT, Patton JM: Exercise therapy for positional vertigo. Neurology 42:1441, 1992

373

Stephen L. Hauser

DISEASES OF THE SPINAL CORD

Diseases of the spinal cord are frequently devastating. They can produce quadriplegia, paraplegia, and sensory deficits far beyond the damage they would inflict elsewhere in the nervous system, because the spinal cord contains, in a small cross-sectional area, almost the entire motor output and sensory input systems of the trunk and limbs. Many spinal cord diseases are reversible if recognized and treated at an early stage (Table 373-1); thus, they are among the most critical of neurologic emergencies. The efficient use of diagnostic procedures, guided by a working knowledge of the relevant anatomy and clinical features of common spinal cord diseases, is often the key to a successful outcome.

Approach to the Patient

Spinal Cord Anatomy Relevant to Clinical Signs The spinal cord is a thin, tubular extension of the central nervous system contained within the bony spinal canal. It originates at the medulla and continues caudally to terminate at the filum terminale, a fibrous extension of the conus medullaris that terminates at the coccyx. The adult spinal cord is approximately 18 inches long, oval or round in shape, and enlarged in the cervical and lumbar regions, where neurons that innervate the upper and lower extremities, respectively, are located. The white matter tracts containing ascending sensory and descending motor pathways are located peripherally, whereas nerve cell bodies are clustered in an inner region shaped like a four-leaf clover that surrounds the central canal (anatomically an extension of the fourth ventricle). The membranes that cover the spinal cord—the pia, arachnoid, and dura—are continuous with those of the brainstem and cerebral hemispheres.

The spinal cord is somatotopically organized, consisting of 31 segments, each containing an exiting ventral motor root and entering dorsal sensory root (Fig. 373-1). During embryologic development, growth of the cord lags behind that of the vertebral column, and in the adult the spinal cord ends at approximately the first lumbar vertebral body. The lower spinal nerves take an increasingly downward course to exit via the appropriate intervertebral foramina. The first seven pairs of cervical spinal nerves exit above the same-numbered vertebral bodies, whereas all the subsequent nerves exit below the same-numbered vertebral bodies; this situation is due to the presence of eight cervical spinal cord segments but only seven cervical vertebrae. The approximate relationship between spinal cord segments and the corresponding vertebral bodies is shown in Table 373-2. These relationships assume importance for localization of lesions that cause spinal cord compression; a T10 spinal cord level, for example, indicates involvement of the cord adjacent to the seventh or eighth thoracic vertebral body.

LEVEL OF THE LESION The presence of a *level* below which sensory, motor, and/or autonomic function is disturbed is a hallmark of spinal cord disease. A sensory level is sought by asking the patient to identify as sharp a pinprick stimulus or as cool a cold stimulus (a dry tuning fork after immersion in cold water) applied to the low back and sequentially moved up toward the neck on each side. In general, a sensory level to pinprick or temperature, indicating damage to the spinothalamic tract, is located one to two segments below the actual level of a unilateral spinal cord lesion, but it may be at the level of

Table 373-1

Some Treatable Spinal Cord Disorders
Compressive
Epidural, intradural, or intramedullary neoplasm
Epidural abscess
Epidural hemorrhage
Cervical spondylosis
Herniated disc
Posttraumatic compression by fractured or displaced vertebra or hemorrhage
Vascular
Arteriovenous malformation
Inflammatory
Transverse myelitis
Multiple sclerosis
Infectious
Herpes simplex virus type 2 infection
Parasitic or bacterial infection
Developmental
Syringomyelia
Metabolic
Subacute combined degeneration

Table 373-2

Spinal Cord Levels Relative to the Vertebral Bodies

Spinal Cord Level	Corresponding Vertebral Body
Upper cervical	Same as cord level
Lower cervical	1 level higher
Upper thoracic	2 levels higher
Lower thoracic	2 to 3 levels higher
Lumbar	T10–T12
Sacral	T12–L1
Coccygeal	L1

the lesion when bilateral. That is because sensory fibers enter the cord at the dorsal root, synapse in the dorsal horn, and then ascend ipsilaterally for several segments before crossing just anterior to the central canal to join the opposite spinothalamic tract. Lesions that disrupt descending corticospinal and bulbospinal tracts cause paraplegia or quadriplegia, with increased muscle tone, exaggerated deep tendon reflexes, and extensor plantar signs. Such lesions also typically produce autonomic disturbances, with disturbed sweating and bladder, bowel, and sexual dysfunction. A sweat level may be determined by drawing a spoon up the torso. There will be little resistance to movement of the spoon along the dry, nonsweating skin; at the level at which sweating begins, resistance will suddenly increase.

The uppermost level of a spinal cord lesion is often localized by attention to *segmental signs* corresponding to disturbed motor or sensory innervation by an individual cord segment. A band of altered sensation (hyperalgesia or hyperpathia) at the upper end of the sensory disturbance, fasciculations or atrophy in muscles innervated by one or several segments, or a single diminished or absent deep tendon reflex may be noted. These signs may also occur with focal root or peripheral nerve disorders; thus, segmental signs are most useful when they occur with other signs of cord disease. With severe and acute transverse lesions, there may be flaccidity of the limbs rather than spasticity (so-called spinal shock). This state may last for several days, rarely for weeks, and may be initially mistaken for extensive damage to many segments of the cord (as in ascending necrotic myelopathy associated with cancer) or as polyneuropathy. Brief clonic or myoclonic movements of the limbs often precede paralysis in acute transverse lesions, particularly those due to cord infarction.

PATTERNS OF SPINAL CORD DISEASE The location of the major ascending and descending pathways of the spinal cord are shown in Fig. 373-1. Most fiber tracts—including the posterior columns and the spinocerebellar and pyramidal tracts—travel ipsilateral to the side of the body they innervate. As noted above, afferent fibers mediating pain and temperature sensation are unusual in that they ascend contralaterally as the spinothalamic tract. The anatomic relationships of these various fiber tracts and nuclei produce distinctive clinical syndromes that are pathognomonic of spinal cord disease and that often provide clues to the underlying disease process.

Brown-Sequard hemicord syndrome This syndrome consists of ipsilateral weakness (pyramidal tract) and loss of joint position and vibratory sense (posterior column), with contralateral loss of pain and temperature sense (spinothalamic tract) below the lesion. The sensory level for pain and temperature is one or two levels below the lesion. Segmental signs, such as radicular pain, muscle atrophy, or loss of a deep tendon reflex, when they occur, are unilateral. Pure examples of hemicord syndromes are rare; partial or bilateral forms are more common. Partial syndromes may involve the dorsal (posterior) quadrant, producing ipsilateral loss of vibration and position sense, or ventral (anterior) quadrant with ipsilateral paralysis and contralateral loss of pain and temperature sense.

Central cord syndrome The central cord syndrome results from disorders of gray matter nerve cells and crossing spinothalamic tracts near the central canal. In the cervical cord, the central cord syndrome produces arm weakness out of proportion to leg weakness and a "dissociated" sensory loss consisting of loss of pain and temperature sense in a cape distribution over the shoulders, lower neck, and upper trunk with intact light touch, joint position, and vibration sense. Trauma, syringomyelia, tumors, and anterior spinal artery ischemia are common causes of the central cord syndrome.

Anterior two-thirds syndrome This syndrome results from extensive bilateral disease of the spinal cord that spares the posterior columns. All spinal cord functions—motor, sensory and autonomic—are lost below the level of the lesion, with the striking exception of intact vibration and position sensation. The etiology is vascular, either thromboembolism of the anterior spinal artery or compression of this vessel by mass lesions within the spinal canal.

Intramedullary and extramedullary syndromes The diagnosis of spinal cord disorders frequently requires that *intramedullary* processes, which arise within the substance of the cord, be distinguished from *extramedullary* processes that compress the spinal cord or its vascular supply. Distinguishing features are relative and serve only as rough guides to clinical decision making. With extramedullary lesions, radicular pain is often prominent, and there is early sacral sensory loss (lateral spinothalamic tract) and spastic weakness in the legs (corticospinal tract) due to the superficial location of these fibers in the lateral spinal cord, which renders them susceptible to external compression. Intramedullary lesions tend to produce poorly localized burning pain rather than radicular pain and spare sensation in the perineal and sacral areas; corticospinal tract signs may appear late. With extramedullary lesions, the distinction between extradural and intradural masses is important, as the former are generally malignant and the latter benign; a long duration of symptoms favors an intradural origin.

SPECIFIC LOCALIZING SIGNS *Cervical cord* High cervical cord lesions are frequently life-threatening, producing quadriplegia and weakness of respiratory muscles innervated by the phrenic nerve (C3-C5). There is diaphragmatic paralysis, and breathing is possible only by use of accessory muscles of respiration. Extensive lesions near the junction of the cervical cord and medulla are usually fatal owing to involvement of adjacent medullary centers, which results in vasomotor and respiratory collapse. Partial lesions in this area, generally due to trauma, may interrupt decussating pyramidal tract fibers destined for the legs, which cross below those of the arms, resulting in a "crural paresis" of

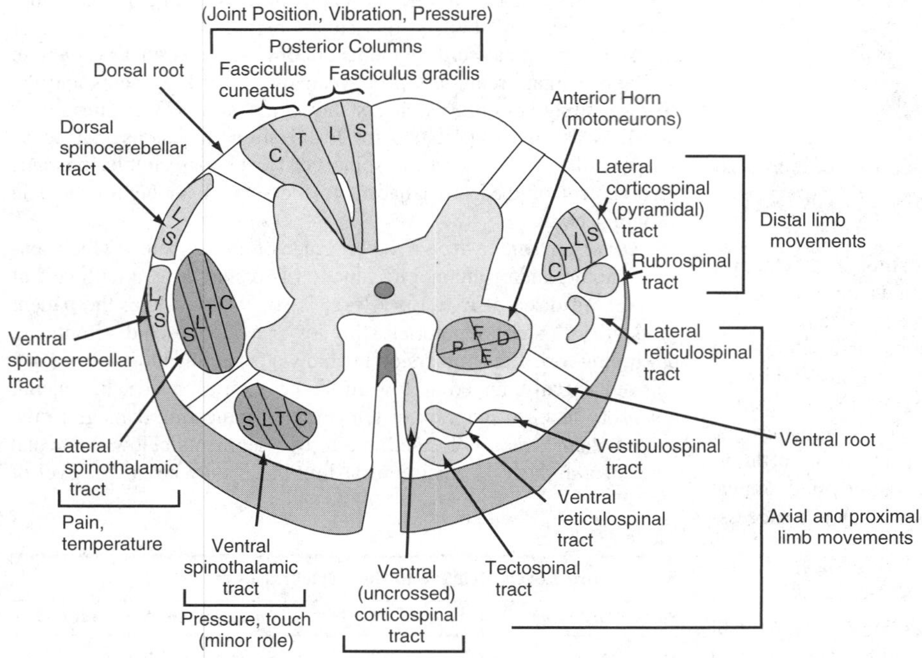

FIGURE 373-1 Transverse section through the spinal cord, composite representation, illustrating the principal ascending (*left*) and descending (*right*) pathways. The lateral and ventral spinothalamic tracts (*dark blue*) ascend contralateral to the side of the body that is innervated. C, cervical; T, thoracic; L, lumbar; S, sacral; P, proximal; D, distal; F, flexors; E, extensors.

the lower limbs. Compressive lesions near the foramen magnum may produce weakness of the ipsilateral shoulder and arm followed by weakness of the ipsilateral leg, then the contralateral leg, and finally the contralateral arm; the patient may complain of suboccipital pain spreading to the neck and shoulders. Lesions at C4-C5 produce quadriplegia with preserved respiratory function. At the midcervical (C5-C6) level, there is relative sparing of shoulder muscles and loss of biceps and brachioradialis reflexes. Lesions at C7 spare the biceps but produce weakness of finger and wrist extensors and loss of the triceps reflex. Lesions at C8 paralyze finger and wrist flexion, and the finger flexor reflex is lost. In general, cervical cord disorders are best localized by the pattern of weakness that ensues, whereas sensory deficits have less localizing value. A Horner's syndrome (miosis, ptosis, and facial hypohidrosis) may also occur ipsilateral to cervical cord lesions at any level.

Thoracic cord Lesions of the thoracic cord are best localized by identification of a sensory level on the trunk. Sensory dermatomes of the body are shown in Fig. 23-1; useful markers are at the nipples (T4) and umbilicus (T10). Weakness of the legs and disturbances of bladder, bowel, or sexual function may also accompany damage to the thoracic cord. The abdominal wall musculature, supplied by the lower thoracic cord, is observed during movements of respiration or coughing or by asking the patient to interlock the fingers behind the head in the supine position and attempt to sit up. Lesions at T9-T10 paralyze the lower, but spare the upper, abdominal muscles, resulting in upward movement of the umbilicus when the abdominal wall contracts (Beevor's sign) and in loss of lower, but not upper, superficial abdominal reflexes (see Chap. 360). With unilateral lesions, attempts to contract the abdominal wall produce movement of the umbilicus to the normal side; superficial abdominal reflexes are absent on the involved side. Midline back pain is a useful localizing sign in the thoracic region.

Lumbar cord The lumbar and sacral cord segments progressively decrease in size, and focal lesions of these segments are less easily localized than in cervical and thoracic regions. Lesions at L2-L4 paralyze flexion and adduction of the thigh, weaken leg extension at the knee, and abolish the patellar reflex. Lesions at L5-S1 paralyze movements of the foot and ankle, flexion at the knee, and extension of the thigh, and abolish the ankle jerk (S1). A cutaneous reflex useful in localization of lumbar cord disease is the cremasteric reflex (see Chap. 360), which is segmentally innervated at L1-L2.

Sacral cord/conus medullaris The conus medullaris is the tapered caudal termination of the spinal cord, comprising the lower sacral and single coccygeal segments. Isolated lesions of the conus medullaris spare motor and reflex functions in the legs. The conus syndrome is distinctive, consisting of bilateral saddle anesthesia (S3-S5), prominent bladder and bowel dysfunction (urinary retention and incontinence with lax anal tone), and impotence. The bulbocavernosus (S2-S4) and anal (S4-S5) reflexes are absent (see Chap. 360). Muscle strength is largely preserved. Lesions of the conus medullaris need to be distinguished from those of the cauda equina, the cluster of nerve roots derived from the lower cord as they descend to their exits in the intervertebral foramina. Cauda equina lesions are characterized by severe low back or radicular pain, asymmetric leg weakness or sensory loss, variable areflexia in the lower extremities, and relative sparing of bowel and bladder function. Mass lesions in the lower spinal canal may produce a mixed clinical picture in which elements of both cauda equina and conus medullaris syndromes coexist. → *Cauda equina syndromes are discussed in Chap. 16.*

ACUTE AND SUBACUTE SPINAL CORD DISEASES

Acute and subacute spinal cord disorders are commonly due to extramedullary compression (tumor, infection, spondylosis, or trauma), infarction or hemorrhage, or inflammation. In this category are some of the most dangerous—and treatable—disorders in clinical practice. Early recognition is the key to successful management. Epidural compression due to malignancy often presents with warning signs, generally neck or back pain, bladder disturbances, or sensory symptoms, that precede the development of paralysis. Infarction, hemorrhage, or spinal subluxation is more likely to produce sudden "strokelike" myelopathy without antecedent symptoms.

NEOPLASTIC SPINAL CORD COMPRESSION Neoplasms of the spinal canal may be extramedullary (epidural or intradural) or intramedullary. In adults, the vast majority of neoplasms are epidural in origin, resulting from metastases to the adjacent vertebral body, spinous or transverse process, or pedicle. Vertebral metastases are essentially bone-marrow metastases, and the propensity of solid tumors to metastasize to the vertebral column probably reflects the high percentage of bone marrow located in the axial skeleton of older individuals. Retroperitoneal neoplasms (especially lymphomas or sarcomas) may enter the spinal canal through the intervertebral foramina; typically they produce radicular pain and other signs of root involvement prior to cord compression. Almost any malignant tumor can metastasize to the spinal canal, although breast, lung, prostate, kidney, lymphoma, and plasma cell dyscrasia are particularly frequent. The thoracic cord is most commonly involved; exceptions are metastases from prostate and ovarian cancer, which occur disproportionately in the sacral and lumbar vertebrae, perhaps resulting from spread through Batson's plexus, a network of veins along the anterior surface of the spinal cord in the epidural space.

Pain is the initial symptom; it may be either aching and localized or sharp and radiating in quality. Pain indicates displacement of pain-sensitive structures, especially periosteum and meninges. The pain worsens with movement, coughing, or sneezing and may awaken patients at night. The recent onset of back pain, particularly if in the thoracic spine (which is uncommonly involved by spondylosis), should prompt consideration of vertebral metastasis. Rarely, pain is mild or absent. Pain typically precedes signs of cord compression by weeks or even months, but once cord compression occurs, it is always progressive and may advance rapidly. Therapy is effective only if administered early, when signs of cord dysfunction are mild or absent; therapy will not reverse fixed paralysis of more than 48 h duration. These realities highlight the importance of prompt recognition and efficient management of epidural metastases.

Plain radiographs of the spine and radionucleotide bone scans have only a limited role in diagnosis because they fail to identify 15 to 20 percent of metastatic vertebral lesions and may miss paravertebral masses that reach the epidural space by growth through the intervertebral foramina. Magnetic resonance imaging (MRI) provides excellent anatomic resolution of the site and extent of the tumor (Fig. 373-2);

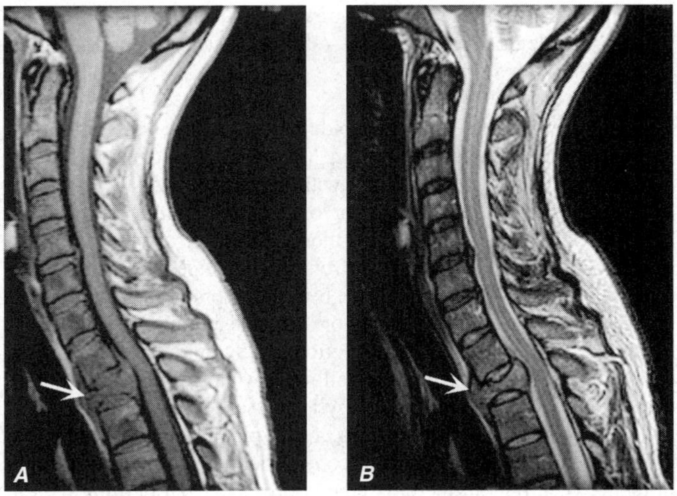

FIGURE 373-2 Epidural spinal cord compression due to breast carcinoma. Sagittal T1-weighted (*A*) and T2-weighted (*B*) MRI scans through the cervicothoracic junction reveal a compression fracture of the second thoracic vertebral body with posterior displacement and compression of the upper thoracic spinal cord. The low-intensity bone marrow signal in *A* signifies replacement by tumor.

at most centers, MRI has largely replaced computed tomography (CT) and myelography in the diagnosis of epidural masses. MRI can often distinguish between malignant lesions and other masses—epidural abscess, tuberculoma, or epidural hemorrhage, among others—that present in a similar fashion. Vertebral metastases are usually hypointense relative to a normal bone marrow signal on T1-weighted MR images; following the administration of gadolinium, contrast enhancement may "normalize" the appearance of the tumor by increasing its intensity to that of normal bone marrow. In contrast to infection, vertebral metastases typically do not cross the disk space. Nonetheless, it can be difficult to distinguish between infection and malignancy by MRI.

Because imaging resources are scarce, and both cancer and back pain are common, it is important to convey to the radiologist an estimate of the urgency of the imaging procedure requested. If signs of spinal cord involvement are present, imaging should be obtained on an emergent basis. If there are radicular symptoms but no evidence of myelopathy, it is usually safe to defer imaging for 24 to 48 h. With back or neck pain only, imaging studies should be obtained within a few days. Finally, up to 40 percent of patients who present with symptomatic disease at one level are found to have asymptomatic epidural disease elsewhere; thus, the entire spine should be imaged in all patients with epidural malignancy.

℞ TREATMENT

Management includes glucocorticoids to reduce interstitial edema, local radiotherapy (initiated as early as possible) to the symptomatic lesion, and specific therapy for the underlying tumor type. Glucocorticoids (dexamethasone, 40 mg daily) can be administered prior to the imaging study if the clinical suspicion is strong, and continued at a lower dose (20 mg daily in divided doses) until radiotherapy (a total of 3000 cGy administered in 15 daily fractions) is completed. Radiotherapy appears to be as effective as surgery, even for classically radioresistant metastases. Biopsy of the epidural mass is usually unnecessary in patients with known preexisting cancer, but biopsy is indicated if a history of underlying cancer is lacking. Surgery, either decompression or vertebral body resection, should be considered when signs of cord compression worsen despite radiotherapy, when the maximum tolerated dose of radiotherapy has been delivered previously to the site, or when a vertebral compression fracture contributes to cord compression. A good response to radiotherapy can be expected in individuals who are ambulatory at presentation; new weakness is prevented, and some recovery of motor function occurs in approximately half of treated patients. Fixed motor deficits—paraplegia or quadriplegia—do not usually respond to either radiotherapy or surgery.

In contrast to tumors of the epidural space, most intradural mass lesions are slow-growing and benign. Meningiomas and neurofibromas account for most of these lesions, with occasional cases representing chordoma, lipoma, dermoid, or sarcoma. Meningiomas (Fig. 373-3) are often located posterior to the thoracic cord or near the foramen magnum, although they can arise from the meninges anywhere along the spinal canal. Neurofibromas are benign tumors of the nerve sheath that typically arise near the posterior root; when multiple, neurofibromatosis (Chap. 375) is the likely etiology. Symptoms usually begin with radicular sensory symptoms followed by an asymmetric, progressive spinal cord syndrome. Therapy is surgical resection.

Primary intramedullary tumors of the spinal cord are uncommon. They typically present as central cord or hemicord syndromes, often in the cervical region; there may be poorly localized burning pain in the extremities and sparing of sacral sensation. In adults, most of these lesions are either ependymomas, hemangioblastomas, or low-grade astrocytomas (Fig. 373-4). Complete resection of an intramedullary ependymoma is often possible using microsurgical techniques. Debulking of an intramedullary astrocytoma can also be helpful, as these are often slowly growing lesions; the value of adjunctive radiotherapy is uncertain. Secondary (metastatic) intramedullary tumors are rare.

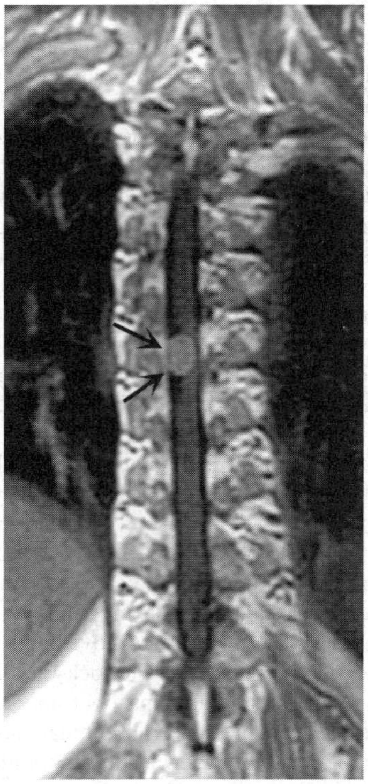

FIGURE 373-3 MRI of a thoracic meningioma. Coronal T1-weighted postcontrast image through the thoracic spinal cord demonstrates intense enhancement of a well-circumscribed extramedullary mass (*arrows*) which displaces the spinal cord to the left, widening the cistern adjacent to the mass.

SPINAL CORD INFARCTION The spinal cord is supplied by three arteries that course vertically over its surface, a single anterior spinal artery, and paired posterior spinal arteries. At each segment, paired penetrators branching from the anterior spinal artery supply the anterior two-thirds of the spinal cord; the posterior spinal arteries, which often become less distinct below the midthoracic level, supply the posterior columns. Rostrally, the spinal arteries arise from the vertebral arteries. During embryogenesis, arterial feeders arise at each

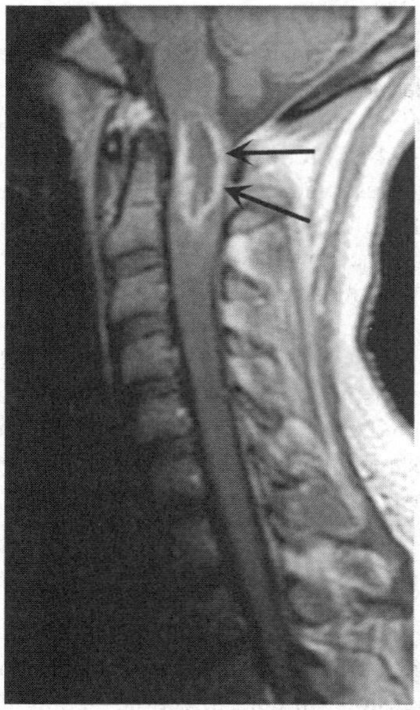

FIGURE 373-4 MRI of an intramedullary astrocytoma. Sagittal T1-weighted postcontrast image through the cervical spine demonstrates expansion of the upper cervical spine by a mass lesion emanating from within the spinal cord at the cervicomedullary junction. Irregular peripheral enhancement occurs within the mass (*arrows*).

segmental level, but most involute before birth; generally, between three and eight major feeders remain, arising from the vertebral, subclavian, intercostal (off the aorta), iliac, and sacral arteries. In addition to the vertebral arteries, in adults, anterior spinal artery feeders often occur at C6, at an upper thoracic level, and at T11-L2 (artery of Adamkiewicz). Feeders from the aorta are more likely to arise from the left side.

Spinal cord ischemia can occur at any level. The signs are determined by the level of the lesion and by the individual vascular anatomy, including areas of watershed flow and potential for anastomosis. The anterior spinal artery is discontinuous in some individuals, increasing the importance of feeders to the lower cord. With systemic hypotension, cord infarction occurs at the level of greatest ischemic risk, often T3-T4, and also at boundary zones between the anterior and posterior spinal artery territories. The latter may result in an acute—or more commonly progressive—syndrome of weakness and spasticity with little sensory change resembling amyotrophic lateral sclerosis (ALS).

Acute infarction in the territory of the anterior spinal artery produces paraplegia or quadriplegia, dissociated sensory loss affecting pain and temperature sense but sparing vibration and position sense, and loss of sphincter control. Onset may be sudden and dramatic or progressive over minutes or hours. Sharp midline or radiating back pain localized to the area of ischemia is frequently noted. Partial infarction of one anterior hemicord (hemiplegia or monoplegia and crossed pain and temperature loss) may also occur. Areflexia due to spinal shock is often present initially; with time, hyperreflexia and spasticity appear.

The acute onset of pain, sparing of posterior column function, and sharply demarcated spinal cord level distinguish anterior spinal artery infarction from epidural spinal cord compression, in which pain is often chronic, posterior column sense is impaired, and a cord level is indistinct. An exception to this rule is when epidural tumors compress or invade vascular structures, resulting in an anterior spinal artery syndrome. Infarction in the territory of the posterior spinal arteries, resulting in loss of posterior column function, also occurs and may be underrecognized as a cause of loss of position and vibration sense.

Spinal cord infarction is associated with aortic atherosclerosis, dissecting aortic aneurysm (chest or back pain with diminished pulses in legs), or hypotension from any cause. Cardiogenic emboli, vasculitis related to collagen vascular disease, and surgical clipping of aortic aneurysms are other predisposing conditions. Occasional cases develop either during pregnancy or following acute back trauma or exercise that by an unknown mechanism leads to embolism of nucleus pulposus material into spinal vessels. In a substantial number of cases, no cause can be found, and thromboembolism in arterial feeders is suspected.

MRI is often normal but is useful to exclude other causes of acute myelopathy, in particular epidural compression, spinal cord hemorrhage (hematomyelia), infectious myelitis, or transverse myelitis. Lumbar puncture is indicated whenever the underlying cause has not been clarified by MRI. Other useful laboratory studies include a sedimentation rate to search for an underlying vasculitis, Venereal Disease Research Laboratories test, and evaluation for aortic or cardiac disease or for a hypercoagulable state.

Therapy is directed at treatment of any predisposing condition. In cord infarction due to presumed thromboembolism, anticoagulation is probably not indicated, with the exception of the unusual transient ischemic attack or incomplete infarction with a stuttering or progressive course.

HEMATOMYELIA Hemorrhage into the substance of the spinal cord is rare. It may result from trauma, an intraparenchymal vascular malformation (see below), vasculitis due to polyarteritis nodosa or lupus erythematosus, bleeding disorders, or spinal cord infection or neoplasm. Hematomyelia presents as an acute painful transverse myelopathy. With large lesions, extension into the subarachnoid space may occur, resulting in subarachnoid hemorrhage (Chap. 366). Diagnosis is best made by MRI. Therapy is supportive, and surgical intervention is generally not useful. An exception is hematomyelia due to an underlying vascular malformation; in such cases, selective spinal angiography may be indicated, followed by acute surgical intervention to evacuate the clot and remove the underlying vascular lesion.

Hemorrhage into the subdural or epidural space can compress the spinal cord or roots. Presenting symptoms are the acute onset of focal or radicular pain followed by variable signs of a spinal cord or conus medullaris disorder. Trauma, tumor, or blood dyscrasias are predisposing conditions; rare cases complicate lumbar puncture or epidural anesthesia. MRI confirms the clinical suspicion and can delineate the extent of the bleed. Extrinsic spinal cord compression from any cause is a medical emergency, and appropriate treatment consists of prompt recognition, reversal of any underlying clotting disorder, and emergency surgical decompression. Surgery may be followed by substantial recovery, especially in patients with some preservation of motor function preoperatively. Because of the risk of hemorrhage, lumbar puncture should be avoided whenever possible in patients with thrombocytopenia or other coagulopathies (including those due to therapeutic anticoagulation) until the underlying bleeding disorder is reversed.

EPIDURAL ABSCESS Spinal epidural abscess presents as a clinical triad of pain, fever, and rapidly progressive weakness. Prompt recognition of this distinctive and treatable medical emergency will in most cases prevent severe and permanent sequelae. Epidural abscesses can form anywhere along the spinal canal. Pain is almost always present, either midline along the spine or radicular in type. The duration of pain prior to presentation is generally two weeks or less, but in some chronic cases it may be several months or longer. Fever is common, often accompanied by an elevated white blood cell count or sedimentation rate. As the abscess expands, spinal cord injury results from venous congestion and thrombosis, thrombophlebitis of the epidural space, spinal artery disease, or cord compression. Once weakness and other signs of myelopathy appear, progression is often rapid, although it may be gradual.

Risk factors include impaired immune status (diabetes mellitus, renal failure, alcoholism, malignancy), intravenous drug abuse, and infections of the skin or other tissues. Two-thirds of epidural infections result from hematogenous spread from the skin (furunculosis), soft tissue (pharyngeal or dental abscesses), or deep viscera (bacterial endocarditis). One-third result from direct extension of a local infection to the subdural space; examples of local predisposing conditions are vertebral osteomyelitis, decubitus ulcers, or iatrogenic complications of lumbar puncture, epidural anesthesia, or spinal surgery.

Most cases are due to *Staphylococcus aureus*; gram-negative bacilli, *Streptococcus*, anaerobes, and fungi can also cause epidural abscesses. Tuberculosis from an adjacent vertebral source remains an important cause in the underdeveloped world. As the population ages and the number of immunosuppressed individuals increases, an increase in the incidence of spinal epidural abscess (currently 2 per 1000 hospital admissions) has been noted.

MR images (Fig. 373-5) localize the abscess and exclude a primary intraparenchymal lesion, for example, transverse myelitis or hematomyelia. Lumbar puncture is often not required but may be indicated if encephalopathy or other clinical signs raise the question of associated meningitis, which is present in fewer than 25 percent of cases. In such situations, the level of the tap should be planned carefully to minimize the risk of inducing either meningitis by passage of the needle through infected tissue or herniation from decompression below an area of obstruction to the flow of cerebrospinal fluid (CSF). A high cervical tap is often the safest approach. CSF abnormalities in subdural abscess consist of pleocytosis with a preponderance of polymorphonuclear cells, an elevated protein level, and a reduced glucose level. Blood cultures are positive in fewer than 25 percent of cases.

℞ TREATMENT

Treatment is emergency decompressive laminectomy with debridement combined with long-term antibiotic treatment. Surgical evacuation will prevent development of paralysis and may improve or reverse paralysis in evolution, but it is unlikely to improve fixed

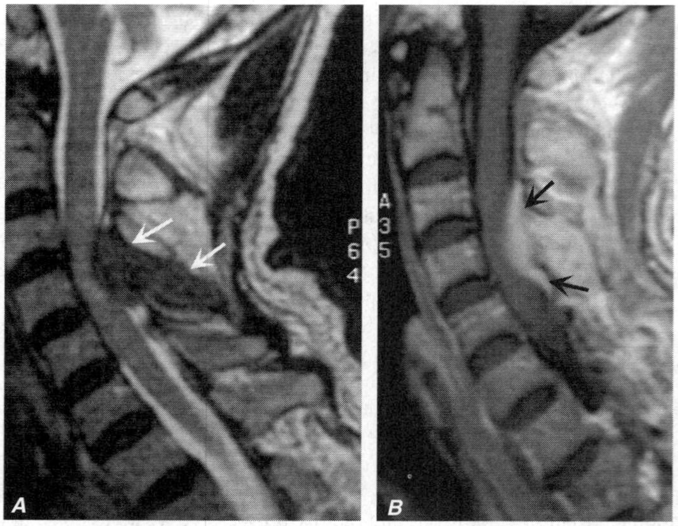

FIGURE 373-5 MRI of a spinal epidural abscess due to tuberculosis. *A.* Sagittal T2-weighted free spin-echo MR sequence. A hypointense mass replaces the posterior elements of C3 and extends epidurally to compress the spinal cord (*arrows*). *B.* Sagittal T1-weighted image following contrast administration reveals a diffuse enhancement of the epidural process (*arrows*) with extension into the epidural space.

neurologic deficits. Antibiotics should be started empirically before surgery, modified on the basis of culture results, and usually continued for at least 4 weeks. If surgery is contraindicated or if there is a fixed paraplegia or quadriplegia that is unlikely to improve following surgery, long-term administration of systemic and oral antibiotics can be used; in such cases, coverage may be guided by results of positive blood cultures. In medically treated patients, paralysis may develop or progress during antibiotic therapy; thus, initial surgical management remains the treatment of choice.

TRANSVERSE MYELITIS Transverse myelitis is an acute or subacute, generally monophasic, inflammatory disorder of the spinal cord. The initial symptom is focal neck or back pain, followed by various combinations of paresthesia, sensory loss, motor weakness, and sphincter disturbance evolving within hours to several days. There may be mild sensory symptoms only, or a devastating functional transection of the cord. Partial forms may selectively involve posterior columns, anterior spinothalamic tracts, or one hemicord. Dysesthesias may begin in the feet and ascend either symmetrically or asymmetrically, earlier in one leg than in the other; these symptoms may initially raise a question of Guillain-Barré syndrome, but involvement of the trunk with a sharply demarcated spinal cord level indicates the myelopathic nature of the process. In severe cases, areflexia indicating spinal shock may be present, but hyperreflexia soon supervenes; persistent areflexic paralysis indicates necrosis over multiple segments of the spinal cord.

Up to 40 percent of cases are associated with an antecedent infection or recent vaccination. Many infectious agents have been implicated, including influenza, measles, varicella, rubeola, mumps, and Epstein-Barr virus and cytomegalovirus, as well as *Mycoplasma.* As in the related disorder acute disseminated encephalomyelitis (Chap. 376), transverse myelitis often begins as the patient appears to be recovering from the infection, and infectious agents have not been isolated from the nervous system of affected individuals. These features suggest that transverse myelitis results from an autoimmune response triggered by infection and not from direct infection of the spinal cord.

Multiple sclerosis (MS) (see below) may present initially as transverse myelitis. MS-associated transverse myelitis usually is not associated with an antecedent infection or vaccination. Devic's disease (Chap. 376) is a demyelinating disorder common in Asians that presents as transverse myelitis associated with optic neuritis that is typically bilateral. Transverse myelitis, at times recurrent, has also been associated with systemic lupus erythematosus and other collagen-vascular diseases, Sjögren's syndrome, and Behçet's disease; sarcoidosis may produce a subacute transverse myelopathy with severe cord swelling.

MRI findings in transverse myelitis consist of variable swelling of the cord and diffuse or multifocal areas of abnormal bright signal on T2-weighted sequences, often extending over several cord segments. Contrast enhancement, indicating disruption in the blood-brain barrier associated with perivenous inflammation, is also present in acute cases. MRI is also useful to exclude cord compression. A brain MRI should also be obtained in all cases to assess the likelihood that the transverse myelitis represents an initial attack of MS. A normal scan indicates that the risk of evolution to MS is low—approximately 5 percent over 3 to 5 years; by contrast, the finding of multiple periventricular T2-bright lesions indicates a risk of 50 percent or greater over the same time period. CSF findings in transverse myelitis may be normal, but more often there is pleocytosis, with up to several hundred mononuclear cells per microliter; in severe or rapidly evolving cases, polymorphonuclear cells may be present. CSF protein levels are normal or at most mildly elevated; oligoclonal banding is a variable finding but, when present, is associated with future evolution to MS.

There are no prospective trials of therapy. Glucocorticoids, consisting of intravenous methylprednisolone followed by oral prednisone (Table 376-4), is employed for treatment of moderate to severe symptoms.

ACUTE INFECTIOUS MYELOPATHIES These inflammatory disorders result from direct invasion of the spinal cord by infectious agents. Poliomyelitis is the prototypic virus that produces acute infection of the spinal cord. Herpes zoster is currently the most common viral cause of acute myelitis; cytomegalovirus, herpes simplex virus type 1, Epstein-Barr virus, and rabies virus have been identified in occasional cases. Herpes simplex virus type 2 may produce a recurrent sacral myelitis, which could be mistaken for MS, in association with outbreaks of genital herpes. → ***Viral infections of the spinal cord are discussed in Chap. 379.***

Schistosomiasis (Chap. 224) is an important cause of parasitic myelitis worldwide. The myelitis is intensely inflammatory and granulomatous in nature, caused by a local response to tissue-digesting enzymes produced by ova from the parasite. Toxoplasmosis (Chap. 219) rarely causes a focal myelopathy, and this diagnosis should be considered in patients with AIDS owing to the high frequency of nervous system toxoplasmosis in this population.

CHRONIC MYELOPATHIES

SPONDYLITIC MYELOPATHY Cervical spondylosis and related degenerative diseases of the spine are discussed in Chap. 16. Neck and shoulder pain with stiffness are early symptoms; pressure on nerve roots results in radicular arm pain, most often in a C5 or C6 distribution. Compression of the cervical cord produces a slowly progressive spastic paraparesis, at times asymmetric, and often accompanied by paresthesia in the feet and hands. Vibratory sense is frequently diminished in the legs, and occasionally there is a sensory level for vibration on the upper thorax. Coughing or straining often produces leg weakness or radiating arm or shoulder pain. Dermatomal sensory loss in the arms, atrophy of intrinsic hand muscles, increased deep tendon reflexes in the legs, and extensor plantar responses are common. Urinary urgency or incontinence occur in advanced cases. Reflexes in the arms are often diminished at some level, often the biceps (C5-C6). In individual cases, radicular, myelopathic, or combined signs may predominate. The diagnosis should be considered in cases of progressive cervical myelopathy, paresthesia of the feet and hands, or wasting of the hands. Spondylitic myelopathy is also one of the most common causes of gait difficulty in the elderly.

Diagnosis is best made by MRI. Extrinsic compression is appreciated on axial views, and T2-weighted sequences may reveal abnormal areas of high signal intensity within the cord adjacent to the site of compression. Definitive therapy consists of surgical relief of the compression, generally by posterior laminectomy. When that is not feasible, an anterior approach with resection of the protruded disc material may be required.

Cervical spondylosis is both an under- and overdiagnosed disease. Many patients with intramedullary cord processes, particularly ALS (Chap. 370), have had cervical laminectomies in the incorrect belief that spondylosis might have been responsible.

VASCULAR MALFORMATIONS Although uncommon, these are important lesions because they represent a treatable cause of progressive myelopathy. Arteriovenous malformations (AVMs) are most often located posteriorly, within the dura or along the surface of the cord, at or below the midthoracic level. The typical presentation is a middle-aged man with a progressive myelopathy. The myelopathy may worsen slowly or rapidly or may have periods of apparent remission with superimposed worsenings resembling MS. Acute deterioration due to hemorrhage into the spinal cord or subarachnoid space may occur but is uncommon. At presentation, most patients have sensory, motor, and bladder disturbances. The motor disorder may predominate and produce a mixture of upper and lower motoneuron signs, simulating ALS. Pain, either dysesthesias or radicular pain, is also common. Other symptoms suggestive of AVM include intermittent claudication (symptoms that appear with exercise and are relieved by rest), or an effect of posture, menses, or fever on symptoms. A rare AVM syndrome presents as a progressive thoracic myelopathy with paraparesis developing over weeks or several months, associated with abnormally thick, hyalinized vessels (Foix-Alajouanine syndrome).

AVMs located at cervical or upper thoracic levels are distinctive; they occur equally in males and females, tend to be located anterior rather than posterior to the cord, often have an intramedullary component to the malformation, and may bleed (see "Hematomyelia," above).

A careful examination of the skin overlying the spine may reveal a vascular lesion, lipoma, or area of altered pigmentation, all clues to a spinal cord AVM. Bruits are rare but should be sought at rest or after exercise. High-resolution MRI with contrast administration will detect the vast majority of AVMs (Fig. 373-6). A small number of AVMs not detected by MRI may be visualized by CT myelography as enlarged vessels along the surface of the cord. Definitive diagnosis requires selective spinal angiography, which will also define the vascular feeders and extent of the malformation. Embolization with occlusion of the major feeding vessels may stabilize a progressive neurologic deficit or produce a gradual recovery.

RETROVIRUS-ASSOCIATED MYELOPATHIES The myelopathy associated with the human T cell lymphotropic virus type I (HTLV-I) presents as a slowly progressive spastic paraparesis with variable sensory and bladder disturbance. The myelopathy is typically thoracic. Approximately half of patients have back or leg pain. Signs may be asymmetric, may lack a well-defined sensory level, and may spare upper extremity function, although hyperreflexia in the arms is common. Onset is generally insidious, and the tempo of progression is variable, but most patients are nonambulatory within 10 years of onset. This presentation may resemble primary progressive MS or a thoracic AVM. Diagnosis is made by demonstration of HTLV-I–specific antibody in serum by enzyme-linked immunosorbent assay (ELISA), confirmed by radioimmunoprecipitation or Western blot analysis of specific antibody directed against protein products of the viral *gag* and *env* genes. There is no effective treatment; symptomatic therapy for spasticity and bladder symptoms may be helpful. → ***HTLV-I infections of the nervous system are discussed in Chap. 379.***

A progressive myelopathy may also occur in AIDS, characterized by vacuolar degeneration of the posterior and lateral tracts resembling subacute combined degeneration (see below).

SYRINGOMYELIA Syringomyelia is a cavitary expansion of the spinal cord that may produce a progressive myelopathy. Syrinxes commonly occur in the lower cervical/high thoracic region or in the high cervical region, where they may extend rostrally to the medulla or pons (syringobulbia). Less commonly, the lumbar cord or the entire spinal cord may be involved. Syringomyelia may result from developmental disorders of the posterior fossa and foramen magnum or from acquired disorders. More than half of all cases are associated with Chiari malformations. In the Chiari type 1 malformation, there is protrusion of the cerebellar tonsils through the foramen magnum and into the cervical spinal canal; when this abnormality is associated with protrusion of meninges (meningocele) or meninges and cord (meningomyelocele) through a spinal canal that has incompletely closed, it is designated a Chiari type 2 (or Arnold-Chiari) malformation. Other developmental disorders associated with syringomyelia are basilar skull impression (platybasia), atresia of the foramen of Magendie, or cysts of the posterior fossa (Dandy-Walker syndrome). Acquired cases result from intramedullary spinal cord tumors, trauma, or chronic arachnoiditis due to tuberculosis or other inflammatory conditions. Occasional cases are idiopathic.

Syringomyelia has been proposed to result from interference with the normal outflow of CSF from the fourth ventricle to the subarachnoid space due to obstruction of the foramina of Luschka and Magendie. This blockage leads to downward pressure on the cervical spinal cord and progressive syrinx formation. However, syringomyelia may occur without foraminal obstruction, indicating that other factors, for example, interference with normal upward CSF flow in the spinal canal, may also be important. Syrinxes associated with Chiari type 1 malformations generally communicate freely with the subarachnoid space, and the syrinx fluid resembles normal CSF; by contrast, in many acquired cases the syrinx cavities do not communicate, and the fluid is proteinaceous. The older literature distinguished between "true" syringomyelia, in which the cavity was separate from the central canal, and hydromyelia due to a primary enlargement of the central canal; this distinction is less useful than determination of whether the cavity communicates freely with the subarachnoid space.

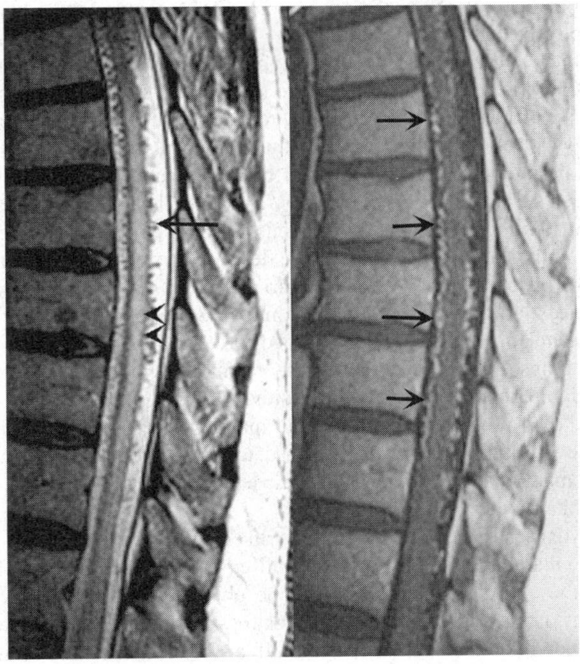

FIGURE 373-6 Arteriovenous malformation. Sagittal MR scans of the thoracic spinal cord: T2 fast spin-echo technique (*left*) and T1 post-contrast image (*right*). On the T2-weighted image (*left*), abnormally high signal intensity is noted in the central aspect of the spinal cord (*arrowheads*). Numerous punctate flow voids indent the dorsal and ventral spinal cord (*arrow*). These represent the abnormally dilated venous plexus supplied by a dural arteriovenous fistula. Following contrast administration (*right*), multiple, serpentine, enhancing veins (*arrows*) on the ventral and dorsal aspect of the thoracic spinal cord are visualized, diagnostic of arteriovenous fistula. This patient was a 54-year-old man with a 4-year history of progressive paraparesis.

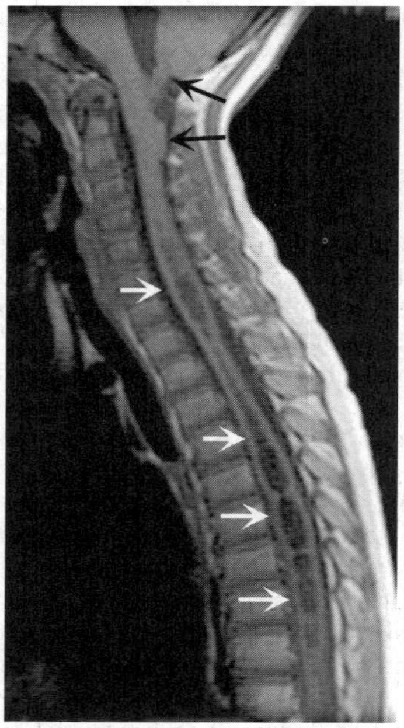

FIGURE 373-7 MRI of syringomyelia associated with Chiari malformation. Sagittal T1-weighted image through the cervical and upper thoracic spine demonstrates descent of the cerebellar tonsils and vermis below the level of the foramen magnum (*black arrows*). Within the substance of the cervical and thoracic spinal cord, a CSF collection dilates the central canal (*white arrows*).

The classic presentation is a central cord syndrome with dissociated sensory loss and areflexic weakness in the upper limbs. The sensory deficit consists of loss of pain and temperature sensation which is "suspended" over the nape of the neck, shoulders, and upper arms in a cape distribution or is in the hands; vibration and position sensation is largely preserved. Most cases begin asymmetrically with unilateral sensory loss. Muscle wasting in the lower neck, shoulders, arms, and hands with asymmetric or absent reflexes reflects extension of the cavity to the anterior horns. As the lesion enlarges, spasticity and weakness of the legs, bladder and bowel dysfunction, and, in some cases, a Horner's syndrome appear. Thoracic kyphoscoliosis is a frequent additional finding. Some patients develop numbness and sensory loss on the face from damage to the descending tract of the trigeminal nerve (C2 level or above). With Chiari malformations, cough headache, and neck, arm, or facial pain are common. Syringobulbia may present as palatal or vocal cord paralysis, dysarthria, horizontal or vertical nystagmus, episodic dizziness, and/or tongue weakness.

Symptoms typically begin insidiously in adolescence or early adulthood, progress irregularly, and may undergo spontaneous arrest for several years. Onset or sudden deterioration may follow trauma, neck manipulation or extension, or severe cough. Symptoms of syringobulbia may progress rapidly.

MRI scans accurately identify syrinx cavities and associated spinal cord enlargement (Fig. 373-7). In all cases, MRI scans of the brain and the entire spinal cord should be obtained to delineate the full extent of the syrinx, assess posterior fossa structures, and determine whether hydrocephalus is present. If a Chiari malformation is not found, a contrast-enhanced MRI scan should be obtained to search for abnormal enhancement from an associated spinal cord tumor.

℞ TREATMENT

Treatment is surgical. Syringomyelia associated with tonsillar herniation is treated with posterior fossa decompression, generally consisting of suboccipital craniectomy, upper cervical laminectomy, and placement of a dural graft. If obstruction of fourth ventricular outflow is present, flow is reestablished by enlargement of the opening. If the syrinx cavity is large, some surgeons recommend direct decompression of the fluid cavity, but the added benefit of this procedure is uncertain, and morbidity may occur. With Chiari malformations, shunting of hydrocephalus should generally precede any attempt to correct the syrinx. Surgical results are often excellent, with stabilization of the neurologic deficit in most cases; some patients have improvement postoperatively. Syringomyelia secondary to trauma or infection is treated with a decompression and drainage procedure in which a small shunt is inserted between the syrinx cavity and the subarachnoid space. Finally, syringomyelia due to an intramedullary spinal cord tumor is managed by resection of the tumor if feasible; decompression of the cyst cavity may produce temporary relief, but recurrence is common.

MULTIPLE SCLEROSIS The primary progressive form of MS may present as a progressive myelopathy. Involvement is typically asymmetric with resulting motor, sensory, and autonomic dysfunction. The diagnosis is made by recognition of other symptoms or signs typical for MS, by characteristic findings on brain MRI scans, by CSF analysis, and by exclusion of other conditions. Therapeutic efforts to reverse neurologic deficits or to stabilize the course of isolated progressive myelopathy due to MS have been disappointing. → *MS is discussed in Chap. 376.*

SUBACUTE COMBINED DEGENERATION (VITAMIN B_{12} DEFICIENCY) This treatable myelopathy presents with parasthesia in the hands and feet, early loss of vibration and position sensation, and a progressive spastic and ataxic weakness. Loss of reflexes due to a superimposed peripheral neuropathy, present in many cases, is an important diagnostic clue. Optic atrophy and irritability and other mental changes may be prominent in advanced cases and on occasion are the presenting symptom (megaloblastic madness). The myelopathy of subacute combined degeneration tends to be diffuse rather than focal; signs are generally symmetric and reflect predominant involvement of the posterior and lateral tracts, and no focal spinal cord level is present. The diagnosis is confirmed by the finding of a low serum B_{12} concentration and a positive Schilling test (Chap. 380).

TABES DORSALIS Tabes dorsalis and meningovascular syphilis of the spinal cord are presently rare but must be considered in the differential diagnosis of spinal cord syndromes, in particular those that arise in individuals infected with human immunodeficiency virus (HIV). The most common symptoms of tabes are characteristic fleeting and repetitive, lancinating pains, which occur mostly in the legs and less commonly in the back, thorax, abdomen, arms, and face. Ataxia of the legs and gait due to loss of position sense occurs in half of patients. Paresthesia, bladder disturbances, and acute abdominal pain with vomiting (visceral crisis) occur in 15 to 30 percent. The cardinal signs of tabes are loss of reflexes in the legs, impaired position and vibratory sense, Romberg's sign, and bilateral Argyll Robertson pupils, which fail to constrict to light but react with accommodation.

FAMILIAL SPASTIC PARAPLEGIA Occasional cases of progressive myelopathy occur on a familial basis. Most present with progressive spasticity and weakness in the legs. Sphincter disturbances and mild degrees of sensory loss may also be present. On examination, a sharply defined spinal cord level is not detected, in contrast to many focal spinal cord disorders. In some families, whose condition is referred to as "complicated" familial spastic paraplegia (FSP), additional neurologic signs, for example, nystagmus, ataxia, or optic atrophy, occur. Onset may be as early as the first year of life or as late as middle adulthood. The genetic basis of some forms of FSP is now known (Table 373-3). Adrenoleukodystrophy should be treated with steroid replacement if hypoadrenalism is present, and bone marrow transplantation, although experimental, has been attempted for this condition. No disease-modifying therapy exists for other forms of FSP.

→ *Traumatic spinal cord lesions are discussed in Chap. 374.*

MEDICAL REHABILITATION OF SPINAL CORD DISORDERS

Following an acute spinal cord lesion, the prospects for significant recovery fade after approximately 4 months. There are currently no effective means to promote repair of injured spinal cord tissue; promising experimental approaches include the use of factors that influence reinnervation by axons of the corticospinal tract or nerve graft bridges that promote reinnervation across spinal cord lesions. The disability associated with irreversible spinal cord damage is determined primarily by the level of the lesion and by whether the disturbance in function is complete or incomplete (Table 373-4). Even complete high cervical cord lesions may be compatible with a productive life. Development of a rehabilitation plan framed by realistic expectations, and attention to the neurologic, medical, and psychological complications that commonly arise, are primary goals of treatment.

Table 373-3

Inherited (Monogenic) Myelopathies*

Designation	Clinical Presentation	Genetics
Autosomal recessive	Early onset (age 1–20), progressive spasticity of legs, mild loss of vibration & position sense, bladder symptoms	Linked to chromosome 8; gene unknown
Autosomal dominant	Most common form; families have either early or late onset (before or after age 35)	Linkage to chromosome 2p for both early and late onset. Second locus at 14q.
X-linked	Early childhood onset as pure spastic paraplegia or "complicated" with nystagmus, ataxia, or other neurologic signs	"Complicated" form due to mutation of proteolipid protein gene (Xq21); differs from the dysmyelinating disorder Pelizaeus-Merzbacher disease in that the allelic protein DM20, essential for oligodendrocyte development, is normal
X-linked	Pure or "complicated"	Mutations in neural cell adhesion molecule L1CAM. Allelic disorders X-linked hydrocephalus and MASA syndrome (mental retardation, aphasia, shuffling gait, adducted thumbs).
X-linked	Adrenoleukodystrophy; may present as pure FSP beginning in early adulthood. Rare heterozygote females may present as FSP.	Accumulation of long-chain fatty acids due to defective peroxysomal degradation; linkage to Xq17-28

* See also Chap. 363.

ABBREVIATION: FSP, familial spastic paraplegia.

The usual symptoms associated with medical illnesses may be lacking, because of the destruction of afferent pain pathways in the cord. Unexplained fever, worsening of spasticity, or deterioration in neurologic function should prompt search for an underlying cause such as infection, thrombophlebitis, or an intraabdominal pathology; these etiologies are far more likely to be responsible than primary neurologic events such as meningitis, secondary syringomyelia or chronic arachnoiditis. The loss of normal thermoregulation and inability to maintain normal body temperature can produce recurrent fever (*quadriplegic fever*), although most episodes of fever are due to infection of the urinary tract, lung, skin, or bone.

Bladder dysfunction generally results from loss of supraspinal innervation of the detrusor muscle of the bladder wall and the sphincter musculature. Detrusor spasticity is treated with anticholinergic drugs (oxybutinin, 2.5 to 5 mg qid) or tricyclic antidepressants with anticholinergic properties (imipramine, 25 to 200 mg/d). Failure of the sphincter muscle to relax during bladder emptying (urinary dyssynergia) may be managed with the alpha-adrenergic blocking agent terazosin hydrochloride (1 to 2 mg tid or qid), with intermittent catheterization, or, if that is not feasible, by use of a condom catheter in men or a permanent indwelling catheter. Surgical options include the creation of an artificial bladder by isolating a segment of intestine that can be catheterized intermittently (enterocystoplasty) or can drain continuously to an external appliance (urinary conduit). Bladder areflexia due to acute spinal shock or conus lesions is best treated by catheterization. The underlying pathophysiology of a bladder disorder correlates poorly with specific symptoms experienced by the patient, so urodynamic evaluation at intervals is required to assess detrusor and sphincter function.

Bladder dysfunction predisposes the patient to urinary tract infection. Bacteriuria due to asymptomatic colonization is extremely common and is generally not treated. Prophylaxis with antiseptics or antibiotics are of little value. Urinary tract infections may present only as foul-smelling urine or a change in voiding pattern; the development of high fever or other systemic signs often indicates pyelonephritis. Bowel regimens and disimpaction are necessary in most patients to ensure at least biweekly evacuation and avoid colonic distention or obstruction.

High cervical cord lesions cause various degrees of mechanical respiratory failure requiring artificial ventilation. In cases of incomplete respiratory failure, chest physical therapy is useful, and a negative-pressure cuirass may alleviate atelectasis, particularly if the major lesion is below C4. With severe respiratory failure, tracheal intubation, followed by tracheotomy, provides tracheal access for ventilation and suctioning. Phrenic nerve pacing may be useful in some patients with lesions at C5 or above.

Patients with acute cord injury are at high risk for venous thrombosis and pulmonary embolism. During the first two weeks, use of calf-compression devices and anticoagulation with heparin (5000 U subcutaneously every 12 h) or warfarin (INR, 2 to 3) are recommended. In cases of persistent paralysis, anticoagulation should probably be continued for 3 months.

Prophylaxis against decubitus ulcers should involve frequent changes in position in a chair or bed, the use of special mattresses, and cushioning of areas where pressure sores often develop, such as the sacral prominence and heels. Early treatment of ulcers with careful cleansing, surgical or enzyme debridement of necrotic tissue, and appropriate dressing and drainage may prevent infection of adjacent soft tissue or bone.

Spasticity (Chap. 21) is often a late manifestation of spinal cord disease, occurring weeks or even months after the initial insult. Stretching exercises are useful to maintain mobility of joints. Drug treatment is effective but may result in reduced function, as some patients use their spasticity as an aid to stand, transfer, or walk. Baclofen (20 to

Table 373-4

Expected Neurologic Function Following Complete Cord Lesions

Level	Self-Care	Transfers	Maximum Mobility
High quadriplegia (C1-C4)	Dependent on others; requires respiratory support	Dependent on others	Motorized wheelchair
Low quadriplegia (C5-C8)	Partially independent with adaptive equipment	May be dependent or independent	May use manual wheelchair, drive an automobile with adaptive equipment
Paraplegia (below T1)	Independent	Independent	Ambulates short distances with aids

SOURCE: Adapted from Ditunno and Formal.

240 mg/d in divided doses) is the most effective drug available; it acts by facilitating GABA-mediated inhibition of motor reflex arcs. Diazepam acts by a similar mechanism and is useful for leg spasms that interrupt sleep (2 to 4 mg at bedtime). For nonambulatory patients, the direct muscle inhibitor dantrolene (25 to 100 mg qid) may be used, but it is potentially hepatotoxic. In severe cases, intrathecal baclofen administered via an implanted pump, botulinum toxin injections, or dorsal rhizotomy may be required to control spasticity.

Paroxysmal autonomic hyperreflexia may occur following lesions above the major splanchnic sympathetic outflow at T6. Headache, flushing, and diaphoresis above the level of the lesion, and hypertension with bradycardia or tachycardia, are the major symptoms. The trigger is typically a noxious stimulus—for example, bladder or bowel distention, a urinary tract infection, or a decubitus ulcer—below the level of the cord lesion. Ascending sensory fibers are thought to activate, via interneurons, sympathetic neurons of the intermediolateral nuclei in the thoracic spinal cord, producing vasoconstriction, tachycardia, and systemic hypertension. Reflex pathways, activated by carotid and aortic baroreceptors and projecting to the CNS via the vagus and glossopharyngeal nerves, then inhibit sympathetic activity above the cord lesion, producing vasodilation, but below the lesion, descending pathways are blocked and sympathetic hyperactivity continues. Treatment consists of removal of offending stimuli; ganglionic blocking agents (mecamylamine, 2.5 to 5 mg) or other short-acting antihypertensive drugs are useful in some patients (see review by Colachis).

BIBLIOGRAPHY

Blaivas JG: Bladder function in the SCI patient. J Neurol Rehab 8:47, 1994

Colachis SC: Autonomic hyperreflexia with spinal cord injury. J Am Paraplegia Soc 15(3):172, 1992

Cristante L, Herrmann H-D: Surgical management of intramedullary spinal cord tumors: Functional outcome and sources of morbidity. Neurosurgery 35:69, 1994

Darouiche RO et al: Bacterial spinal epidural abscess: Review of 43 cases and literature survey. Medicine 71:369, 1992

Ditunno JF, Formal CS: Chronic spinal cord injury. N Engl J Med 330:550, 1994

Jeffery DR et al: Transverse myelitis. Retrospective analysis of 33 cases, with differentiation of cases associated with multiple sclerosis and parainfectious events. Arch Neurol 50:532, 1993

Small JA, Sheridan PH: Research priorities for syringomyelia: A National Institute of Neurologic Disorders and Stroke workshop summary. Neurology 46:577, 1996

Young RR, Woolsey RM: *Diagnosis and Management of Disorders of the Spinal Cord.* Philadelphia, Saunders, 1995

374

Allan H. Ropper

TRAUMATIC INJURIES OF THE HEAD AND SPINE

Head injuries are frequent in industrialized countries, affecting many patients in the prime of life. The medical and social magnitude of this problem can be appreciated by recognizing that almost 10 million head injuries occur annually in the United States alone, about 20 percent of which are serious enough to cause brain damage. Among men under 35 years old, accidents, usually motor vehicle collisions, are the chief cause of death, and over 70 percent of these involve head injury. Minor head injuries are so common that almost all physicians encounter patients requiring immediate care or suffering from various sequelae. Traumatic spinal cord injuries often occur in conjunction with head injury. The two are best considered together in the context of trauma to the nervous system.

Declining mortality from head and spinal cord injuries can be attributed mainly to public health measures, such as use of seat belts and motorcycle helmets, and the development of ambulance systems with trained personnel. A systematic approach to the evaluation of patients with head and spine trauma, beginning at the scene of the accident, has improved outcome. Understanding of the pathologic lesions produced by trauma, essential for diagnosis and management, has been revolutionized by the wide availability of computed tomography (CT).

TYPES OF HEAD INJURIES

SKULL FRACTURES A blow to the skull causes fractures if the elastic tolerance of the bone is exceeded. Significant intracranial lesions accompany two-thirds of skull fractures, and the presence of a skull fracture increases manyfold the chances of an underlying subdural or epidural hematoma. Consequently, fractures are important primarily as markers of the site and severity of injury. They also cause cranial nerve injuries and produce entry pathways to the cerebrospinal fluid (CSF) for bacteria (meningitis) and air (pneumocephalus) or for leakage of CSF. Fractures are classified as *linear*, *basilar*, *compound*, or *depressed*; linear fractures account for 80 percent of all skull fractures and are most often associated with subdural or epidural hematomas. Linear fractures usually extend from the point of impact toward the base of the skull.

Basilar skull fractures are often extensions of adjacent fractures over the convexity of the skull but may occur independently owing to stresses on the floor of the middle cranial fossa or occiput. They are usually located parallel to the petrous bone or along the sphenoid bone toward the sella turcica and ethmoidal groove. Most are uncomplicated, but they may cause CSF leakage, pneumocephalus, or cavernous-carotid fistula. Fractures of the basal skull bones are often accompanied by signs of hemotympanum (blood behind the tympanic membrane), delayed ecchymosis over the mastoid process (Battle's sign), or periorbital ecchymosis ("racoon sign"). Because routine x-ray examination can fail to disclose basilar fractures, they should be suspected if these clinical signs are present. Cerebrospinal fluid also may leak through the cribriform plate or the adjacent sinus and present as a watery discharge from the nose (CSF rhinorrhea). Persistence of rhinorrhea or recurrent meningitis is an indication for surgical repair of torn dura underlying the fracture. The site of the leak is often difficult to determine, but useful diagnostic tests include the instillation of water-soluble contrast into the CSF followed by CT, and injection of radionuclide compounds or fluorescein into the CSF followed by assessment of uptake by absorptive nasal pledgets. The site of intermittent leaks is rarely delineated, and most such leaks resolve spontaneously. Sellar fractures are sometimes radiologically occult, even ones associated with serious neuroendocrine dysfunction. Occasionally, fractures of the dorsum sella cause sixth or seventh nerve palsies or optic nerve damage. An air-fluid level in the sphenoid sinus suggests a fracture of the sellar floor.

About 20 percent of petrous bone fractures, usually ones oriented along the long axis of the bone, are associated with facial palsy. Disruption of ear ossicles and CSF otorrhea are other complications. Transverse petrous fractures are less common; they damage the cochlea or labyrinths almost always and the facial nerve often. External bleeding from the ear can result from petrous bone fractures, although local laceration of the external canal from abrasions is more common. Frontal bone fractures are often depressed, involving the frontal and paranasal sinuses and the orbits; anosmia results if the olfactory filaments in the cribriform plate are disrupted.

Depressed skull fractures are typically compound, but they are neurologically asymptomatic because the impact energy is dissipated in breaking the bone; however, some are associated with brain contusions and focal neurologic signs caused by damage to the underlying cortical area. Prompt debridement and exploration are required in order to avoid infection.

CRANIAL NERVE INJURIES Cranial nerves liable to injury with basilar skull fractures are the olfactory, optic, oculomotor, and trochlear nerves; the first and second branches of the trigeminal nerve; and the facial and auditory nerves. Anosmia and an apparent loss of taste (actually a loss of perception of aromatic flavors, with elementary tastes retained) occurs in approximately 10 percent of persons with serious head injuries, particularly with falls on the back of the head. This sequela results from displacement of the brain and shearing of the olfactory nerve filaments. Recovery usually occurs, leaving residual hyposmia, but if bilateral anosmia persists for several months, the prognosis is poor. Fractures of the sphenoid bone may bruise or transect the optic nerve, resulting in unilateral partial or complete blindness and an unreactive pupil, usually equal in size to that of the other side, with a preserved consensual light response. Partial optic nerve injuries from closed trauma result in blurring of vision, central or paracentral scotomas, or sector defects. Direct orbital injury may cause short-lived blurred vision for close objects because of reversible iridoplegia. Diplopia only on looking down, which suggests trochlear nerve damage from fracture of the lesser sphenoid wing, occurs as an isolated problem from minor injury and may be delayed for several days. Patients report that the diplopia can be corrected by tilting the head away from the affected eye. Direct facial nerve injury by a basal fracture is present immediately in 3 percent of severe injuries; it also may be delayed 5 to 7 days. Petrous fractures, particularly the less common transverse type, are liable to produce this injury. Delayed facial palsy has a good prognosis; its mechanism is not known. Injury to the eighth cranial nerve with fractures of the petrous bone causes loss of hearing, vertigo, and nystagmus immediately after injury; the nystagmus is frequently positional. Deafness due to nerve injury must be distinguished from that due to rupture of the eardrum, blood in the middle ear, or disruption of the ossicles from fracture through the middle ear. A high-tone hearing loss occurs with direct cochlear concussion.

CONCUSSION *Concussion* refers to an immediate but transient loss of consciousness, often described as dazed or "star struck," associated with a short period of amnesia. It typically occurs after a blunt impact to, or deceleration of, the frontal or occipital areas that creates a sudden movement of the brain within the skull. In severe cases, a brief convulsion or autonomic symptoms and signs such as facial pallor, bradycardia, faintness with mild hypotension, or sluggish pupillary reaction may occur, but most patients are neurologically normal. Higher primates are particularly susceptible to concussion; in contrast, billy goats, rams, and woodpeckers can tolerate impact velocity and deceleration a hundred times greater than that experienced by humans. The mechanism of loss of consciousness in concussion is believed to be a transient electrophysiologic dysfunction of the reticular activating system in the upper midbrain caused by rotation of the cerebral hemispheres on the relatively fixed brainstem. The mechanism of the associated amnesia is not known. Gross and light microscopic changes in the brain are usually absent after concussion, but biochemical and ultrastructural changes, such as mitochondrial ATP depletion and local disruption of the blood-brain barrier, suggest that complex abnormalities occur. The CT and magnetic resonance imaging (MRI) scans are usually normal. Approximately 3 percent of patients who have had concussions have an intracranial hemorrhage (subdural, epidural, or parenchymal); the presence of a skull fracture increases this risk.

Amnesia after concussion typically follows a few moments of unresponsiveness. Rarely, there is no loss of consciousness. The memory loss spans the time of, and moments before, mild impact injuries but may encompass previous weeks (rarely months) in cases of more severe trauma. Any anterograde amnesia is usually brief and disappears rapidly in alert patients. The extent of retrograde amnesia has been suggested as a rough measure of the severity of injury. Improvement usually occurs in an orderly progression from most distant to recent memories, with islands of amnesia occasionally remaining in severe cases. Hysterical posttraumatic amnesia is not uncommon and should be suspected when abnormalities of behavior occur, such as a tendency to recount events that cannot be recalled on later testing, bizarre affect, forgetting one's own name, or an anterograde deficit that is excessive in comparison with the degree of injury.

A single, uncomplicated head injury infrequently produces permanent neurobehavioral changes in patients who are free of preexisting psychiatric problems and substance abuse. However, there has been increasing attention to minor problems in memory and concentration that may have an anatomic correlate in small shearing or other microscopic lesions (see below).

CONTUSION, BRAIN HEMORRHAGES, AND SHEARING LESIONS **Hemispheral Lesions** Contusions on the surface of the brain and deeper hemorrhages result from mechanical forces that move the hemispheres relative to the skull. Deceleration of the brain against the inner skull causes contusions, either under a point of impact (coup lesion) or in the antipolar area (contrecoup lesion). Trauma sufficient to cause prolonged unconsciousness usually produces contusions varying from small superficial cortical petechiae to hemorrhagic and necrotic destruction of large portions of a hemisphere. Because the motion of the hemispheres brings them into contact with the prominences of the sphenoid and other frontal basal bones, blunt impact, as from an automobile dashboard or from falling forward while drunk, typically causes contusions on the orbital surfaces of the frontal lobes and the anterior and basal portions of the temporal lobes. With lateral forces, as from the doorframe of a car, contusions occur on the convexity of the hemispheres.

Contusions are visible on CT and MRI scans, appearing early as inhomogeneous hyperdensity on CT and hyperintensity on MR from scattered cortical and subcortical blood (Fig. 374-1); there is often an associated mass effect that distorts adjacent sulci and the lateral ventricles. In almost all cases there is also some degree of subarachnoid bleeding, which may be detected by scans or lumbar puncture. After several hours, the edematous tissue surrounding a contusion appears as a ring of lower density. Confluent, roughly spherical contusions can be distinguished from cerebral hemorrhages because they extend to the cortical surface. After a week, some contusions have a surrounding ringlike contrast enhancement that may be mistaken for tumor or abscess. Glial and macrophage reactions begin within 2 days and result years later in scarred, hemosiderin-stained depressions on the surface (*plaques jaunes*) that are one source of posttraumatic epilepsy.

The clinical signs produced by contusions vary with the location and size of the lesions; most often a hemiparesis or gaze preference is seen, similar to that caused by a middle cerebral artery stroke. Bilateral large contusions produce coma with extensor posturing; when contusions are limited to the frontal lobes, an abulic-taciturn state or inappropriate jocularity and indifference occur. Contusions of the

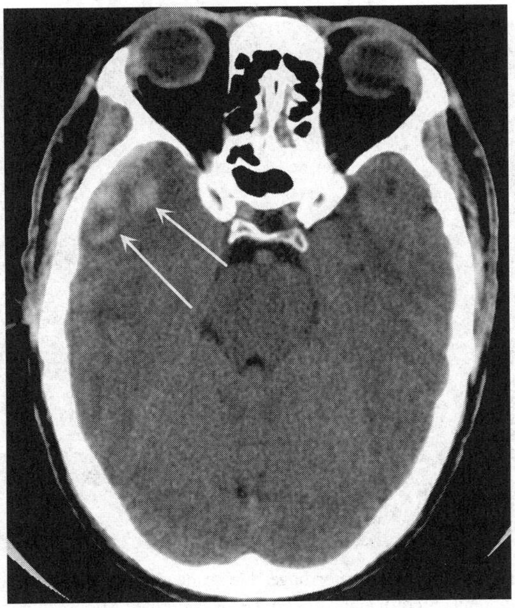

FIGURE 374-1 Temporal lobe contusion. Noncontrast CT scan demonstrates a hyperdense region in the anterior temporal lobe consistent with a hemorrhagic cerebral contusion, which typically occurs in the anterior temporal, frontal, and occipital regions.

temporal lobes may cause an aggressive, combative syndrome, described below. With large contusions, the secondary effect of progressive edema is the most threatening aspect of the injury. Coma and signs of secondary brainstem compression (pupillary enlargement) then dominate. Seizures soon after trauma are rare with contusions, as indeed they are for several weeks after most acute head injuries.

Deep hemorrhages in the central white matter may result from confluent contusions in the depths of a sulcus. However, ganglionic, diencephalic, and other deep hematomas due to torsion or shearing forces in the brain may occur independently of surface damage. The areas around these hematomas can become edematous, resulting in neural dysfunction in the affected region and progressively raised intracranial pressure. Large single hemorrhages after minor trauma may occur in patients with a bleeding diathesis or in the elderly, sometimes related to cerebrovascular amyloidosis. Another type of white matter, or "shearing," lesion consists of widespread acute disruption of axons at the time of impact. The affected areas of white matter are replaced by glial proliferation over a period of several months. In these cases, there are characteristically small areas of tissue disruption in the corpus callosum and dorsolateral pons, but these areas may not be appreciated in scans. There is apparently a continuum of traumatic deep tissue disruption that extends from the limited microscopic shearing lesions to large circumscribed clots within damaged tissue. The presence of widespread axonal shearing lesions in the deep white matter of both hemispheres, called *diffuse axonal injury*, has been proposed as the explanation of persistent coma or vegetative state, but small hemorrhages in the midbrain and low diencephalon are as often the cause. Only severe shearing lesions containing blood are visualized by CT, usually in the corpus callosum and centrum semiovale, but within days of the injury, MRI is able to show them throughout the white matter (Fig. 374-2) especially with the use of gradient echo MR sequences.

On occasion, especially in children, head trauma causes diffuse brain swelling within a few hours after injury, although CT fails to reveal focal lesions or hemorrhage. The swelling creates a mass effect with disastrous consequences. This problem is probably due to microvascular disruption and greatly increased cerebral blood flow.

Deep cerebral hemorrhages may be delayed until several days after severe injury. Sudden neurologic deterioration in an already comatose patient, or a sudden and unexplained rise in intracranial pressure, should therefore prompt a CT scan.

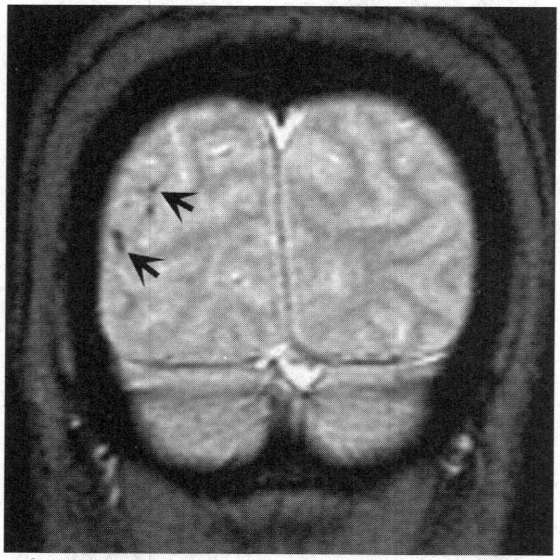

FIGURE 374-2 Shear hemorrhage due to head trauma following a motor vehicle accident. A coronal T2 gradient echo-weighted MRI scan demonstrates several foci of hypointense signal representing small shear hemorrhages at the gray/white junction in the right hemisphere (*arrows*). Foci punctate hemorrhages occur at zones of shearing forces between the gray and white matter of the brain.

Residual symptoms and signs of primary or secondary compressive brainstem hemorrhages or ischemic lesions include cerebellar tremor, pupillary enlargement, eye movement abnormalities, or the "locked-in" syndrome (see Chap. 24). Midbrain or diencephalic hemorrhages are the only well-defined direct traumatic brainstem lesions responsible for coma. Most other lesions causing coma and subsequent persistent vegetative state that are unexplained by CT are probably due to diffuse axonal shearing injuries in the cerebral hemispheres or severe anoxia-ischemia at the time of trauma.

SUBDURAL AND EPIDURAL HEMATOMAS In severe head injury, hemorrhages beneath the dura (subdural) or between the dura and skull (epidural) may be combined with contusions and other injuries, making it difficult to determine their relative contribution to the clinical state. However, subdural and epidural hematomas often occur as the primary lesion, each with a characteristic clinical and radiologic appearance. Because the mass effect of the hemorrhage and the rise in intracranial pressure may be life-threatening, it is important to make an immediate diagnosis by CT or MRI scan (Fig. 374-2) and to carry out surgical evacuation.

Acute Subdural Hematoma Acute subdural hematomas become symptomatic minutes or hours after injury. Up to one-third of patients have a lucid interval before coma supervenes, but most are drowsy or comatose from the moment of injury. Arousable patients complain of unilateral headache and frequently have a slightly enlarged pupil on that side. Stupor or coma and unilateral pupillary enlargement are the major signs in larger hematomas. Pupillary dilation is usually ipsilateral, but 5 to 10 percent are contralateral to the hematoma. Signs such as a hemiparesis are also helpful but occasionally are ipsilateral to the clot. The CT scan shows the clot, allowing early evacuation. The degree of midline shift is often disproportionately greater than the apparent size of the clot in one axial CT scan, but, in general, the rules relating shift to the level of consciousness outlined in Chap. 24 remain useful. In an acutely deteriorating patient with diminished alertness and with pupillary enlargement, burr holes or an emergency craniotomy are appropriate at times without prior radiographic confirmation of subdural hematoma. A subacute syndrome with drowsiness, headache, confusion, or mild hemiparesis occurring days to 2 weeks after injury is seen in alcoholics and in the elderly.

Direct cranial trauma is not required for acute subdural hemorrhage to occur; acceleration forces alone, as from whiplash, are adequate, especially in the elderly. Most subdural hematomas are crescentic collections over the hemispheral convexity, adjacent to a variable degree of surface hemorrhagic contusion. Larger clots are thought to be primarily venous in origin, although additional arterial bleeding sites are often found, and some, when explored surgically, appear to be exclusively arterial. Most are located over the frontotemporal region, less often in the inferior middle fossa or over the occipital poles. Less common instances of interhemispheric, posterior fossa, or bilateral convexity clots are difficult to diagnose clinically, although drowsiness and the signs expected for each region can be detected. Small subdural hematomas may be asymptomatic and usually do not require therapy.

Acute Epidural Hematoma Epidural hematomas evolve more rapidly than subdural hematomas and therefore can be more treacherous. They occur in 1 to 3 percent of all head injuries, in up to 10 percent of severe cases, and are less often associated with underlying cortical damage than are subdural hematomas. Most patients are unconscious when first seen. A "lucid interval" of several minutes to hours before coma supervenes is said to be most characteristic of epidural hemorrhage, although it is not common, and epidural hemorrhage by no means is the only cause of this temporal profile.

The location of an epidural hematoma overlying the lateral temporal convexity is explained by its origin from torn dural vessels, most commonly the middle meningeal artery. Most patients have fractures of the squamous portion of the temporal bone, through the path of the torn vessel. Frontal, inferior temporal, or occipitoparietal epidural hematomas are less frequent, occurring when fractures disrupt branches of the middle meningeal artery. Epidural hematomas strip the tightly attached dura from the inner table of the skull, producing a characteristic lenticular clot on CT. They may be less frequent in the elderly because of the tighter attachment of dura to skull that occurs with aging. Posterior fossa epidural hematomas are rare and difficult to detect clinically; most result from surgery, such as resection of an acoustic neuroma.

Chronic Subdural Hematoma In chronic subdural hematoma, a preceding traumatic cause is less often clear; 20 to 30 percent of patients fail to give a history of injury, particularly elderly patients or those with a bleeding diathesis. The causative injury may be trivial (striking the head against the branch of a tree, a sudden stop in a car with lurching forward, or minor head contact during a fall or faint) and is often forgotten because it was remote in time. A period of weeks, or even months, follows when headaches (common but not invariable), slowed thinking, confusion, changes in personality, seizures, or a mild hemiparesis emerges. The headache typically fluctuates in severity, often with positional changes. Many chronic subdural hematomas are bilateral and give misleading clinical syndromes. The initial clinical impression is often of a stroke, brain tumor, or drug intoxication or of a depressive, senile, or other type of dementia, the latter because drowsiness, inattentiveness, or incoherence of thought is more prominent than focal signs such as hemiparesis. Hemianesthesia or hemianopsia is seldom observed, probably because the anatomic structures subserving these functions are deep and not easily compressed. The diagnosis should be considered in dementias of rapid onset, particularly if headache is present.

Occasionally a chronic hematoma causes brief episodes of hemiparesis or aphasia, lasting more than 10 min, that are indistinguishable from transient ischemic attacks. Patients with undetected small bilateral subdural hematomas seem to have a low tolerance for surgery, anesthesia, and drugs that depress the nervous system, often remaining drowsy or confused for long periods postoperatively.

Skull x-rays are usually normal except for a shift of a calcified pineal body to one side or an occasional unexpected fracture. CT without contrast infusion typically shows a low-density mass over the convexity of the hemisphere, but between 2 to 6 weeks after the initial bleeding, CT may show only a shift of the midline structures and compression of the lateral ventricles because the clot is isodense to adjacent brain. Bilateral chronic hematomas may be missed because of the absence of lateral tissue shifts. A "hypernormal" CT scan with full cortical sulci and small ventricles in an older patient should suggest the diagnosis of bilateral isodense hematomas. Contrast infusion demonstrates a vascular fibrous capsule surrounding the clot. MRI is reliable in identifying a subacute or chronic clot (Fig. 374-3). Lumbar puncture is not recommended for diagnosis because of risk of worsening tissue shifts but, if performed, shows xanthochromia and a variable number of red blood cells. Chronic subdural hematomas can expand gradually and then behave clinically like a tumor. Treatment with glucocorticoids alone is sufficient in some cases, but surgical evacuation is most often successful. Fibrous membranes (pseudomembranes) that grow from the dura and encapsulate the region require surgical resection to prevent recurrent fluid accumulation. Small hematomas are largely resorbed, leaving only the organizing membranes, which become calcified after many years.

PENETRATING INJURIES, COMPRESSIONS, AND LACERATIONS Tangential scalp wounds from bullets can produce neurologic signs or delayed seizures due to small hemorrhages or contusions, even in the absence of missile penetration. Bullets entering the brain cause considerable damage because of tremendous kinetic energy. A cylindrical area of necrosis surrounds the bullet track. Injuries differ for different projectiles; soft civilian bullets typically shatter on impact and leave a track of metallic fragments with moderate parenchymal damage, whereas military bullets, because of their high velocity and energy, disrupt tissue at great distances from the track and produce massive brain destruction.

Penetrating bullet injuries cause a rapid increase in intracranial pressure for several minutes followed by a drop depending on the volume of secondary hemorrhage and the degree of developing edema. Infection is a risk mainly from shell fragments, shrapnel, grenades, and mines, because such small projectiles carry surface bacteria and dirt into the brain. Most neurosurgeons administer systemic antibiotics prophylactically and perform local debridement for all types of penetrating injuries. Traumatic aneurysms can form as a result of disruption of vessel walls from the shock wave of the projectile; facial-orbital entrance wounds have the highest incidence of this complication. The aneurysms have an unpredictable course, but most that rupture do so in the first month. The prognosis for survival after missile injuries is good if consciousness is preserved and poor if coma is present from the outset.

Intracranial foreign bodies in injuries caused by knives, picks, studguns, or high-speed tool bits may be missed unless skull x-rays are taken after minor penetrating injuries. Surgical removal, debridement, and extensive exploration for hemorrhage and necrotic tissue are required.

TRAUMATIC VASCULAR OCCLUSION AND DISSECTION Minor, sometimes unnoticed, head or neck trauma can produce dissection (stripping of the intima or the media) of the internal carotid or vertebral arteries. Chiropractic neck manipulation accounts for some cases. Severe blunt trauma to the neck can initiate a dissection several centimeters above the origins of the internal carotid or vertebral arteries. In awake patients there is usually local neck pain over the affected carotid artery, a Horner's syndrome, and headache over the ipsilateral anterior cranium. Some patients with carotid dissection subsequently have large middle cerebral artery strokes with hemiplegia. In drowsy or comatose patients, evidence of dissection or subsequent stroke is difficult to determine, but its presence is suggested by unexplained hemiplegia, unilateral miosis, or appearance of cerebral infarction on CT scan. Angiography demonstrates either the typical "string sign," characterized by an elongated, narrowed lumen extending over 5 to 10 cm, or complete occlusion of the carotid artery beginning several centimeters distal to the bifurcation.

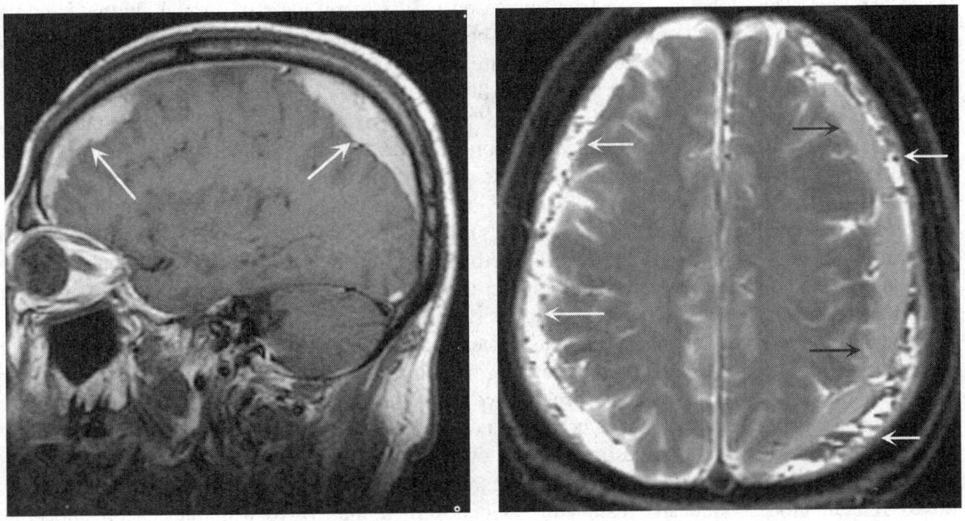

A B

FIGURE 374-3 Acute and subacute subdural hematomas. *A.* Sagittal T1-weighted MRI scan of the brain without contrast demonstrates large fluid collections (*white arrows*) consistent with large subacute subdural hematomas. *B.* Axial T2-weighted MRI scan reveals hyperintense signal (*white arrows*) representing subacute blood and a hypointense signal (*black arrows*) representing more recent subdural hematoma.

Traumatic vertebral artery dissection can produce vertigo, vomiting, suboccipital or supraorbital headache, and other signs of lateral medullary or cerebellar ischemia. These symptoms may be attributed erroneously to vestibular concussion. In comatose patients, the only indication of vertebral artery occlusion may be inferior cerebellar infarction on the CT scan. Vasospasm from traumatic subarachnoid blood may also be involved in the development of infarction after head injury.

Cavernous sinus arteriovenous fistulas are serious complications in patients surviving severe head injury. They are first evident as a self-audible bruit (many are also audible to the examiner), proptosis, conjunctival injection, or visual impairment. Angiography shows early filling of the cavernous sinus and its draining tributaries. The fistula enlarges, causing increasingly severe local changes around the eye and orbit and decreased chances of visual recovery. About 10 percent, mostly small fistulas, resolve spontaneously. Many surgical approaches have been tried, including ligation of the carotid artery and direct obliteration of the fistula or cavernous sinus, but a detachable balloon technique has proved successful in many cases and is currently favored.

INTRACRANIAL PRESSURE AND CEREBRAL BLOOD FLOW

The regulation of intracranial pressure (ICP) and its relationship to cerebral blood flow (CBF), which are relevant to many pathologic processes including cerebral hemorrhage, encephalitis, and brain edema after stroke, is best presented and understood in the context of head trauma. The components of the intracranial compartment are brain, CSF, and blood. Because the skull limits the total intracranial volume, these compartments are compromised by expanding lesions within the cranial cavity. The brain is virtually incompressible; therefore, CSF and blood serve as the main buffers of increasing intracranial volume. The relationship between increments in intracranial volume and the associated rises in ICP, termed *compliance*, approximates an exponential function. ICP is normally between 2 and 12 mmHg. Raised ICP in the range 15 to 40 mmHg, while not harmful by itself, can rapidly progress to a state that causes secondary damage by precipitously decreasing cerebral perfusion when ICP approaches blood pressure (BP). As this is occurring, there are shifts of brain tissue due to compartmentalization of pressure between dural restrictions. These tissue shifts, not the raised ICP per se, compress the upper brainstem and account for the classic neurologic signs of an intracranial mass (see Chap. 24). The global damage from increased ICP is therefore ischemic in nature and related to the difference between ICP and BP in the major cerebral arteries. When this pressure difference, termed *cerebral perfusion pressure* (CPP), is below 20 to 30 mmHg, raised ICP becomes detrimental; therapy is therefore directed toward maintaining perfusion above this range. The rationale for keeping CPP even higher (i.e., bringing ICP below 15 to 20 mmHg) is to afford a margin of safety should transient increases in ICP occur. Physiologic changes or medications that increase BP do not necessarily improve CPP, because increased vascular pressures can exacerbate brain edema in damaged areas and raise cerebral blood volume, thereby resulting in further increases in ICP that ultimately lower perfusion.

The most important secondary nervous system complication of head injury is raised intracranial pressure arising from the added volume of contusions, hematomas, and the progressive edema surrounding them. At least 50 percent of patients who die as a result of head injury do so because of uncontrolled rises in ICP, and outcome is inversely related to the level of ICP after acute injury. Aggressive treatment of raised ICP in modern intensive care units is believed to improve survival after severe head injury, but the role of direct monitoring of ICP to guide therapy and improve outcome is controversial.

Resting ICP, CPP, and compliance are spontaneously interrupted by rises in ICP termed *plateau waves*. These may be precipitated by iatrogenic maneuvers such as suctioning, physical therapy, excess fluid administration, or pain. They are appreciated best by continuous trend recordings of ICP. Plateau waves are apparently due to a loss of cerebrovascular tone with a resultant increase in cerebral blood volume. Some spontaneous plateau waves are provoked by mild, often unnoticed hypotension that causes cerebrovascular dilation. Such episodes (lasting 1 to 10 min and ranging from 25 to 60 mmHg) are most pronounced in patients with diminished intracranial compliance. Signs of transtentorial herniation, such as pupillary enlargement, may occur after plateau waves (although more often they do not), and, occasionally, brain death ensues.

For several minutes to an hour after acute head injury, cerebral blood flow increases in some patients, although metabolic demands and oxygen consumption are diminished. Autoregulation—the ability of the cerebral vasculature to keep blood flow constant in response to decreased or increased perfusion pressure—is also impaired in damaged regions. Vascular factors have been found to account for approximately two-thirds of the rise in ICP after severe head injury. The blood-brain barrier also becomes more permeable after head injury in badly damaged regions, making edema formation more likely. Other secondary systemic phenomena after severe head injury cause brain damage and alter outcome.

CLINICAL SYNDROMES AND TREATMENT OF HEAD INJURY

MINOR INJURY A patient who is fully alert and attentive after head injury and has one or more symptoms of headache, faintness, nausea, a single episode of emesis, difficulty with concentration, or slight blurring of vision has a good prognosis with little risk of subsequent deterioration. Such patients have sustained a concussion and have a brief amnestic epoch surrounding the moment of impact. Occasionally, vasovagal syncope occurs several minutes to an hour after the injury and causes concern. Constant generalized or frontal headache is common in the days following trauma; it is often throbbing or hemicranial in nature, like migraine. Children and young adults are particularly prone to drowsiness, vomiting, and irritability, which is sometimes delayed for several hours after apparently minor injuries. After several hours of observation, arrangements may be made for the patient to be accompanied home to be observed by family or friends. Most patients with a minor syndrome do not have a skull fracture on skull x-ray or hemorrhage on CT. The decision to perform these tests depends largely on clinical signs suggesting that the impact was severe (e.g., prolonged concussion, periorbital or mastoid hematoma, repeated vomiting).

Persistent severe headache and repeated vomiting in the context of normal alertness and no focal neurologic signs are usually benign, but radiologic studies should be obtained. Skull fractures increase the likelihood of a subdural or epidural hematoma. Patients with these exaggerated signs, even if they follow minor injury, deserve observation in the hospital. Clinical judgment, the presence of associated noncranial injuries, the availability of others at home, and the examiner's certainty of a normal neurologic examination should guide the decision regarding further surveillance.

INJURY OF INTERMEDIATE SEVERITY Patients who are not comatose but who have persistent confusion, behavioral changes, subnormal alertness, extreme dizziness, or focal neurologic signs such as hemiparesis should be admitted to the hospital and soon thereafter have a CT scan. Usually a contusion or hematoma is found. The clinical syndromes most common in this group, in addition to postconcussive headache, dizziness, and vomiting of minor injury, include (1) delirium with a disinclination to be examined or moved, expletive speech, and resistance if disturbed (often associated with anterior temporal lobe contusions); (2) a quiet, disinterested, slowed mental state (abulia) with dull facial appearance and slight irascibility if bothered, the patient lying quietly with eyes closed when undisturbed (seen with inferior and frontopolar frontal contusions); (3) memory loss with poor retrograde and anterograde performance (from medial temporal lobe contusions or diffuse injury); (4) a focal deficit such as aphasia or mild hemiparesis (suggesting subdural hematoma or convexity contusion, or, rarely, stroke due to carotid artery dissection); (5) confusion with inattention, poor performance on simple mental tasks, and fluctuating or slightly erroneous orientation (associated with several types of injuries, including the first two described above as well as medial frontal contusions and interhemispheric subdural hematoma); (6) repetitive vomiting, nystagmus, drowsiness, and unsteadiness (usually from a labyrinthine concussion, but occasionally due to a posterior fossa subdural hematoma or vertebral artery dissection); and (7) diabetes insipidus with or without a frontal-temporal lobe syndrome (from damage to the median eminence or pituitary stalk and adjacent medial cortex). Many intermediate injuries are complicated by drug or alcohol intoxication.

Close clinical observation in a well-staffed setting is advisable to detect increasing drowsiness and a change in respiratory pattern or pupillary enlargement and to ensure restriction of free water (unless there is diabetes insipidus). Fully awake or slightly drowsy patients with small subdural hematomas may be treated with glucocorticoids and fluid restriction; those with larger clots, especially if there is fluctuating or worsening alertness, require surgery. Epidural hematomas causing compression of adjacent brain should be evacuated in patients who have a reasonable chance of recovery from other injuries. Free water intake should generally be limited, allowing serum osmolarity to rise spontaneously toward 290 mosmol/L. Fever must be treated assiduously with antipyretics or a cooling blanket, and its source (usually aspiration) must be identified. So-called central fever is rare. The routine administration of phenytoin is controversial; the best randomized trial has shown no benefit beyond the first week of drug administration. Glucocorticoids are of limited usefulness even if there is a contusion or edema on the CT scan; they complicate management and should be omitted.

Most patients with intermediate injury improve over 1 to 6 weeks. During the first week, alertness, irascibility, memory, and mental performance fluctuate. Behavioral changes such as agitation are most evident at night and sometimes seem to be worsened by large doses of glucocorticoids or drugs that depress the central nervous system. Haloperidol is useful when used sparingly. Subtle abnormalities of intellectual function, particularly attention, spontaneity, and memory, tend to return toward normal later, and sometimes do so abruptly. Persistent intellectual difficulties are discussed below.

SEVERE HEAD INJURY AND COMA Patients who are stuporous or comatose from the outset require immediate neurologic attention and, often, resuscitation. Persistent unresponsiveness is a grave sign. After the patient is intubated and the BP is stabilized, attention is given to life-threatening noncranial injuries, followed by a survey neurologic examination. The possibility of cervical injuries should not be overlooked, and the cervical spine must be immobilized during the initial assessment. The depth of coma and the size of the pupils are most important. Extensor limb posturing and bilateral Babinski signs, combined with apparently purposeful movements, are common. Asymmetry in limb posture, limb movement, or gaze preference suggests a subdural or epidural hematoma or a large contusion.

As soon as vital functions permit and cervical spine x-rays and a CT scan have been obtained, the patient should be taken to a critical care unit. The finding of an epidural or subdural hematoma or large intracerebral hemorrhage is usually an indication for surgery and intracranial decompression. In one large series, the time between injury and evacuation of acute subdural hematomas was the major determinant of outcome. If such lesions are not present and the patient is still comatose and critically ill, attention is directed toward treating raised ICP. Patients with abnormal CT scans showing contusions, hemorrhages, or tissue shifts are the best candidates for direct monitoring of ICP. The practice in many head injury treatment centers is to use one of several devices inserted intracranially. The pressure can be monitored continuously; disturbances in compliance and falling cerebral perfusion pressure can be identified; and the appearance of plateau waves can be noted.

The treatment of raised ICP is best guided by direct measurement but may proceed on a presumptive basis using clinical status and CT scan as guides. All potentially exacerbating factors must be eliminated. Hypoxia, hyperthermia, hypercarbia, awkward head positions, and high mean airway pressures from mechanical ventilation all increase cerebral blood volume and ICP. Many, but not all, patients will have lower ICP when the head and trunk are elevated. Active management of raised ICP includes induced hypocarbia to an initial level of 28 to 33 mmHg P_{CO_2} and hyperosmolar dehydration with 20% mannitol (0.25 to 1 g/kg every 3 to 6 h), preferably using directly measured ICP as a guide. Otherwise, a serum osmolality of 300 to 310 mosmol/L is desirable.

A persistently raised ICP after inception of this conservative therapy generally indicates a poor outcome. Although the addition of high-dose barbiturates may further lower ICP there is no beneficial effect on overall outcome. In many instances, barbiturates cause a parallel reduction in ICP and BP without resulting in net improvement in cerebral perfusion. Systolic BP should be maintained above 100 mmHg by vasopressor agents, if necessary. Mean BP levels above 110 to 120 mmHg may exaggerate brain edema, but some neurosurgeons allow the BP to rise above normal on the basis that this may abort plateau waves. A more conventional approach is to treat hypertension with diuretics and beta-adrenergic blocking agents, angiotensin-converting enzyme inhibitors, or intermittent doses of barbiturates. A number of other antihypertensive drugs, including some calcium-channel blockers, are relatively contraindicated because they raise ICP. Fluid must be administered cautiously, and free water intake should be limited. Antacids administered by nasogastric tube or direct-acting drugs should be given to keep gastric pH above 3.5 and prevent gastrointestinal bleeding. The use of large doses of glucocorticoids in severe head injury does not improve outcome. Several studies suggest that early nutritional support results in earlier neurologic recovery from head injury. If the patient remains comatose, it is worthwhile to repeat the CT or MRI scan to exclude a delayed surface or intracerebral hemorrhage. Intensive care salvages some critically ill head-injured patients by concentrating efforts on simple treatments that avoid medical complications, particularly pneumonia and sepsis and preventable increases in ICP. Whether more assiduous control of ICP and CPP produces better results remains to be proved.

ASSOCIATED DERANGEMENTS OCCURRING WITH SEVERE HEAD TRAUMA Injuries outside the cranium should be searched for at the outset, because they are likely to be forgotten if not initially noted. In particular, associated spinal, long bone, and abdominal injuries may cause delayed difficulties in management. However, secondary medical complications dominate the intermediate-term intensive care of head trauma patients.

Fluids and Electrolytes Over half of patients who persist in coma for 24 h after head injury develop abnormalities of electrolytes or fluid balance. Frequently these are a consequence of therapy, but the metabolic responses to head trauma are similar to those produced by trauma elsewhere and are important in planning treatment. Diabetes insipidus should be suspected if urine output increases and urine specific gravity is low. Replacement of water losses suffices for mild cases, but vasopressin may be required. Serum osmolality above approximately 320 mosmol/L should be avoided because of the associated decrease in cardiac output. Secretion of aldosterone and antidiuretic hormone (vasopressin, AVP) in response to stress favor the retention of sodium and free water, respectively. The latter usually predominates, leading to mild hypervolemic hyponatremia in untreated patients, but it is obscured by concomitant administration of osmotic agents. Severe hyponatremia results from excessive AVP secretion, which may occur with raised ICP, basilar skull fractures, and after prolonged mechanical ventilation.

Respiratory Complications Some patients with head injuries have hypoxia acutely after injury without obvious pulmonary infiltrates. Aspiration pneumonia presents a great risk; lung injury from aspirated gastric contents, infection, and atelectasis may combine to produce the adult respiratory distress syndrome (ARDS) and severe arteriovenous shunting. There is some evidence that gastric coating agents, such as sucralfate, are associated with less aspiration pneumonia than are conventional prophylactic agents for gastric bleeding. ARDS also can occur owing to disseminated intravascular coagulopathy, fat embolism, or, rarely, "neurogenic" pulmonary edema (see below). Treatment is similar to that for ARDS in other settings, with positive end-expiratory pressure (PEEP) to allow lowered inspired oxygen concentrations and to prevent further atelectasis. The effect of PEEP on ICP is complex, but PEEP should not be withheld if necessary for oxygenation.

Atelectasis is common in all poorly responsive patients and is treated with chest physical therapy and adequate ventilator tidal volumes. Pulmonary embolism is also a major threat to bedridden patients, and intermittent pneumatic calf compression or modest doses of subcutaneous heparin may be useful prophylaxis. The latter has not predisposed to intracerebral or gastrointestinal bleeding. Early recognition of deep leg vein thrombosis and aggressive treatment by occlusion of the inferior vena cava may prevent later emboli.

Fat Embolism Patients with severe long bone injuries are subject to widespread cerebral fat embolism. This complication is seen less often than previously, perhaps owing to better fluid replacement. In the typical case, head injury is a minor part of the overall trauma; in a few, severe cranial injury masks the syndrome. Several days after the bone fractures occur, restlessness, delirium, or drowsiness progressing to coma in severe cases, seizures, generalized brain edema, and hypoxia develop. About half the patients have retinal and conjunctival punctate hemorrhages or visible fat in retinal vessels. A petechial rash, prominent in the anterior axillary folds and supraclavicular fossae, diffuse interstitial infiltrates on the chest x-ray, fat in the urine, and/or renal failure occurs in some patients. Severe reduction in arterial oxygen content is common from widespread lung injury (ARDS). Cerebral fat embolism causes a cerebral purpura, mainly in the white matter, due to capillary occlusion by fat globules. There is evidence that patients in whom this complication is recognized and treated early have a better prognosis. Massive doses of glucocorticoids and administration of positive-pressure ventilation with high end-expiratory pressures have been claimed to be useful. Heparin or intravenous alcohol are no longer recommended.

Gastrointestinal Hemorrhage Most patients with severe head injuries develop gastric erosions, but only a few have clinically significant hemorrhages. Gastrointestinal bleeding usually occurs in the first days to 1 week after injury. Unlike most patients in shock or with stress ulceration, head-trauma patients often have elevated gastric acidity. The synergistic effect of glucocorticoids in causing upper tract hemorrhage has been questioned, but the incidence of viscus perforation, particularly of the cecum, is elevated. Prophylactic treatment with gastric coating agents, as discussed above, with H_2 receptor blockers, or with frequent antacid administration to keep gastric pH high probably reduces gastric hemorrhage in other stress states and is commonly used in head trauma.

Cardiovascular Changes Acute head trauma may cause transient apnea and cardiac arrest. In the absence of overwhelming brain damage, recovery from the arrest is the rule. Subsequently, a sympathoadrenal discharge or raised ICP may cause systemic hypertension, either with the classically associated bradycardia (Cushing response) or, almost as frequently, with tachycardia. Cardiac arrhythmias are common, most notably sinus bradycardia, supraventricular tachycardias, nodal rhythm, and heart block. T-wave inversion and alterations in the ST segment may simulate subendocardial ischemia.

Neurogenic pulmonary edema is a form of ARDS in which the alveoli fill with fluid as they would in congestive heart failure, but left ventricular end-diastolic pressure (measured by pulmonary capillary wedge pressure) is normal. A pulmonary vascular leak may be produced when a sudden shift of intravascular volume occurs from the systemic to the pulmonary circulation, as occurs transiently with suddenly raised ICP, or there may be a direct neurogenic influence of hypothalamic function on the pulmonary microvasculature. Once the pulmonary vasculature has been damaged, an alveolar capillary leak may continue despite return of pulmonary vascular pressure to normal. The result is pulmonary edema with normal central venous and wedge pressures after the initial injury.

Hematologic Complications A large number of patients demonstrate a mild coagulopathy, and 5 to 10 percent have various degrees of disseminated intravascular coagulation, a harbinger of poor outcome. A correlation may exist between the severity of injury and the level of increased fibrin degradation products in blood. One cause of the coagulopathy is thought to be the release of highly thromboplastic material into the systemic circulation from the damaged brain.

PROGNOSIS Extensive work by Jennet's group in Glasgow and from the Traumatic Coma Data Bank has provided data on the outcome in severe head injury (Table 374-1). Verbal output, eye opening, and the best motor response are important predictors of ultimate outcome. Eighty-five percent of patients with aggregate Glasgow Coma Scale scores of 3 or 4 die 24 h after injury. Yet a number of patients with a poor initial prognosis, including absent pupillary light responses, survive, suggesting that aggressive management is justified in virtually all patients. Patients younger than approximately 20 years, particularly children, may make remarkable recoveries after having grave early neurologic signs. In one large study of severe head injury, 55 percent of children had a good outcome at 1 year, compared with 21 percent of adults. Increased intracranial pressure, older age, and signs of cisternal compression and midline shift on CT scan are all poor prognostic signs.

Evoked potentials also have prognostic value in head injury, similar to their use in ischemic-hypoxic brain injury, and their accuracy probably exceeds that of purely clinical methods. Somatosensory evoked potentials are the most useful, with bilaterally absent cortical potentials (with more caudal potentials present) being predictive of death or a vegetative state in 85 to 95 percent of patients. Prediction of a good functional outcome in the presence of normal or mildly abnormal test results is less certain.

NEUROPSYCHOLOGICAL OUTCOME AFTER HEAD INJURY

Traumatic damage and cognitive sequelae of head injury both constitute a continuum, but most patients recover to normal after mild injury. There is probably a high rate of temporary inattention and memory and other subtle deficits after all but the mildest injuries. Attention has recently been directed toward a structural basis for the fatigue, dizziness, headache, and difficulty in concentration after mild injury, termed the *postconcussion syndrome*. Based on experimental models,

Table 374-1

Glasgow Coma Scale for Head Injury

Eye opening (E)	
Spontaneous	4
To loud voice	3
To pain	2
Nil	1
Best motor response (M)	
Obeys	6
Localizes	5
Withdraws (flexion)	4
Abnormal flexion posturing	3
Extension posturing	2
Nil	1
Verbal response (V)	
Oriented	5
Confused, disoriented	4
Inappropriate words	3
Incomprehensible sounds	2
Nil	1

NOTE: Coma score = E + M + V. Patients scoring 3 or 4 have an 85 percent chance of dying or remaining vegetative, while scores above 11 indicate 5 to 10 percent likelihood of death or vegetative state and 85 percent chance of moderate disability or good recovery. Intermediate scores correlate with proportional chances of patients recovering.

some investigators believe that subtle axonal shearing lesions or biochemical alterations account for these symptoms despite normal findings on brain imaging, normal evoked potentials, and a normal electroencephalogram. In moderate and severe trauma, neuropsychological changes are found routinely; however, formal testing often shows deficits that are not important in daily functioning. This is partly due to the type of testing and the nature of the control groups. Test scores tend to improve rapidly during the first 6 months after injury, then more slowly for years.

SPINAL CORD TRAUMA

Approximately 10,000 patients a year in the United States, mostly young and otherwise healthy, become paraplegic or quadriplegic because of spinal cord injuries. There are an estimated 200,000 quadriplegics in the country. Most spinal cord injuries in civilian life result from damage to the surrounding vertebral column from fracture, dislocation, or both. Vertical compression with flexion is the main mechanism of injury in the thoracic cord, and hyperextension or flexion is the main cause of injury in the cervical cord. Preexisting spondylosis, a congenitally narrowed spinal canal, hypertrophied ligamentum flavum (see Chap. 373), and instability of the apophyseal joints of adjacent vertebrae from diseases such as rheumatoid arthritis predispose to severe spinal cord damage after minor degrees of injury.

PATHOPHYSIOLOGY AND PATHOLOGY OF SPINAL CORD INJURY Much damage to the spinal cord is due to secondary phenomena occurring in the minutes and hours following injury. Even when a complete transverse myelopathy is evident immediately after impact, some secondary changes are avoidable, and the resultant damage may be reversible. The immediate injury causes pericapillary hemorrhages that coalesce and enlarge, particularly in the gray matter. Infarction of gray matter and early white matter edema are evident within 4 h of experimental blunt injury. Eight hours after injury, there is global infarction at the injured level, and only at this point does necrosis of white matter and paralysis below the level of the lesion become irreversible. The necrosis and central hemorrhages enlarge to occupy one or two levels above and below the point of primary impact. Gliosis in these regions results in necrotic areas over several months and may cavitate causing a progressive syringomyelic syndrome.

The early phases of injury are associated with reduced regional blood flow from direct capillary damage and a more prolonged secondary ischemia. A number of interventions, including administration of opiate antagonists or thyrotropin-releasing hormone, local cord cooling, dextran infusion, adrenergic blockade, and hyperbaric oxygen, have been of uncertain clinical usefulness. A randomized trial has shown the benefit of high doses of methylprednisolone administered within 8 h of injury. This effect may result from inhibition of lipid peroxidation rather than from a direct anti-inflammatory action. The critical factor for recoverable function is the time from injury to institution of any therapy. Complete axonal disruption from the immediate trauma or from secondary phenomena precludes recovery.

TYPES OF SPINAL CORD INJURY AND THEIR MANAGEMENT Any patient with severe head injury potentially has an associated instability of the spinal column. The care of such patients begins at the scene of the accident. The neck should be immobilized to prevent spinal cord damage, and care should be taken during transport and during the physical and radiologic examinations to avoid extension or rotation of the neck and to prevent torsion-rotation of the thoracic spine. Most patients can be intubated, if necessary, by blind nasotracheal technique without neck extension. High thoracic or cervical cord trauma regularly causes mild hypotension and bradycardia because of functional sympathectomy, which responds to infusion of crystalloid or colloid (often corroborated by bilateral ptosis and miosis—Horner's syndrome). As noted, a study has demonstrated that acute administration of high doses of glucocorticoids improves functional outcome slightly, and this tactic has been adopted into practice.

The neurologic examination in the awake patient focuses on neck or back pain, diminished limb power, a sensory level on the trunk, and deep tendon reflexes, usually absent below the level of an acute spinal cord injury. Injuries above C5 cause quadriplegia and respiratory failure. At C5 and C6 the biceps are also weak, and at C4 and C5 the deltoid and the supra- and infraspinatus are weak. C7 injuries cause weakness of the triceps, wrist extensors, and forearm pronators. Injuries at T1 and below cause paraplegia; the precise level can be determined from the level of sensory loss. Compression in the low thoracic and lumbar region causes a conus medullaris or cauda equina syndrome (see Chap. 373). Cauda equina injuries are usually incomplete, involving peripheral nerves rather than spinal cord, and therefore are surgically remediable for longer periods after injury than spinal cord compression. In a comatose patient, absent reflexes, especially with small pupils or paradoxical breathing, signify a high cervical cord injury.

The next priority is to exclude a surgically remediable and potentially reversible cord compression due to dislocation of a vertebral body. Many traumatic myelopathies have no clearly associated fracture or dislocation. If x-rays suggest any aberration in the position of vertebrae, then reduction should be undertaken quickly. The role of myelography is controversial, but many neurosurgeons instill a few drops of water-soluble contrast medium into the spinal subarachnoid space to demonstrate a block to the flow of CSF by CT or conventional myelography. Examination by MRI, when available, can be more useful. Decompression within 2 h of severe injury may lead to some recovery of spinal cord function. With incomplete myelopathies, especially if the limbs are becoming progressively weaker, early decompression is strongly recommended, even many hours after injury. The surgical approaches to decompressing the spinal column depend on the specific nature of the injury. In complete transverse myelopathies beyond 6 to 12 h after injury, decompressive laminectomies are usually unsuccessful in restoring function.

The concerns with spinal column fractures, with or without myelopathy, are threefold: (1) detection of vertebral dislocations causing cord compression, (2) instability caused by fractures that will lead to misalignment and cord compression in the future, and (3) the proper treatment of fractures through the pedicles, facets, or vertebral bodies. Some fractures heal with immobilizaton and time, usually 2 to 3 months; others require surgical fusion to ensure stability.

Atlantoaxial dislocations can cause immediate death from respiratory failure, an event that may occur with no other neurologic signs. Rheumatoid arthritis predisposes to this injury. Atlantooccipital dislocations occur predominantly in children and are almost always fatal. "Jefferson's fractures" are burst fractures of the ring of the atlas resulting from a force descending on the vertex of the skull as in diving accidents; they are usually asymptomatic. "Hangman's fractures" are produced by hyperextension and longitudinal distraction of the upper cervical spine, as occurs with penal hanging or striking the chin on a steering wheel in a head-on collision. These are usually fractures through the pedicles of C2 with subluxation anteriorly of C2 on C3. Traction reduction and immobilization allow proper healing.

Hyperflexion dislocation of the cervical vertebrae commonly causes traumatic quadriplegia. Occasionally, a markedly displaced injury is unassociated with neurologic dysfunction, presenting only with neck pain. In most cases, however, minor subluxation is associated with a severe neurologic deficit. Ligamentous disruption presumably allows compression of the cord at the moment of impact, but the vertebral bodies return closer to their original stations afterward. Therefore, any degree of subluxation must be treated as potentially unstable.

Compression fractures of the cervical spine can cause neurologic damage if a bone fragment is driven backward (burst fracture) into the spinal cord. "Teardrop fractures" with crushing of a vertebral body, leaving a fragment of bone anteriorly, are usually associated with ligamentous disruption and spinal instability. Single compression fractures of the thoracic spine are usually stable because the thoracic cage provides support, but they may be associated with anterior spinal cord compression and require decompression and stabilization with the insertion of metal rods.

Mild hyperextension injuries may cause only disruption of supporting ligamentous structures and can be well tolerated. More severe injuries cause vertebral displacement and cord compression. The "central cord syndrome" is produced by brief compression of the cervical cord and disruption of the central gray matter, and usually occurs in patients with an already narrow spinal canal, either congenitally or from cervical spondylosis. There is weakness of the arms, often with pinprick loss over the arms and shoulders, and relative sparing of leg power and sensation on the trunk and legs. Abnormality of bladder function is variable. The prognosis for recovery is good.

Thoracolumbar fractures are produced by impact in the high or middle back, usually while the patient is bent over. Impingement on the spinal canal results in a complex combination of cauda equina and conus medullaris dysfunction. Pure lumbar fractures produce cauda equina compression. Myelography, MRI, or CT allows precise localization, and surgical decompression is usually recommended, even with complete deficits, because the potential for recovery of peripheral nerves is great.

The subsequent care of patients with spinal cord injury is best undertaken in specialized centers. → *General principles of medical and urologic management are discussed in Chap. 373.*

BIBLIOGRAPHY

Adams JH et al: Diffuse brain damage of the immediate impact type. Brain 100:489, 1977

Dacey RG et al: Neurosurgical complications after apparently minor head injury. J Neurosurg 65:203, 1986

Eisenberg HM et al: Report of the Traumatic Coma Data Bank. J Neurosurg 75(Suppl)S1, 1991

Goldstein M: Traumatic brain injury: A silent epidemic. Ann Neurol 27:327, 1990

Langfitt TW, Genarelli TA: Can the outcome from head injury be improved? J Neurosurg 56:19, 1982

Levin HS et al: Neurobehavioral outcome following minor head injury: A three center study. J Neurosurg 66:234, 1987

Reinus WR et al: Practical selection criteria for noncontrast cranial computed tomography in patients with head trauma. Ann Emerg Med 22:1148, 1993

Ropper AH (ed): *Neurological and Neurosurgical Intensive Care*, 3d ed. New York, Raven, 1993

Rosner MJ et al: Cerebral perfusion pressure: Management protocol and clinical results. J Neurosurg 83:949, 1995

Ruff RM et al: Predictors of outcome following severe head trauma: Follow-up data from the Traumatic Coma Data Bank. Brain Inj 7:101, 1993

Stein SC et al: Delayed and progressive brain injury in closed-head trauma: Radiological demonstration. Neurosurgery 32:25, 1993

375

Stephen M. Sagar, Mark A. Israel

TUMORS OF THE NERVOUS SYSTEM

Primary cancer of the brain and central nervous system (CNS) occurred in approximately 18,000 individuals and accounted for an estimated 13,300 deaths in the United States in 1996, a mortality rate of 2.6 per 100,000. Overall, CNS cancer is estimated to comprise 1.1 percent of newly occurring malignant tumors. CNS cancer is second only to leukemia as a cause of cancer-related deaths in children and young adults; it is the third leading cause between ages 15 and 34 and the fourth leading cause of cancer-related deaths in males aged 35 to 54. In older individuals, other diseases—especially cardiovascular and cerebrovascular disease and cancer of other organ systems—vastly exceed CNS tumors in prevalence. Among CNS tumors glial tumors are the most common, accounting for 50 to 60 percent of primary brain tumors. Meningiomas account for about 25 percent, schwannomas for about 10 percent, and all other CNS tumors for the remainder. An increase in the incidence of gliomas in the elderly has been reported in recent years. It is unclear if this apparent increase is real or is the result of more frequent use of modern neuroimaging techniques.

Tumors that metastasize to the brain and vertebrae are more prevalent than primary CNS tumors. These tumors pose a major problem in the management of systemic cancer. About 15 percent of patients who die of cancer (80,000 individuals each year) have symptomatic brain metastases; an additional 5 percent suffer spinal cord involvement.

BRAIN TUMORS

Approach to the Patient

Clinical Features Brain tumors usually present with one of three syndromes: (1) subacute progression of a focal neurologic deficit; (2) seizure; or (3) nonfocal neurologic disorder such as headache, dementia, personality change, or gait disorder. The presence of systemic symptoms such as malaise, weight loss, anorexia, or fever suggests a metastatic rather than a primary brain tumor.

Focal neurologic deficits result from compression of neurons and white matter tracts by expanding tumor and accompanying edema. Although the mechanism of edema is unknown, tumor cells and infiltrating inflammatory cells may secrete cytokines and other factors that produce edema and may also directly affect neuronal and glial function. Venous or arterial compression may produce focal brain ischemia.

Seizures may result from stimulation of excitatory circuits or interference with inhibitory mechanisms by abnormal tissue. Tumors that invade or compress the cerebral cortex are more likely to be associated with seizures than subcortical neoplasms. Even small meningiomas that compress adjacent cerebral cortex may present with seizures.

Nonfocal neurologic dysfunction usually reflects increased intracranial pressure, hydrocephalus, or diffuse tumor spread. Multiple metastases or diffuse infiltration of the brain by glioma or lymphoma may present as dementia or a decline in level of alertness. Tumors arising in some areas of the brain may produce subtle deficits; for example, frontal lobe tumors may present with personality change or depression.

Headache may result from focal irritation or displacement of pain-sensitive structures (see Chap. 15), or from a generalized increase in intracranial pressure. In the former situation, the headache is typically localized and of constant intensity and may be strikingly positional. A headache that worsens rather than abates with recumbency is suggestive of a mass lesion. The headache of increased intracranial pressure has a characteristic pattern. Early on, as long as the elevated intracranial pressure is intermittent, headaches are primarily associated with *plateau waves* of increased intracranial pressure. These headaches are usually holocephalic and episodic, occurring more than once a day. They typically develop rapidly over several minutes, persist for 20 to 40 min, and subside quickly. They may awaken the patient from a sound sleep, generally 60 to 90 min after retiring, or may be precipitated by coughing, sneezing, or straining. Vomiting may occur with severe headaches. As elevated intracranial pressure becomes sustained, the headache becomes continuous but varying in intensity. The recent onset of a constant headache may require neuroimaging studies to distinguish brain tumor from benign etiologies, including the headache of depression. Elevated intracranial pressure may cause papilledema (see Chap. 28), although it is often not observed in patients over 55 years old.

Less commonly, brain tumor may present with a strokelike onset and focal neurologic deficit. This may be caused by hemorrhage into the tumor, but often no hemorrhage can be demonstrated and the mechanism is obscure. Tumors that often cause hemorrhage include high-grade astrocytomas and metastatic melanoma and choriocarcinoma. Rare brain tumor presentations include anosmia from a meningioma arising near the cribriform plates and olfactory tracts, and unilateral hearing loss from schwannomas of the eighth cranial nerve. Asymptomatic brain tumors, most often meningiomas, are commonly discovered incidentally on scans obtained for unrelated purposes.

The Karnofsky performance scale is useful in assessing and following brain tumor patients (see Chap. 81). A score of 70 or greater indicates that the patient is ambulatory and independent in self-care activities; it has often been taken as a level of function justifying aggressive therapy.

Laboratory Examination Primary brain tumors typically do not produce the serologic abnormalities such as an elevated sedimentation rate or tumor-specific antigens associated with other cancers. Metastases to the nervous system, depending on the type and extent of the primary tumor, may be associated with systemic features of malignancy (see Chap. 85). Lumbar puncture may precipitate brain herniation in patients with mass lesions; thus its indications are limited to the suspicion of meningitis or meningeal metastasis. Cerebrospinal fluid (CSF) findings in primary and metastatic nervous system tumors may include raised opening pressure, elevated protein level, and a mild lymphocytic pleocytosis. Astrocytomas that extend to the ventricular surface, or the rupture of an epidermoid cyst, can occasionally produce intense CSF inflammation simulating infectious meningitis. The CSF rarely contains malignant cells, with certain exceptions such as leptomeningeal metastases and primitive neuroectodermal tumors, including medulloblastoma.

Neuroimaging Computed tomography (CT) and magnetic resonance imaging (MRI) reveal mass effect and contrast enhancement. Mass effect reflects the volume of neoplastic tissue as well as surrounding edema. Brain tumors typically produce a *vasogenic* pattern of edema, with accumulation of excess water in white matter. Contrast enhancement reflects a breakdown in the blood-brain barrier, permitting leakage of intravascular contrast agent into the parenchyma. The normal blood-brain barrier results from tight junctions between endothelial cells and between endothelia and astrocytes that prevent entry of most charged molecules into the nervous system. Endothelia associated with malignant gliomas and other CNS tumors lack normal tight junctions and have abnormal passive diffusion and vesicular transport characteristics, all contributing to entry of solutes and edema. In planning therapy for malignant gliomas, the volume of enhancement observed following the intravenous administration of a contrast agent is assumed to represent the major tumor mass, but tumor cells typically extend beyond this boundary. Low-grade astrocytomas typically do not exhibit contrast enhancement.

Positron emission tomography (PET) scanning and single-photon emission tomography (SPECT) have ancillary roles in the imaging of brain tumors, primarily in distinguishing tumor recurrence from tissue necrosis that can occur following irradiation (see below). Electroencephalography (EEG) has a role in the evaluation of patients with possible seizures. Functional imaging with PET, MRI, or magnetoencephalography may be employed in surgical or radiosurgical planning to define the anatomic relationship of the tumor to critical brain regions such as the primary motor cortex.

Rx TREATMENT

Symptomatic Glucocorticoids decrease the volume of edema surrounding brain tumors and improve neurologic function; dexamethasone (12 to 20 mg/d in divided doses orally or intravenously) is employed because it has relatively little mineralocorticoid activity.

Tumors that involve the cerebral cortex or hippocampus may produce epilepsy and frequently present as a seizure. *Anticonvulsants* are therefore employed therapeutically and prophylactically; phenytoin, carbamazepine, and valproic acid are equally effective (Chap. 365). If the tumor is subcortical in location, prophylactic anticonvulsants are unnecessary.

Gliomas are associated with an increased risk for deep vein thrombosis and pulmonary embolism, probably because gliomas secrete procoagulant factors into the systemic circulation. Whether this risk extends to other brain tumors is unknown. Hemorrhage within gliomas is a frequent histopathologic finding, yet patients appear to be at no increased risk for intracranial bleeding following anticoagulation. Anticoagulation with low-dose subcutaneous heparin should be considered in glioma patients, especially those with lower limb weakness.

PRIMARY BRAIN TUMORS

ETIOLOGY Exposure to ionizing radiation is the only well-documented environmental risk factor for the development of brain tumors. A number of heritable syndromes, including several known to be caused by specific genetic alterations, are associated with an increased risk of brain tumors (Table 375-1). Genes that contribute to the development of brain tumors, as well as other malignancies, fall into two general classes. The first class, known as *tumor-suppressor genes*, functions physiologically to restrain cell proliferation. An *inactivating mutation* of a tumor-suppressor gene passed through the germline can predispose to the development of cancer. A single functioning copy of a tumor-suppressor gene is often sufficient to maintain normal function of the genetic locus; loss of both normal alleles is necessary to promote neoplasia. The second class of genes, *proto-oncogenes*, can contribute to tumor development by enhancing cellular proliferation. *Activating mutations* convert proto-oncogenes to oncogenes, which have a variety of functions that can promote the neoplastic phenotype. Proto-oncogenes typically encode proteins such as growth factors or growth factor receptors, mediators of signaling pathways, or regulators of gene expression. Epidermal growth factor receptor (*EGFR*) and c-*myc* are among the oncogenes that may be important for the development of brain tumors (Table 375-2).

Cytogenetic examination of chromosomes within brain tumor cells often reveals characteristic changes (Table 375-2). In astrocytic tumors, DNA is commonly lost on chromosomes 17p, 13q, and 9. In meningiomas portions of 22q are often lost. Less frequently there is evidence of amplification of specific genes, for example *EGFR* in some astrocytomas.

The particular constellation of genetic alterations varies among individual tumors, even those that appear to be histologically indistinguishable, particularly in astrocytomas. The accumulation of mutations is associated with increasingly aggressive malignant behavior.

ASTROCYTOMAS Tumors derived from astrocytes are the most com-

Table 375-1

Selected Hereditary Syndromes Associated with Brain Tumors

Syndrome	Gene	Chromosomal Location	Neoplastic Pathology of the CNS
von Hippel–Lindau syndrome*	VHL	3p	Retinal angioma, cerebellar hemangioblastoma
Li-Fraumeni syndrome*	P53	17p13	Glial tumors, medulloblastoma
Multiple endocrine neoplasia 1* (Werner's syndrome)	NK†	11q13	Pituitary adenomas, malignant schwannoma
von Recklinghausen's disease (neurofibromatosis type 1)*	NF1	17q	Neuroma, schwannoma, meningioma, optic glioma
Neurofibromatosis type 2*	NF2	22q12	Glial tumors
Retinoblastoma*	RB	13q14	Retinoblastoma, pinealoblastoma
Tuberous sclerosis	TSC1	9q	Astrocytoma
	TSC2	16p13	Astrocytoma
Turcot syndrome	APC	5q21	Astrocytomas, medulloblastoma
Werner's syndrome	WRN	8p12	Meningioma

* Genetic testing possible.
† Not known.

Table 375-2

Cytogenetic and Genetic Alterations in Brain Tumors

Tumor Type	Chromosomal Alteration	Genetic Changes
Astrocytoma	$1p^-$, $9p^-$, del10, $13q^-$, $17p^-$, $17q^-$, 19q, $22q^-$, DMs*	P53, RB1, NF1, PTEN, *EGFR*, c-*ros*, *met*, *gli*, c-*myc*, *cdk*4, *neu*, *ras*
Medulloblastoma	17p,$^-$ $6q^-$, 16q, DMs	
Meningioma	$22q^-$	NF2
Oligodendroglioma	$1p^-$, $9p^-$, $19q^-$	

* DMs, double minute chromosomes.

mon primary intracranial neoplasms (Fig. 375-1). Their neuropathologic appearance is highly variable, and numerous attempts have been made to devise histologic grading systems that accurately predict their clinical course. The traditional grading system of Kernohan and Sayre divided astrocytic tumors into grades I to IV, grade IV being the most malignant. Because of a number of limitations, this grading system has been abandoned in favor of two derivative systems, the most widely used of which is the World Health Organization (WHO) four-tiered grading system. Grade I is reserved for special histologic variants of astrocytoma that have an excellent prognosis following surgical excision. These include *juvenile pilocytic astrocytoma*, *subependymal giant cell astrocytoma* (which occurs in patients with tuberous sclerosis), and *pleiomorphic xanthroastrocytoma*. At the other extreme is grade IV, *glioblastoma multiforme*, a clinically aggressive tumor. In between are *astrocytoma* (grade II) and *anaplastic astrocytoma* (grade III). The defining features associated with aggressive behavior are hypercellularity, nuclear and cytoplasmic atypia, endothelial proliferation, mitotic activity, and necrosis. Endothelial proliferation and necrosis are widely regarded as important predictors of a tumor's potential for rapid growth and aggressive invasion of normal surrounding tissue. The WHO classification includes parallel grading systems for oligodendroglial and ependymal tumors. Another widely used grading system for astrocytic tumors, the Saint Anne–Mayo system, assigns a point for each of four histologic features: nuclear atypia, mitoses, endothelial proliferation, and necrosis. This produces a four-tiered grading scheme

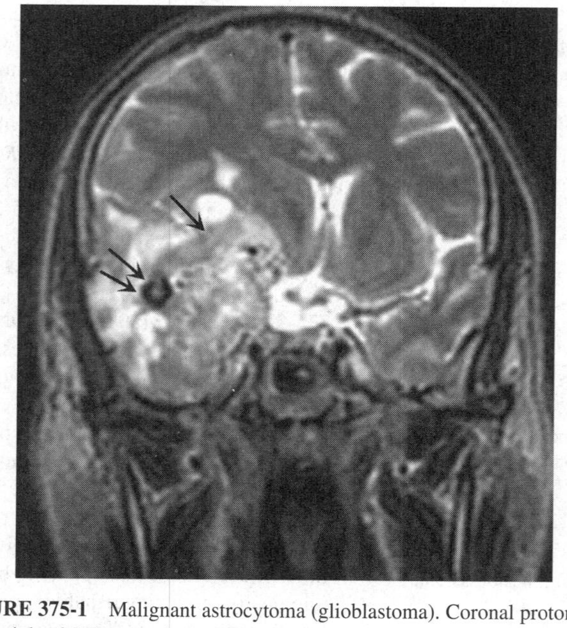

FIGURE 375-1 Malignant astrocytoma (glioblastoma). Coronal proton density-weighted MR scan through the temporal lobes demonstrates a heterogeneous right temporal lobe mass (*arrows*) compressing the third and lateral ventricles. The area of hypointense signal (*double arrows*) indicates either hemorrhage or calcification. Heterogeneous MR signal intensity is typical of glioblastoma.

that correlates well with prognosis. A limitation of all grading schemes, especially when applied to a single biopsy, is that astrocytic tumors are histologically variable from region to region, and their histopathology may change over time. It is common for low-grade astrocytomas to recur with a higher histopathologic grade and more aggressive clinical course.

Quantitative measures of mitotic activity also correlate with clinical course. The *proliferation index* can be determined by measuring the uptake of the thymidine analogue bromodeoxyuridine (BUdR) into tumor tissue. BUdR is administered intravenously prior to surgery, and its uptake into the nuclei of tumor cells is assessed in biopsy specimens using a BUdR-specific monoclonal antibody. This provides a measure of DNA synthesis. Other methods of estimating mitotic activity include immunohistochemical staining with antibodies to the proliferating cell nuclear antigen (PCNA) or with a monoclonal antibody termed *Ki-67*, which recognizes a histone protein expressed in proliferating but not quiescent cells. These measures all correlate with malignant clinical behavior of the tumor.

The overall prognosis for patients with astrocytoma is poor. In a representative Finnish population, employing the WHO grading system, the median survival was 93.5 months for patients with grade I or II astrocytomas, 12.4 months for patients with grade III (anaplastic astrocytoma), and 5.1 months for patients with grade IV (glioblastoma) tumors. In the United States, the median survival of patients with high-grade brain tumors is approximately 12 months. In addition to histopathology, features that correlate with poor prognosis include age over 65 and a poor functional status, as defined by the Karnofsky performance scale (Table 81-2), at presentation.

Low-Grade Astrocytoma Low-grade astrocytomas are more common in children than adults. Pilocytic astrocytoma of the cerebellum, named for its characteristic spindle-shaped cells, is the most common childhood brain tumor. Typically, this tumor is histologically benign, is well demarcated from adjacent brain, and may be cystic. Surgical excision is indicated, and long-term, disease-free survival is the rule.

The optimal management of other low-grade astrocytomas is controversial. For patients who are symptomatic, either from a focal neurologic deficit or poorly controlled epilepsy, surgical excision is the treatment of choice. Whether postoperative radiation should be administered routinely is uncertain. Although radiation may delay tumor recurrence, it is possible that radiation is best reserved for tumor recurrence, at which time the tumor may display a more malignant phenotype. When only a biopsy or partial resection is possible, postoperative external beam radiation therapy is usually administered. For patients who are asymptomatic or minimally symptomatic at presentation, a diagnostic biopsy should be performed or the tumor may be resected. There is no evidence that delaying definitive surgery and radiation therapy until the patient becomes more symptomatic is harmful. No role for chemotherapy in the management of low-grade astrocytoma has been defined.

High-Grade Astrocytoma The overwhelming majority of astrocytomas arising in adults are high grade, supratentorial, and do not have a clear margin separating neoplastic and normal tissue. In such high-grade tumors, neoplastic cells migrate away from the main tumor mass and infiltrate otherwise-normal brain, often tracking along white matter fiber pathways. Imaging studies do not indicate the full extent of the tumor. These tumors are usually fatal, although prolonged survival occurs in a small minority of patients. Unlike systemic cancer, which is generally fatal when complications of metastases arise, gliomas cause fatal effects by local growth. Late in their course, gliomas, especially those located in the posterior fossa, can metastasize along CSF pathways to the spine. Metastases outside the CNS are rare.

High-grade astrocytomas are managed with glucocorticoids, surgery, radiation therapy, and chemotherapy. Therapy with dexamethasone is generally instituted at the time of diagnosis and continued for the duration of radiation therapy. After completion of radiotherapy, the dose is tapered to the lowest tolerated dose.

Because astrocytomas infiltrate adjacent normal tissue, total surgical resection is not possible. Surgery is indicated to obtain tissue for pathologic diagnosis and to control mass effect. In general, accessible astrocytomas are resected aggressively in patients younger than 65 years old who are in good general medical condition and in selected elderly patients. This practice is supported by retrospective studies demonstrating that the extent of tumor removal, as estimated by comparing preoperative and postoperative neuroimaging studies, correlates with survival. The extent to which selection bias influences these data is unknown. It is possible that younger, healthier patients in good neurologic condition are more likely to be offered aggressive surgery than older, sicker patients.

Postoperative radiation therapy prolongs survival and improves the quality of life of patients with high-grade astrocytomas, although the duration of benefit is only a few months. Treated with dexamethasone alone, the mean survival of patients under 65 years of age with glioblastoma is 7 to 9 months. Survival is prolonged to 11 to 13 months with radiation therapy. Focal brain irradiation is less toxic and as effective as whole-brain radiation in the treatment of primary glial tumors. It is generally administered to the tumor mass, as defined by contrast enhancement on a CT or MRI scan, plus a 3- to 4-cm margin. A total dose of 5000 to 7000 cGy is administered in 25 to 35 equal fractions, 5 days per week.

The roles of stereotaxic radiosurgery and interstitial brachytherapy are uncertain. *Stereotaxic radiosurgery* refers to the administration of a single, highly focused dose of radiation to a precisely defined volume of tissue. There are three methods of stereotaxic radiosurgery. The *gamma knife* is a series of gamma radiation sources arranged in a hemisphere around the patient's head. By controlling the dose administered from each source, a high dose of radiation can be administered to irregularly shaped tumors in a single sitting, with very low exposure of surrounding normal brain. Similar effects can be achieved with a modified linear accelerator or with a heavy particle source by rotating either the patient or the source. The latter are extremely expensive and available in only a few centers. Stereotaxic radiosurgery potentially can achieve tumor ablation without a craniotomy, and the entire procedure may be carried out in a single day. A major limitation of stereotaxic radiosurgery is that it can be used for only relatively small tumors, generally less than 3 cm in maximum diameter. *Interstitial brachytherapy*, the stereotaxic implantation of radioactive beads into the tumor mass, is generally reserved for tumor recurrence because of its associated toxicity—in particular, necrosis of normal brain tissue.

Chemotherapy is marginally effective in the treatment of high-grade astrocytoma and is often used as an adjuvant following surgery and radiation therapy. Nitrosoureas, including carmustine (BCNU) and lomustine (CCNU), are the most effective available agents. Since a typical glioma infiltrates normal brain where the blood-brain barrier is relatively intact, lipid-soluble agents such as the nitrosoureas, which cross the blood-brain barrier, may reach more malignant cells than water-soluble agents. Experimental approaches include intraarterial infusion of chemotherapy, administration of chemotherapy following osmotic disruption of the blood-brain barrier, and intensive chemotherapy regimens supported by autologous bone marrow transplantation.

Gliomatosis cerebri is a rare form of astrocytoma in which there is diffuse infiltration of the brain by malignant astrocytes without a focal enhancing mass. It generally presents as a multifocal CNS syndrome or a more generalized disorder including dementia, personality change, or seizures. Neuroimaging studies are often nonspecific, and biopsy is required to establish the diagnosis. Gliomatosis is treated with whole-brain radiation therapy and, in selected patients, systemic chemotherapy.

OLIGODENDROGLIOMAS Oligodendrogliomas have a more benign course and are more responsive to treatment than astrocytomas. Five-year survival is greater than 50 percent, and 10-year survival is 25 to 34 percent.

Oligodendrogliomas occur chiefly in supratentorial locations; in adults about 30 percent are calcified (Fig. 375-2). Many gliomas contain mixtures of cells with astrocytic and oligodendroglial features. If this mixed histology is prominent, the tumor is termed a *mixed glioma* or an *oligoastrocytoma*. The greater the oligodendroglial component, the more benign the clinical course. As a rule, oligodendrogliomas are less infiltrative than astrocytomas, permitting more complete surgical excision. The histologic features of mitoses, necrosis, and nuclear atypia are associated with a more aggressive clinical course. If these features are prominent, the tumor is termed a *malignant oligodendroglioma*.

The optimal management of oligodendrogliomas has not been defined. Surgery, which may be limited to a stereotaxic biopsy, is necessary to establish a diagnosis. Many oligodendrogliomas are amenable to total surgical resection. In addition, oligodendrogliomas may respond dramatically to systemic combination chemotherapy with procarbazine, lomustine and vincristine administered before or after surgery. Chemotherapy may be employed as initial treatment, and residual tumor can be surgically excised or treated with stereotaxic radiosurgery. An alternative approach is to excise the accessible tumor mass initially, administer systemic chemotherapy following surgery, and employ stereotaxic radiosurgery or external beam radiation for residual tumor.

EPENDYMOMAS These tumors are derived from ependymal cells and occur in characteristic locations. In children, they occur within the ventricles, most often the fourth ventricle. Histologically, childhood tumors are highly cellular and may exhibit diagnostic ependymal rosettes. In adults they are located more often in the spinal canal, especially in the lumbosacral region, arising from the filum terminale of the spinal cord. Ependymomas arising in the sacral region of adults often have a *myxopapillary* histology, with a papillary arrangement of cells and mucin production. There is no generally accepted grading system for ependymomas, but ependymomas with his-

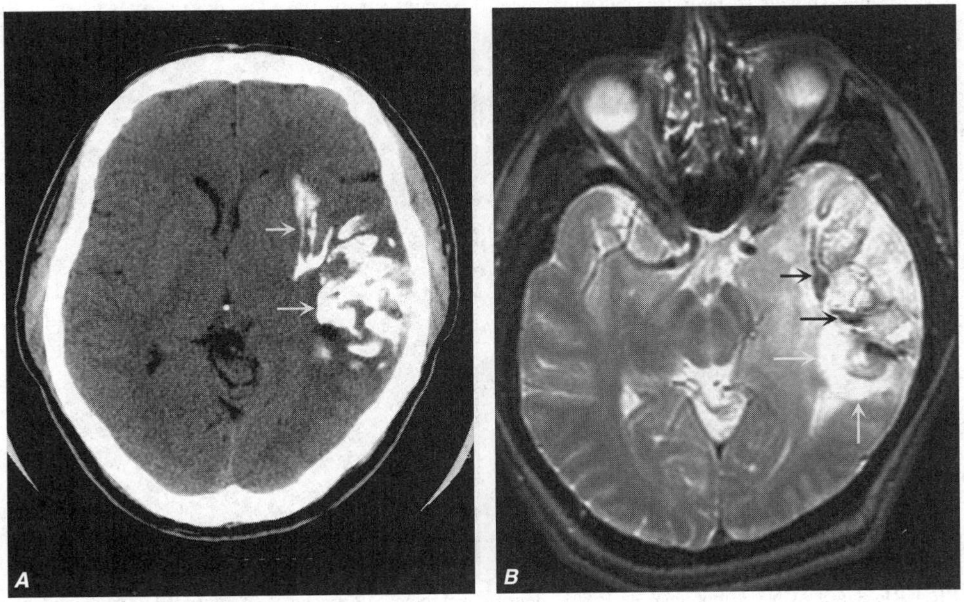

FIGURE 375-2 Oligodendroglioma. *A.* Noncontrast CT scan reveals a calcified mass involving the left temporal lobe (*arrows*) associated with mild mass effect but little edema. *B.* An MR T2-weighted image demonstrates a heterogeneous mass with hypointense signal (*black arrows*) surrounded by a zone of higher signal intensity (*white arrows*), consistent with a calcified temporal lobe mass. The tumor extends into the left medial temporal lobe and compresses the midbrain.

tologic signs of malignancy, including cellular atypia, frequent mitotic figures, or a high labeling index, virtually always recur. CT or MRI scans identify ependymomas as uniformly enhancing masses relatively well demarcated from adjacent neural tissue. Ependymomas may metastasize via CSF pathways: brain tumor metastases that spread to the spinal cord by this means are termed *drop metastases*.

Following total excision of an ependymoma the prognosis is excellent. The 5-year disease-free survival is over 80 percent. However, many ependymomas cannot be totally excised. In this situation, postoperative focal external beam radiation or stereotaxic radiosurgery is most often employed. Whether focal radiation is adequate or whether the entire neuraxis needs to be treated is not resolved. Prolonged survival is the rule, although the tumors generally recur.

GERMINOMAS These tumors most commonly present during the second decade of life, generally at sites within or adjacent to the third ventricle including the pineal region. Germinomas are the most frequent variety of *germ cell tumor*, a tumor type arising in midline structures and including *teratoma*, yolk sac tumor (*endodermal sinus tumor*), *embryonal carcinoma*, and *choriocarcinoma*. Germinomas of the CNS may be benign but are more often aggressive and invasive. Due to their location, patients frequently present with hypothalamic-pituitary dysfunction including diabetes insipidus, visual field deficits, disturbances of memory or mood, or hydrocephalus (see Chap. 328). On neuroimaging studies, germinomas are uniformly enhancing masses with or without well-defined borders. The treatment of choice is complete surgical resection. For unresectable tumors, a stereotaxic biopsy is performed for diagnosis, and focal radiation is given as primary therapy. When the extent of disease or very young age precludes the effective use of radiotherapy, platinum-based chemotherapeutic regimens can provide control, followed by irradiation of residual disease or irradiation of the tumor should it recur. Prognosis depends on the histology and surgical resectability of the tumor; these tumors are generally radiosensitive and chemosensitive, and 5-year survival is greater than 85 percent.

MEDULLOBLASTOMAS AND PRIMITIVE NEUROECTODERMAL TUMORS (PNET) These highly cellular malignant tumors are thought to arise from neural precursor cells. Medulloblastomas of the posterior fossa are the most frequent malignant brain tumor in children. If the tumor is not disseminated at presentation, prognosis is favorable; subsets of pediatric patients have 70 percent survival at 5 years, although fewer than 50 percent of children with medulloblastoma survive to adulthood. PNET is a term applied to tumors histologically indistinguishable from medulloblastoma but occurring either in adults or supratentorially in children. In adults, more than 50 percent present in the posterior fossa, but these tumors frequently disseminate along CSF pathways.

If possible, these tumors should be surgically excised, although outcome is not related to the extent of surgery. In children, the optimal use of radiation therapy and chemotherapy is currently under study; chemotherapy appears of benefit to children with high- but not low-stage disease. In adults, surgical excision of a PNET should be followed by chemotherapy and irradiation of the entire neuraxis, with a boost in radiation dose to the primary tumor. Aggressive treatment can be effective and may result in prolonged survival, although half of adult patients relapse within 5 years of treatment.

CNS LYMPHOMA **Primary CNS Lymphoma** This presents within the neuraxis without evidence of systemic lymphoma. While accounting for only a small proportion of total lymphomas, the incidence of primary CNS lymphoma is increasing in both immunocompetent and immunocompromised patients and may become the most common primary CNS tumor by the year 2000. Leptomeningeal involvement is present in approximately 15 percent of patients at presentation and in 50 percent at some time during the course of the illness. Histologically, primary CNS lymphomas are B cell malignancies of intermediate to high grade. They occur most frequently in immunosuppressed individuals, most often organ transplant recipients or AIDS patients (see Chap. 308). In these settings, CNS lymphomas are invariably associated with latent Epstein-Barr virus (EBV) infection of the tumor cells. Chromosomal translocations involving the c-*myc* gene occur in EBV-associated lymphomas that occur outside the CNS (Chap. 113) but not in primary CNS lymphoma.

In immunocompetent patients, neuroimaging studies most often reveal a uniformly enhancing mass lesion. In immunosuppressed patients, primary CNS lymphoma is likely to be multicentric and exhibit ring enhancement or to arise in the meninges (Fig. 375-3). Stereotaxic needle biopsy can be used to establish the diagnosis.

Prognosis is poor compared to histologically similar disease occurring elsewhere. Many patients experience a transient, at times dramatic, clinical and radiographic response to glucocorticoids. Radiotherapy is the mainstay of treatment, and systemic combination chemotherapy can provide additional benefit. Despite aggressive therapy, over 90 percent of patients develop recurrent CNS disease. In patients who do not receive systemic chemotherapy, intrathecal chemotherapy with

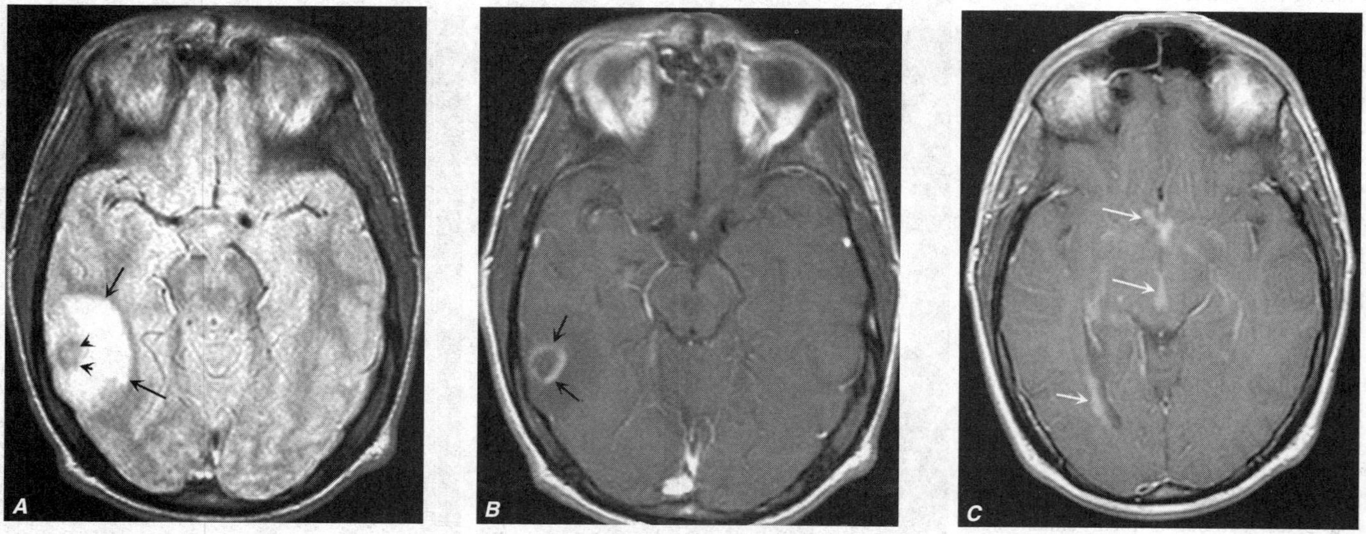

FIGURE 375-3 CNS lymphoma. *A.* Proton density–weighted MR image through the temporal lobe demonstrates a low signal intensity nodule (*small arrows*) surrounded by a ring of high signal intensity edema (*larger arrows*). *B.* Axial postcontrast T1-weighted MRI demonstrates ring enhancement surrounded by a nonenhanced rim of edema. In this patient with AIDS, a solitary lesion of this type suggests either lymphoma or toxoplasmosis; the presence of multiple lesions favors toxoplasmosis. *C.* In a different patient with lymphomatous meningitis, an axial postcontrast T1-weighted MRI through the midbrain demonstrates multiple areas of abnormal enhancement in periventricular and subependymal regions (*arrows*). Lymphoma tends to spread subependymally at interfaces of CSF and brain parenchyma.

methotrexate should be used if leptomeningeal disease is suspected. Historically, the survival of immunocompetent patients with CNS lymphoma has been approximately 18 months, and may now be longer with the use of systemic chemotherapy. In organ transplant recipients, reversal of the immunosuppressed state can improve outcome. AIDS-related primary CNS lymphoma has a very poor prognosis, generally 3 months or less; pretreatment performance status, the degree of immunosuppression, and the extent of CNS dissemination at diagnosis all appear to influence outcome.

Secondary CNS Lymphoma This almost always occurs in association with progressive systemic disease, generally in adults with B cell lymphoma or B cell leukemia who have tumor involvement of bone, bone marrow, testes, or the cranial sinuses. Leptomeningeal lymphoma is detected with contrast-enhanced CT or gadolinium-enhanced MRI of the brain and spine and by CSF examination. Treatment consists of systemic chemotherapy, intrathecal methotrexate, and CNS irradiation. It is usually possible to clear the leptomeningeal disease, although the overall prognosis is determined by the course of the systemic lymphoma.

PITUITARY ADENOMAS See Chap. 328.

MENINGIOMAS Meningiomas are derived from cells of the arachnoid granulations. These usually benign tumors are attached to the dura and may invade the skull but almost never invade the brain. They frequently occur along the sagittal sinus and over the cerebral convexities, in the cerebellar-pontine angle, and along the dorsum of the spinal cord. They are more frequent in women than men, with a peak incidence in middle age.

Meningiomas may be found incidentally on a CT or MRI scan or may present with a focal seizure, a slowly progressive focal deficit, or symptoms of raised intracranial pressure. The radiologic image of a dural-based, extraaxial mass with dense, uniform contrast enhancement is essentially diagnostic, although a dural metastasis must also be considered (Fig. 375-4). A meningioma may have a "dural tail," a streak of dural enhancement flanking the main tumor mass; however, this finding is not specific.

Total surgical resection of benign meningiomas is curative. If a total resection cannot be achieved, local external beam radiotherapy reduces the recurrence rate to less than 10 percent. For meningiomas that are not surgically accessible, targeted radiosurgery with the gamma knife or heavy particle radiation should be considered. Small asymptomatic, incidentally discovered meningiomas can safely be followed radiologically; these tumors grow at an average rate of only 0.24 cm in diameter per year and only rarely become symptomatic.

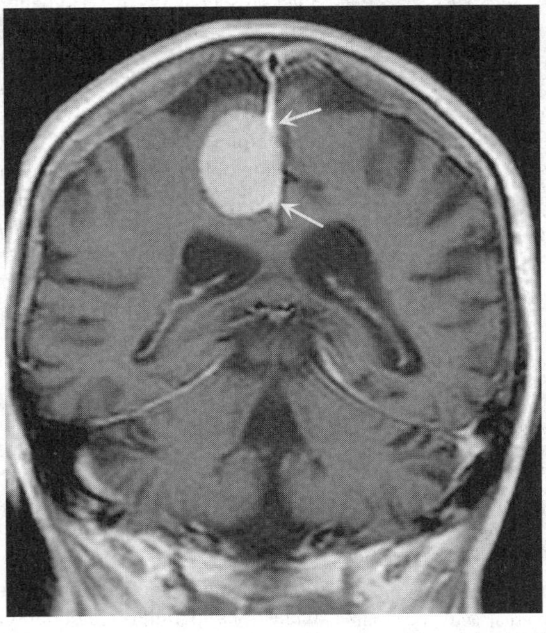

FIGURE 375-4 Meningioma. Coronal postcontrast T1-weighted MR image demonstrates an enhancing extraaxial mass arising from the falx cerebri (*arrows*).

Rare meningiomas have histologic evidence of malignancy such as nuclear pleomorphism and cellular atypia. A high mitotic index, as defined by BUdR labeling, is also predictive of aggressive behavior. *Hemangiopericytoma* is a morphologic variant of meningioma with an especially aggressive behavior. Meningiomas with features of aggressiveness, even if totally excised by gross inspection, should receive postoperative radiotherapy; chemotherapy has no benefit, and these tumors typically recur.

SCHWANNOMAS These tumors are also called *neuromas*, *neurinomas*, or *neurolemmomas*. They arise from Schwann cells of nerve roots, most frequently in the eighth cranial nerve (acoustic schwannoma). The fifth cranial nerve is the second most frequent site; however, schwannomas may arise from any cranial or spinal root, except the optic and olfactory nerves—myelinated by oligodendroglia rather than Schwann cells. Neurofibromatosis (NF) type II (see below) strongly predisposes to acoustic schwannoma, and schwannomas of spinal nerve roots are also seen in these patients.

Acoustic schwannomas are misnamed because they typically arise from the vestibular division of the eighth nerve rather than the acoustic division. Nevertheless, because the vestibular system adapts to slow destruction of the vestibular nerve, acoustic schwannomas characteristically present as progressive unilateral hearing loss rather than with dizziness or other vestibular symptoms. Unexplained unilateral hearing loss always merits evaluation, including audiometry and either brainstem auditory evoked potentials or an MRI scan (see Chap. 29). As an acoustic schwannoma grows, it can compress the cerebellum, pons, or facial nerve, producing corresponding symptoms. Schwannomas are with rare exceptions histologically and clinically benign. They are densely and uniformly enhancing on MRI (Fig. 375-5). Acoustic schwannomas enlarge the internal auditory meatus, an imaging feature that helps distinguish them from other cerebellopontine angle masses.

Whenever possible, schwannomas should be surgically excised. With small tumors, it is usually possible to preserve hearing in the involved ear. With large tumors, the patient is frequently deaf at presentation; nonetheless, surgery is indicated to prevent further compression of posterior fossa structures. Gamma knife treatment is also effective for acoustic schwannoma but is equivalent in cost and complication rate to surgery. Moreover, the long-term consequences of stereotaxic radiosurgery, including the possibility of secondary radiation-induced neoplasms, are unknown.

OTHER BENIGN BRAIN TUMORS *Epidermoid tumors* are thought to arise from embryonic epidermal rests within the cranium. They occur extraaxially near the midline, in the middle cranial fossa, the suprasellar region, or the cerebellopontine angle. Epidermal rests form cystic structures with the proliferative epidermal cells at the periphery, giving rise to more mature epidermal cells that migrate towards the center of the cyst. The mature cells desquamate into the liquid center of the cyst. If the cyst ruptures into the subarachnoid space, an intense chemical meningitis results. Epidermoid cysts are well-demarcated lesions that are amenable to complete surgical excision. Postoperative radiation therapy is unnecessary.

Dermoid cysts are thought to arise from embryonic rests of skin tissue trapped within the CNS during closure of the neural tube. The most frequent locations are in the midline supratentorially or at the cerebellopontine angle. Histologically, they are composed of all elements of the dermis, including epidermis, hair follicles, and sweat glands; they frequently calcify. Treatment is surgical excision.

Craniopharyngiomas are thought to arise from remnants of Rathke's pouch, the mesodermal structure from which the anterior pituitary gland is derived (see Chap. 328). Craniopharyngiomas typically present as suprasellar masses. Histologically, craniopharyngiomas resemble epidermoid tumors; they are usually cystic and in adults 80 percent are calcified. Because of their location, they may present as growth failure in children, endocrine dysfunction in adults, or visual loss in either age group. Treatment is surgical excision;

postoperative external beam radiation or stereotaxic radiosurgery is added if total surgical removal cannot be achieved.

Colloid cysts are benign tumors of unknown cellular origin that occur within the third ventricle. They can obstruct CSF flow. Intermittent obstruction can result in recurrent episodes of acute hydrocephalus, with headache and altered consciousness; sudden death rarely has been reported. Total surgical excision of a colloid cyst is usually possible.

Rare benign primary brain tumors include neurocytomas, subependymomas, and pleomorphic xanthoastrocytomas. Surgical excision is the primary treatment.

NEUROCUTANEOUS SYNDROMES

This group of genetic disorders, also known as the *phakomatoses*, produces a variety of developmental abnormalities that frequently involve skin, along with an increased risk of nervous system tumors (Table 375-1). These disorders are inherited as *autosomal dominant* conditions with variable penetrance.

NEUROFIBROMATOSIS TYPE 1 (VON RECKLINGHAUSEN'S DISEASE) NF1 is characterized by benign tumors of the peripheral nerves called *neurofibromas*, composed of Schwann cells and fibroblasts, and by pigmented lesions of the skin called *café au lait spots*. Neurofibromas frequently involve cutaneous nerves and present as multiple, palpable, rubbery, cutaneous tumors. They are generally asymptomatic; however, if they grow in an enclosed space, e.g., the intervertebral foramen, they may produce a compressive radiculopathy or neuropathy. The presence of at least six café au lait spots of more than 1.5 cm in diameter is diagnostic of NF1. Other features include hamartomas of the iris (*Lisch nodules*), axillary freckling, and pseudoarthrosis of the tibia. Hydrocephalus from aqueductal stenosis, scoliosis, short stature, hypertension, epilepsy, and mental retardation may also occur.

Mutation of the NF1 gene causes von Recklinghausen's disease. The NF1 gene on chromosome 17 encodes a protein, *neurofibromin*, which is a GTPase that modulates signal transduction through the *ras* pathway. NF1 is a tumor-suppressor gene. Patients with NF1 are at increased risk of developing nervous system neoplasms, including plexiform neurofibromas, optic gliomas, pheochromocytomas, ependymomas, meningiomas, and astrocytomas. Neurofibromas may undergo secondary malignant degeneration and become sarcomas.

NEUROFIBROMATOSIS TYPE 2 NF2 is characterized by the development of bilateral acoustic schwannomas in over 90 percent of gene carriers. Patients with NF2 have a predisposition for the development of meningiomas, gliomas, and schwannomas of cranial and spinal nerves. In addition, a characteristic type of cataract—juvenile posterior subcapsular lenticular opacity—occurs in NF2. Multiple café au lait spots and peripheral neurofibromas occur rarely.

In NF2 patients, acoustic schwannomas usually present with progressive unilateral deafness early in the third decade of life. At presentation, bilateral acoustic schwannomas may be detected on MRI (Fig. 375-5). Surgical management, designed to treat the underlying tumor and preserve hearing as long as possible, is difficult.

The NF2 gene on chromosome 22q has at different times been called *neurofibromin 2*, *schwannomin*, or *merlin*, with homology to a family of cytoskeletal proteins that includes moesin, ezrin, and radixin.

TUBEROUS SCLEROSIS (BOURNEVILLE'S DISEASE) Tuberous sclerosis is characterized by cutaneous lesions, seizures, and mental retardation. The cutaneous lesions include adenoma sebaceum (facial angiofibromas), ash leaf–shaped hypopigmented macules (best seen under ultraviolet illumination with a Wood's lamp), shagreen patches (yellowish thickenings of the skin over the lumbosacral region of the back), and depigmented nevi. Rhabdomyomas of the myocardium and angiomyomas of the kidney, liver, adrenals, and pancreas may also occur. Neurologic features may include epilepsy, mental retardation, and hydrocephalus. On neuroimaging studies, the presence of subependymal nodules, which may be calcified, is characteristic. Gene carriers are at increased risk of developing ependymomas and childhood astrocytomas, of which over 90 percent are *subependymal giant cell astrocytomas*. These are benign neoplasms that may develop in the retina or along the border of the lateral ventricles. They may obstruct the foramen of Monro and produce hydrocephalus.

Treatment is symptomatic. Anticonvulsants for seizures, shunting for hydrocephalus, and behavioral and educational strategies for mental retardation are the mainstays of management. Severely affected individuals generally die before age 30.

Mutations at both 9q (TSC-1) and 16p (TSC-2) are associated with tuberous sclerosis. The mutated genes code for *tuberins*, proteins that modulate the GTPase activity of other cellular proteins.

VON HIPPEL–LINDAU SYNDROME This syndrome consists of retinal angiomas and cerebellar hemangioblastomas, which are slowly growing cystic tumors that may present at any age. Hemangioma of the spinal cord; hypernephroma; renal cell carcinoma; pheochromocytoma; and cysts of the kidneys, pancreas, epididymis, or liver may also occur. Erythropoietin production by cerebellar hemangioblastomas may result in polycythemia. The von Hippel–Lindau (VHL) tumor suppressor gene has been identified on chromosome 3p; the normal VHL gene encodes a protein that appears to suppress transcription elongation by RNA polymerase II.

TUMORS METASTATIC TO BRAIN

MECHANISMS OF BRAIN METASTASES The large majority of brain metastases probably arise by hematogenous spread via the arterial circulation. The anatomic distribution of brain metastases parallels regional cerebral blood flow, with a predilection for the gray matter–white matter junction and for the border zone between middle cere-

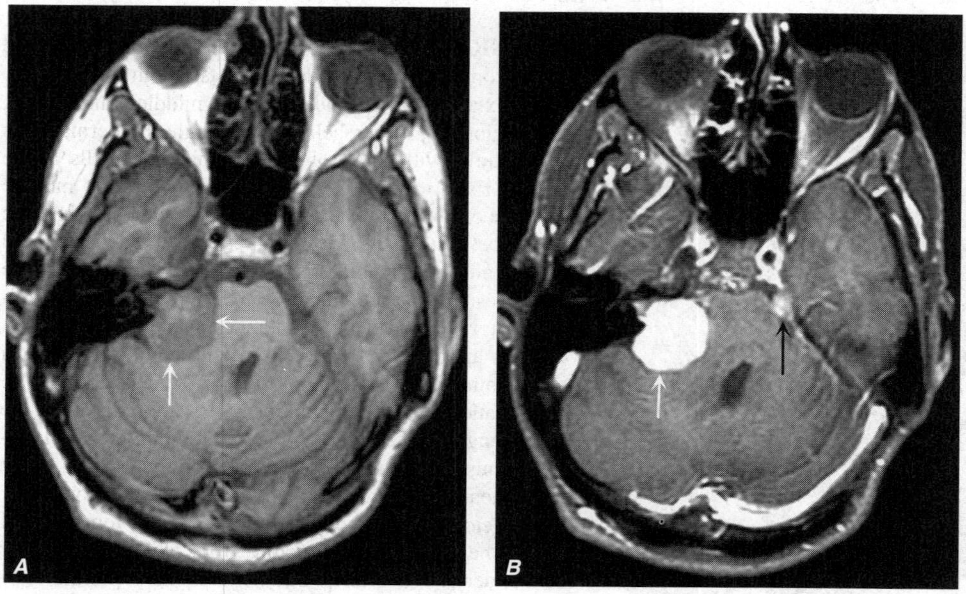

FIGURE 375-5 Acoustic schwannoma (neuroma). *A.* Axial noncontrast T1-weighted MR scan through the cerebellopontine angle demonstrates an extraaxial mass that extends into a widened internal auditory canal, displacing the pons (*arrows*). *B.* Postcontrast T1-weighted image demonstrates intense enhancement of the acoustic schwannoma (*white arrow*). Abnormal enhancement of the left fifth nerve (*black arrow*) most likely represents another schwannoma in this patient with neurofibromatosis type II.

bral and posterior cerebral artery distributions. The lung is the most common origin of brain metastases; both primary lung cancer and cancers metastatic to the lung can metastasize to the brain. Breast cancer has a propensity to metastasize to the cerebellum and the posterior pituitary gland. This propensity could be explained by patterns of retrograde venous flow from the thorax into the skull or by an especially hospitable environment for breast cancer cells provided by the cerebellum and pituitary (the "seed and soil" hypothesis).

Invasion of the brain by a skull metastasis is rare. Although the skull is one of the most frequent bony sites of metastasis from systemic solid tumors, the dura is an effective barrier to tumor invasion of the brain. This same dural barrier also resists invasion by head and neck cancers. Skull metastases, however, can produce neurologic symptoms by compression of adjacent brain tissue or cranial nerves as they pass through skull foramina. They may also obstruct venous sinuses. Slow occlusion of venous sinuses by tumor growth may produce intracranial hypertension; however, hemorrhagic infarction of the brain generally does not occur as it does with acute venous sinus thrombosis (see Chap. 366).

In addition to lung cancer (adenocarcinoma and small cell lung cancer) and breast cancer (especially ductal carcinoma), gastrointestinal malignancies, and melanoma are other common tumors that metastasize to brain (Table 375-3). This reflects in part the high prevalence of these malignancies in the general population. Certain tumors, however, have a special propensity to metastasize to brain, including small cell lung cancer, melanoma, germ cell tumors, and thyroid cancer. By contrast, prostate cancer, ovarian cancer, and Hodgkin's disease rarely metastasize to the brain. Moreover, breast cancer that metastasizes to bone tends not to metastasize to the brain. Therefore, the cellular environment of the brain is hospitable to only a subset of systemic cancers. Parenchymal spinal cord metastases are rare.

EVALUATION OF METASTASES FROM KNOWN CANCER MRI scans reveal brain metastases as well-demarcated, approximately spherical lesions that are hypointense or isointense relative to brain on T1-weighted images, are bright on T2-weighted images, and enhance with gadolinium (Fig. 375-6). The administration of three times the usual dose of gadolinium is more sensitive than the standard protocol for detection of brain metastases. Small metastases often enhance uniformly. Larger metastases typically produce ring enhancement, representing extravasation of gadolinium through tumor vessels that lack a blood-tumor barrier, while the central area of nonenhancement represents a core of necrosis as the metastasis outgrows its blood supply. Metastases are variably surrounded by edema. Blood products may also be seen, reflecting hemorrhage of abnormal tumor vessels.

Table 375-3

Frequency of Primary Tumors that Metastasize to the Nervous System

Site of Primary Tumor	Brain Metastases, %	Leptomeningeal Metastases, %	Spinal Cord Compression, %
Lung	40	24	18
Breast	19	41	24
Melanoma	10	12	4
Gastrointestinal tract	7	13	6
Genitourinary tract	7		18
Other	17	10	30

The radiologic appearance of a brain metastasis is not specific. The differential diagnosis of ring-enhancement lesions includes brain abscess, radiation necrosis, toxoplasmosis, granulomas (tuberculosis, sarcoidosis), demyelinating lesions, primary brain tumors, primary CNS lymphoma, stroke, hemorrhage, and trauma. Prolonged focal seizures may produce MRI features of edema and contrast enhancement (resembling metastasis) at the site of the seizure focus. The contrast enhancement of a benign seizure focus, however, is generally patchy and not dense, only rarely forms a well-defined ring, and resolves 2 to 3 weeks after the seizures are brought under control.

Contrast-enhanced CT scanning is less sensitive than MRI for the detection of brain metastases. Moreover, in the presence of leaky tumor vessels there is some risk of precipitating a seizure by iodinated contrast material used for CT scanning. Pretreatment with intravenous diazepam (10 mg), or lorazepam (4 mg), 10 min before contrast administration may lessen the chance of provoking a seizure.

Cytologic examination of the CSF is not indicated, since intraparenchymal brain metastases almost never shed cells into CSF. Tumor markers such as carcinoembryonic antigen (CEA) are rarely helpful in management.

BRAIN METASTASES WITHOUT A KNOWN PRIMARY TUMOR In general hospital populations, up to one-third of patients presenting with brain metastases do not have a known underlying cancer. Lung cancer, particularly small cell lung cancer, and melanoma are the most frequent primary tumors responsible. No primary tumor can be identified even after extensive evaluation in 30 percent of patients.

The patient generally presents with either a seizure or a progressive neurologic deficit. Neuroimaging studies demonstrate one or multiple ring-enhancement lesions. In individuals who are not immunocompro-

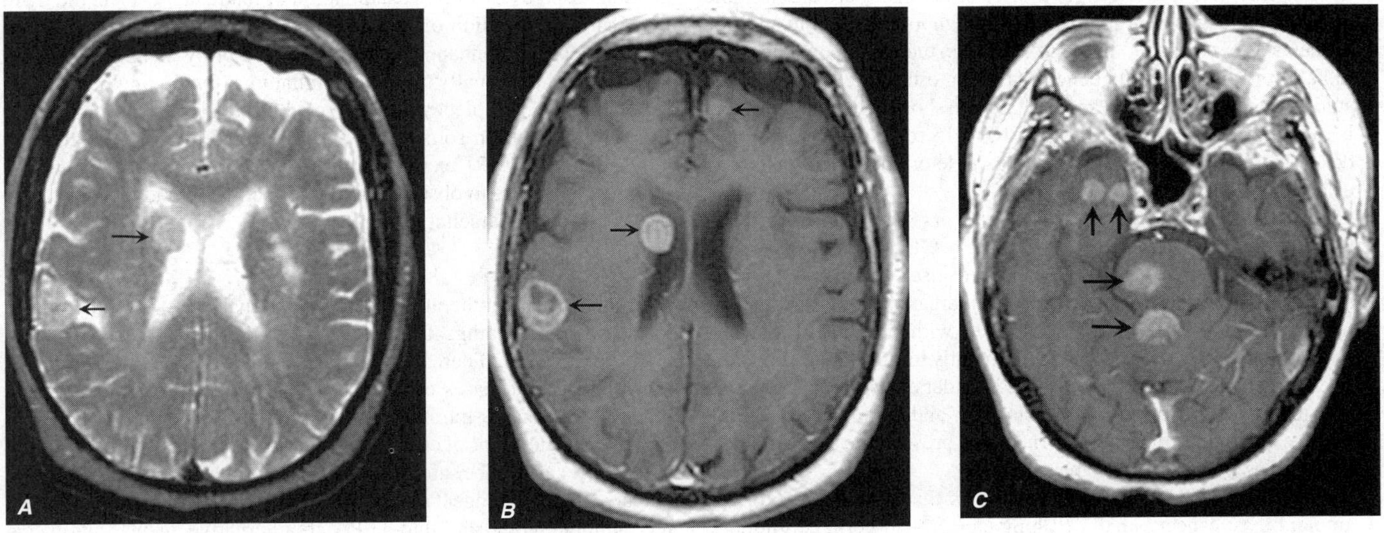

FIGURE 375-6 Brain metastasis. *A.* Axial T2-weighted MRI through the lateral ventricles reveals two isodense masses, one in the subependymal region and one near the cortex (*arrows*). *B.* Postcontrast T1-weighted image at the same level as *A* reveals enhancement of the two masses seen on the T2-weighted image as well as a third mass in the left frontal lobe (*arrows*). *C.* Postcontrast T1-weighted axial image through the pons reveals at least four other enhancing metastatic lesions. Metastatic disease may not always produce vasogenic edema and may only be visible on postcontrast T-1 weighted images.

mised and not at risk for brain abscesses, this radiologic pattern is most likely due to brain metastasis. Diagnostic evaluation begins with a search for the primary tumor. Blood tests should include CEA and liver function tests. A careful examination of the skin for melanoma and the thyroid gland for masses should be carried out. Since most brain metastases arise from either lung cancer or malignancies that have metastasized to the lungs, a chest x-ray is the most important screening test. If the x-ray is negative, a CT scan of the chest is indicated. If these tests are still unrevealing, CT scan of the abdomen and pelvis should be obtained. If these are all negative, further imaging studies, including bone scan, other radionuclide scans, and upper and lower gastrointestinal series, are unlikely to be productive.

A tissue diagnosis is essential. After the above studies are completed, a decision must be made concerning the best site to biopsy. As a rule, the primary tumor will be more accessible to biopsy than any brain lesion. If a single brain lesion is found in a surgically accessible location without a primary tumor being discovered or with a primary tumor in a location difficult to biopsy, the brain metastasis should be approached surgically.

Rx TREATMENT

Once a systemic cancer metastasizes to the brain it is, with rare exception, incurable. Therapy is therefore palliative, designed to prevent disability and suffering and, if possible, to prolong life. Published outcome studies have focused on survival as the primary end point, leaving questions regarding quality of life unanswered. There is, however, widespread agreement that glucocorticoids, anticonvulsants, and radiation therapy improve the quality of life for many patients. The value of surgery and chemotherapy is less well established.

General Measures High-dose glucocorticoids frequently ameliorate symptoms of brain metastases. Improvement is often dramatic, occurs within 6 to 24 h, and is sustained with continued administration, although the toxicity of glucocorticoids is cumulative. Therefore, if possible, a more definitive therapy for metastases should be instituted to permit withdrawal of glucocorticoid therapy.

One-third of patients with brain metastases have one or more seizures. Anticonvulsants are empirically used for seizure prophylaxis when supratentorial metastases are present. There is a small risk of serious allergic reactions to phenytoin in patients undergoing cranial irradiation.

Specific Measures *RADIATION THERAPY* This is the primary treatment for brain metastases. It is assumed that there are multiple microscopic deposits of tumor cells throughout the brain in addition to metastases visualized by neuroimaging studies, thus whole-brain radiation is employed. Its benefit has been established in controlled studies, but no clear dose response has been shown. Standard protocol is to administer a total of 30 Gy in 10 to 15 fractions; an additional dose ("boost") of focal radiation to a single or large metastasis may also be administered.

SURGERY Up to 40 percent of patients with brain metastases have only a single tumor mass identified by CT scanning. Accessible single metastases are usually surgically excised as a palliative measure. Metastases are often sharply demarcated from surrounding normal brain, so they can be removed with minimal damage to functional nervous tissue. Patients frequently improve neurologically after surgery. If the systemic disease is under control, total resection of a brain lesion may improve survival and minimize disability. These expectations have been borne out in prospective and retrospective studies of lung cancer metastases.

CHEMOTHERAPY Some solid tumors that metastasize, for example, breast cancer, small cell lung cancer, and germ cell tumors, are potentially responsive to systemic chemotherapy. Although metastases frequently do not respond as well as the primary tumor, dramatic responses to systemic cytotoxic chemotherapy or hormonal therapy may occur in some cases. In patients who are neurologically stable and in whom there is reason to expect the tumor to be sensitive to systemic therapy, hormonal therapy or two to four cycles of cytotoxic chemotherapy may be administered initially to reduce bulk disease and render the residual tumor more amenable to focal radiation therapy. Even if a complete radiologic remission is achieved, whole-brain radiation should then be administered.

EXPERIMENTAL THERAPIES These include stereotaxic radiosurgery, gene therapy, immunotherapy, intraarterial chemotherapy, and the chemotherapy administered with osmotic disruption of the blood-brain barrier.

LEPTOMENINGEAL METASTASES

Leptomeningeal metastases are also called *carcinomatous meningitis*, *meningeal carcinomatosis*, and, in the cases of specific tumors, *leukemic meningitis* and *lymphomatous meningitis*. Pathologically, three patterns of tumor involvement may be seen: (1) a diffuse coating of the leptomeninges by a thin layer of tumor cells, (2) nodular growth of macroscopic tumor metastases in meninges and on nerve roots, or (3) plaquelike metastases in the leptomeninges with many cells in the subarachnoid space and extension of tumor into Virchow-Robin spaces. Leptomeningeal metastases may coexist with parenchymal CNS metastases.

Cancers usually metastasize to the meninges via the bloodstream. Alternatively, a superficially located parenchymal metastasis may shed cells directly into the subarachnoid space. Some tumors, including squamous cell carcinoma of the skin and some non-Hodgkin's lymphomas, have a propensity to grow along peripheral nerves and may seed the meninges by that route.

Clinical evidence of leptomeningeal metastases is present in 8 percent of patients with metastatic solid tumors; at necropsy, the prevalence is as high as 19 percent. Among solid tumors, adenocarcinomas of the breast and lung and melanoma are most often responsible (Table 375-3). In one-quarter of patients the systemic cancer is under control; thus effective control of leptomeningeal disease can improve the quality and duration of life.

CLINICAL FEATURES Leptomeningeal metastases present with signs and symptoms at multiple levels of the nervous system, often in a setting of known systemic malignancy. Hydrocephalus, encephalopathy, or focal neurologic deficits from coexisting intraparenchymal metastases may occur. Cranial nerve, spinal root, or spinal cord involvement may signify compression by bulky meningeal disease. Typically neurologic signs exceed the symptoms described by the patient.

LABORATORY EVALUATION Leptomeningeal metastases are diagnosed by cytologic examination of malignant cells in the CSF, by MRI demonstration of nodular tumor deposits in the meninges or diffuse meningeal enhancement (Fig. 375-7), or by meningeal biopsy. CSF findings are usually those of an inflammatory meningitis, consisting of lymphocytic pleocytosis, elevated protein levels, normal or low CSF glucose, and in some cases an oligoclonal increase of IgG.

A complete MRI examination of the neuraxis may demonstrate hydrocephalus due to obstruction of CSF pathways and identify bulky disease in the subarachnoid space.

Rx TREATMENT

Intrathecal chemotherapy and focal external beam radiotherapy to sites of leptomeningeal disease are the mainstays of management. Approximately 20 percent of patients aggressively treated for leptomeningeal metastases can expect a sustained response of approximately 6 months. Intrathecal therapy exposes meningeal tumor to high concentrations of chemotherapy with minimal systemic toxicity. Methotrexate can be safely administered intrathecally and is effective against leptomeningeal metastases from a variety of solid tumors and lymphoma; ara-C and thio-TEPA are alternative agents. Intrathecal chemotherapy may be administered either by repeated lumbar puncture or through an indwelling Ommaya reservoir, which consists of a catheter in one lateral ventricle attached to a reservoir implanted under the scalp.

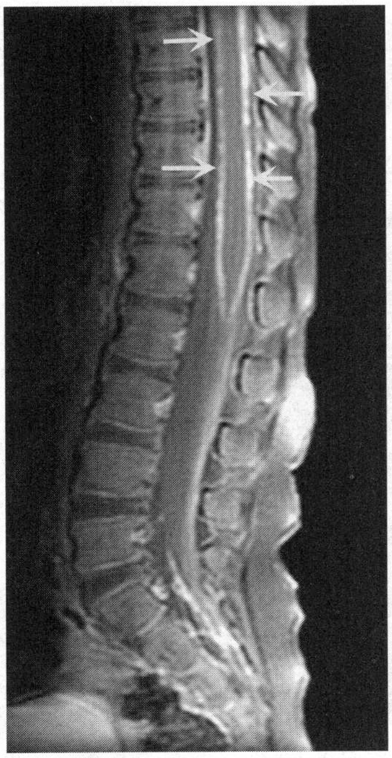

FIGURE 375-7 Carcinomatous meningitis. Sagittal postcontrast MRI through the lower thoracic region demonstrates diffuse pial enhancement along the surface of the spinal cord (*arrows*), typical of CSF spread of neoplasm.

Large deposits of tumor on the meninges or along nerve roots are unlikely to respond to intrathecal chemotherapy, as the barrier to diffusion is too great. Therefore, external beam radiation is employed. Hydrocephalus is treated with a ventriculoperitoneal shunt; although seeding of the peritoneum by tumor is possible, it is rare in clinical practice.

MALIGNANT SPINAL CORD COMPRESSION

Spinal cord compression from solid tumor metastases usually results from expansion of a vertebral metastasis into the epidural space. Primary tumors that frequently metastasize to bone include lung, breast, and prostate cancer (Table 375-3). *Back pain* is usually the first symptom and is prominent at presentation in 90 percent of patients. The pain is typically dull, aching, and may be associated with localized tenderness. If a nerve root is compressed, radicular pain is also present. The neurologic signs that accompany spinal cord compression are determined by the level of the lesion; the thoracic cord is most often affected. Weakness, followed by *sensory loss* and *autonomic dysfunction* (urinary urgency and incontinence, fecal incontinence, and sexual impotence in men) are the hallmarks. Once signs of spinal cord compression appear they tend to progress rapidly. It is thus essential to recognize and treat this devastating complication of malignancy at the earliest possible time in order to prevent irreversible neurologic deficits. → ***Diagnosis and management are discussed in Chap. 373.***

METASTASES TO THE PERIPHERAL NERVOUS SYSTEM

Systemic cancer may compress or invade peripheral nerves. Compression of the brachial plexus may occur by direct extension of Pancoast's tumors (cancer of the apex of the lung) or by extension of local lymph node metastases of breast or lung cancer or lymphoma. The lumbosacral plexus may be compressed by the retroperitoneal spread of prostate or ovarian cancer or lymphoma. Skull metastases may compress cranial nerve branches as they pass through the skull, and pituitary metastases may extend into the cavernous sinus. The epineurium generally provides an effective barrier to invasion of the peripheral nerves by solid tumors, but certain tumors have a special propensity to invade and spread along peripheral nerves. Squamous cell carcinoma of the skin may spread along branches of the trigeminal nerve and extend intracranially. Non-Hodgkin's lymphoma may be neurotrophic and cause a syndrome resembling mononeuropathy multiplex. If the tumor is not sensitive to systemic chemotherapy or hormonal therapy, focal external beam radiation may reduce pain, prevent irreversible loss of peripheral nerve function, and possibly restore function.

In cancer patients with brachial or lumbosacral plexopathy, it may be difficult to distinguish tumor recurrence from radiation injury. High radiation dose or the presence of myokymia (rippling contractions of muscle) suggests radiation injury, whereas pain suggests tumor recurrence. Radiographic imaging studies may be equivocal, and surgical exploration is sometimes required.

COMPLICATIONS OF THERAPY

RADIATION TOXICITY The nervous system is vulnerable to injury by therapeutic radiation, although DNA synthesis, a primary target of radiation, occurs infrequently. The precise mechanism of injury is unknown, but the peroxidation of lipids in myelin and neuronal cell membranes following radiation-induced free radical production is probably contributory. Histologically, there is demyelination, hyaline degeneration of small arterioles, and eventually brain infarction and necrosis. However, radiation injury can occur without vasculopathy, suggesting that ischemia is a late manifestation and does not entirely account for the tissue damage.

Radiation injury to the brain is classified by the time of its occurrence. *Acute radiation injury* occurs during or immediately following therapy. It is rarely seen with current protocols of external beam radiation but may occur following stereotaxic radiosurgery. Manifestations include headache, sleepiness, and worsening of preexisting neurologic deficits. *Early delayed radiation injury* occurs within 4 months of therapy. It is associated with increased white matter T2 signal on MRI scans. In children, a common form of early delayed radiation injury is the *somnolence syndrome*, in which somnolence and ataxia develop after whole-brain radiation. Radiation to the cervical spine may cause Lhermitte's phenomenon, an electricity-like sensation evoked by neck flexion (see Chap. 373). Acute and early delayed radiation injury are steroid-responsive and self-limited disorders and do not appear to increase the risk of late radiation injury.

Late delayed radiation injury produces permanent damage to the nervous system. It occurs more than 4 months (generally 8 to 24 months) after completion of therapy; onset 15 years after therapy has been described. Following whole-brain irradiation, progressive dementia occurs, sometimes accompanied by gait apraxia. White matter signal abnormalities are present on MRI studies (Fig. 375-8). Following focal brain irradiation, radiation necrosis occurs within the radiation field, producing a contrast-enhanced mass, frequently with ring enhancement (Fig. 375-9). MRI or CT scans are often unable to distinguish radiation necrosis from recurrent tumor, but PET scans may demonstrate that glucose metabolism is increased in tumor tissue but decreased in radiation necrosis. Biopsy is frequently required to establish the correct diagnosis. *Peripheral nerves*, including the brachial and lumbosacral plexuses, may also develop late delayed radiation injury over a time span similar to that observed in the CNS.

If untreated, radiation necrosis of the CNS usually acts as an expanding mass lesion, although it may resolve spontaneously or after steroid treatment. Progressive radiation necrosis is best treated with surgical resection if the patient has a life expectancy of at least 6 months and a good Karnofsky performance score. There are anecdotal reports that anticoagulation with heparin or coumadin may be beneficial. Radiation injury also accelerates the development of atherosclerosis in large arteries, but an increase in the risk of stroke becomes significant only years following radiation treatment.

Endocrine dysfunction frequently follows exposure of the hypothalamus or pituitary gland to therapeutic radiation. Growth hormone is

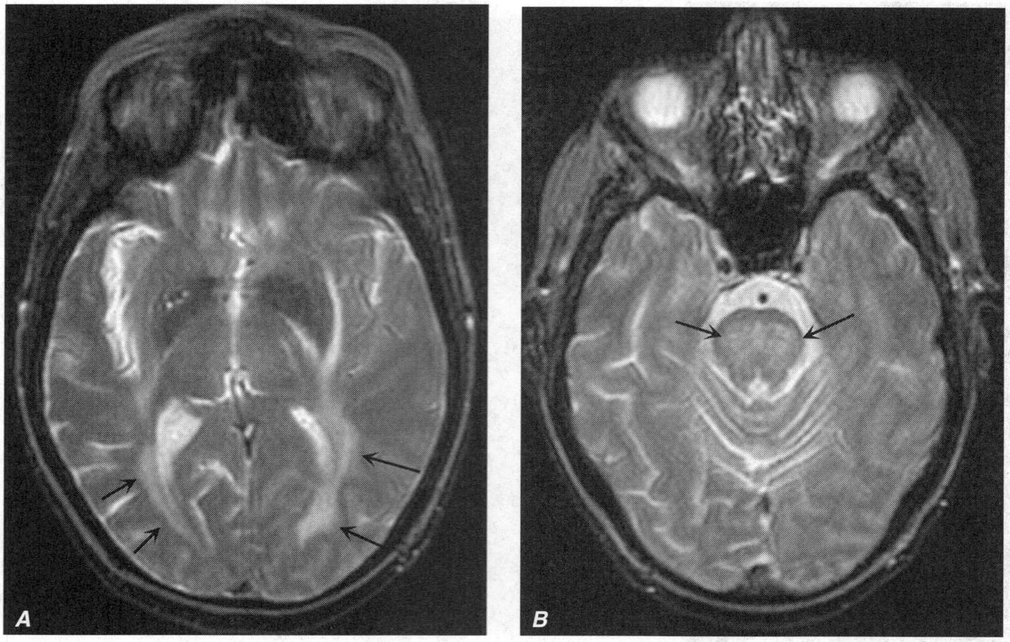

FIGURE 375-8 Late delayed radiation injury 1 year following whole-brain radiation (5500 cGy). *A*. T2-weighted MRI image at the level of the temporal lobes reveals high signal intensity abnormality in periventricular white matter (*arrows*). *B*. Diffuse high signal intensity in pontine white matter (*arrows*) indicating demyelination or small vessel ischemic injury.

the pituitary hormone most sensitive to radiation therapy, and thyroid-stimulating hormone is the least sensitive; ACTH, prolactin, and the gonadotropins have an intermediate sensitivity.

Development of a second neoplasm is another risk of therapeutic radiation that generally occurs many years after radiation exposure. Depending on the radiated field, the risk of gliomas, meningiomas, sarcomas, and thyroid cancer is increased. With most high-grade gliomas and nervous system metastases, patients generally do not survive to experience these late complications of radiation therapy.

COMPLICATIONS OF CHEMOTHERAPY Chemotherapy regimens used for primary brain tumors are generally based on a nitrosourea and are well tolerated. Infrequently, nitrosoureas and other drugs used for CNS neoplasms cause altered mental states (e.g., confusion, depression), ataxia, and seizures. Chemotherapy employed for systemic malignancy is a more frequent cause of nervous system toxicity. Cisplatin commonly produces tinnitus and high-frequency bilateral hearing loss, especially in younger patients. At cumulative doses exceeding 450 mg/m^2, cisplatin can produce a symmetric, large fiber axonal neuropathy. Fluorouracil can cause cerebellar dysfunction that resolves following discontinuation of therapy; paclitaxel (Taxol) produces a similar picture. Vincristine, which is commonly used to treat lymphoma, may cause an acute ileus that requires discontinuation of the drug and is frequently associated with development of a progressive distal, symmetric sensory-motor neuropathy with foot drop and paresthesia.

BIBLIOGRAPHY

BIGNER SH: Cerebrospinal fluid cytology: Current status and diagnostic applications. J Neuropath Exp Neurol 51:235, 1992

BYRNE TN: Spinal cord compression from epidural metastases. N Engl J Med 327:614, 1992

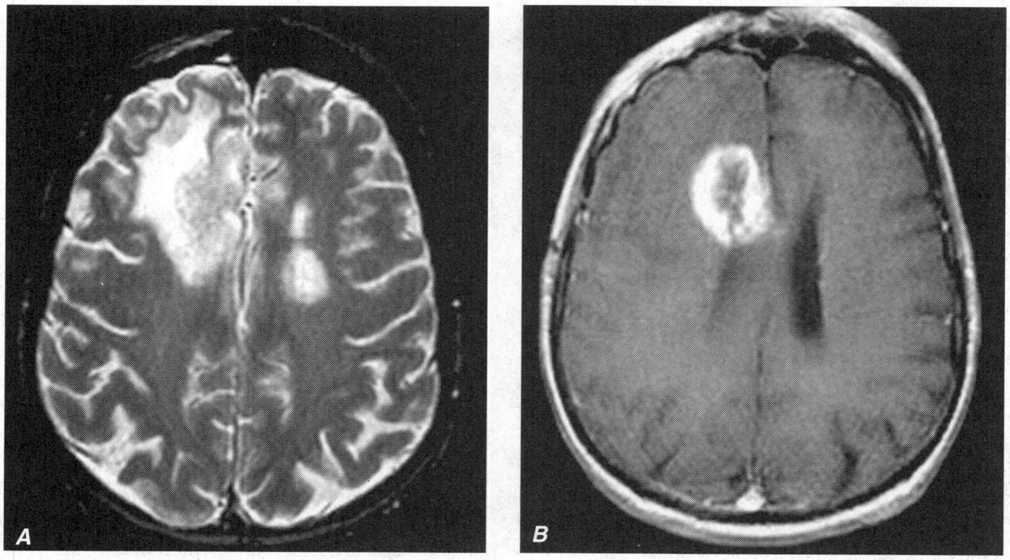

FIGURE 375-9 Focal radiation necrosis 3 years after radiotherapy (7000 cGy) for carcinoma of the nasopharynx. *A*. Axial T2-weighted MRI demonstrates a mass in the right frontal lobe with surrounding vasogenic edema. Abnormal signal changes are also present on the left. *B*. T1-weighted postcontrast MRI reveals a heterogeneously enhancing mass in the right cingulate gyrus.

GLANTZ MJ et al: Treatment of radiation-induced nervous system injury with heparin and warfarin. Neurology 44:2020, 1994
KORI SH et al: Brachial plexus lesions in patients with cancer: 100 cases. Neurology 31:45, 1981
LI J et al: *PTEN*, a putative protein tyrasine phosphatase gene mutated in human brain, breast, and prostate cancer. Science 275:1943, 1997
LUNDBERG N: Continuous recording and control of ventricular pressure in neurosurgical practice. Acta Psychiatr Scand 36(Suppl 149):1, 1960
MCKUSICK VA (ed): *Online Mendelian Inheritance in Man*. URL: http://www3.ncbi.nlm.nih.gov80/Omim/. Washington, DC, National Library of Medicine, 1996
MECKLING S et al: Malignant supratentorial glioma in the elderly: Is radiotherapy useful? Neurology 47:901, 1996
MORANTZ RA, WALSH JW: *Brain Tumors*. New York, Marcel Dekker, 1994
PATCHELL RA et al: A randomized trial of surgery in the treatment of single metastases to the brain. N Engl J Med 322:494, 1990
PORTENOY RK et al: Back pain in the cancer patient: An algorithm for evaluation and management. Neurology 37:134, 1987
POSNER JB: *Neurologic Complications of Cancer*. Philadelphia, FA Davis, 1995
RUSSELL DS, RUBINSTEIN LJ: *Pathology of Tumors of the Nervous System*, 5th ed. Baltimore, Williams & Wilkins, 1989
SKLAR CA, CONSTINE LS: Chronic neuroendocrinological sequelae of radiation therapy. Int J Radiation Oncol Biol Phys 31:1113, 1995
WASSERSTROM WR et al: Diagnosis and treatment of leptomeningeal metastases from solid tumors. Cancer 49:759, 1982
WILSON CB: Meningiomas: Genetics, malignancy, and the role of radiation in induction and treatment. J Neurosurg 81:666, 1994

376

Stephen L. Hauser, Donald E. Goodkin

MULTIPLE SCLEROSIS AND OTHER DEMYELINATING DISEASES

The demyelinating diseases occupy a unique place in neurology owing to their frequency; their tendency to strike young adults; their diversity of manifestations, which challenges the most skilled clinician; and the range of fundamental questions in neurobiology, immunology, virology, and genetics that arise regarding their pathogenesis. These disorders share the common features of inflammation and selective destruction of central nervous system (CNS) myelin. Their course may be chronic (multiple sclerosis) or acute (acute disseminated encephalomyelitis and acute hemorrhagic leukoencephalitis). The peripheral nervous system (PNS) is generally spared. No specific tests for the demyelinating diseases exist, and diagnosis is based on recognition of the distinctive clinical patterns of CNS injury they produce.

MULTIPLE SCLEROSIS

Multiple sclerosis (MS) is characterized by chronic inflammation, demyelination, and gliosis (scarring). Lesions of MS are classically said to be disseminated in time and space. MS affects 350,000 Americans and is, with the exception of trauma, the most frequent cause of neurologic disability commencing in early to middle adulthood. Indirect evidence supports an autoimmune etiology for MS, likely triggered by an environmental exposure in a genetically susceptible host. As in other chronic inflammatory disorders, the manifestations of MS are variable and range from a benign illness to a rapidly evolving and incapacitating disease. Complications from MS may affect multiple body systems and require profound adjustments in life-style and goals for patients and their families; hence, a multidisciplinary approach is necessary to optimize clinical care.

PATHOLOGIC FEATURES MS derives its name from the multiple scarred areas visible on macroscopic examination of the brain. These lesions, termed *plaques*, are well-demarcated gray or pink areas easily distinguished from surrounding white matter. Occasionally, plaques are also present in gray matter. Plaques vary in size from 1 or 2 mm to several centimeters. The acute MS lesion, rarely found at autopsy, is characterized by perivenular cuffing and tissue infiltration by mononuclear cells, predominantly T lymphocytes and macrophages. B cells and plasma cells are rarely found. The inflammatory infiltrates are associated with dissolution of the multilamellated myelin sheaths that surround axon cylinders. As the lesion evolves, large numbers of macrophages and microglial cells (specialized CNS phagocytes of bone marrow origin) scavenge the myelin debris, and proliferation of astrocytes (gliosis) occurs. Proliferation of oligodendrocytes, the myelin-producing cells, also occurs initially in some MS lesions, but these cells appear to be destroyed as the infiltration and gliosis progress. As a general rule, gliosis is more severe in MS lesions than in other neuropathologic conditions. Chronic MS lesions consist of complete or nearly complete demyelination, dense gliosis, and loss of oligodendroglia. In some plaques (chronic active lesions), gradations in histologic findings from the center to the lesion edge suggest that lesions expand by gradual concentric outward growth.

Lesions of MS are typically more numerous than anticipated on the basis of clinical criteria. Selective demyelination with sparing of axon cylinders is the hallmark of the disease, yet partial or total axonal destruction, and in extreme cases cavitation, may occur. Although partial remyelination (resulting in shadow plaques) is present in some lesions, more often significant remyelination does not occur. The correspondence between number and size of plaques ("plaque burden") and the severity of clinical symptoms is imprecise. Hence an extensive plaque burden may be associated with mild symptoms, or, conversely, seemingly minor pathologic changes may be present in some severely disabled individuals. Occasional cases either are clinically silent or produce "nonspecific" isolated symptoms such as facial pain, and evidence of MS is found unexpectedly at autopsy.

PATHOPHYSIOLOGY Experimental studies indicate that demyelination may have either negative or positive effects on axonal conduction. Negative conduction abnormalities consist of slowed axonal conduction, variable conduction block that occurs in the presence of high- but not low-frequency trains of impulses, or complete conduction block. Conduction block in demyelinated fibers also may occur in response to raised temperature or with metabolic changes in the extracellular milieu of axons. Positive conduction abnormalities include ectopic impulse generation, spontaneously or following mechanical stress, and abnormal "crosstalk" between demyelinated axons. Conduction block may account for the fluctuations in function that vary from hour to hour and from day to day in MS and for the worsening that follows elevation in core body temperature. Ectopic impulse generation or "crosstalk" might give rise to Lhermitte's symptom, paroxysmal symptoms, or paresthesia (see below). Experimental therapies based on postulated conduction abnormalities in MS have included the use of calcium channel blockers to reduce the threshold for impulse generation and pharmacologic blockade (with 4-aminopyridine) of voltage-dependent potassium channels that are exposed in the internodal axon membrane following myelin loss.

PATHOGENESIS **Epidemiology** MS is approximately twice as common in females as in males. MS is unusual before adolescence; its incidence rises steadily from the teens to age 35 and declines gradually thereafter. The age of onset is slightly later in men than in women. MS beginning as early as age 2 or as late as the eighth decade of life is rare but well documented.

Different populations and ethnic groups have a markedly different prevalence of MS. The highest known prevalence (250 per 100,000) occurs in the Orkney islands, located north of the mainland of Scotland, and MS is also common in Scandinavia and throughout northern Europe. In the United States, the prevalence of MS is higher in Caucasians than in other racial groups, consistent with observations in other parts of the world. MS is extremely rare in Japan (2 per 100,000) and is essentially unknown in black Africans, yet Japanese Americans and African Americans are at significant risk of developing MS, with respective prevalence rates estimated at one-quarter and one-third that of Caucasian Americans.

MS is in general a disease of temperate climates. In both hemispheres, its prevalence increases with distance from the equator. Comparison of North American and European populations reveals similar prevalence rates and north-south gradients. Migration data in well-defined ethnic populations also support an effect of environment on risk. Numerous studies suggest that the prevalence of MS may be increasing, but it is possible that this finding represents an artifact due to improvements in diagnosis. Other evidence for an environmental effect on MS is derived from possible point epidemics that have occurred, e.g., the cluster of MS cases that appeared in the Faeroe Islands off the coast of Denmark following the British occupation during World War II.

Genetics Evidence for genetic susceptibility to MS has been identified in studies of ethnic groups and in family, adoption, and twin studies. Differences in the prevalence of MS among ethnic groups that reside in the same environment support an underlying genetic predisposition. Familial aggregation is also known to occur in MS, and first-, second-, and third-degree relatives of patients are at increased risk for the disease. Siblings of affected individuals have a lifetime risk for MS of 2 to 5 percent, whereas the risk for parents or to children of affected individuals is somewhat lower. Recent adoption and half-sibling studies from Canada support the concept that familial aggregation in MS is determined by genetics rather than environment. Perhaps the most compelling evidence for a genetic effect on MS is derived from twin studies, which demonstrate concordance rates of 25 to 30 percent in monozygotic twins and of only 2 to 5 percent in dizygotic twins.

A simple genetic model for the inheritance of MS is unlikely to be valid. A single-gene hypothesis is at odds with concordance estimates in twin and family studies and with the observed nonlinear decrease in disease risk as the genetic distance from the MS proband is increased. It is likely that susceptibility is determined by multiple independent genetic loci (polygenic inheritance), each with a relatively small contribution to the overall risk. It is also possible that different genetic causes of susceptibility to MS (genetic heterogeneity) may exist. Linkage and association studies have identified the major histocompatibility complex (MHC) on chromosome 6 as one genetic determinant for MS. This complex encodes the histocompatibility antigens (the HLA system) that present peptide antigens to T cells. The class II (HLA-D) region of the MHC is most strongly associated with MS, and susceptibility appears to result from the presence of the DR2 allele and its corresponding haplotype, defined by molecular criteria as DRB1 *1501, DQA1*0102, DQB1*0602. Attempts to further localize a susceptibility gene within the DR-DQ region have not provided consensus, owing to strong linkage disequilibrium across this region. In addition to the HLA region, some studies have implicated other genes, including the T cell receptor (TCR) β chain region on chromosome 7, the immunoglobulin heavy chain locus on chromosome 19, and, in a Finnish MS population but not other populations, a gene linked to myelin basic protein on chromosome 18.

Immunology MS appears to be an autoimmune disease mediated, at least in part, by T lymphocytes. In the laboratory model experimental allergic encephalomyelitis (EAE), an autoimmune disease resembling MS is induced by immunization with CNS antigens. Depending on the strain of animal or the immunization regimen used, antigens that can elicit EAE are the quantitatively major myelin proteins myelin basic protein (MBP) and proteolipid protein (PLP), the quantitatively minor protein myelin oligodendrocyte glycoprotein (MOG), and other myelin proteins or neural antigens. The sequence of immunopathogenic events in EAE is as follows. (1) Neural antigens are processed by antigen-presenting cells (APCs) in regional lymph nodes and presented to T cells capable of recognizing them. (2) Small numbers of sensitized memory T cells migrate to the CNS, where they are reactivated by antigen presented by macrophages or microglial cells. (3) Proinflammatory cytokines, including interleukin (IL) 1, tumor necrosis factor (TNF) α, RANTES, and interferon (IFN) γ, are secreted that enhance expression of adhesion molecules by vascular endothelium, alter the permeability of the blood-brain barrier, and induce a second wave of inflammatory cell recruitment to the site. (4) Multiple effector mechanisms may contribute to the formation of EAE lesions, including autoantibodies, cytotoxicity mediated by T cells or natural killer cells, and cytokine-mediated injury to oligodendrocytes or myelin. In EAE, disease-inducing T cells most often recognize MBP or PLP, whereas autoantibodies appear to recognize MOG preferentially. The localization of MOG on the external surface of the myelin membrane probably facilitates its targeting by pathogenic antibody.

In MS, MBP-reactive T cells that carry mutations in a marker gene can be isolated from the peripheral blood. Presumably, these mutations result from chronic stimulation of MBP reactive T cells in vivo, and this finding appears to be specific for MS. The frequency of T cells reactive against either MBP or PLP is also higher in cerebrospinal fluid (CSF) than in peripheral blood in MS patients, indicating selective homing of autoreactive T cells to the CNS. Direct evidence that MBP reactive T cells are also present in MS lesions has been suggested based upon sequence analysis of the antigen-binding domain of TCR molecules expressed in brain lesions.

The diversity of the T cell response against MBP has been of considerable interest in MS. In rodents, EAE-inducing T cells recognize limited regions of the MBP molecule, termed *immunodominant regions*. These disease-inducing T cells may also express a limited repertoire of TCR genes. The limited heterogeneity of the T cell response in EAE has been exploited for therapeutic purposes, for example, by administration of synthetic peptides that resemble disease-inducing fragments of MBP but do not activate disease-inducing T cells or by immunization (vaccination) with synthetic peptides corresponding to TCR sequences present on pathogenic T cells. While effective against EAE, the usefulness of these and related approaches for the treatment of MS is uncertain. In MS, the repertoire of T cells capable of reacting against proteins of myelin appears to be heterogeneous as a rule, although immunodominant regions can be identified in some patients; for example, the region of MBP spanning amino acids 89 to 101 appears to be preferentially recognized in DR2-positive individuals.

Elevated levels of immunoglobulin in the CNS are also characteristic of MS. Membrane attack complexes can be detected in the CSF of MS patients, suggesting a role for complement-mediated antibody damage. Oligoclonal antibody—derived from expansion of a small number of different molecules—is also present in most cases. Oligoclonal Ig is also detected in other chronic inflammatory responses, including infections, and thus is not specific to MS. It is synthesized locally, and the specific pattern or fingerprint is unique to each patient. Attempts to identify an antigen against which most oligoclonal Ig is directed have been unsuccessful.

It is probable that cytokines regulate many of the cellular interactions that operate in MS. A large number of proinflammatory cytokines [IL-1, IL-2, IL-6, RANTES, macrophage inhibitory protein (MIP)-1α, TNFα, TNFβ, IFNγ] and regulatory cytokines [(IL-10, IL-4), transforming growth factor β (TGF-β)] have been detected in brain, CSF, and peripheral blood of MS patients. TNFα or IFNγ may contribute directly to tissue damage by injuring oligodendrocytes or the myelin membrane.

Patients with MS may experience relapses following nonspecific upper respiratory infections, suggesting that molecular mimicry between virus and myelin antigens may trigger attacks, or that some viruses may function as superantigens capable of activating disease-inducing T cells in MS.

Virology As noted above, epidemiologic evidence supports the role of an environmental exposure in MS. MS risk also correlates with high socioeconomic status, which may reflect improved sanitation and delayed initial exposures to infectious agents. Some viruses, e.g., poliomyelitis and measles viruses, produce neurologic sequelae that are more common when the age of initial infection is delayed.

Higher antibody titers against many viruses, including measles, herpes simplex, varicella, rubella, Epstein-Barr, and influenza-C viruses and some parainfluenza virus strains, have been detected in serum and CSF samples of MS patients compared to control individuals. In addition, a number of viruses or viral sequences have been recovered from MS tissues and fluids; recently, human herpes virus type 6 (HHV-6) antigen was reported to be commonly expressed in MS plaques. To date, no virus has been isolated consistently, nor viral material identified uniquely, from MS patients. In animals, the most widely studied model of virus-induced demyelinating disease has been infection with Theiler virus, a murine coronavirus similar to measles virus and canine distemper virus. Infection with some Theiler strains results in a chronic infection of oligodendrocytes with multifocal perivascular lymphocytic infiltration and demyelination.

CLINICAL MANIFESTATIONS (See Table 376-1) The onset of MS may be dramatic or so mild as not to cause a patient to seek medical attention. In most published series, the most common initial symptoms were weakness in one or more limbs, visual blurring due to optic neuritis, sensory disturbances, diplopia, and ataxia.

Weakness of the limbs may appear insidiously as fatigue with exertion, a disturbance of gait, or loss of dexterity. Patients may report injury and stubbing of the great toe due to a subtle foot drop. At an early stage of the disease, weakness may not be detectable on testing. Increased motor tone (spasticity), hyperreflexia, an extensor plantar response, a Hoffmann reflex, and absence of the superficial abdominal reflex, all indicative of pyramidal tract disease, may be present. Occasionally, a tendon reflex, e.g., a triceps jerk, may be lost owing to a focal lesion in the dorsal root entry zone through which the afferent fibers of the motor reflex arc pass, simulating a radiculopathy.

Sensory symptoms include paresthesia (tingling, "pins and needles," or painful burning) or hypesthesia (numbness or a "dead" feeling). Sensory symptoms often begin in a focal area of a limb, the torso, or the head and spread over hours or days to adjacent ipsilateral or contralateral areas of the body. Involvement of segmental areas of the trunk with a "cord level" is diagnostically helpful because it distinguishes the spinal cord origin of the sensory attack from peripheral neuropathy due to the Guillain-Barré syndrome or other causes. In patients with established sensory deficits, complaints of unpleasant feelings of "swollen," "wet,", "raw", or "tightly wrapped" body parts are common.

Cerebellar involvement results in ataxia of gait and limbs. In advanced MS, cerebellar dysarthria (scanning speech) is common. In individual patients, the contribution of cerebellar involvement to specific symptoms may be difficult to define when motor and sensory deficits are also present.

Optic neuritis, common in MS, produces variable visual loss. It usually begins as blurring of the central visual field, which may remain mild or progress to severe visual loss, or, rarely, to complete loss of light perception. In mild cases, the patient may complain only of a subjective loss of brightness in the affected eye. Symptoms are generally monocular, but attacks may be bilateral. Pain, localized to the orbit or supraorbital area, is frequently present and may precede visual loss. The pain typically worsens with eye movement. Diminished visual acuity can usually be documented on routine examination, and a scotoma (a focal area of visual loss) may be found. An afferent pupillary response (pupillodilation on exposure to direct light following constriction in response to indirect light) may be detected by a swinging flashlight test. In severe cases, the pupil on the affected side may be enlarged or irregular. Funduscopic examination may be normal or reveal swelling of the optic disc (papillitis). Venous sheathing of retinal vessels, due to the transendothelial migration of lymphocytes, is present in approximately 25 percent of cases. Pallor of the optic disc (optic atrophy) commonly follows bouts of optic neuritis. Rarely, uveitis also is present.

Table 376-1

Initial Symptoms of MS

Symptom	Percent of Cases	Symptom	Percent of Cases
Weakness	35	Lhermitte	3
Sensory loss	37	Pain	3
Paresthesias	24	Dementia	2
Optic neuritis	36	Visual loss	2
Diplopia	15	Facial palsy	1
Ataxia	11	Impotence	1
Vertigo	6	Myokymia	1
Paroxysmal attacks	4	Epilepsy	1
Bladder	4	Falling	1

SOURCE: After WB Matthews et al, *McAlpine's Multiple Sclerosis,* New York, Churchill Livingstone, 1991.

Visual blurring in MS may result from optic neuritis or diplopia. These two causes are distinguished by asking the patient to cover each eye sequentially and observing whether the visual difficulty clears. Diplopia in MS is often due to an internuclear ophthalmoplegia (INO) or to a sixth nerve palsy; ocular muscle palsies due to involvement of the third or fourth cranial nerve are rare. An INO consists of a delay or complete loss of adduction on attempted horizontal gaze to one side accompanied by nystagmus in the abducting eye. Convergence is preserved, which distinguishes INO from medial rectus palsy. An INO results from involvement of the crossed medial longitudinal fasciculus that connects contralateral third and sixth cranial nerve nuclei; involvement is usually on the side of the adducting eye. The finding of bilateral INO in an awake patient is highly suggestive of MS. Other gaze deficits include horizontal gaze palsy due to ipsilateral lesions of the lateral pontine tegmentum and the "one and a half" syndrome, consisting of a horizontal gaze palsy to one direction and an INO to the other.

Trigeminal neuralgia is a lancinating shocklike facial pain. In patients over 50 years of age, idiopathic trigeminal neuralgia is common and is only rarely due to MS (see Chap. 372). In patients with trigeminal neuralgia, clinical features that raise a question of underlying MS include onset at a young age, bilateral occurrence, objective facial sensory loss, and constant rather than paroxysmal pain.

Facial paralysis, resembling idiopathic Bell's palsy, may be due to MS. In MS, facial palsy is usually not associated with ipsilateral loss of taste sensation or retroaural pain, two characteristics of Bell's palsy. Chronic flickering contractions of the facial musculature, termed *facial myokymia*, is common in MS; it is thought to arise from involvement of corticobulbar tracts and deafferentation of the facial nucleus. Less commonly, facial hemispasm may occur.

Vertigo may appear suddenly and in dramatic fashion with gait unsteadiness and vomiting, resembling acute labyrinthitis. A brainstem rather than end-organ origin of vertigo is suggested by the presence of "neighborhood" signs, including trigeminal or facial nerve involvement, vertical nystagmus, or type 3 nystagmus on Bárány testing (i.e., no latency, no direction reversal, and no fatigue). Hearing loss also may occur in MS but is unusual.

Urinary bladder urgency, hesitancy, incomplete emptying, or incontinence occurs at some time in most MS patients and may be present at onset. Constipation, fecal urgency, or bowel incontinence also occur, especially in advanced MS.

Cognitive dysfunction is common in advanced MS and may also develop at an early stage or even at the onset of disease. Memory loss, impaired attention, problem-solving difficulties, slowed information processing, and difficulty in shifting between cognitive tasks are the most frequent cognitive changes observed. Impaired judgment or inappropriate jocularity may also be present. Pseudobulbar palsy consists of emotional lability, usually presenting as episodes of uncontrollable laughter or crying, associated with hyperactive facial reflexes, spastic dysarthria, and dysphagia. Depression is also common in MS.

Ancillary Symptoms Lhermitte's symptom is a momentary electric-like sensation evoked by neck flexion, other neck movements, or coughing. The symptom typically is experienced as a shooting phenomenon that travels down the spine and into the legs. Variants of Lhermitte's symptom include other tingling or painful sensations induced by neck movements, spread of the symptoms to the arms, and induction of the symptoms by movements of the lumbar spine. Lhermitte's symptom is common in MS but also occurs with many other disorders of the cervical spinal cord.

Heat sensitivity, i.e., the appearance or worsening of symptoms upon exposure to heat (typically a hot shower), occurs in most patients with MS. One characteristic form of heat sensitivity is Uhthoff's symptom, in which transient visual blurring, generally monocular, occurs with exercise or heat exposure.

Fatigue occurs in most MS patients. Fatigue is typically present in midafternoon and may consist of increased motor weakness, mental fatigue, or lassitude and sleepiness.

Paroxysmal attacks are brief, stereotyped, recurrent phenomena that frequently occur at the onset of MS or early in its course. Typical is the "tonic seizure," an unpleasant tingling or other sensation associated with tonic contraction of a limb, face, or trunk. Others consist of paroxysmal dysarthria and ataxia, diplopia, or transient unilateral paralysis, paresthesia, or pain. Attacks may be momentary or persist for 30 s or longer. They generally begin in clusters, occurring many times daily, and the patient may identify precipitating factors, such as hyperventilation or particular movements.

DISEASE COURSE The various clinical courses of MS, illustrated in Fig. 376-1, may be grouped into four general categories. The first, *relapsing-remitting MS*, is characterized by unpredictable recurrent attacks of neurologic dysfunction. MS attacks generally evolve over days to weeks and may be followed by complete, partial, or no recovery. Recovery from attacks generally occurs within weeks to several months from the peak of symptoms, although rarely some recovery may continue for 2 or more years. Patients with a relapsing-remitting course experience no progression of neurologic impairment between attacks. This pattern characterizes the early course of the disease in most patients. In the second clinical pattern, *secondary progressive MS*, the disease has a relapsing-remitting pattern at first but evolves to be progressive. The progressive phase may begin shortly after disease onset or be delayed for several years or decades. The secondary progressive phase is distinguished from the relapsing-remitting phase by gradual progression of disability between attacks or gradual progression of disability after attacks are no longer evident.

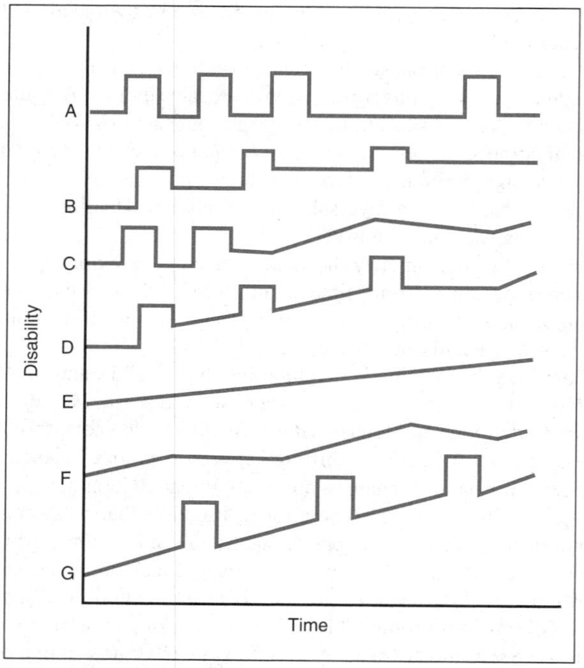

FIGURE 376-1 Clinical patterns of MS. A, B, relapsing-remitting; C, D, secondary-progressive; E, F, primary-progressive; G, progressive-relapsing.

A third pattern of MS, *primary progressive MS*, is characterized by gradual progression of disability from the onset of the disease. In some patients, periods of apparent clinical stability may occur, but there are no distinct relapses. *Primary progressive MS* affects fewer than 15 percent of all patients but is the most common form of MS in late-onset cases (i.e., after age 40). Occasionally, patients who appear to have primary progressive MS will experience superimposed relapses. This uncommon clinical course is known as *progressive-relapsing MS*.

Although the clinical course of MS is highly variable, some clinical and magnetic resonance imaging features appear to have prognostic value. Favorable prognostic factors include early onset (excluding childhood), visual or sensory symptoms alone at presentation, a relapsing-remitting course, and minimal neurologic impairment 5 years after onset. By contrast, poor prognosis is associated with truncal ataxia, severe action tremor, and a primary progressive disease course. In relapsing-remitting MS, disability results from poor or incomplete recovery from attacks in approximately half of patients and from an evolution to secondary progressive MS in the other half. In secondary or primary progressive MS, disability results from progressive spasticity, limb weakness, sphincter dysfunction, visual loss, or cognitive impairment. In general, the longer a cohort is followed, the smaller is the proportion of patients with mild disease. Fifteen years after diagnosis, approximately 20 percent of MS patients have no functional limitation, 70 percent are limited or unable to perform major activities of daily living, and 75 percent are not employed. In 1994, it was estimated that the total economic burden of MS in the United States was more than $9.7 billion.

In patients who experience a *first attack* of isolated optic neuritis, brainstem signs, or acute myelopathy, magnetic resonance imaging (MRI) of the head has been found to yield findings with some prognostic value. These patient groups are at high (50 to 65 percent) risk of developing clinically definite MS within 5 years if their brain MRI shows evidence of multiple T2-weighted lesions shortly after symptom onset. By contrast, patients with no evidence of disseminated disease by MRI at presentation have a low (5 percent) risk of developing MS over a 5 year period.

DIAGNOSIS The diagnosis of MS is usually easily made in a young adult with relapsing and remitting symptoms referable to different areas of CNS white matter. Diagnosis is more difficult in a patient with the recent onset of neurologic complaints or with a primary progressive clinical course. In such situations, the patient should be questioned carefully for a history of prior attacks that may not be recalled initially. Other presentations that may cause diagnostic uncertainty include symptoms with a rapid or even explosive onset, suggesting a cerebrovascular accident; progressive brainstem syndromes, raising a question of brainstem glioma; cervical myelopathy in the setting of degenerative disk disease; or mild symptoms (for example sensory symptoms) unaccompanied by objective signs on examination. Rarely, a mass lesion resulting from intense inflammation and swelling may occur in MS and falsely suggest a primary or metastatic tumor.

Examination reveals evidence of neurologic disease in the great majority of patients. Abnormal signs are often more widespread than expected from the interview. For example, an MS patient may present with symptoms in one leg and signs in both. This type of finding is helpful when it permits exclusion of a single focal lesion as the source of a patient's symptoms. Other MS patients may experience symptoms unaccompanied by objective neurologic signs. They are frequently misdiagnosed as suffering from a conversion reaction, a label that should be avoided unless rigid diagnostic criteria for that condition are met.

The differential diagnosis of MS will vary depending on the specific clinical situation. Numerous diagnostic formulas have been proposed (Table 376-2); while they are useful, they cannot replace sound clinical judgment. No clinical sign or diagnostic test finding is unique to MS. However, the presence of features that are uncommon or rare in MS should call the diagnosis into question. These include aphasia, extrapyramidal syndromes suggesting Parkinson's disease, chorea, isolated dementia, amyotrophy with fasciculations, peripheral neuropathy, seizures, and coma. In patients with mild symptoms, there is often little to be gained by making a diagnosis of definite MS, and a wise course of action may be to exclude other, potentially treatable causes of the presenting symptoms.

Systemic lupus erythematosus (SLE) rarely produces a relapsing or progressive CNS disorder that mimics MS. Other signs of SLE are usually present, including an elevated erythrocyte sedimentation rate (ESR), autoantibodies, and evidence of systemic disease. Behçet's syndrome may produce a chronic illness with optic neuropathy and myelopathy but more often presents as an acute or subacute multifocal CNS disorder; the characteristic oral and genital lesions, associated uveitis, and elevated ESR are distinguishing features. Relapsing-remitting CNS disease also has been described in Sjögren's syndrome. Sarcoidosis may produce cranial nerve palsies (particularly of the seventh nerve), progressive optic atrophy, or myelopathy; lymphadenopathy, pulmonary or hepatic involvement, an elevated level of angiotensin-converting enzyme, and hypercalcemia may be present. Lyme borreliosis may involve the optic nerve, brainstem, or spinal cord in the absence of characteristic rash, fever, or meningoradiculitis. Other chronic infections, notably meningovascular syphilis, infection with human immunodeficiency virus (HIV) type 1, and infection with opportunistic pathogens, may need to be considered.

Human T lymphotropic virus (HTLV) type I–associated myelopathy (HAM; tropical spastic paraparesis) is characterized by back pain, progressive spasticity affecting predominantly the lower limbs, and bladder symptoms (see Chap. 379). Diagnosis is based on identification of specific antibody to HTLV-I in serum and CSF and by direct virus isolation. Infection with the HTLV-II retrovirus may cause a progressive myelopathy similar to that caused by HTLV-I.

Table 376-2

Diagnostic Criteria for MS

1. Examination must reveal *objective* abnormalities of the CNS.
2. Involvement must reflect predominantly disease of white matter long tracts, usually including (a) pyramidal pathways, (b) cerebellar pathways, (c) medial longitudinal fasciculus, (d) optic nerve, and (e) posterior columns.
3. Examination or history must implicate involvement of two or more areas of the CNS.
   a. MRI may be used to document a *second* lesion when only one site of abnormality has been demonstrable on examination. A confirmatory MRI must have either four lesions involving the white matter or three lesions if one is periventricular in location. Acceptable lesions must be greater than 3 mm in diameter. For patients older than 50 years, two of the following criteria must also be met: (a) lesion size >5 mm; (b) lesions abut the bodies of the lateral ventricles, and (c) lesion(s) present in the posterior fossa.
   b. Evoked response testing may be used to document a *second* lesion not evident on clinical examination.
4. The clinical pattern must consist of (a) two or more separate *episodes* of worsening involving different sites of the CNS, each lasting at least 24 h and occurring at least 1 month apart, or (b) gradual or stepwise *progression* over at least 6 months if accompanied by increased CSF IgG synthesis or two or more oligoclonal bands.
5. Age of onset between 15 and 60 years.
6. The patient's neurologic condition could not better be attributed to another disease. Laboratory testing that may be advisable in certain cases includes (a) CSF analysis, (b) MRI of the head or spine, (c) serum vitamin B_{12} level, (d) human T cell lymphotropic virus type I (HTLV-I) titer, (e) erythrocyte sedimentation rate, (f) rheumatoid factor, antinuclear, anti-DNA antibodies (SLE), (g) serum VDRL, (h) angiotensin-converting enzyme (sarcoidosis), (i) *Borrelia* serology (Lyme disease), (j) very long chain fatty acids (adrenoleukodystrophy), and (k) serum or CSF lactate, muscle biopsy, or mitochondrial DNA analysis (mitochondrial disorders).

DIAGNOSTIC CATEGORIES

1. *Definite MS:* All six criteria fulfilled.
2. *Probable MS:* All six criteria fulfilled except (a) only one objective abnormality despite two symptomatic episodes or (b) only one symptomatic episode despite two or more objective abnormalities.
3. *At risk for MS:* All six criteria fulfilled except only one symptomatic episode and one objective abnormality.

As noted above, the acute onset of a focal CNS disturbance in a previously healthy individual may suggest a stroke or migraine. Progressive focal deficits should always prompt consideration of a compressive lesion. Primary CNS lymphoma may produce solitary or multiple lesions that show contrast enhancement on MRI and may resemble acute lesions of MS. A progressive or relapsing brainstem disturbance may be due to a vascular malformation in the posterior fossa. Pontine glioma is distinguished from MS by its tendency to produce progressive deficits that involve contiguous structures. Chiari malformations presenting in adulthood may cause cerebellar ataxia, nystagmus, and spastic weakness of the limbs; headache, lower cranial nerve palsies, and a syringomyelic syndrome are useful distinguishing features. Progressive myelopathies may result from cervical spondylosis, spinal cord tumor, or arteriovenous malformation (see Chap. 373).

Subacute combined degeneration and two related inherited defects—cobalamin G mutation and plasma R binder deficiency—may produce MS-like syndromes in the absence of megaloblastic anemia. If a screening serum vitamin B_{12} level is low, biologically significant vitamin B_{12} deficiency is suggested by the finding of elevated serum methylmalonic acid and homocysteine levels. Mitochondrial disorders, including subacute necrotic encephalopathy (Leigh's disease), mitochondrial encephalopathy with acidosis and stroke (MELAS), and Leber's hereditary optic neuropathy, can be excluded by measurement of blood and CSF lactate levels, by muscle biopsy, and by biochemical or DNA identification of the specific deficit. Heredity ataxias produce progressive symmetric involvement of posterior columns and corticospinal and spinocerebellar tracts, with or without involvement of the peripheral nervous system. Other single-gene disorders that may resemble MS include the autosomal recessive disorders metachro matic leukodystrophy and Krabbe disease and the X-linked disorders Fabry disease and adrenoleukodystrophy. The latter is of particular interest because it is associated with an intense CSF inflammatory response.

Neuromyelitis optica (Devic's syndrome) is characterized by acute bilateral optic neuritis, followed within days to weeks by transverse myelitis. On occasion, optic neuritis may be unilateral or occur following an initial bout of myelitis. This form of demyelinating disease is unusual in Caucasians and is more common in Asians. CNS lesions may be necrotizing and severe. CSF findings may consist of polymorphonuclear pleocytosis and an increase in the protein content. Neuromyelitis optica is often a self-limited syndrome but may occur as an initial manifestation of MS or in association with SLE, or Behçet's disease.

Laboratory Diagnosis CSF abnormalities consist of mononuclear cell pleocytosis, an elevation in the level of total Ig, and the presence of oligoclonal Ig. In one large series, CSF mononuclear pleocytosis (>5 cells/μL) was present in 25 percent of MS patients. CSF cell counts are generally less than 20/μL in MS, and counts above 50/μL are unusual but may occur at the onset of disease. Pleocytosis of >75 cells/μL or a finding of polymorphonuclear leukocytes in CSF makes the diagnosis of MS unlikely. Pleocytosis is more common in young patients with relapsing-remitting MS than in older patients with progressive forms of MS. In approximately 80 percent of patients, CSF IgG is increased with a normal total protein level, due to the selective production of IgG within the CNS. Occasional MS patients exhibit mild elevations in the total CSF protein content. Various formulas are employed to distinguish local synthesized IgG from serum IgG that may have entered the CNS passively across a disrupted blood-brain barrier. One useful formula expresses the ratio of IgG to albumin in the CSF divided by the ratio in the serum ("the CSF IgG index").

Oligoclonal banding of CSF IgG is detected by agarose gel electrophoresis techniques. Two or more oligoclonal bands are found in 75 to 90 percent of MS patients. Oligoclonal banding may be absent at the onset of MS, and in individual patients the number of bands present may increase with time. It is important that paired serum samples be studied to exclude a systemic origin of the oligoclonal bands.

Paraclinical tests for MS include evoked response testing and MRI. Evoked response testing may detect slowed or abnormal conduction in visual, auditory, somatosensory, or motor pathways. These tests employ computer averaging techniques to record the electrical response evoked in the nervous system following repetitive sensory or motor stimuli. One or several evoked responses are abnormal in 80 to 90 percent of patients with MS. Testing is of greatest value when it provides evidence of a second lesion in a patient with a single clinically apparent lesion or when it demonstrates an objective abnormality in a patient with subjective complaints and normal findings on neurologic examination. Slowing of evoked response latencies in MS is thought to result from loss of saltatory conduction along the course of demyelinated axons. Nonetheless, these changes are etiologically nonspecific and are also present in other conditions, including vascular disease, in which selective demyelination does not occur.

Widespread availability of MRI has revolutionized the diagnostic approach to the patient with suspected MS. Disease-related changes are detected by MRI in more than 90 percent of patients who otherwise meet diagnostic criteria for definite MS (Fig. 376-2 and 376-3). On inversion-recovery or T1-weighted imaging sequences, the brain may appear normal or show darkened (hypointense) punctate foci in the white matter. Characteristic changes of MS are best appreciated with spin-echo (T2-weighted) and proton-density sequences, in which abnormal hyperintense areas stand out brightly from the surrounding brain substance. Some foci that are hyperintense on T2-weighted images may appear to extend outward from the ventricular surface, corresponding to a pattern of perivenous demyelination that is observed pathologically in MS (Dawson's fingers). Lesions are also commonly found within the brainstem, cerebellum, and spinal cord. The presence of lesions in the corpus callosum may also be useful, as the corpus callosum is frequently involved in MS but not in most vascular disorders.

Following administration of the contrast agent gadolinium DPTA, foci of white matter enhancement may be present, due to extravasation of the injected substance across a disrupted blood-brain barrier. New T2-weighted lesions are generally preceded or accompanied by transient gadolinium enhancement on T1-weighted scans, and histopathologic data indicate that gadolinium leakage in MS correlates with perivenous inflammation. Focal lesions that appear during or after gadolinium enhancement on T2-weighted and proton-density images are not histopathologically specific; they may reflect edema, inflammation, demyelination, gliosis, or axonal loss.

Serial MRI studies indicate that new abnormal foci appear far more frequently than anticipated by clinical criteria, suggesting that flares of subclinical disease activity occur commonly in MS. There is only a limited correlation between the total volume of lesions visible on

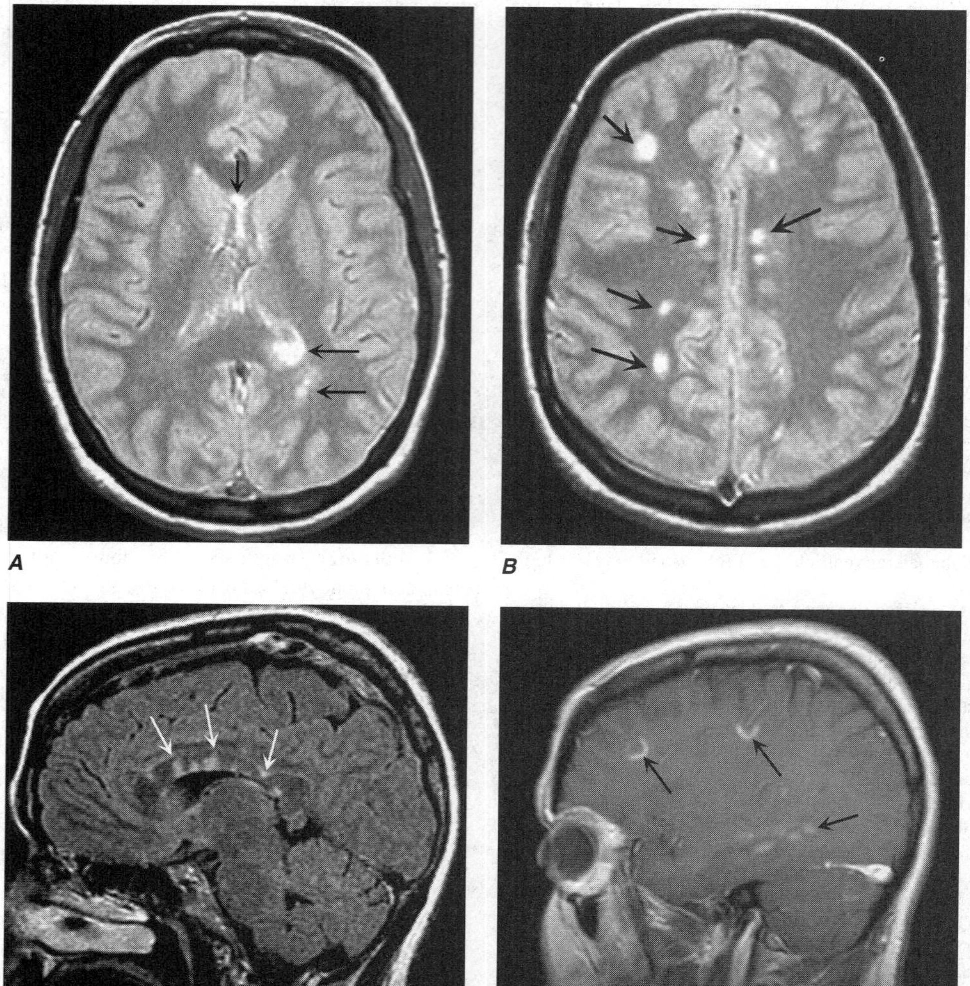

FIGURE 376-2 MRI findings in MS. *A, B.* Axial first-echo images from T2-weighted sequences demonstrate multiple bright signal abnormalities in white matter, typical for MS. *C.* Sagittal T2-weighted FLAIR (fluid attenuated inversion recovery) image in which the high signal of CSF has been suppressed. CSF appears dark, while areas of brain edema or demyelination appear high in signal as shown here in the corpus callosum (*arrows*). *D.* Sagittal T1-weighted image obtained after the intravenous administration of gadolinium DTPA reveals focal areas of blood-brain barrier disruption, identified as high-signal-intensity regions (*arrows*).

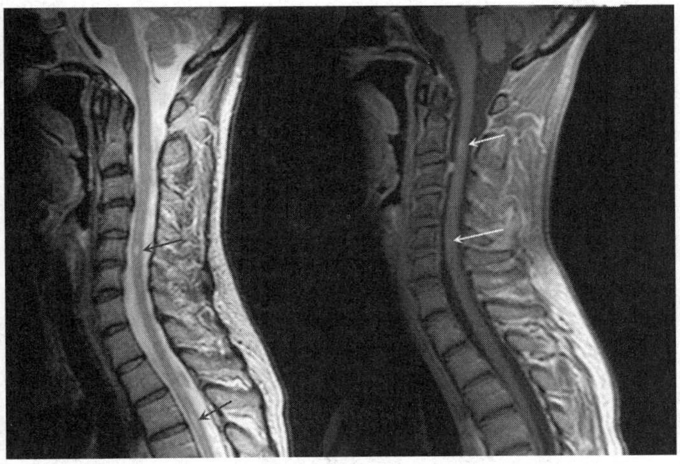

FIGURE 376-3 Spinal cord imaging in MS. Sagittal T2-weighted MRI scan (*left*) reveals multiple areas of bright signal abnormality (*black arrows*) within the spinal cord. In a T1 sequence (*right*), two discrete areas of contrast enhancement (*white arrows*) are present following administration of gadolinium EDTA.

T2-weighted scans and the clinical status of the patient. The correlation between MRI measures and clinical status may be improved by emerging imaging techniques, including magnetization transfer imaging, proton-magnetic resonance spectroscopy, and diffusion-weighted imaging, which better distinguish edema, demyelination, and axonal loss.

Criteria for use of MRI in support of a diagnosis of MS have been proposed. On T2-weighted or proton-density MRI brain scans, a finding of four or more focal lesions ≥3 mm in diameter or of three lesions of which one or more are periventricular in location strongly supports a diagnosis of definite MS in patients younger than 50 years. For patients older than 50 years, acceptable sensitivity and specificity are maintained by adding two of the following criteria: (1) lesion diameter greater than 5 mm, (2) the presence of lesion(s) abutting the bodies of the lateral ventricles, and (3) the presence of lesion(s) in the posterior fossa.

℞ TREATMENT

The treatment of MS may be divided into two categories: (1) treatment designed to arrest the disease process and (2) symptomatic management. The importance of longitudinal scoring of the functional consequences of MS cannot be overemphasized as an aid to decisions regarding therapy. The Kurtzke Expanded Disability Status Scale (EDSS) is the most widely used measure of neurologic impairment and disability in MS. It is based on composite scores of pyramidal, cerebellar, brainstem, sensory, bowel and bladder, visual, and mental functions (Table 376-3).

Disease Modifying Therapy (See Fig. 376-4) ***PROPHYLAXIS AGAINST RELAPSES*** Three treatments are available for patients with relapsing forms of MS: (1) IFNβ1b (Betaseron), (2) IFNβ1a (Avonex), and (3) copolymer 1 (Copaxone). There is a notion that patients with secondary progressive MS who experience frequent exacerbations may also benefit from these treatments. IFNβ1b, 8.0 million international units (MIU), is administered by subcutaneous injection every other day. IFNβ1a, 6.0 MIU, is administered by intramuscular injection once every week. Copolymer 1, 20 mg, is administered by subcutaneous injection every day. The mechanism of action of these treatments is not certain. IFNβ1b and -1a may act by down regulating the following: (1) the expression of MHC molecules on the surface of antigen presenting cells, (2) the actions of proinflammatory cytokines and, (3) the expression of vascular endothelial adhesion molecules that appear to mediate trafficking of activated lymphocytes and macrophages into the CNS. Copolymer 1 may act by (1) induction of antigen-specific suppressor T cells as a result of shared determinants between copolymer 1 and myelin basic protein and, (2) competitive binding to the MHC molecule on the surface of antigen-presenting cells. When compared to results in placebo recipients, each of these therapies reduces annual exacerbation rates by approximately one-third and IFNβ1b and -1a reduce the number of new lesions that are detected by monthly gadolinium-enhanced MRI scans. Of the three treatment options, IFNβ1a most convincingly delays the time to onset of sustained progression of disability. IFNβ1b and -1a and copolymer 1 are generally well tolerated. Erythematous injection site reactions are commonly experienced by IFNβ1b and copolymer 1 recipients. Approximately 15 percent of copolymer 1 recipients experience one or more episodes of flushing, chest tightness, dyspnea, palpitations, and anxiety following injection. This systemic reaction is unpredictable and generally lasts less than 1 h. Approximately 40 percent of IFNβ1b recipients and approximately 20 percent of IFNβ1a recipients develop neutralizing antibodies within 12 months of initiating therapy, and these patients may experience a return to their pretreatment attack rate. Treatment should probably be discontinued in IFNβ1b, -1a, and copolymer 1 recipients who continue to experience frequent attacks or gradual progression of disability for 6 or more months. It is unknown whether patients who fail treatment with one of these interventions will respond favorably to one of the alternatives or to combination therapy. Recently, intravenous immunoglobulin was also reported to be effective as prophylaxis against relapses, but confirmatory studies will be required before a role for this potential therapy is established.

ACUTE RELAPSES Acute relapses may be treated with a short course of intravenous methylprednisolone (MePDN) followed by oral prednisone (PDN) (Table 376-4). This combination has largely

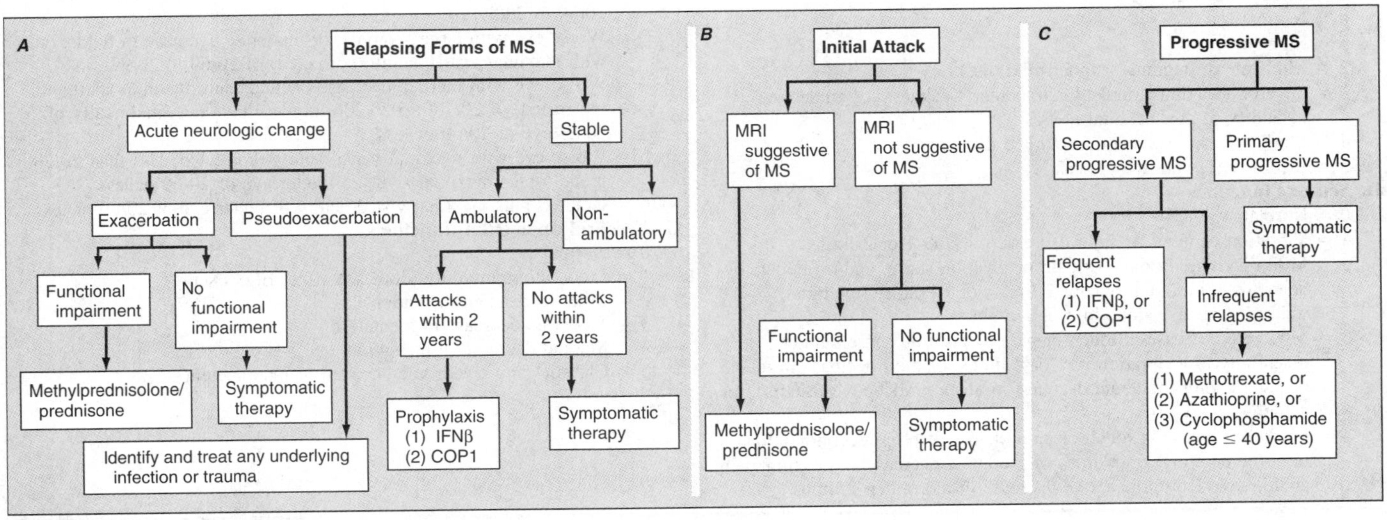

FIGURE 376-4 Therapeutic decision making for MS.

replaced adrenocorticotropic hormone (ACTH) as the mainstay of treatment, but courses of ACTH may still be used in selected patients or in cases of MePDN/PDN treatment failure. Pulse therapy with these agents speeds recovery from acute relapses and may modestly improve the degree of recovery occurring over a short follow-up period.

MePDN/PDN is generally used to treat moderate or severe attacks that result in functional disability that can be measured by changes on the EDSS. Severe attacks that jeopardize patient safety are best treated in the hospital with intravenous methylprednisolone or intramuscular ACTH and coordinated efforts by experts in multidisciplinary rehabilitation. Mild attacks, for example, subjective sensory symptoms unaccompanied by objective changes on examination, Lhermitte's symptom, or worsening of bladder function, are generally not treated.

When neurologic worsening occurs in patients with relapsing MS, it is useful to consider whether it reflects new inflammatory lesions in the CNS or whether it is a nonspecific consequence of infection (commonly a viral infection or urinary tract infection) or other intercurrent illness. MS typically worsens transiently following exposure of the patient to heat, stress, or infection. These "pseudoexacerbations" may consist only of recrudescences of old symptoms and may be short-lived (e.g., less than 48 h in duration). Patients with relapsing MS experience on average fewer than 1.0 true relapses per year.

Common side effects of short-term glucocorticoid therapy include fluid retention, potassium loss, weight gain, gastric distur-

Table 376-3

Scoring Systems for MS

KURTZKE EXPANDED DISABILITY SCORE (EDSS)

- 0.0 = Normal neurologic exam [all grade 0 in functional status (FS)]
- 1.0 = No disability, minimal signs in one FS (i.e., grade 1)
- 1.5 = No disability, minimal signs in more than one FS (more than one grade 1)
- 2.0 = Minimal disability in one FS (one FS grade 2, others 0 or 1)
- 2.5 = Minimal disability in two FS (two FS grade 2, others 0 or 1)
- 3.0 = Moderate disability in one FS (one FS grade 3, others 0 or 1) or mild disability in three or four FS (three/four FS grade 2, others 0 or 1) though fully ambulatory
- 3.5 = Fully ambulatory but with moderate disability in one FS (one grade 3) and one or two FS grade 2; or two FS grade 3; or five FS grade 2 (others 0 or 1)
- 4.0 = Ambulatory without aid or rest for ≥ 500 m
- 4.5 = Ambulatory without aid or rest for ≥ 300 m
- 5.0 = Ambulatory without aid or rest for ≥ 200 m
- 5.5 = Ambulatory without aid or rest for ≥ 100 m
- 6.0 = Unilateral assistance required to walk about 100 m with or without resting
- 6.5 = Constant bilateral assistance required to walk about 20 m without resting
- 7.0 = Unable to walk beyond about 5 m even with aid; essentially restricted to wheelchair; wheels self and transfers alone
- 7.5 = Unable to take more than a few steps; restricted to wheelchair; may need aid to transfer
- 8.0 = Essentially restricted to bed or chair or perambulated in wheelchair, but out of bed most of day; retains many self-care functions; generally has effective use of arms
- 8.5 = Essentially restricted to bed much of the day; has some effective use of arm(s); retains some self-care functions
- 9.0 = Helpless bed patient; can communicate and eat
- 9.5 = Totally helpless bed patient; unable to communicate or eat
- 10.0 = Death due to MS

FUNCTIONAL STATUS (FS) SCORE

A. Pyramidal functions
- 0 = Normal
- 1 = Abnormal signs without disability
- 2 = Minimal disability
- 3 = Mild or moderate paraparesis or hemiparesis, or severe monoparesis
- 4 = Marked paraparesis or hemiparesis, moderate quadriparesis, or monoplegia
- 5 = Paraplegia, hemiplegia, or marked quadriparesis
- 6 = Quadriplegia

B. Cerebellar functions
- 0 = Normal
- 1 = Abnormal signs without disability
- 2 = Mild ataxia
- 3 = Moderate truncal or limb ataxia
- 4 = Severe ataxia all limbs
- 5 = Unable to perform coordinated movements due to ataxia

C. Brainstem functions
- 0 = Normal
- 1 = Signs only
- 2 = Moderate nystagmus or other mild disability
- 3 = Severe nystagmus, marked extraocular weakness, or moderate disability of other cranial nerves
- 4 = Marked dysarthria or other marked disability
- 5 = Inability to swallow or speak

D. Sensory functions
- 0 = Normal
- 1 = Vibration or figure-writing decrease only, in 1 or 2 limbs
- 2 = Mild decrease in touch or pain or position sense, and/or moderate decrease in vibration in 1 or 2 limbs, or vibratory (c/s figure writing) decrease alone in 3 or 4 limbs
- 3 = Moderate decrease in touch or pain or position sense, and/or essentially lost vibration in 1 or 2 limbs, or mild decrease in touch or pain, and/or moderate decrease in all proprioceptive tests in 3 or 4 limbs
- 4 = Marked decrease in touch or pain or loss of proprioception, alone or combined, in 1 or 2 limbs or moderate decrease in touch or pain and/or severe proprioceptive decrease in more than 2 limbs
- 5 = Loss (essentially) of sensation in 1 or 2 limbs or moderate decrease in touch or pain and/or loss of proprioception for most of the body below the head
- 6 = Sensation essentially lost below the head

E. Bowel and bladder functions
- 0 = Normal
- 1 = Mild urinary hesitancy, urgency, or retention
- 2 = Moderate hesitancy, urgency, retention of bowel or bladder, or rare urinary incontinence
- 3 = Frequent urinary incontinence
- 4 = In need of almost constant catheterization
- 5 = Loss of bladder function
- 6 = Loss of bowel and bladder function

F. Visual (or optic) functions
- 0 = Normal
- 1 = Scotoma with visual acuity (corrected) better than 20/30
- 2 = Worse eye with scotoma with maximal visual acuity (corrected) of 20/30 to 20/59
- 3 = Worse eye with large scotoma, or moderate decrease in fields, but with maximal visual acuity (corrected) of 20/60 to 20/99
- 4 = Worse eye with marked decrease of fields and maximal acuity (corrected) of 20/100 to 20/200; grade 3 plus maximal acuity of better eye of 20/60 or less
- 5 = Worse eye with maximal visual acuity (corrected) less than 20/200; grade 4 plus maximal acuity of better eye of 20/60 or less
- 6 = Grade 5 plus maximal visual acuity of better eye of 20/60 or less

G. Cerebral (or mental) functions
- 0 = Normal
- 1 = Mood alteration only (does not affect EDSS score)
- 2 = Mild decrease in mentation
- 3 = Moderate decrease in mentation
- 4 = Marked decrease in mentation
- 5 = Chronic brain syndrome—severe or incompetent

SOURCE: After JF Kurtzke, Neurology 33:1444, 1983.

Table 376-4

Therapeutic Regimens for Exacerbations of MS

Methylprednisolone-Prednisone

Inpatient administration: Methylprednisolone, 250 mg, is mixed in 250 mL D_5W and administered over 1–2 h IV q 6 h for 3 days, followed by oral prednisone (1 mg/kg/d as single A.M. dose) on days 4–17, 20 mg on day 18, and 10 mg on days 19–21

Outpatient administration: Methylprednisolone, 1000 mg slow IV push daily for 3 days, followed by oral prednisone (1 mg/kg/d) on days 4–17, 20 mg on day 18, and 10 mg on days 19–21

ACTH

1. Aqueous ACTH (20 U/mL), 80 U administered in 500 mL D_5W over 6–8 h for 3 days, followed by
2. ACTH gel (40 U/mL), 40 U administered IM bid for 7 days, followed by
3. ACTH gel (40 U/mL), tapered as follows: 35 U bid for 3 days; 30 U bid for 3 days; 50 U qd for 3 days; 40 U qd for 3 days; 30 U qd for 3 days; 20 U qd for 3 days; 20 U every other day for 3 doses

bances, acne, and emotional lability. Salt and fluid retention are managed with a low-salt, potassium-rich diet and avoidance of potassium-wasting diuretics. In patients who have heart disease or require concurrent diuretic therapy, oral potassium supplementation is advised. Lithium carbonate (300 mg orally bid) may provide effective prophylaxis for patients who experience emotional lability and insomnia associated with glucocorticoid therapy. In patients with a history of peptic ulcer disease, cimetidine (400 mg bid) or ranitidine (150 mg bid) is advised.

TREATMENT OF AN INITIAL ATTACK A modified approach is employed for treatment of an initial attack of demyelinating disease. In this setting, MS may be a diagnostic possibility, but recurrent signs and symptoms, required for a diagnosis of definite MS, have not occurred. In cases of moderate to severe acute optic neuritis, MePDN/PDN modestly speeds recovery but has little effect on the ultimate degree of recovery. It may also protect against evolution to clinically definite MS over a 2-year period in patients who have disseminated abnormalities detected by brain MRI. Oral PDN alone should probably not be used for treatment of uncomplicated optic neuritis, as its use in one study was associated with an increase in the frequency of subsequent relapses.

Treatment of other acute demyelinating disorders—including transverse myelitis and isolated brainstem syndromes—is largely empirical. It is reasonable to perform brain MRI on patients with all monosymptomatic presentations of demyelinating disease and to treat moderate to severe symptoms, or presumptive disseminated disease detected by MRI, with MePDN/PDN.

CHRONIC PROGRESSION There is a limited role for chronic immunosuppression in the specific treatment of progressive MS symptoms. These treatments should be administered only with the understanding that they carry both short- and long-term risks and that their efficacy in MS is modest. Monotherapy with either methotrexate or azathioprine given orally is a reasonable initial approach.

Methotrexate, 7.5 mg administered orally once each week for up to 2 years, reduces both disease activity as assessed by MRI and sustained progression of disability as measured by standardized tests of upper extremity function. An important practical advantage of methotrexate is the simplicity of a weekly dosing schedule. Most patients experience few or no side effects from low-dose methotrexate therapy. Nausea, diarrhea, headache, myalgia, or fever may require discontinuation of the drug, or these side effects may be treated symptomatically. Laboratory monitoring should include a complete blood count and tests of hepatic and renal function at 8-week intervals.

Chronic azathioprine therapy also has a small beneficial effect on the course of MS. It is administered orally as a single daily dose of 2 to 3 mg/kg. A complete blood count and tests of liver function should be performed initially at monthly intervals and then bimonthly in patients who receive azathioprine. In patients who experience a fall in the white blood cell count (WBC), the dosage is adjusted to maintain the WBC between 3.5×10^3 and 4.0×10^3 cells/μL. The most frequent side effects of azathioprine therapy are nausea and abdominal pain that may require a lowering of the dose or cessation of therapy. The most serious long-term consequence of azathioprine is the development of hepatic toxicity, and liver function thus must be monitored closely. Other possible adverse effects include skin rash, susceptibility to opportunistic infection, and a possible increase in the frequency of non-Hodgkin's lymphoma.

Pulse therapy with the alkylating agent cyclophosphamide may slow disease progression in patients with secondary progressive MS. Benefits appear to be restricted to patients younger than 40 years who experience rapid progression of neurologic impairment. The side effects associated with treatment include nausea, hair loss, hemorrhagic cystitis, and temporary profound immunosuppression.

2-Chlorodeoxyadenosine (2-CDA; Cladribine) appears to reduce MRI activity and progression of disability in chronic progressive MS. 2-CDA is well tolerated when administered at a dose of 0.1 mg/kg body weight intravenously each day for 1 week each month for 4 months. Sustained lymphopenia, thrombocytopenia, and eruptions of herpes zoster are significant risks of this therapy. Uncontrolled studies suggest similar benefits when 2-CDA is administered subcutaneously at a dose of 0.07 mg/kg body weight for 5 consecutive days each month for 5 months. The results of a phase-III study of 2-CDA in patients with chronic progressive MS are expected in 1997 and will help clarify the role of this promising therapy.

The clinical efficacy of immunosuppression for progressive MS is modest and does not justify its use in all patients with progressive disease. Relative contraindications include age greater than 60 years, nonambulatory status, or a primary progressive course. Patients with secondary progressive MS who also experience frequent relapses may be best treated with IFNβ as initial therapy. If immunosuppression is undertaken, a yearly reevaluation of its value—its beneficial and deleterious effects—is required.

OTHER THERAPEUTIC CLAIMS Purported therapies of no proven value include megadose vitamins, calcium orotate, bee stings, cow colostrum, hyperbaric oxygen, and chelation. Patients should be discouraged from seeking out costly or potentially hazardous therapies carried out by well-meaning but naive practitioners. The National Multiple Sclerosis Society remains the best source for information on therapeutic options for MS.

Symptomatic Therapy Spasticity with stiffness, flexor spasms, and clonus can be disabling and painful. Acute worsening of spasticity may occur with underlying infection (frequently of the urinary tract), obstipation, bedsores, other painful lesions, or injuries. These precipitants should be sought out and treated specifically. All medications for spasticity have limited efficacy and may produce symptomatic worsening in patients who require stiffness in order to ambulate. Baclofen (15 to 80 mg/d in divided doses) is the most useful drug available. In refractory cases, oral baclofen in higher doses (up to 240 mg/d) or intrathecal administration via an indwelling catheter may be effective. Diazepam (2 mg bid or tid) is useful in patients who tolerate its sedative effect, and a single bedtime dose may be especially effective for nocturnal spasms. Cyclobenzaprine hydrochloride (5 to 10 mg bid or tid), clonazepam (0.5 to 1.0 mg tid, including a bedtime dose), tizanidine (2 to 8 mg tid, including a bedtime dose), and clonidine hydrochloride (0.1 to 0.2 mg tid, including a bedtime dose) may be useful in patients who fail to respond to baclofen. Dantrolene may produce unacceptable weakness, and its use is reserved for nonambulatory patients. A course of glucocorticoids may be given in exceptional cases where other agents have failed, but benefits seldom last more than 2 to 3 weeks.

Pain, including trigeminal neuralgia and painful dysesthesias, may respond to carbamazepine (100 to 1200 mg/d in divided, escalating doses), phenytoin (300 mg/d), or amitriptyline (50 to 200 mg/d). It may be difficult to distinguish dysesthesias due to MS from radiculopathy due to lumbar disk disease in patients with unilateral leg pain; nonsurgical therapy is justified in the absence of convincing signs of nerve root compression.

Paroxysmal symptoms respond to carbamazepine (up to 1200 mg in divided doses) or acetazolamide (125 to 250 mg tid). Although no treatment for tremor is satisfactory, slight improvement is occasionally seen with clonazepam (0.5 to 1.0 mg bid or tid), primidone (125 to 250 mg bid or tid), ondansetron (4 to 8 mg bid or tid), and isoniazid (up to 1200 mg in divided doses). Stereotaxic thalamotomy may be considered in rare cases of disabling tremor in which a unilateral reduction in symptoms is required, but the combined experience with this procedure has been disappointing.

Because specific symptoms of bladder dysfunction correlate poorly with physiologic findings, urodynamic evaluation is often required. The pathophysiology of abnormal micturition also may change over time in MS. Bladder hyperreflexia is treated with anticholinergics (oxybutynin, 5 mg bid or tid, or propantheline, 7.5 to 15 mg qid). Urinary retention due to bladder hyporeflexia may respond to the cholinergic drug bethanecol (10 to 50 mg tid or qid). Dyssynergia between detrusor and external sphincter muscles may be treated effectively with a combination of anticholinergic medication to decrease bladder contractions and intermittent catheterization. Terazosin hydrochloride (1 to 5 mg at bedtime) ameliorates dyssynergia but may result in urinary incontinence in occasional patients. Supravesical urinary diversion or a chronic indwelling catheter may be required in cases of severe bladder disturbance. Ascorbic acid may reduce the risk of urinary tract infections.

Bowel dysfunction, including constipation and urge incontinence, can be ameliorated by regimentation of bowel function with laxatives and enemas. A low-fiber diet to decrease bulk may be advised for incontinence. Sexual dysfunction may be treated in males by implantation of a penile prosthesis, or erections may be achieved pharmacologically using papaverine and phentolamine injections in the corpora cavernosa. Women may experience vaginismus, which may respond to antispasticity medications, or decreased vaginal lubrication leading to dyspareunia, which may be simply treated with lubricants.

Afternoon fatigue may benefit from a shift to an early work schedule or by a regular afternoon nap. Amantadine (100 mg bid), pemoline (37.5 mg bid), or fluoxetine hydrochloride (20 mg qd or bid) may prove useful in some patients with disabling fatigue. Emotional lability often responds to amitriptyline (25 to 75 mg/d) or fluoxetine (20 mg/d). It is essential to be vigilant for clinical evidence of depression, since suicide is an important cause of death in MS. Occupational counseling and other support services may assist patients and their families in coping with the effects of the disease. Health maintenance should be emphasized, including stress reduction, a balanced diet, avoidance of rapid weight loss, and adequate rest. There is little evidence linking vaccination with relapses of MS, yet it would be prudent to avoid unnecessary immunizations. Swimming is an ideal form of exercise for many patients because of the buoyant support and hypothermia that is achieved.

Pregnancy may affect the course of MS. Compared with nonpregnant MS patients, pregnant patients experience fewer attacks during gestation but more attacks in the first 3 months after parturition. The two effects appear to be roughly similar in magnitude; thus, no effect of pregnancy on disability or on the overall disease course has been identified. It is possible that high levels of prolactin induced in the postpartum period and maintained by breast feeding result in immune stimulation that predisposes to relapses of MS, but one retrospective study found no effect of breast feeding on attack frequency. The advisability of childbearing should be determined primarily by the patient's physical state and available family support.

ACUTE DISSEMINATED ENCEPHALOMYELITIS

DEFINITION AND PATHOGENESIS In contrast to the chronic disorder MS, acute disseminated encephalomyelitis (ADEM) is distinguished by a monophasic course and a frequent association with antecedent immunization (postvaccinal encephalomyelitis) or infection (postinfectious encephalomyelitis). The pathologic hallmark of ADEM is the presence of widely scattered small foci of perivenular inflammation and demyelination. The illness is sudden in onset and may be neurologically devastating or self-limited.

Postvaccinal encephalomyelitis may follow the administration of smallpox and certain rabies vaccines. Rabies vaccine complications result from the Semple vaccine, which uses phenol-inactivated virus propagated in brains of adult animals. The likelihood of ADEM from this vaccine has been variously estimated at between 1 in 400 and 1 in 5000. The introduction of rabies vaccine grown in duck embryo or human diploid tissue has largely eliminated this complication in developed countries, but use of the Semple vaccine continues in some parts of the world. ADEM also may complicate smallpox vaccination, but the worldwide disappearance of smallpox has eliminated the need for prophylaxis.

Postinfectious encephalomyelitis is most frequently associated with the viral exanthems of childhood. The neurologic syndrome generally begins late in the course of the viral illness as the exanthem is fading. Natural infection with measles virus is the most common antecedent (1 in 1000 cases). Worldwide, measles encephalomyelitis remains a common illness, but in developed countries, use of the live measles vaccine has dramatically reduced its incidence. An ADEM-like illness rarely follows vaccination with live measles vaccine (1 to 2 in 10^6 immunizations). ADEM is now most frequently associated with varicella-chickenpox infections (1 in 4000 to 10,000). It also may follow infection with rubella, mumps, influenza, parainfluenza, and infectious mononucleosis viruses and with *Mycoplasma*. In some patients, a nonspecific upper respiratory infection or no known antecedent illness is present.

An autoimmune response to MBP can be detected in the CSF from many patients with ADEM. This has been most clearly established following rabies vaccination and infection with measles virus. With measles infection, induction of immune responses to a variety of CNS antigens may occur, but only the response to MBP correlates with development of ADEM. As noted earlier, many cases of postvaccinal encephalomyelitis almost certainly result from sensitization with brain material that contaminates the viral vaccines. Many attempts to demonstrate direct viral invasion of the CNS have been unsuccessful. The molecular mechanism responsible for virus-induced triggering of an autoimmune response to MBP is not known but may include molecular mimicry due to antigens shared between the virus and host determinants or to virus-mediated CNS injury with secondary sensitization to MBP.

CLINICAL MANIFESTATIONS The severity of ADEM is variable. In severe cases, the onset is abrupt, and progression is rapid (hours to days). In postinfectious ADEM fever that may have faded reappears, and headache, meningismus, and lethargy progressing to coma may develop. Seizures are common. Signs of disseminated neurologic disease are consistently present. Motor findings may include hemiparesis or quadriparesis and extensor plantar responses. Tendon reflexes may be lost initially, later to become hyperactive. Variable degrees of sensory loss and of brainstem involvement may occur. In ADEM due to complications from chickenpox, cerebellar involvement is often prominent. CSF protein is modestly elevated (50 to 150 mg/dL). Lymphocytic pleocytosis, generally 200 cells per microliter or less, occurs in 80 percent of cases. Occasional patients have higher counts or a mixed polymorphonuclear-lymphocytic pattern during the initial days of the illness. Transient CSF oligoclonal banding has been reported in some patients. MRI scanning may reveal extensive gadolinium enhancement of white matter in brain and spinal cord. Electrophysiologic studies indicate involvement of the peripheral nervous system in a proportion of patients.

The prognosis reflects the severity of the underlying acute illness. Measles encephalomyelitis is associated with an estimated mortality of 5 to 20 percent, and most survivors have permanent neurologic sequelae. Children may recover but have persistent seizures and behavioral and learning disorders.

DIAGNOSIS The diagnosis is easily established when there is a history of recent vaccination or exanthematous illness. In severe cases with predominantly cerebral involvement, acute encephalitis due to infection with herpes simplex or other viruses may be difficult to exclude. In the absence of a specific viral prodrome or of immunization, it may not be possible to distinguish ADEM from acute MS. The simultaneous onset of disseminated symptoms and signs indicating optic nerve, brain, and spinal cord involvement is common in ADEM and rare in MS. Similarly, meningismus, drowsiness or coma, or seizures suggest ADEM. Optic nerve involvement is generally bilateral in ADEM and unilateral in MS, and transverse myelopathy is usually complete in the former and partial in the latter. The CSF protein level is normal in the great majority of MS patients; lymphocyte counts are rarely above 50 cells/μL, and polymorphonuclear leukocytes are not present. MRI findings that may support a diagnosis of ADEM include extensive and relatively symmetric white matter abnormalities and diffuse gadolinium enhancement of all abnormal areas, indicating active disease and a monophasic course. It is worth emphasizing that MS occasionally has an explosive presentation, particularly in children. The clinician is often best advised to classify such cases as acute demyelinating disease, reflecting this uncertainty.

℞ TREATMENT

Treatment consists of intravenous methylprednisolone or methylprednisolone-prednisone as employed for MS (Table 376-4). Uncontrolled studies have found ACTH and plasmapheresis also to be of benefit. Occasional patients show evidence of relapse shortly after termination of therapy, and in such cases, reinstitution of therapy may be useful.

ACUTE HEMORRHAGIC LEUKOENCEPHALITIS

Acute hemorrhagic leukoencephalitis (AHL) of Weston Hurst is a rare, devastating, and hyperacute demyelinating disorder. CNS lesions of AHL are characterized by perivenous demyelination and intense infiltration by mononuclear and especially polymorphonuclear inflammatory cells. Vasculitis results in necrosis of the walls of venules, fibrin deposition, and innumerable small hemorrhages scattered throughout the white matter of the hemisphere, brainstem, and spinal cord. Large necrotic foci may form by coalescence of smaller lesions.

The clinical course resembles that of severe forms of ADEM but may be even more explosive in onset and progression. The CSF profile consists of marked pleocytosis (up to 3000 cells/μL), a variable number of red blood cells, and an elevated protein content. Peripheral blood may show an elevated ESR and leukocytosis. Occasional cases display mixed features of both ADEM and AHL or evolve from one form to the other during the course of the acute illness. As in ADEM, immune sensitization to MBP has been described in AHL. Thus, AHL may represent a form of ADEM in which a hyperacute inflammatory response is superimposed on lymphocyte-mediated perivenular demyelination.

The differential diagnosis of AHL includes viral encephalitis, acute bacterial cerebritis, venous thrombosis, and multiple embolic infarctions. The prognosis is generally poor, and death may occur within 2 to 4 days of onset. Therapy for AHL consists of methylprednisolone or methylprednisolone-prednisone regimens (see Table 376-4).

BIBLIOGRAPHY

BECK RW et al: A randomized, controlled trial of corticosteroids in the treatment of acute optic neuritis. N Engl J Med 326:581, 1992

FAZEKAS F et al: Randomized placebo-controlled trial of monthly intravenous immunoglobulin therapy in relapsing-remitting multiple sclerosis. Lancet 349:589, 1997

GOODKIN DE, RUDICK RA (eds): *Treatment of Multiple Sclerosis: Advances in Trial Design, Results and Future Perspectives*. London, Springer-Verlag, 1996

IFNβ MULTIPLE SCLEROSIS STUDY GROUP: Interferon beta-1b is effective in relapsing-remitting multiple sclerosis. I. Clinical results of a multicenter, randomized, double-blind, placebo-controlled trial. Neurology 43:655, 1993

JACOBS LD et al: Intramuscular interferon beta-1a for disease progression in relapsing multiple sclerosis. Ann Neurol 39:285, 1996

JOHNSON KP et al: Copolymer I reduces relapse rate and improves disability in relapsing-remitting multiple sclerosis. Results of a phase III multicenter, double-blind, placebo-controlled trial. Neurology 45:1268, 1995

JOHNSON RT et al: Measles encephalomyelitis: Clinical and immunologic studies. N Engl J Med 310:137, 1984

MATTHEWS WB et al: *McAlpine's Multiple Sclerosis*. New York, Churchill Livingstone, 1991

PATY DW et al: Interferon beta-1b is effective in relapsing-remitting multiple sclerosis. II. MRI analysis results of a multicenter, randomized, double-blind, placebo-controlled trial. Neurology 43:662, 1993

THE MULTIPLE SCLEROSIS GENETICS GROUP: A complete genomic screen for multiple sclerosis underscores a role for the major histocompatibility complex. Nature Genet 13:469, 1996

WAXMAN SG: Clinical course and electrophysiology of multiple sclerosis. Adv Neurol 47:1, 1988

377

W. Michael Scheld

BACTERIAL MENINGITIS, BRAIN ABSCESS, AND OTHER SUPPURATIVE INTRACRANIAL INFECTIONS

ACUTE BACTERIAL MENINGITIS

DEFINITION Bacterial meningitis may be defined as an inflammatory response to bacterial infection of the pia-arachnoid and the cerebrospinal fluid (CSF) of the subarachnoid space. Since the subarachnoid space is continuous over the brain, spinal cord, and optic nerves, infection in this space extends throughout the cerebrospinal axis unless there is obstruction of the subarachnoid space. Ventriculitis is nearly uniformly present in patients with bacterial meningitis.

EPIDEMIOLOGY Bacterial meningitis remains a common disease worldwide. Although precise figures are unavailable, the incidence of bacterial meningitis is between 3 and 5 per 100,000 people per year in the United States. More than 2000 deaths due to bacterial meningitis are reported annually in the United States. The disease is even more common in developing countries. The relative frequency

Table 377-1

Bacterial Etiologic Agents of Meningitis, by Patient Age

Organism	Neonates (≤1 month), %	Children (1 month to 15 years), %	Adults (>15 years), %
H. influenzae	0–3	40–60	1–3
S. pneumoniae	0–5	10–20	30–50
N. meningitidis	0–1	25–40	10–35
Gram-negative bacilli	50–60	1–2	1–10
Streptococci	20–40*	2–4	5
Staphylococci	5	1–2	5–15
Listeria species	2–10	1–2	5

* Nearly all isolates are group B streptococci.

SOURCE: After KL Roos et al: Acute bacterial meningitis in children and adults, in *Infections of the Central Nervous System,* WM Scheld et al (eds). New York, Raven Press, 1991, pp 335–409.

of isolation of various bacterial species as a cause of meningitis varies with age (Table 377-1). Gram-negative bacilli (principally *Escherichia coli*, of the K1 capsule type), other enteric bacilli, *Pseudomonas* sp., *Listeria monocytogenes*, and group B streptococci are the major causative agents during the neonatal period. *Haemophilus influenzae* and *Neisseria meningitidis* are the major causes in children beyond 1 month of age worldwide, although the proportion due to *H. influenzae* has declined dramatically in many geographic regions. Meningitis in adults is due primarily to meningococci and pneumococci, although disease due to aerobic gram-negative bacilli is observed with increasing frequency, especially in the elderly. *N. meningitidis* is the only major cause of epidemics of bacterial meningitis. Recent trends indicate an increase in the proportion of cases due to gram-negative bacilli and *L. monocytogenes*. The overall incidence per 100,000 population per year in the United States during 1986 was 2.9, 1.35, and 1.0 for meningitis due to *H. influenzae* (with significant variability by geographic region), *N. meningitidis*, and *Streptococcus pneumoniae*, respectively (Table 377-2). These most recent figures are derived from a prospective laboratory-based surveillance project in an area with a population of 34 million, 14 percent of the United States population. A similar overall incidence for neonatal meningitis of 2.8 cases per 100,000 population per year was observed in western Sweden during a comparable time period. A continued high incidence of *H. influenzae* meningitis was documented in a recent 3-year prospective nationwide study in Israel: 67.1 per 100,000 in the first year of life and 18.5 per 100,000 in children less than 5 years old. Nevertheless, there has been a profound reduction (by 76 to 90 percent) in the incidence of invasive *H. influenzae* infections in the United States in the past decade. This remarkable achievement has been attributed, in part, to the widespread use of *H. influenzae* conjugate vaccines, now licensed for use in children beginning at 2 months of age. Similar results have been observed in other areas, for example, Finland (from a peak of 43 cases per 100,000 population per year in the early 1970s to zero cases in 1991 in the greater Helsinki area) and in the United Kingdom (87 percent decline in cases between 1991 and 1993).

Meningitis is a major international health problem, as is evident by the recent experience in Africa and South America: explosive and highly fatal outbreaks may occur. At least 30 countries worldwide, including the United States, have reported serious outbreaks of meningococcal meningitis in recent years. More than 70,000 cases were reported from Africa in 1989 alone. During one decade (1973–1982), 4100 patients with meningitis were admitted to a single hospital in Salvador, Brazil, and this disease accounted for 27 percent of all admissions in this interval. The differences in etiology among various studies performed on four different continents are shown in Table 377-3. Worldwide, the three major meningeal pathogens (*H. influenzae*, *N. meningitidis*, and *S. pneumoniae*) account for approximately 75 to 80 percent of cases, but the proportion due to each organism varies among geographic regions.

ETIOLOGY Nearly all cases of *H. influenzae* meningitis occur in children under 6 years of age, and more than 90 percent are due to capsular type b strains (see Chap. 152). Meningitis usually follows nasopharyngeal acquisition of a virulent organism with subsequent systemic invasion. *H. influenzae* accounts for only about 0.5 percent of total CSF isolates in patients older than 6 years, and isolation of this organism in such a patient should suggest the presence of certain predisposing factors, such as sinusitis, epiglottitis, pneumonia, otitis media, head trauma with a CSF leak, diabetes mellitus, alcoholism, splenectomy or other asplenic states, and immune deficiency (including hypogammaglobulinemia and AIDS).

Table 377-2

Bacterial Meningitis in Five States and Los Angeles County, 1986

Organism	Percent of Total Cases	Case-Fatality Rate, %
H. influenzae	45	3
S. pneumoniae	18	19
N. meningitidis	14	13
Group B streptococci	5.7	12
L. monocytogenes	3.2	22
Other	15	18

SOURCE: After Wenger et al.

Meningitis due to *N. meningitidis* is most often encountered in children and young adults and may occur in epidemics (Chap. 149). Epidemic meningococcal meningitis is usually due to serogroups A or C, although the potential for epidemic spread of any serogroup exists. Type B strains are isolated most frequently in sporadic cases, accounting for approximately 50 percent of all isolates in the United States. A recent increase in the incidence of serogroup C meningococcal disease has been noted in North America, largely due to a clonal strain (ET-15) and related strains, which are associated with an increased number of outbreaks and a higher case-fatality rate. Type Y strains are associated with pneumonia. The meningococcus is isolated from approximately 20 percent of all patients with bacterial meningitis in the United States. Nasopharyngeal carriage of virulent organisms also can account for the initiation of infection. Infection is more likely in patients who have deficiencies in the terminal complement components (C5 to C8, and perhaps C9), the so-called membrane attack complex. Persons with these deficiencies have an 8000-fold increased risk of *Neisseria* infections, although the mortality rates appear to be lower than in patients with an intact complement system. Meningococcal meningitis also may occur in properdin-deficient individuals.

Pneumococcal meningitis is the most common type of meningitis in adults over age 30; it is much less common in children than in adults over age 60. It accounts for approximately 15 percent of the total cases of meningitis in the United States (see Chap. 141). In a recent review of 262 cases of community-acquired meningitis in adults reported from 1962 through 1988, the most common identified pathogens were *S. pneumoniae* (37 percent), *N. meningitidis* (13 percent) and *L. monocytogenes* (10 percent). Mortality rates for pneumococcal meningitis remain high in adults, in the 19 to 30 percent range. Pneumococcal infection of the meninges is often associated with distant foci such as pneumonia, otitis media, mastoiditis, sinusitis, or endocarditis. Serious pneumoccocal infections may be observed in patients with predisposing conditions, including splenectomy or asplenic states, multiple myeloma, hypogammaglobulinemia, alcoholism, cirrhosis, and the Wiskott-Aldrich syndrome. *S. pneumoniae* is the most common meningeal isolate in head trauma patients who have suffered a basilar skull fracture with subsequent CSF leak.

Although *L. monocytogenes* represents only a small minority of cases of bacterial meningitis in the United States, mortality remains high (see Table 377-2). *Listeria* infection is more likely in neonates, the elderly, alcoholics, diabetics, cancer patients, and immunosuppressed adults (e.g., renal transplant patients and patients with AIDS). The incidence of *Listeria* meningoencephalitis may be declining in renal transplant populations owing to the frequent use of trimethoprim-sulfamethoxazole prophylaxis. However, up to 30 percent of adults and 50 percent of children with listeriosis have no apparent underlying condition. Serious *Listeria* infections have been associated with several food-borne outbreaks involving contaminated cole slaw, milk, and cheese.

Meningitis due to aerobic gram-negative bacilli is unusual except at the extremes of life. *E. coli* is isolated from 30 to 50 percent of neonates with bacterial meningitis. *Klebsiella* sp., *E. coli*, and *Pseudomonas aeruginosa* also may be isolated following head trauma or neurosurgical procedures, in the elderly, in immunosuppressed patients, and in patients with gram-negative bacteremia or strongyloidiasis. Despite the relative low frequency of meningitis due to this group of microorganisms, the mortality rates remain high. Many of these infections are nosocomial in origin, although community-acquired gram-negative bacillary meningitis appears to be increasing in frequency, particularly among the elderly and in debilitated, alcoholic, or diabetic adults. Staphylococcal meningitis is rare except in patients with indwelling CSF shunts, in whom *Staphylococcus epidermidis* is the most common organism. Meningitis due to *Staphylococcus aureus* is unusual and accounts for about 1 to 8 percent of cases in various surveys. *S. aureus* is the second most common cause of CSF shunt infections and is also a nosocomial pathogen. Although secondary meningitis in the setting of infective endocarditis is relatively uncommon, most of these infections are due to *S. aureus*. Other important associated conditions include head trauma, abscesses in other organs, neurosurgical procedures, sinusitis, osteomyelitis, pneumonia, cellulitis, decubitus ulcers, and infected intravascular grafts or shunts. Many patients have concomitant conditions, including diabetes mellitus, malignancy, renal failure, and immunosuppression. The mortality rate for staphylococcal meningitis remains high (about 50 percent in adults), although the prognosis for CSF shunt infections is more favorable.

Group B streptococci are an important cause of neonatal meningitis. These infections may occur either as early-onset septicemia associated with premature rupture of the membranes and low birth-weight or as late-onset meningitis appearing more than 7 days after birth. The early-onset form is acquired from the maternal genital tract, whereas the source of the group B streptococci in late-onset disease is more controversial; at least 40 percent of infected infants are born to culture-negative mothers. Rare cases of group B streptococcal meningitis have been reported in adults, including postpartum women after vaginal delivery. Bacteremic infections, unrelated to pregnancy, usually in older adults, occur in the setting of underlying risk factors: diabetes mellitus, malignancy, liver failure or a history of alcoholism, neurologic impairment, renal failure, collagen-vascular diseases, congestive heart failure, use of intravenous catheters, glucocorticoid administration, asplenia, and AIDS. Nevertheless, meningitis due to this organism is a rare disease in adults.

Meningitis due to anaerobic bacteria is rare, accounting for less than 1 percent of pyogenic cases. Recovery of anaerobic bacteria from CSF should suggest intraventricular rupture of a brain abscess. Most other cases arise from spread of infection secondary to a contiguous focus of disease and are seen in patients predisposed to focal suppurative intracranial processes.

A plethora of microorganisms have been documented as the cause of meningitis in isolated case reports or in small numbers of patients. Meningitis due to *Flavobacterium meningosepticum* may be a problem in certain neonatal intensive care units, and nosocomial meningitis due to other gram-negative bacilli or *Acinetobacter* sp. appears to be increasing in frequency. Polymicrobial bacterial meningitis, with simultaneous recovery of two or more bacterial species from CSF, is unusual, accounting for less than 1 percent of cases. Most cases occur in adults, and there is a wide spectrum of etiologic agents. Many patients have had either tumors close to the neuraxis, rectal carcinoma, or a fistulous communication with the central nervous system (CNS). Simultaneous isolation of viruses and bacteria from the CSF is rare. Nevertheless, CSF samples are not often cultured for both groups of microorganisms, so the number of reported cases may grossly underestimate the actual problem.

PATHOGENESIS AND PATHOPHYSIOLOGY Since most cases of bacterial meningitis are hematogenous in origin, pathogenesis involves sequential steps related to the expression of several different bacterial virulence factors that overcome host defense mechanisms and allow the pathogen to reach, invade, and replicate in the CSF. These pathogenic steps include (1) nasopharyngeal colonization, (2) nasopharyngeal epithelial cell invasion, (3) bloodstream invasion, (4) bacteremia with intravascular survival, (5) crossing of the blood-brain barrier and entry into CSF, and (6) survival and replication in the subarachnoid space.

Colonization and invasion of the nasopharyngeal mucosa by meningeal pathogens require evasion of secretory IgA, avoidance of ciliary clearance mechanisms, adhesion to the apical epithelial cell membrane, and passage to the basolateral side of the cell. Virtually all clinical isolates of the three major meningeal pathogens secrete IgA proteases that cleave the hinge region of IgA and render it nonfunctional, thereby facilitating bacterial adhesion to the epithelium. Studies using a human nasopharyngeal organ culture model have elucidated the distinct mechanisms of adhesion and invasion by the human pathogens *H. influenzae* and *N. meningitidis*. Infection of human nasopharyngeal organ cultures with either organism results in injury to ciliated epithelial cells, with ciliostasis and selective adherence to nonciliated epithelial cells. Meningococcal binding is dependent on expression of cell-surface pili, and the organism interacts with epithelial cell microvilli. Meningococci enter nonciliated epithelial cells by an endocytotic process and proceed to the abluminal side by a transcellular route within membrane-bound vacuoles. *H. influenzae*, in contrast, creates separations between apical tight junctions of columnar epithelial cells and invades primarily via an intercellular route. After adhesion to and invasion of the nasopharyngeal epithelium, pathogenic bacteria must enter and survive within the intravascular space before penetrating the CNS. Evasion of the host's alternative complement pathway is an important strategy of meningeal pathogens for intravascular survival; this virulence property depends largely on expression of capsular polysaccharide. The actual molecular basis of this complement evasion strategy differs among the major meningeal pathogens. It has been attributed to the capsular sialic acid in group B streptococci, meningococci of serogroups B and C, and *E. coli*. The *H. influenzae* type b polysaccharide capsule (polyribosoyl ribose phosphate) helps evade complement by a somewhat different mechanism.

Once bacteremia occurs, the bacterial pathogens must invade the CNS. The site and mechanism of meningeal invasion by bacteria, however, are poorly understood. Early studies in an experimental infant rat model of *H. influenzae* meningitis suggested that the dural venous sinuses were the major route of CNS invasion. More recent studies, however, suggest that a nonspecific sterile focal inflammation above the cribriform plate facilitates CNS invasion at this site. Experimental studies also have demonstrated that bacteria may enter the CSF via the choroid plexus, a fact related to the exceptional high rate of blood flow and fenestrated capillaries of this structure. Three hypotheses are proposed to account for the observed neurotropism of meningeal pathogens and for their entry into the CNS: (1) Meningitis is secondary to a sustained bacteremia that must be of sufficient duration and magnitude; (2) adhesion to critical blood-brain barrier components may mediate CNS invasion, supported by the potential role of adhesion of *E. coli* strains to the luminal surface of microvascular cerebral endothelium and the epithelial lining of the choroid plexus and ventricles; and (3) microorganisms are carried in macrophages or other phagocytic cells, which enter the CNS by normal cellular trafficking pathways (as occurs in the case of *Streptococcus suis*).

Once bacteria cross the blood-brain barrier and enter the CNS, host humoral defense mechanisms, particularly those dependent on

Table 377-3

Etiology of Bacterial Meningitis in Four Geographic Areas (Percent of Total Cases)

Organism	United States, 1978–1981	United Kingdom, 1980–1984	Dakar, Senegal, 1970–1979	Salvador, Brazil, 1973–1982
H. influenzae	48	29	20	23
S. pneumoniae	13	20	29	17
N. meningitidis	20	25	11	32
Group B streptococcus	3	7	4	2
L. monocytogenes	2	2	<0.5	—
Other	8	16	9	8
Unknown	6	—	26	19

SOURCE: After KL Roos et al: Acute bacterial meningitis in children and adults, in *Infections of the Central Nervous System,* WM Scheld et al (eds). New York, Raven Press, 1991, pp 335–409.

immunoglobulin and complement activity, are virtually absent, so the pathogen has a significant advantage. Since opsonic activity is often undetectable even in infected CSF, phagocytosis of encapsulated bacterial pathogens in the fluid medium of the CSF is inefficient. Thus, bacterial meningitis represents an infection in an area of impaired host resistance; the bacteria commonly reach very high densities in CSF, and the use of bactericidal agents is a mandatory part of therapy.

Once bacteria enter and replicate in the CSF, the subarachnoid space becomes inflamed. This inflammation is largely responsible for the pathophysiologic consequences that contribute to the clinical syndrome of bacterial meningitis, including increased permeability of the blood-brain barrier, cerebral edema (vasogenic, interstitial, and cytotoxic in origin), increased outflow resistance to CSF, cerebral vasculitis, increased intracranial pressure, decreased cerebral blood flow and/or loss of autoregulation of cerebral blood flow, cortical hypoxia, and CSF acidosis.

CSF neutrophilic pleocytosis is a hallmark of subarachnoid-space inflammation. Nevertheless, the pathway by which neutrophils enter the CSF is largely unknown. Adhesion of neutrophils to vascular endothelial cells is a prerequisite. Pretreatment of endothelial cells in tissue culture with various inflammatory cytokines induces the formation of specific adhesion molecules [e.g., endothelial leukocyte adhesion molecule 1 (ELAM-1)], although some of these adhesion molecules have yet to be demonstrated in cerebral endothelium. Leukocyte endothelial cell adhesion is mediated by specific transmembrane glycoproteins expressed on the endothelial cells that interact with specific counterparts on neutrophils. Three families of adhesion molecules may mediate these important interactions: the immunoglobulin superfamily [e.g., intercellular adhesion molecules (ICAMs) 1 and 2], the integrin family (e.g., the CD11/CD18 subfamily), and the selectin family (ELAM-1). The complex interrelationships among these three families, including the inducibility of neutrophil adhesion, and the participation of multiple glycoproteins in diapedesis and the induction of inflammation are considered in greater detail in Chap. 120. In experimental animal models of meningitis, there is evidence that CSF pleocytosis is reduced by interventions designed to block the adhesion of neutrophils to endothelium—specifically, by the systemic administration of a monoclonal antibody (e.g., IB4) against the CD11/CD18 family of receptors, of monoclonal antibodies directed against ICAM-1, of peptides derived from *Bordetella pertussis* filamentous hemagglutinin (which mimic selectins), or of fucoidin, a homopolymer of sulfated L-fucose known to inhibit leukocyte "rolling receptor" L-selectin. These interventions prevent CSF pleocytosis from developing after challenge with live microorganisms or cell-wall components. Combination treatment with dexamethasone and monoclonal antibody IB4 is more effective than either agent alone in the prevention of CSF pleocytosis. Early in the disease, the adherence of leukocytes to cerebromicrovascular endothelium appears to occur preferentially in pial venules.

Subarachnoid-space inflammation is induced by constituents of bacteria. Capsular polysaccharides are remarkably noninflammatory, although the capsule is crucial for the survival of meningeal pathogens in the bloodstream and the subarachnoid space. Experimental animal studies have documented that the cell wall of gram-positive microorganisms and the endotoxin [lipopolysaccharide (LPS) or lipooligosaccharide] of gram-negative organisms induce subarachnoid space inflammation. In the case of pneumococcus, intracisternal injection of the major components of the cell wall—teichoic acid and peptidoglycan—induces inflammation. In gram-negative meningitis, the lipid A region of LPS is responsible for the induction of inflammation. Inflammatory changes in CSF are also elicited by the intracisternal inoculation of *H. influenzae* type b outer membrane vesicles, which may play a relevant role as a nonreplicating vehicle for the delivery of the toxic moieties of LPS to host cells in vivo. Pneumococcal cell wall and the LPS of *H. influenzae* type b elicit subarachnoid-space inflammation through the release of various inflammatory mediators within the CNS. Both interleukin (IL) 1 and tumor necrosis factor (TNF) appear rapidly in CSF following the intracisternal inoculation of pneumococcal cell wall or of LPS from gram-negative bacteria. These proinflammatory cytokines induce subarachnoid-space inflammation independently and appear to act synergistically in this effect. In addition, increased concentrations of TNF in CSF may be specific for bacterial meningitis, as they are found in bacterial but not viral meningitis in both experimental animals and humans. The role of other inflammatory cytokines in the induction of subarachnoid-space inflammation is less clear. Although IL-6 and platelet-activating factor (PAF) are present in increased concentrations in the CSF during the disease, their role in the CNS is unknown. PAF appears to contribute directly to subarachnoid space inflammation during pneumococcal meningitis but to play only a supporting role when the inflammation is induced by *H. influenzae* LPS. Nevertheless, higher CSF concentrations of TNF and PAF are associated with more severe disease in children. IL-8 and IL-10 are also detected in the CSF of patients with bacterial meningitis; IL-10 may downregulate the inflammatory response in this disease.

One of the major pathophysiologic consequences of bacterial meningitis is an increase in the permeability of the blood-brain barrier, which leads to vasogenic cerebral edema. In experimental meningitis induced in animals by the intracisternal inoculation of bacterial pathogens, the cerebral capillary endothelium exhibits a uniform response, which is characterized morphologically by an early and sustained increase in pinocytotic vesicle formation and a progressive separation of intercellular tight junctions. These morphologic alterations correlate with the penetration of a marker protein (albumin) across the blood-brain barrier. CSF leukocytes augment these changes in permeability late in the disease course. When inoculated intracisternally, pneumococcal cell walls, *H. influenzae* type b LPS, outer membrane vesicles prepared from *H. influenzae,* and various proinflammatory cytokines all induce increased blood-brain permeability in vivo. Encapsulation of *H. influenzae* is not essential for blood-brain barrier injury, but it promotes this process in vivo by allowing the organism to escape host clearance mechanisms in the CSF. Studies that use in situ perfusion of albumin–colloidal gold as a tracer, as well as studies using complementary immunogold detection of perfused monomeric albumin, have identified the postcapillary venules as the site at which albumin enters the subarachnoid space during bacterial meningitis. Albumin crosses the blood-brain barrier primarily by a paracellular pathway through open intercellular junctions in venular segments, since transcytosis to the abluminal side of the endothelium is minimal. Although other gram-negative cell-wall components besides LPS (e.g., peptidoglycan) may induce subarachnoid-space inflammation, their effect is minimal compared to that of LPS. The primary and secondary messengers governing alterations in blood-brain barrier permeability and the paracellular leakage of albumin remain unknown, but ongoing development of in vitro systems of isolated cerebral microvascular endothelial cells may help in the delineation of the cellular mechanisms involved. Furthermore, the recent demonstration of elevated concentrations of excitatory amino acids in CSF during meningitis suggests that these substances may play a role in altered CNS homeostasis.

Another important pathophysiologic consequence of subarachnoid-space inflammation is an increase in intracranial pressure (ICP). This increase is caused primarily (but not exclusively) by cerebral edema, which may be vasogenic, cytotoxic, and/or interstitial in origin. Vasogenic cerebral edema results primarily from increased blood-brain barrier permeability. Cytotoxic cerebral edema results from the swelling of brain cells, most likely owing to the release of toxic factors from neutrophils and/or bacteria. Interstitial cerebral edema occurring during meningitis is due largely to obstruction of normal CSF pathways, with a resulting increase in the resistance to CSF outflow. Cerebral edema is always found in experimental animal models of meningitis, as measured by increased brain water content. The finding that administration of glucocorticoids to animals with experimental meningitis attenuated the cerebral edema, the increased ICP, and the increased CSF outflow resistance led to a reexamination of the potential adjunctive role of glucocorticoids in the treatment of this disease (see below). Cerebral blood flow alterations also have been found by multiple techniques in animal models and in patients with bacterial meningitis. In an infant rhesus monkey model of *H. influenzae* meningitis, certain areas of the cortex (postcentral, temporal, and occipital) were hypoperfused relative to the hypothalamus and midbrain, while the brainstem was hyperperfused. These findings suggest that cerebral cortical hypoperfusion with resulting relative cerebral anoxia may be an early physiologic change during *H. influenzae* meningitis. Loss of cerebral autoregulation has been documented in an experimental rabbit model of pneumococcal meningitis. It has been suggested that even minor fluctuations of mean arterial blood pressure may have adverse consequences for patients with meningitis, since autoregulation may be lost, resulting in an increased risk of brain injury from transient hypotension or hypertension. The blood flow alterations may lead to regional hypoxia, increased brain lactate concentrations secondary to utilization of glucose by anaerobic pathways, and CSF acidosis, which may be a precursor to encephalopathy. It is likely that the generation of reactive oxygen or nitrogen intermediates in the microvasculature potentiates these changes in regional cerebral blood flow. Infusion of superoxide dismutase, catalase, or deferoxime modifies the early alterations in cerebral blood flow in experimental models of pneumococcal meningitis. Elevated CSF concentrations of nitrite, a major metabolite of nitric oxide, have been observed in experimental animal models and patients with bacterial meningitis. Regional cerebral blood flow alterations, cerebral edema, blood-brain barrier permeability, and CSF pleocytosis are often reduced in animals receiving nitric oxide synthase inhibitors.

PATHOLOGY The pathologic hallmark of bacterial meningitis is an exudate in the subarachnoid space. On gross examination, the exudate has a typical grayish yellow or yellowish green appearance. It is most abundant in the cisterns at the base of the brain and over the convexities of the cerebral hemispheres in the rolandic and sylvian fissures. Purulent exudate accumulates in the basal cisterns and also, in the absence of obstruction, extends along the spinal cord and nerve sheaths and into the ventricular system. Microscopic examination of the subarachnoid exudate in the early stages of disease demonstrates large numbers of neutrophils and bacteria. Within 2 to 3 days of infection, evidence of inflammation in the wall of the small and medium-sized subarachnoid blood vessels appears. Subintimal infiltration of arterial walls by lymphocytes and neutrophils is relatively unique to infection of the meninges. The meningeal veins become distended and develop mural infection, which may be complicated by focal necrosis of the vessel wall, mural thrombus formation in the lumen, or involvement of the dural sinuses. Hemorrhagic cortical infarction may be the result of cortical venous and dural sinus thrombosis. By the end of the first week of meningeal inflammation, the cellular composition of the subarachnoid exudate changes. Neutrophils begin to degenerate and are removed by macrophages, which are derived from meningeal histiocytes. The nuclei of affected neurons and glial cells become shrunken, pyknotic, and darkly staining. Further infiltration of subependymal tissues and perivascular spaces by neutrophils and lymphocytes occurs. Blockage of normal CSF pathways, particularly of the midline foramen of Magendie and the lateral foramina of Luschka in the fourth ventricle, may result in noncommunicating or obstructive hydrocephalus. The absorption of CSF by the arachnoid villi may be impeded by accumulation of the fibrinopurulent exudate. Diffuse cerebral edema and/or increased ICP may lead to life-threatening brain herniation. Cranial and spinal nerve deficits, focal neurologic deficits, seizure disorders, encephalopathy, and subdural effusions are all recognized complications of meningitis.

CLINICAL MANIFESTATIONS The classic clinical presentation of adults with bacterial meningitis includes headache, fever, and meningismus, often with signs of cerebral dysfunction; these manifestations are found in more than 85 percent of patients. Nausea, vomiting, rigors, profuse sweating, weakness, myalgias, and photophobia are also common. The meningismus may be subtle or marked, accompanied by Kernig's and/or Brudzinski's signs. These signs are elicited in only about 50 percent of adults with bacterial meningitis, and their absence does not rule out this diagnosis. Cerebral dysfunction is manifested primarily by confusion, delirium, or a declining level of consciousness ranging from lethargy to coma. Cranial nerve palsies, especially palsies involving cranial nerves IV, VI, and VII, are found in 10 to 20 percent of cases, occasionally in concert with focal neurologic deficits such as visual field defects, dysphasia, and hemiparesis. Seizures occur in about 40 percent of cases. Recurrent seizure activity and focal neurologic deficits are more common in the early stages of pneumococcal meningitis than in *H. influenzae* or meningococcal disease. The presence of bilateral sixth nerve palsies, manifested as weakness of the lateral rectus muscles, suggests a raised ICP. Papilledema is rare (<1 percent of patients) and should suggest a different diagnosis, such as an intracranial mass lesion. Later in the disease course, patients may develop other signs of increased ICP, including coma, hypertension, bradycardia, and third nerve palsy; these findings are ominous prognostic signs. Focal neurologic deficits, seizure activity, and encephalopathy may arise from cortical and/or subcortical ischemia and/or infarction, from increased ICP, or from the development of a subdural effusion.

Certain symptoms and/or signs may suggest a specific etiologic diagnosis in patients with meningitis. Meningococcemia with or without meningitis presents with a prominent rash, principally of the extremities, in about 50 percent of patients. Early in the disease process, the rash is often erythematous and macular, but typically it evolves quickly into a petechial phase with further coalescence into a purpuric form with gunmetal-gray necrosis in the center of the purpuric regions. This rash often matures rapidly, sometimes with the appearance of new petechial lesions during the performance of the physical examination. A similar rash may be seen in other forms of meningitis (e.g., meningitis due to echovirus type 9, *S. aureus*, *Acinetobacter* sp., and, rarely, *S. pneumoniae* or *H. influenzae*), in Rocky Mountain spotted fever and other rickettsioses, in *S. aureus* endocarditis, in rapid, overwhelming sepsis due to encapsulated bacteria in splenectomized patients, and in some noninfectious disorders such as vasculitis or thrombotic thrombocytopenic purpura. An additional suppurative focus of infection, typically otitis media, sinusitis, or pneumonia, is seen in approximately 30 percent of patients with pneumococcal or *H. influenzae* meningitis. Patients in whom meningitis develops in the wake of a CSF leak may have rhinorrhea or otorrhea due to a persistent defect.

Conversely, certain subgroups of patients may not manifest many of the classic signs and/or symptoms of bacterial meningitis. Meningismus and/or fever are commonly absent in neonates, and the only clinical clues may be listlessness, high-pitched crying, refusal to feed, irritability, or other nonspecific manifestations. In elderly patients, meningitis often has an insidious onset with lethargy or obtundation and with variable signs of meningeal inflammation and no fever. In this subgroup of patients, an altered mental status should not be ascribed to other causes until bacterial meningitis has been excluded by examination of CSF. Many of the signs of bacterial meningitis, including alteration in consciousness, are present in patients following neurosurgery or head trauma. Meningitis is difficult to spot in this situation, and the physician should have a low threshold for performing CSF examination if any clinical deterioration occurs.

DIAGNOSIS The diagnosis of bacterial meningitis rests on examination of the CSF, which is usually obtained by lumbar puncture. When papilledema and/or focal neurologic findings suggestive of an intracranial mass lesion are present, lumbar puncture should be deferred until computed tomography (CT) or magnetic resonance imaging (MRI) is performed. Nevertheless, if meningitis seems likely, blood should be drawn for culturing and empirical antimicrobial therapy started while the neuroimaging study is being carried out. Although empirical antibiotic therapy may render the CSF sterile (as determined by culturing), the CSF profile will still be suggestive of bacterial meningitis.

The typical CSF findings in acute bacterial meningitis consist of an elevated opening pressure, neutrophilic pleocytosis, elevated protein concentration, and hypoglycorrhachia. The opening pressure is elevated in virtually all cases. Values exceeding 600 mmH_2O suggest cerebral edema, communicating hydrocephalus, or the presence of intracranial suppurative foci. The gross appearance of the fluid may be cloudy or turbid if the white cell count is elevated. Occasionally, the fluid may appear turbid owing to the presence of microorganisms in the absence of significant CSF pleocytosis; this is an ominous prognostic sign. If the lumbar puncture is traumatic, the CSF may be bloody at first, but it should clear as flow continues. Although xanthochromia can occur during meningitis, this finding should suggest the possibility of subarachnoid hemorrhage, and in patients with heart valve disease it raises the possibility of ruptured mycotic aneurysm. The leukocyte concentration in CSF usually is elevated in untreated bacterial meningitis, with counts ranging from 1×10^3 to $>1 \times 10^6$/L. Values in the latter range are found in 60 to 70 percent of cases. The leukocytosis shows a neutrophilic predominance. A very low CSF white cell concentration in bacterial meningitis often has been associated with a poor outcome. Therefore, Gram's stain and culture should be performed on all CSF specimens, even in the absence of CSF pleocytosis. The CSF protein concentration is elevated in virtually all cases of bacterial meningitis, sometimes to an extreme degree when spinal block is present, presumably owing to disruption of the blood-brain barrier and/or generation of protein by leukocytes and/or microorganisms in the subarachnoid space. The CSF glucose concentration is less than <2.2 mmol/L (40 mg/dL) in approximately 60 percent of patients with bacterial meningitis, and the CSF-to-serum ratio of glucose concentrations is less than 0.31 in about 70 percent of patients. The CSF glucose concentration must be compared with a simultaneous serum glucose concentration for proper evaluation. A recent analysis found that each of the following criteria predicted the presence of bacterial as opposed to viral meningitis with a certainty of 99 percent or better: a CSF glucose level of less than 1.9 mmol/L (34 mg/dL), a CSF to blood glucose concentration ratio of less than 0.23, a CSF protein level of greater than 2.2 g/L (220 mg/dL), and more than 2000 $\times 10^6$ leukocytes per liter of CSF or more than 1180 $\times 10^6$ neutrophils per liter of CSF.

Gram's staining should always be used in examining CSF, as it permits rapid and accurate identification of the etiologic agent in approximately 60 to 90 percent of cases of bacterial meningitis (the overall sensitivity is approximately 75 percent). The probability that the organism will be detected varies with the concentration of bacteria in CSF. False-positive findings may be caused by contamination of collection tubes or staining reagents. Negative CSF Gram's stains are usually related to prior antimicrobial therapy and low CSF concentrations of microorganisms. The CSF culture is positive in approximately 70 to 85 percent of patients with bacterial meningitis. The probability of identifying an organism decreases in patients who have received prior antimicrobial therapy. Blood cultures also should be obtained, because they are positive in a variable proportion of patients with bacterial meningitis, depending on the pathogen.

Many other rapid diagnostic tests have been developed to aid in the diagnosis of bacterial meningitis when Gram's staining gives negative results. Countercurrent immunoelectrophoresis (CIE) may be helpful in the detection of specific microbial antigens in CSF with a sensitivity of approximately 62 to 95 percent and with high specificity. Nevertheless, newer techniques employing staphylococcal coagglutination or latex agglutination are more rapid and sensitive than CIE, being able to detect bacterial antigen concentrations in CSF of approximately 1 ng/mL. It must be emphasized that a negative test result does not rule out infection with a particular meningeal pathogen. The limulus lysate test is highly sensitive at detecting LPS in CSF, although it does not distinguish among gram-negative organism, and its results often do not affect decisions regarding therapeutic regimen. Other tests may be useful in selected patients. Failure to find elevated CSF concentrations of C-reactive protein is strong evidence against bacterial meningitis. As noted above, increased CSF levels of TNF suggest a bacterial, not viral, etiology. The polymerase chain reaction (PCR) has been used to amplify bacterial DNA in CSF as an aid in the diagnosis of meningitis caused by *H. influenzae*, meningococci, streptococci, and *Listeria*. Although problems with false-positive results have been noted, the specificity and sensitivity are both ~90 percent, and further refinements may facilitate diagnosis in cases that give negative results on Gram's staining and culture.

Neuroimaging techniques such as CT and MRI have little role in the diagnosis of acute bacterial meningitis, but they may detect complications and/or a parameningeal source of infection. CT or MRI may be useful in patients in whom fever still persists several days after initiation of antimicrobial therapy or who have prolonged obtundation or coma in the presence of new or recurrent seizure activity, signs of increased ICP, or focal neurologic deficits. MRI is more sensitive than CT for the evaluation of subdural effusions, cortical infarction, and cerebritis but is more difficult to perform in a critically ill patient. The vast majority of patients with suspected or proven bacterial meningitis do not require a neuroimaging study; if one is performed, its results usually will not affect decisions concerning therapy.

Most patients with suspected bacterial meningitis should undergo initial evaluation in an intensive care setting. Multiple complications may develop, including shock, disseminated intravascular coagulation, and the syndrome of inappropriate secretion of vasopressin (antidiuretic hormone). In addition to frequent monitoring, blood cultures and tests for coagulation factors and electrolytes, including indicators of renal function, are essential. A chest x-ray may reveal coexisting pneumonia. Staining of material from petechiae or purpuric lesions reveals intracellular cocci in approximately 70 percent of meningococcemia cases. In the presence of frank arthritis, arthrocentesis with culture and staining may reveal the etiologic agent.

DIFFERENTIAL DIAGNOSIS A variety of infectious and noninfectious processes can produce an acute meningitis syndrome and may be confused with acute bacterial meningitis. These entities include parameningeal foci of infection (e.g., brain abscess, subdural empyema, and epidural abscess; see below), viral meningitis or encephalitis, CNS syphilis, the neurologic manifestations of Lyme disease, tuberculous meningitis, fungal meningitis, bacterial endocarditis, rickettsial infections such as Rocky Mountain spotted fever, CNS neoplasms, cerebral vasculitis, granulomatous angiitis, sarcoidosis, cyst-related meningitis, subarachnoid hemorrhage, neuroleptic malignant syndrome, chemical meningitis due to drugs, radiocontrast agents or anesthetics, and various poorly understood chronic or recurrent meningeal syndromes.

℞ TREATMENT

Antimicrobial Therapy The initial procedure in a patient with suspected bacterial meningitis is a lumbar puncture to obtain CSF for analysis (Fig. 377-1). Patients should receive emergent empirical antimicrobial therapy based on age and underlying disease status if no etiologic agent is identified by Gram's staining or rapid diagnostic tests and if the diagnosis of bacterial meningitis is likely. In the few patients who present with focal signs on neurologic examination, a CT scan should be obtained prior to lumbar puncture. However, if meningitis is a strong possibility, empirical antimicrobial therapy should be instituted immediately after obtaining two blood samples for culturing. The empirical regimens for presumed bacterial meningitis are based primarily on the age of the host and the likely infecting pathogens. For neonates under 1 month of age, the most likely pathogens are *E. coli*, *Streptococcus agalactiae*, and *L. monocytogenes*. Empirical therapy commonly consists of ampicillin plus a third-generation cephalosporin, which is usually cefotaxime owing to the concerns of albumin binding by ceftriaxone and bilirubin metabolism in this age group. An alternative treatment regimen is ampicillin plus an aminoglycoside. In older infants (aged 4 to 12 weeks), infections with either *H. influenzae* or *S. pneumoniae* join the typical neonatal bacterial meningitides, and the regimen of choice is ampicillin plus a third-generation cephalosporin. From ages 3 months to 6 years, empirical therapy with a third-generation cephalosporin (and perhaps also with vancomycin; see below) may be used. Some authorities still recommend the use of ampicillin plus chloramphenicol or of chloramphenicol alone in this age group, but cefuroxime should be avoided. In young adults, most cases of meningitis are due to *N. meningitidis* or *S. pneumoniae*, and cefotaxime or ceftriaxone is often used. Because of the prevalence of gram-negative aerobic bacilli in older adults (over 50 years old) and the possibility of *L. monocytogenes* infection, the empirical regimen should consist of ampicillin in combination with a third-generation cephalosporin (and perhaps also with vancomycin). In postneurosurgical patients or in those with CSF shunts or foreign bodies in place, the likely infecting organisms include staphyloccocci, diphtheroids, and gram-negative bacilli, including *P. aeruginosa*. Empirical antimicrobial therapy in these situations should consist of vancomycin plus ceftazidime until culture results are available.

Once the infecting microorganism has been isolated in culture (or identified by other means), antimicrobial therapy can be modified on the basis of susceptibility results. For bacterial meningitis due to *N. meningitidis*, penicillin G or ampicillin remain the drugs of choice. The treatment of meningitis presumed or proved to be caused by *S. pneumoniae* has been markedly compromised by the global spread of penicillin-resistant pneumococci in recent years; penicillin alone can no longer be recommended as empirical therapy in any age group. Furthermore, before using penicillin against pneumococci, it is mandatory to test for susceptibility to this agent using pneumococcal isolates from sterile body fluids. Penicillin resistance is classified as being *relative* or *intermediate* if the minimum inhibitory concentration (MIC) is 0.1 to 1.0 μg/mL and as being *high* if the MIC is ≥2 μg/mL. While some areas (e.g., Spain, Hungary, and South Africa) reported a high proportion of penicillin-resistant isolates in the 1980s, in the United States, as of this writing, ~25 percent of pneumococcal isolates display intermediate resistance to penicillin, and ~5 to 7 percent display high-level resistance. Chloramphenicol is best avoided as an alternative, despite in vitro tests suggesting susceptibility to this agent. Cefotaxime or ceftriaxone alone is recommended when relatively resistant strains are suspected or proved to be present. In contrast, in areas known to harbor isolates highly resistant to penicillin or to have a high proportion of isolates resistant to third-generation cephalosporins, the following regimens have been proposed: vancomycin plus either a third-generation cephalosporin or rifampin, or a third-generation cephalosporin with either ampicillin, vancomycin, or rifampin. No regimen has proven superiority. Care must be exercised when giving vancomycin to a patient who is also being treated with dexamethasone, as the latter agent reduces the penetrance of vancomycin into the CSF. Pending further data, the use of vancomycin plus a third-generation cephalosporin is reasonable. Repeat analysis of CSF after 24 to 48 h is also appropriate, especially if the patient is also receiving dexamethasone.

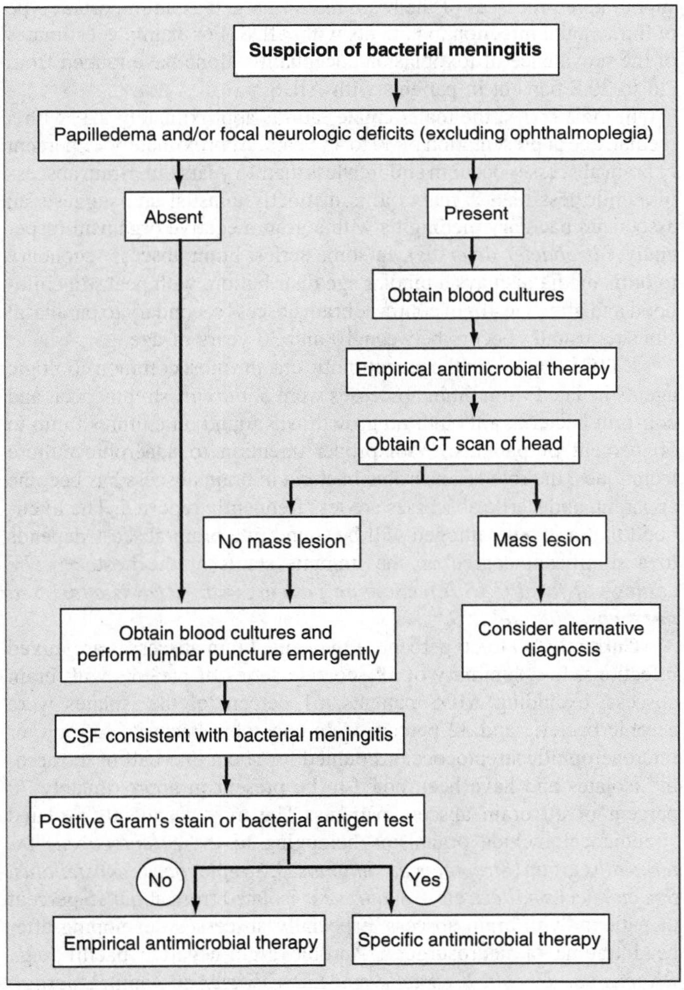

FIGURE 377-1 Algorithm for the initial management of patients with acute bacterial meningitis.

Meningococcal strains that are relatively resistant to penicillin also have been reported from several areas, particularly Spain, but patients harboring these strains have recovered with standard penicillin therapy. Penicillin resistance among meningococci remains stable at extremely low levels in the United States. Approximately 33 percent of *H. influenzae* isolates in the United States produce β-lactamase and are resistant to ampicillin. Fortunately, chloramphenicol resistance is rare in the United States, but it is found in more than 50 percent of CSF isolates in some countries.

The American Academy of Pediatrics has endorsed the use of the third-generation cephalosporins as empirical therapy in children with bacterial meningitis. Ceftriaxone is clearly superior to cefuroxime in this age group. The third-generation cephalosporins have revolutionized the treatment of gram-negative enteric bacillary meningitis. Cure rates of 78 to 94 percent have been achieved with these agents, and one, ceftazidime, may be used alone or as part of combination regimens for the care of patients with *Pseudomonas* meningitis. Intrathecal or intraventricular aminoglycoside administration should be considered for patients with gram-negative aerobic bacillary meningitis if there is no response to systemic therapy alone. The quinolone agents (e.g., ciprofloxacin, pefloxacin, and ofloxacin) have been used in some patients with gram-negative meningitis but should only be considered for adult patients with meningitis due to multidrug-resistant gram-negative bacilli or in patients failing conventional therapy. The third-generation cephalosporins are, however, inactive against *L. monocytogenes*; therefore, ampicillin is often added empirically for treatment of this organism. In documented *Listeria* meningitis, consideration should be given to a combination of an aminoglycoside and ampicillin to achieve synergy in vivo. In the penicillin-allergic patient, systemic trimethoprim-sulfamethoxazole, which is bactericidal against *Listeria* in vitro, can be used. Patients with *S. aureus* meningitis should be treated with nafcillin, oxacillin, or vancomycin. Since *S. epidermidis* is the most likely isolate in patients with a CSF shunt infection, vancomycin is the drug of choice; rifampin may be added if the patient fails to improve. Removal of the shunt often is necessary to optimize therapy.

The duration of therapy for bacterial meningitis is based largely on tradition, as rigorous scientific data are lacking. In general, the following treatment durations are recommended: for *N. meningitidis*, 7 days; for *H. influenzae*, 7 to 10 days; for *S. pneumoniae*, 10 to 14 days; and for gram-negative aerobic bacilli, 3 weeks. Therapy should be individualized and based on the clinical response; some patients require longer courses of treatment.

ADJUNCTIVE THERAPY Despite the availability of bactericidal antimicrobial therapy, the morbidity and mortality from bacterial meningitis remain unacceptably high. Recent studies have focused on the pathogenesis and pathophysiology of bacterial meningitis, since the simple introduction of newer antimicrobial agents may not improve the situation. However, rapid killing of bacteria—the desired effect of therapy with antimicrobial agents—may accelerate the release of proinflammatory bacterial cell-wall components into the CSF. Treatment with bacteriolytic agents in experimental meningitis often results in an increase in CSF leukocyte concentration. Antibiotic therapy also results in higher concentrations of free LPS in the CSF of children with *H. influenzae* meningitis during the first day of treatment. However, anti-inflammatory agents, particularly glucocorticoids, have been shown to decrease the inflammatory response in the subarachnoid space in experimental models of infection (as assessed by CSF pleocytosis), with resulting improvement in many of the pathophysiologic consequences, including increased permeability of the blood-brain barrier, cerebral edema, and increased ICP, On the basis of these studies and the known effects of glucocorticoids on cytokine generation, the use of glucocorticoids in patients with bacterial meningitis has been reevaluated. Several prospective, double-blind, randomized clinical trials have now evaluated dexamethasone as an adjunctive agent for children with meningitis. Most trials found no change in mortality rate, but CSF inflammatory indices normalized faster, fever disappeared more rapidly, and the incidence of moderate to severe bilateral sensorineural hearing loss and/or overall neurologic sequelae was reduced. Dexamethasone also reduced mortality in adults and children with pneumococcal meningitis in one Egyptian trial. Hearing impairment was reduced in children with pneumococcal meningitis in one recent trial reported from Turkey. Although concerns have been raised about the routine use of dexamethasone in all patients with bacterial meningitis, and virtually no information exists on the use of this treatment in neonates or older adults, adjunctive dexamethasone therapy is potentially beneficial in children, particularly those with proven or suspected *H. influenzae* disease. Close monitoring of the hematocrit and stool guaiac test for blood loss is essential during therapy. The mechanism of the beneficial effect of dexamethasone is not completely clear, but CSF concentrations of IL-1β fall more rapidly in children receiving dexamethasone than in children receiving a placebo. If dexamethasone is used, it should be administered shortly before or simultaneously with the first dose of antimicrobial agent to maximally attenuate the CSF inflammatory response. The recommended dose of dexamethasone is 0.15 mg/kg administered four times daily (a total of 0.6 mg/kg per day) for 4 days. Shorter courses of dexamethasone therapy (e.g., 2 days) may be appropriate, pending further data. The role of adjunctive dexamethasone in neonates and adults is unclear.

Other adjunctive treatments may be useful in critically ill patients with bacterial meningitis. Patients with signs of increased ICP may benefit from the insertion of an intracranial pressure monitoring device and vigorous treatment of raised ICP. Elevation of the head of the bed to 30°, hyperventilation to a Pa_{CO_2} of 27 to 30 mmHg, administration of hyperosmolar agents such as mannitol, use of intravenous lidocaine to reduce transient increases in ICP during endotracheal suctioning, and administration of glucocorticoids may be tried alone or in combination (see Chap. 374). Glycerol, which can be administered orally, may reduce auditory and/or neurologic sequelae regardless of dexamethasone use, but further data are needed before its routine use can be recommended in the care of patients with bacterial meningitis. To avoid status epilepticus, seizures should be treated promptly with appropriate agents, such as lorazepam or diazepam and/or phenytoin. Barbiturates occasionally are necessary to control seizure activity. Treatment of shock and/or disseminated intravascular coagulation may be necessary (see Chap. 124). Plasma exchange or plasmapheresis has proved life-saving in some patients with fulminant meningococcemia, but this treatment must be considered experimental.

PROGNOSIS Table 377-2 shows the overall case-fatality rates for meningitis caused by the major meningeal pathogens encountered in the United States in 1986. The mortality rate for *H. influenzae* meningitis is less than 5 percent, although it exceeds 20 to 25 percent in some developing countries. Meningococcemia without meningitis carries a worse prognosis than meningococcal meningitis alone. Pneumococcal meningitis has the highest mortality rate of the three major types of bacterial meningitis. Gram-negative aerobic bacillary meningitis is often refractory to therapy, and relapses may occur. Permanent neurologic sequelae occur in approximately one-third to one-half of survivors of bacterial meningitis. The major sequelae include hearing loss or language delay, mental retardation, cerebral palsy, seizures, and behavioral problems. Prospective studies have documented persistent sensorineural hearing loss in approximately 10 percent of survivors of bacterial meningitis (and in approximately 31 percent of survivors of pneumococcal meningitis), a finding with critical implications for growth and educational development. Despite an apparent recent decline in the incidence of severe neurologic sequelae among children surviving bacterial meningitis, as measured by learning patterns upon school entry, the worldwide public health problems resulting from this disease are significant.

BRAIN ABSCESS

DEFINITION A brain abscess is a focal suppurative process in the brain parenchyma; the pathogenesis and etiology of the condition are diverse.

EPIDEMIOLOGY The incidence of brain abscess has remained relatively stable in the antibiotic era; nevertheless, it is generally regarded as a rare disease, with large autopsy series reporting an occurrence rate of 0.18 to 1.3 percent. It has been estimated that brain abscess accounts for approximately 1 out of every 10,000 general hospital admissions, and about 4 to 10 cases are seen yearly on active neurosurgical services in hospitals of developed countries. Although some series have noted a slightly increased incidence in recent years, this change may be an artifact due to more sensitive diagnostic techniques. In addition, brain abscess remains a significant problem in the developing world, particularly in children living in poverty. Focal suppurative processes of the brain have emerged as an important type of intracranial infection in patients with AIDS. For example, estimates of the prevalence of toxoplasma encephalitis alone have ranged from 2.6 to 30.8 percent in patients with AIDS.

In most series, the male/female ratio is approximately 2:1, with a median age at presentation of 30 to 45 years. Approximately 25 percent of brain abscesses occur in children less than 15 years old. Brain abscess in a child less than 2 years old is distinctly unusual and suggests an associated bacillary meningitis with a gram-negative organism (especially *Citrobacter diversus*). In some series, brain abscess secondary to otitis media displays a bipolar age distribution, with peaks in childhood and after age 40. In contrast, brain abscess secondary to paranasal sinusitis usually occurs between 10 and 30 years of age.

ETIOLOGY In the preantibiotic era, the most common etiologic agents isolated from brain abscesses were *S. aureus*, streptococci, and coliform bacteria, although no growth was found on cultures in up to 50 percent of patients. With proper attention to anaerobic culture techniques, the role of anaerobic bacteria in brain abscess has become apparent, and sterile abscesses are less frequently reported. The likelihood that a given pathogen will be found in a brain abscess depends to a significant degree on the immune status of the host. → *The etiology of focal CNS infections in patients with AIDS is addressed in Chaps. 308 and 379.*

Currently, 30 to 60 percent of pyogenic brain abscesses are mixed infections. In a summary of 12 separate series of patients with brain abscess, excluding AIDS patients, 61 percent of the isolates were aerobic bacteria and 32 percent were anaerobic bacteria. Aerobic or microaerophilic streptococci accounted for about one-half of the aerobic isolates and have been noted to be present in approximately 70 percent of all brain abscess patients. The most frequently isolated streptococci include organisms belonging to the *Streptococcus intermedius* group (*Streptococcus anginosus*, *Streptococcus constellatus*, *Streptococcus milleri*, etc.). *S. aureus* is isolated from about 15 percent of patients with brain abscess, especially abscesses developing after head trauma or neurosurgery. Aerobic gram-negative bacilli (e.g., *Proteus* sp., *E. coli*, *Klebsiella* sp., *Enterobacter* sp., and *P. aeruginosa*) have been observed with increased frequency in recent studies, often in mixed culture, and are isolated from 23 to 33 percent of patients. *Haemophilus* species other than *H. influenzae* are isolated in 5 to 10 percent of cases; *Haemophilus aphrophilus* is the most common of these. The anaerobes most recently encountered include *Bacteroides* sp. (including *Bacteroides fragilis*), *Fusobacterium* sp., *Prevotella* sp., anaerobic streptococci, and *Clostridium* sp. Anaerobic bacteria are particularly common pathogens in the setting of underlying chronic otitis or pulmonary disease.

The location of a brain abscess and its cause often suggest the most likely etiologic agent(s). Frontal lobe abscesses resulting from a preexisting sinusitis often yield an organism of the *S. intermedius* group in pure culture. Furthermore, brain abscess in association with chronic sinusitis is often a mixed infection, having an aerobic/anaerobic ratio of approximately 1 to 1.5 in most series. Posttraumatic or postoperative brain abscesses are usually caused by staphylococci. Temporal lobe abscesses are often a complication of otitis media and almost always yield multiple agents on culture, including streptococci, *Bacteroides* sp., and gram-negative aerobic bacilli. Approximately 33 percent of chronically infected ears yields anaerobes on culture. In contrast to the role of *S. pneumoniae*, *H. influenzae*, and *Moraxella catarrhalis* in acute otitis media, other streptococci, gram-negative aerobes including *P. aeruginosa*, anaerobic cocci, and *Bacteroides* sp. are the most common isolates from cases of chronic otitis media and its intracranial complications. Pneumococci, meningococci, and *H. influenzae* very rarely cause brain abscess, even in association with a purulent meningitis. Diagnosis of pneumococcal brain abscess should prompt consideration of infection with human immunodeficiency virus (HIV) as a predisposing factor.

In addition, the microbiology of a brain abscess is fundamentally influenced by the immune status of the host. Immunocompromised patients may develop brain abscess due to fungi, and *Toxoplasma gondii* is a major cause of focal CNS lesions in patients with AIDS. Brain abscess in neutropenic patients is usually due to aerobic gram-negative bacteria, *Candida* sp., *Aspergillus* sp., or zygomycosis. Approximately 50 percent of brain abscesses developing after bone marrow transplantation are due to *Aspergillus* sp.; survival is rare. Conversely, focal brain abscess in patients with abnormal cell-mediated immunity is commonly due to *T. gondii*, *Nocardia asteroides*, *L. monocytogenes*, *Mycobacterium* sp., or *Cryptococcus neoformans*. *Pseudallescheria boydii* abscess may follow a near-drowning episode. Multiple other fungi, protozoa, and helminths may cause brain abscess. *Xylohypha bantianum*, the most common agent of cerebral phaeohyphomycosis, shows a strong proclivity for causing brain abscesses.

PATHOGENESIS AND PATHOPHYSIOLOGY Most brain abscesses originate in association with one of three clinical settings: (1) the presence of a contiguous focus of infection, particularly otitis, sinusitis, or a dental infection; (2) the presence of a distant focus of infection (especially chronic pyogenic lung disease) with hematogenous spread; and (3) prior cranial trauma or surgery. The predisposing factor remains undefined in approximately 15 to 20 percent of cases.

A review of multiple series encompassing more than 3500 cases of brain abscess in the past half century reveals that about 45 percent of cases were associated with a contiguous focus of infection (predominantly otitis or sinusitis). Recent data suggest that otogenic brain abscesses are decreasing in frequency, perhaps owing to the availability and common use of antimicrobial agents for upper respiratory tract infections. Frequent but inadequate courses of antimicrobial agents for ear or sinus infections have, however, altered the natural history of brain abscess, resulting in puzzling or more subtle clinical presentations, often in association with cholesteatoma. Otogenic brain abscesses are most commonly located in the temporal lobe or cerebellum; conversely, 85 to 95 percent of cerebellar abscesses are associated with ear or mastoid infections. Usually these lesions are solitary. Sinusitis as a cause of brain abscess also appears to be decreasing in incidence. Rhinogenic abscesses are rare in children and in adults over the age of 60 years. Most brain abscesses in the setting of sinusitis are localized in the frontal lobe. Sphenoid sinusitis is notable for the frequency and severity of its intracranial complications. This form of sinusitis is often difficult to diagnose, which may lead to delay in instituting therapy. Cocaine inhalation is an additional risk factor for sphenoid sinusitis and subsequent brain abscess development. Dental infections, often overlooked as a cause of brain abscess, have been implicated in about 10 percent of patients with brain abscess. Periapical abscesses surrounding the teeth are often detected in patients with "cryptogenic brain abscess." Brain abscesses rarely complicate the course of bacterial meningitis in adolescents or adults. However, the presence of a brain abscess should be strongly considered in neonates with gram-negative meningitis, particularly meningitis due to *Citrobacter* or *Proteus* sp.

Brain abscess is a rare complication of neurosurgical procedures or cranial trauma. CNS infections occur in only 0.6 to 1.7 percent of clean neurosurgical procedures, and brain abscess accounts for only 10 percent of these infections. Brain abscess may, however, complicate penetrating cranial injuries and is especially common in the setting of gunshot wound complications. Retained bone fragments have been noted consistently as an important risk factor.

About 25 percent of cases of brain abscess arise by hematogenous spread from a distant focus of infection. These lesions are associated most often with pulmonary infections and share the following characteristics: (1) location in the distribution of the middle cerebral artery, (2) initial location at the gray matter–white matter junction, (3) poor encapsulation, and (4) a higher rate of mortality than from other types of brain abscess. Hematogenous brain abscesses are most likely to present as multiple lesions. Multiple brain abscesses were reported in only 1 to 15 percent in older series; however, with the advent of CT scanning, multiple lesions are now detected in 10 to 50 percent of patients. Important preceding processes have included chronic lung infections (lung abscess, bronchiectasis, and empyema), osteomyelitis, cholecystitis, intraabdominal infection, and/or pelvic sources. Brain abscess has been observed following endoscopic sclerosis of esophageal varices or dilatation of esophageal strictures. Although a transient bacteremia may follow these procedures and is instrumental in the development of a brain abscess, macroscopic CNS lesions are rare as complications of bacterial endocarditis. *S. aureus* is the most common cause of endocarditis complicated by intracranial involvement. Hereditary hemorrhagic telangiectasia is an important risk factor for brain abscess, especially in affected patients with clubbing, cyanosis, and/or polycythemia. This condition (Osler-Rendu-Weber syndrome), as well as unrecognized asymptomatic pulmonary arteriovenous malformations, may be underrecognized in patients with brain abscess. Cyanotic heart disease is recognized in 3 to 14 percent of brain abscess cases and may be the most common underlying process found with brain abscess in children. Tetralogy of Fallot is the most commonly cited anomaly; however, brain abscess may complicate patent foramen ovale, ventricular septal defect, and transposition of the great vessels. The presence of a right-to-left shunt and hypoxia appears to be critical for the development of brain abscess in these patients.

Brain abscess development in any of the above-described clinical settings appears to require a compromised area of brain as the final common pathway. Experimental data suggest that the brain is remarkably resistant to infection. The development of a brain abscess from an area of contiguous infection usually occurs by one of two major mechanisms: (1) direct extension through areas of associated osteitis or osteomyelitis and (2) retrograde thrombophlebitic spread via diploic or emissary veins into the intracranial compartment. The polycythemia and systemic hypoxia observed in patients with cyanotic congenital heart disease and hereditary hemorrhagic telangiectasia increase blood viscosity, which may, in concert with a reduction in brain capillary blood flow, result in microinfarction or reduced tissue oxygenation in brain, which could serve as a nidus for ensuing infection.

PATHOLOGY A solitary brain abscess involves the following brain regions in approximate decreasing order of frequency: frontal $\geq$ temporal $\geq$ frontoparietal $>$ parietal $>$ cerebellar $>$ occipital. This distribution reflects the associated, often contiguous foci of infection. Brainstem, intrasellar, basal ganglia, and thalamic abscesses are rare.

The pathologic evolution of brain abscess has been documented most convincingly in experimental models of infection and appears to involve four histopathologic stages. Importantly, the histopathologic features may correlate with specific findings on CT, a fact that has direct implications for subsequent therapy. The four stages are (1) early cerebritis (days 1 to 3 following intracerebral inoculation of animals), which is characterized by a perivascular inflammatory response surrounding a developing necrotic center, with profound edema; (2) late cerebritis, in which the well-formed necrotic center reaches its maximum size and fibroblasts and neovascularity appear in its periphery; (3) early capsule formation (days 10 to 13 following intracerebral inoculation of experimental animals), characterized by a well-developed layer of fibroblasts with persistent cerebritis, neovascularity, and reactive astrocytosis; and (4) late capsule formation, with thickening of the capsule and an abundance of reactive collagen. It should be noted, however, that this sequence is somewhat idealized; it is best described for abscesses following infection with alpha-hemolytic streptococci and may not represent the course of events in abscesses caused by other microorganisms. Encapsulation is frequently more complete on the cortical side of the abscess than on the ventricular side and is often less extensive in abscesses resulting from hematogenous spread than in those arising from a contiguous focus of infection. These observations may explain the propensity of abscesses to rupture medially into the ventricular system rather than peripherally into the subarachnoid space. Brain abscess formation represents a continuum from cerebritis to a well-encapsulated necrotic focus. The maturity of a given lesion depends on multiple factors, including local oxygen concentration, the offending microorganism, and the host immune response.

CLINICAL MANIFESTATIONS (See Table 377-4) The clinical course of a patient with a brain abscess may range from indolent to fulminant; however, the duration of symptoms is 2 weeks or less in about 75 percent of patients. In most cases, the prominent clinical manifestations of brain abscess reflect the expanding intracerebral mass rather than systemic signs of infection. Furthermore, the clinical manifestations are often nonspecific and depend on several variables (e.g., the virulence of the infecting organisms, the patient's immune status, the location of the abscess or abscesses, and the presence or absence of associated meningitis or ventricular rupture). Only a minority of patients display the classic triad of fever, headache, and focal neurologic deficits. Headache is most consistently observed (70 percent of patients). Fever is reported in only one-half of patients overall, but ≥80 percent of children are febrile. Focal neurologic deficits are encountered in about half the cases. The specific deficits present depend on the number and location of the brain abscesses and may include hemiplegia, hemianopia, cranial nerve abnormalities, and others. Cerebellar abscess often results in nystagmus, ataxia, vomiting, and dysmetria, whereas frontal lobe abscess is often dominated by headache, drowsiness, inattention, and a generalized deterioration in mental function. Hemiparesis with unilateral motor signs and/or a speech disorder are frequent findings. Seizures are observed in 25 to 45 percent of patients and, when present, are usually generalized. The presence of nausea and vomiting correlates to some degree with the ICP. A change in mental status (lethargy to coma) occurs in most patients, but frank coma on presentation is now infrequent, a change that may reflect the availability of improved diagnostic modalities such as CT. Papilledema is observed with varying frequency; it does not correlate with the size of the abscess but appears to be associated closely with the presence of headache and vomiting. Nuchal rigidity (about 25 percent of patients) is observed more commonly with a shorter duration of illness and may lead to confusion with bacterial meningitis. Intrasellar abscess often simulates a pituitary tumor, presenting with headache, visual field defects, and endocrine disturbances.

Table 377-4

Clinical Manifestations of Brain Abscess

Symptom or Sign	Percent
Headache	50–75
Triad of fever, headache, focal deficit	<50
Fever	40–50
Focal neurologic deficit	~50
Seizures	25–40
Nausea/vomiting	22–50
Nuchal rigidity	~25
Papilledema	~25

NOTE: Other symptoms and signs are dependent on location.
SOURCE: After Wispelwey and Scheld.

Since the clinical presentation may be nonspecific and fever is often absent, brain abscess may be confused with several other processes, and the following should be considered in the differential diagnosis: pyogenic meningitis, subdural empyema, epidural abscess, encephalitis, mycotic aneurysm, complicated migraine headache, intracerebral or subarachnoid hemorrhage, cerebral infarction, cerebral venous sinus thrombosis, primary or metastatic malignancies of the CNS, and rarely, multiple sclerosis.

DIAGNOSIS Routine studies of the blood and urine are rarely helpful in the diagnosis of a brain abscess. A moderate peripheral blood leukocytosis may be present, but 40 percent of patients display a completely normal peripheral leukocyte count. The erythrocyte sedimentation rate is often elevated, but it may be normal in the setting of cyanotic congenital heart disease. The serum concentration of C-reactive protein has been used to differentiate brain abscess from intracranial neoplasms but is inadequate for this purpose. Blood cultures are only occasionally (≤10 percent) positive in patients with a brain abscess.

Although the CSF is often abnormal in patients with brain abscess, the findings are nonspecific, and lumbar puncture is usually contraindicated in a patient with a suspected parenchymal abscess. The diagnostic yield is poor, and the risk of herniation after the procedure has been reported to be as high as 20 percent. The poor diagnostic yield and significant morbidity of lumbar puncture in the presence of a brain abscess necessitate that this procedure be delayed in patients with a febrile CNS disorder with focal neurologic signs. However, if pyogenic meningitis is also a strong consideration, blood cultures should be obtained and appropriate antimicrobial agents started parenterally before a neuroradiologic study is performed. Although abnormalities may be noted, skull roentgenograms, electroencephalograms, arteriography, ventriculography, and/or technetium-99m brain scans are rarely necessary in the evaluation of a patient with a suspected brain abscess. Radionuclide brain scans are, however, useful in facilities lacking CT and MRI technology.

The introduction of CT and MRI has revolutionized the diagnostic and therapeutic approach to brain abscess. CT scans of the paranasal sinuses, mastoids, middle ear, and brain should be obtained, along with a chest roentgenogram, in all patients with suspected brain abscess. CT is sensitive (>95 percent) in the detection of a brain abscess, and it can give additional crucial information such as the extent of the surrounding edema, the presence of hydrocephalus and/or a midline shift, and the precise site of the lesion. On CT with contrast administration, a brain abscess typically appears as a hypodense lesion surrounded by a uniformly enhancing ring. A variable, hypodense area of edema extends beyond the ring. Unfortunately, this CT appearance is not specific for a brain abscess, and other processes, including neoplasm, granuloma, cerebral infarction, and resolving hematoma, may have similar appearance on CT. Furthermore, glucocorticoid use may alter the typical appearance on CT; only 40 to 60 percent of brain abscesses in patients receiving glucocorticoid therapy reveal ring enhancement on CT scan. Indium 111–labeled leukocyte scintigraphy may prove complementary to CT in the diagnosis of abscesses in the CNS. However, necrotic tumors may be confused with brain abscess by this technique, and the concomitant use of glucocorticoids also may produce a false-negative scan. A potentially exciting nuclear medicine modality in the evaluation of cerebral mass lesions was developed recently. Thallium-201 single photon emission CT (SPECT) may per-

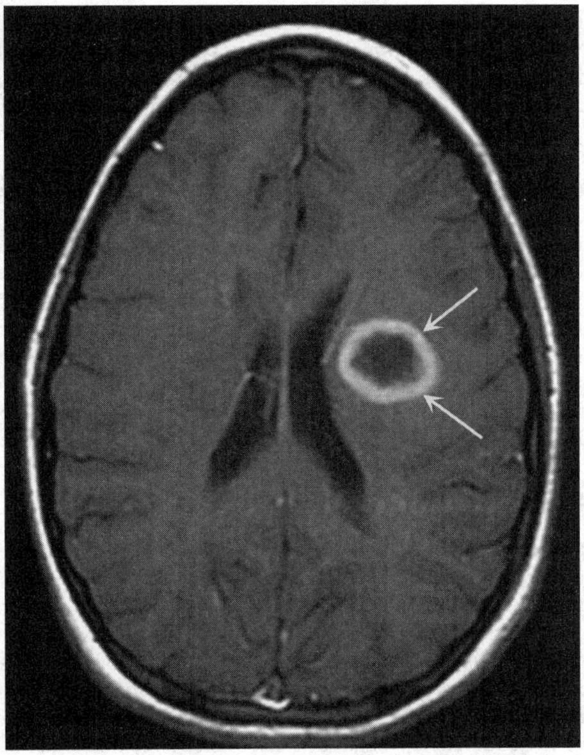

FIGURE 377-2 MRI of brain abscess. Coronal T1-weighted spin-echo image following gadolinium-DTPA enhancement demonstrating large necrotic right frontal lobe mass with intense peripheral enhancement and surrounding edema. Multiple complications are also evident: ependymal enhancement in the lateral and third ventricles and enhancement of the subarachnoid space reflecting ventricular rupture, ventriculitis, and meningitis, and a mass effect with midline shift. Aspiration revealed pus and *S. milleri* in pure culture.

mit differentiation of CNS lymphoma from toxoplasmic encephalitis in AIDS patients (see Chap. 308), but its role in suspected pyogenic abscess is unsettled.

Data on the usefulness of MRI in the diagnosis and evaluation of patients with brain abscess continue to accumulate. MRI permits multiplanar imaging, is better than CT at distinguishing between gray and white matter, and affords a variety of imaging techniques to elucidate pathologic changes. In addition, bony artifact, which may hinder the interpretation of CT scans, is not a problem with MRI. MRI appears to be more sensitive than CT at detecting brain abscess in the cerebritis phase of its development as well as at detecting associated cerebral edema. Therefore, MRI may detect early satellite lesions not demonstrated by CT and is often more useful than CT for demonstration of extraparenchymal extension of an abscess (i.e., ventricular rupture) (Fig. 377-2). The lack of ionizing radiation, better tissue characterization, lack of bony artifact, increased sensitivity in follow-up evaluations, and less toxic contrast agents (e.g., gadolinium-DTPA) make MRI the procedure of choice in the evaluation of a patient with suspected brain abscess.

℞ TREATMENT

The optimal management of most patients with a bacterial brain abscess involves both administration of antimicrobial agents and surgical intervention. CT or MRI should be performed without delay in the patient with neurologic complaints and a predisposing condition suggesting brain abscess, as described above. Results in animal models and humans suggest that focal bacterial infections of the brain parenchyma can be "staged" by sequential CT scanning. Cerebritis is characterized by an area of low density surrounded by ring enhancement (often thick and diffuse) that is undecayed on repeat scans obtained 1 h later. In contrast, an encapsulated abscess is characterized by a faint ring on the unenhanced scan and ring enhancement that is decayed on the repeat CT scan. These parameters may prove useful in planning a combined medical-surgical approach. Since 1971, it has been recognized that early antimicrobial therapy alone, in the absence of surgical intervention, could cure cerebritis and prevent the development of an encapsulated abscess. Subsequent cases in which the cure of an encapsulated abscess was claimed share many of the following features: (1) sequential CT scans were used to diagnose brain abscess and to follow the resolution of the lesion(s); aspiration biopsy and histopathologic analysis usually were not done; (2) prolonged courses (e.g., ≥8 weeks) of high-dose antibiotic therapy were administered; and (3) evidence of encapsulation often was lacking. Based on experimental animal models of brain abscess and the well-defined CT appearance of the cerebritis stage, medical "cures" of established brain abscess may represent successful resolution of bacterial cerebritis. In general, close cooperation between medical and surgical specialists is essential for the optimal management of a patient with suspected brain abscess.

The antimicrobial regimens recommended for the empirical (and specific) therapy of a brain abscess reflect considerations of the microbiology as well as evidence from both animal and human studies evaluating the penetration of a given antimicrobial agent into brain parenchyma and/or brain abscess pus. Unfortunately, no prospective, randomized clinical trials exist to guide the clinician in the choice of an optimal antimicrobial regimen. If CT suggests cerebritis and the patient is neurologically stable, antibiotics can be started and the patient observed. Since the early 1960s, a combination of penicillin G (20 to 24 million units per day intravenously) plus chloramphenicol (1.0 to 1.5 g intravenously every 6 h) has been advocated in adults. Penicillin remains a mainstay of therapy because of (1) excellent activity against streptococci, including the *S. intermedius* group, complicating contiguous foci of infection and pyogenic lung disease; (2) activity against most anaerobes encountered in brain abscess patients; (3) favorable results obtained in experimental animal models of brain abscess; and (4) a marked reduction in brain abscess mortality observed after the introduction of penicillin in the 1940s. Cefotaxime in high doses (e.g., 3 g intravenously every 8 h) is an acceptable substitute for penicillin in empirical combination regimens that include an antianaerobic agent, e.g., metronidazole. Chloramphenicol often has been administered concurrently with penicillin in the past because of its high lipid solubility, which results in brain tissue concentrations that often exceed the levels in plasma, and its good activity against anaerobic bacteria, including *B. fragilis*. The use of metronidazole for the therapy of brain abscess has increased greatly in recent years, and this agent has generally supplanted chloramphenicol because (1) metronidazole is bactericidal against *B. fragilis*, whereas chloramphenicol may be bacteriostatic; (2) metronidazole attains reproducibly excellent concentrations in brain abscess pus; (3) concomitant steroid treatment does not affect the entry of metronidazole into brain abscess pus, in contrast to its effect on several other antibiotics; (4) chloramphenicol may be degraded by desacetylation in pus, as shown in experimental intraabdominal abscess; and (5) use of metronidazole may reduce mortality rates, as suggested by several recent retrospective studies. Although use of metronidazole instead of chloramphenicol may lead to more rapid healing and a lower mortality rate, these two agents have never been compared in a prospective, randomized clinical trial. Nevertheless, an antianaerobic agent such as metronidazole (or, perhaps, ampicillin-sulbactam) is indicated for the treatment of brain abscess complicating otitis media, mastoiditis, or pyogenic lung abscess because anaerobes are often present. Metronidazole should never be used alone to treat a patient with suspected brain abscess. Antianaerobic therapy may not be necessary in addition to penicillin for patients with frontal or ethmoidal sinusitis and brain abscess, because *B. fragilis* is an uncommon isolate; however, empirical therapy with at least two agents is mandatory prior to culture confirmation. When the presence of staphylococci is proven or suspected, as in posttraumatic or postneurosurgical brain abscess, nafcillin or oxacillin (1.5 to 2 g intravenously every 4 h) is indicated. Vancomycin may be substituted if either the patient is allergic to penicillin or a methicillin-resistant strain is isolated. Fusidic acid is frequently employed in Europe, but it is not available in the United States. The frequent isolation of aerobic gram-negative bacilli from brain abscesses of otitic origin prompts many physicians to add a third-generation cephalosporin or trimethoprim-sulfamethoxazole to the antimicrobial regimen while awaiting culture results. Since *P. aeruginosa* is encountered in this setting of chronic middle ear infection, ceftazidime is a logical empirical choice. Recent data suggest that cefotaxime may be adequate for most streptococcal isolates as well, thereby replacing penicillin as the standard regimen (i.e., cefotaxime plus metronidazole as empirical therapy). It is unclear whether instillation of antibiotics into the abscess cavity during aspiration provides additional benefit.

The question of whether to use aspiration alone or total excision of a brain abscess in an individual patient remains problematic. Given the availability of stereotactic CT-guided aspiration, its low morbidity, and the chance it gives to obtain an accurate microbiologic and pathologic diagnosis, operative therapy should remain the definitive approach for most patients with brain abscess. If CT or MRI suggests the presence of cerebritis and the patient is neurologically stable, antibiotic therapy as previously outlined should be initiated and the patient observed. If the patient remains stable and the abscess or abscesses are accessible, CT-guided aspiration is then desirable to facilitate a specific pathologic and microbiologic diagnosis. This approach is advocated even if multiple lesions are present. Although this delay may render subsequent cultures negative, aspiration during the cerebritis stage may be associated with an unacceptable risk of hemorrhage, especially in children. If the lesion appears encapsulated by CT, antibiotic therapy should be started and aspiration for diagnosis and drainage performed immediately. Subsequent management will depend on both clinical and radiologic assessments. Multiple aspirations may be required to drain the abscess successfully, and this is a potential disadvantage relative to total excision. Neurologic deterioration, gas in the abscess cavity, or failure of the lesion to resolve on follow-up imaging studies is an indication for further surgery, often excision if feasible. The duration of antimicrobial therapy is empirical and also may relate to the initial surgical procedure used. Lesions treated by total excision may require a shorter duration of antimicrobial therapy than those treated with aspiration only. In general, most authorities recommend that patients be treated with at least 4 to 6 weeks of parenteral therapy. Metronidazole therapy may be an exception to this rule, because the high oral bioavailability of this agent facilitates the use of oral regimens. If a suitable oral agent or agents is available, a prolonged course of oral therapy, continuing for 2 to 6 months after the end of parenteral therapy, is often given, but it is of no proven benefit when compared with shorter treatment regimens. A cured brain abscess may continue to exhibit contrast enhancement on CT scans for from 4 to 10 weeks to up to 6 to 9 months after completion of successful therapy. The management of a focal CNS process in an HIV-infected patient requires a different approach and is discussed in Chap. 379. Empirical therapy for toxoplasmosis is often started if the CT appearance is characteristic in a seropositive patient. Brain biopsy for diagnosis may be considered in patients with a negative toxoplasmosis serology, atypical findings on CT, or evidence of a disseminated process due to another pathogen.

Adjunctive glucocorticoids are often employed during management of patients with brain abscess, but their role remains controversial. Glucocorticoids may reduce antibiotic entry into the CNS; they may decrease collagen formation and glial response and thereby lessen the degree of encapsulation of the brain abscess; and they may alter the CT appearance of ring enhancement as inflammation subsides, which may obscure information from sequential CT studies for the assessment of cure. Experimental animal models do not suggest that glucocorticoids alter the mortality rate. Glucocorticoids should be employed in patients with proven or suspected elevation of ICP. In this circumstance, ICP monitoring may be advisable, and elevation may be controlled with steroids, hyperventilation, mannitol, or a combination of these methods. Anticonvulsants are frequently administered empirically to patients with suspected brain abscess.

PROGNOSIS The mortality rate of brain abscess was about 40 to 60 percent in the preantibiotic era and has remained high until relatively recently. The major reduction of the mortality rate (to about 10 percent) coincides with the advent of CT. The incidence of neurologic sequelae, however, ranges between 30 and 55 percent, and late seizures have been documented in as many as 90 percent of survivors. The relative uses of medical and surgical approaches for the individual patient continue to be elucidated. Earlier diagnosis through improved technology and an aggressive medical-surgical approach remain essential for the successful management of this unforgiving CNS infection.

SUBDURAL EMPYEMA

DEFINITION Subdural empyema is a collection of pus in the space between the dura mater and the arachnoid membrane. Subdural empyema accounts for about 20 percent of all localized intracranial infections. Prior to the advent of antimicrobial therapy, the disease was almost always fatal, but with current methods of diagnosis and treatment, mortality rates range from 10 to 40 percent.

EPIDEMIOLOGY Although precise incidence figures are unavailable, subdural empyemas are most often a complication of otorhinologic infection. Male patients predominate by a ratio of approximately 3:1, and about 70 percent of patients are in the second or third decade of life.

ETIOLOGY In most cases, a single microorganism is responsible for subdural empyema, but many cultures obtained at surgery are sterile because patients are often receiving antimicrobial therapy. In addition, the precise role of anaerobic bacteria in this infection has not been studied carefully because anaerobic techniques are often inadequate or not performed at surgery. Nevertheless, the major pathogens include aerobic and anaerobic streptococci (about 50 percent), staphylococci (about 12 to 16 percent), aerobic gram-negative bacilli (3 to 10 percent), and other anaerobic bacteria (about 5 percent). As with brain abscess, the causative organism is somewhat predictable based on the anatomic focus of contiguous infection. Otorhinogenic subdural empyemas are usually caused by streptococci (including members of the *S. intermedius* group), whereas staphylococci and anaerobes are unusual. Infections arising from head trauma, surgery, or indwelling foreign devices commonly involve staphylococci and/or aerobic gram-negative bacilli. Subdural empyema rarely complicates meningitis, but cases due to *S. pneumoniae* or *H. influenzae* have been described. Rare etiologic agents include *Salmonella* sp., *Campylobacter fetus*, *N. meningitidis*, *Pasteurella* sp., and *Actinomyces* sp.

PATHOGENESIS AND PATHOPHYSIOLOGY The subdural space, normally a potential rather than an actual space, is divided anatomically into several large compartments by the foramen magnum, tentorium cerebelli, base of the brain, and falx cerebri. Since these spaces are confined anatomically, a developing empyema can quickly evolve into a fatal expanding mass lesion. The pathogenesis usually involves spread of infection to the subdural space via valveless emissary veins in association with thrombophlebitis or by extension of an osteomyelitis of the skull with accompanying epidural abscess. Paranasal sinusitis predominates overwhelmingly as the precipitating factor. The frontal sinuses are almost always involved, often with other sinuses as well. The incidence of subdural empyema following frontal sinusitis is 1 to 2 percent. The frontal and sphenoid sinuses are intimately associated with the dura mater and are often separated from it by only a thin bony layer. Only about 10 percent of subdural empyemas are found infratentorially. The lesion may communicate with the contralateral side via the inferior free margin of the falx cerebri. The mastoid or middle ear is the source of subdural empyema in 10 to 20 percent of patients, especially in geographic areas (e.g., Sri Lanka) where delay in therapy of otitis media may be complicated by this event. Otitis or mastoiditis may extend directly into the subdural space via erosion of the tegmen tympani or bone adjacent to the dura mater and air cells or may spread indirectly by way of a progressive thrombophlebitis of the perforating veins. Otitis-induced subdural empyema is localized initially on or around the tentorium. Bacterial meningitis in adults is a very unusual cause of subdural empyema. Nevertheless, this lesion complicates about 2 percent of bacterial meningitis cases in infants and may follow an initially sterile subdural effusion. Other predisposing conditions include cranial trauma, use of cranial traction devices, neurosurgical or nasal procedures, and infection of a preexisting subdural hematoma. Subdural empyema is metastatic in origin in a small minority of cases (about 5 percent), arising principally from chronic infection in the chest. Once infection develops in the subdural space, spread along the falx and over the convexities may occur. Septic thrombophlebitis of the cortical veins and/or dural venous sinuses may evolve and lead to hemorrhage, cerebral infarction, brain edema, and fatal transtentorial herniation.

CLINICAL MANIFESTATIONS Subdural empyema may present as a rapidly progressive life-threatening condition. The symptoms and signs relate to the presence of increased ICP, meningeal irritation, or focal cortical inflammation. In addition, most patients (60 to 90 percent) have evidence of their antecedent infection (e.g., sinusitis or otitis). In general, patients often have a nonspecific illness for days to weeks prior to an acutely ill presentation. The most common symptoms and signs include headache, fever, stiff neck, and focal neurologic deficits. Headache, initially localized to the infected sinus or ear, is a prominent complaint and can become generalized as the infection progresses. Vomiting is common as ICP rises. Early during the course, about one-half of patients have altered mental status, which can progress to obtundation and/or coma in the absence of treatment. Fever above 39°C is present in most cases. Focal neurologic findings appear after 24 to 48 h of illness and progress rapidly to involvement of the entire cerebral hemisphere. Hemiparesis or hemiplegia is the most common focal finding; ocular palsy is common, and dysphasia, homonymous hemianopia, cerebellar signs, dilated pupils, and other focal presentations also have been observed. Seizures, either focal or generalized, are found in more than 50 percent of cases. Meningeal irritation (particularly meningismus) is found in 70 to 80 percent of patients, although Kernig's and/or Babinski's signs are less frequently noted. In the absence of treatment, neurologic deterioration occurs rapidly with signs of increased ICP and cerebral herniation. Papilledema develops in less than 50 percent of patients. Parafalcine subdural empyema characteristically produces contralateral leg symptoms, including weakness and focal seizures. This fulminant picture may not be seen in several clinical settings, including subdural empyema following cranial surgery and/or trauma, where the presentation may be subacute and subtle; subdural empyema affected by prior antimicrobial therapy; subdural empyema resulting from infection of a subdural hematoma; and metastatic infection of the subdural space from a chronic focus elsewhere. The clinical manifestations of subdural empyema in infants are similar to those found in adults, except that a bulging anterior fontanelle is a common finding.

DIAGNOSIS As with brain abscess, routine studies of blood, urine, and CSF are of limited value in the evaluation of patients with suspected subdural empyema. Most patients have a peripheral blood leukocytosis, and plain films of the skull may be useful in the demonstration of sinusitis or mastoiditis. Since a high degree of clinical suspicion and rapid diagnosis of this condition are critical for a successful outcome, subdural empyema should be suspected in any patient with a CNS syndrome with fever and focal neurologic findings. Lumbar puncture is contraindicated in this setting because of the risk of cerebral herniation. When it is performed, CSF findings are nonspecific and include an elevated opening pressure, a moderate neutrophilic pleocytosis, and an increased protein concentration. Unless the course is complicated by coexisting bacterial meningitis, Gram's staining and cultures of CSF are negative. Cerebral arteriography was the diagnostic procedure of choice prior to the development of CT.

Currently, CT with contrast enhancement and MRI are the diagnostic procedures of choice in patients with suspected subdural empyema. The typical CT appearance is a crescentic or elliptical area of hypodensity below the cranial vault or adjacent to the falx cerebri. Loculations may be seen, and associated mass effect with displacement of midline structures is common. After the administration of contrast material, a fine, intense line of enhancement is seen between the subdural collection and the cerebral cortex. Gyral enhancement also is common. However, false-negative CT scans have been reported; MRI provides greater clarity for morphologic detail and may detect empyema not seen clearly on CT. MRI is of particular value in identifying subdural empyema located at the base of the brain, along the falx cerebri, or in the posterior fossa. On the basis of signal intensity, extraaxial empyemas can be differentiated from sterile effusions and/or chronic hematomas more readily by MRI than by CT. MRI is also better than CT for differentiating subdural empyema from epidural abscess and in delineating brain parenchymal abnormalities.

Both CT and MRI can be useful for the demonstration of sinusitis and otitis, although CT is better than MRI for bone imaging and should be used in cases of penetrating injury or when osteomyelitis is a consideration. Cerebral arteriography should be employed on an emergent basis when MRI is unavailable and subdural empyema is strongly suspected despite a normal CT appearance. Arteriography may establish the presence of a subdural avascular mass and detect spread of the lesion to the contralateral or parafalcine subdural space. As stated above, subdural empyema shows a striking predilection for young men in the second and third decades of life and should be strongly considered when a patient in this group has appropriate clinical findings.

℞ TREATMENT

Subdural empyema is a surgical emergency. While the patient is awaiting operative intervention, antibiotics should be chosen based on the suspected source of infection, the known organisms associated with that focus of infection, and the host immune status. A combined medical-surgical approach is optimal for the management of these patients. As with brain abscess, no controlled clinical trials have evaluated different antimicrobial regimens for the treatment of subdural empyema. Empirical therapy often includes penicillin G and/or chloramphenicol in the same doses as used for brain abscess (see above). If staphylococci are suspected, a β-lactamase–stable penicillin (e.g., nafcillin, 1.5 g intravenously every 4 h) should be used, with vancomycin (about 1 g intravenously every 12 h in adults) reserved for patients allergic to penicillin or when the presence of methicillin-resistant *S. aureus* is suspected. Metronidazole is often substituted for chloramphenicol at a loading dosage of 15 mg/kg, followed by 7.5 mg/kg intravenously every 6 h. Many authorities also add a third-generation cephalosporin (often cefotaxime or ceftriaxone) until culture results are available. Ceftazidime is useful in patients in whom *P. aeruginosa* is a consideration (e.g., in cases following neurosurgery or trauma). The duration of therapy is empirical; however, parenteral antibiotics should be continued for 3 to 4 weeks after drainage, depending on the patient's clinical response. Longer periods of intravenous therapy and/or continuation as an oral regimen may be required if an associated osteomyelitis is present.

Although case reports have suggested that subdural empyema may respond to antimicrobial agents alone, the optimal approach involves surgical drainage. The comparative efficacy of multiple burr holes versus an open craniotomy has not been subjected to rigorous clinical trial. All cases should involve close cooperation with a neurosurgical service. Previous reports of a lower mortality rate in studies of patients undergoing craniotomy may merely reflect the treatment of a larger percentage of gravely ill patients with burr hole drainage alone because of the greater surgical risk associated with an open craniotomy. Unfortunately, burr holes may be inadequate due to the thickened pus during the course of the infection. Craniotomy is often essential for posterior fossa subdural empyemas and is also needed in the 10 to 20 percent of patients who are initially treated with trephination. When craniotomy is performed, wide exposure should be obtained to allow adequate exploration of all areas where subdural pus is suspected. Although antibiotic irrigation at the time of surgery has become common, there are no data on the benefits of this practice. Drains or catheters are often left in the subdural space after the initial drainage, but this practice may increase the risk of nosocomial superinfection. Finally, surgical correction of the antecedent otorhinologic infection also may be necessary on an emergent basis. Adjunctive measures to control raised ICP are also essential. Preoperative use of mannitol, dexamethasone, and/or hyperventilation may be effective in controlling ICP. Glucocorticoids should, however, be tapered rapidly after surgical therapy because of the risk of secondary infection. Anticonvulsants are indicated in patients with seizures.

PROGNOSIS The overall mortality rate from subdural empyema averages 15 to 25 percent, with severe neurologic sequelae (chiefly disabling hemiparesis or aphasia) found in 5 to 25 percent of survivors. Seizures are documented on follow-up in 8 to 46 percent of patients. The presence of severe neurologic sequelae and of a more profound depression of consciousness at the time of presentation and/or initiation of therapy correlates directly with a higher mortality rate, a fact that underscores the need for rapid definitive diagnosis.

SPINAL SUBDURAL EMPYEMA This rare condition, with fewer than 50 cases reported in the literature, is far less common than spinal epidural abscess. The signs and symptoms include fever, back pain, and subsequent manifestations of spinal cord compression, but tenderness to palpation or percussion along the spine is often absent, in contrast to spinal epidural abscess. Most cases occur following hematogenous dissemination from a distant site of infection, and *S. aureus* is the most common etiologic agent. The presentation may resemble that of transverse myelitis. MRI is the diagnostic procedure of choice for suspected spinal subdural empyema, since it defines the extent of the lesion better than does CT. Spinal CT with metrizamide contrast is also useful in the diagnosis of this condition. Myelography should be performed when MRI and CT are not available. Myelography may not detect the entire length of the empyema if complete blocks are present in the spinal canal at multiple levels. Treatment should consist of empirical antibiotics directed initially at *S. aureus*. streptococci, and gram-negative enteric bacilli in association with prompt laminectomy for drainage of the empyema. The antimicrobial regimen is commonly administered for 2 to 4 weeks following surgical drainage.

EPIDURAL ABSCESS

SPINAL EPIDURAL ABSCESS This type of abscess possesses unique clinical features and constitutes an important neurologic and neurosurgical emergency. It is discussed in Chap. 373.

INTRACRANIAL EPIDURAL ABSCESS An *epidural abscess* is defined as a suppurative infection in the epidural space. This space is located between the dura mater and the overlying bone. Cranial epidural abscess often crosses the cranial dura along the emissary veins, so subdural empyema is also often present. Therefore, the etiology, pathogenesis, and bacteriology of intracranial abscess are usually similar to those described for subdural empyema, with an initial focus of infection in the paranasal sinuses, middle ear, or mastoids. The overall incidence of cranial epidural abscess is unknown. In general, it is the third most common localized intracranial infection, following brain abscess and subdural empyema in frequency. Only about 10 percent of all epidural abscesses arise in the intracranial epidural space. Unlike the striking sex and age distribution of subdural empyema, intracranial abscesses are rare in young children and have been reported over a wide age range, with a median in the sixth decade. Above the foramen magnum, the epidural space is only a potential space, since the dura is essentially adherent to the inner lining of the skull. Infections of the intracranial epidural space result primarily from an extension of a contiguous focus of infection, such as sinusitis, mastoiditis, scalp or orbital cellulitis, and rhinocerebral mucormycosis, or as a result of an intracranial defect caused by a skull fracture or neurosurgical procedure, or as a complication of fetal monitoring. The risk of epidural abscess is increased if there has been more than one prior neurosurgical procedure or implantation of foreign material. In general, an epidural abscess is a slowly growing mass, a fact that accounts for its typically insidious clinical presentation. Intracranial abscesses rarely dissect beyond the base of the skull. As with subdural empyema, the organisms responsible for intracranial epidural abscesses depend on the underlying mechanism. Aerobic and microaerophilic streptococci predominate in cases derived from paranasal sinus infections, whereas *S. aureus* or *S. epidermidis* and aerobic gram-negative bacilli and/or anaerobes are associated with cranial trauma. Many other organisms have been isolated from localized intracranial abscesses, including *Salmonella* sp., *Eikenella corrodens*, *Aspergillus* sp., and the agents of mucormycosis. The onset of symptoms is often insidious and may be overshadowed by the primary focus of infection (e.g., sinusitis or otitis). Headache is a usual complaint, but the patient may otherwise be asymptomatic unless the clinical course is complicated by the development of subdural empyema or involvement of deeper intracranial structures, because the epidural abscess usually enlarges slowly and does not produce sudden major neurologic deficits unless complicated by deep extension. However, focal neurologic signs and/or focal generalized seizures, nausea, and vomiting may develop ultimately. Without treatment, papilledema or other signs of increased ICP develop as the abscess enlarges. An epidural abscess localized near the petrous bone may present as Gradenigo's syndrome, characterized by involvement of cranial nerves V and VI with unilateral facial pain and weakness of the lateral rectus muscle. If cranial osteomyelitis is present, edema and cellulitis of the face and/or scalp may be present. Attention may be focused on the primary process, such as sinusitis, cellulitis, or skull fracture, allowing a developing intracranial abscess to remain undetected. Thus, the striking manifestations of the complications, including an alteration in mental status and a declining level of consciousness (including coma and/or meningismus), may be the first indication of an intracranial process. Hyponatremia is found in ≥ 30 percent of cases. As with patients with suspected subdural empyema, CT scanning and MRI are the diagnostic procedures of choice for the detection of intracranial epidural abscess. Both studies usually demonstrate a superficial, circumscribed area of diminished density, often with a rim of contrast enhancement. This rim enhancement is usually thicker and more irregular with an epidural abscess than with subdural empyema. Subgaleal or subperiosteal abscesses, calvarial osteomyelitis, and frontal sinusitis are often associated with intracranial abscesses. MRI offers several advantages over CT scanning in the evaluation of patients with suspected intracranial epidural abscess. Small collections are often identified more accurately with MRI, and streak artifacts from bone are absent. In addition, MRI readily differentiates postoperative and posttraumatic abscesses from sterile effusions and/or chronic extraaxial hematomas; CT is far less accurate at making this distinction.

Rx TREATMENT

As is the case with other focal suppurative infections of the CNS, a combined medical-surgical therapeutic approach is optimal for management of intracranial epidural abscess. In adults, where 60 to 90 percent of intracranial abscesses are a direct result of extension from paranasal sinusitis or mastoiditis, empirical antimicrobial therapy should be directed against aerobic streptococci, staphylococci, and anaerobic bacteria and commonly involves a combination of agents. When cranial defects are suspected or proven, an antistaphylococcal agent such as a penicillinase-resistant penicillin or vancomycin should be added in the dosages discussed above. All intracranial epidural collections should be drained surgically. Furthermore, appropriate stains and cultures should be obtained at the time of surgery, including investigation for acid-fast bacteria and/or fungi if clinically warranted. The actual procedure employed, e.g., burr holes versus craniotomy or craniectomy, depends on the extent of the lesion and involvement of overlying bone. Dural grafting may be necessary if the dura has been breached by infection, and communications between sinus cavities and the epidural space may require surgical closure later. Perhaps owing to the insidious clinical presentation of intracranial epidural abscess, the high diagnostic accuracy of CT and MRI, and the availability of potent antimicrobial agents, the rates of morbidity and mortality from this condition are low. However, the prognosis is inversely related to the degree of encephalopathy at presentation.

SUPPURATIVE INTRACRANIAL THROMBOPHLEBITIS

EPIDEMIOLOGY AND ETIOLOGY Suppurative intracranial thrombophlebitis is defined by the simultaneous presence of venous thrombosis and suppuration in the intracranial compartment. The process may begin in veins and/or venous sinuses following infection of the paranasal sinuses, middle ear, mastoid, facial skin, or oropharynx and may involve additional vessels by propagation of clot or discontinuous spread. Septic intracranial thrombophlebitis also may complicate the presence of epidural abscess, subdural empyema, or bacterial meningitis. Occasionally, but rarely, metastatic spread of infection from a distant site leads directly to suppurative intracranial thrombophlebitis. Conditions that increase blood viscosity or coagulability, including dehydration, pregnancy, oral contraceptive use, sickle cell disease, polycythemia, malignancy, and trauma, all increase the likelihood of intracranial thrombosis and suppurative complications. Intracranial venous sinus thrombosis depends, to a large extent, on the close proximity of the dural venous sinuses to other structures involved by antecedent conditions. The usual predisposing conditions for the development of cavernous sinus thrombosis are paranasal sinusitis (especially of the frontal, ethmoidal, or sphenoidal sinuses) or infections of the face or mouth. The most common bacterial pathogens depend on the initial source of infection; with sinusitis, they are staphylococci, aerobic and/or microaerophilic streptococci, gram-negative bacilli, and/or anaerobes, whereas *S. aureus* predominates when a facial infection is the source. Otitis media or mastoiditis may be complicated by the development of lateral sinus thrombosis and/or infection of the superior and inferior petrosal sinuses. Infections of the face, scalp, subdural space, epidural space, or meninges are associated with suppurative thrombophlebitis of the superior sagittal sinus. Again, the most likely infecting microorganisms depend on the associated primary condition. *S. aureus* is the most important associated pathogen in patients with cavernous sinus thrombosis and is isolated in more than two-thirds of cases. This predominance reflects the importance of this organism in the associated infections of the face and scalp and in acute sphenoid sinusitis. Less common isolates in patients with cavernous sinus thrombosis include streptococci, pneumococci, gram-negative bacilli, and *Bacteroides* sp.

CLINICAL MANIFESTATIONS Not unexpectedly, the clinical presentation of suppurative cortical thrombophlebitis depends on the location of involvement. In addition, if the cortical venous system is involved, the likelihood of neurologic deficits depends on the adequacy of collateral venous drainage. Patients with inadequate collateral flow present with impairment of consciousness, focal or generalized seizures (often alternating in character), symptoms of increased ICP, and various focal neurologic findings (e.g., hemiparesis). Aphasia is common when the dominant cerebral hemisphere is involved. The most common complaints in patients with cavernous sinus thrombosis include periorbital swelling (73 percent) and headache (52 percent). Headache is more common when the antecedent condition is sinusitis rather than a facial cellulitis. Other prominent symptoms include diplopia, tearing, photophobia, drowsiness, and ptosis. Fever is present in over 90 percent of patients with cavernous sinus thrombosis. Upon examination, proptosis, chemosis, periorbital edema, and weakness of the extraocular muscles due to involvement of cranial nerves III, IV, or VI are common. Since the abducens nerve is the only cranial nerve traversing the inferior portion of the cavernous sinus, a lateral gaze palsy may be an early neurologic finding. Papilledema and/or retinal hemorrhages, and venous engorgement with a change in mental status, are observed in approximately 65 and 55 percent of patients, respectively. Meningitis is present in about 40 percent of cases and often creates diagnostic confusion; it is usually secondary to retrograde spread of thrombophlebitis. About 25 percent of patients also have dilated or sluggishly reactive pupils, decreased visual acuity (frequently progressing to blindness), and dysfunction of cranial nerve V. With spread of the infection to the opposite cavernous sinus, these findings may be duplicated in the opposite eye. In addition, septic cavernous sinus thrombosis may present in two ways. In the acute presentation, the delay in onset between the primary infection (usually a facial cellulitis) and cavernous sinus thrombosis is less than 1 week. The patient appears seriously ill, with a rapid development of symptoms and signs described above and progression to bilateral eye signs. In contrast, some patients present with a more indolent form of cavernous sinus thrombosis, usually secondary to dental infections, otitis media, or paranasal sinusitis. The orbital manifestations are less impressive, and involvement of the contralateral eye is a late and inconsistent finding. Headache is the most prominent finding (>80 percent of cases) in patients with septic lateral sinus thrombosis, but earache, vomiting, nausea, and vertigo are often present, since otitis media is a common predisposing condition. Fever and abnormal ear findings are observed in most patients (about 80 and 98 percent, respectively); facial pain, altered facial sensation, papilledema, mild nuchal rigidity, and/or a sixth nerve palsy also may be present. Thrombosis of the superior sagittal sinus produces an abnormal mental status progressing to coma, motor deficits (bilateral leg weakness progressing to arm weakness), nuchal rigidity, and papilledema. Seizurs occur in more than 50 percent of patients. The onset may be subacute, particularly in patients with sinusitis. Involvement of the inferior petrosal sinus may produce ipsilateral facial pain and lateral rectus muscle weakness (Gradenigo's syndrome).

DIAGNOSIS MRI is the diagnostic procedure of choice for the evaluation of patients with suspected suppurative intracranial thrombophlebitis. MRI is far superior to CT in differentiating thrombosis from normally flowing blood and can be improved by use of magnetic resonance angiography. MRI also can reveal the evolution and resolution of the entire venoocclusive process. CT scanning, with and without intravenous contrast enhancement, also permits diagnosis of venous sinus thrombosis, but it is considerably less sensitive and reliable than MRI. The CT appearance usually consists of unilateral or bilateral multiple irregular filling defects in the enhancement of the cavernous sinus with or without orbital inflammatory changes. Both MRI and CT can reliably evaluate the paranasal sinuses and provide information concerning subdural and epidural infection, cerebral infarction, cerebritis, hemorrhage, and/or cerebral edema. In the unusual case in which MRI and CT are negative but suspicion of thrombophlebitis is high, carotid arteriography with venous phase studies should be performed. Arteriography reveals narrowing of the intracavernous segment of the carotid artery in cavernous sinus thrombosis. Orbital venography also may be useful and is the most definitive method of demonstrating cavernous sinus thrombosis. As with other focal suppurative intracranial processes, the lumbar puncture usually demonstrates a mild pleocytosis and an elevated protein concentration. In septic thrombosis of the superior sagittal sinus, however, the CSF findings may be consistent with a frank meningitis, and the causative organism is often isolated on CSF culture. Blood cultures may be positive, especially in patients with a rapidly progressing course. Chest radiographs may reveal evidence of septic pulmonary emboli following propagation of thrombus into the inferior petrosal sinus and the jugular vein.

℞ TREATMENT

As for subdural empyema and epidural abscess, empirical therapy should be directed at gram-positive organisms, including staphylococci, aerobic gram-negative bacilli, and anaerobes. In cavernous sinus thrombosis, a potent antistaphylococcal agent should always be included in the antimicrobial regimen. Nafcillin should be used, with vancomycin reserved for the penicillin-allergic patient and when methicillin-resistant organisms are suspected or proven. Combination regimens including nafcillin or vancomycin plus metronidazole plus a third-generation cephalosporin are often used. Surgical intervention may be required for optimal therapy. Surgical drainage of infected sinuses is necessary when antimicrobial therapy alone is ineffective. Operative intervention is often used for patients with cavernous sinus thrombosis, especially in the setting of sphenoid sinusitis. Internal jugular vein ligation and thrombectomy have been used in patients with lateral sinus vein thrombosis, but the efficacy of these procedures is poorly defined. Surgical therapy also may be necessary for other contiguous foci of infection, e.g., dental abscess. The role of anticoagulation is controversial. Although anticoagulation may prevent the spread of the thrombus, this benefit is most apparent when anticoagulation is started early in the course of disease. However, the hazards of intracranial hemorrhage, including bleeding from sites of cortical venous infarction, must be recognized. In the absence of definitive data and specific contraindications, anticoagulation is most likely to be useful early in the course of cavernous sinus thrombosis or when overt embolization has occurred. Anticoagulation is not recommended for septic lateral sinus thrombophlebitis, because the cortical veins overlying the infected mastoid may become occluded, resulting in small venous hemorrhagic infarcts and leading to intracerebral hemorrhage. The efficacy and safety of thrombolytic therapy (e.g., with urokinase), internal jugular vein ligation, or thrombectomy have not been determined for suppurative intracranial thrombophlebitis.

BIBLIOGRAPHY

BRADLEY JS, SCHELD WM: The challenge of penicillin-resistant *Streptococcus pneumoniae:* Current antibiotic therapy of meningitis in the 1990s. Clin Infect Dis 24 (Suppl 2):5213, 1997

DILL SR et al: Subdural empyema: Analysis of 32 cases and review. Clin Infect Dis 20:372, 1995

DINUBILE MJ et al: Septic cortical thrombophlebitis. J Infect Dis 161:1216, 1990

DURAND ML ET AL: Acute bacterial meningitis in adults. A review of 493 episodes. N Engl J Med 328:21, 1993

GELLIN BG et al: Epidural abscess, in *Infections of the Central Nervous System,* 2d ed, WM Scheld et al (eds). New York, Lippincott-Raven, 1997, pp 507–522

GREENLEE JE: Suppurative intracranial phlebitis, in *Mandell, Douglas and Bennett's Principles and Practices of Infectious Diseases,* 4th ed, Mandell GL et al (eds). New York, Churchill Livingstone, 1995, pp 907–909

HAGENSEE ME et al: Brain abscess following marrow transplantation: Experience at the Fred Hutchinson Cancer Research Center, 1984–1992. Clin Infect Dis 19:402, 1994

HELFGOTT DC et al: Subdural empyema, in *Infections of the Central Nervous System,* 2d ed, WM Scheld et al (eds). New York, Lippincott-Raven, 1997, pp 495–506

HLAVIN ML et al: Intracranial suppuration: A modern decade of postoperative subdural empyema and epidural abscess. Neurosurgery 34:974, 1994

LEBELL MH et al: Dexamethasone therapy for bacterial meningitis: Results of two double-blind, placebo-controlled trials. N Engl J Med 319:964, 1988

LEVY RM: Brain abscess and subdural empyema. Curr Opin Neurol 7:223, 1994

MAMELAK AN et al: Improved management of multiple brain abscesses: A combined surgical and medical approach. Neurosurgery 36:76, 1995

ODIO CM et al: The beneficial effects of early dexamethasone administration in infants and children with bacterial meningitis. N Engl J Med 324:1525, 1991

PARIS M et al: Management of meningitis caused by penicillin-resistant *Streptococcus pneumoniae.* Antimicrob Agents Chemother 39:2171, 1995

PFISTER HW et al: Spectrum of complications during bacterial meningitis in adults—results of a prospective clinical study. Arch Neurol 50:575, 1993

——— et al: Mechanisms of brain injury in bacterial meningitis: Workshop summary. Clin Infect Dis 19:463, 1994

PINNER RW et al: Meningococcal disease in the United States—1986. J Infect Dis 164:368, 1991

QUAGLIARELLO V, SCHELD WM: Bacterial meningitis: Pathogenesis, pathophysiology, and progress. N Engl J Med 327:864, 1992

———, ———: Drug therapy: Treatment of bacterial meningitis. N Engl J Med 336:708, 1997

ROOS KL et al: Acute bacterial meningitis in children and adults, in *Infections of the Central Nervous System,* 2d ed, WM Scheld et al (eds). New York, Lippincott-Raven, 1997, pp 335–402

ROSENFELD EA, BOWLEY AH: Infectious complications of sinusitis, other than meningitis in children: 12 year review. Clin Infect Dis 18:750, 1994

SAEZ-LLORENS X et al: Molecular pathophysiology of bacterial meningitis: Current concepts and therapeutic implications. J Pediatr 116:671, 1990

SEYDOUX CH, FRANCIOLI P: Bacterial brain abscesses: Factors influencing mortality and sequelae. Clin Infect Dis 15:394, 1992

SJOLIN J et al: Treatment of brain abscess with cefotaxime and metronidazole: Prospective study of 15 consecutive patients. Clin Infect Dis 17:857, 1993

SPANOS A et al: Differential diagnosis of acute meningitis. JAMA 262:2700, 1989

STEPHENS DS, FARLEY MM: Pathogenetic events during infection of the human nasal pharnyx with *Neisseria meningitidis* and *Haemophilus influenzae.* Rev Infect Dis 13:22, 1991

TOWNSEND GC, SCHELD WM: Clinically important trends in bacterial meningitis. Infect Dis Clin Pract 4:423, 1995

TUNKEL AR, SCHELD WM: Pathogenesis and pathophysiology of bacterial meningitis. Ann Rev Med 44:103, 1993

———, ———: Acute bacterial meningitis. Lancet 346:1675, 1995

——— et al: Bacterial meningitis: Recent advances in pathophysiology and treatment. Ann Intern Med 112:610, 1990

WENGER JD et al: Bacterial meningitis in the United States, 1986: Report of a multistate surveillance study. J Infect Dis 162:1316, 1990

WISPELWEY B, SCHELD WM: Brain abscess, in *Infections of the Central Nervous System,* 2d ed, WM Scheld et al (eds). New York, Lippincott-Raven, 1997, pp 463–494

378

Walter J. Koroshetz, Morton N. Swartz

CHRONIC AND RECURRENT MENINGITIS

Chronic inflammation of the meninges (pia, arachnoid, and dura) can produce profound neurologic disability and may be fatal if not successfully treated. The condition is most commonly diagnosed when a characteristic neurologic syndrome exists for longer than 4 weeks and is associated with a persistent inflammatory response in the cerebrospinal fluid (CSF) (white blood cell count $>5/\mu L$). The causes are varied, and appropriate treatment depends on identification of the etiology. Five categories of disease account for most cases of chronic meningitis: (1) meningeal infections, (2) malignancy, (3) noninfectious inflammatory disorders, (4) chemical meningitis, and (5) parameningeal infections.

CLINICAL PATHOPHYSIOLOGY Neurologic manifestations of chronic meningitis (Table 378-1) are determined by the anatomic location of the inflammation and its consequences. Persistent headache with or without stiff neck and hydrocephalus, cranial neuropathies, radiculopathies, and cognitive or personality changes are the

Table 378-1

Symptoms and Signs of Chronic Meningitis

Symptoms	Signs
Chronic headache	+/− Papilledema
Neck or back pain	Brudzinski's or Kernig's sign of meningeal irritation
Change in personality	Altered mental status—drowsiness, inattention, disorientation, memory loss, frontal release signs (grasp, suck, snout), perseveration
Facial weakness	Peripheral seventh CN palsy
Double vision	Palsy of CNs III, IV, VI
Visual loss	Papilledema, optic atrophy
Hearing loss	Eighth CN palsy
Arm or leg weakness	Myelopathy or radiculopathy
Numbness in arms or legs	Myelopathy or radiculopathy
Sphincter dysfunction	Myelopathy or radiculopathy Frontal lobe dysfunction
Clumsiness	Ataxia

cardinal features. These can occur alone or in combination. When they appear in combination, widespread dissemination of the inflammatory process along CSF pathways has occurred. In some cases, the presence of an underlying systemic illness points to a specific agent or class of agents as the probable cause. The diagnosis of chronic meningitis is usually made when the clinical presentation prompts the astute physician to examine the CSF for signs of inflammation.

CSF is produced by the choroid plexus of the cerebral ventricles, exits through narrow foramina into the subarachnoid space surrounding the brain and spinal cord, circulates around the base of the brain and over the cerebral hemispheres, and is resorbed by arachnoid villi projecting into the superior sagittal sinus. CSF flow provides a pathway for rapid spread of infectious and malignant processes over the brain, spinal cord, and cranial and spinal nerve roots. Spread from the subarachnoid space into brain parenchyma may occur via the arachnoid cuffs that surround blood vessels that penetrate brain tissue (Virchow-Robin spaces).

Intracranial Meningitis Nociceptive fibers of the meninges (Chap. 15) are stimulated by the inflammatory process, resulting in headache, or neck or back pain. Obstruction of CSF pathways at foramina or arachnoid villi may produce hydrocephalus and symptoms of raised intracranial pressure, including headache, vomiting, apathy or drowsiness, gait instability, papilledema, visual loss, impaired upgaze, or palsy of the seventh cranial nerve (CN) (Chap. 28). Cognitive and behavioral changes during the course of chronic meningitis may also result from vascular damage, which may similarly produce seizures, stroke, or myelopathy.

Inflammatory deposits seeded via CSF circulation are often prominent around the brainstem and cranial nerves and along the undersurface of the frontal and temporal lobes. Such cases, termed *basal meningitis*, often present as multiple cranial neuropathies, with visual loss (CN II), facial weakness (CN VII), hearing loss (CN VIII), diplopia (CNs III, IV, and VI), sensory or motor abnormalities of the oropharynx (CNs IX, X, and XII), decreased olfaction (CN I), or facial sensory loss and masseter weakness (CN V).

Spinal Meningitis Injury may occur to motor and sensory roots as they traverse the subarachnoid space and penetrate the meninges. These cases present as multiple radiculopathies with combinations of radicular pain, sensory loss, motor weakness, and sphincter dysfunction. Meningeal inflammation can encircle the cord, resulting in myelopathy. Patients with slowly progressive involvement of multiple cranial nerves and/or spinal nerve roots are likely to have chronic meningitis. Electrophysiologic testing (electromyography, nerve conduction studies, and evoked response testing) may be helpful in determining whether there is involvement of cranial and spinal nerve roots.

Systemic Manifestations In some patients, evidence of systemic disease provides clues to the underlying cause of chronic meningitis. A careful history and physical examination is essential before embarking on a diagnostic workup, which may be costly, prolonged, and associated with risk from invasive procedures. A complete history of travel, sexual practice, and exposure to infectious agents should be sought. Infectious causes are often associated with fever, malaise, anorexia, and signs of localized or disseminated infection outside the nervous system. Infectious causes are of major concern in the immunosuppressed patient, especially in patients with AIDS, in whom chronic meningitis may present without headache or fever. Noninfectious inflammatory disorders often produce systemic manifestations, but meningitis may be the initial manifestation. Carcinomatous meningitis may or may not be accompanied by clinical evidence of the primary neoplasm.

Approach to the Patient

The occurrence of chronic headache, hydrocephalus, cranial neuropathy, radiculopathy, and/or cognitive decline in a patient should prompt consideration of a lumbar puncture for evidence of meningeal inflammation. On occasion the diagnosis is made when an imaging study [computed tomography (CT) or magnetic resonance imaging (MRI)] shows contrast enhancement of the meninges, always an abnormal finding except after a recent neurosurgical procedure. Once chronic meningitis is confirmed by CSF examination, effort is focused on identifying the cause (Tables 378-2 and 378-3) by (1) further analysis of the CSF, (2) diagnosis of an underlying systemic infection or noninfectious inflammatory condition, or (3) pathologic examination of meningeal biopsy specimens.

Two clinical forms of chronic meningitis exist. In the first, the symptoms are chronic and persistent, whereas in the second there are recurrent, discrete episodes of illness. In the latter group, all symptoms, signs, and CSF parameters of meningeal inflammation resolve completely between episodes without specific therapy. In such patients, the likely etiologies include infection with herpes simplex virus (HSV) type 2; chemical meningitis due to leakage into CSF of contents from an epidermoid tumor, craniopharyngioma, or cholesteatoma; primary inflammatory conditions, including Vogt-Koyanagi-Harada syndrome, Behçet's syndrome, Mollaret's meningitis, and systemic lupus erythematosus; and drug hypersensitivity with repeated administration of the offending agent. The duration of chronic meningitis may also be of value in diagnosis; for example, an untreated patient with tuberculous meningitis is unlikely to survive beyond 4 to 6 weeks.

The epidemiologic history is of considerable importance and may provide direction for selection of laboratory studies. Pertinent features include a history of tuberculosis or exposure to a likely case; past travel to areas endemic for fungal infections (the San Joaquin Valley in California and southwestern states for coccidioidomycosis; midwestern states for histoplasmosis, southeastern states for blastomycosis); travel to the Mediterranean region or ingestion of imported unpasteurized dairy products (*Brucella* infection); time spent in areas endemic for Lyme disease (e.g., Connecticut, New York, Massachusetts); exposure to sexually transmitted disease (syphilis); exposure of an immunocompromised host to pigeons and their droppings (*Cryptococcus*; Fig. 378-1); gardening (*Sporothrix schenkii*); ingestion of poorly cooked meat or contact with a household cat (*Toxoplasma gondii*); residence in Thailand or Japan (*Gnathostoma spinigerum*) or the South Pacific (*Angiostrongylus cantonensis*); rural residence and raccoon exposure (*Baylisascaris procyonis*); and residence in Latin America, the Philippines, or Southeast Asia when eosinophilic meningitis is present (*Taenia solium*).

The presence of focal cerebral signs in a patient with chronic meningitis suggests the possibility of a brain abscess or other parameningeal infection; identification of a potential source of infection (chronic draining ear, sinusitis, right-to-left cardiac or pulmonary shunt, chronic pleuropulmonary infection) supports this diagnosis. In some cases, diagnosis may be established by recognition and biopsy of unusual skin lesions (Behçet's syndrome, cryptococcosis, blastomycosis, lupus erythematosus, Lyme disease, intravenous drug use, sporotrichosis, trypanosomiasis) or enlarged lymph nodes [lymphoma, tuberculosis, sarcoid, infection with human immunodeficiency virus (HIV), secondary syphilis, or Whipple's disease]. A careful ophthalmologic examination may reveal uveitis [Vogt-Koyanagi-Harada syndrome, sarcoid, or central nervous system (CNS) lymphoma], keratoconjunctivitis sicca (Sjögren's syndrome), or iridocyclitis (Behçet's syndrome) and is essential to assess visual loss from hydrocephalus. Aphthous oral lesions, genital ulcers, and hypopyon suggest Behçet's syndrome. Hepatosplenomegaly suggests lymphoma, sarcoid, tuberculosis, or brucellosis. Herpetic lesions in the genital area or on the thighs suggests HSV-2 infection. A breast nodule, a suspicious pigmented skin lesion, or an abdominal mass directs attention to possible carcinomatous meningitis.

Imaging Once the clinical syndrome is recognized as a potential manifestation of chronic meningitis, proper analysis of the CSF is essential. However, if the possibility of raised intracranial pressure exists, a brain imaging study should be performed before lumbar puncture. In patients with communicating hydrocephalus caused by impaired resorption of CSF, lumbar puncture is safe and may lead to temporary improvement. However, if intracranial pressure is elevated because of a mass lesion or a block in ventricular CSF outflow (obstruc-

Table 378-2

Infectious Causes of Chronic Meningitis

Causative Agent	CSF Formula	Helpful Diagnostic Tests	Risk Factors and Systemic Manifestations
COMMON BACTERIAL CAUSES			
Partially treated suppurative meningitis	Mononuclear or mixed mononuclear-polymorphonuclear cells	CSF culture and Gram's stain	History consistent with acute bacterial meningitis and incomplete treatment
Parameningeal infection	Mononuclear or mixed mononuclear-polymorphonuclear cells	Contrast-enhanced MRI or CT to detect parenchymal, subdural, epidural, or sinus infection	Otitis media, pleuropulmonary infection, right-to-left cardiopulmonary shunt for brain abscess, focal neurologic signs; neck, back, ear, or sinus tenderness
Mycobacterium tuberculosis	Mononuclear cells except polymorphonuclear cells in early infection (leukocytes commonly <500/μL); low CSF glucose, elevated protein	Tuberculin skin test may be negative; AFB culture of CSF (sputum, urine, gastric contents if indicated); tuberculostearic acid detection in CSF; identify tubercle bacillus on acid-fast stain of CSF or protein pellicle; PCR	Exposure history; previous tuberculous illness; immunosuppressed or AIDS; young children; fever, meningismus, night sweats, miliary TB on x-ray or liver biopsy; stroke due to arteritis
Lyme disease (Bannwarth's syndrome): *Borrelia burgdorferi*	Mononuclear cells; elevated protein	Serum Lyme antibody titer; western blot confirmation; (patients with syphilis may have false-positive Lyme titer)	History of tick bite or appropriate exposure history; erythema chronicum migrans skin rash; arthritis, radiculopathy, Bell's palsy, meningoencephalitis–multiple sclerosis-like syndrome
Syphilis (secondary, tertiary): *Treponema pallidum*	Mononuclear cells; elevated protein	CSF VDRL; serum VDRL (or RPR); FTA or MHA-TP; serum VDRL may be negative in tertiary syphilis	Appropriate exposure history; HIV seropositive individuals at increased risk of aggressive infection; "dementia"; cerebral infarction due to endarteritis
UNCOMMON BACTERIAL CAUSES			
Actinomyces	Polymorphonuclear cells	Anaerobic culture	Parameningeal abscess or sinus tract (oral or dental focus); pneumonitis
Nocardia	Polymorphonuclear cells; occasionally mononuclear cells; often low glucose	Isolation may require weeks; weakly acid fast	Associated brain abscess may be present
Brucella	Mononuclear cells (rarely polymorphonuclear); elevated protein; often low glucose	CSF antibody detection; serum antibody detection	Intake of unpasteurized dairy products; exposure to goats, sheep, cows; fever, arthralgia, myalgia, vertebral osteomyelitis
Whipple's disease: *Tropherema whippelii*	Mononuclear cells	Biopsy of small bowel or lymph node; CSF PCR for *T. whippelii*; brain and meningeal biopsy (with PAS stain and EM examination)	Diarrhea, weight loss, arthralgias, fever; dementia, ataxia, paresis, ophthalmoplegia, oculomasticatory myoclonus
RARE BACTERIAL CAUSES			
Leptospirosis (occasionally if left untreated may last 3–4 weeks); *Pseudoallescheria boydii* (neutrophilic pleocytosis)			
FUNGAL CAUSES			
Cryptococcus neoformans	Mononuclear cells; count not elevated in some patients with AIDS	India ink or fungal wet mount of CSF (budding yeast); blood and urine cultures; antigen detection in CSF	AIDS and immunosuppression; pigeon exposure; skin and other organ involvement due to disseminated infection
Coccidioides immitis	Mononuclear cells (sometimes 10–20% eosinophils); often low glucose	Antibody detection in CSF and serum	Exposure history—southwestern US; increased virulence in dark-skinned races
Candida sp.	Polymorphonuclear or mononuclear cells	Fungal stain and culture of CSF	IV drug abuse; recent surgery; prolonged intravenous therapy; disseminated candidiasis
Histoplasma capsulatum	Mononuclear cells; low glucose	Fungal stain and culture of large volumes of CSF; antigen detection in CSF, serum, and urine; antibody detection in serum, CSF	Exposure history—Ohio and central Mississippi River Valley; AIDS; mucosal lesions
Blastomyces dermatitidis	Mononuclear cells	Fungal stain and culture of CSF; biopsy and culture of skin, lung lesions; antibody detection in serum	Midwestern and southeastern US; usually systemic infection; abscesses, draining sinus, ulcers
Aspergillus sp.	Mononuclear or polymorphonuclear cells	CSF culture	Sinusitis; granulocytopenia or immunosuppression
Sporothrix schenckii	Mononuclear cells	Antibody detection in CSF and serum; CSF culture	Traumatic inoculation; IV drug use; ulcerated skin lesion
RARE FUNGAL CAUSES			
Cladophialophora bantiana (formerly *Cladosporium trichoides*) and other dark-walled (dematiaceous) fungi such as *Curvularia* and *Drechslera*; *Mucor*			

(continued)

Table 378-2—*(continued)*

Infectious Causes of Chronic Meningitis

Causative Agent	CSF Formula	Helpful Diagnostic Tests	Risk Factors and Systemic Manifestations
PROTOZOAL CAUSES			
Toxoplasma gondii	Mononuclear cells	Biopsy or response to empirical therapy in clinically appropriate context (including presence of antibody in serum)	Usually with intracerebral abscesses; common in HIV-seropositive patients
Trypanosomiasis *Trypanosoma gambiense*, *Trypanosoma rhodesiense*	Mononuclear cells, elevated protein level	Elevated CSF IgM; identification of trypanosomes in CSF and blood smear	Endemic in Africa; chancre, lymphadenopathy; prominent sleep disorder
RARE PROTOZOAL CAUSES			
Acanthamoeba sp. causing granulomatous amebic encephalitis and meningoencephalitis in immunocompromised and debilitated individuals			
HELMINTHIC CAUSES			
Cysticercosis (infection with cysts of *Taenia solium*)	Mononuclear cells; may have eosinophils; glucose level may be low	Indirect hemagglutination assay in CSF; ELISA immunoblotting in serum	Usually with multiple cysts in basal meninges and hydrocephalus; cerebral cysts, muscle calcification
Gnathostoma spinigerum	Eosinophils, mononuclear cells	Peripheral eosinophilia	History of eating raw fish; common in Thailand and Japan; subarachnoid hemorrhage; painful radiculopathy
Angiostrongylus cantonensis	Eosinophils, mononuclear cells	Recovery of worms from CSF	History of eating raw shellfish; common in tropical Pacific regions; often benign
Baylisascaris procyonis (raccoon ascarid)	Eosinophils, mononuclear cells		Infection follows accidental ingestion of *B. procyonis* eggs from raccoon feces; fatal meningoencephalitis
RARE HELMINTHIC CAUSES			
Trichinella spiralis (trichinosis); *Echinococcus* cysts; *Schistosoma* sp. The first may produce a lymphocytic pleocytosis, whereas the latter two may produce an eosinophilic response in CSF associated with cerebral cysts (*Echinococcus*) or granulomatous lesions of brain or spinal cord			
VIRAL CAUSES			
Mumps	Mononuclear cells	Antibody in serum	No prior mumps or immunization; may produce meningoencephalitis; may persist for 3–4 weeks
Lymphocytic choriomeningitis	Mononuclear cells	Antibody in serum	Contact with rodents or their excreta; may persist for 3–4 weeks
Echovirus	Mononuclear cells; may have low glucose	Virus isolation from CSF	Congenital hypogammaglobulinemia; history of recurrent meningitis
HIV (acute retroviral syndrome)	Mononuclear cells	p24 antigen in serum and CSF; high level of HIV viremia	HIV risk factors; rash, fever, lymphadenopathy; lymphopenia in peripheral blood; syndrome may persist long enough to be considered chronic meningitis; or chronic meningitis may develop in later stages (AIDS) due to HIV
Herpes simplex	Mononuclear cells	PCR for HSV DNA; CSF antibody	Recurrent meningitis due to HSV-2 (rarely HSV-1) often associated with genital recurrences

ABBREVIATIONS: ELISA, enzyme-linked immunosorbent assay; EM, electron microscopy; FTA, fluorescent treponemal antibody absorption test; IV, intravenous; MHA-TP, microhemagglutination assay-*Treponema pallidum*; PAS, periodic acid–Schiff; PCR, polymerase chain reaction; RPR, rapid plasma reagin test; TB, tuberculosis.

tive hydrocephalus), then lumbar puncture carries the potential risk of brain herniation. Obstructive hydrocephalus usually requires direct ventricular drainage of CSF.

Contrast-enhanced MRI or CT studies of the brain and spinal cord can identify meningeal enhancement, parameningeal infections (including brain abscess), encasement of the spinal cord (malignancy or inflammation and infection), or nodular deposits on the meninges or nerve roots (malignancy or sarcoidosis). Imaging studies are also useful to localize areas of meningeal disease prior to meningeal biopsy.

Cerebral angiography may be indicated in patients with chronic meningitis and stroke to identify cerebral arteritis (granulomatous angiitis, infectious arteritis).

Cerebrospinal Fluid Analysis The CSF pressure should be measured and samples sent for bacterial culture, cell count and differential, Gram's stain, and measurement of glucose and protein. In cases without a known cause, CSF should be sent for the Venereal Disease Research Laboratories (VDRL) test, acid-fast bacillus (AFB) stain and culture, fungal wet mount and India ink preparation and culture, culture for fastidious bacteria and fungi, assays for cryptococcal antigen and oligoclonal immunoglobulin bands, and cytology. Other specific CSF tests (Tables 378-2 and 378-3) or blood tests and cultures should be ordered as indicated on the basis of the history, physical examination, or preliminary CSF results (i.e., eosinophilic, mononuclear, or polymorphonuclear meningitis).

In most categories of chronic (not recurrent) meningitis, mononuclear cells predominate in the CSF. When neutrophils predominate after 3 weeks of illness, the principal etiologic considerations are *Nocardia asteroides*, *Actinomyces israelii*, *Brucella*, *Mycobacterium tuberculosis* (5 to 10 percent of early cases only), various fungi [*Blastomyces dermatitidis*, *Candida albicans*, *Histoplasma capsulatum*, *Aspergillus* species, *Pseudallescheria boydii*, *Cladophialophora bantiana*] and noninfectious causes [systemic lupus erythematosus (SLE), exogenous chemical meningitis]. When eosinophils predominate or are present in limited numbers in a primarily mononuclear cell response in the CSF, the differential diagnosis includes parasitic diseases (*A. cantonensis*, *G. spinigerum*, *B. procyonis*, or *Toxocara canis* infection, cysticercosis, schistosomiasis, echinococcal disease, *T. gondii* infection), fungal infections (6 to 20 percent eosinophils along with a predominantly lymphocyte pleocytosis, particularly with coccidioidal meningitis), neoplastic disease (lymphoma, leukemia, metastatic carcinoma), or other inflammatory processes (sarcoidosis, hypereosinophilic syndrome).

It is often necessary to broaden the number of diagnostic tests if the initial workup does not reveal the cause. In addition, repeated samples of large volumes of CSF may be required to diagnose certain infectious and malignant causes of chronic meningitis. For instance, lymphomatous or carcinomatous meningitis may be diagnosed by examination of sections cut from a cell block formed by spinning down the sediment from a large volume of CSF. The diagnosis of fungal meningitis may require large volumes of CSF for culture of sediment. If standard lumbar puncture is unrewarding, a cervical cisternal tap to sample CSF near to the basal meninges may be fruitful.

Laboratory Investigation In addition to the CSF examination, an attempt should be made to uncover pertinent underlying illnesses. Tuberculin skin test, chest radiograph, urine analysis and culture, blood count and differential, renal and liver function tests, and measurement of electrolytes (including calcium and phosphate), sedimentation rate, antinuclear antibody, and serum angiotensin-converting enzyme level are often indicated. Liver or bone marrow biopsy may be diagnostic in some cases of miliary tuberculosis, disseminated fungal infection, sarcoidosis, or metastatic malignancy. Abnormalities discovered on chest radiograph or chest CT can be pursued by bronchoscopy or transthoracic needle biopsy.

Meningeal Biopsy A diagnostic meningeal biopsy should be strongly considered in patients who are severely disabled, who need chronic ventricular decompression, or whose illness is progressing

Table 378-3

Noninfectious Causes of Chronic Meningitis

Causative Agents	CSF Formula	Helpful Diagnostic Tests	Risk Factors and Systemic Manifestations
Malignancy	Mononuclear cells, elevated protein, low glucose	Repeated cytologic examination of large volumes of CSF; CSF exam by polarizing microscopy; clonal lymphocyte markers; deposits on nerve roots or meninges seen on myelogram or contrast-enhanced MRI; meningeal biopsy	Metastatic cancer of breast, lung, stomach, or pancreas; melanoma, lymphoma, leukemia; meningeal gliomatosis; meningeal sarcoma; cerebral dysgerminoma; meningeal melanoma or B cell lymphoma
Chemical compounds	Mononuclear cells or PMNs, low glucose, elevated protein; xanthochromia from subarachnoid hemorrhage in week prior to presentation with "meningitis"	Contrast-enhanced CT scan or MRI; cerebral angiogram to detect aneurysm	History of recent injection into the subarachnoid space; history of sudden onset of headache; recent resection of acoustic neuroma or craniopharyngioma; epidermoid tumor of brain or spine, sometimes with dermoid sinus tract; pituitary apoplexy
Primary inflammation CNS sarcoidosis	Mononuclear cells; elevated protein; often low glucose	Serum and CSF angiotensin-converting enzyme levels; biopsy of extraneural affected tissues or brain lesion/meningeal biopsy	CN palsy, especially of CN VII; hypothalamic dysfunction, especially diabetes insipidus; abnormal chest radiograph; peripheral neuropathy or myopathy
Vogt-Koyanagi-Harada syndrome	Mononuclear cells		Recurrent meningoencephalitis with uveitis, retinal detachment, alopecia, lightening of eyebrows, and lashes, dysacusis, cataracts, glaucoma
Isolated granulomatous angiitis of the nervous system	Mononuclear cells, elevated protein	Angiography or meningeal biopsy	Subacute dementia; multiple cerebral infarctions; recent zoster ophthalmicus
Systemic lupus erythematosus	Mononuclear or polymorphonuclear cells	Anti-DNA antibody, antinuclear antibodies	Encephalopathy; seizures; stroke; transverse myelopathy; rash; arthritis
Behçet's syndrome	Mononuclear or polymorphonuclear cells, elevated protein		Oral and genital aphthous ulcers; iridocyclitis; retinal hemorrhages; pathergic lesions at site of skin puncture
Chronic benign lymphocytic meningitis	Mononuclear cells		Recovery in 2–6 months, diagnosis by exclusion
Mollaret's recurrent meningitis	Large endothelial cells and polymorphonuclear cells in first hours, followed by mononuclear cells	PCR for herpes; MRI/CT to rule out epidermoid tumor or dural cyst	Recurrent meningitis; exclude HSV-2; rare cases due to HSV-1; occasional case associated with dural cyst
Drug hypersensitivity	Polymorphonuclear cells; occasionally mononuclear cells or eosinophils		Exposure to ibuprofen, sulfonamides, isoniazid, tolmetin, ciprofloxacin, pyridium; improvement after discontinuation of drug; recurrent episodes with recurrent exposure
Wegener's granulomatosis	Mononuclear cells	Chest and sinus radiographs; urinalysis; ANCA antibodies in serum	Associated sinus, pulmonary, or renal lesions; CN palsies; skin lesions; peripheral neuropathy
Other: multiple sclerosis, Sjögren's syndrome, and rarer forms of vasculitis (e.g., Cogan's syndrome)			

ABBREVIATIONS: ANCA, anti-neutrophil cytoplasmic antibodies; PMN, polymorphonuclear neutrophil; PCR, polymerase chain reaction.

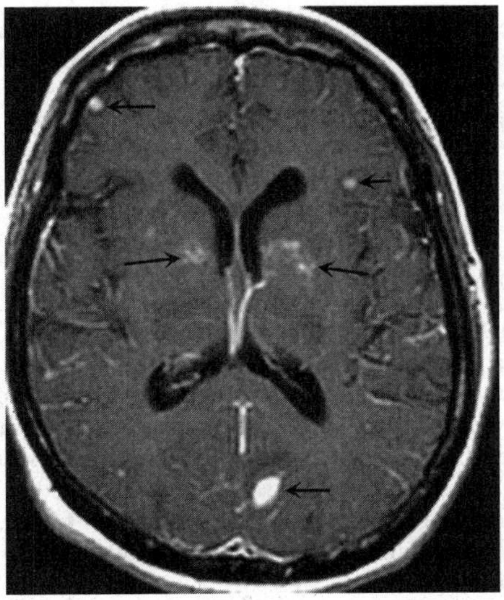

FIGURE 378-1 Cryptococcal disease. A 46-year-old woman presented with altered mental status, fever, and headache. She had many pigeons as pets and frequently cleaned their cage. CSF examination showed elevated protein and a lymphocytic pleocytosis. Cryptococcal antigen test was positive. Axial postcontrast T1-weighted MR image reveals multiple foci of abnormal contrast enhancement in the basal ganglia, internal capsule, and other sites (*arrows*).

rapidly. The activities of the surgeon, pathologist, microbiologist, and cytologist should be coordinated so that a large enough sample is obtained and the appropriate cultures and histologic and molecular studies, including electron microscopic and polymerase chain reaction studies, are performed. The diagnostic yield of meningeal biopsy can be increased by targeting regions that enhance with contrast on MRI or CT. With current microsurgical techniques, most areas of the basal meninges can be accessed for biopsy via a limited craniotomy. In a series from the Mayo Clinic reported by Cheng et al., MRI demonstrated meningeal enhancement in 47 percent of patients undergoing meningeal biopsy. Biopsy of an enhancing region was diagnostic in 80 percent of cases; biopsy of nonenhancing regions was diagnostic in only 9 percent; sarcoid (31 percent) and metastatic adenocarcinoma (25 percent) were the most common conditions identified.

Approach to the Enigmatic Case In approximately one-third of cases, the diagnosis is not known despite careful evaluation of CSF and potential extraneural sites of disease. A number of the organisms that cause chronic meningitis may take weeks to be identified by cultures. In enigmatic cases several options are available, determined by the extent of the clinical deficits and rate of progression. It is prudent to wait until cultures are finalized if the patient is asymptomatic or symptoms are mild and not progressive. Unfortunately, in many cases progressive neurologic deterioration occurs, and rapid treatment is required. Ventricular-peritoneal shunts may be placed to relieve hydrocephalus, but the risk of disseminating the undiagnosed inflammatory process into the abdomen must be considered.

Empirical Treatment Diagnosis of the causative agent is essential because effective therapies exist for many etiologies of chronic meningitis, but if the condition is left untreated, progressive damage to the CNS and cranial nerves and roots is likely to occur. Occasionally, empirical therapy must be initiated when all attempts at diagnosis fail. In general, empirical therapy in the United States consists of antimycobacterial agents, amphotericin for fungal infection, or glucocorticoids for noninfectious inflammatory causes. It is important to direct empirical therapy of lymphocytic meningitis at tuberculosis, particularly if the condition is associated with hypoglycorrhachia and sixth and other CN palsies, since untreated disease is fatal in 4 to 8 weeks. In the Mayo Clinic series, the most useful empirical therapy was administration of glucocorticoids rather than antituberculous therapy. Carcinomatous or lymphomatous meningitis may be difficult to diagnose initially, but the diagnosis becomes evident with time.

THE IMMUNOSUPPRESSED PATIENT Chronic meningitis is not uncommon in the course of HIV infection. Pleocytosis and mild meningeal signs often occur at the onset of HIV infection, and occasionally low-grade meningitis persists. Toxoplasmosis commonly presents as intracranial abscesses and may also be associated with meningitis. Other important causes of chronic meningitis in AIDS include infection with *Cryptococcus, Nocardia,* or other fungi; syphilis; and lymphoma. Toxoplasmosis, cryptococcosis, nocardiosis, and other fungal infections are important etiologic considerations in individuals with immunodeficiency states other than AIDS, including those due to immunosuppressive medications. Because of the increased risk of chronic meningitis and the attenuation of clinical signs of meningeal irritation in immunosuppressed individuals, CSF examination should be performed for any persistent headache or unexplained change in mental state.

BIBLIOGRAPHY

Anderson NE, Willoughby EW: Chronic meningitis without predisposing illness. A review of 83 cases. Q J Med 63:283, 1987

Bouza E et al: Coccidioidal meningitis. Medicine 60:139, 1981

——— et al: Brucellar meningitis. Rev Infect Dis 9:810, 1987

Bross JE, Gordon G: Nocardial meningitis. Rev Infect Dis 13:160, 1991

Cheng TM et al: Chronic meningitis: The role of meningeal or cortical biopsy. Neurosurgery 34:590, 1994

Ellner JJ, Bennett JE: Chronic meningitis. Medicine 55:341, 1976

Hopkins AP, Harvey PK: Chronic benign lymphocytic meningitis. J Neurol Sci 18:443, 1973

Mayer SA et al: Biopsy proven isolated sarcoid meningitis. J Neurosurgery 78:994, 1993

Peacock JE et al: Persistent neutrophilic meningitis. Medicine 63:379, 1984

Phillips ME et al: Neoplastic versus inflammatory meningeal enhancement with Gd-DTPA. J Comput Assisted Tomogr 14:536, 1990

Reik L et al: Granulomatous angiitis presenting as chronic meningitis and ventriculitis. Neurology 33:1609, 1983

Scheld WM et al: *Infections of the Central Nervous System*. New York, Raven Press, 1991

Smith JE, Aksamit AJ: Outcome of chronic idiopathic meningitis. Mayo Clinic Proc 69:548, 1994

Swartz MN: "Chronic meningitis"—many causes to consider. N Engl J Med 317:957, 1987

Wheat LJ et al: Histoplasma capsulatum infections of the central nervous system. Medicine 69:244, 1990

379

Kenneth L. Tyler

ASEPTIC MENINGITIS, VIRAL ENCEPHALITIS, AND PRION DISEASES

Hundreds of viruses have been reported to produce acute infection and injury to the central or peripheral nervous systems. Many aspects of the clinical characteristics of these diseases are determined by whether the infection is limited primarily to the meninges (*meningitis*) or extends to involve the parenchyma of the brain (*encephalitis*) and/or spinal cord (*myelitis*). Although there are a number of similarities in the basic epidemiology and diagnostic approaches to these disorders, they are discussed separately. Viruses also can produce chronic or persistent infections of the central nervous system (CNS). These disorders are sufficiently different from acute viral infections and from each other as to merit separate consideration. Special emphasis is given to infection of the nervous system by human immunodeficiency virus (HIV), both because of its obvious epidemiologic importance and because of its capacity to produce myriad neurologic syndromes as it attacks virtually every part of the nervous system. An additional group of neurologic disorders, commonly discussed in the context of viral infections, are the human prion diseases. Recent evidence indicates that these disorders are caused by the accumulation and/or aberrant metabolism of abnormal isoforms of the prion protein.

ACUTE VIRAL INFECTIONS

VIRAL MENINGITIS **Clinical Manifestations** The syndrome of viral meningitis consists of fever, headache, and meningeal irritation coupled with an inflammatory cerebrospinal fluid (CSF) profile typically consisting of a lymphocytic pleocytosis, a slightly elevated protein level, and a normal glucose level. Fever may be accompanied by malaise, myalgia, anorexia, nausea and vomiting, abdominal pain, and/or diarrhea. It is not uncommon to see a mild degree of lethargy or drowsiness. The presence of more profound alterations in consciousness, such as stupor, coma, or marked confusion, should prompt consideration of alternative diagnoses. Similarly, the presence of seizures, cranial nerve palsies, or other focal neurologic signs or symptoms suggests parenchymal involvement and is not typical of uncomplicated viral meningitis. The headache associated with viral meningitis is typically frontal or retroorbital in location and often associated with photophobia and pain on moving the eyes. Nuchal rigidity is present in most cases but may be mild and present only near the limit of neck anteflexion. Evidence of severe meningeal irritation, such as Kernig's and Brudzinski's signs, are generally absent.

Etiology Using routine serologic and culture techniques, a specific viral cause can be found in 30 to 70 percent of cases of viral meningitis. CSF polymerase chain reaction studies (see below) indicate that at least two-thirds of the cases of CSF culture-negative aseptic meningitis are due to enteroviruses, making this viral group by far the most important cause of viral meningitis (Table 379-1).

Epidemiology It is impossible to determine the exact incidence of viral meningitis in the United States, since most cases go unreported to public health authorities. There is a striking increase in cases during the summer months, reflecting the seasonal predominance of enterovirus and arbovirus infections, with a peak monthly incidence of about 1 reported case per 100,000 population. The striking seasonal predilections of some of the viruses causing meningitis can provide a valuable clue to diagnosis (Table 379-2), although it is important to recognize that seasonal distributions are relative rather than absolute indicators of frequency.

Laboratory Diagnosis *CSF examination* The most important laboratory test in the diagnosis of meningitis is examination of the CSF. The typical profile in cases of viral meningitis is a lymphocytic pleocytosis, slightly elevated protein level, and normal glucose level. Organisms *cannot* be seen on Gram's or acid-fast stained smears or india ink wet mounts of CSF. Polymorphonuclear neutrophils (PMNs) may predominate in the first 48 h of illness, especially in some enteroviral infections, and may last longer when infection is due to echovirus 9 or Eastern equine virus. Patients with suspected viral meningitis and a PMN pleocytosis should have a follow-up CSF examination after 8 to 12 h to look for a shift toward mononuclear cells. The presence of a PMN pleocytosis always should prompt consideration of bacterial meningitis or parameningeal infections. The total CSF cell count per microliter in viral meningitis rarely exceeds 1000. The CSF glucose level is typically normal in viral infections, although it may be decreased in cases due to mumps (10 to 30 percent), lymphocytic choriomeningitis virus (LCMV) and, less frequently, echovirus and other enteroviruses, herpes simplex virus (HSV) type 2, or varicella-zoster virus (VZV). As a rule, a lymphocytic pleocytosis with a low glucose level (≤25 mg/dL) should suggest the presence of fungal, listerial, or tuberculous meningitis or of noninfectious disorders (e.g., sarcoid, neoplastic meningitis).

A number of tests measuring levels of various CSF proteins, enzymes, and mediators, including C-reactive protein, lactic acid, lactate dehydrogenase, neopterin, quinolinate, interleukin (IL) 1β, IL-6, soluble IL-2 receptor, β_2-microglobulin, and tumor necrosis factor (TNF), have been proposed as potential discriminators between viral and bacterial meningitis or as markers of specific types of viral infection (e.g., infection with HIV), but are in limited general use. Patients with HIV CNS infection often have elevated CSF levels of p24 antigen, and this may be useful in diagnosis.

CSF culture The overall results of CSF culture for the diagnosis of viral infection are disappointing (Table 379-3), presumably because of the generally low concentration of infectious virus present and the need to customize isolation procedures for individual viruses. For viral isolation, 2 mL of CSF should be obtained and brought promptly to the microbiology laboratory, where it should be refrigerated and processed as speedily as possible. As a general rule, CSF specimens for viral isolation should never be stored in a freezer (−20°C), since viruses are often unstable at this temperature, and most modern freezers have "frostfree" warmup cycles that are detrimental to viral stability. Storage for more than 24 h is probably best done in a −70°C freezer.

Other sources for viral isolation It is important to remember that viruses also may be isolated from sites and body fluids other than CSF. Enteroviruses and adenoviruses may be found in feces; arboviruses, some enteroviruses, and LCMV, in blood; mumps and cytomegalovirus (CMV), in urine; and enteroviruses, mumps, and adenoviruses, in throat washings. During enteroviral infections, viral shedding in stool may persist for several weeks. The presence of enterovirus in stool is not diagnostic and may result from residual shedding from a previous enteroviral infection; it also occurs in some asymptomatic individuals during enteroviral epidemics.

Nucleic acid amplification Amplification of viral-specific DNA or RNA from CSF using polymerase chain reaction (PCR) amplification has become an important method for diagnosing CNS viral infection. HSV-1 DNA is frequently amplified from the CSF of patients with herpes simplex encephalitis and recurrent (Mollaret) meningitis even when standard culture techniques are negative. PCR is also routinely used to diagnose CNS viral infections caused by CMV, Epstein-Barr virus (EBV), and VZV. Genomic amplification and detection of picornavirus (coxsackie, polio, echo, enterovirus) RNA in the

Table 379-1

Viruses Causing Aseptic Meningitis

Common	Less Common	Rare
Enteroviruses	HSV-1	Adenoviruses
Arboviruses	LCMV	CMV
HIV	Mumps virus	EBV
HSV-2		Influenza A, B; measles; parainfluenza; rubella; VZV

ABBREVIATIONS: CMV, cytomegalovirus; EBV, Epstein-Barr virus; HIV, human immunodeficiency virus; HSV, herpes simplex virus; LCMV, lymphocytic choriomeningitis virus; VZV, varicella-zoster virus.

Table 379-2

Seasonal Prevalence of Viruses Commonly Causing Meningitis

Summer and Early Fall	Fall and Winter	Winter and Spring	Nonseasonal
Arboviruses Enteroviruses	LCMV	Mumps	HIV HSV

ABBREVIATIONS: As in Table 379-1.

Table 379-3

Possibility of Culturing Specific Viruses from CSF

Excellent	Fair	Poor or None
Coxsackievirus, echovirus, LCMV, mumps virus	HIV, adenovirus, arboviruses (most), HSV-2, VZV, rabies virus	Poliovirus, HSV-1, EBV, CMV

ABBREVIATIONS: As in Table 379-1.

CSF of patients with meningitis is now the diagnostic procedure of choice for this group of viruses.

Serologic studies In many cases, diagnosis of viral infection depends on documentation of seroconversion between acute-phase and convalescent sera (typically obtained after 2 to 4 weeks). Antiviral antibodies also may be measured in CSF (see below). The timing of the antibody response often means that serologic data are useful mainly for the retrospective establishment of a specific diagnosis, and their value in initial diagnosis and management is limited. Most viral infections of the CNS are associated with intrathecal synthesis of antiviral antibody. This results in an elevation in the CSF/serum antibody index, which can be calculated using the following formula:

$$\frac{\text{(CSF organism-specific Ig)/(CSF total Ig)}}{\text{(Serum organism-specific Ig)/(Serum total Ig)}}$$

An index value of ≥ 1.5 is suggestive of CSF infection, as it indicates that the CSF contains a relatively higher proportion of Ig specific for a particular organism than does the serum. This finding strongly suggests that CNS infection has resulted in intrathecal synthesis of organism-specific antibodies. Elevations in CSF Ig may occur as a result of breakdown in the blood-brain barrier, but this development typically is associated with elevation in the CSF/serum albumin ratio. Obtaining paired samples of CSF and serum for serologic testing may provide additional evidence that an antibody response is the result of CNS infection. The sensitivity of CSF/serum antibody index studies may be enhanced by correcting for breakdown of the blood-brain barrier using the CSF/serum albumin ratio or using CSF/serum antibody indexes of other viruses as controls. Although use of CSF/serum antibody index determinations may enhance the sensitivity of diagnosis, the technique still suffers from the delay between onset of infection and appearance of the host's antibody response.

Agarose electrophoresis or isoelectric focusing of CSF gamma globulins may reveal the presence of oligoclonal bands. These bands have been found in association with a number of viral infections, including infections with HIV, human T cell leukemia virus (HTLV) type I, and VZV, mumps, subacute sclerosing panencephalitis, and progressive rubella panencephalitis. The associated antibodies are often directed against viral proteins. The finding of oligoclonal bands may be of some diagnostic utility, since typically they are not seen with arbovirus, enterovirus, or HSV infections. It is important to recognize that oligoclonal bands are commonly encountered in certain noninfectious neurologic diseases (e.g., multiple sclerosis) and may be found in nonviral infections (e.g., syphilis, Lyme borreliosis).

Other laboratory studies All patients with suspected viral meningitis should have a complete and differential blood count, a platelet count, liver function tests, and measurement of the hematocrit, erythrocyte sedimentation rate (ESR), blood urea nitrogen (BUN), and the plasma levels of electrolytes, glucose, creatinine, creatine kinase, aldolase, amylase, and lipase. Abnormalities in specific test results may suggest particular etiologic diagnoses. Magnetic resonance imaging (MRI), computed tomography (CT), electroencephalography (EEG), evoked response studies, electromyography (EMG), and nerve conduction studies are not necessary in most cases. They are best used selectively when atypical presentations or unusual features of particular cases present diagnostic problems.

Differential Diagnosis Perhaps the most important issue in the differential diagnosis is the exclusion of nonviral causes that can mimic viral meningitis or encephalitis. The major categories of disease that should always be considered and excluded are (1) parameningeal infections or partially treated bacterial meningitis, (2) nonviral infectious meningitides where cultures may be negative (e.g., fungal, tuberculous, parasitic, or syphilitic disease), (3) infection with certain pathogens whose clinical presentation can resemble encephalitis (e.g., *Listeria, Brucella, Coxiella, Mycoplasma*, and *Rickettsia*), (4) neoplastic meningitis, and (5) meningitis secondary to noninfectious inflammatory diseases such as sarcoid, Behçet's disease, and the uveomeningitic syndromes. Although the diagnosis of a specific viral etiology in a particular case of viral meningitis can rarely be made on clinical grounds alone, proper attention to epidemiologic, clinical, and laboratory features may substantially narrow the diagnostic possibilities. Statistically, *enteroviruses* (see Chap. 195) are the most common cause of viral meningitis (>80 percent of cases with etiology identified) and should be considered the leading candidates when a typical case occurs in the summer months, especially in a child (<15 years of age) (Table 379-4). However, despite their summer prevalence, it is important to recognize that sporadic cases of enteroviral CNS infection are seen year-round. The physical examination should include a careful search for exanthemata, hand-foot-mouth disease, herpangina, pleurodynia, myopericarditis, and hemorrhagic conjunctivitis, which may be stigmata of enterovirus infections. PCR amplification of enteroviral RNA from CSF has become the diagnostic procedure of choice for these infections.

Mumps (see Chap. 198) should be considered when meningitis occurs in the late winter or early spring, especially in males (male/female ratio 3:1). With the widespread use of the live attenuated mumps vaccine in the United States since 1967, the incidence of mumps meningitis has fallen by more than 95 percent. Rare cases of mumps vaccine–associated meningitis have been reported, but they are not usually seen after vaccination with the attenuated Jeryl-Lynn strain of virus used in the United States. The presence of orchitis, oophoritis, parotitis, or pancreatitis or elevations in serum lipase and amylase are suggestive but can be found with other viruses, and their absence does not exclude the diagnosis. Clinical meningitis occurs in 5 percent of patients with parotitis, but only 50 percent of patients with meningitis have associated parotitis. Mumps infection confers lifelong immunity, so a documented history of previous infection excludes this diagnosis. The presence of hypoglycorrhachia (10 to 30 percent) may be an additional diagnostic clue, once other causes have been excluded (see above). Up to 25 percent of patients may have a PMN-predominant CSF pleocytosis, and CSF abnormalities may persist for months. Diagnosis is typically made by isolation of virus from CSF and/or demonstration of seroconversion between acute-phase and convalescent sera.

Development of meningitis in the late fall or winter associated with a history of exposure to house mice (*Mus musculus*), pet or laboratory rodents (e.g., hamsters), or their excreta should suggest the possibility of *LCMV infection* (see Chap. 201). Some patients have an associated rash, pulmonary infiltrates, alopecia, parotitis, orchitis, or myopericarditis. Laboratory clues to the diagnosis may include the presence of leukopenia, thrombocytopenia, abnormal liver function tests, or pulmonary infiltrates. Some cases present with a marked CSF pleocytosis (>1000 cells per microliter) and hypoglycorrhachia (<30 percent).

HSV-2 meningitis (see Chap. 184) occurs in approximately 35 percent of women and 11 percent of men at the time of an initial (primary) episode of genital herpes. Of these patients, 20 percent go on to have recurrent attacks of meningitis. Although HSV-2 can be cultured from CSF during a first episode of meningitis, cultures are invariably negative during recurrent episodes of HSV-2 meningitis. Diagnosis depends on amplification of HSV-2 DNA from CSF by PCR. Almost all cases of recurrent HSV meningitis are due to HSV-2, although rare cases due to HSV-1 have been reported. Most cases of benign recurrent lymphocytic meningitis, including those

Table 379-4

Serotypes of Enteroviruses Causing CNS Infections

Frequency as Cause of CNS Infections	Poliovirus	Coxsackievirus	Echovirus	Enterovirus
Frequent	—	B5	7, 9, 11, 30	70, 71
Common	—	A9, B3, B4	4, 6, 18	—
Rare	1–3	B1, B6	2, 3, 12, 22	—

SOURCE: After Rotbart.

meeting accepted diagnostic criteria for Mollaret's meningitis, appear to be due to HSV. Genital lesions may not be present, and most patients give no history of genital herpes. CSF cultures are negative, but HSV DNA can be amplified from CSF by PCR during attacks of meningitis but not during symptom-free intervals. *Epstein-Barr virus infections* also may produce aseptic meningitis, with or without accompanying evidence of the infectious mononucleosis syndrome. The diagnosis may be suggested by the presence of atypical lymphocytes in the CSF or an atypical lymphocytosis in peripheral blood. The demonstration of IgM antibody to viral capsid antigen (VCA), antibody to the diffuse (D) component of early antigen (EA), and a rising titer of antibody to nuclear antigen (EBNA) are indicative of acute EBV infection. EBV is almost never cultured from CSF, but nested PCR amplification of EBV DNA from CSF may be positive. HIV-infected patients may have positive CSF PCR for EBV DNA in the presence of primary CNS lymphoma, even when EBV-related meningoencephalitis is not present. *VZV meningitis* should be suspected in the presence of concurrent chickenpox or shingles. Some patients develop a distinctive syndrome of acute cerebellar ataxia. This typically occurs in children and presents with the abrupt onset of limb and truncal ataxia. VZV DNA can be amplified from CSF by PCR in many cases of meningitis and myelitis. The diagnosis of a VZV-related CNS infection is also supported by the demonstration of a VZV-specific intrathecal antibody response, or less frequently by positive culture of VZV from CSF. A similar syndrome occurs less commonly in association with EBV and enteroviral infection.

Arbovirus infections typically occur in the summer months, have clear geographic localization, and occur in epidemics, all factors reflecting the ecology of their transmission through infected insect vectors (see Fig. 379-1 and Table 379-6; see also Chap. 200). Arboviral meningitis should be considered when clusters of meningitis cases occur in a restricted geographic region during the summer or early fall. A history of tick exposure or travel or residence in the appropriate geographic area should suggest the possibility of Colorado tick fever virus or Powassan virus infection, although nonviral diseases producing meningitis (e.g., Lyme disease) or headache with meningismus (e.g., Rocky mountain spotted fever) also may present this way.

HIV infection is discussed more fully below and in Chap. 308. HIV meningitis should be suspected in any patient with known or identified risk factors for HIV infection. Aseptic meningitis is a common manifestation of primary exposure to HIV and occurs in 5 to 10 percent of cases (see Chap. 308). In some patients, seroconversion may be delayed for several months, and in seronegative patients, serology should be repeated after 3- and 6-month intervals. HIV can be cultured from CSF in some patients. Cranial nerve palsies are more common in HIV meningitis than in other viral infections, most commonly involving cranial nerves V, VII, or VIII.

Rx TREATMENT

In the usual case of viral meningitis, treatment is symptomatic, and hospitalization is not required. Exceptions to this rule include patients with deficient humoral immunity, neonates with overwhelming infection, and patients in whom the clinical or CSF profile suggests the possibility of a bacterial or other nonviral cause of infection. Patients with suspected bacterial meningitis should receive appropriate empirical therapy pending culture results (see Chap. 377). Patients with deficient humoral immunity should receive a trial of intravenous gamma globulin. Oral or intravenous acyclovir may help patients with meningitis caused by HSV-1 or HSV-2 and in cases of severe EBV or VZV infection. Zidovudine (AZT), didanosine (formerly dideoxyinosine; ddI) or dicalcitrine presumably would be of value in the treatment of HIV meningitis, although no clinical trials have been performed. Patients usually prefer to rest undisturbed in a quiet, darkened room. Analgesics can be used to relieve headache, which is often reduced by the initial diagnostic lumbar puncture. Antipyretics may help to reduce fever, which rarely exceeds 40°C. Hyponatremia may develop as a result of the syndrome of inappropriate vasopressin secretion (SIADH), so fluid and electrolyte status should be monitored. Repeat lumbar puncture is only indicated in patients whose fever and symptoms fail to resolve after a few days or if there is doubt about the initial diagnosis. Vaccination is an effective method of preventing the subsequent development of meningitis and other neurologic complications associated with poliovirus, mumps, and measles infection. A live attenuated VZV vaccine (Varivax) is now approved in the United States. Clinical studies indicate an effectiveness rate of 70 to 90 percent for this vaccine. Reduction in primary VZV infection would be expected to reduce the frequency and/or severity both of primary neurologic complications of varicella and of the consequences of later reactivation (e.g., shingles).

Prognosis In adults, the prognosis for full recovery from viral meningitis is excellent. Rare patients complain of persisting headache, mild mental impairment, incoordination, or generalized asthenia for weeks to months. The outcome in infants and neonates (<1 year of age) is less certain. Intellectual impairment, learning disabilities, hearing loss, and other lasting neurologic sequelae have been reported in some but not all studies; however, their frequency is uncertain.

VIRAL ENCEPHALITIS Definition In distinction to meningitis, where the infectious process and associated inflammatory response is limited largely to the meninges, in encephalitis the brain parenchyma also is involved.

Clinical Manifestations In addition to the acute febrile illness with evidence of meningeal involvement characteristic of meningitis, the patient with encephalitis commonly has an altered level of consciousness, an abnormal mental state, and evidence of either focal or diffuse neurologic signs and symptoms. All degrees of altered consciousness may occur, ranging from mild lethargy to deep coma. A patient with encephalitis is not mentally alert and is frequently confused, delirious, and disoriented. Mental aberrations may include hallucinations, agitation, personality change, behavioral disorders, and, at times, a frankly psychotic state. Focal or generalized seizures occur in more than 50 percent of patients with severe encephalitis. Virtually every possible type of focal neurologic disturbance has been reported in viral encephalitis, the signs and symptoms reflecting the sites of infection and inflammation. The most commonly encountered focal findings are aphasia, ataxia, hemiparesis (with hyperactive tendon reflexes and extensor plantar responses), involuntary movements (e.g., myoclonic jerks), and cranial nerve deficits (e.g., ocular palsies, facial weakness). Involvement of the hypothalamic-pituitary axis may result in temperature dysregulation, diabetes insipidus, or the development of SIADH. Despite the clear neuropathologic evidence that viruses differ in the regions of the CNS they injure, it is often impossible to reliably distinguish on clinical grounds alone one type of viral encephalitis (e.g., that caused by HSV) from others (see "Differential Diagnosis," below).

Etiology The number of viruses reported to cause encephalitis is legion. In the United States, there are approximately 20,000 reported cases per year. The same organisms responsible for aseptic meningitis are also responsible for encephalitis, although their relative frequencies differ (Table 379-5, Fig. 379-1).

Laboratory Diagnosis *CSF examination* CSF examination should be performed in all patients with suspected viral encephalitis unless contraindicated by the presence of severely increased intra-

Table 379-5

Viruses Causing Encephalitis

Common	Less Common	Rare
Arboviruses, enteroviruses, HSV-1, mumps	CMV, EBV, HIV, measles, VZV	Adenoviruses, CTFV, influenza A, LCMV, parainfluenza, rabies, rubella

ABBREVIATIONS: As in Table 379-1; also, CTFV, Colorado tick fever virus.

cranial pressure (ICP). The characteristic CSF profile is indistinguishable from that of viral meningitis and consists of a lymphocytic pleocytosis, a mildly elevated protein level, and a normal glucose level. A CSF pleocytosis (>5 cells per microliter) occurs in more than 95 percent of patients with documented viral encephalitis, and its absence should prompt a careful search for other causes of an encephalopathy. In rare cases, a pleocytosis may be absent on the initial lumbar puncture but present subsequently. Patients who are severely immunocompromised by radiation, chemotherapy, or certain lymphoreticular malignancies may fail to mount a CSF inflammatory response. The cell count exceeds 500/μL in only about 10 percent of patients. Infections with certain arboviruses (Eastern equine encephalitis or California encephalitis), mumps, and LCMV occasionally may result in more than 1000 cells per microliter, but this degree of pleocytosis should suggest the possibility of nonviral infections or other inflammatory processes. Atypical lymphocytes in the CSF may be seen in EBV infection and less commonly with other viruses, including CMV and HSV. The presence of substantial numbers of PMNs after the first 48 h should prompt consideration of bacterial infection, leptospirosis, amebic infection, and noninfectious processes such as acute hemorrhagic leukoencephalitis; however, large numbers of PMNs in the CSF are occasionally present with Eastern encephalitis, echovirus 9 infection, and other enteroviral infections. About 20 percent of patients with encephalitis will have a significant number of red blood cells (>500/μL) in the CSF in a nontraumatic tap. The pathologic correlate of this may be the presence of a hemorrhagic encephalitis of the type seen with HSV, Colorado tick fever virus, and occasionally California encephalitis virus. A decreased CSF glucose level is distinctly unusual in viral encephalitis and should suggest the possibility of fungal, tuberculous, parasitic, leptospiral, syphilitic, sarcoid, or neoplastic meningitis. Rare patients with mumps, LCMV, or advanced HSV encephalitis may have hypoglycorrhachia.

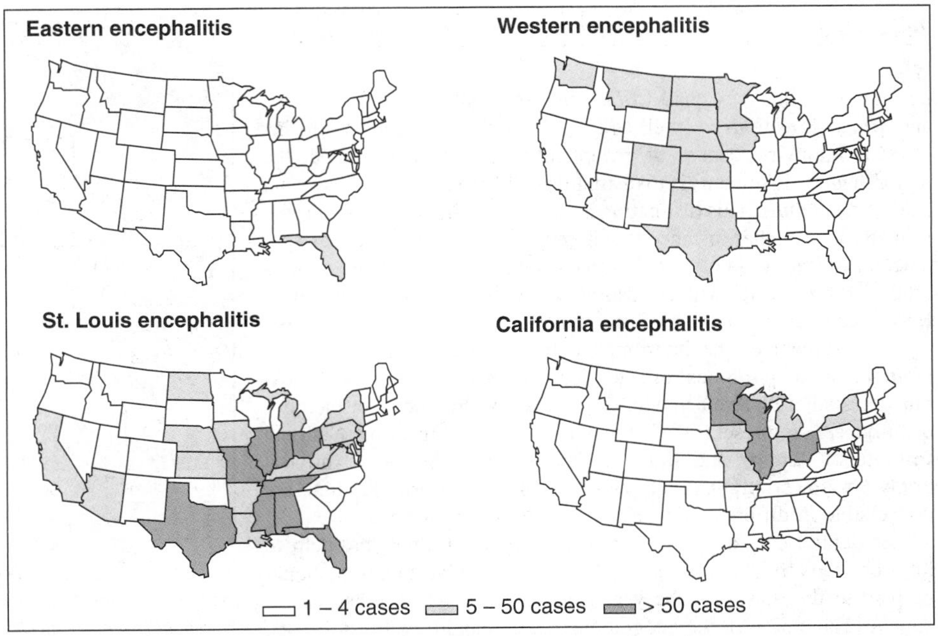

FIGURE 379-1 Geographic distributions of the most commonly encountered arbovirus encephalitides in the United States. *(From Johnson, with permission.)*

CSF culture Attempts to culture viruses from the CSF in cases of encephalitis are often disappointing (see Table 375-3). In particular, it should be noted that cultures are invariably negative in cases of HSV-1 encephalitis.

CSF nucleic acid amplification PCR amplification of viral nucleic acid has become the diagnostic procedure of choice for many types of viral encephalitis. Recent studies with HSV encephalitis indicate that the sensitivity and specificity of CSF PCR equals or exceeds that of brain biopsy. Although less detailed specificity and sensitivity data are available, PCR is now widely used as the primary diagnostic test for CNS infections caused by CMV, EBV, VZV, and enteroviruses (see "Viral Meningitis," above).

Serologic studies and antigen detection The basic approach to the serodiagnosis of viral encephalitis is identical to that discussed earlier for viral meningitis. In the case of HSV encephalitis, attention has focused on the detection of HSV antibodies in the CSF. In one large series, antibodies to HSV-1 glycoprotein B were found in 97 percent of biopsy-proven cases of HSV encephalitis. The specificity was 100 percent if the assay was corrected for leakage across the blood-brain barrier using adenovirus antibodies as a marker. In another study, virus glycoprotein antigens (gB, gC, gD, and gE) were found in the CSF of 92 percent of patients with biopsy-proven cases of HSV encephalitis and had a specificity of 82 percent. Unfortunately, the best results with these types of assays occur after the first week of illness. This limits their utility to retrospective diagnostic confirmation rather than acute diagnosis.

CT, MRI, EEG Patients with suspected encephalitis almost invariably undergo structural imaging studies and often EEG. The utility of these tests is to identify or help exclude alternative diagnoses and to help establish the existence of a focal, as opposed to a diffuse, encephalitic process. The presence of focal findings should always raise the possibility of HSV encephalitis. These are (1) periodic focal spikes on a background of slow or low-amplitude ("flattened") activity with a temporal predominance of EEG; (2) temporoparietal areas of low absorption, mass effect, and contrast enhancement on CT; or (3) areas of increased signal intensity in the frontotemporal, cingulate, or insular regions of the brain on T2-weighted spin-echo MRI images.

Brain biopsy Prior to the availability of PCR amplification of HSV DNA from CSF, the isolation of HSV from brain tissue obtained at biopsy was considered the gold standard for the diagnosis of HSV encephalitis. The need for brain biopsy to diagnose HSV and other forms of viral encephalitis has declined greatly with the widespread availability of CSF PCR diagnostic tests for HSV and many other viruses. When biopsy is performed, the tissue is cultured for virus and examined histopathologically and ultrastructurally. The biopsy is typically carried out under general anesthesia through a craniectomy. Tissue should be taken from a site that appears to be significantly involved on the basis of clinical and laboratory criteria. The sensitivity of brain biopsy exceeds 95 percent, and its specificity is probably greater than 99 percent. Although brain biopsy is not an innocuous procedure, the mortality rate is low (<0.2 percent). Potential morbidity, in addition to that related to general anesthesia, includes local bleeding and edema, the development of a seizure focus, and wound dehiscence or infection. From a practical viewpoint, the incidence of serious morbidity appears to be between 0.5 and 2 percent.

Patients suspected of having HSV encephalitis should be started on acyclovir (see below), and their CSF should be assayed for the presence of HSV DNA by PCR. A negative PCR test effectively excludes the diagnosis of HSV encephalitis and, except in rare circumstances, is sufficiently sensitive to allow discontinuation of acyclovir.

Differential Diagnosis The initial step in diagnosis is to exclude nonviral causes of encephalitis, including both infections and noninfectious diseases. Some of the most common illnesses masquerading as viral encephalitis, as identified in multicenter clinical trials using brain biopsy as a diagnostic standard, were vascular diseases; abscess and empyema; fungal, parasitic, rickettsial, and tuberculous infections; tumors; Reye's syndrome; toxic encephalopathy; subdural hematoma; and systemic lupus erythematosus. Of the nonviral infections, particular attention should be paid to *Listeria*, *Mycoplasma*, *Cryptococcus*, and *Mucor* infections, as well as to toxoplasmosis and tuberculosis.

Once nonviral causes of encephalitis have been excluded, the major diagnostic impetus is to distinguish HSV from other viruses that cause encephalitis. This distinction is particularly important because in virtually every other instance the therapy is supportive, whereas specific and effective antiviral therapy is available for HSV, and its efficacy is enhanced when it is instituted early in the course of infection. HSV encephalitis should be considered when clinical features suggesting involvement of the inferomedial frontotemporal regions of the brain, including prominent olfactory or gustatory hallucinations, anosmia, unusual or bizarre behavior or personality alterations, or memory disturbance, are present. Unfortunately, the results from the National Institute of Allergy and Immune Diseases–Collaborative Antiviral Study Group (NIAID-CASG) suggest that clinical criteria alone are not reliable in differentiating HSV and non-HSV encephalitis.

Epidemiologic factors may provide important clues that help to limit or focus the diagnostic possibilities. Particular attention should be paid to the season of the year (see Table 379-2), the age of the patient (Table 379-6), the geographic location and travel history (see Fig. 379-1 and Table 379-6), and possible exposure to animal bites, rodents, and ticks. *Morbidity and Mortality Weekly Reports* provides regular information about the prevalence of particular viruses causing encephalitis by season and region of the country. State public health authorities provide another valuable resource concerning isolation of particular agents in individual regions.

℞ TREATMENT

Specific antiviral therapy should be initiated when appropriate (Fig. 379-2, and see below). Vital functions, including respiration and blood pressure, should be monitored continuously and supported as required. In the initial stages of encephalitis, many patients will require care in an intensive care unit. Basic management and supportive therapy should include careful monitoring of ICP, fluid restriction and avoidance of hypotonic intravenous solutions, and suppression of fever. Seizures should be treated with standard anticonvulsant regimens, and prophylactic therapy is probably indicated in view of the high frequency of seizures in severe cases of encephalitis (>50 percent). Like all seriously ill, immobilized patients with altered consciousness, encephalitis patients are at risk for aspiration pneumonia, stasis ulcers and decubiti, contractures, deep venous thrombosis and its complications, and infections of indwelling lines and catheters.

Acyclovir (ACV) is of benefit in the treatment of HSV encephalitis and is also useful in selected cases of severe encephalitis due to infection with EBV or VZV (see Chap. 183). These viruses encode an enzyme, deoxypyrimidine (thymidine) kinase, that phosphorylates acyclovir to produce acyclovir-5′-monophosphate. Host cell enzymes then phosphorylate this compound to form a triphosphate derivative. It is the triphosphate that acts as an antiviral agent by inhibiting viral DNA polymerase and by causing premature termination of nascent viral DNA chains. The specificity of action of acyclovir depends on the fact that uninfected cells do not phosphorylate significant amounts of acyclovir to acyclovir-5′-monophosphate. A second level of specificity is provided by the fact that the acyclovir triphosphate is a more potent inhibitor of viral DNA polymerase than of the analogous host cell enzymes.

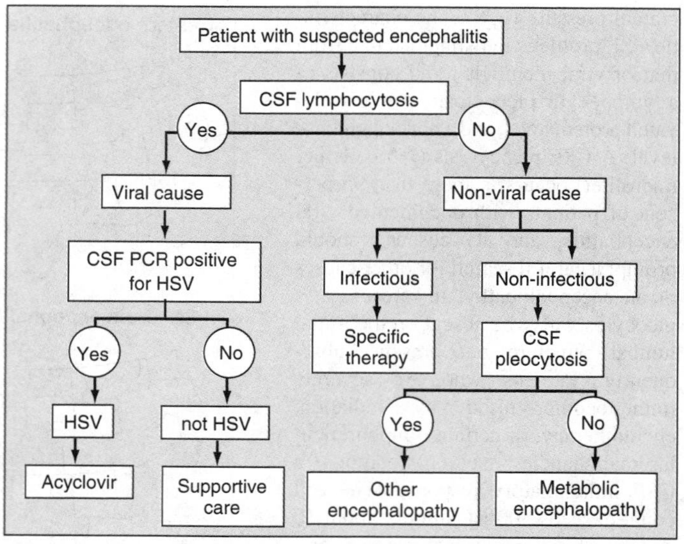

FIGURE 379-2 Scheme for the treatment of patients with suspected encephalitis. HSV, herpes simplex virus. *[Modified from DF Hanley et al: Viral encephalitis and related conditions, in TP Beck (ed): Atlas of Infectious Diseases. New York, Churchill Livingstone, 1995.]*

Patients should receive a dose of 10 mg/kg of acyclovir intravenously every 8 h for a 14-day course. The drug should be diluted to a concentration not exceeding 7 mg/mL. (A 70-kg person would receive a dose of 700 mg, which would be diluted in a volume ≥100 mL.) Each dose should be infused slowly over 60 min rather than by rapid or bolus infusion, to minimize the risk of renal dysfunction. Care should be taken to avoid extravasation or intramuscular or subcutaneous administration. The alkaline pH of acyclovir can cause local inflammation and phlebitis (9 percent). Dose adjustment is required in patients with impaired renal glomerular filtration. Penetration into CSF is excellent, with average drug levels approximately 50 percent of serum levels. Complications of therapy include elevations in BUN and creatinine levels (5 percent), thrombocytopenia (6 percent), gastrointestinal toxicity (nausea, vomiting, diarrhea) (7 percent), and neurotoxicity (lethargy or obtundation, disorientation, confusion, agitation, hallucinations, tremors, seizures) (1 percent). Acyclovir resistance may be mediated by changes in either the viral deoxypyrimidine kinase or DNA polymerase. To date, acyclovir-resistant isolates have not been a significant clinical problem in immunocompetent individuals. However, there has been an increasing number of reports of clinically virulent acyclovir-resistant HSV isolates from immunocompromised individuals, including those with AIDS.

Table 379-6

Features of Selected Arbovirus Encephalitides

	Virus				
Feature	**WEE**	**EEE**	**VEE**	**SLE**	**CE**
Region	West, midwest	Atlantic and Gulf	South	All	East and north-central
Age	Infants, adults >50 years	Children	Adults	Adults >50 years	Children
Deaths	5–15 percent	50–75 percent	1 percent	2–20 percent	<1 percent
Sequelae	Low to moderate	80 percent	Rare	20 percent	Rare
Vector	Mosquito	Mosquito	Mosquito	Mosquito	Mosquito
Animal host	Birds	Birds	Horses, small mammals	Birds	Rodents

ABBREVIATIONS: CE, California encephalitis virus; EEE, Eastern equine encephalitis virus; SLE, St. Louis encephalitis virus; VEE, Venezuelan equine encephalitis virus; WEE, Western equine encephalitis virus.

SOURCE: After Whitley.

Both ganciclovir and foscarnet have been shown to be effective in the treatment of CMV-related CNS infections. Ganciclovir is a synthetic nucleoside analogue of 2′-deoxyguanosine. The drug is preferentially phosphorylated by virus-induced cellular kinases. Ganciclovir triphosphate acts as a competitive inhibitor of the CMV DNA polymerase, and its incorporation into nascent viral DNA results in premature chain termination. Following intravenous administration, CSF concentrations of ganciclovir are 25 to 70 percent of coincident plasma levels. The usual dose for treatment of severe neurologic illnesses is 5 mg/kg every 12 h given intravenously at a constant rate over 1 h. Induction therapy is followed by maintenance therapy of 5 mg/kg every day for an indefinite period. Doses need to be adjusted in patients with renal insufficiency. Treatment is often limited by the development of granulocytopenia and thrombocytopenia, which may require reduction in or discontinuation of therapy.

Foscarnet is a pyrophosphate analogue that inhibits viral DNA polymerases by binding to the pyrophosphate binding site. Following intravenous infusion, CSF concentrations are typically 15 to 100 percent of coincident plasma levels. The usual dose for serious CMV-related neurologic illness is 60 mg/kg every 8 h administered by constant infusion over 1 h. Induction therapy for 14 to 21 days is followed by maintenance therapy (60 to 120 mg/kg per day). Many patients develop renal impairment during treatment, which is reversible following discontinuation of therapy in most, but not all, cases. Reduction in serum calcium, magnesium, and potassium occur in approximately 15 percent of patients and may be associated with symptoms of tetany, cardiac rhythm disturbances, or seizures.

Sequelae There is considerable variation in the incidence and severity of sequelae in patients surviving viral encephalitis. In the case of Eastern equine encephalitis virus infection, nearly 80 percent of survivors have severe neurologic sequelae. At the other extreme are infections due to EBV, California encephalitis virus, and Venezuelan equine encephalitis virus, where sequelae are extremely rare. Detailed information about sequelae in patients with HSV encephalitis treated with ACV are available from the NIAID-CASG trials. Of 32 ACV-treated patients, 26 survived (81 percent). Of the 26 survivors, 12 (46 percent) had no or only minor sequelae, 3 (12 percent) were moderately impaired (gainfully employed but not functioning at their previous level), and 11 (42 percent) were severely impaired (requiring continuous supportive care). The incidence and severity of sequelae were directly related to the age of the patient and the level of consciousness at the time of initiation of therapy. Patients with severe neurologic impairment (Glasgow coma score $\leq$ 6) at initiation of therapy either died or survived with severe sequelae. Young patients ($\leq$30 years old) with good neurologic function at initiation of therapy did substantially better (100 percent survival, 62 percent with no or mild sequelae) compared with their older counterparts ($\geq$30 years); (64 percent survival, 57 percent no or mild sequelae).

MYELITIS AND RADICULITIS

The prototypical viral myelitis is the syndrome of acute anterior poliomyelitis caused by polioviruses and rarely by other enteroviruses and possibly EBV and mumps virus. A distinctive syndrome is produced by enterovirus 70. Patients develop acute hemorrhagic conjunctivitis, followed days to weeks later by a poliomyelitis-like syndrome (see below). Some cases of rabies present with an acute ascending paralysis with areflexia which can resemble poliomyelitis or the Guillain-Barré syndrome. Paralytic polio (see Chap. 195) is a rarity in the United States (<20 cases per year), although it remains a major problem in some other regions of the world. Most cases of paralytic polio in the United States occur as a result of the exceedingly rare reversion of vaccine strains to virulence. The cases are divided among those recently vaccinated and unvaccinated nonimmune adults exposed to recently vaccinated children. Occasional outbreaks have occurred in nonimmunized populations such as the Amish in Pennsylvania. Illness typically begins with prodromal symptoms, including fever, headache, myalgia, pharyngitis, nausea and vomiting, and meningeal signs. These are associated with the typical CSF profile of aseptic meningitis. In some patients these symptoms are followed by the development of muscle weakness. The incidence, severity, and pattern of weakness are age-dependent, with more severe disease being seen with increasing age. Young children often develop weakness of one leg, older children weakness of both legs, and adults asymmetric quadriparesis often with associated urinary retention. Weakness is associated with fasciculations, loss of deep and superficial reflexes, and the development of atrophy. Involvement of the brainstem (bulbar polio) can result in dysphagia, dysarthria, respiratory impairment, and vasomotor disturbances. Although some patients complain of paresthesia, objective sensory loss is not present.

Viruses also may affect both the anterior and posterior portions of the spinal cord over a considerable longitudinal extent, producing the syndrome of "transverse" myelitis. The clinical syndrome is one of acutely developed muscle weakness, which may be of the flaccid hyporeflexic type initially but usually develops into spastic paralysis with hyperreflexia and extensor plantar responses. Sensory loss is almost invariably present and typically involves both pain-temperature and position-vibration, producing a sensory level. Urinary symptoms (retention, overflow incontinence, or in milder cases, hesitancy or decreased voiding sensation) and constipation or even fecal incontinence are present in virtually all patients. Although this syndrome can be caused by a variety of viruses, most cases are due to HSV-2, CMV, VZV, or EBV. Pathologic evidence of myelitis is commonly encountered in severe cases of St. Louis, Eastern, and Western encephalitis. A milder form of the syndrome may be encountered in patients with episodes of herpes genitalia. Especially during the primary outbreak, patients may develop an aseptic meningitis syndrome associated with urinary retention or other symptoms; dysesthesia, paresthesia, or neuralgia in the legs, buttocks, or genital area; and weakness in one or both legs. A chronic viral myelitis is associated with infection by HIV (vacuolar myelopathy) and by HTLV-I (tropical spastic paraparesis and HTLV-I–associated myelopathy) (see Chaps. 192 and 308).

HERPES ZOSTER (See Chap. 185) A distinctive clinical syndrome consisting of paresthesia or dysesthesia in a dermatomal distribution followed by a localized cutaneous eruption ("shingles," "zoster") is commonly associated with VZV infection and rarely may be produced by HSV. Zoster occurs in patients previously infected with chickenpox (varicella). During the initial varicella infection, virus in the skin travels up the sensory nerves to become latent in the sensory ganglia. The mechanisms that account for maintenance of latency and subsequent reactivation remain unknown. Reactivation results in active viral replication in sensory ganglia followed by spread of virus through nerves to the skin, where a dermatomal vesicular eruption occurs. The incidence of zoster increases with age and is higher in patients with compromised cellular immunity. The typical history is one of several days of itching, tingling, burning, or pain in a dermatomal distribution that is followed by a vesicular eruption consisting of clear vesicles on an erythematous base. The vesicles become cloudy, dry, and crust over after 1 to 2 weeks. The lesions are most commonly found in the thoracic dermatomes, with T5-T10 accounting for approximately two-thirds of cases. Most patients will have hypalgesia and hypesthesia in the affected dermatome. About 5 percent of patients develop motor weakness and atrophy (zoster paresis) in the associated myotome.

Three antiviral drugs, acyclovir, famciclovir, and valacyclovir, are available for treatment of herpes zoster (shingles). Both drugs result in more rapid resolution of cutaneous lesions and decreased duration of viral shedding compared to placebo if therapy is started within 72 h of rash onset (and preferably earlier). Antiviral treatment of herpes zoster has not been shown to result in a significant decrease in the incidence of postherpetic neuralgia. However, recent studies suggest that famciclovir may accelerate resolution of postherpetic neuralgia by a mean of twofold, reducing the duration of this debilitating problem by an average of 2 months. Adverse effects of typical oral doses of famciclovir (500 mg three times daily for 7 days), valacyclovir (1 g three times daily for 7 days), or acyclovir (800 mg five times daily for 7 to 10 days) are minor, with headache and nausea being reported in about 8 to 20 percent of recipients. Patients with renal insufficiency require reduction in dosing.

Forty-five percent of patients over age 50 who develop shingles will experience pain persisting for more than 6 weeks after disappearance of the rash, i.e., *postherpetic neuralgia*. Postherpetic neuralgia is almost never seen in children who develop zoster and is rare (6 percent) in adults younger than 50. Patients with postherpetic neuralgia may benefit from topical therapy with capsaicin ointment as well as from systemic therapy with amitriptyline and carbamazepine.

Characteristic syndromes result from zoster eruptions involving the trigeminal and geniculate distribution. In 10 to 15 percent of cases, reactivation of virus in the trigeminal ganglia results in a rash in the distribution of the ophthalmic division of the trigeminal nerve (ophthalmic zoster). Vesicular eruption may be conjoined with conjunctivitis, keratitis, ocular muscle palsies, ptosis, and mydriasis. In rare cases, an attack is followed by the development of cerebral angiitis involving the ipsilateral carotid and/or middle cerebral arteries. Vascular compromise may lead to hemiplegia, aphasia, or other focal deficits contralateral to the side of the facial eruption. Reactivation of virus in the geniculate ganglion is reported to produce the Ramsay Hunt syndrome, consisting of facial palsy often associated with loss of taste in the anterior tongue, tinnitus, hearing loss, and vertigo. Zoster eruptions are found in the external auditory meatus.

HIV AND OTHER VIRAL NEUROPATHIES Isolated virus-induced peripheral or cranial neuropathies or plexopathies are unusual, with the exception of those associated with HIV infection (see below). CMV has been reported to produce both peripheral neuropathy and brachial plexus neuropathy. A similar syndrome may be seen with EBV. The incidence of CMV neuropathy is clearly increased in patients with AIDS. In some cases there has been evidence for direct viral infection, whereas in others the mechanism appears to be one of virus-induced segmental demyelination. CMV, HSV, EBV, VZV, mumps virus, and hepatitis B virus (HBV) also have been associated with Guillain-Barré syndrome. An almost identical syndrome can be seen in association with HIV infection, although these patients typically have a CSF pleocytosis rather than the classic albuminocytologic dissociation (elevated protein, no or few cells). Isolated cranial nerve palsies, especially of the facial nerve (Bell's palsy), have been attributed to VZV (Ramsay Hunt syndrome), HIV, EBV, enteroviruses, mumps virus, and HSV, although in many cases the etiologic relationship appears rather tenuous. Mumps, measles, and VZV may produce unilateral or bilateral nerve deafness. Seroepidemiologic studies also suggest a possible role for parainfluenza viruses, adenoviruses, and HSV in acute hearing loss.

CHRONIC AND PERSISTENT VIRAL CNS DISEASE

GENERAL CONSIDERATIONS From a practical point of view, chronic and persistent CNS viral diseases can be divided into those caused by conventional viruses and those caused by altered metabolism or accumulation of prions (Table 379-7).

HIV A complete discussion of the virologic aspects of HIV infection, of specific complications of HIV infection such as associated opportunistic infections, and of HIV therapy can be found in Chap. 308. We will focus here on the consequences for the central and peripheral nervous system of direct HIV infection.

Neurologic manifestations of HIV infection differ at different stages of illness (Fig. 379-3). Primary HIV infection can be associated with aseptic meningitis and more rarely with an acute encephalopathy. No clinical features clearly differentiate HIV aseptic meningitis from other viral meningitides, although the diagnosis should be strongly considered in patients with known risk factors for HIV infection. The syndrome is characterized by fever, headache, meningeal signs, and in some patients cranial nerve palsies (of nerves V, VII, VIII). The CSF shows a mononuclear pleocytosis, elevated protein level, and normal glucose level. HIV can be isolated from CSF, and p24 core protein may be present, which establishes the diagnosis. More commonly, the diagnosis is established by documenting HIV antibody seroconversion and intrathecal HIV antibody synthesis. In suspected cases, follow-up HIV serology should be obtained at 1, 2, and 3 months, because seroconversion may be delayed.

Persisting CSF pleocytosis also has been found in otherwise asymptomatic HIV-seropositive individuals. Seropositive individuals also may develop Guillain-Barré syndrome (GBS), chronic inflammatory demyelinating polyneuropathy (CIDP), or myopathy. HIV-associated GBS appears to be clinically indistinguishable from the syndrome that occurs in non-HIV-infected individuals. Patients present with acute onset of progressive extremity weakness, which may progress to respiratory failure. Bifacial weakness is common. Sensory symptoms may occur, but sensory signs are far less conspicuous than motor findings. All patients are areflexic or severely hyporeflexic. Findings in CIDP are similar but generally progress chronically rather than acutely and are not typically as severe. A diagnostic clue to HIV-associated GBS or CIDP may be the presence of a CSF pleocytosis in place of the typical albuminocytologic dissociation (no or few cells, elevated protein) seen in non-HIV cases. Electrophysiologic studies are consistent with demyelination (slowed conduction velocities, prolonged or absent F responses, and distal motor latencies, etc.). Extensive controlled trials of therapy in HIV-associated GBS and CIDP are not available. Plasmapheresis is the standard therapy for non-HIV-associated CIDP and GBS. Recent studies suggest that intravenous high-dose immunoglobulin may also be effective and associated with

Table 379-7

Chronic and Persistent CNS Diseases Caused by Viruses and Prions

Disease	Agent	Disease	Agent
Progressive multifocal leukoencephalopathy	JC virus	Creutzfeldt-Jakob disease	Prion
Subacute sclerosing panencephalitis	Measles virus	Gerstmann-Straussler-Scheinker disease	Prion
Progressive rubella panencephalitis	Rubella virus	Kuru	Prion
Tropical spastic paraparesis	HTLV-I	Fatal familial insomnia	Prion
AIDS	HIV	Alper's disease	Prion?

ABBREVIATIONS: HIV, human immunodeficiency virus; HTLV-I, human T cell leukemia virus, type I.

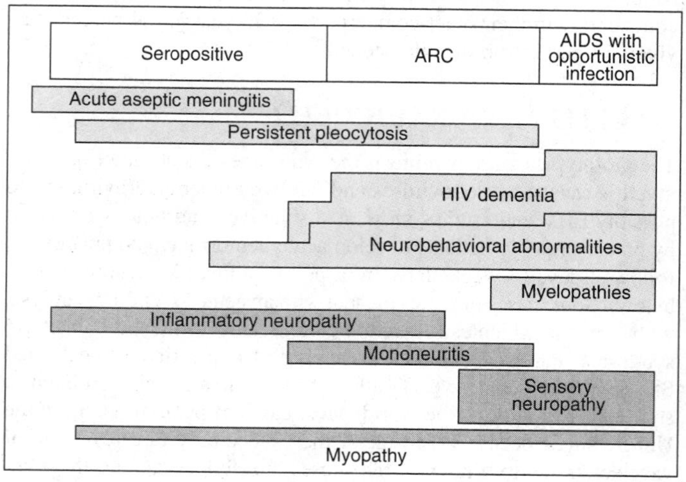

FIGURE 379-3 The relative frequency and timing of major neurologic complications of direct HIV infection. Diseases that affect the CNS are shaded in blue; those that affect the peripheral nervous system are shaded in gray. The height of the boxes is a relative indicator of the frequency of each type of disease. *(From RT Johnson et al, FASEB J 2:2970, 1988, with permission.)*

few side effects, although some patients relapse following treatment. Both these treatments should be considered in HIV-positive individuals.

Progression of HIV infection from the asymptomatic state to more clinically advanced disease is associated with an increased incidence of neuropsychological abnormalities, including the development of HIV encephalopathy and dementia, also referred to as *AIDS-dementia complex* or *HIV-associated cognitive/motor complex*. Common early symptoms of cognitive impairment include difficulty concentrating, memory loss, slowness of thought, apathy, depression, social withdrawal, and personality changes. In distinction to "cortical" dementias such as Alzheimer's disease, aphasia, apraxia, and agnosia are uncommon, leading some investigators to classify HIV encephalopathy as a "subcortical dementia." At least 50 percent of patients will have associated signs or symptoms of motor dysfunction, including leg weakness, balance difficulty, ataxia, tremor, or pyramidal tract signs (hyperreflexia, extensor plantar responses). The illness progresses slowly over months, although mean survival time from the onset of severe dementia rarely exceeds 6 months. Laboratory studies are helpful in excluding or diminishing the possibility of other treatable processes. Twenty percent of patients will have CSF lymphocytic pleocytosis (<50 cells/μL), and 60 percent will have an elevated protein level. Hypoglycorrhachia is rare. CSF concentrations of β_2-microglobulin, neopterin, and quinolinate appear to correlate with the severity of HIV encephalopathy and may serve as useful markers of disease progression or response to antiviral therapy. CT and MRI typically show evidence of diffuse cerebral atrophy with widened sulci and ex vacuo ventricular enlargement. T2-weighted MRI spin-echo images show either patchy or diffuse white matter lesions. EEG findings are nonspecific, although some degree of generalized slowing is almost invariably present.

The neuropathologic hallmarks of AIDS encephalopathy are the presence of multinucleated giant cells seen throughout the cortex and white matter, microglial nodules, white matter pallor, and reactive gliosis. The multinucleated giant cells have been shown to contain HIV particles by electron microscopy and copious amounts of viral antigen and genome by immunocytochemistry and in situ hybridization. They appear to arise by syncytial fusion of infected monocyte-macrophage-microglial cells. These cells contain the bulk of HIV antigen and genome found in brain material. Endothelial cells and oligodendroglia may be found to contain HIV antigen or genome; neurons are rarely, if ever, positive. Neuronal dysfunction is not the result of productive infection with subsequent cell destruction. The mechanism by which HIV infection indirectly produces neuronal injury has not yet been established. Neurons may be injured as a result of cytokines, excitatory neurotoxins, or other soluble factors released by infected immune cells, macrophages, or glia. Alternatively, binding of gp120 or other viral proteins to neurons may result in alterations in ion channel conductance (e.g., of Ca^{2+}) or neurotransmitter levels, leading to cell injury (see also Chap. 308).

No definitive therapy for HIV dementia is available. Both zidovudine and didanosine have been reported to lead to improvement in some patients, although didanosine's limited CSF penetration may limit its usefulness. Some studies suggest that patients receiving higher doses of zidovudine (e.g., 1000 mg/d) do better than those receiving lower doses. Studies are under way to test the efficacy of calcium channel blockers, including nimodipine and memantine, in HIV dementia.

Symptomatic HIV-infected patients also may develop CIDP or mononeuropathy multiplex. Mononeuropathy multiplex typically presents with asymmetric multifocal peripheral and/or cranial nerve lesions. These may appear acutely as isolated regions of sensory loss or weakness in a peripheral nerve distribution. The pathogenesis appears to be ischemic injury to nerves resulting from arteritis of the vasa nervorum. In distinction to CIDP, the electrophysiologic studies suggest an axonal rather than a demyelinating lesion.

A distal symmetric painful sensory neuropathy is the most common form of neuropathy encountered in patients with clinically advanced AIDS and is present in at least one-third of patients. Most patients complain of painful distal paresthesia in the feet ("burning feet"), which are often induced in causalgia-like fashion by pressure or contact. Walking may be difficult or impossible, and even minimal contact with blankets or sheets can produce severe discomfort. Findings on examination include a stocking-type sensory loss to pinprick, temperature, and touch sensation and loss of ankle reflexes. The knee jerks are usually intact. Motor changes (weakness, atrophy) are mild compared with the sensory signs and symptoms and are usually limited to weakness of the intrinsic foot muscles. Trophic changes, including atrophy of the skin, loss of hair, nail abnormalities, edema, and vasomotor disturbances, may be found. Patients with advanced HIV infection also may develop an autonomic neuropathy characterized by diarrhea, postural hypotension, and cardiac arrhythmias. Electrophysiologic studies are indicative of a distal sensorimotor axonopathy, which is consistent with findings on nerve biopsy. Conduction velocities and distal latencies are normal, but compound muscle action potentials in the legs and the sural sensory action potential are diminished in amplitude. HIV has been isolated from nerve biopsy specimens, although the source of virus (Schwann cells, axons, inflammatory cells) has not been established definitively.

Patients with advanced HIV infection may also develop CMV polyradiculopathy. This typically begins with involvement of the lumbosacral roots, resulting in pain and sensory loss in the feet and legs. Many patients have associated signs and symptoms of myelitis. The CSF shows a polymorphonuclear pleocytosis, and CMV DNA can be detected by CSF PCR. CMV antigen and genome can be detected in some biopsy specimens by immunocytochemistry, in situ hybridization, or PCR. Patients receiving either didanosine or dideoxycytidine also may develop neuropathic symptoms, and this possibility should be considered in the differential diagnosis. No adequate therapy exists. Patients with evidence of CMV infection should be treated with ganciclovir or foscarnet (see above). Analgesics, tricyclic antidepressants, anticonvulsants (including phenytoin and carbamazepine), and topical capsaicin ointment may be useful in the control of pain. Mineralocorticoids such as fludrocortisone may help control postural hypotension in patients with autonomic neuropathy.

A chronic progressive myelopathy affecting the posterior and lateral columns of the spinal cord is seen in 10 to 25 percent of AIDS patients. Patients develop a spastic ataxic paraparesis with diminished position and vibratory sense and urinary incontinence. Tibial somatosensory evoked responses are abnormal in virtually all patients. The clinical features resemble those seen in subacute combined degeneration secondary to vitamin B_{12} deficiency and those of nitrous oxide–induced myelopathy. Most patients (>90 percent) have associated HIV encephalopathy or dementia. Pathologic changes consist of vacuolar degeneration of the white matter of the lateral and posterior columns, typically maximal in the thoracic cord. The vacuolar areas result from severe edema within the myelin sheaths of nerve fibers and contain axonal spheroids and lipid-laden macrophages. HIV has been isolated from the spinal cord of affected individuals, and HIV genome has been found by in situ hybridization, although the role of direct viral infection versus indirect mechanism(s) of injury has not been established. No definitive therapy is available, and treatment with either zidovudine or didanosine is generally of little benefit.

In addition to vacuolar myelopathy, a variety of other myelopathic syndromes may occur in HIV-infected individuals. Ganglionitis of the lumbar and sacral dorsal root ganglia can result in secondary degeneration of the fasciculus gracilis within the posterior column of the spinal cord. The resulting clinical syndrome includes paresthesia and sensory loss (vibration, position sense) in the legs. Transverse myelitis also may result from infection with HSV, CMV, HSV plus CMV, or VZV, or from toxoplasmosis. Infection with HIV and HTLV-I together can occur, with the latter producing a spastic myelopathy (see next section).

Patients at any stage of HIV infection may develop myopathy. This is typically characterized by slowly progressive polymyositis-like proximal muscle weakness, myalgia, elevated muscle enzymes [creatine kinase, aldolase, lactate dehydrogenase, serum glutamic-oxaloacetic transaminase (SGOT)], and a myopathic pattern (brief low-amplitude motor unit potentials) on EMG testing. Muscle biopsy may show inflammation and/or myofiber degeneration and necrosis. Some patients have additional histologic changes, including nemaline rod and cytoplasmic bodies, mitochondrial abnormalities, and ragged red fibers. The pathogenesis of the syndrome has not been established. Direct HIV infection of muscle has not been detected, although HIV-infected monocytes, macrophages, and multinucleated giant cells may surround muscle fibers.

HIV-associated myopathy should be distinguished from myopathy as a complication of zidovudine therapy. Most patients with zidovudine myopathy have been receiving the drug for 6 months or more and often have higher enzyme levels and more pain than patients with non-zidovudine myopathy. Biopsy may help with the differential diagnosis, since zidovudine-related cases show more muscle fiber necrosis and less inflammation than patients with HIV myopathy. Discontinuation of zidovudine results in resolution of symptoms. Concurrent glucocorticoid therapy may allow continuation of zidovudine treatment.

TROPICAL SPASTIC PARAPARESIS AND HTLV-I–ASSOCIATED MYELOPATHY These two disorders are characterized by the development of slowly progressive spastic paraparesis, often associated with a neurogenic bladder (see Chap. 192). Symptoms typically appear during the third or fourth decades, and women are affected far more frequently than men. Most reported cases have been from Japan (HTLV-I–associated myelopathy), the Caribbean basin, parts of South America (Panama, Colombia, Peru, Brazil), the Seychelles Islands, and western Africa. Isolated cases have occurred in the southeastern United States and in many other locations. Neurologic examination shows a spastic paraparesis or paraplegia with hyperactive tendon reflexes, clonus, and extensor plantar responses. Although some patients have paresthesia, dyesthesia, or pain in the legs, sensory findings are usually mild (e.g., mild diminution in vibratory sense), and a true sensory level is only rarely found. Additional findings are seen in 5 to 20 percent of cases and can include brisk reflexes in the upper extremities, frontal release responses, cranial nerve abnormalities (optic neuropathy, deafness, nystagmus, diplopia, facial paresis), and cerebellar signs (tremor, dysmetria).

Tropical spastic myelopathies are multifactorial in nature and may be caused by a wide variety of toxic and nutritional factors. Several epidemiologic studies have unequivocally shown that infection with HTLV-I is the cause of an important subset of this disorder. Infection appears to be acquired through blood transfusion, sexual contact, intravenous drug use, and vertical transmission from mother to fetus. HTLV-I–associated cases are characterized by the presence of anti-HTLV-I antibodies in serum and CSF. The CSF/serum antibody index is elevated, indicative of intrathecal antibody synthesis. HTLV-I–specific CSF oligoclonal bands are often present. Between 25 and 60 percent of patients have a mild lymphocytic pleocytosis (<50 cells per microliter), and a higher percentage have a mild elevation in protein. HTLV-I genome can be found in CSF and peripheral blood lymphocytes using Southern blot hybridization or PCR amplification. Virus also can be isolated from the CSF and blood of affected individuals.

A number of abnormalities may be found on laboratory tests, although specific diagnosis requires viral isolation or positive serology. MRI of the spinal cord may show evidence of demyelination, and similar findings are occasionally found in the periventricular white matter in the cerebrum. Somatosensory evoked response studies may show evidence of posterior column dysfunction, even when clinical findings are mild or absent. Some patients have evidence of a demyelinating peripheral neuropathy with slowed conduction velocities, increased distal latencies, and slow or absent F waves. Pathologic examination of the spinal cord typically shows symmetric degeneration of the lateral columns encompassing the corticospinal tracts. Degenerative changes also may involve the posterior columns and spinocerebellar and spinothalamic tracts. There is an associated inflammatory infiltrate in the spinal leptomeninges, cord parenchyma, and surrounding vessels. Myelin destruction at times resembles the vacuolar myelopathy seen in association with AIDS.

The pathogenesis of the spinal cord disease has not been completely established. Both direct viral injury and immune-mediated processes may play a role. Recent evidence suggests that HTLV-I–specific cytotoxic T lymphocytes may be important in the production of immune-mediated spinal cord injury.

Currently there is no definitive therapy. Many patients benefit from oral prednisolone or equivalent glucocorticoid therapy. Zidovudine would be expected to be beneficial in limiting viral replication and associated direct cell injury.

PROGRESSIVE MULTIFOCAL LEUKOENCEPHALOPATHY As the name implies, progressive multifocal leukoencephalopathy (PML) is a progressive disorder characterized pathologically by multifocal areas of demyelination, which vary greatly in size and are scattered throughout the CNS. In addition to demyelination, there are characteristic cytologic alterations in both astrocytes and oligodendrocytes. Astrocytes are tremendously enlarged and contain hyperchromatic, deformed, and bizarre nuclei and frequent mitotic figures. Oligodendrocytes have enlarged, densely staining nuclei that contain viral inclusions formed by crystalline arrays of JC virus particles. Patients often present with visual deficits (45 percent), typically a homonymous hemianopia, and mental impairment (38 percent) (dementia, confusion, personality change). Motor weakness may not be present early but eventually occurs in 75 percent of cases.

CT and MRI remain the most valuable diagnostic studies in suggesting the diagnosis of PML. CT shows hypodense nonenhancing white matter lesions without associated edema or mass effect. Lesions are typically located periventricularly, in the centrum semiovale, in the parietal-occipital region, and in the cerebellum. MRI is more sensitive than CT and reveals hyperintense signal in the white matter on T2-weighted spin-echo images. MRI shows multifocal asymmetric, coalescing white matter lesions with a predilection for the occipital and parietal lobes. These lesions are generally nonenhancing on T1-weighted images following administration of Gd-DTPA or related contrast agents. EEG almost always shows focal or diffuse slowing, and abnormalities may occasionally precede those seen by CT. The CSF is typically normal, although mild elevation in protein and/or IgG may be found. Pleocytosis occurs in less than 25 percent of cases, is predominantly mononuclear, and rarely exceeds 25 cells per microliter. Recently, PCR amplification of JC virus DNA from CSF has shown promise as a diagnostic test for PML. The test has high specificity, but sensitivity has varied among studies. Rare cases of positive CSF PCR for JC virus DNA in the absence of clinical or radiographic evidence of PML have been described in HIV-infected patients. It remains to be established whether these results are false positive or are indicative of preclinical PML. The presence of oligoclonal bands, a substantial pleocytosis, or PMNs or red cells in the CSF should suggest such possibilities as acute multiple sclerosis, acute hemorrhagic leukoencephalitis, HIV-associated leukoencephalomyelopathy, multifocal VZV leukoencephalitis, or postinfectious or vaccinal immune-mediated encephalomyelitis.

Almost all patients (>95 percent) have an underlying immunosuppressive disorder. Prior to the HIV epidemic, common associated diseases included lymphoproliferative disorders, immune deficiency states, myeloproliferative disease, and chronic infectious or granulomatous diseases. Since 1984, the importance of these associated disorders has been dwarfed by that of AIDS. According to some recent estimates, more than 60 percent of currently diagnosed PML cases occur in patients with AIDS. Conversely, it has been estimated that nearly 1 percent of AIDS patients will develop PML. Early indications suggest that the basic clinicopathologic features of AIDS-associated PML do not differ significantly from those of non-AIDS-associated PML. Some patients with AIDS-associated PML have shown significant spontaneous improvement in the absence of therapy. Unfortunately, this appears to be the exception rather than the rule, and most cases pursue the same relentless downhill course to death that characterizes almost all reported cases of non-AIDS-associated PML.

Definitive diagnosis depends on identification of the characteristic neuropathologic abnormalities at biopsy or necropsy. The presence of JC virus antigen and genomic DNA can be confirmed by immunocytochemistry, in situ hybridization, and PCR amplification on brain tissue. However, detection of JC virus antigen or genomic material is not diagnostic of PML unless accompanied by characteristic pathologic changes, since both antigen and genomic material can be found in the brains of normal patients. Between 80 and 90 percent of the population is seropositive for JC virus by middle adult life. Virus may remain latent in brain or other tissues and be reactivated during immunosuppression. PML also may result from primary exposure to JC virus in an immunocompromised host, since 10 to 20 percent of individuals are seronegative at the time of disease diagnosis. As discussed above, PCR amplification of JC virus DNA from CSF appears to be a promising new diagnostic tool.

No effective therapy for PML is currently available. Anecdotal reports have described clinical and radiographic stabilization and in some cases improvement in sporadic patients treated with intravenous or intrathecal cytarabine alone or in combination with α-interferon. A multicenter trial supported by the National Institutes of Health that compared antiretroviral therapy alone to antiretroviral therapy plus either intravenous or intrathecal cytarabine in biopsy-documented HIV-associated PML failed to show any significant benefit from cytarabine treatment.

SUBACUTE SCLEROSING PANENCEPHALITIS This is a rare disease, with fewer than 10 cases per year reported in the United States. The incidence has declined substantially since the introduction of a measles vaccine. Most patients give a history of primary measles infection at an early age ($\leq$2 years), which is followed after a latent interval of 6 to 8 years by the development of a progressive neurologic disorder. Eighty-five percent of patients are between 5 and 15 years old at diagnosis. Initial manifestations include poor school performance and mood and personality changes. As the disease develops, these nonspecific symptoms give way to progressive intellectual deterioration, focal and/or generalized seizures, myoclonus, ataxia, and visual disturbances. In the late stage of the illness, patients are unresponsive, quadriparetic, and spastic, with hyperactive tendon reflexes and extensor plantar responses. The EEG shows a characteristic periodic pattern with bursts every 3 to 8 s of high-voltage, sharp slow waves, followed by periods of attenuated ("flat") background. The CSF pattern may be diagnostic. The fluid is acellular with a normal or mildly elevated protein level and a markedly elevated gamma globulin level (>20 percent of total CSF protein). CSF antimeasles antibody levels are invariably elevated, and oligoclonal antimeasles antibodies are often present. CT and MRI show evidence of multifocal white matter lesions, cortical atrophy, and ex vacuo ventricular enlargement. Measles virus can be cultivated from brain tissue using special cocultivation techniques. Viral antigen can be identified immunocytochemically, and viral genome can be detected by in situ hybridization or PCR amplification. No definitive therapy is currently available. Treatment with Inosiplex (isoprinosine) (100 mg/kg per day) remains controversial but has been reported to prolong survival and produce clinical improvement in some patients.

PROGRESSIVE RUBELLA PANENCEPHALITIS This is an extremely rare disorder that affects mainly children with congenital rubella syndrome, although isolated cases have been reported following childhood rubella. All the approximately 20 cases reported to date have been in male children. After a latent period of 8 to 19 years, patients develop progressive neurologic deterioration. The initial manifestations are similar to those seen in SSPE and include decline in school performance, behavioral alterations, and seizures. These are followed by severe progressive dementia, prominent ataxia, pyramidal signs (spasticity, hyperreflexia, extensor plantar responses), and visual deterioration. Myoclonus may be present but is less prominent than in SSPE, whereas cerebellar signs are a great deal more prominent. In the terminal stages of the illness, patients are globally demented, mute, and quadriparetic, often with associated ophthalmoplegia. CSF shows a mild lymphocytic pleocytosis (<40 cells/μL), slightly elevated protein level [<1.5 g/L (<150 mg/dL)], markedly increased gamma globulin level (35 to 50 percent of total protein), and oligoclonal bands. The oligoclonal antibodies are specific for rubella virus antigens. The CSF/serum antirubella antibody index is markedly elevated, indicating high levels of intrathecal antirubella antibody synthesis. CT scans show ex vacuo ventricular enlargement with associated cortical atrophy. There may be hypodensity in the white matter, especially in the centrum semiovale. Cerebellar atrophy and associated fourth ventricle enlargement may be especially prominent. The EEG is nondiagnostic but is almost invariably abnormal with diffuse slowing. A few patients have a burst-suppression pattern similar to that encountered in SSPE. Biopsy or autopsy material shows perivascular lymphocytic and plasma cell cuffing in the white matter, leukomalacia of the centrum semiovale, and the atrophic and ex vacuo ventricular changes described above. Virus particles are not seen by electron microscopy, although rubella virus has been isolated from explant and cocultivation cultures of brain biopsy material in one reported case. The pathogenesis of the disease remains unclear. No therapy is currently available. Isoprinosine and amantadine are of no benefit. Universal prevention of both congenital and childhood rubella through the use of the available live attenuated rubella vaccine would be expected to eliminate the disease.

PRION DISEASES

Kuru, Creutzfeldt-Jakob disease (CJD), Gerstmann-Straussler-Scheinker (GSS) syndrome, and fatal familial insomnia, although traditionally included in discussions of viral CNS diseases, are due to the abnormal accumulation and/or metabolism of prion proteins. Prion proteins are encoded by a single-copy host gene (designated *PRNP*) present on the short arm of chromosome 20. The function of the normal cellular isoform of the *PRNP* gene (PrP^c) is unknown, although both membrane-associated and secreted forms exist. Neurons contain high concentrations of PrP^c, which is developmentally regulated.

A modified form, PrP^{Sc}, which is resistant to proteolytic digestion and spontaneously aggregates to produce rodlike or fibrillary particles (scrapie-associated fibrils, prion rods) can be identified by immunostaining in brains of animals and humans with prion diseases. The exact mechanism by which the normal cellular protein (PrP^c) is modified to its pathologic isoform (PrP^{Sc}), the method by which PrP^{Sc} replicates itself, and the way PrP^{Sc} accumulation leads to neuronal degeneration remain unknown.

Epidemiologic and clinical studies indicate that human prion diseases can be sporadic (CJD), infectious (kuru, rare cases of CJD), or genetic (GSS syndrome, familial CJD, fatal familial insomnia) in origin. The basic clinical features of each of these diseases are discussed below.

KURU This disease was previously endemic among members of the Fore linguistic tribal group of the Eastern Highlands area of Papua New Guinea. At its peak, the disease affected close to 1 percent of the population, although currently fewer than 10 cases per year are reported. The cardinal features of the illness were severe cerebellar ataxia with associated involuntary movements, including choreoathetosis, myoclonus, and tremor. These were associated with the subsequent development of mental impairment and frontal release signs. Brain material from affected individuals transmits the disease to primates. No new cases of the disease have been reported among individuals born since the cessation of ritual cannibalism in the affected areas. It has been suggested that ingestion of infected brain material during these rituals was responsible for disease transmission.

CREUTZFELDT-JAKOB DISEASE Most cases are sporadic, although 5 to 15 percent are familial with an autosomal dominant pattern of inheritance. Regions of high incidence and prevalence resulting from the presence of families with CJD, are scattered throughout the world, most prominently in parts of Libya and North Africa and in Slovakia. CJD is not contagious, but person-to-person spread of the disease has occurred following transplantation of corneas or dural grafts obtained from infected individuals. Isolated cases also have been attributed to improperly decontaminated neurosurgical instruments and stereotactic intracerebral depth electrodes. Approximately 50 cases have been reported in patients with panhypopituitarism who received supplemental cadaveric human growth hormone therapy and in patients who received cadaveric human gonadotropins for treatment of infertility.

CJD typically presents as a rapidly progressive dementia with prominent associated myoclonus. Clinical manifestations are protean and often include combinations of severe and progressive dementia, pyramidal and extrapyramidal motor disturbances, and signs and symptoms of cerebellar dysfunction. Clinical and pathologic subtypes with predominant involvement of specific regions of the brain have been described (e.g., occipital, thalamic, and cerebellar types). Early signs of mental impairment may be manifested as slowness in thinking, difficulty concentrating, impaired judgment, and memory loss. Mood changes and emotional lability may be combined with visual or other types of hallucinations. About a third of patients present initially with prominent cerebellar or visual disturbances, which may initially overshadow the mental impairment. Myoclonus occurs in more than 90 percent of patients and may be provoked or aggravated by startle. Additional motor signs and symptoms can include tremor, clumsiness, and choreoathetosis. As the disease progresses, about two-thirds of patients develop a parkinsonian extrapyramidal syndrome with hypokinesia and rigidity. Hyperreflexia, spasticity, and extensor plantar responses occur in about half of patients. The clinical presentation of CJD associated with use of cadaveric human pituitary hormone therapy differs from that of classic CJD. Patients are typically younger and often present with a kuru-like illness, in which cerebellar features may be more prominent initially than dementia.

Laboratory tests are helpful in excluding other causes of rapidly progressing dementia. The CSF is typically unremarkable, although the protein level may be mildly elevated. A pleocytosis is unusual and should prompt a thorough search for other processes. It has been suggested recently that two-dimensional isoelectric focusing of CSF proteins may show abnormal protein species, two of which (proteins designated 130 and 131) may be typical of Creutzfeldt-Jakob disease. These proteins appear to be identical to a brain protein designated 14-3-3. An immunoassay on CSF has been developed for this protein, which has been found in CSF from >90 percent of sporadic CJD cases. Approximately 4 percent of patients with other types of dementia, 50 percent of patients with viral encephalitis, and some patients with recent strokes may also have a positive CSF immunoassay for 14-3-3 protein. Further studies are needed to establish the utility of this test for noninvasive diagnosis of CJD. CT and MRI may show evidence of generalized cortical atrophy, but more typically the degree of clinical dementia appears disproportionate to the amount of tissue loss seen on CT and MRI. In some patients MRI has shown areas of high T2 signal intensity in the striatum. In some patients, sequential studies performed at biweekly or monthly intervals may show rapidly progressing loss of brain tissue and ex vacuo ventricular enlargement. The EEG may be quite useful in suggesting the diagnosis. The typical pattern of periodic sharp wave complexes consists of a generalized slow background interrupted by bilaterally synchronous sharp wave complexes occurring at intervals of 0.5 to 2.5 s and lasting for 200 to 600 ms. The classic EEG pattern is found in 75 to 95 percent of cases, although it may not be present very early or in the terminal stages of the disease. Sequential EEG studies may be useful if the initial recording fails to reveal the typical pattern.

The pathologic hallmarks of CJD are spongiform changes (small round vacuoles) within the neuropil, neuronal loss, hypertrophy and proliferation of glial cells, and absence of significant inflammation or white matter involvement. Pathologic changes are strongest in the cortex but are often prominent in the basal ganglia, cerebellum, and thalamus. The brainstem and spinal cord are usually spared. Recent studies indicate that the demonstration by immunostaining of protease-resistant prion proteins in brain material is a sensitive and specific marker for prion diseases. The finding of prion rods or scrapie-associated fibrils, which may be seen in electron micrographs of prepared brain material, also appears to be pathognomonic for prion diseases.

A recent summary of 300 cases of prion disease studied at the National Institutes of Health found that 79 percent of sporadic CJD cases were transmissible, 79 percent involved spongiform neuropathologic changes, and in 83 percent, protease-resistant prion proteins were detected in western immunoblots of brain tissue extracts. All iatrogenic CJD cases and all kuru cases were transmissible and had spongiform changes and positive immunoblots. Cases of familial CJD, GSS syndrome, and fatal familial insomnia showed more variable results. Taken together as a group, only 50 to 60 percent of these cases were transmissible or had positive immunoblots, although 71 percent involved spongiform changes.

CJD is invariably fatal, and no specific therapy is available. A number of drugs, including amantadine, have been reported to slow disease progression in isolated anecdotal case reports; however, the results have not been consistently reproducible.

Recent molecular genetic studies have established an unequivocal linkage between mutations in the *PRNP* gene and familial cases of CJD. Several mutations have been described, which may correlate with variations in the clinical phenotype of the disease in individual familial clusters. These include point mutations in codons 178, 200, and 210. Octarepeat inserts in the *PRNP* gene also occur in several families with CJD. No consistent *PRNP* gene mutation has been identified in cases of sporadic CJD. Some recent reports suggest that homozygosity at a polymorphic amino acid residue at codon 129 of the *PRNP* gene occurs more often than expected in patients with sporadic and iatrogenic CJD and kuru, although this possibility requires further confirmation.

Approximately a dozen cases of a variant form of CJD have been identified in the United Kingdom. It has been suggested that these cases are linked to bovine spongiform encephalopathy (BSE), perhaps as a result of human consumption or other exposure to BSE-infected bovine tissues. Patients have ranged in age from 19 to 41 years and developed a progressive illness leading to death within 7 to 23 months after onset. The clinical features included early and prominent behavioral disturbances and ataxia. Myoclonus and progressive dementia occurred in most patients as later features. The typical periodic EEG pattern usually associated with CJD did not occur. Neuropathologic features included spongiform change and prion protein (PrP) plaques. The PrP plaques resembled those seen in kuru and were often surrounded by a zone of spongiform change. PrP plaques were extensively distributed throughout the cerebrum and cerebellum.

GERSTMANN-STRAUSSLER-SCHEINKER SYNDROME This is a rare hereditary syndrome of spinocerebellar degeneration. Patients develop signs and symptoms of progressive cerebellar dysfunction in midlife, evidenced by unsteadiness, clumsiness, incoordination, and progressive gait difficulty. As the illness progresses, the cerebellar findings become increasingly severe and include ataxia, dysarthria, and nystagmus. Some patients have additional findings, which can include parkinsonian, pyramidal, and extrapyramidal findings; deafness; blindness; and gaze palsies. In distinction to their prominence in CJD, dementia and myoclonus are either absent or minor and are overshadowed by the cerebellar dysfunction.

Molecular genetic studies of GSS syndrome families have consistently demonstrated mutations in the PRNP gene, including point mutations at codons 102, 105, 117, 145, 180, 198, and 217. Although the clinical material is limited because of the rarity of the disease, it appears that ataxia is the dominant feature of the disease in families with the codon-102 mutation, whereas ataxia, dementia, and parkinsonism are seen in those with the codon-198 mutations.

FATAL FAMILIAL INSOMNIA Fatal familial insomnia (FFI) is a rapidly progressive autosomal dominant disease of middle or later life characterized by intractable insomnia, sympathetic hyperactivity and other autonomic and endocrine disturbances, dysarthria, and motor system abnormalities, including myoclonus, tremor, ataxia, hyperreflexia, and spasticity. Dementia is not prominent, although mild memory and attention deficits are common. Patients often experience complex hallucinations with the characteristics of "enacted dreams." A variety of endocrine abnormalities also may occur, including loss of the normal circadian fluctuations in melatonin, prolactin, and growth hormone secretion; decreased secretion of adrenocorticotropic hormone; and elevated cortisol secretion. Pathologic changes include atrophy and gliosis of specific thalamic nuclei and of the cerebellar cortex and inferior olives. One patient has been described who had spongiform changes in the involved areas and periodic sharp wave complexes on EEG, but this appears exceptional rather than typical. Sequencing of the *PRNP* gene from patients in two families with FFI has shown an Asp→Asn mutation in codon 178, similar to that reported in some cases of familial CJD. Brain material from patients in these two families was found to contain the protease-resistant PrP^{Sc} isoform. There have been no reports to date of successful transmission of the disease from brain material of infected cases.

PUTATIVE PRION DISEASES There is one reported case of transmission of a scrapie-like disease to rodents using brain material from a 2½-year-old child diagnosed as having Alper's disease (progressive infantile poliodystrophy). This result has not been confirmed, and no molecular genetic studies on the *PRNP* gene have been reported from patients with Alper's disease.

BIBLIOGRAPHY

BALE JF: Viral encephalitis. Med Clin North Am 77:25, 1993

BERGER JR, CONCHA M: Progressive multifocal leukoencephalopathy: The evolution of a disease once considered rare. J Neurovirol 1:5, 1995

———, LEVY RM: *AIDS and the Nervous System,* 2d ed. New York, Lippincott-Raven, 1997

BOOSS J, ESIRI MM: *Viral Encephalitis.* Oxford, Blackwell Scientific, 1986

BROWN P et al: Human spongiform encephalopathy: The National Institutes of Health series of 300 cases of experimentally transmitted disease. Ann Neurol 35:513, 1995

CONNOLLY KJ, HAMMER SM: The acute aseptic meningitis syndrome. Infect Dis Clin North Am 4:599, 1990

FONG IW, TOMA E: The natural history of progressive multifocal leukoencephalopathy in patients with AIDS. Clin Infect Dis 20:1305, 1995

GESSAIN A, GOUT O: Chronic myelopathy associated with human T-lymphotropic virus type 1 (HTLV-1). Ann Intern Med 117:933, 1992

GILLESPIE SM et al: Progressive multifocal leukoencephalopathy in persons infected with human immunodeficiency virus, San Francisco 1981–1989. Ann Neurol 30:597, 1991

HARRISON MJG, MCARTHUR JC: *AIDS and Neurology.* Edinburgh, Churchill Livingstone, 1995

JEFFERY DR et al: Transverse myelitis—retrospective analysis of 33 cases, with differentiation of cases associated with multiple sclerosis and parainfectious events. Arch Neurol 50:532, 1993

JOHNSON RT: *Viral Infections of the Nervous System.* New York, Raven Press, 1982

LAKEMAN FD et al: Diagnosis of herpes simplex encephalitis: Application of polymerase chain reaction to cerebrospinal fluid from brain-biopsied patients and correlation with disease. J Infect Dis 171:857, 1995

MCKENDALL RR (ed): *Handbook of Clinical Neurology,* vol 56/12: *Viral Disease.* Amsterdam, North-Holland, 1989

PRICE RW: Neurological complications of HIV infection. Lancet 348:445, 1996

PRUSINER SB: Inherited prion diseases. Proc Natl Acad Sci USA 91:4611, 1994

———, DEARMOND SJ: Prion diseases and neurodegeneration. Annu Rev Neurosci 17:311, 1994

———, HSIAO KK: Human prion diseases. Ann Neurol 35:385, 1994

ROOS KL (ed): Central nervous system infections. Semin Neurol 12:155, 1992

ROTBART HA: Enteroviral infections of the central nervous system. Clin Infect Dis 20:971, 1995

SIMPSON DA, TAGLIATI M: Neurologic manifestations of HIV infection. Ann Intern Med 121:769, 1994

SCHELD WM et al: *Infections of the Central Nervous System,* 2d ed. New York: Lippincott-Raven, 1997

TSAI TF: Arboviral infections in the United States. Infect Dis Clin North Am 5:73, 1991

TYLER KL, MARTIN JB (eds): Contemporary Neurology Series, vol 41: *Infectious Diseases of the Central Nervous System.* Philadelphia, FA Davis, 1993

WEBER T et al: Clinical implications of nucleic acid amplification methods for the diagnosis of viral infections of the nervous system. J Neurovirol 2:175, 1996

WHITLEY RJ: Viral encephalitis. N Engl J Med 323:242, 1990

WILL R et al: A new variant of Creutzfeldt-Jakob disease in the UK. Lancet 347:921, 1996

WOOD M, ANDERSON M: *Major Problems in Neurology,* vol 16: *Neurological Infections.* London, Saunders, 1988

380 *M. Flint Beal, Joseph B. Martin**

NUTRITIONAL AND METABOLIC DISEASES OF THE NERVOUS SYSTEM

Nutritional and metabolic diseases of the central nervous system (CNS) can be divided into two groups: acquired and inherited. Most metabolic disturbances in adults, such as hypoxia, hypoglycemia, hepatic encephalopathy, uremia, and electrolyte abnormalities, are acquired disorders. Nutritional diseases, many of which have prominent neurologic manifestations, remain prevalent, particularly those associated with chronic alcoholism. Inherited metabolic diseases of late onset are relatively infrequent, but some are important because they are prototypical and have been explored at the genetic and biochemical levels. This is particularly true of late-onset mitochondrial diseases. Other rare inherited metabolic disorders, such as lipid storage disease, may also present in late life.

ACQUIRED METABOLIC DISORDERS OF THE NERVOUS SYSTEM

The acquired metabolic disorders of the nervous system include anoxic-ischemic encephalopathy, hypoglycemia, hyperglycemic encephalopathy, hepatic encephalopathy, uremic encephalopathy, and electrolyte or endocrine disturbances (see Chaps. 49 and 335).

EXCITOTOXIC CELL DEATH *Excitotoxicity* refers to neuronal death caused by activation of excitatory amino acid receptors. Direct evidence for the role of excitatory amino acids in human neurologic disease arose from observations concerning the neurotoxicity of domoic acid, a potent agonist of the kainic acid subtype of excitatory amino acid receptors. Following consumption of mussels contaminated with domoic acid, individuals can develop encephalopathy with complex partial seizures and memory disturbance. When death occurs, a loss of neurons in the hippocampus can be demonstrated at necropsy.

Further compelling evidence for a role of excitotoxicity in hypoxia-ischemia is derived from observations in experimental animals. Animal models of stroke are associated with increased glutamate in the extracellular fluid, and neuronal damage is attenuated by glutamatergic denervation or the administration of glutamate receptor antagonists. The distribution of cells sensitive to ischemia corresponds closely with that of *N*-methyl-D-aspartate (NMDA) receptors (except for cerebellar Purkinje cells, which are vulnerable to hypoxia-ischemia but lack NMDA receptors). Both competitive and noncompetitive NMDA antagonists are effective in preventing focal ischemia. In diffuse generalized hypoxia-ischemia, non-NMDA receptors (kainic acid and AMPA) are activated. Antagonists to these receptors appear to be protective. Hypoglycemia-induced brain damage is also attenuated by NMDA antagonists.

Excitotoxicity causes an influx of calcium into the cell, and much of the calcium is sequestered in mitochondria rather than in the cytoplasm. Increased mitochondrial calcium causes metabolic dysfunction and free radical generation. It also activates protein kinases, phospholipases, nitric oxide synthase, proteases, and endonucleases, and inhibits

* The authors acknowledge the contribution of Maurice Victor to this chapter in the 13th edition of this book.

protein synthesis. Activation of nitric oxide synthase generates nitric oxide (NO·), which can react with superoxide (O_2·) to generate peroxynitrite ($ONOO^-$) (see Chap. 71), which may play a direct role in neuronal injury. Mice with knockout mutations of neuronal nitric oxide synthase and mice overexpressing superoxide dismutase are resistant to focal ischemia.

ANOXIA-ISCHEMIA Anoxic-ischemic encephalopathy is due to lack of delivery of oxygen to the brain because of hypotension or respiratory failure. The most common causes are myocardial infarction, cardiac arrest, shock, asphyxiation, paralysis of respiration, and carbon monoxide or cyanide poisoning. In some circumstances, hypoxia may predominate. Carbon monoxide and cyanide poisoning are termed *histotoxic hypoxia* since they cause a direct impairment of the respiratory chain.

Clinical Manifestations Mild degrees of hypoxia, such as occur at high altitudes, cause impaired judgment, inattentiveness, motor incoordination, and, at times, euphoria. With more severe hypoxia, such as occurs with circulatory arrest, consciousness is lost within seconds, but if circulation is restored within 3 to 5 min, a full recovery ensues. If anoxia persists beyond 3 to 5 min, cerebral damage is permanent. It is difficult to judge clinically the precise degree of hypoxia-ischemia. Some patients make a relatively full recovery after even 8 to 10 min of cerebral anoxia. A P_{O_2} as low as 2.7 kPa (20 mmHg) can be well tolerated if it develops gradually and normal blood pressure is maintained. The prognosis is better for patients with intact brainstem function, as indicated by normal pupillary light responses, intact doll's-head eye movements, and intact oculovestibular and corneal reflexes. Absence of these reflexes and the presence of persistently dilated pupils that do not react to light are grave prognostic signs. Long-term consequences of hypoxic-ischemic encephalopathy include persistent coma or stupor, dementia, visual agnosia, parkinsonism, choreoathetosis, cerebellar ataxia, myoclonus, and the Korsakoff amnestic state, which may be a consequence of selective damage to the hippocampus.

With severe hypoxia-ischemia, brain death is characterized by dilated, unresponsive pupils, absence of brainstem reflexes and respiration, and an isoelectric electroencephalogram (EEG). This diagnosis must be made with caution and in the absence of evidence of drug intoxication or hypothermia. Less severe anoxic damage can lead to the persistent vegetative state (see Chap. 24).

Pathologic Findings The principal histologic findings are extensive multifocal or diffuse laminar cortical necrosis, with almost invariable involvement of the hippocampus. The hippocampal CA1 neurons are the most vulnerable to even brief episodes of hypoxia-ischemia. Selective persistent memory deficits may occur after brief cardiac arrest. Scattered small areas of infarction or neuronal loss may be present in the deep forebrain nuclei, hypothalamus, or brainstem. In some cases, extensive bilateral thalamic scarring may affect thalamic and extrathalamic pathways that mediate arousal. The persistent vegetative state is thought to result from a complex interplay of discrete cortical and subcortical damage. A specific form of hypoxic-ischemic encephalopathy, so-called watershed infarcts (parieto-occipital), occur at the distal territories between the major cerebral arteries and can cause both cognitive deficits and weakness that is greater in proximal than in distal muscle groups.

DELAYED POSTANOXIC ENCEPHALOPATHY Delayed postanoxic encephalopathy is an uncommon phenomenon in which patients appear to make an initial recovery after a brief episode of cardiac arrest or strangulation, but then develop a relapse characterized by apathy, confusion, and agitation. Progressive neurologic deficits may include shuffling gait, diffuse rigidity and spasticity, persistent parkinsonism, and on occasion coma and death after 1 to 2 weeks. Widespread cerebral demyelination may be present. Carbon monoxide or cyanide intoxication causes delayed damage in both the putamen and the globus pallidus. Little clinical impairment is evident when the patient first regains consciousness, but a parkinsonian syndrome characterized by akinesia and rigidity with no tremor may develop. Symptoms can worsen over months, accompanied by increasing evidence of damage in the basal ganglia as shown by both computed tomography (CT) and magnetic resonance imaging (MRI).

Diagnosis Diagnosis depends on the history of a hypoxic-ischemic event such as cardiac arrest; blood pressures below 70 mm systolic and $Pa_{O_2} < 40$ mmHg are typical. Carbon monoxide intoxification can be confirmed by measurements of carboxyhemoglobin and is suggested by a cherry red color of the skin.

Rx TREATMENT

Treatment is directed at restoration of normal cardiorespiratory function. Initial management is to secure a clear airway and institute artificial respiration. Cardiopulmonary resuscitation and the use of a cardiac defibrillator or pacemaker may be needed. Although neuroprotective agents are undergoing clinical investigation, none has demonstrated efficacy in improving neurologic outcome. Severe carbon monoxide intoxication is treated with hyperbaric oxygen. Seizures should be controlled by anticonvulsants. Posthypoxic myoclonus may respond to oral administration of clonazepam at doses of 1.5 to 10 mg daily.

HYPOGLYCEMIC ENCEPHALOPATHY (See Chaps. 334 and 335) Hypoglycemia typically causes confusion, seizures, stupor, coma, and occasionally hemiparesis or other focal neurologic findings. Blood glucose concentrations are typically <1.4 mmol/L (<25 mg/dL). Persistent hypoglycemia depletes cerebral energy supplies and can lead to irreversible neuronal damage. This process has been shown to involve excitotoxic mechanisms in animal studies.

Etiology Hypoglycemic encephalopathy is typically caused by accidental or deliberate overdoses of insulin or antidiabetic agents, insulin-secreting islet cell tumors or retroperitoneal sarcoma, protracted ethanol intoxication (in rare cases), or Reye's syndrome (in childhood).

Clinical Manifestations The symptoms of hypoglycemia may occur as three syndromes. In the acute syndrome, the initial symptoms are those of adrenergic activation and consist of nervousness, hunger, tachycardia and palpitations, anxiety, sweating, and tremor. These symptoms are frequently recognized by the patient and respond quickly to oral or parenteral glucose. If the syndrome progresses, patients develop increasing confusion, drowsiness, motor restlessness, myoclonic twitching, and seizures. Blood glucose levels of approximately 1 m*M*/L are associated with deep coma, dilated pupils, shallow respirations, and atonia. Subacute hypoglycemia is associated with an absence of adrenergic activation, and patients show slowing of thought processes and a gradual blunting of consciousness with retention of awareness. Hypothermia is commonly encountered in this form of the disorder. Chronic hypoglycemia, which typically occurs with islet cell tumors, is rare and is characterized by insidious changes in personality, memory, and behavior which may be construed as dementia. Some of these patients develop ataxia and, rarely, lower motor neuron involvement.

Pathology The neuropathologic effects of hypoglycemia are similar to those of anoxic injury. There is diffuse neuronal loss in the cerebral cortex and hippocampus, but Purkinje neurons are relatively spared.

Rx TREATMENT

Rapid correction of hypoglycemia is critical to prevent neurologic damage. A 50% dextrose solution is administered initially. Blood glucose is then followed closely and maintained between 8 and 11 m*M*/L by constant infusion of a glucose-containing solution. Glucose levels must be monitored carefully to prevent the development of hypoglycemia in diabetics and to prevent recurrence of hypoglycemia in all subjects. Patients with acute or subacute hypoglycemia show rapid improvement. In patients with chronic hypoglycemia, glucose administration does not promptly relieve symptoms, suggesting the presence of neuronal injury. Clinical improvement after removal of the source of exogenous insulin is gradual and may extend over a period as long as a year.

Differential Diagnosis Episodes of hypoglycemia typically develop more slowly than those of hypoxia, and disturbances in cerebral function may not be apparent for 30 to 60 min, rather than within seconds or minutes. Large overdoses of insulin, however, can cause rapid onset of seizures and coma. Subacute and chronic hypoglycemia, as can occur with islet cell tumors, may masquerade as an episodic confusional state, dementia, or a seizure disorder. The diagnosis is established by demonstrating low blood glucose and elevated levels of insulin.

HYPERGLYCEMIC COMA Hyperglycemia is associated with two coma-producing syndromes in diabetics: hyperglycemia with ketoacidosis and hyperosmolar nonketotic hyperglycemia (see Chap. 334).

HYPERCARBIC ENCEPHALOPATHY Chronic emphysema, pulmonary fibrosis, and occasionally impaired central respiratory drive can lead to chronic respiratory acidosis with elevation of P_{CO_2} and a reduction in arterial P_{O_2}. Common sequelae are secondary polycythemia and "cor pulmonale."

Clinical Manifestations Manifestations include generalized or bilateral frontal headache, which is often intense and persistent, papilledema, mental dullness, drowsiness, confusion, stupor, and coma. At advanced stages a fast-frequency action tremor, as well as myoclonic twitching of the muscles, may be present. Interruption of voluntary movement characteristically causes brief lapses of sustained muscle contraction, known as asterixis. Patients frequently show indifference and inattention to the environment.

Pathogenesis The cerebral disorder is thought to be due to CO_2 narcosis, which causes cerebrovasodilation and leads to increased intracranial pressure. The P_{CO_2} may exceed 75 mmHg, and the oxygen saturation of blood ranges from 80 to 85 percent. The EEG frequently shows slowing in the theta and delta ranges.

℞ TREATMENT

Treatment consists of ventilation with an intermittent positive-pressure respirator. Cor pulmonale is treated with diuretics and agents to lower vascular resistance, as described in Chap. 233. It is imperative to avoid administering narcotics or other sedatives that can blunt the respiratory drive. Oxygen can also be dangerous, because it blunts the hypoxic respiratory drive. Oxygen should be administered only to raise the arterial oxygen level to the range of 50 to 55 mmHg. → *Respiratory failure is discussed in detail in Chap. 266.*

Differential Diagnosis Hypercapnia does not usually cause prolonged coma and does not result in irreversible brain damage. Asterixis is a feature of other metabolic encephalopathies as well, in particular of hepatic encephalopathy. Hypercapnia can be mistaken for a confusional psychosis or occasionally a chronic extrapyramidal syndrome that causes myoclonus or chorea.

HEPATIC ENCEPHALOPATHY (See Chap. 299) Chronic hepatic insufficiency, which is most frequently due to cirrhosis of the liver, results in portacaval shunting of blood and is often punctuated by episodes of stupor, coma, and other neurologic symptoms, termed *hepatic coma* or *portasystemic encephalopathy*. This condition is frequently triggered by gastrointestinal bleeding. In addition, hereditary hyperammonemic syndromes may cause episodic coma with or without seizures in infants (and rarely adults). Reye's syndrome is a hepatic encephalopathy that occurs in association with viral illnesses in children and involves acute brain swelling in conjunction with fatty infiltration of the liver and elevation of serum levels of liver enzymes and ammonia.

Clinical Features Chronic hepatic encephalopathy initially causes mental confusion and decreased motor activity, followed by progressive drowsiness, stupor, and coma. Brain edema, which can be visualized by MRI, may occur with acute hepatic encephalopathy. There are frequently lapses of sustained muscle contraction (asterixis). Characteristic EEG abnormalities in the earliest stages of the confusional state consist of bilaterally synchronous delta waves, which are frequently triphasic and prominent in frontal regions. Fluctuating rigidity of the extremities, as well as grimacing, sucking, grasp reflexes, palmomental reflexes, Babinski's signs, and focal or generalized seizures, may be present.

The syndrome usually evolves slowly over days to weeks with drowsiness, confusion, and asterixis. In its mild form it needs to be distinguished from other confusional states. Recurrent hepatic encephalopathy can lead to persistent dementia and extrapyramidal syndromes, as described below.

Pathology and Pathogenesis The characteristic neuropathologic feature in patients who die in hepatic coma is an increase in the number and size of protoplasmic astrocytes (Alzheimer type II astrocytes) in the deep layers of the cerebral cortex and in the basal ganglia.

The pathogenesis of hepatic encephalopathy remains poorly understood. The disorder may be a consequence of elevated ammonia concentrations, which can cause a number of disturbances of intermediary metabolism. Elevated levels of glutamine in cerebrospinal fluid (CSF) levels are present in most patients with severe hepatic encephalopathy, possibly owing to the reaction of ammonia with α-ketoglutarate. This may impair the function of the Krebs cycle, leading to energy impairment. In animals, hepatic encephalopathy is accompanied by reductions in ATP concentrations. Much of the ammonia appears to arise from the action of urease-containing bacteria in the bowel, which can split urea. Ammonia is absorbed into the portal circulation, where it fails to serve as a substrate for nitrogen fixation because of either hepatocellular disease, portasystemic shunting of blood, or both.

℞ TREATMENT

The standard mode of treatment is to attempt to prevent elevated ammonia concentrations by dietary restriction of protein, mechanical cleansing of the colon, administration of antibiotics such as neomycin (1 g orally tid) to suppress or eliminate urease-producing organisms in the bowel, and administration of lactulose (30 to 50 mL orally tid), an osmotic laxative that acidifies the colonic contents. Liver transplantation has been successful in some patients and can reverse hepatic coma. → *See Chap. 298 for additional methods of treatment.*

CHRONIC ENCEPHALOPATHY (ACQUIRED HEPATOCEREBRAL DEGENERATION) Clinical manifestations of this disorder are now less common owing to the widespread use of liver transplantation. Previously, patients would survive one or more episodes of hepatic coma and be left with residual neurologic abnormalities such as tremor of the head and arms, asterixis, grimacing, chorea, dysarthria, ataxia, and cognitive dysfunction. Some patients with chronic hepatic failure develop a slowly evolving syndrome of ataxia, choreoathetosis, and mild dementia characterized by slowness and indifference.

Pathology Chronic hepatocerebral degeneration is seen with all varieties of chronic liver disease. It is characterized neuropathologically by widespread hyperplasia of protoplasmic astrocytes in the cerebral and cerebellar cortices and in the thalamic and lenticular nuclei. Nerve cells often appear swollen and chromatolytic, accounting for the so-called Opalski cells. The protoplasmic astrocytes may contain periodic acid–Schiff (PAS)-positive glycogen granules.

CENTRAL PONTINE MYELINOLYSIS This disorder typically presents in a devastating fashion as quadriplegia and pseudobulbar palsy. Predisposing factors include severe underlying medical illness or nutritional deficiency; most cases are associated with hyponatremia, which is rapidly corrected by intravenous NaCl, or with other hyperosmolar states. The pathology consists of demyelination without inflammation in the base of the pons, with relative sparing of axons and nerve cells. Experimentally, central pontine myelinolysis can be reproduced by rapid correction of hyponatremia. MRI scans are useful in establishing the diagnosis (Fig. 380-1) and may also identify partial forms that present as confusion, dysarthria, and/or disturbances of conjugate gaze without quadriplegia. Therapeutic guidelines for the restoration of severe hyponatremia should aim for gradual correction, i.e., by no more than 10 mmol/L (10 meq/L) within 24 h and 20 mmol/L (20 meq/L) within 48 h.

HEREDITARY METABOLIC DISEASES OF LATE ONSET

MITOCHONDRIAL DISORDERS When glucose is used by the electron transport chain, it is converted into CO_2 and H_2O and produces 36 high-energy phosphates. In contrast, when glucose is converted to lactate by glycolysis, only 2 high-energy phosphates are produced. The brain has very high energy requirements and a limited capacity to use other substrates for ATP synthesis (see Chap. 335). The brain requires energy for basic housekeeping functions common to all cells and for specific functions such as maintaining ionic gradients. As much as 40 percent of all oxygen consumption in the brain is used to maintain the sodium-potassium gradient across the cell membrane. The energy reserves of the CNS are small, and irreversible cellular damage occurs after a brief deprivation of either glucose or oxygen.

The primary sites of oxidative phosphorylation are the mitochondria. Each mitochondrion has an outer membrane that is permeable to large molecules and an inner membrane that is relatively impermeable and contains the electron transport complexes. The electron transport complexes use both NADH and FADH, each of which is produced by the Krebs cycle and each of which donates electrons through transport enzymes on the inner mitochondrial membrane. The enzymes are designated complexes I through V. Complexes I and II collect electrons and transfer them to ubiquinone (coenzyme Q_{10}). The electrons then move sequentially to complex III, cytochrome c, complex IV, and finally to oxygen, the terminal electron acceptor. Concurrently, ejection of protons across the inner mitochondrial membrane results in an electrochemical proton gradient that stores potential energy. Complex V uses energy stored in the proton gradient to condense ADP with inorganic phosphate into ATP, which is then exchanged with ADP across the inner mitochondrial membrane by the adenine nucleotide translocase.

Kearns-Sayre Syndrome (See also Chap. 383) The first direct evidence that mitochondrial DNA is involved in human disease arose from the finding of large deletions in mitochondrial DNA from patients with myocardial myopathies and the detection of a missense mutation in mitochondrial DNA from patients with Leber's hereditary optic neuropathy. Subsequently, the molecular basis has been elucidated in other mitochondrial encephalomyopathies. Kearns-Sayre syndrome is characterized by progressive external opthalmoplegia, pigmentary retinopathy, and one or more of the following: heart block, cerebellar ataxia, and cerebrospinal fluid protein concentration above 1.0 g/L (100 mg/dL). Onset is usually before age 20, and the prognosis is poor. CSF lactate and pyruvate levels are elevated. Muscle biopsy specimens typically show ragged red fibers. Large deletions of mitochondrial DNA are present. The course is progressively downhill, and most patients die in their third or fourth decade. Most cases appear to be sporadic mutations.

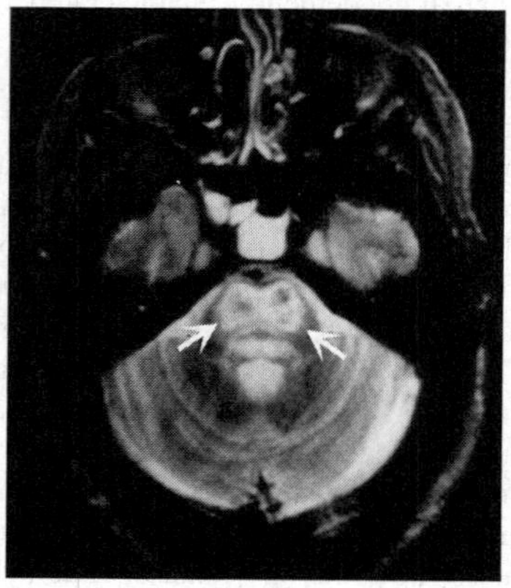

FIGURE 380-1 Central pontine myelinolysis. Axial T2-weighted MR scan through the pons reveals a symmetric area of abnormal high signal intensity within the basis pantis (*arrows*).

MERRF Myoclonic epilepsy with ragged red fibers (MERRF) is characterized by myoclonus, seizures, cerebellar ataxia, and mitochondrial myopathy. Onset is often in childhood or early adult life. Serum and CSF lactate and pyruvate levels are increased, and muscle biopsy specimens show ragged red fibers. The course of this illness is progressively downhill, and most patients die in the third or fourth decade with severe mental deterioration. Maternal relatives may be asymptomatic or have partial clinical syndromes. The pathogenic mutations have been demonstrated at nucleotide positions 8344 and 8356 in the lysine transfer RNA gene.

MELAS Mitochondrial encephalomyopathy, lactic acidosis, and strokelike episodes (MELAS) constitute another maternally inherited disorder characterized by recurrent strokelike episodes, migraine headaches, vomiting, seizures, and lactic acidosis. In most cases there is a point mutation at nucleotide position 3243 in the leucine transfer RNA gene.

Leigh Syndrome Maternally inherited Leigh syndrome is usually a disorder of infancy or childhood, rarely of early adulthood. These patients typically show psychomotor regression, seizures, dystonia, ataxia, optic atrophy, ophthalmoplegia, tremor, pyramidal signs, and respiratory abnormalities. CT or MRI scans show bilateral symmetric areas of signal abnormalities in the basal ganglia and brainstem. Lactic acidosis is common. These patients typically show a progressive downward course. In some families, mitochondrial point mutations have been described at position 8993 in the ATPase 6 gene.

Leber's Disease Leber's hereditary optic neuropathy was the first human disease linked to inherited point mutations in mitochondrial DNA. The phenotype is painless, subacute, bilateral visual loss with central scotomas and abnormal color vision. The mean age of onset is 23 years. Three to four times as many men as women are affected, for unclear reasons. Mitochondrial DNA mutations have been identified in at least eight genes, most encoding subunits of complex I but a few encoding subunits of complex IV. A small number of families with this disorder have degeneration in the basal ganglia with dystonia.

Rx TREATMENT

Many mitochondrial encephalomyopathies follow an episodic course. The most common therapy is to administer agents to stimulate residual electron transport enzyme activity, to supply precursors of coenzymes, or to administer artificial electron acceptors. Coenzyme Q_{10}, an essential component of the electron transport chain that may enhance ATP production and serve as an antioxidant, has been used in patients with mitochondrial disorders, but evidence for efficacy is limited. In a number of case reports, this treatment has been demonstrated to reduce lactate concentrations and to improve visual function. Other approaches have been to use vitamin K_3, nicotinamide, thiamine, riboflavin, and carnitine.

LIPID STORAGE DISORDERS (Inherited metabolic disorders of late life include the lipid storage disorders)

Metachromatic Leukodystrophy (See Chap. 346) Metachromatic leukodystrophy (MLD) may occur in adulthood (25 percent of cases) or in early childhood (75 percent). The mode of inheritance is autosomal recessive. Onset is insidious, and the disease course is progressive. The major clinical manifestation is cognitive deterioration, including forgetfulness, poor scholastic or job performance, and changes in personality. The possibility of psychiatric illness is frequently considered, but eventually mild cerebellar findings appear, with pyramidal signs, masked facies, and strange postures. The diagnosis is established by demonstrating diminished arylsulfatase A activity in white blood cells, serum, or urine; increased excretion of sulfatides in the urine; slowed nerve conduction velocity; and metachromatic material in nerve biopsy samples. No treatment is available, and deterioration progresses until the patient is demented, mute, and bedridden.

Adrenoleukodystrophy This inherited metabolic disorder is characterized by both a lipid storage abnormality and adrenal insufficiency and may present either with a progressive myelopathy or with cognitive findings, homonymous hemianopia, cortical blindness, hemiparesis, aphasia, or dementia. Typically, signs are asymmetric initially and progress intermittently, leading to diagnostic confusion. The diagnosis is usually made by finding low blood cortisol levels or deficient response to cosyntropin stimulation. Patients may develop either a progressive spastic paraparesis or a demyelinating polyneuropathy. There is increased urinary excretion of C22 to C26 fatty acids. The symptoms of adrenal insufficiency are treated by glucocorticoid replacement, but no effective treatment is available.

GM_2 Gangliosidosis GM_2 gangliosidosis (hexosaminidase A deficiency) can occur in young adults. The mode of inheritance is autosomal recessive, and both sexes are equally affected. Patients often develop progressive ataxia with mild signs of corticospinal disease and may have generalized seizures. The fundi are typically normal, but characteristic cherry red spots occur. In some cases the initial manifestations consist of motor neuron involvement with progressive weakness and muscle cramps, mimicking amyotrophic lateral sclerosis (see Chap. 370). The diagnosis is established by visualizing cytoplasmic bodies by electron microscopy or by detecting reduced hexosaminidase A activity in white blood cells. Gaucher's, Niemann-Pick, and Krabbe's diseases also occur rarely in adult life (see Chap. 346).

Ceroid Lipofuscinosis The Kufs type of ceroid lipofuscinosis is a lipid storage disease that can occur in either adolescence or early to mid-adult life. The disease is characterized by mental deterioration with seizures, ataxia, apoptosis, and spasticity. Diagnosis is made by skin or conjunctival biopsies that show lipofucsin storage material and characteristic abnormalities by electron microscopy.

NUTRITIONAL DISEASES

The vitamin deficiency diseases consist of the following neurologic diseases: (1) Wernicke's disease and Korsakoff's psychosis, (2) alcoholic cerebellar degeneration, (3) nutritional polyneuropathy, (4) pellagra, (5) deficiency amblyopia (nutritional optic neuropathy), (6) Strachan's syndrome, consisting of amblyopia, painful neuropathy, and orogenital dermatitis, (7) subacute combined degeneration of the spinal cord, (8) folic acid deficiency, and (9) vitamin E deficiency.

WERNICKE'S DISEASE OR ENCEPHALOPATHY Wernicke's encephalopathy is a common and preventable disorder due to a deficiency of thiamine (see Chap. 79). In the United States, alcoholics account for most cases, but patients are also at risk with malnutrition due to hyperemesis, starvation, renal dialysis, cancer, or acquired immunodeficiency syndrome. The characteristic clinical triad is that of ophthalmoplegia, ataxia, and global confusion. However, only one-third of patients with acute Wernicke's encephalopathy present with the classic clinical triad. Most patients are profoundly disoriented, indifferent, and inattentive, although rarely they have an agitated delirium related to ethanol withdrawal. If the disease is not treated, stupor, coma, and death may ensue. Ocular motor abnormalities include horizontal nystagmus on lateral gaze, lateral rectus palsy (usually bilateral), conjugate gaze palsies, and rarely ptosis. Gait ataxia probably results from a combination of polyneuropathy, cerebellar involvement, and vestibular paresis. The pupils are usually spared, but they may become miotic with advanced disease. Parenteral administration of thiamine in the early stages results in dramatic improvement in ocular motility, but horizontal nystagmus may persist.

Wernicke's disease is usually associated with other manifestations of nutritional disease, such as polyneuropathy, which is seen in 80 percent of patients (see Chap. 386). Rarely, amblyopia or spinal spastic ataxia occur. Tachycardia and postural hypotension may be related to impaired function of the autonomic nervous system or to the coexistence of cardiovascular (wet) beriberi. Patients who recover show improvement in ocular palsies within hours after the administration of thiamine. Ataxia improves more slowly than the ocular motor abnormalities. Approximately half the patients recover incompletely and are left with a slow, shuffling, wide-based gait and an inability to walk tandem. Apathy, drowsiness, and confusion improve more gradually. As these symptoms recede, an amnestic state with impairment in recent memory and learning may become more apparent (Korsakoff's psychosis; see Chap. 386). Korsakoff's psychosis is a part of Wernicke's disease and may occur together with the other components of the illness (Wernicke-Korsakoff syndrome). Korsakoff's psychosis is frequently persistent; the residual mental state is characterized by gaps in memory, confabulation, and disordered temporal sequencing.

Pathology Lesions in the periventricular regions of the diencephalon, midbrain, and brainstem as well as the superior vermis of the cerebellum consist of symmetric discoloration of structures surrounding the third ventricle, aqueduct, and fourth ventricle, with petechial hemorrhages in occasional acute cases and atrophy of the mamillary bodies in most chronic cases. There is frequently endothelial proliferation, demyelination, a loss of neuropil, and some neuronal loss. These changes can be detected in some cases by MRI scanning (Fig. 380-2). The amnestic defect is related to lesions in the medial dorsal nuclei of the thalamus.

Etiology and Pathogenesis The specific factor responsible for the Wernicke-Korsakoff syndrome is a deficiency of thiamine. Thiamine is a cofactor of several enzymes, including transketolase, pyruvate dehydrogenase, and α-ketoglutarate dehydrogenase. Thiamine deficiency produces a diffuse decrease in cerebral glucose utilization and results in mitochondrial damage. Glutamate accumulates owing to impairment of α-ketoglutarate dehydrogenase activity and, in combination with the energy deficiency, may result in excitotoxic cell damage. Electron microscopy shows disintegrating mitochondria, chromatin clumping, and swelling of degenerating neurons in the diencephalic nuclei of thiamine-deficient rats, consistent with excitotoxicity. Cell degeneration can be blocked by an antagonist of the NMDA glutamate receptor.

Rx TREATMENT

Wernicke's disease is a medical emergency and requires immediate administration of thiamine, in a dose of 50 mg either intravenously or intramuscularly. The dose should be given daily until the patient resumes a normal diet and should be begun prior to treatment with

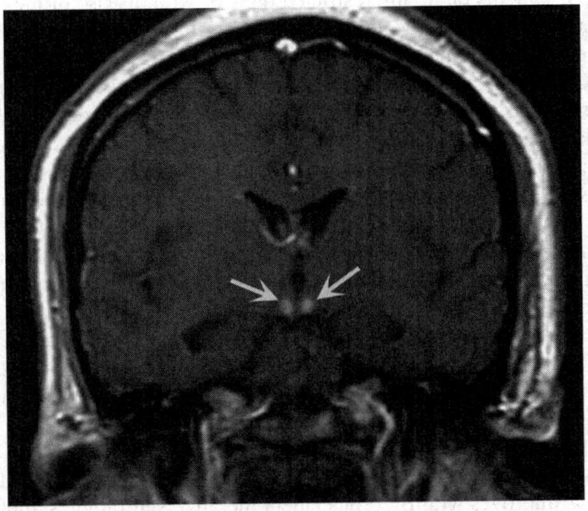

FIGURE 380-2 Wernicke's disease. Coronal T1-weighted postcontrast MR image reveals abnormal enhancement of the mammillary bodies (*arrows*), typical of acute Wernicke's encephalopathy.

intravenous glucose solutions. Glucose infusions may precipitate Wernicke's disease or acute cardiovascular beriberi in a previously unaffected patient or cause a rapid worsening of an early form of the disease. For this reason, thiamine should be administered to all alcoholic patients requiring parenteral glucose. The cardiovascular status of each patient should be carefully monitored.

NUTRITIONAL POLYNEUROPATHY (See also Chaps. 79 and 381) Nutritional polyneuropathy is usually associated with alcoholism. It is present in most patients with Wernicke-Korsakoff syndrome. The neuropathy is identical to that seen with beriberi. The treatment is administration of B vitamins, including thiamine, pyridoxine, pantothenic acid, vitamin B_{12}, and folic acid.

ALCOHOLIC CEREBELLAR DEGENERATION Cerebellar degeneration occurs frequently in chronic alcoholics. The symptoms usually evolve in a subacute fashion over several weeks to months. The cerebellar dysfunction predominantly affects the stance and the gait, which is wide-based. Legs are involved more severely than arms. Nystagmus and dysarthria occur infrequently. The pathologic changes consist of degeneration of neurons in the anterior and superior cerebellar vermis with loss of Purkinje cells. CT or MRI confirms cerebellar vermis atrophy. Abstinence, dietary replenishment, and supplemental B vitamins may produce moderate improvement in the gait ataxia as peripheral neuropathy resolves.

PELLAGRA (See Chap. 79) Pellagra is a result of niacin deficiency. The neurologic symptoms consist of both an encephalopathy and a peripheral neuropathy. Early nonspecific symptoms consist of insomnia, fatigue, anxiety, nervousness, irritability, and depression. With advancing illness, there may be slowing of mental processes and impairment of memory. In some cases there is a spastic spinal syndrome consisting of spastic weakness of the legs, increased tendon reflexes, clonus, and extensor plantar responses.

Pathologic Features The major neuropathologic changes in pellagra are swelling, chromatolysis, and loss of Nissl staining in neurons, particularly the large Betz cells of the motor cortex. The same changes are seen to a lesser extent in smaller pyramidal cells of cerebral cortex and in cells of the basal ganglia, cranial motor nuclei, dentate nuclei, and anterior horns of the spinal cord. The spinal cord lesions consist of symmetric degeneration of the dorsal columns and to a lesser extent the corticospinal tracts.

SUBACUTE COMBINED DEGENERATION OF THE SPINAL CORD (See Chap. 373) This spinal cord disease due to vitamin B_{12} deficiency is typically associated with an acquired defect in intestinal absorption of vitamin B_{12} due to an intrinsic factor deficiency. Rarely, patients on highly restricted diets or with disease of the small intestine or gastric resection manifest the illness. Occasionally, the cause is an abnormal vitamin B_{12} binding protein.

Clinical Manifestations Neurologic symptoms are present in most patients with B_{12} deficiency. The initial symptoms are generalized weakness and paresthesia consisting of tingling and "pins-and-needles" feelings. The paresthesia tends to persist and to cause distress. As the illness progresses, loss of vibration sense is more pronounced in the legs than the arms. Position sense is involved to a lesser extent. The motor defects are usually limited to the legs and include weakness, spasticity, increased deep tendon reflexes, clonus, and extensor plantar responses. At an early stage, the patellar and Achilles reflexes may be diminished, increased, or absent. The gait is initially ataxic but later becomes both spastic and ataxic.

Mental symptoms include irritability, apathy, somnolence, suspiciousness, confusional psychosis, and intellectual deterioration. Personality change and dementia may be the only manifestations. Optic neuropathy with impaired acuity and central scotomas often but not always improves with B_{12} replacement therapy. Neurologic symptoms may occur in the absence of anemia.

Pathology and Pathogenesis The pathologic features consist of swelling of myelin sheaths followed by demyelination and astrocytic gliosis. The changes commence in the posterior columns of the lower cervical and upper thoracic region and spread up and down the spinal cord, followed by involvement of the lateral columns. In the optic nerves there is degeneration of myelinated fibers in the territory of the papillomacular bundles.

The pathogenesis is poorly understood. Vitamin B_{12} deficiency impairs the function of methionine synthetase and methylmalonyl CoA mutase. Impairment of the latter enzyme may lead to the production of abnormal fatty acids, which alters the production of myelin. The major defect, however, may result from impairment of methionine synthase activity, since hereditary cases of cobalamin deficiency have been described in which methylmalonyl CoA mutase activity was normal in the presence of neurologic abnormalities. Interestingly, dentists and others who have overexposure to nitrous oxide may develop neurologic symptoms identical to those in B_{12} deficiency. Prolonged exposure of rats to nitrous oxide inactivates methionine synthetase but has no effects on methylmalonyl CoA mutase. Methylation of myelin basic protein can stabilize its insertion in the myelin sheath, which could play a role in pathogenesis.

Diagnosis Patients are typically screened by measurements of serum vitamin B_{12} levels. Rare patients become symptomatic with serum B_{12} concentrations in the low normal range. Intrinsic factor deficiency can be confirmed by a Shilling test (see Chap. 108). The presence of anti-intrinsic factor or anti-parietal cell antibodies confirms the diagnosis of pernicious anemia. In the rare instances in which these tests are inconclusive, documentation of elevated serum levels of methylmalonic acid and total serum homocysteine may substantiate the diagnosis, but these tests are expensive and are only performed in specialized laboratories. Their role in the screening of patients with nonspecific neuropsychiatric symptoms remains to be established.

℞ TREATMENT

Treatment consists of administration of cobalamin at a dosage of 1 mg (1000 μg) intramuscularly each day for 5 to 10 days, then weekly for a month, and then monthly for life. Folate administration may cause neurologic deterioration in vitamin B_{12}–deficient patients. Therefore, if folate therapy is indicated, it should not be given until cobalamin stores have been repleted for 1 to 2 weeks. The most important factor influencing the response to treatment is the duration of symptoms. Recovery is often complete if therapy is instituted within a few weeks of their onset. For this reason, treatment should be instituted on an emergent basis. If symptoms have been present for several months, the best that can be expected is arrest of progression of the disease.

FOLIC ACID DEFICIENCY Folic acid deficiency occurs frequently, yet its role in the pathogenesis of nervous system disease is not firmly established. Neuropathies associated with some chronic malabsorption syndromes and accompanying chronic administration of phenytoin have been attributed to folate deficiency. Rare cases of subacute combined degeneration have been attributed to folic acid deficiency and have resolved after the institution of folate therapy.

VITAMIN E DEFICIENCY (See Chap. 79) Vitamin E is a fat-soluble vitamin, and deficiency states occur with chronic malabsorption syndromes, such as in abetalipoproteinemia, following surgical resection of the intestine, and with hepatobiliary disease. Vitamin E deficiency also occurs in patients with mutations in the gene for the α-tocopherol transfer protein, which incorporates α-tocopherol into very low density lipoproteins in the liver. Three different mutations have been identified in families suffering from ataxia with vitamin E deficiency. The manifestations include peripheral neuropathy, ataxia, and proximal muscle weakness and resemble those of spinocerebellar degeneration. Pathologic features consist of degeneration of posterior columns, spinocerebellar tracts, posterior columns, dorsal root ganglia, and sensory roots. The pathogenesis of the lesions is of great interest, since vitamin E is known to be a major lipid-soluble antioxidant. It is therefore hypothesized that vitamin E deficiency leads to increased free radical generation and oxidative damage. Treatment consists of supplementation with 60 to 75 U of vitamin E. In patients with malabsorption, it may be necessary to administer other fat-soluble vitamins as well.

DEFICIENCY AMBLYOPIA Deficiency amblyopia (nutritional optic neuropathy, tobacco-alcohol amblyopia) is a form of visual impairment that complicates nutritional deficiency. The symptoms consist of dimness or blurring of vision and impairment of color vision, which then progresses insidiously over days to weeks. On examination, patients show reduced visual acuity and have bilateral and roughly symmetric central or centrocecal scotomas. Pallor of the temporal portion of the optic disc may be present.

Deficiency amblyopia, which was common among prisoners of war in the Far East, has also been associated with some cases of beriberi (due to thiamine deficiency) and pellagra (due to niacin deficiency). In the United States, most cases occur in heavy smokers who also consume alcohol. These cases of so-called tobacco-alcohol amblyopia are thought to be largely of nutritional origin. It has been hypothesized that smoking may contribute to optic nerve toxicity because of the cyanide in tobacco smoke. Cyanide may be detoxified by vitamin B_{12}–dependent mechanisms involving sulfated amino acids. Some cases of tobacco-alcohol amblyopia respond to vitamin B_{12} supplementation. Treatment otherwise consists of administration of a balanced diet, supplementation with vitamins, and restriction of alcohol when it is the cause of nutritional deficiency.

AMBYLOPIA, PAINFUL NEUROPATHY, AND OROGENITAL DERMATITIS (STRACHAN'S SYNDROME) The syndrome of amblyopia, painful neuropathy, and orogenital dermatitis (Strachan's syndrome), originally referred to as Jamaican neuritis, occurs among the undernourished populations of many tropical countries. The disorder occurred in the besieged population in Madrid during the Spanish Civil War and in prisoners of war during World War II in both the Middle and Far East, and an outbreak has occurred in Cuba. In the United States, this syndrome occurs occasionally in alcoholic patients.

The optic neuropathy is characterized by subacute onset of decreased visual acuity and color vision, central scotomas, pallor of the optic disc, and loss of papillomacular bundle fibers. The peripheral neuropathy consists of painful dysesthesia, areas of hyperesthesia, diminished ankle reflexes, decreased sensitivity to vibration, pinprick, and light touch, and rarely high-frequency hearing loss. A few patients have developed a myopathy with decreased posterior column sensation as well as mild spasticity with heightened reflexes, extensor plantar responses, and a spastic bladder.

An epidemic of optic and peripheral neuropathy affected more than 50,000 people in Cuba from 1991 to 1993. This outbreak was associated with tobacco use, particularly cigar smoking, and the risk was reduced with higher dietary intakes of thiamine, vitamin B_{12}, riboflavin, and niacin. In addition, higher serum concentrations of antioxidant carotenoids appear to be protective. Improved nutrition and supplementation with multivitamins have resulted in the disappearance of the syndrome.

BIBLIOGRAPHY

BEAL MF: Aging, energy and oxidative stress in neurodegenerative diseases. Ann Neurol 38:357, 1995

BECK WS: Neuropsychiatric consequences of cobalamin deficiency. Adv Intern Med 36:33, 1991

BUTTERWORTH RF: Pathophysiology of cerebellar dysfunction in the Wernicke-Korsakoff syndrome. Can J Neurol 20(Suppl 3):123, 1993

——— et al: Ammonia: Key factor in the pathogenesis of hepatic encephalopathy. Neurochem Pathol 6:1, 1987

CHARNESS MD et al: Ethanol and the nervous system. N Engl J Med 321:442, 1989

CHOI DW, ROTHMAN SM: The role of glutamate neurotoxicity in hypoxic-ischemic neuronal death. Annu Rev Neurosci 13:171, 1990

DININGER MN: Management of sodium abnormalities in patients with CNS disease. Clin Neuropharmacol 15:427, 1992

FRANCIS GS et al: Metachromatic leukodystrophy: Multiple nonfunctional and pseudodeficiency alleles in a pedigree: Problems with diagnosis and counseling. Ann Neurol 34:212, 1993

GOTODA T et al: Adult-onset spinocerebellar dysfunction caused by a mutation in the gene for the α-tocopherol-transfer protein. N Engl J Med 333:1313, 1995

JOHNS DR: Mitochondrial DNA and disease. N Engl J Med 333:638, 1995

KINNEY HC et al: Neuropathological findings in the brain of Karen Ann Quinlan. N Engl J Med 330:1469, 1994

LAURENO R: Central pontine myelinolysis following rapid correction of hyponatremia. Ann Neurol 13:232, 1983

LEE MS, MARSDEN CD: Neurological sequelae following carbon monoxide poisoning: Clinical course and outcome according to the clinical types and brain computed tomography scan findings. Movement Disord 9:550, 1994

LIEBER CS: Medical disorders of alcoholism. N Engl J Med 333:1058, 1995

OUHCHI K et al: Ataxia with isolated vitamin E deficiency is caused by mutations in the α-tocopherol transfer protein. Nat Genet 9:141, 1995

REYNOLDS EH et al: Subacute combined degeneration with high serum vitamin B_{12} level and abnormal vitamin B_{12} binding protein. Arch Neurol 50:739, 1993

ROMÁN GC: An epidemic in Cuba of optic neuropathy, sensorineural deafness, peripheral sensory neuropathy and dorsolateral myeloneuropathy. J Neurol Sci 127:11, 1994

RIZZO JF, LESSELL S: Tobacco amblyopia. Am J Ophthalmol 116:84, 1993

SERDARU M et al: The clinical spectrum of alcoholic pellagra encephalopathy. Brain 111:829, 1988

SHEVELL MI, ROSENBLATT DS: The neurology of cobalamin. Can J Neurol Sci 19:472, 1990

THE CUBA NEUROPATHY FIELD INVESTIGATION TEAM: Epidemic optic neuropathy in Cuba—clinical characterization and risk factors. N Engl J Med 333:1176, 1995

THE MULTI-SOCIETY TASK FORCE ON PVS: Medical aspects of the persistent vegetative state. N Engl J Med 330:1499, 1994

VICTOR M: Alcoholic dementia. Can J Neurol Sci 21:88, 1994

——— et al: *The Wernicke-Korsakoff Syndrome and Related Disorders Due to Alcoholism and Malnutrition.* Philadelphia, Davis, 1989

ZIEVE L: Pathogenesis of hepatic encephalopathy. Metab Brain Dis 2:147, 1987

SECTION 3

DISORDERS OF NERVE AND MUSCLE

381

Arthur K. Asbury

DISEASES OF THE PERIPHERAL NERVOUS SYSTEM

Peripheral neuropathy is a general term indicating peripheral nerve disorders of any cause; the manifestations of such a disorder may be so bewildering and complex that it is difficult for the physician to know where to begin and how to proceed. Therefore, an assessment scheme is set forth to guide the examiner to correct diagnoses and management decisions (Fig. 381-1).

GENERAL DESCRIPTION Polyneuropathy is a common and important type of peripheral neuropathy. The prototypical picture of polyneuropathy occurs with acquired toxic or metabolic neuropathic states. The first symptoms tend to be sensory and consist of tingling, prickling, burning, or bandlike dysesthesias in the balls of the feet or tips of the toes, or in a general distribution over the soles (see Chap. 23). Symptoms and findings are usually symmetric and graded distally, but occasionally dysesthesias appear in one foot shortly before the other or are more pronounced in one foot. Some care and judgment is needed to avoid confusion with mononeuropathy multiplex. If the polyneuropathy remains mild, no objective motor or sensory signs may be detectable.

With progression, pansensory loss is usually found over both feet, ankle jerks are lost, and weakness of dorsiflexion of the toes, best demonstrated in the great toe, may be present. In some instances, the process begins with weakness in the feet, without sensory symptoms. As worsening occurs, sensory loss moves centripetally in a graded "stocking" fashion, and the patient may complain that the feet have a numb or "wooden" feeling or may say "I feel as though I'm walking on stumps." Patients have difficulty walking on their heels during examination and their feet may slap while walking. Later, the knee jerk reflex disappears, and foot drop becomes more apparent. By the time sensory disturbance has reached the upper shin, dysesthesias are usually noticed in the tips of the fingers. The degree of spontaneous pain varies but is often considerable. Light stimuli to hypesthetic areas, once perceived, may be experienced as extremely uncomfortable (hyperpathia). Unsteadiness of gait may be out of proportion to muscle weakness because of proprioceptive loss.

Worsening is more severe in the legs than in the arms and proceeds in a centripetal, symmetrically graded manner with pansensory loss, areflexia, and muscle atrophy; motor weakness is usually greater in the extensor muscles than in corresponding flexor groups. When the sensory disturbance reaches the elbows and mid-thighs, a tent-shaped area of hypesthesia often may be demonstrated on the lower abdomen. This area will grow broader, and its apex will extend rostrally toward the sternum as the neuropathy worsens. By this time, patients generally cannot stand or walk or hold objects in their hands.

In the most extreme cases, ventilatory capacity is impaired along with sphincteric function. Hyperesthesia at the crown of the scalp may be present and may spread radially into both the trigeminal and the C2 distribution. Overall, nerve fibers are affected according to length of their axon, without regard to root or nerve trunk distribution—hence the aptness of the term *stocking-glove* to describe the pattern of sensory deficit. In general, the motor deficit is also graded, distal, and symmetric.

Variations in disease manifestations are common and explain the diversity of clinical syndromes encountered. Variations occur in the rate of disease evolution, in whether progression is steady or fluctuating, in the eventual degree of severity, in the presence or absence of positive motor and sensory symptoms, in the symmetry of features and their distribution (proximal versus distal, arms versus legs, and motor versus sensory), in the relative proportions of dysfunction attributable to deficits in large and to small fibers, and in the relative importance of axonal and demyelinating processes (as assessed mainly by electrodiagnostic examination).

ASSESSMENT AND DIAGNOSIS OF NEUROPATHY Clues to the diagnosis of specific peripheral neuropathies often lie in unnoticed or forgotten events occurring weeks or months prior to the onset of symptoms. Inquiry should be made about recent viral illnesses; other systemic symptoms; institution of new medications; exposures to solvents, pesticides, or heavy metals; the occurrence of similar symptoms in family members or coworkers; habits concerning alcohol; and the presence of known preexisting medical disorders. It is also useful to ask patients if they would feel well if free of their neuropathic symptoms, to obtain an idea of the presence or absence of an underlying systemic illness.

How did symptoms first appear? Even with distal polyneuropathies, symptoms may appear in the sole of one foot a few days or a week before the other, but usually the patient will describe a distal graded disturbance that moves evenly and symmetrically in centripetal fashion. Symptoms that first appear in the distribution of individual digital nerves, involving only half of a digit at a time, and then gradually spread and coalesce suggest a multifocal process (mononeuropathy multiplex), as might occur with a systemic vasculitis or cryoglobulinemia.

The evolution of neuropathy ranges from rapid worsening over a few days to an indolent process lasting many years. Polyneuropathies

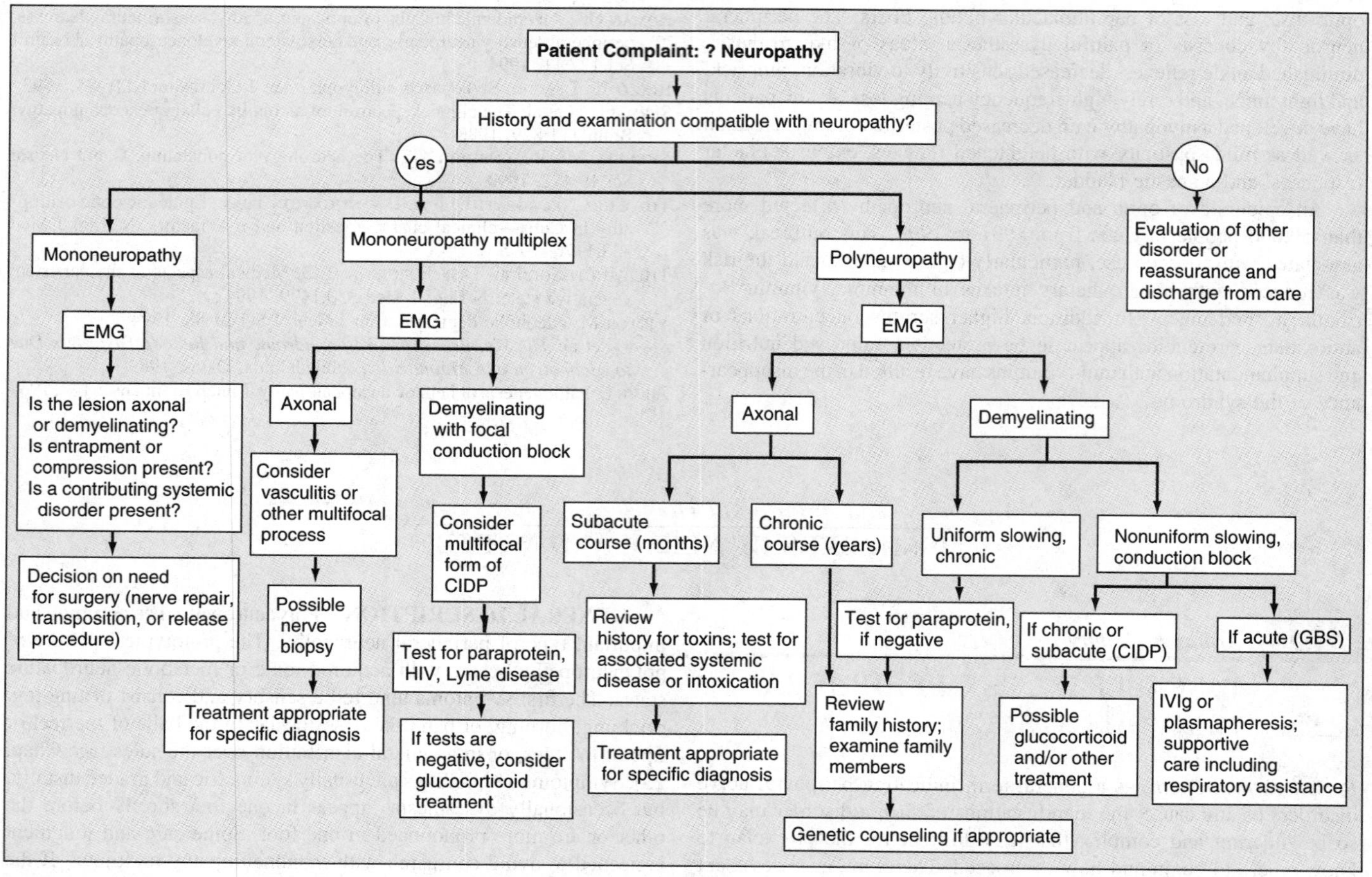

FIGURE 381-1 Approach to the evaluation of peripheral neuropathies. CIDP, chronic inflammatory demyelinating polyneuropathy; EMG, electromyography; GBS, Guillain-Barré syndrome; HIV, human immunodeficiency virus; IVIg, intravenous immunoglobulin. *(After Asbury.)*

that progress slowly, over more than 5 years, are most likely to be genetically determined, particularly if the major manifestations are distal atrophy and weakness with few or no positive sensory symptoms. Diabetic polyneuropathy and paraproteinemic neuropathies also progress insidiously over 5 to 10 years. Axonal degeneration of toxic or metabolic origin tends to evolve over several weeks to a year or more, and the rate of progression of demyelinating neuropathies is highly variable, ranging from a few days in Guillain-Barré syndrome to many years in others.

Major fluctuations in the course of neuropathy raise two possibilities: (1) relapsing forms of neuropathy and (2) repeated toxic exposures. Slow fluctuation in symptoms taking place over weeks or months (reflecting changes in the activity of neuropathy) should not be confused with day-to-day variation or diurnal undulation of symptoms. The latter are common to all neuropathic disorders. An example is carpal tunnel syndrome, in which dysesthesia may be prominent at night but absent during the day.

Palpation of the nerve trunk to detect enlargement is a frequently forgotten part of the neurologic examination. In mononeuropathies, the entire course of the nerve trunk in question should be explored manually for focal thickening, for the presence of neurofibroma, point tenderness, or Tinel's phenomenon (generation of a tingling sensation in the sensory territory of the nerve by tapping along the course of the nerve trunk), and for pain elicited by stretching of the nerve trunk. In leprous neuritis, fusiform thickening of nerve trunks is frequent, and beading of nerve trunks may be encountered in amyloid polyneuropathy. In genetically determined hypertrophic neuropathies, uniform thickening of all nerve trunks may occur, often to the caliber of a clothesline or larger.

Most neuropathies involve nerve fibers of all sizes, but damage sometimes is restricted to either large or small fibers. In a polyneuropathy affecting mainly small fibers, diminished pinprick and temperature sensation, often with painful, burning dysesthesias, may predominate along with autonomic dysfunction, but with relative sparing of motor power, balance, and tendon jerks. Some cases of amyloid and distal diabetic polyneuropathies fall into this category. In contrast, large-fiber polyneuropathy is characterized by areflexia, sensory ataxia, relatively minor cutaneous sensory deficit, and variable but often severe motor dysfunction.

For patients with polyneuropathy or mononeuropathy multiplex, standard tests should include a complete blood count and measurement of erythrocyte sedimentation rate, urinalysis, chest x-ray, postprandial blood glucose determination, and serum protein electrophoresis. Further tests should be dictated by the combined results of the history and the physical and electrodiagnostic examination (see Fig. 381-1).

Electrodiagnosis Electrodiagnostic examination is a key procedure in all patients with suspected neuropathy (see Fig. 380-1). It is not generally possible to make the distinction between axonal and demyelinating disorders by clinical examination alone; here electrodiagnostic analysis is particularly useful. Electrodiagnostic features of demyelination are slowing of nerve conduction velocity (NCV), dispersion of evoked compound action potentials, conduction block (major decrease in amplitude of muscle compound action potentials on proximal stimulation of the nerve, as compared to distal stimulation), and marked prolongation of distal latencies (see Chap. 361). In contrast, axonal neuropathies are characterized by a reduction in amplitude of evoked compound action potentials with relative preservation of NCV. The distinction between a primarily demyelinating neuropathy and an axonal neuropathy is crucial because of the differing approaches to diagnosis and management.

Electrodiagnosis also helps to determine the presence or absence of a sensory involvement when that is not clear by clinical examination alone. It provides information about the distribution of subclinical findings, thus sharpening the diagnostic focus. The issues on which the clinician may ask the electrodiagnostician for clarification include the following:

1. The distinction between disorders primary to nerve and to muscle (neuropathy versus myopathy).
2. The distinction between root or plexus involvement and more distal nerve trunk involvement.
3. The distinction between generalized polyneuropathic processes and widespread multifocal nerve trunk involvement.
4. The distinction between upper and lower motor neuron weakness.
5. The distinction, in a given generalized polyneuropathic process, between primary demyelinating neuropathy and axonal degeneration.
6. The assessment, in both primary axonal and demyelinating neuropathies, of many factors bearing on the nature, activity, and likely prognosis of the neuropathy.
7. The assessment, in mononeuropathies, of the site of the lesion and its major effect on nerve fibers, especially the distinction between demyelinating conduction block and wallerian degeneration.
8. The characterization of disorders of the neuromuscular junction.
9. The identification, often in muscle of normal bulk and strength, of important features such as chronic partial denervation, fasciculations, and myotonia.
10. The analysis of cramp, and its distinction from physiologic contracture.

If in a particular instance of progressive polyneuropathy of subacute or chronic evolution the electrodiagnostic findings are those of an axonopathy, a long list of metabolic states and exogenous toxins comes under consideration (see Tables 381-1 and 381-2). If the course is protracted over several years, it raises the likelihood of the neuronal (axonal) form of peroneal muscular atrophy [hereditary motor and sensory neuropathy (HMSN) type II]; family members must be examined and additional attention given to the family history. If the electrodiagnostic findings indicate primary demyelination of nerve, on the other hand, the approach is entirely different. The possibilities then include acquired demyelinating neuropathy, thought to be immunologically mediated, and genetically determined neuropathies, some of which are marked by uniform and drastic slowing of nerve conduction velocities.

The flowchart in Fig. 381-1 summarizes the clinical and electrodiagnostic approach to evaluation and management of a neuropathic disorder. Using this scheme, the clinician determines for each patient the tempo, distribution, and severity of the disease, the functional impairment of the patient, and other features previously discussed, making a clinical judgment as to whether the problem represents a mononeuropathy, a mononeuropathy multiplex, or a polyneuropathy. Often this distinction is obvious. With the sum of clinical and electrodiagnostic information in hand, the differential diagnostic possibilities and management options will have been narrowed to only a few. The remainder of this chapter deals with the details of this formulation.

Nerve Biopsy The sural nerve at the ankle is the preferred site for cutaneous nerve biopsy. There are few indications to employ this invasive technique. The main one is in asymmetric and multifocal neuropathic disorders producing a clinical picture of mononeuropathy multiplex, the basis of which is still unclear after other laboratory investigations are complete. Diagnostic considerations include vasculitis, multifocal demyelinating neuropathies, amyloidosis, leprosy, and occasionally sarcoidosis. Nerve biopsy is also helpful when one or more cutaneous nerves are palpably enlarged. Another clinical application is in establishing the diagnosis in some genetically determined childhood disorders such as metachromatic leukodystrophy, Krabbe's disease, giant axonal neuropathy, and infantile neuroaxonal dystrophy. In all of these recessively inherited diseases, both the central nervous system (CNS) and the peripheral nervous system (PNS) are affected.

There is a tendency to carry out sural nerve biopsy in distal symmetric polyneuropathies of subacute or chronic evolution. This practice is discouraged because its yield is low. Nerve biopsy in this situation may be useful as part of an approved research protocol when the biopsy will provide crucial information not otherwise obtainable.

Table 381-1

Polyneuropathy Associated with Systemic Diseases

Systemic Disease (Occurrence)	Axonal* Acute	Axonal* Subacute	Axonal* Chronic	Demyelinating* Acute	Demyelinating* Subacute	Demyelinating* Chronic	Sensory vs. Motor†	Autonomic*	Comment
Diabetes mellitus (common)	−	±	+	−	±	+	S, SM, rarely M	± to +	See Table 381-4
Uremia (sometimes)	±	+	+	−	−	−	SM	±	Controllable with proper dialysis; curable with successful renal transplant
Porphyria (3 types) (rare)	+	±	−	−	−	−	M or SM	± to +	May be proximal > distal and may have atypical proximal sensory deficits
Hypoglycemia (rare)	±	+	±	−	−	−	M	−	Usually with insulinoma; arms often > legs
Vitamin deficiency, excluding B_{12} (sometimes)	−	+	+	−	−	−	SM	±	Involves thiamine, pyridoxine, folate, pantothenic acid, and probably others
Vitamin B_{12} deficiency (sometimes)	−	±	+	−	−	−	S	−	Neuropathy overshadowed by myelopathy
Critical illness (sepsis) (common)	−	+	±	−	−	−	M > S	−	Sepsis patients severely ill, often on ventilator
Chronic liver disease (sometimes)	−	−	−	−	−	+	S or SM	−	Usually mild or subclinical
Primary biliary cirrhosis (rare)	−	±	+	−	−	−	S	−	Intraneural xanthomas
Primary systemic amyloidosis (rare)	−	±	+	−	−	−	SM	+	Also in amyloidosis with myeloma or macroglobulinemia
Hypothyroidism (rare)	−	−	−	−	±	+	S	−	May respond to thyroid replacement
Chronic obstructive lung disease (rare)	−	±	+	−	−	−	S or SM	−	Severe pulmonary insufficiency
Acromegaly (rare)	−	−	+	−	−	−	S	−	Carpal tunnel syndrome also frequent
Malabsorption (sprue, celiac disease) (sometimes)	−	±	+	−	−	−	S or SM	±	Basis for neuropathy unclear; deficiency?
Carcinoma (sensory) (rare)	−	+	+	−	−	−	Pure S	−	Due to ganglionitic neuronopathy; mostly small cell lung or breast carcinoma; paraneoplastic
Carcinoma (sensorimotor) (sometimes)	−	+	+	−	−	−	SM	±	Sensorimotor axonal neuropathy; mostly with lung carcinoma
Carcinoma (late) (common)	−	+	+	−	−	−	S > M	±	Mild, probably related to weight loss and wasting
Carcinoma (demyelinating) (sometimes)	−	−	−	+	+	±	SM	−	Acute or relapsing demyelinating neuropathy
HIV infection (sometimes)	−	±	+	−	−	−	S >> M	−	Late stages of AIDS; other neuropathies occur; see text
Lyme disease (sometimes)	−	±	+	−	−	−	S > M	−	Variable picture; see text
Lymphoma, including Hodgkin's (sometimes)	−	+	+	+	+	±	See above	±	Same as with carcinomatous types
Polycythemia vera (rare)	−	±	+	−	−	−	S	−	Also many CNS manifestations; often shooting pains in limbs
Multiple myeloma, lytic type (sometimes)	−	±	+	−	−	−	S, M, or SM	±	Symptomatic neuropathy uncommon; subclinical neuropathy frequent
Multiple myeloma, osteosclerotic or solitary plasmacytoma type‡ (sometimes)	−	−	±	−	±	+	SM	−	May show severe slowing of nerve conduction velocity
Benign monoclonal gammopathy (sometimes):									
IgA	−	±	+	−	−	−	SM	−	IgM_κ (or occasionally IgM_λ) may bind to myelin-associated glycoprotein or glycolipids
IgG	−	±	+	−	−	−	SM	−	
IgM	−	−	−	−	±	+	SM or S	−	
Cryoglobulinemia (rare)	−	±	+	−	−	−	SM	−	May be mononeuropathy multiplex in presentation

* +, Usually; ±, sometimes; −, rare, if ever.
† S, sensory; M, motor; SM, sensorimotor.
‡ Some cases associated with POEMS syndrome (see text).

Table 381-2

Polyneuropathy Associated with Drugs and Environmental Toxins

	Axonal*			Demyelinating*						
	Acute	Subacute	Chronic	Acute	Subacute	Chronic	Sensory vs. Motor†	Autonomic*	CNS*	Comment
DRUGS‡										
Amiodarone (antiarrhythmic)	−	−	+	−	−	+	SM	−	−	Dose-dependent neuropathy, reversible by decreasing dose
Aurothioglucose (antirheumatic)	±	±	−	+	+	−	SM	−	−	Idiosyncratic reaction; ? immune-mediated
Cisplatin (antineoplastic)	−	+	+	−	−	−	S	−	−	Severe sensory neuropathy, also ototoxicity; dose-related
Dapsone (dermatologic agent; used, e.g., for leprosy)	−	±	+	−	−	−	M	−	−	Dose-related pure motor neuropathy
Disulfiram (antialcoholism agent)	±	+	+	−	−	−	SM	−	±	Usually occurs after months of treatment
Hydralazine (antihypertensive)	−	±	+	−	−	−	S > M	−	−	A pyridoxine antagonist
Isoniazid	−	±	+	−	−	−	SM	±	−	A pyridoxine antagonist; neurotoxic in slow acetylators
Metronidazole (antiprotozoal)	−	−	±	−	−	−	S or SM	−	+	Dose-related central-peripheral distal axonopathy
Misonidazole (radiosensitizer)	−	±	+	−	−	−	S or SM	−	+	Neurotoxicity is the limiting factor
Nitrofurantoin (urinary antiseptic)	−	±	+	−	−	−	SM	−	−	Generally total dose-related; renal failure enhances toxicity
Nucleoside analogues (ddC, ddI, d4T) (antiretroviral agents)	±	+	+	−	−	−	S >> M	−	?	Dose-related; painful
Phenytoin (anticonvulsant)	−	−	+	−	−	−	S > M	−	−	After 20–30 years of phenytoin use
Pyridoxine (vitamin)	−	±	+	−	−	−	S	−	−	Occurs with large intake (>300 mg/d)
Suramin (antineoplastic)	+	+	−	+	+	−	M > S	−	−	Related to serum levels >350 mg/mL
Taxol (antineoplastic)	±	+	±	±	+	±	S > M	−	−	Dose-related
Vincristine (antineoplastic)	−	+	+	−	−	−	S > M	−	−	Sensory symptoms common, hands > feet; motor signs ominous; should stop treatment
TOXINS‡										
Acrylamide (flocculant; grouting agent)	−	±	+	−	−	−	S > M	±	+	Large-fiber neuropathy; sensory ataxia
Arsenic (herbicide; insecticide)	±	+	+	−	−	−	SM	±	±	Skin changes, Mees' lines in nails; painful; systemic effects
Diphtheria toxin	−	−	−	+	+	−	SM	−	−	Clinically very rare; can be confused with GBS
γ-Diketone hexacarbons (solvents)	−	±	+	−	−	+	SM	±	+	Neurofilamentous swelling of axons; these solvents now in restricted use
Inorganic lead	−	−	+	−	−	−	M > S or M	−	±	Selective motor neuropathy with prominent wrist drop
Organophosphates	−	±	+	−	−	−	SM	−	+	Brain and spinal cord also affected, the latter irreversibly
Thallium (rat poison)	−	+	+	−	−	−	SM	−	+	Also alopecia, Mees' lines in nails; painful

* +, Usually; ±, sometimes; −, rare, if ever.
† S, sensory; M, motor; SM, sensorimotor.
‡ The following drugs and environmental toxins are also neurotoxic, mainly to the peripheral nervous system:
Drugs: Amitriptyline, chloramphenicol, colchicine, ethambutol, nitrous oxide, perhexiline maleate, sodium cyanate, thalidomide, L-tryptophan
Environmental toxins: Allyl chloride, buckthorn berry, carbon disulfide, dimethylaminoproprionitrile, (DMAPN), ethylene oxide, metallic mercury, methyl bromide, polychlorinated biphenyls, styrene, trichlorethylene, vacor

POLYNEUROPATHY Although *polyneuropathy* connotes a widespread symmetric process, usually distal and graded, polyneuropathies are very diverse because of the extreme variability of tempo, severity, mix of sensory and motor features, and presence or absence of positive symptoms. The patient with a fulminant, severely dysesthetic sensory polyneuropathy and alopecia who is in the early phases of thallium intoxication bears little similarity to the patient with a 40-year history of insidiously progressive clumsiness of gait whose findings are foot drop, lower leg atrophy, pes cavus, and minimal asymptomatic distal sensory deficit (i.e., peroneal muscular atrophy, either type I or II; see Table 381-3). These two patients fall near opposite ends of the spectrum of polyneuropathy.

The classification of peripheral neuropathies has become increasingly complex as the capacity to discriminate new subgroups and identify new associations with toxins and systemic disorders improves. Further, our grasp of the pathophysiologic basis of the clinical phenomena observed in neuropathy has increased rapidly. But these advances are primarily descriptive; little progress has been made in understanding the fundamental pathogenic events in nervous tissue that eventuate in any of the polyneuropathies.

The important features of each major grouping of polyneuropathies are summarized below, and key aspects of specific polyneuropathies are given in Tables 381-1 to 381-5.

Acute Axonal Polyneuropathy In this setting, the term *acute* means evolution over days. Acute axonal polyneuropathies are relatively uncommon. Included are porphyric neuropathy and massive intoxications, often suicidal or homicidal in intent. For example, an individual receiving a large dose of arsenic (e.g., 100 mg of arsenous oxide) will become violently ill in a few hours with vomiting, diarrhea, and circulatory collapse. In 1 to 3 days, serious renal and liver failure will ensue, and between 14 and 21 days, painful polyneuropathy will appear, often as the systemic disorder abates. The polyneuropathy worsens over 2 to 3 weeks and then enters a plateau phase; recovery requires months.

Subacute Axonal Polyneuropathy Many instances of toxic and metabolic polyneuropathy are *subacute*, meaning they evolve over weeks, although even more of these may be chronic in evolution (months to years). Tables 381-1 and 381-2 offer many diagnostic possibilities. Management in almost all instances involves eliminating contact with the offending agent or treating the associated systemic order.

Chronic Axonal Polyneuropathy This category includes many more types of polyneuropathy, in part because the term *chronic* subsumes neuropathies that have progressed over periods from 6 months to 60 years. As a rough approximation, slow worsening for more than 5 years, absence of positive symptoms, deficits that are mainly motor, and absence of systemic disorder all favor a genetically determined neuropathy. Although these disorders are mostly autosomal dominant in inheritance, recessively inherited and X- linked varieties also occur (Table 381-3).

Acute Demyelinating Polyneuropathy For all practical purposes, this category is synonymous with Guillain-Barré syndrome (GBS). This acute, frequently severe, and fulminant polyneuropathy occurs at a rate of one case per million population per month, or approximately 3500 cases per year in the United States and Canada. Incidence patterns are similar worldwide. In over two-thirds of cases, an infection, either clinically overt or evidenced by serum titer rise, precedes the onset of neuropathy by 1 to 3 weeks. Herpesvirus infections (cytomegalovirus, Epstein-Barr virus) account for a large proportion of virus-triggered cases. Other cases appear to be triggered by *Campylobacter jejuni* gastroenteritis. A small proportion, less than 5 percent, occur within 1 to 4 weeks of a surgical procedure. GBS occurs on a background of lymphoma, including Hodgkin's disease, and in lupus erythematosus more frequently than can be attributed to chance alone.

Although the weight of evidence indicates that GBS is immune-mediated, the immunopathogenesis remains obscure. In 1976 to 1977, a flurry of some 500 cases followed the national swine flu vaccination program in the United States. This exceeded by severalfold the baseline incidence expected in this period in those vaccinated. The epidemiologic features of this outbreak resembled a point-source epidemic with an "incubation" period of 1 to 6 weeks. The reason why swine flu vaccine triggered GBS in 1976 to 1977 has never been discovered. In subsequent annual flu vaccine programs in the United States, no excess cases of GBS have been identified.

The clinical features of GBS include areflexic motor paralysis with or without sensory disturbance coupled with an acellular rise of total protein in the cerebrospinal fluid by the end of the first week of symptoms. Several subtypes of GBS are recognized. Approximately 80 percent of cases encountered in North America and Europe are demyelinating and inflammatory. An unusual variant, the Fisher syndrome, presents with ataxia, areflexia, and external ophthalmoplegia, but weakness often appears later in its course. Other variants are notable for an axonal pattern of electrodiagnostic findings and axonal pathology with little inflammation. Most patients with GBS are hospitalized, and about 30 percent require ventilatory assistance at some point during the illness. The prognosis is good; approximately 85 percent of patients make a complete or nearly complete recovery. The mortality rate is 3 to 4 percent. Management consists mostly of supportive care, but plasmapheresis also is important. Large, multicenter, controlled trials in North America and Europe have demonstrated a beneficial effect of plasmapheresis if initiated in the first 2 weeks of illness. Intravenous administration of high-dose immunoglobulin (2 g/kg body weight given over 5 days) is as effective as plasmapheresis, and is more easily administered. In contrast, glucocorticoid treatment has not been shown to be effective.

Other acute demyelinating polyneuropathies are rare and include buckthorn berry intoxication and diphtheritic polyneuritis (see Table 381-2).

Subacute Demyelinating Polyneuropathy Neuropathies in this category are heterogeneous in origin, although all are acquired. Most common is a relapsing and remitting neuropathy that has many clinical features in common with GBS but differs from GBS in tempo, course, and absence of discernible triggering events (see "Acquired Demyelinating Neuropathies," below). Previously mentioned toxins (buckthorn berry, diphtheria toxin, aurothioglucose) may also induce a picture of widespread subacute demyelination of peripheral nerves (see Table 381-2).

Chronic Demyelinating Polyneuropathy Although more common than the subacute neuropathies, chronic polyneuropathy with demyelinating features encompasses a wide diversity of disorders, including hereditary neuropathies, inflammatory neuropathies, and other acquired neuropathies associated with diabetes mellitus, dysproteinemias, other metabolic states, and some chronic intoxications. To complicate matters, many of these disorders present an electrodiagnostic picture of mixed axonal-demyelinative findings. Frequently it is difficult to determine which process—axonal degeneration or demyelination—is the primary event. Aspects of many of these neuropathies are included in Table 381-1 to 381-5 and in the sections below.

SPECIAL CATEGORIES OF NEUROPATHY **Hereditary Neuropathies** The major characteristics of this highly variegated group of disorders are summarized in Table 381-3. With the exception of the porphyric neuropathies, the onset of neuropathic dysfunction is insidious, and progression is indolent, occurring over years or decades. Most of these diseases are rare, with the striking exception of the dominantly inherited peroneal muscular atrophies (HMSN-I and HMSN-II; see Table 381-3). The prevalence of these disorders is roughly 1 case per 3000 to 6000 population. In peroneal muscular atrophy, phenotypic expression is often variable, so affected family members of a propositus may have no symptoms and minimal neurologic findings but (in HMSN-I) may still show severe reduction of nerve conduction velocity. Advances in molecular genetics have had a major impact on defining hereditary neuropathies. Two recent reviews are cited in the references, and Tables 362-1 and 380-3 outline what is known.

Table 381-3

Genetically Determined Neuropathies

Genetic Disorder	Inheritance/ Gene Location	Age of Onset	Basic Process	Other Features*	Other Systems Involved	Genetic Mutation	Comment
Charcot-Marie-Tooth (CMT) disease type 1A	AD 17p11.2-12	Decades 2–3	Demyelinating	Hypertropic change with onion bulbs; marked ↓ NCV	Rare; bony defects	Mutation in peripheral myelin protein gene (*PMP-22*)	Pes cavus, motor deficit predominates (see Chap. 363)
CMT disease type 1B	AD 1q22-23	Decades 2–3	Demyelinating	Hypertropic change with onion bulbs; marked ↓ NCV	—	Mutation in P_O gene	See Chap. 363
CMT disease type 2	AD 1p35-36 3q 7	Decades 3–5	Axonal	Marked ↓ NAP; slight ↓ NCV	—	Unknown	Genetic heterogeneity
Hereditary amyloid polyneuropathies	AD 18q11.2-12.1 9q33 11q23-24	Decades 3–6	Axonal	Small-fiber involvement; endoneurial amyloid deposition	In some families: cornea, kidneys, heart	Point mutations in transthyretin gene in most families	Dysautonomia often prominent
Hereditary sensory neuropathy type I (HSN-I)	AD Unknown	Decades 1–3	Neuronopathic	DRG neurons selectively involved	Sensorineural deafness (some families)	Unknown	Frequent distal mutilation—hands and feet
Porphyric neuropathy	AD 11q23-qter 14q	Adult life	Axonal	Neuropathy part of attacks; may be recurrent	Widespread cellular abnormality	Enzyme defects in porphyrin pathway	Acute intermittent porphyria, coproporphyria, and variegate porphyria
Hereditary liability to pressure palsy	AD 17p11.2-12	Decades 2–3	Demyelinating	Tomaculous changes in myelin	—	*PMP-22* gene deletions	Mostly ulnar, peroneal, and brachial plexus
Fabry's disease	X, R Xq21.33-22	Young males	Neuronopathic	Sensory neuronopathy, small DRG neurons	Kidney, skin, lung	Defect of α-galactosidase A	Neuropathy painful; often die of renal failure
CMT disease type 1, X-linked	D Xq13.1	Infancy to 2d decade	Demyelinating	Heterozygote females have symptoms	—	Defective gap junction protein (connexin 32)	—
Adrenomyeloneuropathy	X, R Xq28	Young males	? Axonal	Mild neuropathy, spastic paraparesis, baldness, hypogonadism	Adrenal cortex, cerebral white matter, spinal cord	Mutation in adrenoleukodystrophy (ALD) protein gene, a peroxisomal membrane transporter	See Chap. 363
Hereditary sensory neuropathy type II (HSN-II)	AR Unknown	Decades 1–3	Neuronopathic	DRG neurons selectively involved	—	Unknown	May be less severe than HSN-I
Déjerine-Sottas neuropathy, types A and B (HMSN-III)	Sporadic 1q22-23 17p11.2-12	1st decade	Demyelinating	Hypertrophic change with onion bulb formation	May be mentally retarded	*PMP-22* and P_O gene mutations	Marked nerve trunk enlargement (see Chap. 362)
CMT disease type 4A	AR 8q13-21.1	1st decade	Demyelinating	Hypomyelination; marked ↓ NCV	—	Unknown	—
Refsum's disease	AR Unknown	Decade 1 or 2	Demyelinating	Hypertropic change with onion bulb formation	Retinitis pigmentosa, ichthyosis, sensorineural deafness	Defect in α-oxidation of β-methylated fatty acids	Therapy consists of low-phytanate diet, plasmapheresis
Ataxia-telangiectasia	AR 11q22.1-22.3	Decade 1 or 2	Axonal	Neuropathy moderate	Cell nuclear aneuploidy, skin and scleral telangiectasia, cerebellar atrophy, immunopathy	Mutations in *ATM* gene	High incidence of early neoplasia (see Chap. 363)
Abetalipoproteinemia	AR Unknown	Decade 1 or 2	Neuronopathic	Large DRG neurons	Retinitis pigmentosa, acanthocytosis of red blood cells	Mutations in microsomal triglyceride transfer protein (*MTP*) gene	Proprioceptive disturbance marked; minimal small-fiber deficit (see Chap. 363)

(continued)

Table 381-3—*(continued)*

Genetically Determined Neuropathies

Genetic Disorder	Inheritance/ Gene Location	Age of Onset	Basic Process	Other Features*	Other Systems Involved	Genetic Mutation	Comment
Giant axonal neuropathy	AR Unknown	1st decade	Axonal	Massive segmented accumulation of neurofilaments in axons	Slowly progressive encephalopathy with Rosenthal fibers	Generalized disorder of 10-nm filaments	Intermediate filament masses in other cell types
Metachromatic leukodystrophy	AR 22q13.3-qter	1st decade	Demyelinating	Schwannopathy with cerebroside accumulation	Cerebral white matter disease predominates	Defect of arylsulfatase A	Infantile, juvenile, and adult-onset forms
Friedreich's ataxia	AR 9q13-21	1st decade	Axonal	Spinocerebellar and corticospinal tracts involved; also 1° sensory neuron	Cardiomyopathy (usual cause of death)	Controversial	Ataxia is both sensory and cerebellar

ABBREVIATIONS: A, autosomal; D, dominant; R, recessive; X, X chromosome; DRG, dorsal root ganglia; NAP, nerve action potential; NCV, nerve conduction velocity; CMT, Charcot-Marie-Tooth disease; HMSN, hereditary motor-sensory neuropathy; HSN, hereditary sensory neuropathy; PMP, peripheral myelin protein.

Table 381-4

Classification of Diabetic Neuropathies

Symmetric

1. Distal, primarily sensory polyneuropathy
   a. Mainly large fibers affected
   b. Mixed*
   c. Mainly small fibers affected*
2. Autonomic neuropathy
3. Chronically evolving proximal motor neuropathy*†

Asymmetric

1. Acute or subacute proximal motor neuropathy*†
2. Cranial mononeuropathy†
3. Truncal neuropathy*†
4. Entrapment neuropathy in the limbs

* Often painful.
† Recovery, partial or complete, is likely.

Acquired Demyelinating Neuropathies These disorders fall into two major groups, the acute form called Guillain-Barré syndrome and more chronic forms, usually referred to as *chronic inflammatory demyelinating polyradiculoneuropathy* (CIDP). The acquired demyelinating neuropathies account for a significant proportion of all cases of polyneuropathy and share a distinctive clinical, electrophysiologic, and pathologic pattern. The diagnosis rests on recognition of the clinical pattern and other features, including an elevated protein level in cerebrospinal fluid (CSF) not accompanied by pleocytosis, and electrophysiologic changes (marked slowing of conduction velocities, delayed late responses, prolonged distal latencies, dispersion of evoked responses, and evidence of conduction block). The course of GBS is acute and monophasic, whereas the more chronic forms pursue either a slowly progressive or a relapsing course. Cases with an intermediate course occur frequently enough to blur the distinction between GBS and CIDP.

This group of neuropathies is generally agreed to be immune-mediated, but the specific antigens involved, the crucial events of the immune response, and the reason it is activated are uncertain. Also unknown is whether GBS and CIDP share a common immunopathogenesis.

Management of CIDP involves a judicious mix of glucocorticoid therapy, plasmapheresis, administration of immunosuppressants such as azathioprine, cyclophosphamide, or cyclosporine, and administration of high-dose intravenous immunoglobulin. These powerful agents are used only if the disorder is severe enough to threaten walking.

Multifocal motor neuropathy is also a chronic acquired demyelinating neuropathy. It may mimic the lower-motor-neuron form of amyo-

Table 381-5

Sensory Neuropathies

Cause or Association	Course	Fiber Size Affected: Small	Fiber Size Affected: Large	Neuronopathy	Comment
TOXINS/DRUGS					
Cisplatin (antineoplastic)	Sub/Chr	+	+ +	+	Dose-related
Pyridoxine (vitamin, in megadose amounts)	Sub/Chr	+	+ +	+/−	Dose-related
Taxol (antineoplastic)	Acu/Sub	+ +	+	−	NGF may be protective
SYSTEMIC DISEASES					
Paraneoplastic	Sub	+	+ +	+ +	Most SCLC and breast
Sjögren's syndrome	Sub/Chr	+/−	+	+ +	Variable presentation
Dysproteinemia (mainly IgM_{κ})	Chr	+	+ +	−	Demyelinating; may bind to MAG
IDIOPATHIC					
Acute sensory neuronopathy	Acu	+/−	+ +	+ +	Poor recovery; persistent deficit
Chronic ataxic neuropathy	Chr	+/−	+ +	Prob.	Gradual progression
HEREDITARY					
Many varieties (see Table 381-3)	Chr	Variable		Some	Progressive

ABBREVIATIONS: + +, most; +, some; ±, occasionally; Prob, probable; Acu, acute; Sub, subacute; Chr, chronic; NGF, nerve growth factor; MAG, myelin-associated glycoprotein; SCLC, small cell lung carcinoma.

tropic lateral sclerosis because of its features of weakness and atrophy without sensory disturbance. In many patients it is responsive to periodic high-dose intravenous immunoglobulin treatment.

Diabetic Neuropathies The neuropathies of diabetes mellitus are classified in Table 381-4. A limitation of this classification is that most patients do not fit neatly into any single category but instead have overlapping clinical features of several. For instance, many diabetics with distal, primarily sensory polyneuropathy also can be shown to have autonomic dysfunction, usually in the form of vasomotor disturbance in the limbs and abnormalities of sweating. Similarly, patients who develop a proximal motor syndrome may have dysautonomic features (including sexual impotence in males) and some degree of distal sensory polyneuropathy. To compound matters, such patients appear at risk of developing a cranial mononeuropathy. Pain is a frequent feature of diabetic neuropathies (see Table 381-4) but is variable in incidence and degree. The term *diabetic amyotrophy* should be avoided because of its ambiguity.

Diabetic neuropathies tend to occur in the setting of long-standing hyperglycemia (decades), whether the diabetes is insulin-dependent or not. By far the most common neuropathies related to diabetes mellitus are the diffuse sensory and autonomic types (categories 1 and 2 under "Symmetric" in Table 381-4). Sensory and autonomic polyneuropathy, chronic and indolent in evolution, may first be noticed in the third or fourth decade in patients with juvenile-onset diabetes but tends to occur after age 50 in patients with adult-onset diabetes. Focal and multifocal types of neuropathy are less common but quite dramatic (categories 1, 2, and 3 under "Asymmetric" in Table 381-4). They rarely occur before the age of 45 and are usually subacute or acute in onset. Cranial mononeuropathies are isolated sixth or third nerve palsies. The latter spares the pupil in three-fourths of cases, and some local pain or headache occurs in one-half. Truncal (thoracoabdominal) neuropathy is painful, involves one or more intercostal or lumbar nerves unilaterally, and frequently coexists with the asymmetric proximal motor neuropathy. The most evident features of asymmetric proximal motor neuropathy are weakened muscles innervated by the femoral and obturator nerves (quadriceps femoris, iliopsoas, adductor magnus) and ipsilateral loss of the knee jerk reflex. Sensory deficit is minor, but pain in the hip and anterior thigh may be prominent. In all these multifocal and focal neuropathies, the pain usually subsides within weeks to a year, and function is usually partly or completely recovered. The same is true for symmetric proximal motor neuropathy (category 3 under "Symmetric" in Table 381-4).

Focal and multifocal diabetic neuropathies are considered to be ischemic in origin, and ischemia may also underlie symmetric polyneuropathies, which are thought by some to involve abnormality of nerve metabolism.

Management of diabetic neuropathies is directed toward optimal control of hyperglycemia and symptomatic pain suppression. In the long-term Diabetes Control and Complications Trial completed recently in North America, patients who controlled their diabetes meticulously showed significantly less neuropathy. The role of aldose reductase inhibitors in preventing or reversing diabetic complications, including neuropathy, remains unclear. Entrapment neuropathies are frequently amenable to surgical decompression.

Neuropathies with Dysproteinemia An association between polyneuropathy and both multiple myeloma and macroglobulinemia has been recognized for many years. In the commonly encountered type of multiple myeloma, which has either lytic or diffuse osteoporotic bone lesions, clinically overt polyneuropathy is relatively infrequent, occurring in approximately 5 percent of patients. These neuropathies are sensorimotor, may be severe, and generally do not reverse with successful suppression of the myeloma. In most cases, electrodiagnostic and pathologic features are consistent with a process of axonal degeneration.

In contrast, myeloma with osteosclerotic features, although representing only 3 percent of all myelomas, is associated with polyneuropathy in almost one-half of cases. These neuropathies, which may also occur with solitary plasmacytoma, seem to be different from those linked to the lytic type of multiple myeloma in that they (1) often

respond to radiation therapy or removal of the primary lesion, (2) are more frequently demyelinating in character, (3) are associated with different monoclonal proteins and light chains (almost all lambda as opposed to mostly kappa in the lytic type of multiple myeloma), and (4) frequently occur in association with other systemic findings. These include skin thickening, hyperpigmentation, hypertrichosis, organomegaly, endocrinopathy, anasarca, papilledema, and clubbing of fingers (POEMS syndrome: *p*olyneuropathy, *o*rganomegaly, *e*ndocrinopathy, *M* protein, and *s*kin changes). A great deal of attention has been paid to this curious syndrome in Japan, where it is more common, but the underlying mechanism remains unknown, other than the association with lambda light chains.

Benign monoclonal gammopathy with an IgM serum spike, and usually with kappa light chains, is described in association with demyelinating polyneuropathy, which often follows a protracted course and indolent progression. In about one-half of cases, the monoclonal serum protein binds to normal human peripheral myelin, specifically to myelin-associated glycoprotein. Treatment with high-dose intravenous immunoglobulin and potent immunosuppressants (chlorambucil, cyclophosphamide, or fludarabine) has been advocated.

Neuropathies with HIV Infection Neuropathies are common in infection with human immunodeficiency virus (HIV), but different types of neuropathy are seen according to the stage of the disease. GBS or CIDP are the neuropathies likely to occur following conversion to seropositivity and during the asymptomatic phase of HIV infection. Treatment is the same as for HIV-negative patients. In later, symptomatic stages, subacute to chronic mononeuritis multiplex, axonal in nature, can occur. In some cases, vasculitis of the vasa nervorum has been demonstrated.

The most common neuropathy is a distal, symmetric, mainly sensory polyneuropathy, which evolves slowly in the late symptomatic stages of HIV infection and frequently coexists with symptomatic encephalopathy and myelopathy (see Table 381-1 and Chap. 308). Improvement of this polyneuropathy with zidovudine treatment has been claimed. Also in the late stages, a severe, destructive, subacute, asymmetric polyradiculopathy involving the cauda equina may be seen; it is caused by an opportunistic infection of the nerve roots with cytomegalovirus. Ganciclovir, started early, can arrest the disorder.

Neuropathies with Lyme Disease A focal or multifocal radiculoneuropathy may occur weeks, months, or even years after primary infection by the tick-borne spirochete *Borrelia burgdorferi*. Although usually sensory and either dysesthetic or painful, the neuropathy is variable in distribution, affecting cranial nerves and spinal roots or nerves in a patchy, asymmetric fashion. Neuropathy is often chronic and persistent; CSF pleocytosis is the rule. In many, improvement occurs spontaneously, but the course is shortened by treatment with antibiotics, usually intravenous ceftriaxone (see Chap. 178).

Autonomic Neuropathy The autonomic nervous system regulates the visceral organs and vegetative functions (see Chap. 371). Many pharmacologic agents modify specific autonomic functions, but autonomic neuropathy (dysautonomia) with structural changes in pre- and postganglionic neurons can also occur. Usually autonomic neuropathy is a manifestation of a more generalized polyneuropathy also affecting somatic peripheral nervous function, as in diabetic neuropathy, GBS, and alcoholic polyneuropathy, but occasionally syndromes of pure pandysautonomia are encountered. Symptoms of dysautonomia are mainly negative (i.e., loss of function) and include postural hypotension with faintness or syncope, anhidrosis, hypothermia, bladder atony, obstipation, dry mouth and dry eyes from failure of salivary and lacrimal glands to secrete, blurring of vision from lack of pupillary and ciliary regulation, and sexual impotence in males. Positive phenomena (hyperfunction) may also occur and include episodic hypertension, diarrhea, hyperhidrosis, and either tachycardia or bradycardia. Autonomic neuropathies have many and diverse causes, and the classification is complex.

Pure Motor Neuropathy Disorder affecting any level of the motor unit—anterior horn cell, motor axon, or neuromuscular junction—can result in a purely lower motor syndrome without sensory disturbance. Distinguishing anterior horn cell disorders (motor neuronopathies) from motor axonopathies may be difficult clinically because they share manifestations (weakness, muscle denervation atrophy, hypo- or areflexia, fasciculations). Electrodiagnostic examination may also fail to localize the primary site of the lesion (neuropathic versus neuronopathic) unless the lesion is demyelinating in nature, in which case it is by definition neuropathic.

Examples of motor neuronopathies include the lower-motor form of amyotrophic lateral sclerosis, poliomyelitis, hereditary spinal muscular atrophies, and adult variant of hexosaminidase A deficiency. Motor neuropathies may be seen with lead or dapsone intoxication, occasionally with porphyria, and also with multifocal motor neuropathy. The latter is a chronic asymmetric disorder of mid-life that may be associated with high titers of antiganglioside antibodies (particularly anti-GM_1), persistent conduction block on electrodiagnostic examination, or both. Neuromuscular junction disorders (e.g., Lambert-Eaton myasthenic syndrome, tick bite paralysis, other types of toxic neuromuscular blockade) can be recognized and localized electrodiagnostically. Some motor-sensory polyneuropathies have predominant motor symptoms and signs, such as hereditary motor-sensory neuropathies, GBS, and CIDP, but the subclinical sensory component is readily demonstrated electrodiagnostically or by quantitative sensory testing.

Pure Sensory Neuropathy Clinical presentations involving primary sensation only (see Chap. 23) are not uncommon. Manifestations may (1) reflect mainly large afferent fiber involvement with deficits of vibratory and proprioceptive sense, areflexia, and sensory ataxia with or without tingling dysesthesias; (2) reflect mainly small afferent fiber involvement with numbness and cutaneous hypesthesia to pinprick and temperature stimuli, often with painful burning dysesthesias; or (3) be pansensory, with both large and small fiber manifestations. The pattern of distribution, although variable, is often distal and symmetric, particularly for large-fiber neuropathies.

The most severe and widespread of these pure sensory syndromes exhibit poor or no recovery, suggesting irreversible lesions of nerve cell bodies in dorsal root and trigeminal ganglia. These are frequently called *sensory neuronopathies*. With sensory neurotoxins, moderate doses lead to potentially reversible neuropathy, but high doses appear to cause neuronopathy (see Table 381-5).

Plexopathy This term refers to disorders of either the brachial or the lumbosacral plexus. Lesions of the brachial plexus are characterized by motor and sensory signs different from those expected in either mononeuropathies of the upper limb or polyneuropathies. The usual causes are direct trauma to the plexus, idiopathic brachial neuritis (also called *neuralgic amyotrophy*), cervical rib or band, infiltration by malignant tumor, or prior radiation therapy. When the upper parts of the brachial plexus, arising from cervical roots 5 through 7, are affected, weakness and atrophy of shoulder girdle and upper arm muscles occur. Injuries to the lower brachial plexus, arising from the eighth cervical and first thoracic roots, produce distal arm weakness, atrophy, and focal sensory deficit in the forearm and hand. In general, idiopathic brachial neuritis, irradiation with greater than 60 Gy (6000 rad), and particular types of trauma (arm jerked downward) result in damage to the upper portions of the brachial plexus. In contrast, infiltration by malignant tumor, cervical rib or band, and certain other types of trauma (arm jerked upward) cause damage to the lower brachial plexus. Lumbosacral plexopathies are less common; they may be due to idiopathic lumbosacral plexitis, retroperitoneal hemorrhage, or malignant tumor infiltration or may occur in association with long-standing diabetes mellitus.

Miscellaneous Causes of Neuropathy Ischemia of nerve severe enough to produce clinical symptoms has as its basis the widespread compromise of blood flow in the vasa nervorum. Typically, this is the result of small-vessel disease involving the vasa nervorum directly, as occurs with vasculitis, rather than large-vessel disease, such as atherosclerosis. Clinically, widespread disease of the vasa nervorum produces mononeuropathy multiplex, which electrodiagnostically has the features of a patchy axonal process.

Cold exerts direct deleterious effects on peripheral nerve, independent of ischemia. Cold injury to nerve occurs after prolonged exposure, usually of a limb, to moderately low temperatures, as with immersion of the feet in seawater; actual freezing of tissue is not required. Axonal degeneration of myelinated fibers is the pathologic expression of cold injury. Frequently, limbs affected by cold injury to nerve show sensory deficit and dysesthesias, cutaneous vasomotor instability, pain, and marked sensitivity to minimal cold exposure, which persist for many years. The pathophysiology of these phenomena is uncertain.

Trophic changes in severe neuropathy The array of observable changes in completely denervated muscle, bone, and skin, including hair and nails, is well known, if incompletely understood. It is unclear what portion of the changes is due purely to denervation versus that caused by disuse, immobility, lack of weight bearing, and particularly recurrent, unnoticed, painless trauma. Considerable evidence favors the view that ulceration of skin, poor healing, tissue resorption, neurogenic arthropathy, and mutilation are the result of repeated heedless injury to insensitive parts. This sequence of events is avoidable with proper attention to and care of the insensitive parts by both patient and physician.

RECOVERY FROM NEUROPATHY In contrast to axons in the CNS, peripheral nerve fibers have an excellent ability to regenerate under proper circumstances. The process of regeneration following axonal degeneration may take from 2 months to more than a year, depending on the severity of the neuropathy and the length of regeneration required. Whether regeneration takes place depends on whether the cause of the neuropathy has been eliminated, as by removal of a neurotoxic substance or correction of an abnormal metabolic state. A deficit secondary to demyelination may recover rapidly, since intact axons may remyelinate in just a few weeks. For example, a patient with GBS, in whom demyelination but no secondary axonal degeneration has occurred, may recover to normal strength from bedfastness and paralysis of arms and legs in as little as 3 to 4 weeks.

MONONEUROPATHY MULTIPLEX (MULTIFOCAL NEUROPATHY) This term refers to simultaneous or sequential involvement of individual noncontiguous nerve trunks, either partially or completely, evolving over days to years. Since the disease process underlying mononeuropathy multiplex involves peripheral nerves in a multifocal and random fashion, progression of the disease involves a tendency for the neurologic deficit to become less patchy and multifocal and more confluent and symmetric. Some patients present with a distal symmetric neuropathy. Attention to the pattern of early symptoms is therefore important in making the judgment that a particular neuropathy is indeed a mononeuropathy multiplex.

Once that issue is settled, the next question is whether the process is primarily axonal or demyelinating. Almost one-third of all adults with the clinical syndrome of mononeuropathy multiplex have a clear-cut picture of a demyelinating disorder, often with multiple foci of persistent conduction block found by electrodiagnostic examination. Multifocal demyelinating neuropathy represents part of the spectrum of chronic acquired demyelinating neuropathy, that is, CIDP. Management of this multifocal subgroup is the same as for CIDP (see "Acquired Demyelinating Neuropathies," above).

The remaining two-thirds of patients with mononeuropathy multiplex have a picture by electrodiagnostic examination of axonal involvement that is heterogeneously distributed. Although ischemia should be suspected as the basis of neuropathy in these patients, only about one-half can be shown to have disease, usually vasculitis, affecting the vasa nervorum. Management of those with proven vasculitis of vasa nervorum is the same as treatment for systemic vasculitis (see Chap. 319). The cause of neuropathy remains undiagnosed in the remaining patients even on follow-up. Management in this group is conservative; in many patients the disease will stabilize or reverse, at least partially.

In individuals in whom vasculitic change in vasa nervorum can be demonstrated, any of a large number of underlying disorders may be responsible. The primary vasculitides of the polyarteritis nodosa group are the most frequent basis, followed closely by the vasculitis syndrome occurring in the course of other connective tissue disorders. In descending order of frequency, the latter are rheumatoid arthritis, systemic lupus erythematosus, and mixed connective tissue disease. Other rarer causes of mononeuropathy multiplex due to nerve ischemia from occlusion of vasa nervorum include mixed cryoglobulinemia, Sjögren's syndrome, Wegener's granulomatosis, progressive systemic sclerosis, Churg-Strauss allergic granulomatosis, and hypersensitivity angiitides (Chap. 319). Management of the neuropathy in each case depends on treatment of the responsible disease.

Mononeuropathy multiplex syndrome may also be seen as a manifestation of leprosy, sarcoidosis, certain types of amyloidosis, hypereosinophilia syndrome, cryoglobulinemia, and multifocal types of diabetic neuropathy.

MONONEUROPATHY *Mononeuropathy* refers to focal involvement of a single nerve trunk and therefore implies a local cause. Direct trauma, compression, and entrapment are the usual causes. Ulnar neuropathies, due to lesions either at the ulnar groove or in the cubital tunnel, and median neuropathy due to compression in the carpal tunnel constitute the great majority of mononeuropathies encountered in clinical practice. These are described below, and other common mononeuropathies are listed in Table 381-6.

In the absence of a history of trauma to the nerve trunk, factors favoring conservative management of a mononeuropathy include sudden onset, no motor deficit, few or no sensory findings (even though pain and sensory symptoms may be present), and no evidence of axonal degeneration by electrodiagnostic criteria. Factors favoring surgical intervention include chronicity and worsening neurologic deficit on examination, particularly if motor, and electrodiagnostic evidence that the lesion has produced a degree of wallerian degeneration.

Ulnar Neuropathy Complete ulnar paralysis results in a characteristic claw-hand deformity owing to wasting and weakness of many of the small hand muscles and hyperextension of the fingers at the metacarpophalangeal joints and flexion at the interphalangeal joints. The flexion deformity is most pronounced in the fourth and fifth fingers. Sensory loss occurs over the fifth finger, the ulnar aspect of the fourth finger, and the ulnar border of the palm. The superficial location of the nerve at the elbow makes it a common site of pressure palsy. The ulnar nerve may also become entrapped just distal to the elbow in the cubital tunnel formed by the aponeurotic arch linking the two heads of the flexor carpi ulnaris. Also, prolonged pressure on the base of the palm, as occurs with use of hand tools or bicycle riding, may result in damage to the deep palmar branch of the ulnar nerve, causing weakness of the small hand muscles but no sensory loss. See also Table 381-6.

Carpal Tunnel Syndrome The median nerve in the carpal tunnel lies in close quarters with nine tendons. Entrapment of the nerve at the wrist (*carpal tunnel syndrome*) may be secondary to excessive use of the wrist, tenosynovitis with arthritis, or local infiltration, for example, by a thickening of connective tissue as in acromegaly or by deposit of amyloid or by one of the mucopolysaccharidoses. Other systemic diseases associated with an increased incidence of carpal tunnel syndrome are hypothyroidism, rheumatoid arthritis, and diabetes mellitus, but underlying diseases account for only a small fraction of all cases. The main symptoms of carpal tunnel syndrome are nocturnal paresthesia of thumb, index, and middle fingers. With worsening, numbness demonstrable by pin examination occurs in that distribution, and eventually weakness and atrophy of the abductor pollicis brevis (thenar eminence) becomes evident. Treatment of carpal tunnel syndrome is surgical section of the carpal ligament to relieve entrapment. Incomplete lesions of the median nerve between the axilla and wrist may result in causalgia (a particularly severe type of burning pain; see Chap. 12). See also Table 381-6.

Tarsal Tunnel Syndrome The distal tibial nerve, along with several tendons and the posterior tibial artery, lies in the tarsal tunnel just posterior to the medial malleolus. Because of its superficial site, the distal tibial nerve is subject to compression or to direct trauma. Causes include sprain or fracture of the ankle, ill-fitting footwear, posttraumatic fibrosis, cysts, or ganglia adjacent to the nerve, arthritis, or tenosynovitis. Symptoms characteristically are pain in the ankle and the sole of the foot with paresthesia, particularly upon walking. On examination, the tibial nerve trunk in the tarsal tunnel is usually tender to palpation, sensory deficit should be demonstrable on the sole of the foot, and weakness of the toe plantar-flexor muscles may be noted. Electrodiagnostic examination and nerve block are useful in establishing the diagnosis. Definitive treatment is extensive surgical decompression of the tibial nerve in the tarsal tunnel. Tarsal tunnel syndrome, in terms of its pathophysiology and management, is similar to carpal tunnel syndrome, but it is much less common (see also Table 381-6).

OTHER FOCAL NEUROPATHIES **Peripheral Nerve Tumors** These tumors are mostly benign and can arise on any nerve trunk or twig. Although peripheral nerve tumors can occur anywhere in the body, including the spinal roots and cauda equina, many are subcutaneous in location and present as a soft swelling, sometimes with a purplish discoloration of the skin. Two major categories of peripheral nerve tumors are recognized: neurilemmoma (schwannoma) and neurofibroma. Neurilemmomas are usually solitary and grow in the nerve sheath, rendering the tumor relatively easy to dissect free. In contrast, neurofibromas tend to be multiple, grow in the endoneurial substance, which renders them difficult to dissect, may undergo malignant changes, and are the hallmark of von Recklinghausen's neurofibromatosis (NF1). This disease is characterized by an autosomal dominant inheritance pattern, any number of neurofibromas from one to thousands, five or more café au lait–pigmented skin lesions greater than 1.5 cm in diameter (80 percent of patients), axillary freckles (93 percent of patients), an increased incidence of seizure disorder and mental retardation, and an exceptionally high rate of spontaneous mutation. The gene for NF1 is on chromosome 17, and its protein product, neurofibromin, is a large, widely expressed protein that appears to regulate the proto-oncogene *ras*.

Herpes Zoster This is a sensory neuritis due to infection with varicella-zoster virus and is characterized by acute inflammation of one or more dorsal root ganglia. Lancinating pain and hyperalgesia over the skin surface supplied by the affected roots occur for 3 to 4 days, followed by the appearance in the same segment of a herpetic eruption characterized by painful raised blisters on reddened bases. Pain usually subsides in a few weeks. If the inflammatory process spreads to involve related motor roots, segmental motor weakness and wasting appear. Paralysis of the oculomotor nerves may occur in conjunction with involvement of the ophthalmic division of the trigeminal ganglion (ophthalmoplegic zoster). Facial paralysis may occur with involvement of the geniculate ganglion and herpetic eruption on the ipsilateral tympanic membrane or external ear canal (Ramsay Hunt syndrome).

In less than 5 percent of patients, neuropathic pain persists in the dermatomal distribution of the affected ganglia. This pain, known as *postherpetic neuralgia*, is intense, burning, hyperpathic, and unrelenting; it often dominates the lives of those affected. Advancing age is a risk factor for this outcome. In some patients, blunting of the pain to tolerable levels is achieved by use of carbamazepine or a tricyclic antidepressant such as desipramine (see also Chap. 12).

Leprous Neuritis This is a major worldwide cause of neuropathy. *Mycobacterium leprae* organisms readily invade Schwann cells in cutaneous nerve twigs, particularly those associated with unmyelinated nerve fibers. *M. leprae* thrives best in the coolest tissues in the body. Two major forms of leprous neuritis are recognized, tuberculoid and lepromatous, which actually represent the ends of a spectrum of disease, the middle of which is called dimorphous leprosy (patchy and multifocal involvement of skin and nerve). The treatment of a given case depends on where it falls in this spectrum (see Chap. 172). Tuberculoid (high-resistance) leprosy consists of a single patch of hypesthetic or anesthetic skin in any location. The skin patch is frequently thickened, reddened, or hypopigmented. If a superficially placed nerve trunk, typically a cutaneous nerve, courses just beneath the area of affected skin, it may be engulfed in the inflammatory reaction, resulting in an associated mononeuropathy. Such a nerve may be palpably enlarged and beaded. Lepromatous (low-resistance) leprosy is marked by immunologic tolerance and widespread skin thickening, cutaneous anesthesia, and anhidrosis, which spare only the warmest parts of the body, notably the axilla, the groin, and beneath the scalp hair. Motor signs (focal weakness and atrophy) result from damage to mixed nerves lying close to the skin, particularly the median, ulnar, peroneal, and facial nerves.

Bell's Palsy This seventh nerve palsy is due to inflammation of the facial nerve in the facial canal, the basis for which remains obscure. Edema may play a part in causing compression of nerve fibers, with resulting acute unilateral paralysis of facial muscles (see Chap. 372).

Sarcoidosis This may involve single or multiple peripheral nerves, producing asymmetric mononeuritis or polyneuritis. Unilateral or bilateral facial paralysis is described in association with parotitis and uveitis (Heerfordt's syndrome).

Table 381-6

Some Common Mononeuropathies

Nerve	Origin (Spinal Segments)	Muscles Innervated	Usual Site of Lesion	Clinical Features	Comments
UPPER EXTREMITY					
Suprascapular	C5, C6	Supraspinatus Infraspinatus	Suprascapular notch of scapula	Weakness of lateral rotation of the humerus	No sensory deficit
Long thoracic	C5–C7	Serratus anterior	Variable	Winging of scapula	No sensory deficit
Axillary	C5, C6	Deltoid, teres minor	Near shoulder joint	Weakness of shoulder abduction; atrophy of shoulder	Sensory deficit similar to C5 dorsal root lesion (see Figs. 23-2 and 23-3)
Radial	C5–T1	Triceps, brachioradialis, wrist, finger, and thumb extensors	Spiral groove of humerus	Wrist drop most obvious, also finger and thumb extensors paralyzed	Saturday night palsy (acute compression) is frequent cause
Posterior interosseous branch	C7, C8	Finger and thumb extensors	Edge of supinator muscle below elbow	Finger drop; wrist relatively spared	No sensory deficit
Ulnar	C8, T1	Ulnar flexor of the wrist, long flexors of 4th and 5th digits, and most intrinsic hand muscles	Ulnar groove at the elbow	Weakness of finger adduction and abduction and thumb adduction (see text); interosseous atrophy, claw-hand	May be acute or insidious; sensory symptoms/signs are distinctive (Figs. 23-2 and 23-3); see also text
			Cubital tunnel	Same as above	Often pain over medial proximal forearm (cubital tunnel)
			Medial base of palm	Intrinsic hand muscles only, interosseous atrophy	No sensory deficit
Median	C6–T1	Abductor pollicis brevis; more proximal muscles include forearm pronator, long finger and thumb flexors	Carpal tunnel	Characteristic sensory symptoms and deficit and inability to make a circle with thumb and index finger	Sensory deficit as per Figs. 23-2 and 23-3 (see text); known as carpal tunnel syndrome
Anterior interosseous branch	C7–T1	Long flexors of thumb and index and middle fingers	Anterior interosseus branch below the elbow	Weakness of pinch; pain in volar forearm	No sensory deficit
LOWER EXTREMITY					
Femoral	L2–L4	Iliopsoas (hip flexor) and quadriceps femoris (knee extensor)	Proximal to inguinal ligament	Knee buckling; absent knee jerk; weak anterior thigh muscles with atrophy	Association with diabetes mellitus; sensory disturbance as per Fig. 23-2
Lateral femoral cutaneous branch	L2, L3	None	Inguinal ligament	Dysesthetic hyperpathia of lateral thigh	Known as meralgia paresthetica
Obturator	L3, L4	Thigh adductors	Intrapelvic or at pubis	Weakness of hip adduction	Sensory deficit on medial thigh
Sciatic	L4–S3	Hamstring muscles, hip abductor, and all muscles below the knee	Near sciatic notch	Severe lower leg and hamstring weakness; flail foot; severe disability	Uncommon except from war wounds
Posterior tibial	L5–S2	Calf muscles (proximally), toe flexors and other intrinsic foot muscles	Tarsal tunnel, near medial malleolus	Pain and numbness of sole, weak toe flexors	Known as tarsal tunnel syndrome
Peroneal	L4–S1	Dorsiflexors of toes and foot, evertors of foot	At neck of fibula	Foot drop and weakness of foot eversion	Sensory deficit is similar in distribution to L5, S1 sensory roots

Polyneuritis Cranialis This is a relapsing and remitting mononeuropathy multiplex restricted to cranial nerves (see Chap. 372). It is usually associated with indolent tuberculous cervical adenitis (scrofula) or sarcoidosis. Treatment of the underlying condition will halt the cranial nerve palsies.

BIBLIOGRAPHY

ASBURY AK: New aspects of disease of the peripheral nervous system, in *Harrison's Textbook of Internal Medicine, Update IV.* New York, McGraw-Hill, 1983, pp 211–229

———, THOMAS PK: *Peripheral Nerve Disorders*, 2d ed. Oxford, Butterworth-Heinemann, 1995

BOLTON CF: The changing concepts of Guillain-Barré syndrome. N Engl J Med 333:1415, 1995

CHANCE PF, FISCHBECK KH: Molecular genetics of Charcot-Marie-Tooth disease and related neuropathies. Hum Mol Genet 3:1503, 1994

DAWSON DM et al: *Entrapment Neuropathies*, 2d ed. Boston, Little, Brown, 1991

DIABETES CONTROL AND COMPLICATIONS TRIAL RESEARCH GROUP: The effect of intensive treatment of diabetes on the development and progression of long-term complications in insulin-dependent diabetes mellitus. N Engl J Med 329:977, 1993

DYCK PJ et al (eds): *Diabetic Neuropathy*. Philadelphia, Saunders, 1987

———: *Peripheral Neuropathy*, 3d ed. Philadelphia, Saunders, 1992

GRIFFIN JW et al: Guillain-Barré syndrome in Northern China. The spectrum of neuropathological changes in clinically defined cases. Brain 118:577, 1995

LAYZER RB: *Neuromuscular Manifestations of Systemic Disease*, vol 25: *Contemporary Neurology Series.* Philadelphia, Davis, 1984

MAX MB et al: Effects of desipramine, amitriptyline, and fluoxetine on pain in diabetic neuropathy. N Engl J Med 326:1250, 1992

REES JH et al: *Campylobacter jejuni* infection and Guillain-Barré syndrome. N Engl J Med 333:1374, 1995

ROPPER AH et al: *Guillain Barré Syndrome*. Philadelphia, FA Davis, 1991

STEWART JD: *Focal Peripheral Neuropathies*. 2d ed. New York, Raven Press, 1993

SUTER U, SNIPES GJ: Biology and genetics of hereditary motor and sensory neuropathies. Annu Rev Neurosci 18:45, 1995

382

Daniel B. Drachman

MYASTHENIA GRAVIS AND OTHER DISEASES OF THE NEUROMUSCULAR JUNCTION

Myasthenia gravis (MG) is a neuromuscular disorder characterized by weakness and fatigability of skeletal muscles. The underlying defect is a decrease in the number of available acetylcholine receptors (AChRs) at neuromuscular junctions due to an antibody-mediated autoimmune attack. Treatment now available for MG is highly effective, although a specific cure has remained elusive.

PATHOPHYSIOLOGY In the neuromuscular junction (Fig. 382-1), acetylcholine (ACh) is synthesized in the motor nerve terminal and stored in vesicles (quanta). When an action potential travels down a motor nerve and reaches the nerve terminal, ACh from 150 to 200 vesicles is released and combines with AChRs that are densely packed at the peaks of postsynaptic folds. Channels in the AChRs open, permitting the rapid entry of cations, chiefly sodium, which produces depolarization at the end-plate region of the muscle fiber. If the depolarization is sufficiently large, it initiates an action potential that is propagated along the muscle fiber, triggering muscle contraction. This process is rapidly terminated by hydrolysis of ACh by acetylcholinesterase (AChE) and by diffusion of ACh away from the receptor.

In MG, the fundamental defect is a decrease in the number of available AChRs at the postsynaptic muscle membrane. In addition, the postsynaptic folds are flattened, or "simplified." These changes result in decreased efficiency of neuromuscular transmission. Therefore, although ACh is released normally, it produces small end-plate potentials which may fail to trigger muscle action potentials. Failure of transmission at many neuromuscular junctions results in weakness of muscle contraction.

The amount of ACh released per impulse *normally* declines on repeated activity (termed *presynaptic rundown*). In the myasthenic patient, the decreased efficiency of neuromuscular transmission combined with the normal rundown results in the activation of fewer and fewer muscle fibers by successive nerve impulses and hence increasing weakness, or *myasthenic fatigue*. This mechanism also accounts for the decremental response to repetitive nerve stimulation seen on electrodiagnostic testing.

The neuromuscular abnormalities in MG are brought about by an autoimmune response mediated by specific anti-AChR antibodies. The anti-AChR antibodies reduce the number of available AChRs at neuromuscular junctions by three distinct mechanisms: (1) accelerated turnover of AChRs by a mechanism involving cross-linking and rapid endocytosis of the receptors; (2) blockade of the active site of the AChR, i.e., the site that normally binds ACh; and (3) damage to the postsynaptic muscle membrane by the antibody in collaboration with complement.

How the autoimmune response is initiated and maintained in MG is not completely understood. However, the thymus appears to play a role in this process. The thymus is abnormal in approximately 75 percent of patients with MG; in about 65 percent the thymus is "hyperplastic," with the presence of active germinal centers, while 10 percent of patients have thymic tumors (thymomas). Muscle-like cells within the thymus (myoid cells), which bear AChRs on their surface, may serve as a source of autoantigen and trigger the autoimmune reaction within the thymus gland.

CLINICAL FEATURES Myasthenia gravis is not rare, having a prevalence of at least 1 in 7500. It affects individuals in all age groups, but peaks of incidence occur in women in their twenties and thirties and in men in their fifties and sixties. Overall, women are affected more frequently than men, in a ratio of approximately 3:2. The cardinal features are *weakness* and *fatigability* of muscles. The weakness increases during repeated use (fatigue) and may improve following rest or sleep. The course of MG is often variable. Exacerbations and remissions may occur, particularly during the first few years after the onset of the disease. Remissions are rarely complete or permanent. Unrelated infections or systemic disorders often lead to increased myasthenic weakness and may precipitate "crisis" (see below).

The distribution of muscle weakness has a characteristic pattern. The cranial muscles, particularly the lids and extraocular muscles, are often involved early, and diplopia and ptosis are common initial complaints. Facial weakness produces a "snarling" expression when the patient attempts to smile. Weakness in chewing is most noticeable after prolonged effort, as in chewing meat. Speech may have a nasal timbre caused by weakness of the palate or a dysarthric "mushy" quality due to tongue weakness. Difficulty in swallowing may occur as a result of weakness of the palate, tongue, or pharynx, giving rise to nasal regurgitation or aspiration of liquids or food. In approximately 85 percent of patients, the weakness becomes generalized, affecting the limb muscles as well. The limb weakness in MG is often proximal and may be asymmetric. Despite the muscle weakness, deep tendon reflexes are preserved. If weakness of respiration becomes so severe as to require respiratory assistance, the patient is said to be in *crisis*.

DIAGNOSIS AND EVALUATION (Table 382-1) The diagnosis is suspected on the basis of weakness and fatigability in the typical distribution described above, without loss of reflexes or impairment of sensation or other neurologic function. The suspected diagnosis should always be confirmed definitively before treatment is undertaken; this is essential because (1) other treatable conditions may closely resemble MG and (2) the treatment of MG may involve surgery and the prolonged use of drugs with adverse side effects.

Anticholinesterase Test Drugs that inhibit the enzyme AChE allow ACh to interact repeatedly with the limited number of AChRs, producing improvement in the strength of myasthenic muscles. Edrophonium is used most commonly, because of the rapid onset (30 s) and short duration (about 5 min) of its effect. An objective end-point must be selected to evaluate the effect of edrophonium. The examiner should focus on one or more unequivocally weak muscle groups and evaluate their strength objectively. For example, weakness of extraocular muscles, impairment of speech, or the length of time that the patient can maintain the arms in forward abduction may be useful measures. An initial dose of 2 mg of edrophonium is given intravenously. If definite improvement occurs, the test is considered positive and is terminated. If there is no change, the patient is given an additional 8 mg intravenously. The dose is administered in two parts because some patients react to edrophonium with unpleasant side effects such as nausea, diarrhea, salivation, fasciculations, and rarely syncope. Atropine (0.6 mg) should be at hand for intravenous administration if these symptoms become troublesome.

False-positive tests occur in occasional patients with other neurologic disorders, such as amyotrophic lateral sclerosis, and in placebo-reactors. False-negative or equivocal tests also may occur. In some cases it is helpful to use a longer-acting drug such as neostigmine (15 mg given orally), since this permits more time for detailed evaluation of strength. In virtually all instances, it is desirable to carry out further testing to establish the diagnosis of MG definitively.

Electrodiagnostic Testing *Repetitive nerve stimulation* often provides helpful diagnostic evidence of MG. Anticholinesterase medication is stopped 6 to 24 h before testing. It is best to test weak muscles or proximal muscle groups. Electric shocks are delivered at a rate of two or three per second to the appropriate nerves, and action potentials are recorded from the muscles. In normal individuals, the amplitude of the evoked muscle action potentials does not change at these rates of stimulation. However, in myasthenic patients there is a rapid reduction in the amplitude of the evoked responses of more than 10 to 15 percent. As a further test, a single dose of edrophonium may be given to prevent or diminish this decremental reaction.

Antiacetylcholine Receptor Antibody As noted above, anti-AChR antibodies are detectable in the serum of approximately 80 percent of all myasthenic patients, but in only about 50 percent of patients with weakness confined to the ocular muscles. The presence of anti-AChR antibodies is virtually diagnostic of MG, but a negative test does not exclude the disease. The measured level of anti-AChR antibody does not correspond well with the severity of MG in different patients. However, in an individual patient, a treatment-induced fall in the antibody level often correlates with clinical improvement.

Table 382-1

Diagnosis of Myasthenia Gravis

History
Diplopia, ptosis, weakness
Weakness in characteristic distribution
Fluctuation and fatigue: worse with repeated activity, improved by rest
Effects of previous treatments
Physical examination
Ptosis, diplopia
Motor power survey: quantitative testing of muscle strength
Forward arm abduction time (5 min)
Vital capacity
Absence of other neurologic signs
Laboratory testing
Anti-AChR radioimmunoassay: ~90% positive in generalized MG; 50% in ocular MG; definite diagnosis if positive; negative result does not exclude MG
Edrophonium chloride (Tensilon) 2 mg + 8 mg IV; highly probable diagnosis if *unequivocally* positive
Repetitive nerve stimulation; decrement of >15% at 3 Hz: highly probable
Single-fiber electromyography: blocking and jitter, with normal fiber density; confirmatory, but not specific
For ocular or cranial MG: exclude intracranial lesions by CT or MRI

SOURCE: From Drachman.

Differential Diagnosis Other conditions that cause weakness of the cranial and/or somatic musculature include drug-induced myasthenia, Lambert-Eaton myasthenic syndrome (LEMS), neurasthenia, hyperthyroidism, botulism, intracranial mass lesions, and progressive external ophthalmoplegia. Treatment with *penicillamine* (used for scleroderma or rheumatoid arthritis) may result in true MG, but the weakness is usually mild, and recovery occurs within weeks or months after discontinuing its use. *Aminoglycoside antibiotics* in very large doses and *procainamide* can cause neuromuscular weakness in normal individuals or exacerbation of weakness in myasthenic patients.

The *Lambert-Eaton myasthenic syndrome* is a presynaptic disorder of the neuromuscular junction that can cause weakness similar to that of MG. The proximal muscles of the lower limbs are most commonly affected, but other muscles may be involved as well. Cranial nerve findings, including ptosis of the eyelids and diplopia, occur in up to 70 percent of patients and resemble features of MG. However, the two conditions are readily distinguished, since patients with Lambert-Eaton syndrome have depressed or absent reflexes, show autonomic changes such as dry mouth and impotence, and show incremental responses on repetitive nerve stimulation. It is now known that Lambert-Eaton syndrome is caused by autoantibodies directed against P/Q type calcium channels at the motor nerve terminals, resulting in impaired release of ACh, which can be detected in approximately 85 percent of LEMS patients. A majority of patients with this syndrome have an associated malignancy, most commonly small cell carcinoma of the lung, which is thought to trigger the autoimmune response. The diagnosis of Lambert-Eaton syndrome may signal the presence of the tumor long before it would otherwise be detected, permitting early removal. Treatment of the neuromuscular disorder involves plasmapheresis and immunosuppression, as for MG.

Neurasthenia may present with weakness and fatigue, but muscle testing usually reveals the "jerky release" characteristic of nonorganic disorders, and the complaint of fatigue in these patients means tiredness or apathy rather than decreasing muscle power on repeated effort. *Hyperthyroidism* is readily diagnosed or excluded by tests of thyroid function, which should be carried out routinely in patients with suspected MG. Abnormalities of thyroid function (hyper- or

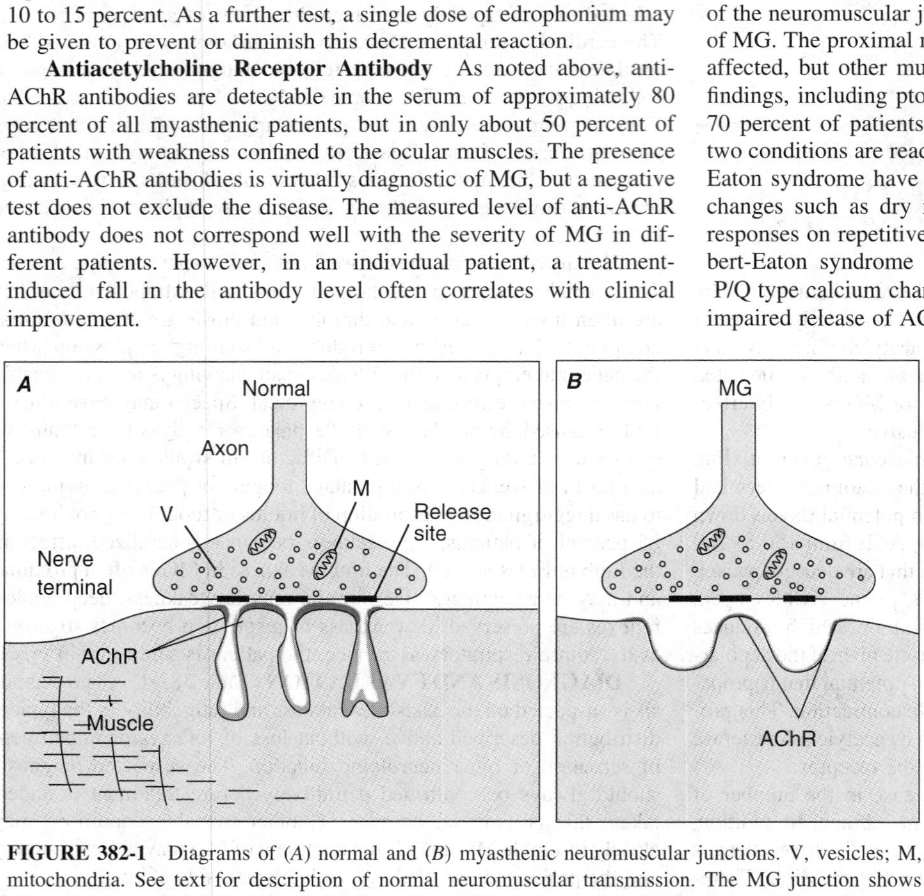

FIGURE 382-1 Diagrams of (*A*) normal and (*B*) myasthenic neuromuscular junctions. V, vesicles; M, mitochondria. See text for description of normal neuromuscular transmission. The MG junction shows reduced number of AChRs (stippling); flattened, simplified postsynaptic folds; a widened synaptic space; and a normal nerve terminal.

hypothyroidism) may increase myasthenic weakness. *Botulism* can cause myasthenic-like weakness, but the pupils are often dilated, and repetitive nerve stimulation gives an *incremental* rather than decremental response. Diplopia that mimics the symptoms of MG may occasionally be due to an *intracranial mass lesion* that compresses nerves to the extraocular muscles (e.g., sphenoid ridge meningioma), but magnetic resonance imaging (MRI) of the head and orbits usually reveals the lesion.

Progressive external ophthalmoplegia is a rare condition resulting in weakness of the extraocular muscles, which may be accompanied by weakness of the proximal muscles of the limbs, and a variety of other systemic features that are beyond the scope of this chapter. Most patients with this condition have mitochondrial disorders that can be detected on muscle biopsy (see Chap. 383).

Search for Associated Conditions (Table 382-2) Myasthenic patients have an increased incidence of several associated disorders. *Thymic abnormalities* occur in approximately 75 percent of patients, as noted above. Neoplastic change (thymoma) may produce enlargement of the thymus, which is detected by computed tomography (CT) or MRI scanning of the anterior mediastinum. Enlargement of the thymus in a patient over 40 years of age is highly suspicious of thymoma. *Hyperthyroidism* occurs in 3 to 8 percent of patients and may aggravate the myasthenic weakness. Tests of thyroid function should be obtained. Because of the *association of MG with other autoimmune disorders*, blood tests for rheumatoid factor and antinuclear antibodies should be carried out in all patients. Chronic infection of any kind can exacerbate MG and should be sought carefully. Finally, measurements of *ventilatory function* are valuable because of the frequency and seriousness of respiratory impairment in myasthenic patients.

Because of the side effects of glucocorticoids and other immunosuppressive agents used in the treatment of MG, a thorough medical investigation should be made, searching specifically for evidence of chronic or latent infection (such as tuberculosis or hepatitis), hypertension, diabetes, renal impairment, and glaucoma.

MEDICAL AND SURGICAL THERAPY (Fig. 382-2) The prognosis has improved strikingly as a result of advances in treatment; virtually all myasthenic patients can be returned to full productive lives with proper therapy. The most important methods used in the treatment of MG include anticholinesterase medications, immunosuppressive agents, thymectomy, and plasmapheresis or intravenous immunoglobulin.

Table 382-2

Disorders Associated with Myasthenia Gravis and Recommended Laboratory Tests

Associated disorders
- *Disorders of the thymus:* thymoma, hyperplasia
- *Other autoimmune disorders:* thyroiditis, Graves' disease, rheumatoid arthritis, lupus erythematosus, skin disorders, family history of autoimmune disorder
- *Disorders or circumstances that may exacerbate myasthenia gravis:* hyperthyroidism or hypothyroidism, occult infection, medical treatment for other conditions (aminoglycoside antibiotics, quinine, antiarrhythmic agents)
- *Disorders that may interfere with therapy:* tuberculosis, diabetes, peptic ulcer, gastrointestinal bleeding, renal disease, hypertension, asthma, osteoporosis

Recommended laboratory tests or procedures
- MRI or CT of mediastinum
- Tests for lupus erythematosus, antinuclear antibody, rheumatoid factor, antithyroid antibodies
- Thyroid-function tests
- Tuberculin test
- Chest radiography
- Fasting blood glucose measurement
- Pulmonary-function tests
- Bone densitometry in older patients

SOURCE: From RT Johnson, JW Griffin (eds): *Current Therapy in Neurologic Disease*, 4th ed. St. Louis, Mosby Year Book, 1993, p 379.

Anticholinesterase Medications Anticholinesterase medication produces at least partial improvement in most myasthenic patients, although improvement is complete in only a few. There is no substantial difference in efficacy among the various anticholinesterase drugs; oral pyridostigmine is the one most widely used in the United States. As a rule, the beneficial action of oral pyridostigmine begins within 15 to 30 min and lasts for 3 to 4 h, but individual responses vary. Treatment is begun with a moderate dose, e.g., 60 mg three to five times daily. The frequency and amount of the dose should be tailored to the patient's individual requirements throughout the day. For example, patients with weakness in chewing and swallowing may benefit by taking the medication before meals so that peak strength coincides with mealtime. Long-acting pyridostigmine tablets may help to get the patient through the night but should never be used for daytime medication because of their variable absorption. The maximum useful dose of pyridostigmine rarely exceeds 120 mg every 3 h during daytime. Overdosage with anticholinesterase medication may cause increased weakness and other side effects. In some patients, muscarinic side effects of the anticholinesterase medication (diarrhea, abdominal cramps, salivation, nausea) may limit the dose tolerated. In these cases,

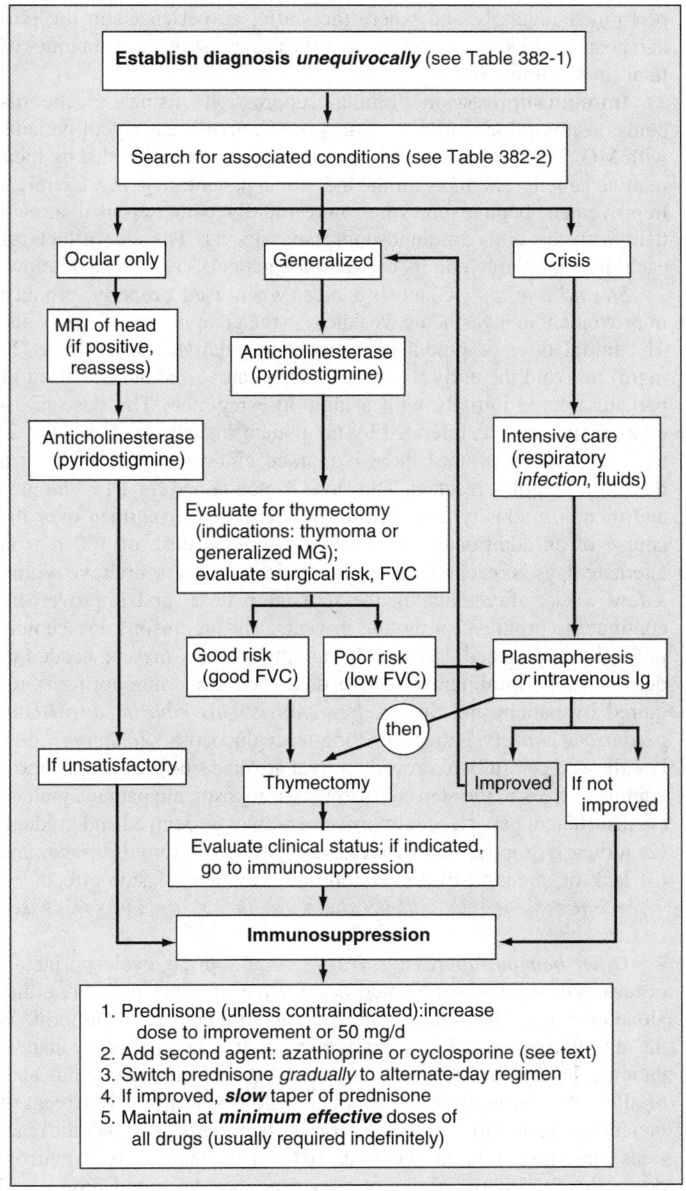

FIGURE 382-2 Algorithm for the management of myasthenia gravis. FVC, forced vital capacity.

propantheline bromide may be used to block the autonomic side effects without altering the beneficial effects on skeletal muscle. Loperamide is useful for the treatment of diarrhea.

Thymectomy Two separate issues should be distinguished: surgical removal of thymoma, and thymectomy as a treatment for myasthenia gravis. Surgical removal of a thymoma is necessary because of the possibility of local tumor spread, although most thymomas are benign. In the absence of a tumor, the available evidence suggests that up to 85 percent of patients experience improvement after thymectomy, and, of these, about 35 percent achieve drug-free remission. However, the improvement is typically delayed for months to years. The advantage of thymectomy is that it offers the possibility of long-term benefit, in some cases diminishing or eliminating the need for continuing medical treatment. In view of these potential benefits and of the negligible risk in skilled hands, thymectomy has gained widespread acceptance in the treatment of MG. It is the consensus that thymectomy should be carried out in all patients with generalized MG between the ages of puberty and at least 55 years. Whether thymectomy should be recommended in children, in adults over 55 years of age, and in patients with weakness limited to the ocular muscles is still a matter of debate. Thymectomy must be carried out in a hospital where it is performed regularly and where the staff is experienced in the pre- and postoperative management, anesthesia, and surgical techniques of total thymectomy.

Immunosuppression Immunosuppression using glucocorticoids, azathioprine, and other drugs is effective in nearly all patients with MG. The choice of which drugs to use should be guided by their relative benefits and risks for the individual patient. In general, clinical improvement begins somewhat more rapidly with steroid treatment than with the other immunosuppressive agents. The side effects of each drug may preclude its use in some patients, as indicated below.

Steroid therapy Glucocorticoids, when used properly, produce improvement in myasthenic weakness in the great majority of patients. The initial dose of prednisone should be relatively low (15 to 25 mg/d) to avoid the early weakening that occurs in about one-third of patients treated initially with a high-dose regimen. The dose is increased stepwise, as tolerated by the patient (usually by 5 mg/d at 2- to 3-day intervals), until there is marked clinical improvement or a dose of 50 mg/d is reached. This dose is maintained for 1 to 3 months and then is gradually modified to an alternate-day regimen over the course of an additional 1 to 2 months, until a dose of 100 mg on alternate days is reached. Generally, patients begin to improve within a few weeks after reaching the maximum dose, and improvement continues to progress for months or years. The prednisone dosage may gradually be reduced, but usually months or years may be needed to determine the minimum effective dose, and close monitoring is required by patient and doctor. *Few patients are able to do without prednisone entirely*. Patients on long-term glucocorticoid therapy must be followed carefully to prevent or treat adverse side effects. The most common errors in the steroid treatment of myasthenic patients include (1) insufficient persistence; improvement may be delayed and gradual; (2) too early, too rapid, or excessive tapering of steroid dosage; and (3) lack of attention to prevention and treatment of side effects. → ***The management of patients treated with glucocorticoids is discussed in Chap. 332.***

Other immunosuppressive drugs Azathioprine, cyclosporine, or occasionally cyclophosphamide is effective in many patients, either alone or in combination with glucocorticoid therapy. Azathioprine is the most widely used of these drugs because of its relative safety in most patients. Its therapeutic effect may add to that of glucocorticoids and/or allow the steroid dose to be reduced. However, up to 10 percent of patients are unable to tolerate azathioprine because of idiosyncratic reactions consisting of flulike symptoms of fever and malaise, bone marrow depression, or abnormalities of liver function. An initial dose of 50 mg/d should be used to test for adverse side effects. If this dose is tolerated, it is increased gradually until the white blood count falls to approximately 3000/μL. In patients who are receiving steroids concurrently, leukocytosis precludes the use of this measure. A reduction of the lymphocyte count below 1000/μL and/or an increase of the mean corpuscular volume may be used as indications of adequacy of azathioprine dosage. The typical dosage range is 2 to 3 mg/kg total body weight (including fat in obese patients). The beneficial effect of azathioprine takes at least 3 to 6 months to begin and even longer to peak.

Cyclosporine is approximately as effective as azathioprine and is being used increasingly in the management of MG. Its beneficial effect appears more rapidly than that of azathioprine. It may be used alone but usually is used as an adjunct to steroids, to permit reduction of the steroid dose. The usual dose of cyclosporine is 4 to 5 mg/kg per day, given in two divided doses (to minimize side effects). Side effects of cyclosporine include hypertension and nephrotoxicity, which must be closely monitored. "Trough" blood levels of cyclosporine are measured 12 h after the evening dose. The therapeutic range, as measured by radioimmunoassay, is 150 to 200 ng/L. Cyclophosphamide is reserved for patients refractory to the other drugs, because of its relatively high risk of adverse side effects, including late development of malignancies.

Plasmapheresis and Intravenous Immunoglobulin Administration In view of the antibody-mediated pathogenesis of MG, plasmapheresis has been used therapeutically. The plasma, which contains the pathogenic antibodies, is mechanically separated from the blood cells, which are returned to the patient. Plasmapheresis produces a short-term reduction in anti-AChR antibodies, with clinical improvement in many patients. It is useful as a temporary expedient in seriously affected patients or to improve the patient's condition prior to surgery (e.g., thymectomy).

The indications for the use of intravenous immunoglobulin are the same as those for plasma exchange: to produce rapid improvement to help the patient through a difficult period of myasthenic weakness, or prior to surgery. This treatment has the advantages of not requiring special equipment or large-bore venous access. The usual dose is 400 mg/kg per day for five successive days (total dose = 2 g/kg). Improvement occurs in about 70 percent of patients, beginning about 4 to 5 days after treatment and continuing for weeks to months. The mechanism of action of intravenous immunoglobulin is not known; the treatment has no consistent effect on the measurable amount of circulating AChR antibody. Adverse reactions are uncommon, but include headache, fluid overload, and rarely renal shutdown.

The long-term treatment of myasthenic patients requires other methods of therapy outlined earlier in this chapter.

Management of Myasthenic Crisis Myasthenic crisis is defined as an exacerbation of weakness sufficient to endanger life; usually it consists of respiratory failure caused by diaphragmatic and intercostal muscle weakness. Treatment should be carried out in an intensive care unit staffed with physicians experienced in the management of myasthenia gravis, respiratory insufficiency, infectious disease, and fluid and electrolyte therapy. The possibility that the deterioration could be due to excessive anticholinesterase medication ("cholinergic crisis") is best excluded by temporarily stopping anticholinesterase drugs. The most common cause of crisis is intercurrent infection. This should be treated *immediately*, because the mechanical and immunologic defenses of the patient can be assumed to be compromised. The myasthenic patient with fever and early infection should be treated like other immunocompromised patients. Early and effective antibiotic therapy, respiratory assistance, and pulmonary physiotherapy are essentials of the treatment program. As discussed above, plasmapheresis is frequently helpful in hastening recovery.

BIBLIOGRAPHY

Drachman DB: Myasthenia gravis; medical progress. N Engl J Med 330:1797, 1994

Gajdos P: Intravenous immune globulin in myasthenia gravis. Clin Exp Immunol 197:49, 1994

Lennon V: Serologic diagnosis of myasthenia gravis and the Lambert Eaton myasthenic syndrome, in *Handbook of Myasthenia Gravis and Myasthenic Syndromes*, RP Lisak (ed). New York, Marcel Dekker, 1994, p 149

Sanders DB: *Myasthenia Gravis and Myasthenic Syndromes*. Philadelphia, Saunders, 1994

383 DISEASES OF MUSCLE

Jerry R. Mendell, Robert C. Griggs, Louis J. Ptáček

The muscle disorders discussed in this chapter include diseases that cause acute, subacute, or chronic muscle weakness. Some cause pain in addition to or instead of weakness. → *Dermatomyositis and polymyositis are discussed in Chap. 315.*

HEREDITARY MYOPATHIES

Muscular dystrophy refers to a group of hereditary progressive diseases. Each type of muscular dystrophy has unique phenotypic and genetic features (Table 383-1).

DUCHENNE MUSCULAR DYSTROPHY This X-linked recessive disorder, sometimes also called *pseudohypertrophic muscular dystrophy*, occurs with an incidence of about 30 per 100,000 liveborn males.

Clinical Features Duchenne dystrophy is present at birth, but the disorder usually becomes apparent between ages 3 and 5. The boys fall frequently and have difficulty keeping up with their friends when playing. Running, jumping, and hopping are invariably abnormal. By age 5, muscle weakness is obvious by muscle testing. On getting up from the floor, the patient uses his hands to climb up himself (Gowers' maneuver). In younger children, the calf muscles are usually enlarged from true muscle hypertrophy; later calf enlargement is appropriately called *pseudohypertrophy* since muscle is replaced by fat and connective tissue. Contractures of the heel cords and iliotibial bands become apparent by age 6, when toe walking is associated with a lordotic posture. Loss of muscle strength is progressive, with predilection for proximal limb muscles and the neck flexors; leg involvement is more severe than arm involvement. Between ages 8 and 10 walking may require the use of braces; joint contractures and limitations of hip flexion, knee, elbow, and wrist extension are made worse by prolonged sitting. By age 12, most patients are confined to a wheelchair. Contractures become fixed, and a progressive scoliosis often develops which may be associated with pain. The chest deformity associated with scoliosis impairs pulmonary function, which is already diminished by muscle weakness. By age 16 to 18, patients are predisposed to serious, sometimes fatal pulmonary infections. Other causes of death include aspiration of food and acute gastric dilation.

A cardiac cause of death is uncommon despite the presence of a cardiomyopathy in almost all patients. Congestive heart failure seldom occurs except with severe stress such as pneumonia. Cardiac arrhythmias are rare. The typical electrocardiogram (ECG) shows an increase net RS in lead V_1; deep, narrow Q waves in the precordial leads; and RSR′ or polyphyasic R waves in V_1. Intellectual impairment in Duchenne dystrophy is common; the average intelligence quotient (IQ) is approximately one standard deviation below the mean. Impairment of intellectual function appears to be nonprogressive and affects verbal ability more than performance. IQs of Duchenne patients are lower than those of children with comparably disabling and chronic disorders, indicating that the mental subnormality in Duchenne dystrophy is not solely a reflection of physical limitations. The basis for intellectual impairment in Duchenne dystrophy has not been established.

Laboratory Investigation Serum creatine phosphokinase (CK) levels are invariably elevated to between 20 and 100 times normal. The levels are abnormal at birth but decline late in the disease because of inactivity and loss of muscle mass. Electromyography (EMG) demonstrates features typical of myopathy. The muscle biopsy shows muscle fibers of varying size as well as small groups of necrotic and regenerating fibers. Connective tissue and fat replace lost muscle fibers.

Table 383-1

Progressive Muscular Dystrophies

Type of Muscular Dystrophy	Genetics	Clinical Features	Other Organ System Involvement
Duchenne	X-linked recessive; mutation of dystrophin gene	Onset before age 5 Progressive weakness of girdle muscles Inability to walk after age 12 Kyphoscoliosis Respiratory failure in 2d or 3d decade	Cardiomyopathy Mental impairment
Becker	X-linked recessive; mutation of dystrophin gene	Onset in early to late childhood Progressive weakness of girdle muscles Still able to walk at age 15 Respiratory failure after 4th decade	Cardiomyopathy
Limb-girdle (see Table 383-2)	Autosomal recessive; includes several disorders with linkage to chromosomes 2p, 4q, 5q, 13q, 17q, 15q; *also* Autosomal dominant; includes more than one disorder; one form maps to chromosome 5q	Onset in early childhood Slowly progressive weakness of shoulder and hip girdle muscles	Cardiomyopathy
Congenital	Autosomal recessive; includes disorders with linkage to chromosomes 6q and 9q	Onset at birth or in the first few months Hypotonia, contractures, delayed motor milestones Progression to respiratory failure in some; static course in others	Central nervous system abnormalities (hypomyelination and malformations) Eye abnormalities
Myotonic	Autosomal dominant; expansion of unstable triplet repeat at chromosome 19q13.3	Onset usually in 2d decade (but in infancy if born to affected mother) Slowly progressive weakness of eyelids, face, neck, distal limb muscles Myotonia	Cardiac conduction defects Mental impairment Cataracts Frontal baldness Gonadal atrophy Hypertension Deafness
Facioscapulohumeral	Autosomal dominant; maps to chromosome 14q	Onset before age 20 Slowly progressive weakness of face, shoulder girdle, foot dorsiflexion	Hypertension Deafness Coats' (eye) diseaes
Oculopharyngeal	Autosomal dominant; maps to chromosome 14q	Onset in 5th to 6th decade Slowly progressive weakness of extraocular, pharyngeal, and limb muscles	—

A definitive diagnosis of Duchenne dystrophy can be established on the basis of dystrophin deficiency in biopsied muscle tissue or mutation analysis on peripheral blood leukocytes as discussed below.

Genetics Duchenne dystrophy is caused by a mutation of the gene responsible for producing dystrophin. The latter is a 427-kDa protein localized to the inner surface of the sarcolemma of the muscle fiber. The dystrophin gene, estimated at 2000 kb in size, is one of the largest identified human genes. It is localized to the short arm of the X chromosome at Xp21. At present, mutations of the gene can be identified (in approximately two-thirds of Duchenne patients) using a battery of cDNA probes. Deletions are not uniformly distributed over the gene, but rather are most common near the beginning (5′ end) and middle of the gene. Deletion size does not correlate with severity of disease. Less often, Duchenne dystrophy is caused by a gene duplication or point mutation. Identification of a specific mutation allows for an unequivocal diagnosis and makes possible accurate testing of potential carriers. Identification of such a mutation in amniotic fluid cells or chorionic villi permits prenatal diagnosis. In families without deletions or duplications, linkage analysis using probes recognizing restriction fragment length polymorphisms is also available.

Dystrophin determination of muscle tissue represents an accurate method of diagnosis of Duchenne dystrophy. The amount and alteration in the size of dystrophin can be determined by western blot analysis of muscle biopsy specimens. In addition, immunocytochemical staining of muscle with dystrophin antibodies can be used to demonstrate absence or deficiency of dystrophin localizing to the sarcolemmal membrane. Carriers of the disease may demonstrate a mosaic pattern, but dystrophin analysis of muscle biopsy specimens for carrier detection is not reliable.

Pathogenesis Dystrophin is part of a large complex of sarcolemmal proteins and glycoproteins (Fig. 383-1). In relation to human muscular dystrophies, it is useful to consider the constituents of the complex falling into three groups. *Group 1* includes dystrophin and the dystroglycans, α and β. Dystrophin binds to F-actin at its amino terminus and to β-dystroglycan at the carboxy terminus. β-dystroglycan in turn binds to α-dystroglycan, and extracellular glycoprotein. In the basal lamina, α-dystroglycan binds to laminin. *Group 2* is composed of the sarcoglycans, which have four transmembrane constituents: α-sarcoglycan (formerly called adhalin), β-sarcoglycan (previously called A3b), γ-sarcoglycan, and δ-sarcoglycan (the newest member to be identified). *Group 3* is composed of laminin, an integral component of the basal lamina, designated laminin 2 in skeletal muscle. It has a heterotrimeric molecular structure arranged in the shape of a cross with one heavy α chain and two light chains, β1 and γ1. The laminin heavy α chain of skeletal muscle is designated lamina α2.

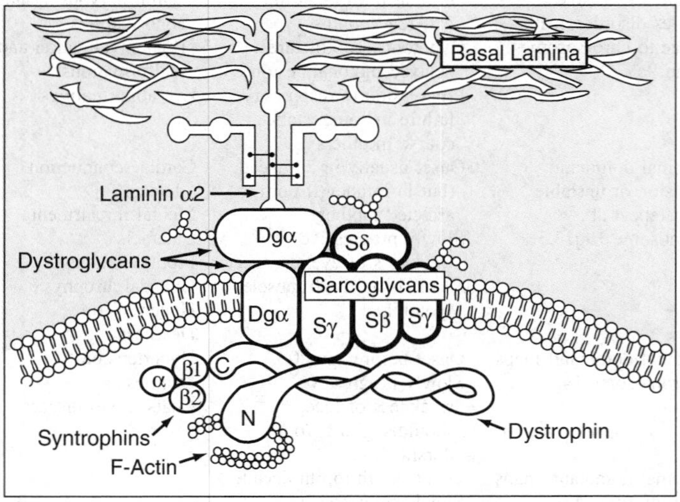

FIGURE 383-1 Dystrophin localizes to the cytoplasmic face of the membrane in a subsarcolemmal location. The syntrophin complex, composed of α, β1, and β2, is shown in its presumed place in relation to the dystrophin-glycoprotein complex. See text for further explanation.

The function of each individual component of the dystrophin-glycoprotein complex is still under study. Nevertheless, important observations indicate that the dystrophin-glycoprotein complex confers stability to the sarcolemma. Furthermore, deficiency of one member of the complex causes loss of other components of the dystrophin-glycoprotein complex. For example, deficiency of dystrophin (Duchenne dystrophy) of α-sarcoglycan (limb-girdle dystrophy, see below) weakens the sarcolemma, causing membrane tears and a cascade of events leading to mucle fiber necrosis. This train of events happens repeatedly during the life of a muscular dystrophy patient.

℞ TREATMENT

Prednisone in a dose of 0.75 mg/kg per day has been shown to significantly alter the progression of Duchenne dystrophy for up to 3 years. Despite these favorable results, some patients clearly cannot tolerate glucocorticoid therapy. The weight gain represents a significant deterrent for some boys. Treatment must be tailored to the individual.

BECKER MUSCULAR DYSTROPHY This less severe form of X-linked recessive muscular dystrophy was described by Becker and Keiner in 1955. It is often called the benign form of pseudohypertrophic muscular dystrophy. Until recently, it was not known whether Duchenne and Becker muscular dystrophies were genetically distinct disorders. Molecular genetic studies now indicate that these dystrophies result from allelic defects of the same gene. Becker muscular dystrophy is approximately 10 times less frequent than Duchenne, with an incidence of about 3 per 100,000.

Clinical Features The pattern of muscle wasting in Becker muscular dystrophy closely resembles that seen in Duchenne. Proximal muscles, especially of the lower extremities, are prominently involved. As the disease progresses, weakness becomes more generalized. Significant facial muscle weakness is not a feature. Hypertrophy of muscles, particularly in the calves, is an early and prominent finding.

Most Becker patients first experience difficulties between ages 5 and 15 years, although onset in the third or fourth decade or even later can occur. By definition, Becker patients ambulate beyond age 15, allowing for a clinical distinction between Becker and Duchenne dystrophy. Becker dystrophy patients have a reduced life expectancy, but most survive into the fourth or fifth decade.

Mental retardation may be seen in Becker dystrophy, but it is not as common as in Duchenne. Cardiac involvement occurs in Becker dystrophy and may result in heart failure.

Laboratory Features The findings from serum CK measurement, EMG, and muscle biopsy closely resemble those in Duchenne dystrophy. The diagnosis of Becker muscular dystrophy requires western blot analysis of muscle biopsy samples demonstrating dystrophin of reduced amount or abnormal size. In addition, in Becker dystrophy, mutation analysis of DNA from peripheral blood leukocytes recognizes deletions and duplications of the dystrophin gene in approximately the same number of patients (65 percent) as in Duchenne. In both Becker and Duchenne dystrophies, the size of the DNA deletion does not predict clinical severity; however, in about 95 percent of Becker dystrophy patients, the DNA deletion does not alter the translational reading frame of messenger RNA. These "in-frame" mutations allow for production of some dystrophin, which accounts for the presence of altered rather than absent dystrophin on western blot analysis.

℞ TREATMENT

The use of prednisone has not been adequately studied in Becker dystrophy and other mild dystrophin-deficiency disorders.

LIMB-GIRDLE DYSTROPHY This term was introduced in 1954 in the Walton and Natrass revision of the classification of the muscular dystrophies. From the outset, it was apparent that limb-girdle dystrophy represented more than one disorder.

Clinical Features Muscle weakness affects both males and females, with onset ranging from late in the first decade to the fourth decade. Most limb-girdle muscular dystrophies are progressive and affect the pelvic and shoulder girdle muscles. Respiratory insufficiency from diaphragm weakness may occur. The distribution of weakness and rate of progression vary from family to family. In some patients, cardiac involvement results in congestive heart failure or arrhythmias; occasional patients present with a cardiomyopathy. Intellectual function remains normal.

Laboratory Features An elevated serum CK level, myopathic EMG findings, and muscle biopsy features indicative of myopathy represent the characteristic changes in limb-girdle dystrophy. Careful attention to exclude phenotypically similar disorders, such as spinal muscular atrophy and metabolic and inflammatory myopathies, is required. The availability of western blot analysis for dystrophin sarcoglycans allows limb-girdle dystrophies to be distinguished unequivocally from Becker and Duchenne muscular dystrophies.

Genetics Limb-girdle dystrophy continues to refer to more than one disease transmitted by autosomal dominant and autosomal recessive inheritance. In a newly proposed genetic classification, *LGMD1* refers to the dominantly inherited cases, while *LGMD2* indicates recessive transmission. Presently, genetic linkage has established only a single, dominantly inherited disorder, LGMD1A. In contrast, the recessively inherited forms of LGMD now number six. In each case genetic linkage has been established, and the specific protein deficiency is known for most forms (Table 383-2 and Fig. 383-1). In LGMD2A the defect lies in a muscle-specific calcium-activated neutral protease, calpain 3. The sarcoglycans, α, β, γ, δ, are deficient in LGMDs 2C–F. In the latter deficiencies, the dystrophin-glycoprotein complex is affected, weakening the muscle membrane in a manner similar to Duchenne muscular dystrophy.

Rx TREATMENT

Supportive care, but not specific treatment, can be offered. Long leg braces are seldom helpful for adults. Wheelchairs may be essential or may be used to help preserve energy for work or recreational activities. Cardiac or respiratory muscle involvement may require individualized treatment.

CONGENITAL MUSCULAR DYSTROPHY This rare autosomal recessive disorder includes four subgroups with overlapping clinical features. Variable involvement of brain and eyes can help differentiate these conditions; two have been mapped to specific chromosomes, with a specific defect identified in one of these.

Clinical Features All the forms of congenital muscular dystrophy present at birth or in the first few months of life with hypotonia and proximal limb weakness. Varying degrees of joint contractures at the elbows, hips, knees, and ankles are seen in most patients. Contractures present at birth are referred to as *arthrogryposis*. Weakness of facial muscles may occur, but other cranial nerve musculature is spared. Severity varies greatly, but about half of affected individuals never achieve the ability to stand independently. Death may ensue because of respiratory insufficiency early in life. Some patients learn to walk, although difficulty in motor activities (e.g., running) persists.

Table 383-2

The Limb-Girdle Muscular Dystrophies Caused by Defects in Proteins Associated with the Muscle Membrane

Disease	Protein	Size	Chromosomal Localization
LGMD1A	Unknown	Unknown	5q31–33
LGMD2A	Calpain 3	95 kDa	15q15.1–15.3
LGMD2B	Unknown	Unknown	2p13.3
LGMD2C	γ-sarcoglycan	35 kDa	13q12
LGMD2D	α-sarcoglycan	50 kDa	17q12–21.33
LGMD2E	β-sarcoglycan	43 kDa	4q12
LGMD2F	δ-sarcoglycan	35 kDa	5q33–34

NOTE: LGMD, limb-girdle muscular dystrophy. Type 1A is autosomal dominant; types 2A–F are autosomal recessive.

One variant of congenital muscular dystrophy has only the muscle features just described; three others have central nervous involvement. In patients with deficiency of laminin α2 (formerly called merosin) diffuse white matter changes typical of hypomyelination are seen by magnetic resonance imaging. There is no accompanying cerebral atrophy, ventricular dilation, or cerebellar hypoplasia. The clinical manifestation of the cerebral hypomyelination is mild, with learning disability as the most severe problem. In *Fukuyama congenital muscular dystrophy*, found mainly in Japan, patients are severely disabled and mentally retarded; most have seizures and die by age 20. Microcephaly and enlarged ventricles occur. Micropolygyria is common. In *cerebroocular-dysplasia muscular dystrophy*, the clinical features are like those of Fukuyama dystrophy, with the addition of eye abnormalities, including corneal defects, cataracts, retinal dysplasia, and hypoplasia of the optic nerve.

Laboratory Features Serum CK levels range from normal to 10 times normal. The EMG shows a myopathic pattern, and muscle biopsy samples demonstrate dystrophic features. In laminin α2 deficiency, the muscle lacks this protein.

Genetics The gene for laminin α2 maps to chromosome 6q22-23; specific mutations of the gene have been identified in some patients with this form of congenital muscular dystrophy. Deficiency of laminin α2 can adversely affect the dystrophin-glycoprotein complex (Fig. 383-1).

The gene for Fukuyama congenital muscular dystrophy has not been identified but has been mapped to the long arm of chromosome 9. The gene causing cerebroocular-dysplasia muscular dystrophy has not been mapped. In cases of congenital muscular dystrophy without brain or eye involvement, no candidate genes have been identified.

Rx TREATMENT

Supportive care and especially stretching to improve joint range of motion is important for congenital muscular dystrophies. Infants and very young children require special wheelchair modifications and adaptive seating to maximize functional capabilities.

MYOTONIC DYSTROPHY This disorder has an incidence of 13.5 per 100,000 live births and affects males and females equally. It is the most common adult muscular dystrophy.

Clinical Features The clinical expression of myotonic dystrophy varies widely and involves many systems other than muscle. Myotonic dystrophy patients have a typical "hatchet-faced" appearance due to temporalis, masseter, and facial muscle atrophy and weakness. Neck muscles, including the flexors and sternocleidomastoids, become involved early, as do distal limb muscles. Weakness of wrist extensors, finger extensors, and intrinsic hand muscles impairs function. Ankle dorsiflexor weakness may cause footdrop. Proximal muscles remain stronger throughout the course, although preferential atrophy and weakness of quadriceps muscles occur in many patients. Palatal, pharyngeal, and tongue involvement produce a dysarthric speech, nasal voice, and swallowing problems. Some patients have diaphragm and intercostal muscle weakness, resulting in respiratory insufficiency.

Myotonia, which usually appears by age 5, is demonstrable by percussion of the thenar eminence, the tongue, and wrist extensor muscles. Myotonia causes a slow relaxation of hand grip following a forced voluntary closure. Advanced muscle wasting makes myotonia more difficult to detect.

Congenital myotonic dystrophy is a more severe form of the disease and occurs in approximately 25 percent of infants of affected mothers. It is characterized by severe facial and bulbar weakness and neonatal respiratory insufficiency. Most patients will recover from respiratory distress. Congenital myotonic dystrophy patients usually have impaired intelligence.

Cardiac disturbances occur in most patients with myotonic dystrophy. Electrocardiographic abnormalities are common, including first-degree heart block and more extensive conduction system involvement. Complete heart block and sudden death can occur. Congestive heart failure occurs infrequently but may result from cor pulmonale secondary to respiratory failure. Mitral valve prolapse also occurs commonly in myotonic dystrophy patients.

Other features associated with myotonic dystrophy include intellectual impairment, hypersomnia, posterior subcapsular cataracts, frontal baldness, gonadal atrophy, insulin resistance, and decreased esophageal and colonic motility.

Laboratory Features The diagnosis of myotonic dystrophy can usually be made on the basis of clinical findings. Serum CK levels may be normal or mildly elevated. EMG evidence of myotonia will be found readily in most cases. Muscle biopsy shows muscle atrophy, which selectively involves type 1 fibers in 50 percent of cases. Typically, increased numbers of central nuclei can be seen. Necrosis of muscle fibers and increased connective tissue, common in other muscular dystrophies, do not usually occur in myotonic dystrophy.

Genetics Myotonic dystrophy is an autosomal dominant disorder. Evidence indicates that new mutations do not contribute to the pool of affected individuals. The disorder is transmitted by a mutation consisting of an unstable expansion of a CTG trinucleotide repeat sequence in a gene at 19q13.3. An increase in the severity of the disease phenotype in successive generations (genetic anticipation) is accompanied by an increase in the number of trinucleotide repeats. A similar type of mutation has been identified in fragile X syndrome (see Chap. 363). The unstable triplet repeat in myotonic dystrophy can be used for prenatal diagnosis. Congenital disease occurs almost exclusively in infants born to affected mothers; it is possible that sperm with greatly expanded triplet repeats do not function well.

The protein encoded by the region adjacent to the unstable repeat has a predicted amino acid composition homologous to a protein kinase (referred to as myotonin-protein kinase). Other genes may also be affected by the enlarged repeat.

A subset of patients with multisystemic disease features similar to myotonic dystrophy do not have the diagnostic expansion of trinucleotide repeats. Their weakness tends to be proximal rather than distal. This condition has been termed *pro*ximal *m*yotonic *m*yopathy (PROMM). At least a proportion of PROMM cases may be caused by a mutation at a different chromosome locus from that causing myotonic dystrophy.

Rx TREATMENT

The myotonia in myotonic dystrophy rarely warrants treatment. Phenytoin is the preferred agent for the occasional patient who requires an antimyotonia drug; other agents, particularly quinine and procainamide, may worsen cardiac conduction. Cardiac pacemaker insertion should be considered for patients with unexplained syncope or advanced conduction system abnormalities with evidence of second-degree heart block, or trifascicular conduction disturbances with marked prolongation of the PR interval. Molded ankle-foot orthoses will help prevent footdrop in patients with distal lower extremity weakness.

FACIOSCAPULOHUMERAL MUSCULAR DYSTROPHY This form of muscular dystrophy has an incidence of approximately 1 in 20,000. It is distinct from a somewhat similar disorder known as scapuloperoneal dystrophy.

Clinical Features The condition typically has an onset in childhood and young adulthood. In most cases, facial weakness is the initial manifestation, appearing as an inability to smile, whistle, or fully close the eyes. Weakness of the shoulder girdles, rather than the facial muscles, usually brings the patient to medical attention. Loss of scapular stabilizer muscles makes arm elevation difficult. Scapular winging becomes apparent with attempts at abduction and forward movement of the arms. Biceps and triceps muscles may be severely affected, with relative sparing of the deltoid muscles. Weakness is invariably worse for wrist extension than for wrist flexion, and weakness of the anterior compartment muscles of the legs may lead to footdrop.

In most patients, the weakness remains restricted to facial, upper extremity, and distal lower extremity muscles. In 20 percent of cases, weakness progresses to involve the pelvic girdle muscles, and severe functional impairment and possible wheelchair confinement result.

Characteristically, patients with facioscapulohumeral dystrophy do not have involvement of other organ systems, although labile hypertension is common, and there is an increased incidence of nerve deafness. Coats' disease, a disorder consisting of telangiectasia, exudation, and retinal detachment, also occurs.

Laboratory Features The serum CK level may be normal or mildly elevated. EMG usually indicates a myopathic pattern. The muscle biopsy shows nonspecific features of a myopathy. A prominent inflammatory infiltrate, which is often multifocal in distribution, is present in some biopsy samples. The cause or significance of this finding is unknown.

Genetics An autosomal dominant inheritance pattern with almost complete penetrance has been established, but each family member should be examined for the presence of the disease, since approximately 30 percent of those affected are unaware of involvement. Facioscapulohumeral dystrophy has been linked to chromosome 4q35, but neither the gene nor the product is known. Nevertheless, deletions of telomeric heterochromatin at 4q35 are proved to be disease-causing with a great deal of certainty. In addition, there is a significant correlation between disease severity and the size of the 4q35-associated deletion. Carrier detection and prenatal diagnosis are possible. Most sporadic cases represent new mutations. Genetic heterogeneity has been documented for facioscapulohumeral dystrophy; in occasional families, the disease is not linked to chromosome 4q.

Rx TREATMENT

No specific treatment is available; ankle-foot orthoses are helpful for patients with footdrop. Scapular stabilization procedures improve scapular winging but may not improve function.

OCULOPHARYNGEAL DYSTROPHY This form of muscular dystrophy represents one of several disorders characterized by *progressive external ophthalmoplegia*, which consists of slowly progressive ptosis and limitation of eye movements with sparing of pupillary reactions for light and accommodation. Patients usually do not complain of diplopia, in contrast to patients having conditions with a more acute onset of ocular muscle weakness (e.g., myasthenia gravis).

Clinical Features This is a late-onset form of muscular dystrophy. Oculopharyngeal muscular dystrophy usually presents with ptosis and/or dysphagia in the fourth to sixth decade. The extraocular muscle impairment is less prominent in the early phase but may be severe later. The swallowing problem may become debilitating and result in pooling of secretions and repeated episodes of aspiration. Mild neck and extremity weakness also occur.

Laboratory Features The serum CK level may be two to three times normal. Myopathic EMG findings are typical. On biopsy, muscle fibers are found to contain vacuoles, which by electron microscopy are shown to contain membranous whorls, accumulations of glycogen, and other nonspecific debris related to lysosomes. A distinct feature of oculopharyngeal dystrophy is the presence of tubular filaments, 8.5 nm in diameter, in muscle cell nuclei.

Genetics Oculopharyngeal dystrophy has an autosomal dominant inheritance pattern with complete penetrance. The incidence is high in French-Canadians and in Spanish-American families of the southwest United States. A large Jewish kindred of eastern European background has been reported. The gene for oculopharyngeal muscular dystrophy maps to the region on chromosome 14q containing the genes for the α and β heavy chains of cardiac myosin.

TREATMENT

Dysphagia can cause inanition and makes oculopharyngeal muscular dystrophy a potentially life-threatening disease. Cricopharyngeal myotomy may improve swallowing, although it does not prevent aspiration. Eyelid crutches can improve vision in patients in whom ptosis obstructs vision; candidates for ptosis surgery must be carefully selected; those with severe facial weakness are not suitable.

DISTAL MYOPATHIES Patients with predominantly distal weakness usually have a disease of peripheral nerve or anterior horn cells rather than of muscle. There is, however, a heterogeneous group of uncommon disorders of this type in which there is histopathologic and electrophysiologic evidence of myopathy. These distal myopathies can be separated into two types with onset in late adulthood and two types with onset in early adulthood.

The most familiar late adult–onset form was described by Welander. It is inherited as an autosomal dominant condition with onset in the fifth decade. Weakness begins in the hands, and distal anterior-compartment leg muscle involvement occurs later in the course. The serum CK level is either normal or mildly increased. Muscle biopsy shows vacuolated muscle fibers.

Another late adult–onset form of distal myopathy, also inherited as an autosomal dominant trait, was first recognized in non-Scandinavian patients and also occurs in Finland. Weakness begins in the anterior compartment of the distal lower extremities. The serum CK level is normal or mildly elevated. Muscle fibers often have vacuoles.

Both of the distal myopathies with onset in early adulthood have autosomal recessive inheritance. In one type, the weakness usually begins in the anterior compartment of the distal lower extremities, although in some cases it begins in the hands. The serum CK level is moderately elevated (less than 10 times normal), and muscle biopsies reveal a myopathy with many fibers showing vacuoles. The other form of early adult–onset distal myopathy (Miyoshi myopathy) is distinguished by weakness beginning in the posterior compartment, i.e., the gastrocnemius muscle. The serum CK level is markedly elevated (>10-fold), and biopsy shows a myopathy without vacuolated fibers. Miyoshi myopathy has been linked to chromosome 2p12-14.

CONGENITAL MYOPATHIES

These rare disorders are distinguished from muscular dystrophies by the presence of specific histochemical and structural abnormalities in muscle. Three major types are described: *central core disease*, *nemaline (rod) myopathy*, and *centronuclear (myotubular) myopathy*. Other rare types, such as multicore disease, fingerprint body myopathy, and sarcotubular myopathy, are not discussed here (see Griggs et al).

CENTRAL CORE DISEASE Clinical Features Patients with central core disease may have decreased fetal movements and breech presentation. Hypotonia and delay in motor milestones, particularly in walking, are common. Later in childhood, patients develop problems with stair climbing, running, and getting up from the floor. On examination, there is mild facial, neck-flexor, and proximal-extremity muscle weakness. Legs are more affected than arms. Skeletal abnormalities include congenital hip dislocation, scoliosis, and pes cavus; clubbed feet also occur. Most cases are nonprogressive, but exceptions are well documented.

Laboratory Features The serum CK level is usually normal. Needle EMG demonstrates a myopathic pattern. Muscle biopsy shows fibers with single or multiple central or eccentric discrete zones (cores) devoid of oxidative enzymes. Cores occur preferentially in type 1 fibers and represent poorly aligned sarcomeres associated with Z disk streaming.

Genetics Autosomal dominant inheritance is characteristic; sporadic cases also occur. The disease is caused by point mutations of the ryanodine receptor gene on chromosome 19q, encoding the calcium release channel of the sarcoplasmic reticulum of skeletal muscle; mutations of this gene also account for some cases of inherited malignant hyperthermia (see Chap. 363).

TREATMENT

Specific treatment is not required, but establishing a diagnosis of central core disease is extremely important, because these patients have a known predisposition to *malignant hyperthermia* during anesthesia.

NEMALINE MYOPATHY The term *nemaline* refers to the distinctive presence in muscle fibers of rods or threadlike structures (Greek *nema*, "thread").

Clinical Features Nemaline myopathy is clinically heterogeneous. A severe neonatal form presents with hypotonia and feeding difficulties leading to early death. Most commonly, nemaline myopathy presents in infancy or childhood with delayed motor milestones. The course is nonprogressive or slowly progressive. The physical appearance may be striking because of the long, narrow facies, high-arched palate, and open-mouthed appearance due to a prognathous jaw. Other skeletal abnormalities include pectus excavatum, kyphoscoliosis, pes cavus, and clubfoot deformities. Facial and generalized muscle weakness are common. These two early childhood forms of nemaline myopathy are referred to as *congenital nemaline myopathy*, in contrast to an adult-onset disorder with progressive proximal weakness. Myocardial involvement is occasionally present in both the congenital and adult-onset forms of the disease.

Laboratory Features The serum CK level is usually normal or slightly elevated. The EMG in weak muscles demonstrates a myopathic pattern with occasional fibrillation potentials. Muscle biopsy demonstrates clusters of small rods (nemaline bodies), which occur preferentially, but not exclusively, in type 1 muscle fibers. The muscle often shows type 1 muscle fiber predominance. Rods originate from the Z disk material of the muscle fiber. In the severe neonatal variant, rods are commonly observed in the nucleus of muscle fibers.

Genetics Nemaline myopathy shows at least two patterns of inheritance: autosomal recessive and autosomal dominant with incomplete penetrance. Sporadic cases also occur. A gene for autosomal dominant nemaline myopathy maps to chromosome 1p, and a missense mutation in the α-tropomyosin gene (TPM3) has been found.

TREATMENT

No specific treatment exists for this condition; some patients require bracing or surgery for the scoliosis as well as ankle-foot orthoses for distal lower extremity weakness.

CENTRONUCLEAR MYOPATHY Clinical Features Three distinct variants of the disease occur. A *neonatal form of centronuclear myopathy* presents with severe hypotonia and weakness at birth. Respiratory assistance may be required, and swallowing difficulties may necessitate a feeding tube. This form of the disease carries a poor prognosis and often results in death. The *late infancy–early childhood form of centronuclear myopathy* presents with delayed motor milestones. Later, difficulty with running and stair climbing becomes apparent. A marfanoid, slender body habitus, long narrow face, and high-arched palate are typical. Scoliosis and clubbed feet may be present. Most patients exhibit progressive weakness, some requiring wheelchairs. Progressive external ophthalmoplegia with ptosis and varying degrees of extraocular muscle impairment are characteristic of both the neonatal and the late-infantile forms.

A third variant, the *late childhood–adult type of centronuclear myopathy*, has an onset in the second or third decade. Patients have full extraocular muscle movements and rarely exhibit ptosis. There is mild, nonprogressive limb weakness and no associated skeletal abnormalities.

Laboratory Features Normal or slightly elevated CK levels occur in each of the forms of centronuclear myopathy. EMG studies often give distinctive results, showing positive sharp waves and fibrillation potentials, complex and repetitive discharges, and rarely myotonic discharges. Muscle biopsy specimens in longitudinal section demonstrate rows of central nuclei, often surrounded by a halo. In transverse sections, central nuclei are found in 25 to 80 percent of muscle fibers.

Genetics The gene for the neonatal form of centronuclear myopathy has been localized to Xq28, permitting identification of carriers and prenatal diagnosis. Inheritance pattern for the late infancy–early childhood disorder is probably autosomal recessive and for the late childhood–adult form, autosomal dominant.

℞ TREATMENT

Patients with the neonatal form of centronuclear myopathy require respiratory support and gastric feeding. For patients with the late infancy–early childhood disorder, ambulatory aids and orthotic devices and, less often, wheelchairs may be necessary. Occasional patients require scoliosis surgery.

DISORDERS OF MUSCLE ENERGY METABOLISM

Skeletal muscle uses two principal sources of energy—fatty acids and glucose. Abnormalities in either glucose or lipid utilization can be associated with distinct clinical presentations. The clinical presentation can range from an acute, painful syndrome with rhabdomyolysis and myoglobinuria to a chronic progressive muscle weakness simulating muscular dystrophy.

GLYCOGEN STORAGE AND GLYCOLYTIC DEFECTS These disorders can be divided into those that cause exercise intolerance, particularly intermittent muscle pain and myoglobinuria, and those in which fixed muscle weakness is the predominant clinical feature. The latter can mimic limb-girdle muscular dystrophy or inflammatory myopathies.

Disorders of Glycogen Storage Causing Fixed Muscle Weakness Three clinical forms of acid maltase deficiency (*type II glycogenosis*) can be distinguished, all of which have autosomal recessive inheritance. The gene for acid maltase is found on the long arm of chromosome 17. *Infantile acid maltase deficiency* is the most common, with onset of symptoms in the first 3 months of life. Infants develop severe muscle weakness, cardiomegaly, hepatomegaly, and respiratory insufficiency. Glycogen accumulation in motor neurons of the spinal cord and brainstem contributes to muscle weakness. Death usually occurs by 1 year of age. In *childhood acid maltase deficiency*, the picture resembles muscular dystrophy. Delayed motor milestones result from proximal limb muscle weakness and involvement of respiratory muscles. The heart may be involved, but the liver and brain are unaffected. The *adult form of acid maltase deficiency* begins in the third or fourth decade. Respiratory failure and diaphragmatic weakness are often initial manifestations heralding progressive proximal muscle weakness. The heart and liver are not involved.

In all forms of acid maltase deficiency, the serum CK level is 2 to 10 times normal. EMG examination demonstrates a myopathic pattern, but other features are especially distinctive, including myotonic discharges, trains of fibrillation and positive waves, and complex repetitive discharges. EMG discharges are very prominent in the lumbosacral paraspinal muscles. The muscle biopsy shows vacuoles containing glycogen and the lysosomal enzyme acid phosphatase. Electron microscopy reveals membrane-bound and free tissue glycogen. Definitive diagnosis is established by enzyme determination in muscle.

No satisfactory treatment exists for acid maltase deficiency. A high-protein diet has been advocated, but efficacy has not been documented. Intravenous enzyme replacement has not shown benefit.

In *debranching enzyme deficiency (type III glycogenosis)*, a slowly progressive form of muscle weakness can develop after puberty. Rarely, myoglobinuria may be seen. Patients are usually diagnosed in infancy, however, because of hypotonia and delayed motor milestones, hepatomegaly, growth retardation, and hypoglycemia. *Branching enzyme deficiency (type IV glycogenosis)* is a rare and fatal glycogen storage disease characterized by failure to thrive and hepatomegaly. Hypotonia and muscle wasting may be present, but the skeletal muscle manifestations are minor compared to liver failure.

Disorders of Glycolysis Causing Exercise Intolerance Five glycolytic defects are associated with recurrent myoglobinuria: *myophosphorylase deficiency (type V glycogenosis), phosphofructokinase deficiency (type VII glycogenosis), phosphoglycerate kinase deficiency (type IX glycogenosis), phosphoglycerate mutase deficiency (type X glycogenosis),* and *lactate dehydrogenase deficiency (glycogenosis type XI).* The features of these conditions are summarized in Table 383-3. Myophosphorylase deficiency, also known as McArdle's disease, is by far the most common of the glycolytic defects associated with exercise intolerance. All are inherited as autosomal recessive traits, except for phosphoglycerate kinase deficiency, which is X-linked recessive. These five glycolytic defects result in a common failure to support energy production at the initiation of exercise, although the exact site of energy failure remains controversial.

Clinical manifestations in these five conditions usually begin in adolescence. Symptoms are precipitated by brief bursts of high-intensity exercise, such as running or lifting heavy objects. A history of myalgia and muscle stiffness usually precedes the intensely painful muscle contractures, which may be followed by myoglobinuria. Acute renal failure accompanies significant pigmenturia. Exercise tolerance can be enhanced by a slow induction phase (warm-up) or brief periods of rest allowing for the start of the "second-wind" phenomenon (switching to utilization of fatty acids).

Certain features help distinguish some enzyme defects. Varying degrees of hemolytic anemia accompany deficiencies of both phosphofructokinase (mild) and phosphoglycerate kinase (severe). In phosphoglycerate kinase deficiency, the usual clinical presentation is a seizure disorder associated with mental retardation; exercise intolerance is an infrequent manifestation.

In all of these conditions, the serum CK levels fluctuate widely and may be elevated even during symptom-free periods. CK levels over 200 times normal are expected accompanying myoglobinuria. All patients with suspected glycolytic defects leading to exercise intolerance should undergo a forearm exercise test (see Griggs et al. for details). Impaired rise in venous lactate is highly indicative of a glycolytic defect. In lactate dehydrogenase deficiency, venous levels of lactate will not increase, but pyruvate will rise to normal, after forearm exercise. In all glycolytic defects, a definitive diagnosis is made by analysis of muscle removed by biopsy.

Training may enhance the second-wind phenomenon, but attempts to raise blood glucose or to modify these disorders through diet have not been shown to be beneficial.

DISORDERS OF LIPID METABOLISM

Lipid is an important muscle energy source during rest and during prolonged, submaximal exercise. Fatty acids are derived from circulating very low density lipoprotein (VLDL) in the blood or from triglycerides stored in muscle fibers. Oxidation of fatty acids occurs in the mitochondria. To enter the mitochondria, a fatty acid must first be converted to an "activated fatty acid," acyl-CoA. The acyl-CoA must be linked with carnitine by the enzyme carnitine palmitoyltransferase (CPT) I for transport into the mitochondria. CPT 1 is present on the inner side of the outer mitochondrial membrane. Carnitine is removed by CPT II, an enzyme attached to the inside of the inner mitochondrial membrane, allowing transport of acyl-CoA into the mitochondrial matrix for β-oxidation.

CARNITINE DEFICIENCY Deficiency of this important substrate results in a myopathic and a systemic disorder.

Myopathic carnitine deficiency is associated with generalized muscle weakness, usually beginning in childhood. The clinical features overlap with those of muscular dystrophy and polymyositis. Patients develop progressive, painless proximal weakness. A severe cardiomyopathy may be present. Serum CK levels may be mildly to markedly (greater than 10-fold) elevated. The muscle biopsy shows striking lipid accumulation. Serum carnitine is normal. The cause for decreased muscle carnitine is not understood. Most cases are sporadic, but the inheritance pattern is thought to be autosomal recessive. Some patients respond to oral carnitine supplementation; this treatment should be tried in all cases. Other patients have responded to prednisone, riboflavin, or propranolol. A diet substituting medium-chain for long-chain triglycerides has been helpful in some cases.

Systemic carnitine deficiency usually presents in infancy and early childhood and is characterized by progressive weakness and episodes of hepatic encephalopathy with nausea, vomiting, confusion, coma, and early death. Carnitine levels are reduced in muscle, liver, kidney, and heart, but the low serum carnitine levels are especially useful in distinguishing this condition from the myopathic form. No single cause has been identified to explain the low serum carnitine levels. Decreased hepatic synthesis explains some cases, while increased urinary excretion is seen in others. Serum CK levels may be slightly elevated. The muscle biopsy may show lipid storage. In some cases, the liver, heart, and kidney show increased lipid. Treatment with oral carnitine supplementation or glucocorticoid administration has helped some, but not all, patients.

Table 383-3

Glycolytic Defects Causing Exercise Intolerance

Enzyme Deficiency	Genetics	Clinical Features	Laboratory Features
Myophosphorylas deficiency (McArdle's disease)	Autosomal recessive; maps to chromosome 11	Exercise intolerance; myoglobinuria; male predominance	Elevated serum CK level No lactate rise on forearm exercise test Muscle weakness in 30%
Phosphofructokinase deficiency (Tarui's disease)	Autosomal recessive; maps to chromosome 1	Exercise intolerance; myoglobinuria; male predominance	Elevated serum CK level No lactate rise on forearm exercise test Mild hemolytic anemia
Phosphoglycerate kinase deficiency	X-linked recessive	*Most common presentation:* seizures, mental retardation, hemolytic anemia *Less commonly,* presentation includes exercise intolerance, myoglobinuria	Elevated serum CK level No lactate rise on forearm exercise test Hemolytic anemia
Phosphoglycerate mutase deficiency	Autosomal recessive	Exercise intolerance; myoglobinuria	Elevated serum CK level No lactate rise on forearm exercise test
Lactate dehydrogenase deficiency	Autosomal recessive, maps to chromosome 11	Exercise intolerance; myoglobinuria	Elevated serum CK level No lactate rise on forearm exercise test, *but* normal pyruvate rise

Secondary carnitine deficiency accompanies a variety of disorders in which carnitine deficiency is caused by decreased synthesis (cirrhosis), insufficient intake (parenteral nutrition), or excessive loss (renal dialysis, Fanconi's syndrome, or organic acidemia). Carnitine deficiency may also be seen in the muscular dystrophies, where it is thought to be a nonspecific result of loss of muscle tissue. Carnitine treatment has not been shown to clearly benefit patients with these secondary syndromes.

CARNITINE PALMITYOLTRANSFERASE DEFICIENCY This disorder is the most common recognizable cause of recurrent myoglobinuria, more common than the glycolytic defects.

Clinical Features This disorder usually has its onset in the teenage years or early twenties. Muscle pain and myoglobinuria occur after prolonged exercise. Fasting predisposes to the development of symptoms. In contrast to disorders caused by defects in glycolysis, in which muscle cramps follow short, intense bursts of exercise, the muscle pain in CPT deficiency does not occur until the limits of utilization have been exceeded and muscle breakdown has already begun. Episodes of rhabdomyolysis may produce severe weakness. In contrast to carnitine deficiency, strength is normal between attacks.

Laboratory Findings Serum CK levels and EMG findings are both usually normal between episodes. A normal rise of venous lactate during forearm exercise distinguishes this condition from glycolytic defects, especially phosphorylase deficiency. Muscle biopsy does not show lipid accumulation and is usually normal between attacks. The diagnosis requires direct measurement of muscle CPT.

Genetics CPT deficiency is much more common in men than women (5:1); nevertheless, all evidence indicates autosomal recessive inheritance. A mutation in the gene for CPT II causes the disease in some individuals.

℞ TREATMENT

It has been suggested that frequent meals and a low-fat, high-carbohydrate diet can prolong exercise tolerance. Others suggest substituting medium-chain triglycerides in the diet. Neither approach has proven benefits.

MYOADENYLATE DEAMINASE DEFICIENCY The muscle enzyme myoadenylate deaminase converts adenosine 5′-monophosphate (5′-AMP) to inosine monophosphate (IMP) with liberation of ammonia. Myoadenylate deaminase may play a role in regulating adenosine triphosphate (ATP) levels in muscles. Most subjects with myoadenylate deaminase deficiency have no symptoms. Many questions have been raised about the clinical effects of myoadenylate deaminase deficiency, and specifically its relationship to exertional myalgia and fatigability, but there is no consensus. There have been a few reports of patients with this disorder who have exercise-exacerbated myalgia and myoglobinuria. The full clinical significance of myoadenylate deaminase deficiency has not been established.

MITOCHONDRIAL MYOPATHIES

In 1972, Olson and colleagues recognized that muscle fibers with significant numbers of abnormal mitochondria could be highlighted using the modified trichrome stain; the term "ragged red fibers" was coined. By electron microscopy, the mitochondria in ragged red fibers are enlarged and often bizarrely shaped and have crystalline inclusions. Since that seminal observation, the understanding of these disorders of muscle (and other tissues, e.g., Leber's hereditary optic atrophy) has expanded (see also Chap. 380).

Mitochondria play a key role in energy production. Oxidation of the major nutrients derived from carbohydrate, fat, and protein leads to the generation of reducing equivalents (2H). The latter are transported through the respiratory chain in the process known as oxidative phosphorylation. The energy generated by the oxidation-reduction reactions of the respiratory chain is stored in an electrochemical gradient coupled to ATP synthesis.

A novel feature of mitochondria is their genetic composition. Each mitochondrion possesses a DNA genome that is distinct from that of the nuclear DNA. Human mitochondrial DNA (mtDNA) consists of a double-stranded, circular molecule comprising 16,569 base pairs. It codes for 22 transfer RNAs, 2 ribosomal RNAs, and 13 polypeptides of the respiratory chain enzymes. The genetics of mitochondrial diseases differs from those of chromosomal disorders. The DNA of mitochondria is directly inherited from the cytoplasm of the gametes, mainly from the oocyte. The sperm contributes very little of its mitochondria to the offspring at the time of fertilization. Thus, mitochondrial genes are derived almost exclusively from the mother, accounting for maternal inheritance of some mitochondrial disorders.

mtDNA DISORDERS OF MUSCLE Many different classifications of mitochondrial myopathies are possible. A convenient scheme allows for disorders to be grouped by the type of mtDNA mutation: deletions or point mutations (see also Chap. 380).

Disorders Associated with mtDNA Deletions The *Kearns-Sayre syndrome* (KSS) is a sporadic, noninherited disorder with onset before age 20. The characteristic findings include a triad of clinical features: progressive external ophthalmoplegia, pigmentary degeneration of the retina, and heart block. Some patients have only extraocular manifestations. KSS patients may also have short stature, ataxia, dementia, sensorineural hearing loss, diabetes, and hypothyroidism. In KSS, two populations of mtDNA, wild-type and mutant, are present in the same cell; the mutations in the latter consist of *single mtDNA deletions*. Heteroplasmy can be recognized on Southern blot analysis. The highest percentage of deleted mtDNA can be detected in postmitotic tissues, especially skeletal muscle. Other tissues can harbor the mutation (e.g., peripheral blood leukocytes, brain, liver, and fibroblasts). The absence of mutant mtDNA reflects both mitotic segregation early in embryogenesis and selection against a mutant cell line in a rapidly dividing tissue. KSS is not inherited, since mutations leading to an affected individual take place in the fertilized ovum.

Patients with *Pearson's marrow-pancreas syndrome*, a disorder of infancy characterized by refractory sideroblastic anemia and exocrine pancreatic dysfunction, may develop features of KSS in adolescence. Single mtDNA deletions account for Pearson's marrow-pancreas syndrome.

An *autosomal dominant disorder with progressive external ophthalmoplegia and proximal weakness* shares clinical features with KSS: hearing loss, ataxia, peripheral neuropathy, mental retardation, and hypoparathyroidism. Some of these patients also exhibit weakness of respiratory muscles, exercise intolerance, cataracts, and early death. The patients have ragged red fibers on muscle biopsy and *multiple mtDNA deletions*, rather than single deletions as in KSS. The mutation accounting for the autosomal dominant inheritance occurs in a *nuclear gene* that encodes a protein involved in the control of mtDNA replication. A failure or disruption of binding of this nuclear-encoded protein during mtDNA replication results in multiple deletions.

Disorders Associated with mtDNA Point Mutations *Myoclonic epilepsy and ragged red fibers*, called the *MERRF syndrome*, consists of mitochondrial myopathy, myoclonus, generalized seizures, intellectual deterioration, ataxia, and hearing loss. Extraocular movements are normal in MERRF. As with other mitochondrial disorders, individuals display varying manifestations of the disease. MERRF syndrome is maternally inherited. Most often, point mutations in the lysine transfer RNA gene of mtDNA can be found. This abnormality can be detected in mtDNA isolated from peripheral blood leukocytes or skeletal muscle and is useful for clinical diagnosis and genetic counseling. These mutations alter the normal conformation of the transfer RNA, impairing translation probably at the ribosomal level.

Mitochondrial myopathy, encephalopathy, lactic acidosis, and stroke-like episodes are referred to by the acronym *MELAS*. This disorder is a multisystem mitochondrial encephalomyopathy that begins in childhood after normal birth and early development. Patients have stunted growth and recurrent stroke-like episodes manifesting as hemiparesis, hemianopia, or cortical blindness. Episodic vomiting may occur, and some patients have hearing loss. Focal or generalized seizures and myoclonic epilepsy may be present. Full expression of the disease leads to dementia, a bedridden state, and death often before age 20. Lactic acidosis may be present. MELAS can be maternally inherited, but sporadic cases are common. No large pedigrees have been reported. In 80 to 90 percent of patients, a point mutation of the leucine transfer RNA gene of mtDNA has been identified at nucleotide 3243. Some patients with this same mutation have only diabetes mellitus and hearing loss. Rarely, an mtDNA mutation of subunit 4 of complex I (ND4) of the respiratory chain causes MELAS. Mutation analysis provides a specific diagnostic test that can be performed on peripheral blood leukocytes or skeletal muscle.

A clinical syndrome with combined features of *skeletal and cardiac myopathies associated with lactic acidosis* that is distinct from MELAS has been described with a point mutation at nucleotide 3260 of the leucine transfer RNA gene of mtDNA.

ENDOCRINE AND METABOLIC MYOPATHIES

Many endocrine disorders cause weakness. Muscle fatigue is more common than true weakness. The cause of weakness in these disorders is not well defined. It is not even clear that weakness results from disease of muscle as opposed to another part of the motor unit since the serum CK level is often normal (except in hypothyroidism), and the muscle histology is characterized by atrophy rather than destruction of muscle fibers. Nearly all endocrine myopathies respond to treatment.

THYROID DISORDERS (See Chap. 331) Abnormalities of thyroid function can cause a wide array of muscle disorders. These conditions relate to the important role of thyroid hormones in regulating the metabolism of carbohydrates and lipids as well as the rate of protein synthesis and enzyme production. Thyroid hormones also stimulate calorigenesis in muscle, increase muscle demand for vitamins, and enhance muscle sensitivity to circulating catecholamines.

Hypothyroidism Hypothyroid patients have frequent muscle complaints, and proximal muscle weakness occurs in about one-third of patients. Muscle cramps, pain, and stiffness occur commonly. Features of slow muscle contraction and relaxation occur in 25 percent of patients, and the relaxation phase of muscle stretch reflexes is characteristically prolonged. The serum CK level is often elevated (up to 10 times normal), even when there is minimal clinical evidence of muscle disease. In both children and adults, a distinct syndrome has been described. Severely hypothyroid children, especially boys, may have the Debré-Kocher-Sémélaigne syndrome, characterized by weakness, slowness of movement, and striking muscle hypertrophy, causing an "infant Hercules appearance." In adult hypothyroidism, Hoffman's syndrome results in prominent muscle enlargement and weakness with muscle stiffness. The cause of muscle enlargement in these two syndromes has not been determined. The muscle biopsy shows only muscle atrophy.

Hyperthyroidism Thyrotoxic patients commonly have proximal muscle weakness and atrophy on examination, but they rarely complain of the deficit. Muscle stretch reflexes are preserved and often brisk. Bulbar, respiratory, and even esophageal muscles may occasionally be affected, causing dysphagia, dysphonia, and aspiration. When bulbar involvement occurs, it is usually accompanied by chronic proximal limb weakness, but occasionally it presents in the absence of generalized thyrotoxic myopathy. Other neuromuscular disorders occur in association with hyperthyroidism, including periodic paralysis, myasthenia gravis, and a progressive ocular myopathy associated with proptosis (Graves' ophthalmopathy). Serum CK levels are low in thyrotoxic myopathy. The muscle histology usually shows only atrophy of muscle fibers.

PARATHYROID DISORDERS (See Chap. 354) **Hyperparathyroidism** Muscle weakness is an integral part of primary and secondary hyperparathyroidism. Proximal muscle weakness, muscle wasting, and brisk muscle stretch reflexes are the main features of this endocrinopathy. Serum CK levels are usually normal or slightly elevated. Serum calcium and phosphorus levels show no correlation with the clinical neuromuscular manifestations. Muscle biopsies show only varying degrees of atrophy without muscle fiber degeneration.

Hypoparathyroidism An overt myopathy due to hypocalcemia is rarely seen. Neuromuscular symptoms are usually related to localized or generalized tetany. Serum CK levels may be increased secondary to muscle damage following tetany. Hyporeflexia or areflexia is usually present and contrasts with the hyperreflexia seen in hyperparathyroidism.

ADRENAL DISORDERS (See Chap. 332) Conditions associated with glucocorticoid excess cause a myopathy and, in fact, steroid myopathy is the most commonly diagnosed endocrine muscle disease. Steroid excess, either endogenous or exogenous (see "Toxic Myopathies," below), produces varying degrees of proximal limb weakness. Muscle wasting may be striking. A cushingoid appearance invariably precedes or accompanies clinical signs of myopathy. Histologic sections demonstrate muscle fiber atrophy rather than degeneration or necrosis of muscle fibers. Adrenal insufficiency commonly causes muscle fatigue. Objective weakness occurs less often and is typically mild.

In primary hyperaldosteronism, or Conn's syndrome, neuromuscular complications are due to potassium depletion. The clinical picture is one of persistent muscle weakness. Long-standing hyperaldosteronism may lead to proximal limb weakness and wasting. Serum CK levels may be elevated, and a muscle biopsy may demonstrate degenerating fibers, some with vacuoles. These changes relate to hypokalemia and are not a direct effect of aldosterone on skeletal muscle.

PITUITARY DISORDERS (See Chap. 328) Patients with acromegaly usually show mild proximal weakness without muscle atrophy. Muscles often appear enlarged, but they have decreased forced generation. The duration of acromegaly, rather than the serum growth hormone levels, correlates with the degree of myopathy.

DIABETES MELLITUS (See Chap. 334) Neuromuscular complications of diabetes mellitus are most often related to neuropathy with cranial and peripheral nerve palsies or distal sensorimotor polyneuropathy. "Diabetic amyotrophy" is now known to be a neuropathy affecting the proximal major nerve trunks and lumbosacral plexus. More appropriate terms for this disorder include *diabetic proximal neuropathy* and *lumbosacral plexopathy*.

The only notable myopathy of diabetes mellitus is ischemic infarction of thigh muscles. This condition occurs in patients with poorly controlled diabetes and presents with acute onset of pain, tenderness, and edema of one thigh with a palpable mass. The muscles most often affected include the vastus lateralis, thigh adductors, and biceps femoris. Computed tomography or magnetic resonance imaging can demonstrate focal abnormalities in the affected muscle. Imaging of the muscle may render muscle biopsy unnecessary.

VITAMIN DEFICIENCY Vitamin D deficiency causes the only myopathy that occurs as an integral part of a vitamin deficiency. Vitamin D deficiency (see Chaps. 79 and 353) due to either decreased intake, decreased absorption, or impaired vitamin D metabolism (as occurs in renal disease) may lead to chronic muscle weakness. Pain reflects the underlying bone disease (osteomalacia). It has not been established that deficiency of other vitamins causes a myopathy.

MYOPATHIES OF SYSTEMIC ILLNESS Systemic illnesses such as chronic respiratory, cardiac, or hepatic failure are frequently associated with severe muscle wasting and complaints of weakness. Strength testing often demonstrates mild weakness in such patients. Lack of endurance is a more significant problem.

Myopathy may be a manifestation of chronic renal failure, independent of the better known uremic polyneuropathy. Abnormalities of calcium and phosphorus homeostasis and bone metabolism in chronic renal failure result from a reduction in 1,25-dihydroxyvitamin D, leading to decreased intestinal absorption of calcium. Hypocalcemia, further accentuated by hyperphosphatemia due to decreased renal phosphate clearance, leads to secondary hyperparathyroidism. Renal osteodystrophy results from the compensatory hyperparathyroidism, which leads to osteomalacia from reduced calcium availability and to osteitis fibrosa from the parathyroid hormone excess. The clinical picture of the myopathy of chronic renal failure is identical to that of primary hyperparathyroidism and osteomalacia. There is proximal limb weakness with bone pain.

Gangrenous calcification represents a separate, rare, and sometimes fatal complication of chronic renal failure. In this condition, widespread arterial calcification occurs and results in ischemia. Extensive skin necrosis may occur along with painful myopathy and even myoglobinuria.

TOXIC MYOPATHIES

The classification of toxic myopathies is shown in Table 383-4. Drugs and chemicals may produce focal or generalized damage of skeletal muscle.

The most common cause of focal damage is the injection of narcotic analgesics. Three agents in particular—pentazocine, meperidine, and heroin—may cause a severe fibrotic reaction in muscle. Common injection sites include deltoid, triceps, gluteus maximus, and quadriceps muscles. The muscles become indurated and may have local abscess formation. Cutaneous ulcerations and depressions may occur. Severe joint contractures may develop.

Other drugs may induce generalized muscle weakness, particularly affecting the proximal muscles. In most cases the exact mechanism of drug toxicity is poorly understood. D-Penicillamine induces a condition simulating the clinical and pathologic picture of polymyositis. A similar condition has been reported with cimetidine. Procainamide may cause myositis as part of a systemic lupus–like reaction. Chloroquine administration may cause a vacuolar myopathy.

Zidovudine, used in the treatment of AIDS, produces proximal weakness and pain. On muscle biopsy, zidovudine myopathy demonstrates a distinctive pathologic alteration of skeletal muscle, affecting mitochondria and resembling ragged red fibers. In some patients, reintroduction of zidovudine in lower doses may be tolerated.

The cholesterol-lowering agents, including clofibrate, lovastatin, pravastatin, gemfibrozil, and niacin, have all been implicated as causes of myopathy. The hydroxymethylglutaryl-CoA (HMG-CoA) inhibitors, either alone or in combination with gemfibrozil, have caused rhabdomyolysis and myoglobinuria. Emetine hydrochloride (used for treatment of amebiasis), ϵ-aminocaproic acid (an antifibrinolytic agent), and perhexiline (used for angina pectoris) have all been observed to cause muscle weakness and muscle fiber necrosis following several weeks of therapy.

Drug-induced myopathy accompanied by proximal weakness occurs with glucocorticoid therapy. Glucocorticoid drugs fluorinated in the 9α-position, such as triamcinolone, dexamethasone, and betamethasone, are most likely to cause weakness, but chronic administration of any glucocorticoid, including prednisone, causes weakness. Divided-dose, as opposed to single-morning-dose, regimens produce more severe weakness. A single-dose, alternate-day regimen is yet less toxic. The clinical diagnosis of steroid-induced muscle weakness can be difficult if the medication is being used to treat an underlying inflammatory myopathy. The presence of a normal serum CK level, minimal or no changes of myopathy on EMG, and type 2 muscle fiber atrophy on biopsy are helpful in suggesting steroid-induced weakness.

Excess alcohol intake causes acute muscle weakness with rhabdomyolysis and myoglobinuria by several different mechanisms, including prolonged obtundation, seizures, hypokalemia, and hypophos-

Table 383-4

Toxic Myopathies

Causes of focal myopathies
Pentazocine, meperdine, heroin
Causes of generalized myopathies
Myotonia: propranolol, cyclosporine, iodides, clofibrate, penicillamine
Elevated serum creatinine kinase without weakness: clofibrate, lovastatin
Inflammatory: cimetidine, penicillamine, procainamide
Muscle weakness and myalgias: chloroquine, clofibrate, colchicine, cyclosporine, emetine, ϵ-aminocaproic acid, glucocorticoids, labetalol, niacin, perhexilline, propranolol, vincristine, zidovudine
Rhabdomyolysis and myoglobinuria: alcohol, amphetamine, barbiturates, clofibrate, cocaine, ϵ-aminocaproic acid, gemfibrozil, heroin, lovastatin, phencyclidine
Malignant hyperthermia: ethyl chloride, ethylene, diethyl ether, gallamine, halothane, lidocaine, mepivacaine, methoxylflurane, trichloroethylene, succinylcholine

phatemia. The existence of a chronic myopathy causing slowly progressive weakness in this setting is controversial. Alcoholics often have chronic weakness resulting from neuropathy and poor nutrition.

A very serious drug-induced condition, *malignant hyperthermia*, occurs in susceptible individuals following exposure to certain general anesthetic and depolarizing muscle relaxants (Table 383-4). The local anesthetic amides, including lidocaine and mepivacaine, have also been implicated as precipitating agents.

PERIODIC PARALYSIS

Recent discoveries of the molecular defects in the primary periodic paralyses provide insight into their pathogenesis and form the basis for their classification. The major disorders constituting this group have some features in common (Table 383-5). Onset is usually early in life; episodic weakness *beginning* after age 25 is almost never due to periodic paralysis. Attacks typically occur after rest or sleep and almost never in the midst of vigorous activity, although antecedent exercise often provokes weakness. Patients remain alert during the attacks. Early in the course of these disorders, interattack strength is normal. After many years of attacks, interictal weakness develops and may be progressive. These disorders are amenable to treatment, and progressive weakness can be prevented and even reversed. Diagnosis is based on patient history and confirmed by appropriate evaluation of serum electrolytes during attacks, by evaluation of the response of strength to provocative testing with glucose, insulin, potassium, and cold, or by DNA analysis of the appropriate gene (Table 383-5).

CALCIUM CHANNEL DISORDERS OF MUSCLE Hypokalemic Periodic Paralysis Hypokalemic periodic paralysis (hypoKPP) causes episodic weakness, which usually affects proximal limb muscles more than distal ones; rarely, ocular, bulbar, or respiratory muscles are affected. Respiratory muscle weakness may prove fatal. Meals high in carbohydrate or sodium can provoke attacks. Reflexes become hypoactive, and cardiac arrhythmias may occur during attacks owing to low serum potassium. Men are more often affected because of decreased penetrance in women.

Diagnosis is established by demonstrating a low serum potassium level during a paralytic attack and by excluding secondary causes of hypokalemia. The molecular defect in the calcium channel can be defined in many patients. Muscle biopsy often shows the presence of single or multiple centrally placed vacuoles. Patients whose attacks are too infrequent for study of a spontaneous attack to be feasible require provocative testing with glucose and insulin administration. Provocative tests are potentially hazardous and require careful monitoring.

The pathogenesis of paralytic attacks in hypoKPP is incompletely understood, even though mutations in the skeletal muscle calcium channel have been identified. The contractile apparatus is normal. The effects of insulin on potassium uptake in muscle suggest that an abnormality of the muscle membrane is involved. Weakness is often severe at levels of serum potassium that do not affect normal individuals. Moreover, attacks may occur when insulin levels are low.

The acute paralysis improves following the administration of potassium salts. Oral KCl (0.2 to 0.4 mmol/kg) should be given to patients with severe weakness and repeated at 15- to 30-min intervals depending on the response of the ECG, serum potassium, and muscle strength. Milder attacks usually resolve spontaneously. When patients are unable to swallow or are vomiting, intravenous therapy may be necessary. Small, repeated boluses of KCl (0.1 mmol/kg) may be administered over 5 to 10 min with careful monitoring of the ECG and serum potassium. If potassium is administered as a dilute solution (20 to 40 mmol/L) in 5% glucose or in physiologic saline solution, serum potassium may decline, and weakness may worsen. Mannitol is the preferred vehicle for administered intravenous potassium in such situations, since it facilitates rapid return of serum potassium to normal and will not cause the lowering of serum potassium that may occur when glucose or saline solutions are given.

The goal of therapy is to eliminate attacks, which also prevents interattack weakness. Before effective means of attack prevention became available, chronic progressive interattack weakness frequently caused serious disability. Prophylactic administration of potassium salts, even in large doses, does not prevent attacks, but acetazolamide (125 to 1000 mg/d in divided doses) abolishes attacks in most cases. The metabolic acidosis induced by acetazolamide may underlie the beneficial effect. Paradoxically, acetazolamide lowers the serum potassium level; to achieve an adequate response in some patients, it may be necessary to give supplementary potassium along with acetazolamide and to avoid high-carbohydrate meals. Chronic acetazolamide treatment may be associated with renal calculi, and patients should be monitored for this complication. In occasional patients, attacks may not respond to or may even be worsened by acetazolamide. In such patients, triamterene (25 to 100 mg/d) or spironolactone (25 to 100 mg/d) may prevent attacks.

SODIUM CHANNEL DISORDERS OF MUSCLE Hyperkalemic Periodic Paralysis Hyperkalemic periodic paralysis (hyperKPP) causes episodic weakness of limb muscles; cranial and respiratory muscles are rarely involved. The term "hyperkalemic" is misleading, since patients are often normokalemic during attacks. It is the fact that attacks are precipitated by potassium administration that best defines the disorder. Paresthesia and muscle pain are present during many attacks.

Diagnosis is suggested by a modest elevation of serum potassium during attacks in nearly half of patients; at times, however, the serum potassium is normal or even low. The so-called hyperkalemic and normokalemic forms of this disorder are not separate entities. Intravenous glucose-insulin loading does not precipitate weakness, but potassium-loading tests (0.05 to 0.15 g/kg) will induce weakness in such patients. Potassium-loading tests are potentially hazardous and are contraindicated in patients with renal disease and diabetes. Random serum potassium measurements may suggest the diagnosis, since potassium elevations are frequent during attack-free intervals. Electromyographic evidence

Table 383-5

Disorders Causing Periodic Paralysis

Feature	Hypokalemic Periodic Paralysis	Hyperkalemic Periodic Paralysis	Paramyotonia Congenita
Mode of inheritance	Autosomal dominant (67%) or sporadic (33%)	Autosomal dominant	Autosomal dominant
Myotonia	Eyelid only	Usually	Yes
Age of onset	Teens (invariably <30 years)	Infancy	Infancy
Attack frequency	Daily to yearly	Ranges from twice to thrice daily	With cold exposure; spontaneous attack rate <1/month
Attack duration	2–12 h (rarely longer)	1–2 h (occasionally longer)	2–24 h
Serum K^+ level during attack	Decreased	Normal or increased (rarely low)	Normal or decreased (rarely elevated)
Effect of K^+ loading	No change	Weakness	No change (occasionally weakness)
Effect of muscle cooling	No change	No change	Weakness
Fixed weakness occurs	Yes	Yes	Yes
Site of molecular defect	Calcium channel	Sodium channel	Sodium channel

of myotonia and the finding of vacuoles on muscle biopsy provide supporting data.

Paramyotonia Congenita Paramyotonia congenita (PC) causes attacks of paralysis either spontaneously or with cold provocation. PC with periodic paralysis is similar to hyperKPP except that it is characterized by paradoxical myotonia (i.e., myotonia worsening with activity) and objective cold sensitivity. Mutations in the skeletal muscle voltage-gated sodium channel SCN4A cause hyperKPP and PC (Fig. 383-2). In vitro study of these mutations demonstrates increased sodium conductance through the channels, which is consistent with findings in patient muscle samples.

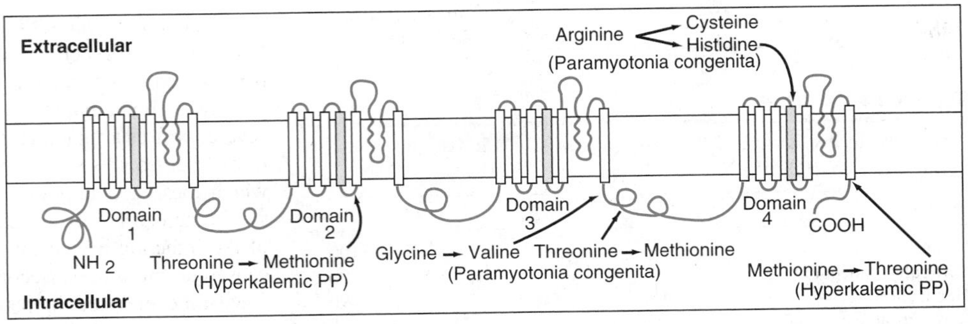

FIGURE 383-2 The sodium channel is depicted here as a molecule containing four homologous domains. Each domain contains six putative membrane-spanning segments. The fourth segment of each domain is thought to act together as the "voltage sensor" for the channel and is cross-hatched in the figure. The tertiary structure of the protein in the membrane and the association of these segments is thought to form a pore through which ions could pass. Mutations that have been identified are shown along with the phenotype that they confer.

In PC, attacks of weakness are seldom severe enough to require emergency treatment and are never fatal. Oral administration of glucose or other carbohydrate hastens recovery. Since interattack weakness may develop after repeated attacks, prophylactic treatment is usually indicated in PC. Thiazide diuretics (e.g., chlorothiazide, 250 to 1000 mg/d) are reported to be effective.

DISORDERS OF UNKNOWN PATHOGENETIC MECHANISM **Thyrotoxic Periodic Paralysis** This disorder is clinically indistinguishable from hypoKPP. It is common in young Latin American and Asian men, among whom up to 10 percent of thyrotoxic patients may have this condition. The thyrotoxicosis may be overlooked for many months. Occasionally, the only indication of thyrotoxicosis is a depressed level of thyroid-stimulating hormone. Acute attacks respond to potassium administration. Treatment of the underlying thyrotoxicosis abolishes attacks. Beta-adrenergic blocking agents are useful for reducing the frequency and severity of attacks while measures to control thyrotoxicosis are instituted. Acetazolamide is not helpful in preventing attacks. The pathogenesis of thyrotoxic periodic paralysis is uncertain, but there is evidence for a decrease in the activity of the calcium pump.

Andersen's Syndrome This is a rare disorder in which patients manifest periodic paralysis (hyperkalemic or hypokalemic), cardiac dysrhythmias (even when normokalemic), and dysmorphic features. Treatment of the episodic weakness is the same as for the other periodic paralyses, although cardiac status must be considered as well.

BIBLIOGRAPHY

Barohn RJ: Distal myopathies and dystrophies. Semin Neurol 13:247, 1993

Britton CH et al: Human liver mitochondrial carnitine palmitoyltransferase I: Characterization of its cDNA and chromosomal localization and partial analysis of the gene. Proc Natl Acad Sci USA 92:1984, 1995

Campbell KP: Adhalin gene mutations and autosomal recessive limb-girdle muscular dystrophy. Ann Neurol 38:353, 1995

Cannon SC: Ion-channel defects and aberrant excitability in myotonia and periodic paralysis. Trends Neurosci 19:3, 1996

DiMauro S: Mitochondrial encephalomyopathies, in *The Molecular and Genetic Basis of Neurologic Disease*, RN Rosenberg et al (eds). Boston, Butterworth-Heinemann, 1993

Dubowitz V: The congenital myopathies, in *Muscle Disorders*, 2d ed, V Dubowitz (ed). London, Saunders, 1995

Elbaz A et al: Hypokalemic periodic paralysis and the dihydropyridine receptor (CACNL1A3): Genotype/phenotype correlations for two predominant mutations and evidence for the absence of a founder effect in 16 Caucasian families. Am J Hum Genet 56:374, 1995

Griggs RC et al: The muscular dystrophies, in *Evaluation and Treatment of Myopathies*, RC Griggs et al (eds). Philadelphia, FA Davis, 1995

Helbling-Leclerc A et al: Mutations in the laminin alpha$_2$-chain gene (LAMA2) cause merosin deficient congenital muscular dystrophy. Nat Genet 11:216, 1995

Kissel JT et al: Endocrine myopathies, in *Handbook of Clinical Neurology*, vol 19, LP Rowland, S DiMauro (eds). New York, Elsevier, 1992

Mendell JR et al: The childhood muscular dystrophies: Diseases sharing a common pathogenesis of membrane instability. J Child Neurol 10:150, 1995

Prior TW et al: Spectrum of small mutations in the dystrophin coding region. Am J Hum Genet 57:22, 1995

Ptáček LJ et al: Sodium channel mutations in acetazolamide-responsive myotonia congenita, paramyotonia congenita and hyperkalemic periodic paralysis. Neurology 44:1500, 1994

Quane KA et al: Mutations in the ryanodine receptor gene in central core disease and malignant hyperthermia. Nat Genet 5:51, 1993

Tawil R et al: Andersen's syndrome: Potassium-sensitive periodic paralysis, ventricular ectopy and dysmorphic features. Ann Neurol 35:326, 1994

Varderio E et al: Carnitine palmitoyltransferase II deficiency: Structure of the gene and characterization of two novel disease-causing mutations. Hum Mol Genet 4:19, 1995

SECTION 4

CHRONIC FATIGUE SYNDROME

384 CHRONIC FATIGUE SYNDROME

Stephen E. Straus

DEFINITION *Chronic fatigue syndrome* is the current name for a disorder characterized by debilitating fatigue and a variety of associated physical, constitutional, and neuropsychological complaints (Table 384-1). The medical literature of the past three centuries informs us that this is not a new type of syndrome. Certain individuals, who were labeled in the past with diagnoses such as the vapors, neurasthenia, effort syndrome, hyperventilation syndrome, chronic brucellosis, epidemic neuromyasthenia, myalgic encephalomyelitis, hypoglycemia, multiple chemical sensitivity syndrome, chronic candidiasis, chronic mononucleosis, chronic Epstein-Barr virus infection, and postviral fatigue syndrome, probably had what we now call chronic fatigue syndrome. The U.S. Centers for Disease Control and Prevention (CDC) developed in 1988 and revised recently a case definition based predominantly on symptoms and on the exclusion of other illnesses (Table 384-2).

EPIDEMIOLOGY Patients with chronic fatigue syndrome are twice as likely to be women as men and are generally 25 to 45

Table 384-1

Approximate Percentage of Patients with the Chronic Fatigue Syndrome Reporting the Specific Symptoms

Symptom	Percentage
Fatigue	100
Difficulty concentrating	90
Headache	90
Sore throat	85
Tender lymph nodes	80
Muscle aches	80
Joint aches	75
Feverishness	75
Difficulty sleeping	70
Psychiatric problems	65
Allergies	55
Abdominal cramps	40
Weight loss	20
Rash	10
Rapid pulse	10
Weight gain	5
Chest pain	5
Night sweats	5

SOURCE: From SE Straus: The chronic mononucleosis syndrome. J Infect Diseases 157:405, 1988.

years old, although cases in childhood and in middle age have been described.

Cases are recognized in many developed countries. Most arise sporadically, but over 30 clusters of similar illness have been reported. The most famous of such "outbreaks" occurred in Los Angeles County Hospital in 1934; in Akureyri, Iceland, in 1948; in the Royal Free Hospital, London, in 1955; in Punta Gorda, Florida, in 1956; and in Incline Village, Nevada, and surrounding communities in 1985. While these clustered cases suggest a common environmental or infectious cause, none has been identified.

The prevalence of chronic fatigue syndrome is difficult to ascertain, since its estimate depends entirely on case definition. Chronic fatigue itself is a ubiquitous symptom, occurring in as many as 20 percent of patients attending a general medical clinic; the chronic fatigue syndrome is far less common. The CDC estimated that its original case definition for chronic fatigue syndrome is met by 2 to 7 individuals per 100,000 population. The revised case definition eliminated many of the ambiguities and some of the restrictions of the original definition. Although this definition will be easier for the clinician to apply, a slightly greater percentage of fatigued people will fulfill the revised criteria.

PATHOGENESIS The diverse names for the syndrome reflect the equally numerous and controversial hypotheses about its etiology.

Table 384-2

Revised CDC Criteria for Chronic Fatigue Syndrome

A case of chronic fatigue syndrome is defined by the presence of:

1. Clinically evaluated, unexplained, persistent or relapsing fatigue that is of new or definite onset; is not the result of ongoing exertion; is not alleviated by rest; and results in substantial reduction of previous levels of occupational, educational, social, or personal activities; and
2. Four or more of the following symptoms that persist or recur during six or more consecutive months of illness and that do not predate the fatigue:
   - Self-reported impairment in short-term memory or concentration
   - Sore throat
   - Tender cervical or axillary nodes
   - Muscle pain
   - Multijoint pain without redness or swelling
   - Headaches of a new pattern or severity
   - Unrefreshing sleep
   - Postexertional malaise lasting ≥24 h

SOURCE: Adapted from Fukuda et al.

Several common themes underlie attempts to understand the disorder: It is often postinfectious, it is associated with immunologic disturbances, and it is commonly accompanied by depression.

Some contemporary workers in the field espouse one or more of several viruses as potential etiologic agents. Among these are lymphotropic herpesviruses, retroviruses, and enteroviruses. The data on which these presumptions rest are as follows: First, chronic fatigue syndrome can be precipitated by a variety of acute infections. Some of the infecting organisms have the ability to persist in humans and cause chronic illness. Second, titers of antibodies to many infectious agents are elevated in patients with chronic fatigue. Included are antibodies to most herpesviruses, measles virus, rubella virus, and coxsackievirus B. Third, there are claims of increased levels of some viral antigens and nucleic acids in patients, although these assertions are not based on firm experimental evidence. While experience suggests that viruses can precipitate the syndrome, it is unlikely that they actually contribute to its long-term features. Common, persisting viruses may simply have a greater likelihood to reactivate because of inadequate immune restraints on them, while causing no symptoms.

Numerous subtle immunologic disturbances have been reported in patients with chronic fatigue syndrome. In addition to the elevated viral antibody titers mentioned above, there are also mild, nonspecific elevations in titers of antinuclear antibodies, modest immunoglobulin subclass reductions, mild deficiencies in mitogen-induced lymphocyte proliferation in vitro and in ensuing cytokine release, reduced natural killer cell activity, and shifts in lymphocyte phenotypes to greater than normal proportions of T cells expressing activation or differentiation markers. None of the immune findings appear in all patients, nor have any been correlated, as yet, with the severity of illness. None are specific for chronic fatigue syndrome; thus they remain nondiagnostic. An immune disturbance of some type, though, is in line with one favored theory that many of the symptoms of chronic fatigue syndrome derive from excessive cytokine release.

Recent controlled studies of patients with chronic fatigue syndrome documented abnormalities in endocrine function consistent with reduced production of corticotropin-releasing hormone in the hypothalamus. Mean serum cortisol concentrations were lower in patients than in controls; levels of adrenocorticotropic hormone (ACTH) were correspondingly high. Hypothetically, these neuroendocrine abnormalities could contribute to the impaired energy and mood of patients. Whatever their importance, these changes further indicate the complex and multifactorial nature of chronic fatigue syndrome.

Mild to moderate depression is evident in about two-thirds of patients. Much of this depression may be reactive, but the prevalence exceeds that seen in other chronic medical illnesses. Thus, some propose that chronic fatigue syndrome is fundamentally a psychiatric disorder and that the various neuroendocrine and immune disturbances arise secondarily.

MANIFESTATIONS The typical case of chronic fatigue syndrome arises suddenly in a previously active individual. An otherwise unremarkable flulike illness or some other acute stress is recalled with great clarity as the triggering event. Unbearable exhaustion is left in the wake of this incident. Other symptoms, such as headache, sore throat, tender lymph nodes, muscle and joint aches, and frequent feverishness, lead to the belief that an infection persists, and medical attention is sought. Over several weeks, the impact of reassurances proffered during that initial evaluation fades as other features of the syndrome become evident—disturbed sleep, difficulty in concentration, and depression (see Table 384-1).

Depending on the dominant symptoms and the beliefs of the patient, additional consultations may be sought from allergists, rheumatologists, infectious disease specialists, psychiatrists, ecologic therapists, homeopaths, or other professionals, frequently with unsatisfactory results. Once the pattern of illness is established, the symptoms may fluctuate somewhat. Many patients report that diverse complaints are linked—that during periods of greatest fatigue they perceive the most pain and difficulty with concentration. Patients also commonly assert that excessive physical or emotional stress may exacerbate their symptoms.

Most patients remain capable of balancing their limited resources to accommodate the obligations of family, work, or community. The discretionary activities are abandoned first. Some feel unable to engage in any gainful employment. A minority of individuals require help with the activities of daily living.

Ultimately, isolation, pathetic resignation, and frustration can mark the protracted course of illness. Patients may become angry at physicians for failing to acknowledge or resolve their plight. Fortunately, the chronic fatigue syndrome does not appear to progress. On the contrary, many patients experience gradual improvement, and a minority recover fully.

DIAGNOSIS Physical examination and routine laboratory tests are required to rule out other possible causes of the patient's symptoms. Prominent findings argue strongly in favor of other processes. No laboratory test, however esoteric or exotic, can diagnose this condition or measure its severity. Elaborate, expensive workups should therefore be avoided except in research settings. The great dilemma for patient and clinician alike is that chronic fatigue syndrome has no pathognomonic features and remains a constellation of symptoms and a diagnosis of exclusion.

Rx TREATMENT

The primary responsibility of a physician confronted with a chronically fatigued patient is to address the cause by taking a thorough history, conducting a complete physical examination, judiciously using the laboratory, and, throughout this process, considering the differential diagnosis. If other illnesses are excluded, there are several points to address in the long-term care of a patient with chronic fatigue.

First, the patient should be informed about the illness and what is truly known of its pathogenesis; its potential impact on the physical, psychological, and social dimensions of life; and its prognosis. Patients are relieved when their complaints are taken seriously.

Second, periodic reassessment is appropriate to identify a possible underlying process that is late in declaring itself and to address intercurrent problems that must not be neglected as yet another subjective complaint.

Third, many symptoms of chronic fatigue syndrome respond to treatment. Nonsteroidal anti-inflammatory drugs alleviate headache, diffuse pain, and feverishness. Allergic rhinitis and sinusitis are common in patients with chronic fatigue syndrome; antihistamines or decongestants may be helpful. Although patients are often averse to psychiatric diagnoses, depression is a prominent symptom that should be confronted. Expert psychiatric assessment is sometimes advisable. Nonsedating antidepressants improve mood and disordered sleep and thereby attenuate the fatigue somewhat. Even modest improvements in symptoms can make an important difference in the patient's degree of self-sufficiency and ability to appreciate life's pleasures.

Fourth, practical advice should be given regarding lifestyle. The consumption of heavy meals with alcohol and caffeine at night can make it harder to sleep, compounding fatigue. Total rest is harmful. It leads to further deconditioning and the self-image of being an invalid. Exacerbation of exhaustion by strenuous exertion leads to total avoidance of exercise, so a moderate, carefully graded regimen needs to be encouraged.

Fifth, unproven treatments should be avoided. Controlled trials have established that acyclovir and intramuscular liver extract–folic acid–cyanocobalamin injections are of no value. Despite one encouraging study, other studies and clinical experience argue that high-dose intravenous immunoglobulin therapy is of no value. Countless anecdotes circulate regarding other traditional or nontraditional therapies. It is important to guide patients, flexibly, away from those therapeutic modalities which are most toxic, expensive, and unreasonable.

The physician should promote the patient's efforts toward improvement. A clinical trial in England showed behavioral therapy to be helpful. The therapy was aimed at dispelling cognitive distortions that lead to inactivity and despair. For chronic fatigue syndrome, as for many conditions, a comprehensive approach to physical, psychological, and social aspects is in order.

BIBLIOGRAPHY

ACHESON ED: The clinical syndrome variously called benign myalgic encephalomyelitis, Iceland disease and epidemic neuromyasthenia. Am J Med 26:569, 1959

BOCK GR, WHELAN J (eds): Ciba Found Symp 173, 1993

FUKUDA K et al: The chronic fatigue syndrome: A comprehensive approach to its definition and study. Ann Intern Med 121:953, 1994

HOLMES GP et al: Chronic fatigue syndrome: A working case definition. Ann Intern Med 108:387, 1988

STRAUS SE (ed): *Chronic Fatigue Syndrome*. New York, Marcel Dekker, 1994

SECTION 5

PSYCHIATRIC DISORDERS

385

Victor I. Reus

MENTAL DISORDERS

The term "mental disorders," as defined in the 4th edition of the standard psychiatric Diagnostic and Statistical Manual (DSM-IV), encompasses a broad range of conditions characterized by patterns of abnormal behavioral and psychological signs and symptoms that result in dysfunction. The implication that mental disorders lack a physical cause is unfortunate and incorrect, and the term survives only for want of a better substitute. Mental disorders are highly prevalent in medical practice, although frequently unrecognized and untreated, and may present as either a primary disorder or as a comorbid condition. Physicians must be prepared to initiate prompt diagnosis and treatment planning of mental disorders to ensure that their patients receive appropriate medical services and that they have the best outcome possible.

The current nosologic system is multiaxial and assesses the presence or absence of a major mental disorder (axis I), any underlying personality disorder (axis II), general medical condition (axis III), psychosocial and environmental problems (axis IV), and overall rating of general psychosocial functioning (axis V). Given our current limited understanding of the etiology of most mental disorders, DSM-IV emphasizes phenomenology and is thus both empirical and atheoretical. The DSM-IV emphasis on strict operational criteria has resulted in high reliability for psychiatric diagnoses and in improved treatment and management.

Current changes in health care delivery underscore the need for primary care physicians to assume responsibility for the initial diagnosis and treatment of the most common mental disorders. Valid patient-based questionnaires have been developed that systematically probe for signs and symptoms associated with the most prevalent psychiatric diagnoses and guide the clinician into a more targeted historical assessment. Prime MD (from Roerig/Pfizer, New York) and the Symptom-Driven Diagnostic System for Primary Care (SDDS-PC) (from Pharmacia-Upjohn, Kalamazoo, MI) are inventories that require only 10 min to complete, in which patient responses can be linked to the formal diagnostic criteria of anxiety, mood, somatoform, and eating disorders, and alcohol abuse or dependence.

This chapter surveys the most commonly encountered conditions in general medical practice and focuses on illnesses whose treatment is likely to be the responsibility of the primary care practitioner rather than the specialist. A physician who refers patients to a psychiatrist must know not only when doing so is appropriate but also how to do it, since societal misconceptions and the stigma of mental illness impede the process. Primary care physicians should base referrals to a psychiatrist on the presence of the signs and symptoms of a mental disorder, and not simply on the absence of physical elements for a patient's complaint. Education of the patient and formation of an alliance are crucial to the success of treatment. Although some of the conditions and states discussed are outside the scope of primary care practice, their prompt recognition is often essential to avoid significant morbidity. When physicians encounter evidence of psychotic symptoms, mania, severe depression or anxiety, dissociative symptoms, suicidal or homicidal preoccupation, or a failure to respond to first-order treatment, consultation with a psychiatrist or transfer of care must be initiated. → *Eating disorders are discussed in Chap. 76.*

ANXIETY DISORDERS

Anxiety disorders, the most prevalent psychiatric illnesses in the general community, are present in 15 to 20 percent of medical clinic patients. Anxiety, defined as a subjective sense of unease, dread, or foreboding, can indicate a primary psychiatric condition, or it can be a component of, or reaction to, a primary medical disease. The primary anxiety disorders are classified according to their duration and course and the existence and nature of precipitants.

When evaluating the anxious patient, the clinician must first determine whether the anxiety antedates or postdates a medical illness or is due to a medication side effect. Approximately one-third of medical patients presenting with anxiety have an organic etiology for their psychiatric symptoms, but an anxiety disorder can also present with somatic symptoms in the absence of a diagnosable medical condition.

PANIC DISORDER Clinical Manifestations Panic disorder is defined by the presence of recurrent and unpredictable panic attacks, which are distinct episodes of intense fear and discomfort associated with a variety of physical symptoms, including palpitations, sweating, trembling, shortness of breath, chest pain, and dizziness, and a fear of impending doom or death (Table 385-1). Paresthesia, gastrointestinal distress, and feelings of unreality are also common. Panic attacks have a sudden onset, developing within 10 min and usually resolving over the course of an hour, and they occur in an unexpected fashion. The frequency and severity of panic attacks varies, ranging from once a week to clusters of attacks separated by months of well-being. The first attack is usually outside the home. Onset is usually in late adolescence to early adulthood. In some individuals, anticipatory anxiety develops over time and results in a generalized fear and a progressive avoidance of places or situations in which a panic attack might recur. *Agoraphobia*, which occurs commonly in patients with panic disorder, is an acquired irrational fear of being in places where one might feel trapped or unable to escape (Table 385-2). Typically it leads the patient into a progressive restriction in life-style and, in a literal sense, in geography. Because patients develop embarrassment about being housebound and dependent on the company of others to go out into the world, physicians may under-recognize the syndrome if they do not pursue direct questioning.

Differential Diagnosis A diagnosis of panic disorder is made after an organic etiology for the panic attacks has been ruled out (Fig. 385-1). A variety of cardiovascular, respiratory, endocrine, and neurologic conditions can present with anxiety as the chief complaint, and patients with true panic disorder will often focus on one specific feature to the exclusion of others. Twenty percent of patients who present with syncope as a primary medical complaint, for example, have a primary mood, anxiety, or substance-abuse diagnosis, the most common being panic disorder. The differential diagnosis of panic disorder is complicated by a high rate of comorbidity with other psychiatric conditions, especially alcohol and benzodiazepine abuse, which patients initially use in an attempt at self-medication. Seventy-five percent of panic disorder patients will also satisfy criteria for major depression at some point in their illness.

When the history of present illness is nonspecific, physical examination and focused laboratory testing must be used to rule out organic anxiety states, such as those resulting from pheochromocytoma, thyrotoxicosis, or hypoglycemia. Electrocardiogram and echocardiogram may detect cardiovascular conditions associated with panic, such as paroxysmal atrial tachycardia and mitral valve prolapse, but in other conditions, such as hyperdynamic beta-adrenergic state, it is difficult to make a meaningful distinction between the independent psychiatric and cardiologic diagnoses. In two studies, panic disorder was the primary diagnosis in 43 percent of patients with chest pain who had normal coronary angiograms and was present in 9 percent of all outpatients referred for cardiac evaluation. Panic disorder has also been diagnosed in many patients referred for pulmonary function testing or having symptoms of irritable bowel syndrome.

Table 385-1

Diagnostic Criteria for Panic Attack

A discrete period of intense fear or discomfort, in which four (or more) of the following symptoms developed abruptly and reached a peak within 10 min:

1. Palpitations, pounding heart, or accelerated heart rate
2. Sweating
3. Trembling or shaking
4. Sensations of shortness of breath or smothering
5. Feeling of choking
6. Chest pain or discomfort
7. Nausea or abdominal distress
8. Feeling dizzy, unsteady, lightheaded, or faint
9. Derealization (feelings of unreality) or depersonalization (being detached from oneself)
10. Fear of losing control or going crazy
11. Fear of dying
12. Paresthesia (numbness or tingling sensations)
13. Chills or hot flushes

SOURCE: *Diagnostic and Statistical Manual of Mental Disorders,* 4th ed.

Table 385-2

Diagnostic Criteria for Agoraphobia

1. Anxiety about being in places or situations from which escape might be difficult (or embarrassing) or in which help may not be available in the event of having an unexpected or situationally predisposed panic attack or panic-like symptoms. Agoraphobic fears typically involve characteristic clusters of situations that include being outside the home alone; being in a crowd or standing in a line; being on a bridge; and traveling in a bus, train, or automobile.

   Note: Consider the diagnosis of specific phobia if the avoidance is limited to one or only a few specific situations, or social phobia if the avoidance is limited to social situations.
2. The situations are avoided (e.g., travel is restricted) or else are endured with marked distress or with anxiety about having a panic attack or panic-like symptoms, or require the presence of a companion.
3. The anxiety or phobic avoidance is not better accounted for by another mental disorder, such as social phobia (e.g., avoidance limited to social situations because of fear of embarrassment), specific phobia (e.g., avoidance limited to a single situation like elevators), obsessive-compulsive disorder (e.g., avoidance of dirt in someone with an obsession about contamination), posttraumatic stress disorder (e.g., avoidance of stimuli associated with a severe stressor), or separation anxiety disorder (e.g., avoidance of leaving home or relatives).

SOURCE: *Diagnostic and Statistical Manual of Mental Disorders,* 4th ed.

Etiology and Pathophysiology The etiology of panic disorder is unknown but appears to involve a genetic predisposition, altered autonomic responsivity, and social learning. Panic disorder shows familial aggregation, although the estimate of concordance in monozygotic twins is only 30 percent. Acute panic attacks appear to be associated with increased noradrenergic discharge in the locus ceruleus. Intravenous infusion of sodium lactate evokes an attack predictably in two-thirds of panic disorder patients, as do the alpha$_2$-adrenergic antagonist yohimbine and carbon dioxide inhalation. It is hypothesized that each of these stimuli activates a neural circuit involving noradrenergic neurons in the locus ceruleus and serotonergic neurons in the dorsal raphe. Although the noradrenergic theory of panic attacks has proved empirically useful, a number of contradictory findings exist. For example, increases in noradrenergic metabolites are not consistently observed during provocative challenge testing. A serotonergic contribution is better established; infusion of the serotonin (5HT) agonist *m*-chlorophenylproperazine induces anxiety in panic-disorder patients but not in control subjects, and agents that block serotonin reuptake are therapeutic in preventing attacks. It is likely that panic-disorder

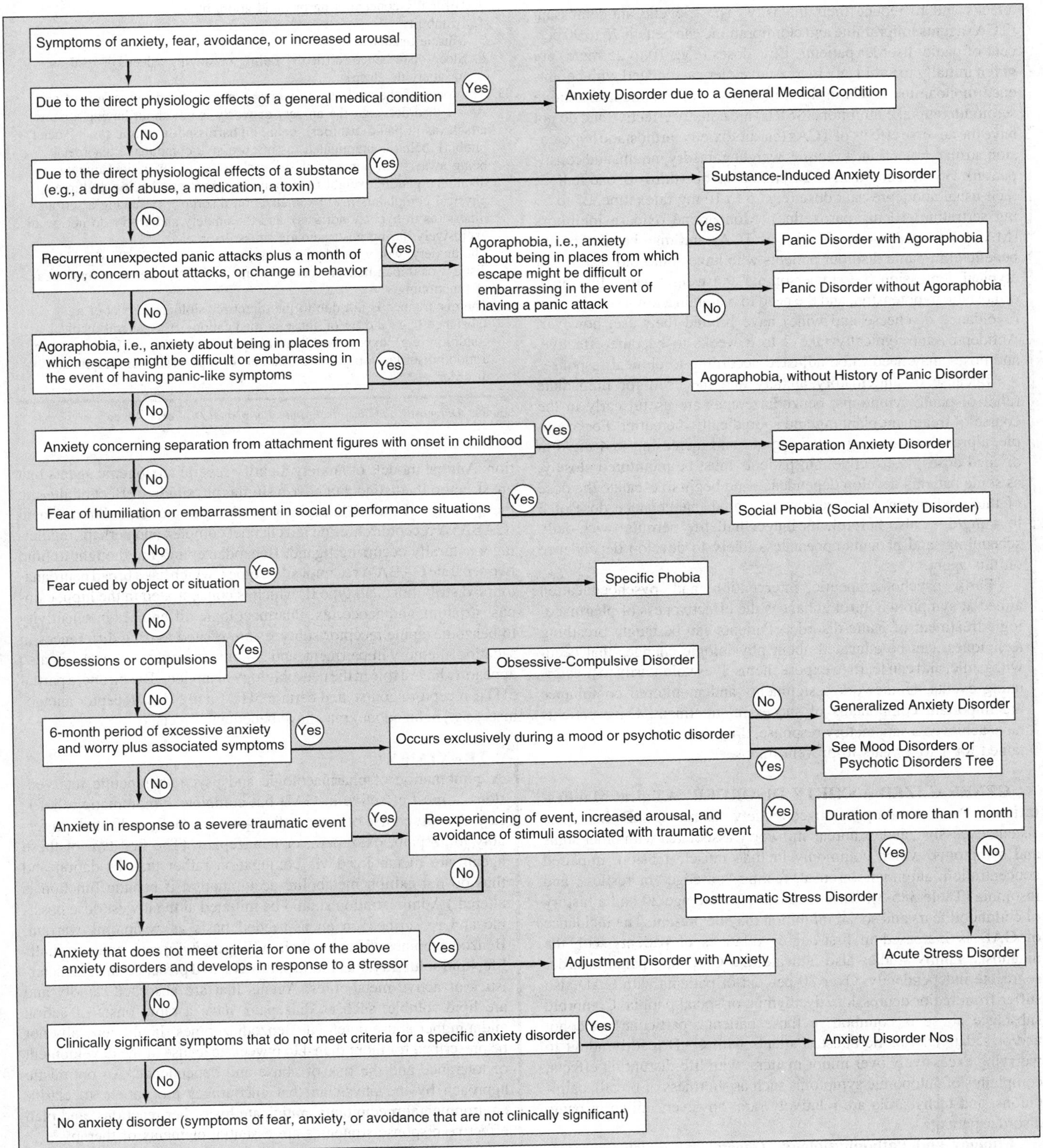

FIGURE 385-1 Differential diagnosis of anxiety disorders. NOS, not otherwise specified. *(From Diagnostic and Statistical Manual of Mental Disorders, 4th ed.)*

patients have a heightened sensitivity to somatic symptoms, which results in positive feedback to control autonomic systems and triggers increasing arousal, setting off the "panic attack" mechanism. Accordingly, successful therapeutic intervention involves altering the patient's cognitive interpretation of anxiety-producing experiences as well as preventing the attack itself.

Rx TREATMENT

Achievable goals of treatment are to decrease the frequency of panic attacks and to reduce their intensity. The tricyclic antidepressant (TCA) agents imipramine and clomipramine can benefit 75 to 90 percent of panic-disorder patients. Low doses (e.g., 10 to 25 mg/d) are given initially to avoid any increased anxiety associated with heightened monoamine levels in the initial stages of treatment. Selective serotonin reuptake inhibitors (SSRIs) are equally effective and do not have the adverse effects of TCAs (cardiotoxicity, orthostatic hypotension, urinary retention, sweating, weight gain, dry mouth, and constipation). SSRIs should also be started at one-third to one-half of their usual antidepressant dose (e.g., 5 to 10 mg fluoxetine, 25 to 50 mg sertraline, 10 mg paroxetine). Monoamine oxidase inhibitors (MAOIs) are at least as effective as TCAs and may be specifically beneficial in panic disorder patients who have comorbid features of atypical depression (i.e., hypersomnia and weight gain). Insomnia, orthostatic hypotension, and the need to maintain a low-tyramine diet (avoidance of cheese and wine) have limited their use, however. Antidepressants typically take 2 to 6 weeks to become effective, and doses may need to be adjusted according to clinical response.

Because of anticipatory anxiety and the need for immediate relief of panic symptoms, benzodiazepines are useful early in the course of treatment planning and sporadically thereafter. For example, alprazolam, starting at 0.5 mg qid and increasing to 4 mg/d in divided doses, is effective, but patients must be monitored closely, as some patients develop dependence and begin to escalate the dose of this medication. Clonazepam, at a final maintenance dose of 2 to 4 mg/d, is also helpful; its longer half life permits twice-daily scheduling, and patients appear less likely to develop dependence on this agent.

Early psychotherapeutic intervention and pyschoeducation aimed at symptom control enhances the effectiveness of pharmacologic treatment of panic disorder. Patients can be taught breathing techniques, can be educated about physiologic changes that occur with panic, and can learn to expose themselves voluntarily to precipitating events. Homework assignments and monitored compliance are important components of successful treatment. Once patients have achieved a satisfactory response, drug treatment must be maintained for 1 to 2 years to prevent relapse.

GENERALIZED ANXIETY DISORDER Clinical Manifestations Patients with generalized anxiety disorder (GAD) have persistent, excessive, and/or unrealistic worry associated with other signs and symptoms, which commonly include muscle tension, impaired concentration, autonomic arousal, feeling "on edge" or restless, and insomnia (Table 385-3). Onset is usually before age 20 and a history of childhood fears and social inhibition may be present. The incidence of GAD is increased in first-degree relatives of patients with the diagnosis; family studies also indicate that GAD and panic disorder segregate independently. Over 80 percent of patients with GAD also suffer from major depression, dysthymia, or social phobia. Comorbid substance abuse is common in these patients, particularly alcohol and/or sedative/hypnotic abuse. Patients with GAD readily admit to worrying excessively over minor matters, with life-disrupting effects; complaints of autonomic symptoms such as shortness of breath, palpitations, and tachycardia are relatively rare, however, unlike in panic disorder patients.

Etiology and Pathophysiology Generalized anxiety disorders are thought to result from aberrations in benzodiazepine receptor regulation. Animal models of anxiety identify several anxiogenic agents that are structurally distinct but have a similar physiologic effect of altering the binding of benzodiazepines to the gamma-aminobutyric acid (GABA) A receptor/chloride ion channel complex and perhaps regulating a naturally occurring ligand. Benzodiazepines are thought to bind two separate GABA A receptor sites: type I, which has a broad neuroanatomic distribution, and type II, which is concentrated in the hippocampus, striatum, and neocortex. Pharmacologic differences in sensitivity to benzodiazepine receptor subtypes are related to drug differences in sedation, memory impairment, and antianxiety efficacy. Serotonin also appears to have a role in the neurobiology of anxiety. Buspirone, a partial $5HT_{1A}$ receptor agonist, and certain $5HT_{2A}$ and $5HT_{2C}$ receptor antagonists (e.g., nefazodone) may have beneficial effects.

Table 385-3

Diagnostic Criteria for Generalized Anxiety Disorder

A. Excessive anxiety and worry (apprehensive expectation), occurring more days than not for at least 6 months, about a number of events or activities (such as work or school performance).
B. The person finds it difficult to control the worry.
C. The anxiety and worry are associated with three (or more) of the following six symptoms (with at least some symptoms present for more days than not for the past 6 months). **Note:** Only one item is required in children.
   1. Restlessness or feeling keyed up or on edge
   2. Being easily fatigued
   3. Difficulty concentrating or mind going blank
   4. Irritability
   5. Muscle tension
   6. Sleep disturbance (difficulty falling or staying asleep, or restless unsatisfying sleep)
D. The focus of the anxiety and worry is not confined to features of an Axis I disorder, e.g., the anxiety or worry is not about having a panic attack (as in panic disorder), being embarrassed in public (as in social phobia), being contaminated (as in obsessive-compulsive disorder), being away from home or close relatives (as in separation anxiety disorder), gaining weight (as in anorexia nervosa), having multiple physical complaints (as in somatization disorder), or having a serious illness (as in hypochondriasis), and the anxiety and worry do not occur exclusively during posttraumatic stress disorder.
E. The anxiety, worry, or physical symptoms cause clinically significant distress or impairment in social, occupational, or other important areas of functioning.
F. The disturbance is not due to the direct physiologic effects of a substance (e.g., a drug of abuse, a medication) or a general medical condition (e.g., hyperthyroidism) and does not occur exclusively during a mood disorder, a psychotic disorder, or a pervasive developmental disorder.

SOURCE: *Diagnostic and Statistical Manual of Mental Disorders,* 4th ed.

Rx TREATMENT

A combination of pharmacologic and psychotherapeutic interventions is most effective in GAD but complete symptomatic relief is rare. A short course of a benzodiazepine is usually indicated, preferably lorazepam, oxazepam, or temazepam. (The first two of these agents are metabolized via conjugation rather than oxidation and thus do not exhibit metabolite accumulation if hepatic function is altered.) Administration should be initiated at the lowest dose possible and prescribed on an as-needed basis as symptoms warrant. Benzodiazepines differ in their milligram/kilogram potency, half-life, lipid solubility, metabolic pathways, and presence and characteristics of active metabolites. Agents that are absorbed rapidly and are lipid soluble, such as diazepam, have a rapid onset of action and a higher abuse potential. Benzodiazepines should generally not be prescribed for more than 4 to 6 weeks because of the development of tolerance and the risk of abuse and dependence. An optimistic approach by the physician that encourages the patient to clarify environmental precipitants, anticipate his or her reactions, and plan effective response strategies are essential elements of therapy.

The adverse effects of benzodiazepines generally parallel their relative half lives. Longer-acting agents, such as diazepam, chlordiazepoxide, flurazepam, clorazepate, halazepam, and prazepam, tend to show accumulation of active metabolites, with sedation, impairment of cognition, and psychomotor performance, while use of shorter-acting compounds, such as alprazolam and oxazepam, can result in daytime anxiety, early morning insomnia, and rebound anxiety and insomnia with discontinuation. Although patients develop tolerance to the sedative effects of benzodiazepines, they are less likely to habituate to the adverse psychomotor effects. It is generally easier to withdraw patients from the longer-half-life benzodiazepines. Withdrawal can be accomplished through gradual, stepwise dose reduction (by approximately 10 percent every 1 to 2 weeks) over a period of 6 to 12 weeks. It is usually much more difficult to taper patients off shorter-acting benzodiazepines. Physicians may need to switch the patient to a benzodiazepine with a longer half life or use an adjunctive medication, such as a beta blocker or carbamazepine, before attempting to discontinue the benzodiazepine. Withdrawal reactions vary in severity and duration; they can include depression, anxiety, delirium, lethargy, diaphoresis, tinnitus, autonomic arousal, unusual neuromuscular movements, and, rarely, seizures.

Buspirone, an azaspirone, is a nonbenzodiazepine anxiolytic agent. It is nonsedating, does not lead to tolerance or dependence, does not interact with benzodiazepine receptors or alcohol, and has no abuse or disinhibition potential. However, it requires several weeks to take effect and requires thrice-daily dosing (occasionally up to 20 mg tid). An extended release version of the drug has recently been introduced and may result in increased treatment adherence. Patients who were previously responsive to a benzodiazepine are unlikely to rate the drug as being equally effective. Patients with head injury or dementia who have symptoms of anxiety and/or agitation may do well with this agent.

Administration of benzodiazepines to geriatric patients requires special care. Such patients have increased drug absorption, decreased hepatic metabolism, protein binding, renal excretion, and an increased volume of distribution, which, together with the likely presence of comorbid medical illnesses and medication, dramatically increase the likelihood of toxicity. Iatrogenic psychomotor impairment can result in falls and fractures, confusional states, or motor vehicle accidents. If used, agents in this class should be started at the lowest possible dose, and results should be monitored closely. Benzodiazepines are contraindicated during pregnancy and lactation.

PHOBIC DISORDERS Clinical Manifestations The cardinal feature of phobic disorders is a marked and persistent fear of objects or situations, exposure to which results in an immediate anxiety reaction. The patient avoids the phobic stimulus, and this avoidance usually impairs occupational or social functioning. Panic attacks may be triggered by the phobic stimulus or may emerge spontaneously during the course of the illness. Unlike patients with other anxiety disorders, individuals with phobias experience anxiety only in specific and identifiable situations. Common phobias include fear of closed spaces (claustrophobia), fear of blood, and fear of flying. Social phobia is distinguished by a specific fear of social or performance situations in which the individual is exposed to unfamiliar individuals or to possible examination and evaluation by others. Examples include having to converse at a party, use public restrooms, and meet strangers. In each case, the affected individual is aware that the experienced fear is excessive and unreasonable given the circumstance. The specific content of a phobia may vary across gender, ethnic, and cultural boundaries.

Phobic disorders are common, with a 1-year prevalence rate of 9 percent and a lifetime rate of 10 to 11 percent. The onset is in childhood to early adulthood, and familial aggregation may occur. In female twins, concordance rates for agoraphobia, social phobia, and animal phobia of 23 percent for monozygotic twins and 15 percent for dizygotic twins are reported. Full criteria for diagnosis are usually evident first in adults, but behavioral avoidance in infancy of unfamiliar people, situations, or objects is common in the history of patients.

Rx TREATMENT

Recent controlled trials have documented the efficacy of several pharmacologic agents in the treatment of phobic disorders. Beta blockers are particularly effective in the treatment of "performance anxiety" (but not general social phobia) and appear to achieve their benefit by preventing the occurrence of peripheral manifestations of anxiety, such as perspiration, tachycardia, palpitations, and tremor. MAOIs alleviate social phobia independently of their antidepressant activity, and SSRIs appear to be effective also. Benzodiazepines can be helpful in reducing fearful avoidance, but the chronic nature of phobic disorders limits their usefulness.

Behaviorally focused psychotherapy is an important component of treatment, as relapse rates are high when medication is used as the sole treatment. Cognitive-behavioral strategies are the keystone of treatment and derive from the finding that patients' distorted perceptions and interpretations of fear-producing stimuli play a major role in perpetuation of phobias. Individual and group therapy sessions teach the patient to identify specific negative thoughts associated with the anxiety-producing situation, and help to reduce the patient's fear of loss of control. In desensitization therapy, hierarchies of feared situations are constructed and the patient is encouraged to pursue and master gradual exposure to the anxiety-producing stimuli.

Patients with social phobia, in particular, have a high rate of comorbid alcohol abuse, as well as of other psychiatric conditions (e.g., eating disorders), necessitating the need for parallel management of each disorder if anxiety reduction is to be achieved.

STRESS DISORDERS Clinical Manifestations Patients may develop significant anxiety after exposure to extreme trauma, defined as an event associated with either actual or threatened death or injury to oneself or another. The reaction may occur shortly after the traumatic exposure, (*acute stress disorder*) or be delayed in time and subject to recurrence (*posttraumatic stress disorder*, PTSD) (Table 385-4). In both syndromes, individuals experience associated symptoms of detachment and loss of emotional responsivity. The patient may feel depersonalized and unable to recall specific aspects of the trauma, though typically it is reexperienced through intrusions in thought, dreams, or flashbacks, particularly when cues of the original event are present. Accordingly, patients often actively avoid stimuli that precipitate recollections of the trauma and demonstrate a resulting increase in vigilance, arousal, and startle response. Patients with stress disorders are at increased risk for the development of other anxiety, mood, and substance-related disorders. Between 5 and 10 percent of Americans will at some time in their life satisfy the full criteria for PTSD with women more likely to be affected than men.

Risk factors for the development of PTSD include a past psychiatric history and personality characteristics of high neuroticism and extroversion. Studies of monozygotic and dizygotic twins showed a substantial influence of genetics on all symptoms associated with PTSD, with no evidence for an environment effect.

Etiology and Pathophysiology It is hypothesized that in PTSD there is impaired alpha$_2$-adrenergic receptor feedback inhibition to stress-induced release of norepinephrine from the locus ceruleus, with a progressive behavioral sensitization and generalization to stimulus cues associated with the original trauma. Increased noradrenergic activity at locus ceruleus projection sites in hippocampus and amygdala theoretically facilitates encoding of fear-based memories which persist and resist extinction. In clinical studies, diminished serotonergic effects, reduction in cortisol release, and increased sensitivity of cortisol to dexamethasone inhibition distinguish patients with PTSD from control subjects. Greater sympathetic responses to cues associated with trauma are shown by laboratory findings of increased release of norepinephrine in response to challenge. Altered alpha$_2$- and beta-adrenergic receptor binding and a lowered activity of platelet adenylate cyclase have also been reported.

Table 385-4

Diagnostic Criteria for Posttraumatic Stress Disorder

A. The person has been exposed to a traumatic event in which both of the following were present:
   1. The person experienced, witnessed, or was confronted with an event or events that involved actual or threatened death or serious injury, or a threat to the physical integrity of self or others.
   2. The person's response involved intense fear, helplessness, or horror. **Note:** In children, this may be expressed instead by disorganized or agitated behavior.

B. The traumatic event is persistently reexperienced in one (or more) of the following ways:
   1. Recurrent and intrusive distressing recollections of the event, including images, thoughts, or perceptions. **Note:** In young children, repetitive play may occur in which themes or aspects of the trauma are expressed.
   2. Recurrent distressing dreams of the event. **Note:** In children, there may be frightening dreams without recognizable content.
   3. Acting or feeling as if the traumatic event were recurring (includes a sense of reliving the experience, illusions, hallucinations, and dissociative flashback episodes, including those that occur on awakening or when intoxicated). **Note:** In young children, trauma-specific reenactment may occur.
   4. Intense psychological distress at exposure to internal or external cues that symbolize or resemble an aspect of the traumatic event.
   5. Physiologic reactivity on exposure to internal or external cues that symbolize or resemble an aspect of the traumatic event.

C. Persistent avoidance of stimuli associated with the trauma and numbing of general responsiveness (not present before the trauma), as indicated by three or more of the following:
   1. Efforts to avoid thoughts, feelings, or conversations associated with the trauma
   2. Efforts to avoid activities, places, or people that arouse recollections of the trauma
   3. Inability to recall an important aspect of the trauma
   4. Markedly diminished interest or participation in significant activities
   5. Feeling of detachment or estrangement from others
   6. Restricted range of affect (e.g., unable to have loving feelings)
   7. Sense of a foreshortened future (e.g., does not expect to have a career, marriage, children, or a normal life span)

D. Persistent symptoms of increased arousal (not present before the trauma), as indicated by two (or more) of the following:
   1. Difficulty falling or staying asleep
   2. Irritability or outbursts of anger
   3. Difficulty concentrating
   4. Hypervigilance
   5. Exaggerated startle response

E. Duration of the disturbance (symptoms in criteria B, C, and D) is more than 1 month

F. The disturbance causes clinically significant distress or impairment in social, occupational, or other important areas of functioning.

SOURCE: *Diagnostic and Statistical Manual of Mental Disorders,* 4th ed.

℞ TREATMENT

Acute stress reactions are usually self-limited, and treatment typically involves only the short-term use of benzodiazepines and supportive/expressive psychotherapy. The chronic and recurrent nature of PTSD, however, requires a more complex approach employing drug and behavioral treatments. TCAs such as imipramine and amitriptyline, the MAOI phenelzine, and the SSRIs (fluoxetine, sertraline, paroxetine) can all reduce anxiety, symptoms of intrusion, and avoidance behaviors. Trazodone, a sedating antidepressant, is frequently used at night to help with symptoms of insomnia (50 to 150 mg qid). Carbamazepine, valproic acid, or alprazolam have also independently produced symptomatic improvement in some patients in uncontrolled trials. There is frequent comorbidity with substance abuse, especially of alcohol.

Psychotherapeutic strategies are used in treatment of PTSD to help the patient overcome avoidance behaviors and demoralization and master fear of recurrence of the trauma; therapies that encourage the patient to dismantle avoidance behaviors through stepwise focusing on the experience of the traumatic event are the most effective.

OBSESSIVE-COMPULSIVE DISORDER **Clinical Manifestations** Obsessive-compulsive disorder (OCD) was previously considered a relatively rare condition, but recent epidemiologic data indicate a lifetime prevalence of 2 to 3 percent worldwide. OCD is characterized by obsessive thoughts and compulsive behaviors that impair everyday functioning. Fears of contamination and germs are common, as are handwashing, counting behaviors, and having to check and re-check such actions as whether a door is locked. The degree to which the disorder is disruptive for the individual varies, but in all cases obsessive-compulsive activities take up more than 1 h/d and are undertaken to relieve the anxiety triggered by the core fear. Patients often conceal their symptoms, usually because they are embarrassed by the content of their thoughts or the nature of their actions. Physicians must ask specific questions regarding recurrent thoughts and behaviors, particularly if physical clues such as chafed and reddened hands or patchy hair loss (from repetitive hair pulling, or *trichotillomania*) are present. Tics are sometimes associated with OCD. OCD usually has a gradual onset, beginning in early adulthood, but childhood onset is not rare. The disorder usually has a waxing and waning course, but some cases may show a steady deterioration in psychosocial functioning.

Etiology and Pathophysiology A genetic contribution to OCD is suggested by a higher monozygotic than dizygotic concordance rate and the fact that familial studies show an aggregation with Tourette's disorder. OCD is more common in males and in first-born children.

The anatomic-physiologic disturbance in obsessive-compulsive behavior is thought to involve an alteration in a frontal-subcortical neural circuit involving the orbital frontal cortex, caudate nucleus, and globus pallidus. Neuroimaging studies have demonstrated a decrease in caudate nucleus volume, abnormalities in frontal lobe white matter, and increases in glucose metabolism in the orbital cortex of the frontal lobes and the head of the caudate nucleus. The caudate nucleus seems particularly involved in the acquisition and maintenance of habit and skill learning, and interventions that are successful in reducing obsessive-compulsive behaviors are paralleled by a comparable decrease in caudate glucose metabolic rate.

℞ TREATMENT

Clomipramine, fluoxetine, and fluvoxamine are approved for the treatment of OCD. Clomipramine is a TCA that is often tolerated poorly owing to significant anticholinergic and sedative side effects at the doses required to treat the illness (150 to 250 mg/d). Its efficacy in OCD is unrelated to its antidepressant activity. Fluoxetine (40 to 60 mg/d) and fluvoxamine (100 to 300 mg/d) are as effective as clomipramine and show a more benign side-effect profile. Fluvoxamine, a structurally unique SSRI, is metabolized through the hepatic P450 microsomal system (as is fluoxetine); it appears to inhibit the III A4 isoenzyme specifically and should not be given with other drugs that act on III A4, such as terfenadine and astemizole, because life-threatening cardiac arrhythmias may result. Only 50 to 60 percent of patients with OCD show an acceptable degree of improvement with pharmacotherapy alone. In treatment-resistant cases, augmentation with other serotonergic agents, such as buspirone, or with a neuroleptic or benzodiazepine may be beneficial. When a therapeutic response is achieved, long-duration maintenance therapy is usually indicated.

Drug treatment by itself is seldom sufficient. For many individuals, particularly those with time-consuming compulsions, behavior therapy will result in as much improvement as that afforded by medication. Effective techniques include having patients gradually increase their exposure to stressful situations, having them keep a diary to clarify stressors, and having them perform homework assignments where they substitute new activities for their compulsive behavior.

MOOD DISORDERS

Mood disorders are characterized by a disturbance in the regulation of mood, behavior, and affect. Mood disorders are subdivided into (1) depressive disorders, (2) bipolar disorders, and (3) depression in association with medical illness or alcohol and substance abuse (see Chaps. 386 through 388) (Fig. 385-2). Depressive disorders are differentiated from bipolar disorders by the absence of a manic or hypomanic episode. The etiopathogenic relationship between pure depressive syndromes and bipolar disorders is not well understood; depression occurs at increased frequency in families of bipolar individuals, but the reverse is not true, suggesting that depressive disorders are etiologically heterogeneous. Because of their common occurrence in general medical practice, mood disorders secondary to medical illness will be discussed first.

DEPRESSION IN ASSOCIATION WITH MEDICAL ILLNESS Depression occurring in the context of medical illness is difficult to evaluate. Depressive symptomatology may reflect the psychological stress of coping with the disease, may be caused by the disease process itself or by the medications used to treat it, or may simply coexist in time with the medical diagnosis.

Virtually every class of *medication* includes some agent that can induce depression. Antihypertensive drugs, anticholesterolemic agents, and antiarrhythmic agents are commonly-used classes of medications that can trigger depressive symptoms. Among the antihypertensive agents, beta-adrenergic blockers and, to a lesser extent, calcium channel blockers are the most likely to cause depressed mood. Iatrogenic depression should be considered in patients receiving, corticosteroids, antimicrobials, systemic analgesics, antiparkinsonian medications, and anticonvulsants. To decide whether a causal relationship exists between pharmacologic therapy and a patient's change in mood, it is necessary to examine the chronology of symptoms and sometimes ultimately to undertake an empirical trial of an alternative medication.

Twenty to thirty percent of *cardiac patients* manifest a depressive disorder; an even higher percentage endorse depressive symptomatology when self-reporting scales are used. Depressive symptoms following myocardial infarction have a negative effect on rehabilitation and predict a higher rate of mortality and medical morbidity. Depressed patients often show decreased variability in heart rate (an index of reduced parasympathetic nervous system activity), and this has been proposed as one mechanism by which depression may predispose individuals to ventricular arrhythmia and increased morbidity. Although TCAs have been used to treat depression in individuals with cardiac disease for a number of years, and although the quinidine-like effect of tricyclics may be useful in patients with preexisting arrhythmias, TCAs are contraindicated in patients with preexisting bundle branch block. They may also paradoxically precipitate arrhythmias in a subset of patients. Tricyclic-induced tachycardia is an additional concern in patients with congestive heart failure. Even though experience with the SSRIs is more limited, thus far they appear not to induce electrocardiographic changes or adverse cardiac events. SSRIs may interfere with hepatic metabolism of anticoagulants, however, resulting in an increase in the blood level of those drugs and in the bleeding time.

Epidemiologic surveys of depression in patients with *cancer* show a wide variability in prevalence, as might be predicted by differences in tumor site, severity of illness, and type of medical or surgical intervention. There is an overall mean prevalence of 25 percent, but depression occurs in 40 to 50 percent of patients with cancers of the pancreas or oropharynx. Assessment of the validity of prevalence rates is complicated by the fact that extreme cachexia may be misinterpreted as part of the symptom complex of the psychiatric diagnosis. The higher prevalence of depression in patients with pancreatic cancer nevertheless persists when patients are stratified and compared to others with advanced gastric cancer. Initiation of antidepressant medication in cancer patients has been shown to improve quality of life as well as mood. Psychotherapeutic approaches, particularly group therapy, may have some effect on short-term depression, anxiety, and pain symptoms and on recurrence rates and long-term survival. In a study of female patients with metastatic breast cancer, patients in group therapy had longer survival than control patients.

Depression occurs frequently in patients with *neurologic disorders*, particularly cerebrovascular disorders, Parkinson's disease, multiple sclerosis, and traumatic brain injury. Left-hemisphere strokes, particularly those involving the dorsal lateral frontal cortex, are most likely to cause depression. Both tricyclic and SSRI antidepressants are effective in the treatment of depression secondary to stroke, as are stimulant compounds and, in some patients, MAOIs.

The reported prevalence of depression in patients with *diabetes mellitus* varies from 8.5 to 27.3 percent, with the severity of the mood state correlating with the physical symptoms of illness and the degree of hyperglycemia. Pharmacologic treatment of depression is complicated by the fact that different antidepressants have different effects on blood glucose level. MAOIs can induce hypoglycemia and weight gain, while TCAs can lead to hyperglycemia and carbohydrate craving. SSRIs, like MAOIs, may cause a reduction in fasting plasma glucose, but they are easier to use. SSRIs result in better dietary and medication compliance.

Clinical hypothyroidism is frequently associated with features of depression, most commonly depressed mood and memory impairment. Hyperthyroid states may also present in a similar fashion, usually in geriatric populations. Improvement in mood usually follows normalization of thyroid function, but adjunctive antidepressant medication is sometimes required. Patients with more subtle thyroid dysfunction, such as subclinical hypothyroidism, can also experience symptoms of depression and cognitive difficulty that respond to thyroid replacement.

DEPRESSIVE DISORDERS **Clinical Manifestations** *Major depression* is defined as depressed mood on a daily basis for a minimum duration of 2 weeks (Table 385-5). An episode may be characterized by sadness, indifference or apathy, or irritability and is usually associated with change in a number of neurovegetative functions, including sleep patterns and appetite and weight, motor agitation or retardation, fatigue, impairment in concentration and decision making, feelings of shame or guilt, and thoughts of death or dying. Patients with endogenous depression have a profound loss of pleasure in all enjoyable activities, exhibit early morning awakening, feel that the dysphoric mood state is qualitatively different from sadness, and often notice a diurnal variation in mood (worse in morning hours). Paradoxically, these more severe features predict a good response to antidepressant treatment.

Approximately 15 percent of the general population experiences a major depressive episode at some point in life, and 6 to 8 percent of all outpatients in primary care settings satisfy diagnostic criteria for the disorder. Depression is often undiagnosed, however, and, even more frequently, it is treated inadequately. If a physician suspects the presence of a major depressive episode, the initial task is to determine whether it represents unipolar or bipolar depression or is one of the 10 to 15 percent of cases that are secondary to general medical illness or substance abuse. Physicians should also assess the risk of suicide by direct questioning, as patients are often reluctant to verbalize such thoughts without prompting. If specific plans are uncovered or if significant risk factors exist (e.g., a past history of suicide attempts, profound hopelessness, concurrent medical illness, substance abuse, or social isolation), the patient must be referred to a mental health specialist for immediate care. Nearly 15 percent of patients whose depressive illness goes untreated will commit suicide; most of these patients will have sought help from a physician within 1 month of their death.

In some depressed patients, the mood disorder does not appear to be episodic and is not as clearly associated with either psychosocial dysfunction or change from the individual's usual experience in life. *Dysthymic disorder* consists in a pattern of chronic (at least 2 years), ongoing, mild depressive symptoms that are less severe and less disabling than those found in major depression; the two conditions are sometimes difficult to separate, however, and can occur together ("double depression"). Interestingly, many patients who exhibit a profile of pessimism, disinterest, and low self-esteem respond to antidepressant treatment. Dysthymic disorder exists in approximately 5 percent of primary care patients.

Studies of various cultures have shown that external manifestations of depression differ but the core symptoms remain the same. The

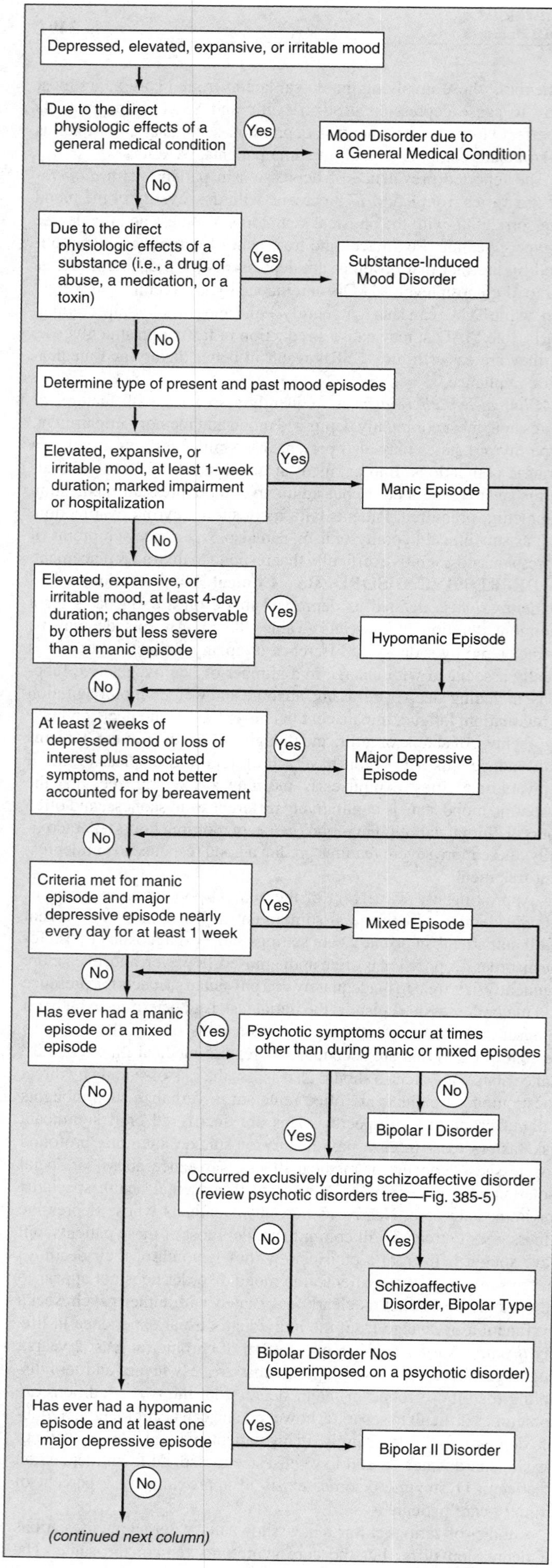
Depressed, elevated, expansive, or irritable mood
Due to the direct physiologic effects of a general medical condition
Yes
Mood Disorder due to a General Medical Condition
No
Due to the direct physiologic effects of a substance (i.e., a drug of abuse, a medication, or a toxin)
Yes
Substance-Induced Mood Disorder
No
Determine type of present and past mood episodes
Elevated, expansive, or irritable mood, at least 1-week duration; marked impairment or hospitalization
Yes
Manic Episode
No
Elevated, expansive, or irritable mood, at least 4-day duration; changes observable by others but less severe than a manic episode
Yes
Hypomanic Episode
No
At least 2 weeks of depressed mood or loss of interest plus associated symptoms, and not better accounted for by bereavement
Yes
Major Depressive Episode
No
Criteria met for manic episode and major depressive episode nearly every day for at least 1 week
Yes
Mixed Episode
No
Has ever had a manic episode or a mixed episode
Yes
Psychotic symptoms occur at times other than during manic or mixed episodes
No
Bipolar I Disorder
Yes
Occurred exclusively during schizoaffective disorder (review psychotic disorders tree—Fig. 385-5)
No
Yes
Schizoaffective Disorder, Bipolar Type
Bipolar Disorder Nos (superimposed on a psychotic disorder)
No
Has ever had a hypomanic episode and at least one major depressive episode
Yes
Bipolar II Disorder
No
(continued next column)

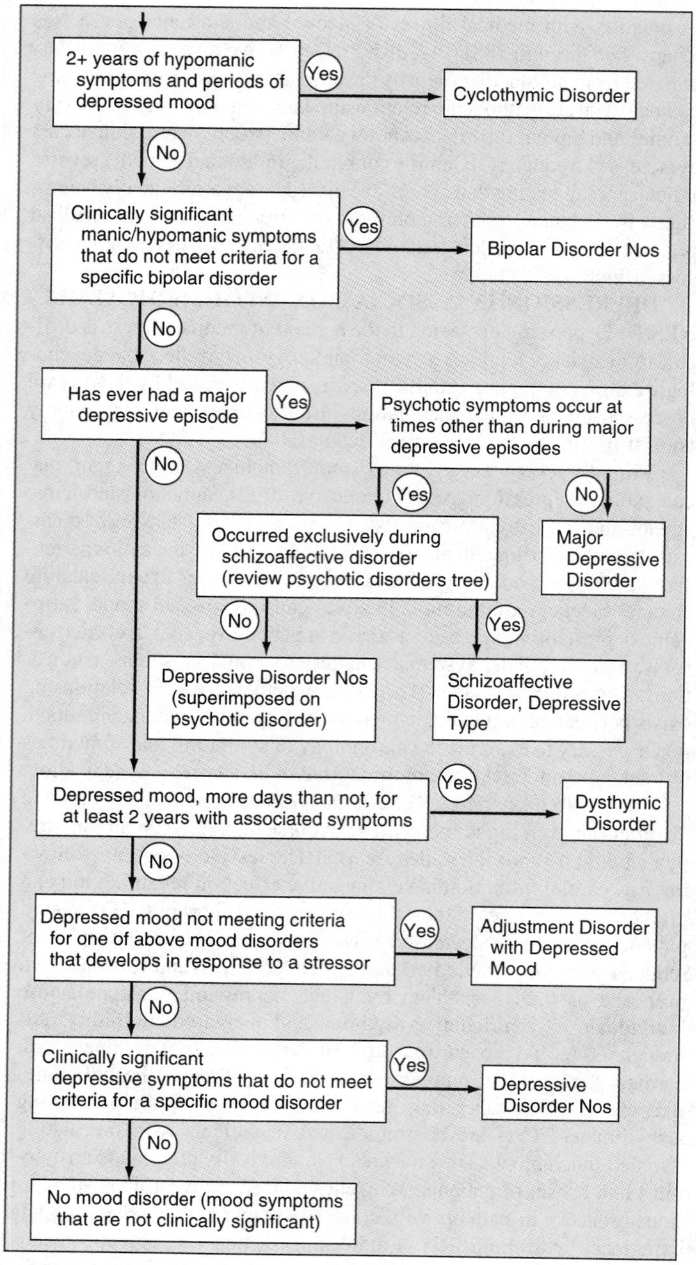
2+ years of hypomanic symptoms and periods of depressed mood
Yes
Cyclothymic Disorder
No
Clinically significant manic/hypomanic symptoms that do not meet criteria for a specific bipolar disorder
Yes
Bipolar Disorder Nos
No
Has ever had a major depressive episode
Yes
Psychotic symptoms occur at times other than during major depressive episodes
No
Yes
No
Occurred exclusively during schizoaffective disorder (review psychotic disorders tree)
Major Depressive Disorder
No
Yes
Depressive Disorder Nos (superimposed on psychotic disorder)
Schizoaffective Disorder, Depressive Type
Depressed mood, more days than not, for at least 2 years with associated symptoms
Yes
Dysthymic Disorder
No
Depressed mood not meeting criteria for one of above mood disorders that develops in response to a stressor
Yes
Adjustment Disorder with Depressed Mood
No
Clinically significant depressive symptoms that do not meet criteria for a specific mood disorder
Yes
Depressive Disorder Nos
No
No mood disorder (mood symptoms that are not clinically significant)

FIGURE 385-2 Differential diagnosis of mood disorders. NOS, not otherwise specified. *(From Diagnostic and Statistical Manual of Mental Disorders, 4th ed.)*

incidence of depression increases with age; the disorder is approximately twice as prevalent in women as in men, regardless of age. These gender differences were previously believed to reflect sociocultural factors, but recent longitudinal twin studies indicate that the liability to major depression in adult women is largely genetic in origin, and that the effect of environmental factors is transitory and does not affect lifetime prevalence. The relationship between psychological stress, negative life events, and the onset of depressive episodes remains unclear. Certainly, negative life events can precipitate and contribute to depression, but depression itself can be the source of stressful experiences as well.

Unipolar depressive disorders usually have their onset in early adulthood, and recurrences over the course of a lifetime are likely. The best predictor of future risk is the number of past episodes, making a prediction after a single episode unreliable; 50 to 60 percent of patients who have a first episode have at least one or two more episodes. Some patients experience multiple episodes that become more severe and frequent over time. The duration of an untreated episode varies greatly, ranging from a few months to 1 or more years. The pattern of

Table 385-5

Criteria for Major Depressive Episode

A. Five (or more) of the following symptoms have been present during the same 2-week period and represent a change from previous functioning; at least one of the symptoms is either (1) depressed mood or (2) loss of interest or pleasure.

Note: Do not include symptoms that are clearly due to a general medical condition, or mood-incongruent delusions or hallucinations.

1. Depressed mood most of the day, nearly every day, as indicated by either subjective report (e.g., feels sad or empty) or observation made by others (e.g., appears tearful). **Note:** In children and adolescents, can be irritable mood.
2. Markedly diminished interest or pleasure in all, or almost all, activities most of the day, nearly every day (as indicated by either subjective account or observation made by others).
3. Significant weight loss when not dieting or weight gain (e.g., a change of more than 5% of body weight in a month), or decrease or increase in appetite nearly every day. **Note:** In children, consider failure to make expected weight gains.
4. Insomnia or hypersomnia nearly every day.
5. Psychomotor agitation or retardation nearly every day (observable by others, not merely subjective feelings of restlessness or being slowed down).
6. Fatigue or loss of energy nearly every day.
7. Feelings of worthlessness or excessive or inappropriate guilt (which may be delusional) nearly every day (not merely self-reproach or guilt about being sick).
8. Diminished ability to think or concentrate, or indecisiveness, nearly every day (either by subjective account or as observed by others).
9. Recurrent thoughts of death (not just fear of dying), recurrent suicidal ideation without a specific plan, or a suicide attempt or a specific plan for committing suicide.

B. The symptoms do not meet criteria for a mixed episode.

C. The symptoms cause clinically significant distress or impairment in social, occupational, or other important areas of functioning.

D. The symptoms are not due to the direct physiologic effects of a substance (e.g., a drug of abuse, a medication) or a general medical condition (e.g., hypothyroidism).

E. The symptoms are not better accounted for by bereavement; i.e., after the loss of a loved one, the symptoms persist for longer than 2 months or are characterized by marked functional impairment, morbid preoccupation with worthlessness, suicidal ideation, psychotic symptoms, or psychomotor retardation.

SOURCE: *Diagnostic and Statistical Manual of Mental Disorders,* 4th ed.

recurrence and clinical progression in a developing episode is variable. Within an individual, there is often long-term stability in phenotype (presenting symptoms, and frequency and duration of episodes). In a minority of patients, the severity of the depressive episode may progress to psychotic symptomatology. A seasonal pattern of depression, called *seasonal affective disorder*, may manifest with onset and remission of episodes at predictable times of the year. This disorder is more common in women, whose symptoms are anergy, fatigue, weight gain, hypersomnia, and episodic carbohydrate craving. The prevalence increases with distance from the equator, and mood improvement can be accomplished with chronobiologic alteration of light exposure.

Etiology and Pathophysiology The neurobiology of unipolar depression is poorly understood. Although evidence for genetic transmission is not as strong as in bipolar disorder, monozygotic twins have a higher concordance rate (46 percent) than dizygotic siblings (20 percent), with little evidence for effect of a shared family environment. Parallels between the affective, motor, and cognitive dysfunctions seen in unipolar depression and those observed in diseases of the basal ganglia have suggested that neural networks involving prefrontal cortex and the basal ganglia may be primary sites of deficit. This hypothesis is supported by positron emission tomography (PET) studies of brain glucose metabolism that show a decrease in metabolic rate in the caudate nuclei and frontal lobes in depressed patients that returns to normal with recovery. Single photon emission computed tomography (SPECT) studies show comparable changes in blood flow. Magnetic resonance imaging (MRI) findings include in some patients an increased frequency of subcortical white matter lesions. However, because these findings are more prevalent in patients with late onset of depressive illness, their significance remains unproven. A number of studies document increased ventricle-to-brain ratios in patients with recurrent depression, but whether this finding is state-dependent or represents true cerebral atrophy is controversial. Postmortem examination of brains of suicide victims suggest altered noradrenergic activity, including increased binding to $alpha_1$-, $alpha_2$-, and beta-adrenergic receptors in the cerebral cortex and a decreased total number and density of noradrenergic neurons in the locus ceruleus.

Involvement of the serotonin system is suggested by findings of lower plasma tryptophan levels, a decreased cerebrospinal fluid level of 5-hydroxyindolacetic acid (the principal metabolite of serotonin in brain), and decreased platelet serotonergic transporter binding. An increase in brain 5HT receptors in suicide victims is also reported, as are neuroendocrine changes consistent with either a pre- or postsynaptic dysfunction in the serotonin neuron. Depletion of blood tryptophan, the amino acid precursor of serotonin, rapidly reverses the antidepressant benefit in depressed patients who have been successfully treated. However, a decrement in mood after tryptophan reduction is considerably less robust in untreated patients, indicating that, if presynaptic serotonergic dysfunction occurs in depression, it likely plays a contributing rather than a directly causal role. Evidence suggests that reduced serotonergic activity in the central nervous system actually correlates with temperament, impulsivity, and aggression better than with mood state or diagnosis per se.

Neuroendocrine abnormalities that are consistent with the neurovegetative signs and symptoms of depression include (1) increased cortisol secretion, (2) an increase in adrenal size, (3) a decreased inhibitory response of glucocorticoids to dexamethasone, and (4) a blunted response of thyroid-stimulating hormone (TSH) level to infusion of thyroid releasing hormone (TRH). Less convincing evidence exists for (1) an alteration in the pituitary response to corticotropin-releasing hormone (CRH), (2) a decrease in growth hormone secretion and responsivity to growth hormone–releasing hormone (GHRH), and (3) a diminished gonadotropin response to gonadotropin-releasing hormone (GNRH). Changes in hypothalamic-pituitary-adrenal regulation suggest that depression may represent an adaptive dysregulation of the stress response that is either genetically mediated or secondary to exposure to significant stress during critical neuroendocrine encoding periods in early development. Rats stressed as pups by maternal separation have increased hypothalamic levels of CRH as adults and significantly greater release of adrenocorticotropic hormone (ACTH) and corticosterone in response to foot shock than do control animals. Interestingly, antidepressant treatment leads to normalization of pituitary-adrenal abnormalities in patients with depression, and amitriptyline and other antidepressants reduce CRH mRNA and increase glucocorticoid receptor mRNA in a time frame compatible with the onset of the clinical response.

Diurnal variations in symptom severity and alterations in circadian rhythmicity of a number of neurochemical and neurohumoral factors suggest that biologic differences may be secondary to a primary defect in regulation of biologic rhythms. Patients with major depression show consistent findings of a decrease in rapid eye movement (REM) sleep onset (REM latency), an increase in REM density, and in some subjects a decrease in stage IV delta slow wave sleep.

Although antidepressant drugs result in a blockade of neurotransmitter uptake within hours, their therapeutic effects typically emerge over several weeks, implicating neuroadaptive changes in second messenger systems, such as the G proteins, as a possible mechanism of action.

Rx TREATMENT

Treatment planning requires coordination of short-term symptom remission with longer term continuation and maintenance strategies designed to prevent relapse and recurrence. The most effective intervention for achieving remission and preventing relapse is medication, but combined treatment, incorporating psychotherapy to help the patient cope with decreased self-esteem and demoralization, demonstrably improves outcome (Fig. 385-3). Forty percent of primary care patients with depression drop out of treatment and discontinue medication if symptomatic improvement is not noted within a month, unless additional support is provided. Outcome improves with (1) increased intensity and frequency of visits during the first 4 to 6 weeks of treatment, (2) supplemental educational materials, and (3) psychiatric consultation as indicated. Despite the widespread acceptance and use of SSRIs, there is no convincing evidence that this class of antidepressant is more efficacious than TCAs. Sixty to seventy percent of all depressed patients respond to any drug chosen, if it is given in a sufficient dose for 6 to 8 weeks (Table 385-6). There is no ideal antidepressant; no current compound combines rapid onset of action, moderate half-life, a meaningful relationship between dose and blood level, a low side effect profile, minimal interaction with other drugs, and safety in overdose. A rational approach to selecting which antidepressant to use involves knowledge of differences in pharmacokinetic activity and matching of the patient's preference and medical history with the metabolic and side effect profile of the drug considered (Table 385-7). A previous response, or a family history of a positive response, to a specific antidepressant would suggest that that drug be tried first. Before initiating antidepressant therapy, the physician should evaluate the possible contribution of comorbid illnesses and consider their specific treatment. In individuals with suicidal ideation, particular atten tion should be paid to choosing a drug with a low toxicity if taken in overdose. The SSRIs and other newer antidepressant drugs are distinctly safer in this regard; nevertheless, the advantages of TCAs have not been completely superseded. The existence of generic equivalents make them relatively cheap, and for several tricyclics, particularly nortriptyline, imipramine, and desipramine, relationships among dose, plasma level, and therapeutic response have been defined and make more specific individual treatment planning possible. The steady-state plasma level achieved for a given drug dose

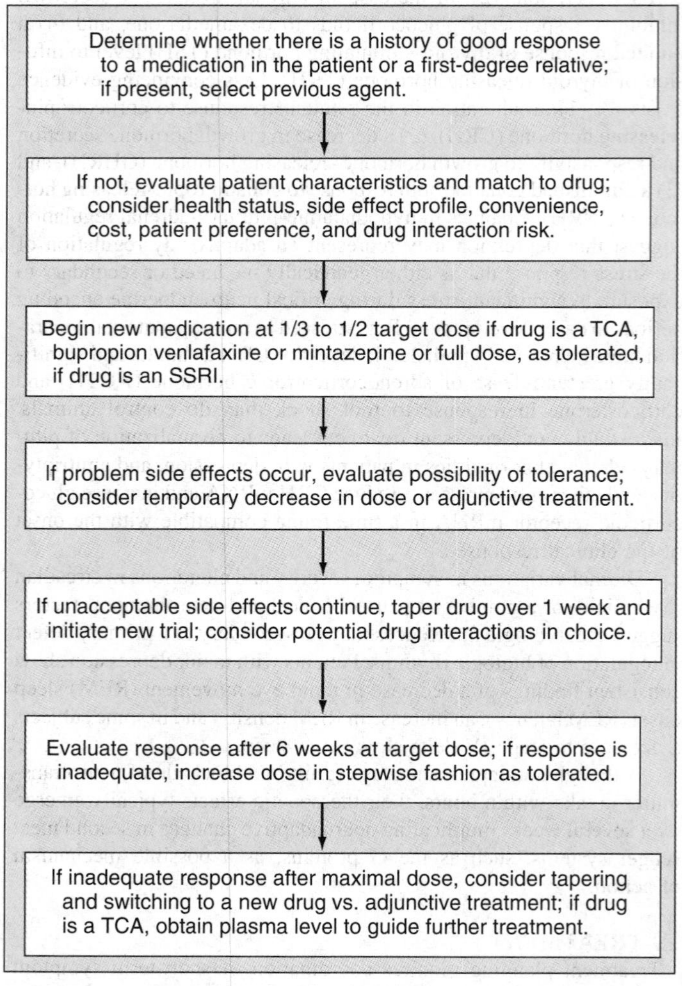
Determine whether there is a history of good response to a medication in the patient or a first-degree relative; if present, select previous agent.
If not, evaluate patient characteristics and match to drug; consider health status, side effect profile, convenience, cost, patient preference, and drug interaction risk.
Begin new medication at 1/3 to 1/2 target dose if drug is a TCA, bupropion venlafaxine or mintazepine or full dose, as tolerated, if drug is an SSRI.
If problem side effects occur, evaluate possibility of tolerance; consider temporary decrease in dose or adjunctive treatment.
If unacceptable side effects continue, taper drug over 1 week and initiate new trial; consider potential drug interactions in choice.
Evaluate response after 6 weeks at target dose; if response is inadequate, increase dose in stepwise fashion as tolerated.
If inadequate response after maximal dose, consider tapering and switching to a new drug vs. adjunctive treatment; if drug is a TCA, obtain plasma level to guide further treatment.

FIGURE 385-3 A guideline for the medical management of major depressive disorder. SSRI, selective serotonin reuptake inhibitor; TCA, tricyclic antidepressant.

Table 385-6

Some Commonly Used Antidepressant Medications

Agent	Usual Daily Oral Therapeutic Dose Range, mg*
Imipramine	150–300
Amitriptyline	150–300
Desipramine	150–300
Nortriptyline	50–150
Doxepin	150–300
Protriptyline	15–60
Trimipramine	150–300
Maprotiline	150–200
Amoxapine	150–450
Trazodone	150–300
Bupropion	250–450
Chlomipramine	100–250
Fluoxetine	20–60
Sertraline	50–200
Paroxetine	20–60
Fluvoxamine	100–300
Nefazadone	300–500
Venlafaxine	125–375
Mirtazapine	15–45
Monoamine oxidase inhibitors	
Phenelzine	45–90
Tranylcypromine	30–50

* After titration; starting doses should be at or below the lowest dosage shown.

Table 385-7

Management of Antidepressant Side Effects

Symptoms	Comments and Management Strategies
Gastrointestinal	
Nausea, loss of appetite	Usually short-lived and dose-related; consider temporary dose reduction or administration with food and antacids
Diarrhea	Famotidine, 20–40 mg/d
Constipation	Wait for tolerance; try diet change, stool softener, exercise; avoid laxatives
Sexual dysfunction	Consider dose reduction; drug holiday
Anorgasmia/impotence; impaired ejaculation	Bethanechol, 10–20 mg, 2 h before activity, or cyproheptadine, 4–8 mg 2 h before activity, or bupropion, 100 mg bid or amantadine, 100 mg bid/tid
Orthostasis	Tolerance unlikely; increase fluid intake, use calf exercises/support hose; fludrocortisone, 0.025 mg/d
Anticholinergic	Wait for tolerance
Dry mouth, eyes	Maintain good oral hygiene; use artificial tears, sugar-free gum
Tremor/"jitteriness"	Antiparkinsonian drugs not effective; use dose reduction/slow increase; lorazepam, 0.5 mg bid, or propranolol, 10–20 mg bid
Insomnia	Schedule all doses for the morning; trazodone, 50–100 mg qhs
Sedation	Caffeine; schedule all dosing for bedtime; buproprion, 75–100 mg in afternoon
Headache	Evaluate diet, stress, other drugs; try dose reduction; amitriptyline, 50 mg/d
Weight gain	Decrease carbohydrates; exercise; consider fluoxetine
Loss of therapeutic benefit over time	Related to tolerance? Increase dose or drug holiday; Add amantadine, 100 mg bid, or buspirone, 10 mg tid

can vary more than tenfold between individuals. Plasma levels may help in understanding resistance to treatment and/or paradoxical drug toxicity. The principal disadvantages of TCAs are antihistamine side effects (sedation) and anticholinergic side effects (constipation, dry mouth, urinary hesitancy, and blurred vision). Severe cardiac toxicity due to conduction block or arrhythmias can also occur but is uncommon at therapeutic levels. Tricyclic agents are lethal in overdose, with desipramine carrying the greatest risk. Prescribing only a 10-day supply may be judicious. Most patients require a daily dose of 150 to 200 mg of imipramine or amitriptyline or its equivalent to achieve a therapeutic blood level of 150 to 300 ng/mL and a satisfactory remission; some patients show a partial effect at lower doses. Ethnic differences in drug metabolism are significant, with Hispanic, Asian, and African American patients generally requiring lower doses to achieve a comparable blood level than Caucasians.

Second-generation antidepressants include amoxapine, maprotiline, trazodone, and bupropion. Amoxapine is a dibenzoxazepine derivative that blocks norepinephrine and serotonin reuptake and has a metabolite that shows a degree of dopamine blockade. Long-term use of this drug carries a risk of tardive dyskinesia. Maprotiline is a potent noradrenergic reuptake blocker that has little anticholinergic effect but may produce seizures. Bupropion is a novel antidepressant whose mechanism of action is thought to involve enhancement of noradrenergic function. It has no specific anticholinergic, sedating, or orthostatic side effects and has a low incidence of impairment of sexual performance. It may, however, be associated with aversive stimulant-like side effects, may lower seizure threshold, and has an exceptionally short half-life, requiring multiple dosing.

SSRIs such as fluoxetine, sertraline, and paroxetine cause a lower frequency of anticholinergic, sedating, and cardiovascular side effects but a possibly greater incidence of gastrointestinal complaints, sleep impairment, and sexual dysfunction than do TCAs (Table 385-8). Akathisia, involving an inner sense of restlessness and anxiety, may also be more common, particularly during the first week of treatment. A serious concern, aside from drug interaction, is the risk of "serotonin syndrome," thought to result from hyperstimulation of brainstem $5HT_{1A}$ receptors and characterized by myoclonus, agitation, abdominal cramping, hyperpyrexia, hypertension, and potentially death. Combinations of serotonergic agonists should be monitored closely for this reason. Choice among the SSRIs relates principally to differences in half-life and issues of improved compliance versus increased risk of toxicity over time, and to variance in the risk of incurring adverse drug-drug interactions. Fluoxetine and its principal active metabolite, norfluoxetine, for example, have a combined half-life of almost 7 days, meaning that it takes 5 weeks to achieve steady-state levels and a similar period for the drug to leave the body once its use is discontinued. All the SSRIs may impair sexual function, resulting in diminished libido, impotence, or difficulty in achieving orgasm. Sexual dysfunction frequently results in noncompliance, and should be asked about specifically in patients using SSRIs. Sexual dysfunction can sometimes be ameliorated by lowering the dose, by instituting drug holidays over the weekend (two or three times a month), or by treatment with amantadine (100 mg tid), bethanechol (25 mg tid), or buspirone (10 mg tid). Paroxetine appears to be more anticholinergic than either fluoxetine or sertraline, and sertraline carries a lower risk of producing an adverse drug interaction than the other two. Rare side effects of SSRIs include vasospastic angina and alterations of prothrombin time.

Table 385-8

Possible Drug Interactions with Selective Serotonin Reuptake Inhibitors

Agent	Effect
Monoamine oxidase inhibitors	Serotonin syndrome—absolute contraindication
Serotonergic agonists, e.g., tryptophan, fenfluramine	Potential serotonin syndrome
Drugs that are metabolized by P450 isoenzymes: tricyclics, other SSRIs, antipsychotics, beta blockers, codeine, terfenadine, astemizole, triazolobenzodiazepines, calcium channel blockers	Delayed metabolism resulting in increased blood levels and potential toxicity—possible fatality secondary to QT prolongation with terfenadine or astemizole
Drugs that are bound tightly to plasma proteins, e.g., warfarin, coumadin	Increased bleeding secondary to displacement
Drugs that inhibit the metabolism of SSRIs by P450 isoenzymes, e.g., quinidine	Increased SSRI side effects

Venlafaxine, like imipramine, blocks the reuptake of both norepinephrine and serotonin, but it produces relatively little in the way of traditional tricyclic side effects. Unlike the SSRIs, it has a relatively linear dose-response curve. Patients should be monitored for a possible increase in diastolic blood pressure, and multiple daily dosing is required because of the drug's short half-life. Nefazadone is a selective $5HT_2$ receptor antagonist that also inhibits the presynaptic reuptake of serotonin and norepinephrine. Its side effects are similar to those of the SSRIs, and twice-daily dosing produces a steady state within 4 to 5 days. The drug is related structurally to trazodone, which is currently used more for its sedative than its antidepressant properties. Nefazadone appears to produce a lower incidence of sexual side effects than do the SSRIs. Mirtazapine is a recently introduced tetracyclic antidepressant that has a comparatively unique spectrum of activity. It increases noradrenergic and serotonergic neurotransmission through a blockade of central $alpha_2$-adrenergic auto- and heteroreceptors and postsynaptic $5HT_2$ and $5HT_3$ receptors. It is also strongly antihistaminic and, as such, may produce sedation at lower doses.

Each of the SSRIs, as well as nefazadone, may inhibit one or more cytochrome P450 enzymes (Table 385-8). Depending on the specific isoenzyme involved, the metabolism of a number of concomitantly administered medications can be dramatically affected. Fluoxetine and paroxetine, for example, by inhibiting 2D6, can cause dramatic increases in the blood level of type 1C antiarrhythmics, while sertraline and nefazadone, by acting on 3A4, may alter blood levels of terfenadine, carbamazepine, and astemizole. Because many of these compounds have a narrow therapeutic window and can cause iatrogenic ventricular arrhythmias when present at toxic levels, the possibility of an adverse drug interaction should be considered before initiation of therapy and at any time during the course of therapy when patient deterioration is noted.

Other treatment options include the MAOIs and electroconvulsive therapy. The MAOIs are highly effective, particularly in the treatment of atypical depression, but the risk of hypertensive crisis following intake of tyramine-containing food or sympathomimetic drugs makes them inappropriate as first-line agents. Common side effects include orthostatic hypotension, weight gain, insomnia, and sexual dysfunction. MAOIs should not be used in close temporal proximity with SSRIs because of the risk of serotonin syndrome. Electroconvulsive therapy is at least as effective as medication, but its use is reserved for treatment-resistant cases and delusional depressions.

Treatment response should be evaluated after approximately 2 months of therapy. Three-quarters of patients show an adequate response by this time, but if remission is inadequate, the patient should be questioned about medication compliance, and an increase in dose should be considered if side effects are not troublesome. Patients with an inadequate response to the higher dose should be offered an alternative medication. There are no data to guide predictably the choice of a second drug, although drugs of a significantly different class or structure may be recommended on theoretical grounds. However, individual patient responses vary even within a class of similar drugs. If the second medication trial fails, consultation with or referral to a mental health specialist is advised. Strategies for treatment then include combinations of antidepressants and/or adjunctive treatment with other classes of drugs, including lithium, thyroid hormone, and dopamine agonists. Patients whose response to an SSRI disappears over time may benefit from the addition of buspirone (10 mg tid) or pindolol (2.5 mg tid) or small amounts of a tricyclic antidepressant such as desipramine (25 mg bid or tid). Once significant remission is achieved, drug treatment should be continued for at least 6 to 9 months to prevent relapse. In patients who have had two or more episodes of depression, indefinite maintenance treatment should be considered.

It is essential to counsel patients about depression and the medications they are receiving. An educational approach is best, describing what is known about the depressive syndrome and how the medications may help. Advice about side effects, and expected length of treatment and cautions about alcohol use are helpful. It is important that patients be given time to describe their experience and the impact it has had on them, their family, and their outlook. Occasional empathic silence may be as helpful for the treatment alliance as verbal reassurance.

BIPOLAR DISORDER Clinical Manifestations Bipolar disorder is common, affecting approximately 3 million persons in the United States, but often difficult to diagnose. It is characterized by unpredictable swings in mood from mania (or hypomania) to depression. Some patients suffer only from recurrent attacks of *mania*, which in its pure form is associated with increased psychomotor activity, excessive social extroversion, decreased need for sleep, impulsivity and impairment in judgment, and expansive, grandiose, and sometimes irritable mood (Table 385-9). In severe mania, patients may experience delusions and paranoid thinking indistinguishable from that associated with schizophrenia. About half of all patients with bipolar disorder present with a mixture of psychomotor agitation and activation with dysphoria, anxiety, and irritability. It may be difficult to distinguish *mixed mania* from *agitated depression*. In some bipolar patients (*bipolar II disorder*), the full criteria for mania are lacking, and recurrent depressions are separated by periods of mild activation and increased energy (hypomania). In *cyclothymic disorder*, there are numerous hypomanic periods, usually of relatively short duration, alternating with clusters of depressive symptoms that fail to meet the criteria of major depression, either in severity or duration. The mood fluctuations are chronic and should be present for at least 2 years before the diagnosis is made.

Manic episodes typically emerge over a period of days to weeks, but onset within hours is possible, usually in the early morning hours. An untreated episode of either depression or mania can last as short as several weeks or as long as 8 to 12 months, and rare patients have an unremitting chronic course. The term "rapid cycling" is used for patients who have four or more episodes of either depression or mania in a given year. This pattern occurs in 15 percent of all patients, almost all of whom are women. In some cases, rapid cycling is linked to an underlying thyroid dysfunction and, in others, iatrogenically triggered by prolonged antidepressant treatment.

Although bipolar illness is associated with frequent episodic recurrence, it was once thought to have a favorable prognosis and outcome. More recent data, however, show that approximately half of patients with the disorder have sustained difficulties in work performance and psychosocial functioning. The most frequent age of onset for bipolar disorder is between 20 and 30 years of age, but many individuals report premorbid symptoms in late childhood or early adolescence. The prevalence is similar for men and women, but there are gender differences in course, with women likely to have more depressive and men more manic episodes over a lifetime.

Differential Diagnosis The differential diagnosis of mania includes ruling out activation by stimulant and sympathomimetic compounds as well as secondary mania induced by hyperthyroidism, AIDS, or neurologic disorders, such as Huntington's or Wilson's disease, or cerebrovascular accidents. This distinction may be difficult to make, because comorbidity with alcohol and substance abuse is common, either because of poor judgment and increased impulsivity or because of an attempt at self-medication.

Etiology and Pathophysiology Evidence for a genetic predisposition to bipolar disorder is significant. The concordance rate for monozygotic twin pairs approaches 80 percent, and segregation analyses are consistent with autosomal dominant transmission. Several chromosomal locations for the gene have been proposed in the last decade on the basis of linkage analysis in affected families. None has yet received independent confirmation. Two independent groups reported the results of complete genome scans. One reported weak evidence for linkage to loci on chromosomes 6, 13, and 15, while the other found a major gene locus and haplotype on 18q22-23 in two large Costa Rican pedigrees.

The pathophysiologic mechanisms underlying the profound and recurrent mood swings of bipolar disorder remain unknown. Cellular models of changes in membrane Na^+ and K^+ activated ATPase and proposals of disordered signal transduction mechanisms involving either the phosphoinositol system or guanine nucleotide binding proteins have received the most attention. Lithium reduces the supply of free inositol used to maintain the lipid precursors involved in intracellular signaling and blocks stimulation-induced increases in GTP binding capacity. Reduction of GTP and downstream effects on protein kinase C are being investigated as possible explanations for the therapeutic effects of the drug.

Neurophysiologic studies suggest that bipolar patients have altered circadian rhythmicity. A possible phase advance induced by desynchronization among controlling circadian oscillators is consistent with a finding that lithium increases period length and may exert its therapeutic benefit through a resynchronization of intrinsic rhythms keyed to the light/dark cycle (see Chap. 27). Neuroimaging techniques have also identified a higher rate of subcortical white matter abnormalities in bipolar patients than in age matched controls.

Rx TREATMENT

Lithium carbonate remains the mainstay of treatment in bipolar disorder, although sodium valproate is equally effective in acute mania. Carbamazepine is also efficacious (Table 385-10). The response rate to lithium carbonate is 70 to 80 percent in acute mania,

Table 385-9

Criteria for a Manic Episode

A. A distinct period of abnormally and persistently elevated, expansive, or irritable mood, lasting at least 1 week (or any duration if hospitalization is necessary).
B. During the period of mood disturbance, three (or more) of the following symptoms have persisted (four if the mood is only irritable) and have been present to a significant degree:
   1. Inflated self-esteem or grandiosity
   2. Decreased need for sleep (e.g., feels rested after only 3 hours of sleep)
   3. More talkative than usual or pressure to keep talking
   4. Flight of ideas or subjective experience that thoughts are racing
   5. Distractibility (i.e., attention too easily drawn to unimportant or irrelevant external stimuli)
   6. Increase in goal-directed activity (either socially, at work or school, or sexually) or psychomotor agitation
   7. Excessive involvement in pleasurable activities that have a high potential for painful consequences (e.g., engaging in unrestrained buying sprees, sexual indiscretions, or foolish business investments)
C. The symptoms do not meet criteria for a mixed episode.
D. The mood disturbance is sufficiently severe to cause marked impairment in occupational functioning or in usual social activities or relationships with others, or to necessitate hospitalization to prevent harm to self or others, or there are psychotic features.
E. The symptoms are not due to the direct physiologic effects of a substance (e.g., a drug of abuse, a medication, or other treatment) or a general medical condition (e.g., hyperthyroidism).

Note: Manic-like episodes that are clearly caused by somatic antidepressant treatment (e.g., medication, electroconvulsive therapy, light therapy) should not count toward a diagnosis of bipolar I disorder.

SOURCE: *Diagnostic and Statistical Manual of Mental Disorders*, 4th ed.

with beneficial effects appearing in 1 to 2 weeks. A prophylactic effect in prevention of recurrent mania, and, to a lesser extent, in the prevention of recurrent depression is documented. A simple cation, lithium is rapidly absorbed from the gastrointestinal tract and remains unbound to plasma or tissue proteins. Ninety-five percent of a given dose is excreted unchanged through the kidneys within 24 h.

Serious side effects from lithium administration are rare, but minor complaints such as gastrointestinal discomfort, nausea, diarrhea, polyuria, weight gain, skin eruptions, alopecia, and edema are common. Over time, urine concentrating ability may be decreased, but changes in function do not result in significant nephrotoxicity. In a small subset of patients in whom excessive polyuria occurs (>3000 mL per 24 h), dose or schedule adjustments or the adjunctive use of diuretics should be considered. Lithium exerts an antithyroid effect by interfering with the synthesis and release of thyroid hormones. Approximately 5 percent of patients taking lithium for 18 months or longer develop hypothyroidism, with women more likely to be affected than men. Iatrogenic hypothyroidism should be ruled out in any patient who experiences recurrence of depressive symptomatology during lithium treatment. More serious side effects include tremor, interference with concentration and memory, ataxia, dysarthria, and incoordination. Electrocardiographic (ECG) changes of T wave flattening and conduction delays may occur (see Table 385-2). There is suggestive but not conclusive, evidence that lithium is teratogenic, inducing cardiac malformations in the first trimester.

In the treatment of acute mania, lithium is initiated at 300 mg bid or tid, and the dose is then increased by 300 mg every 2 to 3 days to achieve blood levels of 0.8 to 1.2 mEq/L. Because the therapeutic effect of lithium may not appear until 7 to 10 days of treatment, adjunctive usage of lorazepam (1 to 2 mg every 4 h) or clonazepam (0.5 to 1 mg every 4 h), may be beneficial to control agitation. Antipsychotics are warranted in patients with severe agitation and who respond only partially to benzodiazepines. These agents should be discontinued in the transition to maintenance lithium therapy. Patients using lithium should be monitored closely, since the blood levels required to achieve a therapeutic benefit are close to those associated with neurotoxicity. Risk factors for neurotoxicity include concomitant medical illness, decrease in salt intake, or concurrent use of medications that may increase the serum level of lithium (neuroleptics, diuretics, and calcium channel blockers).

Valproic acid is an alternative in patients who cannot tolerate lithium or respond poorly to it. Valproic acid may be better than lithium for patients who have a rapid-cycling course (i.e., more than four episodes a year) or who present with a mixed or dysphoric mania. Valproic acid is usually started at 500 to 750 mg/d bid or tid. The dose is increased every several days to achieve blood levels in the range of 50 to 100 μg/mL, which typically are achieved at a dose of 1000 to 2500 mg/d. The most serious adverse effect of valproic acid is hepatoxicity, which may be fatal. Such cases are fortunately rare, but regular monitoring of liver enzymes, particularly during the first 90 days of treatment and periodically thereafter, is indicated.

Carbamazepine, although not formally approved by the Food and Drug Administration (FDA) for bipolar disorder, has clinical efficacy in the treatment of acute mania. Carbamazepine is initiated at 400 to 600 mg/d in divided doses, and the dose is increased to achieve a blood level of 4 to 12 mg/L. Carbamazepine may induce a benign leukopenia, but the risk of aplastic anemia is minimal. Nevertheless, it is wise to obtain a complete blood count (CBC) periodically.

The recurrent nature of bipolar mood disorder necessitates maintenance treatment. Maintenance of at least 0.8 mg/L blood lithium levels is important to achieve optimal prophylaxis. Antidepressant medications are sometimes required for the treatment of severe breakthrough depressions, but their use should generally be avoided during maintenance treatment because of the possible risk of precipitating mania or accelerating the cycle frequency. Loss of efficacy over time may be observed with any of the mood-stabilizing agents. In such situations, an alternative agent or combination therapy usually restores the therapeutic benefit.

Table 385-10

Clinical Pharmacology of Mood Stabilizers

Agent and Dosing	Side Effects and Other Effects
Lithium Starting dose: 300 mg bid or tid Therapeutic blood level: 0.8–1.2 mEq/L	*Common side effects:* nausea/anorexia/diarrhea, fine tremor, thirst, polyuria, fatigue, weight gain, acne, folliculitis, neutrophilia, hypothyroidism Blood level is increased by thiazides, tetracyclines, and NSAIDs Blood level is decreased by bronchodilators, verapamil, and carbonic anhydrase inhibitors *Rare side effects:* Neurotoxicity, renal toxicity, hypercalcemia
Carbamazepine Starting dose: 200 mg bid Therapeutic blood level: 4–12 μg/mL	*Common side effects:* Nausea/anorexia, sedation, rash, dizziness/ataxia Induces hepatic metabolism of other medications *Rare side effects:* Hyponatremia, agranulocytosis, Stevens-Johnson syndrome
Valproic acid Starting dose: 250 mg tid Therapeutic blood level: 50–125 μg/mL	*Common side effects:* Nausea/anorexia, weight gain, sedation, tremor, rash, alopecia Inhibits hepatic metabolism of other medications *Rare side effects:* Pancreatitis, hepatoxicity, Stevens-Johnson syndrome

ABBREVIATION: NSAID, nonsteroidal anti-inflammatory drug.

SOMATOFORM DISORDERS

CLINICAL MANIFESTATIONS Patients with multiple somatic complaints that cannot be explained by a known medical condition or by the effects of alcohol or of recreational or prescription drugs are seen commonly in primary care practice; one survey indicates a prevalence of 5 percent. The somatoform disorders include a variety of conditions that differ in the symptoms present and in whether the symptoms are intentionally produced (Fig. 385-4). In *somatization disorder*, the patient presents with multiple physical complaints derived from different organ systems (Table 385-11). Onset is usually before age 30, and the disorder is persistent. Formal diagnostic criteria require the recording of at least four pain, two gastrointestinal, one sexual, and one pseudoneurologic symptom. Patients with somatization disorder often present with dramatic complaints, but the complaints are inconsistent. Symptoms of comorbid anxiety and mood are common and may be the result of drug interactions due to regimens initiated independently by different physicians. Patients with somatization disorder may be impulsive and demanding and frequently qualify for a formal comorbid psychiatric diagnosis. In *conversion disorder*, the symptoms focus on deficits that involve voluntary motor or sensory function and on psychological factors that initiate or exacerbate the medical presentation. Like somatization disorder, the deficit is not intentionally produced or simulated, as is the case in factitious disorder (malingering). In *hypochondriasis*, the essential feature is a belief of serious medical illness that persists despite reassurance and appropriate medical evaluation. As with somatization disorder, patients with hypochondriasis have a history of poor relationships with physicians stemming from their sense that they have been evaluated and treated inappropriately or inadequately. Hypochondriasis can be disabling in intensity and is persistent, with waxing and waning symptomatology.

In *factitious illnesses*, the patient consciously and voluntarily produces physical symptoms of illness. The term *Munchausen's syndrome* is reserved for individuals with particularly dramatic, chronic, or severe

Table 385-11

Diagnostic Criteria for Somatization Disorder

A. A history of many physical complaints beginning before age 30 years that occur over a period of several years and result in treatment being sought or significant impairment in social, occupational, or other important areas of functioning.
B. Each of the following criteria must have been met, with individual symptoms occurring at any time during the course of the disturbance:
   1. *Four pain symptoms:* a history of pain related to at least four different sites or functions (e.g., head, abdomen, back, joints, extremities, chest, rectum, during menstruation, during sexual intercourse, or during urination)
   2. *Two gastrointestinal symptoms:* a history of at least two gastrointestinal symptoms other than pain (e.g., nausea, bloating, vomiting other than during pregnancy, diarrhea, or intolerance of several different foods)
   3. *One sexual symptom:* a history of at least one sexual or reproductive symptom other than pain (e.g., sexual indifference, erectile or ejaculatory dysfunction, irregular menses, excessive menstrual bleeding, vomiting throughout pregnancy)
   4. *One pseudoneurologic symptom:* a history of at least one symptom or deficit suggesting a neurologic condition not limited to pain (conversion symptoms such as impaired coordination or balance, paralysis or localized weakness, difficulty swallowing or lump in throat, aphonia, urinary retention, hallucinations, loss of touch or pain sensation, double vision, blindness, deafness, seizures; dissociative symptoms such as amnesia; or loss of consciousness other than fainting)
C. Either of the following:
   1. After appropriate investigation, each of the symptoms in criterion B cannot be fully explained by a known general medical condition or the direct effects of a substance (e.g., a drug of abuse, a medication)
   2. When there is a related general medical condition, the physical complaints or resulting social or occupational impairment are in excess of what would be expected from the history, physical examination, or laboratory findings
D. The symptoms are not intentionally produced or feigned (as in factitious disorder or malingering).

SOURCE: *Diagnostic and Statistical Manual of Mental Disorders,* 4th ed.

factitious illness. In true factitious illness, the sick role itself is gratifying. A variety of signs, symptoms, and diseases have been either simulated or caused by factitious behavior, the most common including chronic diarrhea, fever of unknown origin, intestinal bleeding or hematuria, seizures, and hypoglycemia. Factitious disorder is usually not diagnosed until 5 to 10 years after its onset, and it can produce significant social and medical costs. In *malingering*, the fabrication derives from a desire for some external reward, such as a narcotic medication or disability reimbursement.

℞ TREATMENT

Patients with somatization disorders are frequently subjected to multiple diagnostic testing and exploratory surgeries in an attempt to find their "real" illness. Such an approach is doomed to failure and does not address the core issue. Successful treatment is best achieved through behavior modification, in which access to the physician is tightly regulated and adjusted to provide a sustained and predictable level of support that is less clearly contingent on the patient's level of presenting distress. Visits can be brief and should not be associated with a need for a diagnostic or treatment action. Although the literature is limited, some patients with somatization disorder may benefit from antidepressant treatment. Fluoxetine and MAOIs have been found independently to be useful in reducing obsessive ruminations, dysphoria, and anxious preoccupation in patients with multiple somatic complaints.

The treatment of factitious disorder is complicated in that any attempt to confront the patient usually only creates a sense of humiliation and causes the patient to abandon treatment from that care giver. A better strategy is to introduce psychological causation as one of

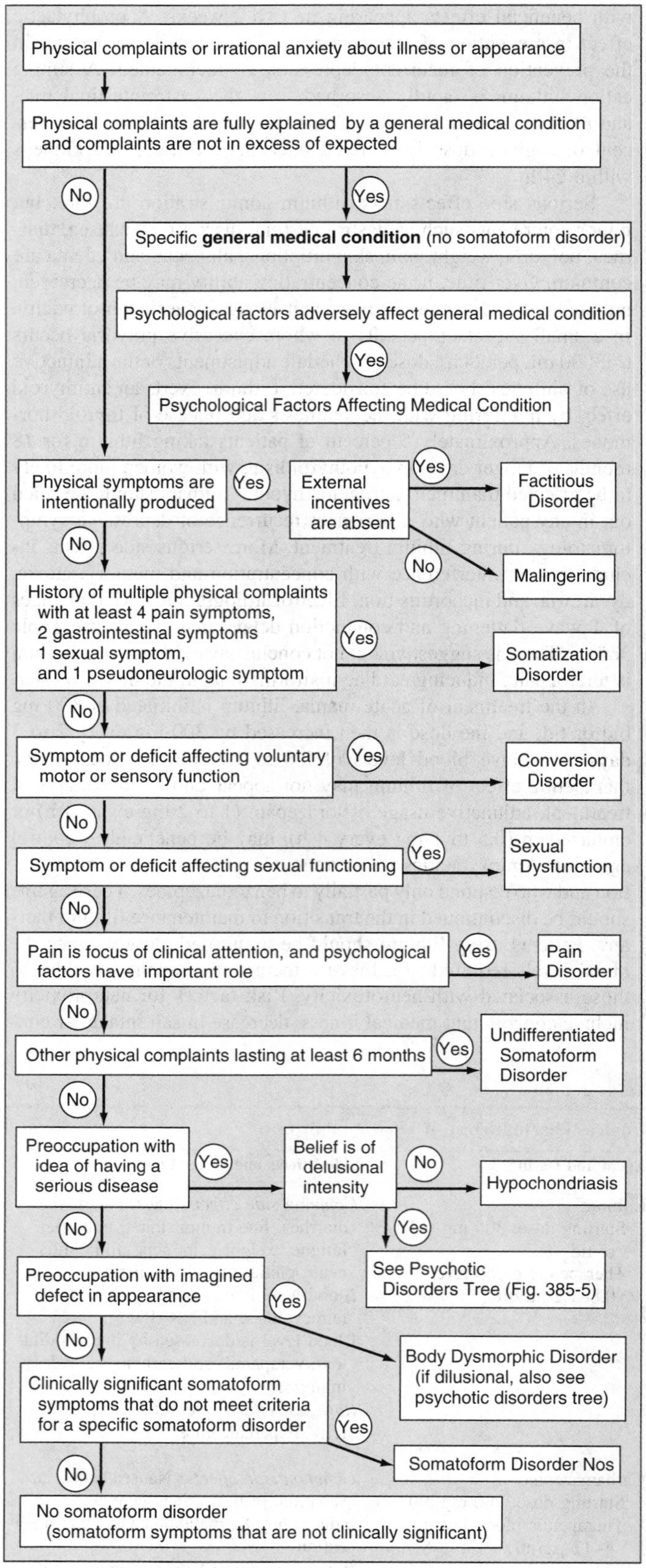

FIGURE 385-4 Differential diagnosis of somatoform disorders. NOS, not otherwise specified. *(From Diagnostic and Statistical Manual of Mental Disorders, 4th ed.)*

a number of possible explanations and to include factitious illness as an option in the differential diagnoses that are discussed. Without directly linking the treatment to the diagnosis, the patient can be offered a face-saving means by which the pathologic relationship with the health care system can be examined and alternative approaches to life stressors developed.

PERSONALITY DISORDERS

CLINICAL MANIFESTATIONS Personality disorders are characteristic patterns of thinking, feeling, and interpersonal behavior that are relatively inflexible and cause significant functional impairment or subjective distress for the individual. To qualify for the formal diagnosis, the observed behaviors should not be secondary to another mental disorder, nor should they be precipitated by substance abuse or a general medical condition. This distinction is often difficult to make in clinical practice, as personality change may be the first sign of serious neurologic, endocrine, or other medical illness. Patients with frontal lobe tumors, for example, can present with changes in motivation and personality while the results of the neurologic examination remain within normal limits. Personality traits are stable over time and environmental situation and are recognizable in adolescence or early adult life. Although DSM-IV portrays personality disorders as qualitatively distinct categories, there is an alternative perspective that personality characteristics vary as a continuum between normal functioning and formal mental disorder.

Personality disorders have been grouped into three clusters that share similar attributes. *Cluster A* includes paranoid, schizoid, and schizotypal personality disorders. It includes individuals who are odd and eccentric and who maintain an emotional distance from others. Individuals have a restricted emotional range and remain socially isolated. Patients with schizotypal personality disorder frequently have unusual perceptual experiences and express magical beliefs about the external world. The essential feature of paranoid personality disorder is a pervasive mistrust and suspiciousness of others to an extent that is unjustified by available evidence. *Cluster B* disorders include antisocial, borderline, histrionic, and narcissistic types and describe individuals whose behavior is impulsive, excessively emotional, and erratic. *Cluster C* incorporates avoidant, dependent, and obsessive-compulsive personality types, whose enduring traits are anxious or fearful in nature. These divisions have not been validated but are useful for understanding some patients whose psychological problems interfere with diagnosis and treatment. The boundaries between cluster types are to some extent artificial, and many patients who meet criteria for one personality disorder also meet criteria for aspects of another. In addition, the risk of a comorbid major mental disorder is increased in patients who qualify for a diagnosis of personality disorder.

℞ TREATMENT

Historically, recommended treatment for personality disorders was long-term psychotherapy, in which the pathologic patterns of interaction with the world at large could be relived and examined through the corrective emotional experience of the controlled therapeutic relationship. More recently, the recognition that personality derives in part from biologically determined components of temperament has given rise to the empirical use of drugs to treat specific symptom clusters as well as any coexisting major mental disorder. To this end, antidepressant medications and low-dose antipsychotic drugs have some efficacy in cluster A personality disorders, while anticonvulsant mood-stabilizing agents and MAOIs may be considered for patients with cluster B diagnoses who show marked mood reactivity, behavioral dyscontrol, and/or rejection hypersensitivity. Anxious or fearful cluster C patients often have a response to medication that parallels that for patients with axis I anxiety disorders. In all cases, it is important for both the physician and the patient to have reasonable expectations as to the possible effect of the medication and any associated side effects. Beneficial responses may be subtle and observable only over a span of time that affords an adequate sampling of life experience.

SCHIZOPHRENIA

CLINICAL MANIFESTATIONS Schizophrenia is no longer considered a single disease, but rather a group of illnesses that are phenomenologically and etiologically heterogeneous (Fig. 385-5). Schizophrenia is characterized by perturbations of language, perception, thinking, social activity, affect, and volition, but there are no pathognomonic features. The syndrome commonly begins in late adolescence, has an insidious onset, and, classically, a poor outcome, progressing from social withdrawal and perceptual distortions to a state of chronic delusions and hallucinations. Patients with schizophrenic syndrome may present with positive symptoms (such as conceptual

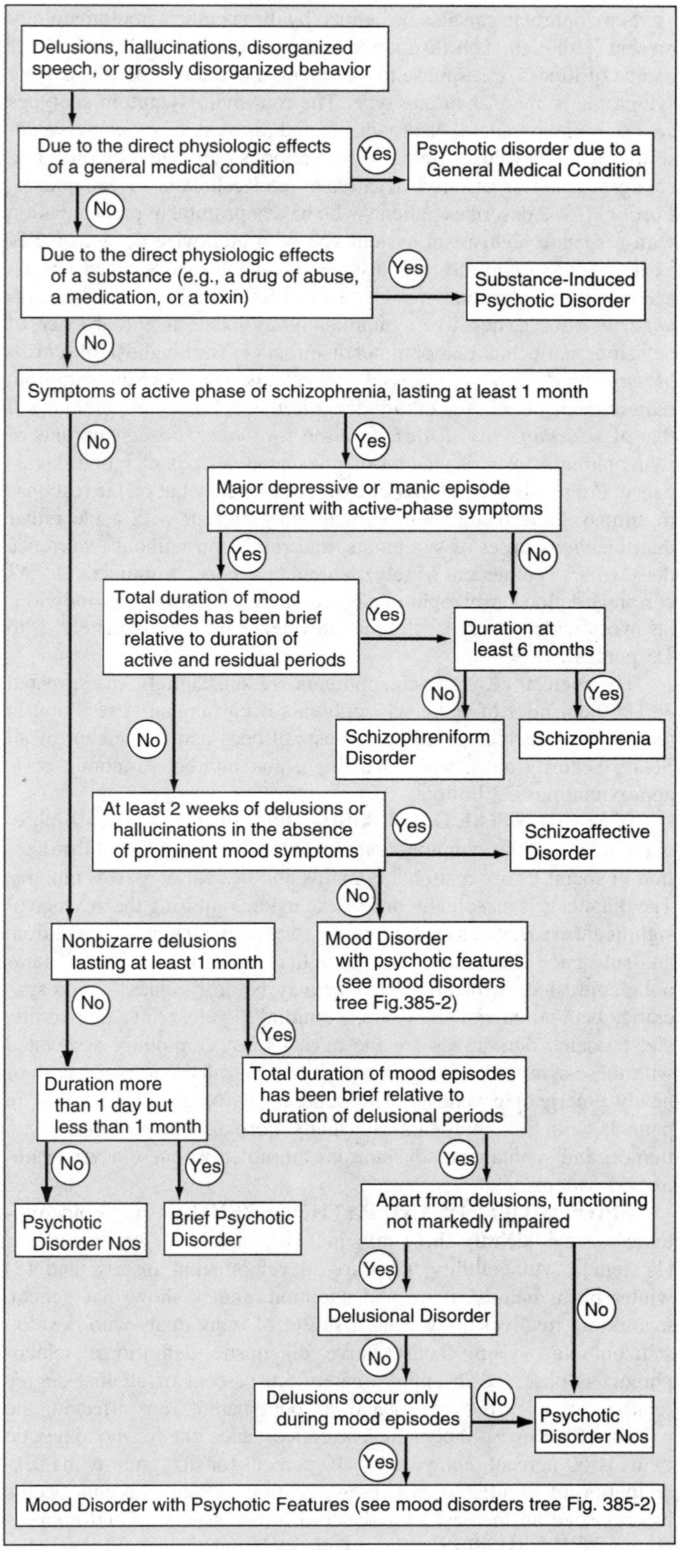

FIGURE 385-5 Differential diagnosis of psychotic disorders. NOS, not otherwise specified. *(From Diagnostic and Statistical Manual of Mental Disorders, 4th ed.)*

disorganization, delusions, or hallucinations) or negative symptoms (loss of function, anhedonia, decreased emotional expression, impaired concentration, and diminished social engagement). "Negative" symptoms predominate in one-third of the schizophrenic population and are associated with a poor long-term outcome and a poor response to drug treatment. However, marked variability in the course and individual character of symptoms is typical.

Schizophrenia can also be defined by the specific symptomatology present, although such distinctions do not correlate well with either course of illness or response to treatment, and many individuals have symptoms of more than one type. The four main symptom subtypes are catatonic, paranoid, disorganized, and residual. *Catatonic-type* describes patients whose clinical presentation is dominated by profound changes in motor activity, negativism, and echolalia or echopraxia. *Paranoid-type* describes patients who have a prominent preoccupation with a specific delusional system and who otherwise do not qualify as having *disorganized-type* disease, in which disorganized speech and behavior are accompanied by a superficial or silly affect. In *residual-type* disease, negative symptomatology exists in the absence of delusions, hallucinations, or motor disturbance. The diagnosis of *schizophreniform disorder* is reserved for patients who meet the symptom requirements but not the duration requirements for schizophrenia, and that of *schizoaffective disorder* is used for those whose symptoms of schizophrenia are independent of associated periods of mood disturbance. Prognosis depends not on symptom severity but on the response to antipsychotic medication. Patients may present with acute rather than insidious onset of symptoms, and remission without recurrence does occur. Ten percent of schizophrenic patients commit suicide. As currently defined, schizophrenia is present in 0.85 percent of individuals worldwide. Overall, lifetime prevalence is approximately 1 to 1.5 percent.

The societal costs of schizophrenia are substantial. An estimated 300,000 episodes of acute schizophrenia occur annually, resulting in the use of 25 percent of all U.S. hospital beds and 20 percent of all Social Security days, with total direct and indirect economic costs approximating $33 billion.

DIFFERENTIAL DIAGNOSIS For a diagnosis of schizophrenia to be made, the symptom complex must cause significant dysfunction in social or occupational domains and last for at least 6 months. The diagnosis is principally one of exclusion, requiring the absence of significant associated mood symptoms, any relevant medical condition, and substance abuse. Drug reactions that cause hallucinations, paranoia, confusion, or bizarre behavior may be dose-related or idiosyncratic; beta-adrenergic blockers, clonidine, cycloserine, quinacrine, and procaine derivatives are the agents most commonly associated with these symptoms. Drug causes should be ruled out in any case of newly emergent psychosis. The general neurologic examination in patients with schizophrenia is usually normal, but motor rigidity, tremor, and spontaneous dyskinesias are noted in one-quarter of untreated patients.

EPIDEMIOLOGY AND PATHOPHYSIOLOGY Epidemiologic surveys identify three principal risk factors for schizophrenia: (1) genetic vulnerability, (2) early developmental insults, and (3) winter birth. Family, twin, and adoption studies show that genetic factors are involved in at least a subset of individuals who develop schizophrenia. Using conservative diagnostic definitions, schizophrenia is observed in approximately 6.6 percent of all first-degree relatives of an affected proband. If both parents are affected, the risk for offspring is 40 percent. The concordance rate for monozygotic twins is 50 percent, compared to 10 percent for dizygotic twins. Examination of families in which aggregation of schizophrenia occurs has revealed an increased incidence of other psychotic and nonpsychotic psychiatric disorders as well, including schizoaffective disorder and *schizotypal* and *schizoid personality disorders*, the latter terms designating individuals who show a lifetime pattern of social and interpersonal deficits characterized by an inability to form close interpersonal relationships, eccentric behavior, and mild perceptual distortions.

There is increasing evidence that environmental influences modulate genetic factors in the expression of schizophrenia, and, in sporadic cases, may serve as a sufficient cause. Gestational and birth complications, including Rh factor incompatibility, prenatal exposure to influenza during the second trimester, and prenatal nutritional deficiency have been implicated. Studies of monozygotic twins discordant for schizophrenia have profiled neuroanatomic and morphologic differences between affected and unaffected siblings, supporting a "two-strike" etiology involving both genetic susceptibility and an environmental insult.

The proposed pathophysiology involves localized hypoxia during critical stages of neuronal migration and maturation. Neuroimaging and postmortem studies have identified a number of structural and functional abnormalities, including (1) enlargement of the lateral and third ventricles with associated cortical atrophy and sulcal enlargement, (2) volumetric reductions in the amygdala, hippocampus, right prefrontal cortex, and thalamus, (3) altered asymmetry of the planum temporale, and (4) decreases in neuronal metabolism in the thalamus and prefrontal cortex. Some, but not all, prospective studies record progressive reduction in hemispheric volume over years. Cytoarchitectural investigations reveal alterations in the size, orientation, and density of cells in the hippocampus and, in the prefrontal cerebral cortex, decreases in neuronal number and the density of interneurons in layer II as well as an increased density of pyramidal cells in layer V. These observations suggest that schizophrenia results from a disturbance in a cortical striatal–thalamic circuit resulting in deficits in sensory filtering and attentional behavior. Although the formal diagnostic requirements for schizophrenia are not usually met until early adult life, children who eventually develop the disorder may exhibit subtle deficits in motor function, cognition, and emotional expression from an early age.

The hypothesized alterations in cortical neuronal circuitry are paralleled clinically by impairments in attention and cortical information processing, autonomic nervous system activation, and habituation. Schizophrenic individuals are highly distractible and demonstrate a relative deficit in perceptual-motor speed, ability to shift attention, and filtering out of background stimuli. Event-related evoked potential studies of schizophrenia have defined a specific reduction in P300 amplitude to a novel stimulus, which implicates an impairment in cognitive processing, since earlier, more sensory-based components are unaffected. Impaired information processing aggregates in family members of schizophrenic probands.

Despite evidence for a genetic causation, the results of molecular genetic linkage studies in schizophrenia are inconclusive. Single reports of linkage of schizophrenia to loci on chromosomes 5, 11, and other regions have not been replicated. However, four separate groups, using 430 families from diverse populations worldwide, have identified an extended region on the short arm of chromosome 6 that appears to be linked to the disorder, while several others have reported a locus on chromosome 22.

The *dopamine hypothesis* of schizophrenia is based on the serendipitous discovery that agents that diminish dopaminergic activity have beneficial effects in reducing the acute symptoms and signs of psychosis, specifically agitation, anxiety, and hallucinations. Amelioration of delusions and social withdrawal is less dramatic. Thus far, however, evidence for increased dopaminergic activity is indirect. An increase in the activity of nigrostriatal and mesolimbic systems and a relative decrease in mesocortical tracts innervating the prefrontal cortex is hypothesized, although it is likely that other neurotransmitters, including serotonin, acetylcholine, glutamate, and GABA also contribute to the pathophysiology of the illness. Involvement of excitatory amino acids is postulated, based on the finding that NMDA receptor antagonists and channel blockers, such as phencyclidine (PCP) and ketamine, produce characteristic signs of schizophrenia in many normal individuals. These effects can be blocked by "atypical" neuroleptics like clozapine and olanzapine. NMDA receptors are located in high density in the frontal cortex, hippocampus, limbic system, and striatum regions suspected to be involved in schizophrenia. Levels of aspartate and glutamate are decreased in the brains of schizophrenics, while a co-localized neuropeptide antagonist compound, *N*-acetyl-aspartyl glutamate (NAAG), is increased. Evidence for reduced GABA transmission derives from decreased gene expression of glutamic acid decarboxylase in the dorsolateral prefrontal cortex of schizophrenic patients; such a deficit could be responsible for a loss of inhibition over dopaminergic activity in the basal ganglia.

TREATMENT

Antipsychotic agents remain the cornerstone of acute and maintenance treatment of schizophrenia and are effective in the treatment of hallucinations, delusions, and thought disorders, regardless of etiology. The exact mechanism of action remains incompletely understood, but dopaminergic receptor blockade in the limbic system and basal ganglia appears to be an essential element, since the clinical potencies of traditional antipsychotic drugs parallel their affinities for the D_2 receptor, and even the newer "atypical" agents exert some degree of D_2 receptor blockade. All neuroleptics induce expression of the immediate-early gene c-*fos* in the nucleus accumbens, a dopaminergic site connecting prefrontal and limbic cortices. The clinical efficacy of newer atypical neuroleptics, however, may involve D_1, D_3, and D_4 receptor blockade, $alpha_1$ and $alpha_2$ noradrenergic activity, and/or the relationship between $5HT_2$ and D_2 receptor activity as well. In experimental investigations of a proposed glutaminergic deficiency model of schizophrenia, high-dose glycine therapy also shows encouraging evidence of efficacy.

Conventional neuroleptics differ in their potency and side-effect profile. Older agents, such as chlorpromazine and thioridazine, are more sedating and anticholinergic and more likely to cause orthostatic hypotension, while higher potency antipsychotics, such as haloperidol, perphenazine, and thiothixene, carry a higher risk of inducing extrapyramidal side effects. The model atypical antipsychotic agent is clozapine, a dibenzoazepine derivative that has a greater potency in blocking the $5HT_2$ than the D_2 receptor and a much higher affinity for the D_4 than the D_2 receptor. Its principal disadvantage is risk of blood dyscrasia, requiring regular monitoring of the CBC. Unlike other antipsychotics, clozapine does not cause a rise in prolactin level. Approximately 30 percent of patients have a better antipsychotic response to these agents than to traditional neuroleptics, suggesting that they will increasingly displace the older-generation drugs. *Clozapine* increases the activity of the immediate-early gene c-*fos* in the prefrontal cortex, the neuroanatomic region having the highest concentration of D_4 receptors and an area thought to mediate the specific executive functions that are prominently impaired in schizophrenia. *Risperidone*, a benzisoxazole derivative, is more potent at $5HT_2$ than D_2 receptor sites, like clozapine, but it also exerts significant $alpha_2$ antagonism, a property that may contribute to its perceived ability to improve mood and increase motor activity. Risperidone is not as effective as clozapine in treatment-resistant cases but does not carry a risk of blood dyscrasia.

Conventional antipsychotic agents are effective in approximately 70 percent of patients presenting with a first episode. Improvement may be observed within hours or days, but full remission usually requires 6 to 8 weeks. Since no antipsychotic drug is clearly superior to any other in efficacy (with the exception of clozapine in treatment-resistant groups), the choice of agent depends principally on the side-effect profile or on a past personal or family history of a favorable response to the drug in question. Equivalent treatment response can usually be achieved through relatively low doses of any drug selected, i.e., 4 to 6 mg/d of haloperidol, 400 mg/d of chlorpromazine, or 4 to 6 mg/d of risperidone. Doses in this range result in greater than 80 percent D_2 receptor blockade, and there is little evidence that higher doses increase either the rapidity or degree of response. Titration of the dose should proceed slowly, particularly with risperidone, for which 2 weeks to 1 month usually is required to arrive at an optimal level. Maintenance treatment requires careful attention to the possibility of relapse and monitoring for the development of a movement disorder. Intermittent drug treatment is less effective than regular dosing, but gradual dose reduction is likely to improve social functioning in many schizophrenic patients who have been maintained at high doses. If medications are completely discontinued, however, the relapse rate is about 60 percent within 6 months. Long-acting injectable preparations (haloperidol decanoate and fluphenazine decanoate) are considered when noncompliance with oral therapy leads to relapses. In treatment-resistant patients, a transition to clozapine usually results in rapid improvement, but a prolonged delay in response in some cases necessitates a 6- to 9-month trial for maximal benefit to occur.

Antipsychotic medications can cause a broad range of side effects, including lethargy, weight gain, postural hypotension, constipation, and dry mouth. Extrapyramidal symptoms such as dystonia, akathisia, and akinesia are also frequent with traditional agents and may contribute to poor compliance if not specifically addressed. Anticholinergic and Parkinsonian symptoms respond well to trihexyphenidyl, 2 mg bid, or benztropine mesylate, 1 to 2 mg bid. Akathisia may respond to beta blockers. In rare cases, more serious and occasionally life-threatening side effects may emerge, including ventricular arrhythmias, gastrointestinal obstruction, retinal pigmentation, obstructive jaundice, and neuroleptic malignant syndrome (characterized by hyperthermia, autonomic dysfunction, muscular rigidity, and elevated creatinine phosphokinase levels). The most serious adverse effects of clozapine are agranulocytosis, which has an incidence of 1 percent, and induction of seizures, which has an incidence of 10 percent. Weekly white blood cell counts are required, particularly during the first 3 months of treatment.

A severe side effect of long-term use of the classic antipsychotic agents is *tardive dyskinesia*, characterized by repetitive, involuntary, and potentially irreversible movements of the tongue and lips (bucco-linguo-masticatory triad), and, in approximately half of cases, choreoathetoid movements of the limbs (see Chap. 21). Tardive dyskinesia occurs in one-quarter to one-half of all patients who are maintained on neuroleptics for longer than 6 months. The prevalence increases with age and with total dose and duration of drug administration, but as yet unknown individual factors play the greatest part in determining risk. The cause of tardive dyskinesia is unknown, but evidence suggests that chronic neuroleptic treatment increases the formation of free radicals and perhaps damages mitochondrial energy metabolism. Vitamin E may reduce abnormal involuntary movements if given early in the development of the syndrome. Other strategies for treatment include use of reserpine and anticholinergics, in addition to very gradual dose reduction. The higher efficacy of clozapine and risperidone in treating negative symptoms, together with their lower risk of tardive dyskinesia, has stimulated the development of additional atypical antipsychotic agents that are likely to revolutionize the treatment of schizophrenia. Quetiapine, olanzapine, ziprasidone, and sertindole promise to have a therapeutic efficacy comparable to that of clozapine without the latter's risk of causing agranulocytosis.

ASSESSMENT AND EVALUATION OF VIOLENCE

Primary care physicians may, in the course of routine medical practice, encounter situations in which familial, domestic, or societal violence is discovered or suspected. Depending on local laws, such an awareness can carry legal and moral obligations. Recent surveys document that child, spousal, and elder abuse is relatively common and that physicians are frequently the first point of contact for both victim and abuser. Between 1 and 2 million older Americans and 1.5 million U.S. children are thought to experience some form of physical maltreatment each year. Spousal abuse is thought to be even more prevalent. A recent broad-based survey of primary care internal medicine practices found that 5.5 percent of all female patients had experienced domestic violence in the previous year, and that these individuals were more likely to suffer from depression, anxiety, somatization disorder, and substance abuse and to have attempted suicide. When domestic violence is suspected, direct but nonjudgmental questioning should be pursued with each party separately—"Do you feel safe at home," and "If there's a disagreement or a conflict between the two of you, how is it worked out?" In addition to obvious and suggestive physical injury, individuals who are abused frequently express low self-esteem, vague somatic symptomatology, social isolation, and a passive feeling of loss of control. Although it is essential to treat these elements in the victim, the first obligation is to ensure that the perpetrator has taken responsibility for preventing any further violence. Substance abuse and/or dependence and serious mental illness in the abuser may contribute to the risk of harm and require direct intervention. Depending on the individual situation, law enforcement agencies, community resources such as support groups and shelters, and individual and family counseling can be appropriate components of a treatment plan. A safety plan should be formulated with the victim, in addition to the provision of information about abuse, its likelihood of recurrence, and its tendency to increase in severity and frequency. Antianxiety and antidepressant medications may sometimes be useful in treating the acute symptoms, but they should only be used if independent evidence for an appropriate psychiatric diagnosis exists. Antidepressants are generally not indicated when the diagnosis is linked to the social situation, such as an adjustment disorder with depressed mood. The most important element in treatment is the development of a supportive doctor-patient relationship that avoids further blame of the victim.

In certain circumstances, a significant potential for societal violence may be discovered. Sympathetic, but direct, questioning of potential violent impulses, access to weapons, recreational drug use, and specific homicidal ideation is necessary for appropriate evaluation and is sometimes therapeutic in its own right. The existence and possible contribution of such medical conditions as delirium and/or intoxication should be evaluated. Available disposition options for potentially violent patients include police custody, psychiatric hospitalization, and referral to home care, with involvement of family, friends, and care givers. In deciding which treatment option is most appropriate, clinicians should endeavor to establish an empathic interaction with the patient, while avoiding interventions or stimuli that might precipitate or increase the risk of violent behavior. Formal verbal limit setting may be necessary if the patient reveals the existence of a weapon or becomes increasingly agitated or verbally abusive. Use of the least restrictive intervention is generally the best approach during the initial evaluation.

MENTAL HEALTH PROBLEMS IN THE HOMELESS

There is increasing recognition of a high prevalence of mental disorders and substance abuse among homeless and impoverished populations. The total number of homeless individuals in the United States is estimated at 2 to 3 million, one-third of whom qualify as having a serious mental disorder. Poor hygiene and nutrition, substance abuse, psychiatric illness, physical trauma, and exposure to the elements combine to make the provision of medical care a challenging enterprise. Only a minority of individuals receive formal mental health care; the main points of contact are outpatient medical clinics and emergency departments. Primary care settings represent a critical site in which housing needs, treatment of substance dependence, and evaluation and treatment of psychiatric illness can most efficiently take place. Successful intervention is dependent on breaking down traditional administrative barriers to health care and recognizing the physical constraints and emotional costs imposed by homelessness. Simplifying health care instructions and follow-up, allowing frequent visits, and dispensing medications in limited amounts that require ongoing contact are possible techniques for establishing a successful therapeutic relationship. Child neglect, resulting in developmental delay and emotional difficulty in addition to other health problems, is unfortunately common and necessitates an effort to independently evaluate the well being of any offspring.

BIBLIOGRAPHY

GENERAL

American Psychiatric Association: Diagnostic and Statistical Manual of Mental Disorders, 4th ed. Washington DC, American Psychiatric Association, 1994

Broadhead WE et al: Development and validation of the SDDS-PC screen for multiple mental disorders in primary care. Arch Fam Med 4:211, 1995

Hyman SE, Nestler EJ: Initiation and adaptation: A paradigm for understanding psychotropic drug action. Am J Psychiatry 153:151, 1996

Lachs M, Pillemer K: Abuse and neglect of elderly persons. N Engl J Med 332:437, 1995

McCauley J et al: The "battering syndrome": Prevalence and clinical characteristics of domestic violence in primary care internal medical practices. Ann Intern Med 123:737, 1995

Oldham JM et al: Comorbidity of axis I and axis II disorders. Am J Psychiatry 152:571, 1995

PSYCHOLOGICAL FACTORS IN MEDICAL ILLNESS

Buckley RA: Differentiating medical and psychiatric illness. Psychiatr Ann 24:584, 1994

Linden W et al: Psychosocial interventions for patients with coronary artery disease. Arch Intern Med 156:745, 1996

McDaniel JS et al: Depression in patients with cancer. Arch Gen Psychiatry 52:89, 1995

ANXIETY DISORDERS

Brown C et al: Treatment outcomes for primary care patients with major depression and lifetime anxiety disorders. Arch Gen Psychiatry 153:1293, 1996

Goldberg RJ: Diagnostic dilemmas presented by patients with anxiety and depression. Am J Med 98:278, 1995

Lydiard B et al: Panic disorder and gastrointestinal symptoms: Findings from the NIMH epidemiologic catchment area project. Am J Psychiatry 151:64, 1994

Magee WJ et al: Agoraphobia, simple phobia, and social phobia in the national comorbidity survey. Arch Gen Psychiatry 53:159, 1996

Marshall RD, Klein DF: Pharmacotherapy in the treatment of posttraumatic stress disorder. Psychiatr Ann 25:588, 1995

MOOD DISORDERS

Burvill PW: Recent progress in the epidemiology of major depression. Epidemiol Rev 17:21, 1995

Depression Guideline Panel: *Depression in Primary Care,* vol 1: *Detection and Diagnosis.* Clinical Practice Guideline no 5. Rockville, MD, US Department of Health & Human Services, AHCPR Publication 93-0550, 1993

———: *Depression in Primary Care,* vol 2: *Treatment of Major Depression.* Clinical Practice Guideline no 5. Rockville, MD, US Department of Health & Human Services, AHCPR Publication 93-0551, 1993

Hirschfeld RMA: Algorithm for the evaluation and treatment of suicidal patients. Prim Psychiatry 3:26, 1996

Katon W et al: Collaborative management to achieve treatment guidelines. JAMA 13:1026, 1995

Kupfer DJ: Sleep research in depressive illness: Clinical implications—a tasting menu. Biol Psychiatry 38:391, 1995

Price LH, Henninger GR: Lithium in the treatment of mood disorders. N Engl J Med 331:591, 1994

Sherbourne CD et al: Subthreshold depression and depressive disorder: Clinical characteristics of general medical and mental health specialty outpatients. Am J Psychiatry 151:1777, 1994

Solomon DA et al: Course of illness and maintenance treatments for patients with bipolar disorder. J Clin Psychiatry 56:5, 1995

Sturm R, Wells KB: How can care for depression become more cost-effective? JAMA 273:51, 1995

SOMATOFORM DISORDERS, PERSONALITY AND BEHAVIORAL DISORDERS

Davis JM et al: Psychopharmacotherapy of the personality-disordered patient. Psychiatr Ann 25:614, 1995

NOYES R JR et al: Somatization. Diagnosis and management. Arch Fam Med 4:790, 1995

SCHIZOPHRENIA

ANDREASEN NC et al: Symptoms of schizophrenia. Arch Gen Psychiatry 52:341, 1995

CARPENTER WT JR, BUCHANAN RW: Schizophrenia. N Engl J Med 330:681, 1994

——— et al: Patient response and resource management: Another view of clozapine treatment of schizophrenia. Am J Psychiatry 152:827, 1995

KANE JM: Schizophrenia. N Engl J Med 334:34, 1996

KETY SS et al: Mental illness in the biological and adoptive relatives of schizophrenic adoptees. Arch Gen Psychiatry 51:442, 1994

WYATT RJ: Neurodevelopmental abnormalities and schizophrenia. Arch Gen Psychiatry 53:11, 1996

SECTION 6

ALCOHOLISM AND DRUG DEPENDENCY

386

Marc A. Schuckit

ALCOHOL AND ALCOHOLISM

Ninety percent of people drink alcohol, 40 to 50 percent of men have temporary alcohol-induced problems, and 10 to 20 percent of men and 3 to 10 percent of women develop pervasive and persistent alcohol-related problems (alcohol dependence or abuse—alcoholism). The usual alcoholic has a family and a job; only about 5 percent live on "skid row." Even light drinking may adversely interact with other medications; temporary heavier drinking can exacerbate most medical illnesses; and alcoholism can masquerade as many different medical disorders and psychiatric syndromes. The following sections describe the pharmacology and clinical effects of alcohol and identify circumstances in which drinking may cause a major medical or psychiatric problem or exacerbate a preexisting disorder.

PHARMACOLOGY OF ETHANOL: ABSORPTION AND METABOLISM Ethanol is a weakly charged molecule that moves easily through cell membranes, rapidly equilibrating between blood and tissues. The effects of drinking depend in part on the amount of ethanol consumed per unit of body weight; the level of alcohol in the blood is expressed as milligrams or grams of ethanol per deciliter (e.g., 100 mg/dL or 0.1000 g/dL). In round figures, 340 mL (12 oz) of beer, 115 mL (4 oz) of nonfortified wine, and 43 mL (1.5 oz) (a shot) of 80-proof beverage each contain approximately 10 g of ethanol; 1 pint of 86-proof beverage contains approximately 160 g, and 1 L of wine contains approximately 80 g of ethanol. Congeners found in alcoholic beverages may contribute to body damage with heavy drinking; these include low-molecular-weight alcohols (e.g., methanol and butanol), aldehydes, esters, histamine, phenols, tannins, iron, lead, and cobalt.

Ethanol is a central nervous system (CNS) depressant that decreases activity of neurons, although some behavioral stimulation is observed at low blood levels. This drug has cross-tolerance and shares a similar pattern of behavioral problems with other brain depressants, including the benzodiazepines and barbiturates. Alcohol is absorbed from mucous membranes of the mouth and esophagus (in small amounts), from the stomach and large bowel (in modest amounts), and from the proximal portion of the small intestine (the major site). The rate of absorption is *increased* by rapid gastric emptying, by the absence of proteins, fats, or carbohydrates (which interfere with absorption), by the absence of congeners, by dilution to a modest percentage of ethanol (maximum absorption is seen at about 20 percent by volume), and by carbonation (e.g., champagne).

Between 2 percent (at low blood alcohol concentrations) and about 10 percent (at high blood alcohol concentrations) of ethanol is excreted directly through the lungs, urine, or sweat, but the greater part is metabolized to acetaldehyde in the liver. At least two metabolic routes, each with different optimal concentrations of ethanol (K_m), result in the metabolism of approximately one drink per hour. The *first* and clinically most important pathway occurs in the cell cytosol via alcohol dehydrogenase (ADH), with a K_m of about 2 mmol. This reaction produces acetaldehyde, which is then rapidly destroyed by aldehyde dehydrogenase (ALDH) in the cytosol and mitochondria. Each of these steps requires nicotinamide adenine dinucleotide (NAD) as a cofactor, and it is the increased ratio of the reduced cofactor (NADH) to NAD (NADH:NAD) that is responsible for many of the metabolic derangements observed after drinking. *Second,* microsomes of the smooth endoplasmic reticulum (the microsomal ethanol-oxidizing system, or MEOS), with a K_m of about 10 mmol, may be responsible for 10 percent or more of ethanol oxidation at high blood alcohol concentrations. Increased activity of this system can be induced by repeated exposure to ethanol.

The specific clinical significance of the first metabolite of alcohol, acetaldehyde, is not fully known, but low levels of this substance may cause stimulation and behavioral reinforcement. Accumulation of higher levels in liver, brain, or other body tissues may cause organ damage.

BEHAVIORAL EFFECTS, TOLERANCE, AND DEPENDENCE The behavioral and physiologic effects of any drug depend on the dose, its rate of increase in plasma, the concomitant presence of other drugs or medical problems, and the past experience with the agent. With alcohol, an additional factor is whether blood alcohol levels are rising or falling; the effects of alcohol are more intense during the former period.

Even though "legal intoxication" requires a blood alcohol concentration of at least 80 to 100 mg/dL, behavioral, psychomotor, and cognitive changes are seen at levels as low as 20 to 30 mg/dL (i.e., after one to two drinks). Narcosis or deep sleep is induced in many people at twice the legal intoxication level, and even in the absence of concomitant medications, death can occur with levels between 300 and 400 mg/dL. Ethanol, either alone or in combination with agents such as benzodiazepines, is probably responsible for more toxic overdose deaths than any other agent.

Ethanol produces simultaneous changes in many neurotransmitters and also increases the fluidity of neuronal cell membranes. After repeated exposure to the drug, the body compensates in at least three ways to tolerate higher ethanol levels. *First,* after 1 to 2 weeks of daily drinking, the liver can increase the rate of ethanol metabolism by as much as 30 percent; i.e., there is *metabolic or pharmacokinetic tolerance.* This alteration disappears almost as rapidly as it develops. *Second, cellular or pharmacodynamic tolerance* probably occurs through complex neurochemical changes and alterations in cell membranes—adjustments that may contribute to physical dependence. *Third,* even at the same blood alcohol concentrations and level of neuronal adaptation, organisms can learn to adapt their behavior so as to function better than expected under drug influence *(behavioral tolerance).*

Once the cells have adapted to chronic ethanol exposure, the structural or biochemical changes may not return to normal for several weeks or more. In the face of these adjustments, the neurons require ethanol to function optimally; i.e., the person is physically addicted. This physical condition is distinct from psychological dependence, a concept indicating that the person is psychologically uncomfortable without the drug.

NUTRITIONAL FACTORS One gram of ethanol has approximately 29.7 kJ (7.1 kcal) of energy, and a drink contains between 293.0 and 418.6 kJ (70 and 100 kcal) from ethanol and other carbohydrates. Therefore, 8 to 10 drinks can yield over 4186 kJ (1000 kcal) per day, but these are "empty" of nutrients such as minerals, proteins, and vitamins.

Any vitamin absorbed through the small intestine by active transport or stored in the liver may be deficient in even apparently well-nourished alcoholics. These include folate (folacin or folic acid), pyridoxine (B_6), thiamine (B_1), nicotinic acid (niacin, B_3), and vitamin A. Thiamine deficiency causes Wernicke's and Korsakoff's syndromes (see Chap. 380).

Low blood levels of potassium, magnesium, calcium, zinc, and phosphorus can occur as a consequence of dietary deficiency and acid-base imbalances during excess alcohol ingestion or withdrawal. Hypokalemia can lead to periodic muscle paralysis and areflexia. Deficiencies in magnesium can add to a clouded sensorium and other neurologic symptoms; hypocalcemia can cause tetany and weakness; low levels of zinc are speculated to contribute to gonadal dysfunction, anorexia, problems with wound healing, and immune deficiencies; and low phosphate levels can contribute to myocardial failure, brain dysfunction, weakness of muscles (including those of respiration), and white blood cell and platelet dysfunction.

An ethanol load in a fasting, healthy individual is likely to produce transient hypoglycemia within 6 to 36 h, secondary to the acute actions of ethanol on gluconeogenesis. This impairment is exacerbated by poor diet and by liver and pancreatic disease. As a result, glucose intolerance may be marked until the alcoholic has abstained for 2 to 4 weeks. Alcohol ketoacidosis, probably reflecting a decrease in fatty acid oxidation coupled with poor diet or recurrent vomiting, should not be misdiagnosed as diabetic ketosis. With the former, patients show an increase in serum ketones along with a mild increase in glucose but a large anion gap, a mild to moderate increase in serum lactate, and a β-hydroxybutyrate/lactate ratio of between 2:1 and 9:1 (with normal being 1:1).

THE EFFECTS OF ETHANOL ON BODY SYSTEMS

This overview of acute and chronic effects of alcohol on body systems outlines signs and symptoms that can aid in the recognition of the hidden alcoholic.

CENTRAL NERVOUS SYSTEM In addition to acute behavioral effects, an evening of heavy drinking can result in an alcoholic *blackout*, i.e., an episode of forgetting all or part of what occurred during drinking. This problem is experienced by 30 to 40 percent of men in their late teens and early 20s, most of whom do not go on to develop more serious and pervasive alcohol-related problems. Even after only a few drinks, alcohol acutely decreases *sleep* latency (helping people to fall asleep) and depresses rapid eye movement (REM) sleep early in the night, sometimes followed by later REM rebound associated with bad dreams. The consequence is to "fragment" sleep, causing a more rapid than normal alternation between sleep stages and a deficiency in deep sleep. The overall effect is likely to be repeated awakenings and a sense of restless sleep even in moderate drinkers.

Chronic intake of high doses of ethanol causes *peripheral neuropathy* in 5 to 15 percent of alcoholics (see Chap. 380), which is possibly related to thiamine deficiency. Patients complain of bilateral limb numbness, tingling, and paresthesia; symptoms are more pronounced distally than proximally. The treatment is abstinence and thiamine supplementation.

Wernicke's and Korsakoff's syndromes (alcohol-induced persisting amnestic disorder) are the result of thiamine deficiency in vulnerable individuals (possibly owing to interaction with a genetic transketolase deficiency). Korsakoff's syndrome presents with profound anterograde amnesia (inability to learn new material) and a milder retrograde amnesia, along with possible impairment in visuospatial, abstract, and conceptual reasoning but with a normal intelligence quotient (IQ). While most patients demonstrate an acute onset of Korsakoff's syndrome in association with the neurologic stigmata seen with Wernicke's syndrome (e.g., sixth nerve palsy and ataxia), some individuals have a more gradual development of symptoms. Wernicke's syndrome responds rapidly to oral thiamine replacement (50 to 100 mg followed by 50 to 100 mg/d). However, only one-quarter of Korsakoff's patients achieve full recovery, one-half experience partial recovery, and one-quarter show no improvement with thiamine even after many months of supplementation.

About 1 percent of alcoholics with long histories of associated malnutrition develop *cerebellar degeneration*, a syndrome of progressive unsteady stance and gait often accompanied by mild nystagmus (see Chap. 380). Cerebellar atrophy is seen on computed tomography (CT) or magnetic resonance imaging (MRI), but the cerebrospinal fluid is usually normal. The major cause is probably nutritional, and identical symptoms can be seen with some forms of severe malnutrition alone. Treatment consists of abstinence and multiple vitamin supplementation, although improvement is often minimal.

Alcoholics can show severe *cognitive* problems and impairment in recent and remote memory for weeks to months after an alcoholic binge. Increased size of the brain ventricles and cerebral sulci are seen in up to 50 percent of chronic alcoholics, but these changes are often reversible, returning toward normal after a year or more of abstinence. Permanent CNS impairment (alcohol-induced persisting dementia) can develop and accounts for up to 20 percent of chronically demented patients. There is no single alcoholic dementia syndrome; rather, this label is used to describe patients who have apparently irreversible cognitive changes (possibly from diverse causes) in the midst of chronic alcoholism (see also Chap. 380).

Finally, almost every psychiatric syndrome can be seen during heavy drinking or subsequent withdrawal. These include intense *sadness* lasting for days to weeks in the midst of heavy drinking, which is classified as an alcohol-induced mood disorder in the Fourth Diagnostic and Statistical Manual of the American Psychiatric Association (DSM-IV); severe *anxiety* during alcohol withdrawal, often persisting for many months after cessation of drinking (alcohol-induced anxiety disorder); and auditory *hallucinations* and/or *paranoid delusions* in the absence of any obvious signs of withdrawal—a state now called alcohol-induced psychotic disorder. Whatever the cause, the treatment of alcohol-induced psychopathology includes abstinence and supportive care, with the likelihood of full recovery within several days to 6 weeks. Alcohol intake is an important part of the differential diagnosis of *any* patient with one of these psychological symptoms.

THE GASTROINTESTINAL SYSTEM Esophagus and Stomach Acute alcohol intake can result in inflammation of the esophagus (possibly secondary to reflux of gastric contents) and stomach (resulting from damage to the gastric mucosal barrier). Esophagitis can cause epigastric distress, and gastritis, the most frequent cause of gastrointestinal bleeding in heavy drinkers, can present with anorexia and abdominal pain. Chronic heavy drinking, if associated with violent vomiting, can produce a longitudinal tear in the mucosa at the gastroesophageal junction—a Mallory-Weiss lesion. Although many gastrointestinal problems are reversible, two complications of chronic alcoholism, esophageal varices secondary to cirrhosis-induced portal hypertension and atrophy of gastric cells, may be irreversible. → *See Chap. 283.*

Small Bowel Acutely, ethanol can cause hemorrhagic lesions of the duodenal villi and diarrhea secondary to increased small-bowel motility and decreased water and electrolyte absorption. Chronic alcoholism can contribute to diarrhea through its effects on the pancreas. → *See Chaps. 285 and 304.*

Pancreas Alcoholics commonly develop acute or chronic pancreatitis. → *See Chap. 304.*

Liver Ethanol absorbed from the small bowel is carried directly to the liver, where it becomes the preferred fuel; NADH accumulates and oxygen utilization escalates; gluconeogenesis is impaired (with a resulting fall in the amount of glucose produced from glycogen); lactate production increases; and there is a decreased oxidation of fatty acids in the citric cycle with an increase in fat accumulation within liver cells. In the healthy individual taking no medications, these changes are reversible, but with repeated exposure to ethanol, more severe changes in liver functioning are likely to occur. These include, in overlapping stages, fatty accumulation, alcohol-induced hepatitis, perivenular sclerosis, and cirrhosis. → *See Chap. 298.*

Increased Cancer Risk Cancer is the second leading cause of death in alcoholics (after cardiovascular disease); alcoholics have a rate of carcinoma 10 times higher than that in the general population. The sites with the greatest increase over expected rates include the head and neck, esophagus, cardia of the stomach, liver, pancreas, and, according to recent data, breast.

HEMATOPOIETIC SYSTEM Ethanol exerts multiple reversible acute and chronic effects on all blood cells. Alcohol alters acutely the production of red blood cells (RBC), and this effect reaches clinical significance after days to weeks of heavy drinking. The most common finding is an increase in RBC size (mean corpuscular volume, MCV), most often without anemia. This change appears to reflect the effect of alcohol on stem cells. If heavy drinking is accompanied by folic acid deficiency, there also can be hypersegmented neutrophils, reticulocytopenia, and hyperplastic bone marrow, and, if malnutrition is present, sideroblastic changes can be observed.

Chronic heavy drinking also can decrease production of most white blood cells (WBCs), decrease granulocyte mobility and adherence, and impair the delayed hypersensitivity response to new antigens (with a possible false-negative tuberculin skin test). While the changes in WBCs are usually temporary, they may contribute to the risk of infections and liver damage and perhaps to the increased risk of cancers in alcoholics. Alcohol also can cause toxic granulocytosis.

Many alcoholics present with mild thrombocytopenia (rarely associated with hemorrhage) due to a decrease in platelet survival and altered function; hypersplenism may occur as a complication of cirrhosis. Alcohol may decrease platelet aggregation and inhibit release of thromboxane A_2. These problems usually return toward normal within a week of abstinence.

CARDIOVASCULAR SYSTEM Modest doses of alcohol can have both deleterious and beneficial effects in individuals with normal cardiovascular status who take no medications. Ethanol acutely decreases myocardial contractility and causes peripheral vasodilation, resulting in a mild drop in blood pressure and a compensatory increased heart rate and cardiac output. Exercise-induced increases in cardiac oxygen consumption are higher after alcohol. A maximum of one to two drinks per day over long periods may decrease the risk of cardiovascular death, perhaps through an increase in high-density lipoprotein (HDL) cholesterol or changes in clotting mechanisms.

Although ethanol in low doses causes a mild acute drop in blood pressure, the consumption of three or more drinks per day results in a dose-dependent increase in blood pressure, which returns to normal within weeks of abstinence. As a result, heavy drinking is an important contributor to mild to moderate hypertension. Chronic heavy drinking can cause cardiomyopathy with symptoms ranging from unexplained arrhythmias in the presence of left ventricular impairment to heart failure with dilation of all four heart chambers and hypocontractility of heart muscle. Mural thrombi can form in the left atrium or ventricle, while heart enlargement exceeding 25 percent can cause mitral regurgitation. Finally, there is an association between cerebrovascular accidents and alcoholism, especially within 24 h of heavy drinking. Atrial or ventricular arrhythmias, especially paroxysmal tachycardia, also can occur after a binge in individuals showing no other evidence of heart disease—a syndrome known as the "holiday heart."

GENITOURINARY SYSTEM CHANGES, SEXUAL FUNCTIONING, AND FETAL DEVELOPMENT Acutely, modest ethanol doses (e.g., blood alcohol concentrations of 100 mg/dL or even less) can increase sexual drive in men. However, modest ethanol doses may simultaneously decrease erectile capacity. Even in the absence of liver impairment, a significant minority of chronic alcoholic men may show irreversible testicular atrophy with concomitant shrinkage of the seminiferous tubules and loss of sperm cells (see Chap. 336).

The repeated ingestion of high doses of ethanol by women can result in amenorrhea, a decrease in ovarian size, absence of corpora lutea with associated infertility, and spontaneous abortions. Heavy drinking during pregnancy results in the rapid placental transfer of both ethanol and acetaldehyde, which may have serious consequences for fetal development. The *fetal alcohol syndrome* can include a mixture of any of the following: facial changes with epicanthal eye folds, poorly formed concha, and small teeth with faulty enamel; cardiac atrial or ventricular septal defects; an aberrant palmar crease and limitation in joint movement; and microcephaly with mental retardation. The specific amount of ethanol and/or specific time of vulnerability during pregnancy have not been defined, making it advisable for pregnant women to abstain completely.

OTHER EFFECTS OF ETHANOL Heavy drinking can produce an acute *alcoholic myopathy* characterized by painful and swollen muscles, high levels of serum creatine phosphokinase (CK), and, rarely, myoglobinemia and myoglobinuria. Effects on the *skeletal system* include alterations in calcium metabolism with an increased risk for fractures and osteonecrosis of the femoral head. *Hormonal* changes include an increase in cortisol levels, which can remain elevated during heavy drinking; inhibition of vasopressin secretion at rising blood alcohol concentrations and the opposite effect at falling blood alcohol concentrations (with the final result that most alcoholics are likely to be slightly overhydrated); a modest and reversible decrease in serum thyroxine (T_4); and a more marked decrease in serum triiodothyronine (T_3).

ALCOHOLISM (ALCOHOL ABUSE OR DEPENDENCE)

Because many drinkers occasionally imbibe to excess, temporary alcohol-related pathology is common in nonalcoholics. The time of heaviest drinking is usually the late teens to the late twenties, when between one-third and one-half of male drinkers experience some isolated (although potentially dangerous) alcohol-related social, occupational, or driving difficulty. These include alcohol-related blackouts, a single drunk driving arrest, and arguments with friends. This prevalent alcohol-related morbidity, however, is temporary and is a separate problem from alcohol dependence. The following sections describe diagnostic criteria for alcoholism, offer suggestions for identifying the usual (i.e., middle-class) alcoholic in everyday medical practice, review evidence that alcoholism is a biologic and genetically influenced disorder, and offer advice on intervention, detoxification, and rehabilitation of alcoholics.

DEFINITIONS AND EPIDEMIOLOGY DSM-IV defines alcohol dependence as repeated alcohol-related difficulties in at least three of seven areas of functioning. These include any combination of tolerance, withdrawal, taking larger amounts of alcohol over longer periods than intended, an inability to control use, spending a great deal of time associated with alcohol use, giving up important activities to drink, and continued use of alcohol despite physical or psychological consequences. This constellation of symptoms is likely to occur in both men and women, in individuals of all socioeconomic strata, and in people of all racial backgrounds. It also predicts a course of recurrent problems with the use of alcohol, and the consequent shortening of the life span by a decade or more. In the absence of alcohol dependence, an individual can be given a diagnosis of *alcohol abuse* if he or she demonstrates *repetitive* problems with alcohol in any one of four life areas, including an inability to fulfill major obligations, use in hazardous situations such as driving, legal problems, or use despite social or interpersonal difficulties.

Thus, the clinical diagnosis of alcohol abuse or dependence rests on the documentation of a pattern of *difficulties associated with alcohol use* and is *not* based on the quantity and frequency of alcohol consumption. This approach is used because an individual's pattern of drinking is difficult to establish and because the amount of alcohol associated with high blood levels differs with a person's age, sex, weight, percent body fat, and concomitant use of other medications. Thus, in screening for alcohol abuse or dependence in a clinical setting, it is important to probe for life problems and then attempt to tie in use of alcohol or another substance. A patient's pattern of life difficulties is important for a clinician to understand, and thus information regarding marital or job problems, legal difficulties, histories of accidents, medical problems, evidence of tolerance, etc., are important components of all evaluations and yield information that is of use even for nonalcoholic individuals.

The lifetime risk for alcohol dependence in most western countries is about 10 percent for men and 3 to 5 percent for women. When alcohol abuse is also considered, the rates double. The average alcoholic (just like the average person) is a blue-collar or white-collar worker or homemaker. Homeless or skid row alcoholics represent only 5 percent or less of the total.

GENETICS OF ALCOHOLISM Alcoholism is a multifactorial disorder in which biologic and genetic factors interact. The importance of genetic factors in alcoholism is supported by family, twin, and adoption studies. Close relatives of alcoholics who themselves have no other psychiatric disorder have an approximately fourfold increased risk for alcoholism but are not significantly more vulnerable to other psychiatric illnesses. The risk for the identical twin of an alcoholic is higher than for the fraternal twin of an alcohol-dependent person. Finally, adoption studies reveal that the fourfold increased risk for children of alcoholics is true even if they were adopted away at birth and raised without knowledge of the problems of their biologic parents.

The evidence supporting genetic influences in alcoholism has stimulated studies attempting to identify possible trait markers of a vulnerability toward the disorder before alcoholism appears. A 10-year follow-up of 453 men originally studied at age 20 has shown that subjects with alcoholic fathers demonstrated relatively lower levels of response to alcohol, including less intense subjective feelings of intoxication, less alcohol-related impairment in cognitive and psychomotor tests, and less intense alcohol-related changes in prolactin and cortisol secretion. This low level of response to alcohol at around age 20 was a powerful predictor of alcoholism a decade later. Taken as a whole, these data underscore the probability that alcoholism is biologically influenced and not related to a lack of "moral fiber." It is not surprising that the average alcoholic may continue to work, has a family, and may be difficult to identify if the physician persists with old stereotypes.

NATURAL HISTORY For the "average" alcoholic, the age of first drink and first minor problems (e.g., an argument with a friend while drunk or an alcoholic blackout) are similar to those in the general population. However, by the early to mid-twenties, most men and women moderate their drinking (perhaps learning from minor problems), whereas difficulties for alcoholics are likely to escalate, with the first major life problem from alcohol appearing in the mid-twenties to early forties. Once established, the course of alcoholism is likely to be one of exacerbations and remissions. As a rule there is remarkably little difficulty in stopping alcohol use when problems develop, and this step often is followed by days to months of carefully controlled drinking. Unfortunately, these periods are almost inevitably followed by escalations in alcohol intake and subsequent problems. The course is not hopeless, because a fifth or more of alcoholics achieve permanent abstinence without formal treatment or aid from self-help groups such as Alcoholics Anonymous (AA). However, should the alcoholic continue to drink, the life span is shortened by an average of 15 years, with the leading causes of death, in decreasing order, being heart disease, cancer, accidents, and suicide.

IDENTIFICATION OF THE ALCOHOLIC AND INTERVENTION Physicians even in affluent areas should recognize that 20 percent or so of patients have alcoholism. Therefore, it is important to pay attention to physical findings and laboratory tests that are likely to be abnormal in the alcoholic. These include a high-normal or slightly elevated MCV (e.g., 91 fL or higher), γ-glutamyl transferase (GGT) (30 or more units), serum uric acid [greater than 416 μmol/L (7 mg/dL)], carbohydrate-deficient transferrin (CDT) (20 g/L or more), and triglycerides [2.0 mmol/L (180 mg/dL) or more]. Mild and fluctuating levels of hypertension (e.g., 140/95), repeated infections such as pneumonia, and otherwise unexplained cardiac arrhythmias all suggest that the patient might be an alcoholic. Certain specific clinical findings also should raise suspicions, including cancer of the head and neck, esophagus, or cardia of the stomach as well as cirrhosis, unexplained hepatitis, pancreatitis, bilateral parotid gland swelling, and peripheral neuropathy.

Once the likelihood of alcoholism is established, only a few moments are needed to gather the history of alcohol-related life problems. The patient *and the spouse* or another close family member should be asked about patterns of accidents, marital difficulties, problems on the job, and driving-related difficulties, after which the role played by alcohol should be identified. All physicians should be able to take the time needed to gather such information. In addition, a simple 25-item form to be answered by the patient, the Michigan Alcohol Screening Test (MAST), is available to aid in identifying alcoholics. However, this is only a screening tool, and a careful face-to-face interview is still required for a meaningful diagnosis. The CAGE, which consists of asking about alcohol-related trouble *c*utting down, being *a*nnoyed by criticisms, *g*uilt, or use of an *e*ye-opener, can also be helpful as an initial screen.

After alcoholism is identified, the diagnosis must be shared with the patient. The presenting complaint can be used as an entrée to the alcohol problem. For instance, the patient complaining of insomnia or hypertension could be told that these are clinically important symptoms and that laboratory tests and physical findings indicate that alcohol appears to have contributed to the complaints and is increasing the risk for further medical and psychological problems. The physician should share information about the course of alcoholism and explore possible avenues of attacking the problem. Some patients and family members will benefit from the opportunity to read additional material, and several items are suggested in the reading list.

The process of intervention is rarely accomplished in one session. It is helpful to let patients know that they are responsible for their own actions and that the decision to quit drinking rests with them. For the person who refuses to stop drinking at the first intervention, a logical step is to "keep the door open," establishing future meetings so that help is available as problems escalate. In the meantime the family may benefit from counseling or referral to self-help groups such as Alanon (the Alcoholics Anonymous group for family members) and Alateen (for teenage children of alcoholics).

Those patients who refuse to stop but who want to "cut down" should be reminded that the average alcoholic successfully cuts back scores of times but that sooner or later drinking again escalates. The patient who refuses to stop might be offered a guideline of drinking no more than two drinks [115 mL (4 oz) of wine, 340 mL (12 oz) of beer, or 43 mL (1.5 oz) of 80-proof beverage amounts to one drink] in any 24-h period, but it is very unlikely that this measure will be effective for an extended period. This is another way of keeping the door open in the hope that the patient will return as drinking escalates.

TREATMENT OF THE ALCOHOL-RELATED WITHDRAWAL SYNDROME **The Clinical Syndrome** In the presence of ethanol-induced cellular tolerance, any sudden decrease in ethanol intake may lead to symptoms of withdrawal from the CNS-depressant effects. As with most syndromes, most patients do not develop every symptom, and the usual clinical picture is mild, resembling a mild to severe hangover that lasts several days. Features include a tremor of the hands (shakes or jitters); autonomic nervous system dysfunction such as increases in pulse, respiratory rate, and body temperature; insomnia, possibly accompanied by bad dreams; feelings of generalized anxiety or panic attacks; and gastrointestinal upset. Symptoms begin within 5 to 10 h of decreasing ethanol intake (addicted patients are likely to awaken in the morning with some signs of withdrawal), peak in intensity on day 2 or 3, and improve by day 4 or 5. Anxiety, insomnia, and mild levels of autonomic dysfunction may persist for 6 months or more as a protracted abstinence syndrome, which may contribute to the tendency to return to drinking.

Only 5 percent or fewer of alcoholics in withdrawal show severe symptoms such as delirium tremens (DTs), a state of confusion sometimes accompanied by visual, tactile, or auditory hallucinations. The likelihood of developing severe withdrawal symptoms increases with concomitant infections or medical problems, a prior history of withdrawal seizures or DTs, and higher quantity and frequency of drinking. These symptoms disappear as the mental state becomes clearer over a period of several days and are distinct from a temporary alcohol-induced psychotic disorder, which usually occurs with a clear sensorium as described earlier in this chapter.

A small percentage of alcoholics also demonstrate one or two generalized seizures ("rum fits"), usually within 48 h of stopping drinking. These are rarely focal in nature (unless there is underlying neuropathology), and electroencephalographic abnormalities are mild and usually return to normal within several days. There is no evidence that withdrawal seizures represent "latent" epilepsy.

℞ TREATMENT

The *first* and most important step is to perform a *thorough* physical examination in all alcoholics who are considering stopping drinking. It is necessary to evaluate organ systems likely to be impaired, including a search for evidence of liver failure, gastrointestinal bleeding, cardiac arrhythmia, and glucose or electrolyte imbalance.

The *second* step in treating withdrawal for even the typical well-nourished alcoholic is to give patients adequate nutrition and rest. All patients should be given oral multiple B vitamins, including 50 to 100 mg of thiamine daily for a week or more. Most patients enter withdrawal with normal levels of body water or mild overhydration, and intravenous fluids should be avoided unless there is evidence of hypotension or a history of recent excessive bleeding, vomiting, or diarrhea. Usually medications can be administered orally.

The *third* step in treatment is to recognize that the CNS symptoms were caused by rapid removal of the brain-depressant effects of ethanol. Symptoms can be alleviated by administering another CNS depressant and gradually decreasing the levels of the drug over a 3- to 5-day period. While many CNS depressants are effective, the *benzodiazepines* have the highest margin of safety and are, therefore, the preferred class of drugs in the treatment of alcohol withdrawal. Benzodiazepines with short half-lives (see Chap. 385) are especially useful for patients with serious liver impairment or evidence of preexisting encephalopathy or brain damage. On the other hand, short-half-life benzodiazepines, e.g., oxazepam or lorazepam, result in rapidly changing drug blood levels; administration every 4 h is required to avoid abrupt fluctuations in blood levels that may increase the risk for seizures. Therefore, most clinicians use drugs with longer half-lives, such as diazepam or chlordiazepoxide. The goal is to administer enough drug on day 1 to alleviate most of the symptoms of withdrawal (e.g., the tremor and elevated pulse), and then to decrease the dose by 20 percent on successive days over a period of 3 to 5 days. The approach is flexible; the dose is increased if signs of withdrawal escalate, and the medication is withheld if the patient is sleeping or shows signs of increasing orthostatic hypotension. The average patient requires 25 to 50 mg of chlordiazepoxide or 10 mg of diazepam given orally every 4 to 6 h on the first day.

The most effective treatment of delirium tremens remains controversial. Most clinicians use benzodiazepines, but despite as much as 300 mg or more per day of chlordiazepoxide, a patient might still remain awake and agitated. Since it is probable that the confused, agitated state will persist for 3 to 5 days regardless of the pharmacologic intervention used, drugs are given to control behavior rather than to change the course of the syndrome. Antipsychotic medications such as thioridazine or haloperidol are sometimes used, although they must be prescribed with care because they might lower the seizure threshold. The antipsychotic drugs have no place in the treatment of mild withdrawal symptoms.

The generalized seizures rarely require aggressive pharmacologic intervention beyond that given to the usual patient undergoing withdrawal, i.e., adequate doses of benzodiazepines. There is little evidence that phenytoin is effective in drug-withdrawal seizures, and the risk of seizures usually has passed by the time effective drug levels are reached. The rare patient with status epilepticus can be treated initially with intravenous diazepam. If anticonvulsants are used for alcohol-withdrawal seizures, they should be stopped within 5 to 7 days unless a cause for a persisting seizure disorder is documented.

While alcohol withdrawal is often treated in a hospital, efforts at reducing costs have resulted in experimentation with outpatient detoxification for alcoholics with mild abstinence syndromes. This outpatient approach is appropriate for patients in good physical condition who demonstrate mild signs of withdrawal despite low blood alcohol concentrations and for those without prior history of DTs or withdrawal seizures. Such individuals still require careful physical examination, evaluation of blood tests, and treatment with vitamin supplementation. Benzodiazepines can be given *in a 1- to 2-day supply* to be administered to the patient by a spouse or other family member four times a day. Patients are asked to *return daily* for evaluation of vital signs, and to come to the emergency room if signs and symptoms of withdrawal escalate.

REHABILITATION OF ALCOHOLICS After completing alcoholic rehabilitation, 60 percent or more of middle-class alcoholics maintain abstinence for at least a year, and many for a lifetime. There is no single best way to rehabilitate the alcoholic, and therapeutic approaches center on general supports that meet commonsense guidelines. Considering the lack of evidence for the superiority of any specific treatment type, it is best to keep interventions as simple, safe, and inexpensive as possible.

Maneuvers in rehabilitation fall into two general categories. *First* are attempts to help the alcoholic achieve and maintain a high level of motivation toward abstinence. These include educating the patient about alcoholism and teaching the family and/or friends to stop protecting the alcoholic from the problems caused by alcohol. The *second* series of maneuvers helps the patient to readjust to life without alcohol and to reestablish a functional lifestyle through personal counseling, vocational rehabilitation, family support, and sexual counseling.

There is no convincing evidence that inpatient rehabilitation is always more effective for the average alcoholic than is outpatient care. The decision to hospitalize can be made if (1) the patient has medical problems that are difficult to treat outside a hospital; (2) depression, confusion, or psychosis interferes with outpatient care; (3) the patient has such a severe life crisis that it is difficult to get his or her attention as an outpatient; (4) outpatient treatment has failed; or (5) the patient lives too far from the treatment center. If inpatient care is needed, free-standing treatment programs, units that are divisions of general hospitals, and those in psychiatric hospitals are all equally effective. The characteristics of the patient predict outcome more than any specific attribute of the program.

Whether the treatment begins in an inpatient or an outpatient setting, subsequent outpatient contact should be maintained for a minimum of 6 months and preferably a full year after abstinence is achieved. Counseling with an individual physician or through groups focuses on day-to-day living—emphasizing areas of improved functioning in the absence of alcohol (i.e., why it is a good idea to continue to abstain) and helping the patient to deal with free time without alcohol, develop a nondrinking peer group, and handle stresses on the job without alcohol.

The physician serves an important role in identifying the alcoholic, treating associated medical or psychiatric syndromes, overseeing detoxification, referring the patient to rehabilitation programs, and providing counseling. The physician also must regulate the use of medications during alcoholism rehabilitation. Once acute detoxification is complete (an average of 3 to 5 days), there is *no place* for hypnotics or antianxiety drugs in the treatment of most alcoholics. The patient has already demonstrated an inability to moderate the use of one brain depressant, alcohol, and is at considerable risk for abusing sleeping pills or antianxiety drugs. Anxiety and insomnia can be treated with behavior modification such as relaxation training, meditation, and exercise or through increased activity in hobbies or religion. For example, regarding insomnia, patients should be reassured that insomnia is normal after alcohol withdrawal and will improve over the subsequent weeks and months. They should then follow a rigid bedtime and awakening schedule and avoid any naps or the use of caffeine in the evenings. The sleep pattern will improve rapidly.

One medication that has been used in alcohol rehabilitation is disulfiram, usually given as 250 mg/d. This drug inhibits aldehyde dehydrogenase, causing very high levels of acetaldehyde to accumulate after alcohol is consumed. The disulfiram-ethanol reaction includes tremor, hypertension or hypotension, nausea and sometimes severe vomiting, and diarrhea. Disulfiram must not be given to persons for whom such a reaction could be dangerous, including patients with portal hypertension, diabetes mellitus, heart disease, or a history of stroke. Unfortunately, there is little convincing evidence from carefully controlled studies that disulfiram is significantly more effective than than placebo. As result, this drug should not be routinely prescribed.

Two medications, naltrexone and acamprosate, are reported to either decrease the amount of alcohol consumed or to shorten the period during which alcohol is used if a relapse occurs. While the mechanisms of action are not understood and the number of subjects on whom data are available is limited for naltrexone, both drugs may have a role in the future in alcohol rehabilitation. However, more data are required before routine clinical use can be justified.

Finally, an inexpensive, readily available, and dedicated additional support for all alcoholics is available in almost every community. Alcoholics Anonymous is a self-help group of recovering alcoholics (men and women who have stopped drinking, perhaps many years ago) that offers an effective model of abstinence, provides a sober peer group, and makes crisis intervention available when the urge to drink escalates. No matter what type of rehabilitation program is planned, the alcoholic should be offered the option of joining Alcoholics Anonymous.

BIBLIOGRAPHY

KENDLER KS et al: The structure of the genetic and environmental risk factors for six major psychiatric disorders in women. Arch Gen Psychiatry 52:374, 1995

LIEBER C: *Medical and Nutritional Complications of Alcoholism*. New York, Plenum, 1992

———: Medical disorders of alcoholism. N Engl J Med 333:1058, 1995

LITTEN RZ et al: Pharmacotherapies for alcoholism. Alcohol Clin Exp Res 15:620, 1991

PROJECT MATCH RESEARCH GROUP: Matching alcoholism treatments to client heterogeneity. J Stud Alcohol 58:7, 1997

SASS H et al: Relapse prevention by acamprosate. Arch Gen Psychiatry 53:673, 1996

SCHUCKIT MA: *Drug and Alcohol Abuse: A Clinical Guide to Diagnosis and Treatment*, 4th ed. New York, Plenum, 1995

———: *Educating Yourself About Alcohol and Drugs: A People's Primer*. New York, Plenum, 1995

———, SMITH TL: An 8-year follow-up of 450 sons of alcoholic and control subjects. Arch Gen Psychiatry 53:302, 1996

——— et al: The time course of development of alcohol-related problems in men and women. J Stud Alcohol 56:218, 1995

YERSIN B et al: Screening for excessive alcohol drinking. Comparative value of carbohydrate-deficient transferrin, gamma-glutamyltransferase, and mean corpuscular volume. Arch Intern Med 155:1907, 1995

387 OPIOID DRUG ABUSE AND DEPENDENCE

Marc A. Schuckit, David S. Segal

The principal effects of the opioids (opiate-like drugs) are a significant damping of pain perception along with modest levels of sedation and euphoria. Drugs in this category range from heroin, morphine, and codeine to many nonsteroidal prescription analgesics and many antitussive agents. Thus, the following comments have wide application in medicine and go far beyond the classical opiate-dependent person on the street.

Tolerance to any one opioid is likely to generalize to the others (i.e., cross-tolerance is likely), and all share a similar pattern of drug-related problems. Each of these substances is capable of producing dependence as defined in the *Fourth Diagnostic and Statistical Manual* of the American Psychiatric Association (DSM-IV), including evidence of physical addiction (and thus they all have some legal restrictions). The abstinence syndrome from any of the substances can be treated with administration of any of the others.

PHARMACOLOGY The prototypic opiates, morphine and codeine (3-methoxymorphine), are taken directly from the milky juice of the poppy *Papaver somniferum*. The semisynthetic drugs produced from the morphine or thebane molecules include hydromorphone, diacetylmorphine (heroin), and oxycodone. The purely synthetic opioids, sharing many of the basic properties of opium and morphine, include meperidine, propoxyphene, diphenoxylate, fentanyl, buprenorphine, methadone, and pentazocine. Despite claims to the contrary, all these substances (including almost all prescription analgesics) are capable of producing euphoria as well as psychological and physical dependence when taken in high enough doses over prolonged periods.

The opioids produce their effects by binding to different types of opioid receptors throughout the body, including the central nervous system. Endogenous opioid peptides (i.e., enkephalins, endorphins, dynorphin, and others) have been identified that appear to be natural ligands for opioid receptors. These peptides have a distinct distribution in the central nervous system (CNS). Recent evidence suggests that the receptors with which opioid peptides interact may be differentially engaged in production of the various opiate effects, such as analgesia, respiratory depression, constipation, and euphoria, but the data are not definitive. Substances capable of antagonizing one or more of these actions include nalorphine, levallorphan, cyclazocine, butorphanol, buprenorphine, and pentazocine, each of which has mixed agonist and antagonist properties, as well as naloxone and naltrexone, which are pure opiate antagonists. All antagonist drugs (including those with mixed agonist properties), if administered to a patient addicted to other narcotics, can precipitate opiate withdrawal symptoms. The availability of relatively specific antagonists has helped identify different receptor subtypes, including the μ_1 and μ_2 subtypes, which are thought to affect some of the more classical opioid actions such as pain control, constipation, and respiration; κ receptors, with possible similar functions along with sedation and effects on hormones; and δ receptors, thought to relate mostly to analgesia.

Opiate tolerance, dependence, and withdrawal are considered to be related phenomena and may share some common underlying mechanisms. Perhaps reflecting the actions of different classes of receptors, tolerance to various opiate actions may develop at different rates, and these same mechanisms may contribute to the diverse signs and symptoms characteristic of withdrawal. Biochemical systems that might contribute to the development of tolerance and dependence include alterations in neurotransmitters, including acetylcholine, serotonin, gamma-aminobutyric acid (GABA), and the catecholamines norepinephrine and dopamine. Behavioral conditioning also plays a role in maintaining dependence in at least some individuals.

All the opioid drugs are absorbed from the gastrointestinal system, the lungs, and/or the muscles. The most rapid and pronounced effects occur following intravenous administration, with only slightly less efficient absorption after smoking or inhaling the vapor ("chasing the dragon"), and the least intense actions are seen after absorption from the digestive tract. Most of the metabolism of opiates occurs in the liver, primarily through conjugation with glucuronic acid, and only small amounts are excreted directly in the urine or feces. The plasma half-lives of these drugs range from 2.5 to 3 h for morphine to more than 22 h for methadone and even longer for levomethadyl acetate (LAAM).

Street heroin typically contains only 5 to 10 percent of the opiate. The remainder consists of materials such as lactose and fruit sugars, quinine, powdered milk, phenacetin, caffeine, antipyrine, and strychnine, which are used to "cut" the drug and increase the profit margin. Any marked, unexpected increase in the purity of street drugs is likely to cause unintentional lethal overdoses in users expecting less effect from a "hit."

THE ACUTE AND CHRONIC EFFECTS OF OPIOID DRUGS ON BODY SYSTEMS With the exception of overdose conditions and changes associated with physical addiction, most opiate actions are relatively benign and rapidly reversible. A major danger, however, comes through the use of contaminated needles by intravenous users. This practice is responsible for increased risks for hepatitis B and C, bacterial endocarditis, and infection with the human immunodeficiency virus (HIV), a major cause of mortality in injection drug users and their sexual partners (see Chap. 308).

Effects on Body Systems Acute changes in the *gastrointestinal (GI) system* are the result of decreased GI motility with resulting constipation and anorexia. Chronic GI problems in opiate-dependent people typically occur as a consequence of hepatitis in injection drug users.

The direct effects on opiate receptors in the CNS can result in intoxication-induced nausea and vomiting (medulla), decreased pain perception (spinal cord, thalamus, and periaqueductal gray region), euphoria (limbic system), and sedation (reticular activating system and striatum). The adulterants added to street drugs may contribute to some of the more permanent nervous system damage, including peripheral neuropathy, amblyopia, myelopathy, and leukoencephalopathy. Whether from the opiate, adulterants, or the consequences of dirty needles, at least one recent study revealed CNS defects in both computed tomographic and cognition evaluations of opiate-dependent people. Acute opiate administration results in decreases in luteinizing hormone (LH), with a subsequent decrease in testosterone, which might contribute to the decreased sex drive reported by most opiate-dependent people. Other hormonal changes include a decrease in the release of thyrotropin as well as increases in prolactin and possibly in growth hormone (see Chap. 328).

Acute changes in the *respiratory system* include respiratory depression, which results from a decreased response of the brainstem to carbon dioxide tension, a component of the drug overdose syndrome described below. At even low drug doses, this effect can be clinically significant in individuals with compromised lung activity. *Cardiovascular* changes tend to be relatively mild, with no direct opiate effect on heart rhythm or myocardial contractility, but there is a potential problem from orthostatic hypotension, probably secondary to dilation of peripheral vessels. Bacterial infections of both the lungs and heart valves can occur from contaminated needles; the latter can result in emboli and thus an increased risk for stroke.

The Toxic Reaction or Overdose Syndrome High doses of opiates taken intentionally (in a suicide attempt) or by a user who has misjudged the potency of the substance can result in a toxic reaction or overdose syndrome with a potentially lethal consequence. While toxic reactions are seen with all opiates, the more potent drugs such as fentanyl (80 to 100 times more powerful than morphine) are especially dangerous. The typical syndrome, which occurs immediately with intravenous overdose, includes shallow respirations at a rate of two to four per minute, pupillary miosis (with mydriasis once brain anoxia develops), bradycardia, a decrease in body temperature, and a general absence of responsiveness to external stimulation. If this medical emergency is not treated rapidly, symptoms can progress to cyanosis, and death can ensue from respiratory depression and cardiorespiratory arrest. Postmortem examination reveals few specific changes except for diffuse cerebral edema. An "allergic-like" reaction to intravenous heroin, apparently at least in part related to adulterants, also can occur and is characterized by decreased alertness, a frothy pulmonary edema, and an elevation in the blood eosinophil count.

The first step in treating any overdose is to support the vital signs through a respirator and other emergency procedures. The preferred, more definitive treatment for the typical opiate overdose is the intravenous or intramuscular administration of the narcotic antagonist naloxone in an initial dose of 0.2 mg (0.5 mL of the 10 mL vial) or more; this dose can be repeated in 3 to 10 min if no response occurs. It is important to titrate the dose relative to the patient's symptoms. Because the effects of this drug diminish within 2 to 3 h, the individual must be monitored for at least 24 h after a heroin overdose and 72 h after an overdose of a longer-acting drug such as methadone. If there is little response to naloxone alone, the possibility of a concomitant overdose with a benzodiazepine should be considered and a challenge with intravenous flumazenil, 0.2 to 0.5 mg/min up to a maximum of 3 mg, might be used. Patients who are physically addicted to an opioid are likely to experience a precipitous onset of an abstinence syndrome within 2 to 8 h after administration of the opioid antagonist, but aggressive treatment of this syndrome is not appropriate until all vital signs are relatively stable.

As with any drug overdose, treatment of either the typical or the "allergic" type of opiate toxic reaction often requires continued support of vital signs until the body detoxifies the substance. Patients may require a respirator (especially one using oxygen and positive-pressure breathing for the "allergic" type of overdose), intravenous fluids perhaps accompanied by pressor agents, to support blood pressure, and gastric lavage to remove any remaining drug, with care taken to use a cuffed endotracheal tube to prevent aspiration if the patient is not alert. It is important to evaluate and treat any possible anaphylactic reactions. Cardiac arrhythmias and/or convulsions, especially likely to be seen with codeine, propoxyphene, or meperidine, also need to be treated.

DIAGNOSIS AND NATURAL HISTORY OF OPIOID ABUSE AND DEPENDENCE Repeated use of opiates to the point of developing multiple problems is a good indicator of the likelihood of future problems with the drug. The approach uses the same DSM-IV criteria for dependence as discussed for alcohol (see Chap. 386). Here, the patient develops repeated difficulties in any three of the criterion areas in any given year, showing a mixture of tolerance, withdrawal, use of greater amounts of opiates than intended, use despite consequences, and so on. Patients who do not have dependence but demonstrate repeated difficulties with the law, impaired ability to meet obligations, use in hazardous situations, or continued use despite problems can be labeled as having abuse.

Natural History Dependence on or abuse of opiates can be seen in at least three types of patients. First, evidence suggests that a minority of people with *chronic pain syndromes* (e.g., back, joint, and muscle disorders) misuse their prescribed drugs at various times. Of course, these comments deal with non-life-threatening chronic pain, not terminal illness, for which high doses of opiates can be important. If physical dependence is established, abstinence syndromes can then intensify the pain, promoting continued drug intake. A few precautions can help the physician to avoid contributing to physical dependence in chronic pain patients, particularly those who have demonstrated a history of misusing opioids. (1) The goal is to minimize the debilitating effects of pain with the understanding that discomfort may not be completely eliminated (see Chap. 12). (2) All possible efforts must be made to get the patient actively involved in and committed to improvement. (3) Analgesic medication should be only one component of treatment and limited to the oral administration of the least potent analgesic that is able to "take the edge off" the pain (e.g., ibuprofen or, if needed, propoxyphene). All such drugs should be coordinated through one physician. (4) Behavior modification techniques, such as muscle relaxation and meditation, and carefully selected exercises should be used as appropriate to help increase function and decrease pain. (5) Finally, nonmedicinal approaches, including electrical transcutaneous neurostimulation for muscle and joint disease, can be applied (see also Chap. 12).

The second group at high risk are *physicians, nurses,* and *pharmacists,* primarily because of their easy access to substances of abuse. Physicians may begin to use opiates to help them sleep or to reduce stress or physical aches and pains. These groups appear to be at especially high risk for developing dependence on the highly potent drugs such as fentanyl. Because of the growing awareness of these problems, impaired physician programs have been established in many hospitals and by most state medical societies. These groups attempt to identify and aid substance-impaired physicians, giving them peer support and education so as to help them achieve abstinence before problems escalate to the point of licensure revocation. In general, doctors are advised never to prescribe opiates for themselves or for members of their family—physicians deserve the same level of care and protection from future problems as their patients.

The third and most obvious group are those who buy their drugs on the street to get high. While some of these men and women have prior histories of severe antisocial problems, most have a relatively high level of premorbid functioning. The typical person begins using opiates occasionally, often after experimenting with tobacco, then alcohol, then marijuana, and then brain depressants or stimulants. Occasional opiate use, or "chipping," might continue for some time, and some individuals never escalate their intake to the point of developing dependence. Another pattern of temporary or intermittent abuse is represented by the experiences of Vietnam soldiers, most of whom had little or no prior experience with opiates and who found themselves in a situation of high stress and readily available drugs. Under these circumstances, as many as one-half tried opiates and, although many became physically addicted, those who had not misused drugs before Vietnam tended to return to drug-free status when back in their home communities.

Of course, opiate-dependent individuals are likely to continue to have experience with many other drugs. At least two of these often remain as problems during the course of opiate dependence. First, alcohol intake is classically used to moderate withdrawal problems, to enhance the opiate high, and as a substitute when the preferred drug is not readily available, including during methadone and other treatments. This pattern of problematic drinking, often meeting criteria for alcohol dependence, is seen in the course of opiate dependence in perhaps 50 percent of opiate-dependent persons. The second drug, cocaine, appears to be taken for many of the same reasons as alcohol and is often administered intravenously with the opiate in a mixture known as a "speedball." Dependence on these as well as other drugs must be addressed during opiate detoxification and rehabilitation.

Once persistent opiate use is established, the outcome is often extremely serious. At least 25 percent of such opiate abusers are likely to die within 10 to 20 years of active abuse, with death resulting from suicide, homicide, accidents, and infectious diseases such as tuberculosis, serum hepatitis, or AIDS. The mortality rate has escalated in recent years in response to the epidemic of AIDS among injection drug users, with an estimated 60 percent of these men and women carrying HIV (see Chap. 208). As many as 50 percent of male and 25 percent of female opiate-dependent persons turn to alcohol when their primary drug is not available, and many meet the criteria for secondary alcohol dependence. The prevalence of alcohol misuse is higher in drug treatment dropouts than in those who stay with therapy, and also in individuals who had alcohol problems before they developed opiate-related difficulties.

Rx TREATMENT

The key to diagnosis is to discard the erroneous stereotype that opiate-dependent men and women are always street people. Abuse or dependence is possible in any patient who demonstrates symptoms of what might be opiate withdrawal; anyone who has a chronic pain syndrome; physicians, nurses, and pharmacists or others with easy access to opiates; and all patients who repeatedly seek out prescription analgesics. The diagnosis is established by reviewing areas of life problems where opiates might be involved, beginning with the DSM-IV items for abuse and dependence.

Identification of the Patient, and Intervention The first step in treatment is identification of the opiate-dependent person—an especially difficult step with middle-class medical patients or physicians with an iatrogenic addiction. Therefore, it is important to take the time with *every* patient, especially those with complaints of pain, to gather a clinical history that includes the patterns of opiate use and the list of doctors and clinics from which they have received prescriptions. If the chronic use of opiates is suspected, gathering further data from an additional informant such as a spouse can be essential. Another indicator of an enhanced risk for opiate dependence is a history of pervasive antisocial problems beginning in the preteen years. Blood and urine screens can be used to identify opiates in patients in whom misuse is suspected, and clinicians should search for physical stigmata of misuse (e.g., needle marks).

After identifying opiate dependence, the next step is intervention. The need for active treatment of the abstinence syndrome can be presented, and the availability of help in establishing a drug-free life-style can be emphasized. The final decision, of course, rests with the patient. Much of this approach is presented in relation to alcoholism in Chap. 386.

The Symptoms of Withdrawal The withdrawal symptoms tend to be opposite to the acute effects of the drug and include nausea and diarrhea, coughing, lacrimation, mydriasis, rhinorrhea, profuse sweating, twitching muscles, and piloerection, or "goose bumps"; mild elevations in body temperature, respiratory rate, and blood pressure are also observed. In addition, sensations of diffuse body pain, insomnia, and yawning occur, along with intense drug craving. Drugs with a short half-life, such as morphine or heroin, cause symptoms typically within 8 to 16 h of the last dose (thus, many dependent individuals awake in mild withdrawal every morning); symptom intensity peaks within 36 to 72 h after discontinuation of the drug, and the acute syndrome disappears within 5 to 8 days. However, a protracted abstinence phase of mild symptoms (e.g., slight changes in pupillary size, autonomic dysfunction, changes in sleep pattern) may persist for 6 or more months. These lingering symptoms, which can be relieved by administering an opiate, probably contribute to relapse.

Treatment of the Withdrawal Syndrome Patients *must* receive a thorough physical examination, which includes an assessment of liver and neurologic function as well as identification of local and systemic infections, especially abscesses. Proper nutrition and rest must be initiated as soon as possible.

Effective treatment of withdrawal, however, also requires readministration of sufficient opiate medication on day 1 to decrease symptoms, followed by a more gradual withdrawal of the drug, usually over 5 to 10 days. Any opiate will work (they all have some level of cross-tolerance), but for ease of administration, many physicians prefer to use a long-acting drug such as methadone. In estimating the first day's dose from the patient's history, 1 mg of methadone is approximately equivalent to 3 mg of morphine, 1 mg of heroin, or 20 mg of meperidine. Most patients require between 10 and 25 mg of methadone orally given twice on day 1, with higher doses given if prominent symptoms of withdrawal are not dampened. After several days of a stabilized drug dose, the opiate is then decreased by 10 to 20 percent of the original day's dose each day.

Most states have restrictions on the prescription of opiates to dependent persons, and, in the absence of special permits, detoxification with opiates is often proscribed or limited to 1 month or less. Thus, pharmacologic treatments are often limited to symptomatic medication of diarrhea with kaopectate or a similar nonopiate, of "sniffles" with decongestants, and pain with nonopiate analgesics (e.g., ibuprofen). Another relatively successful nonopiate approach to the treatment of withdrawal is the use of the $alpha_2$-adrenergic agonist clonidine, used in part to decrease sympathetic nervous system overactivity. Given at doses of approximately 5 μg/kg (up to 0.3 mg given two to four times a day), clonidine decreases autonomic nervous system dysfunction in most patients undergoing opiate withdrawal. Opiates are more effective in relieving discomfort and pain, however, and clonidine is often not well tolerated because it produces high levels of sedation and orthostatic hypotension. Therefore, under most circumstances, opiates are the treatment of choice.

A special case of opiate withdrawal is seen in the newborn passively addicted by the mother's drug misuse during pregnancy. Some level of addiction develops in 50 to 90 percent of children of heroin-dependent mothers. As few as 25 percent of infants of methadone maintenance–addicted mothers show clinically relevant withdrawal symptoms, probably because of the longer half-life of this drug. The syndrome consists of irritability, crying, a tremor (in 80 percent), increased reflexes, increased respiratory rate, diarrhea, hyperactivity (in 60 percent), vomiting (40 percent), and sneezing/yawning/hiccuping (in 30 percent). The child usually has a low birth weight but may be otherwise unremarkable until the second day, when symptoms are likely to begin.

The treatment follows the same general steps used in the treatment of the physically addicted adult. The child must be carefully evaluated to rule out medical problems such as hypoglycemia, hypocalcemia, infections, and trauma; general support in a warm, quiet environment and regulation of electrolytes and glucose are also required. The infant with moderate to severe symptoms can be treated with any of the following: paregoric (0.2 mL orally every 3 to 4 h), methadone (0.1 to 0.5 mg/kg per day), phenobarbital (8 mg/kg per day), or diazepam (1 to 2 mg/kg every 8 h). Medication should be given in decreasing levels for 10 to 20 days. It is also possible to help treat the addicted infants of mothers on methadone maintenance by having the mother breast feed the infant while continuing to take methadone.

Rehabilitation of Opiate-Dependent Persons Despite some differences in demographics, the same general rules for rehabilitation apply to opiate-dependent persons as to alcoholics. The basic strategy includes beginning detoxification and general family support, and the process can benefit from the use of readings or referral to self-help groups. It is also important to establish realistic patient goals and a program of counseling and education to increase motivation toward abstinence. A long-term commitment to rebuilding a life-style without the substance is essential for preventing recidivism.

Most rehabilitation approaches have common elements, regardless of the drug involved. As described in several recent texts, patients are educated about their responsibility for improving their lives, and *motivation for abstinence* is increased by providing information about the medical and psychological problems that can be expected if addiction continues. Patients and families are helped to *establish an opiate-free life-style* by being educated about dealing with chronic pain and developing realistic vocational planning (e.g., for pharmacists, physicians, and nurses). The dependent person also should be encouraged to establish a drug-free peer group and to participate in self-help groups such as Narcotics Anonymous. Much of this advice and counseling can be given by the physician, but many clinicians refer patients to more formal drug programs, including methadone maintenance clinics, programs using narcotic antagonists, and therapeutic communities. Long-term follow-up of treated patients shows that approximately one-third of participants are completely drug free in the year before the follow-up interview and that a total of 60 percent are off opiates, although some are abusing other substances. Individuals who stay in methadone maintenance or in therapeutic communities show significant decreases in police and social problems and increases in job functioning. In general, the best prognosis is for those who are employed, who have higher levels of school completion, and who remain in treatment for at least 2 months. Dependence among health care deliverers, such as physicians, is treated with similar approaches. In addition, a closely supervised "diversion" procedure is usually instituted and carried out for 1 to 2 years or more.

METHADONE MAINTENANCE Maintenance programs with methadone and the even longer-acting agent LAAM should only be used along with education and counseling. It is important to note that drug maintenance is not aimed at "curing" opiate addiction; rather, it provides a substitute drug that is legally accessible, safer, can be taken orally, and has a long half-life so that it can be taken once a day. The goal is to help persons who have repeatedly failed in drug-free programs to improve functioning within the family and job, to decrease legal problems, and to improve health.

Methadone is a long-acting opiate that possesses almost all the physiologic properties of heroin. The recipient, who has been carefully screened to rule out prior psychiatric disorders, may be maintained on a relatively low dose (e.g., 30 to 40 mg/d); a better approach is to use a higher dose (100 to 120 mg/d), which may be more effective in blocking heroin-induced euphoria. There is some evidence that the higher methadone doses result in greater retention in treatment and consequently in lower levels of arrest and readdiction to street drugs. Three-quarters or more of patients, especially those receiving the higher doses, are likely to remain heroin-free for 6 months or longer. Methadone is administered in an oral liquid given once a day at the program center, with weekend portions taken by the patient at home. The longer-acting analogues, such as LAAM, can be given two or three times a week, with the dose of LAAM increased to as high as 80 mg three times a week if needed. After a period of maintenance (usually 6 months to 1 year or longer), the clinician should work closely with the patient to regulate the rate of drug decrease (by about 5 percent per week).

In the past, the British have used heroin maintenance with similar goals and following similar guidelines as those used for methadone. There is no evidence that heroin maintenance has any advantages over methadone maintenance, but the heroin approach does add the risk that the drug will be sold on the streets. These factors have contributed to the virtual abandonment of the heroin maintenance approach. Treatment with mixed agonists-antagonists such as buprenorphine has been proposed, especially to help the individual who is also using cocaine. However, at present these must be considered experimental.

OPIATE ANTAGONISTS The opiate antagonists (e.g., naloxone) compete with heroin and other opiates for opioid receptors, reducing the effects of the opiate agonists. Administered over long periods with the intention of blocking the "high" produced if the patient takes opiates, these drugs can be useful as part of an overall treatment approach that includes counseling and support. The most widely used antagonist in rehabilitation is naltrexone, which is effective for about 24 h and has few side effects. A dose of 50 mg of naltrexone per day will block 15 mg of heroin for 24 h, and higher doses (125 to 150 mg) are capable of blocking the effects of 25 mg of intravenous heroin for up to 3 days. Naltrexone is free of agonist properties and produces no known withdrawal symptoms when stopped, and its side effects tend to be mild. Patients should be free of opiates for a minimum of 5 days before beginning treatment with this medication, to avoid precipitating a withdrawal syndrome. In addition, they must be given a thorough physical examination and should be challenged with 0.4 or 0.8 mg of the shorter-acting agent naloxone to be certain they are able to tolerate the long-acting antagonist. Following this procedure, a test dose of 10 mg of naltrexone can be given, with the expectation that any withdrawal symptoms will be seen in 0.5 to 2 h. Several variations of this approach can be used with methadone maintenance, including a fairly rapid, medically supervised scheme. Over the next 10 days, the daily dose should be increased to about 100 mg on Mondays and Wednesdays and 150 mg on Fridays. Unfortunately, despite the apparent advantages of this treatment approach, patients demonstrate great resistance to continuing care. In one study, only about 60 percent of the patients completed 6 days of naltrexone induction, and only 10 percent remained in the program at the end of 6 months.

DRUG-FREE PROGRAMS Most existing halfway houses and recovery centers for opiate-dependent persons use some variant of the therapeutic community approach. This is an exception to the general preference for short-term inpatient rehabilitation, since care lasts up to a year while the person is taken out of the street culture and given a new life within the group. In this structure, members, including leaders who are themselves in the process of recovery, help participants gain insights into more successful life-styles for coping with problems.

As is true for treatments of all substance-use disorders, it is likely that counseling, behavioral treatments, and relatively simple approaches to psychotherapy add significantly to a positive outcome. Most approaches focus on teaching participants to handle stress better, enhancing their understanding of personality attributes, teaching better cognitive styles, and, through the process of relapse prevention, addressing issues that might contribute to increased craving, easy access to drugs, or periods of decreased motivation. A combination of these therapies with the approaches described above appears to give the best results.

Finally, it is important to briefly discuss prevention. Except for the terminally ill, physicians need to carefully monitor opiate drug use in their patients, keeping the doses as low as is practical and administering them over as short a period as the level of pain would warrant in the average person. Physicians must also be vigilant regarding their own risk for opiate abuse and dependence, *never* prescribing these drugs for themselves. For the nonmedical intravenous drug–dependent person, all possible efforts must be made to prevent AIDS, hepatitis, bacterial endocarditis, and other consequences of contaminated needles through methadone maintenance and by considering needle-exchange programs.

BIBLIOGRAPHY

American Psychiatric Association: Practical guidelines for the treatment of substance use disorders. Am J Psychiatry 52(Suppl):1, 1995

Ball J, Ross A: *The Effectiveness of Methadone Maintenance Treatments*. New York, Springer-Verlag, 1991

Bonner A, Waterhouse J: *Addictive Behaviour: Molecules to Mankind; Perspective on the Nature of Addiction*. New York, St. Martin's Press, 1996

Committee on Opportunities in Drug Abuse Research: Pathways of Addiction. Washington DC, National Academy Press, 1995, pp 56–93

Finnegan LP: Neonatal abstinence syndrome: Assessment and pharmacotherapy, in *Neonatal Therapy: An Update*, FF Rubaltelli, B Granati (eds). New York, Elsevier, 1986

Hughes PH et al: Prevalence of substance use among US physicians. JAMA 267:2333, 1992

Keene J et al: Evaluation of syringe-exchange for HIV prevention among injecting drug users in rural and urban areas of Wales. Addiction 88:1063, 1993

Manfredini R et al: Emergency admissions of opioid drug abusers for overdose: A chronobiological study of enhanced risk. Ann Emerg Med 24:615, 1994

Schuckit MA: *Drug and Alcohol Abuse: A Clinical Guide to Diagnosis and Treatment*, 4th ed. New York, Plenum, 1995

———: *Educating Yourself about Alcohol and Drugs: A People's Primer*. New York, Plenum, 1995

Weiss RD et al: The significance of a coexisting opioid use disorder in cocaine dependence: An empirical study. Am J Drug Alcohol Abuse 22:173, 1996

388

Jack H. Mendelson, Nancy K. Mello

COCAINE AND OTHER COMMONLY ABUSED DRUGS

Although there has been a decline in the occurrence of drug abuse–related problems, particularly among youths, the prevalence of drug abuse in the United States remained at epidemic levels during the mid-1990s and is believed to exceed that of other industrial nations. The primary data resources for assessing the scope and extent of drug abuse in the United States are the High School Senior Survey, the National Household Survey on Drug Abuse, and the Drug Abuse Warning Network (DAWN) supported by the National Institute on Drug Abuse (NIDA). During 1993, the National Household Survey on Drug Abuse revealed that 4.5 million persons in the United States used cocaine. Approximately 1.3 million persons (0.6 percent of the American population) stated that they self-administered cocaine on a frequent, monthly basis. The Drug Abuse Warning Network reported in 1993 that 30,900 cocaine-related emergency room visits occurred during the later part of 1992. Illnesses that prompted cocaine-related emergency room visits included cocaine-induced gastrointestinal, cardiovascular, and cerebrovascular disorders. Although there has been an encouraging trend of decreased cocaine abuse by young persons, the National Institute on Drug Abuse 1995 report *Epidemiologic Trends in Drug Abuse* noted that "the oldest age groups generally comprised the largest and fastest growing percentages of cocaine fatality." The report also highlighted that "cocaine (including crack) remains the nation's most serious drug problem." There is also increasing evidence that crack cocaine is frequently smoked with marijuana. A recent study indicated that a major cause of death of young adults in New York City was fatal injury associated with cocaine abuse.

Chronic drug abuse can be associated with a number of adverse health consequences, ranging from pulmonary disease to reproductive dysfunctions. Preexisting disorders such as hypertension and cardiac disease may be exacerbated by drug abuse, and the combined use of two or more drugs may accentuate medical complications associated with the abuse of one of them. The adverse health consequences of drug abuse are further complicated by AIDS, and drug abuse also increases the risk of exposure to the human immunodeficiency virus (HIV). Drug abuse contributes to the recent AIDS epidemic through HIV infection transmitted by needle-sharing by intravenous drug users and by adverse immunomodulatory effects of abused drugs. During 1993–1994, persons who self-administered drugs intravenously represented the largest single group with HIV infection in several major metropolitan areas in the United States, as well as urban areas in Scotland, Italy, Spain, Thailand, and China. Over 30 countries throughout Europe, North America, South America, Asia, Australia, and Africa have reported AIDS or HIV infection among intravenous drug users.

The initiation and continuation of drug abuse is determined by a complex interaction of the pharmacologic properties and relative availability of each drug, the personality and expectations of the user, and the environmental context in which the drug is used. Polydrug abuse—the concurrent use of several drugs with different pharmacologic effects—is increasingly common among individuals from all socioeconomic strata. There has been an alarming increase in a particularly dangerous form of polydrug abuse, the combined use of heroin and cocaine intravenously, called "speedballing." There is no simple explanation for this change in polydrug use patterns. Sometimes drug abusers attempt to attenuate one drug effect with another, as when heroin or alcohol is used to modulate the cocaine high. Sometimes one drug is used to enhance the effects of another, as with benzodiazepines and methadone, or cocaine plus heroin in methadone-maintained patients. Toxic drug interactions associated with polydrug abuse also contribute to adverse health consequences. This chapter discusses cocaine, marijuana, two hallucinogens [phencyclidine (PCP) and lysergic acid diethylamide (LSD)], and polydrug abuse. → ***Alcohol and alcoholism are discussed in Chap. 386 and opioid drug abuse in Chap. 387.***

COCAINE Cocaine is a stimulant and local anesthetic with potent vasoconstrictor properties. The leaves of the coca plant (*Erythroxylon coca*) contain approximately 0.5 to 1 percent cocaine. The drug produces physiologic and behavioral effects when administered orally, intranasally, intravenously, or via inhalation following pyrolysis (smoking). It is now recognized that cocaine has potent pharmacologic effects on dopamine, norepinephrine, and serotonin neurons in the central nervous system. These effects include alteration and blockade of cellular membrane transport and prevention of the reuptake of biogenic amines. It has been postulated that cocaine-induced euphoria is due to cocaine-induced blockade of dopamine reuptake, but chronic cocaine use may cause dopamine depletion and impairment of dopaminergic function in the brain.

Prevalence of Cocaine Use Cocaine has become more widely available throughout the United States since its cost (relative to disposable income) has decreased considerably. Cocaine is no longer considered a "status" drug, since cocaine abuse occurs in virtually all social and economic strata of society. The prevalence of cocaine abuse in the general population has also been associated with an increase in cocaine abuse by heroin-dependent persons, including those in methadone maintenance programs. Intravenous cocaine is often used concurrently with intravenous heroin (the speedball)—a combination that purportedly attenuates the postcocaine "crash" and substitutes a cocaine "high" for the heroin "high" blocked by methadone. Intravenous use of cocaine plus heroin may further increase risk for HIV infection, both through needle sharing and through the combined immunosuppressive effects of the drugs.

Acute and Chronic Cocaine Intoxication Although cocaine is commonly self-administered by inhalation (snorting), there has been an increase in both intravenous administration and inhalation of pyrolyzed material via smoking. Following intranasal administration, changes in mood and feeling states are perceived within 3 to 5 min, and peak effects occur at 10 to 20 min. The effects rarely last more than 1 h following intranasal administration. Inhalation of pyrolyzed materials include smoking coca paste, a product produced by extracting cocaine preparations with flammable solvents, and cocaine free-base smoking. Coca paste is frequently contaminated with toxic solvents used in its preparation. Free-base cocaine, including the free base prepared with sodium bicarbonate (crack), is becoming increasingly popular because of the relative high potency of the compounds and their rapid onset of action (8 to 10 s following smoking).

Cocaine produces a brief, dose-related stimulation and enhancement of mood and dose-related increases in cardiac rate and blood pressure. Body temperature usually increases following cocaine administration, and high doses of cocaine may induce lethal pyrexia or hypertension. Because cocaine inhibits reuptake of catecholamines at adrenergic nerve endings, the drug potentiates sympathetic nervous system activity. Cocaine has a short plasma half-life of approximately 1 h. In humans, cocaine is primarily metabolized by plasma esterases, and cocaine metabolites are excreted in urine. The very short duration of euphorigenic effects of cocaine observed in chronic abusers is probably due to both acute and chronic tolerance. Frequent self-administration of the drug (two to three times per hour) is often reported by chronic cocaine abusers. Alcohol is used to modulate both the cocaine "high" and the dysphoria associated with the abrupt disappearance of cocaine's effects. A metabolite of cocaine, cocaethylene, has been detected in blood and urine of persons who concurrently abuse alcohol and cocaine. Cocaethylene induces changes in cardiovascular function similar to those of cocaine alone, and the pathophysiologic consequences of alcohol abuse plus cocaine abuse may be additive when both are used together.

The prevalent assumption that cocaine use is relatively safe is challenged by reports of death from respiratory depression, cardiac arrhythmias, and convulsions after cocaine snorting and intravenous administration. Disorders of cerebral blood flow and perfusion in cocaine-dependent persons have been detected with studies using single photon emission computed tomography (SPECT). Severe pulmonary disease may develop in individuals who smoke coca paste; this effect is attributed both to the direct effects of cocaine and to residual solvent contaminants in the smoked material. Hepatic necrosis has also been reported to occur in coca paste smokers. Although men and women who abuse cocaine may report that the drug enhances libidinal drive, chronic cocaine use causes significant loss of libido and adversely affects reproductive function. Impotence and gynecomastia have been observed in male cocaine abusers, and these abnormalities often persist for long periods following cessation of drug use. Women who abuse cocaine have reported major derangements in menstrual cycle function, including galactorrhea, amenorrhea, and infertility. Chronic cocaine abuse may cause persistent hyperprolactinemia as a consequence of cocaine-induced disorders of dopaminergic regulation of prolactin secretion by the pituitary. Cocaine abuse, particularly the smoking of crack by pregnant women, has been implicated as causing an increased risk of congenital malformations and of perinatal cardiovascular and cerebrovascular disease in the mother. However, cocaine abuse per se is probably not the sole cause of these perinatal disorders, since many problems associated with maternal cocaine abuse, including poor nutrition and health care status as well as polydrug abuse, also contribute to the risk for perinatal disease.

Numerous clinical reports, dating from the late nineteenth century, strongly suggest that protracted cocaine abuse may cause paranoid ideation and visual and auditory hallucinations, a state that resembles alcoholic hallucinosis. Psychological dependence on cocaine, as manifested by inability to abstain from frequent compulsive use, also has been reported. Although the existence of withdrawal syndromes involving psychomotor agitation and autonomic hyperactivity remains controversial, severe depression ("crashing") following cocaine intoxication may accompany drug withdrawal.

Rx TREATMENT

Treatment of cocaine overdose is a medical emergency that involves resuscitation in an intensive care unit. Cocaine toxicity produces hypertension, tachycardia, tonic-clonic seizures, dyspnea, and ventricular arrhythmias. Intravenous diazepam in doses up to 0.5 mg/kg administered over an 8-h period has been shown to be effective for control of seizures. The systemic concomitants of a hypermetabolic state produced by cocaine toxicity with concurrent ventricular arrhythmias have been managed successfully by administration of 0.5 to 1.0 mg of propranolol intravenously. Since many instances of cocaine-related mortality have been associated with concurrent use of other illicit drugs (particularly heroin), the physician must be prepared to institute effective emergency treatment for multiple drug toxicity.

Treatment of chronic cocaine abuse requires combined efforts by family physicians, psychiatrists, and psychosocial care providers. Early abstinence from cocaine use is often complicated by symptoms of depression and guilt, insomnia, and anorexia, which may be as severe as those observed in major affective disorders. Individual and group psychotherapy, family therapy, and peer group assistance programs are often useful for inducing prolonged remission from drug use. A number of medications currently available for the treatment of various medical and psychiatric disorders have been administered to reduce the duration and severity of cocaine abuse and dependence. However, survey reports obtained from physicians specializing in the practice of addiction medicine indicate that no available medication is both safe and highly effective for either cocaine detoxification or maintenance of abstinence. A variety of psychotherapeutic and behavioral treatments for cocaine abuse have been attempted, and although some psychotherapeutic interventions are occasionally effective, no specific form of psychotherapy or behavioral modification has been determined to be uniquely beneficial for many persons who abuse or are dependent on cocaine.

MARIJUANA AND CANNABIS COMPOUNDS *Cannabis sativa* contains over 400 compounds in addition to the psychoactive substance, delta-9-tetrahydrocannabinol (THC). Marijuana cigarettes are prepared from the leaves and flowering tops of the plant, and a typical marijuana cigarette contains 0.5 to 1 g of plant material. Although the usual THC concentration varies between 5 and 20 mg, concentrations as high as 100 mg per cigarette have been detected. Hashish is prepared from concentrated resin of *Cannabis sativa* and contains a THC concentration of between 8 and 12 percent by weight. "Hash oil," a lipid- soluble plant extract, may contain a THC concentration of 25 to 60 percent, and it may be added to marijuana or hashish to enhance the THC concentration. Smoking is the most common mode of marijuana or hashish self-administration. During pyrolysis, over 150 compounds in addition to the THC are released in the smoke. Although most of these compounds are not psychoactive, they do have potential physiologic effects.

THC is quickly absorbed from the lungs into blood and is then rapidly sequestered in tissues. It is metabolized primarily in the liver, where it is converted to 11-hydroxy-THC, a psychoactive compound, and more than 20 other metabolites. Most THC metabolites are excreted through the feces at a rate of clearance that is relatively slow in comparison to that of most other psychoactive drugs.

Prevalence of Marijuana Use The National Institute on Drug Abuse 1995 report states that marijuana use, particularly by adolescents, is increasing significantly throughout the United States. Drug-related emergency department admissions increased greatly throughout the United States between 1992 and 1993. Most of these patients were males between the ages of 18 and 25. Marijuana-related emergency department admissions for males between the ages of 12 and 17 escalated by almost 100 percent during 1991 to 1993. Marijuana-filled cigars from which tobacco was removed ("blunts") were increasingly smoked by young adults in urban and some rural areas.

Acute and Chronic Marijuana Intoxication Acute intoxication from marijuana and cannabis compounds is related to both the dose of THC and the route of administration. THC is absorbed more rapidly from marijuana smoking than from orally ingested cannabis compounds. Acute marijuana intoxication usually consists of a subjective perception of relaxation and mild euphoria resembling mild to moderate alcohol intoxication. This condition is usually accompanied by some impairment in thinking, concentration, and perceptual and psychomotor functions. Higher doses of cannabis may produce behavioral effects analogous to severe alcohol intoxication. Although the effects of acute marijuana intoxication are relatively benign in normal users, the drug can precipitate severe emotional disorders in individuals who have antecedent psychotic or neurotic problems. As with other psychoactive compounds, both set (user's expectations) and setting (environmental context) are important determinants of the type and severity of behavioral intoxication.

As is true of alcoholics, chronic marijuana abusers may lose interest in common socially desirable goals and devote steadily more time to drug acquisition and use. However, it should be emphasized that THC does not cause a specific and unique "amotivational syndrome." The range of symptoms sometimes attributed to marijuana use is difficult to distinguish from mild depression and the maturational dysfunctions often associated with protracted adolescence. Chronic use of marijuana has also been reported to increase the probability of exacerbation of psychotic symptoms in individuals with a past history of schizophrenia.

Physical Effects of Marijuana Conjunctival injection and tachycardia are the most frequent immediate physical concomitants of smoking marijuana. Tolerance for marijuana-induced tachycardia develops rapidly among regular users; angina may be precipitated by marijuana smoking in persons with a history of coronary insufficiency. Exercise-induced angina may be increased after marijuana use to a greater extent than after tobacco cigarette smoking. Patients with cardiac disease should be strongly advised not to smoke marijuana or use cannabis compounds.

Significant decrements in pulmonary vital capacity have been found in regular daily marijuana smokers. Because marijuana smoking typically involves deep inhalation and prolonged retention of marijuana smoke, marijuana smokers may develop pulmonary disease such as chronic bronchial irritation. Impairment of single-breath carbon monoxide diffusion capacity (DL_{CO}) is greater in persons who smoke both marijuana and tobacco than in tobacco smokers. Despite the well-documented association between tobacco smoking and lung cancer, at present there is no direct evidence that marijuana smoking induces lung cancer. However, heavy marijuana use among Americans may be too recent to permit detection of this problem.

Although marijuana has also been associated with adverse effects on a number of other systems, many of these studies await replication and confirmation. For example, the reported correlation between marijuana use and decreased testosterone levels in males has not been confirmed. Decreased sperm count and sperm motility and morphologic abnormalities of spermatozoa following marijuana use have also been reported. Administration of high doses of marijuana to female rhesus monkeys has revealed significant marijuana-induced suppression of pituitary gonadotropins and gonadal steroids. Carefully conducted prospective studies demonstrated a significant correlation between impaired fetal growth and development and heavy marijuana use during pregnancy. Marijuana also has been implicated in derangements of the immune response system, in chromosomal abnormalities, and in inhibition of DNA, RNA, and protein synthesis, but these findings have not been confirmed or related to any specific physiologic effect in humans. One report of cannabis-induced brain atrophy in young adults has not been confirmed in computed tomography studies of young men with histories of heavy marijuana smoking.

Tolerance and Physical Dependence Habitual marijuana users rapidly develop tolerance to the psychoactive effects of marijuana and often smoke more frequently and try to secure more potent cannabis compounds. Tolerance for physiologic effects of marijuana develops at different rates; e.g., tolerance for marijuana-induced tachycardia develops rapidly, but tolerance for marijuana-induced conjunctival injection develops more slowly. Tolerance to both behavioral and physiologic effects of marijuana decreases rapidly upon cessation of marijuana use.

Withdrawal signs and symptoms have been reported in chronic cannabis users, with the severity of symptoms related to dosage and duration of use. These include tremor, nystagmus, sweating, nausea, vomiting, diarrhea, irritability, anorexia, and sleep disturbances. Withdrawal signs and symptoms observed in chronic marijuana users are usually relatively mild in comparison to those observed in heavy opiate or alcohol users and rarely require medical or pharmacologic intervention. Somewhat more severe and protracted abstinence syndromes may occur after sustained use of high-potency cannabis compounds for long periods.

LYSERGIC ACID DIETHYLAMIDE (LSD) The serendipitous discovery of the psychedelic effects of LSD in 1947 culminated in an epidemic of LSD abuse during the 1960s. Imposition of stringent legal and regulatory constraints on the manufacture and distribution of LSD [classified as a Schedule I substance by the Food and Drug Administration (FDA)], as well as public recognition that the psychedelic experiences induced by LSD were a health hazard, has resulted in a significant reduction in LSD abuse. Although relatively few instances of LSD abuse have been reported, the drug still retains some popularity among adolescents and young adults. There are recent indications that the prevalence of LSD use among young persons has been accelerating in some communities in the United States.

LSD is a very potent drug; oral doses as low as 20 μg may induce profound psychological and physiologic effects. Tachycardia, hypertension, pupillary dilation, tremor, and hyperpyrexia occur within minutes following oral LSD ingestion in doses of 0.5 to 2 μg/kg. A variety of bizarre and often conflicting perceptual and mood changes, including visual illusions, synesthesias, and extreme lability of mood, usually occur within one-half hour after LSD intake. The action of LSD may persist for 12 to 18 h, even though the half-life of the drug is only 3 h.

Tolerance develops rapidly for LSD-induced changes in psychological function when the drug is used one or more times per day over a course of 4 days or more. Abrupt abstinence following continued use does not produce withdrawal signs or symptoms. To date there have been no clinical reports of death caused by the direct effects of LSD.

The most frequent acute medical emergency associated with LSD use is panic episodes, which may persist for up to 24 h (the "bad trip"). This problem is best managed by supportive reassurance ("talking down") and, if necessary, administration of small doses of anxiolytic drugs. Adverse consequences of chronic LSD use include enhanced risk for schizophreniform psychosis and derangements in memory function, problem solving, and abstract thinking. Treatment of these disorders is best carried out in specialized psychiatric facilities.

PHENCYCLIDINE (PCP) Phencyclidine, a cyclohexylamine derivative, is widely used in veterinary medicine to briefly immobilize large animals and is sometimes described as a dissociative anesthetic. PCP is easily synthesized, and its abusers are primarily young people and polydrug users. The true extent of PCP abuse is unknown, but recent national surveys indicate an increase in frequency of use.

Phencyclidine is taken orally, by smoking, or by intravenous injection. It is also used as an adulterant in illicitly sold THC, LSD, amphetamine, and cocaine. The most common street preparation, "angel dust," is a white granular powder which contains 50 to 100 percent of the drug. Low doses (5 mg) produce agitation, excitement, impaired motor coordination, dysarthria, and analgesia. Users may have horizontal or vertical nystagmus, flushing, diaphoresis, and hyperacusis. Behavioral changes include distortions of body image, disorganization of thinking, and feelings of estrangement. Higher doses of PCP (5 to 10 mg) may produce hypersalivation, vomiting, myoclonus, fever, stupor, or coma. PCP doses of 10 mg or more cause convulsions, opisthotonus, and decerebrate posturing which may be followed by prolonged coma.

The diagnosis of PCP overdose is difficult because the patient's initial symptoms may suggest an acute schizophrenic reaction. Confirmation of PCP use is possible by determination of PCP levels in serum or urine. PCP analysis is currently available at most toxicologic centers. Large quantities of PCP remain in urine for 1 to 5 days following high-dosage PCP intake.

PCP overdose requires prompt life-support measures, including treatment of coma, convulsions, and respiratory depression in a hospital intensive care unit. There is no specific antidote or antagonist for PCP. Excretion of PCP from the body can be enhanced by acidification of urine and gastric lavage. Death from PCP overdose may occur as a consequence of some combination of pharyngeal hypersecretion, hyperthermia, respiratory depression, severe hypertension, seizures, hypertensive encephalopathy, and intracerebral hemorrhage.

Acute psychosis associated with PCP use should be considered a psychiatric emergency, since patients may be at high risk for suicide or extreme violence toward others. Phenothiazines should not be used for treatment of acute PCP psychosis because they potentiate PCP's anticholinergic effects. Haloperidol (5 mg intramuscularly) has been administered on an hourly basis to suppress psychotic behavior. PCP, like LSD and mescaline, produces vasospasm of cerebral arteries at relatively low doses. Chronic PCP use has been shown to induce insomnia, anorexia, severe social and behavioral changes, and, in some cases, chronic schizophrenia.

POLYDRUG ABUSE Although drug abusers often report a preference for a particular drug, such as alcohol or opiates, the concurrent use of other drugs is common. Multiple drug use often involves substances having pharmacologic effects different from those of the preferred drug. Concurrent use of such dissimilar compounds as stimulants and opiates or stimulants and alcohol is not unusual. The diversity of reported drug use combinations suggests that achieving some perceptible change in state, rather than any particular direction of change (stimulation or sedation), may be the primary reinforcer in polydrug use and abuse. There is also evidence that intoxication with alcohol or opiates is associated with increased tobacco smoking, but marijuana smoking does not increase during alcohol intoxication. At present, there is relatively little systematic information available about drug interactions. However, it is known that the combined use of cocaine, heroin, and alcohol carries higher risks for toxic effects and adverse medical consequences than the use of a single drug.

A practical determinant of polydrug use patterns is the relative availability and cost of the drugs. There are many examples of situationally determined drug use patterns. For example, soldiers who became dependent on heroin in Vietnam seldom continued heroin use after leaving military service; but a significant proportion of them abused alcohol and became alcohol-dependent when they returned to the United States. Alcohol abuse, with its attendant medical complications, is one of the most serious problems encountered in former heroin addicts participating in methadone maintenance programs.

The physician must recognize that perpetuation of polydrug abuse and drug dependence is not necessarily a symptom of an underlying emotional disorder. Neither alleviation of anxiety nor reduction of depression accounts for the initiation and perpetuation of polydrug abuse. Severe depression and anxiety as frequently result from as precede polydrug abuse. There is also evidence that some of the most adverse consequences of drug use may reinforce continued polydrug abuse.

Adequate treatment of polydrug abuse, as well as other forms of drug abuse, requires innovative and eclectic programs of intervention. The first step in successful treatment is detoxification, a process which may be difficult because the patient has abused several drugs with different pharmacologic actions (e.g., alcohol, opiates, and cocaine). Since patients may not recall or may deny simultaneous multiple drug use, diagnostic evaluation should always include urinalysis for qualitative detection of psychoactive substances and their metabolites. Treatment of polydrug abuse requires hospitalization or inpatient residential care during detoxification and the initial phase of drug abstinence. When possible, specialized facilities for the care and treatment of chemically dependent persons should be used. Outpatient detoxification of polydrug abuse patients is likely to be ineffective and may be dangerous.

As in the treatment of alcohol abuse, no single therapeutic modality has been shown to be uniquely effective in inducing remission. Polydrug abuse is a chronic disorder with an unpredictable pattern of remission and recrudescence. Therapeutic management of chronic disorders such as cardiac or neoplastic disease should serve as a model for helping the person with polydrug abuse problems. Even temporary remissions with attendant physical, social, and psychological improvements are preferable to the continuation or progressive acceleration of polydrug abuse and its adverse medical and interpersonal consequences. In polydrug abuse, as in most chronic disorders, definitive "cures" are rare. The concerned physician should continue to assist polydrug abuse patients throughout the cyclic oscillations of this complex behavior disorder, recognizing that resumption of drug use may be the rule rather than the exception.

BIBLIOGRAPHY

Carroll KM et al: Psychotherapy and pharmacotherapy for ambulatory cocaine abusers. Arch Gen Psychiatry 51:177, 1994

Cregler LL, Mark H: Medical complications of cocaine abuse. N Engl J Med 315:1495, 1986

Das G: Cocaine abuse in North America—A milestone in history. J Clin Pharmacol 33:296, 1993

Foltin RW, Fischman MW: Smoked and intravenous cocaine in humans: Acute tolerance, cardiovascular and subjective effects. J Pharmacol Exp Ther 257:247, 1991

Gawin FH: Cocaine addiction: Psychology and neurophysiology. Science 251:1580, 1991

———, Ellinwood EH Jr: Cocaine and other stimulants. Actions, abuse, and treatment. N Engl J Med 318:1173, 1988

Halikas J et al: 1990–1991 Survey of pharmacotherapies used in the treatment of cocaine abuse. J Addict Dis 12:129, 1993

Hollander JE: The management of cocaine-associated myocardial ischemia. N Engl J Med 333:1267, 1995

Holman BL et al: Brain perfusion is abnormal in cocaine-dependent polydrug users: A study using technetium-99m-HMPAO and ASPECT. J Nucl Med 32:1206, 1991

Johanson CE, Fischman MW: The pharmacology of cocaine related to its abuse. Pharmacol Rev 41:3, 1989

Jones RT: The pharmacology of cocaine smoking in humans, in *Research Findings on Smoking of Abused Substances*, NIDA Research Monograph vol. 99, CN Chiang, RL Hawks (eds). Washington, DC, U.S. Government Printing Office, 1990, pp 30–41

Levin JM et al: Gender differences in cerebral perfusion in cocaine abuse: Technetium-99m-HMPAO SPECT study of drug- abusing women. J Nucl Med 35:1902, 1994

MARZUK PM et al: Fatal injuries after cocaine use as a leading cause of death among young adults in New York City. N Engl J Med 332:1753, 1995
MCCANCE EF et al: Cocaethylene: Pharmacology, physiology and behavioral effects in humans. J Pharmacol Exp Ther 274:215, 1995
MENDELSON JH, MELLO NK (eds): *Medical Diagnosis and Treatment of Alcoholism.* New York, McGraw-Hill, 1992
———, ———: Management of cocaine abuse and dependence. N Engl J Med 334:965, 1996
——— et al: Acute effects of cocaine on plasma adrenocorticotropic hormone, luteinizing hormone and prolactin levels in cocaine-dependent men. J Pharmacol Exp Ther 263:505, 1992
MOLITERANO DJ et al: Coronary-artery vasoconstriction induced by cocaine, cigarette smoking, or both. N Engl J Med 330:454, 1994
NAJAVITS LM, WEISS RD: The role of psychotherapy in the treatment of substance-use disorders. Harvard Rev Psychiatry 2:84, 1994
NATIONAL INSTITUTE ON DRUG ABUSE: *Epidemiologic Trends in Drug Abuse,* vol 1: *Highlights and Executive Summary.* NIH Publication 95-3990, 1995
OM A et al: Management of cocaine-induced cardiovascular complications. Am Heart J 125:469, 1993
SUBSTANCE ABUSE AND MENTAL HEALTH SERVICES ADMINISTRATION OFFICE OF APPLIED STUDIES: *The 1993 National Household Survey on Drug Abuse.* US Department of Health and Human Services Public Health Service, 1993
SUBSTANCE ABUSE AND MENTAL HEALTH SERVICES ADMINISTRATION OFFICE OF APPLIED STUDIES: *Preliminary Estimates from the Drug Abuse Warning Network (DAWN).* Advance Report no. 2, 1993
WOODS JH, WINGER G: Phencyclidine and related substances, in *Drug Abuse and Drug Abuse Research: The Third Triennial Report to Congress from the Secretary, Department of Health and Human Services.* Washington, DC: U.S. Government Printing Office, 1991, p 145

389

John H. Holbrook

NICOTINE ADDICTION

Cigarette smoking is the principal cause of preventable disease, disability, and premature death in the United States. Nonetheless, each year more than one million American children and teenagers start smoking, and most established smokers have great difficulty in quitting. The addictive effects of nicotine account for most of this persistent personal and public health dilemma. Recognition of tobacco use as an addiction and of nicotine as the addictive drug is essential for effective patient management.

The primary criteria for defining drug addiction are compulsive use, psychoactive effects, and drug-reinforced behavior. Nicotine use fulfills these criteria because it produces a compelling urge to smoke, provides pleasurable alterations in mood, and motivates chronic tobacco-seeking and tobacco-using behavior. Tolerance and physical dependence, manifested by an abstinence-mediated withdrawal syndrome, contribute to the strong control exerted by nicotine on smoking behavior.

Smokers regulate their nicotine dose to obtain desired effects; these include both positive effects, such as pleasure and enhanced vigilance, and avoidance of the withdrawal syndrome. This syndrome is characterized by craving for tobacco products, depressed mood, insomnia, irritability, anxiety, difficulty concentrating, restlessness, and an increased appetite. Most of these symptoms peak in 1 to 2 days and return to baseline within 3 to 4 weeks of quitting; however, craving for tobacco products and hunger may persist for extended periods.

The use of tobacco products is a complex, learned behavior that is woven into the fiber of daily living and is linked to how the smoker deals with the world. Numerous daily activities, thoughts, and emotions serve as powerful cues to smoke. Such conditioned ties become paired with positive neuroregulatory effects of nicotine to reinforce the addictive process. Personal characteristics such as educational level, belief in one's ability to change, and coping skills are determinants of tobacco use. Similarly, environmental factors such as the level of acceptance of smoking in the home, peer group, workplace, and community norms influence smoking behavior.

PHYSICOCHEMICAL PROPERTIES OF CIGARETTE SMOKE Cigarette smoke is a heterogeneous aerosol produced by incomplete combustion of the tobacco leaf. It is composed of a gas phase in which particulate matter is dispersed. Mainstream smoke emerges from the mouthpiece during puffing. Sidestream smoke is emitted between puffs at the burning cone and from the mouthpiece. In the presence of the intense heat of combustion some tobacco constituents undergo thermic decomposition (pyrolysis). Volatile substances are distilled directly into the smoke. Unstable molecules recombine to generate new compounds (pyrosynthesis). Concentration of smoke constituents occurs as the smoke is filtered by unburnt tobacco and is redistilled by the burning cone. Some substances found in tobacco pass unchanged into cigarette smoke.

Approximately 92 to 95 percent of the total weight of mainstream smoke is present in the gas phase. Nitrogen, oxygen, and carbon dioxide account for 85 percent of the smoke's weight. The remaining gases and particulate matter are the substances of medical importance (Table 389-1) A variety of additives are used in the manufacturing of cigarettes; the influence of these substances on the composition and biologic activity of cigarette smoke is not known.

PHARMACOLOGY OF CIGARETTE SMOKE More than 4000 substances have been identified in cigarette smoke, including some that are pharmacologically active, antigenic, cytotoxic, mutagenic, and carcinogenic; these diverse biologic effects provide a framework for understanding the multiple adverse consequences of smoking. A pack-a-day cigarette smoker puffs more than 70,000 times a year, and, consequently, the membranes of the mouth, nose, pharynx, and tracheobronchial tree are exposed repetitively to tobacco smoke. Some constituents act directly on the membranes, while others are absorbed into the blood or are dissolved in saliva and swallowed.

Tissue and organ system responses to cigarette smoke inhalation are multiple and complex. Most studies in humans have dealt with exposure to whole smoke or to selected constituents thought to pose the greatest risk to health, such as nicotine and carbon monoxide.

Table 389-1

Selected Cigarette Smoke Constituents

Substance	Effect(s)
PARTICULATE PHASE	
"Tar"*	Carcinogen
Polynuclear aromatic hydrocarbons	Carcinogens
Nicotine	Neuroendocrine stimulant and depressant; addicting drug
Phenol	Cocarcinogen and irritant
Cresol	Cocarcinogen and irritant
β-Naphthylamine	Carcinogen
N-Nitrosonornicotine	Carcinogen
Benzo[a]pyrene	Carcinogen
Trace metals (e.g., nickel, arsenic, polonium 210)	Carcinogens
Indole	Tumor accelerator
Carbazole	Tumor accelerator
Catechol	Cocarcinogen
GAS PHASE	
Carbon monoxide	Impairs oxygen transport and utilization
Hydrocyanic acid	Ciliotoxin and irritant
Acetaldehyde	Ciliotoxin and irritant
Acrolein	Ciliotoxin and irritant
Ammonia	Ciliotoxin and irritant
Formaldehyde	Ciliotoxin and irritant
Oxides of nitrogen	Ciliotoxin and irritant
Nitrosamines	Carcinogen
Hydrazine	Carcinogen
Vinyl chloride	Carcinogen

* The aggregate of particulate matter in cigarette smoke after subtracting nicotine and moisture.

Relatively little is known about the individual effects and interactions of other potentially toxic smoke constituents that are present in low concentrations.

Nicotine is a highly toxic alkaloid that is both a ganglionic stimulant and depressant. Many of its complex effects are mediated by catecholamine release. Nicotine also increases serum concentrations of glucose, cortisol, free fatty acids, vasopressin, and β-endorphin.

Carbon monoxide interferes with oxygen transport and utilization. Because cigarette smoke contains 2 to 6 percent carbon monoxide, smokers inhale concentrations as high as 400 parts per million (ppm) and develop elevated carboxyhemoglobin (COHb) levels. The range of COHb found in smokers is 2 to 15 percent, while levels for nonsmokers are near 1 percent. The average COHb level of moderate cigarette smokers is 5 percent. Chronic, mild elevations of COHb due to smoking are a common cause of mild polycythemia and may produce subtle impairment of central nervous system function.

Cigarette smoke and its condensate are carcinogenic in several species of animals. The major identified carcinogens in cigarette smoke are polynuclear aromatic hydrocarbons, aromatic amines, and nitrosamines (Table 389-1). Cocarcinogens present in cigarette smoke, such as catechol, greatly enhance its carcinogenicity.

Potent pulmonary irritants and ciliotoxins are found in cigarette smoke (Table 389-1). These substances increase bronchial mucus secretion and mediate acute and chronic decreases in pulmonary and mucociliary function.

EPIDEMIOLOGY Data from large prospective studies of populations in several countries have shown that cigarette-smoking men have 70 percent higher overall death rates than nonsmokers. About half of all regular cigarette smokers will eventually die because of smoking. The effect on mortality is proportionately greatest in younger age groups. The excess mortality of female smokers has been somewhat less than that of male smokers, but it has increased. Cigarette smoking is the largest single health risk in the United States and is responsible for an estimated 430,000 premature deaths each year; this is equivalent to approximately one out of every five deaths. Coronary heart disease (CHD) and lung cancer are the chief contributors to smoking-related excess mortality. In the United States, cigarette smokers also experience more disability due to chronic illness and report significantly more days absent from work than do nonsmokers. Cigarette smoking causes immeasurable personal loss and suffering.

A strong dose-response relationship exists between cigarette smoking and excess mortality, as measured by the age at onset of smoking, the number of cigarettes smoked, the number of years of smoking, and the depth of inhalation. Cessation of smoking is associated with a decrease in the excess mortality. These observations together with clinical, experimental, and pathologic studies indicate that smoking, per se, causes the excess mortality.

CHARACTERISTICS OF SMOKERS Demographic, anthropometric, physiologic, and laboratory features that distinguish cigarette smokers from nonsmokers are due both to baseline differences between these groups and to the effects of smoking. Smokers drink more alcohol, coffee, and tea than do nonsmokers. Their weight and blood pressure are slightly less and their heart rate is slightly faster than those of nonsmokers. In women, the menopause comes earlier in smokers than in nonsmokers. Smokers have impaired maximum exercise performance and impaired immune systems compared to nonsmokers. A markedly increased number of pulmonary alveolar macrophages is present in smokers, and the function and metabolism of these cells are abnormal. When compared with nonsmokers, smokers show small increases in hematocrit, total white blood cell count, and platelet count, as well as small decreases in leukocyte vitamin C levels, serum uric acid, and albumin. In smokers, the ratio of high-density lipoprotein cholesterol to low-density lipoprotein cholesterol is reduced.

CLINICAL CORRELATIONS Large population studies have shown a strong association between cigarette smoking and several diseases. Atherosclerotic cardiovascular disease, cancer, and chronic obstructive pulmonary disease account for most of the excess mortality and morbidity due to smoking.

Individual patient risks due to cigarette smoking vary widely. Factors that influence these risks include the duration, intensity, and type of smoke exposure; genetically mediated susceptibility; occupational and environmental exposures; use of medication; and coexisting risk factors and diseases.

Cardiovascular Disease Cigarette smoking is a major cause of coronary heart disease, and premature CHD is one of its most important medical consequences (see Chap. 244). Approximately 20 percent of the 500,000 CHD deaths occurring each year in the United States is attributable to smoking. Cigarette smoking, hypertension, and hypercholesterolemia are the three major CHD risk factors. Smoking acts both independently of and synergistically with these other CHD risk factors. There is a dose-response relationship between CHD risk and cigarette smoking. CHD death rates are 60 to 70 percent greater in male smokers than nonsmokers. Sudden death may be the first manifestation of CHD, and it is two to four times more likely to occur in younger male cigarette smokers than in nonsmokers. Women cigarette smokers are also at greater risk of developing CHD than nonsmokers, and the use of both cigarettes and oral contraceptives increases this risk approximately tenfold. Those who continue to smoke after an acute myocardial infarction are more likely to die from CHD than are those who quit smoking. Smokers who undergo coronary artery bypass surgery have increased perioperative mortality compared to nonsmokers. Cigarette smoking contributes to both coronary atherosclerosis and acute ischemic, thrombotic, and arrhythmic coronary events. Cigarette smoking may interfere with the efficacy of medications used to treat CHD, such as propranolol.

Cigarette smoking is an important cause of cerebrovascular disease and accounts for an estimated 15 percent of the 150,000 stroke deaths that occur each year in the United States. Large epidemiologic studies in men and women have shown an increased risk of stroke among smokers compared to nonsmokers, a dose-response relationship between smoking and stroke risk, and a decrease in stroke risk with smoking cessation. Among women, subarachnoid hemorrhage is more likely to occur in smokers than nonsmokers, and the use of both cigarettes and oral contraceptives greatly increases this risk.

Cigarette smoking is the most powerful risk factor for arteriosclerosis obliterans and thromboangiitis obliterans. It also aggravates peripheral ischemia and may adversely affect peripheral bypass grafts. The mortality rate for atherosclerotic aortic aneurysm is greater in male smokers than nonsmokers.

Cigarette smoking is not a risk factor for the development of hypertension; however, hypertensives who smoke are at a greater risk of developing malignant hypertension and of dying from hypertension. Because of the association with chronic obstructive pulmonary disease, cigarette smoking is an important factor leading to chronic pulmonary heart disease.

Cancer Cigarette smoking is the single most important cause of cancer mortality in the United States, accounting for 30 percent of all cancer deaths. In spite of the well-documented cause-and-effect relationship between cigarette smoking and lung cancer, more Americans continue to die from this cancer than from any other tumor (see Chap. 90). In 1991, an estimated 143,000 lung cancer deaths occurred in the United States; 85 percent of these deaths were attributable to cigarette smoking. The risk of developing lung cancer is quantitatively related to cigarette smoke exposure. Men who smoke one pack a day increase their risk tenfold compared with nonsmokers; men who smoke two packs a day may increase their risk more than 25 times compared with nonsmokers. Asbestos workers who smoke cigarettes are at especially high risk for developing lung cancer. Cigarette consumption by women increased rapidly in the United States during the past 50 years, and lung cancer mortality among smokers is currently increasing faster in women than in men. Lung cancer has become the leading cause of cancer death among American women.

Cigarette smoking is a cause of laryngeal, oral, pharyngeal, esophageal, and bladder cancer in men and women. Cigarette smoking is an important contributory factor for the development of kidney and pancreatic cancer; it is associated with cancer of the stomach and uterine cervix. Cigarette smoking may also be associated with leukemia, hepatoma, nonmelanoma skin cancer, and cancer of the anus and vulva.

Respiratory Disease Cigarette smoking is the major cause of chronic obstructive pulmonary disease (COPD), that is, chronic bronchitis and emphysema (see Chap. 258). Of the estimated 80,000 deaths from COPD in the United States in 1991, 82 percent were attributable to smoking, and many of these deaths were preceded by prolonged respiratory disability. There is a dose-response relationship between COPD death rates and cigarette smoking. Depending upon the extent of smoke exposure, the mortality rate due to COPD is 4 to 25 times higher in male cigarette smokers than in nonsmokers. Although the death rate from COPD among female smokers is somewhat lower than among male smokers, it is increasing much more rapidly in female than in male smokers. Chronic cough, sputum production, and breathlessness are much more common in smokers. Smokers are more likely than nonsmokers to show abnormalities in a number of pulmonary function tests, including measurements of elastic recoil, airflow in large and small airways, and diffusing capacity. Mild airflow obstruction in small airways may be present even in teenage smokers.

Cigarette smoking has been associated with an increased incidence of respiratory infections and deaths from pneumonia and influenza. Postoperative respiratory complications and spontaneous pneumothorax are also more common in smokers. Because tobacco smoke may increase airway obstruction, asthmatics should be urged not to smoke. Chronic stomatitis and chronic laryngitis occur more frequently in smokers than in nonsmokers.

Pregnancy Smoking may delay conception, and smoking during pregnancy may affect the fetus adversely. Infants whose mothers smoked during pregnancy weigh, on average, 170 g less than infants whose mothers did not smoke. This effect probably results from impaired uteroplacental circulation. Maternal smoking during pregnancy increases the risk of spontaneous abortion, fetal death, neonatal death, and the sudden infant death syndrome. This increased risk may be much greater in pregnancies already at high risk owing to other factors. Smoking during pregnancy may also adversely affect the long-term physical growth and intellectual development of the child.

Gastrointestinal Disorders Gastric and duodenal ulcer disease is more prevalent in male and female cigarette smokers than in nonsmokers and causes more deaths in male smokers than in nonsmokers. Smoking impairs spontaneous and drug-induced healing of peptic ulcers, increases the likelihood of duodenal ulcer recurrence, inhibits pancreactic bicarbonate secretion, and decreases the pressure of esophageal and pyloric sphincters. Smoking also prevents the inhibition of nocturnal gastric secretion by histamine H_2-receptor antagonists.

Other Conditions Cigarette smoking is a risk factor for premature facial wrinkling, osteoporosis in women, and sexual dysfunction in men. It may also be associated with Graves' disease, cataracts, macular degeneration, degenerative disk disease, and sleep disturbances.

Depression Recent studies indicate that the prevalence of cigarette smoking is increased among those who have had a major depressive disorder. Furthermore, smoking cessation rates are lower among depressed smokers compared to nondepressed smokers. What role antidepressants could play in such individuals who are attempting to quit smoking remains to be determined.

Involuntary Smoke Inhalation Indoor atmospheres and other confined spaces are often contaminated by tobacco smoke, which is inhaled involuntarily by both smokers and nonsmokers. Most of the atmospheric pollutants arise from sidestream smoke. It contains greater concentrations of many smoke constituents than does mainstream smoke, but since sidestream smoke is diluted in a large volume of air, the smoke exposure from involuntary inhalation is less than that associated with smoking.

Initially, involuntary or passive smoking was thought to cause primarily an irritant effect such as ocular burning. It is now recognized as a cause of lung cancer in nonsmokers. Parental smoking in the home is associated with an increased risk of acute respiratory illnesses, middle-ear effusions, chronic respiratory symptoms, and slightly impaired lung function in children. Involuntary smoke inhalation may also cause CHD.

Drug Effects Tobacco smoke constituents induce hepatic microsomal enzyme systems that are important in the metabolism of several drugs. For example, cigarette smoking increases the metabolism of propranolol, propoxyphene, and theophylline. Hence, changes in smoking behavior may cause significant alterations of serum drug levels that may result in either drug toxicity or failure of drug treatment.

TYPES OF SMOKING Filter-tipped cigarettes and lower-tar and -nicotine cigarettes now account for more than 95 and 55 percent of sales, respectively. Lung cancer and laryngeal cancer are the only tobacco-related diseases for which the use of lower-tar and -nicotine cigarettes has been shown to result in risk reduction, compared with the use of higher-tar and -nicotine cigarettes; however, compared with not smoking or quitting, the benefits are minimal. Consumers who choose lower-tar and -nicotine cigarettes and then smoke a larger number of cigarettes or inhale more frequently or deeply may actually increase their exposure to harmful substances.

Cigar and pipe smokers usually inhale less smoke than cigarette smokers, presumably because the alkaline pH of cigar and pipe tobacco makes it more irritating to the respiratory tract. The smoke exposure and overall mortality rates of pipe and cigar smokers in the United States are substantially less than those of cigarette smokers; however, death rates of cigarette, cigar, and pipe smokers are approximately equal for carcinoma of the oral cavity, larynx, and esophagus, sites where exposures to cigarette, cigar, and pipe smoke are similar. The mortality rates of most cigar and pipe smokers for cancer at other sites, CHD, and COPD are not greatly elevated above the rates of nonsmokers, but cigar and pipe smokers who inhale consistently may experience adverse health effects comparable with those of cigarette smokers.

The use of chewing tobacco and snuff may produce plasma nicotine levels comparable to those of cigarette smokers and lead to nicotine dependence or addiction. The use of such smokeless tobacco products also increases the risk for oral cancer.

CESSATION OF SMOKING In the United States between 1965 and 1991, the prevalence of smoking in adults declined from 52 to 28 percent of men and 34 to 23 percent of women. Each year in the United States, approximately 1.3 million smokers stop smoking. In 1991 there were an estimated 46.3 million current adult smokers and 43.5 million former smokers. In recent years, the smoking prevalence among senior high school students has leveled off at about 20 percent. The rate of decline in smoking prevalence among the least educated Americans lags behind other groups.

Benefits Smoking cessation produces immediate and long-term physical, psychological, and economic benefits. Within days of quitting the sense of smell and taste may improve. One year after quitting there is a substantial decrease in risk for a myocardial infarction. Total mortality among former smokers decreases almost to that of nonsmokers 15 years after quitting. When chronic smoking produces permanent damage, as it does in the case of emphysema, the benefits of cessation are more modest, such as a slowing in the rate of decline of pulmonary function. The U.S. Surgeon General summarized the major and immediate health benefits of cessation that are valid for men and women of all ages and for those with and without smoking-related disease. Former smokers live, on the average, longer than continuing smokers. Cessation reduces the risk for tobacco-related cancers, myocardial infarction, cerebrovascular disease, and chronic obstructive pulmonary disease. Women who quit smoking prior to pregnancy, or during the first trimester, eliminate the risk of delivering a low-birth-weight baby. The health benefits of quitting smoking far exceed the risks of the average 2.3- to 6.8-kg (5- to 15-lb) weight gain or any adverse psychological effects that may occur after quitting.

Cessation Process Most American smokers would like to quit. Eighty percent have attempted to stop smoking during their lifetime, and 30 percent have stopped for at least one day during the previous year. Most of these attempts to quit are only temporarily successful. Smoking cessation is a dynamic, cyclic process that leads to overcoming an addictive behavior. Smokers move through a series of stages in their attempts to quit, including thinking about quitting, deciding to quit, attempting to quit, and maintaining the ex-smoker status. Most successful quitters relapse and recycle through these stages three or four times before attaining long-term abstinence. Fewer than 5 percent of smokers move directly to the confirmed ex-smoker status without experiencing relapses. Factors encouraging long-term cessation include decreased social acceptability of smoking, increased concern about the health consequences of active and passive smoking, and increased costs of tobacco products. Factors contributing to relapse include craving for nicotine, weight gain, social pressures, and attempts to cope with negative feelings and interpersonal conflicts.

Cessation Methods More than 90 percent of confirmed ex-smokers quit without formal assistance. Quitting "cold turkey" is the method used by more than 80 percent of successful ex-smokers. However, heavy smokers and those most addicted to nicotine may benefit from participation in a cessation program. Organized programs employ a variety of approaches, including self-help, physician advice and counseling, use of medication, group therapy, and behavioral training. With such methods 20 to 30 percent 1-year abstinence rates are commonly reported.

Recent meta-analyses of approximately 300 controlled clinical trials document the effectiveness of smoking cessation treatments. The three modalities that are especially effective are nicotine replacement therapy, social support through clinician-provided encouragement and assistance, and skills training on techniques to achieve and maintain smoking cessation. The most effective programs offer multiple treatment modalities, involvement of physician and nonphysician health personnel, and a clear nonsmoking message presented in a variety of formats over time.

Physician Guidelines Physicians have unique opportunities and effective tools to promote smoking cessation. Seventy percent of American smokers visit a physician at least once a year. Some of these visits occur when the patient is experiencing symptomatic illness. In such settings, patients may be especially responsive to cessation messages, and quit rates may be substantially enhanced. Even brief, physician-delivered stop-smoking messages may double the spontaneous smoking cessation rate. Treatment of nicotine addiction is at least as cost-effective as treating other common medical problems such as hypertension and hypercholesterolemia.

Nicotine addiction should be viewed as a chronic medical problem requiring long-term commitment and management skills. Each patient's smoking status should be noted on the problem list. The primary goal for each clinic visit should be to assist the smoker to move one step closer to quitting. The three essential phases for physician management are assessment, intervention, and follow-up (Table 389-2). During the assessment phase, data are collected on health status, nicotine addiction, quitting experience, and interest in quitting. If the patient doesn't want to stop smoking, the clinician should review the risks of smoking, recommend quitting, and defer further action until the next clinic visit. Most patients are interested in quitting and progress to the intervention phase. Smokers are taught about the benefits of quitting and the cyclical cessation process. The smoker is advised to choose a quit date and to go "cold turkey." When possible, the recommendation to stop smoking is related to the patient's unique needs and risk factors. A cessation method(s) is chosen and implemented. Physicians often provide educational material, counseling, and nicotine replacement therapy. Both nicotine chewing gum and transdermal patches improve cessation rates. Transdermal nicotine doubles smoking cessation rates and should be the pharmacotherapy of choice for most smokers; this effect is independent of the intensity of psychosocial interventions. The proper uses, contraindications, and side effects of these products should be understood. For example, nicotine replacement therapy should not be used when the patient is still smoking. The likelihood of success with any cessation method is enhanced when the clinician responds to individual concerns such as weight gain and helps the smoker to develop practical strategies to avoid relapse. The final phase, follow-up, involves assessing progress, providing support, and dealing with relapse. The last should not be viewed as failure but as part of the cyclic process leading to cessation. Follow-up discussions may focus on alternative cessation methods or referral to a smoking cessation specialist.

Table 389-2

Physician Guidelines for Managing Nicotine Addiction

Assessment	
1. Smoking history	4. Quitting experience
2. Level of nicotine addiction	5. Interest in quitting
3. Health status	
Intervention	
1. Education	3. Selection of cessation method(s)
a. Benefits of cessation	a. Self-help
b. Cessation process	b. Physician-assisted
c. Withdrawal syndrome	c. Nicotine replacement
2. Giving advice to quit	d. Behavioral training
a. Personalized message	e. Group therapy
b. Quit date	4. Implementation of method
c. "Cold turkey"	5. Meeting of special needs
Follow-up	
1. Measurement of progress	4. Consideration of alternative methods
2. Provision of support	5. Consideration of referral
3. Dealing with relapse	

Political, social, and cultural forces play a critical role in the individual decision to start or stop smoking. For this reason, physicians should lead and support efforts to increase tobacco excise taxes, to eliminate all tobacco advertisements and promotional activities, and to ban smoking in public places.

PREVENTION In the United States, more than 90 percent of cases of first tobacco use occurs before high school graduation. The average age of first smoking a cigarette is 14.5 years and of becoming a daily smoker is 17.7 years. Approximately 40 percent of teenage smokers who experiment with a few cigarettes become regular smokers. Even though most adolescent smokers want to quit, they are unable to do so because of nicotine addiction. Because few people start to smoke after the age of 18 years, primary smoking prevention in the pediatric and adolescent age groups is an essential step to reduce the toll of tobacco use. Young people who have been trained to resist social pressures, who appreciate the difficulty of quitting, and who understand the health consequences of smoking are less likely to start smoking.

BIBLIOGRAPHY

American Psychiatric Association: Practice guideline for the treatment of patients with nicotine dependence. Am J Psychiatry 153:1, 1996

Doll R et al: Mortality in relation to smoking: 40 years' observations on male British doctors. BMJ 309:901, 1994

Gries JM et al: Chronopharmacokinetics of nicotine. Clin Pharmacol Ther 60:385, 1996

Henningfield JE: Nicotine medications for smoking cessation. N Engl J Med 333:1196, 1995

Kessler DA: Nicotine addiction in young people. N Engl J Med 333:186, 1995

US Department of Health and Human Services: *The Health Consequences of Smoking: Nicotine Addiction. A Report of the Surgeon General.* DHHS (CDC) Publication 88-8406, 1988

———: *Preventing Tobacco Use Among Young People. A Report of the Surgeon General.* DHHS (CDC), National Center for Chronic Disease Prevention and Health Promotion, Office on Smoking and Health, 1994

———: *Smoking Cessation and Prevention.* Clinical Practice Guideline Number 18, Agency for Health Care Policy and Research Publication No. 96-0692, Public Health Service, DHHS, 1996

PART FIFTEEN

ENVIRONMENTAL AND OCCUPATIONAL HAZARDS

390

Howard Hu, Frank E. Speizer

SPECIFIC ENVIRONMENTAL AND OCCUPATIONAL HAZARDS

It cannot be overemphasized that an appropriate environmental/occupational history is an essential part of the medical workup of many chronic diseases. The general approach to the patient whose illness may have been caused or exacerbated by environmental or occupational hazards is detailed in Chap. 5.

As stated in Chap. 5, the term *hazards* in this context is generally synonymous with *toxins* and *toxic exposures* and encompasses chemical factors as well as other risks posed by the physical environment and by selected natural phenomena. These hazards may exist in the general environment or in the workplace. Strictly speaking, smoking, alcohol ingestion, nutritional factors, and infectious agents can also be considered chemical or environmental hazards.

Once a specific hazard has been identified as a factor in the pathogenesis of an illness or as an imminent threat, the clinical approach must include the development of a strategy for preventing further exposure and for treating the specific manifestations of the illness, using antidotes and supportive measures. In the following chapters, specific hazards are considered, including acute poisoning and drug overdose; heavy metal poisoning; disorders caused by venoms, bites, and stings; drowning and near-drowning; electrical injuries; and radiation injury. The health effects of ambient air pollution, occupational respiratory exposures, passive smoking, and assorted toxic air pollutants are discussed briefly in Chap. 254. Space does not allow specific discussion in this text of many other important categories of hazards, such as organic solvents; chemicals used in the plastics, synthetic textiles, and rubber industries; and pesticides. The reader should consult other detailed texts or electronic information sources for clinical data on these topics. In this volume, however, brief attention is focused on several selected issues in light of recent developments in research that have enhanced our understanding of the way these hazards may interact with human behavior and consequently pose increased risks to both individuals and society.

HAZARDOUS WASTE AND GROUNDWATER CONTAMINATION The term *hazardous waste* embodies toxic chemicals, radioactive materials, and biologic or infectious wastes. In many communities, hazardous waste has emerged as a major public health concern. In the United States, some 50,000 sites (defined by specific criteria) have been estimated to contain hazardous chemicals; 1000 or so of these have been included as "Superfund sites" on a National Priority List drawn up by the Environmental Protection Agency (EPA). New or unrecognized sites are likely to exist as well. These sites may require long-term remedial action. The spectrum of substances contained at the sites is wide and theoretically may include any of some 30,000 chemicals that are commonly used in commerce. However, the EPA keeps fewer than 200 chemicals on a special hazardous substance list in light of their toxicity, the frequency with which they are encountered, and other factors. One difficulty in anticipating risks associated with hazardous waste sites is that the substances are usually present in mixtures whose composition is seldom fully known. In addition, with respect to toxicity, chemicals may interact with one another in an additive, protective, or synergistic fashion, and little knowledge exists on which to base predictions regarding the interactions of these complex mixtures.

Waste-site employees and the surrounding community can incur hazardous exposures through the inhalation of toxic vapors or dusts emanating directly from a waste site or an on-site incinerator; the ingestion of water contaminated by surface runoff or by material leaching through soil into surface water or groundwater; the ingestion of contaminated plants, fish, or other wildlife; or direct contact. This last risk is particularly likely for children, who may enter a poorly secured site. Perhaps the exposure of greatest concern to community residents has been the contamination of groundwater by volatile organic compounds or solvents (VOCs); together, the widespread detection of low levels of VOCs in groundwater and the several studies suggesting an association between heavy VOC contamination of drinking water and cancer probably account for the high priority given in public opinion polls to avoiding cancer risks. A 1983 study found that 11 of the 20 chemicals most commonly detected at National Priority List waste sites were VOCs (Table 390-1).

Current regulatory policy rests on the assumption that there is no threshold below which a carcinogen exerts no effect or risk. Thus, once a substance is identified as a probable carcinogen (see below), it is regulated to a concentration that is believed to be accompanied by an acceptable level of risk. Clearly, great uncertainty exists regarding methods used to classify drinking-water carcinogens and to extrapolate the risks related to exposure to these substances. Regardless, VOC contamination in groundwater is likely to continue to be a high-priority issue in the public arena.

ENVIRONMENTAL CARCINOGENS Based on studies and reviews of the literature by the International Agency for Research on Cancer, enough evidence exists to classify around 50 substances and processes as probably or definitely carcinogenic in humans (Table 390-2). Some processes are deemed carcinogenic on the basis of epidemiologic evidence, even though the specific causative agent cannot always be clearly identified. Tumor promoters are not distinguished from tumor initiators in this listing, and the chemical structures and modes of action are diverse. Around 150 additional agents and processes have been designated as possibly carcinogenic on the basis of studies of bacteria and animals as well as human epidemiologic studies. The extent to which inferences can be made from nonhuman studies is controversial but certainly depends on minimal standards in the execution of such studies. For example, the Interagency Regulatory Liaison Group recommends that for a carcinogen assay to be considered positive, the test must have been performed on at least 50 animals of each sex in two different species with at least three dose groups (control and two dose levels) over the lifetime of the animals.

BUILDING-RELATED ILLNESSES Reports of discomfort and symptoms in relation to office environments began in the United

Table 390-1

Volatile Organic Compounds Most Frequently Detected in 1983 at National Priority List Hazardous Waste Sites (in Order of Frequency and Detection) and (When Known) Associated Cancer Risks

Chemical	Risk Level*
Trichloroethylene	3.0
Toluene	
Benzene	1.0
Chloroform	0.43
Tetrachloroethylene	0.7
1,1,1-Trichloroethane	
Ethylbenzene	
Trans-1,2-dichloroethane	0.4
Xylene	
Dichloromethane	
Vinyl chloride	0.02

* Concentration in water (μg/L) equivalent to a lifetime cancer risk of 1×10^{-6}. Risk estimates used in these calculations were derived from the U.S. Environmental Protection Agency (1990).

States in the 1970s. Research has led to the recognition that some building-related illnesses have a clear etiology; these illnesses include hypersensitivity diseases, infections, and exacerbations of asthma due to airborne irritants. However, the majority of such complaints, particularly those of mucous membrane irritation, fatigue, and headache, have no clear etiology. Terms such as *sick-building syndrome* (SBS; also called *tight-building syndrome*) have been used to designate this constellation of symptoms, which have been found in most investigations to occur most often in sealed buildings with centrally controlled mechanical ventilation. Early characterizations of SBS as mass psychogenic illness have not been borne out in the majority of cases by subsequent epidemiologic investigations. Since indoor air-exchange rates were sharply reduced in the 1970s to conserve energy, current hypotheses focus on inadequate dilution of irritants arising from building materials (such as formaldehyde-containing particle board), office supplies (such as carbonless copy paper and photocopy developer solution), and personal care products used by occupants as risk factors for SBS. Confirmation of these hypotheses and further characterization of SBS await additional research.

MULTIPLE-CHEMICAL SENSITIVITY The multiple-chemical sensitivity (MCS) syndrome is a diagnosis that has increasingly been given to patients with a wide variety of symptoms that they attribute to exposure at very low levels to a number of commonly encountered chemicals. The syndrome usually begins after a well-defined environmental event, such as a reaction to a more clearly toxic dose of an organic solvent, pesticide, or respiratory irritant. Some cases of MCS begin as SBS. Affected persons commonly report symptoms such as fatigue, malaise, headache, dizziness, lack of concentration, memory loss, and "spaciness"—symptoms that overlap somewhat with those of other diagnoses of uncertain etiology, such as chronic fatigue syndrome. The pathogenesis of MCS is obscure, and no proven methods exist for its diagnosis, evaluation, and treatment. Case series suggesting a high prevalence of affective disorders indicate that psychological factors may play a role in causing MCS and/or in determining its severity; however, evidence does not support MCS as a purely psychogenic illness. Some patients have debilitating symptoms that are precipitated by incidental exposures to substances as common as perfumes, motor vehicle exhaust, and paint vapors. Other than the ruling out of other treatable conditions and the avoidance of exacerbating exposures, no specific recommendations for the management of MCS patients can yet be made. A recent panel of European scientists convened by the World Health Organization recommended that the designation MCS be replaced by the term *idiopathic environmental illness* (IEI).

GLOBAL CLIMATIC CHANGES An increasing body of evidence indicates that human activities are responsible for global climatic changes, which, in turn, may be directly or indirectly increasing human exposure to environmental hazards. The depletion of stratospheric ozone by chlorinated fluorocarbons, with a consequent increase in ultraviolet radiation exposure, has been firmly established. Increased risks of skin cancers and cataracts are accepted as results of this phenomenon. Less clear is whether the immunosuppressive effects of ultraviolet radiation detected in animals and in vitro have significant clinical impacts on human resistance to infection. Although uncertainties in climate modeling persist, an increasing if not overwhelming amount of evidence indicates that anthropogenic greenhouse gases are fostering global warming. A prominent concern is that global warming can abet the introduction and dissemination of serious infectious diseases, such as mosquito-borne infections (malaria, dengue, and viral encephalitis) and waterborne infectious and toxin-related illnesses (cholera, shellfish poisoning). The World Health Organization has identified global warming as one of the largest public health challenges facing the twenty-first century.

Table 390-2

Substances and Processes Classified as Definitely or Probably Carcinogenic by the International Agency for Research on Cancer

Aflatoxins	Estrogen, nonsteroidal
Aluminum production	Estrogen, steroidal
4-Aminobiphenyl	Furniture and cabinet working
Analgesic mixtures containing phenacetin	Hematite mining, underground, with exposure to radon
Arsenic and arsenic compounds	Iron and steel founding
Asbestos	Isopropyl alcohol manufacture, strong-acid process
Auramine manufacture	Magenta manufacture
Azathioprine	Melphalan
Benzene	8-Methoxypsoralen (Methoxsalen) plus ultraviolet radiation
Benzidine	Mineral oils, untreated and mildly treated
Betel quid with tobacco	MOPP (combined therapy with nitrogen mustard, vincristine, procarbazine, and prednisone) and other combined chemotherapy including alkylating agents
N,N-bis(2-chloroethyl)-2-naphthylamine (Chlornaphazine)	Mustard gas (sulfur mustard)
Bis(chloromethyl)ether and chloromethyl methyl ether (technical-grade)	2-Naphthylamine
Boot and shoe manufacture and repair	Nickel and nickel compounds
1,4-Butanediol dimethanesulfonate (Myleran)	Oral contraceptives, combined
Chlorambucil	Oral contraceptives, sequential
1-(2-Chloroethyl)-3-(4-methylcyclohexyl)-1-nitrosourea (methyl-CCNU)	Rubber industry
Chromium compounds, hexavalent	Shale oils
Coal gasification	Soots
Coal-tar pitches	Talc-containing asbestiform fibers
Coal tars	Tobacco products, smokeless
Coke production	Tobacco smoke
Cyclophosphamide	Treosulfan
Diethylstilbestrol	Vinyl chloride
Erionite	
Estrogen replacement therapy	

BIBLIOGRAPHY

Bourbeau J et al: Prevalence of sick building syndrome symptoms in office workers before and after being exposed to a building with an improved ventilation system. Occup Environ Med 53:204, 1996

Goldberg MS et al: Incidence of cancer among persons living near a municipal solid waste landfill site in Montreal, Quebec. Arch Environ Health 50:416, 1995

Jeevan A, Kripke ML: Ozone depletion and the immune system. Lancet 342:1159, 1993

Patz JA et al: Global climate change and emerging infectious diseases. JAMA 275:217, 1996

Sparks PJ et al: Multiple chemical sensitivity syndrome: A clinical perspective. I. Case definition, theories of pathogenesis, and research needs. II. Evaluation, diagnostic testing, treatment, and social considerations. J Occup Med 36:718, 1994

US Environmental Protection Agency: *Health Effects Assessment Summary Tables*, first/second quarters, FY-1990. Washington, DC, Office of Solid Waste and Emergency Response, 1990

World Health Organization: *Climate Change and Human Health*. Geneva, World Health Organization, 1996

391

Christopher H. Linden, Frederick H. Lovejoy, Jr.

POISONING AND DRUG OVERDOSAGE

Poisoning refers to the development of harmful effects following exposure to chemicals. In a sufficient dose, substances that are usually innocuous, such as oxygen and water, can cause poisoning. Conversely, in small amounts, poisons such as arsenic and cyanide can be consumed without ill effect. Hence, a given substance may or may not be harmful depending on the conditions of exposure. *Overdosage* is exposure to excessive amounts of a substance normally intended for consumption and does not necessarily imply poisoning

Poisoning may be local (limited to the eyes, skin, lungs, or gastrointestinal tract), systemic, or both, depending on dose, absorption, distribution, potency, and host susceptibility. Absorption and distribution are influenced by properties of the substance (molecular size, degree of ionization, lipid and water solubility, protein binding) and of the biologic barriers (membrane composition, pore size, chemical transport systems) through which it penetrates.

Local poisoning results from nonspecific chemical reactions such as oxidation, protein denaturation, desiccation, and solvent activity. Its severity and reversibility depend on the dose (concentration), contact time, potency of the chemical, and type and condition of the exposed surface. The nature, extent, severity, and reversibility of systemic poisoning depend on the dose, potency, and metabolic disposition of the chemical, the functional reserve of the individual, and the presence of secondary complications (shock, hypoxia). Other variables that influence toxicity include coexisting illnesses, previous chemical exposure (e.g., enzyme induction or inhibition, tolerance), and individual differences in biologic response, tissue concentration (pharmacodynamics), and/or absorption, distribution, metabolism, and elimination (pharmacokinetics). *The effects of an overdose begin sooner, peak later, and last longer than those of therapeutic doses.*

EPIDEMIOLOGY

In the United States, chemical exposures result in over 5 million requests for medical advice or treatment each year. The common routes of exposure are ingestion (74 percent), dermal exposure (87 percent), inhalation (5 percent), ophthalmic exposure (6 percent), bites and stings (3 percent), and parenteral injections (0.3 percent). Exposures most frequently involve cleaning agents, analgesics, cosmetics, plants, cough and cold preparations, and hydrocarbons. Most exposures are acute, accidental, occur in the home, result in minor or no toxicity, and involve children under 6 years of age. Pharmaceuticals are involved in 41 percent of exposures and 75 percent of serious or fatal poisonings.

Accidental exposures can result from the improper use of chemicals at work or play, product mislabeling, label misreading, mistaken identification of unlabeled chemicals, uninformed self-medication, and dosing errors by nurses, parents, pharmacists, physicians, and the elderly. Excluding the recreational use of ethanol, attempted suicide is the most common reason for intentional exposure. Unintended poisonings may result from the intentional use of drugs for psychotropic effects (abuse) or excessive self-dosing (misuse).

About 5 percent of victims of chemical exposure require hospitalization. They account for 5 to 10 percent of all ambulance transports, emergency room visits, and intensive care unit admissions, and up to 30 percent of psychiatric admissions are prompted by attempted suicide via overdosage. Suicide attempts also account for most serious or fatal poisonings. Most deaths are due to carbon monoxide poisoning and occur before arrival at a hospital. Most drug-related fatalities are due to analgesics, antidepressants, sedative-hypnotics, stimulants and street drugs, cardiovascular drugs, asthma medications, and antihistamines. Nonpharmaceutical agents implicated in fatal poisoning include alcohols and glycols, automotive products, inorganic chemicals, hydrocarbons, and cleaning agents.

DIAGNOSIS

Although poisoning can mimic other illnesses, the correct diagnosis usually can be established by the history, physical examination, routine and toxicologic laboratory evaluations, and clinical course. The *history* should include the time, route, duration, and circumstances (location, surrounding events, and intent) of exposure; the name and amount of each drug, chemical, or ingredient involved; the time of onset, nature, and severity of symptoms; the time and type of first aid measures provided; and the medical and psychiatric history.

In many cases the victim is confused, comatose, unaware of an exposure, or unable or unwilling to admit to one. Suspicious circumstances include unexplained illness in a previously healthy person; a history of psychiatric problems (particularly depression); recent changes in health, economic status, or social relationships; and onset of illness while working with chemicals or after ingesting food, drink (especially ethanol), or medications. Patients who become ill soon after arriving from a foreign country or after arrest for criminal activity should be suspected of having illicit drugs concealed in body cavities (the gastrointestinal tract). Family, friends, paramedics, police, pharmacists, physicians, and employers should be questioned regarding habits, hobbies, behavior changes, available medications, and antecedent events. A search of the clothes, belongings, and place of discovery may reveal a suicide note or a container of drugs or chemicals. The imprint code on pills and the label on chemical products may be used to identify the ingredients and potential toxicity of a suspected poison by consulting a reference text, a computerized chemical database, the manufacturer, or a regional poison information center.

The *physical examination* should focus initially on the vital signs and cardiopulmonary and neurologic status. The physiologic state can be characterized as excited, depressed, discordant, or normal on the basis of the pulse, blood pressure, respiratory rate, temperature, and mental status. A differential diagnosis can then be formulated (Table 391-1). Examination of the eyes (for nystagmus, pupil size, and pupil reactivity), abdomen (for bowel activity and bladder size), and skin (for burns, bullae, color, warmth, moisture, pressure sores, and puncture marks) may narrow the diagnosis to a particular disorder. Grading the severity of poisoning (Table 391-2) is useful for assessing the clinical course and response to treatment.

The patient also should be examined for evidence of trauma and underlying illnesses. Except in the case of carbon monoxide, theophylline, and drugs that cause hypoglycemia or hypoxia, seizures and neurologic dysfunction due to poisoning are nonfocal. Hence, focal findings should prompt evaluation for a structural central nervous system (CNS) lesion. When the history is unclear, all orifices should be examined for the presence of chemical burns and drug packets. The odor of breath or vomitus and the color of nails, skin, or urine may provide diagnostic clues.

Laboratory assessment may be helpful in the differential diagnosis of poisoning (Fig. 391-1). An anion-gap metabolic acidosis can be caused by a number of substances (Table 391-1); it is characteristic of methanol, ethylene glycol, and salicylate intoxication but can occur in any poisoning that results in hypoxia, hypotension, or seizures. The serum lactate concentration is low (less than the anion gap) in the former and high (nearly equal to the anion gap) in the latter. An abnormally low anion gap can be due to poisoning with bromide, iodine, lithium, or nitrate or to hypercalcemia or hypermagnesemia. An osmolal gap—the difference between the measured serum osmolality and the calculated osmolality [from the serum sodium, glucose, and blood urea nitrogen (BUN)]—of more than 10 mmol/L indicates the presence of a low-molecular-weight solute such as an alcohol, glycol, or ketone or an unmeasured electrolyte or sugar. Such a gap can also be due to diabetic ketoacidosis or lactic acidosis. The osmolal gap provides an estimate of the amount of anion present (Table 391-3). Ketosis can be due to acetone, isopropyl alcohol, and salicylate. Hypoglycemia may be due to poisoning with beta-adrenergic blocking agents, quinine, ethanol, oral hypoglycemic agents, and salicylates, whereas hyperglycemia suggests poisoning with acetone, a beta-adrenergic agonist, a calcium channel–blocking agent, iron, or theophylline. Hypokalemia can be caused by barium, a beta-adrenergic agonist, a diuretic, theophylline, or toluene; hyperkalemia suggests poisoning with an alpha-adrenergic agonist, a beta-adrenergic blocker, digitalis, or fluoride. Poisons that cause specific signs, symptoms, and other laboratory abnormalities are listed in the bibliography.

Pulmonary edema (adult respiratory distress syndrome, or ARDS) can be caused by poisoning with carbon monoxide, cyanide, an opioid, paraquat, phencyclidine, a sedative-hypnotic, or salicylate; by inhalation of irritant gases, fumes, or vapors (ammonia, metal oxides, mercury); or by prolonged anoxia, hyperthermia, or shock. Aspiration pneumonia is common in patients with coma, seizures, and petroleum distillate ingestion. Radiopaque densities may be visible on abdominal x-rays following the ingestion of calcium salts, chloral hydrate, chlorinated hydrocarbons, heavy metals, illicit drug packets, iodinated compounds, potassium salts, psychotherapeutic agents, lithium, phenothiazines, enteric-coated tablets, or salicylates.

Table 391-2

Severity of Stimulant and Depressant Poisoning and Drug Withdrawal

Severity	Signs and Symptoms
STIMULANT POISONING	
Grade 1	Diaphoresis, flushing, hyperreflexia, irritability, mydriasis, tremors
Grade 2	Confusion, fever, hyperactivity, hypertension, tachycardia, tachypnea
Grade 3	Delirium, mania, hyperpyrexia, tachyarrhythmias
Grade 4	Coma, convulsions, cardiovascular collapse
DEPRESSANT POISONING	
Grade 1	Lethargic but arousable; able to answer questions and follow commands
Grade 2	Comatose; withdraws from pain; brainstem and deep tendon reflexes intact
Grade 3	Comatose; no response to pain; most reflexes absent; respiratory depression
Grade 4	Comatose; no response to pain; reflexes absent; respiratory and cardiovascular depression

Bradycardia and atrioventricular (AV) block may occur in patients poisoned by antiarrhythmic agents, beta blockers, calcium channel blockers, cholinergic agents (carbamate and organophosphate insecticides), digitalis, lithium, phenylpropanolamine, or tricyclic antidepressants. QRS- and QT-interval prolongation may be caused by hyperkalemia and by membrane-active drugs (Table 391-1). Ventricular

Table 391-1

Differential Diagnosis of Poisoning Based on Physiologic Status as Determined by Vital Signs and CNS Activity

Excited	Depressed	Discordant	Normal
Sympathomimetic syndrome	**Sympatholytic syndrome**	**Asphyxiants**	**Agents with slow absorption**
Amphetamines	Alpha-adrenergic blockers	Carbon monoxide	Carbamazepine
Bronchodilators (beta$_2$-adrenergic agonists)	Angiotensin converting enzyme inhibitors	Cyanide	Digitalis preparations
Caffeine	Antiarrhythmics	Hydrogen sulfide	Dilantin Kapseals
Cocaine	Antidepressants (tricyclic)	Inert gases	Enteric-coated pills
Decongestants (alpha-adrenergic agonists)	Beta-adrenergic blockers	Irritant fumes, gases, vapors	Lomotil
Ergot alkaloids	Calcium channel blockers	Methemoglobinemia	Salicylates
MAO inhibitors	Clonidine	Nitrophenol herbicides	Sustained-release preparations
Theophylline	Decongestants (imidazolines)	**Central nervous system syndromes**	**Agents with slow distribution**
Thyroid hormones	Digitalis	Disulfiram	Digitalis preparations
Anticholinergic syndrome	**Cholinergic syndrome**	Dystonic/extrapyramidal reactions	Heavy metals
Antidepressants (tricyclic)	Bethanechol	Isoniazid	Lithium
Antihistamines	Carbamate insecticides	Neuroleptic malignant syndrome	Salicylates
Antiparkinsonian agents	Echothiophate	Serotonin syndrome	**Agents that are activated metabolically**
Antispasmodics (GI, GU)	Myasthenia gravis drugs (e.g., pyridostigmine)	Strychnine	Acetaminophen
Belladonna alkaloids	Organophosphate insecticides	Volatile hydrocarbon inhalation	Chloramphenicol
Cyclobenzaprine	Physostigmine	**Membrane-active agents**	Chlorinated hydrocarbons
Mydriatics (topical)	Pilocarpine	Amantadine	Ethylene glycol
Orphenadrine	Urecholine	Antiarrhythmic agents	L-thyroxine
Plants/mushrooms	**Opioid syndrome**	Antidepressants (cyclic)	Methanol
Phenothiazines	Analgesics	Beta-adrenergic blockers	Paraquat
Hallucinogenic syndrome	Antidiarrheal agents	Fluorides	Certain methemoglobin inducers
LSD and its analogues	Antispasmodics (GI)	Heavy metals	**Inhibitors of metabolic pathways**
Marijuana	Heroin	Lithium	Disulfiram
Mescaline and its analogues	Opium	Local anesthetics	Inhibitors of thyroid hormone synthesis
Phencyclidine	**Sedative-hypnotic syndrome**	Meperidine	Monoamine oxidase inhibitors
Withdrawal syndrome	Alcohols	Neuroleptic agents	Salicylates
Antidepressants	Anticonvulsants	Propoxyphene	**Inhibitors of nucleic acid synthesis**
Beta-adrenergic blockers	Barbiturates	Quinine and related antimalarial agents	Anticancer agents
Clonidine	Benzodiazepines	**Metabolic acidosis (low lactate; high anion gap)**	Antiviral agents
Ethanol	Bromide	Alcoholic ketoacidosis	Immunosuppressive drugs
Opioids	Ethchlorvynol	Ethylene glycol	Mushrooms (amatoxins)
Sedative-hypnotics	γ-Hydroxybutyrate	Methanol	Podophylline
	Hydrocarbons	Metformin/phenformin	**Nontoxic exposure**
	Glutethimide	Paraldehyde	**Psychogenic illness**
	Methyprylon	Salicylate	
	Muscle relaxants	Sulfur/sulfate	
		Toluene	

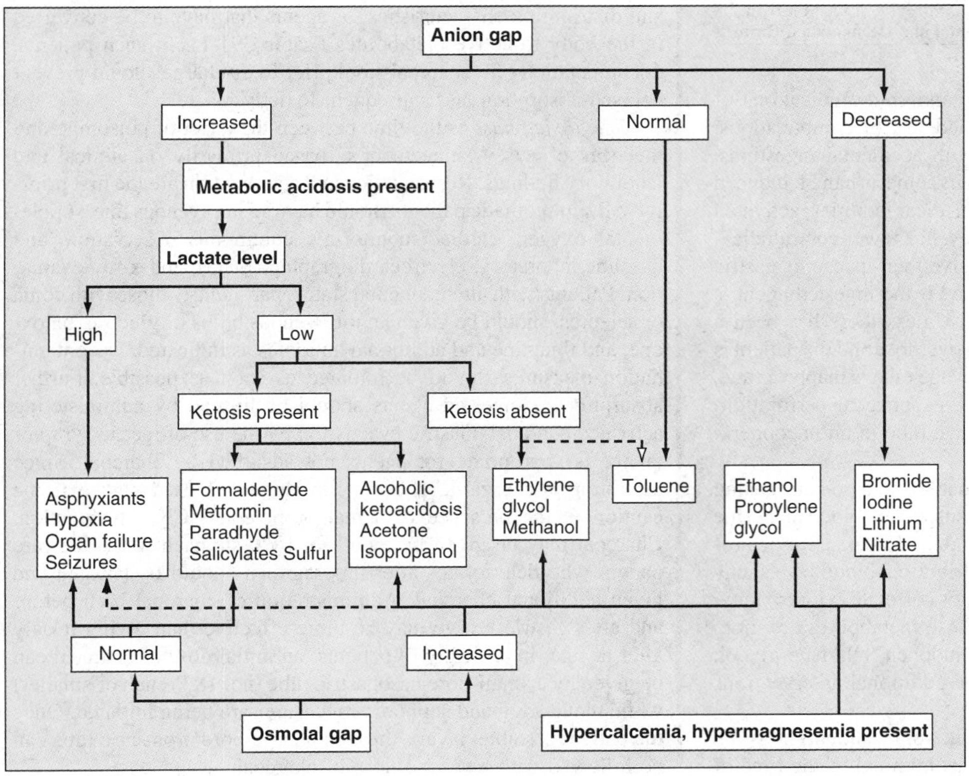

FIGURE 391-1 Differential diagnosis of poisoning based on the results of routine laboratory tests. Dashed lines indicate possible pathways.

Although some rapid screening tests are available, comprehensive screening tests require 2 to 6 h for completion, and immediate management must be based on the history, physical examination, and routine ancillary tests. In addition, when the patient is asymptomatic or when the clinical picture is consistent with the reported history, qualitative screening is neither clinically useful nor cost-effective. It is of greatest value in patients with severe or unexplained toxicity such as coma, seizures, cardiovascular instability, metabolic or respiratory acidosis, and nonsinus cardiac rhythms. Quantitative analysis is useful for poisoning with acetaminophen, acetone, alcohol (including ethylene glycol), antiarrhythmics, antiepileptics, barbiturates, digoxin, heavy metals, lithium, salicylate, and theophylline and for carboxyhemoglobinemia and methemoglobinemia. Results can often be available within an hour.

The *response to antidotes* may be assessed for diagnostic purposes. Resolution of altered mental status and abnormal vital signs within minutes of intravenous administration of dextrose, naloxone, or flumazenil is virtually diagnostic of hypoglycemia, narcotic poisoning, and benzodiazepine intoxication, respectively. The prompt reversal of acute dystonic (extrapyramidal) reactions following an intravenous dose of benztropine or diphenhydramine confirms the diagnosis of a drug etiology. Vin rosé urine color following a diagnostic dose of deferoxamine can be used to confirm iron poisoning when measurements of serum iron and total iron-binding capacity are not immediately available. Although reversal of both central and peripheral manifestations of anticholinergic poisoning by physostigmine is diagnostic, physostigmine may cause arousal in patients with CNS depression of any etiology.

tachyarrhythmias may be seen in poisoning with digitalis, membrane-active drugs, sympathomimetics, or agents that potentiate the effects of endogenous catecholamines such as chloral hydrate and aliphatic or halogenated hydrocarbons.

Analysis of urine and blood (and occasionally of gastric contents and chemical samples) may be useful to confirm or rule out suspected poisoning. Interpretation of laboratory data requires knowledge of the tests used for screening and confirmation (thin-layer, gas-liquid, or high-performance liquid chromatography; colorimetric and fluorometric assays; enzyme-multiplied and radioimmunoassays; gas chromatography; mass spectrometry), their sensitivity (limit of detection) and specificity, the best type of biologic specimens for analysis, and the best time to obtain such specimens. Personal communication with the laboratory is essential. A negative result on a screen may mean the poison is not detectable by the test used or that its concentration is too low for detection at the time of sampling. In the latter case, repeating the test at a later time may yield a positive result.

Table 391-3

Solute Effects on Serum Osmolality

Agent	Approximate Serum Concentrations (mg/dL) of Solute That Will Increase the Serum Osmolality by 1 mmol/kg
Alcohols	
Ethanol	4.6
Isopropanol	6.0
Methanol	2.6
Glycols	
Ethylene glycol	5.2
Propylene glycol	7.6
Ketones	
Acetone	5.8
Electrolytes	
Calcium	4 (2 mmol/L)
Magnesium	2.4 (2 mmol/L)
Sugars	
Mannitol	18
Sorbitol	18

In the absence of a history of chemical exposure the *clinical course* may suggest a diagnosis of poisoning. Poisoning typically evolves and resolves more rapidly than other disorders. Signs and symptoms characteristically develop within an hour of acute exposure, peak within several hours, and resolve over hours to days. However, the absence of signs and symptoms soon after an overdose does not rule out a poisoning.

℞ TREATMENT

General Principles Treatment goals include support of vital signs, prevention of further poison absorption, enhancement of poison elimination, administration of specific antidotes, and prevention of reexposure (Table 391-4). The treatment depends on the identity of the poison, the route and amount of exposure, the time of presentation relative to the time of exposure, and the severity of poisoning. Knowledge of toxin pharmacokinetics and pharmacodynamics is essential.

During the *pretoxic phase*, prior to the onset of manifestations, decontamination is the highest priority, and treatment is based solely on the history. The maximum potential toxicity based on the greatest possible exposure should be assumed. When appropriate, gastrointestinal decontamination to minimize absorption and decrease the severity of toxicity is the first priority. Since decontamination is more effective the sooner performed, the initial history should be focused, and the physical examination should be brief. It is also advisable to establish intravenous access and initiate cardiac monitoring, particularly in patients with potentially serious ingestions or unclear histories. The choice of decontamination procedure depends on the predicted toxicity; the availability, efficacy, and contraindications of the procedure; and the nature, severity, and risk of complications. For the home management of patients with accidental ingestions, reliable histories, and mild predicted toxicity, emesis can be induced with ipecac syrup. For patients treated in medical facilities, activated charcoal has comparable or greater efficacy, has fewer contraindications and complications, and is less invasive than ipecac or gastric lavage. Alternative methods should be used if the ingested agent is not well adsorbed by activated charcoal. Unless there has been a witnessed ingestion of a potentially severe overdose and the patient is comatose, the use of a large-bore gastric lavage tube is inappropriate, since serious complications (aspiration or esophageal perforation) may result from the forcible use of a lavage tube in an uncooperative patient.

When an accurate history is not obtainable and a poison causing delayed toxicity or irreversible damage is suspected, blood and urine should be sent for toxicologic screening and, if indicated, for quantitative analysis. During absorption and distribution, blood levels may be greater than those in tissue and may not correlate with toxicity. However, high blood levels of agents whose metabolites are more toxic than the parent compound (acetaminophen, ethylene glycol, or methanol) may indicate the need for additional interventions (antidotes, dialysis).

After evaluation and decontamination, some patients may be sent home because the predicted toxicity is minimal or the time of expected maximal toxicity has passed without incident. Observation for at least 4 to 6 h after gastrointestinal tract decontamination ensures that most patients who remain asymptomatic can be discharged safely. However, longer observation may be necessary for patients who have ingested agents that slow gastric emptying and intestinal motility and thus will have slowed dissolution, absorption, and distribution characteristics, or agents that have to be converted in the body to active metabolites (Table 391-1). In such patients, documentation of a charcoal stool prior to discharge should prevent delayed absorption and subsequent toxicity.

Table 391-4

Fundamentals of Poisoning Management

SUPPORTIVE CARE	
Airway protection	Treatment of seizures
Oxygenation/ventilation	Correction of temperature abnormalities
Treatment of arrhythmias	Correction of metabolic derangements
Hemodynamic support	Prevention of secondary complications
PREVENTION OF FURTHER POISON ABSORPTION	
Gastrointestinal decontamination	Decontamination of other sites
Syrup of ipecac-induced emesis	Eye decontamination
Gastric lavage	Skin decontamination
Activated charcoal	Body cavity evacuation
Whole bowel irrigation	
Catharsis	
Dilution	
Endoscopic/surgical removal	
ENHANCEMENT OF POISON ELIMINATION	
Multiple-dose activated charcoal	Extracorporeal removal
Forced diuresis	Peritoneal dialysis
Alteration of urinary pH	Hemodialysis
Chelation (see Chap. 397)	Hemoperfusion
	Hemofiltration
	Plasmapheresis
	Exchange transfusion
	Hyperbaric oxygenation
ADMINISTRATION OF ANTIDOTES	
Neutralization by antibodies	Metabolic antagonism
Neutralization by chemical binding	Physiologic antagonism
PREVENTION OF REEXPOSURE	
Adult education	Notification of regulatory agencies
Child-proofing	Psychiatric referral

The *toxic phase* is the time between the onset of poisoning and the peak effects. Management is based primarily on clinical and laboratory findings. Resuscitation and stabilization are the first priority. All symptomatic patients should have an intravenous line, supplemental oxygen, cardiac monitoring, continuous observation, and baseline laboratory, electrocardiographic (ECG), and x-ray evaluation. Patients with altered mental status, particularly those with coma or seizures, should be given an intravenous bolus of glucose, naloxone, and thiamine and additional antidotes as indicated. Decontamination measures should be initiated as soon as possible. Further absorption of ingested agents should be limited by administering activated charcoal. Gastric evacuation by the use of ipecac syrup or lavage is appropriate for agents not adsorbed by charcoal. Since aspiration is a hazard, ipecac syrup should be used with extreme caution in the presence of actual or potential CNS dysfunction. Charcoal may be given by mouth or by a stomach tube. The rare patient who deteriorates after this regimen should be lavaged and given additional charcoal. Administration of charcoal both before and after gastric lavage may be more effective than giving it only after lavage. In critically ill patients, an initial dose of charcoal can be given by a small-bore nasogastric tube (no. 18 French or smaller) while monitoring and supportive measures are being initiated. Once the patient is stable, lavage through a large-bore orogastric tube can be followed with a second dose of charcoal.

Measures that enhance poison elimination may shorten the duration of toxicity and lessen its severity. However, the risks must be weighed against the benefits. Diagnostic certainty (usually via laboratory confirmation) is generally a prerequisite. Intestinal dialysis with repetitive doses of activated charcoal is generally safe and can enhance the elimination of many poisons. Diuresis and chelation therapy are effective in enhancing the elimination of a relatively small number of poisons, and their use is associated with potential complications. Extracorporal methods are effective in removing many poisons, but the expense and risk make their use reasonable only in patients who would otherwise not have a favorable outcome.

Patients with severe poisoning (coma, respiratory depression, hypotension, cardiac conduction abnormalities, cardiac arrhythmias, hypothermia or hyperthermia, seizures), those needing close monitoring or antidotes or enhanced elimination therapy, those showing progressive clinical deterioration, and those with significant underlying medical problems should be admitted to an intensive care unit. Patients with mild to moderate toxicity can be managed on a general medical service, intermediate care unit, or emergency department observation area, depending on the anticipated duration and level of monitoring needed (intermittent clinical observation versus continuous clinical, cardiac, and respiratory monitoring). Patients who have attempted suicide require continuous observation until they are thought unlikely to make further attempts.

During the *resolution phase* of poisoning, supportive care should continue until the patient is alert and laboratory and ECG abnormalities are resolved. Repeat charcoal dosing may prevent rebound toxicity when depressed gastrointestinal function improves and the substances still in the gut are absorbed or when active metabolites are formed. Since chemicals are eliminated from the blood before tissues, blood levels are generally lower than tissue levels during this phase and once again may not correlate with toxicity. This is particularly true when extracorporal elimination procedures are used. Because of redistribution, a rebound increase in blood level and clinical relapse may occur after the termination of such procedures. When a metabolite is responsible for toxic effects, continued treatment of an asymptomatic patient may be necessary because of a blood level predictive of subsequent toxicity (acetaminophen, ethylene glycol, and methanol).

Supportive Care The goal of supportive therapy is to maintain physiologic homeostasis until detoxification is accomplished and to prevent and treat secondary complications such as aspiration, bedsores, cerebral and pulmonary edema, pneumonia, rhabdomyolysis, renal failure, sepsis, thromboembolic disease, and generalized organ dysfunction due to prolonged hypoxia or shock.

Respiratory care is an important component of supportive care. In addition to those needing endotracheal intubation for mechanical ventilation, many patients require semielective endotracheal intubation for protection against aspiration of gastrointestinal contents and of the poison itself. The gag reflex alone is not a reliable indicator of the need for intubation. Since patients may maintain airway patency while being stimulated but not if left unattended, those who cannot respond to voice or who are unable to sit and drink fluids without assistance are best managed by prophylactic intubation. Patients with severe excitation also may require intubation for airway protection (due to the risk or existence of seizures) and sedation or paralysis for control of agitation and prevention of hyperthermia, acidosis, and rhabdomyolysis. Since clinical assessment of respiratory function is often inaccurate, the need for oxygenation and ventilation is best determined by oximetry or analysis of arterial blood gases.

Drug-induced pulmonary edema is usually noncardiac rather than cardiac in nature. Profound CNS depression and cardiac conduction abnormalities suggest the latter etiology. Measurement of pulmonary artery pressure may be necessary to establish etiology and direct appropriate therapy. Extracorporeal membrane oxygenation may be appropriate for severe but reversible respiratory failure.

Cardiovascular manifestations include arrhythmias caused by direct cardiotoxicity, abnormal cardiovascular reflexes, or metabolic derangements. Supraventricular tachycardia associated with hypertension and CNS excitation is almost always due to agents that cause general excitation (see Table 391-1). Most cases are mild or moderate in severity and require only observation or nonspecific sedation with a benzodiazepine. For cases that are severe or associated with hemodynamic instability, with chest pain, or with ECG evidence of ischemia, specific therapy is indicated. Hypoxia, hypoglycemia, and other metabolic causes of sympathetic stimulation also should be ruled out. For patients with sympathetic hyperactivity, treatment with a combined alpha and beta blocker (labetalol), a calcium channel blocker (verapamil or diltiazem), or a combination of a beta blocker and a vasodilator (esmolol and nitroprusside) is preferred. For those with anticholinergic poisoning, physostigmine is the treatment of choice. Supraventricular tachycardia without hypertension is generally secondary to vasodilation or hypovolemia and responds to fluid administration.

Lidocaine and phenytoin are generally safe for ventricular tachyarrhythmias, but beta blockers can be hazardous unless the arrhythmia is clearly due to sympathetic hyperactivity. In poisoning with tricyclic antidepressants (and probably in poisoning with all membrane-active agents (Table 391-1) quinine and procainamide are contraindicated (because of similar electrophysiologic effects), but sodium bicarbonate may be therapeutic. Magnesium sulfate and overdrive pacing (by isoproterenol or a pacemaker) may be useful in patients with torsade de pointes and prolonged QT intervals. Magnesium and antidigoxin antibodies are used in patients with severe digitalis poisoning. Invasive (esophageal or intracardiac) ECG recording may sometimes be necessary to determine the origin (ventricular or supraventricular) of wide-complex tachycardias (see Chap. 231). If the patient is hemodynamically stable, however, it may be prudent to observe rather than to treat with another potentially harmful cardioactive agent. Arrhythmias may be resistant to drug therapy until underlying acid-base and electrolyte derangements, hypoxia, and hypothermia are corrected.

Bradyarrhythmias associated with hypotension generally should be treated as described in Chap. 230. In beta-blocker and calcium channel–blocker poisoning, the administration of glucagon and calcium, respectively, may be effective. Antibody therapy may be indicated for digitalis poisoning. The management of hypotension is described in Chap. 38. If hypotension is unresponsive to volume expansion, norepinephrine or high-dose dopamine may be necessary. Intraaortic balloon pump counterpulsation or full cardiopulmonary bypass pump circulatory support should be considered for severe but reversible cardiac failure.

Central nervous system manifestations are an important component of poisoning. Drug-induced seizures may be due to direct or indirect CNS neuroreceptor stimulation (or inhibition), neuronal membrane destabilization, ischemia, edema, or metabolic abnormalities. Seizures due to excessive stimulation of catecholamine receptors (sympathomimetic or hallucinogen poisoning and drug withdrawal) or decreased activity of gamma-aminobutyric acid (GABA) (isoniazid poisoning) or glycine (strychnine poisoning) are best treated with enhancers of GABA effects such as benzodiazepines or barbiturates. Since benzodiazepines and barbiturates act by slightly different mechanisms (the former increases the frequency and the latter increases the duration of chloride channel opening in response to GABA), therapy with both may be effective when neither is effective alone. Seizures caused by isoniazid, which inhibits the synthesis of GABA, may not respond to GABA-enhancer therapy until GABA synthesis is restored, because enhancers cannot work in the absence of GABA. High doses of pyridoxine, which facilitates the synthesis of GABA, are often necessary to terminate such seizures. For poisons with central dopaminergic effects (phencyclidine), an agent with opposing activity, such as haloperidol, may be useful. Seizures resulting from membrane destabilization (beta-blocker or cyclic antidepressant poisoning) may require a membrane-active agent such as phenytoin as well as a GABA agonist. In rare cases (anticholinergic or cyanide poisoning), specific antidotal therapy may be necessary.

The treatment of seizures secondary to ischemia, edema, or metabolic abnormalities should include correction of the underlying cause. Since prolonged convulsions can lead to rhabdomyolysis and severe acidosis, neuromuscular paralysis is indicated in refractory cases. Electroencephalographic (EEG) monitoring and continuing treatment of seizures are necessary to prevent permanent neurologic damage.

Temperature extremes; metabolic, hepatic, and renal abnormalities; and secondary complications should be treated by standard measures.

Prevention of Poison Absorption GASTROINTESTINAL DECONTAMINATION *Activated charcoal*, as a suspension in water either alone or with a cathartic, is given orally via a nippled bottle (for infants), or via a cup, straw, or small-bore nasogastric tube. The recommended dose is 1 to 2 g/kg body weight, using 8 mL of diluent per gram of charcoal if a premixed formulation is not available. Palatability may be increased by adding a sweetener (sorbitol) or a flavoring agent (cherry, chocolate, or cola syrup) to the suspension. Charcoal adsorbs ingested poisons within the gut lumen, allowing the charcoal-toxin complex to be evacuated with stool. The complex also can be removed from the stomach by induced emesis or lavage. In vitro, charcoal adsorbs 90 percent or more of most poisons when given in a tenfold ratio to the toxin. Charged (ionized) chemicals such as mineral acids, alkalis, and highly dissociated salts of cyanide, fluoride, iron, lithium, and other inorganic compounds are not well adsorbed by charcoal. Experimentally, charcoal decreases the absorption of other chemicals by an average of 73 percent when given within 5 min of administration, 51 percent when given at 30 min, and 36 percent at 60 min. Charcoal is as or more effective as ipecac syrup or gastric lavage. Lavage followed by charcoal is more effective than charcoal alone, and charcoal before and after lavage is more effective than charcoal alone or charcoal after lavage. In general, treatment with charcoal alone gives a better clinical outcome than treatment with ipecac followed by charcoal or lavage followed by charcoal. Side effects of charcoal include nausea, vomiting, and diarrhea or constipation. Charcoal also may prevent the absorption of orally administered therapeutic agents. Complications include mechanical obstruction of the airway, aspiration, vomiting, and bowel obstruction and infection caused by inspissated charcoal.

Charcoal is contraindicated in patients who have ingested corrosives because it obscures endoscopy.

Gastric lavage is performed using a no. 28 French orogastric tube in children and a no. 40 French tube in adults with volumes of about 5 mL fluid per kilogram of body weight. Except for infants, tap water is acceptable. The patient should be placed in Trendelenburg and left lateral decubitus positions to prevent aspiration (even if an endotracheal tube is in place). Experimentally, lavage decreases chemical absorption by an average of 52 percent if performed within 5 min of ingestion, 26 percent if performed at 30 min, and 16 percent if performed at 60 min. Its efficacy is similar to that of ipecac. Significant amounts of ingested drug are recovered in one-tenth of patients. As with ipecac, its effect on the clinical outcome of poisoned patients is not known. Aspiration is a common complication (occurring in up to 10 percent of patients), especially when lavage is improperly performed. Serious complications (tracheal lavage, esophageal and gastric perforation) occur in approximately 1 percent of patients. For this reason, only a physician should insert the lavage tube, and the patient must be restrained (with pharmacologic sedation if necessary) during the procedure. Gastric lavage is contraindicated in patients who have ingested corrosives or petroleum distillate hydrocarbons because of the risk of aspiration-induced hydrocarbon pneumonitis and gastroesophageal perforation.

Syrup of ipecac is administered orally in a dose of 30 mL for adults, 15 mL for children, and 10 mL for small infants. Clear liquids also should be given. Ipecac irritates the stomach and stimulates the central chemoreceptor trigger zone. Vomiting usually occurs approximately 22 min after administration. The dose may be repeated if vomiting does not occur. Experimentally, ipecac decreases chemical absorption by an average of 60 percent if given within 5 min of ingestion, 32 percent if given at 30 min, and 30 percent if given at 60 min. Because there are no suitable control groups, its efficacy in overdose patients is not established. Side effects include lethargy in children (12 percent) and protracted vomiting (8 to 17 percent). Chronic ipecac use (by patients with anorexia nervosa or bulimia) may cause electrolyte and fluid abnormalities, cardiac toxicity, and myopathy. Except for aspiration, serious complications are rare. Isolated cases of gastric and esophageal tears and perforations and stroke have been reported. Ipecac is contraindicated in patients with recent gastrointestinal surgery, CNS depression, or seizures, and in those who have ingested corrosives or rapidly acting CNS poisons (camphor, cyanide, tricyclic antidepressants, propoxyphene, strychnine).

Whole-bowel irrigation is performed by administering a bowel-cleansing solution containing electrolytes and polyethylene glycol (Golytely, Colyte) orally or by gastric tube at a rate of up 0.5 L/h in children and 2.0 L/h in adults until rectal effluent is clear. The patient must be in a sitting position. Although data are limited, whole-bowel irrigation may be as or more effective than the previously discussed procedures and may be particularly useful in patients who have ingested foreign bodies, drug packets, slow-release medications, and agents that are poorly adsorbed by charcoal.

Cathartic salts (disodium phosphate, magnesium citrate and sulfate, sodium sulfate) or *saccharides* (mannitol, sorbitol) promote the rectal evacuation of gastrointestinal contents. The most effective cathartic is sorbitol in a dose of 1 to 2 g/kg of body weight. Alone, cathartics do not prevent poison absorption. Their primary use is to prevent constipation following charcoal administration. Abdominal cramps, nausea, and occasional vomiting are side effects. Complications of repeated dosing include hypermagnesemia and excessive diarrhea. The agents are contraindicated in patients who have ingested corrosives and in those with preexisting diarrhea. Magnesium-containing cathartics should not be used in patients with renal failure.

Dilution is accomplished by having the patient drink 5 mL/kg of body weight of water or another clear liquid as soon as possible after the ingestion of a corrosive (acids, alkali). Dilution also may be used as an adjunct to ipecac syrup administration. Otherwise, it is not indicated because it may increase the dissolution rate (and hence absorption) of capsules, tablets, and other solids.

Endoscopic or surgical removal of poisons may be useful in rare situations, such as ingestion of a potentially toxic foreign body that fails to transit the gastrointestinal tract, a potentially lethal amount of a heavy metal (arsenic, iron, mercury, thallium), or agents that have coalesced into gastric concretions or bezoars (barbiturates, gluthethimide, heavy metals, lithium, meprobamate, sustained-release preparations). Patients who ingest multiple packets of cocaine and then become toxic owing to packet leakage or rupture require immediate surgical intervention.

DECONTAMINATION OF OTHER SITES Immediate, copious flushing with water, saline, or another available clear, drinkable liquid is the initial treatment for topical exposures (particularly with corrosives and solvents). Saline is preferred for eye irrigation. A triple wash (water, then soap, then more water) may be best for dermal decontamination. Inhalational exposures should be treated initially with fresh air or oxygen. The removal of liquids from body cavities such as the vagina or rectum is best accomplished by irrigation. Solids (drug packets, pills) should be removed manually with visual guidance.

Enhancement of Poison Elimination Although the elimination of most poisons can be accelerated by therapeutic interventions, pharmacokinetic efficacy (removal of drug at a rate greater than that accomplished by intrinsic elimination) and the resulting clinical benefits (in terms of a shortened duration of toxicity or improved outcome) are often more theoretical than proven. Hence the decision to use such a procedure should be based on the actual or predicted toxicity and the potential efficacy, cost, and risks of therapy.

MULTIPLE-DOSE ACTIVATED CHARCOAL Repeated oral dosing with charcoal (with sorbitol as needed to enhance gastrointestinal motility) can enhance the elimination of some chemicals. A dose of 1 g/kg body weight every 2 to 4 h, adjusted downward to avoid regurgitation in patients with decreased gastrointestinal motility, is generally recommended. Experimentally, this treatment enhances the elimination of most drugs and chemicals tested (carbamazepine, dapsone, diazepam, digoxin, glutethimide, meprobamate, methotrexate, phenobarbital, phenytoin, salicylate, theophylline, valproic acid). The efficacy approaches that of hemodialysis for some agents (theophylline). Multiple-dose therapy is not effective in accelerating elimination of chlorpropamide, imipramine, or agents that adsorb poorly to charcoal.

FORCED DIURESIS AND ALTERATION OF URINARY pH Diuresis and ion trapping via alteration of urine pH may prevent the renal reabsorption of poisons that undergo excretion by glomerular filtration and active tubular secretion. Since membranes are more permeable to nonionized molecules than to their ionized counterparts, acidic (low-pK_a) poisons are ionized and trapped in an alkaline urine, and basic poisons are ionized and trapped in an acid urine. Saline diuresis can enhance the renal excretion of alcohols, bromide, calcium, fluoride, lithium, meprobamate, potassium, and isoniazid. Alkaline diuresis (a urine pH of 7.5 or greater and a urine output of 3 to 6 mL/kg body weight per hour) enhances the elimination of chlorphenoxyacetic acid herbicides, chlorpropamide, diflunisal, fluoride, methotrexate, phenobarbital (and probably other long-acting barbiturates), sulfonamides, and salicylates. Contraindications include congestive heart failure, renal failure, and cerebral edema. Acid-base, fluid, and electrolyte parameters should be monitored carefully. Saline diuresis may enhance the excretion of bromide, calcium, fluoride, lithium, meprobamate, potassium, and isoniazid. Acid diuresis enhances the renal elimination of amphetamines, chloroquine, cocaine, local anesthetics, phencyclidine, quinidine, quinine, strychnine, sympathomimetics, tricyclic antidepressants, and tocainide. Its use, however, has been largely abandoned because risks are significant and clinical efficacy has not been established.

EXTRACORPOREAL REMOVAL Peritoneal dialysis, hemodialysis, charcoal or resin hemoperfusion, hemofiltration, plasmapheresis, and exchange transfusion are capable of removing any toxin from the bloodstream. The toxins most amenable to enhanced elimination by dialysis have low molecular mass (<500 Da), high water solubility, low protein binding, small volumes of distribution (<1 L/kg body weight), prolonged elimination (long half-life), and high dialysis clearance relative to total-body clearance. The efficacy of the other forms of extracorporeal removal is not limited by molecular weight, water solubility, or protein binding.

Dialysis should be considered in cases of severe poisoning due to barbiturates, bromide, chloral hydrate, ethanol, ethylene glycol, isopropyl alcohol, lithium, methanol, procainamide, theophylline, salicylate, and possibly heavy metals. Although hemoperfusion may be more effective in removing some of these poisons, it does not correct associated acid-base and electrolyte abnormalities. Hemoperfusion should be considered in cases of severe poisoning due to chloramphenicol, disopyramide, and hypnotic-sedatives (barbiturates, ethchlorvynol, glutethimide, meprobamate, methaqualone), phenytoin, procainamide, and theophylline. Both techniques require central venous access and systemic anticoagulation and often result in transient hypotension. Hemoperfusion also may cause hemolysis, hypocalcemia, and thrombocytopenia. Peritoneal dialysis and exchange transfusion are less effective but may be used when other procedures either are not available, are contraindicated, or are technically difficult (e.g., in infants). Exchange transfusion removes poisons affecting red blood cells (as in methemoglobinemia or arsine-induced hemolysis). The efficacy of other extracorporeal elimination procedures has not been defined.

Candidates for these invasive treatments include patients with severe toxicity who deteriorate despite aggressive supportive therapy; those with potentially prolonged, irreversible, or fatal toxicity; those with dangerous blood levels of toxins; those who lack the capacity for self-detoxification because of liver or renal failure; and those with a serious underlying illness or complication that will adversely affect recovery.

OTHER TECHNIQUES The elimination of heavy metals can be enhanced by chelation and urinary excretion of the metal-chelator complex, and the elimination of carbon monoxide can be increased by hyperbaric oxygenation, as discussed in the sections on the specific poisons.

Administration of Antidotes Antidotes counteract the effects of poisons by neutralizing them (e.g., antibody-antigen reactions, chelation, chemical binding) or by antagonizing their physiologic effects (e.g., activation of opposing nervous system activity, provision of competitive metabolic or receptor substrate). Antidotes can significantly reduce morbidity and mortality, but most antidotes are potentially toxic. Poisons or conditions with specific antidotes include acetaminophen, anticholinergic agents, anticoagulants, benzodiazepines, beta blockers, calcium channel blockers, carbon monoxide, cholinergic agents, cyanide, digitalis, drugs that cause dystonic reactions, ethylene glycol, fluoride, heavy metals, hydrogen sulfide, hypoglycemic agents, isoniazid, methemoglobinemia, narcotics, sympatomimetics, and Vacor. Since the safe use of antidotes requires correct identification of a specific poisoning or syndrome, antidotal therapy is discussed with the conditions for which they are indicated.

Prevention of Reexposure Poisoning is a preventable illness. Unfortunately, some adults and children are poison-prone, and recurrences are common. Adults with accidental exposures should be instructed regarding the safe use of medications and chemicals (according to labeling instructions). Confused patients may need assistance with the administration of medications. Errors in dosing by health care providers require special educational efforts. Patients should be advised to avoid circumstances that result in chemical exposure or poisoning. Appropriate agencies and health departments should be notified in cases of environmental or workplace exposure. The best approach with young children and patients with intentional overdose is to limit access to poisons. In households where children live or visit, alcoholic beverages, medications, household products (automotive, cleaning, fuel, pet-care, toiletry products), nonedible plants, and vitamins should be kept out of reach or in locked or child-proof cabinets. Depressed or psychotic patients should receive psychiatric assessment, disposition, and follow-up. They should be given prescriptions for a limited supply of drugs and with a limited number of refills and be monitored for compliance and response to therapy.

SPECIFIC POISONS

The poisons discussed in this section are common, produce life-threatening toxicity, or require unique therapeutic interventions. Poisons not mentioned here are described in the referenced texts. → *Alcohol, cocaine, hallucinogens, and opioids are discussed in Chaps. 386 to 388, and heavy metal poisoning is discussed in Chap. 397.*

ACETAMINOPHEN At therapeutic doses, acetaminophen is metabolized to sulfate and glucuronide conjugates that are excreted in the urine. Minor amounts are excreted unchanged or as mercapturic acid after conjugation with hepatic glutathione. Following an acute overdose of ≥140 mg/kg body weight, the sulfate and glucuronide pathways become saturated, resulting in an increased fraction of acetaminophen metabolized to mercapturic acid. Once hepatic glutathione is depleted, reactive metabolites are formed that bind covalently to hepatocytes and cause cell lysis. Acetaminophen is absorbed rapidly from the stomach and small bowel and has a volume of distribution of 1 L/kg body weight. Plasma concentrations range from 160 to 660 μmol/L (0.5 to 2.0 mg/dL) following therapeutic doses. The plasma half-life is usually 2 to 4 h but may be prolonged if hepatotoxicity develops.

Clinical Toxicity Early manifestations of poisoning are nonspecific and not predictive of subsequent hepatotoxicity. Within 2 to 4 h of ingestion, nausea, vomiting, diaphoresis, and pallor develop. CNS depression is absent unless depressant drugs are coingested. Within 24 to 48 h, hepatotoxicity is evidenced by right upper quadrant tenderness and mild hepatomegaly. Renal function also may be impaired. Laboratory evidence of hepatic toxicity includes prolongation of the prothrombin time and elevation of serum bilirubin and transaminase activity (aspartate transaminase, alanine transaminase). Severe poisoning may cause hepatic failure. A twofold prolongation of prothrombin time and/or a serum bilirubin level greater than 68 μmol/L (4 mg/dL) on the third to fifth day after ingestion indicate hepatotoxicity. Histologic evidence of liver damage varies from cytolysis to centrilobular necrosis. In patients who recover, liver function returns to normal within 1 week, and liver histology returns to normal within 3 months.

Diagnosis A serum acetaminophen level above the lower line on the Rumack Matthew nomogram (Fig. 391-2) between 4 and 24 h after ingestion indicates possible hepatotoxicity and the need for antidote therapy.

℞ TREATMENT

In patients who present within 4 h of ingestion, initial treatment involves gastrointestinal decontamination. Activated charcoal should be administered. (Charcoal does not interfere significantly with acetylcysteine therapy.) In patients with a potentially toxic acetaminophen level, acetylcysteine is given at a loading dose of 140 mg/kg body weight, followed by a maintenance dose of 70 mg/kg body weight every 4 h for 17 additional doses. Treatment is most effective if started within 8 to 10 h of an overdose. Side effects include nausea, vomiting, and epigastric discomfort. If treatment is started before the serum level is known and if the level is subsequently shown to be below the toxic level, therapy may be discontinued.

ACIDS AND ALKALI Common alkaline products include industrial-strength bleach, drain cleaners (sodium hydroxide), surface cleaners (ammonia, phosphates), laundry and dishwasher detergents (phosphates, carbonates), disk batteries, denture cleaners (borates, phosphates, carbonates), and Clinitest tablets (sodium hydroxides). Acids are used in toilet bowl cleaners (hydrofluoric, phosphoric, and

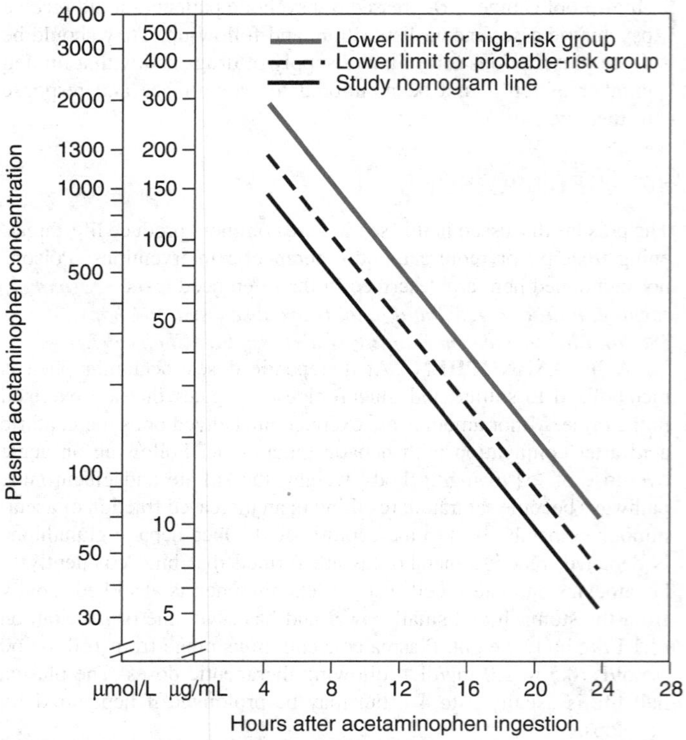

FIGURE 391-2 Nomogram to define risk according to initial plasma acetaminophen concentration. *(After BH Rumack, H Matthew, Pediatrics 55:871, 1975.)*

sulfuric acids), soldering fluxes (hydrochloric acid), antirust compounds (hydrofluoric and oxalic acids), automobile battery fluid (sulfuric acid), and stone cleaners (hydrofluoric and nitric acids).

Alkalis produce liquefactive necrosis with rapidly penetrating tissue burns and a higher risk of perforation of the esophagus and stomach than do acids. Acids produce coagulative necrosis. Both may burn the mouth, esophagus, and stomach. The lack of oral involvement does not rule out esophageal or gastric injury. Liquids tend to produce superficial, often circumferential burns over a larger surface area, while solids and tablets cause localized but deeper burns. The severity of the burn relates to the contact time, the amount ingested, and the pH (especially if <2 or >12) of the ingested product. Corrosives other than acids and bases that cause similar toxicity include household bleach (sodium hypochlorite), hydrogen peroxide, hydrazine, and phenol.

Clinical Toxicity Burns of the mouth result in excess salivation, pain, dysphonia, and dysphagia and are manifested by erythema, edema, ulceration, and necrosis. Deep burns may destroy mucosal nerve endings and produce anesthesia. Esophageal symptoms and signs include drooling, painful swallowing, retrosternal pain, and neck tenderness. Vomiting of blood and mucus may occur. Esophageal perforation following alkali ingestion is suggested by increased severity of chest pain, often with respiratory distress. Epigastric pain, vomiting, and tenderness may occur with burns to the stomach. Aspiration of acids and alkalis may cause fulminant tracheitis and bronchial pneumonia. In severe cases, hypotension, shock, metabolic acidosis, liver and renal dysfunction, hemolysis, and disseminated intravascular coagulation may be seen. Deep burns, particularly if extensive or circumferential, may be followed by fibrosis with stricture formation and obstruction of the esophagus (alkalis) or of the gastric outlet (acids).

Diagnosis Symptoms, history, and physical findings usually suggest the diagnosis. Endoscopy, best performed 12 to 24 h after ingestion in all symptomatic patients, documents the anatomic site and often the severity of the injury. Chest and abdominal x-rays and routine laboratory values should be obtained to evaluate for aspiration, perforation, and organ dysfunction. Residual effects of the ingestion can be assessed by barium swallow.

℞ TREATMENT

Treatment consists of immediate dilution with milk or water. Weak acid or basic solutions should not be used because the heat of neutralization may cause thermal burns and increase tissue injury. Glucocorticoids and Silastic esophageal stents have traditionally been used for alkali burns to prevent esophageal stricture formation. Their efficacy is not proven. Animal studies suggest that glucocorticoids should be begun immediately on presentation. If used, a dose of 1 to 2 mg of prednisone per kilogram every 4 to 6 h for at least 2 weeks is suggested. Prophylactic broad-spectrum antibiotic use is also recommended. Glucocorticoids are not useful for acid burns. Antacids should be used for burns of the stomach. Esophageal stricture or gastric outlet obstruction may require subsequent dilatation and bougienage or surgical reconstruction.

ANTIARRHYTHMIC DRUGS Only drugs that act by blocking myocardial cell-membrane sodium channels are discussed here. These agents can be divided into three subclasses: class IA (disopyramide, procainamide, and quinidine), class IB (lidocaine, mexiletine, phenytoin, and tocainide), and class IC (encainide, moricizine, propafenone, and flecainide). The pharmacology is presented in Chap. 231. Because of toxicity, some agents have been withdrawn from the market but are still available for compassionate use. Antiarrhythmic drugs are rapidly absorbed (except for disopyramide and sustained-release formulations), have volumes of distribution ranging from 1 to 10 L/kg, have half-lives of 3 to 16 h, and are eliminated mainly by hepatic metabolism.

Clinical Toxicity The acute ingestion of more than twice the usual daily dose is potentially toxic. Onset of toxicity occurs within 1 h, and the effects peak within several hours. Toxicity also may develop during chronic therapeutic use. Manifestations include nausea, vomiting, and diarrhea, followed by lethargy, confusion, ataxia, bradycardia, hypotension, and cardiovascular collapse. Anticholinergic effects (blurred vision, dry mucosae) may be seen in disopyramide poisoning. Quinidine and class IB agents may cause agitation, dysphoria, and seizures. Nonspecific ECG findings include bradycardia with AV block and QRS-interval prolongation. Ventricular tachycardia, ventricular fibrillation (including the polymorphous form, torsade de pointes), and QT-interval prolongation are characteristics of poisoning due to class IA and IC drugs. Depressed myocardial contractility and arrhythmias may lead to decreased cardiac output and pulmonary edema. Hypoglycemia and mild hypokalemia may be seen with disopyramide and quinidine intoxication, respectively.

Diagnosis Toxicology screening will detect most of these agents. Measurement of serum levels may confirm an overdose and indicate the need for monitoring.

℞ TREATMENT

Treatment consists of gastrointestinal decontamination and supportive therapy. Hypotension, bradyarrhythmias, and seizures are treated with standard measures. Patients with persistent hypotension and bradycardia require monitoring of pulmonary arterial pressure. Cardiac pacing, intraaortic balloon pump counterpulsation, and cardiopulmonary bypass may be necessary. Ventricular tachyarrhythmias that cause hemodynamic instability should be treated with lidocaine and bretylium. Sodium bicarbonate or sodium lactate (1 mmol/kg by intravenous bolus) may be effective for tachyarrhythmias due to class IA or IC agents. Mild hypokalemia may be protective, and potassium levels that do not fall below 3.0 mmol/L may be best treated by close monitoring. For torsade de pointes (polymorphous or atypical ventricular tachycardia), magnesium sulfate (4 g or 40 mL of a 10% solution given intravenously as an initial dose) and overdrive pacing (with isoproterenol or electricity) may be effective. Hemodialysis and hemoperfusion may enhance the elimination of disopyramide, the active procainamide metabolite *N*-acetylprocainamide, and possibly other agents.

ANTICHOLINERGIC AGENTS Agents with anticholinergic properties include antihistamines (H_1 receptor blockers and over-the-counter hypnotics), belladonna alkaloids and related agents (atropine, glycopyrrolate, homatropine, hyoscine, ipratropium, scopolamine), drugs for Parkinson's disease (benztropine, biperiden, trihexyphenidyl), mydriatics (cyclopentolate, tropicamide), phenothiazines, skeletal muscle relaxants (cyclobenzaprine, orphenadrine), smooth muscle relaxants (clidinium, dicyclomine, isometheptene, oxybutynin), tricyclic antidepressants, and a variety of plants (such as *Datura stramonium* and jimson weed) and mushrooms. More properly called *antimuscarinics*, these agents are competitive inhibitors of acetylcholine only at CNS and parasympathetic postganglionic muscarinic neuroreceptors. They are absorbed efficiently, but absorption can be delayed following an overdose. The antihistamines, belladonna agents, Parkinson's drugs, and smooth muscle relaxants are weak bases (pK_a 8–9), exhibit variable binding to plasma proteins (18 to 98 percent), and have moderate volumes of distribution (2 to 6 L/kg). They are eliminated primarily by hepatic metabolism and have half-lives of 2 to 12 h.

Clinical Toxicity Manifestations usually begin within an hour of acute overdosage and 1 to 3 days after beginning treatment in the case of chronic poisoning. Toxic doses are only slightly greater than therapeutic doses. CNS manifestation include agitation, ataxia, confusion, delirium, hallucinations, and movement disorders (choreoathetoid and picking movements). Lethargy, respiratory depression, and coma may occur. Peripheral nervous system findings include decreased or absent bowel sounds, dilated pupils, dry skin and mucosal surfaces, urinary retention, and increases in pulse rate, blood pressure, respiratory rate, and temperature. The first-generation H_1 blockers (diphenhydramine and probably others) can also cause tricyclic antidepressant–like cardiotoxicity and seizures, and the second-generation H_1 blockers (astemizole, terfenadine) can cause QT-interval prolongation with subsequent ventricular tachyarrhythmias, especially torsade de pointes.

Diagnosis The diagnosis is suggested by the characteristic manifestations and supported by demonstrating the presence of the agents in the urine. Serum assays are not generally available. The diagnosis can be confirmed by demonstrating resolution of anticholinergic toxicity in response to physostigmine.

℞ TREATMENT

Treatment involves gastrointestinal decontamination, supportive measures, and, in severe cases, therapy with physostigmine. Activated charcoal adsorbs these agents effectively. Agitation may respond to benzodiazepines, and comatose patients may require intubation and mechanical ventilation. Cardiovascular toxicity and arrhythmias should be treated as described for antiarrhythmics, phenothiazines, or tricyclic antidepressants. Physostigmine, an acetylcholinesterase inhibitor, reverses anticholinergic toxicity. It is indicated primarily for uncontrolled agitation and hallucinations. The dose is 1 to 2 mg given intravenously over 2 min; the dose can be repeated if there is an incomplete response or recurrent toxicity. If signs of cholinergic poisoning occur (see "Organophosphate and Carbamate Insecticides," below), they can be reversed by atropine in half the amount of physostigmine given. Physostigmine should not be given for seizures or for coma; its arousal effects are nonspecific and cannot be used for diagnostic purposes. Physostigmine is contraindicated in the presence of cardiac conduction defects or ventricular arrhythmias because it can cause asystole in such patients.

BARBITURATES Barbiturates bind to the GABA receptor and prolong the opening of the chloride channels in response to GABA, thereby inhibiting excitable cells of the CNS and other tissues. Long-acting barbiturates are effective for 6 to 12 h and include mephobarbital, barbital, phenobarbital, and primidone. Agents with intermediate (3 to 6 h), short (1 to 3 h), and ultrashort (<30 min) durations of action include amobarbital, aprobarbital, butabarbital, butalbital; hexobarbital, pentobarbital, and secobarbital; and methohexital, thiamylal, and thiopental, respectively.

Barbiturates are well absorbed from the stomach and the small bowel. With therapeutic doses, plasma concentrations generally peak in 1 to 4 h (earlier for short-acting agents than for long-acting ones). Barbiturates are weak acids with pK_a values ranging from 7.2 to 8.5, volumes of distribution of 0.8 to 1.5 L/kg of body weight, and 45 to 70 percent protein binding in the plasma. Most barbiturates are primarily metabolized by the liver. Some long-acting agents are converted to active metabolites: mephobarbital to barbital, and primidone to phenobarbital and phenylethylmalonamide (PEMA). In contrast to short-acting agents, long-acting ones also undergo significant renal excretion: 95 percent for barbital, 25 to 33 percent for phenobarbital, 15 to 42 percent for primidone, and 95 percent for PEMA. Half-lives range from 1 h for ultrashort-acting agents to 6 d for long-acting ones.

Clinical Toxicity Barbiturates cause CNS depression ranging from confusion and lethargy to deep coma. Hypothermia, hypotension, pulmonary edema, and cardiac arrest may occur in severe cases. Pupils are generally constricted but may dilate in terminal phases. Pressure sores and bullous skin lesions can develop with prolonged coma. Maximal toxicity usually occurs within 4 to 6 h but may be delayed to 10 h or more after overdosage with long-acting barbiturates.

Diagnosis Signs of toxicity usually appear when serum concentrations of long-acting barbiturates exceed 170 μmol/L (4 mg/dL) and those of short-acting barbiturates exceed 88 μmol/L (2 mg/dL). Because of tolerance, the degree of CNS depression relative to ingested dose is dependent on prior exposure to the drug.

℞ TREATMENT

Initial management involves gastrointestinal decontamination. Barbiturates are well adsorbed by activated charcoal. Hemodynamic and respiratory support and correction of temperature and electrolyte derangements may be necessary. Since short-acting barbiturates are predominantly metabolized by the liver, diuresis is ineffective. Renal elimination of phenobarbital (and probably other long-acting agents) is enhanced by alkalinization of urine to a pH of 8 (by giving intravenous sodium bicarbonate) and by saline diuresis. Elimination can also be enhanced by repeated doses of activated charcoal. Hemodialysis and hemoperfusion are effective in removing both long- and short-acting barbiturates, but their use is seldom necessary.

BENZODIAZEPINES Benzodiazepines potentiate the inhibitory effect of GABA on CNS neurons by binding to GABA receptors and increasing the frequency of opening of chloride channels in response to GABA stimulation.

Long-acting benzodiazepines include chlordiazepoxide, clonazepam, clorazepate, diazepam, flurazepam, prazepam, and quazepam. Short-acting agents include alprazolam, lorazepam, and oxazepam; ultrashort-acting agents include estazolam, midazolam, temazepam, and triazolam. All benzodiazepines are well absorbed from the gastrointestinal tract, exhibit 85 to 99 percent protein binding in the plasma, are lipid soluble, and have an apparent volume of distribution of 0.3 to 2 L/kg body weight. They are weak acids with pK_a values ranging from 1.3 to 6.2. Benzodiazepines are eliminated mainly by hepatic metabolism, and some have pharmacologically active metabolites. Metabolites are generally excreted in the urine, whereas only a small amount of the parent compound is excreted unchanged by the kidneys. Half-lives range from as little as 2 h for short-acting agents to up to 8 days for long-acting ones.

Clinical Toxicity Effects are evident within 30 min of an overdose and include weakness, ataxia, and drowsiness. Coma and respiratory depression are rare but can occur with ultrashort-acting agents and when benzodiazepines are combined with other CNS depressants. Paradoxical excitation may occur early in the course of poisoning.

Diagnosis The diagnosis can sometimes be confirmed by identification of metabolites in urine. However, routine screening tests do not detect many benzodiazepines so that a negative result does not exclude the diagnosis. A response to flumazenil is a more sensitive diagnostic test.

TREATMENT

Initial management includes gastrointestinal decontamination with single-dose as well as repeated-dose activated charcoal. Respiratory support should be provided as necessary. Flumazenil, a competitive benzodiazepine receptor antagonist, can reverse CNS and respiratory depression and obviate the need for endotracheal intubation. It is administered intravenously in incremental doses of 0.2, 0.3, and 0.5 mg at 1-min intervals until the desired effect is achieved or a cumulative dose of 3 to 5 mg has been given. Since flumazenil has a relatively short duration of action, patients must be monitored carefully for relapse. Should relapse occur, treatment can be repeated (at intervals of 20 min with a maximum dose of 3 mg/h). Failure to respond to flumazenil suggests that benzodiazepines are not the cause of poisoning. Flumazenil can cause seizures in patients who have coingested stimulants and tricyclic antidepressants and in patients who are physically dependent on benzodiazepines as a result of chronic high-dose use. A starting dose of 0.1 mg should be used in patients at risk for withdrawal. Extracorporeal drug removal is not of clinical benefit.

BETA-ADRENERGIC BLOCKING AGENTS Beta-adrenergic blocking agents include acebutolol, atenolol, betaxolol, bisoprolol, carteolol, esmolol, labetalol, metoprolol, nadolol, penbutolol, pindolol, propranolol, sotalol, and timolol. These drugs act by competitively blocking beta-adrenergic neurohumoral receptors. At therapeutic doses, some beta blockers act predominantly on $beta_1$ receptors and are "cardioselective" (acebutolol, atenolol, betaxolol, metoprolol), some have partial agonist or sympathomimetic activity (acebutolol, carteolol, pindolol, timolol, and possibly penbutolol), and some have quinidine-like antiarrhythmic effects (acebutolol, metoprolol, pindolol, propranolol, sotalol, and possibly betaxolol). Antiarrhythmic effects are due to a reduction of sodium and calcium influx during membrane depolarization (phase 0) as a consequence of decreased production of cyclic AMP by adenylate cyclase. This activity defines beta blockers as class II antiarrhythmics. Beta blockers decrease cardiac contractility by directly inhibiting the release of calcium from sarcoplasmic reticulum.

Beta blockers are absorbed rapidly and well, exhibit variable protein binding (5 to 93 percent), and have low water solubility and variable volumes of distribution (0.23 to 10.0 L/kg body weight). Most beta blockers are eliminated predominantly by hepatic metabolism. Atenolol, carteolol, nadolol, and sotalol are eliminated primarily by renal excretion, and esmolol is metabolized by serum esterases.

Clinical Toxicity Effects usually begin within 1/2 h following an overdose and peak within 2 h. Common findings include nausea, vomiting, and diarrhea, followed by bradycardia, hypotension, and CNS depression. However, agents with sympathomimetic activity can cause hypertension and tachycardia. CNS effects vary from lethargy and confusion to coma and seizures and tend to be more pronounced with highly lipophilic agents (acebutolol, metoprolol, pindolol, propranolol, and timolol). The skin is often pale and cool. Bronchospasm and pulmonary edema are uncommon unless there is a history of asthma, chronic obstructive pulmonary disease, or congestive heart failure. Metabolic abnormalities include hyperkalemia and hypoglycemia (as a direct result of beta-adrenergic receptor blockade) and metabolic acidosis (due to seizures, shock, or respiratory depression). ECG manifestations include all degrees of AV block, bundle branch block, prolonged QRS duration, and asystole. Sotalol may cause QT-interval prolongation with ventricular tachycardia, ventricular fibrillation, and torsade de pointes. Patients with mild poisoning usually recover within 6 to 12 h, whereas those with severe poisoning may be symptomatic for 24 to 48 h.

Diagnosis The diagnosis is made on the basis of the history and clinical presentation. A toxicology screen may identify the presence of beta blockers, but blood levels are not generally available nor helpful in guiding therapy.

TREATMENT

Treatment includes gastrointestinal decontamination, nonspecific supportive measures, and the administration of glucagon and calcium. Because gastric emptying procedures may produce vagal stimulation and exacerbate bradyarrhythmias, monitoring should be instituted first. Treatment of bradycardia and hypotension should begin with atropine, isoproterenol, and vasopressors (dopamine, dobutamine, epinephrine, and norepinephrine have been used with variable success, alone or in combination). With severe poisoning, these agents may be ineffective, and glucagon, calcium, cardiac pacing (external or internal), and intraaortic balloon pump support may be necessary. Glucagon, which stimulates adenylate cyclase by a nonadrenergic mechanism, should be given at an initial dose of 5 to 10 mg. Patients who respond favorably should then be given an infusion of 1 to 5 mg/h. Calcium, which may reverse nonadrenergic negative inotropic effects, should be given in the same initial dose as described for calcium channel blocker poisoning. Patients with altered mental status also should have a bedside glucose determination or be given an intravenous bolus of glucose. Bronchospasm may be treated with an inhaled beta agonist, subcutaneous epinephrine, and intravenous aminophylline. Lidocaine, magnesium (as for antiarrhythmic poisoning), or overdrive pacing may be used for sotalol-induced ventricular tachyarrhythmias. Extracorporeal elimination procedures are probably not of benefit, with the possible exceptions of atenolol, carteolol, metoprolol, nadolol, and sotalol.

CALCIUM CHANNEL BLOCKERS Calcium channel blockers include amlodipine, bepridil, diltiazem, felodipine, flunarizine, isradipine, lacidipine, nicardipine, nifedipine, nimodipine, nisoldipine, nitrendipine, and verapamil. These agents act by decreasing the influx of calcium across slow calcium channels in the membranes of myocardial and vascular smooth-muscle cells during phases 2 (plateau) and 4 (spontaneous depolarization) of the action potential. Electrophysiologic effects include decreases in cardiac contractility, heart rate [sinoatrial (SA) node rate], and AV nodal conduction. These actions define calcium channel blockers as class IV antiarrhythmics. At therapeutic doses, diltiazem and verapamil have significant effects on cardiac conduction and contractility. Bepridil also has class I antiarrhythmic activity. All calcium channel blockers cause vasodilation.

Calcium channel blockers are absorbed rapidly and exhibit high (80 to 99 percent) protein binding in the plasma. Most have distribution volumes ranging from 1 to 8 L/kg body weight. They are eliminated mainly by hepatic metabolism, and the half-lives typically range from 1 to 24 h.

Clinical Toxicity Effects begin within 1/2 to 1 h of ingestion of amounts 5 to 10 times the usual therapeutic dose. Toxicity may be delayed for many hours following overdoses of sustained-release preparations. Clinical manifestations include bradycardia, hypotension, and CNS depression. Invasive monitoring almost invariably reveals a low peripheral vascular resistance and normal or increased cardiac output. Mental status changes range from confusion and drowsiness to coma and seizures and are due both to direct membrane effects and to cerebral hypoperfusion. Hypotension may precipitate myocardial ischemia, and depression of cardiac function may lead to pulmonary edema. ECG findings include all degrees of AV block, prolonged QRS and QT intervals (mainly with verapamil), evidence of ischemia or infarction, and asystole. Metabolic acidosis (secondary to shock) and hyperglycemia (resulting from the inhibition of insulin release) may be present. Serum calcium levels, however, remain normal.

Diagnosis The diagnosis is based primarily on the clinical presentation. These agents can be detected by appropriate screening tests. Serum levels are not generally available but can be useful in confirming overdosage when the history is inconclusive.

TREATMENT

Gastrointestinal tract decontamination should be accomplished as soon as possible. Symptomatic bradycardia should be treated with atropine, calcium, isoproterenol, glucagon, and electrical (external or internal) pacing. Calcium, as a 10% chloride or gluconate salt solution, is given in a dose of 0.2 mL/kg body weight (up to 10 mL) intravenously over 5 min. This dose may be repeated up to four times in patients with a partial, transient, or absent response, provided that serum calcium levels are monitored. A continuous calcium infusion (0.2 mL/kg body weight per hour up to a maximum of 10 mL/h) may be appropriate when relapse occurs after an initial bolus. Although electrical pacing is often required, glucagon, in the same dose as for beta-blocker poisoning, should be tried first. Hypotension that persists despite resolution of bradycardia should be treated with fluids and vasopressors. Amrinone, dopamine, dobutamine, glucagon, and norepinephrine, alone or in combination, have been used. Restoring perfusion is particularly important in patients with organ ischemia. Intraaortic balloon pump support should be used in patients unresponsive to the preceding measures. Patients with mild toxicity usually recover within a few hours, whereas those with severe toxicity or overdose with sustained-release preparations may remain symptomatic for 24 h or longer. Extracorporeal removal techniques are unlikely to be of benefit.

CARBON MONOXIDE Carbon monoxide is produced in large amounts in industrial processes as well as by gasoline engines, home appliances, and the incomplete combustion of wood, natural gas, and tobacco products. In addition, methylene chloride, a solvent in paint removers, is metabolized to carbon monoxide.

Carbon monoxide is absorbed rapidly through the lungs and binds to hemoglobin (forming carboxyhemoglobin) with an affinity 210 times that of oxygen. This binding reduces oxygen transportation by hemoglobin and also decreases the release of oxygen to tissues (the oxygen dissociation curve shifts to the left). Carbon monoxide also binds to myoglobin, decreasing its oxygen-carrying capacity, and to mitochondrial cytochrome oxidase, inhibiting cellular respiration. The net effect is profound tissue hypoxia, anaerobic metabolism, and lactic acidosis. Once carbon monoxide exposure is discontinued, dissociation of the hemoglobin–carbon monoxide complex occurs, and carbon monoxide is excreted through the lungs. In room air, the carboxyhemoglobin half-life is 4 to 6 h; the half-life decreases to 40 to 80 min when breathing 100% oxygen and to 15 to 30 min with hyperbaric oxygen therapy. The apparent half-life after methylene chloride exposure is considerably longer.

Clinical Toxicity Manifestations of carbon monoxide poisoning include shortness of breath, dyspnea, tachypnea, headache, emotional lability, confusion, impaired judgment, clumsiness, and syncope. Nausea, vomiting, and diarrhea also may occur. Cerebral edema, coma, respiratory depression, and pulmonary edema occur with severe poisoning. Cardiovascular manifestations include ischemic chest pain, arrhythmias, heart failure, and hypotension. In comatose patients, blisters and bullae may develop over pressure points. Myoglobinuria secondary to muscle necrosis may result in renal failure. A cherry red color of skin and mucous membranes is rare, and cyanosis is usual. Visual field defects, blindness, and venous engorgement with papilledema or optic atrophy may be noted. Measurement of arterial blood gases reveal metabolic acidosis, a normal P_{O_2}, decreased oxygen saturation (by co-oximetry but not when calculated or measured by pulse oximetry), and a variable P_{CO_2}.

After brief exposure, carboxyhemoglobin fractions of 15 to 20 percent are associated with mild symptoms, of 20 to 40 percent with moderate symptoms, and of 40 to 50 percent with severe symptoms. Fractions above 60 percent are often fatal. With prolonged exposure, toxicity occurs at lower percentages. Serum creatine phosphokinase (CK) and lactate dehydrogenase (LHD) levels may be elevated.

Patients with loss of consciousness are at risk for developing neuropsychiatric sequelae 1 to 3 weeks after exposure. Manifestations vary from subtle personality changes and intellectual impairment to gross neurologic deficits such as blindness, deafness, incoordination, and parkinsonism.

Diagnosis The diagnosis is confirmed by determining the carboxyhemoglobin fraction. If this cannot be measured, the difference between the oxygen saturation calculated from the P_{O_2} and that measured by co-oximetry can be used to estimate the carboxyhemoglobin fraction.

TREATMENT

The patient should be removed from the site of exposure. In conscious patients, oxygen should be administered by a non-rebreather mask at 10 L/min until carbon monoxide levels are less than 10 percent and all symptoms have resolved. Infants and pregnant women require treatment for several more hours, because fetal hemoglobin has a high affinity for carbon monoxide. Endotracheal intubation and mechanical ventilation with 100% oxygen are indicated in patients with coma, significant CNS dysfunction, or cardiovascular instability. Arrhythmias and hypotension are treated by usual measures. Patients with coma, syncope, or seizures and those with less severe signs or symptoms of neurologic or cardiovascular dysfunction that do not resolve with oxygen and supportive therapy are candidates for hyperbaric oxygen therapy. Hyperbaric oxygenation shortens the duration of toxicity and may prevent delayed sequelae.

CYANIDE Hydrogen cyanide is used as a fumigant rodenticide and in chemical syntheses. Cyanide salts are used in photography, metallurgy, electroplating, metal cleaning, and ore refining. Organic cyanide compounds (nitriles) are used in the synthetic rubber industry, artificial nail removers, and rodenticides. Cyanogenic glycosides are present in the seeds of the chokeberry, cherry, plum, peach, apricot, pear, bean, apple, and crabapple.

Cyanide inhibits mitochondrial cytochrome oxidase and hence blocks electron transport, resulting in decreased oxidative metabolism and oxygen utilization. Lactic acidosis occurs as a consequence of anaerobic metabolism. Cyanide is rapidly absorbed from the stomach, lungs, mucosal surfaces, and unbroken skin. In the stomach it reacts with hydrochloric acid, liberating hydrocyanic acid, which is absorbed as cyanide ion. Cyanide is 60 percent protein-bound, is concentrated in red cells, and has a volume of distribution of 1.5 L/kg body weight. Cyanide is metabolized by the mitochondrial enzyme rhodanase, which mediates the transfer of sulfur from thiosulfate to the cyanide ion, producing thiocyanate, which in turn is excreted in the urine.

Clinical Toxicity The potentially lethal dose of potassium or sodium cyanide is 200 to 300 mg and of hydrocyanic acid is 50 mg. Effects begin within seconds of inhalation and within 30 min of ingestion. Initial manifestations of cyanide poisoning include headache, faintness, vertigo, excitement, anxiety, a burning sensation in the mouth and throat, dyspnea, tachycardia, and hypertension. Nausea, vomiting, and diaphoresis are common. A bitter almond odor may be detected on the breath. Later effects include coma, convulsions, opisthotonus, trismus, paralysis, respiratory depression, pulmonary edema, arrhythmias, bradycardia, and hypotension. A rough correlation exists between blood cyanide levels and symptoms: Levels less than 8 μmol/L (0.02 mg/L) are associated with no symptoms; 20 to 40 μmol/L (0.05 to 0.1 mg/dL) with flushing and tachycardia; 40 to 100 μmol/L (0.1 to 0.25 mg/dL) with obtundation; 100 to 200 μmol/L (0.25 to 0.3 mg/dL) with coma and respiratory depression; and levels greater than 120 μmol/L (0.3 mg/dL) with death. With significant poisoning, lactic acidosis and narrowing of the arteriovenous oxygen saturation difference may be present. ECG abnormalities include both tachyarrhythmias and bradyarrhythmias, such as nodal or idioventricular rhythm, AV dissociation, and progressive slowing of heart rate.

Diagnosis Although measurement of the whole-blood cyanide level will confirm the diagnosis, cyanide assays are not routinely available. The diagnosis and treatment decisions must therefore be based on clinical findings.

TREATMENT

Initial management involves general supportive measures and gastrointestinal decontamination. Antidotal therapy using amyl nitrite, sodium nitrite, and sodium thiosulfate (the Lilly cyanide antidote kit) coupled with high-dose oxygen should be administered as soon as possible to patients with altered mental status, abnormal vital signs, or metabolic acidosis. The rationale for antidotal therapy is as follows. Nitrites induce methemoglobinemia. Methemoglobin has a higher affinity for cyanide than does cytochrome oxidase and thus promotes its dissociation from this enzyme. Thiosulfate reacts with the cyanide as the latter is slowly released from cyanomethemoglobin, forming the relatively nontoxic thiocyanate, which is excreted in the urine. Oxygen reverses the binding of cyanide to cytochrome oxidase sites and enhances the efficacy of sodium nitrite and sodium thiosulfate, in addition to acting as a substrate for metabolism.

Amyl nitrite is administered for 30 s of each minute. The ampule is broken between two pads of gauze and placed over the airway while the patient breathes spontaneously or is ventilated by a bag-mask unit. A new ampule should be used every 3 min. This process is continued while sodium nitrite is being prepared, but it may be omitted if endotracheal intubation has been performed. Sodium nitrite is administered intravenously as a 3% solution at a rate of 2.5 to 5.0 mL/min up to a total dose of 10 to 15 mL (300 to 450 mg). Sodium thiosulfate is then administered intravenously as a 25% solution at a dose of 50 mL (12.5 g) given over 1 to 2 min. With recurrent or persistent symptoms, half or full doses of both sodium nitrite and sodium thiosulfate are administered. Hyperbaric oxygen therapy should be considered in patients who fail to respond to antidotal therapy.

DIGOXIN Poisoning with digitalis (cardiac glycoside) occurs most often during therapeutic or suicidal use of digoxin and on occasion with plant (oleander) ingestion. Cardiac glycosides act by inhibiting the enzyme sodium-potassium ATPase, leading to increased intracellular levels of Na^+ and Ca^{2+} and decreased intracellular K^+ levels. Digoxin is slowly absorbed and slowly distributed. Serum levels may not correlate with pharmacologic effects for up to 8 h following a therapeutic oral dose. Digoxin is 25 to 30 percent protein-bound in the plasma, has a large volume of distribution of 5 to 6 L/kg body weight, and is localized in skeletal muscle, liver, and heart. Elimination is primarily by renal excretion. The half-life ranges between 36 and 45 h, is prolonged in hepatic failure and in renal failure, and may be shortened in overdose. Approximately 60 percent of a dose is excreted unchanged by the kidneys, and the remainder is metabolized by the liver to inactive metabolites. Therapeutic serum concentrations range from 0.6 to 2.5 nmol/L (0.5 to 2.0 ng/mL).

Clinical Toxicity Symptoms of toxicity include vomiting, confusion, delirium, and occasionally hallucinations, blurred vision, photophobia, scotomata, and disturbed color perception. Cardiac manifestations include sinus arrhythmia, sinus bradycardia, and all degrees of atrioventricular block. Premature ventricular contractions, bigeminy, ventricular tachycardia, and fibrillation also occur. The combination of supraventricular tachyarrhythmia and AV block is highly suggestive of digitalis toxicity. While bradyarrhythmias and hypokalemia are common with chronic intoxication, tachyarrhythmias and hyperkalemia are generally seen with acute poisoning. Similarly, serum digoxin levels may be minimally elevated or even therapeutic in chronic toxicity, whereas they are usually markedly elevated following acute overdose. Clinical toxicity occurs with digoxin levels in excess of 3.8 to 6.4 nmol/L (3 to 5 ng/mL), and levels as high as 64 to 77 nmol/L (50 to 60 ng/mL) have been seen following acute overdose.

Diagnosis The diagnosis is confirmed by finding an elevated serum digoxin level. Since toxicology screening tests do not detect cardiac glycosides, a quantitative drug level must be ordered specifically.

TREATMENT

Gastrointestinal decontamination should be accomplished as soon as possible. Since emesis and gastric intubation may cause vagal stimulation and worsen existing conduction block, activated charcoal is preferred. Repeated doses should be administered because this therapy also can enhance elimination of digoxin. Diuresis, hemodialysis, and hemoperfusion are ineffective, however. Potassium, magnesium, and calcium abnormalities should be corrected. Electrical pacing may be necessary when sinus bradycardia and second- and third-degree heart block result in hypotension and fail to respond to atropine, isoproterenol, or antibody therapy. Magnesium sulfate (as for antiarrhythmic poisoning), phenytoin, and lidocaine may be useful in the treatment of ventricular tachyarrhythmias. Digoxin-specific Fab-fragment antibodies should be administered to patients with potentially life-threatening toxicity not immediately responsive to the above. Following antibody administration, cardiac arrhythmias and hyperkalemia are generally corrected within an hour; the antibodies are given intravenously over 30 min, unless cardiac arrest has occurred, in which case the solution is given as a bolus. The drug-antibody complex is excreted in the urine with a half-life of 16 to 20 h. In patients with renal failure, the drug-antibody complex is metabolized over a period of days to weeks. Although free digoxin levels decrease rapidly to zero following antibody administration, routine methods used to measure digoxin do not differentiate between bound and unbound drug, so that drug levels do not correlate with toxicity after antibody therapy. Antibodies cross-react with other cardiac glycosides, but larger doses may be needed for toxicity not involving digoxin.

Each 40 mg vial of antibody can neutralize 0.6 mg of digoxin. Formulas and tables for calculating the dose of antibody based on body weight and post-distribution serum digoxin level or the amount of drug acutely ingested are available in the package insert. Unfortunately, toxicity may occur before distribution is complete or before levels are available. In addition, the amount of an acute overdose may be unknown, and calculated doses often exceed the effective dose (leading to costly overtreatment). The following doses are therefore suggested. With chronic digoxin intoxication, when total-body drug load only slightly exceeds the therapeutic amount and when patients may be dependent on digoxin for its inotropic effects, an antibody dose of 1 to 2 vials is usually sufficient. In acute poisoning drug levels are generally higher, and 5 to 10 vials are usually required. These doses can be repeated as necessary.

ETHYLENE GLYCOL Ethylene glycol is a colorless, odorless, sweet-tasting, water-soluble liquid that is used as a solvent for paints, plastics, and pharmaceuticals and in the manufacture of explosives, fire extinguishers, foams, hydraulic fluids, windshield cleaners, radiator antifreeze, and de-icer preparations.

Ethylene glycol is absorbed rapidly, and levels peak approximately 2 h after ingestion. Ethylene glycol has a volume of distribution of 0.6 to 0.8 L/kg body weight. It is oxidized by alcohol dehydrogenase to glycoaldehyde, which is metabolized successively to glycolic acid, glyoxylic acid, and oxalic acid. As much as 20 percent is excreted unchanged in the urine. The half-life ranges from 3 to 8 h. Since alcohol dehydrogenase has a higher affinity for ethanol than for ethylene glycol, ethanol is metabolized preferentially when both alcohols are present, and the half-life of ethylene glycol is then prolonged to about 17 h.

Ethylene glycol and its metabolites produce CNS depression. Ethylene glycol is more potent than ethanol in this respect. The glycolic acid metabolite is even more toxic than ethylene glycol. It causes a metabolic acidosis with an increased anion gap and interstitial and tubular damage to the kidney. Glyoxylic acid is more toxic still, but it is metabolized rapidly to oxalic acid and contributes little to the organ toxicity. Oxalic acid may precipitate as calcium oxalate crystals in the brain, heart, kidney, lung, pancreas, and urine and cause hypocalcemia.

Clinical Toxicity As little as 120 mg/kg body weight or 0.1 mL/kg body weight (one swallow) of pure ethylene glycol can result in a potentially toxic blood concentration of 3 mmol/L (20 mg/dL). Effects of the parent compound begin 30 min after ingestion and include nausea, vomiting, slurred speech, ataxia, nystagmus, and lethargy. A faint, sweet aromatic odor may be detected on the breath. Coma, seizures, respiratory depression, cardiovascular collapse, and death may occur. Effects caused by metabolites begin 4 to 12 h after ingestion. At this stage, the patient appears more ill than intoxicated. Manifestations include tachypnea, hypotension, agitation, confusion, lethargy, coma, and seizures. Hypocalcemia occurs in one-third of patients. Leukocytosis is present in most. In severe cases, adult respiratory distress syndrome, cyanosis, pulmonary edema, and cardiomegaly may be seen. Laboratory findings include metabolic acidosis, an increased anion gap (low bicarbonate and chloride), and abnormal urinalysis (crystalluria). Acute tubular necrosis manifested by proteinuria, oliguria, and anuria typically becomes evident 12 to 24 h following ingestion. Renal failure may be permanent but typically lasts days to weeks.

Diagnosis The diagnosis is established by measuring ethylene glycol and glycolic acid levels. In the absence of a history of exposure, the diagnosis is suggested by the finding of an ethanol-like intoxication with an elevated serum osmolality early in the course and with an increased-anion-gap metabolic acidosis and oxalate crystals in the urine later in the course. In the absence of ethanol, signs of intoxication occurs with ethylene glycol levels >8 mmol/L (50 mg/dL).

Rx TREATMENT

Gastrointestinal lavage and activated charcoal should be administered. Supportive measures include protection of the airway, ventilatory and circulatory support, and anticonvulsants for seizures. Hypocalcemia is treated with intravenous calcium salts. Metabolic acidosis should be corrected with sodium bicarbonate; large doses may be required. Alkalinization of the urine enhances the excretion of acid metabolites. Fluids and diuretics may reverse oliguria but do not increase the rate of elimination of ethylene glycol. Indications for ethanol therapy include an elevated osmolal gap or an increased anion gap in a symptomatic patient, a history or strong suspicion of ethylene glycol ingestion and a low or undetectable ethanol level, or an ethylene glycol concentration greater than 3 mmol/L (20 mg/dL). A serum ethanol level of at least 20 mmol/L (100 mg/dL) is required to inhibit the metabolism of ethylene glycol (higher levels may be needed with very high ethylene glycol concentrations). The loading dose of ethanol is 10 mL/kg of 10 percent ethanol intravenously or 1 mL/kg of 95 percent ethanol by mouth; the maintenance dose is 1.5 ml/kg per hour of 10 percent ethanol intravenously or 3 mL/kg per hour of 10 percent ethanol intravenously during hemodialysis. Serum ethanol and ethylene glycol concentrations should be monitored frequently. Therapy should be continued until the ethylene glycol level in blood falls below 1.5 mmol/L (10 mg/dL). Because they are cofactors in the pathway of ethylene glycol metabolism, supplemental folate (50 mg qid), pyridoxine (50 mg qid), and thiamine (100 mg qid) may be beneficial. Hemodialysis enhances the elimination of ethylene glycol and its toxic metabolites. Indications for hemodialysis include metabolic acidosis not readily correctable with bicarbonate and ethanol therapy, lack of clinical improvement despite treatment, ethylene glycol concentrations greater than 8 mmol/L (50 mg/dL), or any detectable level of blood ethylene glycol in the presence of renal failure.

HYDROCARBONS Hydrocarbons exist in a number of forms, including aromatic hydrocarbons, such as xylene and toluene, halogenated hydrocarbons, such as carbon tetrachloride and trichlorethane, and petroleum distillate hydrocarbons, such as gasoline, lacquer thinner, mineral seal oil, kerosene, and lighter fluid.

All hydrocarbons are CNS depressants and irritants of the gastrointestinal and pulmonary systems. They are absorbed rapidly following inhalation or pulmonary aspiration. Aromatic and halogenated hydrocarbons are also absorbed following ingestion and are toxic to the heart, liver, and kidneys. Aromatic hydrocarbons also can cause bone marrow suppression and skeletal muscle damage. Petroleum distillate hydrocarbons are poorly absorbed following ingestion.

Clinical Toxicity Hydrocarbons produce CNS excitation in low doses and depression in high doses. Rarely, coma and seizures occur. Psychosis, cerebral and cerebellar atrophy, encephalopathy, and peripheral neuropathy can result from chronic inhalation. Other effects include nausea, vomiting, abdominal pain, hepatitis, renal tubular acidosis, acute hepatic or renal failure, and rhabdomyolysis. Sudden death due to myocardial irritability and ventricular fibrillation may occur following hydrocarbon sniffing. After ingestion, hydrocarbons cause burning of the mouth and throat with subsequent nausea, vomiting, and diarrhea. Aspiration into the lungs may occur with ingestion or as a result of vomiting and cause pneumonia. Following aspiration, chest x-ray abnormalities include infiltrates, atelectasis, effusions, pneumothorax, and pneumatoceles. Renal tubular acidosis with decreased serum bicarbonate, calcium, phosphate, and potassium and increased serum chloride may result from chronic aromatic hydrocarbon inhalation.

Diagnosis The diagnosis is based on the clinical presentation. Assays for assessing hydrocarbons in blood are not routinely available.

Rx TREATMENT

The ingestion of aromatic and halogenated hydrocarbons requires prompt gastric lavage. More than one episode of ipecac-induced emesis is contraindicated, and the role of activated charcoal is controversial. Since the ingestion of other types of hydrocarbons is unlikely to result in systemic toxicity and since the risk of aspiration during gastric decontamination is greater than the potential benefit, decontamination is contraindicated for these ingestions. Supportive therapy includes oxygen, respiratory support, and monitoring of liver, renal, and myocardial function. Metabolic abnormalities should be corrected, and patients with aspiration paneumonitis should be monitored for superimposed bacterial infection. Glucocorticoids are ineffective.

HYDROGEN SULFIDE Hydrogen sulfide is a rapidly acting, malodorous ("rotten eggs"), colorless, irritating gas. It is encountered in the petroleum and mining industries, tanning of leather, vulcanization of rubber, the production of synthetic fabrics, metal refining, the production of heavy water for atomic reactors, and glue and felt manufacturing. It is also found in sewers, sulfur springs, and the holds of fishing vessels, and as a byproduct of manure storage.

The hydrogen sulfide anion inhibits electron transport in the cytochrome oxidase system, thereby inhibiting aerobic metabolism with resultant cellular anoxia and lactic acidosis. Hydrogen sulfide is detoxified to sulfate products, which are excreted principally by the kidneys.

Clinical Toxicity Exposure to low concentrations of hydrogen sulfide results in rhinitis, conjunctivitis, and pharyngitis. Inhalation of large amounts causes headache, vertigo, nausea, vomiting, confusion, seizures, and coma. Hypoventilation, hypoxia, cyanosis, metabolic acidosis, pneumonia, and pulmonary edema can occur.

Diagnosis The diagnosis is based on the characteristic clinical features, including the breath odor, the setting, and the rapidity of onset.

Rx TREATMENT

Treatment begins with prompt removal of the victim from the site of exposure. The airway should be cleared, ventilation should be assisted when indicated, and 100% oxygen should be administered. The use of amyl and sodium nitrite should be considered when patients fail to respond rapidly to oxygen. Nitrites promote the dissociation of sulfide ions from cytochrome oxidase by providing an alternative binding site (methemoglobin). They also enhance detoxification by acting as a catalyst for sulfide oxidation. Except for cardiac arrest, no clear-cut indications for nitrite administration exist. For optimal effectiveness, they must be used immediately in symptomatic patients (sulfide oxidation is so rapid that the amount of sulfide bound to cytochrome is minimal by the time the patient presents for treatment). The dose schedule is the same as for cyanide poisoning (thiosulfate is not necessary). Hyperbaric oxygen should be considered in patients who do not respond to the preceding measures.

IRON Iron preparations contain ferrous salts that vary in elemental iron content (20 percent in the sulfate salt, 33 percent in the fumarate, 12 percent in the gluconate, and 35 percent in the succinate). Ingestion of 20 mg/kg body weight of elemental iron typically produces gastrointestinal symptoms, and 60 mg/kg body weight may cause systemic toxicity.

Ferrous iron is absorbed into mucosal cells of the duodenum and jejunum and is oxidized to ferric iron and bound to ferritin. It is then slowly released into the plasma, where it is bound to transferrin, an iron-specific binding globulin, and transported to tissues. Iron levels in serum usually peak 4 to 6 h after overdosage (later for delayed-release formulations). Iron bound to transferrin is nontoxic. With overdosage, free iron that exceeds the iron-binding capacity of transferrin and high ferritin levels cause tissue damage and lead to the release of vasoactive substances such as serotonin and histamine. Increased capillary permeability, vasodilation, and fluid loss result in hypotension and metabolic acidosis. Free iron also injures mitochondria, causes lipid peroxidation, and may result in renal, hepatic, myocardial, and pulmonary injury.

Clinical Toxicity Initial manifestations include vomiting and diarrhea (often bloody). X-rays may reveal iron tablets in the stomach or small bowel. A positive x-ray, fever above 38.5°C, hyperglycemia greater than 8.5 mmol/L (150 mg/dL), and leukocytosis (white blood cell count greater than 15,000/μL) are associated with serum iron levels above 50 μmol/L (300 μg/dL) and the potential for systemic toxicity. Systemic effects occur later and include lethargy, hypotension, and metabolic acidosis and, with severe poisoning, seizures, coma, pulmonary edema, and vascular collapse. Jaundice, elevated hepatic enzyme levels, prolongation of prothrombin time, and hyperammonemia are indicative of liver injury. Proteinuria and cells in the urine indicate renal injury. Pulmonary edema and hemorrhage are seen with severe overdose. In the recovering patient, gastric ulcerations and scars may cause outlet obstruction. Overgrowth of *Yersinia enterocolitica* with sepsis is a rare complication of iron overload.

Diagnosis A serum iron concentration above 50 μmol/L (300 μg/dL) is potentially toxic. Serious poisoning is generally associated with levels above 80 μmol/L (500 μg/dL). A positive urine deferoxamine provocative challenge test (see below) is also diagnostic.

℞ TREATMENT

Ingested iron is best removed by either ipecac-induced emesis or a large orogastric tube. An x-ray film following gastric lavage will show the success of the decontamination procedure. Whole-bowel irrigation, endoscopic removal, or gastrostomy may be necessary for large quantities of iron tablets or when concretions form. Activated charcoal is ineffective. Although bicarbonate lavage may cause the formation and removal of the insoluble ferrous carbonate salt, its effectiveness is not proven. Oral deferoxamine may bind the iron remaining in the stomach and form the less toxic ferrioxamine. Since the amount of the deferoxamine that would be required for the typical overdosage is prohibitively large, this therapy is rarely useful. Intravenous sodium bicarbonate should be used to correct metabolic acidosis. Hypotension may respond to volume expansion. Coagulation abnormalities should be treated with vitamin K or blood products.

When the serum iron level or the clinical findings indicate potential systemic toxicity, parenteral deferoxamine should be administered. If levels are not immediately available, or if the patient has mild clinical toxicity, deferoxamine can be given intramuscularly in a challenge dose of 50 mg/kg up to 2 g. A vin rosé urine color indicates the presence of ferrioxamine and means that free iron is present in the circulation. In those with a positive challenge test or with significant clinical toxicity, deferoxamine should be given intravenously at a rate of 10 to 15 mg/kg per hour. When iron levels exceed 180 μmol/L (1000 μg/dL), larger deferoxamine doses (up to 30 mg/kg per hour) can be given initially. Once the patient is asymptomatic or improved, deferoxamine therapy should be discontinued. Exchange transfusion or plasmapheresis to remove the iron-desferal (ferrioxamine) complex should be reserved for patients with renal failure or for those who fail to respond to the preceding therapy.

ISONIAZID Toxic doses of isoniazid decrease the synthesis of the inhibitory CNS neurotransmitter GABA by competing with pyridoxal-5-phosphate, a cofactor for the enzyme glutamic acid decarboxylase. Decreased GABA can result in seizures and consequently in increased lactate production by muscle. Since isoniazid also inhibits the metabolism of lactate to pyruvate, intractable lactic acid acidosis may occur. Isoniazid is rapidly absorbed, mainly from the small intestine. Serum concentrations peak within 1 to 2 h. The volume of distribution is approximately 0.6 L/kg body weight. Serum protein binding is slight. Isoniazid is eliminated primarily by acetylation to acetylisoniazid followed by hydrolysis to isonicotinic acid. Approximately 15 percent of an ingested dose of isoniazid is excreted unchanged by the kidneys. The serum half-life of isoniazid in overdose is approximately 1 to 4 h.

Clinical Toxicity Effects begin within 30 min of ingestion of doses greater than 20 mg/kg body weight. Symptoms include nausea, vomiting, dizziness, slurred speech, lethargy, and confusion. The major manifestations include coma, respiratory depression, generalized seizures, and lactic acid acidosis. Seizures are protracted and relatively unresponsive to standard anticonvulsant therapy. Acidosis does not occur when seizures are prevented.

Diagnosis The diagnosis is confirmed by measuring isoniazid in blood; the assay must be ordered specifically, since routine screening tests do not detect the drug. Toxicity occurs with concentrations as low as 15 μmol/L (2 mg/L). Significant symptoms are seen with serum concentrations greater than 30 to 35 μmol/L (4 to 5 mg/L).

℞ TREATMENT

Initial therapy consists of prompt gastrointestinal decontamination and supportive measures. Ipecac-induced vomiting should be avoided, because of the high incidence of seizures. Isoniazid is well adsorbed by activated charcoal. Seizures can sometimes be treated with benzodiazepines and barbiturates. Administration of pyridoxine (vitamin B_6), which reverses isoniazid-induced enzyme inhibition, is usually necessary for treating seizures. Diazepam is synergistic with pyridoxine. Bicarbonate may be necessary to correct acidosis. Pyridoxine should be given intravenously in an amount equal to the ingested dose of isoniazid. When the ingested dose is not known, 5 g of pyridoxine should be administered. Pyridoxine should be given over 5 min to patients with seizures but over 30 min in the absence of seizures. Cessation of seizures and correction of metabolic acidosis are prompt, but the patient may not awake for several hours. The dose may be repeated if the response is partial or if symptoms recur. Saline diuresis enhances the excretion of isoniazid, and the drug is efficiently removed by hemodialysis. These therapies are rarely necessary because of the efficacy of pyridoxine.

ISOPROPYL ALCOHOL Isopropyl alcohol is a component of rubbing alcohol, solvents, aftershave lotions, antifreeze, and window cleaners. Its metabolite, acetone, is found in cleaners, solvents, and nail polish removers. It is absorbed rapidly from the stomach and the lungs but only minimally through skin. It is distributed in body water and has a volume of distribution of 0.6 L/kg body weight. Its half-life ranges from 3 to 6 h. Isopropyl alcohol is metabolized to acetone in the liver by the enzyme alcohol dehydrogenase, and the acetone is excreted by the kidneys and lungs with a half-life of 20 to 30 h. Up to 20 percent of isopropyl alcohol is excreted unchanged through the kidneys. Isopropyl alcohol and acetone are about twice as potent as ethanol as CNS depressants.

Clinical Toxicity Effects begin within 30 min of ingestion and include vomiting, abdominal discomfort, and sometimes hematemesis. A characteristic smell of rubbing alcohol may be noted. CNS manifestations include headache, dizziness, confusion, and excitation. With severe ingestion, obtundation, coma, respiratory depression, hypothermia, and hypotension may occur. Hypoglycemia may be seen. Isopropyl alcohol can cause a falsely elevated serum creatinine level. A mild anion-gap acidosis, ketonemia, and increased serum osmolality may be present.

Diagnosis Measurement of the serum level must be ordered specifically, since routine screening tests do not detect isopropyl alcohol or acetone. Isopropyl alcohol levels of 8 to 17 mmol/L (50 to 100 mg/dL) produce lethargy; concentrations greater than 25 to 33 mmol/L (150 to 200 mg/dL) are associated with coma; and concentrations greater than 66 to 84 mmol/L (400 to 500 mg/dL) are potentially fatal.

℞ TREATMENT

Gastrointestinal decontamination must be instituted soon after ingestion. Gastric lavage will suffice. Activated charcoal is ineffective. Supportive measures should include intravenous fluids and bicarbonate to correct dehydration, shock, and acidosis. Isopropyl alcohol and acetone are removed efficiently by hemodialysis, which should be considered in patients who have high serum levels and do not respond to conservative therapy.

LITHIUM Lithium is most commonly available as the carbonate or the citrate salt. Lithium may substitute for cellular cations (K^+ and Na^+), thereby interfering with adenylate cyclase activation, inhibiting neurotransmitter (norepinephrine) release, and reducing the activity of Na^+,K^+-ATPase.

The drug is absorbed rapidly from the gastrointestinal tract and reaches peak levels within 2 to 4 h of ingestion (later with overdosage and with sustained-release preparations). It has negligible plasma protein binding and a volume of distribution of approximately 0.6 L/kg body weight. Removal from the body is primarily (95 percent) by glomerular filtration, with significant reabsorption (80 percent) by the proximal tubules. Lithium clearance is increased by alkalinization of the urine and decreased by hypovolemia and hyponatremia. The serum half-life ranges from 18 to 36 h; therapeutic levels range from 0.6 to 1.2 mmol/L.

Clinical Toxicity Effects begin 1 to 4 h after acute overdosage, but the onset can be insidious with chronic poisoning. Gastrointestinal effects include nausea, vomiting, and diarrhea; neuromuscular effects include weakness, fasciculations, and twitching; CNS effects include ataxia, tremor, myoclonus, choreoathetosis, seizures, confusion, and coma; and cardiovascular effects include arrhythmias and hypotension. Hyperthermia may occur. Laboratory abnormalities include leukocytosis, hyperglycemia, albuminuria, glycosuria, and nephrogenic diabetes insipidus. ECG changes include sinus tachycardia or bradycardia, flattened or inverted T waves, atrioventricular block, and a prolonged QT interval. In chronic intoxication signs and symptoms occur at lower serum levels than with acute intoxication.

Diagnosis Lithium is not detected by routine screening tests, so measurement of the serum level must be requested specifically. In chronic poisoning, serum levels between 3 and 4 mmol/L may be associated with severe toxicity. In acute poisoning, serum levels may exceed 8 mmol/L despite minimal symptoms. Serum levels should be measured serially because absorption may be prolonged following overdosage.

℞ TREATMENT

Within 2 to 4 h following ingestion, gastrointestinal decontamination is indicated. Lithium is poorly adsorbed by activated charcoal. Since most patients vomit spontaneously, lavage and bowel irrigation are the treatments of choice, particularly for sustained-release formulations. Supportive therapy includes standard treatments for seizures, CNS depression, hypotension, and arrhythmias. Symptomatic patients with serum concentrations greater than 2 mmol/L require intravenous saline to correct dehydration and achieve a normal urine output. Diuresis and alkalinization of the urine are recommended to enhance renal excretion of lithium. Hemodialysis is indicated for severe intoxication when the serum lithium level is >3 mmol/L. It may need to be repeated or prolonged to prevent serum levels from rebounding when it is stopped.

METHANOL Methanol is a component of shellacs, varnishes, paint removers, Sterno, windshield-washer solutions, and copy machine fluid. It is also a denaturant used to make ethanol unfit for consumption. Methanol, a slightly less potent CNS depressant than ethanol, is metabolized to formaldehyde and formic acid, which in turn causes metabolic acidosis and injury to the retina.

Methanol is absorbed rapidly and completely from the gastrointestinal tract, and levels peak within 1 to 2 h of ingestion. It is distributed throughout body water, with a volume of distribution of 0.7 L/kg body weight. Its protein binding is negligible. Elimination occurs mainly by hepatic metabolism, with up to 10 percent excreted unchanged by the lungs and kidneys. Elimination follows first-order kinetics with a half-life of about 3 h at low serum levels (less than about 15 mmol/L or 50 mg/dL) and converts to zero-order kinetics with an elimination rate of 3 mmol/L per hour (10.5 mg/dL per hour) at higher levels. The half-life of elimination at low serum levels is approximately 14 to 20 h, and at high serum levels it is 24 to 30 h. Ethanol competes with methanol for metabolism by alcohol dehydrogenase and increases the elimination half-life of methanol to 30 to 35 h.

Clinical Toxicity Onset is variable and may be delayed. Absence of signs and symptoms soon after ingestion should not be equated with absence of subsequent toxicity. Early manifestations are caused by methanol itself, and late manifestations are due to the metabolite formic acid. Initially, nausea, vomiting, abdominal pain, headache, vertigo, and an ethanol-like intoxication occur. An increased osmolal gap may be present. Late manifestations include coma, seizures, an increased anion gap, metabolic acidosis, and retinal injury. Ophthalmologic manifestations occur 15 to 19 h or later after ingestion and include clouding and diminished vision, dancing and flashing spots, dilated or fixed pupils, hyperemia of the disk, retinal edema, and blindness. These changes are potentially reversible with prompt institution of therapy. With severe poisoning, myocardial depression, bradycardia, and shock may occur.

Diagnosis Early in the course, the diagnosis is suggested by ethanol-like intoxication and an elevated serum osmolality and is confirmed by measurement of the serum methanol level [usually greater than 6 mmol/L (20 mg/dL)]. Later, the diagnosis is suggested by an increased-anion-gap metabolic acidosis and elevated serum methanol or formate levels.

℞ TREATMENT

Gastrointestinal decontamination is indicated soon after ingestion. Gastric aspiration is the treatment of choice. Supportive measures should include volume replacement, respiratory care, and treatment of seizures. Acidosis should be corrected with sodium bicarbonate; large amounts may be required. Alkalinization of the urine enhances the elimination of formic acid. Supplemental thiamine and folate, which enhance the metabolism of formic acid, are recommended in the same doses as for ethylene glycol toxicity. Ethanol therapy is indicated in patients who are symptomatic or who have an increased osmolar gap, increased-anion-gap metabolic acidosis, or a methanol level exceeding 6 mmol/L (20 mg/dL) and a low or undetectable ethanol level. The loading and maintenance doses of ethanol are the same as for ethylene glycol. Ethanol levels must be monitored frequently to document that they are in the therapeutic range of 20 to 30 mmol/L (100 to 150 mg/dL). Therapy should be continued until the serum methanol level falls below 3 mmol/L (10 mg/dL) and all signs of toxicity are resolved. Hemodialysis enhances the elimination of methanol and formic acid and is indicated when methanol levels exceed 15 mmol/L (50 mg/dL), for patients with visual signs or elevated formic acid levels, and when clinical or metabolic abnormalities are unresponsive to the preceding therapy.

METHEMOGLOBINEMIA Methemoglobinemia results from exposure to chemicals that oxidize the iron in hemoglobin from its ferrous (Fe^{2+}) to its ferric (Fe^{3+}) state. Concomitant oxidation of hemoglobin protein may cause its precipitation (as Heinz bodies) and a hemolytic anemia (with bite cells seen on peripheral blood smear). Oxidizing agents include aniline and its derivates, aminophenols, aminophenones, chlorates, dapsone, local anesthetics such as benzocaine, nitrites, nitrates, naphthalene, nitrobenzene and related chemicals, oxides of nitrogen, phenazopyridine, primaquine and related antimalarials, and sulfonamides.

Methemoglobin (ferric hemoglobin) cannot carry oxygen and, when present in excess, results in a functional anemia. It also shifts the oxygen-dissociation curve to the left, limiting the release of oxygen to tissues. Symptoms are due to hypoxia and anaerobic metabolism.

Various systems normally operate to keep methemoglobin at physiologic levels (1 percent of the total hemoglobin concentration). Oxidant inactivation systems utilize ascorbic acid and sulfhydryl agents such as glutathione. Mechanisms for converting methemoglobin back to oxyhemoglobin include NADH-methemoglobin reductase (responsible for 95 percent of baseline reducing capacity), NADPH-methemoglobin reductase, and the ascorbic acid and glutathione systems. When supplied with the cofactor methylene blue, the capacity of the NADPH-methemoglobin reductase is greatly increased. Because this enzyme is dependent on NADPH, individuals with glucose-6-phosphate dehydrogenase deficiency have profound impairment in the ability to reduce methemoglobin after oxidant exposure.

Clinical Toxicity Cyanosis that is unresponsive to oxygen and may have a gray-brown hue occurs with methemoglobin levels greater than 15 percent (15 g/L or 1.5 g/dL absolute methemoglobin). Patients are otherwise asymptomatic, however, until methemoglobin levels exceed 20 to 30 percent, at which point fatigue, headache, tachycardia, dizziness, and weakness develop. At levels greater than 45 percent, dyspnea, bradycardia, hypoxia, acidosis, seizures, coma, and cardiac arrhythmias may occur. Levels greater than 70 percent are rapidly fatal. Hemolytic anemia may cause hyperkalemia and renal failure.

Diagnosis The diagnosis is confirmed by measuring the methemoglobin level by co-oximetry, a feature of some arterial blood gas analyzers. If co-oximetry is not available, methemoglobin levels can be estimated as the difference between the oxygen saturation calculated from the P_{O_2} and that measured directly. Oxygen saturation measured by pulse oximetry may be falsely normal. Blood with high levels of methemoglobin is chocolate colored when placed on filter paper and compared with normal blood. The chocolate color does not revert to pink when oxygen is bubbled through a tube of blood but does return to normal when 10% potassium cyanide is added. Finally, the toxic screen on blood or urine may identify the drug or chemical that served as the oxidizing agent.

℞ TREATMENT

The toxin, if recently ingested, should be removed by gastrointestinal decontamination. Most oxidizing agents are eliminated by metabolism, making diuresis ineffective. Supplemental oxygen should be administered. Dialysis may be useful, depending on the specific compound. Methylene blue is indicated for methemoglobin levels above 30 percent (cyanosis alone is not an indication for methylene blue therapy). In patients with anemia or cardiovascular disease, methylene blue may be indicated at lower levels when manifestations of hypoxia are present. Methylene blue is given at a dose of 1 to 2 mg/kg body weight as a 1% solution over 5 min. If a clinical response is not observed within 1 h, the dose may be repeated. A methemoglobin level of 40 g/L can be expected to decrease by half in 1 to 2 h. As long as the oxidizing agent remains in the body, methemoglobin will be generated, and additional doses may be necessary. Side effects of methylene blue include precordial pain, dyspnea, restlessness, apprehension, and tremor; a transient blue color to the skin and urine; and the induction of methemoglobinemia at doses greater than 7 mg/kg of body weight. Methylene blue is contraindicated in patients with glucose-6-phosphate dehydrogenase deficiency because it can cause hemolysis. If the methemoglobin level is very high, if the patient is refractory to methylene blue, or if the patient is deficient in glucose-6-phosphate dehydrogenase, exchange transfusion may be indicated.

MONOAMINE OXIDASE INHIBITORS Monoamine oxidase (MAO) inhibitors include furazolidone, isocarboxazid, nialamide, pargyline, phenelzine, procarbazine, and tranylcypromine. These agents block monoamine oxidase, thus inhibiting a major pathway for catabolism of neurotransmitters such as dopamine, norepinephrine, and serotonin. Toxicity results from accumulation of neurotransmitters and hence potentiation of their actions.

MAO inhibitors are absorbed efficiently from the gastrointestinal tract. The volume of distribution is not known but is probably large. These drugs are eliminated mainly by hepatic metabolism, and less than 5 percent is excreted unchanged in the urine. The plasma half-life of phenelzine and tranylcypromine at therapeutic doses is 24 h.

Clinical Toxicity Effects may not begin until 6 to 12 h after ingestion and may not peak until 24 h after ingestion. Initial effects include dilated pupils, hyperpyrexia, tachycardia, hypertension, and tachypnea. Nausea and vomiting also may occur. Agitation, hyperactivity, and confusion may be coupled with fasciculations, twitching, tremor, and rigidity. Cardiovascular collapse and CNS depression are late effects in severe poisoning.

Diagnosis The diagnosis is made on the basis of the clinical presentation. Toxic levels of MAO inhibitors have not been established, and no assay methods are commonly available.

℞ TREATMENT

Gastrointestinal decontamination should be performed as soon as possible. Benzodiazepines should be given for neuromuscular hyperactivity. Hyperthermia should be treated with external cooling and sedation and in severe cases with neuromuscular paralysis. Severe hypertension and tachycardia should be treated with nitroprusside and propranolol, respectively. Hypotension should be treated with volume expanders, and pressor therapy should begin at lower than normal initial doses because of the possibility of an exaggerated response. In fact, before any drug is given, potential adverse interactions with MAO inhibitors should be researched. Arrhythmias can be treated by usual measures. Diuresis, hemodialysis, and hemoperfusion are not effective. No specific antidote exists. Because of persistence of MAO inhibition, drug therapy and diet should be carefully controlled for 7 to 10 days after stopping the agents.

MUSCLE RELAXANTS Muscle relaxants include orphenadrine, methocarbamol, baclofen, chlorphenesin, cyclobenzaprine, chlorzoxazone, and carisoprodol. Muscle relaxants have some direct effects on muscle but act mainly as CNS depressants. They also depress spinal synaptic reflexes, prolong synaptic recovery time, and reduce repetitive discharges. Baclofen enhances the effects of GABA, and cyclobenzaprine and orphenadrine have anticholinergic activity. Muscle relaxants are absorbed rapidly and completely, and blood levels peak 1 to 2 h after ingestion. The half-lives of these drugs vary; most have half-lives between 2 and 6 h. Most muscle relaxants are metabolized by the liver to derivatives that are generally inactive and are excreted by the kidneys. Baclofen, an exception, is largely excreted unchanged in the urine.

Clinical Toxicity Effects of carisoprodol, chlorphenesin, chlorzoxazone, and methocarbamol include nausea, vomiting, dizziness, headache, nystagmus, hypotonia, and central nervous system depression. Cyclobenzaprine and orphenadrine may cause agitation, hallucinations, tachycardia, mydriasis, hyperthermia, and dry skin and mucosa. Orphenadrine can also cause ventricular tachyarrhythmias. Baclofen causes CNS depression, hypothermia, excitability, delirium, myoclonus, seizures, cardiac conduction abnormalities, tachycardia, bradycardia, and hypotension.

Diagnosis The diagnosis is supported by detecting the drugs on comprehensive urine screening. Quantitative measurements of serum levels are not routinely available.

℞ TREATMENT

Initial management includes prompt gastrointestinal decontamination. Muscle relaxants are well adsorbed by a single dose of activated charcoal. Repetitive charcoal administration may be used for baclofen. Diuresis is ineffective. The efficacy of hemodialysis or hemoperfusion is not established. Physostigmine (1 to 2 mg intravenously over 2 to 5 min) will reverse the anticholinergic effects of orphenadrine and cyclobenzaprine but should be reserved for patients with severe hallucinations and hyperactivity.

NONSTEROIDAL ANTI-INFLAMMATORY DRUGS Nonsteroidal anti-inflammatory drugs (NSAIDs) include diclofenac, diflunisal, etodolac, fenoprofen, flurbiprofen, ibuprofen, indomethacin, ketoprofen, ketorolac, meclofenamate, mefenamic acid, naproxen, oxaprozin, piroxicam, phenylbutazone, sulindac, and tolmetin. NSAIDs inhibit prostaglandin synthesis by blocking cyclooxygenase. They are absorbed rapidly, and blood concentrations peak 1 to 2 h after ingestion. They are highly bound (greater than 90 percent) to plasma protein and have volumes of distribution of less than 1.0 L/kg body weight. The pK_a ranges from 3.5 to 6.3. They are metabolized mainly by conjugation, oxidation, and hydroxylation. A small portion (1 to 15 percent) is eliminated unchanged by the kidneys. Half-lives vary from 1 to 16 h except in the case of phenylbutazone, which has a half-life of 2 to 4 days.

Clinical Toxicity Effects are usually mild and include nausea, vomiting, abdominal pain, drowsiness, headache, glycosuria, hematuria, and proteinuria. Acute renal failure and hepatitis are rare. Diflunisal may produce hyperventilation, tachycardia, and sweating. Ibuprofen sometimes causes metabolic acidosis, coma, and seizures. Seizures are relatively common in mefenamic acid and phenylbutazone poisoning and occur rarely with ketoprofen and naproxen. Coma, respiratory depression, and cardiovascular collapse or arrest can occur with mefenamic acid and phenylbutazone. Metabolic acidosis is relatively common in phenylbutazone poisoning and occurs rarely with naproxen.

Diagnosis Comprehensive toxicology screening will identify these drugs in the urine, but quantitative analysis is not useful.

℞ TREATMENT

Therapy for NSAID poisoning includes gastrointestinal decontamination and supportive care. Repeated doses of activated charcoal may be of benefit for indomethacin, phenylbutazone, and piroxicam. Renal excretion is not increased by diuresis, and protein binding limits the efficacy of hemodialysis. Although experience with hemoperfusion is limited, this method might be useful in patients with hepatic or renal failure and severe clinical toxicity.

ORGANOPHOSPHATE AND CARBAMATE INSECTICIDES Organophosphorus insecticides include chlorpyrifos, phosphorothioic acid (Diazinon), dichlorvos, fenthion, malathion, and parathion, and carbamate insecticides include aldicarb, propoxur (Baygon), carbaryl, and bendiocarb (Ficam). (Numerous others are available.) The nerve gas sarin is an organophosphate, and therapeutic carbamates include ambenonium, neostigmine, physostigmine, and pyridostigmine. Organophosphorus insecticides irreversibly inhibit acetylcholinesterase and cause accumulation of acetylcholine at muscarinic and nicotinic synapses and in the CNS. Carbamates reversibly inhibit this enzyme. Organophosphates are absorbed through the skin, lungs, and gastrointestinal tract, are distributed widely in tissues, and are slowly eliminated by hepatic metabolism. The oxidative metabolites of parathion and malathion (paraoxon, malaoxon) are the active forms of the agents. Subsequent hydrolysis produces inactive metabolites. Carbamates are eliminated rapidly by serum and liver enzymes.

Clinical Toxicity The time from exposure to the onset of toxicity varies from minutes to hours but usually is between 30 min and 2 h. Muscarinic effects include nausea, vomiting, abdominal cramps, urinary and fecal incontinence, increased bronchial secretions, cough, wheezing, dyspnea, sweating, salivation, miosis, blurred vision, lacrimation, and urinary frequency and incontinence. In severe poisoning, bradycardia, conduction block, hypotension, and pulmonary edema may occur. Nicotinic signs include twitching, fasciculations, weakness, hypertension, tachycardia, and in severe cases paralysis and respiratory failure. CNS effects include anxiety, restlessness, tremor, convulsions, confusion, weakness, and coma. Toxicity due to carbamates is shorter in duration and usually less severe than that due to organophosphates. Most patients recover within 24 to 48 h, but fat-soluble organophosphates may cause effects for weeks to months. Death is most often due to pulmonary toxicity.

Diagnosis A reduction of cholinesterase activity in plasma and in red blood cells to less than 50 percent of normal confirms the diagnosis. A reduction in red blood cell cholinesterase activity is more specific; however, this test is less readily available, and some organophosphates inhibit only one type of cholinesterase. With carbamate insecticides, depression in plasma or red blood cell cholinesterase levels is transient because of the rapid reversibility of the inhibition. Since cholinesterase assays are not routinely or rapidly available, the initial diagnosis is clinical. Insecticides may be identified in urine by specific testing.

℞ TREATMENT

Contaminated clothing should be removed, and the skin should be washed with soap and water. The patient should be removed from the site of inhalation exposure, and in the case of ingestion, gastrointestinal decontamination should include use of activated charcoal. Supportive measures include oxygen administration, ventilatory assistance, and treatment of seizures. Atropine, a muscarinic receptor antagonist, should be administered for muscarinic effects. A dose of 0.5 to 2 mg of atropine is given intravenously every 15 min until bronchial and other secretions have dried. Pupil size and heart rate cannot be used as end-points. Repeated doses or a constant atropine drip may be necessary for several days. Pralidoxime (2-PAM), an oxime that reactivates cholinesterases, is indicated for nicotinic symptoms due to organophosphate poisoning. The dose is 1 to 2 g intravenously over 5 to 20 min. The dose may be repeated every 4 to 6 h. Neither atropine nor pralidoxime is particularly effective at reversing CNS effects. The use of pralidoxime in carbamate poisoning is controversial. It is usually unnecessary, but its use is safe, particularly if it is administered in conjunction with atropine.

PHENOTHIAZINES Phenothiazines include chlorpromazine, fluphenazine, mesoridazine, perphenazine, prochlorperazine, promazine, promethazine, thioridazine, and trifluoperazine derivatives. Haloperidol, loxapine, pimozide, and thiothixene differ structurally but have similar pharmacologic activity. The principal mechanism of action of these agents is related to inhibition of dopaminergic neurotransmission in the CNS, but they also block some alpha-adrenergic, histaminergic, muscarinic, and serotonergic actions. Some phenothiazines have a quinidine-like effect on the heart. These agents are absorbed efficiently from the gastrointestinal tract, exhibit 90 to 95 percent protein binding in plasma, and have large apparent volumes of distribution (10 to 40 L/kg body weight). They are eliminated slowly by hepatic metabolism with half-lives of 20 to 40 h. Only 1 percent is excreted unchanged in the urine. Most metabolites are inactive.

Clinical Toxicity Effects begin within 30 to 60 min of ingestion and include lethargy, obtundation, respiratory depression, hypotension, hypothermia, and coma. Pupils are often constricted, and the skin is usually warm and dry. Other anticholinergic effects may be evident (see "Anticholinergic Agents," above). Cardiac effects include supraventricular tachycardia, atrioventricular block, and atrial and ventricular arrhythmias. Torsade de pointes, prolonged PR, QRS, and QT intervals, and U- and T-wave abnormalities may be seen with thioridazine and its metabolite mesoridazine. The neuroleptic malignant syndrome (see Chap. 18) rarely, if ever, occurs following acute overdose. In acute dystonic reactions, sustained muscle contractions may result in abnormal posturing of the eyes, face, tongue, jaw, neck, back, abdomen, and pelvis, but the patient remains alert. These reactions are idiosyncratic rather than dose-related.

Diagnosis The diagnosis is supported by detecting the presence of these agents on toxicologic screening of the urine. Quantitative measurement is not helpful.

℞ **TREATMENT**

Gastrointestinal decontamination should be accomplished as soon as possible. Treatment is supportive. Diuresis and dialysis are ineffective. Seizures should be treated with anticonvulsants, and hypotension should be managed with volume expanders and pressor agents. Arrhythmias are treated by standard agents. Quinidine and procainanide, however, should be avoided. Sodium bicarbonate and magnesium may be useful for ventricular tachyarrhythmias associated with intraventricular conduction delays and prolonged QT intervals, respectively. Physostigmine is sometimes useful for anticholinergic toxicity (see "Anticholinergic agents," above).

Acute dystonic reactions respond rapidly to intravenous diphenhydramine (1 mg/kg body weight given over 2 min) or benztropine (1 to 2 mg). Doses may be repeated in 20 min if the response is incomplete. Treatment is generally continued with an oral formulation for 2 to 3 days to prevent recurrence of symptoms.

SALICYLATES All salicylates have pharmacologic activity similar to that of the NSAIDs, and aspirin also inhibits platelet aggregation. Following overdosage, salicylates increase the sensitivity of respiratory centers in the brain to changes in P_{O_2} and P_{CO_2}, resulting in an increased rate and depth of respiration. Later, salicylates uncouple oxidative phosphorylation and increase the metabolic rate, oxygen consumption, glucose utilization, and heat production. They also inhibit the Krebs cycle and block carbohydrate and lipid metabolism, resulting in ketoacidosis. Salicylates inhibit the synthesis of clotting factors in the liver and cause prolongation of the prothrombin time.

Salicylates are well absorbed both from the stomach and the small bowel, but absorption may continue for 24 h or longer following an overdose. Therapeutic blood levels range from 0.7 to 1.4 mmol/L (10 to 20 mg/dL). In the plasma, 50 to 80 percent of drug is bound to albumin. These drugs have a small volume of distribution (0.2 L/kg body weight), which increases with the dose and duration of poisoning. Because salicylate is a weak acid with a pK_a of 3, the unbound portion in the serum exists mainly in an ionized state. Acidosis increases the un-ionized fraction and promotes the distribution of salicylate into brain, liver, and other tissues. Salicylates are eliminated by both hepatic metabolism and renal excretion. The half-life is 2 to 3 h after a single therapeutic dose. Saturation of hepatic metabolic pathways results in a prolonged half-life (20 to 36 h) following overdose. Alkalinization of the urine to a pH of 8 enhances renal excretion by causing the un-ionized drug in the lumen of the renal tubules to ionize; the ionized drug cannot be reabsorbed.

Clinical Toxicity Manifestations begin 3 to 6 h after overdosage and include vomiting, sweating, tachycardia, hyperpnea, fever, tinnitus, lethargy, confusion, respiratory alkalosis, and an alkaline urine (pH >6). Vomiting, diaphoresis, and hyperventilation may lead to dehydration and acute renal failure. An increased-anion-gap metabolic acidosis with an acidic urine (pH <6) may develop. In cases of severe poisoning, convulsions, coma, respiratory depression, and cardiovascular collapse may ensue. Other complications include cerebral and pulmonary edema and myocardial failure. Elevation of the hematocrit, white blood cell count, and platelet count; hypernatremia; hyperkalemia; hypoglycemia; and prolongation of the prothrombin time may be seen. Acid-base disturbances include respiratory alkalosis coupled with metabolic acidosis (40 to 50 percent), respiratory alkalosis (20 percent), metabolic acidosis (20 percent), and mixed respiratory and metabolic acidosis (5 to 10 percent). Lactic and other organic acids are responsible for an increased anion gap.

Diagnosis Salicylates are identified by a positive ferric chloride test in urine. This test is usually included in routine screening procedures. If not, specific serum measurement must be ordered. In the case of an acute single ingestion, a peak level of less than 3 mmol/L (40 mg/dL) is associated with no symptoms, one of 3 to 7 mmol/L (40 to 100 mg/dL) with mild to moderate manifestations, and one of greater than 7 mmol/L (100 mg/dL) with severe toxicity. Because of delayed and prolonged absorption, levels should be assayed serially. In chronic poisoning, symptoms may occur at levels only slightly above the therapeutic range.

℞ **TREATMENT**

Gastrointestinal decontamination is indicated if an ingested dose is greater than 150 mg/kg body weight. Because of delayed absorption, decontamination may be helpful 12 to 24 h after ingestion. If serum salicylate levels rise, whole-bowel irrigation and/or endoscopic removal of bezoars should be considered. Elimination may be increased by repeated administration of activated charcoal. Parenteral fluids should be given to replace fluid losses and to produce a brisk urine flow. Supplemental glucose and oxygen should be given. Electrolyte and metabolic abnormalities should be corrected. Prolongation of prothrombin time should be corrected with intravenous vitamin K. Seizures should be controlled with benzodiazepines or barbiturates. Myocardial failure should be treated with standard therapy. In symptomatic patients treatment should include saline diuresis and alkalinization of the urine to a pH of 8 to enhance urinary excretion. Depending on severity, one to three ampules (44 to 131 mmol) of bicarbonate and 20 to 60 mmol of potassium should be added to a liter of intravenous fluid containing dextrose and administered at a rate of 2 to 6 mL/kg per hour. Electrolytes, calcium, acid-base status, urine pH, and fluid balance must be monitored carefully during such therapy. When acidosis is present, bicarbonate increases the serum pH and limits the tissue uptake of salicylates. If cerebral or pulmonary edema is present, alkalinization is contraindicated. Salicylates are effectively removed by hemodialysis, which should be considered with severe overdose, cerebral edema, failure of conventional therapy, or compromised renal or hepatic function.

STIMULANTS Amphetamines, bronchodilators such as albuterol and metaproterenol, and decongestants such as ephedrine, pseudoephedrine, phenylephrine, and phenylpropanolamine stimulate alpha- and beta-, beta-, and alpha-adrenergic receptors, respectively. These agents are absorbed rapidly from the gastrointestinal tract, reaching peak plasma levels 1 to 2 h after ingestion. They are weak bases with pK_a values ranging from 8 to 10 and a volume of distribution of 2 to 6 L/kg body weight. These agents are eliminated by a combination of hepatic metabolism and renal excretion of unchanged drug. Excretion is enhanced in an acid urine and slowed in an alkaline urine. Half-lives range from 2 to 8 h to 6 to 34 h, depending on urine flow and pH.

Clinical Toxicity Effects are seen within 30 to 60 min after ingestion and include nausea, vomiting, diarrhea, and abdominal cramps. Talkativeness, irritability, confusion, delirium, headache, combativeness, auditory and visual hallucinations, tremors, tachycardia, palpitations, hypertension, and hyperreflexia are common. Other findings may include dilated pupils, dry mouth, pallor, and tachypnea. Hyperpyrexia, seizures, rhabdomyolysis, hypertensive crisis, intracranial hemorrhage, cardiac arrhythmias, and cardiovascular collapse may occur in cases of severe overdose. Bronchodilators may cause hypotension as a result of beta-adrenergic-mediated vasodilation, and decongestants may cause reflex bradycardia secondary to alpha-adrenergic-mediated hypertension.

Diagnosis This diagnosis is supported by finding these agents in the urine by toxicology screening. Quantitative measurement is not useful.

TREATMENT

Gastrointestinal decontamination should be accomplished as soon as possible. Supportive care includes treatment of agitation and seizures with benzodiazepines or barbiturates; of hypertension with labetalol, nifedipine, or phentolamine; of hyperpyrexia with cooling blankets; and of agitation with sedatives, and, if necessary, with paralyzing agents. Lidocaine and propranolol are preferred for the treatment of ventricular tachyarrhythmias. Although theoretically effective for enhancing drug elimination, acid diuresis is not recommended, owing to lack of documented clinical efficacy and risks of side effects such as worsening of acidosis and triggering of myoglobinuric renal failure.

THEOPHYLLINE Theophylline causes the release of endogenous catecholamines and prolongs their effects by inhibiting the degradation of cyclic AMP by phosphodiesterase. Theophylline is absorbed rapidly from the stomach and upper small bowel. Following overdose, serum levels peak 1 to 2 h after ingestion of liquid preparations, 2 to 4 h after ingestion of tablets, and 6 to 24 h after ingestion of sustained-release preparations. Theophylline is approximately 60 percent bound to albumin and has a low volume of distribution (0.6 L/kg body weight). Therapeutic serum levels are 55 to 110 μmol/L (10 to 20 mg/L). Theophylline is eliminated primarily by hepatic metabolism, which is saturable at levels in the high therapeutic range. The serum half-life, normally 4 to 6 h, is therefore prolonged in overdoses. Only 5 percent of the theophylline is excreted unchanged by the kidneys. Theophylline elimination is also decreased with impaired liver function, congestive heart failure, viral infections, and concomitantly administered drugs such as cimetidine, erythromycin, and quinolone antibiotics.

Clinical Toxicity Effects begin 30 min to 2 h following overdose and include nausea, vomiting, restlessness, irritability, agitation, tachypnea, tachycardia, and muscle tremors. Coma, hypotension, respiratory depression, generalized tonic-clonic and focal convulsions, and rhabdomyolysis may occur in cases of severe poisoning. Convulsions are often protracted, repetitive, and resistant to therapy. Cardiovascular effects include atrial arrhythmias, multifocal premature ventricular contractions, idioventricular rhythms, ventricular tachycardia, and ventricular fibrillation. Metabolic abnormalities include ketosis, metabolic acidosis, increased serum amylase levels, hyperglycemia, and decreased serum levels of potassium, calcium, and phosphorus. Toxicity occurs at lower theophylline levels with chronic than with acute poisoning, and mortality rates are higher after chronic ingestion.

Diagnosis Theophylline is not detected by routine urine screening; measurement of its level in serum must be requested specifically. Cardiac arrhythmias and seizures occur following chronic ingestion at serum levels of 200 to 300 μmol/L (40 to 60 mg/L). Similar toxicity, along with hypotension, hypokalemia, and metabolic abnormalities, generally occurs at levels above 400 to 500 μmol/L (80 to 100 mg/L) following acute overdose. Because of prolonged and delayed absorption after overdosage, levels should be measured serially to determine the peak concentration.

TREATMENT

Initial therapy involves prompt gastrointestinal decontamination. Theophylline is well adsorbed by activated charcoal. With sustained-release forms, decontamination should be considered up to 12 to 24 h following ingestion. Repeated doses of charcoal shorten the serum half-life by approximately 50 percent. Metoclopramide and ondansetron may be necessary for controlling theophylline-induced vomiting. Extreme tachycardia should be treated with propranolol or esmolol. Hypotension is treated with volume expansion or propranolol. Benzodiazepines and barbiturates are useful for convulsions and hyperactivity. Phenytoin is ineffective. Treatment of ventricular tachyarrhythmias should include propranolol as well as standard antiarrhythmics. Diuresis is ineffective for enhancing removal of theophylline. Hemodialysis and hemoperfusion are effective in removing theophylline and are indicated in patients with severe toxicity or with a serum level greater than 500 μmol/L (100 mg/L) after acute overdosage and greater than 300 μmol/L (60 mg/L) with chronic poisoning.

TRICYCLIC ANTIDEPRESSANTS Commonly available tricyclic compounds include amitriptyline, imipramine, chlomipramine, desipramine, doxepin, nortriptyline, protriptyline, and trimipramine. Related agents include amoxapine, bupropion, maprotiline, and trazodone. These agents block reuptake of synaptic transmitters such as norepinephrine, dopamine, and serotonin in the CNS. In addition, they have anticholinergic activity, alpha-adrenergic blocking activity, and quinidine-like effects on the heart. Antidepressants that selectively inhibit the reuptake of serotonin (fluoxetine, paroxetin, sertraline) or norepinephrine and serotonin (venlafaxine) do not cause a toxicity similar to that produced by the tricyclics; CNS depression is mild, and cardiotoxicity is virtually nonexistent.

Tricyclics are well absorbed from the gastrointestinal tract, and serum levels peak within 2 to 6 h of an overdose. In rare cases, anticholinergic effects result in prolonged absorption and delayed peak levels (6 to 12 h following ingestion). Tricyclics exhibit high protein binding in the plasma. They have large volumes of distribution, in the range of 20 to 40 L/kg body weight. Elimination is mainly by hepatic metabolism, with an initial demethylation sometimes generating pharmacologically active metabolites. Subsequent steps of metabolism result in metabolites of increasing polarity, which are then excreted by the kidneys. Less than 5 percent of the parent compound is excreted unchanged in urine. The half-lives of tricyclics and their metabolites range from 25 to 30 h but may be longer in the overdose setting.

Clinical Toxicity Effects generally develop within 30 min of overdose and peak in 2 to 6 h. In cases of low overdose, anticholinergic effects predominate (see "Anticholinergic Agents," above). In cases of high overdose, marked CNS depression is coupled with cardiotoxicity, seizures, and hypotension. Ventricular tachyarrhythmias, atrioventricular and intraventricular conduction delays, terminal bradycardia, and decreased cardiac output may occur. Aspiration pneumonia and pulmonary edema also may develop. In fatal cases death usually occurs either within 6 h of ingestion or much later from multiple organ failure or pulmonary complications. Prolongation of the QRS complex (greater than 100 ms) is a characteristic feature. Increasing duration of the QRS complex correlates with an increased risk of cardiac arrhythmias and seizures. A terminal QRS right-axis deviation and a R wave greater than the S wave in lead AVR of the ECG are sensitive indicators of cardiotoxicity.

Diagnosis The diagnosis is supported by the presence of these drugs in the urine on routine screening tests. Serum levels are diagnostic and generally correlate with severity. Serum levels of active metabolites should be summed with that of the parent compound when estimating the serum concentration. Levels less than about 1000 nmol/L (300 ng/mL) are therapeutic. Levels over 3300 nmol/L (1000 ng/mL) indicate serious poisoning.

TREATMENT

Ipecac-induced emesis is contraindicated with tricyclic ingestions. Gastric lavage is indicated for comatose patients with recent ingestion. Activated charcoal in single and repeated doses should be administered. Treatment includes support of respiration and volume expansion and norepinephrine or high-dose dopamine for hypotension. Seizures should be treated with benzodiazepines and barbiturates. Phenytoin is of uncertain benefit. Acidosis worsens the likelihood of arrhythmias and should be corrected. Sodium bicarbonate should be given as a bolus following a seizure and as an infusion to maintain a serum pH of 7.40 to 7.50 in patients with QRS prolongation. Treatment of ventricular tachyarrhythmias should include sodium bicarbonate (0.5 to 1 mmol/kg of body weight), lidocaine, and bretyllium. Phenytoin is often recommended, but its efficacy is not established. Beta-adrenergic blockers and class 1A antiarrhythmics (quinidine, procainamide, and disopyramide) should be avoided. Cardiac pacing and invasive hemodynamic support may be necessary for severe cardiovascular depression. Physostigmine (see "Anticholinergic Agents," above) will reverse low-dose anticholinergic effects and may be administered in cases of mild poisoning if the ECG is normal and deterioration has been excluded by a suitable period of observation.

BIBLIOGRAPHY

GENERAL ASPECTS

AMDUR MO et al (eds): *Casarett and Doull's Toxicology: The Basic Science of Poisons*, 5th ed. New York, McGraw-Hill, 1996

EPIDEMIOLOGY

LITOVITZ TL et al: 1994 annual report of the American Association of Poison Control Centers Toxic Exposure Surveillance System. Am J Emerg Med 13:551, 1995

DIAGNOSIS

AABAKKEN et al: Osmollal and anion gaps in patients admitted to an emergency medical department. Hum Exp Toxicol 13:131, 1994

BRADBERRY SM, VALE JA: Disturbances of potassium homeostasis in poisoning. Clin Toxicol 33:295, 1995

BRETT AS: Implication of discordance between clinical impression and toxicology analysis in drug overdose. Arch Intern Med 148:437, 1988

COUNCIL OF SCIENTIFIC AFFAIRS, AMERICAN MEDICAL ASSOCIATION: Scientific issues in drug testing. JAMA 257:3110, 1987

HEPLER BR et al: Role of the toxicology lab in the treatment of acute poisoning. Med Toxicol 1:61, 1986

HOFFMAN RS, GOLDFRANK LR: The poisoned patient with altered consciousness. Controversies in the use of the "coma cocktail." JAMA 274:562, 1995

KELLERMANN AL et al: Impact of drug screening in suspected overdose. Ann Emerg Med 16:1206, 1987

OLSON KR et al: Physical assessment and differential diagnosis of the poisoned patient. Med Toxicol 2:52, 1987

OSTER JR et al: Use of the anion gap in clinical medicine. South Med J 81:229, 1988

TREATMENT

ALBERTSON TE et al: Superiority of activated charcoal alone compared with ipecac and activated charcoal in the treatment of acute toxic ingestions. Ann Emerg Med 18:56, 1989

BRETT AS et al: Predicting the clinical course of intentional drug overdose: Implications for utilization of the intensive care unit. Arch Intern Med 147:133, 1987

COOMEY DO: *Activated Charcoal in Medical Applications*. New York, Marcel Dekker, 1995

CURTIS RA et al: Efficacy of ipecac and activated charcoal/cathartic: Prevention of salicylate absorption in a simulated overdose. Arch Intern Med 144:48, 1984

GARRETTSON LK, GELLER RJ: Acid and alkaline diuresis: When are they of value in the treatment of poisoning? Drug Safety 5:220, 1990

GOLDBERG MJ et al: An approach to the management of the poisoned patient. Arch Intern Med 146:1381, 1986

KING WD: Syrup of ipecac: A drug review. Clin Toxicol 17:353, 1980

KORNBERG AE, DOLGIN J: Pediatric ingestions: Charcoal alone versus ipecac and charcoal. Ann Emerg Med 20:648, 1991

KRENZELOK EP et al: Gastrointestinal transit times of cathartics combined with charcoal. Ann Emerg Med 14:1152, 1985

KULIG K et al: Management of acutely poisoned patients without gastric emptying. Ann Emerg Med 14:562, 1985

LITOVITZ TL: The anecdotal antidotes. Emerg Med Clin North Am 2:145, 1984

MANNO BR, MANNO JE: Toxicology of ipecac: A review. Clin Toxicol 10:221, 1977

MCCARRON MM, WOOD JD: The cocaine "body packer" syndrome: Diagnosis and treatment. JAMA 250:1417, 1983

MERRIGIAN KS et al: Prospective evaluation of gastric emptying in the self-poisoned patient. Am J Emerg Med 8:479, 1990

MINOCHA A, SPYKER DA: Acute overdose with sustained-release drug formulations: Perspectives in treatment. Med Toxicol 1:300, 1986

NEUVONEN PJ: Clinical pharmacokinetics of oral activated charcoal in acute intoxications. Clin Pharmacokinet 7:465, 1982

———, OLKKOLA KT: Oral activated charcoal in the treatment of intoxications: Role of single and repeated doses. Med Toxicol 3:33, 1988

PARK GD et al: Expanded role of charcoal in the poisoned and overdosed patient. Arch Intern Med 146:969, 1986

PETERSON RG, PETERSON LN: Cleansing the blood: Hemodialysis, peritoneal dialysis, exchange transfusion, charcoal hemoperfusion, forced diuresis. Pediatr Clin North Am 33:675, 1986

POND SM: Diuresis, dialysis and hemoperfusion: Indications and benefits. Emerg Med Clin North Am 2:29, 1984

ROSENBERG J et al: Pharmacokinetics of drug overdose. Clin Pharmacokinet 6:161, 1981

SHANNON M et al: Carthartics and laxatives: Do they still have a place in management of the poisoned patient? Med Toxicol 1:247, 1986

SPYKER DA, MINOCHA A: Toxicodynamic approach to the management of the poisoned patient. J Emerg Med 6:117, 1988

STEAD AH, MOFFAT AC: A collection of therapeutic, toxic and fatal blood drug concentrations in man. Hum Toxicol 3:437, 1983

STEWART JJ: Effects of emetic and cathartic agents on the gastrointestinal tract and the treatment of toxic ingestion. Clin Toxicol 20:199, 1983

TENEBEIN M: Whole bowel irrigation as a gastrointestinal decontamination procedure after acute poisoning. Med Toxicol 3:77, 1988

——— et al: Efficacy of ipecac-induced emesis, orogastric lavage, and activated charcoal for acute drug overdose. Ann Emerg Med 16:838, 1987

WHEELER-USHER DH et al: Gastric emptying: Risk versus benefit in the treatment of acute poisoning. Med Toxicol 1:142, 1986

ZACCARA G et al: Clinical features, pathogenesis, and management of drug-induced seizures. Drug Safety 5:109, 1990

REFERENCE TEXTS

BASENT RC, CRAVEY RH: *Disposition of Toxic Drugs and Chemicals in Man*, 4th ed. Foster City, CA, Chemical Toxicity Institute, 1995

BLOCK JB: *The Signs and Symptoms of Chemical Exposure*. Springfield, IL, Charles C Thomas, 1980

CLAYTON GD, CLAYTON FE (eds): *Patty's Industrial Hygiene and Toxicology*, 4th ed. New York, Wiley, 1993

DANGAARD J: *Symptoms and Signs in Occupational Disease: A Practical Guide*, Copenhagen, Year Book Medical Publishers, 1978

ELLENHORN MJ, BARCELOUX DG: *Medical Toxicology: Diagnosis and Treatment of Human Poisoning*. New York, Elsevier, 1988

GOLDFRANK LR et al (eds): *Goldfrank's Toxicologic Emergencies*, 5th ed. Norwalk, CT, Appleton and Lange, 1994

GOSSELIN RE: *Clinical Toxicology of Commercial Products: Acute Poisoning*, 5th ed. Baltimore, Williams & Wilkins, 1984

HADDAD LM, WINCHESTER JF: *Clinical Management of Poisoning and Drug Overdose* 2d ed. Philadelphia, Saunders, 1990

HAYES WJ, LAW ER: *Handbook of Pesticide Toxicology*. San Diego, Academic Press, 1991

LAMPE KF, MCCANN MA (eds): *AMA Handbook of Poisonous and Injurious Plants*. Chicago, American Medical Association, 1985

RUMACK BH (eds): *Poisindex Information System* (updated quarterly). Denver, Micromedex

SULLIVAN JB, KRIEGER GR: *Hazardous Materials Toxicology: Clinical Principles of Environmental Health*. Baltimore, Williams & Wilkins, 1992

SPECIFIC POISONS

ACETAMINOPHEN

FLANAGAN RJ: The role of acetylcysteine in clinical toxicology. Med Toxicol 2:93, 1987

PRESCOTT LF: Paracetamol overdose. Drugs 25:290, 1983

SMILKSTEIN MJ et al: Efficacy of oral *N*-acetylcysteine in the treatment of acetaminophen overdose. N Engl J Med 319:1558, 1988

ACIDS AND ALKALIS

ANDERSON KD et al: Controlled trial of corticosteroids in children with corrosive injury of the esophagus. N Engl J Med 323:637, 1990

FRIEDMAN EM, LOVEJOY FH JR: The emergency management of caustic ingestions. Emerg Med Clin North Am 2:77, 1984

HOWELL JM et al: Steroids for the treatment of corrosive esophageal injury: A statistical analysis of past studies. Am J Emerg Med 10:421, 1992

WASON S: The emergency management of caustic ingestions. J Emerg Med 2:175, 1984

ANTIARRHYTHMIC DRUGS

DUNBAR DN, PENTEL PR: Antiarrhythmic drug toxicity, in *Intensive Care Medicine*, 3d ed, JM Rippe et al (eds). Boston, Little, Brown, 1995

Freedman MD et al: Extracorporeal pump assistance—a novel treatment for acute lidocaine poisoning. Eur J Clin Pharmacol 22:129, 1982
Hruby K, Misslivetz J: Poisoning with oral antiarrhythmic drugs. Int J Clin Pharmacol 23:253, 1985
Stratman HG, Kennedy HL: Torsade de pointes associated with drugs and toxins: Recognition and management. Am Heart J 113:1470, 1987

BARBITURATES

Boldy DAR et al: Treatment of phenobarbitone poisoning with repeat oral administration of activated charcoal. Q J Med 235:997, 1986
Matthew H: Barbiturates. Clin Toxicol 8(5):495, 1975
McCarron MM et al: Short-acting barbiturate overdosage: Correlation of intoxication score with serum barbiturate concentration. JAMA 248:55, 1982

BENZODIAZEPINES

Hojer J et al: Diagnostic utility of flumazenil in coma with suspected poisoning: A double-blind, randomized controlled study. BMJ 301:1308, 1990
Kulka PJ, Lauven PM: Benzodiazepine antagonists: An update of their role in the emergency care of overdose patients. Drug Safety 7:381, 1992
The Flumazenil in Benzodiazepine Intoxication Study Group (Bayer MJ et al): Treatment of benzodiazepine overdose with flumazenil. Clin Ther 14:978, 1992

BETA BLOCKERS

Critchley JA, Ungar A: The management of acute poisoning due to beta-adrenoreceptor antagonists. Med Tox Adverse Drug Exp 4:32, 1989
Heath A: β-Adrenoceptor blocker toxicity: Clinical features and therapy. Am J Emerg Med 2:518, 1984
Weinstein RS: Recognition and management of poisoning with beta-adrenergic blocking agents. Ann Emerg Med 13:1123, 1984

CALCIUM CHANNEL BLOCKERS

Herrington DM et al: Nifedipine overdose. Am J Cardiol 81:344, 1986
McMillan R: Management of acute severe verapamil intoxication. J Emerg Med 6:193, 1988
Snover SW, Bocchino V: Massive diltiazem overdose. Ann Emerg Med 15:1221, 1986

CARBON MONOXIDE

Dolan MC: Carbon monoxide poisoning. Can Med Assoc J 133:392, 1985; Symposium—carbon monoxide poisoning—mechanism of damage, late sequelae and therapy. Clin Toxicol 23:247, 1985
Mofenson HC et al: Carbon monoxide poisoning. Am J Emerg Med 2:254, 1984
Tibbles PM, Perrotta PL: Treatment of carbon monoxide poisoning: A critical review of human outcome studies comparing normobaric oxygen with hyperbaric oxygen. Ann Emerg Med 24:269, 1994

CYANIDE

Caraveti M, Litovitz T: Pediatric cyanide intoxication and death from acetonitrile-containing cosmetic. JAMA 260:3740, 1988
Graham DL et al: Acute cyanide poisoning complicated by lactic acidosis and pulmonary edema. Arch Intern Med 137:1051, 1977
Hall AH et al: Clinical toxicology of cyanide: North American clinical experiences, in *Clinical and Experimental Toxicology of Cyanides*, B Ballantyne, TC Marrs (eds). Bristol, Wright, 1987, p 312

DIGOXIN

Smith TW et al: Digitalis glycosides: Mechanisms and manifestations of toxicity. Prog Cardiovasc Dis 26:413, 1984 (part I); 26:495, 1984 (part II); 27:26, 1984 (part III)
Taboulet P et al: Clinical features and management of digitalis poisoning—rationale for immunotherapy. Clin Toxicol 31:247, 1993
Wenger TL et al: Treatment of 63 severely digitalis-toxic patients with digoxin-specific antibody fragments. J Am Coll Cardiol 5:118A, 1985

ETHYLENE GLYCOL

Gabow PA et al: Organic acids in ethylene glycol intoxication. Ann Intern Med 105:16, 1986
Jacobsen D, McMartin KE: Methanol and ethylene glycol poisonings: Mechanism of toxicity, clinical course, diagnosis and treatment. Med Toxicol 1:309, 1986
Parry MF, Wallach R: Ethylene glycol poisoning. Am J Med 57:143, 1974

HYDROCARBONS

Anas N et al: Criteria for hospitalizing children who have ingested products containing hydrocarbons. JAMA 246:840, 1981
Streichen M et al: Syndromes of solvent sniffing in adults. Ann Intern Med 94:785, 1981
Truempier E et al: Clinical characteristics, pathophysiology and management of hydrocarbon ingestion: Case report and review of the literature. Pediatr Emerg Care 3:187, 1987

HYDROGEN SULFIDE

Hoidal CR et al: Hydrogen sulfide poisoning from toxic inhalations of roofing fumes. Ann Emerg Med 15:826, 1986
Smith RP: Management of acute sulfide poisoning. Arch Environ Health 31:166, 1976
Whitecraft DD et al: Hydrogen sulfide poisoning treated with hyperbaric oxygen. J Emerg Med 3:23, 1985

IRON

Banner W et al: Iron poisoning. Pediatr Clin North Am 33:393, 1986
Proudfoot AT et al: Management of acute iron poisoning. Med Toxicol 1:83, 1986
Tenebein M et al: Myocardial failure and shock in iron poisoning. Hum Toxicol 7:281, 1988

ISONIAZID

Orlowski JP et al: Treatment of potentially lethal dose isoniazid ingestion. Ann Emerg Med 17:73, 1988
Wason S et al: Single high-dose pyridoxine treatment for isoniazid overdose. JAMA 246:1102, 1981
Yarbrough B, Wood J: Isoniazid overdose treated with high-dose pyridoxine. Ann Emerg Med 12:303, 1983

ISOPROPYL ALCOHOL

Lacouture PG et al: A review of acute isopropyl alcohol intoxication: Diagnosis and management. Am J Med 75:680, 1983
Natowicz M et al: Pharmacokinetic analysis of a case of isopropyl intoxication. Clin Chem 31:326, 1985

LITHIUM

Amdisen A: Clinical features and management of lithium poisoning. Med Toxicol 3:18, 1988
Dyson EH et al: Self-poisoning and therapeutic intoxication with lithium. Human Toxicol 6:326, 1987

MAO INHIBITORS

Kaplan RF et al: Phenelzine overdose treated with dantrolene sodium. JAMA 255:642, 1986
Linden CH: Monoamine oxidase inhibitor overdose. Ann Emerg Med 13:1137, 1984

METHANOL

Jacobsen D, McMartin KE: Methanol and ethylene glycol poisoning: Mechanism of toxicity, clinical course, diagnosis and treatment. Med Toxicol 1:309, 1986
Osterloh JD et al: Serum formate concentrations in methanol intoxication as a criterion for hemodialysis. Ann Intern Med 104:200, 1986
Swartz RD et al: Epidemic methanol poisoning: Clinical and biochemical analysis of a recent episode. Medicine 60:373, 1981

METHEMOGLOBINEMIA

Curry S: Methemoglobinemia. Ann Emerg Med 11:214, 1982
Hall AH et al: Drug and chemical-induced methaemoglobinaemia. Med Toxicol 1:253, 1986
Harvey JW, Keitt AS: Studies of the efficacy and potential hazards of methylene blue therapy in aniline-induced methaemoglobinaemia. Br J Haematol 53:29, 1983

MUSCLE RELAXANTS

Bailey DN: Meprobamate ingestion: A five-year review of cases with serum concentrations and clinical findings. Am J Clin Pathol 75:102, 1981
Cohen MD et al: Atropine in the treatment of baclofen overdose. Am J Emerg Med 4:552, 1986

NONSTEROIDAL ANTI-INFLAMMATORY DRUGS

Court H, Volans GN: Poisoning after overdose with nonsteroidal anti-inflammatory drugs. Adverse Drug React Acute Poisoning Rev 3:1, 1984

HALL AH et al: Ibuprofen overdose: 126 cases. Ann Emerg Med 15:1308, 1986
VALE JA, MEREDITH TJ: Acute poisoning due to nonsteroidal anti-inflammatory drugs: Clinical features and management. Med Toxicol 1:11, 1986

ORGANOPHOSPHATE AND CARBAMATE INSECTICIDES

MINTON NA, MURRAY VSG: A review of organophosphate poisoning. Med Toxicol 3:350, 1988
NAMBA T et al: Poisoning due to organophosphate insecticides. Am J Med 50:475, 1971
SENANAYAKE N, KARALLIEDDE L: Neurotoxic effects of organophosphorus insecticides: An intermediate syndrome. N Engl J Med 316:761, 1987

PHENOTHIAZINES

BARRY D et al: Phenothiazine poisoning: A review of 48 cases. Calif Med 118:1, 1983
BENOWITZ NL et al: Cardiopulmonary catastrophes in drug-overdosed patients. Med Clin North Am 63:267, 1979
BORYS DJ et al: Acute fluoxetine overdose: A report of 234 cases. Am J Emerg Med 10:115, 1992
LEE A: Treatment of drug-induced dystonic reactions. J Am Coll Emerg Phys 8:453, 1979

SALICYLATES

BRENNER BE, SIMON RR: Management of salicylate intoxication. Drugs 24:335, 1987
GAUDREAULT P et al: The relative severity of acute vs chronic salicylate poisoning in children: A clinical comparison. Pediatrics 70:566, 1982
TEMPLE AR: Acute and chronic effects of aspirin toxicity and their treatment. Arch Intern Med 141:364, 1981
THISTED B et al: Acute salicylate poisoning in 177 consecutive patients treated in an ICU. Acta Anaesthesiol Scand 31:312, 1987

STIMULANTS

AARON CK: Sympathomimetics. Emerg Med Clin North Am 8:513, 1990
LINDEN CH et al: Amphetamines. Top Emerg Med 7:18, 1985
PENTEL P: Toxicity of over-the-counter stimulants. JAMA 252:1898, 1984

THEOPHYLLINE

GAUDREAULT P, GUAY J: Theophylline poisoning. Med Toxicol 1:169, 1986
OLSON KR et al: Theophylline overdose: Acute single ingestion versus chronic repeated overmedication. Am J Emerg Med 3:386, 1985
PARK GD et al: Use of hemoperfusion for treatment of theophylline intoxication. Am J Med 74:961, 1983
SHANNON MW, LOVEJOY FH JR: The influence of age versus peak concentration on life-threatening events after chronic theophylline intoxication. Arch Intern Med 150:2045, 1990

TRICYCLIC ANTIDEPRESSANTS

BOEHNERT MT, LOVEJOY FH JR: Value of QRS duration versus the serum drug level in predicting seizures and ventricular arrhythmias after an acute overdose of tricyclic antidepressants. N Engl J Med 313:474, 1985
CROME P: Poisoning due to tricyclic antidepressant overdose. Med Toxicol 1:261, 1986
FROMMER DA et al: Tricyclic antidepressant overdose: A review. JAMA 257:521, 1987
LIEBETT EL et al: ECG lead a VR versus QRS in predicting seizures and arrhythmias in acute tricyclic antidepressant toxicity. Ann Emerg Med 26:195, 1995

392

Robert L. Norris, Scott Oslund, Paul S. Auerbach

DISORDERS CAUSED BY REPTILE BITES AND MARINE ANIMAL ENVENOMATIONS

Few topics in medicine are as controversial or as influenced by tradition as the management of bites and stings from venomous creatures. Because the incidence of serious bites and stings is relatively low in developed nations, there is a paucity of relevant clinical research and literature, and therapeutic decision-making is often based on anecdotal information. Furthermore, the different responses of different species to various toxins make it difficult to extrapolate data from animal studies to clinical application. This chapter outlines general principles for the evaluation and management of victims of venom poisoning by certain reptiles and marine creatures and presents a clinical approach to these emergencies.

VENOMOUS SNAKEBITE

EPIDEMIOLOGY The venomous snakes of the world are classified in Table 392-1. A number of snakes in the family Colubridae (traditionally thought of as harmless snakes) can be dangerous to humans because of toxic salivary secretions. The incidence of venomous snakebites is low in most developed countries, but in regions of the world where people are engaged in manual agriculture, often with exposed lower extremities, attack rates are higher. About 30,000 to 40,000 persons die each year from venomous snakebite; incomplete reporting in disadvantaged regions probably makes this range an underestimate.

ANATOMY The typical snake-venom apparatus consists of paired venom glands—one on each side of the head, below and behind the eye—connected by ducts to hollow, anterior maxillary teeth. In viperids, these teeth are large, mobile fangs that retract against the roof of the mouth when the animal is at rest. In elapids and sea snakes, the fangs are only slightly enlarged and are fixed in an erect position. For reasons that are unclear but may be related to the venom apparatus itself, venomous snakes can bite without injecting any venom. Approximately 20 percent of pit viper bites and an even higher percentage of bites inflicted by some other snake families (up to 75 percent for sea snakes) are "dry."

Differentiation of venomous from nonvenomous snake species can be difficult unless one is familiar with local fauna. Viperids are characterized by somewhat triangular heads (a feature shared with many harmless snakes); elliptical pupils (also seen in the nonvenomous boas and pythons as well as some colubrids); enlarged maxillary fangs; subcaudal scalation that involves a single scale running the full width of the ventral surface of the tail for several rows just distal to the anal plate (as opposed to the two scales in each subcaudal row in most nonvenomous snakes); and, in the case of the pit vipers, the heat-sensing pits (foveal organs) for which they are named, located slightly inferior and anterior to the eyes on each side. Color pattern is notoriously unhelpful in identifying most venomous snakes except for the coral snakes, whose other body characteristics are similar to those of harmless colubrids. The American coral snakes can be identified by red, yellow (or white), and black bands completely encircling the body; a few species have red and black bands only. North of Mexico City, the immediate contiguity of red and yellow bands is fairly reliable for distinguishing a coral snake from one of its harmless colubrid mimics. Further south, differentiation by color pattern is less reliable.

Immunodiagnostic techniques have been developed for species identification of the snakes involved in bites. An enzyme-linked immunoassay (ELISA) can be used to identify a specific type of snake venom in a victim's blood, wound aspirate, or urine, and this method is finding clinical application around the world. However, no commercial ELISA kit is currently available in the United States.

VENOMS AND CLINICAL MANIFESTATIONS Snake venoms are complex mixtures of enzymes, low-molecular-weight polypeptides, glycoproteins, and metal ions. The enzymes and polypeptides affect the human body in a multisystem fashion. Among the deleterious components are hemorrhagins that render the vasculature leaky and thus cause both local and systemic bleeding; various proteolytic enzymes that cause local tissue necrosis, affect the coagulation pathway at various steps, or impair organ function; myocardial depressant factors that reduce cardiac output; and neurotoxins that act either pre- or postsynaptically to inhibit peripheral nerve impulses. Most snake venoms can adversely affect multiple organs.

℞ TREATMENT

Field Management First-aid or "field" measures to be used in the management of venomous snakebite should focus on delivery of the victim to definitive medical care as quickly as possible; the victim should be as inactive as is feasible to limit systemic spread of the venom. Beyond this, any measure employed should at least do no further harm.

After viperid bites, local mechanical suction may be beneficial if applied to the puncture wounds within 3 to 5 min. A useful device is the Extractor (Sawyer Products, Safety Harbor, FL), which delivers one atmosphere of negative pressure to the wound. Suction should be continued for at least 30 min. Mouth suction should be avoided as it inoculates the wound with oral flora and theoretically can also result in the absorption of venom by the rescuer through lesions of the upper digestive tract. A proximal lymphatic-occlusive constriction band may limit the spread of venom if applied within 30 min. To avoid compounding of tissue necrosis, however, the band should not be allowed to interrupt arterial flow. A bitten extremity should be splinted if possible and kept at approximately heart level. Incisions into the bite site should never be made, and no form of cooling or electric shock is advantageous.

For elapid or sea snake bites, the Australian pressure-immobilization technique, in which the entire bitten extremity is wrapped with an elastic or crepe bandage and then splinted, is highly beneficial. The bandage is applied as tightly as it would be to treat a sprained ankle. This technique greatly restricts the absorption and circulation of venom from the bite site. However, an assessment of the potential utility of this method in viperid poisoning requires further research, as it may compound local tissue damage following these bites.

Hospital Management Once in the hospital, the victim should be closely monitored (vital signs, cardiac rhythm, and oxygen saturation) while a history is quickly obtained and a brief but thorough physical examination is performed. The level of erythema/swelling in a bitten extremity should be marked and the circumferences measured in several locations every 15 min until swelling has stabilized. Large-bore intravenous access in unaffected extremities should be obtained in the event that hypotension develops. Early hypotension is due to pooling of blood in the pulmonary and splanchnic vascular beds; hours later, hemolysis and loss of intravascular volume into soft tissues may play important roles. Fluid resuscitation with normal saline or Ringer's lactate should be initiated for clinical shock. If the blood pressure response is inadequate after the administration of 20 to 40 mL/kg body weight, then a trial of 5% albumin (10 to 20 mL/kg) is in order. If volume resuscitation fails to improve tissue perfusion, vasopressors (e.g., dopamine) should be administered. Invasive hemodynamic monitoring (central venous and/or pulmonary arterial pressures) can be helpful in such cases. Central access must be obtained with extra caution if coagulopathy is evident.

Blood should be drawn for laboratory evaluation (including determination of blood type and cross-matching) as soon as possible, before the effects of circulating venom interfere with typing. Also important are a complete blood count to evaluate the degree of hemorrhage or hemolysis, studies of renal and hepatic function, coagulation studies to identify signs of consumptive coagulopathy, and testing of urine for blood or myoglobin. In severe cases or in the face of significant comorbidity, arterial blood gas studies, electrocardiography, and chest radiography may be necessary.

Attempts to locate a source of appropriate antivenin should begin early in all cases of known venomous snakebite, regardless of symptoms. If signs or symptoms develop, they may progress rapidly, making any delay in the administration of antivenin dangerous for the victim. Antivenins rarely offer cross-protection against snake species other than those used in their production unless the species are closely related. An example of good cross-protection is in the use of Australian tiger snake (*Notechis scutatus*) antivenin for sea snake bites (see below). The package insert accompanying a particular antivenin should be consulted for information regarding the spectrum of coverage. In the United States, assistance in finding antivenin can be obtained 24 hours a day from the University of Arizona Poison and Drug Information Center (520-626-6016).

Rapidly progressive and severe local findings (soft tissue swelling, ecchymosis, petechiae, etc.) or manifestations of systemic toxicity (signs and symptoms or laboratory abnormalities) are indications for the administration of intravenous antivenin. The package insert outlines techniques for reconstitution of antivenin (when necessary), skin-testing procedures (for potential allergy), and appropriate starting doses. Most antivenins are of equine origin and carry a risk of anaphylactic, anaphylactoid, and delayed-hypersensitivity reactions. Skin testing does not always reliably predict which patients will have an allergic reaction to equine antivenin; a skin test can be either false negative or false positive. Before antivenin infusion, the patient should receive appropriate loading doses of intravenous antihistamines (e.g., diphenhydramine, 1 mg/kg to a maximum of 100 mg; and cimetidine, 5 to 10 mg/kg to a maximum of 300 mg) in an effort to limit acute reactions. Expanding the patient's intravascular volume with crystalloids may also be beneficial in this regard (unless contraindicated by the patient's cardiac status). Epinephrine should be immediately available, and the antivenin dose to be administered should be diluted (e.g., in 1000 mL of normal saline, Ringer's lactate, or 5% dextrose in water for adults or in 20 mL/kg for children). This volume can be decreased if necessary for the treatment of patients with compromised cardiovascular reserve. The antivenin infusion should be started slowly, with the physician at the bedside to intervene in the event of an acute reaction. The rate of infusion can be increased gradually in the absence of allergic phenomena until the total starting dose has been administered (over a period of 1 to 4 h). Further antivenin may be necessary if clinical abnormalities worsen. Laboratory values should be rechecked hourly, particularly if abnormal, until stability is ensured.

The management of a life-threatening envenomation in a victim with an apparent allergy to antivenin requires significant expertise. Consultation with a poison specialist, an intensive care specialist, or an allergist is recommended. Often, antivenin can still be adminis-

Table 392-1

Venomous Snakes of the World

Family	Subfamily	Representative Species	Remarks
Viperidae	Crotalinae	Rattlesnakes (*Crotalus* and *Sistrurus* species), water moccasins and copperheads (*Agkistrodon* species), lancehead vipers (*Bothrops* species)	New World and Asian pit vipers
	Viperinae	Russell's viper (*Vipera russelli*), saw-scaled viper (*Echis carinatus*), puff adder (*Bitis arietans*)	European, Asian, African vipers
Elapidae		Cobras (*Naja* species), mambas (*Dendroaspis* species), taipan (*Oxyuranus scutellatus*)	Temperate and tropical New and Old World; all venomous terrestrial snakes of Australia
Hydrophiidae		Pelagic sea snake (*Pelamis platurus*)	Pacific and Indian oceans
Atractaspididae		Burrowing asps (*Atractaspis* species)	Africa, Middle East
Colubridae		Boomslang (*Dispholidus typus*), twig snake (*Thelotornis kirtlandii*)	Rear-fanged snakes with toxic salivary secretions

tered in these situations under closely controlled conditions and with intensive premedication (e.g., with epinephrine, antihistamines, and steroids).

Care of the bite wound should include application of a dry sterile dressing and splinting of the extremity with padding between the digits. Because of the risk of central spread of venom, an extremity should be elevated only when antivenin is available. Tetanus immunization should be updated as appropriate. The use of prophylactic antibiotics is controversial, as the incidence of secondary infection following venomous snakebite appears to be low. Many authorities, however, prescribe a broad-spectrum antibiotic (such as ampicillin or a cephalosporin) for the first few days.

If swelling in the bitten extremity raises concern that subfascial muscle edema may be impeding tissue perfusion (muscle-compartment syndrome), intracompartmental pressures should be checked by any minimally invasive technique (e.g., the wick catheter). If pressures are elevated, prompt surgical consultation for possible fasciotomy should be obtained while antivenin administration continues. Compartment syndromes, however, are quite rare after snakebites.

Whether or not antivenin is given, any patient with signs of venom poisoning should be admitted to the hospital for observation for at least 24 h. A patient with an apparently "dry" bite should be watched for at least 6 to 8 h before discharge. An occasional viperid "dry" bite progresses to significant toxicity after a delay of several hours, and the onset of systemic symptoms is commonly delayed for a number of hours after bites by several of the elapids (especially the coral snakes) and sea snakes. Patients bitten by these reptiles should be observed in the hospital for 24 h.

MORBIDITY AND MORTALITY The overall mortality rates for venomous snakebite are low in areas of the world with rapid access to medical care and appropriate antivenin. In the United States, for example, the mortality rate is <1 percent for victims who receive antivenin. Eastern and western diamondback rattlesnakes (*Crotalus adamanteus* and *Crotalus atrox*, respectively) are responsible for most snakebite deaths in the United States. Snakes responsible for large numbers of deaths in other regions of the world include the cobras (*Naja* species) of Asia and Africa, the carpet and saw-scaled vipers of the Middle East and Africa (*Echis* species), Russell's viper (*Vipera russelli*) of the Middle East and Asia, the large African vipers (*Bitis* species), and the lancehead pit vipers of Central and South America (*Bothrops* species).

The incidence of morbidity in terms of permanent functional loss in a bitten extremity is difficult to estimate but is probably substantial. Such loss may be due to muscle, nerve, or vascular injury or to scar contracture. In the United States, such loss due to snakebite tends to be much more common and severe after rattlesnake bites than after bites by copperheads or water moccasins.

LIZARD BITES

Bites from the two species of venomous lizards (the gila monster, *Heloderma suspectum*, of the southwestern United States and the Mexican beaded lizard, *Heloderma horridum*) are infrequent and usually follow attempts to capture or handle these creatures. The wounds are characterized by soft tissue trauma with surrounding local edema and occasionally local cyanosis and ecchymosis. Broken teeth may be embedded in the wounds. The venom contains proteases and phospholipases, and systemic effects may include hypotension, weakness, dizziness, and diaphoresis.

First-aid measures for these bites best follow the guidelines listed above for viperid bites. If the biting lizard is still attached to the victim, mechanical opening of its jaws may be required for its removal.

The sparseness of the data on the pathophysiologic effects of helodermatid venom precludes specific recommendations regarding laboratory evaluation, but routine studies (complete blood count, coagulation studies, electrolyte analysis, blood typing and cross-matching, urinalysis, and electrocardiography) are prudent in anything other than a trivial envenomation. Wounds should be cleansed thoroughly and irrigated when possible. Tetanus immunization should be updated as indicated. Soft tissue radiography of the bite site and sterile probing under local anesthesia may identify retained teeth. An extremity should be splinted and elevated, but antibiotic treatment is not usually required. Systemic care is supportive (e.g., use of intravenous normal saline or Ringer's lactate for hypotension). No commercial antivenin exists. Pain due to local venom effects and mechanical trauma can be treated with opiates and regional nerve blocks. The mortality rate is extremely low.

MARINE ENVENOMATIONS

Management of venom poisoning by marine creatures is similar to that of venomous snakebite in that much of the treatment administered is supportive in nature. A few specific marine antivenins can be used when appropriate.

INVERTEBRATES Hydroids, fire coral, jellyfish, Portuguese man-of-war, and sea anemones possess specialized stinging cells called nematocysts. The venoms from these organisms are mixtures of proteins, carbohydrates, and other components. The clinical syndrome following envenomation by any of these species is similar but of variable severity. Victims usually report immediate prickling or burning, pruritus, paresthesia, and painful throbbing with radiation. A legion of neurologic, cardiovascular, respiratory, rheumatologic, gastrointestinal, renal, and ocular symptoms have been described. Victims in unstable condition with hypotension or respiratory distress should be treated supportively. During stabilization, the skin should be immediately decontaminated with a forceful jet of vinegar (5% acetic acid) or rubbing alcohol (40% to 70% isopropyl alcohol), which inactivates nematocysts. For the venomous box-jellyfish (*Chironex fleckeri*), vinegar should be used. Perfume, aftershave lotion, and high-proof ethanol are less efficacious and may in fact be detrimental. Shaving the skin helps remove remaining nematocysts. Freshwater irrigation and rubbing lead to further stinging by adherent nematocysts and should be avoided. After decontamination, application of anesthetic ointments (lidocaine, benzocaine), antihistamine creams (diphenhydramine), or steroid lotions (hydrocortisone) may be helpful. Persistent pain following decontamination may be treated with morphine or meperidine. Muscle spasms may respond to 10% calcium gluconate (5 to 10 mL) or diazepam (5 to 10 mg) given intravenously. An antivenin is available from Commonwealth Serum Laboratories (see last section of this chapter) for stings from the venomous box-jellyfish found in Australian waters.

Touching of a sea sponge may result in dermatitis. If contact occurs, the skin should be gently dried and adhesive tape used to remove embedded spicules. Vinegar should be applied immediately and then for 10 to 30 min three or four times a day. Rubbing alcohol may be used if vinegar is unavailable. After spicule removal and skin decontamination, a steroid or antihistamine cream may be applied to the skin. Severe vesiculation should be treated with a 2-week course of systemic glucocorticoids.

Annelid worms (bristleworms) possess rows of soft, cactus-like spines capable of inflicting painful stings. Contact results in symptoms similar to those of nematocyst envenomation. Without treatment, pain usually subsides over several hours, but inflammation may persist for up to a week. Victims should resist the urge to scratch, since scratching may fracture retrievable spines. Visible bristles should be removed with forceps and adhesive tape, a commercial facial peel, or a thin layer of rubber cement. Use of vinegar, rubbing alcohol, or dilute ammonia or a brief application of unseasoned meat tenderizer (papain) may provide additional relief. Local inflammation should be treated with topical or systemic glucocorticoids.

Sea urchins possess either hollow, venom-filled, calcified spines or triple-jawed, globiferous pedicellariae with venom glands. Their venom contains several toxic components, including steroid glycosides, hemolysins, proteases, serotonin, and cholinergic substances.

Contact with either of the venom apparatuses produces immediate and intensely painful stings. The affected part should be immersed immediately in hot water (see below). Accessible embedded spines should be removed but may break off and remain lodged in the victim. Residual dye from the surface of a spine remaining after the spine's removal may mimic retained spines but is otherwise of no consequence. Soft tissue radiography or magnetic resonance imaging can confirm the presence of retained spines; this finding may warrant referral for attempted surgical removal if the spines are located near vital structures (e.g., joints, neurovascular bundles). Retained spines may cause the formation of granulomas that are amenable to excision or to intralesional injection with triamcinolone hexacetonide (5 mg/mL).

Cone shells are predatory, carnivorous mollusks. The most dangerous of these creatures are found in the Indian and Pacific oceans. A neurotoxic venom comprising multiple peptides is delivered through harpoon-like darts propelled from an extensible proboscis. Clinically, the sting is like that of a bee. The victim may report wound, perioral, and generalized paresthesia. Bulbar dysfunction and systemic muscular paralysis indicate severe envenomation. The sting of the geographer cone (*Conus geographus*) can cause cerebral edema, coma, and death due to respiratory or cardiac failure. Immediately after envenomation, a circumferential pressure-immobilization dressing 15 cm wide should be applied over a gauze pad measuring approximately 7 cm by 7 cm by 2 cm that has been placed directly over the sting. The dressing should be applied at venous-lymphatic pressure with the preservation of distal arterial pulses. Once the victim has been transported to the nearest medical facility, the bandage can be released. Provision should be made for cardiovascular and respiratory support.

Serious envenomations and deaths have followed bites of the Australian blue-ringed octopuses (*Octopus maculosus* and *Octopus lunulata*). Although these animals rarely exceed 20 cm in length, their venom contains a potent neurotoxin (maculotoxin) that inhibits peripheral nerve transmission by blocking sodium conductance. Within several minutes of a serious envenomation, oral and facial numbness develops and rapidly progresses to total flaccid paralysis, including failure of respiratory muscles. If respirations are assisted, the victim may remain awake although completely paralyzed. Since there is no antidote, treatment is supportive. Immediately after envenomation, attempts should be made to limit the dispersion of venom by application of a pressure-immobilization or a venous-lymphatic pressure dressing. Hot-water immersion and cryotherapy are ineffective. Artificial respiration should be provided. Even with serious envenomations, significant recovery often takes place within 4 to 10 h. Sequelae are uncommon unless related to hypoxia.

VERTEBRATES A number of marine vertebrates, including stingrays, scorpionfish, catfish, surgeonfish, and weeverfish, are capable of envenoming humans. The management of most of these stings is similar.

A stingray injury is both an envenomation and a traumatic wound. The venom, which contains serotonin, 5′-nucleotidase, and phosphodiesterase, causes immediate and intense pain that may last up to 48 h. Systemic effects include weakness, diaphoresis, nausea, vomiting, diarrhea, dysrhythmias, syncope, hypotension, muscle cramps, fasciculations, paralysis, and (in rare cases) death.

The designation *scorpionfish* encompasses members of the family Scorpaenidae and in fact includes not only scorpionfish but also lionfish and stonefish. A complex venom with neuromuscular toxicity is delivered through 12 or 13 dorsal, two pelvic, and three anal spines. Pectoral spines do not contain venom. The severity of envenomation depends on the species of fish, the number of stings, and the amount of venom released. In general, the sting of a stonefish is regarded as the most serious (severe to life-threatening); that of the scorpionfish is of intermediate seriousness; and that of the lionfish is the least serious. Like that of a stingray, the sting of a scorpionfish is immediately and intensely painful. Pain from a stonefish envenomation may last for days. The systemic manifestations are similar to those of stingray envenomations but may be more pronounced, particularly in the case of a stonefish sting. The rare deaths following stonefish envenomation usually occur within 6 to 8 h.

Two species of marine catfish, *Plotosus lineatus* (the oriental catfish) and *Galeichthys felis* (the common sea catfish), as well as several species of freshwater catfish are capable of stinging humans. Venom is delivered through a single dorsal spine and two pectoral spines. Clinically, a catfish sting is comparable to that of a stingray, although marine catfish envenomations are generally more severe than those of their freshwater counterparts. Surgeonfish (doctorfish, tang), weeverfish, and horned venomous sharks have also been implicated in human envenomations.

The stings of stingrays, scorpionfish (lionfish, scorpionfish, stonefish), catfish, weeverfish, venomous horned sharks, and surgeonfish are treated in a similar fashion. Except for stonefish and serious scorpionfish envenomations (see below), no antivenin is available. The affected part should be immersed immediately in nonscalding hot water (113°F/45°C) for 30 to 90 min or until there is significant relief of pain. This measure also helps to inactivate the heat-labile components of the venoms. Recurrent pain may respond to repeated hot-water treatment. Cryotherapy is contraindicated. Opiates will help alleviate the pain, as will local wound infiltration or regional nerve block with 1% lidocaine, 0.5% bupivacaine, and sodium bicarbonate mixed in a 5:5:1 ratio. After soaking and anesthetic administration, the wound must be explored and debrided. Radiography may be helpful in the identification and location of foreign bodies. After exploration and debridement, the wound should be vigorously irrigated with warm sterile water, saline, or 1% povidone-iodine in solution. Unless immediate wound closure is necessary for hemostasis, wounds should be left open to heal by secondary intention or to undergo delayed primary closure. Tetanus immunization should be updated. Antibiotic treatment should be considered for serious wounds and for envenomation in immunocompromised hosts. The initially administered antibiotics should cover *Staphylococcus* and *Streptococcus* species. If the victim is immunocompromised or an infection develops, antibiotic coverage should be broadened to include *Vibrio* species.

SOURCES OF ANTIVENINS AND OTHER ASSISTANCE An antivenin for stonefish (and severe scorpionfish) envenomation made in Australia by the Commonwealth Serum Laboratories (CSL; 45 Poplar Road, Parkville, Victoria, Australia 3052; 61-3-389-1911; fax: 61-3-389-1434) is available in the United States through the pharmacies of Sharp Cabrillo Hospital Emergency Department, San Diego, CA, at (619) 221-3429, and Community Hospital of Monterey Peninsula (CHOMP) Emergency Department, Monterey, CA, at (408) 625-4900.

Polyvalent sea snake antivenin is available from CSL or CHOMP. If sea snake antivenin is unavailable, tiger snake (*N. scutatus*) antivenin should be used.

Divers Alert Network, a nonprofit organization designed to assist in the care of injured divers, may also help with the treatment of marine injuries. The network can be reached 24 h a day at (919) 684-8111 or on the Internet at http://www.dan.ycg.org.

BIBLIOGRAPHY

SNAKES AND LIZARDS

Dart RC et al: Validation of a severity score for the assessment of crotalid snakebite. Ann Emerg Med 27:321, 1996

Kunkel DB et al: Reptile envenomations. J Toxicol Clin Toxicol 21:503, 1983–1984

Minton SA, Norris RL: Non-North American venomous reptile bites, in *Wilderness Medicine: Management of Wilderness and Environmental Emergencies,* 3d ed, PS Auerbach (ed). St. Louis, Mosby, 1995, pp 710–730

Russell FE: *Snake Venom Poisoning.* New York, Scholium International, 1983

Sullivan JB et al: North American venomous reptile bites, in *Wilderness Medicine: Management of Wilderness and Environmental Emergencies,* 3d ed, PS Auerbach (ed). St. Louis, Mosby, 1995, pp 680–709

Swaroop S, Grab B: Snakebite mortality in the world. Bull World Health Org 10:35, 1954

MARINE CREATURES

AUERBACH PS: Marine envenomation, in *Wilderness Medicine: Management of Wilderness and Environmental Emergencies,* 3d ed, PS Auerbach (ed). St. Louis, Mosby, 1995, pp 1327–1374

———: Marine envenomations. N Engl J Med 325:486, 1991

BROWN CK, SHEPHERD SM: Marine trauma, envenomations, and intoxications. Emerg Med Clin North Am 10:385, 1992

HALSTEAD BW, AUERBACH PS: *Dangerous Aquatic Animals of the World: A Color Atlas: With Prevention, First Aid, and Emergency Treatment Procedures.* Princeton, Darwin Press, 1992, 29–124, 241–252

MEIER J, WHITE J (eds): *Handbook of Clinical Toxicology of Animal Venoms and Poisons.* Boca Raton, FL, CRC Press, 1996, pp 89–176

393

James H. Maguire, Andrew Spielman

ECTOPARASITE INFESTATIONS AND ARTHROPOD BITES AND STINGS

Ectoparasites are arthropods or helminths that *infest* the skin of other animals from which they derive sustenance. They may penetrate beneath the surface of the host or attach superficially by their mouthparts. These organisms damage their hosts by inflicting direct injury, by eliciting a hypersensitivity reaction, or by inoculating toxins or pathogens. The main medically important ectoparasites are arachnids (including mites and ticks), insects (including lice, fleas, and flies), pentastomes (tongue worms), and leeches. Arthropods may also harm humans through brief encounters in which they take a blood meal or attempt to defend themselves by biting, stinging, or inoculating venoms. Various arachnids (spiders, scorpions), insects (including bees, hornets, wasps, ants, flies, bugs, caterpillars, and beetles), millipedes, and centipedes produce ill effects in this manner. More people in the United States die each year as a consequence of arthropod stings than from poisonous snake bites.

ECTOPARASITE INFESTATIONS

SCABIES The human itch mite, *Sarcoptes scabiei*, which infests some 300 million persons each year, is one of the most common causes of itching dermatoses throughout the world. Gravid female mites measuring 0.3 to 0.4 mm in length burrow superficially beneath the stratum corneum for a month, depositing two or three eggs a day. Nymphs that hatch from these eggs mature in about 2 weeks through a series of molts and then emerge as adults to the surface of the skin, where they mate and subsequently reinvade the skin of the same or another host. Transfer of newly fertilized female mites from person to person occurs by intimate personal contact and is facilitated by crowding, uncleanliness, and sexual promiscuity. Medical practitioners are at particular risk of infestation. Transmission via sharing of contaminated bedding or clothing is infrequent because these mites cannot survive much more than a day without host contact. In the United States, scabies may account for 2 to 5 percent of visits to dermatologists; involved particularly often are children, immigrants from developing countries, and close household contacts. Outbreaks occur in nursing homes, mental institutions, and hospitals.

The itching and rash associated with scabies derive from a sensitization reaction directed against the excreta that the mite deposits in its burrow. For this reason, an initial infestation remains asymptomatic for 4 to 6 weeks, and a reinfestation produces a hypersensitivity reaction without delay. Scratching generally destroys the burrowing mite, but symptoms remain even in its absence. Burrows become surrounded by infiltrates of eosinophils, lymphocytes, and histiocytes, and a generalized hypersensitivity rash later develops in remote sites. By destroying these pathogens, immunity and associated scratching limit most infestations to fewer than 15 mites per person. Hyperinfestation with thousands or millions of mites, a condition known as *crusted* (or *Norwegian*) *scabies*, may result from glucocorticoid use, immunodeficiency diseases (including AIDS), and neurologic and psychiatric illnesses that interfere with itching and scratching.

Patients with scabies report intense itching that worsens at night and after a hot shower. Typical burrows may be difficult to find because they are few in number and may be obscured by excoriations. Burrows appear as dark wavy lines in the epidermis that measure 3 to 15 mm and end in a small pearly bleb that contains the female mite. Such lesions generally develop on the volar wrists, between the fingers, on the elbows, and on the penis. Small papules and vesicles, often accompanied by eczematous plaques, pustules, or nodules, are symmetrically distributed in these sites and in skin folds under the breasts and around the navel, axillae, belt line, buttocks, upper thighs, and scrotum. Except in infants, the face, scalp, neck, palms, and soles are spared. Burrows and other typical lesions may be sparse in persons who wash frequently, and topical glucocorticoid treatment and bacterial superinfection may alter the appearance of the rash. Superinfection with nephritogenic strains of streptococci has led to acute glomerulonephritis. Crusted scabies resembles psoriasis in its typical widespread erythema, thick keratotic crusts, scaling, and dystrophic nails. Characteristic burrows are not seen in crusted scabies, and patients usually do not itch, although their infestations are highly contagious and have been responsible for outbreaks of classic scabies in hospitals. Bacteremia occurs frequently in AIDS patients with crusted scabies and prominent fissures. Persons with massive infestations occasionally present with diffuse pruritus and generalized papules or with minimal or no cutaneous signs.

A diagnosis of scabies should be considered in patients with pruritus and symmetric polymorphic skin lesions in characteristic locations, particularly if there is a history of household contact with a case. Burrows should be sought and unroofed with a sterile needle or scalpel blade, and the scrapings should be examined microscopically for the mite, its eggs, and its fecal pellets. A drop of mineral oil facilitates removal of the sample. Biopsies or scrapings of papulovesicular lesions also may be diagnostic. In the absence of identifiable mites or mite products, the diagnosis is based on clinical presentation and history. The possibility of other sexually transmitted diseases should be excluded in adults with scabies.

For the treatment of scabies, 5% permethrin cream is less toxic than the once commonly used 1% lindane preparations and is effective against lindane-tolerant infestations. Both scabicides are applied thinly but thoroughly behind the ears and from the neck down after bathing and are removed 8 h later with soap and water. Lindane is absorbed through the skin, and its overuse has led to seizures and aplastic anemia. It should not be applied to pregnant women or infants. Alternatives include topical crotamiton cream, benzyl benzoate, and sulfur ointments. Successful treatment of crusted scabies requires the application first of a keratolytic agent such as 6% salicylic acid (to improve the penetration of scabicides) and then of scabicides to the scalp, face, and ears (with care to avoid the eyes). Repeated treatments or the sequential use of several agents may be necessary. A single oral dose of ivermectin (200 μg/kg) effectively treats scabies in otherwise healthy persons. Patients with crusted scabies may require two or more doses of ivermectin.

Although effectively treated scabies infestations become noninfectious within a day, itching and rash due to hypersensitivity frequently persist for weeks or months. Unnecessary retreatment of the affected patients may provoke contact dermatitis. Antihistamines, salicylates, and calamine lotion relieve itching during treatment, and topical glucocorticoids are useful for the pruritus that lingers after effective treatment. An oral antibiotic may be necessary for bacterial superinfections that fail to resolve with antiscabietic therapy. To prevent reinfestations, bedding and clothing should be washed in hot water, and close contacts, even if asymptomatic, should be treated simultaneously.

SARCOPTIC MANGE (ANIMAL SCABIES) Persons who have close contact with dogs may become transiently infested by the mites responsible for zoonotic scabies; such infestation less often follows contact with cats and horses. Zoonotic mites are unable to propagate on the human host or to produce their elongate burrows, and the characteristic pruritic papulovesicular rash is self-limited.

CHIGGER AND OTHER MITE INFESTATIONS Chiggers are the larvae of trombiculid (harvest) mites that normally feed on mice in grassy or brush-covered sites in the tropics, subtropics, and (less frequently) in temperate areas during warm months. They wait for hosts on low vegetation and attach themselves to passing animals or to people. The larva then pierces the skin of its host and deposits a tubelike structure in the dermis through which it imbibes lymph and tissue juices. This highly antigenic "stylostome" serves as the focus of an exceptionally pruritic papule that may be 2 cm in diameter and that develops within hours of attachment in persons previously sensitized to mite antigen. Scratching invariably destroys the body of a mite attached to a person. These lesions generally vesiculate and develop a hemorrhagic base. Itching and burning last for weeks. The rash is most common on the ankles or near tight-fitting clothes that obstruct the mites' movements. Chiggers are the vectors of scrub typhus in tropical and subtropical parts of Asia. Repellents are useful for preventing chigger bites.

Certain mesostigmatid mites that infest the nests of mice or birds feed on human beings when their usual hosts have been displaced. For example, intense episodes of itching dermatitis in humans may follow the removal of trash from a human residence or the departure of pigeons that have been nesting on a window air-conditioner. Other mites that infest grain, straw, cheese, or other animal products occasionally produce similar episodes. Mouse mites are the vectors of rickettsialpox in cities of the northeastern United States. Although sanitary measures effectively prevent rickettsialpox, removal of accumulated refuse may result in a transient period of elevated risk.

Diagnosis of mite-induced dermatitides (including those caused by chiggers) relies heavily on a history of exposure to the source of the mite, since the tiny mite may escape notice or may already have fallen off or been scratched off the lesions. Antihistamines or topical steroids effectively reduce mite-induced pruritus.

Species of *Demodex*, the follicle mite, live in hair follicles and sebaceous glands of the face and ears. The worm-like mites measure up to 0.4 mm in length and, if carefully sought, can be found on almost all persons. They appear not to cause disease, although their density is high in persons with rosacea. House dust mites of the genus *Dermatophagoides* infest houses throughout the world, living on furniture and rugs and feeding on shed human dander. Exposure to their allergens causes asthma, rhinitis, conjunctivitis, and eczema in persons with house dust allergies. Management includes immunotherapy with mite extracts and environmental interventions such as frequent vacuuming and removal of rugs from bedrooms to reduce mite density.

TICK INFESTATIONS AND TICK PARALYSIS In the United States, hard ticks (Ixodidae) have increased in abundance since the mid-1900s to become the most common carriers of vector-borne diseases. Deer ticks of the genus *Ixodes* transmit the pathogens of Lyme disease, babesiosis, and human granulocytic ehrlichiosis. Other ticks, such as *Dermacentor variabilis* (the dog tick), *Dermacentor andersoni* (the wood tick), and *Amblyomma americanum* (the Lone Star tick), are vectors of tularemia, Rocky Mountain spotted fever, Colorado tick fever, and human monocytic ehrlichiosis. Outside the United States, hard ticks transmit pathogenic rickettsiae and arboviruses as well. Soft ticks (Argasidae) of the genus *Ornithodoros* transmit tick-borne relapsing fever (see Chap. 177). Except in parts of Africa, soft ticks rarely attack human beings, and relapsing fever occurs only sporadically in the United States.

Ticks attach and feed painlessly; blood is their only food. Their secretions, however, produce local reactions, a febrile illness, or paralysis. Local reactions to tick bites vary from small pruritic papules to chronic nodules, or "tick granulomas," that reach several centimeters in diameter and may require surgical excision. Tick-induced fever, associated with headache, nausea, and malaise, usually resolves within 24 to 36 h after the tick is removed. Tick paralysis is an ascending flaccid paralysis believed to be caused by a toxin in tick saliva that causes neuromuscular block and decreased nerve conduction. Throughout the world, this rare complication has followed the bites of more than 40 kinds of tick—most commonly, dog and wood ticks in the United States. Children, especially girls with long hair, are most often affected. Weakness begins in the lower extremities 5 to 6 days after the tick's attachment and ascends symmetrically over several days to result in complete paralysis of the extremities and cranial nerves. Deep tendon reflexes are diminished or lacking altogether, but sensory examination and findings on lumbar puncture are typically normal. Removal of the tick results in improvement within a few hours and usually in complete recovery after several days. Failure to remove the tick may lead to death from aspiration or respiratory paralysis. Diagnosis depends on finding the tick, which often is hidden beneath hair. An antiserum to the saliva of *Ixodes holocyclus*, the usual cause of tick paralysis in Australia, effectively reverses paralysis caused by these ticks. Ticks should be removed by firm traction with a forceps placed near their point of attachment. The site of attachment should be disinfected (e.g., with tincture of iodine). Removal of ticks during the first 48 h of attachment prevents transmission of the agents of Lyme disease and babesiosis. Gentle handling to avoid rupture of ticks and use of gloves may avert accidental contamination with tick fluids containing pathogens. Protective measures against ticks include avoidance of brushy vegetation, use of protective clothing sprayed with 0.5% permethrin, and application of a repellent containing *N,N*-diethyl-*m*-toluamide (DEET). The cuffs of trousers should be tucked inside the socks.

PEDICULOSIS (LOUSE INFESTATIONS) All three species of human louse feed at least once a day on human blood. *Pediculus humanus* var. *capitis* infests the head, *P. humanus* var. *corporis* the clothing, and *Pthirus pubis* mainly the hair of the pubis. Females cement their eggs (nits) firmly to hair or clothing. The saliva of lice produces an intensely irritating maculopapular or urticarial rash in sensitized persons.

Head lice are transmitted directly from person to person and occasionally by shared headgear and grooming implements. The prevalence is highest among school-aged girls who wear long hair; black children are less frequently infested than other children. Excoriations of pruritic lesions on the scalp, neck, and shoulders lead to oozing, crusting, matting of hair, bacterial infections, and regional lymphadenopathy.

Body lice remain in clothing except when feeding and cannot survive more than a few hours away from the human host. It follows, therefore, that *P. humanus* var. *corporis* mainly infests disaster victims or indigent persons who do not change their clothes. Transmission by direct contact or by sharing of clothing and beds is enhanced under crowded conditions. The fact that the body louse leaves febrile persons or corpses as they become cold facilitates the transmission of typhus, louse-borne relapsing fever, and trench fever (see Chap. 179). Pruritic lesions are particularly common around the neckline. Chronic infestations result in the postinflammatory hyperpigmentation and thickening of skin known as *vagabonds' disease*.

The cosmopolitan crab or pubic louse is transmitted mainly by sexual contact but can infest eyelashes, axillary hair, and hair in other sites as well as pubic hair. Intensely pruritic lesions and 2- to 3-mm blue macules (maculae ceruleae) develop at the site of bites. Blepharitis commonly accompanies infestations of the eyelashes.

A suspected diagnosis of pediculosis is confirmed by the finding of nits or adult lice on hairs or in clothing. The preferred treatment is 1% permethrin creme rinse, which kills both lice and eggs and is available without prescription. An alternative, 0.5% malathion, requires a prescription and may not be as effective. Other agents, such as the more toxic 1% lindane and pyrethrins with piperonyl butoxide, are not ovicidal and require a second application 1 week after the first to kill hatching nymphs. Dead or hatched nits, which remain attached to hair sheaths, may falsely suggest an active infection. Lindane-resistant head lice have been reported. After louse infestations have been treated with insecticide, the hair should be combed with a fine-toothed nit comb to remove nits. Combs and brushes should be disinfected in hot water at 65°C for 5 min or soaked in insecticide for 1 h. Body lice can be eliminated by bathing and application of topical pediculicides from head to foot. Clothes and bedding are deloused by heat sterilization in a dryer at 65°C for 30 min or by fumigation. Infestations with pubic lice are treated with topical pediculicides except for eyelid infestations (*phthiriasis palpebrum*), which respond to a coating of petroleum applied for 3 to 4 days or 1% yellow oxide of mercury ointment applied four times daily for 2 weeks.

FLEA INFESTATIONS AND TUNGIASIS Fleas are wingless insects 2 to 4 mm long that feed on the blood of human beings and other warm-bodied animals. Common human-biting fleas include the dog and cat fleas (*Ctenocephalides* species) and the rat flea (*Xenopsylla cheopis*), which inhabit the nests and resting sites of their hosts. Larval fleas feed on pellets of dried host blood that the adult fleas eject from their rectums while feeding. The high-jumping adults attack human beings or other available warm-bodied animals when the usual host abandons or is driven from its nest. The human flea (*Pulex irritans*) infests human bedding and furniture but mainly in relatively humid buildings that lack central heating. Sensitized persons develop erythematous pruritic papules, urticaria, and occasionally vesicles and bacterial superinfection at the site of the bite. Treatment consists of antihistamines and antipruritics.

Fleas transmit plague, murine typhus, the rat and dog tapeworms, and possibly *Bartonella henselae*. Flea infestations are eliminated by frequent cleaning of the nesting sites and bedding of the host or judicious dusting or spraying of insecticides such as pyrethrin, DDT, or malathion.

Human infestations with *Tunga penetrans* (the chigoe flea, sand flea, or jigger) occur in tropical regions of Africa and the Americas. Adults live in sandy soil and burrow under the skin between toes, under nails, or on the soles of bare feet. The fleas engorge on blood and grow from pinpoint to pea size over a 2-week period. The lesions resemble a white pustule with a central black depression and may be pruritic or painful. Occasional complications include tetanus, bacterial infections, and autoamputation of toes. Tungiasis is treated by removal of the intact flea with a sterile needle or scalpel.

MYIASIS *Myiasis* refers to infestations by maggots, mainly due to the larvae of metallic-colored screw-worm flies or botflies. Maggots invade living or necrotic tissue or body cavities and produce different clinical syndromes depending on the species of fly.

Furuncular Myiasis In forested parts of Central and South America, larvae of *Dermatobia hominis* (the human botfly) produce boil-like subcutaneous nodules 2 to 3 cm in diameter. The adult female captures a mosquito or other bloodsucking insect and deposits her eggs beneath its abdomen. When the carrier insect attacks a human or bovine host several days later, the warmth and moisture of the host's surface stimulate the larvae to hatch and penetrate the skin. After 6 to 12 weeks, the larvae mature and drop to the ground, where they pupate. The African tumbu fly, *Cordylobia anthropophaga*, produces similar lesions. Dozens of eggs are deposited on sand or drying laundry that is contaminated with urine or sweat. Larvae hatch on contact with the body, penetrate the skin, and produce boils from which they emerge 8 or 9 days later. A diagnosis of furuncular myiasis is suggested by uncomfortable lesions with a central breathing pore that emits bubbles when submerged in water. Tumbu fly larvae can be removed by manual expression after the air pore is coated with petroleum to suffocate the larvae and induce them to emerge. *Dermatobia* larvae often require surgical excision.

Creeping Dermal Myiasis Maggots of the horse botfly, *Gasterophilus intestinalis*, do not mature after penetrating human skin but migrate for weeks in the epidermis. The resulting pruritic and serpiginous eruption resembles cutaneous larva migrans caused by *Ancylostoma braziliense*. Horseback riders become infested when eggs deposited on the flank of the horse hatch against their bare legs. The black spines of the larvae can be identified after mineral oil is smeared over the lesion. Larva are removed with a needle. The larvae of the cattle botfly (*Hypoderma* species) invade more deeply and produce boil-like swellings.

Wound and Body Cavity Myiasis Certain flies are attracted to blood and pus, and their newly hatched larvae enter wounds or diseased skin. Larvae of species such as *Phaenicia sericata*, the green-bottle fly, remain superficial and confined to necrotic tissue and were used in the past to debride purulent wounds. Other species, including the screw-worms (*Chrysomyia bezziana* in Asia and Africa and *Cochliomyia hominivorax* in Latin America) and the flesh fly (*Wohlfahrtia vigil* in northern North America), invade more deeply into viable tissue and produce large suppurating lesions. Larvae that infest wounds also may infest body cavities such as the mouth, nose, ears, sinuses, anus, vagina, and lower urinary tract, particularly in unconscious or otherwise debilitated patients. The consequences range from harmless colonization to destruction of the nose, meningitis, and deafness. Treatment involves removal of maggots and debridement of tissue.

Other Forms of Myiasis The maggots responsible for furuncular and wound myiasis also may cause ophthalmomyiasis. Sequelae include nodules in the eyelid, retinal detachment, and destruction of the globe. In addition, the adult sheep botfly, *Oestrus ovis*, may deposit larvae in the eyes of persons tending sheep and goats, and the larvae may produce a conjunctival infestation and acute conjunctivitis. True intestinal myiasis occurs when eggs or larvae of the drone fly (*Eristalis tenax*) are ingested with contaminated food, mature in the gut, and cause enteritis. Most instances in which maggots are found in human feces are the result of larviposition by flesh flies on recently passed stools.

PENTASTOMIASIS Pentastomids, or tongue worms, are parasites with characteristics of both helminths and arthropods and are classified in a separate phylum. The wormlike adults inhabit the respiratory passages of reptiles and carnivorous mammals. Human infestation with *Linguatula serrata* is common in the Middle East and occurs in the Sudan following ingestion of encysted larval stages in raw liver or lymph nodes of sheep and goats, the intermediate hosts. The larvae migrate to the nasopharynx and produce an acute self-limiting syndrome known as *halzoun* (*Marrara* in the Sudan), which is characterized by pain and itching of the throat and ears, coughing, hoarseness, dysphagia, and dyspnea. Severe edema may cause obstruction and necessitate tracheostomy, and ocular invasion has been described. Diagnostic larvae measuring 5 to 10 mm in length are found in the copious nasal discharge or vomitus. Human beings become infected with *Armillifer armillatus* by ingesting eggs in contaminated food or drink or after handling the definitive host, the African python. Larvae encyst in various organs but rarely cause symptoms unless they compress vital structures or perforate an organ during migration. Cysts occasionally require surgical removal as they enlarge during molting, but they are usually encountered as an incidental finding at autopsy. There are reports of the cutaneous larva migrans syndrome due to other pentastomes (*Reighardia* and *Sebekia* species) in Southeast Asia and Central America.

LEECH INFESTATIONS Medically important leeches are annelid worms that attach to their hosts with chitinous cutting jaws and draw blood with muscular suckers. The medicinal leech, *Hirudo medicinalis*, is still used occasionally to reduce venous congestion in surgical flaps or replanted body parts. This practice has been complicated by wound infections, myonecrosis, and sepsis due to *Aeromonas hydrophila*, which colonizes the gullets of commercially available leeches.

Ubiquitous aquatic leeches that parasitize fish, frogs, and turtles readily attach to the skin of human beings and avidly suck blood. More notorious are the land leeches (*Haemadipsa*) that live in moist vegetation of tropical rain forests. Attachment is usually painless. Hirudinin, a powerful anticoagulant secreted by the leech, causes continued bleeding after the leech has detached. Healing of the wound is slow, and bacterial infections are not uncommon. Several species of aquatic leeches in Africa, Asia, and southern Europe can enter through the mouth, nose, and genitourinary tract and attach to mucosal surfaces at sites as deep as the esophagus and trachea. Bleeding may be intense. Externally attached leeches are removed by steady gentle traction. Removal is hastened by application of alcohol, salt, vinegar, or a flame to the leech. Internally attached leeches may detach on exposure to gargled saline or may be removed by forceps.

DELUSIONAL INFESTATIONS The groundless conviction that one is infested with arthropods or other parasites is an extremely difficult disorder to treat and unfortunately is not rare. Patients report infestations of their skin, clothing, or homes and describe sensations of something moving in or on their skin. Excoriations often accompany complaints of pruritus or insect bites. Patients bring in as evidence of infestation specimens that are identified microscopically as plant-feeding or peridomestic arthropods, pieces of skin, vegetable matter, or inanimate objects. In suspected cases, it is imperative to rule out true infestations and neuropathies, environmental irritants such as fragments of fiberglass, and other causes of tingling or prickling sensations. Pharmacotherapy with pimozide, which blocks dopamine receptors, has been more helpful than psychotherapy in treating this disorder.

ARTHROPOD BITES AND STINGS

SPIDER BITES Of the more than 30,000 recognized species of spider, only about 100 defend themselves aggressively and have fangs sufficiently long to penetrate human skin. The venom that spiders use to immobilize and digest their prey can cause necrosis of skin and systemic toxicity. While the bites of most spiders are painful but not harmful, envenomations of the brown or fiddle spiders (*Loxosceles* species), widow spiders (*Latrodectus* species), and other species may be life-threatening. Identification of the offending spider should be attempted, since specific treatments exist for bites of widow and brown recluse spiders and since injuries attributed to spiders are frequently due to other causes.

Recluse Spider Bites and Necrotic Arachnidism Severe necrosis of skin and subcutaneous tissue follows envenomation by *Loxosceles reclusa*, the brown recluse spider, and by at least four other species of *Loxosceles* in the southern and midwestern United States. Other spiders that produce necrotic ulceration include the hobo spider (*Tegenaria agrestis*) in the Pacific Northwest, the sac spiders (*Chiracanthium* species) throughout the United States and abroad, the South American brown spider *Loxosceles laeta* in Central and South America, and other *Loxosceles* species in Africa and the Middle East. All these spiders measure 7 to 15 mm in body length and 2 to 4 cm in leg span. Recluse spiders are brown and have a dark violin-shaped spot on their dorsal surface; hobo spiders are brown with gray markings; and sac spiders may be pale yellow, green, or brown.

These spiders are not aggressive toward human beings and bite only if threatened or pressed against the skin. They hide under rocks and logs or in caves and animal burrows, and they emerge at night to hunt other spiders and insects. They invade homes, particularly in the fall, and seek dark and undisturbed hiding spots in closets, in folds of clothing, or under furniture and rubbish in storage rooms, garages, and attics. Bites often occur while the victim is dressing and are sustained primarily to the arms, neck, and lower abdomen.

The clear viscous venoms of these spiders contain an esterase, alkaline phosphatase, protease, and other enzymes that produce tissue necrosis and hemolysis. Sphingomyelinase B, the most important dermonecrotic factor, binds cell membranes and promotes chemotaxis of neutrophils, leading to vascular thrombosis and an Arthus-like reaction. Initially, the bite is painless or produces a stinging sensation. Within the next few hours, the site becomes painful and pruritic, with central induration surrounded by a pale zone of ischemia and a zone of erythema. In most cases, the lesion resolves without treatment over 2 to 3 days. In severe cases, the erythema spreads, and the center of the lesion becomes hemorrhagic and necrotic with an overlying bulla. A black eschar forms and sloughs several weeks later, leaving an ulcer that may be ≥25 cm in diameter and eventually a depressed scar. Healing usually takes place within 3 to 6 months but may take as long as 3 years if adipose tissue is involved. Local complications include injury to nerves and secondary infection. Fever, chills, weakness, headache, nausea, vomiting, myalgia, arthralgia, maculopapular rash, and leukocytosis may develop within 72 h of the bite. In rare instances, acute complications such as hemolytic anemia, hemoglobinuria, and renal failure are fatal.

Initial management includes local cleansing, application of sterile dressings and cold compresses, and elevation and loose immobilization of the affected limb. Analgesics, antihistamines, antibiotics, and tetanus prophylaxis should be administered if indicated. Within the first 48 to 72 h, the administration of dapsone, a leukocyte inhibitor, may halt the progression of lesions that are becoming necrotic. Dapsone is given in oral doses of 50 to 100 mg twice daily after glucose-6-phosphate dehydrogenase deficiency has been ruled out. The efficacy of locally or systemically administered glucocorticoids has not been demonstrated, and a potentially useful *Loxosceles*-specific antivenin has not been approved for use in the United States. Debridement and later skin grafting may be necessary after signs of acute inflammation have subsided, but immediate surgical excision of the wound is detrimental. Patients should be monitored closely for signs of hemolysis, renal failure, and other systemic complications.

Widow Spider Bites The bite of the female widow spider is notorious for the effect of its potent neurotoxin. *Latrodectus mactans*, the black widow, has been found in every state of the United States except Alaska and is most abundant in the southeast. It measures up to 1 cm in body length and 5 cm in leg span, is shiny black, and has a red hourglass marking on the ventral abdomen. Other dangerous North American *Latrodectus* species include *L. geometricus* (the brown widow), *L. bishopi* (the red widow), *L. variolus*, and *L. hesperus*, and there are related species in other temperate and subtropical parts of the world.

Widow spiders spin their webs under stones, logs, plants, or rock piles or in dark spaces in barns, garages, and outhouses. Bites are most common in the summer and early autumn and occur when the web is disturbed or when the spider is trapped or provoked. The buttocks or genitals are sites of bites incurred by humans while sitting in an outdoor privy.

The initial bite goes unnoticed or is perceived as a sharp pinprick. Two small red marks, mild erythema, and edema develop at the fang entrance site. The oily yellow venom that is injected does not produce local necrosis, and some persons experience no other symptoms. However, alpha-latrotoxin, the most active component of the venom, binds irreversibly to nerves and causes release and eventual depletion of acetylcholine, norepinephrine, and other neurotransmitters from presynaptic terminals. Within 30 to 60 min, painful cramps spread from the bite site to large muscles of the extremities and the trunk. Extreme rigidity of the abdominal muscles and excruciating pain may suggest peritonitis, but the abdomen is not tender on palpation. Other features include salivation, diaphoresis, vomiting, hypertension, tachycardia, labored breathing, anxiety, headache, weakness, fasciculations, paresthesia, hyperreflexia, urinary retention, uterine contractions, and premature labor. Rhabdomyolysis and renal failure have been reported, and respiratory arrest, cerebral hemorrhage, or cardiac failure may end fatally, especially in very young, elderly, or debilitated persons. The pain begins to subside during the first 12 h but may recur during several days or weeks before resolving spontaneously.

Treatment consists of local cleansing, application of ice packs, and tetanus prophylaxis. Hypertension that does not respond to analgesics and antispasmodics, such as benzodiazepines or methocarbamol, requires specific antihypertensive medication. Intravenous administration of one or two vials of a widely available equine antivenin rapidly relieves pain and can be life-saving. Because of the risk of anaphylaxis and serum sickness, antivenin should be reserved for severe cases involving respiratory arrest, uncontrollable hypertension, seizures, or pregnancy.

Envenomations by Tarantulas and Other Spiders Tarantulas are long-lived, hairy spiders of which 30 species are found in the United States, primarily in the southwest. The tarantulas that have become popular household pets are usually imported species with bright colors and a leg span of up to 25 cm. Tarantulas bite only when threatened and cause no more harm than a bee sting, but the venom occasionally provokes deep pain and swelling. Several species are covered with urticating hairs that are launched in the thousands when a threatened spider rubs its hind legs across the dorsal abdomen. These hairs penetrate human skin and produce pruritic papules that last for weeks. Treatment of bites includes local washing and elevation of the bitten area, tetanus prophylaxis, and analgesic administration. Antihistamines and topical or systemic glucocorticoids are given for exposure to urticating hairs.

Atrax robustus, the Sydney funnel-web spider of Australia, and *Phoneutria* species, the South American banana spiders, are among the most dangerous spiders in the world because of their aggressive behavior and potent neurotoxins. Envenomation by *A. robustus* causes a rapidly progressive neuromotor syndrome that can be fatal within 2 h. The bite of the banana spiders causes severe local pain followed by profound systemic symptoms and respiratory paralysis that can lead to death within 2 to 6 h. Specific antivenins for envenomation by each of these spiders are available. *Lycosa* species (wolf spiders) are found throughout the world and may produce painful bites and transient local inflammation.

SCORPION STINGS Scorpions are crablike arachnids that feed on ground-dwelling arthropods and small lizards, which they grasp with a pair of frontal pinchers and paralyze by injecting venom from a stinger on the tip of the tail. Painful but relatively harmless scorpion stings need to be distinguished from the potentially lethal envenomations that are produced by about 30 of the approximately 1000 known species and cause more than 5000 deaths worldwide each year. Scorpions feed at night and remain hidden during the day in crevices or burrows or under wood, loose bark, or rocks on the ground. They seek cool spots under buildings and often enter houses, where they get into shoes, clothing, or bedding or enter bathtubs and sinks in search of water. Scorpions sting human beings only when disturbed.

Scorpions of the United States Of the 40 or so scorpion species in the United States, only the bark scorpion (*Centruroides sculpturatus* or *Centruroides exilicauda*) produces a venom that can be lethal. Stings of the other species, such as the common striped scorpion *Centruroides vittatus* and the large *Hadrurus arizonensis*, cause immediate sharp local pain followed by edema, ecchymosis, and a burning sensation. Symptoms typically resolve within a few hours, and skin does not slough. Allergic reactions to the venom sometimes develop.

The deadly *C. sculpturatus* of the southwestern United States and northern Mexico measures about 7 cm in length and is yellow-brown in color. Its venom contains neurotoxins that cause sodium channels to remain open and neurons to fire repetitively. In contrast to the stings of nonlethal species, *C. sculpturatus* envenomations are usually associated with little swelling, but prominent pain, paresthesia, and hyperesthesia can be accentuated by tapping on the affected area (the tap test). These symptoms soon spread to other locations; dysfunction of cranial nerves and hyperexcitability of skeletal muscles develop within hours. Patients present with restlessness, blurred vision, abnormal eye movements, profuse salivation, lacrimation, rhinorrhea, slurred speech, difficulty in handling secretions, diaphoresis, nausea, and vomiting. Muscle twitching, jerking, and shaking may be mistaken for a seizure. Complications include tachycardia, arrhythmias, hypertension, hyperthermia, rhabdomyolysis, and acidosis. Symptoms progress to maximal severity in about 5 h and subside within a day or two, although pain and paresthesia can last for weeks. Fatal respiratory arrest is most common among young children and the elderly.

Other Dangerous Scorpions Envenomations by *Leiurus quinquestriatus* in the Middle East and North Africa, by *Mesobuthus tamulus* in India, by *Androctonus* species along the Mediterranean littoral and in North Africa and the Middle East, and by *Tityus serrulatus* in Brazil cause massive release of endogenous catecholamines with hypertensive crises, arrhythmias, pulmonary edema, and myocardial damage. Acute pancreatitis occurs with stings of *Tityus trinitatis* in Trinidad, and central nervous toxicity complicates stings of *Parabuthus* and *Buthotus* scorpions of South Africa. Tissue necrosis and hemolysis may follow stings of the Iranian *Hemiscorpius lepturus*.

℞ TREATMENT

Identification of the offending scorpion aids in planning therapy. Stings of nonlethal species require at most ice packs, analgesics, or antihistamines. Because most victims of dangerous envenomations (such as those produced by *C. sculpturatus*) experience only local discomfort, they can be managed at home with instructions to return to the emergency department if signs of cranial-nerve or neuromuscular dysfunction develop. Aggressive supportive care and judicious use of antivenin can reduce or eliminate mortality from more severe envenomations. Keeping the patient calm and applying pressure dressings and cold packs to the sting site decrease the absorption of venom. Although narcotics and sedatives can control restlessness and hypertension, these agents interfere with protective airway reflexes and should not be given to patients with neuromuscular symptoms unless endotracheal intubation is planned. Hypertension and pulmonary edema respond to nifedipine, nitroprusside, hydralazine, or prazosin, and bradyarrhythmias can be controlled with atropine.

Commercially prepared antivenins are available in several countries for some of the most dangerous species. A caprine *C. sculpturatus* antivenin[1] is available as an investigational drug only in Arizona. Because of the risk of anaphylaxis or serum sickness following administration of goat serum, use of the antivenin is controversial. Intravenous administration of antivenin rapidly reverses cranial-nerve dysfunction and muscular symptoms but does not affect pain and paresthesia.

Prevention In scorpion-infested areas, shoes, clothing, bedding, and towels should be shaken and inspected before being used. Removal of wood, stones, and debris from yards and campsites eliminates hiding places for scorpions, and household spraying of insecticides can deplete their source of food.

HYMENOPTERA STINGS Insects that sting to defend their colonies or subdue their prey belong to the order Hymenoptera, which includes apids (bees and bumblebees), vespids (wasps, hornets, and yellow jackets), and ants. Their venoms contain a wide array of amines, peptides, and enzymes that are responsible for local and systemic reactions. Although the toxic effect of multiple stings can be fatal, nearly all of the 50 or more deaths due to hymenopteran stings in the United States each year are the result of allergic reactions.

Bee and Wasp Stings Bees lose their venom apparatus in the act of stinging and subsequently die, while vespids can sting numerous times in succession. The familiar honeybees (*Apis mellifera*) and bumblebees (*Bombus* and other genera) attack when a colony is disturbed, but the extremely aggressive Africanized honeybees respond to minimal intrusions rapidly and in large numbers. Since their introduction into Brazil in 1957, these "killer bees" have spread through South and Central America to the southern United States.

The common vespids in the United States include the yellow jacket, notable for the yellow and black bands on its abdomen; the bald-faced hornet, with a black body and a white face; the brown hornet, measuring 2.5 to 3.5 cm in length; and the paper wasps, which have variously colored elongate bodies. Vespids sting in defense of their nests, which they often build near human dwellings and suspend from eaves or shubbery, plaster onto walls, or burrow into wood or soil. Yellow jackets feed on sugary substances and decaying meat and are annoyingly abundant at recreation sites and around garbage, particularly in the late summer and fall.

Venom is produced in glands at the posterior end of the abdomen and is expelled rapidly by contraction of muscles of the venom sac, which has a capacity of up to 0.1 mL in large insects. The venoms

[1] This agent had not been approved by the Food and Drug Administration for this purpose at the time of publication.

of different species of hymenopterans are biochemically and immunologically distinct. Direct toxic effects are mediated by mixtures of low-molecular-weight compounds such as serotonin, histamine, and acetylcholine and several kinins. Polypeptide toxins in honeybee venom include mellitin, which damages cell membranes; mast cell–degranulating protein, which causes histamine release; apamin, a neurotoxin; and adolapin, which has anti-inflammatory action. Enzymes in venom include hyaluronidase, which allows the spread of other venom components, and phospholipases, which may be among the major venom allergens. There appears to be little cross-sensitization between honeybee and wasp venoms.

Uncomplicated stings cause immediate pain, a wheal-and-flare reaction, and local edema and swelling that subside in a few hours. Stings from accidentally swallowed insects may induce life-threatening edema of the upper airways. Multiple stings can lead to vomiting, diarrhea, generalized edema, dyspnea, hypotension, and collapse. Rhabdomyolysis and intravascular hemolysis may cause renal failure. Death from the direct effects of venom has followed 300 to 500 honeybee stings.

Large local reactions that spread ≥10 cm around the sting site over 24 to 48 h are not uncommon. These reactions may resemble cellulitis but are caused by hypersensitivity rather than secondary infection. Such reactions tend to recur on subsequent exposure but seldom are accompanied by anaphylaxis and are not prevented by venom immunotherapy.

An estimated 0.4 to 4.0 percent of the U.S. population exhibits clinical immediate-type hypersensitivity to insect stings, and 15 percent may have asymptomatic sensitization manifested by positive skin tests. Persons who experience severe allergic reactions are likely to have similar reactions after subsequent stings; occasionally, adults who have had mild reactions later experience serious reactions. Mild anaphylactic reactions from insect stings, as from other causes, consist of nausea, abdominal cramping, generalized urticaria, flushing, and angioedema. Serious reactions, including upper airway edema, bronchospasm, hypotension, and shock, may be rapidly fatal. Severe reactions usually begin within 10 min of the sting and only rarely develop after 5 h. Unusual complications, including serum sickness, vasculitis, neuritis, and encephalitis, develop several days or weeks after a sting.

℞ TREATMENT

Stingers embedded in the skin should be scraped or brushed off with a blade or a fingernail but not removed with forceps, which may squeeze more venom out of the venom sac. The site should be cleansed and disinfected and ice packs used to slow the spread of venom. Elevation of the affected site and administration of analgesics, oral antihistamines, and topical calamine lotion relieve symptoms; application of meat tenderizer containing papain is of no proven value. Large local reactions may require a short course of oral therapy with glucocorticoids. Patients with numerous stings should be monitored for 24 h for evidence of renal failure or coagulopathy.

Anaphylaxis is treated with subcutaneous injection of 0.3 to 0.5 mL of epinephrine hydrochloride in a 1:1000 dilution; treatment is repeated every 20 to 30 min if necessary. Intravenous epinephrine (2 to 5 mL of a 1:10,000 solution administered by slow push) is indicated for profound shock. A tourniquet may slow the spread of venom. Parenteral antihistamines, fluid resuscitation, bronchodilators, oxygen, intubation, and vasopressors may be required. Patients should be observed for 24 h for recurrent anaphylaxis.

Prevention Persons with a history of allergy to insect stings should carry a sting kit with a preloaded syringe containing epinephrine for self-administration in case of a sting. These patients should seek medical attention immediately after using the kit. To avoid stings when outdoors, individuals can wear shoes and protective clothing and avoid attracting insects with sweet foods, bright-colored clothes, perfumes, or cosmetics.

Venom Immunotherapy Repeated injections of purified venom produce a blocking IgG antibody response to venom and reduce the incidence of recurrent anaphylaxis from between 50 and 60 percent to less than 5 percent. Honeybee, wasp, yellow jacket, and mixed vespid venoms are commercially available for desensitization and for skin testing. Adults with a history of anaphylaxis should undergo desensitization. Results of skin tests and venom-specific radioallergosorbent tests aid in the selection of patients for immunotherapy and guide the design of such treatment. A 3- to 5-year course of immunotherapy usually eliminates the risk of anaphylaxis.

Stings of Fire Ants and Other Ants All ants that are large enough can bite human beings, and some can secrete repugnant substances when handled. Stinging fire ants are an important medical problem in the United States. The imported fire ants *Solenopsis richteri* and *Solenopsis invicta* were introduced from South America into Alabama in 1918 and now infest urban and rural areas of southern states from Texas to North Carolina, where each year they sting up to 60 percent of the inhabitants of some cities. They excavate open fields and yards to build tall mounds that can harbor 200,000 worker ants. Slight disturbances of the mounds have provoked massive outpourings of ants and as many as 10,000 stings on a single person. Waterborne ants bite on contact during times of flooding.

Red-brown or brown-black fire ants attach to human skin with powerful mandibles and rotate their bodies around their heads while repeatedly injecting venom with posteriorly situated stingers. The alkaloid venom consists of cytotoxic and hemolytic piperidines and several proteins with enzymatic activity. The initial wheal-and-flare reaction, burning, and itching resolve in about 30 min, and a sterile pustule develops within 24 h. The pustule ulcerates over the next 48 h and then heals a week or 10 days later unless it becomes secondarily infected. Large areas of erythema and edema lasting several days are not uncommon and in extreme cases may compress nerves and blood vessels. Anaphylaxis occurs in about 1 to 2 percent of persons, and seizures and mononeuritis have been reported. Stings are treated with ice packs, topical glucocorticoids, and oral antihistamines. Covering pustules with bandages and antibiotic ointment may prevent bacterial infection. Epinephrine and supportive measures are indicated for anaphylactic reactions. Whole-body extracts are available for skin testing and immunotherapy, which appears to lower the rate of anaphylactic reactions.

The western United States is home to harvester ants (*Pogonomyrmex* species) as well as to less aggressive fire ants not yet displaced by the introduced species. The painful local reaction following harvester ant stings often extends to lymph nodes and may be accompanied by anaphylaxis. Large Australian bulldog ants and the aggressive South American *Paranopera* ants deliver extremely painful stings and may cause systemic symptoms. Velvet ants that inhabit sandy beaches in the United States and sting the bare feet of bathers are actually wingless female wasps of the genus *Dasymutilla*.

OTHER ARTHROPOD BITES AND ENVENOMATIONS

Dipteran (Fly) Bites In the process of feeding on vertebrate blood, adults of certain fly species inflict painful bites, produce local allergic reactions, or transmit infectious diseases. Unlike insect stings, insect bites rarely cause anaphylaxis. Mosquitoes are ubiquitous pests and are the vectors of malaria, filariasis, yellow fever, dengue, and viral encephalitides. Their bite typically produces a wheal and later a pruritic papule. In the United States, a similar reaction follows the bite of tiny but aggressive midges known as "no-see-ums," which attack in swarms during warm months, or of other *Culicoides* species that transmit "nonpathogenic" filariae in tropical climates. The bite of the small humpbacked blackfly of the genus *Simulium* leaves a large bleeding puncture and painful and pruritic sores that are slow to heal; regional lymphadenopathy, fever, or anaphylaxis occasionally ensues. Blackflies are common summertime nuisances in the United States and Canada and are vectors of onchocerciasis in Africa and Latin America. The widely distributed tabanids, including deerflies (*Chrysops* species) and horseflies (*Tabanus* species), are stout flies measuring 10 to 25 mm in length that attack during the day and produce large and painful bleeding punctures. Deerflies transmit loiasis in African equatorial rain forests and tularemia in the United States and elsewhere. Tsetse flies of the genus *Glossina* transmit African trypanosomiasis in sub-Saharan Africa. Tiny phlebotomine sand flies are the vectors of leishmaniasis, bartonellosis (Carrión's disease), sand-fly fever, and other arboviral infections in warm climates. *Stomoxys calcitrans*, the stable fly, which resembles a large housefly, is a fierce biter of human beings and domestic animals and a major pest in seacoast areas.

Treatment of fly bites is symptom-based. Topical application of antipruritic agents, glucocorticoids, or antiseptic lotions may relieve the itching and pain. Allergic reactions may require oral antihistamines. Antibiotics may be necessary for large bite wounds that become secondarily infected. Personal protection measures against biting flies include avoidance of infested areas, application of a DEET-containing repellent to exposed skin, and use of protective clothing and bed nets treated with permethrin.

Hemipteran (True Bug) Bites Several true bugs of the family Reduviidae inflict bites that produce allergic reactions and are sometimes painful. The cosmopolitan bedbug (*Cimex* species) hides in mattresses, behind bedboards, and under loose wallpaper during the day and takes its blood meal at night. The bite is painless, but sensitized persons develop erythema, itching, and wheals around a central hemorrhagic punctum. The cone-nose bugs, so called because of their elongated heads, include the assassin and wheel bugs, which feed on other insects and bite human beings only in self-defense, and the kissing bugs, which routinely feed on vertebrate blood. Assassin and wheel bugs inhabit many parts of the world, including the southwestern and southern United States, where they are notorious for their painful bites. The bites of the nocturnally feeding kissing bugs are painless and occur commonly in groups on the face and other exposed parts of the body. Reactions to such bites depend on prior sensitization and include tender and pruritic papules, vesicular or bullous lesions, giant urticaria, fever, lymphadenopathy, and anaphylaxis. *Triatoma infestans* and other species of kissing bug are the vectors of *Trypanosoma cruzi* in South and Central America and Mexico, but transmission of *T. cruzi* to human beings by species indigenous to the United States is exceedingly rare. Bug bites are treated with topical antipruritics or oral antihistamines. Persons with anaphylactic reactions to reduviid bites should keep an epinephrine kit available.

Centipede Bites and Millipede Dermatitis The fangs of centipedes of the genus *Scolopendra* can penetrate human skin and deliver a venom that produces intense burning pain, swelling, erythema, and lymphangitis. Dizziness, nausea, and anxiety are occasionally described, and rhabdomyolysis and renal failure have been reported. Treatment includes washing of the site, application of cold dressings, oral analgesic administration or local lidocaine infiltration, and tetanus prophylaxis. Species of *Scolopendra*, measuring up to 25 cm, occur widely in the southern United States and other areas with warm climates worldwide. The smaller house centipede *Scutigera coleopatrata*, which is common throughout the United States, is harmless.

Millipedes, unlike centipedes, do not bite but rather secrete and in some cases eject defensive fluids that burn and discolor human skin. Affected skin turns brown overnight and may blister and exfoliate. Secretions in the eye cause intense pain and inflammation that may lead to corneal ulceration and blindness. Management includes irrigation with copious amounts of water or saline, use of analgesics, and local care of denuded skin. Millipedes are found throughout the world in leaf litter and under rocks.

Caterpillar Stings and Dermatitis The surface of caterpillars of several moth species is covered with hairs or spines that produce mechanical irritation and may contain or be coated with venom. Contact with these caterpillars causes an immediate burning sensation followed by local swelling and erythema and occasionally by regional lymphadenopathy, nausea, vomiting, and headache; shock, seizures, and coagulopathy are rare complications. In the United States, stings are most often caused by io moth larvae and puss as well as saddleback and brown-tail moth caterpillars as they cling to leaves and branches. Contact with even detached hairs of other caterpillars, such as gypsy moth larvae (*Lymantria dispar*) in the northeastern United States, can produce a pruritic urticarial or papular rash hours later. Spines may be deposited on tree trunks and drying laundry or may be airborne and cause irritation of the eyes and upper airways. Treatment of caterpillar stings consists of repeated application of adhesive or cellophane tape to remove the hairs, which can then be identified microscopically. Local ice packs, topical steroids, and oral antihistamines relieve symptoms.

Beetle Vesication When disturbed, blister beetles extrude cantharidin, a low-molecular-weight toxin that produces thin-walled blisters measuring up to 5 cm in diameter 2 to 5 h after contact with the beetle. The blisters are not painful or pruritic unless broken, and they resolve without treatment in a week to 10 days. Nephritis may follow unusually heavy cantharidin exposure. In the southern United States, blister beetles of several *Epicauta* species are abundant in the summer months. Contact occurs when people sit on the ground, work in the garden, or deliberately handle the beetles. In other countries, different species of beetle produce different vesicants. No treatment is necessary, although ruptured blisters should be kept clean and bandaged until healing is complete.

BIBLIOGRAPHY

AUERBACH PS (ed): *Wilderness Medicine*, 3d ed. St. Louis, Mosby, 1995

BEAUCHER WN, FARNHAM JE: Gypsy-moth-caterpillar dermatitis. N Engl J Med 306:1301, 1982

BURGESS I: *Sarcoptes scabiei* and scabies. Adv Parasitol 33:235, 1994

CENTERS FOR DISEASE CONTROL AND PREVENTION: Necrotic arachnidism—Pacific Northwest, 1988–1996. Morb Mort Week Rep 45:433, 1996

CLARK RF et al: Clinical presentation and treatment of black widow spider envenomation: A review of 163 cases. Ann Emerg Med 21:782, 1992

DESHAZO RD et al: Reactions to the stings of the imported fire ant. N Engl J Med 323:462, 1990

DRABICK JJ: Pentastomiasis. Rev Infect Dis 9:1087, 1987

GODDARD J: *Physician's Guide to Arthropods of Medical Importance*. Boca Raton, FL, CRC Press, 1993

HALL M, WALL R: Myiasis of humans and domestic animals. Adv Parasitol 35:257, 1995

MEINKING TL et al: The treatment of scabies with ivermectin. N Engl J Med 333:26, 1995

MILLIKAN LE: Mite infestations other than scabies. Semin Dermatol 12:22, 1993

PETERS W: *A Colour Atlas of Arthropods in Clinical Medicine*. London, Wolfe, 1992

REISMAN RE: Insect stings. N Engl J Med 331:523, 1994

TAN BB et al: Double-blind controlled trial of effect of house dust-mite allergen avoidance on atopic dermatitis. Lancet 347:15, 1996

WILLIAMS ST et al: Severe intravascular hemolysis associated with brown recluse spider envenomation. A report of two cases and review of the literature. Am J Clin Pathol 104:463, 1995

394 DROWNING AND NEAR-DROWNING

Jerome H. Modell

It is an unexpected tragedy when a previously healthy person dies or is exposed to severe cerebral hypoxia and suffers permanent brain damage. For many years, drowning was considered a "fight for survival": Arms flailing and screaming for help, a person who could not swim struggled to remain on the surface of the water to reach safety. This situation, however, is rarely reported by persons at the scene of aquatic emergencies. Furthermore, no single set of circumstances comprises drowning or near-drowning. It may be a secondary event following such precursors as head or spinal trauma, hypoxia-induced unconsciousness, or unconsciousness due to preexisting cardiovascular disease, sudden cardiac death, or myocardial infarction. The initiating event is usually unknown, so the drowned or near-drowned victim must be treated based on probable physiologic effects of the near-drowning itself. If survival with normal brain function is to occur, a thorough understanding of the pathophysiology of drowning and an organized approach to therapy are imperative.

PATHOPHYSIOLOGY OF DROWNING Approximately 90 percent of drowning victims aspirate fluid into their lungs. In those who do not aspirate fluid, hypoxemia results simply from apnea. In those who do aspirate, the volume and the composition of the fluid determine the physiologic basis of the hypoxemia. Freshwater aspiration alters the surface tension properties of pulmonary surfactant and makes alveoli unstable, which causes a decreased ventilation/perfusion ratio. Some alveoli collapse and become atelectatic, which produces a true or absolute intrapulmonary shunt, while others are poorly ventilated and produce a relative shunt; in either case, significant pulmonary venous admixture occurs. Fresh water in the alveoli is hypotonic and is rapidly absorbed and redistributed throughout the body. While some have proposed that water continues to enter the lungs after death, at autopsy, the lungs of victims who died in the water frequently contain little water. These findings support the premise that active respiration determines the volume of water aspirated.

Hypertonic seawater pulls additional fluid from the plasma into the lungs, and thus the alveoli are fluid-filled but perfused, which causes substantial pulmonary venous admixture. With both types of water, pulmonary edema may occur secondary to events such as fluid shifts, a change in capillary permeability, or cerebral hypoxia, which causes neurogenic pulmonary edema. Regardless of the cause, pulmonary edema adds to the ventilation/perfusion abnormality.

Water that is grossly contaminated with bacteria or that contains particulate matter may complicate the picture. Particulate matter can obstruct the smaller bronchi and respiratory bronchioles. Grossly contaminated water increases the risk of severe pulmonary infection. Neither problem is sufficiently common, however, to justify recommending specific therapy routinely for all victims.

At least 85 percent of near-drowned victims are thought to aspirate 22 mL/kg of water or less, which does not significantly affect blood volume or serum electrolyte concentrations. After resuscitation, by the time blood is analyzed, serum electrolyte concentrations usually are normal or close to normal. Significant changes are documented in only approximately 15 percent of those who cannot be resuscitated and only rarely in those who are resuscitated. These findings suggest that either a small amount of water was aspirated, fluid was rapidly redistributed, or both. Therefore, electrolyte disturbance rarely needs treatment. When a large quantity of water is aspirated, seawater causes hypovolemia, which concentrates extracellular electrolytes, and fresh water causes acute hypervolemia. If enough water is aspirated that plasma becomes severely hypotonic and the patient is hypoxemic, red cell membranes can rupture, and plasma hemoglobin and serum potassium concentrations increase significantly. However, this development has been reported only rarely. With rapid redistribution of fluid and development of pulmonary edema, even freshwater victims frequently demonstrate hypovolemia by the time they reach the hospital.

Hypercarbia, which is associated with apnea and/or hypoventilation, is less often documented by blood gas analysis than is hypoxemia. While hypoxemia due to pulmonary venous admixture persists in all near-drowned victims who aspirate water, hypercarbia is usually corrected sooner with artificial mechanical ventilation and improved minute ventilation and, thus, is reported in only a small percentage of victims evaluated at the hospital. Besides hypoxemia, metabolic acidosis also persists in most patients. Abnormal cardiovascular function, usually ascribed to hypoxemia, is brief with effective, timely therapy. Abnormality in renal function is uncommon, but when it does occur, it too is secondary to hypoxemia, altered renal perfusion, or, in extremely rare circumstances, significant hemoglobinuria.

TREATMENT OF NEAR-DROWNING The first step is retrieving the victim from the water, and, if necessary, performing artificial ventilation and circulation. The American Heart Association recommends that an abdominal thrust not be used routinely in victims of submersion. This recommendation was upheld by a special committee of the Institute of Medicine convened in 1994 specifically to evaluate the efficacy of an abdominal thrust in the treatment of near-drowned victims. In these patients, an abdominal thrust may lead to regurgitation of gastric contents and, thus, to aspiration of the vomitus. Further, an abdominal thrust may delay ventilatory or circulatory resuscitation. Therefore, an abdominal thrust should only be used when the airway is obstructed with a foreign body or when the victim fails to respond to mouth-to-mouth ventilation.

Because emergency services and intensive pulmonary and cardiovascular care have improved during the past two decades, central nervous system depression now presents the major therapeutic challenge in near-drowning. The rate of survival with normal cerebral function varies considerably in retrospective studies. Some factors that adversely influence survival are prolonged submersion, delay in initiation of effective cardiopulmonary resuscitation, severe metabolic acidosis (pH < 7.1), asystole upon arrival to a medical facility, fixed dilated pupils, and a low Glasgow coma score (<5). None of these predictors is absolute, however, and normal survivors have been reported in all of the above categories. Absence of cortical evoked potentials does indicate irreversibility of the cerebral hypoxic lesion; this test, however, cannot be done in the field to guide rescuers. A comparison of outcomes between one institution that added brain preservation techniques to intensive pulmonary and circulatory treatment and another institution that did not found no significant differences.

Hypothermia appears to be protective, but only if it occurs early, at the time of the accident, in which case it increases the victim's chance of cerebral salvage after relatively long periods of acute hypoxia and cardiac arrest. While hypothermia prolongs tolerance to hypoxia, it also can precipitate fatal cardiac arrhythmia; thus, its occurrence can be helpful on the one hand and harmful on the other. The diving reflex produces bradycardia, breath-holding, and circulatory redistribution when the face is submerged in cold water. However, the effect of the diving reflex in explaining cerebral recovery after prolonged immersion has not been specifically documented.

Significant pulmonary venous admixture usually persists even after successful resuscitation; therefore, supplemental oxygen should be administered until arterial blood gas analysis confirms that oxygen is no longer needed. Intravenous access should be established as soon as possible. The trachea should be intubated if necessary for airway maintenance or to facilitate mechanical ventilatory support. Electrocardiographic monitoring will facilitate prompt treatment of cardiac arrhythmia.

Victims should be transported to a hospital for definitive testing of the adequacy of ventilation and blood gas exchange, cardiac activity, and effective circulating blood volume. Other variables, such as serum electrolyte concentrations, renal function, and cerebral status, should be analyzed as indicated.

The single most effective treatment for hypoxemia, regardless of cause, is mechanical ventilatory support including continuous positive airway pressure (CPAP). After freshwater aspiration, improvement in ventilation/perfusion matching is more consistent when CPAP is combined with mechanical inflation of the lung than with spontaneous respiration. The question of whether CPAP should be combined with spontaneous respiration or with mechanical ventilation should be decided by whether the specific patient can perform the necessary work of breathing, adequately eliminate carbon dioxide, and adequately match ventilation/perfusion ratios. Positive airway pressure should be withdrawn gradually as the lungs stabilize and ventilation/perfusion ratio returns toward normal.

The pH in near-drowned victims is commonly significantly acidotic, which, in turn, can depress cardiac function. The metabolic component of the acidosis, if it results in a pH < 7.20, should be corrected pharmacologically, although there is some disagreement on this point. With cardiovascular instability, cannulation of the pulmonary artery with a Swan-Ganz catheter or evaluation by transesophageal echocardiography is indicated. Many patients will be hypovolemic from loss of fluid into the lung as pulmonary edema or from decreased venous return secondary to increased intrathoracic pressure during mechanical ventilatory support.

Because recovery after long periods of submersion under frigid conditions has been reported, body temperature should be taken into account before a decision is made to terminate therapy. The body temperature of victims depends not only on the temperature of the water from which they are retrieved but also on how well they were insulated by clothing. The volume of water actually aspirated is also important, because a large volume, if distributed before cardiac arrest occurs, can produce rapid central cooling. Thus, cold water can be protective when it produces total-body hypothermia, which decreases metabolic oxygen requirement. On the other hand, cold water may also contribute to the accident if hypothermia occurs before total submersion, and severe, or even fatal, cardiac arrhythmia results. Several methods of rewarming hypothermic victims have been advocated, but any technique that increases oxygen utilization, such as shivering, should be avoided.

Regardless of the conditions surrounding a drowning or near-drowning, treatment should adhere to the following sequence of priorities (Fig. 394-1):

1. Remove the victim from the water as soon as possible and stabilize the patient's head and neck if trauma is suspected.
2. Immediately follow the ABCs of cardiopulmonary resuscitation—even in the water if this does not endanger the rescuer.
3. If the patient is unconscious, protect the airway as needed with endotracheal intubation.
4. Establish venous access as soon as possible.
5. Provide supplemental oxygen and ventilatory support until each is no longer needed. This can be judged from analysis of arterial blood for oxygen tension, carbon dioxide tension, and pH.
6. Monitor cardiac rhythm with an electrocardioscope as soon as possible.
7. Monitor body temperature and restore it to normal.
8. If the patient has persistent respiratory insufficiency, provide intensive pulmonary support with CPAP and mechanical ventilation therapy as necessary.
9. If the patient has cardiovascular instability, evaluate cardiac output and effective circulatory volume by invasive monitoring, and measure serum electrolyte concentrations.
10. Evaluate and treat renal function and cerebral status as indicated.

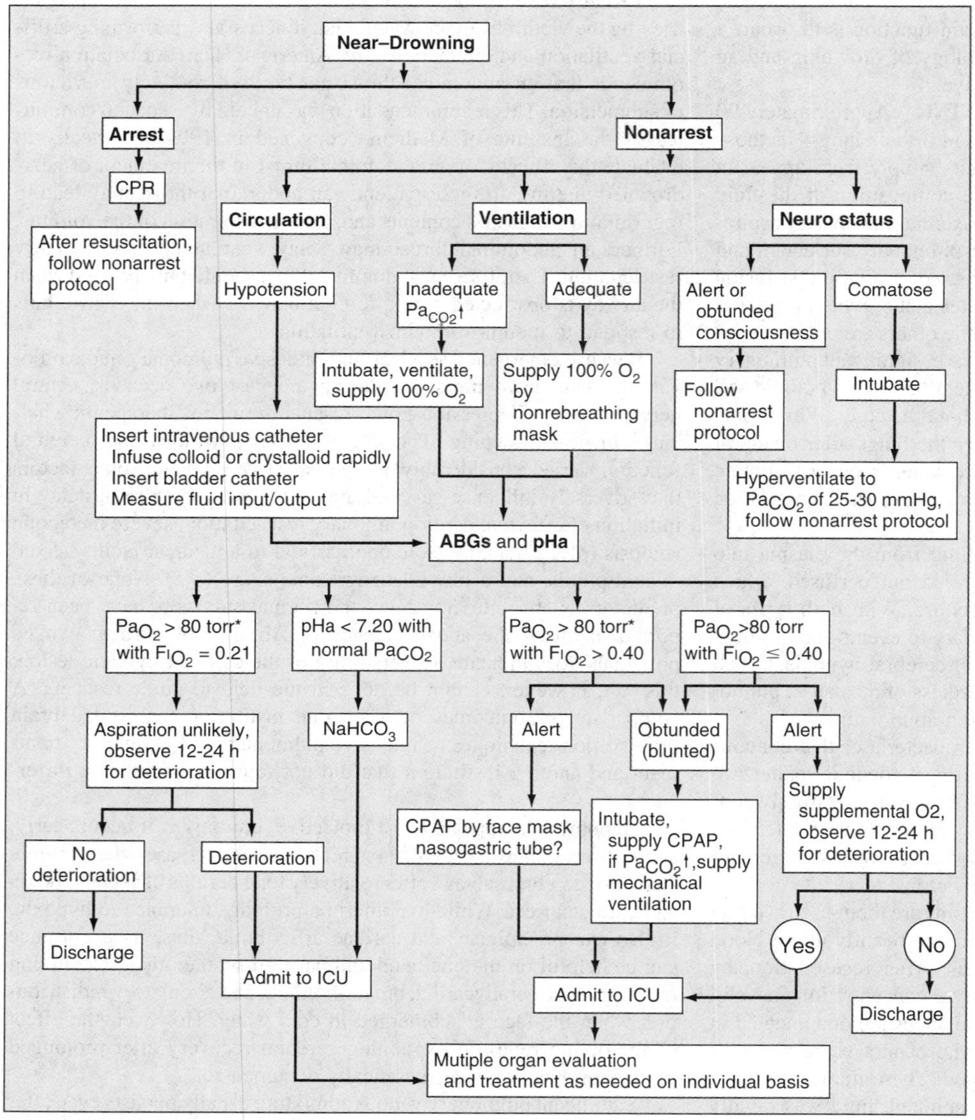

FIGURE 394-1 Treatment of a near-drowned victim should follow a sequence of priorities. *Guidelines only; assumes victim had normal arterial blood gas values (ABGs) before near-drowning. Abbreviations/definitions: CPAP, continuous positive airway pressure; CPR, cardiopulmonary resuscitation; F_{IO_2}, fraction of inspired oxygen; intubate: endoctracheal intubation; ICU, intensive care unit; $NaHCO_3$, bicarbonate; Pa_{O_2}/Pa_{CO_2}, arterial oxygen/carbon dioxide tension; pHa, arterial pH. *(Modified from Graves and Layon.)*

Glucocorticoid therapy, prophylactic antibiotic therapy, and monitoring of intracranial pressure are no longer recommended.

ACCIDENT PREVENTION Because drowning begins as an accident that results in a medical problem, the definitive strategy is to prevent the accident. For those victims in whom the accident is secondary to a medical condition, as in persons susceptible to syncope or seizure, the only way to prevent the accident is to identify those who ought to avoid the water or to encourage them to use the buddy system. For young children, early swimming lessons, vigilant caretakers, and stringent laws governing pool enclosures are needed. Those who teach parenting classes should routinely warn parents about the risk of toddlers' drowning in such household fixtures as toilets, buckets of water, and even washing machines. Preventing accidents during boating, athletics, and other water-related recreational activities requires public education. Rules associated with these activities to maximize safety and judicious, responsible behavior should be portrayed as life-saving measures. Similarly, drinking alcohol, a "ubiquitous catalyst" to drowning, should be portrayed as life-threatening whenever water is nearby.

BIBLIOGRAPHY

American Heart Association: Guidelines for cardiopulmonary resuscitation and emergency cardiac care. JAMA 268:2171, 1992

Bohn DJ et al: Influence of hypothermia, barbiturate therapy, and intracranial pressure monitoring on morbidity and mortality after near-drowning. Crit Care Med 14:529, 1986

Fuller RH: The 1962 Welcome Prize Essay. Drowning and the postimmersion syndrome. A clinicopathologic study. Milit Med 128:22, 1963

Graves SA, Layon AJ: Drowning and near-drowning, in *Emergency Medicine: A Comprehensive Review*, 3d ed, TC Kravis et al (eds). New York, Raven, 1993, pp 689–700

Modell JH: Drowning. N Engl J Med 328:253, 1993

———: *Pathophysiology and Treatment of Drowning and Near-Drowning*. Springfield, IL, Charles C Thomas, 1971

——— et al: Clinical course of 91 consecutive near-drowning victims. Chest 70:231, 1976

Ornato JP: The resuscitation of near-drowning victims. JAMA 256:75, 1986

Rosen P et al (eds): *The Use of the Heimlich Maneuver in Near-Drowning*. Committee on the Treatment of Near-Drowning Victims, Institute of Medicine, Washington, DC, 1994

395

Alan R. Dimick

ELECTRICAL INJURIES

EPIDEMIOLOGY The exact incidence of electrical injury is unknown. Each year in the United States, approximately 1000 deaths, constituting roughly 1 percent of all accidental deaths, are attributed to electric current. The prevalence of electrical technology in modern society has resulted in more people experiencing electrical injury. The current treatment of electrical injury has resulted in a low mortality, ranging from 3 to 15 percent, but the amputation rate remains high, and disfigurement due to extensive soft tissue destruction is frequent. More than 60 percent of the electricity-related fatalities occur in males, with the highest incidence among those 20 to 34 years of age. Approximately one-third of *high-voltage* injuries occur in electrical workers, one-third in construction workers, and the remainder from non-work-related events. One-half of *low-voltage* injuries occur at home, most of them to young children. Burn center referral is usually necessary for electrical burns.

PATHOPHYSIOLOGY Electrical burns result from the conversion of electrical energy into heat. Factors that determine the severity and distribution of injury include the type of current (direct or alternating), the quantity of the current (amperage), the potential of the current (voltage), the resistance offered by the body, the pathway of the current, and the duration of contact. These variables are interrelated, and their interactions produce the varied spectrum of injury seen clinically.

Direct and alternating current have different effects. At low voltages (<1000 V), the low-frequency (40 to 150 Hz) alternating current range, which is used almost exclusively for incandescent lighting and appliances, is three times more dangerous than direct current. Immediate death can result from ventricular fibrillation, central respiratory arrest, or asphyxia due to tetanic respiratory muscle contractions. Tetanic muscle spasms, which freeze the contact point to the power source, tend to increase the flow of current and the severity of injury. Cutaneous burns may be entirely absent or minimal. In contrast, at high voltages, high-frequency alternating current and direct current are equally lethal.

Survivals from electric shocks of greater than 100,000 V and deaths from as little as 50 V have occurred, which underscores the interplay of the variables already noted. Clinically, the severity of injury relates primarily to the voltage. Low-voltage contact, while potentially lethal, does not result in the magnitude of tissue necrosis seen with high-voltage injury. Tissue resistance is an important factor in determining both the initiation of current flow and its subsequent path. A person completing a circuit between two contact points has a resistance that is the sum of the skin resistances at both contact points plus the internal body resistance. If skin resistance is high, there will be considerable local tissue destruction. Conversely, if skin resistance is low, systemic effects, such as those on the heart and brain, predominate. Skin resistance varies widely according to the thickness, cleanliness, and wetness of the skin. The resistance of skin in water is only about 0.1 percent of the resistance of dry skin. The extent of tissue damage can be explained by the differing resistances of various tissues. Listed in the order of increasing magnitude of resistance are nerves, blood vessels, muscle, skin, tendon, fat, and bone.

All tissues and organs can be affected by electrical injury. The cutaneous burns are often limited, with variable deep tissue damage. Appreciation of this special property of electrical wounds is critical in their management. Skin wounds are typically leathery or charred areas of full-thickness skin loss. The entry and exit sites are usually depressed, giving the appearance that current exploded the tissues. The arc burn is produced by current coursing external to the body from contact to ground, favoring a path of least resistance. The flexor surfaces of the wrist, elbow, and axilla are most often involved, because the hand is the most commonly involved body part. After several days, the demarcation between viable and nonviable tissue becomes more obvious. Flame burns of the skin may result from ignition of clothing by electrical arcing and may be full-thickness burns because of the prolonged exposure of the dazed victim to the flame.

The most severe cardiopulmonary manifestations occur at the time of the injury. These include anoxia and ventricular fibrillation, which may cause immediate death due to respiratory or cardiac arrest. Major electrical injury is accompanied by a 3 to 15 percent incidence of acute renal failure, which is greater than the incidence after thermal burns.

Nervous tissue is highly susceptible to electrical injury because of its low resistance. Neurologic deficits can be seen initially or up to 3 years later, and neurologic aberrations are the most frequent nonfatal sequelae of electrical injury. An important diagnostic point is to ask the patient if the details of the accident are remembered. An inability to recall recent events indicates that electricity entered the body, erasing recent memory. This loss of recent memory is used by psychiatrists treating severely depressed people by means of electroshock therapy. Lesions of the central nervous system may cause varying levels of consciousness and respiratory and motor paralysis, which are usually transient; recovery is the rule. If the effects are permanent, they often assume the character of cortical encephalopathy or hemiplegia with or without aphasia. Spinal cord damage is the most common permanent sequela of electrical injury and is seldom complete. Many deficits seen initially resolve spontaneously; others may not develop until 6 to 9 months after the electrical injury. Permanent deficits may not be seen for days to months, are of gradual onset, and progress slowly. Often these disturbances are not noted until the rehabilitative phase of recovery, when gait abnormalities become evident. Peripheral nerves may be burned directly or may be compressed by surrounding edema or scar tissue. Neuropathies also can develop in unburned limbs. Autonomic nervous system dysfunction may be seen in both the acute and recovery phases. Reflex sympathetic dystrophy or causalgia can occur. Late onset of burning pain, frequently associated with vasomotor, trophic, and dermal changes, is characteristic.

Cataracts characteristically occur following high-voltage injuries. The incidence of these lesions, which are usually bilateral, may be as great as 30 percent when electrical contact is made above the clavicles, particularly when the entry wound is on the head. The latent period between the accident and the onset of blurred vision averages 6 months but ranges from a few weeks to 3 years.

Direct vascular injury is more common after electrical injury than after any other type of burn. The blood flow in large arteries and veins is usually sufficient to dissipate the heat generated by the electric current. However, smaller vessels may experience significant heat-related damage, resulting in thrombosis. Direct vascular injury probably contributes to the high amputation rate after high-voltage electrical injury. Delayed hemorrhage from mural necrosis of large blood vessels also may occur.

Associated injury in electrical accidents can be due to falls of considerable distance or to the explosive effects of the current. Fractures of the vertebrae and long bones and dislocations also may result from the violent tetanic muscle contractions.

℞ TREATMENT

At the scene of the accident, the patient must be separated immediately from the electric current, but rescuers must not touch or approach the patient until the current has been shut off to avoid injury to themselves. Flames should then be extinguished.

Cardiopulmonary support must be initiated if necessary and maintained during transport. Aggressive life support is essential, because victims of high-voltage electrical injury may be resuscitated successfully without permanent neurologic damage even after a prolonged cessation of vital functions. Because blunt trauma and skeletal injury may both coexist, a thorough history and careful physical examination are essential. Accurate assessment of the extent and nature of the burns is essential to the determination of subsequent therapy. Neurologic status must be evaluated repeatedly during convalescence because it changes frequently.

Fluid replacement is essential in the initial management. Hypovolemia results from the rapid loss of fluid into damaged tissues. Small entry and exit wounds may lead to underestimation of the underlying injury, so fluid requirements may be grossly underestimated. Ringer's lactate should be infused rapidly (0.5 to 1 mL/kg per hour) as necessary to correct hypovolemia and to maintain urinary output. Large volumes of fluid are necessary in high-voltage injury because the fluid and electrolyte needs are much greater than in patients with thermal burns of equivalent surface area. The adequacy of resuscitation is monitored, with urinary output being the single most reliable indicator of circulatory status. The presence of urinary hemoglobin and myoglobin necessitates treatment with mannitol, and the urine should be made alkaline to prevent precipitation of these pigments in the kidney. When hemoglobinuria and/or myoglobinuria is present, the rate and volume of the crystalloid infusion must be sufficient to maintain a minimum urine output of 100 mL/h. This infusion is continued until the urine is grossly clear of pigment. Acute renal failure, if it occurs, is treated as described in Chap. 270. Red blood cell transfusion, plasma, dextran, or other plasma expanders are unnecessary during the acute resuscitative phase.

Low-Voltage Injury Injuries resulting from low-voltage current, such as those related to household appliances, are usually small and limited to the area of contact. These burns frequently involve the hands, feet, or, in children, the corners of the mouth, lips, and tongue. The evolution of tissue injury and vascular necrosis from the current itself are complete within 7 to 10 days. During this time, the wounds are allowed to slough and heal by contracture. Small but deep contact injuries on the trunk and extremities may be excised and grafted as necessary when the extent of the slough is evident. Early excision and local flap repair are rarely indicated. Delayed bleeding from the lip, seen in one-quarter of these injuries, is usually readily controlled by direct pressure.

High-Voltage Injury High-voltage injuries with devitalized skin, fat, and muscle are fundamentally surgical problems. They usually involve a limited amount of the total body surface, have upper-extremity contact points, and require amputation or other surgical procedures. They may affect any organ system. The ultimate treatment goals are stabilization of the patient, salvage of the limb, debridement of devitalized tissue, wound coverage, and rehabilitation. Prolonged expectant nonsurgical therapy only increases the risk of invasive infection.

The timing of surgical debridement and its aggressiveness are controversial issues. Opinions range from early total excision with primary wound closure to the now outmoded expectant nonsurgical approach. Most surgeons favor an intermediate approach, individualizing according to the amount of tissue destruction and the location and type of the injury. Major amputations and surgical debridement are usually performed 2 to 4 days following injury, when the extent of necrosis is reasonably well defined but the risk of significant infection is small. High-voltage electrical burns frequently produce muscle compartment syndromes requiring fasciotomy. Circumferential deep limb burns due to associated flame or arc burns also may require escharotomy or fasciotomy. Indications for surgical decompression include loss of distal pulses, impaired capillary filling, paresthesia, and rigid muscle compartments. Decompression of the carpal tunnel is especially important owing to the high incidence of electrical injury to hands. If done expeditiously, this procedure may save a hand.

Debridement When possible, formal amputation and major debridement are delayed for 2 to 4 days following injury. During this interval, neurologic and cardiopulmonary abnormalities usually stabilize or resolve, and the demarcation between viable and nonviable tissues becomes more evident. Because these wounds are prone to anaerobic infection, particularly myonecrosis with clostridia, aqueous penicillin is given prophylactically from the time of admission until debridement is complete. Antibiotic administration should be further guided by identification of infecting organisms. Local wound care is started immediately and includes mechanical cleansing followed by the application of topical antibacterial agents and cotton gauze dressings. Silver sulfadiazine cream has excellent antibacterial activity but penetrates only a few millimeters into the tissues. Sulfamylon, a burn cream containing mafenid (a carbonic anhydrase inhibitor that readily penetrates soft tissue), may be advantageous in deep injuries and, therefore, is the topical agent of choice in the prevention and/or treatment of deep-seated infections. However, when absorbed, this drug causes a bicarbonate diuresis resulting in systemic acidosis.

Coverage of open wounds usually requires skin grafting. Deep electrical injuries frequently result in complex soft tissue wounds, which may require skin flaps for coverage. Nutritional support is essential and should be instituted early. As with other types of burns, appropriate splints should be fashioned and applied, and an aggressive program of physical therapy should be formulated and instituted. Psychological counseling is usually beneficial for patients who require a major amputation or other mutilating surgical procedure.

LIGHTNING INJURY

When the difference in potential between the undersurface of a cloud that becomes progressively more negative and the surface of the earth, which is positive, exceeds the insulator strength of air, electrical energy discharges as lightning. There are four mechanisms of lightning strike:

direct strike, flashover phenomenon, side flash, and stride potential. A direct strike consists of a major current flow directly through the victim. It is the most serious type of strike and is facilitated by metal objects such as golf clubs, umbrellas, or tools carried during a thunderstorm. In flashover, the lightning travels on the outside of the body; this type of strike is facilitated by wet garments and sweat. Side flash occurs when the current splashes from a building, tree, or other person and then travels to the victim. Stride potential occurs when the lightning strikes the ground close to a victim with one foot touching the ground closer to the point of the lightning strike than the other foot. In this position, there will be a potential electrical difference between the legs called *stride potential*. The lightning current may enter one leg, pass up and through the victim's body, and exit through the other leg. Stride potential and side-flash strikes can involve several individuals at once and may contribute to the multiple casualties often associated with lightning strike.

The pathophysiology of lightning injury is similar to that described for other electrical injuries. Lightning is direct current. The voltage of lightning may range from 3 million to 200 million volts and may carry a current of between 2000 and 3000 A. Lightning victims have a very short exposure to current because of the brief duration of lightning strike, which usually lasts only 1 to 100 ms. Most of the current may flash over the outside of the body. In contrast, contact with current from high-voltage electrical injuries may be prolonged, since the victim may become frozen to the current source. The injuries resulting from lightning strikes are similar to those from direct current and alternating current, as described above. Thus, treatment is essentially the same as for other types of electrical injury. The best form of treatment is prevention, consisting of avoidance of dangerous situations during rainstorms and electrical storms, such as standing near tall structures and metal poles or beneath metal shelters. It is erroneous to assume that once lightning strikes it is safe to venture into the open; another strike may occur in the same location. Many towers and churches have sustained multiple strikes.

BIBLIOGRAPHY

GROSSMAN AR et al: Auditory and neuropsychiatric behavior patterns after electrical injury. J Burn Care Rehab 14:169, 1993

GRUBE BJ et al: Neurologic consequences of electrical burns. J Trauma 30:254, 1990

HANUMADASS ML et al: Acute electrical burns: A 10-year clinical experience. Burns 12:427, 1986

JORDAN MH et al: Lightning strike to the head. J Trauma 36:113, 1994

LICHTENBERG R et al: Cardiovascular effects of lightning strikes. J Am Coll Cardiol 21:531, 1993

LIFSCHULTZ BD, DONOGHUE ER: Deaths caused by lightning. J Forensic Sci 38:353, 1993

PATTEN BM: Lightning and electrical injuries: A review. Neurol Clin 10:1047, 1992

SAFFLE JR et al: Recent outcomes in the treatment of burn injury in the U.S. J Burn Care Rehab 16:219, 1995

396

L. Chinsoo Cho, Eli Glatstein

RADIATION INJURY

All human beings are constantly exposed to ionizing radiation. The sources of radiation include both the natural environment and man-made products. The natural sources include the cosmic radiation from space and radiation from the ground and from inhaled and ingested materials. Airline travel and mining both increase exposure to the background radiation. For example, air travel at 30,000 ft exposes individuals to a dose equivalent of 0.5 mrem/h. Radiation originating in the body comes mainly from radioactive potassium, which emits beta and gamma rays. Lungs are exposed to irradiation from inhaled air, which contains small amounts of radioactive radon. The cosmic exposure contributes approximately 28 mrem per year. The ground and internal sources contribute approximately 26 and 27 mrem per year, respectively. The most prominent man-made sources of radiation include x-ray equipment, nuclear weapons, and radioactive medications.

TERMINOLOGY AND DEFINITIONS

The first major unit of radiation exposure was the roentgen (R), defined as an amount of x-rays or gamma rays that produces a specific amount of ionization in a unit of air under standard temperature and pressure (Table 396-1); this quantity can be measured directly in an ionization chamber. The rad, or *r*adiation *a*bsorbed *d*ose, is defined as 100 ergs/g of tissue. Thus, the rad represents a net deposition of energy in a three-dimensional volume, because x-rays attenuate as they traverse tissue. The rad has been replaced by the Système Internationale (SI) unit of the gray (Gy), which represents 100 rad. Roentgens and rads can be converted by means of various tables; the relation between them depends on photon energy.

The above definitions reflect physical variables. The unit that reflects the biologic response and that can be used to compare the effects of various types of radiation is the unit of *dose equivalence*, the rem (*r*oentgen *e*quivalent in *m*an). The rem has been replaced by the SI unit, the sievert (Sv). These units reflect the exposure or absorption dose multiplied by a biologic factor that represents the biologic effectiveness of the specific type of radiation (see below).

TYPES OF IONIZING RADIATION

The absorption of energy from radiation in tissue often leads to excitation or ionization. Excitation involves elevation of an electron in an atom or molecule to a higher energy state without actual ejection of the electron. Ionization involves actual ejection of one or more electrons from the atom. Ionizing radiation is subclassified as electromagnetic (photon) or particulate radiation (Table 396-2). X-rays and gamma rays are examples of electromagnetic photon radiation. They differ only in their source: X-rays are produced mechanically, by making electrons strike a target, which causes the electrons to give up their kinetic energy as x-rays, while gamma rays are produced by nuclear disintegration of radioactive isotopes. The wavelength λ of the electromagnetic radiation is related to the frequency ν by the formula $\lambda\nu = c$, where c is the speed of light. Thus, wavelength is inversely proportional to frequency. The wavelength for x-rays is on the order of 10^{-10} m (1 Å).

X-rays can be thought of as packets of energy, or photons. X-rays have no mass or charge, travel in straight lines, and attenuate continuously as they traverse tissue. Gamma rays have similar properties. Each photon contains an amount of energy equal to $h\nu$, where h is Planck's constant. The critical difference between nonionizing and ionizing radiation is the energy of individual photons, not the energy of the total dose. The energy in keV of a particular x-ray or gamma ray can be calculated to be equal to 12.4 divided by the wavelength in angstroms.

Table 396-1

Units and Definitions

Unit	Quantity Measured	Definition
Roentgen (R)	Exposure	Amount of x-rays or gamma rays that produces a specific amount of ionization in a given volume of air
Rad	Dose	100 ergs deposited per gram of tissue
Gray (Gy)	Dose	SI unit of dose; equals 100 rad
Rem	Dose equivalence	Unit that reflects the biologic response. It is used to compare various types of radiation
Sievert (Sv)	Dose equivalence	SI unit of dose equivalence; equals 100 rem

Table 396-2

Common Types of Ionizing Radiation

Type	Mass	Charge	Comment
Electromagnetic			
X-ray	0	0	X-rays and gamma rays do not differ except in the source. Gamma rays are produced intranuclearly, and x-rays are produced extranuclearly (i.e., mechanically).
Gamma ray	0	0	
Particulate			
Electron (e)	9.1×10^{-31} kg	−1	—
Proton (p)	2000 × e	+1	Exhibits a Bragg peak
Neutron (n)	2000 × e	0	Cannot be accelerated by an electrical field
Alpha particle	2p + 2n ~8000 × e	+2	Helium nucleus

Types of *particulate radiation* include electrons, protons, alpha particles, neutrons, negative pi-mesons, and heavy charged ions; these have discrete mass and charge (except for neutrons, which lack charge) (see Table 396-2). *Electrons*, or *beta particles*, are small and negatively charged, and can be accelerated to close to the speed of light. They decelerate fairly rapidly in tissue and penetrate it to only a limited depth. Thus, electron beams are often used to treat superficial problems. *Protons* are positively charged and have a mass about 2000 times that of an electron. Protons stop abruptly, depending on their energy; in the process of sudden deceleration, most of their energy is given up, which tends to cause ionization just before the proton stops. This region of enhanced ionization, sometimes called the Bragg peak, means that proton beams exert their effects in a relatively compact region. *Alpha particles* are helium nuclei, consisting of two protons and two neutrons. The mass and charge are great enough that these particles do not penetrate far through matter unless they have tremendous energy; even a piece of paper is enough to protect against most alpha particles. Because these particles are charged, they can be accelerated in electrical fields.

Neutrons are similar in mass to protons (having an atomic mass of 1), but they are not charged and therefore cannot be accelerated in an electrical field. Neutron beams are produced by colliding charged particles into a suitable target or are emitted as a fission product of heavy radioactive atoms. *Heavy charged ions* are nuclei of heavier elements that have a positive charge owing to the stripping away of some or all of the orbiting electrons.

Equal doses of different types of radiation do not necessarily produce equal biologic effects. One gray of neutrons produces a greater biologic effect than 1 Gy of x-rays. The biologic effects produced by a given dose of radiation can be quantified by the relative biologic effectiveness (RBE) value, which relates them to the effects produced by 250 kV photon radiation as a standard. The RBE value will be greater for more densely ionizing radiation, such as neutrons. In general, the RBE value depends on the linear energy transfer (see below), the dose, the dose rate, and the nature of the biologic system. Gamma rays and x-rays generally have an RBE of approximately 1. Beta radiation (electrons) also has an RBE of approximately 1. The exact RBE value depends on the specific energy. Higher-energy x-rays are associated with a slightly lower RBE value. Neutrons and alpha particles have RBEs of about 3 for most biologic systems.

The linear energy transfer (LET) is the amount of ionization occurring per unit length of the radiation track. It is usually expressed as kilovolts per micron, and it increases with the square of the charge of the incident particle. High-LET radiation is biologically different from low-LET (i.e., conventional) radiation: Hypoxic and oxygenated cells respond similarly to high-LET irradiation, whereas it takes about three times as much low-LET radiation to produce a given killing effect in hypoxic cells as in oxygenated cells. It is thought that low-LET radiation must produce multiple hits on DNA to destroy a cell, whereas high-LET radiation need produce only a single hit on DNA to kill a cell. Representative values of LET and RBE are given in Table 396-3.

There are three major ways in which radiation, especially x-rays, is absorbed and results in ionization: the *photoelectric effect*, the *Compton effect*, and *pair production*. At low energies (30 to 100 keV), as in diagnostic radiology, the photoelectric effect is important. In this process, the incident photon interacts with an electron in one of the outer shells of an atom (typically K, L, or M). If the energy of the photon is greater than the binding energy of the electron, then the electron is expelled from the orbit with a kinetic energy that is equal to the energy of the incident photon minus the binding energy of the electron. The photoelectric effect varies as a function of the cube of the atomic number of the material exposed (Z^3); this fact explains why bone is visualized much better than soft tissue on radiographs.

At higher energies, as used in therapeutic radiology, the Compton effect dominates. In this process, the incident photon interacts with an electron in an orbital shell. Part of the incident photon energy appears as kinetic energy of electrons, and the residual energy continues as a less energetic deflected photon.

At energy levels above 1.02 MeV, the photons may be absorbed through pair production. In this process, both a positron and an electron are produced in the absorbing material. A positron has the same mass as an electron but has a positive instead of a negative charge. The positron travels a very short distance in the absorbing medium before it interacts with another electron. When that happens, the entire mass of both particles is converted to energy, with the emission of two photons in exactly opposite directions.

BIOLOGIC EFFECTS OF RADIATION

Radiation must generally produce double-strand breaks in DNA to kill a cell, owing partly to the high capacity of mammalian cells for repairing single-strand damage. Radiation can also produce effects indirectly by interacting with water (which makes up approximately 80 percent of a cell's volume) to generate free radicals, which can damage the cell. Free radicals are highly reactive chemical entities that lack a stable number of outer-shell electrons. A free radical is not stable and has a life span of a fraction of a second. It is estimated that most x-ray–induced cell damage is due to the formation of hydroxyl radicals, as follows:

$$\text{Ionizing radiation} + H_2O \rightarrow H_2O^+ + e^-$$
$$H_2O^+ + H_2O \rightarrow H_3O^+ + OH\cdot$$
$$OH\cdot \rightarrow \text{Cell damage}$$

Cell killing is the result of radiation damage. The biologic effects on epithelial cell reproduction are typically expressed only when the damaged cells attempt to divide. Another biologic effect is the induction of cancerous growth by mutation many years after radiation exposure. It is clear that patients who receive low doses of radiation in childhood have a significant risk of neoplasm two to three decades after their exposure; this risk is significantly higher than that of the population as a whole.

Table 396-3

LET and RBE Values

Type of Radiation	LET Values, keV/μm
Cobalt-60 gamma rays	0.2
250-keV x-rays	2.0
10 MeV protons	4.7
Type of Radiation	**RBE Values (Quality Factors)**
X-rays, gamma rays, and electrons	1
Neutrons	3–20
Heavy particles	1–20

RADIATION-INDUCED CHROMOSOME ABERRATIONS Chromosome breaks can occur when cells are irradiated. The broken ends of chromosomes can combine with broken ends of different chromosomes. These abnormal combinations are most readily seen during mitosis. Chromosome abnormalities typically occur in cells irradiated in the G1 phase of the cell cycle, before the doubling of genetic material. If cells are irradiated in the G2 phase, chromatid aberrations may result. The frequency of chromosomal aberrations in peripheral circulating lymphocytes correlates with dose received. The dose can be estimated by comparing the chromosomal changes to in vitro cultures exposed to controlled doses of irradiation. The minimum dose that can be detected by peripheral lymphocyte analysis is about 10 to 20 rem. Lymphocyte analysis may provide evidence of recent total-body exposure.

CELL SURVIVAL CURVE The dose-response curve for all mammalian cells appears to have a linear-quadratic relationship. In simple terms, the mathematical model that explains the relationship between the dose and the fraction of surviving cells has both linear and exponential components. The linear component results from double-stranded chromosomal breaks produced by single hits. The exponential component represents breaks produced by multiple hits. Figure 396-1 shows the shape of a typical survival curve for mammalian cells exposed to radiation. The fraction of cells surviving is plotted on a semilogarithmic scale. For alpha particles or low-energy neutrons, the dose-response curve is a straight line from the origin. There appears to be no shoulder, which is thought to represent the accumulation of sublethal events within the cells beyond which one additional hit will cause cell death, and which also reflects the cell's ability to repair sublethal injury. Thus, the survival rate is an exponential function of the dose. In the case of x-rays or gamma rays, the dose-response curve has a shoulder, which is followed by a straight-line curve as the dose is increased.

D_0 represents the straight-line portion of the curve; it is the dose required to reduce the fraction of surviving cells to 37 percent of its previous value. D_0 represents the dose at which each cell receives an average of one lethal hit. The number N is defined by extrapolating the D_0 line directly back to the Y axis and is a measure of the width of the shoulder; presumably it represents the cell's repair capability. D_q is the dose at which the straight portion of the curve intersects a horizontal line drawn through unity; it represents a quasi-threshold dose.

In all mammalian cell lines studied, increases in the radiation dose decrease the survival rate of cells; i.e., there is no absolute radioresistance for mammalian cells, although relative resistance is common. Membrane-based resistance mechanisms, commonly responsible for resistance to chemotherapy, have not been identified with radiation.

Four important processes that occur after radiation exposure can be summarized as the "four R's" of radiobiology. The first is *repair*. Repair is temperature dependent and is thought to represent the enzymatic mechanisms for healing intracellular injury. The second R is *reoxygenation*. Reoxygenation represents a process whereby oxygen (and other nutrients) actually are better distributed to viable cells following radiation injury and cell killing. The third R is *repopulation*, the ability of the cell population to continue to divide and to replace dying and dead cells. The fourth R is *redistribution*, which reflects the variability of a cell's radiosensitivity over the cell cycle. Radiosensitivity can vary through cell cycle by as much as a factor of 3. The G1 phase has the most variable length of all the phases of the cell cycle. For most cell lines, cells that have a short G1 period are most sensitive at the G2/mitosis interface, less sensitive in G1, and most resistant toward the end of the synthesis (S) period.

When radiation works as an anticancer treatment, it works because of differences in the four Rs between tumor cells and normal tissues. Those differences are best exploited by radiotherapy regimens that employ dose fractionation.

CLINICAL FINDINGS RELATED TO FRACTIONATION The clinical radiation response may be related to the interactions of various growth factors and cytokines. For example, radiation can induce growth factors and cytokines such as tumor necrosis factor (TNF), interleukin (IL) 1, and others to be released by irradiated cells. TNF can induce proliferation of fibroblasts and enhance the inflammatory response. TNF and IL-1 have been shown to radioprotect hematopoietic cells in vitro by increasing the D_0 of the cell survival curve. TNF also has been shown to enhance killing of a human tumor cell line when added before irradiation. TNF may produce radioprotection or radiosensitization depending on the cell type, and it remains unclear what degree of sensitization or protection can be derived from TNF. Other factors implicated in the radiation response are basic fibroblast growth factor and platelet-derived growth factor-β, which may be associated with late effects of radiation on vessels. Cytokines are induced by transcriptional activation after exposure to ionizing radiation. Interactions of these factors may modify the clinical response to radiation exposure.

The rate and the length of functional recovery of normal tissues are related to the number of stem cells surviving after irradiation. The volume of the irradiated tissue will also influence the rate of recovery from the radiation as well as the severity of the side effects. If the stem cells are destroyed in the irradiated volume and there is inadequate

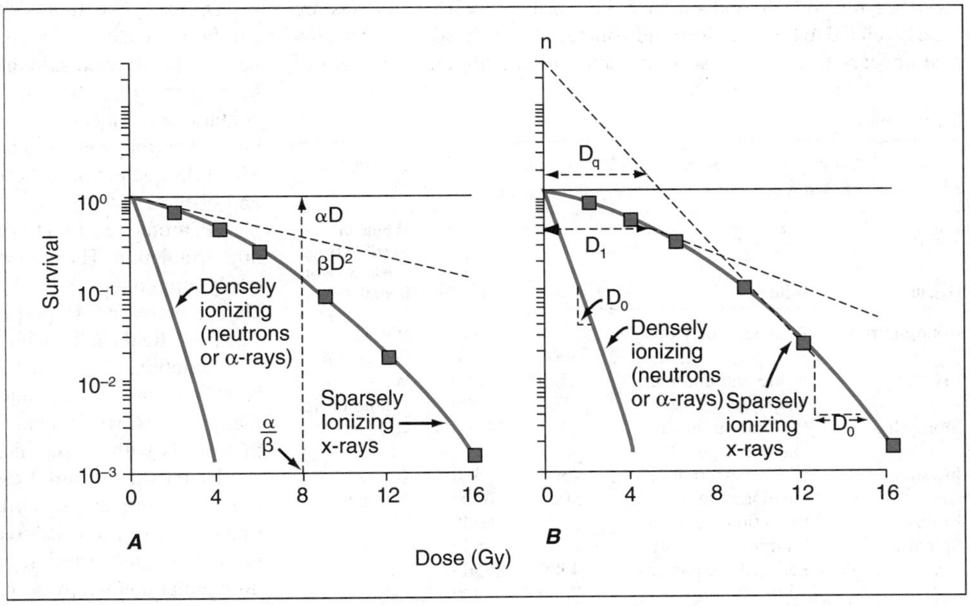

FIGURE 396-1 Shape of survival curve for mammalian cells exposed to radiation. The fraction of cells surviving is plotted on a logarithmic scale against dose on a linear scale. For alpha particles or low-energy neutrons (said to be densely ionizing) the dose-response curve is a straight line from the origin (i.e., survival is an exponential function of dose). The survival curve can be described by just one parameter, the slope. For x-rays or gamma rays (said to be sparsely ionizing), the dose-response curve has an initial linear slope, followed by a shoulder; at higher doses the curve tends to become straight again. *A*. The experimental data are fitted to a linear-quadratic function. There are two components of cell killing: one is proportional to dose (αD), while the other is proportional to the square of the dose (βD^2). The dose at which the linear and quadratic components are equal is the ratio α/β. The linear-quadratic curve bends continuously but is a good fit to experimental data for the first few decades of survival. *B*. The curve is described by the initial slope (D_1), the final slope (D_0), and a parameter that represents the width of the shoulder, either n or D_q. (From Hall, with permission.)

replacement from adjacent tissues, radiation injury will persist. True late effects develop independent of early reactions; they occur despite recovery from acute radiation injury.

Table 396-4 shows the frequency of radiation tolerance seen with fractionated radiotherapy at 5 years of follow-up. These numbers are rough estimates at best. The clinical manifestations of irradiation will depend on the volume of the organ irradiated, the total dose, the dose per fraction, and the length of time taken to deliver the dose. In addition, the cellular consequences of treatment can be progressive over time. Thus, length of follow-up is also crucial in judging clinical sequelae.

Central Nervous System Traditionally, the central nervous system (CNS) has been described as relatively resistant to radiation-induced changes. When the human brain is treated with standard fractionation (1.8 to 2.0 Gy/d), acute reactions are seldom observed.

Subacute CNS reactions to radiation treatment are more common. The clinical manifestations may include Lhermitte's sign, which is a self-limited paresthesia occurring with flexion of the neck. It is believed to be due to transient demyelination of the spinal cord following significant radiation exposure. It can be seen 1 to 3 months after completion of radiation treatment to the spinal cord. The frequency of Lhermitte's sign varies according to the type of radiation therapy and can be as high as 15 percent after the mantle radiation treatments commonly employed to treat Hodgkin's disease. Mild encephalopathy and focal neurologic changes can occur after irradiation limited to the cranium. If radiation treatments to the brain are given at the same time that chemotherapeutic agents are administered, the effects can be more severe, presumably reflecting altered permeability to the drugs. The effect of cranial irradiation is believed to be secondary to radiation effects on the replicating oligodendrocytes and possibly on the microvasculature. Both clinical and radiologic changes may simulate tumor progression and can often pose diagnostic and treatment dilemmas.

Post-irradiation pathology and associated clinical symptoms typically begin 6 to 36 months after radiation therapy. These effects are clearly related to the total dose and volume treated. In addition, fraction size appears to be the most important variable affecting the rate of

Table 396-4

Class 1 Organs: Fatal or Severe Morbidity Following Cumulative Doses of Radiation Delivered with Standard Fractionation

Organ	Injury	$TD_{5/5}$*	$TD_{50/5}$†	Whole or Partial Organ (Field Size or Length)
Bone marrow	Aplasia, pancytopenia	250	450	Whole
		3000	4000	Segmental
Liver	Acute and chronic hepatitis	2500	4000	Whole
		1500	2000	Whole (strip)
Stomach	Perforation, ulcer, hemorrhage	4500	5500	100 cm
Intestine	Ulcer, perforation, hemorrhage	4500	5500	400 cm
		5000	6500	100 cm
Brain	Infarction, necrosis	5000	6000	Whole
Spinal cord	Infarction, necrosis	4500	5500	10 cm
Heart	Pericarditis, pancarditis	4500	5500	60%
		7000	8000	25%
Lung	Acute and chronic pneumonitis	3000	3500	100 cm
		1500	2500	Whole
Kidney	Acute and chronic nephrosclerosis	1500	2000	Whole (strip)
		2000	2500	Whole
Fetus	Death	200	400	Whole

* $TD_{5/5}$ is the minimal tolerance dose—the dose that, when administered to a given patient population under a standard set of treatment conditions, results in a rate of severe complications of 5 percent or less within 5 years of treatment.

† $TD_{50/5}$ is the maximal tolerance dose—the dose that, when administered to a given population of patients under a standard set of treatment conditions, results in a rate of severe complications of 50 percent within 5 years of treatment.

SOURCE: From Rubin et al, 1975.

post-irradiation brain necrosis. Neurocognitive changes can also be seen in children after cranial irradiation. The important pretreatment factors that predict the degree of late CNS effects include the age at which cranial irradiation was given and neurocognitive functional level at the time of treatment.

A unique late effect of cranial irradiation combined with chemotherapy, known as leukoencephalopathy, has been described in some patients. Leukoencephalopathy is a necrotizing reaction usually noted 4 to 12 months after combined treatment with methotrexate and cranial irradiation. Dementia and dysarthria may progress to seizures, ataxia, or death.

Transverse myelitis after radiation treatment is a spinal cord reaction similar to cerebral necrosis. This syndrome consists of progressive and irreversible leg weakness, and loss of bladder function and sensation referrable to a single spinal cord level. Flaccid paralysis eventually occurs. Symptoms can occur as early as 6 months after radiation treatment, but the usual time to onset is 12 to 24 months. There is no known correlation between Lhermitte's sign and transverse myelitis.

Skin Skin reaction can be seen within 2 weeks of fractionated radiotherapy, a delay that correlates with the time required for cells to move from the basal to the keratinized layer of skin. The severity of the reaction depends on the amount of skin dose per fraction and the total dose delivered to an area of skin. Erythema is observed, soon followed by dry desquamation. The skin at this time can be erythematous, warm, and sometimes edematous. There is dilation of the vessels in the upper dermis and an associated inflammatory infiltration with granulocytes, macrophages, eosinophils, plasma cells, and lymphocytes.

Modern high-energy radiotherapy machines often do not produce significant skin reactions. When a severe skin reaction occurs, it is usually located where the beam strikes the skin tangentially. *Moist desquamation* consists of eruption of the epidermal layer. Healing is through re-epithelialization from cells of less affected basal layers. When skin reactions are severe, treatment interruptions are needed to permit healing.

Dry desquamation is treated conservatively. Symptoms of dryness can be alleviated by advising the patient to wear only cotton fabric next to the affected skin and to refrain from the use of irritants of any kind. If treatment becomes necessary, hydrophilic agents that do not contain heavy metals are recommended. Petroleum jellies should not be used, as they may trap bacteria and increase the chance of infection. Moist desquamation is best managed by leaving the affected area dry and open to air.

A chronic reaction to radiation can be seen starting 6 to 12 months after irradiation. The epidermis is usually atrophic, and it may be more easily injured than normal skin. The amount of interstitial fibrosis may also be increased. Hyperpigmentation of irradiated skin outlining the treatment field can be seen within a couple of months after completion of irradiation. This will fade gradually. The skin becomes thin, and hair loss may be permanent. Radiation therapy can induce second malignancies, which tend to be more aggressive than cancers arising in patients without significant radiation exposure.

Heart and Blood Vessels When cardiac disease appears after radiation treatment, it is often difficult to tell to what extent the radiation treatment was causative. The pathogenesis of atherosclerotic heart disease is multifactorial. Exposure of a large heart volume to high-dose radiation therapy probably enhances the development of coronary artery disease. Acute "pericarditis" may result from cardiac irradiation. The symptoms may include chest pain and fever, with or without pericardial effusion. This syndrome is usually self-limited and typically manifests itself a few months after treatment. Asymptomatic pericardial effusion may be the most common manifestation of radiation-induced heart disease. It is usually detected by chest x-ray and confirmed by an echocardiogram.

Most patients with symptomatic radiation-induced constrictive pericarditis will have received more than 40 Gy to a large portion of the heart. The risk increases significantly with cardiac doses greater than 50 Gy.

Chronic cardiac changes may have their onset from 6 months to several years after irradiation. The clinical symptoms may indicate chronic constrictive disease due to pericardial, myocardial, and endocardial fibrosis—a pancarditis. The clinical signs may include dyspnea, chest pain, venous distention, pleural effusion, and paradoxical pulse.

Lung The clinical symptoms of radiation pneumonitis can be separated into early and late phases. During the early phase, clinical manifestations may include dyspnea, cough, and fever. Shortness of breath is relatively infrequent. It is more common to observe only the radiologic changes on a chest x-ray, without clinical symptoms. The clinical signs and symptoms of radiation pneumonitis may appear in 3 to 6 weeks if a large region of lung is irradiated to a dose above 25 Gy. An infiltrate outlining the treatment field may become evident on the chest x-ray. Radiation changes should not occur outside the treated field. Computed tomography can often help in distinguishing radiation pneumonitis from other causes of the infiltrate. The incidence of radiation pneumonitis can be reduced with careful treatment planning designed to lower the total dose given to the treated lung volume. Permanent scarring that results in respiratory compromise may develop if the dose and the volume of lung irradiated are excessive. Dyspnea and cough may be severe and debilitating.

There may be a role for glucocorticoids, especially in patients with hypoxemia. Patients with symptoms of radiation pneumonitis may respond rapidly to glucocorticoids, but the medication has little effect on fibrotic changes. Steroid treatment must be tapered very slowly to avoid rebound exacerbation of symptoms, which can prove lethal for some patients. Prophylactic administration of steroids is of questionable merit. Unless the symptoms are severe, it is preferable to provide supportive care, including bronchodilators and oxygen at the lowest possible FI_{O_2}.

Digestive Tract The limited available human data show that pathologic changes of the epithelial layer occur early during radiation treatments. The underlying submucosa may become edematous, with dilation of capillaries. Recovery from radiation damage can be expected within a few weeks after completion of radiation therapy, provided that sufficient numbers of stem cells are left. The radioresponsiveness of the aerodigestive tract, like that of other strctures, is not uniform but varies according to the location.

Patients often have symptoms from radiation exposure that are similar to other forms of acute gastritis. The clinical signs include epigastric pain, loss of appetite, nausea, and vomiting. Decreased gastric acidity is observed after 15 to 20 Gy of fractionated radiation therapy. The tolerance of the stomach to radiation is also aggravated by addition of systemic chemotherapy, such as therapy with 5-fluorouracil.

The germinal centers of the bowel mucosa are in the crypts of Lieberkühn. Newly formed cells move upward along the walls of the crypts as transitional cells, undergoing maturation. The epithelial lining of the small bowel is the most rapidly renewed system in the human body and it is completely renewed in 3 to 6 days. Within 12 to 24 h after the first dose of radiation therapy, pathologic evidence of dead cells are seen in the mucosal lining. Complete denudation of the mucosal surface rarely occurs during a regular course of radiation treatment because of the high capacity of the mucosa for regeneration. However, a focal area of erosion may be seen. The histologic appearance may be nearly normal within 2 to 3 weeks after radiation therapy.

Clinical manifestations of acute radiation enteropathy are nausea and vomiting, diarrhea, and cramping pain. Relevant factors contributing to the pathogenesis of diarrhea include malabsorption and alterations in the intestinal bacterial flora. The severity of symptoms, as in other anatomic areas, is proportional to the irradiated volume and the total dose.

The symptoms of chronic radiation enteropathy include diarrhea, abdominal cramping, nausea, malabsorption, vomiting, and obstruction. Progressive fibrosis, perforation, fistula formation, and stenosis of the irradiated portion of the bowel can also occur during the chronic phase of radiation enteropathy. Most clinical manifestations of chronic changes occur between 6 months and 5 years after radiation therapy.

Conservative noninvasive treatment can frequently control gastrointestinal symptoms. A low-residue or elemental diet may be beneficial. When nonsurgical treatment fails to relieve severe symptoms, surgical intervention is often indicated.

Bladder Radiation injury to the bladder generally becomes symptomatic 3 to 6 weeks after the start of treatment, and symptoms usually subside 3 to 4 weeks after completion of radiation therapy. Patients often complain of increased frequency and dysuria. Cystoscopy often shows diffuse mucosal changes similar to those of acute cystitis. Sometimes desquamation and ulceration can be seen. Without infection, urinary symptoms are managed symptomatically. Concurrent chemotherapy with cytotoxic agents such as cyclophosphamide increases the severity of the acute bladder reaction.

The late effects of high radiation doses to the bladder may include interstitial fibrosis, telangiectasia, and ulceration. The blood vessels may be dilated and prone to rupture, resulting in painless hematuria. These changes are often difficult to distinguish from tumor recurrence and progression. A contracted bladder may result from doses in excess of 60 Gy.

Testis and Ovaries In general, type B spermatogonia are exquisitely sensitive to the effects of radiation. The type A spermatogonia are thought to be more resistant because their longer cell cycle time allows considerable variation in radiosensitivity among different phases of the cell cycle. Sertoli cells and Leydig cells are less radiosensitive than the spermatogonia. FSH and LH elevation have been observed after as little as 75 cGy. Doses as low as 10 cGy to the testicles may result in injury to the type B spermatogonia. The single dose required for permanent sterilization on normal human males is not clearly established but it is believed to be between 6 and 10 Gy. In normal human males, sperm count recovery requires 9 to 18 months after a fractionated dose of 8 to 100 cGy.

The radiation dose necessary to induce ovarian failure is age dependent. A single dose of 3 to 4 Gy can induce amenorrhea in almost all women over 40 years of age. In young women, oogenesis is much less sensitive to radiation than spermatogenesis in men.

ACUTE TOTAL-BODY IRRADIATION The data regarding the acute effects of total-body irradiation on humans come primarily from Japanese survivors of the atomic bomb, Marshallese exposed to radioactive fall-out in 1954, and persons exposed to radiation from the recent Chernobyl accident. Early symptoms of acute total-body irradiation last for a limited time. This is known as the *prodromal radiation syndrome*. Clinical manifestations depend on the total-body dose. At doses in excess of 100 Gy to the total body, death usually occurs 24 to 48 h later from neurologic and cardiovascular failure. This is known as the *cerebrovascular syndrome*. Because cerebrovascular damage causes death very quickly, the failures of other systems do not have time to develop.

At doses between 5 and 12 Gy, death may occur in a matter of days as a result of the *gastrointestinal syndrome*. The symptoms during this period may include nausea, vomiting, and prolonged diarrhea for several days leading to dehydration, sepsis, and death. A total-body dose of greater than 1000 cGy is uniformly fatal unless supportive therapy (fluid, electrolytes, blood products, and antibiotics) is given. The process of intestinal denudation depends on the dose and may take between 3 and 120 days. Death from intestinal denudation usually occurs before the full effects of radiation on the blood-forming elements are seen.

At total-body doses between 2 and 8 Gy, death may occur several weeks after exposure and is due to effects on the bone marrow, which results in the *hematopoietic syndrome*. The full effect of radiation is not apparent until the mature hematopoietic cells are depleted. Death from the hematologic damage occurs at about 20 to 30 days after exposure, and the risk of death continues over the next 30 days. Clinical symptoms during this period may include chills, fatigue, and petechial hemorrhage. Peripheral blood lymphopenia develops during the first 12 to 48 h after any significant exposure. Beyond 5 to 6 Gy, the rate and magnitude of the drop are not well correlated to radiation exposure. Some stem cells may survive acute exposure to 10 Gy or more. Anemia from red cell depression usually does not occur because of the long half-life of erythrocytes.

It is estimated that the $LD_{50/60}$ (the dose at which 50 percent of the population is dead by 60 days) is around 325 cGy if support is not given. There is considerable variability in the total-body dose tolerated. The very young and the old are more radiosensitive than middle-aged and young adult individuals. Females in general appear to be more tolerant of radiation than males. Persons exposed to less than 2 Gy will require little or no therapy, but they should probably be observed closely with daily blood counts for a few days.

There is a considerable controversy regarding the utility of bone marrow transplantation for patients exposed to acute total body irradiation. At doses less than 800 cGy, the patient is likely to survive with supportive care. Most people exposed to doses higher than 1000 cGy will die from the gastrointestinal syndrome. Therefore, 800 to 1000 cGy may be the dose range in which bone marrow transplantation could have a role, although the Chernobyl experience did not confirm that. It is difficult to estimate the dose received by a given patient after radiation exposure. This is an important point, because bone marrow transplantation is most effective if it is performed within the first 3 to 5 days after exposure. It is, therefore, extremely important to estimate the received dose quickly.

RADIATION AND CANCER INDUCTION Some nonlethal changes in DNA sequences caused by irradiation may cause malignant transformations. Thus, it is not surprising that second neoplasms can be caused by exposure to ionizing radiation. However, paradoxically, this risk is actually less with doses above a certain level. It is unclear whether there is a "safe" dose that will not have any adverse biologic effect. It should be emphasized that the estimates of the risk of developing cancer after low-level exposure to ionizing radiation are often derived by extrapolation from the risks for higher doses and acute exposures. Predicted risks of cancer are, therefore, prone to modification depending on the assumptions made about the data available for analysis.

Throughout the history of human exposure to ionizing radiation, there have been documented cases of increased rates of cancer after exposure to radiation. The populations studied include survivors of the atomic bomb during World War II, radium watch dial painters who shaped their brush tips with their tongue, patients who have undergone multiple fluoroscopic examinations for tuberculosis, patients who received spinal irradiation for ankylosing spondylitis, patients who received breast irradiation for postpartum mastitis, and others. Exposure to ionizing radiation at an earlier age appears to increase the chance of developing radiation-induced carcinomas. However, the radiation-induced cancers have an age of onset similar to that of the native cancers, and the available data argue against radiation as the only cause of the increased incidence of cancers seen after exposure to radiation. Table 396-5 shows examples of cancer observed in specific situations.

Table 396-5

Examples of Radiation-Induced Cancers

Types of Exposure	Types of Cancer Observed
Neck irradiation during infancy for benign conditions	Thyroid carcinoma
Radiation therapy for other malignant tumors	Thyroid carcinoma Breast cancer Gastric cancer Melanoma Lung cancer Sarcomas in the field
Cranial irradiation	Central nervous system tumors
Breast irradiation for postpartum mastitis	Breast cancer
Brush-licking by radium dial painters	Bone sarcomas
Uranium mining	Lung cancer
In utero exposure	Leukemia

Because a safe dose of radiation is unknown at present, it is prudent to avoid routine exposures to ionizing irradiation.

BIBLIOGRAPHY

COX JD: Moss' *Radiation Oncology: Rationale, Technique, Results*, 7th ed. St. Louis, Mosby, 1994

GLATSTEIN E, CARTER SK: The chronic toxicity of cancer treatment, in *Principles of Cancer Treatment*, SK Carter et al (eds). New York, McGraw-Hill, 1982, pp 221–236

HALL EJ: *Radiobiology for the Radiologist*, 4th ed. Philadelphia, Lippincott, 1994

HALLAHAN D et al: The role of cytokines in radiation oncology, in *Important Advances in Oncology 1993*, VT DeVita Jr et al (eds). Philadelphia, Lippincott, 1993

KARAS JS, STANBURY JB: Fatal radiation syndrome from an accidental nuclear excursion. N Engl J Med 272:755, 1965

KHAN FM: *The Physics of Radiation Therapy*, 2d ed. Baltimore, Williams & Wilkins, 1993

LITTLEFIELD LG, LUSHBAUGH CC: Cytogenetic dosimetry for radiation accidents: "The good, the bad, and the ugly," in *The Medical Basis for Radiation Accident Preparedness*, vol 2: *Clinical Experience and Follow-up Since 1979*, RC Ricks, SA Fry (eds). New York, Elsevier, 1990, pp 461–478

METTLER FA JR, UPTON AC: *Medical Effects of Ionizing Radiation*, 2d ed, Philadelphia, Saunders, 1995

PEREZ CP, BRADY LW: *Principles and Practice of Radiation Oncology*, 2d ed, Philadelphia, Lippincott, 1992

RUBIN P et al (eds): *Radiation Biology and Radiation Pathology Syllabus*, set RT 1: *Radiation Oncology*. Chicago, American College of Radiology, 1975

——— et al: Late effects of normal tissues consensus conference. Int J Radiat Oncol Biol Phys 31:5, 1995

SCHWADE JG, LICHTER AS: Management of acute effects of radiation therapy, in *Principles of Cancer Treatment*, SK Carter et al (eds). New York, McGraw-Hill, 1982, pp 212–220

TEPPER JE (ed): Normal tissue effects of radiation therapy. Semin Radiat Oncol 4:2, 1994

397

Howard Hu

HEAVY METAL POISONING

Metals constitute a major category of toxins that pose a significant threat to health through occupational as well as environmental exposures. One indication of their importance relative to other potential hazards is their ranking by the U.S. Agency for Toxic Substances and Disease Registry, which lists all hazards present in toxic waste sites according to their prevalence and the severity of their toxicity. The first, second, third, and sixth hazards on the list are heavy metals: lead, mercury, arsenic, and cadmium, respectively. This chapter offers specific information on the sources and metabolism of each of these metals as well as on the toxic effects produced by each and the appropriate treatment for poisoning by each.

The intrinsic atomic stability of metals allows their relatively easy tracing and measurement in biologic material, although the clinical significance of the levels measured is not always clear. Metals are inhaled primarily as dusts and fumes (the latter defined as tiny particles generated by combustion). Metal poisoning can also result from exposure to vapors (e.g., mercury vapor in the manufacture of fluorescent lamps). When metals are ingested in contaminated food or drink or through hand-to-mouth activity (implicated especially often in children), their gastrointestinal absorption varies greatly with the specific chemical form of the metal and the nutritional status of the host. Once a metal is absorbed, blood is the main medium for its transport, with the precise kinetics dependent on diffusibility, binding forms, rates of biotransformation, availability of intracellular ligands, and other factors. Some organs (such as bone, liver, and kidney) sequester metals in relatively high concentrations for years. Most metals are excreted through renal clearance and gastrointestinal excretion; some proportion is also excreted through salivation, perspiration, exhalation, lactation, skin exfoliation, and loss of hair and nails.

Some metals, such as copper and selenium, are essential to normal metabolic function as trace elements (see Chap. 80) but are toxic at high levels of exposure. Others, such as lead and mercury, are xenobiotic and theoretically are capable of exerting toxic effects at any level of exposure. Indeed, much research is currently focused on the contribution of low-level xenobiotic metal exposure to chronic diseases and to subtle changes in health that may have significant public health consequences.

The most important component of treatment for metal toxicity is the termination of exposure. Another component is the use of *chelating agents*, which are used to bind metals into stable cyclic compounds with relatively low toxicity and to enhance their excretion. The principal chelating agents are dimercaprol (British Anti-Lewisite, BAL), edetate (EDTA), succimer (DMSA, dimercaptosuccinic acid), and penicillamine; their specific use depends on the metal involved and the clinical picture. Activated charcoal does not bind metals and thus is of limited usefulness in cases of acute metal ingestion.

Besides the four metals discussed in detail in this chapter, several others deserve mention. *Aluminum* contributes to the encephalopathy seen in patients with severe renal disease who are undergoing dialysis (see Chap. 354). High levels of aluminum are found in the neurofibrillary tangles in the cerebral cortex and hippocampus of patients with Alzheimer's disease as well as in the drinking water and soil of areas with an unusually high incidence of Alzheimer's disease. The experimental and epidemiologic evidence for the aluminum–Alzheimer's disease link is so far relatively weak, however, and it cannot be concluded that aluminum is a causal agent or a contributing factor in neurodegenerative disease. Hexavalent *chromium* is corrosive and sensitizing. Workers in the chromate and chrome pigment production industries have consistently had an excess risk of lung cancer. The introduction of *cobalt* chloride as a fortifier in beer led to outbreaks of fatal cardiomyopathy among heavy consumers. Occupational exposure (e.g., of some miners, dry-battery manufacturers, and arc welders) to *manganese* can cause a Parkinsonian syndrome within 1 to 2 years, including gait disorders; postural instability; a masked, expressionless face; tremor; and psychiatric symptoms. *Nickel* exposure induces an allergic response, and inhalation of nickel compounds with low aqueous solubility (such as nickel subsulfide and nickel oxide) in occupational settings is associated with an increased risk of cancer of the lung. Overexposure to *selenium* may cause local irritation of the respiratory system and eyes, gastrointestinal irritation, liver inflammation, loss of hair, depigmentation, and peripheral nerve damage. Workers exposed to certain organic forms of *tin* (particularly trimethyl and triethyl derivatives) have developed psychomotor disturbances including tremor, convulsions, hallucinations, and psychotic behavior.

Finally, *thallium*, which is a component of some insecticides, metal alloys, and fireworks, is absorbed through the skin as well as through ingestion and inhalation. Severe poisoning follows a single ingested dose of >1 g or >8 mg/kg. Nausea and vomiting, abdominal pain, and hematemesis precede confusion, psychosis, organic brain syndrome, and coma. Thallium is radiopaque. Induced emesis or gastric lavage is indicated within 4 to 6 h of acute ingestion; Prussian blue prevents absorption and is given orally at 250 mg/kg in divided doses. Unlike other types of metal poisoning, thallium poisoning may be less severe when activated charcoal is used to interrupt its enterohepatic circulation. Other measures include forced diuresis, treatment with potassium chloride (which promotes renal excretion of thallium), and peritoneal dialysis.

LEAD

SOURCE Lead has been mined and used in industry and in household products for centuries. The dangers of lead toxicity, the clinical manifestations of which are known as *plumbism*, have been known since ancient times. The twentieth century has seen both the greatest-ever exposure of the general population to lead and an extraordinary amount of new research on lead toxicity.

Populations are exposed to lead chiefly via paints, cans, plumbing fixtures, and leaded gasoline. The intensity of these exposures, while recently decreased by regulatory actions, remains high in some segments of the population because of the deterioration of lead paint used in the past and the entrainment of lead from paint and vehicle exhaust into soil and house dust. Many other environmental sources of exposure exist, such as leafy vegetables grown in lead-contaminated soil, improperly glazed ceramics, lead crystal, and certain herbal folk remedies. Many industries, such as battery manufacturing, demolition, painting and paint removal, and ceramics, continue to pose a significant risk of lead exposure to workers and surrounding communities.

New research on lead toxicity has been stimulated by advances in toxicology and epidemiology as well as by a shift of emphasis in toxicology away from binary outcomes (life/death; 50 percent lethal dose) to grades of function, such as neuropsychological performance, indices of behavior, blood pressure, and kidney function.

Tests for levels of lead in blood have facilitated both research on lead and surveillance of individuals at risk. Blood lead is now measured with stringent quality controls in commercial laboratories throughout the United States. Measurement of the blood lead levels of children 6 months to 5 years of age is currently mandated by some states, and the U.S. Occupational Safety and Health Administration (OSHA) requires the testing of workers who may be exposed to lead in the course of their jobs.

METABOLISM Elemental lead and inorganic lead compounds are absorbed through ingestion or inhalation. Organic lead (e.g., tetraethyl lead, the lead additive to gasoline) is absorbed to a significant degree through the skin as well. Pulmonary absorption is efficient, particularly if particle diameters are <1 μm (as in fumes from burning lead paint). Children absorb up to 50 percent of the amount of lead ingested, whereas adults absorb only about 10 to 20 percent. Gastrointestinal absorption of lead is enhanced by fasting and by dietary deficiencies in calcium, iron, and zinc; such absorption is minimal, however, for lead in the form of lead sulfide, a common constituent of mining waste. Lead is absorbed into blood plasma, where it equilibrates rapidly with extracellular fluid, crosses membranes (such as the blood-brain barrier and the placenta), and accumulates in soft and hard tissues. In the blood, around 95 to 99 percent of lead is sequestered in red cells, where it is bound to hemoglobin and other components. As a consequence, lead is usually measured in whole blood rather than in serum. The largest proportion of absorbed lead is incorporated into the skeleton, which contains more than 90 percent of the body's total lead burden. Lead is excreted mainly in the urine (in a process that depends on glomerular filtration and tubular secretion) and in the feces. Lead also appears in hair, nails, sweat, saliva, and breast milk. The half-life of lead in blood is approximately 25 days; in soft tissue, about 40 days; and in the nonlabile portion of bone, more than 25 years. Thus, blood lead levels may decline significantly while the body's total burden of lead remains heavy.

The toxicity of lead is probably related to its affinity for cell membranes and mitochondria, as a result of which it interferes with mitochondrial oxidative phosphorylation and sodium, potassium, and calcium ATPases. Lead impairs the activity of calcium-dependent intracellular messengers and of brain protein kinase C. In addition, lead stimulates the formation of inclusion bodies that may translocate the metal into cell nuclei and alter gene expression.

CLINICAL TOXICOLOGY Symptomatic lead poisoning in childhood generally develops at blood lead levels exceeding 3.9 μmol/L (80 μg/dL) and is characterized by abdominal pain and irritability followed by lethargy, anorexia, pallor (resulting from anemia), ataxia, and slurred speech. Convulsions, coma, and death due to generalized cerebral edema and renal failure occur in the most severe cases. Subclinical lead poisoning [blood lead level >1.4 μmol/L (>30 μg/dL)] can cause mental retardation and selective deficits in language, cognitive function, balance, behavior, and school performance despite the lack of discernible symptoms. Epidemiologic studies and meta-analyses of studies regarding lead's effect on the intellectual function of children indicate that cognition is probably impaired in a dose-related fashion at blood lead levels well below 1.4 μmol/L (30 μg/dL) and that no threshold for this effect is likely to exist above the lowest measurable blood lead level of 0.05 μmol/L (1 μg/dL). The impact is greatest when the exposure is of long duration and when it takes place around the age of 2 years.

In adults, symptomatic lead poisoning usually develops when blood lead levels exceed 3.9 μmol/L (80 μg/dL) for a period of weeks and is characterized by abdominal pain, headache, irritability, joint pain, fatigue, anemia, peripheral motor neuropathy, and deficits in short-term memory and the ability to concentrate. Encephalopathy is rare. A "lead line" sometimes appears at the gingiva-tooth border after prolonged high-level exposure. Some individuals develop these symptoms and signs at lower blood lead levels [1.9 to 3.9 μmol/L (40 to 80 μg/dL)] and/or with briefer periods of exposure. Chronic subclinical lead exposure is associated with interstitial nephritis, tubular damage (with tubular inclusion bodies), hyperuricemia (with an increased risk of gout), and a decline in glomerular filtration rate and chronic renal failure. Epidemiologic evidence also suggests that blood lead levels in the range of 0.34 to 1.7 μmol/L (7 to 35 μg/dL) are associated with increases in blood pressure, decreases in creatinine clearance, and decrements in cognitive performance that are too small to be detected as a lead effect in individual cases but nevertheless may contribute significantly to the causation of chronic disease.

An additional issue for both children and adults is whether lead that has accumulated in bone and lain dormant for years can pose a threat later in life, particularly at times of increased bone resorption such as pregnancy, lactation, and senile osteoporosis. Elevation of the bone lead level appears to be a risk factor for anemia and hypertension. Hyperthyroidism has been reported to cause lead toxicity in adults by mobilizing stores of bone lead acquired during childhood.

Genetic polymorphisms of the gene that codes for aminolevulinic acid dehydratase, a critical enzyme in the production of heme, may confer differences in susceptibility to lead retention and toxicity; 15 percent of Caucasians have a variant form of this gene. This issue is the focus of continued research.

LABORATORY FINDINGS In 1991, the Centers for Disease Control and Prevention designated 0.48 μmol/L (10 μg/dL) as the blood lead level of concern in children. A specific set of interventions is recommended when the level exceeds this value. OSHA requires the regular measurement of blood lead in lead-exposed workers and the maintenance of blood lead levels below 1.9 μmol/L (40 μg/dL). Concentrations of heme precursors (such as δ-aminolevulinic acid) in plasma and urine are sometimes increased at blood lead levels as low as 0.73 μmol/L (15 μg/dL). Levels of protoporphyrin (free erythrocyte or zinc) rise—although not consistently—once blood lead levels have exceeded 1.2 μmol/L (25 μg/dL) for several months. Lead-associated anemia is usually normocytic and normochromic and may be accompanied by basophilic stippling. Lead-induced peripheral demyelination is reflected by prolonged nerve conduction time and subsequent paralysis, usually of the extensor muscles of the hands and feet ("wrist and foot drop"). An increased density at the metaphyseal plate of growing long bones ("lead lines") can develop in children and resemble those seen in rickets. Children with high-level lead exposure sometimes develop Fanconi's syndrome, pyuria, and azotemia. Adults chronically exposed to lead can develop elevated serum creatinine levels, decreased creatinine clearance rates, and chronic changes and intranuclear inclusion bodies (detected at renal biopsy). Deficits may be apparent in neuropsychometric tests of both children and adults; these abnormalities by themselves are not pathognomonic. X-ray fluorescence is being investigated as a method for estimating long-term accumulation of lead in bone.

℞ TREATMENT

It is absolutely essential to prevent further exposure of affected individuals to lead. Cases of lead poisoning should be reported to OSHA (if the exposure is occupational) and to local boards of health so that home evaluations can be performed. Pharmacologic treatment for lead toxicity entails the use of chelating agents, principally edetate calcium disodium (CaEDTA), dimercaprol, penicillamine, and succimer, which is given orally and has relatively few side effects. Chelation is recommended for the treatment of all children whose blood lead levels are greater than 2.7 μmol/L (55 μg/dL), with the addition of dimercaprol if lead encephalopathy is found. Chelation is also recommended for children if blood lead levels are between 1.2 and 2.7 μmol/L (25 and 55 μg/dL) and the total amount of lead excreted in urine during the 8 h after a single dose of edetate calcium disodium exceeds 9.7 μmol/L (200 μg/dL). Chelation is recommended for adults if blood lead levels exceed 3.9 μmol/L (80 μg/dL) or if blood lead levels exceed 2.9 μmol/L (60 μg/dL) and symptoms have developed. The ability of chelation to improve subclinical outcomes (such as performance on psychometric testing) at lower levels of blood lead in both children and adults is the subject of current research.

MERCURY

SOURCE Metallic mercury (Hg^0) is used in thermometers, dental amalgams, and some batteries. Mercurous mercury (Hg^+) and mercuric mercury (Hg^{2+}) can be combined with other chemicals, such as carbon, chlorine, or oxygen, to form inorganic or organic mercury compounds. All three forms of mercury are toxic to various degrees. Organic mercury compounds are slowly broken down into inorganic compounds; conversely, inorganic mercury can be converted by microorganisms in soil and water into the organic compound methyl mercury. Fish, particularly tuna and swordfish, can concentrate methyl mercury at high levels; such contamination of fish by industrial runoff and their subsequent ingestion was responsible for the Minamata Bay epidemic of mercury poisoning in Japan in 1955. Occupational exposure to inorganic mercury compounds continues in some chemical, metal-processing, electrical-equipment, automotive, and building industries and in medical and dental services. Environmental exposure probably takes place most commonly through ingestion of contaminated fish and through inhalation of the vapor generated by ordinary dental amalgam, which typically contains about 50 percent metallic mercury. There is also concern about exposure to drinking water contaminated by toxic waste sites included on the National Priority List, almost half of which contain mercury, and about the inhalation of fumes from incinerators burning mercury-contaminated waste products. Whether the latter types of exposure confer a significant risk of toxicity is controversial.

METABOLISM Elemental mercury is not well absorbed by the gastrointestinal tract and is excreted almost entirely in the feces after being ingested; however, when left standing, mercury is volatilized at room temperature into a vapor that is well absorbed by the lungs. Once absorbed, mercury in this form is lipid soluble, crosses the blood-brain barrier and the placenta, and can be oxidized by catalase and hydrogen peroxide into mercuric chloride, which is retained by the kidney and brain for years. Elemental mercury in blood has a half-life of approximately 60 days and is excreted mainly in the urine and feces.

The gastrointestinal and dermal absorption of inorganic mercury is significant. Large overdoses disrupt gastrointestinal barriers, further enhancing absorption. Once absorbed, inorganic mercury breaks down into metallic and mercuric mercury. Relatively little of this mercury crosses the blood-brain barrier; most is excreted in the urine or feces, with a half-life of 40 days, or is retained by the kidneys as mercuric mercury.

Organic mercury, particularly methyl mercury, can evaporate and undergo pulmonary absorption. Forms that are ingested (e.g., in contaminated fish) are well absorbed. Only small amounts are absorbed through the skin. Absorbed organic mercury is lipid soluble, readily crosses the blood-brain barrier and the placenta, appears in breast milk, and concentrates in the kidneys and central nervous system. Methyl mercury is acetylated in the liver, excreted in bile, reabsorbed, and then excreted in urine. Methyl mercury can also be conjugated with cysteine or glutathione. Only 1 percent of organic mercury is excreted unchanged into urine. The half-life of organic mercury compounds is in the range of 70 days.

Exposure to mercury in any form stimulates the kidney to produce metallothionein, a metal-binding protein that affords partial protection against mercury toxicity.

CLINICAL TOXICOLOGY Inhalation of metallic mercury vapor is the form of mercury exposure that has been best studied in terms of toxicity. High levels of exposure are most likely in an occupational setting in which mercury vapors are generated by heat-induced volatilization of metallic mercury. Cough, dyspnea, and tightness or burning pain in the chest are common symptoms that may be accompanied by diffuse infiltrates or a pneumonitis-like appearance on chest x-ray. Respiratory distress, pulmonary edema, lobar pneumonia, fibrosis, and desquamation of the bronchiolar epithelium can occur in relatively severe cases and have sometimes led to death. Acute inhalation of mercury vapor can also cause neurologic toxicity manifested by tremors (beginning in the hands), emotional lability, headaches, and polyneuropathy. Chronic exposure to metallic mercury produces a characteristic intention tremor and mercurial *erethism*, a constellation of findings including excitability, memory loss, insomnia, timidity, and sometimes delirium that was described in workers with occupational exposure in the felt-hat industry—hence the expression "mad as a hatter." Dentists with occupational exposure to mercury score below normal on neurobehavioral tests of motor speed, visual scanning, verbal and visual memory, and visuomotor coordination. Low-level exposure from dental amalgams may also be associated with adverse immunologic reactions in individuals with certain major human leukocyte antigen genotypes; further research is needed in this area.

Acute high-dose ingestion of inorganic mercury causes severe gastrointestinal corrosion with nausea, vomiting, hematemesis, and abdominal pain; acute renal failure, cardiovascular collapse, and shock may ensue. The lethal dose of inorganic mercury is estimated to be in the range of 10 to 42 mg/kg. Lower levels of exposure cause milder forms of gastrointestinal inflammation, gingivitis and loosening of the teeth, increased blood pressure and tachycardia, and the nephrotic syndrome. Symptoms similar to erethism may develop. Skin exposure to mercuric salts can cause exfoliative dermatitis.

Ingestion of organic mercury compounds is followed by diarrhea, tenesmus, and blisters of the upper gastrointestinal tract. The fatal dose of organic mercury is estimated at 10 to 60 mg/kg. People who ingested flour contaminated with *N*-(ethylmercuri)-*p*-toluenesulfonanilide developed bradycardia, QT prolongation, ST-segment depression, and T-wave inversions. The neurotoxicity resulting from organic mercury exposure is characterized by paresthesia; impaired peripheral vision, hearing, taste, and smell; slurred speech; unsteadiness of gait and limbs; muscle weakness; irritability; memory loss; and depression. In general, such symptoms begin at doses above 1.7 mg/kg. Autopsy findings suggest that lesions in the basal ganglia and gray matter of the cortex and cerebellum are chiefly responsible for these symptoms. Organic mercury exposure, primarily through the ingestion of grain treated with mercuric fungicides or of contaminated fish, is also associated with an increased risk of fetal toxicity. After the 1955 mercury poisoning outbreak in Minamata, Japan, exposed mothers gave birth to infants with mental retardation; retention of primitive reflexes; cerebellar symptoms; dysarthria; hyperkinesia; hypersalivation; atrophy of the cerebral cortex, corpus callosum, and cerebellum; and abnormal neuronal cytoarchitecture. This last change may reflect derangement of neuronal migration during fetal development.

Exposure of children to mercury in any of its forms can cause a particular syndrome known as *acrodynia*, or pink disease. This condition is characterized by flushing, itching, swelling, tachycardia, elevated blood pressure, excessive salivation or perspiration, irritability, weakness, morbilliform rashes, and desquamation of the palms and soles.

LABORATORY FINDINGS Levels of mercury in blood and urine should not exceed 180 nmol/L (3.6 μg/dL) and 0.7 μmol/L (15 μg/L), respectively. Symptoms may develop when blood and urine mercury levels exceed 1 μmol/L (20 μg/dL) and 3 μmol/L (60 μg/L), respectively. If a baseline 24-h urinary mercury value is low, repetition of the measurement after a single 2-g oral dose of succimer may be useful in documenting elevated renal mercury burdens in retired mercury-exposed workers; an increase of more than 20 μg in a 24-h urine sample suggests previous exposure. Levels in hair may be used as a dosimeter for chronic organic mercury exposure; neurobehavioral dysfunction in children may occur if the maternal mercury concentration in hair exceeds 30 nmol/g (6 μg/g).

Rx TREATMENT

Acute ingestion of mercuric salts can be treated by induced emesis or gastric lavage. Polythiol resins can be administered orally to bind mercury in the gastrointestinal tract. The most effective chelating agents are dimercaprol, succimer, and penicillamine, which have active mono- or dithiol groups. Acute inorganic mercury poisoning can be treated with dimercaprol at a dose not exceeding 24 mg/kg per day and given intramuscularly in divided doses. Therapy is usually given in 5-day courses separated by several days of rest. The *N*-acetyl form of penicillamine is also useful at a dose of 30 mg/kg per day in divided doses. Peritoneal dialysis, hemodialysis, and extracorporeal regional complexing hemodialysis with succimer have all been used with some success in the treatment of patients with renal failure.

Chronic inorganic mercury poisoning is best treated with *N*-acetyl penicillamine.

ARSENIC

SOURCE Significant exposure to arsenic occurs through both anthropogenic and natural sources. Arsenic is released into the air by volcanoes and is a natural contaminant of some deep-water wells. Occupational exposure to arsenic is common in the smelting industry (in which arsenic is a byproduct of ores containing lead, gold, zinc, cobalt, and nickel) and is increasing in the microelectronics industry (in which gallium arsenide is responsible). Low-level arsenic exposure continues to take place in the general population (as do some cases of high-dose poisoning) through the commercial use of inorganic arsenic compounds in common products such as wood preservatives, pesticides, herbicides, fungicides, and paints; through the consumption of foods and the smoking of tobacco treated with arsenic-containing pesticides; and through the burning of fossil fuels in which arsenic is a contaminant. Arsenic was also a major ingredient of Fowler's solution and continues to be found in some folk remedies.

METABOLISM The toxicity of an arsenic-containing compound depends on its valence state (zero-valent, trivalent, or pentavalent), its form (inorganic or organic), and the physical aspects governing its absorption and elimination. In general, inorganic arsenic is more toxic than organic arsenic, and trivalent arsenite is more toxic than pentavalent and zero-valent arsenic. The normal intake of arsenic by adults occurs primarily through ingestion and averages around 50 μg/d (range, 8 to 104 μg/d). Most (around 64 percent) of this amount is accounted for by organic arsenic from fish, seafood, and algae; the specific arsenic compounds obtained from these sources are arsenobentaine and arsenocholine, which are relatively nontoxic and are rapidly excreted in unchanged form in the urine. After absorption, inorganic arsenic accumulates in the liver, spleen, kidneys, lungs, and gastrointestinal tract. It is then rapidly cleared from these sites but leaves a residue in keratin-rich tissues such as skin, hair, and nails. Arsenite (+5) undergoes biomethylation in the liver to the less toxic metabolites methylarsenic acid and dimethylarsenic acid; biomethylation can quickly become saturated, however, and the result is the deposition of increasing doses of inorganic arsenic in soft tissues. Arsenic, particularly in its trivalent form, inhibits critical sulfhydryl-containing enzymes. In the pentavalent form, the competitive substitution of arsenic for phosphate can lead to rapid hydrolysis of the high-energy bonds in compounds such as ATP.

CLINICAL TOXICOLOGY Acute arsenic poisoning from ingestion results in increased permeability of small blood vessels and inflammation and necrosis of the intestinal mucosa; these changes manifest as hemorrhagic gastroenteritis, fluid loss, and hypotension. Delayed cardiomyopathy accompanied by electrocardiographic abnormalities may develop. Symptoms include nausea, vomiting, diarrhea, abdominal pain, delirium, coma, and seizures. A garlicky odor may be detectable on the breath. Acute tubular necrosis and hemolysis may develop. The reported lethal dose of arsenic ranges from 120 to 200 mg in adults and is 2 mg/kg in children. Arsine gas causes severe hemolysis within 3 to 4 h of exposure and can lead to acute tubular necrosis and renal failure.

In chronic arsenic poisoning, the onset of symptoms comes at 2 to 8 weeks. Typical findings are skin and nail changes, such as hyperkeratosis, hyperpigmentation, exfoliative dermatitis, and Mees' lines (transverse white striae of the fingernails); sensory and motor polyneuritis manifesting as numbness and tingling in a "stocking-glove" distribution, distal weakness, and quadriplegia; and inflammation of the respiratory mucosa. Epidemiologic evidence has linked chronic consumption of water containing arsenic at concentrations in the range of 10 to 1820 ppb with vasospasm and peripheral vascular insufficiency culminating in "blackfoot disease," a gangrenous condition affecting the extremities. Chronic arsenic exposure has also been associated with a greatly elevated risk of skin cancer and possibly of cancers of the lung, liver (angiosarcoma), bladder, kidney, and colon.

LABORATORY FINDINGS When acute arsenic poisoning is suspected, an x-ray of the abdomen may reveal ingested arsenic, which is radiopaque. The serum arsenic level may exceed 0.9 μmol/L (7 μg/dL); however, arsenic is rapidly cleared from the blood. Electrocardiographic findings may include QRS complex broadening, QT prolongation, ST-segment depression, T-wave flattening, and multifocal ventricular tachycardia. Urinary arsenic should be measured in 24-h specimens collected after 48 h of abstinence from seafood ingestion; normally, levels of total urinary arsenic excretion are less than 0.67 μmol/d (50 μg/d). Arsenic may be detected in the hair and nails for months after exposure. Abnormal liver function, anemia, leukocytosis or leukopenia, proteinuria, and hematuria may be detected. Electromyography may reveal features similar to those of Guillain-Barré syndrome.

℞ TREATMENT

Vomiting should be induced with ipecac in the alert patient with acute arsenic ingestion. Gastric lavage may be useful; activated charcoal with a cathartic (such as sorbitol) may be tried, although its efficacy is not clear. Aggressive therapy with intravenous fluid and electrolyte replacement in an intensive-care setting may be lifesaving. Dimercaprol is the chelating agent of choice and is administered intramuscularly at an initial dose of 3 to 5 mg/kg on the following schedule: every 4 h for 2 days, every 6 h on the third day, and every 12 h thereafter for 10 days. (An oral chelating agent may be substituted.) Succimer is sometimes an effective alternative, particularly if adverse reactions to dimercaprol develop (such as nausea, vomiting, headache, increased blood pressure, and convulsions). In cases of renal failure, doses should be adjusted carefully, and hemodialysis may be needed to remove the chelating agent–arsenic complex. Arsine gas poisoning should be treated supportively with the goals of maintaining renal function and circulating red-cell mass. Other than the avoidance of additional exposure, specific treatment is not of proven benefit in chronic arsenic toxicity. Recovery, particularly from the resulting peripheral neuropathy, may take months and may never be complete.

CADMIUM

SOURCE Environmental exposure to cadmium can result from the ingestion of basic foodstuffs, especially grains, cereals, and leafy vegetables, which readily absorb cadmium occurring naturally or in soil contaminated by sewage sludge, fertilizers, and polluted groundwater. Serious cadmium poisoning can follow the contamination of food and water by mining effluents, as took place in the 1946 outbreak of *itai-itai* ("ouch-ouch") disease (so named because cadmium-induced bone toxicity caused painful bone fractures) in the Jintzu River basin in Japan. Airborne cadmium can be released during smelting or during the incineration of municipal waste containing plastics and nickel-cadmium batteries. Cigarette smoke contains cadmium. Occupational exposure takes place in the metal-plating, pigment, battery, and plastics industries.

METABOLISM The normal daily intake of cadmium through ingestion or inhalation is from 20 to 40 μg, although only 5 to 10 percent of this amount is absorbed. Most absorbed cadmium is concentrated in the liver and kidneys. In erythrocytes and soft tissues, cadmium is bound to metallothionein, a low-molecular-weight protein that mitigates the toxicity of the unbound ion. This complex is filtered at the glomerulus but is then reabsorbed by the proximal tubules. The lack of an effective elimination pathway is responsible for cadmium's biologic half-life of 10 to 30 years. The toxicity of cadmium may involve its binding to key cellular sulfhydryl groups, its competition with other metals (zinc and selenium) for inclusion in metalloenzymes, and its competition with calcium for binding sites on regulatory proteins such as calmodulin.

CLINICAL TOXICOLOGY Acute high-dose cadmium inhalation can cause severe respiratory irritation with pleuritic chest pain, dyspnea, cyanosis, fever, tachycardia, nausea, and life-threatening noncardiogenic pulmonary edema. The onset of symptoms may be delayed from 4 to 24 h. Acute exposure through ingestion can cause severe nausea, vomiting, salivation, abdominal cramps, and diarrhea. Single lethal oral doses have reportedly ranged from 350 to 8900 mg. Chronic effects of cadmium exposure are dose-dependent and include anosmia, yellowing of the teeth, emphysema, minor changes in liver function, microcytic hypochromic anemia unresponsive to iron therapy, renal tubular dysfunction characterized by proteinuria and increased urinary excretion of β_2-microglobulin, and (with prolonged poisoning) osteomalacia leading to bone lesions and pseudofractures. In follow-up studies of occupationally exposed workers, β_2-microglobulinuria was found to be irreversible. Associations with hypertension, prostate cancer, and lung cancer have been suggested by some studies but await confirmation.

LABORATORY FINDINGS The daily level of excretion of cadmium by persons without known cadmium exposures is usually below 10 nmol/L (1 μg/L or 1 μg/g of creatinine). This level increases somewhat with age and smoking. Toxicity, including renal dysfunction, is considered unlikely until the urinary cadmium level exceeds 100 nmol/L (10 μg/g of creatinine). Serum cadmium levels reflect recent rather than chronic exposure and generally are below 30 nmol/L (0.3 μg/dL) in unexposed persons. A blood level exceeding 500 nmol/L (5 μg/dL) is considered toxic. An increased urinary concentration of β_2-microglobulin is the most sensitive indicator of an elevated cadmium dose and of nephropathy but may also be detected in other renal diseases, such as chronic pyelonephritis.

℞ TREATMENT

There is no proven effective treatment for cadmium poisoning. Succimer has been used as an antagonist for cadmium intoxication in animals. Although there is no published experience in humans, this drug might be considered for therapy. Chelation therapy is not useful, and use of dimercaprol is contraindicated as this agent may exacerbate nephrotoxicity. Avoidance of further exposure and supportive therapy (including vitamin D if osteomalacia exists) are the mainstays of management.

BIBLIOGRAPHY

GENERAL

Aposhian HV et al: Mobilization of heavy metals by newer, therapeutically useful chelating agents. Toxicology 97:23, 1995

Christensen J: Human exposure to toxic metals: Factors influencing interpretation of biomonitoring results. Sci Total Environ 166:89, 1995

Friberg L, Elinder CG: Biological monitoring of toxic metals. Scand J Work Environ Health 1:7, 1993

Goyer RA: Nutrition and metal toxicity. Am J Clin Nutr 61:646S, 1995

Wennberg A: Neurotoxic effects of selected metals. Scand J Work Environ Health 20:65, 1994

LEAD

Balbus-Kornfeld JM et al: Cumulative exposure to inorganic lead and neurobehavioural test performance in adults: An epidemiological review. Occup Environ Med 52:2, 1995

Goldman R et al: Lead poisoning from mobilization of bone stores during thyrotoxicosis. Am J Ind Med 25:417, 1994

Hu H et al: The relationship between bone lead and hemoglobin. JAMA 272:1512, 1994

——— et al: The relationship of blood and bone lead to hypertension among middle-aged to elderly men. JAMA 275:1171, 1996

Kim R et al: A longitudinal study of low-level lead exposure and renal function in men from the Normative Aging Study. JAMA 275:1177, 1996

Lockitch G: Perspectives on lead toxicity. Clin Biochem 26:371, 1993

Smith MC et al: A polymorphism in the delta-aminolevulinic acid dehydratase gene is a possible modifier of the pharmacokinetics of lead. Environ Health Perspect 103:248, 1995

MERCURY

Clarkson TW: Mercury: Major issues in environmental health. Environ Health Perspect 100:31, 1993

Corbin SB, Kohn WG: The benefits and risks of dental amalgam: Current findings reviewed. J Am Dent Assoc 125:381, 1994

Enestrom S, Hultman P: Does amalgam affect the immune system? A controversial issue. Int Arch Allergy Immunol 106:180, 1995

Harada M: Minamata disease: Methylmercury poisoning in Japan caused by environmental pollution. Crit Rev Toxicol 25:1, 1995

Ngim CH et al: Chronic neurobehavioural effects of elemental mercury in dentists. Br J Ind Med 49:782, 1992

Roels HA et al: Urinary excretion of mercury after occupational exposure to mercury vapour and influence of the chelating agent meso-w,e-dimercaptosuccinic acid (DMSA). Br J Ind Med 48:247, 1991

ARSENIC

Bates MN et al: Arsenic ingestion and internal cancers: A review. Am J Epidemiol 135:462, 1992

Heaven R et al: Arsenic intoxication presenting with macrocytosis and peripheral neuropathy, without anaemia. Acta Haematol 92:142, 1994

Kelafant GA et al: Arsenic poisoning in central Kentucky: A case report. Am J Ind Med 24:723, 1993

CADMIUM

Basinger MA et al: Antagonists for acute oral cadmium chloride intoxication. J Toxicol Environ Health 23:77, 1988.

Lauwerys RR et al: Cadmium: Exposure markers as predictors of nephrotoxic effects. Clin Chem 40:1391, 1994

Staessen J, Lauwerys R: Health effects of environmental exposure to cadmium in a population study. J Hum Hypertens 7:195, 1993

Waalkes MP, Rehm S: Cadmium and prostate cancer. J Toxicol Environ Health 43:251, 1994

APPENDICES

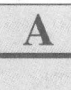

A LABORATORY VALUES OF CLINICAL IMPORTANCE

INTRODUCTORY COMMENTS

All laboratory appendices should be interpreted with caution since normal values differ widely among clinical laboratories. The values given in this Appendix are meant primarily for use with this text. In preparing the Appendix, the editors have taken into account the fact that the system of international units (SI, système international d'unités) is now used in most countries and in most medical and scientific journals.[1] However, clinical laboratories in many countries continue to report values in traditional units. Therefore, both systems are used in the Appendix. Values in SI units appear first, and traditional units appear in parentheses after the SI units. The dual system is also used in the text except for (1) those instances in which the numbers remain the same but only the terminology is changed (mmol/L for meq/L or IU/L for mIU/mL), when only the SI units are given; and (2) most pressure measurements (e.g., blood and cerebrospinal fluid pressures), when the traditional units (mmHg, mmH_2O) are used. In all other instances in the text the SI unit is followed by the traditional unit in parentheses. The SI base units, SI derived units, other units of measure referred to in Appendix A, and SI prefixes are listed in Tables A-1 to A-3 at the end of Appendix A. Conversions from one system to another can be made as follows:

$$\text{mmol/L} = \frac{\text{mg/dL} \times 10}{\text{atomic weight}}$$

$$\text{mg/dL} = \frac{\text{mmol/L} \times \text{atomic weight}}{10}$$

ASCITIC FLUID

See Chapter 46

BODY FLUIDS AND OTHER MASS DATA

Body fluid, total volume: 50 percent (in obese) to 70 percent (lean) of body weight
- Intracellular: 0.3–0.4 of body weight
- Extracellular: 0.2–0.3 of body weight

Blood
- Total volume:
  - Males: 69 mL per kg body weight
  - Females: 65 mL per kg body weight
- Plasma volume:
  - Males: 39 mL per kg body weight
  - Females: 40 mL per kg body weight
- Red blood cell volume:
  - Males: 30 mL per kg body weight (1.15–1.21 L/m^2 of body surface area)
  - Females: 25 mL per kg body weight (0.95–1.00 L/m^2 of body surface area)

[1] Young DS: Implementation of SI units for clinical laboratory data. Ann Intern Med 106:114, 1987

CEREBROSPINAL FLUID[2]

		Conversion Factor (CF) C × CF = SI
Osmolarity	292–297 mmol/kg water (292–297 mOsm/L)	—
Electrolytes:		
Sodium	137–145 mmol/L (137–145 meq/L)	—
Potassium	2.7–3.9 mmol/L (2.7–3.9 meq/L)	—
Calcium	1.0–1.5 mmol/L (2.1–3.0 meq/L)	0.5
Magnesium	1.0–1.2 mmol/L (2.0–2.5 meq/L)	0.5
Chloride	116–122 mmol/L (116–122 meq/L)	—
CO_2 content	20–24 mmol/L (20–24 meq/L)	—
P_{CO_2}	6–7 kPa (45–49 mmHg)	0.1333
pH	7.31–7.34	—
Glucose	2.2–3.9 mmol/L (40–70 mg/dL)	0.05551
Lactate	1–2 mmol/L (10–20 mg/dL)	0.1110
Total protein:	0.2–0.5 g/L (20–50 mg/dL)	0.01
Albumin	0.066–0.442 g/L (6.6–44.2 mg/dL)	0.01
IgG	0.009–0.057 g/L (0.9–5.7 mg/dL)	0.01
IgG index[3]	0.29–0.59	
Oligoclonal bands (OCB)	<2 bands not present in matched serum sample	
Ammonia	15–47 μmol/L (25–80 μg/dL)	0.5872
Creatinine	44–168 μmol/L (0.5–1.9 mg/dL)	88.40
Myelin basic protein	<4 μg/L	—
CSF pressure	50–180 mmH_2O	—
CSF volume (adult)	~150 mL	—
Leukocytes		
Total	<5 per mL	—
Differential:		
Lymphocytes	60–70 percent	—
Monocytes	30–50 percent	—
Neutrophils	None	—

[2] Since cerebrospinal fluid concentrations are equilibrium values, measurements of the same parameters in blood plasma obtained at the same time are recommended. However, there is a time lag in attainment of equilibrium, and cerebrospinal levels of plasma constituents that can fluctuate rapidly (such as plasma glucose) may not achieve stable values until after a significant lag phase.

[3] $$\text{IgG index} = \frac{\text{CSF IgG(mg/dL)} \times \text{serum albumin(g/dL)}}{\text{Serum IgG(g/dL)} \times \text{CSF albumin(mg/dL)}}$$

CHEMICAL CONSTITUENTS OF BLOOD

See also function tests, especially "Metabolic and Endocrine Tests."

	Conversion Factor (CF) $C \times CF = SI$
Acetoacetate, plasma: <100 μmol/L (<1 mg/dL)	97.95
Albumin, serum: 35–55 g/L (3.5–5.5 g/dL)	10.00
Aldolase: 0–100 nkat/L (0–6 U/L)	16.67
$Alpha_1$ antitrypsin, serum: 0.8–2.1 g/L (85–213 mg/dL)	0.01
Alpha fetoprotein (adult), serum: <30 μg/L (<30 ng/mL)	—
Aminotransferases, serum:	
Aspartate (AST, SGOT): 0–0.58 μkat/L (0–35 U/L)	0.01667
Alanine (ALT, SGPT): 0–0.58 μkat/L (0–35 U/L)	0.01667
Ammonia, as NH_3, plasma: 6–47 μmol/L (10–80 μg/dL)	0.5872
Amylase, serum: 0.8–3.2 μkat/L; 60–180 U/L	0.01667
Angiotensin-converting enzyme (ACE): <670 nkat/L (<40 U/L)	16.67
Anticonvulsant drug levels: see Fig. 365-8	
Arterial blood gases:	
$[HCO_3^-]$: 21–28 mmol/L (21–30 meq/L)	—
P_{CO_2}: 4.7–5.9 kPa (35–45 mmHg)	0.1333
pH: 7.38–7.44	—
P_{O_2}: 11–13 kPa (80–100 mmHg)	0.1333
Ascorbic acid (vitamin C), serum: 23–57 μmol/L (0.4–1.0 mg/dL)	56.78
Barbiturates, serum: normal, nondetectable	
Phenobarbital, "potentially fatal" level: approximately 390 μmol/L (9 mg/dL)	43.06
Most short-acting barbiturates, "potentially fatal" levels: approximately 150 μmol/L (35 mg/L)	4.419
β-Hydroxybutyrate, plasma: <300 μmol/L (<3 mg/dL)	96.05
Bilirubin, total, serum (Malloy-Evelyn): 5.1–17 μmol/L (0.3–1.0 mg/dL)	17.10
Direct, serum: 1.7–5.1 μmol/L (0.1–0.3 mg/dL)	17.10
Indirect, serum: 3.4–12 μmol/L (0.2–0.7 mg/dL)	17.10
Calciferols (vitamin D), plasma:	
1,25-dihydroxyvitamin D $[1,25(OH)_2D]$: 40–160 pmol/L (16 to 65 pg/mL)	2.4
25-hydroxyvitamin D [25(OH)D]: 20–200 nmol/L (8–80 ng/mL)	2.496
Calcium, ionized: 1.1–1.4 mmol/L (4.5–5.6 mg/dL)	0.2495
Calcium, plasma: 2.2–2.6 mmol/L (9–10.5 mg/dL)	0.2495
Carbon dioxide content, plasma (sea level): 21–30 mmol/L (21–30 meq/L)	—
Carbon dioxide tension (P_{CO_2}), arterial blood (sea level): 4.7–5.9 kPa (35–45 mmHg)	0.1333
Carbon monoxide content, blood: symptoms with over 20 percent saturation of hemoglobin	
Carotenoids, serum: 0.9–5.6 μmol/L (50–300 μg/dL)	0.01863
Ceruloplasmin, serum: 270–370 mg/L (27–37 mg/dL)	10.00
Chloride, serum (as Cl^-): 98–106 mmol/L (98–106 meq/L)	—
Cholesterol: see Table A-4	
Complement, serum:	
C3: 0.55–1.20 g/L (55–120 mg/dL)	0.01
C4: 0.20–0.50 g/L (20–50 mg/dL)	0.01
Copper, serum: 11–22 μmol/L (70–140 μg/dL)	0.1574

	Conversion Factor (CF) $C \times CF = SI$
Creatine kinase, serum (total):	
Females: 0.17–1.17 μkat/L (10–70 U/L)	0.01667
Males: 0.42–1.50 μkat/L (25–90 U/L)	0.01667
Creatine kinase-MB: 0–7 μg/L	—
Creatinine, serum: <133 μmol/L (<1.5 mg/dL)	88.40
Digoxin serum:	
Therapeutic level: 0.6–2.8 nmol/L (0.5–2.2 ng/mL)	1.281
Toxic level: >3.1 nmol/L (>2.4 ng/mL)	1.281
Ethanol, blood:	
Behavioral changes: >4.3 mmol/L (>20 mg/dL)	0.2171
Legal intoxication: >17 mmol/L (>80 mg/dL)	0.2171
Coma and death: >65 mmol/L (>300 mg/dL)	0.2171
Fatty acids, free (nonesterified), plasma: 180 mg/L (<18 mg/dL)	10.00
Ferritin, serum:	—
Women: 10–200 μg/L (10–200 ng/ml)	
Men: 15–400 μg/L (15–400 ng/ml)	
Fibrinogen, plasma: see "Hematologic Evaluations: Platelets and Coagulation"	—
Fibrinogen split products: see "Hematologic Evaluations: Platelets and Coagulation"	—
Folic acid, red cell: 340–1020 nmol/L cells (150–450 ng/mL cells)	2.266
Folic acid, serum: 7–36 nmol/L cells (3–16 ng/mL cells)	—
Gastrin, serum: 40–200 ng/L (40–200 pg/mL)	—
Glucose (fasting), plasma:	
Normal: 4.2–6.4 mmol/L (75–115 mg/dL)	0.05551
Diabetes mellitus: >7.8 mmol/L [>140 mg/dL (on more than one occasion)]	0.05551
Glucose, 2 h postprandial, plasma:	
Normal: <7.8 mmol/L (<140 mg/dL)	0.05551
Impaired glucose tolerance: 7.8–11.1 mmol/L (140–200 mg/dL)	0.05551
Diabetes mellitus: >11.1 mmol/L on more than one occasion (>200 mg/dL)	0.05551
Hemoglobin, blood (sea level):	
Male: 140–180 g/L (14–18 g/dL)	10.00
Female: 120–160 g/L (12–16 g/dL)	10.00
Hemoglobin A_{1c}: up to 6 percent of total hemoglobin	—
Immunoglobulins, serum:	
IgA: 0.9–3.2 g/L (90–325 mg/dL)	0.01
IgD: 0–0.08 g/L (0–8 mg/dL)	0.01
IgE: <0.00025 g/L (<0.025 mg/dL)	0.01
IgG: 8.0–15.0 g/L (800–1500 mg/dL)	0.01
IgM: 0.45–1.5 g/L (45–150 mg/dL)	0.01
Iron, serum: 9–27 μmol/L (50–150 μg/dL)	0.1791
Iron-binding capacity, serum: 45–66 μmol/L (250–370 μg/dL)	0.1791
Saturation: 0.2–0.45 (20–45 percent)	
Lactate dehydrogenase, serum: 1.7–3.2 μkat/L (100–190 U/L)	0.01667
Lactate dehydrogenase isoenzymes, serum (agarose):	
Fraction 1 (of total): 0.14–0.25 (14–26 percent)	0.01
Fraction 2: 0.29–0.39 (29–39 percent)	0.01
Fraction 3: 0.20–0.25 (20–26 percent)	0.01
Fraction 4: 0.08–0.16 (8–16 percent)	0.01
Fraction 5: 0.06–0.16 (6–16 percent)	0.01
Lactate, venous plasma: 0.6–1.7 mmol/L (5–15 mg/dL)	0.1110
Lead, serum: <1.0 μmol/L (<20 μg/dL)	0.04826
Lipase, serum: 0–2.66 μkat/L (0–160 U/L)	0.01667
Lipids: see Table A-4	—

	Conversion Factor (CF) C × CF = SI
Lipids, triglyceride, serum: see "Triglycerides"	—
Lipoprotein: see Table A-4	—
Lithium, serum:	
Therapeutic level: 0.6–1.2 mmol/L (0.6–1.2 meq/L)	—
Toxic level: >2 mmol/L (2 meq/L)	—
Magnesium, serum: 0.8–1.2 mmol/L (1.8–3 mg/dL)	0.4114
Osmolality, plasma: 285–295 mmol/kg serum water (285–295 mosmol/kg serum water)	—
Oxygen content:	
Arterial blood (sea level): 17–21 volume percent	—
Venous blood, arm (sea level): 10 to 16 volume percent	—
Oxygen percent saturation (sea level):	
Arterial blood: 0.97 mol/mol (97 percent)	0.01
Venous blood, arm: 0.60–0.85 mol/mol (60–85 percent)	0.01
Oxygen tension (P_{O_2}) blood: 11–13 kPa (80–100 mmHg)	0.1333
pH, blood: 7.38–7.44	—
Phenytoin, plasma: See Fig. 365-8	
Phosphatase, acid, serum: 0.90 nkat/L (0–5.5 U/L)	—
Phosphatase, alkaline, serum: 0.5–2.0 nkat/L (30–120 U/L)	—
Phosphorus, inorganic, serum: 1.0–1.4 mmol/L (3–4.5 mg/dL)	0.3229
Potassium, serum: 3.5–5.0 mmol/L (3.5–5.0 meq/L)	—
Protein, total, serum: 55–80 g/L (5.5–8.0 g/dL)	10.00
Protein fractions, serum:	
Albumin: 35–55 g/L [3.5–5.5 g/dL (50–60 percent)]	10.00
Globulin: 20–35 g/L [2.0–3.5 g/dL (40–50 percent)]	10.00
Alpha$_1$: 2–4 g/L [0.2–0.4 g/dL (4.2–7.2 percent)]	10.00
Alpha$_2$: 5–9 g/L [0.5–0.9 g/dL (6.8–12 percent)]	10.00
Beta: 6–11 g/L [0.6–1.1 g/dL (9.3–15 percent)]	10.00
Gamma: 7–17 g/L [0.7–1.7 g/dL (13–23 percent)]	10.00
Pyruvate, venous, plasma: 60–170 μmol/L (0.5–1.5 mg/dL)	113.6
Quinidine, serum:	
Therapeutic range: 4.6–9.2 μmol/L (1.5–3 mg/L)	3.082
Toxic range: 15.4–18.5 μmol/L (5–6 mg/L)	3.082
Salicylate, plasma: 0 mmol/L	
Therapeutic range: 1.4–1.8 mmol/L (20–25 mg/dL)	0.07240
Toxic range: >2.2 mmol/L (>30 mg/dL)	0.07240
Sodium, serum: 136–145 mmol/L (136–145 meq/L)	—
Steroids: see "Metabolic and Endocrine Tests"	—
Transferrin, serum: 2.3–3.9 mg/L (230–390 μg/dL)	10.00
Triglycerides: <1.8 mmol/L (<160 mg/dL)	0.01129
Troponin I, serum: 0–0.4 μg/L (0–0.4 ng/mL)	—
Troponin T, serum: 0–0.1 μg/L (0–0.1 ng/mL)	—
Urea nitrogen, serum: 3.6–7.1 mmol/L (10–20 mg/dL)	0.3570
Uric acid, serum:	
Men: 150–480 μmol/L (2.5–8.0 mg/dL)	59.48
Women: 90–360 μmol/L (1.5–6.0 mg/dL)	59.48
Vitamin A, serum: 0.7–3.5 μmol/L (20–100 μg/dL)	0.03491
Vitamin B$_{12}$, serum: 148–443 pmol/L (200–600 pg/mL)	0.7378
Zinc, serum: 11.5–18.5 μmol/L (75–120 μg/dL)	0.1530

CIRCULATORY FUNCTION TESTS

Arteriovenous oxygen difference: 30–50 mL/L
Cardiac output (Fick): 2.5–3.6 L/m^2 of body surface area per minute
Contractility indexes:
- Maximum left ventricular *dp*/*dt*: 1650 mmHg/s (range, 1320–1880, mmHg/s)
- (*dp*/*dt*)/DP when DP = 40 mmHg: 37.6 ±12.2 s^{-1} (DP, diastolic pressure)
- Mean normalized systolic ejection rate (angiography): 3.32 ± 0.84 end-diastolic volumes per second
- Mean velocity of circumferential fiber shortening (angiography) 1.66 ± 0.42 circumferences per second

Ejection fraction, stroke volume/end-diastolic volume (SV/EDV): normal range: 0.55–0.78; average: 0.67
End-diastolic volume: 75 mL/m^2 (range, 60–88 mL/m^2)
End-systolic volume: 25 mL/m^2 (range, 20–33 mL/m^2)
Left ventricular work:
- Stroke work index: 30–110 (g·m)/m^2
- Left ventricular minute work index: 1.8–6.6 [(kg·m)/m^2]/min
- Oxygen consumption index: 110–150 mL

Maximum oxygen uptake: normal range 20–60 mL/min; average: 35 mL/min
Pulmonary vascular resistance: 20–120 (dyn·s)/cm^5 (2–12 kPa·s/L)
Systemic vascular resistance: 770–1500 (dyn·s)/cm^5 (77–150 kPa·s/L)

GASTROINTESTINAL TESTS

See also "Stool Analysis."

Absorption tests:
- D-Xylose absorption test: After an overnight fast, 25 g xylose is given in aqueous solution by mouth. Urine collected for the following 5 h should contain 33–53 mmol (5–8 g) (or >20 percent of ingested dose). Serum xylose should be 1.7–2.7 mmol (25–40 mg/dL) 1 h after the oral dose.
- Vitamin A absorption test: A fasting blood specimen is obtained and 200,000 units of vitamin A in oil is given by mouth. Serum vitamin A levels should rise to twice fasting level in 3–5 h.

Bentiromide test (pancreatic function): 500 mg bentiromide (chymex) orally; *p*-aminobenzoic acid (PABA) measured in plasma and/or urine
- Plasma: >3.6 (±1.1) μg/mL at 90 min
- Urine: >50 percent recovered as PABA in 6 h

Gastric juice:	Conversion Factor (CF) C × CF = SI
Volume:	
24 h: 2–3 L	
Nocturnal: 600–700 mL	
Basal, fasting: 30–70 mL/h	
Reaction:	
pH: 1.6–1.8	
Titratable acidity of fasting juice: 4–9 μmol/s (15–35 meq/h)	0.261
Acid output:	
Basal:	
Females (mean ± 1 SD): 0.6 ± 0.5 ρmol/s (2.0 ± 1.8 meq/h)	0.2778
Males (mean ± 1 SD): 0.8 ± 0.6 μmol/s (3.0 ± 2.0 meq/h)	0.2778
Maximal (after subcutaneous histamine acid phosphate 0.004 mg/kg body weight and preceded by 50 mg promethazine or after betazole 1.7 mg/kg body wt or pentagastrin 6 μg/kg body wt):	
Females (mean ± 1 SD): 4.4 ± 1.4 μmol/s (16 ± 5 meq/h)	0.2778
Males (mean ± 1 SD): 6.4 ± 1.4 μmol/s (23 ± 5 meq/h)	0.2778

	Conversion Factor (CF) C × CF = SI
Basal acid output/maximal acid output ratio: 0.6 or less	
Gastrin, serum: 40–200 ng/L (40–200 pg/mL)	—
Secretin test (pancreatic exocrine function): 1 unit per kg body wt, intravenously	
Volume (pancreatic juice): >2.0 mL/kg in 80 min	—
Bicarbonate concentration: >80 mmol/L (>80 meq/L)	—
Bicarbonate output: >10 mmol in 30 min (>10 meq in 30 min)	—

METABOLIC AND ENDOCRINE TESTS

	Conversion Factor (CF) C × CF = SI
Adrenocorticotropin (ACTH) plasma, 8 A.M.: 2–11 pmol/L (9–52 pg/mL)	0.2202
Adrenal cortex function tests: see Chap. 332	—
Adrenal medulla function tests: see Chap. 333	—
Adrenal steroids, plasma:	
Aldosterone, 8 A.M.: <220 pmol/L (patient supine, 100 meq Na and 60–100 meq K intake) (<8 ng/dL)	27.74
Cortisol:	
8 A.M.: 140–690 nmol/L (5–25 μg/dL)	27.59
4 P.M.: 80–330 nmol/L (3–12 μg/dL)	27.59
Dehydroepiandrosterone (DHEA): 7–31 nmol/L (2–9 μg/L)	3.467
Dehydroepiandrosterone sulfate (DHEA sulfate): 1.3–6.8 μmol/L (500–2500 μg/L)	0.002714
11-Deoxycortisol (compound S): <30 nmol/L (<1 μg/dL)	28.86
17-Hydroxyprogesterone:	
Women: follicular phase, 0.6–3 nmol/L (0.20–1 μg/L); luteal phase 1.5–10.6 nmol/L (0.5–3.5 μg/L)	3.026 3.026
Men: 0.2–9 nmol/L (0.06–3 μg/L)	3.026
Adrenal steroids, urinary excretion	
Aldosterone: 14–53 nmol/d (5–19 μg/d)	2.774
Cortisol, free: 55–275 nmol/d (20–100 μg/d)	2.759
17-Hydroxycorticosteroids: 5.5–28 μmol/d (2–10 mg/d)	2.759
17-Ketosteroids:	
Men: 20–69 μmol/d (6–20 mg/d)	3.467
Women: 20–59 μmol/d (6–17 mg/d)	3.467
Angiotensin II, plasma, 8 A.M.: 10–30 nmol/L (10–30 pg/mL)	—
Arginine vasopressin (AVP), plasma:	
Random fluid intake: 1.5–5.6 pmol/L (1.5–6 ng/L)	0.92
Calcitonin, plasma: <50 ng/L (<50 pg/mL)	—
Catecholamines, urinary excretion:	
Free catecholamines: <590 nmol/d (<100 μg/d)	5.911
Epinephrine: <275 nmol/d (<50 μg/d)	5.458
Metanephrines: <7 μmol/d (<1.3 mg/d)	5.458
Norepinephrine: 89–473 nmol/d (15–80 μg/d)	5.91
Vanillylmandelic acid (VMA): <40 μmol/d (<8 mg/d)	5.046
Glucagon, plasma: 50–100 ng/L (50–100 pg/mL)	—
Gonadal function tests: see Chaps. 336 and 337	—
Gonadal steroids, plasma:	
Androstenedione:	
Women: 3.5–7.0 nmol/L (1–2 ng/mL)	3.492
Men: 3.0–5.0 nmol/L (0.8–1.3 ng/mL)	3.492

	Conversion Factor (CF) C × CF = SI
Estradiol:	
Women: 70–220 pmol/L (20–60 pg/mL), higher at ovulation	3.671
Men: <180 pmol/L (<50 pg/mL)	3.671
Progesterone:	
Men, prepubertal girls, preovulatory women, and postmenopausal women: <6 nmol/L (<2 ng/mL)	3.180
Women, luteal, peak: 6–60 nmol/L (2–20 ng/mL)	3.180
Testosterone:	
Women: <3.5 nmol/L (<1 ng/mL)	3.467
Men: 10–35 nmol/L (3–10 ng/mL)	3.467
Prepubertal boys and girls: 0.17–0.7 nmol/L (0.05–0.2 ng/mL)	3.467
Gonadotropins, plasma:	
Women, mature, premenopausal, except at ovulation:	
FSH: 1.4–9.6 IU/L (1.4–9.6 mIU/mL)	—
LH: 0.8–26 IU/L (0.8–26 mIU/mL)	—
Ovulatory surge:	
FSH: 2.3–21 IU/L (2.3–21 mIU/mL)	—
LH: 25–57 IU/L (25–57 mIU/mL)	—
Postmenopausal women:	
FSH: 34–96 IU/L (34–96 mIU/mL)	—
LH: 40–104 IU/L (40–104 mIU/mL)	—
Men, mature:	
FSH: 0.9–15 IU/L (0.9–15 mIU/mL)	—
LH: 1.3–13 IU/L (1.3–13 mIU/mL)	—
Children of both sexes, prepubertal:	
LH: 1.0–5.9 IU/L (1.0–5.9 mIU/mL)	
Growth hormone, after 100 g glucose by mouth: <2 μg/L (<2 ng/ml)	—
Human chorionic gonadotropin, β subunit (β-hCG), plasma:	
Men and nonpregnant women: <3 IU/L (<3 mIU/mL)	—
Insulin, serum or plasma, fasting: 43–186 pmol/L (6–26 μU/mL)	7.175
Insulin-like growth factor I (somatomedin C, IGF-1/SM C): see Chap. 329	—
Oxytocin: random 1–4 pmol/L (1.25–5 ng/L)	0.80
Ovulatory peak in women 4–8 pmol/L (5–10 ng/L)	—
Pancreatic islet function tests: see Chap. 334	—
Parathyroid function tests: see Chap. 354	—
Pituitary function tests: see Chaps. 328 to 330	—
Pregnancy tests: see Chap. 337	—
Prolactin, serum: 2–15 μg/L (2–15 ng/mL)	—
Renin-angiotensin function tests: see Chap. 332	—
Semen analysis: see Chap. 336	—
Thyroid function tests:	
Dynamic tests of thyroid function: see Chap. 331	—
Radioactive iodine uptake, 24 h: 5–30 percent (range varies in different areas due to variations in iodine intake)	—
Resin T_3 uptake: 0.25–0.35 (25–35 percent) (varies among laboratories; for calculation of free T4 estimate, see Chap. 331)	0.01
Reverse triiodothyronine (rT_3), plasma: 0.15–0.61 nmol/L (10–40 ng/dL)	0.01536
Thyroid-stimulating hormone (TSH): 0.4–5 mU/L (0.4–5 μU/mL)	—
Thyroxine (T_4), serum radioimmunoassay: 64–154 nmol/L (5–12 μg/dL)	12.86
Triiodothyronine (T_3), plasma: 1.1–2.9 nmol/L (70–190 ng/dL)	0.01536

PULMONARY FUNCTION TESTS

See Table A-9

RENAL FUNCTION TESTS

	Conversion Factor (CF) C × CF = SI
Clearances (corrected to 1.72 m^2 body surface area):	
Measures of glomerular filtration rate:	
Insulin clearance (C1):	
Males (mean ± 1 SD): 2.1 ± 0.4 mL/s (124 ± 25.8 mL/min)	0.01667
Females (mean ± 1 SD): 2.0 ± 0.2 mL/s (119 ± 12.8 mL/min)	0.01667
Endogenous creatinine clearance: 1.5–2.2 mL/s (91–130 mL/min)	0.01667
Urea: 1.0–1.7 mL/s (60–100 mL/min)	0.01667
Measures of effective renal plasma flow and tubular function:	
p-Aminohippuric acid clearance ($C1_{PAH}$):	
Males (mean ± 1 SD): 10.9 ± 2.7 mL/s (654 ± 163 mL/min)	0.01667
Females (mean ± 1 SD): 9.9 ± 1.7 mL/s (594 ± 102 mL/min)	0.01667
Concentration and dilution test:	
Specific gravity of urine:	
After 12-h fluid restriction: 1.025 or more	—
After 12-h deliberate water intake: 1.003 or less	—
Protein excretion, urine: <0.15 g/d (<150 mg/d)	0.01
Males: 0–0.06 g/d (0–60 mg/d)	0.01
Females: 0–0.09 g/d (0–90 mg/d)	0.01
Specific gravity, maximal range: 1.002–1.028	—
Tubular reabsorption, phosphorus: 79–94 percent of filtered load	—

HEMATOLOGIC EVALUATIONS

See also "Chemical Constituents of Blood."

	Conversion Factor (CF) C × CF = SI
Bone marrow: see Table A-6	—
Carboxyhemoglobin:	
Nonsmoker: 0–0.023 (0–2.3 percent)	0.01
Smoker: 0.021–0.042 (2.1–4.2 percent)	0.01
Erythrocyte:	
Count: 4.15–4.90 × 10^{12}/L (4.15–4.90 × 10^6/mm^3)	—
Distribution width: 0.13–0.15 (13–15 percent)	—
Glucose-6-phosphate dehydrogenase: 12.1 ± 2 IU/gHb (WHO)	—
Life span:	
Normal survival: 120 days	—
Chromium-labeled, half-life ($t_{1/2}$): 28 days	—
Mean corpuscular hemoglobin (MCH): 28–33 pg/cell (28–33 pg/cell)	—
Mean corpuscular hemoglobin concentration (MCHC): 320–360 g/L (32–36 g/dL)	10.00
Mean corpuscular volume (MCV): 86–98 fl (86–98 μm^3)	—
Ham's test (acid serum): negative	—
Haptoglobin, serum 0.5–2.2 g/L (50–220 mg/dL)	0.01
Hematocrit	
Males: 0.42–0.52 (42–52%)	—
Females: 0.37–0.48 (37–48%)	—
Hemoglobin:	
Plasma: 0.01–0.05 g/L (1–5 mg/dL)	0.01
Whole blood:	
Males: 8.1–11.2 mmol/L (13–18 g/dL)	—
Females: 7.4–9.9 mmol/L (12–16 g/dL)	—
Hemoglobin A_2 (HbA_2): 0.015–0.035 (1.5–3.5 percent)	0.01
Hemoglobin, fetal (HbF): <0.02 (<2 percent)	0.01
Leukocytes:	
Alkaline phosphatase (LAP): 0.2–1.6 μkat/L (13–100 μ/L)	—
Count: 4.3–10.8 × 10^9/L (4.3–10.8 × 10^3/mm^3)	
Differential:	
Neutrophils: 0.45–0.74 (45–74 percent)	
Bands: 0–0.04 (0–4 percent)	
Lymphocytes: 0.16–0.45 (16–45 percent)	
Monocytes: 0.04–0.10 (4–10 percent)	
Eosinophils: 0–0.07 (0–7 percent)	
Basophils: 0–0.02 (0–2 percent)	
Methemoglobin: <2 mg/L (<2 μg/mL)	—
Osmotic fragility:	
Slight hemolysis: 0.45–0.39 percent	—
Complete hemolysis: 0.33–0.30 percent	—
Platelets and coagulation parameters:	
Alpha$_2$ antiplasmin: 70–130 percent	
Antithrombin III: 80–120 percent	
Bleeding time:	
Simplate: <7 min	
Euglobulin lysis time: >2 h	
Factor II: 60–100 percent	
Factor V: 60–100 percent	
Factor VII: 60–100 percent	
Factor IX: 60–100 percent	
Factor X: 60–100 percent	
Factor XI: 60–100 percent	
Factor XII: 60–100 percent	
Factor XIII: 60–100 percent	
Fibrinogen: 200–400 mg/dL	
Plasminogen: 2.4–4.4 CTA U/mL	
Protein C (antigenic assay): 58–148 percent	
Protein S (antigenic assay): 58–148 percent	
Partial thromboplastin time (activated PTT): comparable to control	
Prothrombin time (quick one-stage): control ± 1 s	
Platelets: 130–400 × 10^9/L (130,000–400,000/mm^3)	
Thrombin time: control ± 3 s	
von Willebrand's antigen: 60–150 percent	
Protoporphyrin, free erythrocyte (FEP): 0.28–0.64 μmol/L of red blood cells (16–36 μg/dL of red blood cells)	0.0177
Red cells: (see "Erythrocytes")	
Schilling test: 7–40 percent of orally administered vitamin B_{12} excreted in urine	
Sedimentation rate:	
Westergren, <50 years of age:	
Males: 0–15 mm/h	
Females: 0–20 mm/h	
Westergren, >50 years of age:	
Males: 0–20 mm/h	
Females: 0–30 mm/h	
Sucrose hemolysis: negative	
Viscosity	
Plasma: 1.7–2.1	
Serum: 1.4–1.8	
White blood cells: (see "Leukocytes")	

STOOL ANALYSIS

	Conversion Factor (CF) C × CF = SI
Bulk:	
Wet weight: <197.5 (115 ± 41) g/d	—
Dry weight: <66.4 (34 ± 15) g/d	—
Alpha$_1$ antitrypsin: 0.98 (±0.17) mg/g dry weight stool	—
Coproporphyrin: 600–1500 nmol/d (400–1000 μg/d)	1.527
Fat (on diet containing at least 50 g fat): <6.0 (4.0 ± 1.5) g/d when measured on a 3-day (or longer) collection	
Percent of dry weight: 0.30 (<30.4 percent)	0.01
Coefficient of fat absorption: >0.95 (>95 percent)	0.01
Fatty acid:	
Free: 0.01–0.10 (1–10 percent of dry matter)	0.01
Combined as soap: 0.005–0.12 (0.5–12 percent of dry matter)	0.01
Nitrogen: <1.7 (1.4 ± 0.2) g/d	—
Protein content: minimal	—
Urobilinogen: 68–470 μmol/d (40–280 mg/d)	1.693
Water: 0.65 (approximately 65 percent)	0.01

URINE ANALYSIS

See also "Metabolic and Endocrine Tests"

	Conversion Factor (CF) C × CF = SI
Acidity, titratable: 20–40 mmol/d (20–40 meq/d)	—
Ammonia: 30–50 mmol/d (30–50 meq/d)	—
Amylase: 35–260 Somogyi units/h	—
Amylase/creatinine clearance ratio [(Cl_{am}/Cl_{cr}) × 100]: 1–5	—
Bentiromide (pancreatic function): 50 percent excreted in 6 h as *p*-amino benzoic acid (PABA) after 500 mg oral bentiromide	—
Calcium (10 meq/d or 200-mg/d calcium diet): <3.8 mmol/d (<7.5 meq/d)	0.5
Catecholamines: see under "Metabolic and Endocrine Tests"	—
Copper: 0–0.4 μmol/d (0–25 μg/d)	0.01574
Coproporphyrins (types I and III): 150–460 nmol/d (100–300 μg/d)	1.527
Creatine, as creatinine:	
Adult males: <380 μmol/d (<50 mg/d)	7.625
Adult females: <760 μmol/d (<100 mg/d)	7.625
Creatinine: 8.8–14 mmol/d (1.0–1.6 g/d)	8.840
Glucose, true (oxidase method): 0.3–1.7 mmol/d (50–300 mg/d)	0.5551
5-Hydroxyindoleacetic acid (5-HIAA): 10–47 μmol/d (2–9 mg/d)	5.230
Lead: <0.4 μmol/d (<80 μg/d)	0.004826
Protein: <0.15 g/d (<150 mg/d)	0.1
Porphobilinogen: none	—
Potassium: 25–100 mmol/d [25–100 meq/d (varies with intake)]	—
Sodium: 100–260 mmol/d [100–260 meq/d (varies with intake)]	—
Urobilinogen: 1.7–5.9 μmol/d (1–3.5 mg/d)	1.693
D-Xylose excretion: 5 to 8 g within 5 h after oral dose of 25 g	—

Table A-1

SI and Other Units

Quantity	Name of Unit	Symbol for Unit	Derivation of Units
SI BASE UNITS			
Length	meter	m	
Mass	kilogram	kg	
Time	second	s	
Thermodynamic temperature	Kelvin	K	
Amount of substance	mole	mol	
SI DERIVED UNITS			
Area	square meter	m^2	
Force	newton	N	$(m \cdot kg)/s^2$
Pressure	pascal	Pa	$N \cdot m^2$
Work, energy	joule	J	N·m
Celsius temperature	degree Celsius	°C	K
OTHER UNITS RETAINED FOR USE			
Time	minute	min	
	hour	h	
	day	d	
Volume	liter	L	

Table A-2

Radiation Derived Units

Quantity	Old Unit	SI Unit	Name for SI Unit (and Abbreviation)	Conversion
Activity	curie (Ci)	Disintegrations per second (dps)	becquerel (Bq)	1 Ci = 3.7 × 10^{10} Bq 1 mCi = 37 mBq 1 μCi = 0.037 MBq or 37 GBq 1 Bq = 2.703 × 10^{-11} Ci
Absorbed dose	rad	joule per kilogram (J/kg)	gray (Gy)	1 Gy = 100 rad 1 rad = 0.01 Gy 1 mrad = 10^{-3} cGy
Exposure	roentgen (R)	coulomb per kilogram (C/kg)	—	1 C/kg = 3876 R 1 R = 2.58 × 10^{-4} C/kg 1 mR = 258 pC/kg
Dose equivalent	rem	joule per kilogram (J/kg)	sievert (Sv)	1 Sv = 100 rem 1 rem = 0.01 Sv 1 mrem = 10 μSv

Table A-3

SI Prefixes and Their Symbols

Factor	Prefix	Symbol for Prefix
10^9	giga	G
10^6	mega	M
10^3	kilo	k
10^2	hecto	h
10^1	deka	da
10^{-1}	deci	d
10^{-2}	centi	c
10^{-3}	milli	m
10^{-6}	micro	μ
10^{-9}	nano	n
10^{-12}	pico	p
10^{-15}	femto	f
10^{-18}	alto	a

Table A-4

Classification of Total Cholesterol, LDL-Cholesterol, and HDL-Cholesterol Values

	Total Plasma Cholesterol	LDL-Cholesterol	HDL-Cholesterol	Conversion Factor (C to SI)
Desirable	<5.20 mmol/L (<200 mg/dL)	<3.36 mmol/L (<130 mg/dL)	>1.55 mmol/L (>60 mg/dL)	0.02586
Borderline	5.20–6.18 mmol/L (200–239 mg/dL)	3.36–4.11 mmol/L (130–159 mg/dL)	0.9–1.55 mmol/L (35–60 mg/dL)	0.02586
Undesirable	≥6.21 mmol/L (≥240 mg/dL)	≥4.14 mmol/L (≥ 160 mg/dL)	<0.9 mmol/L (<35 mg/dL)	0.02586

SOURCE: Modified from the report of the Expert Panel on Detection, Evaluation, and Treatment of High Blood Cholesterol in Adults: Second Report of the National Cholesterol Education Program (NCEP) expert panel on detection, evaluation, and treatment of high blood cholesterol (Adult Treatment Panel II). Circulation 89:1329, 1994.

Table A-5

Normal Values of Doppler Echocardiographic Measurements in Adults

	Range	Mean
RVD (cm)	0.9 to 2.6	1.7
LVID (cm)	3.5 to 5.7	4.7
Posterior LV wall thickness (cm)	0.6 to 1.1	0.9
IVS wall thickness (cm)	0.6 to 1.1	0.9
Left atrial dimension (cm)	1.9 to 4.0	2.9
Aortic root dimension (cm)	2.0 to 3.7	2.7
Aortic cusps separation (cm)	1.5 to 2.6	1.9
Percentage of fractional shortening	34 to 44%	36%
Mitral flow (m/sec)	0.6 to 1.3	0.9
Tricuspid flow (m/sec)	0.3 to 0.7	0.5
Pulmonary artery (m/sec)	0.6 to 0.9	0.75
Aorta (m/sec)	1.0 to 1.7	1.35

NOTE: RVD, right ventricular dimension; LVID, left ventricular internal dimension; LV, left ventricle; IVS, interventricular septum.

SOURCE: From H Feigenbaum, *Echocardiography,* 5th ed, Philadelphia. Lea & Febiger, 1994

Table A-6

Differential Nucleated Cell Counts of Bone Marrow

	Normal, Mean%*	Range, %†		Normal, Mean%*	Range, %†
Myeloid	56.7		Erythroid	25.6	
Neutrophilic series	53.6		Pronormoblasts	0.6	0.2–1.3
Myeloblast	0.9	0.2–1.5	Basophilic normoblasts	1.4	0.5–2.4
Promyelocyte	3.3	2.1–4.1	Polychromatophilic normoblasts	21.6	17.9–29.2
Myelocyte	12.7	8.2–15.7			
Metamyelocyte	15.9	9.6–24.6	Orthochromatic normoblasts	2.0	0.4–4.6
Band	12.4	9.5–15.3	Megakaryocytes	<0.1	
Segmented			Lymphoreticular	17.8	
Eosinophilic series	3.1	1.2–5.3	Lymphocytes	16.2	11.1–23.2
Basophilic series	<0.1	0–0.2	Plasma cells	2.3	0.4–3.9
			Reticulum cells	0.3	0–0.9

* From MM Wintrobe et al, *Clinical Hematology,* 8th ed. Philadelphia, Lea & Febiger, 1981.
† Range observed in 12 healthy men.

Table A-7

Erythrocytes and Hemoglobin: Normal Values at Various Ages

				Corpuscular Values			
Age	Red Blood Cell Count,* 10^{12}/L	Hemoglobin,* g/L (g/dL)	Vol. Packed RBCs,* mL/dL	MCV, fL	MCH, pg	MCHC, g/L (g/dL)	MCD, μm
Days 1–13	5.1 ± 1.0	195 ± 50 (19.5 ± 5)	54.0 ± 10.0	106–98	38–33	340–360 (36–34)	8.6
Days 14–60	4.7 ± 0.9	140 ± 33 (14 ± 3.3)	42.0 ± 7.0	90	30	330 (33)	8.1
3 months to 10 years	4.5 ± 0.7	122 ± 23 (12.2 ± 2.3)	36.0 ± 5.0	80	27	340 (34)	7.7
11–15 years	4.8	131 (13.14)	39.0	82	28	340 (34)	
Adults:							
Females	4.8 ± 0.6	140 ± 20 (14 ± 2)	42.0 ± 5.0	90 ± 7	29 ± 2	340 ± 20 (34 ± 2)	7.5 ± 0.3
Males	5.4 ± 0.9	160 ± 20 (16 ± 2)	47.0 ± 5.0	90 ± 7	29 ± 2	340 ± 20 (34 ± 2)	7.5 ± 0.3

* The range of values represents almost the extremes of observed variations (93 percent or more) at sea level. The blood values of healthy persons should fall well within these mean ± SD figures.

NOTE: MCV, mean corpuscular volume; MCH, mean corpuscular hemoglobin; MCHC, mean corpuscular hemoglobin concentration; MCD, mean corpuscular diameter.

SOURCE: MM Wintrobe et al, *Clinical Hematology,* 8th ed, Philadelphia, Lea & Febiger, 1981.

Table A-8

Normal Leukocyte Count, Differential Count, and Hemoglobin Concentration at Various Ages

Age	Leukocytes, Total	Neutrophils Total	Neutrophils Band	Neutrophils Segmented	Eosinophils	Basophils	Lymphocytes	Monocytes
12 mo	11.4(6.0–17.5)	3.5(1.5–8.5) *31*	0.35 *3.1*	3.2 *28*	0.3(0.05–0.7) *0.4*	0.05(0–0.20) *0.4*	7.0(4.0–10.5) *61*	0.55(0.05–1.1) *4.8*
4 yr	9.1(5.5–15.5)	3.8(1.5–8.5) *42*	0.27(0–1.0) *3.0*	3.5(1.5–7.5) *39*	0.25(0.02–0.65) *2.8*	0.05(0–0.20) *0.6*	4.5(2.0–8.0) *50*	0.45(0–0.8) *5.0*
6 yr	4.3(1.5–8.0)	0.25(0–1.0) *51*	4.0(1.5–7.0) *3.0*	4.0(1.5–7.0) *48*	0.23(0–0.65) *2.7*	0.05(0–0.20) *0.6*	3.5(1.5–7.0) *42*	0.40(0–0.8) *4.7*
10 yr	8.1(4.5–13.5)	4.4(1.8–8.0) *54*	0.24(0–1.0) *3.0*	4.2(1.8–7.0) *51*	0.20(0–0.60) *2.4*	0.04(0–0.20) *0.5*	3.1(1.5–6.5) *38*	0.35(0–0.8) *4.3*
21 yr	7.4(4.5–11.0)	4.4(1.8–7.7) *59*	0.22(0–0.7) *3.0*	4.2(1.8–7.0) *56*	0.20(0–0.45) *2.7*	0.04(0–0.20) *0.5*	2.5(1.0–4.8) *34*	0.30(0–0.8) *4.0*

NOTE: Values are expressed as "cells $\times 10^9$/L." The numbers in italic are percentages.

SOURCE: E Beutler et al (eds), *Williams Hematology*, 5th ed, New York, McGraw-Hill, 1995. By permission.

Table A-9

Summary of Values Useful in Pulmonary Physiology

	Symbol	Typical Values: Man Aged 40, 75 kg, 175 cm Tall	Typical Values: Woman Aged 40, 60 kg, 160 cm Tall
PULMONARY MECHANICS			
Spirometry—volume-time curves:			
Forced vital capacity	FVC	4.8 L	3.3 L
Forced expiratory volume in 1 s	FEV_1	3.8 L	2.8 L
FEV_1/FVC	FEV_1%	76%	77%
Maximal midexpiratory flow	MMF (FEF 25–27)	4.8 L/s	3.6 L/s
Maximal expiratory flow rate	MEFR (FEF 200–1200)	9.4 L/s	6.1 L/s
Spirometry—flow-volume curves:			
Maximal expiratory flow at 50% of expired vital capacity	V_{max} 50 (FEF 50%)	6.1 L/s	4.6 L/s
Maximal expiratory flow at 75% of expired vital capacity	V_{max} 75 (FEF 75%)	3.1 L/s	2.5 L/s
Resistance to airflow:			
Pulmonary resistance	RL (R_L)	<3.0 (cmH_2O/s)/L	
Airway resistance	Raw	<2.5 (cmH_2O/s)/L	
Specific conductance	SGaw	>0.13 cmH_2O/s	
Pulmonary compliance:			
Static recoil pressure at total lung capacity	Pst TLC	25 ± 5 cmH_2O	
Compliance of lungs (static)	CL	0.2 L cmH_2O	
Compliance of lungs and thorax	C(L + T)	0.1 L cmH_2O	
Dynamic compliance of 20 breaths per minute	C dyn 20	0.25 ± 0.05 L/cmH_2O	
Maximal static respiratory pressures:			
Maximal inspiratory pressure	MIP	>90 cmH_2O	>50 cmH_2O
Maximal expiratory pressure	MEP	>150 cmH_2O	>120 cmH_2O
LUNG VOLUMES			
Total lung capacity	TLC	6.4 L	4.9 L
Functional residual capacity	FRC	2.2 L	2.6 L
Residual volume	RV	1.5 L	1.2 L
Inspiratory capacity	IC	4.8 L	3.7 L
Expiratory reserve volume	ERV	3.2 L	2.3 L
Vital capacity	VC	1.7 L	1.4 L
GAS EXCHANGE (SEA LEVEL)			
Arterial O_2 tension	Pa_{O_2}	12.7 ± 0.7 kPa (95 ± 5 mmHg)	
Arterial CO_2 tension	Pa_{CO_2}	5.3 ± 0.3 kPa (40 ± 2 mmHg)	
Arterial O_2 saturation	Sa_{O_2}	0.97 ± 0.02 (97 ± 2%)	
Arterial blood pH	pH	7.40 ± 0.02	
Arterial bicarbonate	HCO_3^-	24 + 2 meq/L	
Base excess	BE	0 ± 2 meq/L	
Diffusing capacity for carbon monoxide (single breath)	DL_{CO}	0.42 mLCO/s/mmHg (25 mL CO/min/mmHg)	
Dead space volume	V_D	2 ml/kg body wt	
Physiologic dead space; dead space-tidal volume ratio	V_D/V_T		
Rest		≤35% V_T	
Exercise		≤20% V_T	
Alveolar-arterial difference for O_2	$P(A - a)_{O_2}$	≤2.7 kPa ≤20 kPa (≤20 mmHg)	

B

INSTRUCTIONS FOR COLLECTION AND TRANSPORT OF SPECIMENS FOR CULTURE

It is absolutely essential that the microbiology laboratory be informed of the site of origin of the sample to be cultured and of the infections that are suspected. This information determines the selection of culture media and the length of culture time.

Type of Culture (Synonyms)	Specimen	Minimum Volume	Container	Other Considerations
BLOOD				
Blood, routine (blood culture for aerobes, anaerobes, and yeasts)	Whole blood	10 mL in each of 2 bottles for adults and children; 5 mL, if possible, in each of 2 bottles for infants; less for neonates	See below.[a]	See below.[b]
Blood for fungi/ *Mycobacterium* spp.	Whole blood	10 mL in each of 2 bottles, as for routine blood cultures, or in Isolator tube requested from laboratory	Same as for routine blood culture	Specify "hold for extended incubation," since fungal agents may require 4 weeks or more to grow.
Blood, Isolator (lysis centrifugation)	Whole blood	10 mL	Isolator tubes	Use mainly for isolation of fungi, *Mycobacterium,* or other fastidious aerobes and for elimination of antibiotics from cultured blood in which organisms are concentrated by centrifugation.
RESPIRATORY TRACT				
Nose	Swab from nares	1 swab	Sterile culturette or similar transport system containing holding medium	Swabs made of calcium alginate may be used.
Throat	Swab of posterior pharynx, ulcerations, or areas of suspected purulence	1 swab	Sterile culturette or similar swab specimen collection system containing holding medium	See below.[c]
Sputum	Fresh sputum (not saliva)	2 mL	Commercially available sputum collection system or similar sterile container with screw cap	*Cause for rejection:* Care must be taken to ensure that the specimen is sputum and not saliva. Examination of Gram's stain, with number of epithelial cells and PMNs noted, can be an important part of the evaluation process. Induced sputum specimens should not be rejected.
Bronchial aspirates	Transtracheal aspirate, bronchoscopy specimen, or bronchial aspirate	1 mL of aspirate or brush in transport medium	Sterile aspirate or bronchoscopy tube, bronchoscopy brush in a separate sterile container	Special precautions may be required, depending on diagnostic considerations (e.g., *Pneumocystis*).
STOOL				
Stool for routine culture; stool for *Salmonella, Shigella,* and *Campylobacter*	Rectal swab or (preferably) fresh, randomly collected stool	1 g of stool or 2 rectal swabs	Plastic-coated cardboard cup or plastic cup with tight-fitting lid. Other leak-proof containers are also acceptable.	If *Vibrio* spp. are suspected, the laboratory must be notified, and appropriate collection/transport methods should be used.
Stool for *Yersinia, E. coli* O157	Fresh, randomly collected stool	1 g	Plastic-coated cardboard cup or plastic cup with tight-fitting lid	*Limitations:* Procedure requires enrichment techniques.
Stool for *Aeromonas* and *Plesiomonas*	Fresh, randomly collected stool	1 g	Plastic-coated cardboard cup or plastic cup with tight-fitting lid	*Limitations:* Stool should not be cultured for these organisms unless also cultured for other enteric pathogens.

(*continued*)

Type of Culture (Synonyms)	Specimen	Minimum Volume	Container	Other Considerations
UROGENITAL TRACT				
Urine	Clean-voided urine specimen or urine collected by catheter	0.5 mL	Sterile, leak-proof container with screw cap or special urine transfer tube	See below.[d]
Urogenital secretions	Vaginal or urethral secretions, cervical swabs, uterine fluid, prostatic fluid, etc.	1 swab or 0.5 mL of fluid	Transwab containing Amies transport medium or similar system containing holding medium for *Neisseria gonorrhoeae;* modified Todd-Hewitt broth for group B *Streptococcus* surveillance cultures	Vaginal swab samples for "routine culture" should be discouraged whenever possible unless a particular pathogen is suspected. For detection of multiple organisms (e.g., group B *Streptococcus, Trichomonas, Chlamydia,* or *Candida* spp.), 1 swab per test should be obtained.
BODY FLUIDS, ASPIRATES, AND TISSUES				
Cerebrospinal fluid (lumbar puncture)	Spinal fluid	1 mL for routine cultures; ≥5 mL for *Mycobacterium*	Sterile tube with tight-fitting cap	Do not refrigerate; transfer to laboratory as soon as possible.
Body fluids	Aseptically aspirated body fluids	1 mL for routine cultures	Sterile tube with tight-fitting cap. Specimen may be left in syringe used for collection if the syringe is capped before transport.	For some body fluids (e.g., peritoneal lavage samples), increased volumes are helpful for isolation of small numbers of bacteria.
Biopsy and aspirated materials	Tissue removed at surgery, bone, anticoagulated bone marrow, biopsy samples, or other specimens from normally sterile areas	1 mL of fluid or a 1-g piece of tissue	Sterile "culturette"-type swab or similar transport system containing holding medium. Sterile bottle or jar should be used for tissue specimens.	Accurate identification of specimen and source is critical. Enough tissue should be collected for both microbiologic and histopathologic evaluations.
Wounds	Purulent material or abscess contents obtained from wound or abscess without contamination by normal microflora	2 swabs or 0.5 mL of aspirated pus	Culturette swab or similar transport system or sterile tube with tight-fitting screw cap. For simultaneous anaerobic cultures, send specimen in anaerobic transport device or closed syringe.	*Collection:* Abscess contents or other fluids should be collected in a syringe (see above) when possible to provide an adequate sample volume and an anaerobic environment.
SPECIAL RECOMMENDATIONS				
Fungi	Specimen types listed above may be used. When urine or sputum is cultured for fungi, a first morning specimen is usually preferred.	1 mL or as specified above for individual listing of specimens. Large volumes may be useful for urinary fungi.	Sterile, leak-proof container with tight-fitting cap	*Collection:* Specimen should be transported to microbiology laboratory within 1 h of collection. Contamination with normal flora from skin, rectum, vaginal tract, or other body surfaces should be avoided.
Mycobacterium (acid-fast bacilli)	Sputum, tissue, urine, body fluids	10 mL of fluid or small piece of tissue. Swabs should not be used.	Sterile container with tight-fitting cap	Detection of *Mycobacterium* spp. is improved by use of concentration techniques. Smears and cultures of pleural, peritoneal, and pericardial fluids often have low yields. Multiple cultures from the same patient are encouraged. Culturing in liquid media shortens the time to detection.
Legionella	Pleural fluid, lung biopsy, bronchoalveolar lavage fluid, bronchial/transbronchial biopsy. Rapid transport to laboratory is critical.	1 mL of fluid; any size tissue sample, although a 0.5-g sample should be obtained when possible	—	—
Anaerobic organisms	Aspirated specimens from abscesses or body fluids	1 mL of aspirated fluid or 2 swabs	An appropriate anaerobic transport device is required.[e]	Specimens cultured for obligate anaerobes should be cultured for facultative bacteria as well.

(*continued*)

Type of Culture (Synonyms)	Specimen	Minimum Volume	Container	Other Considerations
SPECIAL RECOMMENDATIONS *(Continued)*				
Viruses[f]	Respiratory secretions, wash aspirates from respiratory tract, nasal swabs, blood samples (including buffy coats), vaginal and rectal swabs, swab specimens from suspicious skin lesions, stool samples (in some cases)	1 mL of fluid, 1 swab, or 1 g of stool in each appropriate transport medium	Fluid or stool samples in sterile containers or swab samples in viral culturette devices (kept on ice but not frozen) are generally suitable. Plasma samples and buffy coats in sterile collection tubes should be kept at 4 to 8°C. If specimens are to be shipped or kept for a long time, freezing at −80°C is usually adequate.	Most samples for culture are transported in holding medium containing antibiotics to prevent bacterial overgrowth and viral inactivation. Many specimens should be kept cool but not frozen, provided they are transported promptly to the laboratory. Procedures and transport media vary with the agent to be cultured and the duration of transport.

[a] For samples from adults and children, two bottles (smaller for pediatric samples) should be used: one with dextrose phosphate, tryptic soy, or another appropriate broth and the other with thioglycollate or another broth containing reducing agents appropriate for isolation of obligate anaerobes. For special situations (e.g., suspected fungal infection, culture-negative endocarditis, or mycobacteremia), different blood collection systems may be used (Isolator systems; see table).

[b] *Collection:* An appropriate disinfecting technique should be used on both the bottle septum and the patient. Do not allow air bubbles to get into anaerobic broth bottles. *Special considerations:* There is no more important clinical microbiology test than the detection of blood-borne pathogens. The rapid identification of bacterial and fungal agents is a major determinant of patients' survival. Bacteria may be present in blood either continuously (as in endocarditis, overwhelming sepsis, and the early stages of salmonellosis and brucellosis) or intermittently (as in most other bacterial infections, in which bacteria are shed into the blood on a sporadic basis). Most blood culture systems employ two separate bottles containing broth medium: one that is vented in the laboratory for the growth of facultative and aerobic organisms and a second that is maintained under anaerobic conditions. In cases of suspected continuous bacteremia/fungemia, two or three samples should be drawn before the start of therapy, with additional sets obtained if fastidious organisms are thought to be involved. For intermittent bacteremia, two or three samples should be obtained at least 1 h apart during the first 24 h.

[c] Normal microflora includes alpha-hemolytic streptococci, saprophytic *Neisseria* spp., diphtheroids, and *Staphylococcus* spp. Aerobic culture of the throat ("routine") includes screening for and identification of beta-hemolytic *Streptococcus* spp. and other potentially pathogenic organisms. Although considered components of the normal microflora, organisms such as *Staphylococcus aureus, Haemophilus influenzae,* and *Streptococcus pneumoniae* will be identified by most laboratories, if requested. When *Neisseria gonorrhoeae* or *Corynebacterium diphtheriae* is suspected, a special culture request is recommended.

[d] (1) Clean-voided specimens, midvoid specimens, and Foley or indwelling catheter specimens that yield ≥50,000 organisms/mL and from which no more than three species are isolated should have organisms identified. (2) Straight-catheterized, bladder-tap, and similar urine specimens should undergo a complete workup (identification and susceptibility testing) for all potentially pathogenic organisms, regardless of colony count. (3) Certain clinical problems (e.g., acute dysuria in women) may warrant identification and susceptibility testing of isolates present at concentrations of <50,000 organisms/mL.

[e] Aspirated specimens in capped syringes or other transport devices designed to limit oxygen exposure are suitable for the cultivation of obligate anaerobes. A variety of commercially available transport devices may be used. Contamination of specimens with normal microflora from the skin, rectum, vaginal vault, or another body site should be avoided. Collection containers for aerobic culture (such as dry swabs) and inappropriate specimens (such as refrigerated samples; expectorated sputum; stool; gastric aspirates; and vaginal, throat, nose, and rectal swabs) should be rejected as unsuitable.

[f] Laboratories generally use diverse methods to detect viral agents, and the specific requirements for each specimen should be checked before a sample is sent.

INDEX

Bold number indicates the start of the chapter that contains the main discussion of the topic; numbers with "f" and "t" refer to figure and table pages and are listed at the end of the entries.

ISBN 0-07-912013-X
90000
9 780079 120137
SETCODE

ISBN 0-07-020293-1
90000
9 780070 202931
VOL 2

TOPICAL CONTENTS